Bailey & Love's SHORT PRACTICE of SURGERY

28th EDITION

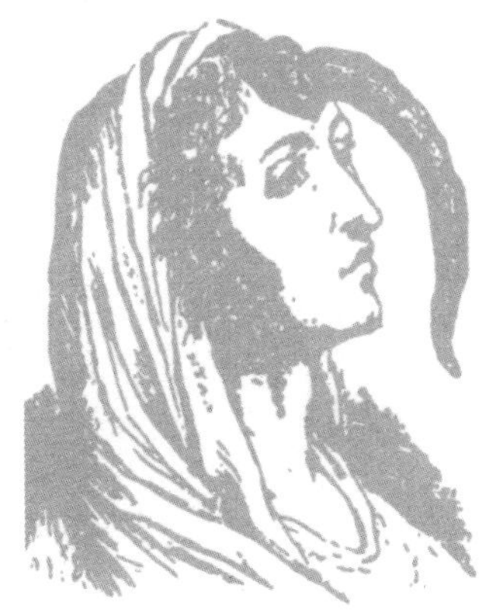

Sebaceous horn

(The owner, the widow Dimanche, sold water-cress in Paris)

A favourite illustration of Hamilton Bailey and McNeill Love, and well known to readers of earlier editions of Short Practice.

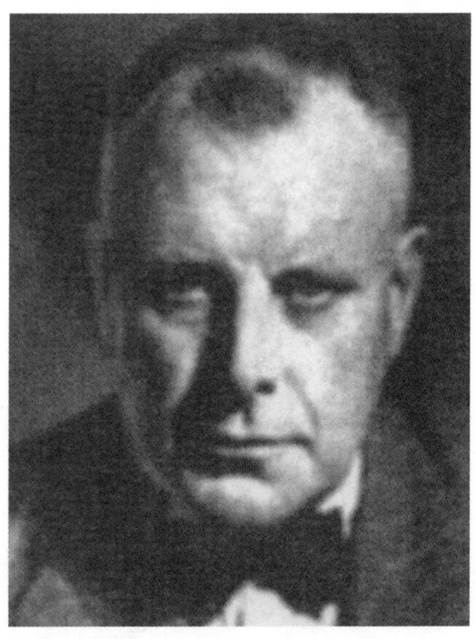

Henry Hamilton Bailey 1894–1961

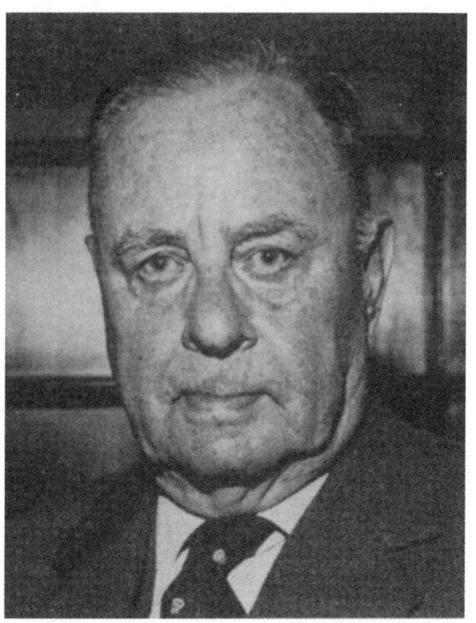

Robert J. McNeill Love 1891–1974

Skilled surgeons, inspirational teachers, dedicated authors

Bailey & Love's SHORT PRACTICE of SURGERY

28th EDITION

Edited by

Professor P. Ronan O'Connell
BA MD FRCSI FRCSGlasg FRCSEd FRCSEng (Hon) FCSHK (Hon)
President, Royal College of Surgeons in Ireland;
President, European Surgical Association;
Emeritus Professor of Surgery, University College Dublin,
Dublin, Ireland

Professor Andrew W. McCaskie
MMus MD FRCSEng FRCS (Tr and Orth)
Professor of Orthopaedic Surgery and Head of Department of Surgery,
University of Cambridge; Honorary Consultant, Addenbrooke's Hospital,
Cambridge University Hospitals NHS Foundation Trust, Cambridge, UK

Professor Robert D. Sayers
MBChB(Hons) MD AFHEA FRCSEng
George Davies Chair of Vascular Surgery,
University of Leicester and Glenfield Hospital, Leicester, UK

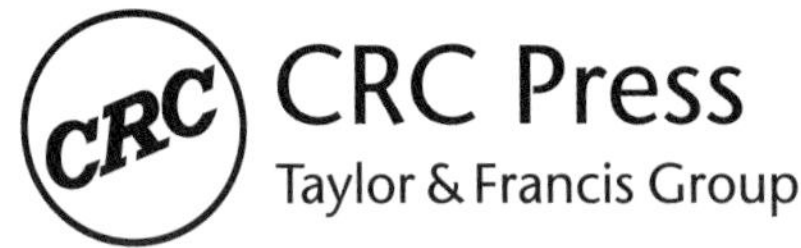

Twenty-eighth edition published 2023
by CRC Press
6000 Broken Sound Parkway NW, Suite 300, Boca Raton, FL 33487-2742

and by CRC Press
4 Park Square, Milton Park, Abingdon, Oxon, OX14 4RN

CRC Press is an imprint of Taylor & Francis Group, LLC

© 2023 Taylor & Francis Group, LLC

First published in Great Britain in 1932

This book contains information obtained from authentic and highly regarded sources. While all reasonable efforts have been made to publish reliable data and information, neither the author[s] nor the publisher can accept any legal responsibility or liability for any errors or omissions that may be made. The publishers wish to make clear that any views or opinions expressed in this book by individual editors, authors or contributors are personal to them and do not necessarily reflect the views/opinions of the publishers. The information or guidance contained in this book is intended for use by medical, scientific or health-care professionals and is provided strictly as a supplement to the medical or other professional's own judgement, their knowledge of the patient's medical history, relevant manufacturer's instructions and the appropriate best practice guidelines. Because of the rapid advances in medical science, any information or advice on dosages, procedures or diagnoses should be independently verified. The reader is strongly urged to consult the relevant national drug formulary and the drug companies' and device or material manufacturers' printed instructions, and their websites, before administering or utilizing any of the drugs, devices or materials mentioned in this book. This book does not indicate whether a particular treatment is appropriate or suitable for a particular individual. Ultimately it is the sole responsibility of the medical professional to make his or her own professional judgements, so as to advise and treat patients appropriately. The authors and publishers have also attempted to trace the copyright holders of all material reproduced in this publication and apologize to copyright holders if permission to publish in this form has not been obtained. If any copyright material has not been acknowledged please write and let us know so we may rectify in any future reprint.

Except as permitted under U.S. Copyright Law, no part of this book may be reprinted, reproduced, transmitted, or utilized in any form by any electronic, mechanical, or other means, now known or hereafter invented, including photocopying, microfilming, and recording, or in any information storage or retrieval system, without written permission from the publishers.

For permission to photocopy or use material electronically from this work, access www.copyright.com or contact the Copyright Clearance Center, Inc. (CCC), 222 Rosewood Drive, Danvers, MA 01923, 978-750-8400. For works that are not available on CCC please contact mpkbookspermissions@tandf.co.uk

Trademark notice: Product or corporate names may be trademarks or registered trademarks and are used only for identification and explanation without intent to infringe.

Library of Congress Cataloging-in-Publication Data
Names: O'Connell, P. Ronan, editor. | McCaskie, A. W., editor. | Sayers, Robert D., editor.
Title: Bailey & Love's short practice of surgery / edited by Professor P. Ronan O'Connell, Professor Andrew W. McCaskie, Professor Robert D. Sayers.
Other titles: Bailey and Love's short practice of surgery
Description: 28th edition. | Boca Raton : CRC Press, Taylor & Francis Group, 2023. | Includes bibliographical references and index. | Summary: "Bailey & Love is the world famous textbook of surgery. Its comprehensive coverage includes the scientific basis of surgical practice, investigation, diagnosis, and pre-operative care. Trauma and Orthopaedics are included, as are the subspecialties of plastic and reconstructive, head and neck, cardiothoracic and vascular, abdominal and genitourinary surgery. The user-friendly format includes photographs, line diagrams, learning objectives, summary boxes, biographical footnotes, memorable anecdotes and full-colour page design. This book's reputation for unambiguous advice make it the first point of reference for student and practising surgeons worldwide"– Provided by publisher.
Identifiers: LCCN 2022037936 (print) | LCCN 2022037937 (ebook) | ISBN 9780367548117 (paperback) | ISBN 9780367618599 (hardback) | ISBN 9781032301518 (paperback) | ISBN 9781003106852 (ebook)
Subjects: MESH: Surgical Procedures, Operative | Perioperative Care
Classification: LCC RD31 (print) | LCC RD31 (ebook) | NLM WO 500 | DDC 617--dc23/eng/20220819
LC record available at https://lccn.loc.gov/2022037936
LC ebook record available at https://lccn.loc.gov/2022037937

ISBN: 9780367618599 (hbk)
ISBN: 9780367548117 (pbk)
ISBN: 9781003106852 (ebk)
ISBN: 9781032301518 (International Student Edition; restricted territorial availability)

DOI: 10.1201/9781003106852

Typeset in Baskerville MT Std
by Evolution Design & Digital Ltd (Kent), UK

Additional resources available at: www.baileyandlove.tandf.co.uk

Bailey & Love Bailey & Love Bailey & Love
Bailey & Love Bailey & Love Bailey & Love

Contents

Bailey & Love

Digital resources to support your surgical training are available at: www.baileyandlove.tandf.co.uk

Bailey & Love

Digital resources to support your surgical training are available at: www.baileyandlove.tandf.co.uk

PART 10: VASCULAR

PART 11: ABDOMINAL

PART 12: GENITOURINARY

PART 13: TRANSPLANTATION

Bailey & Love

Digital resources to support your surgical training are available at: www.baileyandlove.tandf.co.uk

VIDEOS

Bailey & Love

Digital resources to support your surgical training are available at: www.baileyandlove.tandf.co.uk

Preface to 28th Edition

It is a great privilege to have been entrusted with the responsibility of overseeing the 28th edition of Hamilton Bailey and McNeil Love's *Short Practice of Surgery*. When first published in 1932, almost a century ago, surgery was very different. Then, many surgical procedures, now taken for granted, had not been invented, there were no antibiotics available, and anaesthesia was in its infancy. Endoscopy, cross-sectional imaging, automated biochemical and molecular diagnostics had not been conceived, while open heart surgery, joint replacement and transplantation were still decades away. Yet after 28 editions '*Bailey & Love*' continues to find a place in every medical library. It remains a familiar friend, venerated by generations of medical students and surgeons young and old as a rite of passage and a repository of the core knowledge needed for safe surgical practice. The basic principles of careful history taking, observation, deductive reasoning, technical knowledge and postoperative patient care set out in the first edition, remain the cornerstones of safe clinical practice.

In developing the 28th edition, we have tried to retain the heritage and tradition of this great textbook, while ensuring that every chapter has been revised, and the most up-to-date content has been included in a familiar format, accessible to first time medical student readers while serving as an easy reference source for those more experienced and studying for postgraduate surgical examinations.

Conscious of the need to match content with both undergraduate and postgraduate curriculae, we have made every effort to cover core knowledge, highlighted in summary boxes throughout the text, while more senior readers will find links to supplementary materials online and links to core references and guidelines in the Further Reading sections. Throughout the text, we have endeavoured to highlight where major developments in surgical practice have occurred or are likely to transform surgical practice in the next decade. While surgery retains its prowess as a curative or restorative intervention, it increasingly is part of a multidisciplinary care pathway. Thus, throughout the text, there is particular emphasis on the importance of multidisciplinary team meetings and patient engagement in difficult decision making.

There is no more intense environment than an operating theatre, so how a surgical team interacts is crucial to the outcome for a patient undergoing a surgical procedure. In recent years regulation of medical practice has become tighter. Whereas in certain jurisdictions some may feel that this has become stifling, there is no doubt that regulation is here to stay. Needless to say, we should all be aware of our responsibilities to patients, both morally and ethically, and, although most need no reminding, the law is continually changing as test cases are brought before the courts. Hence, we draw the attention of the reader to the chapters on consent, ethics and the law, patient safety, human factors and quality improvement.

We are very conscious that *Bailey & Love* is popular throughout the world with a substantial readership in India, Nepal, Pakistan, Bangladesh, and Sri Lanka. We have consequently ensured that the 28th edition has an authorship reflective of the readership. Our new authors bring a refreshing enthusiasm and perspective while retaining much of the accumulated wisdom of authors from the 27th and earlier editions. We have worked to create a consistent layout and style of tables, graphics and diagrams. Where appropriate we have included algorithms to assist the reader in understanding patient care pathways. Additional material is included in the Digital Learning Resource, including more detailed descriptions of operative techniques, explanatory videos and hyperlinks to other information sources. We have of course kept the biographical details of individual scientists and practitioners, beloved of readers throughout the generations.

A book as comprehensive as this could never have been completed without the dedication and professionalism of our contributors. They have invariably answered our demands appreciating the responsibility that goes with informing the readership of such a respected and established textbook. We are extremely grateful for all their efforts. In bringing in new contributors, we must also say farewell to many who have contributed to previous editions. We are grateful to them for magnanimously stepping down and making way for 'new blood' and none more so than our previous editor-in-chief Professor Sir Norman Williams who has been an editor since the 22nd edition published in 1997. We thank Sir Norman for his 20-year association with *Bailey & Love* and for his wisdom and guidance. We are delighted to welcome Professor Robert Sayers as our new senior editor and associate editors Mr. Anthony D. Lander (General Paediatrics section), Dr. Anand M. Sardesai (Perioperative Care), Mr. Peter J. Conboy (Head and Neck section) and Professor Prokar Dasgupta (Genitourinary section).

Readers of *Bailey & Love* have always been an integral part of the development of the book over the years and the present editorial group appreciate your feedback, which we know from experience will be forthcoming. Such input is vital if the book is to continue to reach the very high standards expected from each new edition. This has been a labour of love for all of us involved and we do hope it fulfils your needs, no matter whether you are an undergraduate student exploring the exciting world of surgical practice for the first time, a postgraduate trainee studying for exams or an established consultant who wishes to refresh his or her memory.

We wish you all well in your careers no matter which specialty you choose to practise, and we very much hope that the 28th and indeed subsequent editions of *Bailey & Love* accompany you on your travels through this most rewarding of professions.

P. Ronan O'Connell
Andrew W. McCaskie
Robert D. Sayers

Associate Editors

PART 2: GENERAL PAEDIATRICS
Anthony D. Lander PhD FRCSEng (Paed.Surg) MBBS DCH
Consultant Neonatal and Paediatric Surgeon
Birmingham Women's and Children's Hospital
Birmingham, UK

PART 3: PERIOPERATIVE CARE
Anand M. Sardesai MBBS MD DA FRCA
Consultant Anaesthetist
Cambridge University Hospitals NHS Foundation Trust
Cambridge, UK

PART 7: HEAD AND NECK
Peter J. Conboy MBChB(Hons) FRCSEd FRCSEng FRCS(ORL-HNS)
Consultant ENT and Head and Neck Surgeon
Leicester Royal Infirmary
University Hospitals of Leicester
Leicester, UK

PART 12: GENITOURINARY
Prokar Dasgupta MSc MD DLS FRCSEd FRCSEng FRCS(Urol) FEBU FLS FKC
King's Health Partners Professor of Surgery
Chair in Robotic Surgery and Urological Innovation
King's College London
Honorary Consultant Urological Surgeon
Guy's and St Thomas' NHS Foundation Trust
London, UK

Contributors

Richard M. Adamson MBBS FRCS(Ed) MSc DMI
Consultant ENT Surgeon
NHS Lothian
Edinburgh, UK

Muaaze Z. Ahmad MBChB FRCR
Consultant Radiologist
The Royal London Hospital
Barts Health NHS Trust
London, UK

Iain D. Anderson MBE MD FRCS FRACS(Hon)
Consultant General Surgeon
Salford Royal NHS Foundation Trust
Salford
University of Manchester
Manchester, UK

Gnaneswar Atturu MS ChM FRCSEd
Consultant Vascular and Endovascular Surgeon
Hyderabad, Telangana, India

Anita Balakrishnan BMedSci(Hons) BMBS PhD FRCS
Consultant Hepatopancreatobiliary Surgeon
Cambridge University Hospitals NHS Foundation Trust
Cambridge, UK

Anusha Balasubramanian MBBS MRCS MMed(ORL-HNS)
Clinical Fellow
The Royal Marsden NHS Foundation Trust
London
Specialty Registrar
Surrey and Sussex NHS Healthcare Trust
Redhill, UK

Christian M. Becker MD
Associate Professor
University of Oxford
Consultant Gynaecologist and Subspecialist in Reproductive Medicine and Surgery
Oxford University Hospitals NHS Foundation Trust
Oxford, UK

Antonio Belli MD FRCS(Neuro.Surg)
Professor of Trauma Neurosurgery
Director of NIHR Surgical Reconstruction and Microbiology Research Centre
University of Birmingham
Birmingham, UK

Alex M.D. Bennett MBBS DLO FRCS(ORL-HNS) MEd DIC FFST(Ed)
Consultant ENT Surgeon
NHS Lothian
Edinburgh, UK

Sarah L. Benyon BSc(Hons) MBBS(Hons) MRCS FRCS(Plast)
Consultant Plastic and Reconstructive Surgeon
Divisional Director
Cambridge University Hospitals NHS Foundation Trust
Cambridge, UK

Satyajit Bhattacharya LVO MB MS MPhil FRCS
Consultant Hepatopancreatobiliary Surgeon
The London Clinic
London, UK

Catherine L. Boereboom MBChB FRCS PhD
Consultant Colorectal Surgeon
Nottingham University Hospitals NHS Trust
Nottingham, UK

Kenneth D. Boffard MBBCh BSc(Hons)(Aerospace Medicine) FRCS FRCS(Ed) FRCS(Glasg) FCSSA FISS FACS(Hon) MAMSE
Specialist Trauma and Critical Care Surgeon
Professor Emeritus
Department of Surgery
University of the Witwatersrand
Trauma Director and Academic Head
Milpark Hospital Academic Trauma Centre
Johannesburg, South Africa

Peter A. Brennan MD PhD FRCS(Eng) FRCSI FRCS FFST(Ed) FDSRCS
Consultant Oral and Maxillofacial Surgeon
Honorary Professor of Surgery
Portsmouth Hospitals University NHS Trust
Portsmouth, UK

Karim Brohi FRCS FRCA
Consultant Trauma Surgeon
Professor of Trauma Sciences
Barts Health NHS Trust
Queen Mary, University of London
London, UK

Steven R. Brown BMedSci MBChB FRCS MD
Professor of Surgery
University of Sheffield
Sheffield, UK

Harry J.C.J. Bulstrode MA(Cantab) BMBCh(Oxon) PhD FRCS
Fellow in Functional Neurosurgery
National Hospital for Neurology and Neurosurgery
London, UK

Andrew Butler MA MBBChir MChir FRCS
Consultant Transplant Surgeon
Addenbrooke's Hospital
Cambridge University Hospitals NHS Foundation Trust
Cambridge, UK

Gordon L. Carlson CBE BSc(Hons) MBChB(Hons) MD FRCS FRCS(Ed)(Ad Hom)
Consultant General and Colorectal Surgeon and Honorary Professor of Surgery
Salford Royal Hospital
Northern Care Alliance NHS Foundation Trust
Salford, UK

Daniel Carradice MBChB FRCS MD(Hons) PGC Med US(Dist) PGD Health Econ
Senior Lecturer
Hull York Medical School
Consultant Vascular and Endovascular Surgeon
Hull University Teaching Hospitals NHS Trust
Hull, UK

James K.-K. Chan MA DPhil FRCS(Plast)
Consultant Hand, Plastic and Reconstructive Surgeon
Buckinghamshire Healthcare NHS Trust
Aylesbury
University of Oxford
Oxford, UK

Serene H.-L. Chang MBBS FRCA MD(Res)UK
Senior Consultant Anaesthesiology
Ng Teng Fong General Hospital
National University Health System
Singapore

Ian C. Chetter MBChB MD FRCS(Eng) FRCS(Gen. Surg)
Chair of Surgery
Hull York Medical School
University of Hull
Honorary Consultant Vascular Surgeon
Hull University Teaching Hospitals NHS Trust
Hull, UK

Stephen C. Clark MBBS DM FACS FRCP FRCS
Professor of Cardiothoracic Surgery and Transplantation
Freeman Hospital
Newcastle upon Tyne Hospitals NHS Foundation Trust
Newcastle upon Tyne, UK

Jon Clasper CBE DSc DPhil DM FRCS(Ed)(Orth)
Consultant Orthopaedic Surgeon (retired)

J. Calvin Coffey MBBCh BAO BSc PhD FRCSI
Professor of Surgery
Head of Department of Surgery
University of Limerick Hospital Group
Foundation Chair of Surgery
School of Medicine
University of Limerick
Limerick, Ireland

Mark G. Coleman MD FRCS
Consultant Colorectal Surgeon
University Hospitals Plymouth NHS Trust
Plymouth, UK

W. Paul Cool MD FRCS(Ed)(Tr and Orth)
Professor of Orthopaedics
Keele University
Keele
Consultant Orthopaedic Surgeon
The Robert Jones and Agnes Hunt Orthopaedic Hospital NHS Foundation Trust
Oswestry, UK

John R. Crawford MA BSc MBBS FRCS FRCS(Orth)
Consultant Orthopaedic Surgeon
Cambridge University Hospitals NHS Foundation Trust
Cambridge, UK

Lindsay L. Damkat-Thomas FRCSI(Plast) MSc MBBCh BAO
Consultant Burns, Plastic and Reconstructive Surgeon
New Zealand National Burn Centre and Plastic Surgery Department
Middlemore Hospital
Counties Manukau District Health Board
Auckland, New Zealand

Ara Darzi OM PC KBE FMedSci FREng(Hon) FRS
Co-Director of the Institute of Global Health Innovation
Imperial College London
Paul Hamlyn Chair of Surgery
Imperial College Hospital NHS Trust
Consultant Surgeon
Royal Marsden NHS Trust
London, UK

Robert S.M. Davies MBChB MMedSci MD FRCS
Consultant Vascular Surgeon
Leicester Vascular Institute
University Hospitals of Leicester NHS Trust
Leicester, UK

Dan Deakin FRCS(Tr and Orth)
Consultant Orthopaedic Trauma Surgeon
Nottingham University Hospital
Nottingham, UK

Sanjay De Bakshi MBBS MS FRCS(Ed) FRCS(Eng)
Consultant Surgeon
Director
Calcutta Chirurgiae Collective
Kolkata, India

Ashley R. Dennison MBChB MD FRCS
Professor of Hepatobiliary and Pancreatic Surgery
University of Leicester
Consultant Hepatobiliary Surgeon
University of Leicester and Leicester General Hospital
University Hospitals of Leicester NHS Trust
Leicester, UK

Mark F. Devlin FRCS(Ed)(OMFS) FRCS(Ed)(CSiG) FRCS(Glasg) FDSRCPS FFST(Ed) PGDipClinEd(RCPSG) MBChB BDS
Consultant Cleft and Maxillofacial Surgeon
Royal Hospital for Children and Young People/Queen Elizabeth University Hospital Glasgow
Glasgow, UK

Anita Dhar MBBS DNB(Surg) PhD
Professor, Department of Surgical Disciplines
All India Institute of Medical Sciences
New Delhi, India

Barbora East MD PhD FEBS AWS
Consultant General and Abdominal Wall Reconstruction Surgeon
First Faculty of Medicine of Charles University and Motol University Hospital
Prague, Czech Republic

Deborah M. Eastwood MB FRCS
Consultant Orthopaedic Surgeon
Great Ormond Street Hospital for Children NHS Foundation Trust
London
Royal National Orthopaedic Hospital NHS Trust
Stanmore, UK

Tim Eisen BSc MBBChir PhD FRCP FMedSci
Professor of Medical Oncology
University of Cambridge
Addenbrooke's Hospital
Cambridge University Hospitals NHS Foundation Trust
Cambridge, UK
Global Franchise Head Genito-Urinary Oncology, Product Development
Roche

Oussama Elhage MD MD(Res) FRCS(Urol)
Consultant Urological Surgeon
Guy's and St Thomas' NHS Foundation Trust
Honorary Senior Lecturer
Faculty of Life Sciences and Medicine
King's College London
London, UK

Jonathan C. Epstein MD FRCS
Consultant General and Colorectal Surgeon
Salford Royal Hospital
Northern Care Alliance NHS Foundation Trust
Salford, UK

Roger M. Feakins MBBCh BAO BA FRCPI FRCPath MD
Consultant Histopathologist and Honorary Professor of Gastrointestinal Pathology
Royal Free London NHS Foundation Trust
London, UK

Nicola S. Fearnhead BMBCh(Oxon) MA(Cantab) DM(Oxon) FRCS FRCS(Ed) FASCRS
Consultant Colorectal Surgeon
Cambridge University Hospitals NHS Foundation Trust
Cambridge, UK

Joshua Franklyn MS FRCS
Senior Fellow in Colorectal Surgery
University Hospitals Plymouth NHS Trust
Plymouth, UK

Brian J.C. Freeman MBBCh BAO DM(Nott) FRCS(Tr and Orth) FRACS(Ortho) FAOrthA
Professor of Spinal Surgery
University of Adelaide
Head of Spinal Services
Royal Adelaide Hospital
Centre for Orthopaedic and Trauma Research
Adelaide, Australia

Peter J. Friend MA MB MD FRCS FMedSci
Professor of Transplantation
Nuffield Department of Surgical Sciences
University of Oxford
Oxford Transplant Centre
Oxford, UK

Elizabeth Gavens BMBS MPhil FRCS(Paed.Surg)
Consultant Paediatric Surgeon
Sheffield Children's Hospital
Sheffield, UK

Craig H. Gerrand MBChB FRCS(Ed)(Tr and Orth) MD
Consultant Orthopaedic Surgeon
Royal National Orthopaedic Hospital NHS Trust
Stanmore, UK

Peter V. Giannoudis BS MBBS MD PhD FACS FRCS(Eng) FRCS(Glasg)
Professor of Trauma and Orthopaedic Surgery
School of Medicine
University of Leeds
Leeds Teaching Hospitals NHS Trust
Leeds, UK

Rondell P. Graham MBBS
Consultant in Gastrointestinal/Liver and Molecular Pathology
Mayo Clinic
Rochester, MN, USA

William P. Gray MB MD FRCSI FRCS(Neuro.Surg)
Professor of Functional Neurosurgery
University Hospital of Wales
Cardiff, UK

Adam R. Greenbaum MBBS MBA PhD FRCS(Plast) FEBOPRAS FACS
Consultant Plastic Surgeon
Cutting Edge Plastic Surgery
Pukekohe, New Zealand

John E. Greenwood AM BSc(Hons) MBChB MD DHlthSc FRCS(Eng) FRCS(Plast) FRACS
Former Director Adult Burns Service
Royal Adelaide Hospital
Central Adelaide Local Health Network
South Australia

Liam M. Grover BMedSc(Hons) PhD FIMMM
Professor of Biomaterials Science
Director of the Healthcare Technologies Institute
University of Birmingham
Birmingham, UK

Mohan S. Gundeti MD MCh FEBU FRCS(Urol) FEAPU
Pediatric Urologist
The University of Chicago Medicine & Biological Sciences
Director Pediatric Urology
Comer Children's Hospital
Chicago, IL, USA

Abdul Rahman Hakeem FRCS PhD SERF FEBS
Consultant Hepatobiliary Surgery and Liver Transplantation Surgeon
Leeds Liver Unit
St James's University Hospital
Leeds, UK

Robert C. Handley BSc MBChB FRSCS
Consultant Trauma and Orthopaedic Surgeon
Oxford University Hospitals NHS Foundation Trust
Oxford, UK

Leanne Harling MBBS BSc PhD FRCS
Consultant Thoracic Surgeon
Guy's and St Thomas' NHS Foundation Trust
Honorary Lecturer in Surgery
Imperial College London
Honorary Senior Lecturer in Surgery
Kings College London
London, UK

Iain F. Hathorn BSc MBChB DOHNS FRCS(Ed)(ORL-HNS) PGCMEd
Consultant Ear, Nose and Throat Surgeon/Rhinologist and Endoscopic Skull Base Surgeon
Honorary Clinical Senior Lecturer
University of Edinburgh
NHS Lothian
Edinburgh, UK

Douglas S. Hay MBBS FRCS FRCS(Orth)
Consultant Orthopaedic Surgeon
Cambridge University Hospitals NHS Foundation Trust
Cambridge, UK

Octavio Herrera MD
The University of Chicago Pritzker School of Medicine
Chicago, IL, USA

James Hill MBChB FRCS ChM
Clinical Professor of Colorectal Surgery
Manchester Royal Infirmary
Manchester, UK

Shervanthi Homer-Vanniasinkam BSc MD FRCSEd FRCS
Consultant Vascular Surgeon, Leeds General Infirmary
Leeds
Founding Director of EXSEL, University of Leeds Medical School
Leeds
Professor of Surgery (Founding), University of Warwick Medical School
& University Hospitals Coventry and Warwickshire NHS Trust
Warwick
Professor of Engineering and Surgery, University College London, UK
Yeoh Ghim Seng Visiting Professor of Surgery
National University of Singapore
Brahm Prakash Visiting Professor, Indian Institute of Science
Visiting Scholar, Harvard University
Cambridge, MA, USA

Ian Hunt BSc MBBS MRCS FRCS(C-Th)
Consultant Thoracic Surgeon
St George's Hospital NHS Foundation Trust
London, UK

James P. Hunter BSc MBChB MD FRCS
Senior Research Fellow in Transplantation and Consultant Transplant Surgeon
University Hospitals Coventry and Warwickshire
Coventry
Nuffield Department of Surgical Sciences
University of Oxford
Oxford Transplant Centre
Oxford, UK

David G. Jayne BSc MBBCh MD FRCS FASCRS
Bowel Cancer UK/Royal College of Surgeons of England Colorectal Research Chair of Surgery
University of Leeds
Leeds, UK

Nitin Kekre MBBS MS DNB(Urol)
Consultant and Head of Department, Urology
Christian Medical College Vellore and Naruvi Hospital
Vellore, India

Mansoor Ali Khan MBBS PhD MBA FRCS FEBS FACS CMgr FCMI AKC
Consultant Oesophagogastric, General and Trauma Surgeon
Honorary Professor of General Surgery
University Hospitals Sussex
Brighton, UK

Wasim S. Khan MBChB MSc MA(Cantab) PhD FRCS(Tr and Orth)
Associate Professor and Honorary Consultant Orthopaedic Surgeon
Addenbrooke's Hospital
Cambridge University Hospitals NHS Foundation Trust
Cambridge, UK

Vikas Khanduja MA(Cantab) MSc PhD FRCS (Tr and Orth)
Consultant Orthopaedic Surgeon and Research Lead
Addenbrooke's Hospital
Cambridge University Hospitals NHS Foundation Trust
Cambridge, UK

Charles H. Knowles MBBChir PhD FRCS FACCRS(Hon)
Professor of Surgery
Barts and the London School of Medicine and Dentistry
Queen Mary, University of London
London, UK

David A. Koppel MBBS BDS FDSRCS FRCS
Associate Professor
McGill University
Montreal, Canada

Sanjay B. Kulkarni MBBS MS FRCS Dip. Urology
Director
Kulkarni Reconstructive Urology Center
Pune, India

Anant Kumar MBBS MS MCh
Chairman, Urology and Kidney Transplantation
Max Super Speciality Hospitals
Delhi, India

Rajeev Kumar MBBS MS MCh FAMS
Professor of Urology
All India Institute of Medical Sciences
New Delhi, India

Pawanindra Lal MBBS MS DNB FRCS(Ed) FRCS(Glasg) FRCS(Eng) FRCSI FACS FAMS
Director Professor of Surgery
Chairman, Division of Minimal Access Surgery
Maulana Azad Medical College and Associated Lok Nayak Hospital
University of Delhi
Executive Director and CEO
National Board of Examinations in Medical Sciences
New Delhi, India

Anthony D. Lander PhD FRCSEng (Paed.Surg) MBBS DCH
Consultant Neonatal and Paediatric Surgeon
Birmingham Women's and Children's Hospital
Birmingham, UK

Christopher B.D. Lavy MD MCh FCS FRCS
Consultant Spine Surgeon
Oxford University Hospitals NHS Foundation Trust
Professor of Orthopaedics and Tropical Surgery
University of Oxford
Oxford, UK

Simon Y.K. Law MBBChir(Cantab) MA(Cantab) MS(HK) PhD(HK) FRCS(Ed) FCSHK FHKAM(Surg) FACS
Cheung Kung-Hai Professor in Gastrointestinal Surgery
Chair and Chief, Division of Esophageal and Upper Gastrointestinal Surgery
The University of Hong Kong
Pokfulam, Hong Kong

David Limb BSc MBBS FRCS(Ed)(Orth)
Consultant Orthopaedic Surgeon
Leeds Teaching Hospitals NHS Trust
Leeds, UK

Anna-May Long DPhil(PhD) FRCS(Paed.Surg) PGDip MBBS IBSc(Hons)
Consultant Paediatric Surgeon
Cambridge University Hospitals NHS Foundation Trust
Cambridge, UK

Guy J. Maddern MBBS PhD MS MD FRACS
RP Jepson Professor of Surgery
University of Adelaide
Director, Division of Surgery
Consultant Hepatobiliary Surgeon
Head, Department of General Surgery
Head, Upper Gastrointestinal Unit
The Queen Elizabeth Hospital
Woodville, South Australia

Manish D. Mair MBBS MS MCh
Consultant, Head and Neck Surgery
University Hospitals of Leicester NHS Trust
Leicester, UK

Andrew W. McCaskie MMus MD FRCSEng FRCS(Tr and Orth)
Professor of Orthopaedic Surgery and Head of Department of Surgery
University of Cambridge
Honorary Consultant
Addenbrooke's Hospital
Cambridge University Hospitals NHS Foundation Trust
Cambridge, UK

Stephen M. McDonnell MBBS BSc MD MA(Cantab) FRCS(Tr and Orth)
Associate Professor
University of Cambridge
Consultant Orthopaedic Surgeon
Addenbrooke's Hospital
Cambridge University Hospitals NHS Foundation Trust
Cambridge, UK

Martin A. McNally MBBCh BAO MD FRCS(Ed) FRCS(Orth)
King James IV Professor
Consultant in Limb Reconstruction Surgery
The Bone Infection Unit
Nuffield Orthopaedic Centre
Oxford University Hospitals NHS Foundation Trust
Oxford, UK

Deborah A. McNamara MB BAO BCh(Hons) FRCSI MD FRCSI(Gen.Surg)
Vice-President, Royal College of Surgeons in Ireland
Consultant General and Colorectal Surgeon
Clinical Professor and
Co-Lead National Clinical Programme in Surgery
Beaumont Hospital and RCSI University of Medicine and Health Sciences
Dublin, Ireland

Sachin Malde MBBS MSc(Urol) FRCS(Urol)
Consultant Urological Surgeon
Guy's and St Thomas' NHS Foundation Trust
London, UK

Keith R. Martin MA BMBCh DM MRCP FRCOphth FRANZCO FARVO FAAPPO ALCM
Ringland Anderson Professor and Head of Ophthalmology
Director, Centre for Eye Research Australia
University of Melbourne
Melbourne, Australia

Matthew Matson MBBS MRCP FRCR
Director of Imaging
Barts Health NHS Trust
London, UK

Kenneth Mealy MD FRCSI
Consultant Gastrointestinal Surgeon
Co-Lead National Clinical Programme in Surgery
Wexford General Hospital
Wexford
RCSI University of Medicine and Health Sciences
Dublin, Ireland

Vivek Mehta MBBS FRCA MD FFPMRCA
Consultant in Pain Medicine
St Bartholomew's Hospital
Barts Health NHS Trust
Honorary Senior Lecturer
Queen Mary, University of London
London, UK

John K. Mellon MD FRCS(Urol)
Consultant Urological Surgeon
University Hospitals of Leicester NHS Trust
Leicester, UK

Peter J. Millett MD MSc
Shoulder, Knee, Elbow and Sports Medicine Surgeon
The Steadman Clinic and Steadman Philippon Research Institute
Vail, CO, USA

Monica Mittal BSc MBBS MRCOG MD
Consultant Gynaecologist and Subspecialist in Reproductive Medicine
St Mary's Hospital
Imperial College Healthcare NHS Trust
London, UK

Chris Moran MD FRCS(Ed)
National Clinical Director for Trauma
NHS England
Professor of Orthopaedic Trauma Surgery
Nottingham University Hospital
Nottingham, UK

Jürgen Mulsow MD FRCSI
Consultant Colorectal, Peritoneal Malignancy and General Surgeon
National Centre for Peritoneal Malignancy
Mater Misericordiae University Hospital
Dublin, Ireland

Deepa Nair MBBS MS DNB
Consultant, Head and Neck Services
Tata Memorial Hospital
Mumbai, India

Michael L. Nicholson MD DSc FRCS
Professor of Transplant Surgery
University of Cambridge
Cambridge, UK

Iain J. Nixon MBChB FRCS(ORL-HNS) PhD
Consultant ENT Surgeon
NHS Lothian
Edinburgh, UK

Karen P. Nugent MA MS MEd FRCS(Eng)
Consultant Colorectal Surgeon
University of Southampton
Southampton, UK

John Edward O'Connell BDS FFD(OSOM) RCSI MB BA BCh BAO FRCSI(OMFS)
Consultant in Oral and Maxillofacial/Head and Neck Surgery
National Maxillofacial Unit
St James Hospital
Dublin, Ireland

P. Ronan O'Connell BA MD FRCSI FRCSGlasg FRCSEd FRCSEng (Hon) FCSHK (Hon)
President, Royal College of Surgeons in Ireland
President, European Surgical Association
Emeritus Professor of Surgery
University College Dublin
Dublin, Ireland

Prathamesh Pai MBBS MS DNB
Consultant, Head and Neck Service
Tata Memorial Hospital
Mumbai, India

Vinidh Paleri MBBS MS FRCS FRCS(ORL-HNS)
Consultant Head and Neck Surgeon
The Royal Marsden NHS Foundation Trust
Professor of Head and Neck Surgery
The Institute of Cancer Research
London, UK

Hemant G. Pandit MBBS FRCS(Tr and Orth) DPhil(Oxon)
Honorary Consultant Orthopaedic Surgeon
Chapel Allerton Hospital
Leeds Teaching Hospitals NHS Trust
Professor of Orthopaedic Surgery
University of Leeds
Leeds, UK

Phill Pearce MBBS PhD FRCS
Registrar in General Surgery
Barts Health NHS Trust
London, UK

Thomas D. Pinkney MBChB MMedEd MD FRCS
George Drexler and Royal College of Surgeons Chair of Surgical Trials
University of Birmingham
Honorary Consultant Colorectal Surgeon
University Hospitals Birmingham
Birmingham, UK

Andrew J. Porteous MBChB(UCT) DipPEC(SA) FRCS(Ed) MSc(Ortho Engin) FRCS(Tr and Orth)
Consultant Orthopaedic Knee Surgeon
North Bristol NHS Trust
Bristol, UK

Dimitri J. Pournaras PhD FRCS
Consultant Upper Gastrointestinal and Bariatric Surgeon
Department of Bariatric/Metabolic Surgery
Southmead Hospital
North Bristol NHS Trust
Bristol, UK

Niall Power MRCPI FRCR
Consultant Radiologist
Barts Health NHS Trust
London, UK

Ramkrishna Y. Prabhu MBBS MS DNBE(Surg Gastroenterol) FICS
Associate Professor, Surgical Gastroenterology
Seth G S Medical College and K E M Hospital
Mumbai, India

Ruth S. Prichard MB BAO BCh MCh FRCSI
Consultant Endocrine and Breast Surgeon
St Vincent's University Hospital
Dublin, Ireland

John N. Primrose MD FRCS(Glasg) FRCS(Eng) FRCS(Ed) FMedSci
Professor of Surgery
University of Southampton and University Hospital Southampton NHS Foundation Trust
Southampton, UK

Aaron J. Quyn MBChB PhD FRCS
Associate Clinical Professor/Honorary Consultant Surgeon
University of Leeds
St James's Hospital
Leeds, UK

Rohit Rao MBBS BSc MRCP
Consultant Gastroenterologist
The Royal London Hospital
Barts Health NHS Trust
London, UK

Mamoon Rashid SE MBBS FRCS(Eng) FCPS(Pak)
Professor of Plastic Surgery
STM University
Section Head and Programme Director
Department of Plastic Surgery
Shifa International Hospital
Islamabad, Pakistan

Jaikirty Rawal MBBS MA FRCS(Tr and Orth)
Consultant Trauma and Orthopaedic Surgeon
Addenbrooke's Hospital
Cambridge University Hospitals NHS Foundation Trust
Cambridge, UK

Zeeshan Razzaq MCh FRCSI(Gen.Surg) FRCS(Eng) FEBS
Cork University Hospital
University College Cork
Cork, Ireland

H. Paul Redmond MCh FRCSI FRCSI(Gen.Surg) FRCS(Eng) FRCS(Glasg)(Hon) FACS
Professor of Surgery
Cork University Hospital
University College Cork
Cork, Ireland

Mohamed Rela MS FRCS DSc
Professor, Chairman and Managing Director
Institute of Liver Disease and Transplantation
Dr. Rela Institute and Medical Centre
Chennai, India

Nobhojit Roy MS(Gen.Surg) MPH PhD
Formerly Professor and Head
WHO Collaborating Centre for Research in Surgical Care Delivery in Low and Middle Income Countries
Department of Surgery
BARC Hospital
HBNI University
Mumbai
The George Institute of Global Health
New Delhi, India

David A. Russell MB ChB MD FRCS (Gen.Surg)
Consultant Vascular Surgeon
Leeds Vascular Institute
Leeds General Infirmary
Leeds, UK

Neil Russell BSc(Hons) MBBChir MChir FRCS
Consultant Transplant Surgeon
Addenbrooke's Hospital
Cambridge University Hospitals NHS Foundation Trust
Cambridge, UK

Kim E. Russon MBChB FRCA
Consultant Anaesthetist and Clinical Lead for Day Surgery
The Rotherham NHS Foundation Trust
Rotherham, UK

Joseph J. Ruzbarsky MD
Shoulder, Knee, Elbow and Hip Preservation Surgeon
The Steadman Clinic and Steadman Philippon Research Institute
Vail, CO, USA

Anand M. Sardesai MBBS MD DA FRCA
Consultant Anaesthetist
Cambridge University Hospitals NHS Foundation Trust
Cambridge, UK

Andrew Schache PhD BDS MBChB(Hons) FDSRCS FRCS(OMFS)
Reader in Head and Neck Surgery
Department of Molecular and Clinical Cancer Medicine
Institute of Systems, Molecular and Integrative Biology
The University of Liverpool Cancer Research Centre
Consultant in Oral and Maxillofacial/Head and Neck Surgery
Liverpool Head and Neck Centre
Liverpool University Hospitals NHS Foundation Trust
Liverpool, UK

David M. Scott-Coombes MBBS FRCS MS FEBS
Consultant Endocrine Surgeon
University Hospital of Wales
Cardiff, UK

Dhananjaya Sharma MBBS MS PhD DSc FRCS(Glasg) FRCSI FRCS(Ed) FRCS(Eng) FCLS(Hon) FRCST(Hon)
Honorary Member Académie Nationale de Chirurgie France
Professor and Head, Department of Surgery
NSCB Government Medical College
Jabalpur, India

Bob Sharp BMBCh(Oxon) MA(Cantab) FRCS(Tr and Orth)
Consultant Orthopaedic Surgeon
Nuffield Orthopaedic Centre
Oxford University Hospitals NHS Foundation Trust
Oxford, UK

Rabindra P. Singh MBChB(Hons) BDS MFDSRCS FHEA FRCS(Eng)
Consultant Maxillofacial/Head and Neck Surgeon
University Hospital Southampton NHS Foundation Trust
Southampton, UK

Anurag Srivastava MBBS MS FRCS(Ed) PhD MPH
Retired Professor and Head, Department of Surgical Disciplines
All India Institute of Medical Sciences
New Delhi, India

Michael J. Stechman MBChB MD FRCS(Gen.Surg)
Consultant Endocrine Surgeon
University Hospital of Wales
Cardiff, UK

Grant D. Stewart BSc MBChB PhD(Ed) MA(Cantab) FRCS(Ed)(Urol)
Professor of Surgical Oncology
Department of Surgery
University of Cambridge
Honorary Consultant Urological Surgeon
Department of Urology
Addenbrooke's Hospital
Cambridge University Hospitals NHS Foundation Trust
Cambridge, UK

Suhani Suhani MBBS MS DNB MRCS(Ed) FACS
Additional Professor, Department of Surgical Disciplines
All India Institute of Medical Sciences
New Delhi, India

Karadi H. Sunil Kumar MBBS MCh(Orth) MFSEM MFST(Ed) FEBOT FRCS(Ed)(Tr and Orth)
Consultant Orthopaedic Surgeon
Addenbrooke's Hospital
Cambridge University Hospitals NHS Foundation Trust
Cambridge, UK

Avinash N. Supe MBBS MS FICS DNBE MHPE
Emeritus Professor, Surgical Gastroenterology
Seth G S Medical College and K E M Hospital
Mumbai, India

Prasanna R. Supramaniam MBChB MSc MRCOG MAcadMEd
Consultant Gynaecologist and Subspecialist in Reproductive Medicine and Surgery
Oxford University Hospitals NHS Foundation Trust
Oxford, UK

Marc C. Swan DPhil FRCS(Plast)
Consultant Plastic and Reconstructive Surgeon
Oxford University Hospitals NHS Foundation Trust
Oxford, UK

Carol Tan MBChB MRCS FRCS(C-Th)
Consultant Thoracic Surgeon
St George's Hospital NHS Foundation Trust
London, UK

Amy J. Thomas MBChB FRCA
Consultant Anaesthetist
Rotherham NHS Foundation Trust
Rotherham, UK

Bruce R. Tulloh MB MS FRCS
Consultant General Surgeon
Royal Infirmary of Edinburgh
Edinburgh, UK

Timothy J. Underwood PhD FRCS(Eng)
Professor of Gastrointestinal Surgery
University of Southampton and University Hospital Southampton NHS Foundation Trust
Southampton, UK

Lee Van Rensburg MBBCh FRCS(Tr and Orth)
Consultant Orthopaedic Surgeon
Addenbrooke's Hospital
Cambridge University Hospitals NHS Foundation Trust
Cambridge, UK

Samuel R. Vollans BSc MBChB FRCS(Orth)
Consultant Trauma and Orthopaedic Surgeon
Leeds Teaching Hospitals NHS Trust
Leeds, UK

Richard Welbourn MD FRCS
Consultant Upper Gastrointestinal and Bariatric Surgeon
Department of Upper Gastrointestinal and Bariatric Surgery
Musgrove Park Hospital
Somerset NHS Foundation Trust
Taunton, UK

Malcolm A. West MD PhD FRCS(Eng)
Consultant Colorectal Surgeon
University of Southampton
Southampton, UK

Robert Wheeler FRCS MS LLB(Hons) LLM
Consultant Paediatric and Neonatal Surgeon
Director, Department of Clinical Law
University Hospital Southampton NHS Foundation Trust
Southampton, UK

Birgit Whitman PhD
Head of Research Governance and Integrity
University of Birmingham
Birmingham, UK

Ian Y.H. Wong MBBS(HK) FRCS(Ed)(Gen.Surg) FCSHK FHKAM(Surg) FACS
Clinical Assistant Professor
Division of Esophageal and Upper Gastrointestinal Surgery
The University of Hong Kong
Pokfulam, Hong Kong

Kai Yuen Wong MA MBBChir FHEA FRSPH FRCS(Plast)
Consultant Plastic and Reconstructive Surgeon
Cambridge University Hospitals NHS Foundation Trust
Cambridge, UK

Philip Woodland MBBS PhD FRCP
Consultant Gastroenterologist
The Royal London Hospital
Barts Health NHS Trust
London, UK

Tet L. Yap MBBChir MA MD FRCS FEBU
Consultant Uro-Andrological Surgeon and Honorary Reader in Urology
Guy's and St Thomas' NHS Foundation Trust and King's College Hospital NHS Foundation Trust
London, UK

Mustafa Zakkar PhD FRCS(C-Th)
Associate Professor
Department of Cardiovascular Sciences
University of Leicester
Honorary Consultant Cardiac Surgeon
Glenfield Hospital
Leicester, UK

Authors Emeritus from the 27th Edition

Derek Alderson
Gina Allen
Jonathan R. Anderson
Hutan Ashrafian
John Andrew Bradley
Christopher L.H. Chan
Kevin C.P. Conlon
Pradip K. Datta
Elias Degiannis
Ian Eardley
Michael John Earley
Jonothan J. Earnshaw
Hiba Fatayer
Pierre Foex
O. James Garden
Sudip J. Ghosh
Fay Gilder
Tim Goodacre
Freddie C. Hamdy
Ian Jackson
Terry M. Jones
Robert P. Jones
Frank B.V. Keane
Peter Lamont
Tom W.J. Lennard
James O. Lindsay
John MacFie
Philippa C. Matthews
Mark McGurk
Douglas McWhinnie
Alastair Munro
David E. Neal
Stephen J. Nixon
Alan Norrish
Graeme J. Poston
Richard C. Sainsbury
Greg Shaw
William P. Smith
Mattias Soop
Robert J.C. Steele
Michael P.H. Tyler
Madha Vanarase-Pandit
Leandros-Vassilios F. Vassiliou

Acknowledgements

In this day and age, it is impossible to produce a book like Bailey and Love without the contribution of numerous individuals. Although it is impractical to mention all those who have played a part in producing the 28th Edition, it would be remiss not to express our gratitude to all those who have made significant contributions in previous editions.

Chapter 1, *Metabolic response to injury*, contains some material from *Metabolic response to injury* by the late Kenneth Fearon. The material has been revised and updated by the current author.

Chapter 3, *Wound healing and tissue repair*, contains some material from *Wounds, healing and tissue repair* by Michael John Earley. The material has been revised and updated by the current authors.

Chapter 4, *Tissue engineering and regenerative therapies*, contains some material from *Tissue engineering and regeneration* by John Andrew Bradley. The material has been revised and updated by the current authors.

Chapter 5, *Surgical infection*, contains some material from *Surgical infection* by Peter Lamont. The material has been revised and updated by the current authors.

Chapter 6, *Tropical infections and infestations*, contains some material from *Tropical infections and infestations* by Pradip K. Datta. The material has been revised and updated by the current authors.

Chapter 9, *Gastrointestinal endoscopy*, contains some material from *Gastrointestinal endoscopy* by James O. Lindsay. The material has been revised and updated by the current authors.

Chapter 10, *Principles of minimal access surgery*, contains some material from *Principles of laparoscopic and robotic surgery* by Hutan Ashrafian. The material has been revised and updated by the current authors.

Chapter 12, *Principles of oncology*, contains some material from *Principles of oncology* by Robert J.C. Steele and Alastair Munro. The material has been revised and updated by the current authors.

Chapter 13, *Surgical audit and research*, contains some material from *Surgical audit and research* by Jonothan J. Earnshaw. The material has been revised and updated by the current authors.

Chapter 15, *Human factors, patient safety and quality improvement*, contains some material from *Human factors, patient safety and quality improvement* by Frank B.V. Keane. The material has been revised and updated by the current authors.

Chapter 16, *Global health and surgery*, contains some material from *Appendix 2: Fundamental principles in the operating theatre and the importance of global health* by Alan Norrish. The material has been revised and updated by the current authors.

Chapter 21, *Preoperative care including the high-risk surgical patient*, contains some material from *Preoperative care including the high-risk surgical patient* by Madha Vanarase-Pandit, Pierre Foex and Anand Sardesai. The material has been revised and updated by the current author.

Chapter 22, *Day case surgery*, contains some material from *Day case surgery* by Douglas McWhinnie and Ian Jackson. The material has been revised and updated by the current author.

Chapter 24, *Postoperative care*, contains some material from *Postoperative care* by Fay Gilder. The material has been revised and updated by the current authors.

Chapter 25, *Nutrition and fluid therapy*, contains some material from *Nutrition and fluid therapy* by John MacFie. The material has been revised and updated by the current author.

Chapter 29, *Torso and pelvic trauma*, contains some material from *Torso trauma* by Elias Degiannis. The material has been revised and updated by the current authors.

Chapter 31, *Maxillofacial trauma*, contains some material from *Maxillofacial trauma* by David A. Koppel. The material has been revised and updated by the current authors.

Chapter 36, *Sports medicine and sports injuries*, contains some material from *Sports medicine and sports injuries* by Gina Allen. The material has been revised and updated by the current authors.

Chapter 43, *Infection of the bones and joints*, contains some material from *Infection of the bones and joints* by Philippa C. Matthews. The material has been revised and updated by the current author.

Chapter 45, *Skin and subcutaneous tissue*, contains some material from *Skin and subcutaneous tissue* by Christopher L.H. Chan. The material has been revised and updated by the current author.

Chapter 46, *Burns*, contains some material from *Burns* by Michael P.H. Tyler and Sudip J. Ghosh. The material has been revised and updated by the current authors.

Chapter 47, *Plastic and reconstructive surgery*, contains some material from *Plastic and reconstructive surgery* by Tim

Goodacre. The material has been revised and updated by the current authors.

Chapter 50, *Developmental abnormalities of the face, mouth and jaws: cleft lip and palate*, contains some material from *Cleft lip and palate: developmental abnormities of the face, mouth and jaws* by William P. Smith. The material has been revised and updated by the current authors.

Chapter 51, *The ear, nose and sinuses*, contains some material from *The ear, nose and sinuses* by Iain J. Nixon. The material has been revised and updated by the current authors.

Chapter 52, *The pharynx, larynx and neck*, contains some material from *Pharynx, larynx and neck* by Terry M. Jones. The material has been revised and updated by the current authors.

Chapter 53, *Oral cavity cancer*, contains some material from *Oral cavity malignancy* by William P. Smith. The material has been revised and updated by the current authors.

Chapter 54, *Disorders of the salivary glands*, contains some material from *Disorders of the salivary glands* by William P. Smith, Mark McGurk and Leandros-Vassilios F. Vassiliou. The material has been revised and updated by the current authors.

Chapter 57, *The adrenal glands and other abdominal endocrine disorders*, contains some material from *The adrenal glands and other abdominal endocrine disorders* by Tom W.J. Lennard. The material has been revised and updated by the current authors.

Chapter 58, *The breast*, contains some material from *The breast* by Richard C. Sainsbury. The material has been revised and updated by the current authors.

Chapter 59, *Cardiac surgery*, contains some material from *Cardiac surgery* by Jonathan R. Anderson. The material has been revised and updated by the current author.

Chapter 61, *Arterial disorders*, contains some material from *Arterial disorders* by Rob Sayers. The material has been revised and updated by the current author.

Chapter 62, *Venous and lymphatic disorders*, contains some material from *Lymphatic disorders* by Gnaneswar Atturu, David A. Russell and Shervanthi Homer-Vanniasinkam. The material has been revised and updated by the current authors.

Chapter 63, *History and examination of the abdomen*, contains some material from *History and examination of the abdomen* by P. Ronan O'Connell. The material has been revised and updated by the current author.

Chapter 64, *The abdominal wall, hernia and umbilicus*, contains some material from *Abdominal wall, hernia and umbilicus* by Stephen J. Nixon. The material has been revised and updated by the current authors.

Chapter 65, *The peritoneum, mesentery, greater omentum and retroperitoneal space*, contains some material from *The peritoneum, omentum, mesentery and retroperitoneal space* by Charles H. Knowles. The material has been revised and updated by the current author.

Chapter 66, *The oesophagus*, contains some material from *The oesophagus* by Derek Alderson. The material has been revised and updated by the current authors.

Chapter 69, *The liver*, contains some material from *The liver* by Robert P. Jones and Graeme J. Poston. The material has been revised and updated by the current authors.

Chapter 70, *The spleen*, contains some material from *The spleen* by O. James Garden. The material has been revised and updated by the current author.

Chapter 71, *The gallbladder and bile ducts*, contains some material from *The gallbladder and bile ducts* by Kevin C.P. Conlon. The material has been revised and updated by the current authors.

Chapter 74, *The small intestine*, contains some material from *The small intestine* by Mattias Soop. The material has been revised and updated by the current authors.

Chapter 77, *The large intestine*, contains some material from *The large intestine* by Gordon Lawrence Carlson and Jonathan Epstein. The material has been revised and updated by the current authors.

Chapter 79, *The rectum*, contains some material from *The rectum* by Hiba Fatayer. The material has been revised and updated by the current authors.

Chapter 82, *The kidney and ureter*, contains some material from *Kidneys and ureters* by J. Kilian Mellon. The material has been revised and updated by the current author.

Chapter 83, *The urinary bladder*, contains some material from *The urinary bladder* by Freddie C. Hamdy. The material has been revised and updated by the current author.

Chapter 84, *The prostate and seminal vesicles*, contains some material from *The prostate and seminal vesicles* by David E. Neal and Greg Shaw. The material has been revised and updated by the current authors.

Chapter 85, *The urethra and penis*, contains some material from *Urethra and penis* by Ian Eardley. The material has been revised and updated by the current author.

Chapter 86, *The testis and scrotum*, contains some material from *Testis and scrotum* by Ian Eardley. The material has been revised and updated by the current author.

Part 13: Transplantation, contains some material from *Transplantation* by John Andrew Bradley. The material has been split into subsections, revised and updated by the current authors.

PART 1 | Basic principles

CHAPTER

1 Metabolic response to injury

Learning objectives

To understand:

- How the body responds to accidental injury and surgery
- Physiological and biochemical changes that occur during injury and recovery
- Mediators and pathways of the metabolic response to injury
- Avoidable factors that compound the metabolic response to injury
- How the metabolic response to injury influences surgical outcomes
- Concepts behind optimal perioperative care

INTRODUCTION

As surgeons we are inextricably linked with tissue injury and its effects, both from the damage which operating inevitably causes and from the treatment of accidental traumatic injury. The body responds to significant local tissue injury, whether surgical or accidental, with a series of systemic changes which affect the functions of vital organs. This surgical stress response is brought about by several pathways involving hormones, inflammation-related cytokines and neural circuits. It leads to alterations in body metabolism, wound healing and immunity and in the function of specific organs. These changes are known collectively as the metabolic response to injury. While these responses are designed to limit damage and begin repair processes, not all the effects are beneficial by any means. They can lead to complications, especially sepsis, which can then amplify and prolong the abnormal processes and lead to or prolong multiple organ dysfunction syndrome (MODS). Given that these metabolic effects of injury can have a significant impact on recovery and survival from many types of surgery and surgical illness, surgeons require an understanding of them in order to care optimally for their patients. Successful management of the metabolic response improves outcomes and forms the basis of modern perioperative care after major surgery as well as the treatment of severely injured and septic patients. This chapter will look primarily at the metabolic responses to injury while shock, fluid balance, sepsis and nutrition are covered in greater depth in *Chapters 2 and 25.*

Homeostasis

Homeostasis is the concept of maintaining a constant internal environment that allows cellular processes to function optimally. Many aspects of surgery, trauma and injury affect homeostasis and can lead to organ dysfunction. Traditionally the metabolic response to injury is divided into an initial period of catabolism (which may include a period of shock) followed by an anabolic phase of repair and tissue healing.

The catabolic phase begins at the time of injury and is characterised by hypovolaemia, decreased basal metabolic rate, reduced cardiac output, hypothermia and lactic acidosis. The main physiological role of this phase is to conserve both circulating volume and energy stores and thus maximise survival chances for future recovery. A series of neurohormonal responses accompany these effects and trigger a systemic inflammatory response syndrome (SIRS), where body stores are mobilised for recovery and repair. The catabolic effects include muscle breakdown, weight loss and hyperglycaemia, which themselves increase the risk of complications, especially sepsis. As the catabolic phase subsides, an anabolic (rebuilding) phase develops, which may last for weeks if extensive recovery and repair are required following serious injury.

Modern surgical care

The role of surgical critical care, including resuscitation and/or organ support, must be to work alongside the metabolic effects of injury while the patient is restored to a situation from which homeostatic mechanisms can achieve a return to normality. The systemic effects of injury still impact heavily on survival and complications through loss of muscle mass, sepsis and MODS. In fact, modern treatment of major trauma can now be so successful that the great majority of hospital deaths in developed countries occur after some days as a result of complex physiological processes, rather than as a direct and rapid consequence of organ damage or blood loss, although it is the initial injury and blood loss that sets the scene for the later systemic effects. Parallel with the catabolic effects introduced above, inflammatory-type processes cause immune suppression. While this inflammation is often initially sterile, the nature of surgery and injury predisposes to infection and sepsis. Impaired immunity as part of the metabolic response compounds this risk and explains why sepsis and MODS/failure is a key part of perioperative care and a leading mode of death among our patients. Even in modern trauma systems, MODS carries a mortality of around 25%.

As a consequence of modern understanding of the metabolic response to injury, elective surgical practice now seeks to actively reduce the need for a homeostatic response by minimising the primary insult via minimal access surgery and by 'stress-free' perioperative care or enhanced recovery after surgery (ERAS). This chapter will review the mediators of the stress response, the physiological and biochemical pathway changes associated with surgical injury and the changes in body composition that occur following surgical injury. Emphasis is placed on why knowledge of these events is important to understand the rationale for modern 'stress-free' perioperative and critical care.

Summary box 1.1

Basic concepts

- Homeostasis is the foundation of normal physiology
- 'Stress-free' perioperative care helps to preserve homeostasis following elective surgery
- Resuscitation, surgical intervention and critical care can return the severely injured patient to a situation in which homeostasis becomes possible once again
- The metabolic response to surgery influences these processes profoundly, particularly through catabolic effects, MODS and impaired immunity

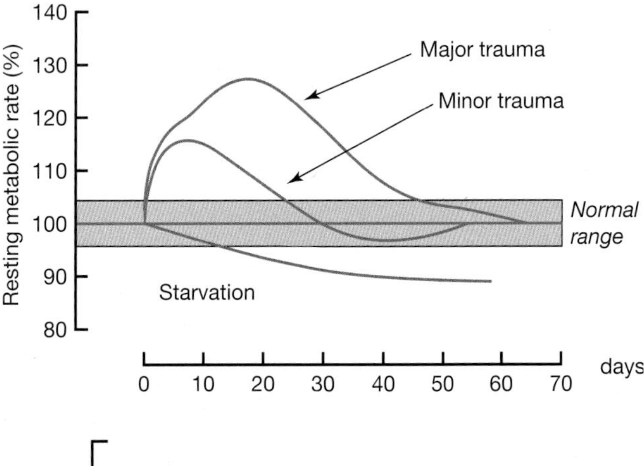

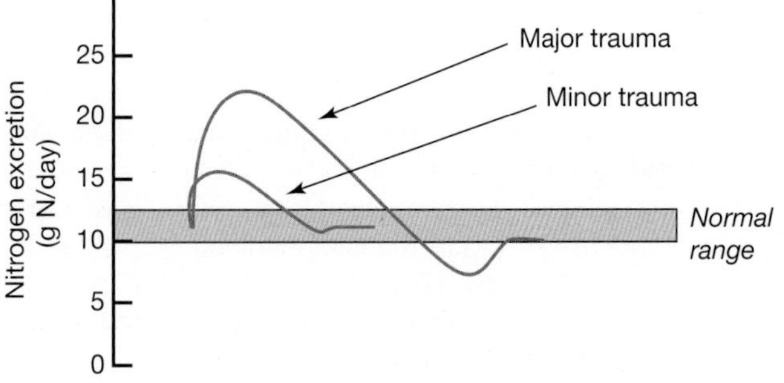

Figure 1.1 Hypermetabolism and increased nitrogen excretion are closely related to the magnitude of the initial injury and show a graded response.

THE MAGNITUDE OF THE INJURY RESPONSE

It is important to recognise that, in general or population terms, the metabolic response to injury is graded: the more severe the injury, the greater the response (***Figure 1.1***). This concept applies not only to physiological and metabolic changes but also to immunological changes and other sequelae. Thus, following major elective surgery, there may be a transient and modest rise in temperature, heart rate, respiratory rate, energy expenditure and peripheral white cell count. Following major trauma, emergency surgery, sepsis or burns, these changes are accentuated, resulting in SIRS, with hypermetabolism, marked catabolism, shock and even MODS. However, genetic variability also plays a key role in determining the intensity of the inflammatory response, with some individual patients responding much more dramatically than others to apparently similar conditions.

MEDIATORS OF THE METABOLIC RESPONSE TO INJURY

Tissue damage and inflammation

Tissue injury is sensed in several ways. Tissue damage causes the release of cellular and other molecular fragments known as damage-associated molecular patterns (DAMPs) or alarmins. These DAMPs are sensed by pattern recognition receptors (PRRs), such as Toll-like receptors and NOD-like receptors (or nucleotide-binding leucine-rich repeat receptors) on cells of the innate immune system, which includes macrophages, neutrophils and dendritic cells. These cells are attracted and activated, triggering the formation of complex intracellular proteins known as inflammasomes. This results in the activation of caspases; these are enzymes that, in turn, activate key inflammatory cytokines including interleukin-1 (IL-1), IL-6 and many others. PRR activation also leads to release of tumour necrosis factor alpha (TNF), interferons, chemokines and other mediators. Thus begins a sterile systemic inflammatory cascade that leads to local inflammation and, when sufficiently severe, to a clinically detectable SIRS. Once activated by DAMPs, inflammasomes also contribute to cell death, tissue damage and immune suppression. DAMPs can activate inflammasome formation in endothelial cells and platelets, resulting in leaky capillaries and coagulopathy; these are changes that can result in the production of more DAMPs owing to local ischaemia from microcirculatory effects. Local inflammation begins the process of tissue repair but SIRS, when uncontrolled or prolonged, becomes a risk factor for acute kidney injury, acute lung injury and coagulopathy, and hence for MODS and organ failure. Within the injured brain, secondary brain injury can occur.

DAMPs thought to be important in tissue trauma include heat shock proteins, high mobility group protein B1 (HMGB1), S100 proteins and fragments of nucleic acids. Commonly, DAMPs can activate several different receptors and pathways. This crossover, or redundancy as it is termed, is a characteristic of inflammation and has been one of the barriers to developing effective therapeutic blockade of these mechanisms. Furthermore, DAMPs can be self-perpetuated during the complicated course of a surgical critical illness, amplifying and prolonging the inflammatory process and related organ dysfunction. Triggers to further release of DAMPs include sepsis, haemorrhage, massive transfusion, acidosis, surgery, crush syndrome and ischaemia–reperfusion. Thus the secondary insults of delayed or ineffective treatment of complications such as ongoing bleeding, ischaemia or sepsis will tend to maintain and amplify the inflammatory process and its resulting immune dysfunction. This can become a prolonged or self-perpetuating process (***Table 1.1***).

Summary box 1.2

Neuroendocrine response to injury/critical illness

The neuroendocrine response to severe injury/critical illness is biphasic:

- **Acute phase** (hours) characterised by elevated counter-regulatory hormones (cortisol, glucagon, adrenaline). Changes are thought to be beneficial for short-term survival
- **Chronic phase** (days) associated with hypothalamic suppression and low serum levels of the respective target organ hormones. Changes may contribute to chronic wasting

TABLE 1.1 Some secondary triggers of the metabolic response to injury.

Secondary triggers of inflammatory pathways in trauma and surgery
• Sepsis
• Haemorrhage
• Massive transfusion
• Acidosis
• Surgery
• Crush syndrome
• Ischaemia–reperfusion
These events can amplify or prolong the catabolic phase, leading to organ failure or immune dysfunction.

Neuroendocrine response to injury

Patients also respond rapidly to injury by the classical neuroendocrine pathways of the stress response, consisting of afferent nociceptive neurones, the spinal cord, thalamus, hypothalamus and pituitary (***Figure 1.2***). Nociceptive neurones are excited by the effects of local inflammation as well as by direct injury. The neurones terminate in the hypothalamus and release corticotropin-releasing factor (CRF). CRF stimulates adrenocorticotropic hormone (ACTH) release from the anterior pituitary, which then acts on the adrenals to increase the secretion of cortisol within hours of injury. Hypothalamic activation of the sympathetic nervous system causes release of adrenaline (epinephrine) and also stimulates release of glucagon. An intravenous infusion of a cocktail of these 'counter-regulatory' hormones (glucagon, glucocorticoids and catecholamines) reproduces many aspects of the metabolic response to injury. The metabolic effects of the acute rise in the levels of these hormones is to liberate glucose from carbohydrate stores and to begin the breakdown of fat and protein as metabolic substrates for energy and repair. There are, however, many other effects, including alterations in insulin release and sensitivity, hypersecretion of prolactin and growth hormone (GH) in the presence of low circulatory insulin-like growth factor-1 (IGF-1) and inactivation of peripheral thyroid hormones and gonadal function. Of note, GH has direct lipolytic, insulin-antagonising and proinflammatory properties.

As described above, the innate immune system (principally macrophages), once activated by DAMPs, interacts in a complex manner with the adaptive immune system (T cells, B cells) in co-generating the metabolic response to injury (***Figure 1.2***). Proinflammatory cytokines including IL-1, TNF alpha (TNFα), IL-6 and IL-8 are produced within the first 24 hours and act directly on the hypothalamus to cause pyrexia. Such cytokines also augment the hypothalamic stress response and act directly on skeletal muscle to induce proteolysis while inducing acute-phase protein production in the liver. Proinflammatory cytokines also play a complex role in the development of peripheral insulin resistance. Other important proinflammatory mediators include nitric oxide ([NO] via inducible nitric oxide synthetase [iNOS]) and a variety of prostanoids (via cyclooxygenase-2 [Cox-2]). Changes in organ function (e.g. renal hypoperfusion/impairment) may be induced by excessive vasoconstriction via endogenous factors such as endothelin-1. Complement and kinin pathways are also activated and processes of programmed cell death and phagocytosis are triggered to clear damaged tissues.

There are many complex interactions among the neuroendocrine, cytokine and metabolic axes. For example, although cortisol is immunosuppressive at high levels, it acts synergistically with IL-6 to promote the hepatic acute-phase response. ACTH release is enhanced by proinflammatory cytokines and the noradrenergic system. The resulting rise in cortisol levels may form a weak feedback loop, attempting to limit the proinflammatory stress response. Finally, hyperglycaemia may aggravate the inflammatory response in the mitochondria, causing the formation of excess oxygen free radicals and also altering gene expression to enhance cytokine production.

At the molecular level, the changes that accompany systemic inflammation are extremely complex. In one study using network-based analysis of changes in mRNA expression in leukocytes following exposure to endotoxin, there were changes in the expression of more than 3700 genes, with over half showing decreased expression and the remainder increased expression. The cell surface receptors, signalling mechanisms and transcription factors that initiate these events are also complex. Although the detailed mechanisms are being steadily identified, specific molecular therapies remain elusive and certainly subservient to optimal clinical care.

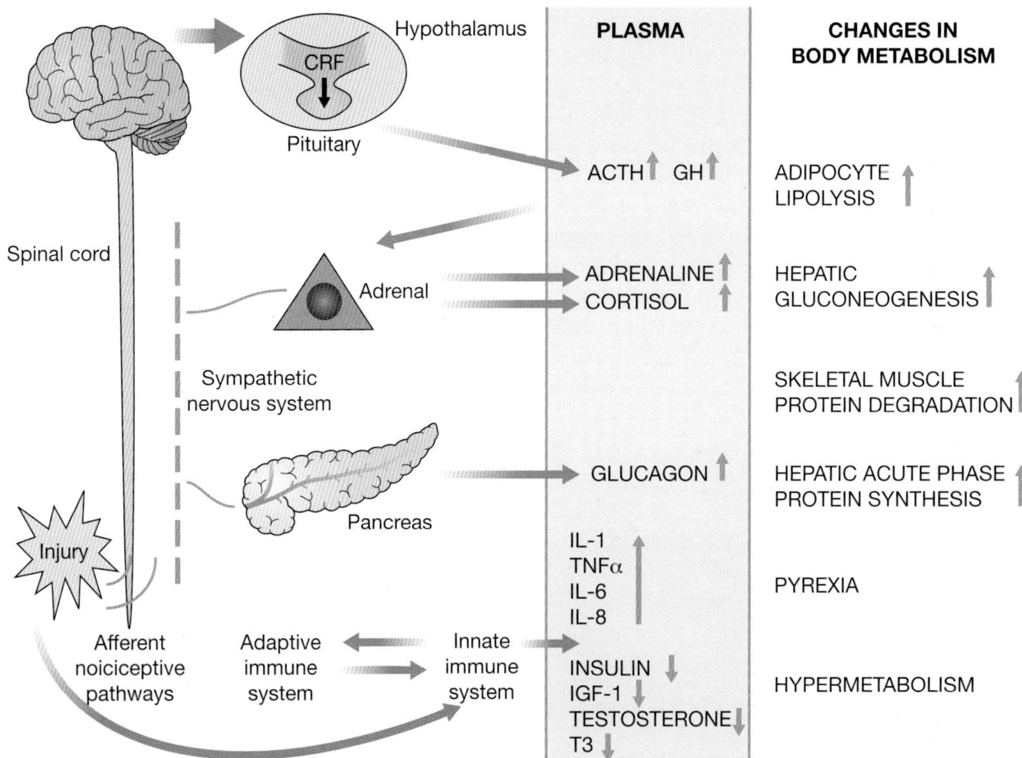

Figure 1.2 The integrated response to surgical injury (first 24–48 hours): there is a complex interplay between the neuroendocrine stress response and the proinflammatory cytokine response of the innate immune system. ACTH, adrenocorticotropic hormone; GH, growth hormone; IGF, insulin-like growth factor; IL, interleukin; T3, triiodothyronine; TNFα, tumour necrosis factor alpha.

Agonists and antagonists: an uncertain balance

Within hours of the upregulation of proinflammatory cytokines, endogenous cytokine antagonists enter the circulation (e.g. interleukin-1 receptor antagonist [IL-1Ra] and TNF-soluble receptors [TNF-sR-55 and 75]) and act to control the initial proinflammatory response and limit any systemic organ damage caused by it. A complex further series of adaptive changes includes the development of a counter-inflammatory response regulated by IL-4, -5, -9 and -13 and transforming growth factor beta (TGFβ). Within inflamed tissue the duration and magnitude of acute inflammation as well as the return to homeostasis are influenced by a group of local mediators known as specialised pro-resolving mediators (SPMs), which include essential fatty acid-derived lipoxins, resolvins, protectins and maresins. These endogenous resolution agonists orchestrate the uptake and clearance of apoptotic polymorphonuclear neutrophils and microbial particles, reduce proinflammatory cytokines and lipid mediators as well as enhance the removal of cellular debris. Thus, both at the systemic level (endogenous cytokine antagonists – see earlier) and at the local tissue level, the body attempts to limit the inflammatory response, but further tissue damage, sepsis or other complications challenge these processes of resolution. As with the initial inflammatory response to tissue injury, it appears that the degree of the secondary anti-inflammatory response varies between individuals, probably on a genetic basis. If the anti-inflammatory response dominates or is accentuated and prolonged in critical illness, it is characterised as a compensatory anti-inflammatory response syndrome (CARS), resulting in immunosuppression and an increased susceptibility to opportunistic (nosocomial) infection. Further sepsis, with its associated catabolism, results. CARS can be prolonged by ongoing critical illness as part of an ongoing vicious cycle of chronic critical illness (also known as Persistent Inflammation, Immunosuppression and Catabolism) syndrome. Thus both the initial inflammatory response to tissue injury and the secondary modulating responses can be seen to differing degrees in different individuals or at different stages of the critical illness. Either circumstance can cause harm, and rapid restoration of homeostasis and preventing secondary inflammation or sepsis are key therapeutic principles that influence late outcomes as well as immediate ones.

Summary box 1.3

The metabolic response to surgery and injury: key characteristics

- Rapid onset driven by proinflammatory cytokines (e.g. IL-1, IL-6 and TNFα)
- Broadly related to injury severity; most severe in sepsis, burns and major trauma
- Varies in severity between individuals (genetic)
- Causes catabolism, muscle breakdown, immunosuppression and organ dysfunction/failure
- Counterbalanced by antagonist response but the balance may be imperfect
- Prolonged by sepsis and other secondary insults
- Can become chronic
- Associated with most late deaths from injury or surgery in developed health systems

METABOLIC CHANGES AFTER SURGERY AND TRAUMA

The catabolic phase begins at the time of injury and lasts for approximately 24–48 hours. It may be attenuated by proper resuscitation and is characterised by hypovolaemia, decreased basal metabolic rate, reduced cardiac output, hypothermia and lactic acidosis. The predominant hormones regulating the catabolic phase are catecholamines, cortisol and aldosterone (following activation of the renin–angiotensin system). The magnitude of this neuroendocrine response depends on the degree of tissue damage, blood loss and the stimulation of somatic afferent nerves at the site of injury. The main physiological role of the catabolic phase is to conserve both circulating volume and energy stores for later recovery and repair.

Following resuscitation, the catabolic phase evolves into a hypermetabolic flow phase, which corresponds to SIRS. This phase involves the mobilisation of body energy stores for recovery and repair, and the subsequent replacement of lost or damaged tissue. It is characterised by tissue oedema (from vasodilatation and increased capillary leakage), increased basal metabolic rate (hypermetabolism), increased cardiac output, raised body temperature, leukocytosis, increased oxygen consumption and increased gluconeogenesis.

During the catabolic phase, the increased production of counter-regulatory hormones (including catecholamines, cortisol and glucagon) and inflammatory cytokines (e.g. IL-1, IL-6 and TNFα) results in significant fat and protein mobilisation, leading to significant weight loss and increased urinary nitrogen excretion. During shock, insulin levels do not rise as expected to combat the hyperglycaemia that occurs in response to stress hormone release and plasma insulin can even fall after severe injury. Within a few days, insulin production is increased but is associated with significant insulin resistance and, therefore, injured patients often exhibit poor glycaemic control. Importantly, the combination of pronounced or prolonged catabolism in association with insulin resistance places patients within this phase at increased risk of septic and other complications. Obviously, the development of complications will further aggravate the neuroendocrine and inflammatory stress responses, thus creating a vicious catabolic cycle and management of blood sugar levels remains an important step.

Summary box 1.4

Purpose of neuroendocrine changes following surgery or trauma

The constellation of neuroendocrine changes following surgery or trauma acts to:

- Provide essential substrates for survival from tissue breakdown
- Postpone anabolism
- Optimise host defence

These changes may be helpful in the short term, but may be harmful in the long term, especially to the severely injured or critically ill patient.

MANAGING THE CATABOLIC STRESS RESPONSE

There are several key elements that determine the extent of catabolism and thus govern the metabolic and nutritional care of the surgical patient. It must be remembered that, during the response to injury, not all tissues are catabolic. Indeed, the essence of this coordinated response is to allow the body to reprioritise limited resources away from peripheral tissues (muscle, adipose tissue, skin) and towards key viscera (liver, immune system) and the wound (***Figure 1.3***). However the damage to skeletal muscle can be catastrophic.

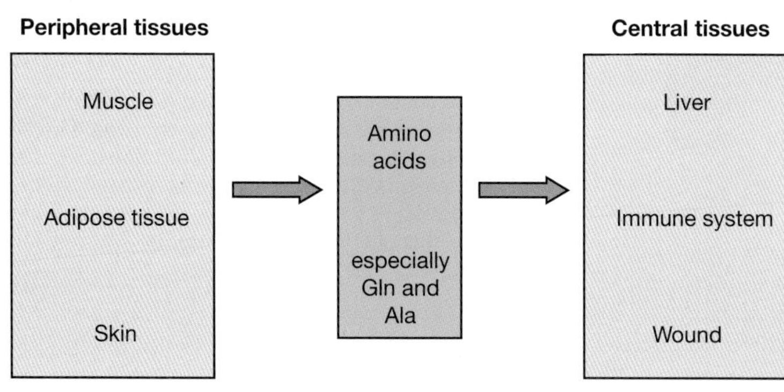

Figure 1.3 During the metabolic response to injury, the body reprioritises protein metabolism away from peripheral tissues and towards key central tissues such as the liver, immune system and wounds. One of the main reasons why the reutilisation of amino acids derived from muscle proteolysis leads to net catabolism is that the increased glutamine and alanine efflux from muscle is derived, in part, from the irreversible degradation of branched chain amino acids. Ala, alanine; Gln, glutamine.

Hypermetabolism

The majority of trauma patients (except possibly those with extensive burns, in whom a greater effect can be seen) demonstrate energy expenditures approximately 15–25% above predicted healthy resting values. The predominant cause appears to be a complex interaction between the central control of metabolic rate and peripheral energy utilisation. In particular, central thermodysregulation (caused by the proinflammatory cytokine cascade), increased sympathetic activity, abnormalities from wound circulation (ischaemic areas produce lactate, which must be metabolised by the adenosine triphosphate [ATP]-consuming hepatic Cori cycle; hyperaemic areas cause an increase in cardiac output), increased protein turnover and nutritional support may all increase patient energy expenditure. Theoretically, patient energy expenditure could rise even higher than observed levels following surgery or trauma, but several features of standard intensive care (including bed rest, paralysis, ventilation and external temperature regulation) limit the hypermetabolic driving forces of the stress response. Furthermore, the skeletal muscle wasting experienced by patients with prolonged catabolism actually limits the volume of metabolically active tissue (see ***Alterations in skeletal muscle protein metabolism***).

Alterations in skeletal muscle protein metabolism

Muscle protein is continually synthesised and broken down with a turnover rate in humans of 1–2% per day. Under normal circumstances, synthesis equals breakdown and muscle bulk remains constant. Physiological stimuli that promote net muscle protein increase include feeding (especially extracellular amino acid concentration) and exercise. Paradoxically, during exercise, skeletal muscle protein synthesis is depressed, but it increases again during rest and feeding.

During the catabolic phase of the stress response, muscle wasting occurs as a result of an increase in muscle protein degradation (via enzymatic pathways), coupled with a decrease in muscle protein synthesis. The major site of protein loss is peripheral skeletal muscle, but it also occurs in the respiratory muscles (predisposing the patient to hypoventilation and chest infections) and in the gut (reducing gut motility). Cardiac muscle appears to be mostly spared. The predominant mechanism involved in the wasting of skeletal muscle is the ATP-dependent ubiquitin–proteasome pathway (***Figure 1.4***), although the lysosomal cathepsins and the calcium–calpain pathway play facilitatory and accessory roles.

Under extreme conditions of catabolism (e.g. major sepsis), urinary nitrogen losses can reach 14–20 g/day; this is equivalent to the loss of 500 g of skeletal muscle per day. Muscle catabolism cannot be inhibited fully by providing artificial nutritional support as long as the stress response continues. Hyperalimentation (excess feeding beyond requirements) was once in vogue to try and match the large losses, but it is now recognised that hyperalimentation represents a metabolic stress in itself and that nutritional support should be at a modest level to attenuate rather than replace energy and protein losses. Treating underlying sepsis adequately is fundamental to limiting protein catabolism and is an essential part of effective nutritional support. This includes searching for and treating recurrent septic episodes in the critically ill.

Clinically, a patient with skeletal muscle wasting will experience weakness, fatigue, reduced functional ability, decreased quality of life and an increased risk of morbidity and mortality. In critically ill patients, muscle weakness may be further worsened by the development of critical illness myopathy, a multifactorial condition that is associated with impaired excitation–contraction coupling.

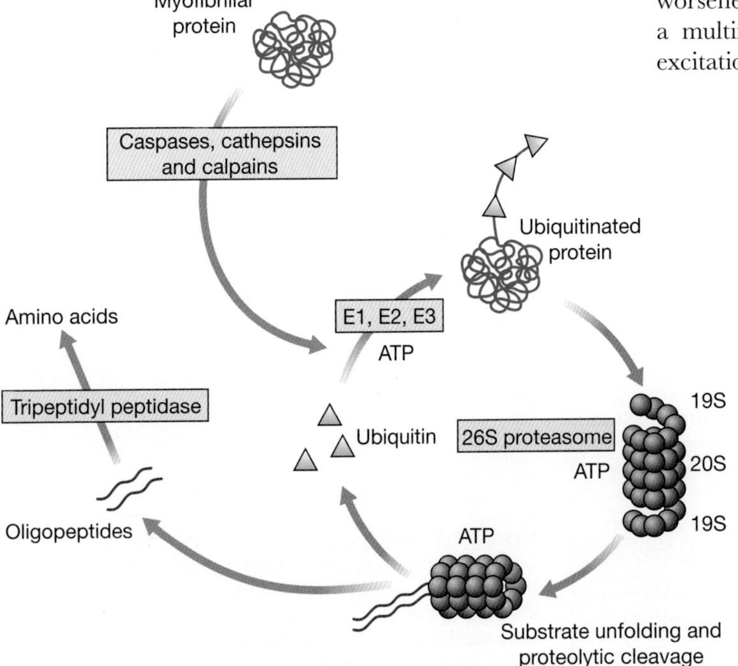

Figure 1.4 The intracellular effector mechanisms involved in degrading myofibrillar protein into free amino acids. The ubiquitin–proteasome pathway is a complex multistep process. ATP, adenosine triphosphate; E1, ubiquitin-activating enzyme; E2, ubiquitin-conjugating enzyme; E3, ubiquitin ligase.

Carl Ferdinand Cori, 1896–1984, and his wife **Gerty Theresa Cori**, 1896–1957, Professors of Biochemistry, Washington University Medical School, St Louis, MI, USA, were awarded a share of the 1947 Nobel Prize for Medicine.

Summary box 1.5

Skeletal muscle wasting

- Provides amino acids for the metabolic support of central organs/tissues
- Is mediated at a molecular level mainly by activation of the ubiquitin–proteasome pathway
- Is inevitable to some degree but is prolonged by sepsis in particular
- Can result in immobility and contribute to prolonged recovery, poor healing, hypostatic pneumonia and death if prolonged and excessive

Alterations in hepatic protein metabolism: the acute-phase protein response

The liver and skeletal muscle together account for >50% of daily body protein turnover. Skeletal muscle has a large mass but a low turnover rate (1–2% per day), whereas the liver has a relatively small mass (1.5 kg) but a much higher protein turnover rate (10–20% per day). Hepatic protein synthesis is divided roughly 50:50 between renewal of structural proteins and synthesis of export proteins. Albumin is the major export protein produced by the liver and is renewed at the rate of about 10% per day. The transcapillary escape rate (TER) of albumin is about 10 times the rate of synthesis, and short-term changes in albumin concentration are most probably due to increased vascular permeability. Albumin TER may be increased threefold following major injury/sepsis. In response to inflammatory conditions, including surgery, trauma and sepsis, proinflammatory cytokines, including IL-1, IL-6 and TNFα and in particular IL-6, promote the hepatic synthesis of positive acute-phase proteins, e.g. fibrinogen and C-reactive protein (CRP). The acute-phase protein response represents a 'double-edged sword' for surgical patients as it provides proteins important for recovery and repair but only at the expense of valuable lean tissue and energy reserves. In contrast to the positive acute-phase reactants, the plasma concentrations of other liver export proteins (the negative acute-phase reactants) fall acutely following injury, e.g. albumin. However, rather than representing a reduced hepatic synthesis rate, the fall in plasma concentration of negative acute-phase reactants is thought principally to reflect increased transcapillary escape, secondary to an increase in microvascular permeability.

Summary box 1.6

Hepatic acute-phase response

The hepatic acute-phase response represents a reprioritisation of body protein metabolism towards the liver and is characterised by:

- **Positive** reactants (e.g. CRP): plasma concentration ↑
- **Negative** reactants (e.g. albumin): plasma concentration ↓

Insulin resistance

Following surgery or trauma, postoperative hyperglycaemia develops as a result of increased glucose production combined with decreased glucose uptake in peripheral tissues. Decreased glucose uptake is a result of insulin resistance, which is temporarily induced within the stressed patient. Suggested mechanisms for this phenomenon include the action of proinflammatory cytokines and the decreased responsiveness of insulin-regulated glucose transporter proteins. The degree of insulin resistance is proportional to the magnitude of the injurious process. Following routine upper abdominal surgery for example, insulin resistance may persist for approximately 2 weeks but this period will extend with prolonged sepsis. Postoperative patients with insulin resistance behave in a similar manner to individuals with type 2 diabetes mellitus. In intensive care, the mainstay of management of insulin resistance is intravenous insulin infusion, which is used to keep blood glucose level within reasonable limits on the basis that this will reduce both morbidity and mortality. However, unduly tight control can increase the risk of significant hypoglycaemia. It should be noted that patients with diabetes whose glycaemic control has been poor prior to their critical illness pose a particular challenge.

CHANGES IN BODY COMPOSITION FOLLOWING INJURY

The average 70 kg male can be considered to consist of fat (13 kg) and fat-free mass (or lean body mass: 57 kg). In such an individual, the lean tissue is composed primarily of protein (12 kg), water (42 kg) and minerals (3 kg) (***Figure 1.5***). The protein mass can be considered as two basic compartments: skeletal muscle (4 kg) and non-skeletal muscle (8 kg), which includes the visceral protein mass. The water mass (42 litres) is divided into intracellular (28 litres) and extracellular (14 litres) spaces. Most of the mineral mass is contained in the bony skeleton.

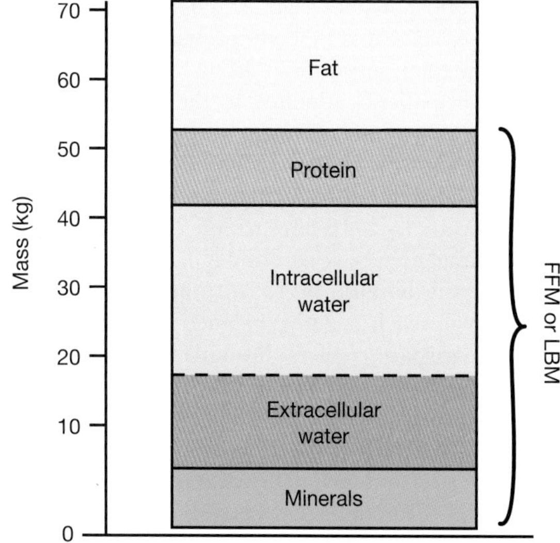

Figure 1.5 The chemical body composition of a normal 70 kg male. FFM, fat-free mass; LBM, lean body mass.

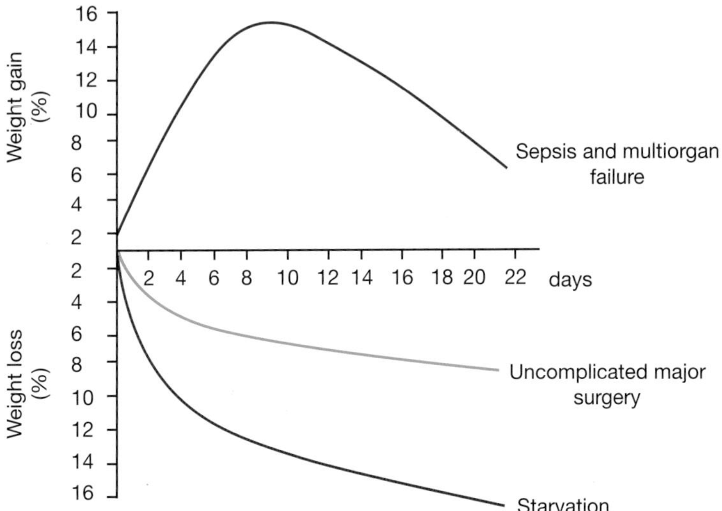

Figure 1.6 Changes in body weight that occur in serious sepsis, after uncomplicated surgery and in total starvation.

The main labile energy reserve in the body is fat, and the main labile protein reserve is skeletal muscle. While fat mass can be reduced without major detriment to function, loss of protein mass results not only in skeletal muscle wasting but also in depletion of visceral protein status. Within lean tissue, each 1 g of nitrogen is contained within 6.25 g of protein, which is contained in approximately 36 g of wet weight tissue. Thus, the loss of 1 g of nitrogen in urine is equivalent to the breakdown of 36 g of wet weight lean tissue. Protein turnover in the whole body is of the order of 150–200 g per day. A normal human ingests about 70–100 g protein per day, which is metabolised and excreted in urine as ammonia and urea (i.e. approximately 14 g N/day). During total starvation, urinary loss of nitrogen is rapidly attenuated by a series of adaptive changes. Loss of body weight follows a similar course (***Figure 1.6***), thus accounting for the survival of hunger strikers for a period of 50–60 days. Following major injury, and particularly in the presence of ongoing septic complications, this adaptive change fails to occur and there is a state of 'auto-cannibalism', resulting in continuing urinary nitrogen losses of 10–20 g N/day (equivalent to 500 g of wet weight lean tissue per day). As with total starvation, once loss of body protein mass has reached 30–40% of the total, survival is unlikely.

Critically ill patients admitted to the intensive care unit with severe sepsis or major blunt trauma undergo massive changes in body composition (***Figure 1.7***). Body weight increases immediately on resuscitation with an expansion of extracellular water by 6–10 litres within 24 hours. Thereafter, even with optimal metabolic care and nutritional support, total body protein will diminish by 15% in the next 10 days, and body weight will reach negative balance as the expansion of the extracellular space resolves. In marked contrast, it is now possible to maintain body weight and nitrogen equilibrium following major elective surgery. This can be achieved by blocking the neuroendocrine stress response with epidural analgesia/other related techniques and providing early oral/enteral feeding. Moreover, the early fluid retention phase can be avoided by careful intraoperative management of fluid balance, with avoidance of excessive administration of intravenous saline.

Summary box 1.7

Changes in body composition following major surgery/critical illness

- Catabolism leads to a decrease in fat mass and skeletal muscle mass
- Body weight may paradoxically increase because of expansion of fluid within the extracellular fluid space

AVOIDABLE FACTORS THAT COMPOUND THE RESPONSE TO INJURY

There are several factors that prolong the acute-phase response to injury (***Table 1.1***) and keep the patient in a catabolic state. Other factors can exacerbate or compound the metabolic stress response both in elective surgery and in the emergency setting. These include anaesthesia, dehydration, starvation (including preoperative fasting), acute medical illness, frailty, chronic diseases or even severe psychological stress (***Figure 1.7***). Attempts to limit or control these factors can also be beneficial to the patient.

Summary box 1.8

Avoidable factors that compound the metabolic response to injury during elective surgery

- Continuing haemorrhage/volume loss
- Hypothermia
- Tissue oedema
- Tissue underperfusion
- Starvation
- Immobility

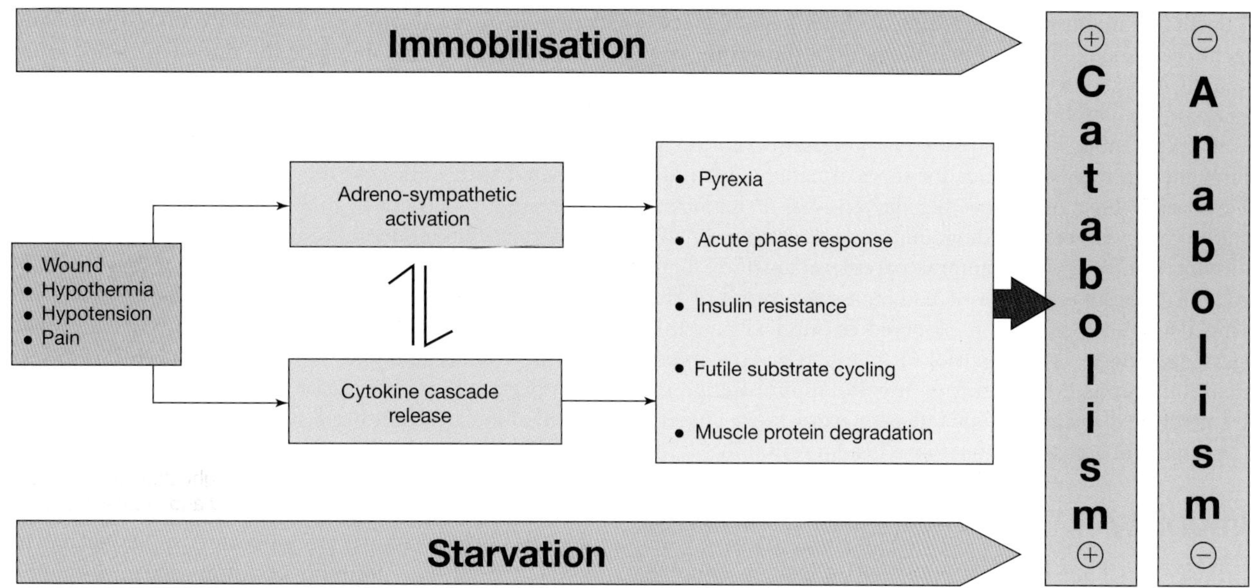

Figure 1.7 Factors that exacerbate the metabolic response to surgical injury include hypothermia, uncontrolled pain, starvation, immobilisation, sepsis and medical complications.

Volume loss

During simple haemorrhage, baroreceptors in the carotid artery and aortic arch and volume receptors in the wall of the left atrium initiate afferent nerve input to the central nervous system, resulting in the release of both aldosterone and antidiuretic hormone (ADH). Pain can also stimulate ADH release. ADH acts directly on the kidney to cause fluid retention. Decreased pulse pressure stimulates the juxtaglomerular apparatus in the kidney and directly activates the renin–angiotensin system, which in turn increases aldosterone release.

Aldosterone causes the renal tubule to reabsorb sodium (and consequently conserve water). ACTH release also augments the aldosterone response. The net effects of ADH and aldosterone result in the natural oliguria observed after surgery and conservation of sodium and water in the extracellular space. The tendency towards water and salt retention is exacerbated by resuscitation with saline-rich fluids. Salt and water retention can result in not only peripheral oedema but also visceral oedema (e.g. in the stomach). Such visceral oedema has been associated with reduced gastric emptying, delayed resumption of food intake and prolonged hospital stay. Careful limitation of intraoperative administration of balanced crystalloids so that there is no net weight gain following elective surgery has been proven to reduce postoperative complications and length of stay.

Hypothermia

Hypothermia results in increased production of adrenal steroids and catecholamines. When compared with normothermic controls, even mild hypothermia results in a two- to threefold increase in postoperative cardiac arrhythmias and increased catabolism. Randomised trials have shown that maintaining normothermia during surgery by an upper body forced-air heating cover reduces wound infections, cardiac complications and bleeding and transfusion requirements.

Tissue oedema

During systemic inflammation, fluid, plasma proteins, leukocytes, macrophages and electrolytes leave the vascular space and accumulate in the tissues as oedema. The oedema can diminish the alveolar diffusion of oxygen and may also impair renal function. Increased capillary leak is mediated by a wide variety of mediators, including cytokines, prostanoids, bradykinin and nitric oxide. Cellular hypoxia and dysfunction can occur. Intracellular volume decreases, and this provides part of the volume necessary to replenish intravascular and extravascular extracellular volume.

Systemic inflammation and tissue underperfusion

The vascular endothelium controls vasomotor tone and microvascular flow and regulates trafficking of nutrients and biologically active molecules. When endothelial activation is excessive, compromised microcirculation and subsequent cellular hypoxia contribute to the risk of organ failure. Controlling the blood sugar appropriately with insulin infusion during critical illness has been proposed to protect the endothelium, probably, in part, via inhibition of excessive iNOS-induced NO release.

Starvation

During starvation, the body is faced with an obligate need to generate glucose to sustain cerebral energy metabolism (100 g of glucose per day). This is achieved in the first 24 hours by mobilising glycogen stores and thereafter by hepatic gluconeogenesis from amino acids, glycerol and lactate. The energy metabolism of other tissues is sustained by mobilising fat from adipose tissue. Such fat mobilisation is mainly dependent on a fall in circulating insulin levels. Eventually, accelerated loss of lean tissue (the main source of amino acids for hepatic gluconeogenesis) is reduced as a result of the liver converting free fatty acids into ketone bodies, which can serve as a substitute for glucose for cerebral energy metabolism. Provision of 2 litres of intravenous 4% dextrose/0.18% sodium chloride as maintenance intravenous fluids for surgical patients who are fasted provides 80 g of glucose per day and has a significant protein-sparing effect. Avoiding unnecessary fasting in the first instance and early oral/enteral/parenteral nutrition form the platform for avoiding loss of body mass as a result of the varying degrees of starvation observed in surgical patients. Modern guidelines on fasting prior to anaesthesia allow intake of clear fluids up to 2 hours before surgery. Administration of a carbohydrate drink at this time reduces perioperative anxiety and thirst and decreases postoperative insulin resistance.

Immobility

Immobility has long been recognised as a potent stimulus for inducing muscle wasting. Inactivity impairs the normal meal-derived amino acid stimulation of protein synthesis in skeletal muscle. Avoidance of unnecessary bed rest and active early mobilisation are essential measures to avoid muscle wasting as a consequence of immobility. Pre-habilitation programmes provide a better starting point before surgery.

ENHANCED RECOVERY AFTER SURGERY

Modern understanding of the metabolic response to surgical injury and the mediators involved has led to a complete reappraisal of traditional perioperative care and the process known as ERAS. ERAS is evidence based on the strong scientific rationale for avoiding unmodulated exposure to stress, prolonged fasting and excessive administration of intravenous (saline) fluids (***Figure 1.8***). ERAS principles are now applied by protocol to many types of major surgery, bringing considerable benefit in terms of improved outcomes. Reductions in length of hospital stay after surgery of 30–50% are common, with associated savings in healthcare costs. ERAS depends on a multimodal approach where the combined effects of several interventions achieve significant benefits. The widespread adoption of minimal access (e.g. laparoscopic) surgery is a key change in surgical practice that can reduce the magnitude of surgical injury and enhance the rate of patients' return to homeostasis and recovery. Modulating the stress/inflammatory response at the time of surgery may have long-term sequelae over periods of months or longer. For example, β-blockers are associated with improved short- and long-term survival after major surgery, perhaps by modulating the effects of the hyperadrenergic state induced by surgical stress. Equally, in 'open' surgery the use of epidural analgesia to reduce pain, block the cortisol stress response and attenuate postoperative insulin resistance may, via effects on the body's protein economy, favourably affect many of the patient-centred outcomes that are important to postoperative recovery. However, because of the reduction in wound size and tissue trauma, it should be noted that epidural analgesia is no longer recommended for laparoscopic surgery. Patient-controlled analgesia is usually sufficient and avoids the fluid shifts and hypotension seen with epidurals. Adjuncts such as 'one-shot' spinal diamorphine and/or a 6–12-hour infusion of intravenous lidocaine have been suggested to be opiate sparing, to improve gut function and to enhance overall recovery.

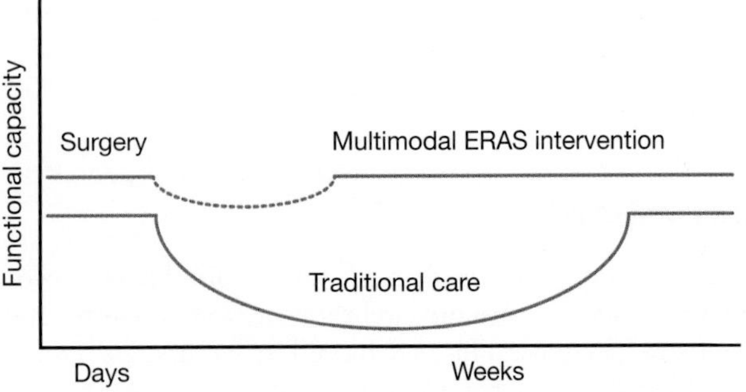

Figure 1.8 Enhanced recovery after surgery (ERAS) programmes use multimodal techniques to limit pain, fluid shifts and tissue damage and to enhance nutrition and rehabilitation in order to minimise the stress response. They have been hugely successful in improving outcomes.

Summary box 1.9

A proactive ERAS approach to prevent unnecessary aspects of the surgical stress response

- Minimal access techniques
- Blockade of afferent painful stimuli (e.g. epidural analgesia, spinal analgesia, wound catheters)
- Minimal periods of starvation
- Early mobilisation

FURTHER READING

Ahl R, Matthiessen P, Sjölin G *et al.* Effects of betablocker therapy on mortality after elective colon cancer surgery: a Swedish nationwide cohort study. *BMJ Open* 2020; **10**: e036164.

Bortolotti P, Faure E, Kipnis E. Inflammasomes in tissue damages and immune disorders after trauma. *Front Immunol* 2018; **9**:1900.

Cole E, Gillespie S, Vulliamy P *et al.* Multiple organ dysfunction after trauma. *Br J Surg* 2020; **107**: 402–12.

Fearon KCH, Ljungqvist O, von Meyenfeldt M *et al.* Enhanced recovery after surgery: a consensus review of clinical care for patients undergoing colonic resection. *Clin Nutr* 2005; **24**: 466–77.

Huber-Lang M, Lambris JD, Ward PA. Innate immune responses to trauma. *Nat Immunol* 2018; **19**(4): 327–41.

Ljungqvist O. Insulin resistance and outcomes in surgery. *J Clin Endocrinol Metab* 2010; **95**: 4217–19.

Ljungqvist O, Scott M, Fearon KCH. Enhanced recovery after surgery: a review. *JAMA Surg.* 2017; **152**(3): 292–8.

Mira J, Cuschieri J, Ozrazgat-Baslanti T *et al.* The epidemiology of chronic critical illness after severe traumatic injury at two level-one trauma centers. *Crit Care Med* 2017; **45**(12): 1989–96.

Vanhorebeek O, Langounche L, Van den Berghe G. Endocrine aspects of acute and prolonged critical illness. *Nat Clin Pract Endocrinol Metab* 2006; **2**: 20–31.

Vourc'h M, Roquilly A, Asehnoune K. Trauma-induced damage-associated molecular patterns-mediated remote organ injury and immunosuppression in the acutely ill patient. *Front Immunol* 2018; **9**: 1330.

Wilmore DW. From Cuthbertson to fast-track surgery: 70 years of progress in reducing stress in surgical patients. *Ann Surg* 2002; **236**: 643–8.

CHAPTER 2

Shock, haemorrhage and transfusion

Learning objectives

To understand:

- The pathophysiology of shock
- The different patterns of shock and the principles and priorities of resuscitation
- Appropriate monitoring and end points of resuscitation
- Recognition and management of bleeding
- Use of blood and blood products, the benefits and risks of blood transfusion

INTRODUCTION

Shock is the most common cause of death of surgical patients. Death may occur rapidly because of a profound state of shock or may occur later because of the consequences of organ ischaemia and reperfusion injury. It is important therefore that every surgeon understands the pathophysiology, diagnosis and priorities in management of shock and haemorrhage.

SHOCK

Shock is a systemic state of low tissue perfusion that is inadequate for normal cellular respiration. With insufficient delivery of oxygen and glucose, cells switch from aerobic to anaerobic metabolism. If perfusion is not restored in a timely fashion, cell death ensues.

Pathophysiology

Cellular

As perfusion to the tissues is reduced, cells are deprived of oxygen and must switch from aerobic to anaerobic metabolism. The product of anaerobic respiration is not carbon dioxide but lactic acid. When enough tissue is underperfused the accumulation of lactic acid in the blood produces a systemic metabolic acidosis.

As glucose within cells is exhausted, anaerobic respiration ceases and there is failure of sodium/potassium pumps in the cell membrane and intracellular organelles. Intracellular lysosomes release autodigestive enzymes and cell lysis ensues. Intracellular contents, including potassium, are released into the bloodstream.

Microvascular

As tissue ischaemia progresses, changes in the local milieu result in activation of the immune and coagulation systems. Hypoxia and acidosis activate complement and prime leukocytes, resulting in the generation of oxygen free radicals and cytokine release. These mechanisms lead to injury of the capillary endothelial cells. These, in turn, further activate the immune and coagulation systems. Damaged endothelium loses its integrity and becomes 'leaky'. Spaces between endothelial cells allow fluid to leak out and tissue oedema ensues, exacerbating cellular hypoxia.

Ischaemic cell death releases potassium into the circulation, leading to systemic hyperkalaemia and acidosis, as well as further damage to molecules that systemically activate the immune system.

Systemic

Cardiovascular

As preload and afterload decrease, there is a compensatory baroreceptor response, resulting in increased sympathetic activity and release of catecholamines into the circulation. This results in tachycardia and systemic vasoconstriction (except in sepsis – see ***Distributive shock***).

Respiratory

The metabolic acidosis and increased sympathetic response result in an increased respiratory rate and minute ventilation to increase the excretion of carbon dioxide (and so produce a compensatory respiratory alkalosis).

Renal

Decreased perfusion pressure in the kidney leads to reduced filtration at the glomerulus and a decreased urine output. The renin–angiotensin–aldosterone axis is stimulated, resulting in further vasoconstriction and increased sodium and water reabsorption by the kidney.

Endocrine

As well as activation of the adrenal and renin–angiotensin systems, vasopressin (antidiuretic hormone) is released in response to decreased preload and results in vasoconstriction and resorption of water in the renal collecting system. Cortisol is also released from the adrenal cortex, contributing to the sodium and water resorption and sensitising cells to catecholamines.

Classification of shock

There are numerous ways to classify shock, but the most common and most clinically applicable is one based on the initiating mechanism. All states are characterised by systemic tissue hypoperfusion, and different states may coexist within the same patient.

Summary box 2.1

Classification of shock

- Haemorrhagic/hypovolaemic shock
- Cardiogenic shock
- Obstructive shock
- Distributive shock
- Endocrine shock

Haemorrhagic and hypovolaemic shock

Hypovolaemic shock is due to a reduced circulating volume. Hypovolaemia may be due to haemorrhagic or non-haemorrhagic causes. Non-haemorrhagic causes include poor fluid intake (dehydration), excessive fluid loss due to vomiting, diarrhoea, urinary loss (e.g. diabetes), evaporation or 'third-spacing', where fluid is lost into the gastrointestinal tract and interstitial spaces, as for example in bowel obstruction or pancreatitis.

Hypovolaemia is the most common form of shock, and to some degree is a component of all other forms of shock. Absolute or relative hypovolaemia must be excluded or treated in the management of the shocked state, regardless of cause.

Cardiogenic shock

Cardiogenic shock is due to primary failure of the heart to pump blood to the tissues. Causes of cardiogenic shock include myocardial infarction, cardiac dysrhythmias, valvular heart disease, blunt myocardial injury and cardiomyopathy. Cardiac insufficiency may also be due to myocardial depression caused by endogenous factors (e.g. bacterial and humoral agents released in sepsis) or exogenous factors, such as pharmaceutical agents or drug abuse. Evidence of venous hypertension with pulmonary or systemic oedema may coexist with the classical signs of shock.

Obstructive shock

In obstructive shock there is a reduction in preload owing to mechanical obstruction of cardiac filling. Common causes of obstructive shock include cardiac tamponade, tension pneumothorax, massive pulmonary embolus or air embolus. In each case, there is reduced filling of the left and/or right sides of the heart, leading to low cardiac output.

Distributive shock

Distributive shock describes the pattern of cardiovascular responses characterising a variety of conditions, including septic shock, anaphylaxis and spinal cord injury. Inadequate organ perfusion is accompanied by vascular dilatation with hypotension, low systemic vascular resistance, inadequate afterload and a resulting abnormally high cardiac output.

In anaphylaxis, vasodilatation is due to histamine release, while in high spinal cord injury there is failure of sympathetic outflow and adequate vascular tone (neurogenic shock). The cause in sepsis is less clear but is related to the release of bacterial products (endotoxin) and the activation of cellular and humoral components of the immune system. There is maldistribution of blood flow at a microvascular level, with arteriovenous shunting and dysfunction of cellular utilisation of oxygen.

In the later phases of septic shock there is hypovolaemia from fluid loss into interstitial spaces and there may be concomitant myocardial depression, complicating the clinical picture (***Table 2.1***).

Endocrine shock

Endocrine shock may present as a combination of hypovolaemic, cardiogenic or distributive shock. Causes of endocrine shock include hypo- and hyperthyroidism and adrenal insufficiency. Hypothyroidism causes a shock state similar to that of neurogenic shock due to disordered vascular and cardiac responsiveness to circulating catecholamines. Cardiac output falls as a result of low inotropy and bradycardia. There may also be an associated cardiomyopathy. Thyrotoxicosis may cause a high-output cardiac failure.

Adrenal insufficiency leads to shock due to hypovolaemia and a poor response to circulating and exogenous

TABLE 2.1 Cardiovascular and metabolic characteristics of shock.

	Hypovolaemic	Cardiogenic	Obstructive	Distributive
Cardiac output	Low	Low	Low	High
Systemic vascular resistance	High	High	High	Low
Venous pressure	Low	High	High	Low
Mixed venous saturation	Low	Low	Low	High
Base deficit	High	High	High	High

catecholamines. Adrenal insufficiency may be due to preexisting Addison's disease or be a relative insufficiency due to a pathological disease state, such as systemic sepsis.

Clinical consequences of shock

Unresuscitatable shock

Patients who are in profound shock for a prolonged period of time become 'unresuscitatable'. Cell death follows from cellular ischaemia and the ability of the body to compensate is lost. In the heart there is myocardial cell death from poor coronary perfusion and myocardial depression from severe acidaemia and hyperkalaemia. This leads to poor cardiac output and limited response to fluids or inotropic therapy. Peripherally there may also be loss of the ability to maintain systemic vascular resistance and further hypotension ensues. The peripheries no longer respond appropriately to vasopressor agents. Once patients enter this stage of systemic ischaemic injury, death is inevitable.

Ischaemia-reperfusion and the systemic inflammatory response syndrome (SIRS)

During the period of systemic hypoperfusion, cellular and organ damage progresses owing to the direct effects of tissue hypoxia and local activation of inflammation. Further injury occurs once normal circulation is restored to these tissues. The acid and potassium load that has built up can lead to direct myocardial depression, vascular dilatation and further hypotension. Molecules released from the interior of cells are released into the circulation. These are sensed by and activate leukocytes. These, together with cellular and humoral elements activated by the hypoxia (complement, neutrophils, microvascular thrombi), overwhelm the local anti-inflammatory response and are flushed back into the systemic circulation, where they cause injury to distant organs such as the lungs and the kidneys. This leads to acute lung injury, acute renal injury, cerebral oedema, multiple organ failure and death. Reperfusion injury can currently only be attenuated by reducing the extent and duration of tissue hypoperfusion.

Multiple organ failure

As techniques of resuscitation have improved, more and more patients are surviving shock. Where intervention is timely and the period of shock is limited, patients may make a rapid, uncomplicated recovery. However, the result of prolonged systemic ischaemia and reperfusion injury is end-organ damage and multiple organ failure.

Multiple organ failure is defined as two or more failed organ systems. There is no specific treatment for multiple organ failure. Management is support of organ systems, with ventilation, cardiovascular support and haemofiltration/dialysis until there is recovery of organ function. Multiple organ failure currently carries a mortality of 60%; thus, prevention is vital by early aggressive identification and reversal of shock.

Summary box 2.2

Effects of organ failure

- Cardiac: Cardiovascular failure
- Lung: Acute respiratory distress syndrome
- Kidney: Acute renal insufficiency
- Liver: Liver failure and coagulopathy
- Brain: Cerebral swelling and dysfunction

Recognition and diagnosis of shock

Shock may be profound and easily recognised or it may be subtle and only diagnosed with directed clinical examination and cardiovascular and metabolic monitoring.

Compensated shock

As shock progresses, the body's cardiovascular and endocrine compensatory responses reduce flow to non-essential organs to preserve preload and flow to the lungs and brain. In compensated shock, there is adequate cardiovascular compensation to maintain central blood volume and preserve flow to the kidneys, lungs and brain. Apart from a tachycardia and cool peripheries (vasoconstriction, circulating catecholamines), there may be no other clinical signs of hypovolaemia.

However, this cardiovascular state is only maintained by reducing perfusion to the skin, muscle and gastrointestinal tract. These organs are underperfused: their cells are respiring anaerobically and sustaining ischaemic damage. There is systemic metabolic acidosis and both local and systemic activation of humoral and cellular inflammation.

Although clinically occult, this state will lead to multiple organ failure and death if prolonged. Patients with occult hypoperfusion (metabolic acidosis despite normal urine output and cardiorespiratory vital signs) for more than 12 hours have a significantly higher mortality, infection rate and incidence of multiple organ failure (see ***Multiple organ failure***).

Decompensation

Further loss of circulating volume overloads the body's compensatory mechanisms and there is progressive renal, respiratory and cardiovascular decompensation. In general, loss of around 15% of the circulating blood volume is within normal compensatory mechanisms. Blood pressure is usually well maintained and only falls after 30–40% of circulating volume has been lost.

Mild (compensated) shock

Initially there is tachycardia, tachypnoea, a mild reduction in urine output and the patient may exhibit mild anxiety. Blood pressure is maintained, although there is a decrease in pulse pressure. The peripheries are cool and sweaty with prolonged capillary refill times (except in septic distributive shock).

Thomas Addison, 1799–1860, physician, Guy's Hospital, London, UK, described the effects of disease of the suprarenal capsules in 1849.

TABLE 2.2 Clinical features of shock.

	Compensated	Uncompensated	
	Mild	Moderate	Severe
Lactic acidosis	+	++	+++
Urine output	Normal	Reduced	Anuric
Conscious level	Mild anxiety	Drowsy	Comatose
Respiratory rate	Increased	Increased	Laboured
Pulse rate	Increased	Increased	Increased
Blood pressure	Normal	Mild hypotension	Severe hypotension

Moderate shock

As shock progresses, renal compensatory mechanisms fail, renal perfusion falls and urine output dips below 0.5 mL/kg/hour. There is further tachycardia, and now the blood pressure starts to fall. Patients become drowsy and mildly confused.

Severe shock

In severe shock, there is profound tachycardia and hypotension. Urine output falls to zero and patients are unconscious with laboured respiration.

Clinical features

The classic cardiovascular responses described (***Table 2.2***) are not seen in every patient. It is important to recognise the limitations of the clinical examination and to recognise patients who are in shock despite the absence of classic signs.

Capillary refill

Most patients in hypovolaemic shock will have cool, pale peripheries, with prolonged capillary refill times. However, the actual capillary refill time varies so much in adults that it is not a specific marker of whether a patient is shocked, and patients with short capillary refill times may be in the early stages of shock. In distributive (septic) shock, the peripheries will be warm and capillary refill will be brisk, despite profound shock.

Tachycardia

Tachycardia may not always accompany shock. Patients who are on β-blockers or who have implanted pacemakers are unable to mount a tachycardia. A pulse rate of 80 in a fit young adult who normally has a pulse rate of 50 is very abnormal. Furthermore, in some young patients with penetrating trauma, where there is haemorrhage but little tissue damage, there may be a paradoxical bradycardia rather than tachycardia accompanying the shocked state.

Blood pressure

It is important to recognise that hypotension is one of the last signs of shock. Children and fit young adults are able to maintain blood pressure until the final stages of shock by dramatic increases in stroke volume and peripheral vasoconstriction. These patients can be in profound shock with a normal blood pressure.

Elderly patients who are normally hypertensive may present with a 'normal' blood pressure for the general population but be hypovolaemic and hypotensive relative to their usual blood pressure. β-blockers or other medications may prevent a tachycardic response. The diagnosis of shock may be difficult unless one is alert to these pitfalls.

HAEMORRHAGE

Uncontrolled bleeding will lead to a hypovolaemic shock state, or haemorrhagic shock. While haemorrhage and shock often coexist, they are not the same. Patients who are actively bleeding may not yet be in shock. Conversely, patients may be in shock as a consequence of haemorrhage, but they may no longer be actively bleeding.

Resuscitation is very different if patients are actively bleeding or if they are not bleeding. In patients who are bleeding, the priority is to stop bleeding. In patients who are not bleeding, the priority shifts to normalising end-organ perfusion (correcting the shock state). Thus it is vital to recognise patients who are actively bleeding, and this is different from recognising that a patient is in shock.

Haemorrhage must be recognised and managed rapidly and decisively to reduce the severity and duration of shock. Haemorrhage is treated by arresting the bleeding – not by fluid resuscitation or blood transfusion. Although necessary as supportive measures to maintain organ (especially cardiac) perfusion, repeated volume resuscitation of patients who have ongoing haemorrhage will lead to physiological exhaustion (profound coagulopathy, acidosis and hypothermia) and subsequently death.

Pathophysiology

In trauma and surgery, the combination of tissue trauma and hypovolaemic shock leads to the development of an endogenous coagulopathy called acute traumatic coagulopathy (ATC). Up to 25% of all trauma patients develop ATC within minutes of injury and it is associated with a fourfold increase in mortality. ATC is characterised by systemic hyperfibrinolysis, low fibrinogen levels and platelet dysfunction.

ATC evolves into a more complex, multifactorial 'trauma-induced coagulopathy' owing to further derangements induced by resuscitation (***Figure 2.1***). Fluid and red blood cell transfusions lead to dilution of coagulation factors, which worsens the pre-existing coagulopathy. Underperfused muscle is unable to generate heat and hypothermia ensues, again worsened by cold fluid or blood transfusion. Further heat is lost by opening

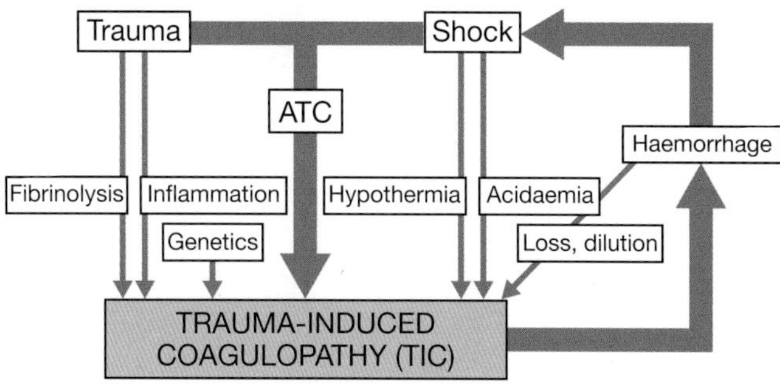

Figure 2.1 Trauma-induced coagulopathy. ATC, acute traumatic coagulopathy.

body cavities during surgery. Severe acidosis and hypothermia both inhibit coagulation proteases and reduce coagulation function. These then lead to further bleeding and a downward spiral, leading to physiological exhaustion and death.

Definitions

Revealed and concealed haemorrhage

Haemorrhage may be revealed or concealed. Revealed haemorrhage is obvious external haemorrhage, such as exsanguination from an open arterial wound or from massive haematemesis from a duodenal ulcer.

Concealed haemorrhage is contained within the body cavity and must be suspected, actively investigated and controlled. In trauma, haemorrhage may be concealed within the chest, abdomen, pelvis, retroperitoneum or in the limbs with contained vascular injury or associated with long-bone fractures. Examples of non-traumatic concealed haemorrhage include occult gastrointestinal bleeding or ruptured aortic aneurysm.

Primary, reactionary and secondary haemorrhage

Primary haemorrhage is haemorrhage occurring immediately as a result of an injury (or surgery).

Reactionary haemorrhage is delayed haemorrhage (within 24 hours) and is usually due to dislodgement of a clot by resuscitation, normalisation of blood pressure and vasodilatation. Reactionary haemorrhage may also be due to technical failure, such as slippage of a ligature.

Secondary haemorrhage is due to sloughing of the wall of a vessel. It usually occurs 7–14 days after injury and is precipitated by factors such as infection, pressure necrosis (such as from a drain) or malignancy.

Surgical and non-surgical haemorrhage

Surgical haemorrhage is due to a direct injury and is amenable to surgical control (e.g. suture ligation) or other techniques such as angioembolisation.

Non-surgical haemorrhage is general bleeding from raw surfaces and mucous membranes due to coagulopathy and cannot be stopped by surgical means (except packing). Treatment requires correction of the coagulation abnormalities.

Diagnosis of active bleeding: response to fluid therapy

The mode of resuscitation is determined by whether patients are actively bleeding, which requires a dynamic assessment of the blood pressure response to volume infusion. Patients who are 'non-responders' or 'transient responders' are still bleeding and must have the site of haemorrhage identified and controlled.

Responder

There is a good and sustained improvement in blood pressure in response to a bolus transfusion.

Transient responder

There is an improvement in the blood pressure but this is not sustained. The rate of haemorrhage is less than the rate of volume administration.

Non-responder

There is no improvement in the blood pressure to a bolus transfusion. The rate of haemorrhage is greater than the rate of volume administration.

Degree of haemorrhage and classification

The adult human has approximately 5 litres of blood (70 mL/kg for children and adults, 80 mL/kg for neonates). Estimation of the amount of blood that has been lost is difficult, inaccurate and usually underestimates the actual value.

External haemorrhage is obvious, but it may be difficult to estimate the actual volume lost. In the operating theatre, blood collected in suction apparatus can be measured and swabs soaked in blood weighed.

The haemoglobin level is a poor indicator of the degree of haemorrhage because it represents a concentration and not an absolute amount. In the early stages of rapid haemorrhage, the haemoglobin concentration is unchanged (as whole blood is lost). Later, as fluid shifts from the intracellular and interstitial spaces into the vascular compartment, the haemoglobin and haematocrit levels will fall.

TABLE 2.3 Traditional classification of haemorrhagic shock.

	Class			
	1	2	3	4
Blood volume lost as percentage of total	<15%	15–30%	30–40%	>40%

The amount of haemorrhage is historically classified into classes 1–4 based on the estimated blood loss required to produce certain physiological compensatory changes (***Table 2.3***). Although conceptually useful, this classification system is never applied clinically, and indeed is difficult if not impossible to determine. There is variation in clinical response across ages (the young compensate well, the old very poorly), variation among individuals (e.g. athletes versus the obese) and variation owing to confounding factors (e.g. concomitant medications, pain).

HAEMORRHAGE RESUSCITATION

The conduct and goals of resuscitation change depending on whether the patient is actively bleeding. In this case, the resuscitation focuses on achieving rapid haemostasis and maintaining the ability of the blood to clot. This paradigm is called damage control resuscitation (see ***Damage control resuscitation***).

If the patient is not actively bleeding, has stopped bleeding or the cause of shock is not haemorrhage, then resuscitation is directed at correcting the shock state and restoring perfusion to end organs.

Identify haemorrhage

External haemorrhage may be obvious, but the diagnosis of concealed haemorrhage may be more difficult. Any shock should be assumed to be hypovolaemic until proven otherwise and, similarly, hypovolaemia should be assumed to be due to haemorrhage until this has been excluded.

Once haemorrhage has been identified, the institution's major haemorrhage protocol should be activated, which will specify the approach to damage control resuscitation. Immediate resuscitative measures include the assessment of airway and breathing and control of life-threatening issues as necessary. Large-bore intravenous access should be instituted and blood drawn for cross-matching (see ***Cross-matching***). Transfusion should start with emergency (type O) blood (see ***Transfusion***).

Once haemorrhage has been considered, the site of haemorrhage must be rapidly identified. Note that this is not to identify the exact location definitively, but rather to define the next step in haemorrhage control (operation, angioembolisation, endoscopic control). Clues may be in the history (previous episodes, known aneurysm, non-steroidal therapy for gastrointestinal bleeding) or examination (nature of blood – fresh, melaena; abdominal tenderness, etc.). For shocked trauma patients, the external signs of injury may suggest internal haemorrhage, but haemorrhage into a body cavity (thorax, abdomen) must be excluded with rapid investigations (chest and pelvis radiographs, abdominal ultrasound).

Investigations for blood loss must be appropriate to the patient's physiological condition. Rapid bedside tests such as ultrasound are more appropriate for profound shock and exsanguinating haemorrhage than investigations such as computed tomography. Patients who are not actively bleeding can have a more methodical, definitive work-up.

Damage control resuscitation

Damage control resuscitation (DCR), also known as haemostatic resuscitation, is a paradigm that prioritises haemorrhage control in patients who are still actively bleeding. The rationale is that no aspect of the shock state – end-organ perfusion, blood pressure, temperature, lactic acidosis – can be corrected

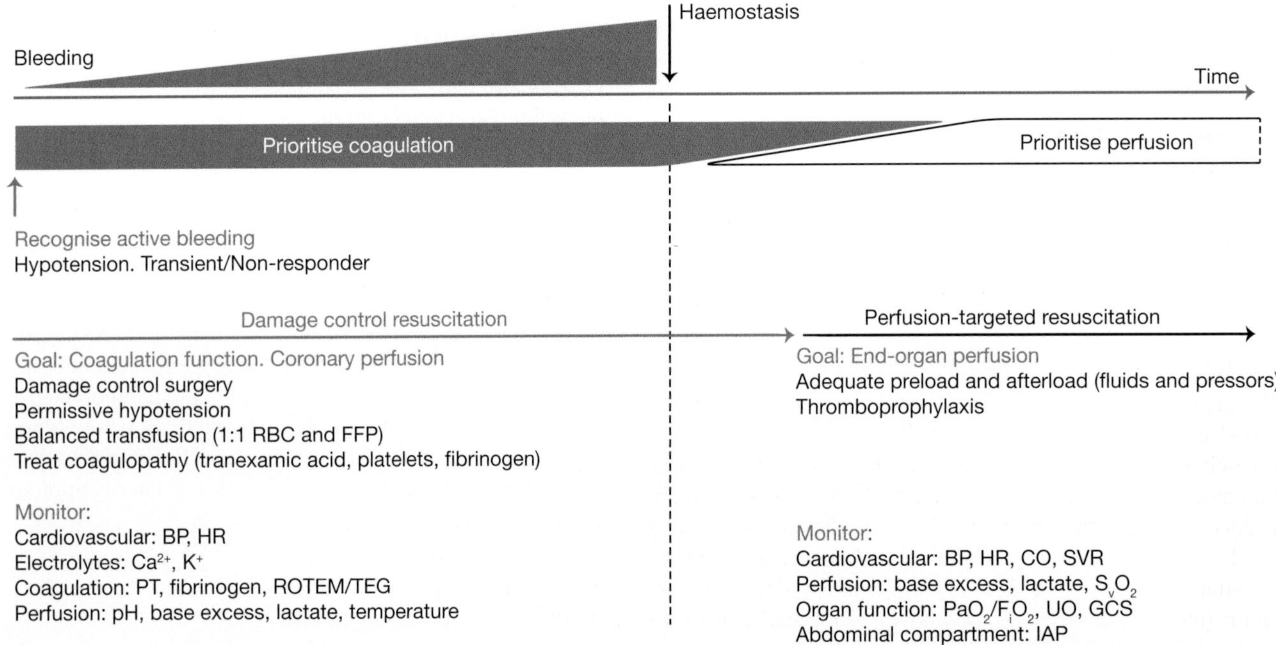

Figure 2.2 Haemorrhage resuscitation. BP, blood pressure; CO, cardiac output; FFP, fresh-frozen plasma; F_iO_2, fraction of inspired oxygen; GCS, Glasgow Coma Scale score; HR, heart rate; IAP, intra-abdominal pressure; PaO_2, arterial oxygen tension; PT, prothrombin time; RBC, red blood cells; ROTEM, rotational thromboelastometry; SVR, systemic vascular resistance; S_vO_2, mixed venous oxygen saturation; TEG, thromboelastography; UO, urine output.

while patients are bleeding, and repeated cycles of volume resuscitation will exacerbate coagulopathy, hypothermia and metabolic derangements (acidosis, hyperkalaemia, hypocalcaemia). The introduction of DCR has been associated with substantial reductions in mortality from haemorrhagic shock in the last decade.

DCR applies only while patients are bleeding and is based on four key principles – rapid haemorrhage control; permissive hypotension; avoiding dilutional coagulopathy; and treating existing coagulation deficits (***Figure 2.2***).

Rapid haemorrhage control

At all times, control of bleeding is the priority. Direct pressure should be placed over the site of external haemorrhage. Temporary bleeding control should be achieved with tourniquets, balloon occlusion or other techniques. Intracavitary haemorrhage should be suspected and searched for, and the pathway should actively move patients forwards to the operating theatre or interventional radiology room to achieve this.

The damage control approach is extended to the conduct of surgery to prioritise rapid bleeding control. In damage control surgery, surgical intervention is limited to the minimum necessary to stop bleeding and control sepsis, in order to avoid additional tissue damage, bleeding and physiological stress. More definitive repairs can be delayed until the patient is haemodynamically stable and physiologically capable of sustaining the procedure. Thus the operation is tailored to match the patient's physiology, and is not focused on reconstructing anatomy. 'Damage control' is a term borrowed from the military: it ensures continued functioning of a damaged ship above conducting complete repairs, which would prevent rapid return to battle.

Summary box 2.3

Damage control surgery

- Arrest haemorrhage
- Control sepsis
- Protect from further injury
- Nothing else

Permissive hypotension

Permissive hypotension allows the patient to set their own blood pressure while bleeding and avoids continued volume resuscitation in the vain attempt to normalise perfusion while bleeding. This reduces blood loss from bleeding sites and reduces dilutional coagulopathy and hypothermia induced by fluids. It is important to maintain baseline perfusion of the coronary arteries at minimum, and thus a palpable central pulse (mean arterial pressure above ~50 mmHg) must be maintained by whatever means are available.

Avoid dilutional coagulopathy

Avoid dilutional coagulopathy by avoiding clear fluids (crystalloids or colloids) and by giving a transfusion that approximates whole blood – usually administered as equal volumes of packed red blood cells and plasma.

Treat existing coagulation deficits

Treat existing coagulopathies either empirically or by regular coagulation testing and acting on the results. Tranexamic acid should be given as soon as possible in almost all bleeding patients to stop hyperfibrinolysis. Blood component concentrates should be given to correct existing deficits, such as cryoprecipitate for low fibrinogen levels or platelet transfusions for platelet dysfunctions.

After haemorrhage control

Once haemorrhage is controlled, patients should be definitively resuscitated, warmed and have coagulopathy corrected. Attention should be paid to fluid responsiveness and the end points of resuscitation to ensure that patients are fully resuscitated and to reduce the incidence and severity of organ failure (***Figure 2.2*** and ***Shock resuscitation***).

SHOCK RESUSCITATION

Immediate resuscitation manoeuvres for patients presenting in shock are to ensure a patent airway and adequate oxygenation and ventilation. Once 'airway' and 'breathing' are assessed and controlled, attention is directed to cardiovascular resuscitation. Haemorrhagic shock resuscitation should proceed as damage control resuscitation while bleeding continues (as discussed earlier). After bleeding is controlled, and for all other causes, shock resuscitation is guided by measures of tissue perfusion, as described in ***Monitoring***.

Conduct of resuscitation

Resuscitation should not be delayed in order to definitively diagnose the source of the shocked state. However, the timing and nature of resuscitation will depend on the type of shock and the timing and severity of the insult. Rapid clinical examination will provide adequate clues to make an appropriate first determination, even if a source of bleeding or sepsis is not immediately identifiable. If there is initial doubt about the cause of shock, it is safer to assume the cause is hypovolaemia and begin with fluid resuscitation, and then assess the response.

Correction of shock is important in the pre- and perioperative period for all cases of urgent surgery. For example, a patient with bowel obstruction and hypovolaemic shock must be adequately resuscitated before undergoing surgery. If not, the additional surgical injury and hypovolaemia induced during the procedure will increase the physiological demand on the heart, increasing the risk of myocardial infarction; will exacerbate the inflammatory activation and thus the incidence and severity of organ damage (especially acute kidney injury); will increase susceptibility to infection and venous thromboembolism; and will prolong the period of gut dysfunction and overall recovery from surgery.

Fluid therapy

In all cases of shock, regardless of classification, hypovolaemia and inadequate preload must be addressed before other therapy is instituted. Administration of inotropic or chronotropic agents to an empty heart will rapidly and permanently deplete the myocardium of oxygen stores and dramatically reduce diastolic filling and therefore coronary perfusion. Correction of preload by ensuring adequate volume resuscitation should be prioritised before introducing vasopressors or inotropic agents.

First-line therapy, therefore, is intravenous access and administration of intravenous fluids. Access should be through short, wide-bore catheters that allow rapid infusion of fluids as necessary. Long, narrow lines, such as central venous catheters, have too high a resistance to allow rapid infusion and are more appropriate for monitoring than fluid replacement therapy.

Type of fluids

As a general rule, the ideal replacement fluid is one that approximates the fluid lost by the underlying cause of shock. If blood is being lost, the replacement fluid is whole blood or its equivalent in components – although crystalloid therapy may be required while awaiting blood products. Other causes of shock will require crystalloid resuscitation with appropriate electrolyte supplementation.

In most studies of shock resuscitation there is no overt difference in response or outcome between crystalloid solutions (normal saline, Hartmann's solution, Ringer's lactate) and colloids (albumin or commercially available products). Furthermore, there is less volume benefit to the administration of colloids than had previously been thought, with only 1.3 times more crystalloid than colloid administered in blinded trials. On balance, there is little evidence to support the administration of colloids, which are more expensive and have worse side-effect profiles.

Hypotonic solutions (e.g. dextrose) are poor volume expanders and should not be used in the treatment of shock unless the deficit is free water loss (e.g. diabetes insipidus) or patients are sodium overloaded (e.g. cirrhosis).

Vasopressor and inotropic support

Vasopressor or inotropic therapy is not indicated as first-line therapy in hypovolaemia. Administration of these agents in the absence of adequate preload rapidly leads to decreased coronary perfusion and depletion of myocardial oxygen reserves.

Vasopressor agents (phenylephrine, noradrenaline [norepinephrine]) are indicated in distributive shock states (sepsis, neurogenic shock) where there is peripheral vasodilatation and a low systemic vascular resistance, leading to hypotension despite a high cardiac output. Where the vasodilatation is resistant to catecholamines (e.g. absolute or relative steroid deficiency), vasopressin may be used as an alternative vasopressor.

In cardiogenic shock, or where myocardial depression has complicated a shock state (e.g. severe septic shock with low cardiac output), inotropic therapy may be required to increase cardiac output and therefore oxygen delivery. The inodilator dobutamine is the agent of choice.

Monitoring

The **minimum** standard for monitoring of the patient in shock is continuous heart rate and oxygen saturation monitoring, frequent non-invasive blood pressure monitoring and hourly urine output measurements. Most patients will need more aggressive invasive monitoring, including central venous pressure (CVP) and invasive blood pressure monitoring.

Summary box 2.4

Monitoring for patients in shock

Minimum	Additional modalities
• ECG	• Central venous pressure
• Pulse oximetry	• Invasive blood pressure
• Blood pressure	• Cardiac output
• Urine output	• Base deficit and serum lactate

Cardiovascular

Cardiovascular monitoring at minimum should include continuous heart rate (electrocardiogram, oxygen saturation and pulse waveform and non-invasive blood pressure). Patients whose state of shock is not rapidly corrected with a small amount of fluid should have CVP monitoring and continuous blood pressure monitoring through an arterial line.

Central venous pressure

There is no 'normal' CVP for a shocked patient, and reliance cannot be placed on an individual pressure measurement to assess volume status. Some patients may require a CVP of 5 cmH_2O, whereas some may require a CVP of 15 cmH_2O or higher. Further, ventricular compliance can change from minute to minute in the shocked state, and CVP is a poor reflection of end-diastolic volume (preload).

CVP measurements should be assessed dynamically as the response to a fluid challenge. A fluid bolus (250–500 mL) is infused rapidly over 5–10 minutes.

The normal CVP response is a rise of 2–5 cmH_2O, which gradually drifts back to the original level over 10–20 minutes. Patients with no change in their CVP are empty and require further fluid resuscitation. Patients with a large, sustained rise in CVP have high preload and an element of cardiac insufficiency or volume overload.

Alexis Frank Hartmann, 1898–1964, paediatrician, St Louis, MO, USA, described the solution; should not be confused with the name of Henri Albert Charles Antoine Hartmann, French surgeon, who described the operation that goes by his name.
Sidney Ringer, 1835–1910, Professor of Clinical Medicine, University College Hospital, London, UK.

Cardiac output

Cardiac output monitoring allows assessment of not only the cardiac output but also the systemic vascular resistance and, depending on the technique used, end-diastolic volume (preload) and blood volume. Use of invasive cardiac monitoring with pulmonary artery catheters is becoming less frequent as new non-invasive monitoring techniques, such as Doppler ultrasound, pulse waveform analysis and indicator dilution methods, provide similar information without many of the drawbacks of more invasive techniques.

Measurement of cardiac output, systemic vascular resistance and preload can help distinguish the types of shock present (hypovolaemia, distributive, cardiogenic), especially when they coexist. The information provided guides fluid and vasopressor therapy by providing real-time monitoring of the cardiovascular response.

Measurement of cardiac output is desirable in patients who do not respond as expected to first-line therapy or who have evidence of cardiogenic shock or myocardial dysfunction. Early consideration should be given to instituting cardiac output monitoring for patients who require vasopressor or inotropic support.

Systemic and organ perfusion

Ultimately, the goal of treatment is to restore cellular and organ perfusion. Ideally, therefore, monitoring of organ perfusion should guide the management of shock. The best measure of organ perfusion and the best monitor of the adequacy of shock therapy remains the urine output. However, this is an hourly measure and does not give a minute-to-minute view of the shocked state. The level of consciousness is an important marker of cerebral perfusion, but brain perfusion is maintained until the very late stages of shock and hence is a poor marker of adequacy of resuscitation (*Table 2.4*).

Currently, the only clinical indicators of perfusion of the gastrointestinal tract and muscular beds are the global measures of lactic acidosis (lactate and base deficit) and the mixed venous oxygen saturation.

Base deficit and lactate

Lactic acid is generated by cells undergoing anaerobic respiration. The degree of lactic acidosis, as measured by serum lactate level and/or the base deficit, is sensitive for both diagnosis of shock and monitoring the response to therapy. Patients with a base deficit of more than 6 mmol/L have a much higher morbidity and mortality than those with no metabolic acidosis. Furthermore, the length of time in shock with an increased base deficit is important, even if all other vital signs have returned to normal (see occult hypoperfusion below under ***End points of resuscitation***).

These parameters are measured from arterial blood gas analyses, and therefore the frequency of measurements is limited and they do not provide minute-to-minute data on systemic perfusion or the response to therapy. Nevertheless, the base deficit and/or lactate should be measured routinely in these patients until they have returned to normal levels.

Mixed venous oxygen saturation

The percentage saturation of oxygen returning to the heart from the body is a measure of the oxygen delivery and extraction by the tissues. Accurate measurement is via analysis of blood drawn from a long central line placed in the right atrium. Estimations can be made from blood drawn from lines in the superior vena cava, but these values will be slightly higher than those of a mixed venous sample (as there is relatively more oxygen extraction from the lower half of the body). Normal mixed venous oxygen saturation levels are 50–70%. Levels below 50% indicate inadequate oxygen delivery and increased oxygen extraction by the cells. This is consistent with hypovolaemic or cardiogenic shock.

High mixed venous saturations (>70%) are seen in sepsis and some other forms of distributive shock. In sepsis, there is disordered utilisation of oxygen at the cellular level and

TABLE 2.4 Monitors for organ/systemic perfusion.

	Clinical	Investigational
Systemic perfusion		Base deficit
		Lactate
		Mixed venous oxygen saturation
Organ perfusion		
Muscle	–	Near-infrared spectroscopy
		Tissue oxygen electrode
Gut	–	Sublingual capnometry
		Gut mucosal pH
		Laser Doppler flowmetry
Kidney	Urine output	–
Brain	Conscious level	Tissue oxygen electrode
		Near-infrared spectroscopy

Christian Johann Doppler, 1803–1853, Professor of Experimental Physics, Vienna, Austria, enunciated the Doppler principle in 1842.

arteriovenous shunting of blood at the microvascular level. Therefore, less oxygen is presented to the cells, and those cells cannot utilise what little oxygen is presented. Thus, venous blood has a higher oxygen concentration than normal.

Patients who are septic should therefore have mixed venous oxygen saturations above 70%; below this level, they are not only in septic shock but also in hypovolaemic or cardiogenic shock. Although the S_vO_2 level is in the 'normal' range, it is low for the septic state, and inadequate oxygen is being supplied to cells that cannot utilise oxygen appropriately. This must be corrected rapidly. Hypovolaemia should be corrected with fluid therapy, and low cardiac output due to myocardial depression or failure should be treated with inotropes (dobutamine) to achieve a mixed venous saturation greater than 70% (normal for the septic state).

New methods for monitoring regional tissue perfusion and oxygenation are becoming available, the most promising of which are muscle tissue oxygen probes, near-infrared spectroscopy and sublingual capnometry. While these techniques provide information regarding perfusion of specific tissue beds, it is as yet unclear whether there are significant advantages over existing measurements of global hypoperfusion (base deficit, lactate).

End points of resuscitation

It is much easier to know when to start resuscitation than when to stop. Traditionally, patients have been resuscitated until they have a normal pulse, blood pressure and urine output. However, these parameters are monitoring organ systems whose blood flow is preserved until the late stages of shock. A patient therefore may be resuscitated to restore central perfusion to the brain, lungs and kidneys and yet continue to underperfuse the gut and muscle beds. Thus, activation of inflammation and coagulation may be ongoing and lead to reperfusion injury when these organs are finally perfused, and ultimately multiple organ failure.

This state of normal vital signs and continued underperfusion is termed 'occult hypoperfusion'. With current monitoring techniques, it is manifested only by a persistent lactic acidosis and low mixed venous oxygen saturation. The time spent by patients in this hypoperfused state has a dramatic effect on outcome. Patients with occult hypoperfusion for more than 12 hours have two to three times the mortality of patients with a limited duration of shock. Resuscitation algorithms directed at correcting global perfusion end points (base deficit, lactate, mixed venous oxygen saturation) rather than traditional end points have been shown to improve mortality and morbidity in high-risk surgical patients.

However, it is also clear that aggressive crystalloid resuscitation regimens can lead to tissue oedema and organ failure, especially acute respiratory distress syndrome, abdominal compartment syndrome and cerebral oedema. Some patients cannot be resuscitated to normal parameters within 12 hours by fluid resuscitation alone and care must be taken with all patients to be judicious in the approach to all therapies as end points are approached.

TRANSFUSION

The transfusion of blood and blood products has become commonplace since the first successful transfusion in 1818. Although the incidence of severe transfusion reactions and infections is now very low, in recent years it has become apparent that there is an immunological price to be paid for the transfusion of heterologous blood, leading to increased morbidity and decreased survival in certain population groups (trauma, malignancy). Supplies are also limited, and therefore the use of blood and blood products must always be judicious and justifiable for clinical need (***Table 2.5***).

TABLE 2.5 History of blood transfusion.

1492	Pope Innocent VIII suffers a stroke and receives a blood transfusion from three 10-year-old boys (paid a ducat each). All three boys died, as did the pope later that year
1665	Richard Lower in Oxford conducts the first successful canine transfusions
1667	Jean-Baptiste Denis reports successful sheep–human transfusions
1678	Animal–human transfusions are banned in France because of the poor results
1818	James Blundell performs the first successful documented human transfusion in a woman suffering postpartum haemorrhage. She received blood from her husband and survived
1901	Karl Landsteiner discovers the ABO system
1914	The Belgian physician Albert Hustin performed the first non-direct transfusion, using sodium citrate as an anticoagulant
1926	The British Red Cross instituted the first blood transfusion service in the world
1939	The rhesus system was identified and recognised as the major cause of transfusion reactions

Blood and blood products

Blood is collected from donors who have been previously screened before donating to exclude any donor whose blood may have the potential to harm the patient or to prevent possible harm that donating a unit of blood may have for the donor. In the UK, up to 450 mL of blood is drawn, a maximum of three times each year. Each unit is tested for evidence of hepatitis B, hepatitis C, human immunodeficiency virus (HIV)-1, HIV-2 and syphilis. Donations are leukodepleted as a precaution against variant Creutzfeldt–Jakob disease (this may also reduce the immunogenicity of the transfusion).

Karl Landsteiner, 1868–1943, Professor of Pathological Anatomy, University of Vienna, Austria. In 1909 he classified the human blood groups into A, B, AB and O. For this he was awarded the Nobel Prize in Physiology or Medicine in 1930.
Hans Gerhard Creutzfeldt, 1885–1946, neurologist, Kiel, Germany.
Alfons Maria Jakob, 1884–1931, neurologist, Hamburg, Germany.

The ABO and rhesus D blood groups are determined, as well as the presence of irregular red cell antibodies. The blood is then processed into subcomponents.

Whole blood

Whole blood is now rarely available in civilian practice because it has been seen as an inefficient use of the limited resource. However, whole blood transfusion has significant advantages over packed cells as it is coagulation factor rich and, if fresh, more metabolically active than stored blood.

Packed red cells

Packed red blood cells are spun-down and concentrated packs of red blood cells. Each unit is approximately 330 mL and has a haematocrit of 50–70%. Packed cells are stored in a SAG-M (saline–adenine–glucose–mannitol) solution to increase shelf life to 5 weeks at 2–6°C. (Older storage regimes included storage in CPD [citrate–phosphate–dextrose] solutions, which have a shelf life of 2–3 weeks.)

Fresh-frozen plasma

Fresh-frozen plasma (FFP) is rich in coagulation factors and is removed from fresh blood and stored at −40°C to −50°C with a 2-year shelf life. It is the first-line therapy in the treatment of coagulopathic haemorrhage (see ***Management of coagulopathy***). Rhesus D-positive FFP may be given to a rhesus D-negative woman, although it is possible for seroconversion to occur with large volumes owing to the presence of red cell fragments and Rh-D immunisation should be considered.

Cryoprecipitate

Cryoprecipitate is a supernatant precipitate of FFP and is rich in fibrinogen, factor VIII and factor XIII. It is stored at −30°C with a 2-year shelf life. It is given in low-fibrinogen states or factor VIII deficiency.

Platelets

Platelets are supplied as a pooled platelet concentrate and contain about 250 × 10^9/litre. Platelets are stored on a special agitator at 20–24°C and have a shelf life of only 5 days. Platelet transfusions are given to patients with thrombocytopenia or with platelet dysfunction who are bleeding or undergoing surgery.

Patients are increasingly presenting on antiplatelet therapy such as aspirin or clopidogrel for reduction of cardiovascular risk. Aspirin therapy rarely poses a problem but control of haemorrhage on the more potent platelet inhibitors can be extremely difficult. Patients on clopidogrel who are actively bleeding and undergoing major surgery may require almost continuous infusion of platelets during the course of the procedure. Arginine vasopressin or its analogues (DDAVP) have also been used in this patient group, although with limited success.

Prothrombin complex concentrates

Prothrombin complex concentrates are highly purified concentrates prepared from pooled plasma. They contain factors II, IX and X. Factor VII may be included or produced separately. It is indicated for the emergency reversal of anticoagulant (warfarin) therapy in uncontrolled haemorrhage.

Autologous blood

It is possible for patients undergoing elective surgery to pre-donate their own blood up to 3 weeks before surgery for re-transfusion during the operation. Similarly, during surgery blood can be collected in a cell saver, which washes and collects red blood cells that can then be returned to the patient.

Indications for blood transfusion

Blood transfusions should be avoided if possible, and many previous uses of blood and blood products are now no longer considered appropriate. The indications for blood transfusion are as follows:

- Acute blood loss, to replace circulating volume and maintain oxygen delivery;
- Perioperative anaemia, to ensure adequate oxygen delivery during the perioperative phase;
- Symptomatic chronic anaemia, without haemorrhage or impending surgery.

Transfusion trigger

Historically, patients were transfused to achieve a haemoglobin >10 g/dL. This has now been shown not only to be unnecessary but also to be associated with an increased morbidity and mortality compared with lower target values. A haemoglobin level of 6 g/dL is acceptable in patients who are not actively bleeding, those who are not about to undergo major surgery and those who are not symptomatic. There is some controversy as to the optimal haemoglobin level in some patient groups, such as those with cardiovascular disease, sepsis and traumatic brain injury. Although, conceptually, a higher haemoglobin level improves oxygen delivery, there is little clinical evidence at this stage to support higher levels in these groups (***Table 2.6***).

TABLE 2.6 Perioperative red blood cell transfusion criteria.

Haemoglobin level (g/dL)	Indications
<6	Probably will benefit from transfusion
6–8	Transfusion unlikely to be of benefit in the absence of bleeding or impending surgery
>8	No indication for transfusion in the absence of other risk factors

Blood groups and cross-matching

Human red cells have on their cell surface many different antigens. Two groups of antigens are of major importance in surgical practice – the ABO and rhesus systems.

ABO system

These proteins are strongly antigenic and are associated with naturally occurring antibodies in the serum. The system consists of three allelic genes – A, B and O – which control synthesis of enzymes that add carbohydrate residues to cell surface glycoproteins. A and B genes add specific residues while the O gene is an amorph and does not transform the glycoprotein.

TABLE 2.7 ABO blood group system.

Phenotype	Genotype	Antigens	Antibodies	Frequency (%)
O	OO	O	Anti-A, anti-B	46
A	AA or AO	A	Anti-B	42
B	BB or BO	B	Anti-A	9
AB	AB	AB	None	3

The system allows for six possible genotypes although there are only four phenotypes. Naturally occurring antibodies are found in the serum of those lacking the corresponding antigen (***Table 2.7***).

Blood group O is the universal donor type as it contains no antigens to provoke a reaction. Conversely, group AB individuals are 'universal recipients' and can receive any ABO blood type because they have no circulating antibodies.

Rhesus system

The rhesus D (Rh(D)) antigen is strongly antigenic and is present in approximately 85% of the population in the UK. Antibodies to the D antigen are not naturally present in the serum of the remaining 15% of individuals, but their formation may be stimulated by the transfusion of Rh-positive red cells or they may be acquired during delivery of a Rh(D)-positive baby.

Acquired antibodies are capable, during pregnancy, of crossing the placenta and, if present in a Rh(D)-negative mother, may cause severe haemolytic anaemia and even death (hydrops fetalis) in a Rh(D)-positive fetus *in utero*. The other minor blood group antigens may be associated with naturally occurring antibodies, or may stimulate the formation of antibodies on relatively rare occasions.

Transfusion reactions

If antibodies present in the recipient's serum are incompatible with the donor's cells, a transfusion reaction will result. This usually takes the form of an acute haemolytic reaction. Severe immune-related transfusion reactions due to ABO incompatibility result in potentially fatal complement-mediated intravascular haemolysis and multiple organ failure. Transfusion reactions from other antigen systems are usually milder and self-limiting.

Febrile transfusion reactions are non-haemolytic and are usually caused by a graft-versus-host-response from leukocytes in transfused components. Such reactions are associated with fever, chills or rigors. The blood transfusion should be stopped immediately. This form of transfusion reaction is rare with leukodepleted blood.

Cross-matching

To prevent transfusion reactions, all transfusions are preceded by ABO and rhesus typing of both donor and recipient blood to ensure compatibility. The recipient's serum is then mixed with the donor's cells to confirm ABO compatibility and to test for rhesus and any other blood group antigen–antibody reaction.

Full cross-matching of blood may take up to 45 minutes in most laboratories. In more urgent situations, 'type-specific' blood is provided; this is only ABO/rhesus matched and can be issued within 10–15 minutes. Where blood must be given in an emergency, group O (universal donor) blood is given (O– to females, O+ to males).

When blood transfusion is prescribed and blood is administered, it is essential that the correct patient receives the correct transfusion. Two healthcare personnel should check the patient's details against the prescription and the label of the donor blood. In addition, the donor blood serial number should also be checked against the issue slip for that patient. Provided these principles are strictly adhered to, the number of severe and fatal ABO incompatibility reactions can be minimised.

Complications of blood transfusion

Complications from blood transfusion can be categorised as those arising from a single transfusion and those related to massive transfusion.

Complications from a single transfusion

Complications from a single transfusion include:

- incompatibility haemolytic transfusion reaction;
- febrile transfusion reaction;
- allergic reaction;
- infection:
  - bacterial infection (usually due to faulty storage);
  - hepatitis;
  - HIV;
  - malaria;
- air embolism;
- thrombophlebitis;
- transfusion-related acute lung injury (usually from FFP).

Complications from massive transfusion

Complications from massive transfusion include:

- coagulopathy;
- hypocalcaemia;
- hyperkalaemia;
- hypokalaemia;
- hypothermia.

In addition, patients who receive repeated transfusions over long periods of time (e.g. patients with thalassaemia) may develop iron overload. (Each transfused unit of red blood cells contains approximately 250 mg of elemental iron.)

Management of coagulopathy

Correction of coagulopathy is not necessary if there is no active bleeding and haemorrhage is not anticipated (not due for surgery). However, coagulopathy will occur during major haemorrhage and should be anticipated and managed actively.

Prevention of dilutional coagulopathy is central to the damage control resuscitation of patients who are actively bleeding. This is the prime reason for delivering balanced transfusion regimes that deliver a resuscitation which approximates that of whole blood. In most practice this means delivering matched units of red blood cells, plasma and platelets in a 1:1:1 ratio. Crystalloids and colloids should be avoided if at all possible.

The balanced transfusion approach will not correct an established coagulopathy. Most bleeding patients are hyperfibrinolytic, and should be empirically given tranexamic acid, an antifibrinolytic agent, as quickly as possible.

Low fibrinogen levels are very common, and fibrinogen is vital to clot formation and stabilisation. Cryoprecipitate can be given empirically or guided by laboratory or point-of-care tests of clotting (e.g. thromboelastometry). Similarly platelet concentrates are given for low platelet counts or observed platelet dysfunction. Clotting function should be assayed frequently during haemorrhage and acted upon until bleeding has been controlled.

Blood substitutes

Blood substitutes are an attractive alternative to the costly process of donating, checking, storing and administering blood, especially given the immunogenic and potential infectious complications associated with transfusion.

There are several oxygen-carrying blood substitutes under investigation in experimental animal or early clinical trials. Blood substitutes are either biomimetic or abiotic. Biomimetic substitutes mimic the standard oxygen-carrying capacity of the blood and are haemoglobin based. Abiotic substitutes are synthetic oxygen carriers and are currently primarily perfluorocarbon based.

Haemoglobin is seen as the obvious candidate for developing an effective blood substitute, and one free haemoglobin solution is available in some countries where blood components are not readily available. Various other engineered molecules are under clinical trials and are based on human, bovine or recombinant technologies. Second-generation perfluorocarbon emulsions are also showing potential in clinical trials.

FURTHER READING

Cole E, Weaver A, Gall L *et al.* A decade of damage control resuscitation: new transfusion practice, new survivors, new directions. *Ann Surg* 2019; **273**(6): 1215–20.

Duchesne JC, McSwain NE Jr, Cotton BA *et al.* Damage control resuscitation: the new face of damage control. *J Trauma* 2010; **69**: 976–90.

Glen J, Constanti M, Brohi K; Guideline Development Group. Assessment and initial management of major trauma: summary of NICE guidance. *BMJ* 2016; **353**: i3051.

Harris T, Thomas GO, Brohi K. Early fluid resuscitation in severe trauma. *BMJ* 2012; **345**: e5752.

Nguyen HB, Jaehne AK, Jayaprakash N *et al.* Early goal-directed therapy in severe sepsis and septic shock: insights and comparisons to ProCESS, ProMISe, and ARISE. *Crit Care* 2016; **20**(1): 160.

Pearse RM, Ackland GL. Perioperative fluid therapy. *BMJ* 2012; **344**: e2865.

Semler MW, Rice TW. Sepsis resuscitation: fluid choice and dose. *Clin Chest Med* 2016; **37**: 241–50.

Sihler KC, Nathans AB. Management of severe sepsis in the surgical patient. *Surg Clin N Am* 2006; **86**: 1457–81.

Spahn DR, Bouillon B, Cerny V *et al.* The European guideline on management of major bleeding and coagulopathy following trauma: fifth edition. *Crit Care* 2019; **23**: 98.

CHAPTER 3 Wound healing and tissue repair

Learning objectives

To understand:

- Normal wound healing and how it can be adversely affected
- Types of healing and how to classify wounds
- The principles of wound management
- The principles of scar management

INTRODUCTION

Wound healing is a complex and dynamic biological process. In human adults, the normal response to injury across all organ systems typically results in fibrosis and scar formation. Fibrotic healing causes tissue dysfunction and its potential impact on patients is often underappreciated. This contrasts with early gestation when fetal tissues can remarkably heal without fibrosis. Regenerative medicine is therefore an exciting field of research. A better understanding of the mechanisms involved can potentially help reduce the global burden of disease associated with wound healing. This chapter describes the pathophysiology of wound healing, the types of healing and how to classify wounds. Clinical judgement is crucial in managing wounds. A framework is provided to better understand the key principles of wound and scar management.

NORMAL WOUND HEALING IN SKIN

Classically, wound healing has been arbitrarily described in three overlapping but distinct stages, including inflammation, proliferation and remodelling (***Figure 3.1***). An additional stage, haemostasis, is often described as the immediate phase occurring before inflammation.

Haemostasis

Disruption of the vascular endothelium following injury causes vasoconstriction and exposure of the subendothelial extracellular matrix. This encourages platelets to adhere, activate and aggregate, resulting in a platelet plug, which also helps limit further blood loss.

Platelet adhesion results in their activation and release of granules. Alpha granules contain hundreds of proteins, including cytokines and growth factors; for example, transforming growth factor beta, platelet-derived growth factor, fibroblast growth factor, epidermal growth factor and vascular endothelial growth factor. These are involved in the deposition of extracellular matrix, chemotaxis, epithelialisation and the formation of new blood vessels (angiogenesis).

Platelet aggregation occurs once platelets become activated. At the same time, tissue factor at the site of injury initiates the coagulation cascade (***Figure 3.2***), resulting in the formation of thrombin. Thrombin performs various functions, including fibrin generation, which helps to stabilise the platelet plug and form a scaffold for infiltrating cells.

Inflammation

In the early inflammatory phase (days 1–2), platelet activation causes an influx of inflammatory cells led by polymorphonuclear leukocytes, particularly neutrophils. The latter are important for minimising bacterial contamination of the wound. Platelets and the local injured tissue also release vasoactive amines such as histamine and serotonin, which increase vascular permeability, thereby aiding infiltration of inflammatory cells.

During the late inflammatory phase (days 2–3) monocytes appear in the wound and differentiate into macrophages. Macrophages play a vital role in wound healing. They function as phagocytic cells and release proteolytic enzymes to help debride the wound. They are also the primary producer of cytokines and growth factors promoting fibroblast proliferation and angiogenesis.

Historically, this phase has been described by *rubor* (redness), *tumor* (swelling), *calor* (heat) and *dolor* (pain).

Proliferation

The proliferative phase starts around day 3 and lasts for 2–4 weeks. It consists mainly of fibroblast activity with the production of ground substance (glycosaminoglycans and proteoglycans), collagen, angiogenesis and re-epithelialisation of the wound.

The wound tissue formed in the early part of this phase is called granulation tissue. It has a pink and granular appearance. In the later part of this phase, there is an increase in the

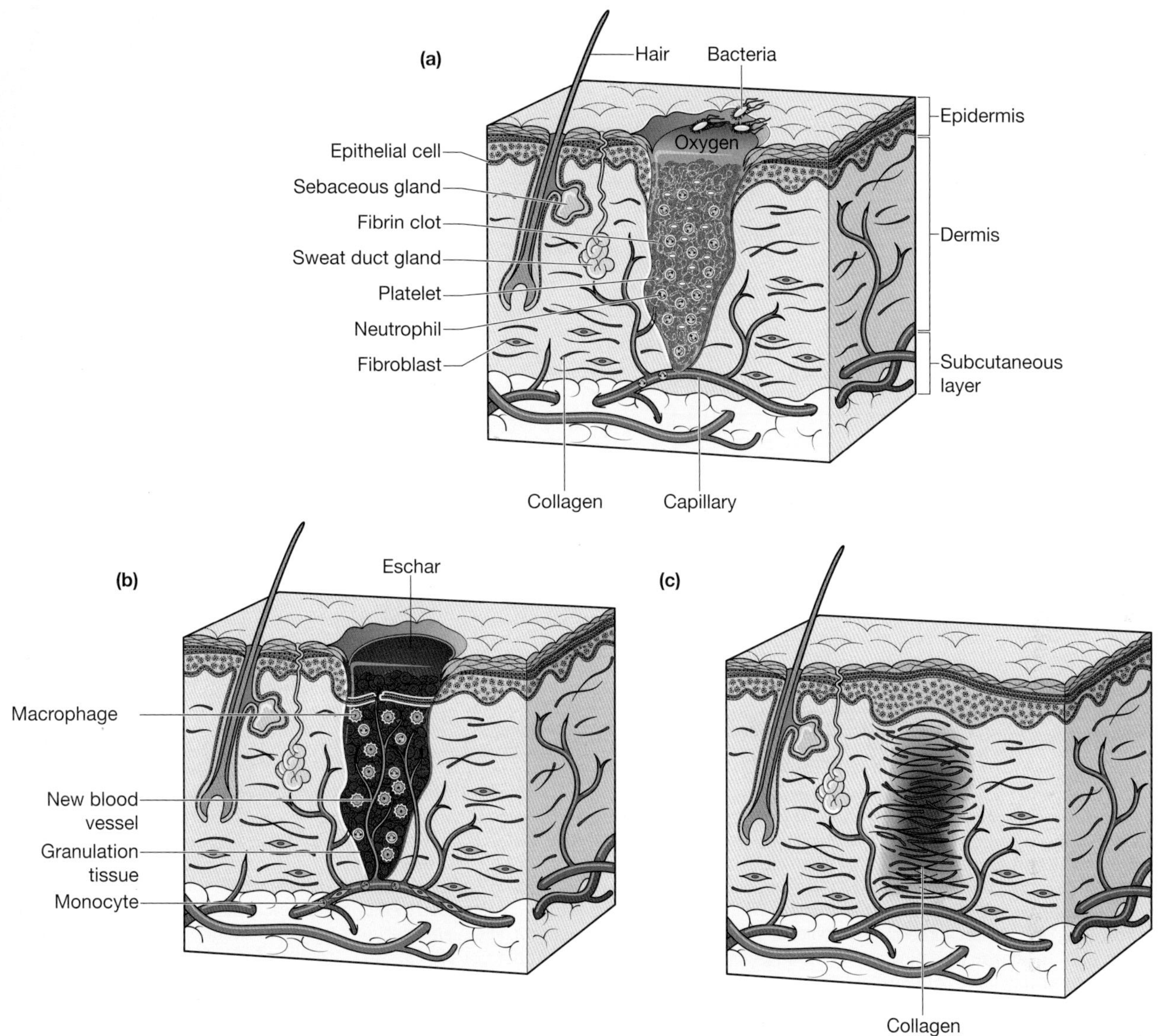

Figure 3.1 Classic stages of wound healing. (a) Inflammation. (b) Proliferation. (c) Remodelling. (Adapted by permission from Springer: Gurtner G, Werner S, Barrandon Y *et al*. Wound repair and regeneration. *Nature* 2008; **453**: 314–21. 2008).

tensile strength of the wound as a result of increased collagen synthesised by fibroblasts. Some fibroblasts differentiate into myofibroblasts, which are contractile cells. These play an important role in contraction to bring the edges of the wound together.

Remodelling

The remodelling phase begins 2–3 weeks after injury and lasts for a year or more. This phase is characterised by maturation of collagen. Type III collagen, which is prevalent during proliferation, is replaced by stronger type I collagen until the normal skin ratio of 4:1 type I to type III collagen is re-established. The collagen becomes more cross-linked and uniformly aligned. This maturation of collagen leads to increased tensile strength in the wound, which is maximal 12 weeks post injury and represents approximately 80% of the uninjured skin strength.

NORMAL HEALING IN OTHER SPECIFIC TISSUES

Bone

Bone healing occurs in similar phases to those for skin but with some differences (***Figure** 3.3*). Most fractures heal by callus formation, which involves intramembranous and endochondral ossification. This is known as indirect or secondary bone healing and typically occurs in non-operative fracture management. A haematoma forms at the fracture site and there is an inflammatory response. The fracture haematoma is gradually replaced by a soft callus. This fibrocartilage callus then undergoes endochondral ossification to form hard callus, which is woven bone helping to stabilise the fracture. Intramembranous ossification also occurs directly adjacent to the distal and proximal fracture ends. Hard callus formation is

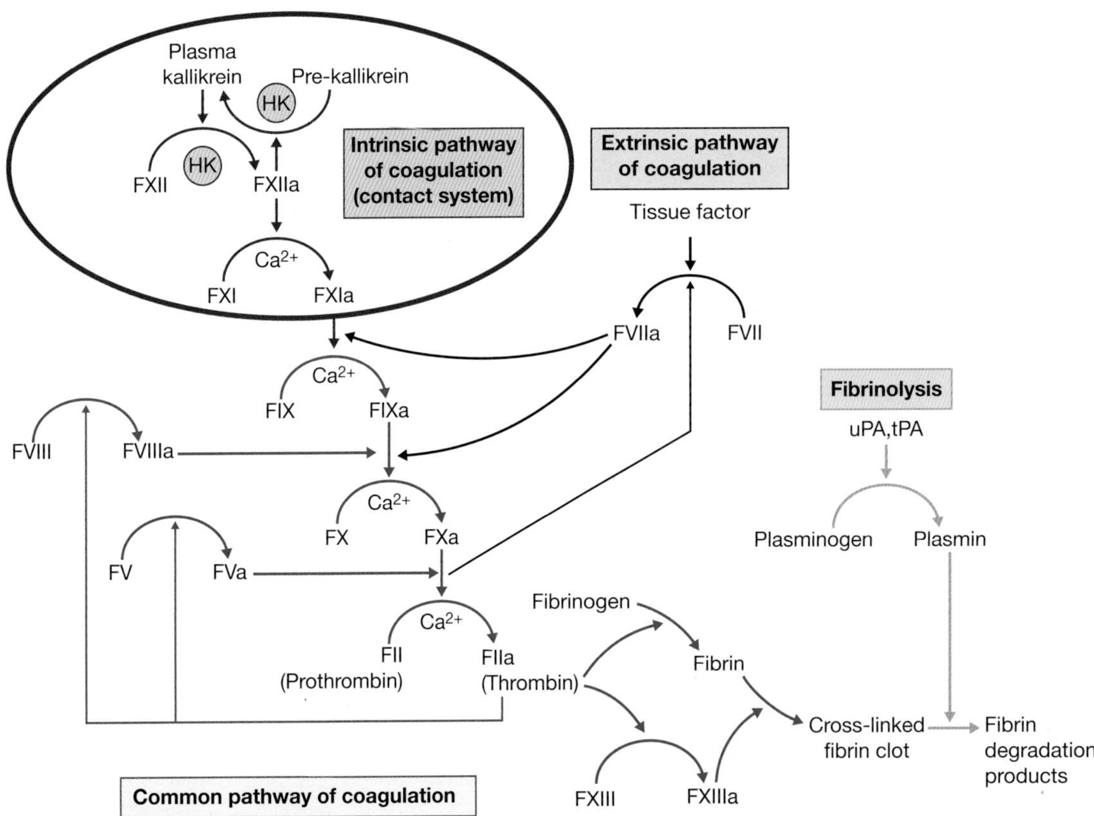

Figure 3.2 Schematic representation of the coagulation cascade and the fibrinolytic system. The coagulation cascade (blue arrows) can be activated during haemostasis via the intrinsic pathway (contact system; red arrows) or the extrinsic pathway (black arrows), which ultimately converge on the common pathway of coagulation. Both pathways lead to the activation of factor X and subsequently of thrombin, which is required for the conversion of fibrinogen into fibrin and for activation of factor XIII. The fibrin clot is cross-linked and stabilised by factor XIII. Fibrinolysis (green arrows) is activated at the same time as the coagulation system but operates more slowly and is important for the regulation of haemostasis. During fibrinolysis, plasminogen is converted into plasmin, which degrades the fibrin network. Coagulation factors are indicated by 'F' followed by a roman numeral; an additional 'a' denotes the activated form. HK, high-molecular-weight kininogen; tPA, tissue plasminogen activator; uPA, urokinase plasminogen activator. (Adapted with permission from Loof TG, Deicke C, Medina E. The role of coagulation/fibrinolysis during *Streptococcus pyogenes* infection. *Front Cell Infect Microbiol* 2014; **4**: 128. 2014. http://creativecommons.org/licenses/by/4.0/)

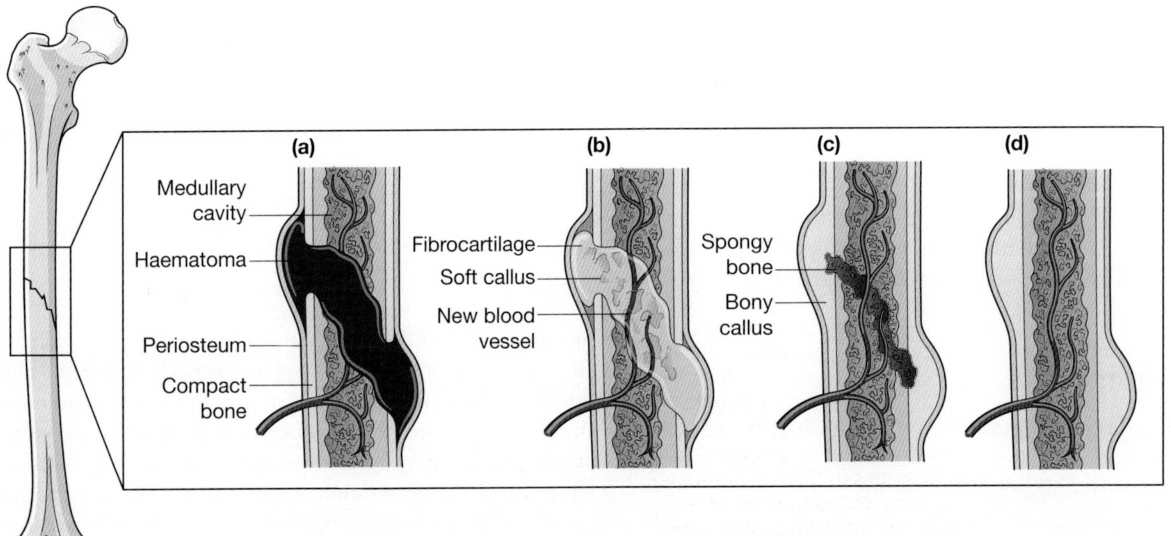

Figure 3.3 Common stages of bone healing. (a) At the fracture site, haematoma formation and inflammation lead to (b) soft callus formation. (c) Hard callus formation from osteoblasts forming woven bone. (d) Remodelling proceeds with osteoclasts and osteoblasts facilitating the conversion of woven bone into lamellar bone and eventually recreating the appropriate anatomical shape. (Adapted with permission from Li J, Kacena MA, Stocum DL. Fracture healing. In: Burr DB, Allen MR (eds). *Basic and applied bone biology*, 2nd edn. London: Academic Press, 2019: 235–53.)

followed by bony remodelling, where woven bone is replaced by lamellar bone.

Primary bone healing is a direct bone union process involving intramembranous ossification without callus formation. It does not commonly occur in the natural process of healing since it requires fracture ends to be directly apposed and rigidly fixed with absolute stability. If a gap exists, then secondary healing may lead to delayed union, non-union or malunion. Primary healing is therefore the aim of open reduction and internal fixation surgery. (See also *Chapter 32*) .

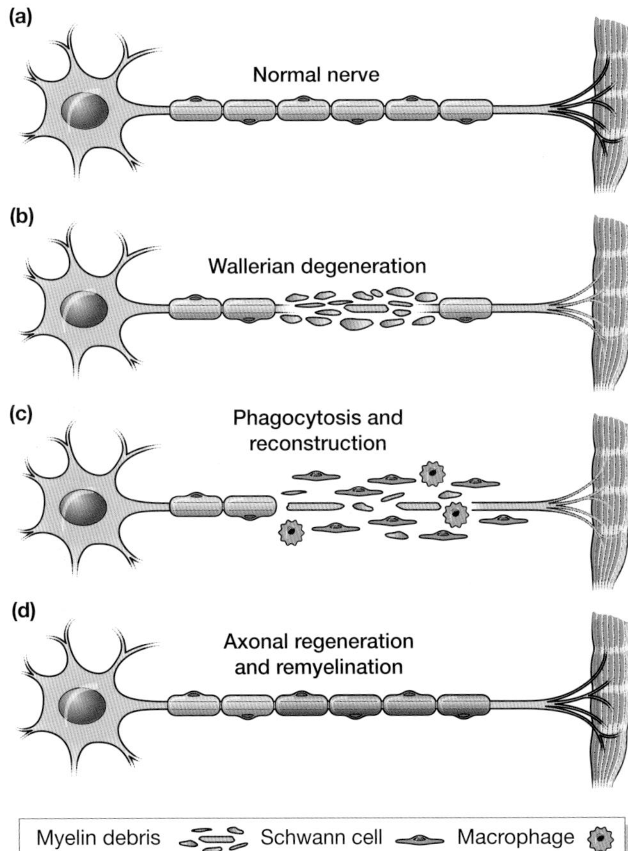

Figure 3.4 Schematic diagram illustrating the process of degeneration and regeneration after peripheral nerve injury. When normal nerves (a) suffer a physical injury, the portion of the lesion site and its distal stump undergo destruction and break down to produce myelin debris. This degenerative process is called Wallerian degeneration (b). Then, Schwann cells (SCs) recruit macrophages to scavenge degenerated myelin fragments (c). Meanwhile, SCs proliferate and migrate alone to the basal lamina to form bands of Büngner, which guide the axon to reinnervate towards the corresponding target (d). (Adapted from Li R, Li DH, Zhang HY *et al*. Growth factor-based therapeutic strategies and their underlying signaling mechanisms for peripheral nerve regeneration. *Acta Pharmacol Sin* 2020; **41**: 1289–300. 2020. http://creativecommons.org/licenses/by/4.0/)

Nerve

Peripheral nerve degeneration and regeneration are summarised in ***Figure 3.4***. Distal to nerve injury (neurotmesis), Wallerian degeneration occurs. Proximally, the nerve suffers degeneration as far as the nearest node of Ranvier. The regenerating nerve fibres are attracted to their receptors by neurotropism, which is mediated by growth factors, hormones and the extracellular matrix. Injury of the perineurium and inflammation can lead to neuroma formation, where the disorganised nerve regeneration leads to a painful lump.

Tendon

Although repair follows the normal pattern of wound healing, there are two main mechanisms whereby nutrients, cells and new vessels reach the severed tendon. Intrinsic healing consists of vincular blood flow and synovial diffusion. Extrinsic healing depends on the formation of fibrous adhesions between the tendon and the tendon sheath. Early active mobilisation following tendon repairs prevents adhesions limiting the range of motion and therefore promotes the more desired intrinsic healing. At the same time, tendon repairs must be protected by splintage to avoid rupture.

ABNORMAL WOUND HEALING

Various factors can adversely affect wound healing (***Summary box 3.1***). Some wounds fail to heal in a timely and orderly manner, resulting in chronic non-healing wounds, significant morbidity and poor cosmesis. On the other hand,

Summary box 3.1

Local and systemic factors influencing wound healing

- Local
  - Skin tension
  - Hypoxia and ischaemia
  - Vascular insufficiency
  - Lymphoedema
  - Contamination
  - Infection
  - Presence of foreign bodies
  - Radiotherapy
- Systemic
  - Advancing age
  - Obesity
  - Malnutrition
  - Smoking
  - Diseases (e.g. diabetes mellitus, connective tissue diseases)
  - Immunocompromised (e.g. acquired immunodeficiency syndrome)
  - Medications (e.g. steroids, immunosuppressants, chemotherapy)

Augustus Volney Waller, 1816–1870, general practitioner of Kensington, London, UK (1842–1851), subsequently worked as a physiologist in Bonn, Germany; Paris, France; Birmingham, UK; and Geneva, Switzerland.

Louis Antoine Ranvier, 1835–1922, physician and histologist who was a professor in the College of France, Paris, France, described these nodes in 1878.

aberrations of normal wound healing such as prolonged inflammation can result in excessive scar tissue, for example hypertrophic and keloid scars. These abnormal scars contain excess collagen, which is arranged in a disorganised pattern in keloid scars as opposed to a parallel pattern in hypertrophic scars.

Hypertrophic scars do not extend beyond the boundary of the original incision or wound and eventually regress. They are more common in areas of increased tension, wounds crossing tension lines, deep dermal burns and wounds left to heal by secondary intention (longer than 3 weeks).

Keloid scars extend beyond the boundaries of the original incision or wound (***Figure 3.5***), do not spontaneously regress and are difficult to treat. The aetiology is unknown but genetic predisposition is implicated. They often occur as a result of relatively minor trauma and mainly in those with darker skin pigmentation.

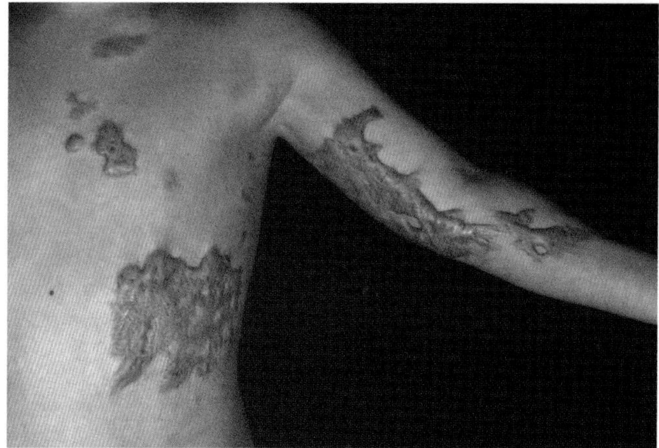

Figure 3.5 Multiple keloid scars.

TYPES OF WOUND HEALING

There are different types of healing (***Summary box 3.2***). Primary healing is also known as healing by first intention. This occurs when there is direct approximation of the wound edges and is the aim of treatment. When there are no adverse influences, these wounds heal well and leave the best scar. Delayed primary healing occurs when the wound edges are not opposed immediately, which may be necessary in contaminated or untidy wounds. After debridement of non-viable tissue and when the wound is clean, the wound edges may be surgically approximated. This is also called healing by tertiary intention.

Secondary healing or healing by secondary intention occurs in wounds that are left open and allowed to heal by granulation, contraction and re-epithelialisation.

Summary box 3.2

Classification of wound closure and healing

- Primary
  - Wound edges apposed
  - Normal healing
  - Minimal scar
- Secondary
  - Wound left open
  - Heals by granulation, contraction and re-epithelialisation
  - Increased inflammation and proliferation
  - Poor scar
- Tertiary (delayed primary)
  - Wound initially left open
  - Edges apposed later when healing conditions favourable

CLASSIFICATION OF WOUNDS

Wounds are diverse and there is no standard classification system that incorporates all relevant aspects for different clinical contexts. A wide variety of classifications (***Summary box 3.3***) are used and descriptors from more than one system are required to accurately describe a given wound.

A widely accepted wound classification was first introduced in 1964 by the US National Research Council[1] to describe the degree of bacterial load or contamination of surgical wounds at the time of surgery. It was subsequently adapted by the US Centers for Disease Prevention and Control[2] to classify wounds as clean, clean–contaminated, contaminated and dirty (***Table 3.1***). Although the simplicity of this classification has led to its widespread use, the definitions are not entirely clear and low interobserver reliability has been reported.[3,4]

Various grading and scoring systems exist for specific conditions such as pressure ulcers and diabetic ulcers. The National Nosocomial Infections Surveillance (NNIS) score is commonly used to predict surgical site infections (SSIs). It was established in recognition of the effectiveness of infection surveillance in reducing SSIs.[5] The NNIS score stratifies surgical wound infection rates by risk factors. This risk index score ranges from 0 (lowest SSI risk) to 3 (highest SSI risk) with a point allocated for the presence of each of the following risk factors:

TABLE 3.1 US Centers for Disease Prevention and Control surgical wound classification.[2]

Class I *Clean*	Uninfected operative wounds No inflammation is encountered Respiratory, alimentary, genital or uninfected urinary tracts are not entered Primarily closed and, if necessary, drained using a closed system
Class II *Clean–contaminated*	Respiratory, alimentary, genital or urinary tracts are entered under controlled conditions and without unusual contamination No evidence of infection or major break in technique is encountered
Class III *Contaminated*	Open, fresh, accidental wounds Operations with major breaks in sterile technique (e.g. open cardiac massage) or gross spillage from the gastrointestinal tract Incisions in which acute, non-purulent inflammation is encountered
Class IV *Dirty*	Old traumatic wounds with retained devitalised tissue and those that involve existing clinical infection or perforated viscera

- contaminated or dirty wound;
- American Society of Anesthesiologists score ≥3;
- operative time longer than the expected duration for similar procedures (>75th percentile).

Summary box 3.3

Synopsis of wound classification systems

- Aetiology
  - Clean, surgical
  - Shearing or degloving
  - Crush
  - Blast
  - Burn (thermal, electrical, chemical, radiation, mechanical)
  - Cold injury
  - Avulsion or traction
  - Low or high energy
  - Bite
- Depth
  - Epidermal
  - Dermal (superficial or deep)
  - Full thickness
- Contamination
  - Clean
  - Clean–contaminated
  - Contaminated
  - Dirty
  - Implant or non-implant
- Complexity
  - Simple
  - Complex
    - Significant soft-tissue loss
    - Open fracture or joint
    - Visceral involvement
  - Complicated
    - Infection
    - Necrosis
    - Haematoma
    - Gas gangrene
    - Compartment syndrome
- Chronic
  - Vascular ulcers (venous or arterial)
  - Pressure ulcers
  - Diabetic ulcers

WOUND MANAGEMENT

Assessment

Wound management is guided by the timing and mechanism of injury as well as factors affecting healing (***Summary box 3.1***). It is also important to assess the patient's ideas, concerns and expectations. Patient outcomes also rely on good postoperative compliance.

Assess the patient using Advanced Trauma Life Support principles to first identify and treat life- and then limb-threatening conditions. Some wounds require a multidisciplinary approach; for example, the involvement of orthopaedic surgeons and plastic surgeons in managing complex open lower limb fractures.[6]

Assess the site, size, geometry and nature of any wounds. Look for signs of contamination, infection, swelling and pulsatile bleeding. Deformities may suggest underlying fractures or dislocations. Has there been skin loss or degloving? What structures are visible? Thorough irrigation of wounds will allow better visualisation.

It is important to correlate the clinical examination with the mechanism of injury as seemingly innocuous wounds can lead to underestimation of tissue damage. For example, high-pressure injection injuries of the hand can cause significant mechanical and chemical tissue damage with risk of amputation. The injected substances can track proximally into the forearm. Urgent surgical exploration and debridement is required.

Before palpation, ensure that the patient has adequate analgesia or a local anaesthetic block. When possible, it is important to assess motor and sensory function before any local anaesthesia. Unless there are obvious muscle injuries, the purpose of testing specific muscle groups is to evaluate potential nerve or tendon injuries. Imaging is useful to exclude foreign bodies, fractures or dislocations where appropriate.

Principles

Clinical judgement is crucial in managing wounds. Some general principles of wound management are summarised in ***Table 3.2***. Antibiotic prophylaxis is needed for clean–contaminated, contaminated and dirty wounds. It may also be used in clean wounds when there is a high risk of infection or when the sequelae of infection are potentially disastrous. Tetanus prophylaxis should be given based on the type of wound (***Table 3.3***) and immunisation status (***Figure 3.6***).

TABLE 3.2 Principles of wound management.

Preparation	Antibiotic prophylaxis Tetanus prophylaxis Adequate analgesia/anaesthesia Wound irrigation
Wound	Early debridement and irrigation Exploration Repair structures Haemostasis
Closure	Skin closure without tension Consider reconstruction options Suture choice Consider drains Optimal dressings
Follow-up	Removal of sutures/splints Physiotherapy Monitoring for complications Scar management

TABLE 3.3 Tetanus-prone wounds.[7]

Tetanus-prone wounds	High-risk tetanus-prone wounds
• Puncture-type injuries in a contaminated environment • Bites • Compound fractures • Containing foreign bodies • Wounds or burns with systemic sepsis	Any tetanus-prone wound with: • Heavy contamination, e.g. soil or manure • Wound requiring surgery with >6-hour delay • Extensive devitalised tissue

Adapted from https://www.gov.uk/government/publications/tetanus-prone-wounds-posters.

Debridement is essential to remove any devitalised tissue and foreign material from the wound. Non-viable tissue must be excised until healthy bleeding occurs at the wound edges. The importance of thorough debridement is often

Post exposure management for Tetanus Prone Wounds

Immunisation Status	Immediate treatment					Later treatment
	Clean wound[1]	Tetanus prone		High risk tetanus prone		
Those aged 11 years and over, who have received an adequate priming course of tetanus vaccine[1] with the last dose within 10 years	None required	None required		None required		Further doses as required to complete the recommended schedule (to ensure future immunity)
Children aged 5-10 years who have received priming course and pre-school booster						
Children under 5 years who have received an adequate priming course						
Received adequate priming course of tetanus vaccine[3] but last dose more than 10 years ago	None required	Immediate reinforcing dose of vaccine		Immediate reinforcing dose of vaccine	One dose of human tetanus immunoglobulin[2] in a different site	
Children aged 5-10 years who have received an adequate priming course but no pre-school booster						
(Includes UK born after 1961 with history of accepting vaccinations)						
Not received adequate priming course of tetanus vaccine[3] (Includes uncertain immunisation status and/or born before 1961)	Immediate reinforcing dose of vaccine	Immediate reinforcing dose of vaccine	One dose of human tetanus immunoglobulin[2] in a different site	Immediate reinforcing dose of vaccine	One dose of human tetanus immunoglobulin[2] in a different site	

1 Clean wounds are defined as wounds less than six hours old, non-penetrating with negligible tissue damage.

2 If TIG is not available, HNIG may be used as an alternative.

3 At least three doses of tetanus vaccine at appropriate intervals. This definition of "adequate course" is for risk assessment of tetanus-prone wounds only. The full UK schedule is five doses of tetanus containing vaccine.

Patients who are severely immunosuppressed may not be adequately protected against tetanus, despite having been fully immunised and additional booster doses or treatment may be required.

Figure 3.6 Postexposure management for tetanus-prone wounds. (Redrawn with permission from https://www.gov.uk/government/publications/tetanus-prone-wounds-posters. © Crown copyright 2019. 2019TET02 10K OCT 2019 (APS).

underappreciated and is not as simple as is often perceived. The end points of surgical debridement can sometimes be difficult to determine. Healthy subcutaneous fat is yellow and soft. Muscle viability is judged by its colour, capacity to bleed and contractility. Contaminated, complex and complicated wounds often require more than one surgical debridement before definitive repair and closure; for example, blast injuries and necrotising fasciitis (see ***Part 4***). Other types of debridement are summarised in ***Table 3.4***.

TABLE 3.4 Types of debridement.

Surgical	Excision of non-viable tissue using surgical instruments such as a scalpel, curette, scissors or rongeur until healthy bleeding occurs at the wound edges
Mechanical	Non-selective debridement such as using irrigation, wet-to-dry dressings and hydrotherapy. Both non-viable and viable tissue may be removed
Autolytic	Using dressings such as hydrocolloids or transparent films to retain moisture and allow wound enzymes to selectively liquefy non-viable tissue
Enzymatic	Chemically liquefy necrotic tissue with enzymes using topical agents such as collagenase or papain–urea
Biological	Medical-grade larvae of *Lucilia sericata* release proteolytic and antimicrobial substances to remove necrotic tissue. They also directly promote wound healing

All wounds should be irrigated at the first available opportunity to reduce bacterial contamination. This also allows better visualisation for wound assessment. Warm normal saline

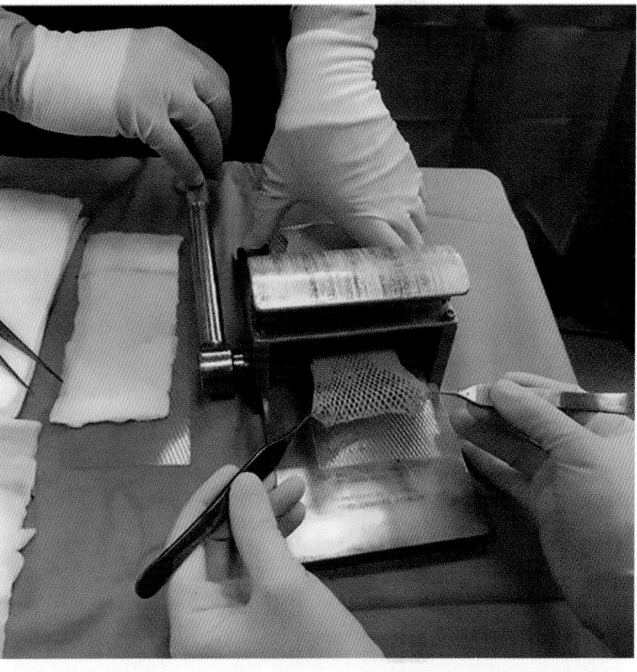

Figure 3.7 Meshing a split-thickness skin graft. (Reproduced with permission of MA Healthcare Limited from Hili S, Wong KY, Stephens P. Pretibial lacerations. *Br J Hosp Med* 2017; **78**: C162–6.)

is typically used, although other irrigation fluids are available such as water and antiseptic solutions. Irrigation can also be performed with a soft brush or sponge to clear particulate matter prior to preoperative application of skin antiseptic preparation.

Wounds should be explored to determine the extent of injury, including any damage to underlying neurovascular structures, tendons, joints and bones. Careful tissue handling and meticulous technique are important throughout. Repair of all damaged structures may be attempted once the wounds are clean. Repair of nerves and vessels should be performed under magnification using loupes or a microscope.

Skin closure should always be without tension. Direct closure is not always possible and other reconstruction methods should be considered. Historically, the reconstructive ladder and its variants such as the reconstructive elevator[8] have been used as a framework to consider the simplest means to achieve wound closure for the desired goal. Advances in technology and surgical techniques have led to ongoing adjustments of these frameworks. Although these frameworks do not guide the selection of a particular technique over another, they provide a useful reminder of the options available (***Summary box 3.4***).

A skin graft has no inherent blood supply and is dependent on a well-vascularised recipient site for survival and wound healing. Split-thickness skin grafts (***Figure 3.7***) consist of the epidermis and a small portion of dermis whereas full-thickness skin grafts consist of the epidermis and the majority of the dermis.

A flap contains tissue with its intrinsic blood supply that is transferred from one part of the body (donor) to another (recipient). The blood supply of the flap therefore does not rely on the recipient site like a skin graft. A free flap contains tissue with its vascular pedicle that is surgically detached and transferred from its original location to a distant recipient site (***Figure 3.8***). A microscope is used to perform microvascular anastomoses to connect the blood vessels in the free flap to blood vessels close to the recipient site.

Since its development in the 1990s, negative-pressure wound therapy (NPWT) is now widely used. It is not a replacement for definitive wound closure but is a useful adjunct

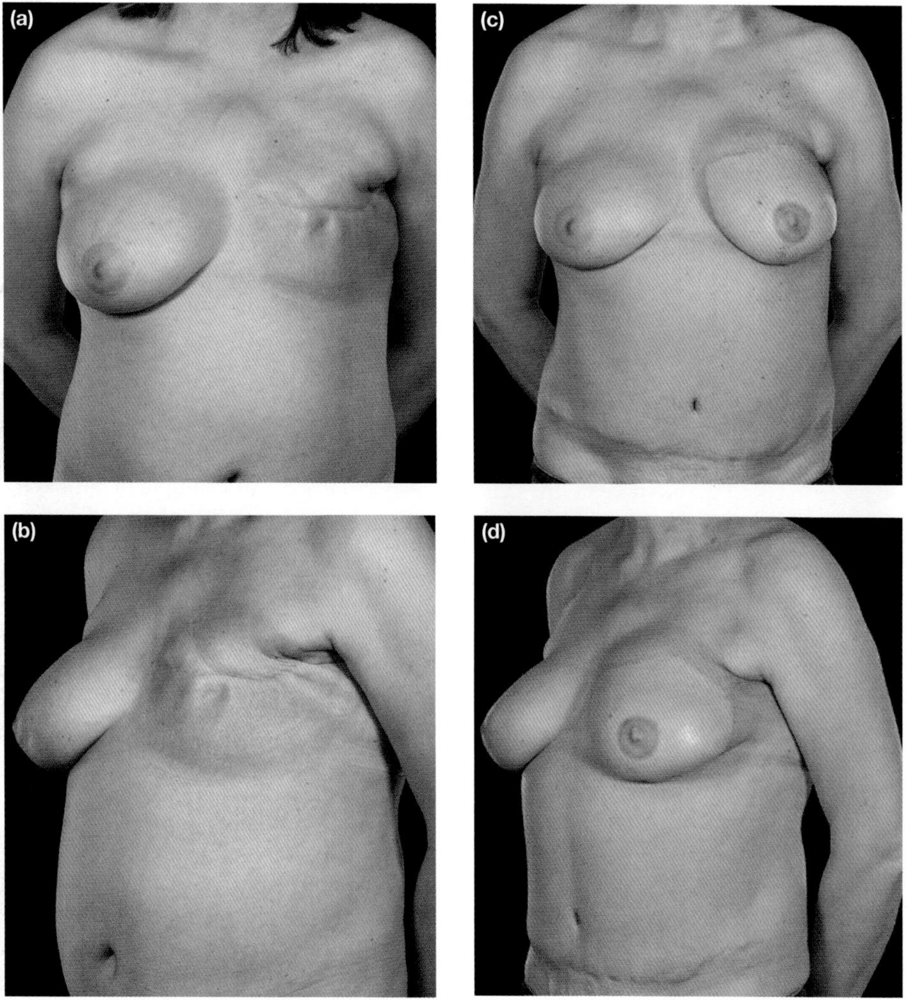

Figure 3.8 Left mastectomy (a, b) and delayed left breast reconstruction with a deep inferior epigastric artery perforator free flap and nipple reconstruction (c, d) (©Addenbrookes Hospital).

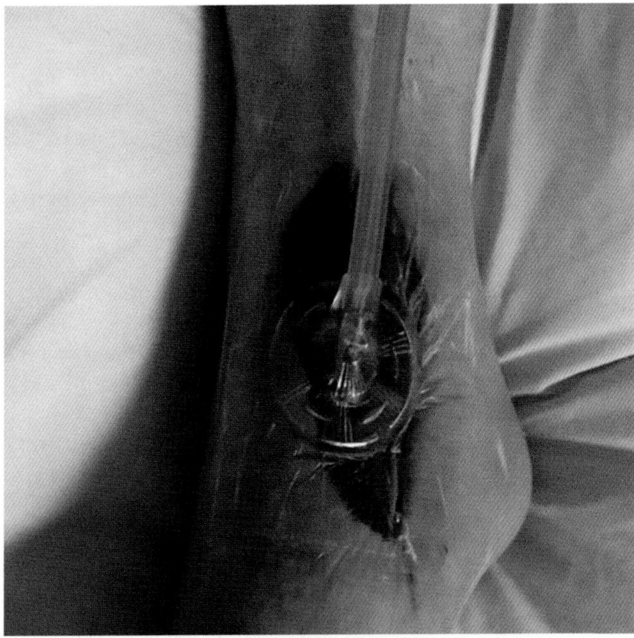

Figure 3.9 Negative-pressure wound therapy for a lower limb wound. (Reproduced with permission of MA Healthcare Limited from Hili S, Wong KY, Stephens P. Pretibial lacerations. *Br J Hosp Med* 2017; **78**: C162–6.)

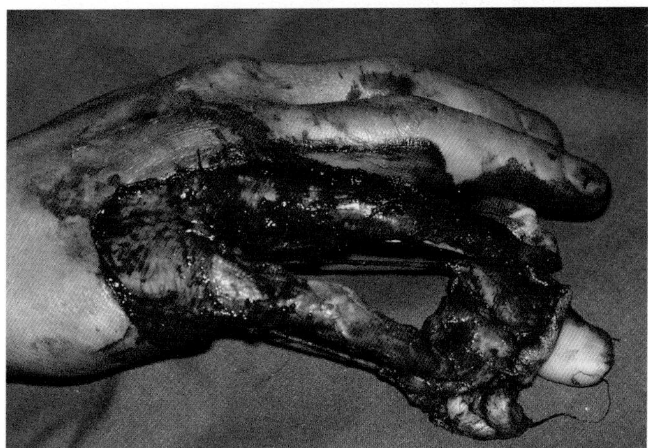

Figure 3.10 Degloving injury of the right little and ring fingers.

(*Figure 3.9*). Negative pressure helps draw the wound edges together, remove exudate, reduce oedema and promote granulation tissue formation. NPWT is not recommended in the setting of exposed vessels, malignancy, untreated osteomyelitis, necrotic tissue or non-enteric and unexplored fistulae.

ACUTE WOUNDS

Bites

Most bites involve either puncture wounds or avulsions. Wounds over the metacarpophalangeal joint should be treated as a human bite following a punch to the mouth until proven otherwise. Joint infections are a surgical emergency as they can result in articular cartilage destruction. They present as hot, swollen and tender joints with a limited range of motion.

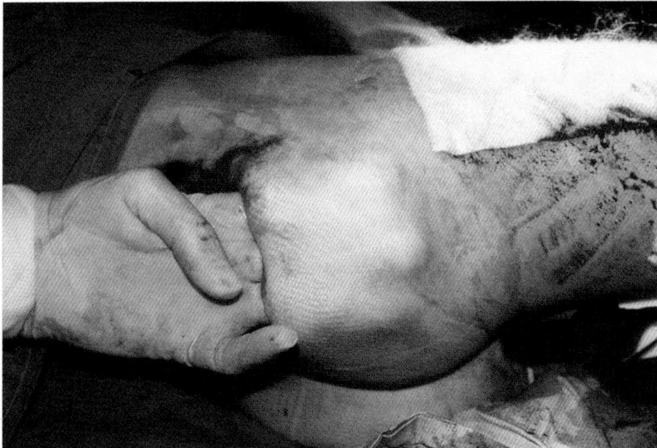

Figure 3.11 Degloving buttock injury.

Summary box 3.4

Reconstruction options for wound closure

- Primary closure
- Secondary closure
- Tertiary (delayed primary) closure
- NPWT
- Split-thickness skin graft
- Full-thickness skin graft
- Dermal matrices
- Local, regional or pedicled flap
- Tissue expansion
- Free flap

Degloving

Degloving is the avulsion of skin and subcutaneous fat from the underlying fascia, muscle or bone. A degloving injury may be open or closed. An example of an open degloving is a finger avulsion injury with loss of skin (*Figure 3.10*).

Closed degloving injuries result from shearing forces, which may occur with motor vehicle collisions. The extent of these injuries is often underappreciated and much of the skin may be non-viable (*Figure 3.11*). Disruption of perforating vascular and lymphatic vessels may result in a characteristic haemolymphatic collection between the fascial planes called a Morel-Lavallée lesion (*Figure 3.12*). Although these lesions were originally described as occurring over the greater trochanter the term is also used now for similar lesions in other anatomical locations.

Assessing the viability of degloved tissue can be difficult and may therefore require more than one surgical exploration and debridement before definitive reconstruction. Non-viable skin may show fixed staining and thrombosis of subcutaneous veins. Most surgeons serially excise the degloved skin until punctate dermal bleeding is seen from viable tissue. Intravenous fluorescein may also help delineate non-viable tissue, but

Victor-Auguste-François Morel-Lavallée, 1811–1865, surgeon who first described this lesion in 1863.

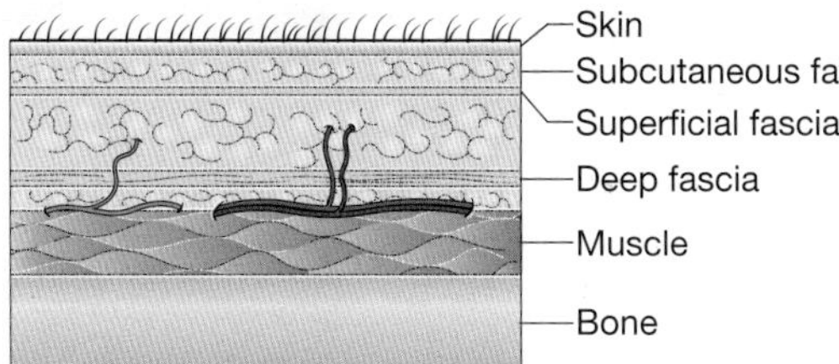

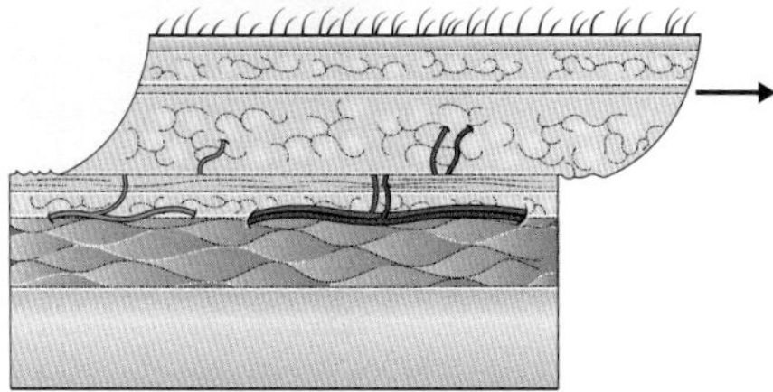

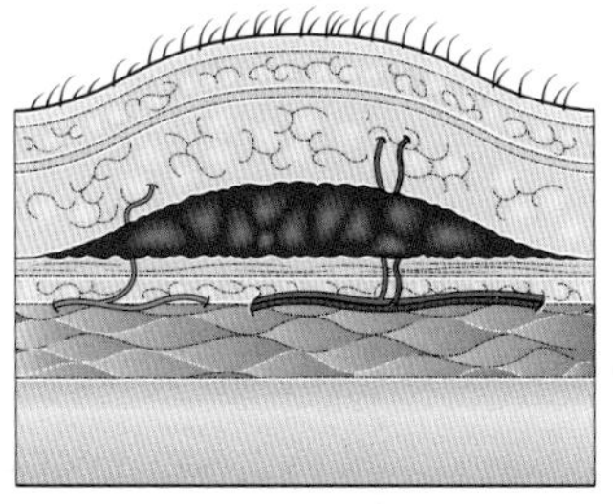

Figure 3.12 Mechanism of injury for Morel-Lavallée lesions. Cross-sectional illustrations of the layers of tissue from the skin to the bone demonstrate how a shearing force can cause the comparatively mobile subcutaneous tissues to move relative to the comparatively fixed underlying deep fascia, causing shearing of perforating arteries (red), veins (blue) and lymphatics (green) and ultimately leading to the formation of a haemolymphatic collection in this potential space. (Adapted with permission from Bonilla-Yoon I, Masih S, Patel DB *et al*. The Morel-Lavallée lesion: pathophysiology, clinical presentation, imaging features, and treatment options. *Emerg Radiol* 2014; **21**(1): 35–43.)

it requires specialist equipment and there is a small risk of anaphylaxis. More recently, the use of indocyanine green fluorescence has been reported.

A useful classification system to help guide management describes four patterns of degloving (***Summary box 3.5***).

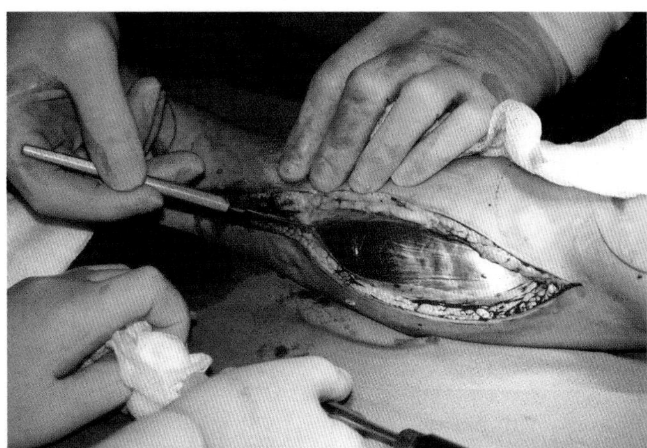

Figure 3.13 Fasciotomy of the leg.

It may be appropriate to offer primary amputation in cases of severe multiplanar degloving.

Summary box 3.5

Classification of degloving injuries in limb trauma[9]

1. Limited degloving with abrasion or avulsion
2. Non-circumferential degloving
3. Circumferential single plane degloving
4. Circumferential multiplanar degloving

Acute compartment syndrome

Acute compartment syndrome occurs when there is increased interstitial pressure within a closed osteofascial compartment, which results in microvascular compromise. It is a surgical emergency as delayed treatment may lead to irreversible muscle ischaemia and significant long-term morbidity.

Compartment syndrome most commonly occurs after lower limb fractures, both open and closed (see ***Chapter 32***). It also occurs in the upper limb, buttock and abdomen. Other causes include soft-tissue trauma, arterial injuries, burns and prolonged compression. It is characterised by pain out of proportion to the injury, particularly with passive movement of the affected compartment muscles. Paraesthesia is another early sign. Absent pulses are uncommon and suggest the possibility of vascular injury.

Compartment syndrome is generally a clinical diagnosis. It can be difficult to diagnose in the presence of impaired consciousness, in children and in patients with regional nerve blocks. Monitoring intracompartment pressures (ICPs) can sometimes help to guide management. A pressure of ≤30 mmHg between the diastolic pressure and ICP has been recommended as the threshold for fasciotomy.

Fasciotomy involves incising the skin and deep fascia with long axial incisions (***Figure 3.13***). If the compartment pressure was high, the muscle will then be seen bulging out through the fasciotomy opening. The lower limb is reliably decompressed via two incisions. A medial longitudinal incision 1–2 cm posterior to the medial border of the tibia decompresses the superficial and deep posterior compartments. A lateral longitudinal incision 2 cm lateral to the anterior tibial border decompresses the peroneal and anterior compartments.

Late diagnosis of compartment syndrome is a management dilemma as a late fasciotomy may result in rhabdomyolysis, infection, need for amputation and even death.

Necrotising fasciitis

This is a severe, rapidly progressing infection of the soft tissue and fascia associated with significant morbidity and mortality (***Figure 3.14***). Reported mortality rates vary widely but a Danish nationwide cohort study including over 1500 patients found 30-day and 1-year mortality rates of up to 26% and 40%, respectively.[10] The infection is commonly polymicrobial but monomicrobial presentation with *Streptococcus pyogenes* (group A streptococcus) is also frequent. Examples of other

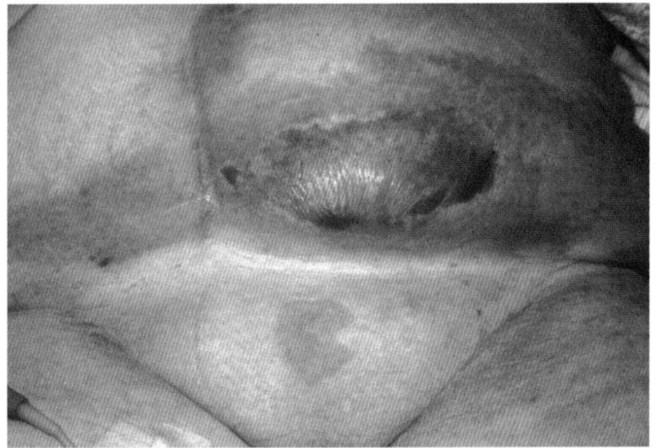

Figure 3.14 Necrotising fasciitis of the anterior abdominal wall.

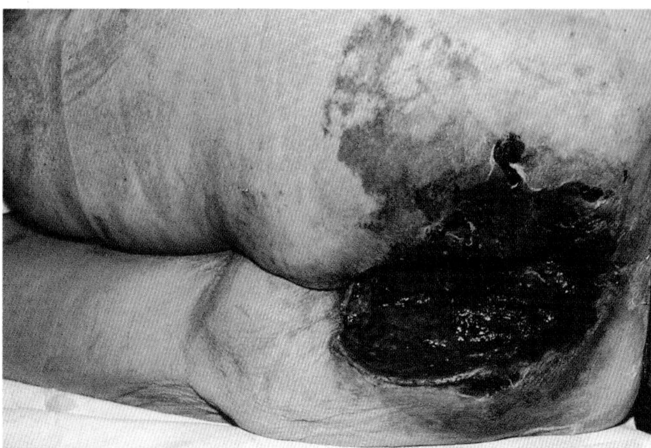

Figure 3.15 Pressure ulcer.

organisms include *Staphylococcus aureus*, *Escherichia coli*, *Pseudomonas*, *Clostridium* and *Bacteroides*.

There is usually a history of trauma or surgery with wound contamination. Diabetes mellitus is the most common comorbidity, although up to 30% of patients may not have any comorbidities.[10,11] Clinical features are shown in ***Summary box 3.6***. A scoring system to aid clinical decision making has been developed, but its performance remains questionable.[12] It remains primarily a clinical diagnosis and surgical treatment should not be delayed if suspicion is high.

Treatment consists of appropriate intravenous antibiotics with urgent radical surgical debridement. A *second look* operation is usually planned in 24–48 hours depending on clinical response. Multiple debridements may be required.

Summary box 3.6

Signs and symptoms of necrotising fasciitis

- Local
  - Unusual pain
  - Erythema, oedema, warmth
  - Crepitus
  - Blisters, bullae
  - Greyish drainage ('dishwater pus')
  - Fixed staining
  - Necrosis, gangrene
- Systemic
  - Fever, tachycardia, tachypnoea
  - Shock
  - Coagulopathy
  - Multiorgan failure

CHRONIC WOUNDS

These wounds fail to progress through the normal stages of wound healing in a timely manner. They are often characterised by a prolonged inflammatory phase and persistent infections. The management of chronic wounds therefore often involves debridement (***Table 3.4***), control of infection and inflammation and appropriately selected dressings to correct moisture imbalances. Chronic wounds can be categorised into vascular ulcers (venous or arterial), diabetic ulcers and pressure ulcers.

Leg ulcers

In developed countries, the most common chronic wounds are leg ulcers. An ulcer can be defined as a break in the epithelial continuity. A prolonged inflammatory phase leads to overgrowth of granulation tissue and attempts to heal by scarring leave a fibrotic margin. Necrotic tissue, often at the ulcer centre, is called slough. The more common aetiologies are listed in ***Summary box 3.7***.

A chronic ulcer that is unresponsive to dressings and simple treatments should be biopsied to rule out neoplastic change, a squamous cell carcinoma known as a Marjolin's ulcer being the most common. Effective treatment of any leg ulcer depends on treating the underlying cause, and diagnosis is therefore vital. Arterial and venous circulation should be assessed, as should sensation throughout the lower limb. Surgical treatment is only indicated if non-operative treatment has failed.

Summary box 3.7

Aetiology of leg ulcers

- Vascular (venous, arterial, mixed)
- Trauma (bites, self-inflicted, burns)
- Infection (bacterial, fungal, mycobacterial, syphilis)
- Metabolic disorders (diabetes mellitus, gout, calciphylaxis)
- Autoimmune disorders (vasculitis, systemic sclerosis, rheumatoid arthritis)
- Neoplastic (squamous cell carcinoma, basal cell carcinoma)

Pressure ulcers

Pressure ulcers occur over a bony prominence or under a medical or other device (***Figure 3.15***). A number of similar classifications exist. The US National Pressure Injury Advisory

Jean-Nicholas Marjolin, 1780–1850, surgeon, Paris, France, described the development of carcinomatous ulcers in scars in 1828.

Panel has replaced the term 'pressure ulcer' with 'pressure injury' in its staging system (*Table 3.5*) to provide a more accurate description of injuries to both intact and ulcerated skin.[13]

Pressure injuries should be regarded as preventable. There is a higher incidence in those who are severely ill, those who have impaired mobility or those with a significant loss of sensation. The most common sites are listed in *Summary box 3.8*.

TABLE 3.5 US National Pressure Injury Advisory Panel staging of pressure injuries.[13]

Stage	Description
1	Non-blanchable erythema of intact skin
2	Partial-thickness skin loss with exposed dermis
3	Full-thickness skin loss
4	Full-thickness skin and tissue loss
Unstageable full-thickness pressure injury	Obscured full-thickness skin and tissue loss
Deep tissue pressure injury	Persistent non-blanchable, deep red, maroon or purple discoloration

Summary box 3.8

Common sites for pressure injuries and ulcers

- Ischium
- Greater trochanter
- Sacrum
- Heel
- Malleolus
- Occiput

Prevention starts with assessing risk using a validated score to support clinical judgement such as the Braden scale, Waterlow score or Norton risk assessment scale. Patients at risk of developing pressure injuries should have a skin assessment, regular repositioning every 2–4 hours and the use of pressure-redistributing devices as appropriate. Patients should receive education on self-care and risk factors need to be addressed, such as providing nutritional support for any deficiencies.

The treatment of pressure ulcers should focus on patient optimisation especially any aspects of poor nutrition and ongoing poorly managed medical problems to address any risk factors. Preventative measures are used and debridement may be appropriate (*Table 3.4*). Dressings should be chosen to create an optimum wound-healing environment and appropriate antibiotics given if there are signs of infection. Surgery is not first-line treatment and is only considered when the above measures have been fully implemented. Patients must also be well motivated and able to fully comply with postoperative preventative measures.

Surgical management of pressure sores follows some of the same principles described for wound management in *Table 3.2*. Primary closure and skin grafting should be avoided as they are likely to fail. In suitable patients, successful reconstruction options include the use of large fasciocutaneous or musculocutaneous flaps. If possible, use a flap that can be advanced further if there is recurrence and that does not interfere with the planning of neighbouring flaps that may be used in the future.

SCAR MANAGEMENT

Principles

The remodelling and maturation phase of wound healing results in scar formation. The immature scar is at first pink, hard, raised and often itchy. As the collagen matures, the scar becomes almost acellular as the fibroblasts and blood vessels reduce. The external appearance of the scar becomes paler, while the scar becomes softer, flattens and its itchiness diminishes. Most of these changes occur over the first 3 months but a scar will continue to mature over 1–2 years, and sometimes more. Tensile strength will continue to increase but would not be expected to exceed around 80% that of normal skin.

There is well-established evidence for managing scars with pressure/compression therapy, silicone sheets and gels, intralesional corticosteroid injection and surgery.[14] Other treatment modalities include massage therapy, psychological counselling, laser therapy, radiotherapy, cryosurgery and intralesional injection of other products.

Prevention of adverse scar formation is better than treatment, so it is important to correctly manage wounds (*Table 3.2*). Optimal surgical management starts with careful planning, tissue handling and meticulous technique. For example, placing incisions along relaxed skin tension lesions where possible, and avoiding straight-line incisions across flexion creases. Early debridement reduces the risk of infection and allows for earlier wound closure. Dirt-ingrained (tattooed) scars are usually preventable by proper initial scrubbing and cleansing of the wound (*Figure 3.16*). It is important to recognise normal

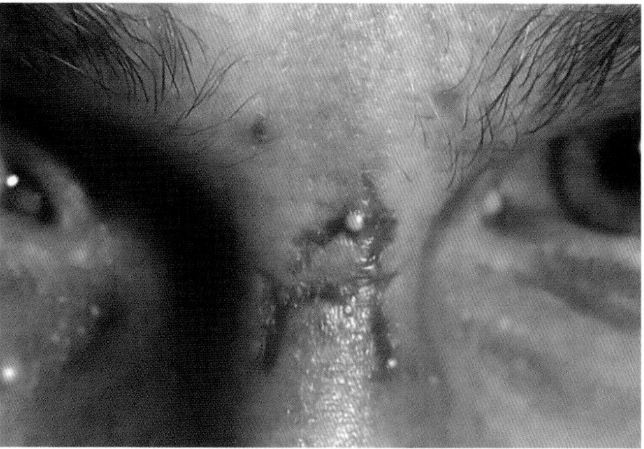

Figure 3.16 Dirt-ingrained scar.

Barbara Braden, contemporary, developed the Braden scale with Nancy Bergstrom in 1987.
Judy Waterlow, contemporary, developed the Waterlow score in 1985.
Doreen Norton, 1922–2007, nurse, developed the Norton risk assessment scale in 1962.

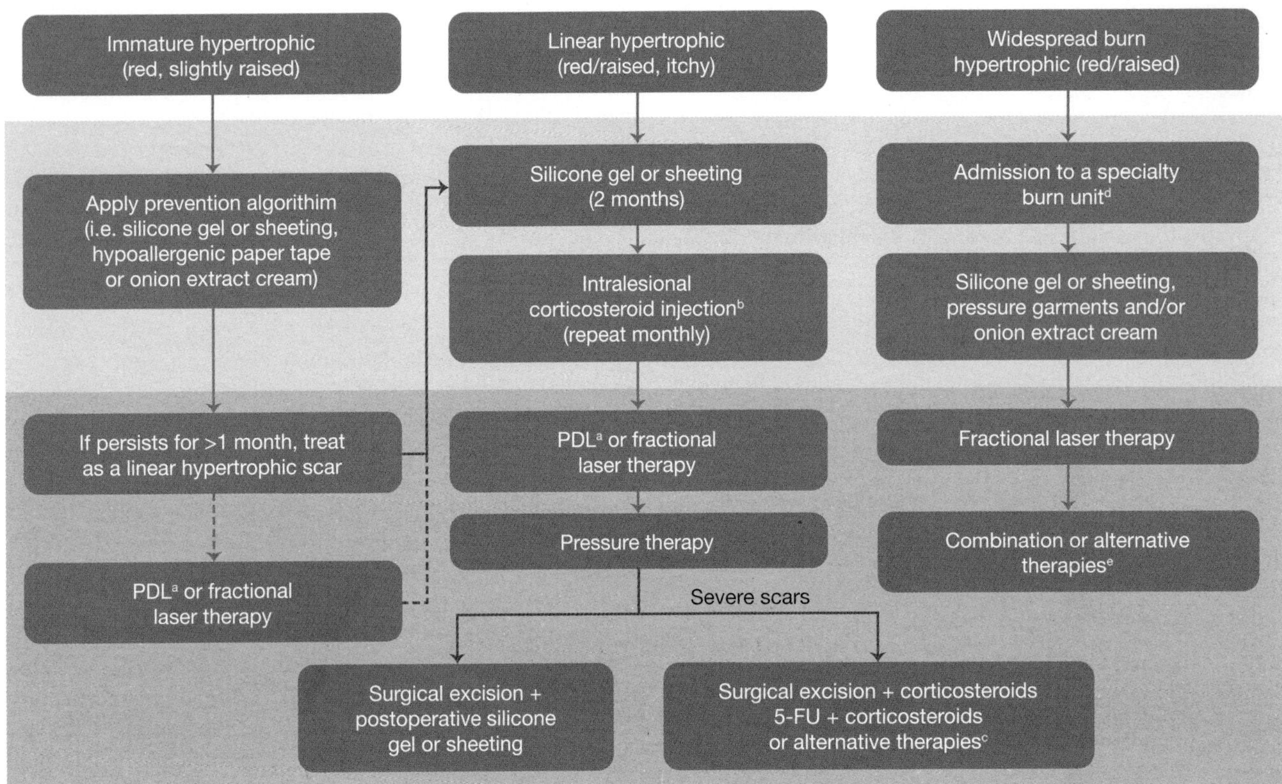

Figure 3.17 Management algorithm for hypertrophic scars. Light grey indicates initial management strategies; dark grey indicates secondary management options. [a]Preferred initial option. [b]2.5–20 mg/mL (face); 20–40 mg/mL (body). [c]Alternative therapy options for severe lesions include bleomycin, mitomycin C, laser therapy and cryotherapy. [d]Scar prevention and treatment should not begin before epithelium and wound stabilisation. [e]Combination and alternative therapies include massage, physical therapy, corticosteroids, tension-relieving surgical intervention, excision, grafting or flap coverage, hydrocolloid dressings, antihistamines and laser therapy. 5-FU, 5-fluorouracil; PDL, pulsed-dye laser. (Redrawn with permission from Gold MH, McGuire M, Mustoe TA *et al*. Updated international clinical recommendations on scar management: part 2–algorithms for scar prevention and treatment. *Dermatol Surg* 2014; **40**(8): 825–31.)

anatomical landmarks to avoid misaligned scars, such as at the lip vermilion border where even a 1-mm discrepancy is noticeable at a distance. Skin closure should be without tension and allow for postoperative oedema typically associated with injury and healing. Wounds should be sutured in layers unless they are very small. Deep dermal absorbable sutures hold the skin edges together to allow subsequent subcuticular or skin sutures. Large and deep wounds also require closure of the fascial layer, for example Scarpa's fascia in the abdomen. Subcuticular suturing avoids skin suture marks. If skin sutures are used, suture marks may be minimised by using monofilament sutures that are removed in a timely fashion depending on anatomical location. For example, sutures are typically removed by 5 days in the face versus 10–14 days in the lower limb.

Following wound closure, scar prevention measures include tension relief, taping, hydration and ultraviolet protection.[14] Silicone sheeting or gel is widely accepted as the first-line prophylactic and treatment option for hypertrophic and keloid scars. The management of hypertrophic and keloid scars is difficult and international recommendations from 2014 are summarised in ***Figures 3.17 and 3.18***.[15]

Later scar treatment includes intralesional corticosteroid injections, typically using triamcinolone acetonide 10–40 mg/mL every 4–6 weeks until the scar has flattened. Revisional scar surgery may be appropriate. For example, for correcting alignment of scars.

Contractures

Scar contractures can cause severe functional, psychological and aesthetic problems (***Figure 3.19***). Contractures across joints may restrict the range of movement, leading to deformity, impairment and disability. Contractures may also result from the differential growth pattern between scar and surrounding tissues.

Surgical contracture release and reconstruction can be an effective treatment option. A key principle is the replacement of scar tissue with healthy tissue. A wide range of reconstructions are described (***Summary box 3.4***) and typically involve skin grafts or flaps (more information can be found in ***Part 6***). Local flaps such as Z-plasty (***Figure 3.20***) and its variants can be used to lengthen and transpose the scar. Many other local flaps have been described, including Y–V, V–Y and W-plasty. Free flaps may be required for resurfacing severe contractures. In general, flaps are preferable to skin grafts because of graft contracture. When skin grafts are used, full thickness is preferred to split thickness as they have a better texture and contract less during healing.

Antonio Scarpa, 1747–1832, Professor of Anatomy, Pavia, Italy.

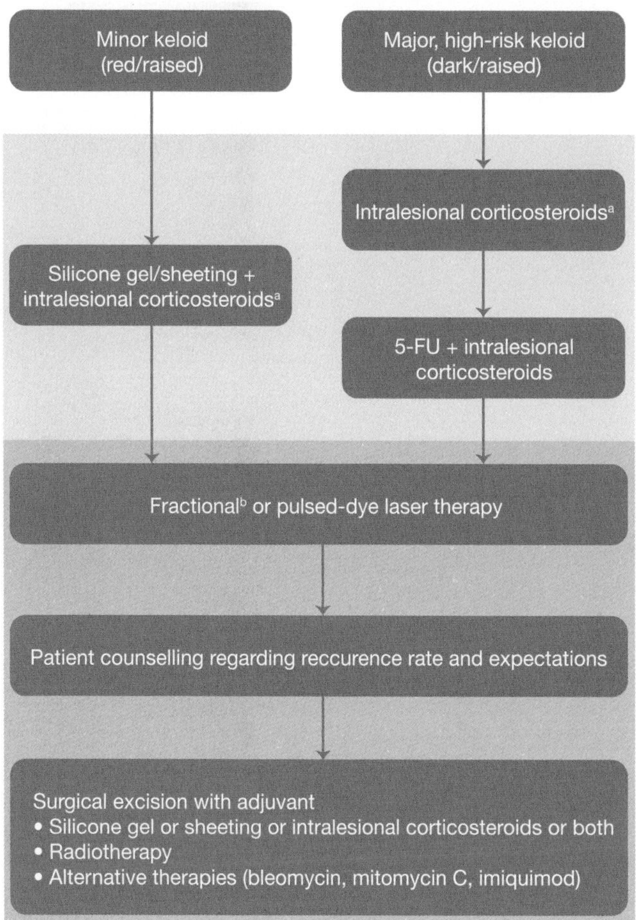

Figure 3.18 Management algorithm for keloids. Light grey indicates initial management strategies; dark grey indicates secondary management options. [a]Cryotherapy may be used in conjunction with intralesional corticosteroids, depending on physician experience and comfort with its application. [b]Ablative fractional lasers are the preferred initial laser therapy option for patients with minor keloids. 5-FU, 5-fluorouracil. (Redrawn with permission from Gold MH, McGuire M, Mustoe TA *et al*. Updated international clinical recommendations on scar management: part 2–algorithms for scar prevention and treatment. *Dermatol Surg* 2014; **40**(8): 825–31.)

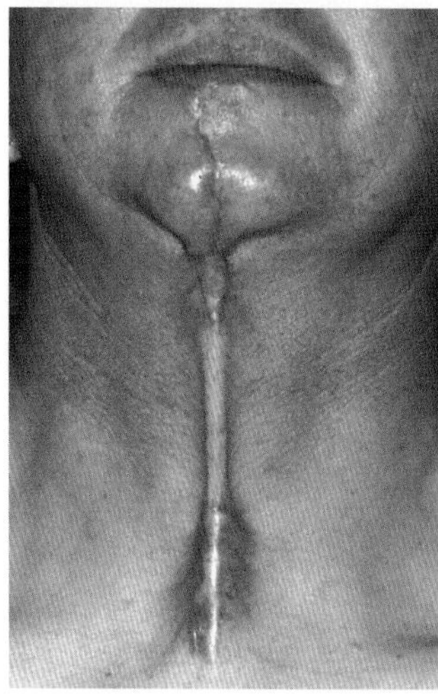

Figure 3.19 Midline neck contracture from a chainsaw injury.

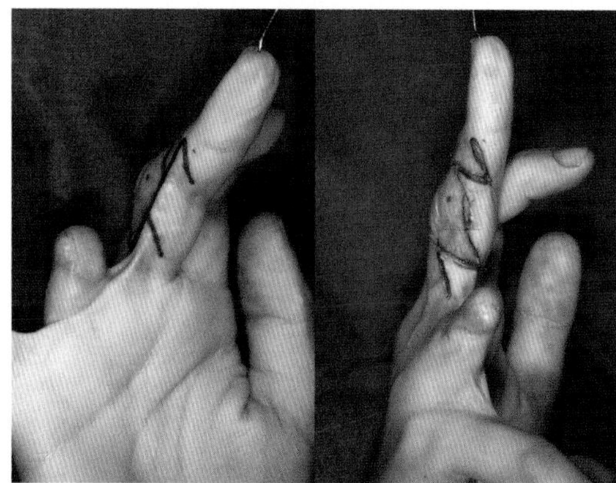

Figure 3.20 Multiple Z-plasty release of finger contracture.

REFERENCES

1 Berard F, Gandon J. Postoperative wound infections: the influence of ultraviolet irradiation of the operating room and various other factors. *Ann Surg 1964;* **160**(Suppl): 1–192.

2 Garner JS. CDC guideline for prevention of surgical wound infections, 1985. *Infect Control* 1986; **7**(3): 193–200.

3 Levy SM, Holzmann-Pazgal G, Lally KP *et al.* Quality check of a quality measure: surgical wound classification discrepancies impact risk-stratified surgical site infection rates in pediatric appendicitis. *J Am Coll Surg* 2013; **217**(6): 969–73.

4 Onyekwelu I, Yakkanti R, Protzer L *et al.* Surgical wound classification and surgical site infections in the orthopaedic patient. *J Am Acad Orthop Surg Glob Res Rev* 2017; **1**(3): e022.

5 Haley RW, Culver DH, White JW *et al.* The efficacy of infection surveillance and control programs in preventing nosocomial infections in US hospitals. *Am J Epidemiol* 1985; **121**: 182–205.

6 Eccles S, Handley B, Khan U *et al. Standards for the management of open fractures*. Oxford: Oxford University Press, 2020.

7 Public Health England. *Post exposure management for tetanus prone wounds*, 2019. Available from https://www.gov.uk/government/publications/tetanus-prone-wounds-posters (accessed 29 January 2021)

8 Gottlieb LJ, Krieger LM. From the reconstructive ladder to the reconstructive elevator. *Plast Reconstr Surg* 1994; **93**(7): 1503–4.

9 Arnez ZM, Khan U, Tyler MP. Classification of soft-tissue degloving in limb trauma. *J Plast Reconstr Aesthet Surg* 2010; **63**(11): 1865–9.

10 Hedetoft M, Madsen MB, Madsen LB *et al.* Incidence, comorbidity and mortality in patients with necrotising soft-tissue infections, 2005–2018: a Danish nationwide register-based cohort study. *BMJ Open* 2020; **10**: e041302.

11 Madsen MB, Skrede S, Perner A *et al.* Patient's characteristics and outcomes in necrotising soft-tissue infections: results from a Scandinavian, multicentre, prospective cohort study. *Intensive Care Med.* 2019; **45**(9): 1241–51.

12 Fernando SM, Tran A, Cheng W *et al.* Necrotizing Soft tissue infection: diagnostic accuracy of physical examination, imaging, and LRINEC score: a systematic review and meta-analysis. *Ann Surg* 2019; **269**(1): 58–65.

13 Edsberg LE, Black JM, Goldberg M *et al.* Revised National Pressure Ulcer Advisory Panel pressure injury staging system: revised pressure injury staging system. *J Wound Ostomy Continence Nurs* 2016; **43**(6): 585–97.

14 Monstrey S, Middelkoop E, Vranckx JJ *et al.* Updated scar management practical guidelines: non-invasive and invasive measures. *J Plast Reconstr Aesthet Surg* 2014; **67**(8): 1017–25.

15 Gold MH, McGuire M, Mustoe TA *et al.* Updated international clinical recommendations on scar management: part 2—algorithms for scar prevention and treatment. *Dermatol Surg* 2014; **40**(8): 825–31.

CHAPTER 4 Tissue engineering and regenerative therapies

Learning objectives

To understand:

- The potential opportunities afforded by tissue engineering and regenerative therapy
- The nature of stem cells, including somatic and adult stem cells, embryonic stem cells and induced pluripotent stem cells
- The role and range of materials and scaffolds for tissue engineering
- The role and range of molecules and their delivery
- The main challenges, safety issues and future directions

INTRODUCTION

Tissue engineering and regenerative medicine are relatively new but rapidly expanding multidisciplinary fields relevant to surgery that have the potential to transform the treatment of a wide range of human diseases. The ability of tissues to undergo spontaneous repair and regeneration is highly variable and, in most cases, limited. This has driven the development of approaches that harness the biology at the site of tissue damage to mediate regeneration through the localised delivery of cells, materials and molecules. The continuing improvement in our understanding of how tissues are formed and how they heal underpins the continuous development of novel approaches. As these technologies improve, translate and build up clinical evidence of effectiveness, the prospect of actual tissue regeneration, not just repair, will establish clinical utility. In this chapter, we explore the development of the tissue engineering paradigm (***Figure 4.1***) and the constituent processes that have been used to enhance tissue healing by considering cells, materials and molecules and the interplay between them, alongside key exemplars. We further highlight the opportunities, challenges and likely future directions for the field.

OPPORTUNITIES

The potential impact of tissue engineering and regenerative therapies is so far-reaching that practising surgeons should be aware of the resulting opportunities to improve patient management. Several conditions that could benefit from this approach are of particular relevance to surgeons because they are closely involved in assessment and treatment (***Table 4.1***). Selected examples include the repair or replacement of injured or diseased cartilage, skin, pancreatic islets, bladder, intestine, heart tissue, arteries, larynx and bronchus. A longer term goal in tissue engineering is the replacement of diseased whole organs such as the liver and kidney, although the technical challenges here are enormous.

Surgeons are integral to many of the multidisciplinary research teams currently undertaking translational research in this field and will play a vital role in the future delivery and

TABLE 4.1 Examples of tissues created by tissue engineering and conditions they may be used to treat.

Tissue	Conditions treated
Skin	Burns and skin defects after excision or trauma
Eye	Retinal and corneal disease
Cardiac muscle	Heart failure
Heart valves	Congenital and acquired valvular heart disease
Cartilage and bone	Degenerative and traumatic bone and joint disorders
Trachea and bronchus	Congenital and acquired stenosis and resection for malignancy
Bladder	Congenital bladder malformation and cystectomy
Anal/bladder sphincter	Incontinence
Pancreatic islets	Insulin-dependent diabetes
Large blood vessels	Atheromatous, aneurysmal and traumatic arterial disease
Oesophagus	Benign stenosis and resection for malignancy
Small intestine	Intestinal failure after surgical resection for Crohn's disease, cancer or ischaemia

Burrill Bernard Crohn, 1884–1983, gastroenterologist, Mount Sinai Hospital, New York, NY, USA, described regional ileitis in 1932.

evaluation of resulting treatments. In addition to its direct therapeutic application, tissue engineering also has the potential to provide *in vitro* tissues that can be used to model human disease and to test therapeutic drugs for efficacy and toxicity. However, it is important to emphasise that, while the potential benefit of cell therapy and tissue engineering is undeniable, there are many technical, regulatory and safety issues to be addressed for it to have wide clinical impact.

Summary box 4.1

Tissue engineering and regenerative therapies

These have potential to provide:

- Treatment for a wide range of diseases
- Clinical applications – underpinned by translational research, delivery strategies and clinical evidence
- Models to test therapeutic efficacy and toxicity

KEY AREAS OF UNDERPINNING SCIENCE

Advances in tissue engineering and more broadly regenerative medicine are underpinned by developments in both the physical and biological sciences, building on the classical tissue engineering paradigm (***Figure 4.1***). An improved understanding of developmental biology and the cues that direct stem cell fate have been key to advancement of the field. A better understanding of the stem cell niche has enabled scientists to propose changes to molecular and mechanical properties that could bring about modified cell behaviour. This has been realised by advances in materials science, which have been critical in the development of structures (scaffolds), onto and into which cells can be grown and where delivery vehicles can be used to localise cells and molecules to a specific site within the body. Notwithstanding the potential offered by these therapies, it should be emphasised that the whole field is still at a relatively early stage of development. Although there are examples where tissue engineering and regenerative therapies have already been introduced into clinical practice, for example the repair of damaged cartilage, most potential regenerative therapies have not yet entered routine surgical practice as there are considerable barriers to be overcome before this translational step can be achieved. We have divided the chapter into sections relating to cells, materials and molecules, while recognising the interplay and composite therapeutic solutions that ultimately arise.

CELLS

Although both fully differentiated cells (somatic cells) and stem cells are being used and developed for tissue engineering and regenerative therapy, most of the focus is on the use of stem cells, particularly somatic stem cells (SSCs) and induced pluripotent stem cells (iPSCs). The major features of the different cell types are listed in ***Table 4.2***.

Somatic cells

Fully differentiated specialised cells (somatic cells) obtained from normal tissues have been used for tissue engineering and regenerative therapy with some degree of success. For example, skin has been engineered using cultured epithelial cells grown *in vitro* and used to treat patients with burn injuries. Chondrocytes have been isolated, expanded *in vitro* and implanted into areas of deficient cartilage in a procedure called autologous chondrocyte implantation. Bladder wall has

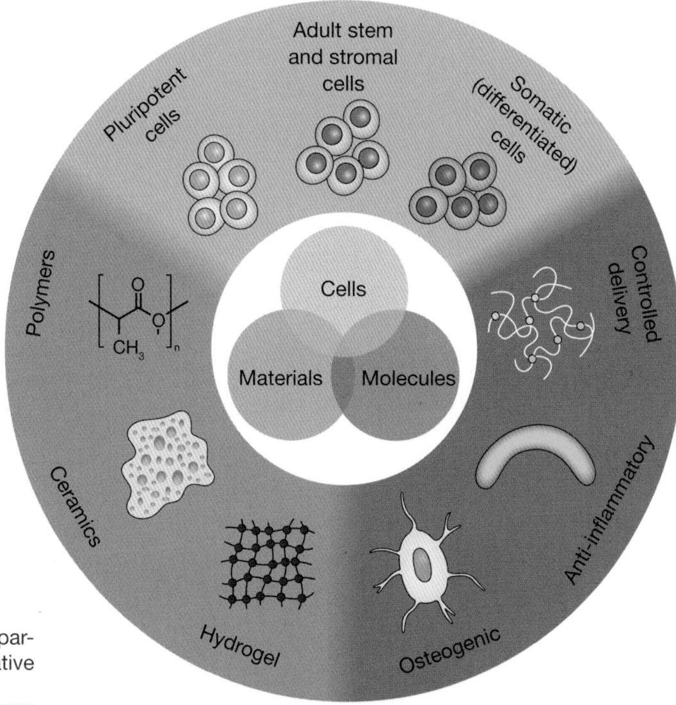

Figure 4.1 The tissue engineering paradigm in the context of regenerative therapies.

TABLE 4.2 Cells used in tissue engineering and regenerative therapy.

Cell type	Somatic cells	SSCs	hESCs	Fetal cells	iPSCs
Ease of availability	Limited	Good	Moderate	Moderate	Good
Expansion *in vitro*	Limited	Good	Excellent	Good	Excellent
Potency	No	Limited	Excellent	Limited	Excellent
Ethical concerns	No	No	Yes	Yes	Yes[a]
Risk of malignancy	None	Low	Moderate	Moderate	Moderate
Autologous	Yes	Yes	No	No	Yes
Anticipated future use	Limited	High	Limited	Limited	High

hESCs, human embryonic stem cells; iPSCs, induced pluripotent stem cells; SSCs, somatic stem cells. [a]Note that iPSCs avoid some of the ethical issues associated with hESCs.

also been engineered using a combination of smooth muscle cells and uroepithelial cells expanded *in vitro* and grown on a scaffold before reimplantation. Such tissues can be grown using cells obtained from the intended recipient by tissue biopsy (autologous cells) or using cells obtained from unrelated donors (allogeneic cells). The major advantage of the former source is that, after implantation, they are not rejected by the recipient's immune system; hence there is no requirement for immunosuppression (see ***Chapter 88***).

For other indications, the use of fully differentiated specialised cells is not practical in most situations because such cells are not readily available in sufficient numbers and they have only limited proliferative ability *in vitro*, which means that their numbers cannot be readily expanded to sufficient levels. To overcome these limitations, the major focus in the field of cell therapy has been on the use of stem cells.

Stem cells

Stem cells are undifferentiated or non-specialised cells that are able, through cell division, to renew themselves indefinitely (self-renewal). Crucially, they are also able, when provided with appropriate stimuli, to differentiate into one or more of the different types of specialised cell found in tissues and organs (potency). Because of their unique ability to undergo self-renewal when cultured *in vitro* and to be directed to differentiate into specialised cell types, they have enormous potential for use as cell-based therapies or, by way of their different characteristics, to otherwise contribute to regenerative medicine.

Stem cells can be classified in different ways, for example by using their characteristic level of potency such as pluripotent and multipotent (***Figure 4.2***) or with reference to the tissue from which they are derived, for example the early embryo

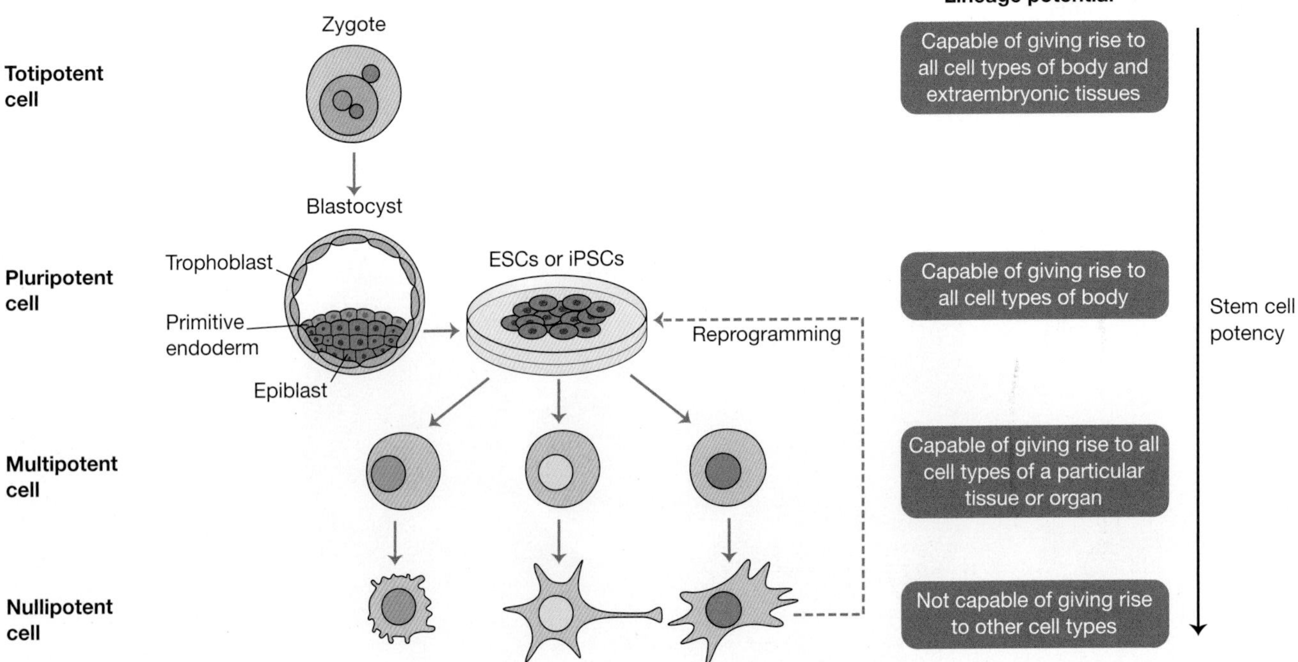

Figure 4.2 Hierarchy of cells according to potency, ranging from stem cells to specialised differentiated cells. ESC, embryonic stem cell; iPSC, induced pluripotent stem cell. (Adapted with permission from Tewary M, Shakiba N, Zandstra PW. Stem cell bioengineering: building from stem cell biology. *Nat Rev Genet 2018*; **19**: 595–614.)

(embryonic stem cells [ESCs]), later in development (SSCs) or whether they are derived by reprogramming adult specialised cells to a pluripotent state (iPSCs).

Adult tissue resident or somatic stem cells

Stem cells resident in the different tissues and organs are responsible for providing replacements for specialised cells that have reached the end of their functional lifespan either through natural attrition or because of damage and disease. In certain tissues and organs, notably the bone marrow and gut, stem cells regularly divide and differentiate into specialised cells to replace senescent or damaged cells in the blood and the gastrointestinal mucosa, respectively. Stem cells in other organs, such as the heart or central nervous system, are less able to effect repair or replacement. SSCs have the capacity to differentiate into a limited number of specialised cell types (multipotent); among the best characterised types are haematopoietic stem cells. In tissue engineering and regenerative medicine, mesenchymal stem or stromal cell (MSC) populations are widely described but have been more difficult to characterise, particularly in terms of stem cell attributes relating to clinical use.

Mesenchymal stem and stromal cells

Building on earlier observations in the 1960s[1] relating to bone marrow-derived cell populations, in the 1990s the term 'mesenchymal stem cell' (MSC) was used in relation to therapy, based on observations that some of these cells, under the right conditions, could differentiate into cell types relating to musculoskeletal, adipose and other tissues.[2] In 2005 the International Society for Cellular Therapy (now the International Society for Cell and Gene Therapy; ISCT) proposed that these cells be termed multipotent 'mesenchymal stromal cells' with the same abbreviation MSC, and that the term mesenchymal stem cell should be 'reserved for a subset of these (or other) cells that demonstrate stem cell activity by clearly stated criteria'.[3] They went on to describe minimum criteria in 2006[4]: adherence to plastic, expression of certain surface markers (CD105, CD73 and CD90) but a lack of expression of others (CD45, CD34, CD14 or CD11b, CD79α or CD19 and HLA-DR) and, finally, the ability to differentiate into osteoblasts, adipocytes and chondroblasts *in vitro*, often described by authors as trilineage differentiation.

The importance of nomenclature relates to the mechanism by which such cells might achieve a clinical effect. The earlier term mesenchymal 'stem' cell implies that cells directly contribute to repair and regeneration by differentiation, whereas using the term 'stromal' can encompass paracrine and secretory behaviour, in which cells are envisaged to work with other cells to influence the outcome of repair and regeneration (***Figure 4.3***). As a consequence, the term mesenchymal 'stem' cell has been highlighted as a cause of potential confusion, whereby patients might wrongly infer that the cell constitutes a 'stem cell therapy'.[5,6] In 2019, the ISCT gave continued support for the term mesenchymal stromal cell but recommended that it be: supplemented with the tissue source of the cell; intended unless rigorous evidence for stemness exits; associated with robust functional assays demonstrating properties.[7]

A further consideration is the manufacture and delivery of such cells. MSCs can be isolated from bone marrow (iliac crest aspiration) or from subcutaneous fat (liposuction/lipoaspiration). Cells can be delivered at the point of care, using bedside systems, or isolated *in vitro* on the basis of their adherence to plastic and subsequently further characterised. Therefore, they can be used shortly after extraction or after expansion of their numbers by *in vitro* culture. Furthermore, MSCs can be differentiated into the desired lineage *in vitro* by addition of suitable growth factors and chemicals.

The wide variety of cell type, source and manufacturing process represent important opportunities for treatment.

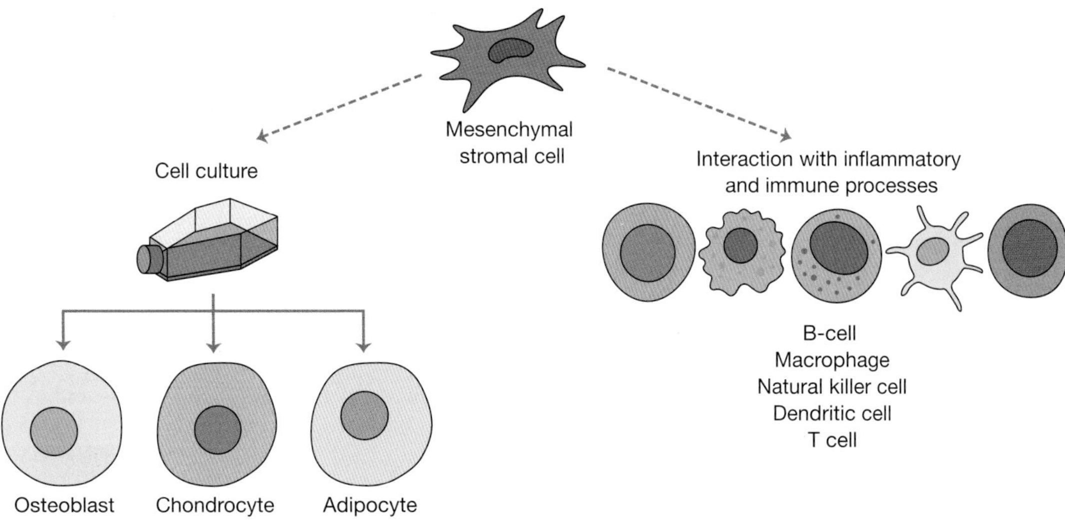

Figure 4.3 Proposed characteristics of mesenchymal stromal cells relevant to tissue engineering and regenerative medicine.

However, they also demonstrate considerable heterogeneity, the understanding of which will be greatly improved by molecular biology techniques and functional assay. In terms of agreed nomenclature, a report on consensus has described key parameters in the abbreviation DOSES: D – donor, O – origin tissue, S – separation method, E – exhibited characteristics, S – site of delivery.[8]

The relative ease of cell acquisition has meant that autologous MSCs have been used in clinical settings and they represent a great opportunity for new treatment development. Before widespread adoption, more translational research is required to understand and refine the therapeutic mechanism of action and conduct well-designed clinical trials to establish the evidence of effectiveness.

Embryonic stem cells

In the embryo, stem cells are able to give rise to all of the different cell types of the body at the gamete stage (totipotent) and nearly all cell types (pluripotent) when at the blastocyst stage (***Figure 4.1***). ESCs can be obtained from the inner cell mass of the early human blastocyst (days 4–5), using embryos that have been created through *in vitro* treatment of infertility and are surplus to those needed for reimplantation. The technique for isolating and growing human ESCs in culture was developed by James Thomson in 1998.[9]

ESCs have proliferative ability and possess key characteristics of self-renewal and pluripotency. However, their use in the clinic has major limitations, one of which is ethical. The surplus embryos used for derivation of ESCs would otherwise be discarded but, because they need to be destroyed to obtain ESCs, the approach has raised major ethical and political debate. The dominant view in many countries, including the UK, is that the potential therapeutic benefits of ESCs justify their use but there are very strict guidelines for their derivation; to date their clinical use has been limited. Cells from ESCs would be allogeneic and therefore be at risk of immunological rejection.

Induced pluripotent stem cells

The discovery in 2006 by Shinya Yamanaka,[10] building on the earlier work of John Gurdon,[11] that certain types of specialised adult cells could be reprogrammed using genetic manipulation to become embryonic-like iPSCs was a major breakthrough. Using retroviral or lentiviral transfection to introduce a combination of transcription factors (OCT3/4, SOX2 and either Kruppel-like factor and C-MYC [together designated the OSKM reprogramming factors] or NANOG and LIN28), it was shown that specialised somatic cells can be reprogrammed to become stem cells. Moreover, iPSCs proliferate *in vitro* as efficiently as ESCs and are pluripotent, thereby circumventing concerns about the use of human embryos. Importantly, the development of iPSCs also means that, at least in principle, an intended recipient of stem cell therapy can themselves provide a source of stem cells (e.g. from a skin biopsy or blood sample) that can then be directed to differentiate into the desired specialised cell type for therapy; because such cells would be autologous they would not provoke an immunological rejection response (***Figure 4.4***). Alternatively, iPSCs could be obtained from a number of volunteer donors selected on the basis of their HLA type and stored to create a national or international tissue bank of iPSCs. Lines of iPSCs could then be chosen from the bank to provide a fully or partially matched cell transplant for recipients, eliminating or reducing the need for immunosuppression to prevent immunological rejection.

One of the problems of reprogramming somatic cells to become iPSCs using retroviruses is that genomic integration of the virus may lead to activation of oncogenic genes, causing tumorigenesis. To reduce this risk, non-retroviral vectors have been used (such as adenovirus and Sendai virus vectors, which do not insert their own genes into the host cell genome) or plasmids, episomal vectors and synthetic RNA. There has also been much recent progress in identifying combinations of small molecules, growth factors and chemicals that mimic the effect of viral transfection with transcription factors and obviate the need for viral vectors altogether. The production process from sourcing cells (e.g. skin fibroblasts or peripheral blood mononuclear cells) to obtaining an adequate number of validated iPSCs may take several weeks.

In vitro differentiation of stem cells to specialised tissue cells

There is an enormous research effort aimed at better understanding the factors responsible for cell fate decisions and establishing effective and reproducible protocols that can be used to differentiate stem cells *in vitro* into the desired type of specialised cell. Typically, such protocols use culture in chemically defined media containing cocktails of small molecules that stimulate or inhibit key signalling pathways, along with cytokines, growth factors and chemicals. It is becoming increasingly clear that exposure to certain biomaterials and the physical attributes of a scaffold, including its surface characteristics, also promote stem cell differentiation along a particular lineage. Mechanical stress also influences cell fate decisions. After stem cells have been subjected to *in vitro* differentiation, it is essential that the purity of the differentiated cells and the absence of undifferentiated stem cells are confirmed to reduce the risk of tumour transmission. The cells must also be fully characterised and their function confirmed before they are used for therapeutic purposes.

Exemplars: cells as a therapy

The delivery of cells into damaged tissues has long been used to facilitate enhanced regeneration. The first modern example of successful cell therapy was bone marrow transplantation for the treatment of leukaemia, which was successfully performed in 1956. Since then, cells have been used for the regeneration

---

James Thomson, b. 1958, Professor and Director of Regenerative Biology, Morgridge Institute for Research, University of Wisconsin-Madison, Madison, WI, USA.
Shinya Yamanaka, b. 1962, Japanese stem cell researcher, winner of the Nobel Prize in Physiology or Medicine in 2012.
Sir John Bertrand Gurdon, b. 1933, British developmental biologist, winner of the Nobel Prize in Physiology or Medicine in 2012 with Shinya Yamanaka.

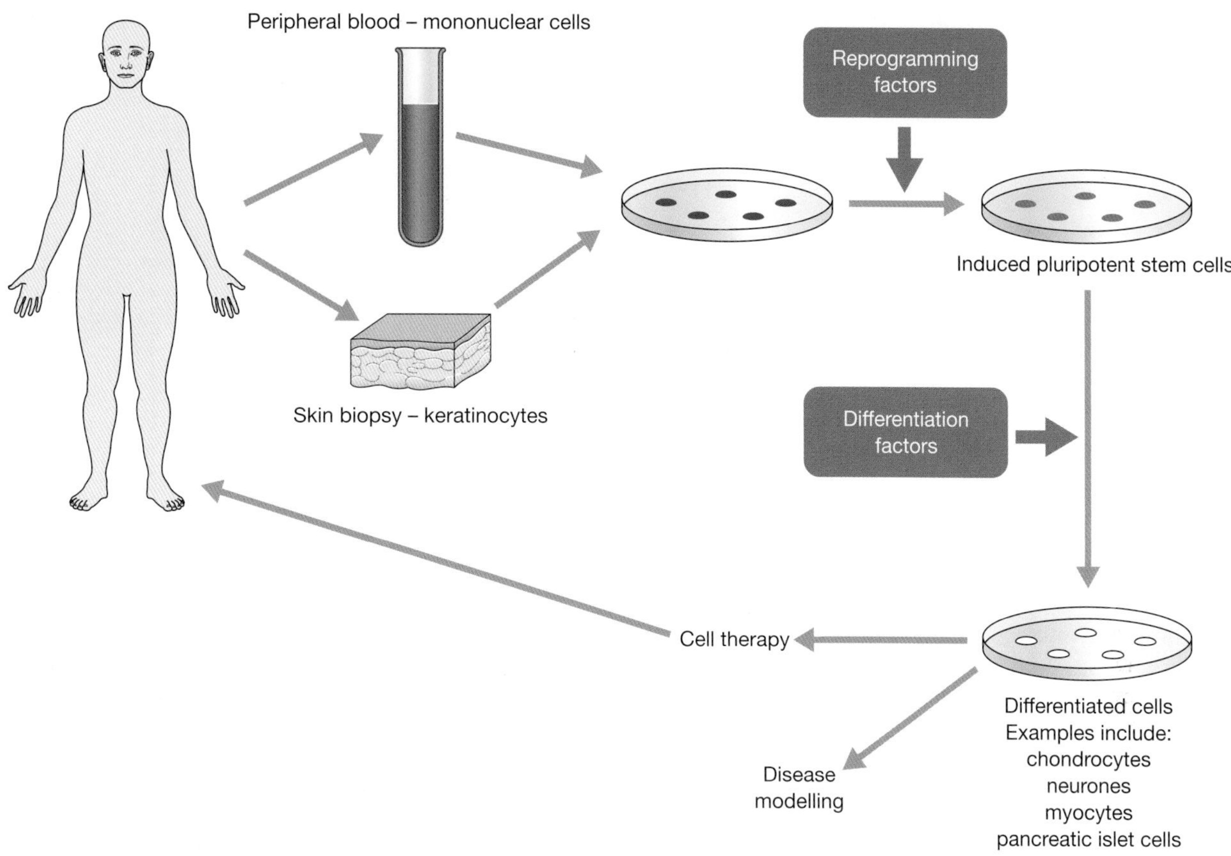

Figure 4.4 Schematic diagram showing the principles of induced pluripotent stem cell (iPSC) therapy. Mononuclear cells from peripheral blood or keratinocytes from a skin biopsy are cultured *in vitro* and then reprogrammed to become iPSCs by addition of reprogramming factors. The iPSCs are then expanded and selected differentiation factors added to promote differentiation of iPSCs into the desired specialised cell type for use as therapy.

of a range of different tissues. The following section details exemplars of the use of cells as therapeutic agents, for the regeneration of skin and cartilage (articular and auricular).

Skin

The tissue that was one of the first regenerated using human cells was skin. The pioneering work of Rheinwald and Green in this area led to the identification of optimal conditions for the growth and maintenance of keratinocytes harvested from skin in culture. The first tissue engineered skin consisted of a layer of keratinocytes grown on a collagenous membrane, which could be directly applied to a healing wound. In the original skin tissue engineering process, the keratinocytes were grown onto a membrane and were cultured in the same system as a layer of confluent but (unable to divide) fibroblasts. The fibroblasts are required in this culture because they provide a series of paracrine factors that allow for the keratinocytes to maintain their phenotype and also mature when lifted to the air–liquid interface. The fibroblasts had to be mitotically inhibited because they tend to proliferate at a greater rate than the keratinocytes and can consequently overtake the complex culture. As a consequence of the need for multiple steps and cell types, in addition to the air-lift required for stratification of the epidermal keratinocyte layer to occur, the process is relatively slow (requiring up to a month). This means that the burn wound to be resurfaced using this process needs to be closed and protected prior to application. This process has been refined over the years and has resulted in the development of a range of technologies, some of which are still on the market. Despite a reasonable level of integration, the skin itself lacks many of the features of normal human skin, for example coloration, and is not in widespread use in the clinic.

Articular cartilage regeneration

Microfracture or microdrilling (***Figure 4.5***) into subchondral bone at the base of a chondral defect creates a communication between the intra-articular and subchondral spaces, allowing blood, containing bone marrow stromal cells, to arrive at the defect. Used clinically for more than 30 years, the formation of the clot creates an environment that allows for the reformation of cartilage within the defect, which subsequently provides a level of mechanical function. Although widely used in the clinic with success, the cartilage formed is typically fibrocartilage, which is mechanically inferior to the native articular cartilage and lacks longer term durability.

James George Rheinwald, b. 1948, American research scientist.
Howard Green, 1925–2015, George Higginson Professor of Cell Biology, Harvard Medical School, Boston, MA, USA, pioneer in the science of skin regeneration.

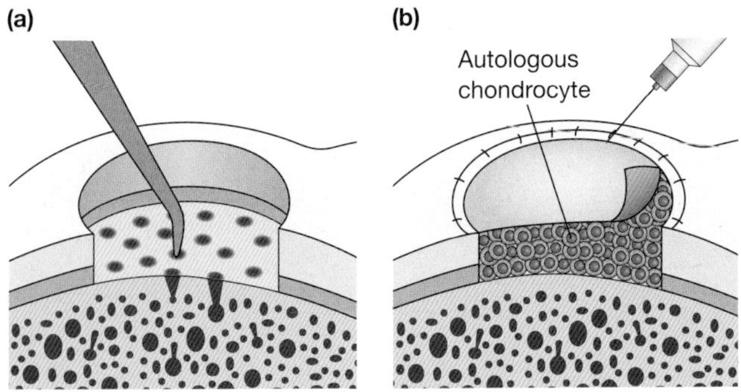

Figure 4.5 Examples of (a) endogenous cell targeting (microfracture) and (b) cells being used as a therapy (autologous chondrocyte implantation). (Adapted with permission from Makris E, Gomoll A, Malizos K *et al*. Repair and tissue engineering techniques for articular cartilage. *Nat Rev Rheumatol* 2015; **11**, 21–34.)

To overcome these limitations, research has focused on ways to create an environment in the chondral defect that is more conducive to the formation of articular or hyaline cartilage. Autologous chondrocyte implantation (ACI) is one such method (***Figure 4.5***). In the first step a small number of cells are harvested from healthy cartilage within a patient's joint, for example the knee. The cells are then expanded, to increase the cell number, in a laboratory (with good manufacturing practice [GMP] quality standards). In a second procedural step, cells are reintroduced into the defect, classically with a surgically positioned 'roof' or patch over the defect, prior to injection of the cells below. In 2017, following the evaluation of evidence, the UK's National Institute for Health and Care Excellence (NICE) recommended ACI for use in the National Health Service (NHS). The recommendation was for defined patients who have symptomatic articular cartilage defects of the knee, with a cost-effectiveness estimate thought likely to be less than £20 000 per quality-adjusted life year (QALY) gained.

MATERIALS

A large number of materials have been used in tissue engineering and regenerative medicine, either as delivery vehicles or as scaffolds; it is beyond the scope of this chapter to describe them extensively (see ***Further reading***). In simple terms, materials can be either natural or synthetic and further characterised by their mechanical properties, which will often need to take account of porosity. A further layer of complexity relates to specific molecules within and upon the material and the intended targeting or seeding with cells. In this section, we will focus on synthetic polymers, hydrogels and osteoinductive ceramics such as Bioglass®. These materials have been selected because of their broad relevance in tissue engineering and regenerative medicine.

Exemplars: materials in development

Synthetic and engineered polymers

Synthetic polymers are those made from chemical processing of natural components or from complex synthesis from precursors such as fossil fuels. There are a great many synthetic polymers that are used in the body, including polymethyl methacrylate

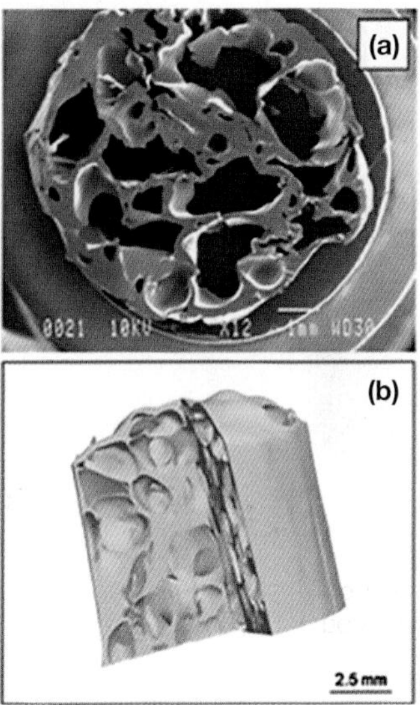

Figure 4.6 Electron micrograph of a poly(lactic acid) scaffold foamed using supercritical carbon dioxide (a) with pore structure assessed using micro-computed tomography (b). (Adapted with permission from Collins NJ, Leeke GA, Bridson RH *et al*. The influence of silica on pore diameter and distribution in PLA scaffolds produced using supercritical CO_2. *J Mater Sci: Mater Med* 2008; **19**: 1497–502.)

(PMMA), which is used to make intraocular lenses and as a cement in joint replacement; Dacron™ (Terylene™), used in vascular grafts; and a range of resorbable materials, including poly(caprolactone) (PCL), poly(lactic acid) (PLA), poly(glycolic acid) (PGA) and copolymers thereof (PLGA). These resorbable polymers have been used in the body for some time as sutures and in other degradable structures. Moreover, they have become widely used in regenerative medicine for the production of scaffolds, on which cells can be seeded and grown prior to, during or after implantation into the body. Synthetic materials can be processed in a range of different ways in order to provide a structure optimised to the intended purpose. Porous monoliths can be produced by foaming processes, which can include but are not limited to infiltration and then expansion of supercritical carbon dioxide in order to create a foamed structure. The pore sizes of such structures may be tailored by modifying process conditions or material compositions (***Figure 4.6***).

Such polymers can also be formed as spheres by using emulsion processing or they can be processed into a mat of fibres using a process known as electrospinning, whereby charged threads of polymer are drawn using an electric field and subsequently deposited onto a surface (***Figure 4.7***). Manufactured in this way, the materials tend to have a very high surface area and can exhibit structural features across the same length scales as the fibrous components of the extracellular matrix. As a consequence, electrospun patches have been designed for the repair of anatomical structures such as the rotator cuff and have even been used to explore how modifications in matrix geometry may result in pathology.

Bioceramics

A range of ceramics have been used for the delivery of compounds that can trigger the regeneration of mineralised tissues.

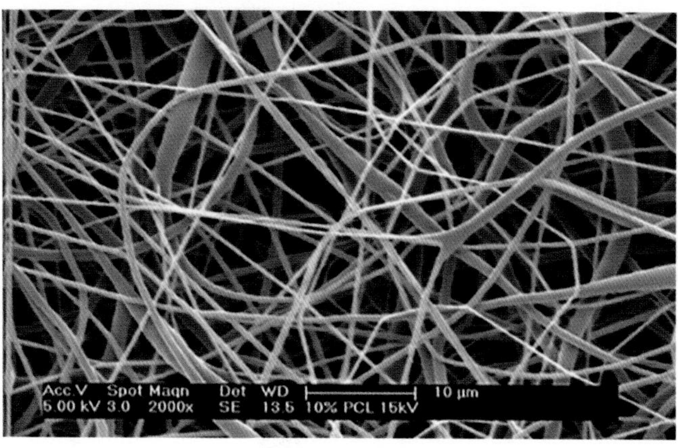

Figure 4.7 Electrospun poly(caprolactone) fibres intended for use in tendon reconstruction (courtesy of Dr Anita Ghag).

The most widely used such material is Bioglass®, a glassy material (a ceramic with no crystal structure) containing calcium, silicate and phosphate ions ($Na_2O–CaO–P_2O_5–SiO_2$). When placed into an aqueous environment, such as within body fluids, the surface of the ceramic material can break down, releasing the component ions into the surrounding liquid. This can result in the deposition of a bone-like mineral across the surface of the material itself, which can encourage the material to bond to surrounding hard and soft tissues. In addition, the eluted ions can trigger specific biological responses that include the recruitment and differentiation of mesenchymal cell populations. Bioglass® has been used in a range of medical products and has recently been widely applied in remineralising toothpaste formulations (as Novamin®). The incorporation of other ions, such as strontium and lithium, into the glassy matrix can drive specific biological processes, enhancing the process of bone formation. Bioglass® can be manufactured as a foamed structure and as a monolith. It is most frequently supplied in the form of granules and incorporated into polymer matrices to drive the process of bone integration.

Hydrogels

Hydrogels are an emerging and increasingly researched class of materials in regenerative medicine. They consist of hydrophilic polymers that are typically dispersed in an aqueous component to form a hydrocolloid. Interactions between the individual polymer chains can then be formed by modifying the temperature, adding ions or adding a chemical cross-linking agent. The resulting network retains water and forms a solid but highly hydrated structure (typically *c.* 99wt% water). The high water content of these materials means that nutrients, oxygen and metabolic by-products can diffuse through them. As a consequence, they have been widely used for the encapsulation of cells, typically allowing the maintenance of high levels of viability. Alginate, a seaweed-derived polysaccharide blend, for example, has been used to protect pancreatic islets from immunological attack. In recent years, this approach has been refined to allow for pancreatic islets to be shipped between medical centres (***Figure 4.8***). Other materials that form gels include chitosan, gellan, collagen and hyaluronic acid. In addition to these biologically derived materials, hydrogels may also be formed from synthetic polymers, including poly(ethylene glycol), and these can be chemically modified to provide specific biological stimuli to entrapped cells.

Additive layer manufacturing and hydrogels

As described above, hydrogels have been used for cell encapsulation. The potential to modify both the chemical and mechanical properties exhibited by these materials makes them perfect candidates for the growth of tissues outside the body, prior to eventual implantation into a defect site inside the body. As a consequence, hydrogel-based structures have provided scaffolding for many different engineered tissues, ranging from bone through to brain. However, a major issue

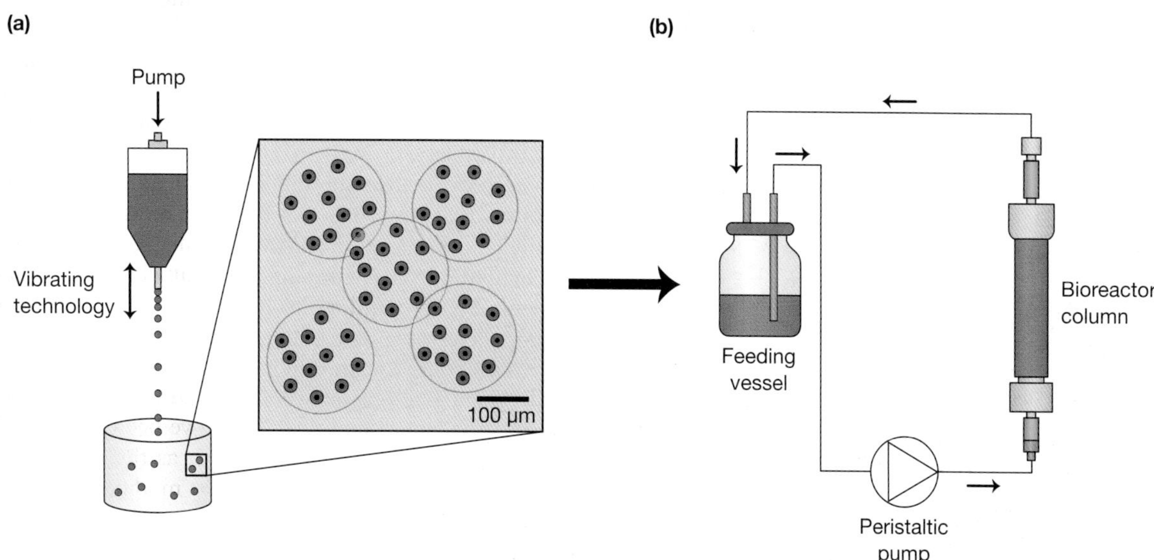

Figure 4.8 Schematic of (a) pancreatic β-cell encapsulation and (b) bioreactor cultivation. (Adapted with permission from Nikravesh N, Cox SC, Ellis MJ, Grover LM. Encapsulation and fluidization maintains the viability and glucose sensitivity of beta-cells. *ACS Biomater Sci Eng* 2017; 3(8): 1750–7.)

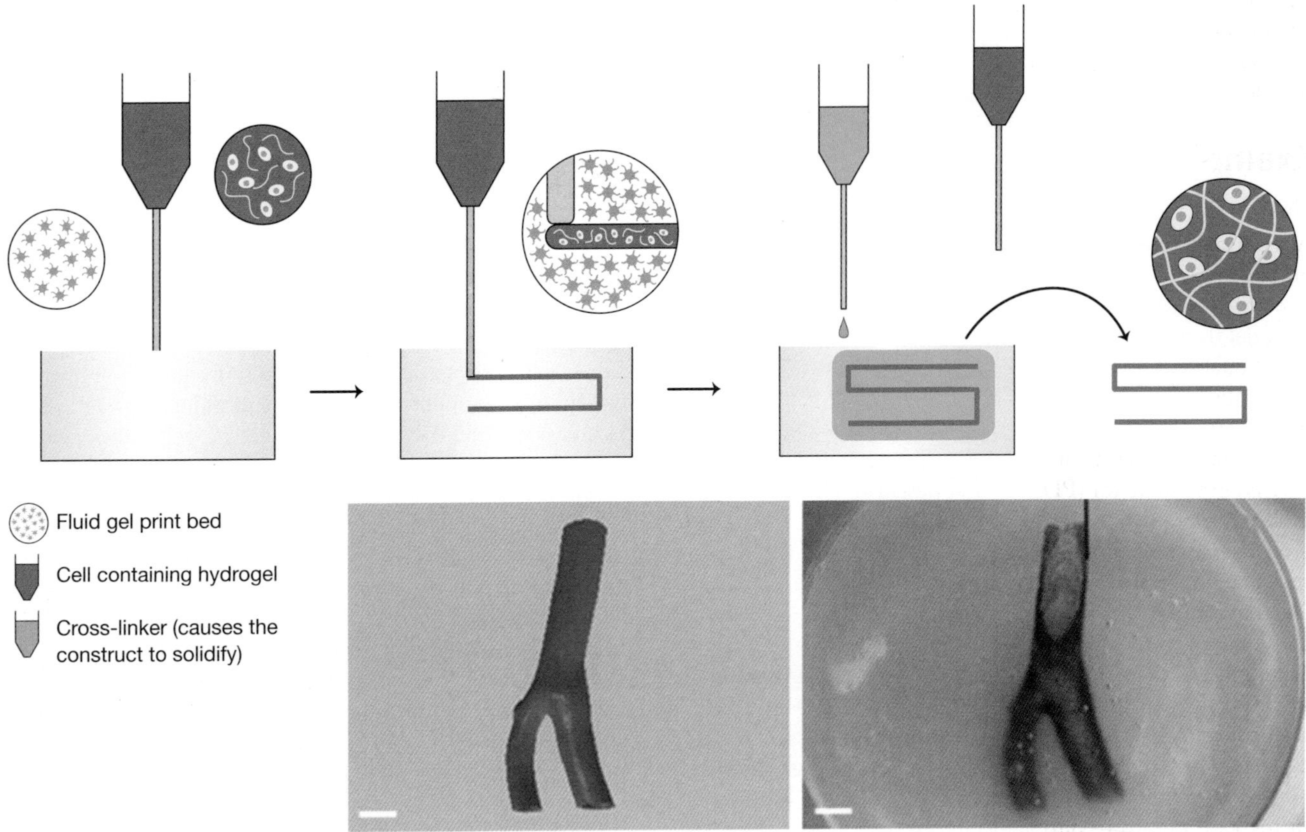

Figure 4.9 Schematic showing the formation of complex hydrogel structures using a suspended manufacturing process where a cell containing hydrogel is deposited into a supportive bed. This process allows for the production of hydrogels in complex geometries such as the carotid arteries shown here. (Adapted with permission from Senior JJ, Cooke ME, Grover LM, Smith AM. Fabrication of complex hydrogel structures using suspended layer additive manufacturing (SLAM). *Adv Funct Mater* 2019; **29**: 1904845.)

with hydrogels is that they are normally extremely weak during the gelation process, meaning that they will slump and lose their shape when cast. In order to get around this major issue, printed structures may be suspended in a secondary (often shear thinning) medium that provides both a level of support during the printing process and time for the hydrogel to develop sufficient mechanical integrity to support its own weight. Once this point has been reached, the structure can be removed from the supporting medium and washed prior to onward culturing. A wide range of substances have been used to provide support, including Pluronic® and agarose; however, the most widely used method currently is known as free-form reversible embedding of suspended hydrogels (FRESH), which uses gelatin. The FRESH method utilises a macerated gelatin-based support matrix. The particulate nature of the gelatin means that the printed hydrogel (which may or may not contain cells) can be deposited within the bed and will be supported while the mechanical properties exhibited by the as-deposited hydrogel become fully developed. The supporting matrix can then be melted (at 37°C) to leave the complex hydrogel structure. Other suspended printing methods have been developed that do not require the use of an animal-derived support medium (and that are therefore compatible with translation to the clinic) or the elevation of temperature to remove the supporting phase. One such method, suspended layer additive manufacturing (SLAM), uses a supportive matrix formed from hydrogel particulate systems that shear thin but exhibit rapid elastic recovery; this allows for the production of high-resolution prints that can be removed from the supporting bed by the application of a simple wash with water. This method enables the production of structures exhibiting complex morphology, such as the carotid artery (***Figure 4.9***), and can even be used to produce structures formed or modified from multiple material types, meaning that structures can be tailored with high resolution. With clinical relevance, SLAM has been used to manufacture osteochondral plugs containing both bony and cartilaginous regions. At present, these technologies are most likely to have an impact on disease modelling and drug candidate evaluation, but in the longer term they may emerge as key technologies facilitating tissue regeneration.

MOLECULES

Modification of the tissue environment during healing can be achieved by the delivery of molecules that are selected and able to specifically modify biological responses at the site of injury. In terms of tissue regeneration, these molecules can modulate the inflammatory environment, either by enhancement or by inhibition of specific biological response pathways, such as angiogenesis. This approach has been used to optimise tissue regeneration across several applications, with specific examples, for the skin and the eye, described below.

Exemplars: molecules in action

Healing skin without scarring

All tissues in the body, when damaged, are subject to a conserved process by which cells are recruited to the wound to remove damaged tissue fragments and then deposit and subsequently remodel the tissue (see ***Chapter 3***). In the case of the skin, the initial damage results in bleeding into the wound followed by haemostasis and, when the platelets within the clot degranulate, the secretion of proinflammatory factors. The tumour necrosis factor alpha (TNFα), interleukin (IL) 1 and IL-6, platelet-derived growth factor (PDGF), fibroblast growth factor (FGF), insulin-like growth factor 1 (IGF-1) and vascular endothelial growth factor (VEGF) recruit monocytes and endothelial cells into the wound bed to begin the wound-healing process. These cells release further cytokines, such as transforming growth factor beta 1 (TGFβ1), that mediate the formation of new extracellular matrix (normally initially collagen III in skin). Over time, the collagen III is remodelled and replaced with collagen I, which is normally deposited in a basket weave pattern. This process very efficiently closes wounds and, when not too severe, healing can be with minimal scar formation. In the case of severe damage or infection, the inflammatory response can 'overshoot', resulting in the overproduction of cytokines such as TGFβ1, which drive the recruitment of excess myofibroblasts to the wound site. This leads to the deposition and subsequent overcontraction of collagen matrix, which can result in the classic appearance of a scar.

A number of interventions have targeted this process with the aim of preventing the formation of a scar on the skin. Of note was the identification and isolation of TGFβ3, which plays a role in regulating extracellular matrix formation. This molecule was shown to regulate wound healing by blocking the TGFβ1 and -2 receptors on the cell surface and by modulating the penetration of cells in a newly forming tissue. TGFβ3 was subsequently developed as a therapeutic agent for use within the skin, with the aim of preventing scar formation. As TGFβ3 is a large, protein-based drug it was challenging to manufacture and purify and so was expensive in comparison with small-molecule drugs. Although this molecule had significant potential as an antiscarring agent in phase I and II trials, ultimately it was not adopted. This is an exemplar of a translational approach, working from a proposed mechanism through to stepwise clinical trials to test effectiveness.

Molecular delivery to prevent ocular fibrosis

Another example of the function of a tissue being significantly impaired by fibrosis is the eye. When the cornea is damaged, as long as the wound is kept clean, re-epithelialisation of the surface can occur relatively quickly with full restoration of the corneal surface within 7 days or so. However, if there is an infection on the surface of the eye there can be a potent inflammatory response that results in the rapid and disordered deposition of collagenous tissue across the ocular surface. If the surface of the eye becomes cloudy as a consequence, the patient can become blind. Recent work to create a therapeutic agent to prevent ocular scarring has focused on the localised delivery of a TGFβ1 antagonist called decorin. Decorin is a proteoglycan with a high affinity for collagen I, which it decorates the surface of in normal extracellular matrix. When free in solution, decorin also has an affinity to seven different cytokine molecules, one of which is TGFβ1, and has been shown to modulate fibrosis. A decorin-containing eye drop is able to deliver a sustained dose of decorin to the surface of the cornea following damage and subsequent infection. The drop has been shown to be effective in preclinical models of ocular fibrosis, facilitating the restoration of a transparent ocular surface with a significant reduction in markers that are usually indicative of scar formation (***Figure 4.10***).

Challenges to the delivery of molecules

Despite the opportunities afforded by molecules in tissue regeneration, major challenges remain that relate to getting the therapeutic agent to the right part of the body at the right time. Small molecules tend to diffuse rapidly through excipient (delivery) materials and so are rapidly released into the tissue environment, meaning that a strategy for sustained delivery is a necessity if repeat administration of the drug molecule is to be avoided. A number of implantable materials exist that allow for the slow localised release of molecules at the desired site of application. The majority of these are dense, degradable polymers that can be implanted locally and allowed to degrade, thus enabling sustained release of the therapeutic agent. The issues are potentially even more significant for large biomolecules such as proteins, which tend to be very sensitive to local environmental changes, with associated reductions in bioactivity. They can also have extremely high activities at very low concentrations and can be extremely expensive. In addition, excipients for these therapeutic products must be chosen very carefully so that potency is maintained and storage time maximised.

SAFETY CONCERNS

The major safety concerns of cell-based therapy and tissue engineering are listed in ***Table 4.3***. One of the most serious concerns is that of tumour formation and malignant transformation. The risk of tumour formation varies according to the cell type used, the genetic modification strategy used to transform the stem cells, the site of transplantation and whether the cells are autologous or allogeneic. The direct risk of tumour formation by the transplanted cells relates specifically to ESCs and iPSCs and there appears to be little risk with SSCs. The ability of stem cells to form teratomas is one of the hallmarks

TABLE 4.3 Risks of cell-based therapy.

- Tumour formation
- Genetic and epigenetic abnormalities
- Transmission of infection
- Poor viability and loss of function
- Differentiation to undesired cell types
- Rejection (allogeneic cells)
- Side effects of immunosuppression (allogeneic cells)

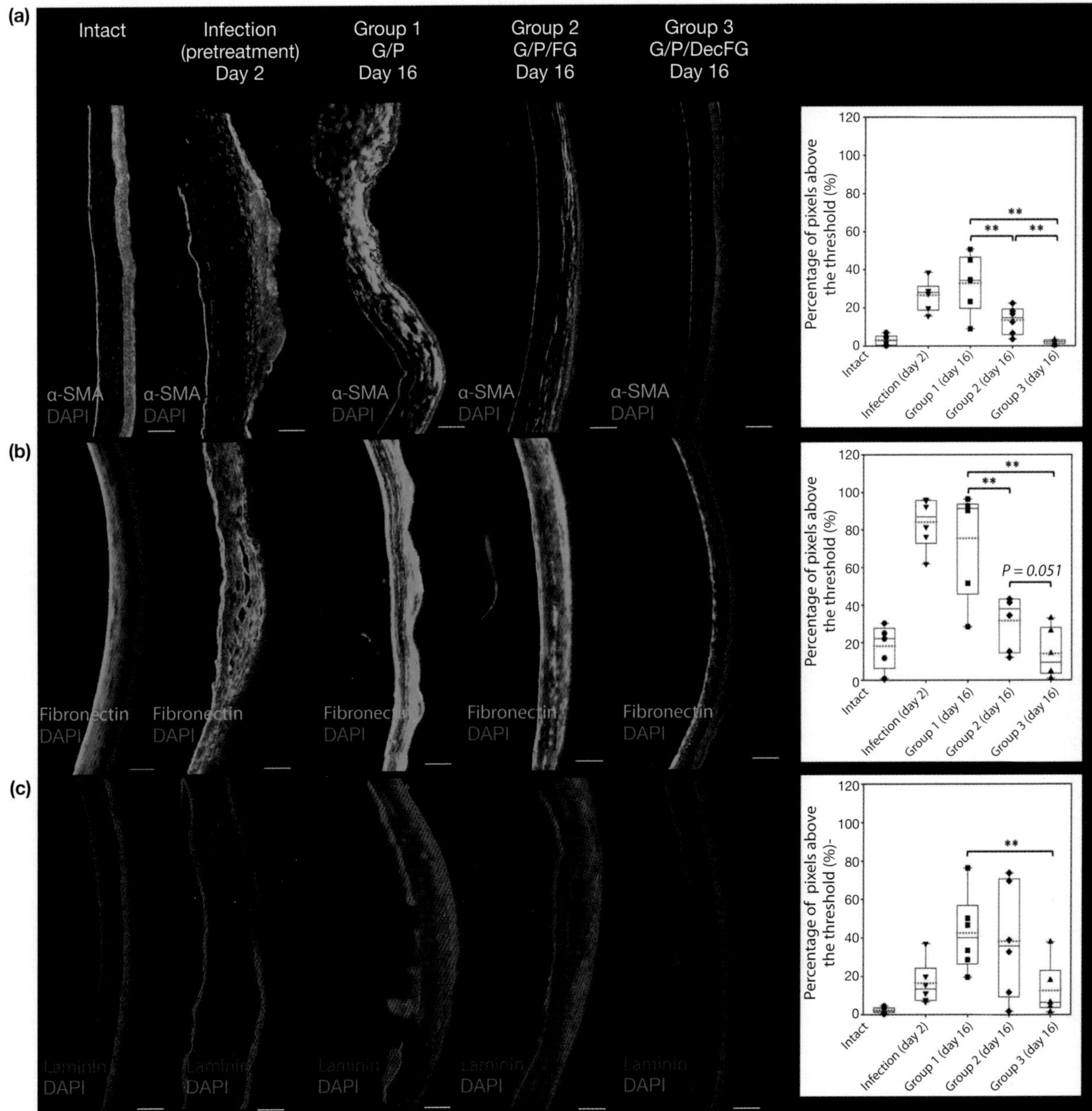

Figure 4.10 Stained sections through a mouse cornea before (left) and after (second column) injury and subsequent treatment with standard of care (gentamicin [G] and prednisolone [P]; group 1), standard of care plus a novel fluid gel carrier (FG) (group 2) and standard of care plus the carrier and decorin (Dec) (group 3). Sections are stained for markers of scarring: (a) α-smooth muscle actin (α-SMA), (b) fibronectin and (c) laminin. Importantly, the use of the slow-release decorin resulted in rapid restoration of the corneal structure with a significant reduction in scar markers. DAPI, 4′,6-diamidino-2-phenylindole (fluorescent stain that binds strongly to adenine-/thymine-rich regions in DNA). (Adapted with permission from Hill LJ, Moakes RJA, Vareechon C *et al*. Sustained release of decorin to the surface of the eye enables scarless corneal regeneration. *npj Regen Med* 2018; 3: 23.)

of pluripotency, and the risk of this happening following stem cell therapy may be reduced by ensuring that only cells that have been fully differentiated *in vitro*, and not those that are still pluripotent, are used for therapy. The risk of malignancy may also be reduced by the choice of *in vitro* strategy used to differentiate stem cells prior to use: the use of viral vectors that do not integrate into the genome or of non-viral approaches to differentiation reduces the risk of malignant transformation. There is also interest in developing techniques for directly reprogramming somatic cells to adopt the function of a different cell type without having to make them first revert back to the pluripotent state – so-called transdifferentiation.

Another major concern is that of transmitting infection. It is essential that if allogeneic stem cells are used they are screened to exclude infection and that cells and engineered tissues are prepared according to GMP guidelines to avoid bacterial infection during *in vitro* culture prior to use. Moreover, if allogeneic cells are used for tissue engineering and regenerative therapy, they may be susceptible to graft rejection and immunosuppressive therapy may be necessary.

FUTURE DIRECTIONS

Tissue engineering and regenerative strategies hold out great hope for effectively repairing or replacing tissues in a wide number of human diseases. The field is moving rapidly, underpinned by new developments in the relevant science in stem cells, materials and molecules. New emerging areas of technology include therapeutic signalling by way of extracellular vesicles (EVs) and gene editing of cells using CRISPR-Cas9, and gene therapies. All will require the use of a translational approach, whereby the hypothesised mechanism is developed and translated to the clinic, building up robust clinical evidence of efficacy, by way of well-designed and well-conducted clinical trials before widespread adoption.

It is likely that patient stratification will further refine therapy options. The ability to phenotype, genotype and profile patients at a molecular level will allow more detailed characterisation of patient subgroups and staging of disease. In addition to clinical studies and evidence, the rapid pace of therapy development will need to be accompanied by the development of new regulatory frameworks, for example in point-of-care manufacturing.

REFERENCES

1 Friedenstein AJ, Piatetzky-Shapiro II, Petrakova KV. Osteogenesis in transplants of bone marrow cells. *J Embryol Exp Morphol* 1966; **16**: 381–90.
2 Caplan AI. Mesenchymal stem cells. *J Orthop Res* 1991; **9**(5): 641–50.
3 Horwitz EM, Le Blanc K, Dominici M *et al.*; International Society for Cellular Therapy. Clarification of the nomenclature for MSC: The International Society for Cellular Therapy position statement. *Cytotherapy* 2005; **7**(5): 393–5.
4 Dominici M, Le Blanc K, Mueller I *et al.* Minimal criteria for defining multipotent mesenchymal stromal cells. The International Society for Cellular Therapy position statement. *Cytotherapy* 2006; **8**(4): 315–17.
5 Caplan AI. Mesenchymal stem cells: time to change the name! *Stem Cells Transl Med* 2017; **6**: 1445–51.
6 Sipp D, Robey PG, Turner L. Clear up this stem-cell mess. *Nature* 2018; **561**: 455–7.
7 Viswanathan S, Shi Y, Galipeau J *et al.* Mesenchymal stem versus stromal cells: International Society for Cell & Gene Therapy (ISCT®) Mesenchymal Stromal Cell committee position statement on nomenclature. *Cytotherapy* 2019; **21**(10): 1019–24.
8 Murray IR, Chahla J, Safran M *et al.* International expert consensus on a cell therapy communication tool: DOSES. *J Bone Joint Surg* 2019; **101**(10): 904–11.
9 Thomson JA, Itskovitz-Eldor J, Shapiro SS *et al.* Embryonic stem cell lines derived from human blastocysts. *Science* 1998; **282**(5391): 1145-7. Erratum in: *Science* 1998; **282**(5395): 1827.
10 Takahashi K, Yamanaka S. Induction of pluripotent stem cells from mouse embryonic and adult fibroblast cultures by defined factors. *Cell* 2006; **126**(4): 663-76.
11 Gurdon JB. The developmental capacity of nuclei taken from intestinal epithelium cells of feeding tadpoles. *J Embryol Exp Morphol* 1962; **10**: 622-40.

FURTHER READING

Fisher S. *Handbook of regenerative medicine and tissue engineering.* New York: Hayle Medical, 2015.
Wagner WR, Sakiyama-Elbert SE, Zhang G, Yaszemski MJ. *Biomaterials science: an introduction to materials in medicine*, 4th edn. Oxford: Academic Press, 2020.

CRISPR-Cas9, clustered regularly interspaced short palindromic repeats and associated protein 9. Resulted in the Nobel Prize in Chemistry being awarded to Emmanuelle Charpentier and Jennifer A. Doudna in 2020.

CHAPTER 5 Surgical infection

Learning objectives

To understand:

- The characteristics of the common surgical pathogens and their sensitivities
- The factors that determine whether a wound will become infected
- The classification of sources of infection and their severity
- The clinical presentation of surgical infections
- The indications for and choice of prophylactic antibiotics
- The spectrum of commonly used antibiotics in surgery and principles of therapy
- The misuse of antibiotic therapy with the risk of resistance to antibiotics (such as methicillin-resistant *Staphylococcus aureus* [MRSA]) and emergence of resistant strains (such as *Clostridium difficile* enteritis)

To learn:

- Koch's postulates
- The management of abscesses
- The Surviving Sepsis Campaign, sepsis bundle and Sepsis Six
- Surgical implications of the COVID-19 pandemic

To appreciate:

- The importance of aseptic and antiseptic techniques and delayed primary or secondary closure in contaminated wounds

To be aware of:

- The causes of reduced resistance to infection (host response)

To know:

- The definitions of infection, particularly at surgical sites
- What basic precautions to take to avoid surgically relevant hospital-acquired infections

HISTORY OF SURGICAL INFECTION

Background

Surgical infections have always been a major complication related to surgery and trauma and have been documented for 4000–5000 years. Egyptians popularised some concepts about infection, as they were able to prevent putrefaction using their skills in mummification. Their medical papyruses also describe the use of salves and antiseptics to prevent surgical site infections (SSIs). This 'prophylaxis' had also been known earlier by the Assyrians, although it is less well documented. It was described again independently by the Greeks.

The Hippocratic teachings described the use of antimicrobials, such as wine and vinegar, which were widely used to irrigate open, infected wounds before delayed primary or secondary wound closure. A belief common to all these civilisations, and indeed even later to the Romans, was that whenever pus was localised in an infected wound it needed to be drained.

Galen recognised that this localisation of infection (suppuration) in wounds inflicted in the gladiatorial arena often heralded recovery, particularly after drainage (*pus bonum et laudabile*). Theodoric of Cervia, Ambroise Paré and Guy de Chauliac observed that clean wounds, closed primarily, could heal without infection or suppuration.

Koch's postulates

An understanding of the causes of infection came in the nineteenth century. Microbes had been seen under the microscope, but Koch laid down the first definition of infective disease (Koch's postulates; see ***Summary box 5.1***).

The Austrian obstetrician Ignaz Semmelweis showed that puerperal sepsis could be reduced from an incidence of over

---

Hippocrates of Kos, Greek physician and surgeon, and by common consent 'the father of medicine', was born on the island of Kos, off Turkey, about 460 BCE and probably died in 375 BCE.

Galen, 130–200, Roman physician, commenced practice as Surgeon to the Gladiators at Pergamum (now Bergama in Turkey) and later became personal physician to the Emperor Marcus Aurelius. As a prolific writer in anatomy, medicine, pathology and philosophy, his work affected medical thinking for 15 centuries after his death. (Gladiator is Latin for 'swordsman'.)

Theodoric of Cervia, 1210–1298, Bishop of Cervia, published a book on surgery ca. 1267.

Ambroise Paré, 1510–1590, French military surgeon, also worked at the Hotel Dieu, Paris, France.

Guy de Chauliac, 1298–1368, physician and chaplain to Pope Clement VI at Avignon, France, and the author of *Chirurgia Magna*, which was published about 1363.

Robert Koch, 1843–1910, Professor of Hygiene and Bacteriology, Berlin, Germany, stated his 'Postulates' in 1882.

Ignaz Semmelweis, 1818–1865, Professor of Obstetrics, Budapest, Hungary.

Summary box 5.1

Koch's postulates proving whether a given organism is the cause of a given disease

- It must be found in every case
- It should be possible to isolate it from the host and grow it in culture
- It should reproduce the disease when injected into another healthy host
- It should be recovered from an experimentally infected host

10% to under 2% by the simple act of handwashing between cases, particularly between postmortem examinations and the delivery suite.

Louis Pasteur recognised through his germ theory that microorganisms were responsible for infecting humans and causing disease. Joseph Lister applied this knowledge to the reduction of colonising organisms in compound fractures by using antiseptics. The principles of antiseptic surgery were soon enhanced with aseptic surgery at the turn of the twentieth century. As well as killing the bacteria on the skin before surgical incision (antiseptic technique), the conditions under which the operation was performed were kept free of bacteria (aseptic technique). This technique is still employed in modern operating theatres (***Figure 5.1***).

Discovery of antibiotics

The concept of a 'magic bullet' (*Zauberkugel*) that could kill microbes but not their host became a reality with the discovery of sulphonamide chemotherapy in the mid-twentieth century. The discovery of the antibiotic penicillin is attributed to Alexander Fleming in 1928, but it was not isolated for clinical use until 1941, by Florey and Chain. The first patient to receive penicillin was Police Constable Alexander in Oxford. Since then there has been a proliferation of antibiotics with broad-spectrum activity and antibiotics today remain the mainstay of antimicrobial therapy.

Misuse of antibiotic therapy with the risk of resistance

Many staphylococci today have become resistant to penicillin. Often bacteria develop resistance through the acquisition of β-lactamases, which break up the β-lactam ring present in the molecular structure of many antibiotics. The acquisition of extended-spectrum β-lactamases (ESBLs) is an increasing concern in some Gram-negative organisms that cause urinary tract infections because it is difficult to find an antibiotic effective against them. In addition, there is increasing concern about the rising resistance of many other bacteria to antibiotics, in particular the emergence of methicillin-resistant *Staphylococcus aureus* (MRSA), which is very relevant in general surgical practice.

The introduction of antibiotics for prophylaxis and for treatment, together with advances in anaesthesia and critical care medicine, has made possible surgery that would not previously have been considered. Faecal peritonitis is no longer inevitably fatal, and incisions made in the presence of such contamination can heal primarily without infection in over 90% of patients with appropriate antibiotic therapy. Despite

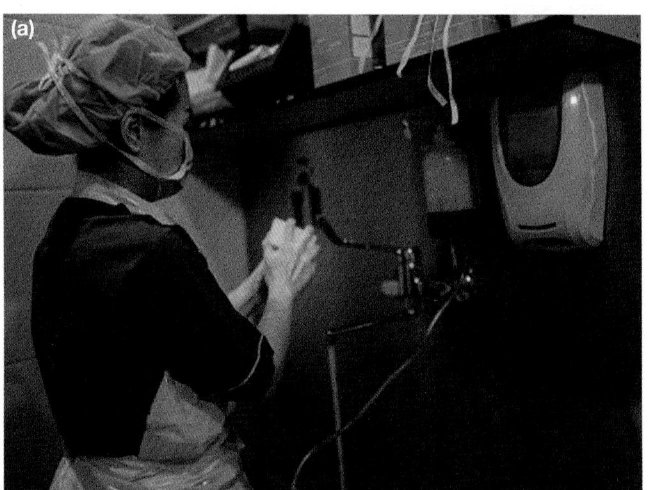

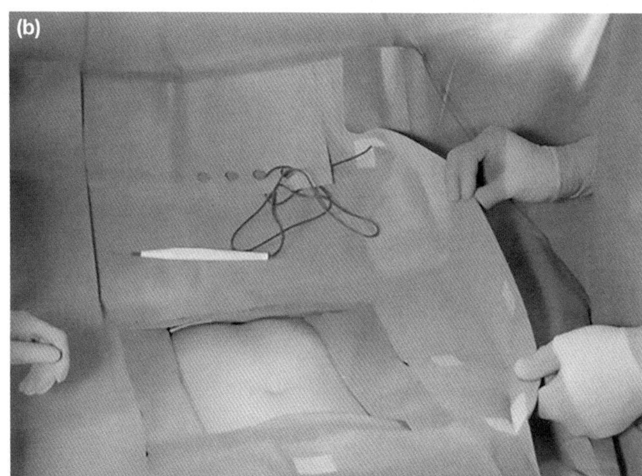

Figure 5.1 Aseptic techniques of scrubbing and draping in a modern operating theatre.

Louis Pasteur, 1822–1895, French chemist, bacteriologist and immunologist, Professor of Chemistry at the Sorbonne, Paris, France.
Lord Joseph Lister, 1827–1912, Professor of Surgery, Glasgow, Scotland (1860–1869), Edinburgh, Scotland (1869–1877) and King's College Hospital, London, England (1877–1892).
Sir Alexander Fleming, 1881–1955, Professor of Bacteriology, St Mary's Hospital, London, England, discovered *Penicillium notatum* in 1928.
Howard Walter Florey (Lord Florey of Adelaide), 1898–1968, Professor of Pathology, the University of Oxford, Oxford, England.
Sir Ernst Boris Chain, Professor of Biochemistry, Imperial College, London, England. Fleming, Florey and Chain shared the 1945 Nobel Prize in Physiology or Medicine for their work on penicillin.
Hans Christian Joachim Gram, 1853–1938, Professor of Pharmacology (1891–1900) and of Medicine (1900–1923), Copenhagen, Denmark, described this method of staining bacteria in 1884.

this, it is common practice in many countries to delay wound closure in patients in whom the wound is known to be contaminated or dirty. Waiting for the wound to granulate and then performing a delayed primary or secondary closure may be considered a better option in such cases (***Summary box 5.2***).

> **Summary box 5.2**
>
> Advances in the control of infection in surgery
>
> - Aseptic operating theatre techniques have enhanced the use of antiseptics
> - Antibiotics have reduced postoperative infection rates after elective and emergency surgery
> - Delayed primary, or secondary, closure remains useful in heavily contaminated wounds

SSI in patients who have contaminated wounds, who are immunosuppressed or who are undergoing prosthetic surgery is now the exception rather than the rule since the introduction of prophylactic antibiotics. The evidence for this is of the highest level. The use of prophylactic antibiotics in clean, non-prosthetic surgery is of less value as infection rates are low and the indiscriminate use of antibiotics simply encourages the emergence of resistant strains of bacteria.

MICROBIOLOGY OF SURGICAL INFECTION

Common bacteria involved in surgical infections

Streptococci

Streptococci form chains and are Gram positive on staining (***Figure 5.2a***). The most important is the β-haemolytic *Streptococcus*, which resides in the pharynx of 5–10% of the population. In the Lancefield A–G carbohydrate antigens classification, it is the group A *Streptococcus*, also called *Streptococcus pyogenes*, that is the most pathogenic. It has the ability to spread, causing cellulitis, and to cause tissue destruction through the release of enzymes such as streptolysin, streptokinase and streptodornase.

Streptococcus faecalis is an enterococcus in Lancefield group D. It is often found in synergy with other organisms, as are the γ-haemolytic *Streptococcus* and *Peptostreptococcus*, which is an anaerobe.

Both *Streptococcus pyogenes* and *Streptococcus faecalis* may be involved in wound infection after bowel surgery, but the α-haemolytic *Streptococcus viridans* is not associated with wound infections.

All the streptococci remain sensitive to penicillin and erythromycin. The cephalosporins are a suitable alternative in patients who are allergic to penicillin.

Staphylococci

Staphylococci form clumps and are Gram positive (***Figure 5.2b***). *Staphylococcus aureus* is the most important pathogen in this group and is found in the nasopharynx of up to 15% of the population. It can cause suppuration in wounds and around implanted prostheses. Some strains are resistant to many common antibiotics (especially MRSA) and so are difficult to treat. MRSA can be found in the nose of asymptomatic carriers among both patients and hospital workers, a potential source of infection after surgery. In parts of northern Europe, the prevalence of MRSA infections has been kept at very low levels using 'search and destroy' methods, which use screening techniques to look for MRSA in patients before they come in to hospital for elective surgery so that any carriers can be treated before their admission for surgery. Local policies on the management of MRSA depend on the prevalence of MRSA, the type of hospital, the clinical specialty and the availability of facilities. Widespread swabbing, ward closures, isolation of patients and disinfection of wards by deep cleaning must all be carefully considered.

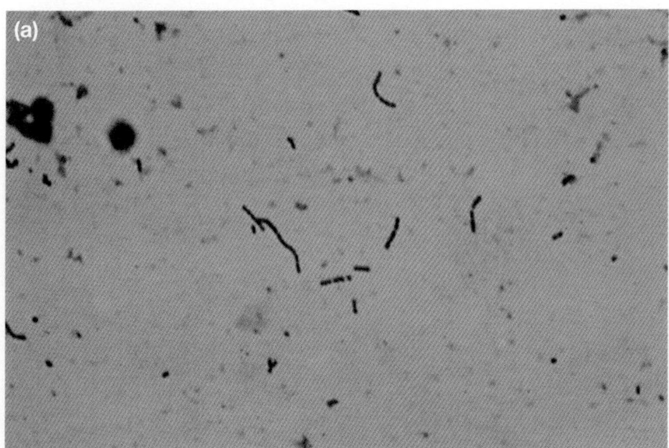

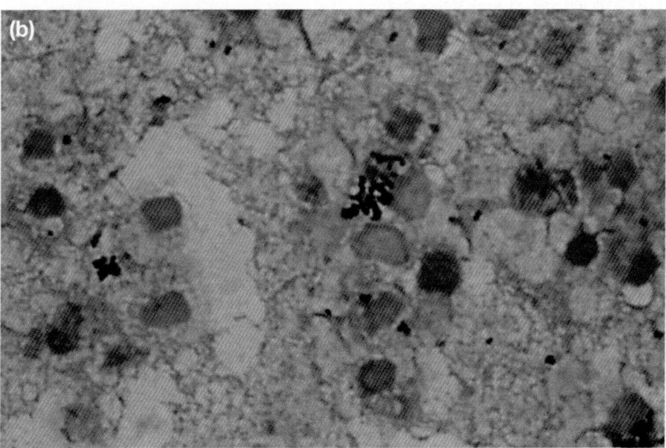

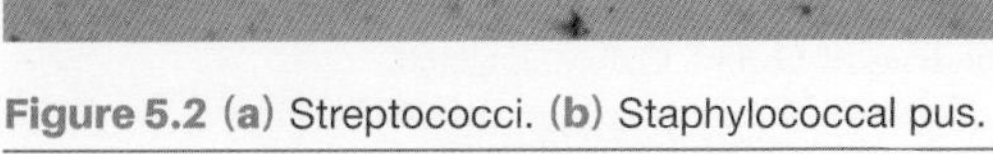

Figure 5.2 (a) Streptococci. (b) Staphylococcal pus.

Rebecca Graighill Lancefield, 1895–1981, American bacteriologist, classified streptococci in 1933.

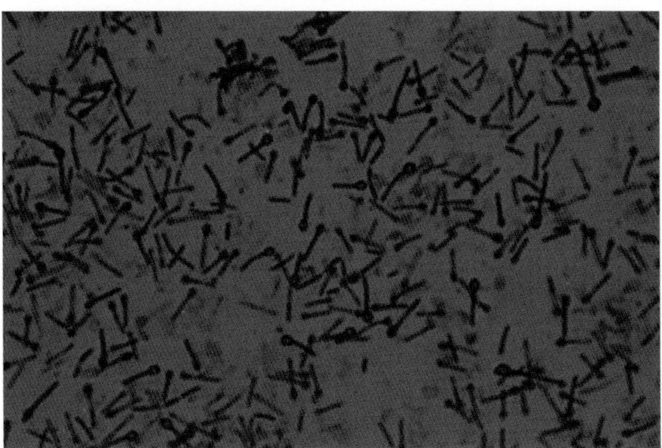

Figure 5.3 *Clostridium tetani* (drumstick spores).

Staphylococcal infections are usually suppurative and localised. Most hospital *Staphylococcus aureus* strains are now β-lactamase producers and so are resistant to penicillin, but many strains remain sensitive to flucloxacillin, vancomycin, aminoglycosides and some cephalosporins. Nowadays, several novel and innovative antibiotics have become available that have high activity against resistant strains. Some have the advantage of good oral activity (linezolid), some have a wide spectrum (teicoplanin), some have good activity in bacteraemia (daptomycin) but all are relatively expensive, and some have side effects involving marrow, hepatic and renal toxicity. Their use is justified but needs to be controlled by tight local policies and guidelines that involve clinical microbiologists.

Staphylococcus epidermidis (previously *Staphylococcus albus*), also known as coagulase-negative *Staphylococcus*, was regarded as a non-pathogenic commensal organism commonly found on the skin, but is now recognised as a major threat in vascular and orthopaedic prosthetic surgery and in indwelling vascular cannulae/catheters. The bacteria form biofilms that adhere to prosthetic surfaces and limit the effectiveness of antibiotics.

Clostridia

Clostridial organisms are Gram-positive, obligate anaerobes that produce resistant spores (***Figure 5.3***). *Clostridium perfringens* is the cause of gas gangrene, and *Clostridium tetani* causes tetanus.

Clostridium difficile (*C. diff.*) is the cause of pseudomembranous colitis, in which destruction of the normal colonic bacterial flora by antibiotic therapy allows an overgrowth of the normal gut commensal *C. diff.* to pathological levels. Any antibiotic may cause this phenomenon, although the quinolones such as ciprofloxacin seem to be the highest risk, especially in elderly or immunocompromised patients. In its most severe form, the colitis may lead to perforation and the need for emergency colectomy with an associated high mortality. Treatment involves resuscitation and antibiotic therapy. The fibrinous exudate is typical and differentiates the colitis from other inflammatory diseases.

Rapid testing for *C. diff.* is now available in the form of testing either *C. diff.* glutamate dehydrogenase (GDH) antigen or *C. diff.* toxin A/B. The *Clostridium difficile* GDH Ag Rapid test qualitatively detects for the presence of *C. diff.* GDH antigen in faeces. On the other hand, the *Clostridium difficile* Toxin A/B rapid test qualitatively detects for the presence of *C. diff.* toxins A and B in faeces. These rapid tests apply lateral flow immunochromatography and are for professional *in vitro* diagnostic use. Results are usually returned from this rapid testing in less than 30 minutes. Empirical treatment with metronidazole or vancomycin is recommended while awaiting results.

Aerobic Gram-negative bacilli

These bacilli are normal inhabitants of the large bowel. *Escherichia coli* and *Klebsiella* spp. are lactose fermenting; *Proteus* is non-lactose fermenting. Most organisms in this group act in synergy with *Bacteroides* to cause SSIs after bowel operations (in particular, appendicitis, diverticulitis and peritonitis). *Escherichia coli* is a major cause of urinary tract infection, although most aerobic Gram-negative bacilli can be involved, particularly in relation to urinary catheterisation. There is increasing concern about the development of ESBLs in many of this group of bacteria, which confer resistance to many antibiotics, particularly cephalosporins.

Pseudomonas spp. tend to colonise burns and tracheostomy wounds, as well as the urinary tract. Once *Pseudomonas* has colonised wards and intensive care units (ICUs), it may be difficult to eradicate. Surveillance of cross-infection is important in outbreaks. Hospital strains become resistant to β-lactamase as resistance can be transferred by plasmids. Wound infections need antibiotic therapy only when there is progressive or spreading infection with systemic signs. The aminoglycosides and the quinolones are effective, but some cephalosporins and penicillin may not be. Many of the carbapenems (e.g. meropenem) are useful in severe infections.

Bacteroides

Bacteroides are non-spore-bearing, strict anaerobes that colonise the large bowel, vagina and oropharynx. *Bacteroides fragilis* is the principal organism that acts in synergy with aerobic Gram-negative bacilli to cause SSIs, including intra-abdominal abscesses after colorectal or gynaecological surgery. They are sensitive to the imidazoles (e.g. metronidazole) and some cephalosporins (e.g. cefotaxime).

Sources of infection

The infection of a wound can be defined as the invasion of organisms into tissues following a breakdown of local and systemic host defences, leading to cellulitis, lymphangitis, abscess formation or bacteraemia. The infection of most surgical wounds is referred to as superficial surgical site infection (SSSI). The other categories include deep SSI (infection in the deeper musculofascial layers) and organ space infection (such

Theodor Escherich, 1857–1911, Professor of Paediatrics, Vienna, Austria, discovered the Bacterium coli commune in 1886.
Theodor Albrecht Edwin Klebs, 1834–1913, Professor of Bacteriology successively at Prague, Czechoslovakia, Zurich, Switzerland and The Rush Medical College, Chicago, IL, USA.

as an abdominal abscess after an anastomotic leak or pelvic abscess after a perforated appendicitis).

Pathogens resist host defences by releasing toxins, which favour their spread, and this is enhanced in anaerobic or frankly necrotic wound tissue. *Clostridium perfringens*, which is responsible for gas gangrene, releases proteases such as hyaluronidase, lecithinase and haemolysin, which allow it to spread through the tissues. Resistance to antibiotics can be acquired by previously sensitive bacteria by transfer through plasmids.

The human body harbours approximately 10^{14} organisms. They can be released into tissues before, during or after surgery, contamination being most severe when a hollow viscus perforates (e.g. faecal peritonitis following a diverticular perforation). Any infection that follows surgery may be termed endogenous or exogenous, depending on the source of the bacterial contamination. Endogenous organisms are present on or in the patient at the time of surgery, whereas exogenous organisms come from outside the patient. In modern hospital practice, endogenous organisms colonising the patient are by far the most common source of infection (***Summary box 5.3***).

Summary box 5.3

Classification of sources of infection

- **Endogenous**: present in or on the host, e.g. SSSI following contamination of the wound from a perforated appendix
- **Exogenous**: acquired from a source outside the body, such as the operating theatre (inadequate air filtration, poor antisepsis) or the ward (e.g. poor handwashing compliance). The cause of hospital-acquired infection (HAI)

Microorganisms are normally prevented from causing infection in tissues by intact epithelial surfaces, most notably the skin. These surfaces are broken down by trauma or surgery. In addition to these mechanical barriers, there are other protective mechanisms, which can be divided into:

- **chemical**: low gastric pH;
- **humoral**: antibodies, complement and opsonins;
- **cellular**: phagocytic cells, macrophages, polymorphonuclear cells and killer lymphocytes.

All of these natural mechanisms may be compromised by surgical intervention and treatment.

The chance of developing an SSI after surgery is also determined by the pathogenicity of the organisms present and by the size of the bacterial inoculum. The more virulent the organism or the larger the extent of bacterial contamination, the more likely is wound infection to occur. Host factors are also important, so a less virulent organism or a lower level of wound contamination may still result in a wound infection if the host response is impaired (***Summary box 5.4***). Devitalised tissue, excessive dead space or haematoma, which are all the results of poor surgical technique, increase the chances of infection. The same applies to foreign materials of any kind, including sutures and drains. These principles are important to an understanding of how best to prevent infection in surgical practice (***Summary box 5.5***).

Summary box 5.4

Factors that determine whether a wound will become infected

- Host response
- Virulence and inoculum of infective agent
- Vascularity and health of tissue being invaded (including local ischaemia as well as systemic shock)
- Presence of dead or foreign tissue
- Presence of antibiotics during the 'decisive period'

Summary box 5.5

Risk factors for increased risk of wound infection

- Malnutrition (obesity, weight loss)
- Metabolic disease (diabetes, uraemia, jaundice)
- Immunosuppression (cancer, acquired immunodeficiency syndrome [AIDS], steroids, chemotherapy and radiotherapy)
- Colonisation and translocation in the gastrointestinal tract
- Poor perfusion (systemic shock or local ischaemia)
- Foreign body material
- Poor surgical technique (devitalised tissue, dead space, haematoma)

The decisive period

There is up to a 4-hour interval before bacterial growth becomes established enough to cause an infection after a breach in the tissues, whether caused by trauma or by surgery. This interval is called the 'decisive period' and strategies aimed at preventing infection from taking a hold become ineffective after this time period. It is therefore logical that prophylactic antibiotics should be given to cover this period and that they could be decisive in preventing an infection from developing before bacterial growth takes a hold. The tissue levels of antibiotics during the period when bacterial contamination is likely to occur should be above the minimum inhibitory concentration (MIC90) for the expected pathogens.

Reduced resistance to infection

Reduced resistance to infection has several causes, particularly those that impair the inflammatory response. Host response is weakened by malnutrition associated with a low or high body mass index. Metabolic diseases such as diabetes mellitus, uraemia and jaundice, disseminated malignancy and acquired immunodeficiency syndrome (AIDS) are other contributors to infection and a poor healing response, as are iatrogenic causes including the immunosuppression caused by radiotherapy, chemotherapy and drugs such as steroids and methotrexate (***Figures 5.4 and 5.5***).

When enteral feeding is suspended during the perioperative period, and particularly with underlying disease such as cancer, immunosuppression, shock or sepsis, bacteria (particularly aerobic Gram-negative bacilli) tend to colonise the normally sterile upper gastrointestinal tract. They may then translocate

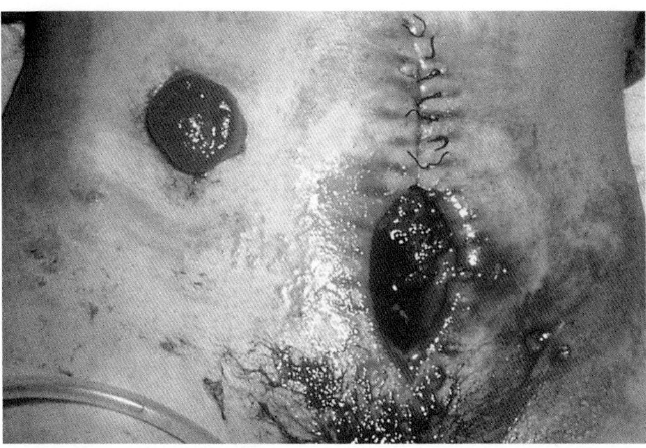

Figure 5.4 Major wound infection and delayed healing presenting as a faecal fistula in a patient with Crohn's disease on steroid treatment.

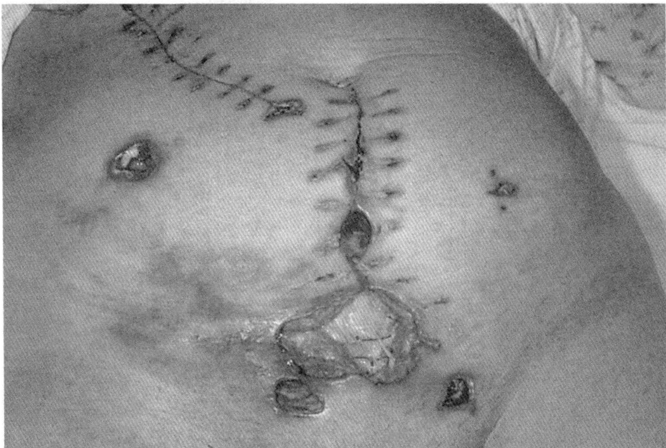

Figure 5.5 Delayed healing relating to infection in a patient on high-dose steroids.

to the mesenteric nodes and cause the release of endotoxins (lipopolysaccharide in bacterial cell walls), which can be one cause of a harmful systemic inflammatory response through the excessive release of proinflammatory cytokines and activation of macrophages (*Figure 5.6*). In the circumstances of reduced host resistance to infection, microorganisms that are not normally pathogenic may start to behave as pathogens. This is known as opportunistic infection. Opportunistic infection with fungi is an example, particularly when prolonged and changing antibiotic regimes have been used.

PRESENTATION OF SURGICAL INFECTION

Major and minor surgical site infection (SSI)

Infection acquired from the environment or the staff following surgery or admission to hospital is termed hospital-acquired infection (HAI). There are four main groups: respiratory infections (including ventilator-associated pneumonia), urinary tract infections (mostly related to urinary catheters),

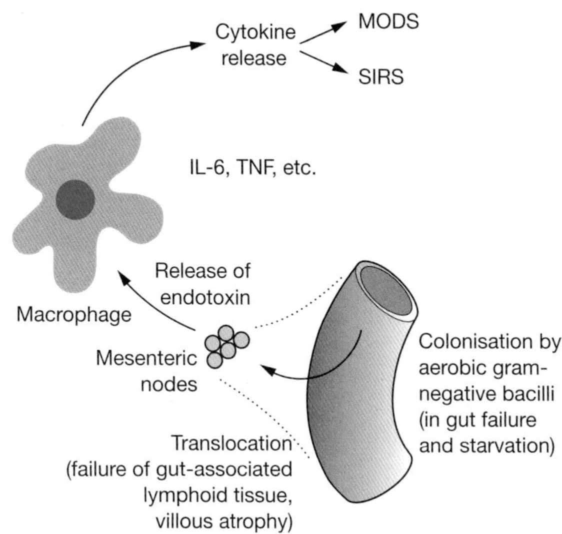

Figure 5.6 Gut failure, colonisation and translocation related to the development of systemic inflammatory response syndrome (SIRS) and multiple organ dysfunction syndrome (MODS). IL, interleukin; TNF, tumour necrosis factor.

bacteraemia (mostly related to indwelling vascular catheters) and SSIs.

A major SSI is defined as a wound that either discharges significant quantities of pus spontaneously or needs a secondary procedure to drain it (*Figure 5.4*). The patient may have systemic signs such as tachycardia, pyrexia and a raised white cell count (*Summary box 5.6*).

Summary box 5.6

Major wound infections

- Significant quantity of pus
- Delayed return home
- Patients are systemically ill

Minor wound infections may discharge pus or infected serous fluid but are not associated with excessive discomfort, systemic signs or delay in return home (*Figure 5.7*).

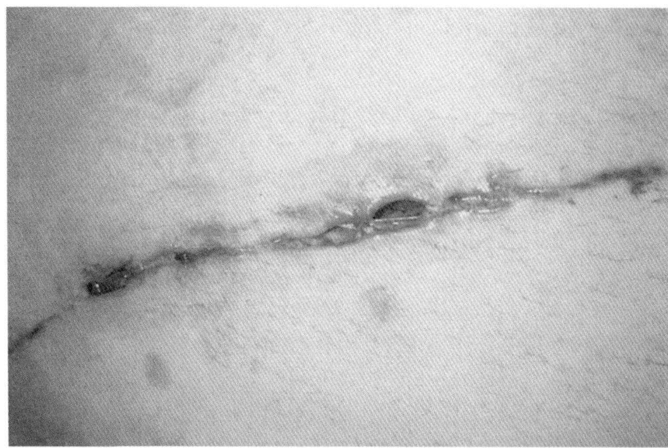

Figure 5.7 Minor wound infection that settled spontaneously without antibiotics.

Localised infection

Abscess

An abscess presents all the clinical features of acute inflammation originally described by Celsus: *calor* (heat), *rubor* (redness), *dolor* (pain) and *tumor* (swelling). To these can be added *functio laesa* (loss of function: if it hurts, the infected part is not used). Abscesses usually follow a puncture wound of some kind, which may have been forgotten, as well as surgery, but can be metastatic in all tissues following bacteraemia.

Pyogenic organisms, predominantly *Staphylococcus aureus*, cause tissue necrosis and suppuration. Pus is composed of dead and dying white blood cells, predominantly neutrophils, that have succumbed to bacterial toxins. An abscess is surrounded by an acute inflammatory response composed of a fibrinous exudate, oedema and the cells of acute inflammation. Granulation tissue (macrophages, fibroblasts and new blood vessel proliferation) forms later around the suppurative process and leads to collagen deposition. If it is not drained or resorbed completely, a chronic abscess may result. If it is partly sterilised with empirical antibiotics, an antibioma may form.

Abscesses contain hyperosmolar material that draws in fluid. This increases the pressure and causes pain. If they spread, they usually track along planes of least resistance and point towards the skin. Wound abscesses may discharge spontaneously by tracking to a surface but may need drainage through a surgical incision. Most abscesses relating to surgical wounds take 7–10 days to form after surgery. As many as 75% of SSIs present after the patient has left hospital and may thus be overlooked by the surgical team.

Abscess cavities need cleaning out after incision and drainage and are traditionally encouraged to heal by secondary intention. When the cavity is left open to drain freely, there is no need for antibiotic therapy as well. Antibiotics should be used if the abscess cavity is closed after drainage, but the cavity should not be closed if there is any risk of retained loculi or foreign material. Thus a perianal abscess can be incised and drained, the walls curetted and the skin closed with good results using appropriate antibiotic therapy, but a pilonidal abscess has a higher recurrence risk after such treatment because a nidus of hair may remain in the subcutaneous tissue adjacent to the abscess. Some small breast abscesses can be managed by simple needle aspiration of the pus and antibiotic therapy (***Summary box 5.7***).

Persistent chronic abscesses may lead to sinus or fistula formation. In a chronic abscess, lymphocytes and plasma cells are seen. There is tissue sequestration and later calcification may occur. Certain organisms are associated with chronicity and with sinus and fistula formation. Common ones are *Mycobacterium* and *Actinomyces*. They should not be forgotten when these complications occur and persist.

Perianastomotic contamination may be the cause of an abscess but, in the abdomen, abscesses are more usually the result of anastomotic leakage. An abscess in a deep cavity such as the pleura or peritoneum may be difficult to diagnose or locate even when there is strong clinical suspicion that it is present (***Figure 5.8***). Plain or contrast radiographs may not be helpful, but ultrasonography, computed tomography (CT), magnetic resonance imaging (MRI) and isotope-labelled white cell scans are all useful and may allow image-guided aspiration and drainage of intra-abdominal abscesses without the need for surgical intervention.

Summary box 5.7

Abscesses

- Abscesses need drainage
- Modern imaging techniques may allow guided needle aspiration, e.g. ultrasound-guided drainage of breast abscesses
- Antibiotics are indicated if the abscess cavity is not left open to drain freely
- An open abscess cavity heals by secondary intention

Cellulitis and lymphangitis

Cellulitis is a non-suppurative, invasive infection of tissues, which is usually related to the point of injury. There is poor localisation in addition to the cardinal signs of spreading inflammation. Such infections presenting in surgical practice are typically caused by organisms such as β-haemolytic streptococci (***Figure 5.9***), staphylococci (***Figure 5.10***) and *Clostridium perfringens*. Tissue destruction, gangrene and ulceration may follow, which are caused by release of proteases.

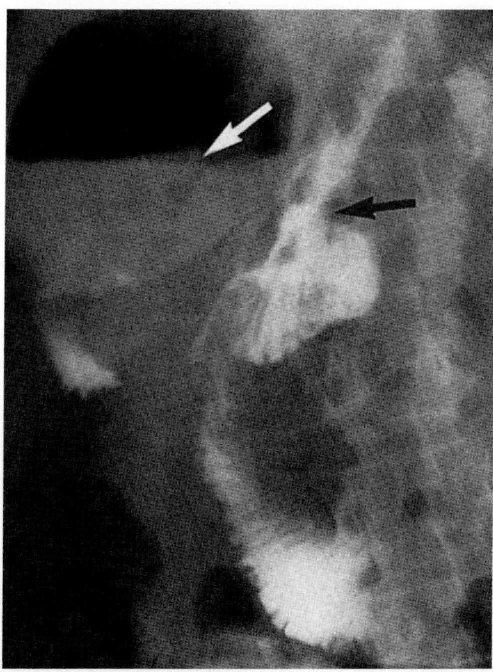

Figure 5.8 Plain radiograph showing a subphrenic abscess with a gas/fluid level (white arrow). Gastrografin is seen leaking from the oesophagojejunal anastomosis (after gastrectomy) towards the abscess (black arrow).

Aulus Aurelius Cornelius Celsus, 25 BCE–50 CE, Roman surgeon and the author of *De Re Medico Libri Octo*.

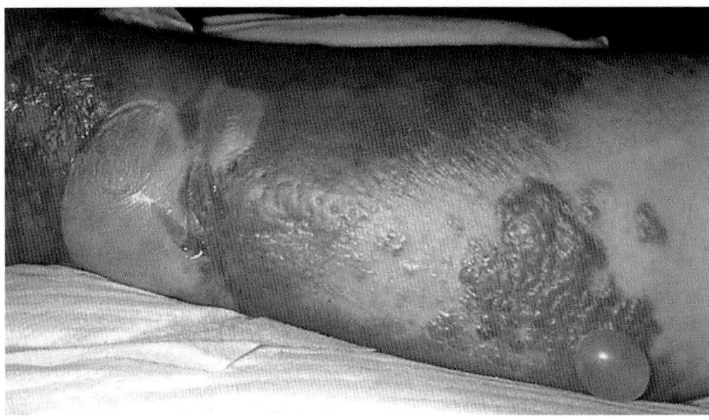

Figure 5.9 Streptococcal cellulitis of the leg following a minor puncture wound.

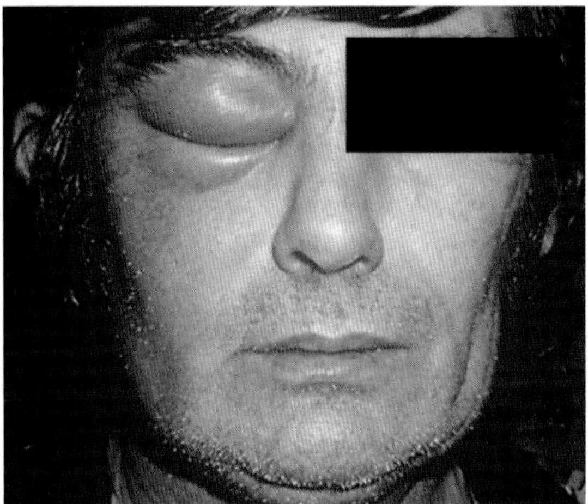

Figure 5.10 Staphylococcal cellulitis of the face and orbit following severe infection of an epidermoid cyst of the scalp.

Systemic signs (the old-fashioned term is toxaemia) are common, with chills, fever and rigors. These events follow the release of toxins into the circulation, which stimulate a cytokine-mediated systemic inflammatory response even though blood cultures may be negative.

Lymphangitis is part of a similar process and presents as painful red streaks in affected lymphatics draining the source of infection. Lymphangitis is often accompanied by painful lymph node groups in the related drainage area, e.g. cervical, axillary or inguinal (***Summary box 5.8***).

Summary box 5.8

Cellulitis and lymphangitis

- Non-suppurative, poorly localised
- Commonly caused by streptococci, staphylococci or clostridia
- Blood cultures are often negative

Specific local wound infections

Gas gangrene

Gas gangrene is caused by *Clostridium perfringens*. These Gram-positive, anaerobic, spore-bearing bacilli are widely found in nature, particularly in soil and faeces. Patients who are immunocompromised, diabetic or have malignant disease are at greater risk, particularly if they have wounds containing necrotic or foreign material, resulting in anaerobic conditions. Military wounds provide an ideal environment as the kinetic energy of high-velocity missiles or shrapnel causes extensive tissue damage. The cavitation which follows passage of a missile through the tissues causes a 'sucking' entry wound, leaving clothing and environmental soiling in the wound in addition to devascularised tissue. Gas gangrene wound infections are associated with severe local wound pain and crepitus (gas in the tissues, which may also be visible on plain radiographs). The wound produces a thin, brown, sweet-smelling exudate, in which Gram staining will reveal bacteria. Oedema and spreading gangrene follow the release of collagenase, hyaluronidase, other proteases and alpha toxin. Early systemic complications with circulatory collapse and organ failure follow if prompt action is not taken (***Summary box 5.9***).

Antibiotic prophylaxis should always be considered in patients at risk, especially when amputations are performed for peripheral vascular disease with open necrotic ulceration. Once gas gangrene infection is established, large doses of intravenous penicillin and aggressive debridement of affected tissues are required.

Summary box 5.9

Gas gangrene

- Caused by *Clostridium perfringens*
- Gas and smell are characteristic
- Immunocompromised patients are most at risk
- Antibiotic prophylaxis is essential when performing amputations to remove dead tissue

Clostridium tetani

This is another anaerobic, terminal spore-bearing, Gram-positive bacterium, which can cause tetanus following implantation into tissues or a wound. The spores are widespread in soil and manure. The signs and symptoms of tetanus are mediated by the release of the exotoxin tetanospasmin; these include spasms in the distribution of the short motor nerves of the face followed by the development of severe generalised motor spasms including opisthotonus, respiratory arrest and death. Prophylaxis with tetanus toxoid is the best preventative treatment but, in an established infection, minor debridement of the wound may need to be performed and antibiotic treatment with benzylpenicillin provided in addition. Relaxants may also be required and the patient will require ventilation in severe forms, which are associated with a high mortality.

Synergistic spreading gangrene (synonym: subdermal gangrene, necrotising fasciitis)

This is a rare but serious bacterial infection that affects and spreads via the deep fascia; hence, it is termed fasciitis. A mixed pattern of organisms is responsible for this serious condition: coliforms, staphylococci, *Bacteroides* spp., anaerobic streptococci and peptostreptococci have all been implicated, acting in synergy. Often, aerobic bacteria destroy the living tissue, allowing anaerobic bacteria to thrive. Severe wound pain, signs of spreading inflammation with crepitus and odour are all signs of the infection spreading. Untreated, it will lead to widespread local gangrene and systemic multisystem organ failure. Abdominal wall infections are known as Meleney's synergistic gangrene and scrotal infections as Fournier's gangrene (***Figure 5.11***). Patients are almost always immunocompromised, with conditions such as diabetes mellitus. The wound initiating the infection may have been minor, but severely contaminated wounds are more likely to be the cause.

The subdermal spread of gangrene is always much more extensive than appears from initial examination. The finger test can be used in the diagnosis of patients who present with suspected necrotising fasciitis. The area of suspected involvement is first infiltrated with local anaesthesia. A 2-cm incision is made in the skin down to the deep fascia. Lack of bleeding is a sign of necrotising fasciitis. On some occasions, a dishwater-coloured fluid is noticed seeping from the wound. A gentle, probing manoeuvre with the index finger covered by a sterile glove is then performed at the level of the deep fascia. If the tissues dissect with minimal resistance, the finger test is positive. Tissue biopsies are then sent for frozen section analysis. The characteristic histological findings are obliterative vasculitis of the subcutaneous vessels, acute inflammation and subcutaneous tissue necrosis. If either the finger test or rapid frozen section analysis is positive, or if the patient has progressive clinical findings consistent with necrotising fasciitis, immediate operative treatment must be initiated.

Broad-spectrum antibiotic therapy must be combined with aggressive circulatory support. Locally, there should be wide excision of necrotic tissue and laying open of affected areas. The debridement may need to be extensive, and patients who survive may need large areas of skin grafting later.

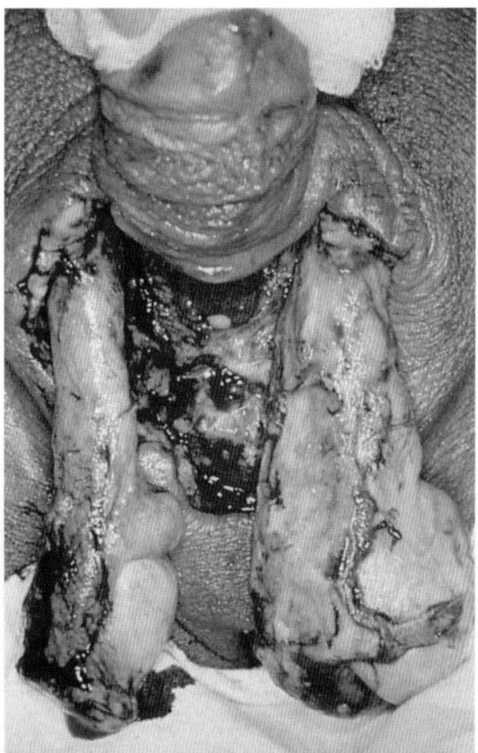

Figure 5.11 A classic presentation of Fournier's gangrene of the scrotum with 'shameful exposure of the testes' following excision of the gangrenous skin.

Systemic infection

Bacteraemia

Bacteraemia is unusual following superficial SSIs, which tend to drain through the wound, but common after deep space SSIs, such as following an intestinal anastomotic breakdown. It is usually transient and can follow procedures undertaken through infected tissues (particularly instrumentation in infected bile or urine). It may also occur through bacterial infection of indwelling intravenous cannulae, which should be replaced regularly to avoid colonisation. Bacteraemia is important when a prosthesis has been implanted, as infection of the prosthesis can occur through haematogenous spread. Aerobic Gram-negative bacilli are often responsible, but *Staphylococcus aureus* and fungi may be involved (***Summary box 5.10***).

Summary box 5.10

Bacteraemia

- Common after anastomotic breakdown
- Dangerous if the patient has a prosthesis, which can become infected
- May be associated with systemic organ failure

Systemic inflammatory response syndrome

Systemic inflammatory response syndrome (SIRS) is a systemic manifestation of sepsis (***Table 5.1***), although the syndrome may also be caused by multiple trauma, burns or pancreatitis without infection. Serious infection, such as secondary peritonitis, may lead to SIRS through the release of lipopolysaccharide endotoxin from the walls of dying Gram-negative bacilli (mainly *Escherichia coli*) or other bacteria or fungi. This and other toxins stimulate the release of cytokines from macrophages (***Figure 5.6***). SIRS should not be confused with bacteraemia, although the two may coexist.

Frank Lamont Meleney, 1889–1963, Professor of Clinical Surgery, Columbia University, New York, NY, USA.
Jean Alfred Fournier, 1832–1915, syphilologist, the founder of the Venereal and Dermatological Clinic, Hôpital Saint-Louis, Paris, France.

TABLE 5.1 Definitions of systemic inflammatory response syndrome (SIRS) and sepsis

SIRS is ***Presence of two out of three of the following:*** • Hyperthermia (>38°C) or hypothermia (<36°C) • Tachycardia (>90/min, no β-blockers) or tachypnoea (>20/min) • White cell count >12 × 10^9/litre or <4 × 10^9/litre
Sepsis is SIRS with a documented source of infection
Severe sepsis or sepsis syndrome is sepsis with evidence of failure of one or more organs: respiratory (acute respiratory distress syndrome), cardiovascular (septic shock follows compromise of cardiac function and fall in peripheral vascular resistance), renal (usually acute tubular necrosis), hepatic, blood coagulation systems or central nervous system

Septic manifestations and multiple organ dysfunction syndrome (MODS) in SIRS are mediated by the release of pro-inflammatory cytokines such as interleukin-1 (IL-1) and tumour necrosis factor alpha (TNFα). These cytokines normally stimulate neutrophil adhesion to endothelial surfaces adjacent to the source of infection and cause them to migrate through the blood vessel wall by chemotaxis, where they can attack the bacterial invasion. A respiratory burst occurs within such activated neutrophils, releasing lysosomal enzymes, oxidants and free radicals, which are involved in killing the invading bacteria but which may also damage adjacent cells. Coagulation, complement and fibrinolytic pathways are also stimulated as part of the normal inflammatory response. This response is usually beneficial to the host and is an important aspect of normal tissue repair and wound healing. On occasions, this response may become harmful to the host if it occurs in excess, when it is known as the systemic inflammatory response syndrome or SIRS. There are high circulating levels of cytokines and activated neutrophils that stimulate fever, tachycardia and tachypnoea. The activated neutrophils adhere to vascular endothelium in key organs remote from the source of infection and damage it, leading to increased vascular permeability, which in turn leads to cellular damage within the organs, which become dysfunctional and give rise to the clinical picture of multiple organ dysfunction syndrome or MODS. In its most severe form, MODS may progress into multiple system organ failure (MSOF). Respiratory, cardiac, intestinal, renal and liver failure ensue in combination with circulatory failure and shock. In this state, the body's resistance to infection is reduced and a vicious cycle develops where the more organs that fail, the more likely it becomes that death will follow despite all that a modern ICU can do for organ support (*Summary box 5.11*).

Summary box 5.11

Definitions of infected states

- SSI is an infected wound or deep organ space
- SIRS is the body's systemic response to severe infection
- MODS is the effect that SIRS produces systemically
- MSOF is the end stage of uncontrolled MODS

Surviving Sepsis Campaign/sepsis bundle/ Sepsis Six

The European Society of Intensive Care Medicine (ESICM) alongside the Society of Critical Care Medicine (SCCM) spearheaded the Surviving Sepsis Campaign (SSC) in 2002 with several aims, including the development of guidelines for the diagnosis, treatment and post-ICU care of sepsis and a reduction in mortality from sepsis. The Surviving Sepsis Campaign continually develops and updates resources and implementation tools to further its mission of reducing sepsis and septic shock.

The **sepsis bundle**, also known as the resuscitation bundle, is a combination of evidence-based objectives that must be completed within 6 hours for patients presenting with severe sepsis, septic shock and/or lactate >4 mmol/L.

The **Sepsis Six** is the name given to a bundle of medical therapies designed to reduce mortality in patients with sepsis. Drawn from international guidelines that emerged from the Surviving Sepsis Campaign, the Sepsis Six was developed by the UK's Sepsis Trust. The components of the Sepsis Six are:

- **give three to patients:** (1) intravenous fluid challenge, (2) intravenous antibiotics, (3) oxygen and monitor urine output;
- **take three from patients:** (4) blood cultures, (5) full blood count, (6) lactate.

Viral infections relevant to surgery

Hepatitis

Both hepatitis B and hepatitis C carry risks in surgery as they are blood-borne pathogens that can be transmitted both from the patient to the surgeon and vice versa. The usual mode of transmission is blood-to-blood contact through a needle-stick injury or a cut. Many cases of hepatitis B are asymptomatic and a surgeon may carry the virus without being aware of it. As there is an effective vaccine against hepatitis B, surgeons should know their immune status to hepatitis B and be vaccinated against it. Hepatitis C infection often becomes chronic with the risk of significant liver damage but is potentially curable with interferon-alpha and ribavirin treatment, so surgeons who are exposed to an infection risk should seek medical advice and antibody measurement.

Human immunodeficiency virus

The type I human immunodeficiency virus (HIV) is one of the viruses of surgical importance because it can be transmitted by body fluids, particularly blood. It is a retrovirus that has become increasingly prevalent through sexual transmission (both homo- and heterosexual), intravenous drug addiction and in infected blood products used to treat patients with haemophilia in particular. The risk in surgery is mostly through needle-stick injury during operations.

The risk of opportunistic infections (such as *Pneumocystis carinii* pneumonia, tuberculosis and cytomegalovirus) and neoplasms (such as Kaposi's sarcoma and lymphoma) is thereby increased.

Moritz Kaposi, 1837–1902, Professor of Dermatology, Vienna, Austria, described pigmented sarcoma of the skin in 1872.

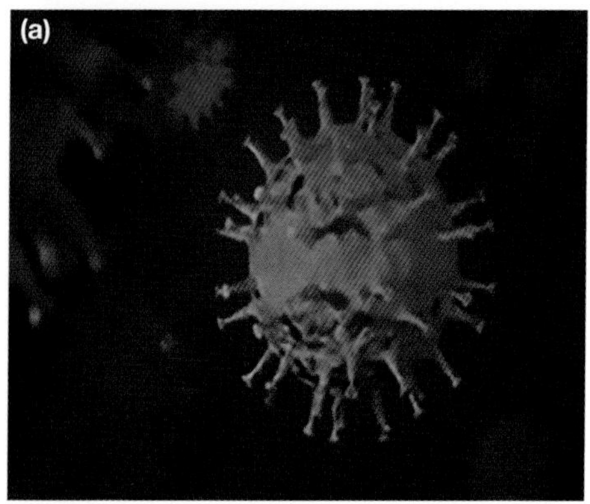

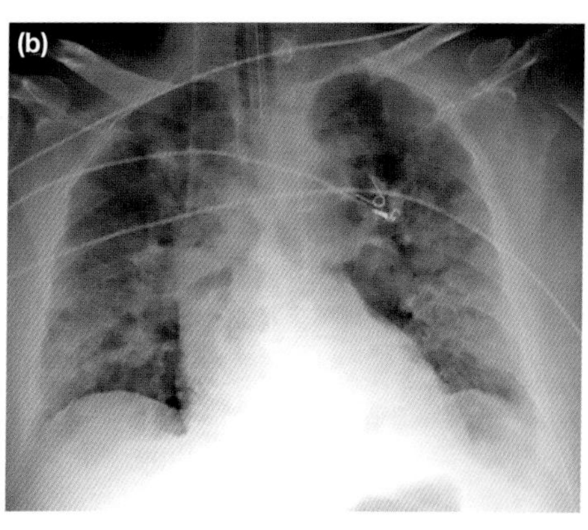

Figure 5.12 (**a**) Severe acute respiratory syndrome coronavirus 2 (SARS-CoV-2). (**b**) Chest radiograph showing coronavirus disease 2019 (COVID-19) pneumonia changes.

In the early weeks after HIV infection, there may be a flu-like illness and, during the phase of seroconversion, patients present the greatest risk of HIV transmission. It is during these early phases that drug treatment, highly active antiretroviral therapy (HAART), is most effective through the ability of these drugs to inhibit reverse transcriptase and protease synthesis, which are the principal mechanisms through which HIV can progress. These drugs suppress the virus but do not clear it completely from the body and treated patients can still transmit the virus to others. Within 2 years, untreated HIV can progress to acquired immunodeficiency syndrome (AIDS) in 25–35% of patients.

Universal precautions

Patients may present to surgeons for operative treatment if they have a surgical disease and they are known to be infected or 'at risk', or because they need surgical intervention related to their illness for vascular access or a biopsy when they are known to have hepatitis, HIV infection or AIDS. Particular care should be taken when there is a risk of splashing/aerosol formation, particularly with power tools. Universal precautions have been drawn up by CDC in the USA and largely adopted by the NHS in the UK. In summary, these are:

- use of a full face mask ideally, or protective spectacles;
- use of fully waterproof, disposable gowns and drapes, particularly during seroconversion;
- boots to be worn, not clogs, to avoid injury from dropped sharps;
- double gloving needed (a larger size on the inside is more comfortable);
- allow only essential personnel in theatre;
- avoid unnecessary movement in theatre;
- respect is required for sharps, with passage in a kidney dish;
- slow meticulous operative technique is needed with minimised bleeding.

After contamination

Needle-stick injuries are commonest on the non-dominant index finger during operative surgery. Hollow needle injury carries the greatest risk of viral transmission. The injured part should be washed under running water and the incident reported. Local policies dictate whether postexposure antiretroviral treatment should be given. Occupational health advice is required after high-risk exposure, together with the need for hepatitis/HIV testing and the option for continuation in a non-operative specialty.

COVID-19 pandemic

The global pandemic of coronavirus disease 2019 (COVID-19) was announced by the World Health Organization on 11 March 2020. As of 16 August 2021, more than 207 million cases and more than 4.36 million deaths had been reported in 210 countries.* The rapid spread of the outbreak has had short-term implications for global healthcare systems, including the field of surgery. Many hospitals were forced to stop or postpone elective surgical interventions during the first wave in early to mid-2020. However, emergency surgery and time-sensitive surgery, i.e. cancer surgery, continued with relevant precautions, including the use of personal protective equipment.

COVID-19 is a contagious respiratory and vascular disease. The aetiology is severe acute respiratory syndrome coronavirus 2 (SARS-CoV-2) (***Figure 5.12a***), which is a specific type of coronavirus. Common symptoms include fever, cough, fatigue, shortness of breath or breathing difficulties as well as loss of smell and taste. The incubation period may range from 1 to 14 days. While most people have mild symptoms, some people develop acute respiratory distress syndrome (ARDS), possibly precipitated by a cytokine storm; multiorgan failure; septic shock; and hypercoagulable states. Longer term damage to organs (in particular, the lungs and heart) has been observed.

Complications in postoperative surgical patients infected with COVID-19 in either an elective or emergency setting may include pneumonia (***Figure 5.12b***), ARDS, multiorgan failure, septic shock and death. Measures to control COVID-19-related morbidity and mortality have thus been implemented by many countries, including a mandatory preoperative cocooning of elective surgical patients 10–14 days prior to surgery and preoperative COVID-19 swab testing 2–3 days prior to elective surgery. Like many other viral infections, there is no definite pharmacological cure for this infection, although there has been some evidence for supportive care, e.g. with hydroxychloroquine and dexamethasone. Multiple vaccines were made available at the end of 2020 and, currently, the majority of countries have most of their population vaccinated.

*Data from: COVID-19 dashboard by the Center for Systems Science and Engineering (CSSE) at Johns Hopkins University (accessed 16 August 2021).

PREVENTION OF SURGICAL INFECTION

Preoperative preparation

A short preoperative hospital stay lowers the risk of acquiring MRSA, multidrug-resistant coagulase-negative staphylococci and other antibiotic-resistant organisms from the hospital environment. Medical and nursing staff should always wash their hands after any patient contact. Hand gels containing at least 70% alcohol can act as a substitute for handwashing, but do not destroy the spores of *C. diff.*, which may cause pseudo-membranous colitis, especially in immunocompromised patients or those whose gut flora is suppressed by antibiotic therapy. Although the need for clean hospitals, emphasised by the media, is logical, the 'clean your hands campaign', particularly in the COVID-19 era, is beginning to result in falls in the incidence of HAIs. Staff with open, infected skin lesions should not enter the operating theatres. Ideally, neither should affected patients, especially if they are having a prosthesis implanted. Antiseptic baths (usually chlorhexidine) are popular in Europe, but there is no hard evidence for their value in reducing wound infections. Preoperative skin shaving should be undertaken in the operating theatre immediately before surgery as the SSI rate after clean wound surgery may be doubled if shaving is performed the night before because minor skin injury enhances superficial bacterial colonisation.

Scrubbing and skin preparation

When washing the hands prior to surgery, dilute alcohol-based antiseptic hand soaps such as chlorhexidine or povidone–iodine should be used, and the scrub should include the nails (***Figure 5.1***).

One application of a more concentrated alcohol-based antiseptic is adequate for skin preparation of the operative site. This leads to a >95% reduction in bacterial count but caution should be taken not to leave a pool of alcohol-based fluid on the skin as it could ignite with diathermy and burn the patient (***Figure 5.1***).

Theatre technique and discipline also contribute to low infection rates. Numbers of staff in the theatre and movement in and out of theatre should be kept to a minimum. Careful and regular surveillance is needed to ensure the quality of instrument sterilisation, aseptic technique and theatre ventilation. Laminar flow systems direct clean, filtered air over the operating field, with any air potentially contaminated as it passes over the incision then directed away from the patient. Operator skill in gentle manipulation and dissection of tissues is much more difficult to audit, but dead spaces and haematomas should be avoided. There is no evidence that drains, incision drapes or wound guards help to reduce wound infection. There is a high level of evidence that both the perioperative avoidance of hypothermia and the use of supplemental oxygen during recovery significantly reduce the rate of SSIs.

Prophylactic antibiotics

Prophylactic antibiotics are used when there is a risk of wound contamination with bacteria during surgery. The theoretical degree of contamination, proposed by the National Research Council (USA) over 40 years ago, relates well to infection rates (***Table 5.2***). The value of antibiotic prophylaxis is low in non-prosthetic clean surgery, with most trials showing no clear benefit because infection rates without antibiotics are so low. The exception to this is where a prosthetic implant is used, as the results of infection are so catastrophic that even a small risk of infection is unacceptable. There is undisputed evidence that prophylactic antibiotics are effective in reducing the risk of infection in clean-contaminated and contaminated operations. When wounds are heavily contaminated or when an incision is made into an abscess, a 5-day course of therapeutic antibiotics may be justified on the assumption that the wound is inevitably infected and so treatment is needed rather than prophylaxis.

TABLE 5.2 Surgical site infection rates relating to wound contamination with and without using antibiotic prophylaxis

Type of surgery	Infection rate with prophylaxis (%)	Infection rate without prophylaxis (%)
Clean (no viscus opened)	1–2	1–2
Clean-contaminated (viscus opened, minimal spillage)	3	6–9
Contaminated (open viscus with spillage or inflammatory disease)	6	13–20
Dirty (pus or perforation, or incision through an abscess)	7	40

If antibiotics are given to prevent infection after surgery or instrumentation, they should be used before bacterial growth becomes established (i.e. within the decisive period). Ideally, maximal blood and tissue levels should be present at the time at which the first incision is made and before contamination occurs. Tissue levels of the antibiotic should remain high throughout the operation and antibiotics with a short tissue half-life should be avoided. Intravenous administration at induction of anaesthesia is therefore optimal, as unexpected delays in the timing of surgery may occur before then and antibiotic tissue levels may fall off before the surgery starts. In long operations or when there is excessive blood loss, or when unexpected contamination occurs, antibiotics may be repeated at 4-hourly intervals during the surgery because tissue antibiotic levels often fall faster than serum levels. There is no evidence that further doses of antibiotics after surgery are of any value in prophylaxis against infection and the practice can only encourage the development of antibiotic resistance. The choice of an antibiotic depends on the expected spectrum of organisms likely to be encountered, which will depend on the site and type of surgery and whether the patient has any antibiotic allergies. Hospitals in the UK and across Europe now have standardised antibiotic prophylaxis policies that take account of the above factors and are only deviated from with microbiological advice.

Patients with known valvular disease of the heart (or with any implanted vascular or orthopaedic prosthesis) should have prophylactic antibiotics during dental, urological or open viscus surgery to prevent bacterial colonisation of the valve or prosthesis during the transient bacteraemia which can occur during such surgery (***Summary box 5.12***).

Summary box 5.12

Antibiotic prophylaxis

- Not required in clean surgery unless a prosthesis is implanted
- Use antibiotics that are effective against expected pathogens within local hospital guidelines
- Plan for single-shot intravenous administration at induction of anaesthesia
- Repeat only during long operations or if there is excessive blood loss
- Patients with heart valve disease or a prosthesis should be protected from bacteraemia caused by dental work, urethral instrumentation or visceral surgery

Postoperative wound infections

The majority of wound infections arise from endogenous sources within the patient, but exogenous SSIs may also occur from bacteria present in the ward or on staff and so can be related to poor hospital standards. Strict attention to ward cleanliness, gloving before touching patient wounds and hand-washing between all patient contacts are important preventive measures. An outbreak of wound infections on the ward with bacteria having the same antibiotic sensitivity profile implies an exogenous source of infection, which needs to be investigated by swabbing all staff and work surfaces. It may need temporary ward closure and a deep clean to eradicate the infection source.

Now that patients are discharged more quickly after surgery and many procedures are performed as day cases, many SSIs are missed by the surgical team unless they undertake a prolonged and carefully audited follow-up with primary care doctors. Suppurative wound infections take 7–10 days to develop, and even cellulitis around wounds caused by invasive organisms (such as β-haemolytic *Streptococcus*) takes 3–4 days to develop. Major surgical infections with systemic signs (***Figure 5.13***), evidence of spreading infection, cellulitis or bacteraemia need treatment with appropriate antibiotics. The choice may need to be empirical initially but is best based on culture and sensitivities of isolates harvested at surgery or from culture of wound fluids or wound swabs. Although the identification of organisms in surgical infections is necessary for audit and wound surveillance purposes, it is usually 2–3 days before sensitivities are known (***Figures 5.14 and 5.15***). It is illogical to withhold antibiotics until results are available but, if clinical response is poor by the time sensitivities are known, then antibiotics can be changed. Such changes are unusual if the empirical choice of antibiotics is sensible; change of antibiotics promotes resistance and risks complications, such as *C. diff.* enteritis.

If an infected wound is under tension, or there is clear evidence of suppuration, sutures or clips need to be removed, with curettage if necessary, to allow pus to drain adequately. In severely contaminated wounds, such as an incision made for drainage of an abscess, it is logical to leave the skin open. Delayed primary or secondary closure can be undertaken when the wound is clean and granulating (***Figures 5.16 and 5.17***). Some heavily infected wounds may be left to heal by secondary intention, with no attempt at closure, particularly where there is a loss of skin cover and healthy granulation tissue develops

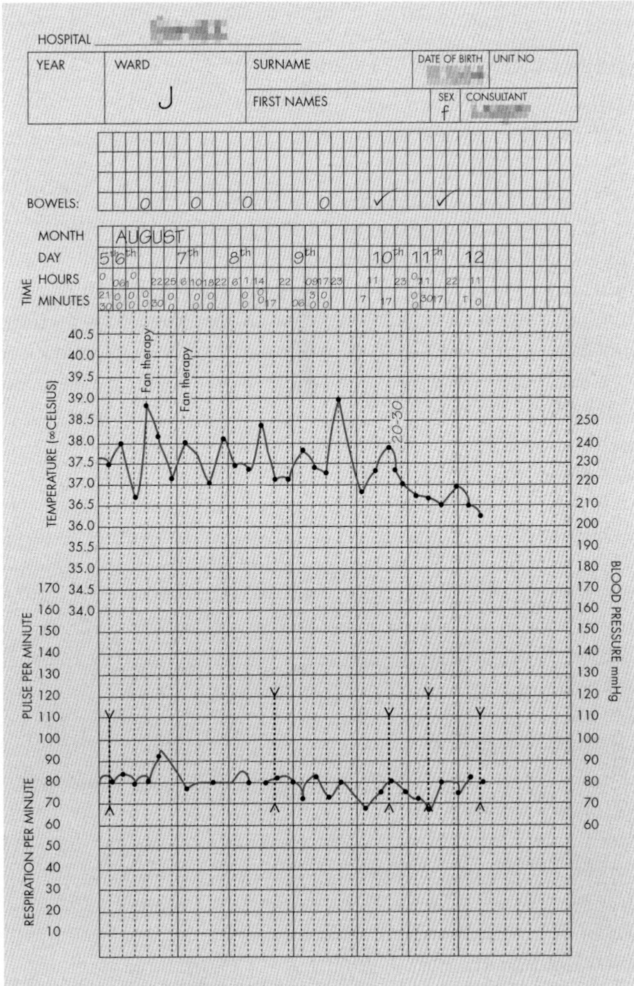

Figure 5.13 Classic swinging pyrexia related to a perianastomotic wound abscess that settled spontaneously on antibiotic therapy.

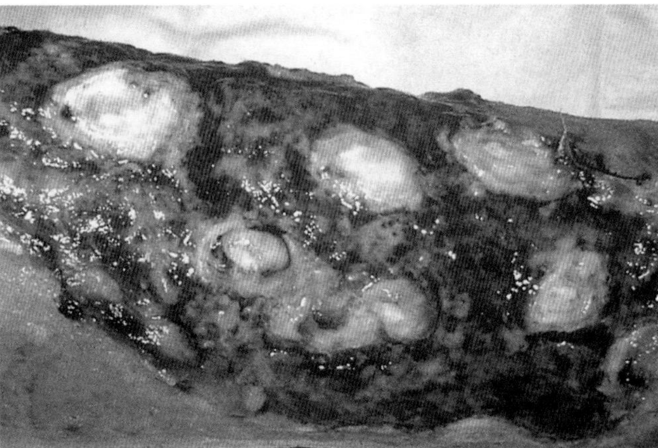

Figure 5.14 Mixed streptococcal infection of a skin graft with very poor 'take'.

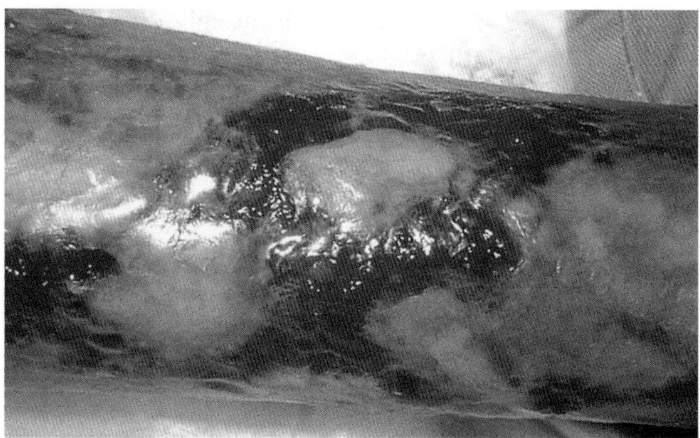

Figure 5.15 After 5–6 days of antibiotics, the infection shown in ***Figure 5.14*** is under control, and the skin grafts are clearly viable.

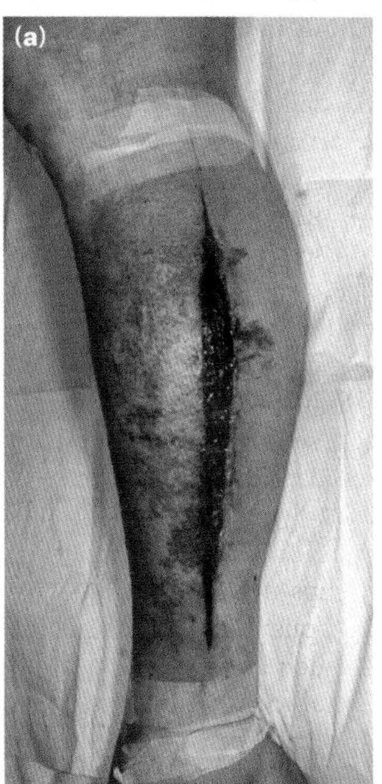

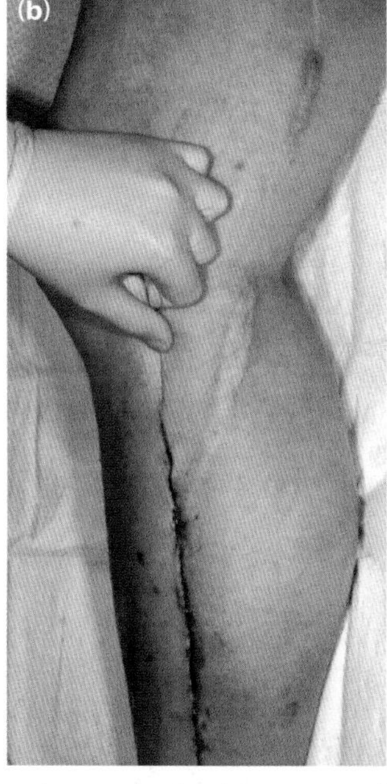

Figure 5.16 (a, b) Delayed primary closure of a fasciotomy wound after 3–5 days.

(*Figure 5.18*). While the end result may be excessive scarring, that can always be revised with plastic surgery under clean surgical conditions at a later stage (***Summary box 5.13***).

Summary box 5.13

Surgical incisions through infected or contaminated tissues

- When possible, tissue or pus for culture should be taken before antibiotic cover is started
- The choice of antibiotics is empirical until sensitivities are available
- Heavily contaminated wounds are best managed by delayed primary or secondary closure

When taking pus from infected wounds, specimens should be sent fresh for microbiological culture. Swabs should be placed in transport medium, but the larger the volume of pus sent, the more likely is the accurate identification of the organism involved. Providing the microbiologist with as much information as possible and discussing the results with them gives the best chance of the most appropriate antibiotic treatment. If bacteraemia is suspected, but results are negative, then repeat specimens for blood culture and an immediate Gram stain.

Topical antiseptics should only be used on heavily contaminated wounds for a short period to clear infection as they inhibit epithelial ingrowth and so impair wound healing.

ANTIMICROBIAL TREATMENT OF SURGICAL INFECTION

Principles

Antimicrobials may be used to prevent or treat established surgical infection.

The use of antibiotics for the treatment of established surgical infection ideally requires recognition and determination of the sensitivities of the causative organisms. Antibiotic therapy

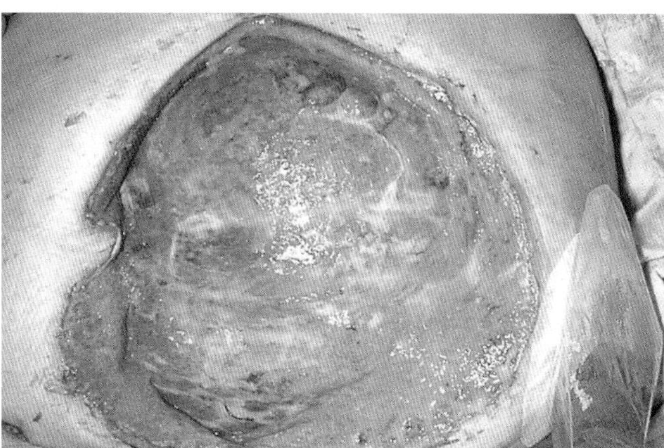

Figure 5.17 Skin layers left open to granulate after laparotomy for faecal peritonitis, ready for skin grafting.

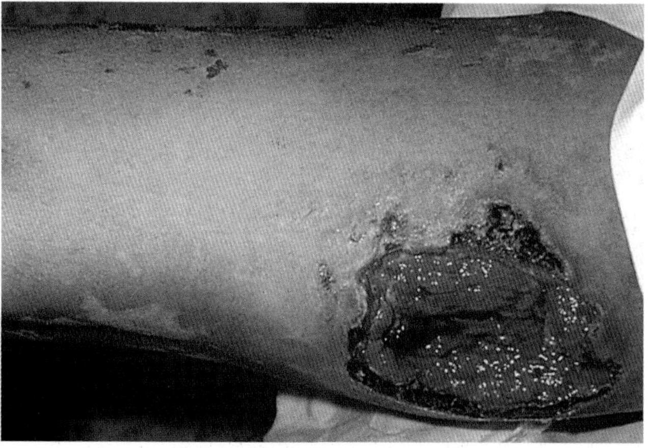

Figure 5.18 Infected animal bite/wound of the upper thigh, treated by open therapy following virulent staphylococcal infection.

should not be held back if it is indicated, the choice being empirical and later modified depending on microbiological findings on culture and sensitivity. Once antibiotics have been administered, it may not be possible to grow bacteria from the wound and so the opportunity to ascertain the most appropriate antibiotic sensitivities is lost if a patient's condition does not improve on empirical antibiotic therapy. Antibiotics alone are rarely sufficient to treat SSIs, which may also need open drainage and debridement (***Summary box 5.14***).

Summary box 5.14

Principles for the use of antibiotic therapy

- Antibiotics do not replace surgical drainage of infection
- Only spreading infections or signs of systemic infection justify the use of antibiotics
- Whenever possible, the organism and sensitivity should be determined

There are two approaches to antibiotic treatment:

A **narrow-spectrum antibiotic** may be used to treat a known sensitive infection; for example, MRSA (which may be isolated from pus) is usually sensitive to vancomycin or teicoplanin, but not flucloxacillin.

Combinations of broad-spectrum antibiotics can be used when the organism is not known or when it is suspected that several bacteria, acting in synergy, may be responsible for the infection. For example, during and following emergency surgery requiring the opening of perforated or ischaemic bowel, any of the gut organisms may be responsible for subsequent peritoneal or bacteraemic infection. In this case, a broad-spectrum antibiotic such as teicoplanin or meropenem, which are effective against a wide range of aerobic bacteria, is combined with metronidazole, which is effective against anaerobic bacteria. Alternatively, triple therapy is used with amoxicillin, gentamicin and metronidazole. The use of such broad-spectrum antibiotic strategies should be guided by specialist microbiological advice. If clinical response is poor after 3–4 days, there should be a re-evaluation with a review of available culture and sensitivity results and further investigations requested to exclude the development or persistence of infection such as a collection of pus.

In surgical units in which resistant *Pseudomonas* or other Gram-negative species (such as *Klebsiella*) have become 'resident opportunists', it may be necessary to rotate anti-pseudomonal and anti-Gram-negative antibiotic therapy (***Summary box 5.15***).

Summary box 5.15

Treatment of commensals that have become opportunist pathogens

- They are likely to have multiple antibiotic resistance
- It may be necessary to rotate antibiotics

Antibiotics used in treatment and prophylaxis of surgical infection

Antimicrobials may be produced by living organisms (antibiotics) or by synthetic methods. Some are bactericidal, e.g. penicillins and aminoglycosides, and others are bacteriostatic, e.g. tetracycline and erythromycin. In general, penicillins act upon the bacterial cell wall and are most effective against bacteria that are multiplying and synthesising new cell wall materials. The aminoglycosides act at the ribosomal level, preventing or distorting the production of proteins required to maintain the integrity of the enzymes in the bacterial cell. Hospital and formulary guidelines should be consulted for doses and monitoring of antibiotic therapy.

Penicillin

Benzylpenicillin has proved most effective against Gram-positive pathogens, including most streptococci, the clostridia and some of the staphylococci that do not produce β-lactamase. It is still effective against *Actinomyces,* which is a rare cause of chronic wound infection. It may be used specifically to treat spreading streptococcal infections. Penicillin is valuable even if other antibiotics are required as part of multiple therapy for a mixed infection. Some serious infections, e.g. gas gangrene, require high-dose intravenous benzylpenicillin.

Flucloxacillin

Flucloxacillin is resistant to β-lactamases, and is therefore of use in treating infections with penicillinase-producing staphylococci that are resistant to benzylpenicillin, but it has poor activity against other pathogens. It has good tissue penetration and therefore is useful in treating soft-tissue infections and osteomyelitis.

Ampicillin, amoxicillin and co-amoxiclav

Ampicillin and amoxicillin are β-lactam penicillins and can be taken orally or may be given parenterally. Both are effective against Enterobacteriaceae, *Enterococcus faecalis* and the majority of group D streptococci, but not species of *Klebsiella* or *Pseudomonas.* Clavulanic acid has no antibacterial activity itself, but it does inactivate β-lactamases, so can be used in conjunction with amoxicillin. The combination is known as co-amoxiclav and is useful against β-lactamase-producing bacteria that are resistant to amoxicillin on its own. These include resistant strains of *Staphylococcus aureus, Escherichia coli, Haemophilus influenzae, Bacteroides* and *Klebsiella.*

Piperacillin and ticarcillin

These are ureidopenicillins with a broad spectrum of activity against a broad range of Gram-positive, Gram-negative and anaerobic bacteria. Both are used in combination with β-lactamase inhibitors (tazobactam with piperacillin and clavulanic acid with ticarcillin). They are not active against MRSA but are used in the treatment of septicaemia, hospital-acquired pneumonia and complex urinary tract infections, where they are active against *Pseudomonas* and *Proteus* spp. and have a synergistic effect when used with aminoglycosides such as gentamicin.

Cephalosporins

There are several β-lactamase-susceptible cephalosporins that are of value in surgical practice: cefuroxime, cefotaxime and ceftazidime are widely used. The first two are most effective in intra-abdominal skin and soft-tissue infections, being active against *Staphylococcus aureus* and most Enterobacteriaceae. As a group, the enterococci (*Streptococcus faecalis*) are not sensitive to the cephalosporins. Ceftazidime, although active against the Gram-negative organisms and *Staphylococcus aureus*, is also effective against *Pseudomonas aeruginosa*. These cephalosporins may be combined with an aminoglycoside, such as gentamicin, if Gram-negative cover is needed, and an imidazole, such as metronidazole, if anaerobic cover is needed.

Aminoglycosides

Gentamicin and tobramycin have similar activity and are effective against Gram-negative Enterobacteriaceae. Gentamicin is effective against many strains of *Pseudomonas*, although resistance has been recognised. All aminoglycosides are inactive against anaerobes and streptococci. Serum levels immediately before and 1 hour after intramuscular injection must be taken and repeated at 48 hours after the start of therapy, and dosage should be modified to satisfy peak and trough levels. Ototoxicity and nephrotoxicity may follow sustained high toxic levels and therefore single, large doses may be safer.

Vancomycin and teicoplanin

These glycopeptide antibiotics are most active against Gram-positive aerobic and anaerobic bacteria and have proved to be effective against MRSA, so are often used as prophylactic antibiotics when there is a high risk of MRSA. They are ototoxic and nephrotoxic, so serum levels should be monitored. They are effective against *C. diff.* in cases of pseudomembranous colitis.

Carbapenems

Meropenem, ertapenem and imipenem are members of the carbapenems. They are stable to β-lactamase, have useful broad-spectrum anaerobic as well as Gram-positive activity and are effective for the treatment of resistant organisms, such as ESBL-resistant urinary tract infections or serious mixed-spectrum abdominal infections (peritonitis).

Metronidazole

Metronidazole is the most widely used member of the imidazole group and is active against all anaerobic bacteria. It is particularly safe and may be administered orally, rectally or intravenously. Infections caused by anaerobic cocci and strains of *Bacteroides* and *Clostridia* can be treated, or prevented, by its use. Metronidazole is useful for the prophylaxis and treatment of anaerobic infections after abdominal, colorectal and pelvic surgery and in the treatment of *C. diff.* pseudomembranous colitis.

Ciprofloxacin

Quinolones, such as ciprofloxacin, have a broad spectrum of activity against both Gram-positive and Gram-negative bacteria but are particularly useful against *Pseudomonas* infections. Many UK and European hospitals have restricted their use as a preventive measure against the development of *C. diff.* enterocolitis.

FURTHER READING

Fraise AP, Bradley C. *Ayliffe's control of healthcare associated infection: a practical handbook.* London: Hodder Arnold, 2009.

Fry DE. *Surgical infections.* London: JP Medical Ltd, 2013.

Sawyer RG, Hedrick TL. *Surgical infections, an issue of surgical clinics.* New York: Elsevier –Health Sciences Division, 2014.

Thomas WEG, Reed MWR, Wyatt MG. *Oxford textbook of fundamentals of surgery.* Oxford: Oxford University Press, 2016.

Torok E, Moran E, Cooke F. *Oxford handbook of infectious diseases and microbiology*, 2nd edn. Oxford: Oxford University Press, 2016.

CHAPTER 6 Tropical infections and infestations

Learning objectives

To be able to list:
- The common surgical infections and infestations that occur in the tropics

To appreciate:
- That many patients do not seek medical help until late in the course of the disease because of socioeconomic reasons

To be able to describe:
- The emergency presentations of the various conditions, as patients may not seek treatment until they are very ill

To be able to:
- Diagnose and treat these conditions, particularly as emergencies. The ease of global travel has connected areas where tropical infections are common to areas where they are not. Patients with such an infection who are recently returned from the tropics will mostly present as emergencies

To realise:
- That the ideal management involves a multidisciplinary approach between the surgeon, physician, radiologist, pathologist and microbiologist. In case of doubt, in a difficult situation, there should be no hesitation in seeking help from a specialist centre

INTRODUCTION

Most surgical conditions in the tropics (regions of the Earth surrounding the equator) are associated with parasitic infestations and infections related to poor hygienic conditions. With the ease of international travel, diseases that are common in the tropics may present in areas of the world where they are not commonly seen, especially as emergencies.

This chapter deals with the conditions that a surgeon might occasionally see when working in an area where such diseases are uncommon. Typically the patient would be a visitor from a tropical climate or a local resident who has visited the tropics either on holiday or to work. The life cycles of the parasites will not be described. The principles of surgical treatment are dealt with in the appropriate sections although, for operative details, referral to a relevant textbook is advised.

AMOEBIASIS

Introduction

Amoebiasis is caused by *Entamoeba histolytica*. The disease is common in the Indian subcontinent, Africa and parts of Central and South America, where almost half the population is infected. The majority remain asymptomatic carriers. The mode of infection is via the faecal–oral route and the disease occurs as a result of substandard hygiene and sanitation; therefore, the population from the poorer socioeconomic strata are more vulnerable. The prevalence of *E. histolytica* in stool samples in high-endemic zones such as South East Asia averages 10%; the incidence of amoebic liver abscesses in such populations, however, can be as high as 21 per 100 000 population.

Pathogenesis

The organism enters the gut through food or water contaminated with the cyst. In the small bowel, the cysts hatch and a large number of trophozoites are released and carried to the colon, where flask-shaped ulcers form in the submucosa. The trophozoites multiply, ultimately forming cysts, which either enter the portal circulation or are passed in the faeces as an infective form that infects other humans as a result of insanitary conditions.

Having entered the portal circulation, the trophozoites are filtered and trapped in the interlobular veins of the liver. They multiply in the portal triads, causing focal infarction of hepatocytes and liquefactive necrosis as a result of proteolytic enzymes produced by the trophozoites. The areas of necrosis eventually coalesce to form the abscess cavity. The term 'amoebic hepatitis' is used to describe the microscopic picture in the absence of macroscopic abscess, a differentiation only in theory because the medical treatment is the same.

The right lobe is involved in 80% of cases, the left in 10% and the remainder are multiple. One possible explanation for the more common involvement of the right lobe of the liver is that blood from the superior mesenteric vein runs on a straighter course through the portal vein into the larger lobe. The abscesses are most common high in the diaphragmatic surface of the right lobe. This may cause pulmonary symptoms and chest complications. The abscess cavity contains chocolate-coloured, odourless, 'anchovy sauce'-like fluid that is a mixture of necrotic liver tissue and blood. There may be secondary infection of the abscess, which causes the pus to smell. While pus in the abscess is sterile unless secondarily infected, trophozoites may be found in the abscess wall in a minority of cases. Untreated abscesses are likely to rupture.

Chronic infection of the large bowel may result in a granulomatous lesion along the large bowel, most commonly seen in the caecum, called an amoeboma.

Summary box 6.1

Amoebiasis: pathology

- *E. histolytica* is the most common pathogenic amoeba in humans
- The vast majority of carriers are asymptomatic
- Insanitary conditions and poor personal hygiene encourage transmission of the infection
- In the small intestine, the parasite hatches into trophozoites, which invade the submucosa to produce flask-shaped ulcers in the colon
- In the portal circulation, the parasite causes liquefactive necrosis in the liver, producing an abscess, the commonest extraintestinal manifestation
- The majority of abscesses occur in the right lobe of the liver
- A mass in the course of the large bowel may indicate an amoeboma

Clinical features

The typical patient with an amoebic liver abscess is a young adult male with a history of insidious onset of non-specific symptoms, such as abdominal pain, anorexia, fever, night sweats, malaise, cough and weight loss. These symptoms gradually progress to more specific symptoms of pain in the right upper abdomen and right shoulder tip, hiccoughs and a non-productive cough. A past history of bloody diarrhoea or travel to an endemic area raises the index of suspicion.

Examination reveals a patient who is toxic and anaemic. The patient will have upper abdominal rigidity, tender hepatomegaly, often with tender and bulging intercostal spaces and overlying skin oedema, a pleural effusion and basal pneumonitis – the last feature is usually a late manifestation. Occasionally, a tinge of jaundice or ascites may be present. Rarely, the patient may present as an emergency owing to the effects of rupture of an abscess into the peritoneal, pleural or pericardial cavity.

Amoeboma

This is a chronic granuloma arising in the large bowel, most commonly seen in the caecum. It is prone to occur in long-standing amoebic infection that has been treated intermittently with drugs without completion of a full course, a situation that arises from indiscriminate self-medication, particularly in resource-poor countries. Hence this is more often seen in such countries.

This can easily be mistaken for a carcinoma. An amoeboma should be suspected when a patient from an endemic area with generalised ill health and pyrexia has a mass in the right iliac fossa with a history of blood-stained mucoid diarrhoea. Such a patient is highly unlikely to have a carcinoma because altered bowel habit is not a feature of right-sided colonic carcinoma. While iron deficiency anaemia is a classical elective presentation of a caecal carcinoma, the same is present in an amoeboma because of chronic malnutrition.

Investigations

The haematological and biochemical investigations reflect the presence of a chronic infective process: anaemia, leukocytosis, raised inflammatory markers – erythrocyte sedimentation rate (ESR) and C-reactive protein (CRP) – hypoalbuminaemia and deranged liver function tests, particularly elevated alkaline phosphatase.

Serological tests are more specific, with the majority of patients showing antibodies in serum. These can be detected by tests for complement fixation, indirect haemagglutination (IHA), indirect immunofluorescence, counter-immunoelectrophoresis and enzyme-linked immunosorbent assay (ELISA). These tests are extremely useful in detecting acute infection in non-endemic areas. IHA has a very high sensitivity in acute amoebic liver abscess in non-endemic regions and remains elevated for some time. The persistence of antibodies in a large majority of the population in endemic areas precludes its use as a diagnostic investigation in those locations. A combination of serological tests detecting antibodies in combination with detection of the parasite by antigen detection or DNA polymerase chain reaction is likely to be more beneficial in such cases, though with the limitation of cost and accessibility in developing nations.

While amoebiasis may affect the entire colon, it has a predilection for the caecum and ascending colon. A colonoscopy may reveal discrete exudate-covered areas of ulceration with normal areas in between.

Imaging techniques

On ultrasonography, an abscess cavity in the liver is seen as a hypoechoic or anechoic lesion with ill-defined borders; internal echoes suggest necrotic material or debris (***Figure 6.1***). The investigation is very accurate and is used for aspiration, both diagnostic and therapeutic. When there is doubt about the diagnosis, a computed tomography (CT) scan may be helpful (***Figure 6.2***).

Diagnostic aspiration is of limited value except for establishing the typical colour of the aspirate, which is sterile and odourless unless it is secondarily infected.

A CT scan may show a raised right hemidiaphragm, a pleural effusion and evidence of pneumonitis (***Figure 6.3***).

An 'apple-core' deformity on barium enema would arouse suspicion of a carcinoma. A colonoscopy with biopsy is mandatory because the radiological and macroscopic appearance may be indistinguishable from a carcinoma. In doubtful cases, vigorous medical treatment is given and the patient undergoes colonoscopy again in 3–4 weeks, as these masses are known to

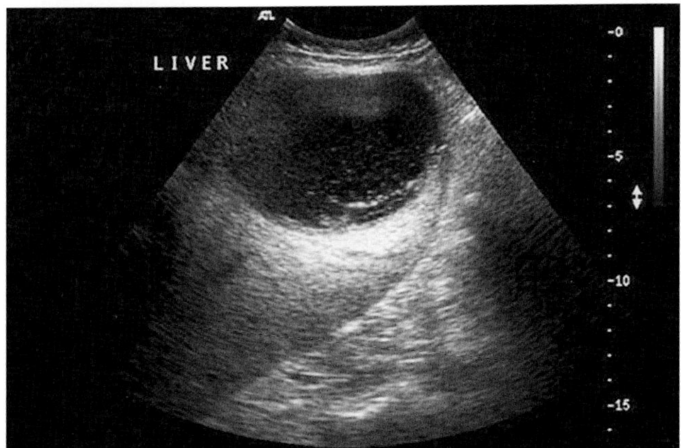

Figure 6.1 Ultrasound of the liver showing a large amoebic liver abscess with necrotic tissue in the right lobe.

regress completely on a full course of drug therapy. If symptoms persist even partially following full medical treatment in a patient who has recently returned from an endemic area, a colonic carcinoma must be excluded forthwith. This is because a dormant colonic carcinoma may become apparent as a result of infestation with amoebic dysentery causing 'traveller's diarrhoea'. However, it must be borne in mind that an amoeboma and a carcinoma can coexist.

Summary box 6.2

Diagnostic pointers for infection with *Entamoeba histolytica*

- Bloody mucoid diarrhoea in a patient from an endemic area or following a recent visit to such a country
- Upper abdominal pain, fever, cough, malaise
- In chronic cases, a mass in the right iliac fossa may be an amoeboma but caecal cancer must be excluded by colonoscopy and biopsy
- Sigmoidoscopy shows typical ulcers – biopsy and scrapes may be diagnostic
- Serological tests are highly sensitive and specific outside endemic areas
- Ultrasonography and CT scans are the imaging methods of choice

Treatment

Medical treatment is very effective and should be the first choice in the elective situation, with surgery being reserved for complications. Metronidazole and tinidazole are the effective drugs. After treatment with metronidazole and tinidazole, diloxanide furoate, a luminal amoebicide that is not effective against hepatic infestation, is used for 10 days to destroy any intestinal amoebae.

Aspiration is carried out when imminent rupture of an abscess is expected, especially when involving the left lobe. Pigtail catheter drainage may be considered in those patients who are not responding to intravenous metronidazole in the first 48–72 hours to improve antibiotic penetration. If there is evidence of secondary infection, appropriate drug treatment is added. The threshold for draining a left liver lobe abscess should be low, given its propensity for rupture into either the peritoneal, pleural or pericardial cavity.

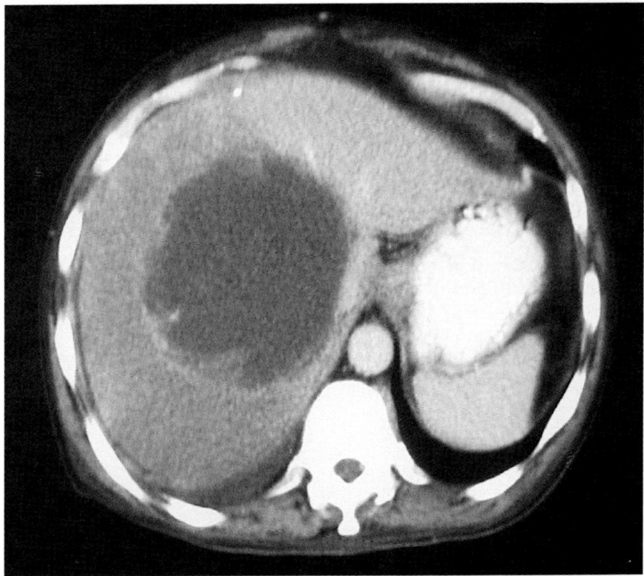

Figure 6.2 Computed tomographic scan showing an amoebic liver abscess in the right lobe.

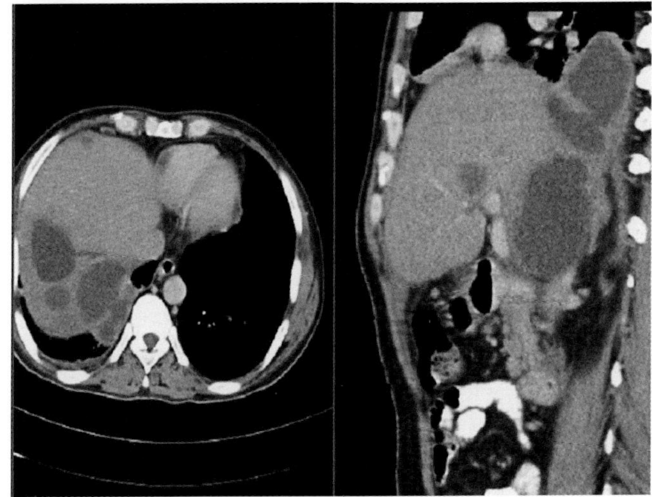

Figure 6.3 Computed tomographic scans showing multiple amoebic liver abscesses with extension into the chest.

Surgical treatment should be reserved for the complications of rupture into the pleural (usually the right side), peritoneal or pericardial cavities. Resuscitation, drainage and appropriate lavage with vigorous medical treatment are the key principles. In the large bowel, severe haemorrhage and toxic megacolon are rare complications. In these patients, the general principles of a surgical emergency apply, the principles of management being the same as for any toxic megacolon. Resuscitation is followed by resection of bowel with exteriorisation. Then the patient is given vigorous supportive therapy. All such cases are managed in the intensive care unit, as would any patient with toxic megacolon whatever the cause.

An amoeboma that has not regressed after full medical treatment should be managed with colonic resection, particularly if cancer cannot be excluded.

Summary box 6.3

Amoebiasis: treatment

- Medical treatment is very effective
- For large abscesses, repeated aspiration or pigtail catheter drainage is combined with drug treatment
- Surgical treatment is reserved for complications, such as rupture into the pleural, peritoneal or pericardial cavities
- Acute toxic megacolon and severe haemorrhage are intestinal complications that are treated with intensive supportive therapy followed by resection and exteriorisation: subtotal colectomy with terminal ileostomy and closure of the rectal stump
- When an amoeboma is suspected in a colonic mass, cancer should be excluded by appropriate imaging and biopsy

ROUNDWORM (*ASCARIS LUMBRICOIDES*)

Introduction

Ascaris lumbricoides, commonly called the roundworm, is the commonest intestinal nematode to infect humans and affects a quarter of the world's population. The parasite causes pulmonary symptoms as a larva and intestinal symptoms as an adult worm.

Pathology and life cycle

The fertilised eggs can survive in a hostile environment for a long time. The hot and humid conditions in the tropics are ideally suited for the eggs to turn into embryos. The fertilised eggs are present in soil contaminated with infected faeces, becoming infective in about 3 weeks. Faecal–oral contamination causes human infection.

The eggs are ingested and the larvae are released in the jejunum, from where they travel to the liver via the portal system and the lymphatics. The larvae reach the lungs via the systemic circulation, where they undergo maturation for 2 weeks.

The developed larvae reach the alveoli, are coughed up, swallowed and continue their maturation in the small intestine. Sometimes, the young worms migrate from the tracheobronchial tree into the oesophagus, thus finding their way into the gastrointestinal tract, from where they can migrate to the common bile duct or pancreatic duct. The mature female, once in the small bowel, produces innumerable eggs that are fertilised and thereafter excreted in the stool to perpetuate the life cycle. Eggs in the biliary tract can form a nidus for a stone.

Clinical features

The larval stage in the lungs causes pulmonary symptoms – dry cough, chest pain, dyspnoea and fever – referred to as Loeffler's syndrome. The adult worm can grow up to 45 cm long. Its presence in the small intestine causes malnutrition, failure to thrive, particularly in children, and abdominal pain. Worms that migrate into the common bile duct can produce ascending cholangitis and obstructive jaundice, while features of acute pancreatitis may be caused by a worm in the pancreatic duct.

Small intestinal obstruction can occur, particularly in children, owing to a bolus of adult worms incarcerated in the terminal ileum. This is a surgical emergency. Rarely, perforation of the small bowel may occur from ischaemic pressure necrosis from the bolus of worms.

A high index of suspicion is necessary so as not to miss the diagnosis. If a person from a tropical country, or one who has recently returned after spending some time in an endemic area, presents with pulmonary, gastrointestinal, hepatobiliary and pancreatic symptoms, ascariasis should be high on the list of possible diagnoses.

Investigations

As with most parasitic infestations, an increase in the eosinophil count is common. Stool examination may show ova. Sputum or bronchoscopic washings may show Charcot–Leyden crystals or the larvae.

Chest radiograph may show fluffy exudates in Loeffler's syndrome. A barium meal and follow-through may show a bolus of worms in the ileum or lying freely within the small bowel (***Figure** 6.4*). Ultrasonography may show a worm in the gallbladder, the common bile duct (***Figure** 6.5*) or pancreatic duct. On magnetic resonance cholangiopancreatography (MRCP), an adult worm may be seen in the common bile duct in a patient presenting with features of obstructive jaundice (***Figure** 6.6*). In patients with intestinal obstruction, plain abdominal radiograph may show tubular structures within dilated small bowel, denoting the presence of worms, which would also show up on a contrast CT scan as curvilinear structures.

Summary box 6.4

Ascariasis: pathogenesis

- It is the commonest intestinal nematode affecting humans
- Typically found in a humid atmosphere and poor sanitary conditions, hence is seen in the tropics and resource-poor countries
- Larvae cause pulmonary symptoms; adult worms cause gastrointestinal, biliary and pancreatic symptoms
- Distal ileal obstruction is due to a bolus of worms; ascending cholangitis and obstructive jaundice are due to infestation of the common bile duct
- Acute pancreatitis occurs when a worm is lodged in the pancreatic duct
- Perforation of the small bowel is rare

Wilhelm Loeffler, 1887–1972, Professor of Medicine, Zurich, Switzerland.
Jean Martin Charcot, 1825–1893, French neurologist and Professor of Pathology at Hôpital Universitaire la Pitié-Salpêtrière, Paris, France.
Ernst von Leyden, 1832–1910, Professor of Medicine, Berlin, Germany.

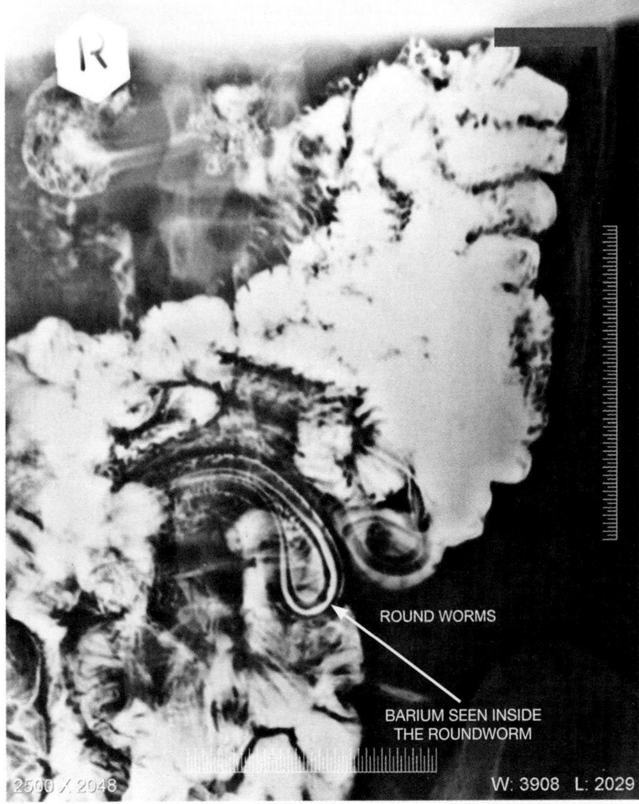

Figure 6.4 Barium meal and follow-through showing roundworms in the course of the small bowel with barium seen inside the worms in an 18-year-old patient who presented with bouts of colicky abdominal pain and bilious vomiting, which settled with conservative management (courtesy of Dr PP Bhattacharyya, Kolkata, India).

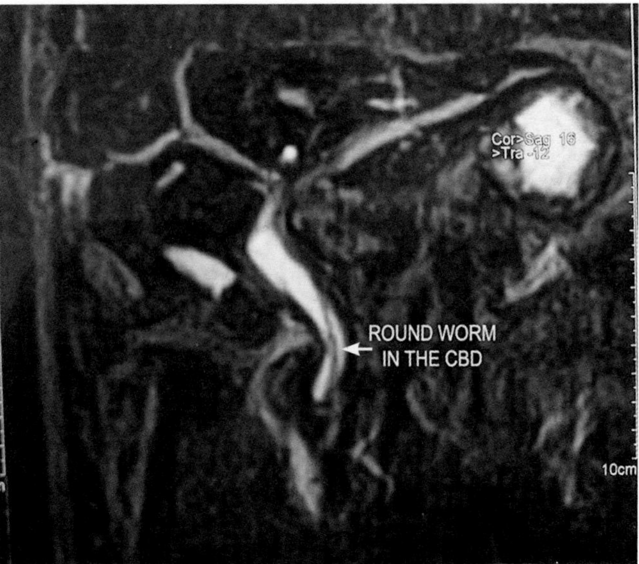

Figure 6.6 Magnetic resonance cholangiopancreatography showing a roundworm in the common bile duct (CBD). The worm could not be removed endoscopically. The patient underwent an open cholecystectomy and exploration of the CBD (this can also be addressed laparoscopically in some centres).

Treatment

The pulmonary phase of the disease is usually self-limiting and requires symptomatic treatment only. For intestinal disease, patients should ideally be under the care of a physician for treatment with anthelminthic drugs. Certain drugs may cause rapid death of the adult worms and, if there are many worms in the terminal ileum, the treatment may actually precipitate acute intestinal obstruction from a bolus of dead worms. Children who present with features of intermittent or subacute obstruction should be given a trial of conservative management in the form of intravenous fluids, nasogastric suction and hypertonic saline enemas. The last of these helps to disentangle the bolus of worms and also increases intestinal motility.

Surgery is reserved for complications, such as intestinal obstruction that has not resolved on a conservative regime, or when perforation is suspected. At laparotomy, the bolus of worms in the terminal ileum is milked through the ileocaecal valve into the colon for natural passage in the

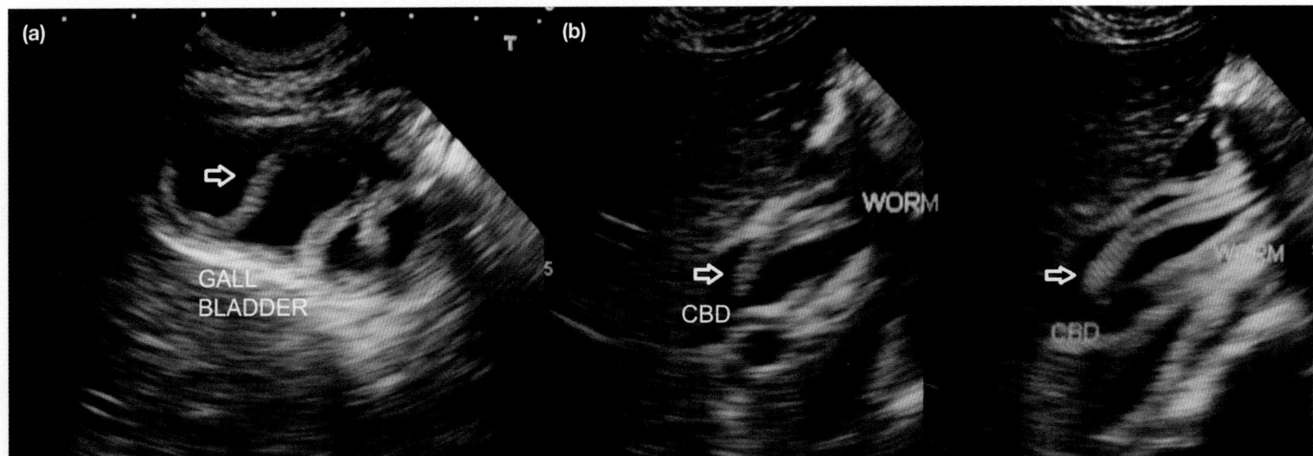

Figure 6.5 Ultrasound scan showing a live worm (arrow) in the gallbladder (a) and the common bile duct (CBD) (b) (courtesy of Dr A Bhattacharyya, Kolkata, India).

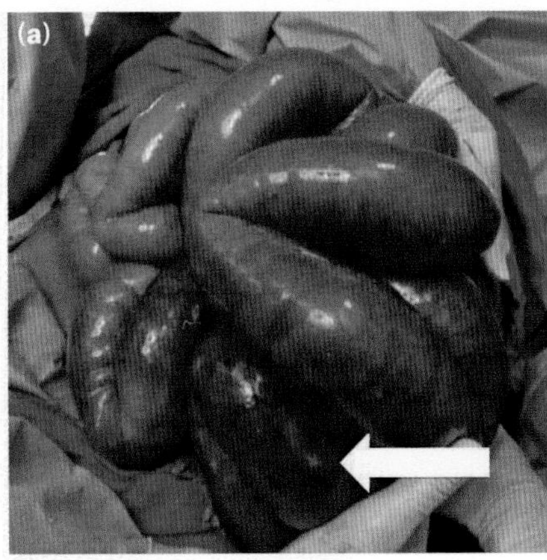
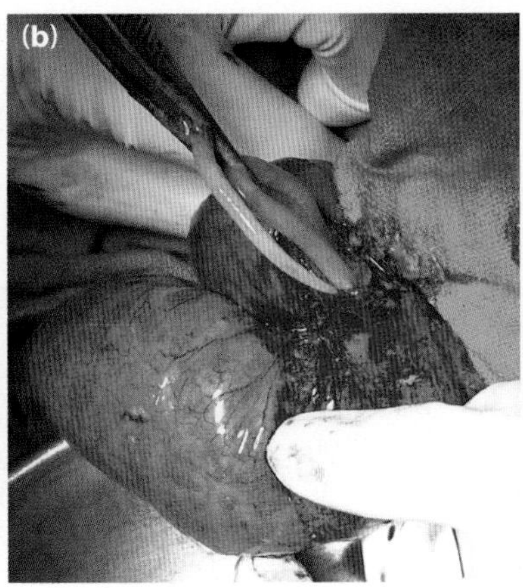
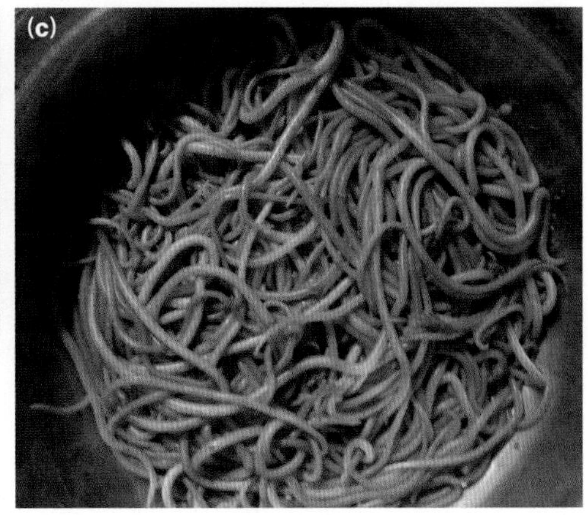

Figure 6.7 (a) Roundworms seen through the bowel wall (arrowed). (b) Roundworm being removed through enterotomy. (c) Removed roundworms.

stool. Postoperatively, hypertonic saline enemas may help in the extrusion of the worms. Strictures, gangrenous areas or perforations need resection and anastomosis. If the bowel wall is healthy, enterotomy and removal of the worms may be performed (***Figure 6.7***).

Rarely, when perforation occurs as a result of roundworm, the parasites may be found lying free in the peritoneal cavity. It is safer to bring out the site of perforation as an ileostomy because, in the presence of a large number of worms, the closure of an anastomosis may be at risk of breakdown from the activity of the residual worms in the bowel.

When a patient is operated upon as an emergency for a suspected complication of roundworm infestation, the actual diagnosis at operation may turn out to be acute appendicitis, typhoid perforation or a tuberculous stricture and the presence of roundworms is an incidental finding. Such a patient requires the appropriate surgery depending upon the primary pathology.

Common bile duct or pancreatic duct obstruction from a roundworm can be treated by endoscopic removal at endoscopic retrograde cholangiopancreatography (ERCP), failing which laparoscopic or open exploration of the common bile duct is necessary. Cholecystectomy is also carried out. A full course of antiparasitic treatment must follow any surgical intervention.

Summary box 6.5

Ascariasis: diagnosis and management

- Barium meal and follow-through will show worms scattered in the small bowel
- Ultrasonography may show worms in the common bile duct and pancreatic duct
- Plain abdominal radiograph and contrast CT scan will show the worms as tubular or curvilinear structures
- Conservative management with anthelminthics is the first line of treatment even in obstruction
- Surgery is a last resort for acute abdomen – various options are available

ASIATIC CHOLANGIOHEPATITIS

Introduction

This disease, also called oriental cholangiohepatitis, is caused by infestation of the hepatobiliary system by a trematode, *Clonorchis sinensis*. It has a high incidence in the tropical regions of South East Asia, particularly among those living in the major sea ports and near river estuaries. The organism, which is a type of liver fluke, develops in snails that act as an intermediate host. Free swimming from snails, the cercariae penetrate the flesh of freshwater fish, crabs and crayfish, which also act as an intermediate host. Ingestion of infected fish, crabs and crayfish, when eaten raw or improperly cooked, causes the infection in humans and other fish-eating mammals, which are the definitive hosts. Two other parasites, *Opisthorchis*, which has the same life cycle as *Clonorchis*, and *Fasciola*, the metacercariae of which colonise vegetation, can cause similar damage to the biliary channels.

Pathology

In humans, the parasite matures into the adult worm in the intrahepatic biliary radicles, where it may reside for many years. The intrahepatic bile ducts are dilated, with epithelial hyperplasia and periductal fibrosis. These changes may lead to dysplasia, causing cholangiocarcinoma – the most serious and dreaded complication of this parasitic infestation.

The eggs or dead worms may form a nidus for stone formation in the gallbladder or common bile duct, which becomes thickened and much dilated in the late stages. Intrahepatic bile duct stones are also caused by the parasite producing mucin-rich bile. The dilated intrahepatic bile ducts may lead to cholangitis, liver abscess and hepatitis.

Diagnosis

The disease may remain dormant for many years. Clinical features are non-specific and include fever, malaise, anorexia and upper abdominal discomfort. The complete clinical picture can consist of fever with rigors due to ascending cholangitis, obstructive jaundice, biliary colic and pruritus from stones in the common bile duct. Acute pancreatitis may occur because of obstruction of the pancreatic duct by an adult worm. Particularly when presenting in non-endemic areas, it should be noted that if a person from an endemic area complains of symptoms of biliary tract disease, *Clonorchis* infestation should be high in the differential diagnosis.

In advanced cases, liver function tests are abnormal. Confirmation of the condition is by examination of stool or duodenal aspirate, which may show the eggs or adult worms. Ultrasonography findings may be characteristic, showing uniform dilatation of small peripheral intrahepatic bile ducts with only minimal dilatation of the common hepatic and common bile ducts, although the latter are much more dilated when the obstruction is caused by stones. The thickened duct walls show increased echogenicity and non-shadowing echogenic foci in the bile ducts, representing the worms or eggs. ERCP will confirm these findings.

Summary box 6.6

Asiatic cholangiohepatitis: pathogenesis and diagnosis

- Occurs in Far Eastern tropical zones
- The causative parasite is *Clonorchis sinensis*, *Opisthorchis* or *Fasciola*
- Produces bile duct hyperplasia, intrahepatic duct dilatation and stones
- Increases the risk of cholangiocarcinoma
- May remain dormant for many years
- When active, there are biliary tract symptoms in a generally unwell patient
- Stool examination for eggs or worms is diagnostic
- Ultrasonography of the hepatobiliary system and ERCP is also diagnostic

Treatment

Praziquantel and albendazole are the drugs of choice. However, the surgeon faces a challenge when there are stones not only in the gallbladder but also in the common bile duct. Cholecystectomy with exploration of the common bile duct is performed when indicated; currently, both procedures are performed laparoscopically as a single-stage procedure. Repeated washouts are necessary during the exploration of the common bile duct as there are stones, biliary debris, sludge and mud in the dilated duct. This should be followed by choledochoduodenostomy. As this is a disease with a prolonged and relapsing course, some surgeons prefer to do a choledochojejunostomy to a Roux loop. The Roux loop is brought up to the abdominal wall, referred to as 'an access loop', which allows the interventional radiologist to deal with any future stones.

As a public health measure, people who have emigrated from an endemic area should be offered screening for *Clonorchis* infestation in the form of ultrasonography of the hepatobiliary system. This condition can be diagnosed and treated, and even cured, when it is in its subclinical form. Most importantly, the risk of developing the dreadful disease of cholangiocarcinoma is eliminated.

Summary box 6.7

Asiatic cholangiohepatitis: treatment

- Medical treatment can be curative in the early stages
- Surgical treatment is cholecystectomy, exploration of the common bile duct and some form of biliary–enteric bypass
- Prevention: consider offering hepatobiliary ultrasonography as a screening procedure to recently arrived migrants from endemic areas

FILARIASIS

Introduction

Filariasis is mainly caused by the parasite *Wuchereria bancrofti*, which is transmitted by the mosquito. Variants of the parasite called *Brugia malayi* and *Brugia timori* are responsible for causing the disease in about 10% of those infected. The condition affects more than 120 million people worldwide, two-thirds of whom live in India, China and Indonesia. According to the World Health Organization (WHO), after leprosy, filariasis is the most common cause of long-term disability.

Once the host has been bitten by the mosquito, the matured eggs enter the human circulation to hatch and grow into adult worms; the process of maturation takes almost a year. The adult worms mainly colonise the lymphatic system.

Diagnosis

It is mainly males who are affected because females generally cover a greater part of their bodies with clothing, thus making them less prone to mosquito bites. In the acute presentation, there are episodic attacks of fever with lymphadenitis and lymphangitis.

Occasionally, adult worms may be felt subcutaneously. Chronic manifestations appear after repeated acute attacks over several years. The adult worms cause lymphatic obstruction, resulting in massive lower limb oedema. Obstruction to the cutaneous lymphatics causes skin thickening, not unlike the *peau d'orange* appearance in breast cancer, thus exacerbating the limb swelling. Secondary streptococcal infection is common. Recurrent attacks of lymphangitis cause fibrosis of the lymph channels, resulting in a grossly swollen limb with thickened skin, producing the condition of elephantiasis (***Figure 6.8***). Bilateral lower limb filariasis is often associated with scrotal and penile elephantiasis. Early on, there may be a hydrocele underlying scrotal filariasis (***Figure 6.9***).

César Roux, 1857–1934, Professor of Surgery and Gynaecology, Lausanne, Switzerland, described this method of forming a jejunal conduit in 1908.
Otto Eduard Heinrich Wucherer, 1820–1873, German physician who practised in Brazil.
Joseph Bancroft, 1836–1894, English physician who worked in Australia.
Peau d'orange is French for 'orange peel skin'.

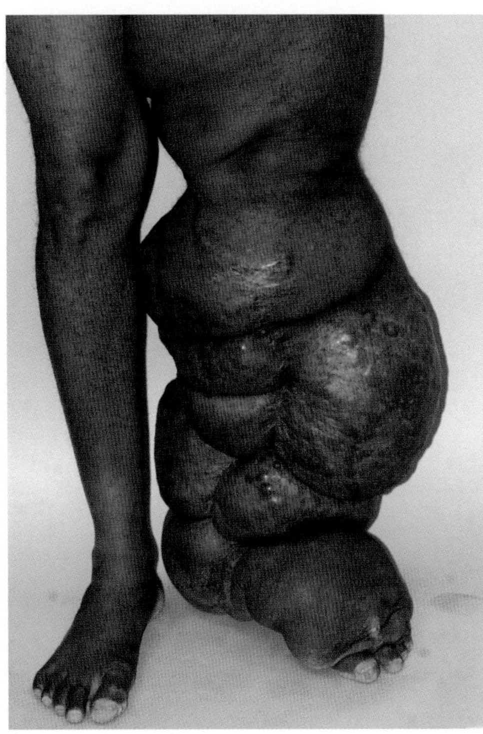

Figure 6.8 Left lower limb filariasis – elephantiasis (courtesy of Professor Ahmed Hassan Fahal, FRCS MD MS, Khartoum, Sudan).

Chyluria and chylous ascites may occur. A mild form of the disease can affect the respiratory tract, causing dry cough, and is referred to as tropical pulmonary eosinophilia. The condition of filariasis is clinically very obvious, and thus investigations in the full-blown case are superfluous. Eosinophilia is common and a nocturnal peripheral blood smear may show the immature forms, or microfilariae. The parasite may also be seen in chylous urine, ascites and hydrocele fluid.

Treatment

Medical treatment with diethylcarbamazine is very effective in the early stages before the gross deformities of elephantiasis have developed. In the early stages of limb swelling, intermittent pneumatic compression helps, but the treatment has to be repeated over a prolonged period.

Summary box 6.8

Filariasis

- Caused by *Wuchereria bancrofti*, which is carried by the mosquito
- Lymphatics are mainly affected, resulting in gross limb swelling
- Eosinophilia occurs; immature worms may be seen in a nocturnal peripheral blood smear
- Gross forms of the disease cause a great deal of disability and misery
- Early cases are very amenable to medical treatment
- Intermittent pneumatic compression gives some relief
- The value of various surgical procedures is largely unproven and hence they are rarely performed

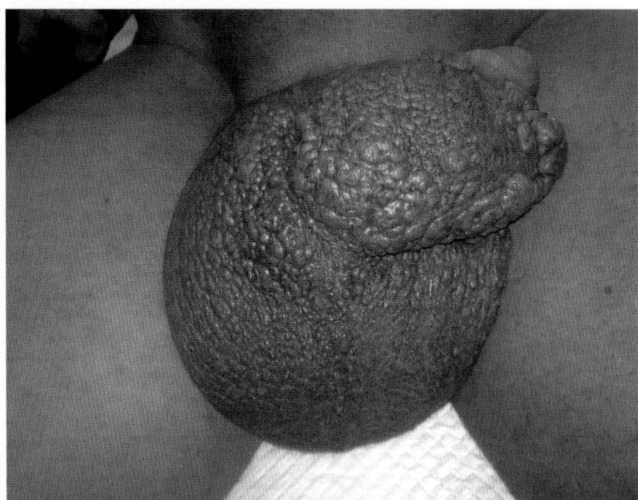

Figure 6.9 Filariasis of the scrotum and penis (courtesy of Professor Ahmed Hassan Fahal, FRCS MD MS, Khartoum, Sudan).

A hydrocele is treated by the usual operation of excision and eversion of the sac with, if necessary, excision of redundant scrotal skin. Operations for reducing the size of the limb are hardly ever done these days because the procedures are so rarely successful.

HYDATID DISEASE

Introduction and pathology

Hydatid disease is caused by *Echinococcus granulosus*, commonly called the dog tapeworm. The disease is globally distributed and, while it is common in the tropics, it is much less common in other countries; for example, in the UK the occasional patient may come from a rural sheep-farming community.

The dog is the definitive host and is the commonest source of infection transmitted to the intermediate hosts – humans, sheep and cattle. In the dog, the adult worm reaches the small intestine and the eggs are passed in the faeces. These eggs are highly resistant to extremes of temperature and may survive for long periods. In the dog's intestine, the cyst wall is digested, allowing the protoscolices to develop into adult worms. Close contact with an infected dog causes contamination by the oral route, with the ovum thus gaining entry into the human gastrointestinal tract.

The cyst is characterised by three layers: an outer **pericyst**, which is derived from compressed host organ tissues; an intermediate hyaline **ectocyst**, which is non-infective; and an inner **endocyst**, which is the germinal membrane and contains viable parasites that can separate, forming daughter cysts. A variant of the disease occurs in colder climates caused by *Echinococcus multilocularis*, in which the cyst spreads from the outset by actual invasion rather than expansion.

Classification

In 2003, the WHO Informal Working Group on Echinococcosis (WHO-IWGE) proposed a standardised ultrasound classification based on the status of activity of the cyst (*Table 6.1*). This is universally accepted, particularly because it helps to decide on the appropriate management. Three groups have been recognised:

- Group 1: Active group – cysts larger than 2 cm and often fertile.
- Group 2: Transition group – cysts starting to degenerate and entering a transitional stage because of host resistance or treatment but may contain viable protoscolices.
- Group 3: Inactive group – degenerated, partially or totally calcified cysts; unlikely to contain viable protoscolices.

Clinical features

As the parasite can colonise virtually every organ in the body, the condition can be protean in its presentation. When a sheep farmer who is otherwise healthy complains of a gradually enlarging painful mass in the right upper quadrant with the physical findings of a liver swelling, a hydatid liver cyst should be considered. The liver is the organ most often affected. The lung is the next most common. The parasite can affect any organ (*Figures 6.10 and 6.11*) or several organs in the same patient (*Figure 6.12*).

The disease may be asymptomatic and discovered coincidentally at postmortem or when an ultrasonography or CT scan is done for some other condition. Symptomatic disease presents with a swelling causing pressure effects. Thus, a hepatic lesion causes dull pain from stretching of the liver capsule, and a pulmonary lesion, if large enough, causes dyspnoea. Daughter cysts may communicate with the biliary tree, causing obstructive jaundice and all the usual clinical features associated with it in addition to symptoms attributable to a parasitic infestation (*Figure 6.13*). Features of raised intracranial pressure or unexplained headaches in a patient from a sheep-rearing community should raise the suspicion of a cerebral hydatid cyst.

The patient may present as an emergency with severe abdominal pain following minor trauma, when the CT scan may be diagnostic (*Figure 6.14*). Rarely, a patient may present as an emergency with features of anaphylactic shock without any obvious cause. Such a patient may subsequently cough up white material that contains scolices that have travelled into the tracheobronchial tree from rupture of a hepatic hydatid on the diaphragmatic surface of the liver.

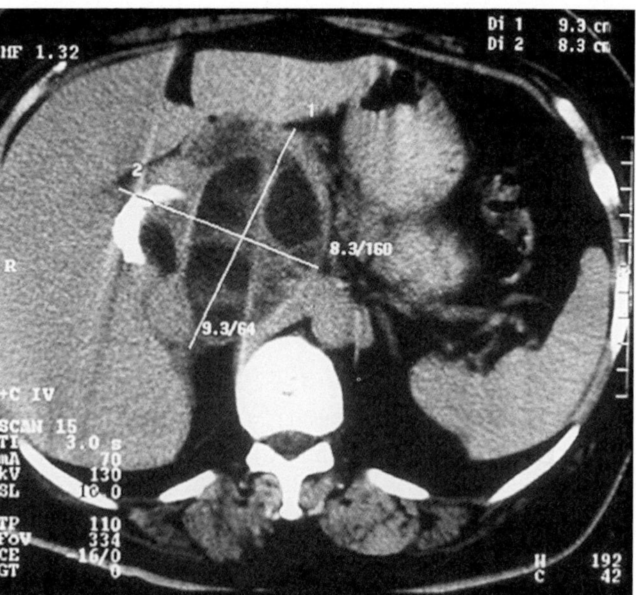

Figure 6.10 Computed tomographic scan showing a hydatid cyst of the pancreas. A differential diagnosis of hydatid cyst or a tumour was considered. At exploration, the patient was found to have a hydatid cyst, which was excised. This was followed by 30 months of treatment with albendazole. The patient remains free of disease.

Diagnosis

There should be a high index of suspicion. Investigations show a raised eosinophil count; serological tests, such as ELISA and immunoelectrophoresis, point towards the diagnosis. Ultrasonography and CT scan are the investigations of choice. The CT scan shows a smooth space-occupying lesion with several septa. Ultrasonography of the biliary tract may show abnormality in the gallbladder and bile ducts, when hydatid infestation of the biliary system should be suspected. An MRCP may even show multiple cysts communicating with the biliary tree (*Figure 6.13*). Ultimately, the diagnosis is made by a combination of good history and clinical examination supplemented by serology and imaging.

TABLE 6.1 Classification of hepatic hydatid cyst

Stage	Description
CL (cystic lesion)	Unilocular anechoic cystic lesion without internal echoes or septations
CE (cystic echinococcosis) 1	Uniformly anechoic cyst with fine internal echoes that represent protoscolices after rupture of a vesicle, called 'hydatid sand'
CE 2	Cyst with internal septation representing the walls of the daughter cyst described as multivesicular, honeycomb, cartwheel or rosette formation
CE 3 (transitional stage) description of daughter cyst	3A: daughter cysts with detached laminated membrane
	3B- daughter cysts inside a solid matrix
CE 4 (inactive/degenerative)	Daughter cysts can no longer be seen Mixture of hypoechoic and hyperechoic features – like a bag of wool
CE 5 (inactive/degenerative)	Calcification of the wall; either partial or complete

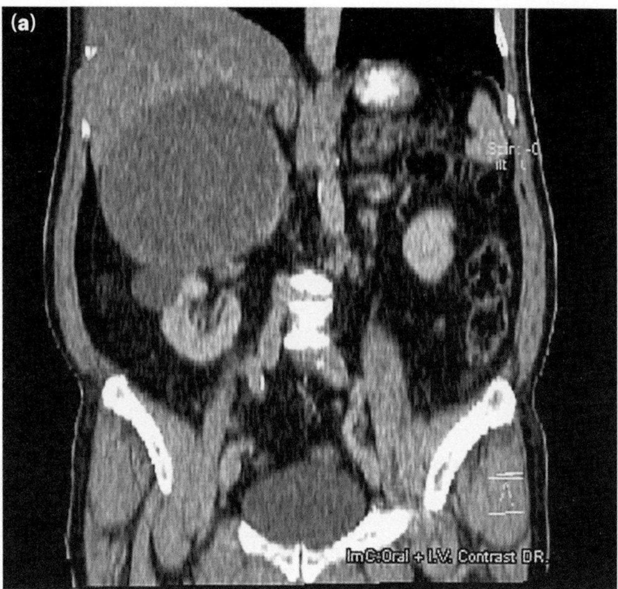

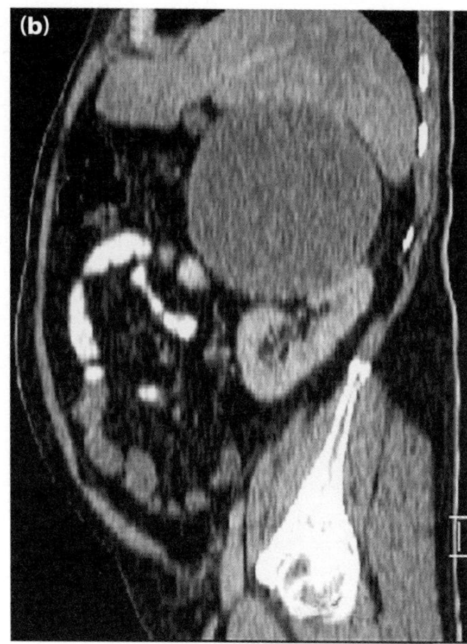

Figure 6.11 Anteroposterior (a) and lateral (b) views of computed tomographic scans showing a large hydatid cyst of the right adrenal gland. The patient presented with a mass in the right loin and underwent an adrenalectomy (courtesy of Dr PP Bhattacharyya, Kolkata, India).

Summary box 6.9

Hydatid disease: diagnosis

- In the UK, the usual sufferer is a sheep farmer
- While any organ may be involved, the liver is by far the most commonly affected
- Elective clinical presentation is usually in the form of a painful lump arising from the liver
- Anaphylactic shock due to rupture of the hydatid cyst is the emergency presentation
- CT scan is the best imaging technique – the diagnostic feature is a space-occupying lesion with a smooth outline with septa

Treatment

Here, the treatment of hepatic hydatid is outlined because the liver is most commonly affected, but the same general principles apply whichever organ is involved.

These patients should be treated in a tertiary unit where good teamwork between an expert hepatobiliary surgeon, an experienced physician and an interventional radiologist is available. Surgical treatment by minimal access therapy is best summarised by the mnemonic PAIR (puncture, aspiration, injection and reaspiration). This is done after adequate drug treatment with albendazole, although praziquantel has

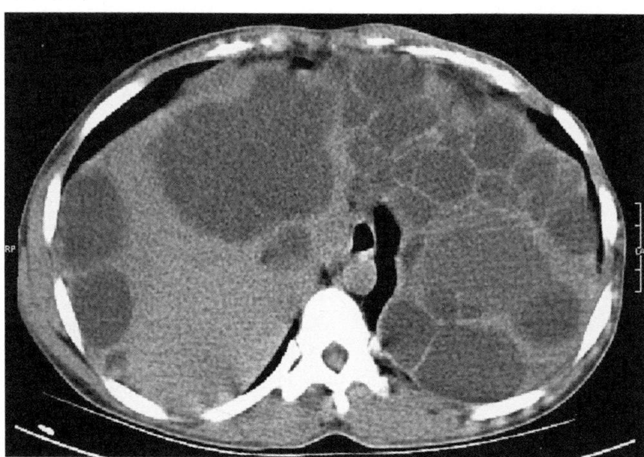

Figure 6.12 Computed tomographic scan showing disseminated hydatid cysts of the abdomen. The patient was started on albendazole but was lost to follow-up (courtesy of Dr PP Bhattacharyya, Kolkata, India).

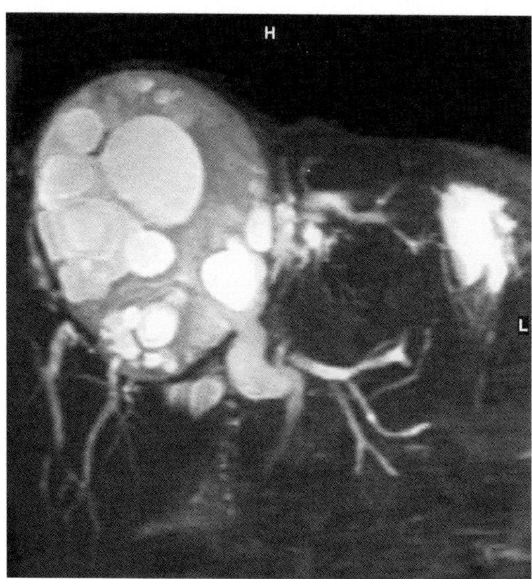

Figure 6.13 Magnetic resonance cholangiopancreatography showing a large hepatic hydatid cyst with daughter cysts communicating with the common bile duct, causing obstruction and dilatation of the entire biliary tree (courtesy of Dr B Agarwal, New Delhi, India).

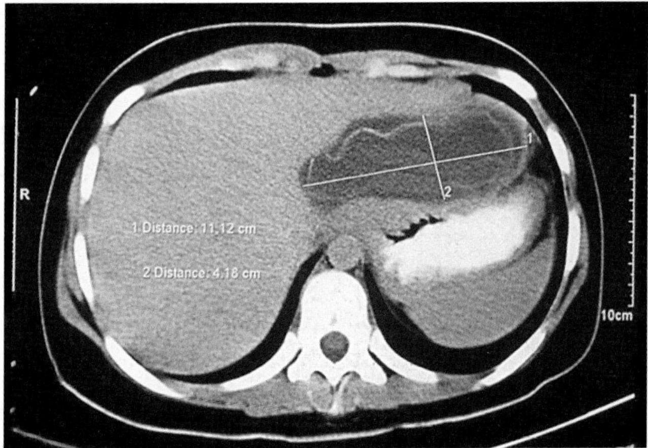

Figure 6.14 Computed tomographic (CT) scan of the upper abdomen showing a hypodense lesion of the left lobe of the liver; the periphery of the lesion shows a double edge. This is the lamellar membrane of the hydatid cyst that separated after trivial injury. The patient was a 14-year-old girl who developed a rash and pain in the upper abdomen after dancing. The rash settled down after a course of antihistamines. The CT scan was performed 2 weeks later for persisting upper abdominal pain.

also been used, both of these drugs being available only on a 'named patient' basis.

Whether the patient is treated only medically or in combination with surgery will depend upon the clinical group (which gives an idea as to the activity of the disease), the number of cysts and their anatomical position. Radical total or partial pericystectomy with omentoplasty or hepatic segmentectomy (especially if the lesion is in a peripheral part of the liver) are some of the surgical options. During the operation, scolicidal agents are used, such as hypertonic saline (15–20%), ethanol (75–95%) or 5% povidone–iodine (although some use a 10% solution). This may cause sclerosing cholangitis if biliary radicles are in communication with the cyst wall. A laparoscopic approach to these procedures is being tried (see next section, ***Laparoscopic management***).

Obviously, cysts in other organs need to be treated in accordance with the actual anatomical site, along with the general principles described. An asymptomatic cyst that is inactive (group 3) may be left alone.

Summary box 6.10

Hydatid cyst of the liver: treatment

- Ideally managed in a tertiary unit by a multidisciplinary team of hepatobiliary surgeon, physician and interventional radiologist
- Leave asymptomatic and inactive cysts alone – monitor size by ultrasonography
- Active cysts should first be treated by a full course of albendazole
- Several procedures are available – PAIR, pericystectomy with omentoplasty and hepatic segmentectomy; appropriate management is customised according to the particular patient and organ involved
- Increasingly, a laparoscopic approach is being tried

Laparoscopic management

Currently, surgeons trained in minimal access surgery perform hydatid surgery using minimal access. Laparoscopic marsupialisation of the cyst (deroofing), consisting of removal of the cyst containing the endocyst along with daughter cysts, is the most common procedure. In the initial steps, the cyst is aspirated, taking care not to spill any contents, using povidone–iodine or hypertonic saline as a scolicidal agent. Any communication with the biliary tree is oversewn and pedicled omentum is sutured to the margins of the cyst.

If the cyst is small and superficial, a cystopericystectomy is performed at centres experienced enough to do more advanced surgery, removing the entire cyst intact.

Pulmonary hydatid disease

The lung is the second commonest organ affected after the liver. The size of the cyst can vary from very small to a considerable size. The right lung and lower lobes are slightly more often involved. The cyst is usually single, although multiple cysts do occur and concomitant hydatid cysts in other organs, such as the liver, are not unknown. The condition may be silent and found incidentally. Symptomatic patients present with cough, expectoration, fever, chest pain and sometimes haemoptysis. Silent cysts may present as an emergency because of rupture or an allergic reaction.

Uncomplicated cysts present as rounded or oval lesions on chest radiography. Erosion of the bronchioles results in air being introduced between the pericyst and the laminated membrane and gives a fine radiolucent crescent, the 'meniscus' or 'crescent' sign (***Figure 6.15***). This is often regarded as a sign of impending rupture. When the cyst ruptures, the crumpled collapsed endocyst floats like a lily on the residual fluid, giving rise to the 'water-lily' sign on CT scan (***Figure 6.16***). Rupture into the pleural cavity results in pleural effusion. CT scan defines the pathology in greater detail.

The mainstay of treatment of pulmonary hydatid is surgery. Medical treatment is less successful and considered when surgery is not possible because of poor general condition or diffuse disease affecting both lungs, or recurrent or ruptured cysts. The principle of surgery is to preserve as much viable lung tissue as possible. The exact procedure can vary: cystotomy, capitonnage, pericystectomy, segmentectomy or occasionally pneumonectomy.

Summary box 6.11

Pulmonary hydatid disease

- The second most common organ involved
- Size of the cyst has a wide variation
- May present as an incidental finding
- Clinical presentation may be elective or as an emergency because of rupture
- Plain radiograph shows 'meniscus' or 'crescent' sign; CT shows 'water-lily' sign
- Ideal treatment is surgical – various choices are available

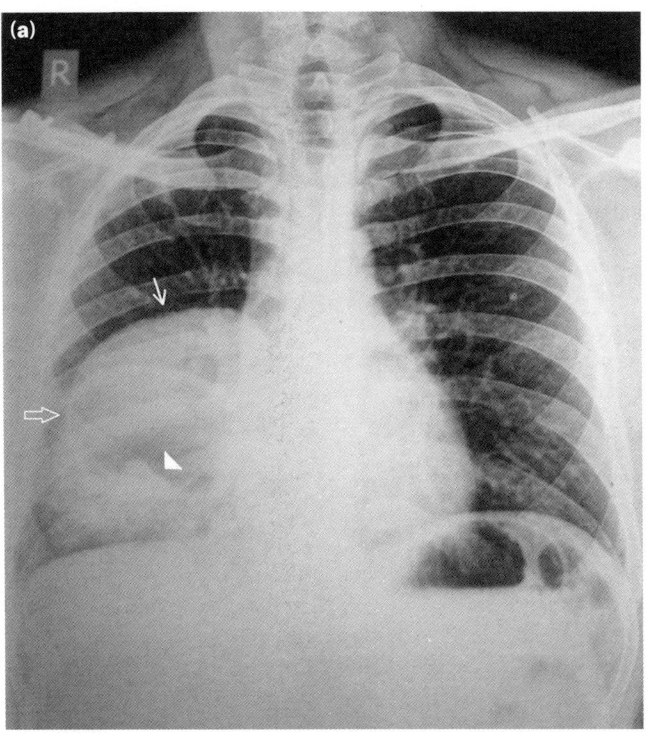

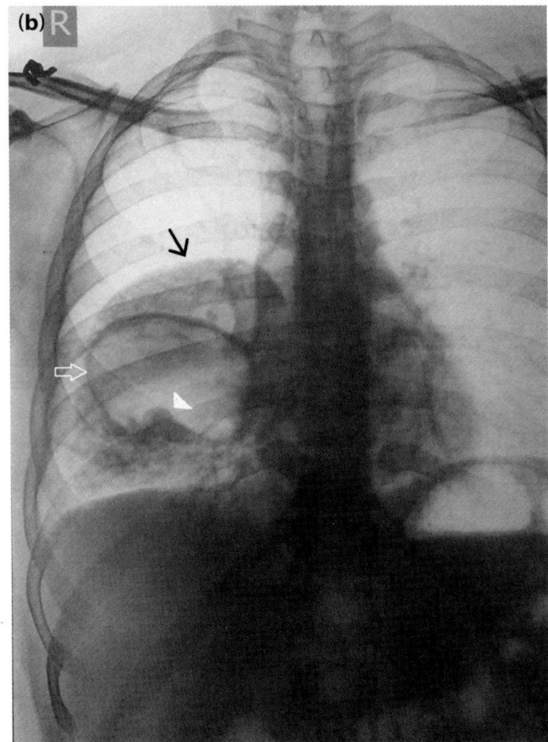

Figure 6.15 Hydatid cysts of the lung, one intact (solid arrow), one ruptured (hollow arrow) showing the lamellar membrane floating like a water lily (solid arrowhead) (courtesy of Professor Saibal Gupta, MS, FRCS, Professor of Cardiovascular Surgery, Kolkata, India and Dr Rupak Bhattacharya, Kolkata, India).

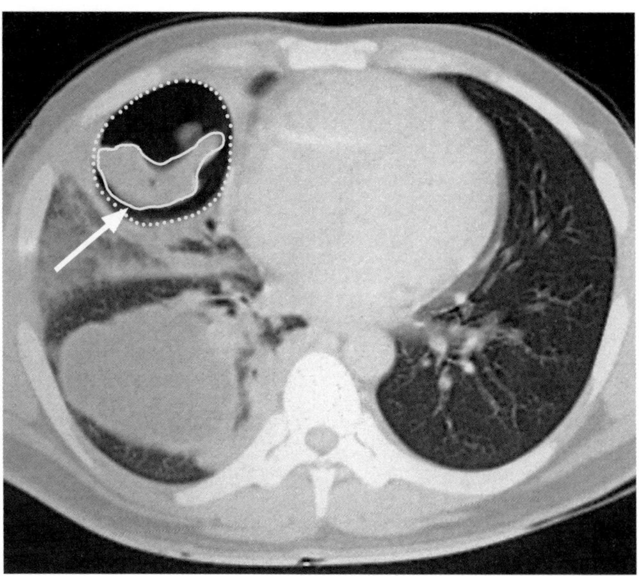

Figure 6.16 Computed tomographic scan showing the 'water-lily' sign (arrow). While on a high-altitude trip a young mountaineer complained of sudden shortness of breath, cough and copious expectoration consisting of clear fluid and flaky material. At first thought to be due to pulmonary oedema, it turned out to be ruptured hydatid cyst, successfully treated by surgery (courtesy of Professor Saibal Gupta, MS, FRCS, Professor of Cardiovascular Surgery, Kolkata, India and Dr Rupak Bhattacharya, Kolkata, India).

LEPROSY

Introduction

Leprosy, also called Hansen's disease, is a chronic infectious disease caused by an acid-fast bacillus, *Mycobacterium leprae,* that is widely prevalent in the tropics. Globally, India, Brazil, Nepal, Mozambique, Angola and Myanmar account for 91% of all cases; India alone accounts for 78% of the world's disease. Patients suffer not only from the primary effects of the disease but also from social discrimination, sadly compounded by use of the word 'leper' for one afflicted with this disease.

Close contact over a long duration (several years) is required for disease transmission. Ignorance of this fact on the part of the general public results in ostracism and social stigma. History records that in the distant past sufferers were made to wear cow bells so that other people could avoid them. The use of the term 'leper', still used metaphorically to denote an outcast, does not help to break down the social barriers that continue to exist against the sufferer.

Pathology

The bacillus inhabits the colder parts of the body; hence, it is found in the nasal mucosa and skin in the region of the ears,

Owing to the stigma attached to the word 'leper', RG Cochrane suggested that the best name for leprosy is 'Hansen's disease'.
Robert Greenhill Cochrane, 1899–1985, medical missionary who became an international authority on leprosy; he devoted his time to leprosy patients in South East Asia, particularly India.
Gerhard Henrik Armauer Hansen, 1841–1912, physician in charge of a leper hospital near Bergen, Norway.

thus involving the facial nerve as it exits from the stylomastoid foramen. The disease is transmitted from the nasal secretions of a patient, the infection being contracted in childhood or early adolescence. After an incubation period of several years, the disease presents with skin, upper respiratory or neurological manifestations. The bacillus is acid fast but weakly so when compared with *Mycobacterium tuberculosis*.

The disease is broadly classified into two groups: lepromatous and tuberculoid. In lepromatous leprosy, there is widespread dissemination of abundant bacilli in the tissues, with macrophages and few lymphocytes. This is a reflection of the poor immune response, resulting in depleted host resistance from the patient. In tuberculoid leprosy, on the other hand, the patient shows a strong immune response with scant bacilli in the tissues, epithelioid granulomas, numerous lymphocytes and giant cells. The tissue damage is inversely proportional to the host's immune response. There are various grades of the disease between the two main spectra called dimorphous or borderline variant.

Summary box 6.12

Mycobacterium leprae: pathology

- Leprosy is a chronic curable infection caused by *M. leprae*
- It occurs mainly in tropical regions and resource-poor countries
- The majority of cases are located in the Indian subcontinent
- Transmission is through nasal secretions, the bacillus inhabiting the colder parts of the body
- It is attributed to poor hygiene and insanitary conditions
- The incubation period is several years
- The initial infection occurs in childhood
- Lepromatous leprosy denotes a poor host immune reaction
- Tuberculoid leprosy occurs when host resistance is stronger than the virulence of the organism

Clinical features and diagnosis

The disease is slowly progressive and affects the skin, upper respiratory tract and peripheral nerves. In tuberculoid leprosy, the damage to tissues occurs early and is localised to one part of the body, with limited deformity of that organ. Neural involvement is characterised by thickening of the nerves, which are tender. There may be asymmetrical well-defined anaesthetic hypopigmented or erythematous macules with elevated edges and a dry and rough surface – lesions called leprids. In lepromatous leprosy, the disease is symmetrical and extensive. Cutaneous involvement occurs in the form of several pale macules that form plaques and nodules called lepromas. The deformities produced are divided into primary, which are caused by leprosy or its reactions, and secondary, resulting from effects such as anaesthesia of the hands and feet. Nodular lesions on the face in the acute phase of the lepromatous variety are known as 'leonine facies' (looking like a lion). Later, there is wrinkling of the skin, giving an aged appearance to a young individual. There is loss of the eyebrows and destruction of the lateral cartilages and septum of the nose with collapse of the nasal bridge and lifting of the tip of the nose (***Figure 6.17***). There may be paralysis of the branches of the facial nerve in the bony canal or of the zygomatic branch. Blindness may be attributed to exposure keratitis or iridocyclitis. Paralysis of the orbicularis oculi causes incomplete closure of the eye, epiphora and conjunctivitis (***Figure 6.18***). The hands are typically clawed (***Figure 6.19***) because of involvement of the ulnar nerve at the elbow and the median nerve at the wrist. Anaesthesia of the hands makes these patients vulnerable to frequent burns and injuries. Similarly, clawing of the toes (***Figure 6.20***) occurs as a result of involvement of the posterior tibial nerve. When the lateral popliteal nerve is affected, it leads to foot drop, and the nerve can be felt to be thickened behind the upper end of the fibula. Anaesthesia of the feet predisposes to trophic ulceration (***Figure 6.21***), chronic infection, contraction and autoamputation. Involvement of the testes causes atrophy, which in turn results in gynaecomastia (***Figure 6.22***). Confirmation of the diagnosis is obtained by a skin smear or skin biopsy, which shows the classical histological and microbiological features.

Summary box 6.13

Leprosy: diagnosis

- Typical clinical features and awareness of the disease should help to make a diagnosis
- The face has an aged look, with collapse of the nasal bridge and ocular changes
- Thickened peripheral nerves, patches of anaesthetic skin, claw hands, foot drop and trophic ulcers are characteristic
- Microbiological examination of the acid-fast bacillus and typical histology on skin biopsy are confirmatory

Treatment

A herbal derivative from the seeds of *Hydnocarpus wightianus* (Chaulmoogra) was the mainstay of treatment, with some success, until the advent of dapsone (diamino-diphenyl sulphone). Dapsone, one of the principal drugs, was a derivative of prontosil red and was discovered by Domagk. This is used according to the WHO guidelines along with rifampicin and clofazimine. During treatment, the patient may develop acute manifestations. These are controlled with steroids. Multiple drug therapy for 12 months is the key to treatment. A team approach between an infectious diseases specialist, plastic surgeon, ophthalmologist, and hand or orthopaedic surgeon is important.

Surgical treatment is indicated in advanced stages of the disease for functional disability of limbs, cosmetic disfigurement of the face and visual problems. These entail major reconstructive surgery, which is the domain of the plastic surgeon.

Gerhard Domagk, 1895–1964, German physician, Lecturer in Pathologic Anatomy, University of Munster, Germany, discovered prontosil in 1935, for which he was awarded the Nobel Prize in Physiology or Medicine in 1939.

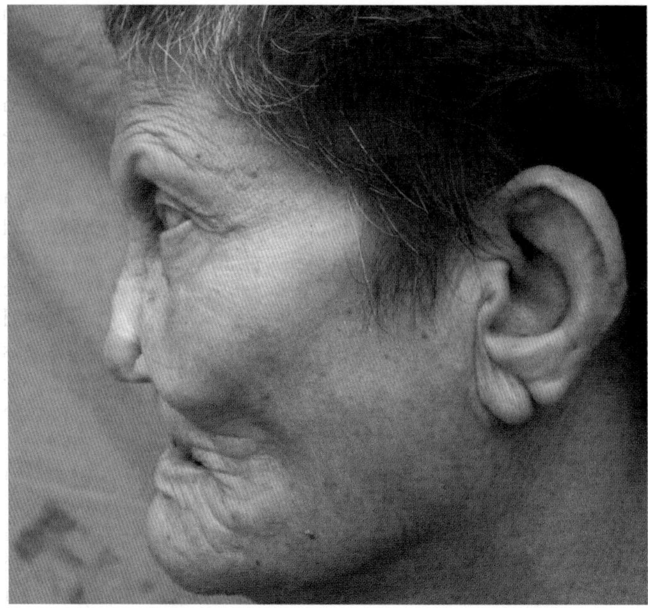

Figure 6.17 Lateral view of the face showing collapse of the nasal bridge due to destruction of nasal cartilage by leprosy.

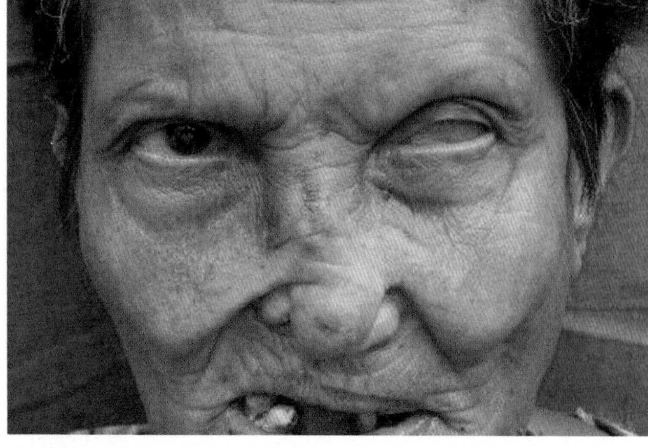

Figure 6.18 Frontal view of the face showing eye changes in leprosy: paralysis of orbicularis oculi and loss of eyebrows.

Surgery for deformities in the hand is aimed at returning the ability to achieve a grasp and a pinch grip. Tendon transfers (pioneered by Brand and Tovey) are used to recreate the function of the lumbricals that have been lost due to damage to the ulnar nerve. In the foot, damage to the common peroneal nerve leads to a foot drop due to paralysis of tibialis

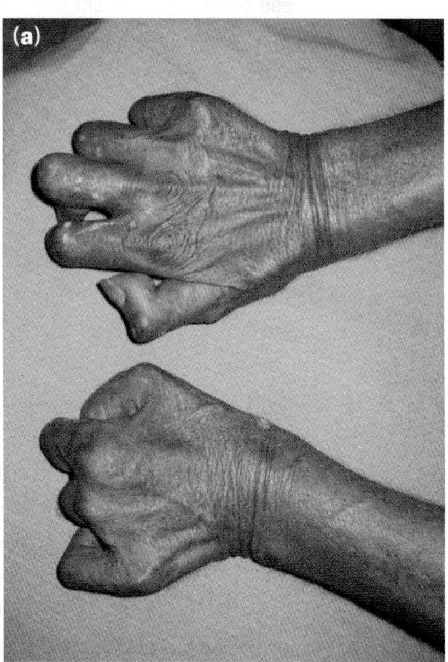

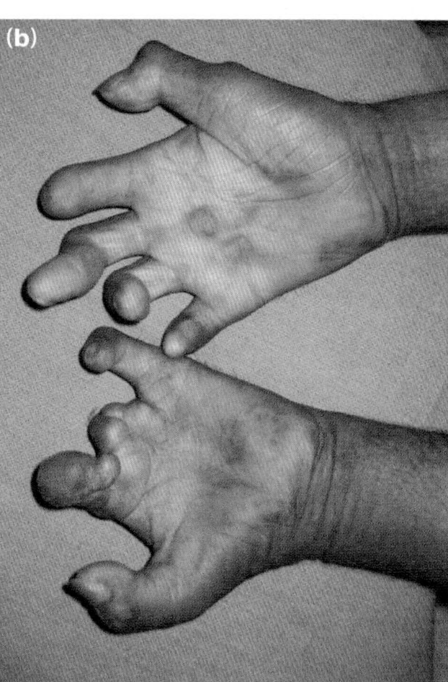

Figure 6.19 (a, b) Typical bilateral claw hand from leprosy due to involvement of the ulnar and median nerves.

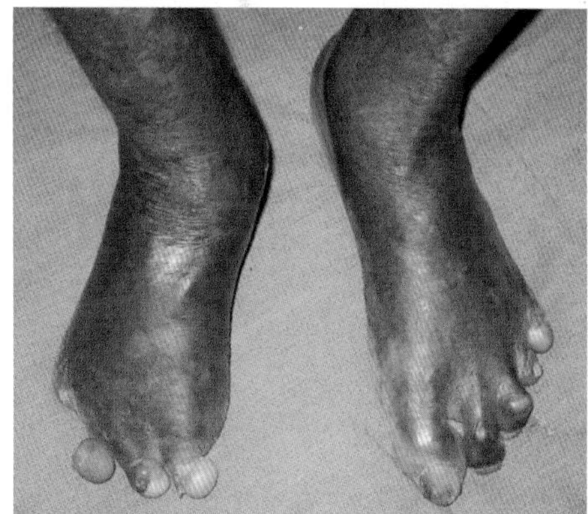

Figure 6.20 Claw toes from involvement of the posterior tibial nerve by leprosy; also note autoamputation of toes of the right foot.

Paul Wilson Brand CBE, FRCS, 1914–2003, was born to missionary parents in Southern India, and qualified in London in 1943. He himself was a dedicated missionary who was 'An extraordinary gifted orthopaedic surgeon who straightened crooked hands and unravelled the riddle of leprosy.' As a pioneer in tendon transfer techniques, he established and practised initially in New Life Center, Vellore, South India and Schieffelin Leprosy Research Centre, Karigiri, South India. Initially he trained as a carpenter and builder and maintained that his training as a carpenter helped him in his expertise in tendon transplantation. When he was awarded the CBE, his wife, Margaret, came to know about it when she found a letter from Her Majesty's Government informing him of the award while emptying the pockets of his trousers before they were put into the wash. He later moved to Louisiana State University, Baton Rouge, LA, where he continued his work, and finally to Seattle as Emeritus Professor of Orthopaedics at the University of Washington, Seattle, USA.

Margaret Brand, alongside her husband, Paul Brand, also contributed immensely to the health of leprosy patients by concentrating on research to prevent blindness in leprosy. She became known as 'the woman who first helped lepers to see'.

Frank Tovey OBE, 1921–2019, another English surgeon at about the same time (1951–1967), also performed extensive tendon transfers and facial and other reconstructive surgery on patients with leprosy in southern India in the State of Mysore. In this he was helped by his wife, Winifred, who organised the physiotherapy and rehabilitation of the patients and established village diagnostic and treatment centres.

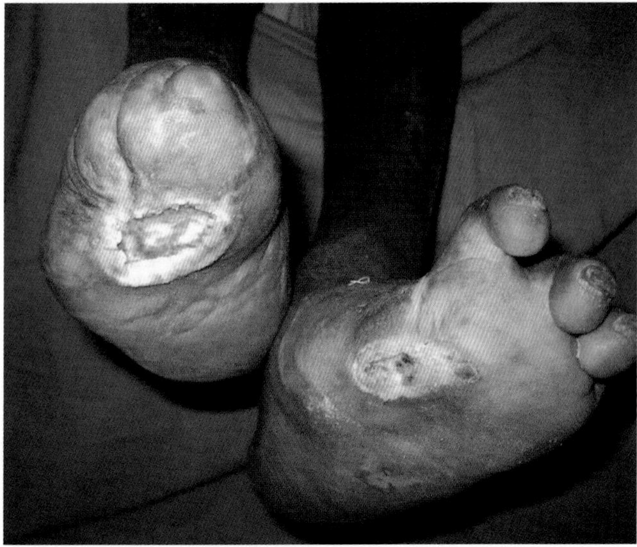

Figure 6.21 Bilateral trophic ulceration of the feet due to anaesthesia of the soles resulting from leprosy; also note claw toes on the left foot.

anterior. If a foot-drop splint is not adequate, then once again a tendon transfer (tibialis posterior into the dorsum of the foot) will improve function. Ulcers resulting from an insensate foot should be completely debrided followed by protection with a plaster cast.

The general surgeon may be called upon to treat a patient when the deformity is so advanced that amputation is required or an abscess needs drainage as an emergency.

All surgical procedures obviously need to be done under antileprosy drug treatment. This is best achieved by a team approach. Educating patients about the dreadful sequelae of the disease so that they seek medical help early is important. It is also necessary to educate the general public that patients suffering from the disease should not be made social outcasts.

Summary box 6.14

Leprosy: treatment

- Multiple drug therapy for a year
- Team approach
- Surgical reconstruction requires the expertise of a hand surgeon, orthopaedic surgeon and plastic surgeon
- Education of the patient and general public should be the keystone in prevention

MYCETOMA

Introduction

Mycetoma is a chronic, specific, granulomatous, progressive, destructive inflammatory disease that involves the skin, subcutaneous tissues and deeper structures. The causative organism may be true fungi, when the condition is called eumycetoma; when caused by bacteria it is called actinomycetoma.

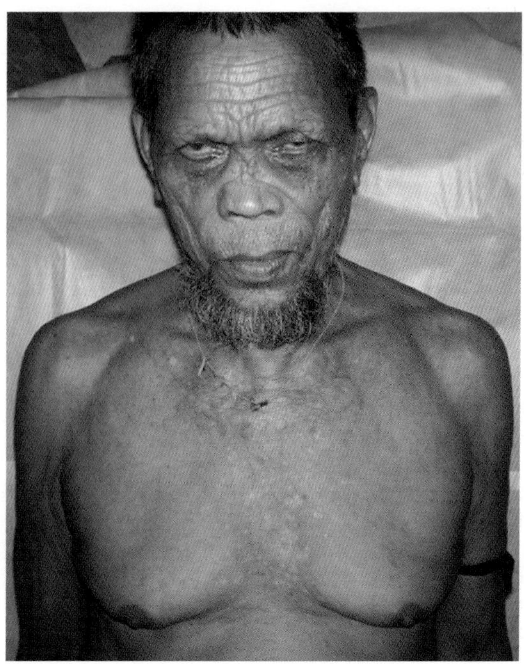

Figure 6.22 Typical leonine facies and gynaecomastia in leprosy.

The pathognomonic feature is the triad of painless subcutaneous mass, multiple sinuses and seropurulent discharge. It causes tissue destruction, deformity and disability, and death in extreme cases.

Epidemiology and pathogenesis

The condition predominantly occurs in the 'mycetoma belt' that lies between latitudes 15° south and 30° north, comprising the countries of Sudan, Somalia, Senegal, India, Yemen, Mexico, Venezuela, Columbia, Argentina and a few others. The route of infection is inoculation of the organism that is resident in the soil through a traumatised area. Although in the vast majority there is no history of trauma, the portal of entry is always an area of minor unrecognised trauma in a bare-footed individual walking in a terrain full of thorns. Hence the foot is the commonest site affected. Mycetoma is not contagious.

Once the granuloma forms it increases in size, and the overlying skin becomes stretched, smooth, shiny and attached

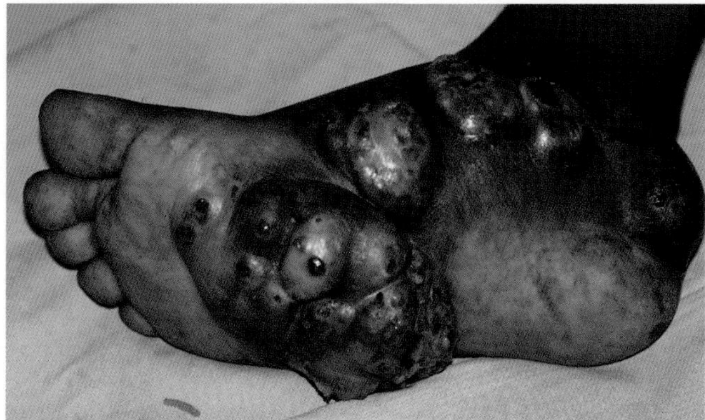

Figure 6.23 Mycetoma of the foot.

to the lesion. Areas of hypo- or hyperpigmentation sometimes develop. Eventually it invades the deeper structures. This is usually gradual and delayed in eumycetoma. In actinomycetoma, invasion to deeper tissues occurs earlier and is more extensive. The tendons and nerves are spared until late in the disease. This may explain the rarity of neurological and trophic changes even in patients with longstanding disease. Trophic changes are rare because the blood supply is adequate.

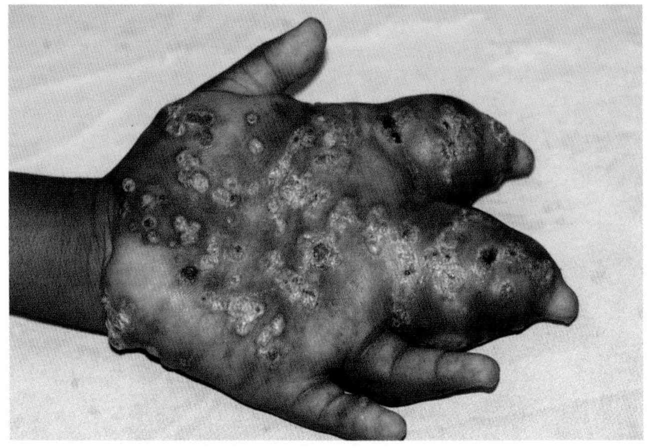

Figure 6.24 Mycetoma of the hand.

Summary box 6.15

Mycetoma: pathogenesis

- Mostly occurs in the 'mycetoma belt'
- There are two types – eumycetoma and actinomycetoma
- Caused by fungi or bacteria entering through a site of trauma, which may not be apparent; hence the foot is most commonly affected
- Produces a chronic, specific, granulomatous, progressive, destructive inflammatory lesion
- Results in tissue destruction, deformity, disability and sometimes death

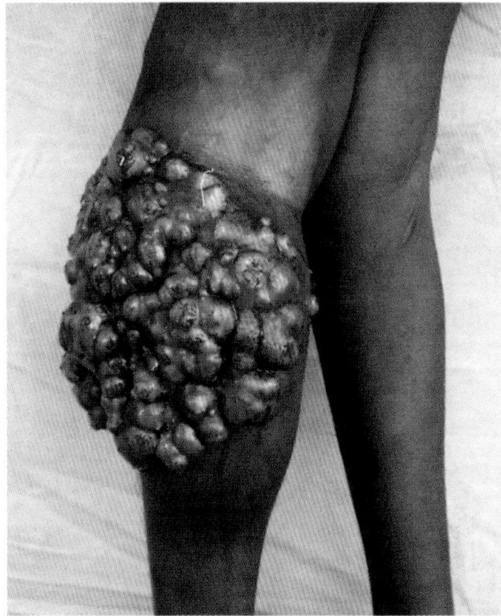

Figure 6.25 Mycetoma of the knee.

Clinical presentation

As mycetoma is painless, presentation is late in the majority. It presents as a slowly progressive, painless, subcutaneous swelling commonly at the site of presumed trauma. The swelling is variable in its physical characteristics: firm and rounded, soft and lobulated, rarely cystic and often mobile. Multiple secondary nodules may evolve; they may suppurate and drain through multiple sinus tracts. The sinuses may close transiently after discharge during the active phase of the disease. Fresh adjacent sinuses may open while some of the old ones may heal completely. They coalesce and form abscesses, the discharge being serous, serosanguineous or purulent. During the active phase of the disease the sinuses discharge grains, the colour of which can be black, yellow, white or red depending upon the organism. Pain supervenes when there is secondary bacterial infection.

The common sites affected are those that come into contact with soil during daily activities: the foot in 70% (***Figure 6.23***) and the hand in 12% (***Figure 6.24***). In endemic areas the knee (***Figure 6.25***), arm, leg, head and neck (***Figure 6.26***), thigh and perineum (***Figure 6.27***) can be involved. Rare sites are the chest, abdominal wall, facial bones, mandible, testes, paranasal sinuses and eye.

In some patients there may be areas of local hyperhidrosis over the lesion. This may be due to sympathetic overactivity or increased local temperature due to raised arterial blood flow caused by the chronic inflammation. In the majority of patients, the regional lymph nodes are small and shotty. Lymphadenopathy is common. This may be due to secondary bacterial infection, lymphatic spread of mycetoma or a local immune response to the disease.

The condition remains localised; constitutional disturbances are a sign of secondary bacterial infection. Cachexia and anaemia from malnutrition and sepsis may be seen in late cases. It can be fatal, especially in cases of cranial mycetoma.

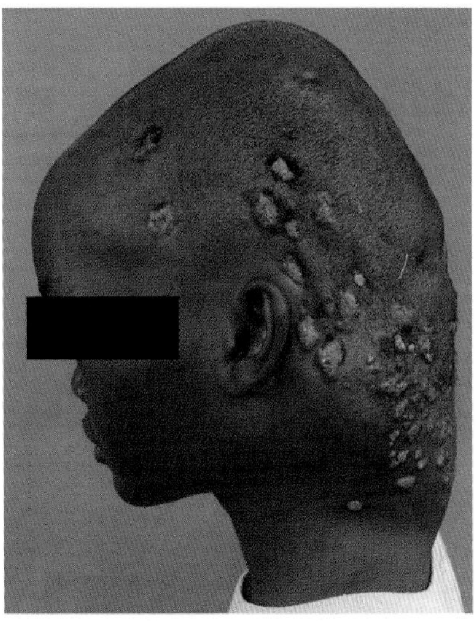

Figure 6.26 Actinomycetoma of the head and neck.

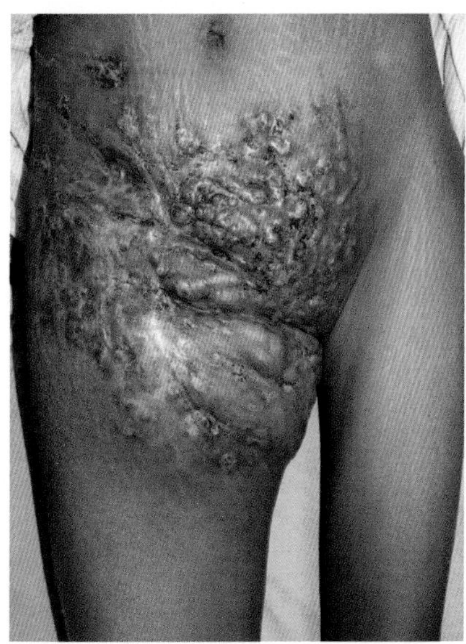

Figure 6.27 Extensive satellite inguinal actinomycetoma from a primary foot lesion involving the anterior abdominal wall and perineum.

Spread

Local spread occurs predominantly along tissue planes. The organism multiplies to form colonies that spread along the fascial planes to skin and underlying structures. Lymphatic spread, more common in actinomycetoma, occurs to the regional lymph nodes, and increases with repeated inadequate surgical excision procedures. During the active phase of the disease, these lymphatic satellites may suppurate and discharge; lymphadenopathy may also be due to secondary bacterial infection. Spread via the bloodstream can occur.

The apparent clinical features of mycetoma are not always a reliable indicator of the extent and spread of the disease. Some small lesions with few sinuses may have many deep connecting tracts, through which the disease can spread quite extensively. Therefore, surgery in mycetoma under local anaesthesia is contraindicated.

Differential diagnosis

Mycetoma should be distinguished from Kaposi's sarcoma, malignant melanoma, fibroma and foreign body (thorn) granuloma. A radiograph that demonstrates the presence of bone destruction in the absence of sinuses is suggestive of tuberculosis. The radiological features of advanced mycetoma are similar to those of primary osteogenic sarcoma. Primary osseous mycetoma is to be differentiated from chronic osteomyelitis, osteoclastoma, bone cysts and syphilitic osteitis. In endemic areas the dictum should be 'any subcutaneous swelling must be considered a mycetoma until proven otherwise'.

Diagnosis

Several imaging techniques are available to confirm the diagnosis: plain radiography, ultrasonography, CT and magnetic resonance imaging (MRI).

Plain radiograph

In the early stages, soft-tissue shadows (often multiple) with calcification and obliteration of the fascial planes may be seen. As the disease progresses, the cortex may be compressed from the outside by the granuloma, leading to bone scalloping. Periosteal reaction with new bone spicules may create a sun-ray appearance and Codman's triangle, not unlike an osteogenic sarcoma (*Figure 6.28*). Late in the disease, there may be multiple punched-out cavities throughout the bone.

Ultrasonography

This can differentiate between eumycetoma and actinomycetoma as well as between mycetoma and other conditions. In eumycetoma, the grains produce numerous sharp bright hyper-reflective echoes. There are multiple thick-walled cavities with absent acoustic enhancement. In actinomycetoma, the findings are similar but the grains are less distinct. The size and extent of the lesion can be accurately determined ultrasonically, a finding useful in planning surgical treatment.

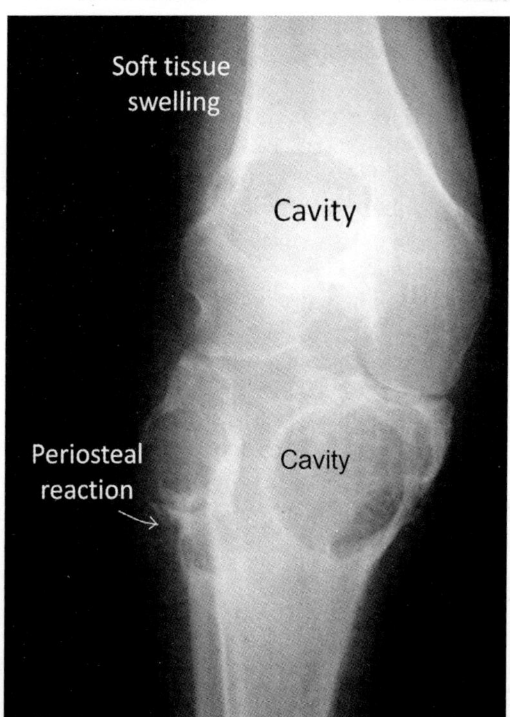

Figure 6.28 Plain radiograph of the knee showing multiple large cavities involving the lower femur, upper tibia and fibula, with well-defined margins and periosteal reaction typical of eumycetoma.

Moritz Kaposi, 1837–1902, Hungarian-born Professor of Dermatology, University of Vienna, Austria, described pigmented sarcoma of the skin in 1872. The viral cause was discovered in 1994.

Ernest Codman, 1869–1940, American surgeon. Codman's triangle can be seen in osteosarcoma, Ewing's sarcoma, subperiosteal abscess and haematoma.

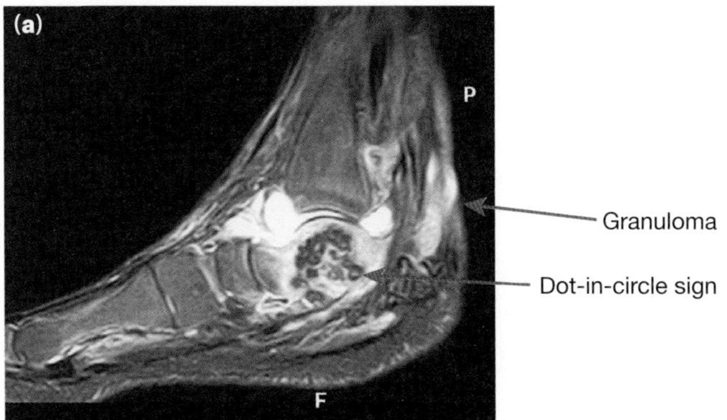

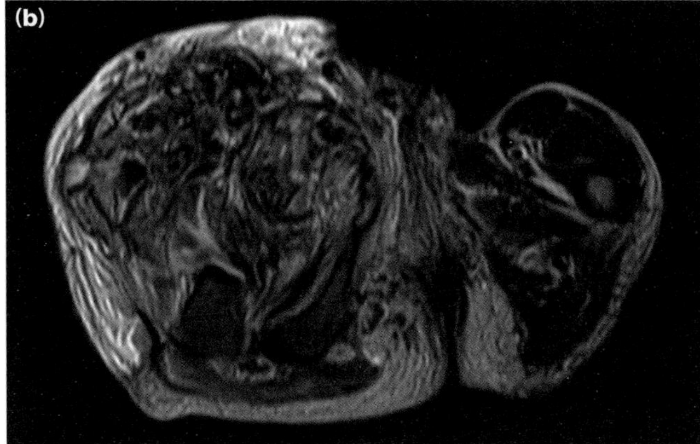

Figure 6.29 (a) Magnetic resonance imaging (MRI) of the foot showing multiple lesions of high signal intensity, which indicates granuloma, interspersed within a low-intensity matrix, which is the fibrous tissue and the 'dot-in-circle' sign, which indicates the presence of grains. (b) MRI showing massive upper thigh and lower abdominal actinomycetoma.

Magnetic resonance imaging

This helps to assess bone destruction, periosteal reaction and particularly soft-tissue involvement (***Figure 6.29***). MRI usually shows multiple 2- to 5-mm lesions of high signal intensity, which indicates the granuloma, interspersed within a low-intensity matrix denoting the fibrous tissue. The 'dot-in-circle' sign, which indicates the presence of grains, is highly characteristic.

Computed tomography

CT findings in mycetoma are not specific but are helpful to detect early bone involvement.

Histopathological diagnosis

Deep biopsy is obtained under general or regional anaesthesia, although the chance of local spread is high. The biopsy should be adequate, contain grains and should be fixed immediately in 10% formal saline.

Three types of host tissue reaction occur against the organism.

- **Type I:** the grains are usually surrounded by a layer of polymorphonuclear leukocytes. The innermost neutrophils are closely attached to the surface of the grain, sometimes invading the grain and causing its fragmentation. The hyphae and cement substance disappear and only remnants of brown pigmented cement are left behind. Outside the zone of neutrophils there is granulation tissue containing macrophages, lymphocytes, plasma cells and few neutrophils. The mononuclear cells increase in number towards the periphery of the lesion. The outermost zone of the lesion consists of fibrous tissue.
- **Type II:** the neutrophils largely disappear and are replaced by macrophages and multinucleated giant cells that engulf the grain material. This consists largely of pigmented cement substance although hyphae are sometimes identified.
- **Type III:** this is characterised by the formation of a well-organised epithelioid granuloma with Langhans-type giant cells. The centre of the granuloma will sometimes contain remnants of fungal material.

Fine-needle aspiration cytology

Fine-needle aspiration cytology (FNAC) can yield an accurate diagnosis and helps in distinguishing between eumycetoma and actinomycetoma. The technique is simple, rapid and sensitive.

Culture

A variety of microorganisms are capable of producing mycetomata that can be identified by their textural description, morphology and biological activities in pure culture. Deep surgical biopsy is always needed to obtain the grains that are the source of culture. The grains extracted through the sinuses are usually contaminated and not viable and hence should be avoided. Several media may be used to isolate and grow these organisms.

In the absence of the classical triad of mycetoma, the demonstration of significant antibody titres against the causative organism may be of diagnostic value and aid follow up. The common serodiagnostic tests are immunoelectrophoresis and ELISA.

Summary box 6.16

Mycetoma: diagnosis

- Usually presents late as it is painless
- Triad of painless subcutaneous mass, multiple sinuses and seropurulent discharge
- Clinical picture may be deceptive as there may be deep-seated extension
- May spread to lymph nodes
- Can be confused with Kaposi's sarcoma
- Radiologically can be mistaken for osteosarcoma
- MRI shows typical 'dot-in-circle' sign
- Open biopsy and FNAC are confirmatory

Theodor Langhans, 1839–1915, Professor of Pathological Anatomy, University of Berne, Switzerland.

Management

Ideally this should be a combined effort between the physician and the surgeon. In actinomycetoma, combined drug therapy with amikacin sulphate and co-trimoxazole in the form of cycles is the treatment of choice. Amoxicillin–clavulanic acid, rifampicin, sulphonamides, gentamicin and kanamycin are used as a second line of treatment. Long-term drug treatment can have serious side effects.

In eumycetoma, ketoconazole, itraconazole and voriconazole are the drugs of choice. They may need to be used for up to a year. Use of these drugs should be closely monitored for side effects. While not curative, these drugs help to localise the disease by forming thickly encapsulated lesions that are then amenable to surgical excision. Medical treatment for both types of mycetoma must continue until the patient is cured and also in the postoperative period.

Surgical treatment

Surgery is indicated for small, localised lesions, resistance to medical treatment or for a better response after medical treatment in patients with massive disease. Excision may need to be much more extensive than suggested at first on clinical appearance because the disease may extend to deeper planes that are not clinically apparent. The surgical options are wide local and debulking excisions and amputations. Amputation, used as a life-saving procedure, is indicated in advanced mycetoma refractory to medical treatment with severe secondary bacterial infection. The amputation rate is 10–25%.

Postoperative medical treatment should continue for an adequate period to prevent recurrence. The recurrence rate varies from 25% to 50%. This can be local or distant, to regional lymph nodes. Recurrence is usually due to inadequate surgical excision, use of local anaesthesia, lack of surgical experience, non-compliance with drugs for financial reasons and lack of health education.

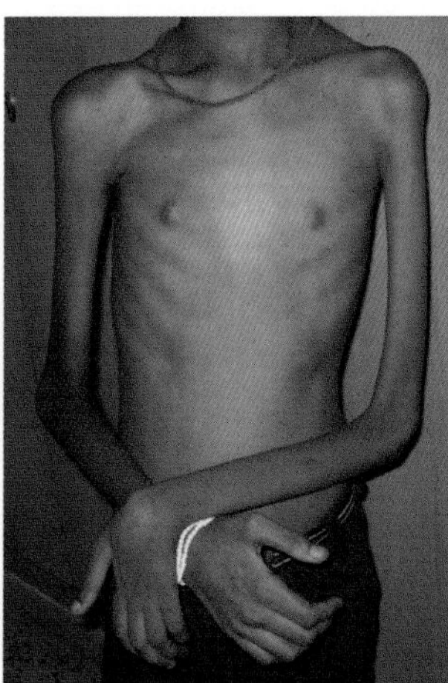

Figure 6.30 Polio affecting predominantly the upper limb muscles with wasting of the intercostal muscles.

Summary box 6.17

Mycetoma: management

- Ideally combined management by physician and surgeon
- Medical treatment with appropriate long-term antibiotics
- In large lesions medical treatment to reduce the size followed by excision
- Beware of serious drug side effects
- Surgery in the form of wide excision and amputation as a life-saving procedure
- High recurrence rate

POLIOMYELITIS

Introduction

Poliomyelitis is an enteroviral infection that sadly still affects children in certain parts of the world – this is in spite of effective vaccination having been universally available for several decades. The virus enters the body by inhalation or ingestion. Clinically, the disease manifests itself in a wide spectrum of symptoms – from a few days of mild fever and headache to the extreme variety consisting of extensive paralysis of the bulbar form that may not be compatible with life because of involvement of the respiratory and pharyngeal muscles.

Diagnosis

The disease targets the anterior horn cells, causing lower motor neurone paralysis. Muscles of the lower limb are affected twice as frequently as those of the upper limb (***Figures 6.30 and 6.31***). Fortunately, only 1–2% of sufferers develop paralytic symptoms but, when they do occur, the disability causes much misery (***Figure 6.32***). When a patient develops fever with muscle weakness, Guillain–Barré syndrome needs to be excluded. The latter has sensory symptoms and signs. Cerebrospinal fluid analysis should help to differentiate the two conditions.

Management

Surgical management is directed mainly towards the rehabilitation of the patient who has residual paralysis, the operations being tailored to the particular individual's disability. Children especially may show improvement in their muscle function for up to 2 years after the onset of the illness. Thereafter, many patients learn to manage their disability by incorporating various manoeuvres ('trick movements') into their daily life. The surgeon must be cautious in considering such a patient for any form of surgery.

Surgical treatment in the chronic form of the disease is the domain of a highly specialised orthopaedic surgeon who needs

Georges Guillain, 1876–1961, Professor of Neurology, The Faculty of Medicine, Paris, France.
Jean Alexandre Barré, 1880–1967, Professor of Neurology, Strasbourg, France.
Guillain and Barré described the condition in a joint paper in 1916 while serving as Medical Officers in the French Army during the First World War.

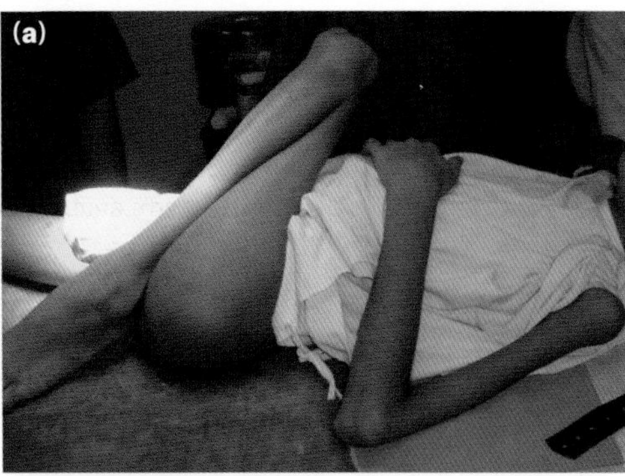
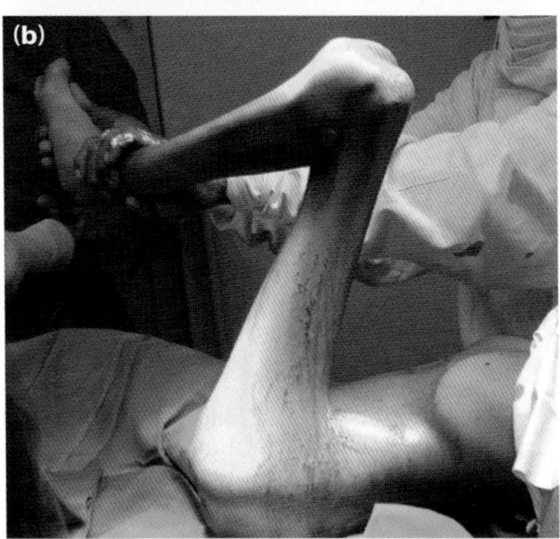

Figure 6.31 (a, b) A 12-year-old patient with polio showing marked wasting of the left upper arm muscles with flexion contractures of the left knee and hip; there is equinus deformity of the foot (courtesy of Dr SM Lakhotia, MS and Dr PK Jain, MD, DA, Kolkata, India).

to work closely with the physiotherapist both in assessing and in rehabilitating the patient. Operations are only considered after a very careful and detailed assessment of the patient's needs. A multidisciplinary team, consisting of the orthopaedic surgeon, neurologist, physiotherapist, orthotist and the family, should decide upon the need for and advisability of any surgical procedure.

A description of the operations for the various disabilities is beyond the scope of this book. The reader should therefore seek surgical details in a specialist textbook. In 2012, WHO declared India a polio-free country.

Summary box 6.18

Poliomyelitis

- A viral illness that is preventable
- Presents with protean manifestations of fever, headache and muscular paralysis without sensory loss, more frequently affecting the lower limbs
- Treatment is mainly medical and supportive in the early stages
- Surgery should only be undertaken after very careful assessment as most patients learn to live with their disabilities
- Surgery is considered for the various types of paralysis in the form of tendon transfers and arthrodesis, which is the domain of a specialist orthopaedic surgeon

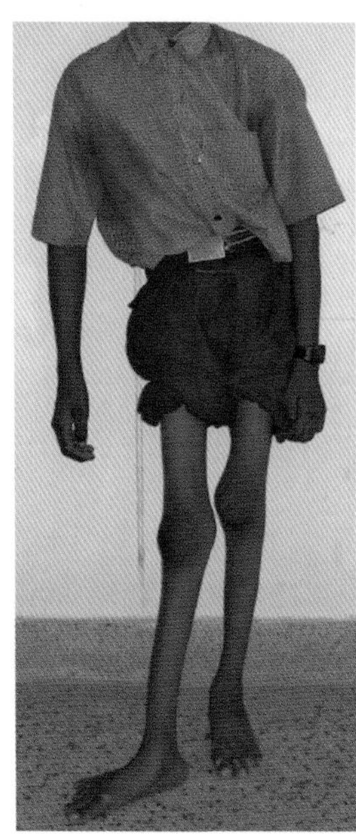

Figure 6.32 A young patient with polio showing paralysis of the lower limb and paraspinal muscles causing marked scoliosis and a deformed pelvis.

TROPICAL CHRONIC PANCREATITIS

Introduction

Tropical chronic pancreatitis is a disease affecting the younger generation from poor socioeconomic strata in resource-poor countries, seen mostly in southern India. The aetiology remains obscure, with malnutrition, dietary, familial and genetic factors being possible causes. Alcohol ingestion does not play a part in the aetiology.

Aetiology and pathology

Cassava (tapioca) is a root vegetable that is readily available and inexpensive and is therefore consumed as a staple diet by people from a poor background. It contains derivatives of cyanide that are detoxified in the liver by sulphur-containing amino acids. The less well off among the population lack such amino acids in the diet. This results in cyanogen toxicity, causing the disease. Several members of the same family have been known to suffer from this condition; this strengthens the theory that cassava toxicity is an important cause because family members eat the same food.

Macroscopically, the pancreas is firm and nodular with extensive periductal fibrosis, with intraductal calcium carbonate stones of different sizes and shapes that may show branches and resemble a staghorn. The ducts are dilated. Microscopically, intralobular, interlobular and periductal fibrosis is the predominant feature, with plasma cell and lymphocyte infiltration. There is a high incidence of pancreatic cancer in these patients.

Summary box 6.19

Pathology of tropical chronic pancreatitis

- Almost exclusively occurs in resource-poor countries and is due to malnutrition; alcohol is not a cause
- Cassava ingestion is regarded as an aetiological factor because of its high content of cyanide compounds
- Dilatation of pancreatic ducts with large intraductal stones
- Fibrosis of the pancreas as a whole
- A high incidence of pancreatic cancer in those affected by the disease

Diagnosis

The patient, usually male, is almost always below the age of 40 years and from a poor socioeconomic background. The clinical presentation is abdominal pain, thirst, polyuria and features of gross pancreatic insufficiency causing steatorrhoea and malnutrition. The patient looks ill and emaciated.

Initial routine blood and urine tests confirm that the patient has type 1 diabetes mellitus. This is known as fibrocalculous pancreatic diabetes, a label that is aptly descriptive of the typical pathological changes. Serum amylase is usually normal; in an acute exacerbation, it may be elevated. A plain abdominal radiograph shows typical pancreatic calcification in the form of discrete stones in the duct (***Figure 6.33***). Ultrasonography and CT scanning of the pancreas confirm the diagnosis. An ERCP, as an investigation, should only be done when the procedure is also being considered as a therapeutic manoeuvre for removal of ductal stones in the pancreatic head by papillotomy.

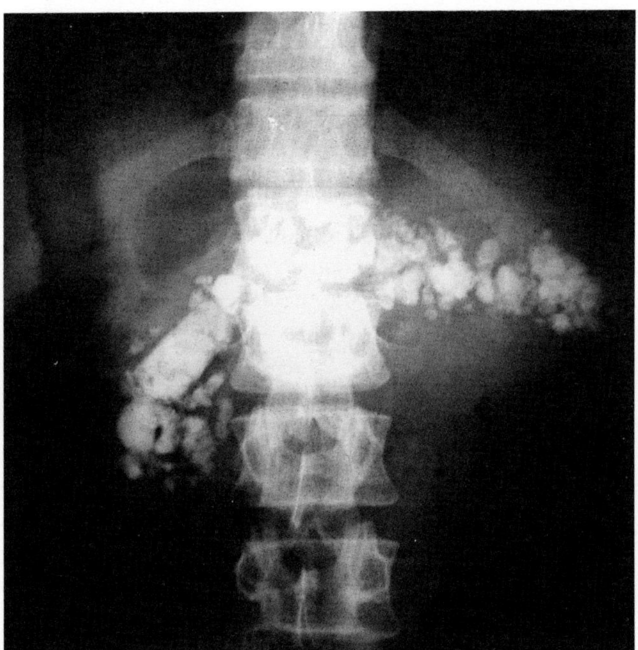

Figure 6.33 Plain radiograph of the abdomen showing large stones along the main pancreatic duct typical of tropical chronic pancreatitis (courtesy of Dr V Mohan, Chennai, India).

Summary box 6.20

Diagnosis of tropical chronic pancreatitis

- The usual sufferer is a type 1 diabetic under 40 years of age
- Serum amylase may be elevated in an acute exacerbation
- Plain radiograph shows stones along the pancreatic duct
- Ultrasonography and CT scan of the pancreas confirm the diagnosis
- ERCP should be used as an investigation only when combined with a therapeutic procedure

Treatment

The treatment is mainly medical, with exocrine support using pancreatic enzymes, treatment of diabetes with insulin and the management of malnutrition. Treatment of pain should be along the lines of the usual analgesic ladder: non-opioids, followed by weak and then strong opioids and, finally, referral to a pain clinic.

Surgical treatment is necessary for intractable pain, particularly when there are stones in a dilated duct. Removal of the stones, with a side-to-side pancreaticojejunostomy to a Roux loop, is the procedure of choice. As most patients are young, pancreatic resection is only very rarely considered, and only as a last resort, when all available methods of pain relief have been exhausted.

Summary box 6.21

Treatment of tropical chronic pancreatitis

- Mainly medical – pain relief, insulin for diabetes and pancreatic supplements for malnutrition
- Surgery is reserved for intractable pain when all other methods have been exhausted
- Operations are side-to-side pancreaticojejunostomy; resection in extreme cases

TUBERCULOSIS

Although tuberculosis can affect all systems in the body, in the tropical world the surgeon is most often faced with tuberculosis affecting the cervical lymph nodes and the small intestine. Therefore, in this chapter tuberculous cervical lymphadenitis and tuberculosis of the small bowel will be described.

TUBERCULOUS CERVICAL LYMPHADENITIS

Introduction

This is common in the Indian subcontinent. A young person who has recently arrived from an endemic area, presenting with cervical lymphadenopathy, should be diagnosed as having tuberculous lymphadenitis unless otherwise proven. With acquired immune deficiency syndrome (AIDS) being globally prevalent, this is not as rare in the West in the indigenous population as it used to be.

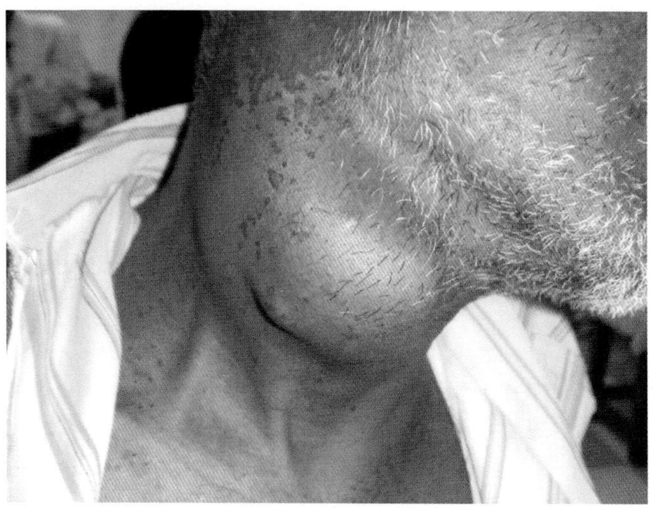

Figure 6.34 Cervical tuberculous: cold abscess about to burst.

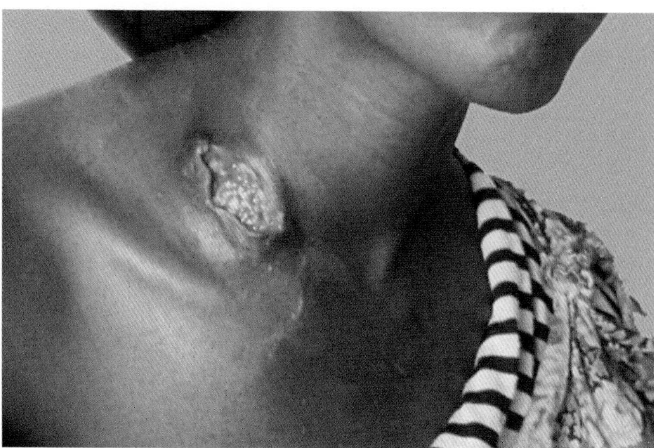

Figure 6.35 Cervical tuberculous ulcer with typical overhanging edges (courtesy of Professor Ahmed Hassan Fahal, FRCS MD MS, Khartoum, Sudan).

Diagnosis

Any of the cervical group of lymph nodes (jugulodigastric, submandibular, supraclavicular, posterior triangle) can be involved. The patient has the usual general manifestations of tuberculosis: evening pyrexia, cough (maybe from pulmonary tuberculosis) and malaise; if the sufferer is a child, failure to thrive is a significant finding. Locally there will be regional lymphadenopathy where the lymph nodes may be matted; in late stages a cold abscess may form – a painless, fluctuant, mass which is not warm; significantly there are no signs of inflammation (*Figure 6.34*), hence it is called a 'cold abscess'. This is a clinical manifestation of underlying caseation.

Left untreated, the cold abscess, initially deep to the deep fascia, bursts through into the space just beneath the superficial fascia. This produces a bilocular mass with cross-fluctuation. This is called a 'collar-stud' abscess. Eventually this may burst through the skin, discharging pus and forming a tuberculous sinus and eventually might ulcerate (*Figure 6.35*). The latter typically has watery discharge with undermined edges as the tubercle bacilli destroy the subcutaneous tissue faster than the rest and thrive in the relatively anoxic environment.

Summary box 6.22

Tuberculous cervical lymphadenitis

- This is a common condition at any age
- A matted lymph nodal mass is the typical clinical feature
- In later stages the mass may be cystic, denoting an abscess
- The abscess denotes underlying caseation and does not show any features of inflammation – hence called a cold abscess
- Ultimately the abscess may burst, forming a sinus
- Diagnosis is clinched by culture of pus and biopsy of the lymph node
- Involvement of other systems must be excluded
- Treatment is mainly medical

Investigations

Raised ESR and CRP, low haemoglobin and a positive Mantoux test are usual, although the last is not significant in a patient from an endemic area. The Mantoux test (tuberculin skin test), although in use for over a hundred years, has now been superseded by interferon-gamma (IFN-γ) release assays. This is an *in vitro* blood test of cellular immune response. Antigens unique to *M. tuberculosis* are used to stimulate and measure T-cell release of IFN-γ. This helps to earmark patients who have latent or subclinical tuberculosis and thus will benefit from treatment.

Sputum for culture and sensitivity (the result may take several weeks) and staining by the Ziehl–Neelsen method for acid-fast bacilli (the result is obtained much earlier) should be carried out.

Specific investigations would include aspiration of the pus from a cold abscess for culture and sensitivity. If the mass is still in the early stages of adenitis, excision biopsy should be done. Here, part of the lymph nodes should be sent fresh and unfixed to the laboratory, which should be warned of the arrival of the specimen so that the tissue can be appropriately processed immediately.

Treatment

This must be combined management between the physician and the surgeon. Tuberculous infection at other sites must

A collar-stud abscess is so-called because it resembles a collar stud (which has two parts) used in shirts with detachable collars, now largely out of fashion.
Charles Mantoux, 1877–1947, physician, Le Cannet, Alpes Maritimes, France, described the intradermal tuberculin skin test in 1908.
Franz Heinrich Paul Ziehl, 1857–1926, German bacteriologist and professor in Lübeck, Germany. With pathologist **Friedrich Neelsen**, he developed the Ziehl–Neelsen stain, also known as the acid-fast stain, which is used to identify acid-fast bacteria.
Friedrich Carl Adolf Neelsen, 1854–1898, pathologist and professor at the Institute of Pathology, University of Rostock, Germany.

be excluded and suitably managed. Medical treatment is the mainstay. The reader is asked to look up details of medical treatment in an appropriate source.

TUBERCULOSIS OF SMALL INTESTINE

Introduction

Infection by *M. tuberculosis* is common in the tropics. In these days of international travel and increased migration, tuberculosis in general and intestinal tuberculosis in particular are no longer clinical curiosities in non-endemic countries. Any patient, particularly one who has recently arrived from an endemic area and who has features of generalised ill health and altered bowel habit, should arouse suspicion for intestinal tuberculosis. The increased prevalence of human immunodeficiency virus (HIV) infection worldwide has also made tuberculosis more common. The infection is transmitted by swallowing of infected sputum in a patient with pulmonary tuberculosis, by drinking infected unpasteurised milk or by a haematogenous route.

Pathology

There are two types: ulcerative and hyperplastic. In both types, there may be marked mesenteric lymphadenopathy.

- **Ulcerative type:** The organism colonises the lymphatics of the terminal ileum, causing transverse ulcers with typical undermined edges. The serosa is usually studded with tubercles. Histology shows caseating granuloma with giant cells (*Figure 6.36*). This pathological entity, referred to as the ulcerative type, denotes a severe form of the disease in which the virulence of the organism overwhelms host resistance. The ulcers heal by fibrosis and transverse ulcers lead to multiple strictures that may present later with luminal narrowing and intestinal obstruction.
- **Hyperplastic type:** This occurs when host resistance has the upper hand over the virulence of the organism. There is a marked inflammatory reaction causing hyperplasia and thickening of the terminal ileum because of its abundance of lymphoid follicles, thus resulting in narrowing of the lumen and obstruction. Macroscopically, this type may be confused with Crohn's disease. Ileocaecal tuberculosis (*Figure 6.37*) may present with a right iliac fossa mass and features of intestinal obstruction. As a result of fibrosis, there is shortening of the bowel with the caecum being pulled up into a subhepatic position with resultant widening of the ileocaecal angle beyond 90°.

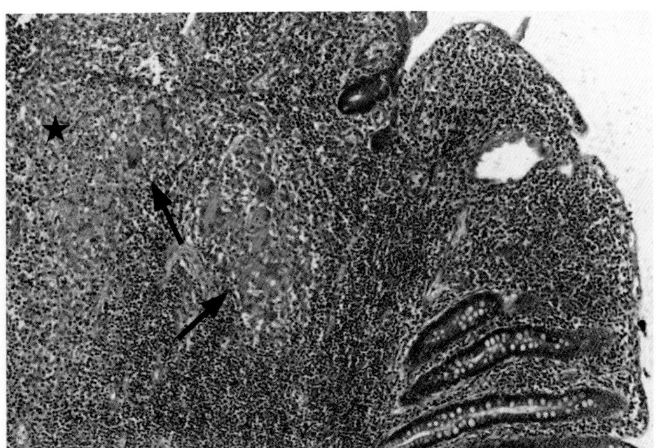

Figure 6.36 Histology of ileocaecal tuberculosis showing epithelioid cell granuloma (black arrows) with caseation (star) (courtesy of Dr AK Mandal, New Delhi, India).

Summary box 6.23

Tuberculosis: pathology

- Increasingly being seen in non-endemic areas, mostly among immigrants from endemic areas
- Two types are recognised – ulcerative and hyperplastic
- The ulcerative type occurs when the virulence of the organism is greater than the host defence and forms strictures
- The opposite occurs in the hyperplastic type and presents with a mass
- Small bowel strictures are common in the ulcerative type, presenting with obstructive symptoms, while the hyperplastic type mainly affects the ileocaecal area and presents with a right iliac fossa mass and obstructive symptoms
- In peritoneal tuberculosis, the parietal and visceral peritoneum is studded with tubercles
- Localised areas of ascites (loculated) depicts peritoneal involvement
- Encasement of bowel in a fibrotic sac (cocoon) may be seen in the plastic type of peritoneal tuberculosis, which presents with obstruction
- The lungs and other organs, particularly of the genitourinary system, may also be involved simultaneously

Clinical features

Patients present electively with weight loss, chronic cough, malaise, evening rise in temperature with sweating, vague abdominal pain with distension and alternating constipation and diarrhoea. As an emergency, they present with features of distal small bowel obstruction from strictures of the small bowel, particularly the terminal ileum. Rarely, a patient may present with features of peritonitis from perforation of a tuberculous ulcer in the small bowel (*Figure 6.37*).

Examination shows a chronically ill patient with a 'doughy' feel to the abdomen from areas of localised ascites. In the hyperplastic type, a mass may be felt in the right iliac fossa. In addition, some patients may present with fistula-*in-ano*, which is typically multiple with undermined edges and watery discharge.

Burrill Bernard Crohn, 1884–1983, gastroenterologist, Mount Sinai Hospital, New York, NY, USA, described regional ileitis in 1932 along with Leon Ginzburg and Gordon Oppenheimer.

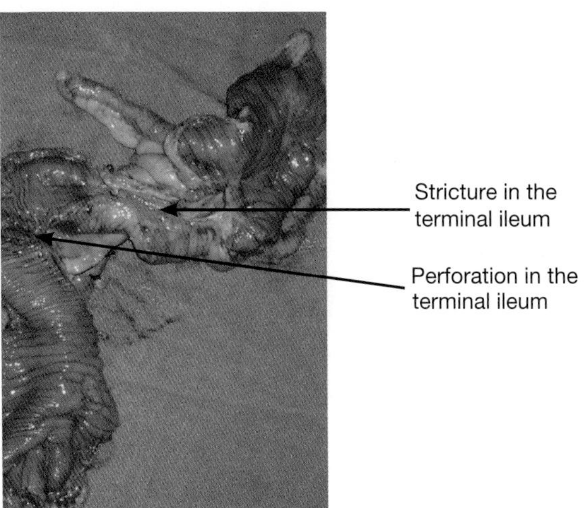

Figure 6.37 Emergency limited ileocolic resection: specimen showing a tuberculous stricture in the terminal ileum and perforation of a transverse ulcer just proximal to the stricture.

As this is a disease mainly seen in certain resource-poor countries, patients may present late as an emergency from intestinal obstruction. Abdominal pain and distension, constipation and bilious and faeculent vomiting are typical of such a patient, who is usually *in extremis*.

There may be involvement of other systems, such as the genitourinary tract, when the patient complains of frequency of micturition. Clinical examination does not show any abnormality. The genitourinary tract should then be investigated.

Summary box 6.24

Tuberculosis: clinical features

- Intestinal tuberculosis should be suspected in any patient from an endemic area who presents with weight loss, malaise, evening fever, cough, alternating constipation and diarrhoea and intermittent abdominal pain with distension
- The abdomen has a doughy feel; a mass may be found in the right iliac fossa
- The emergency patient presents with features of distal small bowel obstruction – abdominal pain, distension, bilious and faeculent vomiting
- Peritonitis from a perforated tuberculous ulcer in the small bowel can be another emergency presentation, though rare

Investigations

General investigations are the same as those for suspected tuberculosis anywhere in the body. They have been detailed in the previous section under investigations for tuberculous cervical adenitis.

A barium meal and follow-through (or small bowel enema) shows strictures of the small bowel, particularly the ileum, typically with a high subhepatic caecum with the narrow ileum entering the caecum directly from below upwards in a straight line rather than at an angle (***Figures 6.38 and 6.39a***). Laparoscopy reveals the typical picture of tubercles on the bowel serosa, multiple strictures, a high caecum, enlarged lymph nodes, areas of caseation and ascites. Culture of the ascitic fluid may be helpful. A chest radiograph is essential (***Figure 6.39b***) as there may be features of pulmonary tuberculosis.

If the patient complains of urinary symptoms, urine is sent for microscopy and culture; the finding of sterile pyuria should alert the clinician to the possibility of tuberculosis of the urinary tract, when the appropriate investigations should be done. A flexible cystoscopy would be very useful in the presence of sterile pyuria. A contracted bladder ('thimble' bladder) with ureteric orifices that are in-drawn ('golf-hole' ureter) may be seen; these changes are due to fibrosis.

In the patient presenting as an abdominal emergency, urea and electrolytes may show evidence of gross dehydration. A plain abdominal radiograph shows typical small bowel obstruction – valvulae conniventes (concertina effect) of dilated jejunum and featureless ileum with evidence of fluid between the loops.

Summary box 6.25

Intestinal tuberculosis: investigations

- Raised inflammatory markers, anaemia and positive sputum culture
- IFN-γ release assays for subclinical infection
- Ultrasonography of the abdomen may show localised areas of ascites
- Chest radiograph shows pulmonary infiltration
- Barium meal and follow-through shows multiple small bowel strictures particularly in the ileum, with a subhepatic caecum
- If symptoms warrant, the genitourinary tract is also investigated

Treatment

On completion of medical treatment, the patient's small bowel is reimaged to look for significant strictures. If the patient has features of subacute intermittent obstruction, bowel resection, in the form of limited ileocolic resection with anastomosis between the terminal ileum and ascending colon for ileocolic hyperplastic disease, strictureplasty for single ileal stricture, bowel resection for multiple closely placed strictures or right hemicolectomy for extensive ileocolic disease precluding limited resection, is performed as deemed appropriate. The surgical principles and options in the elective patient are very similar to those for Crohn's disease, where resections should be kept as conservative as possible.

The emergency patient presents a great challenge. Such a patient is usually from a poor socioeconomic background, hence the late presentation of acute, distal, small bowel obstruction. The patient is extremely ill from dehydration, malnutrition, anaemia and probably active pulmonary tuberculosis. Vigorous resuscitation should precede the operation. At laparotomy, the minimum life-saving procedure is carried out, such as a resection of diseased segment with proximal ileostomy and distal ileal or colonic mucus fistula to avoid anastomosis, which has a high chance of leaking in the presence of active infection and poor general condition. If, however, the general condition of the patient permits, a one-stage resection and anastomosis may rarely be performed.

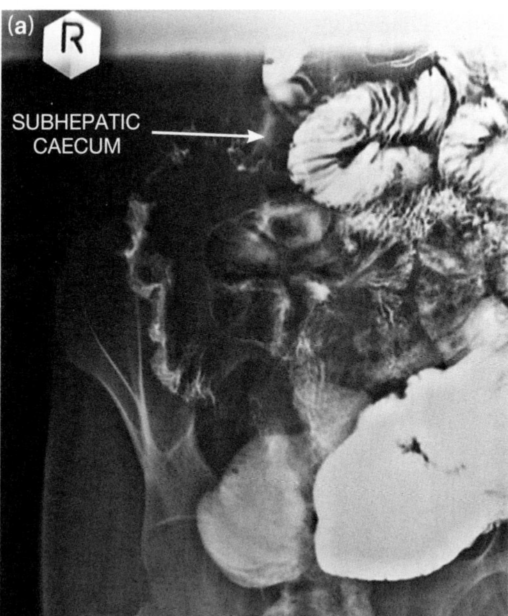

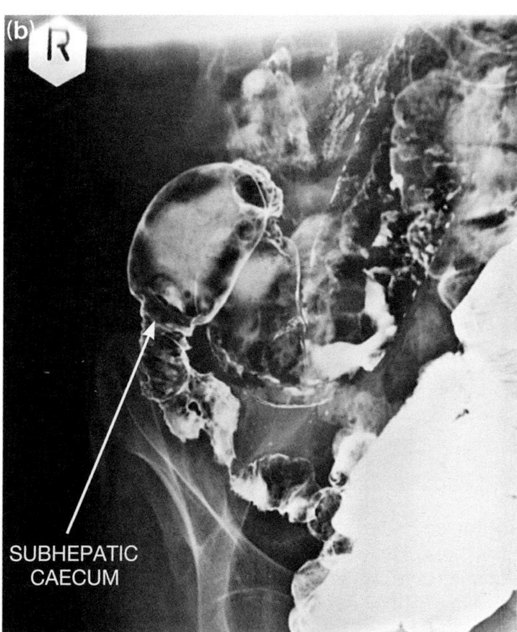

Figure 6.38 (a, b) Series of a barium meal and follow-through showing strictures in the ileum, with the caecum pulled up into a subhepatic position.

Thereafter, the patient should ideally be under the combined care of the physician and surgeon for a full course of standard multidrug antitubercular chemotherapy (intensive and maintenance phases) and improvement in nutritional status, which may take up to 6–12 months. The patient who had a simple bypass procedure is reassessed and, when the disease is no longer active (as evidenced by return to normal inflammatory markers, weight gain, negative sputum culture), an elective right hemicolectomy is done to remove the blind loop. This may be supplemented with strictureplasty for short strictures at intervals or resection of a segment with several strictures.

Perforation is treated by thorough resuscitation followed by resection of the affected segment. Anastomosis is performed, provided it is regarded as safe to do so, when peritoneal

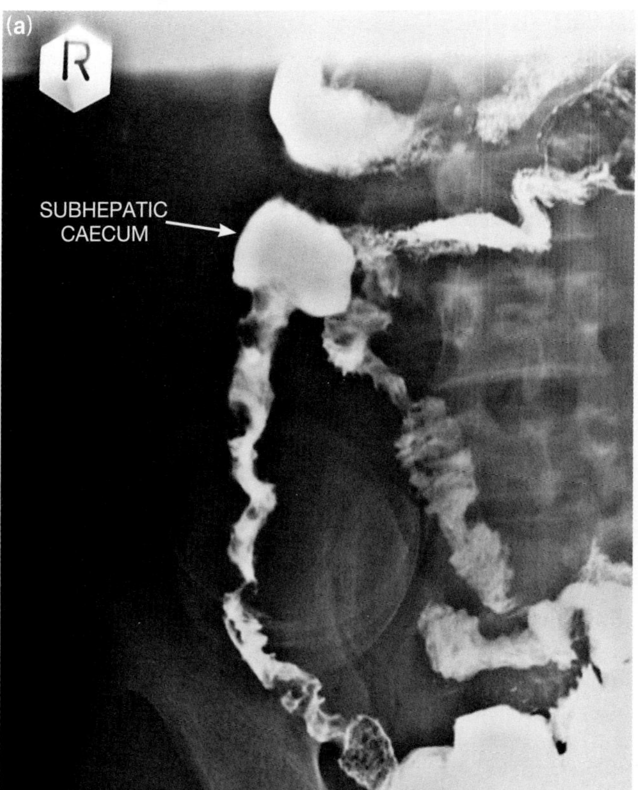

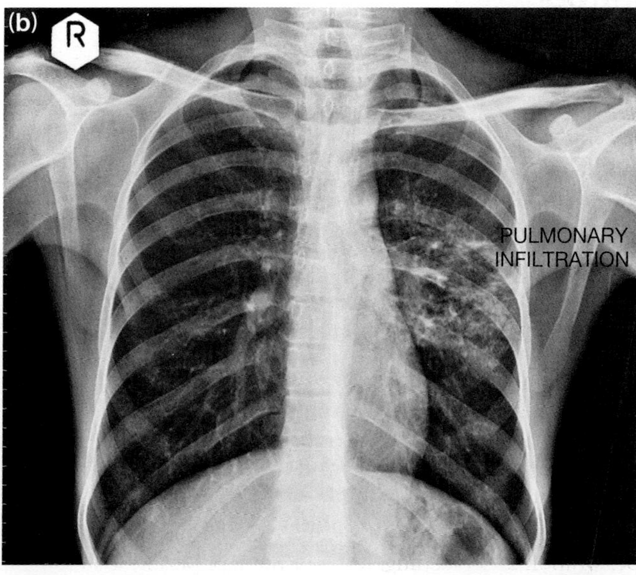

Figure 6.39 Barium meal and follow-through (a) and chest radiograph (b) in a patient with extensive intestinal and pulmonary tuberculosis, showing ileal strictures with high caecum and pulmonary infiltration.

contamination is minimal and widespread disease is not encountered; otherwise, as a first stage, resection and ileostomy are performed followed by restoration of bowel continuity as a second stage later on after a full course of antitubercular chemotherapy and improvement in nutritional status.

Summary box 6.26

Tuberculosis: treatment

- Patients should ideally be under the combined care of a physician and surgeon
- Vigorous supportive and full drug treatment are mandatory in all cases
- Symptomatic strictures are treated by the appropriate resection, e.g. local ileocolic resection or strictureplasty or resection as an elective procedure once the disease is completely under control
- Acute intestinal obstruction from distal ileal stricture is treated by thorough resuscitation followed by resection with ileostomy or primary anastomosis
- One-stage resection and anastomosis can rarely be considered if the patient's general condition permits
- Perforation is treated by appropriate local resection and anastomosis or ileostomy if the condition of the patient is very poor; this is later followed by restoration of bowel continuity after the patient has fully recovered with antitubercular chemotherapy

TYPHOID

Introduction

Typhoid fever is caused by *Salmonella* Typhi, also called the typhoid bacillus, a Gram-negative organism. Like most infections occurring in the tropics, the organism gains entry into the human gastrointestinal tract as a result of poor hygiene and inadequate sanitation. It is a disease normally managed by physicians, but the surgeon may be called upon to treat the patient with typhoid fever because of perforation of a typhoid ulcer.

Pathology

Following ingestion of contaminated food or water, the organism colonises the Peyer's patches in the terminal ileum, causing hyperplasia of the lymphoid follicles followed by necrosis and ulceration. The microscopic picture shows erythrophagocytosis with histiocytic proliferation (***Figure 6.40***). If the patient is left untreated or inadequately treated, the ulcers may lead to perforation and bleeding. The bowel may perforate at several sites, including the large bowel.

Diagnosis

A typical patient is from an endemic area or has recently visited such a country and suffers from a high temperature for 2–3 weeks. The patient may be toxic with abdominal distension from paralytic ileus and may have melaena due to haemorrhage from a typhoid ulcer; this can lead to hypovolaemia.

Blood and stool cultures confirm the nature of the infection and exclude malaria. Although obsolete in some parts of the world, the Widal test is still done on the Indian subcontinent. The test looks for the presence of agglutinins to O and H antigens of *Salmonella* Typhi and Paratyphi in the patient's serum. In endemic areas, laboratory facilities may sometimes be limited. Certain other tests have been developed that identify sensitive and specific markers for typhoid fever. Practical and cheap kits are available for their rapid detection that need no special expertise and equipment. These are MultiTest Dip-S-Ticks to detect immunoglobulin G (IgG), Tubex to detect immunoglobulin M (IgM) and TyphiDot to detect IgG and IgM. These tests are particularly valuable when blood cultures are negative (as a result of prehospital treatment or self-medication with antibiotics) or facilities for such an investigation are not available.

In the second or third week of the illness, if there is severe generalised abdominal pain, this indicates a perforated typhoid ulcer unless otherwise proven. The patient, who is already very ill, deteriorates further with classical features of peritonitis. An erect chest radiograph or a lateral decubitus film (in the very ill, as they usually are) will show free gas in the peritoneal cavity. In fact, any patient being treated for typhoid fever who shows a sudden deterioration accompanied by abdominal signs should be considered to have a typhoid perforation until proven otherwise.

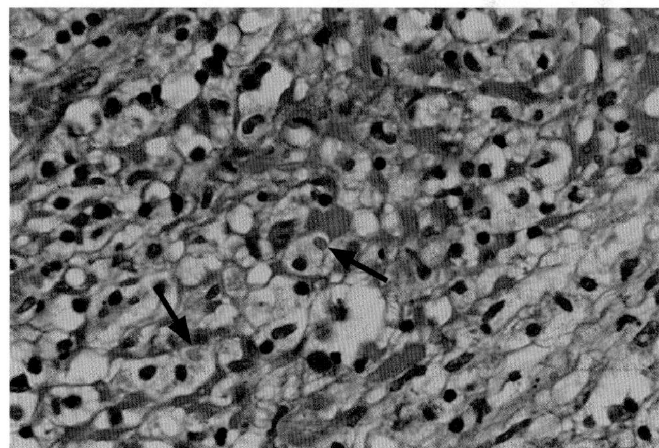

Figure 6.40 Histology of enteric perforation of the small intestine showing erythrophagocytosis (arrows) with predominantly histiocytic proliferation (courtesy of Dr AK Mandal, New Delhi, India).

Daniel Elmer Salmon, 1850–1914, veterinary pathologist, Chief of the Bureau of Animal Industry, Washington, DC, USA.
Johann Conrad Peyer, 1653–1712, Professor of Logic, Rhetoric and Medicine, Schaffhausen, Switzerland, described the lymph follicles in the intestine in 1677.
Georges Fernand Isidore Widal, 1862–1929, Professor of Internal Pathology, and later of Clinical Medicine, The Faculty of Medicine, Paris, France.

Summary box 6.27

Diagnosis of bowel perforation secondary to typhoid

- The patient presents in, or has recently visited, an endemic area
- The patient has persistent high temperature and is very toxic
- Positive blood or stool cultures for *Salmonella* Typhi and the patient is already on treatment for typhoid
- After the second week, signs of peritonitis usually denote perforation, which is confirmed by the presence of free gas seen on a radiograph

Treatment

Vigorous resuscitation with intravenous fluids and antibiotics in an intensive care unit gives the best chance of stabilising the patient's condition. Metronidazole, cephalosporins and gentamicin are used in combination. Chloramphenicol, despite its potential side effect of aplastic anaemia, is still used occasionally in resource-poor countries. Laparotomy is then carried out.

Several surgical options are available, and the most appropriate operative procedure should be chosen judiciously depending upon the general condition of the patient, the site of perforation, the number of perforations and the degree of peritoneal soiling. The alternatives are closure of the perforation (***Figure 6.41***) after freshening the edges, wedge resection of the ulcer area and closure, resection of bowel with or without anastomosis (exteriorisation), closure of the perforation and side-to-side ileotransverse anastomosis, ileostomy or colostomy where the perforated bowel is exteriorised after refashioning the edges.

After closing an ileal perforation, the surgeon should look for other sites of perforation or necrotic patches in the small or large bowel that might imminently perforate, and deal with them appropriately. Thorough peritoneal lavage is essential. The linea alba is closed, leaving the rest of the abdominal wound open for delayed closure, as wound infection is almost inevitable and dehiscence not uncommon. In the presence of rampant infection, laparostomy may be a good alternative.

When a typhoid perforation occurs within the first week of illness, the prognosis is better than if it occurs after the second or third week because, in the early stages, the patient is less nutritionally compromised and the body's defences are more robust. Furthermore, the shorter the interval between diagnosis and operation, the better the prognosis.

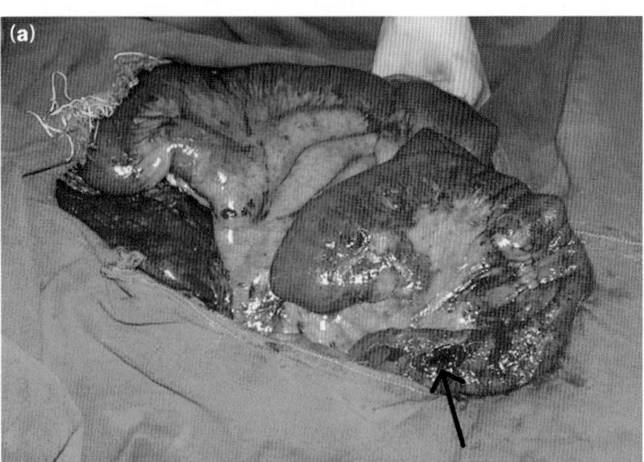

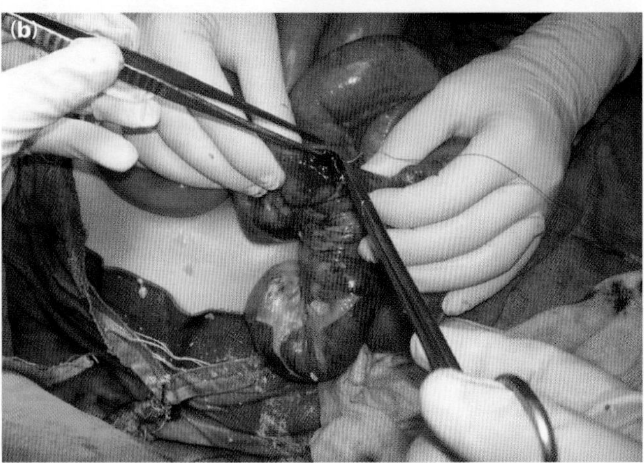

Figure 6.41 (a, b) Typhoid perforation of the terminal ileum (arrow in (a)).

Summary box 6.28

Treatment of bowel perforation from typhoid

- Manage in intensive care
- Resuscitate and give intravenous antibiotics
- Laparotomy – choice of various procedures
- Commonest site of perforation is the terminal ileum
- Having found a perforation, always look for others
- In the very ill patient, consider some form of exteriorisation
- Close the peritoneum and leave the wound open for secondary closure

ACKNOWLEDGEMENT

The authors acknowledge the contribution of Professor Ahmed Hassan Fahal MBBS, FRCS, FRCSI, FRCSG, MD, MS, FRCP (London), Professor of Surgery, University of Khartoum, Khartoum, Sudan, in the section relating to Mycetoma.

FURTHER READING

AMOEBIASIS

Barnes SA, Lillemore KD. Liver abscess and hydatid disease In: Zinner NJ, Schwartz I, Ellis H (eds). *Maingot's abdominal operations*, 10th edn, vol. 2. New York: Appleton and Lange, McGraw-Hill, 1997: 1527–45.

Blessmann J, Van Linh P, Nu PA *et al.* Epidemiology of amebiasis in a region of high incidence of amebic liver abscess in central Vietnam. *Am J Trop Med Hyg* 2002; **66**(5): 578–83.

Bruns BR, Scalea TM. Complex liver abscess. In: Diaz JJ, Efron DT (eds). *Complications in acute care surgery.* Cham: Springer International Publishing, 2017: 189–97.

Shirley D-AT, Watanabe K, Moonah S. Significance of amebiasis: 10 reasons why neglecting amebiasis might come back to bite us in the gut. *PLoS Negl Trop Dis* 2019; **13**(11): e0007744.

Tanyuksel M, Petri Jr WA. Laboratory diagnosis of amebiasis. *Clin Microbiol Rev* 2003; **16**(4): 713–29.

ASCARIASIS

Carrero JC, Reyes-Lopez M, Serrano-Luna J, Shibayama M, Unzueta J, Leon-Sicairos N, de la Garza M. Intestinal amoebiasis: 160 years of its first detection and still remains as a health problem in developing countries. *Int J Med Microbiol* 2020; **310**(1): 151358.

Das AK. Hepatic and biliary ascariasis. *J Global Infect Dis* 2014; **6**(2): 65.

Steinberg R, Davies J, Millar AJ *et al.* Unusual intestinal sequelae after operations for *Ascaris lumbricoides* infestation. *Paediatr Surg Int* 2003; **19**(1–2): 85–7.

Wani RA, Parray FQ, Bhat NA *et al.* Non-traumatic terminal ileal perforation. *World J Emerg Surg* 2006; **10**: 1–7.

ASIATIC CHOLANGIOHEPATITIS

Choi BI, Han JK, Hong ST, Lee KH. Clonorchiasis and cholangiocarcinoma: etiologic relationship and imaging diagnosis. *Clin Microbiol Rev* 2004; **17**(3): 540–52.

Verweij KE, van Buuren H. Oriental cholangiohepatitis (recurrent pyogenic cholangitis): a case series from the Netherlands and brief review of the literature. *Neth J Med* 2016; **74**(9): 401-5.

FILARIASIS

Lim KH, Speare R, Thomas G, Graves P. Surgical treatment of genital manifestations of lymphatic filariasis: a systematic review. *World J Surg* 2015; **39**(12): 2885–99.

Manjula Y, Kate V, Ananthakrishnan N. Evaluation of sequential intermittent pneumatic compression for filarial lymphoedema. *Natl Med J India* 2002; **15**(4): 192–4.

HYDATID DISEASE

Barnes SA, Lillemore KD. Liver abscess and hydatid disease. In: Zinner NJ, Schwartz I, Ellis H (eds). *Maingot's abdominal operations*, 10th edn, vol. 2. New York: Appleton and Lange, McGraw Hill, 1997: 1527–45.

Botezatu C, Mastalier B, Patrascu T. Hepatic hydatid cyst–diagnose and treatment algorithm. *J Med Life* 2018; **11**(3): 203.

Chiodini P. Parasitic infections. In: Russell RCG, Williams NS, Bulstrode CJK (eds). *Bailey & Love's short practice of surgery*, 24th edn. London: Arnold, 2004: 146–74.

WHO Informal Working Group. International classification of ultrasound images in cystic echinococcosis for application in clinical and field epidemiological settings. *Acta Trop* 2003; **85**(2): 253–61.

LEPROSY

Anderson GA. The surgical management of deformities of the hand in leprosy. *Bone Joint J* 2006; **88**(3): 290–4.

MYCETOMA

Fahal AH. Management of mycetoma. *Expert Rev Dermatol* 2010; **5**(1): 87–93.

Hassan MA, Fahal AH. Mycetoma. In: Kamil R, Lumby J (eds). *Tropical surgery*. London: Westminster Publications Ltd, 2004: 786–90.

TROPICAL CHRONIC PANCREATITIS

Barman KK, Premlatha G, Mohan V. Tropical chronic pancreatitis. *Postgrad Med J* 2003; **79**: 606–15.

TYPHOID

Aziz M, Qadir A, Aziz M, Faizullah. Prognostic factors in typhoid perforation. *J Coll Physicians Surg Pak* 2005; **15**(11): 704–7.

Olsen SJ, Pruckler J, Bibb W *et al.* Evaluation of rapid diagnostic tests for typhoid fever. *J Clin Microbiol* 2004; **42**(5): 1885–9.

CHAPTER

7 Basic surgical skills

Learning objectives

To understand:

- The importance of safe patient positioning
- The steps involved in surgical site preparation
- The principles of surgical exposure and laparoscopic access
- Surgical craft and wound closure
- Haemostasis and electrosurgery
- The role of drains in surgery

INTRODUCTION

Successful outcomes in surgery depend on knowledge, skills and judgement. While this chapter focuses on technical skills, the importance of surgical preparedness in the form of appropriate safety checks, correct positioning and non-technical skills such as communication and teamwork cannot be overstated.

Patient safety and transfer to the operating table

Patient safety is of paramount importance. The safe transfer and positioning of the patient is a responsibility that is shared by the anaesthetist, surgeon, nurse and operating department practitioners. The anaesthetist managing the airway usually coordinates the transfer of the patient by calling the count. The transfer of the patient is a critical moment during which there is a significant risk of falls and injuries, not to mention injury to operating theatre personnel. Additional care and specialised equipment may be required when transferring patients who are obese or emaciated and those at extremes of age.

POSITIONING ON THE OPERATING TABLE

Summary box 7.1

Objectives of correct surgical positioning

- Facilitate safe anaesthesia and surgery
- Reduce adverse physiological insults
- Optimise surgical exposure and ergonomics
- Maintain patient's dignity by avoiding unnecessary exposure

Summary box 7.2

Pre-positioning planning

- Final checks of the operating table and accessories
- Optimum positioning of laparoscopic stacks, electrosurgical unit, surgical ancillaries and nursing trolley
- Passive diathermy leads and underbody heating blankets placed appropriately
- Age, body habitus and joint mobility to be considered
- Compromise between perfect surgical positioning and physiologically permissible positioning needs to be reached

Supine position

This is the most common position for general surgical procedures. The patient's arms may be placed by their side or extended to afford access to intravenous and arterial cannulae. This is a versatile position and can be modified as follows:

- Rose's position: slight neck extension for head and neck surgery.
- Shoulder and arm extended: to assist in axillary and breast surgery.
- Trendelenburg position: the head end of the table is tilted down on an incline with the patient's knees slightly flexed. This is often used in pelvic procedures and when resuscitating a patient in shock (***Figure 7.1***).
- Reverse Trendelenburg position: the head end of the table is tilted up, thereby placing the head higher than the feet (***Figure 7.2***).

In advanced laparoscopic surgery, exaggerated and frequent position changes during the course of the operation are used to enhance surgical exposure. An excellent example

Friedrich Trendelenburg, 1844–1924, Professor of Surgery successively at Rostock (1875–1882), Bonn (1882–1895), Leipzig (1895–1911), Germany. The Trendelenburg position was first described in 1885.

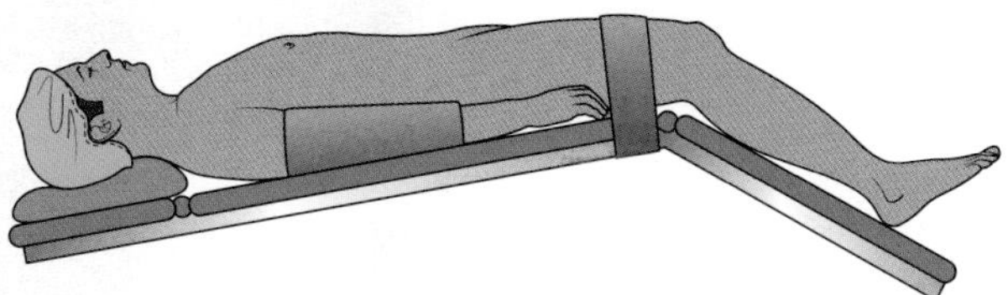

Figure 7.1 Trendelenburg position.

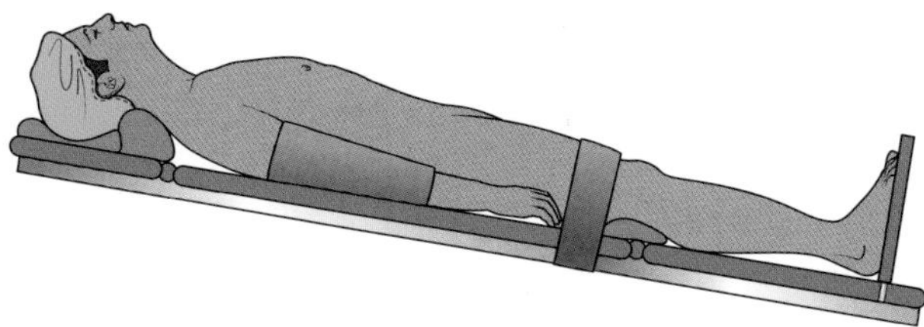

Figure 7.2 Reverse Trendelenburg position.

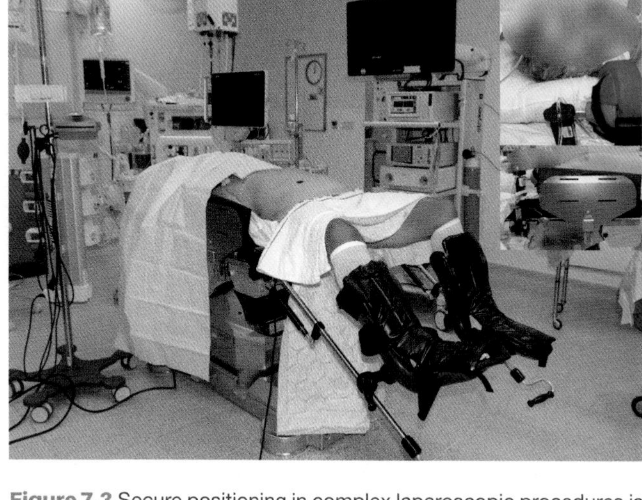

Figure 7.3 Secure positioning in complex laparoscopic procedures is aided with shoulder and side supports, straps and stirrups.

would be in laparoscopic resection of the rectum, wherein the table is tilted to the right to aid in left colon mobilisation; a neutral or reverse Trendelenburg position is used to mobilise the transverse colon; and pelvic dissection is completed with a steep Trendelenburg position. This can only be achieved if the patient is well positioned and secured (***Figure 7.3***).

Straps and supports to secure the patient

- The safety belt to prevent the patient from sliding off the table is placed 5 cm above the knee and never over the abdomen.
- Shoulder supports are used if the Trendelenburg position is necessary.
- Side supports to prevent lateral displacement of the patient are essential if the table needs to be tilted laterally.
- Foot support is required for the reverse Trendelenburg position.
- Alternatively, vacuum-activated positioning systems that gently conform to the contours of the patient's body can be used.

Potential complications specific to supine positioning

- Ulnar, axillary, peroneal and brachial neuropraxia.
  - To reduce the risk of brachial plexus injury, the arm should not be hyperextended (abducted by greater than 90°). Pronation of the extended arm causes traction of the brachial plexus and also causes pressure on the ulnar nerve.
- Pressure necrosis of the heels, shoulder, sacral region and scalp.
- Steep Trendelenburg position can cause respiratory compromise and raise intracranial and intraocular pressure.

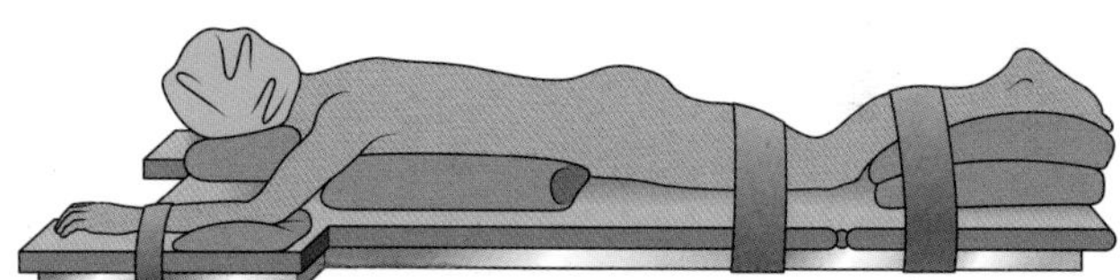

Figure 7.4 Prone position. Padded material is placed under the axillae and extends down to the iliac crest to facilitate breathing.

Prone position

In the prone position (***Figure 7.4***), the patient is intubated and then log-rolled onto the operating bed with the assistance of at least four members of the team. This position is used in spinal surgery and in certain general surgical procedures, e.g. extralevator abdominoperineal excision for rectal cancer.

A common modification of the prone position is the jackknife position, which offers excellent access to the perineum.

Key points

- Axillary and lateral chest rolls are essential to aid in the movement of the chest, abdomen and diaphragm.
- Female breasts and male genitalia have to be carefully positioned.
- Arms may be placed by the side of the head by reversing the arm boards with care taken to avoid shoulder dislocation.
- Toes should be elevated off the bed by placing pads under the shins.
- Specially designed pillows with a hollow to accommodate the face and endotracheal tube, while gently supporting the forehead and chin, are also used.

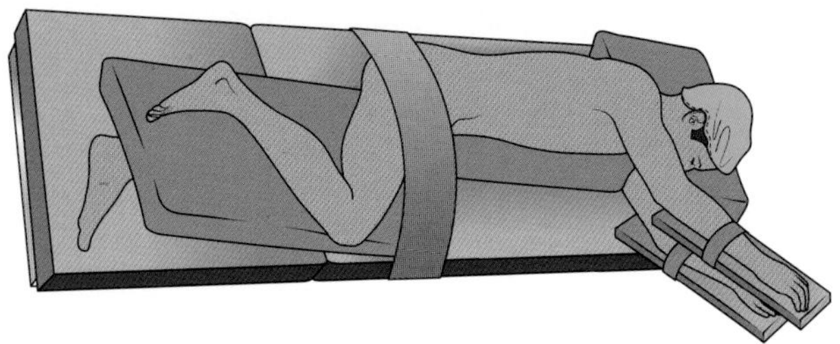

Figure 7.5 Left lateral position with the patient safely stabilised using stirrups and straps.

Potential complications

- Brachial plexus injury and shoulder dislocation.
- Facial trauma, including blindness secondary to vascular congestion of the eye.
- Pressure necrosis of the breasts, external genitalia and pressure-bearing bony prominences.
- Displacement of the endotracheal tube

Lateral position

Left or right lateral positioning (***Figure 7.5***) are useful alternatives to prone positioning in many circumstances, such as the drainage of perianal or pilonidal abscesses. The lateral position also allows for good access to the thorax when performing a lateral thoracotomy. A modified lateral position, commonly referred to as the 'kidney position', can aid in urological and retroperitoneal procedures by increasing the distance between the costal margin and the iliac bone. This is achieved by 'breaking the table' or angulating the table with the summit near the middle of the table and the two ends sloping away.

Key points

- The lower leg is slightly flexed at the knee, a pillow is placed between both the legs and the upper leg is flexed in a more exaggerated position.
- The arms are usually placed in stirrups.
- Maintaining cervical alignment of the head is very important.

Potential complications

- Respiratory complications secondary to preferential ventilation of one lung over the other and accidental endobronchial migration of the tube.
- Traction injury of the brachial plexus and ulnar nerve injury.
- Corneal abrasions and ocular trauma.

Lithotomy and Lloyd-Davies position

This is commonly employed for gynaecological, perineal and urological procedures. The patient is positioned supine with the legs flexed at the hip and knee and placed in stirrups. In the lithotomy position the hips are flexed to 90°; however, the degree of hip and knee flexion can be controlled depending upon the type of procedure performed (***Figure 7.3***). The Lloyd-Davies position is a modification of the lithotomy position with hips minimally flexed to around 15° with a 30° head-down tilt.

Key points

- Both legs are simultaneously placed in the stirrups.
- The fingers should not extend past the edge of the table as they can be crushed or even amputated accidentally.
- The legs should not be externally rotated or unduly abducted.
- Sequential compression devices may be useful to prevent venous stasis, especially in major operations.

Potential complications

- Venous and arterial insufficiency in long procedures can lead to limb ischaemia and compartment syndrome, besides having a higher chance of deep venous thrombosis.
- Digital amputation at the edge of the bed.
- Hyperflexion can cause damage to the sciatic nerve.
- Saphenous and peroneal neuropraxia when legs are placed in the stirrups.

PREPARATION OF THE SURGICAL SITE

Correct skin preparation can reduce surgical site infection (SSI). The steps involved in preparing the skin prior to making an incision are described below.

Removal of metals and other foreign bodies

Removal of piercings and rings from the surgical site is important as they often act as a nidus for infection; metallic objects could also potentially lead to thermal injury when diathermy is used. In addition, finger rings or toe rings can cause digital vascular compromise if there is postoperative oedema following operations on the extremities.

Hair removal from the surgical site

Hair is removed from the surgical site when it is deemed to interfere with the operation; it also makes postoperative plaster or dressing changes relatively pain free. However, removal of hair causes microabrasions and can potentially cause cellulitis and SSI.

Timing of hair removal

The ideal time and place for hair removal is on the operating table after a dose of prophylactic antibiotic is given. Preoperative removal of hair outside the confines of the operating room is discouraged.

Method of hair removal

Skin clippers with disposable blades are preferred as they are safe and result in the fewest SSIs. Shaving using a razor blade is discouraged as unintended microincisions caused by the blade often result in exaggerated skin infection and inflammation.

Skin antisepsis

Skin antisepsis removes transient organisms and dirt, thereby preventing SSI. The principles involved in skin antisepsis are as follows.

- The use of alcohol-based antiseptic solution is recommended. The World Health Organization recommends the use of chlorhexidine alcohol; however, the clinical difference between povidone–iodine and chlorhexidine is marginal and therefore the use of any alcohol-based antiseptic solution is acceptable.
- Extensions of the main incision, additional incisions and drain placement have to be factored in when planning the preparation of the surgical site.
- A slender cotton-tipped swab can be used to clean the umbilicus when preparing for an abdominal procedure.
- In contaminated or dirty wounds it is advisable to start from an area of lower bacterial contamination and move towards a region with greater contamination. However, in clean procedures, starting from the area where skin incision is likely to be made and working towards the periphery is advised.
- Using concentric circles, horizontal or vertical lines do not make a difference in preventing SSI.
- It is important to allow the antiseptic solution to dry and to avoid dripping of the solution onto the diathermy electrodes or pooling under the patient.

Draping

Draping is the process of forming a sterile perimeter around the operating site using disposable or reusable sterile sheets. The drape sheets ideally serve to form a fluid-resistant barrier; they are antistatic, flame resistant, lint free and, although waterproof, are porous enough to prevent heat build-up.

Each procedure has a unique method of draping; this is beyond the scope of this chapter. However, a few practical considerations are discussed below.

- The drapes are usually placed over the periphery of the area that has been painted, once the antiseptic solution has dried. This can be aided by dabbing the perimeter with a sterile cloth or waiting for the antiseptic solution to dry.
- It is advisable to stand an arm's length away from the operating table and spread the drapes with arms extended.
- Avoid reaching across the operating table to drape.
- Sharp towel clips pierce the drapes and thereby contaminate the sterile field; they should be avoided if possible.
- If there is any doubt that there could be a breach in sterile technique, then it is advisable to redo the process or at least replace/cover the offending drape.
- Draping non-disposable equipment such as laparoscopic cords, ultrasonic devices, image intensifiers and light handles may be required. Prefabricated, customised drapes are preferred where possible.
- The routine use of transparent adhesive skin drapes (with or without antibiotic impregnation) over the surgical site cannot be recommended based on the available literature.

Summary box 7.3

Salient features in preparing the operative area

- Remove metal rings and piercings from the surgical field
- Hair removal is advised only if it interferes with surgery
- Hair clippers are preferred to razor blades
- Alcohol-based povidone–iodine or chlorhexidine solution for skin antisepsis
- Drape the perimeter of the operative field using sterile drapes

SURGICAL EXPOSURE AND WOUND APPROXIMATION

Skin incisions

Skin incisions (***Figure 7.6***) are made using a scalpel with the blade pressed firmly down at right angles to the skin and then drawn gently across the skin in the desired direction to create a clean incision. It is important not to incise the skin obliquely as such a shearing mechanism can lead to necrosis of the undercut edge. The incision is facilitated by tension being applied across the line of the incision by the fingers of the non-dominant hand, but the surgeon must ensure that at no time is the scalpel blade directed at their own fingers as any slip may result in a self-inflicted injury. Blades for skin incisions usually have a curved cutting margin, while those used for an arteriotomy, abscess drainage or drain site insertion have a sharp tip (***Figure 7.7***). Scalpels should at all times be passed in a kidney dish rather than by a direct hand-to-hand process as this can lead to a needle stick-like injury.

When planning a skin incision a few factors should be considered:

1. **Skin tension lines and cosmesis**. Langer's lines (representing the orientation of dermal collagen fibres) have been used to guide skin incision placement; however, the clinical relevance of these lines has been questioned. The use of relaxed skin tension lines (RSTLs), which follow creases formed when the skin is pinched and relaxed, have increasingly been employed to guide skin incision placement, especially in the head and neck. In practice, placing incisions based on natural body creases and wrinkles can reduce tension on the suture line and camouflage scars.

Karl Ritter von Edenberg Langer, 1819–1887, Professor of Anatomy, Vienna, Austria, described these lines in 1862.

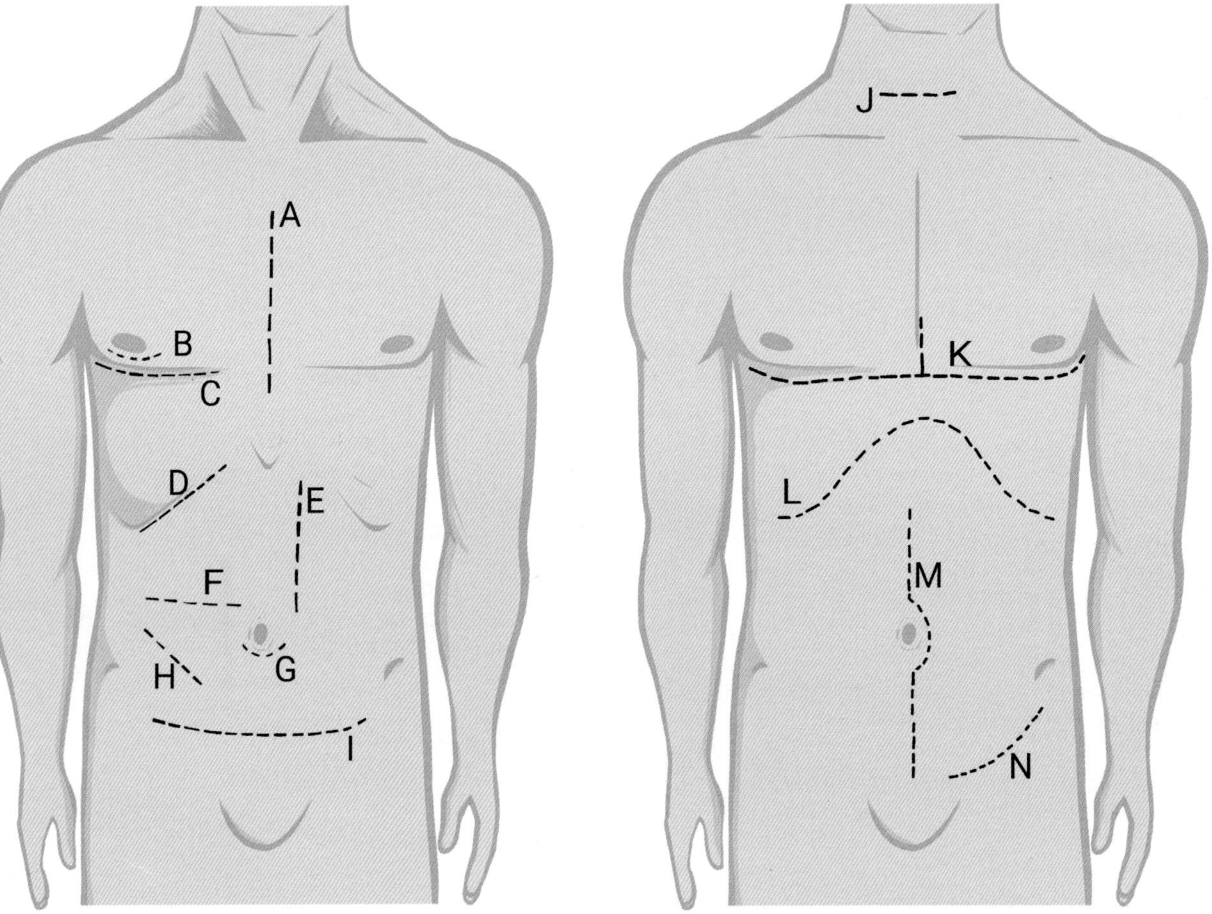

Figure 7.6 Skin incisions in general surgery. A, sternotomy; B, periareolar; C, inframammary; D, subcostal; E, paramedian; F, transverse; G, periumbilical; H, McBurney's; I, Pfannenstiel; J, Kocher's incision for thyroidectomy; K, clamshell thoracotomy; L, chevron incision; M, midline incision; N, inguinal incision (courtesy of Dr Vinay Timothy Kuruvilla).

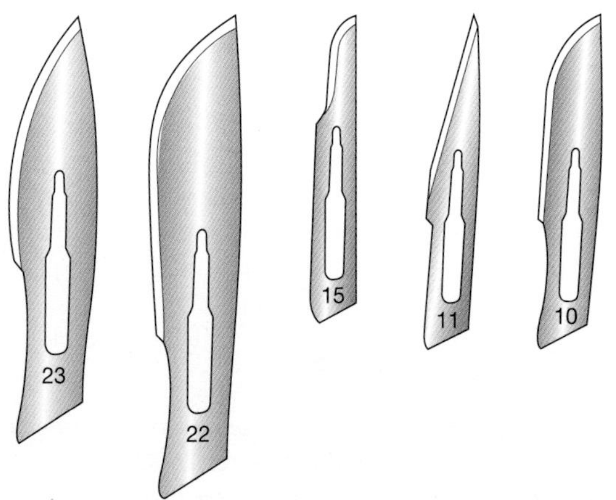

Figure 7.7 Scalpel blade sizes and shapes. The 22-blade is often used for abdominal incisions, the 11-blade for arteriotomy and abscess drainage and the 15-blade for minor surgical procedures.

2 **Anatomical structure**. Incisions should avoid bony prominences and take into consideration underlying structures, such as nerves and vessels. Surface landmarks, previous operations and body habitus also need to be considered.
3 **Adequate access for the procedure**. The incision must be functionally effective as any compromise purely on cosmetic grounds may render the operation ineffective or even dangerous.

Occasionally, it may be necessary to excise a circular skin lesion. An elliptical rather than a circular incision is preferred to enhance tension-free, aesthetic tissue approximation, remembering the rule of thumb that 'an elliptical incision must be at least three times as long as it is wide for the wound to heal without tension'. Occasionally, 'dog ears' remain in the corner of elliptical incisions despite adequate care having been

Charles McBurney, 1854–1913, Professor of Surgery, Columbia College of Physicians and Surgeons, New York, NY, USA. In 1889 McBurney published a paper on appendicitis in which he stated 'I believe that in every case the seat of greatest pain "determined by the pressure of one finger" has been very exactly between an inch and a half and two inches from the anterior spinous process of the ilium on a straight line drawn from that process to the umbilicus.'
Hermann Johann Pfannenstiel, 1862–1909, gynaecologist, Breslau, Germany (now Wrocław, Poland), described this incision in 1900.
Emil Theodor Kocher, 1841–1917, Professor of Surgery, Berne, Switzerland. In 1909, he was awarded the Nobel Prize in Physiology or Medicine for his work on the thyroid.

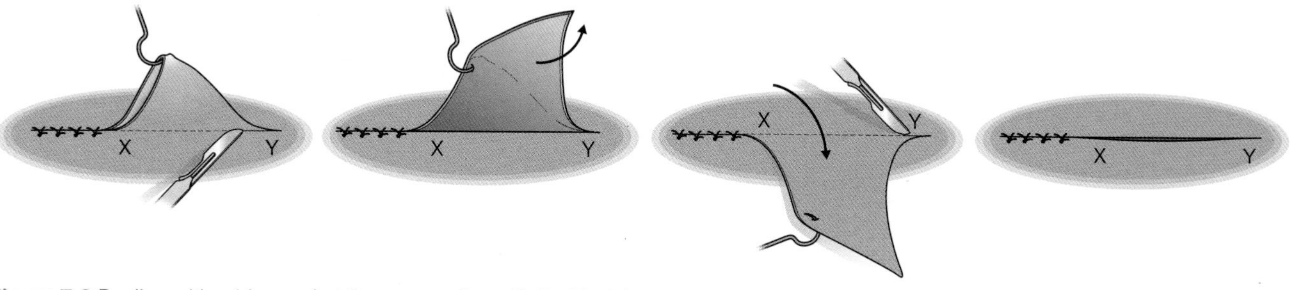

Figure 7.8 Dealing with a 'dog ear' at the corner of an elliptical incision.

taken during the formation and primary closure of an elliptical wound. In these situations, it is advisable to pick up the 'dog ear' with a skin hook and excise it as shown in *Figure 7.8*. This allows for a satisfactory cosmetic outcome.

Surgical access to the abdomen in general surgery

Access to the abdominal cavity can be achieved in many ways and the exposure required will depend on the surgical pathology anticipated, procedure performed and expertise of the surgeon (*Summary box 7.4*).

> **Summary box 7.4**
>
> Surgical exposure of the abdomen
>
> **Open surgical exposure**
> - Intraperitoneal access
>   - Longitudinal
>   - Transverse
>   - Oblique
>   - Pelvic
> - Retroperitoneal access – flank incision
> - Multicompartment access – thoracoabdominal incisions
>
> **Laparoscopic exposure**
> - Multiport, single port, hand-assisted laparoscopy

Scalpel versus diathermy?

Abdominal incisions can be made using a scalpel or diathermy. Recent data suggest that there is no difference with regards to SSI, blood loss or operative time between the two; however, using diathermy resulted in a lower requirement for postoperative analgesia. Usually, it is down to the surgeon's preference as there appears to be no clinically discernible difference.

Transverse versus longitudinal?

Transverse incisions result in less pain, better pulmonary function and fewer incisional hernias but have higher wound infection rates. However, as a rule of thumb, the midline laparotomy is preferred for most emergency procedures as this is quicker to perform and is more versatile.

The steps in performing a midline laparotomy are detailed below. Every incision should be made with closure in mind and based on the suspected site of pathology: an upper midline, lower midline or mid-midline laparotomy incision can be made and extended as required.

1 The first step is to make a skin incision using landmarks such as the xiphisternum, umbilicus and pubic symphysis as reference (*Figure 7.9a*).
2 The subcutaneous tissue is then dissected away, exposing the rectus and the linea alba (*Figure 7.9b*).
3 The linea alba is longitudinally incised close to the umbilical cicatrix to prevent straying into the rectus sheath on either side, thereby exposing the pre-peritoneal fat (*Figure 7.9c*).
4 The pre-peritoneal fat is divided carefully and the peritoneum is picked up between two haemostats and incised using scissors (*Figure 7.9d*).
5 Once the peritoneum is entered, the surgeon's fingers are usually inserted into the peritoneal cavity and the desired length of the peritoneal cavity is opened (*Figure 7.9e*).

Re-entry incisions

Avoid railroading and criss-crossing incisions as they can lead to skin necrosis; it is better to make an incision through the previous scar or excise the scar in total. Extending the skin incision past the previous scar to enter the peritoneal cavity at a virgin plane may help avoid inadvertent injury to the underlying viscera, which may be adherent to the scar.

Laparoscopic access and port placement

There are two fundamental ways to access the abdomen laparoscopically:

1 the open technique (Hasson's or modified Hasson's)
2 the closed technique (Veress needle and/or visual entry trocar).

The advantages and complication rates of each of these techniques are not significantly different; therefore, the technique that the surgeon is most accustomed to should be used.

Harrith Hasson, 1931–2012, Professor of Gynaecology, Chicago, IL, USA.
Janos Veress, 1903–1979, surgeon, Hungary.

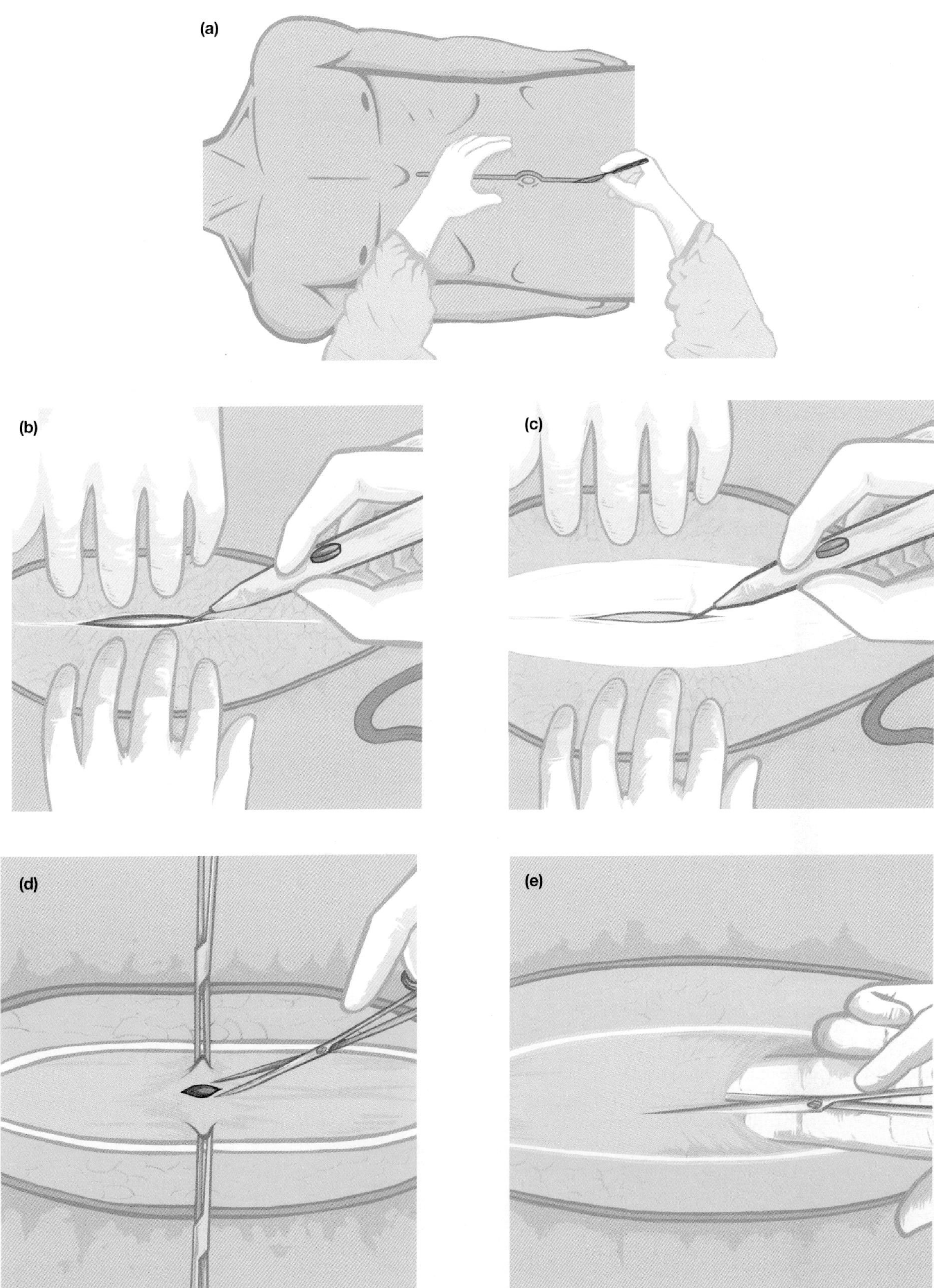

Figure 7.9 Midline laparotomy incision. **(a)** Skin incision; **(b)** subcutaneous fat is incised; **(c)** linea alba is opened to expose peritoneum; **(d)** peritoneum is picked up between haemostats and incised; **(e)** peritoneal cavity opened (courtesy of Dr Vinay Timothy Kuruvilla).

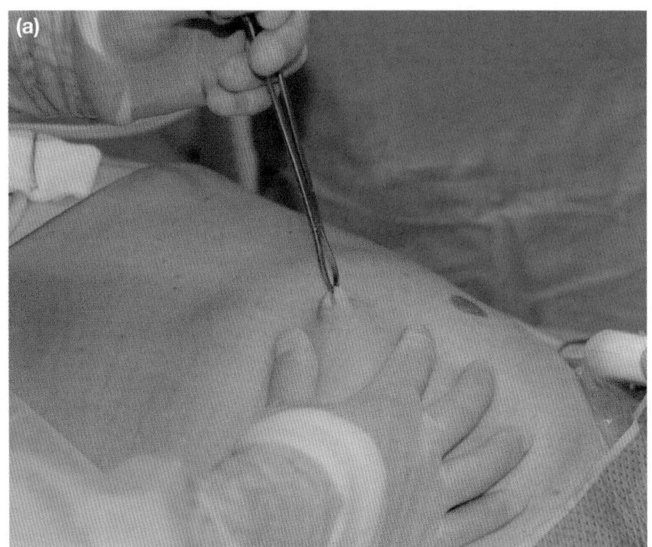

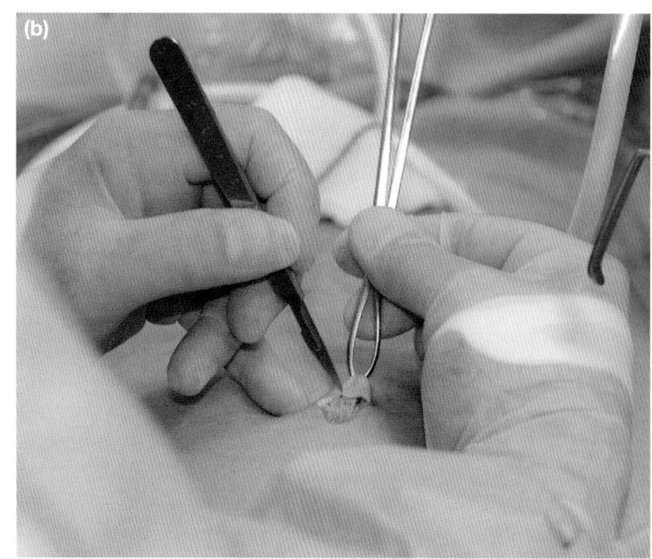

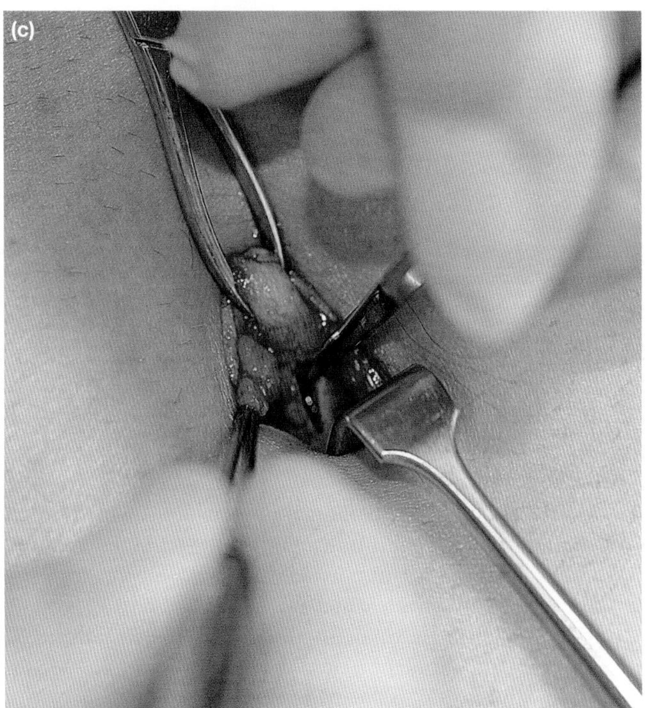

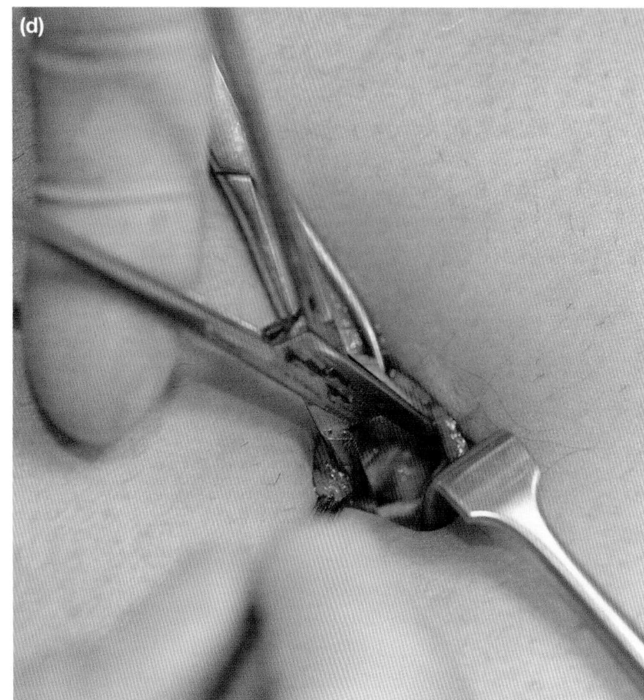

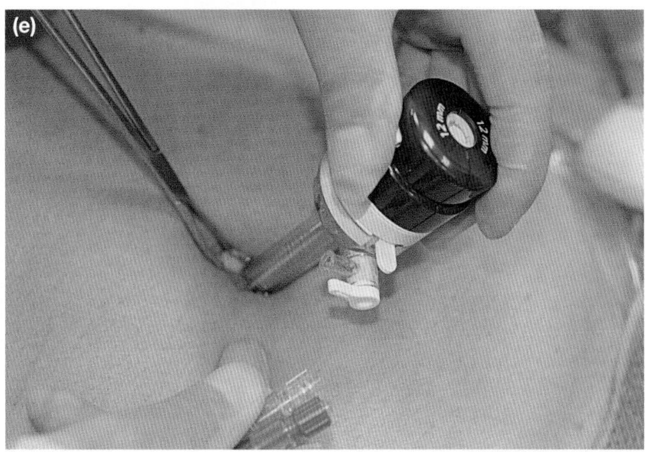

Figure 7.10 Laparoscopic access to the abdomen using the modified Hasson's technique. **(a)** Umbilicus everted, revealing the stalk of the umbilicus. **(b)** Periumbilical skin incision. **(c)** The junction of the umbilicus and linea alba is identified and opened longitudinally. **(d)** A curved haemostat used to break the peritoneum, which is then stretched open. **(e)** A blunt-tipped primary trocar is inserted.

However, a competent laparoscopic surgeon should be familiar with both techniques to provide access as directed by circumstances such as pregnancy, scars from previous operations or as dictated by disease pathology.

Blind trocar insertion with or without Veress needle insufflation is avoided.

Open Hasson's technique for laparoscopic primary trocar insertion

In most cases, the umbilicus is the preferred site for a 10–12-mm initial port placement (*Figure 7.10a–e*).

1 The umbilical cicatrix is everted with a toothed tissue-grasping forceps. It is important to grasp the cicatrix directly as this is closest to the adherent peritoneum. Counter-traction is maintained throughout the subsequent steps until the primary trocar is inserted.
2 The umbilical stalk is palpated inferior to the everted cicatrix while maintaining cephalad traction.
3 A curved 10–12-mm transverse incision is made inferior to the cicatrix.
4 The umbilical stalk is exposed with sharp and blunt dissection to reveal the decussation (crossing) of fibres just above its junction with the linea alba.
5 A 5-mm vertical incision is made through the decussation with an 11-blade scalpel, taking care only to incise the fascia at this point and not to enter the peritoneum.
6 A blunt haemostat angled away from the bowel and major vessels is then pushed through the pre-peritoneal fat and peritoneum; the surgeon will feel a 'pop' as the instrument enters the peritoneal cavity.
7 A blunt-tipped 10- or 12-mm trocar is pushed through the same point of insertion of the haemostat and in the same direction.
8 The laparoscopic camera is used to confirm successful placement in the peritoneal cavity before insufflation with CO_2 gas.
9 CO_2 gas insufflation is commenced at low flow (1–4 litres per minute) and increased to a maximum pressure of 15 mmHg and with a maximum flow rate of 20 L/min.
10 For the patient with scars from previous abdominal surgery, the safest technique is an open approach at Palmer's point, 3 cm below the left subcostal margin in the mid-clavicular line. Adequate lighting and good assistance with retraction are essential.

Veress needle and optical entry

A Veress needle is a spring-loaded needle that consists of an outer sharp bevel that cuts through tissue. Once the needle enters the peritoneal cavity, owing to the loss of resistance the spring-loaded blunt inner stylet deploys and prevents inadvertent injury to the bowel or blood vessels. The Veress needle can be inserted in the umbilical region or in other regions of the abdomen, such as Palmer's point.

The steps involved in Veress needle insertion are as follows (*Figure 7.11*).

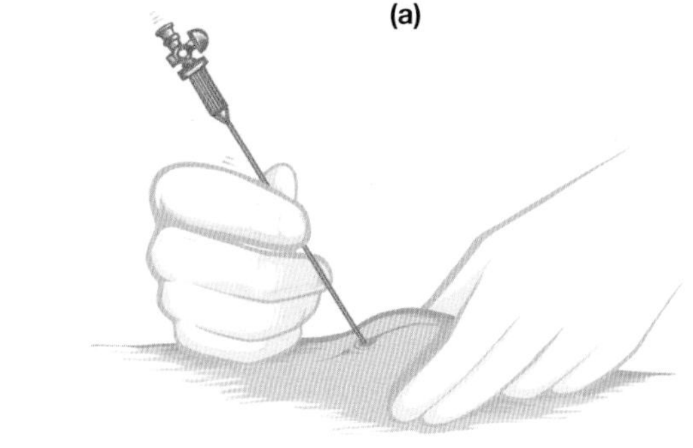

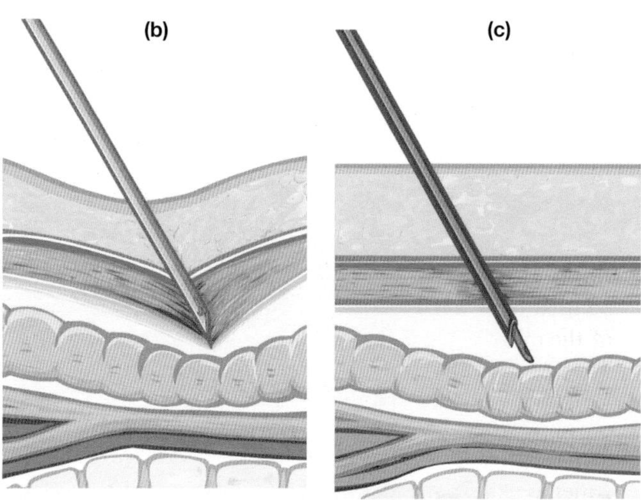

Figure 7.11 Veress needle to establish pneumoperitoneum (courtesy of Dr Vinay Timothy Kuruvilla).

1 A 10-mm incision in Palmer's point (3 cm below the left costal margin, in the mid-clavicular plane) is the location preferred by many surgeons for Veress needle insertion.
2 The needle is advanced until it reaches the muscle. The abdominal wall is then lifted and the needle advanced through the oblique muscles.
3 Classically, a 'pop' is heard and a 'give' felt on successful insertion into the peritoneal cavity.
4 The intraperitoneal placement is confirmed using a combination of the following techniques.
   - The hanging drop method, wherein a drop of water is placed in the hub of the needle; on elevating the abdominal wall the resultant loss of intra-abdominal pressure would result in the drop emptying into the abdominal cavity.
   - Free flow of saline into the peritoneal cavity and no return of bowel content or blood on aspiration.
   - Abdominal pressure reading of less than 10 mmHg.
5 Once the position is confirmed CO_2 insufflation at a slow pace is commenced until the target pressure is reached. The needle is now removed.

Raol Palmer, 1904–1945, gynaecologist, France.

6 Optical primary port placement after Veress needle insufflation:
- The primary port is placed by following the Veress needle track. A visual entry port is recommended as it allows for a more controlled entry under vision. This technique involves the placement of a 0° laparoscope through a transparent optical port, which is tunnelled into the abdomen under vision. The port is advanced with a twisting motion while the camera is held steady.
- The layers of the abdominal wall musculature are seen. When the peritoneal cavity (distended beforehand using the Veress needle) is entered the omentum and intra-abdominal viscera are seen and a gush of air is heard and felt. The 0° camera is subsequently replaced with an appropriate 30° camera if required.
- It is also common practice to use the optical entry method without prior insufflation using a Veress needle.

The basic principles of secondary port (trocar) placement in laparoscopic surgery are as follows:

1 All secondary trocars should be inserted under direct vision to avoid damage to bowel, bladder and blood vessels. A two-handed or controlled single-handed technique should be used to avoid sudden movement, resulting in plunging of the trocar intraperitoneally.
2 Trocars should always be inserted perpendicular to the abdominal wall. Oblique insertion results in increased pressure or torque while instruments are used, which causes fatigue for the surgeon and increased trauma to the patient's abdominal wall. This is of particular relevance in obese patients.
3 A hand's breadth (the patient's hand) either side of the midline represents the extent of the rectus sheath, which contains the epigastric vessels. By placing non-midline trocars lateral to the rectus sheath, usually in the midclavicular line, the epigastric vessels can be avoided.
4 Where possible, smaller diameter trocars should be used as they are associated with less postoperative pain, a lower incidence of port site incisional hernia and better cosmesis. All port sites above 5 mm in diameter should undergo suture closure of the fascial layers to reduce the possibility of port site hernia.
5 All secondary trocars should be removed under direct vision to observe for port site bleeding.

Summary box 7.5

The benefits of laparoscopic surgery
- Less postoperative pain
- Better cosmesis
- Earlier return to normal physiology
- Shorter hospital stays
- Fewer intraoperative adhesions created
- Better perception of anatomy as image is often magnified

WOUND CLOSURE AND SUTURING TECHNIQUE

The suturing of an incision or wound needs to take into consideration the site and tissues involved. There is no ideal wound closure technique that would be appropriate for all situations, and the ideal suture has yet to be produced, although many of the desired characteristics are listed in ***Summary box 7.6***.

Summary box 7.6

Suture material: desired characteristics
- Easy to handle
- Predictable behaviour in tissues
- Predictable tensile strength
- Sterile
- Glides through tissues easily
- Secure knotting ability
- Inexpensive
- Minimal tissue reaction
- Non-capillary
- Non-allergenic
- Non-carcinogenic

Clean wounds with a good blood supply heal by primary intention and so closure simply requires accurate apposition of the wound edges. However, if a wound is left open, it heals by secondary intention through the formation of granulation tissue, which is tissue composed of capillaries, fibroblasts and inflammatory cells. Wound contraction and epithelialisation assist in ultimate healing, but the process may take several weeks or months. Delayed primary closure or tertiary intention is utilised when there is a high probability of the wound being infected. The wound is left open for a few days and if the infective process is resolved then the wound is closed to heal by primary intention. Skin grafting is another form of tertiary intention healing.

Summary box 7.7

Types of wound healing
- Primary intention – clean wounds that are often sutured together
- Secondary intention – healthy granulation tissue filling up an open wound
- Tertiary intention – delayed closure or skin grafting

Suture characteristics

There are five characteristics of any suture material that need to be considered:

1 **Physical structure**: monofilament or multifilament.
- Monofilament sutures are smooth and tend to slide through tissues easily, but are more difficult to knot effectively. Such material can be easily damaged by gripping it with a needle holder and this can lead to fracture of the suture.
- Multifilament or braided sutures are much easier to knot but have a surface area of several thousand times that of monofilament sutures and thus have a capillary

action and interstices where bacteria may lodge and be responsible for persistent infection or sinuses. To overcome some of these problems, certain materials are produced as a braided suture that is coated with silicone to make it smooth.

2 **Strength**: the strength of a suture depends upon its constituent material, thickness and its response to various tissues and circumstances. Suture material thickness is classified according to its diameter in tenths of a millimetre. The tensile strength of a suture can be expressed as the force required to break it when pulling the two ends apart. Absorbable sutures show decay of this strength with time. Although the material may last in the tissues for the stated period in the manufacturer's product profile, its tensile strength cannot be relied on *in vivo* for this entire period.

   Materials such as catgut (no longer in use in the UK) have a tensile strength of only about a week while polydioxanone sulphate (PDS) will remain strong in the tissues for several weeks. However, even non-absorbable sutures do not necessarily maintain their strength indefinitely. Non-absorbable materials of synthetic origin, such as polypropylene, probably retain their tensile strength indefinitely, whereas non-absorbable materials of biological origin, such as silk, will fragment with time and lose their strength, and such materials should never be used in vascular anastomoses for fear of late fistula formation.

3 **Tensile behaviour**: suture materials behave differently depending upon their deformability and flexibility. Some may be 'elastic', in which case the material will return to its original length once any tension is released, while others may be 'plastic', in which case this phenomenon does not occur. Many synthetic materials demonstrate 'memory', which means they keep curling up in the shape that they adopted within the packaging. A sharp but gentle pull on the suture material helps to diminish this memory, but the more memory a suture material has, the less is the knot security.

4 **Absorbability**: suture materials may be non-absorbable (***Table 7.1***) or absorbable (***Table 7.2***).

5 **Biological behaviour**: the biological behaviour of suture materials within the tissues depends upon the constituent raw material. Biological or natural sutures, such as catgut, are proteolysed, but this involves a process that is not entirely predictable and can cause local irritation; therefore, such materials are seldom used. Man-made synthetic polymers are hydrolysed and their disappearance in the tissues is more predictable. The presence of pus, urine or faeces influences the final result and renders the outcome more unpredictable.

Needles

Most needles in present practice are eyeless, or 'atraumatic', with the suture material embedded within the shank of the needle. The needle has three main parts:

1 shank;
2 body;
3 point.

The needle should be grasped by the needle holder approximately one-third of the way back from the rear of the needle, avoiding both the shank and the point.

The body of the needle is either round, triangular or flattened. Round-bodied needles gradually taper to a point, while triangular needles have cutting edges along all three sides. The point of the needle can be round with a tapered end, conventional cutting, which has the cutting edge facing the inside of the needle's curvature, or reversed cutting, in which the cutting edge is on the outside.

Round-bodied needles are designed to separate tissue fibres rather than cut through them and are commonly used in intestinal and cardiovascular surgery. Cutting needles are used where tough or dense tissue needs to be sutured, such as skin and fascia. Blunt-ended needles are now being advocated in certain situations, such as the closure of the abdominal wall, to diminish the risk of needle-stick injuries in this era of virally transmitted disorders. The choice of needle shape tends to be dictated by the accessibility of the tissue to be sutured, and the more confined the operative space, the more curved the needle. Hand-held straight needles may be used on skin, although today it is advocated that needle holders should be used in all cases to reduce the risk of needle-stick injuries.

Half-circle needles are commonly utilised in the gastrointestinal tract, while J-shaped needles, quarter-circle needles and compound curvature needles are used in special situations such as the laparoscopic port site closure, eye and oral cavity, respectively. The size of the needle tends to correspond with the gauge of the suture material, although it is possible to get similar sutures with differing needle sizes (***Figure 7.12***).

When choosing suture materials, there are certain specific requirements depending on the tissue to be sutured.

- Vascular anastomoses require smooth, non-absorbable, non-elastic material.
- Biliary anastomoses require an absorbable material that will not promote tissue reaction or stone formation.
- When using absorbable material, always be mindful that certain tissues require wound support for longer than others; for example, muscular aponeuroses compared with subcutaneous tissues.
- Bowel anastomosis is usually performed using polyglactin, PDS or polypropylene based on the surgeon's preference.
- The size of the needle and suture size used depends on the tissue that is approximated (***Table 7.3***).

TABLE 7.3 Size of suture material.

Metric (EurPh)	Range of diameter (mm)	USP ('old')
1	0.100–0.149	5–0
1.5	0.150–0.199	4–0
2	0.200–0.249	3–0
3	0.300–0.349	2–0
3.5	0.350–0.399	0
4	0.400–0.499	1
5	0.500–0.599	2

TABLE 7.1 Non-absorbable suture materials.

Suture	Silk	Linen	Surgical steel	Nylon	Polyester	Polypropylene
Frequent uses	Ligation and suturing when long-term tissue support is necessary. For securing drains externally	Ligation and suturing in gastrointestinal surgery. No longer in common use in most centres	Closure of sternotomy wounds. Previously found favour for tendon and hernia repairs	General surgical use, e.g. skin closure, abdominal wall mass closure, hernia repair, plastic surgery, neurosurgery, microsurgery, ophthalmic surgery	Cardiovascular, ophthalmic, plastic and general surgery	Cardiovascular surgery, plastic surgery, ophthalmic surgery, general surgical subcuticular skin closure
Contraindications	Not for use with vascular prostheses or in tissues requiring prolonged approximation under stress. Risk of infection and tissue reaction makes silk unsuitable for routine skin closure	Not advised for use with vascular prostheses	Should not be used in conjunction with prosthesis of different metal	None	None	None
Tissue reaction	Moderate to high Not recommended. Consider suitable absorbable or non-absorbable	Moderate	Minimal	Low	Low	Low
Absorption rate	Fibrous encapsulation in body at 2–3 weeks. Absorbed slowly over 1–2 years	Non-absorbable. Remains encapsulated in body tissues	Non-absorbable. Remains encapsulated in body tissues	Degrades at approximately 15–20% per year	Non-absorbable: remains encapsulated in body tissues	Non-absorbable: remains encapsulated in body tissues
Tensile strength	Loses 20% when wet; 80–100% lost by 6 months. Because of tissue reactions and unpredictability, silk is increasingly not recommended	Stronger when wet. Loses 50% at 6 months; 30% remains at 2 years	Infinite (>1 year)	Loses 15–20% per year	Infinite (>1 year)	Infinite (>1 year)
Raw material	Natural protein. Raw silk from silkworm	Long staple flax fibres	An alloy of iron, nickel and chromium	Polyamide polymer	Polyester (polyethylene terephthalate)	Polymer of propylene
Types	Braided or twisted multifilament. Dyed or undyed. Coated (with wax or silicone) or uncoated	Twisted	Monofilament or multifilament	Monofilament or braided multifilament. Dyed or undyed	Monofilament or braided multifilament. Dyed or undyed. Coated (polybutylate or silicone) or uncoated	Monofilament. Dyed or undyed
Common name	Silk	Linen	Steel	Ethilon®, Dafilon®	Ethibond®	Prolene®, Premilene®

TABLE 7.2 Absorbable suture materials.

Suture	Catgut	Catgut	Polyglactin	Polydioxanone (PDS)	Polyglycaprone
Frequent uses	Ligate superficial vessels, suture subcutaneous tissues. Stomas and other tissues that heal rapidly	As for plain catgut	General surgical use where absorbable sutures required, e.g. gut anastomoses, vascular ligatures. Has become the 'workhorse' suture for many applications in most general surgical practices, including undyed for subcuticular wound closures. Ophthalmic surgery	Uses as for other absorbable sutures, in particular where slightly longer wound support is required	Subcuticular in skin, ligation, gastrointestinal and muscle surgery
Contraindications	Not for use in tissues that heal slowly and require prolonged support. Synthetic absorbables are superior	As for plain catgut. Synthetic absorbables are superior	Not advised for use in tissues that require prolonged approximation under stress	Not for use in association with heart valves or synthetic grafts, or in situations in which prolonged tissue approximation under stress is required	No use for extended support
Tissue reaction	High	Moderate	Mild	Mild	Mild
Absorption rate	Phagocytosis and enzymatic degradation within 7–10 days	Phagocytosis and enzymatic degradation within 90 days	Hydrolysis minimal until 5–6 weeks. Complete absorption 60–90 days	Hydrolysis minimal at 90 days. Complete absorption at 180 days	90–120 days
Tensile strength retention *in vivo*	Lost within 7–10 days. Marked patient variability Unpredictable and not recommended	Lost within 21–28 days. Marked patient variability. Unpredictable and not recommended	Approximately 60% remains at 2 weeks. Approximately 30% remains at 3 weeks	Approximately 70% remains at 2 weeks. Approximately 50% remains at 4 weeks. Approximately 14% remains at 8 weeks	21 days maximum
Raw material	Collagen derived from healthy sheep or cattle	Collagen derived from healthy sheep or cattle. Tanned with chromium salts to improve handling and to resist degradation in tissue	Copolymer of lactide and glycolide in a ratio of 90:10, coated with polyglactin and calcium stearate	Polyester polymer	Copolymer of glycolite and caprolactone
Types	Plain	Chromic	Braided multifilament	Monofilament. Dyed or undyed	Monofilament
Common name	Catgut	Chromic catgut	Vicryl®, Novosyn®	PDS	Monocryl®, Monosyn®

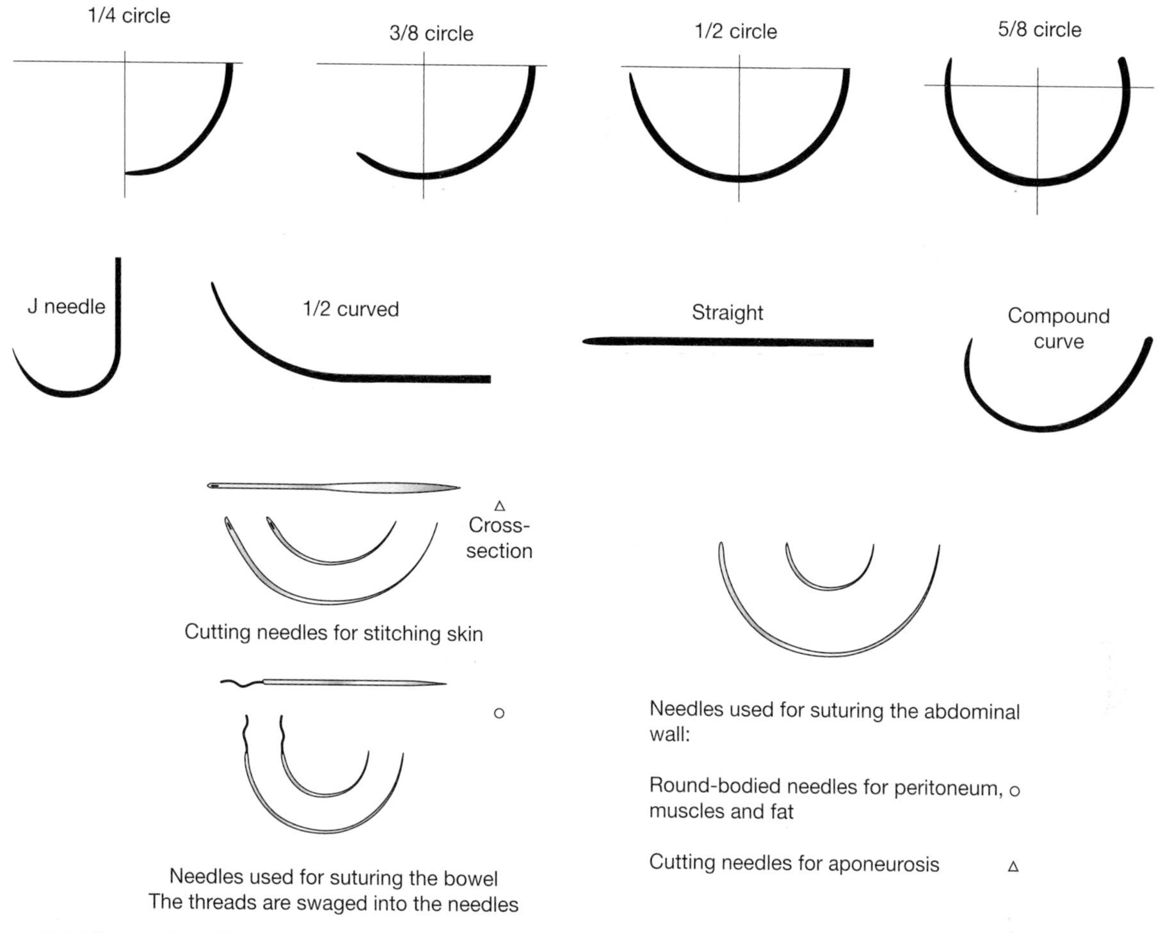

Figure 7.12 Types of needle.

Suture techniques

There are four frequently used suture techniques.

1 **Interrupted sutures**. Interrupted sutures require the needle to be inserted at right angles to the incision and then to pass through both aspects of the suture line and exit again at right angles (*Figure 7.13a*). The needle needs to be rotated through the tissues rather than to be dragged through for fear of enlarging the needle hole. As a guide, the distance from the point of the needle to the edge of the wound should be approximately the same as the depth of the tissue being sutured, and each successive suture should be placed at twice this distance apart (*Figure 7.13b*). Each suture should reach into the depths of the wound and be placed at right angles to the axis of the wound. In linear wounds, it is sometimes easier to insert the middle suture first and then to complete the closure by successively inserting sutures, halving the remaining deficits in the wound length.
2 **Continuous sutures**. For a continuous suture, the first suture is inserted in an identical manner to an interrupted suture, but the rest of the sutures are inserted in a continuous manner until the far end of the wound is reached (*Figure 7.14*). Each throw of the continuous suture should be inserted at right angles to the wound and this will mean that the externally observed suture material will usually lie diagonal to the axis of the wound. It is important to have an assistant who will follow the suture, keeping it at the same tension to avoid either purse stringing the wound by too much tension or leaving the suture material too slack. There is more danger of producing too much tension by using too little suture length than there is of leaving the suture line too lax. Postoperative oedema will often take up any slack in the suture material. At the far end of the wound, this suture line should be secured either by using an Aberdeen knot or by tying the free end to the loop of the last suture to be inserted.
3 **Mattress sutures**. Mattress sutures may be either vertical or horizontal and tend to be used to produce either eversion or inversion of a wound edge (*Figure 7.15*). The initial suture is inserted as for an interrupted suture, but then the needle moves either horizontally or vertically and traverses both edges of the wound once again. Such sutures are very useful in producing an accurate approximation of wound edges, especially when the edges to be anastomosed are irregular in depth or disposition.
4 **Subcuticular suture**. This technique is used in skin where a cosmetic appearance is important and where the skin edges may be approximated easily (*Figure 7.16*). The suture material used may be either absorbable or

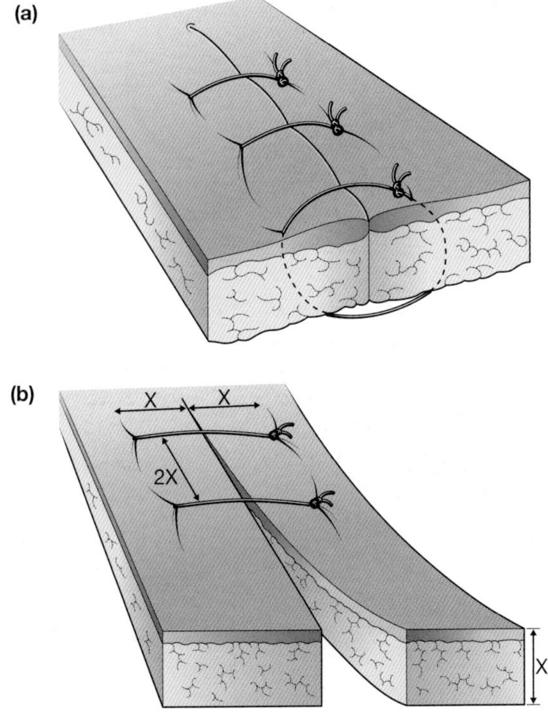

Figure 7.13 (a) Interrupted suture technique. Reproduced with permission from Royal College of Surgeons of England. (b) The siting of sutures. As a rule of thumb, the distance of insertion from the edge of the wound should correspond to the thickness of the tissue being sutured (×). Each successive suture should be placed at twice this distance apart (2×).

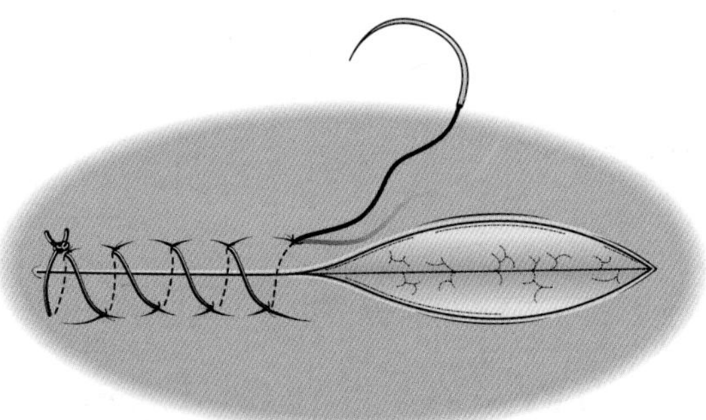

Figure 7.14 Continuous suture technique.

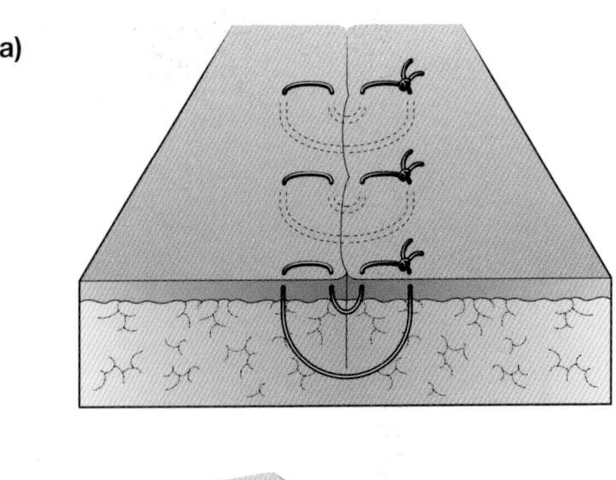

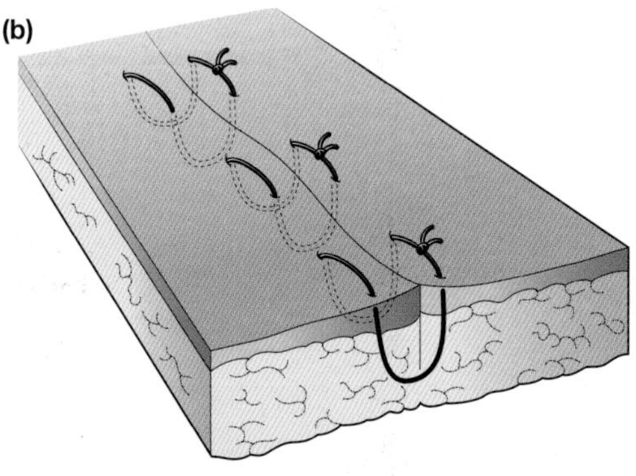

Figure 7.15 Mattress suture techniques.

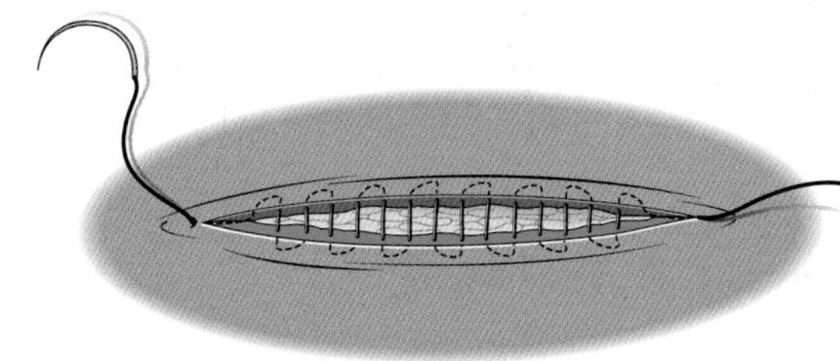

Figure 7.16 Subcuticular suture technique.

non-absorbable. For non-absorbable sutures, the ends may be secured using a collar and bead, or tied loosely over the wound. When absorbable sutures are used, the ends may be secured using a buried knot. Small bites of the subcuticular tissues are taken on alternate sites of the wound and then gently pulled together, thus approximating the wound edges without the risk of the cross-hatched markings of interrupted sutures.

Knotting techniques

Knot tying is one of the most fundamental techniques in surgery and a poorly constructed knot may jeopardise an otherwise successful surgical procedure. The general principles behind knot tying are as follows:

- The knot must be tied firmly, but without strangulating the tissues.
- The knot must be as small as possible to minimise the amount of foreign material.
- The knot must be tightened without exerting any tension or pressure on the tissues being ligated, i.e. the knot should be bedded down carefully, only exerting pressure against counter-pressure from the index finger or thumb.
- The suture material must not be 'sawed' as this weakens the thread and cuts through delicate tissue like a cheese wire.
- The suture material must be laid square during tying; otherwise, tension during tightening may cause breakage or fracture of the thread.
- When tying an instrument knot, the thread should only be grasped at the free end, as gripping the thread with the needle holder can damage the material, resulting in breakage or fracture.
- The standard surgical knot is the reef knot with a third throw for security, although with monofilament sutures six throws are required for security.
- When added security is required, a surgeon's knot using a two-throw technique is advisable to prevent slippage.

- When using a continuous suture technique, an Aberdeen knot may be used for the final knot.
- When the suture is cut after knotting, the ends should be left about 1–2 mm long to prevent unravelling. This is particularly important when using monofilament material.

Abdominal wall closure and laparoscopic port closure

Abdominal wound closure technique

The surgical technique involved in abdominal wall closure varies from hospital to hospital with practice heavily influenced by local opinion and training exposure. The objective of abdominal wall closure is to provide a tension-free closure with adequate strength to prevent early dehiscence or an incisional hernia in the long term.

Most abdominal incisions are closed such that the rectus sheath or linea alba is approximated in a continuous manner using delayed absorbable or non-absorbable sutures employing a five-eighths circle, round-bodied, blunt-tipped needle. However, despite a plethora of meta-analyses certain controversies abound.

- **Layered versus mass closure of the abdomen.** Abdominal wounds can be closed either by closing all layers of the abdomen (musculoaponeurotic layers avoiding skin) together or by closing individual layers of the rectus sheath. An alternative would be to approximate only the anterior rectus sheath in situations where mass closure is not feasible (***Figure 7.17***).
- **Continuous versus interrupted sutures.** Simple continuous sutures theoretically seem to be better than interrupted sutures as the tension is evenly distributed, resulting in less ischaemia; in addition, they are quicker to perform. The literature supporting this practice is, however, sparse.
- **Absorbable versus delayed absorbable versus non-absorbable suture material.** Delayed absorbable monofilament material such as PDS is usually the suture material of choice. In patients with multiple previous operations, non-absorbable material such as nylon or polypropylene may be an alternative.
- **Big bites, big needle versus small bites, small needle.** Abdominal closure is commonly performed by placing the sutures 1 cm apart from each other and 1 cm from the fascial edge. Recent studies have shown decreased incisional hernia when the interval between sutures is reduced to 0.5 cm and performed using a smaller sized needle (2.0 PDS as opposed to the much larger 1 PDS). It is argued that the larger needle causes buttonhole defects when compared with the entry point of a narrow needle and thread. This, coupled with the increased distance between bites, causes the suture to act like a cheese wire through the tissue, thereby slackening the stitch and resulting in hernia.

(a)

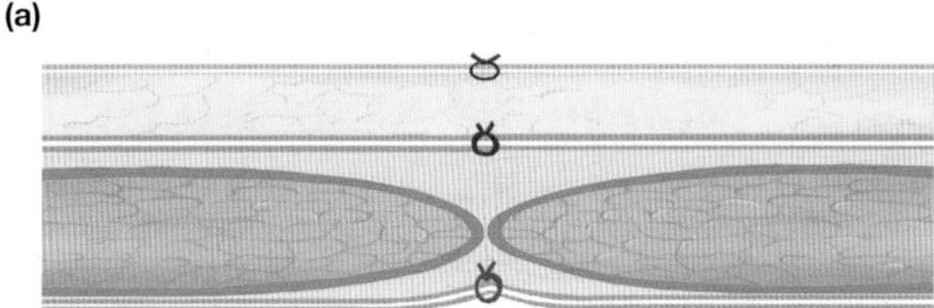

(b)

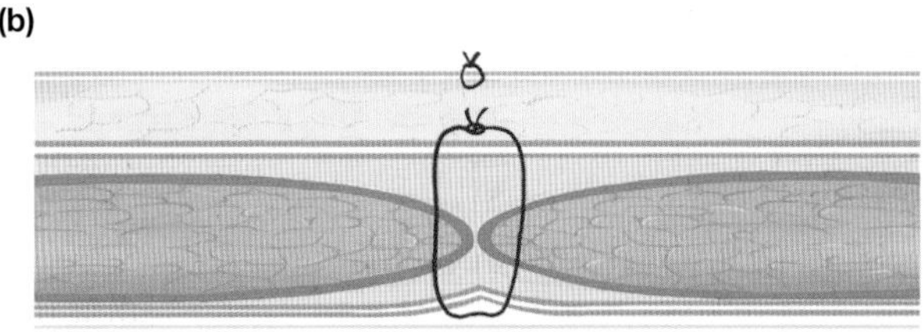

Figure 7.17 Abdominal closure techniques. (**a**) Layered closure. (**b**) Mass closure of all musculoaponeurotic layers (courtesy of Dr Vinay Timothy Kuruvilla).

Despite these variations in practice it is important to provide a tension-free approximation, to avoid subcutaneous fat (as the fat is likely to necrose) and, if employing a continuous suturing technique, to start from the inferior and superior ends with two separate sutures and meet in the middle to aid in better visualisation of the final stitches.

Alternatives to sutures

Skin adhesive strips

Self-adhesive tapes may be used where there is no tension and the wound is clean; for example, adhesive strips are used following clean procedures on the face.

Tissue glue

Tissue glue can be used as a means of primary tissue apposition or as an adjunct to sutures. Some specific uses have been described such as closing a laceration on the forehead of a fractious child in Accident and Emergency, thus dispensing with local anaesthetic and sutures.

Staples

There is a wide range of mechanical devices that can be used to staple skin, bowel or even major vascular pedicles. Most of these devices are disposable and relatively expensive, but their cost is offset by the saving of operative time.

Removal of skin staples or sutures

The timing of removal of non-absorbable sutures depends on the anatomic location, tension with which the wound was closed and the operation performed. It is customary for the operating surgeon to specify the time of suture removal in the operative notes.

While early removal can minimise unsightly scars and prevent sutures from being embedded in the skin, removing them prematurely can result in wound dehiscence.

As a rule, facial sutures are removed in 3–5 days after the operation, neck sutures in 5–7 days and abdominal sutures between 10 and 14 days.

Basic haemostatic methods and the principles of electrosurgery

Bleeding encountered during an operation can be arterial, venous or capillary. Surgical haemorrhage is categorised as primary (during the operation), reactionary (24–48 hours postoperatively) or secondary (days to weeks postoperatively).

Reactionary haemorrhage is usually a consequence of a slipped ligature or when a vessel injury is missed with bleeding temporarily stopped owing to a combination of vasoconstriction and hypotension. In the postoperative period, once blood pressure improves bleeding will ensue. Secondary haemorrhage is often a manifestation of a deep-seated infection eroding into a blood vessel.

As depicted in ***Summary box 7.8***, it is obvious that there is a plethora of devices and techniques to help control surgical bleeding; however, there can be no substitute for adequate preoperative preparation, careful management of antiplatelets and anticoagulants and meticulous surgical technique.

When establishing haemostasis, care should be taken to avoid damage to adjacent nerves and organs, prevent unintentional vascular thrombosis and avoid adjacent tissue injury. Plunging clamps and suturing blindly in pools of blood may cause more damage than serving any purpose.

The appropriate use of different techniques to control haemorrhage will depend on the site of bleeding, the extent of bleeding and the surgical pathology encountered.

Summary box 7.8

Common haemostatic technique used intraoperatively

Mechanical

- Digital pressure
- Ligatures
- Haemostatic clamps and ligating clips
- Vascular stapling devices
- Wound packing
- Bone wax
- Image-guided embolisation

Thermal

- Electrosurgery
- Cryosurgery
- Argon beam coagulation
- Vessel sealing devices

Chemical or topical haemostatic agents

- Physical: absorbable collagen, gelatin, oxidised cellulose
- Biological: topical thrombin, fibrin sealant, tranexamic acid

ELECTROSURGERY

Electrosurgery employs high-frequency electrical current to assist in making surgical incisions, dissection of tissue and achieving haemostasis. Its widespread use in open, laparoscopic and intraluminal endoscopic surgery such as transurethral resection of the prostate have made it an indispensable part of the surgeon's armamentarium.

Despite its uses many avoidable accidents have occurred. It is therefore vital for a surgeon to have a sound understanding of the principles of electrosurgery to facilitate safe surgery (***Summary box 7.9***).

Summary box 7.9

Safe electrosurgery

- Always check diathermy setting before use
- Use the safest, lowest diathermy current setting
- Be careful when diathermy is used near other metallic instruments
- Employ the diathermy intermittently and for brief spells
- Use bipolar diathermy and advanced vessel-sealing devices where appropriate
- Smoke extractors to remove bio-aerosolised particles are essential

The principles of electrosurgery

Electric current is defined as the flow of charged particles through a circuit. Alternating current (AC), a type of current wherein current periodically changes direction, is solely employed in electrosurgery. The time taken to complete one positive and one negative alternation is called one cycle. Frequency, measured in Hertz (Hz), denotes the number of such cycles in 1 second; the more the cycles, the higher the frequency.

Electrosurgical units (ESUs) work by converting electrical frequencies from the wall outlet (50–60 Hz) to high frequencies ranging from 500 000 to 3 000 000 Hz. When current passes through a conductor at such high frequencies, energy is converted to heat, which is used to cut or coagulate tissue.

It is important to bear in mind that human muscle and nerves are stimulated at frequencies below 10 000 Hz; therefore, ESUs must convert electrical frequency to a much higher frequency.

Monopolar and bipolar diathermy

In monopolar surgery (***Figure 7.18a***), the electrical current created in the ESU passes through a single electrode (diathermy pencil) to the tissue, causing the desired tissue effect (cut or coagulation). To complete the cycle, the current then passes through the tissues and returns via a very large surface plate (the indifferent electrode or dispersive cable) back to the earth pole of the generator.

In bipolar diathermy (***Figure 7.18b***), the two active electrodes are usually represented by the limbs of a pair of diathermy forceps, blades of scissors or graspers. Both forceps ends are therefore active and current flows between them and only the tissue held between the limbs of the forceps heats up. This form of diathermy is used when working in sensitive areas (e.g. near the recurrent laryngeal nerve in thyroid surgery) or in patients with implantable electrical devices, as current can interfere with these devices. A separate return electrode (the indifferent electrode) to return current is not needed.

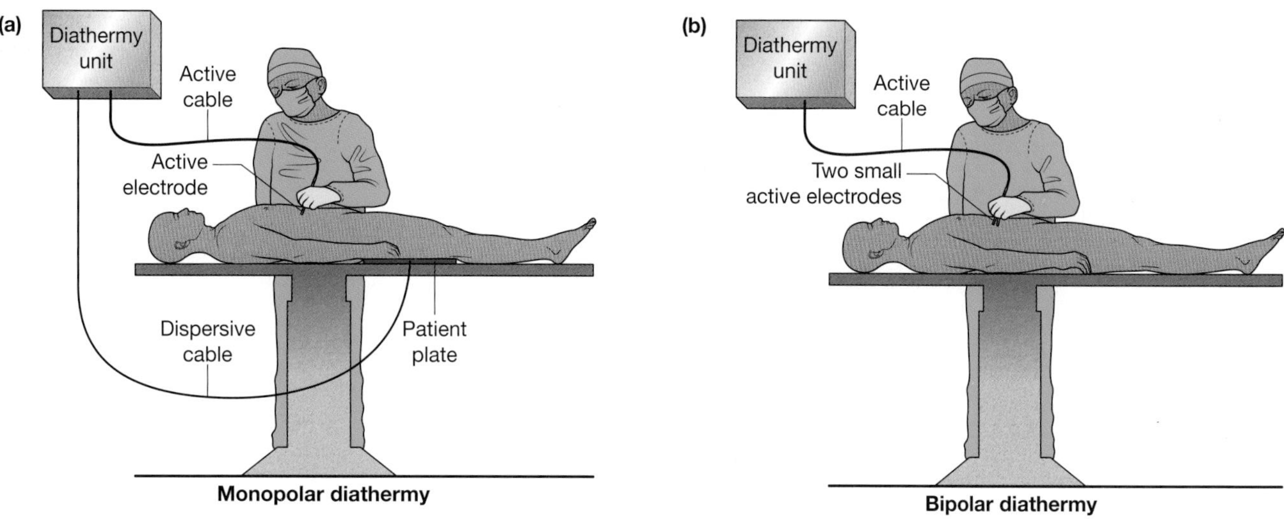

Figure 7.18 The principles of diathermy. (**a**) Monopolar diathermy. (**b**) Bipolar diathermy.

TABLE 7.4 Comparison of cutting and coagulation of tissue using diathermy.

Cutting	Coagulation
Lower voltage current	Higher voltage current
Continuous (current is 'on' 100% of the time when used)	Interrupted (current flows 6% of the time and off for the remaining 94%)
Energy concentrated over a small area	Energy dispersed over a large area
Tissue is heated rapidly and to a higher temperature, causing vaporisation of tissue and thereby resulting in 'cutting' tissue	The modulated current allows the tissue to cool slightly, so tissue heating is slower than with cutting mode. This causes a dehydration effect (loss of cellular fluid and protein denaturation), resulting in coagulation of tissue. Dehydration is not as effective as vaporisation for cutting tissue but is ideal for haemostasis. Bleeding is stopped by a combination of the distortion of the walls of the blood vessel, coagulation of the plasma proteins and stimulation of the clotting cascade
Minimal lateral spread and collateral damage	Extensive lateral spread
Cutting divides tissue by generating sparks, which arc to the tissue; this is most efficient when the tip is held just above the tissue	Similar to cutting and works best when held just above the tissue, with no contact or minimal contact with tissue
Uses: clean cut of tissue To be used to dissect and divide tissue and not just to make skin incisions	Uses: coagulation and achieving haemostasis

The effects of diathermy

Diathermy (***Figure 7.19***) can be used for two basic purposes (***Table 7.4***):

1 coagulation: to achieve haemostasis;
2 cutting: incision and dissection of tissues during surgery.

Several 'blend' options are also available, combining various proportions of the two main modalities.

Hazards of diathermy

Burns

These are the most common type of diathermy accidents and occur when the current flows in some way other than that which the surgeon intended; they are far more common in monopolar than bipolar diathermy. Diathermy can also cause thermal injury to the surgeon and theatre staff.

These may occur as a result of:

- Faulty application of the indifferent electrode (footplate) with an inadequate contact area.
- The patient being earthed by touching any metal object, e.g. the Mayo table, the bar of an anaesthetic screen or a leg touching the metal stirrups used in maintaining the lithotomy position.
- Faulty insulation of the diathermy leads.
- Inadvertent activity such as the accidental activation of the diathermy or accidental contact of the active electrode with other metal instruments, such as retractors or towel clips.

A hole in the glove can also result in burns to the fingers, double gloving may help prevent this.

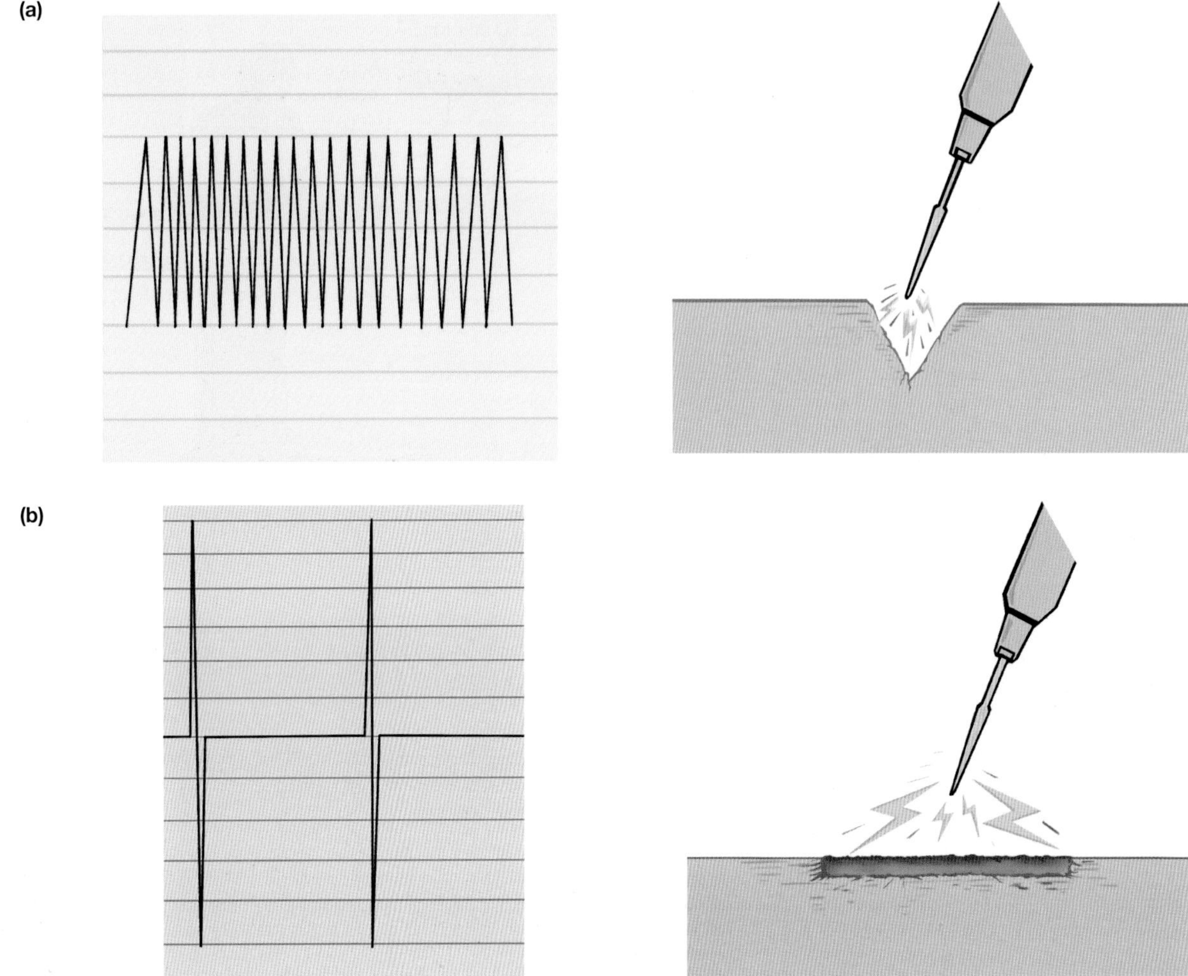

Figure 7.19 **(a)** Cutting and **(b)** coagulation of tissue using monopolar diathermy (courtesy of Dr Vinay Timothy Kuruvilla).

Electrocution

Today, diathermy machines are manufactured to very high safety standards, which minimise the risk. However, as with any electrical instrument, there must be regular and expert servicing.

Explosion

Sparks from the diathermy unit can ignite volatile or inflammable gas or fluid within the theatre. Alcohol-based skin preparation can catch fire if allowed to pool on or around the patient. It may be difficult to detect these flames early on as they may be invisible under the bright operating theatre lights.

Channelling

Channelling of current happens when current is applied to tissues that have a narrow stalk, resulting in a 'bottleneck' causing current to concentrate and thereby damage or char tissue. Channelling is also used to describe a phenomenon wherein distant tissues may be affected if current contacts and then travels through tissue, resulting in unintentional coagulation of distant tissue. For example:

- coagulation of the penis in a child undergoing circumcision;
- coagulation of the spermatic cord when the electrode is applied to the testis.

In such situations, diathermy should not be used; if it is necessary, then bipolar diathermy should be employed.

Interference with implantable electronic devices

Diathermy currents can interfere with the working of a gastric or cardiac pacemaker, implantable cardioverter defibrillator, cochlear implants, etc. The use of an ultrasonic scalpel and bipolar diathermy are relatively safer; it may be prudent to liaise with the cardiology team and the anaesthetist pre-emptively in such circumstances.

Occupational hazard from surgical smoke

Viral particles, bacteria, respiratory and ophthalmic irritants and carcinogens have been identified in surgical smoke from diathermy devices. Universal precautions, smoke evacuation systems or simple suction devices can be used to minimise the risk to theatre personnel.

Laparoscopic surgery and diathermy injuries

Diathermy burns are a particular hazard in laparoscopic surgery owing to a relative lack of visibility of the entire instrument. Such burns may occur by:

- faulty insulation of any of the laparoscopic instruments or equipment;
- intraperitoneal contact of the diathermy with another metal instrument while activating the pedal (direct coupling);
- inadvertent activation of the pedal while the diathermy tip is out of the vision of the camera;
- retained heat in the diathermy tip touching susceptible structures, such as the bowel.

Advanced vessel-sealing devices

Advanced laparoscopic procedures have driven a parallel explosion in novel technologies that facilitate the performance of such procedures. This is particularly the case for vessel-sealing devices. Monopolar diathermy still plays a vital and effective role in laparoscopic surgery, but has limitations in terms of sealing larger blood vessels and is accompanied by the risks outlined above. Therefore surgeons have increasingly used advanced energy devices to facilitate dissection and to seal and divide blood vessels up to 7 mm in diameter.

Furthermore, it is suggested that the use of advanced vessel-sealing devices reduces operative time and thus recovery is enhanced.

There are three main types of advanced energy devices: bipolar electrosurgery, ultrasonic electrosurgery and combination devices. In all cases, the surgeon needs to be aware of the characteristics of these devices and their capacity to cause thermal injury in order to use them safely.

Bipolar electrosurgery devices

Advanced bipolar tissue fusion technology is a vessel-sealing system that is used in both open and laparoscopic surgery by fusing the vessel walls to create a permanent seal. It uses a combination of pressure and energy to create vessel fusion that can withstand up to three times the normal systolic pressure. New technology such as the LigaSure™ system (Medtronic) involves advanced bipolar technology that uses the body's collagen and elastin to both seal and divide, allowing surgeons to reduce instrument handling when dissecting, ligating and grasping – a valuable asset particularly during laparoscopic surgery. The feedback-sensing technology incorporated in the instrument is designed to manage the energy delivery in a precise manner and results in automatic discontinuation of energy once the seal is complete, thus removing any concern that the surgeon has to use guesswork as to when the seal is complete. The newer instruments actively monitor tissue impedance and provide a real-time adjustment of the energy being delivered. Using this technology, LigaSure can seal vessels of up to 7 mm diameter, with an average seal time of 2–4 seconds, as well as pedicles, tissue bundles and lymphatics with a consistent controlled and predictable effect on tissue, including less desiccation.

Ultrasonic energy devices

The harmonic scalpel is an instrument that uses ultrasound technology to cut tissues while simultaneously sealing them. It utilises a hand-held ultrasound transducer and scalpel that is controlled by a hand switch or foot pedal. During use, the scalpel vibrates in the 20 000–50 000-Hz range and cuts through tissues, effecting haemostasis by sealing vessels and tissues by means of protein denaturation caused by vibration rather than heat (in a similar manner to whisking an egg white). It provides cutting precision, even through thickened scar tissue, and visibility is enhanced because less smoke is created by this system during use compared with routine electrosurgery.

Currently, the harmonic scalpel is in common use during laparoscopic procedures, as well as open surgery, such as thyroidectomy, and several plastic surgery operations, e.g. cosmetic breast surgery. There are several such devices on the market, which vary in form and function.

Combination energy devices

In the last 5 years, technology has evolved concerning both harmonic and bipolar advanced energy devices. One product, the Thunderbeat STM (Olympus), has combined both modalities in a single device. By simultaneously using ultrasonic vibration and bipolar diathermy, this device can seal and divide arteries and veins up to 7 mm in diameter in a shorter amount of time with no smoke or mist.

TOPICAL HAEMOSTATIC AGENTS

Physical or biological topical haemostatic agents are considered adjuncts to traditional mechanical and electrosurgical techniques. The physical agents commonly used are absorbable gelatin, absorbable collagen and oxidised cellulose and function by providing a scaffold that encourages fibrin deposition and accelerates clot formation; they can also soak up as much as 40 times their weight in blood, providing tamponade and compression.

Biological topical haemostatic agents such as thrombin and fibrin sealants encourage clot formation and are often injected or sprayed over the bleeding site. A combination of the above can also be used.

DRAINS IN SURGERY

In 1887 Lawson Tait suggested 'when in doubt drain!'. This edict has been criticised and the value of routine drain placement has been scrutinised.

Drains are inserted to allow fluid that might collect in a body cavity to drain freely to the surface. The fluid to be drained may include blood, serum, pus, urine, faeces, bile, lymph or air. Drains may also be used for wound irrigation in certain circumstances. Their use can be regarded as prophylactic or therapeutic, depending on the circumstance warranting their insertion. Abdominal drains are usually placed in the pelvis to drain collections as this is the most dependent area. Other locations are usually dictated by the pathology and procedure performed.

Robert Lawson Tait, 1845–1899, surgeon, Birmingham, UK.

Classification of drains

- **Open drains** (*Figure 7.20a*). These aid in passive drainage of a cavity based on gravity by forming a channel between the body and the external environment. They are often unsightly, require frequent dressing changes and may act as a conduit that enhances bacterial colonisation. The Penrose and corrugated drains are examples of an open drain used in debrided wounds and abscess cavities.
- **Closed drains:**
  - **Suctioned (active)** (*Figure 7.20b*). These maintain negative pressure, thereby actively suctioning out fluid and/or obliterating dead space and preventing fluid accumulation. Caution must be exercised when used adjacent to vital structures. A suction drain is often used after ventral hernia repair, following axillary dissections and in head and neck surgery.
  - **Non-suctioned (passive)** (*Figure 7.20c*). Use capillary action and gravity to drain fluid. The most common examples are urinary catheters, nasogastric drainage systems and a Robinson's drain, which is used within the abdominal cavity to help to evacuate fluid without sucking viscera or omentum.

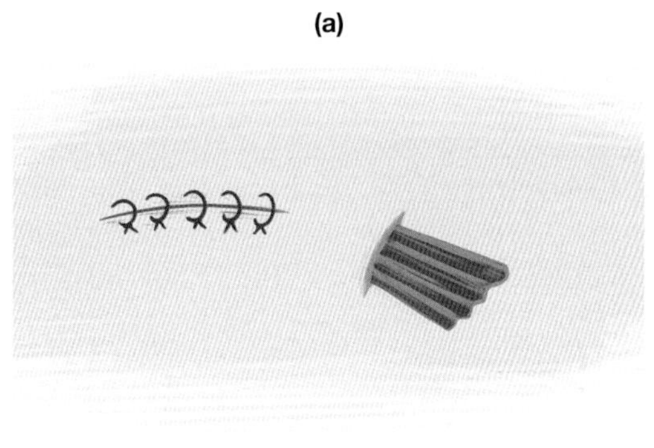

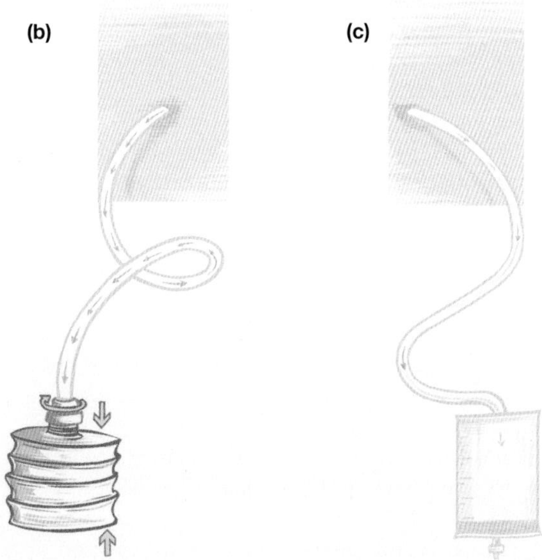

Figure 7.20 Drains in surgery. **(a)** Open drainage of a wound using a corrugated drain. **(b)** A closed suction drain using a vacuum-assisted drainage system. **(c)** A closed, non-suction drain commonly used to drain the abdominal cavity (courtesy of Dr Vinay Timothy Kuruvilla).

The role of drains in modern surgery

The routine use of surgical drains has generated much controversy. Protagonists suggest that the use of drains may:

- help remove the collection of purulent material, blood, serous fluid, bile, chyle, pancreatic or intestinal secretions;
- act as a signal for postoperative haemorrhage or anastomotic leakages
- provide a track for long-term drainage.

However, detractors claim that the presence of a drain may:

- increase intra-abdominal and wound infections by introducing skin bacteria into the peritoneal cavity;
- delay recovery and increase hospital stay;
- increase abdominal pain;
- decrease pulmonary function;
- falsely reassure the clinician that there is no intra-abdominal collection, when in fact the drain is blocked.

In reality, the use of drains depends on the surgeon's individual preference and surgical philosophy. However, there is reasonable consensus regarding the role of drains in certain surgical procedures, as elucidated in ***Summary boxes 7.10 and 7.11***.

Summary box 7.10

Current role of drain placement in non-gastrointestinal surgery

Avoid routine drain placement

- Thyroid surgery
- Breast lumpectomy
- Inguinal hernia repair

Consider routine drain placement

- Radical and modified radical neck dissection
- Parotid surgery
- Axillary dissection with or without mastectomy
- Inguinal lymphadenectomy
- Ventral hernia repair in obese patients

Charles Bingham Penrose, 1862–1925, Professor of Gynecology, The University of Pennsylvania, Philadelphia, PA, USA.

Summary box 7.11

Current role of drain placement in gastrointestinal surgery

Avoid routine drain placement following
- Colonic surgery
- Small bowel resections
- Hepatic resections
- Cholecystectomy

Consider routine drain placement following
- Oesophageal surgery
- Major pancreatic resection

Selective use of drains following
- Rectal surgery
- Gastric resections

Emergency gastrointestinal surgery and drains

While there seems to be some anecdotal evidence advising against drainage following appendicular perforation, duodenal perforation and bowel pathology leading to localised or generalised peritonitis, a less dogmatic approach is more realistic. Patients with four-quadrant peritoneal contamination usually benefit from routine drainage, whereas a more selective approach can be tailored in patients with localised peritoneal contamination.

The decision to avoid drain placement in emergency surgery needs to be contextualised, taking into account the patient's clinical state and comorbid illnesses as well as the healthcare and hospital setting, including access to round-the-clock interventional radiologists.

Specialist use of drains

Nasogastric drainage

The role of nasogastric tube placement in the surgical patient has been steeped in dogma. There is no doubt that selective use of nasogastric tubes have a vital place in the perioperative management of patients; however, there is a trend to move away from routine placement of nasogastric tubes and from keeping them in place for protracted lengths of time when inserted. Most enhanced recovery after surgery (ERAS) pathways forbid the prophylactic use of nasogastric tubes in the elective setting, except following procedures in the upper aerodigestive tract. The indications and potential problems associated with nasogastric drainage have been detailed in ***Summary boxes 7.12 and 7.13***.

T-tube drains

A T-tube (***Figure 7.21***) may be inserted after exploration of the common bile duct and stone retrieval or following repair of a damaged common bile duct. The principle is to allow bile to

Summary box 7.12

Indications for placement of the nasogastric tube

Drainage purposes
- Conservative management of postoperative paralytic ileus
- Conservative management of bowel obstruction (adhesional or partial)
- Decompression of the stomach before an emergency operation
- Prophylactically, when postoperative ileus is anticipated following extensive bowel handling

Feeding purposes
- Following procedures in the upper aerodigestive tract (nasogastric or nasoenteral)
- In patient with motor neurone disease or stroke

Summary box 7.13

Placement of nasogastric tubes

Contraindications
- Suspected or proven base of skull fracture as this may result in inadvertent cranial injury
- Oesophageal stricture or recent oesophageal surgery (unless under vision)

Complications
- Upper airway damage – pressure necrosis of the nasal ala owing to the placement of an oversized tube or following prolonged placement
- Reflux oesophagitis
- Pulmonary aspiration due to impaired function of the lower gastro-oesophageal sphincter
- Inadvertent placement into the lungs
- Traumatic placement causing bleeding and perforation

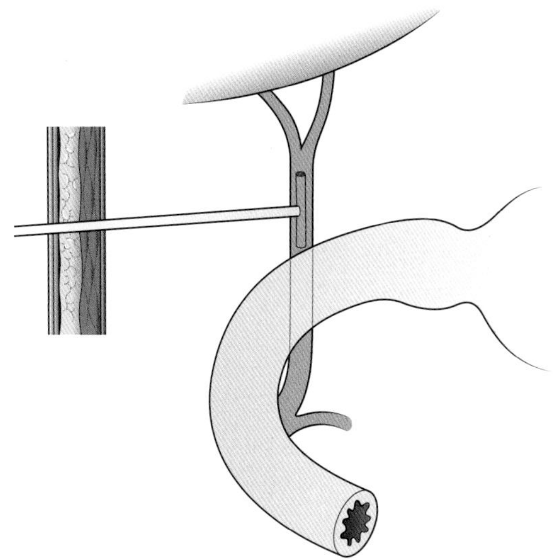

Figure 7.21 T-tube.

drain while the sphincter of Oddi is in spasm postoperatively and to act as a safety valve if there are any stones retained in the distal common bile duct. Despite its perceived uses, the T-tube is not without problems; a recent Cochrane analysis concluded that it is associated with increased bile leakage and increased hospital stay and cost with minimal benefits.

Once inserted, a T-tube should remain in place for at least 2–3 weeks to encourage fistulous tract formation, thereby minimising the risk of biliary peritonitis after removal of the T-tube. Before removal, a T-tube cholangiogram should demonstrate the free flow of bile into the duodenum with no retained stones or bile leak. The T-tube is then clamped for 24 hours and removed. The T-tube is clamped to allow preferential drainage of bile to the duodenum; if there is no distal obstruction the patient will be asymptomatic. Once the T-tube is removed, there will be minimal bile leakage through the fistulous tract for a few days. This should stop as a fistula will close if there is no distal obstruction.

Removal of drains

A drain should be removed as soon as it has served its purpose. It is important to define the objective of each drain and to ensure that, once that objective has been met, the drain is removed rather than waiting for an arbitrary drain volume amount.

- Drains placed to signal perioperative bleeding may usually be removed after 24 hours.
- Drains put in because of infection should be left until the infection is subsiding or the drainage is minimal.
- Drains placed following routine bowel anastomoses should be removed at 3–5 days. However, it should be stressed that in no way does a drain prevent an intestinal anastomotic leak, but merely may assist any such leakage to drain externally rather than producing life-threatening peritonitis.
- A suction drain should have the suction taken off before removal of the drain.
- During removal of a chest drain, the patient should be asked to breathe in and hold their breath, thus doing a Valsalva manoeuvre. In this way, no air is sucked into the pleural cavity as the tube is removed. Once the drain is out, a previously inserted purse-string suture should be tied.

FURTHER READING

Kirk RM. *Basic surgical techniques*, 6th edn. Edinburgh: Churchill Livingstone 2010.

Pignata G, Bracale U, Fabrizio Lazzara F (eds). *Laparoscopic surgery: key points, operating room setup and equipment.* Berlin: Springer, 2016.

Royal College of Surgeons of England. *Intercollegiate basic surgical skills course (participant handbook)*, 4th edn. London: Royal College of Surgeons of England, 2007.

Soper NJ, Scott-Conner CEH (eds). *The SAGES manual. Volume 1: basic laparoscopy and endoscopy.* New York: Springer, 2012.

CHAPTER 8 Diagnostic imaging

Learning objectives

To understand:

- The advantages of good working relationships and close collaboration with the imaging department in planning appropriate investigations
- The basic principles of radiation protection and know the law in relation to the use of ionising radiation
- The principles of different imaging techniques and their advantages and disadvantages in different clinical scenarios
- The role of imaging in directing treatment in various surgical scenarios

INTRODUCTION

Appropriate surgical management of the patient relies on correct diagnosis. While clinical symptoms and signs may provide a firm diagnosis in some cases, other conditions will require the use of supplementary investigations including imaging techniques. The number and scope of imaging techniques available to the surgeon have dramatically increased within a generation, from a time when radiographs alone were the mainstay of investigation. The development of ultrasound and colour Doppler, computed tomography (CT) and magnetic resonance imaging (MRI) has enabled the surgeon to make increasingly confident diagnoses and has reduced the need for diagnostic surgical techniques such as explorative laparotomy.

As a basic principle, the simplest, cheapest test should be chosen hoping that it will answer the clinical question. This necessitates knowledge of the potential complications and diagnostic limitations of the various methods. For example, in a patient presenting with the clinical features of biliary colic, an ultrasound examination alone may give enough information to enable appropriate surgical management. In more complex cases, it may be more efficient to opt for a single, more expensive investigation, such as CT, rather than embarking on multiple simpler and cheaper investigations that may not yield the answer. The choice of technique is often dictated by equipment availability, expertise and cost, as well as the clinical presentation. However, it must be emphasised that, not infrequently, the most valuable investigation is prior imaging; this not only reduces the cost and the amount of radiation a patient receives but very often improves patient care.

REQUESTING IMAGING

Best practice depends on close collaboration between the radiologist and the referrer and must take into account local expertise and access to facilities. When requesting imaging, consider what it is that you want to know from the investigation. Give a provisional diagnosis or state the clinical problem. If there is uncertainty over the best method to answer the clinical problem, then discussion with a radiologist is always worthwhile, informally or within the context of a clinic–radiological meeting or a multidisciplinary team (MDT) meeting.

As well as the basic demographic information stored on the radiology information system, it is important to provide relevant past medical history, e.g. diabetes, epilepsy, renal failure, allergies and anticoagulation, all of which can affect which contrast agent can be given safely, and the date of the last menses in women of childbearing potential.

INTERPRETING IMAGES

While the role of the imaging department is to provide radiological reports for imaging examinations performed, it is nevertheless good clinical practice to be able to evaluate your patients' examinations, and a systematic approach is encouraged.

The systematic approach to examining a radiograph varies according to the part of the body being imaged. For instance, for a radiograph of an extremity, the alignment, the cortices and the medullary cavity of the individual bones, the joints and the soft tissues all need to be assessed on each view.

Christian Johann Doppler, 1803–1853, Professor of Experimental Physics, Vienna, Austria, enunciated the 'Doppler principle' in 1842.

Summary box 8.1

A simple system for checking radiographs

Label	Name of patient
Site	Date of examination
Side (check marker)	
	What part is the film centred on?
	Does the film cover the whole area required?
	Is there more than one view?
Quality	Is the penetration appropriate?
Compare	How have the appearances changed from previous images?
Conclude	Is the diagnosis clear?
	Is further imaging needed?

HAZARDS OF IMAGING

Contrast media

There has been a dramatic increase in the use of contrast agents in recent years, mainly related to the increasing use of CT. Potential problems include allergic reaction and nephrotoxicity. Reactions are rare: serious reactions occur in about 1:2500 cases and life-threatening reactions in fewer than 1:100 000 cases. The risk of sudden death, however, has not changed with the new agents. Local policies for dealing with patients at increased risk vary between departments and, indeed, between countries. Premedication with steroids given at least 6 hours before the contrast can reduce the incidence and severity of anaphylactoid reactions but there is no evidence it reduces the risk of death. Low-osmolality contrast media (LOCMs) or iso-osmolar media are up to 10 times safer than the older ionic media. Most serious reactions occur shortly after injection, so observation of the patient for 30 minutes after injection with the intravenous cannula still *in situ* is recommended for higher risk individuals.

In patients with diabetes or renal impairment, a recent creatinine level should be available. The risks of contrast-induced acute kidney injury are highest in patients with severe renal impairment (estimated glomerular filtration rate [eGFR] <30 mL/min/1.73 m^2), whereas in patients with normal renal function (eGFR >60 mL/min/1.73 m^2) or even moderately impaired stable renal function (eGFR 45 mL/min/1.73 m^2) the risk is zero to minimal.

Contrast should never be withheld if the benefits to the patient of making the diagnosis are felt to be justified by the referring surgeon and radiologist. But in patients with severe renal impairment the risks and benefits of contrast administration need to be carefully assessed and, if contrast is given, the patient should be well hydrated and the lowest dose of an LOCM should be given. The evidence for the use of *N*-acetylcysteine or sodium bicarbonate for renal protection is mixed, and their use is not recommended.

Concerns have been raised about giving contrast to patients taking metformin. Latest recommendations are that it appears safe to continue the metformin if the eGFR is above 30 mL/min/1.73 m^2 for intravenous administration or above 45 mL/min/1.73m^2 for intra-arterial injections. Any decision to stop metformin should be made with the radiologist and the physician managing the patient's diabetes.

Gadolinium-containing contrast agents are used in MRI examinations. Allergic reactions to these agents are very rare, occurring in less than 0.1% of administrations. However, they can be nephrotoxic in patients with renal failure. In addition, they are associated with a risk of nephrogenic systemic fibrosis (NSF), an extremely rare but serious life-threatening condition whereby connective tissue forms in the skin causing it to become coarse and hard. NSF may also affect other organs, including joints, muscle, liver and heart. High-risk gadolinium-containing contrast agents are contraindicated in severe renal failure, in neonates and in the perioperative period of liver transplantation, and are not recommended in pregnancy. However, lower risk gadolinium preparations are available that may be used with caution.

Liver-specific contrast agents for MRI, selectively taken up by hepatocytes, are increasingly used to characterise liver lesions and in cancer staging.

HAZARDS OF IONISING RADIATION

The majority of ionising radiation comes from natural sources on Earth and cosmic rays, and this makes up the background radiation. However, medical exposure accounts for around 15% of the total received by humans. The effects of ionising radiation can be broadly divided into two groups. The first group comprises predictable, dose-dependent tissue effects and includes, for example, the development of cataracts in the lens of the eye. These effects are important for those chronically exposed to radiation, including those using image intensifiers regularly. The second group comprises the all-or-nothing effects such as the development of cancer (termed stochastic). These effects are not dose dependent, but increase in likelihood with increased radiation dose.

The risk of radiation-induced cancer for plain films of the chest or extremities is very small, of the order of 1:1 000 000. However, that risk rises considerably for high-dose examinations such as CT of the abdomen or pelvis, where the estimated lifetime excess risk of cancer increases to the order of 1:1000. Use of CT has increased dramatically in the last 20 years, with a 12-fold increase in the UK, and it has been estimated that up to 30% of these examinations may be unnecessary. Obviously, the risk of such examinations has to be balanced against the benefit to the patient in terms of increased diagnostic yield, and must also be viewed in the context that the lifetime risk of cancer for people generally is about 1:3. Nevertheless, the increased risk is important since it is iatrogenic and applied to a large population. Therefore, techniques that do not use ionising radiation, such as ultrasound and MRI, should be carefully considered as alternatives, particularly in children and young people.

CURRENT LEGISLATION

In the UK, the Ionising Radiation (Medical Exposure) Regulations (IR(ME)R) introduced in 2000, and amended in 2006, impose on the radiologist the duty to the patient to make sure that all studies involving radiation (plain radiographs, CT and nuclear medicine) are performed appropriately and to the highest standards. Inappropriate use of radiation is a criminal offence, so investigations involving radiation need careful consideration in order to prevent wasteful use of radiology.

Summary box 8.2

Criteria for useful investigations

A useful investigation is one in which the result – positive or negative – will inform clinical management and/or add confidence to the clinician's diagnosis. A significant number of radiological investigations do not fulfil these aims and may add unnecessarily to irradiation of patients. To avoid the wasteful use of radiology, the important questions to be asked are as follows.

1. **Has it been done already**? Repeating investigations that have already been done: such as at another hospital, in an outpatient department or in an emergency department. Every attempt should be made to obtain previous images and reports. Transfer of digital data through electronic links will assist in this respect. Although guidelines may not directly address this question, there are other initiatives that do
2. **Is it needed**? Undertaking investigations when results are unlikely to affect patient management or over-investigating: because the anticipated positive finding is usually irrelevant – for example, degenerative spinal disease – or because a positive finding is unlikely. Some clinicians and patients tend to rely on investigations more than others for reassurance
3. **Is it needed now**? Investigating too early: for example, before the disease could have progressed or resolved, or before the results could influence treatment. The need for investigation and treatment should be reviewed at a more appropriate time
4. **Is this the best investigation**? Doing the wrong investigation: imaging techniques undergo rapid change. It is often helpful to discuss an investigation with a specialist in clinical radiology or nuclear medicine before it is requested
5. **Has the problem been properly explained**? Failing to provide appropriate clinical information and questions that the imaging investigation should answer: deficiencies here may lead to the use of the wrong technique, or the report being poorly focused on the clinical problem. In some clinical situations firm guidelines have been established

There are special considerations for portable and fluoroscopy units. The longer an operator keeps the fluoroscopy unit running, the higher the dose of radiation to all in the vicinity. Portable x-ray machines and fluoroscopic imaging equipment use much more radiation to achieve the same result. The staff, and patients in the next bed, are at risk when portable equipment is used. The result is also of lower quality, so portable x-ray machines should not be used unless absolutely necessary. When using the image intensifier, lead aprons, thyroid shields, lead glasses and radiation badges should always be worn. Pregnancy in the female patient or staff must be excluded.

Summary box 8.3

Responsibilities of the radiologist and referrer

- Radiologists have a legal responsibility to keep imaging as safe as possible
- The referrer has a duty to balance risk against benefit
- The referrer must provide adequate clinical details to allow justification of the examination
- Avoid using portable (mobile) x-ray machines whenever practical
- Take all precautions when using an image intensifier
- The gonads, eyes and thyroid are especially vulnerable to radiation and should be protected

The UK's Royal College of Radiologists produces an evidence-based guidance tool, called iRefer, which is widely available on line and shows radiation doses for common procedures (***Table 8.1***).

TABLE 8.1 Band classification of the typical doses of ionising radiation from common imaging procedures.

Symbol	Typical effective dose (mSv)	Examples	Lifetime additional risk of cancer induction /exam
None	0	US; MRI	0
☢	<1	CXR; XR limb, pelvis, lumbar spine; mammography	<1:20 000
☢☢	1–5	IVU; NM (e.g. bone); CT head and neck	1:20 000–1:4000
☢☢☢	5.1–10	CT KUB; NM (e.g. cardiac)	1:4000–1:2000
☢☢☢☢	>10	Extensive CT studies, some NM studies (e.g. some PET/CT)	>1:2000

CT, computed tomography; CXR, chest x-ray; IVU, intravenous urography; KUB, kidneys, ureters and bladder; MRI, magnetic resonance imaging; NM, nuclear medicine; PET, positron emission tomography; US, ultrasound; XR, x-ray.

Source: https://www.rcr.ac.uk/sites/default/files/documents/irefer_introductoryiaea.pdf.

DIAGNOSTIC IMAGING

Basic principles of imaging methods

Conventional radiography

Although it is over 120 years since the discovery of x-rays by Roentgen in 1895, conventional radiography continues to play a central role in the diagnostic pathway of many acute

Wilhelm Conrad Roentgen, 1845–1923, Professor of Physics, Würzburg (1888–1900), and then at Munich, Germany. He was awarded the Nobel Prize in Physics in 1901 for his work on x-rays.

surgical problems and particularly in chest disease, trauma and orthopaedics.

X-rays emitted from an x-ray source are absorbed to varying degrees by different materials and tissues and therefore cause different degrees of blackening of radiographic film, resulting in a radiographic image. This differential absorption is dependent partly on the density and the atomic number of different substances. In general, higher density tissues result in a greater reduction in the number of x-ray photons and reduce the amount of blackening caused by those photons. In terms of conventional radiographs, a large difference in tissue structure and density is required before an appreciable difference is manifested radiographically. The different densities visible consist of air, fat, soft tissue, bone and mineralisation, and metal. Different soft tissues cannot be reliably distinguished as, in broad terms, they possess similar quantities of water (***Figure 8.1***). Manipulation of x-ray systems and x-ray energies, as used in circumstances such as mammography, may allow better differentiation between some soft-tissue structures. Despite this inherent lack of soft-tissue contrast, conventional radiography has many advantages. It is cheap, universally available, easily reproducible and comparable with prior examinations and, in many instances, has a relatively low dose of ionising radiation in contrast to more complex examinations. However, injudicious repeat radiography, particularly of the abdomen, pelvis and spine, can easily result in doses similar to CT.

The lack of soft-tissue contrast allows little assessment of the internal architecture of many abdominal organs. To obviate this problem, techniques employing the administration of contrast material combined with radiography have long been used. These techniques include intravenous urography (IVU) and barium examinations (***Figure 8.2***). IVU involves a series of radiographs taken before and after contrast injection, but has been largely superseded by CT urography, which is more accurate in detecting and defining pathology (***Figure 8.3***). A further modification of conventional x-rays uses fluorescent screens to allow real-time monitoring of organs and structures as opposed to the 'snapshot' images obtained with radiographs. This is used to follow the passage of barium through the bowel, obtaining dedicated images at specific points of interest only. Motility of the bowel can also be assessed in this way. Fluoroscopy is used extensively in interventional radiology, allowing the operator to guide catheters and wires into the patient while monitoring their position in real time.

Naturally, with the more sustained use of ionising radiation, the cumulative doses tend to be greater than when obtaining a conventional radiograph.

Ultrasound

Ultrasound is the second most commonly used method of imaging. It relies on high-frequency sound waves generated by a transducer containing piezoelectric material. The generated sound waves are reflected by tissue interfaces and, by ascertaining the time taken for a pulse to return and the magnitude and direction of a pulse, it is possible to form an image. Medical ultrasound uses frequencies in the range 3–20 MHz. The higher the frequency of the ultrasound wave, the greater the resolution of the image, but the less depth of view from the skin. Consequently, abdominal imaging uses transducers with

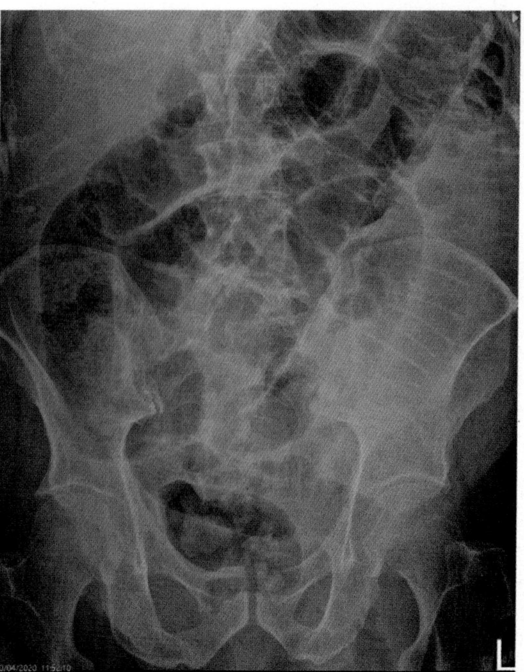

Figure 8.1 Supine abdominal radiograph of a patient with small bowel obstruction demonstrates multiple dilated small bowel loops. The different densities visible are air (within the bowel), bones, soft tissues and fat. The different soft tissues, subcutaneous and intra-abdominal, cannot be differentiated.

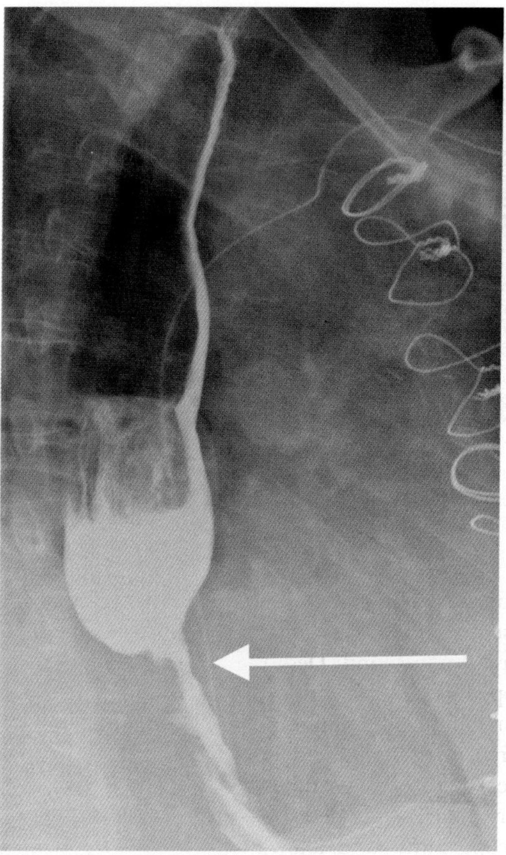

Figure 8.2 Barium swallow examination showing a malignant stricture (arrow) due to an oesophageal carcinoma.

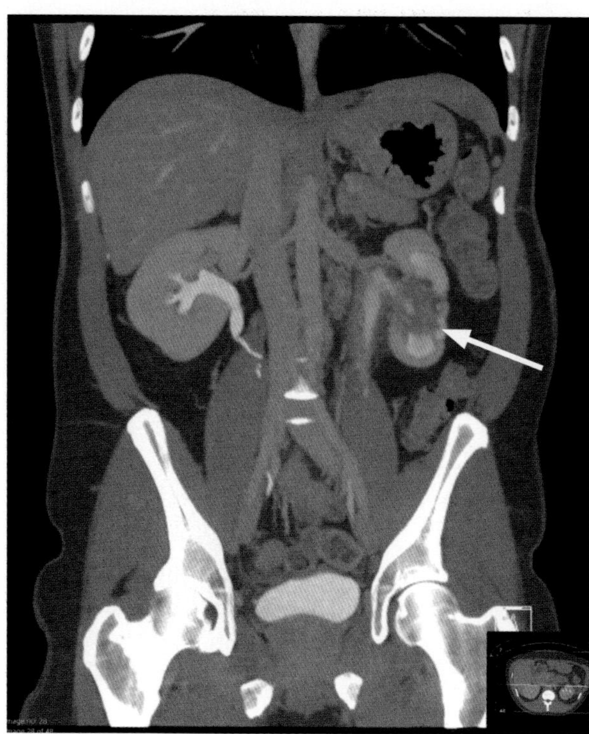

Figure 8.3 Coronal maximum intensity projection image from a computed tomography intravenous urogram shows a transitional cell carcinoma in the left renal pelvis (arrow) with normal excretion of contrast on the right.

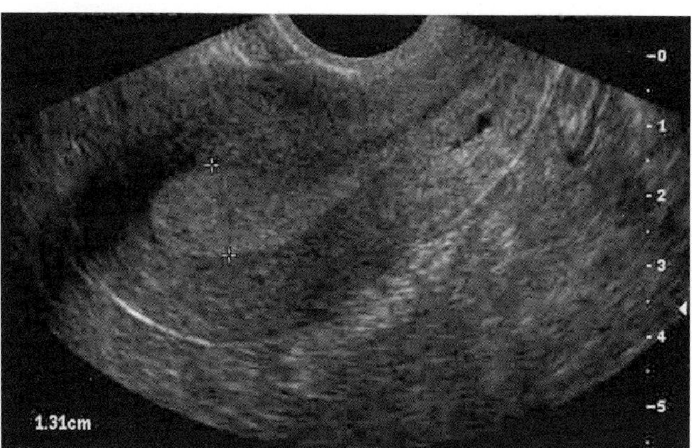

Figure 8.4 Longitudinal transvaginal ultrasound scan of the uterus demonstrates thickening of the endometrium in a patient during the secretory phase of the menstrual cycle.

a frequency of 3–7 MHz, while higher frequency transducers are used for superficial structures, such as musculoskeletal and breast ultrasound. Dedicated transducers have also been developed for endocavity ultrasound, such as transvaginal scanning and transrectal ultrasound of the prostate, allowing high-frequency scanning of organs by reducing the distance between the probe and the organ of interest (*Figure 8.4*). A further application of dedicated probes has been in the field of endoscopic ultrasound, allowing exquisite imaging of the wall of a hollow viscus and the adjacent organs such as the biliary tree and pancreas.

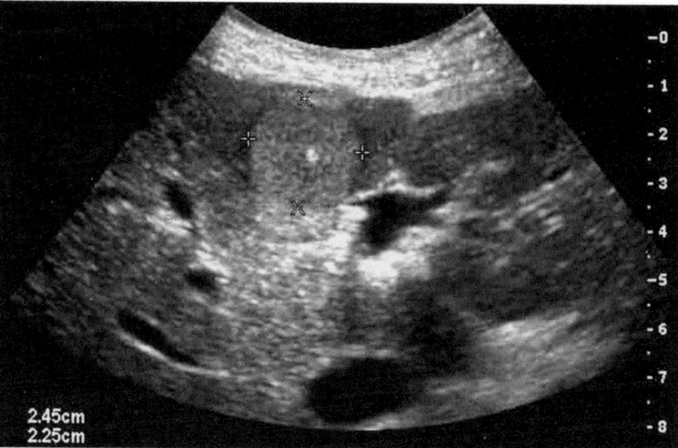

Figure 8.5 Transverse ultrasound image of the liver in a patient with colorectal cancer shows a solitary liver metastasis.

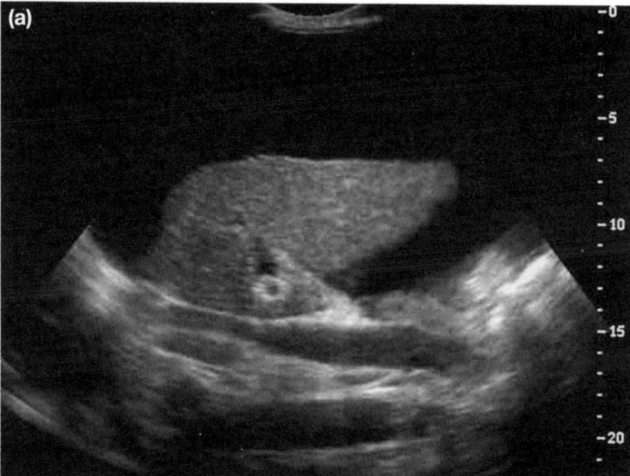

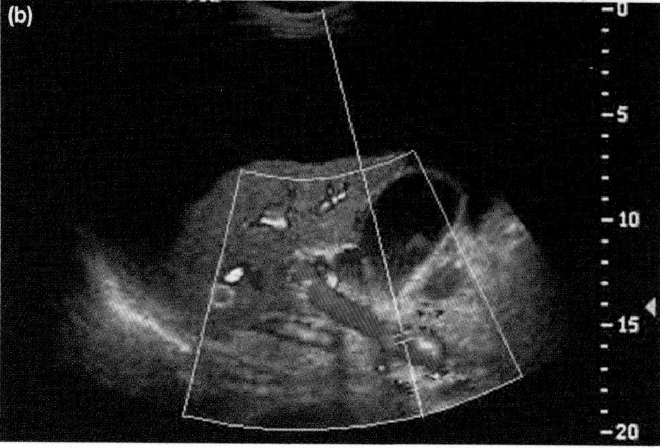

Figure 8.6 Sagittal ultrasound image of the liver (a) in a patient with cirrhosis demonstrates nodularity of the liver surface and extensive ascites. Doppler ultrasound (b) illustrates portal vein flow with a normal direction.

Reflection of an ultrasound wave from moving objects such as red blood cells causes a change in the frequency of the ultrasound wave. By measuring this frequency change, it is possible to calculate the speed and direction of the movement. This principle forms the basis of Doppler ultrasound, whereby velocities within major vessels, as well as smaller vessels in organs such as the liver and the kidneys, can be measured.

Doppler imaging is widely used in the assessment of arterial and venous disease, in which stenotic lesions cause an alteration in the normal velocity. Furthermore, diffuse parenchymal diseases, such as cirrhosis, may cause an alteration in the normal Doppler signal of the blood vessels of the affected organ.

The advantages of ultrasound are that it is cheap and easily available. It is the first-line investigation of choice for assessment of the liver, the biliary tree and the renal tract (***Figures 8.5 and 8.6***). Ultrasound is also the imaging method of choice in obstetric assessment and gynaecological disease. High-frequency transducers have made ultrasound the best imaging technique for the evaluation of thyroid and testicular disorders, in terms of both diffuse disease and focal mass lesions. It is also an invaluable tool for guiding needle placement in interventional procedures such as biopsies and drainages, allowing direct real-time visualisation of the needle during the procedure. Ligament, tendon and muscle injuries are also probably best imaged in the first instance by ultrasound (***Figure 8.7***). The ability to stress ligaments and to allow tendons to move during the investigation gives an extra dimension, which greatly improves its diagnostic value. The use of 'panoramic' or 'extended field of view' ultrasound (***Figure 8.8***) provides images that are more easily interpreted by an observer not performing the examination, and are of particular assistance to surgeons planning a procedure. Ultrasound will demonstrate most foreign bodies in soft tissues, including those that are not radio-opaque.

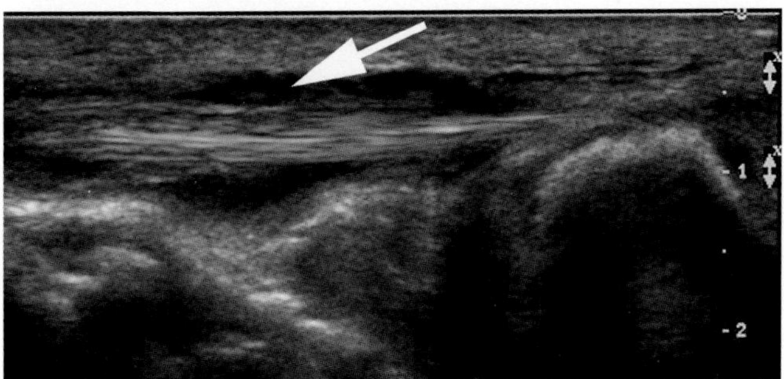

Figure 8.7 Ultrasound of the dorsal surface of the wrist shows the normal fibrillar pattern of the extensor tendons. There is increased fluid (arrow) within the tendon sheath in this patient with extensor tenosynovitis.

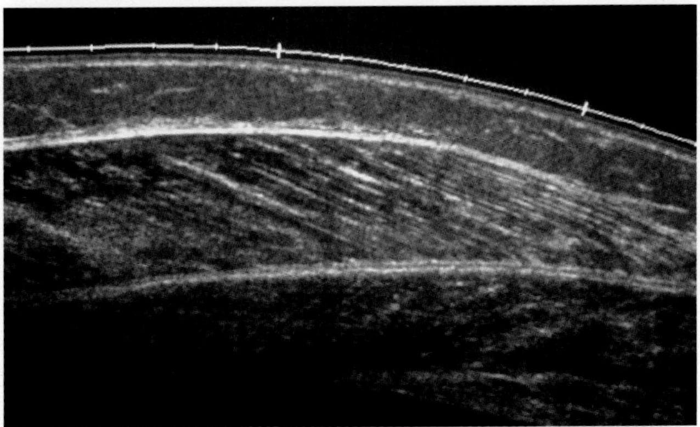

Figure 8.8 Panoramic ultrasound of the calf. The normal muscle fibres and the fascia can be identified over an area measuring approximately 12 cm.

The disadvantages of ultrasound are that it is highly operator dependent, and most of the information is obtained during the actual process of scanning as opposed to reviewing the static images. Another drawback is that the ultrasound wave is highly attenuated by air and bone and, thus, little information is gained with regard to tissues beyond bony or air-filled structures; alternative techniques may be required to image these areas.

Summary box 8.4

Ultrasound

Strengths

- No radiation
- Inexpensive
- Allows interaction with patients
- Superb soft-tissue resolution in the near field
- Dynamic studies can be performed
- First-line investigation for hepatic, biliary and renal disease
- Endocavity ultrasound for gynaecological and prostate disorders
- Excellent resolution for breast, thyroid and testis imaging
- Good for soft tissue, including tendons and ligaments
- Excellent for cysts and foreign bodies
- Doppler studies allow assessment of blood flow
- Good real-time imaging to guide interventional biopsies and drainages

Weaknesses

- Interpretation only possible during the examination
- Visualisation of structures can be hampered by overlying gas and bone, and body habitus may also impact on the scan
- Long learning curve for some areas of expertise
- Resolution dependent on the machine available
- Images cannot be reliably reviewed away from the patient

Computed tomography

There has been a great deal of development in CT technology over the last 30 years from the initial conventional CT scanners through to helical or spiral scanners and the current multidetector machines. CT scanners consist of a gantry containing the x-ray tube, filters and detectors, which revolve around the patient, acquiring information at different angles and projections. This information is then mathematically reconstructed to produce a two-dimensional grey-scale image of a slice through the body. This technique overcomes the problem of superimposition of different structures, which is inherent in conventional radiography. Improvements in gantry design, development of more sensitive detectors and an increase in the number of detectors have resulted in an increase in spatial resolution, as well as the speed at which the images are acquired. In early CT scanners, the table on which the patient was positioned moved in between the gantry revolution to allow imaging of an adjacent slice. Modern scanners allow for continuous movement of the table and the patient during the gantry revolution, thus greatly reducing the scan time. With

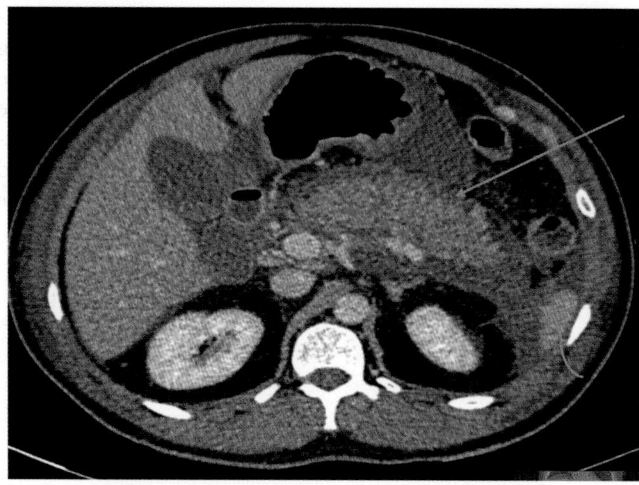

Figure 8.9 Axial computed tomography scan of a patient with acute pancreatitis demonstrates a swollen oedematous pancreas (arrow) with extensive peripancreatic free fluid (curly arrow).

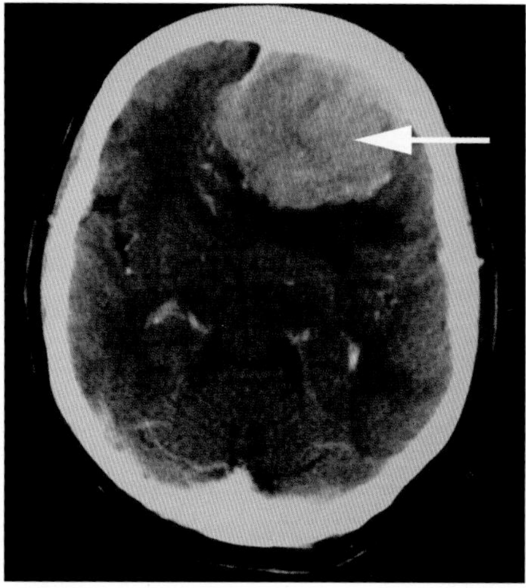

Figure 8.10 Axial computed tomography scan of the head following intravenous contrast demonstrates a large mass lesion in the left frontal region (arrow) in a patient with a large left frontal meningioma.

modern equipment, it is now not only possible to obtain images of the chest, abdomen and pelvis in under 10 seconds but these axial images can also be reformatted in multiple planes with practically no degradation in image quality.

In addition, CT has a far higher contrast resolution than plain radiographs, allowing the assessment of tissues with similar attenuation characteristics. As with radiographs, the natural contrast of tissues is further augmented by the use of intravenous iodinated contrast medium. Rapid scanning of a volume of tissue also allows the scans to be performed at different phases of enhancement, which is advantageous in identifying different diseases. For instance, very early scanning during the arterial phase is ideally suited to the examination of the arterial tree and hypervascular liver lesions, whereas scanning performed after a delay may be better suited to the identification of other solid organ pathology such as renal masses. More delayed scans, for example at 5–10 minutes post contrast injection, can be used to assess the ureters and bladder (***Figure 8.3***). Furthermore, it is possible to obtain scans during several phases including the arterial and venous phases in the same patient, which may aid in the identification and characterisation of lesions.

CT is widely used in thoracic, abdominal (***Figure 8.9***), neurological (***Figure 8.10***), musculoskeletal (***Figure 8.11***) and trauma imaging. The thinner collimation and improved spatial resolution have also resulted in the development of newer techniques such as CT angiography, virtual colonoscopy and virtual bronchoscopy. Furthermore, three-dimensional images can be reconstructed from the raw data to aid in surgical planning and to provide virtual endoluminal views in virtual colonoscopy for example. The disadvantage of CT compared with ultrasound and conventional radiography lies largely in the increased costs and the far higher doses of ionising radiation. For instance, a CT scan of the abdomen and pelvis has a radiation dose equivalent to approximately 500 chest radiographs.

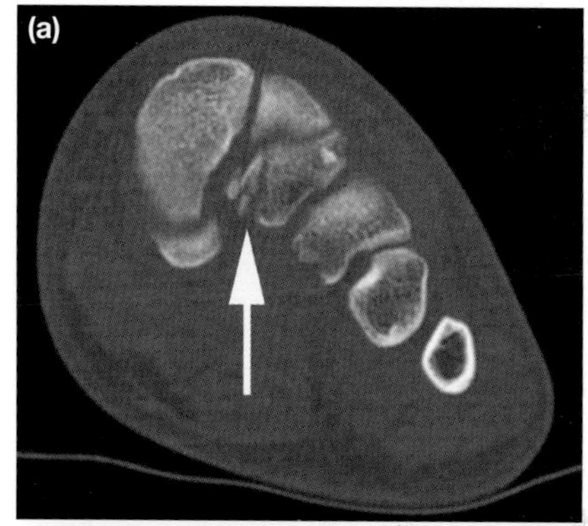

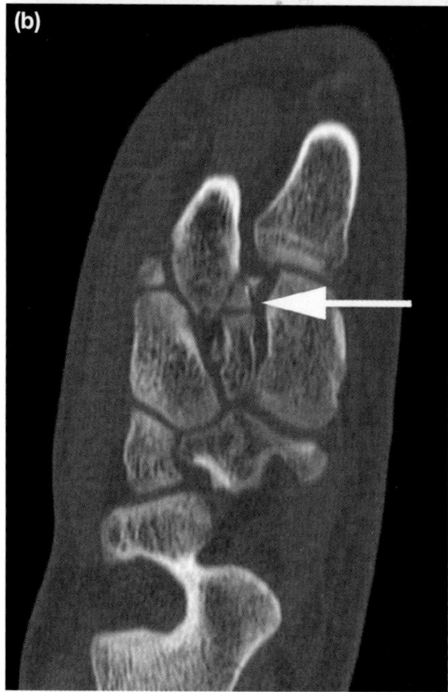

Figure 8.11 Coronal computed tomography (a) and axial reformats (b) of the foot in a patient involved in a road traffic accident demonstrates Lisfranc fracture dislocation with a comminuted fracture of the base of the second metatarsal (arrows).

Jacques Lisfranc de St. Martin, 1790–1847, Professor of Surgery and Operative Medicine, Paris, France.

Summary box 8.5

Computed tomography

Strengths

- High spatial and contrast resolution
- Contrast resolution enhanced by ability to image in multiple phases, including arterial, venous and delayed
- Rapid acquisition of images in one breath-hold
- Imaging of choice for the detection of pulmonary masses
- Allows global assessment of the abdomen and pelvis
- Excellent for liver, pancreatic, renal and bowel pathology
- Three-dimensional reconstruction allows complex fracture imaging
- Multiplanar reconstruction and three-dimensional imaging, e.g. CT angiography and colonoscopy
- Ability to guide intervention such as percutaneous biopsy and drainage

Weaknesses

- High radiation dose
- Poor soft-tissue resolution of the peripheries and superficial structures
- Patient needs to be able to lie flat and still
- Less readily available than plain films and ultrasound

Magnetic resonance imaging

Over the last 20 years, MRI has become an integral part of the imaging arsenal with ever-expanding indications. MRI relies on the fact that nuclei containing an odd number of protons have a characteristic motion in a magnetic field (precession) and produce a magnetic moment as a result of this motion. In a strong uniform magnetic field such as an MRI scanner, these nuclei align themselves with the main magnetic field and result in a net magnetic moment. A brief radiofrequency pulse is then applied to alter the motion of the nuclei. Once the radiofrequency pulse is removed, the nuclei realign themselves with the main magnetic field (relaxation) and in the process emit a radiofrequency signal that can be recorded, spatially encoded and used to construct a grey-scale image. The specific tissue characteristics define the manner and rate at which the nuclei relax. This relaxation is measured in two ways, referred to as the T1 and T2 relaxation times. The relaxation times and the proton density determine the signal from a specific tissue.

There are a large number of imaging sequences that can be used by applying radiofrequency pulses of different strengths and durations. The image characteristic and signal intensity from different tissues are governed by the pulse sequence employed and whether it is T1 weighted or T2 weighted. For instance, fat, methaemoglobin and mucinous fluid are bright on T1-weighted images, whereas water and thus most pathological processes, which tend to increase tissue water content, are bright on T2-weighted images. Cortical bone, air, haemosiderin and ferromagnetic materials are of very low signal on all pulse sequences. In general, T1-weighted images are superior in the delineation of anatomy, while T2-weighted images tend to highlight pathology better. For added tissue contrast, intravenous gadolinium may be administered. Other more specific contrast media are also available for liver, bowel and lymph node imaging.

MRI's exquisite contrast resolution, coupled with a lack of ionising radiation, is very attractive in imaging, particularly of tissues that have relatively little natural contrast. MRI also has the advantage of multiplanar imaging, as images can be acquired in any plane prescribed. It has traditionally been used extensively in the assessment of intracranial, spinal and musculoskeletal disorders (***Figures 8.12, 8.13 and 8.14***), allowing a global assessment of bony and soft-tissue structures. More recent developments have resulted in new indications and applications. Today, MRI is commonly used in oncological imaging, such as staging of rectal carcinoma and gynaecological malignancies, identification and characterisation of hepatic

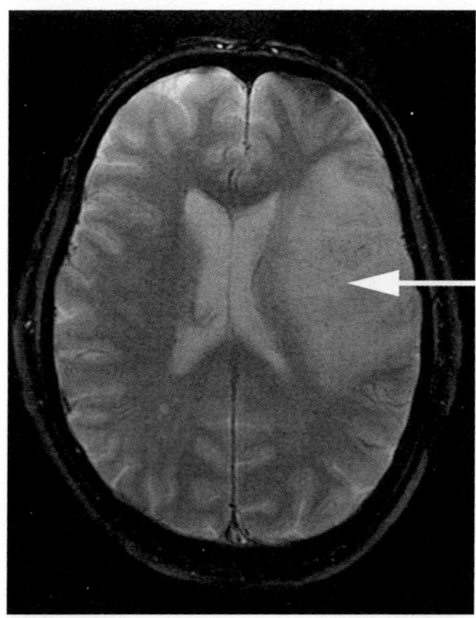

Figure 8.12 T2-weighted axial magnetic resonance imaging scan of the head in a patient with a large left-sided oligodendroglioma (arrow).

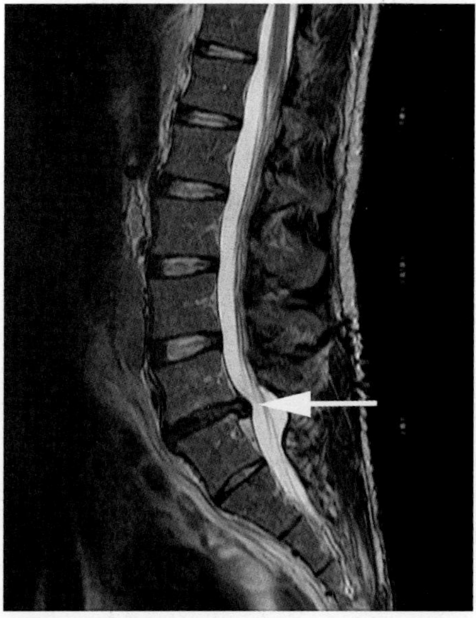

Figure 8.13 Sagittal T2-weighted magnetic resonance imaging scan of the lumbar spine demonstrates disc herniation (arrow) in a patient with acute back pain.

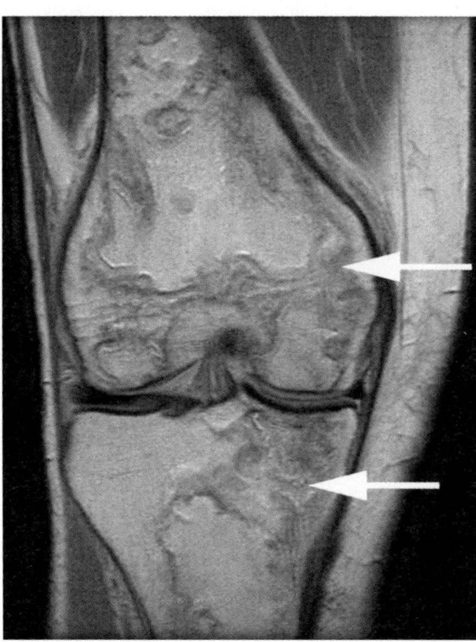

Figure 8.14 Coronal magnetic resonance imaging scan of the knee demonstrates extensive serpiginous areas of altered signal intensity in the distal femur and proximal tibia (arrows) in a patient with bone infarcts secondary to oral corticosteroids.

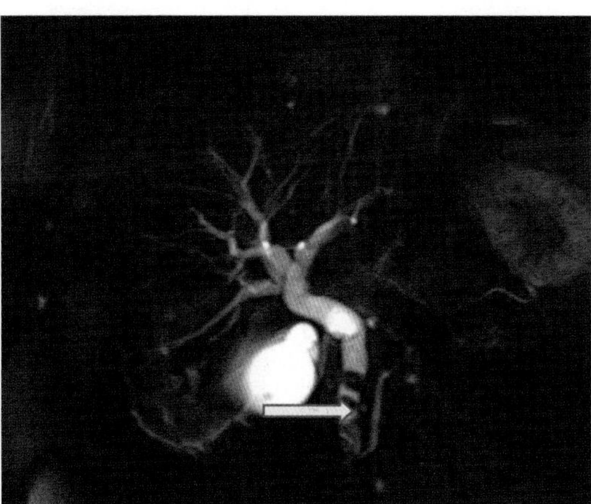

Figure 8.15 Magnetic resonance cholangiopancreatography image demonstrates dilated intrahepatic ducts and proximal common bile duct (CBD) secondary to multiple calculi in the distal CBD (arrow). This type of imaging has the potential to alter cholecystectomy surgical planning.

masses and assessment of the biliary tree (magnetic resonance cholangiopancreatography [MRCP]; ***Figure 8.15***). MRI has become increasingly important in imaging of the small bowel, for example in Crohn's disease, where repeated imaging with ionising radiation can incur a significant radiation dose over time. Magnetic resonance (MR) angiographic techniques allow non-invasive angiographic assessment of the cranial and peripheral circulation (***Figure 8.16***) and cardiac imaging.

Diffusion-weighted imaging is a relatively new type of MRI sequence that exploits the different rates of Brownian motion between different tissues. Tissues with greater cellular density have lower rates of diffusion of water molecules, and this difference can be exploited to distinguish benign and malignant or inflammatory lesions in a variety of organs as malignant or inflammatory lesions tend to have greater density of cells.

However, the availability of MRI is still relatively limited in comparison with other imaging techniques, and it is time-consuming with respect to image acquisition and interpretation. Images are easily degraded by motion, including respiratory and cardiac motion. The use of respiratory and cardiac gating can minimise this, although bowel peristalsis can still be a problem. The long acquisition times require a cooperative patient who can lie very still, which can be difficult especially in claustrophobic individuals or those in pain. Furthermore, because of the use of high-strength magnetic fields, patients with some metallic implants, such as some aneurysm clips and prosthetic heart valves, and those with implanted electronic devices, such as pacemakers and defibrillators, cannot be examined. Some newer implants may, however, be MRI compatible, and patients with joint replacements can be studied safely.

Summary box 8.6

Magnetic resonance (MR) imaging

Strengths
- No ionising radiation
- Excellent soft-tissue contrast
- Best imaging technique for
  - Intracranial lesions
  - Spine
  - Bone marrow and joint lesions

Other uses
- Staging
- MRCP
- MR angiography
- Breast malignancy
- Pelvic malignancy
- Cardiac imaging
- MR enterography
- Diffusion-weighted imaging

Weaknesses
- Absolute contraindications
  - Ocular metallic foreign bodies
  - Cochlear implants
  - Cranial aneurysm clips
- Relative contraindications
  - Pacemakers
  - First trimester of pregnancy
  - Claustrophobia
- Long scan times so patients may not be able to keep still, especially if in pain
- Limited availability
- Expensive

Nuclear medicine

In other imaging techniques using ionising radiation such as CT and conventional radiography, the individual is exposed to ionising radiation from an external source and the radiation transmitted through the patient is recorded. In nuclear medicine, however, a radioactive element or radionuclide such

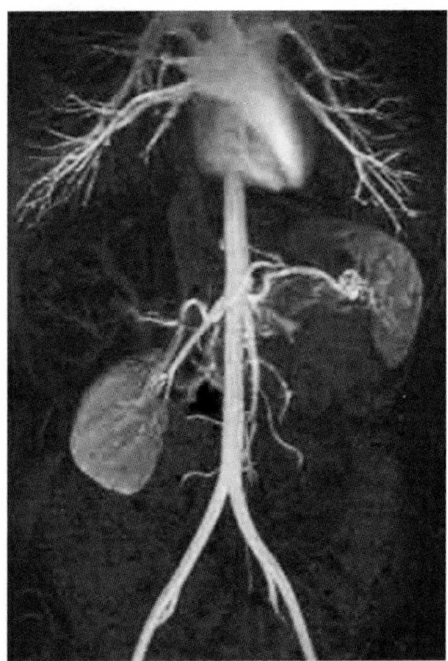

Figure 8.16 Maximum intensity projection image from a magnetic resonance angiogram demonstrates the abdominal aorta, common and external iliac arteries as well as parts of the pulmonary, mesenteric and renal vasculature.

as technetium, gallium, thallium or iodine is administered to the patient as part of a radiopharmaceutical agent, and a detector such as a gamma camera is then used to record and localise the emission from the patient, thus forming the image. The radionuclide is chosen and coupled with other compounds such that it is distributed and taken up in the tissues of interest. Therefore, a variety of radionuclides are required for imaging of different tissues. Nuclear medicine also differs from other means of imaging, which are largely anatomically based, as it also provides functional information.

Radionuclide imaging is widely used in bone imaging with very high sensitivity for assessing metastatic disease, metabolic bone disease, established arthropathies and occult infection and traumatic injuries (***Figure 8.17***), although many of these applications are being replaced by MRI. In genitourinary disease, dynamic imaging can be performed to assess renal perfusion and function including obstruction, to investigate renovascular hypertension and to evaluate renal transplants. Radionuclide imaging is also commonly used in thyroid and parathyroid disorders, ischaemic cardiac disease, detection of pulmonary emboli and assessment of occult infection and inflammatory bowel disease.

Positron emission tomography (PET) is an extension of nuclear medicine, in which a positron-emitting substance such as ^{18}F is tagged and used to assess tissue metabolic characteristics. The most commonly used radiolabelled tracer is ^{18}F-2-fluoro-2-deoxy-D-glucose (FDG), although other tracers can also be used in order to assess metabolic functions such as oxygen and glucose consumption and blood flow. Radioisotope decay causes the emission of a positron, which subsequently, within a few millimetres, collides with and annihilates an electron to produce a pair of annihilation photons. The drawbacks have been high cost, very limited availability and relatively low spatial resolution. The last of these has been addressed by PET/CT systems combining simultaneous PET imaging and CT, allowing the two sets of images to be registered so that the anatomical location of the abnormality can be localised more precisely. This modality has significantly improved the accuracy of cancer staging for a range of malignancies and is also useful in inflammatory conditions and imaging pyrexia of unknown origin.

Summary box 8.7

Radionuclide imaging

Strengths

- Allows functional imaging
- Allows imaging of the whole body
- Bone scan has a high sensitivity for metastatic bone disease, fractures and infection
- PET scanning is valuable in the detection of metastatic cancer

Weaknesses

- Specific agents are required for specific indications
- Often non-specific and an abnormal result may require further imaging
- Generally poor spatial resolution

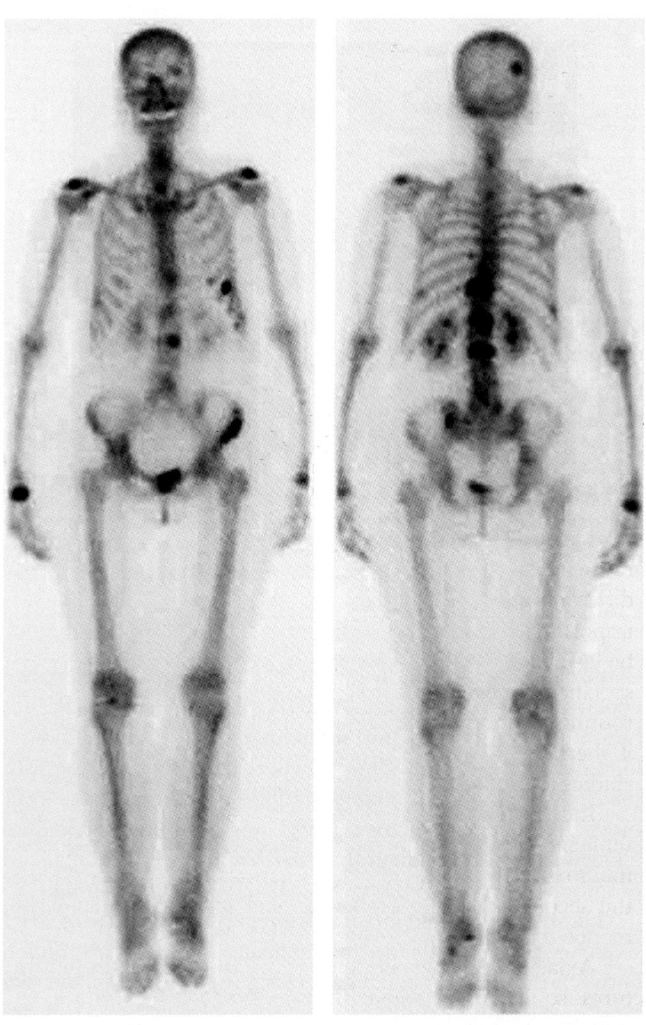

Figure 8.17 Bone scintigraphy in a patient with carcinoma of the breast illustrates bony metastatic deposits involving multiple vertebrae, the skull, pelvis and ribs.

IMAGING IN ORTHOPAEDIC SURGERY

Introduction

Imaging is an integral part of musculoskeletal diagnosis. Image-guided, minimally invasive techniques also play a major role in treatment. In broad terms, radiographs are the best method of looking for bony lesions or injuries, MRI shows bone marrow disease, muscle, tendon and soft-tissue disorders and ultrasound has better resolution than MRI for small structures, with the added advantage of showing dynamic changes. CT enables visualisation of the fine detail of bony structures, clarifying abnormalities seen on plain radiographs.

There are occasions when a combination of techniques will be important, and due consideration should be given to reducing the ionising radiation burden to the patient, using ultrasound and MRI as primary investigations whenever appropriate.

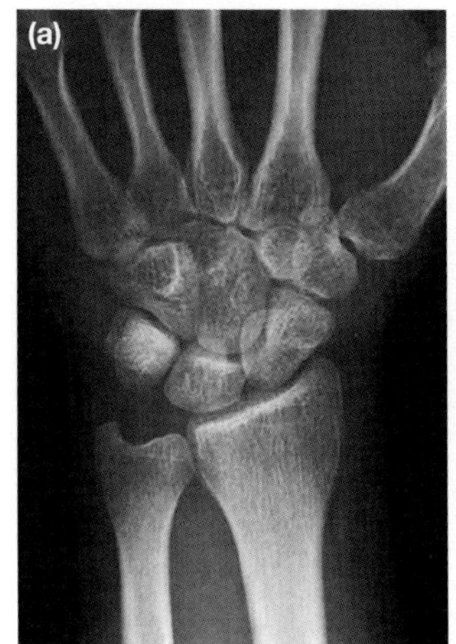

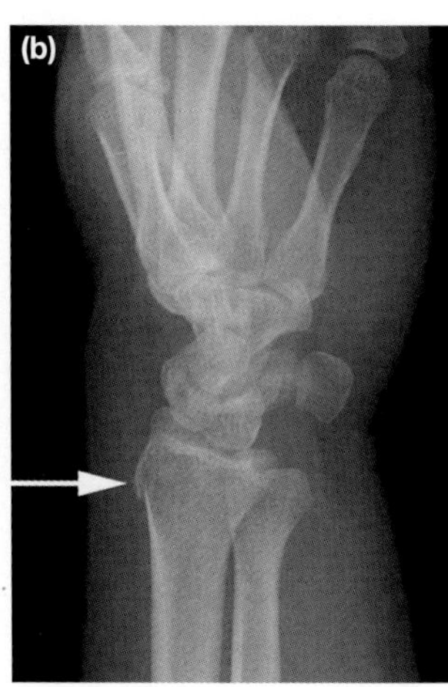

Figure 8.18 Anteroposterior radiograph of the wrist (a) in a patient following a fall does not show an acute bony injury. It is only on the second view (b) that a fracture of the dorsal cortex of the distal radius is visualised (arrow).

Summary box 8.8

Imaging in musculoskeletal conditions

- Radiographs are the best first-line test for bone lesions and fractures
- MRI is good for diagnosing bone marrow disease, occult fractures and tendon and soft-tissue disorders
- CT enables visualisation of the fine detail of bony structures
- CT gives the best three-dimensional information on fractures
- Ultrasound has better resolution in accessible soft tissues and can be used dynamically
- Ultrasound is the best method of distinguishing solid from cystic lesions
- Ultrasound is the only method for locating non-metallic foreign bodies
- Ultrasound is the best method for detecting muscle hernias

Skeletal trauma

Musculoskeletal trauma is best imaged by an initial plain radiograph. All skeletal radiographs should be taken from two different angles, usually at right angles to each other. This is important in trauma because a fracture or dislocation may not be visible on a single view (***Figure 8.18***). Occasionally, and in specific locations such as the scaphoid, more than two views are routinely performed. If this fails to make a clear diagnosis, or if there is suspicion of soft-tissue injuries, then cross-sectional studies are indicated.

Increasingly in the assessment of spinal trauma, CT is replacing radiographs as the first-line investigation for two main reasons: the first is that the sensitivity of CT is superior, the second is that it is quicker, enabling treatment to commence sooner.

Axial CT images alone may fail to diagnose some fractures, so three-dimensional reformatting is important to prevent errors. Sections should be thin, but care must be taken not to cover too wide an area, as the radiation burden may be excessive, particularly with multislice CT.

Summary box 8.9

Trauma imaging

- Initial imaging is either radiography or CT
- At least two views are needed for radiographs
- Use CT for spine, intra-articular or occult fractures

Degenerative disease

Synovitis

Radiographs are usually the first-line imaging investigation performed for the examination of joints. Typical changes of a degenerative or an erosive arthropathy are well known and understood. However, early arthropathy will be missed on radiographs and, with the advent of disease-modifying drugs, it is important to detect early synovitis before it is even apparent on clinical examination. Gadolinium diethyl triamine penta-acetic (DTPA)-enhanced MRI is the most sensitive method for detecting synovial thickening of numerous joints, but ultrasound is also sensitive, albeit more laborious to perform. Ultrasound shows effusions and synovial thickening clearly, and shows the increased blood flow around the affected joints without the use of contrast agents (***Figures 8.19 and 8.20***).

Articular cartilage damage

Articular surface disease is difficult to detect using non-invasive techniques. MRI is probably the best method, although it is not sensitive to early chondral changes (***Figure 8.21***). Higher field strength magnets (3 tesla and above) with dedicated surface coils provide more precise assessment; however, MR arthrography is currently the imaging 'gold standard'. A dilute quantity of

Nikola Tesla, 1856–1943, American physicist and electrical engineer who worked for the Westinghouse Electric and Manufacturing Company. A tesla is the SI unit of magnetic flux density.

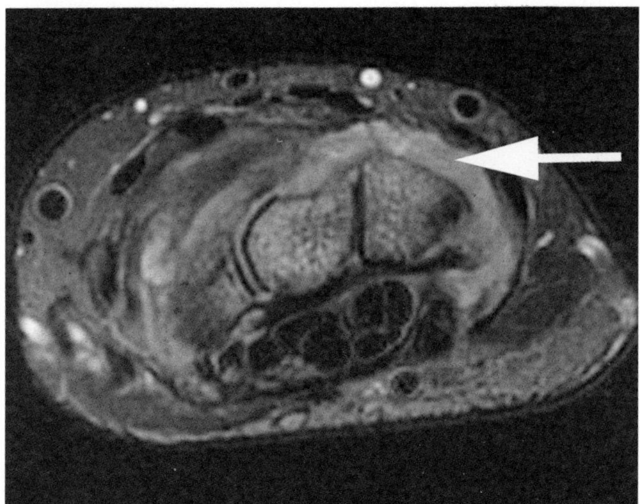

Figure 8.19 Axial T2-weighted fat-suppressed image of the wrist in a patient with rheumatoid arthritis demonstrates synovitis manifested as increased signal dorsal to the carpal bones (arrow).

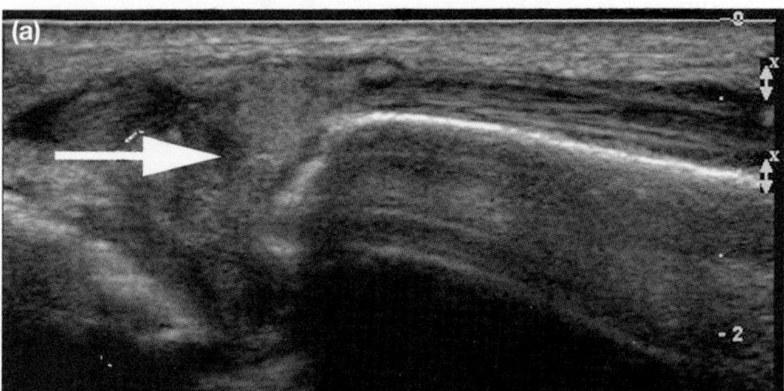

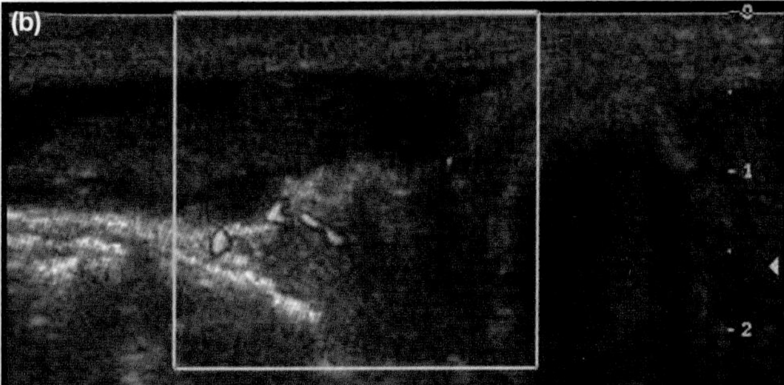

Figure 8.20 Ultrasound of the wrist (a) shows thickening of tissues on the dorsal aspect of the radiocarpal joint (arrow). (b) There is increased flow on power Doppler ultrasound in this patient with wrist synovitis and rheumatoid arthritis.

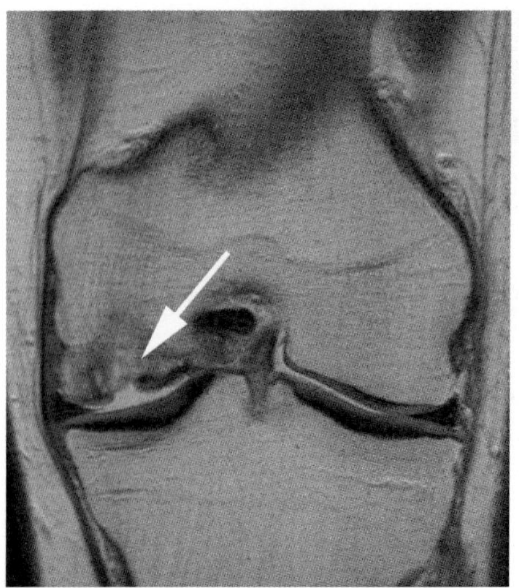

Figure 8.21 Coronal magnetic resonance imaging of the knee demonstrates a focal osteochondral abnormality of the medial femoral condyle, with full-thickness loss of the articular cartilage and abnormality of the subchondral bone (arrow).

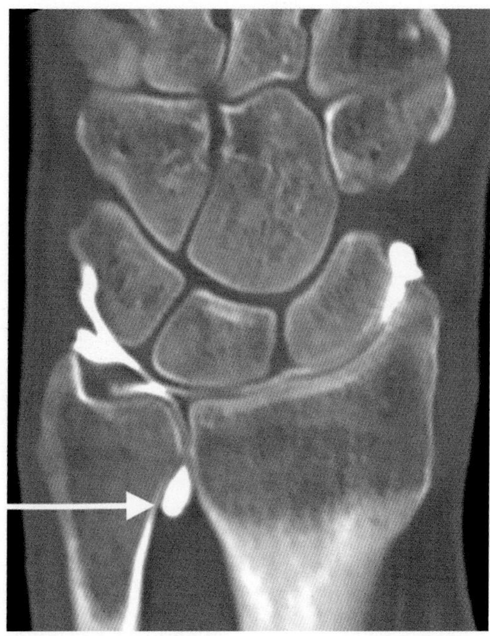

Figure 8.22 Coronal computed tomography arthrogram of the wrist showing a central perforation of the triangular fibrocartilage with contrast extending into the distal radioulnar joint (arrow) and radiocarpal articulation.

gadolinium DTPA is introduced into the joint by needle puncture under fluoroscopic, CT or ultrasound guidance, which is followed by an MRI examination. Using this technique, more subtle changes in the articular surface can be seen, including thinning, fissuring and ulceration. However, early softening of articular cartilage will not be visible. MR arthrography is also useful for detecting labral tears in the shoulder or hip, and in the assessment of patients who have undergone a previous meniscectomy. The triangular fibrocartilage of the wrist is also difficult to assess fully without MR or CT arthrography (*Figure 8.22*).

In the shoulder, rotator cuff trauma and degenerative changes can be studied using ultrasound or MRI. In experienced hands, ultrasound has a higher accuracy rate because image resolution is better and because the mechanical integrity of the cuff can be tested by dynamically stressing it (*Figure 8.23*). MRI has the advantage of being able to show abnormalities in the subcortical bone.

In the majority of arthropathies and degenerative disorders, serial imaging is useful. Changes in films taken weeks or months apart are far easier to see and interpret than a single snapshot study.

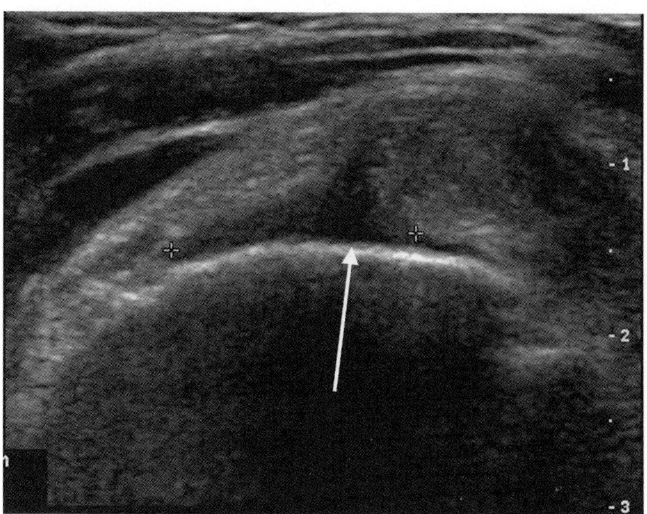

Figure 8.23 Ultrasound of the supraspinatus tendon identifies a partial tear of the tendon (arrow), which is predominantly articular sided but with a component that is nearly full thickness.

Summary box 8.10

Imaging techniques for joint disease

- Radiographs are good for assessing established articular disease
- Synovitis can be detected using ultrasound or contrast-enhanced MRI
- Early damage to articular cartilage is difficult to image by conventional methods
- Rotator cuff lesions are best studied using ultrasound or MRI
- Destructive lesions are best studied first on plain radiographs
- MRI is best for staging tumours
- Biopsy can be guided by fluoroscopy, CT or ultrasound

Aggressive bone disease

The radiograph is the first imaging technique for destructive lesions in bones. There is considerable experience required in the interpretation of these films, especially with regard to whether the lesion is benign or malignant (***Figure 8.24***).

Radiographs are also vital in the assessment of soft-tissue calcification in tumours of muscle, tendon and subcutaneous fat. When a lesion is detected, there needs to be an early decision as to whether this is benign or malignant. If there is a suspicion of malignancy on the radiograph, or any uncertainty, then local staging is indicated. This is best performed by MRI for both bone and soft-tissue lesions (***Figure 8.25***). At this stage, it is likely that a biopsy will be indicated, and preferably under image guidance. Soft-tissue and bone biopsy needles may be guided by CT, ultrasound or interventional MRI systems. The route of puncture should avoid vital structures and must be agreed with the surgeon, who will perform local excision if the lesion proves to be malignant. Care should be taken to avoid contaminating other compartments. In all circumstances, samples are best sent for both histopathological and microbiological examination. It may be difficult to tell on imaging whether or not a lesion is infected, and histology often provides a clear diagnosis in inflammatory conditions. Bone scintigraphy is useful in detecting whether a lesion is solitary or multiple, although whole-body MRI is becoming available.

Summary box 8.11

Imaging of aggressive lesions in bone

- Plain radiographs are important as a first investigation
- MRI is best for local staging
- Bone scintigraphy or whole-body MRI for solitary or multiple lesion determination
- CT detects lung metastases
- Fluoroscopy, CT, MRI or ultrasound can be used to guide the biopsy

Mass lesions

Mass lesions in muscle and soft tissue are examined by ultrasound, which can be diagnostic in the majority of cases, thereby avoiding the need for further imaging. This is most often the case when a lesion is purely cystic and, as most soft-tissue masses are cysts, ultrasound is a very effective screening test. There are occasions when no mass lesion is found at the site of

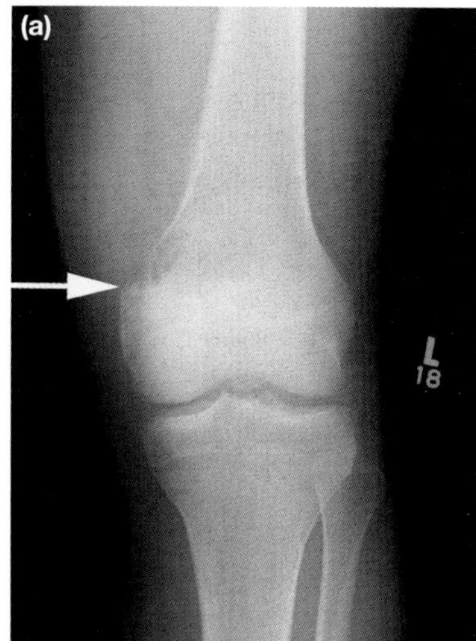

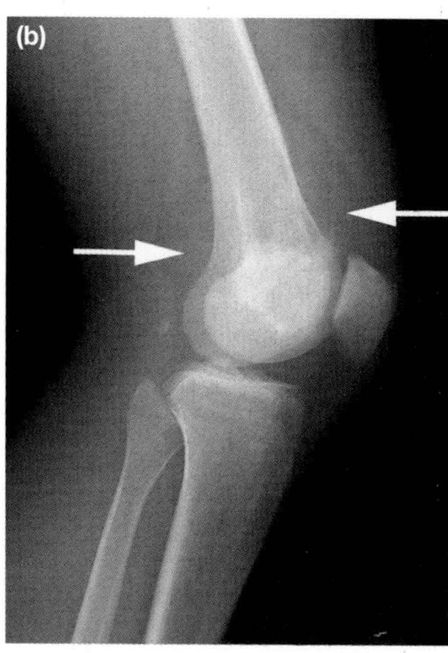

Figure 8.24 Anteroposterior (a) and lateral (b) radiographs of the left knee in a young patient with knee pain. There is a mixed lucent and sclerotic lesion of the distal femur with breach of the cortex medially and soft-tissue extension seen anteriorly and posteriorly (arrows). The location and appearances are consistent with osteosarcoma.

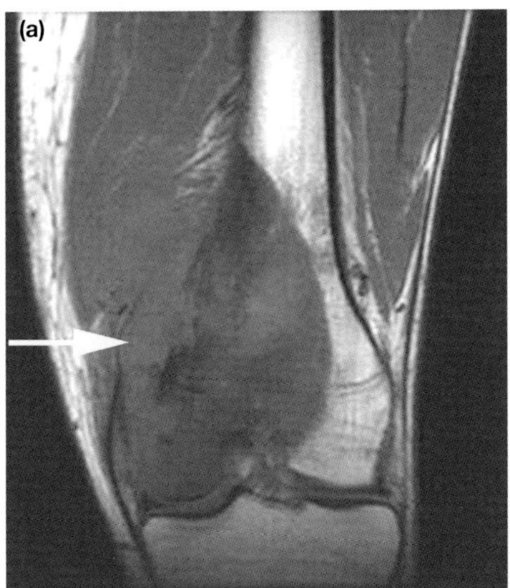

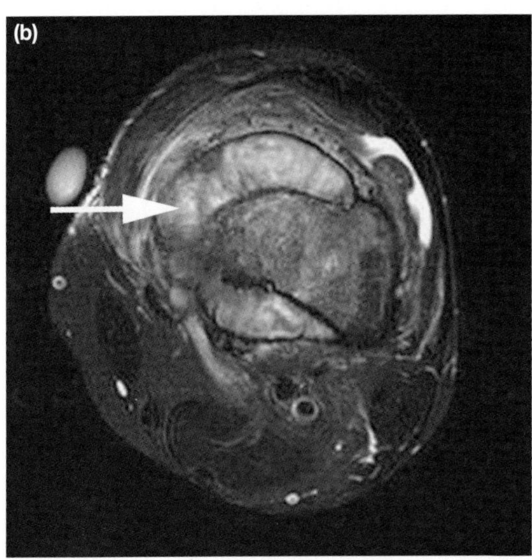

Figure 8.25 Coronal T1- (a) and axial T2-weighted fat-suppressed (b) images through the distal femur of the patient in **Figure 8.24** illustrates the bony area involved, the soft-tissue extent of the tumour and the relationship of the neurovascular structures to the mass (arrows).

concern, and then reassurance can be offered. If the ultrasound examination is normal, this effectively excludes soft-tissue neoplasia. A reasonable protocol is to perform ultrasound on all palpable 'lesions' to exclude cysts, and on patients without any identifiable mass, and to proceed to MRI only when there is a solid or partly solid element to an unidentifiable lesion. Tumour vascularity is best assessed by Doppler ultrasound. It can be studied by intravenous gadolinium DTPA-enhanced MRI; however, this is a more expensive and invasive technique, providing no more information than Doppler ultrasound.

Summary box 8.12

Imaging of soft-tissue lesions

- Ultrasound is the best for screening; it is often the only imaging required
- MRI is best for local staging and follow-up
- Doppler ultrasound can assess vascularity cheaply and effectively
- Ultrasound is useful for biopsy

Infection

In the early stages of joint infection, the plain films may be normal, but they should still be performed to exclude bony erosions in case a painful joint is the first sign of an arthropathy. Ultrasound examination is the easiest and most accurate method of assessing joint effusions, although, when an effusion is identified, it is not possible to discriminate between blood and pus. Aspiration guided by ultrasound is the best method of making this distinction. MRI may be required to assess early articular cartilage and bone involvement.

Radiographs should also be used to examine patients with suspected osteomyelitis. Although they may not detect early infection, they will demonstrate or exclude bony destruction, calcification and sequestrum formation. CT may be needed to give a cross-sectional view, in order to assess the extent of bony sequestrum.

MRI is perhaps the most sensitive method for detecting early disease and is the preferred technique to define the activity and extent of infection, as it shows not only the bony involvement but also the extent of oedema and soft-tissue involvement (***Figure 8.26***). Abscesses may be detected or excluded, and subperiosteal oedema is readily visible. MRI can be used as a staging procedure to plan treatment, including surgical intervention. Serial examinations can be used to follow the response to intravenous antibiotics and are very useful in the management of complex osteomyelitis. In cases of negative or equivocal MRI, nuclear medicine techniques such as bone scintigraphy can be very sensitive, and specialised studies using tracers such as gallium citrate or indium-labelled white cells increase specificity.

Summary box 8.13

Imaging of potentially infected bone and joint

- Plain radiographs may be needed to exclude bone erosion
- Ultrasound is sensitive for an effusion, periosteal collections and superficial abscesses and can be used for guided aspiration
- CT is useful in established infection to look for sequestrum
- MRI is useful to define the activity of osteomyelitis, early infection and soft-tissue collections
- Bone scans are sensitive but of low specificity
- Complex nuclear medicine studies are useful in negative MR examinations or equivocal cases

Metabolic bone disease

Plain radiographs should be the first images of patients with metabolic bone disease. They may detect the subperiosteal erosions in hyperparathyroidism or, more commonly, the osteopenia in osteoporosis, but they cannot be used to quantify osteoporosis. The apparent density of the bone on the film is linked to the penetration of the rays, among other variables, as well as to the bone density. If a quantitative method is needed, however, bone mineral density using dual x-ray absorptiometry (DEXA) is the most accurate and practical. However, fractures will cause erroneously high readings, and they tend to occur in the vertebrae used for DEXA measurements. Quantitative CT is an alternative technique, although this is less readily available. Ultrasound transmission measurement in the extremities has its advocates, as it arguably measures factors that better represent the strength of bone rather than its density. Its limitations are that it cannot be used to study the vertebrae or hip, and these are the sites where osteoporotic fractures occur most frequently. MRI may be useful in detecting fractures and is an essential prerequisite to percutaneous vertebroplasty.

IMAGING IN MAJOR TRAUMA

Introduction

Trauma remains a major cause of mortality and morbidity in all age groups. Presented with a multiply injured patient, rapid and effective investigation and treatment are required to maximise the chances of survival and to reduce morbidity. Imaging plays a major role in this assessment and in guiding treatment. As with the clinical assessment, imaging is carried out according to the principles of primary and secondary surveys, identifying major life-threatening injuries of the airway, respiratory system

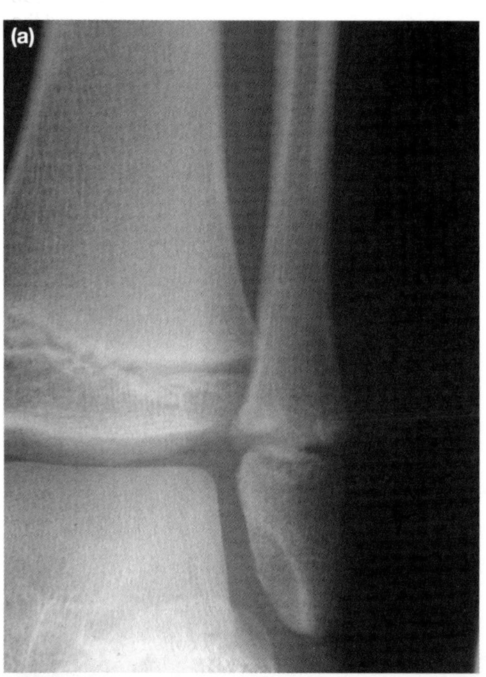

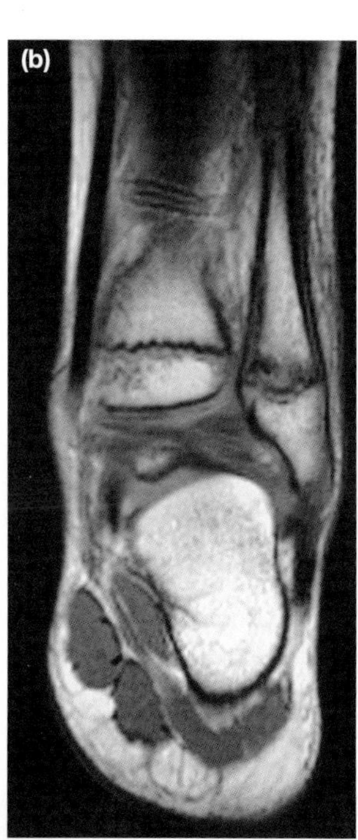

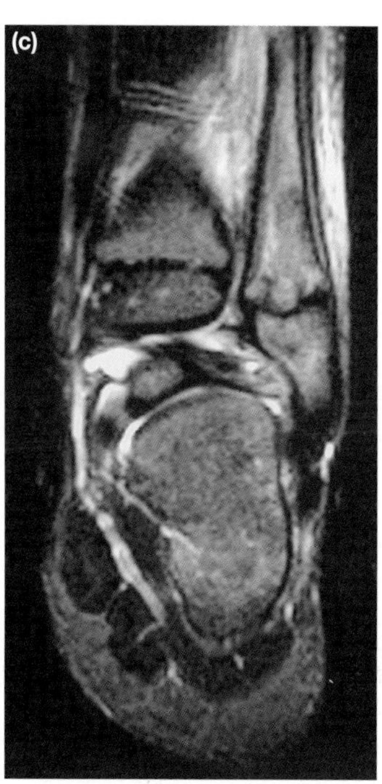

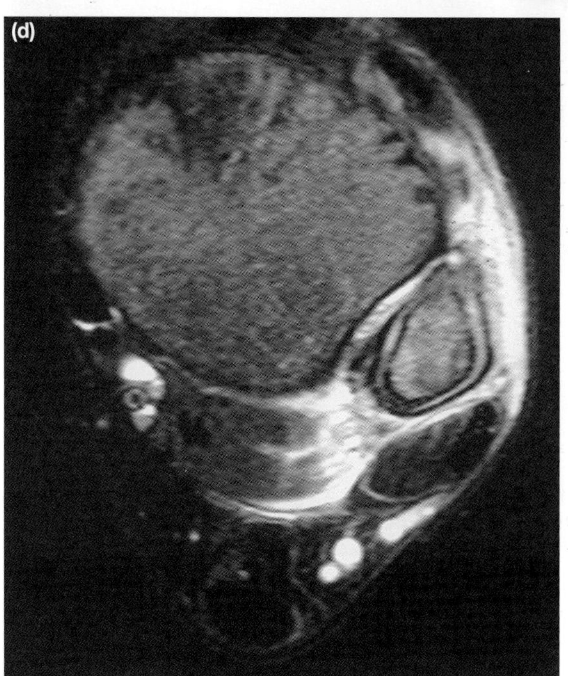

Figure 8.26 (a) The plain films of this 13-year-old are close to normal. On close inspection, there is a fine periosteal reaction on the fibula. (b) The coronal T1-weighted magnetic resonance image shows little more, but (c) the coronal fast short tau inversion recovery (STIR) images and (d) axial T2 fast spin echo with fat suppression show the oedema in bone as white and the extensive periosteal fluid with soft-tissue inflammation. The diagnosis is acute osteomyelitis.

and circulation before a more detailed and typically time-consuming assessment of other injures. At no point should imaging delay the treatment of immediately life-threatening injuries. As in other settings, the quickest and least invasive examinations should be performed first. A radiologist present in the trauma room at the time of patient assessment is able to evaluate the radiographs rapidly, relay this information back to the team and guide further imaging, which may include further plain films, CT, ultrasound and MRI.

Plain radiographs

Conventional radiography allows rapid assessment of the major injuries and can be carried out in the trauma room while the patient is clinically assessed and treated. Despite the time constraints, the number of staff involved and the restricted mobility of the patient, high-quality images can be routinely obtained with due care and attention. Increasingly plain films are being replaced by whole-body CT. In many centres CT scanners are immediately available in the emergency department and indeed in some departments patients are assessed and treated on the scanning table.

There is no routine set of radiographs to be obtained, and the decision is based on the mechanism of injury, the stability of the patient's condition and whether the patient is intubated. The most commonly performed initial radiographs are a chest radiograph, a single anteroposterior view of the pelvis and a cervical spine series.

The supine chest radiograph should encompass an area from the lung apices to the costophrenic recesses and include the ribs laterally. Chest radiographs give valuable information in both blunt and penetrating trauma. Evaluation of the radiograph should be undertaken in a systematic manner to minimise the chances of missing an injury. In the first instance, the position of lines and tubes, including the endotracheal tube, should be assessed, followed by assessment of the central airways. Following this, the lungs should be evaluated for abnormal focal areas of opacification, which may represent aspiration, haemorrhage, haematoma or oedema, as well as more diffuse opacification reflecting a pleural collection. Alternatively, relative focal or unilateral lucency may reflect a pneumothorax in the supine position. Evaluation of the mediastinum should include its position, which may be altered by tension pneumothoraces or large collections, as well as its contour, an alteration of which may reflect a mediastinal haematoma due to aortic or spinal injury. Finally, the skeleton and the soft tissue should be carefully examined for rib, vertebral, scapular and limb fractures, as well as evidence of surgical emphysema and paraspinal haematomas (***Figure 8.27***).

Pelvic radiographs are also commonly performed to screen for, and assess, fractures of the bony pelvis. The image should include the iliac crests in their totality and extend inferiorly to below the lesser trochanters. When assessing the film, the alignment of the sacroiliac joints and the symphysis pubis should be carefully examined, as some fractures, especially those of the sacral arcades, can be very subtle on the pelvic radiograph. The presence of pubic fractures raises the possibility of urethral injury and should alert clinicians to exercise caution with bladder catheterisation (***Figure 8.28***).

The utility of cervical spine x-rays depends on the consciousness level of the patient and the presence of distracting injuries. In fully conscious patients with an isolated neck injury, clinical assessment can be used to guide the need for x-rays. In patients with distracting injuries and/or altered consciousness, including intubated patients, CT is preferred (***Figure 8.29***).

Further radiographs of the thoracic and lumbar spine and the peripheral skeleton may be required, depending on the clinical setting. As with all skeletal radiographs, two

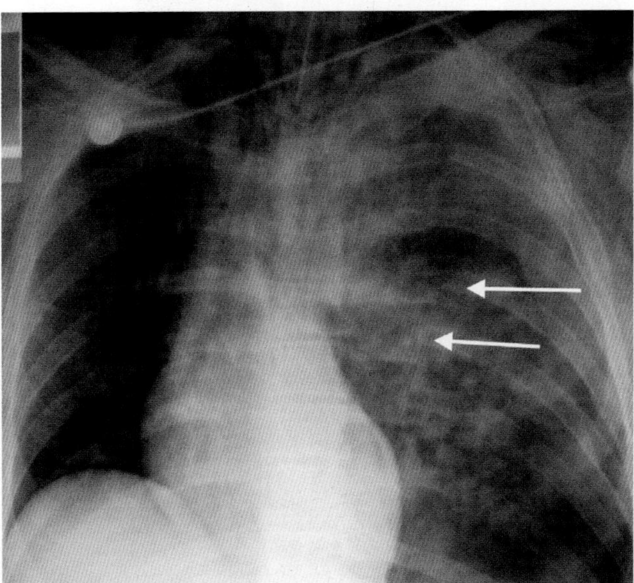

Figure 8.27 Supine chest radiograph of a patient involved in a road traffic accident. The patient is intubated. There are multiple left-sided rib fractures (arrows) and extensive surgical emphysema. Depression of the left hemidiaphragm and mediastinal shift to the right suggest that there is a tension pneumothorax present.

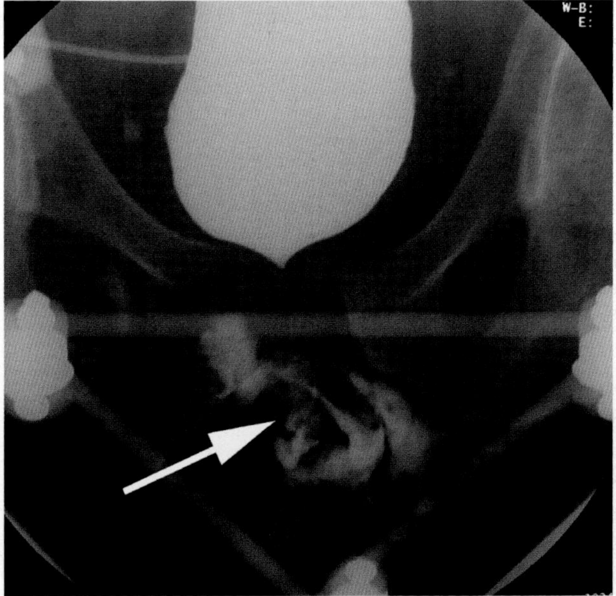

Figure 8.28 Retrograde urethrogram in a patient who sustained extensive pelvic fractures following a fall. The pelvic injuries have been stabilised using an external fixation device. The urethrogram identifies extensive injury to the urethra with extravasation of contrast (arrow).

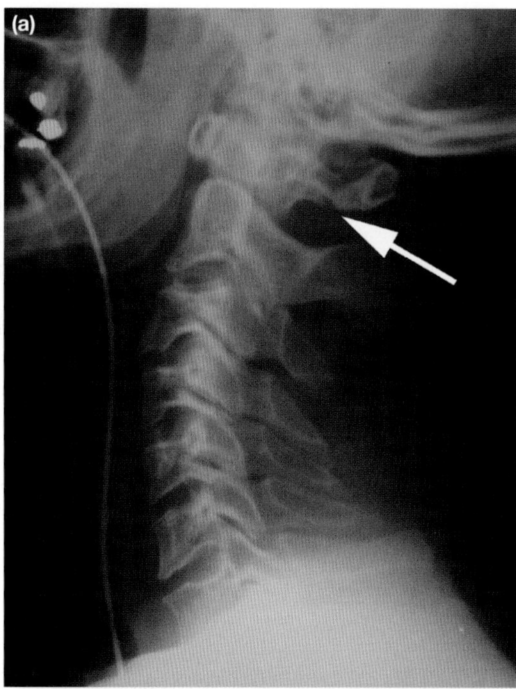

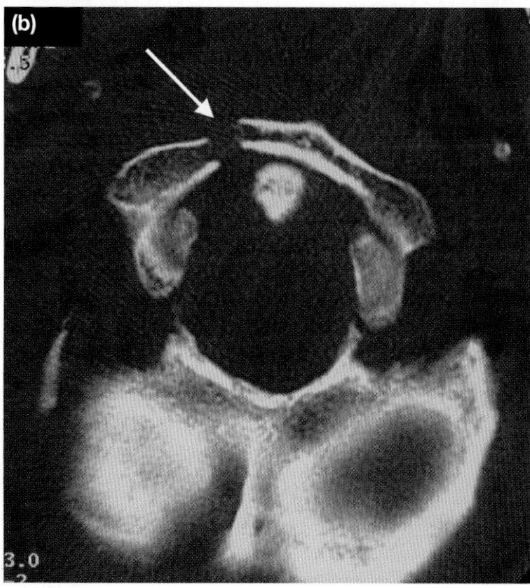

Figure 8.29 Lateral view of the cervical spine (a) fails to demonstrate the cervicothoracic junction. In addition, there appears to be a break in the posterior arch of C1 (arrow). Computed tomography of the cervical spine (b) demonstrates a fracture of the anterior arch as well as the posterior arch of C1 (arrow).

perpendicular views are required for adequate assessment. However, with the increasing use of CT in assessment of the torso the need for plain films is diminishing.

Radiographs of the skull or facial bones have no role in the immediate assessment of the multitrauma individual, except for immediate localisation of a penetrating object.

Ultrasound

Ultrasound has an evolving role in the assessment of acutely traumatised patients. The main current roles of ultrasound include the assessment of intraperitoneal fluid and haemopericardium (focused assessment with sonography for trauma [FAST]), the evaluation of pneumothoraces in supine patients and in guiding intervention.

FAST ultrasound is a limited examination directed to look for intraperitoneal fluid or pericardial injury as a marker of underlying injury. This avoids the invasiveness of diagnostic peritoneal lavage. In the presence of free intraperitoneal fluid and an unstable patient, the ultrasound allows the trauma surgeon to explore the abdomen as a cause of blood loss. In the presence of fluid and a haemodynamically stable individual, further assessment by way of CT can be performed. However, it is important to realise that ultrasound has limitations in the identification of free fluid. This includes obscuration of fluid by bowel gas or extensive surgical emphysema. More organised haematoma may be more difficult to visualise. It must also be emphasised that the principal role of ultrasound is not to identify the primary solid organ injury, although this may be visualised. Occasionally, a second ultrasound scan may show free fluid in the presence of an initially negative FAST scan.

The detection of a pneumothorax on a supine radiograph can be very difficult. Ultrasound examination may be used to identify a radiographically occult pneumothorax. With a high-resolution linear probe, the pleura can be visualised as an echogenic stripe, and its motion with respiration can also be assessed. In the presence of a pneumothorax, the sliding motion of the pleura is lost. Ultrasound may also be used to detect a haemothorax or haemopericardium.

Finally, ultrasound may be of value in guiding the placement of an intravascular line by direct visualisation of the vessels. This can be especially advantageous in shocked patients.

Computed tomography

CT is the main imaging method for the investigation of intracranial and intra-abdominal injuries and vertebral fractures. With current multidetector scanners a comprehensive examination of the head, spine, chest, abdomen and pelvis can be completed in less than 5 minutes. Traditionally the CT scanner was referred to as 'the doughnut of death', as imaging could lead to delays in emergency treatment. However, as the availability of scanners and the speed of scanning has dramatically increased, it has become standard practice to use CT early in the assessment of trauma patients. Emergency departments have CT scanners co-located to the resuscitation or trauma bays or patients can be assessed and treated while on the CT table.

CT examination of the head is accurate in identifying treatable intracranial injuries (***Figures 8.30 and 8.31***) and should not be delayed by radiography of peripheral injuries, as there is declining success in cases of intracranial collection when treated after the initial 3–4 hours. In comparison, identification of more widespread injuries, such as diffuse axonal injury, is relatively poor. Examination of facial injuries and cervical spine fractures can also be carried out at the same time as this only adds seconds to the examination. There is evidence that CT of the abdomen and pelvis is of benefit in multiple trauma when there is a head injury, as it often shows unexpected abnormalities; this may affect the immediate management, especially if the patient deteriorates.

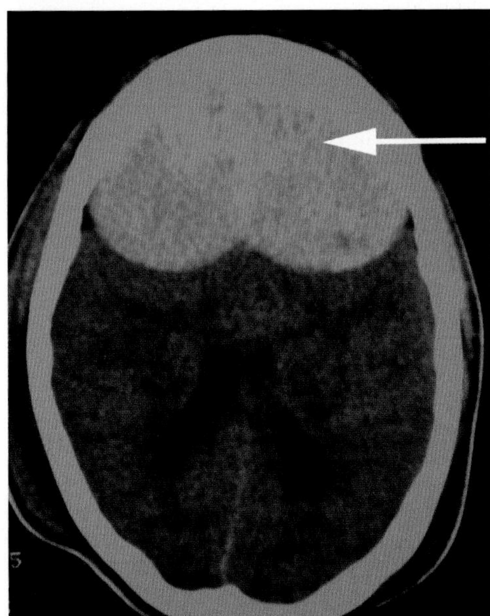

Figure 8.30 Computed tomography of the head in a patient with head injury shows bilateral large frontal extradural collections (arrow).

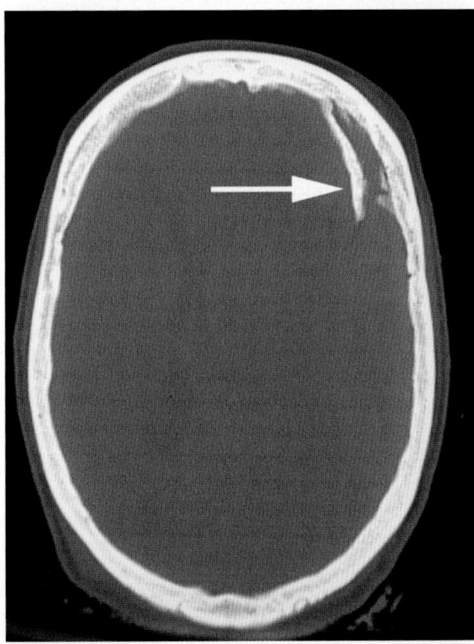

Figure 8.31 Computed tomography of the head following head trauma shows a skull fracture with a large depressed component (arrow).

Chest CT with intravenous contrast agent is valuable in identifying vascular and lung injuries and is the most accurate way of demonstrating haemothorax and pneumothorax. The position of chest drains can be identified, allowing adjustment of position if necessary. Abdominal and pelvic CT is usually undertaken as an extension to the chest CT. If an abdominal examination is performed, the pelvis should be included to avoid missing pelvic injuries and free pelvic fluid. CT is an excellent means of identifying hepatic, splenic (***Figure 8.32***) and renal injuries. Delayed examination after the administration of intravenous contrast agents allows assessment of the pelvicalyceal system in cases of renal trauma. Pancreatic and duodenal injuries may also be identified, but detection of these injuries may be more problematic. Using CT, the accuracy of detection of bowel or mesenteric injuries is less than it is for solid organ injury, and these injuries should be suspected when there is free intraperitoneal fluid without an identifiable cause (***Figure 8.33***). Close clinical follow-up and early repeat scanning with oral contrast can often reveal the bowel or mesenteric injury in patients with free fluid with no other cause identified.

The image data may be reconstructed into thinner slices for the diagnosis of injuries to the thoracic and lumbar spine and for the better delineation of pelvic and acetabular fractures. Complex intra-articular fractures of the peripheral skeleton, such as calcaneal and tibial plateau fractures, may be usefully examined by dedicated thin-section studies provided this does not delay the treatment of other more serious injuries (***Figure 8.34***). CT angiography may be used to demonstrate vascular injuries in the limbs in those with penetrating injuries or complex displaced fractures.

Magnetic resonance imaging

The value of immediate MRI in trauma is relatively limited and is largely confined to the imaging of spinal injuries (***Figure 8.35***).

Access to urgent MRI is not widely available, and there are major practical problems in imaging patients who require ventilation or monitoring. MRI is therefore only practical in stable patients. All monitoring equipment must be MRI compatible, and ventilation support should be undertaken by staff skilled and experienced in these techniques as applied to the MRI environment. MRI may be used to diagnose injuries of the spinal cord and associated perispinal haematomas in patients with neurological signs or symptoms. MRI can supplement CT in spinal injuries by imaging soft-tissue injuries to the longitudinal and interspinous ligaments. MRI is mandatory in patients in whom there is facetal dislocation if surgical reduction is being considered, to minimise the risk of displacing soft-tissue or disc material into the spinal canal during reduction procedures. Subtle fractures may be difficult to identify, particularly if they are old, but an acute injury is normally identified by the surrounding oedema. Bony abnormalities should be reviewed using CT as fracture lines are hard to identify with MRI and unstable injuries may be overlooked. In the less acute setting, MRI may also be used to assess diffuse axonal injuries, with an accuracy exceeding CT.

Vascular interventional radiology

With the development and refinement of CT angiography techniques, the diagnostic role of formal angiography has become limited. CT angiography is the first-line investigation for aortic trauma and for penetrating and non-penetrating peripheral vascular trauma.

Endovascular techniques play an important role in the treatment of acute solid organ injuries, and the interventional radiologist should be consulted early in the decision-making

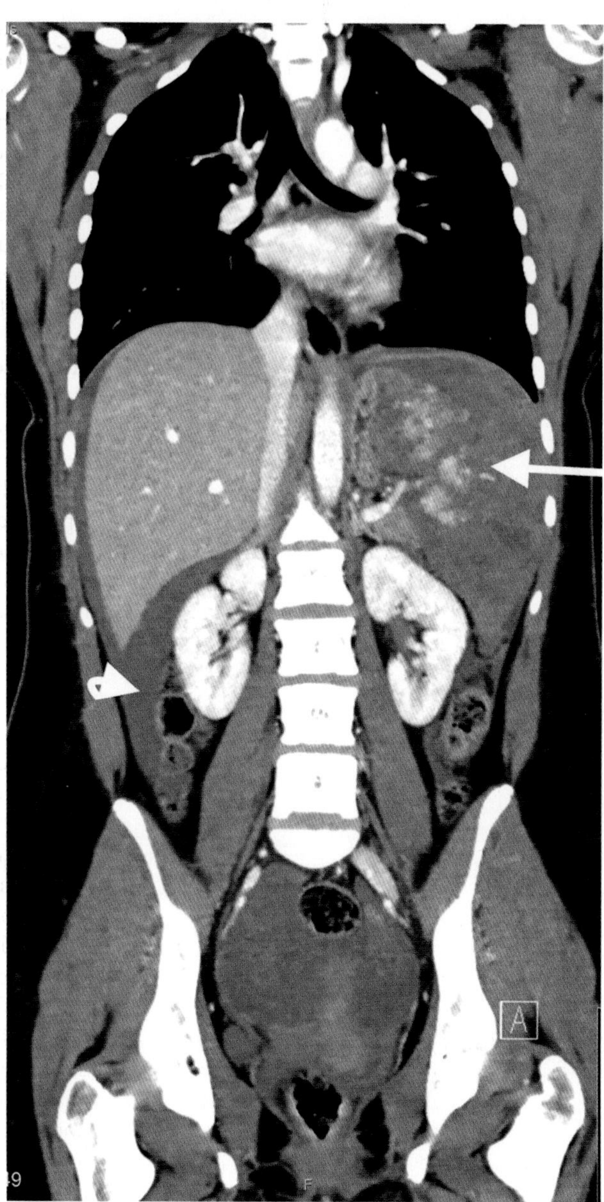

Figure 8.32 Coronal computed tomography image of the body shows a grade V splenic injury ('shattered spleen'; arrow) with vascular injury at the hilum and free fluid around the spleen and liver (arrowhead).

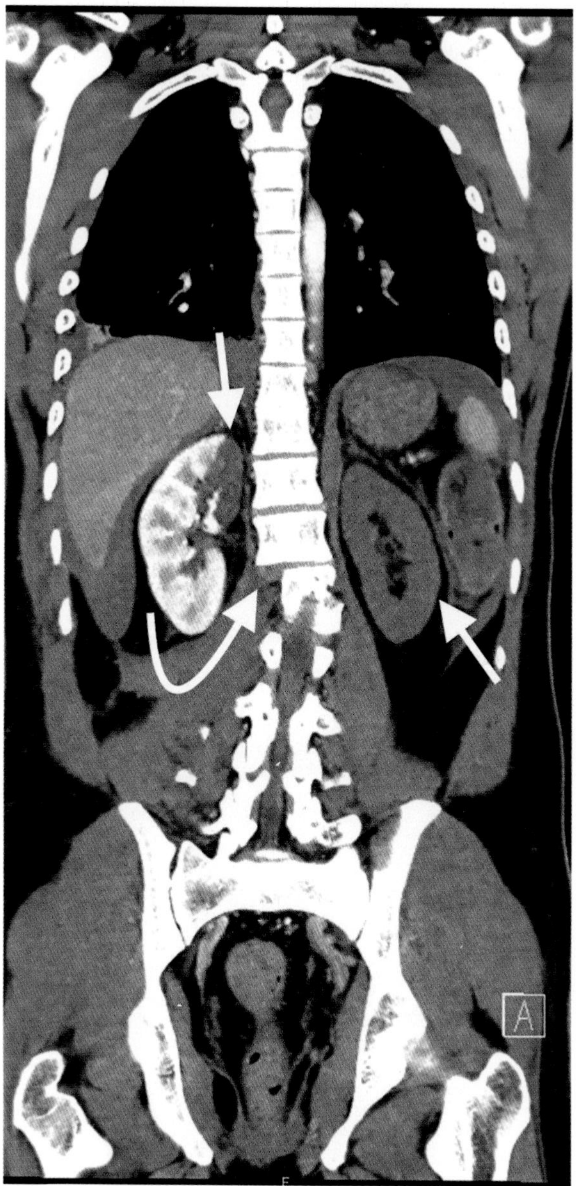

Figure 8.33 Coronal computed tomography demonstrating free fluid around the liver. The upper pole of the right kidney and whole left kidney demonstrate no contrast uptake in keeping with acute vascular injury (arrows). In addition there is a distraction injury with lateral dislocation of the T11–T12 intervertebral junction (curved arrow).

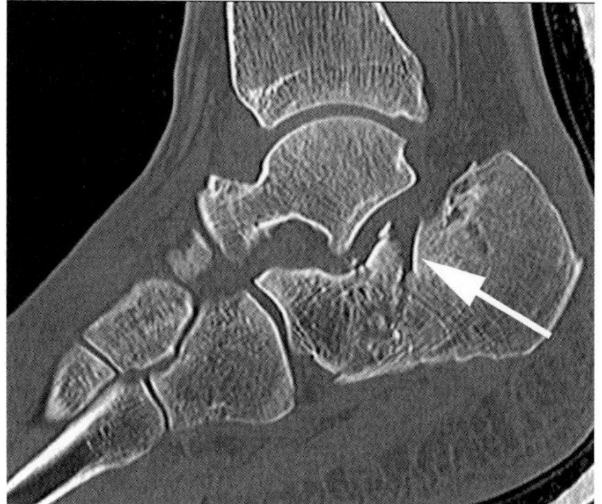

Figure 8.34 Sagittal reformats of computed tomography of the calcaneus in a patient following a fall illustrate a comminuted calcaneal fracture with intra-articular extension into the posterior facet of the subtalar joint (arrow).

process. Using coaxial catheter systems and a variety of available embolic agents such as soluble gelatin sponge and microcoils, selective embolisation and reduction of blood flow to the injured segment can be achieved without causing infarction. Selective embolisation techniques are also suitable for the treatment of patients with pelvic fractures with ongoing blood loss and volume issues. With penetrating and non-penetrating extremity trauma, balloon occlusion and embolisation may be employed to control haemorrhage, while the application of stent grafts can aid in re-establishing the circulation to the affected extremity.

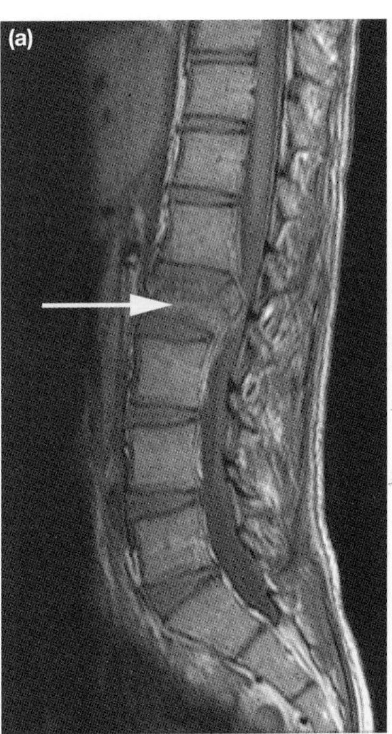

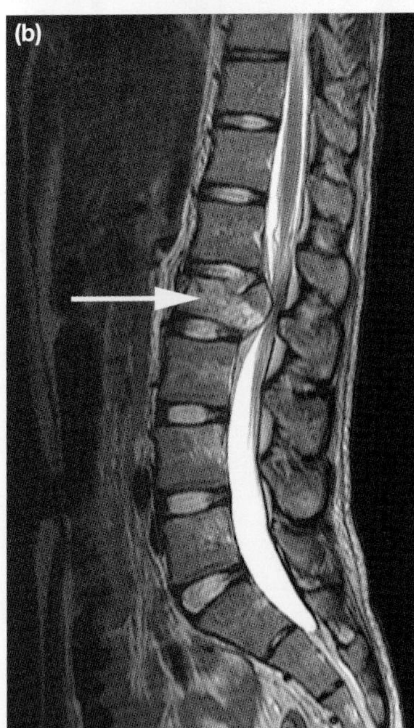

Figure 8.35 Sagittal T1-weighted (a) and T2-weighted (b) magnetic resonance imaging of the spine demonstrate a burst fracture of L2 causing neural compression (arrows).

IMAGING IN ABDOMINAL SURGERY

The acute abdomen

The term 'acute abdomen' encompasses many diverse entities.

IMAGING IN COMMON SURGICAL CLINICAL SCENARIOS

In this section the roles of different radiological modalities in common surgical scenarios are discussed, with a brief rationale behind their use and typical appearances of various pathological processes.

Bowel obstruction

The plain abdominal radiograph is a useful tool in diagnosing bowel obstruction. Small bowel obstruction can generally be distinguished from large bowel obstruction by virtue of the following: the small bowel lies centrally in the abdomen while the large bowel lies peripherally; the valvulae conniventes (folds) of the small bowel traverse the entire width of the lumen while the haustra of the large bowel do not; and the calibre of the small bowel is typically less than the large, even when obstructed (typical measurements in obstruction: small bowel 3.5–5 cm, large bowel 5–8 cm).

However, it must be stressed that a normal plain radiograph does not exclude an obstruction – if there is persistent concern, further imaging is indicated; CT is the modality of choice, having largely superseded the contrast follow-through or enema, particularly in the acute setting. The key to diagnosis of a mechanical obstruction of either small or large bowel on CT, and differentiation from paralytic ileus, is identification of a transition zone from dilated proximal bowel to collapsed distal bowel. In small bowel obstruction if no obvious cause such as a mass, volvulus or intussusception is identified, then the most likely aetiology is adhesional. There is no need to give oral contrast for a suspected bowel obstruction CT as fluid in the lumen is a natural contrast agent and, in any case, oral contrast may well not reach the point of obstruction by the time of the scan. CT is also invaluable to diagnose complications of bowel obstruction such as perforation and ischaemia. If there is ongoing uncertainty after CT as to whether the diagnosis is mechanical obstruction or a paralytic ileus, delayed plain abdominal radiographs obtained 1 and 4 hours after ingestion of dilute Gastrografin (typically 75 mL Gastrografin mixed with 75 mL water) can be useful to assess if contrast reaches the colon. Gastrografin also has an osmotic effect that can, on occasion, be therapeutic.

Closed loop obstruction, where the bowel is obstructed at two points, often in close proximity to each other and frequently related to an internal hernia or adhesional band, is a particular type of small bowel obstruction prone to developing ischaemia. It should be suspected at CT if the bowel is dilated distal to a transition point with a further transition point more distally (*Figure 8.36*).

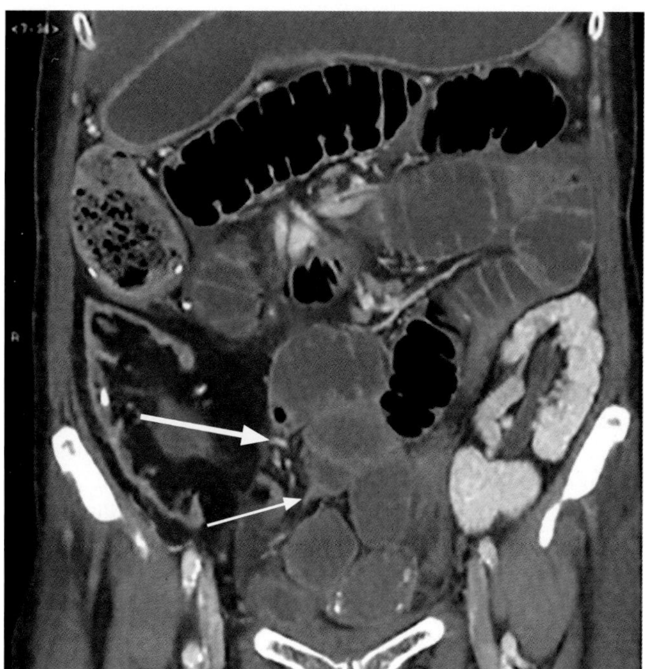

Figure 8.36 Coronal computed tomography showing a failed renal transplant in the right iliac fossa and second transplant in the left iliac fossa. There has also been a right hemicolectomy. There is proximal small bowel obstruction with dilated fluid-filled small bowel loops. Distal to the first point of obstruction (large arrow) there are dilated thick-walled fluid-filled loops in the pelvis with some adjacent free fluid, which could be followed to a second point of obstruction (small arrow). Laparotomy confirmed a closed loop obstruction secondary to an adhesive band with ischaemia in the segment of small bowel between the points of obstruction.

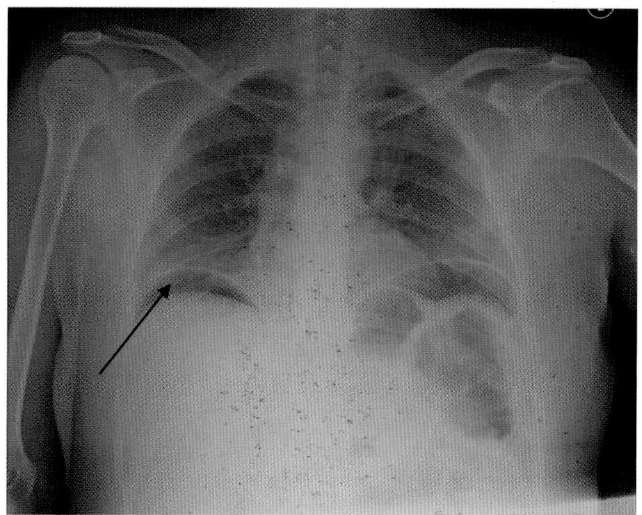

Figure 8.37 Erect chest radiograph showing subdiaphragmatic free gas (arrow) consistent with hollow organ perforation.

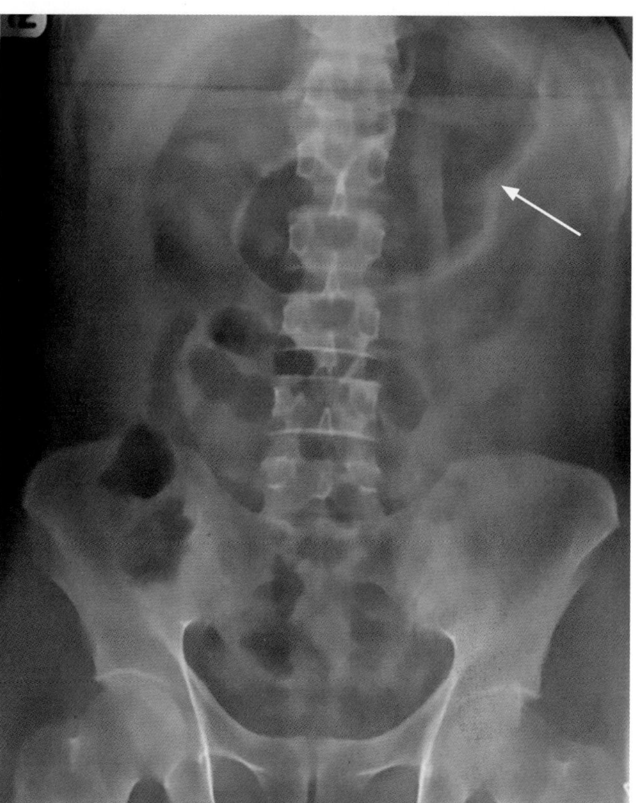

Figure 8.38 Plain abdominal radiograph showing an abnormal appearance to the gastric wall, which is very clearly visualised owing to the presence of gas both inside the lumen and outside the lumen (arrow). This is Rigler's sign of hollow organ perforation, in this case due to a duodenal ulcer.

Perforation

The erect chest x-ray (CXR) is the ideal first test for hollow organ perforation and as little as 10–20 mL of free air can be detected under the diaphragm (***Figures 8.37 and 8.38***). About 10 minutes should be left between sitting the patient upright and taking the film to allow time for air to rise; the free air must be sought under the right hemidiaphragm to prevent misinterpretation of the gastric air bubble; and the reviewer must be able to recognise Chilaiditi's syndrome, the harmless and asymptomatic interposition of large bowel between the liver and diaphragm. Caution must also be exercised in interpreting any free air in the context of recent abdominal surgery, as postoperative air can persist for up to 5–7 days in the peritoneal cavity.

If the erect CXR is equivocal or a possible walled-off perforation is suspected, a CT is the optimal modality, which may show tiny quantities of free air but may also show the cause, e.g. peptic ulcer, diverticulitis or a neoplastic lesion. As with suspected obstruction, oral or rectal contrast is unnecessary if perforation is suspected as making the diagnosis should prompt appropriate management even if the precise site of perforation is not identified. Also, it cannot be overstressed that if there is any possibility of a leak from the gastrointestinal tract (GIT)

Leo George Rigler, 1896–1979, American radiologist, described the double-wall sign in pneumoperitoneum.
Demetrius Chilaiditi, 1883–1975, Greek radiologist.

(including an anastomotic leak after surgery), then the use of barium is absolutely contraindicated as it can induce a serious and potentially fatal peritonitis.

Ischaemia/infarction

The most useful test when bowel ischaemia or infarction is suspected is a CT scan. Intravenous contrast administration is essential to look for thrombus/embolus in the mesenteric vessels, though ischaemia due to low-flow states can still occur in their absence. Ischaemia can be a difficult diagnosis to make radiologically but is suspected, in the appropriate clinical context, by bowel wall thickening, submucosal oedema and free fluid between the folds of the mesentery (particularly if haemorrhagic). Ischaemia must be strongly suspected if these findings are seen in association with a closed loop obstruction or strangulated hernia. Ischaemic colitis typically affects the 'watershed area', which is the junction of the areas supplied by the superior and inferior mesenteric arteries, typically in the region of the splenic flexure.

When bowel wall ischaemia proceeds to transmural infarction, the diagnosis is usually more straightforward with evidence of pneumatosis (air in the bowel wall) typically identified. The air in the bowel wall can then track into mesenteric veins and thence to the portal vein, a CT sign of grave prognostic significance in an adult as it implies widespread and relatively longstanding bowel infarction.

Gastrointestinal haemorrhage

The aetiology of acute gastrointestinal (GI) haemorrhage varies between the upper GIT (common causes including peptic ulcer disease, varices and Mallory–Weiss tears) and the lower GIT (common causes including angiodysplasia, diverticular haemorrhage and neoplastic lesions). While endoscopy is a useful first-line investigation for both, in refractory or occult GI haemorrhage radiology can also contribute to diagnosis and management. Nuclear medicine scans using radioisotope-labelled red blood cells are useful when bleeding is intermittent, but for patients suspected of active bleeding the best investigation is a CT mesenteric angiogram. Non-contrast scans to look for bright blood in the bowel lumen should be supplemented with scans in the arterial phase to assess for a blush due to active extravasation and the portal venous phase to optimise detection of wall thickening and masses and to look for sites of venous bleeding. If non-invasive imaging is effective, catheter angiography can be used to embolise a bleeding point.

Inflammatory processes

Appendicitis

Historically, a straightforward clinical diagnosis of appendicitis obviated any need for imaging, but with the proven accuracy of available modalities imaging has become increasingly popular to reduce negative appendicectomy rates and to make alternative diagnoses. While a plain radiograph may demonstrate a calcified appendicolith in the right iliac fossa, it is insufficiently sensitive or specific to be reliable. In children, who typically have a favourable body habitus, ultrasound is the best test as it reduces radiation exposure. This also applies to females of childbearing age, again to reduce radiation exposure, but also because the symptoms may be mimicked by gynaecological pathology, such as ectopic pregnancy, haemorrhagic ovarian cyst and tubo-ovarian abscess, all diagnoses that are best made with ultrasound. The definitive exclusion of appendicitis, however, hinges on the identification of a normal appendix, measuring less than 6 mm in diameter. Retrocaecal appendicitis can readily escape detection with ultrasound, and thus CT is the next modality of choice; indeed, frequently it is the first requested in most adults (***Figure 8.39***). The diagnosis of appendicitis on CT requires the identification of a thickened appendix (>7 mm), with periappendiceal inflammatory change as evidenced by stranding in the surrounding fat. Other signs that may be sought include free fluid, thickening of the caecal pole, possible localised small bowel ileus and right iliac fossa lymphadenopathy. Both CT and ultrasound can also identify collections if an inflamed appendix ruptures, and can be used to guide percutaneous drainage as a bridge to definitive surgery.

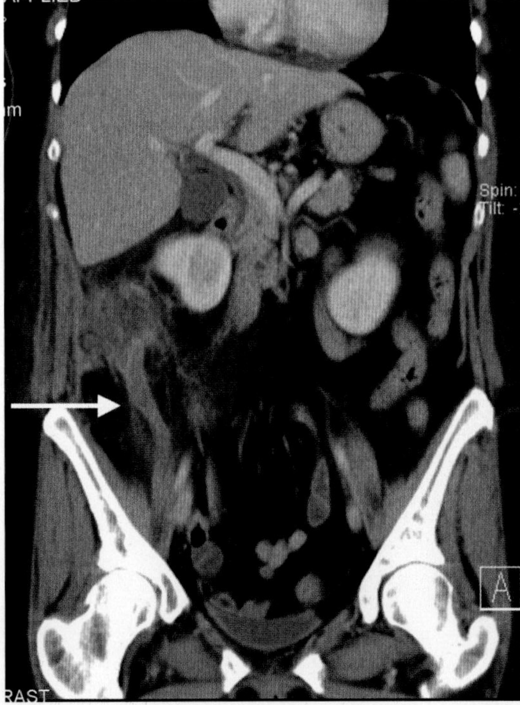

Figure 8.39 Acute appendicitis. Contrast-enhanced computed tomography scan reconstructed in the coronal plane demonstrates a thickened appendix in the right iliac fossa (arrow) with inflammatory changes in the surrounding fat and reactive thickening of the caecal pole.

George Kenneth Mallory, 1900–1986, Professor of Pathology, Boston University, Boston, MA, USA.
Soma Weiss, 1898–1942, Professor of Medicine, Harvard University Medical School, Boston, MA, USA.

Diverticulitis

Inflammation of an obstructed diverticulum typically presents with left iliac fossa pain and pyrexia (***Figure 8.40***). While some authors have promoted the use of focused ultrasound for this indication, in general it is best diagnosed with a CT scan. The typical CT appearance is of pericolic inflammatory change around a diverticulum, most commonly in the sigmoid colon. Complications of diverticulitis include perforation, abscess formation, fistulation to adjacent structures and strictures in the bowel. CT is also the modality of choice to identify these; as with appendicitis, it can be used to guide percutaneous abscess drainage as a bridge to definitive surgery.

Inflammatory bowel disease

The diagnosis of inflammatory bowel disease is made histologically. Radiologically, the diagnosis and monitoring of inflammatory bowel disease has changed significantly in recent years. Previously a barium study of the small bowel, either a follow-through (where barium is ingested orally) or enteroclysis (where dilute barium is infused via a nasojejunal tube) was used as a screening tool if symptoms are vague. If the diagnosis of Crohn's disease is established, barium studies can still be useful to demonstrate the extent of disease, particularly to demonstrate the length and number of strictures if surgery is planned. Increasingly, however, the role of barium studies has been superseded by cross-sectional imaging, particularly MRI enterography, which entails an abdominopelvic MRI scan after ingestion of an agent such as lactulose or mannitol to distend the small bowel. The other obvious advantage of MRI is the lack of radiation, which is particularly relevant in young patients with Crohn's disease, who often undergo multiple imaging studies over their lifetime; for this reason it is gaining in popularity for inflammatory bowel disease follow-up.

An acute flare-up may also require imaging, and an ultrasound is usually a good first test to look for dilated bowel loops and any abscess, though CT may ultimately be required as gas-filled bowel loops can obscure visualisation of an abscess on ultrasound. MRI is the imaging modality of choice to assess perianal fistulae and abscesses.

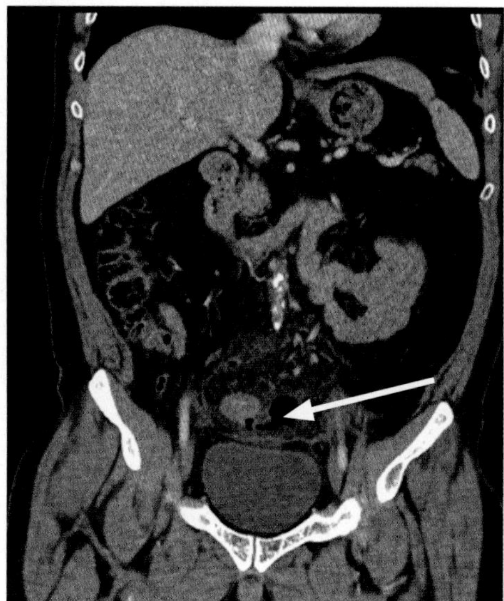

Figure 8.40 Coronal computed tomography reformatted images showing a diverticular perforation. There is stranding around the sigmoid colon with an extraluminal track of gas (arrow). Because of surrounding inflammatory changes diverticular perforation usually leads to pericolic localised gas collections rather than generalised pneumoperitoneum.

Acute pancreatitis

As with acute appendicitis, when the diagnosis is straightforward clinically there may be no need for imaging, though increasingly it is used to confirm the diagnosis, to assess the severity of the process and to look for complications. While ultrasound may show gallstones and can demonstrate an enlarged pancreas with peripancreatic fluid and inflammatory changes, the optimal modality is CT. CT performed too early in the course of the attack, e.g. in the first 12 hours, can be equivocal and the optimal timing of imaging is 48–72 hours.

In mild acute pancreatitis, CT may be normal or may show an enlarged oedematous gland, but in more severe attacks other findings which should be sought include peripancreatic fluid collections, vascular complications such as arterial pseudoaneurysm formation or venous thrombosis and necrosis, either of the gland itself or of the surrounding fat. Necrosis typically develops 48–72 hours after the onset of symptoms and is manifest on CT as lack of enhancement of the necrotic areas. CT with intravenous contrast is therefore essential to look for necrosis, which is potentially catastrophic, particularly if it becomes infected. While CT is not always reliable to diagnose infected necrosis, it is suggested by bubbles of air in the necrotic segment. As with other intra-abdominal inflammatory processes, either ultrasound or more usually CT can be used to guide percutaneous drainage of inflammatory fluid collections.

Acute cholecystitis/biliary colic/jaundice

While acute cholecystitis is usually due to mechanical obstruction of the cystic duct or gallbladder neck by a gallstone, acute acalculous cholecystitis can occur in critically ill patients from a number of causes. In any case ultrasound is the modality of choice should this diagnosis be suspected, and the classic diagnostic features are of gallbladder distension with wall thickening (>3 mm). A gallstone obstructing the gallbladder neck or cystic duct may be visualised; alternatively, in acalculous cholecystitis sludge may be seen layering in the gallbladder lumen. Associated signs include pericholecystic fluid and hyperaemia on Doppler examination. Ultrasonographic Murphy's sign refers to tenderness over the gallbladder when

Burrill Bernard Crohn, 1884–1983, gastroenterologist, Mount Sinai Hospital, New York, NY, USA, described regional ileitis in 1932 along with Leon Ginzburg and Gordon Oppenheimer.

John Benjamin Murphy, 1857–1916, Professor of Surgery, Northwestern University, Chicago, IL, USA, described his sign in 1903. He was the son of Irish immigrants fleeing the potato famine in Ireland, and was known as the 'Stormy Petrel' of American surgery, demonstrating the benefit of appendicectomy over conservative treatment among many things.

pressure is applied while scanning and is a supportive finding in making the diagnosis. As a second-line investigation CT is also accurate for this condition, demonstrating similar signs of gallbladder distension and wall thickening with surrounding inflammatory changes. CT is also useful to diagnose complications such as gangrenous cholecystitis, gallbladder perforation and emphysematous cholecystitis, which may necessitate emergency cholecystectomy. If cross-sectional studies are equivocal, hepatobiliary scintigraphy can be useful, with the diagnosis of acute cholecystitis suggested by non-visualisation of the gallbladder 3 hours after radioisotope administration.

A frequent limitation of ultrasound is failure to visualise the common bile duct throughout its length owing to overlying bowel gas, and elective cholecystectomy was typically accompanied by bile duct imaging or exploration to look for duct calculi. Increasingly, however, MRCP has been shown to be highly accurate in excluding bile duct calculi before surgery.

Ultrasound is also a useful first-line investigation for jaundice of unknown cause as it can demonstrate duct dilatation and gallstones. If a definitive cause is not shown with ultrasound, or a mass is identified but its precise nature and extent is uncertain, CT is indicated to look for common causes, including stones, cholangiocarcinoma and pancreatic carcinoma. CT can not only identify malignant lesions but also demonstrate the extent of local infiltration, including the very important assessment of vascular involvement if surgery is considered, and the presence of metastases to determine potential resectability. If the ducts are of normal calibre in a jaundiced patient, liver biopsy should be considered.

Renal colic

The historical methods of imaging for renal colic all have their limitations. Plain film radiography may not demonstrate all calculi, will not show renal tract obstruction and is unreliable for alternative diagnoses. IVU necessitates the administration of intravenous contrast and, if a level of obstruction is sought, delayed films up to 8 hours after injection may be required; it also will not provide alternative diagnoses. Ultrasound will demonstrate hydronephrosis and hydroureter, and calculi in the kidneys and either the proximal or distal ureters can usually be identified as echogenic foci with posterior acoustic shadowing; however, the ureter from just below the kidneys to the pelvis is usually obscured by bowel gas, which significantly impairs stone detection.

For these reasons the optimal investigation is now CT of the kidneys, ureters and bladder, a non-contrast, low-dose (2–3 MSv if a low mA scan is performed, equivalent to the dose from a limited IVU series) scan from the upper poles of the kidneys to the pubic symphysis. Contrast administration, either orally or intravenously, is not employed as it does not aid stone detection and may even impair it. Stones are readily identified as high-attenuation (typically calcific) foci, and the secondary signs of acute ureteric obstruction may also be seen, including hydronephrosis and hydroureter, renal enlargement and perinephric fat stranding. The most common sites for stones to be seen are at the areas of ureteric narrowing, namely the pelviureteric junction, the pelvic brim and vesicoureteric junction. CT also offers unrivalled capability for making alternative diagnoses when compared with other modalities.

Abdominal aortic aneurysm

If a pulsatile mass is felt in the abdomen and the diagnosis of a possible abdominal aortic aneurysm (AAA) is suspected, ultrasound is a useful modality; provided the aorta is not obscured by bowel gas, an aneurysm can usually reliably be excluded. If, however, ultrasound visualisation is suboptimal and the diagnosis is as a result equivocal, or if an aneurysm is identified and information regarding the extent and exact size is required, for example for surgical or endovascular repair planning, CT angiography is indicated, with the aorta typically scanned from the arch to the pubic symphysis in the arterial phase after intravenous contrast. MR angiography is a useful alternative if iodinated contrast is contraindicated.

In the case of suspected aneurysm rupture, provided the patient is sufficiently haemodynamically stable to undergo CT, CT angiography should be urgently performed; a supplementary non-enhanced initial scan is useful to look for retroperitoneal haematoma, which is typically of relatively high attenuation compared with the blood in the lumen on a non-contrast scan.

IMAGING IN ONCOLOGY

Modern surgical treatment of cancer requires an understanding of tumour staging systems, as in many instances the tumour stage will define appropriate management. The development of stage-dependent treatment protocols involving neoadjuvant chemotherapy and preoperative radiotherapy relies on the ability of imaging to determine stage accurately before surgical and pathological staging. The importance of accurate cancer staging is reflected in the central role of the radiologist in most MDT meetings.

Once a diagnosis of cancer has been established, often by percutaneous or endoscopic biopsy, new imaging techniques can considerably improve the ability to define the extent of tumour, although the pathological specimen remains the 'gold standard'. Many staging systems are based on the tumour–node–metastasis (TNM) classification.

Tumour

In most published studies, cross-sectional imaging techniques (CT, ultrasound, MRI) are more accurate in staging advanced (T3, T4) than early (T1, T2) diseases, and the staging of early disease remains a challenge. In gut tumours, endoscopic ultrasound is more accurate than CT or MRI in the local staging of early disease (T1, T2) by virtue of its ability to demonstrate the layered structure of the bowel wall and the depth of tumour penetration (***Figure 8.41***). Developments in MRI may also improve the staging accuracy of early disease. MRI is extremely valuable in bone and soft-tissue tumour staging and in intracranial and spinal disease.

Nodes

Accurate assessment of nodal involvement remains a challenge for imaging. Most imaging techniques rely purely on size criteria to demonstrate lymph node involvement, with

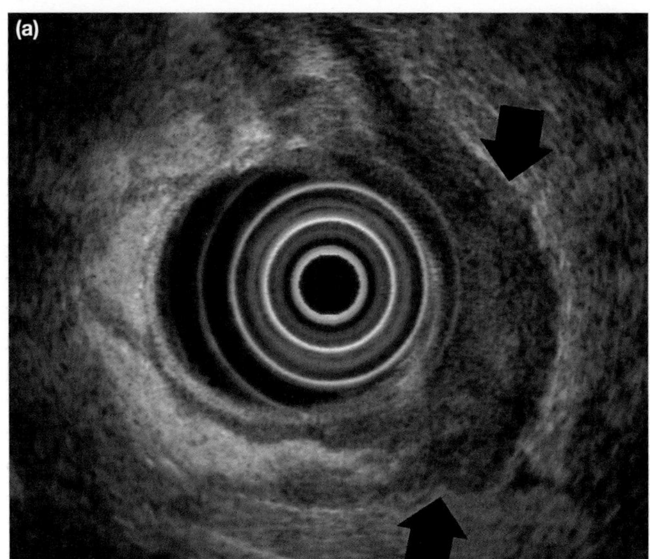

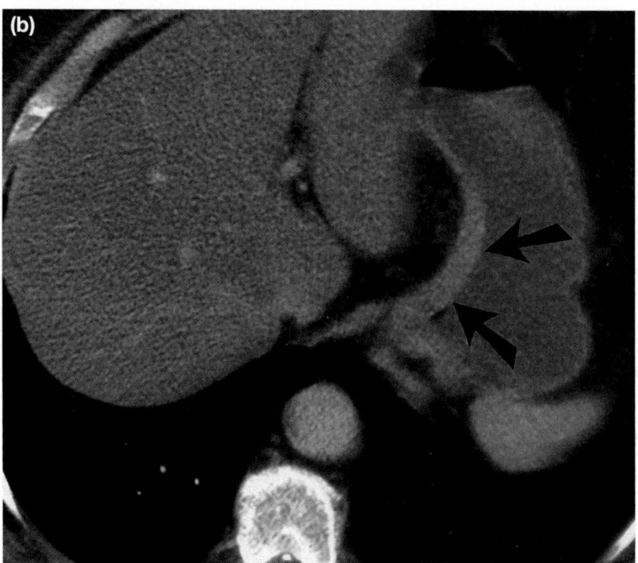

Figure 8.41 (a) Endoscopic ultrasound in gastric cancer. The hypoechoic tumour (arrows) is infiltrating the layered structure of the gastric wall and extending out beyond the serosa. (b) Computed tomography scan demonstrates thickening and enhancement of the gastric wall in the same area (arrows). The stomach is distended with water to provide low-density contrast.

no possibility of identifying micrometastases in normal-sized nodes. A size criterion of 8–10 mm is often adopted, but it is not usually possible to distinguish benign reactive nodes from infiltrated nodes. This is a particular problem in patients with intrathoracic neoplasms, in whom enlarged benign reactive mediastinal nodes are common. The echo characteristics of nodes at endoscopic ultrasound have been used in many centres to increase the accuracy of nodal staging, and nodal sampling is possible via either mediastinoscopy or transoesophageal biopsy under endoscopic ultrasound control. PET/CT is of increasing use in detecting nodal metastases from a wide range of malignancies, with the capacity to co-register the area of increased FDG uptake with a precise anatomical location. Novel MRI contrast agents may help in the identification of non-enlarged tumour-infiltrated nodes.

Metastases

The demonstration of metastatic disease will usually significantly affect surgical management. Modern cross-sectional imaging has greatly improved the detection of metastases, but occult lesions will be overlooked in between 10% and 30% of patients. CT is the most sensitive technique for the detection of lung deposits, although the decision to perform CT will depend on the site of the primary tumour, its likelihood of intrapulmonary spread and the effect on staging and subsequent therapy of the demonstration of intrapulmonary deposits.

Ultrasound and CT are most frequently used to detect liver metastases. Contrast-enhanced CT can detect most lesions greater than 1 cm, although accuracy rates vary with the technique used and range from 70% to 90%. Recent studies suggest that MRI may be more accurate than CT in demonstrating metastatic disease. Preoperative identification of the segment of the liver involved can be determined by translation of the segmental surgical anatomy, as defined by Couinaud, to the cross-sectional CT images (***Figure 8.42***).

The technique of PET/CT with FDG, an analogue of glucose, is becoming a powerful tool in oncological imaging. This functional and anatomical imaging technique reflects tumour metabolism and allows the detection of otherwise occult metastases. The most common indications for PET/CT have been staging of lymphoma, lung cancer, particularly non-small cell lung cancer, and preoperative assessment of potentially resectable liver metastases, such as colorectal carcinoma metastases (***Figure 8.43***).

Intraoperative ultrasound is an additional method of staging that provides superb high-resolution imaging of subcentimetre liver nodules that may not be palpable at surgery. This is often used immediately prior to resection of liver metastases.

Claude Couinaud, 1922–2008, French surgeon and anatomist, described the segmental anatomy of the liver in his seminal book *Le Foie: Études anatomiques et chirurgicales.*

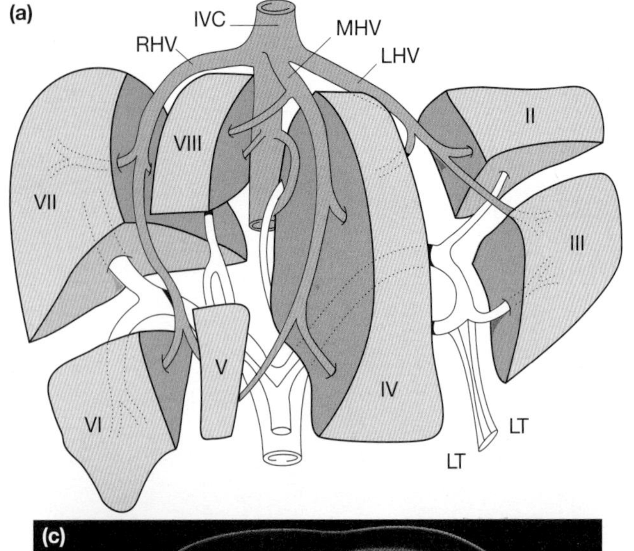

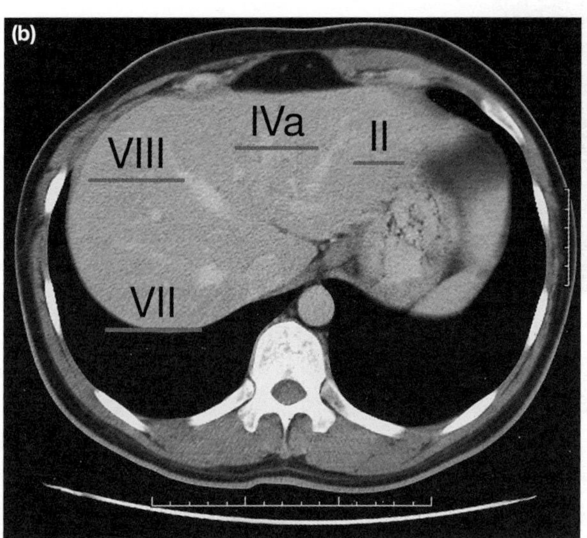

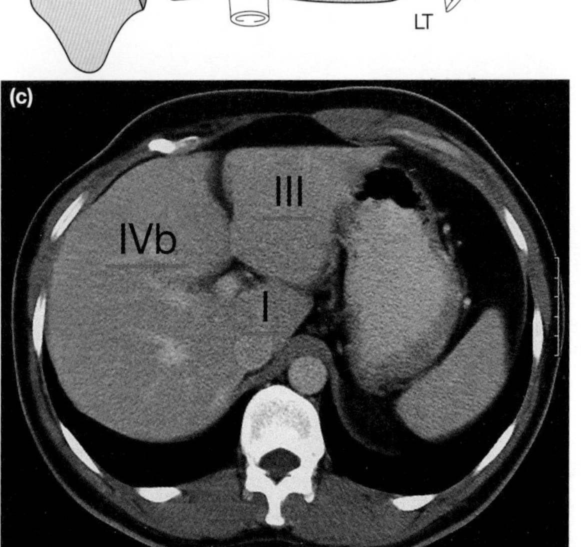

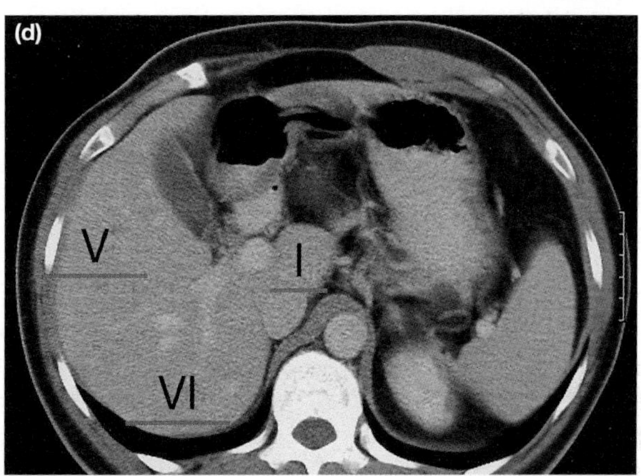

Figure 8.42 (a) Surgical lobes of the liver (after Couinaud). IVC, inferior vena cava; LHV, left hepatic vein; LT, ligamentum teres; MHV, middle hepatic vein; RHV, right hepatic vein. (b) Segmental anatomy on computed tomography scan at the level of the hepatic veins. (c) Segmental anatomy at the level of the portal veins. (d) Segmental anatomy below the level of the portal veins.

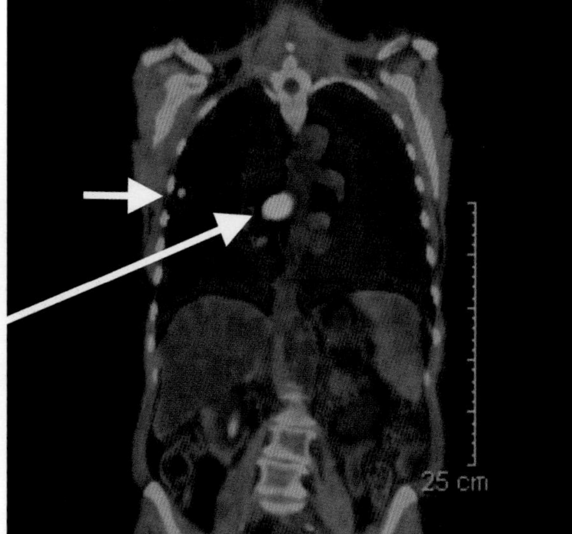

Figure 8.43 Positron emission tomography shows fluorodeoxyglucose uptake in a carcinoma of the lung (short arrow) and mediastinal lymph nodes (long arrow).

FURTHER READING

Adam A, Dixon AK (eds). *Grainger and Allison's diagnostic radiology: a textbook of medical imaging*, 7th edn. London: Elsevier, 2020.

iRefer Guidelines. *Making the best use of clinical radiology*, 8th edn. London: Royal College of Radiologists, 2017.

Krishnam MS, Curtis J (eds). *Emergency radiology*. New York: Cambridge Medicine, 2010.

Pope T, Bloem HL, Beltran J *et al*. *Musculoskeletal imaging*, 2nd edn. Oxford: Saunders, 2015.

Rockall AG, Hatrick A, Armstrong P, Wastie M. *Diagnostic imaging*, 7th edn. Oxford: Wiley-Blackwell, 2013.

The Royal Australian and New Zealand College of Radiologists. *Iodinated contrast media guideline*. Sydney: RANZCR, 2018.

CHAPTER 9 Gastrointestinal endoscopy

Learning objectives

To gain an understanding of:

- The role of endoscopy as a diagnostic and therapeutic tool
- The basic organisation of an endoscopy unit and its equipment
- Consent and safe sedation
- Special situations: the key points in managing endoscopy in at-risk patients
- The indications for diagnostic and therapeutic endoscopic procedures including endoscopic ultrasound
- The recognition and management of complications
- Novel techniques for endoscoping the small bowel
- Advances in diagnostic ability

INTRODUCTION

The gastrointestinal tract has a myriad of functions, such as digestion, absorption and excretion, as well as the synthesis of an array of hormones, growth factors and cytokines. In addition, a complex enteric nervous system has evolved to control its function and communicate with the central and peripheral nervous systems. Finally, as the gastrointestinal tract contains the largest sources of foreign antigens to which the body is exposed, it houses well-developed arms of both the innate and acquired immune systems. Therefore, it is not surprising that malfunction or infection of this complex organ results in a wide spectrum of pathology. However, its importance in disease pathogenesis is matched only by its inaccessibility to traditional examination.

Few discoveries in medicine have contributed more to the practice of gastroenterology than the development of diagnostic and therapeutic endoscopy. Although spectacular advances in radiology have occurred recently with the introduction of multislice spiral computed tomography (CT) and magnetic resonance imaging (MRI), the ability to take targeted mucosal biopsies remains a unique strength of endoscopy. Historically, radiological techniques were required to image areas of jejunum and ileum inaccessible to the standard endoscope; however, the introduction of both capsule endoscopy and single-/double-balloon enteroscopy allows both diagnostic and therapeutic access to the entire gastrointestinal tract. Image enhancement with techniques such as chromoendoscopy, magnification endoscopy and narrow band imaging allows increased resolution at the mucosal level and increases diagnostic yield. Endoscopic ultrasound (EUS) can examine all layers of the intestinal wall as well as extraintestinal structures. Finally, experimental techniques such as confocal laser endomicroscopy give resolution at a level compatible with standard histology. The advances in the diagnostic accuracy of endoscopy lend themselves to disease surveillance for specific patient groups as well as population screening for gastrointestinal malignancy. Likewise, there has been a rapid expansion in the therapeutic capability of endoscopy with both luminal and extraintestinal surgery being performed via endoscopic access.

As in all areas of interventional practice, competent endoscopists must match a thorough grounding in anatomy and physiology with a clear understanding of the capabilities and limitations of the rapidly advancing techniques available. Perhaps most importantly they must appreciate all aspects of patient care, including preprocedural management, communication before and during the procedure and the management of endoscopic complications. This chapter aims to guide the reader through these areas in addition to introducing the breadth of procedures that are currently performed.

HISTORY OF ENDOSCOPY

Over the last 50 years, endoscopy has become a powerful diagnostic and therapeutic tool. However, its development required two obvious but formidable barriers to be overcome. First, the gastrointestinal tract is rather long and tortuous and, second, no natural light shines through the available orifices! Therefore, successful visualisation of anything beyond the distal extremities requires a flexible instrument with an intrinsic light source that can transmit images to the operator.

The breakthrough was the discovery that images could be transmitted using flexible quartz fibres. Although this was first described in the late 1920s, it was not until 1954 that Hopkins built a model of a flexible fibre imaging device. The

Harold Horace Hopkins, 1918–1994, Professor of Applied Optics, The University of Reading, Reading, UK.

TABLE 9.1 Historical landmarks of gastrointestinal endoscopy.

1958	Development of fibreoptic gastroscope
1968	Endoscopic retrograde pancreatography
1969	Colonoscopic polypectomy
1970	Endoscopic retrograde cholangiography
1974	Endoscopic sphincterotomy (with bile duct stone extraction)
1979	Percutaneous endoscopic gastrostomy
1980	Endoscopic injection sclerotherapy
1980	Endoscopic ultrasonography
1983	Electronic (charge-coupled device) endoscope
1985	Endoscopic control of upper gastrointestinal bleeding
1990	Endoscopic variceal ligation
1996	Introduction of self-expanding metal stents
2008	Endomicroscopy delivers histological mucosal definition

availability of highly transparent optical quality glass led to the development in 1958 of the first flexible fibreoptic gastroscope by Larry Curtiss, a graduate student in physics, and Basil Hirschowitz, a trainee in gastroenterology.

Over the next 30 years, the fibrescope evolved to allow examination of the upper gastrointestinal tract, the biliary system and the colon. In parallel with advances in diagnostic ability, a range of therapeutic procedures was developed (*Table 9.1*). Although the fibreoptic endoscope has been the workhorse of many endoscopy units over the last three decades, its obsolescence was guaranteed by the invention of the charge-coupled device (CCD) in the 1960s, which allowed the creation of a digital electronic image, permitting endoscopic images to be processed by a computer and transmitted to television screens. Thus, the modern endoscope was born (*Figure 9.1*).

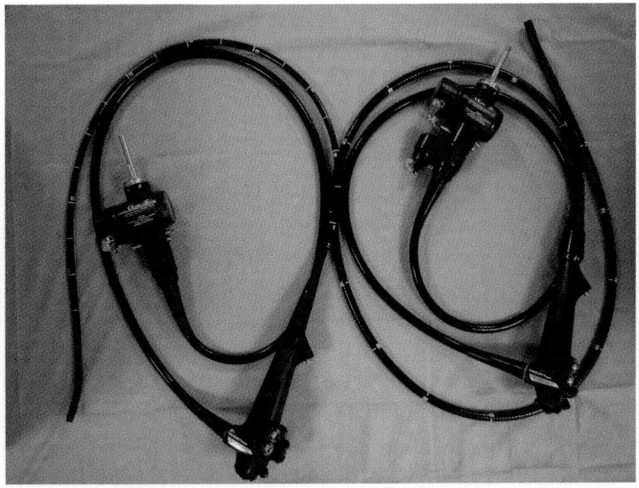

Figure 9.1 Photograph of a standard gastroscope and colonoscope.

History does not sit still, and endoscopic evolution will continue with the replacement of much diagnostic endoscopy with capsule endoscopy and virtual imaging. Enhanced resolution with high-definition operating systems, dye and digital chromoendoscopy and even histological-grade images have increased the diagnostic yield of surveillance procedures. EUS allows diagnosis and therapy to extend beyond the mucosal surface of the intestine. Endoscopy has become increasingly therapeutic and historical divisions between medicine, radiology and surgery will become progressively blurred. As the complexity of the procedures increases, the distinction between specialist and general endoscopists will become more definite. This reinforces the need for all endoscopic practitioners to have a detailed understanding of the units in which they work and the instruments that they use.

THE MODERN ENDOSCOPY UNIT

Organisation

A well-designed endoscopy unit staffed by trained endoscopy nurses and dedicated administrative staff is essential to support good endoscopic practice and training. Clinical governance with regular appraisal and assessment of performance should be embedded within the unit's philosophy. Endoscopist training demands particular attention, with a transparent process of skills- and theory-based education centred on practical experience and dedicated training courses. Experienced supervision of all trainees is essential until competency has been obtained and assessed by an appropriately validated technique, such as direct observation of practical skills (DOPS) and review of procedure logbooks. All endoscopists should record diagnostic and therapeutic procedure numbers and markers of competency such as colonoscopy completion rates, polyp detection rates, mean sedation use and complication rates. Central to this is an efficient data management system that provides outcome analysis for all aspects of endoscopy, including adherence to guidelines, near misses, patient satisfaction, decontamination processes and scope tracking, as well as the more obvious completion and complication rates.

In the UK the Joint Advisory Group (JAG) provides guidance for endoscopist competence assessment and operates a certification system of individual endoscopic competencies, based on procedure numbers, key performance indicators (e.g. caecal intubation rate, adenoma detection, sedation levels, complications), course attendance and peer assessment.

Equipment

A full description of all available endoscopic equipment is beyond the scope of this chapter. However, each unit should have a sufficient range of endoscopes, processors and accessories as dictated by the local case mix and sufficient endoscope numbers to ensure smooth service provision. These should include both forward- and lateral-viewing gastroscopes, an enteroscope for proximal small bowel visualisation and a

Larry E Curtiss, physicist, University of Michigan, Ann Arbour, MI, USA.
Basil I Hirschowitz, 1925–2013, Professor of Medicine, University of Alabama, Birmingham, AL, USA.

range of adult and paediatric colonoscopes to aid examination of both redundant and fixed colons. Dedicated small bowel centres require capsule endoscopy and a single-/double-balloon enteroscope for ileojejunal visualisation and therapeutics. Larger centres will require linear and radial EUS, particularly if they specialise in gastrointestinal and hepatobiliary malignancy. An electrosurgical unit is the cornerstone of many therapeutic procedures, and this may be supplemented by argon plasma coagulation (APC), laser units and radiofrequency ablation for advanced therapeutics.

Instrument decontamination

Endoscopes will not withstand steam-based autoclaving and therefore require high-level disinfection between cases to prevent transmission of infection. Although accessories may be autoclaved, best practice requires the use of disposable single-use items whenever possible. All equipment should be decontaminated to an identical standard whether for use on immunocompromised/infected patients or not. This process involves two equally important stages: first, removal of physical debris from the internal and external surfaces of the instrument and, second, chemical neutralisation of all microbiological agents. A variety of agents are available and endoscopists should familiarise themselves with the agent in use in their department. In 2020 the British Society of Gastroenterology updated its guidelines for decontamination of endoscopes (see Further reading). Care should be applied to the decontamination of duodenoscopes because of reports of transmission of multiresistant bacteria (*Summary box 9.1*).

Summary box 9.1

Disinfection of endoscopes

- All channels must be brushed and irrigated throughout the disinfection process
- All instruments and accessories should be traceable to each use, patient and cleaning cycle
- All staff should be trained and protected (particularly if glutaraldehyde is used in view of its immune-sensitising properties)
- Regular monitoring of disinfectant power and microbiological contamination should be performed

There are currently no reliable means of decontaminating scopes from contact with prion-associated conditions such as variant Creutzfeldt–Jakob disease (vCJD), although risk of transmission of this is considered very low. If an 'invasive' procedure (where gut mucosa is breached and an unsheathed accessory withdrawn through the endoscope working channel) is conducted in a patient with known or possible vCJD, the endoscope needs to be quarantined after use. The performance of an invasive procedure in a patient at risk of vCJD owing to receipt of pooled plasma concentrates is no longer deemed to confer a high risk of endoscope contamination. A single quality assured decontamination cycle is considered sufficient, but the endoscope should be decontaminated separately from others with a single-use disinfectant. There is no longer a requirement to quarantine the endoscope provided that routine traceability data can be demonstrated.

CONSENT IN ENDOSCOPY

Approximately 1% of medical negligence claims in the USA relate to the practice of endoscopy. Many of these could have been avoided by a careful explanation of the procedure, including an honest discussion of the risks and benefits. Therefore, obtaining informed consent is a cornerstone of good endoscopic practice. It preserves a patient's autonomy, facilitates communication and acts as a shield against future complaints and claims of malpractice.

The most important aspect of the consent procedure is that a patient understands the nature, purpose and risk of a particular procedure, in addition to potential alternatives. Current guidelines would suggest that a patient should be informed of minor adverse events with a risk of more than 10% and serious events with an incidence of more than 0.5%. The key risks of endoscopy are summarised in *Summary box 9.2*. British Society of Gastroenterology Guidelines for Consent have been published (see Further reading).

Summary box 9.2

The risks of endoscopy

- Sedation-related cardiorespiratory complications
- Damage to dentition
- Aspiration
- Perforation or haemorrhage after endoscopic dilatation/therapeutic EUS
- Perforation, infection and aspiration after percutaneous endoscopic gastrostomy insertion
- Perforation or haemorrhage after flexible sigmoidoscopy/colonoscopy with polypectomy
- Pancreatitis, cholangitis, perforation or bleeding after endoscopic retrograde cholangiopancreatography

SAFE SEDATION

If performed competently the majority of diagnostic endoscopies and colonoscopies can be performed without sedation or with pharyngeal anaesthesia alone. However, therapeutic procedures may cause pain and patients are often anxious; thus, in most countries sedation and analgesia are offered to achieve a state of conscious sedation (not anaesthesia). Medication-induced respiratory depression in elderly patients or those with comorbidities is the greatest cause of endoscopy-

---

Hans Gerhard Creutzfeldt, 1885–1964, neurologist, Kiel, Germany.
Alfons Marie Jakob, 1884–1931, neurologist, Hamburg, Germany.

related mortality and, therefore, safe sedation practices are essential. The involvement of anaesthetists to advise on appropriate protocols is recommended. Endoscopy in certain situations (particularly paediatric endoscopy) requires a general anaesthetic – this should only be undertaken by appropriately trained staff with adequate equipment available.

Summary box 9.3

Sedation in endoscopy

- Pharyngeal anaesthesia may increase the risk of aspiration in more heavily sedated patients
- Comorbidities must be identified so that sedation can be individualised
- All sedated patients require secure intravenous access
- Benzodiazepines reach their maximum effect 9–20 minutes after administration – doses should be titrated carefully, particularly in the elderly or those with comorbidities
- Coadministration of opiates and benzodiazepines has a synergistic effect; opiates should be given first and doses need to be reduced
- The use of supplementary oxygen is essential in all sedated patients
- Sedated patients require pulse oximetry to monitor oxygen saturation; high-risk patients or those undergoing high-risk procedures also require blood pressure and electrocardiogram monitoring
- A trained assistant should be responsible for patient monitoring throughout the procedure
- Resuscitation equipment and sedation reversal agents must be readily available
- The use of anaesthetic agents such as propofol for complex procedures requires specialist training
- The half-life of benzodiazepines is 4–24 hours – appropriate recovery and monitoring is essential. Postprocedural consultations may not be remembered, and patients must be advised not to drink alcohol or drive for 24 hours

ENDOSCOPY IN PATIENTS WITH DIABETES

As approximately 2% of the population has diabetes, managing glycaemic control before and after endoscopy is an essential aspect of endoscopic practice. Each unit should develop a policy for managing diabetic control during endoscopy. Factors influencing management include the type of diabetes, the procedure that is planned, the preparation/recovery time and the history of diabetes control in the individual patient. Thus, a patient with poorly controlled insulin-dependent diabetes undergoing colonoscopy will require more input than a patient with type 2 diabetes on oral hypoglycaemic medication undergoing upper gastrointestinal endoscopy. All patients should bring their own medication to the unit and should be advised not to drive in case there is an alteration in their glycaemic control. Most patients can be managed using clear protocols on an outpatient basis; however, elderly patients and those with brittle control should be admitted. In general, patients with diabetes should be endoscoped first on the morning list. In complex cases the diabetes team should be involved.

ANTIBIOTIC PROPHYLAXIS

The majority of endoscopies can be performed safely without the need for routine antibiotic prophylaxis. However, given that certain endoscopic procedures are associated with a significant bacteraemia (***Table 9.2***), there are several specific situations where antibiotic cover is required to prevent either bacterial endocarditis, infection of surgical prostheses or systemic sepsis. In general, the risk of infection relates to the level of bacteraemia and the risk of the underlying medical condition. Traditionally, patients with a previous history of endocarditis or a metallic heart valve received antibiotic prophylaxis for all endoscopic procedures, and some national guidelines still reflect this. However, in 2009 UK guidelines changed in response to the low reported incidence of infective endocarditis in this patient group undergoing endoscopy. Patients with severe neutropenia may also require antibiotic prophylaxis for endoscopy. The antibiotic regime used will depend on local guidelines.

TABLE 9.2 Approximate incidence of bacteraemia in immunocompetent individuals following various procedures involving the gastrointestinal tract.

Procedure	Incidence of bacteraemia (%)[a]
Rectal digital examination	4
Proctoscopy	5
Barium enema	11
Tooth brushing	25
Dental extraction	30–60
Colonoscopy	2–4
Diagnostic upper gastrointestinal endoscopy	4
Sigmoidoscopy	6–9
ERCP (no duct occlusion)	6
ERCP (duct occluded)	11
Oesophageal varices band ligation	6
Oesophageal varices sclerotherapy	10–50[b]
Oesophageal dilatation/prosthesis	34–54
Oesophageal laser therapy	35
EUS +/– fine-needle aspirate	0–6

ERCP, endoscopic retrograde cholangiopancreatography; EUS, endoscopic ultrasound.
[a] Summary of published data.
[b] Higher after emergency than after elective management.

Procedures such as endoscopic percutaneous gastrostomy are associated with a significant incidence of wound or stoma infection, particularly if inserted for malignancy. Antibiotic prophylaxis reduces this complication and a single intravenous injection of co-amoxiclav should be administered before the procedure. Antibiotics are routinely used during endoscopic manipulation of an obstructed biliary tree in which it is unlikely that complete drainage will be achieved or there is significant comorbidity. When cystic cavities are aspirated at EUS, a one-off dose of a broad-spectrum antibiotic (e.g. co-amoxiclav) is recommended to prevent cyst infection.

ANTICOAGULATION IN PATIENTS UNDERGOING ENDOSCOPY

Many patients undergoing endoscopy may be taking a medication that interferes with normal haemostasis, such as warfarin, heparin, direct oral anticoagulants, clopidogrel or aspirin. The key points to remember when managing anticoagulants in patients undergoing endoscopy are given in ***Summary box 9.4***.

Summary box 9.4

Managing anticoagulants in patients undergoing endoscopy

It is important to recognise and understand:

- The risk of complications related to the underlying gastrointestinal disease from anticoagulant therapy
- The risk of haemorrhage related to an endoscopic procedure in the setting of anticoagulant therapy
- The risk of a thromboembolic/ischaemic event related to interruption of anticoagulant therapy

Urgent endoscopy for gastrointestinal bleeding in the anticoagulated patient

The risk of clinically significant gastrointestinal bleeding in patients on warfarin is increased, particularly in patients with a past history of similar events, if the international normalised ratio (INR) is above the therapeutic range or if the patient is taking concomitant aspirin/non-steroidal anti-inflammatory drugs (NSAIDs). In these situations, the risk of reversing the anticoagulation must be weighed against the risk of ongoing haemorrhage. If complete reversal is not appropriate, correction of the INR to approximately 1.5 is usually sufficient to allow endoscopic diagnosis and therapy. Anticoagulation can often be resumed 24 hours after successful endoscopic therapy (***Figure 9.2***).

Elective endoscopy in patients on anticoagulants and antiplatelet agents

Endoscopic procedures vary in their potential to produce significant or uncontrolled bleeding. Diagnostic oesophagogastroduodenoscopy (OGD), colonoscopy, enteroscopy, diagnostic EUS and endoscopic retrograde cholangiopancreatography (ERCP) without sphincterotomy are considered low risk, as is mucosal biopsy. High-risk procedures include polypectomy, endoscopic sphincterotomy, stent placement and procedures with the potential to produce bleeding that is inaccessible or uncontrollable by endoscopic means, such as dilatation of benign or malignant strictures, percutaneous gastrostomy insertion and EUS-guided fine-needle aspiration. Likewise, the probability of a thromboembolic complication during temporary cessation of anticoagulant or antiplatelet therapy depends on the underlying medical condition (***Table 9.3***).

TABLE 9.3 The risk of a thromboembolic event varies according to the underlying medical condition.

Condition	Risk
Atrial fibrillation with valvular heart disease	High
Mechanical mitral valve	High
Mechanical valve and previous thromboembolic event	High
Deep vein thrombosis	Low
Uncomplicated atrial fibrillation	Low
Bioprosthetic valve	Low
Mechanical aortic valve	Low

Aspirin

Aspirin and NSAIDs inhibit platelet cyclo-oxygenase, resulting in suppression of thromboxane A_2-induced platelet aggregation. Limited published data do not suggest an increased bleeding risk in patients taking standard doses and, therefore, there is no need to discontinue therapy before endoscopic procedures.

UPPER GASTROINTESTINAL ENDOSCOPY

OGD is the most commonly performed endoscopic procedure. Excellent visualisation of the oesophagus, gastro-oesophageal junction, stomach, duodenal bulb and second part of the duodenum can be obtained. Retroversion of the gastroscope in the stomach is essential to obtain complete views of the gastric cardia and fundus (***Figure 9.3***). Traditional forward-viewing endoscopes do not adequately visualise the ampulla, and a side-viewing scope should be used if this is essential. Likewise, although it is possible to reach the third part of the duodenum with a standard 120-cm instrument, a longer enteroscope is required if views beyond the ligament of Treitz are required. In addition to clear mucosal views, diagnostic endoscopy allows mucosal biopsies to be taken, which may either undergo processing for histological examination or be used for near-patient detection of *Helicobacter pylori* infection using a commercial urease-based kit. In addition, brushings may be taken for cytology and aspirates for microbiological culture.

Indications for oesophagogastroduodenoscopy

A full assessment of the role of OGD is outside the scope of this chapter. It will vary with local circumstances and the availability of alternative diagnostic techniques. OGD is usually appropriate when a patient's symptoms are persistent despite appropriate empirical therapy or are associated with warning signs such as intractable vomiting, anaemia, weight loss, dysphagia or bleeding. It is also part of the diagnostic work-up for patients with anaemia, symptoms of

Wenzel Treitz, 1819–1872, Professor of Pathology, Prague, Czech Republic.

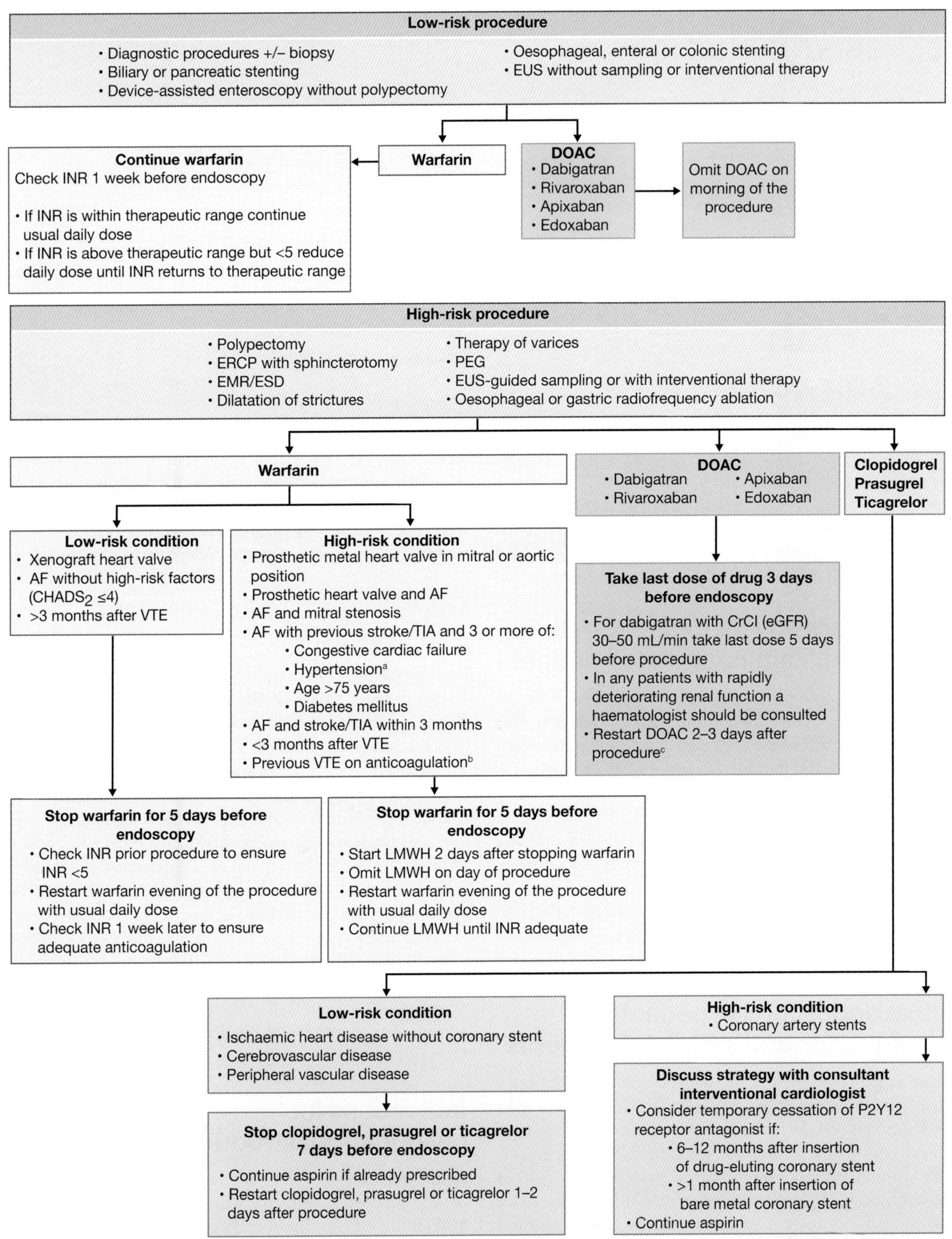

Figure 9.2 British Society of Gastroenterology and European Society of Gastrointestinal Endoscopy 2021 guidelines for management of endoscopy in patients on antiplatelet or anticoagulant therapy. AF, atrial fibrillation; CHADS, score for stroke risk assessment in atrial fibrillation; DOAC, direct oral anticoagulant; eGFR, estimated glomerular filtration rate; EMR, endoscopic mucosal resection; ERCP, endoscopic retrograde cholangiopancreatography; ESD, endoscopic submucosal dissection; EUS, endoscopic ultrasound; INR, international normalised ratio; LMWH, low molecular weight heparin; PEG, percutaneous endoscopic gastroenterostomy; TIA, transient ischaemic attack; VTE, venous thromboembolism. [a]Blood pressure >140/90 mmHg or on antihypertensive medication. [b]Previous VTE on anticoagulation and target INR now 3.5. [c]Depends on haemorrhagic and thrombotic risk; consider extending interval for ESD. (Adapted from Veitch *et al.* 2021.)

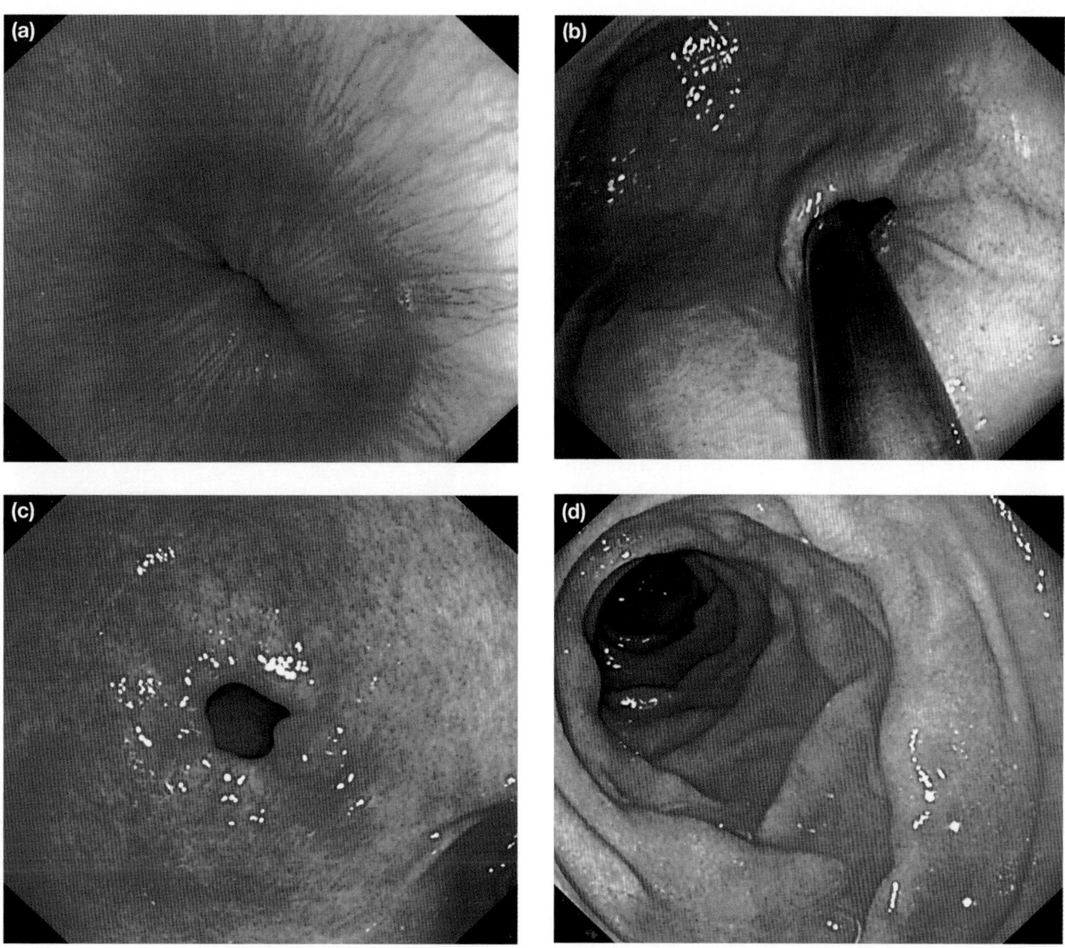

Figure 9.3 A normal upper gastrointestinal endoscopy showing the gastro-oesophageal junction (a), the gastric fundus in the 'J' position (b), the gastric antrum (c) and the second part of the duodenum (d).

malabsorption and chronic diarrhoea. However, increasing ease of access to OGD with the availability of 'open access' endoscopy has resulted in a significant number of unnecessary procedures being performed in young patients with dyspepsia or gastro-oesophageal reflux disease (GORD). This has led to a number of international gastroenterology societies proposing guidelines for the management of dyspepsia and GORD, including the empirical use of acid suppression and non-invasive *H. pylori* tests, such as urease breath tests and stool antigen assay (e.g. the National Institute for Health and Care Excellence guidelines on dyspepsia: https://www.nice.org.uk/guidance/cg184/chapter/1-recommendations). In addition

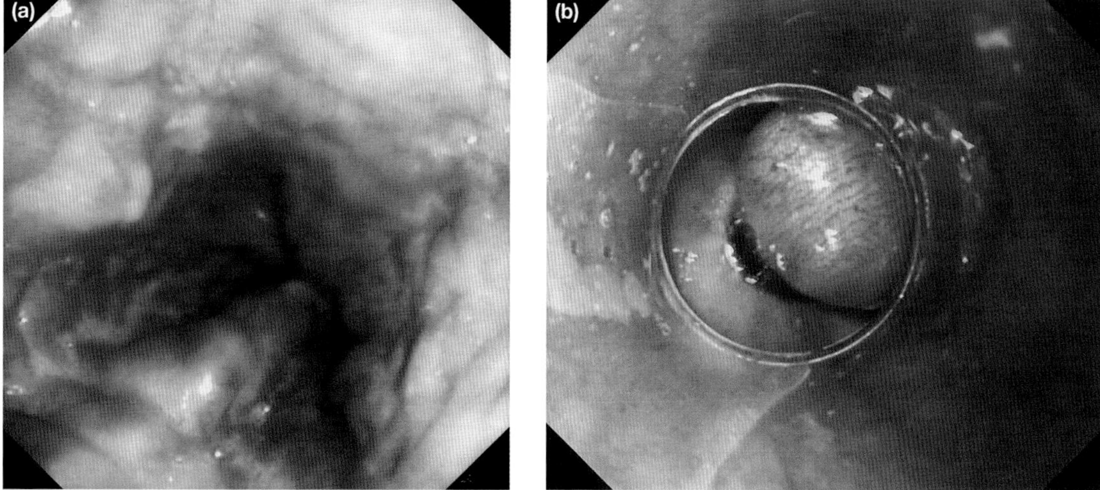

Figure 9.4 Grade 2 oesophageal varices (a), which can be treated by the application of bands to ligate the vessel and reduce blood flow (b).

to the role of OGD in diagnosis, it is also commonly used in the surveillance of neoplasia development in high-risk patient groups, such as those with genetic conditions such as familial adenomatous polyposis and premalignant conditions such as Barrett's oesophagus (see *Chapter 66*).

Therapeutic oesophagogastroduodenoscopy

Appropriate patient selection and monitoring are essential to minimise complications. The most common therapeutic endoscopic procedure performed as an emergency is the control of upper gastrointestinal haemorrhage of any aetiology. Band ligation has replaced sclerotherapy in the management of oesophageal varices (*Figure 9.4*), whereas sclerotherapy using thrombin-based glues can be used to control blood loss from gastric and duodenal varices. Injection therapy with adrenaline (epinephrine) coupled with a second haemostatic technique such as thermal coagulation or endoclip application is the technique of choice for a peptic ulcer with active bleeding or high-risk stigmata of haemorrhage (*Figure 9.5*). Such high-risk bleeds should be followed by 72 hours of intravenous proton pump inhibition. Chronic blood loss from angioectasia is most safely treated with APC because of the controlled depth of burn compared with alternative thermal techniques (*Figure 9.6*). Haemostatic powders provide a further way to arrest bleeding; these work best for diffuse bleeding or as salvage therapy.

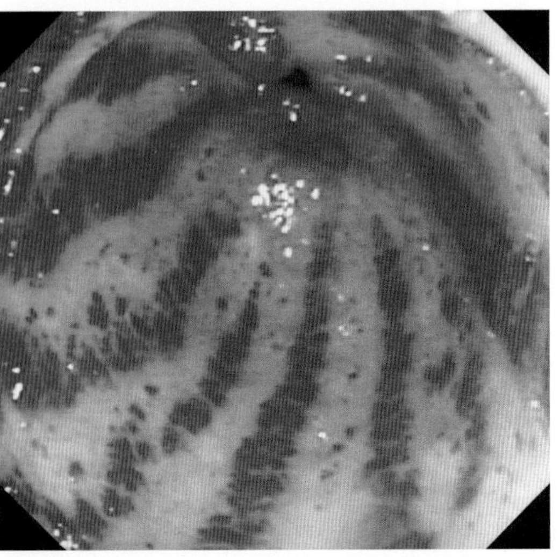

Figure 9.6 The classic appearance of gastric antral vascular ectasia, which is often treated with argon plasma coagulation.

Benign oesophageal and pyloric strictures may be dilated under direct vision with through-the-scope (TTS) balloon dilators or the more traditional guidewire-based systems such as Savary–Gilliard bougie dilators (*Figure 9.7*). On occasion, more difficult benign strictures can be treated by the insertion of a fully covered removable stent, or with a biodegradable stent. Likewise, the non-relaxing lower oesophageal sphincter associated with achalasia can be treated by pneumatic balloon

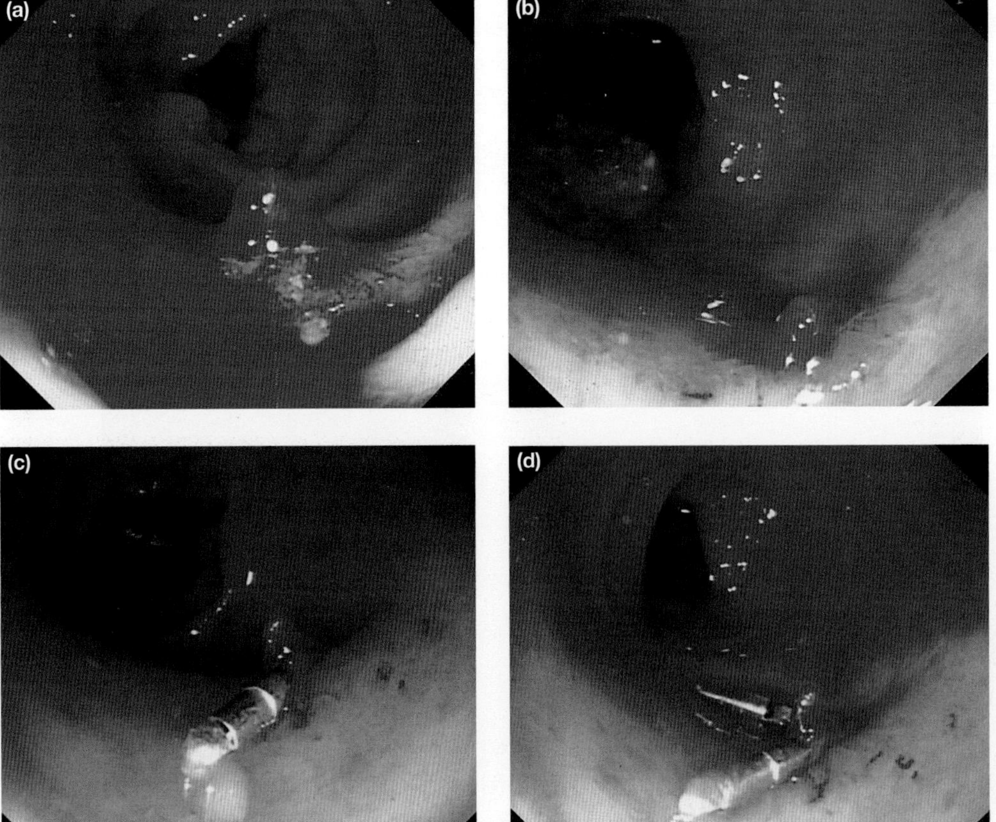

Figure 9.5 A gastric ulcer with active bleeding (a) is initially treated with adrenaline injection to achieve haemostasis (b). Two haemoclips are then applied to prevent rebleeding (c and d).

Norman Rupert Barrett, 1903–1979, surgeon, St Thomas's Hospital, London, UK.

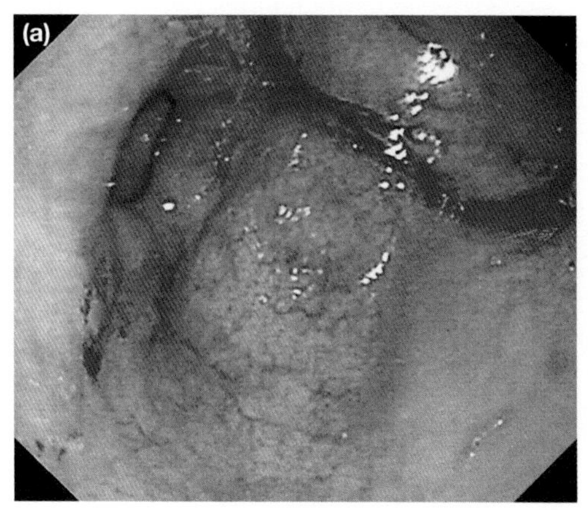

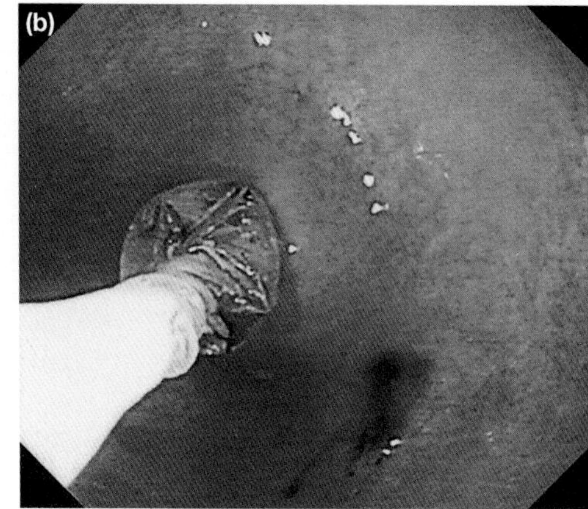

Figure 9.7 A pyloric stricture (a) can be dilated using a through-the-scope balloon under direct vision to minimise complications (b).

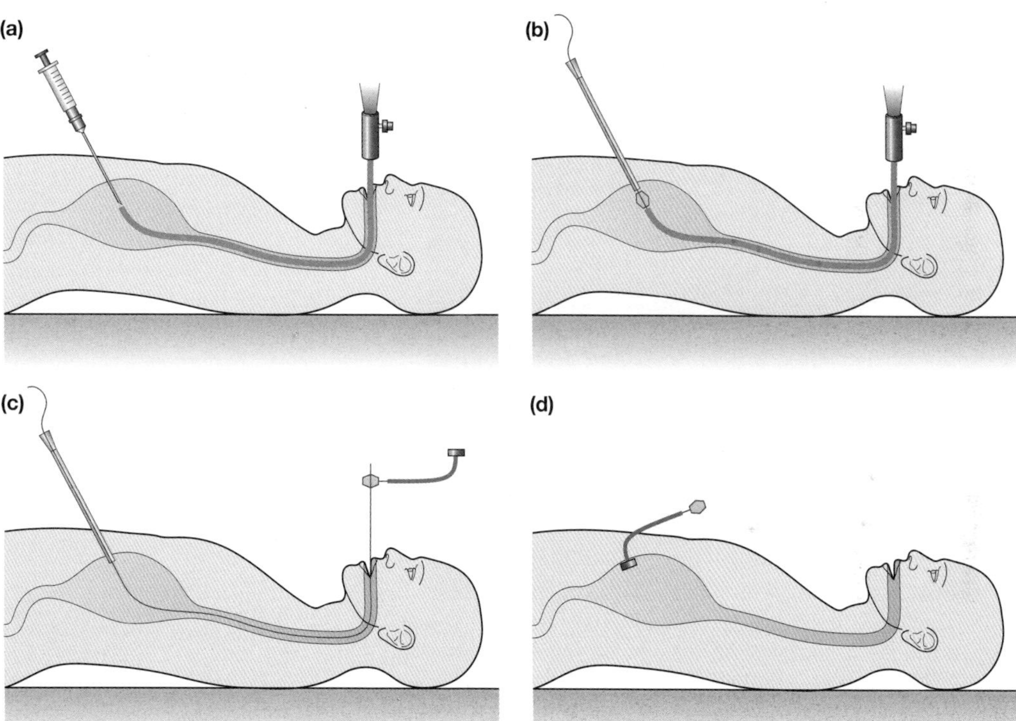

Figure 9.8 A schematic diagram of percutaneous endoscopic gastrostomy insertion. A standard endoscopy is performed to ensure that there are no contraindications to gastrostomy insertion. The stomach is insufflated with air and a direct percutaneous needle puncture made at a point where the stomach abuts the abdominal wall. Lignocaine is infused on withdrawal (a). A trocar is inserted and a wire passed into the stomach, which can be caught with a snare (b). The scope is withdrawn, pulling the wire out through the mouth, at which point it is attached to the gastrostomy tube (c). The gastrostomy is pulled through into the stomach and out through the track created by the trocar insertion (d).

dilatation with a 30- to 40-mm balloon. Endoscopic dissection techniques (see ***Therapeutic colonoscopy***) are now being employed to treat achalasia by natural orifice myotomy (peroral endoscopic myotomy; POEM) with good follow-up results. An alternative in unfit patients is injection of botulinum toxin into the lower oesophageal sphincter, although this has a limited (3–6 months) duration of benefit.

There are a limited number of endoscopic techniques available to reduce gastro-oesophageal reflux, which rely on tightening the loose gastro-oesophageal junction by plication, by the application of radiofrequency ablation or by mucosal resection techniques. These may have a role in some patients but are yet to demonstrate benefit over surgical fundoplication.

Endoscopic bariatric therapies, such as intragastric balloons, sleeve gastroplasty and duodenal resurfacing, may all provide alternatives to more established surgical options. In contrast, there is clear evidence that the insertion of a percutaneous endoscopic gastrostomy (PEG) tube enhances nutritional and functional outcome in patients unable to maintain oral nutritional intake (***Figure 9.8***). PEG insertion is often a prelude to treatment of complex orofacial malignancy and may be used to support nutrition in patients with alternative malignant, degenerative or inflammatory diseases.

The deployment of self-expanding metal stents with or without a covering sheath inserted over a stiff guidewire leads to a significant improvement in symptomatic dysphagia and quality of life in patients with malignant oesophageal and gastric outlet obstruction (***Figure 9.9***). Covered stents are the mainstay of treatment for benign or malignant tracheo-oesophageal fistulae.

It is now possible to endoscopically manage early oesophageal and gastric neoplasia with endoscopic mucosal resection (EMR) or endoscopic submucosal dissection (ESD). These techniques require specialist training but have allowed

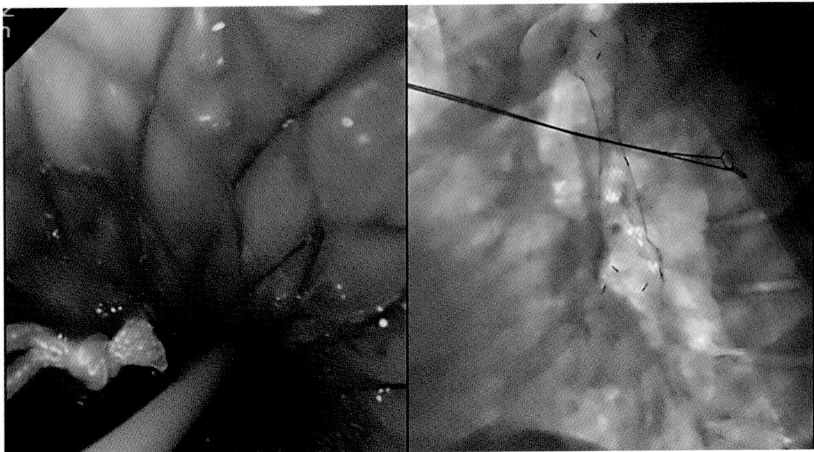

Figure 9.9 A self-expanding metal stent may alleviate symptoms relating to malignant oesophageal strictures. (Left) An endoscopic view of a deployed stent, and (right) the radiographic image.

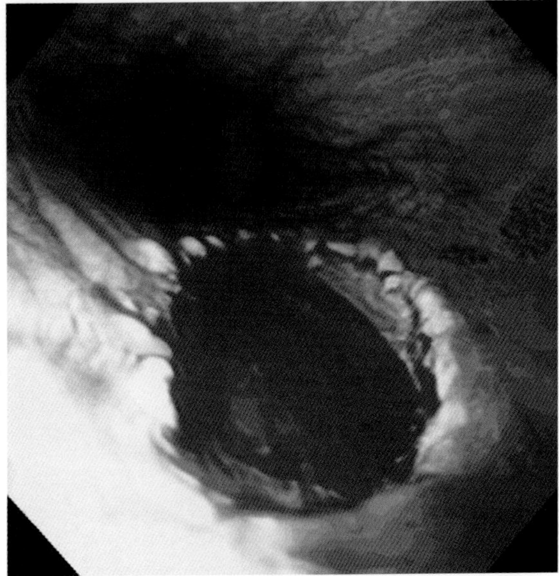

Figure 9.10 Novel upper gastrointestinal therapeutic uses of oesophagogastroduodenoscopy include the use of endoscopic mucosal resection to remove early gastric cancer leaving a clean base.

endoscopic management of mucosal lesions that were previously subject to surgical intervention (***Figure 9.10***). A prime example has been improved endoscopic treatment of Barrett's high-grade dysplasia and early oesophageal adenocarcinoma. Destruction of residual Barrett's epithelium in cases of low- or high-grade dysplasia is possible with endoscopic ablation, and has been shown to reduce risk of progression to cancer. The most commonly used technique for this purpose is radiofrequency ablation, where 360° ablation can be achieved with a balloon catheter, or more focused ablation with smaller probes. Cryotherapy and APC can also be used for ablation, but photodynamic therapy is now used much less often.

Complications of diagnostic and therapeutic oesophagogastroduodenoscopy

Diagnostic upper gastrointestinal endoscopy is a safe procedure with minimal morbidity as long as appropriate patient selection and safe sedation practices are embedded in the unit's policy. The rate of serious complications is approximately 1:10 000. The majority of adverse events relate to sedation and patient comorbidity. Particular caution should be exercised in patients with recent unstable cardiac ischaemia and respiratory compromise. Perforation can occur at any point in the upper gastrointestinal tract, including the oropharynx. It is rare during diagnostic procedures and is usually associated with inexperience. Perforation is more common in therapeutic endoscopy, particularly oesophageal dilatation and EMR/ESD for early malignancy. Early diagnosis significantly improves outcome and can potentially be managed endoscopically with clips or endoscopic suturing.

Prompt management includes radiological assessment using CT/water-soluble contrast studies, strict nil by mouth, intravenous fluids and antibiotics and early review by an experienced upper gastrointestinal surgeon.

Summary box 9.5

Symptoms of endoscopic oesophageal perforation

- Neck/chest pain
- Increasing tachycardia
- Dysphagia/drooling saliva
- Hypotension
- Abdominal pain
- Surgical emphysema

ENDOSCOPIC ASSESSMENT OF THE SMALL BOWEL

Introduction and indications

The requirement to visualise, biopsy and treat the small bowel is far less than in the stomach, biliary tree or colon, resulting in a time lag in technological advances. The most frequent indication is investigation of gastrointestinal blood loss, which may present with either recurrent iron deficiency anaemia (occult haemorrhage) or recurrent overt blood loss per rectum (cryptic haemorrhage) in a patient with normal OGD (with duodenal biopsies) and colonoscopy. Other indications include the investigation of malabsorption; the exclusion of cryptic small bowel inflammation such as Crohn's disease in patients with diarrhoea/abdominal pain and evidence of an inflammatory response; targeting lesions seen on radiological investigations; and surveillance for neoplasia in patients with inherited polyposis syndromes.

A standard enteroscope is able to reach and biopsy lesions detected in the proximal small bowel; however, even in the most experienced hands this is limited to approximately 100 cm distal to the pylorus, although the use of a stiffening overtube may increase this somewhat. The procedure takes approximately 45 minutes and may be uncomfortable, requiring high doses of sedation with the attendant increased risk of perforation and sedation-related morbidity.

Therefore, until recently, barium follow-through or enteroclysis were the most effective imaging modalities to visualise the distal duodenum, jejunum and ileum. Obviously, these techniques do not give true mucosal views, and outside specialist centres their decreasing use has led to diminished expertise and a reduced diagnostic yield. There have been rapid advances in axial radiological techniques such as MRI and CT enterography, which demonstrate excellent diagnostic accuracy in this area (see ***Chapter 8***). However, although these techniques may yield information about vascularity and bowel wall thickening, they do not allow direct mucosal views, have no biopsy capability and have limited scope in terms of therapeutics. Historically, if an area of interest was outside the reach of a standard enteroscope, direct access via enterotomy under either laparoscopic or open surgery was required. Two major clinical advances have revolutionised small bowel diagnosis and therapeutics. First, the development of the capsule endoscope allows diagnostic mucosal views of the entire small bowel to be obtained with minimal discomfort in unsedated patients. Second, the novel technique of single-/double-balloon enteroscopy allows endoscopic access to the entire small bowel for biopsy and therapeutics (***Table 9.4***).

TABLE 9.4 Comparison of the advantages and disadvantages of the currently available modalities to endoscope the small intestine.

Technique	Advantages	Disadvantages
Conventional enteroscopy	Simple technique with wide availability Full range of therapeutics available Performed under sedation	Some discomfort Can only access proximal small bowel
Capsule endoscopy	Able to visualise the entire small bowel Preferable for patients No sedation Painless	No biopsies Not controllable and no accurate localisation Variable transit Incomplete studies owing to battery life Not suitable for patients with strictures Large capsule to swallow
Double-/single-balloon enteroscopy	Able to visualise the entire small bowel Full range of therapeutics	Requires admission Specialist centres only Complications include perforation

Capsule endoscopy

The prototype capsule endoscope was developed at the Royal London Hospital in the UK by Professor Paul Swain. Several companies have developed different systems for routine clinical use, but the basic principles remain identical. The technique requires three main components: an ingestible capsule, a portable data recorder and a workstation equipped with image-processing software. The capsule consists of an optical dome and lens, two light-emitting diodes, a processor, a battery, a transmitter, and an antenna encased in a resistant coat the size of a large vitamin pill (***Figure 9.11***). It acquires video images during natural propulsion through the digestive system that it transmits via a digital radiofrequency communication channel to the recorder unit worn outside the body; this also contains sensors that allow basic localisation of the site of image capture within the abdomen. Upon completion of the examination, the physician transfers the accumulated data to the workstation for interpretation via a high-capacity digital link. The workstation is a modified personal computer required for off-line data storage, interpretation and analysis of the acquired images and report generation.

The small bowel capsule provides good visualisation from mouth to colon with a high diagnostic yield. It compares favourably with other techniques for localisation of occult gastrointestinal bleeding and the diagnosis of small bowel Crohn's disease. Use of the capsule endoscope is contraindicated in patients with known small bowel strictures in which it may impact, resulting in acute obstruction and requiring retrieval at laparotomy or via laparoscopy. Severe gastroparesis and pseudo-obstruction are also relative contraindications to its use. Some units advocate a barium follow-through or small bowel MRI to exclude stricturing disease in all patients before capsule endoscopy. However, there are well-reported episodes of capsule impaction in a stricture that was not visualised on prior imaging. Therefore, a 'dummy' patency capsule that can be tracked via a handheld device or conventional radiology as it passes through the intestine should be used in all patients in whom there is a possibility of stricturing disease. The patency capsule will dissolve after 40 hours if it becomes impacted. Technology in this field is rapidly advancing, with capsule systems now available to image the colon.

Single-/double-balloon enteroscopy

This technique allows the direct visualisation of and therapeutic intervention for the entire small bowel and may be attempted via either the oral or rectal route. Double-balloon enteroscopy involves the use of a thin enteroscope and

Christopher Paul Swain, b. 1943, gastroenterologist, The Royal London Hospital, London, UK.
Burrill Bernard Crohn, 1884–1983, gastroenterologist, Mount Sinai Hospital, New York, NY, USA, described regional ileitis in 1932.

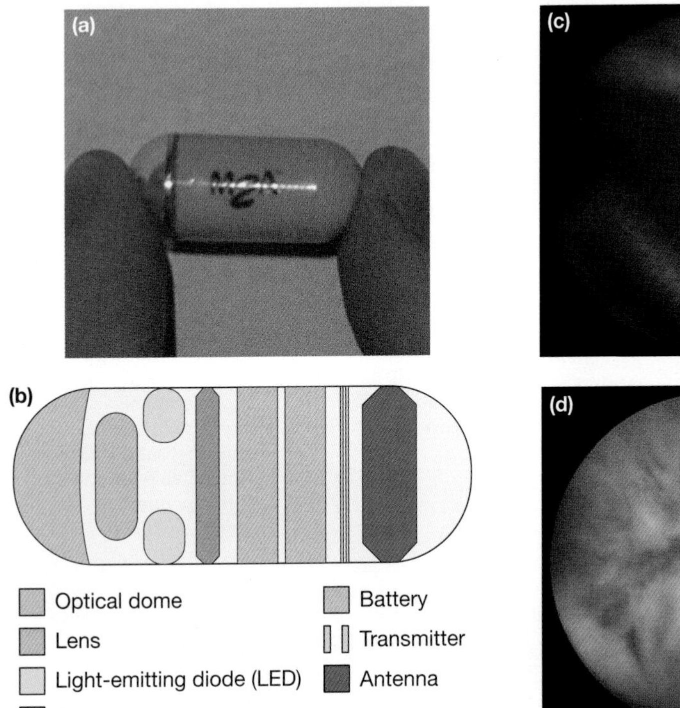

Figure 9.11 Complete diagnostic visualisation of the small bowel can be achieved with capsule endoscopy (a). The structure of the capsule is shown in (b). Clear mucosal pictures can be achieved, here showing angioectasias (arrow) (c) and small bowel Crohn's disease (d).

an overtube, which are both fitted with a balloon. The procedure is usually carried out under general anaesthesia but may be undertaken with the use of conscious sedation. The enteroscope and overtube are inserted through either the mouth or anus and steered to the proximal duodenum/terminal ileum in the conventional manner. Following this the endoscope is advanced a small distance in front of the overtube and the balloon at the end is inflated. Using the assistance of friction at the interface between the enteroscope and intestinal wall, the small bowel is accordioned back to the overtube. The overtube balloon is then deployed and the enteroscope balloon is deflated.

The process is then continued until the entire small bowel is visualised (*Figure 9.12*). In single-balloon enteroscopy, developed more recently, an enteroscope and overtube are used, but only the overtube has a balloon attached. A full range of therapeutics including diagnostic biopsy, polypectomy, APC and stent insertion are available for balloon enteroscopy. Some experts advocate routine capsule endoscopy before balloon enteroscopy in an attempt to localise any lesions and plan whether oral or rectal access is more appropriate. The indications for single-/double-balloon endoscopy are given in *Summary box 9.6*.

Summary box 9.6

Current established indications for single-/double-balloon endoscopy

- Bleeding from the gastrointestinal tract of obscure cause
- Iron deficiency anaemia with normal colonoscopy and gastroscopy
- Visualisation of and therapeutic intervention for abnormalities seen on traditional small bowel imaging/capsule endoscopy

ENDOSCOPIC RETROGRADE CHOLANGIOPANCREATOGRAPHY

This procedure involves the use of a side-viewing duodenoscope, which is passed through the pylorus and into the second part of the duodenum to visualise the papilla. This is then cannulated, either directly with a catheter or with the help of a guidewire (*Figure 9.13*). Occasionally a small precut is required to gain access. By altering the angle of approach one can selectively cannulate the pancreatic duct or biliary tree, which is then visualised under fluoroscopy after contrast injection. The significant range of complications associated with this procedure and improvements in radiological imaging using magnetic resonance cholangiopancreatography (MRCP) have rendered much diagnostic ERCP obsolete, and thus most procedures are currently performed for therapeutic purposes. There is still a role for accessing cytology/biopsy specimens.

Therapeutic endoscopic retrograde cholangiopancreatography

It is essential to ensure that patients have appropriate assessment prior to therapeutic ERCP, which is associated with a significant morbidity and occasional mortality. All patients require routine blood screening including a clotting screen. Both cardiac and oxygen saturation monitoring are required during the procedure because of the high level of sedation that is often required.

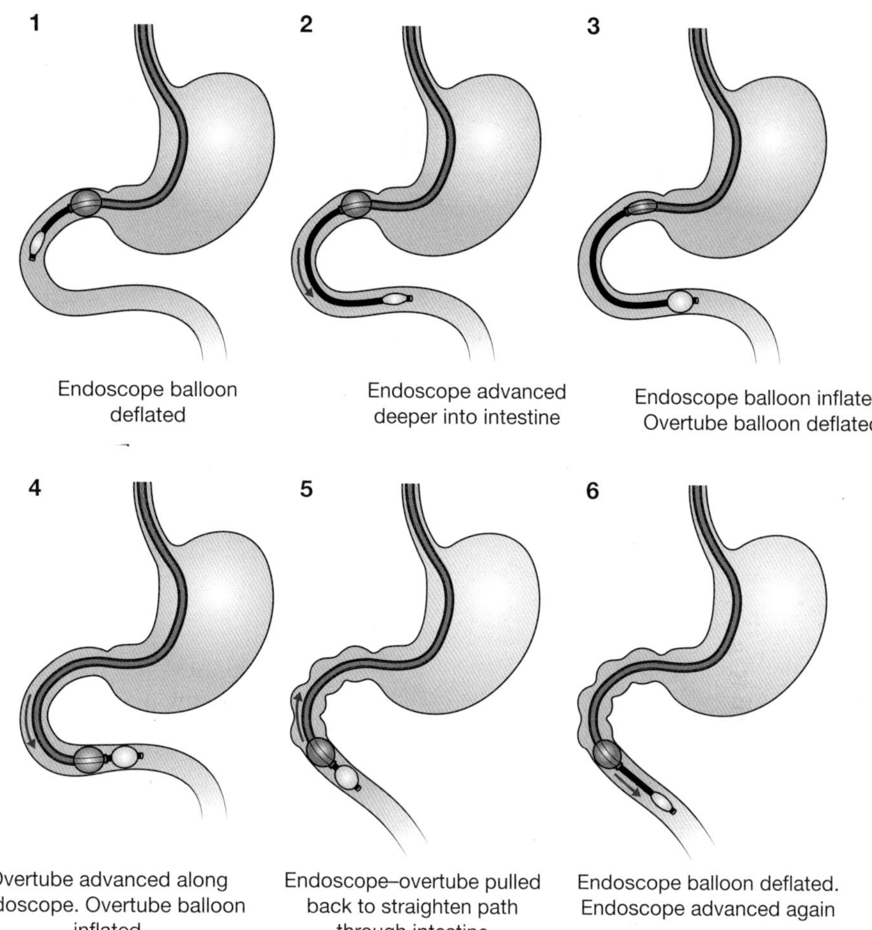

Figure 9.12 The technique of double-balloon enteroscopy is performed with an adapted enteroscope and overtube, both of which have inflatable balloons at their tip.

The most common indication for therapeutic ERCP is relief of biliary obstruction due to gallstone disease or benign or malignant biliary strictures. The preprocedural diagnosis can be confirmed by contrast injection, which will clearly differentiate the filling defects associated with gallstones and the luminal narrowing of a stricture. If there is likely to be a delay in relieving an obstructed system, percutaneous drainage may be required.

The cornerstone of gallstone retrieval is an adequate biliary sphincterotomy, which is normally performed over a well-positioned guidewire using a sphincterotome connected to an electrosurgical unit. Most gallstones <1 cm in diameter will pass spontaneously in the days and weeks following a sphincterotomy, but most endoscopists prefer to ensure duct clearance at the initial procedure to reduce the risk of impaction, cholangitis or pancreatitis. This can be achieved by trawling the duct using a balloon catheter or by extraction using a wire basket. If standard techniques fail, large or awkwardly placed stones can be crushed using mechanical lithotripsy. If adequate stone extraction cannot be achieved at the initial ERCP it is imperative to ensure biliary drainage with the placement of a removable plastic stent while alternative options are considered. These include surgery, endoscopically directed shockwaves under direct choledochoscopic vision and extracorporeal shockwave lithotripsy with subsequent ERCP to remove stone fragments.

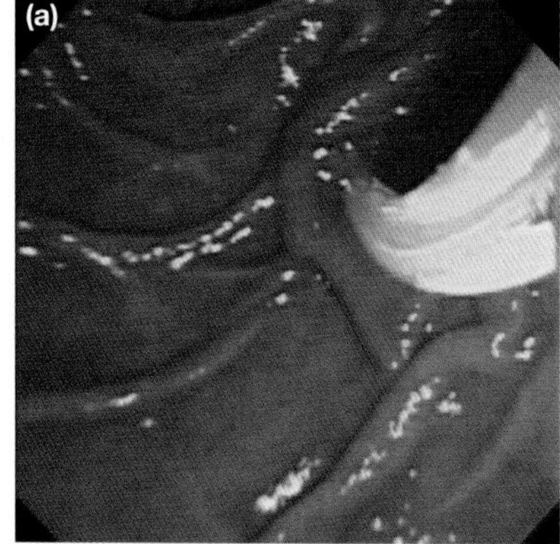

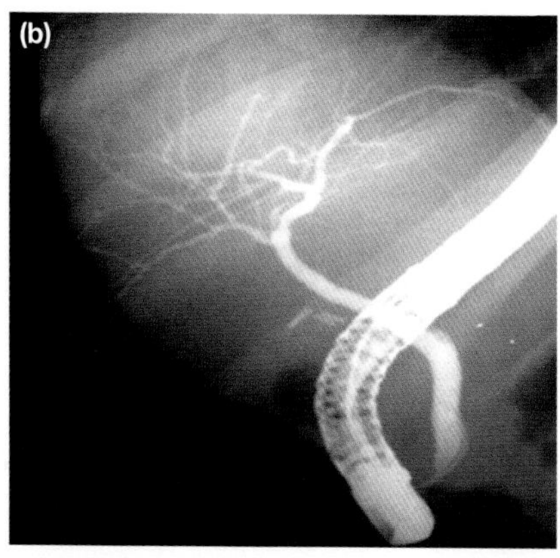

Figure 9.13 During endoscopic retrograde cholangiopancreatography a side-viewing duodenoscope is positioned opposite the papilla, which can then be cannulated using either a catheter or a guidewire (a). Contrast is injected to achieve a cholangiogram (b).

Dilation of benign biliary strictures uses balloon catheters similar to those used in angioplasty inserted over a guidewire under fluoroscopic control. It is traditional to insert a temporary plastic stent to maintain drainage as several attempts at dilatation may be required. Self-expanding metal stents are most commonly used for the palliation of malignant biliary obstruction and are also normally inserted after a modest sphincterotomy. Correct stent placement can normally be confirmed by a flow of bile after release and by the presence of air in the biliary tree on follow-up plain abdominal radiographs. Stent malfunction, associated with recurrent or persistent biochemical cholestasis, may be due to poor initial stent position, stent migration, blockage with blood clot or debris or tumour ingrowth. A repeat procedure is required to assess the cause, which can usually be remedied by the insertion of a second stent through the original one.

In addition to the standard techniques discussed above, ERCP is also used for pancreatic disease and the assessment of biliary dysmotility (sphincter of Oddi dysfunction) using manometry in specialist centres. Indications include pancreatic stone extraction, the dilatation of pancreatic duct strictures and the transgastric drainage of pancreatic pseudocysts. To minimise the risks of subsequent pancreatitis, pancreatic sphincterotomy is most safely performed after the placement of a temporary pancreatic stent to prevent stasis within the pancreatic duct.

Visualisation and sampling of biliary lesions is becoming easier and more effective with the development of newer through-the-duodenoscope cholangioscopes that allow direct visualisation and instrumentation of the biliary and pancreatic ducts.

Complications associated with endoscopic retrograde cholangiopancreatography

The same risks associated with other endoscopic procedures also apply to patients undergoing ERCP, but risks may be increased because of the increased patient frailty and high sedation levels required. Complications specific to ERCP include duodenal perforation (1.3%), haemorrhage (1.4%) after sphincterotomy, pancreatitis (4.3%) and sepsis (3–30%); the mortality rate approaches 1%. It is important to remember that postsphincterotomy complications may be retroperitoneal and CT scanning should be performed in patients with pain, tachycardia or hypotension post procedure.

Although normally mild, post-ERCP pancreatitis can be severe with extensive pancreatic necrosis and is associated with a significant mortality rate (***Table 9.5***). Where there is no contraindication, patients undergoing ERCP should receive per-rectal indometacin or diclofenac immediately before or after the procedure to reduce the risk of post-ERCP pancreatitis.

TABLE 9.5 Risk factors for post-ERCP pancreatitis.

Definite	Suspected SOD
	Young age
	Normal bilirubin
	Prior ERCP-related pancreatitis
	Difficult cannulation
	Pancreatic duct contrast injection
	Pancreatic sphincterotomy
	Balloon dilatation of biliary sphincter
Possible	Female sex
	Low volume of ERCPs performed
	Absent CBD stone

CBD, common bile duct; ERCP, endoscopic retrograde cholangiopancreatography; SOD, sphincter of Oddi dysfunction.

COLONSCOPY

Early attempts at colonoscopy were hindered by poor technique and limitations of available instruments. The ability to steer an endoscope around the entire colon and into the terminal ileum was made possible by the development of fully flexible colonoscopes with >90° angulation of the tip. Advances in bowel preparation have enhanced mucosal visualisation. Understanding two key technical aspects of colonoscopy allows a greater caecal intubation rate and ileal intubation with minimal discomfort using light sedation. The first is that continued inward pressure of the endoscope results in loop formation within the mobile sigmoid and transverse colon, which in turn leads to paradoxical movement and loss of fine tip control. The second is that pulling back the scope regularly with appropriate torque to ensure a straight passage through the sigmoid colon and around the splenic flexure greatly aids the completion of right-sided examination.

Endoscopic navigation systems such as Scope Guide (Olympus) and Scope Pilot (Pentax) can help to characterise the nature of the loop, allowing for more accurate loop resolution techniques. Increasing the stiffness of the colonoscope, targeted abdominal pressure and regular patient position change are also important aids to successfully reaching the caecum. It is expected that the caecum should be reached in at least 90% of colonoscopies and is confirmed by the presence of the appendiceal orifice, the triradiate fold, the ileocaecal valve and preferably terminal ileal intubation (***Figure 9.14***). Historically, air was used to insufflate the bowel, but carbon dioxide is now preferred owing to better patient tolerance and lower risk of perforation. Recent evidence has suggested that using water alone to distend the colon may reduce patient discomfort further.

The ability to take mucosal biopsies and resect polyps ensures that colonoscopy is the most appropriate investigation for the majority of patients. In selected groups, CT colonography

Ruggero Oddi, 1866–1913, anatomist and physiologist, Perugia, Italy, wrote about the structure and function of the ampullary sphincter in 1887, when still a student. He struggled in later life with drug addiction.

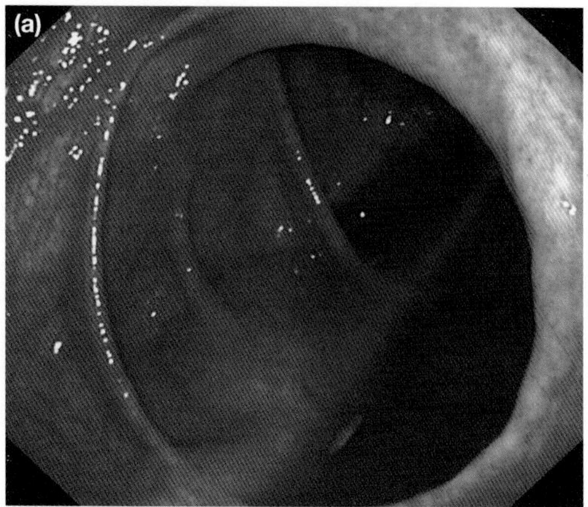

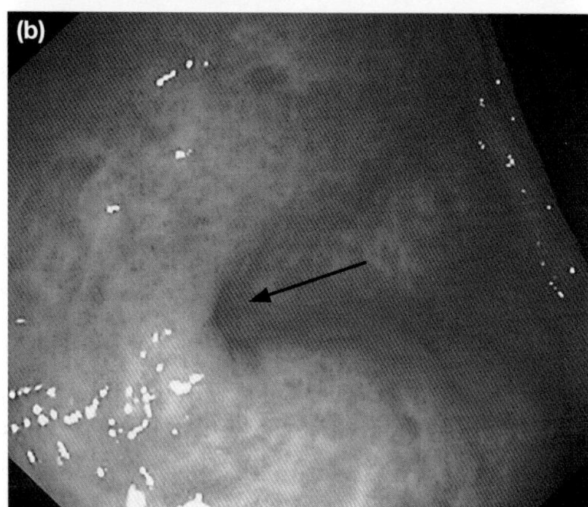

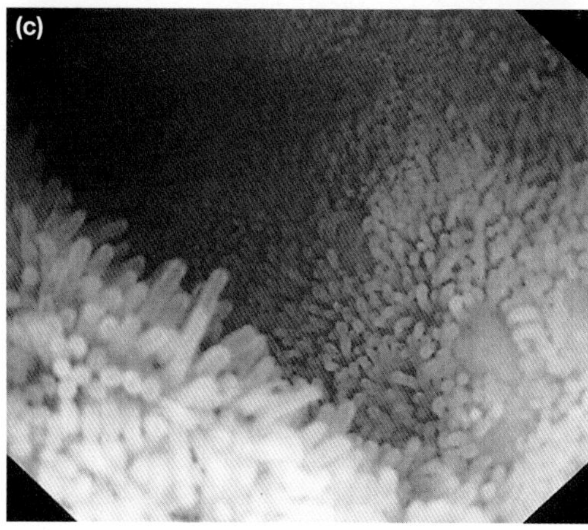

Figure 9.14 The caecal pole may not be easy to identify (a) and, therefore, the endoscopist should confirm complete colonoscopy by visualising the appendix orifice (b) (arrow) or preferably intubating the terminal ileum (c), which demonstrates villi and Peyer's patches.

and colon capsule endoscopy provide an alternative route for investigating colonic pathology, though these are limited by the inability to acquire tissue. Accordingly, colonoscopy remains the cornerstone of most colorectal cancer (CRC) screening programmes globally, whether it is used as the initial screening modality or following a faecal immunochemical test (FIT). The goal is to increase the number of early-stage CRCs detected and hence decrease mortality, as well as to identify and remove adenomatous polyps prior to the development of overt cancer. Higher adenoma detection rates (ADRs) are associated with lower rates of interval cancers and, as such, the ADR is an important indicator of colonoscopy quality. ADRs can be improved with measures such as a longer time taken on withdrawal from the caecum, optimal bowel preparation, patient position changes and a 'second look' of the right colon by changing patient position or by retroflexing the colonoscope. Distal attachments, such as a transparent cap or an Endocuff Vision™, can improve ADRs further.

Summary box 9.7

Indications for colonoscopy

- Rectal bleeding unexplained after proctoscopy/sigmoidoscopy (see *Chapter 77*)
- Abdominal pain related to bowel actions
- Iron deficiency anaemia (combined with OGD)
- Right iliac fossa mass if imaging suggestive of colonic origin
- Unexplained alteration in bowel habit
- Chronic diarrhoea (>6 weeks) after sigmoidoscopy/rectal biopsy and negative coeliac serology
- Follow-up of CRC and polyps
- Screening of patients with a family history of CRC
- Assessment/removal of a lesion seen on radiological examination
- Assessment of ulcerative colitis/Crohn's extent and activity
- Surveillance of inflammatory bowel disease
- Surveillance in patients with acromegaly or following ureterosigmoidostomy

Optical diagnosis and image enhancement

With the assistance of advanced imaging techniques, endoscopists are now able to characterise colorectal polyps with high diagnostic accuracy. This begins with a white light assessment: polyps larger than 2 cm with a large sessile component or a depressed region have the highest risk of containing cancer. Application of advanced imaging techniques can improve diagnostic accuracy further (***Figure 9.15***).

Dye-based chromoendoscopy involves topical application of stains or pigments to improve mucosal characterisation. Several agents have been described, which can broadly be categorised as absorptive (vital) stains, such as methylene blue, and contrast (reactive) stains, such as crystal violet and indigo carmine. These highlight the mucosal pits, which can aid optical diagnosis; different lesions demonstrate specific pit patterns. Dye chromoendoscopy is still widely used and remains the recommended method of dysplasia detection in inflammatory bowel disease.

Narrow band imaging (NBI; Olympus) relies on optical filter technology that radically improves the visibility of

Johann Conrad Peyer, 1653–1712, Professor of Logic, Rhetoric and Medicine, Schaffhausen, Switzerland, described the lymph follicles in the intestine in 1677.

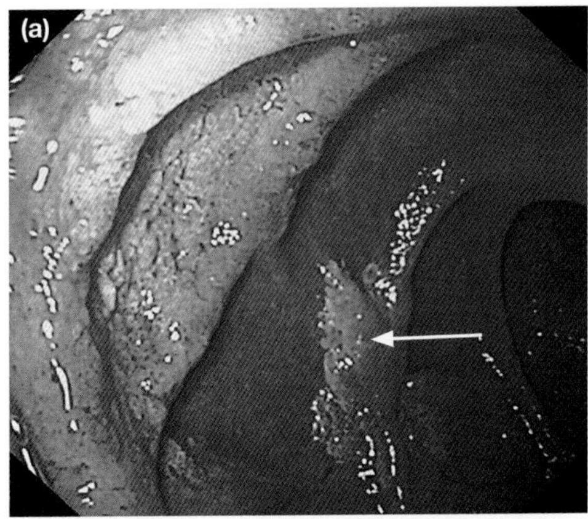

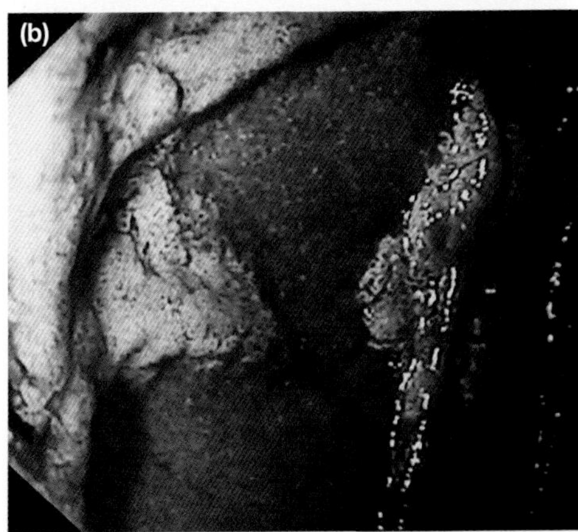

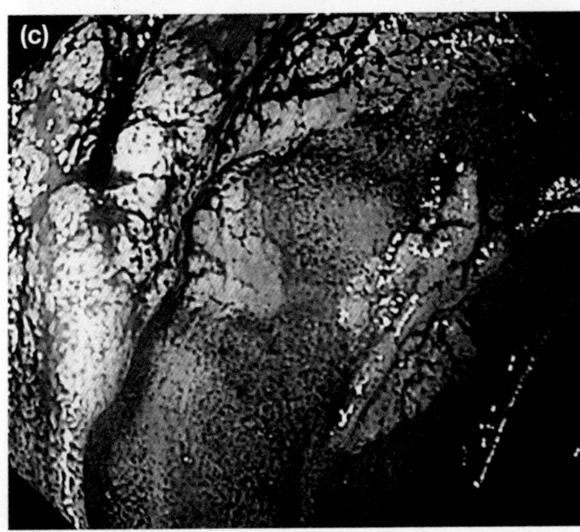

Figure 9.15 Endoscopic diagnostic accuracy can be improved by novel endoscopic techniques. This duodenal adenoma can be seen with conventional white light (a) (arrow), but its full extent is more clearly delineated using narrow band imaging (b) or chromoendoscopy with indigo carmine (c).

capillaries, veins and other subtle tissue structures by optimising the absorbance and scattering characteristics of light. NBI uses two discrete bands of light: one blue at 415 nm and one green at 540 nm. Narrow band blue light displays superficial capillary networks, whereas green light displays subepithelial vessels; when combined they offer an extremely high contrast image of the tissue surface. Similar modalities such as i-Scan (Pentax) and Blue Light Imaging (BLI; Fujifilm) are also available.

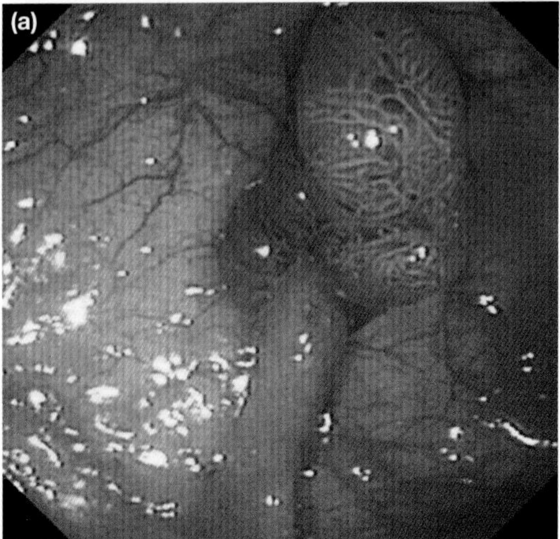

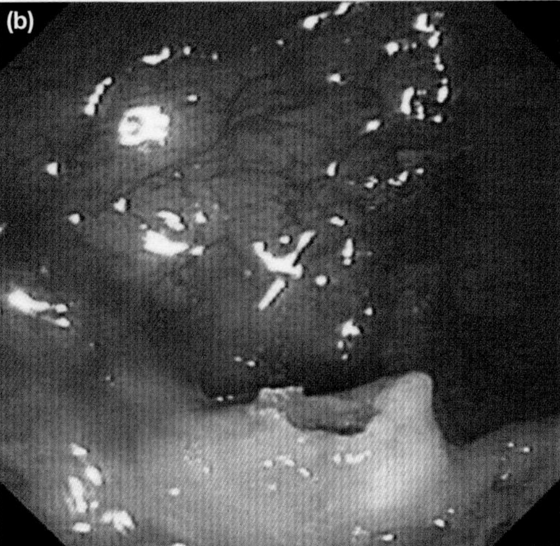

Figure 9.16 Colonoscopy is the most appropriate investigation to detect colonic polyps (a), which can be removed by snare polypectomy during the same procedure, leaving a clean polyp base (b).

Dye-based and digital enhancement, particularly when combined with magnification endoscopy, can differentiate between hyperplastic, serrated, adenomatous and malignant pathology. Combining this with a detailed white light assessment allows endoscopists to determine endoscopic resectability, avoiding more extensive surgery in some cases.

Therapeutic colonoscopy

The most common therapeutic procedure performed at colonoscopy is resection of colonic polyps (***Figure 9.16***). Retrieved specimens can be assessed for risk factors for neoplastic progression and an appropriate surveillance strategy determined (https://www.bsg.org.uk/wp-content/uploads/2019/09/201.full_.pdf). Non-pedunculated polyps up to 15 mm should be removed by cheese wiring with a dedicated 'cold' snare. Stalked polyps can be resected using 'hot' snare polypectomy. Here, diathermy is used with either a 'cut', 'coagulation' or a blended current. Postpolypectomy bleeding can be prevented by preinjection of the stalk with adrenaline, or with application of endoclips or an Endoloop®.

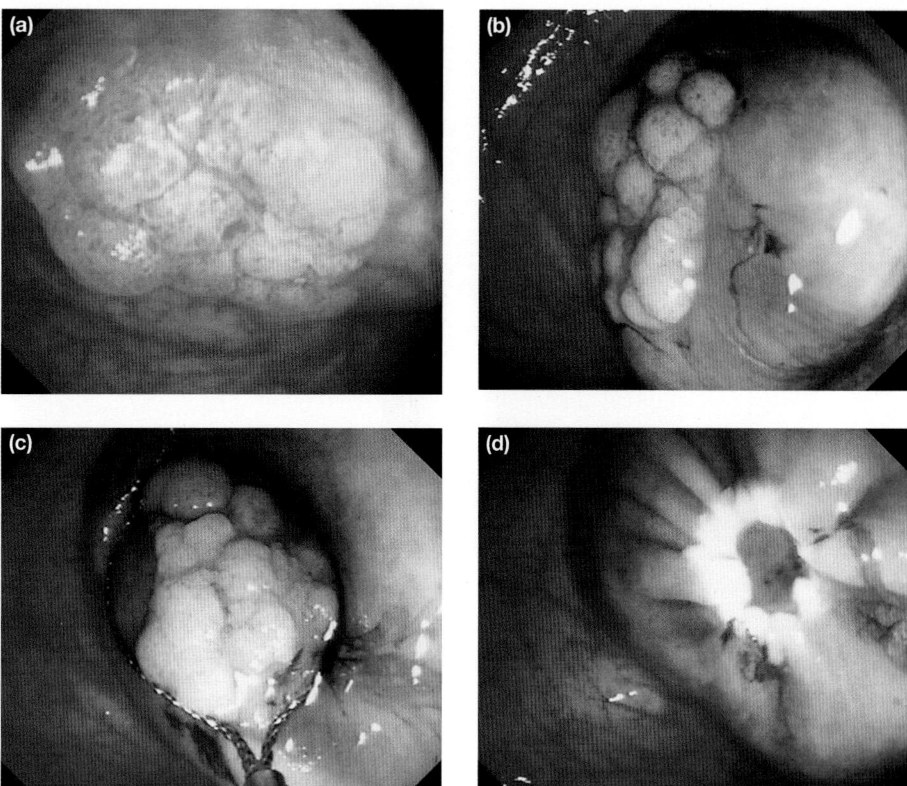

Figure 9.17 Large sessile polyps (a) can be removed by endoscopic mucosal resection. First the polyp is raised on a bed of injected saline containing dye (b). This ensures that there is no submucosal invasion and protects from transmural perforation. A snare is closed around the polyp (c), which is then resected leaving a clean excision base (d).

Non-pedunculated polyps of between 10 and 19 mm can be removed en bloc by EMR, which involves lifting the polyp from the muscularis propria with a submucosal injectate to prevent iatrogenic perforation (***Figure 9.17***). Lesions >20 mm can be removed with piecemeal EMR (pEMR); on completion, thermal ablation (with either APC or coagulation) is applied to the edge of the resection site to prevent adenoma recurrence. An alternative to pEMR is ESD, which is typically performed with a knife rather than a snare. This technique involves the injection of a submucosal solution, followed by a circumferential incision and submucosal dissection, with coagulation of blood vessels that are encountered. This enables an en bloc resection of large polyps and superficial submucosal cancers. Although technically challenging with a steep learning curve, benefits include a more accurate histopathological assessment and lower adenoma recurrence rates.

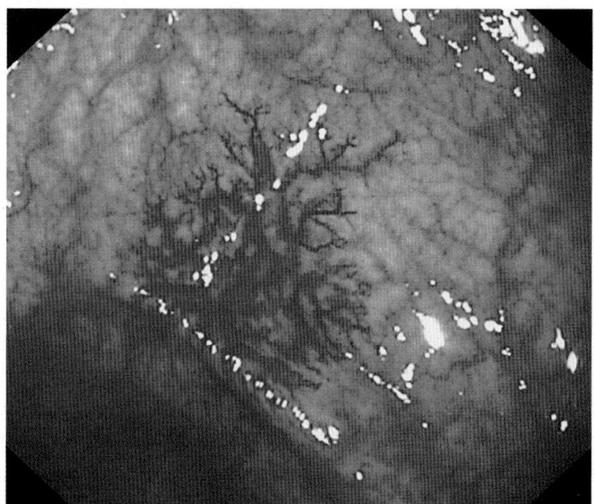

Figure 9.18 A large angioectasia of the colon. If this results in symptomatic anaemia, it should be obliterated with argon plasma coagulation.

APC and alternative thermal therapies such as heater probes are also used in the treatment of symptomatic angioectasias of the colon (***Figure 9.18***). Laser photocoagulation may be used to debulk colonic tumours not suitable for resection. As with benign oesophageal strictures, TTS balloons can be used to dilate short (<5 cm) colonic strictures. The dilatation of surgical anastomoses gives the most durable benefit as inflammatory strictures tend to recur even if intramucosal steroids are injected at the time of the dilatation. Finally, the colonoscopic placement of self-expanding metal stents may provide excellent palliation of inoperable malignant strictures (***Figure 9.19***) and may also play an invaluable role in decompressing an obstructed colon to allow planned as opposed to emergency surgery.

Complications of colonoscopy

Complications during routine diagnostic colonoscopy are rare when performed by an experienced endoscopist. Extensive diverticulosis, diverticulitis and severe colitis are risk factors for perforation during colonoscopy. In the case of colitis, an unprepared flexible sigmoidoscopy is usually sufficient for diagnostic purposes. Polypectomy is associated with an increased rate of perforation (0.1%) and haemorrhage (0.3%). Immediate haemorrhage can be managed with endoclips or snare-tip

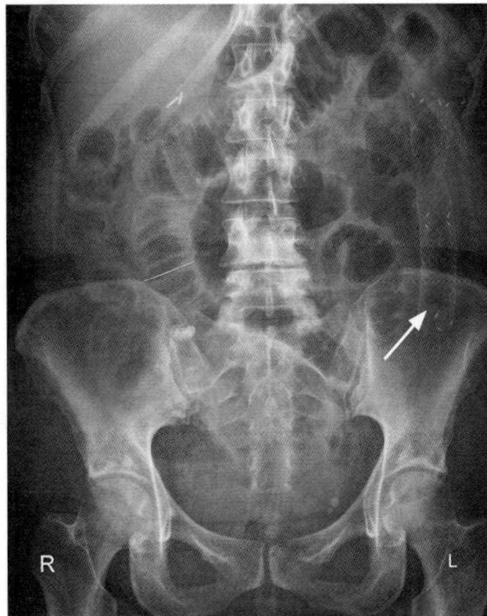

Figure 9.19 Malignant colonic obstruction can be palliated or temporarily relieved by insertion of a self-expanding metal stent (arrow).

coagulation. Delayed haemorrhage may occur 1–14 days post polypectomy and can normally be managed by conservative observation. Transfusion may occasionally be required, and a repeat colonoscopy may be necessary. If recognised at the time of polypectomy, small perforations should be closed using endoclips and the patient may need a period of observation. Symptoms of abdominal pain and cardiovascular compromise after a polypectomy raise the possibility of a delayed perforation and faecal contamination. Patients should be kept nil by mouth and receive intravenous resuscitation and antibiotics. Prompt assessment with a CT scan will often distinguish between a frank perforation and a transmural burn with associated localised peritonitis (the postpolypectomy syndrome). Assessment by an experienced colorectal surgeon is essential, as surgery is often the most appropriate course of action.

ENDOSCOPIC ULTRASOUND

One disadvantage of conventional endoscopy is that examination is limited to the mucosal surface, and it is not possible to diagnose submucosal or extraintestinal pathology. These limitations can be overcome using EUS, which combines the traditional mucosal image with a separate ultrasound view that clearly depicts the intestinal layers and proximate extraintestinal structures. Its use has revolutionised the staging and management of upper gastrointestinal and hepatobiliary malignancy.

There are two main types of echoendoscope: the radial echoendoscope has a radially arranged ultrasound probe and a forward-viewing lens. This is used for diagnostic work such as local tumour staging in the oesophagus and stomach. The linear echoendoscope is a side-viewing scope with a working channel much like an ERCP scope, and a linearly arranged ultrasound probe. This conformation allows ultrasound assessment and ultrasound-guided sampling of tissues to be performed (***Figures 9.20 and 9.21***). Sampling of paraoesophageal and coeliac lymph nodes and pancreatic, biliary and other solid abdominal lesions as well as drainage of peripancreatic abscess or pseudocysts can be performed. Using TTS Cystotomes™ it is possible to perform EUS cystgastrostomy and stent placement, and increasingly biliary interventional procedures are being performed with EUS assistance.

EUS requires dedicated training, in both scope manipulation and radiographic interpretation. Owing to the width and lack of flexibility of the endo-ultrasound scope as well as the duration of complex therapeutic procedures, sedation is normally required, and some units perform tests using propofol-based anaesthesia. The main indications for EUS are listed in ***Table 9.6***. All patients undergoing therapeutic EUS require a normal coagulation screen. Complications include oversedation and oesophageal perforation during diagnostic procedures and haemorrhage/perforation during therapeutic procedures.

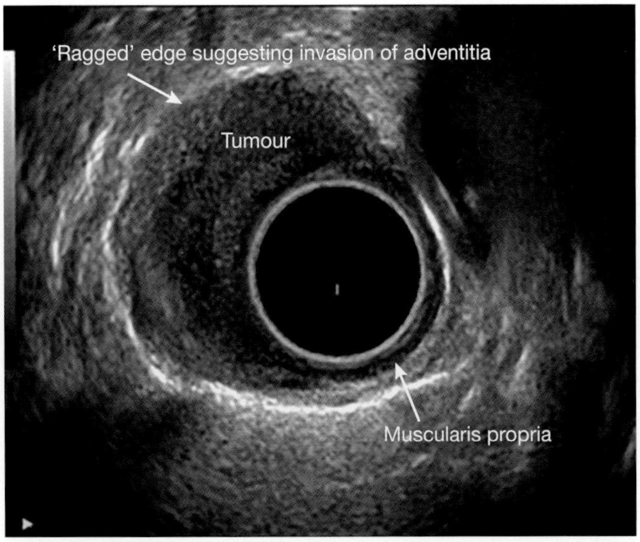

Figure 9.20 Endoscopic ultrasound image of an oesophageal tumour invading into the wall.

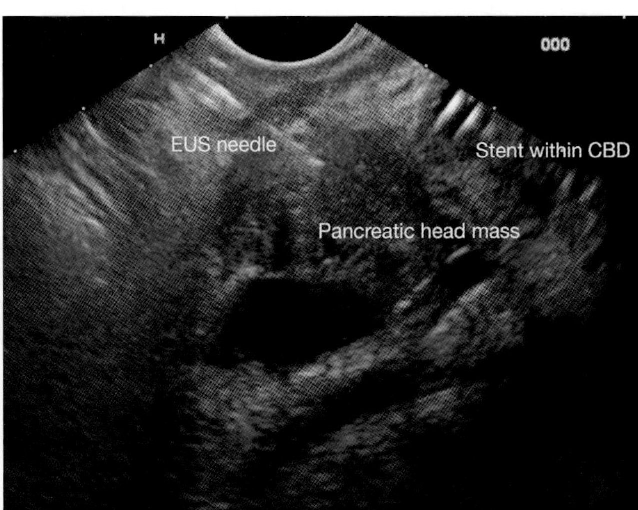

Figure 9.21 Endoscopic ultrasound (EUS)-guided fine-needle aspiration of a pancreatic head mass. CBD, common bile duct.

TABLE 9.6 Indications for endoscopic ultrasound.

Diagnostic	Staging of oesophageal/gastric malignancy
	Staging of hepatobiliary malignancy
	Diagnosis of choledochal microlithiasis
Therapeutic	Biopsy of paraoesophageal lymph nodes
	Biopsy of submucosal upper gastrointestinal lesions
	Biopsy of pancreaticobiliary mass
	Biopsy of portal lymphadenopathy
	Biopsy of left adrenal and left liver masses
	Transgastric drainage of pancreatic pseudocyst
	Coeliac plexus block

CONCLUSIONS

Over the last 30 years endoscopy has become an integral part of the diagnostic work-up of patients with gastrointestinal disease. Whereas advances in radiology and capsule studies may obviate the need for some diagnostic procedures, the ability to take mucosal biopsies will ensure that it retains a vital role. Ongoing developments in technology such as magnifying endoscopy and chromoendoscopy give near-histological quality definition and there is considerable interest in the role of artificial intelligence to augment near-patient diagnosis. There have also been major advances in the range of conditions that are amenable to endoscopic therapy; such therapy may have substantially lower associated morbidity rates than traditional surgical approaches. However, as the scope of procedures widens and the age range/comorbidities of the patients increases, it is beholden on the endoscopist to ensure that he or she adheres to appropriate governance/consent and sedation practice to minimise complications.

FURTHER READING

Allison MC, Sandoe JAT, Tighe R *et al.* Antibiotic prophylaxis in gastrointestinal endoscopy. *Gut* 2009; **58**: 869–80.

Everett SM, Griffiths H, Nandasoma U *et al*, Guideline for obtaining valid consent for gastrointestinal endoscopy procedures *Gut* 2016; **65**(10): 1585–601.

Ferlitsch M, Moss A, Hassan C *et al.* Colorectal polypectomy and endoscopic mucosal resection (EMR): European Society of Gastrointestinal Endoscopy (ESGE) Clinical Guideline. *Endoscopy* 2017; **49**: 270–97.

Hawes RH, Fockens P, Varadarajulu S. *Endosonography*, 3rd edn. Philadelphia: Saunders, 2014.

Haycock A, Cohen J, Saunders BP *et al. Cotton and Williams' practical gastrointestinal endoscopy*, 7th edn. Oxford: Wiley-Blackwell, 2014.

Members of the British Society of Gastroenterology Endoscopy Section Committee Working Party on Decontamination of Equipment for Gastrointestinal Endoscopy. *BSG guidance for decontamination of equipment for gastrointestinal endoscopy*, 2020. Available from https://www.bsg.org.uk/wp-content/uploads/2021/02/BSG-Decontamination-guidance-2020-update.pdf

Rees CJ, Thomas Gibson S, Rutter MD *et al.* UK key performance indicators and quality assurance standards for colonoscopy. *Gut* 2016; **65**: 1923–29.

Rutter MD, East J, Rees CJ, *et al.* British Society of Gastroenterology/Association of Coloproctology of Great Britain and Ireland/Public Health England post-polypectomy and post-colorectal cancer resection surveillance guidelines. *Gut* 2020; **69**: 201–23.

Veitch AM, Radaelli F, Alikhan R *et al.* Endoscopy in patients on antiplatelet or anticoagulant therapy: British Society of Gastroenterology (BSG) and European Society of Gastrointestinal Endoscopy (ESGE) guideline update. *Gut* 2021; **70**: 1611–1628.

CHAPTER 10 Principles of minimal access surgery

Learning objectives

To understand:

- The principles of minimal access surgery
- The advantages and disadvantages of minimal access approaches
- The safety issues and indications for minimal access surgery
- The perioperative assessment of patients undergoing minimal access surgery
- Novel advances in minimal access surgery and its adjuncts
- The application of artificial intelligence to minimal access surgery

DEFINITION

Minimal access surgery is a product of modern technology and surgical innovation that aims to accomplish surgical therapeutic goals with minimal somatic and psychological trauma. This type of surgery has reduced wound access trauma and is less disfiguring than conventional techniques. It can offer cost-effectiveness to both health services and employers by shortening operating times, shortening hospital stays, improving operative precision compared with open surgery in some (but not all) cases and allowing faster recuperation.

History of minimal access surgery

The first experimental laparoscopic procedure was performed by Kelling in 1901. Jacobaeus performed the first thoracoscopy in 1910, again using a cystoscope; however, it took another 70 years before Steptoe in the UK developed laparoscopy for treatment of infertility and Mouret performed the first video-laparoscopic cholecystectomy in 1987. Since laparoscopic techniques became widely adopted in the mid-1990s, minimal access surgery has developed into a multidisciplinary approach that crosses all traditional specialty boundaries and serves the patient as a whole and not specific organ systems.

MINIMAL ACCESS APPROACHES

Laparoscopy

A rigid endoscope is introduced through a port into the peritoneal cavity. Full details of laparoscopy including the principles of pneumoperitoneum can be found in *Chapter 7*.

Thoracoscopy

A rigid endoscope is introduced through an incision placed between the ribs to gain access to the thorax. In the majority of cases, specialist anaesthetic support is required to ensure isolation of the lung on the side of surgery, enabling the patient to be ventilated only on the non-operative side. This is achieved through the use of right- or left-sided double lumen endotracheal tubes that comprise both a bronchial and a tracheal lumen. Usually there is no requirement for gas insufflation as the operating space is held open by the rigidity of the thoracic cavity. In specific cases, such as mediastinal tumour resection and diaphragmatic surgery, gas insufflation at low pressure (5–8 mmHg) may be applied. Further information on the general principles of thoracoscopy are found in *Chapter 60*.

Single-incision minimal access surgery

Single-incision minimal access surgery has varied in popularity with both strong advocates and others who are sceptical of any advantages. Single-incision laparoscopic surgery (SILS) involves insertion of all instrumentation through a multiple channel port via a single incision at the umbilicus. The benefits are that the incision, through a natural scar (the umbilicus), is virtually 'scarless' and that fewer port sites potentially reduces pain and lessens the risks of port site bleeding and the potential for port site hernia.

SILS requires specially manufactured multichannel ports and often roticulating instruments. It has most commonly been adopted in gallbladder and hernia surgery, although more

Georg Kelling, 1866–1945, surgeon, Dresden, Germany, performed the first 'celioscopy' on a dog in 1901 using air insufflation and a Nitze-cystoscope.
Hans Christian Jacobaeus, 1879–1937, physician, Karolinska Institutet, Sweden.
Patrick Christopher Steptoe, 1913–1988 gynaecologist, Oldham, UK, a pioneer of *in vitro* fertilisation.
Phillippe Mouret, 1938–2008, surgeon, Lyon, France.

complex colon and rectal surgery can be performed. There remains debate as to whether the increased procedural difficulty, steep learning curve and increased direct costs in terms of devices, instruments and operating time can be offset by significant clinical benefit.

Uniportal thoracic surgery requires less specialist equipment; many minor thoracic procedures are commonly performed using this technique. More complex resectional procedures are less commonly performed, largely because of technical complexity when compared with multiport techniques, which are on the whole very well tolerated.

Endoluminal endoscopy and natural orifice surgery

Flexible or rigid endoscopes are introduced into hollow organs or systems, such as the urinary tract, upper or lower gastrointestinal tract and the respiratory and vascular systems. Advances in endoluminal technology now enable more complex procedures to be completed endoscopically where previous transabdominal or transthoracic surgical resection would have been advocated. Examples include endoscopic submucosal resection of complex colonic polyps, transanal endoscopic microsurgery and endobronchial laser resection of tracheal pathology.

Natural orifice translumenal endoscopic surgery (NOTES) offers the opportunity for 'scar-free' surgery by performing entire procedures via natural body orifices. While these techniques have been applied in the pelvis, abdomen and thorax, technical limitations and safety concerns have limited adoption. Concern over closure of the visceral puncture site is the principal issue that has prevented widespread uptake, as transgastric and transcolonic closure of peritoneal entry sites in a safe manner remains problematic. In addition, there are significant cost and training implications that have limited more widespread adoption.

Perivisceral endoscopy

Body planes can be accessed even in the absence of a natural cavity. Examples are mediastinoscopy, retroperitoneoscopy and retroperitoneal approaches to the kidney, aorta and lumbar sympathetic chain. Some of these approaches have been in place for many years (cervical mediastinoscopy was first performed in 1959); however, the availability of novel videoscopes has enhanced visualisation, thus improving the safety and accuracy of dissection.

Extraperitoneal approaches to the retroperitoneal organs, as well as hernia repair, are now commonplace, further decreasing morbidity associated with manipulation of the visceral peritoneum. Other examples include subfascial endoscopic perforator surgery for ligation of incompetent perforating veins in varicose vein surgery and endoscopic harvesting of the saphenous vein for use in coronary artery bypass grafting.

Arthroscopy and intra-articular joint surgery

Arthroscopy was one of the earliest applications of endoscopic techniques, first being applied in the knee as early as the 1930s. In the 1950s Watanabe developed arthroscopic techniques that have evolved such that shoulder, wrist, elbow and hip arthroscopy is now commonplace. Novel approaches to smaller joints such as the temporomandibular and metatarsal joints are being developed.

Hybrid minimal access surgery

Hybrid surgery may utilise a combination of flexible and straight stick endoscopic approaches or a combination of open and endoscopic surgery.

Totally endoscopic hybrid approach

The diseased organ is visualised and treated by an assortment of endoluminal and extraluminal endoscopes and other imaging devices. In the abdomen, examples include the combined laparo-endoscopic approach for the management of biliary lithiasis, colonic polyp excision and several urological procedures, such as pyeloplasty and donor nephrectomy. In the thorax, navigational bronchoscopy with placement of fiducial markers has been employed as a means of marking lung nodules that can then be resected via a minimal access video-assisted approach. Cardiovascular surgeons have for some time employed hybrid technologies to facilitate catheter-based placement of cardiac valves, atrial devices and intravascular stents.

Hybrid techniques offer improved visualisation, facilitating the primary procedure to be carried out either via a smaller incision or a minimal access approach where otherwise open surgery would have been necessary. Such approaches may necessitate the availability of 'hybrid' theatre facilities, limiting this approach to tertiary centres where such technology is available (***Figure 10.1***).

Open and endoscopic hybrid approach

Hand-assisted laparoscopic surgery (HALS) is a well-developed technique. It involves the intra-abdominal placement of a

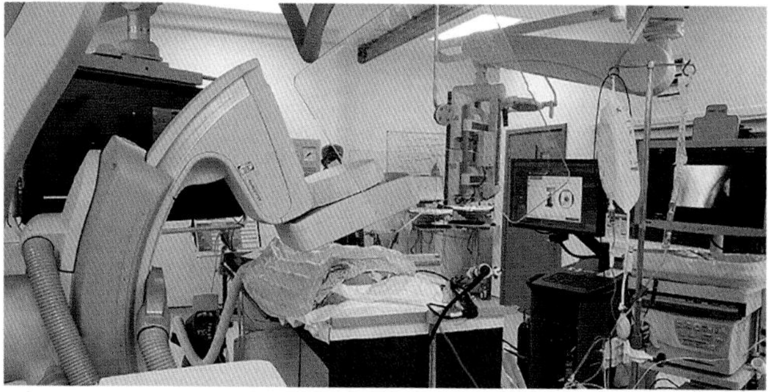

Figure 10.1 Modern hybrid theatre set-up (courtesy of Mr Kelvin Lau, Barts Thorax Centre, London, UK).

Masaki Watanabe, 1911–1995, orthopaedic surgeon, Tokyo, Japan, known as the 'founder of modern arthroscopy'.

hand or forearm through a minilaparotomy incision, while pneumoperitoneum is maintained. In this way, the surgeon's hand can be used as in an open procedure. It can be used to palpate organs or tumours, reflect organs atraumatically, retract structures, identify vessels, dissect bluntly along a tissue plane and provide finger pressure to bleeding points, while proximal control is achieved. This approach has been suggested to offer technical and economic efficiency when compared with a totally laparoscopic approach, in some instances reducing both the number of laparoscopic ports and the number of instruments required. Indeed, some advocates argue that if such an incision is necessary for extraction of the final specimen then HALS does not significantly increase surgical trauma over totally laparoscopic approaches. Furthermore, for those trained in open surgery it may be easier to learn and perform than totally laparoscopic approaches, subsequently improving patient safety. With the new generation of surgeons training in totally laparoscopic surgery it is likely that use of HALS will diminish, although it should remain part of the minimally invasive surgeon's armamentarium.

SURGICAL TRAUMA IN OPEN, MINIMALLY INVASIVE AND ROBOTIC SURGERY

Most of the trauma of an open procedure is inflicted because the surgeon must have a wound that is large enough to give adequate exposure for safe dissection at a target site. The wound is often the cause of morbidity, including infection, dehiscence, bleeding, herniation and nerve entrapment. Wound pain prolongs recovery time and, by reducing mobility, contributes to an increased incidence of pulmonary atelectasis, chest infection, paralytic ileus and deep venous thrombosis.

Mechanical and human retractors cause additional trauma. Body wall retractors can inflict localised damage that may be as painful as the wound itself. In contrast, during laparoscopy, the retraction is provided by the low-pressure pneumoperitoneum, giving a diffuse force applied gently and evenly over the whole body wall, causing minimal trauma.

Exposure of any body cavity to the atmosphere also causes morbidity through cooling and fluid loss by evaporation. The incidence of postsurgical adhesions is reduced by use of minimally invasive approaches because there is less damage to delicate serosal coverings. In the manual handling of intestinal loops, the surgeon and assistant disturb the peristaltic activity of the gut and provoke adynamic ileus.

While minimal access methods were initially established in elective surgery, the advantages have led to increased uptake for a number of emergency surgical procedures, including perforated viscus repair, such as omental patch repair of a peptic ulcer perforation, lavage of localised perforation of diverticular disease, intrathoracic debridement of empyema and pneumothorax and haemothorax surgery. More recently, some experienced surgeons have chosen to employ minimal access approaches to trauma situations for initial assessment and treatment in stable patients.

Summary box 10.1

Advantages of minimal access surgery

- Decrease in wound size
- Reduction in wound infection, dehiscence, bleeding, herniation and nerve entrapment
- Decrease in wound pain
- Improved mobility
- Decreased wound trauma
- Decreased heat loss
- Improved visualisation

LIMITATIONS OF MINIMAL ACCESS SURGERY

Minimal access surgery has limitations. A number of these have been addressed with advances in instrumentation and endoscopic systems; however, the basic principles remain. Surgical robots further address a number of these limitations but present novel challenges.

Endoscopic surgery

Lack of three-dimensional vision

To perform minimal access surgery with safety, the surgeon must operate using an imaging system that provides a two-dimensional (2D) representation of the operative site. The endoscope offers a whole new anatomical landscape, which the surgeon must learn to navigate without the usual 'open approach' clues that make it easy to judge depth. The instruments are longer and sometimes more complex to use than those commonly used in open surgery. This results in the novice being faced with significant problems of hand–eye coordination. There is a well-described learning curve for novice surgeons and experienced 'open' surgeons when adopting the minimally invasive approach. Simulation training and mentoring are required to attain competence.

Three-dimensional (3D) imaging systems are available but are expensive and currently are not commonplace. Many surgeons feel that endoscopic 3D technology does not yet offer the technical enhancement necessary to improve safety. Indeed, 3D technology has been associated with ergonomic problems such as headache without quantifiable benefit in terms of accuracy and time to perform directed tasks. Future improvements in these systems carry the potential to enhance manipulative ability in critical procedures, such as knot tying and dissection of closely overlapping tissues. There are, however, some drawbacks, such as reduced display brightness and interference with normal vision because of the need to wear specially designed glasses for some systems. It is likely that brighter projection displays will be developed; however, the need to wear glasses is not easily overcome. These factors currently limit stereoscopic straight stick endoscopic surgery, which has largely been superseded by the development of robotic technology incorporating 3D vision.

Increased operative time

Minimal access surgery can be more technically demanding and slower to perform than conventional open surgery. On occasion, a minimally invasive operation is so technically demanding that both patient and surgeon would be better served by conversion to an open procedure. Prolonged anaesthetic and operative times may negate a number of the beneficial effects of minimal access surgery and increase the risk of respiratory and wound complications as well as compression neuropathy and venous thromboembolism. It is vital for surgeons and patients to appreciate that the decision to convert to an open operation is not a complication but, instead, usually implies sound surgical judgement in favour of patient safety.

Control of bleeding and haemostasis

Haemostasis may be difficult to achieve endoscopically because blood may obscure the field of vision with reduced image quality owing to light absorption. Experienced surgeons may be able to manage a degree of bleeding via an endoscopic approach; however, this requires a significant degree of experience and skill to be achieved safely. Such scenarios are also reliant on an experienced assistant able to reduce visual loss through optimal camera positioning. It should be remembered that a situation of controlled conversion can easily become uncontrolled, negating any benefit a minimally access approach would have achieved.

Advanced electrosurgery/diathermy and laser technology have improved dissection precision and haemostatic efficacy in endoscopic surgery. Ultrasonic dissection and tissue fusion devices continue to evolve with incremental technical improvements and surgeons are increasingly familiar with their use. Some devices now combine the functions of three or four separate instruments, reducing the need for instrument exchanges during a procedure. This flexibility, combined with the ability to provide a clean, smoke-free field, facilitates dissection, improves haemostasis and reduces operating times.

Loss of tactile feedback

Minimal access surgery is associated with some loss of tactile feedback, although this is less with straight stick endoscopy than with robotic procedures. This is an area of ongoing research in haptics and biofeedback systems. Early work suggested that laparoscopic ultrasonography might be a substitute for the need to 'feel' in intraoperative decision-making. Rather than producing tactile feedback, endoscopic ultrasound provides a visual representation of structures that in open surgery would rely on palpation for accurate localisation and appraisal. Widely used examples include appraisal of nodal disease in cancer surgery and biliary tract exploration.

Tissue extraction

Large pieces of tissue, such as the lung or colon, may have to be extracted from the body cavity following resection. In some circumstances this significantly increases the surgical trauma of the procedure that could otherwise be carried out via two or three small port incisions. Although tissue 'morcellators, mincers and liquidisers' can be used in some circumstances, they have the disadvantage of disrupting gross specimen morphology and cannot be used in surgery for malignancy. Typically, extraction is performed by enlarging one incision so as to facilitate removal without disruption to the specimen. Strategies to reduce surgical trauma have been considered. These include removal of lung via a subxiphoid approach so as to reduce intercostal neuropraxia or natural orifice extraction of abdominal resection specimens. However, such approaches are themselves associated with different complications such as herniation and injury to structures outside the direct operative field.

While tumour implantation and localisation at port sites initially raised important questions about the future of the laparoscopic treatment of malignancy, large-scale trials have shown concerns to be minimised by appropriate tissue handling, separating any tumours by bagging, irrigation and protecting the extraction site.

Cost

Initially high consumable costs and factors such as surgical learning curve and high conversion rates led to increased costs of minimal access approaches compared with their open equivalents. This is now largely no longer the case for straight stick endoscopic surgery such as laparoscopy and thoracoscopy. Indeed, despite higher direct consumable costs, improvements in outcomes, hospital stay and general upscaling of the procedural volume have resulted in improved cost-effectiveness for many minimal access procedures.

Future reductions in the costs of image-processing technology will result in a wide range of transformed presentations becoming available. It should ultimately be possible for a surgeon to access any view of the operative region accessible to a camera and present it stereoscopically in any size or orientation, superimposed on past images taken in other modalities. Such augmented reality systems continue to improve and are discussed in more detail below.

Summary box 10.2

Limitations of minimal access surgery

- Lack of 3D vision
- Loss of tactile feedback
- Haemostasis
- Extraction of large specimens
- Learning curve and increased operative time
- Cost
- Reliance on new technologies

ROBOTIC SURGERY

A robot is a mechanical device that performs automated physical tasks according to direct human supervision, a predefined program or a set of general guidelines, using artificial intelligence (AI) technology. In surgery, robots can be used to assist surgeons to perform operative procedures, primarily in the form of automated camera systems and telemanipulator systems, thus resulting in the creation of a human–machine interface. Reduced degrees of freedom of movement and difficult ergonomic positioning for the surgeon can limit the application of straight stick endoscopy to a number of specialties owing to a loss in surgical precision. This has driven the uptake of robotic surgical systems, currently existing as two main categories:

- **Teleoperated (master–slave) systems:** a surgeon performs an operation via a robot and its robotic instruments through a televisual computerised platform (where the surgeon is the master, i.e. the operator, and the robot is the slave). This may be via onsite connections or remotely through the internet or other digital channels – hence the publicity of 'operating on a patient from another country' (such 'remote' operations are currently rarely performed but their existence is established).
- **Active or semiactive systems: these are typically image-guided or pre-programmed.** In active systems, a surgical robot completes a pre-programmed surgical task. This is guided by preoperative imaging and real-time anatomical constraints and cues through the application of in-built navigation systems. In semiactive systems, the robotic device may be in part pre-programmed and in part surgeon driven.

History of robotic surgery

The first documented clinical robotic procedure was a computed tomography (CT)-guided brain biopsy performed in 1985 utilising the PUMA (Programmable Universal Machine for Assembly) 560 system. This was followed by the ROBODOC, a pre-programmed active robot that enabled precise preparation of the femoral implant cavity during hip replacement. The benefit of such a device was the ability to perform tasks to a high degree of accuracy, thus minimising error and variation. While this and other active surgical robots demonstrated a number of advantages, they were largely superseded by the advent of wider laparoscopy and thoracoscopy, which became increasingly commonplace across during the 1990s and 2000s.

In 1992, Computer Motion developed the AESOP (Automated Endoscopic System for Optimal Positioning) system, which mounted the endoscopic camera on a single robotic arm, allowing the surgeon to control it remotely via voice command. The system was widely used in cholecystectomy and hernia surgery and for harvesting the mammary conduit in coronary artery bypass. This was followed by the development of the ZEUS robot in 1996, a master–slave teleoperated system that provided three robotic arms, one for the voice-controlled endoscope and two further instrument arms. The surgeon was positioned at a remote console and the device was capable of motion scaling and tremor correction, facilitating its use for microsurgical procedures. ZEUS was used for the first fully endoscopic robotic surgical procedure, the reanastomosis of a Fallopian tube in 1998. The first remote surgical procedure was performed in 2001, also utilising the ZEUS system. Here a cholecystectomy was performed on a patient in Paris by a surgeon in New York, demonstrating the feasibility of remote operating. ZEUS was discontinued in 2003 after the merger of Computer Motion with Intuitive Surgical.

The current era of surgical robots is dominated by the da Vinci® surgical system, which was first approved for clinical use in 2000. The system offers a number of advantages, including 3D surgical vision, EndoWrist® precision instruments, tremor reduction, motion scaling and improved ergonomics. The initial system was released in 1999 and provided three robotic arms, one of which held the endoscope. This was upgraded to the da Vinci S (2006), the da Vinci Si (2009) and subsequently the da Vinci Xi in 2014 (***Figure 10.2***). With each iteration came improvements in vision and instrumentation, along with which came integrated fluorescence imaging. More recently, novel technologies include the development of a single port system (da Vinci SP), which combines multijointed wristed instrumentation with a wristed camera through a single port to further improve dexterity and minimise surgical trauma.

(a)
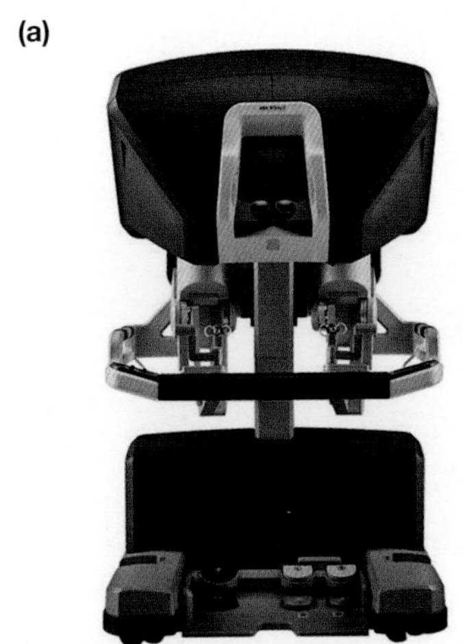
(b)
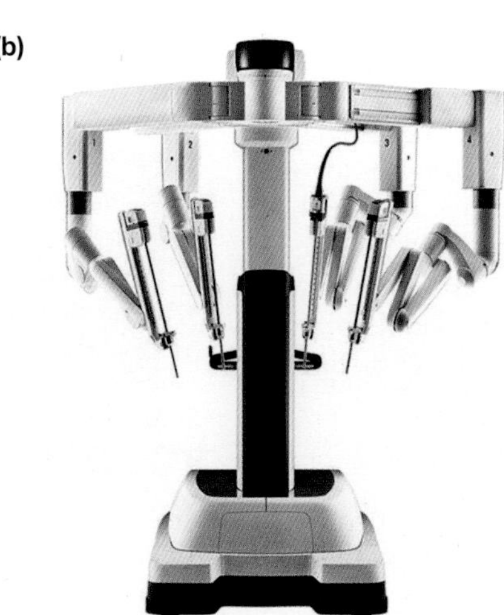
(c)
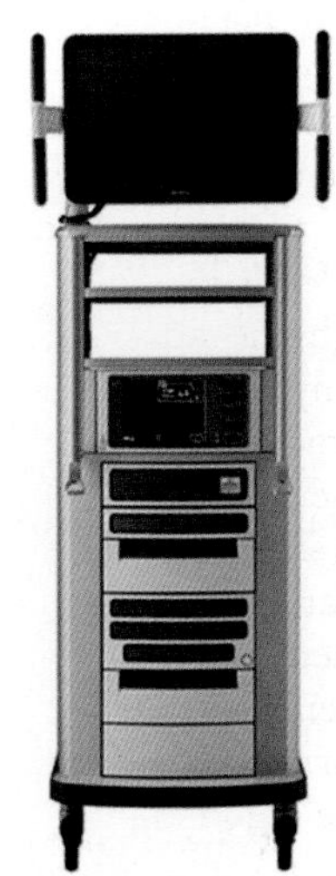

Figure 10.2 The da Vinci Xi system: **(a)** surgeon console; **(b)** da Vinci Xi robot; **(c)** vision cart (courtesy of Intuitive Surgical).

Advantages of robotic surgery

Surgical robots have been considered to offer many benefits, which have arisen as a result of new technology in lenses, cameras and computer software. Just as laparoscopic surgery benefited from advances in light technology allowing the targeted transmission of light down tubing, robotic surgery benefits from computer integration of mechanical (surgical) arms that have paved the way for computer-integrated surgery.

Vision

Modern robotic camera systems offer 3D high-definition imaging, providing stereoscopic vision with true depth perception that enhances the visualisation of tissue planes and key structures. Multiport systems typically employ a rigid endoscope with or without angulation. As with conventional endoscopes, angulation to 30° allows for a wider range of vision through manipulation of the camera position, which, in the case of robotic surgery, can be controlled by the surgeon at the console or, if required, by the assistant at the bedside. A reference horizon is commonly provided to the surgeon at the console system so as to maintain orientation throughout the procedure. More recently, modern single-port systems such as the da Vinci SP employ a wristed camera system that, in combination with fully wristed instruments, may allow for operative triangulation while at the same time maintaining a small, single skin incision.

Manoeuvrability, motion scaling and tremor suppression

Improved manoeuvring as a result of the 'robotic wrist' in some systems allows for up to seven degrees of freedom, thus improving dexterity for the surgeon. This has particular benefits in fields with significant space restraints such as transoral surgery, where conventional laparoscopy has limited applicability. Furthermore, the increased dexterity of surgical robots may facilitate a minimal access approach to more complex procedures where the technical difficulty of applying conventional laparoscopy may be prohibitive. As the motion of the surgeon's hand is translated to the 'slave' motion of the robotic arm, modern surgical robots are able to scale down large external movements of the surgical hands to limited internal movements. At the same time, the computer may filter out tremor in the surgeon's hands, thus ensuring stability of the instrument tips and enhancing surgical precision.

Ergonomics

Although the advent of straight stick laparoscopic surgery had many advantages for the patient, for the surgeon there was a trade-off in terms of operative ergonomics. Increased operative time in addition to unergonomic positioning can result in significant physical discomfort for the surgeon. This is particularly true in specialties such as bariatric surgery, where the patient's body habitus and the use of long, fulcrumed instruments puts further strain on the surgeon's back, neck and upper arms. The advent of robotic surgery vastly improves upon the ergonomic environment for the surgeon; in the case of many of the current master–slave systems, allowing for the surgeon to be seated at a console remote from the operating table (***Figure 10.3***). The console positioning can be optimised to fit the individual profile of the operator, thus reducing physical stress and fatigue. The enclosed console system of many robotic systems also provides the advantage of surgical isolation from external distractions that may impact on the operator's concentration. The disadvantage is reduced awareness of non-verbal communication, thus highlighting the importance of team training and regular verbal cues.

Motion compensation

Although not commonplace in current clinical practice, robotic surgical systems may in future provide motion compensation to facilitate surgery on a moving target. Examples where this may be beneficial are in beating heart cardiac surgery, such as coronary artery bypass grafting and mitral valve repair. In this setting, the increased dexterity of robotic surgery combined with removing the need for cardioplegia and cross-clamping may be particularly beneficial in terms of reducing the post-operative inflammatory response and improving its associated morbidity.

Disadvantages of robotic surgery

Cost

Robotic surgery remains more costly than minimally invasive alternatives. Through upscaling of use between surgical specialties, the direct costs of purchasing a novel robotic system can be partially offset; however, consumable costs remain high. When compared with open techniques, robotic surgical procedures can reduce hospital stay, thus in part offsetting this expenditure; however, it remains difficult to demonstrate significant improvement in length of stay or clinical outcomes when compared with other minimally invasive alternatives. Another consideration is the increased operating time and overall learning curve requirement when establishing a robotic surgical programme. While some specialties have reported shorter learning curves than in the early days of laparoscopic surgery, this is highly heterogeneous, across both specialties and practitioners. Furthermore, although shared interspecialty

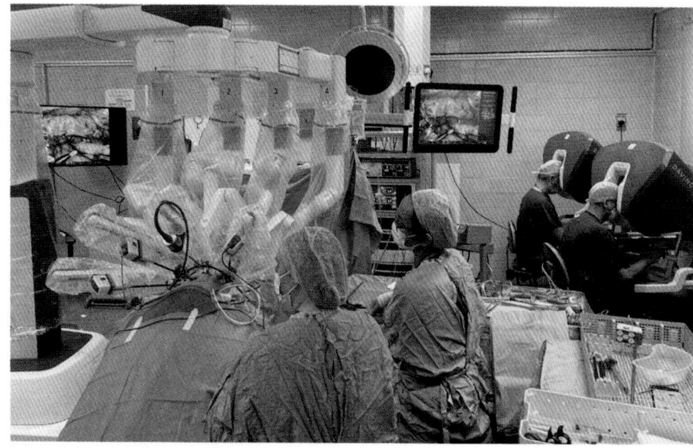

Figure 10.3 Robotic theatre set-up demonstrating the da Vinci Xi system. The surgeon and trainee surgeon are positioned at joint consoles remote from the operating table with the surgical assistant and scrub nurse at the bedside (courtesy of Mr Tom Routledge, Guy's and St Thomas' NHS Foundation Trust, London, UK).

use increases cost-effectiveness for the institution, it also consequently reduces the access opportunities for each individual user, potentially prolonging the learning curve.

Uptake of robotic surgery

Many surgical specialties have embraced robot-assisted techniques, including general surgery, cardiothoracic surgery, urology, orthopaedics, ear, nose and throat surgery, gynaecology and paediatric surgery. Specialties that use microsurgical techniques also benefit from this technology. Current robotic systems were designed to offer multifunctionality, including multianatomy and specialty capability in both operating theatre and remote environments. Currently, despite a small number of reports of remote surgical procedures, robotic surgery remains focused on in-house operating.

New entrants

In 2017, Intuitive Surgical released the da Vinci X, a low-cost entry point in its robotic surgical portfolio that includes features of the Xi while sacrificing some flexibility in terms of multi-quadrant surgery. In the same year, Korean company Meere gained a licence for the use of its surgical robot, the REVO-I, by the local Ministry for Food and Drug Safety. Similar to the da Vinci, this four-arm robot is mounted on a single cart. The surgeon is seated at an open vision cart and, by use of 3D glasses, can achieve three-dimensional high-definition (3D-HD) vision. In March 2019, CMR Surgical received a European CE mark for its novel modular robot, the Versius (***Figure 10.4***). This system incorporates individual cart-mounted modular robotic arms that can be configured to fit the procedure and the operating room environment. The design differs from other robotic arms in that it aims to more closely mimic a human arm, improving freedom of port placement. Its vision cart similarly allows for ergonomic operating with 3D-HD vision, through the use of 3D glasses.

Bridging the gap between laparoscopic and robotic surgery the Senhance® robotic system received its CE mark in 2016. In order to reduce cost and sustain familiarity with conventional laparoscopy, the system uses independent robotic arms mounted on separate carts that can be placed in accordance with the procedure required. The system utilises reusable non-wristed instruments that can be inserted through standard laparoscopic trocars so as to reduce consumable cost. This system also creates familiarity with conventional laparoscopy and facilitates hybrid techniques where this may be beneficial. Surgery is enhanced though a 3D-HD system with the use of 3D glasses and eye-tracking camera control.

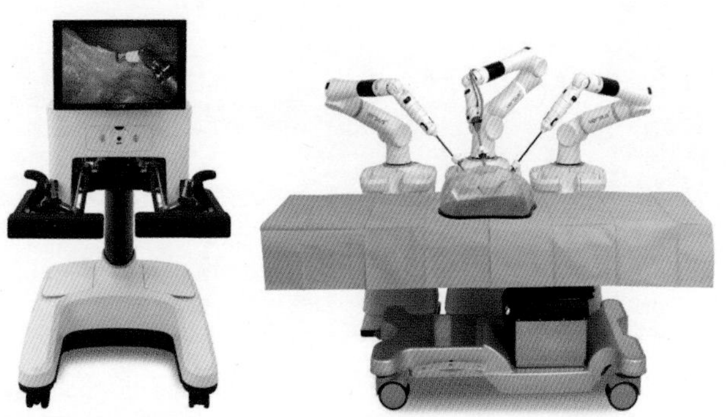

Figure 10.4 The Versius robotic system (courtesy of CMR Surgical).

As the field of robotic surgery continues to expand and innovate, there also remain a number of systems in development that are not yet approved for clinical use. Examples similar to existing technologies include the Medtronic Hugo Robotic-Assisted Surgery (RAS) system, which was launched in late 2019. This modular system aims to provide a lower cost alternative by means of a more readily upgradeable model that may be used flexibly across surgical specialties and procedures. Moving forward, companies such as Verb Surgical strive to build on the currently dominant master–slave model, incorporating robotic autonomy and machine learning. While this may in time revolutionise robotic surgery, such technologies remain in the early phase of development.

Direct robotic systems and hybrid robotic surgery

In addition to the remote master–slave platform design, direct robot systems also exist. Each of these systems offers different advantages to the operating surgeon, ranging from reducing the need for assistants and providing better ergonomic operating positions to providing experienced guidance from surgeons not physically present in the operating theatre. Examples include:

- tremor suppression robots;
- active guidance systems;
- articulated mechatronic devices;
- force control systems;
- haptic feedback devices.

PERIOPERATIVE PLANNING FOR MINIMAL ACCESS SURGERY

Preparation of the patient

Although the patient may be in hospital for a shorter period, careful preoperative management is essential to minimise morbidity. Recognition of patient- or procedure-related factors that may in turn complicate a minimal access approach is vital to optimise outcomes.

History

Patients must be fit for general anaesthesia and open operation if necessary. Potential coagulation disorders are particularly dangerous in minimal access surgery where options for haemostasis may be more limited. A prior history of surgical intervention in the same area is vitally important and should be carefully documented, so as to best predict factors such as adhesions that may preclude a minimal access approach. Previous oncological treatment can also create a more hostile surgical environment and an appropriate threshold for conversion to open access should be set prior to the procedure and communicated clearly with the patient.

Summary box 10.3

Preparation for minimal access surgery

- Overall fitness: cardiac arrhythmia, lung function, medications, allergies
- Previous surgery or oncological intervention: scars, adhesions
- Body habitus: obesity, skeletal deformity
- Normal coagulation
- Thromboprophylaxis
- Informed consent
- Operative difficulty is predicted when possible with appropriate risk model
- Appropriate theatre time and facilities are available (especially important for robotic cases)

Examination

Routine preoperative physical examination is required as for any major operation. Although, in general, minimal access surgery allows quicker recovery, it may involve longer operating times and carbon dioxide insufflation in both the chest and abdomen may provoke cardiac arrhythmias. Severe chronic obstructive airways disease and ischaemic heart disease may be contraindications to a minimal access approach. Moderate obesity does not increase operative difficulty significantly, but morbid obesity may require specialist instrumentation and trocars. Patients with a particularly low body mass index and small body habitus may present separate challenges in terms of port placement, particularly when adopting a robotic approach. Severe spinal deformity including kyphosis and scoliosis may present problems in terms of positioning as well as impact on overall recovery if there are associated problems with sputum clearance and mobility.

Prophylaxis against thromboembolism

Venous stasis induced by the reverse Trendelenburg position during laparoscopic surgery coupled with prolonged duration of operation are risk factors for deep vein thrombosis. Subcutaneous low-molecular-weight heparin and antithromboembolic stockings should be used routinely in addition to pneumatic calf compression during the operation. Patients already taking anticoagulation should have this stopped temporarily or, where appropriate, be converted to intravenous or subcutaneous heparin, depending on the underlying condition and local thromboprophylaxis protocols. In most cases patients can continue on aspirin when the benefits outweigh the slight increase in bleeding potential.

Urinary catheters and nasogastric tubes

In the early days of minimal access surgery, routine bladder catheterisation and nasogastric intubation were advised. Most surgeons now omit these in favour of enhanced recovery, which has demonstrated benefits in terms of both length of stay and morbidity outcomes. It remains essential to check that the patient has fasted and has recently emptied their bladder, particularly before creating pneumoperitoneum for minimal access surgery approaches to the abdomen.

Informed consent

It is essential that the patient understands the nature of the procedure, the risks involved and, when appropriate, the alternatives that are available. A locally prepared explanatory booklet concerning the minimal access procedure to be undertaken is extremely useful (***Chapter 14***). The patient should understand that the procedure may be converted to an open operation. Common complications should be mentioned, such as shoulder tip pain and minor surgical emphysema, as well as rare but serious complications, such as inadvertent visceral injury from trocar insertion or diathermy. Patients may also have specific questions or requests in terms of the application of minimal access surgery. It is important to be considerate and address these. Some patients remain concerned about the application of technology, particularly robotics, to their care and it is important to ensure they understand and agree with the proposed surgical approach.

THEATRE SET-UP AND TOOLS

Operating theatre design is key to efficiency. Modern theatres are designed with moveable booms for video, diathermy and laparoscopic equipment with at least two high-resolution, high-definition (HD) or ultra-high-definition (4K) monitors, a carbon dioxide supply and flow monitor and appropriate audiovisual kit (***Figure 10.1***).

Image quality is vital to the success of minimal access surgery. New camera and lens technology allows the use of smaller cameras while maintaining excellent resolution. Automatic focusing and charge-coupled devices (CCDs) are used to detect different levels of brightness and adjust for the best image possible.

Efficient teamwork is crucial for high-quality surgery and quick yet safe turnover. This is particularly important in robotic surgery, where verbal interaction between all team members is paramount throughout the procedure. The robotic team must carefully rehearse protocols for both controlled and uncontrolled conversion in the event of emergency.

GENERAL INTRAOPERATIVE PRINCIPLES

Many minimal access procedures have a unique set of procedural steps that may often be in a distinctly different sequence from those of the open alternative.

Methods for creating a pneumoperitoneum are described in ***Chapter 7***. Preoperative evaluation is necessary to assess the type and location of surgical scars and potential for perivisceral adhesions. In the setting of redo surgery, trocar insertion may be complex and should be performed by an open approach with direct visualisation on entry to the body cavity (abdomen

---

Friedrich Trendelenburg, 1844–1924, Professor of Surgery successively at Rostock (1875–1882), Bonn (1882–1895), Leipzig (1895–1911), Germany. The Trendelenburg position was first described in 1885.

or thorax). Before trocar insertion, the introduction of a fingertip helps to ascertain penetration into the body cavity and allows adhesions to be gently removed from the entry site. The endoscopic camera may be used as a blunt dissector to tease adhesions gently away and form a tunnel towards the quadrant where the operation is to take place. With experience, the surgeon learns to differentiate visually between thick adhesions that should be avoided and thin adhesions that would lead to a window into a free area.

In obese patients the location of some of the ports may need to be modified and, in some instances, larger and longer instruments may be necessary. It is important to recognise this preoperatively to ensure that adequate measures are put in place to ensure safe and efficient surgery when the patient arrives. It is also important to consider the weight and dimension restrictions of the operating table. In some cases, specialist operating tables will be required (***Chapter 68***).

Operative problems

Intraoperative perforation of a viscus or vascular injury

Perforation of any viscus, such as bowel, is a potential hazard that may occur inadvertently and go unrecognised or be of a severity that may require emergency conversion. The added time required for this to take place may result in increased blood loss and haemodynamic instability that would not have occurred should the same injury have occurred in an open setting. With surgical experience, education, preparation and patient selection many of these emergencies and their resultant complications can be avoided. It is vital for the surgical team to both recognise its own limitations and continually reflect throughout the procedure on the surgical progress and operative difficulty.

Bleeding

Bleeding is the most common cause of conversion to open surgery. The impact of light absorption is particularly important in robotic surgery, and regular haemostasis is paramount to facilitate dissection and surgical progress. Risk factors that predispose to increased bleeding include:

- liver disease impacting on the production of vitamin K-dependent clotting factors, e.g. cirrhosis, autoimmune liver disease;
- inflammatory conditions (acute cholecystitis, diverticulitis);
- patients on anticoagulants;
- coagulation defects: these may be contraindications to both open and minimal access surgery and require thorough discussion with haematology colleagues to determine, where possible, how to optimise the patient for surgery.

Damage to a large vessel requires immediate assessment of the magnitude and type of bleeding. It is paramount that as soon as bleeding is identified this is communicated clearly to all members of the theatre and anaesthetic team. There should be a relatively low threshold for early conversion; however, this will depend on the expertise of the operating team. It is pertinent to achieve early control by whatever means necessary. When the bleeding vessel can be identified and grasped, control may be achieved by clipping, stapling or use of an energy device, depending on vessel size. Occasionally suturing may be possible; however, this may be significantly more complex via a minimal access approach. When the vessel is not identified, compression should be applied immediately with a blunt instrument, a cotton swab or with the adjacent organ. Good suction and irrigation are of utmost importance. Once the area has been cleaned, pressure should be released gradually to identify the site of bleeding. Insertion of an extra port may be required. There should be no delay in converting to an open procedure when necessary. This is of particular importance in robotic surgery as some or all of the robotic arms may need to be urgently undocked to facilitate the surgeon gaining bedside access to the patient. The bedside assistant should be confident to perform this process. It is sometimes appropriate for a single robotic arm to be left in place to help maintain pressure on the bleeding vessel while direct access is achieved. Alternatively, pressure may be maintained via an assistant port (if present), allowing the robot to be undocked completely and removed from the surgical field.

Bleeding from organs encountered during surgery

Excessive retraction can tear a visceral surface, resulting in bleeding. This is particularly so in robotic surgery, where instrument graspers have a small surface area, increasing the potential for injury to retracted tissue. Here rolled swabs may be inserted into the surgical field and held within the grasper, producing a larger surface for retraction and reducing tissue injury. Surgicel® (absorbable fibrillar oxidised cellulose polymer) or other clot-promoting strips, tissue glues or other haemostatic agents may also be used to aid haemostasis, e.g. from the gallbladder bed during cholecystectomy.

Bleeding from a trocar site

Bleeding from the trocar sites is usually treated by localised diathermy or applying upwards and lateral pressure with the trocar itself. Considerable bleeding may occur if a vessel such as the inferior epigastric or intercostal artery is injured. Haemostasis can be accomplished either by pressure or by suturing the bleeding site. Devices such as the EndoClose™ may also be used to apply transabdominal sutures under direct laparoscopic view to close port sites that bleed.

When a bleeding vessel cannot be easily identified, mass ligation of the vessel around the port site can be performed. This manoeuvre is accomplished by extending the skin incision by 3 mm at both ends of the bleeding trocar site wound. Two figure-of-eight sutures are placed in the path of the vessel at both ends of the wound (***Figure 10.5***). Alternatively, pressure can be applied using a Foley balloon catheter. The catheter is introduced into the abdominal cavity through the bleeding trocar site wound, the balloon is inflated and traction is placed on the catheter, which is bolstered in place to keep it under tension. The catheter is left *in situ* for 24 hours and then removed.

If significant continuous bleeding from the falciform ligament occurs, haemostasis is achieved by percutaneously inserting a large, straight needle at one side of the ligament. A monofilament suture attached to the needle is passed into the abdominal cavity and the needle is exited at the other side of the ligament using a grasper. The loop is suspended and compression is achieved. Maintaining compression throughout the procedure usually suffices. After the procedure has been completed, the loop is removed under direct laparoscopic visualisation to ensure complete haemostasis.

Evacuation of blood clots

Careful haemostasis is important as even small, localised pools of blood or clot absorb light and can significantly impair the surgical view. Carefully directed suction is usually sufficient in open cases; however, suction may be problematic in laparoscopic and robotic procedures that are reliant on carbon dioxide insufflation to maintain the surgical field. It is important that suction is applied below a fluid level, or, if used in the operative field, only in short bursts as required. Should tissue be inadvertently sucked into the end of the suction device, the tubing can be kinked to allow the tissue to drop away before removing. Rolled swabs or sponges can be used to remove blood from the surgical field without need for suction (***Figure 10.6***). These can also be used for gentle retraction, minimising tissue damage and thus further reducing blood loss. Such swabs may be inserted and removed via a 15-mm assistant port or in some cases a 12-mm robotic trocar with the port cap removed. Care should be taken to avoid carbon dioxide loss during extraction. Finally, the surgeon may choose to use a specially designed robotic sucker that integrates with the robotic system. Alternatively, non-wristed suction can be provided via an assistant port if included in the operative set-up.

Principles of electrosurgery during laparoscopic surgery

Inadvertent electrosurgical injuries during minimal access surgery are potentially serious and are often unrecognised at the time. The vast majority occur following the use of monopolar diathermy. For conventional laparoscopy, the overall incidence is thought to be between one and two cases per 1000 operations. Injuries can occur through inadvertent touching or grasping of tissue during current application; direct coupling between tissue and a metal instrument that is touching the activated probe; insulation breaks in the laparoscopic or robotic instruments; direct sparking from the diathermy probe; or current passage from recently coagulated, electrically isolated tissue. Bipolar diathermy is safer and should be used in preference to monopolar diathermy, especially in anatomically crowded areas. If monopolar diathermy is to be used, important safety measures include attainment of a perfect visual image, avoiding excessive current application and meticulous attention to insulation. Alternative methods of performing dissection, such as the use of ultrasonic devices, may improve safety.

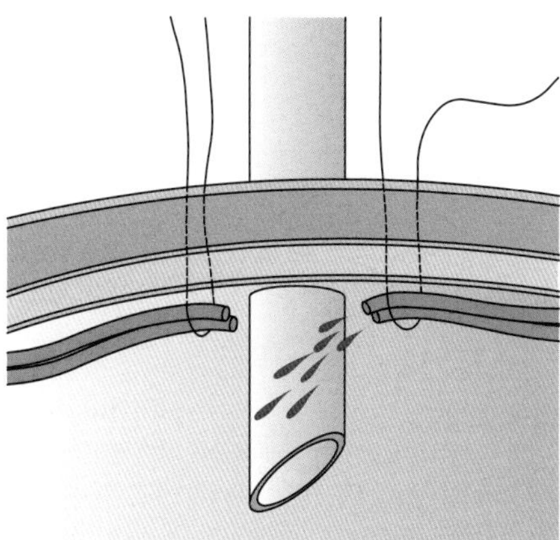

Figure 10.5 Management of bleeding from a surgical trocar site.

POSTOPERATIVE CARE

The postoperative care of patients after minimal access surgery is generally straightforward, with a low incidence of pain or other problems when compared with their open counterparts. It is a good general rule that if the patient develops a fever or tachycardia, or complains of severe pain at the operation site, something is wrong and close observation or intervention is necessary (see also ***Chapter 24***).

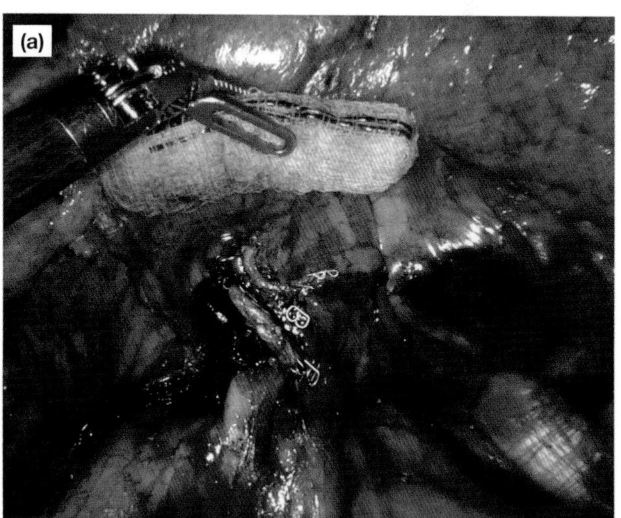

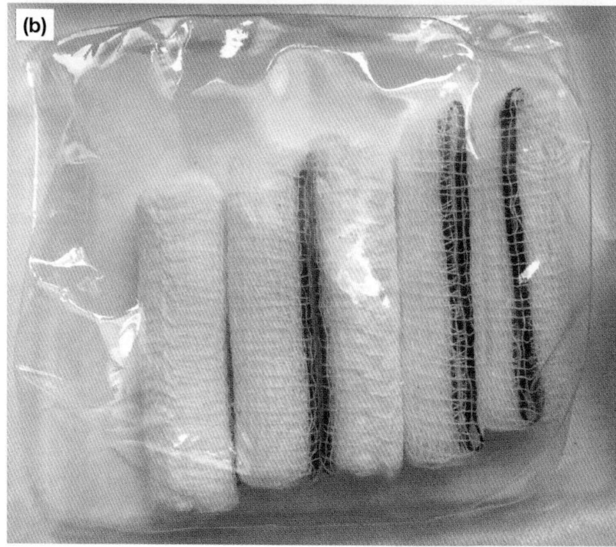

Figure 10.6 Use of rolled swabs for retraction of the lung during pulmonary lobectomy (courtesy of Mr Tom Routledge, Guy's and St Thomas' NHS Foundation Trust, London, UK).

Nausea

About half of patients experience some degree of nausea after minimal access surgery. It usually responds to an antiemetic, such as ondansetron, and settles within 12–24 hours. It is made worse by opiate analgesics and these should be rationalised or avoided where at all possible.

Shoulder tip pain

Patients should be warned about this preoperatively and informed that the pain is referred from the diaphragm and that it is not due to a local problem in the shoulders. It can be at its worst 24 hours after the operation. It usually settles within 2–3 days and is relieved by simple analgesics, such as paracetamol.

Port site pain and numbness

Pain in one or other of the port site wounds is not uncommon and is worse if there is haematoma formation. It usually settles very rapidly. In the case of thoracoscopy, intercostal nerve pain may be more common in those with smaller intercostal spaces. Nerve blockade by means of directed local anaesthesia is effective at reducing pain and the need for opiate medication in the immediate postoperative period. Increasing pain after 2–3 days may be a sign of infection and, with concomitant signs, antibiotic therapy is occasionally required. Occasionally, herniation through a port may account for localised pain and should be considered, particularly if occurring late with a relevant preceding history (e.g. coughing). Failure of a patient to follow the expected recovery pathway should prompt senior review with appropriate imaging and relook surgery if considered necessary.

Analgesia

The type and extent of analgesic requirement will depend on both the patient and procedural factors. Prior experience of opiate analgesia may increase patient tolerance to similar agents, necessitating larger doses. There is also evidence to suggest that those patients struggling with chronic pain preoperatively often present a more complex postoperative analgesic problem. The extent and region of surgery will also dictate the analgesic regimen. For example, even minimal access thoracic surgical procedures commonly require patient-controlled opiate analgesia with or without local nerve blockade (intercostal or paravertebral) in the initial 48 hours after surgery. This may be avoided for some abdominal surgery by careful use of non-steroidal agents and paracetamol. Opiate analgesics cause nausea, impair gut motility and should be avoided unless the pain is very severe. When pain is disproportionate to the presenting problem, suspect a complication (see also *Chapter 23*).

Orogastric or nasogastric tube

An orogastric or nasogastric tube may be placed for some abdominal surgery if the stomach is distended and obscuring the view. It is not necessary in all cases and is very rarely used in other minimal access surgery. Where possible, it should be removed as soon as the operation is over and before the patient regains consciousness. This is most commonly used in bariatric and oesophagogastric surgery, where a larger (32F or 34F) tube is used.

Oral fluids

There is no significant ileus after minimal access surgery, except in abdominal resectional procedures, such as colectomy or small bowel resection. Patients may resume oral fluids as soon as they are conscious; they usually do so 4–6 hours after the end of the operation.

Oral feeding

Provided that the patient has an appetite, a light meal can be taken 4–6 hours after the operation. Some patients remain slightly nauseated at this stage, but almost all eat a normal breakfast on the morning after surgery. Subsequently a balanced diet is recommended in most cases and where specific procedural recommendations are needed these should be clearly communicated to both the patient and relatives with appropriate dietetic referral made.

Urinary catheter

The requirement for a urinary catheter depends on the operation. In shorter (<4 hours) minimal access procedures a urinary catheter is not usually required. If a urinary catheter has been placed in the bladder during an operation with likely short stay, it can be removed before the patient regains consciousness if the procedure has been uneventful. Postoperatively it is important to check that the patient has been able to pass urine and empty their bladder without difficulty. When there is uncertainty point-of-care bladder scanning can assess residual bladder volume.

Drains

The use of postoperative drains depends on the operation performed. Drain output should initially be documented at least hourly or more regularly in the event of concern regarding high drain output. Given the heterogeneity of drainage systems available it is paramount that nursing staff are familiar with the system used. The exact location and size of any drains should be clearly documented in the operation notes and the tubing labelled accordingly. This avoids inadvertent removal of the wrong drain or confusion for the ward team. Continued blood loss from a drain is an indication for re-exploration and should be immediately highlighted to the operating surgeon.

DISCHARGE FROM HOSPITAL

The discharge of patients is based on clinical indicators and the patient's fitness for recuperating in a non-hospital environment. One of the core drivers for the application of minimally invasive surgery is an earlier recovery and therefore discharge from hospital. Patients should not be discharged until they are comfortable, have passed urine and are eating and drinking

Summary box 10.4

Principles of minimal access surgery

- Meticulous care in the creation of a pneumoperitoneum
- Controlled dissection of adhesions
- Adequate exposure of operative field
- Avoidance and control of bleeding
- Avoidance of organ injury
- Avoidance of diathermy damage
- Vigilance in the postoperative period

satisfactorily. They should be told that if they develop worsening pain or other severe symptoms they should return to the hospital or to their general practitioner. Even for more major cases, some units have demonstrated safe and feasible protocols for a 23-hour stay.

Skin sutures

If non-absorbable sutures or skin staples have been used, they can be removed from the port sites after 7–10 days.

Mobility and convalescence

Patients can get out of bed to go to the toilet as soon as they have recovered from the anaesthetic and they should be encouraged to do so. Such movements are remarkably pain free when compared with the mobility achieved after an open operation. Similarly, patients can cough actively and clear bronchial secretions, and this helps to diminish the incidence of chest infections.

FURTHER DEVELOPMENTS

Augmented reality and minimal access surgical adjuncts

The future of minimal access surgery will almost certainly feature more advanced applications of adjuncts to facilitate anatomical recognition and the localisation of pathology. These are becoming commonplace in both video-assisted and robotic-assisted procedures.

Augmented reality

Augmented reality by definition comprises the fusion of projected computerised images with a real environment. In surgery, this involves the application of real-time imaging or other data overlaid via computer processing software onto the surgical field. Such technology may be particularly beneficial in minimal access surgery where the localisation of pathology and identification of anatomy may be more difficult than in open surgery because of the lack of digital palpation of the relevant structures. At an elementary level, examples include the use of indocyanine green for immunofluorescent localisation of tumours as well as vascular, bronchial or lymphatic structures. When bound to plasma proteins, indocyanine green emits light with a peak wavelength of around 820–830 nm on illumination with near-infrared light. Through use of a specifically designed HD camera and software system with imposed pseudo-colour, areas of differential tissue density and vascular supply can be detected clearly without the need for digital palpation, thus facilitating complete resection and clear surgical margins. Its use is now well established in procedures such as minimal access liver, lung, renal and prostatic resections, and its role in other specialties such as colorectal surgery is also under investigation. The technology can be integrated into both video-assisted and robotic-assisted surgical procedures and is available within the da Vinci Xi and X robotic surgical systems as the Firefly® mode, which can be turned on as required from the surgical console (***Figure 10.7***).

Another role for augmented reality in minimal access surgery is the overlay of imaging beside or directly onto the surgical field, 'navigating' the surgeon to the site of interest without the need to look away from the patient to review imaging. Such navigational techniques originated in image-guided diagnostics, enabling identification of pathology in areas more difficult to reach anatomically. Through increasing adoption of hybrid theatre complexes, these approaches may be utilised for both diagnosis and treatment in a single setting. An example is the use of navigational bronchoscopy to identify, diagnose and treat difficult to reach or small lung nodules. Preoperative planning CT scan is reconstructed by specialist software. The result is a 3D 'road map' of the bronchial tree and a side-by-side picture of real-time endobronchial images with those from the imaging system (***Figure 10.8***). The surgeon is then guided directly along the airway to the lesion of interest that can be biopsied with on-site frozen section. Where the lesion is resectable but difficult to localise, a fiducial marker may be placed to enable localisation under fluoroscopy guidance in a second-stage procedure performed in a hybrid theatre (***Figure 10.9***). Where resection is not possible, ablation or other treatment may be offered in the same setting, both reducing surgical invasiveness and increasing the provision of curative surgery to patients who may not otherwise be candidates for resection.

An area of interest is the application of head-mounted displays and eyeglasses to minimal access surgery. Although the majority of applications remain in the realm of simulation and training, the promise of real-time image guidance by means of multiplanar or imaging overlay of the surgeon's view is particularly attractive. Head-mounted displays may also provide data display or communication tools, reducing the need for the surgeon to look away from the operative field and allow real-time guidance by a trainer or proctor. To date, clinical application is limited owing to time lag, the need for high-speed wireless Internet or Bluetooth connection and device weight and battery life; application to minimal access surgery remains under development.

THE FUTURE

Minimal access surgery has changed surgical practice; however, it has not changed the nature of disease. The basic principles of good surgery still apply, including appropriate case selection, excellent exposure, adequate retraction and a high level of technical expertise. Endoscopic and robotic surgery training is

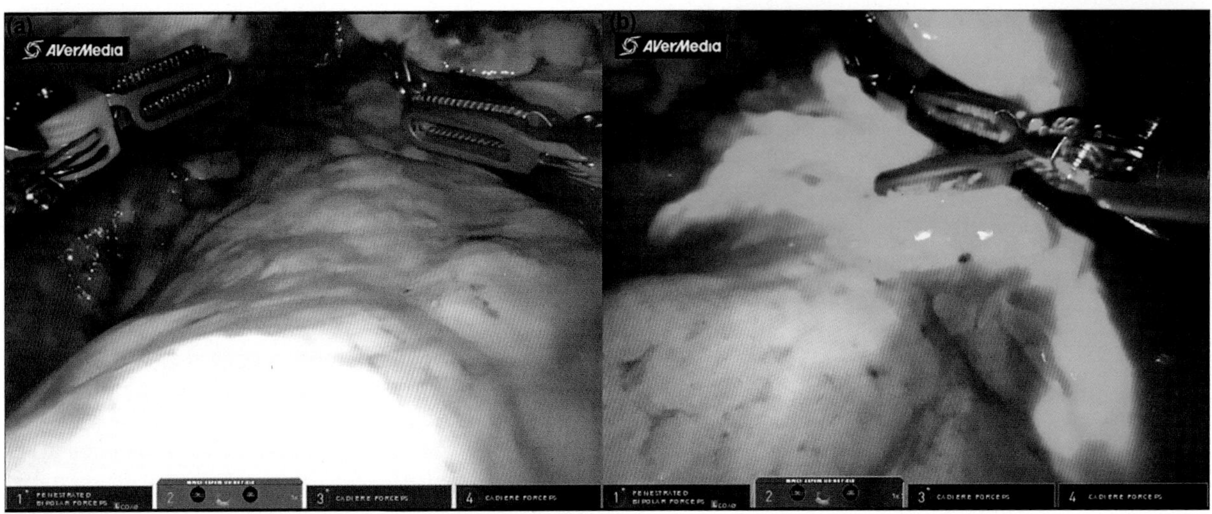

Figure 10.7 Robotic-assisted lung segmentectomy utilising indocyanine green administered endobronchially to highlight the segment for resection. (a) Robotic dissection of the superior (S6) segment. (b) Indocyanine green immunofluorescence of the marked segment, enabling clear identification of the area for resection.

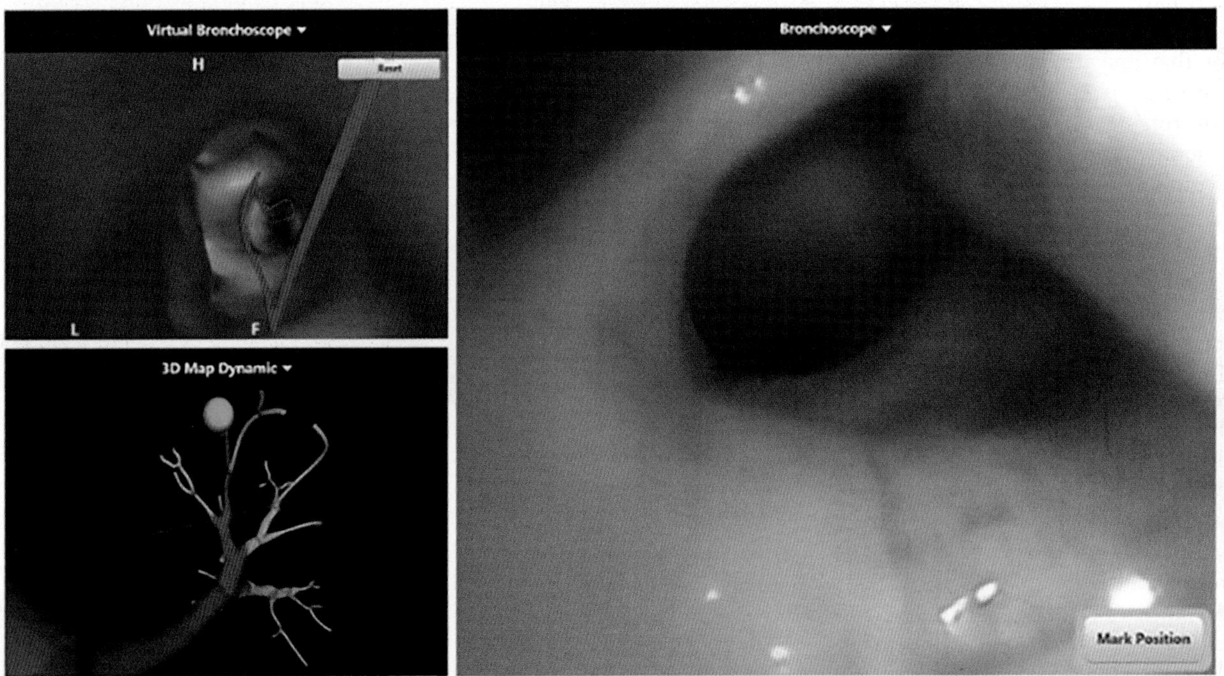

Figure 10.8 Navigational bronchoscopy. Split screen image demonstrating real-time endobronchial imaging adjacent to a virtual bronchoscope image and a three-dimensional map of the lesion and bronchial tree (courtesy of Mr Kelvin Lau, Barts Thorax Centre, London, UK).

key to allow the specialty to progress. The pioneers of yesterday have to teach the surgeons of tomorrow not only the technical and dexterous skills required but also the decision-making and innovative skills necessary for the field to continue to evolve. Training is often perceived as difficult, as trainers have less control over the trainees at the time of surgery and caseloads may be smaller, especially in centres where laparoscopic and robotic procedures are not common. However, trainees now rightly expect exposure to these procedures, and training systems should be adaptable for international exposure so that these techniques can be disseminated worldwide.

The predominant video and digital component of these new techniques opens the door for simulation approaches for training in these modalities, which have demonstrated benefits in reducing learning curves and in turn are aimed at improving patient outcomes. The ultimate goal for this educational approach is to develop expert surgeons through the 'totally safe' and 'risk-free' environment of simulation before they

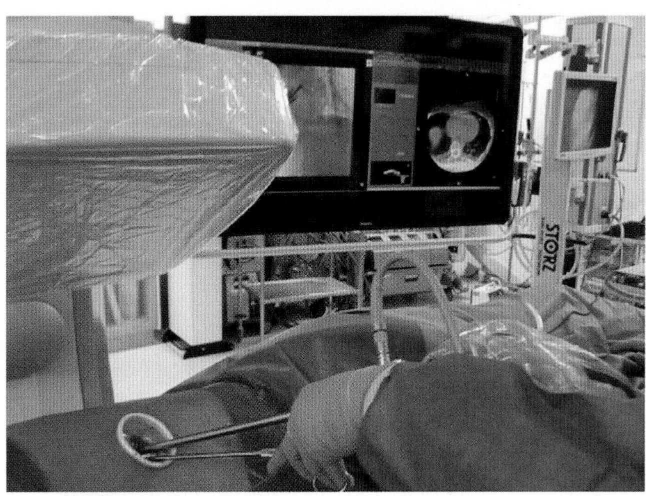

Figure 10.9 Image-guided video-assisted thoracoscopic surgery with the use of a navigationally placed fiducial marker to guide tumour resection (courtesy of Mr Kelvin Lau, Barts Thorax Centre, London, UK).

actually have to operate on patients. Indeed, both videoscopic and robotic platforms now have established simulation programs that are a prerequisite for surgical trainees. Modern robotic simulation modules are able to create an environment that mirrors console use (face validity) and subsequently provide hierarchical training compatible with the user's expertise. The combination of simulation with proficiency-based 'mastery' training may be the key to optimising the impact that simulation may have on the surgical learning curve and remains the subject of research in a range of surgical specialties.

With widespread uptake of minimal access surgery, trainees are now facing a new problem owing to lack of experience in open surgery. Surgeons must have sufficient open surgical experience to feel comfortable converting cases in the event of difficulty or emergency. A minimal access approach to a particular procedure may differ significantly in the order of operative steps and dissection technique. It is therefore vital that the new generation of surgeons continues to receive training in open surgery so that they can apply either technique as appropriate.

Advances in robotic surgery lend themselves to further AI integration, with potential advantages such as providing enhanced clinical decision support, warning of deviations from optimal workflow or detecting and overlaying potentially at-risk structures. In this way, artificially intelligent systems may streamline procedural technique, reduce error and improve patient outcomes. Intelligent operating theatres may provide automated optimisation of a wide range of ergonomic features such as table positioning, lighting and temperature, further facilitating procedural efficiency and effectiveness. In turn, more advanced artificial systems may also develop a degree of supervised autonomy whereby basic surgical procedures can be independently performed by the robotic system. Indeed, in a preclinical setting, the STAR (Smart Tissue Autonomous Robot) robotic system has demonstrated superiority over human surgeons in porcine bowel anastomosis.

Translation of such laboratory-based experiments to real-world surgery is not simple. Application requires detailed understanding of surgical workflow and integration of complex data. To provide a fully comprehensive, annotated training data set on which deep learning may be established, all devices and systems in the dynamic operating environment must be integrated, including operating room set-up, tool and camera usage and the variable patient and procedural factors. In addition there are complex questions in terms of data protection and confidentiality, not to mention the ethical considerations and accountability of autonomous or semi-autonomous robotic surgeons. The most promising elements of AI integration into minimal access surgery remain enhanced object detection, speech recognition, video characterisation and integration with next-generation technologies. Real-time metabolic profiling and tissue-level diagnosis may differentiate between cancerous and non-cancerous tissues on the basis of their metabolic signature. An example is the iKnife, which uses a rapid evaporative ionisation mass spectrometric (REIMS) technique to report tissue histology in real time by analysing aerosolised tissue during electrosurgical dissection.

Artificially intelligent systems also hold potential to dramatically improve the fidelity of simulation training in minimal access surgery, through the creation of a 'real-world' training environment based on the vast data accrued in their development. Such data may be used to create a dynamic simulation environment for any procedure, much more akin to that of 'real-life' surgery. This holds potential for a stepwise tutorial system similar to that of bedside teaching, with objective feedback provided against standardised proficiency benchmarks that can be easily integrated into national training programmes.

One major obstacle for minimally invasive technology remains the cost efficiency and device financing in an increasingly rationed global healthcare environment; this is an issue that will require surgical liaison with hospital management and national policy providers. Surgeons need to continue to have a dialogue, discussing their experiences and ideas in order to effectively progress minimal access surgery and continue to adopt novel technology. As technological advancements are adopted, carefully designed outcomes research is required to provide a clear evidence base to support changes to clinical practice. In this way the comparative effectiveness of novel minimal access technologies will be better understood in terms of both clinical outcomes and cost-effectiveness, allowing selection of those with the greatest potential to provide lasting improvements in patient care.

> The cleaner and gentler the act of operation, the less the patient suffers, the smoother and quicker his convalescence, the more exquisite his healed wound.
>
> Berkeley George Andrew Moynihan (1920)

Berkeley George Andrew Moynihan (Lord Moynihan), 1865–1936, Professor of Clinical Surgery, Leeds, UK. Moynihan felt that English surgeons knew little about the work of their colleagues both at home and abroad. Therefore, in 1909, he established a small travelling club which in 1929 became the Moynihan Chirurgical Club. It still exists today. He took a leading part in founding the *British Journal of Surgery* in 1913 and became the first chairman of the editorial committee until his death.

FURTHER READING

Athanasiou T, Ashrafian H, Rao C *et al.* The tipping point of robotic surgery in healthcare: from master–slave to flexible access bio-inspired platforms. *Surg Technol Int* 2011; **21**: 28–34.

Bhandari M, Zeffiro T, Reddiboina M. Artificial intelligence and robotic surgery: current perspective and future directions. *Curr Opin Urol* 2020; **30**(1): 48–54.

Bodenstedt S, Wagner M, Müller-Stich BP *et al.* Artificial intelligence-assisted surgery: potential and challenges. *Visc Med* 2020; **36**(6): 450–5.

Brodie A, Vasdev N. The future of robotic surgery. *Ann R Coll Surg Engl* 2018; **100**(Suppl 7): 4–13.

Hussain I, Cosar M, Kirnaz S *et al.* Evolving navigation, robotics, and augmented reality in minimally invasive spine surgery. *Global Spine J* 2020; **10**(2 Suppl): 22S–33S.

St John ER, Balog J, McKenzie JS *et al.* Rapid evaporative ionization mass spectrometry of electrosurgical vapours for the identification of breast pathology: towards an intelligent knife for breast cancer surgery. *Breast Cancer Res* 2017; **19**(1): 59.

Tan A, Ashrafian H, Scott AJ *et al.* Robotic surgery: disruptive innovation or unfulfilled promise? A systematic review and meta-analysis of the first 30 years. *Surg Endosc* 2016; **30**(10): 4330–52.

CHAPTER

11 Tissue and molecular diagnosis

Learning objectives

To understand:

- The value and limitations of tissue diagnosis
- Approaches to tissue processing

To be aware of:

- The principles of microscopic diagnosis
- The features of neoplasia
- The importance of clinicopathological correlation
- The role of additional techniques, including special stains, immunohistochemistry and molecular pathology

INTRODUCTION

Pre-nineteenth century tissue diagnosis depended on naked eye examination of autopsy material and of a small selection of surgical specimens. The development of the light microscope allowed closer examination of tissue from autopsies and surgical procedures, with visualisation of cells, nuclei and tissue structure. Microscopic diagnosis was initially controversial, partly as a result of the 'Kaiser's cancer' (a histological diagnosis by Virchow of a non-malignant laryngeal lesion, after which Kaiser Friedrich III died of laryngeal malignancy), but the medical and surgical community eventually accepted its value.

Tissue analysis is now an integral and routine element of clinical practice. It is heavily dependent on microscopic assessment, although newer methods of tissue analysis will increasingly provide additional information. Assessment of tissue is usually the responsibility of a histopathologist/cellular pathologist (a medically qualified practitioner), who depends on support from technical staff. In the UK, the staff responsible for tissue processing and the production of sections on glass slides are known as biomedical scientists (BMSs). The specialty variably known as Histopathology, Anatomic Pathology or Cellular Pathology encompasses histopathology, cytopathology, autopsy work and molecular tissue diagnosis.

Developments and changes in cellular pathology are continuous. The volume of biopsies continues to increase as a result of increasing clinical demands, expectations of greater diagnostic precision, widespread flexible endoscopy and an ageing population with a higher prevalence of cancer and other illnesses. Cancer screening programmes also have an impact as they often depend heavily on cellular pathology. New techniques to refine histological assessment require additional resources. There is an increasing obligation to comply with national or international standards of reporting, e.g. for cancer, and participation by pathologists in multidisciplinary team meetings is now routine rather than occasional. Other developments may reduce activity. Newer, less invasive methods may replace tissue analysis, e.g. human papilloma virus (HPV) testing for cervical pre-neoplastic lesions is replacing cytological assessment. New methods in imaging may reduce the need for tissue analysis.

The location of a modern cellular pathology department is usually within or near a medium-sized or large hospital or in a purpose-built off-site centre. Typically, more than 80% of specimens are from the gastrointestinal tract, gynaecological tract, skin or urological system. In line with clinical services, highly specialised work such as neuropathology takes place in major regional centres. Consolidation of clinical services may result in reconfiguration of relevant pathology services and molecular testing facilities.

REASONS FOR ASSESSMENT OF TISSUE

The contributions that tissue analysis makes to clinical management include diagnosis, staging, prediction of outcome and assistance with selection of therapy. These are often interrelated. The process of tissue assessment may make a new diagnosis or may confirm or refute a suspected or existing clinical diagnosis. There may be pointers towards a cause. Analysis may also reveal additional diagnoses that may be unsuspected.

As an example, pathological assessment of an appendicectomy specimen most often confirms a suspected clinical diagnosis of acute appendicitis. However, the appendix sometimes contains an incidental neuroendocrine neoplasm, mucinous

Rudolf Ludwig Carl Virchow, 1821–1902, pathologist, Charité Hospital, Berlin, Germany, known as the 'father of modern pathology'.

neoplasm or carcinoma. Sometimes, an inflamed appendix contains granulomas, raising the possibility of Crohn's disease or infection. Also, a specific cause of abdominal pain other than appendicitis, e.g. endometriosis, may be apparent in the appendiceal tissue. Absence of any histological abnormality raises the possibility of an extra-appendiceal cause. Similarly, biopsies from a patient with inflammatory bowel disease may confirm the diagnosis but may sometimes reveal or suggest an alternative cause of intestinal inflammation such as tuberculosis, amoebiasis, ischaemia or mucosal prolapse.

Summary box 11.1

Reasons for analysis of tissue

- Diagnosis
  - Confirmation/rejection of a clinical diagnosis
  - Additional diagnoses
  - Classification of neoplasia
  - Classification of non-neoplastic disease
- Staging of malignancy
- Prognosis
- Management
  - Selection of therapy
  - Assessment of response to treatment
- Cancer screening programmes and related programmes
  - Cervical, bowel, breast, inflammatory bowel disease, Barrett's oesophagus
- Clinical trial support
- Audit

Tissue analysis also helps, increasingly, to determine or refine treatment and prognosis. For example, the assessment of a breast, lung, colorectal or other major cancer resection specimen helps to confirms the diagnosis but, more importantly, provides crucial information about features such as tumour stage, vascular invasion, perineural invasion and resection margin involvement, which in turn help to predict clinical outcome and determine postoperative treatment. The degree of tumour regression in a resection after neoadjuvant therapy may also have prognostic value. Additionally, pathological assessment of resections helps surgeons and radiologists to audit their accuracy and performance.

Molecular pathological analysis of cancer tissue (see ***Diagnostic molecular pathology***) increasingly contributes to management, including diagnostic categorisation, prognostic predictions and selection of drug therapy. The molecular test or group of tests that an oncologist chooses depends on patient status, tumour location, tumour morphology and stage, among other factors. The identification of a particular biomarker may provide an indication for targeted therapy. For example, detection of high microsatellite instability (MSI) in metastatic colorectal carcinoma (CRC) may predict responsiveness to immune checkpoint inhibition.

Of course, a tissue sample does not represent the entire patient. Correlation with the clinical picture and the macroscopic findings enhances the interpretation of pathological changes considerably. Therefore, absence of relevant details may cause unnecessary delays and even errors. For example, radiation therapy can have profound effects on tissue morphology, including mimicry of other inflammatory conditions or neoplasia. Accordingly, a request form with adequate information should accompany all specimens. Examples of important details include site of biopsy/resection, clinical setting, reasons for the procedure, patient details, medications, relevant risk factors and past medical and surgical history, including previous chemotherapy and radiotherapy. A request form stating 'cancer' or 'Crohn's' is better than a form with no details but is clearly not sufficient.

For small and large resection specimens, good quality macroscopic assessment and sampling is an important precursor to microscopic assessment (see ***Specimen processing***).

TISSUE SPECIMENS

Routine tissue specimens received by a histopathology department include those intended for histopathological analysis and those for cytopathological assessment. These may overlap, and 'cytology' preparations sometimes undergo reprocessing to become histological specimens.

Histology

Specimens for histology are classified as biopsies and resections, although strictly speaking all samples are biopsies. The reasons for taking small biopsies include diagnosis, further assessment and prognostic prediction. Types of small biopsy include punch biopsy, needle core biopsy and mucosal biopsy (***Summary box 11.2***).

The purpose of a resection is usually treatment of a lesion (e.g. a tumour) by removing it. Other reasons for a resection exist, e.g. sleeve gastrectomy for obesity or creation of an ileostomy or colostomy. The pathologist's approach depends on the reason for surgery. For example, assessment of a cancer resection has multiple purposes, including confirmation of the diagnosis, classification, grading, staging, determination of further management and prediction of outcome.

An excision biopsy is larger than the common types of small biopsy and serves as both a diagnostic biopsy and as a resection. For example, excision of a small skin lesion achieves its removal and also allows histological diagnosis and classification.

Ultrasound-guided and computed tomography (CT)-guided biopsies of focal and less accessible lesions have become more common and may pose challenges to the pathologist because of limited sample size.

Material from biopsies or resections is usually suitable for molecular analysis. Increasingly, the role of pathologists includes the identification of appropriate material for various

Burrill Bernard Crohn, 1884–1983, gastroenterologist, Mount Sinai Hospital, New York, NY, USA.
Norman Rupert Barrett, 1903–1979, surgeon, St Thomas's Hospital, London, UK.

Summary box 11.2

Common types of tissue sample

Histology

- Formalin-fixed tissue
  - Biopsy
    - Mucosal, e.g. gastrointestinal, bronchial, oral
    - Punch, e.g. skin
    - Needle (core), e.g. liver
    - Curettings, e.g. endometrium, prostate
    - Excision biopsy
  - Resection
- Fresh tissue
  - Frozen section diagnosis
  - Research
  - Tissue banking
  - Occasional special stains that require fresh tissue

Cytology

- Cervical
- Washings, brushings, scrapes
- Fine-needle aspirate
- Fluids, e.g. ascites, pleural fluid
- Sputum

molecular tests and assessment of tissue suitability for molecular testing. For example, some tumour biopsies may contain insufficient tumour for molecular testing. Of course, correct diagnosis and grading are essential before molecular testing occurs, and attempts to bypass this step and take tissue for molecular testing without including the step of histological assessment run many unnecessary risks such as absence of tumour in the sample or the presence of a tumour that is different from that expected clinically.

All samples for routine histology are immediately placed in a fixative, usually formalin (10% formaldehyde), by the surgical team or by other clinical staff to preserve morphology. This usually happens before delivery to the pathology laboratory.

Cytology

There are various approaches to the procurement of a cytology sample. Some samples are easy to obtain, e.g. urine and sputum, whereas others require more intervention. A conventional cervical smear is obtained by sampling the cervical transformation zone with a brush/broom. Bronchial aspirates and washings and bronchial, gastrointestinal and biliary brushings sample a relatively wide area and may therefore be useful for the diagnosis of malignancy.

Fine-needle aspiration (FNA) cytology may sample accessible sites such as the breast, thyroid and superficial lymph nodes, while ultrasound or CT guidance assists FNA from deeper and less accessible structures, e.g. liver, pancreas, kidney and lung. Ultrasound-guided transbronchial FNA may allow sampling of mediastinal masses and transmucosal FNA may be appropriate for submucosal gastrointestinal lesions or perivisceral lesions. A biopsy taken at the same procedure may accompany FNA cytology samples. Fluids may be submitted directly to the laboratory for cytological assessment.

Fresh tissue

The most common indication for submission of a fresh tissue sample (i.e. without the usual formalin or any other fixative) is rapid frozen section diagnosis, usually done intraoperatively. Other indications are microbiological assessment, electron microscopy, chemical analyses (e.g. quantification of iron in the tissue), research work, tissue banking and some types of molecular pathological analysis.

RISK MANAGEMENT

Safety and risk management are priorities in the laboratory. The use of warning labels helps to reduce the risk of contamination by transmissible infection, e.g. hepatitis B virus or human immunodeficiency virus (HIV). This is especially important when submitting and handling fresh (unfixed) tissue. Formalin kills many microorganisms, but a risk of transmissible infection still requires notification. Also, formalin itself is toxic to the eyes and skin. Accordingly, laboratory staff and indeed any staff should discard leaking or faulty specimen containers and deal immediately with formalin spillages. Patient details should be present on all specimen containers so as to avoid errors of identity (***Figure 11.1***). Rigorous systems are in place to avoid interchange of specimens or confusion between different patients' samples.

Figure 11.1 Sections on glass slides stained with haematoxylin and eosin. Each slide has a unique specimen identifying number (06S022081), a letter corresponding to the biopsy site (A–F) and a site label (e.g. DUOBX for duodenal biopsy).

SPECIMEN PROCESSING

Histology specimen

On arrival in the pathology laboratory, specimens receive a unique identification number, usually with a barcode. They proceed to macroscopic assessment and sampling (colloquially known as 'cut up'). The largest specimens require initial opening (e.g. gastrointestinal tract) or slicing (e.g. uterus, pancreas, breast) to allow further and adequate fixation in formalin, usually over 24–48 hours (***Figure 11.2***). When fixation is complete and the specimen is in a suitable condition for cutting and sampling, a pathologist or BMS describes the appearances and lists the method of sampling. Specimens a few millimetres

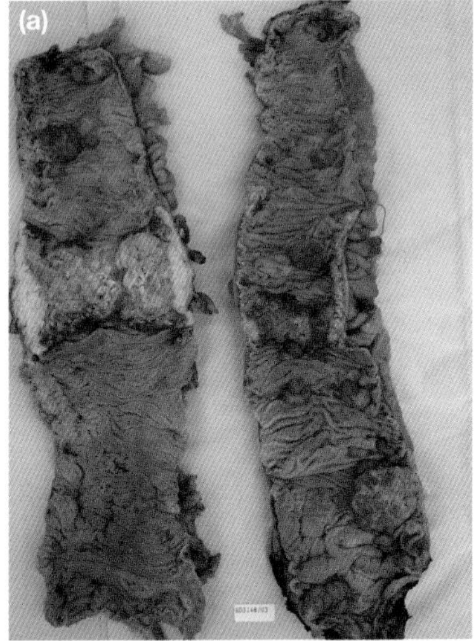

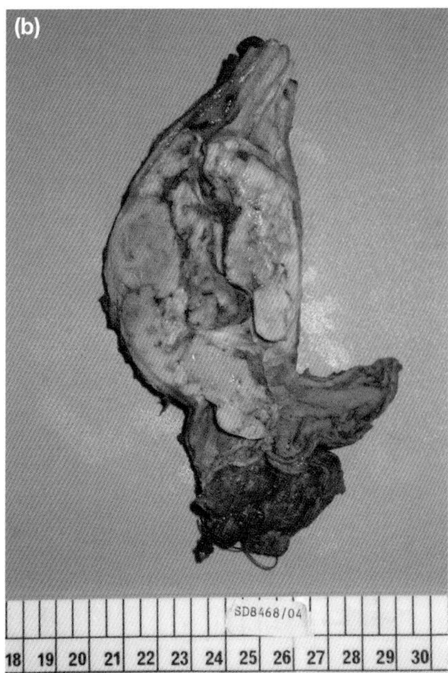

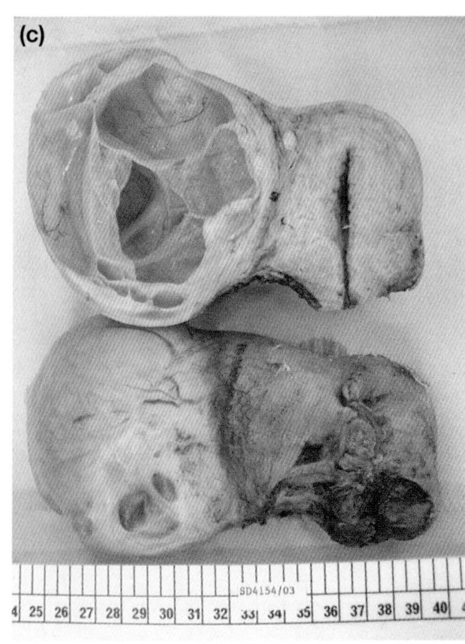

Figure 11.2 (a) A colon from a patient with familial adenomatous polyposis has been opened longitudinally, and the brown appearance reflects adequate fixation. Numerous polyps and a carcinoma are apparent. (b) An oesophagogastrectomy containing a distal oesophageal tumour after opening. In this example, there is less fixation, as a result of which the mucosa in the lower part of the picture remains red rather than brown. (c) A uterus and an adjacent cystic lesion after slicing to allow fixation (all figures courtesy of Dr J Chin Aleong, Barts Health NHS Trust, London, UK).

in size such as endoscopic biopsies are suitable for submission in their entirety. Small resections, e.g. skin excision biopsies, may be suitable for slicing into two or more pieces and, again, submission in their entirety. For any specimen that is too large for these approaches, the prosector takes representative samples of areas of interest or relevance (*Figure 11.3*). This is traditionally the remit of the histopathologist, but BMSs or other non-medical staff with specific training increasingly contribute.

In the UK and many other countries, there is often adherence to a regional, national or international guideline that includes a protocol for sampling. For example, samples from most types of cancer should include tumour, resection margins, lymph nodes, non-neoplastic tissue and any other abnormal areas. Inks of various colours help to identify resection margins and surfaces during microscope assessment as they remain in place after processing (*Figure 11.4*).

The prosector places specimens, or samples from specimens, in plastic cassettes (*Figure 11.5*). BMSs/technical staff then embed the tissue in paraffin wax while in the cassette to produce a tissue block (*Figure 11.6*). BMSs then cut sections with a thickness of approximately 5 μm from the block using a microtome (*Figure 11.7*), place the sections on a glass slide and stain them with haematoxylin and eosin (H&E) (*Figure 11.1*). These steps require training and skill. A poor quality section may have various artefacts, such as lines, folds and shatter effect, which impede accurate assessment.

H&E remains by far the most common initial stain for histopathology assessment, probably because it is inexpensive, safe, fast, reliable, familiar and informative. There is a wider variety of stains for cytology preparations including H&E and Giemsa.

Traditionally, a pathologist examines stained sections with a microscope (*Figure 11.8*) and correlates the appearances with the clinical details and the macroscopic description. After completion of any additional studies such as special stains, immunohistochemistry and molecular analysis, the pathologist enters a report onto a computer system and allocates specific topography and morphology codes that will facilitate future searches. Recent improvements in technology and information technology (IT) mean that some laboratories use scanning machines to create digital images of the glass slides that pathologists and others can then access locally or remotely at any time (see ***Digital pathology and artificial intelligence***).

Summary box 11.3

Histological processing: sequence of events

- Receipt of specimen
- Macroscopic (gross) description
- Sampling of specimen (unless small enough to submit in its entirety)
- Specimen or samples placed in cassette(s)
- Production of paraffin wax block(s)
- Cutting of 5-μm sections with microtome
- Sections placed on glass slides
- Sections stained with H&E
- Histopathologist examines slides, taking clinical and macroscopic findings into account
- Further studies on tissue, if necessary
- Entry of report onto computer system
- Authorisation of report by pathologist

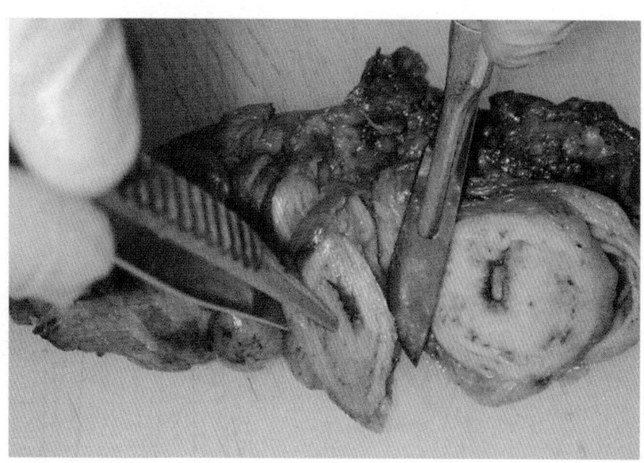

Figure 11.3 A pathologist takes a sample from a resection specimen with a scalpel and forceps.

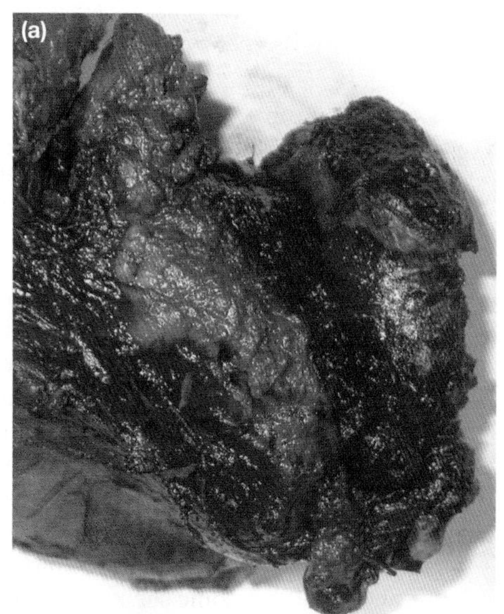

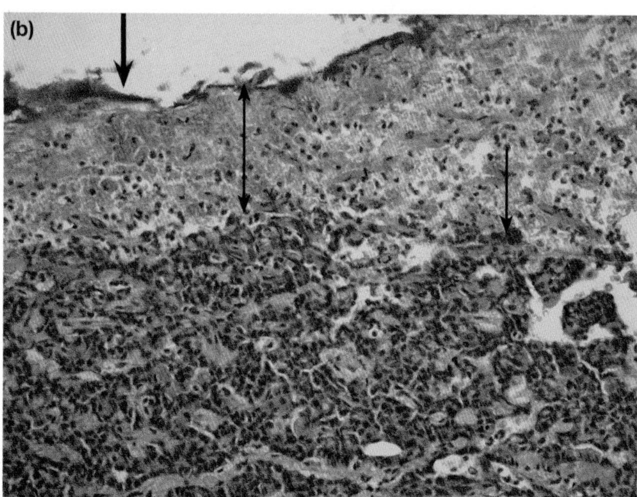

Figure 11.4 (a) An unopened pancreatoduodenectomy specimen (posterior view). Four inks of different colours have been painted onto separate margins and surfaces. (b) Yellow ink on the edge of a histology section (thick arrow). Tumour (thin arrow) lies close to the surface. The pathologist can measure the distance between the tumour and a surface or a resection margin (double-headed arrow).

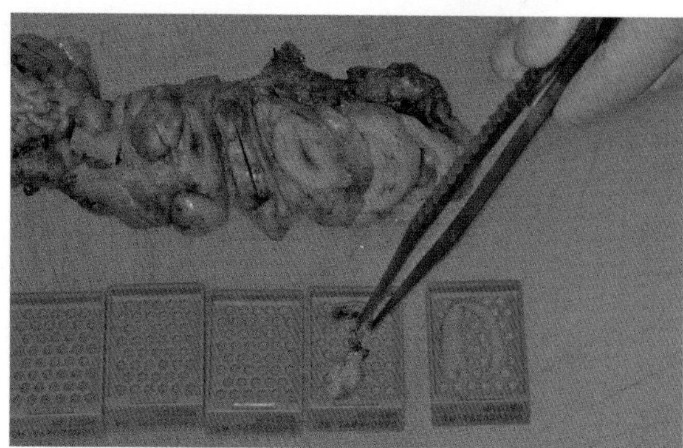

Figure 11.5 A pathologist places a tissue sample from a resection specimen in a cassette.

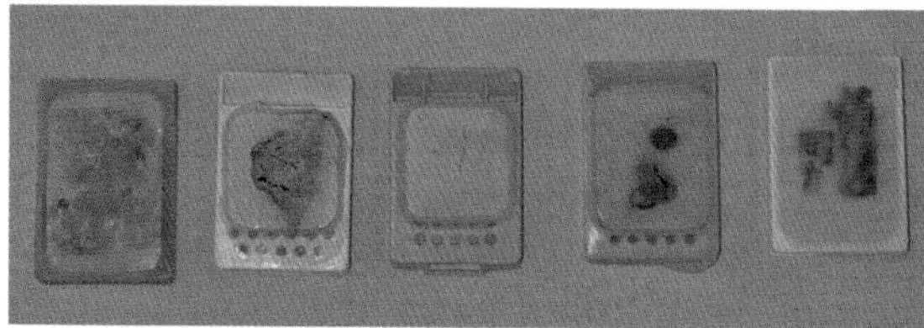

Figure 11.6 Paraffin wax blocks. Cassettes of different colours allow the organisation of samples and specimens into groups, e.g. according to specialty or degree of urgency.

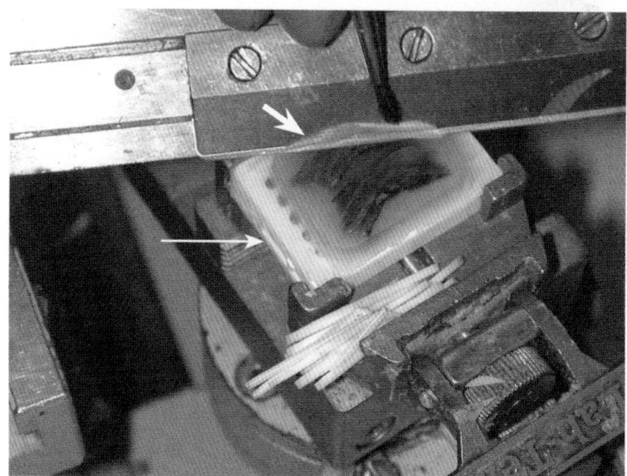

Figure 11.7 A section (thick arrow) being cut from a paraffin wax block (thin arrow) with a microtome.

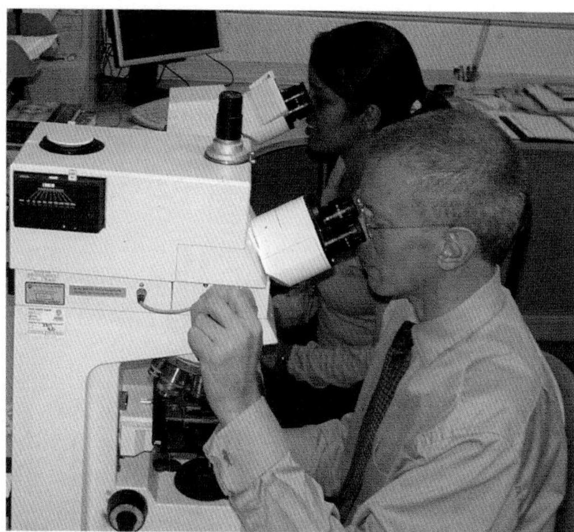

Figure 11.8 A double-headed microscope allows a consultant histopathologist and a trainee to view a slide simultaneously.

Frozen section specimen

Frozen section diagnosis is useful when a very rapid answer is necessary. Surgeons are the main users. The surgeon supplies a small representative fresh tissue sample of the area of interest. A BMS freezes the tissue quickly in the pathology laboratory and can produce sections for microscopic examination within several minutes. There are a few disadvantages in comparison with routine processing: fresh tissue carries a higher risk of infection; the quality is inferior to that of routine material, resulting in a potential reduction in diagnostic accuracy and precision; small but representative samples are necessary; certain types of tissue (e.g. fat) are difficult to process; and the process is time-consuming and disruptive (*Summary box 11.4*).

Summary box 11.4

Frozen section: advantages and disadvantages

Advantages
- Quick diagnosis

Disadvantages
- Poorer quality sections
- Potential reduction in accuracy and precision of histological diagnosis
- Labour intensive
- Disruptive
- Risk of infection
- Small sample required
- Some tissue types difficult to process

Cytology specimen

Samples for cytology can be smeared immediately onto glass slides, fixed (usually in alcohol) or air dried and stained immediately or later. The process usually produces several slides, some of which are stained with a Papanicolaou (Pap) stain and some with another method such as May–Grünwald–Giemsa (MGG), H&E or Romanowsky (*Figure 11.9*). Liquid-based thin-layer technology is now replacing older methods. For liquid-based cytology, the sampling device is usually washed in a liquid medium and the material obtained is then processed in the laboratory using purpose-built equipment.

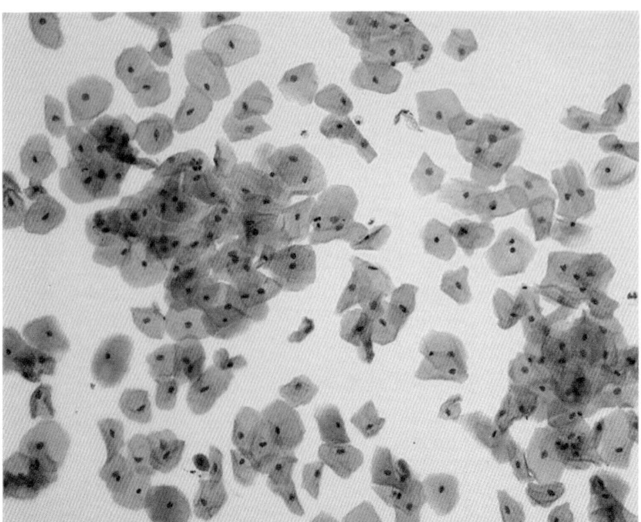

Figure 11.9 A cervical smear stained with a Papanicolaou stain. Numerous cells are present (courtesy of Professor MT Sheaff, Barts Health NHS Trust).

Storage

Resection specimens are generally stored for about 4–6 weeks. Tissue blocks and slides are retained for as long as space permits. Fresh tissue can be frozen for future clinical review, teaching, audit or research. Many countries now have formal tissue-banking processes that allow construction of an archive of cases. In many countries, the storage, transport and subsequent use of tissue is subject to many legal constraints.

PRINCIPLES OF MICROSCOPIC DIAGNOSIS

Diagnosis of malignancy

Neoplasia is a broad term that includes benign and malignant tumours and precursors of malignancy. The word 'cancer' is not precise, derives from observations of the similarities between crabs and tumours by ancient Greek physicians such as Hippocrates and usually refers to all malignancies (rather than carcinoma alone). Classification of a tumour as malignant implies that it can behave aggressively. The main features of malignancy are metastasis and invasion and there are characteristic architectural and cytological abnormalities. However, the criteria for a diagnosis of malignancy differ between anatomical sites and between tumour types. Sometimes, the traditional concept of benign and malignant is not applicable and instead there is a classification that identifies a spectrum of tumours from well differentiated to poorly differentiated or from low grade to high grade depending on known clinical behaviour.

George Nicholas Papanicolaou, 1883–1962, Professor of Anatomy, Cornell University, New York, NY, USA.
Richard May, 1863–1936, Professor of Medicine, Munich, Germany.
Ludwig Grünwald, 1863–1927, otolaryngologist, Munich, Germany.
Gustav Giemsa, 1867–1948, chemist and bacteriologist, Hamburg, Germany.
Dmitri Leonidovich Romanowsky, 1861–1921, Professor of Medicine, St Petersburg, Russia.
Hippocrates of Kos, Greek physician and surgeon, and by common consent 'the father of medicine', was born on the island of Kos, off Turkey, about 460 BCE and probably died in 375 BCE.

Summary box 11.5

Microscopic features of malignancy

- Metastasis
- Invasion
  - Of surrounding tissue
  - Vascular (intraluminal tumour and/or tumour in blood vessel wall)
  - Perineural
- Architectural abnormalities
- Necrosis
- Numerous mitotic figures
- Atypical mitotic figures
- Nuclear abnormalities
  - Pleomorphism
  - Enlargement
  - Hyperchromaticity
  - Chromatin clumping
- Nucleolar enlargement and multiplicity

Microscopic evidence of aggressive behaviour by the tumour is usually sufficient for a malignant label. For example, metastasis to another organ such as lymph nodes or liver is diagnostic of malignancy. Invasion of surrounding structures, perineural invasion (***Figure 11.10***) and vascular spread or invasion (***Figure 11.11***) strongly suggest malignancy.

Other microscopic features that are typical of malignancy include derangement of the usual tissue architecture, an increase in the number of mitotic figures, atypical mitotic figures and necrosis (tissue death) (***Figure 11.12***). Changes in the appearances of individual cells, i.e. cytological changes, include nuclear enlargement, an increase in the nuclear: cytoplasmic ratio, nuclear pleomorphism (variation in nuclear appearance) and nuclear hyperchromasia (dark colour) (***Figure 11.13a***). Multiplicity, irregularity and enlargement of nucleoli may also be apparent (***Figure 11.13b***). However, none of these features is diagnostic of malignancy in isolation.

The criteria for a histological diagnosis of malignancy vary according to the site and type of tissue. Carcinoma is by far the most common type of malignancy, and in many settings is diagnosable when epithelial cells invade beyond their normal boundaries. However, the categorisation of some types of non-epithelial proliferations (e.g. lymphoid or mesenchymal) as malignant may rely on cytological and/or architectural features rather than on invasiveness. In some cases, e.g. phaeochromocytoma, reliable histological distinction between benign and malignant is not possible. In other cases, e.g. gastrointestinal stromal tumours (GISTs), there are risk categories based on combinations of histological features that help to predict the likelihood of aggressive behaviour rather than benign or malignant designations. Additional techniques such as immunohistochemistry and clonality studies occasionally help to confirm or support a diagnosis of neoplasia or malignancy (see ***Immunohistochemistry: tumour pathology*** and ***Diagnostic molecular pathology***).

The term 'dysplasia' usually indicates that microscopic features similar to those of carcinoma are present but that there is no invasion. The term 'intraepithelial neoplasia' is analogous to dysplasia. Examples include cervical intraepithelial neoplasia (CIN) and gastrointestinal dysplasia (***Figure 11.14***). Grading of dysplasia may be as low grade/high grade or as mild/moderate/severe while grading of intraepithelial neoplasia may be numerical (e.g. CIN 1, CIN 2 and CIN 3).

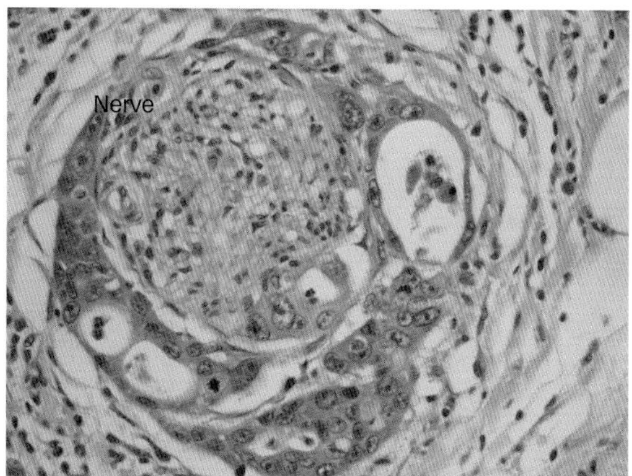

Figure 11.10 Perineural invasion. A nerve is almost surrounded by adenocarcinoma.

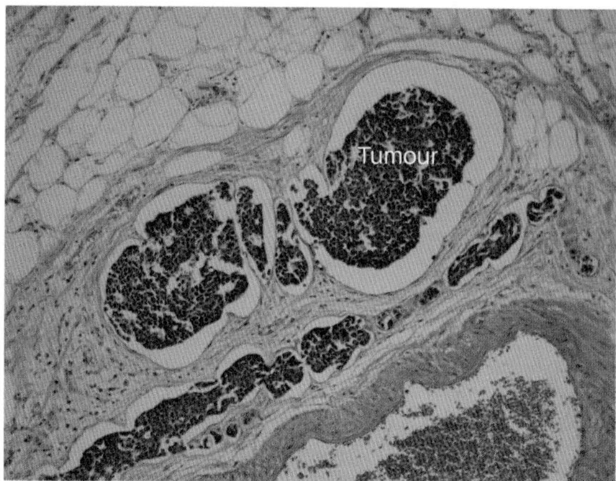

Figure 11.11 Vascular invasion. Aggregates of carcinoma cells are present within blood vessels. The tumour is poorly differentiated.

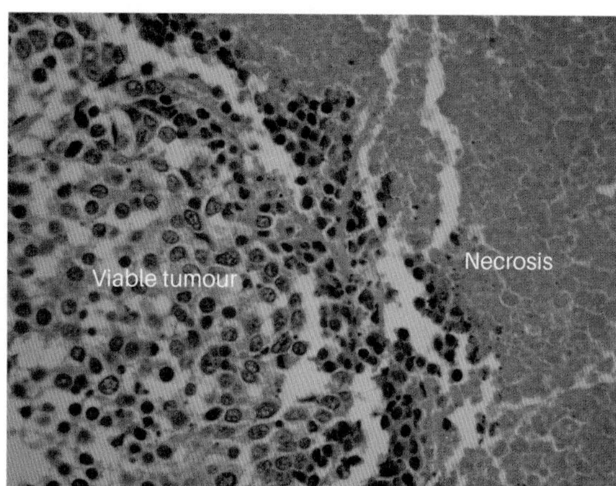

Figure 11.12 An area of necrosis in a poorly differentiated carcinoma.

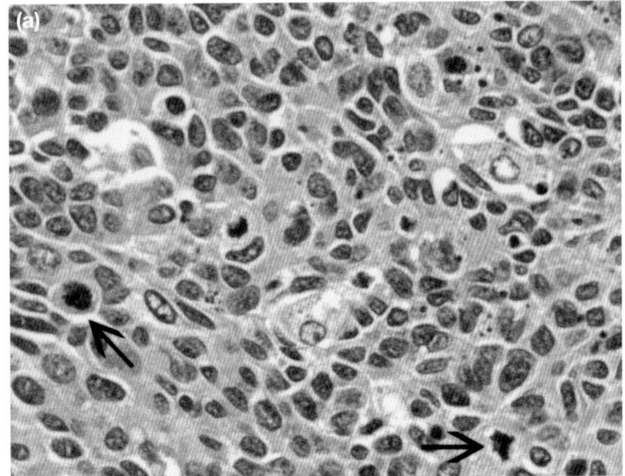

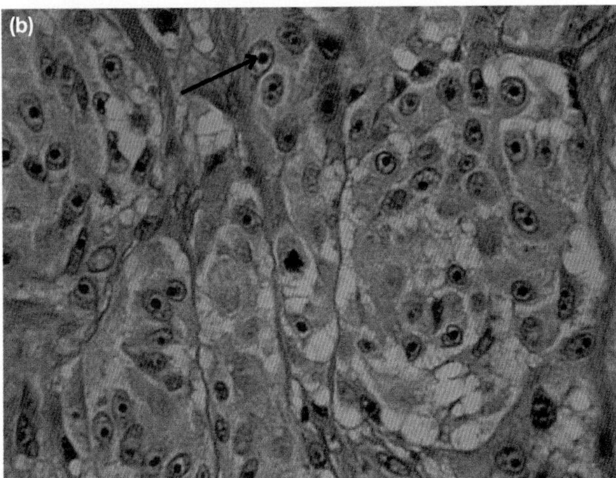

Figure 11.13 Cellular features of malignancy. (a) A neuroendocrine carcinoma showing nuclear pleomorphism (variation in shape) and variation in nuclear size. There are several mitotic figures (arrows). (b) A malignant melanoma showing nuclear pleomorphism and prominent nucleoli (arrow) (courtesy of Dr E Husain, Aberdeen Royal Infirmary, Aberdeen, UK).

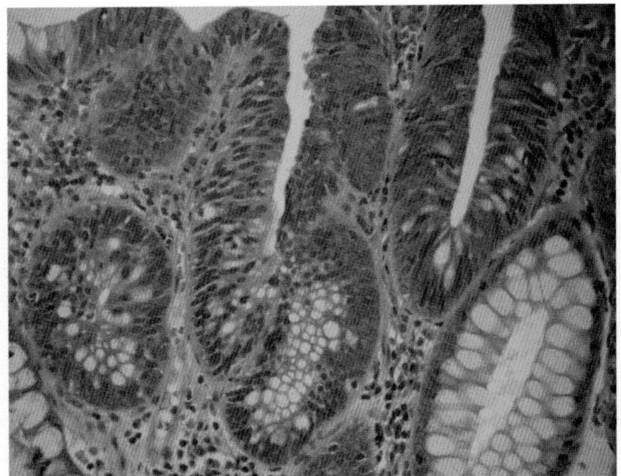

Figure 11.14 A colonic biopsy from a tubular adenoma with low-grade dysplasia. A non-dysplastic crypt is apparent at lower right. The remaining crypts mostly show features of dysplasia, including nuclear stratification (multilayering), nuclear enlargement and nuclear hyperchromaticity (dark colour).

There are various causes of a false-positive diagnosis of malignancy. These include contamination of a specimen with tumour from elsewhere, interchanging of specimens, observer error and histological mimicry. A false-negative diagnosis, i.e. a failure to diagnose malignancy when present, may reflect absence of tumour in the specimen or failure of the pathologist to recognise the changes as neoplastic.

Several conditions can resemble malignancy histologically. For example, radiation effect can produce cytological atypia that mimics malignancy, and the epithelial changes in regenerating tissue adjacent to a mucosal ulcer may show features reminiscent of neoplasia. The risk of interpretative error by the histopathologist is likely to be lower if there is thorough training of pathologists, regular updating of knowledge, discussion of difficult cases with colleagues and avoidance of excessive workloads. The surgeon also helps to minimise errors by supplying good clinical details.

Summary box 11.6

Causes of false-positive diagnoses of malignancy

- Interchanged samples
- Contamination
- Interpretative error
- Treatment-induced change, e.g. radiotherapy
- Ulceration

Histological types of malignancy

A malignant tumour showing features of epithelial differentiation, and typically arising in an epithelial layer, is a carcinoma. Other important types of malignancy include malignant melanoma (melanocytes) (***Figure 11.13b***), lymphoma (lymphoid cells) and sarcoma (mesenchymal cells). Further subclassification is often appropriate and necessary. For example, categories of carcinoma include squamous cell carcinoma (with evidence of keratinisation) (***Figure 11.15***), adenocarcinoma (with evidence of glandular differentiation and/or mucin production) (***Figure 11.16***) or neuroendocrine carcinoma (***Figure 11.13a***) (usually requiring immunohistochemical confirmation of neuroendocrine differentiation). Some carcinomas have a pattern that raises a certain differential diagnosis, e.g. clear cell carcinoma (***Figure 11.17***). There are many other morphological types of carcinoma.

Prognostic factors for malignant tumours

Tissue assessment is important for cancer prognosis. Stage is generally the most important prognostic factor for carcinomas. The internationally accepted Union for International Cancer Control (UICC)/American Joint Committee on Cancer (AJCC) staging schemes depend heavily on the histopathological TNM (Tumour Node Metastasis) category (pTNM), although the overall stage and in particular the M category are also evaluated clinically and on imaging and the final stage is derived from a combination of clinical, imaging, pathological and other assessments. The degree of differentiation may also be prognostic and is usually determined microscopically. As a

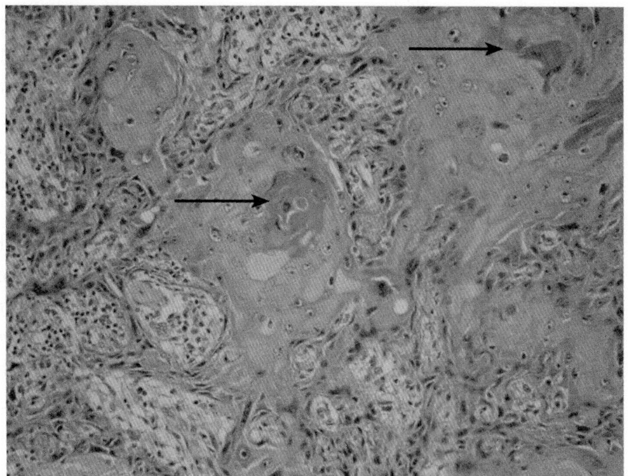

Figure 11.15 A well-differentiated squamous cell carcinoma. Irregular nests of squamous cells are present. They include foci of keratinisation (arrows).

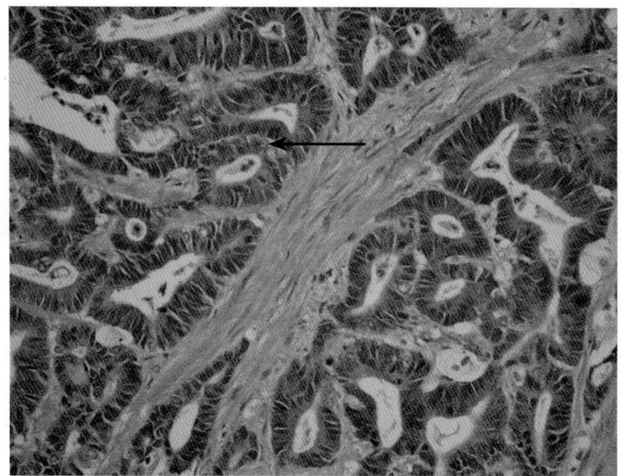

Figure 11.16 A well-differentiated adenocarcinoma. Gland formation (arrow) is obvious.

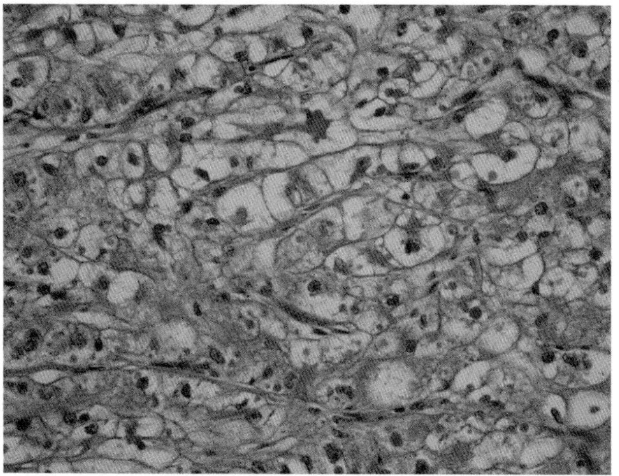

Figure 11.17 A metastatic clear cell carcinoma composed of sheets of cells with clear cytoplasm. A tumour with this appearance is most likely to be of renal origin but could have other sources such as liver, parathyroid gland, gynaecological tract and gastrointestinal tract.

rule, well-differentiated tumours recapitulate the appearances of their non-neoplastic tissue counterparts (***Figures 11.15 and 11.16***), whereas poorly differentiated tumours do not (***Figures 11.11 and 11.12***). Other histological features associated with a worse prognosis include vascular invasion (***Figure 11.11***), perineural invasion (***Figure 11.10***) and positive resection margins. The prognostic value of these factors differs between tumour types and sites.

There is an increasing number of potential prognostic factors for a wide range of malignancies and preneoplastic lesions. These include immunohistochemical tests and molecular tests that may aim to detect underlying genetic changes such as mutations or amplifications or may help to refine grading. For example, immunohistochemistry for the proliferation marker Ki67 is now essential for grading and prediction of behaviour of well-differentiated neuroendocrine neoplasms. Screening for mismatch repair (MMR) gene abnormalities using immunohistochemistry helps to predict response to therapy, outcome and the need for genetic testing for familial disease.

Although controversial, immunohistochemical staining might help to predict the behaviour of preneoplastic lesions such as Barrett's oesophagus (p53 staining) or cervical/anal intraepithelial neoplasia (p16 staining).

Non-neoplastic and inflammatory conditions

The diagnosis, assessment and management of non-neoplastic disease generates numerous pathology specimens. Examples include appendectomy for appendicitis, cholecystectomy for gallstone disease, hysterectomy for fibroids, skin excision for various lesions such as sebaceous cysts and prostatic chippings from glands with hyperplasia. Thorough histological examination helps to confirm or refute the provisional clinical diagnosis and also to exclude other conditions, some of which may be entirely incidental, e.g. neoplasia of the gallbladder, malignant change in uterine fibroids or carcinoma in prostatic chippings. Surgical and medical teams also generate a very large number of biopsies with the purpose of diagnosing and assessing non-neoplastic disease. In this setting, correlation with the clinical picture may be very important. For example, clinical details are essential for meaningful interpretation of inflammatory bowel disease biopsies, inflammatory skin biopsies, renal biopsies and medical liver biopsies.

Microscopic features of inflammation

Acute inflammation is characterised histologically by neutrophils (polymorphonuclear leukocytes), erosion or ulceration (***Figure 11.18***) and chronic inflammation by lymphocytes and plasma cells. Other inflammatory cells include eosinophils (***Figure 11.19***), mast cells and histiocytes. Granulomas (collections of epithelioid histiocytes) (***Figure 11.20a***) raise the possibility of mycobacterial infection (***Figure 11.20b***), fungal infection, parasites, sarcoidosis, Crohn's disease or a reaction to foreign material, among numerous other possible causes. Eosinophils in large numbers may reflect parasitic infection or allergy. Interpretation depends heavily on the site and clinical setting.

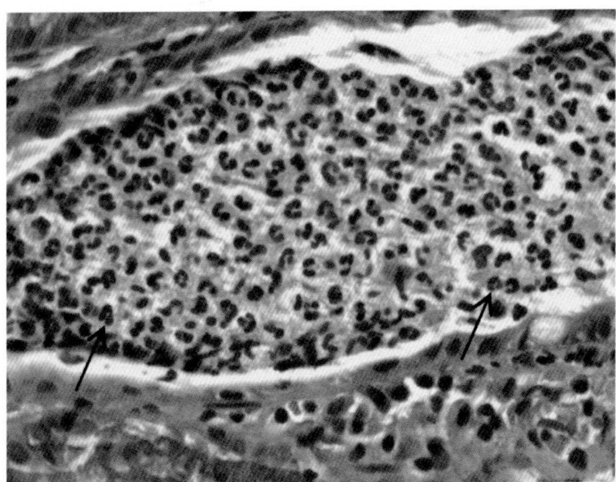

Figure 11.18 An acute inflammatory process characterised by numerous neutrophils. Note the typical multilobated nuclei (arrows).

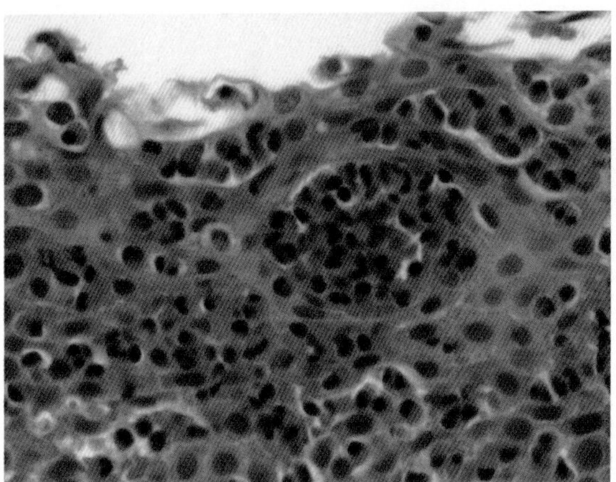

Figure 11.19 Oesophageal mucosa infiltrated by numerous eosinophils with bright red cytoplasm, many of which are forming clusters. Eosinophils may reflect allergy, parasitic infection or a wide variety of other causes. In this example, the clinicopathological diagnosis was eosinophilic oesophagitis.

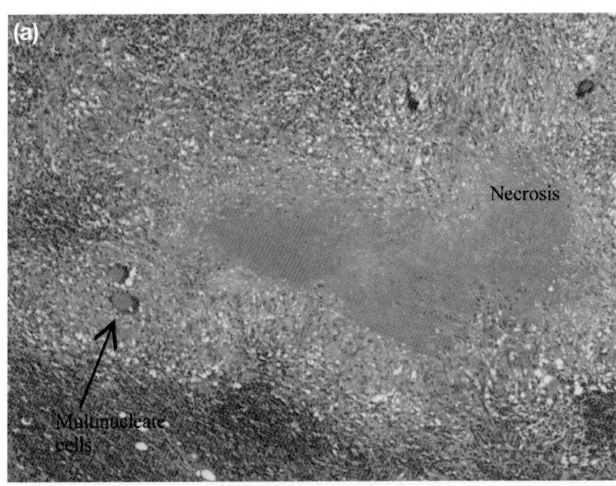

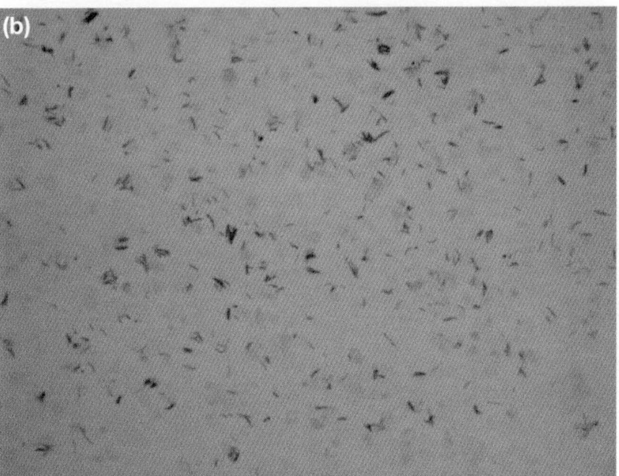

Figure 11.20 (a) A granuloma with necrosis, suggesting tuberculosis. Multinucleate giant cells of Langhans type are also present (arrow). (b) A Ziehl–Neelsen stain (from a different case) shows numerous pink acid-fast rod-shaped bacilli, confirming mycobacterial infection.

Other terms

Other specific tissue abnormalities are also detectable by microscopy. Histopathologists may use specific terms. Some examples are as follows.

- Hyperplasia: an increase in cell number.
- Hypertrophy: an increase in cell size.
- Atrophy: may refer to a reduction in cell number or cell size or a diminution in size of a structure (e.g. a duodenal villus undergoing atrophy in coeliac disease).
- Metaplasia: a change from one mature cell type to another, e.g. columnar metaplasia in the oesophagus (Barrett's oesophagus), whereby metaplastic gastric or intestinal-type epithelium replaces normal squamous epithelium.
- Necrosis: cell or tissue death, typically because of factors external to the cell, and associated with cell swelling, inflammation and eventual disappearance of cells (*Figure 11.20*).
- Apoptosis: a process of programmed cell death that occurs because of internal signals, and on histological examination typically manifests as cell shrinkage and nuclear chromatin condensation.

ASSESSMENT

Light microscopy

Most tissue assessment depends on conventional light microscopy. Microscopes have several lenses with various powers of magnification, typically ranging from ×20 to ×400 or more. A low-power lens allows scanning of a sample and assessment of overall architecture, while a higher power lens allows a

Theodor Langhans, 1839–1915, Professor of Pathological Anatomy, University of Bern, Bern, Switzerland.
Franz Heinrich Paul Ziehl, 1859–1926, neurologist, Lübeck, Germany.
Friedrich Carl Adolf Neelsen, 1854–1894, pathologist, prosector, the Stadt-Krankenhaus, Dresden, Germany.

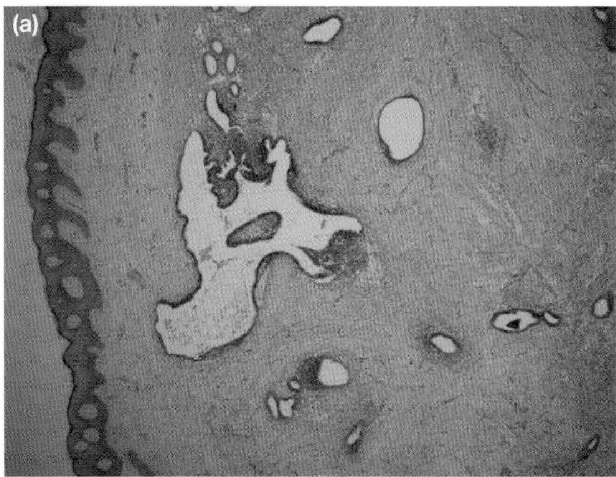

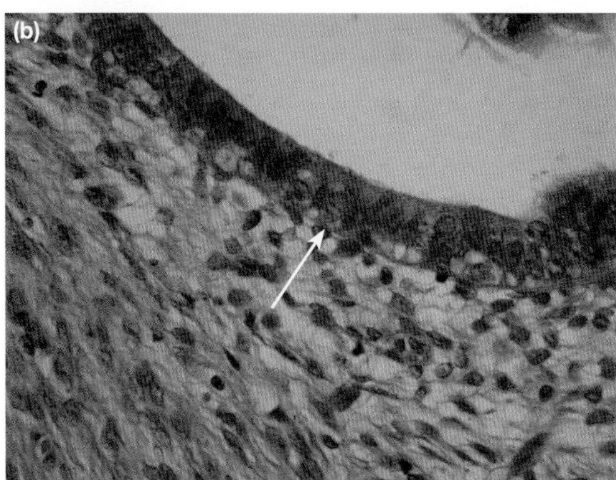

Figure 11.21 (a) Low-power view of an umbilical nodule. Glands are distributed irregularly through the tissue. (b) High-power view shows benign columnar epithelium lining the glands (arrow), indicating endometriosis rather than carcinoma.

closer view with more detail (*Figure 11.21*). Attachment of one or more teaching arms, a camera and other accessories are possible for many microscopes (*Figure 11.8*). Polarisation assists with detection of some types of foreign material (e.g. sutures) or to assess a special stain (e.g. Congo red for amyloid deposition).

Histological assessment

In a histological preparation, the microscopic structure of the tissue remains intact, allowing direct visualisation of tissue architecture. Accordingly, the pathologist can see not only the characteristics of the cells that form the tissue, but also the way in which these cells relate to one another and the structure and arrangement of the various tissue compartments.

Cytological assessment

A cytological preparation consists of a sample of cells only. Assessment of architecture is not usually possible because intact tissue is absent or sparse (*Figures 11.9 and 11.22*). Therefore, assessment relies on the characteristics of the individual cells. Accordingly, diagnosis of malignancy is often difficult because the pathologist cannot assess certain features that support a diagnosis of malignancy such as invasiveness. However, cytology has several potential advantages over a biopsy. Obtaining a specimen may be easier and less traumatic. The area of sampling may be wider. Processing times are usually shorter and costs lower. Also, the ability of non-medical staff to report a proportion of cases reduces costs.

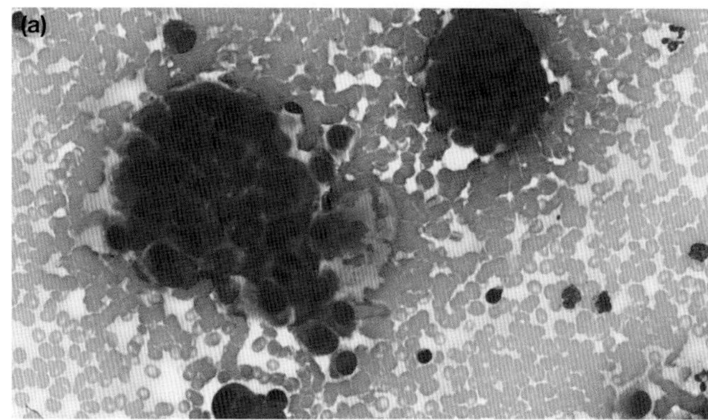

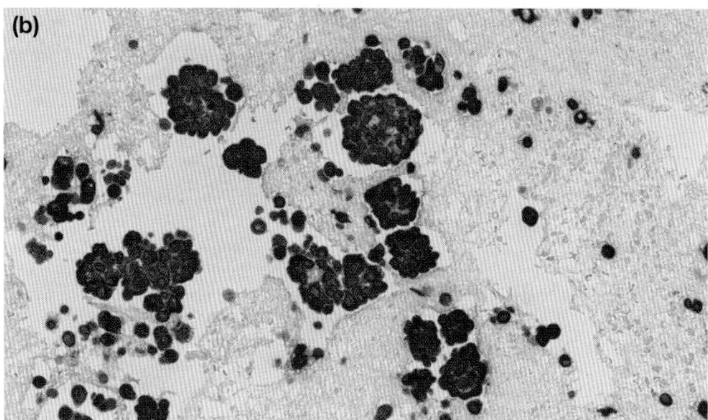

Figure 11.22 (a) A cytology preparation of a pleural effusion. Numerous cells with atypical features are present, forming closely packed groups of overlapping cells. (b) Immunohistochemistry shows positive staining for carcinoembryonic antigen, favouring carcinoma over mesothelioma.

Summary box 11.7

Cytology compared with histology

Advantages

- Wider area of sampling in some cases
- Often less invasive
- Fast
- Cheap

Disadvantages

- Cannot assess tissue architecture
- Less amenable to further tissue studies

Sodium diphenylbisazobisnaphthylamine sulphonate is a red dye marketed in 1884 by the AGFA company of Berlin, Germany, using the name '**Congo red**'. It is no longer used as a cloth dye owing to the carcinogenic risks of the benzidine moiety.

Screening

Screening programmes aim to detect and treat premalignant tissue changes (dysplasia/intraepithelial neoplasia) or early-stage malignancy for which treatment is likely to be curative. The programmes may rely on clinical assessment, imaging and/or pathological assessment. The cervical cancer programme traditionally relied on cytology, with biopsy and histology follow-up if appropriate, but the alternative of HPV testing is increasingly available. The breast cancer screening programme relies on imaging and may use cytology and/or histology to assess possible lesions. The bowel cancer screening programme relies initially on a non-tissue-based test followed, if appropriate, by lower gastrointestinal endoscopy with or without biopsy of abnormal areas. Screening for neoplasia in ulcerative colitis and in Barrett's oesophagus relies on endoscopic assessment and biopsy.

Specimen adequacy

There are many reasons for an inadequate specimen. The operator may fail to sample the target organ or lesion or may take a sample that is too small to include or reveal a heterogeneous abnormality. A sample from the centre of a necrotic or ulcerated lesion might include no viable tissue. Superficial biopsies from a carcinoma may fail to distinguish dysplasia (***Figure 11.14***) from invasive carcinoma. Cautery and crush artefact are sometimes severe enough to impede assessment. Suboptimal laboratory processing can also cause problems with interpretation.

Summary box 11.8

Reasons for an inadequate sample

Histology and cytology

- Failure or inability to sample the intended area
- Sample too small
- Sample unrepresentative
- Non-viable tissue, e.g. ulcer or necrosis

Histology

- Sample too superficial to detect deeper layers
- Cautery artefact
- Crush artefact

Deeper levels and extra blocks

The pathologist may request 'deeper levels', whereby the BMS cuts further into the paraffin block to obtain further sections that may provide more information. For example, deeper levels of an atypical but non-invasive epithelial lesion might show foci of invasion, allowing a definite diagnosis of carcinoma. Further sampling of tissue from a resection specimen (extra blocks) is sometimes necessary, e.g. if the number of lymph nodes in a cancer case is insufficient for accurate staging.

FURTHER WORK

Pathologists request further stains or other tests on a significant minority of histology specimens. This includes special stains, immunohistochemistry, *in situ* hybridisation and various molecular pathology techniques. Electron microscopy may assist with renal biopsy assessment. Some of these additional investigations are also applicable to cytology specimens (***Figure 11.22***). Sufficient tissue is again important for accurate interpretation of some tests, e.g. molecular testing and quantitative immunohistochemical methods.

Special stains

A 'special stain' is a stain that is not routine, i.e. not an H&E stain. Immunohistochemical stains are conventionally separate from this category. Some special stains demonstrate normal substances in increased quantities or in abnormal locations. The periodic acid–Schiff (PAS) stain demonstrates both glycogen and mucin, whereas a diastase PAS (D-PAS) stain demonstrates mucin, e.g. in an adenocarcinoma. Perls Prussian blue stain demonstrates iron accumulation (***Figure 11.23***), e.g. in haemochromatosis. A reticulin stain helps to demonstrate fibrosis (***Figure 11.24***). Elastic stains also show fibrosis and can highlight blood vessels by outlining their elastic laminae. Special stains can also reveal the accumulation of abnormal substances, e.g. a Congo red stain for amyloid.

Summary box 11.9

Additional techniques for assessing tissue

- Special stains
- Immunohistochemistry
- Electron microscopy
- *In situ* hybridisation, including fluorescence *in situ* hybridisation (FISH)
- Molecular pathology techniques (including single biomarker polymerase chain reaction [PCR] and next-generation sequencing [NGS])

Summary box 11.10

Common special stains

- PAS: glycogen, fungi
- D-PAS: mucin
- Perls Prussian blue: iron
- Reticulin: reticulin fibres, fibrosis
- van Gieson: collagen
- Congo red: amyloid
- Ziehl–Neelsen: mycobacteria

Hugo Schiff, 1834–1915, German biochemist who worked in Florence, Italy.
Max Perls, 1843–1881, pathologist, Giessen, Germany.
Ira Thompson van Gieson, 1866–1913, American neuropathologist, described this stain in 1889.

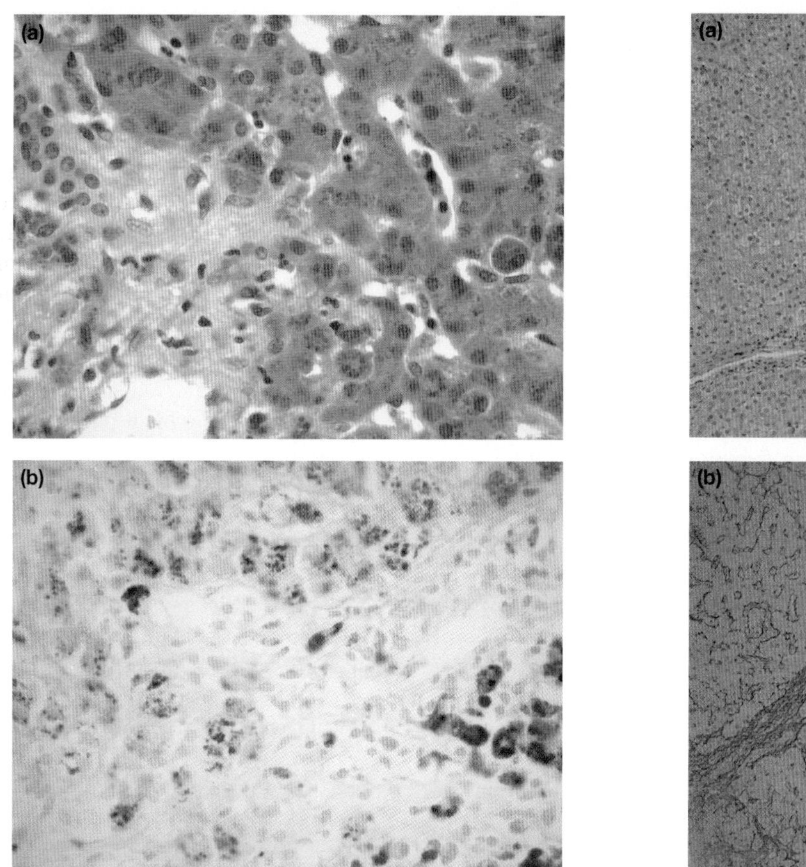

Figure 11.23 (a) Brown pigment in a biopsy. (b) A Perls stain is positive, indicating that the pigment is iron.

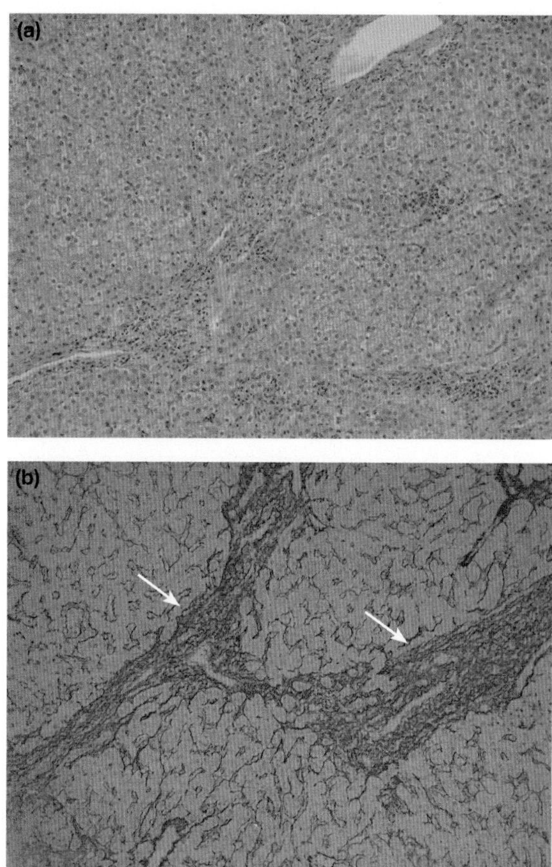

Figure 11.24 (a) A liver biopsy stained with haematoxylin and eosin in which the severity of fibrosis cannot be determined. (b) A reticulin stain demonstrates fibrous bridges (arrows).

Special stains are also useful for the diagnosis of infection. Some microorganisms are not visible on routine H&E slides but are demonstrable with a stain. For example, a Ziehl–Neelsen stain demonstrates acid-fast bacilli, particularly mycobacteria, by staining them bright red on a blue background (***Figure 11.20***). Other microorganisms may be detectable on H&E but are easier to see with a special stain, e.g. fungi (PAS or Grocott stain), protozoa (Giemsa stain) and spirochaetes (Warthin–Starry stain). Immunohistochemistry and *in situ* hybridisation also help to detect some microorganisms (see ***Immunohistochemistry: infections and other applications*** and ***In situ hybridisation***).

Electron microscopy

Electron microscopy allows visualisation of tissue at very high magnification, e.g. ×1000 to ×500 000. It may help to decide the lineage of a non-neoplastic or neoplastic cell and may help to determine the nature of abnormal deposits, e.g. in renal disease. However, it is time-consuming, labour intensive and expensive and consequently has limited applications.

Immunohistochemistry

Immunohistochemistry emerged in the 1970s and has had a major impact on histopathological diagnosis. The technique detects a specific antigen using an antibody. The antibody is labelled with a dye and after binding to its target antigen is visible in the tissue section as a coloured stain, often brown (***Figure 11.25***). This allows the pathologist to confirm or exclude the presence of an antigen as well as determine its tissue distribution and cellular localisation. Quantification may also be possible. For example, Ki67 is a cell cycle marker that allows the pathologist to calculate a proliferative index, which in turn has prognostic value for neuroendocrine neoplasms and other lesions. Immunohistochemistry is applicable to fixed and frozen tissue and to cytological preparations (***Figure 11.22b***). It is safe, quick and relatively inexpensive and is often specific. However, false-positive results can result from non-specific staining or from cross-reaction with similar antigens. Excessive reliance on immunohistochemistry can lead to errors.

Alfred Scott Warthin, 1866–1931, Professor of Pathology, The University of Michigan, Ann Arbor, MI, USA.
Allen Chronister Starry, 1890–1973, American pathologist.

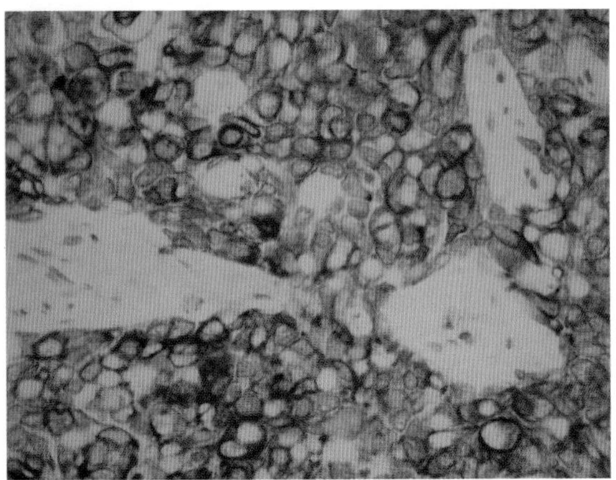

Figure 11.25 Diffuse immunohistochemical staining (brown) for a pancytokeratin marker in a malignancy, favouring carcinoma over other tumours.

Immunohistochemistry: tumour pathology

Immunohistochemistry has multiple applications in tumour pathology, including elucidation of site of origin and determination of cell type/direction of differentiation. Immunohistochemistry may also help to confirm neoplasia, determine the selection of treatment, refine prognostic predictions and screen for known underlying genetic changes.

Numerous immunohistochemical stains help to determine cell type in tumours. Epithelial cells express cytokeratins. Therefore, cytokeratin positivity, though not diagnostic, favours carcinoma (***Figure 11.25***) over other types of malignancy. Lymphoid markers include the panlymphoid marker CD45, the T-lymphocyte marker CD3 and the B-lymphocyte marker CD20. Markers of melanocytic differentiation include S100, MelanA and HMB45. Chromogranin, synaptophysin and CD56 help to confirm neuroendocrine neoplasia. A GIST typically expresses CD117 (***Figure 11.26***) and DOG-1. Endothelial cell markers include CD31, which may confirm a diagnosis of vascular neoplasia or highlight vascular invasion by tumours.

H&E appearances may indicate or suggest the anatomical site of origin of a metastatic tumour. For example, an adenocarcinoma has several possible sources such as gastrointestinal tract, pancreatobiliary system, bronchus, breast and gynaecological tract. A clear cell carcinoma (***Figure 11.17***) is often of renal origin but could be from the liver, pancreas, parathyroid or endometrium, among other sites. Immunohistochemical stains often provide valuable further information about anatomical origin. Some are highly specific for a particular site, e.g. prostate-specific antigen (PSA) and thyroglobulin. Others are somewhat less specific, e.g. thyroid transcription factor-1 (TTF-1), a marker of bronchogenic or thyroid origin; hepatocyte-specific antigen, suggesting hepatocellular origin; and cytokeratin 20, typically expressed by colorectal epithelium. Carcinoembryonic antigen (CEA) is present in several types of carcinoma (***Figure 11.22b***). In practice, pathologists encountering a neoplasm of uncertain origin or uncertain phenotype usually request a panel of markers relevant to the clinical setting and to the H&E appearances. Some malignancies, especially poorly differentiated examples, do not conform to the

Summary box 11.11

Some immunohistochemical stains used for tumours

- Cell type/site of origin
  - Epithelial (carcinoma): cytokeratins
  - Lymphoid (lymphoma): CD45, CD3 (T cells), CD20 (B cells)
  - Melanocytic (melanoma): S100, HMB45, Melan A
  - Neuroendocrine: synaptophysin, chromogranin
  - Vascular: CD31
  - Myoid: desmin, actin
- Site of origin/cell type
  - Prostate: prostate-specific antigen (PSA)
  - Lung: thyroid transcription factor-1 (TTF-1)
  - Thyroid: thyroglobulin
  - Colorectum: cytokeratin 20 (CK20), CDX2
  - Liver: hepatocyte-specific antigen (HSA)
  - Gastrointestinal stromal tumour (GIST): CD117, DOG-1
- Prognosis and treatment
  - Breast carcinoma and gastric carcinoma: HER-2
  - Neuroendocrine tumours: Ki67 proliferation index
- Screening for mutations
  - Colorectal carcinoma: mismatch repair proteins (MLH1, MSH2, MSH6, PMS2)

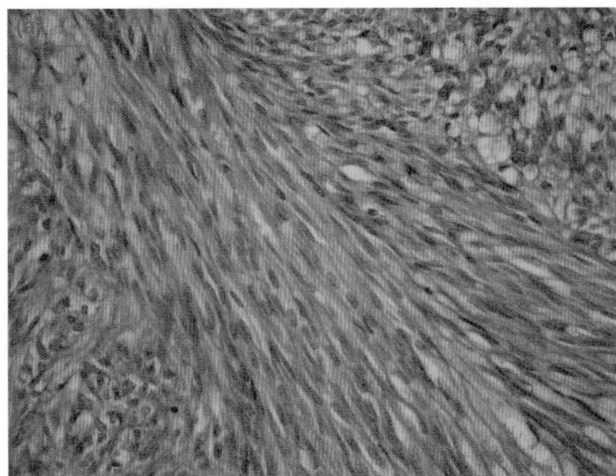

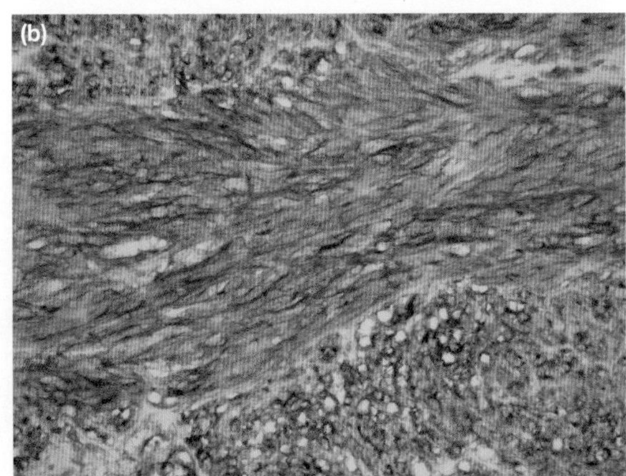

Figure 11.26 (a) A metastatic tumour composed of spindle cells. The clinical team suspected a diagnosis of gastrointestinal stromal tumour (GIST). **(b)** Positive immunohistochemistry for CD117, supporting a diagnosis of GIST.

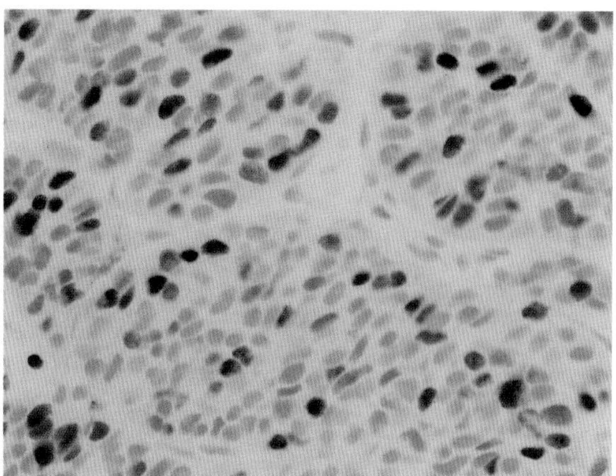

Figure 11.27 Immunohistochemistry for Ki67. The proliferative index is approximately 35% in this field.

typical immunohistochemical profiles. In all circumstances, interpretation takes place in the light of the clinical picture and imaging findings.

Less often, immunohistochemistry helps to confirm malignancy. For example, kappa or lambda light chain restriction (expression of only one immunoglobulin light chain) in lymphoid proliferations suggests clonality and, in turn, neoplasia rather than a reactive process. In general, immunohistochemistry does not distinguish well between benign and malignant.

Immunohistochemistry also plays a role in the selection of treatment and in predicting prognosis. For example, assessment of oestrogen receptor (ER) and human epidermal growth factor receptor-2 (HER2) status is routine for carcinomas of the breast (see ***Immunohistochemistry: tumour pathology***), while lymphomas are typically subjected to a comprehensive panel of markers that help determine treatment and prognosis. Ki67 proliferative index is an important prognostic factor for neuroendocrine neoplasms (***Figure 11.27***).

Immunohistochemistry: infections and other applications

There are antibodies to many infective agents, including cytomegalovirus (CMV), Epstein–Barr virus (EBV), herpes simplex virus, human herpes virus 8 (HHV8), hepatitis B virus and *Helicobacter pylori*. Some of these organisms, e.g. *H. pylori* and CMV, may be obvious or suspected on H&E examination, while others, e.g. EBV and HHV8, always require immunohistochemistry or other techniques for their detection.

Immunohistochemistry can also detect immunoglobulin and complement expression (e.g. in lymphomas or renal biopsies); confirm the abnormal accumulation of various proteins such as alpha-1-antitrypsin (A1AT); and help to characterise amyloid.

Newer immunohistochemical markers that detect specific gene mutations are appearing and may become useful in clinical practice in the future. An important example is screening for MMR gene mutations in most gastrointestinal carcinomas and endometrial carcinomas. Immunohistochemistry for *BRAF* V600E can replace mutational analysis in some settings. The major advantages of immunohistochemistry over other molecular tests for detecting genetic alterations are lower cost and faster turnaround.

Summary box 11.12

Uses of immunohistochemistry

- Cell type
- Neoplasia
  - Direction of differentiation/phenotype
  - Determination of anatomical site of origin
  - Confirmation of neoplasia
  - Grading
  - Selection of treatment
  - Detection of/screening for mutations
  - Prognosis
- Microorganisms – detection
- Other
  - Amyloid
  - Immunoglobulins
  - Complement

DIAGNOSTIC MOLECULAR PATHOLOGY

The broad heading of diagnostic molecular pathology refers to multiple tests that assess molecules (proteins, ribonucleic acid [RNA] and deoxyribonucleic acid [DNA]) in tissue. The information that they provide may be useful for diagnosis, classification of tumours, prognostic predictions, identifying patients with a hereditary cancer risk, determining treatment and identifying residual disease after treatment. Immunohistochemistry is conventionally separate from this category.

Basic methods in diagnostic molecular pathology

In situ hybridisation

In situ hybridisation (ISH) uses a labelled oligonucleotide probe that targets a specific sequence of RNA or DNA. It allows visualisation of the presence or absence and location of a particular RNA or DNA sequence *in situ* in tissue sections. Visualisation may depend on autoradiography, fluorescence microscopy or bright-field microscopy. Chromogenic *in situ* hybridisation (CISH) combines ISH and immunohistochemistry for the detection of specific nucleic acid sequences and is a common alternative to fluorescence *in situ* hybridisation (FISH) for the detection of *HER2* amplification. Viral genomes, e.g. EBV (***Figure 11.28***), CMV and high-risk HPV types are detectable using this approach. ISH plays an important role in tissue diagnostics and the management of tumours.

Sir Michael Anthony Epstein, b.1921, Professor of Pathology, University of Bristol, Bristol, UK.
Yvonne Barr, 1931–2016, Irish born virologist who emigrated to Australia. Epstein and Barr discovered this virus in 1964.

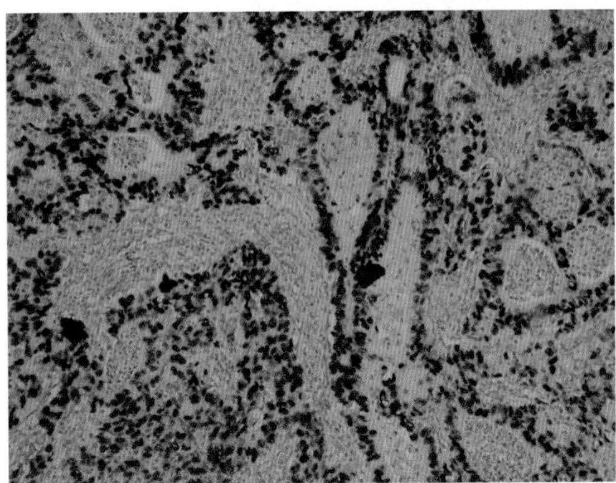

Figure 11.28 *In situ* hybridisation for Epstein–Barr virus (EBV) showing extensive nuclear positivity (black nuclei) in an EBV-positive gastric adenocarcinoma.

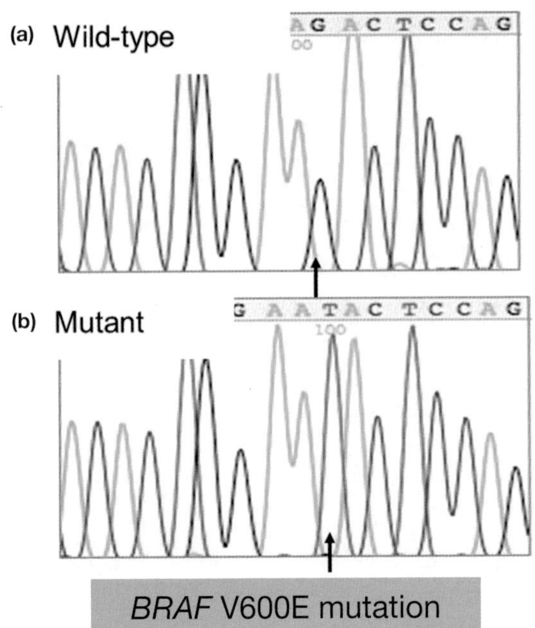

Figure 11.29 Sanger sequencing showing wild-type *BRAF* (a) and a *BRAF* V600E mutation (b) (courtesy of Dr M Rodriguez-Justo, UCL-AD, Cancer Institute, London, UK).

Polymerase chain reaction

The polymerase chain reaction (PCR) amplifies DNA, yielding millions of copies from a single copy of a selected target. Amplification of RNA is also possible, using the technique of reverse transcriptase PCR (RT-PCR). It is worth noting that real-time PCR (RTPCR) is a different method, typically used for quantification, with a very similar abbreviation. PCR is fast and safe and can be performed on homogenised fresh or formalin-fixed tissue. PCR-based methods have numerous applications in oncology (see ***Detection of clinically relevant abnormalities in genes***), including mutational analysis (***Figure 11.29***), testing for clonality, detection of fusion transcripts resulting from cytogenetic changes, detection of amplifications, demonstration of MSI and detection of gene hypermethylation. PCR-based methods can also detect microorganisms in tissue but this is not a common application because of the risk of false positives.

Cytogenetics and fluorescence in situ hybridisation

Conventional cytogenetics is the microscopic study of chromosomal changes in individual cells. Newer techniques, including FISH, array comparative genomic hybridisation, RT-PCR and next-generation sequencing (NGS) are increasingly replacing conventional cytogenetics. Cytogenetic tests seek alterations such as gene amplification, loss of segments of chromosomal material, loss of whole chromosomes (e.g. in renal cell carcinoma) and translocations with associated fusion genes (e.g. *EWSR1-FLI1* in Ewing's sarcoma).

Flow cytometry

Flow cytometry is a laser-based or impedance-based technique used for cell counting, cell sorting, biomarker detection and protein engineering. Cells are suspended in a stream of fluid and passed by an electronic detection apparatus. It is useful for detecting antigens in haematological neoplasms, usually in blood samples, and for determining ploidy, i.e. the number of sets of chromosomes in the nucleus of a cell. Although traditional flow cytometry is of limited value for tissue analysis, new applications of image cytometric DNA analysis allow detection of aneuploidy in tissue sections of gastrointestinal cancers.

Genomic changes in tumours

In normal circumstances, there is precise control of the division and proliferation of human cells. For example, various growth factors influence division by binding to specific cell surface tyrosine kinase receptors, resulting in the initiation of a complex intracellular cascade of changes. Damaged cells may undergo apoptosis, a carefully regulated process of programmed cell death.

Tumours require loss of control of cell proliferation. Abnormalities of numerous genes can affect proliferation and facilitate tumour development. The relevant genes fall into two main categories, i.e. proto-oncogenes (which stimulate cell proliferation) and tumour suppressor genes (which inhibit proliferation) but the picture is not always so straightforward. Activation of proto-oncogenes by genetic changes may induce or accelerate cell proliferation, while inhibition of tumour suppressor genes may remove the controls that normally prevent or retard proliferation. When a proto-oncogene contributes to cancer development, it is usually known as an oncogene. Other genetic changes can also facilitate tumorigenesis.

James Ewing, 1866–1943, Professor of Pathology, Cornell University Medical College, New York, NY, USA, described this type of sarcoma in 1921.
Frederick Sanger, 1918–2013, biochemist, Cambridge University, Cambridge, UK, awarded the Nobel Prize in Chemistry twice: once in 1958 for work on the structure of proteins and again in 1980 for work on base sequences of nucleic acids.

Abnormalities occur at various points during tumorigenesis. The classical model for this process is the 'adenoma–carcinoma sequence' of Fearon and Vogelstein, whereby the accumulation of mutations such as *APC*, *KRAS* and *TP53* in the colorectal mucosa corresponds broadly to the transformation of non-neoplastic mucosa into a colorectal adenoma and subsequently a carcinoma. Current models show that the picture is often very complex and differs between tumours and that a simple sequence does not operate consistently.

Several types of genetic abnormality can occur during tumorigenesis. The main categories of abnormalities are point mutations, fusion genes and copy number changes. Point mutations are single changes in the sequence of nucleotides in DNA and can be germline, i.e. inherited from a parent and accordingly present in every cell in the body, or somatic, i.e. acquired at some point during life and affecting only the tumour cells. Deletions and insertions (indels) of nucleotides result in a frameshift mutation. Examples include *TP53* tumour suppressor gene mutations, causing production of an abnormal p53 protein that lacks suppressor function; and mutation of the *KIT* gene, causing ligand-independent activation of a growth factor receptor.

Fusion genes may be formed by several mechanisms, including translocations and deletions. The translocation t(14:18) in follicular lymphoma results in juxtaposition of the anti-apoptotic *BCL2* to a regulatory region of an immunoglobulin heavy chain gene, with subsequent bcl-2 overexpression. Fusion genes can result from various chromosomal changes, e.g. *TMPRSS2-ERG* gene fusion in prostate adenocarcinoma can occur as a result of a chromosomal deletion and causes abnormal oncogenic activation of *ERG*.

Gene amplification refers to an increase in copy number, resulting in overexpression of the gene, and can variably result from abnormalities in DNA replication, chromosomal structure or telomeres. An example is *HER2* amplification, resulting in overexpression of the growth factor in carcinomas of breast and stomach.

These many types of abnormality in the genome may ultimately interfere with the function of proteins involved in regulatory processes: *TP53* and *KRAS* mutations are among the most common. Genetic changes can disrupt various pathways, including signal transduction (e.g. various growth factors and growth factor receptors, intracellular components such as *RAS* genes, *APC* gene), cell cycle regulators (e.g. *p16*, *RB*), DNA repair pathways (e.g. MMR genes, *BRCA1* mutations in breast carcinoma) and apoptosis (e.g. *BCL2*, an inhibitor of apoptosis).

DNA MMR genes play a vital role in correcting replication errors and other errors. Abnormalities of MMR genes cause instability of short tandem repeated sequences of DNA known as microsatellites, resulting in MSI. Tumours with this characteristic are MSI-H (high level of MSI). The relevant genes are *MLH1*, *MSH2*, *MSH6* and *PMS2*. MSI is a feature of around 15% of CRCs and can result either from a germline mutation in the MMR gene (Lynch syndrome) or, more often, from sporadic methylation of the *MLH1* gene (see ***Mismatch repair gene abnormalities in tumours***).

Epigenetic changes and methylation

Epigenetic factors are external to the gene sequence and can switch it on or off. The latter is known as epigenetic silencing and can result from DNA methylation (addition of a methyl group to DNA), modifications of histones and RNA-associated silencing. Loss of methylation with gene activation can occur in tumours. Conversely, hypermethylation of tumour suppressor genes or of the MMR gene *MLH1* can reduce or halt their activity, favouring malignancy.

Detection of clinically relevant abnormalities in genes

There are two broadly related areas of clinical practice that rely on molecular analysis. First, analysis of tumour DNA may improve diagnostic precision, enhance treatment plans and help predict clinical outcome. Second, it may suggest or detect germline mutations that are characteristic of an inherited disease. This can confirm non-neoplastic conditions, such as cystic fibrosis, or be used to diagnose a hereditary predisposition to cancer, e.g. Lynch syndrome.

Mutational analysis requires extraction of DNA from tissue (or from other sources such as blood) and often includes sequencing-based screening methods (e.g. Sanger sequencing, pyrosequencing) (***Figure 11.29***), screening methods comparing mutated with normal DNA and targeted mutation detection methods.

NGS (***Figure 11.30***) emerged relatively recently. The term NGS encompasses several platforms, each of which performs massively parallel sequencing, allowing simultaneous examination of millions of fragments of DNA for molecular alterations. It is applicable to formalin-fixed tissue, allows evaluation of many DNA regions in a single assay and displays increased analytical sensitivity (i.e. the ability to detect low-frequency alleles) compared with Sanger sequencing or conventional PCR. Widely clinically used targeted NGS panels can identify multiple known mutations and other variants in 20–500 genes of interest in a single test.

New powerful platforms can detect not only point mutations but also copy number variants and gene fusions in more than 100 genes involved in human oncogenesis with minimal nuclear acid (DNA and RNA) sample input.

Adequate amounts of good quality tumour DNA are necessary for the success of these techniques. Histology samples usually include both non-neoplastic tissue and tumour. The pathologist plays a crucial role in assessing the suitability of tissue samples for molecular analysis by analysing tumour cell content as a percentage of all cells, cellularity and degree of necrosis. Microdissection of the area of interest using conventional techniques or laser-assisted approaches improves yields of tumour-derived DNA.

Eric R Fearon, contemporary, Professor of Oncology, University of Michigan, Ann Arbor, MI, USA.
Bert Vogelstein, b. 1949, Professor of Oncology and Pathology, Johns Hopkins Medical School, Baltimore, MD, USA.
Henry Thompson Lynch, 1928–2019, Chair of Preventative Medicine, Creighton University, Omaha, NE, USA.

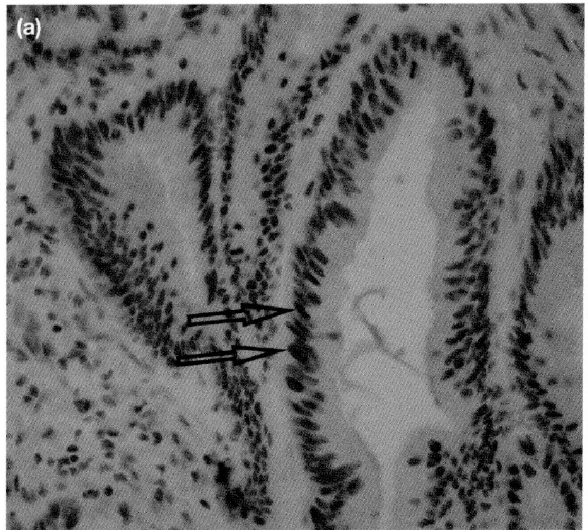

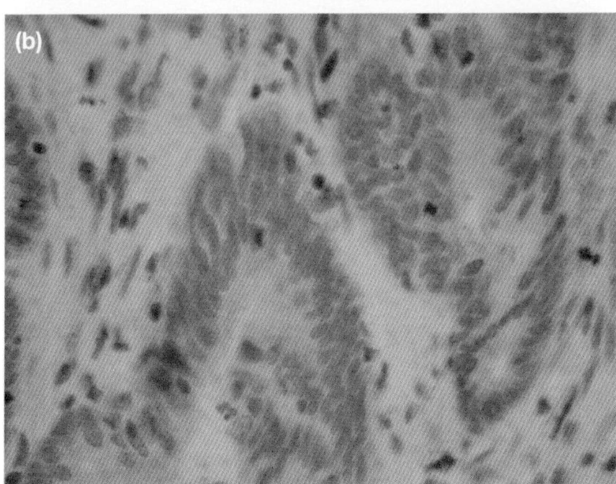

Figure 11.30 Immunohistochemical screening for mismatch repair gene abnormalities in a carcinoma. **(a)** There is retention of nuclear MLH1 expression (arrows showing positively staining brown neoplastic nuclei). **(b)** In contrast, there is loss of MSH2 expression (no staining in neoplastic nuclei), suggesting a mismatch repair gene abnormality.

Summary box 11.13

Genes and carcinogenesis

Genes

- (Proto-) oncogenes
  - *KRAS*
  - *BRAF*
  - *EGFR*
  - *BCL2*
- Tumour suppressor genes
  - *TP53*
  - *BRCA1/2*

Pathways

- Proliferation and signal transduction
- Cell cycle control
- DNA repair
- Apoptosis

Summary box 11.14

Indications for molecular analysis of tumour tissue

- Diagnosis and classification
- Selection of therapy
- Prognosis
- Staging
- Monitoring disease burden
- Screening for germline mutations
- Confirmation of neoplasia (e.g. clonality)

Summary box 11.15

Detection methods for main molecular changes

- Point mutations and small insertions and deletions: NGS, PCR
- Fusions: FISH, NGS, PCR
- Amplifications: FISH, NGS
- Tumour mutation burden: NGS
- Immunohistochemistry may be a very useful initial test, and is often sufficient

Molecular changes and drug therapy

An increasingly common reason for molecular testing and related immunohistochemistry is the prediction of the response of advanced malignant tumours to specific drugs whose target is usually known ('theranostics'). For example, tumours with tyrosine kinase gene fusions that result in activation of the kinase are more likely than their counterparts to respond to tyrosine kinase inhibitors. A newer class of drugs known collectively as immune checkpoint inhibitors (ICIs) is highly successful for the treatment of a variety of advanced malignancies. Detection of any of several biomarkers may predict responsiveness to ICIs.

HER2 gene amplification

HER2 status influences the selection of therapy for breast cancer and metastatic gastric adenocarcinoma. Tumours with *HER2* amplification may be treated with the monoclonal antibodies trastuzumab or pertuzumab, often in combination with other drugs. Recent data suggest that *HER2* amplification may be a relevant therapeutic target in metastatic CRCs that are microsatellite stable.

Summary box 11.16

Tumour types that may respond to immune checkpoint inhibitor drugs

- Breast carcinoma
- Urothelial carcinoma
- Non-small cell lung cancer
- Small cell lung cancer
- Hepatocellular carcinoma
- Malignant melanoma

Translocations

Translocations can produce novel fusion genes that either produce a chimeric protein, e.g. *BCR-ABL* t(9:22) in chronic myeloid leukaemia, or may place an active promoter next to a proto-oncogene, causing its activation, e.g. t(14:18) *IGH-BCL2* in follicular lymphoma. Translocations that activate tyrosine kinases can result in drug responsiveness, e.g. *ALK*, *RET*, *NTRK*, *ROS* and *FGFR2*.

Tumour mutation burden

Tumour mutation burden (TMB) is a recently recognised biomarker. A higher number of mutations within the tumour corresponds to a higher TMB. High levels of TMB can predict response to ICIs. PD-L1 immunohistochemistry and detection of MSI-H are also used for this purpose.

Mismatch repair gene abnormalities in tumours

High levels of microsatellite instability (MSI-H), also known as deficient mismatch repair (D-MMR), occur as a result of germline mutations or acquired somatic events in the MMR genes (*MLH1*, *MSH2*, *MSH6* and *PMS2*). The former is referred to as Lynch syndrome (previously known as hereditary non-polyposis colorectal carcinoma) and is an autosomal dominant condition with predisposition to colorectal, gynaecological and other tumours (often at an early age).

Summary box 11.17

Microsatellite instability and mismatch repair genes

- Microsatellite instability (MSI)
  - Regulated by four main genes: *MLH1, PMS2, MSH2, MSH6*
- Genetic changes responsible for MSI
  - Sporadic hypermethylation of *MLH1* (more common; 85%)
  - Germline mutation, i.e. Lynch syndrome (less common)
- Microsatellite unstable (MSI-H) tumours
  - 15% of colorectal carcinoma (CRC)
  - 30% of endometrial carcinoma
- Tests
  - Immunohistochemistry
    - Recommended for all newly diagnosed CRCs
    - The preferred initial test in most centres
  - PCR-based microsatellite testing
  - NGS
- Clinicopathological correlation: MSI-H CRC
  - Typically right sided
  - More likely to have mucinous element histologically
  - Likely to have *BRAF* V600E mutation
- Clinical value
  - Phenotypic classification, e.g. medullary CRC is typically MSI-H
  - Prognosis, e.g. MSI-H better prognosis overall
  - Selection of drug therapy, e.g. MSI-H CRC responds better to ICIs and has no response to 5-fluorouracil
  - Screening for germline mutation, i.e. Lynch syndrome

Immunohistochemistry is the usual screening method for MMR mutations, although some centres use PCR-based microsatellite testing for screening. Loss of immunohistochemical staining by neoplastic cells is a marker for a gene defect, an indication for further testing and may lead to genetic testing for Lynch syndrome (***Figure 11.30***). In most patients, a detectable MMR abnormality is sporadic and does not represent Lynch syndrome.

MMR gene defects in CRC also identify sporadic tumours with different phenotypic and genetic characteristics. For example, *BRAF* V600E mutations are frequent in these cases and such cancers develop via the serrated polyp pathway rather than from adenomas (see ***Chapter 77***). MMR abnormalities generally predict lower recurrence rates, better survival rates and a lack of need for 5-fluorouracil.

Prognosis

Tests that help determine the selection of therapy for tumours may also have additional prognostic value. For example, a *BRAF* mutation in metastatic CRC is associated with a very poor prognosis. Commercially available multiple molecular marker tests may provide prognostic information (see ***Chapter 58***).

Cancer 'precision medicine'

This refers to the development of individualised cancer care plans, partly on the basis of molecular abnormalities in a tumour. Germline and somatic mutations may be taken into consideration, with the aim of tailoring treatments and targeting cancer cells precisely. With NGS, analysis of a single sample of tumour tissue for multiple known mutations that may predict treatment response is possible. In addition, many assays can detect mutations affecting as few as 5% of neoplastic cells. Other techniques may be used at the same time to detect abnormalities in the proteome (protein), transcriptome (mRNA), metabolome (metabolites) or epigenome, sometimes referred to as 'omics' assays. Such plans may, inevitably, be very complex (see ***Chapter 12***).

Molecular profile: examples of specific tumours

Colorectal carcinoma

In CRC, the anti-EGFR monoclonal antibodies cetuximab and panitumumab are used in combination with chemotherapy for metastatic disease. These drugs are less likely to be effective if *KRAS* or *NRAS* mutations are present than if a tumour is 'wild type' (i.e. has no *RAS* mutation). Various other genetic changes assist with selection of therapy and making prognostic predictions (***Summary boxes 11.17 and 11.18***).

Summary box 11.18

Molecular analysis in colorectal carcinoma

- Mismatch repair gene abnormalities
  - Multiple considerations (see *Summary box 11.17*)
- *KRAS or NRAS* mutation
  - Predicts resistance to EGFR inhibitors
- Tumour mutation burden
  - Predicts response to ICI therapy
- *BRAF* V600E mutation
  - Poor prognosis in metastatic CRC
  - Predictive of response to therapy
- *NTRK* fusion
  - Uncommon (<1% CRC)
  - Usually MSI-H
  - Poor prognosis
  - Specific therapy available: tyrosine kinase inhibitors

Bronchial (lung) carcinoma

In non-small cell lung cancer, specific *EGFR* mutations occur in a minority of lesions and identification predicts a response to the anti-EGFR tyrosine kinase inhibitor gefitinib, while *ALK* gene rearrangement predicts a response to the anaplastic lymphoma kinase (ALK) inhibitor crizotinib (see ***Chapter 60***). ***Summary box 11.19*** shows other relevant molecular changes.

Summary box 11.19

Molecular and related changes in non-small cell lung carcinoma

Prediction of response to tyrosine kinase therapy

- Mutations
  - *EGFR*
  - *KRAS*
  - *BRAF* V600E
- Fusions
  - *ALK*
  - *RET*
  - *NTRK*

Prediction of response to immune checkpoint inhibitors

- PD-L1 expression (in a subgroup)

Gynaecological carcinoma

MMR status is increasingly important for the classification and management of ovarian and endometrial carcinomas. Other molecular changes that are important for prognosis and selection of therapy in endometrial cancer include polymerase ε (POLε) and *TP53* abnormalities. *HER2* amplification and PD-1 expression may be relevant in some settings. Classification into categories such as serous, mucinous and endometrioid influences prognostic predictions and now depends not only on traditional histology but also on a number of molecular changes (many of which are detectable using immunohistochemistry) (see ***Chapter 87***).

Breast carcinoma

The most important ancillary tests for breast carcinoma remain ER immunohistochemistry and HER2 testing. As for many advanced malignancies, ICIs may be useful and accordingly PD-L1 immunostaining (with the appropriate antibody clone) may help predict outcome (see ***Chapter 58***).

Lymphoma

The distinction between benign and malignant lymphoid proliferations is sometimes difficult. Clonal immunoglobulin heavy chain (IgH) gene rearrangements in B-cell proliferations and clonal T-cell receptor gene rearrangements in T-cell proliferations favour lymphoma over reactive proliferations. Identification of characteristic cytogenetic abnormalities plays an important role in diagnosis, classification and management of several haematological neoplasms. PCR-based tests help detect minimal residual disease after therapy.

Gastrointestinal stromal tumour, soft-tissue tumours and malignant melanoma

Most GISTs have either a *KIT* gene mutation or a *PDGFRA* gene mutation, more often the former. A few have defects in succinate dehydrogenase (*SDH*), *BRAF* or *NF1* genes. Identification of known mutations helps confirm the diagnosis. Mutational profile also helps predict clinical outcome and response to chemotherapy. For example, imatinib, a tyrosine kinase inhibitor, is a useful drug for advanced GIST but is ineffective in those with *SDH* mutations.

Molecular testing assists the diagnosis and classification of many types of soft-tissue tumour. Examples include Ewing's sarcoma and alveolar rhabdomyosarcoma, in which specific fusion genes are diagnostic. FISH testing detects characteristic cytogenetic changes.

In metastatic malignant melanoma, specific *BRAF* mutations predict response to the BRAF kinase inhibitor vemurafenib.

Table 11.1 outlines the clinical applications of some biomarkers in tumours.

DIGITAL PATHOLOGY AND ARTIFICAL INTELLIGENCE

The term 'digital pathology' usually refers to the examination of digitised slides on a workstation (computer) or another device. Uses include education, quality assurance, surveys, research and expert consults. With the development of high-quality scanners, histopathology departments can scan all slides and store them so that pathologists can access them anywhere.

Advantages include more flexible on-site and remote reporting, easy sharing, a reduction in costs and better recruitment. Disadvantages include the expense of set-up, maintenance and IT and repetitive strain injury. Additionally, diagnostic

TABLE 11.1 Clinical applications of selected biomarkers in tumours.

Biomarker	Examples of tumours where relevant	Application	Methodology for assessment
Mismatch repair genes	CRC Gynaecological carcinomas Other digestive system carcinomas	See *Summary box 11.17*	IHC PCR NGS
HER2	Breast carcinoma Gastric/oesophageal adenocarcinoma CRC (emerging evidence)	Amplification predicts response to anti-HER2 therapy, e.g. trastuzumab, pertuzumab	IHC FISH/CISH NGS
PD-L1	Lung carcinoma Gastric carcinoma Bladder/urological carcinoma Malignant melanoma Breast carcinoma Endometrial carcinoma	Predicts response to immune checkpoint inhibitors	IHC (not required for melanoma)
EGFR mutation	Lung carcinoma	Predicts response to tyrosine kinase inhibitors	PCR NGS
BRAF mutation	Malignant melanoma CRC	Predicts response to anti-BRAF therapy Prognosis	PCR NGS
KRAS mutation	CRC	Predicts resistance to EGFR inhibitors	PCR NGS
NTRK fusions	CRC	Predicts response to tyrosine kinase inhibitors	NGS
ALK fusion	Non-small cell lung carcinoma Renal cell carcinoma	Predicts response to tyrosine kinase inhibitors	IHC screen FISH NGS
FGFR fusions	Bladder carcinoma	Predicts response to tyrosine kinase inhibitors	NGS
Tumour mutation burden	Various	Predicts response to immune checkpoint inhibitors	NGS

CISH, chromogenic *in situ* hybridisation; CRC, colorectal carcinoma; FISH, fluorescence *in situ* hybridisation; IHC, immunohistochemistry; NGS, next-generation sequencing; PCR, polymerase chain reaction.

accuracy may be slightly lower than with glass slides. Some pathologists, particularly cytopathologists, dislike the loss of a three-dimensional image, and detection of very small items such as microorganisms can be difficult.

AUTOPSY

In the past, autopsies (postmortems) allowed physicians and scientists to improve their knowledge of the human body and various diseases. The main reason for an autopsy is to confirm the cause of death, but autopsies remain very useful for medical education and audit. In the UK there are two main types. The first is the coroner's autopsy, when the coroner decides that there is a legal requirement to establish the cause of death, e.g. unexpected death or death during surgery or soon afterwards. Consent from relatives is not necessary. The second type is the hospital autopsy, which requires relatives' consent. For various reasons hospital autopsies are considerably less common than in the past.

ACKNOWLEDGEMENTS

The authors are very grateful to the following contributors for assistance with previous versions of the chapter and for providing images: Professor Mike Sheaff, London, UK; Dr Manuel Rodriguez-Justo, London, UK.

FURTHER READING

Brierley JD, Gospodarowicz MK, Wittekind C. *TNM classification of malignant tumours*, 8th edn. Oxford: Wiley-Blackwell, 2017.

Cardesa A, Zidar N, Alos L *et al.* The Kaiser's cancer revisited: was Virchow totally wrong? *Virchows Arch* 2011; 458(6): 649–57.

Feakins RM, Allen D, Campbell F *et al. Tissue pathways for gastrointestinal and pancreatobiliary pathology*, 2nd edn. London: Royal College of Pathologists, 2011.

Goldblum JR, Lamps LW, McKenney JK, Myers JL. *Rosai and Ackerman's surgical pathology*, 11th edn. Cambridge, MA: Elsevier, 2017.

Kumar V, Abbas AK, Aster JC. *Robbins and Cotran. Pathologic basis of disease*, 10th edn. Philadelphia, PA: Elsevier, 2020.

Loughrey MB, Quirke P, Shepherd NA. *Dataset for colorectal cancer*, 4th edn. London: Royal College of Pathologists, 2018.

World Health Organization Classification of Tumours Editorial Board. *Digestive system tumours*, 5th edn. Lyon: International Agency for Research on Cancer, 2019.

CHAPTER 12 Principles of oncology

Learning objectives

To understand:

- The biological nature of cancer
- That curative treatment is only one component in the overall management of cancer
- The principles of cancer prevention, early detection and screening
- The principles underlying non-surgical treatments for cancer

To appreciate:

- The principles of cancer aetiology and the major causative factors
- The multidisciplinary management of cancer
- The distinction between palliative care and end-of-life care
- The principles of palliative care

WHAT IS CANCER?

History

The word 'cancer' is credited to Hippocrates (460 BCE–370 BCE), who is widely agreed to be the father of medicine, and comes from the Greek word for a crab, referring to the finger-like projections of a cancer from a central mass, which have similarities to a crab's claws and legs.

The study of cancer has long been a part of clinical medicine: theories have moved from divine intervention and are now firmly based on the molecular origins of cancer. Rudolf Virchow was the first to demonstrate that cancer is a disease of cells and that the disease progresses as a result of abnormal proliferation, encapsulated by his dictum *omnes cellula e cellula* (every cell from a cell). In 1914, Theodor Boveri pointed out the importance of chromosomal abnormalities in cancer cells and, in the 1940s, Oswald Avery demonstrated that DNA was the genetic material within the chromosomes. In 1953, Watson and Crick described the structure of DNA, which was the key discovery leading to the understanding of the molecular biology of cancer. This understanding has allowed the investigation and understanding of the molecular mechanisms whereby cancer cells are formed and their abnormal behaviours are mediated; in turn, this has allowed modern molecular-based therapies to be developed.

The hallmarks of cancer

Cancer cells are able to proliferate in an uncontrolled fashion; their ability to divide and spread is unbounded. Cancer cell growth destroys first the tissue from which they arise and eventually the person in which they are present.

In order to survive, divide, invade and spread, cancer cells have to acquire a number of characteristics. No one characteristic is sufficient and not all characteristics are absolutely necessary. These features, based on articles by Hanahan and Weinberg, are given in ***Summary box 12.1***.

Establish an autonomous lineage

Cells develop independence from the normal signals that control supply and demand. The healing of a wound is a physiological process; the cellular response is exquisitely coordinated so that proliferation occurs when it is needed and ceases when it is no longer required. The whole process is controlled by a series of

---

Hippocrates, 460 BCE–375 BCE, was a Greek Physician and, by common consent, 'the father of medicine'.
Rudolf Ludwig Carl Virchow, 1821–1902, Professor of Pathology, Berlin, Germany.
Theodor Heinrich Boveri, 1862–1913, Professor of Zoology and Comparative Anatomy, Würzburg, Germany.
Oswald Theodore Avery, 1877–1955, bacteriologist, Rockefeller Institute, New York, NY, USA.
James Dewey Watson, b.1928, American biologist who worked in Cambridge, UK, and later became Director of the Cold Spring Harbor Laboratory, New York, NY, USA.
Francis Harry Compton Crick, 1916–2004, British molecular biologist who worked at the Cavendish Laboratory, Cambridge, UK, and later at the Salk Institute, San Diego, CA, USA. Watson and Crick shared the 1962 Nobel Prize in Physiology or Medicine with ***Maurice Hugh Frederick Wilkins***, 1916–2004, of Kings College, London, UK.
Douglas Hanahan, b.1951, American biologist and director of the Swiss Institute for Experimental Cancer Research (ISREC), Lausanne, Switzerland.
Robert Allan Weinberg, b.1942, The Whitehead Institute of Biomedical Research and Department of Biology, The Massachusetts Institute of Technology, Cambridge, MA, USA.

Summary box 12.1

Features of malignant transformation

- Establish an autonomous lineage
  - Resist signals that inhibit growth
  - Sustain proliferative signalling
- Obtain replicative immortality
- Evade apoptosis
- Acquire angiogenic competence
- Acquire ability to invade, disseminate and implant
- Evocation of inflammation
- Evade detection/elimination
- Loss of specialist cell function
- Develop ability to change energy metabolism

signals telling cells when, and when not, to divide. Cancer cells escape from this normal system of checks and balances: they grow and proliferate in the absence of external stimuli and regardless of signals telling them to desist.

Oncogenes are genes with the potential to cause cancer if mutated and expressed at high levels; they are key factors in carcinogenesis. Most oncogenes are normally involved in physiological processes, i.e. cell growth, but if mutated they can predispose a cell to cancer and in concert with other oncogenes can enable cancer cell survival and development of an established tumour. The implication is that we all carry the seeds of our own destruction: genetic sequences that, through mutation, can turn into active oncogenes and thereby cause malignant transformation. Indeed, through study of the timing of key genetic events in adult cancer development, a handful of cells develop the founder mutations of cancer development several decades prior to diagnosis. If the individual is unfortunate enough to accumulate further mutations in key driver genes, that cell becomes malignant and, if it proliferates, a cancer may develop. Only very rarely is a single mutation sufficient to cause cancer; multiple mutations are usually required. Colorectal cancer provides the classical example of how multiple mutations are necessary for the complete transformation from normal cell to malignant cell. Vogelstein and his colleagues identified the genes implicated and also postulated that it is necessary to have mutations in all the relevant genes; they also noted that these mutations must be acquired in a specific sequence for malignant transformation to occur.

Obtain replicative immortality

According to the Hayflick hypothesis, normal cells are permitted to undergo only a finite number of divisions. For humans this number is between 40 and 60. The limitation is imposed by the progressive shortening of the end of the chromosome (the telomere) that occurs each time a cell divides; eventually the lineage will die out. Cancer cells utilise the enzyme telomerase to rebuild the telomere at each cell division, such that there is no telomeric shortening, and the lineage will never die out. The cancer cell hence develops immortality.

Evade apoptosis

Apoptosis, taken from the Greek for 'leaf fall', is a form of programmed cell death that occurs as the direct result of internal cellular events instructing the cell to die. Unlike necrosis, which is a form of traumatic cell death resulting from acute cellular injury, apoptosis is an orderly and internally driven process. The cell dismantles itself neatly for disposal (***Figure 12.1***). There is minimal inflammatory response. Apoptosis is a physiological process. Cells that are redundant normally die by apoptosis and this is an important self-regulatory mechanism in growth and development, i.e. cells in the web space of the embryo die by apoptosis, or lymphocytes that could react to self. Genes, such as *p53*, that can activate apoptosis function as tumour suppressor genes. Mutation in such genes causes a loss of this inhibitory function, which will contribute to malignant transformation as apoptosis is evaded; this means that the wrong cells can be in the wrong places at the wrong times.

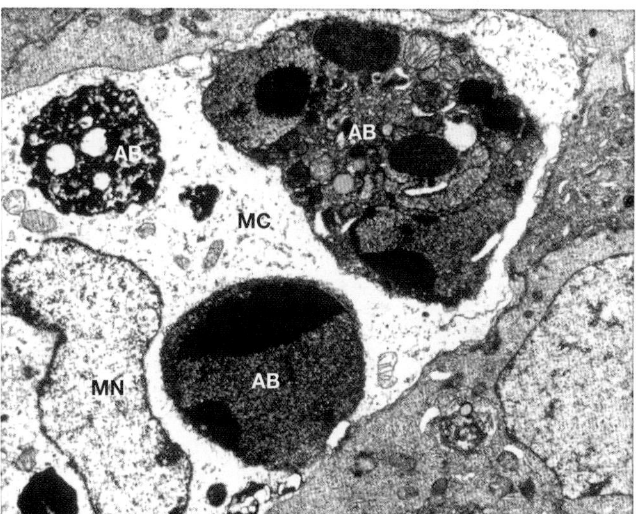

Figure 12.1 Electron micrograph of apoptotic bodies (AB) engulfed by a macrophage. Note the macrophage nucleus (MN) and macrophage cytoplasm (MC).

Acquire angiogenic competence

A mass of cancer cells cannot, in the absence of a blood supply, grow beyond a diameter of about 1 mm. This places a severe restriction on the capabilities of the tumour (note that the word tumour means swelling and does not mean the lesion is malignant, although 'tumour' is often taken by patients to be synonymous with cancer). It cannot grow much larger or spread widely within the body. If, however, the mass of cancer cells is able to attract or to construct a blood supply then it is able to quit its dormant state and behave in a far

Bert Vogelstein, b.1949, molecular biologist, Johns Hopkins Hospital, Baltimore, MD, USA.
Leonard Hayflick, b.1928, while working at the Wistar Institute in Philadelphia in 1962, he noted that normal mammalian cells growing in culture had a limited, rather than an indefinite, capacity for self-replication.

more aggressive fashion. The ability of a cancer to form blood vessels is termed angiogenesis and is a key feature of malignant transformation.

Acquire ability to invade

Cancer cells have no respect for the structure of normal tissues. They acquire the ability to breach the basement membrane and gain direct access to blood and lymph vessels. Cancer cells use three main mechanisms to facilitate invasion: (i) cause a rise in the interstitial pressure within a tissue; (ii) secrete enzymes that dissolve extracellular matrix; and (iii) become mobile. Unrestrained proliferation and a lack of contact inhibition enable cancer cells to exert pressure directly on the surrounding tissue and push beyond the normal limits. They secrete collagenases and proteases that chemically dissolve any extracellular boundaries that would otherwise limit their spread through tissues and, by modulating the expression of cell surface molecules called integrins, are able to detach themselves from the extracellular matrix. The abnormal integrins associated with malignancy can also transmit signals from the environment to the cytoplasm and nucleus of the cancer cells ('outside-in signalling') and these signals can induce increased motility. These processes are similar to those involved in normal development, i.e. in the migration of the neural crest or the formation of the heart. Epithelial cells behave as if they were mesenchymal cells and the process is termed epithelial–mesenchymal transition (EMT). EMT is a crucial step in malignant transformation and many of the genes and proteins implicated in the formation of cancer control processes are involved in EMT, e.g. *Src, Ras,* integrins, *Wnt*/β-catenin, Notch.

Acquire ability to disseminate and implant

Once cancer cells gain access to vascular and lymphovascular spaces, they can be readily distributed systemically throughout the body. This is not, of itself, sufficient to cause tumours to develop at distant sites. The cells also need to acquire the ability to implant. As Paget pointed out over a century ago, there is a crucial relationship here between the seed (the tumour cell) and the soil (the distant tissue). Most of the cancer cells discharged into the circulation probably do not form viable metastases. Circulating cancer cells can be identified in patients who never develop clinical evidence of metastatic disease; presumably these cells die if they cannot implant or they are destroyed by the patient's immune system.

Cancer can spread as individual cells or cell clumps that migrate and implant. Whether spread occurs in groups or as individual cells there is still the problem of crossing the vascular endothelium (and basement membrane) to gain access to the tissue itself. Cancer cells probably implant themselves in distant tissues by exploiting, and subverting, the normal inflammatory response. By expressing inflammatory cytokines, cancer cells can deceive the endothelium of the host tissue into becoming activated and allowing cancer cells access to the extravascular space. Activated endothelium expresses receptors that bind to integrins and selectins on the surface of cells, allowing the cancer cells to move across the endothelial barrier.

Tumour-related inflammation

A malignancy can provoke an inflammatory response and the cytokines and other factors produced as a result of that response may act to promote and sustain malignant transformation. Growth factors, mutagenic reactive oxygen species, angiogenic factors and anti-apoptotic factors may all be produced as part of an inflammatory process and all may contribute to the progression of a cancer.

Evade detection/elimination

Although derived from normal cells ('self') cancer cells are, in terms of their genetic make-up, behaviour and characteristics, foreign ('not self'). As such, they ought to provoke an immune response and be eliminated. It is entirely possible that malignant transformation is a more frequent event than the emergence of clinical cancer. The possible role of the immune system in eliminating nascent cancers was proposed by Paul Ehrlich in 1909 and revisited by both Sir Frank McFarlane Burnet and Lewis Thomas in the late 1950s. Cancer cells, or at least those that give rise to clinical disease, appear to gain the ability to escape detection by the immune system. This may be through suppressing expression of tumour-associated antigens or it may be through actively co-opting one part of the immune system to help the tumour escape detection by other parts of the immune surveillance system. This hallmark has been exploited in recent years in the development of T-cell checkpoint inhibitors, which 'take the brakes' off the immune system to re-enable T-cell killing of cancer cells, e.g. in renal cell carcinoma, lung cancer and melanoma.

Loss of specialist cell function

Cancer cells are geared to excessive proliferation. They do not need to develop or retain those specialised functions that prior to malignant transformation were their physiological function. These cells can therefore afford to repress or permanently lose those genes that control such functions. The longer term disadvantage to this process is that cancer cells are vulnerable to external stressors, which may, in part, explain why some cancer treatments work.

Stephen Paget, 1855–1926, surgeon, The West London Hospital, London, UK. Paget's 'seed and soil' hypothesis is contained in his paper 'The distribution of secondary growths in cancer of the breast', published in the *Lancet* in 1889.

Paul Ehrlich, 1854–1915, Professor of Hygiene, the University of Berlin, and later Director of the Institute for Infectious Diseases, Berlin, Germany. In 1908, he shared the Nobel Prize in Physiology or Medicine with **Elie Metchnikoff**, 1845–1916, 'in recognition of his work on immunity'. Metchnikoff was Professor of Zoology at Odessa in Russia, and later worked at the Pasteur Institute in Paris, France.

Sir Frank McFarlane Burnet, 1899–1985, Australian virologist, Walter and Eliza Hall Institute, Melbourne, Australia. Burnett shared the 1960 Nobel Prize in Physiology or Medicine with **Sir Peter Brian Medawar**, 1915–1987, Jodrell Professor of Zoology, University College, London, UK, 'for their discovery of acquired immunological tolerance'.

Lewis Thomas, 1913–1993, American pathologist and immunologist, who became President of the Sloan Kettering Memorial Institute, New York, NY, USA.

Develop ability to change energy metabolism

Blood flow in malignant tumours is often sporadic and unreliable. As a result, cancer cells may have to spend prolonged periods in low-oxygen states (i.e. relative hypoxia). Compared with the corresponding normal cells, some cancer cells may be better able to survive in hypoxic conditions. This ability may enable tumours to grow and develop despite an impoverished blood supply. Cancer cells can alter their metabolism even when oxygen is abundant; they break down glucose but do not, as normal cells would do, send the resulting pyruvate to the mitochondria for conversion, in an oxygen-dependent process, to carbon dioxide. This is the phenomenon of aerobic glycolysis, or the Warburg effect, and leads to the production of lactate. In an act of symbiosis, lactate-producing cancer cells may provide lactate for adjacent cancer cells, which are then able to use it, via the citric acid cycle, for energy production. This cooperation is similar to that which occurs in skeletal muscle during exercise.

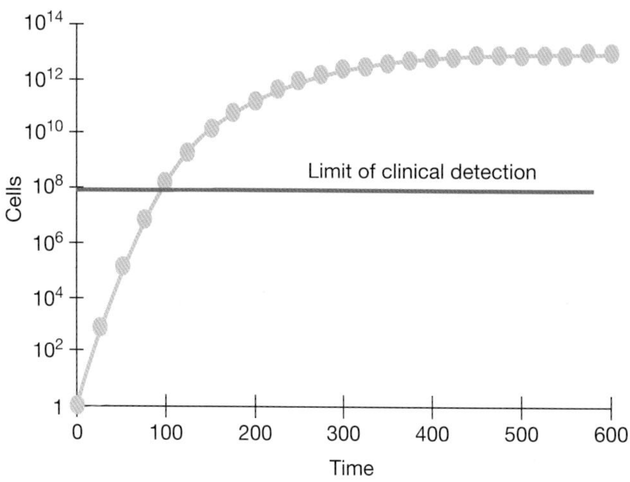

Figure 12.2 The Gompertzian curve describing the growth of a typical tumour. In its early stages, growth is exponential but, as the tumour grows, the growth rate slows. This decrease in growth rate probably arises because of difficulties with nutrition and oxygenation. The tumour cells are in competition: not only with the tissues of the host, but also with each other.

The growth of a cancer

If it is accepted that a cancer starts from a single transformed cell then it is possible, using straightforward arithmetic, to describe the progression from a single cell to a mass of cells large enough to kill the host. The division of a cell produces two daughter cells. The relationship $2n$ will describe the number of cells produced after n generations of division. There are between 10^{13} and 10^{14} cells in a typical human being. A tumour 10 mm in diameter will contain about 10^9 cells. Since $2^{30} = 10^9$ this implies that it would take 30 generations to reach the threshold of clinical detectability and, as $2^{45} = 3 \times 10^{13}$, it will take fewer than 15 subsequent generations to produce a tumour that, through sheer bulk alone, would be fatal. This is an oversimplification because cell loss is a feature of many cancers: for squamous cancers as many as 99% of the cells produced may be lost, mainly by exfoliation. It will, in the presence of cell loss, take many cellular divisions to produce a clinically evident tumour. The growth of a typical human tumour can be described by an exponential relationship, the doubling time of which increases exponentially – so-called Gompertzian growth (***Figure 12.2***).

THE CAUSES OF CANCER

The interplay between nature and nurture

Both inheritance and environment are important determinants of cancer development. Neither influence is completely dominant. The balance between genes and the environment is context specific and not consistent. Two contrasting examples are breast and lung cancer. Although not all smokers develop lung cancer and lung cancer can occur in people who have never smoked, non-small cell lung cancer is much more common in smokers and is such a powerful risk factor that it accounts for approximately 80% of the disease. Conversely, germline *BRCA* gene mutations are highly penetrant and women with a *BRCA1* mutation can have a 60–90% lifetime risk of being diagnosed with breast cancer and 40–60% will develop ovarian cancer.

Knowledge about the causes of cancer can be used to design appropriate strategies for prevention or earlier diagnosis. As we find out more about the genes associated with cancer, genetic testing and counselling play increasingly important roles in the prevention of cancer. These considerations are incorporated into ***Table 12.1***, on the inherited cancer syndromes, and into ***Table 12.2***, on the environmental contribution to cancer.

THE MANAGEMENT OF CANCER

Management is more than treatment

The traditional approach to cancer concentrates on diagnosis and active treatment. This is a very limited view that, in terms of public health, may not have served society well. It implies a fatalistic attitude to the occurrence of cancer and an assumption that, once active treatment is complete, there is little more to be done. Prevention was forgotten and rehabilitation was ignored.

Otto Warburg, 1883–1970, chemist, Director of the Kaiser Wilhelm Institute for Cell Physiology, Berlin-Dahlem, Germany. Awarded the Nobel Prize in Physiology or Medicine in 1931 for 'his discovery of the nature and mode of action of the respiratory enzyme'.

Benjamin Gompertz, 1779–1865, an insurance actuary who described mathematically the relationship between life expectancy and age. The Gompertzian function provides an excellent fit to data points plotting tumour size against time.

TABLE 12.1 Examples of inherited syndromes associated with cancer.

Syndrome	Gene(s) implicated	Inheritance	Associated tumours and abnormalities	Strategies for prevention/ early diagnosis
Familial adenomatous polyposis (FAP)	*APC* gene	D	Colorectal cancer under the age of 25 Papillary carcinoma of the thyroid Cancer of the ampulla of Vater Hepatoblastomas Primary brain tumours (Turcot syndrome) Osteomas of the jaw CHRPE (congenital hypertrophy of the retinal pigment epithelium)	Prophylactic panproctocolectomy
Hereditary non-polyposis colorectal cancer (HNPCC1), Lynch syndrome 1	DNA mismatch repair genes *(MLH1; MSH2; MSH6)*	D	Colorectal cancer (typically in forties and fifties)	Surveillance colonoscopies/ polypectomies Non-steroidal anti-inflammatory drugs
HNPCC2	DNA mismatch repair genes *(MLH1; MSH2; MSH6)*	D	HNPCC associated with other cancers of the gastrointestinal or reproductive system	
Peutz–Jeghers syndrome	*STK11*	D	Bowel cancer; breast cancer; freckles round the mouth	Surveillance colonoscopy; mammography
Cowden[a] syndrome	*PTEN*	D	Multiple hamartomas of skin, breast and mucous membranes Breast cancer Neuroendocrine tumours Endometrial cancer Thyroid cancer	Active surveillance
Retinoblastoma	*RB*	D	Retinoblastoma Pinealoma Osteosarcoma	Surveillance of uninvolved eye
Multiple endocrine neoplasia (MEN) type 1	*Menin*	D	Parathyroid tumours Islet cell tumours Pituitary tumours	Awareness of associations and paying attention to relevant symptoms
MEN type 2A	*RET*	D	Medullary carcinoma of the thyroid Phaeochromocytoma Parathyroid tumours	Regular screening of blood pressure, serum calcitonin and urinary catecholamines Prophylactic thyroidectomy
MEN type 2B	*RET*	D	Medullary carcinoma of the thyroid Phaeochromocytoma Mucosal neuromas Ganglioneuromas of the gut	Regular screening of blood pressure, serum calcitonin and urinary catecholamines Prophylactic thyroidectomy
Li–Fraumeni	*P53*	D	Sarcomas Leukaemia Osteosarcomas Brain tumours Adrenocortical carcinomas	Very difficult, since pattern of tumours is so heterogeneous and varies between patients
Familial breast cancer	*BRCA1; BRCA2*	D	Breast cancer Ovarian cancer Papillary serous carcinoma of the peritoneum Prostate cancer	Screening mammography; pelvic ultrasound PSA (in males) Prophylactic mastectomy; prophylactic oophorectomy
Familial cutaneous malignant melanoma	*CDNK2A; CDK4*	D	Cutaneous malignant melanoma	Avoid exposure to sunlight, careful surveillance

Continued

Abraham Vater, 1684–1751, Professor of Anatomy and Botany, and later of Pathology and Therapeutics, Wittenberg, Germany.
Jacques Turcot, 1914–1977, surgeon, Hôtel-Dieu de Quebec hospital, Quebec, Canada.
Henry Thompson Lynch, 1928–2019, Chair of Preventative Medicine, Creighton University, Omaha, NE, USA.
John Law Augustine Peutz, 1886–1968, Chief Specialist for Internal Medicine, St John's Hospital, The Hague, The Netherlands.
Harold Joseph Jeghers, 1904–1990, Professor of Internal Medicine, The New Jersey College of Medicine and Dentistry, Jersey City, NJ, USA.
Frederick Pei Li, 1940–2015, Professor of Medicine, Harvard University Medical School, Boston, MA, USA.
Joseph F Fraumeni, b.1933, Director of Cancer Epidemiology and Genetics, The National Cancer Institute, Bethesda, MD, USA.

TABLE 12.1 Examples of inherited syndromes associated with cancer – *continued*.

Syndrome	Gene(s) implicated	Inheritance	Associated tumours and abnormalities	Strategies for prevention/ early diagnosis
Basal cell naevus syndrome (Gorlin)	*PTCH*	D	Basal cell carcinomas Medulloblastoma Bifid ribs	Careful surveillance, awareness of diagnosis (look for bifid ribs on x-ray)
von Hippel–Lindau disease	*VHL*	D	Clear cell renal cell carcinoma Phaeochromocytoma Haemangiomas of the cerebellum and retina	Urinary catecholamines
Neurofibromatosis type 1	*NF1*	D	Astrocytomas Primitive neuroectodermal tumours Optic gliomas Multiple neurofibromas	A difficult problem; maintain a high index of suspicion concerning any rapid changes in growth or character of any nodule
Neurofibromatosis type 2	*NF2*	D	Acoustic neuromas Spinal tumours Meningiomas Multiple neurofibromas	
Xeroderma pigmentosum	Deficient nucleotide excision repair (*XPA,B,C*)	R	Skin sensitive to sunlight. Early onset of cutaneous squamous or basal cell carcinomas	Avoidance of sun exposure Active surveillance and early treatment Retinoids for chemoprevention
Ataxia–telangiectasia	*AT*	R	Progressive cerebellar ataxia Leukaemia Lymphoma Breast cancer Melanoma Upper gastrointestinal tumours	Active surveillance
Bloom syndrome	*BLM helicase*	R	Sensitivity to ultraviolet light Leukaemia Lymphoma	Active surveillance

D, dominant; PSA, prostate-specific antigen; R, recessive.
[a]One of the few clinical syndromes named for the patient rather than the clinician. Rachel Cowden was, in 1963, the first patient described with the syndrome. She died from breast cancer at the age of 20.

TABLE 12.2 Environmental causes of cancer (and suggested measures for reducing their impact).

Environmental/behavioural factor		Associated tumours	Strategy for prevention/early diagnosis
Tobacco		Lung cancer Head and neck cancer Bladder cancer	Ban tobacco Ban smoking in public places Punitive taxes on tobacco
Alcohol		Head and neck cancer Oesophageal cancer Hepatocellular carcinoma	Avoid excess alcohol Surveillance of high-risk individuals
Ultraviolet exposure		Melanoma Non-melanoma skin cancer	Avoid excessive sun exposure, use high-factor sunscreen, avoid sunbeds
Ionising radiation		Leukaemia Breast cancer Lymphoma Thyroid cancer	Limit medical exposures to absolute minimum; safety precautions at nuclear facilities; monitor radiation workers
Viral infections	Human papillomavirus	Cervical cancer Penile cancer Head and neck cancer	Avoid unprotected sex Vaccination

Continued

Robert Gorlin, 1923–2006, Professor of Dentistry, The University of Minnesota, Minneapolis, MN, USA.
Eugen von Hippel, 1867–1939, Professor of Ophthalmology, Göttingen, Germany.
Arvid Lindau, 1892–1958, Professor of Pathology, Lund, Sweden.
David Bloom, 1892–1985, dermatologist at the Skin and Cancer Clinic, New York University, New York, NY, USA, described the syndrome in 1954.

TABLE 12.2 Environmental causes of cancer (and suggested measures for reducing their impact) – *continued.*

Environmental/behavioural factor			Associated tumours	Strategy for prevention/early diagnosis
Viral infections – *continued*	Human immunodeficiency virus		Kaposi's sarcoma Lymphomas Germ cell tumours Anal cancer	Avoid unprotected sex
	Hepatitis B		Hepatocellular carcinoma	Avoid contaminated injections/ infusions Vaccination
Other infections	Schistosomiasis		Bladder cancer	Treatment of infection
	Helicobacter pylori		Stomach cancer	Eradication therapy
Inhaled particles	Asbestos		Mesothelioma	Protect workers from inhaled dusts and fibres
	Wood dust		Paranasal sinus cancers	
Chemicals	Environmental pollutants/chemicals used in industry		Angiosarcoma (vinyl chloride) Bladder cancer (aniline dyes, vulcanisation of rubber) Lung, nasal cavity (nickel) Skin (arsenic) Lung (beryllium, cadmium, chromium) All sites (dioxins)	Protection of exposed workers; avoid chemical discharge and spillages
	Medical	Alkylating agents used in cytotoxic chemotherapy	Leukaemia Lymphoma Lung cancer	Avoid over-treatment; only combine drugs with ionising radiation when absolutely necessary
		Immunosuppressive treatment	Kaposi's sarcoma	As low a dose as possible, for as short a period as possible
		Tamoxifen	Endometrial cancer	Biopsy if patient on tamoxifen develops uterine bleeding
Fungal and plant toxins	Aflatoxins		Hepatocellular carcinoma	Appropriate food storage, screen for fungal contamination of foodstuffs
Obesity/lack of physical exercise			Breast Endometrium Kidney Colon Oesophagus	Maintain ideal body weight, regular exercise

A more comprehensive view considers the management of cancer as taking place along two axes: one is an axis of scale, from the individual to the world population; the other is an axis based on the development of the disease, from prevention through to rehabilitation or palliative care (***Figure 12.3***).

Prevention

There is much written on the evidence on the preventable causes of cancer. It is concluded that many cancers could be prevented if people ate sensibly, exercised more and avoided carcinogens such as cigarette smoke. Early identification of premalignant conditions may also prevent certain malignancies developing, e.g. Barrett's oesophagus as a premalignant condition in oesophageal cancer. This advice supplements the preventative measures outlined in ***Table 12.2***.

Screening

Screening involves the detection of disease in an asymptomatic population in order to improve outcomes by early diagnosis of cancer at a curable stage. It follows that a successful screening programme must achieve early diagnosis and that the disease in question has a better outcome when treated at an early stage. The criteria that must be fulfilled for the disease, screening test and the screening programme itself are given in ***Summary box 12.2***. Merely to prove that screening picks up disease at an early stage, and that the outcome is better for patients with screen-detected disease than for those who present with symptoms, is an insufficient criterion for the success of a screening programme. This is because of potential inherent biases of screening (lead time bias, selection bias and length bias), which make screen-detected disease appear to be associated with better outcomes than symptomatic disease.

Moritz Kaposi (originally Kohn), 1837–1902, Professor of Dermatology, Vienna, Austria, described pigmented sarcoma of the skin in 1872.
Norman Rupert Barrett, 1903–1979, surgeon, St Thomas' Hospital, London, UK.

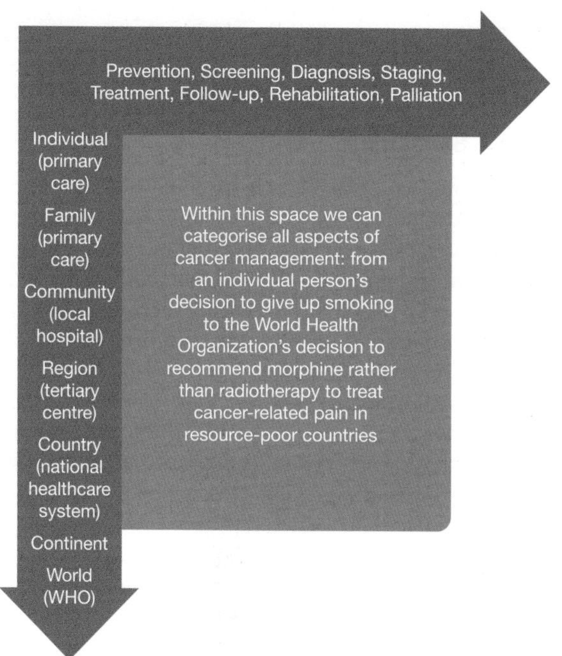

Figure 12.3 The management of cancer spans the natural history of the disease and all humankind, from the individual to the population of the world.

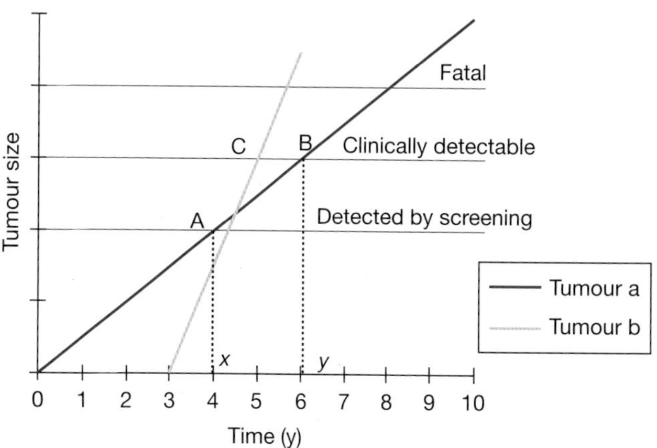

Figure 12.4 An illustration of lead time and length bias. ***Tumour a*** is a steadily growing tumour; its progress is uninfluenced by any treatment. Point A indicates the time at which the tumour would be diagnosed in a screening programme, and point B indicates the time at which the tumour would be diagnosed clinically, i.e. in the absence of any screening programme. If the date of diagnosis is used as the start time for measuring survival, then, in the absence of any effect from treatment, the screening programme will, artefactually, add to the survival time. The amount of 'increased' survival is equal to $y - x$ years, in this example just over 2 years. This artefactual inflation of survival time is referred to as lead time bias. ***Tumour b*** is a rapidly growing tumour; again its progress is uninfluenced by treatment. It grows so rapidly that, in the interval between two screening tests, it can cross both the threshold for detectability by screening and that of clinical detectability (at point C). It will continue to progress rapidly after diagnosis and the measured survival time will be short. This phenomenon, whereby those tumours that are 'missed' by the screening programme are associated with decreased survival, is called length time bias.

Summary box 12.2

Criteria for screening (based on Wilson–Junger criteria for a screening programme)

The disease:

- Recognisable early stage
- Treatment at early stage more effective than at later stage
- Sufficiently common to warrant screening

The test:

- Sensitive and specific
- Acceptable to the screened population
- Safe
- Inexpensive

The programme:

- Adequate diagnostic facilities for those with a positive test
- High-quality treatment for screen-detected disease to minimise morbidity and mortality
- Screening repeated at intervals if disease of insidious onset
- Benefit must outweigh physical and psychological harm

Lead time bias describes the phenomenon whereby early detection of a disease will always prolong survival from the time of diagnosis when compared with disease picked up at a later stage in its development whether or not detection in the screening process has altered the progression of the cancer (***Figure 12.4***). Selection bias describes the finding that individuals who accept an invitation for screening are, in general, healthier than those who do not. It follows that individuals with screen-detected disease will tend to live longer, independently of the condition for which screening is being performed. Length bias occurs because small, slow-growing tumours are likely to be picked up by screening whereas larger, fast-growing tumours are likely to arise and produce symptoms in between screening rounds. Screen-detected tumours will therefore tend to be less aggressive than symptomatic tumours. Because of these biases it is essential to carry out population-based randomised controlled trials and to compare the mortality rate in a whole population offered screening (including those who refuse to be screened and those who develop cancer after a negative test) with the mortality rate in a population that has not been offered screening. This research design has been applied to both breast cancer and colorectal cancer: in both cases there was a reduction in disease-specific mortality. However, in general, clinical trials of screening with the gold-standard endpoint of overall survival have not been undertaken because of the very large number of participants required with long study follow-up periods.

Cancer screening remains a controversial topic with advocates on both sides of the argument. Targeted, risk-based screening approaches, such as computed tomography (CT) scan-based screening of smokers and ex-smokers for lung cancer, are being evaluated as methods of developing more conclusive screening programmes.

James Maxwell Glover Wilson, 1913-2006, Principal Medical Officer at the Ministry of Health in London, England.
Gunnar Jungner, 1914–1982, Chief Clinical Chemistry, Sahlgrenska Hospital, Gothenburg, Sweden.

Diagnosis and classification

Accurate diagnosis is the key to successful management of cancer. Precise diagnosis is crucial to the choice of correct therapy; the wrong operation, no matter how well performed, is useless. An unequivocal diagnosis is also the key to an accurate prognosis. Only rarely can a diagnosis of cancer be confidently made in the absence of tissue for pathological or cytological examination. Cancer is a disease of cells and, for accurate diagnosis, the abnormal cells need to be obtained and visualised by a histopathologist. Different tumours are classified in different ways: most squamous epithelial tumours are classed as well (G1), moderate (G2) or poorly (G3) differentiated. Adenocarcinomas are also often classified as G1, G2 or G3 but prostate cancer is an exception, with widespread use of the Gleason system. The Gleason system grades prostate cancer according to the degree of differentiation of the two most prevalent architectural patterns. The final score is the sum of the two grades and can vary from 6 (3 + 3) to 10 (5 + 5) with the higher scores indicating poorer prognosis.

The ongoing development of molecular classifiers in many cancer types is beginning to profoundly alter our approach to treatment of these malignancies based on genetic mutations and other molecular features identified in individual patients, i.e. in melanoma where patients with *BRAF* gene mutations can be successfully treated with the *BRAF* inhibitors. Molecular characterisation of malignancies and identification of their vulnerabilities have already become standard of care in many cancers (i.e. breast, colorectal and lung cancer) and this list is likely to expand.

Cancer staging

It is not sufficient simply to know what and where a cancer is; its extent must also be known. If it is localised, then locoregional treatments such as surgery and radiation therapy may be curative. If the disease is widespread then, although such local interventions may contribute to cure, they will be insufficient and systemic treatment, for example with drugs or hormones, will also be required.

Staging is the process whereby the extent of disease is mapped out. Staging used to be a fairly crude process based on clinical examination, chest x-ray and occasionally ultrasound; it is now a sophisticated process, reliant on advanced imaging techniques such as CT, magnetic resonance imaging (MRI) and positron emission tomography (PET) scans. These technological advances bring with them the implication that patients staged as having localised disease today are not comparable to patients described in 1985 as having localised disease. Many of these latter patients would, had they been imaged using the technology of today, have had occult metastatic disease detected.

The Union for International Cancer Control (UICC) is responsible for the TNM (tumour, nodes, metastases) staging system for cancer. This system is compatible with, and relates to, the American Joint Committee on Cancer (AJCC) system

TABLE 12.3 Staging of colorectal cancer.

TNM		
TX,	Primary tumour cannot be assessed	
T0,	No evidence of primary tumour	
Tis,	Carcinoma *in situ* or intramucosal carcinoma	
T1,	Tumour invades submucosa	
T2,	Tumour invades muscularis propria	
T3,	The tumour has grown through the muscularis propria and into the subserosa, which is a thin layer of connective tissue beneath the outer layer of some parts of the large intestine, or it has grown into tissues surrounding the colon or rectum	
T4,	Tumour directly invades beyond bowel	a, The tumour has grown into the surface of the visceral peritoneum
		b, The tumour has grown into or has attached to other organs or structures
NX,	Regional lymph nodes cannot be assessed	
N0,	No metastases in regional nodes	
N1a,	Metastases in 1 regional lymph node	
N1b,	Metastases in 2 or 3 regional lymph nodes	
N1c,	There are nodules made up of tumour cells found in the structures near the colon that do not appear to be lymph nodes	
N2a,	Metastases in 4–6 regional lymph nodes	
N2a,	Metastases in ≥7 regional lymph nodes	
MX,	Not possible to assess the presence of distant metastases	
M0,	No distant metastases	
M1a,	The cancer has spread to 1 other part of the body beyond the colon or rectum	
M1b,	The cancer has spread to more than 1 part of the body other than the colon or rectum	
M1c,	The cancer has spread to the peritoneal surface	

Donald F Gleason, 1920–2008, pathologist, The University of Minnesota, Minneapolis, MN, USA.

for stage grouping of cancer. As an example, the TNM clinicopathological staging system for colorectal cancer is shown in *Table 12.3*.

The purpose of staging is twofold: to estimate prognosis and to help select appropriate treatment options. Anatomical staging provides important information as to the surgical resectability of disease and the risk of its recurrence. However, the risk assessment for most cancers is suboptimal and provides a wide confidence interval. Better staging techniques are entering care, such as the determination of circulating tumour DNA (ctDNA) in the blood of postoperative patients. Patients who demonstrate ctDNA postoperatively have a substantially higher risk of relapse than patients who do not. This information may be useful in the future to select patients who should be offered further treatment to eliminate residual tumour cells and, of equal importance, to identify patients with a low chance of relapse who can avoid further treatment.

Therapeutic decision making and the multidisciplinary team

As the management of cancer becomes more complex, it becomes impossible for an individual clinician to have the competence that is necessary to manage all patients presenting with a particular type of tumour. The formation of multidisciplinary teams represents an attempt to make certain that each and every patient with a particular type of cancer is managed appropriately. Teams should not only be multidisciplinary – they should also be multiprofessional. The advantages and disadvantages of multidisciplinary teams are summarised in *Table 12.4*.

The multidisciplinary team needs to answer three basic questions for every patient:

- What is the patient's diagnosis, stage and molecular characteristics of disease?
- What is the goal of treatment for the patient? In simple terms, this can be divided into cure, prolongation of life and palliation of symptoms.
- What treatment options are there to achieve these aims with the fewest possible side effects? Options may include surgery, radiotherapy, anti-cancer systemic (drug) treatment, symptom control measures, a combination of these options and, in some cases, observation.

It is important to realise that the multidisciplinary team makes recommendations, rather than definite treatment decisions. Several other factors must be considered, which can only be done by a clinician making a direct assessment of the patient's health and wishes. The clinician must ascertain the patient's fitness and hence their ability to tolerate treatment. This will be heavily influenced by comorbidities. Patients vary greatly in their willingness to tolerate treatment for a given benefit and particularly how they value quality of life compared with length of life or chance of cure.

There are often several possible treatment plans and the clinical team must take the time to explain the options carefully to the patient and the patient's supporters. In many cancer centres, there will be both standard-of-care and research options available for patients. Explanations should include what is involved in the treatment, what benefits may result and the chance of the patient receiving those benefits. The clinical team must also explain the possible downsides of treatment and the likelihood of experiencing them. Patients are often faced with a large amount of complex and difficult information at a time when they are extremely vulnerable. The clinical team must support patients to reach a decision and this may take time and repeated explanation.

Principles of cancer surgery

For most solid tumours, surgery remains the definitive treatment and the only realistic hope of cure. However, surgery has many roles in cancer treatment from diagnosis, prevention, removal of primary disease, removal of metastatic disease, reconstruction through to palliation of symptoms.

Role in diagnosis and staging

In most, but not all, patients the diagnosis of cancer has been confirmed by biopsy before definitive surgery is carried out; however, occasionally a surgical procedure is required to make the diagnosis, e.g. in renal cell cancer where not all patients with a renal mass will undergo a biopsy, prior to definitive surgery to remove and diagnose the tumour as either malignant or benign. Laparoscopic surgery is used as part of the staging of intra-abdominal malignancy, particularly oesophageal and gastric cancer. By this means it is often possible to diagnose widespread peritoneal disease and small liver metastases that may have been missed on cross-sectional imaging. Laparoscopic

TABLE 12.4 The advantages and disadvantages of the multidisciplinary team.

Advantages	Disadvantages
Open debate concerning management of complex patients with many specialists	Less confident and less articulate members of the team may not be able to express their views, even though their views may be extremely important
Decision making is open, transparent and explicit	May become a rubber-stamping exercise in which the class solutions implied by guidelines are applied to disparate individuals
Team members educate each other	Decisions are made in the absence of patients and their carers
A useful educational experience for trainees and students	Clinicians are able to avoid having to take responsibility for their decisions and their actions – 'corporate responsibility'
Performance can be monitored by managers	Time-consuming and resource intensive: takes multiple busy clinicians away from clinical practice for hours at a time

Summary box 12.3

Potential members of the cancer multidisciplinary team

- Site-specialist surgeon
- Surgical oncologist
- Plastic and reconstructive surgeon
- Clinical oncologist/radiotherapist
- Medical oncologist
- Diagnostic radiologist
- Interventional radiologist
- Palliative care physician
- Pathologist
- Speech therapist
- Physiotherapist
- Prosthetist
- Clinical nurse specialist (rehabilitation, supportive care)
- Clinical trial team representative
- Palliative care nurse
- Social worker/counsellor
- Medical secretary/administrator
- Multidisciplinary team coordinator

ultrasound is a particularly useful adjunct for the diagnosis of intrahepatic metastases. Other examples of when surgery is central to the diagnosis of cancer include orchidectomy, in a patient suspected of testicular cancer; lymph node biopsy in a patient with lymphoma; and sentinel node biopsy in melanoma and breast cancer.

Removal of primary disease

Radical surgery for cancer involves removal of the primary tumour and as much of the surrounding tissue and lymph node drainage as possible in order not only to ensure local control but also to prevent spread of tumour through the lymphatics. Although the principle of local control is still extremely important, it is now recognised that ultra-radical surgery probably has little effect on the development of metastatic disease, as evidenced by the randomised trials of radical versus simple mastectomy for breast cancer. It is important, however, to appreciate that high-quality, meticulous surgery taking care not to disrupt the primary tumour at the time of excision is of the utmost importance in obtaining a cure in localised disease and in preventing local recurrence.

Removal of metastatic disease

Under certain circumstances surgery for metastatic disease may be appropriate. This is particularly true for liver metastases arising from colorectal cancer where successful resection of all detectable disease can lead to long-term survival in about one-third of patients. With multiple liver metastases, it may still be possible to take a surgical approach by using *in situ* ablation with cryotherapy or radiofrequency energy. Another situation in which surgery may be curative in metastatic disease is that of pulmonary resection for isolated lung metastases, particularly from renal cell carcinoma.

Palliation

In many cases surgery is not appropriate for cure but may be valuable for palliation. A good example of this is the patient with a symptomatic primary tumour who also has distant metastases, e.g. a patient with a large, symptomatic renal cell cancer but diffuse metastatic disease. In this case, removal of the primary will increase the patient's quality of life but will have little effect on the ultimate outcome.

Principles underlying the non-surgical treatment of cancer

Medical and clinical (radiation) oncology are rapidly changing fields. Both understanding of cancer and the technology available are expanding at a rapid pace. Nevertheless, there are basic principles that remain constant. These are to ascertain as precisely as possible the diagnosis, stage of disease and molecular characteristics of the tumour and, from this information, assess via the multidisciplinary team the management options for the patient. In general terms, where a local treatment, i.e. surgery or ablation, is as effective as a systemic treatment, the local treatment will be preferred. The range of options will be specific to each tumour type and is constantly evolving. This is most true of the systemic therapy options available to patients.

The purposes of oncology treatment can be conveniently divided into:

- **curative primary**: the effect of non-surgical treatment alone is highly effective, e.g. head and neck cancers (***Table 12.5***);
- **neoadjuvant**: where non-surgical treatment prior to surgery can substantially reduce the morbidity of treatment and increase its chances of success, e.g. radiotherapy to downstage rectal carcinoma prior to surgery;
- **adjuvant**: where non-surgical treatment after surgery can increase the chance of cure, e.g. radiotherapy and chemotherapy after breast cancer;
- **life-prolonging/palliative**: these terms are better separated, especially in the case of life-prolonging treatments in a non-curative setting that may add years to life, e.g. use of olaparib in *BRCA*-mutated ovarian cancer.

Systemic therapies

In recent decades, drug development has evolved from screening large libraries of chemicals for their ability to interfere with cellular processes. Increased understanding of the molecular pathophysiology of cancers has identified key molecules essential to tumour function. Many of these molecules can be inhibited and are termed 'druggable targets'. Three-dimensional characterisation of these targets and synthesis of molecules to inhibit them has produced a large number of highly effective targeted therapies. The pace of change is sufficiently rapid that it is now only possible for an individual clinician to keep abreast of developments in a limited number of cancers.

The following principles are key in decision making over systemic therapy administration to individual patients:

TABLE 12.5 Examples of malignancies that may be cured without the need for surgical excision.

Malignancy	Potentially curative treatment
Leukaemia	Chemotherapy (+/– radiotherapy)
Lymphoma	Chemotherapy (+/– radiotherapy)
Small cell lung cancer	Chemotherapy (+/– radiotherapy)
Tumours of childhood (rhabdomyosarcoma, Wilms' tumour)	Chemotherapy (+/– radiotherapy)
Early laryngeal cancer	Radiotherapy
Advanced head and neck cancer	Chemoradiation (synchronous chemotherapy and radiotherapy)
Oesophageal cancer	Chemoradiation (synchronous chemotherapy and radiotherapy)
Squamous cell cancer of the anus	Chemoradiation (synchronous chemotherapy and radiotherapy)
Advanced cancer of the cervix	Radiotherapy (+/– chemotherapy)
Medulloblastoma	Radiotherapy (+/– chemotherapy)
Skin tumours (BCC, SCC)	Radiotherapy

BCC, basal cell carcinoma; SCC, squamous cell carcinoma.

- Assess the fitness and willingness of the patient to tolerate each of these options.
  Most cancers occur in middle-aged or older patients. The older a patient is, the more likely they are to have comorbidities or be frail. It is important to note that middle-aged patients may be unfit or have serious comorbidities and that older patients may actually be very fit. Organ dysfunction and frailty may substantially increase the risks of treatment and reduce its chance of success. This must be assessed on an individual basis.
- Support the patient to understand the options and choose the most appropriate management approach.
  Discussions about prognosis and treatment options are complex, difficult and any decisions made are often irrevocable. They also take place when the patient and their family are at their most anxious and vulnerable. It is often necessary to provide information in digestible amounts and to do so repeatedly. There are few oncological situations where an immediate decision needs to be taken by the patient.
  The difficulties of drawing a balance between risk and benefit are illustrated by considering adjuvant therapy for a solid malignancy. In the absence of a good test to ascertain individual risk of relapse, it is necessary to treat large numbers of patients to benefit a small proportion, often around 10% (***Figure 12.5***). Although 10% is a small proportion, it represents a small chance of a major benefit, namely cure. If there were a test that could accurately determine patients with no residual disease after resection, then a lower proportion of patients would need to have adjuvant therapy, each of whom would have a higher chance of benefit (***Figures 12.5 and 12.6***).
- Frequently reassess the balance of risk and benefit during treatment.
  For patients receiving repeated cycles of treatment, there are three key questions to consider before proceeding with the next cycle of treatment:

  1. **Is the treatment working**? Where there is measurable disease, this is usually assessed by radiological restaging at intervals of 6–12 weeks. The test for whether the treatment is working will depend on the goals of treatment: if the goal is stabilisation of disease then it may be sufficient that the tumour is not growing; if the goal is elimination of disease then progressive shrinkage of the radiological abnormalities will be necessary.
  2. **Is the patient tolerating treatment?** This can only be discovered by asking the patient what side effects they are experiencing. Clinicians should be used to detecting and managing the side effects of the drugs they are prescribing. In addition to open questions, the clinician should enquire specifically about common or dangerous side effects. If the patient is not tolerating treatment, then it may be necessary to delay the next cycle or to reduce the dose, even though this may be at the expense of reducing the effectiveness of treatment.
  3. **Is it safe to give the next cycle of treatment?** To answer this question, the clinician will have to assess what side effects the patient is experiencing and also ensure that laboratory measures are within acceptable limits. The necessary laboratory tests will commonly include full blood count, urea and electrolytes and liver function tests as well as other tests determined by which treatments are being used.

The range of non-surgical anti-cancer treatments

Radiotherapy

Half of all patients will receive radiotherapy during their cancer journey. The mechanism of action of radiotherapy is that ionising radiation causes single- and double-stranded DNA breaks. Cells most sensitive to radiotherapy are in mitosis or late G2 in the cell cycle. Damage may be caused by the direct effect of the ionising radiation on the DNA. However, the predominant therapeutic effect is indirect, and is achieved by ionising radiation causing the creation of oxygen free radicals, which then damage the DNA. The fact that the indirect damage is predominant explains why hypoxic cells are relatively resistant to radiotherapy. In practice, adequate

Max Wilms, 1867–1918, Professor of Surgery, Heidelberg, Germany.

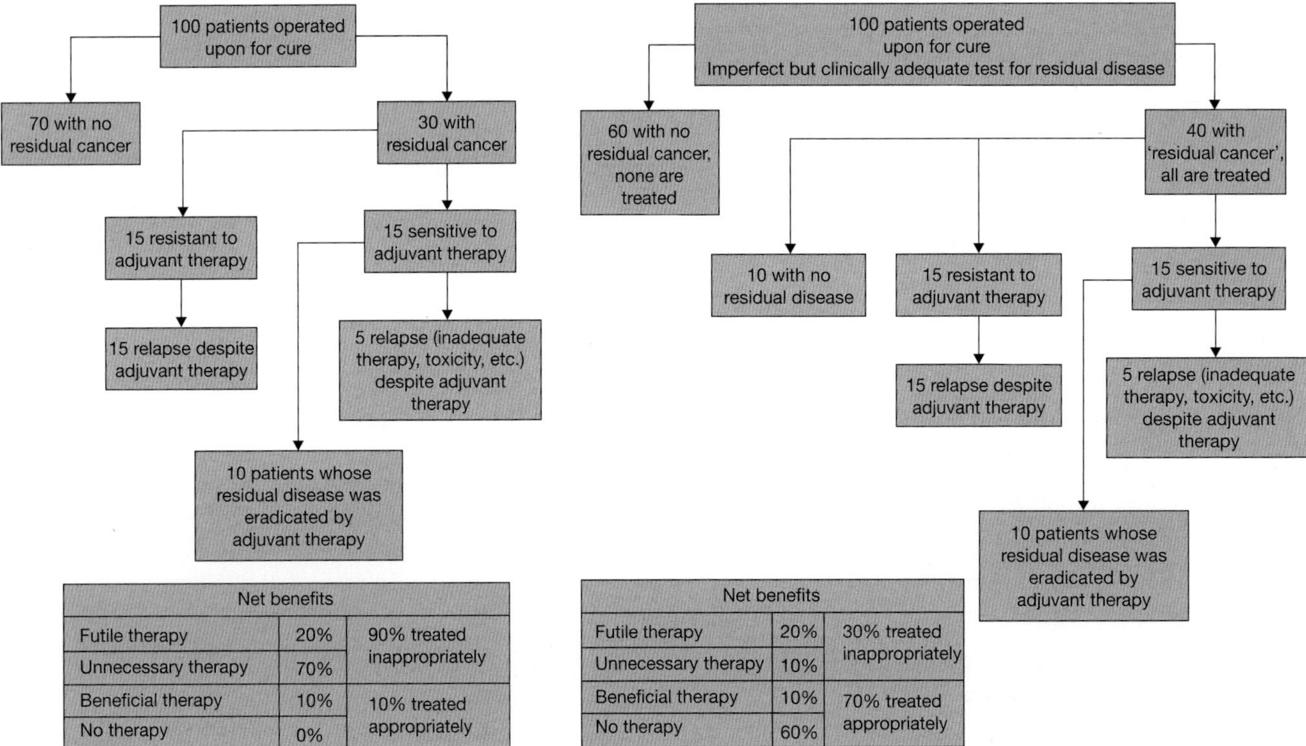

Figure 12.5 The concept of adjuvant chemotherapy.

Figure 12.6 The concept of adjuvant chemotherapy and testing for minimal residual disease.

oxygenation of tissues is assisted by simple measures such as correcting anaemia prior to radiotherapy.

Cancer types differ greatly in their sensitivity to radiotherapy. Similarly, higher doses of radiotherapy are needed to control bulky disease (~70 Gy) than to eliminate residual tumour cells (~50 Gy) or to palliate symptoms (~30 Gy).

Radiotherapy is mainly used as a localised treatment (***Figure 12.7***). The target area is defined by imaging, which will include anatomical imaging, such as CT and MRI, to identify the tumour mass, neighbouring structures and landmarks for radiotherapy planning. Sometimes functional imaging, such as PET, is used to further define structures that should be included in the radiation field such as lymph nodes containing small volumes of tumour, whose metabolic signature is detected by PET. The planning and technical set-up of radiotherapy is a highly specialised subject. Planning can be extremely difficult and time-consuming, e.g. in the treatment of head and neck cancer, where the treatment intent is curative but there are multiple vital and highly sensitive structures close to the target area.

In general terms, the radiotherapy team will aim to provide a uniform therapeutic radiation dose to the target area, while sparing adjacent structures from significant damage. The most common form of treatment is external beam radiotherapy in which x-rays are aimed at the target volume from an external source. Where necessary, modern radiotherapy can employ sophisticated computer programs and algorithms to sculpt the shape of the treatment volume. It is now possible to irradiate irregularly shaped target volumes using techniques such as intensity-modulated radiation therapy (IMRT) and image-guided radiation therapy (IGRT). The ability to give high fractional doses in this way has led to the development of stereotactic ablative radiotherapy (SAbR), in which a small number of fractions can be used to treat primary tumours, or isolated metastases, to curative dose levels.

Other ways of targeting the tumour volume include brachytherapy, in which the radiation source is brought very close to the tumour by insertion of radioactive seeds, and radionuclide therapy, in which a radioactive source is concentrated at the tumour site.

One of the main problems in determining the optimal schedule of radiation is that there is a dissociation between the acute effects on normal tissues and the late damage. The acute reaction is not a reliable guide to the adverse consequences of treatment in the longer term. Since the late effects following irradiation can take over 20 years to develop, this poses an obvious difficulty: if a radiation schedule is changed it will be known within 2 or 3 years whether or not the new schedule has improved tumour control; it may, however, be two decades before it is known, with any degree of certainty, whether or not the new technique is safe.

Anti-cancer drugs

The classes of anti-cancer drugs, their modes of action and clinical indications are summarised in ***Table 12.6***.

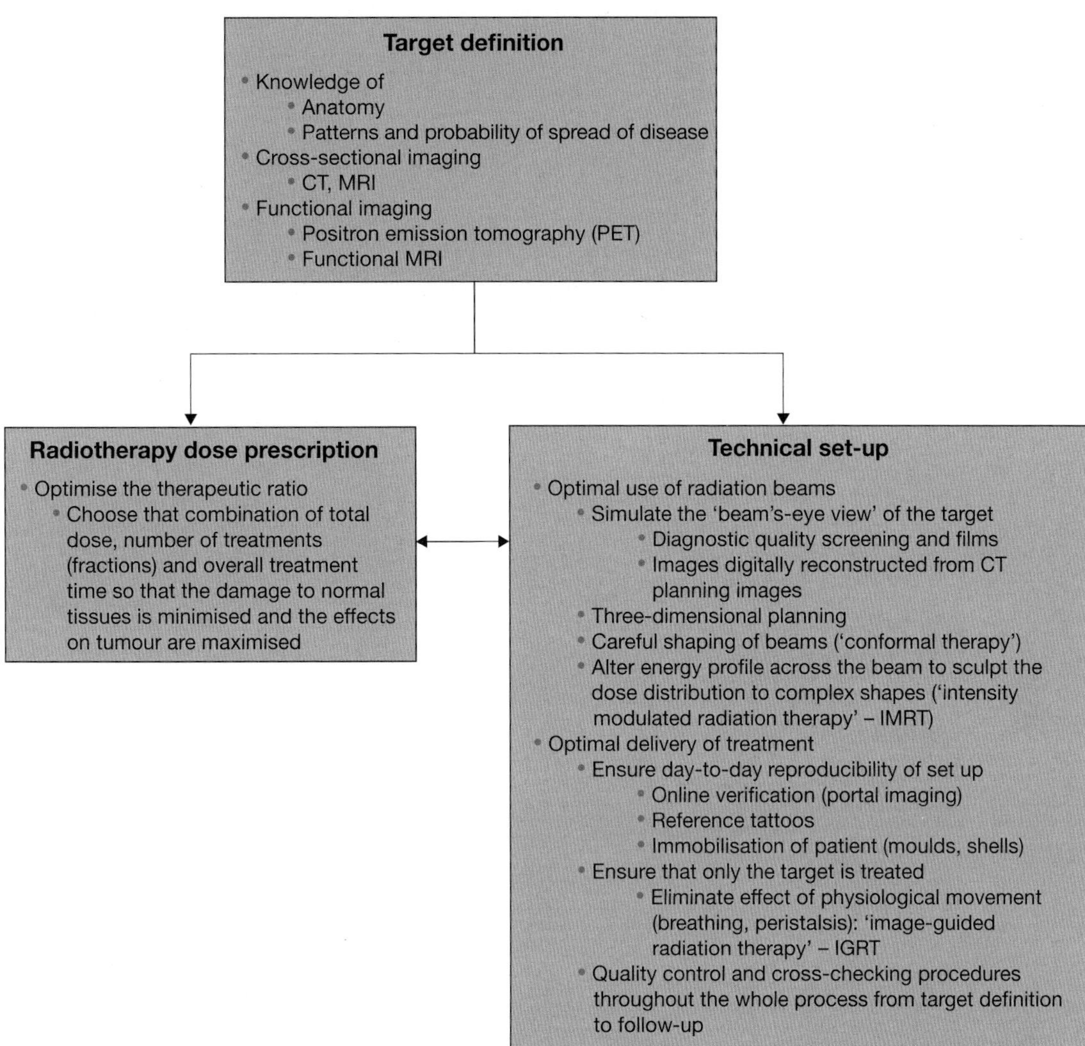

Figure 12.7 The processes involved in clinical radiotherapy. CT, computed tomography; MRI, magnetic resonance imaging.

TABLE 12.6 Examples of anti-cancer drugs currently in use.

Class	Examples	Putative mode of action	Tumour types that may be sensitive to drug
Drugs that interfere with mitosis	Vincristine Vinblastine	Interfere with formation of microtubules: 'spindle poisons'	Lymphomas Leukaemias Brain tumours Sarcomas
	Taxanes: paclitaxel docetaxel cabazitaxel	Stabilise microtubules	Breast cancer Non-small cell lung cancer Ovarian cancer Prostate cancer Head and neck cancer
Drugs that interfere with DNA synthesis (antimetabolites)	5-Fluorouracil Capecitabine	Inhibition of thymidylate synthase, false substrate for both DNA and RNA synthesis	Breast cancer GI cancer
	Methotrexate	Inhibition of dihydrofolate reductase	Breast cancer Bladder cancer Lymphomas Cervical cancer
	6-Mercaptopurine 6-Thioguanine	Inhibit *de novo* purine synthesis	Leukaemias

Continued

TABLE 12.6 Examples of anti-cancer drugs currently in use – *continued*.

Class	Examples	Putative mode of action	Tumour types that may be sensitive to drug
Drugs that interfere with DNA synthesis (antimetabolites) – *continued*	Cytosine arabinoside	False substrate in DNA synthesis	Leukaemias Lymphomas
	Gemcitabine	Inhibits ribonucleotide reductase	Non-small lung cancer Pancreatic cancer
Drugs that directly damage DNA or interfere with its function	Mitomycin C	DNA cross-linking, preferentially active at sites of low oxygen tension (a bioreductive drug)	Anal cancer Bladder cancer Gastric cancer Head and neck cancer Rectal cancer
	Cisplatin Carboplatin	Form adducts between DNA strands and interferes with replication	Germ cell tumours Ovarian cancer Non-small cell lung cancer Head and neck cancer Oesophageal cancer
	Oxaliplatin	Forms adducts between DNA strands and interferes with replication	Colorectal cancer
	Doxorubicin	Intercalates between DNA strands and interferes with replication	Breast cancer Lymphomas Sarcomas Kaposi's sarcoma
	Cyclophosphamide	A prodrug converted via hepatic cytochrome p450 to phosphoramide mustard. Causes DNA cross-links	Breast cancer Lymphomas Sarcomas
	Ifosfamide	Related to cyclophosphamide, causes DNA cross-links	Small cell lung cancer Sarcomas
	Bleomycin	DNA strand breakage via formation of metal complex	Germ cell tumours Lymphomas
	Irinotecan	Inhibits topoisomerase 1, prevents DNA from unwinding and repairing during replication	Colorectal cancer
	Etoposide	Inhibits topoisomerase 2, prevents DNA from unwinding and repairing during replication	Small cell lung cancer Germ cell tumours Lymphomas
	Dacarbazine	A nitrosourea that requires activation by hepatic cytochrome p450. Methylates guanine residues in DNA	Brain tumours Sarcoma
	Temozolomide	A nitrosourea but, unlike dacarbazine, does not require activation by hepatic cytochrome p450. Methylates guanine residues in DNA	Glioblastoma multiforme
	Actinomycin D	Intercalation between DNA strands, DNA strand breaks	Rhabdomyosarcoma Wilms' tumour
DNA damage response inhibitors	Olaparib Niraparib Rucaparib	Inhibit DNA repair by PARP, especially in *BRCA*-mutated cancers	Ovarian cancer Breast cancer Prostate cancer
Hormones	Tamoxifen	Blocks oestrogen receptors	Breast cancer
	Anastrozole Letrozole Exemestane	Aromatase inhibitors that block postmenopausal (non-ovarian) oestrogen production	Breast cancer
	Leuprolide Goserelin Buserelin	Analogues of gonadotropin-releasing hormone, continued use produces downregulation of the anterior pituitary with consequent fall in testosterone levels	Prostate cancer
	Cabergoline	Blocks prolactin release, a long-acting dopamine agonist	Prolactin-secreting pituitary tumours

Continued

TABLE 12.6 Examples of anti-cancer drugs currently in use – *continued*.

Class	Examples	Putative mode of action	Tumour types that may be sensitive to drug
Hormones – *continued*	Bromocriptine	Dopamine agonist, blocks stimulation of anterior pituitary	Pituitary tumours
	Cyproterone acetate Flutamide Nilutamide Bicalutamide	Block the effect of androgens	Prostate cancer
	Abiraterone Cyproterone acetate	Block testosterone production	Prostate cancer
Inhibitors of receptor tyrosine kinases	Osimertinib Erlotinib Afatinib Gefitinib	Inhibit EGFR tyrosine kinase	Non-small cell lung cancer
	Imatinib	Blocks ability of mutant BCR-ABL fusion protein to bind ATP	Chronic myeloid leukaemia
	Imatinib	Inhibition of mutant c-KIT	GISTs
	Erlotinib	Inhibits EGFR tyrosine kinase	Non-small cell lung cancer Pancreatic cancer
	Sunitinib Regorafenib Lenvatinib	Promiscuous tyrosine kinase inhibitors (PDGFR, VEGFR, KIT, FLT)	Renal cancer GIST refractory to Imatinib Colorectal cancer Thyroid cancer
	Lapatinib	Inhibits tyrosine kinases associated with EGFR and HER2	Breast cancer
	Axitinib	Inhibits tyrosine kinase associated with VEGFR	Renal cancer
Cyclin-dependent kinase inhibitors	Palbociclib	Inhibits growth signal	Breast cancer
Protease inhibitors	Bortezomib	Interferes with proteasomal degradation of regulatory proteins, in particular stops NF-κB from preventing apoptosis	Multiple myeloma
Differentiating agents	All-*trans*-retinoic acid	Induces terminal differentiation	Acute promyelocytic leukaemia
Farnesyl transferase inhibitors	Lonafarnib	Inhibition of farnesyl transferase and consequent inactivation of *ras*-dependent signal transduction	Leukaemia
	Tipifarnib	Inhibition of farnesyl transferase and consequent inactivation of *ras*-dependent signal transduction	Acute leukaemia Myelodysplastic syndrome
Antibodies directed to cell surface antigens	Trastuzumab	Antibody directed against HER2 receptor	Breast cancer
	Cetuximab	Antibody directed against EGFR	Colorectal cancer Head and neck cancer
	Bevacizumab	Antibody directed against VEGFR	Colorectal cancer
	Rituximab	Antibody against CD20 antigen	Lymphomas
	Alemtuzumab	Antibody against CD52 antigen	Lymphomas
Antibody drug conjugates	Trastuzumab deruxtecan	Targets chemotherapy to *Her2* expressing tumour	Breast cancer
	Sacituzumab govitecan	Targets chemotherapy to *Trop2* expressing tumour	Breast cancer
	Enfortumab vedotin	Targets chemotherapy to *Nectin4* expressing tumour	Urothelial cancer
Inducers of apoptosis	Arsenic trioxide	Induces apoptosis by caspase inhibition Inhibition of nitric oxide	Acute promyelocytic leukaemia
	Venetoclax	BH3 mimetic	CML AML Lymphoma

Continued

TABLE 12.6 Examples of anti-cancer drugs currently in use – *continued*.

Class	Examples	Putative mode of action	Tumour types that may be sensitive to drug
Immunological mediators	Ipilimumab	Blocks CTLA-4 and thus releases the brakes on the activation of T cells	Melanoma Lung cancer Renal cancer
	Pembrolizumab Nivolumab Atezolizumab Durvalumab	Block the PD-1 signalling on T lymphocytes and thereby prevents the inhibition of T-cell activation	Melanoma Lung cancer Renal cancer Bladder cancer
	Interferon alpha-2b	Activates macrophages, increases the cytotoxicity of T lymphocytes, inhibits cell division (and viral replication)	Hairy-cell leukaemia
	Thalidomide	Anti-inflammatory, stimulates T cells, antiangiogenic	Myeloma
HDAC inhibitors	Panobinostat Vorinostat	Acetylation of histones is associated with increased transcription of genes; inhibiting deacetylation can decrease expression of mutated or dysregulated genes	Cutaneous T-cell lymphoma
	Entinostat	Acetylation of histones is associated with increased transcription of genes; inhibiting deacetylation can decrease expression of mutated or dysregulated genes	Melanoma
PI3K inhibitors	Idelalisib	Inhibits signalling via the PI3K/AKT/mTOR pathway and thereby switch off stimulus to cellular proliferation	B-cell lymphomas
mTOR inhibitors	Temsirolimus Everolimus	Inhibit mTOR, a key component in the PI3K/AKT/mTOR pathway	Renal cancer Neuroendocrine tumours
MEK inhibitors	Trametinib Selumetinib	Inhibit the MAPK pathway	Melanoma Neurofibroma
RAF inhibitors	Dabrafenib Vemurafenib	Inhibit the MAPK pathway	Melanoma

AML, acute myeloid leukaemia; ATP, adenosine triphosphate; CML, chronic myeloid leukaemia; CTLA-4, cytotoxic T-lymphocyte-associated protein 4; EGFR, epidermal growth factor receptor; FLT3, FMS-like tyrosine kinase; GI, gastrointestinal; GIST, gastrointestinal stromal tumour; HDAC, histone deacetylase; HER2, human epidermal growth factor receptor 2; MAPK, mitogen-activated protein kinase; mTOR, mammalian target of rapamycin; NF, nuclear factor; PARP, poly-ADP ribose polymerase; PD-1, programmed cell death protein 1; PDGFR, platelet-derived growth factor receptor; PI3K, phosphoinositide 3-kinase; RAF, rapidly accelerated fibrosarcoma; TKI, tyrosine kinase inhibitor; VEGFR, vascular endothelial growth factor receptor.

Cytotoxic chemotherapy

Selective toxicity is the fundamental principle underlying cytotoxic chemotherapy. Tumour types vary greatly in their sensitivity to cytotoxic chemotherapy and their vulnerability to drugs with specific mechanisms of action. Treatments are often given for a limited number of treatment days during a cycle of treatment lasting typically 3–4 weeks. This allows the tumour to receive an effective dose while providing sufficient time for the patient to recover in time for the next cycle. Many treatment regimens give a limited number of cycles, typically three to six in total. Other regimens are maintenance treatments, in which an unlimited number of cycles are given.

Hormonal treatments

Several tumour types, notably breast cancer and prostate cancer, are stimulated by endogenous hormones. Removal of this stimulus from sensitive tumours will result in their shrinkage. An understanding of the relevant endocrine pathways has identified several points for therapeutic intervention, including interference with hormone receptors and with hormone production.

Targeted treatments

The explosion of knowledge about the molecular biology of cancer has identified multiple therapeutic targets. This has ushered in an era of highly specific treatments that aim to inhibit a target essential for tumour survival while leaving other tissues unaffected. At present, most targeted therapies are not absolutely specific for their primary target and therefore do have unwanted or 'off-target' side effects. In addition, successful inhibition of the target may have inevitable undesirable consequences in addition to the desired effect, so-called 'on-target' side effects. Many targeted treatments are given in continuous cycles and the dosing and toxicity management strategies are therefore of particular importance.

These treatments will only work if a patient's tumour depends on a therapeutic target. The kinase inhibitor vemurafenib will only be effective in patients with melanoma whose tumours have the V600E *BRAF* mutation; cetuximab is only effective in patients with colorectal cancer who have wild-type (non-mutated) *ras*; imatinib is particularly effective in patients with gastrointestinal stromal tumours who have mutations in exon 11 of the *Kit* gene – patients with mutations in exon 9 may still respond to imatinib but will require higher doses and patients without mutations in *Kit* are far less likely to respond to imatinib.

Treatment choice therefore requires a molecular analysis of the patient's tumour. It is this determination of treatment at the individual level that has led to the concept of 'personalised medicine'. Although major advances have been made, important targets such as *ras* remain elusive at present, although several *ras*-targeted molecules are in development.

Immunotherapy

Treatments to activate the immune system against cancer have a long history, stimulated by the observation that up to half of the volume of certain tumours was known to be made up of immune cells, which appeared to be inactive or dead. There is now an appreciation that multiple malignancies activate mechanisms whose normal purpose is to downregulate the immune system after elimination of an infectious organism. These mechanisms are called T-cell checkpoints. Inhibition of these checkpoints can reactivate the immune cells and has had remarkable success in previously virtually untreatable diseases such as metastatic melanoma. This novel form of treatment is generally much better tolerated than cytotoxic chemotherapy but may result in side effects owing to the uncontrolled activation of the immune system. Side effects such as pneumonitis, colitis, adrenal failure and hypophysitis (pituitary inflammation) may be life-changing or life-threatening and are more common when using a combination of checkpoint inhibitors.

Immunotherapy is a very active field of research and it is likely that vaccines and engineered immune cells will increasingly enter treatment protocols in the coming years.

Principles of combined treatment

Non-surgical treatments are often used in combination. For example, radiotherapy and chemotherapy are often given together as an alternative to surgery, e.g. in the treatment of rectal, cervical, head and neck or brain cancers (***Table 12.5***). The rationale behind combination, as opposed to single-modality therapy, is straightforward and is somewhat analogous to that used for combined antibiotic therapy: it is a strategy designed to combat resistance. By the time of diagnosis many tumours will contain cancer cells that, through spontaneous mutation, have acquired resistance to individual modalities of treatment. Unlike antibiotic resistance, there is no need for previous exposure to the treatment. Spontaneous mutation rates are high enough to allow chance to permit the occurrence, and subsequent expansion, of clones of cells resistant to a treatment to which they have never been exposed. If only single-modality treatments were used, then the further expansion of these *de novo* resistant subclones would limit cure. The problem can be mitigated by, from the outset of treatment, combining treatment modalities.

There are three main principles upon which the choice of drugs for combination therapy is based: (i) use drugs active against the diseases in question; (ii) use drugs with distinct modes of action; (iii) use drugs with non-overlapping toxicities. By using drugs with different biological effects, for example by combining an antimetabolite with an agent that actively damages DNA, it may be possible to obtain a truly synergistic effect, i.e. where the effects of the two modalities together are superior to the additive effects of both separately. It is inadvisable to combine drugs with similar adverse effects: combining two highly myelosuppressive drugs may produce an unacceptably high risk of neutropenic sepsis. Where possible, combinations should be based upon a consideration of the toxicity profiles of the drugs concerned.

In considering the combination of radiotherapy and chemotherapy, radiation could be considered as just another drug. There is, in addition to synergy and toxicity, another factor to consider in the combination of drugs and radiation – the concept of spatial cooperation. Chemotherapy is a systemic treatment, radiotherapy is not. Radiotherapy is, however, able to reach sites, such as the central nervous system and testis, that drugs may not reach effectively. This is why, for example in patients treated primarily with chemotherapy for leukaemias, lymphomas and small cell lung cancer, prophylactic cranial irradiation may be part of the treatment protocol.

Summary box 12.4

Principles of combined treatment

- Use effective agents
- Use agents with different modes of action (synergy)
- Use agents with non-overlapping toxicities
- Consider spatial cooperation

Oncological emergencies

There are a limited number of true emergencies in oncology. Those that require immediate recognition and management are:

- **Cord compression**: rapid diagnosis and management to relieve pressure on the spinal cord is essential to obtain the best results for patients. Ideally, treatment should be instituted when cord compression is threatened rather than when it has already occurred. Management is likely to include steroids and either neurosurgery or radiotherapy.
- **Neutropenic sepsis**: rapid diagnosis and antibiotic therapy are essential. There is a strong inverse relationship between the time taken to start antibiotics and the chance of patient survival.
- **Immune side effects** including hypophysitis, adrenal failure and insulin-dependent diabetes.

In contrast, there are many urgent oncological situations that are very unpleasant for the patient or that can rapidly deteriorate if not recognised quickly. These include thrombosis, effusion, superior vena cava obstruction and pain, among many others.

Life after cancer

As early diagnosis becomes more common and treatment outcomes improve, so an increasing number of people are cured of cancer. However, the impact of a cancer diagnosis and its treatment is profound. Organisations such as UK-based Macmillan Cancer Support can provide information and support to patients facing the health, work and financial sequelae of cancer.

Symptom control and palliative care

The distinction between palliative and curative treatment is not always clear-cut and will become increasingly blurred as professional and public attitudes towards the management of cancer change. Twenty years ago cancer was perceived as a disease that was either cured or it was not; patients either lived or died. There was little appreciation that, for many patients, cancer might be a chronic disease. Nowadays, it is appreciated that many patients will have multiple different treatment options during their cancer journey. Five-year survival is not necessarily tantamount to cure. With the development of targeted therapies that regulate, rather than eradicate, cancer this state of affairs is likely to continue. The aim of treatment will be growth control rather than the extirpation of every last cancer cell. Patients will live with their cancers, perhaps for years. They will die with cancer, but not necessarily of cancer.

Patients fear the symptoms, distress and disruption associated with cancer almost as much as they fear the disease itself. Palliative treatment has as its goal the relief of symptoms. Sometimes this will involve treating the underlying problem, as with palliative radiotherapy for bone metastases; sometimes it will not. Sometimes it may be inappropriate to treat the cancer itself, but that does not imply that there is nothing more to be done – it simply means that there may be better ways to assuage the distress and discomfort caused by the tumour. Palliative medicine in the twenty-first century is about far more than optimal control of pain: its scope is wide and its impact immense (***Table 12.7***). The most important factor in the successful palliative management of a patient with cancer is early referral. Transition between curative and palliative modes of management should be seamless.

Common problems that may be effectively palliated include:

- **Cerebral metastases**: stereotactic radiosurgery for small lesions is highly effective, although limited to patients who are likely to survive long enough to benefit.
- **Effusions**: pleural and ascitic drains may control these chronic problems. In the case of pleural effusion pleurodesis may prevent reaccumulation.
- **Thrombosis**: increased coagulability and pressure on blood vessels make this a common problem in oncology.
- **Hypercalcaemia**: bisphosphonates may control the patient's calcium level and regular infusions will be necessary when the underlying tumour process is not controlled by other means.

TABLE 12.7 An outline of the domains and interventions included within palliative and supportive care.

Holistic needs assessment	Pain, anorexia, fatigue, dyspnoea, etc.	
	Treatment-related toxicity	
Symptom relief	Drugs	
	Surgery	
	Radiotherapy	
	Complementary therapies:	Acupuncture
		Homeopathy
		Aromatherapy, etc.
Psychosocial interventions	Psychological support Relaxation techniques Cognitive behavioural therapy Counselling Group therapy Music therapy Emotional support	
Physical and practical support	Physiotherapy Occupational therapy Speech therapy	
Information and knowledge	Macmillan	
	Maggie's centres	
Nutritional support	Dietary advice	
	Nutritional supplements	
Social support	Patients	
	Relatives and carers	
Financial support	Ensure uptake of entitlements	
	Grants from charities, e.g. Macmillan	
Spiritual support		

- **Fatigue**: this is often a difficult symptom, which is partly due to the tumour and partly due to its treatment. Encouraging aerobic exercise, even at a low level, can improve fatigue and also stimulate appetite.
- **Weight loss**: patients often lose their appetite and consequently lose weight. Eating little and often with food supplements as necessary may be effective in mitigating weight loss.
- **Fever**: recurrent fevers are a feature of certain tumours such as lymphoma and renal cell cancer. Tumour fever must be distinguished from infection and this can often only be done by exclusion.
- **Paraneoplastic syndromes**: these are varied and often difficult to recognise. Management of the underlying malignancy may not necessarily resolve the syndrome.

End-of-life care

End-of-life care is distinct from palliative care. Patients treated palliatively may survive for many years; end-of-life care concerns the last few months of a patient's life. Many issues, such as symptom control, are common to both palliative care and end-of-life care but there are also problems that are specific to the sense of approaching death. These include a heightened sense of spiritual need, profound fear and the specific needs of those who are facing bereavement. The concept of a 'good death' has been embedded in many cultures over many centuries. Healthcare professionals deal with many deaths and sometimes forget that the patient who hopes for a good death has only one chance to get it right. This is why end-of-life care is worth considering in its own right and not as a mere appendage to palliative care.

Summary box 12.5

Issues at the end of life

- Appropriateness of active intervention
- Euthanasia
- Physician-assisted suicide
- Living wills
- Bereavement
- Spirituality
- Support to allow death at home
- The problem of the medicalisation of death

FURTHER READING

Allison JP. Immune checkpoint blockade in cancer therapy: the 2015 Lasker–DeBakey Clinical Medical Research Award. *JAMA* 2015; **314**(11): 1113–14.

Atun R, Jaffray DA, Barton MB *et al.* Expanding global access to radiotherapy. *Lancet Oncol* 2015; **16**(10): 1153–86.

Bailar JC 3rd, Gornik HL. Cancer undefeated. *N Engl J Med* 1997; **336**(19): 1569–74.

Doll R. The Pierre Denoix Memorial Lecture: nature and nurture in the control of cancer. *Eur J Cancer* 1999; **35**(1): 16–23.

Hanahan D, Weinberg RA. The hallmarks of cancer. *Cell* 2000; **100**(1): 57–70.

Hanahan D, Weinberg RA. Hallmarks of cancer: the next generation. *Cell* 2011; **144**(5): 646–74.

Martincorena I, Raine KM, Gerstung M *et al.* Universal patterns of selection in cancer and somatic tissues. *Cell* 2017; **171**(5): 1029–41.

Meara JG, Leather AJM, Hagander L *et al.* Global surgery 2030: evidence and solutions for achieving health, welfare, and economic development. *Lancet* 2015; **386**(9993): 569–624.

Murtaza M, Dawson SJ, Tsui D *et al.* Non-invasive analysis of acquired resistance to cancer therapy by sequencing of plasma DNA. *Nature* 2013; **497**(7447): 108–12.

Solda F, Lodge M, Ashley S *et al.* Stereotactic radiotherapy (SABR) for the treatment of primary non-small cell lung cancer; systematic review and comparison with a surgical cohort. *Radiother Oncol* 2013; **109**(1): 1–7.

Tomasetti C, Vogelstein B. Cancer etiology. Variation in cancer risk among tissues can be explained by the number of stem cell divisions. *Science* 2015; **347**(6217): 78–81.

Tree AC, Khoo VS, Eeles RA *et al.* Stereotactic body radiotherapy for oligometastases. *Lancet Oncol* 2013; **14**(1): e28–e37.

Weinberg RA. *The biology of cancer*, 2nd edn. New York, London: Garland Science, 2013.

Wu S, Powers S, Zhu W, Hannun YA. Substantial contribution of extrinsic risk factors to cancer development. *Nature* 2016; **529**(7584): 43–7.

CHAPTER 13 Surgical audit and research

Learning objectives

To understand:
- The planning and conduct of surgical audit and research
- How to write up a project
- How to review a journal article and determine its value

INTRODUCTION

Surgeons are innovators and a key aspect of a surgical career is to constantly adapt, tweak and improve surgical techniques and treatments to provide the best outcomes for those under our care. In addition, few others in the hospital use more technology or devices on a day-to-day basis than surgeons. It is therefore beholden upon all surgeons to be able to critically evaluate both our individual performance and the impact of adaptations in techniques, devices and treatment pathways on the individual and collective outcomes of our patients.

Involvement in research and audit activities will form a stable cornerstone within a long and successful surgical career. The aim of this chapter is to outline both how to undertake a successful audit cycle and how to design and conduct a surgical research study. Key aspects associated with enhanced chances of a successful project are discussed, including how collaboration with others can be crucial.

Large numbers of clinical papers appear in the surgical literature every year. Many are flawed, and it is important that a surgeon has the skills to examine publications critically. The best way to develop a critical understanding of the research and audit undertaken by others is to perform studies of one's own. The hardest part of audit and research is writing it up, and the hardest article to write is the first. This chapter contains the information required to write a surgical paper and to evaluate the publications of others.

AUDIT OR RESEARCH?

Health professionals are expected to undertake audit and service evaluation as part of quality assurance. These usually involve minimal additional risk, burden or intrusion for participants. It is important to determine at an early stage whether a project is audit or research, and sometimes that is not as easy as it seems. The decision will determine the framework in which the study is undertaken. In the UK, the Health Research Authority (HRA) has developed a decision tool to help decide whether your project is classified as research (http://www.hra-decisiontools.org.uk/research/). This tool crystallises the differentiation between audit and research to three overarching questions:

1. Are the participants in your study randomised to different groups?
2. Does your study protocol demand changing treatment/care/services from accepted standards for any of the patients/service users involved?
3. Is your study designed to produce generalisable or transferable findings?

Although the first two questions are simple to comprehend, the third can create some confusion at times. The HRA states that, in this context, 'generalisable' means the findings can be reliably extrapolated from the study to a broader population of patients/service users and/or applied to settings or contexts other than those in which they were tested. The majority of audits can be assumed to be hypothesis generating as they would require subsequent prospective testing in a new population before findings could be considered as new 'evidence' – as such they do not fulfil this generalisability criterion. Finally, in this context, 'transferable' means that the findings of a qualitative study can be assumed to be applicable to a similar context or setting. Most qualitative studies are not usually generalisable but can quite often be considered to be transferable.

Further useful information on classifying your proposed project can be found in the HRA leaflet 'Differentiating clinical audit, service evaluation, research and usual practice/surveillance work in public health' (http://www.hra-decisiontools.org.uk/research/docs/DefiningResearchTable_Oct2017-1.pdf).

AUDIT AND SERVICE EVALUATION

Clinical audit is a process used by clinicians who seek to improve patient care. The process involves comparing aspects of care (structure, process and outcome) against explicit criteria and defined standards. Keeping track of personal outcome data and contributing to a clinical database ensures that a surgeon's own performance is monitored continuously and can be compared with a national data set to ensure compliance with agreed standards. Involvement in active audit processes is also an essential component of revalidation for the individual surgeon in the UK. If care falls short of the guidance standard being compared against, some change in the way that care is organised should be proposed. This change may be required at one of many levels. It might be an individual who needs training or surgical equipment that needs replacing. At times, the change may need to take place at the team level. Sometimes, the only appropriate action is change at an institutional level (e.g. a new antibiotic policy), regional level (provision of a tertiary referral centre) or, indeed, national level (screening programmes and health education campaigns).

There are two main types of audit in common practice – single site/local audits and multisite regional, national or international audits. Both are designed to improve the quality of care. In an ideal world local audits might identify needs closest to the patient, which can then be further investigated in multisite larger scale audits. For example, hospital topics are often identified at departmental morbidity and mortality meetings, where issues relating to patient care are discussed. The reporting process might identify a possible national issue, and a national or international audit could be designed to be delivered by local surgical teams.

Audits are formal processes that require a structure. The following steps are essential to establish an audit cycle:

1. Define the audit question in a multidisciplinary team.
2. Identify the body of evidence and current standards.
3. Design the audit to measure performance against agreed standards based on strong evidence. Seek appropriate advice (local audit department in the UK) and ensure institutions have agreed to undertake the audit.
4. Measure over an agreed interval.
5. Analyse results and compare performance against agreed standards.
6. Undertake gap analysis:
   a. if all standards are reached, reaudit after an agreed interval;
   b. if there is a need for improvement, identify possible interventions such as training, and agree with the involved parties.
7. Reaudit.

A new type of audit that has developed significant traction in surgery over recent years is the 'multicentre snapshot audit', whereby many collaborators across multiple hospitals prospectively collate anonymised patient-level data for a specific condition, presentation or intervention over a short time period of normally around 6–8 weeks. This allows exploration of differences in patients, techniques and management across the cohort to identify areas of practice variability that may result in apparent differences in outcome. These studies generate hypotheses and identify areas where further prospective research is needed. Key advantages of these snapshot audits are their easy accessibility and the fact that they can be conducted at almost zero cost, so they can be an excellent means of bringing a new group together to collaborate and create contemporaneous and 'real-world' data together.

IDENTIFYING A RESEARCH TOPIC

Research is designed to generate new knowledge and might involve testing a new treatment or regimen. Once an idea has been formed, or a question asked, it needs to be transformed into a hypothesis. It is helpful to approach surgeons who regularly publish articles and who have a special interest in the subject area being considered. As ideas are suggested, it is important to consider whether the question posed really matters. Spending time refining the question (hypothesis) is probably the most important part of the process. Choosing the wrong topic can lead to many wasted hours. Once a topic has been identified, it is also important not rush into the study. The worst possible outcome is to find at the end of a long arduous study that the research has already been performed or that the chosen methodology did not support investigation of the primary/secondary outcomes.

The first port of call for information is the Internet (with assistance as needed from a medical librarian). Current articles about the proposed research should be retrieved; review articles and meta-analyses can be particularly helpful. It is very important to learn how to do an accurate and efficient search as early as possible. Collections of reviews are available – the Cochrane Collaboration brings together evidence-based medical information and is available in most libraries. Once information on the subject has been obtained and the relevant literature identified, it is important that these are carefully perused. It is not sufficient to just read the abstract! Further information is given in ***Table 13.1***.

An excellent source of ideas where research is needed can come from reviewing high-quality national guidelines such as those produced by the UK National Institute for Health and Care Excellence (NICE) on a particular area of interest, many of which include a section beneath the headline guidance being made on 'recommendations for research'. This section is populated after the currently available evidence for an intervention or treatment has been reviewed by the expert team and found lacking. Designing a research project to cover one or more of these agreed areas can be easily justified to both funders and clinicians alike.

Finally, there is an increased number of Priority Setting Partnerships across all aspects of surgery, including those formally undertaken by the James Lind Alliance and by others run by surgical associations and their patient–partner groups. These partnerships consist of patients, carers, healthcare professionals and organisations or charities representing people with the particular condition. They focus on identifying and prioritising research gaps or important specific questions for

---

Archibald Leman Cochrane, 1909–1988, Director of the UK Medical Research Council Epidemiology Unit, Cardiff, UK, after whom the Cochrane Collaboration is named.

TABLE 13.1 Electronic information sites.

Database	Producer	Coverage	Availability
PubMed http://www.ncbi.nlm.nih.gov/pubmed	US National Library of Medicine (NLM)	PubMed comprises more than 25 million citations for biomedical literature from MEDLINE, life science journals and online books Citations may include links to full-text content from PubMed Central and publisher websites	Internet
PubMed Central http://www.ncbi.nlm.nih.gov/pmc	US National Institutes of Health (NIH) free digital archive	Full-text archive of biomedical and life sciences journal literature at the US National Institutes of Health's National Library of Medicine	Internet
EMBASE http://embase.com	EMBASE	Providing extensive coverage of peer-reviewed biomedical literature, along with indexing, searching and information management tools	Subscription
CINAHL https://www.ebsco.com/products/research-databases/cinahl-database	CINAHL is owned and operated by EBSCO Publishing	Cumulated index to nursing and allied health literature	Subscription
Cochrane Collaboration and Library http://uk.cochrane.org	Global independent network of researchers, professionals, patients, carers and people interested in health to produce credible, accessible health information that is free from commercial sponsorship and other conflicts of interest	Preparing, updating and promoting the accessibility of Cochrane Reviews published online in The Cochrane Library	Internet

which additional new research is needed to answer them. Again, creating research projects in these areas is likely to be well received; sometimes such studies are also prioritised for funding support.

It is also helpful to seek support from specific networks set up to support health research. In the UK, the National Institute for Health Research (NIHR) runs the Research Design Service (RDS), which provides free and confidential advice on research design, writing funding applications and obtaining public engagement in research for all researchers. There are also a number of training courses available in research methodology and application.

FORMING A TEAM

One of the most common reasons for the failure of an otherwise good research project is failure to involve others. Only the smallest single-centre project can be delivered by an individual researcher working alone; almost any project worth doing will need a team to deliver it. This team can bring the necessary skills and experience to help bring the project to fruition but also, and perhaps more importantly, it can provide the momentum required to keep pushing a project through to completion when the inevitable hurdles are met.

There may be local colleagues who form a natural team for a project, perhaps with the oversight of an experienced trainer or mentor. Another solution can be to get involved in a collaborative research group. Surgery has led the way with collaborative research working over recent years.

The first trainee-level research collaborative in the UK was formed in 2008 when a group of surgical trainees who shared the same frustrations around the challenges of conducting high-quality research while engaged in a full-time training programme came together to create the West Midlands Research Collaborative (WMRC). The premise was simple: to create and conduct prospective research projects that simultaneously collate data from across all of the members' units and to take advantage of the rotation of trainees' postings between units to ensure project longevity and thus enable longer term outcome collection. By achieving a critical mass of engaged members in these projects, the collective momentum ensured completion even if individuals were unable to personally contribute in a consistent manner because of examinations, family life or busy clinical periods. Such research collaboratives can be most effective in undertaking two key types of study: (i) simple randomised controlled trials (RCTs) and (ii) multicentre snapshot audits (see ***Audit and service evaluation***).

The first RCT undertaken by the WMRC was the ROSSINI trial, which explored the clinical effectiveness of a simple wound-edge protection device in reducing wound infections after abdominal surgery. A network of trainees mobilised 21 units for the trial and together they completed the trial 2 months ahead of schedule, having randomised 760 patients over a 23-month period, completing in January 2013. This achievement galvanised the research collaborative model and stimulated other new groups to form.

There are now general surgical research collaboratives in every region of the UK and national collaboratives for each surgical subspeciality area such as neurosurgery and cardiothoracic surgery. Many other countries with rotational surgical training programmes have also formed their own parallel collaboratives, including Australia, Portugal, Italy, The Netherlands and Canada. The collaborative movement has established a new paradigm for evidence-based surgical practice, engaged thousands of surgical trainees and their consultant mentors and created an active network of research active clinicians at many hospitals across the world.

In the UK, trainee collaboratives have, to date, developed at least 10 RCTs and been awarded competitive grant funding worth over £8 million. The model has also extended to medical student collaboratives (STARSurg), and all 42 medical schools in the UK now have an active network student research collaborative. More recently, similar research collaboratives have also formed, utilising the established core principles, in non-surgical specialities such as anaesthetics, gastroenterology and elderly care.

All of these collaborative groups work on a principle of complete inclusivity – any interested person is very welcome to get involved in the collaborative; both in existing projects and in suggesting new ideas. People can join at any stage from medical student to consultant. Anyone interested in surgical research should seek out their local or national surgical research collaborative group and get involved.

PROJECT DESIGN

During the first phase, it is important to keep in the mind some important questions (***Summary box 13.1***).

Summary box 13.1

Questions to answer before undertaking research

- Why do the study?
- Will it answer a useful question?
- Is it practical?
- Can it be accomplished in the available time and with the available resources?
- Will the project benefit from collaboration to increase numbers or make best use of high-technology equipment?
- What findings are expected?
- What are the research governance requirements?
- What are the ethical issues?
- What impact could it have?

There are many different types of scientific study. The design used depends on the study. Time spent carefully designing a potential project is never wasted. An RCT is regarded as one of the best methods of scientific research; however, much surgical practice has been advanced through other different types of study such as those listed in ***Table 13.2***. For example, testing a new type of operation often requires a pilot study to assess feasibility, which is then followed by a formal RCT. The introduction of innovative surgical techniques may require novel handling, and recommendations have been made by the IDEAL collaborators (see ***Further reading***).

Research can be qualitative or quantitative. Quantitative research allows hard facts to speak for themselves. A medical condition is analysed systematically using hard, objective end points such as death or major complications, which should be clearly defined. For example, surgical complications are now classified using the Clavien–Dindo system. In qualitative research, data often come from patient narratives, and the psychosocial impact of the disease and its treatment are analysed; for example, narratives from patients with breast cancer. These kinds of data are often collected using quality-of-life measurements. A variety of different quality-of-life questionnaires exist to suit several different clinical situations. Much of the best research is both quantitative and qualitative. Recently, the importance of outcomes from the patient's perspective has been emphasised: patient-reported outcome measures (PROMs) are now an important component of the evaluation of surgical procedures.

TABLE 13.2 Types of study.

Type of study	Definition
Observational	Evaluation of condition or treatment in a defined population
	Retrospective: analysis of past events
	Prospective: contemporaneous collection of data
Case–control	Series of patients with a particular disease or condition compared with matched control patients
Cross-sectional	Measurements made on a single occasion, not looking at the whole population but selecting a small similar group and expanding results
Longitudinal	Measurements taken over a period of time, not looking at the whole population but selecting a small similar group and expanding results
Experimental	Two or more treatments are compared. Allocation to treatment groups is under the control of the researcher
Randomised	Two or more randomly allocated treatments
Randomised controlled	Includes a control group with standard treatment

Research should be focused according to institutional, national and international strategies. As finances for health care are always limited, it is important to consider including a cost–benefit analysis in any major area of research so that the value of the proposed intervention or change in treatment can be assessed. The NIHR provides the framework through which the Department of Health maintains and manages the research, research staff and research infrastructure of the National Health Service (NHS) in England.

Sample size

Calculating the number of patients required to perform a satisfactory investigation is an important prerequisite to any study. An incorrect sample size is probably the most frequent reason for research being invalid. Often, surgical trials are marred by the possibility of error caused by the inadequate number of patients investigated.

Pierre-Alain Clavien, contemporary, Professor of Surgery, Zurich, Switzerland.
Daniel Dindo, contemporary, surgeon, Zurich, Switzerland.

- **Type I error**. Benefit is perceived when really there is none (false positive).
- **Type II error**. Benefit is missed when it was there to be found (false negative).

Calculating the number of patients required in the study can overcome this bias. Unfortunately, it often reveals that a larger number of patients is needed for the study than can possibly be obtained from available local resources. This usually means expanding enrolment by running a multicentre study – which has the added benefit of improving the external validity of findings. More patients will need to be randomised than the final sample size to take into account patients who die, drop out or are lost to follow-up; this is known as the attrition rate. A longer time from trial entry to primary outcome assessment will result in an increased attrition rate of participants.

The following is an example calculation for a study to recruit patients into two groups. In order to calculate a sample size, it is now common practice to set the level of power for the study at 90% with a 5% significance level. This means that, if there is a difference between study groups, there is a 90% chance of detecting it. Based on previous studies, realistic expectations of differences between groups (i.e. the magnitude of the effect seen from utilising the intervention under study), according to the best available evidence, should be used to calculate the sample size. The formula below uses the results of a reduction in event rate from 30% to 20% (e.g. a new treatment expected to reduce the complication rate such as wound infection from 30% = r to 20% = s).

$$9 \times \frac{[r(100 - r) + s(100 - s)]}{(r - s)^2}$$

$$\text{e.g. } 9 \times \frac{[30(100 - 30) + 20(100 - 20)]}{(30 - 20)^2}$$

$$= 333 \text{ needed in each group}$$

Eliminating bias

It is important to imagine how a study could be invalidated by thinking of things that could go wrong. One way to eliminate any bias inherent in the data collection is to have observers or recorders who do not know which treatment has been used (blinded observer). It might also be possible to ensure that the patient is unaware of the treatment allocation (single blind). In the best randomised studies, neither patient nor researcher is aware of which therapy has been used until after the study has finished (double blind). Randomised trials are essential for testing new drugs. In practice, however, in some surgical trials, randomisation may not be possible or ethical.

Study protocol

Now that the research question has been decided, and it has been checked that sufficient patients should be available to enrol into the study, it is time to prepare the detail of the trial. At this stage, a study protocol should be constructed to define the research plan. It should contain the background of the proposed study, the aims and objectives, a clear methodology, definitions of population and sample sizes and methods of proposed analysis. It should include the patient numbers, inclusion and exclusion criteria and the timescale for the work. The protocol should be detailed enough for another party to come along in the future and theoretically replicate the study. It is useful to construct a flow diagram giving a clear summary of the research protocol and its requirements (***Figure 13.1***). It is helpful to imagine the paper that will be written about the study before the study is performed. This may prevent errors in data collection.

When a study is planned, sufficient time should be reserved at the beginning for fund-raising and obtaining ethical, regulatory and or other approvals (e.g. HRA). Time for data analysis and preparation of publication needs to be included in funding applications. The cost of any non-routine investigations and extra treatments should be identified and covered by the research grant in line with national guidance (in the UK, the Attributing the costs of health and social care Research and Development [AcoRD] guidance; https://www.gov.uk/government/publications/guidance-on-attributing-the-costs-of-health-and-social-care-research).

A data collection form should be designed or a computer collection package developed. If data are collected on a computer, appropriate safeguards for privacy, confidentiality and data quality will be necessary to comply with legislation. At this stage it is important to consider any validation requirements and needs for open access, either in a recognised archive (e.g. the UK Data Archive) or in an institutional repository. Any form of data collection needs to be quality assured. The quality assurance process will include training, standard operating procedures as well as monitoring and checking a certain sample of the data. At the end of data collection and analysis, a final database with all data should be locked and kept for future reference in a safe location. A data-archiving policy with a nominated data custodian should be in place.

Research is no longer confined by institutional or even geographical boundaries. Collaborative research groups in surgery at a national or international level have come together to undertake high-quality surgical research in recent years, aided by online communication and the availability of secure electronic databases such as REDCap™. The SUNRRISE trial shown in ***Figure 13.1*** was undertaken by researchers from two trainee-led research collaborative groups across the UK, in conjunction with a parallel collaborative group in Australia. All patients were included within the same study cohort in real time: the Australian sites were effectively identical to those in the UK because of online electronic randomisation systems and online live data capture via REDCap.

Some publishers require registration of a study at the time it is set up on a publicly available database (e.g. the World Health Organization's recognised registries such as ISRCTN, EudraCT and ClinicalTrials.gov). It is becoming increasingly popular to consider publication of a protocol paper.

Regulatory framework

In the UK, the implementation of the UK Policy Framework for Health and Social Care Research provides a framework

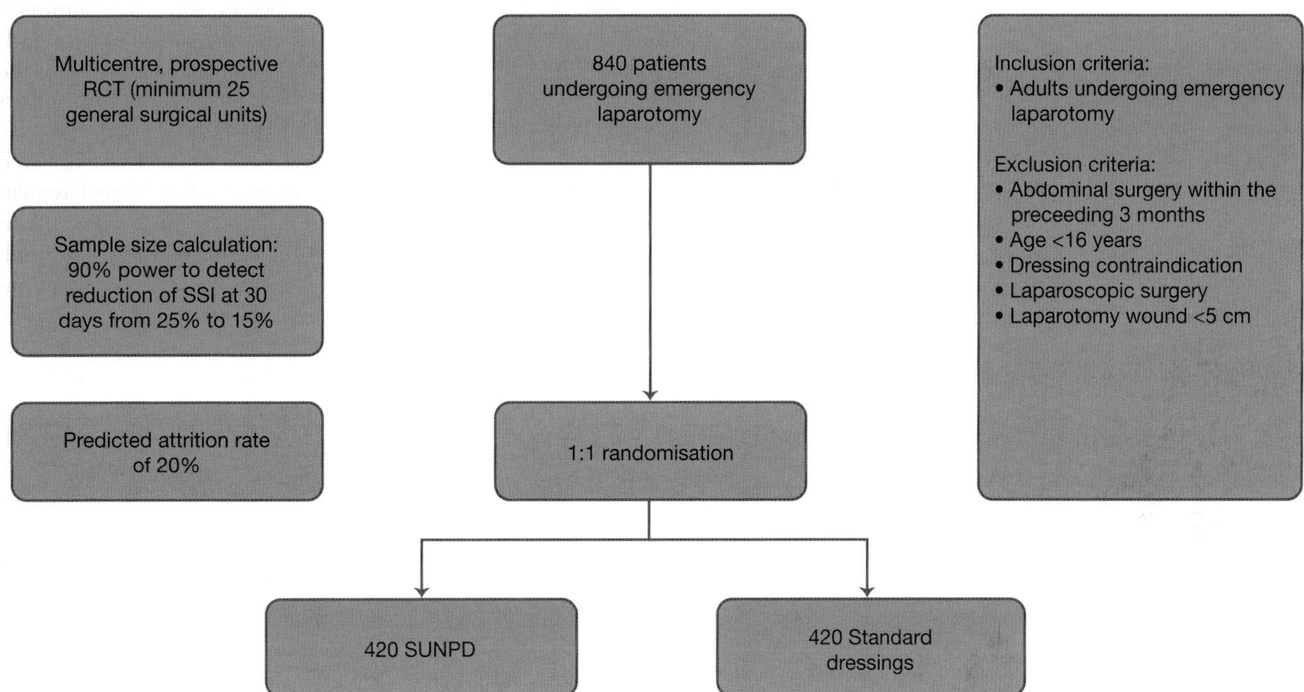

Figure 13.1 SUNRRISE trial: protocol summary and recruitment flowchart. Permission is granted by Birmingham Clinical Trials Unit, University of Birmingham, UK. RCT, randomised controlled trial; SSI, surgical site infection; SUNPD: single-use negative-pressure dressing.

that enhances the integrity of the study and includes requirements for sponsorship by an institution to ensure the following: peer review, independent ethics review, compliance with data protection principles, financial probity, dissemination and management of intellectual property.

Sponsorship is defined by the HRA as the individual, company, institution or organisation that takes on ultimate responsibility for the initiation, management (or arranging the initiation and management) of and/or financing (or arranging the financing) for that research. The sponsor takes primary responsibility for ensuring that the design of the study meets appropriate standards and that arrangements are in place to ensure appropriate conduct and reporting (https://www.hra.nhs.uk/planning-and-improving-research/research-planning/roles-and-responsibilities/#sponsor).

Peer review

Once the protocol is finalised, formal peer review is needed. In the UK, evidence of peer review will be needed before submitting an application to a research ethics committee and for HRA approval. Many funders of research will undertake their own independent peer review. There is usually feedback from this process that can provide valuable advice about the study.

Ethics

In the first instance, common sense is the best guide to whether or not a study is ethical. It is still important to seek advice from an independent research ethics committee whenever research is contemplated.

In the UK the requirement is that an NHS Research Ethics Committee (NHS REC) provides an independent ethical review of all health and social care research if it involves patients and/or carers. The Governance arrangements for Research Ethics Committees (GafREC) provides detailed guidance about NHS REC review requirements. The application for NHS REC review is made using the Integrated Research Application System (IRAS). IRAS enables entry of information about the project once, instead of duplicating information in separate application forms for regulators.

If the study does not require review by an NHS REC, the need for an independent ethical review should still be considered. Universities have developed their own ethical review infrastructure and this will be institute specific and location specific. For collaborative research, local ethical review should be obtained where possible, and developing a local ethics infrastructure should be considered if it does not already exist. Duplication of ethical review should be avoided.

Ethics committee forms may seem long and detailed, but it is important that these are filled in correctly as this helps to prepare the investigators for all practical aspects of the project. All dealings with ethics committees should be intelligent and courteous. It is important to attend the meeting at which the study will be discussed, if invited, as it provides a forum for direct communication in relation to the study. It can save time as possible concerns of the ethics committee can be addressed at the time, avoiding lengthy correspondence.

Regulatory approvals

Interventional clinical or device trials are regulated by the Medicines and Healthcare products Regulatory Agency (MHRA) in the UK. Researchers are encouraged to use an existing and established international register such as ISRCTN or ClinicalTrials.gov to ensure that the public is aware of a trial before recruitment of the first participant. Trials involving sites specifically in EU countries must be registered in the EU Clinical Trials Register. Trials should be registered before applying to the MHRA for a clinical trial authorisation via the MHRA submissions portal and researchers must ensure that the registry is kept up to date and trial results are uploaded in the appropriate timeframe. This can be a complicated and trying process, and support should be sought from the investigators' employing institution. Editors of the major surgical journals now agree that all clinical trials should have been registered before an article relating to a trial can be published.

All studies undertaken with NHS patients and/or carers will need HRA Approval and confirmation of capacity and capability from NHS sites. Studies involving animals require approval from statutory licensing authorities. In the UK this is the Home Office. Animal research should be based on ARRIVE guidelines (Animal Research: Reporting of In Vivo Experiments).

Research integrity

In 2013, Universities UK, in collaboration with major funders of research, developed The Concordat to Support Research Integrity, which sets out key commitments to ensure a high standard in research. It highlights the principles and professional responsibilities of researchers and research institutions that are fundamental to the integrity of research wherever it is undertaken. These centre on:

- honesty in all aspects of research;
- accountability and transparency in the conduct of research;
- professional courtesy and fairness in working with others;
- good stewardship of research.

A study should not under any circumstances commence until appropriate approvals have been granted and compliance with the principles of research integrity is ensured. A helpful international summary of country-specific approval requirements is available from NIH (https://clinregs.niaid.nih.gov).

STATISTICAL ANALYSIS

Both audit and research commonly require statistical analysis. Many surgeons find the statistical analysis of a project the most difficult part. It is also the most commonly criticised part of papers written by clinicians. There are many useful books about statistics (see ***Further reading***); if in any doubt, a statistician will be pleased to give assistance. Statisticians should be consulted before research or audit has been conducted rather than being presented with the data at the end; they often give helpful advice over study design and can be an important part of the project team.

The following terms are frequently used when summarising statistical data:

- **Mean**: the result of dividing the total by the number of observations (the average).
- **Median**: the middle value with equal numbers of observations above and below – used for numerical or ranked data.
- **Mode**: the value with the highest frequency observed – used for nominal data collection.
- **Range**: the largest to the smallest value.

The most important decision for analysis is whether the distribution of the data is normal (i.e. parametric or non-parametric). Normally, distributed data have a symmetrical bell-shaped curve, and the mean, median and mode all lie at the same value. The type of data collected determines which statistical test should be used.

1. Numerical and normally distributed (e.g. blood pressure) – use an unpaired *t*-test to compare two groups or a paired *t*-test to assess whether a variable has changed between two time points.
2. Numerical but not normally distributed (e.g. tumour size) – use a Mann–Whitney *U*-test to compare two groups or a Wilcoxon signed rank test to assess whether a variable has increased/stayed the same/decreased between two time points.
3. Categorical (e.g. admitted or not admitted to an intensive care unit) – a chi-squared test can be used to compare two groups.

(**Note**: the use of these and any other statistical tests may benefit from professional advice.)

Confidence intervals are the best guide to the possible range in which the true differences are likely to lie. A confidence interval that includes zero usually implies a lack of statistical significance.

Scientists usually employ probability (*P*-values) to describe statistical chance. A *P*-value <0.05 is commonly taken to imply a true difference. It is important not to forget that $P = 0.05$ simply means that there is only a 1:20 chance that the differences between the variables would have happened by chance when in fact there is no real difference. If enough variables are examined in any study, significant differences will occur simply

Henry Berthold Mann, 1905–2000, and his student **Donald Ransom Whitney**, 1915–2007, Ohio State University, OH, USA, published their seminal paper 'On a test of whether one of two random variables is stochastically larger than the other' in 1947.
Frank Wilcoxon, 1892–1965, born County Cork, Ireland, American chemist and statistician.

by chance. Trials with multiple end points or variables require more sophisticated analysis to determine the significance of individual risk factors. Univariable or multivariable logistic regression analysis techniques may be appropriate.

Statistics simply deal with the chance that observations between populations are different and should be treated with caution. Clinical results should show clear differences. If statistics are required to demonstrate differences between results, it is likely that they are unlikely to have major clinical significance.

Computer software packages available

Statistical computer packages offer a quick way of analysing descriptive statistics such as mean, median and range, as well as the most commonly used statistical tests such as the chi-squared test. Various packages are available commercially and are useful tools in data analysis.

ANALYSING A SCIENTIFIC ARTICLE

The simplest way to analyse an article from a scientific journal is to look at the checklist of requirements for good scientific research. A group of scientists and editors developed the Consolidated Standards of Reporting Trials (CONSORT) statement to improve the quality of reporting of RCTs. Looking in detail at the study design is often the best way of deciding whether a trial is of value. The CONSORT document includes a checklist for the conduct of good RCTs (***Table 13.3***). Often clinicians overlook biases that others find obvious to detect, which can have a profound influence on the outcome of any study. Even the randomised design does not always guarantee quality, and a core component of systematic review is the grading of trial quality; several scoring systems have been developed (e.g. Jadad score). Recent guidelines have been published formalising the methods of systematic review and meta-analysis (Preferred Reporting Items for Systematic Reviews and Meta-Analyses [PRISMA] guidelines), and also many other types of article. These can be found in the instructions to authors of most surgical journals, which will now only accept articles that follow those rules.

TABLE 13.3 Consolidated Standards of Reporting Trials (CONSORT) checklist for authors.

Heading	Subheading	Descriptor
Title		Identify as randomised trial
Abstract		Structured format
Introduction		Prospectively defined hypotheses, clinical objective
Methods	Protocol	Study population
		Intervention, timing
		Primary and secondary outcome
		Statistical rationale
		Stopping rules
	Assignment	Unit of randomisation
		Method: allocation schedule
	Masking (blinding)	
Results	Participant flow and follow-up	Trial profile, flow diagram
	Analysis	Estimated effect of intervention
		Summary data with appropriate inferential statistics
		Protocol deviation
Comment		Specific interpretation of study
		Sources of bias
		External validity
		General interpretation

From the CONSORT statement: *Journal of the American Medical Association* 1996; 276: 637–9.

PRESENTING AND PUBLISHING AN ARTICLE

There is no point in conducting a research or audit project and then leaving the results unreported. Even when results are negative, they are worth distributing; no project if properly conducted is worthless. Under-reporting of negative outcomes causes a systematic bias in the literature in favour of positive trials. Most studies do not provide dramatic results, and few surgeons publish seminal articles.

The key to both presentation and publication is to decide on the message and then aim for an appropriate forum. Big important randomised studies or national audits merit presentation at national or international meetings and publication in international journals. Small observational studies and audits are more often accepted for presentation at regional meetings and for publication in smaller specialist journals. Help and advice from clinicians familiar with presentation and publication are invaluable at this stage. The most important piece of advice is to follow accurately the instructions for journal submission. Most international meetings will accept presentations eagerly (especially by poster) as this increases the attendance at a conference.

Most surgeons publish research in peer-reviewed journals. The work that is submitted is checked anonymously by other surgeons before publication. If in doubt about whether to submit to a journal, many editors will give advice about the suitability of an article for submission to their journal. It is usually free to publish in surgical journals since the cost of refereeing and editing is borne by the journal subscriber. A second model of publication is becoming more prevalent: open access, in which the author pays. This ensures that all research is visible to anyone, by pushing the costs of the editorial process onto the study budget. It may well become standard in future.

Convention dictates that articles are submitted in IMRAD form: introduction, methods, results and discussion. Increas-

Alejandro R Jadad Bechara, b.1963, Canadian–Colombian physician, University of Toronto, ON, Canada.

ingly, electronic publication and the Internet is changing the face of scientific publication and, in the next decade, these restrictions on style may disappear. For now, the IMRAD format remains inviolable. The length of an article is important: a paper should be as long as the size of the message. Readers of large randomised multicentre trials need to know as much detail about the study as possible; reports on small and simple trials should be brief.

- **Introduction**. This should always be short. A brief background of the study should be presented and then the aims of the trial or audit outlined.
- **Methods**. The methodology and study design should be given in detail. It is important to identify potential biases. New techniques or investigations should be detailed in full; if they are common practice or have been described elsewhere, this should be referenced instead of described.
- **Results**. Results are almost always best shown diagrammatically using tables and figures. Results shown in the form of a diagram need not then be duplicated in the text.
- **Discussion**. It is important not to repeat the introduction or reiterate the results in this section. The study should be interpreted intelligently and any suggestions for future studies or changes in management should be made. It is prudent not to indulge in flights of fantasy or wild imagination about future possibilities; most journal editors will delete these. Recently, a standard format for the discussion section has been promoted, and journals such as the *BMJ* are keen that authors use it.
- **References**. This section should include all relevant papers recording previous studies on the subject in question. The reference section does not usually have to be exhaustive, but should include up-to-date articles. Remember to present the references in the style of the journal of submission.

EVIDENCE-BASED SURGERY

Surgical practice has been considered an art: ask 50 surgeons how to manage a patient and you will probably get 50 different answers. There is so much clinical information available that no surgeon can know it all. Evidence-based surgery is a move to find the best ways of managing patients using clinical evidence from collected studies. It was estimated that sufficient evidence to justify routine myocardial thrombolysis for heart attacks was available years before the randomised clinical studies that finally made it clinically acceptable; no one had gathered all the available information together.

Centres such as the Cochrane Collaboration have been collecting randomised trials and reviews to provide up-to-date information for clinicians. The Cochrane Library presently includes a database of systematic reviews, reviews of surgical effectiveness and a register of controlled trials. The *BJS* has been collecting surgical randomised trials on its website archive for 20 years (www.bjs.co.uk). As evidence accumulates, it is expected that this will gradually smooth out the differences between clinicians as the best way of managing patients becomes more obvious. Collecting published evidence together and analysing it often requires reviews of multiple randomised trials. These meta-analyses involve complex statistical analyses designed to interpret multiple findings and synthesise the results of multiple studies.

FURTHER READING

Altman DG, Machin D, Bryant TN, Gardner MJ. *Statistics with confidence*, 2nd edn. London: BMJ Publishing Group, 2002.

Dindo D, Demartines N, Clavien P-A. Classification of surgical complications: a new proposal with evaluation of a cohort of 6336 patients and the results of a survey. *Ann Surg* 2004; **240:** 205–13.

Greenhalgh T. *How to read a paper: the basics of evidence-based medicine*, 6th edn. Hoboken NJ: Wiley Blackwell, 2019.

Kilkenny C, Browne WJ, Cuthill IC *et al.* Improving bioscience research reporting: the ARRIVE guidelines for reporting animal research. *PloS Biol* 2010; **8**(6): e1000413.

Kirkwood BR *Essentials of medical statistics*, 2nd edn. Oxford: Blackwell Publishing, 2003.

McCulloch P, Altman DG, Campbell WB *et al.* No surgical innovation without evaluation: the IDEAL recommendations. *Lancet* 2009; **374**(9695): 1105–13.

Moher D, Cooke DJ, Eastwood S *et al.* Improving the quality of reports of meta-analyses of randomised controlled trials: the QUORUM statement. *Lancet* 2009; **354:** 1896–900.

Moher D, Liberati A, Tetzlaff J *et al.*, The PRISMA Group. Preferred reporting items for systematic reviews and meta-analyses: the PRISMA Statement. *Open Med* 2009; **3**: 123–30.

Pinkney TD, Calvert M, Bartlett DC *et al.* Impact of wound edge protection devices on surgical site infection after laparotomy: multicentre randomised controlled trial (ROSSINI Trial). *BMJ* 2013; **347**: f4305.

ONLINE RESOURCES

AcoRD: https://www.gov.uk/government/publications/guidance-on-attributing-the-costs-of-health-and-social-care-research
CLAHRC: https://clahrcprojects.co.uk/about
Clinical Evidence: www.clinicalevidence.com
Cochrane Library: www.cochrane.org/index.htm
Concordat to Support Research Integrity: https://ukrio.org/revised-concordat-to-support-research-integrity-published
Consolidated Standards of Reporting Trials: http://www.consort-statement.org
Data Archive: http://www.data-archive.ac.uk
Eudract database: https://www.clinicaltrialsregister.eu
European Code of Conduct: https://allea.org/wp-content/uploads/2017/05/ALLEA-European-Code-of-Conduct-for-Research-Integrity-2017.pdf
GafREC: https://www.hra.nhs.uk/planning-and-improving-research/policies-standards-legislation/governance-arrangement-research-ethics-committees
Health Research Authority: http://www.hra.nhs.uk
Integrated Research Application System: https://www.hra.nhs.uk/about-us/committees-and-services/integrated-research-application-system
ISRCTN: http://www.isrctn.com
MHRA: https://www.gov.uk/government/organisations/medicines-and-healthcare-products-regulatory-agency
National Institute for Health and Care Excellence (NICE): https://www.nice.org.uk
NHS England audits: https://www.england.nhs.uk/clinaudit
REDCap: https://projectredcap.org
Scottish Intercollegiate Guideline Network (SIGN): www.sign.ac.uk
Singapore Statement on Research Integrity: https://wcrif.org/guidance/singapore-statement
Vascular Society: http://www.vascularsociety.org.uk

CHAPTER 14 Ethics and law in surgical practice

Learning objectives

To understand:

- The importance of autonomy in good surgical practice
- The necessity for reasonable disclosure prior to seeking consent for surgery
- Good practice in making decisions about withdrawal of life-sustaining treatment
- The primacy of confidentiality in surgical practice
- The importance of appropriate regulation in surgical research
- The importance of rigorous training and maintenance of good practice standards

INTRODUCTION

This chapter incorporates references to English common and statute law. Nevertheless, these legal and ethical principles have much in common with other jurisdictions across the world.

Surgery, ethics and law go hand in hand. In any other arena of public or private life, if someone deliberately cuts another person, draws blood, causes pain, leaves scars and disrupts everyday activity, then the likely result will be a criminal charge. If the person dies as a result, the charge could be manslaughter or even murder. Self-evidently, the difference between the criminal and the surgeon is that their intentions differ. While a criminal intentionally (or recklessly) inflicts harm, the surgeon's intention is limited to the treatment of illness. Any harm that ensues is either unintentional or is necessary (such as an incision) to facilitate treatment.

Patients submit to surgery because they trust their surgeons. What should 'consent' entail in practice and what should surgeons do when patients need help but are unable or unwilling to agree to it? When patients do consent to treatment, surgeons are provided with a wide discretion. The end result may be cure, but disfigurement, disability and death may also result. How should such surgical 'power' be regulated to reinforce the trust of patients and to ensure that surgeons practise to an acceptable professional standard? Are there circumstances, in the public interest, in which it is acceptable to sacrifice the trust of individual patients through revealing information that was communicated in what patients believed to be conditions of strict privacy?

These questions about what constitutes good professional practice concern medical ethics and law relating to consent, confidentiality and the underlying concept of personal autonomy.

In addition, these principles need to be applied to surgical activities, including professional matters relating to governance, regulation and the process of revalidation in its different guises around the world. Surgical training is starting to embrace the 'basic science' of surgical law to offer surgeons assistance in the resolution of such ethical dilemmas. This chapter is evidence of that process.

RESPECT FOR AUTONOMY

Surgeons have a duty of care towards their patients that goes beyond merely protecting life and health. Their additional duty of care is to respect the autonomy of their patients and their ability to make choices about their treatments, and to evaluate potential outcomes in light of other life plans. Such respect is particularly important for surgeons because, without it, the trust between them and their patients may be compromised, along with the success of the surgical care provided. We are careful enough in everyday life about whom we allow to touch us and to see us unclothed. It is hardly surprising that many people feel strongly about exercising the same control over a potentially hazardous activity, such as surgery.

For all these reasons, there is a wide moral and legal consensus that patients have the right to exercise choice over their surgical care. In this context, a right should be interpreted as a claim that can be made on the surgeon. The surgeon, therefore, accepts the strict duty to respect the patient's choice, regardless of personal preferences. Thus, to the degree that patients have a right to make choices about proposed surgical treatment, it then follows that they should be allowed to refuse treatments that they do not want, even when surgeons think that they are wrong. The right to make an unwise decision was exemplified in a case where a woman with capacity refused renal replacement therapy.[1] The court reminded doctors that, notwithstanding the fact that other citizens might consider her decision unreasonable, illogical or even immoral, none of these criticisms of the decision by themselves provide evidence of a lack of capacity. Patients can refuse surgical treatment that will save their lives, either at present or in the future. The latter, through the formulation of advance decisions or lasting powers of attorney, specify the types of life-saving treatments that patients do not wish to have, notwithstanding that they may later become incompetent to refuse them.

DISCLOSURE PRIOR TO CONSENT

In surgical practice, respect for autonomy translates into the clinical duty to obtain informed consent before the commencement of treatment.

It is easy to underestimate the gap in understanding between a surgeon and his or her patient.[2] How many patients would recognise that unilateral eye surgery might lead to contralateral blindness? The risks and side effects of many operations are not intuitive, and the surgeon is not in a position to guess how the patient's plans for employment, leisure and family life may be inadvertently affected by a foreseeable complication. A budding Olympic gymnast might choose to forego surgery on a quiescent posterior triangle lesion if he or she knew the potential consequences of division of the accessory nerve. That is why patients need to be informed, beforehand, so they can choose whether or not to take the risk.

To establish valid consent to treatment, patients need to be given appropriate and accurate information. In England and Wales, the Department of Health's (DH) *Reference Guide to Consent for Examination or Treatment* (second edition) should be consulted, together with the General Medical Council's (GMC) most recent guidance *Decision Making and Consent* (GMC 2020).

Such information, disclosed during a formal and tangible discussion, must include:

- the condition and the reasons why it warrants surgery;
- the type of surgery proposed and how it might correct the condition;
- the anticipated prognosis and expected side effects of the proposed surgery;
- the unexpected hazards of the proposed surgery;
- any alternative and potentially successful treatments other than the proposed surgery;
- the consequences of no treatment at all.

With such information, patients can link their clinical prospects to the management of other aspects of their lives and the lives of others for whom they may be responsible. Good professional practice dictates that obtaining informed consent should occur in circumstances that are designed to maximise the chances of patients understanding what is said about their condition and the proposed treatment, as well as giving them an opportunity to ask questions and express anxieties.

Where possible:

- a quiet venue for discussion should be found;
- written material in the patient's preferred language should be provided to supplement verbal communication, together with diagrams where appropriate;
- patients should be given time and help to come to their own decision;
- the person obtaining the consent should ideally be the surgeon who will carry out the treatment. It should not be – as is sometimes the case – a junior member of staff who has never conducted such a procedure and thus may not have enough understanding to counsel the patient properly.

Good communication skills go hand in hand with properly obtaining informed consent for surgery. It is not good enough just to go through the motions of providing patients with the information required for considered choice. Attention must be paid to:

- whether or not the patient has understood what has been stated;
- avoiding overly technical language in descriptions and explanations;
- the provision of translators for patients whose first language is not English;
- asking patients if they have further questions.

When there is any doubt about their understanding, patients should be asked questions by their surgeon about what has supposedly been communicated to see if they can explain the information in question for themselves.

Surgeons have a legal as well as a moral obligation to obtain consent for treatment based on appropriate disclosure. Failure to do so could result in one of two civil proceedings, assuming the absence of criminal intent. First, in law, intentionally to touch another person without their consent is a battery, remembering that we are usually touched by strangers as a consequence of accidental contact. Surgeons have an obligation to give the conscious and capacitous patient sufficient information 'in broad terms' about the surgical treatment being proposed and why. If the patient agrees to proceed, no other treatment should ordinarily be administered without further explicit consent.

The second legal action that might be brought against a surgeon for not obtaining appropriate consent to treatment is in the tort (civil wrong) of negligence. Patients may have been given enough information about what is surgically proposed to agree to be touched in the ways suggested. However, surgeons may still be in breach of their professional duty if they do not provide sufficient information about the risks that patients will encounter through such treatment. Although standards of how much information should be provided about risks vary between nations, as a matter of good practice surgeons should inform patients of the hazards that any reasonable person in the position of the patient would wish to know. In UK law, this level and style of disclosure has been most recently reviewed in the case of *Montgomery v Lanarkshire Health Board*.[2]

Finally, surgeons now understand that, when they obtain consent to proceed with treatment, patients are expected to sign a consent form of some kind. The detail of such forms can differ, but they often contain very little of the information supposedly communicated to the patient who signed it. Partly for this reason, the process of formally obtaining consent can become overly focused on obtaining the signature of patients rather than ensuring that appropriate disclosure has been provided and understood.

It is important for surgeons to understand that a signed consent form is not proof that valid consent has been properly obtained. It is simply a piece of evidence that disclosure may have been attempted. Even when they have provided their signature, patients can and do deny that appropriate information has been communicated or that the communication was effective. Surgeons are therefore well advised to make brief notes of what they have said to patients about their proposed treatments, especially information about significant risks. These notes should be placed in the patient's clinical record, perhaps by referring to the disclosure in the letter to the family doctor, copied to the patient. In addition, information sheets describing the generic risks, benefits, complications and alternatives associated with the proposed procedure can be provided. It seems that, soon, a record of dialogue will replace the consent form; see GMC (2020), para. 55.

DUTY OF CANDOUR

Equal consideration should be given to disclosure of information that was generated by the intervention, particularly where 'something went wrong' that caused (or had the potential to cause) harm or distress. The duty to disclose these matters is described as the duty of candour.

Surgeons are accustomed to disclosing to their patients that the proposed operation may go wrong. The disclosures of 'bleeding and infection' are ubiquitous across the land, together with the more specific foreseeable risks, such as damage to contiguous structures, recurrence of the original diagnosis or inadvertent exacerbation of disease. Failure to disclose these foreseeable complications prior to surgery, particularly if they then maim, paralyse or scar the patient, may lead to a claim that the consent was invalid and that the patient, had they known of the risk, either would have never had the operation or would have had it performed by somebody else at another time.

Since all of these misadventures are plainly caught by the GMC's threshold of 'something going wrong', they would need to be reported to the patient by the candid surgeon if they crystallise during surgery. Merely because the division of a ureter during hysterectomy appears as a foreseeable complication on a consent form cannot negate the duty to be candid should it occur; it is plainly an example of something going wrong.

This class of surgical complication must be starkly distinguished from the complications of the disease itself, since these are explicitly excluded from the duty of candour. The patient awaiting surgery for her rectal cancer might present with venous thromboembolism. This is a regrettable complication of her disease, but by itself cannot lead to the deduction that something has gone wrong with surgical management. Accordingly, there would be no duty to be candid.

By contrast, if the same patient, on arriving thrombus-free for her resection, then had a postoperative venous thromboembolism and if the unit's protocol of 28 days of low-molecular-weight heparin was not prescribed, a duty of candour would certainly be owed since something went wrong.

In clinical practice fault is **not** determinative when considering whether to be candid over the occurrence of a complication. Thus clinicians will wish to ensure that the patient is made aware of events to which she may otherwise remain oblivious, since this information may have an effect on her subsequent decision making. Accordingly, if something goes wrong that causes a complication, irrespective of whether the 'thing that went wrong' is indicative of substandard care, our obligation to be candid about the existence of the complication persists. The question of whether fault has occurred, and whether it has caused the complication, is likely to require careful consideration. Clinicians, and those in the hospital who advise them, need to be certain of the facts before being candid to ensure that they do not mislead the patient when fulfilling their duty of candour. It is likely that candour relating to fault and causation, while eventually necessary, may only be possible after an investigation of the event leading to the complication is concluded.

FURTHER PRACTICAL APPLICATIONS OF CLINICAL LAW IN SURGICAL PRACTICE

Thus far, the moral and legal reasons why the duty of surgeons to respect the autonomy of patients translates into the specific responsibility to obtain informed consent to treatment have been reviewed. For consent to be valid, adult patients must:

- have capacity to give it – be able to understand, remember and deliberate over the information disclosed to them about treatment choices, and to communicate those choices;
- not be coerced into decisions that reflect the preferences of others rather than themselves;
- have been given sufficient information for these choices to be based on an accurate understanding of reasons for and against proceeding with specific treatments.

Surgical care would grind to a halt if it were always necessary to obtain explicit informed consent every time a patient is touched in the context of their care. Fortunately, it is an elementary step merely to ask the patient whether they mind being examined – the usual response will be acceptance. This simple transaction illustrates that the legal and ethical 'rules' that govern a surgeon are often no more than an expression of good clinical practice; in this case, politeness.

Some patients will not be able to give consent because of temporary incapacity. This may result from their presenting illness or intoxication, or an unanticipated situation may be encountered midway through a general anaesthetic. The moral and legal rules that govern such situations are clear. The doctrine of medical necessity enables the surgeon, in an emergency, to save life and prevent permanent disability, operating without consent. This has historically been employed daily, where unconscious emergency patients undergo surgery to save 'life and limb'. No consent has been provided and none is required, providing the treatment is in the patient's best interests.

However, if the patient has made a legally valid advance decision refusing treatment of the specific kind required, their decision must be honoured, providing it is applicable to the current clinical situation. Wherever possible, surgery on patients who are temporarily incapacitated should be postponed until their capacity is restored and they are able to give informed consent or refusal for themselves.

Surgeons must take care to respect the distinction between procedures that are necessary to prevent death or irremediable harm and those that are done merely out of convenience. If the patient consents only to a dilatation and curettage, do not consider performing instead a hysterectomy 'in her best interests', simply because she is anaesthetised.

CHILDREN AND YOUNG PEOPLE

In England and Wales, a person is a child until their 18th birthday; older children are distinguished from their younger counterparts, since 16- and 17-year-olds are additionally described as 'young people'. Citizens under 16 years are presumed incompetent, but they may rebut that presumption and establish their competence by demonstrating that they have sufficient maturity – intelligence to understand fully what is proposed – to make the relevant decision. Hence 'Gillick' competence. In the case of incompetent children (or competent children who choose to rely on a proxy), parents or someone with parental responsibility are ordinarily required to provide consent on their behalf. This said, surgeons should:

- take care to explain to children what is being surgically proposed, and why;
- always consult with children about their response;
- where possible, take the child's views into account and note that even young children can be competent to consent to treatment provided that they can 'pass' the Gillick test for the decision in question;
- it is almost always appropriate, in addition, to separately discuss the treatment with their parents, although it should be noted that, if a child is Gillick competent to defend their confidential information, it should not be assumed that they wish to share this with their parents.

When such Gillick competence is present, under English law, children can provide their own consent to surgical care, although they cannot unconditionally refuse it until they are 18 years old. These provisions illustrate the importance of respecting the autonomy of child patients and remembering that, for the purposes of consent to medical treatment, they may be just as capable as adults. If faced with a surgical emergency in a child of 15 for whom no consent is available for life- or limb-saving treatment, and there **really is no time** to seek authority from someone with parental responsibility, the child or the court, then proceed with the operation without consent. So far, in the English common law stretching back 800 years, no case has been brought to court complaining of a child's life being saved using this doctrine of necessity.

ADULTS: PEOPLE 18 AND ABOVE

Capacity in adults is presumed, but this may be challenged on the basis of a reasonable belief that they are incapacitated.

Incapacity in England and Wales is established (in those aged 16 years and over) by a two-stage test. First, the functional test for incapacity is employed: is the person unable to make the relevant decision? If they are **able** to make the decision, the presumption of capacity endures. If they are unable to make the decision, then the second (diagnostic) stage must be employed: is there an impairment or disturbance of the mind or the brain? If so, the two stages in combination result in a conclusion of incapacity. How this assessment is carried out and the entire structure of this area of law is set out in the Mental Capacity Act (MCA) 2005 Code of Practice. This is essential reading, and must be available to clinicians in all UK National Health Service (NHS) hospitals. Capacity is not synonymous with (Gillick) competence, but that is a topic for further reading. Capacity and incapacity are the significant binary measure by which the capability of young people and adults is judged, but be aware of the notion of the **vulnerable** patient, who may possess capacity but risks falling victim to predatory actors.

Capacity may be erased by psychiatric illness, but even in circumstances where patients have been legally detained for compulsory psychiatric care it **by no means** follows that such patients are unable to provide consent for surgical care. Their capacity should be presumed and consent should be sought. Only if it is established that such patients also (in addition to or as a consequence of their mental illness) lack capacity to provide consent for surgery can therapy then proceed in their best interests. However, if possible postpone treatment until, as a result of their psychiatric care, patients become able either to consent or to refuse. If this timely recovery is not predicted, then legal steps using the authority of the MCA 2005 must be taken to make elective surgery lawful. It would be unlikely that treatment for physical illness could be authorised under the Mental Health Act 1983. As with children, respect should always be shown for as much autonomy as is present.

INCAPACITY

Absence of capacity in adults does not vitiate the requirement, where possible, to take into account the patient's sentiments during clinical decision making. In one case, a judge declared that an elderly man with a septic leg, although incapacitated by his mental illness, had feelings, beliefs and values that weighed so heavily in the consideration of his best interests that they outweighed the clinical desire to save his life by amputation.[3] Although an unusual judgement in this context, it reflects the growing determination to give incapacitated adults an opportunity to influence their fate, as best they can.

Elective treatment for less grave complaints can also be provided; in England and Wales this is done under the auspices of the MCA 2005. The associated Code of Practice guides the surgeon in matters of capacity and disclosure, and in dealing with those who have taken steps to influence their treatment, anticipating the time that they will have lost their capacity. These arrangements may manifest either in documentary form, such as Advance Decisions, or in person, in the form of persons appointed with a Lasting Power of Attorney.

It is not possible for relatives of incapacitated adult patients to sign consent forms for surgery on their behalf unless the relative or friend has, very unusually, been appointed as a deputy by the Court of Protection. Indeed, to make such requests can be a disservice to relatives, who may feel an unjustified sense of responsibility if the surgery fails. This said, relatives play a vital role in providing background information about the patient, allowing the clinician to assess and then determine what treatment is in the best interests of the patient.

INCAPACITY IN AN EMERGENCY

It is not lawful to force a capacitous adult to have treatment without their consent.

Since the advent of the MCA 2005, the notion of acting based only on the common law 'doctrine of necessity' has largely become historical. This is because if an adult lacks capacity, and you are treating in their best interests, the Act authorises necessary and proportionate steps to save life and to prevent serious and permanent injury. It is difficult to envisage circumstances where the statute would not be engaged, but the common law doctrine has not been extinguished by the Act, so should give extra reassurance to surgeons acting in emergencies in the best interests of incapacitated patients. Bear in mind that the presently incapacitated patient may yet regain his or her capacity, so if an intervention can safely be deferred to await cognitive recovery it should be, provided that deferral is in your patient's best interests.

DECISIONS IN THE BEST INTERESTS OF INCAPACITATED PATIENTS

We are all well aware that adults with capacity must make their own treatment decisions. There is no justification or need to determine the best interests of such patients since they can (by definition) decide these matters for themselves. Accordingly, their 'best interests' are never explored. Naturally, clinicians will on occasion disagree with a capacitous patient's decision, and they are at liberty to try and persuade the patient to change his or her mind, but the patient with capacity has the last word. This is starkly exemplified by the adult with capacity who chooses to refuse the blood that would otherwise have saved his life. Or the capacitous woman who refuses the caesarean section that alone would allow her child to be born alive.

But for those who lack capacity to make decisions relating to their treatment, clinicians have become accustomed to acting in the patient's **best interests**. Meetings devoted to this subject are a ubiquitous daily occurrence in hospitals across the country. Again, we are all well aware of the general principle standing behind 'best interests'; the incapacitated patient's welfare must be viewed in its widest terms, not simply in the sense of medical but also social and psychological interests. The patient's previously expressed wishes, values, feelings and beliefs must be taken into account. This will involve consideration of the proposed medical treatment, the prospects of success and the likely outcome. That is all very well; how should we achieve this?

A case decided in 2017 provided us with clear, specific guidance concerning Mrs P, who was 72 years old when she suffered the intracranial bleed that left her in a minimally conscious state.[4] It was agreed that there was no prospect of her regaining the capacity to make decisions relating to her health, and it was speculated that her potential life expectancy was in the region of 3–5 years. Nonetheless, she was otherwise relatively healthy and the hospital wished to insert a gastrostomy for hydration and nourishment. She would not tolerate a nasogastric tube, the presence (and frequent replacement) of which distressed her. Mrs P's daughters disagreed with this proposal, explaining that their mother had previously expressed a wish not to be kept alive if severely handicapped, especially if her mental function was severely affected.

Because of this disagreement, the court was approached, the hospital seeking a declaration that the proposed treatment was lawful. The judgement was centred on the notion that, when considering best interests, those making the decisions must try and put themselves in the place of the individual patient and ask what her attitude to the proposed treatment is likely to be. And they must consult those who befriend or look after the patient, in particular to obtain a view on what her attitude to the treatment might be. Factors that should be taken into account would include the views of those who had a close relationship with the patient when she had capacity, and the impact of the patient's fate on those who were closest to her.

The court nevertheless made it crystal clear that what the patient would have done in the circumstances (if her capacity had been preserved) would not automatically be regarded as to be in her best interests. While courts (and clinical decision makers) will strive to recognise and comply with what the patient is likely to have wanted, acting in her best interests remains the paramount objective.

THE ROLE OF THE COURT

The question has arisen regarding the circumstances in England in which clinical decisions relating to withdrawal of treatment should be automatically referred to the court.[5]

Mr Y was an active man in his fifties when he had a cardiac arrest and consequent cerebral hypoxia. He never regained consciousness. He was fed through a gastrostomy, and over the following 3 months his doctors concluded that he had a 'prolonged disorder of consciousness' (a term that courts have accepted as encompassing persistent vegetative and minimally conscious states). It was also concluded that, if he were to regain consciousness, he would have profound disability, both physical and cognitive, and remain dependent on others to care for him. This prognosis was confirmed by a second opinion. His wife and children told the clinicians that Mr Y would not have wished to be kept alive if he had received that prognosis during the time preceding his loss of capacity. Accordingly, the family and clinicians all agreed that it would be in Mr Y's best interests to withdraw his clinically assisted nutrition and hydration (CANH).

The question for the court was whether a court order must **always** be obtained in such situations, or whether, under certain circumstances, these decisions can be taken without the involvement of a court.

Twenty-five years earlier, the courts had considered two very different clinical questions. In *re F* the question related to whether sterilisation to prevent pregnancy (rather than to treat disease) could be performed on an incapacitated woman.[6] In *Bland* it was proposed that CANH in a young man who had been in a persistent vegetative state for 3 years should be withdrawn.[7] The House of Lords had made it clear in both cases that, as a matter of good practice, a court declaration should be obtained (that the proposed treatment was in an incapacitated person's best interests) prior to the actions being taken.

In considering Mr Y's case, the Supreme Court noted that decisions on withdrawing CANH are frequent and ubiquitous, taken consensually every day throughout the country in the best interests of patients with a wide range of neurodegenerative conditions, notably stroke and dementia. There could be no principled or logical reason to demand a court review of the tiny subset of patients with a 'prolonged disorder of consciousness' while blithely accepting the commonplace practice of withdrawal in other patients without recourse to the courts. Similarly, since CANH is seen as medical treatment, there can be no reason why its withdrawal should be seen as 'first among equals', there being no automatic recourse to declarations for withdrawal of antibiotics, ventilation or organ support.

For these and other reasons, the Supreme Court held that, provided the provisions and guidance of the MCA 2005 are followed, and that there is agreement as to what is in the patient's best interests, then life-sustaining treatment, whether this is CANH or any other form of life support, can be withdrawn or withheld without needing to make an application to the court.

Plainly, if there is any hint of lack of agreement or conflict of interest from any quarter, clinical or family, when the withdrawal of life-sustaining treatment is being considered, an application to court must be made. Equally, if in these circumstances at the end of the decision-making process the clinicians or family remain uncertain, because the conclusions on best interests are finely balanced, an application must be made.

This judgement marked a 'handing back' to clinicians of responsibility to make some decisions that for the last 25 years have been exclusively within the control of our courts. This redoubles the responsibility that clinicians bear to ensure that the MCA 2005 is understood and applied assiduously.

DO NOT ATTEMPT RESUSCITATION?

Furthermore, the decision to discontinue life-sustaining treatment may go hand in hand with a decision not to attempt cardiopulmonary resuscitation, in the event of cardiorespiratory arrest. In England, it is settled law that before finally making this 'DNACPR' decision, doctors must discuss it with patients or their relatives.[8] The reason for this insistence is that the patient may have personal circumstances, unbeknown to the surgeon, that might yet influence this final (and for the patient, portentous) decision. The only exclusion to this legal rule is where discussion of this matter with the patient may cause them not merely distress, but harm. The duty to consult a patient prior to deciding to withhold cardiopulmonary resuscitation was subsequently extended to a duty to consult those befriending an incapacitated adult.

DOCTRINE OF DOUBLE EFFECT

Surgeons could find themselves involved in the palliative care of patients whose pain is increasingly difficult to control. There may come a point in the management of such pain when effective palliation is possible only at the risk of shortening a patient's life because of the respiratory effects of the palliative drugs. In such circumstances, surgeons can, with legal justification, administer a dose that might be dangerous (although experts in palliative care are sceptical that this is ever necessary with appropriate training). In any case, the argument employed to justify such action refers to its 'double effect': that both the relief of pain and death might follow from such an action. Intentional killing (active euthanasia) is rejected as criminal malpractice throughout most of the world. A foreseeably lethal analgesic dose is thus regarded as lawful **only when it is solely motivated by palliative intent**, and this motivation has been documented. Recent authority from criminal law indicates that, if an analgesic injection is 'virtually certain' also to kill the patient, a court might deduce that the person giving the injection had an intention to kill. The key to the defence of double effect is the absolute absence of such an intention. It follows that if you are **virtually certain** that a palliative act will end the patient's life, consult widely before embarking upon it.

CONFIDENTIALITY BALANCED AGAINST THE RISK OF SERIOUS HARM

Respect for autonomy does not entail only the right of capacitous patients to consent to treatment. Their autonomous right extends to control over their confidential information, and surgeons must respect their patients' privacy, not communicating information revealed in the course of treatment to anyone else without consent. Generally speaking, such respect means that surgeons must not discuss clinical matters with relatives, friends, employers and other state actors unless the patient explicitly agrees. To do otherwise is regarded by all the regulatory bodies of medicine and surgery as a grave offence, incurring harsh penalties. Breaches of confidentiality are not only abuses of human dignity; they undermine the trust between surgeon and patient on which successful surgery and the professional reputations of surgeons depend. The delicacy of this situation was amply demonstrated in a recent case.

A woman (ABC) had a father (XX) who killed her mother, leading to his detention in a psychiatric facility.[9] His clinicians tested him for Huntington's disease, which proved positive. He had capacity, and agreed to the testing only on the basis that his results were not shared with his family.

In the meantime, ABC fell pregnant. Her father's doctors knew about the pregnancy and wanted to disclose XX's diagnosis to his daughter; from the time of his diagnosis there would have been a window of 2 months during which termination of her pregnancy was feasible. XX refused to disclose, aware that such knowledge might have an impact on his two daughters' reproductive decision making.

ABC discovered her father's diagnosis during a clinical visit when her baby was 4 months old. Shortly afterwards, she decided that her father's diagnosis should not be disclosed to her sister, now in the early stages of her own pregnancy.

Four years later, ABC tested positive for Huntington's. Feeling that it had been unfair to bring a child into the world in these tragic circumstances, she claimed that the doctors should have breached her father's confidentiality and told her of his diagnosis while she had a chance to choose whether she would undergo termination. In making this claim, she asserted that she was owed a duty of care by the doctors who also had a duty to respect her father's confidentiality.

The claimant told the court that the clinicians had a '...duty to balance the claimant's interest in being informed of her risk of a genetic disorder against her father's interest in having the confidentiality of that diagnosis preserved'. The court noted that if on that basis the clinicians properly considered and balanced the conflicting interests, but decided not to disclose, they would have fulfilled their obligation, provided their conclusion not to disclose the information was reasonable. The judge concluded that it was just, fair and reasonable to impose a legal duty to balance ABC's interest in being informed against XX's interest in maintaining his confidentiality relating to both his diagnosis (and the public interest in maintaining medical confidentiality generally).

The decision in ABC reveals that, important as respect for confidentiality is, it is not an absolute right. Surgeons are allowed to communicate private information to other professionals who are part of the healthcare team, provided that the information has a direct bearing on treatment. Here, it is argued that patients have given their 'implied' consent to such communication when they explicitly consent to a treatment plan. Whether implied consent can in any circumstances be valid is a matter for public debate, as government applies these words to tissue donation and access to electronic health records. Academic lawyers are sceptical that it is a species of consent at all, since there is no guarantee of the now-treasured disclosure prior to agreement. Such examples of 'implied' consent are better viewed as mere acquiescence on the behalf of patients, ignorant of and not objecting to decisions made about them, in the absence of personal consultation.

Patients cannot expect strict adherence to the principle of confidentiality if it poses a serious threat to the health and safety of others. There will be some circumstances in which confidentiality either must or may be breached in the public interest. For example, it must be breached as a result of court orders or in relation to the requirements of public health legislation.

SHARING INFORMATION WITH THE POLICE

It is not uncommon to receive a request from the police for patient data. Consider the patient admitted after a fall down the stairs; it is suggested that his partner had caused the fall. The partner is in police custody, awaiting a court's decision on bail the following day.

The patient, at the time of the police enquiry, was intubated and ventilated, lacking capacity to decide whether to consent to the disclosure of his clinical details. What should our position be in these circumstances? Sixty years ago Lord Denning made it clear that there is no general obligation for clinicians to disclose confidential information following a request from the police. Naturally, a constable can always approach a court in the face of clinical refusal; it would be most unlikely that an NHS trust would refuse to comply with a court order to disclose.

The DH suggests that doctors should consider disclosure if, among other considerations, the alleged offence is grave and the prevention or detection of crime would be prejudiced or delayed but for prompt disclosure.

Clinicians must disclose to the police any information identifying a driver alleged of committing a traffic offence; and even in the absence of a police request, their suspicions of a person's involvement in terrorist activities. Less specifically, doctors must disclose to the police the admission of a person wounded by knife or gun, so that at least the constabulary is made aware of an armed assailant in the neighbourhood. Whether the stabbed or shot person allows subsequent disclosure of their identity rather depends on their capacity at the time. Naturally, if the patient consents to disclosure no problem occurs. But some victims of assault may choose to remain silent, perhaps fearing more grievous injury if they become identified as an informer.

The patient who lacks capacity poses a more difficult problem. If it seems likely that they will soon regain the ability to make their own decision, it would be prudent to await that recovery. If there is evidential material that could be lost during the lapse of time, such as clear scars or bruises or footprints, by all means have these images recorded, but await the patient's capacitous consent before handing them to the police. At the other extreme, if the patient is unlikely to recover capacity after an assault, a grave offence may have transpired, making disclosure in the absence of consent more palatable.

If there is a simple stark binary choice between either respecting a person's confidentiality or protecting them from death or serious harm, most clinicians would likely value life and limb over a notion of confidences. Guidance from DH suggests that unlawful killing, rape, treason and child abuse could all cross the 'serious harm' threshold. By contrast, theft, fraud and criminal damage would not.

The leading case is of Dr Egdell, a psychiatrist instructed by W, who had killed five people with extreme violence.[10] W was seeking review of his secure hospital order and hoped that Dr Egdell would provide a favourable report of his mental health. On the contrary, Dr Egdell found that W was highly dangerous, fascinated by high explosives, and that the secure hospital's staff were oblivious to the threat W continued to pose.

Faced with the unhelpful report W's solicitors did not pursue the application to the Mental Health Tribunal, but Dr Egdell felt his report should nonetheless go to the Home Secretary and the medical director of the hospital. W disagreed. In subsequent litigation the Court of Appeal held that this disclosure in the teeth of W's capacitous opposition was justified and in the public interest. The breach in confidentiality was made lawful by the real risk of serious harm to others should W be released.

Frustratingly, the paucity of cases provides us with no further judicial gloss on this clinical dilemma.

TRANSPLANTATION

The law and ethics of organ transplantation require more space than this chapter allows. In common with other nations, the UK has a statutory framework for transplantation, but even among this small group of nations there is no unanimity of legislation, thus rules for deceased and live donor transplants differ. In general, the rules for defining a dead donor, for compensating a living donor and for legitimising a market in organs differ widely. It is strongly recommended that you refer to the rules within your own jurisdiction.

RESEARCH

As part of their duty to protect life and health to an acceptable professional standard, surgeons have a subsidiary responsibility to strive to improve operative techniques through research to assure themselves and their patients that the care proposed is the best that is currently possible. Yet there is moral tension between the duty to act in the best interests of individual patients and the duty to improve surgical standards through exposing patients to the unknown risks that any form of research inevitably entails.

The willingness to expose patients to such risks may be further increased by the professional and academic pressures on many surgeons to maintain a high research profile in their work. For this reason, surgeons (and physicians, who face the same dilemmas) now accept that their research must be externally regulated to ensure that patients give their informed consent, that any known risks to patients are far outweighed by the potential benefits and that other forms of protection for the patient are in place (e.g. proper indemnity) in case they are unexpectedly harmed. The administration of such regulation is through research ethics committees, and surgeons should not participate in research that has not been approved by such bodies. Equally, special provisions will apply to research involving incompetent patients who cannot provide consent to participate, and research ethics committees will evaluate specific proposals with great care.

In practice, it is not always clear as to what constitutes 'research' that should be subjected to regulation, as compared with a minor innovation dictated by the contingencies of a particular clinical situation. Surgeons must always ask themselves in such circumstances whether or not the innovation in question falls within the boundaries of standard procedures in which they are trained. If so, what may be a new technique for them will count not as research but as an incremental improvement in personal practice. Nevertheless, major innovations in operative procedure are scrutinised by national regulatory authorities; in the UK by the National Institute for Health and Care Excellence (NICE). This process of scrutiny has been designed to ensure that the innovation is safe, efficacious and cost-effective. It is regarded (by the NHS) as a mandatory step when introducing a new interventional procedure.

Equally, surgeons know that exigencies of operative surgery sometimes demand a novel and hitherto undescribed manoeuvre to get the surgeon (and the patient) out of trouble. Providing your solution is necessary, proportionate to the circumstances, performed in good faith and would pass the scrutiny of your peers as reasonable, it is unlikely that any subsequent criticism of your actions could be sustained.

If a proposed innovation passes the criteria for research, it should be approved by a research ethics committee. Such surgical research should also be subject to a clinical trial designed to ensure that findings about outcomes are systematically compared with the best available treatment and that favourable results are not the result of arbitrary factors (e.g. unusual surgical skill among researchers) that cannot be replicated (see also *Chapter 12*).

STANDARDS OF EXCELLENCE

To optimise success in protecting life and health to an acceptable standard, surgeons must only offer specialised treatment in which they have been properly trained. To do so will entail sustained further education throughout a surgeon's career in the wake of new surgical procedures. While training, surgery should be practised only under appropriate supervision by someone who has appropriate levels of skill. Such skill can be demonstrated only through appropriate clinical audit, to which all surgeons should regularly submit their results. When these reveal unacceptable levels of success, no further surgical work of that kind should continue unless further training is undergone under the supervision of someone whose success rates are satisfactory. To do otherwise would be to place the interest of the surgeon above that of their patient, an imbalance that is never morally or professionally appropriate.

Surgeons also have a duty to monitor the performance of their colleagues. To know that a fellow surgeon is exposing patients to unacceptable levels of potential harm and to do nothing about it is to incur some responsibility for such harm when it occurs. Surgical teams and the institutions in which they function should have clear protocols for exposing unacceptable professional performance and helping colleagues to understand the danger to which they may expose patients. If necessary, offending surgeons must be stopped from practising until they can undergo further appropriate training and counselling. Too often, such danger has had to be reported by individuals whose anxieties have not been properly heeded and who have then been professionally pilloried rather than acknowledged for their contribution to patient safety. Those who participate in closing ranks, and ostracism, share the moral responsibility for any resulting harm to patients. If something goes wrong with surgical treatment, the UK health regulators unanimously insist that the patient should be told what has happened; in many senses, a similar disclosure to that which occurred during the consent process, but now with the benefit of hindsight. Again, this candid disclosure is designed to put the patient in the same position as the surgeon, with respect to information about their health.[11]

CONCLUSION

Surgeons have combined duties to their patients: to protect life and health and to respect autonomy, both to an acceptable professional standard. The specific duties of surgeons are shown to follow from these: reasonable practice concerning informed consent; confidentiality; decisions not to provide, or to omit, life-sustaining care; surgical research; and the maintenance of good professional standards. The final duty of surgical care is to exercise all these general and specific responsibilities with fairness and justice, and without arbitrary prejudice. Now, at least partly either enshrined in statute or echoed in the English common law, these duties closely reflect the guidance of the GMC.

The conduct of ethical surgery illustrates good citizenship: protecting the vulnerable and respecting human dignity; and equality. To the extent that the practice of individual surgeons is a reflection of such sustained conduct, they deserve the civil respect that they often receive. To the extent that it is not, they should not practise the honourable profession of surgery.

REFERENCES

1 Kings College Hospital v C & V [2015] EWCOP 80
2 Montgomery (Appellant) v Lanarkshire Health Board (Respondent) (Scotland) [2015] UKSC 11
3 Wheeler RA. Tangible Sentiments. Bulletin RCSE, 2016 January 98 44
4 Salford Royal NHSFT v P & Q [2017] EWCOP 23
5 An NHS Trust & Ors v Y [2018] UKSC 46
6 In re F (Mental Patient: Sterilisation) [1990] 2 AC 1
7 Airedale NHST v Bland [1993] AC 789
8 Regina (Tracey) v Cambridge University Hospital NHS Foundation Trust and another [2014] EWCA Civ 822
9 ABC v St George's Healthcare NHST [2020] EWHC 455 QB
10 W v Egdell [1990] Ch 359 (CA)
11 http://www.uhs.nhs.uk/HealthProfessionals/Clinical-law-updates/Clinicallawupdates.aspx

FURTHER READING

Department of Constitutional Affairs. *Mental Capacity Act 2005 Code of Practice.* London: The Stationery Office, 2007.

Department of Health. *Confidentiality: NHS Code of Practice. Supplementary guidance: public interest disclosures.* London: Department of Health, 2010.

General Medical Council. *Confidentiality: protecting and providing information.* Available from https://www.gmc-uk.org/ethical-guidance/ethical-guidance-for-doctors/confidentiality

General Medical Council. *Good medical practice.* London: General Medical Council, 2006.

General Medical Council. *0–18 years: guidance for all doctors.* London: General Medical Council, 2007.

General Medical Council. *Decision making and consent.* London: General Medical Council, 2020.

Mason JK, Laurie GT. *Mason and McCall Smith's law and medical ethics,* 11th edn. Oxford: Oxford University Press, 2019.

Nair R, Holroyd DJ (eds). *Oxford handbook of surgical consent.* Oxford: Oxford University Press, 2012.

Wheeler RA. Presumed or implied; it's not consent. *Clin Risk* 2010; **16**: 1–2.

Wheeler RA. *Clinical law for clinical practice.* London: CRC Press, Taylor & Francis Group, 2020.

Wheeler RA. Gillick or Fraser? A plea for consistency over competence in children. *Br Med J* 2006; **332**: 807.

Woodcock T. Surgical research in the United Kingdom. *Ann R Coll Surg Engl* 2009; **91**: 188–91.

Woodcock T. Law and medical ethics in organ transplantation surgery. *Ann R Coll Surg Engl* 2010; **92**: 282–5.

CHAPTER 15 Human factors, patient safety and quality improvement

Learning objectives

To learn:

- The importance of understanding human behaviour, quality and value in healthcare delivery
- The importance of human factors and teamworking in reducing and rectifying error
- Medical error and its definitions, including adverse events and near misses
- The importance of patient safety, strategies and application in clinical practice
- Quality improvement as an overarching activity
- The need for system thinking and leadership

INTRODUCTION

In recent years, increased emphasis has been placed on the study of healthcare systems to better understand the relationship of how management and administrative systems best support clinical practice and promote quality improvement and patient safety. To some extent this has come about as a consequence of the increasing complexity of healthcare delivery, which, although credited with dramatically improving public health over the last 50 years, has led to the realisation that patient satisfaction and safety is frequently compromised. This issue is multifactorial but includes poor integration of care pathways, poor planning and utilisation of resources and errors in management and clinical care. A disaffected healthcare workforce challenged with excessive administrative and governance workloads compounds these issues and leads to 'burnout', which contributes to poor clinical outcomes and further compounds societal and patient dissatisfaction with patient care.

Understanding healthcare systems, promoting 'value' for both healthcare providers and patients and supporting the healthcare workforce to deliver high-quality and safe care remains the biggest challenge for the healthcare industry in the current decade. This chapter addresses some of these important issues and provides a framework for surgeons to contribute to the design of safe and efficient surgical pathways of care.

Today's healthcare systems face two big challenges: increasing demand because of greater volumes of patients who are older, who often have comorbidities and who often require multidisciplinary care; and an increasing volume of treatment options, often of greater complexity and cost.

Despite the ability of medical science to manage and treat an increasing array of complex medical conditions, not all medical conditions are managed well. Implementing evidence-based care in complex health systems is challenging. Added to this, the financial cost of health care challenges both healthcare recipients and providers and questions how best to drive the 'quality' agenda in healthcare delivery.

According to the Institute of Medicine, patients do not always receive the most suitable care at the best time or in the best place. Its influential report, *Crossing the Quality Chasm: A New Health System for the 21st Century*, emphasises the need to redesign healthcare processes and systems in response to this quality gap.

The concept of 'value' in health care has been developed to provide a focus for both healthcare recipient and provider. Professor Michael Porter, director of the Harvard Business School's Institute for Strategy and Competitiveness, has advocated value-based health care as one of the most important topics in healthcare transformation. Porter proposed six principles that support a value-based approach to health care:

1. Organise care around medical conditions – care should be based upon the medical needs of a community.
2. Measure outcomes and costs for every patient.
3. Align reimbursement with value – to support better outcomes and more efficient care.
4. Systems integration – organise treatment around matching patient, treatment and location.
5. Geography of care – provide centres of excellence for complex care.
6. Information technology – provide integration of the healthcare system.

While value-based care has mainly gained traction within the USA and the private healthcare sector elsewhere, it is interesting to see its conceptual components being taken up by public health systems such as the National Health Service (NHS) in the UK, with an understanding of the need for a universal healthcare number and integrated healthcare information technology (IT) platforms and healthcare initiatives such as

Michael E Porter, b.1947, economist, Harvard Business School, Boston, MA, USA.

'Right care, right time, right place for carers' and 'Choosing Wisely UK', all of which are based on designing healthcare systems that are truly patient-centric and offer quality outcomes that matter to patients.

HUMAN FACTORS

The healthcare setting has become increasingly complex. Patient and societal demands for transparency in defining and justifying treatment decisions impact on all healthcare workers, who need to understand their professional responsibilities when working within complex social and work environments. Healthcare workers must understand that patients are increasingly better informed and wish to be included more fully within the decision-making processes regarding treatment options. Likewise, when performance and clinical outcomes are less than expected, patients and their supporters are entitled to timely and honest appraisal of 'what went wrong' and to be part of the discussion regarding ongoing care.

Therefore, increasingly, surgeons will need to integrate knowledge, technical skills and mastery of complex equipment while participating in a multidisciplinary healthcare setting, in order to deliver safe and effective care. The communication skills required to work in these complex environments and engage effectively with audit, management and quality improvement systems are all dependent on human behaviour.

These complex skill sets are set out in the study of human factors (HF), which examines the behavioural interrelationships between humans, the tools they work with and the environment in which they work. It is a complex area that incorporates knowledge derived from many disciplines. A better understanding of the effects of teamwork, tasks, equipment, workspace, culture and organisation on human behaviour will improve performance in clinical settings. A HF approach to patient safety differs from traditional safety training in that the focus is less with the technical knowledge and skills required to perform specific tasks, but rather with the cognitive and interpersonal skills needed to effectively manage team-based, high-risk activities. With time, HF training has evolved from models describing human interactions within complex environments to more nuanced programmes that modify workers' behaviour and improve patient safety.

HF was originally conceived in the 1940s in the aviation industry to better understand the relationship between a team's behaviour, its technical surroundings and a changing environment. The 'cognitive skills' of the aircraft crew refers to the mental processes used for gaining and maintaining situational awareness, for solving problems and for making decisions, whereas 'interpersonal skills' are the communications and behavioural activities associated with teamwork.

Crew resource management (CRM) training was developed to build effective communication skills and a cohesive environment among team members and to build an atmosphere in which all personnel feel empowered to speak up when they suspect a problem. Team members are trained to cross-check each other's actions, offer assistance when needed and address errors in a non-judgemental fashion. Debriefing and providing feedback are key components of CRM training. It also emphasises the roles of fatigue, perceptual errors (such as misreading monitors or mishearing instructions) and the impact of management styles and organisational cultures.

More recent developments in HF have looked more closely at designing systems better suited to minimising error. Studies examining the hierarchy of intervention effectiveness and concepts based on nudge theory allow for design of healthcare systems that increase safety and give a better understanding of how people make decisions and behave.

The nudge theory, introduced by Richard Thaler and Cass Sunstein, is based on shaping the environment to encourage choice selection along pathways deemed to be beneficial to the individual, an organisation or society. A key feature of nudge theory is to structure the selection of preferred options while allowing individuals to maintain freedom of choice within the decision-making process. One successful example is the adoption of generic medication brands on electronic medical records by the use of a simple opt-out checkbox if the prescriber wishes to use a non-generic medication.

It is now widely recognised that HF need to be considered in every aspect of surgical care if the highest standards in patient safety are to be achieved. However, safety is just one aspect of a wider HF systems approach to equipment, task, environment and organisational design. Better understanding of HF can also significantly contribute to the quality, accessibility and cost of healthcare services and to the recruitment and retention of healthcare staff.

Summary box 15.1

Acknowledging the gap between medical progress and delivery of quality patient care

- Health care is complex with many areas for improvement
- Understanding of the influence of HF among care givers can highlight areas of risk but also potential solutions
- The different factors that impact human behaviour can be identified and influenced in a way that improves health care
- Acknowledge the importance of 'value' for both healthcare provider and patient
- Training in human factors to enhance teamworking is a prerequisite of contemporary health care

PATIENT SAFETY

Medicine will never be risk-free. From the beginning of training, doctors are taught that errors are unacceptable and that the philosophy of *primum non nocere* (first, do no harm) should permeate all aspects of treatment. Yet, worldwide, despite all the improvements in treatment and investment in technologies,

Richard H. Thaler, b.1945, economist, University Chicago, IL, USA, winner of the Sveriges Riksbank Prize in Economic Sciences in Memory of Alfred Nobel 2017 for contributions to behavioural economics.

Cass R Sunstein, b.1954, lawyer, Harvard Law School, Boston, MA, USA, co-authored *Nudge: Improving Decisions about Health, Wealth, and Happiness* with Thaler in 2008.

training and services, there remains the challenge of dealing with unsafe practices, incompetent healthcare professionals, poor governance of healthcare service delivery, errors in diagnosis and treatment and non-compliance with accepted standards.

When errors occur, it is important that there are systems in place to ensure that all those affected are informed and cared for, and that there is a process of analysis and learning to uncover the causes and prevent recurrence of such events. It is equally important to learn more about the characteristics and facilitators of safe, high-quality care. The study of patient safety is now a healthcare discipline in its own right, encompassing patient safety methodologies, health service design, investigation of incidents and related research. The development of risk management strategies within the healthcare setting attempts to address these failings. Comprehensive risk management is not just an exercise in ligation avoidance but aims to develop a cultural awareness and support for all healthcare workers in defining and delivering high-quality clinical care.

A milestone report by the US Institute of Medicine of the National Academy of Sciences (now the National Academy of Medicine), *To Err is Human: Building a Safer Health System*, drew widespread attention to the impact of medical error on healthcare outcomes. The World Health Organization (WHO) estimates that, even in advanced hospital settings, one in 10 patients receiving health care will suffer preventable harm, although measurement of the incidence of suboptimal outcomes remains challenging. In addition to the potential for needless suffering, the financial burden of unsafe care globally is compelling, resulting as it does in prolonged hospitalisation, loss of income, disability and litigation costing many billions of dollars every year. In 2017 the Organisation for Economic Co-operation and Development (OECD) published *The Economics of Patient Safety*, which indicates that this is a problem faced in all healthcare systems, with iatrogenic patient harm being the 15th leading cause of the global disease burden and accounting for 15% of all OECD countries' hospital expenditure.

While the relationship between medical error and litigation is particularly complex, sophisticated healthcare systems understand that effective strategies to promote patient safety and quality improvement must include a whole organisational culture change with both central senior management involvement and active engagement by all those within the organisation. Furthermore, clinical audit, data management and incident reporting must be carried out in a 'blame-free' culture with an emphasis on education and the avoidance of an adversarial culture, which hinders active participation.

PATIENT SAFETY AND RISK MANAGEMENT

Patient safety can only be considered in a broader understanding of risk management. Healthcare risk management has traditionally focused on the important role of patient safety and the reduction of medical error. However, with the increasing complexity of the healthcare environment, which includes not only the increasing complexity of medical care but also the use of new and advanced technologies, IT and cybersecurity risks and the ever-changing legal and regulatory frameworks that health providers work in, a more comprehensive approach to risk management is required.

As comprehensive risk management will increasingly become central to the design and delivery of all aspects of health care, surgeons need to be not only aware of the developments in this area but also willing to contribute to the design, implementation and assessment of risk management systems.

Supporting a safety culture

Adverse events and near misses go unreported for many reasons, including a fear of blame and the potential for litigation. Clinical risk management is an integrated process, based on risk identification, analysis and control of events, carried out within a 'blame-free' environment. Data collected from these episodes should be collated and learnt both institutionally and by uploading to a national database. Doctors should be familiar with the systems that operate within their own working environment.

Complaints from a patient or carer often highlight a problem that, when analysed, provides opportunities for reducing adverse events. Knowing how to manage complaints is an important part of providing better health care. There is wide acceptance for the need for complaints to be made easily and effectively, such that now more and more patient advocacy units provide a range of options for resolving complaints, including the provision of information and mediation and the setting up of conciliation meetings between the parties. Such risk management is complex and involves multiple domains, including operational, legal and financial issues. For the purpose of this chapter the focus is on clinical risk, benchmarking and incident reporting.

Most medical care entails some level of risk to the patient, either from the underlying condition or comorbidity or from the treatment itself, each of which may lead to recognised complications or side effects. These episodes must be differentiated from patient safety incidents, which have been described as preventable events or circumstances that did or could result in unnecessary harm to a patient. These include adverse events that result in actual harm, near-miss events that by chance or intervention cause no harm and no-harm events that reach a patient but result in no harm because of chance or other mitigating circumstance.

The most frequent contributing factors that lead to patient safety incidents are listed in ***Table 15.1***. Of these, inadequate communication between healthcare staff, or between medical staff and their patients or family members, ranks highest in frequency.

UNDERSTANDING PATIENT SAFETY INCIDENTS

Understanding the concepts underlying patient safety incidents is useful because it helps to anticipate situations that are likely to lead to errors and highlights areas where preventative action can be taken. The problem of error can be viewed in two ways – from a person approach or from a system approach.

TABLE 15.1 Factors that contribute to patient safety incidents.

Human factors	• Inadequate patient assessment; delays or errors in diagnosis • Failure to use or interpret appropriate tests • Error in performance of an operation, treatment or test • Inadequate monitoring or follow-up of treatment • Deficiencies in training or experience • Fatigue, overwork, time pressures • Personal or psychological factors (e.g. depression or drug abuse) • Patient or working environment variation • Lack of recognition of the dangers of medical errors
System failures	• Poor communication between healthcare providers • Inadequate staffing levels • Disconnected reporting systems or over-reliance on automated systems • Lack of coordination at handovers • Drug similarities • Environment design, infrastructure • Equipment failure owing to lack of parts or skilled operators • Cost-cutting measures by hospitals • Poor governance structures and inadequate systems to report and review patient safety incidents
Medical complexity	• Advanced and new technologies • Potent drugs, their side effects and interactions • Working environments – intensive care, operating theatres

The person approach

Human performance principles tell us that humans are fallible and that errors can occur through doing the wrong thing – errors of commission; failure to act – errors of omission; or errors of execution – doing the right thing incorrectly. These principles also tell us that, by understanding the reasons why adverse events and near misses occur and by applying the lessons learnt from past events, future errors can be prevented. However, for most errors the person approach on its own tends to blame the individual and restricts learning. For this reason, individual performance may be best assessed by professional appraisal processes and clinical audit, which ensures that performance outcomes are benchmarked across institutional, national and international norms.

The system approach

Health systems add complex organisational structures to human fallibility, thus substantially increasing the potential for errors. A systems approach to error recognises that adverse events rarely have an isolated cause and that they are best addressed by examining why the system failed rather than who made the mistake. This is clearly outlined in the 2013 report by Professor Don Berwick called *A Promise to Learn – A Commitment to Act*, which looked into improving patient safety in the NHS, where the emphasis is on a system-wide approach to patient safety.

However, greater analysis of organisational safety needs to go beyond understanding not only why unanticipated events occur, which has been referred to as safety 1; it also needs to understand the robustness and resilience within systems due to human innovation and adaptability, which frequently prevents untoward events and is referred to as safety 2. Safety 1 places the emphasis on identifying errors after the event and aims to prevent them from occurring or recurring in the future, whereas safety 2 acknowledges that healthcare work is resilient and that everyday performance succeeds much more often than it fails. This is because clinicians constantly adjust what they do to match the conditions. Working flexibly, and actively trying to increase clinicians' capacity to deliver more care more effectively, is key to this new approach. At its heart, proactive safety management focuses on how everyday performance usually succeeds rather than why it occasionally fails, and it actively strives to improve the former rather than simply preventing the latter.

The publication 'From Safety-I to Safety-II: A White Paper' (2015) expands on this concept and stresses the importance of assimilation of these two ways of thinking. Sophisticated healthcare systems need not only to examine what works well but also to examine adverse events and understand and plan for adverse outcomes. Balancing these concepts should be considered an investment not only in safety but also in improving productivity and patient and staff well-being.

The underlying principles to these approaches to risk management stem from theories such as Heinrich's safety pyramid, which proposes that each major injury within a system masks a multiple of minor injuries and near misses. This model stresses the importance of near-miss reporting in order to fully understand the spectrum of patient safety and allow adequate risk management planning.

More recently James Reason proposed the 'Swiss cheese' model of causation to explain the consequences of multiple errors that result in harm, analogous to the holes in a Swiss cheese, which if aligned create a defect that has adverse consequences. For organisational safety to be effective each

Donald Berwick, b.1946, Professor of Pediatrics and Health Care Policy, Harvard Medical School, Boston, MA, USA.
Herbert W Heinrich, 1886–1962, engineer, Hartford, CT, USA, a pioneer in industrial safety.
James T Reason, b.1938, Professor Emeritus of Psychology, University of Manchester, Manchester, UK.

healthcare worker is required to take responsibility for their respective roles in order to avoid the summation of error and resultant harm. Consequently, the more layers of responsibility, the fewer the chances of adverse events occurring.

Summary box 15.2

Understanding patient safety incidents

- Errors can be viewed from a person-centred or a system approach
- The majority of near misses or adverse events are due to system factors
- Understanding why these errors occur and applying the lessons learnt will prevent future injuries to patients
- It is important to report all near misses or adverse events so that we can constantly learn from mistakes
- Error models can help us understand the factors that cause near misses and adverse events
- Examining what works well may be an additional constructive approach to defining safe patient pathways

STRATEGIES FOR PATIENT SAFETY

As safety is everybody's business, building and embedding a safety culture into surgical service delivery is the key to improving patient outcomes. At an institutional level, defining 'best practice' within a robust governance system and benchmarking against national and international norms is required prior to implementation of strategies for improvement. Clearly these strategies will vary depending on local requirements and resources.

International

Since 2009, WHO has embarked on a series of global and regional initiatives to improve surgical outcomes. Much of this work has stemmed from WHO's Second Global Patient Safety Challenge, *Safe Surgery Saves Lives*. One specific strategy that has been shown to be effective is the use of the surgical checklist, which, when properly implemented, has been shown to improve surgical outcomes in both low- and middle-income countries and in wealthier countries.

Checklists

Checklists in the operating theatre environment are now accepted as standard safety protocols since the *Safe Surgery Saves Lives* Study Group at WHO published its results. The use of a perioperative surgical safety checklist in eight hospitals around the world was associated with a reduction in perioperative mortality from 1.5% to 0.7% and major inpatient complications from 11.0% before to 7.0% after the introduction of the checklist. A more recent study from two hospitals in Norway (2015) showed a decrease in complications from 19.9% to 11.5%, a fall in mean length of stay of 2 days and a significant fall in hospital mortality from 1.9% to 0.2% in one hospital.

The surgical safety checklist identifies specific checks to be carried out at three obligatory time points (***Figure 15.1***). The checklist items are not intended to be comprehensive and additions and modifications are encouraged. For example, during the COVID-19 pandemic, the checklist lent itself to including COVID-19-specific checks within this pathway.

The benefits of standardisation of surgical processes need not be limited to the operating theatre. Several studies have shown that the majority of surgical errors (53–70%) occur outside the operating theatre, either before or after surgery, and that a more substantial improvement in safety can be achieved by targeting the entire surgical pathway.

There is no question that checklists are tools that improve outcomes, provided they are correctly implemented. However, there are some important considerations. Checklists are suited to solving specific kinds of problems, but not others. Even in comparison with aviation, managing patients involves an enormous amount of coordinated, time-pressured decision making and potential delays. Checklists are simple reminders of what to do; however, unless they are coupled with attitude change and efforts to remove barriers to actually using them, they will have limited impact. Simply put, if one begins to believe that safety is simple and that all it requires is a checklist, there is a danger of abandoning other important efforts to achieve safer, higher quality care.

Experience has shown, however, that for successful implementation of a checklist considerable attention is required to the following factors:

- early engagement of staff;
- active leadership and identification of local champions;
- extensive discussion, education and training;
- multidisciplinary involvement;
- coaching;
- ongoing feedback;
- local adaptation.

Resource-rich countries

Many countries and professional bodies in resource-rich countries have developed various strategies to improve outcomes in surgical practice. These include:

- regulatory systems for the licensing of physicians and healthcare institutions;
- national/statutory policies for patient safety;
- standard setting by surgical professional bodies;
- national clinical audits and quality improvement programmes;
- statutory reporting of adverse events.

Low- and middle-income countries

Resource-poor countries share many of the aspirations and challenges of resource-rich countries; however, they also face issues that require different strategies. The probability of a patient being harmed in hospital is greater with, for example, a greater risk of healthcare-associated infection and difficulty maintaining medical equipment because of lack of parts or necessary skills. In some countries, the proportion of injections

Surgical Safety Checklist

World Health Organization | Patient Safety
A World Alliance for Safer Health Care

Before induction of anaesthesia → **Before skin incision** → **Before patient leaves operating room**

Before induction of anaesthesia

(with at least nurse and anaesthetist)

Has the patient confirmed his/her identity, site, procedure, and consent?
- ☐ Yes

Is the site marked?
- ☐ Yes
- ☐ Not applicable

Is the anaesthesia machine and medication check complete?
- ☐ Yes

Is the pulse oximeter on the patient and functioning?
- ☐ Yes

Does the patient have a:

Known allergy?
- ☐ No
- ☐ Yes

Difficult airway or aspiration risk?
- ☐ No
- ☐ Yes, and equipment/assistance available

Risk of >500ml blood loss (7ml/kg in children)?
- ☐ No
- ☐ Yes, and two IVs/central access and fluids planned

Before skin incision

(with nurse, anaesthetist and surgeon)

- ☐ **Confirm all team members have introduced themselves by name and role.**
- ☐ **Confirm the patient's name, procedure, and where the incision will be made.**

Has antibiotic prophylaxis been given within the last 60 minutes?
- ☐ Yes
- ☐ Not applicable

Anticipated Critical Events

To Surgeon:
- ☐ What are the critical or non-routine steps?
- ☐ How long will the case take?
- ☐ What is the anticipated blood loss?

To Anaesthetist:
- ☐ Are there any patient-specific concerns?

To Nursing Team:
- ☐ Has sterility (including indicator results) been confirmed?
- ☐ Are there equipment issues or any concerns?

Is essential imaging displayed?
- ☐ Yes
- ☐ Not applicable

Before patient leaves operating room

(with nurse, anaesthetist and surgeon)

Nurse Verbally Confirms:
- ☐ The name of the procedure
- ☐ Completion of instrument, sponge and needle counts
- ☐ Specimen labelling (read specimen labels aloud, including patient name)
- ☐ Whether there are any equipment problems to be addressed

To Surgeon, Anaesthetist and Nurse:
- ☐ What are the key concerns for recovery and management of this patient?

This checklist is not intended to be comprehensive. Additions and modifications to fit local practice are encouraged.

Revised 1 / 2009

© WHO, 2009

Figure 15.1 World Health Organization's surgical safety checklist (https://www.who.int/teams/integrated-health-services/patient-safety/research/safe-surgery/tool-and-resources).

given with syringes or needles reused without sterilisation is as high as 70%. Each year, unsafe injections cause 1.3 million deaths, primarily as a result of transmission of hepatitis viruses and human immunodeficiency virus.

Identifying and addressing patient safety risks in collaboration with colleagues across the world allows progress to be made on a number of important areas of surgical safety as well as supporting improvements in surgical training. International collaborations, often based on personal professional relationships, can be a catalyst to supporting surgical training and surgical safety initiatives worldwide. The WHO surgical safety checklist (*Figure 15.1*) demonstrates that many patient safety initiatives are not resource intensive but require attention to the details of process and care pathways commensurate with the local context.

Hospital level

Clinical governance

Patient safety requires a team approach. Many national and international bodies, professional organisations and medical and academic health centres now realise the importance of leadership training. Motivated and well-prepared healthcare workers trained to work together can reduce risks to patients, themselves and their colleagues, especially if incidents are managed positively and opportunities to learn from adverse events and near misses are used. High-performing institutions consistently develop transparent governance structures to provide robust oversight of not only risk management but also all aspects of business planning and outcome reporting in addition to workforce education and training.

Summary box 15.3

Strategies for patient safety

- WHO has established a number of international initiatives for patient safety, including the surgical safety checklist
- Seek opportunities for certification and accreditation from national and international healthcare quality improvement organisations
- Engage with available national and international audits
- Seek collaboration with recognised training bodies and quality improvement organisations
- Hospitals or institutions that offer the greatest patient safety systems develop clinical governance, leadership and team-building programmes and foster teamworking

SPECIFIC ISSUES IN COMMUNICATION

Professional behaviour and maintaining fitness to practice

Professionalism is an important component of patient safety. This embraces attitudes and behaviours that serve the patient's best interests above and beyond other considerations. Organisations responsible for maintaining ethical standards include professionalism as one of the standards by which healthcare workers are judged (see *Chapter 14*).

Fitness to work or practice – **competence** – refers not just to knowledge and skills but also to the attitudes required to be able to carry out one's duties. Monitoring their own fitness for work is the responsibility of each individual, their employer and professional organisations. Healthcare workers are required to have transparent systems in place to identify, monitor and assist them to maintain their competence. **Credentialing** is one way to ensure that clinicians are adequately prepared to safely treat patients with particular problems or to undertake defined procedures.

Communicating openly with patients and their carers and obtaining consent

A patient-centred approach by medical staff, with involvement of patients and their carers as partners, is now recognised as being of fundamental importance. There are better treatment outcomes and fewer errors when there is good communication, while poor communication is a common reason for patients taking legal actions.

Involving patients in and respecting their right to make decisions about their care and treatment is crucial. Explaining risk is a difficult but important part of good communication. It requires skill to explain the potential for harm of a procedure so that it is fully understood because patients vary in their perception and understanding and it is often difficult to assess the trade-offs between harm and benefit.

Obtaining consent for surgery requires that surgeons provide information to help patients to understand the positives and negatives of their various treatment options (*Table 15.2*). Patients should be allowed to make these informed decisions without coercion or manipulation. Consent should be obtained by someone who is capable of performing the surgery, and this should be taken when the patient is fully aware, especially in the non-urgent situation, well before the surgical procedure (see *Chapter 14*). A failure to provide adequate time for discussion regarding consent and also to understand that consent is a process that frequently requires multiple interactions with a patient are frequent causes of an unsatisfactory consent process.

TABLE 15.2 Information to be provided when seeking consent for surgery.

- The condition and the reasons why it warrants surgery.
- The type of surgery proposed and how it might correct the condition.
- The anticipated prognosis and expected side effects of the proposed surgery.
- The unexpected hazards of the proposed surgery.
- Any alternative and potentially successful treatments other than the proposed surgery.
- The consequences of no treatment at all.

When things go wrong: open disclosure

Communicating honestly with patients after an adverse event, or **open disclosure**, includes a full explanation of what happened, the potential consequences and what will be done to fix the problem. Safe care also involves taking care of the patient after the event, ensuring that the problem does not happen again and sincerely offering regret or an apology, as appropriate. These issues are increasingly reflected in open disclosure policies for healthcare workers; in the UK they are explicitly outlined in the General Medical Council's professional duty of candour and statements by many of the professional bodies. Since 2015, and as a consequence of the Francis report, a duty of candour has been placed on a statutory basis in the UK for all healthcare providers.

Situational awareness: understanding the work environment and working well within it

Nowhere is teamworking more important than in managing the flow of information within health care. Poor communication can lead to misinformation to patients and staff and delays in diagnosis, treatment and discharge as well as in failures to follow up on test results. On the other hand, good teamwork, good communication and continuity of care reduce errors and improve patient care and staff satisfaction within a team.

The nuances of good communication extend beyond the ability to converse with other members of the healthcare team and include specific competencies, namely situational awareness and emotional intelligence. Situational awareness describes an awareness of all individuals within the environment and an appreciation of the importance of change with time. Emotional intelligence, as defined by Peter Salovey and John Mayer, is 'the ability to monitor one's own and other people's emotions, to discriminate between different emotions and label them appropriately, and to use emotional information to guide thinking and behavior'. Experienced clinicians and clinical leaders understand that excellent communication skills are based on both situational awareness and emotional intelligence.

Sir Robert Anthony Francis, b.1950, British barrister, chaired the Stafford Hospital Inquiry.
Peter Salovey, b.1958, social psychologist, President of Yale University, New Haven, CT, USA.
John D Mayer, b. 1953, contemporary, psychologist, University of New Hampshire, NH, USA.

These features of situational awareness and emotional intelligence are important in identifying stress within oneself and other members of the healthcare team. **Stress, tiredness and mental fatigue** in the workplace are significant occupational health and safety risks in health care. There is good evidence linking tiredness with medical errors. Fatigue can also affect well-being by causing depression, anxiety and confusion, all of which negatively impact on clinicians' performance. Increasingly 'burnout' has been identified as a major cause of poor performance in the medical workforce. **Burnout** is characterised by a state of emotional, mental and physical exhaustion caused by prolonged stress. Burnout in the medical workforce has increased in recent years and has been attributed to lack of autonomy within the profession and increased administrative workloads; the latter is compounded by electronic record-keeping and working in an increasingly regulated environment. Doctors suffer from burnout to a greater extent than other professions.

Organisations and those in leadership positions bear responsibility for managing the working environment and work practices to minimise fatigue and stress. While this is widely reflected in legal restriction of working hours, much needs to be done to determine whether reducing resident or trainee hours of work leads to greater patient safety because of the 'trade-off' in requiring additional 'handovers' between clinical teams and subsequent loss of continuity of care.

Prescribing safely

Patients are vulnerable to mistakes made in any one of the many steps involved in the ordering, dispensing and administration of medications. Medication errors are one of the most common errors across all medical specialties. Accuracy requires that all steps are correctly executed. Common medication errors include:

- poor assessment or inadequate knowledge of patients and their clinical conditions;
- inadequate knowledge of the medications;
- dosage calculation errors;
- illegible handwriting;
- confusion regarding the name or the mixing up medications.

PATIENT SAFETY AND THE SURGEON: PROFESSIONAL RESPONSIBILITY

Among medical specialties, surgery is one of the most invasive healthcare interventions that a patient can experience. More than 100 million people worldwide undergo surgical treatment every year. Problems associated with surgical safety in resource-rich countries account for half of the avoidable adverse events that result in death or disability.

The 'more than one cause' theory of accident causation can be aptly applied to many aspects of surgical patient care during the perioperative period. However, irrespective of the safety event or issue, the surgeon as the likely senior team leader will play a key role in reporting and communicating these events with patients and carers, other team members and hospital administration. This is particularly so for those so-called '**coal-face**' errors where patients identify the surgeon as being responsible for a defined episode of care.

Summary box 15.4

Patient safety at the coal face

- Communicating well with patients and their carers
- Understanding situational awareness and emotional intelligence
- Effective teamworking
- Professionalism, as another essential component of patient safety
- System approach to clinical risk management events and patients' complaints

Cuschieri and others have described coal-face errors as those that can potentially be committed by surgeons during the care of their patients and include:

- diagnostic and management errors;
- resuscitation errors;
- prophylaxis errors;
- prescription/parenteral administration errors;
- situation awareness, identification and teamwork errors;
- technical and operative errors.

Situation awareness: identifying teamwork errors

Operating theatres have been described as 'among the most complex political, social and cultural structures that exist, full of ritual, drama, hierarchy and too often conflict'. In such an environment, systems should seek to prevent error by improving workplace preparedness and by incorporating defences that reduce human error or minimise its consequence. Well-recognised and potential errors include:

- the wrong patient in the operating theatre;
- surgery performed on the wrong side or site;
- the wrong procedure performed;
- failure to communicate changes in the patient's condition;
- disagreements about proceeding;
- retained instruments or swabs (***Figure 15.2***).

All these events are catastrophic for the patient and almost invariably occur through a lack of communication (see ***Never events***). This means that all theatre staff should follow protocols and be familiar with the underlying principles supporting a uniform approach to caring for patients.

Technical and operative errors

In surgery, the person rather than systems approach emphasises the accountability of the surgeon, who, unlike colleagues in other medical disciplines, when operating carries specific

Sir Alfred Cuschieri, b.1938, Maltese surgeon and Emeritus Professor of Surgery, Dundee, UK.

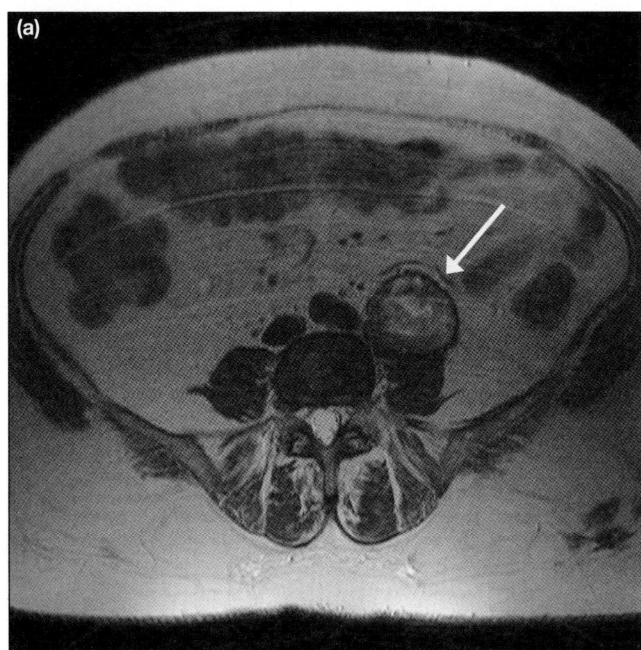

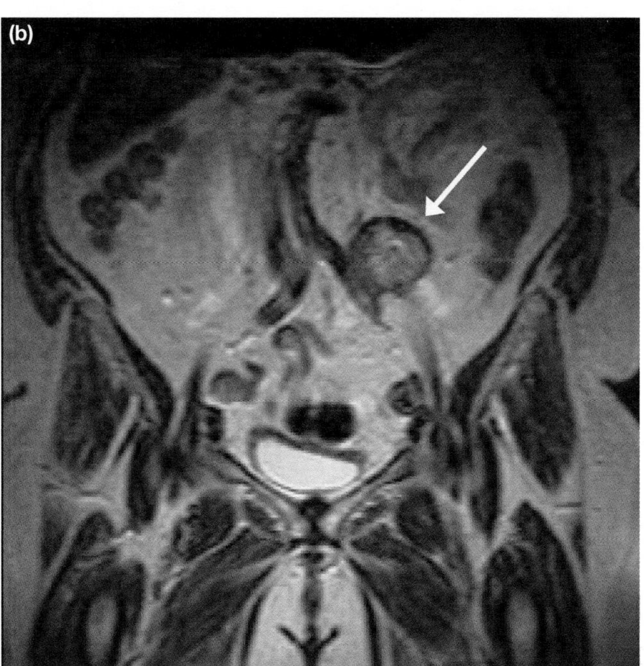

Figure 15.2 Axial (a) and coronal (b) magnetic resonance images demonstrating a well-defined abdominal mass with whorled stripes in a fluid-filled central cavity (arrows). This 60-year-old woman had had an abdominal hysterectomy 10 years previously and presented with pyrexia and flank pain. The cause was due to the late presentation of a retained surgical swab.

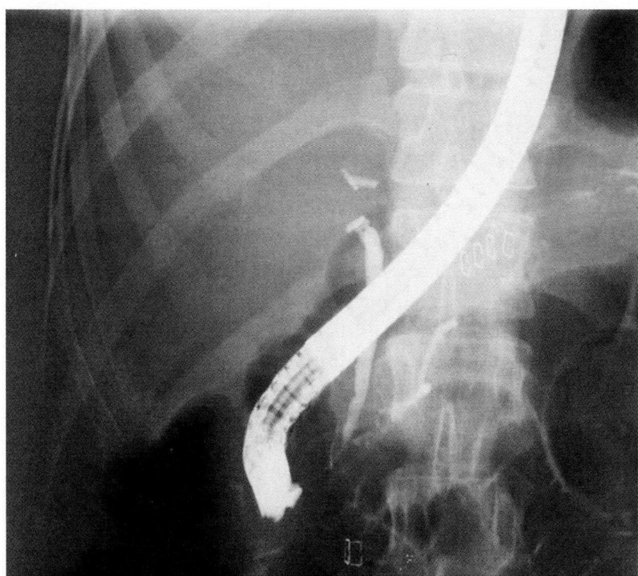

Figure 15.3 Endoscopic retrograde cholangiopancreatography radiograph showing an iatrogenic bile duct injury.

responsibilities. During a surgical procedure, for example, there may be a specific action that, of itself, may be the error, such as inadvertent injury to the common bile duct during a cholecystectomy (*Figure 15.3*). The practical value of this kind of interpretation is that, provided latent conditions are excluded, it gives a sense of responsibility to the surgeon and it may also help to point to the most effective pathway for remediation, by counselling or retraining, as against reassessing the system and putting in place further safeguards.

Central to operative performance is proficiency, an acquired state, honed by sound teaching, practice and repetition, by which a surgeon consistently performs operations with good outcomes. In cognitive psychology, high surgical proficiency is a state of automatic unconscious processing, with the execution being effortless, intuitive and untiring, as opposed to non-proficient execution, which is characterised by conscious control processing, requiring constant attention and resulting in slow, deliberate execution and inducing fatigue. The transition from one state to the other is better known as the 'learning curve' and is reflected in the hierarchal pyramid of competence (*Figure 15.4*). This should not carry negative connotations for trainee surgeons, who might be at the conscious processing stage but still perform a perfectly good operation, although it might take longer and be more tiring.

Failures in operative technique include:

- **cognitive** errors of judgement, such as late conversion of a difficult laparoscopic procedure into an open one;
- **procedural**, when the steps of an operation are not followed or are omitted;
- **executional**, when, for example, too much force is used, which may result in damage that may or may not have consequences;
- **misinterpretation** of anatomy/pathology, which is compounded by minimal access surgery with the limitations of a two-dimensional image;
- **misuse** of instrumentation, such as with energised dissection modalities (e.g. diathermy);
- **missed** iatrogenic injury either at the time of surgery or diagnosed late.

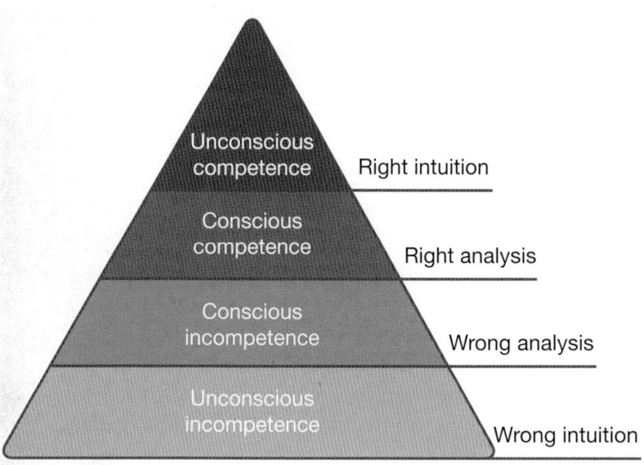

Figure 15.4 Hierarchy of competence.

Never events

Many national health services and institutions now require that all incidents are managed, reported and investigated. Incidents can be defined as events that could have or did result in unintended and/or unnecessary serious harm.

One subset of serious incidents is a **never or serious reportable event**. These events are considered to be wholly preventable; for example, a retained abdominal swab or instrument, where guidance providing strong systemic protective barriers should have been implemented, namely checklists. Each 'never event' type has the potential to cause serious harm to the patient or even death. However, serious harm or death is not required to have occurred for that incident to be categorised as a 'never or serious reportable event'. As previously described clinical incidents of this nature, by definition, mandate an open disclosure process with patients and their carers.

Shouldering the burden of adverse event

As primary care givers and clinical leaders, surgeons will not infrequently find themselves taking an active part in adverse event reporting. The professional responsibilities involved with managing adverse outcomes can be onerous, particularly understanding societal change and patients' expectations, in increasingly litigious societies. The administrative burden and responsibility associated with this need to be recognised. Issues relating to surgeons' well-being and burnout remain a cause for concern: supporting surgeons following adverse events has been increasingly recognised as a responsibility of all within the surgical community. The concept of the 'second victim' has been advanced to acknowledge the effects of adverse outcomes on surgeons' well-being. This is not to denigrate the undoubted harm caused to the 'first victim', or patient. Increasingly, however, comprehensive risk management systems will need not only to be patient-centric but also to acknowledge and support resilience of those working within our health services.

QUALITY IMPROVEMENT

In health care, quality improvement is defined as the continuous and combined efforts of people to make changes that will lead to better patient outcomes, enhanced healthcare system performance and better learning and professional development. Improvements come about through the intentional actions of staff equipped with the skills and data needed to bring about changes in patient care, either directly or indirectly. Such changes require substantial and sustained commitments of time and resources. The field of improvement science provides frameworks and methodologies that help when designing or redesigning healthcare processes and systems, especially when the aim is to ensure more efficient, safe, timely, effective, patient-centred and equitable care. The concept of value is an important adjunct to healthcare improvement. Value takes into account the total cost of health care as compared with the outcomes delivered to patients and helps to place emphasis on health, well-being and preventative care as opposed to exclusively focusing on treatment of illness.

There are large numbers of improvement activities that range from redesigning how teams deliver care in the multiple small clinical groupings (microsystems) that make up healthcare organisations to more large-scale reconfigurations of specialist services such as stroke care and cancer care. Other areas of healthcare improvement focus on areas as diverse as the redesign of training, budgeting processes and information systems. Common to all healthcare improvement is the necessity for doctors and other healthcare staff to reflect on and improve the way they work and to build a culture that both understands and values continuous improvement.

CLINICAL OUTCOMES, AUDIT AND IMPROVEMENT

Clinical audit, a function of clinical governance, is the means by which the health care being provided is compared with accepted standards. It allows care providers and patients to know how their service is doing (known as quality assurance) and to identify where there could be improvements. Clinical audits can look at care nationwide or locally within hospitals and their departments, in GP practices or anywhere health care is provided (***Table 15.3***).

Measuring clinical outcomes as part of a quality improvement cycle can help to:

- improve the quality of clinical care, with shorter hospital stays, better outcomes and fewer complications, reduced readmissions and greater patient satisfaction;
- inform the development of national clinical audits, including driving participation, data completeness and accuracy;
- support shared decision making and empowerment of patients, including their treatment options and choice of provider;
- improve the oversight and management of clinicians, their teams and practises, thus reassuring patients that their clinical care is being actively monitored and improved;
- help medical specialty associations to become increasingly transparent and patient focused;

- support team and individual quality improvement, including providing information for appraisal and revalidation;
- learn from, spread and celebrate best practice.

TABLE 15.3 Four stages of high value quality improvement or clinical audit activity

- Preparation and planning
- Measurement of performance
- Implementation of change
- Sustainment and evaluation of the improvement

QUALITY MEASURES

Measurement is a key principle of quality improvement. Although many changes take place in health care, without measurement it is impossible to determine whether those changes actually result in improved quality. Measurement of improvement requires different methods from those used in research, being concerned more with testing of how best to effectively introduce and replicate best practice rather than determining for the first time what best practice should be. Quality measures are tools that help to quantify the characteristics of high-quality health care and may measure the healthcare process, its outcomes, the patient's experience or the organisational structures or systems that support care delivery. Quality may be measured in terms of structure, process and outcomes.

Structural measures outline the characteristics of the health system that affect the system's ability to meet the healthcare needs of individual patients or a population. Structural measures usually refer to the availability of material, infrastructural or human resources, e.g. the number of surgeons per 100 000 population or the number of staffed operating theatre sessions in a hospital. Structural measures are especially useful in evaluating and improving equity of access to health care. They may include measurement of the availability in a healthcare setting of policies or procedures needed to deliver high-quality care, such as standards for the frequency and nature of clinical observation of postoperative patients.

Process measures assess what the healthcare provider did for the patient and how well it was done. The term process is used to refer to the implementation of procedures and practices by staff when planning, prescribing, delivering and evaluating care. Each surgical patient's journey is a composite of multiple processes, such as preoperative assessment, hospital admission and undergoing an operation, among others. Measurement for improvement most commonly involves tracking processes at the same site over time in an attempt to reduce inappropriate variation. Process improvement measures should be associated with better outcomes of care and, ideally, should be important from a patient's perspective. An example of a clinical process measure might be the starting times of operating lists. Consistently starting the operating day on time reduces delays for patients awaiting surgery and has a number of associated possible benefits, such as shorter fasting times preoperatively and a greater ability to plan the theatre day. Sometimes process measures are used as a management tool, comparing sites or performance against defined thresholds. In this example, starting theatres on time might be part of a wider improvement plan that aims to reduce underutilisation of staffed theatre time.

Outcome measures describe the effects of care on the health status of patients and populations – they are specific, observable and measurable changes that represent the achievement of an outcome of a quality improvement initiative. **Clinical outcome measures** refer specifically to outcomes of healthcare interventions, whether they are to do with diagnosis, treatment or care received by service users. Ideally, they should be outcomes that are important to patients rather than to the healthcare provider (PROM: patient-reported outcome measure), and there should be evidence that they reflect the quality of the interventions and their effect. Outcome measures are what are commonly used in **clinical audit** when outcomes achieved are compared with evidence-based standards of clinical care.

An important principle of healthcare improvement is patient-centred co-design, a process by which healthcare providers work in partnership with the people receiving care to identify and prioritise desirable outcomes. Such outcomes may include factors experienced by people accessing care, such as:

- the speed of their access to reliable health advice;
- the effectiveness of their treatment delivered by trusted professionals;
- the continuity of their care and its smooth transitions;
- the involvement of, and support for, their family and carers;
- the availability of clear, comprehensible information and support for self-care;
- their involvement in decisions and the respect for their preferences;
- the emotional support, empathy and respect provided;
- the attention paid to their physical and environmental needs.

The collection and interpretation of reliable data are of fundamental importance to any quality improvement exercise (***Table 15.4***).

THE PROCESS OF SURGICAL CARE

Patients attend surgeons in many different settings depending on whether they present **electively** (scheduled) or **urgently** (unscheduled). An elective patient's journey is usually predictable and typically starts with referral from primary care for outpatient (ambulatory) consultation and investigation. If a surgical procedure is required, the patient undergoes assessment from both a surgical and anaesthetic perspective prior to admission. Ideally the patient is then admitted in a timely manner to the level of care that best meets their needs, whether as a day case, on the day of surgery, or for as short a time as possible before surgery as an inpatient. Preoperative checking is followed by the theatre journey, which includes reception, anaesthesia, the surgery itself and recovery – each, in their own way, a series of complex interventions. Returning to the ward and recovery demands another set of skills, procedures and processes followed by a final 'discharge from hospital'

TABLE 15.4 Three pioneers of quality improvement and their quotes on data.

William Edwards Deming (1900–1993)	American engineer, statistician, author and management consultant. Pioneered the PDSA (plan–do–study–act) cycle	'In God we trust, all others bring data.'
Peter Ferdinand Drucker (1909–2005)	Austrian-born American management consultant and educator	'What gets measured gets improved.'
Donald Berwick (b.1946)	American paediatrician. Former President and Chief Executive Officer of the Institute for Healthcare Improvement	Sequence of reactions that challenge data: "The data are wrong." "The data are right but it's not a problem." "The data are right; it is a problem but not my problem." "I accept the burden of improvement."

process and transition of care back to the community services if required.

The urgent, emergency or unscheduled patient journey is different because it is unpredictable for each individual, although patterns of presentation do emerge when managing large numbers. The patient commonly presents at the emergency department of a hospital either as a self-referral, as a primary care referral or by ambulance. The journey begins with triage by a team, who assess the severity of the illness and then stream the patient to the most appropriate area for their needs, which might include, for example, a resuscitation unit, a rapid assessment and treatment unit, an acute surgical assessment unit, a minor injuries unit or an ambulatory care unit. The objective is that the patient is seen as soon as possible by a **senior decision maker**, so that the patient can be treated or discharged as expeditiously as possible or, if admission and surgery are required, this too can be expedited. Thereafter, the journey follows a similar course to that of an elective admission.

This simple outline of surgical patients' journeys serves to illustrate the many individual steps or processes in that journey, each with scope for errors, delays and inefficiencies. Opportunities for improvement are almost limitless.

THE QUALITY IMPROVEMENT PATHWAY

Quality improvement can be applied to almost any step, process or activity. The science of improvement is an applied science that prioritises innovation, rapid-cycle testing and spread with the aim of identifying what changes, and in what contexts, will result in improvement. Healthcare Improvement Scotland identifies seven stages when undertaking improvement:

1. **discovering** – is about defining the aims and vision; understanding what the problem is and what data are available;
2. **exploring** – is about defining the present state and visualising the future state;
3. **designing** – is about defining how to move from the present state to the future state and identifying the priorities;
4. **refining** – is about testing change, learning from the data and identifying the benefits;
5. **introducing** – is about managing communications and building the will and culture to change;
6. **spreading** – is about showing the improvements, telling the story and disseminating the message;
7. **closing** – is about capturing and sustaining the learning.

Each step is supported by the use of tools and methodologies that are appropriate to the design and planning of each step, depending on the improvement exercise being undertaken (*Table 15.5*).

TABLE 15.5 Examples of tools used in quality improvement.

Organisational	Graphical
Root cause analysis Benefits realisation planning Demand and capacity planning Process mapping Value stream mapping Kanban and 5 'S'	Driver diagrams Fishbone cause and effect diagrams Spaghetti diagrams Box, frequency and scatter plots Pareto charts Run charts Statistical process control charts

Model for improvement

Based on the teachings of W. Edwards Deming (*Table 15.4*), the model for improvement is a system popularised by the Institute for Healthcare Improvement that asks three questions: 'What are we trying to accomplish?', 'How will we know that a change is an improvement?' and 'What changes can we make that will result in improvement?' The system employs plan–do–study–act (PDSA) cycles to perform and evaluate small, rapid-cycle tests of change.

Lean

Lean improvement methodologies originated in industrial settings among frontline workers and were pioneered in Japan, giving rise to much of the terminology used. *Kaizen* is the Japanese word for improvement. A single 'cycle' of kaizen activity is defined as requiring similar steps to a PDSA cycle. The same application can be used in health care, with many sequential cycles growing to 'continuous improvement'. The essential

TABLE 15.6 Seven types of waste in health care and possible solutions.

Overproduction Example: ordering unnecessary preoperative tests Solution: implementation of evidence-based preassessment pathways
Inventory Example: storing excessive medication or supplies in ward storage with a risk of them going out of date Solution: alphabetically ordered medication cupboards with small amounts of commonly used drugs in conjunction with an efficient replenishment system
Waiting Example: patients waiting long periods to come to theatre Solution: staggered admission times aligned to operating theatre schedule
Waste of transportation Example: using trolleys to bring ambulatory day patients to the operating theatre Solution: better design of the admissions process to enable patients to walk to theatre
Waste of overprocessing Example: using computed tomography scans to assess children with possible appendicitis Solution: consider whether ultrasound could be used instead
Defect Example: patients arriving for surgery with incomplete or inappropriate preoperative paperwork Solution: more robust checking systems before patients come to theatre
Motion Example: frequent searching in theatres and the anaesthetic room to find necessary drugs and equipment Solution: an efficient theatre layout, common to all operating theatres in the hospital, where everything needed is easily available with minimal movement and always in the same place

philosophy behind lean methodologies is the elimination of waste through continuous improvement. Lean identifies seven forms of waste, each of which is relevant to health care (***Table 15.6***). Identifying waste leads inevitably to the need to define value from the perspective of the patient, a factor that is central to the Choosing Wisely initiative (https://www.choosingwisely.org).

Clinical microsystems

A **clinical microsystem** is an interdependent quality improvement unit made up of a small group of people who work together, usually on a regular basis, to provide care. Such groups are typically multidisciplinary. The patients who receive that care can also be recognised as members of a discrete group, such as patients with cancer or people attending an emergency department. Clinical microsystems share clinical and business aims, have linked processes and share information. Each microsystem produces services or care that can be measured as performance outcomes. Microsystems evolve over time and normally form part of a larger macrosystem or organisation.

They are considered 'living adaptive systems' as each microsystem must carry out work, meet staff needs and maintain its coherence as a clinical unit. Clinical microsystems can be assessed on their evidence base, leadership, patient and staff focus, and information systems.

Six Sigma

Six Sigma refers to another business performance methodology that has been adopted for use in health care. The fundamental objective of the Six Sigma methodology is the implementation of a measurement-based strategy that focuses on process improvement and especially on reducing unnecessary variation. One of its sub-methodologies is DMAIC (Define, Measure, Analyse, Improve, Control), which is an improvement system for existing processes that fall below specification and require incremental improvement.

Systems thinking and leadership

In a system as complex as health care, 'systems' thinking allows the whole system and the relationships of the parts to be considered rather than just isolated functions. Health care is a shared resource with many interdependencies; for surgery these include anaesthesia, critical care, nursing and other specialties we work with to manage comorbid patients.

If quality problems exist primarily because of systems problems, solutions are more likely in systems where relationships and integration are considered important and where emphasis is placed on HF such as communication, team building, conflict management, process management and education. Systems work best when there is a non-punitive culture and when they have leaders who understand the complexity of systems and foster a culture of continuous quality improvement. Those leaders should be visible at the front line and be champions of a supportive practice environment.

Improvement in the quality of care does not occur by chance and a programme team, armed with just organisational and graphical tools, will not succeed in producing sustainable change. True change can only happen when supported and driven by front-line staff. The underlying, central and agreed principles must include the creation of value for the patient, a constancy of purpose and systems thinking. These should be enabled by the intentional actions of trained staff supported by humble leadership and respect for individuals. Such a culture adjustment also requires integrated and coherent strategies and a sustained commitment of time, patience and resources.

Health care as a sector has been slow to recognise the important contribution that the theory and practice of quality improvement are able to make in delivering better value care. The experience of a relatively small number of healthcare organisations that have successfully done so, such as the Virginia Mason Medical Centre in Seattle, WA, is a challenge to others to invest in acquiring the necessary skills and capabilities.

A recent report by the Academy of the Medical Royal Colleges of UK and Ireland (2016) has argued that quality improvement should be at the heart of medical training and that there is a pressing need to develop quality improvement learning across the continuum of medical education. Understanding how health systems can be improved and how evidence-based practice can be implemented in complex healthcare settings are important skills for surgeons to master.

Summary box 15.5

Understanding quality improvement and its application in health care

- The definition of quality improvement and its relationship to clinical audit
- The different kinds of quality measures
- The patient's surgical journey and its potential for improvement
- Examples of quality improvement pathways, organisational methodologies and tools
- What systems thinking is and its importance alongside leadership
- The requirement for more education and training in quality improvement

FURTHER READING

Ham C, Berwick D, Dixon J. *Improving quality in the English NHS – a strategy for action.* The Kings Fund, 2016. Available from http://www.kingsfund.org.uk/publications/quality-improvement

Hollnagel E, Wears RL, Braithwaite J. *From Safety-I to Safety-II: A White Paper.* The Resilient Health Care Net, 2015. Available from https://www.england.nhs.uk/signuptosafety/wp-content/uploads/sites/16/2015/10/safety-1-safety-2-whte-papr.pdf

Institute of Medicine. *Crossing the quality chasm: a new health system for the 21st century.* Washington, DC: National Academies Press, 2001.

Jones B, Vaux E, Olsson-Brown A. How to get started in quality improvement. *BMJ* 2019; **364**: k5408.

Kohn LT, Corrigan JM, Donaldson MS (eds). *To err is human – building a safer health system.* Washington, DC: National Academies Press, 2000: 312.

Langley GL, Moen R, Nolan KM *et al. The improvement guide: a practical approach to enhancing organizational performance*, 2nd edn. San Francisco: Jossey-Bass Publishers, 2009.

National Advisory Group on the Safety of Patients in England. *A promise to learn – a commitment to act. Improving the safety of patients in England.* National Advisory Group on the Safety of Patients in England, 2013. Available from https://assets.publishing.service.gov.uk/government/uploads/system/uploads/attachment_data/file/226703/Berwick_Report.pdf

NHS Scotland. *Quality improvement hub.* Available from https://ihub.scot/improvement-resources (accessed 2 September 2021).

Slawomirski L, Auraaen A, Klazinga N. *The economics of patient safety: strengthening a value-based approach to reducing patient harm at national level.* OECD, 2017. Available from https://www.oecd.org/els/health-systems/The-economics-of-patient-safety-March-2017.pdf

Thaler R, Sunstein C. *Nudge: improving decisions about health, wealth, and happiness.* New Haven, CT: Yale University Press, 2008.

CHAPTER 16 Global health and surgery

Learning objectives

To define:
- The term global surgery

To describe:
- The role of a global surgeon

To understand:
- That surgery can be cost-effective
- Concepts of surgery and impoverishment
- How essential surgery can be delivered through surgical healthcare delivery platforms

To appreciate:
- The importance of access to surgical care
- The global surgical workforce
- The importance of global surgical metrics and research

INTRODUCTION AND DEFINITION

Global health is the health of populations in the global context. Global surgery is surgery with an understanding of public health. Surgeons understand the needs of their individual patients, while public health adds the understanding of the surgical operations needed in the population. Global surgery aims to provide equitable and improved surgical care across the world.

Global surgeons are not system-specific surgeons but are 'specialised' in providing the surgical needs of their communities. A practising surgeon can be viewed as a 'retailer' for the individual patient, whereas a global surgeon is typically the 'wholesaler' of the surgical needs of the population. This means that all surgeons working in non-tertiary hospitals who perform life-saving and essential surgeries, guided by the prevalent burden of surgical disease, are global surgeons. There is a misconception that a global surgeon is primarily a high-income country (HIC) surgeon helping low- and middle-income country (LMIC) surgeons periodically or through surgical missions. The HIC surgeons and subspecialist surgeons will be able to mitigate only a very small part of the vast unmet need of surgical disease burden in LMICs. Global surgery focuses on improving surgical health systems in parts of the world with a high surgical burden of disease by the local surgeons in those communities.

SURGERY AS AN ESSENTIAL AND COST-EFFECTIVE INTERVENTION

With the decline in the burden of communicable diseases in the world, one-third of the total disease burden is now due to surgical disease, with the majority being injury and cancers. In 2015, responding to this epidemiological transition, the World Health Organization (WHO) declared surgery to be a part of public health at the World Health Assembly, a meeting of all health ministers. Previously, surgical and anaesthesia care were perceived as too expensive and too complex to be a public health priority in resource-poor settings. The fact that early surgery saves lives and boosts the economy encouraged health planners to put surgery in the essential group of services in any national health strategy. Since then, scaling up surgical and anaesthesia care became a new worldwide movement under the umbrella term of 'global surgery'.

The Disease Control Priorities group of the World Bank has clearly identified surgical procedures that address the substantial needs of populations. In the absence of investments in surgical care, case-fatality rates and lifetime costs to the individual and society are high for common and easily treatable conditions, including appendicitis, hernia, fractures, obstructed labour, congenital anomalies and breast and cervical cancer. Furthermore, the cost-effectiveness of surgery for cataracts, hydrocephalus, limb deformity, general surgery and cleft lip or palate repair is comparable to widely used public health strategies, such as the bacille Calmette–Guérin (BCG) vaccine, and is much greater than other standard public health measures, such as antiretroviral therapy. Surgery becomes more cost-effective when not delivered as isolated interventions, but rather as a group of interventions within a platform of clinical care, such as a district hospital.

ACCESS TO SURGICAL CARE

The Lancet Commission on Global Surgery (2015) estimated that 5 billion out of the 7 billion people on the planet do not have access to surgery (see ***Summary box 16.2***). This is concerning, as access to timely life-saving essential surgery is a fundamental need for all. Although barriers to surgical access appear to be pronounced in LMICs, there are also disadvantaged and vulnerable populations in HICs. Access to

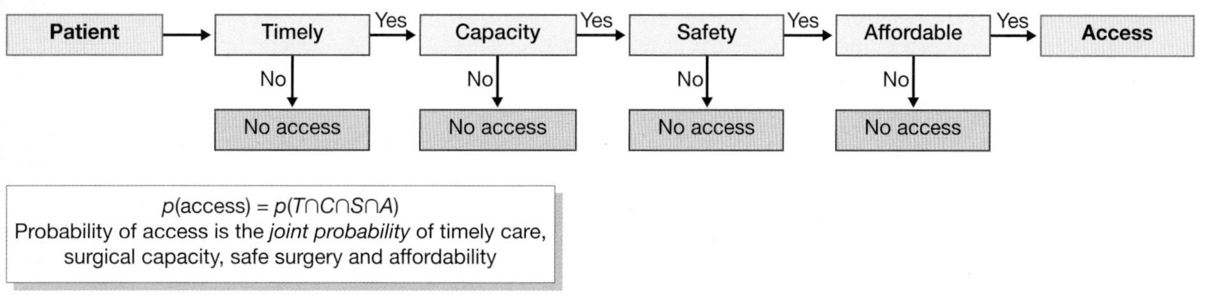

Figure 16.1 Access to surgery: the four dimensions.

surgery can be viewed through four lenses, namely; timeliness, capacity, safety and affordability (***Figure 16.1***).

Geographical access is the ability of a patient to reach a surgical facility within 2 hours, which is the crucial time for life-threatening haemorrhage. Capacity denotes that the facility has the required infrastructure and workforce and is able to perform safe surgery. However, the final barrier is when a patient cannot afford the surgery offered. A staggering nine out of 10 people in LMICs do not have access to surgery. Consequently, patients with acute surgical needs in LMICs do not reach hospital or reach it too late, in advanced stages of cancer, with already infected open fractures, with a perforated bowel or with burn contractures.

The world needs 143 million more surgical operations (unmet need) to be performed each year to save lives and prevent disability. Of the 313 million procedures undertaken worldwide each year, only 6% occur in the poorest countries, where over one-third of the world's population lives (see ***Further reading***). Unmet need is greatest in eastern, western and central sub-Saharan Africa and South Asia. These regions have young mothers dying of physiological conditions such as pregnancy, for want of a caesarean section. The global surgical community hopes to achieve an optimum operative volume of 5000 surgical procedures per 100 000 population across the world by 2030. Currently, there are countries such as Ethiopia which do 150 operations per 100 000 population, while Hungary performs 23 000. However, more than 5000 operations and further expenditure do not bring commensurate health benefits to the population. Low operative volumes are also associated with high case-fatality rates from common, treatable surgical conditions, which include injuries, early cancer and burns.

THE GLOBAL SURGICAL WORKFORCE

A surgeon, anaesthetist and obstetrician (SAO) at the district hospital are considered essential staffing. In many LMICs the SAO density is less than 5 per 100 000 population. As the SAO number increases, there is a dramatic improvement in key indicators, such as the maternal mortality ratio. However, the benefits plateau beyond 20 SAOs per 100 000 population. By 2030, all LMICs are committed to scaling up their surgical workforce to at least 20 SAO providers per 100 000 population. For all countries to reach this benchmark 1.27 million providers will need to be trained by 2030. Where there is a workforce shortage with a high surgical burden of disease, 'task-shifting' is common, whereby appropriate tasks are moved to less specialised health workers. For example, essential life-saving anaesthesia is a short course for medical graduates to address the specialist anaesthetist shortage in rural areas. In countries where there are still too few medical graduates, task-shifting in both anaesthesia and surgery involves appropriately trained non-medically qualified clinicians or midwives.

Ironically, the countries in the world where the fewest children are born have the greatest number of paediatric surgeons. There is much redundancy in human resources and low volumes of surgery in many HICs. In countries with a large burden of surgical disease and large populations, often a single surgeon caters to the surgical needs of many millions of people. However, these global surgical champions have high burnout rates. Healthcare workers, including doctors and nurses, in LMIC settings are often mobile and may choose to migrate overseas, either staying in healthcare or taking up alternative professions (commonly referred to as the 'brain drain'). Twelve per cent of SAOs in HICs have graduated from LMICs and two-thirds of these graduates are from countries with fewer than 20 SAOs per 100 000 population. More surgeons and anaesthetists are needed in LMICs, but the trend cannot be mitigated by simply training more, as the migration rates and the in-country maldistribution of surgeons remain. The answer is starting global surgery units in teaching universities, e-grand rounds, remote specialist support, e-intensive care units, low-cost robotics, online learning platforms, supportive supervision, recognition, peer support and collegiality for upskilling these champions.

A surgical system goes beyond a surgeon and a sterile operating theatre. Clearly, it requires a contribution from many other people to make the surgical ecosystem work, both before and after the patient's visit to the operating theatre. Global surgery includes healthcare workers beyond anaesthetists, obstetricians and all surgical specialities. It encourages a multidisciplinary team approach to the profession and acknowledges the important role of physicians, nurses, public health practitioners, health managers, surgical, laboratory, supply-chain specialists, biomedical engineers, radiology and blood bank technicians. The role of community health workers in reducing delays and facilitating the referral pathway is vital in LMICs. Engaged and caring hospital managers are critical in coordinating this process. Finally, private practitioners constitute a significant portion of the surgical manpower in LMICs and can contribute greatly to achieving the 2030 surgical burden goals, when appropriately incentivised and regulated for quality.

SURGERY AND IMPOVERISHMENT

Surgeons are tasked to operate and, in so doing, aim to successfully treat the surgical condition. A hernia not operated upon in a timely fashion costs the nation (and the individual) more when it becomes incarcerated. A delayed caesarean section puts mother and child at risk of death. In addition to risks associated with timing, the financial implications of a procedure can lead to poverty and catastrophic expenditure (more than 40% of annual household income). The one-time payment for surgery can push vulnerable populations into financial ruin, and those in poverty to extreme poverty. Forty-four per cent of the world's population is at risk of financial catastrophe with a single major operative procedure. In numbers, 33 million people (which is more than the population of Australia) each year will be pushed into poverty by paying for the surgery and anaesthesia that they need. Catastrophic expenditure is greatest for time-critical surgical conditions, such as peritonitis. Surgeons may have at times been less engaged with the patients' economic and social conditions that influence their health status. In many instances those who cannot afford to pay simply do not reach the operating theatre. Furthermore, lay people and policy makers alike can view surgery as an expensive business. This can lead to a problem, in that we can appreciate that everyone needs access to surgery, but commonly only the upper wealth quintiles are privileged to be in this position. When aggregated, the national estimate of out-of-pocket expenses of injury care alone exceeds the total health budget of many LMICs.

GLOBAL SURGICAL METRICS AND RESEARCH

Surgeons are familiar with vital-sign-based scoring systems for individual patients and with hospital metrics for inpatient hospital stay, surgical site infection or ventilator-associated pneumonia. Global surgery requires the addition of population-level metrics for the surgical burden of disease, which are less readily available. Household-level surveys of injury burden, vision care, cancer screening and worldwide metrics such as maternal mortality ratio and caesarean section rates are indicative of the surgical health systems in countries. Demographic surveillance systems and surveys such as the Million Death Study have been used to assess acute abdominal disorders at the national level. Most public health interventions are measured in terms of disability-adjusted life-years (DALYs) averted, which calculates how much it costs to avert 1 year of suffering due to a disability. One-third of all deaths worldwide are the result of conditions needing surgical care, and this surpasses human immunodeficiency virus, malaria and tuberculosis combined.

The core indicators to monitor the realisation of universal access to safe, affordable surgical and anaesthesia care are shown in ***Table 16.1***.

TABLE 16.1 Core indicators to monitor the realisation of universal access to safe, affordable surgical and anaesthesia care.

Preparedness	a	Access to timely essential surgery (proportion of population within 2 hours of a facility that can perform the bellwether procedures)
	b	Density of surgeons, anaesthetists and obstetricians working per 100 000 population
Surgical service delivery	a	Procedures done in an operating theatre, per 100 000 population per year
	b	All-cause death rate before discharge of patients who have undergone a procedure in an operating theatre, divided by the total number of procedures
Affordability of surgery		Proportion of households protected against impoverishment and catastrophic expenditure from direct out-of-pocket payments for surgical care

ESSENTIAL SURGERY THROUGH SURGICAL HEALTHCARE DELIVERY PLATFORMS

The 44 essential surgeries listed by WHO are critical to life, and 29 of them can be done at a district hospital. The bellwether procedures include caesarean sections, laparotomies and treatment of open fractures. These serve as a proxy measure to gauge the functionality of the surgical health system and its ability to perform a broad range of other essential surgical procedures. In places where there are few specialist surgeons, surgical needs are triaged as: 'must-do' procedures (cannot wait for 24 hours), 'should-do' procedures (cannot be delayed beyond a week) and 'can-do' procedures (can wait for more than a week), rather than by specialty.

The suggested core packages for strengthening emergency and essential surgical care and anaesthesia as a component of universal health coverage are shown in ***Summary box 16.1***.

National surgical plans consider country-specific contexts of disease burden, severity of disease, effectiveness of surgical intervention, economic effects and social implications. These plans influence decisions to tailor these procedures, packages and platforms for delivery. National standard treatment guidelines, which are commonplace in HICs, are now being adapted and used in the context of LMICs. They ensure that incentives for hospital management and clinical leadership align with the goal of efficient, system-wide reductions in the burden of surgical disease.

In the interconnected world, HICs can contribute in many important ways to global surgery: in elective and planned surgeries, academic grand rounds, relevant LMIC research

Summary box 16.1

Core packages for strengthening emergency and essential surgical care and anaesthesia

- *Emergency procedures packages* include:
  - Basic trauma package (e.g. fracture treatment, trauma laparotomy, debridement)
  - Basic obstetric package (e.g. caesarean section)
  - Basic emergency general surgical package (e.g. laparotomy, incision and drainage)
- *Planned care packages* can include:
  - General surgical package (e.g. hernia repair, bowel resection)
  - Obstetric and gynaecological package (e.g. hysterectomy)
  - Specialist surgical package (e.g. cataract, clubfoot correction)
  - Palliative surgical package (e.g. diversion colostomy, analgesics)

and research into the burden of surgical disease. Traditionally, mission surgeries for rarer conditions such as cleft lip and palate have contributed to high-quality protocols of safety and standards in surgery (Operation Smile, Smile Train). The critiques and concerns have been around HIC surgeons parachuting into LMICs and a lack of follow-up of their operated patients. Short-term visiting teams can draw resources away from local providers delivering continuous care, creating a perception within the community that visiting teams provide higher quality care. Improved LMIC institutional partnerships, local capacity building and collegiality are key to global surgery collaborative work with HICs. On their part, HICs have learned from LMIC institutions, such as the Aravind Eye Institute, about affordable surgery through remarkable cost reductions in high-volume cataract surgeries. While achieving high-volume surgeries, surgical safety is paramount and is dependent on training and upskilling of human resources in health, health infrastructure, the supply chain and equipment maintenance. Improved connectivity, infrastructure, Internet and wearables as well as low-cost simulation and robotics are remarkable global innovations that may make surgery accessible to those who were previously unable to reach it.

In the future, global surgery will drive surgeons in academic university hospitals to partner with their public health and community medicine colleagues for creating hub-and-spoke models for outreach surgery. Surgical practices will evolve to address the high unmet surgical burden of disease with high-volume and low-profit operations, with enhanced recovery in hospitals and postdischarge follow-ups by community health workers. Surgeons will go beyond the technical aspects of surgical practice to advocate for affordable and equitable surgical care for everyone, without compromising on safety.

Summary box 16.2

Key messages from the Lancet Commission on Global Surgery

- 5 billion out of the 7 billion people on the planet cannot access the surgeons who read this book for safe and affordable surgery
- 143 million more surgical procedures are needed each year in the world
- 33 million people each year will be impoverished because of paying for the surgery and anaesthesia that they need
- Investing in surgery is affordable, saves lives and promotes economic growth
- Surgery is an indivisible, indispensable part of health care. Surgical and anaesthesia care should be an integral component of a national health system in countries at all levels of development

FURTHER READING

Bath M, Bashford T, Fitzgerald JE. What is 'global surgery'? Defining the multidisciplinary interface between surgery, anaesthesia and public health. *BMJ Glob Health* 2019; **4**(5): e001808.

Debas HT, Donkor P, Gawande A *et al.* (eds). *Essential surgery. Disease control priorities*, 3rd edn, vol. 1. Washington, DC: World Bank, 2015.

Meara JG, Leather AJM, Hagander L *et al.* The Lancet Commission on Global Surgery 2030: evidence and solutions for achieving health, welfare and economic development. *Surgery* 2015; **157**(5): 834–5.

Smiley KE, Debas HT, DeVries CR, Price RR. Global surgery. In: Brunicardi F, Andersen DK, Billiar TR *et al.* (eds). *Schwartz's principles of surgery*, 11th edn. McGraw-Hill Education, 2019.

World Health Organization. *Surgical care at the district hospital.* Geneva: World Health Organization, 2003. Available from https://www.who.int/surgery/publications/en/SCDH.pdf.

PART 2 | General paediatrics

CHAPTER 17 Paediatric surgery

Learning objectives

After studying this chapter, you will be able to:
- Outline subspecialisations within children's surgery
- Safely prescribe perioperative fluids in children
- Compare and contrast inguinal hernias and hydroceles
- Discuss the causes and management of the acute scrotum
- Outline the presentation, resuscitation and operation for pyloric stenosis
- Outline causes and management of abdominal pain in children of different ages
- Describe two solid abdominal tumours of childhood

INTRODUCTION

In high-income countries paediatric surgeons have subspecialised, whereas in low-income countries surgeons must maintain diverse skills and knowledge. Some conditions, previously managed by paediatric surgeons, are now managed by others (e.g. clefts in plastic surgery, syndactyly in hand surgery, spina bifida and ventriculoperitoneal shunts in neurosurgery, ligation of patent ductus arteriosus in cardiac surgery and cervical cystic hygromas, thyroglossal cysts, preauricular sinuses and branchial remnants in ear, nose and throat surgery). This new edition recognises specialisation with chapters devoted to neonatal surgery, specialist paediatric urology and paediatric trauma. Those managing the general surgery of childhood in non-specialist hospitals should study the inguinoscrotal conditions described here and the foreskin as outlined in *Chapter 20*.

AGE

Biological domains (e.g. physiology, pathology, pharmacology) change continuously with age, whereas hospital services recognise artificial boundaries often set at 12, 16 or 18. The terminology related to children and young people (CYP) includes **neonate** (<4 weeks) and **infant** (<1 year). The World Health Organization defines **adolescence** as ages 10–19 and **young people** as 10–24. Some anatomical differences between infants and older children appear in *Table 17.1* and *Figure 17.1*. A few conditions described in *Chapter 18* require management throughout childhood and later after handover in transitioning by adult surgeons.

TABLE 17.1 Some examples of differences between infants and older children

Facts	Infants and some young children have a wide abdomen, a broad costal margin and a shallow pelvis
	The edge of the liver comes below the costal margin, and the bladder is partly intra-abdominal
	The ribs are more horizontal and are flexible
	The umbilicus is relatively low lying
Implications	Transverse supraumbilical incisions can give greater access than vertical midline incisions
	Abdominal trauma (including surgical incisions) can easily damage the liver or bladder
	The geometry of the ribs means that ventilation requires more diaphragmatic movement than in adults
	A stoma in the lower abdomen of an infant must be carefully sited for its bag not to interfere with the umbilicus

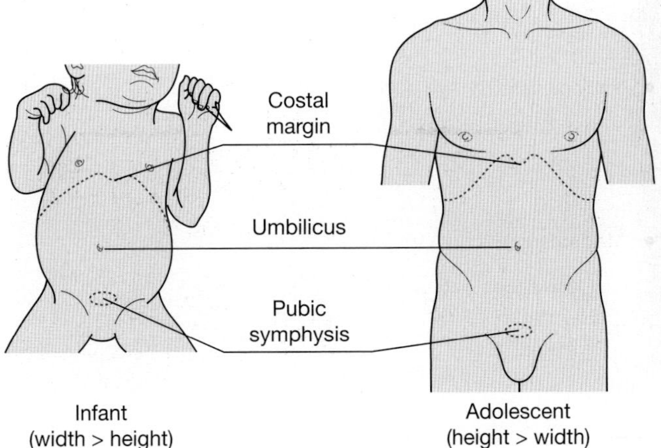

Figure 17.1 Topographical differences in the abdomen.

ENVIRONMENT

Children, especially infants, should be managed in a warm environment. Compared with adults, children lose more heat and fluid with surface area to weight ratios being higher;

consider this in the clinic, emergency room, anaesthetic rooms and theatres. An infant's head accounts for 20% of the surface area compared with 10% in adults. Intravenous infusions are warmed, and respiratory gases are both warmed and humidified. Core temperature is monitored in operations, and warming devices are used (e.g. heated mattresses, warm air blowers).

PERIOPERATIVE FLUIDS

There are four reasons for giving intravenous fluids: acute circulatory support, correction of previous losses, replacing ongoing losses and maintenance fluids (***Summary box 17.1***). Before prescribing fluids, weight, vital signs and fluid requirements are considered (***Table 17.2***). Dehydration as a percentage loss of total body water is difficult to assess; moderate dehydration (5%) causes low urine output, dry mouth and sunken eyes and fontanelle; severe dehydration (>10%) causes drowsiness, tachycardia and slow capillary refill (>2 seconds).

Hyponatraemia (<135 mmol/L) is common, but progression risks an encephalopathy from water movement into the brain. Water diffuses slowly by osmosis, equalising osmotic pressures, or swiftly through aquaporins. Sodium homeostasis maintains intravascular volume through antidiuretic hormone (ADH) and thirst. ADH binds to receptors in the distal nephron, inducing aquaporins and water retention. Increasing plasma osmolarity and hypotension both increase ADH levels.

TABLE 17.2 Basic paediatric data.

Vital signs			
Age (years)	Heart rate (bpm)	Systolic blood pressure (mmHg)	Respiratory rate (b/min)
<1	110–160	70–90	30–40
2–5	90–140	80–100	25–30
5–12	80–120	90–110	20–25
Maintenance fluid requirements			
Weight		Daily fluid requirement (mL/kg/day)	(mL/kg/h)
Neonate		120–150	5
First 10 kg		100	4
Second 10 kg		50	2
Subsequent kg		20	1

Systolic blood pressure = 80 + (age in years × 2) mmHg
Circulating blood volume = 70–80 mL/kg (90–100 mL/kg in preterms)
b/min, breaths per minute; bpm, beats per minute.

Summary box 17.1

Fluids in children

Fluids are given intravenously for four reasons:

- Circulatory support in resuscitating vascular collapse
  - 0.9% saline, Blood, 4.5% albumin, Colloid — Given as a bolus of 10 or 20 mL/kg over periods of up to 20 minutes while monitoring the response. Can be repeated up to 40 mL/kg then seek help
- Replacement of previous fluid and electrolyte deficits
  - 0.9% saline 0.15% KCl, Hartmann's solution — Given over a longer period of up to 48 hours with clinical and biochemical review
- Replacement of ongoing losses
  - 0.9% saline + 0.15% KCl, Hartmann's solution — Or a fluid tailored to the losses, e.g. 4.5% albumin if protein loss is great. Replace losses millilitre for millilitre
- Maintenance outside the neonatal period
  - Plasma-Lyte 148, Hartmann's solution ± glucose, 0.9% saline + 0.15% KCl ± glucose — Hypotonic 0.18% saline should not be used outside the neonatal period

An abundance of free water causes hyponatraemia. Since glucose is metabolised to water, glucose is ignored when calculating tonicity; 0.45% saline in 5% dextrose is considered hypotonic. Hyponatraemia is seen in normovolaemia if ADH rises inappropriately (e.g. surgical stress, trauma, chest infections, head injuries). Clinical problems arise if hypotonic fluids are used to resuscitate or replace losses or if maintenance fluids are given in excess.

Restricting maintenance fluids to 50–70% is appropriate after major surgery, gradually increasing the rate daily if sodium levels are not falling. Urine output naturally decreases after major surgery, but a common pitfall is to increase maintenance fluids, predisposing to hyponatraemia. A postoperative fluid bolus is appropriate in hypovolaemia, hypotension or poor peripheral perfusion, but given simply because urine output is low can be inappropriate. If hyponatraemia is mild and asymptomatic fluids are restricted, if symptomatic with headache, lethargy or seizures and the sodium concentration is <125 mmol/L, intravenous 3% saline is given.

HISTORY AND EXAMINATION

An opportunistic rather than a systematic approach may be needed in the preschool child. Children should be told what to expect from examinations, investigations or procedures in terms they can understand. Fear, anxiety and pain are reduced in a child-friendly environment. Consent is requested from someone with parental responsibility.

OPERATIVE SURGERY

Preoperative fasting should be limited (***Summary box 17.2***). Surgery requires meticulous and gentle tissue handling, strict haemostasis, fine sutures and magnification. Tissues should

Alexis Frank Hartmann, 1898–1964, paediatrician, St Louis, MO, USA, described the solution; should not be confused with Henri Albert Charles Antoine Hartmann, French surgeon, who described the operation that goes by his name.

be well vascularised, tension avoided and contamination minimised. The intestine can be anastomosed with single-layer interrupted or continuous extramucosal sutures. Wounds are closed with absorbable sutures in layers or a mass closure. Establishing a layer of fat between skin and muscle in the malnourished or thin child prevents the skin from adhering to muscle. Toothed forceps may be used when closing the skin, but the skin must not be punctured; epidermal tunnels can form, trapping skin debris and creating a comedo-like blackhead. Clean skin incisions are closed with absorbable subcuticular sutures or skin glue, avoiding staples. Minimally invasive approaches can be used at all ages with appropriate instruments, flow rates and pressures. Postoperatively, children recover swiftly with adequate analgesia.

Summary box 17.2

Fasting instructions

- 1 hour for clear fluids
- 4 hours for breast milk
- 6 hours for solids

INGUINOSCROTAL DISORDERS

Undifferentiated gonads, influenced by the Y chromosome, develop into testes in the posterior abdominal urogenital ridges. An abdominal phase in testicular descent involves migration towards the internal ring guided by the gubernaculum. Descent into the scrotum requires fetal testicular testosterone. The peritoneum preceding the testis through the inguinal canal becomes the processus vaginalis, which usually obliterates after birth; failure of obliteration leads to an indirect inguinal hernia or hydrocele (***Figure 17.2***).

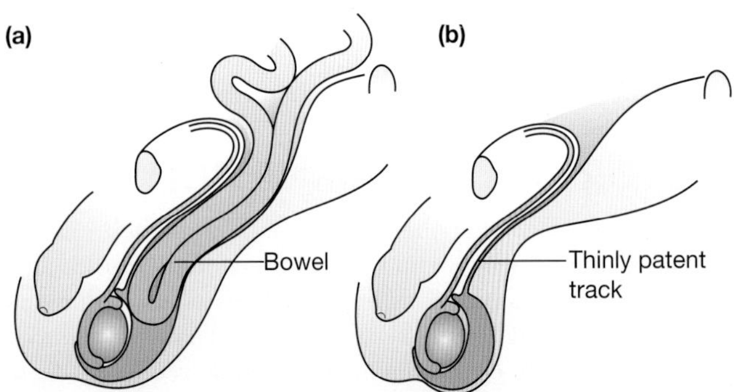

Figure 17.2 (a) Inguinal hernia and **(b)** hydrocele in children are the result of incomplete obliteration of the processus vaginalis.

Inguinal hernias

Inguinal hernias occur in 4% of infants with prematurity, low birth weight and male sex being risk factors (M:F 6:1). Inguinal hernias are twice as common on the right side as on the left, with 10% occurring bilaterally. The hernia may contain omentum, intestine, appendix (Amyand's) or a Meckel's diverticulum (Littre's). An ovary can prolapse and twist in a girl, requiring emergency exploration. Prolapsed ovaries, therefore, need prompt repair. Rarely in phenotypic girls, a testicle is found, suggesting androgen insensitivity (see ***Chapter 20***).

An inguinal hernia presents as an intermittent bulge in the groin extending to the scrotum (***Figure 17.3***) or labia, often exacerbated by crying or straining. Most reduce on lying down or with gentle manipulation. A thickened cord in boys, or round ligament in girls, may be all that is palpable. Reducible inguinal hernias are repaired electively. If the herniated contents become firm, tender and irreducible, there may be oedema and erythema, irritability, vomiting and the passage of some rectal blood. An attempt to reduce an incarceration with sustained gentle pressure may be successful; if unsuccessful, emergency exploration, reduction and repair are required.

Inguinal hernia repair

The herniated contents may reduce after the induction of anaesthesia. If incarcerated, the neck of the sac is found at the external ring. Open repair involves ligating the sac at the external or the internal inguinal ring. In a repair at the internal ring, an incision is made over the inguinal canal, Scarpa's fascia is incised and the fat cleared to expose the external oblique rolling over to form the inguinal ligament. The external

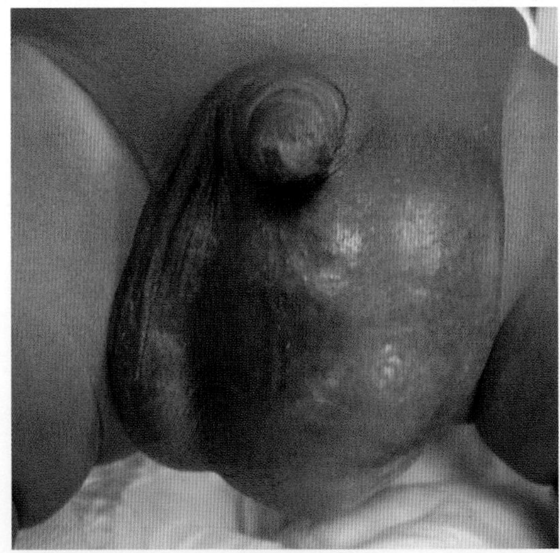

Figure 17.3 A left inguinal swelling. Clinical examination is needed to confidently distinguish a hydrocele from an inguinal hernia.

Claudius Amyand, 1660–1740, French surgeon who performed the first successful appendectomy in 1735. He was first Principal Surgeon to the Westminster Hospital, and founder and first Principal Surgeon to St George's Hospital in London.
Johann Frederick Meckel (the Younger), 1781–1833, Professor of Anatomy and Surgery, Halle, Germany, described his diverticulum in 1809.
Alexis Littre, 1654–1726, surgeon and lecturer in anatomy, Paris, France, described Meckel's diverticulum in a hernial sac in 1700, 81 years before Meckel was born.
Antonio Scarpa, 1752–1832, Italian anatomist and pupil of Morgagni.

oblique is incised to identify the cremaster overlying the sac. The cremaster is opened with fine scissors or blunt dissection. The cord is lifted through the cremaster and a clip passed behind. The sac is mobilised from the testicular vessels and vas deferens. The sac is divided, twisted to reduce any contents and transfixed/ligated at the internal ring. The wound is closed in layers. A laparoscopic approach places an encircling suture at the internal ring.

Hydroceles

A hydrocele is a fluid collection between the parietal and visceral layers of the tunica vaginalis and is usually confined to the scrotum – one can feel the cord above it. Occasionally, it extends into the external ring and one cannot feel the cord. Hydroceles are typically asymptomatic, non-tender and may fluctuate, reducing overnight; they can be bilateral. Infant hydroceles can be tense and uncomfortable, especially if over-examined, causing confusion with an incarcerated inguinal hernia. Although hydroceles transilluminate, this is a flawed test for distinguishing one from an incarcerated inguinal hernia since light easily shines through an infant's intestine.

Surgery is rarely indicated before 2 years because a majority resolve. Occasionally an encysted hydrocele of the cord (or hydrocele of the canal of Nuck in a girl) forms as the processus obliterates; persistence warrants exploration. Occasionally, a febrile boy presents with a viral-like illness and an acute hydrocele. These generally resolve over a few weeks, and only those that remain need exploration. Ligation of a patent processus vaginalis is similar to an inguinal hernia repair.

Teenage boys may have a non-communicating hydrocele with fluid arising from the tunica vaginalis; a plication (Lord's procedure) or excision/eversion of the tunica vaginalis (Jaboulay procedure) are needed.

Undescended testes

A normally descended testis reaches the scrotal floor with a good cord length above it and remains there. Testicular descent is usually complete by the 30th week of gestation. At birth, 4% of full-term and 30% of premature boys have an undescended testis (UDT). Boys should be examined at birth and at 6 weeks; if a UDT is found, they should be seen at 3 months since a testis is unlikely to descend after this time. An orchidopexy is then scheduled for between 6 and 12 months. Occasionally a palpable UDT undergoes torsion and presents as a painful lump in the groin with an empty hemi-scrotum.

Clinical examination distinguishes a normal testis from a palpable or an impalpable UDT. A testis cannot be palpated in the canal; it can only be felt when delivered to the superficial pouch, which is also called Denis Browne's pouch (a pocket between Scarpa's fascia and the external oblique fascia at the external ring). Cremasteric activity may draw a testis into the pouch or the canal. Gentle strokes over the canal, directed towards the scrotum, may deliver a normal scrotal or a palpable UDT. Ectopic testes are found beneath the skin of the medial thigh or lower abdomen; they have a long cord, facilitating easy scrotal placement at operation. If hypospadias is seen with bilateral, impalpable UDTs, then a disorder of sexual differentiation is possible and referral indicated (see ***Chapter 20***).

Retractile testes

A retractile testis is palpable in the groin and can be brought into the scrotum but promptly returns to the groin. Retractile testes are common in infants and most eventually settle in the scrotum; follow-up is needed because some permanently ascend and require an orchidopexy.

Ascending testes

Some scrotal testes in infancy are later found in the high scrotum or groin with ascent attributed to insufficient cord growth; a few were retractile in infancy. An orchidopexy is required. An argument exists for screening all boys for ascending testes in late childhood.

Palpable undescended testes

Palpable UDTs require an orchidopexy at between 6 and 12 months. The canal is opened through an external oblique incision. The testis is mobilised on its vas and vessels, and the gubernaculum is usually divided. Any peritoneal outpocketing is ligated and divided at the internal ring, where dissection adds length to the cord. The testis is placed in a subdartos scrotal pouch. Early orchidopexy, placing the testis in a cooler environment, improves spermatogenesis and may reduce the risk of testicular malignancy.

Impalpable undescended testes

Impalpable UDTs are absent, canalicular or abdominal. Imaging is unreliable. Examination under anaesthesia and laparoscopy is performed at around 1 year. If palpable under anaesthesia, an inguinal orchidopexy is performed. At laparoscopy, a testis is absent if a blind-ending vas is seen. If the vas and vessels enter the inguinal canal, then the groin is explored. A canalicular testis may be amenable to an inguinal orchidopexy, or there may be a remnant to excise. If there is a viable intra-abdominal testis (***Figure 17.4***), a two-stage Fowler–Stephens orchidopexy is performed. In the first stage, testicular vessels are ligated, leaving the testis *in situ*, anticipating survival on the vessels accompanying the vas. Three

Anton Nuck, 1650–1692, Dutch anatomist and surgeon who described the peritoneal outpocketing neighbouring the round ligament of the uterus as it extends to the labia majora.
Peter H Lord, 1925–2017, Consultant General Surgeon, Wycombe General Hospital, High Wycombe, UK.
Mathieu Jaboulay, 1860–1913, Professor of Surgery in Lyon, France.
Sir Denis John Browne KCVO, 1892–1967, the first British surgeon to devote all his care to children.
Robert Fowler, b 1928, retired surgeon, Royal Children's Hospital Melbourne.
Frank Douglas Stephens, 1913–2011, paediatric surgeon who worked in Melbourne, Australia.

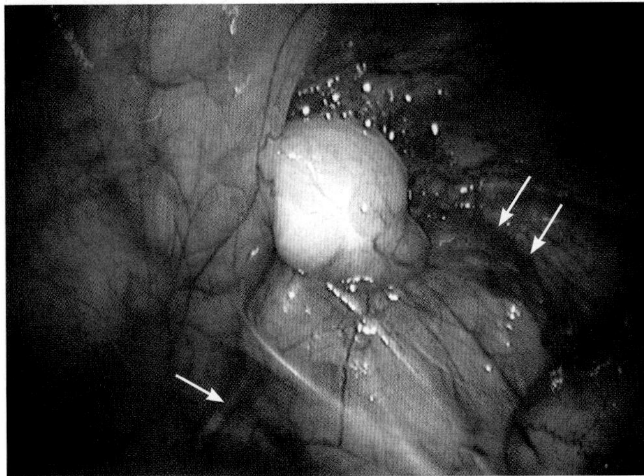

Figure 17.4 Laparoscopic view of a right-sided intra-abdominal testis visible at the internal ring. Vas (single arrow) and testicular vessels (double arrow).

months later a second operation is performed; if the testis has survived, it is brought into the scrotum.

ACUTE SCROTAL DISORDERS

Testicular torsion

Intravaginal (bell clapper) testicular torsion is well recognised in adolescents but may occur at any age. Abnormal posterior anchoring of the testis allows torsion within the tunica vaginalis. Torsion compromises blood flow, causing acute scrotal or abdominal/groin pain, nausea and vomiting. Tenderness, an absent cremasteric reflex and a high testis may be found on examination; oedema and erythema appear later. Sometimes there have been transient episodes (intermittent torsion). Doppler ultrasound may help (***Figure 17.5***). Exploration within 6–8 hours of the onset of symptoms improves the chances of testicular salvage.

At operation, testicular viability is assessed after derotation (***Figure 17.6***). Only gangrenous testes should be excised since some severely compromised testes survive, and those that then atrophy are not harmful. If salvageable, three-point fixation of both testes with non-absorbable sutures is performed or a dartos pouch is fashioned.

Extravaginal torsion is seen in newborns, with 70% occurring prenatally and 30% postnatally; emergency neonatal exploration remains controversial since salvage rates are low.

Torsion of the appendix testis and appendix epididymis

The appendix testis (hydatid of Morgagni) is a remnant of the Müllerian (paramesonephric) duct, whereas the appendix epididymis is a Wolffian (mesonephric) remnant. Both are small and pedunculated and are located on the upper testis or epididymis; they can twist and infarct (***Figure 17.7***). Appendage torsion occurs most commonly between 7 and 14 years. Mild to severe acute scrotal pain is present, usually without vomiting. On examination, a small area just above the testis may be tender; occasionally, a dark mass is visible, known as the blue-dot sign. A Doppler ultrasound can help exclude testicular torsion. Analgesia, and rest, may be sufficient, with exploration reserved for severe pain and equivocal cases.

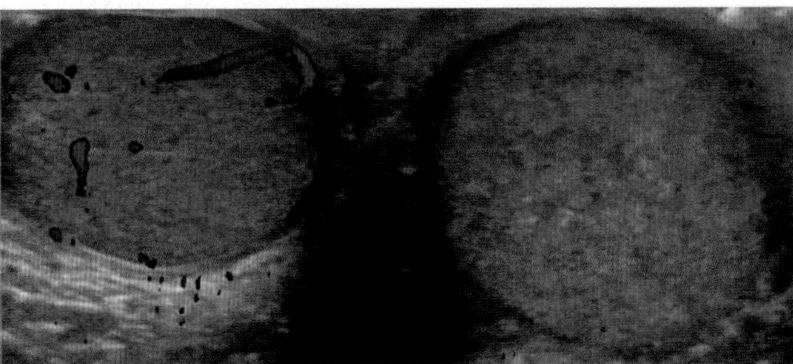

Figure 17.5 The red and blue colour on one testis shows normal blood flow whereas the contralateral testis has no blood supply, consistent with a torsion.

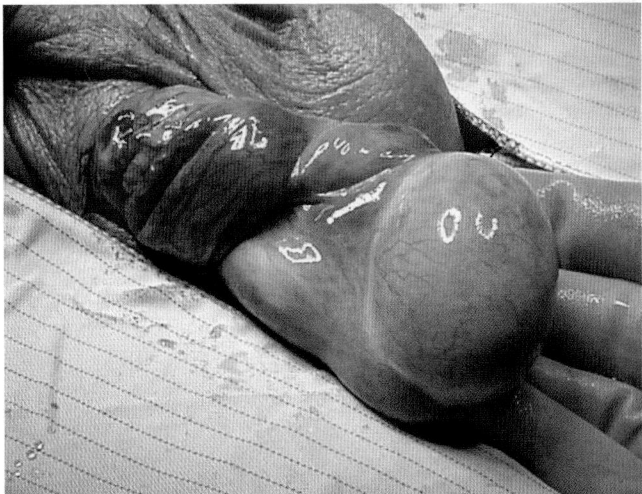

Figure 17.6 Torsion of the right testis with only modest vascular compromise in a boy with a history of intermittent pain.

Epididymo-orchitis

Bacterial or viral inflammation is occasionally found on exploration for suspected torsion. Epididymitis is seen before 6 months and is caused by infected urine travelling up the vas. Epididymo-orchitis (*Chlamydia trachomatis, Neisseria gonorrhoea* and *Escherichia coli*) is seen after puberty in sexually active boys presenting with acute testicular pain, dysuria, frequency, urethral discharge and fever. In addition, there may be scrotal

Giovanni Battista Morgagni, 1682–1771, Italian anatomist, considered the father of modern anatomical pathology.
Johannes Peter Müller, 1801–1858, German physiologist, comparative anatomist, ichthyologist and herpetologist.
Caspar Friedrich Wolff, 1733–1794, German physiologist and one of the founders of embryology.

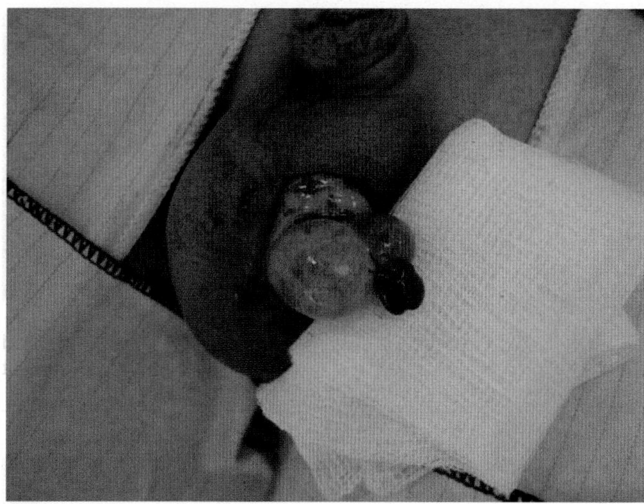

Figure 17.7 Two torted and infarcted hydatids, one arising from the epididymis and one from the testis.

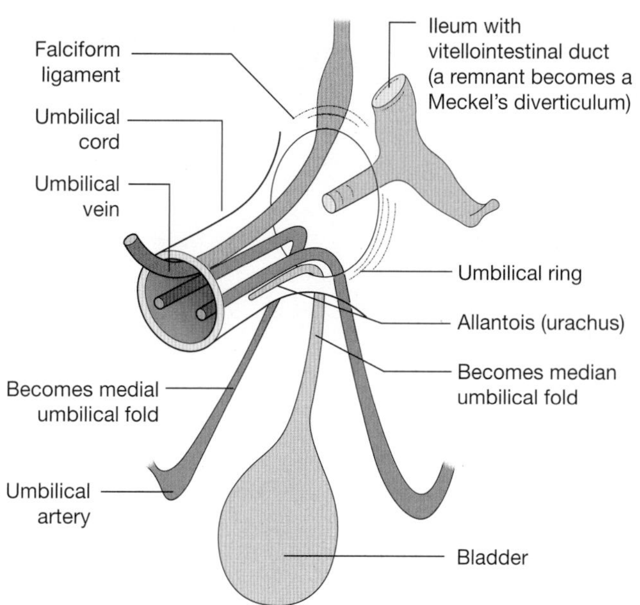

Figure 17.8 Structures at the umbilicus.

erythema and oedema with a normal cremasteric reflex. Pain may subside on elevation of the testis (Prehn's sign). Management includes rest, analgesia, antibiotics and re-evaluation if there is no improvement.

Idiopathic scrotal oedema

Typically, a 5- to 7-year-old boy presents with a swollen hemi-scrotum with erythema extending towards the anus and the groin. The testicle is scrotal and not tender, though the dartos and skin are swollen. Antihistamines may help.

MIDLINE HERNIAS

The embryonic umbilical ring encircles a defect in the ventral abdominal wall transmitting structures connecting the fetus to the placenta (***Figure 17.8***). Umbilical hernias are common following incomplete closure of the umbilical ring, though incarceration is rare. Most umbilical hernias resolve by 4 years. Supraumbilical hernias are defects in the linea alba just above the umbilical ring; these do not close but are still repaired around 4 years. Epigastric hernias are defects higher still that allow a small amount of preperitoneal fat to prolapse; they are repaired if symptomatic.

INFANTILE HYPERTROPHIC PYLORIC STENOSIS

Pyloric stenosis presents with non-bilious projectile vomiting starting between 2 and 6 weeks of age. Its presentation differs from infective causes of vomiting (e.g. meningitis, urinary tract infections [UTIs]) because of postprandial hunger. Once vomiting starts, its frequency and forcefulness increase daily, distinguishing it from gastro-oesophageal reflux (GOR), which waxes and wanes and starts shortly after birth. In the UK, pyloric stenosis affects 1:300 infants with a M:F ratio of 4:1. There is often a maternal family history.

If the presentation is early, clinical findings are unremarkable; if late, weight loss and dehydration requiring resuscitation predominate. The diagnosis is made on a test feed or on abdominal ultrasound showing a thickened and lengthened pylorus. In a test feed, gastric peristalsis is seen passing from left to right across the abdomen, and in a relaxed (feeding) baby, the pyloric 'tumour' is palpable as an 'olive' in the right upper quadrant. Feeds are discontinued, and the stomach is emptied with an 8–10Fr nasogastric tube. Loss of gastric acid causes a hypochloraemic, hypokalaemic alkalosis and correction may take 24–48 hours; 0.9% saline with 0.15% KCl in 5% glucose given at 6–7.5 mL/kg/h provides maintenance and corrects deficits in most babies. As the chloride deficit is replaced, the kidneys correct the pH.

Ramstedt's pyloromyotomy is performed laparoscopically or through a supraumbilical or right upper quadrant incision. A pyloric serosal incision is made, and the 'tumour' spread (***Figure 17.9***), leaving an intact submucosa from the duodenal fornix to gastric antrum. The incision must extend onto the stomach; short incisions cause an early recurrence. Postoperatively, intravenous fluids are continued until feeds are re-established within 24 hours. Early postoperative vomiting usually swiftly resolves, with GOR being more likely than an incomplete myotomy if it persists.

GOR is common and tends to resolve spontaneously with maturity. Persistent symptoms respond to thickened feeds and antireflux medication. Failure to thrive or respiratory problems demand investigation and, in some cases, laparoscopic fundoplication.

Douglas Prehn, 1901–1974, American urologist, Wisconsin, USA.
Wilhelm Conrad Ramstedt, 1867–1963, German surgeon credited with describing the pyloromyotomy.

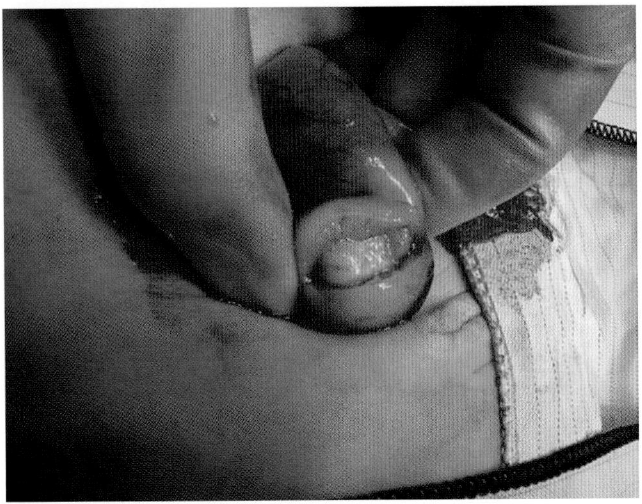

Figure 17.9 Pyloromyotomy for infantile hypertrophic pyloric stenosis.

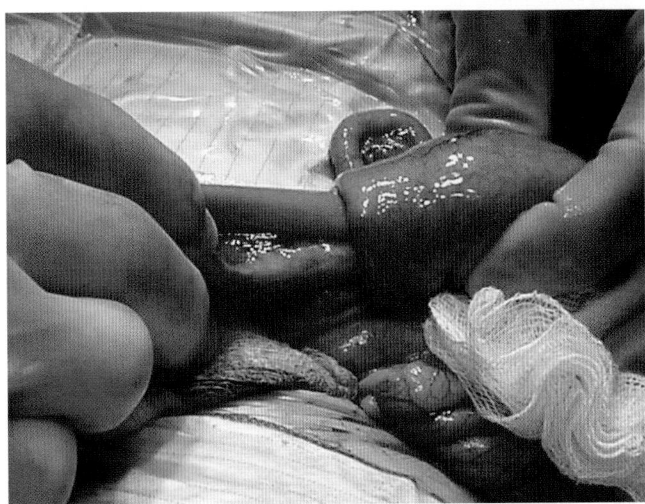

Figure 17.10 Ileocolic intussusception causing small bowel obstruction.

INTUSSUSCEPTION

Most intussusceptions occur between 2 months and 2 years. More than 80% are ileocolic (***Figure 17.10***), beginning proximal to the ileocaecal valve with an apex in the ascending or transverse colon. Strangulation can progress to gangrene and perforation. The lead point is commonly viral-induced hyperplasia in a Peyer's patch, but a few have a pathological lead such as a Meckel's diverticulum, duplication cyst or a small bowel lymphoma. Pathological leads are found more commonly in those over 2 years and in a recurrence.

A previously healthy infant presents with colicky pain, vomiting and drawing up their legs. Between episodes, they initially appear well. Later, they may pass a 'redcurrant jelly' stool. Signs include dehydration, abdominal distension and a palpable right upper quadrant mass.

A plain radiograph shows small bowel obstruction, a mass and a paucity of gas in the right iliac fossa. A concentric target sign is seen on an abdominal ultrasound. An air reduction enema is attempted after resuscitation with intravenous fluids, broad-spectrum antibiotics and nasogastric drainage (***Figure 17.11***). Success is recognised if air flows into the small bowel and symptoms and signs resolve. An air enema is contraindicated if there is peritonitis, perforation or shock. More than 70% are reducible non-operatively. Strangulation and pathological lead points are unlikely to reduce. Colonic perforation during pneumatic reduction is rare. Recurrence occurs in 5% after non-operative reduction. Operative reduction is performed open or laparoscopically. An irreducible intussusception or one complicated by infarction or a pathological lead point requires resection.

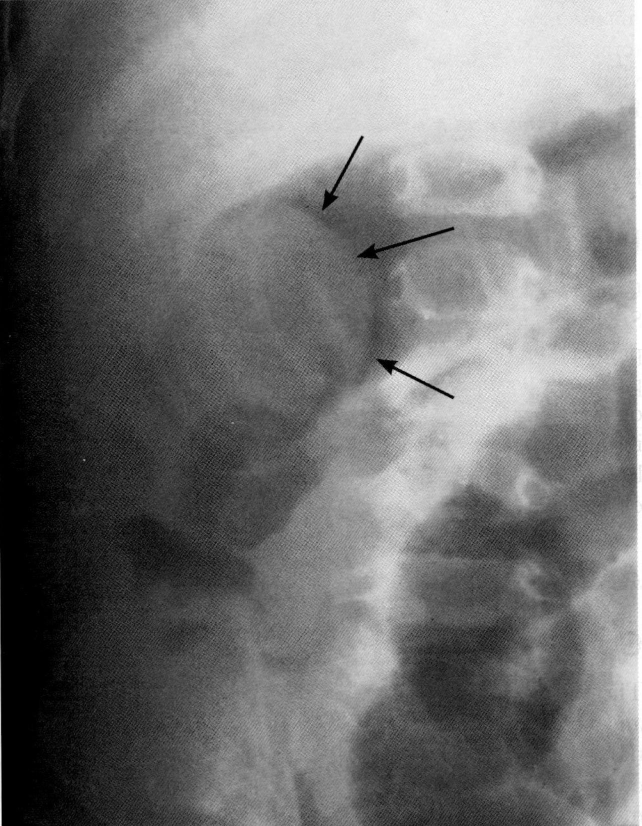

Figure 17.11 Air enema reduction of an intussusception (the arrows mark the soft tissue shadow of the intussusceptum).

ACUTE APPENDICITIS

In early appendicitis, there is a fever of 37.3–38.4°C, anorexia, a few vomits and central abdominal pain settling in the right iliac fossa. Persistent guarding in the right iliac fossa distinguishes it from self-resolving non-specific abdominal pain (NSAP). Investigations and scoring systems may help but neither replace regular clinical review. Treatment starts with intravenous fluids, analgesia and broad-spectrum antibiotics. Early appendicitis is managed laparoscopically, though some mild cases may resolve with antibiotics alone.

Johann Conrad Peyer, 1653–1712, Swiss anatomist.

Complicated appendicitis describes any of the following: perforation, abscess formation, a mass or generalised peritonitis. One pitfall is to diagnose gastroenteritis when there are loose stools, and another is to attribute pain on micturition and pyuria to a UTI; both can occur in pelvic appendicitis with a collection. Referred pain from right lower lobe pneumonia should be considered. Antibiotics given for any reason may mollify signs and delay or complicate a presentation. The diagnosis can be difficult in those under 5 years, with many presenting after a perforation. Before 5 years, the omentum is less well developed and inflammation less well contained. An appendix mass in an unobstructed child may respond to non-operative management with antibiotics. An interval appendicectomy can be considered 6 weeks later but is not mandated.

Non-specific abdominal pain

The clinical features of NSAP are similar to acute appendicitis, but the pain is poorly localised, not aggravated by movement and not accompanied by guarding. The site and severity of maximum tenderness vary on repeated examinations. Symptoms are typically self-limiting. The aetiology is obscure, but viral infections are hypothesised if there is lymphadenopathy. In some children, recurrent abdominal pain can be organic; in others, it is eventually attributed to an underlying psychosocial problem.

Rare causes of abdominal pain

Other causes of acute abdominal pain include Henoch–Schönlein purpura, sickle cell disease, primary peritonitis, acute pancreatitis, biliary colic, testicular torsion, gynaecological pathology (e.g. ovarian cysts and tumours, pelvic inflammatory disease, haematometrocolpos) and urinary stone disease. UTIs in children may be due to a urinary tract abnormality and may lead to renal scarring from ascending infection. Infection and obstruction are particularly hazardous; see *Chapter 20*.

ANORECTAL PROBLEMS

Constipation

The passage of hard or infrequent stools may be secondary to an anal fissure, Hirschsprung's disease, an anorectal malformation, a neuropathic bowel, a mega-rectosigmoid or idiopathic constipation. A detailed history and examination of the abdomen, anus and spine identify most causes. A rectal biopsy may be needed to exclude late presenting Hirschsprung's disease. In the absence of surgical pathology, the child is best managed by a paediatrician.

Rectal prolapse

Rectal mucosal prolapse occurs in toddlers and is exacerbated by straining or squatting on defecation. It is typically intermittent and self-limiting. Underlying constipation should be treated. Rarely, it may be secondary to cystic fibrosis or spinal dysraphism. A rectal polyp can mimic a prolapse. Recurrent symptomatic prolapse may respond to injection sclerotherapy. Rare cases need laparoscopic rectopexy.

Meckel's diverticulum

A 4-year-old presenting with a haemoglobin level of 40 g/L will most likely have bled from an ulcer adjacent to a Meckel's diverticulum containing ectopic gastric mucosa (*Figure 17.12*). A technetium scan may demonstrate ectopic gastric mucosa (*Figure 17.13*). A Meckel's diverticulum may also be complicated by an obstructing band between the diverticulum and the umbilicus, diverticulitis, intussusception, intestinal volvulus or perforation.

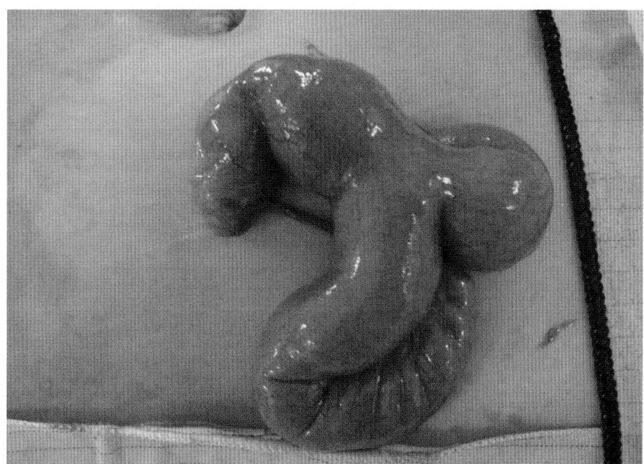

Figure 17.12 Meckel's diverticulum containing ectopic gastric mucosa.

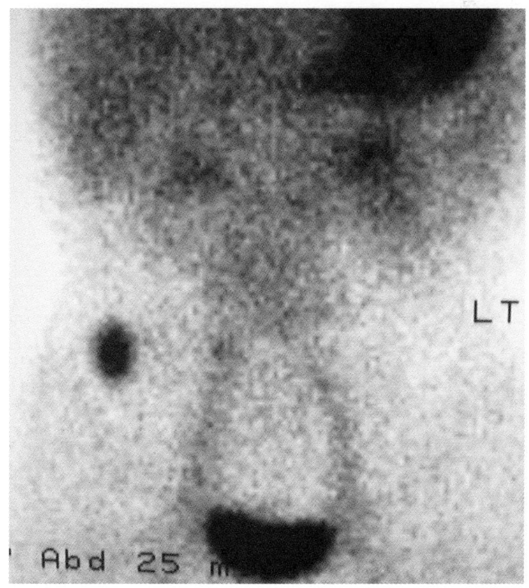

Figure 17.13 A positive Meckel's scan.

Eduard Heinrich Henoch, 1820–1910, Professor of Diseases of Children, Berlin, Germany, described this form of purpura in 1868.
Johann Lucas Schönlein, 1793–1864, Professor of Medicine, Berlin, Germany, published his description of this form of purpura in 1837.
Harald Hirschsprung, 1830–1916, physician, The Queen Louise Hospital for Children, Copenhagen, Denmark, described congenital megacolon in 1887.

Swallowed or inhaled foreign bodies

Coins and other foreign bodies are often swallowed and, if radio-opaque, are seen on a plain radiograph. Oesophageal objects are removed endoscopically under general anaesthesia. Oesophageal button batteries must be removed within hours as they can perforate into the trachea or aorta. Once beyond the cardia, most objects pass in a few days. Batteries in the stomach are removed urgently or followed closely with repeat radiographs. The need to remove sharp objects depends on their size, location and the age of the child. Ingested magnets can cause entero-enteric fistulae when they fix to one another in adjacent loops of bowel.

Inhaled foreign bodies cause sudden-onset coughing and stridor. If there is worsening dyspnoea or hypoxia in an infant they should be given back blows in a head-down position. Abdominal thrusts (Heimlich manoeuvre) are reserved for older children. A foreign body in a bronchus is suggested by a unilateral wheeze, decreased transmitted breath sounds and a hyperinflated lung on an expiratory chest radiograph. Rigid bronchoscopy with a ventilating bronchoscope facilitates removal.

GASTROSTOMY

A gastrostomy may be requested for nutritional support. Options include an open Stamm gastrostomy, a Ponsky–Gauderer percutaneous endoscopic gastrostomy (PEG) or a laparoscopic approach using a Seldinger technique. The Stamm gastrostomy employs two gastric purse-string sutures imbricated to fashion a tunnel. In the PEG technique, a gastroscope illuminates the stomach and abdominal wall, allowing identification of a site through which a needle and wire are passed into the stomach and extracted orally. A gastrostomy tube is then drawn into place. In the Seldinger technique, the stomach is punctured percutaneously with a needle through which a guidewire is advanced, and the needle is then withdrawn. A series of dilators are passed over the guidewire and finally the gastrostomy tube; the guidewire is then withdrawn.

PAEDIATRIC SURGICAL ONCOLOGY

Neuroblastoma and nephroblastoma are two solid abdominal tumours.

Neuroblastomas arise in the adrenal medulla or sympathetic ganglia and present with an abdominal or paravertebral mass. They metastasise to lymph nodes, bone and liver, raising urinary catecholamine levels. Small, localised tumours are excised. Advanced tumours are excised after chemotherapy. Survival exceeds 90% for small, localised tumours but is less than 50% for advanced tumours.

Wilms' tumour (nephroblastoma) is a malignant renal tumour derived from embryonal cells and typically presenting with an abdominal mass between 1 and 4 years. A mutation in the Wilms' tumour suppressor gene (*WT1*) causes some cases. The tumour can extend into the renal vein and vena cava and metastasises to lymph nodes and lungs. Treatment is with chemotherapy and surgery. Survival depends on tumour spread, completeness of excision and histological appearance but exceeds 70% even with advanced tumours.

Henry Judah Heimlich, 1920–2016, thoracic surgeon, Xavier University, Cincinnati, OH, USA.
Martin Stamm, 1847–1918, American gastric surgeon, educated in Germany.
Jeffrey Ponsky, contemporary, endoscopist, Rainbow Babies & Children's Hospital, University Hospitals of Cleveland, Cleveland, OH, USA.
Michael WL Gauderer, contemporary, paediatric surgeon, Greenville, SC, USA.
Sven Ivar Seldinger, 1921–1998, Swedish radiologist, introduced the procedure in 1953.
Carl Max Wilhelm Wilms, 1867–1918, German pathologist and surgeon, died of diphtheria after operating on the larynx of a French prisoner of war.

CHAPTER 18 Neonatal surgery

Learning objectives

To be able to:

- List five aetiological classes underlying structural congenital anomalies
- Give five examples of how neonatal physiology and anatomy influence surgical care
- Describe at least five congenital anomalies managed by neonatal surgeons
- Outline the presentation and management of necrotising enterocolitis
- Describe two newborn tumours
- Explain why adult surgeons need an overview of neonatal surgery

INTRODUCTION

Neonatal surgeons are paediatric surgeons who manage life-threatening non-cardiac congenital anomalies and the acquired condition necrotising enterocolitis (NEC), seen in premature babies. Structural anomalies are associated with gene defects, aneuploidies (abnormal number of chromosomes), infections (e.g. toxoplasmosis, cytomegalovirus, rubella) and teratogens (e.g. drugs, smoking, alcohol). Late mechanical aetiologies are illustrated by ileal volvulus in cystic fibrosis, some lung hypoplasia in congenital diaphragmatic hernias and small intestine loss in closing gastroschisis. Insults acting during gastrulation – when cells are told what to do and where to go – may cause multiple anomalies, e.g. VACTERL syndrome (**v**ertebral, **a**norectal, **c**ardiac, **t**racheo**e**sophageal, **r**enal and **l**imb anomalies) and CHARGE syndrome (**c**oloboma, **h**eart defects, choanal **a**tresia, growth **r**etardation, **g**enital anomalies and **e**ar anomalies). See ***Chapter 44*** for neural tube defects and ***Chapter 59*** for heart defects. See ***Chapter 48*** for the overlap with general surgery of childhood. ***Table 18.1*** illustrates the need for careful examination, imaging and genetic investigations to screen for associations when an anomaly is found. When well-recognised anomalies are identified antenatally, neonatal surgeons, working with fetal medicine specialists and neonatologists, counsel parents about prognosis and postnatal surgical management.

NEWBORN PHYSIOLOGY AND THE PRINCIPLES OF NEONATAL SURGERY

Neonatal physiology can pose challenges when there is a surgical condition (***Table 18.2***). Perioperatively, a newborn needing ventilation is best managed in a surgical unit co-located with a medical neonatal intensive care unit (NICU). Some babies are transferred many miles between units. If a neonatal surgical transfer team is not available, accompanying clinicians should be reminded that neonates with bowel obstruction need a nasogastric tube to decompress the stomach; this should be left on free drainage and regularly aspirated.

Neonates, especially the premature, lose heat and fluid rapidly, have poor nutritional reserves, are susceptible to infection and have an immature blood-brain barrier. Surgery should be efficiently performed in a warm environment with gentle tissue handling and broad-spectrum antibiotic cover. The liver can be fragile, and blood should be available for laparotomies. Sick babies with NEC or an acute volvulus may be best operated upon at the cot side in a NICU. In an unstable infant with an acute abdomen, damage control principles should be applied with a second-look laparotomy and definitive repair following stabilisation. Electrocautery is delivered on the lowest working setting. Avoid the Trendelenburg position in the preterm when placing a diathermy pad as elevation risks intraventricular haemorrhages.

A laparotomy may be performed through a right-sided transverse muscle-cutting incision just above the umbilicus, taking care to avoid the large, fragile liver, or through a midline longitudinal incision, avoiding the bladder, which rises into the abdomen. A muscle-sparing symmetrical supraumbilical

Friedrich Trendelenburg, 1844–1924, Professor of Surgery successively at Rostock (1875–1882), Bonn (1882–1895), Leipzig (1895–1911), Germany. The Trendelenburg position was first described in 1885.

TABLE 18.1 Congenital malformations managed by neonatal surgeons.

Primary abnormality	Incidence/ 100 000 live births	Associations illustrating the need for screening
Oesophageal atresia/ tracheoesophageal fistula	24	VACTERL, CHARGE, aneuploidy/other gene defects, duodenal atresia, anorectal malformations, tracheomalacia, gastroesophageal reflux
Duodenal atresia	13	Trisomy 21, other intestinal atresias, oesophageal atresia/tracheoesophageal fistula, intestinal malrotation
Intestinal atresias	10	Cystic fibrosis, other atresias
Anorectal malformations	26	Oesophageal atresia/tracheoesophageal fistula, VACTERL, Trisomy 21
Hirschsprung's disease	14	Trisomy 21, other chromosomal defects, familial **Structural anomalies:** Cardiac, craniofacial, cleft palate, polydactyly, intestinal atresias/anorectal malformations **Syndromic:** Multiple endocrine neoplasia, Waardenburg–Shah syndrome, congenital hypoventilation syndrome (Ondine's curse)
Biliary atresia	3	Biliary atresia splenic malformation (BASM) syndrome: polysplenia, vascular and cardiac anomalies, defects of situs Cytomegalovirus
Gastroschisis	20	Intestinal atresias, undescended testes
Exomphalos (major and minor)	12	Aneuploidy, chromosomal anomalies, cardiac defects, Beckwith–Wiedemann syndrome
Congenital diaphragmatic hernia	20	Aneuploidy, chromosomal anomalies, CHARGE, malrotation. Syndromic
Congenital pulmonary airway malformations (CPAM)	10	Vertebral/chest wall deformities, intestinal duplications, cardiac anomalies, congenital diaphragmatic hernia

CHARGE, **c**oloboma, **h**eart defects, choanal **a**tresia, growth **r**etardation, **g**enital anomalies and **e**ar anomalies; VACTERL, **v**ertebral, **a**norectal, **c**ardiac, **t**racheoesophageal, **r**enal and **l**imb anomalies.

incision or an omega incision are options with the recti pulled laterally. A left-sided diaphragmatic hernia can be approached through a subcostal incision. The umbilical vein remains patent for many days and is divided between ligatures if the midline is crossed. Gastrointestinal surgery may involve bowel resection with a single layer interrupted or continuously sutured anastomosis or formation of a temporary spouted enterostomy. In stable, well babies, laparoscopy is suitable for some procedures (e.g. duodenal atresia repair, malrotation without acute volvulus, excision of large ovarian cysts). Central venous access is needed for parenteral nutrition (PN) if enteral feeds are likely to be delayed.

NEONATAL GASTROINTESTINAL SURGERY

Oesophageal atresia/ tracheoesophageal fistula (OA/TOF)

Five anatomical variations appear in ***Figure 18.1***. When the oesophagus ends blindly, amniotic fluid cannot be swallowed and polyhydramnios results. If there is no fistula (type A), the stomach may be small or difficult to detect antenatally and is often wrongly referred to as 'absent'. Postnatal presentations are with drooling, aspiration or cyanosis on feeding.

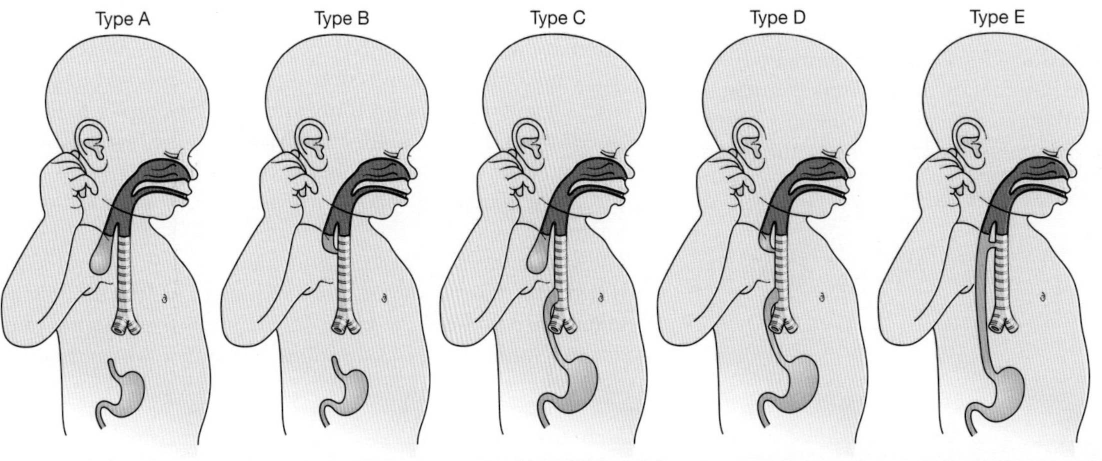

Figure 18.1 Anatomical variations in tracheoesophageal fistula with or without oesophageal atresia. In Type C, the upper pouch ends in the neck or upper chest but occasionally it reaches the fistula where muscle fibres are shared.

Harald Hirschsprung, 1830–1916, first Danish paediatrician, considered Hirschsprung's disease to be developmental.

Table 18.2 Physiological considerations in newborn infants.

Airway

Intubation can be challenging as the occiput flexes the neck, the tongue is large and the epiglottis is long, angulated and positioned high and close to the soft palate.

- A straight blade laryngoscope, an uncuffed tube and a neutral position for the neck

Abdomen

The liver is large and fragile and the bladder rises out of the pelvis. The abdomen must be entered carefully. The umbilical vein is patent for many days after birth and is ligated before being divided.

Respiratory (respiratory distress syndrome [RDS], chronic lung disease)

Preterm delivery, gestational diabetes and birth asphyxia all lower pulmonary surfactant levels, resulting in decreased lung volume and compliance and promoting airway collapse on expiration and atelectasis. Fewer type 1 muscle fibres in the diaphragm and intercostals increases early fatigue. Chronic inflammatory lung disease with scarring is seen in preterm babies from prolonged ventilation, overinflation, high pressures and oxygen toxicity.

- Surfactant, oxygen, continuous positive airway pressure (CPAP) or mechanical ventilation

Cardiovascular

A fall in pulmonary vascular resistance (PVR) at birth helps establish the postnatal circulation.

- In the early postnatal period, hypoxia, stress, high PCO_2 or acidosis may raise PVR; if the ductus arteriosus and foramen ovale are open, blood shunts R→L causing hypoxaemia
- An underdeveloped baroreflex means unchecked blood loss leads rapidly to hypotension

Fluids and electrolytes

Excess total body water and extracellular fluid are excreted after birth in a physiological diuresis. Insensible losses increase with low birth weight and low gestational age. The immature kidney loses sodium, bicarbonate, glucose, amino acids and phosphates. Low glycogen stores at birth promote hypoglycaemia, particularly in the preterm.

- Use local neonatal intensive care unit (NICU) protocols. Maintenance fluids need 10% glucose and appropriate electrolytes
- Watch for hyperglycaemia with hypernatraemia, which increases the risk of intraventricular haemorrhage in the preterm
- Replace nasogastric losses or stoma losses (>15 mL/kg/day) millilitre for millilitre with 0.9% NaCl, 0.15% KCl

Nutrition

Reserves are deficient in the premature and postnatal starvation affects neurological development.

- Start central parenteral nutrition as a matter of urgency

Thermoregulation

A high surface area to bodyweight ratio increases heat loss; particularly during exposure for anaesthesia (exacerbated by vasodilation) and surgery, there is an inability to shiver. Low temperatures promote coagulopathy, which is compounded by the acidosis from poor peripheral perfusion and myocardial depression.

- Warm incubators, limit exposure for procedures, warm theatre, warm fluids

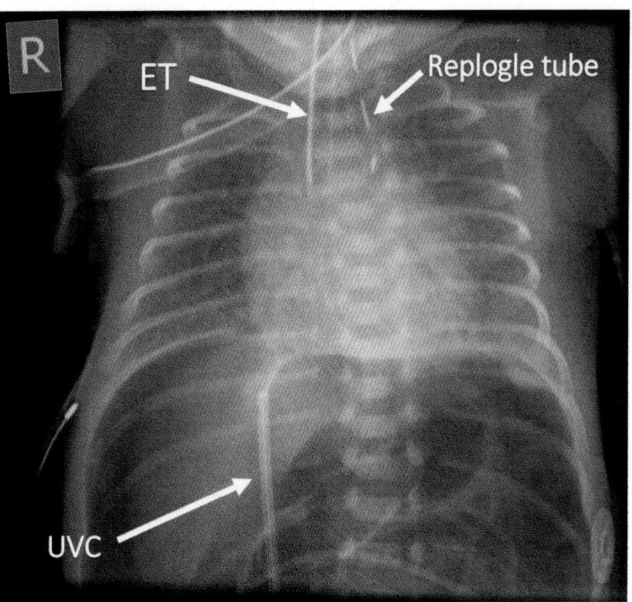

Figure 18.2 Tracheoesophageal fistula/oesophageal atresia with gastric perforation in a 28-week gestation, 1000-g baby. Note the endotracheal tube (ET), Replogle tube in the upper pouch, the umbilical venous catheter (UVC), free abdominal air around the liver and either side of the falciform ligament above the UVC and patchy lung fields of respiratory distress syndrome.

A nasogastric tube coiled in the upper oesophageal pouch on a chest radiograph suggests the diagnosis. A nasal or oral sump Replogle tube is placed to drain saliva and prevent aspiration. Positive airway pressure is avoided as air passing through the fistula causes gastric distension, compromised ventilation, and risks perforation (***Figure 18.2***). If pressure support is needed, perhaps because of RDS, prompt fistula ligation is needed.

Types A and B typically have a long gap and may require oesophageal replacement; options include colonic or jejunal interposition or gastric transposition some months after a cervical oesophagostomy and a gastrostomy. In many cases the ends can be brought together by progressive traction and delayed anastomosis.

In types C and D, the fistula is divided through a right thoracotomy or thoracoscopically. If the neonate is stable and the gap favourable, an anastomosis is fashioned over a trans-anastomotic tube, facilitating early feeding. If a primary anastomosis is not possible, then options include a delayed anastomosis after a few weeks of growth, or the use of traction sutures and an earlier anastomosis, or a much later interposition. Traction sutures can be internal or external. Nutrition is supported through a gastrostomy.

Complications after a repair include anastomotic leaks, oesophageal strictures and refistulation. Minor leaks often settle without intervention, strictures need dilating with a bougie or a balloon, and refistulation needs repair.

Type E is an isolated 'H'-type tracheoesophageal fistula without atresia. The fistula is usually found in the neck on a contrast swallow. Type E presents with recurrent chest infections or coughing after feeds and is usually repaired in the neck.

Robert L Replogle, 1931–2016, Chicago, the last trainee of Robert E Gross.

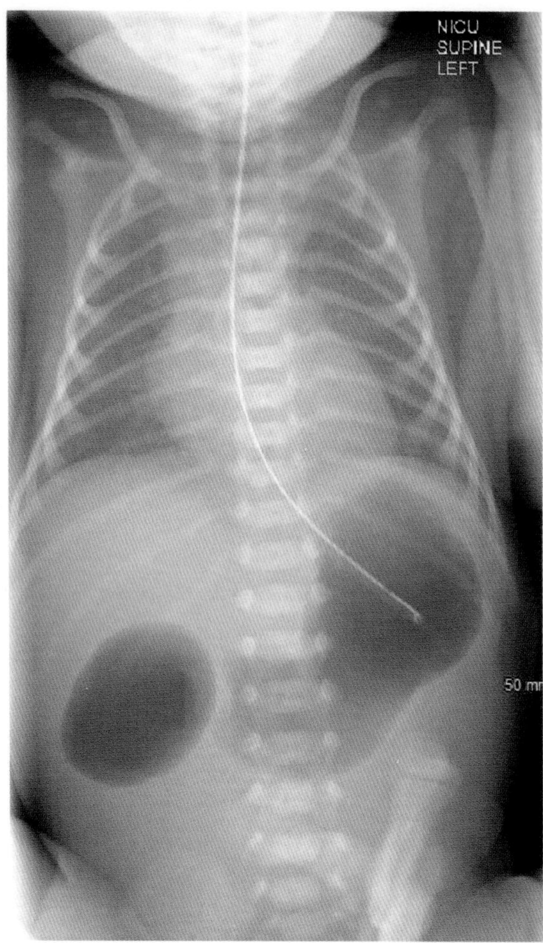

Figure 18.3 Double bubble in duodenal atresia (gastric and first part of the duodenum). Note the umbilical cord and clamp in the lower part of the image.

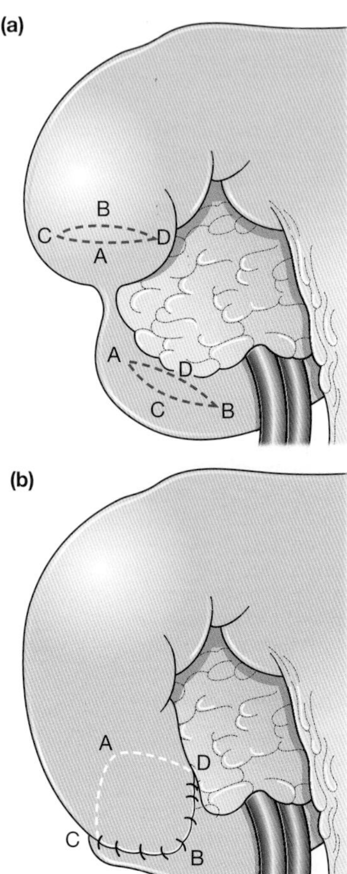

Figure 18.4 (a, b) Duodenal atresia and the incisions used to repair it: a diamond anastomosis is shown.

Duodenal atresia

The obstruction in duodenal atresia usually lies just distal to the ampulla of Vater. The proximal duodenum and pylorus dilate with swallowed amniotic fluid, rendering the pylorus temporarily incompetent. Occasionally, there is a web that may stretch like a windsock. If suspected antenatally, duodenal atresia is confirmed postnatally on an abdominal radiograph, showing a 'double bubble' (***Figure 18.3***); if missed, it presents with bilious vomiting. The hepatopancreatic duct may have openings on either side of the atresia, and a little gas can pass distally. Repair is by open Kimura duodenoduodenostomy (***Figure 18.4***) with or without a trans-anastomotic tube.

Small bowel atresias

Small bowel atresias may be isolated (***Figure 18.5***) or multiple. If seen without other anomalies, they are thought to have been caused by localised vascular events occurring after organogenesis. Rarely multiple intestinal atresias are seen with an immune deficiency related to mutations of the tetratricopeptide gene (TTC7A). A segmental ileal volvulus can cause an atresia; thick meconium in cystic fibrosis is a risk factor. The upstream bowel dilates and becomes dysmotile, while the downstream bowel remains narrow; a primary anastomosis can accommodate up to a 5:1 discrepancy. Resection of the dilated portion is appropriate if this does not sacrifice too much intestine. Otherwise, a temporary stoma and mucous fistula facilitate a staged repair.

Malrotation and volvulus

Complex rotations *in utero* give the small bowel mesentery its broad, stable base, running from the duodenal–jejunal (DJ) flexure in the left upper quadrant to the caecum in the right lower quadrant. Incomplete rotations leave the mesentery with a narrow, unstable base at risk of twisting. Sometimes, fibrous Ladd's bands run between a central upper abdominal caecum and the right lateral abdominal wall, obstructing the duodenum (***Figure 18.6***). A chronic volvulus that spares the vessels may present with protein-losing enteropathy or chylous ascites, while acute luminal obstruction presents with green bilious vomiting and is the harbinger of vascular compromise

Abraham Vater, 1684–1751, Professor of Anatomy and Botany, and later of Pathology and Therapeutics, Wittenberg, Germany.
Ken Kimura, contemporary, paediatric surgeon, Kobe University, Kobe, Japan, and Iowa City, IA, USA.
William E Ladd, 1880–1967, American surgeon, regarded as a founder of paediatric surgery.

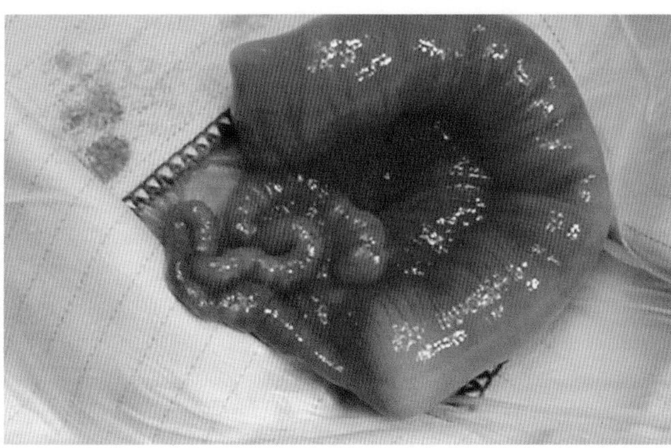

Figure 18.5 Small bowel atresia.

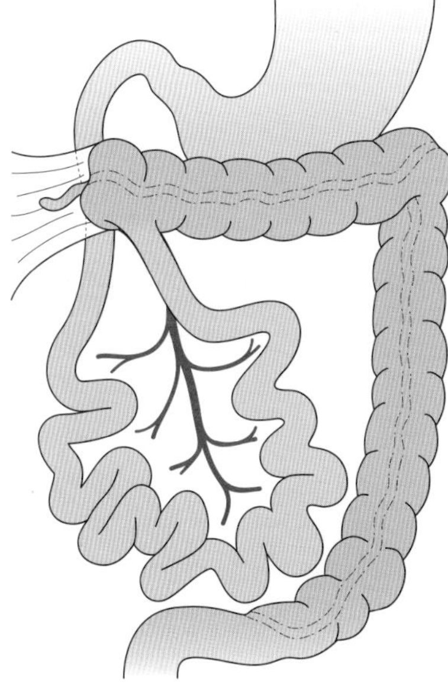

Figure 18.6 The narrow origin of the small bowel mesentery predisposes to midgut volvulus.

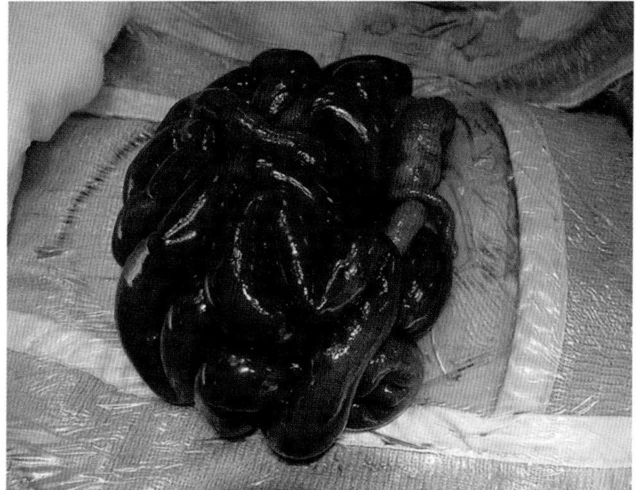

Figure 18.7 An acute small bowel volvulus with vascular compromise: the baby's head is to the right. Note that the terminal ileum, caecum and appendix in the upper central abdomen are well perfused.

(***Figure 18.7***), which can be fatal. An acute small bowel volvulus suspected in an acidotic baby vomiting bile with a gasless abdominal radiograph and a scaphoid abdomen demands an immediate laparotomy. Well babies presenting with bilious vomiting have a contrast study to locate the DJ flexure. If the DJ flexure lies to the left of the vertebral column, at the level of the pylorus, the mesentery is likely to be stable. At operation, the bowel is placed in the non-rotated position and the mesentery is broadened – Ladd's procedure (***Figure 18.8***).

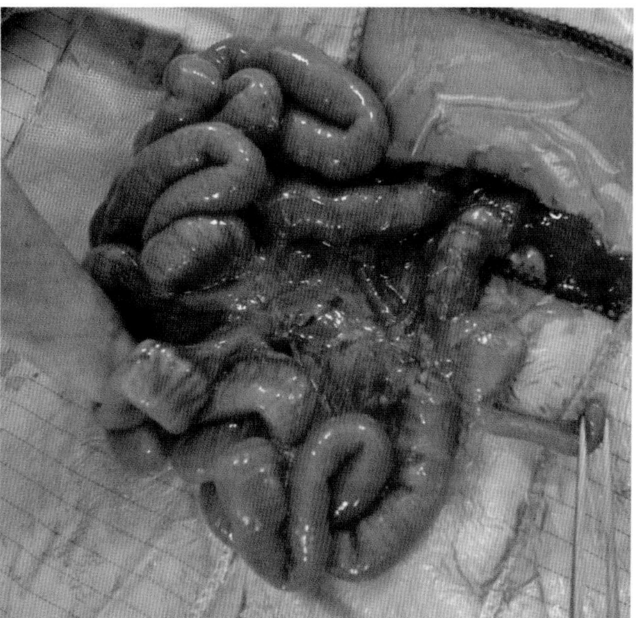

Figure 18.8 Ladd's procedure: the duodenum is placed on the right, the colon on the left and the mesentery is broadened. The duodenum appears to lie near the colon since the wound is small. The appendix may be removed.

Meconium ileus

Inspissated meconium may cause a distal ileal obstruction. A segmental ileal volvulus can follow and create an atresia. If the ileum perforates, it may seal or persist and cause a large meconium pseudocyst. An abdominal radiograph shows obstruction with a ground-glass appearance. Peritoneal calcification indicates an antenatal perforation. Simple cases are managed with a water-soluble hyperosmolar contrast enema (diatrizoate) using fluoroscopy in a well-hydrated neonate (***Figure 18.9***). Complicated cases require a laparotomy and enterotomy for a luminal washout; a temporary stoma may be required. Postoperatively, N-acetylcysteine can be given by nasogastric tube and as enemas to loosen residual meconium. Genetic investigations look for defects in the cystic fibrosis transmembrane conductance regulator (CFTR) protein.

Necrotising enterocolitis

NEC is a patchy haemorrhagic enteritis seen in about 10% of preterm babies on NICUs; all are more than a few days old and have been fed. NEC is less common in breastfed than in

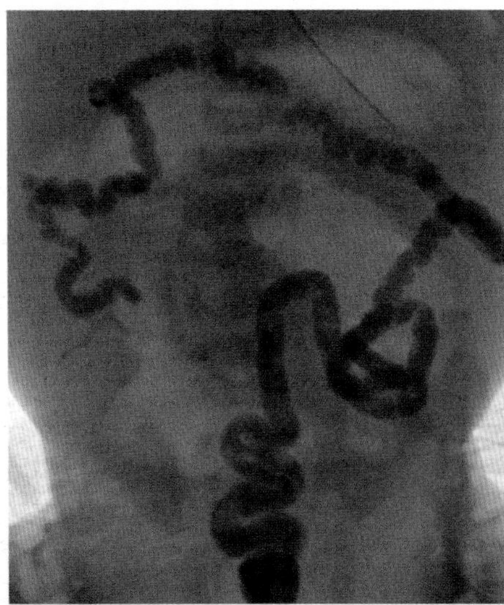

Figure 18.9 Water-soluble contrast in meconium ileus showing a microcolon.

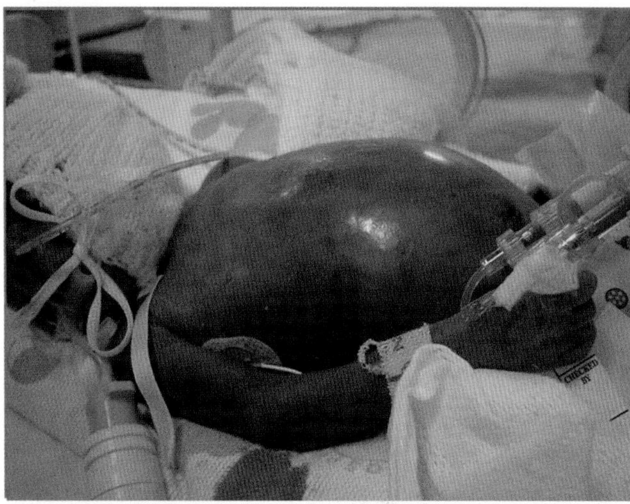

Figure 18.10 A ventilated neonate with an acute abdomen awaiting laparotomy.

formula-fed babies. NEC commonly involves the colon and terminal ileum, less commonly the jejunum and rarely the duodenum. Mild NEC presents with feed intolerance, bilious aspirates, distension and rectal bleeding – gut rest, antibiotics and PN may be sufficient treatment. If tenderness and signs of sepsis are present surgical intervention may be needed, especially if there is a deterioration needing mechanical ventilation and inotropes. Some can be observed closely for a short time. A laparotomy is needed if there is no improvement, a persistent mass, worsening obstruction, perforation, or further deterioration. The sickest babies have a rapidly progressing multiorgan failure with a discoloured abdomen (***Figure 18.10***) and a mortality of around 30%. Radiological signs include pneumatosis intestinalis (***Figure 18.11***), gas in the portal vein and if perforated, a pneumoperitoneum. A peritoneal drain can occasionally be sufficient, but definitive surgery is usually needed. At laparotomy (***Figure 18.12***), bowel resection and anastomosis or a defunctioning stoma are options. In the sickest babies, dead intestine is removed, open bowel ends closed (clip and drop), and the abdomen left open (laparostomy) with a vacuum dressing applied on low suction. Definitive surgery follows stabilisation. Survivors with >40 cm of small intestine usually adapt over a few months, but others may need prolonged admissions or home PN.

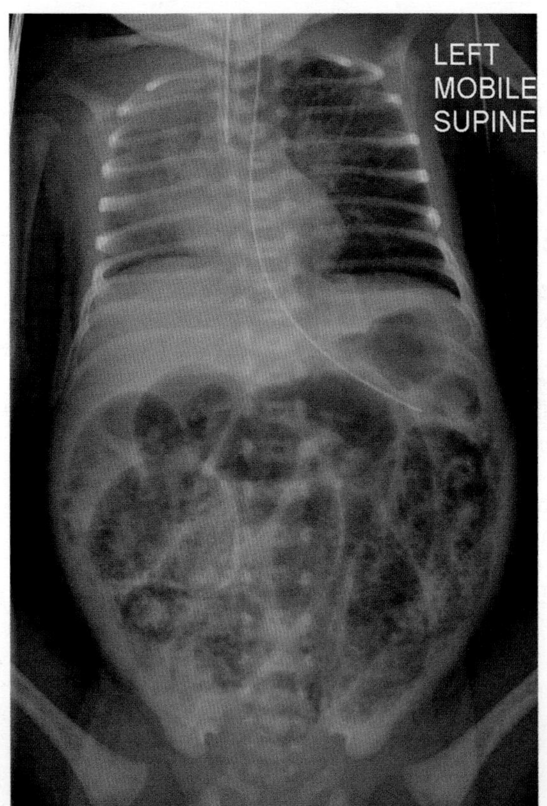

Figure 18.11 Abdominal radiograph showing pneumatosis.

Biliary atresia/choledochal malformation

Congenital or acquired (e.g. cytomegalovirus) extrahepatic biliary atresia is a progressive obliterative cholangiopathy with absent or narrow bile ducts. Type I involves the common bile duct, type II the common hepatic duct, and 80% have the most common type III, involving the proximal bile ducts. Biliary atresia presents with conjugated hyperbilirubinaemia, pale stools and dark urine in the first few weeks of life. If presenting late, there may be malabsorption, growth failure and coagulopathy. Some associations appear in ***Table 18.1***. The diagnosis is confirmed with a radionucleotide hepatobiliary iminodiacetic acid (HIDA) scan. Early diagnosis and avoiding sepsis may prevent irreversible liver fibrosis and death. The Kasai hepatico-portoenterostomy using a jejunal Roux-en-Y loop anastomosed to the portal plate gives drainage for some years,

Morio Kasai, 1922–2008, pioneering Japanese surgeon, trained by C Everett Koop.
César Roux, 1857–1934, Swiss surgeon, assistant to Theodor Kocher.

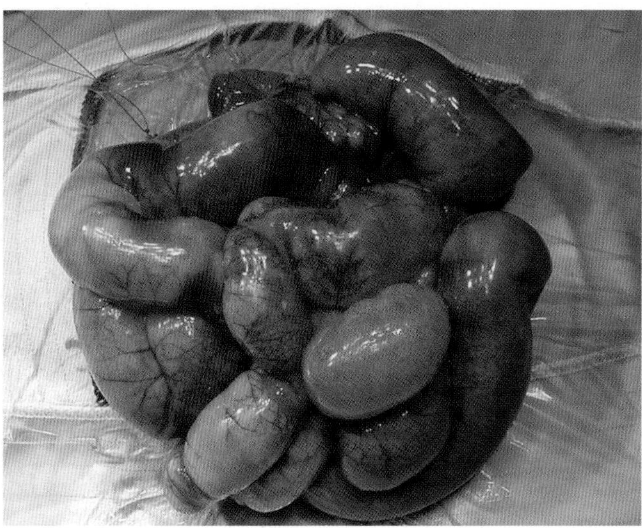

Figure 18.12 Operative appearance of neonatal necrotising enterocolitis.

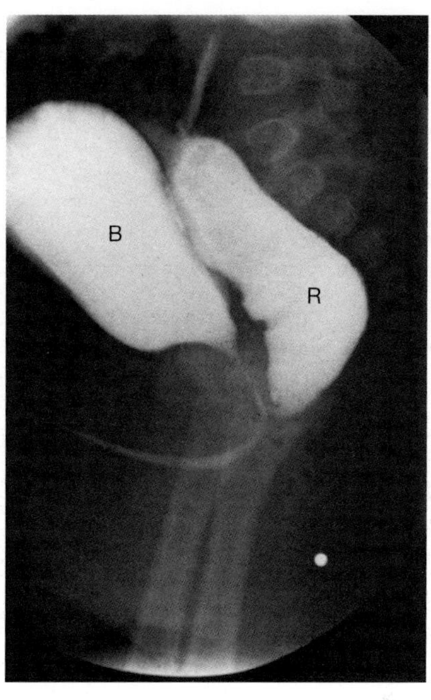

Figure 18.14 A rectourethral fistula, visible on a contrast study performed via a sigmoid colostomy. The bladder is filled with contrast via the fistula and the radio-opaque dot has been placed on the infant's perineum over the normal site of the anus. B, bladder; R, rectum.

but many need liver transplantation. Congenital choledochal malformations manifest as cystic dilatations of the biliary tree and are also managed with resection and portoenterostomy.

Anorectal malformations

In an anorectal malformation, there is usually no opening in boys, and the rectum ends either blindly (notably in aneuploidies) or with a fistula to the bulbar urethra (***Figure 18.13a***), prostate or bladder neck. Occasionally, there is a rectoperineal fistula in a boy. In contrast, there is usually a rectovestibular (***Figure 18.13b***) or rectoperineal fistula in girls; meconium is passed and therefore, many are missed on cursory newborn examinations. In girls, the rectum may join a common channel with the vagina and urethra; this is referred to as a cloaca (***Figure 18.13c***).

In boys, a divided proximal sigmoid colostomy allows feeding. A contrast study is performed through the defunctioned end (***Figure 18.14***). Repair of prostatic and bladder neck fistulae may be approached with a combined laparoscopic and perineal approach, whereas prostatic and bulbar urethral fistulae can both be approached in a posterior sagittal anorectoplasty (PSARP). The stoma is closed at a third stage. Most perineal and some vestibular fistulae can be transposed into the muscle complex without a stoma.

Hirschsprung's disease

Genetic defects (e.g. *RET*, *EDNRB*, *EDN3*) can affect the migration of neural crest-derived intestinal neurones (neurocristopathy), leading to aganglionosis and thickened nerve trunks in the distal bowel. There may be a family history. Aganglionic bowel fails to relax, causing a functional obstruction. Aganglionosis extends from the anus to the sigmoid colon in 75%, the proximal colon in 15%, and the terminal ileum in 10% of cases. A transition zone lies between dilated, proximal, normal bowel and narrow, distal aganglionic bowel. Neonatal Hirschsprung's disease presents with delayed passage of meconium, abdominal distension and bilious vomiting requiring resuscitation, gastric decompression, antibiotics and a bowel washout. The diagnosis is made on a cot-side suction rectal biopsy. A contrast enema may show the narrow aganglionic segment, a cone and dilated proximal bowel (***Figure 18.15***). Daily rectal washouts may allow a period of growth at home before surgery. If decompression fails, a stoma is fashioned using frozen section histopathology to identify ganglionic bowel. Definitive surgery removes the aganglionic segment

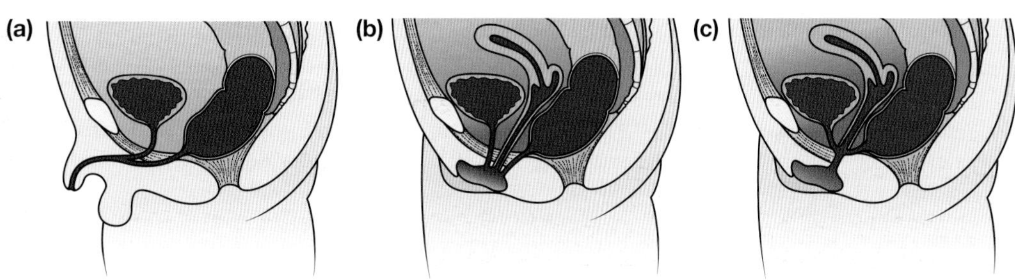

Figure 18.13 (a) Rectobulbar urethral fistula in a boy. (b) Rectovestibular fistula in a girl. (c) Cloaca in a girl.

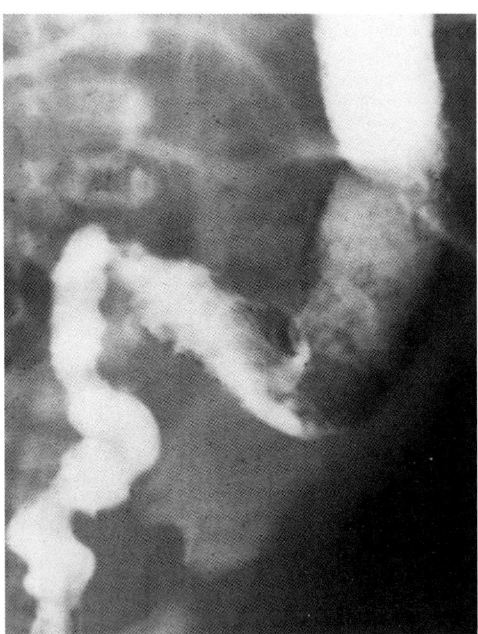

Figure 18.15 Barium enema in an infant, showing a 'transition zone' in the proximal sigmoid colon between the dilated proximal normally innervated bowel and the contracted aganglionic rectum.

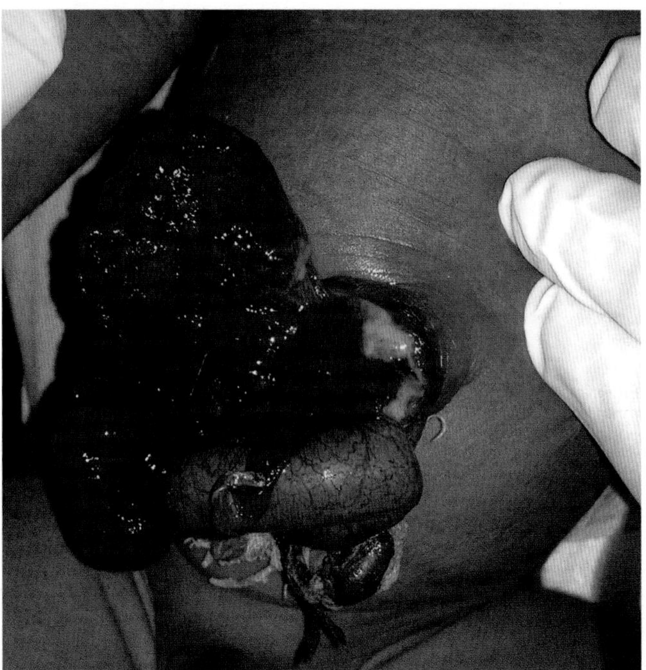

Figure 18.16 Gastroschisis.

and brings ganglionic bowel to the anus; Swenson, Duhamel, Yancey–Soave and transanal 'pull-throughs' are options. Most children achieve reasonable bowel control, but some have residual constipation, incontinence or episodes of enterocolitis.

Gastroschisis

In gastroschisis, an abdominal wall defect lies to the right-hand side of the umbilical cord and transmits the small and large intestine, stomach, bladder and sometimes the ovaries or undescended abdominal testes (***Figure 18.16***). Risk factors include teenage pregnancy, recreational drugs, smoking and genitourinary infection in pregnancy. It is easily diagnosed antenatally, allowing delivery near a surgical unit. Vaginal delivery is appropriate. After birth, twisting or kinking of the mesenteric blood supply must be avoided. The abdomen and viscera are wrapped using a transparent plastic food wrap (e.g. cling film, Saran wrap), a large-bore nasogastric tube is placed, and fluid resuscitation is initiated. The bowel may have a thick wall and be matted together. Sometimes, the defect closes antenatally, causing an atresia and an external length of damaged intestine (***Figure 18.17***). A narrow defect may need to be widened and a sutured silo (silo: structure for storage) created using Silastic sheeting or an empty intravenous fluid bag. Primary closure under general anaesthesia usually requires NICU admission for postoperative ventilation. An alternative is to place a preformed silo at the bedside (***Figure 18.18***), followed by gradual reduction, which sometimes avoids general anaesthesia altogether. PN is needed for around 4 weeks or longer while intestinal motility improves.

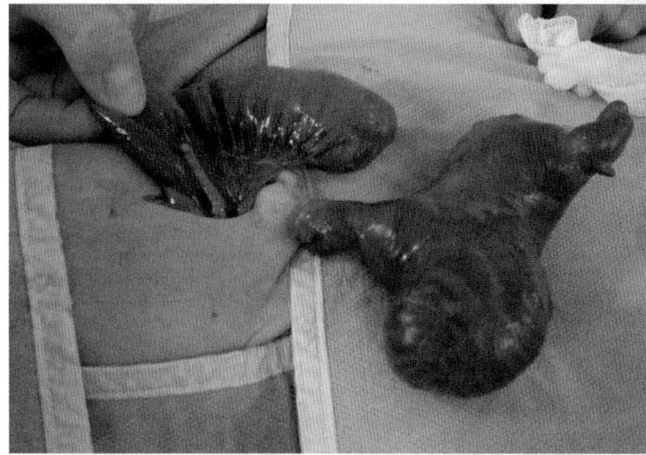

Figure 18.17 Closing gastroschisis: the defect has narrowed and occluded the vessels to a few loops of intestine. Note the atresia found at laparotomy.

Exomphalos

Exomphalos describes a central abdominal wall defect in which prolapsed viscera are covered in a thin, three-layered membrane (peritoneum, Wharton's jelly and amnion) in continuity with the umbilical cord. Exomphalos minor (<5 cm, liver not involved) is commonly associated with other anomalies (***Table 18.1***) and the defect is easily closed. In exomphalos major (***Figure 18.19***) the sac can be dressed with a topical antibacterial agent (e.g. manuka honey, silver sulfadiazine), allowing epithelialisation

Orvar Swenson, 1909–2012, Swedish-born American paediatric surgeon who discovered the cause of Hirschsprung's disease.
Bernard Duhamel, 1917–1996, Professor of Surgery, Hôpital Saint-Denis, Paris, France.
Asa G Yancey, 1916–2013, African-American surgeon who described in 1952 what **Soave** described in 1964.
Thomas Wharton, 1614–1673, English anatomist: 'The description of the glands of the entire body', 1656.

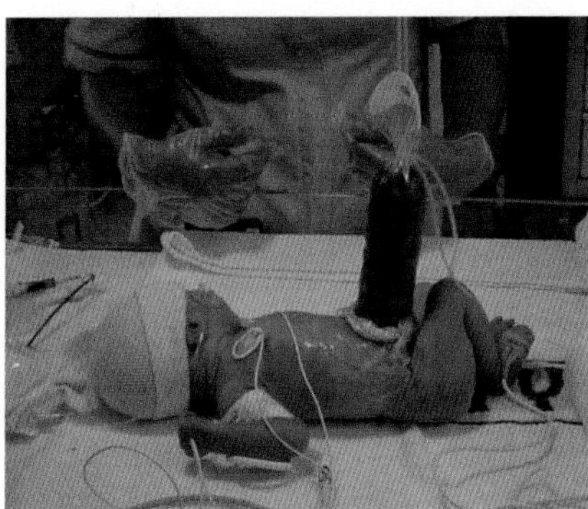

Figure 18.18 Gastroschisis in a preformed silo.

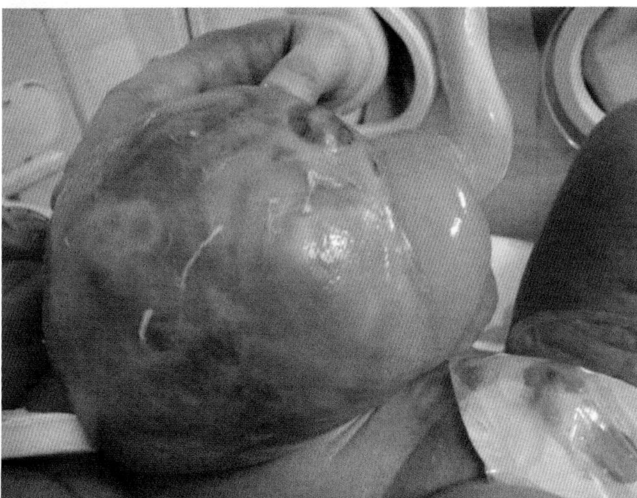

Figure 18.19 Exomphalos major.

and later closure of the ventral hernia. If an early closure of an exomphalos major is attempted, close observation for an abdominal compartment syndrome is mandated.

Summary box 18.1

Neonatal abdominal wall defects

Gastroschisis

- Environmental risk factors (young maternal age, drug use)
- Bowel complications common (atresia, matting, volvulus)
- Associated anomalies rare

Exomphalos

- Frequent association with aneuploidies and other genetic syndromes (e.g. Beckwith–Wiedemann)
- Other structural anomalies common (e.g. cardiac malformations)
- Large defects may contain liver (exomphalos major) and require delayed or staged closure

THORACIC SURGERY

Congenital diaphragmatic hernia

Several genes share roles in diaphragmatic, pulmonary, cardiac and foregut development; consequently, congenital diaphragmatic hernias are associated with lung hypoplasia, pulmonary hypertension, cardiac defects and gastroesophageal reflux, with half having additional anomalies. The pulmonary hypoplasia is partly due to lung compression from herniated abdominal contents (mechanical aetiology) and partly due to genetic causes (e.g. *FOG2, GATA4*). Commonly, there is a left posterolateral or Bochdalek defect, less commonly a ventral or Morgagni defect.

The diagnosis is usually made antenatally. A prognosis based on an observed-to-expected lung–head ratio (ultrasound), total fetal lung volume (magnetic resonance imaging) and whether or not the fetal liver is in the chest informs counselling.

After birth, intubation, muscle relaxation and gentle ventilation aim to maintain pH, and oxygen saturation so avoiding right-to-left shunting. Permissive hypercapnia and high-frequency oscillation may help. Pulmonary hypertension may lead to vascular shunting, hypoxia, hypercapnia and cardiac dysfunction. Cardiac dysfunction, assessed by echocardiography, may respond to nitric oxide, prostaglandin E1, milrinone and inotropes, but severe dysfunction requires extracorporeal life support (ECLS). Repair is offered if the pulmonary circulation stabilises. Unlike in traumatic diaphragmatic hernias, urgently reducing the bowel does not improve gas exchange in a congenital diaphragmatic hernia. The defect can be approached from the abdomen or the chest, either open or minimally invasively. The defect may be small, needing only a few sutures, or larger, needing a conical Silastic or GOR-TEX patch. A hernial sac may be present, which may be removed or plicated.

Pulmonary airway malformations

There are three groups: congenital cystic adenomatoid malformations (CCAMs), bronchopulmonary sequestrations (BPSs) and congenital lobar emphysema (CLE). The sequestrations may be intralobar or extralobar and are accompanied by an aberrant arterial supply from a major vessel, usually the aorta. Hybrid lesions have both a CCAM and a BPS. Some malformations cause respiratory or cardiovascular compromise at birth and require excision, but most are asymptomatic and imaging may be delayed for several months. Cross-sectional computed tomography imaging defines the anatomy and vasculature.

Vincent Alexander Bochdalek, 1801–1883, Professor of Anatomy, Prague, Czech Republic.
Giovanni Battista Morgagni, 1682–1771, Italian anatomist, the father of modern anatomical pathology.
John Bruce Beckwith, 1933, American paediatric pathologist.
Hans-Rudolf Wiedemann, 1915-2006, German paediatrician. Both Beckwith and Wiedemann reported cases of the syndrome independently in 1963 and 1964.

NEWBORN TUMOURS

Sacrococcygeal teratoma

These germ cell tumours arise from the coccyx and are usually diagnosed antenatally. They may have internal and external components or both (***Figure 18.20***). Most are benign mature teratomas, but some contain immature embryonic elements. Complete excision is usually achieved in the prone position and must include removing the coccyx and reconstruction of the pelvic floor. If the intra-abdominal component is large or vascular, the median sacral artery can be ligated through the abdomen. Bladder and bowel function are assessed following the pelvic floor repair. α-Fetoprotein levels are measured to detect recurrence.

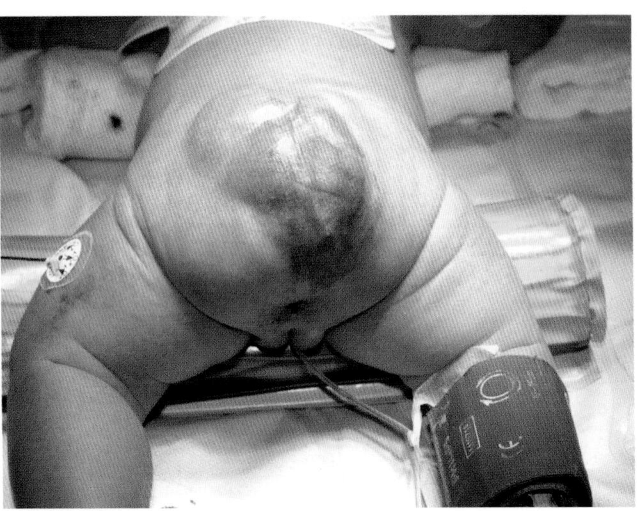

Figure 18.20 Sacrococcygeal teratoma.

Congenital mesoblastic nephroma

This renal tumour may present as a large palpable mass in a newborn with some having hypertension and hypercalcaemia (paraneoplastic syndromes). Cross-sectional imaging distinguishes a tumour from a multicystic dysplastic kidney. A nephroureterectomy is usually curative, but some may recur locally or metastasise.

WHY ADULT SURGEONS NEED AN OVERVIEW OF NEONATAL SURGERY

Rarely, malrotation, congenital diaphragmatic hernias and lung malformations described in this chapter may present for the first time in adulthood. More commonly, adults who had neonatal surgery may present with incidental or related pathology. Children who had anorectal malformations or Hirschsprung's disease need colorectal follow-up, with girls also needing a gynaecologist and obstetrician who understands the pathology; those with oesophageal atresia/tracheoesophageal fistula need an upper gastrointestinal surgeon.

CHAPTER 19 Trauma in children

Learning objectives

To be able to:

- Systematically assess an injured child
- Give examples of how mechanisms of, and responses to, injury differ from those in adults
- Distinguish the elements of the primary and secondary surveys
- Explain when and how to transfuse blood products in children
- Describe some common patterns of injury in children
- Request appropriate investigations for an injured child
- Outline the non-operative management of solid organ injuries
- Outline the principles of the trauma laparotomy and the clamshell thoracotomy
- Explain the principle of damage control surgery

INTRODUCTION

Trauma is the leading cause of death in children over 1 year old, and blunt trauma is the most common mechanism. Prompt, guideline-driven management by a trauma team reduces complications and saves lives. For cranial injuries in children, see ***Chapter 28***; for orthopaedic injuries in children, see ***Part 4, Trauma***.

THE PRIMARY SURVEY

Injured children are assessed using the Advanced Trauma Life Support (ATLS) structured **cABCDE** approach: **c**ontrol of catastrophic bleeding with pressure, **A**irway with C-spine control, **B**reathing with oxygen, **C**irculation with further control of haemorrhage, **D**isability, **E**xposure and Environment. In contrast to managing trauma in adults (see ***Part 4, Trauma***), the following should be considered:

- **A** – overextension of the neck can cause airway obstruction; a neutral position is used for infants and a 'sniffing the morning air' position for older children.
- **B** – hypoxia is usually the cause of cardiac arrest in children; if easily reversed, the cardiac rhythm returns.
- **C** – hypotension occurs comparatively late after 20% of the circulating volume is lost.
- **D** – an age-dependent modified Glasgow Coma Scale (GCS) is used.
- **E** – small children lose heat rapidly, with hypothermia exacerbating any coagulopathy. If their weight in kilograms is unknown, it can be estimated from 2 × (age in years + 4).

In cardiac arrest, the four Hs and four Ts are considered: **H**ypoxia, **H**ypovolaemia, **H**ypothermia/Hyperthermia, **H**yperkalaemia/hypokalaemia, **T**ension pneumothorax, cardiac **T**amponade, **T**oxins, **T**hrombus.

Spinal cord injury without radiological abnormality (SCIWORA)

Cervical hyperextension can occur during a rear impact in a car accident or from a frontal impact to the head. If such a mechanism dissipates a lot of energy, the spinal cord can be damaged even though a cervical radiograph may look normal. Compared with adults, children have a proportionally heavier head and weaker cervical muscles, which together with more elastic spinal ligaments and horizontal facet joints permit displacement without fracture and spontaneous anatomical resolution. A myelopathy can follow a contusion or follow ischaemia from temporary vertebral artery occlusion. If an older child gives a history of transient paraesthesia, numbness or paralysis, cervical immobilisation should be continued, and magnetic resonance imaging obtained. Immobilisation of the cervical spine can be with blocks and tapes or, if tolerated, a collar.

Resuscitation

All children initially receive high-flow oxygen, preferably via a non-rebreathe mask; this can be stopped if there is cardiorespiratory stability after a period of observation. Intubation and ventilation are required if oxygenation is inadequate or if there is a low GCS, combative behaviour, an inability to cooperate, severe burns, prolonged seizures or imminent operative intervention. Ideally, seriously injured children require two large well-secured cannulae. Alongside the antecubital fossa, other suitable veins include the long saphenous at the ankle, the femoral, the external jugular and, in neonates, scalp veins. If intravenous access cannot be established, an intraosseous needle can be placed in the tibia (***Figure 19.1***) or the humeral head, which has the benefit of being easily accessed by an anaesthetist.

Fluid volume resuscitation aims to restore and maintain age-adjusted cardiovascular parameters. Initially, 10 mL/kg of a warmed isotonic fluid is given. Total blood volume (TBV) is around 85 mL/kg in a neonate, rising to 100 mL/kg at 1 month and then falling to 75–80 mL/kg in a child. Major haemorrhage is defined as loss of 50% of TBV in <3 hours, 100% in 24 hours or >20% in <1 hour, but is challenging to assess, especially in blunt trauma. Hospitals should have a major haemorrhage protocol. If the capillary refill is >2 seconds and the child has lost mainly blood, then blood is given, using O rhesus-negative blood until type-specific or cross-matched blood is available. Severe trauma-induced coagulopathy is best managed by correcting specific coagulation factors and using point-of-care testing thromboelastography (TEG) and thromboelastometry (ROTEM), but if these are not available the following are given: packed cells 20 mL/kg, fresh-frozen plasma 20 mL/kg, platelets 10 mL/kg and cryoprecipitate 5 mL/kg, and repeated maintaining these ratios and aiming for a haemoglobin level >80 g/L, platelets >75 × 10^9/L, fibrinogen >1.5 g/L and activated partial thromboplastin time (APTT)/prothrombin time (PT) <1.5 × normal midpoint. If the major haemorrhage occurred within 3 hours, a slow tranexamic acid bolus of 15 mg/kg followed by an infusion (15 mg/kg over 8 hours) should be given.

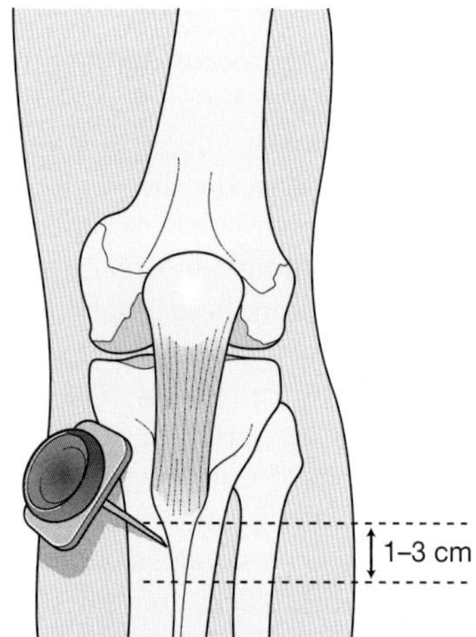

Figure 19.1 The intraosseous needle is inserted into the proximal tibia's medullary cavity about 1–3 cm below the tibial tuberosity.

Trauma-induced coagulopathy

Tissue damage releases factors that encourage coagulation but acidosis and hypothermia prolong it; therefore, blood products should be warmed. For each 1°C fall in temperature, factor activity falls by 10%. Below 34°C clotting times are prolonged, and platelets pool in the spleen and have poor adherence and aggregation. Poor perfusion increases thrombomodulin, which binds to thrombin and activates protein C, so inhibiting cofactors V and VIII. Activated protein C can deplete plasminogen activator inhibitor-1, which results in the formation of plasmin and fibrinolysis. Citrate in blood products can bind to calcium and, if this falls below 0.6 mmol/L, platelets are less effective.

Haemostasis is immature in neonates with procoagulant and anticoagulant proteins, remaining low until 6 months old. Fibrinogen is qualitatively dysfunctional, existing in a fetal form for 6–12 months after birth and contributing to an increased risk of bleeding. Burns can also cause a consumptive coagulopathy with microangiopathic haemolysis.

Children are more susceptible to hypothermia than adults: wet clothes should be removed early and warming blankets used. Children are more likely to become hypoglycaemic after a major injury as they mobilise glycogen poorly – blood sugar should be monitored in the significantly injured child, especially if they are nil by mouth.

A nasogastric tube and a urinary catheter should be considered for children who have had a major abdominal or head injury or are unconscious or ventilated. An orogastric tube is used if there is suspicion of a basal frontal skull fracture and a suprapubic catheter if a urethral injury is suspected.

Injury Severity Score

An Injury Severity Score (ISS) (see ***Chapter 26***) >15 predicts mortality in adults, but children require an ISS >25 for the same prediction; this is because most children have an isolated head or extremity injury. Only around 10% of children have multiple injuries.

- **Head**: in a neonate, the fontanelle or 'soft spot' may not have closed, leading to a bony space that could be confused with a fracture. A bulging fontanelle may suggest raised intracranial pressure, whereas a sunken fontanelle is seen in hypovolaemia.
- **Chest**: a child's rib cage is very compliant and ribs may bend and recover rather than break, leading to lung contusions or mediastinal injuries without fractures. If diagnosed clinically, a tension pneumothorax need not be confirmed with a chest radiograph before needle thoracocentesis and placing a chest drain. Although uncommon, cardiac tamponade should be considered and requires an emergency subxiphoid needle pericardiocentesis; a limited echocardiogram may confirm the diagnosis.
- An emergency department clamshell thoracotomy should be performed for penetrating chest injury where the patient had a witnessed arrest within the last 15 minutes. An incision is made across the chest in the fifth intercostal space. It may be possible to cut the sternum with scissors rather than needing a Gigli saw. The pericardium is opened, blood removed and bleeding controlled. A hole in the heart can be oversewn, taking care to avoid the coronary vessels. If the bleeding appears to be from lung, the lung can either be rotated 180° (lung twist) or the hilum slooped. The aim is not to perform a definitive repair but to buy time, allowing resuscitation, including internal massage until cardiac output returns. The clamshell thoracotomy also allows compression of the aorta just above the diaphragm to aid vascular filling.

Leonardo Gigli, 1863–1908, Florentine surgeon and obstetrician.

- **Abdomen**: the liver and spleen in children are less well protected by the rib cage than they are in adults and are at greater risk of injury from blunt trauma. Signs may be subtle, and tenderness should be investigated with cross-sectional imaging. If there is significant abdominal bleeding, aortic compression may be helpful, and this may be easier to achieve through a thoracotomy than a laparotomy; it can be challenging to reach the aorta above the liver.
- **Extremities**: in comparison with adults, children's bones are more compliant – they may bend or fracture one cortex. Children's bones also remodel as they grow; therefore, the position of an angled distal limb fracture may be accepted in a child when it would be manipulated in an adult. The growth plates in children are not yet fused and a fracture involving the growth plate can limit future limb growth – these fractures should be referred to a paediatric orthopaedic surgeon.

SECONDARY SURVEY

The secondary survey is performed after resuscitation and stabilisation. The history is reviewed and a complete clinical examination is performed to assess for other injuries.

Imaging

The choice of imaging depends on the mechanism of injury and the findings on examination. Cross-sectional imaging can be invaluable, but a head-to-toe computed tomography (CT) scan should only be performed with good reason to limit exposure to ionising radiation.

Plain radiograph

A chest radiograph is mandated in major trauma. The cervical spine is rarely injured, but if the injury mechanism leads to suspicion of cervical damage, then a cervical spine series is requested. Lateral and anteroposterior images must include the base of the skull and the C7–T1 junction. The odontoid or 'peg' projection can be difficult to obtain as the mouth needs to be open for the anteroposterior projection to see C1 (atlas) and C2 (axis). A pelvic radiograph is requested if a pelvic fracture is suspected. Suspected limb fractures initially undergo anteroposterior and lateral radiographs with CT reserved for those that are complex.

CT scans

A head CT scan should be performed within 1 hour if the GCS is <14 at the initial assessment or within 2 hours if the GCS is <15 after the injury. Other indications include a tense fontanelle, suspicion of an open or depressed skull fracture or a basal skull fracture, abnormal pupillary response, abnormal posturing, a focal neurological defect or concern about a non-accidental injury. A head CT scan should also be performed if there are three or more vomiting episodes, a witnessed loss of consciousness for >5 minutes or amnesia >5 minutes.

A CT scan of the chest, abdomen and pelvis is performed if there is abdominal wall bruising (***Figure 19.2***), tenderness, distension, peritonitis, blood per rectum or blood in the nasogastric tube. Some relative indications include an aspartate aminotransferase >200 U/L, amylase >100 U/L or microhaematuria >5 erythrocytes/high-power field. Abdominal and pelvic CT should be single-volume dual-contrast to minimise radiation exposure using the Camp Bastion or Afghan protocol.

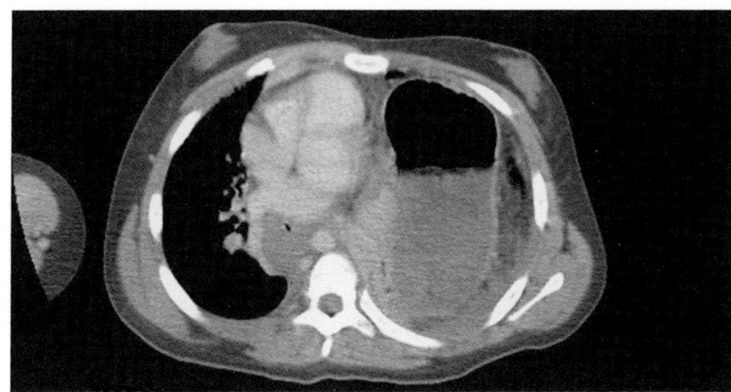

Figure 19.2 Traumatic diaphragmatic rupture found in a child with abdominal wall bruising.

A CT scan of the chest should be performed after a penetrating chest injury or a significant deceleration. However, most blunt chest injuries are detected on a chest radiograph; if the mediastinal silhouette is normal, a chest CT is not usually required.

A focused abdominal sonography trauma (FAST) scan is not helpful in children as the findings can be difficult to interpret.

Patterns of injury

There are some well-recognised patterns of injury in children.

Lap belt

If a child experiences a forced flexion over a lap belt in a car accident, the small bowel or its mesentery or the bladder's abdominal portion may get compressed against the spine. These tissues may fail up to 72 hours after the injury. Lumbar fractures may also be seen. In small children, the pancreas can be compressed by a lap belt.

Handlebar injury

A child who falls onto the end of a bicycle handlebar may crush the pancreas, duodenum, small intestine or its mesentery against the spine. A duodenal haematoma may cause an obstruction, the pancreas may be injured or divided and contused intestine may perforate after a delay of a few days, so a period of observation is required. When this injury pattern is seen in a child under 3 years old, a non-accidental injury must be considered.

Straddle injury

A child typically falls onto the side of a bath or a toy, causing a perineal injury that may involve the urethra or vagina.

Non-accidental injury

Non-accidental injuries should be suspected when the reported mechanism of injury or its timing are unusual. Fractures, abdominal injuries and intracranial haemorrhages in those under 2 years old are often non-accidental. Bruises are remarkably difficult to date, but their shape and pattern may distinguish accidental from abusive bruising if they leave an imprint. Patterned bruises generally do not occur during regular play. Bruises over soft tissues in an immobile infant are suspicious, whereas those over bony prominences such as the knees, elbows and the forehead in a mobile child are not. Bruises on the cheeks, neck, genitals, buttocks and back are unlikely to be accidental. Some benign entities may be confused with abusive bruises, such as Mongolian spots and haemangiomas. Children with idiopathic thrombocytopenic purpura or leukaemia may present with unexplained bruises in different stages of healing.

DEFINITIVE MANAGEMENT

Chest

A small pneumothorax detected on a chest radiograph may be observed rather than drained. Lung contusions require analgesia and chest physiotherapy to prevent secondary infection. Penetrating lung injuries may be assessed at either thoracoscopy or thoracotomy and the underlying lung injury sealed with fibrin glue or by applying a stapler; segmentectomy or lobectomy are rarely required.

Abdomen

Intraperitoneal air mandates a laparoscopy or laparotomy. Penetrating wounds that have not entered the abdominal cavity should be cleaned and closed. The spleen and liver account for 70% of all visceral injuries caused by blunt trauma. In the haemodynamically stable child, most solid organ injuries can be managed without an operation, but if unstable despite appropriate transfusion, or only transiently responding, interventional radiology and embolisation or a laparotomy should be considered. Recurrent instability may reflect an inadequate initial resuscitation, and the need for a second transfusion does not mandate an operation.

Following an abdominal solid organ injury, bed rest is advised until pain free, with mobilisation after a minimum of 1 night for grade I and II injuries and after a minimum of 2 nights for grade >III injuries. High-impact activities and contact sports should be limited for grade IV and V injuries for 6 weeks. However, delayed haemorrhage can arise spontaneously several days after an injury and is thought to occur in a hyperosmolar setting when a haematoma breaks down. Discharged patients need to know to return to the hospital if unwell.

TABLE 19.1 Spleen injury scale.

Grade	Injury type	Description of injury
I	Haematoma	Subcapsular, <10% surface area
II	Laceration	Capsular tear, <1 cm parenchymal depth
	Haematoma	Subcapsular, 10–50% surface area, intraparenchymal, <5 cm in diameter
III	Laceration	Capsular tear, 1–3 cm parenchymal depth not involving a trabecular vessel
	Haematoma	Subcapsular, >50% surface area or expanding; ruptured subcapsular or parenchymal haematoma, intraparenchymal haematoma ≥5 cm or expanding
IV	Laceration	>3 cm parenchymal depth or involving a trabecular vessel
	Laceration	Laceration involving segmental or hilar vessels producing major devascularisation (>25%)
V	Laceration	Completely shattered spleen
	Vascular	Devascularised by a hilar injury

TABLE 19.2 Liver injury scale.

Grade	Injury type	Description of injury
I	Haematoma	Subcapsular, <10% surface area
	Laceration	Capsular tear, <1 cm parenchymal depth
II	Haematoma	Subcapsular, 10–50% surface area, intraparenchymal, <10 cm in diameter
III	Haematoma	Subcapsular, >50% surface area or expanding; ruptured subcapsular or parenchymal haematoma; intraparenchymal haematoma ≥10 cm or expanding
	Laceration	>3 cm parenchymal depth or involving a trabecular vessel
IV	Laceration	Parenchymal disruption involving 25–75% of hepatic lobe or 1–3 Couinaud segments in a single lobe
V	Laceration	Parenchymal disruption involving >75% of hepatic lobe or >3 Couinaud segments within a single lobe
	Vascular	Juxtahepatic venous injuries
VI	Vascular	Hepatic avulsion

Specific considerations

Spleen

There is a risk of splenic pseudoaneurysm after splenic trauma, which is unrelated to the severity of the injury (***Table 19.1***). Therefore, a follow-up ultrasound is recommended.

Liver

The grades of liver trauma are given in ***Table 19.2***. Bile leaks are rare and often resolve after drainage rather than repair but should be discussed with a paediatric liver surgeon.

Claude Couinaud, 1922–2008, French surgeon and anatomist, described the segmental anatomy of the liver.

Pancreas

Pancreatic trauma may lead to a pancreatic pseudocyst, which requires endoscopic drainage into the stomach. For distal lacerations in the pancreatic tail, some surgeons prefer an early distal pancreatectomy rather than non-operative management. Proximal pancreatic duct injuries in older children can be stented.

Renal

After severe renal injuries, hypertension can develop, which may need treatment. A dimercaptosuccinic acid (DMSA) scan is used to assess function in those with hypertension or following grade IV or V injuries (***Table 19.3***).

TABLE 19.3 Renal injury scale.

Grade	Injury type	Description of injury
I	Contusion	Microscopic or gross haematuria. Normal imaging
	Haematoma	Subcapsular, not expanding and without parenchymal laceration
II	Haematoma	Non-expanding peri-renal haematoma confined to the retroperitoneum
	Laceration	<1.0 cm parenchymal depth without extravasation of urine
III	Laceration	>1.0 cm parenchymal depth without collecting system rupture or extravasation of urine
IV	Laceration	Parenchymal laceration extends through the cortex, medulla and collecting system
	Vascular	Main renal artery or vein injury with contained haemorrhage
V	Laceration	Shattered kidney
	Vascular	Avulsion of the renal hilum devascularising the kidney

Duodenum

A duodenal haematoma has a risk of late perforation, which may be retroperitoneal. Therefore, a second abdominal CT scan or a contrast study should be considered if there is deterioration or recovery is particularly slow.

Bowel

There are three mechanisms: the bowel wall may fail instantly if pressure rises rapidly in a trapped loop, it may fail up to 72 hours after a direct crush injury or it may become ischaemic following a mesenteric injury damaging its blood supply.

Urethral injury

In straddle injuries and pelvic fractures there may be blood at the urethral meatus. Urethral catheterisation can aggravate a urethral injury, and so a suprapubic catheter should be placed.

DAMAGE CONTROL SURGERY

Damage control surgery aims to break the 'vicious cycle' of hypothermia, tissue hypoxia, coagulopathy and acidosis before later definitive repair. Anatomy is restored when the physiology is optimised. The principles are in sequence: (i) short operations aiming to control haemorrhage and limit contamination; (ii) ongoing correction of deranged physiology – acidosis, hypothermia, perfusion and organ function on intensive care; (iii) definitive surgical repair.

In a trauma laparotomy, a midline incision is made from the xiphisternum to the pubic symphysis. Large clots are removed and the abdomen is packed in all four quadrants with large swabs to tamponade bleeding. If packing does not control bleeding, it is either inadequate packing, and more should be applied, or there is a significant arterial bleed, and so pressure should be applied to the aorta above the liver. Once bleeding is stemmed and the intravascular volume restored, the packs are removed systematically one quadrant at a time to find the source of the bleeding. Control is by vessel repair, ligation or removal of the organ or reapplication of the packs. Contamination is controlled by either repairing a simple bowel injury with a continuous suture or resection of multiple areas of perforated bowel with a clip-and-drop technique (either stapling or tying off the ends but not attempting primary anastomosis). Bile injuries are managed with a drain, and bladder injuries are oversewn and a urethral catheter placed. The abdomen is left open, allowing transfer to critical care for ongoing physiological correction before returning to theatre in the following days for further procedures.

Summary box 19.1

Paediatric trauma

- Use the Advanced Trauma Life Support (ATLS) guidelines
- Overextension of the neck can compromise the airway
- Cervical spine injury can be present without radiographic signs
- Intraosseous access is helpful in small children
- Lung contusion can occur without rib fractures
- In a stable child, abdominal injuries are best assessed by CT
- Blunt abdominal organ injury can usually be managed non-operatively
- Damage control surgery aims to correct physiology before definitive repair

CHAPTER

20 Paediatric urology

Learning objectives

At the end of this chapter, you will be able to:

- Explain the indications for circumcision in childhood and list the complications
- Describe three levels of urinary tract obstruction and outline their management
- Describe the anomalies of hypospadias and epispadias
- List risk factors for urolithiasis and describe three methods of stone management
- Categorise with examples three differences of sex development (DSD)
- Describe the ileocystoplasty with appendicovesicostomy for managing neuropathic bladders

INTRODUCTION

Paediatric urologists are paediatric surgeons who subspecialise in the conditions outlined in this chapter; they also manage the acute and elective inguinoscrotal pathology described in *Chapter 17*. Surgeons in many specialities are consulted about the foreskin; this is covered in detail here. Specialist paediatric urological conditions include hypospadias, epispadias, bladder exstrophy, vesicoureteral reflux, renal duplications, urolithiasis and urinary tract obstruction. Obstruction occurs at three levels: dysfunction at the ureteropelvic junction, dysfunction at the ureterovesical junction and in the posterior urethra with congenital valves. Obstructions may present with fetal hydronephrosis. Postnatally, obstruction with infection causes renal damage. The relevant embryology and epidemiology are summarised. Choosing the right time to operate, often based on diagnostic imaging, and gentle tissue handling are central to achieving good outcomes with few complications. Diagnostic imaging includes ultrasonography, voiding cystourethrography and the use of the radioisotope technetium-99m (^{99m}Tc) linked to dimercaptosuccinic acid (DMSA) or mercaptoacetyltriglycine (MAG-3). The management of the neuropathic bladder may involve an ileocystoplasty with a continent catheterisable channel. Many specialist paediatric urological conditions require close follow-up and later transfer to specialist adult surgical care.

EMBRYOLOGY

Four areas of developmental biology are relevant: (i) the two stages of testicular descent; (ii) the Weigert–Meyer rule – in a duplex system the ectopic upper pole ureter has an orifice lying inferomedial to the lower pole ureter; (iii) the role of the urethral plate in the tubularisation of the urethra and the aetiology of hypospadias and its relevance to operative repairs; and (iv) morphological differentiation in relation to disorders, or differences, of sex development. These areas are addressed in the recommended further reading.

THE PENIS

Foreskin disorders and circumcision

Surgical referrals for foreskin problems are common in early childhood, and reassurance is often all that is needed after taking a careful history and examination. The foreskin, or prepuce, is a highly innervated, double-layered fold of skin. The inner layer is a mucous membrane and the outer layer is skin, with a mucocutaneous zone where the layers meet. The prepuce has similarities to the eyelids, labia minora, anus and lips. The prepuce provides mucosa and skin to cover the erect penis. The foreskin is adherent to the glans at birth and gradually separates in most boys by the age of 5 years and in the remaining before puberty, allowing the foreskin to become fully retractile. Forceful retraction is not recommended as it can cause tears and scarring. The adhesions are natural and not pathological. The foreskin may balloon on micturition as the plane between glans and prepuce develops. Ballooning is not an indication for circumcision. If spraying of urine on micturition is causing concern, the parent and child can be taught to partially draw back the foreskin so the meatus is unobstructed and spraying is reduced. Occasionally a nodule of entrapped smegma, termed a 'smegma pearl', accumulates in the developing plane between the glans and prepuce, causing parental anxiety. These are harmless collections that discharge on their own when the developing plane finally opens onto the exposed glans.

Carl Weigert, 1845–1904, German pathologist and anatomist known for work on cellular staining.
Robert Meyer, 1864–1947, German pathologist in Berlin, removed from his position for being Jewish, emigrated in 1939 to Minneapolis, MN, USA.

Circumcision, being the removal of the foreskin, is the oldest and most common surgical procedure and is usually performed for cultural reasons. About 40% of males worldwide are circumcised. Circumcision is performed in Judaism, on day 8 of life (brit milah), and in Islam (khitan), at varying ages. In early infancy, circumcision can be performed under local anaesthesia using simple devices like the PlastiBell or Gomco clamp. In older boys under general anaesthesia, the foreskin is removed with a blade or scissors, followed by attention to haemostasis and skin apposition with sutures or glue. Complications include bleeding, dehiscence, infection, cicatrix, adhesion formation, meatal stenosis, the removal of too little or too much tissue, cosmetic concerns and rarely urethral injury or amputation. Medical indications for circumcision include:

- **True phimosis**: the foreskin is non-retractile because of a tight fibrotic preputial ring.
- **Balanitis xerotica obliterans (BXO)**: a chronic, possibly autoimmune, preputial inflammation that may also affect the distal urethra and is rarely seen before 5 years of age. Boys present with progressive phimosis and white, hard preputial skin (***Figure 20.1***), dysuria and ballooning on micturition. Usually, circumcision is required, although some boys respond to topical corticosteroids. Follow-up is required to exclude meatal stenosis.
- **Recurrent balanoposthitis**: an inflammation of the glans penis and its retractile foreskin due to infection, irritation or trauma. Boys may present with pain, itching, rash, dysuria and a non-urethral penile discharge. Most boys have only one or two episodes and need no intervention, but a few have sufficient trouble with recurrence that circumcision is indicated.
- **Recurrent urinary tract infections (UTIs)**: though rare in most boys, UTIs are a particular risk with some anomalies, such as posterior urethral valves, where infection can lead to pyelonephritis, renal scarring and renal insufficiency. In these boys, circumcision may reduce those risks.
- **Paraphimosis**: sometimes, the prepuce retracts back over the glans and cannot be brought forward again; the glans swells and becomes painful. If manipulation fails, an emergency dorsal slit or circumcision is indicated.

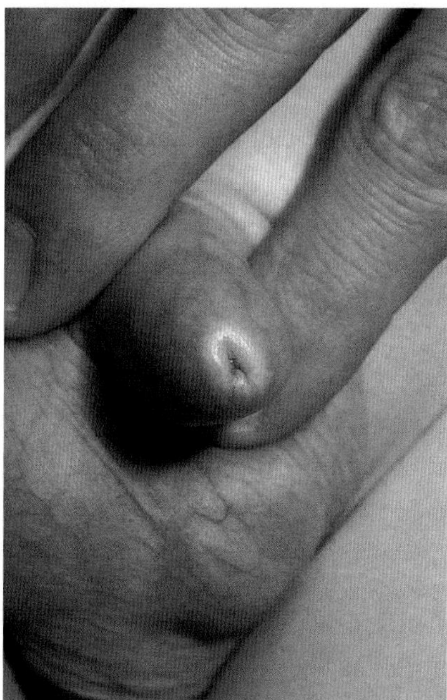

Figure 20.1 Balanitis xerotica obliterans.

Hypospadias

The genital tubercle becomes a penis under the influence of androgens with a tubular urethra arising from the urethral plate. The urethral plate develops a diamond-shaped groove whose edges fold over and fuse in the midline, forming a tube. In girls, the urethral plate's homologue forms the vestibular groove with edges that do not fuse but form the labia minora. Hypospadias is a congenital malformation seen in 1 in 300 boys. The urethral opening lies on the ventral aspect of the penis anywhere from the proximal glans to the perineum in association with a ventral curvature (called a chordee) and a ventrally deficient foreskin leading to a dorsal 'hooded' prepuce. Clinicians should document phallus length, meatal location, glans volume, depth and width of the urethral plate, degree of chordee, foreskin appearance and the testes' presence and location. Circumcision is contraindicated because the foreskin may be needed for the reconstruction. The anomaly should be diagnosed in the newborn examination.

Hypospadias repair aims to achieve the usual meatal location and a straight penis to facilitate micturition and ejaculation. Distal hypospadias, where the opening is on the glans, may be repaired in a single stage, whereas more proximal openings and those with severe curvatures require staged procedures. Many operations have been described. One technique is the tubularised incised plate procedure, which widens and then tubularises the urethral plate (***Figure 20.2***). Staged repairs may use the foreskin as a first-stage graft, followed by tubularisation in a second stage. Complications include urethrocutaneous fistulae, meatal stenosis, glans dehiscence and hypospadias persistence.

Epispadias/bladder exstrophy

Epispadias is a rare dorsal penile defect with an opening whose upper limit lies anywhere from the penopubic junction to the glans (***Figure 20.3***). Epispadias may be part of the bladder exstrophy–epispadias complex in which the bladder and bladder neck are also open on the lower abdominal wall. Ileocaecal exstrophy (cloacal exstrophy) represents the most severe variant, in which there is a small exomphalos with an everted caecum and ileum separating halves of the bladder and, in males, a split penis. If we imagine hypospadias as the anatomy that might result from making an opening with scissors placed with one blade into the urethra and one blade ventrally, then epispadias is akin to making this opening on the dorsal aspect and through the pubis into the bladder for the bladder exstrophy. Children with epispadias have problems with urinary incontinence but are often otherwise healthy. Boys with epispadias and a functioning bladder neck may have a

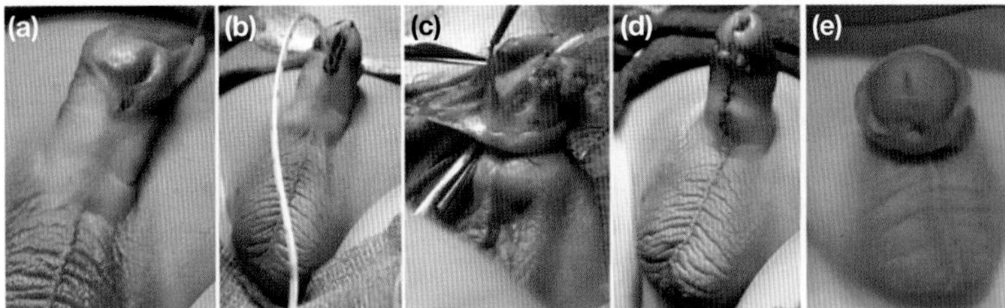

Figure 20.2 **(a)** Subcoronal hypospadias with dorsal hooded prepuce. **(b)** 5-Fr feeding tube in hypospadiac meatus. **(c)** Urethroplasty. **(d)** Creation of a terminal neo-meatus with skin closure. **(e)** Healed penis after hypospadias repair.

penile reconstruction around 2 years of age. Follow-up is required to monitor bladder emptying, continence and the upper urinary tracts, which may deteriorate if reconstruction causes a degree of obstruction.

UROLITHIASIS

The prevalence of urolithiasis in children varies from around 1–5% in Asia, 5–10% in Europe to 15% in North America. Investigations include serum electrolytes, urinalysis, urine culture and stone analysis. Common metabolic risk factors include high oxalate and calcium levels and low levels of citrate in the urine. Therapy aims to alter these levels to reduce recurrence. Approximately 25% of stones are caused by a UTI from urease-producing bacteria, *Proteus mirabilis* or *Klebsiella pneumoniae*. Anatomic anomalies leading to urinary stasis and urolithiasis include ureteropelvic junction obstruction, polycystic kidney and neurogenic bladder. Children may present with flank or abdominal pain, gross haematuria, dysuria, nausea or vomiting. Stones are easily detected with ultrasound. Non-contrast computed tomography scans are very sensitive but involve ionising radiation.

Small stones may pass with generous oral hydration and analgesia. Some stones with associated infection require intravenous hydration and antibiotics. α-Blockers and calcium channel blockers may reduce dysmotile ureteric contractions initiated by a stone while preserving helpful expulsive peristaltic activity. Reimaging may confirm the passage of a stone. Intervention may be required to manage pain, obstruction and treatment-resistant stones. Extracorporeal shock wave lithotripsy (ESWL) can safely and effectively fragment stones smaller than 2 cm using focused, high-energy shock waves delivered under general anaesthesia. Ureteroscopy allows fragmentation and removal of stones smaller than 2 cm from the ureter or kidney but is avoided in those younger than 5 years. Percutaneous nephrolithotomy (PCNL) can be used to extract stones from the kidney through a dilated tract. PCNL is used for stones larger than 2 cm, ESWL-refractory stones smaller than 2 cm and multiple stones.

Summary box 20.1

Urolithiasis

- Children with urolithiasis should be evaluated for metabolic risk factors
- Urological management depends on the size of calculi, age, number of stones and the presence of obstruction, infection or pain

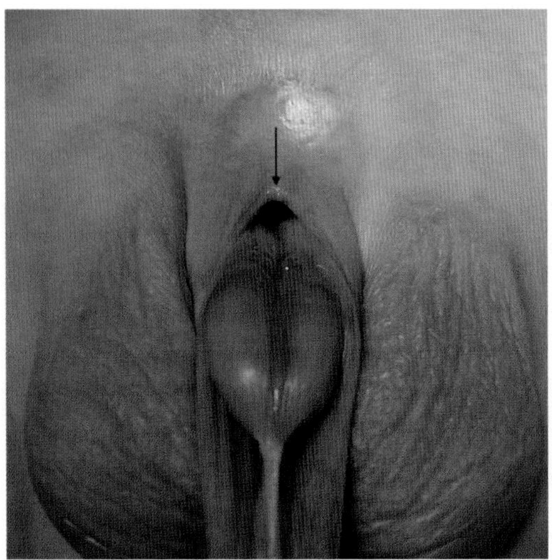

Figure 20.3 Penopubic meatus (arrow) in epispadias in a boy.

URINARY TRACT OBSTRUCTION

Antenatal fetal hydronephrosis

Hydronephrosis – a dilated renal pelvis – is found in 1% of antenatal scans and most commonly it resolves, especially if the dilatation is mild to moderate. Severe dilatation is associated with urinary tract obstruction or vesicoureteral reflux. Antenatal interventions are rarely indicated except in posterior urethral valves (PUVs), but postnatal imaging is needed to confirm resolution or make a diagnosis. Amniotic fluid is principally fetal urine; thus, if there is antenatal bilateral hydronephrosis with decreased amniotic fluid, PUV is a likely cause. If the PUV obstruction is thought to be damaging the kidneys, then there may be a role for an antenatal vesicoamniotic shunt to take the pressure off the upper tracts.

Radioisotope renal imaging

The metastable radioisotope ^{99m}Tc emits gamma rays during an isomeric transition to ^{99}Tc. It has a 6-hour emission half-life and a 1-day biological half-life, so imaging with low exposure is possible. For static imaging, ^{99m}Tc is linked to DMSA and given intravenously; an image is captured after 2–3 hours to assess renal morphology (e.g. agenesis and duplex systems), structure (e.g. renal scarring in reflux nephropathy) and function. For dynamic imaging, ^{99m}Tc is linked to diethylenetriaminepentaacetate (DTPA) or MAG-3 and given intravenously; a series of images capture renal excretion. If the renal blood supply is compromised, the kidney is not imaged; if it is well perfused but partially obstructed, delayed transit is seen. Activity curves and comparison with the contralateral kidney are informative. MAG-3 is preferred to DTPA in neonates and children with impaired function and when an obstruction is suspected since it is more efficiently extracted from the blood by the proximal tubules and clearance correlates with blood flow. After extraction by the proximal tubules, MAG-3 is secreted into the tubular lumen, whereas DTPA is filtered by the glomerulus and provides a measure of the glomerular filtration rate.

Ureteropelvic junction obstruction

Ureteropelvic junction (UPJ) obstruction, also often called pelviureteric junction (PUJ) obstruction, describes an incomplete and intermittent reduction in urine flow from the kidney to the proximal ureter and occurs in 1 in 1000 live births with a male and left-sided predominance. It is the most common cause of serious antenatal hydronephrosis. Commonly a disruption of circular muscle or collagen fibres in the proximal ureter results in an intrinsic narrowing near the renal pelvis. Extrinsic compression is less common and results from an aberrant renal vessel compressing the ureteropelvic junction. Most cases are diagnosed in the postnatal evaluation of an antenatally detected hydronephrosis, although some newborns present with an abdominal or flank mass and a history of urinary tract infection or haematuria. Older children may present with severe intermittent flank or abdominal pain associated with nausea and vomiting, known as Dietl's crisis. MAG-3 imaging confirms the diagnosis, and knowing the differential renal function helps to decide between surgical and non-surgical management (***Figures 20.4 and 20.5***).

In symptomatic children, a pyeloplasty is indicated. In many countries, this is now commonly performed laparoscopically, with some using robotic assistance. A pyeloplasty involves transection at the obstruction and the fashioning of a funnel-like anastomosis; a temporary stent and a drain may be placed. Follow-up with serial ultrasounds and MAG-3 imaging is required.

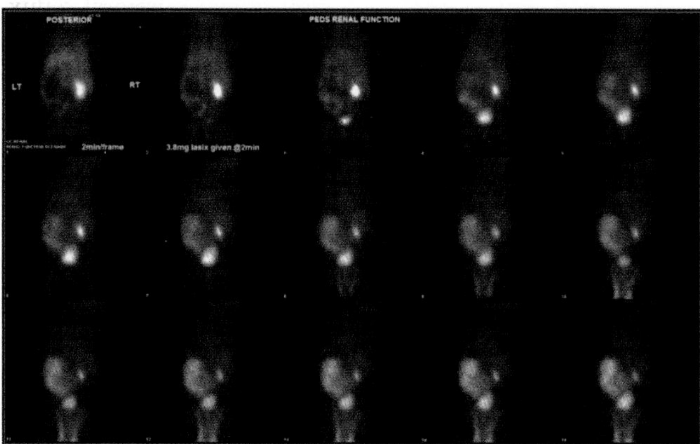

Figure 20.4 Mercaptoacetyltriglycine (MAG-3) renal scan showing poor drainage of a hydronephrotic left kidney due to partial uretero-pelvic junction obstruction. Note that nuclear scans are shown as if looking from behind the patient.

Ureterovesical junction obstruction/ megaureters

Ureterovesical junction (UVJ) obstruction is the second most common cause of antenatal hydronephrosis and arises from an adynamic and stenotic region obstructing the distal ureter near the bladder (***Figure 20.6***). Older children may have a distal ureteric polyp or calculus and present with a UTI, haematuria, abdominal pain or a hydronephrotic mass. Ultrasonography shows ureteric dilation (megaureter), hydronephrosis or both (hydroureteronephrosis). Importantly, obstruction is not the only cause of a dilated ureter. A primary megaureter refers to one that arises from an abnormality at the junction, whereas a secondary megaureter arises from a problem in the bladder or urethra (myelomeningocele/neurogenic bladder, PUV). Although reflux may cause a megaureter, it is also possible to have a refluxing obstructed megaureter, and so a voiding cystourethrogram is needed to look for reflux. A MAG-3 renal scan indicates the severity of obstruction. If intervention is required, ureteric reimplantation is performed.

Vesicoureteral reflux

Vesicoureteral reflux (VUR) is the retrograde flow of urine from the bladder to the upper urinary tracts. Primary VUR occurs because of a congenitally short intravesical ureter, resulting in inadequate closure of the UVJ during bladder contractions, and is seen in 1% of newborns. Secondary VUR follows from elevated intravesical pressure and is typically caused by PUV or

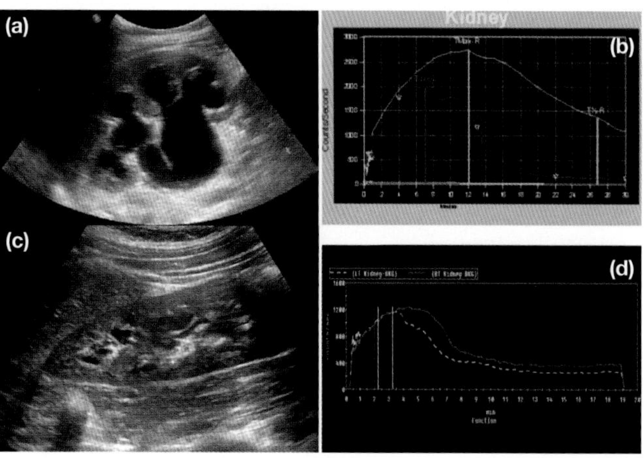

Figure 20.5 (a) Preoperative ultrasound of a right kidney with uretero-pelvic junction obstruction showing hydronephrosis. **(b)** Preoperative mercaptoacetyltriglycine (MAG-3) activity curve showing delayed excretion of the obstructed right kidney with a half-life of 26 minutes. **(c)** Ultrasound image of the right kidney after a pyeloplasty showing resolution of the hydronephrosis. **(d)** Postoperative MAG-3 activity curve graph showing improved excretion with a half-life of 7.6 minutes.

Józef Dietl, 1804–1878, Austrian–Polish physician and Mayor of Kraków, reformed medicine by showing through experiments that bloodletting was not only useless but dangerous.

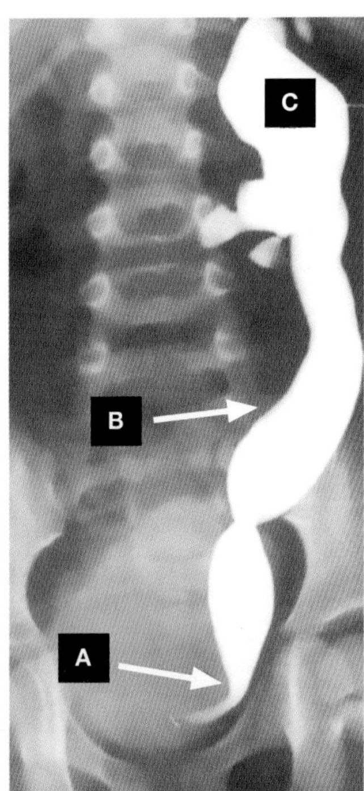

Figure 20.6 A retrograde pyelogram showing a left-sided ureterovesical junction obstruction (A), causing a megaureter (B) and hydronephrosis (C).

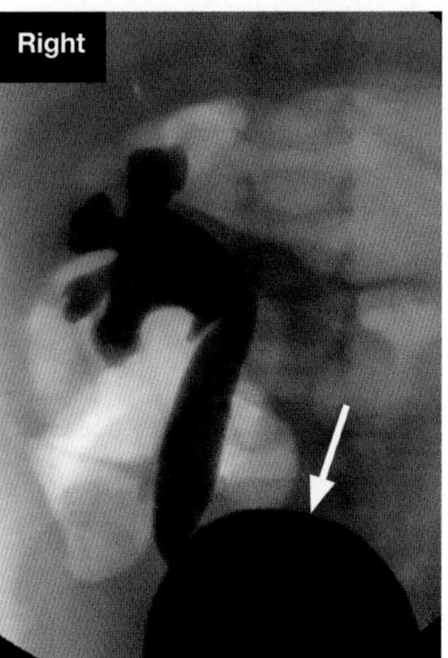

Figure 20.7 Voiding cystourethrogram demonstrating right-sided vesicoureteral reflux. The bladder is full of contrast (arrow).

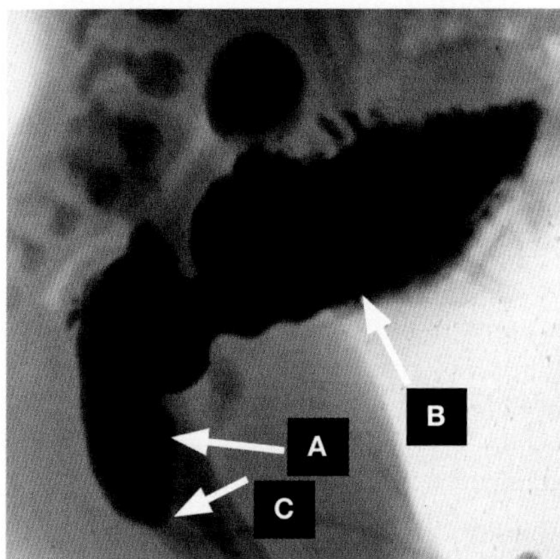

Figure 20.8 Lateral view showing a dilated posterior urethra (A) and trabeculated bladder (B) due to posterior urethral valves (C), seen on a voiding cystourethrogram.

a neurogenic bladder. VUR may be seen with hydronephrosis on an antenatal ultrasound or with a symptomatic UTI postnatally. A voiding cystourethrogram establishes the diagnosis and severity of VUR (***Figure 20.7***). Mild VUR typically resolves spontaneously as the patient grows and the intravesical ureter matures and lengthens. These children are managed with surveillance if toilet-trained or prophylactic antibiotics if they are not. Moderate-to-severe VUR less commonly resolves and recurrent UTIs may lead to pyelonephritis and renal parenchymal loss from scarring. Persistent or severe VUR can be managed with a subureteric Teflon injection (STING), which alters the anatomy at the UVJ and limits reflux, or with ureteric reimplantation. Long-term follow-up is required.

Posterior urethral valves

PUVs are membranous folds that obstruct the lumen of the posterior urethra, affecting about 1 in 4000 live-born boys. Girls are not affected. About one-third are identified antenatally with bilateral hydronephrosis, a dilated bladder and a dilated posterior urethra, which, on imaging, looks like a keyhole. In severe cases, there is oligohydramnios and lung hypoplasia. Postnatal presentations include urinary tract infections, bladder distension and voiding dysfunction. The diagnosis is confirmed on a voiding cystourethrogram, which shows a dilated posterior urethra with a thick-walled bladder (***Figure 20.8***). Ultrasonography looks for hydronephrosis and a thickened bladder. Renal function can be assessed with routine blood tests and glomerular filtration rate or a DMSA scan. The valves are ablated or resected; close follow-up is needed since bladder dysfunction is common and 30% develop renal failure.

Summary box 20.2

Urinary tract obstruction

- Prenatal fetal hydronephrosis often resolves under observation alone
- Severe ureteropelvic junction obstruction warrants a pyeloplasty
- Ureterovesical junction obstruction is one cause of megaureter
- Vesicoureteral reflux: severity is determined by voiding cystourethrography
- Posterior urethral valves lead to renal failure in 30% of affected boys

DUPLEX SYSTEMS

One in a hundred people have an upper renal moiety draining into a duplicated ureter. Both ipsilateral ureters may fuse such that only one ureter enters the bladder, or the duplicated ureter may have an ectopic opening into the bladder, urethra, vagina, vulval vestibule, seminal vesicle or rectum and is a rare cause of wetting. A vesical ectopic ureter may be associated with a dilated and obstructed intravesical length of ureter. Such a structure is known as a ureterocele and may be detected antenatally. The ectopic upper pole ureter typically has an orifice lying inferomedial to the lower pole ureter; an arrangement known as the Weigert–Meyer rule. The upper renal moiety has a ureter that may be obstructed at the bladder, whereas the lower renal moiety has a ureter with a predisposition to reflux.

DISORDERS OR DIFFERENCES IN SEX DIFFERENTIATION

Some, but not all, children with abnormalities of their sex chromosomes, gonads or reproductive anatomy are considered to have a disorder or difference in sex differentiation (DSD). Isolated undescended testes, hypospadias and labial adhesions are excluded. Unfortunately, there is no consensus on the indications, timing, best procedures or how to evaluate DSD surgery. The classification of disorders into groups is complex and controversial. For simplicity, only the following groups are described here: 46-XX DSD, 46-XY DSD and sex-chromosome mosaicism DSD variants. DSD management benefits when the paediatric urologist works in a multidisciplinary team, including a geneticist, endocrinologist, an adolescent gynaecologist and a psychologist.

The **46-XX DSD** group is exemplified by congenital adrenal hyperplasia (CAH), in which gender is usually straightforward (female), except with late diagnoses and severe masculinisation. At birth, the urethra may open on a prominent genital tubercle, appearing like a small phallus and looking similar to a 46-XY boy with severe hypospadias and non-palpable testes. In 46-XX CAH, the vagina opens into the posterior wall of the urethra a variable distance from the bladder neck but not higher than where the verumontanum, a Müllerian structure, is typically located in the male urethra. Genital fold fusion varies from a vulval-like to a scrotal-like appearance.

The **46-XY DSD** group is exemplified by androgen insensitivity syndrome (AIS), 17β hydroxysteroid dehydrogenase (17β HSD) deficiency and 5α reductase deficiency. AIS is complete (CAIS), with a feminine phenotype, or partial (PAIS), in which the external genitals are undermasculinised at birth and undervirilised at puberty. Infants with CAIS (reared as girls) may present with bilateral inguinal hernias or with inguinal testes thought to be prolapsed ovaries. Similarly, those with 17β HSD deficiency and 5α reductase deficiency, having low androgens, may have an external feminine phenotype with palpable inguinal testes undergoing virilisation at puberty. In challenging cases, controversy surrounds gender assignment, sex of rearing and surgery.

One critical issue is the fate of the testicles: should gonads be left alone until the individual can determine their gender for themselves? Or, if female sex rearing is decided on, should they be removed early to avoid virilisation at puberty? If conservative management is chosen, temporarily blocking virilisation with a gonadotropin-releasing hormone analogue is an option until gender identity is determined.

Sex-chromosome mosaicism is exemplified by 45X/46XY DSD. These individuals may have a hemiscrotum containing a testis-like gonad, paired with a labia majora with an inguinal or impalpable streak gonad; a streak gonad has stromal tissue without tubules or follicles. There is usually severe hypospadias.

NEUROPATHIC BLADDER

A myelomeningocele, lipomyelomeningocele, fatty filum or an occult tethered cord can cause a neuropathic bladder that may need lifelong care to protect the kidneys from high urinary pressures and reflux, and support continence and independence where appropriate. If reconstructive surgery is needed, it must follow detailed assessments of (i) the adequacy of the bladder neck/sphincter complex, (ii) bladder capacity, (iii) the need for a cutaneous catheterisable channel, and (iv) any associated faecal continence procedures. Bladder neck procedures include endoscopic injections, slings, reconstructions and bladder neck closure. Bladder capacity and compliance can be increased with a bladder augmentation (e.g. ileocystoplasty), which takes the pressure off the upper tracts. An appendicovesicostomy (Mitrofanoff), using the appendix as a conduit between the skin and the bladder, allows intermittent catheterisation as an alternative to urethral catheterisation (***Figure 20.9***).

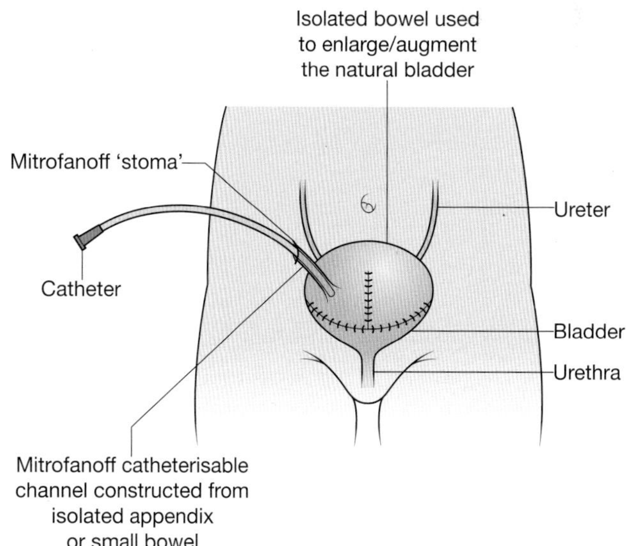

Figure 20.9 Mitrofanoff appendicovesicostomy draining an ileocystoplasty, which augments and converts a high-pressure bladder into a low-pressure system to protect the kidneys in a patient with a neuropathic bladder.

Johannes Peter Müller, 1801–1858, German physiologist and comparative anatomist after whom the paramesonephric duct structures are named.
Paul Mitrofanoff, b. 1934, paediatric surgeon, Rouen, France, devised the appendicovesicostomy in the mid-1970s.

TESTICULAR TUMOURS

Testicular tumours are rare. Most prepubertal tumours arise before 3 years and are benign, allowing testis-sparing surgery. Malignant tumours in older boys require an orchidectomy (performed through the groin) and selective chemotherapy. Germ cell tumours include the teratomas and epidermoid cysts (typically benign) and the malignant yolk sac tumours, seminomas, choriocarcinomas and embryonal carcinomas. Gonadal stromal tumours are typically benign and include Leydig cell tumours, Sertoli cell tumours, juvenile granulosa cell tumours and gonadoblastomas.

FURTHER READING

Grinspon RP, Rey RA. Disorders of sex development. In: Kovacs C, Deal C (eds). *Maternal–fetal and neonatal endocrinology*. San Diego, CA: Academic Press, 2020: 841–67.

Gundeti MS. *Surgical techniques in pediatric and adolescent urology*. Delhi: Jaypee Brothers Medical Publishers, 2019.

Hutson JM, Thorup JM, Beasley SW. *Descent of the testis*. Cham: Springer, 2016.

Franz von Leydig, 1821–1908, German zoologist and comparative anatomist, discovered the Leydig cells.
Enrico Sertoli, 1842–1910, Italian physiologist, discovered the Sertoli cells of the testis.

CHAPTER 21 Preoperative care including the high-risk surgical patient

Learning objectives

To understand preoperative preparation for surgery:
- Surgical, medical and anaesthetic aspects of assessment
- How to optimise patients and identify those at higher risk
- Importance of critical care in management
- Emergency cases

To be able to organise preoperative care and the operating list

INTRODUCTION

The stress of major surgery can lead to increased oxygen demand by up to 40%. Inflammatory changes due to cytokine release, endocrine responses, hypercoagulability and redistribution of fluid between compartments may last several postoperative days. The purpose of careful preoperative planning is to minimise the unwanted effects of these physiological changes.

Systematic history taking, examination and investigation at the preoperative clinic should include not only an assessment of functional reserve but also the formulation of advice on optimisation, to best cope with the anticipated operative stress. Primary care physician records and hospital notes are useful sources of baseline information. Ideally a multidisciplinary team approach, including the primary care physician, specialist nurses, physiotherapist, dietician and perioperative physician, is utilised. This allows optimisation of chronic conditions, facilitates weight reduction and smoking cessation, and allows coordination of prehabilitation and postoperative rehabilitation needs. The anaesthetist and surgeon must plan the safest anaesthetic technique and operation for the patient.

A simple questionnaire can identify risk factors for patients undergoing surgery that will require specific tests or optimisation. Patients with severe comorbidities or undergoing high-risk surgery should be referred to specialists to quantify and reduce perioperative risks. The risks of surgery and anaesthesia and the effects of comorbid conditions should be discussed so that the patient can make an informed decision. Patients should be given advice on preoperative fasting times, adjustments to regular medication and specific premedication at the preoperative visit.

To enable the list to run smoothly on the day, key personnel involved in the list (surgeon, anaesthetist and senior theatre staff) should be involved in planning the list order. The National Patient Safety Agency's adaptation of the World Health Organization's checklist recommends a 'team brief' before the start of each list, which is also a valuable opportunity to share information with the theatre team and improve the safety of anaesthesia and surgery.

Summary box 21.1

Preoperative plan for the best patient outcomes
- Gather and record all relevant information
- Optimise patient condition
- Choose surgery that offers minimal risk and maximum benefit
- Informed consent of the patient (see *Chapter 14*)
- Anticipate and plan for adverse events
- Adequate hydration, nutrition and exercise are advised

PATIENT ASSESSMENT

History taking

A thorough past medical history, surgical history and systemic enquiry should be documented, including important negatives (***Table 21.1***). The history of past surgery and anaesthetic events can reveal the problems one may face during future procedures e.g. intra-abdominal adhesions for planned laparoscopic surgery, a difficult airway or suxamethonium apnoea. The use of recreational drugs and alcohol consumption should be noted as they are known to be associated with adverse outcomes. A full drug history and list of allergies should be documented. Social history, ability to communicate and mobility are important in planning admission, discharge route and rehabilitation after surgery.

Examination

Patients should be treated with respect and dignity, receive a clear explanation of the examination undertaken and be kept as comfortable as possible. A chaperone should be present, especially for intimate examinations. This should be part of a local guideline or policy.

TABLE 21.1 Key conditions in past medical history.

Cardiovascular
- Valvular heart disease
- Ischaemic heart disease: angina, myocardial infarction, coronary stents
- Hypertension
- Heart failure
- Dysrhythmia
- Peripheral vascular disease
- Cardiac devices, i.e. permanent pacemaker

Respiratory
- Chronic obstructive pulmonary disease
- Asthma
- Respiratory infections
- Obstructive sleep apnoea symptoms

Gastrointestinal
- Peptic ulcer disease and gastro-oesophageal reflux
- Liver disease

Genitourinary tract
- Urinary tract infection
- Renal dysfunction
- For females last menstrual period/pregnancy/breastfeeding status

Neurological
- Epilepsy
- Cerebrovascular accidents and transient ischaemic attacks
- Parkinson's disease
- Multiple sclerosis

Psychiatric disorders
- Cognitive function
- Anxiety or depression

Endocrine/metabolic
- Diabetes
- Thyroid dysfunction
- Phaeochromocytoma
- Porphyria

Locomotor system
- Osteoarthritis
- Inflammatory arthropathy, i.e. rheumatoid arthritis
- Disorders of muscle, i.e. muscular dystrophy, myasthenia, myopathy

Haematological
- Bleeding disorders
- Personal or family history of deep vein thrombosis and pulmonary embolism
- Objection to blood product transfusion
- Haemoglobinopathy, i.e. sickle cell disease

Infection
- Human immunodeficiency virus/hepatitis/tuberculosis
- Other, i.e. MRSA/COVID-19/drug-resistant organisms

Previous surgery and anaesthesia
- Problems encountered, i.e. Difficult Airway Society Alert, suxamethonium apnoea
- Family history of problems with anaesthesia, i.e. malignant hyperpyrexia

COVID-19, coronavirus disease 2019; MRSA, methicillin-resistant *Staphylococcus aureus*.

Summary box 21.2

Examination

- General: positive findings, even if not related to the proposed procedure, should be explored further
- Surgery related: type and site of surgery, with reference to imaging and investigations
- Systemic: comorbidities and extent of limitation of each organ's function
- Specific: for example, suitability for positioning during surgery or to plan airway management

Examination is especially important in symptomatic individuals and at a minimum should include cardiorespiratory examination and airway assessment. Specifically, look for signs of heart failure, valvular heart disease, peripheral vascular disease and respiratory disease (***Table 21.2***).

TABLE 21.2 Medical examination.

General	Anaemia, jaundice, cyanosis, frailty, nutritional status, sources of infection (teeth, feet, leg ulcers), height, weight and BMI
Cardiovascular	Pulse rate and rhythm, blood pressure, heart sounds, bruits, jugular venous pressure, peripheral oedema, exercise tolerance
Respiratory	Respiratory rate and effort, chest expansion and percussion note, breath sounds, oxygen saturation at rest and exertion, consider PEFR
Gastrointestinal	Abdominal masses, ascites, bowel sounds, hernia, genitalia
Neurological	Consciousness level, cognitive function, sensation, muscle power, tone and reflexes
Airway assessment	Mouth opening, neck extension, Mallampati score, thyromental distance, jaw protrusion, scarring to mouth or neck, dentition

BMI, body mass index; PEFR, peak expiratory flow rate.

Airway assessment

The difficulty encountered when performing airway manoeuvres, i.e. hand ventilation, intubation and front of neck access, can be predicted to some extent by simple examination. Failure to assess and plan airway management can have fatal consequences.

The patient is assessed for:

- modified Mallampati class (***Table 21.3***);
- mouth opening >3 cm (***Figure 21.1***);
- thyromental distance >6.5 cm;
- thyrosternal distance >12.5 cm;
- ability to protrude the jaw (***Figure 21.2***);
- ability to extend the head at the atlanto-occipital junction (***Figure 21.3***).

James Parkinson, 1755–1824, general practitioner of Shoreditch, London, UK, published *An essay on the shaking palsy* in 1817.
SR Mallampati published the original article suggesting that the size of the base of the tongue is an important factor in determining the degree of difficulty of direct laryngoscopy in the *Canadian Anaesthetists' Society Journal* in 1985. The original Mallampati classification was modified from a total of three to four classes by **GLT Samsoon** and **JRB Young** after reviewing a series of obstetric and general surgical patients who had had difficult intubations.

TABLE 21.3 Airway assessment (Mallampati test as modified by Samsoon and Young).

Grade 1	Fauces, pillars, soft palate and uvula seen
Grade 2	Fauces, soft palate with some part of uvula seen
Grade 3	Soft palate seen
Grade 4	Hard palate only seen

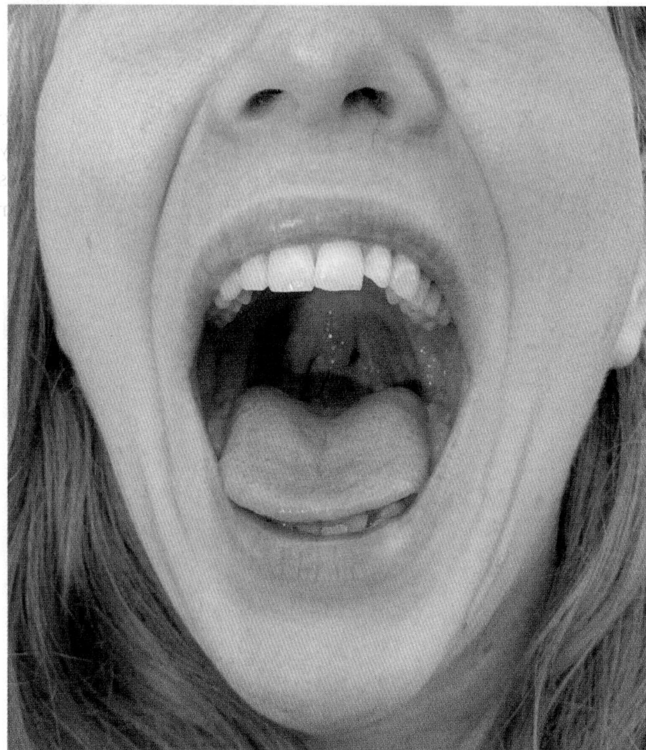

Figure 21.1 Normal mouth opening (>3 cm), demonstrating Mallampati grade 1.

When more than one of the above tests are abnormal, the chances of experiencing difficulty in obtaining and securing the airway become greater. Poor dentition, facial hair, upper airway tumours/scarring/infections, obesity and neck size are also important factors that will affect the airway management plan. Previous anaesthetic charts or alerts carried by patients for a difficult airway are invaluable sources when assessing a patient.

Investigations

Guidelines produced by the UK's National Institute for Health and Care Excellence (NICE) set out the investigations needed for various categories of elective surgery and American Society of Anesthesiologists (ASA) score of the patient. The following are some of the tests done preoperatively, although not all are done routinely or are recommended by NICE.

- **Full blood count (FBC)**. An FBC is needed for major operations, in the elderly and in those with anaemia or pathology with ongoing blood loss and chronic disease.

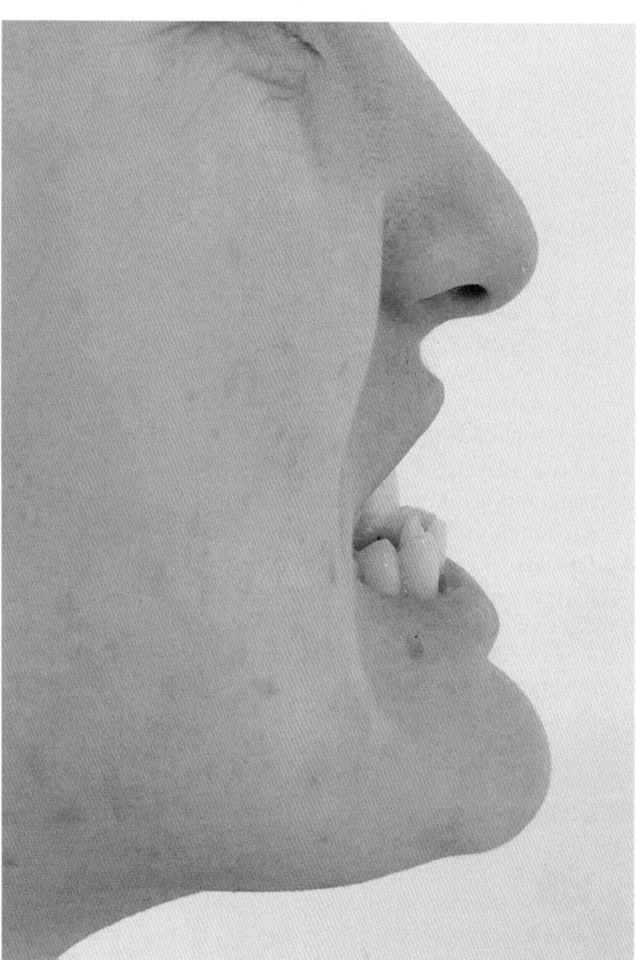

Figure 21.2 Ability to protrude jaw.

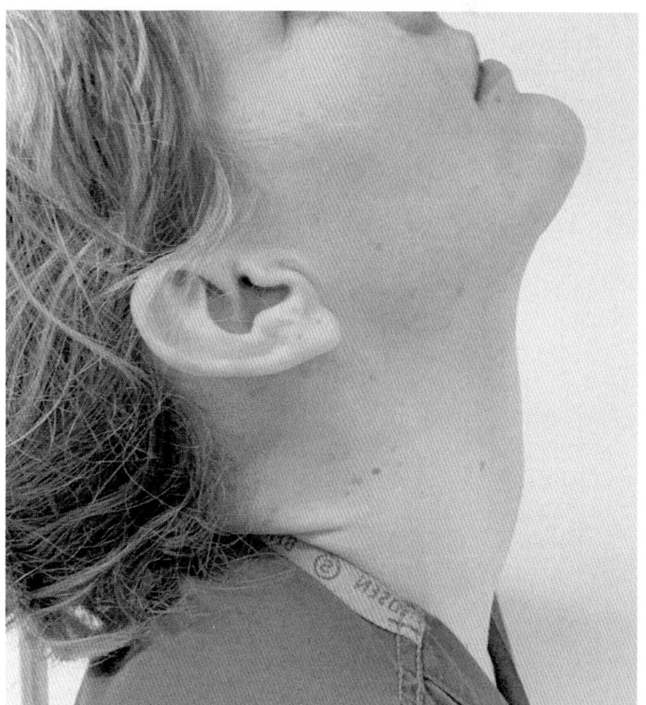

Figure 21.3 Normal head extension.

- **Haemoglobin A1c (HbA1c) level**. This should be measured in patients with diabetes who have not had it measured in the last 3 months.
- **Sickle cell test**. Not routinely offered, but in cases of suspicion of a sickle crisis or a family history of sickle cell disease a sickle cell test is needed.
- **Urea and electrolytes (U&Es)**. U&Es are needed before all major operations, in patients over 65 years of age, in patients with cardiovascular, renal or endocrine disease or if significant blood loss is anticipated. They are also needed in those on medications that affect electrolyte levels, e.g. steroids, diuretics, digoxin, non-steroidal anti-inflammatory drugs, intravenous fluid or nutrition therapy, and in those with endocrine problems.
- **Liver function tests**. These are indicated in patients with jaundice, known or suspected hepatitis, cirrhosis, malignancy, alcohol excess or poor nutritional status.
- **Clotting/coagulation screen**. This is needed if a patient has a history suggestive of a bleeding diathesis, liver disease, eclampsia or cholestasis, is on antithrombotic or anticoagulant agents or has a family history of a bleeding disorder. It should be noted that the effects of antiplatelet agents, low-molecular-weight heparins (LMWHs) and newer agents affecting factor Xa cannot be measured by routine laboratory tests.
- **Electrocardiogram (ECG)**. This is required for patients over 65 years of age or symptomatic patients with a history of rheumatic fever, diabetes or cardiovascular, renal or cerebrovascular disease, with or without severe respiratory problems. It will also depend on whether the surgery is minor/intermediate or major, as described in NICE guidance.
- **Chest radiograph**. Not routinely offered unless there is concern on clinical examination.
- **Echocardiogram (echo)**. Consider in those with heart murmurs who are symptomatic or in those with signs of heart failure.
- **Urine tests**. Only consider microscopy and culture of midstream urine if infection would influence the decision to operate.
- **β-Human chorionic gonadotrophin (pregnancy test)**. Women of childbearing age should be asked sensitively about their pregnancy status as this will affect the surgical plan and consent. Pregnant patients must be consented for the risk to a fetus that surgery and anaesthetic pose, and obstetric advice sought. In addition, on the day of surgery the woman should be consented for a urine/serum pregnancy test.
- **Others**:
  - **Venous bicarbonate**. For patients who have screened as being at high risk for obstructive sleep apnoea (OSA). Followed by formal sleep studies if significant OSA is a concern.
  - **Arterial blood gases**. A low-cost tool that can give quick and vital information in acute or chronic severe respiratory conditions, acid–base disturbances and conditions where there is a changing milieu, e.g. immediately before kidney transplant.
  - **Blood group and cross-match** if expected blood loss >500 mL.
  - **Methicillin-resistant *Staphylococcus aureus* (MRSA)** swabs.
  - **Coronavirus 2019 (COVID-19)** polymerase chain reaction (PCR) swabs.
  - **Spirometry**.
  - **Cardiopulmonary exercise testing** to assess fitness for high-risk surgery.
  - **Specialist radiological views** are sometimes required. If imaging is going to be needed during surgery, this needs to be planned in advance.

COMMON PREOPERATIVE PROBLEMS AND MANAGEMENT

Specific medical problems encountered during preoperative assessment should be corrected to the best possible level. Many patients with severe disease will need to be referred to specialists; the referral letter should contain all the details, including history, examination and investigation results.

Cardiovascular disease

Perioperative cardiovascular complications are frequent. Patients who can climb a flight of stairs without getting short of breath, having chest pain or needing to stop are likely to tolerate a wide range of surgeries with an acceptable risk of perioperative cardiovascular morbidity and mortality. However, at preoperative assessment it is important to identify those patients who have a high perioperative risk of a major adverse cardiovascular event (MACE) and to try to reduce this risk. Patients at high risk are those with ischaemic heart disease (IHD), congestive cardiac failure, arrhythmias, severe peripheral vascular disease, cerebrovascular disease or significant renal impairment, especially if they are undergoing major intra-abdominal or intrathoracic surgery.

Ischaemic heart disease

Patients with angina that is not well controlled should be investigated further by a cardiologist. The indications for coronary revascularisation in patients awaiting surgery are the same as at any other time. Pharmacological protection is indicated. Patients established on β-blockers and statins should have their medication continued perioperatively. Initiating statins preoperatively should be considered if not already prescribed. Most long-term cardiac medications should be continued over the perioperative period. Angiotensin-converting enzyme (ACE) inhibitors and receptor blockers are often omitted 24 hours prior to surgery to prevent intraoperative hypotension, and restarted the next day for most surgery.

In patients with IHD the cardiac and coronary reserve can be evaluated using a stress test (stress ECG, stress echo, myocardial scintigraphy). The tests have a high negative predictive value but a relatively low positive predictive value. If the test is negative, the patient is unlikely to have IHD; conversely, if it is positive the chances of the patient actually having IHD are not necessarily very high, but there is a need

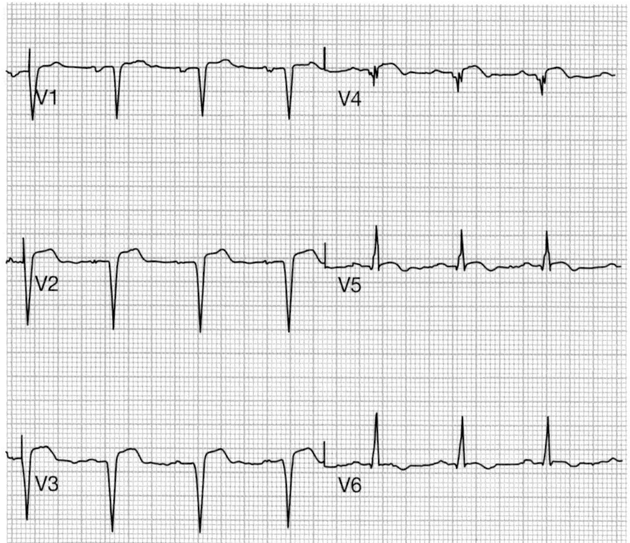

Figure 21.4 Preoperative electrocardiogram of a patient who complained of chest pain the previous day, showing recent transmural anterior myocardial infarction with Q waves and ST elevation.

for further investigation such as coronary angiography or cardiac computed tomography. Recently, measurement of the coronary fractional flow reserve during coronary angiography using a pressure wire has made it possible to identify coronary lesions that have the largest impact on myocardial perfusion.

After a proven myocardial infarction (MI) (*Figure 21.4*), elective surgery should be postponed for 3–6 months to reduce the risk of perioperative reinfarction. Ischaemic changes can be seen on ECG even if the patient is not symptomatic (silent ischaemia/silent MI). These merit discussion with a cardiologist.

Hypertension

Prior to elective surgery blood pressure should be controlled to <160/100 mmHg. If a new antihypertensive agent is introduced, a stabilisation period of at least 2 weeks should be allowed.

Heart failure

Left ventricular failure is the end result of several conditions, including IHD, hypertension, cardiomyopathies and valve dysfunction. Decompensated heart failure puts the patient at risk of multiorgan failure. Those with ejection fractions of less than 35%, and in whom the failure is undiagnosed or its severity underestimated, are at highest risk. The patient's functional capacity needs to be assessed and surgery may have to be delayed for investigations such as an echo and/or for optimisation of medical therapy. B-type natriuretic peptide is a useful marker and can be prognostic.

Drugs used in chronic heart failure can have significant implications for perioperative care, including intraoperative hypotension. β-blockers and probably ACE inhibitors (unless renal perfusion is to be significantly affected) should be continued. A left ventricular ejection fraction of less than 35% should be discussed with a cardiologist and optimised. Cardiac resynchronisation therapy devices may be considered, depending on the QRS duration.

Drug-eluting coronary stents (DES)

Primary percutaneous intervention is the treatment of choice for acute coronary syndromes, and many patients receive stents and are on dual antiplatelet therapy for 12 months. If surgery is absolutely necessary within the period of dual antiplatelet therapy, the management strategy should be decided jointly by the surgeon, cardiologist, anaesthetist and patient, as it is essential to consider the balance of risk of continuing antiplatelet agents (with the risk of increased bleeding) and stopping them (with the risk of stent thrombosis).

Dysrhythmias

In patients with atrial fibrillation (AF), β-blockers, digoxin or calcium channel blockers should be continued in order to control rate. New AF or atrial flutter should be investigated and treated. These patients should be considered for cardioversion as restoring sinus rhythm can improve cardiac output by 15% (*Figure 21.5*). Patients with an abnormal rhythm on ECG, for example tachycardia/bradycardia or heart block, should also be discussed with a cardiologist (*Figure 21.6*). Symptomatic heart blocks and asymptomatic second- (Mobitz II) and third-degree heart blocks, if discovered at the preoperative assessment clinic, will need cardiology consultation and potentially temporary or permanent pacemaker insertion.

Warfarin in patients with AF should be stopped 5 days preoperatively to achieve an international normalised ratio (INR) of 1.5 or less, which is safe for most surgery. The newer anticoagulants such as dabigatran (direct thrombin inhibitor) or rivaroxaban, apixaban and edoxaban (direct factor Xa inhibitors) do not have antagonists and must be stopped preoperatively, generally for 2–3 days in patients with normal renal function and longer when renal function is impaired. Alternative anticoagulation is not required in the perioperative

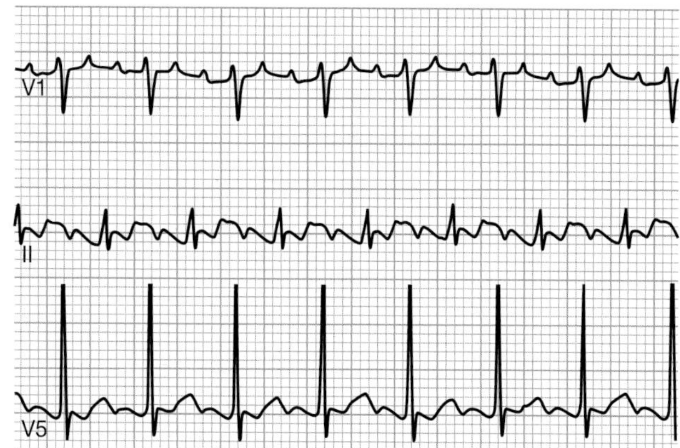

Figure 21.5 Atrial flutter

Woldemar Mobitz, 1889–1951, Russian–German physician, researched atrioventricular dissociation and heart blocks.

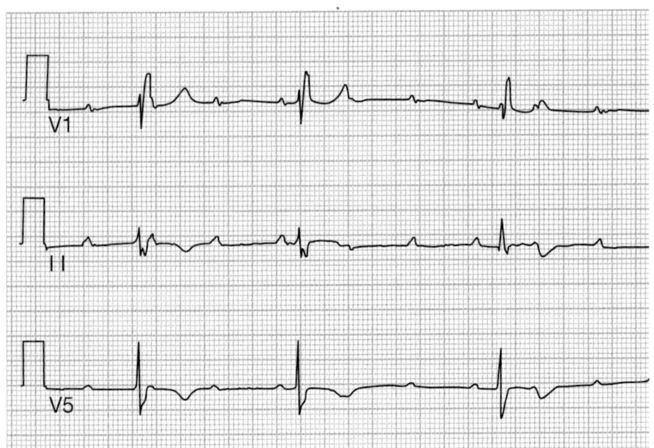

Figure 21.6 Routine preoperative electrocardiogram in an 83-year-old patient with no symptoms other than lethargy for the last 3 months. This shows complete heart block with dissociated P waves and QRS complexes, requiring preoperative pacing.

period unless the risk of stroke is high (assessed using the CHA_2DS_2-VASc [congestive heart failure, hypertension, age ≥75 years, diabetes mellitus, stroke or transient ischemic attack, vascular disease, age 65–74 years, sex category] score). Decisions on bridging therapy should balance the risks of stroke and bleeding.

Implanted pacemakers and cardiac defibrillators

Checks and appropriate reprogramming should be done preoperatively by specialists and advice followed. Monopolar diathermy activity during surgery may be sensed by the pacemaker as ventricular fibrillation or a paced beat. Therefore, cardioversion and over-pace modes must be turned off (and switched back on after surgery) or converted to 'ventricle paced, not sensed with no response to sensing' (VOO) mode. Bipolar diathermy should be made available at surgery.

Valvular heart disease

While anaesthetic management is altered to achieve haemodynamic stability in moderate valvular diseases, patients with severe aortic and mitral stenosis may benefit from valvuloplasty before elective non-cardiac surgery. Appropriate referral to an anaesthetist and cardiologist should be made.

An echo is required in symptomatic patients with a new murmur. Patients with known significant valve pathology may benefit from a recent echo, especially if their clinical status has changed (standard intervals for surveillance echo can be guided by local cardiology policy). Patients with prosthetic valves are normally monitored with surveillance echo at intervals. In patients with mechanical heart valves, warfarin needs to be stopped preoperatively and bridging anticoagulation given to prevent valve thrombosis. Bridging options include unfractionated heparin infusions or LMWHs and should be done under guidance agreed with haematology. Bridging therapy should continue postoperatively until the patient is re-established on warfarin with a therapeutic INR but must be balanced with the postoperative bleeding risk. Thrombin inhibitors and factor Xa inhibitors are not licensed and should not be used in patients with mechanical valves.

Cerebral vascular disease

Patients who have suffered a cerebrovascular accident have been shown to have a higher rate of MACE postoperatively. This is highest in the first 3 months after a stroke. The urgency of surgery needs to be discussed with the surgeon, anaesthetist and a stroke physician. Ideally elective surgery is postponed until MACE risks stabilise after 9 months. The bleeding versus thrombosis risk of continuing dual antiplatelet therapy needs to be considered.

Respiratory disease

Postoperative respiratory complications, such as pneumonia, are a major cause of morbidity and mortality, especially after major abdominal and thoracic surgery. A patient's current respiratory status should be compared with their 'normal state'. Patients with severe disease are at risk of pneumonia and respiratory failure in the postoperative period. Severe disease would include patients with a forced expiratory volume in the first second (FEV_1) of less than 30% of predicted value, dependence on oral steroid treatment, home ventilation or oxygen therapy or a $PaCO_2$ level of greater than 6 kPa.

Patients should continue to use their regular inhalers until the start of anaesthesia. Brittle asthmatics may also need extra steroid cover. Encourage the patients to be compliant with the medications and stop smoking. Information should be provided to indicate perioperative risks associated with smoking. Stopping smoking reduces carbon monoxide levels and offers the patient a better ability to clear sputum. Evidence suggests that preoperative inspiratory muscle training significantly improves respiratory (muscle) function in the early postoperative period, reducing the risk of pulmonary complications.

Regional anaesthetic techniques and less invasive surgical options should be considered in severe cases. Elective surgery should be postponed until acute exacerbations are treated.

The patient should be referred to a respiratory physician if:

- there is a severe disease or significant deterioration;
- major surgery is planned in a patient with significant respiratory comorbidities;
- right heart failure is present – dyspnoea, fatigue, tricuspid regurgitation, hepatomegaly and oedematous feet;
- the patient is young and has severe respiratory problems (may indicate a rare condition).

Gastrointestinal disease

Regurgitation risk

Patients undergoing general anaesthesia or sedation have a risk of regurgitation of stomach contents and aspiration pneumonia. To reduce this risk patients should fast preoperatively. This should be clearly explained to the patient: 6 hours for solids or non-clear fluids (e.g. milk), 2 hours for clear fluids and 4 hours for infants consuming breast milk.

Prolonged fasting is detrimental to the patient so should not be encouraged. Patients with hiatus hernia, obesity, pregnancy or diabetes are at higher risk of pulmonary aspiration, even if they have been fasted appropriately before elective surgery. Clear antacids, H_2-receptor blockers, e.g. ranitidine, or proton pump inhibitors, e.g. omeprazole, may be given at an appropriate time in the preoperative period to reduce stomach acidity.

Liver disease

In patients with liver disease, the cause of the disease needs to be known, as well as any evidence of clotting problems, renal involvement and encephalopathy. Elective surgery should be postponed until any acute episode has settled, e.g. cholangitis. The presence of ascites, oesophageal varices, hypoalbuminaemia or sodium and water retention should be noted, as all can influence the choice and outcome of anaesthesia and surgery. Patients with cirrhosis undergoing major surgery have a very high mortality; the Model for End-stage Liver Disease (MELD) can be used to predict mortality of cirrhotic patients undergoing non-transplant surgery. If alcohol addiction is the aetiology then reduction of alcohol intake should be encouraged but abstinence must be medically supervised to prevent delirium tremens.

Genitourinary disease

Renal failure

Underlying conditions leading to chronic renal failure such as diabetes mellitus, hypertension and IHD should be stabilised before elective surgery. Appropriate measures should be taken to treat acidosis, hypocalcaemia and hyperkalaemia of greater than 6 mmol/L. Arrangements should be made to continue peritoneal dialysis or haemodialysis until a few hours before surgery. After the final dialysis before surgery, a blood sample should be sent for FBC and U&Es.

Patients with chronic renal failure often have chronic anaemia that is well tolerated; therefore, preoperative blood transfusion is often not necessary. Optimisation of the haemoglobin is best guided by the renal team.

Urinary tract infection

Uncomplicated urinary tract infections are common in women, while outflow uropathy with chronically infected urine is common in men. These infections should be treated before embarking on elective surgery where infection carries dire consequences, e.g. joint replacement. For emergency procedures, antibiotics should be started and care taken to ensure that the patient maintains a good urine output before, during and after surgery.

Endocrine and metabolic disorders

Malnutrition

Body mass index (BMI) is weight in kilograms divided by height in metres squared. A BMI of less than 18.5 indicates nutritional impairment and a BMI below 15 is associated with significant hospital mortality. Nutritional support for a minimum of 2 weeks before surgery is required to have any impact on subsequent morbidity. If a patient is unlikely to be able to eat for a significant period postoperatively this can be anticipated and alternative nutritional support must be planned.

Obesity

Morbid obesity can be defined as BMI of more than 35 (other definitions exist) and is associated with an increased risk of postoperative complications. Patients should be made aware of the risks involved and advised on healthy eating and taking regular exercise. If possible, surgery should be delayed until the patient is more active and has lost weight. If this fails, prophylactic measures need to be taken, such as preventative measures for acid aspiration and deep vein thrombosis (DVT).

OSA that is unrecognised has been shown to be associated with a higher incidence of MACE in comorbid patient groups. Identification of those at higher risk by using a clinical scoring system, such as the perioperative sleep apnoea prediction (P-SAP) score, can rationalise referral for formal sleep apnoea studies. Urgency of surgery may preclude full investigation and treatment preoperatively. Patients with severe OSA require 6 weeks of nocturnal continuous positive airway pressure (CPAP) use preoperatively to reduce their risks. Associated risks need to be explained prior to the surgery and an appropriate anaesthetic technique planned with postoperative monitoring.

Diabetes mellitus

Diabetes and associated cardiovascular and renal complications should be controlled to as near a normal level as possible before embarking on elective surgery. Any history of hyper- and hypoglycaemic episodes and hospital admissions should be noted. For elective surgery, an HbA1c of <69 mmol/mol is recommended. Lipid-lowering medication should be started in patients who are in a high-risk group for cardiovascular complications of diabetes.

Patients with diabetes should be first on the operating list and their antidiabetic medication adjusted as per local or national guidance, as they will miss a meal preoperatively. Although tight control of blood sugar is not needed, the patient's blood sugar levels should be checked hourly. Variable rate intravenous insulin infusion (VRIII) should be started for patients with diabetes on insulin undergoing major surgery or if blood sugar is difficult to control for other reasons.

Adrenocortical suppression

Patients receiving oral adrenocortical steroids should be asked about the dose and duration of the medication to determine the need for supplementation with extra doses of steroids perioperatively so as to avoid an Addisonian crisis. A patient taking >5 mg prednisolone equivalent within a month of surgery will require supplementation at induction and postoperatively.

Neuroendocrine tumours, including phaeochromocytoma, carcinoid, gastrinoma, VIPomas and insulinoma, have specific treatments that must be started preoperatively in liaison with specialist endocrinology physicians.

Thomas Addison, 1795–1860, physician, Guy's Hospital, London, UK, described the effects of disease of the suprarenal capsules in 1849.

Haematological disorders

Anaemia and blood transfusion

Patients found to be newly anaemic (haemoglobin <130 g/L), with an expected operative blood loss of >500 mL, should be investigated for the cause of their anaemia. Any vitamin or iron deficiency should be corrected before proceeding for elective surgery. Chronic anaemia is well tolerated in the perioperative period where <500 mL blood loss is expected, but where possible should be corrected. Preoperative transfusion may be considered rarely for elective patients when guided by a haematologist. Local policy should agree which procedures require a preoperative 'group and save' or cross-matched blood sample.

Some patients may refuse blood transfusion, for example a Jehovah's Witness. In such a case, during the consent process discussion should include which blood product and/or device system (e.g. cell salvage, reinfusion from drains) is acceptable. The discussion should extend to other areas, for example whether refusal of transfusion would apply in life-threatening situations. As in all consent processes, the discussion and outcome should be clearly documented.

Thrombophilia

Factor V Leiden and deficiencies in antithrombin III and proteins C and S increase the patient's thrombosis risk. The patient will need special discussion with a haematologist to tailor their venous thromboembolism prophylaxis. For all other patients a DVT risk assessment should be made preoperatively and precautions planned as per local or national guidance. Risk factors are included in ***Table 21.4***.

The progesterone-only contraceptive pill should be continued; however, the risks of continuing the combined pill (slight increased risk of significant thrombosis) should be weighed against the risks of an unplanned pregnancy. Consider stopping oestrogen-containing oral contraceptives or hormone replacement therapy 4 weeks before surgery (NICE guidance; see ***Further reading***).

Bleeding disorders

Bleeding disorders such as haemophilia, von Willebrand disease or thrombocytopenia are best discussed with haematology preoperatively.

Neurological and psychiatric disorders

Anticonvulsants and anti-Parkinson's medication must be continued perioperatively to help early mobilisation of the patient, and patients should be planned early on a theatre list to reduce starvation times. Parenteral medication plans can be set in place preoperatively if there is potential for a prolonged 'nil by mouth' period postoperatively.

Lithium should be stopped 24 hours prior to major surgery but can be continued for minor surgery with careful fluid management and U&Es monitoring. The anaesthetist should be informed if patients are on psychiatric medications, such as tricyclic antidepressants or monoamine oxidase inhibitors (MAOIs), as these may interact with anaesthetic drugs. Case-by-case decisions with a psychiatrist must be undertaken as stopping irreversible MAOIs safely may take many weeks of planning under psychiatric supervision.

TABLE 21.4 Risk factors for thrombosis.

- Age >60 years
- Obesity (BMI >30 kg/m^2)
- Trauma or surgery (especially of the abdomen, pelvis and lower limbs)
- Total anaesthesia time >90 minutes
- Reduced mobility for more than 3 days
- Pregnancy/puerperium
- Varicose veins with phlebitis
- Drugs, e.g. oestrogen contraceptive, HRT, smoking
- Known active cancer or on treatment, significant medical comorbidities, critical care admission
- Family/personal history of thrombosis, e.g. deficiencies in antithrombin III, protein S or C

BMI, body mass index; HRT, hormone replacement therapy.

Musculoskeletal disorders

Muscular disorders have serious implications and require a tailored anaesthetic approach. They include muscular dystrophies, myotonic dystrophy and myasthenia gravis and a personal or family history of malignant hyperpyrexia.

Rheumatoid arthritis can lead to an unstable cervical spine with the possibility of spinal cord injury during intubation. Therefore, flexion and extension lateral cervical spine radiographs should be obtained in symptomatic patients (***Figures 21.7 and 21.8***). Assessment of the severity of renal, cardiac, valvular and pericardial involvement as well as restrictive lung disease should be carried out. Rheumatologists will advise on steroids and disease-modifying drugs so as to balance immunosuppression (chance of infections) against the need to stabilise the disease perioperatively (stopping disease-modifying drugs can lead to flare-up of the disease).

In patients with ankylosing spondylitis, in addition to the problems discussed above, techniques of spinal or epidural anaesthesia are often challenging. Patients with systemic lupus erythematosus may exhibit a hypercoagulable state along with airway difficulties.

PHYSICAL FITNESS

Functional physical fitness can be judged by the ability to tolerate metabolic equivalent tasks (METs) (***Table 21.5***). One MET is equivalent to the oxygen consumption of an adult at rest (~3.5 mL/kg/min). Different tasks are assigned a number of METs. If the patient is able to perform >4 METs (e.g. climbing at least one flight of stairs) they are accepted to proceed for low-risk surgery in the USA and Europe. However this depends on a subjective assessment of the ability of a patient and may be overestimated by them. The Duke Activity Status Index (DASI) is a less subjective patient questionnaire. An estimate of the patient's peak oxygen consumption (VO_2 peak)

Erik Adolf von Willebrand, 1870–1949, physician, Diakonissanstaltens Hospital, Helsinki, (Helsingfors), Finland, described hereditary pseudohaemophilia in 1926.

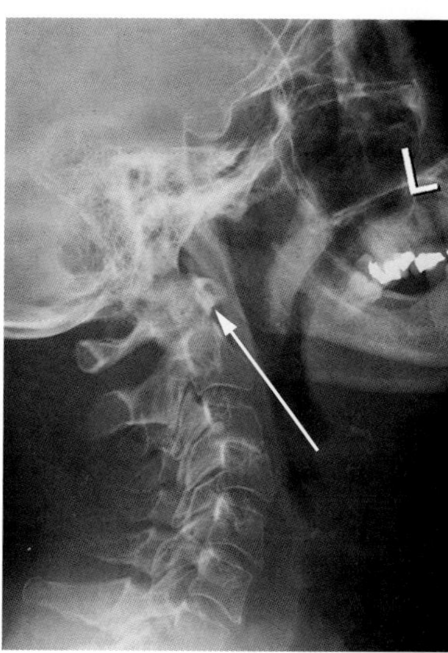

Figure 21.7 Extension view of the cervical spine in a patient with rheumatoid arthritis. Arrow indicates the atlantodens interval.

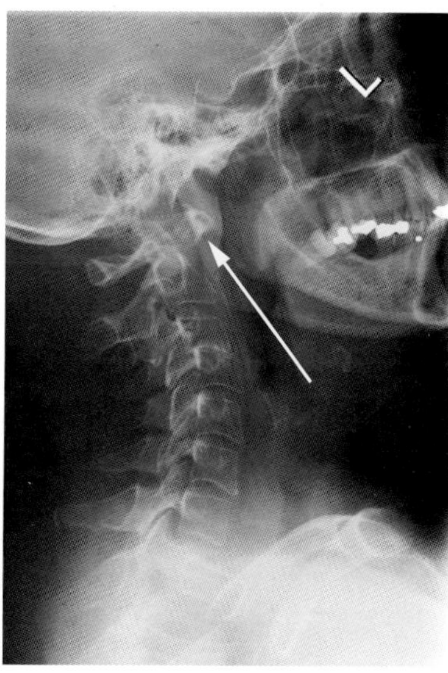

Figure 21.8 Flexion view in the same patient as in *Figure 21.7*. Note the large increase in the atlantodens interval (arrow), implying significant instability at this level.

can be calculated from their point score. Although it correlates with cardiopulmonary exercise testing (CPET), some patients who score poorly on DASI go on to score well on CPET. An objective measure of fitness is required for high-risk surgery.

Cardiopulmonary exercise testing

CPET is the gold standard measurement of a patient's fitness. The oxygen consumption (VO_2) and carbon dioxide production (VCO_2) of the patient are measured while they undergo a 10-minute period of incrementally demanding exercise (usually on a cycle ergometer) up to their maximally tolerated level (***Figure 21.9***).

CPET is based on the principle that, when a subject's delivery of O_2 to active tissues becomes inadequate, anaerobic metabolism begins; lactate is buffered by bicarbonate and the resulting CO_2 increases out of proportion to the escalation in physical difficulty and O_2 consumption. The 'anaerobic threshold' (AT) is the VO_2 in mL/kg/min at which this occurs. Peak oxygen consumption is also measured. This is the end-product of a subject's combined respiratory, cardiac, vascular and musculoskeletal fitness, and subjects with either an AT below 11 mL/kg/min or a VO_2 peak below 15 mL/kg/min are at higher risk of morbidity and mortality after major surgery.

Patients who are found to be unfit can be enrolled in prehabilitation. This involves supervised exercise over 4–6 weeks with the aim of improving the patient's AT and reducing their risk profile.

Where CPET is not available, the low-cost incremental shuttle walk test (ISWT) is an attractive option. It depends on the patient's ability to walk at increasing speed over a flat surface. Patients who fail to achieve 350 metres on the ISWT have been shown to be at higher risk for oesophageal surgery. It correlates well with VO_2 peak but does not identify all low-risk patients as it is subject to patient motivation and is affected by sex, age and height.

TABLE 21.5 Metabolic equivalent tasks (METs).

- 1 MET = 3.5 mL O_2/kg/min (oxygen consumption by a 40-year-old, 70-kg man at rest)
- 1 MET = eating and dressing
- 4 METs = climbing two flights of stairs
- 6 METs = short run
- >10 METs = able to participate in strenuous sport

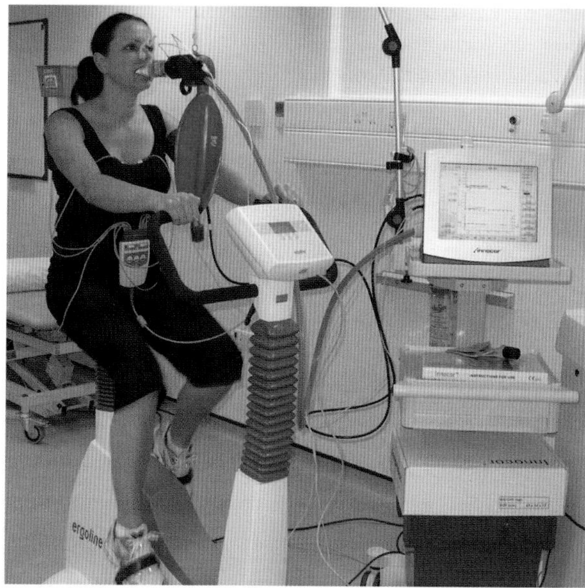

Figure 21.9 Cardiopulmonary exercise testing (CPET).

CONSENT

Consent is a key part of preoperative care. The process of consent has evolved over the years and, in the UK, is determined by relevant Acts of Parliament, legal judgement and the development of specific guidance. Consent is considered in detail in ***Chapter 14***.

ASSESSMENT OF RISK

Despite more comorbid patients presenting for surgery, the perioperative mortality has decreased significantly over the last half century, especially in resource-rich countries. In a published systematic review in *The Lancet* by Bainbridge *et al.* (2012), perioperative mortality has declined from 10 603 per million (95% confidence interval [CI] 10 423–10 784) in the 1970s to 1176 per million (95%CI 1148–1205) in the 1990s to 2000s ($P < 0.0001$). However, there remains a subgroup of patients who are at higher risk of morbidity and mortality after surgery. Patients who have a predicted mortality ≥5% should be considered as 'high risk'. It is estimated that, although the high-risk group accounts for less than 15% of all surgical procedures, they contribute to more than 80% of all perioperative deaths in UK.

What causes these patients to be at a high risk of death and complications after surgery? After surgery tissue destruction, blood loss, fluid shifts and changes in temperature, pain and anxiety result in increased demands for oxygen delivery to the tissues. This demand increases from an average of 110 mL/min/m^2 at rest to 170 mL/min/m^2 in the postoperative period. Most patients meet this increase in demand by increasing their cardiac output and tissue oxygen extraction. Patients who are unable to meet these demands, as a result of a limited cardiorespiratory reserve, are at a risk of oxygen debt. Occult hypovolaemia resulting from fluid shift or blood loss can further impair oxygen delivery. Splanchnic vasoconstriction to compensate for this may result in gut ischaemia. Those with coronary or cerebrovascular disease are also at a higher risk of myocardial ischaemia or stroke.

Factors contributing to risk

Risk is a complex interaction of multiple factors that can be classified into patient and surgical factors. Patient factors are listed in ***Table 21.6***. The elderly, although not independently at higher risk, not only have more cardiac, pulmonary and renal disease but also require surgery four times as often as the rest of the population. Around 10% of the population over 65 are frail, with increasing incidence associated with age. Multiple body systems lose their in-built reserves in the elderly.

The type of surgery contributes independently and is listed in ***Table 21.7***. This risk increases if the surgery is performed as an emergency. Often, the underlying condition requiring surgery itself may be associated with an increased risk of complications. For example, a patient with severe peripheral vascular disease resulting from heavy smoking may need a femoral–popliteal bypass graft and can be expected also to have significant COPD and IHD.

Moreover, when mortality by type of surgery is adjusted for patient risk factors, the apparent hierarchy of surgical risk may change. The average mortality risk for an individual patient undergoing thoracic surgery, for example, is likely to be higher than the average risk for that same patient undergoing vascular surgery. Complications associated with the latter are nevertheless more frequent because vascular patients have greater medical risk factors (***Table 21.8***).

TABLE 21.6 Patient factors that predispose to high risk of morbidity and mortality.

- Previous severe cardiorespiratory illness, e.g. acute myocardial infarction, COPD or stroke
- Late-stage vascular disease involving the aorta
- Age >70 years with limited physiological reserve in one or more vital organs
- Extensive surgery for carcinoma
- Acute abdominal catastrophe with haemodynamic instability (e.g. peritonitis)
- Acute massive blood loss >8 units
- Septicaemia
- Positive blood culture or septic focus
- Respiratory failure: PaO_2 <8 kPa or F_iO_2 >0.4 or mechanical ventilation >48 hours
- Acute renal failure: urea >20 mmol or creatinine >260 mmol/L

COPD, chronic obstructive pulmonary disease; F_iO_2, fraction of inspired oxygen; PaO_2, arterial oxygen partial pressure.

Based on clinical criteria used by Shoemaker and colleagues, modified by Boyd.

TABLE 21.7 Surgery-specific estimates of risk.

High risk (cardiac risk >5%)	Intermediate risk (cardiac risk 1–5%)	Low risk (cardiac risk <1%)
Open aortic	Elective abdominal	Breast
Major vascular	Carotid	Dental
Peripheral vascular	Endovascular	Thyroid
Urgent body cavity	Aneurysm	Ophthalmic
	Head and neck	Gynaecological
	Major neurosurgery	Reconstructive
	Arthroplasty	Minor orthopaedic
	Elective pulmonary	Minor urology
	Major urology	

From Eagle KA, Berger PB, Calkins H *et al.*; American College of Cardiology; American Heart Association. ACC/AHA guideline update for perioperative cardiovascular evaluation for noncardiac surgery: executive summary: a report of the American College of Cardiology/American Heart Association evaluation for noncardiac surgery. *J Am Coll Cardiol* 2002; **39**(3): 542–53.

TABLE 21.8 The effect of adjustment for patient factors on surgery-specific operative mortality.

Type of surgery	Unadjusted 30-day mortality (% (rank))	Adjusted 30-day mortality (%(rank))
Vascular	5.97 (1)	0.98 (5)
Thoracic	3.40 (2)	2.28 (1)
Abdominal	2.73 (3)	1.83 (2)
Cardiac	2.70 (4)	1.13 (4)
Neurosurgery	1.74 (5)	1.60 (3)
Orthopaedic	1.25 (6)	0.49 (7)
Ear–nose–throat	0.85 (7)	0.68 (6)
Urology	0.81 (8)	0.38 (8)
Gynaecology	0.13 (9)	0.17 (9)
Breast	0.07 (10)	0.08 (10)

Modified from Noordzij *et al.* (2010).

TABLE 21.9 Surgical risk scores classified by outcome measures and need for intraoperative information.

	Scores predicting mortality	Scores predicting morbidity
Scores not requiring operative information	ASA APACHE-II Hardman index Glasgow aneurysm score Surgical Outcome Risk Tool (SORT) Boey score Hacetteppe score Physiological POSSUM ACS NSQIP surgical risk score	ASA APACHE-II Revised Cardiac Risk Index (RCRI) Veltkamp score VA respiratory failure score VA pneumonia prediction index ACS NSQIP surgical risk score
Scores requiring operative information	Mannheim peritonitis index NELA score Reiss index Fitness score POSSUM P-POSSUM Cleveland colorectal model Surgical risk scale	POSSUM P-POSSUM

ACS NSQIP, American College of Surgeons National Surgical Quality Improvement Programme; APACHE-II, Acute Physiology and Chronic Health Evaluation II; ASA, American Society of Anesthesiologists; NELA, National Emergency Laparotomy Audit; POSSUM, Physiologic and Operative Severity Score for the enUmeration of Mortality and Morbidity; P-POSSUM, Portsmouth-POSSUM; VA, Veterans Affairs.

Modified from Rix TE, Bates T. Pre-operative risk scores for the prediction of outcome in elderly people who require emergency surgery. *World J Emerg Surg* 2007; **2**: 16.

Risk prediction

The key to managing patients effectively is the identification and accurate quantification of the risk, and subsequent measures taken to minimise it.

Realistic estimates of risk are the cornerstone of informed patient consent and shared decision making. The patient and the surgeon may choose a less extensive or even a non-surgical option when the risks of the definitive procedure are deemed to be too high or unacceptable. The Royal College of Surgeons of England has recommended that patients who are predicted to have >5% mortality risk should have active consultant input in all stages of their management. Surgical procedures in those with predicted mortality of >10% should be conducted under the direct supervision of a consultant surgeon or anaesthetist, unless the consultants are satisfied with the seniority and competence of the staff managing these patients. Moreover, those with a mortality >10% should be managed in the critical care facility postoperatively. The identification of patients who will benefit the most from these interventions is important, not only for the improvement of outcomes but also for the effective allocation of resources.

A number of scoring systems have been developed over the years with the aim of identifying high-risk patients (***Table 21.9***).

American Society of Anesthesiologists system

The ASA scoring system is widely used. Although not designed to be used as a risk prediction score, it has a quantitative association with the predicted percentage of postoperative mortality (***Table 21.10***). However, it does not account for the patient's age or the nature of the surgery and the term 'systemic disease' in ASA grading introduces an element of 'subjectivity'. Examples of each physical status added in 2015 aim to reduce this.

The POSSUM score

The POSSUM (Physiologic and Operative Severity Score for the enUmeration of Mortality and Morbidity) and its modifications (P-POSSUM, CR-POSSUM) are used to predict all-cause mortality in postoperative critical care patients as well as non-cardiac morbidity.

TABLE 21.10 Operative mortality by American Society of Anesthesiologists (ASA) grade.

ASA grade	Description	30-day mortality (%)
I	Healthy	0.1
II	Mild systemic disease, no functional limitation	0.7
III	Severe systemic disease, definite functional limitation	3.5
IV	Severe systemic disease, constant threat to life	18.3
V	Moribund patient unlikely to survive 24 hours with or without operation	93.3
E	Emergency operation	–

From Boyd and Jackson (2005).

Lee Goldman, b. 1948, Dean of Health Sciences and Medicine, Columbia University, New York, NY, USA, since 2006. He developed his index in 1977.

Lee's Revised Cardiac Risk index

Lee's Revised Cardiac Risk index (RCRI) uses objective indices based on weighted scores pertaining to surgery and comorbidity. This stratifies cardiac risk but is not designed to predict mortality (*Table 21.11*).

ACS NSQIP score

The American College of Surgeons (ACS) National Surgical Quality Improvement Program (NSQIP) surgical risk score estimates the chance of a complication or death after surgery for more than a thousand different surgical procedures. It compares the patient's risk with an average person's risk. It is a Web-based tool done preoperatively. The risk is calculated based on surgical procedure and 19 patient-specific preoperative risk factors.

TABLE 21.11 The Revised Cardiac Risk index of Lee.

Risk factors	Risk of major cardiac complications (%)
History of ischaemic heart disease History of compensated or prior heart failure History of cerebrovascular disease Diabetes mellitus Renal insufficiency (creatinine >177 μmol/L) High-risk surgery	Number of factors 0 = 0.4 1 = 0.9 2 = 7.0 3+ = 11.0

Choosing the right operation for the high-risk patient

There are situations in which the selection of one surgical technique over another may be significantly influenced by patient risk factors. Some procedures are not primarily high risk but may become so in unsuitable patients. Laparoscopic surgery, for example, has come of age as a preferred technique for patients predisposed to postoperative respiratory complications, but its effect on cardiac physiology means that the same may not apply to patients at risk of cardiac complications. The expanding demand and indications for minimal access surgery are now pushing the boundaries of intraoperative physiological tolerance. Robotic prostatectomy and some laparoscopic colorectal procedures require a pneumoperitoneum with steep Trendelenburg (head down) positioning for several hours (*Figure 21.10*). This can be associated with adverse cardiovascular and neurological complications, such as myocardial ischaemia and increased intracranial pressure in the high-risk group. This risk may be minimised by attention to patient selection.

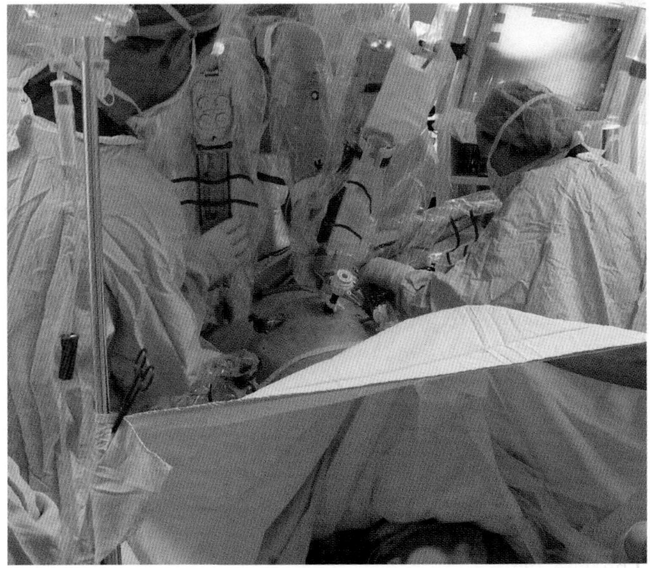

Figure 21.10 Robotic surgery

Role of critical care and outreach services

Reports from the National Confidential Enquiry into Patient Outcome and Death (NCEPOD) show that the majority of postoperative deaths in the UK occur more than 5 days after surgery. Admission to a critical care unit allows for early treatment of complications and a level of care that is difficult to deliver in the ward environment during this crucial period. Common complications include myocardial ischaemia, cardiac, respiratory or renal failure and sepsis.

Perioperative MI is associated with a high mortality (15–25%). Critical care uses invasive cardiac monitoring and vasoactive drugs to help provide cardiac stability postoperatively to minimise ischaemia and guide fluid management to prevent cardiac failure.

Postoperatively, 1.5% of patients develop lower respiratory tract infection after surgery, with a 30-day mortality of >20%. Respiratory failure, which is defined as PaO_2 <8 kPa in air, PaO_2/F_iO_2 (the ratio of arterial oxygen partial pressure to the fraction of inspired oxygen) <40 kPa or the inability to extubate a patient 48 hours after surgery, is by far the most significant of these and is associated with a mortality of 27–40%. Elective non-invasive ventilation, chest physiotherapy and incentive spirometry should be considered for patients at increased risk of respiratory complications. These are commonly delivered on the critical care unit (*Figure 21.11*).

The high-risk surgical population accounts for 80% of postoperative deaths, but only about 15–30% of high-risk surgical patients are admitted to a critical care unit at any time following surgery. Work by the National Emergency Laparotomy Audit in the UK is seeking to standardise treatment of this high-risk group with many recommendations, including admission to critical care where predicted mortality is >5%.

In the last decade, the role of critical care has been expanded to the concept of 'critical care without walls'. The intensive care outreach services (ICORS) grew from a recognition that

Thomas H Lee, Professor of Medicine, Harvard Medical School, Professor of Health Policy and Management, Harvard School of Public Health, Boston, MA, USA.
Friedrich Trendelenburg, 1844–1924, successively Professor of Surgery at Rostock (1875–1882), Bonn (1822–1895) and Leipzig, (1895–1911), Germany. The Trendelenburg position was first described in 1885.

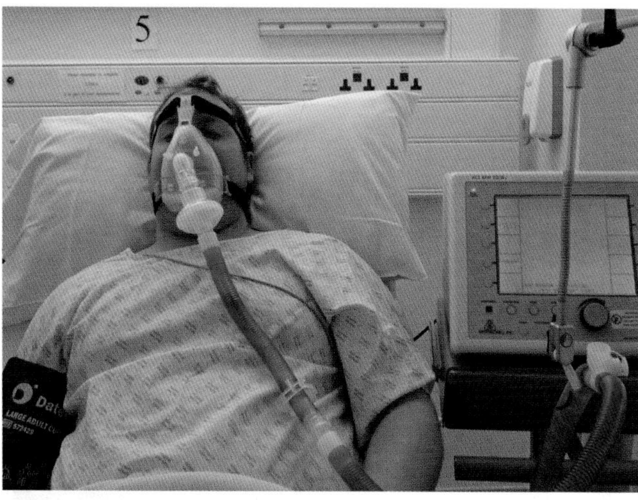

Figure 21.11 A high-risk patient admitted to critical care postoperatively.

there were many patients in hospital who are at risk of being critically ill and that early identification of these patients using 'early warning scores' could allow for early intervention. The outreach team functions to bridge the gap between the critical care unit and ward.

ARRANGING AN ELECTIVE THEATRE LIST

The date, place and time of operation should be matched with the availability of appropriately skilled personnel. Appropriate equipment and instruments should be made available. The operating list should be distributed as early as possible to all staff who are involved in making the list run smoothly (***Table 21.12***). If this is done electronically, familiarity with the computer system is required. A critical care bed should be prearranged for high-risk cases.

Elective list order should prioritise patients who are vulnerable to long starvation times, e.g. children and patients with diabetes. For a prompt theatre start, planning a straightforward case first can utilise time waiting for preprocedure imaging on the second case, e.g. breast wire insertion, or confirmation of a postoperative critical care bed for a high-risk case. List planning using a surgeon's average operation times for a procedure rather than generic estimates leads to better list utilisation. Staggering admission times can improve patient satisfaction but reduces flexibility for 'on the day' changes to list order.

TABLE 21.12 Perioperative teams.

- Ward, theatre and specialist nursing staff
- Anaesthetic and surgical teams
- Radiology and pathology involvement
- Rehabilitation and social care workers
- Administration and scheduling team
- Specific personnel in individual cases, e.g. cardiac devices team

PREOPERATIVE ASSESSMENT FOR EMERGENCY SURGERY

In emergency surgery the principles of preoperative assessment should be the same as in elective surgery, except that the opportunity to optimise the condition of the patient is limited by time constraints. The urgency of surgery should be graded, e.g. by using the NCEPOD classification of intervention, and emergency theatre cases should be prioritised accordingly, i.e. immediate (within minutes), urgent (within hours), expedited (within days) or elective (timing to suit patient, hospital and staff). Medical assessment and treatments should be started even if there is no time to complete them before the start of a time-critical surgical procedure. Some risks may be reduced but some may persist; whenever possible, these need to be discussed with the patient during the consent process. Optimisation before urgent surgery can be more effective in a critical care environment and patients may need to be admitted to critical care preoperatively. The likelihood of a high-risk emergency patient requiring postoperative critical care should be identified and discussed with the duty critical care physician.

Summary box 21.3

Preoperative assessment for emergency surgery

- **Start.** Similar principles to that for elective surgery
- **Constraints.** Time, facilities available
- **Consent.** May not be possible in life-saving emergencies
- **Organisational efforts.** For example, local/national algorithms for the treatment of patients with multiple injuries

FURTHER READING

Bainbridge D, Martin J, Arango M, Cheng D; for the Evidence-based Peri-operative Clinical Outcomes Research (EPiCOR) Group. Perioperative and anaesthetic-related mortality in developed and developing countries: a systematic review and meta-analysis. *Lancet* 2012; **380**(9847): 1075–81.

Barker P, Creasey PE, Dhatariya K *et al.* Peri-operative management of the surgical patient with diabetes. *Anaesthesia* 2015; **70**(12): 1427–40.

Boyd O, Jackson N. How is risk defined in high-risk surgical patient management? *Crit Care* 2005; **9**: 390–6.

Chan MTV, Wang CY, Edwin S *et al.* Association of unrecognized obstructive sleep apnoea with postoperative cardiovascular events in patients undergoing major non cardiac surgery. *JAMA* 2019; **321**(18): 1788–98.

Department of Health. *Mental Capacity Act (MCA). England and Wales.* London: HMSO, 2005.

Duminda N, Wijeysundera W, Beattie S *et al.* Integration of the Duke Activity Status Index into preoperative risk evaluation: a multicentre prospective cohort study. *Br J Anaesth* 2020; **124**(3): 261–70.

Fleisher L, Fleischmann K, Auerback A *et al.* 2014 ACC/AHA guideline on perioperative cardiovascular evaluation and management of patients undergoing noncardiac surgery: a report of the American College of Cardiology/American Heart Association Task Force on Practice Guidelines. *J Am Coll Cardiol* 2014; **64**(22): e77–e137.

General Medical Council. *Decision making and consent*, 2020. Available from https://www.gmc-uk.org/ethical-guidance/ethical-guidance-for-doctors/decision-making-and-consent.

Griffiths R, Beech F, Brown A *et al.* Peri-operative care of the elderly 2014. *Anaesthesia.* 2014; **69**: 81–98.

Griffiths R, Babu S, Dixon S *et al.* Guideline for the management of hip fractures 2020. *Anaesthesia* 2021; **76**: 225–37.

Hartle A, McCormack T, Carlisle J *et al.* The measurement of adult blood pressure and management of hypertension before elective surgery. *Anaesthesia* 2016; **71**(3): 326–37.

Jørgensen ME, Torp-Pedersen C, Gislason GH *et al.* Time elapsed after ischemic stroke and risk of adverse cardiovascular events and mortality following elective noncardiac surgery. *JAMA* 2014; **312**(3): 269–77.

Kristenson SD, Knuuti J, Saraste A *et al.* 2014 ESC/ESA Guidelines on non-cardiac surgery: cardiovascular assessment and management: The Joint Task Force on non-cardiac surgery: cardiovascular assessment and management of the European Society of Cardiology (ESC) and the European Society of Anaesthesiology (ESA). *Eur Heart J* 2014; **35**: 2383–431.

Lee TH, Marcantonio ER, Mangione CM *et al.* Derivation and prospective validation of a simple index for prediction of cardiac risk of major noncardiac surgery. *Circulation* 1999; **100**: 1043–9.

Minto G, Biccard B. Assessment of the high-risk perioperative patient. *BJA Educ* 2014; **14**(1): 12–17.

Munoz M, Acheson G, Auerbach M *et al.* International consensus statement on the perioperative management of anaemia and iron deficiency. *Anaesthesia* 2017; **72**(2): 233–47.

Murray P, Whiting P, Hutchinson S *et al.* Preoperative shuttle walking testing and outcome after oesophagogastrectomy. *Br J Anaesth* 2007; **99**(6): 809–11.

National Confidential Enquiry into Patient Outcome and Death (NCEPOD). *An age-old problem: a review of the care received by elderly patients undergoing surgery*, 2010. Available from https://www.ncepod.org.uk/2010report3/downloads/EESE_fullReport.pdf.

National Confidential Enquiry into Patient Outcome and Death (NCEPOD). *Knowing the risk. A review of the perioperative care of surgical patients*, 2011. Available from https://www.ncepod.org.uk/2011report2/downloads/POC_fullreport.pdf.

National Emergency Laparotomy Audit (NELA) Project Team. *Sixth patient report of the National Emergency Laparotomy Audit*, 2020. Available from https://www.nela.org.uk/reports.

National Institute for Health and Care Excellence. *Routine preoperative tests for elective surgery*. NICE Guideline 45. London: NICE, 2016. Available from https://www.nice.org.uk/guidance/ng45.

National Institute for Health and Care Excellence. *Decision-making and mental capacity*. NICE Guideline 108. London: NICE, 2018. Available from https://www.nice.org.uk/guidance/ng108.

National Institute for Health and Care Excellence. *Venous thromboembolism in over 16s: reducing the risk of hospital-acquired deep vein thrombosis or pulmonary embolism*. NICE Guideline 89. London: NICE, 2019. Available from https://www.nice.org.uk/guidance/ng89.

National Institute for Health and Care Excellence. *Perioperative care in adults*. NICE Guideline 180. London: NICE, 2020. Available from https://www.nice.org.uk/guidance/ng180.

Noordzij PG, Poldermans D, Schouten O *et al.* Postoperative mortality in The Netherlands: a population based analysis of surgery-specific risk in adults. *Anesthesiology* 2010; **112**(5): 1105–15.

Practice guidelines for the perioperative management of patients with obstructive sleep apnea: a report by the American Society of Anesthesiologists Task Force on Perioperative Management of Patients with Obstructive Sleep Apnea. *Anesthesiology* 2006; **104**: 1081–93.

Royal College of Surgeons. *Caring for patients who refuse blood: a guide to good practice for the surgical management of Jehovah's Witnesses and other patients who decline transfusion*, 2016. Available from https://www.rcseng.ac.uk/-/media/files/rcs/library-and-publications/non-journal-publications/caring-for-patients-who-refuse-blood--a-guide-to-good-practice.pdf.

Royal College of Surgeons. *Consent: supported decision making: a guide to good practice*, 2018. Available from https://www.rcseng.ac.uk/standards-and-research/standards-and-guidance/good-practice-guides/consent/.

Shoemaker WC, Appel PL, Kram HB *et al.* Hemodynamic and oxygen transport responses in survivors and non survivors of high risk surgery. *Crit Care Med* 1993; **21**(7): 977–90.

Woodcock T, Barker P, Daniel S *et al.* Guidelines for the management of glucocorticoids during the perioperative period for patients with adrenal insufficiency. *Anaesthesia* 2020; **75**(5): 654–63.

CHAPTER 22 Day case surgery

Learning objectives

To understand:

- The key components of the day surgery pathway
- Which surgical procedures can be done as day surgery
- Patient selection and preparation for day surgery
- Basic principles of anaesthesia and surgery for day surgery
- How to achieve successful discharge after day surgery

DAY SURGERY

In the UK the definition of day surgery is the admission of selected patients to hospital for a planned surgical procedure, returning home on the same day. 'True day surgery' patients are day case patients who require full operating theatre facilities and/or a general anaesthetic, and any day cases not included as outpatients or undergoing endoscopy. Surgery that requires a 23-hour stay, including an overnight stay, is *not* classed as day surgery.

Day surgery offers benefits for patients and hospitals. Patients often prefer to recover in the comfort of their own home, and day surgery may cause less disruption to their domestic situation. It also reduces their risk of a hospital-acquired infection. For the hospital, it can provide greater patient satisfaction and increase the number of inpatient beds available for patients who need to be cared for in hospital.

Successful delivery of day surgery requires the day surgery service to be considered a priority by the hospital, with key enablers in all areas of the pathway providing effective implementation, refinement and progression. There must be a high-quality pathway (***Figure 22.1***) staffed by experienced/expert members of the multidisciplinary team with the equipment and resources they need. This will ensure that there is a well-prepared patient who is in receipt of high-quality day case anaesthesia and surgery and who subsequently has a safe and successful day case discharge.

SELECTION CRITERIA

Surgical

Surgical techniques have progressed significantly and now cause less physiological disruption and stress to patients; therefore, they have a lower postoperative complication profile and a faster recovery rate. The British Association of Day Surgery's (BADS) Directory of Procedures (DOP) lists over 200 procedures that are now considered to be suitable as a day case (***Table 22.1***).

Traditionally day surgery was limited to cases that lasted less than 1 hour but surgical procedures lasting 3–4 hours are now being routinely performed as successful day cases.

Day surgery surgical criteria include the following:

- There must be a low risk of significant immediate postoperative complications, e.g. catastrophic bleeding or airway compromise.
- The patient should be able to eat and drink or take oral nutrition postoperatively.
- Postoperative pain needs to be managed by oral painkillers, which may be in conjunction with local anaesthetic infiltration or peripheral nerve block.
- The patient should be able to mobilise postoperatively with or without aid.

If these criteria are met then the surgeon booking the procedure should add the patient to a day surgery pathway.

TABLE 22.1 Examples from British Association of Day Surgery *Directory of Procedures*, 6th edn (2019).

Specialty	Procedure	Recommended day case rate (%)
Breast	Simple mastectomy	75
Ear–nose–throat	Tonsillectomy	90
General surgery	Laparoscopic cholecystectomy	75
Gynaecology	Vaginal hysterectomy	60
Orthopaedics	Arthroscopy of knee or shoulder	99
Urology	Ureteroscopic extraction of calculus from the ureter	70
Vascular surgery	Transluminal operations on the iliac and femoral arteries	85

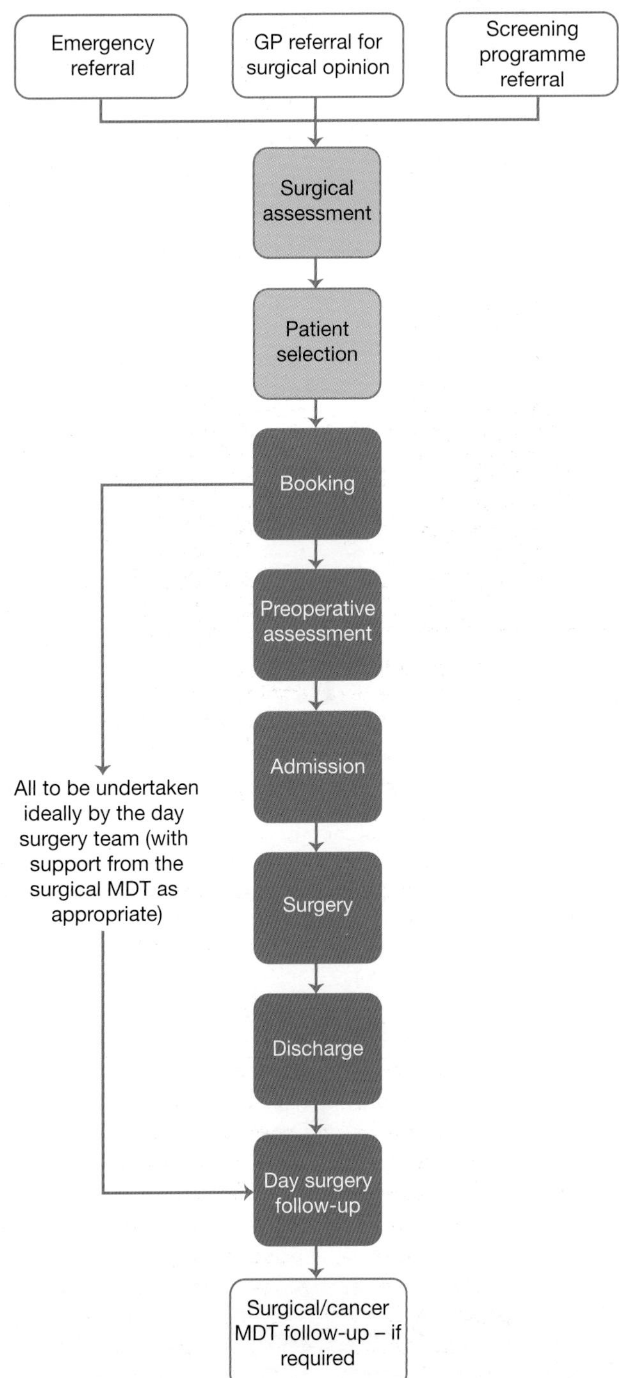

Figure 22.1 Day surgery pathway. GP, general practitioner; MDT, multidisciplinary team.

Medical

With the developments of anaesthesia and surgery, there should be very few restrictions to patients having day surgery (***Table 22.2***). Every effort should be made to optimise a patient's health so that they can be treated as a day case.

There should be no arbitrary cut-offs according to age, weight or criteria specified by the American Society of Anesthesiologists. A patient's suitability for day surgery should be judged on their comorbidities and functional status. Older patients and patients with higher body mass index (BMI) benefit from awake surgery or short-acting anaesthetic agents with a good recovery profile.

TABLE 22.2 Medical exclusions to day surgery.

- Unstable ASA 3
- ASA 4 or 5
- Any poorly controlled abnormality/comorbidity

ASA, American Society of Anesthesiologists.

Diabetes

Patients with diabetes are often better at managing their own diabetes than healthcare professionals. UK national guidance recommends that patients with well-controlled diabetes (haemoglobin A1c [HbA1c] <69 mmol/mol) can be safely managed as a day case. Patients with poorly controlled diabetes have an increased risk of cardiovascular complications and poor wound healing. They should have their surgery delayed until their diabetes is well controlled. If surgery cannot wait or it is thought the underlying disorder (e.g. tooth infection) is causing the diabetes control to be disrupted then diabetic control should be optimised as much as possible prior to surgery.

Epilepsy

Patients with well-controlled epilepsy should not be excluded from day surgery. It is essential that normal medications are not missed. Poorly controlled epilepsy should be optimised prior to any elective surgery.

Obesity

Traditionally there has been caution treating patients who have a higher BMI as a day case. Guidance from the Association of Anaesthetists of Great Britain and Ireland/BADS in 2019 states that 'even morbidly obese patients can be safely managed in expert hands, with appropriate resources'.

Preoperative assessment of patients should routinely include STOP-BANG (Snoring, Tiredness, Observed apnoeas, Pressure [hypertension], Body mass index, Age, Neck circumference, Gender) to identify undiagnosed OSA (obstructive sleep apnoea). The Society for Obesity and Bariatric Anaesthesia (SOBA) Guideline for Anaesthesia of the obese patient identifies a number of risk factors that may make day surgery unsuitable, e.g. poor functional capacity, oxygen saturation <94% on air, STOP-BANG ≥5 (***Figure 22.2***; see also tools.farmacologiaclinica.info, riskcalculator.facs.org/RiskCalculator and www.stopbang.ca). Obese patients considered suitable for day surgery should receive a short-acting anaesthetic, avoiding long-acting opiates, with allowance for the additional time that may be required anaesthetically, surgically and for recovery.

Social

Social criteria for day surgery include:

- Adequate housing conditions such as heating, an inside toilet and access to a phone.

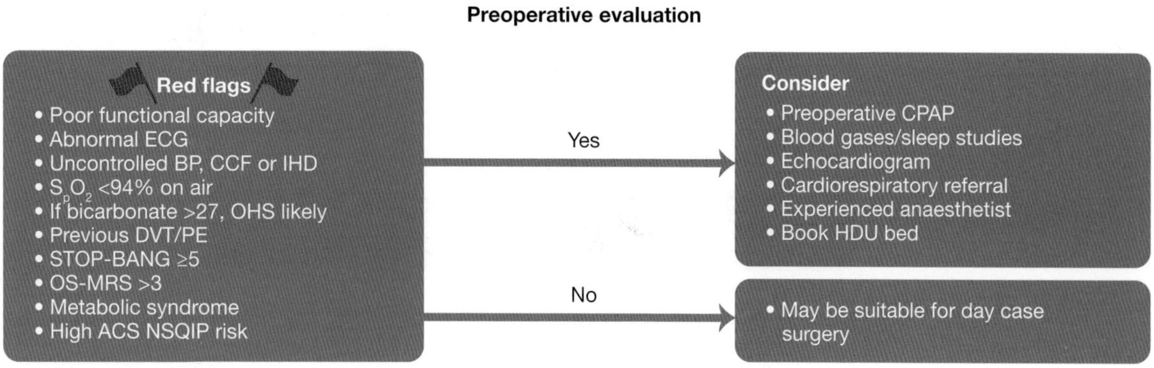

Preoperative evaluation

Red flags		Consider
• Poor functional capacity • Abnormal ECG • Uncontrolled BP, CCF or IHD • S_pO_2 <94% on air • If bicarbonate >27, OHS likely • Previous DVT/PE • STOP-BANG ≥5 • OS-MRS >3 • Metabolic syndrome • High ACS NSQIP risk	Yes →	• Preoperative CPAP • Blood gases/sleep studies • Echocardiogram • Cardiorespiratory referral • Experienced anaesthetist • Book HDU bed
	No →	• May be suitable for day case surgery

Figure 22.2 Society of Bariatric Anaesthesia (SOBA) red flags. BP, blood pressure; CCF, congestive cardiac failure; CPAP, continuous positive airway pressure; DVT, deep vein thrombosis; ECG, electrocardiogram; HDU, high-dependency unit; IHD, ischaemic heart disease; ACS NSQIP, American College of Surgeons National Surgical Quality Improvement Program; OHS, obesity hypoventilation syndrome; OS-MRS, obesity surgery mortality risk score; PE, pulmonary embolism; S_pO_2, oxygen saturation; STOP-BANG, Snoring ,Tiredness, Observed apnoeas, Pressure (hypertensive), Body mass index, Age, Neck circumference, Gender.

- The patient should live within a 1-hour drive of a hospital.
- A responsible adult should be able to stay with the patient for 24 hours after a regional anaesthetic/general anaesthetic.

The first two points are generally achievable as the patient needs to be 1 hour from 'a hospital' that can treat them rather than the hospital where surgery was performed.

With respect to the responsible adult, there have been two solutions introduced for this by centres in the UK:

1. The Torbay and South Devon NHS Foundation Trust model provides carers into the patient's home.
2. Norfolk and Norwich University Hospital model allows some patients home without carers after certain procedures (*Figure 22.3*).

Both pathways have been in place for a number of years with excellent patient satisfaction and no adverse outcomes.

TABLE 22.3 Benefits of dedicated day surgery facilities.

- All members of the multidisciplinary team are focused on day surgery
- Nurses with expertise in day surgery
- Nurses not distracted by inpatients
- Activity can continue even during a time of pressures on inpatient beds
- Fewer cancellations because activity can continue even when there are pressures on inpatient beds
- Can be made a COVID secure area – protected from COVID-positive areas of hospital
- Higher chance of successful day case discharge
- Separation from inpatient activity and so patients are more likely to be motivated to get up and go home if they see this as the 'norm'
- Higher patient satisfaction
- Higher quality outcomes

COVID, coronavirus disease.

DELIVERY OF DAY SURGERY

Facilities

National guidance from the Royal College of Anaesthetists, Royal College of Surgeons and BADS recommends that, ideally, day surgery should be performed in a dedicated unit with its own admission area, operating theatres and discharge ward. As a minimum a dedicated day surgery ward is required. This offers a number of benefits, as listed in *Table 22.3*.

It is important to remember that to deliver high-quality successful day surgery the appropriate equipment, drugs and expertise are essential.

Preoperative assessment

A key component to successful day surgery is a well-informed, well-prepared patient. It is essential that the day surgery message starts at the time of referral by the primary care doctor and continues throughout the pathway by all staff who the patient interacts with.

Preoperative assessment should follow the same principles as for any other patient and should be nurse led (see *Chapter 21*). The anaesthetist should review the patient's notes where appropriate and the suitability of the patient for day case surgery should be discussed with the day surgery lead to optimise day case rates.

Key preassessment considerations specific to day surgery include:

- Can surgery be delayed until the medical condition is optimised and then plan as a day case?
- Can social factors be addressed for the patient to become a suitable day case?

Admission and list planning

Day surgery patients should follow the same starvation guidance as any other elective patient. All patients, but especially day surgery patients, should be encouraged to walk to theatre.

Consider the list order to optimise successful day surgery and therefore put operations with longer recovery times or patients who take longer to recover early on the lists

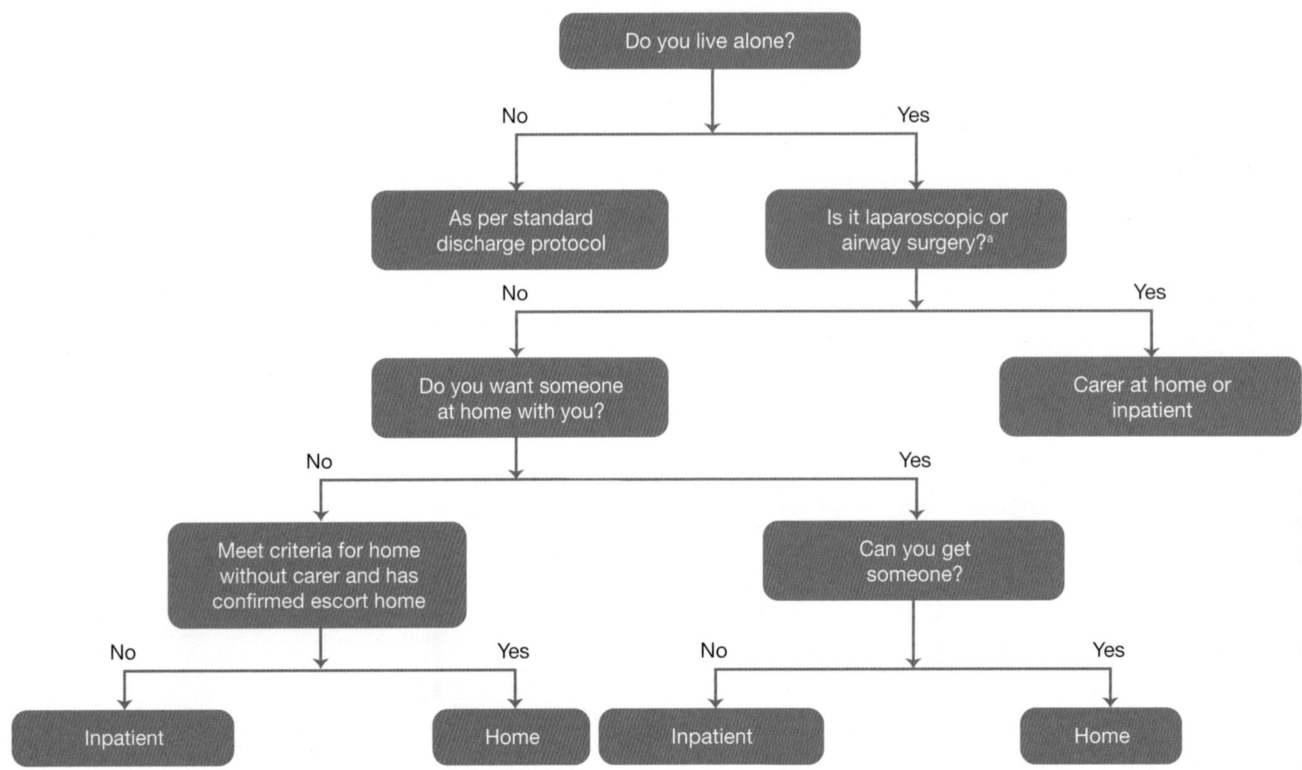

Figure 22.3 The Norfolk and Norwich Day Surgery Home Alone flowchart. (Reproduced with the permission of The Norfolk and Norwich Day Surgery Team.)

(*Table 22.4*). This needs to be balanced with patients who would benefit from being first on the list, such as patients with insulin-dependent diabetes and patients with learning difficulties who would struggle to wait for long periods of time.

Anaesthesia and surgery

It is not expected that there should be any difference in surgical technique. Surgeons should perform their usual operation, which should be appropriate for rapid recovery and should be performed well. Drains should generally be avoided or, if used, clear plans of when they should be removed and by whom made clear. Any specific postoperative care or discharge information should be documented in theatre to avoid delay to discharge.

Appropriate day surgery anaesthesia requires meticulous attention to ensuring good pain relief and avoidance of postoperative nausea and vomiting. This should include premedication and a multimodal approach. Short-acting general anaesthesia agents, day case spinals or regional anaesthesia techniques should be used to enable rapid recovery. Use of long-acting opioids such as intravenous morphine is discouraged because they can delay recovery owing to increased sleepiness or nausea.

TABLE 22.4 List planning.

Operation with potentially longer recovery times	Types of patients who might need longer recovery time
Tonsillectomy	Very elderly
Knee replacement	High BMI
Hip replacement	
Complex laparoscopic cholecystectomy	

BMI, body mass index.

Discharge

The expectation by the patient and healthcare team should be that the patient will be going home the same day. Therefore, unless there has been an unexpected anaesthetic or surgical issue the patient should routinely have a nurse-led discharge. Patients should meet any pre-agreed general criteria (*Table 22.5*) as well as any surgery-specific criteria prior to discharge. In general, there should be no time restriction except for certain procedures, e.g. patients should remain in hospital until 6 hours after tonsillectomy.

TABLE 22.5 Discharge criteria.

- Vital signs stable for at least 1 hour
- Correct orientation as to time, place and person if appropriate
- Adequate pain control with supply of oral analgesia
- Understands how to use oral analgesia supplied
- Ability to dress and walk where appropriate
- Minimal nausea, vomiting or dizziness
- Has taken oral fluids
- Minimal bleeding or wound drainage
- Has passed urine (if appropriate)
- Has a responsible adult to take them home
- Written and verbal instructions given about postoperative care
- Knows when to come back for follow-up (if appropriate)
- Emergency contact number supplied

The patient should receive written and verbal postoperative instructions and a phone number to contact should they have a problem out of hours. This must be a phone with a suitable person to advise and not an answerphone.

Take-home medications should provide adequate pain relief and may include an antiemetic. These should be prescribed when the patient is in theatre and pre-packs of common analgesics should be used to improve the efficiency of prescribing and reduce delays to discharge.

All day surgery patients should be telephoned the day after surgery to provide support and to check that they have no problems. This call can also be used to collect valuable audit data, which can be used to refine the day surgery pathway.

EMERGENCY DAY SURGERY

Many emergency surgical procedures are minor and non-life-threatening. Patients may be considered low priority for surgical intervention and can therefore end up waiting hours or days for a slot on the emergency theatre list, resulting in prolonged starvation times and inpatient stay.

With appropriate planning and preparation these patients could have surgery performed as a day case. This has become reasonably commonplace in orthopaedics for many upper limb traumas and in gynaecology for the evacuation of retained products of conception (ERPC). It has also increasingly been recognised for many other surgical procedures, as listed in the BADS DOP (***Table 22.6***).

For certain procedures that can wait more than 24 hours patients can follow an 'elective pathway'. They can be swabbed and isolate as per current coronavirus 2019 (COVID-19) requirements and then attend via an 'elective green pathway'. Alternatively, they can be discharged home and then return to an acute surgical admission area to be added to a suitable list or be first on the emergency list (priority slot) and discharged the same day.

Contraindications to being discharged must be identified, e.g. systemic sepsis, unstable diabetes, major comorbidities, if parenteral pain relief is needed or if patients are deemed unsafe to mobilise.

TABLE 22.6 Common procedures suitable for an emergency day surgery pathway.

Procedure	Suggested BADS DOP day case rate (%)
Evacuation of retained products of conception	95
Incision and drainage of a perianal abscess	95
Appendicectomy	15
Reduction of a fracture of the zygomatic complex of bones	60
Repair of hand or wrist tendon	95
Primary reduction and open fixation of the ankle	25
Primary reduction and open fixation of the wrist	60

BADS DOP, British Association of Day Surgery *Directory of Procedures*, 6th edn (2019).

FURTHER READING

Bailey CR, Ahuja M, Bartholomew K *et al.* Guidelines for day-case surgery 2019: guidelines from the Association of Anaesthetists and the British Association of Day Surgery. *Anaesthesia* 2019; **74**(6): 778–92.

British Association of Day Surgery. *BADS directory of procedures*, 6th edn, 2019. Available from https://publications.bads.co.uk.

Centre for Perioperative Care. *Guideline for perioperative care for people with diabetes mellitus undergoing elective and emergency surgery*. London: Centre for Perioperative Care, 2021. Available from: https://www.cpoc.org.uk/guidelines-resources-guidelines-resources/guideline-diabetes

Erskine R, Ralph S, Rattenberry W. Spinal anaesthesia for day-case surgery. *Anaesthesia* 2019; **74**(12): 1625.

Russon K, Hinde T. Chapter 5 Day surgery services, raising the standards. In: Chereshneva M, Johnston C, Colvin JR, Peden CJ (eds). *RCoA Quality improvement compendium*, 4th edn. London: Royal College of Anaesthetists, 2020.

Russon K *et al. Chapter 6 Guidelines for the provision of anaesthesia services for day surgery*, 2020. Available from https://rcoa.ac.uk/gpas/chapter-6.

Stocker M *et al. National day surgery delivery pack*, 2020. Available from https://www.gettingitrightfirsttime.co.uk/bpl/day-surgery/.

British Association of Day Surgery booklets (www.bads.co.uk):

Day case breast surgery (2020)

Day case gynaecology (2020)

Day case hip & knee replacement, 2nd edn (2020)

Day case laparoscopic cholecystectomy, 3rd edn (2018)

Managing diabetes in patients having day and short stay surgery, 4th edn (2016)

Nurse led discharge, 2nd edn (2016)

Spinal anaesthesia for day surgery patients: a practical guide, 4th edn (2019)

Surgical same-day emergency care, 2nd edn (2020)

CHAPTER 23 Anaesthesia and pain relief

Learning objectives

To gain an understanding of:

- Techniques of anaesthesia and airway maintenance
- Methods of providing pain relief
- Local and regional anaesthesia techniques
- The management of chronic pain and pain from malignant disease

HISTORY

Anaesthesia, as we know it today, was first successfully demonstrated by William Morton, a local dentist, at the Massachusetts General Hospital, Boston, MA, USA on 16 October 1846 when he administered ether to Gilbert Abbot for an operation on a vascular tumour on his neck. Earlier Horace Wells had used nitrous oxide in 1844 for painless extraction of teeth successfully.

Simpson, at Edinburgh University, overcame some of the technical difficulties of ether administration by introducing chloroform. The benefits of anaesthesia were then universally recognised and antagonism by religious leaders was countered when Queen Victoria accepted chloroform from John Snow during the birth of Prince Leopold in 1853.

KEY PRINCIPLES OF ANAESTHESIA

Optimum patient care is dependent on a collaborative approach by the anaesthetic and surgical teams. The importance of multidisciplinary collaboration has been clearly demonstrated by national audits such as the National Confidential Enquiry into Patient Outcome and Death (NCEPOD) and the Confidential Enquiry into Maternal Deaths in the UK. These audits have led to changes in clinical and non-clinical practice to improve morbidity and mortality.

The use of a safety checklist in operating theatres in the form of the World Health Organization's (WHO) 'WHO Surgical Safety Checklist' has shown a reduction in the incidence of perioperative untoward events.

The role of the modern anaesthetist has evolved from just being responsible for the patient in the operating suite into a 'perioperative physician' who optimises the patient for surgery, assesses and minimises risk, cares for the patient during the operation and then manages both pain and homeostasis in the postoperative period.

Summary box 23.1

Ground rules for anaesthesia

- Safe surgery is achieved by close teamwork between the surgeon and the anaesthetist
- Safety checklists ensure that things are not forgotten
- Risk assessments allow the best strategy to be chosen
- Anaesthetists are extending their care into the pre- and postoperative phases

PREPARATION FOR ANAESTHESIA

A surgeon's role is to carry out, in cooperation with the anaesthetist, a thorough preoperative assessment that recognises medical and anaesthetic risk factors and facilitates the optimisation of the patient's condition (see ***Chapter 21***).

Anaesthesia; the name was suggested by Oliver Wendell-Homes, first appeared in Bailey's *An Universal Etymological English Dictionary* in 1751.
William Thomas Gren Morton, 1819–1868, dentist who practised in Boston, MA, USA.
Horace Wells, 1815–1848, Harvard, CT, USA, dentist who pioneered the use of nitrous oxide anaesthesia to prevent pain during dental procedures.
Sir James Young Simpson, 1811–1870, Professor of Midwifery, Edinburgh, UK.
John Snow, 1813–1858, general practitioner, London, UK, was one of the pioneers of anaesthesia.
Humphrey Davy, 1800, suggested that nitrous oxide inhalation might be used to relieve the pain of surgical operations and named it 'laughing gas'.
Henry Edmund Gaskin Boyle, in 1917, got his gas-oxygen machine, which became the first 'Boyle apparatus'.
The first examination for a **Diploma in Anaesthesia** was held in London in 1935.
The **First Chair in Anaesthesia**: Ralph Waters, Wisconsin, USA, in 1933 and RR Macintosh in Oxford, UK, in 1937.
During the First World War **Sir Ivan Magill** and **Stanley Rowbotham**, while working with Harold Gillies (pioneer of plastic surgery), developed tracheal intubation. Sir Magill is also remembered for his laryngoscope, Magill attachment and laryngeal forceps.

A careful preassessment, multidisciplinary approach and standardised care pathway with a carefully chosen anaesthetic and analgesic technique is the cornerstone of the 'enhanced recovery programmes' that have been introduced recently across the surgical specialties.

GENERAL ANAESTHESIA

General anaesthesia is commonly described as the triad of unconsciousness, analgesia and muscle relaxation.

Summary box 23.2

The general anaesthetic triad

- Amnesia: loss of awareness
- Analgesia: pain relief
- Muscle relaxation

Induction of general anaesthesia is most frequently done by intravenous agents. Propofol has replaced thiopentone as the most widely used induction agent and can be used for maintenance of anaesthesia. Other infrequently used intravenous agents include etomidate and ketamine. Newer agents based on a benzodiazepine receptor agonist, etomidate derivatives and fospropofol are still in the experimental stage.

Inhalational induction using agents such as non-pungent sevoflurane is useful in children, needle-phobic adults and those in whom a difficult airway is anticipated. These patients will have a higher risk of developing airway obstruction. *Figure 23.1* shows a commonly used anaesthetic machine.

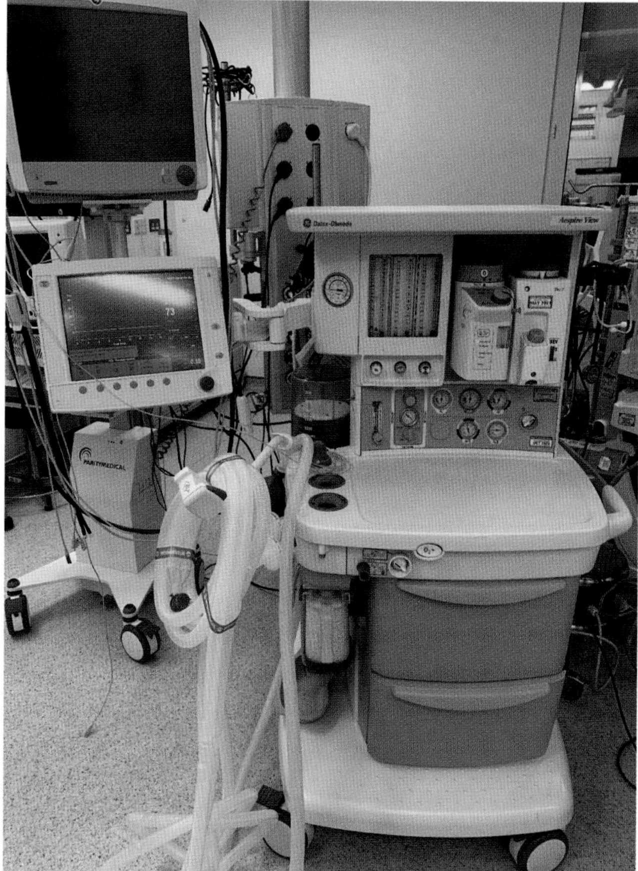

Figure 23.1 Anaesthetic machine.

Summary box 23.3

Key features of commonly used intravenous anaesthetic agents

- **Propofol (di-isopropyl phenol)**: smooth induction, better haemodynamic stability, blunting of autonomic reflexes and ability to use as a continuous infusion
- **Thiopentone (barbiturate)**: rapid induction, myocardial depression. A reduced metabolic rate and lowering of intracranial pressure is useful in neurosurgical patients but the drop in blood pressure can have detrimental effects
- **Etomidate (steroid derivative)**: good haemodynamic stability, brief duration of action, but concern over adrenocortical depression
- **Ketamine (phencyclidine derivative)**: preservation of blood pressure and respiratory reflexes together with excellent analgesia makes it an ideal choice for field anaesthesia. Emergence delirium is associated with administration of ketamine

Rapid sequence induction (RSI) using a predetermined dose of intravenous anaesthetic agent together with a rapidly acting muscle relaxant is used in those with a high risk of regurgitation in order to secure the airway quickly. Commonly needed in emergency surgery, it is also a technique of choice in any non-emergency surgery in a patient with delayed emptying of the stomach.

Total intravenous anaesthesia (TIVA) is becoming popular following the introduction of propofol and the ultra-short-acting opioid remifentanil. The lack of cumulative effect, better haemodynamic stability, excellent recovery profile and concerns over environmental effects of inhalational agents have made TIVA an attractive choice. TIVA is routinely used in neurosurgery, airway laser surgery, during cardiopulmonary bypass and for day case anaesthesia.

Summary box 23.4

Special terms in anaesthesia

- RSI is a technique that allows the airway to be rapidly secured. It is used when there is a high risk of regurgitation that may lead to pulmonary aspiration
- TIVA is becoming increasingly popular

Maintenance of anaesthesia can be done using a continuous infusion of intravenous agent (propofol) or an inhaled vapour such as isoflurane, sevoflurane or desflurane.

The use of nitrous oxide is declining, despite its analgesic and weak anaesthetic properties, because of concerns over postoperative nausea and vomiting. It also increases the size of air bubbles, causing adverse effects, for example, in eye, ear and abdominal surgery. Finally it is possibly mutagenic and is a powerful greenhouse gas.

Management of the airway during anaesthesia

Loss of muscle tone as a result of general anaesthesia means that the patient can no longer keep their airway open. Therefore, patients need their airway to be maintained for them. The use of muscle relaxants will mean that they will also be unable to breathe for themselves and so will require artificial ventilation. Head tilt, chin lift and jaw thrust manoeuvres along with adjuncts such as oropharyngeal airways (***Figure 23.2***) are used to facilitate bag–mask ventilation while induction agents exert their full effect. A laryngeal mask airway or endotracheal tube is then inserted, and the patient is allowed to breathe spontaneously or is ventilated during the procedure.

The addition of a cuff to the endo-tracheal tube facilitates positive pressure ventilation and protects the lungs from aspiration of regurgitated gastric contents.

Supraglottic airways

- **Laryngeal mask airway (LMA)**. Developed by Dr Archie Brain in the UK, the original LMA® is a first-generation supraglottic airway. The mask with an inflatable cuff is inserted via the mouth and produces a seal around the glottic opening, providing a very reliable means of maintaining the airway. Its placement is less irritating and less traumatic to a patient's airway than endotracheal intubation. The technique can be easily taught to non-anaesthetists and paramedics and can be used as an emergency airway management tool. Several varieties of first-generation LMAs are available, including the classic LMA and the flexible LMA. Further advancements have led to the development of second-generation supraglottic devices, such as the ProSeal® LMA and the i-gel® (***Figure 23.3***). These devices usually have an in-built 'bite block' and oesophageal drain tube. They can be used for ventilation of the lungs at higher inflation pressures and are more suitable for patients with a higher body mass index. There are also modified versions of the LMA, including the ILMA (intubating LMA), that allow a blind technique, aiding insertion of a tracheal tube in difficult conditions. There is increasing evidence that second-generation devices have a good safety and efficacy profile and should be replacing all first-generation devices.
- **Difficult intubation**. Endotracheal intubation is feasible in most patients, but in a certain proportion of patients it may be difficult or impossible. However, if it is compounded by an inability to ventilate and therefore maintain oxygenation of the patient by bag–mask, the consequence can be catastrophic hypoxia. Many devices have been developed to aid intubation if difficulty is anticipated (e.g. McGrath® blade, Airtraq®, C-MAC® video laryngoscope) (***Figures 23.4 and 23.5***); similarly, protocols have been created by specialised societies to deal

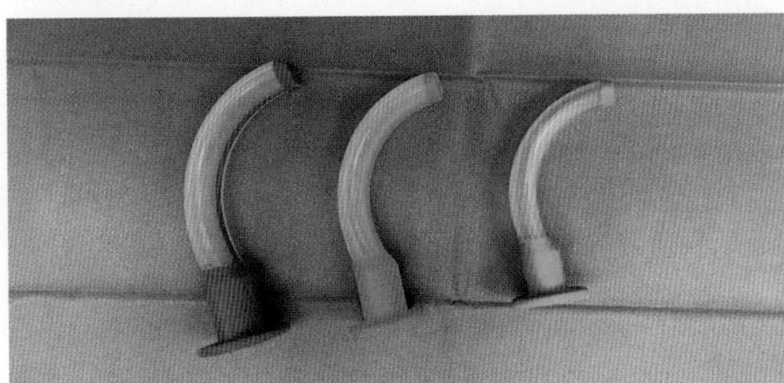

Figure 23.2 Oropharyngeal airways.

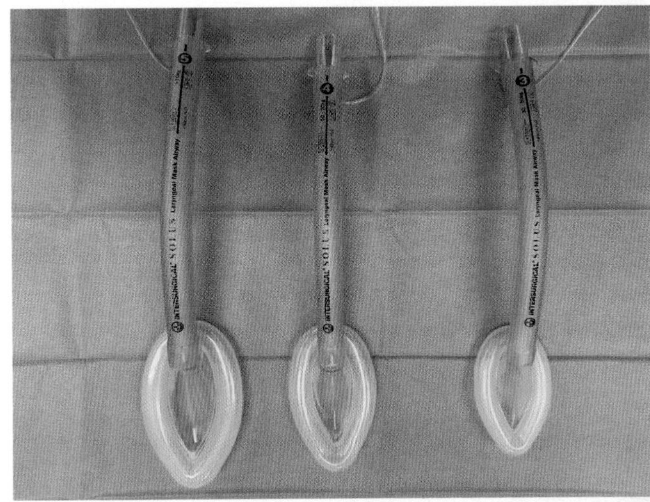

Figure 23.3 i-gel® supraglottic airway.

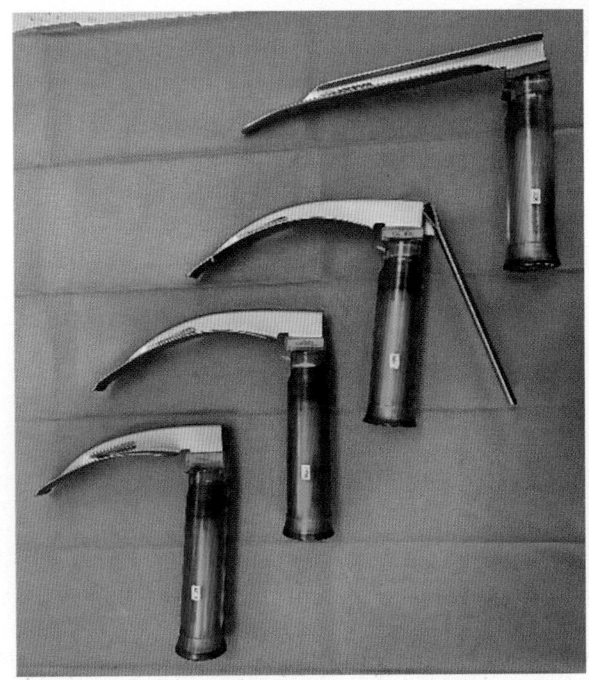

Figure 23.4 Single-use laryngoscope.

Archie Brain, b. 1942, formally an anaesthetist, whose patent application for the laryngeal mask airway was granted in 1982.

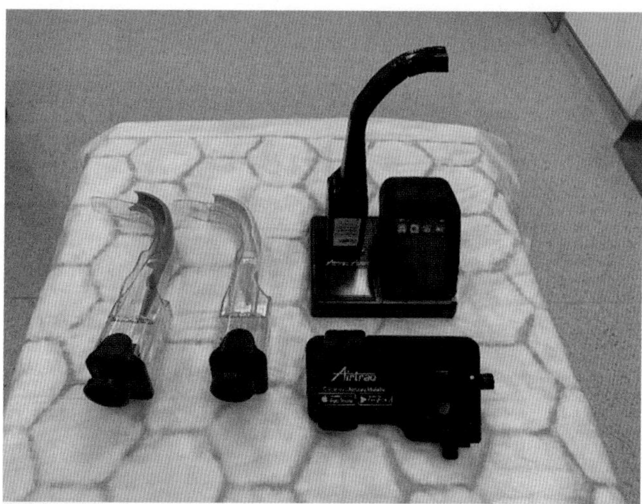

Figure 23.5 Airtraq® intubating device.

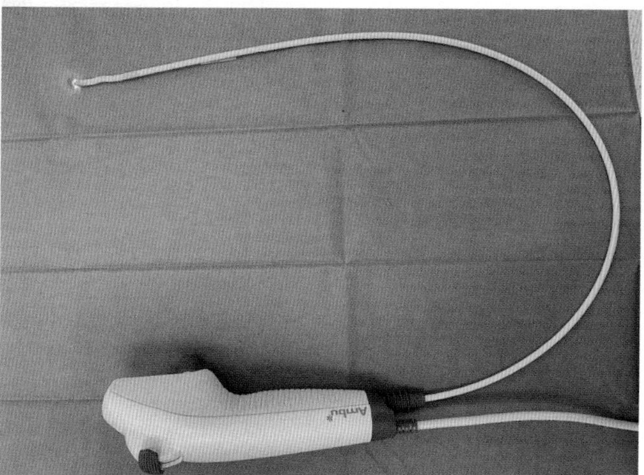

Figure 23.6 Fibreoptic intubating bronchoscope.

with such situations. One specialised method for intubation in difficult situations is the use of the fibreoptic intubating bronchoscope (*Figure 23.6*), facilitated by topical local anaesthetic in awake patients or using general anaesthesia. The anaesthetist places the endotracheal tube in the trachea by threading the tube over the bronchoscope, and so places the tube in the trachea under direct bronchoscopic vision. An awake intubation requires careful patient selection, as it may not be a suitable technique for all patient groups.

Double-lumen tubes and endobronchial tubes are used in procedures such as thoracoscopic, pulmonary and oesophageal surgery to allow collapse of one lung (while ventilating the other) for ease of surgery. Their use is also essential to isolate the healthy lung in empyema and in the case of a bronchopleural fistula.

Ventilating bronchoscopes and endobronchial catheters can be used to maintain oxygenation during laryngotracheal surgery or bronchoscopy by using intermittent jets of oxygen.

Summary box 23.5

Techniques for maintaining an airway

- Chin lift and jaw thrust: suitable for the short term when no aid is available
- Guedel airway: holds the tongue forward but does not prevent aspiration
- Supraglottic device: easy insertion, reliable airway, allows ventilation
- Endotracheal intubation: secure and protected airway

Summary box 23.6

Complications of intubation

- Failed intubation
- Accidental bronchial intubation
- Trauma to teeth, pharynx or larynx
- Aspiration of gastric contents during intubation
- Disconnection, blockage or kinking of tube
- Delayed tracheal stenosis

Muscle relaxation and artificial ventilation

Pharmacological blockade of neuromuscular transmission by neuromuscular blocking agents provides relaxation of muscles, allowing easy surgical access. However, the patient will need artificial ventilation. Neuromuscular blocking agents are broadly classified into depolarising and non-depolarising groups according to their mode of action (*Table 23.1*).

Suxamethonium is the most commonly used depolarising agent. It binds to the nicotinic acetylcholine receptors, resulting in opening of the cation channel, leading to depolarisation and rapid relaxation of muscles. Despite its adverse effects such as hyperkalaemia, muscle pain, anaphylaxis and potentially life-threatening malignant hyperthermia, suxamethonium is still widely used because of its quick onset and short duration of action. These properties are useful when rapid endotracheal intubation is necessary to protect the patient's airway or when short duration surgery is performed.

Non-depolarising muscle relaxants act by competitive blockade of postsynaptic receptors at the neuromuscular junction. They provide longer, predictable activity but require careful monitoring, appropriate timing and reversal of their action by agents such as neostigmine and sugammadex at the end of the procedure. A peripheral nerve stimulator is routinely used to monitor the depth of neuromuscular block and also to confirm satisfactory recovery of muscle power prior to extubation. With the increasing availability and evidence of the use of sugammadex, the non-depolarising muscle relaxant rocuronium is an alternative to suxamethonium in the 'rapid-sequence' induction as it allows reversal of its actions with sugammadex in a rapid manner.

Arthur Ernest Guedel, 1883–1956, Clinical Professor of Anesthesiology, University of Southern California, Los Angeles, CA, USA.

TABLE 23.1 Properties of commonly used muscle relaxants

	Advantages	Disadvantages
Suxamethonium	• Quickest onset, very short duration, spontaneous recovery • Ideal for rapid intubation and for short procedures	• Muscle pain, hyperkalaemia, prolonged apnoea and life-threatening malignant hyperthermia
Vecuronium	• Long acting • Minimal cardiovascular effect and less allergic reaction	• Dependent on hepatic metabolism and renal clearance; hence, caution if hepatic and renal impairment
Atracurium	• Intermediate acting • Non-enzymatic Hofmann degradation • Suitable in renal and hepatic failure	• Histamine release and allergic reactions
Rocuronium	• Rapid onset, intermediate action • Suitable for rapid intubation • Rapid reversal possible using sugammadex	• Allergic reactions • Excreted unchanged via bile and urine

Ventilation during anaesthesia

Mechanical ventilation is required when the patient's spontaneous ventilation is inadequate or when the patient is not breathing because of the effects of the anaesthetic, analgesic agents or muscle relaxants.

In volume control ventilation, a preset volume is delivered by the machine irrespective of the airway pressure. The pressure generated will be, in part, dependent on the resistance and compliance of the airway. In laparoscopic surgery requiring the Trendelenburg position (the patient is positioned head down), morbidly obese patients and those with lung disease, this may result in excessive pressures being developed, which may lead to barotrauma (pneumothorax).

In pressure control mode the ventilator generates flow until a preset pressure is reached. The actual tidal volume delivered is variable and depends on airway resistance, intra-abdominal pressure and the degree of relaxation.

Positive end-expiratory pressure (PEEP) is often applied to help maintain functional residual capacity. This avoids lung collapse by opening collapsed alveoli and maintains a greater area of gas exchange, so reducing vascular shunting.

Monitoring and care during anaesthesia

A minimum basic monitoring of cardiovascular parameters is required during surgery. This includes:

- vascular
  - electrocardiogram (ECG);
  - blood pressure;
- adequacy of ventilation:
  - inspired oxygen concentration;
  - oxygen saturation by pulse oximetry;
  - end-tidal carbon dioxide concentration.

Monitors of temperature, ventilation parameters and delivery of anaesthetic agents are also routinely used, while measurement of urine output and central venous pressure are recommended for major surgery.

Summary box 23.7

Intermittent positive-pressure ventilation

- Volume controlled, which ensures adequate gas entry but risks high-pressure damage
- Pressure controlled, which avoids high-pressure damage but risks inadequate ventilation
- PEEP reduces alveolar collapse and reduces vascular shunting so improving perfusion

LOCAL ANAESTHESIA

Local anaesthetic drugs (***Table 23.2***) may be used to provide anaesthesia and analgesia, as a sole agent or as adjuncts to general anaesthesia. Available techniques include topical anaesthesia, local infiltration, regional nerve blocks and central neuraxial blocks (spinal and epidural anaesthesia).

TABLE 23.2 The common local anaesthetic drugs.

Name	Maximum dose	Comments
Lidocaine	3 mg/kg (7 mg/kg with adrenaline [epinephrine])	Early onset, short acting, good sensory block
Bupivacaine	2 mg/kg	Long lasting, more cardiotoxic, must never be used intravenously
Prilocaine	6 mg/kg (9 mg/kg with adrenaline)	Least systemic toxicity, causes methaemoglobinaemia
Ropivacaine	3–4 mg/kg	Less cardiotoxic, greater sensory–motor separation
Levobupivacaine	2 mg/kg	Isomer of bupivacaine with fewer cardiotoxic properties

Local anaesthesia techniques can lead to complications that may be local, such as infection or haematoma, or systemic, as a result of overdose or accidental intravascular injection.

Friedrich Trendelenburg, 1844–1924, successively Professor of Surgery at Rostock (1875–1882), Bonn (1822–1895) and Leipzig (1895–1911), Germany. The Trendelenburg position was first described in 1885.

The systemic effects of local anaesthetic agents are dose dependent and manifest as cardiovascular (cardiac arrhythmia, cardiac arrest) or neurological (depressed consciousness, convulsions). Prilocaine overdose causes methaemoglobinaemia, whereas bupivacaine overdose causes treatment-resistant ventricular arrhythmia and cardiac arrest.

The addition of adrenaline (epinephrine) to local anaesthetic solutions hastens onset, prolongs the duration of action and permits a higher upper dose limit. The use of adrenaline is contraindicated in patients with cardiovascular disease, those taking tricyclic and monoamine oxidase inhibitors and in end-arterial locations.

Appropriately skilled personnel, resuscitation equipment and oxygen should always be available with local anaesthetic use because of the potential risks of life-threatening complications.

Regional anaesthesia

Regional anaesthesia involves central neuraxial or peripheral nerve or plexus blocks using local anaesthetic drugs. It has a clear advantage when general anaesthesia carries a higher risk of morbidity and mortality, such as in patients with debilitating respiratory and cardiovascular disease and obstetric cases. It also provides excellent pain relief in the postoperative period, reducing the need for analgesics such as opioids.

As with general anaesthesia, venous access should be established and vital parameters should be monitored during regional anaesthesia.

Localising nerves using anatomical landmarks and eliciting paraesthesia alone carries a high risk of nerve damage and intravascular injection and has a lower success rate. The use of nerve stimulators to localise nerves improves the success rate and reduces risks. Ultrasound-guided regional anaesthesia allows the visualisation of nerves and the spread of local anaesthetics, enabling the use of a smaller dose of local anaesthetic agents with improved success rates and safety.

Summary box 23.8

Types of anaesthesia

- General anaesthesia may be more acceptable to patients
- Regional anaesthesia has major advantages in obstetrics and patients with respiratory compromise
- Local blocks have been transformed by nerve stimulators and ultrasound guidance
- All require full resuscitation and monitoring equipment to be available

Common local anaesthesia techniques

Topical anaesthesia

- **EMLA (eutectic mixture of local anaesthetics).** This is a mixture of lidocaine and prilocaine for application to the skin for venepuncture in children.
- **Cocaine.** It may be called Moffett's solution (with an added mixture of adrenaline and sodium bicarbonate) and used in nasal surgery for anaesthesia and vasoconstriction.
- **Lidocaine 2/4/10%.** Spray to anaesthetise the airway during awake fibreoptic intubation.

Nerve blocks

An interscalene approach to brachial plexus for shoulder surgery produces excellent postoperative analgesia. Complications include phrenic nerve block, Horner's syndrome and accidental intravascular and spinal injection. Supraclavicular, infraclavicular or axillary approaches to the brachial plexus can be used as the sole anaesthetic technique for upper limb surgery (***Figure 23.7***). Femoral and sciatic nerve blocks are often used for anaesthesia and analgesia for lower limb surgery.

Local anaesthetic blocks have been described that block the nerves closer to the joint so that motor blockade of the whole lower limb can be minimised. An example of this type of block is the iPACK (infiltration between the popliteal artery and capsule of the knee) block, which targets the genicular nerves supplying the knee joint by using ultrasound-guided injection posterior to the knee joint.

Transversus abdominis plane/quadratus lumborum and erector spinae plane block are examples of fascial plane blocks, which have grown rapidly in popularity. Local anaesthetic is injected in the fascial planes containing the nerves from abdominal or chest wall structures. Transversus abdominis plane (TAP) block has been claimed to provide effective

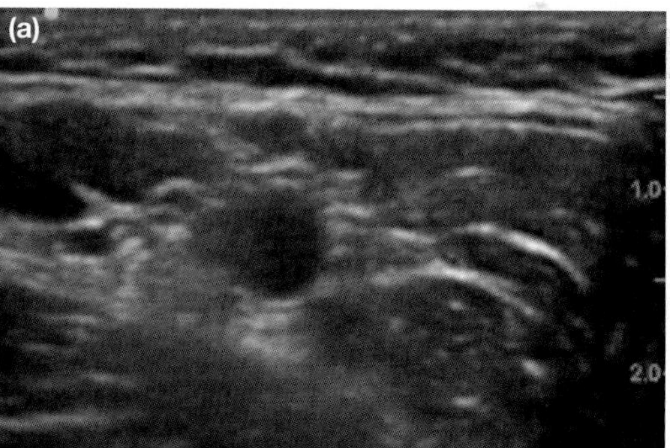

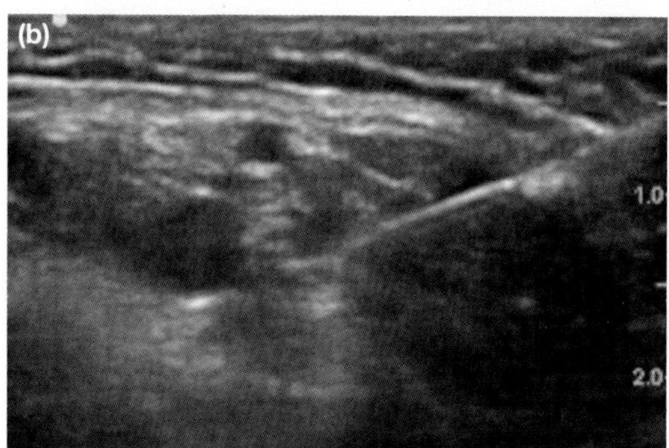

Figure 23.7 (a, b) Ultrasonic picture of brachial plexus block.

Johann Friedrich Horner, 1831–1886, Professor of Ophthalmology, Zurich, Switzerland, described this syndrome in 1869.
Major A. J. Moffett of the Royal Army Medical Corps first described its use in 1941. He modified it in 1946 to include 2 mL of 8% cocaine, 2 mL of 1% sodium bicarbonate, and 1 mL of 1:1000 adrenaline.

analgesia after a wide range of abdominal surgery. The T6–L1 segmental nerves enter the plane between the internal oblique muscle and the transverse abdominis muscle just medial to the anterior axillary line. Injection of local anaesthetic into the fascial plane between the internal oblique and transversus abdominis muscles allows a block of all these nerves, and excellent anaesthesia of the anterior abdominal wall. Quadratus lumborum block also aims to target abdominal nerves as they pass in front of the quadratus lumborum muscle. Erector spinae block aims to block the spinal nerves at various sites, depending on the site of injection. Local anaesthetic is deposited underneath the erector spinae group of muscles as they lie over the transverse process of the vertebra.

Intravenous regional anaesthesia (Bier's block)

Bier's block produces excellent anaesthesia for short surgery, particularly for the upper limb (e.g. carpal tunnel release). In this technique local anaesthetic is injected intravenously to produce anaesthesia of the upper limb. A double tourniquet is used on the side of surgery. An intravenous cannula is sited into a vein on the back of the hand on the side that is being operated on. The upper limb is then exsanguinated using an Esmarch bandage. The proximal cuff of the double tourniquet is inflated, followed by intravenous injection of prilocaine into the cannula. After 20 minutes the distal cuff of the tourniquet is inflated and then the proximal cuff is deflated. Even if surgery is finished, the tourniquet should be left inflated until the local anaesthetic has bound to tissues (20 minutes) so that release of local anaesthetic into the systemic circulation does not occur. Lidocaine can be used with caution (consider the safe dose of lidocaine and the time of tourniquet inflation) but bupivacaine should never be used for Bier's block.

Spinal anaesthesia

Spinal anaesthesia alone or in combination with general anaesthesia or sedation is used extensively for lower limb, obstetric and pelvic surgery. Injection of a 'single-shot' local anaesthetic agent intrathecally produces intense and rapid block for surgery. The addition of opioids provides prolonged postoperative analgesia but carries the risk of late respiratory depression.

Autonomic sympathetic blockade produces hypotension, particularly if the level of block is above the T10 spinal dermatome. Caution is needed in patients with hypovolaemia and cardiovascular disease.

The incidence of dural puncture headache can be minimised by limiting the number of punctures and using fine-bore pencil-tip needles that are designed to split rather than cut the dura.

Epidural anaesthesia

Epidural anaesthesia is slower in onset than spinal but has the advantage of prolonged analgesia by multiple dosing or continuous infusion through a catheter placed in the epidural space. Being slower in onset, the resulting hypotension from sympathetic blockade can be better controlled and can reduce blood loss.

Continuous infusion (with a patient-controlled bolus) of weak local anaesthetic combined with opioids (such as fentanyl) is routinely used for postoperative analgesia. Placement of an epidural catheter in the high thoracic region provides excellent analgesia for a wide variety of upper abdominal and thoracic surgical operations, enabling early mobilisation and reducing respiratory complications.

Epidural anaesthesia is technically more difficult than spinal anaesthesia; it has a higher failure rate and carries the risk of nerve damage, spinal injuries, accidental spinal injection of a large volume of local anaesthetic, infection and epidural haematoma.

Summary box 23.9

Local anaesthetics

- EMLA cream for children needing injections
- Regional and nerve blocks for limb surgery
- Spinal anaesthesia offers a quick onset and a short duration of anaesthesia
- Epidurals are more difficult but can then be topped up postoperatively and used as a continuous infusion

PAIN

Pain is defined as 'An unpleasant sensory and emotional experience associated with, or resembling that associated with, actual or potential tissue damage.' Most patients will experience pain after surgery. This is usually managed by a combination of painkillers and local anaesthetic techniques (multimodal analgesia). The common painkillers that are used are regular paracetamol, non-steroidal anti-inflammatory drugs (NSAIDs) and opioids. Opioids can be weak, such as codeine, or stronger opioids, such as morphine and oxycodone. Opioids are associated with a high incidence of side effects (nausea and vomiting, respiratory depression, itching). By combining opioids with other drugs, the dose of opioid can be minimised, thus side effects can be reduced.

Paracetamol and non-steroidal anti-inflammatory drugs

Paracetamol was first synthesised in 1878 by Morse and was introduced for medical usage in 1883. However, because of misinterpretation of its safety profile, its use was limited until the 1950s, when the chemically similar, and until then preferred analgesic, phenacetin was withdrawn owing to renal toxicity. Paracetamol is probably now the most commonly used drug worldwide; it is available over the counter, used in almost all ages and forms step 1 of the WHO analgesic ladder. It is first-line treatment for pyrexia and pain, plays an important role in multimodal analgesia and is considered to possess a generally excellent safety profile, except in significant overdose, with only a few drug interactions. Oral and rectal administration can produce analgesia within 40 minutes, with maximal effect at

August Karl Gustav Bier, 1861–1949, Professor of Surgery, Bonn (1903–1907) and Berlin (1907–1932), Germany.

1 hour, but because of variability in bioavailabilities (in the range 63–89% for oral and 24–98% for rectally administered preparations) the timing of onset can be unpredictable. The introduction of its intravenously administered preparation within the last decade overcomes this issue.

NSAIDs are used in the treatment of acute pain for their opioid-sparing effects, as part of a multimodal analgesic regimen. However, it is important to recognise that long-term usage and an increase in prescription may be associated with significant morbidities. Increased risk of perioperative bleeding, gastrointestinal bleeding and ulceration, thrombotic events such as myocardial infarction and stroke, renal impairment, fluid retention and exacerbation of asthma are some of the side effects of NSAIDs, suggesting cautious usage.

Intravenous opioids administered as patient-controlled analgesia (PCA) for pain relief is a useful technique. The patient is trained to give a bolus dose of drug by pressing a control button on a machine, the functions of which have been regulated by medical staff. The strength, frequency and total dose of drug in a given time are all limited by computer. This method is popular with patients as they have control and prevents delays in administration of doses.

Chronic pain

Chronic pain is defined as pain that persists or recurs for more than 3 months. In chronic pain syndromes, pain can be the sole or a leading complaint and requires special treatment and care. This could be 'chronic primary pain', which may be conceived of as a disease in its own right, for example in conditions such as fibromyalgia or non-specific low-back pain. In six other subgroups, pain is secondary to an underlying disease: chronic cancer-related pain, chronic neuropathic pain, chronic secondary visceral pain, chronic post-traumatic and postsurgical pain, chronic secondary headache and orofacial pain and chronic secondary musculoskeletal pain. These conditions are summarised as 'chronic secondary pain', in which pain may at least initially be conceived as a symptom.

In surgical practice, patients with chronic pain may present for treatment of the cause (e.g. pancreatitis, malignancy) or concomitant benign pathology. Almost 50 years ago, using gate theory, Melzeck and Wall proposed pain to be not only subjective but also a multidimensional experience that incorporates sensory/discriminative, motivational/affect and cognitive aspects. Recent guidance from the International Association for the Study of Pain highlights that the multidimensional aspect is one of the key components, hence the treatment of chronic pain involves a multidisciplinary multimodal approach.

Mechanistically, chronic pain may be classified into:

- **Nociceptive pain**, which may result from musculoskeletal disorders or cancer activating cutaneous nociceptors (pain receptors). Prolonged ischaemic or inflammatory processes result in sensitisation of peripheral nociceptors and altered activity in the central nervous system, leading to exaggerated responses in the dorsal horn of the spinal cord. The widened area of hyperalgesia and increased sensitivity (allodynia) have been attributed to increased transmission in the central nervous system.
- **Neuropathic (or neurogenic) pain** is dysfunction in the peripheral or central nerves (excluding the 'physiological' pain due to noxious stimulation of the nerve terminals). It is classically of a 'burning', 'shooting' or 'stabbing' type and may be associated with allodynia, numbness and diminished thermal sensation. It is poorly responsive to opioids. Examples include trigeminal neuralgia, postherpetic neuropathy and diabetic neuropathy.

Principles of chronic pain management

Non-pharmacological treatment

This involves a multidisciplinary approach targeting the biopsychosocial model of health (***Figure 23.8***). Early assessment and engagement with physiotherapy and exercise are key contributors in successful management. Psychological interventions such as counselling, cognitive behaviour therapy and mindfulness are recognised strategies for pain control. 'Pain management programmes' lay out a logical structure for this.

Pharmacological treatment

Drugs in chronic non-malignant pain

Paracetamol and NSAIDs are the mainstays of musculoskeletal pain treatment. The tricyclic antidepressant drugs and anticonvulsant agents are often useful for the pain of nerve injury, although side effects can prove troublesome and reduce compliance. Both pregabalin and gabapentin reduce spontaneous neuronal activity by their action on the $\alpha_2\delta$ subunit of the calcium channel. They are now routinely used for managing neuropathic chronic pain. In more severe and debilitating non-malignant chronic pain, opioid analgesic drugs are used in slow release oral preparations (morphine and oxycodone) and transcutaneous patches (fentanyl and buprenorphine).

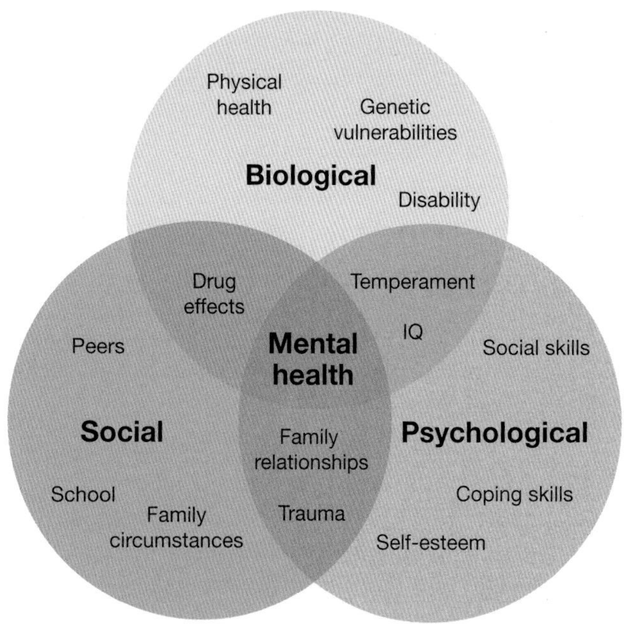

Figure 23.8 Biopsychosocial model of health.

Summary box 23.10

Commonly used terms in chronic pain

Term	Definition
Allodynia	Pain due to a stimulus that does not normally provoke pain. Allodynia involves a change in the quality of a sensation, whether tactile, thermal or of any other sort
Analgesia	Absence of pain in response to stimulation that would normally be painful
Central sensitisation	Increased responsiveness of nociceptive neurones in the central nervous system to their normal or subthreshold afferent input. The net effect is that innocuous stimuli will be interpreted as painful
Epidural space	The space (or potential space) between the ligamentum flavum (or vertebral wall) and the dura, just outside the spinal canal, extending from the foramen magnum to the sacrum. Leads and catheters may be placed in this space via a needle
Hyperalgesia	Abnormally heightened sensitivity to pain. For pain evoked by stimuli that usually are not painful, the term allodynia is preferred, while hyperalgesia is more appropriately used for cases with an increased response at a normal threshold or at an increased threshold
Hypoalgesia	Decreased sensitivity to painful stimuli. Hypoalgesia can be caused by exogenous chemicals such as opioids, as well as by chemicals produced by the body in phenomena such as fear- and exercise-induced hypoalgesia
Intrathecal space	The cerebrospinal fluid-filled space around the spinal cord, protected by the dura mater, into which certain medicines may be delivered to achieve their most potent effect
Nociception	Sensory response to certain harmful or potentially harmful stimuli. Nociception triggers a variety of biological and behavioural responses and may also result in a subjective experience of pain
Neuropathic pain	Neuropathic pain is defined as pain caused by a lesion or disease of the somatosensory nervous system
Nociceptive pain	Pain that arises from actual or threatened damage to non-neural tissue and that is due to the activation of nociceptors
Noxious stimulus	An actual or potential tissue-damaging event
Off-label	When a prescription drug is prescribed for uses other than what Australia's Therapeutic Goods Administration, the USA's Food and Drug Administration or the UK's Medicines and Healthcare products Regulatory Agency has approved and published in the drug's package insert
Pain	An unpleasant sensory and emotional experience associated with actual or potential tissue damage, or described in terms of such damage
Pain threshold	The minimum amount of a stimulus with which pain begins to be felt. It is an entirely subjective phenomenon
Paraesthesia	Abnormal cutaneous sensations such as tingling, tickling, pricking or burning with no apparent physical cause. Often described as 'pins and needles' or of a limb 'falling asleep'
Peripheral neuropathic pain	Pain caused by a lesion or disease of the peripheral somatosensory nervous system

Tapentadol, with its dual action on the opioid and noradrenaline (norepinephrine) selective reuptake inhibition pathway, may provide relief in patients with both a neuropathic and nociceptive element to their pain. Combinations of drugs often prove useful to achieve the optimum of efficacy with minimal side effects.

Treatment of pain dependent on sympathetic nervous system activity

Even minor trauma and surgery (often of a limb) can provoke excessive sympathetic adrenergic activity, inducing vasoconstriction and abnormal nociceptive transmission. This can lead to chronic burning pain, allodynia, trophic changes and resultant disuse.

Management includes antineuropathic pain medications (pregabalin, gabapentin, amitriptyline) as part of multimodal analgesia with a multidisciplinary pain management approach. This includes considerable input from psychological services and targeted physiotherapy. Interventional treatment may include local anaesthetic injection of the stellate ganglion for upper limb symptoms. Percutaneous chemical lumbar sympathectomy with local anaesthetic is used for relief of rest pain in advanced ischaemic disease of the legs.

Interventional pain management for chronic pain

Local anaesthetic and steroid injections can be effective around an inflamed nerve and they reduce the cycle of constant pain transmission with consequent muscle spasm. Transforaminal selective root blocks in the epidural space are used for the pain of nerve root irritation associated with or without minor disc prolapse, followed by active physiotherapy and rehabilitation to promote mobility.

Nerve stimulation procedures such as acupuncture and transcutaneous nerve stimulation increase endorphin production in the central nervous system. Nerve decompression craniotomy rather than percutaneous coagulation of the ganglion is now performed for trigeminal neuralgia.

Spinal cord stimulation (SCS) by dorsal column stimulation is now a recognised and effective management of intractable neuropathic pain (***Figure 23.9***). This involves placement of electrodes in the posterior epidural space to allow dorsal column stimulation through an implantable pulse generator inserted in the body. In the UK this has been recommended by National Institute for Health and Care Excellence (NICE) guidance for intractable neuropathic pain management. Robust evidence exists for its clinical and health economic benefit in failed back surgery syndrome, in which patients have undergone previous spinal surgery. Early use of SCS in surgery-naive patients might lead to better outcomes. National guidelines in the UK do not recommend disc replacements or spinal fusions in patients with lower back pain unless the latter are part of a trial, rendering a large part of the patient population ineligible for surgery. In these instances, SCS could prove to be an effective solution.

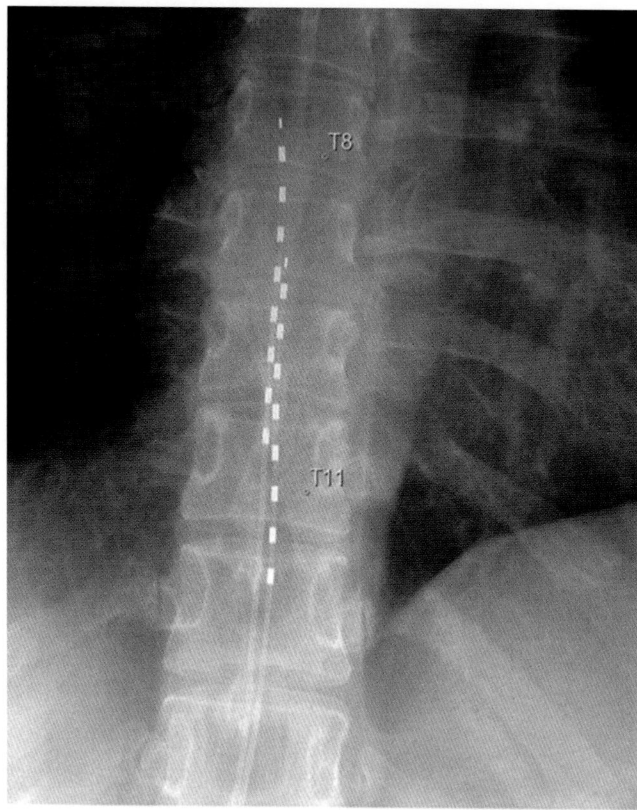

Figure 23.9 Dual-lead spinal cord stimulator in the epidural space.

Pain control in malignant disease

Pain is a common symptom associated with cancer, even more so during the advanced stages. In intractable pain, the underlying principle of treatment is to encourage independence of the patient and an active life in spite of the symptom. WHO advises use of the 'WHO analgesic ladder':

- first step: simple analgesics – paracetamol, NSAIDs, tricyclic drugs or anticonvulsant drugs;
- second step: intermediate-strength opioids – codeine, tramadol;
- third step: strong opioids – morphine (pethidine has now been withdrawn).

Oral opiate analgesia is necessary when the less powerful analgesic agents no longer control pain on movement or enable the patient to sleep. Opioids may exhibit both dependence and addiction with long-term use. It is important to distinguish between addiction and dependence; the former is a psychosocial phenomenon whereas the latter is a purely physiological response to a given drug. Some patients experience 'breakthrough pain' (acute, excruciating and incapacitating), which occurs either spontaneously or in relation to a specific predictable or unpredictable trigger experienced by patients who have relatively stable and adequately controlled background pain. Opioid rotation or switching may be considered if a patient obtains pain relief with one opioid and has severe adverse effects.

Oral morphine, which is often used for chronic pain, can be prescribed in short-acting liquid or tablet form and should be administered regularly every 4 hours until an adequate dose of drug has been titrated to control the pain over 24 hours. Once this is established, the daily dose can be divided into two separate administrations of enteric-coated, slow-release morphine tablets (MST morphine) every 12 hours. Additional short-acting opioids (morphine/fentanyl) can then be used to cover episodes of 'breakthrough pain'. Nausea treated using antiemetic agents does not usually persist, but constipation is a frequent and persistent complication requiring regular prevention by laxatives.

Infusion of subcutaneous, intravenous, intrathecal or epidural opiate drugs

The infusion of an opiate is necessary if a patient is unable to take oral drugs. Subcutaneous infusion of diamorphine is effective and simple to administer. Epidural infusions of diamorphine with an external pump can be used in mobile patients. Intrathecal infusions with pumps programmed by external computers are used; however, there is a possibility of the patient developing an infection with catastrophic effects. Intravenous narcotic agents may be reserved for acute crises, such as pathological fractures.

Neurolytic techniques in cancer pain

These should only be used if life expectancy is limited and the diagnosis is certain. The useful procedures are:

- subcostal phenol injection for a rib metastasis;
- coeliac plexus neurolytic block with alcohol for the pain caused by pancreatic, gastric or hepatic cancer;
- intrathecal neurolytic injection of hyperbaric phenol;

- percutaneous anterolateral cordotomy to divide the spinothalamic ascending pain pathway; this is a highly effective technique in experienced hands, selectively eliminating pain and temperature sensation in a specific limited area.

Alternative strategies include:

- the development of anti-pituitary hormone drugs, such as tamoxifen and cyproterone, has enabled effective pharmacological therapy for the pain of widespread metastases instead of pituitary ablation surgery;
- palliative radiotherapy can be most beneficial for the relief of pain in metastatic disease; adjuvant drugs such as corticosteroids to reduce cerebral oedema or inflammation around a tumour, which may be useful in symptom control; tricyclic antidepressants, anticonvulsants and flecainide are also used to reduce the pain of nerve injury.

Summary box 23.11

Approximate equianalgesic potencies of opioids for oral administration

	Potency	Equivalent dose to 10 mg oral morphine
Codeine phosphate	0.1	100 mg
Dihydrocodeine	0.1	100 mg
Hydromorphone	5	2 mg
Morphine	1	10 mg
Oxycodone	1.5	6.6 mg
Tapentadol	0.4	100 mg

Adapted from the British National Formulary.

FURTHER READING

Chou R, Gordon DB, de Leon-Casasola OA *et al.* Management of postoperative pain: a clinical practice guideline from the American Pain Society, the American Society of Regional Anesthesia and Pain Medicine, and the American Society of Anesthesiologists' Committee on Regional Anesthesia, Executive Committee, and Administrative Council. *J Pain* 2016; **17**(2): 131–57.

Dansie EJ, Turk DC. Assessment of patients with chronic pain. *Br J Anaesth* 2013; **111**(1): 19–25.

Frerk C, Mitchell VS, McNarry AF *et al.* Difficult Airway Society 2015 guidelines for management of unanticipated difficult intubation in adults. *Br J Anaesth* 2015; **115**(6): 827–48.

McLeod GA, McCartney CGL, Wildsmith JAW. *Wildsmith and Armitage's principles and practice of regional anaesthesia*, 4th edn. Oxford: Oxford University Press, 2012.

Rawal N (ed.). *Management of acute and chronic pain.* London: BMJ Books, 1998.

Sneyd JR. Recent advances in intravenous anaesthesia. *Br J Anaesth* 2004; **93**(5): 725–36.

Thompson J, Moppett I, Wiles M. *Smith and Aitkenhead's textbook of anaesthesia*, 7th edn. Edinburgh: Elsevier, 2019.

CHAPTER 24 Postoperative care including perioperative optimisation

Learning objectives

To understand:

- The integrated approach to caring for patients in the perioperative period
- Common postoperative problems seen in the immediate postoperative period
- How to predict, recognise, prevent and treat common postoperative complications
- The principles of enhanced recovery

INTRODUCTION

Perioperative care is integrated care delivered to the patient by a multidisciplinary team before, during and after surgery.

The multidisciplinary perioperative team comprises doctors from various specialties, such as surgery, anaesthesia, acute medicine, care of the elderly and cardiology, along with nurses, physiotherapists and occupational therapists. The aim of this is to bring together the patient and the care team in the perioperative period to improve the patient's outcome and reduce healthcare-related costs. The input from the multidisciplinary team will vary depending on the medical condition of the patient and the complexity of the surgery.

Many patients coming for surgery will have long-term health problems that are at risk of worsening in the perioperative period. The time period between a decision to operate and the actual surgery can be used by the perioperative team to risk assess the patient and identify medical problems and treat them accordingly to ensure an optimal medical state prior to surgery. This will stop deterioration in long-term health problems perioperatively and will prevent a delay in discharge. Risk assessment may involve simple blood tests to identify health problems, e.g. heart or renal failure, or more sophisticated tests, such as cardiopulmonary exercise testing (CPET), to assess the patient's level of fitness. Providing high-quality care during surgery is essential and expected. Preventing harm by medical errors is also important. Checklists, such as the World Health Organization's (WHO) 'Surgical Safety Checklist', are now routinely used to prevent surgical errors. Postoperative pain can delay the patient's recovery, increase the risk of chest complications and chronic pain and contribute to a poor patient experience. A well-trained perioperative team led by an anaesthetist can develop a plan for managing pain.

Increasingly patients are coming for surgery with complex medical problems that require management from the multidisciplinary team of physicians. This role is now taken over by anaesthetists as they have a better understanding of complications occurring in the perioperative setting.

After complex surgery, many patients will need more intensive monitoring of their physiological parameters than is possible on a normal surgical ward, but they do not necessarily need all of the facilities available on an intensive care unit. In such a case, patients are admitted for a period of 24–48 hours to an 'overnight intensive recovery unit' or 'postanaesthesia care unit' (PACU), where this facility can be provided. After this time period patients are transferred to either a surgical ward or critical care unit depending on how they are recovering from surgery or according to the level of cardiac or respiratory support they need.

Hospital beds are a finite and expensive resource. The beds can be utilised efficiently if the patient can be discharged home quickly and safely. Good communication between hospital and care givers in the community will facilitate a smooth transition to home.

PREHABILITATION

The functional capacity of a patient can be reduced following major surgery. This can have a significant negative impact on the recovery of patients with poor functional reserve prior to surgery. Prehabilitation is a process of improving the functional capacity of patients prior to major surgery in order to improve postoperative outcomes.

The time period between the decision to operate and the surgery date itself is used for prehabilitation. The patient is medically optimised by asking them to, for example, stop smoking, reduce their alcohol intake or lose weight. Anaemia should be treated and blood sugar can be effectively controlled in patients with diabetes during this period. Existing medication should be reviewed and modified if necessary to better control

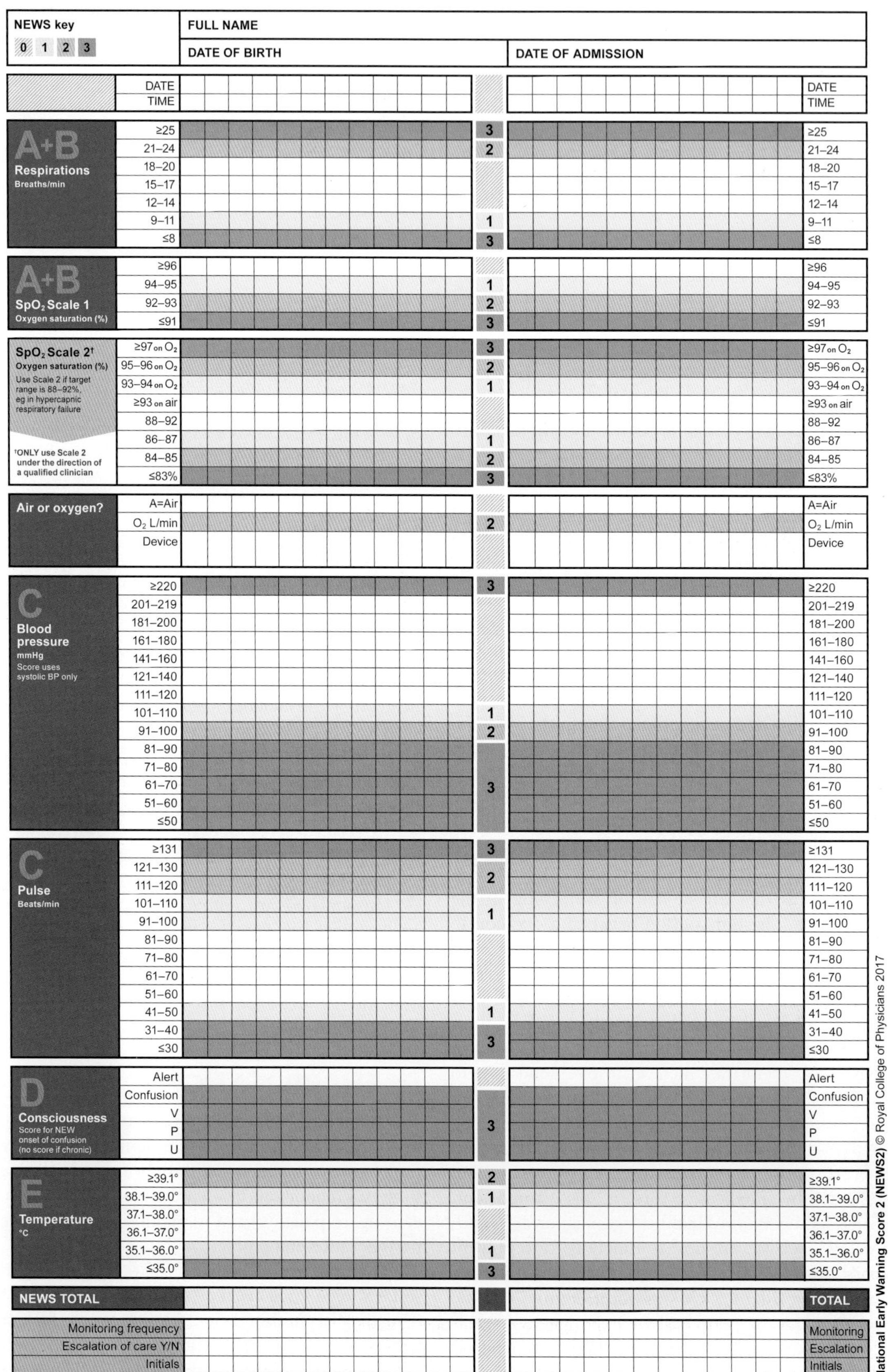

NEWS key: 0 1 2 3

FULL NAME

DATE OF BIRTH | DATE OF ADMISSION

Parameter	Value	Score
	DATE / TIME	
A+B Respirations Breaths/min	≥25	3
	21–24	2
	18–20	
	15–17	
	12–14	
	9–11	1
	≤8	3
A+B SpO₂ Scale 1 Oxygen saturation (%)	≥96	
	94–95	1
	92–93	2
	≤91	3
SpO₂ Scale 2† Oxygen saturation (%) Use Scale 2 if target range is 88–92%, eg in hypercapnic respiratory failure. †ONLY use Scale 2 under the direction of a qualified clinician	≥97 on O_2	3
	95–96 on O_2	2
	93–94 on O_2	1
	≥93 on air	
	88–92	
	86–87	1
	84–85	2
	≤83%	3
Air or oxygen?	A=Air	
	O_2 L/min	2
	Device	
C Blood pressure mmHg Score uses systolic BP only	≥220	3
	201–219	
	181–200	
	161–180	
	141–160	
	121–140	
	111–120	
	101–110	1
	91–100	2
	81–90	3
	71–80	3
	61–70	3
	51–60	3
	≤50	3
C Pulse Beats/min	≥131	3
	121–130	2
	111–120	2
	101–110	1
	91–100	1
	81–90	
	71–80	
	61–70	
	51–60	
	41–50	1
	31–40	3
	≤30	3
D Consciousness Score for NEW onset of confusion (no score if chronic)	Alert	
	Confusion	3
	V	3
	P	3
	U	3
E Temperature °C	≥39.1°	2
	38.1–39.0°	1
	37.1–38.0°	
	36.1–37.0°	
	35.1–36.0°	1
	≤35.0°	3
NEWS TOTAL		
	Monitoring frequency	
	Escalation of care Y/N	
	Initials	

National Early Warning Score 2 (NEWS2) © Royal College of Physicians 2017

Figure 24.1 An example of an early warning system using patient observations: the National Early Warning System (NEWS) from the Royal College of Physicians. (Reproduced from Royal College of Physicians. *National Early Warning Score (NEWS) 2: Standardising the assessment of acute-illness severity in the NHS*. Updated report of a working party. London: RCP, 2017.)

chronic health conditions such as diabetes, asthma and hypertension. Functional capacity can be assessed formally using either CPET or the 6-minute walk test. Patients should be encouraged to undertake strength and aerobic exercises in formal programmes or as far as possible to improve their physical fitness. A poor preoperative nutritional state leads to poorer outcomes, and correcting nutritional imbalances will help the recovery of the patient. Psychological interventions to reduce anxiety prior to surgery and improve the patient's motivation to recover after surgery will benefit the patient greatly.

Preoperative assessment, including assessment of high-risk surgical patients, has been covered in ***Chapter 21***. Anaesthesia and pain relief has been covered in ***Chapter 23***.

The postoperative phase begins at the end of surgery when the patient is transferred to 'recovery' or 'PACU'. At the end of surgery, a 'sign out' is performed as part of the WHO checklist. The theatre team should then formally hand over the care of the patient to the PACU staff. The information provided should include the patient's name and age, the surgical procedure, the anaesthetic and analgesics given, fluid replacement, blood loss, urine output, any surgical/anaesthetic problems encountered or expected, existing medical problems and allergies. A plan for the management of pain and nausea or vomiting should also be conveyed.

POSTOPERATIVE OBSERVATIONS

The patient's vital signs (including pulse, blood pressure and pulse oximetry reading), level of consciousness, pain and hydration status are monitored in the recovery room and supportive treatment is given. In recent years, patient observations have been collated in recording systems designed to provide an early warning of clinical deterioration (***Figure 24.1***). The recording of observations as an 'early warning system' begins in recovery and is continued on the ward until the patient is discharged from the hospital.

The following six simple physiological parameters, which are routinely measured, are used to calculate the score:

1 respiration rate;
2 oxygen saturation;
3 systolic blood pressure;
4 pulse rate;
5 level of consciousness or new-onset confusion, disorientation and/or agitation;
6 temperature.

Each measured parameter is allocated a score depending on how much it varies from a normal value. Two points are added if the patient needs supplemental oxygen. The score is then aggregated. An aggregate score places patients in different risk categories (low to high risk) that trigger an appropriate clinical response, as seen in ***Figure 24.2***. Depending on the risk categories patients may need level 2 or level 3 care. Patients who are in the high-risk category of clinical deterioration will need urgent assessment by staff with critical care experience and airway skills.

Surgery-specific observations, such as Doppler flow for a free flap, regular neurological evaluation and laboratory tests, such as blood gas analysis, should also be performed when necessary.

The patient can be discharged from PACU when they fulfil the following criteria:

- they are fully conscious;
- respiration and oxygenation are satisfactory;
- they are normothermic, not in pain and not nauseous;
- cardiovascular parameters are stable;
- oxygen, fluids and analgesics have been prescribed;
- there are no concerns relating to the surgical procedure.

However, as discussed above, some patients who have had complex surgery or who have severe chronic health conditions will stay for a period of 24–48 hours on PACU or an overnight intensive recovery unit until they are discharged to either a surgical ward or critical care unit.

NEW score	Clinical risk	Response
Aggregate score 0–4	Low	Ward-based response
Red score Score of 3 in any individual parameter	Low–medium	Urgent ward-based response*
Aggregate score 5–6	Medium	Key threshold for urgent response*
Aggregate score 7 or more	High	Urgent or emergency response**

* Response by a clinician or team with competence in the assessment and treatment of acutely ill patients and in recognising when the escalation of care to a critical care team is appropriate.

**The response team must also include staff with critical care skills, including airway management.

Figure 24.2 Risk category from the National Early Warning (NEW) score and response. *Response by a clinician or team with competence in the assessment and treatment of acutely ill patients and in recognising when the escalation of care to a critical care team is appropriate. **The response team must also include staff with critical care skills, including airway management. (Reproduced from Royal College of Physicians. *National Early Warning Score (NEWS) 2: Standardising the assessment of acute-illness severity in the NHS*. Updated report of a working party. London: RCP, 2017.)

Summary box 24.1

Postoperative period
- All anaesthetised patients should be recovered in a dedicated PACU
- All vital parameters should be monitored and documented according to local protocols
- Treat pain and nausea/vomiting
- Observe for complications

POSTOPERATIVE COMPLICATIONS

Postoperative complications are an important cause of morbidity, mortality, extended hospital stay and increased costs. Most patients at increased risk of developing postoperative complications can be identified prior to surgery at the preoperative assessment clinic using a variety of scoring systems (for example the American College of Surgeons National Surgical Quality Improvement Program surgical risk calculator for a patient's risk of postoperative complications [ACS NSQIP], as discussed in ***Chapter 21***). Early identification of risk allows for targeted, appropriate, anticipatory and supportive medical care, which will reduce both the incidence and severity of such complications when they occur.

The Clavien–Dindo classification of postoperative complications (***Table 24.1***) is used to objectively and reproducibly measure the impact of surgical complications on the outcome of the procedure. Complications are graded according to the treatment they require. This eliminates subjective bias and prevents complications from being downgraded.

TABLE 24.1 Clavien–Dindo classification of postoperative complications.

Grade	Definition
I	• Any deviation from the normal postoperative course without the need for pharmacological treatment or surgical, endoscopic or radiological intervention • Acceptable therapeutic regimens are: drugs as antiemetics, antipyretics, analgesics, diuretics and electrolytes and physiotherapy. This grade also includes wound infections opened at the bedside
II	Requiring pharmacological treatment with drugs other than such allowed for grade I complications. Blood transfusions and total parenteral nutrition are also included
III	Requiring surgical, endoscopic or radiological intervention
IIIa	Intervention not under general anaesthesia
IIIb	Intervention under general anaesthesia
IV	Life-threatening complication (including CNS complications, e.g. brain haemorrhage, but excluding TIAs) requiring ICU management
IVa	Single-organ dysfunction (including dialysis)
IVb	Multiorgan dysfunction
V	Death of a patient

CNS, central nervous system; ICU, intensive care unit; TIA, transient ischaemic attack.

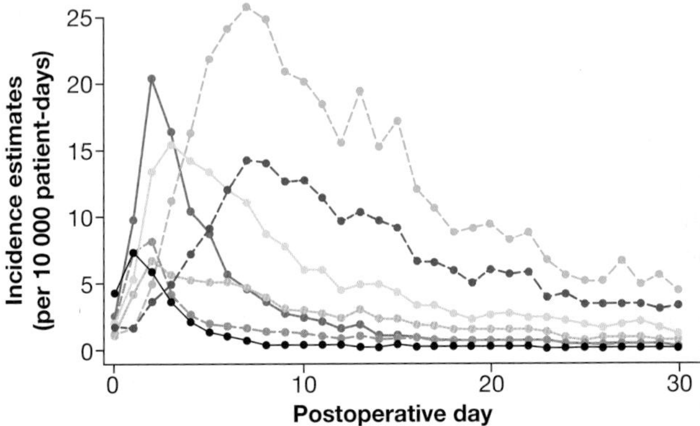

Figure 24.3 Timing and incidence of postoperative complications. Modified from Hyder JA, Wakeam E, Arora V *et al*. Investigating the "Rule of W," a mnemonic for teaching on postoperative complications. *J Surg Educ* 2015; **72**(3): 430-7.

Complications can occur throughout the postoperative period. However, certain complications are more common earlier in the postoperative period than others, as shown in ***Figure 24.3***.

Postoperative complications can be further classified into system-specific and surgery-specific complications.

SYSTEM-SPECIFIC COMPLICATIONS

Respiratory system

Early detection of respiratory complications is facilitated by periodic assessment of airway patency, respiratory rate and routine oxygen saturation measurement, performed during emergence and recovery as described earlier. Postoperative respiratory complications can occur immediately on PACU or later when a patient is on the surgical ward or is discharged home.

Immediate respiratory complications on PACU

Airway

Upper airway obstruction is one of the commonest immediate postoperative complications and can be due to laryngospasm, persisting relaxation of airway muscles, soft-tissue oedema, haematoma, vocal cord dysfunction or a foreign body. Vigilance and early intervention are necessary to prevent harm to the patient. Most interventions are simple and involve manual support of the jaw or insertion of an oral or nasal airway.

Pierre-Alain Clavien, contemporary, professor, University Hospital Zurich, Zurich, Switzerland.
Daniel Dindo, contemporary, surgeon, Centre for Surgery, Zurich, Switzerland.

Hypoventilation

The residual effects of anaesthetic drugs (neuromuscular blockers, anaesthetic agents, opioids) can contribute to reduced or impaired adequacy of ventilation postoperatively. Continuous pulse oximetry and respiratory rate evaluation can identify respiratory compromise and consequent hypoxia early. Supplemental oxygen should be given to all patients on PACU until adequate respiration and oxygenation are restored.

Hypoxaemia

This may occur, in addition to the situations already described above, as a consequence of acute pulmonary oedema (fluid overload, cardiac failure, postobstructive), bronchospasm, pneumothorax (***Figure 24.4***), aspiration and, rarely, pulmonary embolism (PE) (***Figure 24.5***). *De novo* pneumonia is very unusual in the immediate postoperative period. Hypoxaemia develops most quickly in patients with obstructive sleep apnoea (OSA), lung disease and obesity; these patients should therefore be closely observed.

Patients with hypoxaemia should be treated urgently. If the patient is breathing spontaneously, oxygen should be administered at 15 L/min using a non-rebreathing mask. A head tilt, chin lift or jaw thrust should relieve obstruction related to reduced muscle tone. Suctioning of any blood or secretions and insertion of an oropharyngeal airway may be needed. Early anaesthetic intervention may be required.

Vocal cord palsy (as a consequence of recurrent laryngeal nerve injury), neck haematoma and post-tonsillectomy bleeding are recognised as life-threatening complications of head and neck surgery, which need immediate medical attention for safe resolution.

Although the above respiratory complications are more common on PACU, they can occur after discharge from PACU as well.

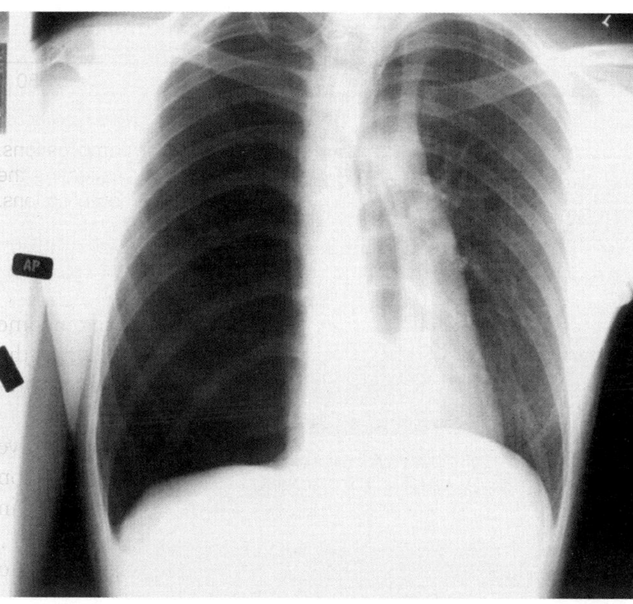

Figure 24.4 Radiograph showing a right tension pneumothorax with tracheal deviation to the left (courtesy of Professor Stephen Eustace, Dublin, Ireland).

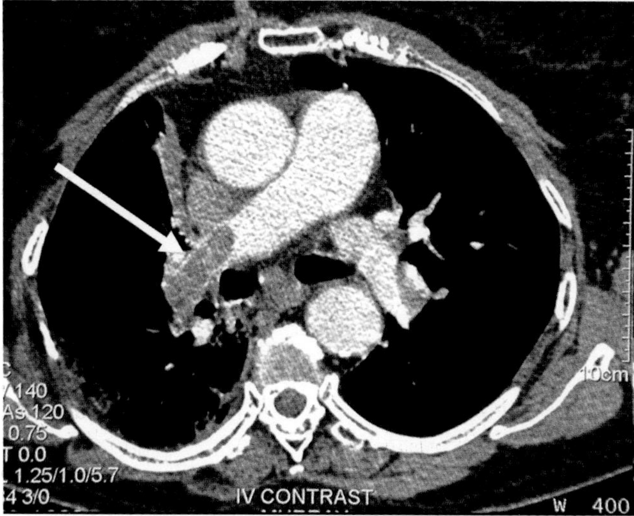

Figure 24.5 Computed tomography scan showing a pulmonary artery blood embolism (arrow) (courtesy of Professor Stephen Eustace, Dublin).

Respiratory complications after discharge from PACU

Postoperative pulmonary complications are a significant cause of postoperative morbidity and mortality (figures vary between 5% and 70%). Complications include fever (due to microatelectasis), cough, dyspnoea, bronchospasm, hypercapnia, atelectasis (***Figure 24.6***), pneumonia (***Figure 24.7***), pleural effusion, pneumothorax and respiratory failure. The risk of each varies with the patient and the type of surgery being performed. Thoracic or abdominal surgery carries the highest risk. The majority of patients at risk (obese, smokers, chronic lung disease, OSA, poor nutritional status) can be identified

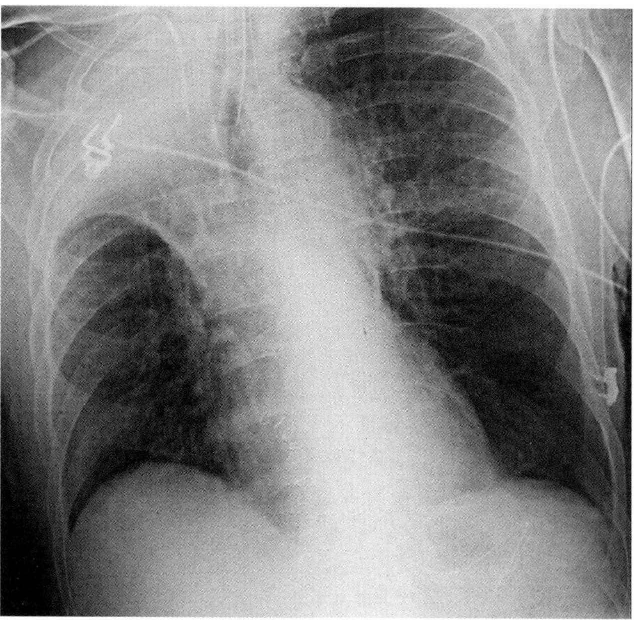

Figure 24.6 Radiograph showing right upper lobe atelectasis (courtesy of Professor Stephen Eustace, Dublin, Ireland).

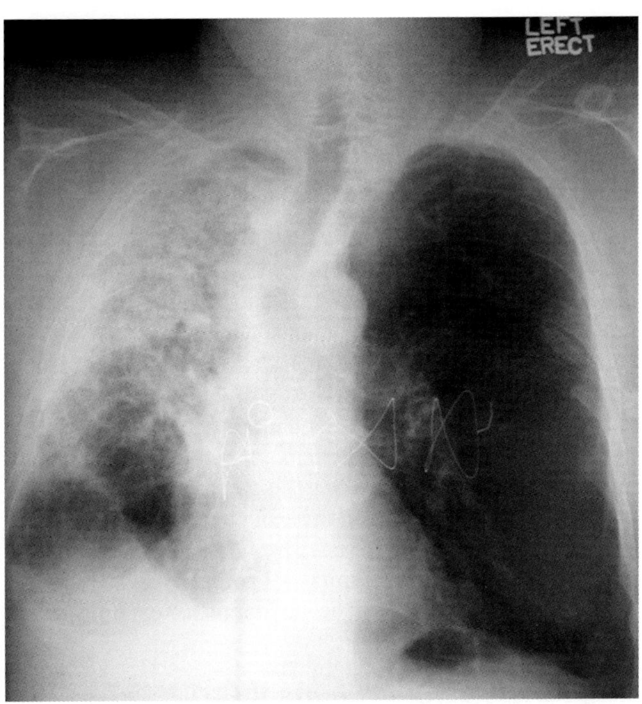

Figure 24.7 Radiograph showing classical Staphylococcus aureus pneumonia (courtesy of Professor Stephen Eustace, Dublin, Ireland).

preoperatively, facilitating the development of strategies that will reduce the impact of surgery on the individual patient.

Table 24.2 shows risk factors for developing a postoperative pulmonary complication.

Summary box 24.2

Respiratory complications

- Respiratory complications can occur either immediately or a few days later on the ward
- Obesity, smoking, chronic lung disease, poor nutritional status and OSA predispose to a higher risk of respiratory complications
- Early intervention and multidisciplinary involvement can prevent life-threatening respiratory complications

Cardiovascular system

Thirty per cent of patients undergoing non-cardiac surgery will have at least one cardiovascular risk factor. In this group 30-day mortality is 0.5–2% as a result of cardiac complications.

Routine pulse, blood pressure and electrocardiogram (ECG) monitoring will detect cardiovascular complications, reduce adverse outcomes and should be recorded during emergence from, and recovery after, anaesthesia. There are certain categories of patient and procedure for which routine cardiovascular monitoring may be required for 24 hours or longer, usually on a PACU or high-dependency unit.

Hypotension

In the immediate postoperative period this is associated with adverse outcomes. Hypotension may be due to hypovolaemia, myocardial impairment or vasodilatation from subarachnoid and epidural anaesthesia. Other causes of hypotension such as

TABLE 24.2 Risk factors for developing a postoperative pulmonary complication.

Patient factors	Procedure-related factors	Laboratory testing
Non-modifiable • Age • Male sex • ASA grade >II • Frailty • Acute respiratory infection within 1 month of surgery • Impaired cognition/sensorium/stroke • Malignancy • Weight loss >10% (within 6 months • Long-term steroid use • Prolonged hospitalisation	Non-modifiable • Type of surgery • Upper abdominal or vascular surgery • Emergency surgery • Long-duration surgery (>2 hours) • Reoperation or multiple surgery	Increased urea and creatinine • Low albumin • Preoperative low saturation (<96%) or abnormal chest radiograph • Preoperative anaemia (<10 g/dL) • FEV_1/FVC <0.7 and FEV_1 <80% predicted
Modifiable • Smoking • COPD/asthma • OSA • BMI <18.5 or >40 • Hypertension • Chronic heart failure • Chronic liver failure/ascites • Renal failure • Diabetes mellitus • Alcohol • GORD • Preoperative sepsis and shock	Modifiable • Use of general anaesthesia versus regional anaesthesia • Use of neuromuscular blocking agents • Mechanical ventilation strategy • Open versus laparoscopic surgery • Intraoperative blood transfusion	

ASA, American Society of Anesthesiologists; BMI, body mass index; COPD, chronic obstructive pulmonary disease; FEV_1, forced expiratory volume in 1 second; FVC, forced vital capacity; GORD, gastro-oesophageal reflux disease; OSA, obstructive sleep apnoea.

Modified from Miskovic A, Lumb AB. Postoperative pulmonary complications. *Br J Anaesth* 2017; **118**(3): 317–34.

surgical bleeding, sepsis, arrhythmias, tension pneumothorax, PE, pericardial tamponade and anaphylaxis should also be considered in the differential diagnosis.

A high prevalence of diastolic dysfunction is seen in middle-aged patients having non-cardiac surgery. These patients are susceptible to exaggerated hypotension following hypovolaemia and pulmonary oedema in response to fluid overloading.

Treatment should be aimed at the cause. Postoperative hypotension leading to end-organ dysfunction (e.g. decreased urine output <0.5 mL/kg/h, decreased level of consciousness, myocardial ischaemia, capillary refill >2 seconds) needs immediate management with fluid and may require the use of vasopressors and inotropes.

Hypertension

Hypertension is also common. It may be due to pain, agitation, anxiety, bladder spasm secondary to urinary catheterisation or pre-existing poorly controlled hypertension. The consequences include bleeding from vascular suture lines, cerebrovascular haemorrhage and myocardial ischaemia or infarction.

Myocardial ischaemia

Patients with a history of cardiovascular disease or with known cardiac risk factors undergoing major surgery are at risk of major adverse cardiac events (MACE). The spectrum of myocardial damage can range from injury (myocardial injury after non-cardiac surgery [MINS]) to ischaemia or infarction. Symptoms can include retrosternal pain radiating into the neck, jaw or arms, nausea, dyspnoea or syncope, but many events in the perioperative period are silent.

ECG changes can include ST elevation in two continuous leads, new left bundle branch block or an arrhythmia. In the case of a non-ST segment myocardial infarction, only a rise in serial troponin levels will clarify the diagnosis. Cardiologists should be involved early and may start coronary reperfusion therapy in the form of primary percutaneous coronary intervention or thrombolysis. These should be discussed with the surgical team because of the risk of bleeding after major surgery.

Arrhythmias

When they occur in the postoperative period, arrhythmias can cause hypotension, myocardial ischaemia and cardiac arrest. Treatment should be guided by the Resuscitation Council UK's peri-arrest guidelines.

Tachycardia (sinus or supraventricular, including atrial fibrillation) may occur as a result of anxiety, pain, myocardial ischaemia or infarction, hypovolaemia, sepsis, electrolyte imbalance or hypoxia in the postoperative period. Consideration should be given to correction of the underlying causes and the rate controlled with β-blockers, amiodarone or cardioversion, depending on the state of the patient.

Sinus bradycardia may be normal in athletes, but it may also be associated with hypoxia, preoperative β-blockers, digoxin and increased intracranial pressure. Pharmacological options include glycopyrrolate or atropine intravenously.

A prolonged QT interval may be seen in the perioperative period. It is multifactorial in origin with most patients having predisposing risk factors, such as long QT syndrome or electrolyte abnormalities.

Summary box 24.3

Cardiovascular complications

- Hypotension and hypertension in the postoperative period can be multifactorial and result in serious morbidity
- Arrhythmias can be prevented and corrected by treating hypotension and electrolyte imbalance
- Arrhythmias, myocardial ischaemia/infarction and stroke will need management with the help of cardiologists and neurologists

Renal and urinary system

Acute kidney injury

Renal failure occurring during the perioperative period is associated with considerable mortality and morbidity. About one-quarter of cases of hospital-acquired renal failure occur in the perioperative period and are associated with high mortality, especially after cardiac and major vascular surgery. Several definitions of acute kidney injury have been proposed that use changes in serum creatinine and urine output to stage kidney injury. One of the more recent examples is KDIGO (Kidney Disease: Improving Global Outcomes), which is shown in ***Table 24.3***.

Certain groups of patients with comorbidities such as diabetes or those undergoing emergency surgery or certain high-risk procedures such as cardiac/transplantation surgeries are more susceptible. ***Table 24.4*** lists the causes of perioperative acute kidney injury.

To prevent acute kidney injury in the perioperative period it is important to identify patients who are more susceptible to it. Normovolaemia and normal blood pressure should be maintained during surgery. Avoiding nephrotoxic agents and unnecessary blood transfusions and treating infections promptly will also help to avoid acute kidney injury.

Urine output is reduced during surgery and does not correlate with renal function. Fluids should not be given excessively to treat oliguria.

TABLE 24.3 KDIGO: Kidney Disease: Improving Global Outcomes.

Stage 1	Increased sCr × 1.5–1.9 of baseline that is known or presumed to have occurred within the preceding 7 days or sCr increase ≥0.3 mg/dL within 48 hours or Urine output <0.5 mL/kg/h for 6–12 hours
Stage 2	Increased sCr × 2–2.9 of baseline or Urine output <0.5 mL/kg/h for ≥12 hours
Stage 3	Increased sCr × 3 of baseline or sCr ≥4 mg/dL or initiation of RRT or GFR decrease to <35 mL/min/1.73 m^2 in patients <18 years old or Urine output <0.3 mL/kg/h for ≥24 hours or anuria for ≥12 hours

GFR, glomerular filtration rate; RRT, renal replacement therapy; sCr, serum creatinine.

TABLE 24.4 Causes of perioperative acute kidney injury.

Prerenal	• Hypovolaemia due to third space losses and bleeding • Sepsis • Cardiac failure • Low cardiac output due to anaesthesia and cardiopulmonary bypass • Increased intra-abdominal pressure • Cirrhosis, hepatorenal syndrome • Aortic cross-clamp
Renal	• Inflammation and sepsis • Chronic kidney disease and comorbidities, e.g. diabetes, obesity • Endogenous (e.g. myoglobin) and exogenous (e.g. radiocontrast dyes) toxins • Blood transfusions • Chloride-rich solution and hydroxyethyl starch
Post renal	• Surgery • Tumour • Benign prostatic hypertrophy • Neurogenic bladder

Urinary retention

Inability to void after surgery is common after anaesthesia and surgery with the incidence ranging from 5% to 70%. Risk factors include age >50 years, male sex, certain surgeries such as hernia, anorectal and pelvic surgery, a history of benign prostatic hypertrophy and neurological disease. Neuraxial anaesthesia and certain drugs given during anaesthesia such as anticholinergic medications, α-/ β-blockers, sedatives and fluids increase the risk. The diagnosis of retention may be confirmed by clinical examination and by using ultrasound imaging. Urinary retention needs treatment as it can cause not only discomfort but also long-term bladder dysfunction. Catheterisation should be performed prophylactically when an operation is expected to last 3 hours or longer, or when large volumes of fluid are administered.

Urinary infection

Urinary infection is one of the most commonly acquired infections in the postoperative period. Patients may present with dysuria and/or pyrexia. Immunocompromised patients, patients with diabetes and those with a history of urinary retention are known to be at higher risk. Treatment involves adequate hydration, proper bladder drainage and antibiotics depending on the sensitivity of the microorganisms.

Summary box 24.4

Renal and urinary complications

- Postoperative renal failure is associated with high mortality
- Prophylactic measures to prevent renal failure should be taken in high-risk cases
- Urinary retention and infection are common problems postoperatively

Central nervous system

Postoperative delirium and postoperative cognitive dysfunction

Postoperative delirium (POD) is characterised by a reduced awareness of the environment and a disturbance in attention accompanied by either hallucinations or disorientation or temporary memory loss.

Postoperative cognitive dysfunction (POCD) refers to deterioration in cognition temporally associated with surgery.

POD can occur during recovery from anaesthesia or a few days after surgery. The overall incidence of POD is 5–50%. It occurs more frequently in elderly orthopaedic patients and those undergoing emergency surgical procedures. Delirium is associated with increased all-cause morbidity, mortality and discharge to a nursing home. There are two types of delirium: hyperactive (restlessness, incoherent speech, agitation, hallucinations) and hypoactive (withdrawn, poorly responsive to the environment, depressed). Preoperative risk factors for POD include pre-existing cognitive impairment, dementia, frailty, Parkinson's disease, severe illness, renal impairment and depression. Precipitating factors include surgery, intraoperative administration of narcotics and benzodiazepines, change of medications, electrolyte and fluid abnormalities, constipation, catheterisation and an unfamiliar environment (***Table 24.5***).

Correcting any reversible cause, involving relatives or friends whom the patient knows and pain control can all contribute to reducing the impact and duration of delirium. As a last option, haloperidol may be given in titrated doses according to local protocols.

TABLE 24.5 Causes of delirium.

Renal	• Renal failure/uraemia • Hyponatraemia and electrolyte disorders • Urinary tract infection • Urinary retention
Respiratory	• Hypoxia, e.g. chest infection • Atelectasis
Cardiovascular	• Pulmonary embolism • Dehydration • Septic shock • Myocardial infarction • Chronic heart failure • Arrhythmia
Drugs	• Opiates including heroin • Hypnotics • Cocaine • Alcohol withdrawal • Hypoglycaemia
Neurological	• Epilepsy • Encephalopathy • Head injury • Cerebrovascular accident
Idiopathic (rare)	• Hypothyroidism • Hyperthyroidism • Addison's disease

James Parkinson, 1755–1824, general practitioner of Shoreditch, London, UK, published *An essay on the shaking palsy* in 1817.
Thomas Addison, 1795–1860, physician, Guy's Hospital, London, UK, described the effects of disease of the suprarenal capsules in 1849.

Stroke

Stroke is a recognised complication of carotid endarterectomy surgery both early (secondary to emboli) and later (secondary to cerebral hyperperfusion syndrome). It is also a recognised consequence of both hypotension and hypertension. Thrombolysis may be indicated but the neurology and surgical teams must discuss together the risks and benefits of such a treatment plan.

Seizures

These are uncommon except in those patients with known poorly controlled epilepsy. They may occur as a complication of neurosurgery.

GENERAL POSTOPERATIVE COMPLICATIONS

Bleeding

Postoperative haemorrhage is most common in the immediate postoperative period. It may be caused by an arterial or venous leak, but also by a generalised ooze or a coagulopathy. Slow bleeds may go undetected for hours and then the patient suddenly decompensates. All patients must have their vital signs (pulse rate, blood pressure, oximetry, central venous pressure, if available, and urine output) monitored regularly. Dressings and drains should be inspected regularly in the first 24 hours after surgery. If haemorrhage is suspected, blood samples should be taken for a full blood count, coagulation profile and cross-match. A large-bore intravenous cannula should be sited and fluid resuscitation commenced. If the source of bleeding is in doubt and the patient is stable, an ultrasound or computed tomography (CT) scan may be required to determine the nature of the bleed (most commonly if a haematoma is suspected in the days following surgery). If the patient's cardiovascular system is unstable or compromised in any way (for example neck haematoma or bleeding tonsil) they should be taken back to the operating theatre immediately.

The treatment of haemorrhage is both to stop the bleeding and supportive. Supportive treatment includes oxygen and fluid resuscitation. It may require correction of coagulopathy. All patients will require close observation. Blood transfusion carries risks (acute haemolytic transfusion reaction, sensitisation, fluid overload, hyperkalaemia, transfusion-related lung injury and transmission of blood-borne infection). There is much published about what is the right transfusion trigger and how to balance the need for adequate tissue perfusion and the risks of transfusion. According to the Joint United Kingdom (UK) Blood Transfusion and Tissue Transplantation Services Professional Advisory Committee transfusion should be considered if the haemoglobin (Hb) level is below 8g/dL. The decision to transfuse should be based on the clinical condition of the patient with acceptance of higher thresholds in individual cases. If the Hb level is below 7g/dL transfusion is usually indicated (see also ***Chapter 2***).

Patients who are symptomatic of anaemia, e.g. having chest pain, orthostatic hypotension or tachycardia unresponsive to fluid resuscitation, or who have congestive heart failure may need transfusion at a higher threshold.

All hospitals should have a 'major haemorrhage protocol' in place. The consultant surgeon, anaesthetist and haematologist should all be involved early on in the care of unstable patients.

Summary box 24.5

Postoperative bleeding

- All hospitals should have a major haemorrhage protocol in place
- The need to transfuse blood in the absence of continued bleeding, guided by the Hb level, should be weighed against the risks

Deep vein thrombosis

Deep vein thrombosis (DVT) is a well-known and, when complicated by pulmonary embolus, potentially fatal complication of surgery (***Table 24.6***). All hospitals must have a process for screening all surgical patients to identify those at risk and for implementing prophylactic measures to avoid this dreaded complication. Risk assessment should occur within 24 hours of admission. Risk should be reviewed if the clinical situation changes. Methods of prevention are guided by the risk score and include the use of compression stockings, calf pumps and pharmacological agents, such as low-molecular-weight heparin. Compression stockings are not offered to patients who have suspected or proven peripheral arterial disease or neuropathy. They are also avoided or used with caution in those with sensitive or broken skin and in those who are allergic to the material used, have severe leg oedema or have a leg deformity.

The symptoms and signs of DVT include calf pain, swelling, warmth, redness and engorged veins. However, most will show no physical signs. On palpation the muscle may be tender and there may be a positive Homans' sign (calf pain on dorsiflexion of the foot), but this test is neither sensitive nor specific. Use the two-level DVT Wells score to assess the probability of DVT (***Table 24.7***).

TABLE 24.6 Stratification of surgical procedure and the associated risk of deep vein thrombosis.

Low
- Maxillofacial surgery
- Neurosurgery
- Cardiothoracic surgery

Medium
- Inguinal hernia repair
- Abdominal surgery
- Gynaecological surgery
- Urological surgery

High
- Pelvic elective and trauma surgery
- Total knee and hip replacement

John Homans, 1877–1954, Professor of Clinical Surgery, Harvard Medical School, Boston, MA, USA.
Philip Wells, contemporary, physician, University of Ottawa, Ottawa, Ontario, Canada.

TABLE 24.7 Two-level deep vein thrombosis (DVT) Wells score.

Clinical features	Points
Active cancer (treatment ongoing, within 6 months or palliative)	1
Paralysis, paresis or recent plaster immobilisation of the lower extremities	1
Recently bedridden for 3 days or more, or major surgery within 12 weeks requiring general or regional anaesthesia	1
Localised tenderness along the distribution of the deep venous system	1
Entire leg swollen	1
Calf swelling at least 3 cm larger than asymptomatic side	1
Pitting oedema confined to the symptomatic leg	1
Collateral superficial veins (non-varicose)	1
Previously documented DVT	1
An alternative diagnosis is at least as likely as DVT	–2
Clinical probability simplified score	**Points**
DVT likely	2 points or more
DVT unlikely	1 point or less

If DVT is suspected, duplex Doppler ultrasound and venography can be used to assess flow and the presence of a thrombosis. If DVT is unlikely by Wells's score then d-dimer testing can be done. A negative d-dimer test makes DVT unlikely; however, patients should be told about the signs and symptoms of PE and how to seek medical help if necessary.

If a significant DVT is found (one that extends above the knee), treatment with parenteral anticoagulation initially, followed by longer term warfarin or a new oral anticoagulant (refer to national guidance, e.g. National Institute for Health and Care Excellence [NICE]; see ***Further reading***) is necessary. In some patients with a large DVT, a caval filter may be required to decrease the possibility of PE.

Pulmonary embolus

PE is not usually an immediate complication but can present in the early postoperative period. Thrombus can arise from DVT in the legs/pelvis, venae cavae or the right atrium. Signs and symptoms depend on the size of the embolus and may range from dyspnoea, cough and pleuritic chest pain to sudden cardiovascular collapse. Diagnosis of PE begins with the history (including risk factors and recent surgery) and a physical examination (which may include signs of DVT). The two-level Wells PE score (***Table 24.8***) can be used to determine the probability of PE.

Depending on the presentation, investigations may include ECG, chest radiograph, blood tests (arterial blood gas and d-dimer) and radiological tests (usually CT pulmonary angiography).

TABLE 24.8 Two-level pulmonary embolism (PE) Wells score.

Clinical features	Points
Clinical signs and symptoms of DVT (minimum of leg swelling and pain with palpation of the deep veins)	3
An alternative diagnosis is less likely than PE	3
Heart rate more than 100 beats per minute	1.5
Immobilisation for more than 3 days or surgery in the previous 4 weeks	1.5
Previous DVT/PE	1.5
Haemoptysis	1
Malignancy (on treatment, treated in the last 6 months or palliative)	1
Clinical probability simplified score	**Points**
PE likely	More than 4 points
PE unlikely	4 points or less

DVT, deep vein thrombosis.

If the presentation includes cardiovascular collapse, resuscitation will be needed. Thrombolysis can be considered with massive PE causing cardiovascular collapse, but this should include senior clinical opinion and would generally follow appropriate guidelines. The patient may need inotropes and admission to the intensive care unit. In less severe cases of PE, supportive measures include oxygen therapy and analgesia. After initial resuscitation, the patient will need anticoagulation – initially parenteral anticoagulation – followed by long-term oral anticoagulation (refer to national guidance, e.g. NICE; see ***Further reading***). A vena cava filter may be needed if anticoagulation is not possible or if the patient has an embolism while anticoagulated (see ***Further reading***).

Fever

About 40% of patients develop pyrexia after major surgery; however, in most cases no cause is found. The inflammatory response to surgical trauma may manifest itself as fever, and so pyrexia does not necessarily imply sepsis. However, in all patients with a pyrexia, a focus of infection should be sought.

The causes of a raised temperature postoperatively include:

- atelectasis of the lung;
- superficial and deep wound infection;
- chest infection, urinary tract infection and thrombophlebitis;
- wound infection, anastomotic leakage, intracavitary collections and abscesses.

The possible causes of pyrexia of a non-infective origin include:

- DVT;
- transfusion reactions;
- wound haematomas;

Christian Johann Doppler, 1803–1853, Professor of Experimental Physics, Vienna, Austria, enunciated the 'Doppler principle' in 1842.

- atelectasis;
- drug reactions.

Patients with a persistent pyrexia need a thorough review. Relevant investigations include full blood count, urine culture, sputum microscopy and blood cultures.

Summary box 24.6

Fever

- A very common problem postoperatively
- Consider infection in the lung, urine and wound

Wound dehiscence

Wound dehiscence is disruption of any or all of the layers in a wound. Dehiscence may occur in up to 3% of abdominal wounds, increases the risk of postoperative mortality and is very distressing to the patient.

Wound dehiscence most commonly occurs from the fifth to the eighth postoperative day when the strength of the wound is at its weakest. It may herald an underlying abscess and usually presents with a serosanguinous discharge. The patient may have felt a popping sensation during straining or coughing. Most patients with a full thickness dehiscence of an abdominal wound will need to return to the operating theatre for resuturing. In patients in whom tissues are suspected to be infected, of poor quality or under excessive tension, it may be appropriate to leave the wound open and treat with dressings or vacuum-assisted closure pumps.

Summary box 24.7

Risk factors in wound dehiscence

General

- Malnourishment
- Diabetes
- Obesity
- Renal failure
- Jaundice
- Sepsis
- Cancer
- Treatment with steroids
- Emergency surgery

Local

- Inadequate or poor closure of wound or closure of a wound under tension
- Poor local wound healing, e.g. because of infection, haematoma or seroma
- Increased intra-abdominal pressure, e.g. in postoperative patients with chronic obstructive airway disease, during excessive coughing

Pressure sores

Patients undergoing surgery for a prolonged period of time are vulnerable to the development of a pressure sore or to worsening of a pre-existing sore as a result of prolonged immobility during, and sometimes after, the operation. Careful positioning and padding of the patient are standard practice intraoperatively to reduce the risk. Pressure sores occur as a result of friction or persisting pressure on soft tissues. They particularly affect the pressure points of a recumbent patient, including the sacrum, greater trochanter and heels. Risk factors are poor nutritional status, dehydration, lack of mobility and nerve block anaesthesia technique. Early mobilisation of the patient and regular inspection of pressure points by the nursing team can act to prevent pressure sores. High-risk patients may be nursed on an air mattress, which automatically relieves the pressure areas.

Pressure ulcers can be graded according to an internationally recognised grading system based on the extent of skin loss. Category 1 ulcers involve non-blanching erythema with intact skin. Category 2 ulcers have partial thickness skin loss and appear as a shallow open ulcer with a red-pink wound bed or an intact or ruptured serum-filled blister. Category 3 ulcers have full thickness skin loss, with subcutaneous fat visible in the wound, but not bone, tendon or muscle. Category 4 ulcers have full thickness loss with exposed bone, tendon or muscle; osteomyelitis may develop at these sites.

Summary box 24.8

Preventing pressure sores

- Recognise patients at risk
- Address nutritional status
- Keep patients mobile or regularly turned if bed-bound

SURGERY-SPECIFIC COMPLICATIONS

This section provides an overview of selected important complications, rather than a comprehensive account of all possible complications. The reader is advised to consult chapters where specific procedures are described in more detail.

Abdominal surgery

The abdomen should be examined daily for excessive distension, tenderness or drainage from wounds or drain sites. In certain operations, such as those for intestinal obstruction or oesophageal and gastric procedures, a nasogastric tube may be required. This is of particular value in those patients with ileus or a marked level of altered consciousness, who are therefore liable to aspirate.

Paralytic ileus

Paralytic ileus may present with nausea, vomiting, loss of appetite, bowel distension and absence of flatus or bowel movements. Following laparotomy, gastrointestinal motility temporarily decreases. Treatment is usually supportive, with maintenance of adequate hydration and electrolyte levels. However, intestinal complications may present as prolonged ileus and so should be actively sought and treated. It is important to note that nutrient absorption from the gut will be impaired in the context of paralytic ileus, and parenteral nutrition will therefore need to be considered in any patient with prolonged ileus.

Return of function of the intestine occurs in the following order: small bowel, large bowel and then stomach. This pattern allows the passage of faeces despite continuing lack of stomach emptying and, therefore, vomiting may continue even when the lower bowel has already started functioning normally.

Localised intra-abdominal infection or anastomotic leakage

Intra-abdominal infection may develop from a complication such as anastomotic leakage or persistent abscess following a laparotomy for a perforated viscus, as well as from less common causes such as iatrogenic perforation of a viscus during an elective operation. Intra-abdominal infection may be localised, presenting with focal tenderness, a spiking fever, raised inflammatory markers and sometimes positive blood cultures and a prolonged ileus. These patients can often be managed by radiological drainage, if accessible, and appropriate antibiotic treatment. In some patients the leak may be more widespread, causing generalised peritonitis and severe sepsis and necessitating urgent laparotomy (see also ***Chapters 64 and 75***).

Bleeding

Postoperative bleeding is a well-recognised complication but can still sometimes be overlooked. Hb levels may not always decrease in patients who are bleeding because of the relative haemoconcentration, and drains may not demonstrate significant blood loss if blocked with clot. It is important to have a high index of suspicion for bleeding and a low threshold for appropriate intervention for any postoperative patient with a drop in blood pressure, tachycardia, demonstrable bleeding in the drains, progressive distension of the abdomen or a drop in Hb.

Summary box 24.9

The main complications after abdominal surgery

- Paralytic ileus
- Localised infection or anastomotic leakage
- Bleeding

Orthopaedic surgery

Neurovascular supply to the extremity

Patients who have undergone extremity surgery, for example open reduction and internal fixation of a fracture, require regular neurovascular observations, both in recovery and on the ward (this will usually follow a local or national guideline). Moreover, if a tourniquet has been used, the restoration of the distal neurovascular supply should be established. Careful documentation of findings before and after surgery will allow comparison. Concern about the neurovascular status requires urgent and experienced surgical review and further management. Circumferential casts can be split and dressings cut down to skin to improve the blood supply to the limb.

Compartment syndrome

Raised pressure in an osseofascial compartment can manifest after surgical intervention to a limb and can prevent adequate tissue perfusion. Patients with compartment syndrome complain of pain that is (i) out of proportion to that expected, (ii) increasing in intensity, and (iii) worse on passive stretching of the muscles in the affected compartment. Other symptoms that relate to pressure on nerves (paralysis, paraesthesia) and blood vessels (pallor and pulselessness) may only be noticed after irretrievable injury to the limb has occurred from the ischaemia. Extreme vigilance and early intervention is necessary to identify and manage compartment syndrome. When suspected, prompt senior input is required. In terms of initial management, circumferential casts can be split, dressings cut down to skin and the limb elevated. Further management will require experienced judgement and may include compartment pressure monitoring and/or fasciotomies. Compartment syndrome is considered more extensively in ***Chapters 3 and 32***.

Summary box 24.10

Compartment syndrome symptoms and signs

- Pain out of proportion to that expected
- Pain that is increasing
- Pain on passive stretching of the muscles in the affected compartment
- Paralysis, paraesthesia, pallor and pulselessness generally occur late

Neck surgery

Patients undergoing neck surgery, e.g. thyroid surgery, must be observed for accumulation of blood in the wound, which may obstruct the airway and cause rapid asphyxia. This potentially life-threatening complication necessitates systems for early detection and prompt evacuation (see guidelines from the Difficult Airway Society, the British Association of Endocrine and Thyroid Surgeons and the British Association of Otorhinolaryngology, Head and Neck Surgery). Another potential but less dangerous complication is damage to the recurrent laryngeal nerve, which can produce voice change (see also ***Chapter 55***).

Thoracic surgery

Careful fluid management is important in patients undergoing a lobectomy or pneumonectomy as they are susceptible to fluid overload in the first 24–48 hours postoperatively. Chest drains require regular review. If the fluid in a chest drain swings then the drain has been correctly inserted into the pleural cavity. Bubbling of the chest drain confirms the release of air from the pleural cavity; however, if the bubbling persists, this may represent a bronchopleural fistula. A haemothorax or pleural effusion will reveal itself as a prolonged loss of blood or fluid, respectively, into the drain. Cardiac patients require continuous ECG monitoring postoperatively (see also ***Chapter 60***).

Neurosurgery

Postoperatively the patient should be kept under close observation. A rise in intracranial pressure may be signalled by a deterioration in the state of consciousness, as well as by neurological signs. Urgent imaging and intervention are likely to be necessary in these cases to avoid the risk of mortality from complications such as an intracranial haematoma. Some patients may have an intracranial monitoring device to allow for more sensitive monitoring.

Vascular surgery

The patency of grafts and anastomoses, for example femoropopliteal bypasses and abdominal aneurysm, needs to be checked by regular clinical assessment of the limbs and by Doppler ultrasound in the postoperative phase.

Plastic surgery

The viability of flaps is crucial and the perfusion needs to be monitored regularly. The blood supply may be compromised by position, dressings or collection of fluids or blood beneath the flap.

Urology

Catheter patency must be checked regularly following urological surgery. In patients who have undergone transurethral resection of the prostate, continuous bladder irrigation may be used. More generalised complications can occur, for example transurethral resection syndrome, and are discussed further in the appropriate section.

GENERAL POSTOPERATIVE PROBLEMS AND MANAGEMENT

This section provides an overview of selected important postoperative problems and the principles of their management. It does not set out to describe such problems relating to the vast array of all surgical techniques and procedures. The reader is advised to consult chapters where specific procedures are described in more detail. Moreover, when considering postoperative problems, the importance of pain control and fluid management should be appreciated, and the reader is directed to ***Chapters 23 and 25***.

Drains

Drains are used to prevent accumulation of blood and serosanguineous or purulent fluid. In clean surgery, such as joint replacement, blood collected in drains can be transfused back into the patient provided that an adequate volume is collected rapidly and that a specifically designed drain and filter system is used.

The use of surgical drains has decreased in recent years as the evidence for their benefits has been questioned. Complications of drains include trauma to surrounding tissues and infection. The quantity and character of drain fluid can be used to identify an abdominal complication such as fluid leakage (e.g. bile or pancreatic fluid) or bleeding.

Drains should be removed as soon as it is considered safe to do so. The timing of drain removal is related to the volume and nature of fluid being evacuated (e.g. a drain may be left longer to evacuate a pancreatic leak, but removed earlier if only serous fluid is draining) and balanced against the risk of leaving the drain in place (such as damage to the surrounding tissues).

Wound care

Within hours of the wound being surgically closed, the dead space fills up with an inflammatory exudate. Within 48 hours of closure a layer of epidermal cells from the wound edge bridges the gap. Consequently, sterile dressings applied in theatre should not be removed before this time.

Wounds should be inspected only if there is a concern about their condition or the dressing needs changing. Inspection of the wound should be performed under sterile conditions. If the wound looks inflamed, a wound swab can be taken and sent for microbiological examination, but this can be unreliable. Infected wounds and haematomas may need treatment with antibiotics or even wound washout. If a surgical procedure is performed it gives an opportunity to collect samples for bacteriology (before any antibiotics, if the patient's general condition allows), to excise dead tissue and to control any bleeding. Depending on location, the wound may require packing if it is contaminated or if non-viable tissue remains. The dressing should then be changed regularly until the wound is clean.

Skin sutures or clips are usually removed between 6 and 10 days after surgery. The period can be shorter in wounds on the face or neck, or longer for tougher tissues such as the back. Wound healing is delayed in patients who are malnourished or in those who have vitamin A and C deficiency. Steroids also inhibit the adequate healing of wounds as they inhibit protein synthesis and fibroblast proliferation. Poorly controlled diabetes delays wound healing and increases the risk of infection at the surgical site (see also ***Chapter 3***).

DISCHARGE OF PATIENTS

Patients discharged home need a 'discharge letter' detailing the postoperative plan. The discharge letter should include details of the final diagnosis, the treatment and any complications that may have occurred. There should be advice for referring the patient back to hospital and indications for readmission if specific problems do occur. The general practitioner (GP) should be informed of the subsequent care plan, including follow-up, physiotherapy and other support needed. Pathology results should be included if available, and the basis of these in the subsequent care plan should be described along with the prognosis if appropriate.

Summary box 24.11

Discharge letter

- Diagnosis
- Treatment
- Laboratory results
- Complications
- Discharge plan
- Support needed
- Follow-up

Follow-up in clinic

Patients should be reviewed in clinic if a key decision on management needs to be made. The findings and the care plan agreed with the patient at the clinic appointment should be included in a letter to the patient's GP, as well as in a clear entry in the notes or electronic patient record. This should include advice on how to recognise the onset of complications and what to do if there is concern. Patients should be discharged from clinic as soon as no further input from the surgical team is required and their GP or they themselves can manage their care.

ENHANCED RECOVERY

Enhanced recovery is an approach to the perioperative care of patients undergoing surgery. It is designed to speed clinical recovery of the patient and reduce both the cost and the length of stay of the patient in the hospital. It is achieved by optimising the health of the patient before surgery through prehabilitation and then delivering evidence-based best care in the perioperative period.

Postoperative strategies advocated by enhanced recovery protocols include:

- early planned physiotherapy and mobilisation;
- early oral hydration and nourishment;
- opioid-sparing analgesia regimens that include the use of regional blocks, regular non-steroidal anti-inflammatory drugs and paracetamol;
- early discharge planning (started even before the patient is admitted to hospital and involving support from stoma care nurses, physiotherapists and other community care workers).

Early mobilisation is encouraged to reduce the risks of DVT, urinary retention, atelectasis, pressure sores and faecal impaction. Telephone follow-up is carried out to make sure that the patient is recovering well.

FURTHER READING

Goren O, Matot I. Perioperative acute kidney injury. *Br J Anaesth* 2015; **115**(Suppl 2): ii3–14.

https://anaesthetists.org/Home/Resources-publications/Guidelines/Immediate-post-anaesthesia-recovery (accessed 27 November 2021).

https://cpoc.org.uk/ (accessed 24 November 2021).

https://www.england.nhs.uk/ourwork/clinical-policy/sepsis/nationalearlywarningscore/ (accessed 24 November 2021).

https://ics.ac.uk/Society/Policy_and_Communications/Patients_and_Relatives/Levels_of_Care/Society/Patients_and_Relatives/Levels_of_Care.aspx?hkey=2a40dba7-a0b8-4669-ac85-cfa224275ca3 (accessed 27 November 2021).

Iliff HA, El-Boghdadly K, Ahmad I *et al.* Management of haematoma after thyroid surgery: systematic review and multidisciplinary consensus guidelines from the Difficult Airway Society, the British Association of Endocrine and Thyroid Surgeons and the British Association of Otorhinolaryngology, Head and Neck Surgery. *Anaesthesia* 2022; **77**: 82-95. https://doi.org/10.1111/anae.15585nae.

Joint United Kingdom (UK) Blood Transfusion and Tissue Transplantation Services Professional Advisory Committee. *Transfusion handbook.* Available from https://www.transfusionguidelines.org/transfusion-handbook/7-effective-transfusion-in-surgery-and-critical-care/7-1-transfusion-in-surgery.pdf.

Miskovic A, Lumb AB. Postoperative pulmonary complications. *Br J Anaesth* 2017; **118**(3): 317–34.

National Institute for Health and Care Excellence. *Acute kidney injury: prevention, detection and management.* NICE Guideline 148. London: NICE, 2019. Available from https://www.nice.org.uk/guidance/ng148.

National Institute for Health and Care Excellence. *Venous thromboembolic diseases: diagnosis, management and thrombophilia testing.* NICE Guideline 158. London: NICE, 2020. Available from https://www.nice.org.uk/guidance/ng158.

Sellers D, Srinivas C, Djaiani G. Cardiovascular complications after non-cardiac surgery. *Anaesthesia* 2018; **73**(Suppl 1): 34–42.

Smetana GW, Lawrence VA, Cornell JE. Preoperative pulmonary risk stratification for non-cardiothoracic surgery: systematic review for the American College of Physicians. *Ann Intern Med* 2006; **144**: 581–95.

CHAPTER 25 Nutrition and fluid therapy

Learning objectives

To understand:

- The importance of assessment of perioperative nutritional status and fluid balance
- The nutritional requirements of surgical patients and the effects of intestinal resection on nutrition
- The causes and complications of malnutrition and their management
- The options for nutritional intervention and the indications for enteral versus parenteral nutritional support

INTRODUCTION

Optimal nutritional status, both pre- and postoperatively, is a key factor in reducing perioperative complications and improving surgical outcomes. However, the pathologies requiring surgical intervention often contribute to malnutrition, and a lack of appreciation of preoperative nutritional status can unnecessarily increase the risk of the operation and compromise recovery from surgery (***Figure 25.1***). Some operations, particularly abdominal operations, can compromise absorption from the gastrointestinal tract, at least temporarily if not permanently. It is therefore imperative that the effects of surgical intervention on the patient's nutritional status are taken into consideration perioperatively, and appropriate intervention taken as early as possible to correct any nutritional deficits.

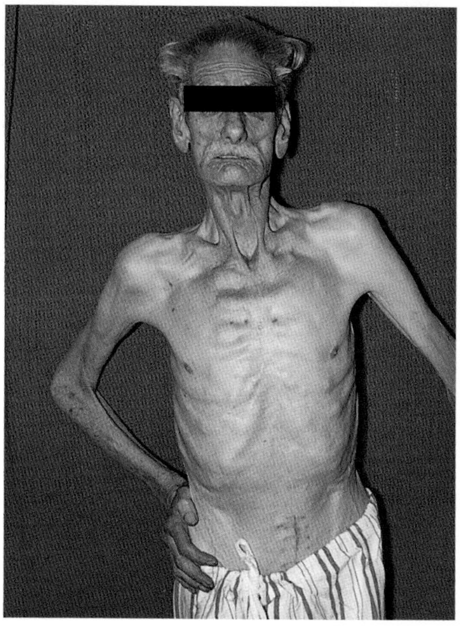

Appreciation of the importance of nutritional status is becoming more widespread within the healthcare profession and many tools have been developed to help identify poor nutritional status. These assessment tools and the availability of improved options for both enteral and parenteral delivery of nutrients allows any nutritional deficiency to be expeditiously identified and corrected until normal intestinal absorption can resume.

Figure 25.1 Severely malnourished patient with evidence of fat and muscle wasting.

PHYSIOLOGICAL RESPONSES TO NUTRITIONAL IMPAIRMENT

Metabolic response to fasting or starvation

The constant need for glucose by metabolically active tissues in the body, such as the brain, red and white blood cells and the renal medulla, necessitates homeostasis of blood glucose levels even during periods of fasting. During short-term fasting periods, when insulin levels fall and glucagon levels rise, glycogenolysis is the main source of glucose, whereby glycogen stores from the liver and skeletal muscle are converted to glucose via lactate (the Cori cycle). After approximately 24–40 hours of fasting, glycogen reserves are depleted and gluconeogenesis (the *de novo* synthesis of glucose from non-carbohydrate precursors such as the amino acids glutamine and alanine, as well as fructose,

Carl Ferdinand Cori, 1896–1984, Professor of Pharmacology and later Biochemistry, Washington University Medical School, St Louis, MI, USA, and his wife **Gerty Theresa Cori**, 1896–1957, also Professor of Biochemistry at the Washington University Medical School. In 1947, the Coris were awarded a share of the Nobel Prize in Physiology or Medicine for their discovery of how glycogen is catalytically converted.

lactate and glycerol) takes over as the predominant source of glucose production. The generation of amino acids occurs from catabolism of skeletal muscle, in amounts of up to 75 g per day for the average-sized individual.

Under conditions of even more prolonged fasting (>48 hours), glucose production is met by the breakdown of fat stores (lipolysis); this provides glycerol, which is then converted to fatty acids and glucose. Fatty acids can be converted to ketones, which can be used as a metabolic substrate by the majority of tissues in circumstances of extended fasting, reducing the need for muscle breakdown.

Resting energy expenditure levels significantly decrease in starvation, related in part to reduced conversion of inactive thyroxine (T_4) to active tri-iodothyronine (T_3). Nevertheless, this reduction is insufficient to obviate the need for metabolic substrates, leaving a glucose requirement of approximately 200 g per day even during conditions of prolonged fasting.

Summary box 25.1

Metabolic response to starvation

- Low plasma insulin
- High plasma glucagon
- Hepatic glycogenolysis
- Protein catabolism
- Hepatic gluconeogenesis
- Lipolysis: mobilisation of fat stores (increased fat oxidation) – overall decrease in protein and carbohydrate oxidation
- Adaptive ketogenesis
- Reduction in resting energy expenditure (from approximately 25–30 kcal/kg per day to 15–20 kcal/kg per day

Metabolic response to trauma and sepsis

This is described in greater detail in ***Chapter 1***, and covered briefly in ***Summary box 25.2***.

It is important to note that the metabolic response to trauma is influenced by the early and rapid rises in sympathetic nervous system activity and circulating catecholamines and elevated levels of glucocorticoids, glucagon and growth hormone, as well as insulin. Energy requirements often remain increased to allow tissue repair and inflammatory cell function. Elevated stress hormone levels can lead to net catabolism of tissue protein and thus a negative nitrogen balance. Ketone body production and utilisation may be impaired in the response to trauma, further exacerbating the catabolic response and protein breakdown.

The effect of the metabolic response to surgery on nutrition

The metabolic response to surgery is affected not only by the induced fasting period but also by the phenomenon of insulin resistance, which has been described in surgery and in other similar stresses, including trauma and burn injuries.

Summary box 25.2

Metabolic response to trauma and sepsis

- Increased counter-regulatory hormones: adrenaline (epinephrine), noradrenaline (norepinephrine), cortisol, glucagon and growth hormone
- Increased energy requirements (up to 40 kcal/kg per day)
- Increased nitrogen requirements
- Insulin resistance and glucose intolerance
- Preferential oxidation of lipids
- Increased gluconeogenesis and protein catabolism
- Loss of adaptive ketogenesis
- Fluid retention with associated hypoalbuminaemia

These stresses elicit combined hormonal and inflammatory responses to the triggers of pain, immobility, acidosis, tissue damage, hypoxia and impairment of homeostasis. Insulin resistance causes hyperglycaemia as a result of increased gluconeogenesis and reduced peripheral glycolysis. This is further worsened by reduced transport of glucose into muscle cells (the main tissue for uptake of insulin-mediated glucose) owing to reduced activation of the glucose transporter protein GLUT4. Instead, muscle protein is broken down to produce amino acids as substrates for gluconeogenesis, inducing a catabolic state with loss of lean muscle mass. The lack of response to insulin means that the catabolic processes induced by fasting or starvation are not resolved with the provision of glucose, and the inappropriate handling of peripheral glucose and breakdown of lean muscle continues for as long as the triggers for insulin resistance persist. Pre-existing comorbidities such as metabolic syndrome, diabetes, cancer and obesity have been shown to contribute to perioperative insulin resistance, which in turn is associated with an increased risk of major complications, in particular severe postoperative infection. Increased awareness of perioperative insulin resistance has led to the incorporation of specific interventions such as preoperative high-carbohydrate drinks to increase insulin sensitivity, adoption of minimally invasive surgery where appropriate (more invasive surgery appears to trigger a greater degree of insulin resistance) and early mobilisation protocols to minimise the impact and duration of insulin resistance on postoperative outcomes and recovery.

NUTRITIONAL ASSESSMENT

The nutritional status of an individual can be assessed by the ABCD of anthropometry, biochemistry, clinical evaluation and dietary assessment.

Anthropometry

Anthropometry uses several different parameters to obtain an estimate of body composition as a surrogate for nutritional status. These parameters can include weight and percentage weight change, body mass index (BMI) (weight [kg]/height^2 [m^2]), mid-upper arm circumference (MUAC), skinfold thickness (TSF) and mid-arm muscle circumference (MAMC), where

MAMC = MUAC (cm) – 3.14 × TSF (cm). These measurements are indirect assessments of energy and protein stores and are not sufficiently accurate to facilitate planning of nutritional support regimens.

BMI, in particular, has often been used as a quick screening measure to identify those who are malnourished. A BMI of less than 18.5 kg/m^2 and unintentional weight loss greater than 10% within the last 3–6 months or a BMI of less than 20 kg/m^2 and unintentional weight loss greater than 5% within the last 3–6 months are indicators of a need for nutrition support. It is important to note, however, that both BMI and body weight can be altered by major changes in fluid balance, and thus may not be reliable indicators of nutritional status in critically ill patients.

Biochemistry

Biochemical tests can be used in conjunction with clinical history, examination, comorbidities and drug history. Albumin, C-reactive protein and white cell counts can be markers of infection or inflammation, which can compromise nutritional status. Hypoalbuminaemia can be associated with malnutrition; however, it is easily affected by fluid balance and is not a reliable parameter of nutritional status in the acute setting.

Haemoglobin levels can indicate the presence of anaemia related to a lack of appropriate vitamins. Glycated haemoglobin can reflect diabetes and blood glucose control. Electrolytes such as sodium and urea can reflect underlying renal function, while calcium and phosphate are useful baseline measurements in anticipation of potential refeeding syndrome (discussed in more detail later in this chapter). Specific micronutrient levels such as vitamin D levels can also be measured in the appropriate clinical contexts.

Clinical evaluation

Clinical assessment of nutritional status should begin by consideration of any important symptoms that may suggest malnutrition. Upper abdominal symptoms such as nausea and vomiting, early satiety, dysphagia, reflux or bloating as well as lower gastrointestinal symptoms of diarrhoea or constipation can all indicate inadequate nutritional intake or absorption.

A thorough assessment of the past medical history and comorbidities is also essential in assessing nutritional status, as conditions such as cancer, gastrointestinal pathologies (e.g. inflammatory bowel disease and liver disease) and neurological conditions (e.g. stroke, Parkinson's disease and dementia) can all contribute to affect nutritional status. Nutrient absorption can be impaired by conditions directly affecting the bowel such as short bowel syndrome, high-output stoma and enterocutaneous fistulae, and also by disorders more proximally in the gastrointestinal tract such as pancreatic insufficiency, in which absorption is impaired because of a lack of pancreatic enzyme secretion into the bowel. These conditions and the appropriate management are dealt with in the relevant chapters in this book.

Dietary assessment tools

The total daily calorie intake of an individual can be estimated via a diary of their food and fluid intake, taking into account the quality of the food or fluid consumed. For patients who are unwell, this needs to take into account any differences in current food and fluid consumption compared with their typical intake when well. Their caloric intake can be assessed against their calculated energy requirements, estimated with the calculation of 25–35 kcal/kg lean body weight and taking into account any metabolic stresses and activity level.

Patients whose caloric intake falls short of their caloric requirements or who are anticipated to eat little or nothing for over 5 continuous days in the near future (e.g. owing to upcoming abdominal surgery) are likely to require nutritional support.

The Malnutrition Universal Screening Tool (MUST), developed by the British Association for Parenteral and Enteral Nutrition (BAPEN), is a rapid screening tool that can be used in both hospitals and the community, and takes into account a combination of the above factors to identify those individuals at risk of malnutrition (***Figure 25.2***). Patients who are found to be likely to be malnourished require referral to a dietician or nutritional support team, with regular reviews to ensure sustained improvement in nutritional status.

FLUID AND ELECTROLYTE REPLACEMENT

Daily fluid balance

Fluid intake consists of liquid ingested in the form of oral fluids as well as fluid released during oxidation of consumed food. ***Table 25.1*** shows the average daily fluid balance for a healthy adult.

It must be noted that insensible losses can increase in conditions of pyrexia, exertion or warm environments. Patients with a tracheostomy can lose a larger amount of fluid via insensible losses, emphasising the importance of humidification of inspired air. In addition, fluid loss via the faecal route will inevitably increase in diarrhoea or more chronic bowel pathologies, such as high-output stoma, short bowel syndrome and enterocutaneous fistulae.

TABLE 25.1 Estimated daily fluid balance for a healthy 70-kg adult in a temperate climate.

Intake (L)		Output (L)	
Water from beverages	1.2	Urine	1.5
Water from food	1.0	Insensible losses (skin and lungs)	0.9
Metabolic processes of oxidation	0.3	Faeces	0.1

James Parkinson, 1755–1824, general practitioner of Shoreditch, London, UK, published *An essay on the shaking palsy* in 1817.

Prescription of maintenance fluids should aim to restore fluid losses and provide sufficient water and electrolytes to maintain the intracellular and extracellular fluid compartments, and to enable the kidneys to excrete waste products. The normal volume of water required for daily maintenance in a healthy 70-kg adult is approximately 2.2 litres or 30 mL/kg per day. Accurate assessment of maintenance fluid volumes requires both intake and output to be taken into account, in addition to the patient's body weight.

Fluid replacement should also encompass replacement of key electrolytes. The approximate daily requirements of the main electrolytes are as follows:

- sodium: 0.9–1.2 mmol/kg per day
- potassium: 1 mmol/kg per day
- calcium: 5 mM per day
- magnesium: 1 mM per day

Replacement of fluid and electrolytes should be by the simplest and safest route of administration. Where feasible the oral route should be used via oral rehydration solutions. In patients whose ability to swallow is impaired, fluid may be replaced via feeding nasogastric tubes or nasojejunal tubes, provided intestinal absorptive function is maintained.

Intravenous fluid replacement solutions

Intravenous fluid replacement may be necessary in conditions of gastrointestinal absorptive impairment or large fluid losses that cannot be quickly replaced via the enteral route. The specific type of fluid replacement therapy will be determined by the individual patient's needs. ***Table 25.2*** shows the composition of some commonly used intravenous fluid replacement solutions, in contrast to the average composition of the same components in plasma.

In addition to the crystalloid fluid solutions above, fluid can also be replaced with colloid solutions, which usually contain a form of modified gelatin. Examples of these include Gelofusine® or Volplex®, which both contain 4% w/v succinylated gelatin, or Voluven®, which contains hydroxyethyl starch. These solutions are often used as plasma expanders as the larger molecules are thought to be slower to diffuse into the extravascular space. Colloids are therefore sometimes used for fluid resuscitation in preference to crystalloids, but they can cause renal failure or coagulopathy. There is ongoing controversy regarding the use of crystalloids or colloids in the setting of fluid resuscitation. Albumin solutions have also been used

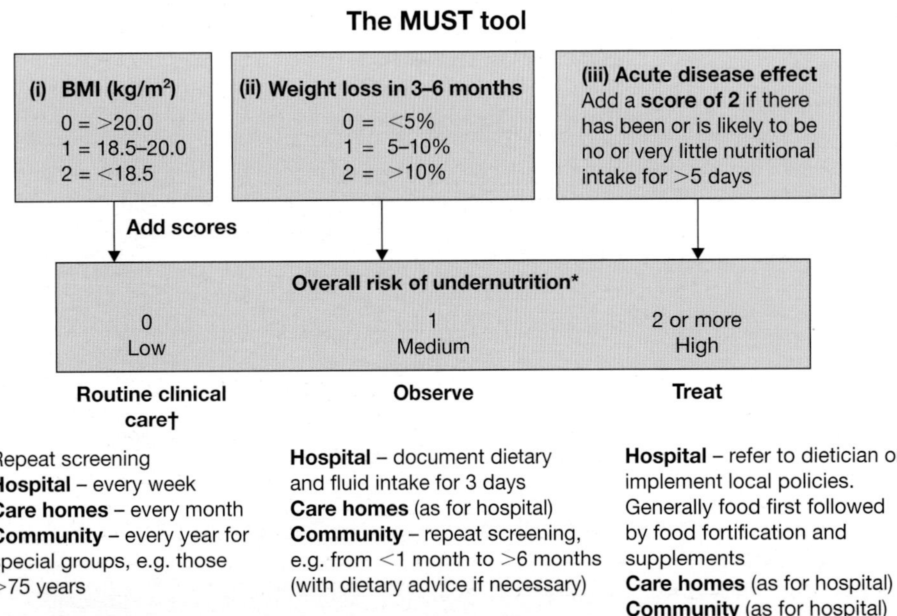

Figure 25.2 The Malnutrition Universal Screening Tool (MUST) for adults. (Adapted from Elia M (ed.). *The MUST Report. Nutritional screening of adults: a multidisciplinary responsibility. Development and use of the 'Malnutrition Universal Screening Tool' ('MUST') for adults.* A report by the Malnutrition Advisory Group of the British Association for Parenteral and Enteral Nutrition. Report no. 152. Redditch: BAPEN, 2003. ISBN 1 899467 70 X.)

TABLE 25.2 Composition of plasma in comparison with commonly used intravenous fluid replacements.

	Plasma	0.9% saline	Hartmann's solution	5% dextrose
Sodium (mmol/L)	135–145	154	131	0
Chloride (mmol/L)	95–105	154	111	0
Potassium (mmol/L)	3.5–5.3	0	5	0
Bicarbonate (mmol/L)	24–32	0	29	0
Calcium (mmol/L)	2.2–2.6	2	2	0
Magnesium (mmol/L)	0.8–1.2	0	0	0
Glucose (mmol/L)	3.5–5.5	0	0	227.8 (50 g)
Lactate (mmol/L)	0.5–1.0	0	29	0
pH	7.35–7.45	4.5–7.0	5.0–7.0	3.5–5.5
Osmolality (mOsmol/L)	275–295	308	273	278

in the past for fluid resuscitation; however, increasing evidence shows no benefit for the use of albumin outside of certain specific indications such as replacement of ascitic fluid losses or in the context of liver insufficiency. It is important to remember that if fluid loss is related to haemorrhage then the best form of fluid replacement is blood.

It must be noted that, as seen in ***Table 25.2***, none of the different intravenous fluid replacement solutions have electrolyte levels that completely mirror plasma levels, and thus there is no single ideal fluid replacement therapy. The specific choice of fluid replacement should take into account the nature of fluid losses and the amount of fluid replacement necessary in a specific patient.

Such an assessment would include:

- measurement of the pulse, blood pressure and, if available, the central venous pressure, as an estimate of intravascular fluid depletion;
- accurate intake and output charts, especially in inpatients in the acute care setting, taking into account urine output as well as losses from drains, fistulae, nasogastric tubes and faecal losses;
- measurement of serum electrolytes and haematocrit.

The choice of fluid replacement will also be guided by the time of gastrointestinal fluid loss, as the composition of gastrointestinal secretions varies with anatomical location (***Table 25.3***).

TABLE 25.3 Composition of gastrointestinal secretions (mmol/L).

	Sodium	Potassium	Chloride	Bicarbonate
Saliva	10	25	10	30
Stomach	50	15	110	–
Duodenum	140	5	100	–
Ileum	140	5	100	30
Pancreas	140	5	75	115
Bile	140	5	100	35

NUTRITIONAL REQUIREMENTS

Patients who are considered to be unable to consume enough nutrition via dietary means will need to be considered for either enteral or parenteral nutrition. Provision of enteral and parenteral nutrition should take into account not only macronutrients, such as carbohydrate, fat and protein, but also vitamins, trace elements, electrolytes and water. Planning of the feeding regimen will require the patient's weight as well as daily energy and protein requirements, which can be calculated based on standard tables. These regimens will need to be assessed on a daily basis and adjusted according to any changes in requirements, as overfeeding is one of the most common causes of complications regardless of the route of nutrient delivery. Regular biochemical monitoring is also mandatory as electrolyte and nutrient requirements can vary based on plasma levels (***Table 25.4***).

TABLE 25.4 Recommended schedule for monitoring feeding regimens.

Daily[a]	Observations including: • pulse, blood pressure and temperature • body weight • fluid balance, including volume of urine and/or urine and intestinal losses • quantity and type of food consumed, if allowed to eat Plasma levels: • sodium, potassium, urea and creatinine • blood glucose • magnesium and phosphate (if at risk of refeeding syndrome) • liver function tests • C-reactive protein
Weekly to fortnightly	Plasma levels: • full blood count • calcium, zinc, copper • plasma proteins including albumin • thiamine • triglycerides • vitamin B12 • folic acid
3–6 monthly	• Ferritin • Selenium, manganese • 25-hydroxyvitamin D

[a]Could be converted to weekly once the patient is established on a stable feeding regimen.

Macronutrient requirements

Total energy intake

In a normal state of health, the basal metabolic rate (BMR) can be calculated using the Harris–Benedict equation:

Men

$$\text{BMR} = (10 \times \text{weight in kg}) + (6.25 \times \text{height in cm}) - (5 \times \text{age in years}) + 5$$

Women

$$\text{BMR} = (10 \times \text{weight in kg}) + (6.25 \times \text{height in cm}) - (5 \times \text{age in years}) - 161$$

In the unwell patient population (acute or chronic disease), a degree of hypermetabolism exists, but no more than 120% of the predicted values. Stable patients with a normal or only moderately increased nutritional need should therefore be provided with a corresponding energy intake of 20–30 kcal for every kilogram of ideal body weight per day. Daily energy expenditure and thus requirements can be severely overestimated in obese patients, hence the ideal body weight should be used in these calculations rather than the actual body weight.

Nutrient requirements may increase to 30 kcal/kg ideal body weight per day under conditions of severe stress. However, the introduction of nutrition should be cautious in these patients as well as in those at risk of refeeding syndrome; nutrition should be started at no more than 50% of the estimated target energy needs. This can be increased to the full requirement over 24–48 hours, according to tolerance. Patients at risk of refeeding syndrome (discussed in more detail in ***Refeeding syndrome***) should have a maximum of 50% of their target requirements for the first 48 hours; this is subsequently increased only if clinical and biochemical monitoring shows no evidence of refeeding syndrome.

Carbohydrate

Glucose is the main substrate for the central nervous system and certain haematopoietic cells, which require the equivalent of 2 g/kg of glucose per day. Dietary guidelines therefore recommend that carbohydrates form 45–65% of the total caloric intake per day.

Protein

In the ill patient population, daily nitrogen requirements increase from approximately 0.15 g/kg per day to 0.25 g/kg per day. This is equivalent to a daily protein intake of 1.5 g/kg ideal body weight or around 20% of total energy requirements, in order to reduce nitrogen losses at times of illness.

Fat

Dietary fat consists of triglycerides of saturated and unsaturated fatty acids. Of these, the unsaturated fatty acids linoleic acid and linolenic acid are particularly notable, as they cannot be synthesised *in vivo* from non-dietary sources and are therefore considered essential fatty acids. Emulsions of long-chain triglycerides are now routinely used in parenteral nutrition, in which a mixture of glucose (a minimum of 100–200 g per day) and fat (100–200 g per week) is delivered. The combination of fat and glucose delivery minimises metabolic complications associated with parenteral nutrition, improves substrate utilisation and reduces fluid retention and carbon dioxide production.

Vitamins, minerals and trace elements

Vitamins B and C are important in optimising recovery from illness, in particular for collagen formation and wound healing. Vitamin C requirement in the postoperative period increases to 60–80 mg per day. It is important to consider the need for supplemental vitamin B12, especially in patients who have undergone gastric surgery and in those with a history of alcohol dependence. Surgical procedures or medical conditions associated with a reduction in pancreatic or biliary enzymes in the intestinal tract (e.g. obstruction of the biliary or pancreatic ducts) will result in malabsorption of the fat-soluble vitamins A, D, E and K. Increased intestinal losses such as in chronic diarrhoea can cause hyponatraemia, hypokalaemia and hypophosphataemia, which will all need monitoring and replacement. Trace elements such as magnesium, zinc and iron are important cofactors in metabolic processes and may be reduced as part of the inflammatory response. Replacement of these elements is necessary to ensure appropriate utilisation of amino acids and avoidance of refeeding syndrome.

EFFECTS OF INTESTINAL RESECTION ON FLUID AND NUTRIENT ABSORPTION

The main role of the intestine is the absorption of fluid, nutrients and electrolytes, and as such it has a large capacity for adaptation to the loss of intestinal length by increasing the absorptive surface area as well as molecular changes increasing nutrient transporter levels. This may be due to either surgical resection or a reduction in functional capacity associated with severe cases of chronic inflammatory intestinal conditions such as Crohn's disease or ulcerative colitis. Patients with reduced functional intestinal length may therefore require supplemental parenteral nutrition, intravenous fluid or both, depending on the site and extent of affected bowel. Resection of the proximal jejunum can be compensated by the ileum and colon adapting to absorb the additional fluid and electrolyte load, hence these patients do not require supplemental nutrition. Resection of the ileum, however, may have more significant consequences. The ileum is responsible for bile salt reabsorption and loss of even 100 cm of ileum may cause steatorrhoea, which can be treated by the administration of cholestyramine for bile salt binding. If greater lengths of ileum are affected, dietary fat restriction may also be necessary. Ileal resection also increases

---

J Arthur Harris, 1880–1930, botanist and biometrician, head of the Department of Botany, University of Minnesota, St Paul, MN, USA (1924–1930).
Francis G Benedict, 1870–1957, American chemist, physiologist and nutritionist, developed a calorimeter and a spirometer used to determine oxygen consumption and measure metabolic rate.
Burrill Bernard Crohn, 1884–1983, gastroenterologist, Mount Sinai Hospital, New York, NY, USA, described regional ileitis in 1932.

gastric motility and intestinal transit, resulting in a greater volume of fluid and electrolytes reaching the colon, causing symptoms of diarrhoea. The greatest consequences of loss of functioning intestinal length occur in patients with remnant small intestine of less than 200 cm. This results in significantly reduced absorptive capacity, with the associated metabolic and nutritional consequences of short bowel syndrome.

Short bowel syndrome (discussed in more detail in ***Chapter 74***) is characterised by symptoms of diarrhoea, malnutrition and dehydration, with variable severity depending on the extent and function of the remaining small bowel. The acute stage of short bowel syndrome occurs in the first few weeks following the insult. It is characterised by high intestinal losses, gastric hypersecretion and hypergastrinaemia and can result in acute renal failure and acid–base imbalances. The subsequent adaptation stage occurs over 1–2 years and is a consequence of the structural and functional changes within the remnant bowel, allowing increased absorptive capacity and ameliorating some of the earlier symptoms. Sufficient recovery may occur in some patients to render parenteral nutrition no longer necessary; however, some features of intestinal insufficiency may still remain, requiring special diets, supplementation of nutrients and some pharmacological treatments. Intestinal rehabilitation programmes have been developed over the last decade to optimise intestinal function in short bowel syndrome as much as possible; however, recovery of function to allow weaning from home parenteral nutrition becomes unlikely beyond 3 years of onset. Intestinal transplantation is an option in those dependent on lifelong parenteral nutrition; this is covered in greater detail in ***Chapter 91***.

Patients who have less than 100 cm of total residual bowel have a particularly severe form of short bowel syndrome as they will lose more water and electrolytes from their bowel than consumed by mouth. Daily bowel losses can exceed 4 litres in a 24-hour period. Consumption of oral fluids with sodium concentrations of less than 90 mmol/L will result in a net efflux of sodium from plasma into the bowel lumen, hence hypotonic fluids should be restricted to less than 1 litre per day and patients should be encouraged to drink glucose and saline replacement solutions such as oral rehydration salts. Fluid balance needs to be carefully monitored; while some of the fluid intake will be covered by parenteral nutrition, further intravenous fluid supplementation may also be necessary in cases of particularly high bowel output.

ARTIFICIAL NUTRITIONAL SUPPORT

Given the importance of adequate nutrition in recovery from illness and surgery, consideration for artificial nutritional support should be given in any patient who has had inadequate nutritional intake for 5 days or more. In patients with pre-existing chronic malnutrition, this should be instituted earlier, and ideally in the preoperative period if feasible. Patients due to undergo major surgery for head and neck or abdominal cancers (such as laryngeal or pharyngeal resections, oesophagectomies, gastrectomies and pancreaticoduodenectomies) are more likely to have difficulty consuming any or sufficient oral nutrition postoperatively because of oedema, obstruction, delayed gastric emptying and paralytic ileus. These patients are also more likely to have nutritional depletion preoperatively owing to the effects of the underlying disease. Forethought should be given preoperatively in these patients regarding the placement of intravenous access, nasojejunal tubes or feeding jejunostomies intraoperatively to facilitate postoperative nutrient delivery (***Figure 25.3***).

Enteral nutrition

Enteral nutrition (the delivery of nutrients into the gastrointestinal tract) should always be the preferred route of administration of nutrition where possible. Benefits of enteral nutrition include preservation of the gut mucosal barrier and immunity and prevention of gut atrophy. The use of enteral nutrition is also associated with reduced infection rates, better wound healing and a reduced length of stay compared with parenteral nutrition. Supplementary enteral nutrition can be in the form of oral supplements as well as via tube-feeding techniques such as feeding gastrostomies or jejunostomies and nasogastric or nasojejunal tubes.

Enteral feeds contain variable nutrient formulations with respect to the content of energy, fat and nitrogen, as well as the osmolarity and nutrient complexity. In general, most feed formulations contain 1–2 kcal/mL and up to 0.6 g/mL protein.

Oral supplements

Many liquid oral supplements are commercially available, supplying around 200 kcal and 2 g of nitrogen per 200-mL carton. These can be used to increase daily caloric intakes in addition to that provided by diet alone, and are useful when weaning patients off tube-feeding regimens.

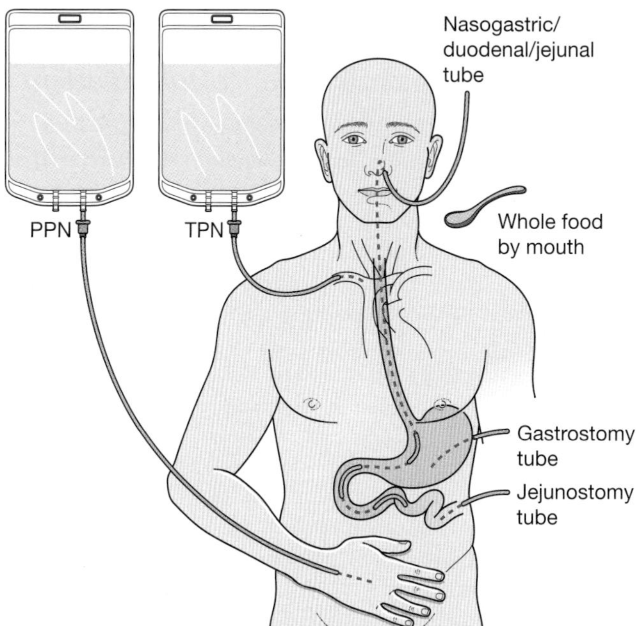

Figure 25.3 Routes available for delivery of artificial nutritional support. PPN, partial parenteral nutrition; TPN, total parenteral nutrition. (Redrawn with permission from Rick Tharp, rxkinetics.com.)

Tube feeding

Patients who are unable to maintain adequate nutritional intake with oral supplements will need administration of enteral feed via tube feeding. This can be prepyloric either via a conventional nasogastric (Ryle's) tube or a fine-bore feeding tube inserted into the stomach or via a surgical or endoscopically placed gastrostomy. Feed can also be delivered beyond the pylorus via a nasojejunal tube or surgical or endoscopic feeding jejunostomy.

The enteral feeding regime is best planned and managed by a trained dietician as administration of enteral feed requires calculation of the patient's nutritional requirements to allow caloric requirements to be met but at a sufficiently gradual rate of increase to prevent the onset of refeeding syndrome in the chronically malnourished patient. The rate of feeding typically starts at 10–20 mL/h and can increase to approximately 75 mL/h if tolerated.

Enteral feeding protocols should include aspiration of the tube, if of sufficiently wide calibre, to reduce the risk of nosocomial aspiration pneumonia by reducing or stopping the administration of enteral feed if aspirate volumes are high. Tube blockage is common and can be prevented by regular flushing with water daily. Specific agents such as chymotrypsin may be used to unblock a partially obstructed tube; however, guidewires should not be used because of the risk of perforation of the tube and thus damage to the lumen of the stomach or bowel. A radio-opaque nasogastric or Ryle's tube can be used for short-term feeding in the majority of patients and provides the advantage of also having a wide enough calibre to allow aspiration; however, the high-grade polyvinylchloride (PVC) material used can become brittle over time and thus should be changed every 2 weeks. For longer term feeding a fine-bore feeding tube (8–12Fr) may be preferable to minimise the risk of rhinitis, pharyngitis and gastric and oesophageal erosions. These tubes are also less likely to interfere with eating and drinking and are often better tolerated by patients.

Techniques for establishment of tube feeding

Insertion of nasogastric and nasojejunal feeding tubes

Nasogastric tubes can usually be inserted in the ward setting; however, in patients in whom there may be any concerns regarding the oropharyngeal or oesophagogastric anatomy, endoscopic insertion under direct visualisation may be needed. Patients are positioned in a semirecumbent position and the distance between the xiphisternum and the tip of the nose measured. The tube is inserted into the chosen nostril and advanced gently to the 10-cm point. Patients are then encouraged to swallow and the tube simultaneously advanced down the oesophagus with successive swallows until the distance measured to the xiphisternum is reached. The position of the nasogastric tube will need to be checked before feed is administered, either by pH testing (pH <5 is considered safe) or with a chest radiograph to confirm that the tip of the nasogastric tube is below the diaphragm and well past the bronchial bifurcation. Fine-bore feeding tubes can be inserted in a manner similar to above, but may require a guidewire within the tube to facilitate insertion; this must be confirmed to have been removed after insertion of the tube (***Figure 25.4***).

Feed can also be delivered directly to the jejunum via either tube feeding or surgically created jejunostomies. The advantage of this is that it bypasses the stomach and can thus overcome problems of delayed gastric emptying without necessitating the use of total parenteral nutrition (TPN). Nasojejunal feeding can also be used in patients who are unable to have a gastrostomy as this is the least invasive form of nutrient delivery into the jejunum. The siting of nasojejunal tubes requires either endoscopic or radiological (fluoroscopic) guidance; therefore, unlike nasogastric tubes, these cannot be inserted in the typical ward setting. Abdominal radiographs can confirm the position of the nasojejunal tube if there is any concern regarding proximal migration or displacement (***Figure 25.5***).

Gastrostomy

Gastrostomy tubes are generally reserved for patients who require longer term feeding. The decision for insertion of these tubes is increasingly discussed in the multidisciplinary context because of the long-term physical, psychological and lifestyle implications. Gastrostomy insertion can be endoscopic (percutaneous endoscopic gastrostomy [PEG]), radiological (radiologically inserted gastrostomy [RIG]) or surgical (***Figure 25.6***).

A PEG involves the insertion of the gastrostomy tube through the abdomen and stomach under vision via an endoscope, avoiding a surgical incision and a general anaesthetic. The endoscopist is able to visualise a cannula entering the

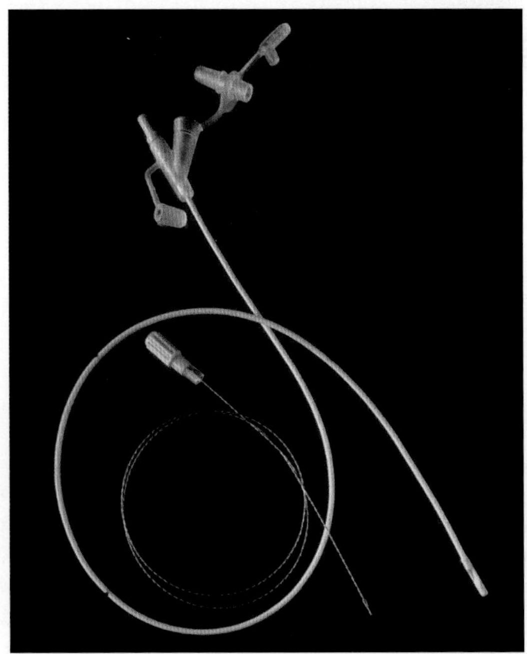

Figure 25.4 A fine-bore feeding tube with its guidewire.

John Alfred Ryle, 1889–1950, Regius Professor of Medicine, University of Cambridge, Cambridge, and later Professor of Social Medicine, University of Oxford, Oxford, UK, introduced the Ryle's tube in 1921.

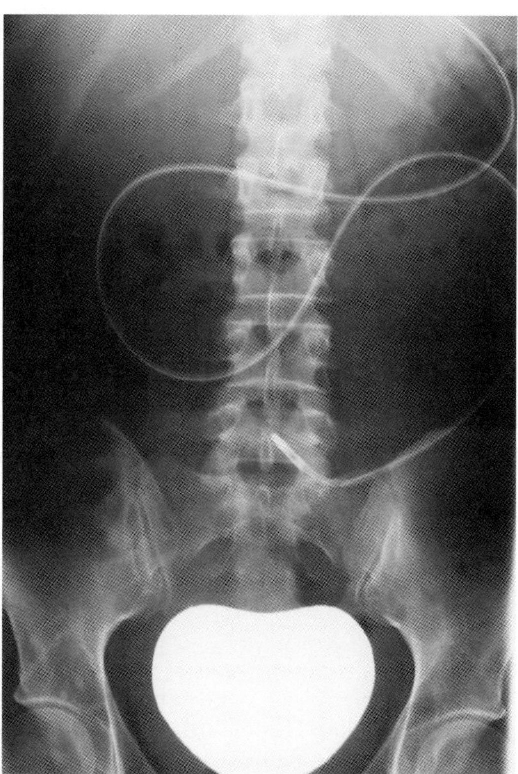

Figure 25.5 Abdominal radiograph confirming that the position of the tip of a nasojejunal feeding tube is past the duodenojejunal flexure.

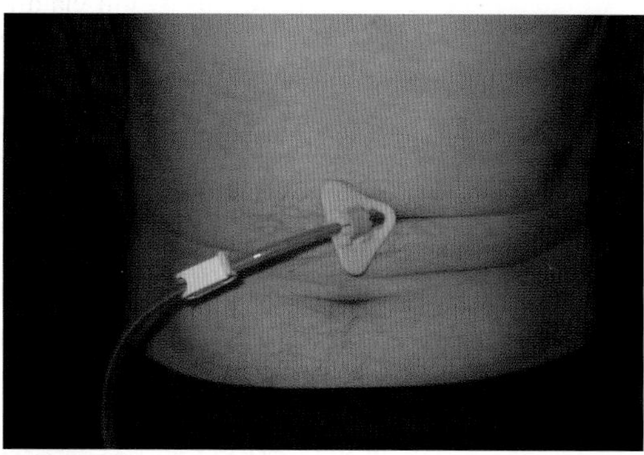

Figure 25.6 Percutaneous endoscopic gastrostomy tube, showing the external bumper and tube clamp

insufflated stomach via the anterior abdominal wall, through which a guidewire is passed. Then either the gastrostomy tube can be inserted through the anterior abdominal wall over the guidewire or the guidewire can be pulled out via the mouth and the tube secured to the guidewire, pulled down into the stomach and then pulled out through the abdominal wall. The stomach wall is pulled up to the anterior abdominal wall and held in place by a cuff, balloon or plastic bumper to minimise the risk of intraperitoneal leakage (***Figure 25.7***).

A RIG is an option in patients who are unable to have a PEG because of difficulty with oesophageal intubation, compromised respiratory function or oropharyngeal anatomy distortion such as from head and neck cancers. A nasogastric tube is inserted to insufflate the stomach and a cannula is

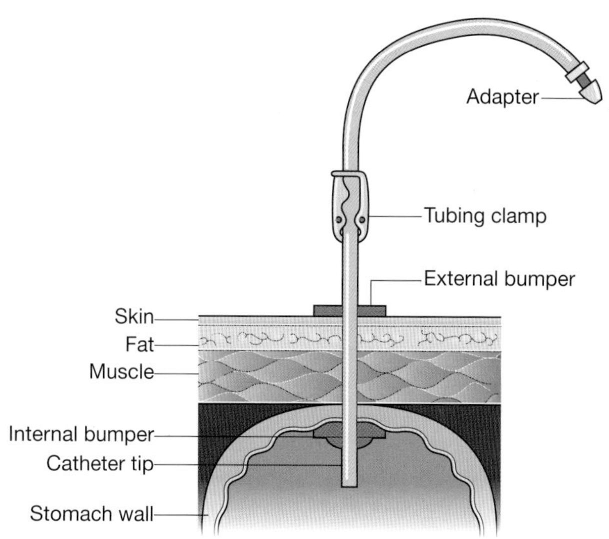

Figure 25.7 Cross-sectional appearance of a percutaneous endoscopic gastrostomy tube *in situ*, showing the abutment of the stomach to the abdominal wall to minimise risk of leakage and peritonitis.

inserted under radiographic guidance to facilitate insertion of the gastrostomy device, which is retained internally via a balloon or a pigtail. Contrast can be administered via the RIG to confirm the correct site of placement.

A surgical gastrostomy may be necessary in patients who are unable to have either a PEG or a RIG, most commonly because of distorted intra-abdominal anatomy, usually from previous surgical intervention. This will require either a laparotomy or a laparoscopy with a small gastrostomy to allow insertion of the feeding tube, which can be held in place either by insufflation of a balloon or by a plastic 'bumper'. The stomach wall is fixed to the anterior abdominal wall with sutures to minimise intraperitoneal leakage. Some gastrostomy devices also allow the fitting of jejunal extensions, thus allowing venting of stomach contents and simultaneous delivery of nutrients into the jejunum.

Complications of a gastrostomy, regardless of the technique of placement, include perforation, bleeding and peritonitis. Localised sepsis around the insertion site is very common and may require systemic antibiotics. Gastrostomies that have been in place for a long period are likely to develop a persistent gastric fistula on removal owing to epithelialisation of the tract, which may require surgical intervention for closure. Tube blockage may occur, as well as tube displacement.

Nasojejunal tubes and jejunostomies

Surgical jejunostomies are often created at the time of resection in patients undergoing major oesophagogastric surgery who are likely to have insufficient oral intake in the immediate postoperative period.

Jejunostomies require a general anaesthetic and either a laparotomy or a laparoscopy, facilitating the insertion of a feeding tube through the anterior abdominal wall into the proximal jejunum. The site of insertion in the jejunum is usually fixed to the anterior abdominal wall to further reduce the risk of leakage. A more recent development is the siting of a jejunostomy via radiological guidance. The jejunum is punctured under image guidance and a guidewire inserted, over which the tract is dilated to allow a feeding jejunostomy tube to be passed. The position of the tube is confirmed with fluoroscopy and the tube anchored to the skin with sutures.

Complications of jejunostomy insertion in the perioperative period include bleeding or tube displacement and leakage causing peritonitis. In the longer term, granulation tissue formation or localised sepsis at the site of insertion is common.

Complications of enteral feeding

The complications of enteral feeding can be divided into three main groups and are outlined in *Summary box 25.3*. The first group is that of complications related to the siting of tubes or creation of gastrostomies or jejunostomies, which have been covered individually in the sections above. The second group are gastrointestinal complications related to ongoing nutrient delivery. Enteral feeding is not appropriate in patients who are not likely to absorb the delivered nutrients. This includes patients who have an insufficient length of functioning intestine as well as patients with mechanical intestinal obstruction or paralytic ileus. These patients will require TPN as enteral nutrient delivery is likely to result in complications such as aspiration and failure to meet nutritional requirements. Enteral feeding can cause bloating and vomiting and is associated with diarrhoea in over 30% of patients, which can compromise nutritional uptake.

The third group refers to the development of metabolic or biochemical complications, and thus the establishment of feeding should be monitored carefully as rapid increases in nutrient delivery in patients with chronic malnutrition can cause electrolyte disorders and refeeding syndrome (see *Refeeding syndrome*).

Summary box 25.3

Complications of enteral feeding

- Tube related
  - Malposition
  - Displacement
  - Blockage
  - Breakage/leakage
  - Local complications (e.g. erosion of skin/mucosa)
- Gastrointestinal
  - Diarrhoea
  - Bloating, nausea, vomiting
  - Abdominal cramps
  - Aspiration
  - Constipation
- Metabolic/biochemical
  - Electrolyte disorders, including refeeding syndrome
  - Vitamin, mineral, trace element deficiencies
  - Drug interactions

Parenteral nutrition

Indications and composition of parenteral nutrition

Nutrition may need to be delivered intravenously in patients in whom adequate feeding through the alimentary tract is not possible. This can be either in addition to enteral feeding (supplemental parenteral nutrition) or the sole source of nutrition (TPN). TPN is indicated in patients who are unable to meet their nutritional requirements via absorption of nutrients from their intestinal tract. The commonest cause for this is in patients with short bowel syndrome related to massive intestinal resection or a significant reduction in functional small bowel, often related to intestinal fistulation. In some cases the establishment of TPN is a temporary endeavour for a few days to minimise nutritional depletion until a route of enteral nutrition is established, e.g. awaiting the siting of a nasojejunal tube in patients with delayed gastric emptying.

Parenteral nutrition formulations have evolved over the years, but are currently commonly provided by the hospital pharmacy in the form of a 3-litre bag containing a lipid emulsion with a mixture of essential and non-essential amino acids, glucose, electrolytes, trace elements and vitamins. The energy content of parenteral nutrition is in the ratio of 150–250 kcal per gram of protein nitrogen, with usually 30–50% of the energy coming from fat. This ensures sufficient energy provision for amino acids to be utilised for tissue maintenance. Folic acid is supplemented in the solution once or twice a week at a dose of 15 mg and other vitamins are given daily. Patients requiring long-term parenteral nutrition (over many months) would also benefit from a single-dose injection of vitamin B12. Phosphate is an essential component of parenteral nutrition regimens: 20–30 mmol phosphate is required daily to ensure phosphorylation of glucose and prevent hypophosphataemia. The specific composition of parenteral nutrition can be changed daily to reflect the patient's needs and tailored to address any electrolyte deficiencies and ongoing energy requirements. This is guided by daily assessments (including weight and electrolytes). In addition, the protein content will differ in patients who are critically ill (requiring more protein) compared with those with chronic renal failure (requiring less protein). Micronutrients such as zinc, copper, selenium, ferritin, folate and vitamins B12 and D will need to be checked in patients on parenteral nutrition for more than 28 days and every 3 months in patients on long-term parenteral nutrition.

Administration of parenteral nutrition

Parenteral nutrition is usually administered directly into the central venous system (the superior vena cava [SVC] or the right atrium) to minimise the risk of venous thrombophlebitis, through either a peripherally inserted central catheter (PICC) or central venous catheter (*Figure 25.8*). PICC lines may be inserted through the basilic (most commonly used), cephalic, brachial or median cubital vein of the arm, and can be used for parenteral nutrition administration over several weeks to months. Femoral lines should be avoided for parenteral nutrition because of the high risk of infection at this site. Chest radiographs should be performed after PICC or central venous catheters are inserted to confirm the correct position of the line tip within the SVC or right atrium prior to commencing the parenteral feed (*Figure 25.9*).

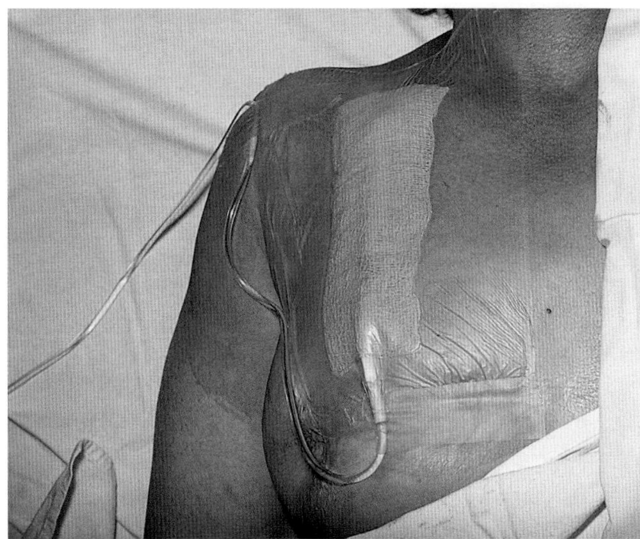

Figure 25.8 An example of a central venous line (in this case a subclavian line) used for administration of parenteral nutrition.

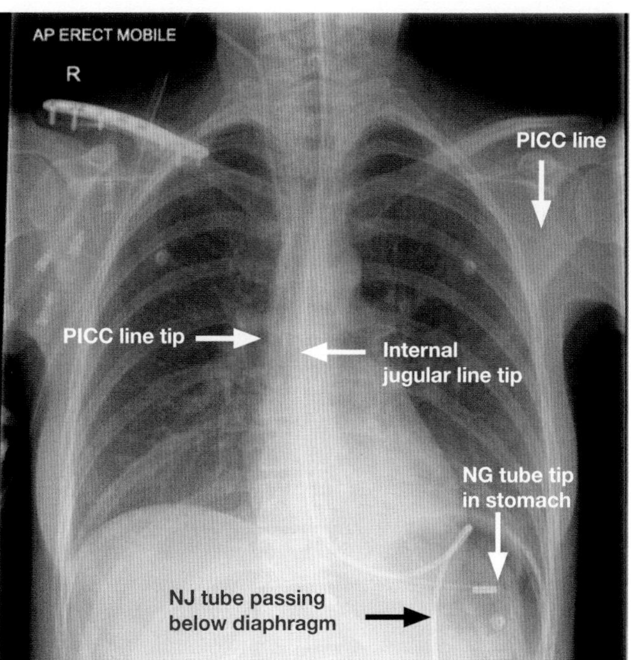

Figure 25.9 A chest radiograph showing correct positioning of the internal jugular and peripherally inserted central catheter lines within the superior vena cava, as well as the tip of the nasogastric (NG) tube in the stomach and the nasojejunal (NJ) tube passing into the abdomen.

In patients who are likely to require long-term parenteral nutrition, an implantable port or a Hickman line may be more appropriate. These are implanted via fluoroscopic or ultrasound guidance with a subcutaneous port or cuff and a catheter attachment sitting within the SVC.

Rarely, parenteral nutrition can be administered through a peripheral venous catheter; however, the high osmolarity of parenteral nutrition produces an increased rate of thrombophlebitis at these sites because of the narrower calibre and low rate of flow in peripheral veins, making it an appropriate option only where the duration of parenteral nutrition administration is less than 14 days. The risk of thrombophlebitis can be reduced to some extent by the use of soft polyurethane paediatric cannulae and using feeds of low osmolarity and neutral pH. The cannulae used will need to be changed every few days.

The parenteral nutrition bag should be covered at all times, including during infusion, with an opaque protective bag to prevent the vitamins from degradation. If the parenteral nutrition infusion is disconnected from the line for any reason during administration the bag will need to be discarded. It is important to remember that parenteral nutrition administration contributes to fluid intake, and thus the volume infused should be carefully recorded on the fluid balance chart to avoid fluid overload. In patients in whom parenteral nutrition is a temporary measure, oral nutritional input or enteral feeding should be monitored, and parenteral nutrition withdrawal planned in a stepwise manner and stopped once the patient is established on adequate oral or enteral support.

Complications of parenteral nutrition

The complications of parenteral nutrition are best considered to fall within one of three categories: insertion complications, line complications and metabolic complications (see *Summary box 25.4*).

Summary box 25.4

Complications of parenteral feeding

- Insertion complications
  - Pneumothorax
  - Misplacement
- Line complications
  - Sepsis
  - Thrombosis
- Metabolic complications
  - Electrolyte disorders, including refeeding syndrome
  - Blood sugar derangement
  - Liver dysfunction
  - Metabolic bone disease
  - Vitamin deficiencies

Insertion complications

The most common complication of line insertion is an inadvertent pneumothorax, which occurs in around 0.5–1% of cases, most commonly during insertion of subclavian lines. It is managed by insertion of a chest drain, which can be removed once the pneumothorax has resolved. Line misplacement can also occur and is diagnosed on chest radiograph, which is mandatory following central line insertion. The line is considered to be in the correct place if the tip is in the inferior third of the SVC or at the atriocaval junction (see ***Figure 25.9***).

Robert O Hickman, 1926–2019, formerly paediatric nephrologist, Seattle Children's Hospital, Seattle, WA, USA.

Line complications

One of the most important line complications is line sepsis, which can occur in up to 15% of patients and is associated with significant morbidity and mortality. Insertion of the line and administration of parenteral nutrition requires strict aseptic technique as line infections can rapidly progress to septicaemia. Catheter entry sites should be checked daily. Patients with suspected line sepsis will need paired blood cultures taken from the line and a separate peripheral site and use of the line should be stopped until culture results are available. Positive cultures will require line removal and commencement of antibiotics. Fungal line infections in particular can be associated with uveitis and bacterial endocarditis.

Line thrombosis is not uncommon and can occasionally occur in major veins in association with line infection, causing serious complications such as SVC occlusion and pulmonary embolism. Treatment is by anticoagulation, rarely requiring fibrinolysis for acute SVC occlusion and endovascular intervention in the longer term. Line blockage is relatively common and can be prevented by regular line flushing after manipulation and the use of a dedicated parenteral nutrition line or, in the case of a multilumen centrally placed catheter, a dedicated lumen. Blocked lines can be unclogged by locking the affected line with heparin–saline or thrombolytic agents.

Metabolic complications

Refeeding syndrome. One of the most significant metabolic complications of both parenteral and enteral feeding is refeeding syndrome. This occurs in the first days after feeding is commenced in patients who have been severely malnourished. Patients due to start nutritional support need to be screened for the risk of refeeding syndrome. The degree of risk is related to their BMI, amount and rate of unintentional weight loss, period of starvation and electrolyte levels (see ***Summary box 25.5***).

The main underlying pathological process is one of hypophosphataemia, resulting in fluid and electrolyte shifts between the intra- and extracellular compartments. Patients may develop arrythmias, muscle weakness, respiratory or cardiac failure, oedema, lethargy or seizures; at its most severe the syndrome can be fatal. Laboratory tests will reveal low levels of phosphate, potassium, calcium and magnesium and a lactic acidosis. Nutritional support in this group of patients should be started at a maximum of 10 kcal/kg per day, aiming to increase levels slowly to meet full needs by 4–7 days. Frequent monitoring and replacement of the electrolytes listed above is essential. Nutritional support should include supplementary thiamine, vitamin B, multivitamins and trace elements.

Summary box 25.5

Refeeding syndrome

Patient is considered to be at risk of developing refeeding syndrome with
EITHER

One or more of the following:

- BMI <16 kg/m^2
- Unintentional weight loss >15% within the last 3–6 months
- Little or no nutritional intake for more than 10 days
- Low potassium, phosphate or magnesium levels prior to feeding

OR

Two of more of the following:

- BMI <18.5 kg/m^2
- Unintentional weight loss >10% within the last 3–6 months
- Little or no nutritional intake for more than 5 days
- History of alcohol abuse or on medication, including insulin, chemotherapy, antacids or diuretics

Blood sugar derangement. In patients with diabetes and those with impaired blood glucose control owing to critical illness, administration of parenteral nutrition should coincide with a variable insulin infusion regimen to avoid hyperglycaemia. Conversely, insulin dosing should be reduced accordingly when parenteral nutrition is interrupted to avoid hypoglycaemia.

Liver dysfunction. Long-term use of parenteral nutrition is associated with derangement of liver function tests in at least 25% of patients. Fatty liver is a common complication. This is worse in children, and the degree can be reduced by modifying the parenteral nutrition solution, such as alternating the use of lipid-free parenteral nutrition solutions. A smaller percentage of patients may subsequently develop liver fibrosis and cirrhosis. Once liver disease is established in these patients the term 'intestinal failure-associated liver disease' (IFALD) is used, as these cholestatic changes in liver function profile are difficult to separate from the effects of short bowel syndrome. Factors such as a lack of colonic continuity, extreme short bowel, lack of enteral intake and high energy and fat content in feed have all been associated with a higher risk of the development of IFALD.

Metabolic bone disease and vitamin deficiencies. Osteoporosis or osteomalacia are both known complications of long-term parenteral nutrition, leading to fractures or kidney stones. Supplementation of calcium, phosphate, vitamin D and sometimes bisphosphonates can both prevent and treat this complication. Excess or deficiency of vitamins or trace elements may occur, manifesting with non-specific symptoms such as anaemia, hair loss or neurological symptoms. Regular measurements and replacement, as well as clinical assessment, can prevent this from occurring.

NUTRITION SUPPORT TEAMS

Multidisciplinary nutrition support teams are essential to ensure that all essential aspects relating to the appropriateness of nutritional support, initiation and maintenance are addressed safely. The team should include doctors, dieticians, specialist nutrition support nurses and pharmacists and may also include other allied healthcare professionals such as speech and language therapists. Specialist nutrition support nurses, in conjunction with ward nurses and dieticians, should aim to minimise complications related to enteral or parenteral feeding, develop and implement protocols for training of ward nurses in administration of enteral and parenteral nutrition, and support transition of feeding into the community setting around the time of discharge from hospital.

SUMMARY

Appropriate and safe assessment and administration of fluid therapy and nutritional support is of key importance in good surgical practice. It is imperative that the preoperative nutritional state of the patient and the impact of any surgical intervention are taken into account when considering nutritional requirements and the mode of nutrient delivery. Appreciation and avoidance of complications of both enteral and parenteral nutrition such as refeeding syndrome are also essential. Nutrient support teams play an important role in ensuring the safe administration and weaning of supplemental nutrition in a challenging area of practice.

FURTHER READING

British Association for Parenteral and Enteral Nutrition. *Parenteral nutrition.* Redditch: BAPEN, 2016. Available from https://www.bapen.org.uk/nutrition-support/parenteral-nutrition/.

National Institute for Health and Care Excellence. *Nutrition support for adults: oral nutrition support, enteral tube feeding and parenteral nutrition.* NICE Clinical Guideline 32. London: NICE, 2017. Available from https://www.nice.org.uk/guidance/cg32/chapter/1-Guidance#parenteral-nutrition-in-hospital-and-the-community/.

CHAPTER 26 Introduction to trauma

Learning objectives

- Become familiar with the timeline concept in trauma management
- Understand how to assess a trauma problem
- Appreciate the importance of observing trends for identification of evolving conditions
- Recognise that specific criteria exist for implementation of different treatment strategies

DEFINITION OF TRAUMA

Trauma can be defined as an injury to any part of the human body as the result of energy transfer from an inflicting source. The forces that can lead to injury include chemical, thermal, ionising radiation and mechanical. The extent and severity of the trauma sustained depends upon the magnitude, nature and duration of the inflicting cause.

Major trauma denotes injuries to more than one body region or organ system. In Part 4, trauma will be examined from a variety of viewpoints, interconnected to different specialties. In this chapter we will examine the facets that bind the whole topic together.

THE MAGNITUDE OF THE PROBLEM

In western industrialised countries, trauma accounts for the largest number of deaths and disability in children and young adults. According to the World Health Organization, there are an estimated 5 million injury fatalities worldwide, representing about 9% of global deaths. This rate is 1.7 times higher than deaths caused by malaria, tuberculosis and human immunodeficiency virus (HIV)/acquired immunodeficiency syndrome (AIDS).

Road traffic accidents (RTAs), falls and intentional violence continue to be the most prevalent causes of trauma fatalities, with a combined rate of 64%. Of note, the major burden of injury is increasing in low- and middle-income countries secondary to industrialisation and increasing motorised transportation. Interestingly, the annual incidence and trends over time show that there is variation from country to country. Information is usually obtained from national statistics organisations that use the International Classification of Diseases, a system that can be limited in providing accurate descriptions of injury severity. In contrast, the Abbreviated Injury Scale dictionary consists of a greater level of detail (including more than 2000 injury codes) and assigns to every injury a severity score between 1 (mild) and 6 (maximum). This can be summated into the so-called injury severity score (ISS), which provides an indication of the anatomical severity of injury suffered by the individual patient. Major trauma is defined as an ISS greater than 15. The majority of patients admitted to hospital with injury have low ISS values, ranging between 4 and 9, with injuries such as an isolated limb fracture and/or isolated mild head injury. Overall, major trauma affects approximately 15% of all injured patients.

According to the UK Department of Transport, in 2019, the overall number of casualties following an RTA reported to the police, including all severities, was 153 158, of whom 25 945 had sustained severe injuries. Overall, 1752 individuals died as a result of their injuries. Across Europe, according to the data presented by the European Transport Safety Council's Performance Index (PIN) report, it appears that the overall number of fatalities was reduced by 3% compared with 2018, and was estimated to be 22 660. In 16 countries, the death rate decreased whereas in 12 it increased, with the four remaining countries registering no change.

As countries do not use the same definition of serious injury, international comparisons are based on road deaths per million inhabitants. In the 27 Member States of the European Union (EU27), the overall level of road mortality was 42 deaths per million inhabitants in 2020 compared with 67 per million in 2010 (***Figure 26.1***). The EU road mortality rate was 51 per million in 2019; the unprecedented drop in mortality between 2019 and 2020 was mainly due to the traffic restrictions to contain the pandemic.

Norway remains the leader among PIN countries with 17 road deaths per million inhabitants, followed by Sweden with 20 deaths per million inhabitants in 2020. In Malta, the UK, Switzerland and Denmark, road mortality is below 27 per million. The highest road mortality is in Romania and Latvia, with 85 and 73 road deaths per million inhabitants, respectively.

A large proportion of severely injured survivors experience long-term or permanent disability as a result of their injuries. Approximately one-third of severely injured survivors sustained life-changing injuries and were unable to return to

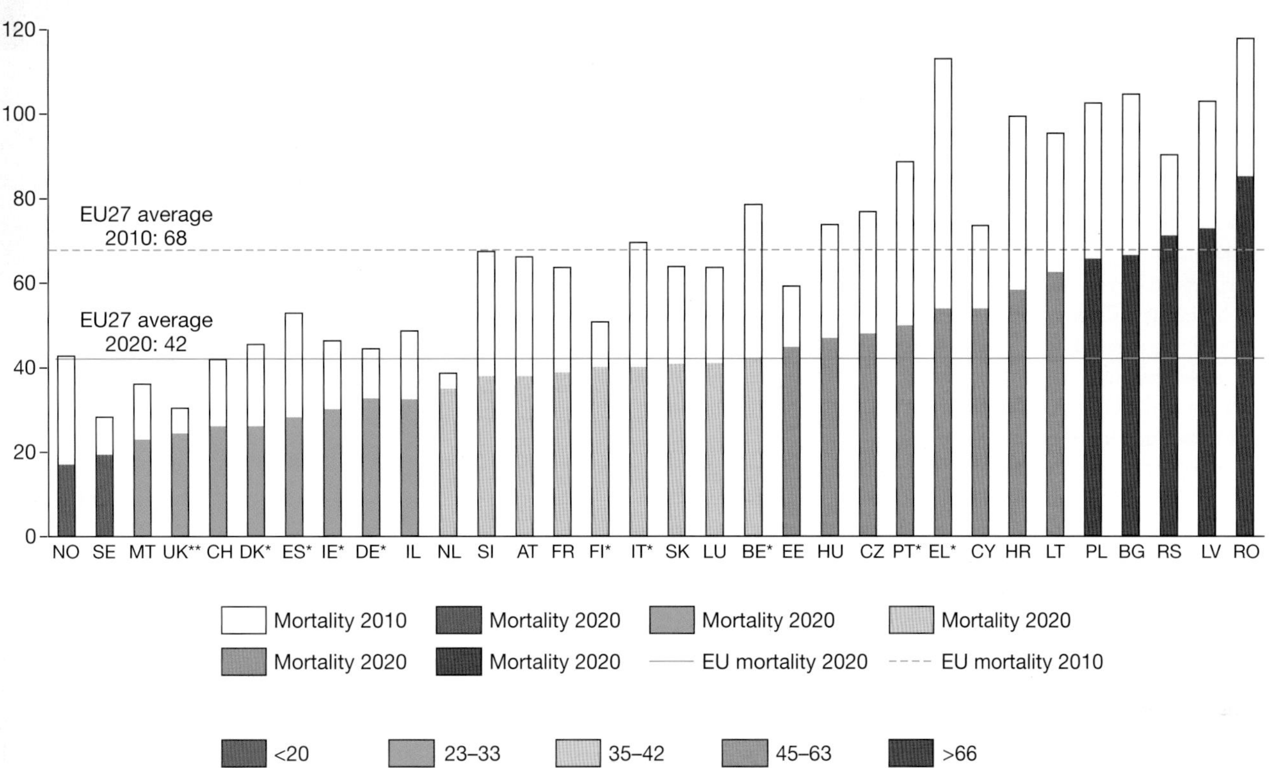

Figure 26.1 Mortality (road deaths per million inhabitants) in 2020 (coloured bars) with mortality in 2010 for comparison (white bars) (courtesy of the European Transport Council). *National provisional estimates used for 2020. The annual number of deaths in LU and MT are particularly small and, therefore, subject to substantial annual fluctuations. **UK data for 2020 are the provisional total for Great Britain for the year ending June 2020 combined with the total for Northern Ireland for the calendar year 2020.

their previous level of function and occupation, undergoing profound lifestyle changes including long-term pain and suffering. It should be emphasised that an injury affects not only the injured person but also everyone who is involved in the injured person's life. The impact of the modern epidemic of RTAs on the universal epidemic of violent injury cannot be overstated. The annual direct medical cost of injuries treated in hospitals and additional care facilities is estimated to be somewhere between £3.5 billion and £4 billion. Moreover, additional indirect costs, due to loss of earnings, loss of productivity and a reduced quality of life, increase the total sum significantly.

Multiple injuries are often thought to occur primarily in younger patients who are involved in incidents with a high energy transfer. Lately, multiple injuries are also seen in the older population as patients live longer, are more active and we have better diagnostics. The last point is particularly important as older adult patients were often underinvestigated, so the full extent of injury was not appreciated.

Recent data published by the UK's National Institute for Health and Care Excellence (NICE) revealed that there are an estimated 500 000 new patients with fragility fractures per year in the UK; approximately 70 000 of these are admitted with proximal femoral fractures, among whom 6.7% of those aged >65 years will die within 30 days of the incident, as reported by the National Hip Fracture Database. Most of the remaining patients with proximal femoral fractures will have diminished independence and functional capacity. It is therefore unsurprising that this particular cohort of patients, the number of whom will increase in coming years owing to the anticipated increase in life expectancy, is thought to represent a huge burden on healthcare services and society in general.

In summary, the overwhelming majority of trauma is not life- or limb-threatening and full recovery with return to preinjury status is usually expected. However, it remains of paramount importance that injuries are detected early in order to properly intervene and therefore achieve a favourable outcome. For instance, one must be vigilant not to miss paediatric non-accidental injury (NAI) (see ***Chapter 44***) or injuries secondary to a chronic underlying disease process rather than the injury itself, for example pathological fractures in older age groups. Of note, it has been shown that, in 66% of cases when children die as a result of abuse, there has been some previous interaction with a health professional or with social services, but the seriousness of the situation was not fully appreciated.

Summary box 26.1

Trauma: the magnitude of the problem

- The vast majority of trauma is not life- or limb-threatening
- Severe trauma continues to be a major cause of death in young patients
- Older adult patients with fragility fractures are a special group posing a further burden to a healthcare system
- Promptly identifying important features of injuries could influence the outcome

THE MANAGEMENT OF TRAUMA

As soon as a severe injury occurs, every second counts, and all aspects of decision making and management are critical for a patient's long-term quality of life and even their survival. The concepts of initial assessment and management have specific goals that are based on practice over a long period of time. In the modern era, new protocols have been formulated that are centred on a profound understanding of the physiology of the host response to an acute threat to homeostasis; these protocols allow clinicians to use standardised measures and to speak a common language. They also reduce delays and expedite patient care, especially when clinicians are under pressure to make a critical decision. However, an understanding of the reasoning behind them remains crucial.

As in other acute conditions, the patient is particularly reliant upon the clinician when trauma occurs. A patient with a chronic condition is familiar with the nature of their problem and the way in which it is progressing. The surgeon may offer a remedy and the patient may consider the potential benefits and choose appropriately whether to accept the remedy. The injured patient does not know what will happen without treatment and so relies on the surgeon to inform them of both the natural history and the potential benefits of any intervention. The implication is that, as surgeons, we have a duty to be aware of both.

The significance of time in the outcome

Injuries can happen at lightning speed. Time point 0 (time 0) is defined as literally the seconds prior to the event, when the patient is at their normal baseline. All subsequent events, including the acute physiological response to injury, the body's internal mechanisms to maintain homeostasis (to compensate for the sequelae of trauma), the healing processes and the actions instigated by health professionals, are associated with a 'timeline'. This 'timeline principle' is crucial to a deeper understanding of how to prioritise assessment, investigation and treatment in what may be a rapidly evolving situation following injury. There is an optimal time window during which an intervention can have a radically positive effect on treatment outcome. Based on this timeline, interventions may be grossly categorised as emergent (life-saving), acute (restoring and maintaining physiological and physical stability) and delayed or semielective (focusing on the treatment of post-fracture fixation complications [non-union, infection and malunion from the orthopaedic trauma point of view]).

In the immediate aftermath of a major trauma, the physiological crisis continues to evolve, the risk of death is increased and less appropriate and prompt interventions are carried out. Potentially rapidly evolving situations, such as airway obstruction, tension haemothorax and haemopericardium, if left untreated, will inevitably have catastrophic consequences and therefore should be given priority in terms of the initial medical response to an injured patient. Thus, the seriousness and the immediate impact of a specific clinical condition should dictate its prioritisation, leading to a systematic approach ('what kills first should be managed first') (*Figure 26.2*).

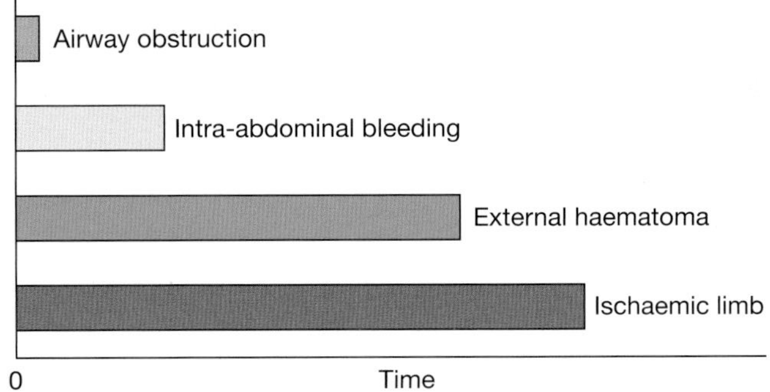

Figure 26.2 Estimated time from incident to death or irretrievable damage for various conditions.

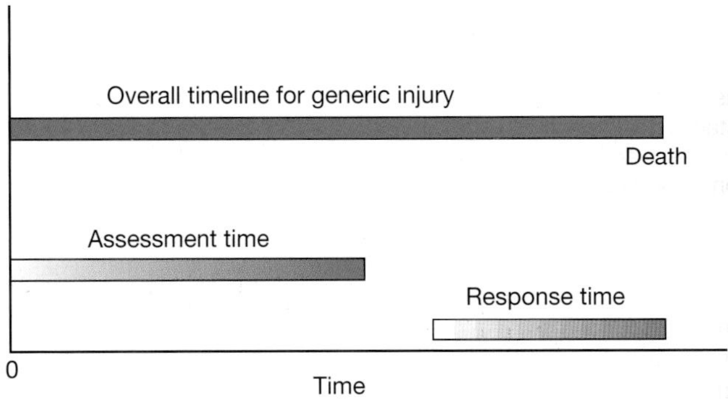

Figure 26.3 Diagrammatic representation of the relationship between assessment and response times. In this example, there is time to assess and respond effectively before death.

The Advanced Trauma Life Support (ATLS) system delineates an order of priorities defined by ABCD; that is, airway, breathing, circulation and disability (neurology). This hierarchy of priorities is based on the 'time dependence' principle. In other words, the time taken to manage an individual problem is the sum of the time taken to identify it and to execute effective treatment (*Figure 26.3*). In such settings, time is critical, so the normal history and physical investigations are not performed during the ATLS primary survey, but the primary focus is on detecting and identifying individual problems, ranking them in order of priority and dealing with them effectively and efficiently in their appropriate timeframes.

The clinician should take into consideration the mechanism of injury and initial clinical findings then promptly request and carry out specific investigations, for example computed tomography (CT) scans. This is to allow rapid and precise identification of injuries that may benefit from early therapeutic intervention and that otherwise might be clinically challenging as the initial signs may be subtle or non-specific. This proactive approach is critical, as the evaluation and diagnosis of an important injury may be difficult before the full-blown and potentially life-threatening presentation of that injury.

A typical example would be an RTA victim with a scalp laceration and a reduced Glasgow Coma Scale (GCS) score of 13/15; such a drop in the GCS could be explained by head

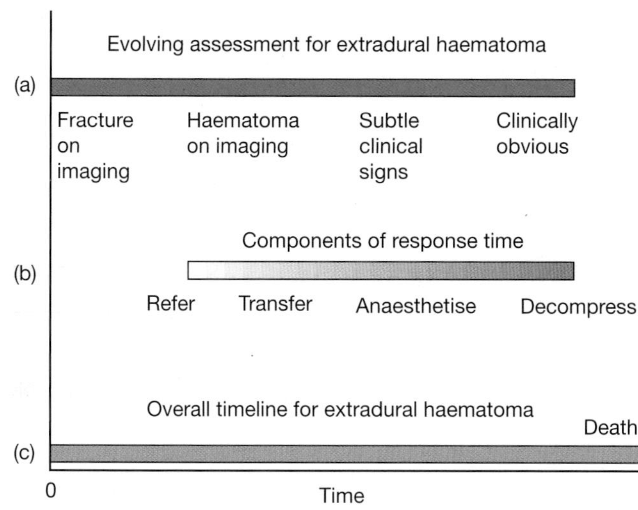

Figure 26.4 Diagrammatic representation of the relationship between assessment and response times for extradural haematoma: (a) the stages of assessment, (b) the components of the response and (c) the overall time from incident to death. It can be seen that relying on obvious clinical signs gives insufficient time to respond effectively.

injury or by the presence of shock and hypoxia. Waiting for the development of overt clinical signs could be dangerous. Should there be any injury such as an extradural haematoma this can be diagnosed with a head CT prior to the presentation of clinical signs. Prompt surgical decompression will result in a reduced risk of morbidity and mortality. In this situation, if the time taken to make the diagnosis were prolonged, such that the clinical signs presented prior to treatment intervention, it may be too late to prevent the death of the patient (*Figure 26.4*). This frequently encountered clinical case scenario demonstrates the principle that we need to introduce a management response even before we have made the definitive diagnosis if we want to save the patient's life. It is clear, therefore, that the 'timeline concept' is critical in the safe management of trauma patients.

Reducing the diagnosis time and response time of our interventions is dependent not only on clinical staff but also on the availability of resources. For the example above, a dedicated trauma team and a CT scanner should be available 24/7. Recently, this 24/7 availability of the trauma team and the designation of regional hospitals to operate as Level I Trauma Centres, with the availability of all disciplines and appropriate equipment on site, has provided the necessary foundation for the development of a unified trauma care system in England. Indeed, the first reports published on its effectiveness in saving lives have been very positive.

The 'timeline concept' that has been discussed in the management of patients with multiple trauma can be applied to patients with isolated injuries. Again, the key issue – irrespective of the number of injuries – is to minimise delays in making the diagnosis and promptly initiate treatment. Such a global approach would save lives, reduce morbidity and make the healthcare system more efficient in terms of resource utilisation, as well as cost-effectiveness.

Summary box 26.2

The importance of time

- A thorough understanding of the 'timeline concept' in trauma is critical
- Assessment should be completed within a set time
- The time to respond is limited
- The goal is for both assessment and response to take place in the time window prior to irreversible damage or death

Most importantly, dealing with a patient in an acute setting is a dynamic situation, which may fluctuate unpredictably along the timeline. Therefore, any observation and analysis may evolve rapidly to an extent that interventions need to be modified accordingly. Thus, ongoing patient evaluation is essential in order to identify and respond to every fluctuation noted in a timely fashion. The initial primary survey, applied according to the ATLS protocol in trauma patients, should be followed by secondary and tertiary clinical assessment, even after the acute phase of treatment has been completed successfully. Ongoing monitoring of vital organ activity, ordering of the necessary biochemical and radiological investigations and recording of all the findings in a single place can allow easier evaluation and identification of trends over time to facilitate prompt intervention. Such a strategy may reduce the risk of having undiagnosed injuries and delays in a patient's treatment. Several studies have been published that report on missed injuries and make some recommendations on how to avoid these.

The timeline following an injury is continuous, and the accumulated documentation may become voluminous, complex and confusing. It is helpful periodically to make the effort to stand back and summarise the situation. In its recent trauma guidelines, NICE refers to this and advises that a plain language summary of the situation directed at the patient's family doctor, but intelligible and available to the patient or carers, should be produced within 24 hours.

ASSESSMENT AND RESPONSE

The assessment of trauma

Traditionally, and especially when learning the theory of the various component parts of the assessment of the injured patient, this is done in a sequential linear fashion. However, when dealing with a severely injured patient in practice, time is of the essence and when resources allow several things may be happening simultaneously – this is so-called horizontal management; while there may be a number of practical activities occurring simultaneously, the coordination, assessment and control of the situation remains as a mental exercise for the 'hands-off' team leader. In particular, acquiring very early definitive diagnoses with CT is increasingly important. To provide such a level of care generally needs a systematic approach to concentrating resources and to preferably bringing the severely injured patient to that resource – a major trauma system.

The objective of assessment of a trauma patient is to form the best understanding possible of the injuries sustained and their consequences. Forming that whole picture is a challenging process. The clinician must make the best use of what they know of the mechanism of injury, pre-existing patient factors and the injuries already found. Synthesising the associations of these three factors will help direct attention to finding other less obvious problems. Sometimes, the pieces of the puzzle do not 'add up'; at that point, the clinician should attempt to think 'outside of the box' as there may be something unexpected, such as an unknown underlying pathology leading to a pathological fracture, or deliberately concealed, such as in NAI.

For instance, a 50-year-old male restrained passenger in a car involved in a head-on collision with another vehicle may sustain rib fractures, a sternal fracture and a thoracic spine fracture but there may also be cardiac contusion and abdominal injuries. Very early CT and echocardiography may decrease the need for clinical acumen, but in many centres it is not available. The clinician then needs to use their knowledge of the mechanism of injury and the obvious rib and sternal fractures to direct their attention to excluding the less obvious but potentially life-threatening abdominal or cardiac injuries. Similarly, when sophisticated investigations and techniques are available, the clinician should not be over-reliant on them and neglect the important logical thought processes required to piece together the information that is available. It remains of value to consider how a clinician can make best use of the available information for the benefit of the patient.

Summary box 26.3

The assessment of trauma

- Appreciate the factors in the relationship: mechanism + patient factors = injuries sustained
- Use this to allow obvious features to lead to the discovery of less obvious injuries
- When the features do not appear to 'add up' this should be an alert for the clinician to think 'outside the box' and connect the dots

Mechanisms

Mechanisms may be broadly classified as blunt, penetrating or even of a combined nature. *Table 26.1* shows examples of how knowledge of the mechanism may help detect more covert injuries. Early definitive imaging may be thought to reduce the need for such considerations, but the clinician can help the radiologist by directing their attention to potential diagnoses. The adage that 'unless you are very fortunate you only find what you look for' is apt. The most common mechanism involves blunt trauma, which may be either direct or indirect. In a direct mechanism, the damage is localised to the initial site of that mechanism. In contrast, in an indirect mechanism the damage occurs at a distant site after transmission of the force exerted. For example, a direct kick to the medial aspect of the mid-shaft of the tibia in a footballer by an opponent may induce an isolated transverse tibial fracture. There will be localised bruising and ecchymosis where the force was applied.

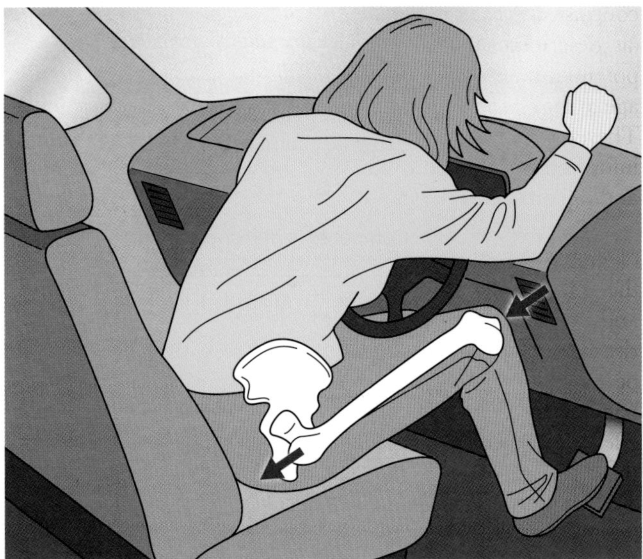

Figure 26.5 The injury force in a car accident can be transmitted from the dashboard to the knee and then to the hip, which is the site of injury.

On the other hand, a fall from a height of 1 metre with a twisting moment as the foot hits the ground can lead to a spiral fracture of the distal tibia. In this situation the force is transmitted through the body's tissues to a location some distance away from its original point of application. In this case, other injuries may have occurred along that line of transmission and should also be sought, such as a remote fibular fracture. Similarly, a motor vehicle crash associated with a point of impact of the knee joint of the driver on the dashboard of the car could induce a fracture dislocation of the acetabulum and hip joint (transmission of force from the knee joint to the hip socket – an indirect blunt mechanism) (*Figure 26.5*).

TABLE 26.1 Examples of patterns of injury.

Mechanism	Obvious features	Covert injuries
Left-sided impact from road traffic accident	• Lateral compression of the pelvis • Left-sided pneumothorax	• Splenic rupture • Extradural haematoma
Flexion distraction (lap belt)	• Chance fracture of the lumbar spine • Dislocated knee • Head injury	• Duodenal rupture • Popliteal artery disruption • Cervical spine fracture
Electrocution	Burn on hand and collapse	Posterior dislocation of the shoulder
Dashboard impact	Knee wound	Posterior dislocation of the hip

The 'timeline concept' previously discussed should not be taken to imply that every injury needs urgent treatment or that every injury of a similar type is of equal urgency. For instance, a tibial fracture that a footballer has sustained may be treated satisfactorily for some time after the moment of injury but, in contrast, a fracture of the acetabulum with a hip dislocation (as described above) represents an emergency owing to the potential development of neurovascular complications (damage to the sciatic nerve; avascular necrosis of the femoral head). Therefore, the clinician's decision-making process should be informed by the peculiarities of the type of injury sustained and the anatomical location involved.

Moreover, it should be appreciated that the conduction of energy in an indirect mechanism, which is transferred via the soft tissues or fluid, can be difficult both to understand and to diagnose (accurately and promptly). For example, the rise in pressure secondary to a lower abdominal force could be passed to the vascular tree (aorta), leading to unexpected haemorrhage and death. Therefore, one can argue that the effects of direct mechanisms are easier to comprehend than those of indirect ones.

Penetrating injuries are caused either by sharp objects or by firearms (see *Chapter 34*). When dealing with sharp objects, it is necessary to take into account their length, surface area and the size of the entry point. For example, a pair of scissors will cause damage to the underlying tissues that they contact (skin, subcutaneous fat, fascia, etc.). Local examination will confirm the extent of the injury and the need for wound exploration. It is critical to be familiar with the relevant anatomy of the area involved to accurately assess peripheral nerve function and tendon and muscle integrity. Here again the 'timeline concept' of prompt assessment and response (treatment) can be crucial in cases where there is vascular injury, a compartment syndrome due to internal bleeding or even joint penetration that could lead to septic arthritis. Knowledge of the anatomical structures at risk is essential to making the right decision in a timely fashion. This is particularly critical for penetrating wounds over the torso (see *Chapter 29*) because it is not always easy to establish the track that the sharp object has followed. In this context, it should not be forgotten that the abdominal structures extend higher than anticipated, and as high as the level of the fifth rib in expiration.

Summary box 26.4

Sharp object injuries

- Length of the sharp object involved is important
- Familiarity with local anatomy is essential
- Crucial point: abdominal structures at risk of injury extend high into the chest

Penetrating injuries caused by firearms are more difficult to understand than incisional injuries caused by sharp objects. A low-velocity projectile may cause similar injuries to a knife, whereas a high-velocity projectile (bullet) causes extensive damage to the tissues as it travels, inducing lateral acceleration far from the point of impact and producing either a permanent or a temporary cavity (see *Chapter 34*). The importance of the temporary cavity is that it lasts for only milliseconds and is usually not evident during the clinical examination. It is important to be aware that this temporary cavity usually extends far from the boundaries of the apparent injury and there may be ingress of foreign material. Awareness of this phenomenon will ensure that the surgeon carries out sufficient exploration and wound excision.

Summary box 26.5

Firearm injuries

- Passage of high-velocity bullets induces permanent and temporary cavitation
- Temporary cavitation can contain foreign material, but disappears after a few seconds and is less evident to the clinician
- Low-velocity bullets induce similar damage to knives

Patient factors

Every patient is different: each possesses a unique profile and medical history and so will respond differently to a given traumatic incident. Of note, age plays an important role in this regard. Children and adults of different ages will sustain different injuries as a result of the same mechanism. For instance, a car hitting a pedestrian will induce different injuries in an adult from those in a child (*Figure 26.6*). It is important to consider the other aspects of the patient's history: past medical history, medication and allergy risk will direct not only the clinical assessment but also the treatment.

Obvious injuries

Some injuries are very obvious and can be identified before details of the mechanism or patient are known. One can take advantage of this, as the presence of an obvious injury can inform and lead to the identification of another that is less obvious. Obvious injuries are usually visible externally. It is therefore unsurprising that at the end of the ABCD protocol there is also an E, referring to exposure and the need to look for other signs of injury. Bruising to the scrotum of a motorcyclist following a collision with a car suggests a pelvic fracture. Contusion over the greater trochanter of the proximal femur in an older patient experiencing difficulty with straight leg raise points to a fracture of the neck of the femur. Finger-shaped bruises on a child's arms or thighs suggest NAI. The presence of a seat belt mark on the lower abdomen of a patient involved in a car crash and who has substantial abdominal pain points to damage inside the abdomen. Thus, exposure of the trauma patient should be routine practice in order to avoid missing the 'obvious'.

Hidden factors

Mechanisms

Sometimes, the formula 'mechanism + patient = injury' does not seem to 'add up'. If this is the case, the clinician should look further as hidden information may be contained in the mechanism. Occasionally, there is a deliberate attempt to misinform. While the majority of alert and orientated patients tell the truth, other patients, in order to protect themselves or others, may fabricate a mechanism. This may mislead the clinician and guide them to look for the wrong pattern of injuries. For instance, a patient in their twenties with a calcaneal fracture

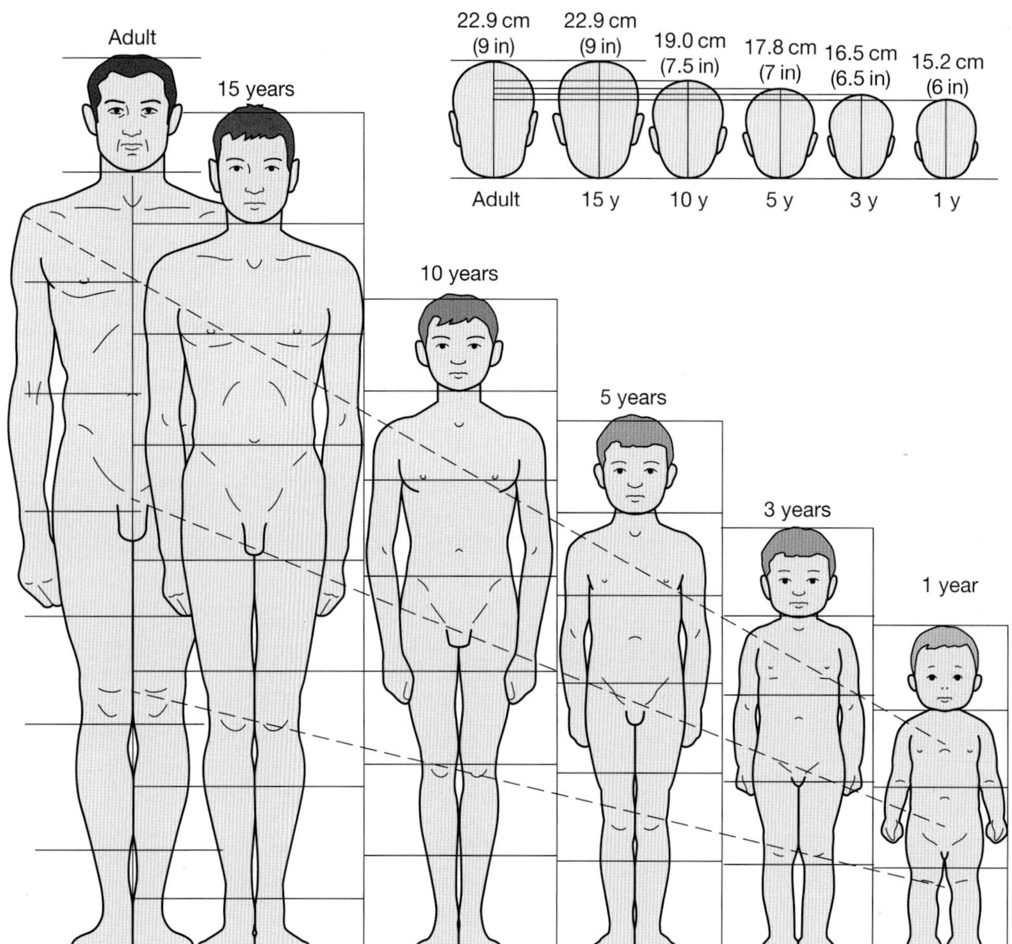

Figure 26.6 Body proportions at various ages and the anatomical location of injuries when hit by a car.

may report that this was the result of a fall into a pothole in the road, when in fact it had occurred during a burglary following a fall from a height of 10 metres. This can delay the accurate diagnosis of the specific injury and may prevent the diagnosis of other important injuries, such as a lumbar spine fracture. Although the patient should be given the chance to tell their story, it should not always be believed, particularly if there are inconsistencies.

A similar situation may arise when a patient is unable to give their history of events, for instance patients who are unconscious. In this scenario, the mechanism of injury is missing. The physically and mentally vulnerable include older patients, perhaps with dementia, and very young children. The difficulty or inability to report the injury is compounded by the fact that it might relate to criminal activity (e.g. NAI). Parameters that should alert the clinician and raise suspicion of NAI include:

- external signs of injuries not consistent with the mechanism reported;
- long bone fractures in a preambulatory child;
- inconsistent or changing history;
- aggressive or unusual behaviour of carers at interview;
- posterior rib injuries.

Summary box 26.6

Hidden mechanisms

- The vast majority of conscious patients will tell the truth
- Patients involved in criminal activity may not tell the truth
- Fear of abuse may prevent vulnerable patients from telling the truth
- Clinicians have the responsibility to take action when NAI is suspected

It is absolutely paramount to make a rapid diagnosis and treat the injuries, but most importantly to protect the patient from further harm, particularly vulnerable individuals (children and older adults). An early sign of abuse that is neglected may lead to further episodes and the potential of serious harm. For these reasons, procedures are usually in place and can be followed by passing on the problem to the appropriate team and professionals (see ***Chapter 44***).

Another important issue is the fact that any obvious injuries may provide important evidence regarding the mechanism, which may be important to a criminal investigation. The clinician must endeavour, without compromising treatment, not to affect such evidence by their medical actions and bear in mind that forensic evidence may be needed for a conviction at a later stage. Furthermore, the importance of this is made more apparent if we consider that the victim of an attack may subsequently be a murder victim.

Patients

Apart from the deliberate circumstances outlined above, where the injury and mechanism are inconsistent, the clinician should consider the possibility that the patient may have an unknown pre-existing condition. For example, when a fracture occurs following what seems to have been an insufficient mechanism, the clinician should suspect that the bone was already susceptible to fracture. Such pathological fractures may be secondary to underlying problems such as metastatic or primary tumour, osteoporosis or congenital disease. One example is the preambulatory child with multiple fractures secondary to osteogenesis imperfecta, which may mimic NAI. Failure to identify a pathological fracture through a primary tumour will lead to inappropriate initial management compromising appropriate cancer treatment. An initial osteoporotic or herald fracture should signal the need for appropriate investigation and, potentially, treatment to prevent further or secondary fractures. Similarly, fractures may be secondary to an undiagnosed or poorly controlled medical condition. For example, a patient presenting with a scalp laceration and a wrist fracture may have fallen as a result of a transient ischaemic attack (a hidden patient factor). In this situation, it is essential to include a medical secondary survey to identify the real cause of the injuries sustained and prevent further trauma.

Injuries

When analysis of the formula 'mechanism + patient = injury' has failed to identify hidden injury, there are two other approaches:

1 the look everywhere approach;
2 the focused exclusion approach.

Look everywhere approach. This represents the secondary and tertiary elements of the ATLS system and involves a detailed secondary survey, from top to bottom and at different time points: soon after the initial treatment phase when measures relating to saving the patient's life have been completed, the day after injury, e.g. during a ward round, or several days after injury, e.g. when the patient first wakes up in the intensive care unit (ICU). The implementation of whole-body CT (WBCT) (scanning the whole body) in all major trauma centres has allowed the clinical team to pick up injuries early. Such injuries would have been missed in the past when reliance was placed on the initial radiographs of the chest, pelvis and cervical spine. The threshold for using more WBCT has been lowered substantially. There is no doubt that WBCT scan algorithms have been shown to accelerate diagnostic work-up, but their effect on survival is controversial. Moreover, concerns have been voiced about the overexposure of patients to radiation with the increasing and often uncritical use of this type of scan. The effective radiation dose to all organs from a single full-body CT is 12–16 millisieverts (mSv). Survivors of the atomic bomb whose radiation dose was in the range 5–100 mSv had a statistically significant increase in the risk of solid cancers. Overall, the risks associated with one scan are relatively modest, approximately 1 in 1250 or 0.08%. However, it has been reported that widespread liberal use of CT is responsible for 1.5–2.0% of all cancers in the USA. Of interest, WBCT equates to 76 chest radiographs or 6 months of background radiation. It has been suggested that it should be requested wisely and that developing a triaging protocol can minimise the criticism of its overuse.

Focused exclusion approach. This is based on the knowledge that some specific injuries are missed on a remarkably regular basis. Such injury patterns include metatarsal and metacarpal fractures, scaphoid fractures, perilunate dislocations and posterior shoulder dislocations. When such injuries are suspected, a detailed focused history, clinical examination and appropriate investigations should be carried out to either confirm or exclude them. A high level of alertness and a high index of suspicion are always required to think beyond the obvious.

Summary box 26.7

Trauma assessment

- Knowledge of timelines for important diagnoses is essential
- Initial assessment should focus on what kills first
- Screen high-risk patients before clinical signs become apparent, as it may be too late to intervene once signs develop

THE RESPONSE TO TRAUMA

Completion of the initial patient evaluation according to the formula (patient + mechanism = injury) should provide the necessary information to formulate and implement a 'response' (treatment). During this stage of management, the response to injury will continue to evolve and decompensation may occur unexpectedly. Vigilance is required throughout treatment to identify the potential exhaustion of biological reserve mechanisms.

The patient's response to injury

Immediately after the traumatic event, physiological reactions are initiated as part of the body's homeostasis mechanisms to preserve vital organ functions and to maintain survival. Initial responses represented by the so-called acute-phase response may be altered as the insult of injury evolves and deterioration of the patient's condition may occur.

It is essential therefore that the timing and nature of interventions should be altered accordingly. Reversal of haemodynamic instability due to ongoing bleeding must be carried out promptly in order to avoid the development of coagulopathy and secondary damage to vital organs (i.e. the brain) due to hypoxia. It is important to monitor the patient's physiological state, including body temperature, degree of oxygenation and organ perfusion. Low body temperature is commonly present as a result of exposure, blood loss and dormancy. Covering the patient with appropriate blankets during transportation, resuscitation and surgery will reduce the risk of hypothermia, coagulation disturbances and ongoing bleeding. Administration of inspired oxygen or ventilation, if required, will improve the patient's degree of oxygenation.

Ongoing blood loss is associated with low blood pressure, reduced perfusion of the extremities (skin discoloration), tachycardia and an altered level of consciousness. Normally, vasoconstriction and endogenous clotting factors are activated to stop the bleeding in order to maintain adequate circulatory volume. A further consideration is that traumatised lung parenchyma cannot tolerate surplus fluid. Therefore, the latest resuscitation guidelines advocate a reduction in crystalloid administration and the early transfusion of blood products. Furthermore, there is a need to quickly identify the source of bleeding and stop loss of blood.

Another important part of the response to injury is activation of the immune–inflammatory system. Acute-phase mediators are released systemically, stimulating polymorphonuclear leukocytes to interact with the endothelium via the expression of surface receptors (integrins). If certain conditions are met extravasation of leukocytes may take place, particularly into the lung parenchyma, causing autodestruction. Clinical decisions should aim to minimise the risk of an exaggerated immune–inflammatory reaction. Surgical procedures, which can act as a second insult, where injury is considered the first, should be carefully timed and selected.

The medical response to injury

Initial management

After initial assessment of the patient's condition at the scene of an accident, paramedics communicate with the nearest hospital, triggering activation of 'the trauma team on call' and allowing personnel to expect the patient's arrival in the resuscitation room. The team leader, according to the ATLS protocol, will assign trained nurses and doctors to specific duties. Protective clothing, such as gloves and lead aprons, is required to protect the personnel from fluids and radiation exposure. Optimum coordination of the trauma team throughout the resuscitation process is essential to avoid careless delays, which may compromise the response time and the patient's condition. Timely involvement of different disciplines in assessing and planning treatment of injuries in different body areas is crucial and may lead to issues around priority in terms of planning and interventions. This situation could lead to confusion and uncertainty: 'Who should go first?' or 'What investigation should be next?' It is the role of the team leader to ensure that this is avoided and that decisions which may be critical for the patient's well-being are executed smoothly.

In situations where the system operates according to locally developed protocols, someone should have the responsibility of overruling the protocol if this is in the best interests of the patient, in order to keep the process moving along.

Following common pathways to manage patients can save time and reduce errors. In this respect the development of the NICE guidelines for the initial assessment and treatment of patients with major trauma can be useful. In addition, short standards documents, such as BOAST (British Orthopaedic Association Standards for Trauma), can be downloaded and printed for display in hospitals and so can support planning and decision making.

The development of local protocols, NICE guidelines and BOAST documents has contributed to the establishment of specific treatment pathways and to improved patient care and outcomes. Nonetheless, caution should prevail as, once a diagnosis (label) has been made, the pathway is set and it may not be in the patient's best interests if the diagnosis is misleading and troublesome. For instance, an older male patient fell in his garden and sustained a wrist fracture. He was given the label of 'accidental fall and wrist fracture', placed in a plaster of Paris back slab and arrangements were made for him to be admitted for fracture stabilisation. However, this patient had a number of medical comorbidities (heart failure, epilepsy, previous myocardial infarction and high blood pressure). Consequently, the label given as 'accidental fall and wrist fracture' may be associated with more severe underlying pathology and injuries. The wrong label may disguise the seriousness of the injuries sustained and the patient's condition may rapidly deteriorate, putting their life at risk. Thus, the first clinician in the diagnostic chain has disproportionate responsibility. Early inappropriate assessment and incorrect labelling could place the patient on the wrong treatment care pathway. This can be avoided by conducting appropriate physiological triage with senior input.

Beyond the first hour

The objective of the first (golden) hour is to reach the end points of resuscitation and completion of the diagnostic procedures identifying the injuries sustained. However, in polytraumatised patients, further interventions are necessary. For example, a spleen laceration, a lung contusion, a vertical shear pelvic fracture, an open right tibial fracture, a left femoral fracture or a distal humerus fracture are injuries necessitating treatment. The spleen laceration may be managed non-operatively or with embolisation, depending on its severity. The timing and priority of fixation of the other skeletal injuries and the type of fixation have been points of much discussion during the past decade.

Two treatment strategies have prevailed: early total care (ETC) and damage control orthopaedic (DCO) surgery. Since the late 1990s the ETC approach (fix all fractures early within 24 hours) revolutionised the management of patients with multiple injuries. This practice became the gold standard of treatment for polytrauma patients. Nonetheless, in specific groups of patients, for example those with severe chest and/or head injuries or those in an extreme physiological state (with ongoing bleeding from different sources such as the abdomen, pelvis and chest), it was observed that the ETC concept led to early complications and mortality.

With the advances made in the fields of molecular medicine, biology, intensive care and immunology the physiological response to injury was better understood. It was appreciated that the trauma sustained at the scene of an accident (first hit) induces an immune–inflammatory reaction that evolves with time and can prime the patient to reach an uncontrolled physiological state. Subsequently, surgical interventions can induce an additional physiological stress (second hit) response, exhausting the biological reserve of the patient and leading to the development of adult respiratory distress syndrome (ARDS), multiple organ dysfunction syndrome (MODS) and mortality. These observations led to the acceptance of the so-called DCO philosophy, which is also called damage control surgery (DCS) in more generalised settings (see later chapters). The stages of DCO are:

- resuscitation;
- haemorrhage control;
- decompression;
- decontamination;
- fracture splintage.

Application of the DCO concept includes temporary stabilisation of long bone fractures and pelvis with external fixators. This approach allows rapid procedures to stabilise the affected bones as part of the resuscitation process. Definitive fixation of the fractures (conversion of the external fixators to intramedullary nailing for the femur and plating of the pelvis) would usually take place 4 days later, when the physiological state of the patient has been normalised, or even later if necessary. The two strategies of fracture fixation – the ETC and DCS – are currently practised on the basis of some specific criteria. The vast majority of polytrauma patients are suitable for ETC (80–90%). Specific criteria are shown in *Table 26.2*.

TABLE 26.2 Criteria for damage control surgery (DCS) and early total care (ETC).

Criteria for DCS	Criteria for ETC
Hypothermia: <34°C	Stable haemodynamics
Acidosis: pH <7.2	No need for vasoactive/ inotropic stimulation
Serum lactate >5 mmol/L	No hypoxaemia, no hypercapnia
Coagulopathy	Serum lactate <2 mmol/L
Blood pressure <70 mmHg	Normal coagulation
Transfusion approaching 15 units	Normothermia
Injury severity score >36	Urinary output >1 mL/kg/h

Lately, other fixation strategies that have been proposed include the Early Appropriate Care, Safe Definitive Surgery and Prompt Individualised Safe Management (PRISM) concepts. The PRISM concept accepts that the decision-making process should be based on the principles of doing no 'further harm to the patient', intervening promptly and utilising the idea of individualised/personalised medicine. It is based on the understanding that every patient responds differently to the same degree of trauma, every individual has a different genetic profile and the fact that each trauma centre may have different resources and staff available to deal successfully with every trauma eventuality.

Irrespective of the treatment strategy selected, it is imperative to be aware that the patient's condition can change and deteriorate quickly. In particular, patients with a high ISS are at risk of decompensating rapidly. Therefore, ongoing evaluation of a patient's physiology is essential, with senior input involvement in order to deal successfully with the unexpected.

Overall, a plan should always be made available to the trauma team to inform them about the details of treatment, particularly in the operating theatre environment. The plan can be recorded on a whiteboard with clear guidance on the alternative pathway to be implemented should the patient's condition deteriorate. Ongoing monitoring of such parameters as core temperature, lactate, base excess and coagulation will provide knowledge of the patient's condition at any time point during care. Appropriate decisions can then be taken to ensure that the safety of the patient has not been compromised. For instance, if the ETC concept has been applied and a polytrauma patient with a head injury and chest trauma is on the operating table waiting to have a femoral fracture stabilised with intramedullary nailing and their condition deteriorates, the ETC plan can be changed to DCO (an external fixator can be applied quickly to stabilise the femoral fracture temporarily). This allows prompt transfer of the patient to the ICU, where resuscitation can continue within a safe environment with ongoing monitoring of vital organ function (lungs and brain).

When injuries involve the input of different disciplines in terms of surgical intervention, for instance a general surgeon for a liver laceration, a neurosurgeon for an intracranial haematoma, an orthopaedic surgeon for a pelvic and femoral fracture and a maxillofacial surgeon for a depressed orbital fracture, the most important intervention should go first. Clearly, communication and prioritisation among the team members is essential. As each procedure nears completion, communication with the anaesthetist will allow a decision as to whether it is safe to go on to the next procedure. Not infrequently, and assuming that it is technically possible, two teams can work simultaneously to significantly shorten the time the patient will spend in the operating theatre and allow subsequent prompt transfer to the ICU for optimisation and ongoing monitoring.

LOCAL PROTOCOLS AND GUIDELINES

While the ATLS protocol has become the standard of care for the initial management of patients with multiple injuries, other protocols and guidelines have also been developed to facilitate the treatment of patients in a more standardised way. Nowadays it is common practice for trauma centres to develop their own local protocols and guidelines, although national guidelines may also exist. However, regional developed guidelines may refer to smaller areas of clinical practice, such as antibiotic prophylaxis for open fractures, mass transfusion, pharmacotherapy for coagulation disturbances, steroids for spinal cord injuries, clearance of the cervical spine and angiographic embolisation of pelvic fractures or abdominal injuries. These protocols can facilitate swifter decision making, eliminating delays and benefiting the patient. They also protect the clinician and care provider with regard to medicolegal issues. An example relating to angiographic embolisation of pelvic fractures is shown in *Figure 26.7*.

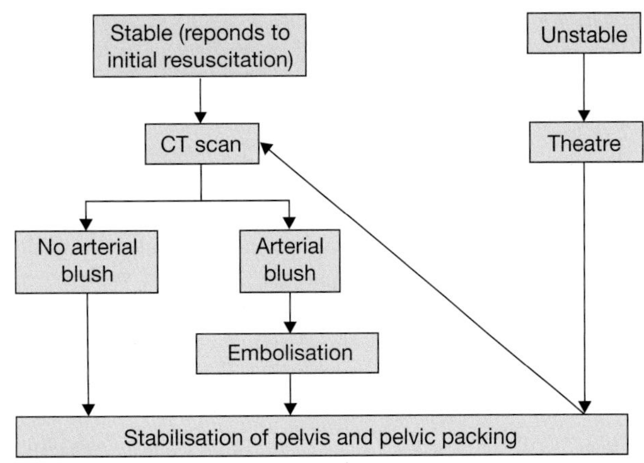

Figure 26.7 Pelvic fracture: angiography protocol. CT, computed tomography.

Local policies focusing on the creation of single charts facilitating daily input of a patient's vital signs and biochemical results are also useful in allowing sequential observation of the results, which can demonstrate important trends. These trends can be useful in identifying, at an early stage, a clinical condition that can be treated within the timeline concept and prior to irreversible damage to the affected organ, at which point any form of intervention will be meaningless. For instance, the clinical evolution of respiratory insufficiency in an individual without pre-existing lung disease secondary to pulmonary embolism is easier to identify by evaluating the trend in the oxygen saturation of inspired oxygen.

Planning an individual operation

Operative procedures in a multiply injured patient in a critical physiological state can be essential for their survival. It is vital to make the right decision the first time. This can be successfully done by studying in detail the history, the patient's condition and any interventions made, followed by appropriate planning and execution of treatment. For example, analysing the biochemical markers, overall physiological state and fracture pattern and deciding factors such as patient positioning, the surgical approach to be used to gain adequate access to a bone for reduction, the type of implant to be used, the correct positioning of the implant, soft-tissue handling and the type of rehabilitation are just some of the parameters for consideration.

Summary box 26.8

The response to trauma

- Rationalise patient management with the development of protocols and guidelines
- Avoid unnecessary delays
- Observe trends and promptly identify evolving conditions

The surgeon should ask themselves (and ensure that they have answered) questions such as: Is it the optimum time to carry out the procedure? Am I the most appropriate person to carry out the procedure? Have I made a contingency plan should the procedure become difficult to complete? What is my plan A, B and C so I am able to successfully finish the procedure? Recording all the important issues on a piece of paper, or suitable alternative, will ensure that no parameter of importance is left out of the planning. In order that the procedure runs smoothly in theatre, the plan can be documented on the whiteboard. Such a practice will allow every member of the surgical team to be aware of the potential issues to be addressed and the plan of action that has been decided. The appropriate surgical equipment for plans A, B and C can be clearly identified and kept in close proximity to the operating theatre. The above strategy will eliminate unnecessary detail and ensure that there will be no surprises, for instance essential equipment being unavailable.

The response to the mechanism of injury (injury prevention)

Not infrequently, two or more patients are seen who have been injured in the same geographical area by the same mechanism. A possible scenario is that, over a period of a few weeks, several patients are noted to present with a fall of 2–3 metres in the same location, for example from a particular bridge. Further investigation might establish that the bridge is easy to access, perhaps because of damage to safety measures. With appropriate steps the damage can be rectified and access to the bridge limited, preventing further harm. In this example, the surgeon is involved in both the treatment and the prevention of injury. Therefore, when a mechanism of injury becomes more frequent and is associated with serious life-threatening trauma, it is essential to take steps either to eliminate the mechanism or to lessen the consequences.

Summary box 26.9

Planning an individual operation

- Adequate preoperative planning is essential to eliminate unnecessary delays
- Document the plan to ensure no important parameter is left out
- A whiteboard can be used to demonstrate the order of plan execution and to act as a means of communication among staff

The issue of injury prevention is an important consideration not only for clinicians but also for other stakeholders, for example politicians (developing appropriate legislation relevant to road safety), manufacturers (optimising the safety of cars) and the construction industry. This accounts for the improvements in safety that can be achieved.

The response to patient factors

Injuries presenting with increased frequency in an individual patient require special attention. Older patients, perhaps with multiple medical problems, can represent such a vulnerable group. The reduced bone mineral density making their

Summary box 26.10

Response to the mechanism of injury

- Be alert to identifying frequent patterns of injury
- Many stakeholders, including clinicians, should engage in injury prevention
- Legislation and education are essential

skeletons 'fragile' is associated with an increased risk of fracture. Hip fractures, wrist fractures, spinal fractures and pelvic fractures are just some of the many results following minimal trauma. The risk of fracture is increased with the presence of comorbidities such as visual impairment, Parkinsonism or transient ischaemic heart attacks. Consequently, knowing the parameters associated with a particular group of patients, attempts can be made to reduce the number of patients requiring treatment. For instance, prescription of bone protection therapy and addressing medical comorbidities early (e.g. cataract surgery) may help to reduce the number and severity of injuries sustained. Development of specific guidelines and protocols can facilitate the much-needed implementation of unified measures allowing easy patient access and treatment.

Summary box 26.11

Response to patient factors

- Older patients may be vulnerable to injury, owing to poor bone stock and other comorbidities
- Bone protection treatment is essential
- Development of local and national guidelines to respond to patient factors is desirable

CONCLUSION

Trauma can affect all patient age groups. The severity of injury depends on the type and nature of the mechanical force applied. The formula 'patient + mechanism = injury' should be kept in mind when dealing with trauma patients. There is a connection among the three components of the formula, all of which should fit together in a coherent way. When no relationship can be made, examine for pre-existing pathology and hidden injuries or consider whether the history given by the patient is at fault (including deliberate attempts to mislead).

Be aware of the timeline concept because there is a minimum response time to initiate and complete treatment in order to deal with a specific condition successfully.

In patients with multiple injuries early assessment and management is performed using the ATLS protocol and other guidelines developed either locally or at a national level. In the early clinical pathway of the patient the objective is to restore haemodynamic stability (save life – prevent uncontrollable bleeding and death) and minimise the risk of developing subsequent complications. Surgical interventions should be short and part of the resuscitation process, executed in a timely manner. Afterwards, treatment for definitive stabilisation can be personalised for optimum outcomes. Existing specific criteria can aid the clinician to make the right decision for the right patient at the right time. Different groups of patients, such as older patients and children, have different demands and should be managed accordingly. While clinicians are focused on treating the injury sustained, they have other responsibilities, including active involvement in preventive measures. Preventive measures should be commissioned when particular mechanisms can be identified as being common or important causes of injury.

Summary box 26.12

Conclusion

- Look for hidden injuries
- Remember the timeline concept
- Different treatment strategies exist, complementing each other
- Specific criteria will decide the fixation strategy: ETC or DCO

FURTHER READING

Department for Transport. *Reported road casualties in Great Britain: 2019 annual report*, 2020. Available from https://assets.publishing.service.gov.uk/government/uploads/system/uploads/attachment_data/file/922717/reported-road-casualties-annual-report-2019.pdf

European Transport Safety Council. *14th Annual road safety performance index (PIN) report*, 2020. Available from https://etsc.eu/14th-annual-road-safety-performance-index-pin-report

Giannoudis PV, Giannoudis VP, Horwitz DS. Time to think outside the box: 'Prompt-Individualised-Safe Management' (PR.I.S.M.) should prevail in patients with multiple injuries. *Injury* 2017; **48**(7): 1279–82.

Moran CG, Lecky F, Bouamra O *et al.* Changing the system – major trauma patients and their outcomes in the NHS (England) 2008–17. *EClinicalMedicine* 2018; **2–3**: 13–21.

National Institute for Health and Care Excellence. *Major trauma: assessment and initial management.* NICE Guideline 39. London: NICE, 2016. Available from https://www.nice.org.uk/guidance/ng39.

National Institute for Health and Care Excellence. *NICEimpact falls and fragility fractures.* London: NICE, 2018. Available from https://www.nice.org.uk/media/default/about/what-we-do/into-practice/measuring-uptake/nice-impact-falls-and-fragility-fractures.pdf

Pape HC, Pfeifer R. Safe definitive orthopaedic surgery (SDS): repeated assessment for tapered application of early definitive care and damage control?: an inclusive view of recent advances in polytrauma management. *Injury* 2015; **46**(1): 1–3.

World Health Organization. *Injuries and violence: the facts 2014*, 2015. Available from https://www.who.int/publications/i/item/9789241508018

James Parkinson, 1755–1824, general practitioner of Shoreditch, London, UK, published *An essay on the shaking palsy* in 1817.

CHAPTER 27

Early assessment and management of severe trauma

Learning objectives

- How to identify and assess the severely injured patient
- Early treatment goals for multiply injured patients
- Understand the role of permissive hypotension, tranexamic acid and massive transfusion protocols
- Understand the principles of damage control surgery (DCS) versus early total care (ETC)

IDENTIFICATION OF SEVERE TRAUMA

The severely injured patient, with multiple injuries to different body systems, poses unique diagnostic and treatment challenges. The early assessment and management of severe trauma begins in the prehospital environment. Many of these patients will be easily identified at the scene of injury. Forewarning the receiving hospital allows the activation of the trauma team to prepare for the patient's arrival. Key information in the pre-alert includes basic demographic information (age and gender), mechanism of injury, injuries identified and vital signs, including respiratory rate, pulse, blood pressure and Glasgow Coma Scale (GCS).

Patients who are identified before reaching hospital as having sustained, or are at high risk of sustaining, severe multisystem trauma should generate trauma team activation in the receiving hospital. It should be noted that not all patients with severe multisystem trauma are immediately obvious. An older adult patient falling down a few steps can easily sustain a hip fracture, multiple rib fractures and a small subdural haemorrhage. At first glance the patient can appear well, but their injury severity score (ISS) and potential mortality could easily exceed those of a younger patient with multiple open long bone fractures. Both patients are critically injured and should be managed with the same principles in mind.

ROLE OF THE TRAUMA TEAM

All hospitals managing severe trauma should have a dedicated trauma team that is available immediately to attend and manage patients presenting with severe trauma. The composition of the team will depend on local policies but it will invariably involve doctors from the emergency department, anaesthetics and/or critical care, trauma and orthopaedics and general surgery. Increasingly, radiology and haematology doctors are contributing to the trauma team, as part of the patient's initial assessment and management. Hospitals managing large volumes of cases of severe multisystem trauma are recognising the need for an enhanced trauma team activation for the most severely injured patients – the so-called 'code red trauma call'. Patients identified before reaching hospital as being haemodynamically unstable or having acute airway compromise may initiate 'code red', triggering the automatic attendance of the most senior clinicians from each discipline prior to the patient's arrival and prehospital activation of massive transfusion protocols.

The role of the trauma team is to apply the principles of Advanced Trauma Life Support (ATLS) to rapidly identify and treat life-threatening injuries during the primary survey. The principal advantage of a trauma team is that this activity can occur concurrently instead of sequentially; while the anaesthetist is assessing and managing the patient's airway, another team member can be assessing and managing the patient's breathing, etc. The importance of the trauma team leader cannot be overemphasised: they brief and prepare the team, coordinate these sequential activities, manage time, interpret findings and plan the next move. Increasing recognition of the importance of this role has led to the development of postgraduate training courses designed to teach both the technical and non-technical skills required. Generally, the trauma team leader and most senior clinicians should be standing back from the patient, looking at the bigger picture, in order to anticipate the next key decisions.

Summary box 27.1

The role of the trauma team

- Allows the simultaneous and efficient application of ATLS principles to rapidly identify and treat life-threatening pathologies
- Should be led by the most senior clinician
- The most senior clinicians from each specialty should attend 'code red trauma calls'
- The team leader should be constantly trying to anticipate the next move

PRIMARY SURVEY

The primary survey aims to identify and manage the most immediately life-threatening pathologies first and follows cABCDE.

c: Exsanguinating external haemorrhage

Experience from war zones over the past 20 years has shown that exsanguinating external haemorrhage from massive arterial bleeding needs to be controlled even before the airway is managed (see *Chapter 34*). Most of these injuries are due to gunshot wounds or blasts and are mainly seen in military practice. However, they are also encountered in civilian practice. Bleeding must be controlled immediately by the application of packs and pressure directly onto the bleeding wound and proximal artery. Haemostatic dressings that contain agents that augment local coagulation are now available. Failure to control bleeding in the limb by direct pressure with surgical dressings should be followed by the application of a tourniquet proximal to the wound. In the field, simple tourniquets can be improvised if pneumatic tourniquets are not available. It is vital to appreciate that once a tourniquet is applied the limb becomes ischaemic; therefore, the length of time for which the tourniquet is applied must be recorded on the patient and the patient requires urgent surgical control of the bleeding in order to reperfuse the limb.

A: Airway with cervical spine control

All trauma patients should have their cervical spine immobilised and protected throughout. An immediate assessment of the patient's airway is made. A compromised airway requires a stepwise progression, first clearing the airway by suctioning secretions or blood, followed by simple airway manoeuvres such as a jaw thrust, chin lift and insertion of an oropharyngeal or nasopharyngeal airway. Advanced airway manoeuvres necessitate the insertion of a cuffed endotracheal tube. This may require an anaesthetic with rapid sequence induction or a surgical airway. Emergency intubation of the severely injured trauma patient is a difficult and demanding skill – standardised and rehearsed procedures should be in place for failure to intubate (*Figure 27.1*). Equipment and expertise for achieving a surgical airway must be readily available.

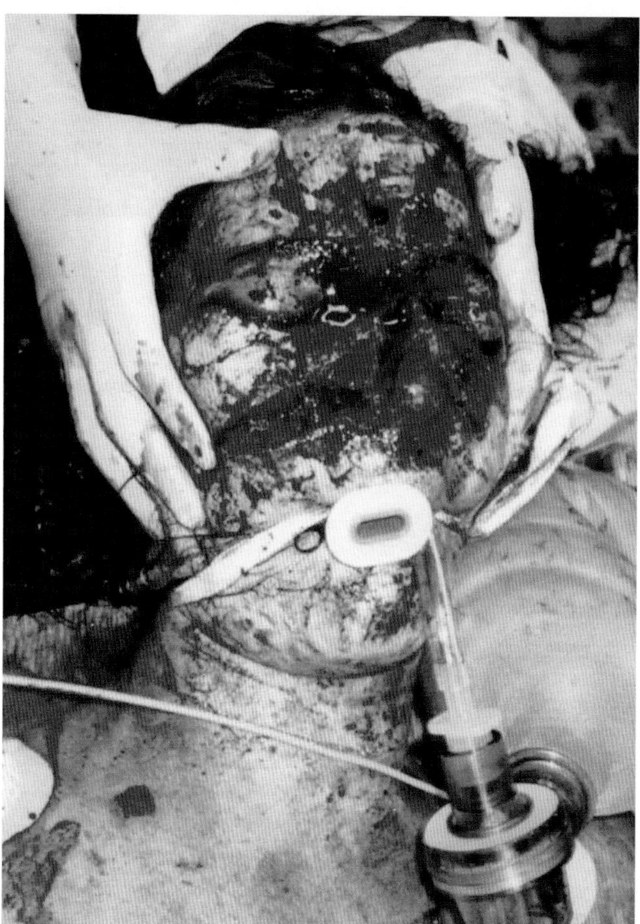

Figure 27.1 Unrestrained driver with severe craniofacial injury (courtesy of Johannesburg Hospital Trauma Unit).

B: Breathing and ventilation

All patients should receive high-flow oxygen. Life-threatening chest pathology such as tension pneumothorax, massive haemothorax and flail segment should be diagnosed and managed immediately. Equipment and expertise for rapid insertion of intercostal chest drains should be available.

C: Circulation and haemorrhage control

All patients require adequate intravenous (IV) access with at least two large-bore IV cannulae. Equipment and expertise for insertion of central or intraosseous venous access should be available where peripheral access is not easily obtainable. Blood should be taken for cross-match and laboratory assessment, including haemoglobin and venous lactate. An assessment of the haemodynamic status should be made to identify shocked patients: the skin may be cool and sweaty, the pulse rate raised to over 100 per minute and the blood pressure low. A pelvic binder should be applied to all haemodynamically unstable patients following blunt trauma and not removed until after a pelvic fracture has been excluded. Hypotensive trauma patients are treated as hypovolaemic until proven otherwise. The priority is simultaneous fluid resuscitation and identification of the source of the haemorrhage.

Permissive hypotension, massive transfusion protocols and tranexamic acid

The initial aim of resuscitation is to maintain the blood supply to the vital organs: the brain, heart and kidneys. For a short time, this can be achieved with a target systolic blood pressure of 70–90 mmHg, although a higher pressure of >90 mmHg should be the target if a head injury is suspected. Small boluses of IV fluids (e.g. 250 mL of O negative blood, or normal saline if blood is not immediately available) should be administered to achieve this target, which should result in a palpable radial pulse. Excessive IV crystalloid or colloid solutions should be avoided because they cause haemodilution, increase coagulopathy and increase the risk of adult respiratory distress syndrome. However, the key to this approach of permissive hypotension is that it is time limited. The primary source of haemorrhage must be identified and controlled as soon as possible.

Severely injured hypovolaemic patients should be resuscitated with blood and blood products, not crystalloid/colloid fluids. These must be warmed. All hospitals managing severe trauma should have a massive transfusion protocol that aims to provide blood and blood products in a ratio of 1 packed red cells : 1 fresh-frozen plasma : 1 platelets.

Tranexamic acid

Tranexamic acid is an antifibrinolytic drug that reduces the risk of mortality from bleeding in both blunt and penetrating trauma. One gram is given intravenously over 10 minutes, followed by a further 1-g dose over 8 hours. Tranexamic acid should be given to all trauma patients suspected to have significant haemorrhage, including those with a systolic blood pressure of <110 mmHg or a pulse of over 110 per minute. It needs to be administered as early as possible and ideally within the first hour from injury; the first dose should not be administered more than 3 hours from injury. In the UK it is normally given by paramedics in the prehospital environment.

Summary box 27.2

Severe hypovolaemia

- Tranexamic acid reduces mortality after trauma
- All traumatised patients suspected of bleeding should receive tranexamic acid as soon as possible after injury
- All trauma centres should have an established massive transfusion protocol
- Severely hypovolaemic trauma patients should be resuscitated using blood and blood products
- The only role for crystalloids in the initial management of severely hypovolaemic patients is for the administration of small quantities to maintain blood pressure while waiting for blood products to become available

Identification and management of haemorrhage

The sites of major haemorrhage in trauma patients are the chest, abdomen, pelvis and long bones, and external haemorrhage (*Figure 27.2*). Blunt trauma patients frequently have multiple sources of haemorrhage. Clinical examination and investigations should aim to rapidly confirm or exclude significant bleeding from each of these sites. Computed tomography (CT) from the head to pelvis with IV contrast, the so-called 'whole-body CT' (WBCT), is the gold standard investigation in patients with signs or symptoms of multiple injury or deranged physiology, but note that WBCT should not be performed on the basis of the mechanism of injury alone (see ***Further reading***). There is no role for scanning selective body systems in the severely injured trauma patient. Wherever possible, WBCT should be performed as soon as possible during the patient's resuscitation. A provisional 'hot report' can be issued within minutes to identify immediate life-threatening pathology to the trauma team. A more detailed definitive report should be available within 30–60 minutes.

Traditionally, chest and pelvis radiographs have been obtained early in the assessment of patients with polytrauma but these investigations are increasingly omitted in favour of obtaining a rapid CT scan, as described above. Most trauma centres now have rapid access to CT scanners located within, or immediately adjacent to, the resuscitation area. This has allowed haemodynamically unstable patients to have a WBCT with resuscitation by the trauma team continuing simultaneously during CT. Identifying which patients are too haemodynamically unstable to scan safely is a difficult decision for the trauma team leader and will be influenced by local factors and facilities.

Some patients will be so haemodynamically unstable on arrival that they need immediate surgical control of their haemorrhage before a CT scan. The most likely sources are abdominal or pelvic bleeding. An immediate chest radiograph will exclude catastrophic intrathoracic haemorrhage. An immediate pelvic radiograph is essential but should not delay transfer to the operating theatre. A focused abdominal sonography for trauma (FAST) scan (if immediately available) may also be useful in this scenario to locate the major source of haemorrhage. All patients undergoing immediate laparotomy in the operating theatre should have a pelvic binder applied and not removed. A correctly positioned pelvic binder at the level of the greater trochanters does not obstruct trauma laparotomy. These patients will invariably require a WBCT scan after surgical control of haemorrhage has been achieved.

Summary box 27.3

Whole-body CT (WBCT)

- WBCT from the head to pelvis with IV contrast is the gold standard investigation of the severely injured adult blunt trauma patient
- There is no role for selective scanning of body systems in these patients
- WBCT scan is a time-critical investigation and should be obtained as early as possible in resuscitation of the severely injured patient
- Any patient undergoing immediate trauma laparotomy after blunt trauma without a WBCT scan should have a pelvic binder applied and not removed until a pelvic fracture is excluded. Such patients should have an immediate pelvic radiograph either in the emergency department or as they arrive in the operating theatre

D: Disability and E: Exposure

On admission, the GCS score should be calculated (***Table 27.1***), the pupils assessed for size and reaction to light and the patient observed to determine whether they are moving all four limbs. The core temperature must be recorded. Patients are managed with cervical spine protection (cervical collar and blocks) and protection of the thoracolumbar spine using standard log roll techniques until a spinal injury has been excluded. Early WBCT scan will rapidly identify the majority of intracranial and spinal pathology.

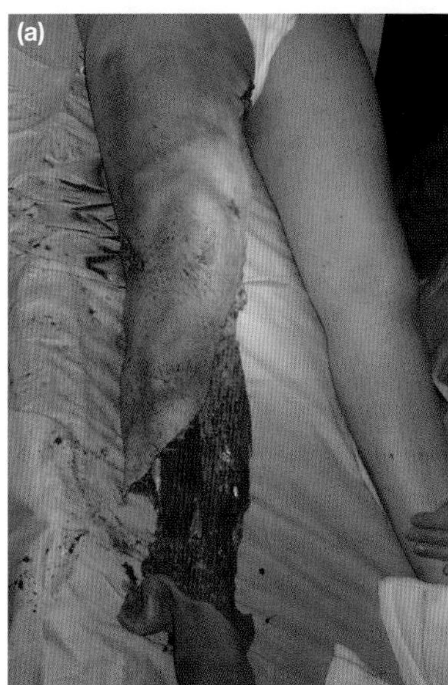

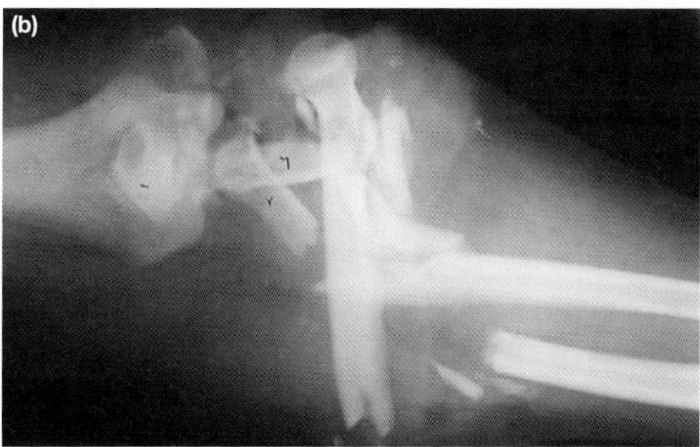

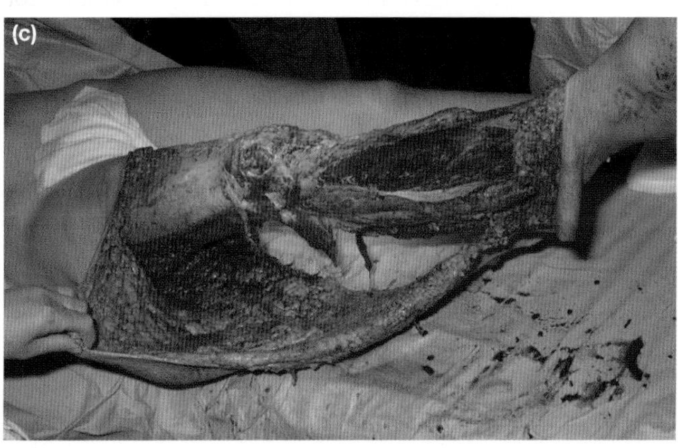

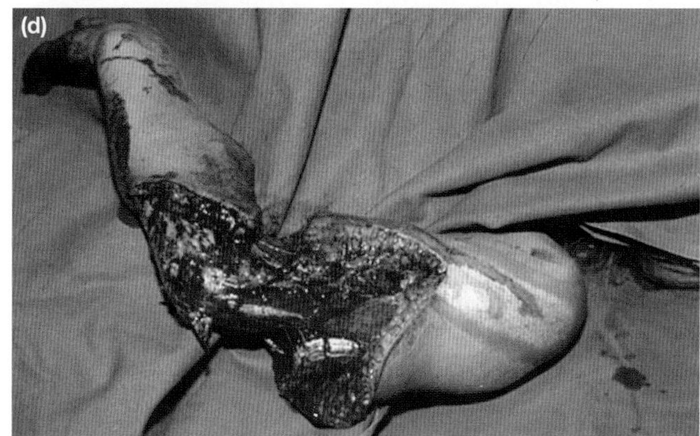

Figure 27.2 (a–d) Severe degloving injuries to the upper and lower limbs following a high-speed road traffic accident. The initial appearance and severity of the injury should not detract from following the important Advanced Trauma Life Support (ATLS) sequence in evaluating and treating immediate life-threatening injuries. Bleeding and severe injuries within the chest, abdomen and pelvis must be actively excluded.

The patient must be adequately exposed to allow a thorough and systematic clinical examination during the secondary survey but they must be kept warm. Trauma patients are frequently hypothermic and this will further increase coagulopathy. Every effort should be made to maintain normal temperature by minimising unnecessary exposure of the patient and by using warmed blankets and trolleys and warmed fluids during resuscitation.

Log-rolling patients with severe pelvic fractures may harm the patient by disturbing established blood clots. Log-rolling should not occur until a pelvic fracture has been radiographically excluded. If patients need to be moved during their primary survey, such as when moving onto the CT scanning gantry, a 20° roll with inline spinal stabilisation should be used. Modern 'scoop stretchers' mean that there is no requirement to roll any patient more than 20° until a pelvic fracture has been excluded.

Formal log-rolling of the blunt trauma patient to examine the back during the primary survey adds minimal useful clinical information, delays the WBCT scan and may cause harm to a patient with a pelvic fracture. It should be deferred until after the primary survey, with the exception of patients

TABLE 27.1 Glasgow Coma Scale.

Best eye response (E)	Best verbal response (V)	Best motor response (M)
4 Eyes opening spontaneously	5 Oriented	6 Obeys commands
3 Eye opening to speech	4 Confused	5 Localises to pain
2 Eye opening in response to pain	3 Inappropriate words	4 Withdraws from pain
1 No eye opening	2 Incomprehensible sounds	3 Flexion in response to pain
	1 None	2 Extension to pain
		1 No motor response

with penetrating trauma, where it is important to identify the presence of a posterior torso wound.

Mechanical testing of the pelvis in the emergency room ('springing the pelvis') adds no useful clinical examination and will disrupt any blood clot that has formed around a pelvic fracture. It should never be performed – a pelvic fracture should always be diagnosed radiographically.

Summary box 27.4

The cABCDE of trauma care

- c – Control of massive external haemorrhage
- A – Airway with cervical spine protection
- B – Breathing and ventilation
- C – Circulation and haemorrhage control: apply a pelvic binder and do not remove until a pelvic fracture is excluded
- D – Disability (neurological status)
- E – Exposure (assess for other injuries)

SECONDARY SURVEY

All severely injured patients require a detailed top-to-toe examination after life-threatening injuries have been identified and managed during the primary survey. Patients may be intubated and unresponsive at this point, limiting the accuracy of clinical examination. Such patients should have a 'tertiary survey' when extubated and alert to identify any missed 'minor' injuries, such as a scaphoid fracture in the wrist or a rotator cuff tear in the shoulder. These injuries have the potential to cause significant long-term disability. It is essential that the findings of the primary, secondary and tertiary surveys are clearly recorded in the patient's case notes.

DAMAGE CONTROL SURGERY VERSUS EARLY TOTAL CARE

As discussed in *Chapter 26*, the concept of damage control surgery (DCS) was developed because severely traumatised patients with impaired physiology have poor outcomes after lengthy and complex surgical reconstructive procedures performed shortly after their trauma. Prolonged procedures result in additional trauma and further immune and physiological derangement; the 'triad of death' – a cycle of acidosis, coagulopathy and hypothermia – may develop and result in multiorgan failure and death.

Consequently, surgical interventions in the trauma patient with physiological abnormality are limited to rapid life- and limb-saving procedures: control of haemorrhage, decompression of cavities (e.g. craniotomy, fasciotomy), revascularisation of ischaemic organs and limbs and removal of contamination. This damage control approach aims to rapidly achieve these objectives and then move the patient to a critical care environment and continue with resuscitation.

Subsequent definitive reconstructive procedures are deferred until the patient is adequately resuscitated and physiologically optimised. DCS in the abdomen is limited to packing and control of haemorrhage, debridement and resection of devitalised tissue and removal of contamination by foreign bodies or faeces. Damage control orthopaedic surgery is limited to debridement of severe open fractures, rapid temporary splintage or stabilisation of long bone fractures and decompression of limb compartment syndrome where required.

Revascularisation of a limb following arterial injury may be appropriate for isolated injuries but in the patient with severe multiple system trauma it may increase the threat to life and therefore amputation may be the better option. Such patients are then transferred to critical care for further resuscitation and physiological stabilisation before definitive surgical procedures can be planned.

The majority of trauma patients respond well to resuscitation, are not physiologically compromised after appropriate resuscitation and are therefore suitable for early total care (ETC). A number of physiological indices are used to evaluate the response to resuscitation, including a pulse rate less than 100 per minute, normal blood pressure and respiratory rate, as well as urine output >30 mL/h. The patient should not have hypothermia (temperature <35°C) nor evidence of acidosis on arterial blood gases and should have a normal coagulation screen.

Lactate levels are also a good indicator of tissue perfusion and should rapidly return to normal. In this situation, it is usually safe for the surgeon to proceed with definitive repair or reconstruction of injured organs.

For musculoskeletal injuries, ETC allows definitive fixation of all unstable long bone, spinal and pelvic fractures within 36 hours of injury. This facilitates nursing care, allows early mobilisation of the patient and reduces pulmonary complications and length of stay on intensive care.

If a sequence of fracture fixations is required, at the conclusion of each procedure the surgeon and anaesthetist should determine whether the patient's physiological status has been maintained sufficiently to allow the next procedure, or whether the patient should return to critical care for a further period of resuscitation.

Summary box 27.5

ETC versus DCS

- ETC describes the definitive management of a patient's injuries within 36 hours of injury after a period of initial resuscitation
- DCS describes simultaneous resuscitation with early rapid life- and limb-saving surgery. Time-consuming definitive surgery is deferred until the patient's physiological status allows
- An ETC approach can be changed to a damage control approach if the patient's physiology deteriorates during definitive surgery

Venous lactate

Venous lactate is a useful marker of resuscitation and physiological state. A normal lactate (<2 mmol/L) is a sign that the patient is probably resuscitated and suitable for ETC. An elevated lactate (>3 mmol/L) suggests the patient is under-resuscitated and should either have a period of further resuscitation or DCS if surgery is urgent. If a patient's lactate is 2–3 mmol/L then the trend (upwards or downwards) should be noted and the other physiological markers considered to determine whether the patient is suitable for definitive surgical procedures.

The identification of patients suitable for ETC versus DCS should be made by senior surgeons and anaesthetists/critical care doctors. This may be an easy decision, for example the haemodynamically unstable patient with intra-abdominal bleeding will always undergo rapid damage control laparotomy. In other cases a careful review of the patient's physiology and coagulation state will be required.

Summary box 27.6

Venous lactate is an essential marker of resuscitation

- <2 mmol/L – ETC
- 2–3 mmol/L – look at the trend (increasing or decreasing)
- >3 mmol/L – may be under-resuscitated; should either have further resuscitation or DCS if surgery is urgent
- >5 mmol/L – DCS (see *Chapters 26 and 29*)

SUMMARY

The early assessment and management of trauma patients should follow established ATLS principles.

A WBCT scan, from the head to the pelvis, with IV contrast is the gold standard investigation for major trauma patients and should be performed early and whenever possible.

Warmed blood and blood products in a 1:1:1 ratio of blood : plasma : platelets should be used with tranexamic acid in the early resuscitation of haemodynamically unstable trauma patients.

Trauma patients requiring surgery should have an early decision made whether a damage control or ETC approach is required. Surgical procedures in physiologically compromised patients should be limited to those required to save the life and/or limb of the patient, while simultaneous resuscitation is continued.

FURTHER READING

Sierink HJC, Treskes K, Edwards MJR *et al.*, for the REACT-2 Study Group. Immediate total-body CT scanning versus conventional imaging and selective CT scanning in patients with severe trauma (REACT-2): a randomised controlled trial. *Lancet* 2016; **388**: 673–83.

CHAPTER

28 Traumatic brain injury

Learning objectives†

To be familiar with:

- The physiology of cerebral blood flow and the pathophysiology of raised intracranial pressure
- The resuscitation, assessment, investigation and continuing care of head-injured patients
- The prevention and detection of secondary intracranial and systemic insults

INTRODUCTION

Head injury accounts for 3–4% of emergency department attendances, with around 1500 cases per 100 000 population per year in the UK. Annual mortality attributable to head injury is estimated at 9 per 100 000, and it remains the leading cause of death and disability from childhood to early middle age, with an estimated 2% of the US population suffering long-term disability as a result of head injury. Road traffic accidents are the leading cause of head injury, responsible for up to 50% of cases. Other common mechanisms of injury include falls and assault. There is significant geographical variation, for example firearms are the third leading cause in the USA.

Traumatic brain injury (TBI) can be considered as the combination of primary injury sustained on impact, and hence not medically modifiable, and secondary injury developing in the following hours and days. Understanding the importance of intracranial pressure (ICP) and related parameters is key to minimising secondary injury and improving outcomes.

INTRACRANIAL PRESSURE

Intracranial pressure and cerebral blood flow

The brain depends on continuous perfusion for oxygen and glucose delivery, and hence survival. Normal cerebral blood flow (CBF) is about 55 mL/min for every 100 g of brain tissue. Ischaemia results when this rate drops below 20 mL/min, and even lower levels will result in infarction unless promptly corrected.

Flow depends on cerebral perfusion pressure (CPP), which is the difference between the mean arterial pressure (MAP) and the intracranial pressure (ICP):

CPP (75–105 mmHg) =
MAP (90–110 mmHg) – **ICP** (5–15 mmHg)

Typical normal values are given in parentheses. In fact, in the normal brain, variations in vascular tone maintain a constant CBF across a range of MAP between 50 and 150 mmHg (or higher in the setting of chronic hypertension) and a corresponding range of CPP – the process of **cerebral autoregulation**. Autoregulation can be impaired in the context of trauma, so that MAP and ICP must be actively regulated in these patients to maintain proper perfusion.

The Monro-Kellie doctrine and herniation syndromes

Alexander Monro observed in 1783 that the cranium is a 'rigid box' containing a 'nearly incompressible brain'. Any expansion in the contents, especially haematoma and brain swelling, may be initially accommodated by exclusion of fluid components, venous blood and cerebrospinal fluid (CSF). Further expansion is associated with an exponential rise in ICP (*Figure 28.1*).

Uncontrolled increases in ICP result in cerebral herniation (*Figure 28.2*). Typically, herniation of the uncus of the temporal lobe over the tentorium results in pupil abnormalities (see *Pupils*), usually occurring first on the side of any expanding haematoma. Cerebellar tonsillar herniation through the foramen magnum compresses medullary vasomotor and

†The learning objectives of this chapter are aligned with the Intercollegiate Surgical Curriculum Programme (ISCP) ST3 Neurosurgery Knowledge Requirements in Cranial Trauma and comprise:

- the resuscitation, assessment, investigation and continuing care of head-injured patients
- the prevention and detection of secondary intracranial and systemic insults.

Alexander Monro (secundus), 1733–1817, Scottish anatomist, physician and medical educator.

George Kellie, 1770–1829, Scottish surgeon and pupil of Alexander Monro (secundus).

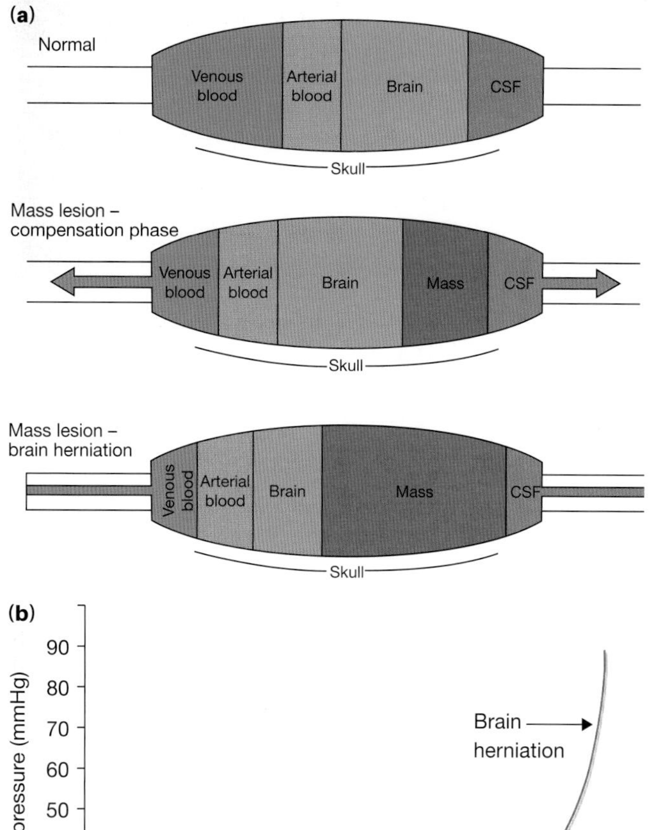

Figure 28.1 The Monro–Kellie doctrine accounts for the ability of the intracranial compartment to accommodate expanding mass lesions, primarily by excluding venous blood and cerebrospinal fluid (CSF), and the rapid rise in pressure associated with exhaustion of this compensation.

respiratory centres, classically producing **Cushing's triad**: hypertension, bradycardia and irregular respiration. The patient is then said to be '**coning**', and brainstem death will result without immediate intervention.

Summary box 28.1

Intracranial pressure

- A continuous supply of oxygenated blood is essential for brain survival
- Raised ICP can compromise cerebral perfusion, resulting in a cycle of secondary brain injury and swelling

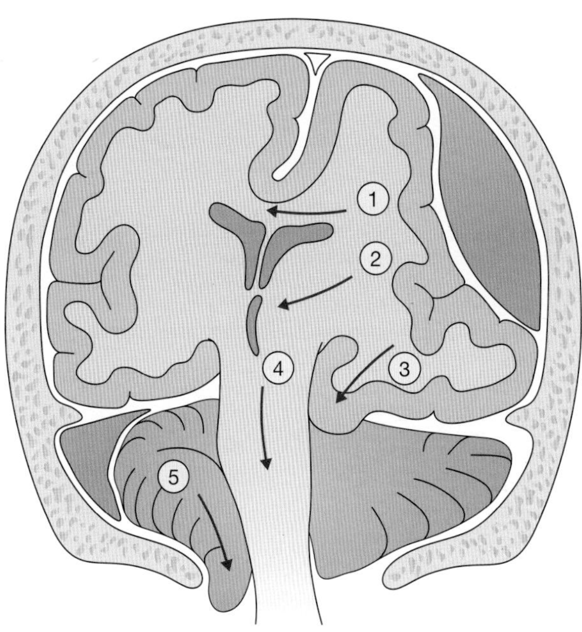

Figure 28.2 Brain herniation. (1) Subfalcine herniation – the cingulate gyrus is herniating under the falx cerebri. (2) Midline shift is evident. (3) Uncal herniation – the temporal lobe is herniating over the tentorium cerebelli, where it can compress the third nerve. (4) Central herniation and (5) tonsillar herniation result in brainstem compromise, manifesting as Cushing's triad.

CLASSIFICATION OF HEAD INJURY

The severity of head injury is classified according to the post-resuscitation Glasgow Coma Scale (GCS) score (***Table 28.1***), as it is the GCS score – and in particular the motor score – that is the best predictor of neurological outcome. In broad terms, significantly obtunded patients have moderate injuries and comatose patients have severe injuries; alcohol and drug effects often complicate the classification.

TABLE 28.1 Head injury severity: clinical classification.

Minor head injury	GCS 15 with no LOC
Mild head injury	GCS 14 or 15 with LOC
Moderate head injury	GCS 9–13
Severe head injury	GCS 3–8

GCS, Glasgow Coma Scale; LOC, loss of consciousness.

MINOR AND MILD HEAD INJURY

After exclusion of associated cervical spine injury, it is important to consider the possibility of a 'lucid interval' that may precede delayed deterioration due to an expanding intracranial haematoma. In general, patients with isolated head injuries and without ongoing deficits can be safely discharged from the emergency department, provided they meet suitable criteria,

Harvey Williams Cushing, 1869–1939, Professor of Surgery, Harvard University Medical School, Boston, MA, USA, considered the founding father of modern neurosurgery.

for instance those provided by the UK National Institute for Health and Care Excellence (NICE) (*Table 28.2*).

TABLE 28.2 UK National Institute for Health and Care Excellence discharge criteria in minor and mild head injury.

- GCS 15/15 with no focal deficits
- Normal CT brain if indicated (see *Table 28.3*)
- Patient not under the influence of alcohol or drugs
- Patient accompanied by a responsible adult
- Verbal and written head injury advice: seek medical attention if:
  - Persistent/worsening headache despite analgesia
  - Persistent vomiting
  - Drowsiness
  - Visual disturbance
  - Limb weakness or numbness

CT, computed tomography; GCS, Glasgow Coma Scale score.

Patients who do not meet all the discharge criteria will need admission for a further period of observation and/or brain imaging. Early computed tomography (CT) imaging is desirable in patients with a persistent reduced conscious level, focal deficits, suspected fractures or risk factors for intracranial bleed (*Table 28.3*). Significant clinical or radiological abnormalities should be discussed with the neurosurgical service. Many of these patients will struggle with features of concussion for a period after their injury, with headaches and somnolence typical. Follow-up by a head injury specialist nurse or equivalent is therefore desirable.

TABLE 28.3 UK National Institute for Health and Care Excellence (NICE) guidelines for computed tomography (CT) in head injury.

Indications for CT imaging in head injury within 1 hour

- GCS <13 at any point
- GCS <15 at 2 hours
- Focal neurological deficit
- Suspected open, depressed or basal skull fracture
- More than one episode of vomiting
- Post-traumatic seizure

Indications for CT imaging within 8 hours

- Age >65
- Coagulopathy (e.g. aspirin, warfarin or rivaroxaban use)
- Dangerous mechanism of injury (e.g. fall from a height, RTA)
- Retrograde amnesia >30 minutes

GCS, Glasgow Coma Scale score; RTA, road traffic accident.

Non-accidental injury

Head injury in children and vulnerable adults may be due to abuse. Significant findings include delayed presentation, injuries of disparate age, retinal haemorrhages, bilateral chronic subdural haematomas, multiple skull fractures and neurological injury without external signs of trauma.

Concussion, second impact syndrome and postconcussive syndrome

Concussion is defined as the alteration of consciousness as a result of closed head injury but is generally used to describe mild head injury without imaging abnormalities: loss of consciousness at the time of injury is not a prerequisite. Key features include confusion and amnesia. The patient may be lethargic, easily distractable, forgetful, slow to interact or emotionally labile. Gait disturbance and incoordination may be seen. While symptomatic following a head injury, patients may exhibit disordered cerebral autoregulation, making them especially vulnerable to repeat impacts. Second impact syndrome following an apparently trivial repeat injury comprises malignant brain swelling that can quickly progress to coma and death. Although the existence of the syndrome is disputed, and it is certainly rare, it should be considered in advice to individuals engaged in sports or activities carrying a risk of further injury: symptomatic players should not return to play.

Postconcussive syndrome is a loosely defined constellation of symptoms persisting for a prolonged period after injury. Patients may report somatic features such as headache, dizziness and disorders of hearing and vision. They may also suffer a variety of neurocognitive and neuropsychological disturbances, including difficulty with concentration and recall, insomnia, emotional lability, fatigue, depression and personality change. Some patients may exaggerate symptoms, seeking secondary gain (compensation).

Summary box 28.2

Minor and mild head injury

- Decisions on imaging and discharge are best made guided by published criteria
- In preverbal children and other vulnerable groups, non-accidental injury must be considered
- Amnesia, confusion, headaches and somnolence are typical features of concussion

MODERATE AND SEVERE TRAUMATIC BRAIN INJURY

Resuscitation and evaluation

Resuscitation is performed according to Advanced Trauma Life Support (ATLS) guidelines, beginning with management of the airway with cervical spine control and proceeding to assess and manage breathing and circulation. The history obtained in parallel is key to shaping ongoing management.

History

Mechanism

In moderate and severe TBI, a history must be obtained from witnesses and paramedics. High-energy mechanisms of injury, including a fall from a height or a high-speed road accident, will require careful clinical and radiological exclusion of associated multisystem and spinal injury (see *Chapters 27 and 30*). In the case of road traffic accidents in particular, extraction time and evidence of hypoxia or haemodynamic instability at the scene is important information to obtain from the paramedics. Falls and crashes are often caused by a primary medical problem such as myocardial infarction, hypoglycaemia or subarachnoid haemorrhage, with crucial implications for management.

Neurological progression

A specific check should be made for any loss of consciousness at the time of injury and its duration. The GCS score and pupil responses should be recorded at the scene, during transfer, at admission and regularly thereafter. A deterioration in the GCS score is an important index of developing a potentially reversible secondary injury. It is also useful to assess the extent of amnesia, retrograde (events prior to the injury) and anterograde (events afterwards). If the patient was intubated at the scene of the accident, it is valuable to know whether the patient was moving all four limbs before this.

Past medical history

Obtain details of the patient's medical background, including allergies and normal medications. Of particular note here are antiplatelet agents, potentially requiring platelet transfusion especially if surgery is required, and anticoagulants, which may need reversal.

Summary box 28.3

History

- Bystanders and paramedics may give vital information on the:
  - Preinjury state (fits, alcohol, chest pain)
  - Mechanism and energy involved in the injury (speed of vehicles, height fallen)
  - Conscious state and haemodynamic stability of the patient after the accident
  - Length of time taken for extrication
- Check the medication history, especially anticoagulants and antiplatelet agents

Examination: primary survey

ATLS guidelines address a fundamental priority: ensuring uninterrupted perfusion of the brain with oxygenated blood. This is especially important after a head injury, given the disturbance to intracranial autoregulation and the sensitivity of the primary injured brain tissue to further insult. Bleeding from scalp lacerations may require management as part of the primary survey as the blood loss can be substantial and ongoing. Check the responsiveness of the pupils and conscious level and check for any gross focal neurological deficits. The blood glucose level should also be measured as early as possible as hypoglycaemia is very dangerous and easily reversible.

Pupils

The pupil size should be recorded in millimetres and the reactivity documented as present, sluggish or absent. Uncal herniation (*Figure 28.2*) can compress the third nerve, compromising the parasympathetic supply to the pupil. Unopposed sympathetic activity produces a sluggish enlarged pupil, progressing to fixed and dilated under continued compression. Established pupil changes may reflect pathology anywhere in the eye or the reflex loop made up by the optic nerve, the oculomotor nerve and the brainstem. Direct ocular trauma or nerve injury in association with a skull base fracture can cause mydriasis (dilated pupil) to be present from the time of injury. Pre-existing discrepancy in the pupil size (anisocoria), as a result of Holmes–Adie pupil or cataracts for example, may also complicate assessment.

Glasgow Coma Scale score

The GCS score is the sum of scores on three components, as detailed in *Table 28.4*. The breakdown of the GCS score into eye opening, verbal and motor components should always be recorded and used when communicating the status to other doctors. Remember that the score represents the best performance elicited, so a patient flexing in response to a painful stimulus on the left and localising on the right scores 'M5'. A sternal or supraorbital rub or trapezius squeeze represents an appropriate painful stimulus.

Neurological deficit

Gross focal neurological deficits, such as paraplegia, may be evident at the primary survey, and an assessment to exclude such a deficit should be carried out, especially if the patient is to be intubated so that subsequent examination will be impossible. Detailed neurological examination is included in the secondary survey.

TABLE 28.4 Glasgow Coma Scale score for head injury.

Eyes open	Spontaneously	4
	To verbal command	3
	To painful stimulus	2
	Do not open	1
Verbal	Normal	5
	Confused	4
	Inappropriate/words only	3
	Sounds only	2
	No sounds	1
	Intubated patient	T
Motor	Obeys commands	6
	Localises to pain	5
	Withdrawal/flexion	4
	Abnormal flexion	3
	Extension	2
	No motor response	1

Sir Gordon Morgon Holmes, 1876–1965, physician, National Hospital for Nervous Diseases, London, UK.
William John Adie, 1886–1935, physician, National Hospital for Nervous Diseases, London, UK.

Summary box 28.4

Primary survey

- Ensure adequate oxygenation and circulation
- Exclude hypoglycaemia
- Check pupil size and response and GCS score as soon as possible
- Check for focal neurological deficits before intubation if possible

Examination: secondary survey

A full secondary survey will be required. Particular attention must be paid to the head, neck and spine.

Head

Examination of the head should include inspection and palpation of the scalp for evidence of subgaleal haematoma and scalp lacerations, which may bleed profusely and potentially overlie fractures. Examine the face for evidence of fractures, especially to the orbital rim, zygoma and maxilla. Clinical evidence of a skull base fracture may include Battle's sign (*Figure 28.3*) and 'racoon' or 'panda' eyes (bilateral periorbital bruising). Haemotympanum, or overt bleeding from the ear if the tympanic membrane has ruptured, and CSF rhinorrhoea or otorrhoea are also highly suggestive of a fracture of the base of the skull.

A complete examination of the cranial nerves will reveal, for example, facial or vestibulocochlear nerve damage associated with skull base fracture. Midbrain or brainstem dysfunction may produce gaze paresis (inability of the eye to look across beyond the midline), dysconjugate gaze (inability of the eyes to work together) or roving eye movements. Inspect the conjunctiva and cornea of the eyes, and the retina using an ophthalmoscope, looking for hyphaema (blood in the anterior chamber of the eye), papilloedema or retinal detachment. Blood in the mouth may be due to tongue-biting at seizure. The GCS score and pupil status, assessed as part of the primary survey, require re-evaluation at the secondary survey and regularly thereafter.

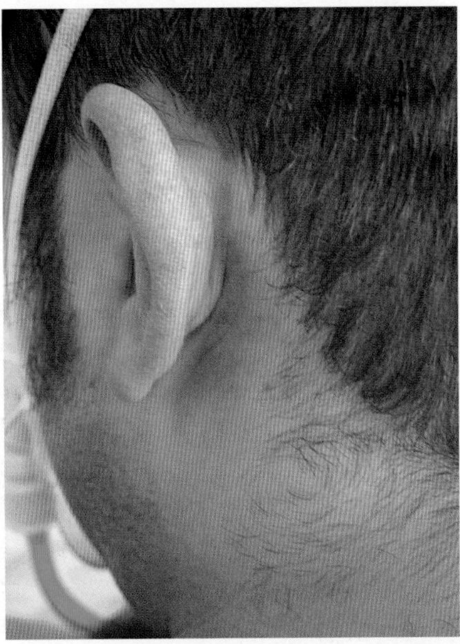

Figure 28.3 Battle's sign. A skull base fracture may be associated with bruising over the mastoid process.

Neck and spine

Studies have demonstrated an incidence of cervical fracture of up to 10% in association with moderate and severe TBI. Cervical spine injury must be presumed in the context of head injury until actively excluded. In a high-energy mechanism such as a road traffic accident or fall from a height, thoracic and lumbar spine injuries must also be excluded. Plain radiographs are of limited value in excluding significant cervical spine injury. Even CT imaging does not exclude the possibility of significant ligamentous injury. Therefore, whenever feasible, these patients should be managed in a hard collar until the neck can be cleared clinically.

A peripheral nerve examination with documentation of limb tone, power, reflexes and sensation needs to be performed early to identify spinal pathology. This is especially important in patients who may subsequently be intubated and ventilated when this assessment will no longer be possible. Obtunded patients should move all four limbs in response to an appropriate painful stimulus.

The patient will need to be log-rolled to palpate for thoracic or lumbar deformity, and any cervical collar should be removed at this stage to allow palpation of the cervical spine before it is then replaced again. If there is associated spinal injury, a thoracic sensory level is much more easily established by sensory examination on the back. A per rectum examination is also performed at log-roll, assessing for anal tone, sensation in the awake patient and anal wink (sphincter seen to contract in response to a pinprick stimulus). Priapism is a strong predictor of severe cord injury even in intubated patients.

Summary box 28.5

Secondary survey

- Battle's sign, periorbital bruising and blood in the ears/nose/mouth may point to a base of skull fracture
- Cervical spine fractures are common and must be actively excluded
- Log-roll to check the whole spine for steps and tenderness and for a per rectum examination

Surgical pathology

Fractures: skull vault

Closed linear fractures of the skull vault are managed conservatively. Open or comminuted fractures should be considered for

William Henry Battle, 1855–1936, surgeon, St Thomas's Hospital, London, UK.

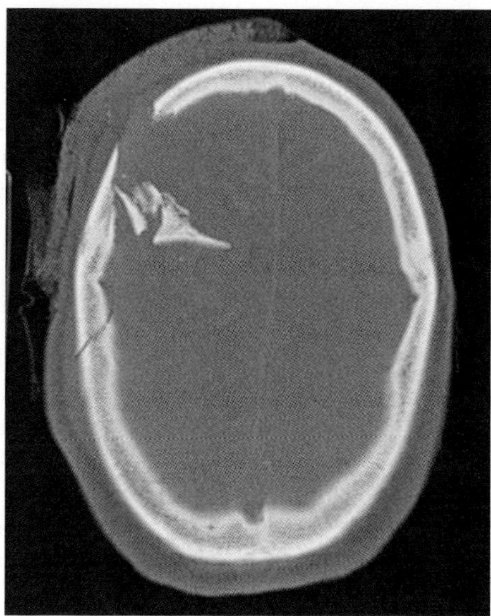

Figure 28.4 A right frontal comminuted depressed skull fracture, with a linear undisplaced fracture of the right parietal bone visible posteriorly.

debridement and prophylactic antibiotic therapy. Depressed skull fractures involve inward displacement of a bone fragment by at least the thickness of the skull (*Figures 28.4 and 28.5*). They occur when small objects hit the skull at high velocity. They are usually compound (open) fractures, and are associated with a high incidence of infection, neurological deficit and late-onset epilepsy. These fractures require exploration and elevation, especially where intracranial air is present, pointing to a breach in the dura mater. Fractures that involve the air sinuses should generally be managed as open fractures, using broad-spectrum antibiotics with or without exploration.

Fractures: skull base

Clinical signs of skull base fracture include bleeding or CSF leak from the ears (otorrhoea) or nose (rhinorrhoea) and bruising behind the ear (*Figure 28.3*) or around the eyes. Skull base fractures may be complicated by pituitary dysfunction, arterial dissection or cranial nerve deficits, with anosmia, facial palsy or hearing loss typical. CSF leak will generally resolve spontaneously but persistent leak can result in meningitis so repair may be required. Blind nasogastric tube placement is contraindicated in these patients.

Extradural haematoma

Extradural haematoma (*Figure 28.6*) is a neurosurgical emergency. It results from rupture of an artery, vein or venous sinus, in association with a skull fracture. The classical injury is a fracture to the thin squamous temporal bone, with associated damage to the middle meningeal artery. Transient loss of consciousness is typical, and the patient may then present in the subsequent lucid interval with headache but without any neurological deficit. As the haematoma expands, compensation is exhausted (see *The Monro–Kellie doctrine and herniation syndromes*) with rapid deterioration. There is contralateral hemiparesis, a reduced conscious level and ipsilateral pupillary

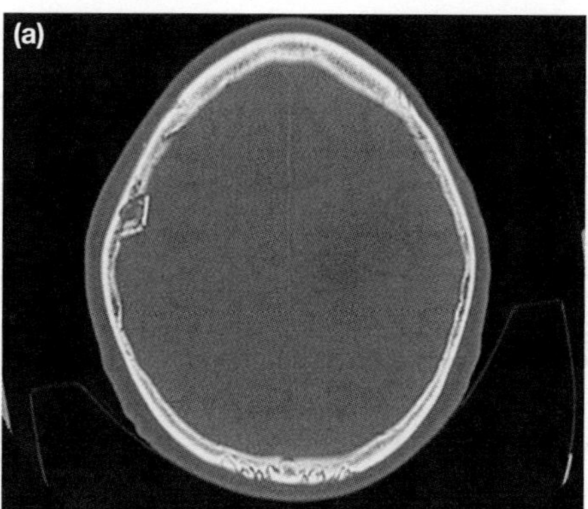

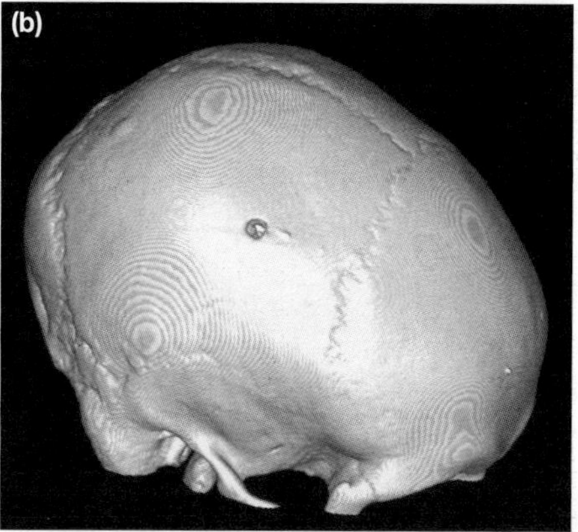

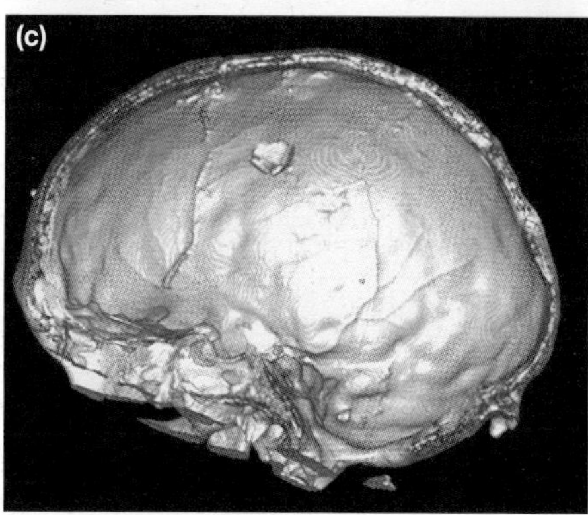

Figure 28.5 (a–c) A small depressed skull fracture of the parietal bone visible on an axial bone window (a), visualised on bone vault reconstructions (b) with an underlying breach of the dura (c).

dilatation, the cardinal signs of brain compression and herniation. Although this '**talk and die**' pattern of deterioration occurs in only one-third of cases, it is critically important to recognise the potential for rapid avoidable secondary brain injury in patients who present neurologically intact.

On CT, extradural haematomas appear as a lentiform (lens-shaped or biconvex) hyperdense lesion between the skull and the brain, constrained by the adherence of the dura to the skull. A mass effect may be evident, with compression of the surrounding brain and midline shift. Areas of mixed density suggest active bleeding. A skull fracture will usually be evident. Significant extradural haematoma mandates urgent transfer to the most accessible neurosurgical facility for immediate evacuation in deteriorating or comatose patients or those with large bleeds and for close observation with serial imaging in other cases. The prognosis for promptly evacuated extradural haematoma, without associated primary brain injury, is excellent.

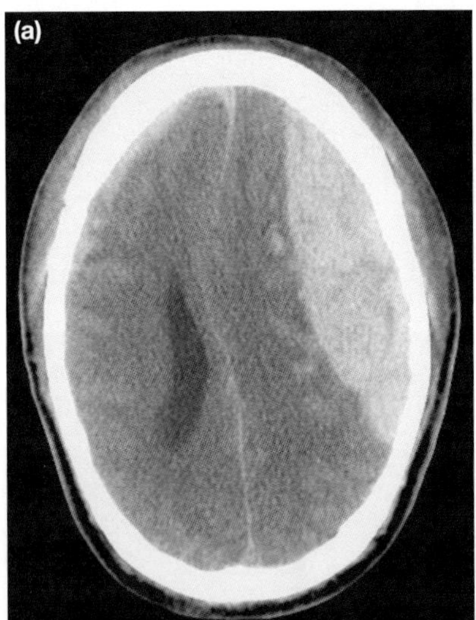

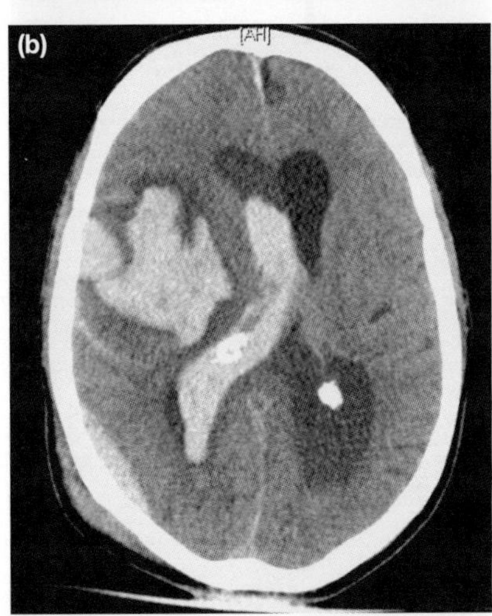

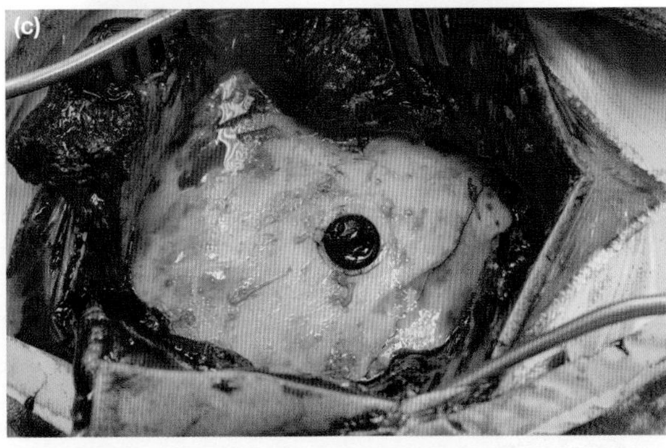

Figure 28.6 (a) A large left extradural haematoma (note the biconvex shape) exerts a mass effect; a smaller right acute subdural haematoma is also evident. (b) Right frontal intracerebral haematoma extending into the lateral ventricle is evident. There is a small right posterior extradural haematoma and traumatic subarachnoid bleeding in the sulci of the right hemisphere. (c) A surgical temporal bone exposure showing a linear skull fracture with underlying extradural haematoma visible through a burr hole.

Summary box 28.6

Extradural haemorrhage

- Can follow relatively minor trauma with brief loss of consciousness
- Followed by a lucid interval and then sudden deterioration
- Lentiform lesion on CT
- Require immediate transfer to a neurosurgical unit for decision on evacuation

Acute subdural haematoma

Acute subdural haematoma (*Figure 28.7*) is encountered in two broadly distinct contexts. First, high-energy injury mechanisms can result in the rupture of cortical surface vessels with significant associated primary brain injury. This results in an expanding haematoma with rapid deterioration and

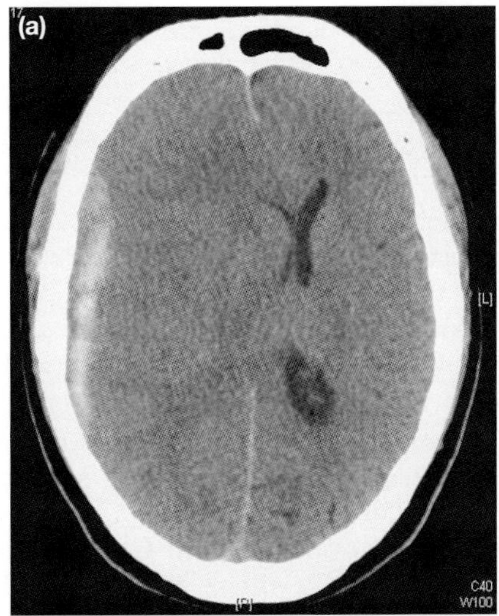

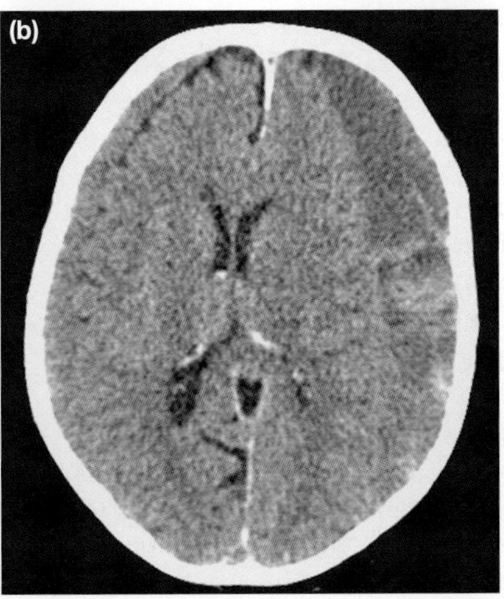

Figure 28.7 (a) Right-sided acute subdural haematoma (hyperdense). The substantial midline shift reflects brain swelling as well as bleeding – this is a high-energy injury. (b) Bilateral subdural haematomas: the left is mixed density, the hypodense material representing old blood and the higher density indicating more recent bleeding, probably loculated so requiring a craniotomy to evacuate. The bleed on the right is isodense, indicating intermediate age.

development of signs of raised ICP reminiscent of extradural haematoma, without the lucid interval. These collections require prompt evacuation, typically by craniotomy or craniectomy.

In a second group of patients, older and often anticoagulated, a lower energy injury leads to venous bleeding around the brain. Depending on the total volume of bleeding, the resulting haematoma may present early as acute subdural haematoma, after delay and osmotic expansion as chronic subdural haematoma or may even remain clinically silent. This last group may present much later with a further 'acute-on-chronic' subdural haematoma. On diagnosis, clotting function should be corrected wherever possible. Bleeds of significant size, with significant associated midline shift or with deteriorating neurology, require urgent evacuation. Smaller bleeds in neurologically stable patients may be managed conservatively, at least initially: liquefaction of the clot over 7–10 days after the bleed may allow for a much less invasive evacuation through burr holes.

Since the dura is not as adherent to the brain as it is to the skull, subdural blood is free to expand across the brain surface, giving a diffuse concave appearance.

Summary box 28.7

Acute subdural haemorrhage

- High-energy injuries, or elderly/anticoagulated
- Generally require urgent evacuation by craniotomy/craniectomy

Chronic subdural haematoma

Chronic subdural haematoma (*Figure 28.7*) is a common cause of acute neurological deterioration in older adults. Cerebral atrophy in this age group results in stretching of the cortical–dural bridging veins, which are then vulnerable to rupture. The resulting haematoma can expand over days or weeks by osmosis, ultimately producing symptoms of raised ICP or focal deficits. There is usually a history of recent injury, but, especially in the context of antiplatelet or anticoagulant medication, even apparently trivial impacts may be responsible.

On presentation it is important to exclude coexisting electrolyte disturbance and infections, which may contribute to clinical impairment. Imaging reveals diffuse hypodensity overlying the brain surface. Recent bleeding may be isodense or hyperdense, and mixed density can indicate an acute-on-chronic subdural haematoma.

Anticoagulation should be reversed, either by administration of vitamin K or urgently by transfusion of recombinant clotting factors in patients who have deteriorated acutely. Conservative management, sometimes with administration of corticosteroids, can be considered for small bleeds without symptoms or with headache alone. For the majority drainage is performed using burr holes. Urgency is dictated by the clinical condition of the patient and imaging evidence of mass effect. If clinically stable, a delay of 7–10 days to allow platelet function to normalise after withdrawal of aspirin/clopidogrel may be considered.

Summary box 28.8

Chronic subdural haemorrhage

- Common in the elderly, especially those on anticoagulants
- Clinical deficits result from osmotic expansion of a degrading clot over days/weeks
- Diffuse hypodense lesion on CT
- Burr hole drainage is usually preferred

Traumatic subarachnoid haemorrhage

Trauma is the commonest cause of subarachnoid haemorrhage (*Figures 28.6b and 28.8*), and this is managed conservatively. It is not usually associated with significant vasospasm, which characterises aneurysmal subarachnoid haemorrhage. The possibility of spontaneous subarachnoid haemorrhage actually leading to collapse and so causing a head injury needs to be borne in mind, and formal or CT angiography may be required to exclude this.

Cerebral contusions

Contusions are common and are found predominantly where the brain is in contact with the irregularly ridged inside of the skull, i.e. at the inferior frontal lobes and temporal poles. '**Coup contre-coup**' contusions refer to brain injury both at the site of impact and distant to this, where the brain impacts on the inside of the skull as the skull and brain accelerate and then decelerate out of synchrony with each other. Contusions appear heterogeneous on CT, reflecting their composition of injured brain matter interspersed with acute blood (*Figure 28.8*). Contusions rarely require surgical intervention but may warrant delayed evacuation to reduce a mass effect.

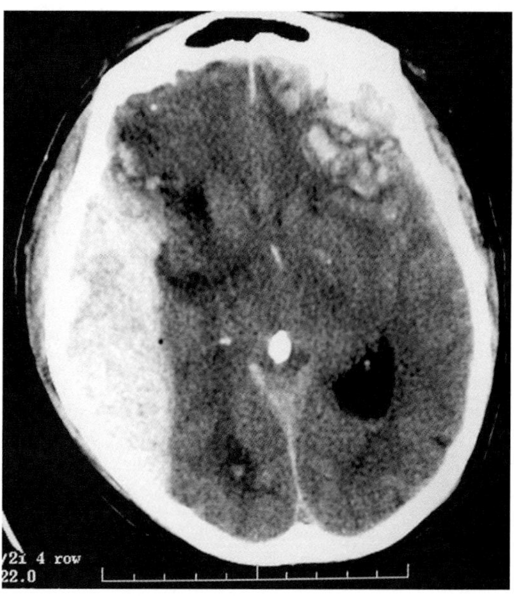

Figure 28.8 A large right extradural haematoma is evident. There are widespread cerebral contusions most prominent in the left frontal lobe. There is traumatic subarachnoid blood in the third and lateral ventricles.

Diffuse axonal injury

This is a form of primary brain injury seen in high-energy accidents that usually renders the patient comatose; it is associated with poor outcomes. It is strictly a pathological diagnosis made at postmortem, but haemorrhagic foci in the corpus callosum and dorsolateral rostral brainstem on CT may be suggestive. Magnetic resonance imaging is more sensitive and is employed to evaluate for diffuse axonal injury in patients who fail to improve neurologically.

Arterial dissection

Cerebral arterial dissection occurs spontaneously or in the context of trauma. In the hours after significant trauma, dissection of the carotid extracranially, or at the skull base in association with fractures, is most common. It presents with headache, neck pain and focal ischaemic deficits due to occlusion by mural haematoma, thrombus and thromboembolism. Intracranial dissection often affects the vertebral artery and may result in subarachnoid bleeding.

Summary box 28.9

Specific injuries

- Traumatic versus primary subarachnoid haemorrhage is an important distinction
- Cerebral contusions arise adjacent to rough bone surfaces
- Diffuse axonal injury results from extreme accelerations of the skull contents
- Arterial dissection is associated with fractures of the skull base

Medical management

From initial resuscitation, through surgical intervention and into the subsequent phase of ICU management, medical management strategies aim to minimise secondary brain injury through avoidance of hypoxia and hypotension and control of ICP. Unchecked, secondary injury leads to a further cycle of deterioration (*Figures 28.2 and 28.9*).

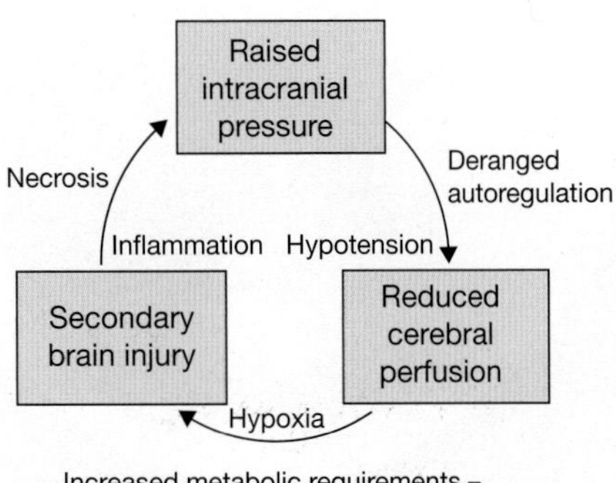

Figure 28.9 Brain swelling and mass lesions contribute to raised intracranial pressure, which compromises perfusion, leading to secondary brain injury and further swelling.

The role of neurosurgical centres

Early discussion of patients and imaging with the regional neurosurgical service is advisable. UK trauma audit and research network data show higher mortality in patients with severe TBI managed in non-neurosurgical centres, and this is reflected in NICE guidelines, which recommend early transfer irrespective of the need for surgery.

Control of intracranial pressure

Intubation and ventilation are required early in the management of severe brain injury for airway control. They are often required in moderate brain injury to facilitate the safe management and transfer of unstable and frequently agitated patients and in order to control ICP. A bolus of mannitol or hypertonic saline may be administered to temporise ICP, for example while scanning and transferring the patient.

Management of the intubated patient, following evacuation of any focal haematomas, is guided by ICP monitoring using a bolt ICP monitor or else an external ventricular drain inserted into the lateral ventricle, which can also contribute to ICP control by permitting CSF drainage. A sustained elevated ICP exceeding 20–25 mmHg is associated with a poor outcome, and maintenance of a CPP of at least 60 mmHg is important in preventing secondary injury.

ICP can be controlled by simple measures, including raising the head of the bed and loosening the collar to improve venous drainage. Seizures and pyrexia should be actively controlled. Medical management titrated to ICP includes escalating doses of sedatives, analgesics and ultimately muscle relaxants. Target ventilatory and circulatory parameters are set out in *Table 28.5*.

TABLE 28.5 Key parameters to maintain in head-injured patients in neurointensive care.

- $PaCO_2$ = 4.5–5.0 kPa
- PaO_2 >11 kPa
- MAP = 80–90 mmHg
- ICP <20 mmHg
- CPP >60 mmHg
- $[Na^+]$ >140 mmol/L
- $[K^+]$ >4 mmol/L

$[K^+]$, plasma potassium concentration; $[Na^+]$, plasma sodium concentration; CPP, cerebral perfusion pressure; ICP, intracranial pressure; MAP, mean arterial pressure; $PaCO_2$, partial pressure of carbon dioxide in arterial blood; PaO_2, partial pressure of oxygen in arterial blood.

Where these measures fail, neurointensivists may seek to control brain swelling using mannitol or hypertonic saline infusions. Where autoregulation is preserved, inducing high CPP may reduce ICP through vasoconstriction. A range of further interventions are effective in controlling ICP, but evidence for long-term outcome benefit is limited or absent. These interventions include induction of therapeutic hypothermia or thiopentone coma and surgical decompressive craniectomy.

Pituitary dysfunction

Electrolyte imbalance is common in TBI and contributes to brain swelling and to causing seizures. Diverse mechanisms are involved. Cerebral salt wasting, a poorly understood form of excretory dysregulation in association with brain insult, leads to volume depletion and hyponatraemia. The syndrome of inappropriate antidiuretic hormone (SIADH) leads to water retention and hyponatraemia in the context of pituitary damage. This is of particular concern in head injury since low serum osmotic pressure can contribute to brain swelling, so hypotonic fluids are avoided in this setting. Conversely antidiuretic hormone secretion may be compromised in the context of trauma, producing diabetes insipidus, resulting in hypernatraemia.

All aspects of pituitary function may be compromised in the setting of TBI. Routine screening of pituitary hormone levels and liaison with endocrinology are important aspects of optimal medical management. Note that routine, rather than directed, administration of corticosteroids in severe head injury is associated with increased mortality and is not recommended.

Seizures

Seizures may occur early (within 7 days) or late. The cumulative probability is between 2% (mild TBI) and 60% (severe TBI with exacerbating features). Risk factors include injury severity, especially the presence of intracerebral haemorrhage, depressed skull fractures and tears of the dura. Antiepileptics, typically phenytoin, are administered prophylactically to patients at high risk of seizures.

Nutrition

Enteral nutrition is preferred to intravenous parenteral nutrition on the grounds of cost and associated complications, and should be commenced within 72 hours of injury. Prokinetics (e.g. metoclopramide, erythromycin) can be administered to promote absorption.

Outcomes and sequelae

The long-term sequelae of moderate and severe TBI include headache and memory and cognitive impairments, contributing to the postconcussive syndrome described above. Rehabilitation represents a complex and prolonged multidisciplinary challenge. The Glasgow Outcome Scale score is used to quantify the degree of recovery achieved after head injury, especially for research purposes, and is detailed in *Table 28.6*. Good recovery implies independence and potential to return to work rather than a full return to previous capacity.

TABLE 28.6 Glasgow Outcome Scale.

Good recovery	5
Moderate disability	4
Severe disability	3
Persistent vegetative state	2
Dead	1

Summary box 28.10

Medical management of head injury

- First line ICP control involves optimising sedation, ventilation and serum sodium levels
- Paralysis and external ventricular CSF drainage are important adjuncts
- There is little evidence for benefit with therapeutic hypothermia, barbiturate coma or decompressive craniectomy
- Check pituitary function, consider seizure prophylaxis, commence enteral nutrition within 72 hours

TRAUMATIC BRAIN INJURY IN THE CHILD

Head injury in children is common and presents specific challenges relating to physiology, assessment, management and safeguarding. Children have large heads compared with the rest of their bodies, predisposing to both head and neck injury. In the case of minor head injury, good assessment depends on winning the trust of child and parent, while identifying risk factors requiring further admission for observation or CT scan (*Table 28.7*). Non-accidental injury should always be considered; for example, it is key to ensure that the reported mechanism of injury is in keeping with the child's developmental stage and to examine for injuries outside the normal distribution for childhood accidents. The Paediatric Glasgow Coma Scale is applied in the under-twos (*Table 28.8*).

Moderate and severe head injury should be managed by a trauma team in a resuscitation room, using paediatric ATLS protocols directed at optimising physiology to prevent secondary brain injury, and with intensive care unit (ICU) involvement for airway management as appropriate. Children with open sutures can lose substantial blood volumes into the head. Palpating the fontanelle allows direct assessment of ICP, and in all cases head and neck CT imaging are key to guiding definitive management.

TABLE 28.7 UK National Institute for Health and Care Excellence criteria for computed tomography scan in children following head injury.

- Suspicion of NAI
- First seizure
- GCS <14 or <15 in under-ones
- GCS <15 2 hours post injury
- Signs of fracture of the base of skull
- Focal neurological deficit
- Bruise/swelling/laceration >5 cm in under-ones
- More than one of:
  - Loss of consciousness >5 minutes
  - Abnormal drowsiness
  - Four or more episodes of vomiting
  - Dangerous mechanism
  - Amnesia >5 minutes

GCS, Glasgow Coma Scale score; NAI, non-accidental injury.

TABLE 28.8 Paediatric Glasgow Coma Scale score.

Eye opening	Spontaneously	4
	To verbal stimulus	3
	To pain	2
	No response	1
Verbal response	Coos/babbles	5
	Irritable cries	4
	Cries in response to pain	3
	Moans in response to pain	2
	No response	1
Motor response	Purposeful/spontaneous movements	6
	Withdraws to touch	5
	Withdraws to pain	4
	Flexes to pain	3
	Extends to pain	2
	No response	1

FURTHER READING

Greenberg MS. *Handbook of neurosurgery*, 9th edn. Stuttgart: Thieme Medical Publishers, 2019.

Samandouras G (ed.). *The neurosurgeon's handbook.* Oxford: Oxford University Press, 2010.

CHAPTER 29 Torso and pelvic trauma

Learning objectives

To understand:
- The importance of physiology over anatomy in the management of trauma
- The gross surgical anatomy of the chest and abdomen
- The pathophysiology of torso injury
- The clinical assessment in the injured patient
- The use of special investigations and their limitations
- The operative approaches to the thoracic cavity
- The special features of an emergency department thoracotomy for haemorrhage control
- The indications for, and techniques of, the trauma laparotomy
- The philosophy of damage control resuscitation
- The management of trauma to the pelvis

INTRODUCTION

Injury seldom respects anatomical boundaries, hence the division of the body into the abdomen and the thorax is artificial. Therefore, injury to the torso with its associated physiological consequences is more appropriate. The torso is generally regarded as the focal point of the human body, consisting of the chest, abdomen and pelvis and not including the head, neck, arms and legs. About 42% of all deaths are the result of brain injury, but some 39% of all trauma deaths are caused by major haemorrhage, usually from torso injury (*Figure 29.1*).

Historically, injury was treated on an anatomical basis; however, it has become clear that physiology should be the over-riding consideration. The driver of successful resuscitation is therefore the preservation of normal physiology. Techniques such as damage control resuscitation and its key component damage control surgery have dramatically improved survival through an understanding of the best techniques required to restore physiological stability (see *Chapters 1, 26 and 27*).

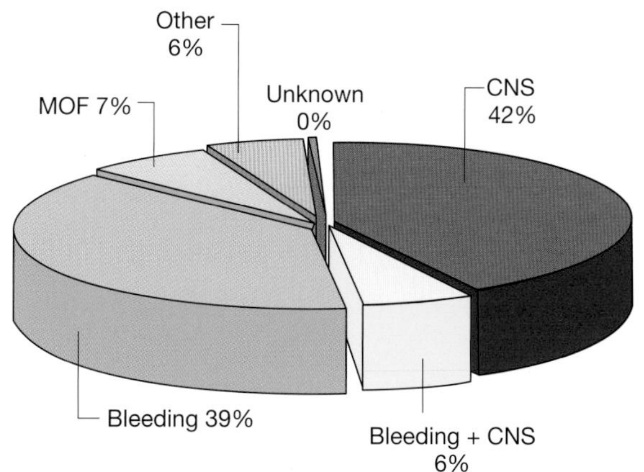

Figure 29.1 Causes of death in trauma. CNS, central nervous system; MOF, multiple organ failure.

INJURY MECHANISMS ASSOCIATED WITH TORSO TRAUMA

Injury consistently traverses different anatomical zones of the body, affecting structures on both sides of traditional anatomical zones. These zones are known as junctional zones.

Junctional zones

The key junctional zones are:

- between the neck and the thorax;
- between the thorax and the upper limbs;
- between the thorax and the abdomen;
- between the abdominopelvic structures and the groin.

These zones represent surgical challenges in terms of both diagnosis of the area of injury and the required surgical approach. Such factors have to be balanced against the physiological stability of the patient.

Root of the neck

Most injuries affecting the base of the neck may also affect the upper mediastinum and thoracic inlet. Choice of access is determined by the need for surgical control of the vascular structures contained within.

The mediastinum

The mediastinum, with its major vessels and the heart, is also an extremely high-risk area for penetrating wounds. Any wound in this region should immediately raise the suspicion of a major vascular or an associated cardiac injury, even in the absence of initial gross physical signs.

Diaphragm

The thorax and abdomen are separated by the diaphragm, which is mainly responsible for breathing, allowing movement during breathing between the fourth and eighth intercostal space. Any penetrating injury below the nipples on the chest may therefore have penetrated the diaphragm and entered the abdomen. Injuries in this junctional zone, therefore, should be investigated as if both cavities had been penetrated (*Figure 29.2*). In blunt trauma, rupture of the diaphragm can result in migration of abdominal viscera into the chest, with left-sided hemidiaphragm rupture being more common.

Pelvic structures

The pelvis contains a large plexus of vessels, both venous and arterial. Should injury occur, control of haemorrhage can prove to be exceptionally difficult and may require control of both arterial inflow and venous outflow. Angioembolisation can be a very useful adjunct to treatment, especially with deep pelvic injuries.

Summary box 29.1

Junctional zones

- Between neck and the thorax
- Between thorax and upper limbs
- Between thorax and the abdomen
- Between the abdominopelvic structures and the groin

CRITICAL PHYSIOLOGY

Resuscitation of all injuries to the chest and abdomen should follow the latest Advanced Trauma Life Support (ATLS) principles (*Table 29.1*; see *Chapters 26 and 27*).

TABLE 29.1 Advanced Trauma Life Support principles of resuscitation.

C	Catastrophic haemorrhage
A	Airway
B	Breathing
C	Circulation
D	Disability (neurology)
E	Environment and exposure

TABLE 29.2 Clinical indicators of potential ongoing bleeding in torso trauma.

Physiological	Increasing respiratory rate
	Increasing pulse rate
	Falling blood pressure
	Rising serum lactate
Anatomical	Visible bleeding
	Injury in close proximity to major vessels
	Penetrating injury with a retained missile

Haemorrhage is the major problem. This may be obvious at the time of evaluation; however, in the young physically fit individual, bleeding may produce no or only minimal changes in vital measures and, therefore, be difficult to assess (*Table 29.2*). Although obvious injury may be present, traditional indicators (such as pulse rate), in isolation, are unreliable.

Bleeding occurs from five major sites – '**one on the floor and four more**':

- external – 'floor';
- chest;
- abdomen (including the retroperitoneum);
- pelvis;
- extremities.

THORACIC INJURY

Thoracic injury accounts for 25% of all severe injuries. In a further 25%, it may be a significant contributor to the subsequent death of the patient. In most of these patients, the cause of death is haemorrhage. In excess of 80% of patients with chest injury can be managed non-operatively. The key to a good outcome is early physiological resuscitation followed by a correct diagnosis.

Investigation

Routine investigation in the emergency department of injury to the chest is based on clinical examination, supplemented by appropriate imaging.

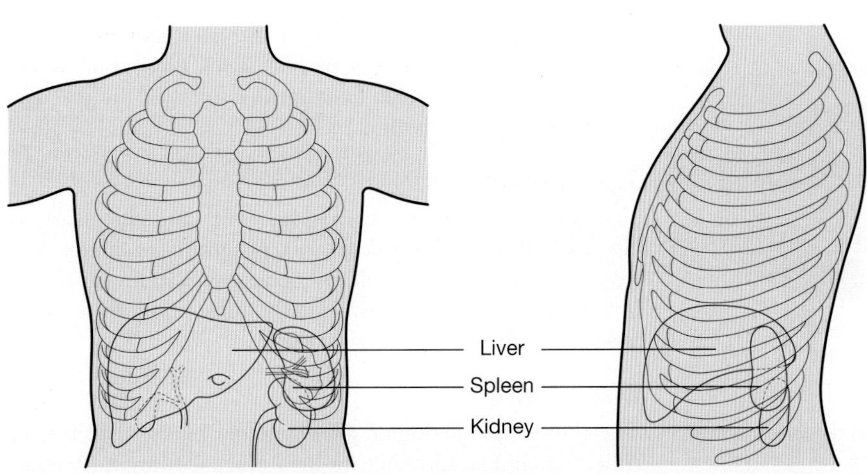

Figure 29.2 The anatomical extent of the abdomen.

Ultrasound – extended focused assessment with sonography for trauma (eFAST)

Ultrasound can be used to differentiate between contusion and the actual presence of blood. Extended focused assessment with sonography for trauma (eFAST) is becoming the most common investigation. The technique uses sonographic assessment in the chest, looking for a cardiac tamponade or free blood and air in the hemithoraces, and assessment for blood in the abdominal cavity, in the paracolic gutters, subdiaphragmatic spaces and pelvis.

Finger thoracostomy

In the physiologically grossly unstable patient, where physical examination is inconclusive and there is no time for radiological investigations, bilateral finger thoracostomy can be a diagnostic procedure as well as a therapeutic one, and the benefits of undertaking it often outweigh the risks. It is undertaken by making a 5-cm skin incision on the fifth rib just anterior to the mid-axillary line. The intercostal muscles are then separated just above the fifth rib and the pleural cavity entered. A finger is then inserted and a pleural sweep made to ensure the pleural cavity has been entered.

Chest radiograph

In those cases where the patient is physiologically non-compromised or the spine is at risk, an anteroposterior (AP) supine chest radiograph is usually the simplest initial investigation. It will provide good information regarding tracheal deviation, lung and mediastinal pathology as well as skeletal injury.

In penetrating injury, it may be more helpful for the radiograph to be performed with the patient positioned erect, as this will best reveal a small pneumothorax, fluid meniscus, air–fluid level or the presence of free gas under the diaphragm, indicating the presence of a hollow abdominal viscus perforation. Note that up to 300 mL of blood may pool behind the domes of the diaphragm, and may not be visible even in the erect view.

The presence of thoracic skeletal injury should alert the clinician to the possibility of adjacent thoracic or abdominal visceral injury. Rupture of the thoracic aorta can be related to fractures of the first and second rib, bilateral clavicular fracture and fracture of the sternum, thoracic spine or scapula. Fracture of the lower ribs can be related to injury of the liver or spleen. Fracture of the ribs, irrespective of site, can be related to injury to the lung parenchyma or thoracic wall vasculature, causing pneumothorax, haemothorax or lung contusion.

Computed tomography scan

The computed tomography (CT) scan with contrast allows for three-dimensional reconstruction of the chest and abdomen, as well as of the bony skeleton. It has become the principal and most reliable examination for major injury in trauma. In blunt chest trauma, the CT scan will allow the definition of fractures, as well as showing haematomas, pneumothoraces and pulmonary contusion. In penetrating trauma, the scan may show the track or presence of the missile and allow the proper planning of definitive surgery. However, although the presence of an isolated rupture of the diaphragm with migration of abdominal contents into the chest can be detected by CT scan, in injury without migration the diagnosis will not be obvious.

The pitfalls of investigation are:

- failure to assess tracheal shift immediately above the sternal notch clinically (deviation of the trachea occurs away from the affected side in tension pneumothorax and towards the affected side in lung collapse);
- failure to percuss and auscultate both front and back in a supine patient (an inflated lung will 'float' on a haemothorax, so auscultation from the front may sound normal);
- failure to pass a nasogastric tube if rupture of the diaphragm is suspected; a chest radiograph will show the nasogastric tube apparently within the chest cavity;
- a supine chest radiograph can show a haemothorax as a homogeneous increase in opacity of the hemithorax – this can cause confusion between the darker side and the lighter side as to which may be a haemothorax (less radiolucent) or a pneumothorax (more radiolucent); look carefully for lung markings and do not drain the wrong side;
- pursuing radiological investigation (radiography or CT scan) instead of resuscitation in the unstable patient.

Summary box 29.2

Investigation of chest injuries

- Directly or indirectly involved in >50% of trauma deaths
- More than 80% can be managed non-operatively
- A chest radiograph is the investigation of first choice
- Finger thoracostomy can be diagnostic and therapeutic
- A pan-CT scan provides rapid diagnosis

Management

In penetrating injury, most patients who have suffered injury to the chest can be managed with appropriate resuscitation and insertion of an intercostal drain.

If a sucking chest wound is present, this should not be fully closed but should be covered with a piece of plastic, closed on three sides to form a one-way valve, and thereafter an underwater chest drain should be inserted remote from the wound. No attempt should be made to close a sucking chest wound until controlled drainage has been achieved, in case a stable patient with an open pneumothorax is converted into an unstable patient with a tension pneumothorax.

In blunt injury, most bleeding occurs from the intercostal or internal mammary vessels and it is relatively rare for these to require surgery. If bleeding does not stop spontaneously, the vessels can be embolised, via an interventional radiological approach, or treated operatively, during which the vessels can be tied off or encircled. In blunt chest compressive injury, particularly in the presence of a flail chest, there can be an associated lung contusion.

The patient in extremis with exsanguinating chest haemorrhage is discussed in ***Emergency department thoracotomy or sternotomy***.

Life-threatening injuries can be remembered as the 'deadly dozen'. Six are immediately life-threatening and should be

Summary box 29.3

Closed management of chest injuries

- More than 80% of chest injuries can be managed with the insertion of an intercostal drain only
- Do not close a sucking chest wound until a drain is in place
- If bleeding persists, the chest will need to be opened and direct haemostatic control is obtained

sought and managed during the primary survey and six are potentially life-threatening and should be detected during the secondary survey (*Table 29.3*). A high index of suspicion must be maintained thereafter to diagnose the potential threats to life, as their symptoms and signs can be very subtle. Early consultation and referral to a trauma centre is advised in cases of doubt.

Immediate life-threatening injuries

Airway obstruction

Early intubation is very important, particularly in cases of neck haematoma or possible airway oedema. Airway distortion can be insidious and progressive and can make delayed intubation more difficult if not impossible.

Tension pneumothorax

A tension pneumothorax develops when a 'one-way valve' air leak occurs either from the lung or through the chest wall. Air is sucked into the thoracic cavity without any means of escape, completely collapsing and then compressing the affected lung. The mediastinum is displaced to the opposite side, decreasing venous return and compressing the opposite lung.

The most common causes are penetrating chest trauma, blunt chest trauma with a parenchymal lung injury and air leak that did not spontaneously close, iatrogenic lung injury (e.g. due to central venepuncture) and mechanical positive-pressure ventilation.

TABLE 29.3 The 'deadly dozen' threats to life from chest injury.

Immediately life-threatening	• Airway obstruction • Tension pneumothorax • Pericardial tamponade • Open pneumothorax • Massive haemothorax • Flail chest
Potentially life-threatening	• Aortic injuries • Tracheobronchial injuries • Myocardial contusion • Rupture of the diaphragm • Oesophageal injuries • Pulmonary contusion

The clinical presentation is dramatic. The patient is increasingly restless with tachypnoea, dyspnoea and distended neck veins (similar to pericardial tamponade). Clinical examination may reveal tracheal deviation; this is a late finding and is not

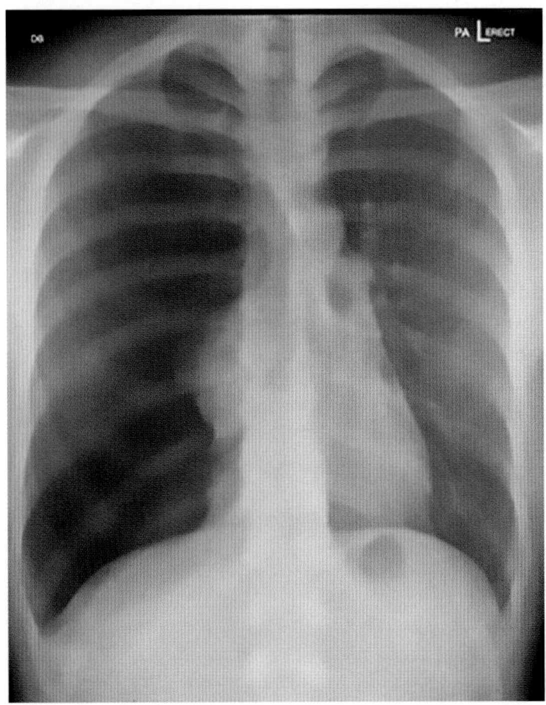

Figure 29.3 Radiological appearance of a tension pneumothorax (courtesy of Dr Elizabeth Dick, Consultant Radiologist, Imperial College Healthcare NHS Trust, London, UK).

necessary to clinically confirm diagnosis. There will also be hyper-resonance and decreased or absent breath sounds over the affected hemithorax. Tension pneumothorax is a clinical diagnosis and treatment should never be delayed by waiting for radiological confirmation. Always treat it with a high index of suspicion of being present (*Figure 29.3*).

Treatment consists of immediate decompression. This was historically taught by rapid insertion of a large-bore cannula into the second intercostal space in the mid-clavicular line of the affected side, followed by insertion of a chest tube through the fifth intercostal space in the anterior axillary line. However, current teaching advocates undertaking decompression in the safe triangle – defined posteriorly by latissimus dorsi, anteriorly by the lateral border of pectoralis major and inferiorly by a line perpendicular to the nipple going to the back, just anterior to the mid-axillary line – or, in extremis, a finger thoracostomy at the same location.

Pericardial tamponade

Pericardial tamponade needs to be differentiated from a tension pneumothorax in the shocked patient with distended neck veins. It is most commonly the result of penetrating trauma. Accumulation of a relatively small amount of blood (50 mL) into the non-distensible pericardial sac can produce compression of the heart and obstruction of the venous return, leading to decreased filling of the cardiac chambers during diastole. All patients with penetrating injury anywhere near the heart plus shock must be considered to have a cardiac injury until proven otherwise. Classically, the presentation consists of central venous pressure elevation, a decline in arterial pressure with tachycardia and muffled heart sounds. However, in cases in which major bleeding from other sites has taken place, the neck veins may be flat. A high index of suspicion and further diagnostic investigations will be needed to make the diagnosis is those cases that are not clinically obvious. These include an eFAST showing fluid in the pericardial sac, which is the most expeditious and reliable diagnostic tool, or chest radiography, looking for an enlarged heart shadow.

In penetrating injury to the heart there is usually a substantial clot in the pericardium, which may prevent aspiration. **Pericardiocentesis has no role in the management of cardiac tamponade secondary to penetrating myocardial injury**. The correct immediate treatment of tamponade is operative, either via a subxiphoid window or by open surgery (sternotomy or left anterolateral thoracotomy), with repair of the heart in the operating theatre if time allows or otherwise in the emergency department.

Summary box 29.4

Pericardial tamponade

- The presentation is similar to a tension pneumothorax – deteriorating cyanosis, tachycardia and agitation
- eFAST is diagnostic and may also detect free fluid in the abdomen or pericardium
- There is no role for pericardiocentesis in traumatic cardiac tamponade. A left anterolateral thoracotomy or sternotomy should be performed with evacuation of the haematoma and repair of the myocardium

Open pneumothorax ('sucking chest wound')

This is due to a large open defect in the chest (>3 cm), leading to immediate equilibration between intrathoracic and atmospheric pressure. If the opening in the chest wall exceeds about two-thirds of the diameter of the trachea, then with each inspiratory cycle air will be preferentially drawn through the defect rather than through the trachea. Air accumulates in the hemithorax (rather than in the lung) with each inspiration, leading to profound hypoventilation on the affected side and hypoxia. If there is a valvular effect, increasing amounts of air in the pleura will result in a tension pneumothorax (see *Tension pneumothorax*).

Initial management consists of promptly closing the defect with a sterile occlusive plastic dressing (e.g. OPSITE◊ or similar product), taped on three sides to act as a flutter-type valve. A chest tube is inserted as soon as possible in a site remote from the injury site.

Massive haemothorax

The most common cause of massive haemothorax in blunt injury is continuing bleeding from torn intercostal vessels or occasionally from the internal mammary artery secondary to fractures of the ribs. In penetrating injury, a variety of viscera, both thoracic and abdominal (with blood leaking through a hole in the diaphragm from the positive pressure abdomen into the negative pressure thorax), may be involved.

Accumulation of blood in a haemothorax can significantly compromise respiratory efforts, compressing the lung and preventing adequate ventilation. Presentation is with haemorrhagic shock, flat neck veins, unilateral absence of breath sounds and dullness to percussion. The initial treatment consists of correcting the hypovolaemic shock, insertion of an intercostal drain and, in some cases, intubation. Initial drainage of more than 1500 mL of blood or ongoing haemorrhage of more than 200 mL/h over 3–4 hours is generally considered an indication for urgent thoracotomy.

Blood in the pleural space should be removed as completely and rapidly as possible to prevent ongoing bleeding, an empyema or fibrothorax later. **There is no role for clamping a chest tube to tamponade a massive haemothorax**.

The following points are important in the management of an open pneumothorax/haemothorax:

- if the lung does not reinflate, the drain should be placed on low-pressure (5 cmH_2O) suction;
- clot occlusion of a chest drainage tube may result in 'no' drainage, even in the presence of ongoing bleeding;
- a second drain is sometimes necessary (but see *Tracheobronchial injuries*);
- a chest radiograph or eFAST can help identify the presence of blood;
- physiotherapy and active mobilisation should begin as soon as possible.

Flail chest

This condition usually results from blunt trauma associated with multiple rib fractures, and is defined as three or more ribs fractured in two or more places. The blunt force typically also produces an underlying pulmonary contusion. The diagnosis is made clinically in patients who are not ventilated, not by radiography. To confirm the diagnosis the chest wall can be observed for paradoxical motion of a chest wall segment. On inspiration, the loose segment of the chest wall is displaced inwards and therefore less air moves into the lungs. On expiration, the segment moves outwards (paradoxical respiration). Voluntary splinting of the chest wall occurs as a result of pain, so mechanically impaired chest wall movement and the associated lung contusion all contribute to the hypoxia. There is a high risk of developing a pneumothorax or haemothorax. The CT scan remains the gold standard for diagnosis of this condition.

Traditionally, mechanical ventilation was used to 'internally splint' the chest but had a price in terms of intensive care unit (ICU) resources and ventilation-dependent morbidity. Currently, treatment consists of oxygen administration, adequate analgesia (including opiates) and physiotherapy. If a chest tube is in place, topical intrapleural local analgesia introduced via the tube can also be used. Ventilation is reserved for patients developing respiratory failure despite adequate analgesia and oxygen. Surgery to stabilise the flail segment using internal fixation of the ribs may be useful in a selected group of patients with isolated or severe chest injury and pulmonary contusion.

◊ Trademark of Smith+Nephew.

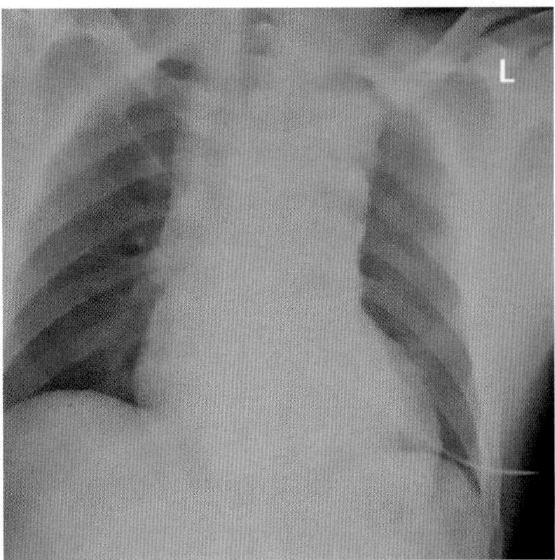

Figure 29.4 Chest radiograph showing a widened mediastinum (courtesy of Dr Elizabeth Dick, Consultant Radiologist, Imperial College Healthcare NHS Trust, London, UK).

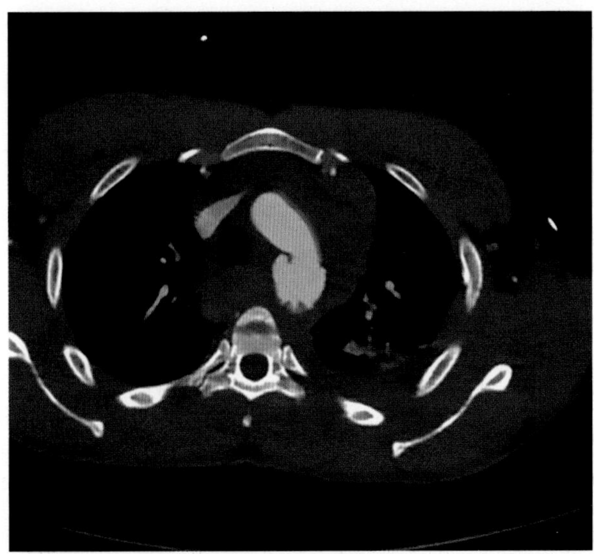

Figure 29.5 Computed tomography scan showing aortic disruption (courtesy of Dr Elizabeth Dick, Consultant Radiologist, Imperial College Healthcare NHS Trust, London, UK).

Potentially life-threatening injuries

Thoracic aortic disruption

Traumatic aortic rupture is a common cause of sudden death after a vehicle collision or fall from a great height. The vessel is relatively fixed distal to the ligamentum arteriosum, just distal to the origin of the left subclavian artery. The shear forces from a sudden impact disrupt the intima and media. If the adventitia is intact, the patient may remain physiologically non-compromised.

Thoracic aortic injury should be clinically suspected in patients with gross asymmetry in systolic blood pressure (between the two upper limbs, or between upper and lower limbs), widened pulse pressure and chest wall contusion. Erect chest radiography can also suggest thoracic aortic disruption, the most common radiological finding being a widened mediastinum (*Figure 29.4*). The diagnosis is confirmed by a CT scan of the mediastinum (*Figure 29.5*). In the hypotensive patient, widening of the mediastinum and aortic injury is not the cause of the hypotension. Invariably, these patients have other injuries causing hypotension as patients with complete aortic disruption rarely, if ever, survive to reach hospital.

In the presence of thoracic aortic injury, initial management consists of control of the systolic arterial blood pressure (to less than 120 mmHg). Thereafter, an endovascular intra-aortic stent (*Figure 29.6*) can be placed, or the tear can be operatively repaired by direct repair or by excision and grafting using a Dacron graft.

Tracheobronchial injuries

Severe subcutaneous emphysema with respiratory compromise can suggest tracheobronchial disruption. A chest drain placed on the affected side will reveal a large air leak and the collapsed lung may fail to re-expand. Bronchoscopy is diagnostic. Treatment involves intubation of the unaffected bronchus followed by operative repair. Referral to a trauma centre is advised.

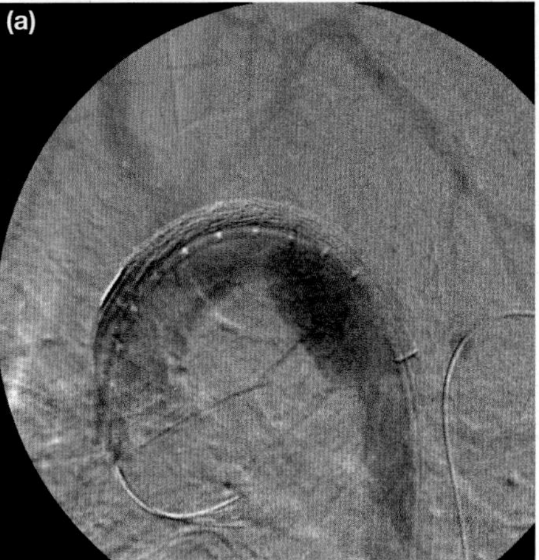

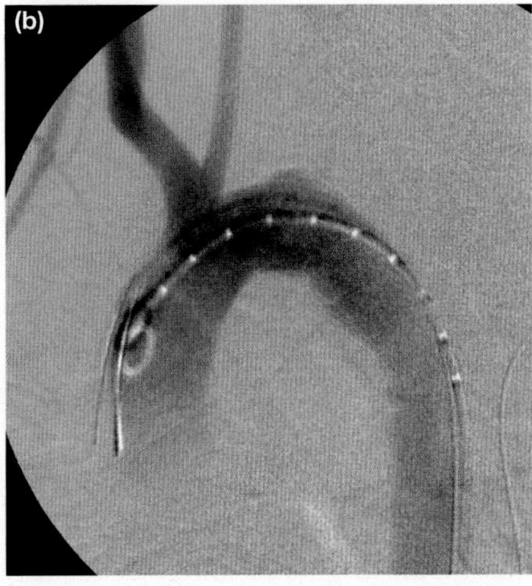

Figure 29.6 (a) Aortic tear showing the presence of a preinflation stent and test run. (b) Aortic tear post inflation of the stent and test run (courtesy of Dr Elizabeth Dick, Consultant Radiologist, Imperial College Healthcare NHS Trust, London, UK).

Blunt myocardial injury

Significant blunt cardiac injury that causes haemodynamic and physiological instability is rare. Blunt myocardial injury should be suspected in any patient sustaining blunt trauma who develops early electrocardiogram abnormalities.

Transthoracic echocardiography may show wall motion abnormalities. A transoesophageal echocardiogram may also be helpful. There is very little evidence that enzyme estimations have any place in diagnosis.

All patients with myocardial contusion diagnosed with conduction abnormalities are at risk of developing sudden dysrhythmias and should be closely monitored.

Diaphragmatic injuries

Any penetrating injury below the fifth intercostal space should raise suspicion of diaphragmatic penetration and, therefore, injury to abdominal contents.

Blunt injury to the diaphragm is usually caused by a compressive force applied to the torso. The diaphragmatic rupture is usually large, with herniation of the abdominal contents into the chest. Diagnosis of diaphragmatic rupture can easily be missed in the acute phase, and may only be discovered at operation or through the presentation of complications.

Most diaphragmatic injuries are silent and the presenting features are those of injury to the surrounding organs. There is no single standard investigation. Historically and in limited resource environments, chest radiography after placement of a nasogastric tube may be helpful (as this may show the stomach herniated into the chest). CT scan and ultrasound scan all lack positive or negative predictive value. The most accurate evaluation is by video-assisted thoracoscopy or laparoscopy, the latter offering the advantage of allowing the surgeon to proceed to a repair and additional evaluation of the abdominal organs.

The thorax is at negative pressure and the abdomen is at positive pressure. A complication of a breach of the diaphragm is herniation of abdominal contents into the chest. This may present much later, and strangulation of any of the contents can then occur, with a high mortality rate. Operative repair is recommended in all cases. All penetrating diaphragmatic injury must be repaired via the abdomen – and not the chest – to rule out penetrating hollow viscus injury.

Oesophageal injury

Most oesophageal injuries result from penetrating trauma; blunt injury is rare but should be suspected in patients exposed to barotrauma. A high index of suspicion is required. The patient can present with odynophagia (pain on swallowing saliva, foods or fluids), subcutaneous or mediastinal emphysema, pleural effusion, air in the perioesophageal space and unexplained fever. Mediastinal and deep cervical emphysema are evidence of an aerodigestive injury until proven otherwise.

The mortality rate rises exponentially if treatment is delayed. A combination of CT with oral contrast and oesophagoscopy confirms the diagnosis in the great majority of cases. The treatment is operative repair of any defect and drainage.

Pulmonary contusion

Pulmonary contusion occurs more frequently following blunt trauma, and is usually associated with a flail segment or fractured ribs. This is a very common, potentially lethal injury and the major cause of hypoxaemia after blunt trauma. Following gunshot wounds, there is an area of contusion from the shock wave of the bullet.

The natural progression of pulmonary contusion is worsening hypoxaemia for the first 24–48 hours. Chest radiographic findings may be typically delayed. Contrast CT scanning can be confirmatory. Haemoptysis or blood in the endotracheal tube is a sign of pulmonary contusion. In mild contusion, the treatment is oxygen administration, pulmonary toilet and adequate analgesia. In more severe cases mechanical ventilation is necessary. Normovolaemia is critical for adequate tissue perfusion and fluid restriction is not advised.

EMERGENCY THORACIC SURGERY

Emergency thoracic surgery is an essential part of the armamentarium of any surgeon dealing with major trauma. A timely surgical intervention for the correct indications can be the key step in saving an injured patient's life.

It is important to make a distinction between:

- immediate thoracotomy in the emergency department for the control of haemorrhage, cardiac tamponade or internal cardiac massage;
- emergency sternotomy for anterior mediastinal structures and the heart;
- planned thoracotomy for definitive correction of the problem – this usually takes place in the more controlled environment of the operating theatre.

The clinical decision as to whether a patient requires surgery in the emergency department or they can be transferred to the operating theatre can be complex. It is far better to perform a thoracotomy in the operating theatre, either through an anterolateral approach or a median sternotomy, with good light and assistance and the potential for autotransfusion or bypass, than it is to attempt heroic emergency surgery in the resuscitation area. However, if the patient is *in extremis* with a falling systolic blood pressure, there is no choice but to proceed immediately with a left anterolateral thoracotomy. In certain circumstances, when care is futile, it may not need to be performed at all. A resuscitation room thoracotomy following blunt trauma has limited indications and is rarely successful.

Emergency department thoracotomy or sternotomy

Emergency department thoracotomy (EDT) should be reserved for those patients with penetrating injury in whom signs of life are still present. Patients who have received cardiopulmonary resuscitation (CPR) in the prehospital phase of their care are unlikely to survive, and electrical activity must be present.

In certain situations, EDT is considered futile:

- CPR for more than 15 minutes (despite endotracheal intubation) in the presence of penetrating thoracic trauma;
- CPR for more than 10 minutes (despite endotracheal intubation) in the presence of blunt thoracic trauma;
- blunt trauma when there have been no signs of life at the scene.

The survival rates for EDT in patients with penetrating trauma in whom the blood pressure is falling despite adequate resuscitation are shown in *Table 29.4*.

TABLE 29.4 Survival rates for thoracotomy in patients with penetrating trauma.

Blood pressure despite resuscitation	Survival
>60 mmHg	60%
>40 mmHg	30%
<40 mmHg	3%

The aim of EDT is to perform:

- internal cardiac massage in the cardiovascularly 'full' patient (no role for internal massage in the 'empty' patient);
- control of haemorrhage from injury to the heart or lung;
- control of intrathoracic haemorrhage from other sources;
- control of massive air leak;
- clamping of the thoracic aorta to preserve the blood supply to the heart and brain, and cutting off the arterial supply distally, in a moribund patient with a major distal penetrating injury.

Planned emergency thoracotomy

Planned emergency thoracotomy implies an emergency thoracotomy performed as a planned procedure in the operating theatre, directed at the management of a specific injury. As such, the approach chosen is dependent on the indication for surgery and the organ injured (*Table 29.5*). Some organs are best approached through a median sternotomy. Otherwise the thoracotomy may be right or left sided, and these may be joined, producing the so-called 'clamshell incision'. This gives excellent exposure for any surgeon who is not routinely entering the chest.

Posterolateral thoracotomy is not used in the emergency situation because of the difficulties in positioning of the patient, except for specific access to certain posterior mediastinal organs.

TABLE 29.5 Different approaches to the contents of the chest cavity.

Approach	Best for
Left anterolateral thoracotomy	• Left lung and lung hilum • Thoracic aorta • Origin of left subclavian artery • Left side of heart • Lower oesophagus
Right anterolateral thoracotomy	• Right lung and lung hilum • Azygos veins • Superior vena cava • Infracardiac inferior vena cava • Upper oesophagus • Thoracic trachea
Median sternotomy	• Anterior aspect of heart • Anterior mediastinum • Ascending aorta and arch of aorta • Pulmonary arteries • Carina of the trachea

ABDOMINAL INJURY

Patients who have suffered abdominal trauma can generally be classified into the following categories based on their physiological condition after initial resuscitation:

- physiologically 'normal' – investigation can be completed before treatment is planned;
- physiologically 'non-compromised' – investigation is more limited; it is aimed at establishing whether the patient can be managed non-operatively, whether angioembolisation can be used or whether surgery is required;
- physiologically 'compromised' – investigations need to be suspended as immediate surgical correction of the bleeding is required.

A trauma laparotomy is the final step in the pathway to delineate intra-abdominal injury. Occasionally it is difficult to determine the source of bleeding in the shocked, multiple injured patient. If doubt still exists, especially in the presence of other injuries, a laparotomy may still be the safest option. The key is to make a decision, as indecision leads to delay in definitive control.

The patient's physiology must be assessed constantly; if there is an indication that the patient is still actively bleeding, the source must be identified unless the patient is unstable and requires immediate surgery. Blood loss into the abdomen can be subtle and there may be no clear clinical signs. Blood is not an irritant and does not initially cause any abdominal pain. Distension is subjective, and a drop in the blood pressure may be a very late sign in a young fit patient. Examination in compromised patients should take place either in the emergency department or in the operating theatre if the patient is deteriorating rapidly.

Investigation

Investigations are driven by the cardiovascular status of the patient. In torso trauma, the best and most sensitive modality is a CT scan with intravenous contrast; however, in the unstable patient, this is generally not possible.

In patients with penetrating injury, metal markers (e.g. bent paper clips) should be placed on all external wounds before plain films are taken, irrespective of the area being radiographed, as this allows an assessment of the trajectory and helps to correlate the number of holes and the number of missiles that can be seen within the patient. This will help determine whether two holes are indicative of one missile passing through the patient, or two missiles, both retained internally (*Figure 29.7*). A single hole implies that the projectile has been retained.

Focused abdominal sonography for trauma and extended FAST (FAST and eFAST)

Focused abdominal sonography for trauma (FAST) is a technique whereby ultrasound (sonography) imaging is used to assess the torso for the presence of free fluid in the abdominal cavity, and is extended into the thoracic cavities and pericardium (eFAST). There should be no attempt to determine the nature or extent of the specific injury. eFAST is usually a

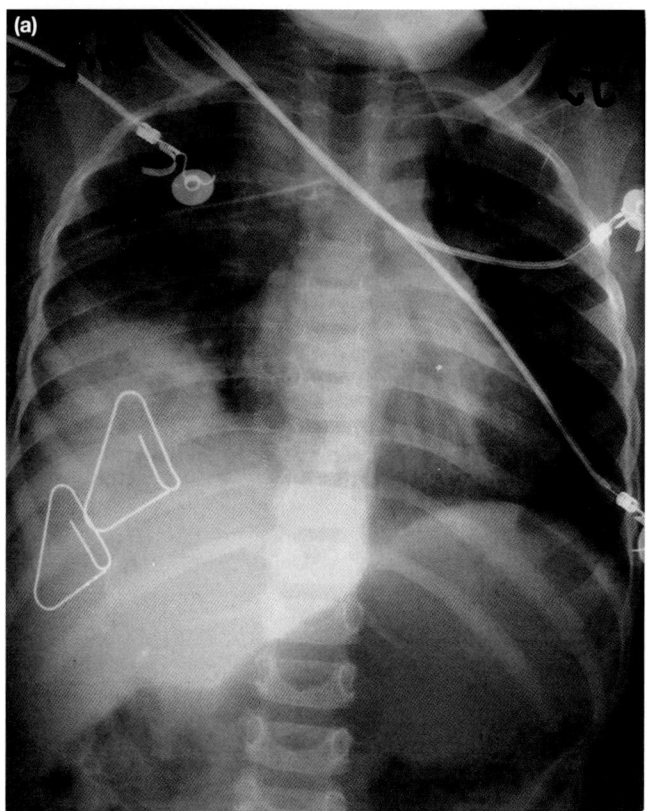

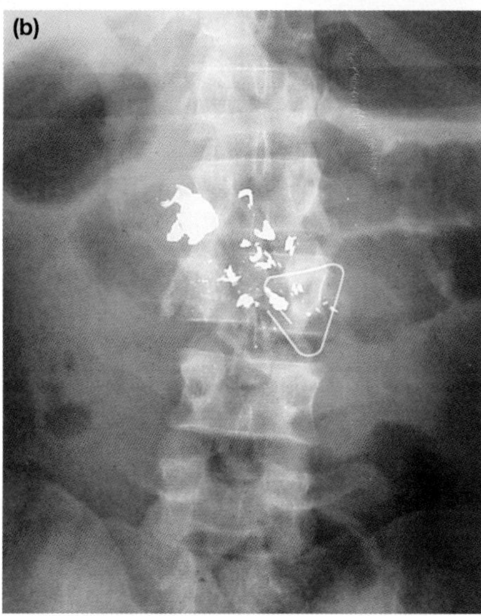

Figure 29.7 (a) Chest radiograph showing a gunshot wound with bullet markers. (b) Abdominal radiograph of a gunshot wound showing bullet markers.

rapid, reproducible, portable and non-invasive bedside test and can be performed at the same time as resuscitation. eFAST is accurate at detecting >100 mL of free blood; however, it is very operator dependent and, especially if the patient is very obese or the bowel is full of gas, it may be unreliable. Hollow viscus injury and solid organ injury are difficult to diagnose, even in experienced hands, as small amounts of gas or fluid are difficult to assess and eFAST has a low sensitivity (29–35%) for organ injury without haemoperitoneum. eFAST is also unreliable for excluding injury in penetrating trauma. If there is doubt, the eFAST examination can be repeated.

Summary box 29.5

Utilisation of eFAST

- Detects free fluid in the abdomen or pericardium
- Will not reliably detect less than 100 mL of free blood
- Does not directly identify injury to hollow viscus
- Cannot reliably exclude injury in penetrating trauma
- May need repeating or supplementing with other investigations
- Is unreliable for assessment of the retroperitoneum

Diagnostic peritoneal lavage

Diagnostic peritoneal lavage (DPL) is a test rarely used in modern-day practice but can be of value in resource-limited settings. It is a test used to assess the presence of blood or contaminants in the abdomen. A nasogastric tube is placed to empty the stomach and a urinary catheter is inserted to drain the bladder.

A cannula is inserted below the umbilicus, directed caudally and posteriorly. The cannula is aspirated for blood (>10 mL is deemed as positive) and, following this, 500 mL of warmed Ringer's lactate solution is allowed to run into the abdomen from a 1-litre bag. The bag, with 500 mL remaining, is placed on the floor and the intra-abdominal fluid is allowed to flow under the influence of gravity – this aids drainage. The presence of frank blood or similar contents to a nasogastric tube or urinary catheter denotes a positive DPL. If time allows and laboratory diagnosis is available, the presence of >100 000 red cells/μL or >500 white cells/μL is deemed positive (this is equivalent to 20 mL of free blood in the abdominal cavity), as is a raised amylase level. In the absence of laboratory facilities, a urine dipstick may be useful. Drainage of lavage fluid via a chest drain indicates penetration of the diaphragm.

Although DPL has largely been replaced by eFAST (see *Focused abdominal sonography for trauma and extended FAST (FAST and eFAST)*), it remains the standard in many institutions where eFAST is not available or is unreliable.

Computed tomography scan

CT has become the 'gold standard' for the intra-abdominal diagnosis of injury in the stable patient. The scan can be performed using intravenous contrast. CT is sensitive for blood and individual organ injury as well as for retroperitoneal injury. An entirely normal abdominal CT is usually sufficient to exclude intraperitoneal injury.

The following points are important when performing CT:

- it remains an inappropriate investigation for physiologically compromised patients;

Sydney Ringer, 1835–1910, Professor of Clinical Medicine, University College Hospital, London, UK.

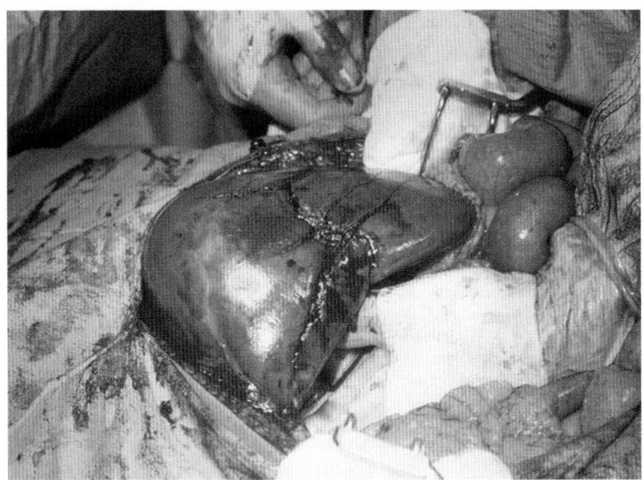

Figure 29.8 Compression injury to the liver, bursting the liver substance.

- if duodenal injury is suspected from the mechanism of injury, oral contrast may be helpful;
- if rectal and distal colonic injury is suspected in the absence of blood on rectal examination, air around the colon may indicate injury; in all cases clinical suspicion supersedes investigation results.

Laparoscopy

Laparoscopy or thoracoscopy may be a valuable screening investigation in physiologically non-compromised patients with penetrating trauma to detect or exclude peritoneal penetration and/or diaphragmatic injury.

Laparoscopy may be divided into:

- screening: used to exclude a penetrating injury with breach of the peritoneum;
- diagnostic: finding evidence of injury to viscera;
- therapeutic: used to repair the injury.

In most institutions, evidence of penetration requires a laparotomy to evaluate organ injury as it is difficult to exclude all intra-abdominal injuries laparoscopically. When used in this role laparoscopy reduces the non-therapeutic laparotomy rate. There is no place for laparoscopy in the unstable patient.

INDIVIDUAL ORGAN INJURY

Liver

Blunt liver trauma occurs as a result of direct injury. The liver is a solid organ and compressive forces can easily burst the liver substance (*Figure 29.8*). The liver is usually compressed between the impacting object and the ribcage or vertebral column. Most injuries are relatively minor and can be managed non-operatively.

Penetrating trauma to the liver is relatively common. Bullets have a shock wave and when they pass through a solid structure such as the liver they cause significant damage some distance from the actual track of the bullet. Not all penetrating wounds require operative management and may stop bleeding spontaneously.

In the physiologically non-compromised patient, CT is the investigation of choice. It provides information on the liver injury itself, as well as on injuries to the adjoining major vascular and biliary structures. Injury in which there is a suggestion of a vascular component should be reimaged, as there is a significant risk of the development of subsequent ischaemia, false aneurysms, arteriovenous fistulae or haemobiliary fistula. It is advised that all patients should be rescanned prior to discharge.

Liver injury can be graded and managed using the American Association for the Surgery of Trauma (AAST) Injury Scoring Scale (ISS) (https://www.aast.org/resources-detail/injury-scoring-scale).

Management

The operative management of liver injuries can be summarised as 'the four Ps':

- Pressure;
- Pringle;
- Plug;
- Pack.

At laparotomy the liver is reconstituted and bleeding is controlled by direct bimanual compression to achieve its normal architecture as best as possible (Pressure). The inflow from the portal triad is controlled by a Pringle's manoeuvre, with direct compression of the portal triad, either digitally or using a soft clamp (*Figure 29.9*). This has the effect of reducing arterial and portal venous inflow into the liver, although it does not control the backflow from the inferior vena cava and hepatic veins. Any holes due to penetrating injury can be plugged directly using silicone tubing or a Sengstaken–Blakemore tube; after controlling any arterial bleeding, the liver can then be packed (see ***Damage control surgery***).

Bleeding points should be controlled locally when possible, and such patients, if required, subsequently undergo angioembolisation. It is not usually necessary to suture penetrating injuries of the liver unless haemostasis cannot be controlled by other means. If there has been direct damage to the hepatic artery, it can be tied off. Damage to the portal vein must be repaired, as tying off the portal vein carries a greater than 50% mortality rate. If it is not technically feasible to repair the vein at the time of surgery, it should be shunted and the patient referred to a specialist centre. A drainage system must be left *in situ* following hepatic surgery. Finally, the liver can be definitively packed, restoring the anatomy as closely as possible. Placing omentum into cracks in the liver is not recommended.

James Hogarth Pringle, 1863–1941, Australian-born surgeon, The Royal Infirmary, Glasgow, UK.

Robert William Sengstaken, 1923–1978, surgeon, Garden City, NY, USA, and **Arthur Hendley Blakemore**, 1897–1970, Associate Professor of Surgery, The College of Physicians and Surgeons, Columbia University, New York, NY, USA, designed a tube with two in-built balloons for the treatment of oesophageal varices. The tube was passed and the distal balloon inflated. The tube was drawn backwards until the distal balloon was held at the oesophageal hiatus. The proximal balloon was inflated, allowing tamponade of any varices in the distal oesophagus.

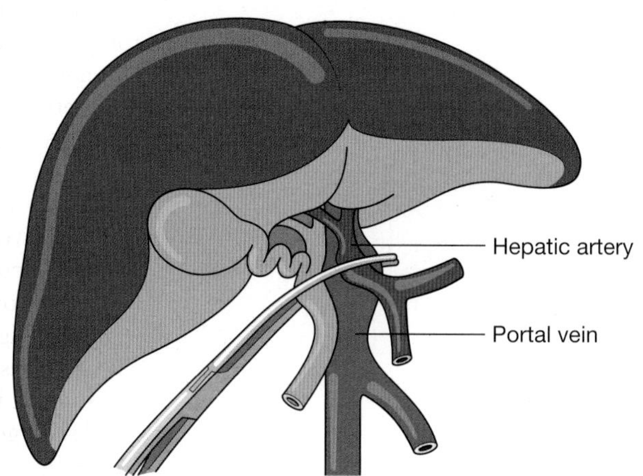

Figure 29.9 The Pringle manoeuvre.

Summary box 29.6

Liver trauma

- Blunt trauma occurs as the result of direct compression
- Penetrating trauma of the upper abdomen or lower thorax can damage the liver
- CT scanning is the investigation of choice in a stable patient
- Surgical management consists of: Pressure, Pringle, Plug and Pack
- The hepatic artery can be tied off but not the portal vein (which should be stented)
- Closed drainage should always be used

Biliary injuries

Isolated traumatic biliary injuries are rare and occur mainly from penetrating trauma, often in association with injuries to other structures that lie in close proximity. The common bile duct can be repaired over a T-tube or drained and referred to appropriate care as part of damage control, or even ligated.

Spleen

Splenic injury occurs from direct blunt trauma. Most isolated splenic injuries, especially in children, can be managed non-operatively. However, in adults, especially in the presence of other injury or physiological compromise, laparotomy should be considered. The spleen can be theoretically packed, repaired or placed in a mesh bag. However, in reality, splenectomy is the safer option, especially in the compromised patient with multiple potential sites of bleeding. In certain situations, selective angioembolisation of the spleen can play a role.

Following splenectomy there are significant, though transient, changes to blood physiology. The platelet and white count rise and may mimic sepsis. Inoculation against *Pneumococcus* is advisable within 2–3 weeks, by which time the patient's immune system has recovered.

Pancreas

Most pancreatic injury occurs as a result of blunt trauma. The major problem is that of diagnosis because the pancreas is a retroperitoneal organ. CT remains the mainstay of accurate diagnosis. Amylase or lipase estimation is insensitive. In penetrating trauma, injury may only be detected during laparotomy.

Classically the pancreas should be treated with conservative surgery and closed, low-suction drainage. Injuries are treated according to the ISS system of the AAST. Injuries to the pancreatic body to the left of the superior mesenteric vessels and to the tail are treated by closed drainage alone, with distal pancreatectomy if the duct is involved. Proximal injuries (to the right of the superior mesenteric artery) are treated as conservatively as possible, although partial pancreatectomy may be necessary. The role of pyloric exclusion remains controversial and remains surgeon dependent. A Whipple's procedure (pancreaticoduodenectomy) is rarely needed and should not be performed in the emergency situation because of the very high associated mortality rate. A damage control procedure with packing and drainage should be performed and the patient referred for definitive surgery once stabilised.

Stomach

Most stomach injuries are caused by penetrating trauma. Blood presence is diagnostic if found in the nasogastric tube, in the absence of bleeding from other sources. Surgical repair is required but great care must be taken to examine the stomach fully, as an injury to the front of the stomach can be expected to have an 'exit' wound elsewhere on the organ.

Duodenum

Duodenal injury is frequently associated with injuries to the adjoining pancreas. Like the pancreas, the duodenum lies retroperitoneally and so injuries are hidden, discovered late or at laparotomy performed for other reasons. CT is the diagnostic modality of choice. The only sign may be gas or a fluid collection in the periduodenal tissue, and leakage of oral contrast, administration of which may improve accuracy of diagnosis.

Smaller injuries can be repaired primarily. The first, third and fourth parts of the duodenum behave like small bowel and can be repaired in the same fashion. The second part of the duodenum is fixed to the head of the pancreas with a common blood supply and may have a poorer blood supply than the remainder. Major trauma, especially if the head of the pancreas is simultaneously injured, should be treated as part of a damage control procedure and be referred for definitive care.

Small bowel

The small bowel is frequently injured as a result of blunt trauma. The individual loops may be trapped, causing high-pressure rupture of a loop or tearing of the mesentery. Penetrating trauma is also a common cause of injury.

Allen Oldfather Whipple, 1881–1963, Valentine Mott Professor of Surgery, The College of Physicians and Surgeons, Columbia University, New York, NY, USA.

Small bowel injuries need urgent repair. Haemorrhage control takes priority and these wounds can be temporarily controlled with simple sutures. In blunt trauma with mesenteric vessel damage, the bowel ischaemia that results will dictate the extent of a resection. Resections should be carefully planned to limit the loss of viable small bowel, but should be weighed against an excessive number of repairs or anastomoses. Haematomas in the small bowel mesenteric border need to be explored to rule out perforation. With low-energy wounds, primary repair can be performed, whereas more destructive wounds associated with military-type weapons require resection and anastomosis. Damage control 'clip and drop' of damaged or resected bowel may be necessary.

Colon

Blunt injuries to the colon are relatively infrequent; penetrating injuries occur more often. If relatively little contamination is present and the viability is satisfactory, such wounds can be repaired primarily. If, however, there is extensive contamination, the patient is physiologically compromised or the bowel is of doubtful viability, then the bowel can be closed off ('clip and drop'). A defunctioning colostomy can be formed later or the bowel reanastomosed once the patient is stable.

Rectum

Approximately 5% of colon injuries involve the rectum. These are generally from a penetrating injury, although occasionally the rectum may be damaged following fracture of the pelvis. Digital rectal examination will reveal the presence of blood, which is evidence of intestinal or rectal injury. These injuries are often associated with bladder and proximal urethral injury.

With intraperitoneal injuries, the rectum is managed as for colonic injuries. Full-thickness extraperitoneal rectal injuries can be managed with primary repair and drainage depending on the type of injury, i.e. suitable for knife wounds but not ballistic trauma. Where there is extensive tissue loss, this should be managed with either a diverting end-colostomy and closure of the distal end (Hartmann's procedure) or a loop colostomy. Presacral drainage is no longer used.

Renal and urological tract injury

In physiologically non-compromised patients, CT scanning with contrast is the investigation of choice. For assessment of bladder injury a cystogram should be performed at the time of CT. A minimum of 300 mL of contrast is instilled into the bladder via a urethral catheter. The large volume is essential because a small volume may not distend the bladder enough to produce a leak from a small bladder injury, once the cystic muscle is contracted.

Generally, renal injury is managed non-operatively unless the patient is physiologically compromised. The kidney can be angioembolised if required.

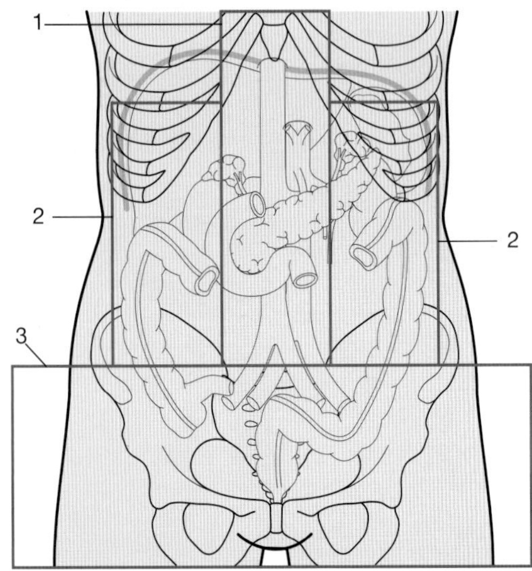

Figure 29.10 The zones of the retroperitoneum. Zone 1, central; zone 2, lateral; zone 3, pelvic.

Ureteric injury is rare and is generally due to penetrating trauma. Most ureters can be repaired or diverted if necessary, or may even be ligated as part of damage control procedures.

Intraperitoneal rupture of the bladder, usually from direct blunt injury, will require surgical repair. Extraperitoneal rupture is usually associated with a fracture of the pelvis and will heal with adequate urine drainage via the transurethral route. Suprapubic drainage is reserved for when this is not possible.

Summary box 29.7

Injuries to structures in the abdomen

- In children, splenic injury can be managed non-operatively in most cases, but not if physiologically compromised
- Duodenal injuries are often associated with pancreatic trauma
- Bowel injuries need urgent definitive repair, or isolation using resection or by stapling
- Rectal injuries are managed depending on whether intra- or extraperitoneal
- Kidney and urinary tract injuries are best diagnosed with contrast CT scanning
- Intraperitoneal bladder tears need formal repair and drainage

Retroperitoneum

Injury to the retroperitoneum is often difficult to diagnose, especially in the presence of other injury, when the signs may be masked. Diagnostic tests (such as ultrasound and DPL) may be negative. The best diagnostic modality is CT, but this requires a physiologically stable patient. The retroperitoneum is divided into three zones (*Figure 29.10*) for the purposes of intraoperative management in blunt trauma:

Henri Albert Charles Antoine Hartmann, 1860–1952, Professor of Clinical Surgery, Faculty of Medicine, University of Paris, Paris, France.

- Zone 1 (central): central haematomas should always be explored, once proximal and distal vascular control has been obtained.
- Zone 2 (lateral): lateral haematomas should only be explored if they are expanding or pulsatile or penetrating injury is present. They are usually renal in origin and can be managed non-operatively, although they may sometimes require angioembolisation.
- Zone 3 (pelvic): as with zone 2, these should only be explored if they are expanding or pulsatile or penetrating injury is present. Pelvic haematomas are exceptionally difficult to control and, whenever possible, should not be opened; they are best controlled with compression or-extraperitoneal packing, or, if the bleeding is arterial in origin, with angioembolisation.

THE PELVIS

Although mortality following severe pelvic fractures has decreased dramatically with better methods of controlling haemorrhage, these patients still represent a significant challenge to every link of the treatment chain. Mortality rates exceeding 40% have recently been reported. Further, pelvic bleeding as one of the 'hidden bleeding sources' is still underestimated or missed, as retrospective chart analyses of potentially preventable deaths have revealed. Extreme force is required to disrupt the pelvic ring, and associated injuries and extrapelvic bleeding sources are common (up to 50% of cases). The haemodynamically unstable patient with severe pelvic fracture has a 90% risk of associated injuries and a 30% risk of intra-abdominal bleeding.

To save these patients, three questions need to be addressed:

- Is the patient at high risk of massive bleeding?
- Where is the source of the bleeding?
- How to stop the bleeding?

Anatomy

The surgical anatomy of the pelvis is key to the understanding of pelvic injuries.

- The pelvic inlet is circular. It is a structure that is immensely strong, but routinely gives way at more than one point should sufficient force be applied to it. Therefore, isolated fractures of the anterior or posterior pelvic ring are uncommon.
- The forces required to fracture the pelvic ring do not respect the surrounding organ systems.
- The pelvis has a rich collateral blood supply, especially across the sacrum and posterior part of the ileum. The cancellous bone of the pelvis also has an excellent blood supply. Most pelvic haemorrhage emanates from venous injury and fracture sites. However, in the haemodynamically unstable patient with severe pelvic injury, arterial bleeding is more frequent. Important for the treatment is that the surgeon has to deal with both arterial and venous bleeding.

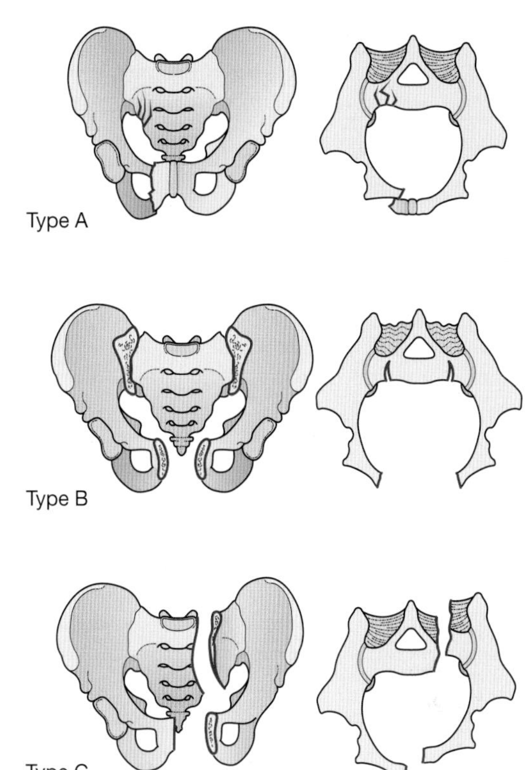

Figure 29.11 Tile classification of fractures of the pelvis.

- Postmortem examination has shown that the extrapelvic peritoneal space can accommodate more than 3000 mL. However, in the case of a severe pelvic fracture where the retroperitoneal compartment is disrupted and the external bony barrier is not stable, haematoma may extend upwards towards the mediastinum ('chimney effect') or downwards into the medial thigh in case of rupture of the pelvic floor.
- All iliac vessels, the sciatic nerve roots (including the lumbosacral nerve) and the ureters cross the sacroiliac joint; disruption of this joint may cause severe haemorrhage and sometimes cause arterial obstruction of the internal iliac artery and sciatic nerve palsy. Injuries to the ureters are rare.
- The pelvic viscera are suspended from the bony pelvis by condensations of the endopelvic fascia. Shear forces acting on the pelvis will transmit these to pelvic viscera, leading to avulsion and shearing injuries.
- The pelvis also includes the acetabulum, a major structure in weight transfer to the leg. Inappropriate treatment will lead to severe disability.

Classification

Pelvic ring fractures can be classified into three types, using the Tile classification (for subtypes and other classifications see ***Further reading***), based on the severity of the fracture (and reflecting the energy required to cause it) (***Figure 29.11***). However, no fracture pattern can exclude significant haemorrhage.

Marvin Tile, b. 1933, orthopaedic surgeon, Sunnybrook Medical Centre, Toronto, Canada.

Type A

Type A are the most common fractures and are completely stable. They result from lateral compression, which causes compression fractures of the pubic rami or compression fracture of the sacrum posteriorly.

Type B

These fractures are partially stable, and there is disruption of the anterior pelvis and partial disruption of the posterior pelvis. The pelvis can open and close 'like a book', but because the sacroiliac ligaments remain intact there is no vertical displacement. Internal or external stabilisation is required. Blood loss can be significant.

Type C

This fracture is completely unstable. Both the anterior pelvis and the entire posterior pelvic complexes are disrupted and the disrupted pelvic bones are free to displace horizontally and vertically. In both type B and type C pelvic injuries, there is a high risk of associated abdominal injuries (bowel perforation or mesenteric laceration) and rupture of the diaphragm.

Clinical examination

Pelvic fractures should be easily identified if ATLS guidelines are followed. There is no role of 'springing' the pelvis. If a binder has not been applied and an 'open book' fracture is suspected, a binder must be immediately applied as the presence of major pelvic fracture is associated with life-threatening blood loss and requires appropriate measures.

Inspection of the skin may reveal lacerations in the groin, perineum or sacral area, indicating an open pelvic fracture, the result of gross deformation. Evidence of perineal injury or haematuria mandates radiological evaluation of the urinary tract from below upwards (retrograde urethrogram followed by cystogram or CT cystogram and an excretory urogram, as appropriate) when the physiology allows. Inspection of the urethral meatus may reveal a drop of blood, indicating urethral damage.

Inspection of the anus may reveal lacerations to the sphincter mechanism. Rectal examination may reveal blood in the rectum and/or discontinuity of the rectal wall, indicating a rectal laceration. In male patients, the prostate is palpated; a high-riding prostate indicates a complete urethral avulsion. A full neurological examination is performed of the perineal area, sphincter mechanism and femoral and sciatic nerves.

Diagnosis

Radiograph

Examination of a plain radiograph of the pelvis requires an understanding of the mechanism of injury and a decision on the stability of the pelvic rim. It is important to note that the vast majority of patients with suspected pelvic fractures may have a pelvic binder in place and hence plain radiograph findings may be normal. FAST may be unreliable as it does not localise intra-abdominal bleeding in these patients. CT is the diagnostic modality of choice in the physiologically non-compromised patient, and CT angiography is particularly helpful in providing details of both the anatomy of the fracture and the origin of the bleeding (venous or arterial).

An open book-type mechanism causes one or both ilia to rotate externally (opening, like a book). A lateral compression mechanism causes the pelvis to collapse. An 'open book fracture' is seen as a widening of the pubic symphysis or widening at the site of a fracture in the pubic ramus. Not only is there disruption of the bony pelvis, but also tearing of the pelvic floor and thus the pelvic venous plexus is at risk. The more unstable the pelvis, the more likely the structures are to be damaged. When the pelvis collapses from a lateral compression injury, the pubic bones usually fracture. Displacement of the anterior pelvis by greater than 2 cm indicates at least partial instability. A vertical shear disruption of the sacroiliac joint with apparent shortening of the limb on the affected side implies significant energy of injury.

Management

The treatment for bleeding is to stop the bleeding!

The priorities for resuscitating patients with pelvic fractures are no different from the standard. These injuries can produce a real threat to the circulation, and management is geared towards controlling this threat. Initial management requires the use of a compression binder or a sheet, applied around the true pelvis at the level of the greater trochanters ('reduce the pelvic volume'), a potentially life-saving procedure that has to be done in the emergency department.

Eighty-five per cent of bleeding originating from the pelvis is of venous origin and can be controlled by non-operative means, including compression either by binding or external fixator or by extraperitoneal pelvic packing (i.e. packing the loose space between the bony wall of the pelvis and the peritoneum) to compress the pelvic veins. If other sources of bleeding have been ruled out, the extraperitoneal pelvic packing is done without entering the peritoneal cavity. This may be combined with external fixation.

If the bleeding is of arterial origin, interventional angioembolisation is the next choice for bleeding control. The techniques for bleeding control (compression, packing, fixation and angioembolisation) do not exclude each other but rather may complement each other. Persistent bleeding after packing may require angioembolisation and vice versa.

Severe pelvic injuries require a multidisciplinary team approach. If adequate orthopaedic experience is unavailable, consideration should be given towards early transfer of this patient to an institution with the necessary expertise.

If the source of the bleeding is in doubt or FAST/CT results are positive, showing a significant amount of blood in the peritoneal cavity, concurrent intra-abdominal injury cannot be excluded and it is wise to perform an exploratory laparotomy to treat or rule out intra-abdominal bleeding.

Summary

In summary, a haemodynamically normal patient can be safely transferred for stabilisation of unstable fractures within hours after injury and following control of the associated damage.

Summary box 29.8

Pelvic injury

- Associated injuries can only be managed once the patient is physiologically non-compromised
- Decision on the stability is of paramount importance
- Procedures for damage control may be the only available option
- External stabilisation of the pelvic ring is the basis of all treatment
- If necessary, further bleeding control can be achieved either by angioembolisation or by extraperitoneal packing

DAMAGE CONTROL

Following major injury, protracted surgery in the physiologically unstable patient can in itself prove fatal. Patients with the 'deadly triad' (hypothermia, acidosis and coagulopathy) are those at highest risk. Damage control or damage limitation surgery is a concept that originated from a naval shipbuilding strategy, whereby ships were designed so that the damage was kept 'local' and only minimal repairs were needed to prevent the ship from sinking while definitive repairs waited until it had reached port. The technique has been adopted following major trauma and includes initial care and resuscitation (damage control resuscitation) and the surgical correction of the injury (damage control surgery).

The minimum amount of surgery needed to stabilise the patient's condition may be the safest course until the physiological derangement can be corrected. Damage control surgery is restricted to only three goals:

- stopping any active surgical bleeding;
- controlling any contamination;
- restoring normal physiology.

Once the first two have been achieved then the operation is suspended and the abdomen temporarily closed to allow for restoration of physiology to occur. The patient's resuscitation then continues in the ICU, where other therapeutic interventions can take place. Once the physiology has been corrected, the patient warmed and the coagulopathy corrected, the patient is returned to the operating theatre for any definitive surgery.

Damage control resuscitation

The concept of damage control has been broadened to include the techniques used in resuscitation as well as in surgery. The time in the emergency department is minimised and the majority of resuscitation of the patient is carried out in the operating theatre and not in the resuscitation bay (*Table 29.6*). Resuscitation is individualised through repeated point-of-care testing of haemoglobin, acidosis (pH and lactate) and clotting, and is therefore directed towards the early delivery of biologically active colloids, clotting products and whole blood in order to buy time. The physiological disturbances that are associated with the downward spiral of acidosis, coagulopathy and hypothermia in these serious injuries are predicted and attempts are made to avoid them rather than react to them.

Damage control surgery

This is a key component of damage control resuscitation. The decision of whether damage control surgery is the appropriate course should be made early (*Table 29.7*) and allows the whole surgical and anaesthetic team to work together to limit the time in surgery and achieve the earliest possible admission of the patient to the ICU. Damage control is a staged process.

The initial focus is haemorrhage control, followed by control and limitation of contamination, which are achieved using a range of abbreviated techniques including simple ligation of bleeding vessels, shunting of major arteries and veins, drainage, temporary stapling of bowel and therapeutic packing.

Following the above, the abdomen is closed in a temporary fashion either by using commercially available products or by using a sheet of plastic (e.g. OPSITE◊ or similar product) over the bowel, an intermediate pack to allow suction and a further sheet of adherent plastic drape to the skin to form a watertight and airtight seal. Suction is applied to the intermediate pack area to collect abdominal fluid. This technique is known as the 'Vac-Pac' or 'OPSITE◊ sandwich' (*Figure 29.12*). As soon as control has been achieved the patient is transferred to the ICU, where resuscitation is continued.

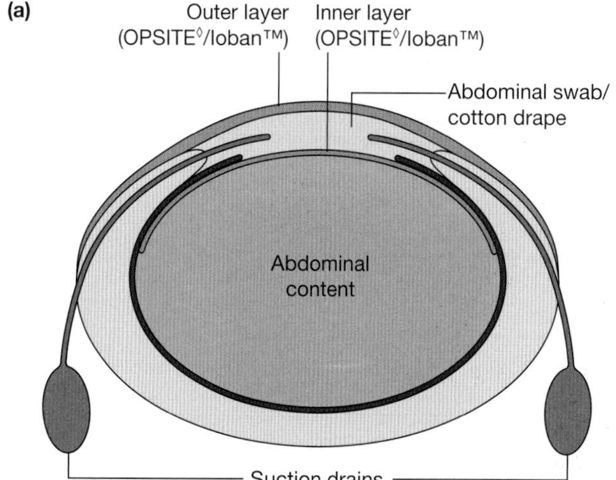

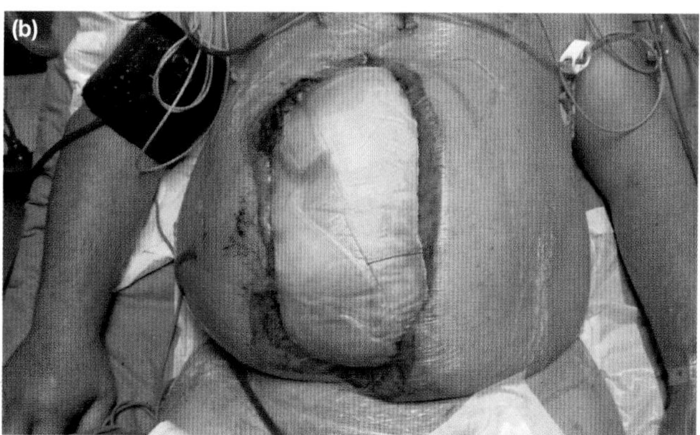

Figure 29.12 (a) Diagram showing temporary skin closure in damage control. (b) Abdominal closure following damage control surgery showing an OPSITE◊ closure.

TABLE 29.6 The stages of damage control surgery.

Stage	Intervention
I	Patient selection
II	Control of haemorrhage and control of contamination
III	Resuscitation continued in the intensive care unit
IV	Definitive surgery
V	Abdominal closure

The next stage following damage control surgery and physiological stabilisation is definitive surgery. The team should aim to perform definitive anastomoses, vascular reconstruction and closure of the body cavity within 24–72 hours of injury. However, this must be individualised to the patient, the response to critical care resuscitation and the progression of injury.

TABLE 29.7 Indications for damage control surgery.

Anatomical	• Inability to achieve haemostasis • Complex abdominal injury, e.g. liver and pancreas • Combined vascular, solid and hollow organ injury, e.g. aortic or caval injury • Inaccessible major venous injury, e.g. retrohepatic vena cava • Demand for non-operative control of other injuries, e.g. fractured pelvis • Anticipated need for a time-consuming procedure
Physiological (decline of physiological reserve)	• Temperature <34°C • pH <7.2 • Serum lactate >5 mmol/L (normal: <2.5 mmol/L) • Prothrombin time >16 s • Partial thromboplastin time >60 s • >10 units blood transfused • Systolic blood pressure <90 mmHg for >60 min
Environmental	• Operating time >60 min (core temperature loss is usually 2°C/h) • Inability to approximate the abdominal incision • Desire to reassess the intra-abdominal contents (directed relook)

The abdomen is closed as soon as possible, bearing in mind the risks of abdominal compartment syndrome (ACS). The closure is not without its own morbidity. Successful closure may require aggressive off-loading of fluid and even haemofiltration to achieve this if the patient will tolerate it. The best situation is closure of the abdominal fascia, or, if this cannot be achieved, then skin closure only. Occasionally, mesh closure can be used, with skin grafting over the mesh and subsequent abdominal wall reconstruction.

Thoracic damage control is conceptually based on the same philosophy. This is that haemorrhage control and focused surgical procedures minimise further surgical insult and lead to improved survival in the unstable trauma patient. The aim is to control bleeding and limit air leaks using the fastest procedures available, such as staplers, to minimise the operative time.

The indications and techniques for emergency thoracic surgery have already been described.

Damage control applies equally to the extremities. In this case, it is shunting of blood vessels, identifying and marking damaged structures such as nerves, fasciotomy and removal of contaminated tissue that are the main tasks. Subsequent definitive management can be carried out at a later stage.

Summary box 29.9

Damage control

- Resuscitation is carried out in the operating theatre using biologically active fluids (i.e. blood) – damage control resuscitation
- The surgery performed is the minimum needed to stabilise the patient
- The aims of surgery are to control haemorrhage and limit contamination
- Secondary surgery is aimed at definitive repair

ABDOMINAL COMPARTMENT SYNDROME AND THE OPEN ABDOMEN

Raised intra-abdominal pressure has far-reaching consequences for the patient; the syndrome that results is known as ACS. ACS is a major cause of morbidity and mortality in the critically ill patient and its early recognition is essential (*Table 29.8*).

In all cases of abdominal trauma in which the development of ACS in the immediate postoperative phase is considered a risk, the abdomen should be left open and managed as for damage control surgery.

TABLE 29.8 Effect of raised intra-abdominal pressure on individual organ function.

System	Effect
Renal	Increase in renal vascular resistance leading to a reduction in glomerular filtration rate and impaired renal function
Cardiovascular	Decrease in venous return resulting in decreased cardiac output because of both a reduction in preload and an increase in afterload
Respiratory	Increased ventilation pressures because of splinting of the diaphragm, decreased lung compliance and increased airway pressures
Visceral effects	Reduction in visceral perfusion
Intracranial effects	Severe rises in intracranial pressures

INTERVENTIONAL RADIOLOGY

Interventional radiology can be useful in the management of torso trauma as both an investigative and a therapeutic tool for patients with vascular injury. Angioembolisation following demonstration of ongoing bleeding in splenic and renal injury is a valuable technique.

NON-OPERATIVE MANAGEMENT

Non-operative management is generally preferred for the management of solid organ injury in physiologically non-compromised children. Non-operative management of solid abdominal organ injury has rapidly gained acceptance in the management of adults as well. A stable patient and accurate CT imaging are prerequisites for this approach. Failure of non-operative management is uncommon and typically occurs within the first 12 hours after injury. Therefore, if correctly selected, the vast majority of these patients will avoid surgery, require less blood transfusion and sustain fewer complications than operated patients.

ANTIBIOTICS IN TORSO TRAUMA

There is no level 1 evidence to recommend the use of antibiotics for the insertion of chest drains. However, prophylactic antibiotics prior to surgery should be used in all cases of penetrating abdominal trauma. Unless there is major contamination, a single dose is sufficient.

FURTHER READING

American Association for the Surgery of Trauma. *Organ injury scaling system*. Available from http://www.aast.org (accessed February 2022).

American College of Surgeons. *Advanced trauma life support course manual for doctors*, 10th edn. Chicago, IL: American College of Surgeons, 2020.

Boffard KD (ed.). *Definitive surgery of trauma care*, 5th edn. London: Taylor and Francis, 2019.

Eastern Association for the Surgery of Trauma. *Guidelines for practice management: evidence-based guidelines*. Available from http://www.east.org (accessed February 2022).

Feliciano DV, Mattox LK, Moore EE (eds). *Trauma*, 9th edn. New York, NY: McGraw Hill, 2020.

Khan MA, McMonagle M (eds). *Trauma: code red: companion to the RCSEng definitive surgical trauma skills course*. Boca Raton, FL: CRC Press, 2018.

Khan MA, Nott D (eds). *Fundamentals of frontline surgery*. Boca Raton, FL: CRC Press, 2021.

Tornetta P, Ricci W, Court-Brown CM *et al. Rockwood and Green's fractures in adults*, 9th edn. Philadelphia, PA: Wolters Kluwer, 2019.

World Society for Abdominal Compartment Syndrome. *Abdominal compartment syndrome*. Available from http://www.wsacs.org (accessed February 2022).

CHAPTER

30 The neck and spine

Learning objectives

To be familiar with:
- The accurate assessment of spinal trauma
- The basic management of spinal trauma and the major pitfalls
- The pathophysiology and types of spinal cord injury
- The prognosis of spinal cord injury, factors affecting functional outcome and common associated complications

ANATOMY OF THE SPINE AND SPINAL CORD

Spinal column anatomy

The vertebral column is composed of a series of motion segments (*Figure 30.1*). A motion segment consists of two adjacent vertebrae, their intervertebral disc and ligamentous restraints (*Figure 30.2*).

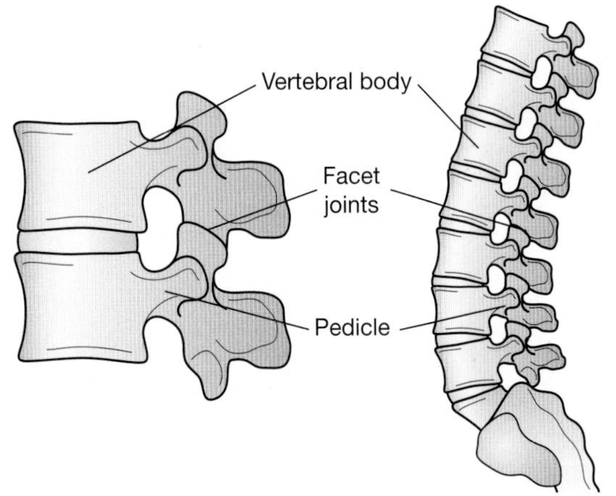

Figure 30.1 The spinal motion segment.

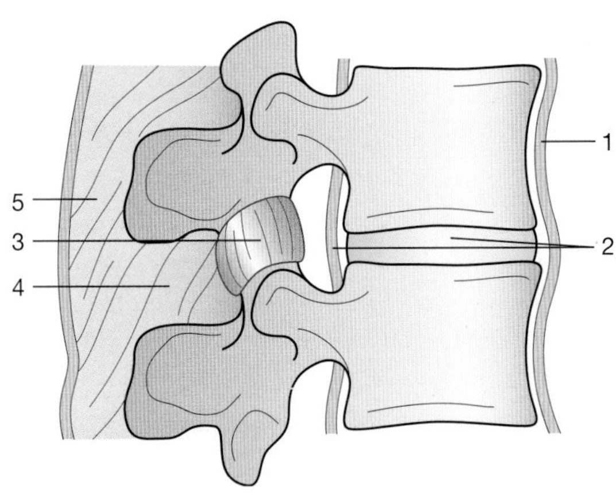

Figure 30.2 Ligamentous spinal restraints. (1) Anterior longitudinal ligament, (2) intervertebral disc and posterior longitudinal ligament, (3) facet joint capsule, (4) interspinous ligament, (5) supraspinous ligament.

Regional variations

Upper cervical spine anatomy is designed to facilitate motion (*Figure 30.3*), and stability here is dependent on ligamentous restraints (*Figure 30.4*). Vertebral anatomy from C3 to C7 is similar. The cervicothoracic (*Figure 30.5*) and thoracolumbar (*Figure 30.6*) junctions are transitional zones where the spine changes from a mobile section (cervical and lumbar) to a more fixed one (thoracic). These two areas are common sites of injury.

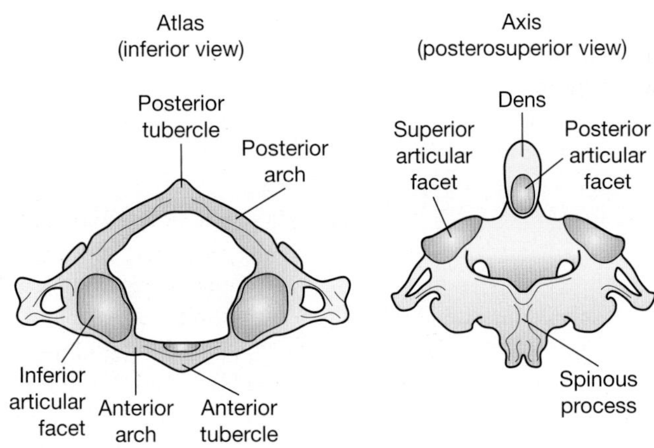

Figure 30.3 Atlantoaxial bony anatomy.

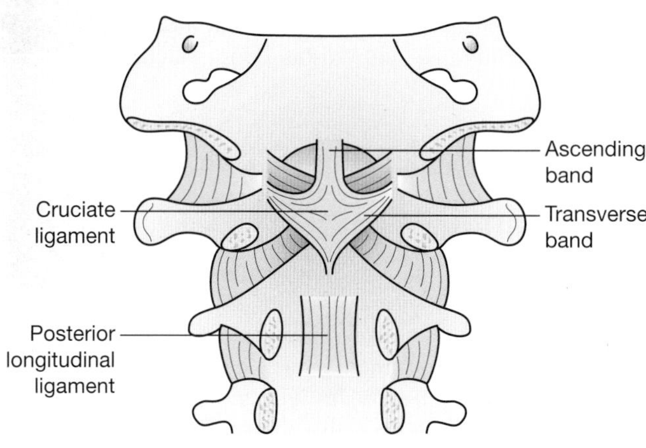

Figure 30.4 Atlantoaxial ligaments.

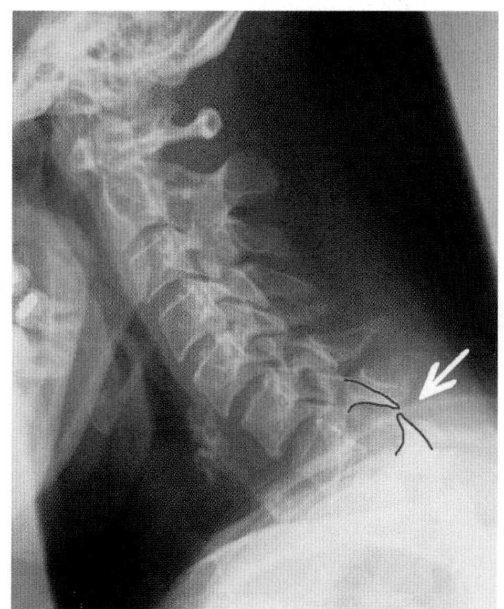

Figure 30.5 Cervicothoracic facet subluxation (arrow) (easily missed with inadequate radiographs).

Spinal stability

Spinal stability is the ability of the spine to withstand physiological loads with acceptable pain, avoiding progressive deformity or neurological deficit. The spine can be divided into three columns: anterior, middle and posterior (*Figure 30.7*). If two or more columns of the spine are injured, it is considered

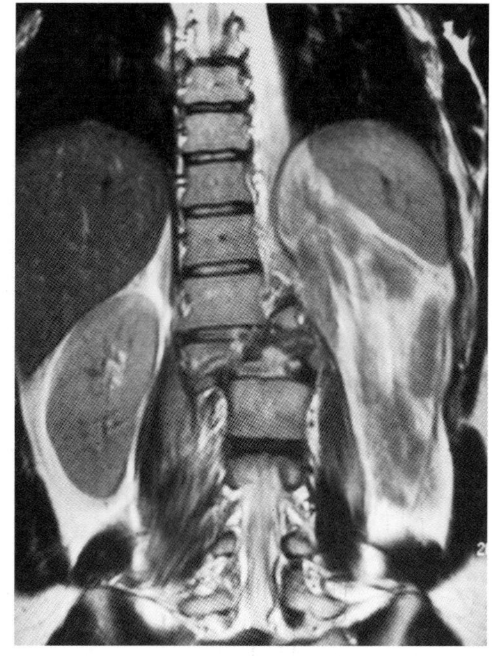

Figure 30.6 Coronal T2-weighted magnetic resonance image demonstrating a fracture dislocation at the thoracolumbar junction.

unstable. The AO classifications (Magerl and AO Spine Subaxial Classification System) are based on the mechanism of injury and are used to assess spinal stability.

Summary box 30.1

Spinal column anatomy

- Upper cervical spine stability is dependent on ligamentous restraints
- The cervicothoracic and thoracolumbar junctions are common sites of injury

Spinal neuroanatomy

The spinal cord extends from the foramen magnum to the L1/L2 level, where it ends as the conus medullaris in adults (lower in children) (*Figure 30.8*). Below this level lies the cauda equina. *Figure 30.9* illustrates a cross-section of the spinal cord.

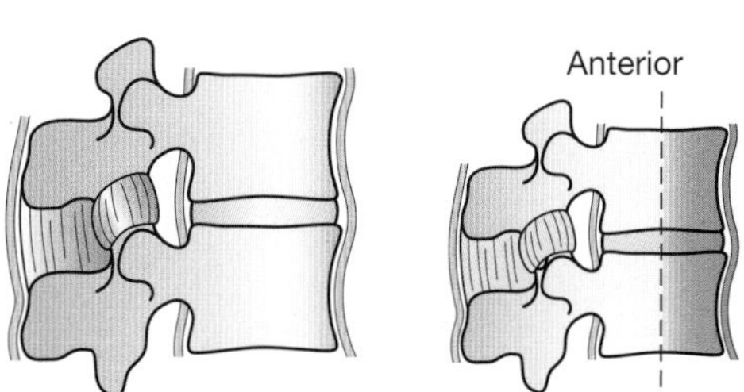

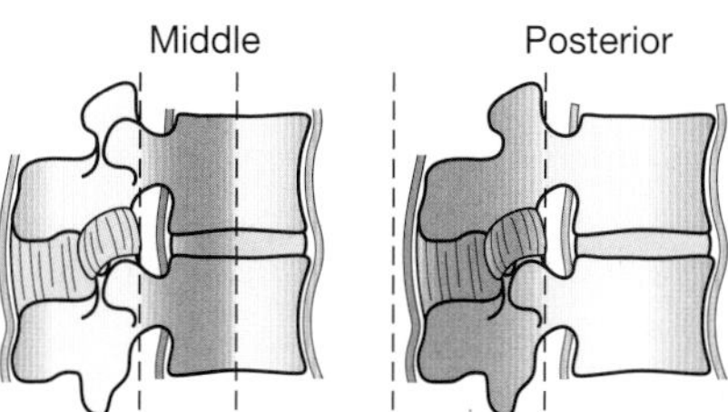

Figure 30.7 The three-column model of spinal stability.

Friedrich Paul Magerl, 1931–2020, Austrian surgeon and pioneer of spinal surgery.
AO, Arbeitsgemeinschaft für Osteosynthesefragen, may be translated from the German as 'Working Party on Problems of Bone Repair'.

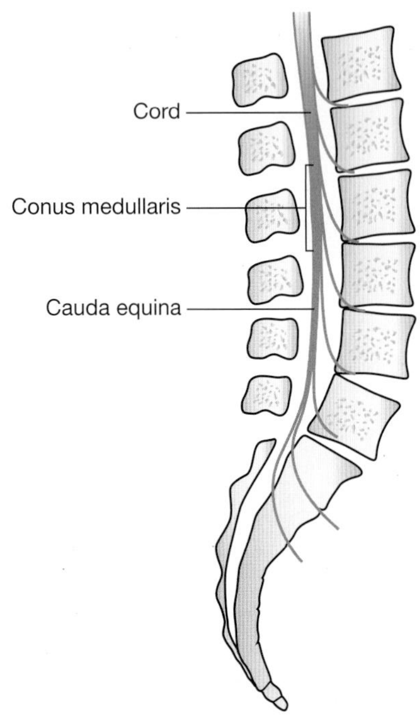

Figure 30.8 The spinal cord ends at L1/L2 at the conus medullaris, which gives rise to the cauda equina.

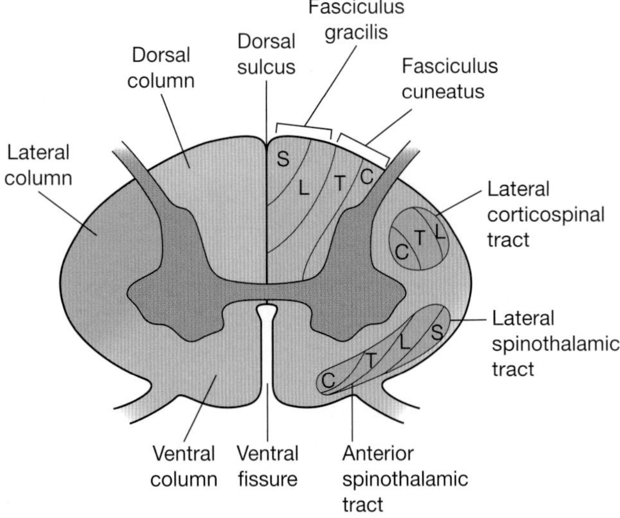

Figure 30.9 A cross-section of the spinal cord. C, cervical; L, lumbar; S, sacral; T, thoracic.

The lateral spinothalamic tracts transmit the sensations of pain and temperature, the lateral corticospinal tracts are responsible for motor function and the posterior columns transmit position, vibration and deep pressure sensation.

The spinothalamic tracts cross to the opposite side of the spinal cord within three levels of entering the cord. In contrast, the corticospinal tracts and the posterior columns decussate proximally at the craniocervical level. The tracts are topographically arranged; proximal body function is represented centrally, with distal body function arranged peripherally.

PATIENT ASSESSMENT

Basic points

The Advanced Trauma Life Support (ATLS) principles apply in all cases (see *Chapters 26 and 27*). The spine should initially be immobilised using full spinal precautions, on the assumption that every trauma patient has a spinal injury until proven otherwise (*Figure 30.10*). The finding of a spinal injury makes it more (not less) likely that there will be a second injury at another level.

Spinal boards lead to skin breakdown in insensate patients, and are very uncomfortable for those with normal sensation (*Figure 30.11*). They should only be used for transferring patients.

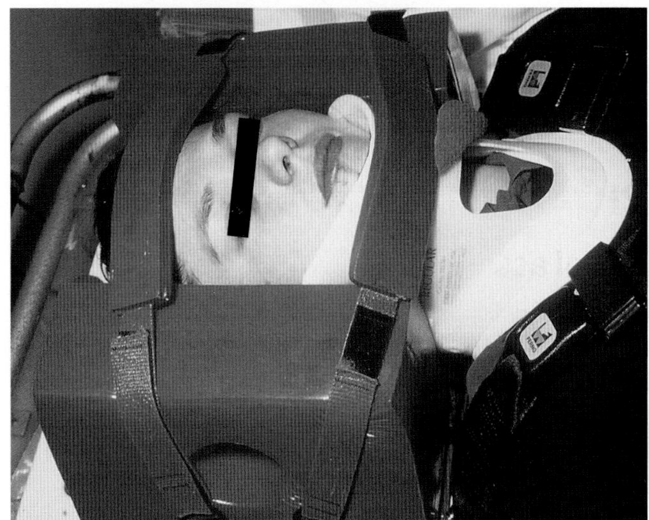

Figure 30.10 Spinal immobilisation.

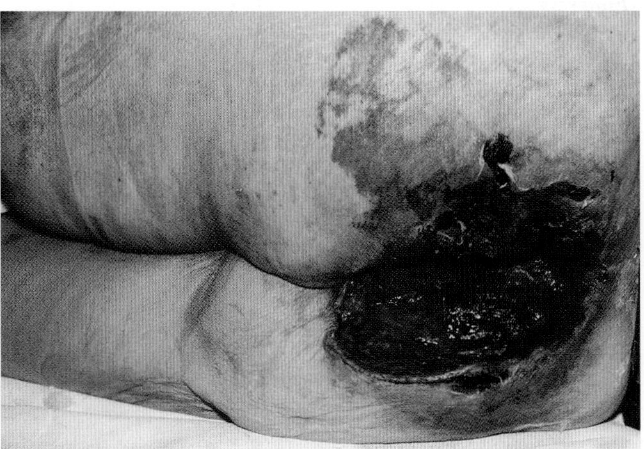

Figure 30.11 Pressure sores may develop rapidly in insensate patients.

The unconscious patient

Definitive clearance of the spine may not be possible in the initial stages; if this is the case, spinal immobilisation should be maintained until magnetic resonance imaging (MRI) or equivalent can be used to rule out an unstable spinal injury.

Summary box 30.2

Patient assessment

- Use ATLS principles in all cases of spinal injury
- In polytrauma cases suspect a spinal injury
- A second spinal injury at a remote level may be present in 10% of cases
- Spinal boards cause pressure sores

PERTINENT HISTORY

The mechanism and velocity of injury should be determined at an early stage. A check for the presence of spinal pain should be made. The onset and duration of neurological symptoms should also be recorded.

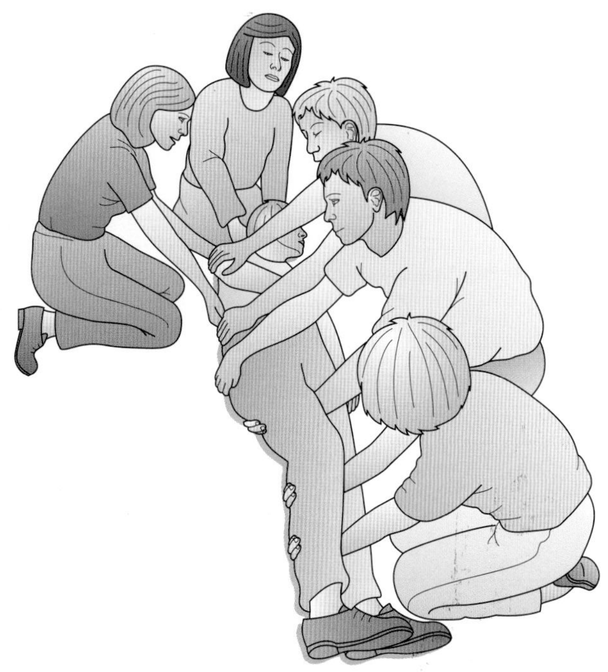

Figure 30.12 Spinal log roll.

PHYSICAL EXAMINATION

Initial assessment

The primary survey always takes precedence, followed by a careful systems examination paying particular attention to the abdomen and chest. Spinal cord injury may mask signs of intra-abdominal injury.

Spinal examination

The overlying skin should be inspected (e.g. for possible penetrating wounds) and the entire spine must be palpated. A formal spinal log roll must be performed to achieve this (*Figure 30.12*). Significant swelling, tenderness, palpable steps or gaps suggest a spinal injury. A rectal examination should be undertaken to assess anal tone and perianal sensation (see *Neurological examination*). Seatbelt marks on the abdomen and chest must be noted, as these suggest a high-energy accident.

Neurological examination

The American Spinal Injury Association (ASIA) neurological evaluation system (*Figure 30.13*) is an internationally accepted method of neurological evaluation.

Motor function is assessed using the Medical Research Council (MRC) grading system (0–5) in key muscle groups (*Figure 30.13*). A motor score can then be calculated (maximum 100).

Sensory function (light touch and pin prick) is assessed using the dermatomal map (*Figure 30.13*). A total sensory score is then calculated.

Rectal examination is performed to assess anal tone, voluntary anal contraction and perianal sensation.

Level of neurological impairment

The extent of spinal cord injury is defined by the American Spinal Injury Association (ASIA) Impairment Scale (modified from the Frankel classification):

- **A:** complete spinal cord injury;
- **B:** sensation present, motor absent;
- **C:** sensation present, motor present but not useful (MRC grade $<3/5$);
- **D:** sensation present, motor useful (MRC grade $\geq 3/5$);
- **E:** normal function.

Summary box 30.3

Physical examination

- The ASIA neurological scoring system should be used
- Functional motor power is MRC grade 3/5 or higher

Hans Ludwig Frankel, b. 1932, Clinical Director, The National Spinal Injuries Centre, Stoke Mandeville, UK.

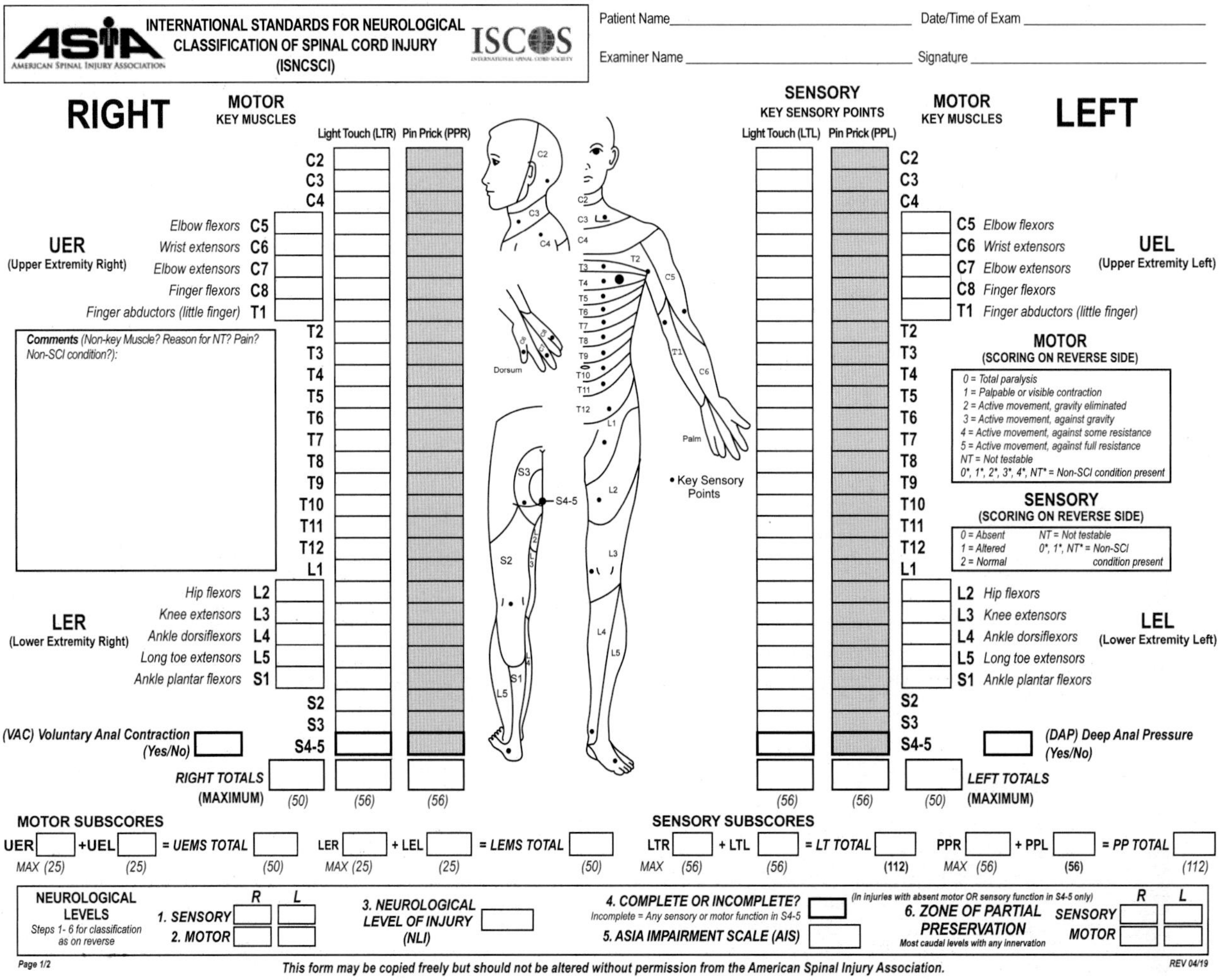

ASIA — AMERICAN SPINAL INJURY ASSOCIATION
INTERNATIONAL STANDARDS FOR NEUROLOGICAL CLASSIFICATION OF SPINAL CORD INJURY (ISNCSCI)
ISCOS — INTERNATIONAL SPINAL CORD SOCIETY

Patient Name ______ Date/Time of Exam ______
Examiner Name ______ Signature ______

RIGHT

MOTOR KEY MUSCLES — SENSORY KEY SENSORY POINTS: Light Touch (LTR) | Pin Prick (PPR)

C2, C3, C4

UER (Upper Extremity Right): Elbow flexors C5; Wrist extensors C6; Elbow extensors C7; Finger flexors C8; Finger abductors (little finger) T1

T2, T3, T4, T5, T6, T7, T8, T9, T10, T11, T12, L1

Comments (Non-key Muscle? Reason for NT? Pain? Non-SCI condition?):

LER (Lower Extremity Right): Hip flexors L2; Knee extensors L3; Ankle dorsiflexors L4; Long toe extensors L5; Ankle plantar flexors S1

S2, S3, S4-5

(VAC) Voluntary Anal Contraction (Yes/No)

RIGHT TOTALS (MAXIMUM) (50) (56) (56)

LEFT

SENSORY KEY SENSORY POINTS: Light Touch (LTL) | Pin Prick (PPL) — MOTOR KEY MUSCLES

C2, C3, C4

UEL (Upper Extremity Left): C5 Elbow flexors; C6 Wrist extensors; C7 Elbow extensors; C8 Finger flexors; T1 Finger abductors (little finger)

T2, T3, T4, T5, T6, T7, T8, T9, T10, T11, T12, L1

MOTOR (SCORING ON REVERSE SIDE)
0 = Total paralysis
1 = Palpable or visible contraction
2 = Active movement, gravity eliminated
3 = Active movement, against gravity
4 = Active movement, against some resistance
5 = Active movement, against full resistance
NT = Not testable
0*, 1*, 2*, 3*, 4*, NT* = Non-SCI condition present

SENSORY (SCORING ON REVERSE SIDE)
0 = Absent; NT = Not testable
1 = Altered; 0*, 1*, NT* = Non-SCI condition present
2 = Normal

LEL (Lower Extremity Left): L2 Hip flexors; L3 Knee extensors; L4 Ankle dorsiflexors; L5 Long toe extensors; S1 Ankle plantar flexors

S2, S3, S4-5

(DAP) Deep Anal Pressure (Yes/No)

LEFT TOTALS (MAXIMUM) (56) (56) (50)

• Key Sensory Points (Dorsum, Palm, C2–S4-5 dermatomes)

MOTOR SUBSCORES
UER __ + UEL __ = UEMS TOTAL __ (MAX (25) (25) (50)); LER __ + LEL __ = LEMS TOTAL __ (MAX (25) (25) (50))

SENSORY SUBSCORES
LTR __ + LTL __ = LT TOTAL __ (MAX (56) (56) (112)); PPR __ + PPL __ = PP TOTAL __ (MAX (56) (56) (112))

NEUROLOGICAL LEVELS (Steps 1-6 for classification as on reverse): 1. SENSORY R L; 2. MOTOR R L
3. NEUROLOGICAL LEVEL OF INJURY (NLI)
4. COMPLETE OR INCOMPLETE? (Incomplete = Any sensory or motor function in S4-5)
5. ASIA IMPAIRMENT SCALE (AIS)
6. ZONE OF PARTIAL PRESERVATION (In injuries with absent motor OR sensory function in S4-5 only) — Most caudal levels with any innervation: SENSORY R L; MOTOR R L

Page 1/2 — This form may be copied freely but should not be altered without permission from the American Spinal Injury Association. — REV 04/19

Figure 30.13 American Spinal Injury Association neurological evaluation. (Reproduced with permission from American Spinal Injury Association: *International standards for neurological classification of spinal cord injury*, revised 2019; Richmond, VA.)

DIAGNOSTIC IMAGING

Plain radiographs

A full cervical spine series includes anteroposterior and lateral radiographs of the whole cervical spine, and open mouth views. Clear visualisation of the cervicothoracic junction is essential in all cases of suspected spinal injury, as this is a common site for injury and often not seen on a plain radiograph. If a spinal fracture is identified then further imaging of the whole spine is required because there is a 15% incidence of a further spinal fracture.

A system for evaluation of the lateral cervical spine radiograph

1 Assess prevertebral soft-tissue swelling (*Figure 30.14*).
2 Assess sagittal alignment using three imaginary lines (*Figure 30.15*).
3 Assess for instability (*Figure 30.16*):
   a 3.5 mm of sagittal translation;
   b sagittal angulation of >11° (compared with the adjacent level).

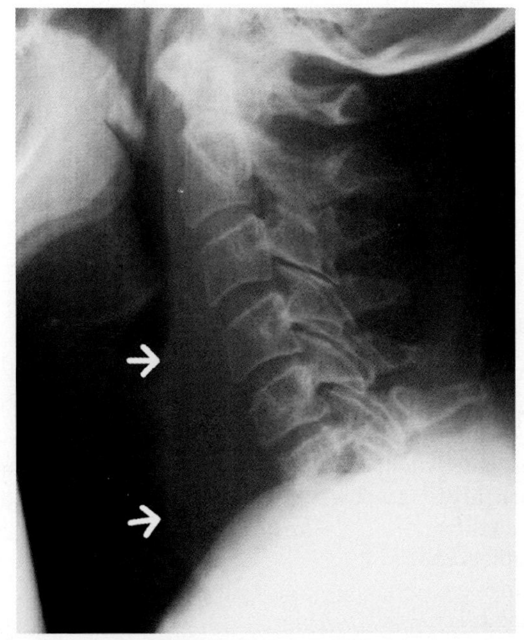

Figure 30.14 Large prevertebral haematoma (arrows).

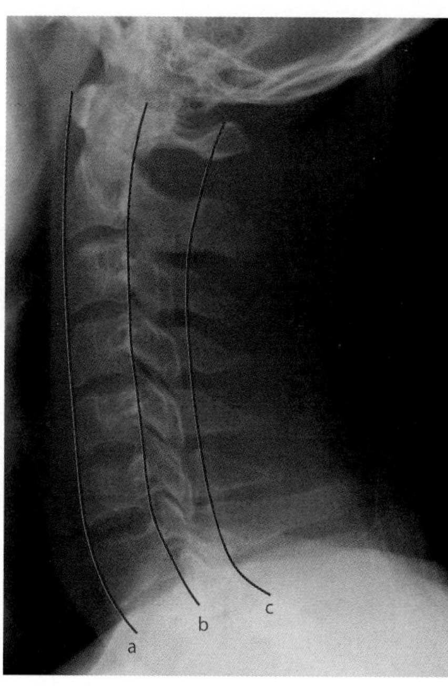

Figure 30.15 The anterior (a), posterior (b) and spinolaminar (c) lines are useful in identifying anterior translation on lateral radiographs of the neck.

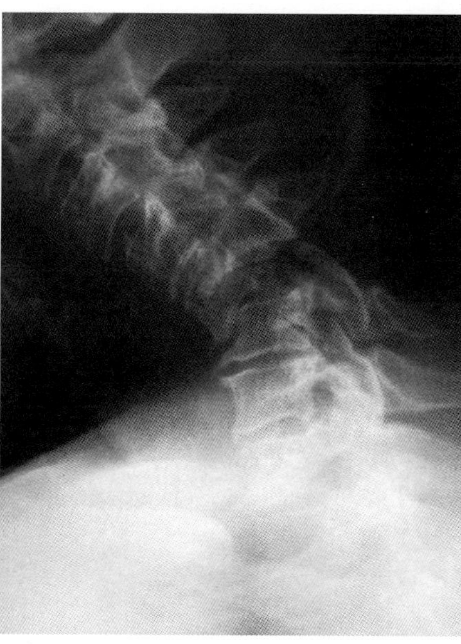

Figure 30.16 Lateral cervical spine radiograph showing obvious spinal instability with marked sagittal angulation and translation. This patient walked into the outpatient department.

Computed tomography

Computed tomography (CT) scanning with two-dimensional reconstruction remains the gold standard in spinal trauma and is indicated for patients with suspected or visible injuries on plain radiographs (*Figure 30.17*). Patients undergoing a head CT scan for closed head injury should also have a cervical screening CT. Often CT scans of the chest and abdomen are performed as part of the assessment of polytrauma patients and will usually include the spine.

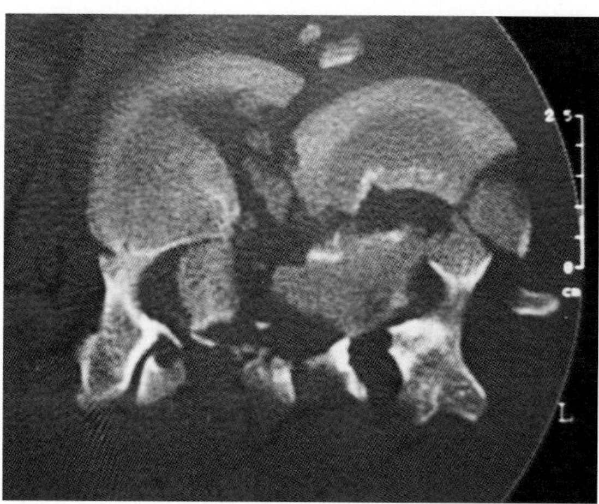

Figure 30.17 Axial computed tomography demonstrating a thoraco-lumbar fracture dislocation.

Magnetic resonance imaging

MRI is indicated in all patients with neurological deficit and where assessment of ligamentous structures is important (*Figure 30.18*).

Dynamic imaging

Lateral flexion–extension radiographs of the cervical spine should not be undertaken acutely, although they can have a role in assessing spinal stability in the longer term.

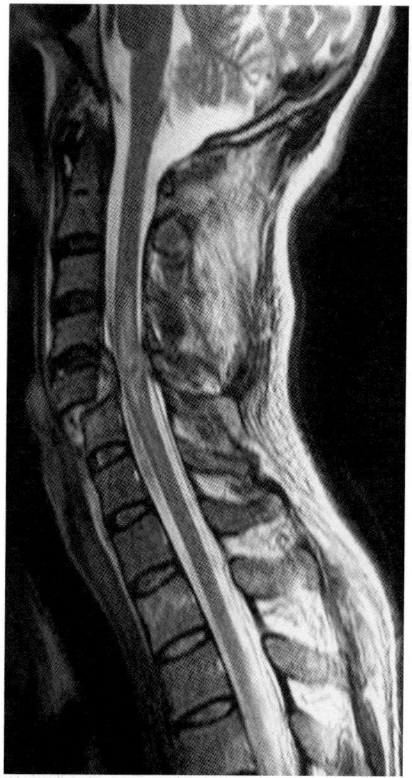

Figure 30.18 Sagittal T2-weighted magnetic resonance imaging scan demonstrating a cervical spine subluxation and spinal cord contusion.

Summary box 30.4

Diagnostic imaging of spinal injuries

- Clear visualisation of the cervicothoracic junction is mandatory
- Plain cervical spine radiographs fail to identity 15% of injuries

CLASSIFICATION AND MANAGEMENT OF SPINAL AND SPINAL CORD INJURIES

Basic management principles

Spinal realignment

In cases of cervical spine subluxation or dislocation, skeletal traction is necessary to achieve anatomical realignment. This is done using skull tongs (*Figure 30.19*).

In many cases of spinal trauma, formal open reduction and stabilisation using internal fixation is also required (*Figure 30.20*).

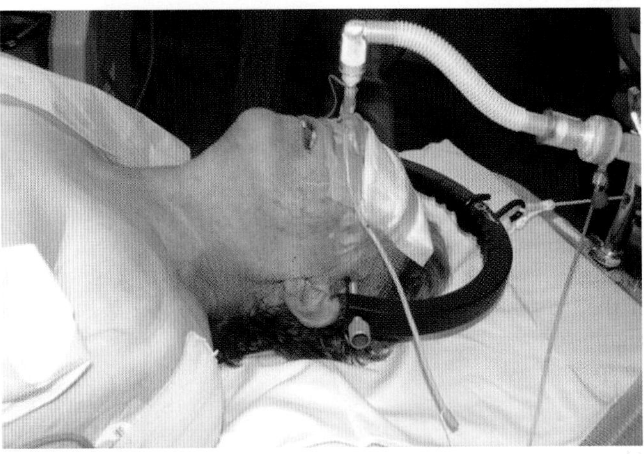

Figure 30.19 Skeletal traction using skull tongs.

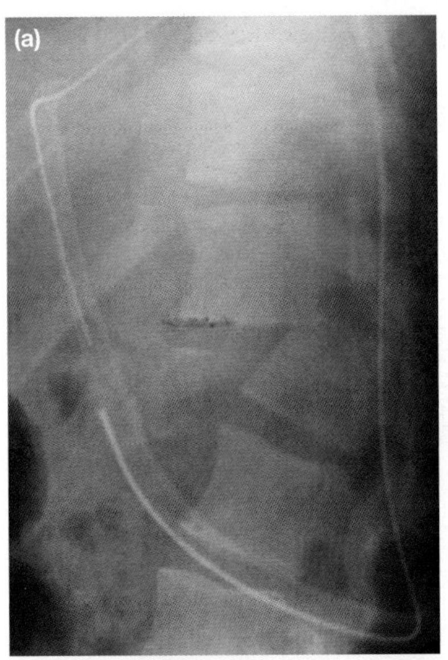

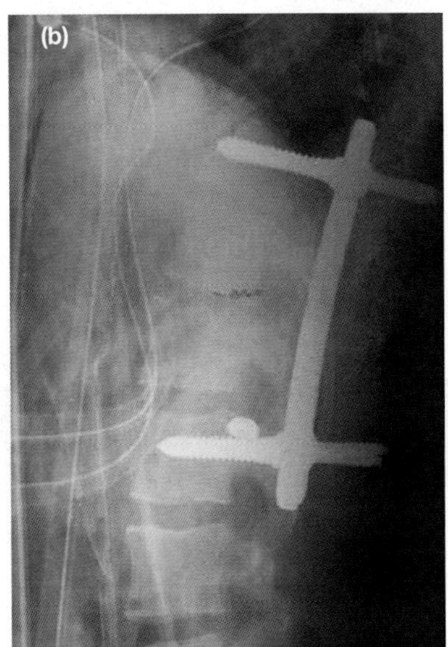

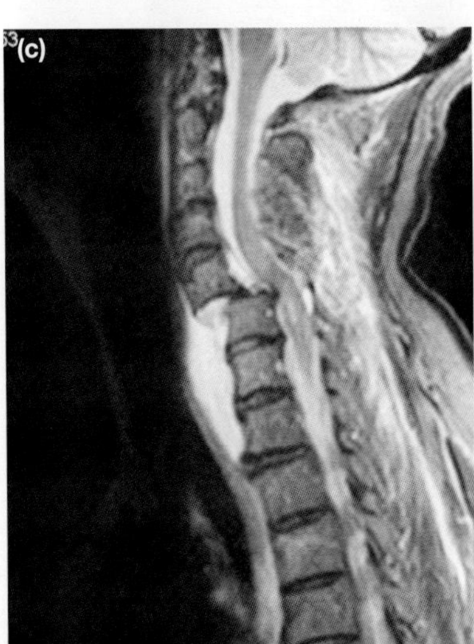

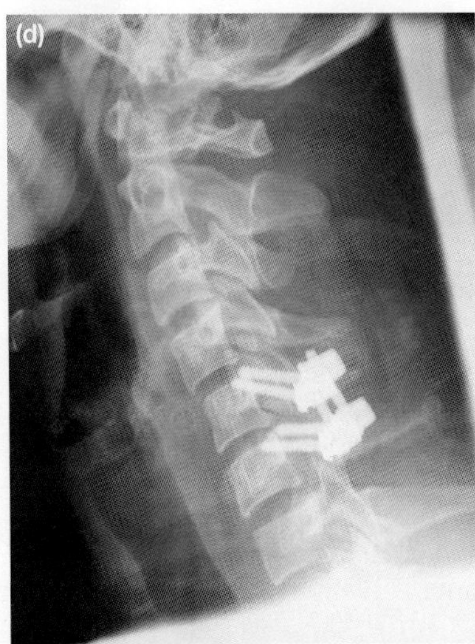

Figure 30.20 (a) Thoracolumbar fracture dislocation, (b) treated with open reduction and posterior fixation. (c) Bifacetal cervical spine dislocation. (d) Posterior stabilisation following closed reduction.

A halo brace can be used to perform a closed realignment and immobilisation of cervical fractures (*Figure 30.21*).

Stabilisation

The indication for operative intervention is influenced by the injury pattern, level of pain, degree of instability and the presence of a neurological deficit. The only absolute indication for surgery in spinal trauma is deteriorating neurological function.

Decompression of the neural elements

Realignment of the spine and correction of the spinal deformity may achieve an indirect decompression. A direct decompression of the neural elements may also be indicated if there are bone fragments causing residual compression or a significant haematoma (*Figure 30.22*). The timing of surgery in spinal cord trauma remains controversial.

Corticosteroids

Corticosteroids are no longer indicated in acute spinal cord injury because of a lack of evidence to support efficacy. Steroids do have a role in non-traumatic spinal cord compression, e.g. malignant spinal cord compression.

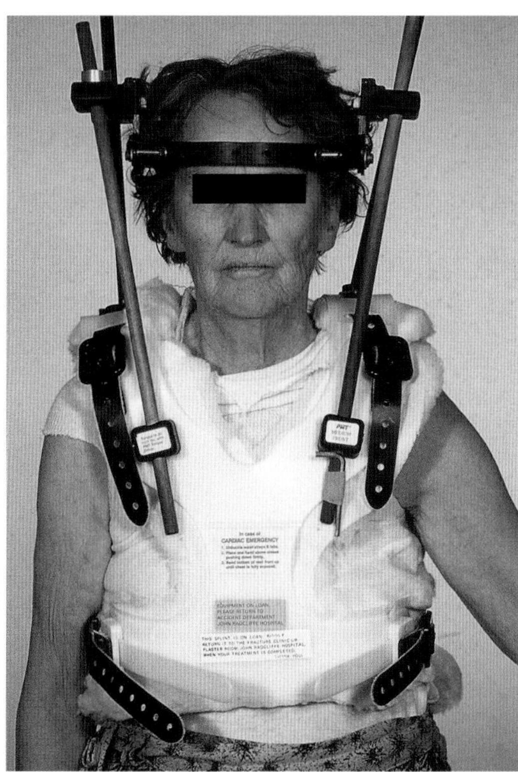

Figure 30.21 External immobilisation using a halo jacket.

> **Summary box 30.5**
>
> Management of spinal trauma
> - Neurological deficit determines management
> - Deteriorating neurological status requires surgical intervention
> - Corticosteroids are ineffective

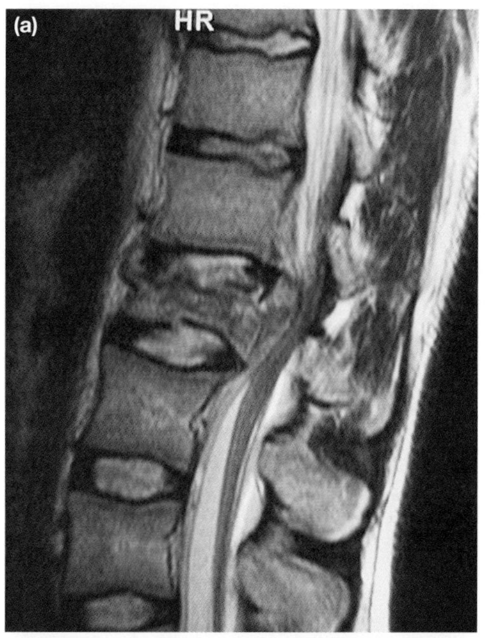

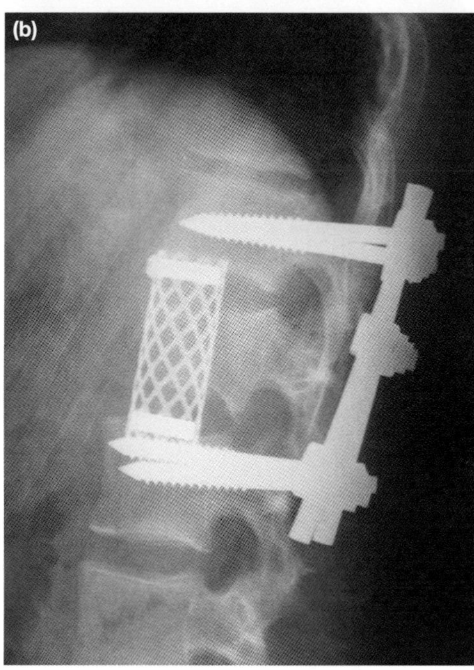

Figure 30.22 (a) Sagittal T2-weighted magnetic resonance imaging scan showing an L1 burst fracture and neural compression; (b) treated with combined anterior and posterior surgery.

SPECIFIC SPINAL INJURIES

Upper cervical spine (skull-C2)

Occipital condyle fracture

This is a relatively stable injury often associated with head injuries and is best treated in a hard collar for 6–8 weeks.

Occipitoatlantal dislocation

This injury is usually caused by high-energy trauma and is often fatal. The dislocation may be anterior, posterior or vertical (*Figure 30.23*). Powers' ratio (*Figure 30.24*) is used to assess skull translation. Treatment is with a halo brace or occipitocervical fixation.

Atlas fracture (Jefferson fracture)

Fracture of the C1 ring is associated with axial loading of the cervical spine and may be stable or unstable (*Figure 30.25a,b*). Associated transverse ligament rupture may occur (*Figure 30.25c*). Most are treated non-operatively in a cervical collar or halo brace.

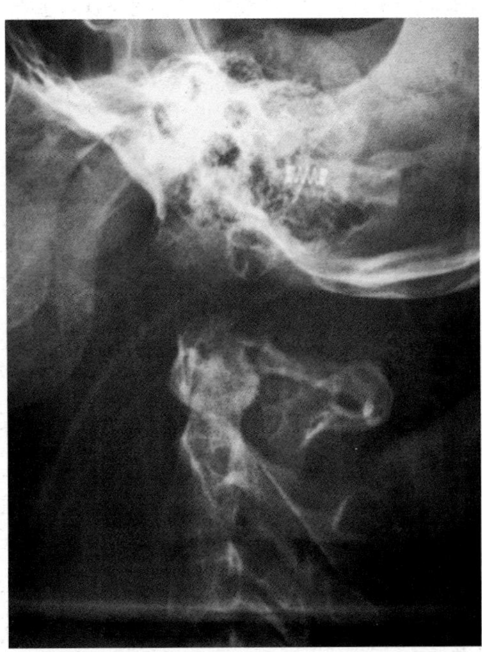

Figure 30.23 Vertical occipitocervical dislocation.

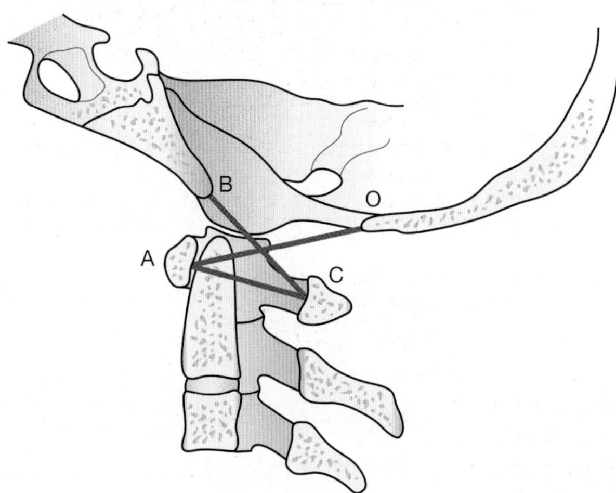

Figure 30.24 Powers' ratio. BC/OA ≥1 indicates anterior translation; ≤0.75 indicates posterior translation.

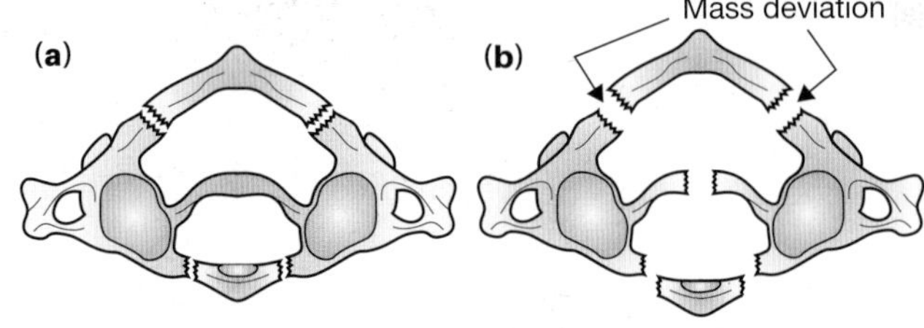

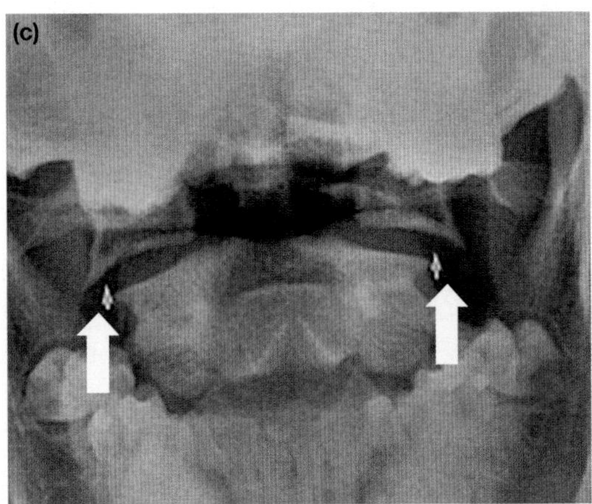

Figure 30.25 Stable (a) versus unstable (b) Jefferson's fracture of C1. (c) Open mouth view of C1/2 demonstrating C1 lateral mass deviation (arrows). Rupture of the transverse ligament is present when the combined lateral mass deviation exceeds 6.9 mm.

Atlantoaxial instability

This is defined as non-physiological movement between C1 and C2. It can be translational or rotatory and resolves either spontaneously or with traction followed by a cervical collar. Isolated, traumatic transverse ligament rupture leading to C1/2 instability is uncommon and is treated with posterior C1/2 fusion (*Figure 30.26*).

Odontoid fractures

There are three types of odontoid peg fracture (*Figure 30.27*). Neurological injury is rare. The majority of acute injuries are treated non-operatively in a hard collar or halo jacket for 3 months. Internal fixation with an anterior compression screw is indicated for displaced fractures (*Figure 30.28*), and a posterior C1/2 fusion is considered in cases of non-union. In the elderly, treatment in a soft collar should be considered on the basis that a relatively stable pseudarthrosis will occur.

Barry Powers, contemporary, Chief and Clinical Professor of Radiology, Duplin General Hospital, Kenansville, NC, USA, described his ratio in 1979.

Sir Geoffrey Jefferson, 1886–1961, Professor of Neurosurgery, University of Manchester, UK, became the UK's first Professor of Neurosurgery in 1939. In 1947 he was elected a Fellow of the Royal Society, a rare distinction for a practising surgeon. Although he became a neurosurgeon, he performed the first successful embolectomy in England in 1925 at Salford Royal Hospital.

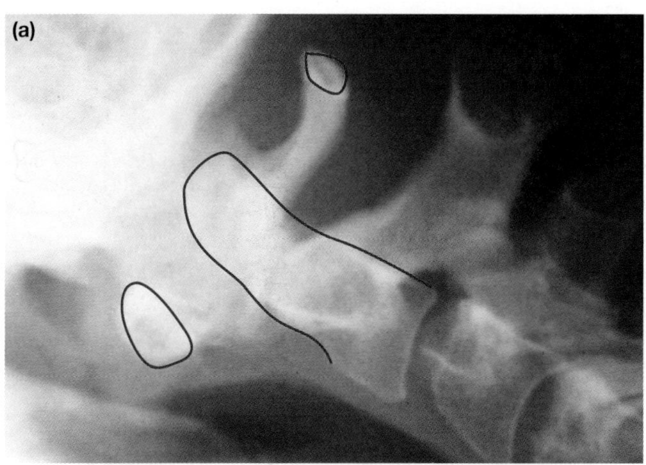

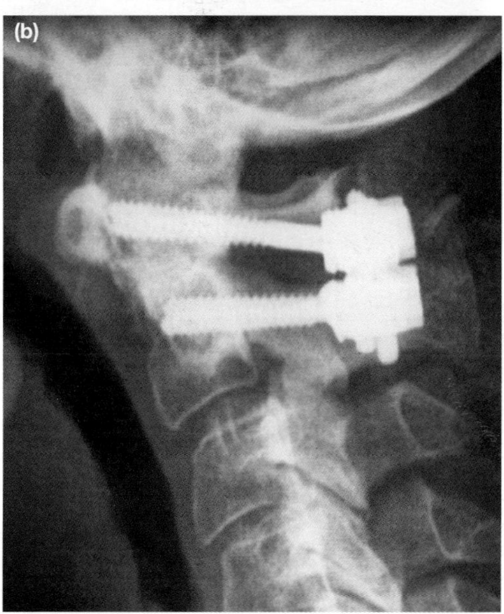

Figure 30.26 (a) Atlantoaxial subluxation. (b) C1/2 posterior fusion using C1 lateral mass and C2 pedicle screws.

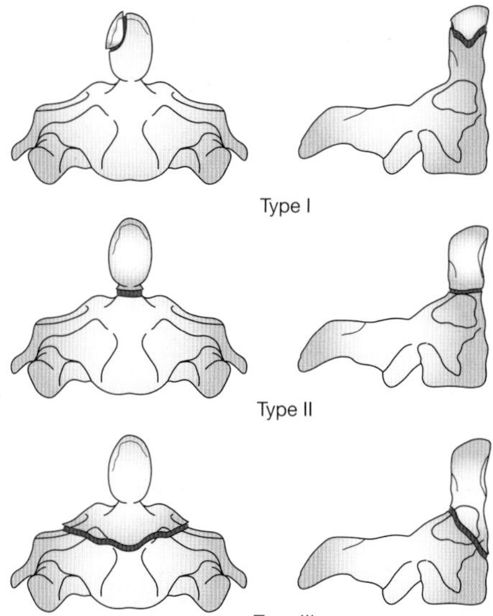

Figure 30.27 Types of odontoid fracture.

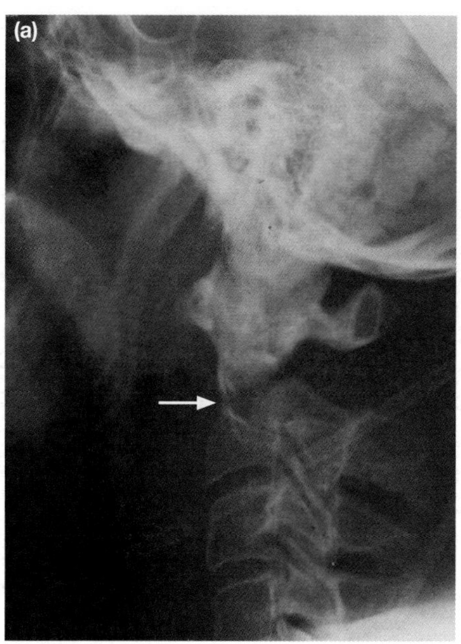

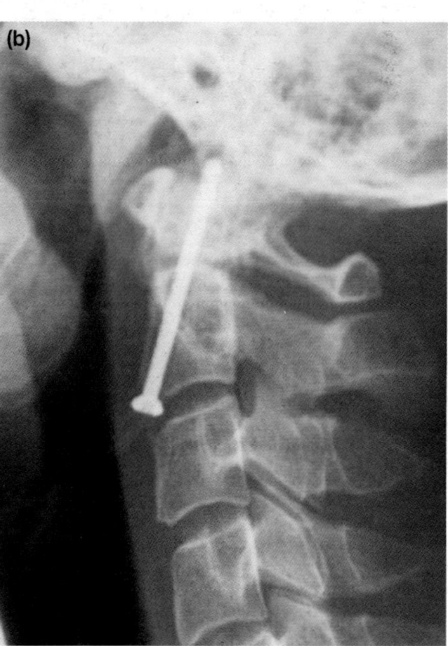

Figure 30.28 (a) Type II odontoid fracture (arrow); (b) treated with an anterior compression screw.

Traumatic spondylolisthesis of the axis (hangman's fracture)

This is a traumatic spondylolisthesis of C2 on C3. There are four types with varying degrees of instability (*Figure 30.29*). Those with significant displacement or associated facet dislocation are treated operatively, usually with posterior stabilisation.

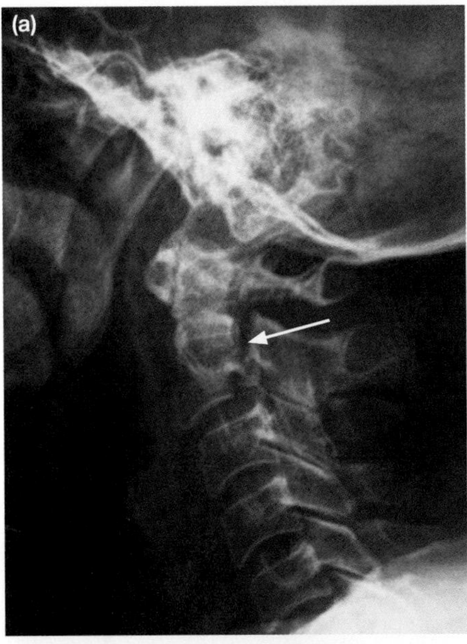

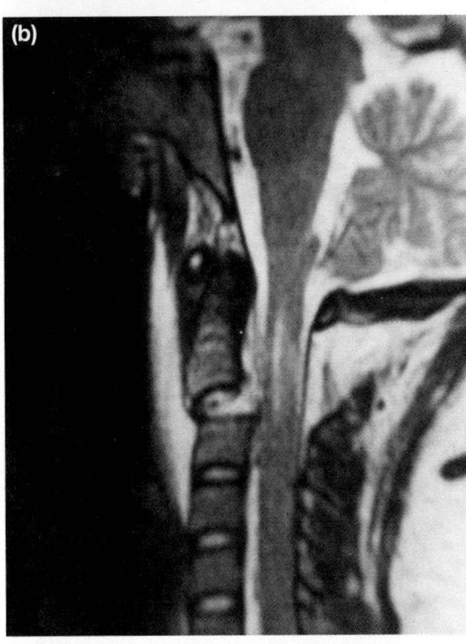

Figure 30.29 (a) Hangman's fractures of C2 with minimal forward translation (arrow). (b) C2/3 subluxation with spinal cord contusion.

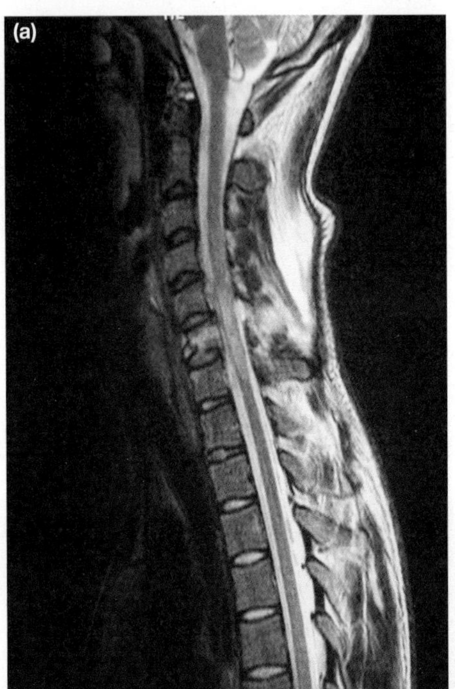

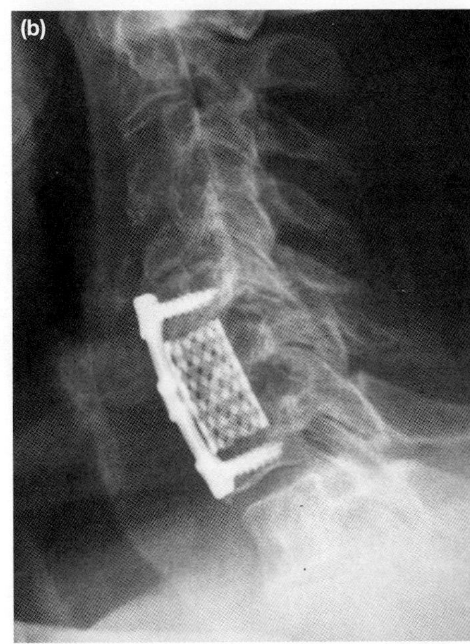

Figure 30.30 (a) Cervical burst fracture with spinal cord contusion; (b) treated with anterior decompression and reconstruction.

Subaxial cervical spine (C3-C7)

The pattern of lower cervical spine injury depends on the mechanism of trauma. These include compression fractures (hyperflexion), burst fractures (axial compression), facet subluxation/dislocation injuries (distraction–flexion), teardrop fractures (hyperextension) and fracture of posterior elements. The more severe injuries may have an associated spinal cord injury (*Figure 30.30a*). Operative intervention may be required to decompress the spinal cord and to stabilise the spine with internal fixation (*Figure 30.30b*).

Facet subluxation/dislocation ranges in severity from minor instability to complete dislocation with spinal cord injury (*Figure 30.31*).

Fractures in patients with ankylosing spondylitis

Ankylosing spondylitis is a seronegative inflammatory disorder that causes autofusion of the spine. These patients have a higher risk of spinal fractures and spinal cord injury than the normal population. Senior advice should be obtained, because application of a cervical collar may be contraindicated, and patients should be managed instead in a position of comfort. Surgical stabilisation is commonly indicated.

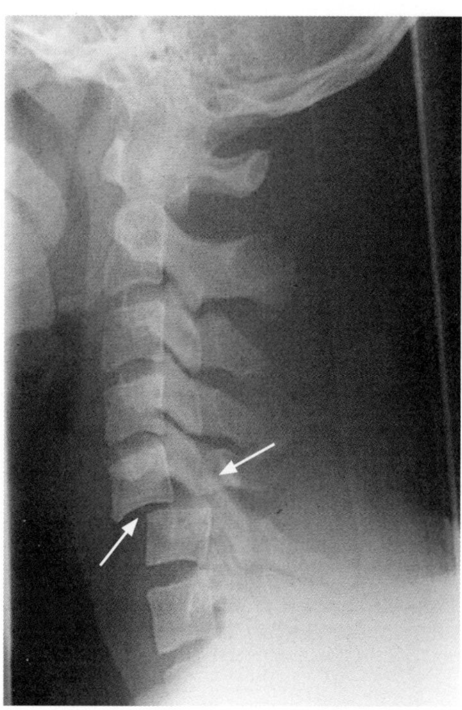

Figure 30.31 C5/6 bifacetal dislocation (arrows).

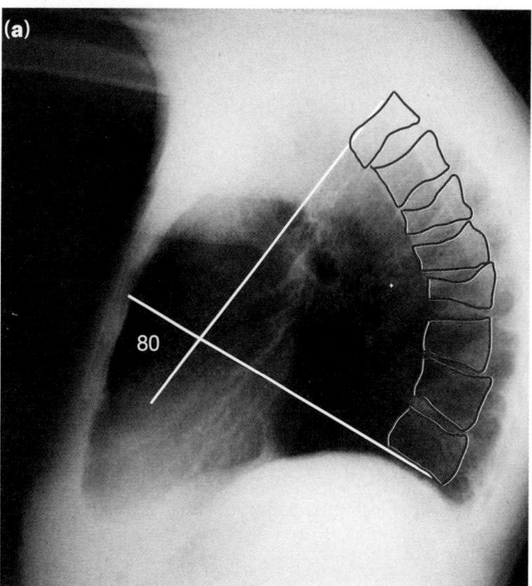

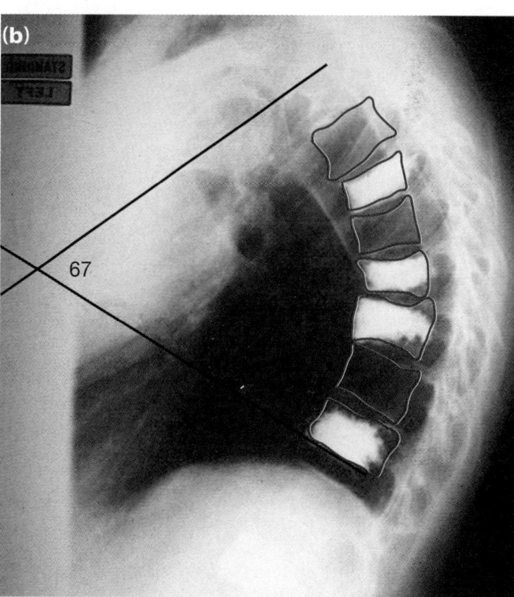

Figure 30.32 (a) Lateral radiograph showing multiple osteoporotic compression fractures. (b) Reduction in thoracic kyphotic deformity following four-level kyphoplasty.

Summary box 30.6

Cervical spine injuries

- The majority of upper cervical spinal injuries are treated non-operatively
- Spinal cord injury is more commonly associated with subaxial cervical spinal injuries

Thoracic and thoracolumbar fractures

The system developed by the AO (Arbeitsgemeinschaft für Osteosynthesefragen) can be used to classify these fractures. There are three main injury types, A, B and C, with increasing instability and risk of neurological injury.

Type A fractures are vertebral body compression fractures. Type B injuries involve distraction of the anterior or posterior elements and type C injuries are rotational and often coexist with type A or type B injuries. The majority of type B and type C injuries require surgical stabilisation.

Thoracic spine (T1–T10)

Osteoporotic wedge compression fractures in older adults are the commonest injury in this group. Most of these fractures heal, but symptomatic fractures can be treated with percutaneous bone cement augmentation, known as vertebroplasty or kyphoplasty (*Figure 30.32*).

In trauma cases, unstable fractures are associated with significant energy transfer to the patient and may be associated with major internal injuries, such as pulmonary contusion and spinal cord injury. The combination of thoracic spine disruption and a sternal fracture (*Figure 30.33*) also carries a significant risk of aortic rupture. Multiple posterior rib fractures and rib dislocations above and below a thoracic spinal injury signify a major rotational injury to the chest and can be associated with vascular injury and significant pulmonary contusion (*Figure 30.34*). Multimodality diagnostic imaging is recommended. Surgery is appropriate for most thoracic injuries if unstable.

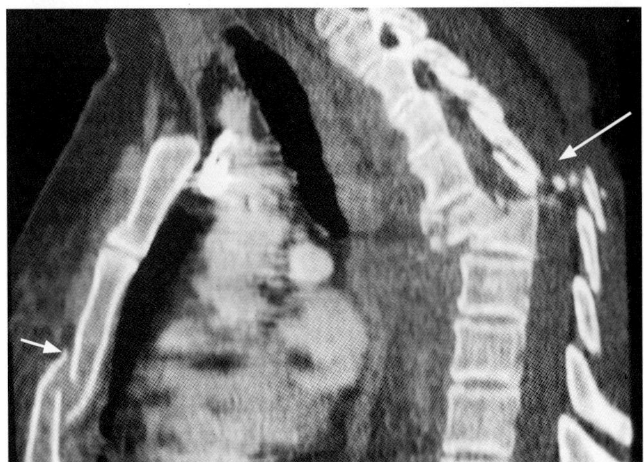

Figure 30.33 Sagittal computed tomography reconstruction showing an upper thoracic spine fracture dislocation (long arrow) and an associated sternal fracture (short arrow).

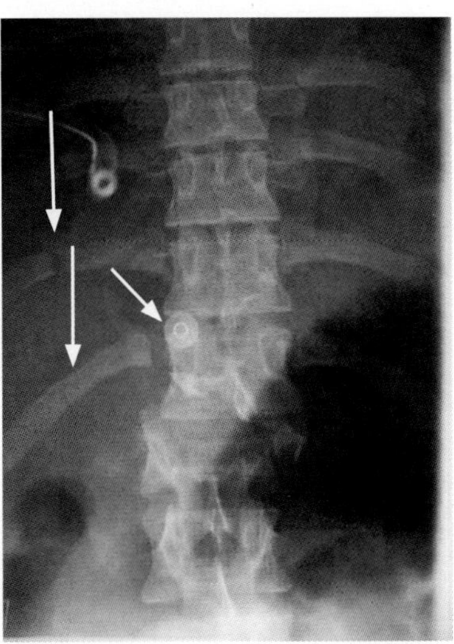

Figure 30.34 Rotational (type C) injury at the thoracolumbar junction. Note rib fractures (long arrows) and dislocation (short arrow), and the presence of a chest tube.

Thoracolumbar spinal fractures (T11-L2)

The thoracolumbar junction is especially prone to injury. This can vary from a minor wedge fracture to spinal dislocation (*Figure 30.35*). Burst fractures are comminuted fractures of the vertebral body. They are characterised by widening of the distance between the pedicles and can be associated with retropulsion of bone fragments into the spinal canal (*Figure 30.36*). Anterior surgery for this type of fracture is now very rarely used and the current treatment principles involve posterior fixation (*Figure 30.37*). Chance fractures

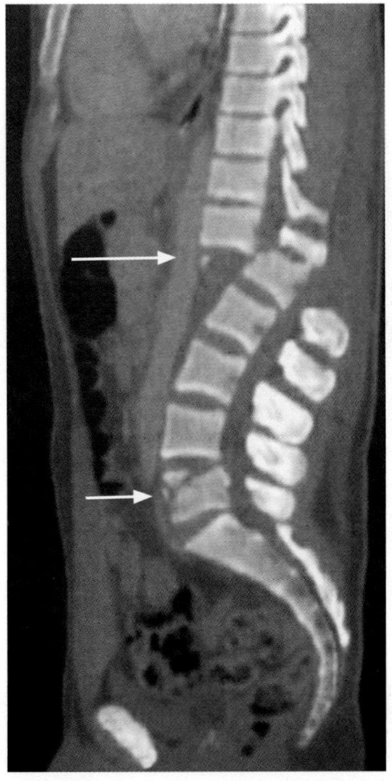

Figure 30.35 Total spinal sagittal computed tomography reconstruction demonstrating a thoracolumbar fracture dislocation (long arrow) and fracture of L5 (short arrow).

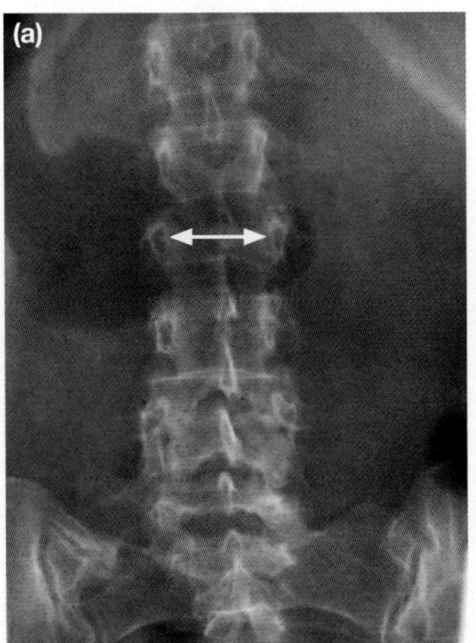

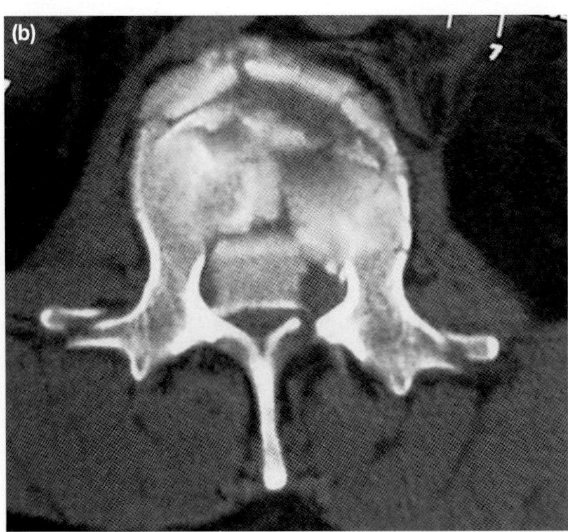

Figure 30.36 Lumbar burst fracture with an increase in the interpedicular distance (a) (arrow) and spinal canal compromise (b).

George Quentin Chance, Director of Diagnostic Radiology, The Derby Group of Hospitals, Derby, UK.

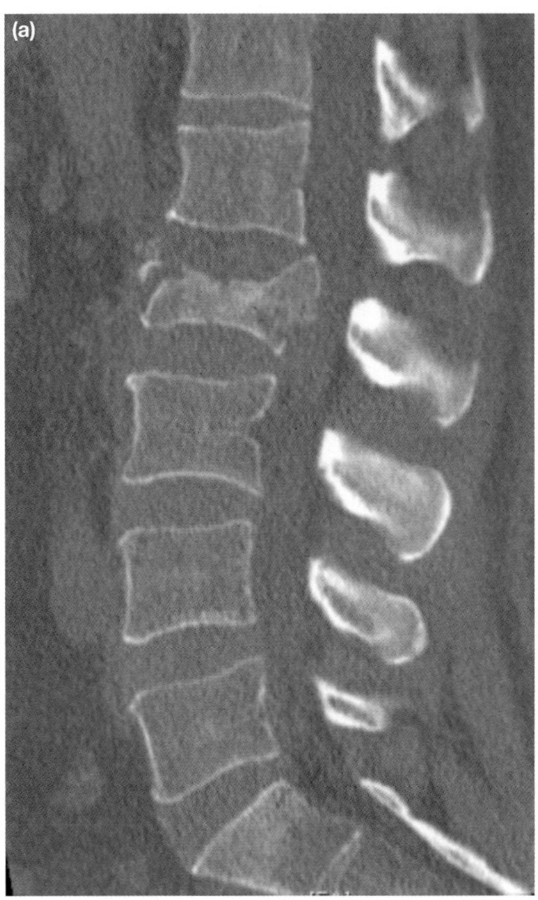

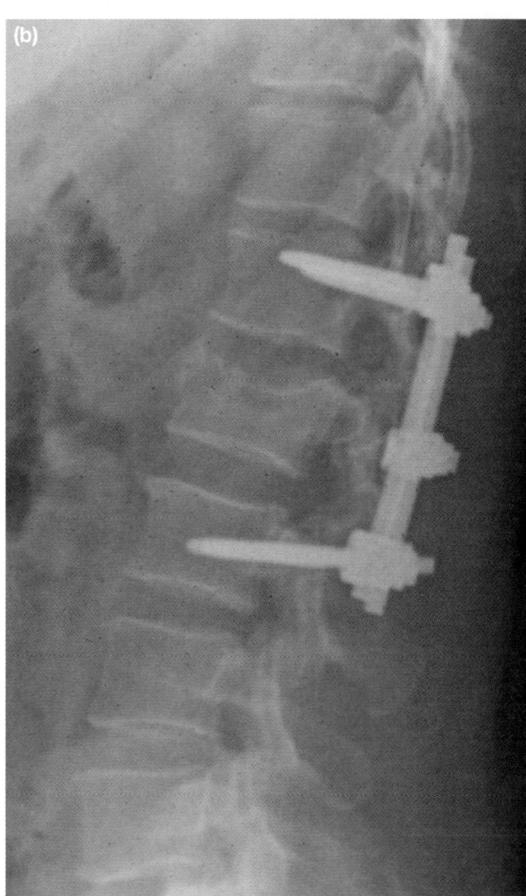

Figure 30.37 Lumbar burst fracture at L2 (a), and posterior instrumentation with indirect reduction (b).

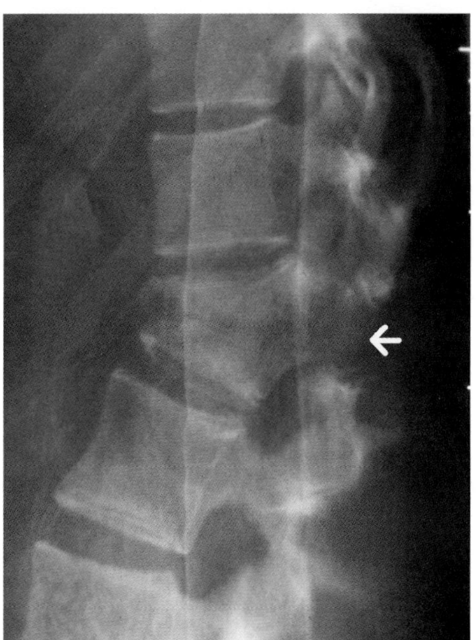

Figure 30.38 A bony Chance fracture at the thoracolumbar junction (arrow) secondary to a lap-belt injury.

are flexion–distraction injuries of the thoracolumbar junction and are classically associated with the use of lap belts (*Figure 30.38*). Duodenal, pancreatic and/or aortic ruptures are also associated with these injuries.

Lumbar spinal fractures (L3-S1)

Most fractures of the lower lumbar spine can be treated non-surgically because the incidence of neurological injury is lower. The neural canal is more capacious at this level (the spinal cord terminates at L1/L2). Owing to the lumbar lordosis, patients with these injuries are less likely to develop a kyphotic deformity than those with injuries at the thoracolumbar junction.

Summary box 30.7

Thoracic and thoracolumbar fractures

- Unstable thoracic spine fractures and thoracolumbar flexion–distraction injuries are commonly associated with vascular and/or visceral injuries

EPIDEMIOLOGY OF SPINAL CORD INJURY

The incidence and causation of spinal cord injury vary globally and reflect the demographics and industrialisation of society. Every year, around the world, between 250 000 and 500 000 people suffer a spinal cord injury according to the World Health Organization in 2013. Road traffic accidents remain the leading cause of spinal cord injuries worldwide. Men in the third decade of life are the most likely group to sustain serious spinal cord injury.

EVOLUTION OF THE MANAGEMENT OF SPINAL CORD INJURY

The development of specialised spinal cord injury centres has dramatically improved the survival rates, health and functional outcomes of individuals with spinal cord injury. The first spinal cord injury centre was established in the USA in 1936 by Dr Donald Munro. In 1944 The National Spinal Injuries Centre was established at Stoke Mandeville, UK, by Sir Ludwig Guttmann.

Summary box 30.8

Spinal cord injury

- The incidence of spinal cord injury remains constant
- The outcome is improved in regional/national spinal cord injury centres

PATHOPHYSIOLOGY OF SPINAL CORD INJURY

The primary injury

This is the direct insult to the neural elements and occurs at the time of the initial injury.

The secondary injury

Haemorrhage, oedema and ischaemia result in a biochemical cascade that causes the secondary injury. This may be accentuated by hypotension, hypoxia, spinal instability and/or persistent compression of the neural elements. Management of spinal cord injury must focus on minimising secondary injury.

Summary box 30.9

Pathophysiology of spinal cord injury

- The spinal cord contains various tracts that are topographically arranged
- Spinal cord injury involves both primary and secondary phases
- Therapeutic strategies are directed at reducing the secondary injury

Identification of shock

Three categories of shock may occur in spinal trauma

- **Hypovolaemic shock**. Hypotension with tachycardia and cold clammy peripheries. This is most often due to haemorrhage. It should be treated with appropriate resuscitation.
- **Neurogenic shock**. This presents with hypotension, a normal heart rate or bradycardia and warm peripheries. This is due to unopposed vagal tone resulting from cervical spinal cord injury at or above the level of sympathetic outflow (T5). It should be treated with inotropic support, and care should be taken to avoid fluid overload.
- **Spinal shock**. Spinal shock is a temporary physiological disorganisation of spinal cord function that starts within minutes following the injury. The length of effect is variable, but it can last 6 weeks or longer. It is characterised by paralysis, decreased tone and hyporeflexia. Once it has resolved the bulbocavernosus reflex (*Figure 30.39*) returns.

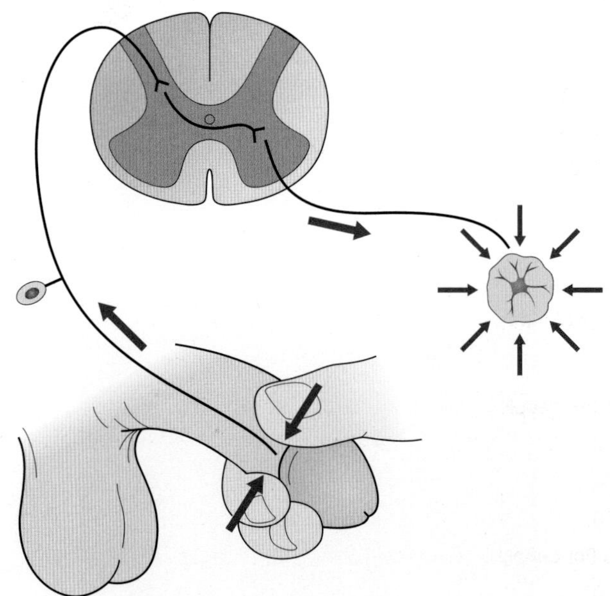

Figure 30.39 The bulbocavernosus reflex (this can be elicited in females by traction on the Foley catheter).

Donald Munro, 1889–1973, established the first spinal cord unit in the USA at the Boston City Hospital, Boston, MD, USA.
Sir Ludwig Guttmann, 1899–1980, considered by many to be the father of spinal cord medicine. He was a leading neurosurgeon in Germany, working at the Jewish Hospital in Breslau. He fled to England in 1939.
Frederic Eugene Basil Foley, 1891–1966, urologist, Ancker Hospital, St Paul, MN, USA.

Level of neurological injury

The level of neurological injury is simply the most caudal neurological level with normal neurological function.

Complete versus incomplete spinal cord injury

A spinal cord injury is incomplete when there is preservation of perianal sensation.

Types of incomplete spinal cord injury

There are several types of incomplete spinal cord injuries.

These include:

- central cord syndrome;
- Brown-Séquard syndrome (hemisection);
- anterior spinal syndrome;
- posterior cord syndrome;
- cauda equina syndrome.

REHABILITATION AND PATIENT OUTCOME

The goal of spinal cord injury rehabilitation is based on a multidisciplinary approach. There is a focus on goal-setting, maximising remaining neurological function and reintegration into employment and society. The level of neurological impairment determines the functional outcome (*Table 30.1*).

Prognosis of spinal cord injury

Despite continuing improvements in patient care, life expectancy remains below normal following spinal cord injury. The median life expectancy is 33 years, but varies considerably (*Table 30.2*).

The prognosis for neurological recovery is strongly influenced by factors such as the level and completeness of the injury, ventilator dependence and the age at presentation.

TABLE 30.1 Expected functional outcome versus level of cervical spinal cord injury.

Level of injury	Functional goal
C3–C4	Power wheelchair with mouth or chin control. Verbalise care, communicate through adaptive equipment. May be ventilator dependent
C5	Power wheelchair, dress upper body, self-feed with aids, wash face with assistance
C6	Propel power wheelchair, possibly push manual wheelchair, transfer with assistance, dress upper body (lower body with assistance), self-groom with aids, bladder/bowel care with assistance, self-feed with splints, able to drive
C7	Manual wheelchair, independent transfer, dressing (with aids), feeding, bathing, self-care. Bladder and bowel care with assistance
C8–T4	Independent with most activities of daily living, and bowel and bladder care
T5–T12	As above but with more ease. Independent with all self-care
L1–L5	Independent. Walk with short or long leg braces
S1–S5	Independent, able to walk if able to push off (S1) (may need brace). Bladder, bowel and sexual function may remain compromised

TABLE 30.2 Life expectancy (years) post injury by severity of injury and age at injury.

Age at injury	No SCI	Motor functional at any level	Paraplegic	Low tetraplegic (C5–C8)	High tetraplegic (C1–C4)	Ventilator dependent at any level
a For people who survive the first 24 hours						
20	58.4	52.8	45.6	40.6	36.1	16.6
40	39.5	34.3	28.0	23.8	20.2	7.1
60	22.2	17.9	13.1	10.2	7.9	1.4
b For people surviving at least 1 year post injury						
20	58.4	53.3	46.3	41.7	37.9	23.3
40	39.5	34.8	28.6	24.7	21.6	11.1
60	22.2	18.3	13.5	10.8	8.8	3.1

SCI, spinal cord injury.

Charles Edward Brown-Séquard, 1817–1894, physiologist and neurologist who held a number of academic posts, among them Physician, the National Hospital for Nervous Diseases, London, UK (1860–1864), Professor of Medicine at Harvard University, Boston, MA, USA (1864–1878), and at the Collège de France, Paris, France (1878–1894). He described his syndrome in 1851.

Complications associated with spinal cord injury

Pressure ulcers

Many are preventable. Patients should be turned regularly on an appropriate mattress to minimise the risk of skin breakdown.

Pain and spasticity

Neurogenic pain is common. Once reflex activity returns following cord injury, spasticity may occur and can be problematic. Intrathecal infusion of baclofen may be required in resistant cases.

Autonomic dysreflexia

This is a paroxysmal syndrome of hypertension, hyperhidrosis (above the level of injury), bradycardia, flushing and headache in response to noxious visceral and other stimuli. It is most commonly triggered by bladder distension or rectal loading from faecal impaction.

Neurological deterioration

Post-traumatic syringomyelia may occur in around 28% of patients with spinal cord injury up to 30 years following injury. Approximately 30% of cases are symptomatic. Clinically, patients present with segmental pain at or above the level of injury, sensory loss, progressive asymmetrical weakness or increased spasticity. This warrants early MRI assessment. Expanding cavities require neurosurgical intervention.

Thromboembolic events

Deep vein thrombosis occurs in 30% of patients with spinal cord injury. Fatal pulmonary embolus is reported in 1–2% of cases. Thromboprophylaxis with compression stockings and low-molecular-weight heparin is indicated, provided there are no contraindications.

Osteoporosis, heterotopic ossification and contractures

Disuse osteoporosis is an inevitable consequence of spinal cord injury and fragility fractures may occur. Heterotopic ossification may affect the hips, knees, shoulders and elbows. It occurs in 25% of patients with spinal cord injury. Surgery is appropriate in selected cases. Soft-tissue contractures around joints may occur as a result of spasticity but can be avoided by appropriate physical therapy, positioning and splinting.

FURTHER READING

American Spinal Injury Association. *International standards for neurological classification of SCI (ISNCSCI) worksheet.* Available from https://asia-spinalinjury.org/international-standards-neurological-classification-sci-isncsci-worksheet/ (accessed July 2022).

Bridwell KH, DeWald RL (eds). *The textbook of spinal surgery*, 4th edn. Philadelphia, PA: Lippincott Williams and Wilkins, 2020.

British Orthopaedic Association. *British Orthopaedic Association standards for trauma: the management of traumatic spinal cord injury*. London: British Orthopaedic Association, 2014.

Cotler JM, Simson MJ, An HS *et al.* (eds). *Surgery of spinal trauma.* Philadelphia, PA: Lippincott Williams and Wilkins, 2000.

Denis F. The three column spine and its significance in the classification of acute thoracolumbar spinal injuries. *Spine* 1983; **8**(8): 817–31.

Dimar JR. Early versus late stabilisation of the spine in the polytrauma patient. *Spine* 2010; **35**(21S): S187–92.

Fehlings MG. *Essentials of spinal cord injury. Basic research to clinical practice.* Stuttgart: Thieme, 2013.

Fehlings MG, Tetreault LA, Wilson JR *et al.* A clinical practice guideline for the management of acute spinal cord injury: introduction, rationale, and scope. *Global Spine J* 2017; **7**(3 Suppl): 84S–94S.

National Institute for Health and Care Excellence. *Spinal injury: assessment and initial management.* NICE Guideline NG41. London: NICE, 2016. Available from https://www.nice.org.uk/guidance/ng41.

Vaccaro AR, Andersson G. Spine trauma focus edition. *Spine* 2006; **31**(11S): S1–104.

CHAPTER

31 Maxillofacial trauma

Learning objectives

- To understand and identify potentially life-threatening injuries to the face, head and neck
- To safely perform a systematic examination of facial injuries, and describe the basic classification of soft-tissue and bony injuries
- To describe the principles of management of facial soft-tissue injuries
- To understand and describe the principles of management of fractures of various facial bones, and appreciate the initial management of dental injuries

EMERGENCY ASSESSMENT AND MANAGEMENT

Maxillofacial injuries that require hospital attendance are common and are most frequently related to trips and falls, road traffic accidents (RTAs), taking part in sports and interpersonal violence. Initial assessment requires a focused history of the mechanism of injury and a general medical and social history, followed by clinical examination. An injury to the body including facial trauma must be managed with an immediate assessment of the airway, breathing and circulation (ABC) in line with the established Advanced Trauma Life Support (ATLS) guidelines. Any visible object obstructing the airway should be removed if possible, and, if indicated, direct pressure should be applied to bleeding points. If the patient has midface bleeding where direct pressure cannot be applied, the conscious patient may sit forwards or be placed on their side in the standard recovery position to minimise the risk of blood obstructing the airway. Care should be exercised if there are concerns of concurrent spinal injury.

In severe injury to the midface skeleton, the maxilla can become detached from the skull base and displaced downwards and backwards (*Figure 31.1*). The patient may present with acute airway compromise if the midface impaction is also combined with a bilateral mandibular fracture, which can displace the tongue backwards. Such injuries are often associated with significant oedema of the soft palate and tongue (*Figure 31.2*). In these situations, the team must be prepared to undertake an endotracheal intubation, a needle cricothyroidotomy or an emergency surgical airway procedure if intubation proves difficult. There are certain techniques that can be used immediately to relieve airway compromise, while preparations are made for definitive airway management. In the obtunded or unconscious patient, the maxilla can be disimpacted and pulled forwards using fingers. The tongue can be pulled and held forwards, with a large suture or a towel clip, to help open up the airway. High-volume suction must be readily available to clear the blood as well as tooth fragments and debris from the oral cavity and upper aerodigestive tract.

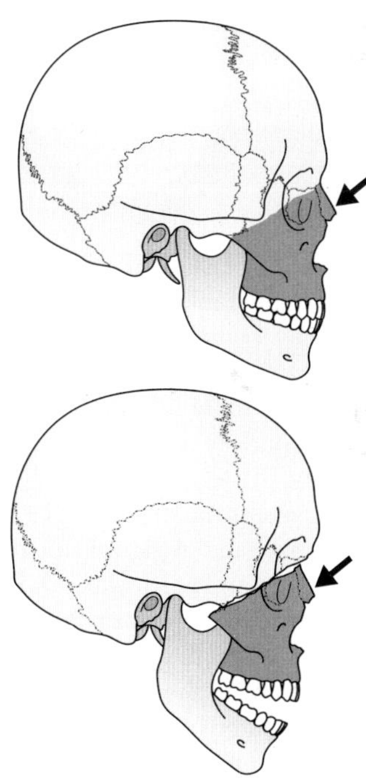

Figure 31.1 A severe blow to the midface may detach the facial skeleton from the base of the skull and push it downwards and backwards.

Torrential life-threatening haemorrhage may be seen in facial trauma that involves large soft-tissue lacerations, penetrating neck injuries or ballistic injuries. The source of such bleeding is likely to be from injury to the maxillary artery or pterygoid venous plexus in the grossly damaged midface, or branches of the external carotid artery or tributaries of the internal jugular vein in penetrating injuries of the neck. The management of severe bleeding may require application of

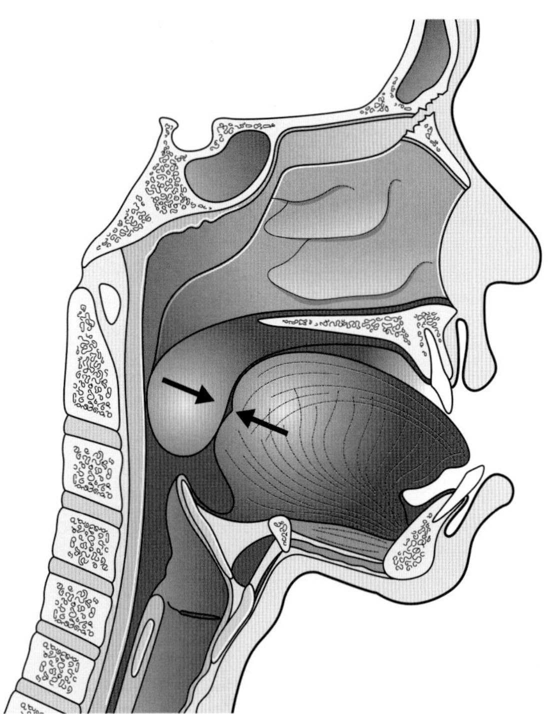

Figure 31.2 Loss of pharyngeal space secondary to oedema of the soft palate and the posteriorly displaced tongue may restrict the airway.

direct digital pressure or placement of anterior and posterior nasal packs. Specific inflatable balloon nasal packs or Foley urinary catheters may be utilised to exert pressure on the bleeding points. An endotracheal intubation or a surgical airway may be required if there is concern regarding extensive soft-tissue swelling secondary to injury or surgical intervention (*Figure 31.3*).

It is important to assess the maxillofacial patient for severe head injury that can result in significant cerebral damage. Patients with facial injury and particularly those with injury due to interpersonal violence are frequently intoxicated because of alcohol or drug abuse, which may mask the symptoms of head injury. Therefore, clinicians should have a low threshold for requesting a brain computed tomography (CT) scan to exclude significant intracranial injury. In such cases, it is prudent to include the facial bones in the CT request if indicated. Injuries to the midface are frequently associated with orbital damage, which can lead to loss of sight if not dealt with urgently. Retrobulbar haemorrhage, which can cause acute compression of the optic nerve if not treated immediately, may lead to loss of vision (see *Orbital fractures*).

Summary box 31.1

Emergency assessment and management

- Immediate management must include assessment of ABC with cervical spine protection, following which a more detailed assessment should ensue
- Life- and sight-threatening facial injuries should be treated immediately
- The clinical team should be prepared for endotracheal intubation or, if required, a surgical airway

CLASSIFICATION OF FACIAL INJURIES

Bony injury

Maxillofacial bone fractures can be divided into several types: simple (isolated single), compound (communicates through the skin or oral/nasal mucosal surfaces), comminuted (multiple fragments), complicated (with neurological or vascular injury), greenstick (includes single cortex) and pathological (through an existing lesion such as neoplastic or inflammatory). Fractures can be further classified into undisplaced, minimally displaced or displaced.

The facial skeleton can be divided vertically into thirds using horizontal lines: upper face (from the level of the canthi upwards), midface (from the maxillary teeth to the canthi) and lower face (mandible and mandibular teeth). The midface can be further divided into central and lateral, with the naso-orbital–ethmoidal complex forming the central and the zygomaticomaxillary complex forming the lateral components. Orbital (eye socket) fractures can occur in isolation or in combination with other fractures. Orbital fractures can be classified into orbital floor, medial and/or lateral walls and the roof of the orbit.

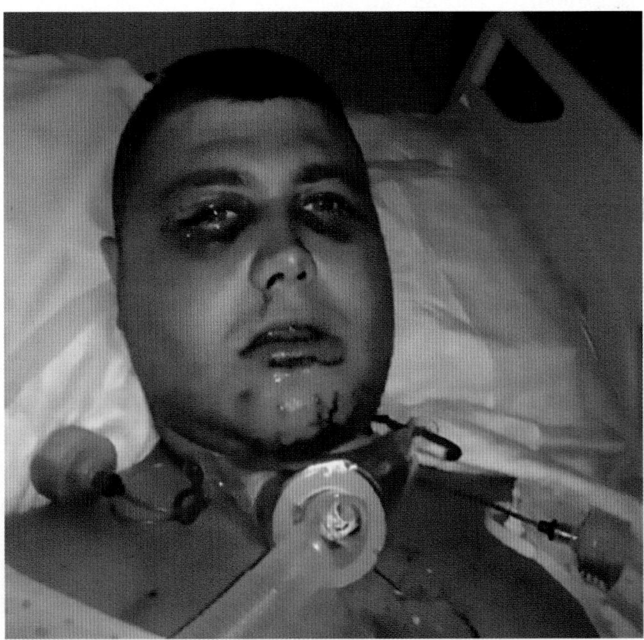

Figure 31.3 Tracheostomy *in situ* perioperatively to protect the airway in a patient with extensive facial fractures secondary to a road traffic accident.

Frederic Eugene Basil Foley, 1891–1966, urologist, Ancker Hospital, St Paul, MN, USA.

Skull fractures including frontal and ethmoidal sinuses, in combination with facial fractures, are termed craniofacial fractures. A joint neurosurgical and maxillofacial approach is necessary in these cases because of the possibility of intracranial injury. Frontal sinus fractures are classified into those involving the anterior or posterior table, with or without damage to the frontonasal duct.

The most severe facial fractures involving bony injury at all levels of the facial skeleton are referred to as panfacial fractures. These usually imply that a significant degree of force has been involved, suggesting significant other injuries such as head, abdominal or chest injuries.

Soft-tissue injury

Lacerations are a result of crushing injuries where the soft tissues are compressed onto the underlying bone, usually by a blunt object. Sharp implements, such as a knife or glass, cause incised wounds. Any soft-tissue injury can present with or without tissue loss. Where the injury results in a communication between the skin and the mucosa of the oral or nasal cavity, the wound is termed 'through and through'. The soft-tissue injury may present with or without damage to the underlying bony structure.

Summary box 31.2

Classification of facial injuries

- There are multiple ways of classifying facial fractures, the simplest way is to divide the face into thirds and describe the specific bone involved
- Assess orbit independently
- Assess soft-tissue injury in terms of loss of tissue and damage to the underlying bone

CLINICAL ASSESSMENT

History

The history should include the mechanism of injury, past medical history and the postinjury events; it should be obtained directly from the patient and from witnesses and the first responding emergency services if required. Knowledge of the mechanism of injury will often help to identify potential occult injuries that may not be readily detectable on first inspection. Factors such as sharp or blunt trauma, wound contamination and energy transfer should be assessed and recorded. The medical history should gain information to indicate the general fitness of the patient for potential treatment under general anaesthesia. It is important to obtain previous tetanus vaccination history, and the vaccine should be given promptly if there is a high risk of contamination.

Examination

Primary survey

The primary survey is aimed at protection of the airway, control of bleeding, restoration and maintenance of the circulation and assessment for neurological deficits, including the Glasgow Coma Scale (GCS) score, with cervical spine control.

The head and neck region should be inspected, with wounds assessed for skin or soft-tissue loss and subsequently dressed appropriately to control any bleeding. The wound size, location and depth should be carefully recorded. Large and obvious foreign bodies should be removed but care should be exercised with penetrating wounds involving large fragments or blades, which can potentially penetrate important deep structures. These should be removed in the operating theatre, under more controlled conditions, after appropriate imaging.

Secondary survey

The secondary survey examination should be conducted in a systematic way, preferably following a top-down approach carefully examining all structures, recording obvious as well as less conspicuous injuries. The surface inspection should include the scalp, posterior neck and ears and then move to the frontal view. A brief cranial nerve examination should be undertaken as guided by the injury site. Particular attention must be paid to cervical spine examination as the patient with facial injury may have concurrent spinal injury, which may have been missed in the primary assessment.

Examination of the eyes should include visualisation of the periorbital tissues and assessment of globe position, visual acuity, diplopia (double vision), intercanthal distance and eye motility. This examination may be difficult if the eyelids are swollen and the eyes are shut. However, such an examination is crucial as inadequate examination may lead to a delay in the diagnosis of serious eye injury that may need urgent intervention to prevent blindness. Examination is possible even in the most swollen of eyes by gently pulling the eyelids apart with dry gauze, a cotton bud/roll or a microbiology swab stick. Gentle pressure on the eyelid for a brief period may reduce oedema, which may facilitate the opening of the eyelids. It may be helpful to ask a colleague to perform the eye examination if one is holding the eyelids apart to facilitate examination.

The facial bones should be palpated for signs of fractures, which may include step deformity, tenderness or bony asymmetry. A systematic approach would include palpation of the supraorbital ridge followed by the lateral orbital wall, inferior orbital rim, zygomatic bone, nasal bones, temporomandibular joint and the rest of the mandible on both sides.

The examination of the oral cavity should include inspection for any soft-tissue lacerations, bruising, haematoma, injury to dentition and assessment of occlusion (bite). Any blood and excessive secretions should be suctioned and a good light source used to facilitate thorough examination. The teeth should be examined and their presence or absence noted. Teeth may be knocked out completely (avulsed), displaced but still attached to soft tissues and/or bone (luxated) or fractured. It is important to account for all missing teeth or tooth fragments as aspiration is a major risk for developing chest infection. If it is unclear about the location of missing teeth, a chest radiograph should be considered.

A key feature of displaced mandibular or maxillary fractures is altered occlusion. The patient may be able to detect even a tiny alteration in their occlusion. If there is a fracture of the mandible, the overlying mucosa is often torn and there

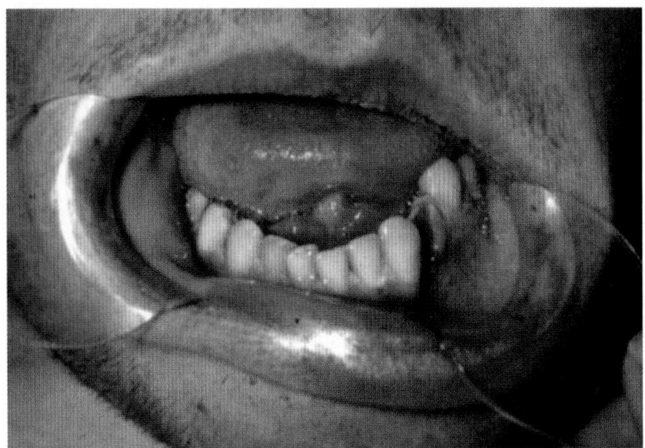

Figure 31.4 Left parasymphyseal fracture of the mandible demonstrating a step deformity that could be confused with a missing tooth in inexperienced eyes.

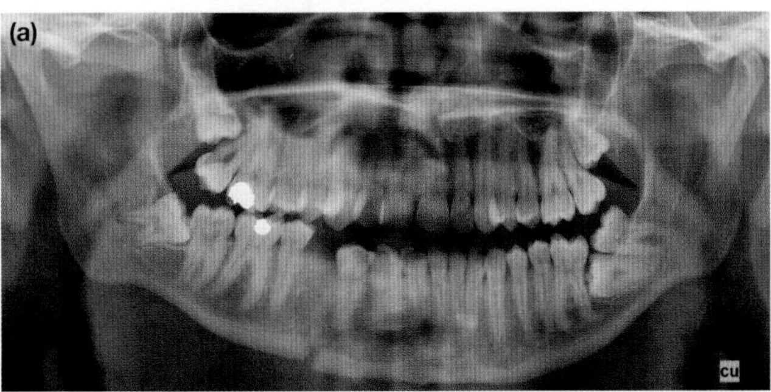

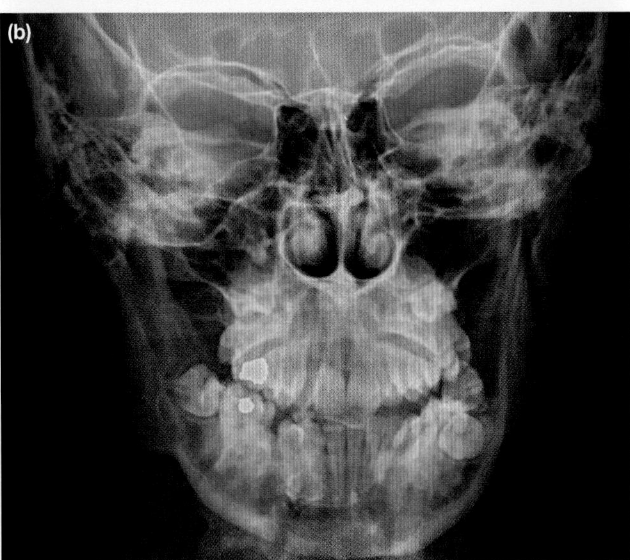

Figure 31.5 (a) Orthopantomogram (OPT) demonstrating a right mandibular body and left condylar fracture. (b) A posteroanterior mandible radiograph reveals the left low condylar fracture more clearly, which may not be as obvious as in the OPT to an inexperienced clinician.

may be an associated haematoma in the floor of the mouth (*Figure 31.4*). If the mandibular fracture is grossly displaced, the patient may have altered sensation in the region of the lip and chin, due to damage to the inferior alveolar nerve running along the canal within the mandible and involvement of the mental nerve, a sensory branch, which emerges from the mental foramen.

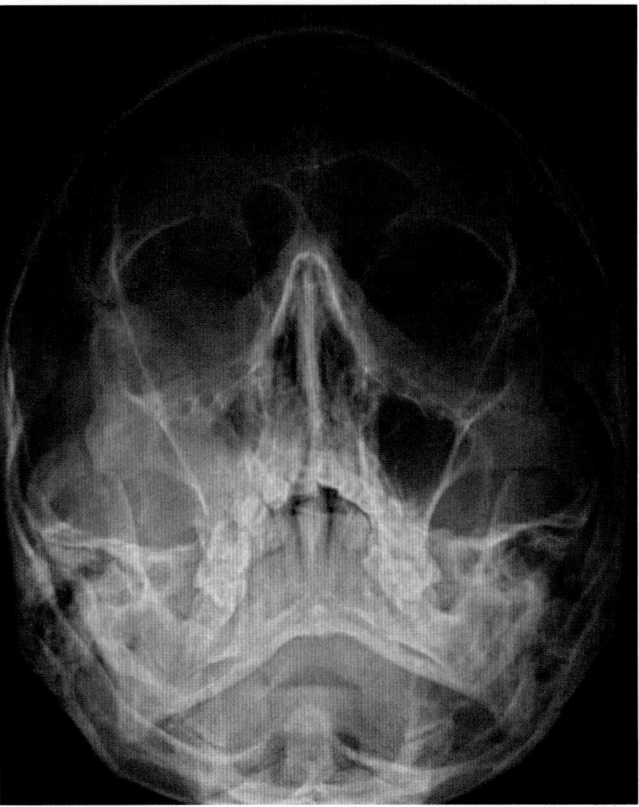

Figure 31.6 Occipitomental radiograph demonstrating a right zygomatic fracture. Note the right maxillary sinus opacification, which is one of the radiological hallmarks of zygomatic fracture due to collection of fluid in the sinus.

Investigations

The nature of the injury sustained will determine the specific investigations required to facilitate diagnosis. Systemic investigations may include routine haematology and biochemistry investigations, and imaging requests such as cervical spine, chest, abdominal or limb radiographs depending on the site of injury.

If a mandibular fracture is suspected, an orthopantomogram (OPT) and a posteroanterior (PA) radiograph of the mandible should be obtained (*Figure 31.5*). It is extremely important to have two views at right angles to each other to avoid missing any fractures. Very occasionally a lateral mandibular view may have to be utilised as a screening radiograph if the patient is unable to cooperate for the OPT (e.g. patients with dementia). For a suspected midface fracture, occipitomental (OM) radiographs at 10° and 30° should be obtained (*Figure 31.6*). A CT of the facial bones would be more suitable if an orbital fracture is suspected or in the case of a high-impact injury; this will provide the gold standard detail of bony structures and, as previously mentioned, should include the brain if there is any suggestion of a head injury. A three-dimensional (3D) reformatting of the CT scan allows for excellent visualisation of the maxillofacial bony structures.

Summary box 31.3

History, examination and investigation

- A detailed history of the mechanism of injury is crucial in any initial assessment
- A systematic approach should be adopted in examination of the craniomaxillofacial structures; a top-down approach is recommended
- The most common radiographs requested in facial fracture investigation are OPT and PA mandible for mandibular fractures, and OM facial views for midface fractures

SPECIFIC INJURIES

Soft-tissue injuries

Lacerations

Soft-tissue injuries of the face are a result of blunt or sharp trauma and should be carefully examined to exclude any associated nerve, parotid duct or underlying bony injury (***Figure 31.7***). These can mostly be repaired under local anaesthesia (LA) and should be treated within 24 hours of injury to avoid poor healing and an unsightly scar. Lacerations in uncooperative children and large contaminated wounds in adults usually require repair under general anaesthesia (GA). Uncomplicated wounds with no tissue loss should be cleaned and closed in layers. If the skin is contaminated with dirt, it should be gently scrubbed with a soft brush to prevent dirt tattoo. Facial skin has a rich blood supply, which contributes to its excellent healing; therefore, wounds should only be debrided of frankly necrotic tissue.

Intraoral wounds heal very well; if small, they can be left to heal by secondary intention, especially in children to avoid treatment under GA. Resorbable 3-0 or 4-0 sutures are placed intraorally and for the deep layers of the skin. The most superficial skin layer should be closed with a 5-0 non-resorbable monofilament suture, except in potentially uncooperative children when 5-0 or 6-0 resorbable sutures can be used. Some surgeons also use resorbable 5-0 or 6-0 skin sutures in adults. For some small superficial clean incised wounds, cyanoacrylate tissue glue can be utilised. This must be avoided in periocular skin because of the risk of spillage into the eye, which can lead to severe corneal damage.

Lacerations involving the eyelid margins and those crossing the vermilion border of the lip need special attention to avoid poor approximation of the skin edges, which can result in a poor cosmetic outcome. If there is tissue loss, adjacent skin can be undermined and mobilised to achieve primary closure, but incisions for local flaps or skin grafts should be avoided in the initial management. Very large areas of tissue loss may require free flap reconstruction if local tissue flaps are inadequate for resurfacing the defect.

Facial nerve

Facial nerve function should be routinely assessed in all facial lacerations. Any nerve injuries are best repaired primarily under high magnification and GA. In general, nerve injuries that lie lateral to the line drawn vertically down from lateral canthus of the eye are repairable, and this should be attempted. A nerve stimulator or monitor may be helpful in identifying the transected nerve ends.

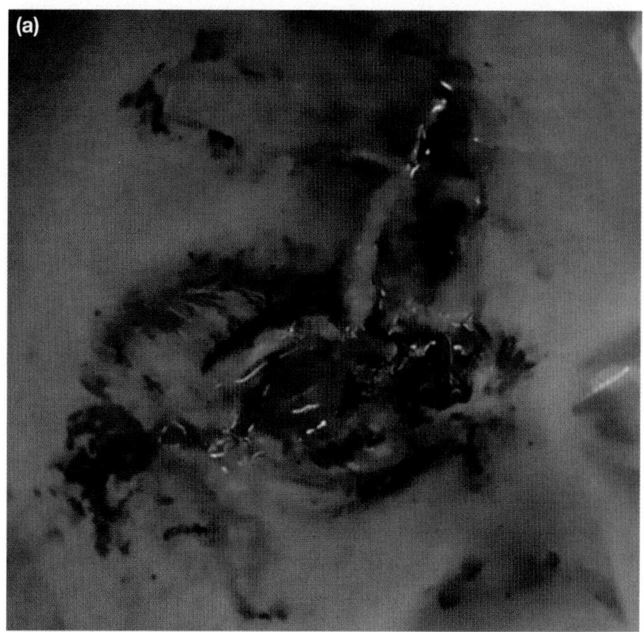

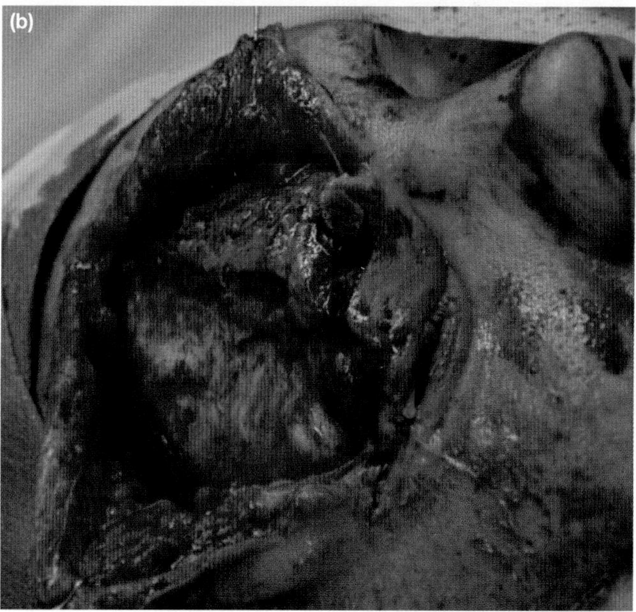

Figure 31.7 (a, b) Extensive soft-tissue laceration, the full extent of which may only be revealed on careful examination. Corneal protection *in situ*.

Parotid duct

The middle third of a line drawn from the tragus of the ear to the midpoint between the upper lip and the alar base represents the surface landmarking of the parotid duct. A careful examination of the wound may reveal saliva leak in the case of a duct injury. Methylene blue solution can be injected through the parotid duct opening intraorally (adjacent to the upper molar teeth) and any leak assessed in the wound bed. The repair is best achieved under high magnification, over a cannula inserted through the duct opening under GA. The buccal branch of the facial nerve that closely follows the duct may also get transected in the injury; this requires careful examination.

Animal and human bites

Facial bites should be cleaned thoroughly and closed primarily in layers. Because of the high risk of wound infection, antibiotics must be prescribed according to local microbiology guidelines. With human bites, consideration should be given to testing the patient for human immunodeficiency virus (HIV) infection, and hepatitis serology is also sensible, if the patient is deemed to be at high risk of being infected as a result of the bite. If there is significant tissue loss, a staged reconstruction may be required.

Summary box 31.4

Soft-tissue injuries

- Examination of the function of both motor and sensory nerves should be conducted prior to the administration of LA
- All animal and human bites must be covered with prophylactic antibiotics
- Tissue loss may require staged reconstruction

Mandibular fractures

Fractures of the mandible are common in the context of facial injury and may frequently involve multiple sites. The commonest fracture patterns are parasymphysis and angle fractures, or parasymphysis and condylar fractures (contralateral sites in both cases). The specific sites in the mandible most prone to fractures are shown in ***Figure 31.8***. It is very important to record the presence or absence of any paraesthesia in the region of the lower lip and chin, which may be the result of damage to the inferior alveolar nerve.

Most displaced mandibular fractures are treated with antibiotics on admission followed by open reduction and internal fixation (ORIF). Typically, titanium miniplates and screws are placed (***Figure 31.9***) under GA with two or three postoperative intravenous antibiotic doses given. Undisplaced fractures may be treated conservatively; this may include antibiotics, analgesia and a soft diet for 4 weeks. These patients need to be monitored closely to exclude failure of conservative management, which will commonly be indicated by increasing pain and a change in occlusion. In general, facial bones heal well after about 4 weeks. Occasionally, if the fractures are severely comminuted and difficult to fix with titanium plates, intermaxillary fixation (IMF) with wires can be considered; however, this is becoming exceedingly rare owing to the advances in osteosynthesis fixation techniques.

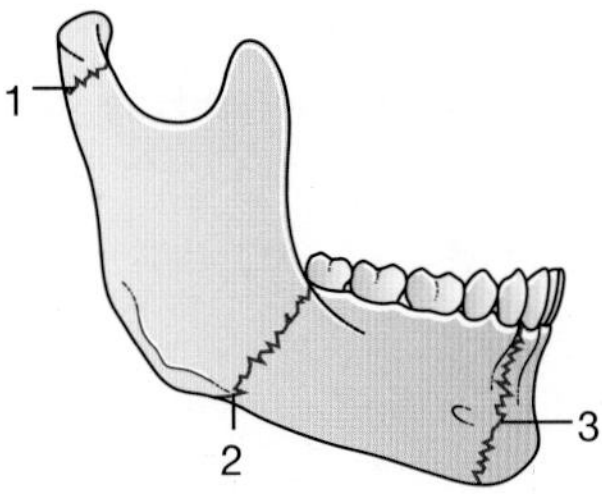

Figure 31.8 Fractures of the mandible. (1) The neck of the condyle is the most common site, followed by (2) the angle of the mandible. (3) The third point of weakness is in the region of the mental foramen.

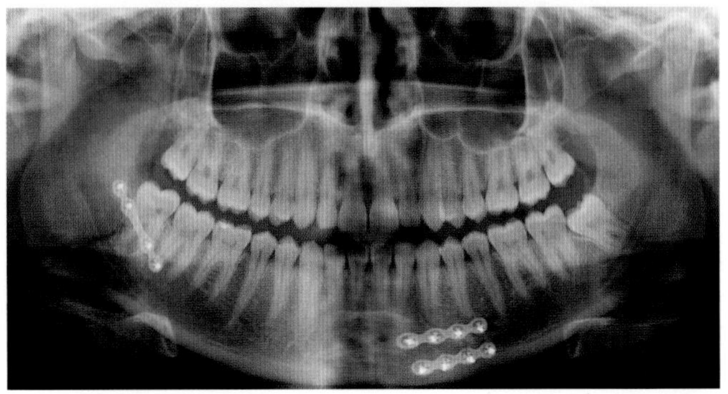

Figure 31.9 Postoperative orthopantomogram demonstrating fixation of a right angle and left parasymphyseal fracture with miniplates and screws.

Simple mandibular fractures treated with the ORIF technique should have two 2-mm-diameter screws on either side of the fracture, engaging a single bone cortex (monocortical). These small plates are load sharing, which indicates that the fractures are reduced and load is shared between the bone and the plate. With more complex or comminuted fractures, heavy profile reconstruction plates and bicortical screws may be placed as a load-bearing fixation technique. In general, different mandibular sites determine the number of miniplates used; for example, a single plate is placed along the line of maximal tension for angle and body of mandible fractures, while two plates are placed 5 mm apart for parasymphyseal fractures to resist the torsional forces of the anterior mandible musculature. A transbuccal approach through a tiny incision in the cheek skin is frequently utilised for angle fractures to allow placement of screws perpendicular to the plate and the bone.

Most condylar fractures can be treated with closed reduction with IMF elastic guidance and a strict soft diet and analgesic regimen. However, displaced condylar neck fractures with significant loss of mandibular height are increasingly treated with ORIF techniques. Various approaches can be adopted depending on the condylar fracture location, although the most common approach is transparotid access with a retromandibular incision. There have been some advances towards endoscopic-assisted fixation of the condylar fractures in some maxillofacial units.

The optimal timing for the repair of a mandibular fracture is within 24–48 hours post injury. For a heavily displaced fracture where there is likely to be delay in taking the patient to theatre, a bridal wire that goes around the teeth to temporarily reduce the fractures may be useful in alleviating pain and facilitating oral intake.

Summary box 31.5

Mandibular fractures

- Always look for a second mandibular fracture as contralateral fractures are common
- It is important to record the presence or absence of paraesthesia in the distribution of the mental nerve
- Most mandibular fractures are treated with ORIF using titanium miniplates and screw fixation, ideally within 24–48 hours of injury

Zygomatic fractures

Zygomatic (cheek/malar) bone fractures are often the result of blunt trauma to the midface, such as from a fist. From a clinical perspective, it is helpful to consider the zygomatic bone as a four-legged stool, as shown in *Figure 31.10*. The four legs comprise the zygomatic arch running anteroposteriorly, the zygomatic process running vertically to join the frontozygomatic (FZ) process of the frontal bone at the FZ suture, the infraorbital rim running horizontally and the maxillary buttress running vertically. Zygomatic fractures may include isolated or multiple fracture lines involving any of these legs, often in combination with orbital wall fracture.

Zygomatic fractures may be difficult to assess in the presence of significant facial swelling; therefore, patients are usually reviewed in clinic 1 week after injury to allow the swelling to subside. There may be periorbital swelling and bruising, step deformity and frequently a subconjunctival haemorrhage with no posterior border or limit (*Figure 31.11*). A concomitant orbital bone fracture also needs to be excluded; if suspected, a CT scan to include the orbits should be obtained.

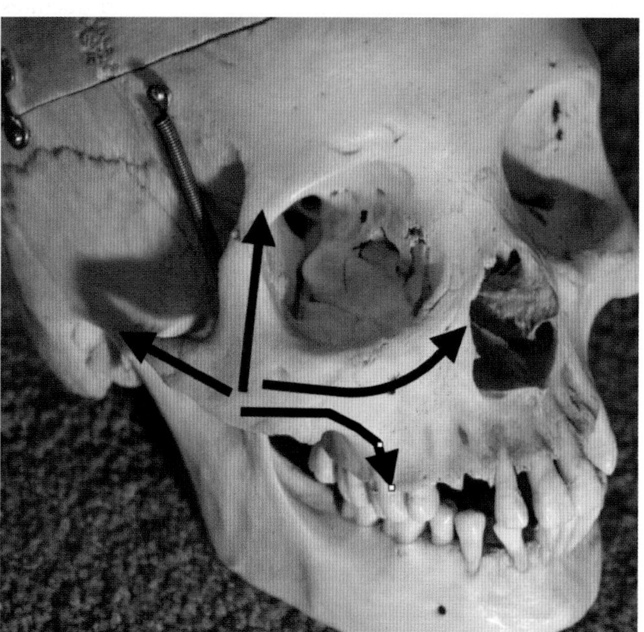

Figure 31.10 The 'four legs of the stool'.

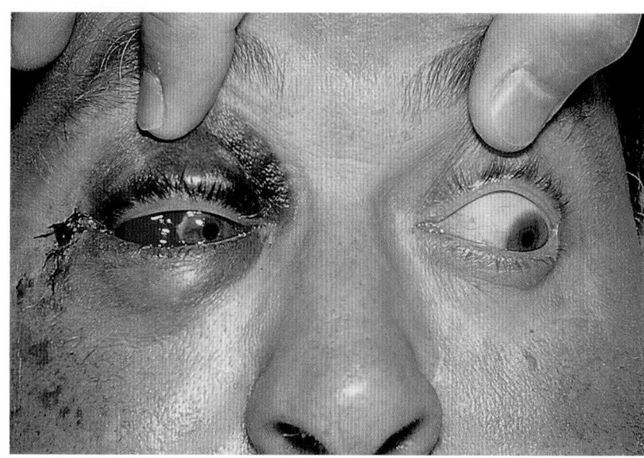

Figure 31.11 Fractures of the zygoma may often be associated with periorbital swelling and subconjunctival haemorrhage without a posterior border or limit.

Undisplaced or minimally displaced zygomatic fractures are often treated conservatively, with patients being told to avoid any excessive pressure on the affected side for a minimum of 3 weeks. The indications for surgical intervention include asymmetrical cheek bone prominence, persistent eye symptoms such as diplopia, orbital deformity and restricted mouth opening due to impingement of the coronoid process by the bone fragment.

There are a variety of transcutaneous (including upper and lower lid) and intraoral surgical approaches for access, determined by the exact location of the fracture. The isolated zygomatic fracture is often reduced by a closed technique involving an incision in the temple (Gillies' lift) or intraorally (Keen's technique). The ORIF of FZ suture fractures and infraorbital rim or maxillary buttress fractures usually includes low-profile 1.5-mm midface titanium plates and screws. The provision for single-, double-, triple- or four-point fixation of the zygomatic fracture is dependent on the stability of the fracture post reduction and the degree of bone comminution.

Summary box 31.6

Fractures of the zygomatic bone

- Fractures of the zygomatic bone often require follow-up 1 week after the injury for the swelling to subside to allow full assessment
- Orbital fractures may occur in combination with zygomatic fractures
- There are a variety of transcutaneous or intraoral surgical approaches that are determined by the exact location of the fracture

Sir Harold Delf Gillies, 1882–1960, born New Zealand, studied medicine at the University of Cambridge, Cambridge, UK, pioneer of plastic surgical techniques during and after the First World War.
William Williams Keen, 1837–1932, pioneer American neurological surgeon.

Maxillary bone fractures

Maxillary fractures are classified according to their anatomical level, as originally described by René Le Fort (***Figure 31.12***). Le Fort I involves a fracture line extending from the pterygoid plates through the lateral wall of the maxillary sinus and piriform aperture of the nose. Le Fort II involves the whole of the dentition-bearing portion of the maxilla and the nasal bones. The fracture line extends from the pterygoid plates to the inferior orbital rim and across the bridge of the nose. Le Fort III fracture essentially is where the whole of the midface is separated from the skull base. The fracture line runs from the pterygoid plates to the base of the zygomatic arch, the lateral walls of the orbit through the FZ suture and the nasal bridge.

The Le Fort classification is simple to describe, but the clinical presentation may not be as clear-cut as the fractures at these levels rarely occur in isolation. There may be significant

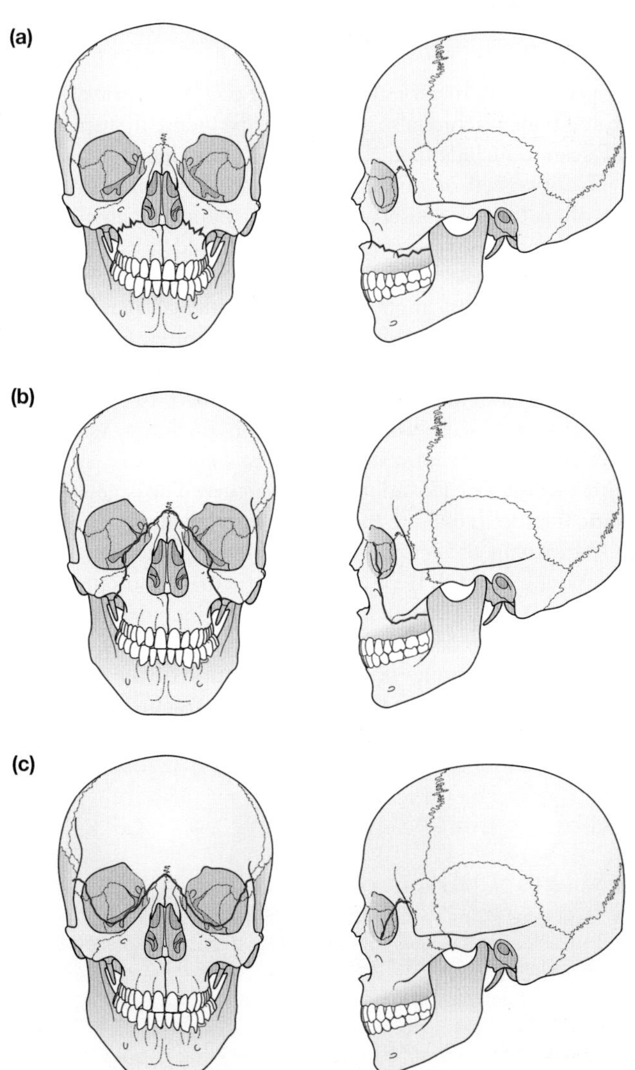

Figure 31.12 Maxillary fractures as classified by Le Fort. (a) Le Fort I; (b) Le Fort II; (c) Le Fort III.

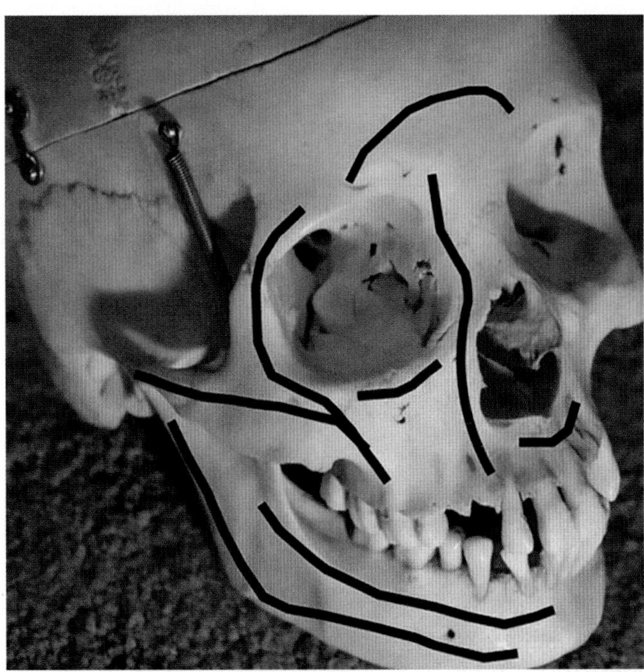

Figure 31.13 The buttresses of the facial bones. These are the strongest part of the facial skeleton and may help with fixation because of good bone quality.

commination owing to the thin composition of the maxillary bone as well as the differing pattern of fracture on two sides.

Undisplaced or minimally displaced factures are best treated conservatively with a soft diet and analgesia. The indications for ORIF include a mobile, unstable maxilla, deranged occlusion such as an anterior open bite and loss of facial projection and width resulting in obvious facial deformity. Fixation is achieved with midface 1.5-mm miniplates and screws, with various surgical approaches for access depending on the location of the fracture. Plates are usually placed along the main facial buttresses, which provide the optimal strength and bone quality to be able to hold the screws (***Figure 31.13***).

Summary box 31.7

Maxillary bone fractures

- Maxillary fractures occur at various levels, which may not follow the typically described Le Fort classification pattern owing to comminution and asymmetry of the fracture
- Maxillary fractures may be associated with significant bleeding (often from the pterygoid plexus), which may require packing of the nasal cavity

Orbital fractures

Orbital fractures may be isolated or more commonly occur in conjunction with zygomatic or maxillary complex fractures. They most frequently involve the orbital floor, followed by the medial wall, lateral wall or the roof, which may present in

René Le Fort, 1869–1951, French surgeon, classified facial fractures after macabre research in which he dropped rocks and other heavy objects onto the faces of cadavers.

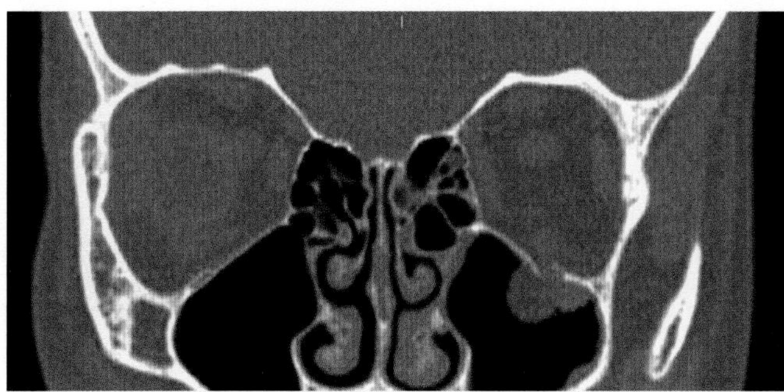

Figure 31.14 Coronal computed tomography (CT) scan demonstrating a left orbital blow-out fracture, with soft-tissue herniation into the maxillary antrum.

combination or as isolated injuries. Isolated orbital injuries are described as 'blow-out' or 'blow-in' fractures. An example of a blow-out fracture is shown in *Figure 31.14*.

Orbital floor fractures may lead to restricted upward gaze owing to trapping of orbital fat and fibrous septae resulting in diplopia on looking upwards. Occasionally, the inferior rectus or inferior oblique muscles may also be trapped. Inferior rectus muscle entrapment in children may present as the oculocardiac reflex: a triad of bradycardia, nausea and syncope. This needs to be treated as an emergency because irreversible damage related to muscle necrosis can occur within hours. In these cases, on imaging, the orbital floor may appear undisplaced or minimally displaced, which means that a trapdoor defect has opened and then closed again, entrapping the muscle. They are also described as a 'white eye' blow-out fracture as children often present with no subconjunctival haemorrhage (*Figure 31.15*). In addition to the restricted eye movement, orbital wall fractures can lead to changes in globe position, with inferior positioning of the globe (hypoglobus) or sinking in of the globe due to an increase in orbital volume (enophthalmos). These globe position changes may only become visible after the initial swelling has subsided; the true extent is only revealed 2–4 weeks after the injury.

The indications for surgical repair of orbital fractures include enophthalmos or persistent diplopia resulting from restricted eye motility as a result of extraocular muscle entrapment within the fracture line. It is important to seek orthoptic assessment; this is helpful in differentiating between muscle entrapment and muscle dysfunction (secondary to inflammation), both of which may cause diplopia. Diplopia secondary to muscle dysfunction is likely to resolve spontaneously with time. Repair of the orbital rim is usually accomplished with ORIF techniques and the orbital walls repaired with preformed or patient-specific titanium implants or less commonly autologous materials such as cranial bone grafts.

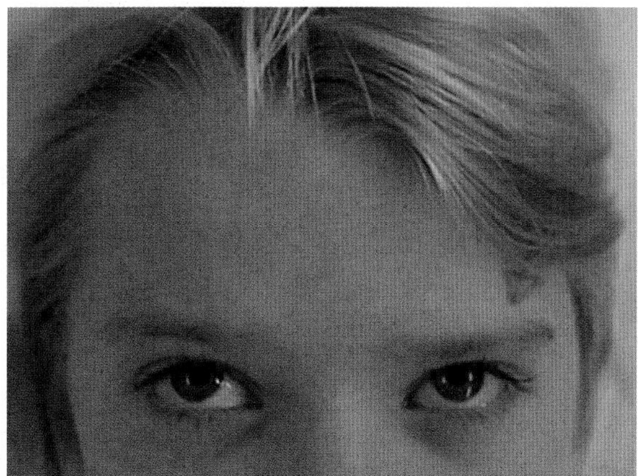

Figure 31.15 This 11-year-old boy presented with an oculocardiac reflex secondary to a 'white eye' blow-out left orbital floor fracture following a rugby injury.

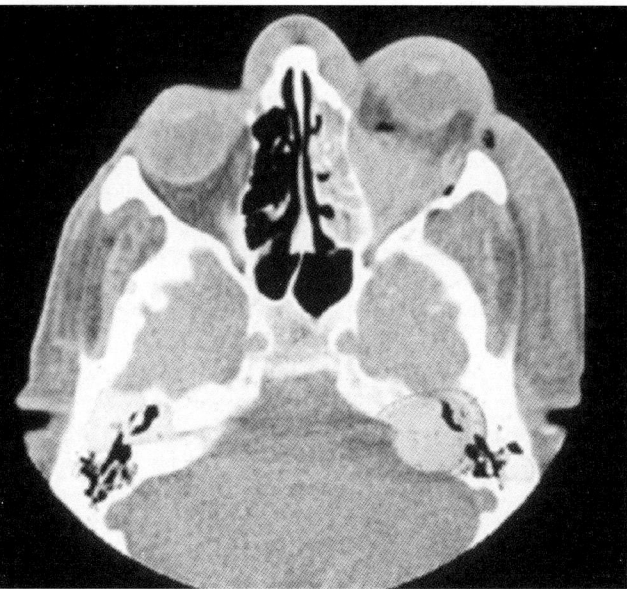

Figure 31.16 An axial CT scan demonstrating left retrobulbar haemorrhage and severe proptosis. This should be a clinical diagnosis and treated immediately, rather than as a finding on the CT scan later.

A retrobulbar haemorrhage is an acute surgical emergency as it can lead to blindness secondary to pressure-induced reduced flow on the retinal artery, leading to ischaemic damage to the optic nerve (*Figure 31.16*). It presents with tense proptosis, increasing pain, reduced visual acuity and loss of the pupillary response. One of the early signs may be altered perception of red colour in the affected eye. If this is suspected, preparation should be made for immediate bedside lateral canthotomy and cantholysis under LA to allow the globe to bulge forwards and relieve the pressure posteriorly. Concomitant medical management should also be initiated with mannitol, acetazolamide and steroids.

Summary box 31.8

Orbital fractures

- Orbital fractures may be isolated or in combination with zygomatic or maxillary fractures
- Children may present with a trapdoor orbital floor fracture that may cause an oculocardiac reflex, requiring urgent surgical intervention to prevent muscle necrosis
- Retrobulbar haemorrhage is a surgical emergency treated with bedside lateral canthotomy and cantholysis under LA to prevent blindness

Frontal sinus fractures

As frontal sinus fracture signifies a large amount of force applied to the cranium, any concomitant intracranial injuries must also be identified and treated appropriately. Frontal sinus fracture may be classified according to whether the anterior, posterior or both tables are involved with or without fracture of the sinus floor, which raises concern for possible injury to the nasofrontal duct (*Figure 31.17*). If combined with a dural tear, there may be cerebrospinal fluid (CSF) rhinorrhoea, which can be confirmed by sending the fluid sample for β_2-transferrin assay.

The aim of fracture management is to achieve a 'safe sinus', which means establishing normal sinus function, protecting intracranial structures and preventing short- and long-term complications such as meningitis, Pott's puffy tumour and mucocele. Minimally displaced (<2 mm) fractures of the anterior or posterior table can be managed conservatively with nasal decongestants and long-term observation to exclude complications. The indications for surgical intervention include anterior table disruption with significant forehead deformity, frontonasal duct involvement/obstruction and significant displacement of the posterior table with underlying neurological injury.

Isolated anterior table fractures are usually accessed via a coronal flap; they are reduced and fixed with low-profile titanium miniplates. Posterior table fractures are jointly treated with neurosurgeons and require cranialisation of the frontal sinus with obliteration of the sinus cavity and frontonasal duct. A pericranial flap is placed between the brain and the cranial vault to add an additional barrier against potential postoperative infection. A CT scan at 6 months to 1 year is recommended to ensure that there are no signs of complications.

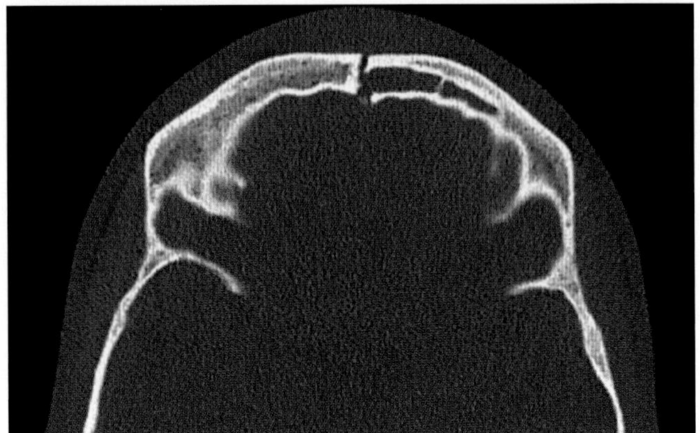

Figure 31.17 An axial CT scan demonstrating a frontal bone fracture through the anterior and posterior table of the frontal sinus.

Summary box 31.9

Frontal sinus fractures

- Frontal sinus fractures may be associated with significant neurological injury because of the significant amount of force directed at the cranium
- The aim of fracture management is to achieve a 'safe sinus'
- Follow-up with a CT scan at 6 months to 1 year is important to exclude long-term complications, which can have severe consequences

Isolated nasal and nasoethmoidal fractures

Isolated nasal bone fractures are common, and the full extent of the deformity may not be apparent for several days after injury. A follow-up appointment 1 week after the initial assessment is important (when the swelling is expected to subside) as it allows for accurate examination. The indications for surgical treatment include a cosmetic defect resulting from deviation and nasal obstruction. Closed reduction with digital manipulation under LA is common, but GA may be required if the nasal bone needs significant disimpaction. A mouldable nasal splint may be utilised to protect the bone reduction from inadvertent force.

Nasoethmoidal fractures occur secondary to significant force transfer across the bridge of the nose and the base of the frontal bone. Comminution is common as the nasal and ethmoidal bones are both thin and delicate. The clinical features of nasoethmoidal fractures include periorbital ecchymosis, a depressed nasal bridge, an upturned nasal tip (piggy nose) and telecanthus (increased distance between the inner corners of the eyelids with a normal interpupillary distance), a result of displacement of the bone where the medial canthal ligament is attached. The nasal septum should be inspected for haematoma and a CSF leak excluded.

It is important to identify and treat nasoethmoidal fracture in the primary setting as the untreated fracture can lead to unsightly deformity, which is extremely difficult to correct later. Treatment is often delayed for 7–10 days post injury to allow for the swelling to subside. The key to successful reduction is accurate repositioning of the medial canthus, which can be technically challenging because of the comminuted nature of the fracture.

Summary box 31.10

Nasoethmoidal fractures

- Nasoethmoidal fracture presents with typical features such as a depressed nasal bridge, an upturned nose and telecanthus
- ORIF can be challenging as it requires repositioning of the medial canthal attachment

Panfacial fractures

Combined fractures involving multiple levels such as the mandible, maxilla, zygoma, orbit or frontal bone are described as panfacial fractures. These are some of the most complex of facial injuries and indicate that a significant amount of force

Percival Pott, 1714–1788, surgeon, St Bartholomew's Hospital, London, UK, described the 'puffy tumour' in 1760.

has been applied to the facial skeleton. Panfacial fractures are often associated with severe intracranial, spinal or other organ injuries. Reformatted 3D CT imaging is helpful in demonstrating the full extent and the nature of these fractures (*Figure 31.18*).

Fractures are treated with ORIF once the patient has been stabilised from other significant injuries, and the soft-tissue swelling has sufficiently resolved, usually at a week from injury. The key to panfacial fracture management is in the 'sequencing' of repair, with individual fractures fixed in a similar way to those already described above. The repair of multiple fractures can be difficult because there may be little normal anatomy or intact bony buttresses to act as a guide. Most surgeons experienced in managing this type of injury would tailor the sequence to the particular fracture pattern, optimising the use of normal or near-normal anatomy as a guide.

One of the most common sequencing techniques is a 'top-down' and 'outside-in' approach. This includes first repairing the frontal bone and zygomatic arch fractures followed by orbital rim, nasoethmoidal and mandible fractures. The Le Fort I level maxillary and orbital floor fractures are repaired last. A tracheostomy is often placed because of difficulty with nasal endotracheal intubation and the need to check occlusion during fracture repair, which means oral intubation is not desirable. Alternatively, a submental intubation technique may be one that allows for the occlusion to be checked during fracture repair.

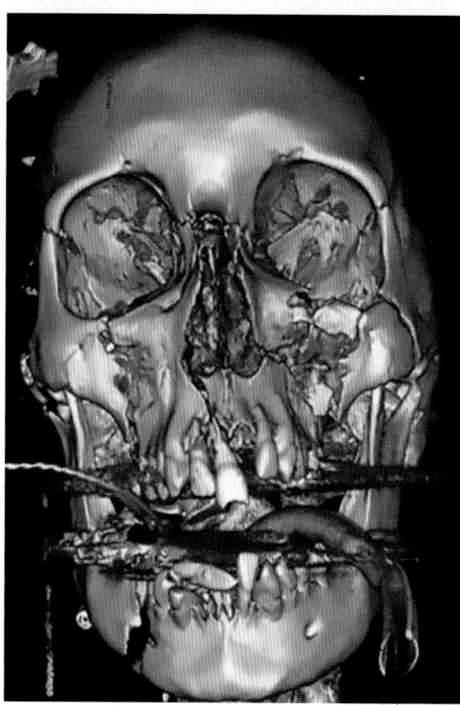

Figure 31.18 A three-dimensional reformatted CT scan demonstrating extensive midface and mandibular fractures (endotracheal and intracranial pressure tubes *in situ*).

Summary box 31.11

Panfacial fractures

- Reformatted 3D CT imaging is very useful in demonstrating the extent and nature of fractures
- Panfacial fracture management requires a 'sequencing' approach, which allows for the fractures to be treated in a systematic way

Dental injuries

The first permanent teeth usually erupt around the age of 6 years; usually lower incisors are followed by upper incisors. Between the ages of 6 and 13, the primary (deciduous) dentition is expected to be exfoliated and replaced by permanent (adult) teeth.

Fractures of the teeth may involve enamel only or enamel in combination with dentine with or without pulp exposure. Exposed dentine and pulp can be exquisitely painful and may benefit from a simple temporary dental dressing.

Avulsed primary teeth should not be reimplanted. Avulsed adult teeth are best reimplanted into the socket immediately after the injury. However, this is generally not possible during prehospital care, and therefore the tooth should ideally be stored in a suitable medium such as milk, saliva or normal saline until expertise is available. The reimplanted tooth needs to be splinted to other teeth with wire and a composite resin material for 2 weeks (sometimes a custom-made splint can be made instead), and the patient treated with antibiotics, chlorhexidine mouthwash and a tetanus vaccine booster as appropriate.

Adult luxated (displaced) teeth mostly require repositing and splinting for 4 weeks. A dentoalveolar fracture (part of the jawbone that includes the teeth) is repositioned and supported with a dental splint for 4 weeks. Luxated primary teeth are generally treated conservatively, or extracted if they are interfering with occlusion.

All dental injuries should be followed up by a dentist for splint removal or monitoring and dental treatment as appropriate.

Summary box 31.12

Dental injuries

- It is important to account for all missing teeth and/or dental fragments – a chest radiograph may be indicated
- An avulsed adult tooth should be reimplanted into the socket as soon as possible or stored in milk, saliva or normal saline
- All dental injuries should be followed up by a dentist

FURTHER READING

Brennan PA, Schliephake H, Ghali GE, Cascarini L. *Maxillofacial surgery*, 3rd edn. London: Elsevier, 2017.

Newlands C, Kerawala C. *Oral and maxillofacial surgery*, 3rd edn. Oxford Specialist Handbooks in Surgery. Oxford: Oxford Medical Publications, 2020.

Perry M, Holmes S. *Atlas of operative maxillofacial trauma surgery: primary repair of facial injuries.* Berlin: Springer, 2014.

CHAPTER 32 Extremity trauma

Learning objectives

To gain an understanding of:
- How to identify whether an injury exists
- The important injuries not to miss
- The principles of the description and classification of fractures
- The range of available treatments
- How to select an appropriate treatment

INTRODUCTION

In several chapters the importance of life-threatening trauma is emphasised, but numerically for every patient who dies following a traumatic event there are three who are left with a lifelong functional impairment. Extremity trauma can be thought of as injury in isolation or in the context of trauma to the whole body. In the latter scenario extremity trauma and the mode in which it is managed may be important, as is the physiological stability of the patient – a concept known as damage control orthopaedic surgery. Furthermore, extremity trauma not only involves the bones, most obviously through a fracture, but also involves the surrounding soft-tissue envelope and thus could describe injury to nerves, other connective tissue and skin.

The goal of extremity trauma management is to return the injured area to optimal function as quickly as possible and therefore return function to the patient. The management of extremity trauma is step-wise and involves initially saving the patient's life by the identification and treatment of life- and limb-threatening injuries, according to the Advanced Trauma Life Support (ATLS) principles. ATLS principles are a useful starting point in the evaluation of extremity trauma. They put the injury into context, attributing to it a priority in the management of all the patient's injuries; for example, a traumatic head injury may require management before operative femoral fracture stabilisation with an intramedullary nail, yet the application of traction to the affected limb, or an external fixator, may reduce the physiological insult to the patient as a whole. Therefore, the context of extremity trauma is extremely important. Applying the principles of ATLS in the initial assessment, followed by damage control orthopaedics in the ongoing surgical management, provides a framework for patient management.

One could summarise this by noting that treatment depends on patient factors, injury-specific factors and surgeon factors, including the resources available.

It is imperative for the clinician to involve the patient in the decision-making process when it comes to the choice of treatment for that individual. Moreover, treatment priorities, functional demands and risk versus benefit vary from individual to individual.

DIAGNOSIS

The diagnosis of extremity trauma begins with the taking of a pertinent history followed by focused physical examination and appropriate special tests.

History

It is important to ascertain the mechanism of injury and the amount of force involved in the injury. Take time to gather sufficient detail in order to do this. The mechanism of injury gives an indication to the clinician of the energy and forces imparted onto the patient. Certain injury mechanisms result in classical injury patterns; for example, electrocution or seizure activity may lead to a posterior dislocation of the shoulder. In your mind translate the mechanism of injury into the common anatomical injury patterns. For example, a head-on collision between two cars each travelling at 40 miles per hour coming to a dead stop should be interpreted by the history taker as a rapid deceleration injury, which then allows anticipation of likely injuries, such as rupture of the aortic arch. Similarly, a fall onto an outstretched hand might be associated with wrist, elbow, shoulder and clavicular injuries.

Following the history of the presenting complaint, it is important to collect information beyond that of the injury. The AMPLE mnemonic is an abbreviated system taught in ATLS that is designed to provide key information quickly in a focused way.

A: Allergies
M: Medication – important to ask about anticoagulant and antiplatelet therapies, corticosteroid use and any possible immunosuppressive treatment
P: Past medical and surgical history – has the patient had an anaesthetic in the past and were there any complications

L: Last time – something to eat or drink
E: Events – events that led to the injury

In the multiply injured patient or patients with altered levels of consciousness, gain as much collateral history as possible. Listen to the account of prehospital personnel; for example, the amount of cabin intrusion in a vehicle or whether a collision was head-on or side-on.

Examination

An initial general examination, including vital signs and general assessment, should be conducted. Is this an isolated injury or do you need to start right at the beginning, considering the A, B, C approach as advocated by ATLS? Examination of the individual extremity only begins once you are sure the patient is stable and life- and limb-threatening conditions have been excluded.

It is crucial to undertake a thorough top-to-toe evaluation in the secondary survey. Often the minor extremity injuries are missed (*Figure 32.1*) and can cause significant long-term problems (*Table 32.1*).

A top-to-toe evaluation is achieved by a systematic approach (see *Chapter 35* and *Apley's system of orthopaedics and fractures [Further reading]*) to the injured extremity:

- look;
- feel;
- move (active and passive);
- special tests;
- special investigations.

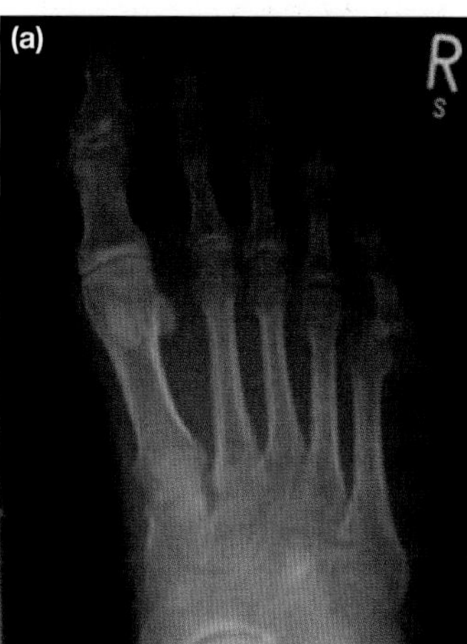

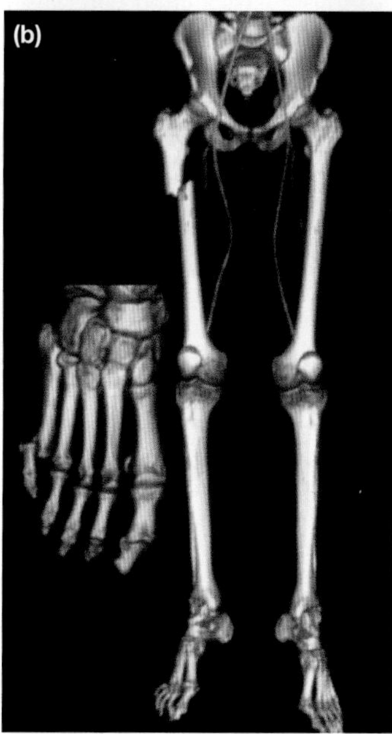

Figure 32.1 (a) Missed dislocation of the metatarsophalangeal joint of the little toe, picked up at 8 weeks. (b) Initial trauma computed tomography angiogram. In retrospect, on close inspection the dislocation is visible on the angiogram; do not be distracted by the obvious femoral shaft fracture.

TABLE 32.1 Extremity injuries that are notorious for being missed.

- Posterior dislocation of the shoulder
- Lateral condylar mass fracture of the distal humerus
- Perilunate dislocation
- Scaphoid fracture
- Tarsometatarsal fracture dislocation
- Compartment syndrome
- Vascular injury with knee dislocation
- Talar neck fracture
- Slipped upper femoral epiphysis
- Achilles tendon rupture

Ensure you examine the joint above and the joint below the site of injury. Consider the events and mechanism of injury and examine the areas that could possibly be affected. For example, a patient who falls from a height may fracture the calcaneus, which is an obvious diagnosis with a very swollen hindfoot and extremely tender heel. The concomitant lumbar spine fracture may not become evident until a few days later when the distracting pain in the heel starts to subside.

Look

It is important to look at the whole limb, back and front, noting any localised swelling, bruising and any obvious deformity. A shortened externally rotated leg in an older patient suggests a fracture of the proximal femur. A slightly flexed, adducted internally rotated leg might suggest a posterior dislocation of the hip.

Any break in the skin or abrasion needs to be noted and the treating orthopaedic surgeon informed, even if you do not think it communicates with the fracture. A graze over the knee in a closed tibial fracture may preclude intramedullary nailing until the wound has healed over, or perhaps an alternative treatment may have to be considered.

Ideally a photograph (with appropriate consent) should be taken to document the injury and obviate the need for repeated manipulation of the dressings (see *Open fractures*).

Achilles, the Greek hero, was the son of Peleus and Thetis. When he was a child, his mother dipped him in the Styx, one of the rivers of the Underworld so that he should be invulnerable in battle. The heel by which she held him did not get wet, and was, therefore, not protected. Achilles died from a wound in the heel received at the siege of Troy.

Note the colour of the limb and the degree of general swelling. A compartment syndrome may still be present even when a limb does not appear to be very swollen (see ***Compartment syndrome***), but if it is grossly swollen, note, document and pass on the information.

Look for pre-existing scars; a scar at the back of the elbow or over the cubital tunnel might signify an anterior transposition of the ulnar nerve. Scars might signify previous metalwork that remains *in situ* or has been removed in the past.

Feel

Start gently examining the limb away from the zone of obvious injury, gaining the patient's trust and gathering as much information as possible beforehand, and without causing the patient pain or discomfort. Feel for bony tenderness and note the degree of swelling and tenseness of the compartments. It should be noted that it is not possible to exclude a compartment syndrome based on how tense the limb feels. The deep posterior compartment of the lower leg cannot be felt when palpating the skin.

The characteristic crepitus of subcutaneous air can be felt in the setting of open fractures, air-jet injuries and around the chest in the presence of a pneumothorax.

The examiner should feel for pulses and assess capillary return (see ***Neurovascular examination***) as well as feeling for temperature changes.

Move

Movement as part of the examination should once again be approached carefully and without causing the patient pain and discomfort. Two types of movement can be assessed:

1 active – active movement is movement initiated and maintained by the patient;
2 passive – passive movement is when the examiner moves the limb.

Special tests

There are often special tests to detect injury in precise anatomical locations and many are described elsewhere in the book; for example, looking for a ruptured Achilles tendon by placing the patient prone with the foot over the edge of the bed and squeezing the calf; plantarflexion of the foot and ankle then suggests the Achilles tendon is intact.

The examiner should be aware of gravity simulating active movements. For example, a leg lying flat, fully extended on the couch does not mean the extensor mechanism of the knee is intact. In all knee injuries make sure the patient can actively straight leg raise and get their leg off the couch.

Similar pitfalls exist in the upper limb with gravity straightening the elbow. In order to assess triceps function and elbow extension, ensure that the patient can actively extend against resistance from the examiner or against gravity.

Beware of trick movements. Patients with a complete rupture of the quadriceps can still walk with the leg locked in full to slight hyperextension by using the iliotibial band. Patients with complete rupture of the Achilles tendon can still actively plantar flex the foot and ankle using the long toe flexors.

Neurovascular examination

This is an important part of extremity examination and summary terms such as 'neurovascularly intact' are best avoided. It is preferable to clearly document the examination performed and its findings, along with a conclusion about the function of the particular neurological or vascular anatomy tested. On occasion you may not be able to examine all movements because of injury or casts.

It is important to examine and document findings before and after any manipulation or cast application to ensure no change. A radial nerve palsy in association with a humeral shaft fracture that occurs at the time of injury may be treated expectantly. If, however, radial nerve function is lost after application of a cast or brace, the nerve should be explored. Most peripheral nerves have a motor and sensory component; document both sensibility and motor function.

Laceration or rupture of major vessels may result in life- and limb-threatening injury and should be dealt with as an emergency (see ATLS principles discussed in ***Chapter 27***). Complete laceration or occlusion of a major vessel is obvious and seldom missed. In contrast, occult vessel injuries must be considered and actively excluded. In 30% of knee dislocations (tibiofemoral dislocation) a vascular injury will occur (***Figure 32.2***).

The presence of palpable pulses does not exclude a significant vascular injury and an intimal flap may develop, progress and thrombose over time. Repeated evaluation is necessary, before and after any intervention, for example a manipulation or cast application.

In injuries commonly associated with vascular injury, such as knee dislocations, occult injury should be actively excluded with an angiogram. If an angiogram is not performed, repeated thorough vascular evaluation of the limb should be undertaken for the first 24–48 hours.

Open fractures also demand attention to the neurological and vascular status of the limb. In the more severe injuries, there may be both neurological and vascular injury requiring immediate surgical attention through rapid spanning of the limb, creation of an arterial shunt to provide urgent inflow and subsequent vascular grafting. Once flow has been restored, usually at the same or another surgical sitting, the fracture can then be stabilised definitively with appropriate soft-tissue cover. Performing the arterial shunt before temporary stability has been achieved can compromise the later arterial reconstruction as length, rotation and alignment would not have been restored, thereby pulling on the graft. Open fractures require multiple specialty input.

Investigations

The mainstay of extremity trauma investigation remains radiography of the affected limb to see if there is a bony injury. However, this is not the sole investigation available.

Haematological investigations

Simple haematological investigations are seldom useful in the evaluation of a single limb injury. In the polytrauma patient a full blood count, serum biochemistry, clotting factor and

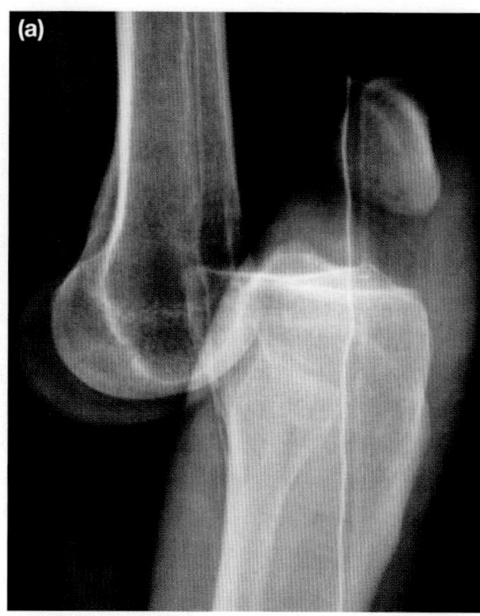

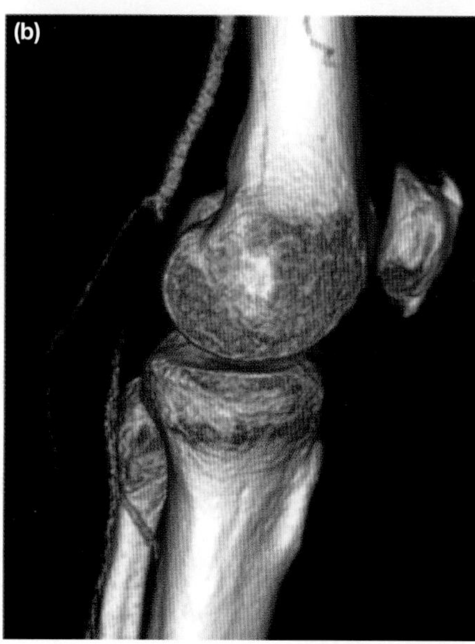

Figure 32.2 (a) Initial anterior tibiofemoral dislocation. (b) Postreduction computed tomography angiogram showing complete blockage of the popliteal artery with reconstitution distally from a collateral blood supply.

creatinine kinase may be useful. A blood gas, including pH, base excess and lactate, can be useful to show the severity of the injury and the response to resuscitation.

Ultrasound

Ultrasound is very useful to define soft-tissue injuries. Fractures of the bones can be visualised on ultrasound but generally it is reserved for the soft tissues. One limitation of ultrasound is the variability depending on the experience of the sonographer.

Radiography

Radiographs are the mainstay in the initial evaluation of suspected extremity trauma. The rule of 2s should be remembered:

- 2 views – ensure acquisition of two views in orthogonal planes to avoid missing a fracture out of plane on the first radiograph view. For shoulder injuries ensure at least an anteroposterior and axillary or modified axillary view (*Figure 32.3*).
- 2 joints – radiographs are required of the joint above and the joint below the fracture.
- 2 occasions – sometimes the fracture may not be initially visible; a second series of radiographs should be undertaken after 10–14 days if suspicion of bony injury persists. The classic injury here is a scaphoid fracture. If initial scaphoid views are normal, consider repeating them 10–14 days later if pain and tenderness in the anatomical snuff box (*Figure 32.4*) persist.
- 2 sides – in paediatric injuries it can be useful to consider a radiograph from the opposite and uninjured side if doubt exists. With improved access to atlases of normal variants this is less important.

Computed axial tomography

Computed axial tomography (CT) is very good for characterising the bony anatomy of injuries, allowing for multiplanar reconstruction of injury anatomy and providing other three-dimensional information. It is very useful for periarticular injuries, where the exact characterisation of the bony injury is essential. A CT with contrast creating a CT angiogram provides very useful information regarding the vascularity and its association with the fracture. The CT angiogram also gives an indication to plastic reconstruction surgeons of reconstructive options for limb trauma.

Surface volume rendering is a useful addition allowing for easier visualisation of the injury (*Figure 32.1b*). CT angiography (*Figure 32.2b*) may be added, providing information on the vascular anatomy. One disadvantage of CT is the dose of radiation involved.

Magnetic resonance imaging

Magnetic resonance imaging (MRI) provides three-dimensional information without the radiation involved in CT. It provides useful information, particularly about the soft tissues. MRI can provide information on the blood supply to the bone; for example, avascular necrosis of the proximal pole of the scaphoid.

One disadvantage of MRI is the time taken to acquire the image; patients suffering from claustrophobia find the experience traumatic. It is essential to ensure patient safety and consideration should be given to potential risks of MRI that may apply, for example with certain implanted devices and metallic foreign bodies, e.g. in the eye (see MHRA guidance in *Further reading*).

MRI angiography can also be performed, providing information about the vascular anatomy.

Nuclear medicine scans

Technetium-99 nuclear medicine scans register osteoblastic activity and may be used to demonstrate occult fractures; for example, an undisplaced scaphoid fracture.

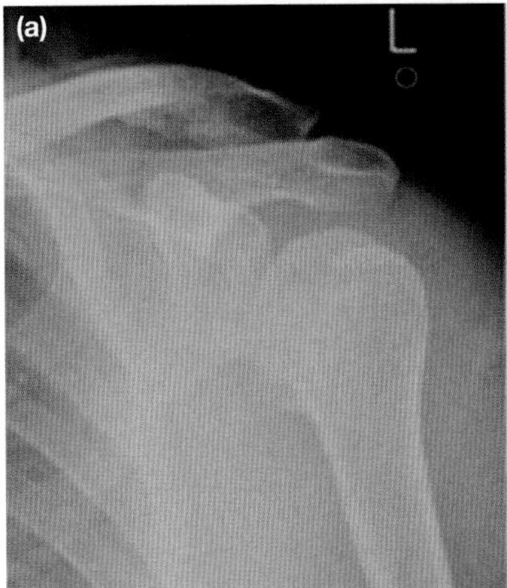

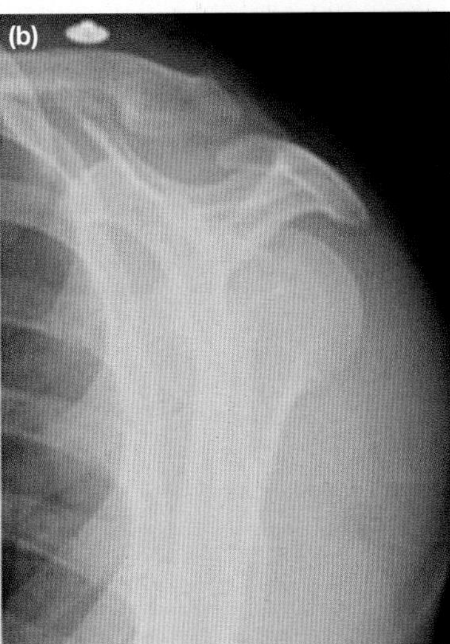

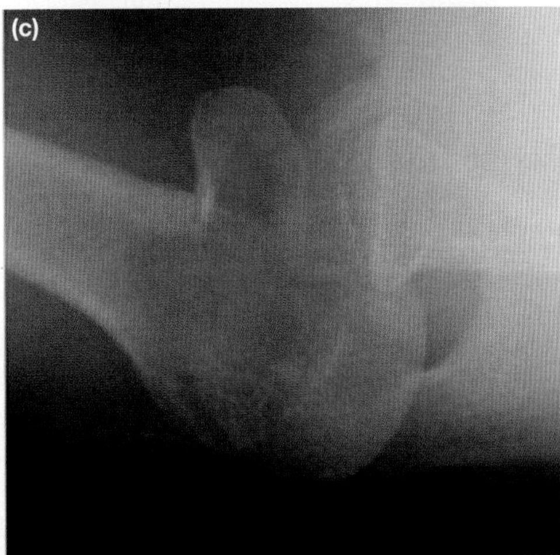

Figure 32.3 Radiographic series of the same patient demonstrating the value of two views in two planes and the true value of the axillary view in shoulder trauma. (a) Anteroposterior radiograph of the shoulder, initially reported as normal. (b) Lateral scapula radiograph, initially reported as normal; humeral head slightly posteriorly directed. (c) Axillary view – true value of the axillary view shown with obvious posterior dislocation of the glenohumeral joint.

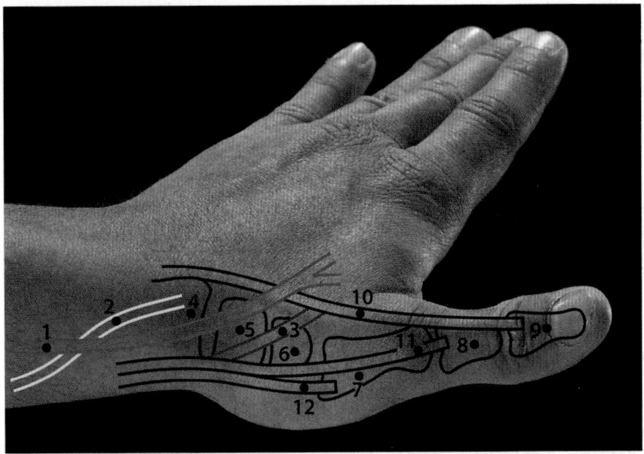

Figure 32.4 Surface anatomy of the anatomical snuffbox: 1, cephalic vein (blue); 2, radial nerve (yellow); 3, radial artery (red); 4, lower end of radius; 5, scaphoid; 6, trapezium; 7, first metacarpal; 8, proximal phalanx; 9, distal phalanx; 10, extensor pollicis longus; 11, extensor pollicis brevis; 12, abductor pollicis longus. (Reproduced with permission from Lumley JSP, Craven JL, Abrahams PH, Tunstall RG. *Bailey & Love's essential clinical anatomy*. Boca Raton, FL: CRC Press, 2019.)

Summary box 32.1

History, examination and investigations

- Follow a systematic approach
- History requires sufficient detail of injury
- History can be organised in the AMPLE format
- Examination follows look, feel, move, special tests approach
- Investigations will include radiographs with the rule of '2s' observed
- Selective use of special investigations can help diagnosis

DESCRIPTION AND CLASSIFICATION OF THE INJURY

Soft-tissue injury

There are several classification systems for soft-tissue injuries: the Tscherne classification for closed injuries, the Gustilo and Anderson for open injuries (*Table 32.2*) and the Ganga classification of severe open injuries.

The first step in soft-tissue injury characterisation is to decide if this is an open or closed fracture – an open fracture being any fracture where the fracture haematoma communicates with a breach in the epithelial lining, not just skin. For example, an open pelvic fracture may communicate with the vagina or rectum and a mandibular fracture through the mucosa of the mouth (see *Open fractures*).

Consider all the soft tissues crossing the zone of injury, as it is possible to get a closed rupture or avulsion of tendons without a break in the skin. Consider the possibility of a neurovascular injury (see *Neurological injury*). Severe soft-tissue injury in the presence or absence of a fracture may still lead to compartment syndrome (see *Compartment syndrome*).

Harald Tscherne, b. 1933, Austrian trauma surgeon, Director of the Trauma Department, Medical Graduate School, Hannover, Germany.
Ramon Balgoa Gustilo, surgeon, Hennepin County Medical Center, Minneapolis, MN, USA.
John T Anderson, surgeon, Hennepin Medical Center, Minneapolis, MA, USA.

TABLE 32.2 Gustilo and Anderson open fracture classification.

Type	
I	A low-energy open fracture with a wound less than 1 cm long and clean
II	An open fracture with a laceration more than 1 cm long without extensive soft-tissue damage, flaps or avulsion
III	Characterised by high-energy injury irrespective of the size of the wound. Extensive damage to soft tissues, including muscles, skin and neurovascular structures, and a high degree of contamination. Multifragmentary and unstable fractures
Subgroups of type III	
A	Adequate soft-tissue cover of a fractured bone after stabilisation
B	Inadequate soft-tissue cover of a fractured bone after stabilisation (i.e. flap coverage required)
C	Open fracture associated with an arterial injury requiring repair

Source: Gustilo RB, Mendoza RM, Williams DN. Problems in the management of type III (severe) open fractures: a new classification of type III open fractures. *J Trauma* 1984; **24**: 742–6.

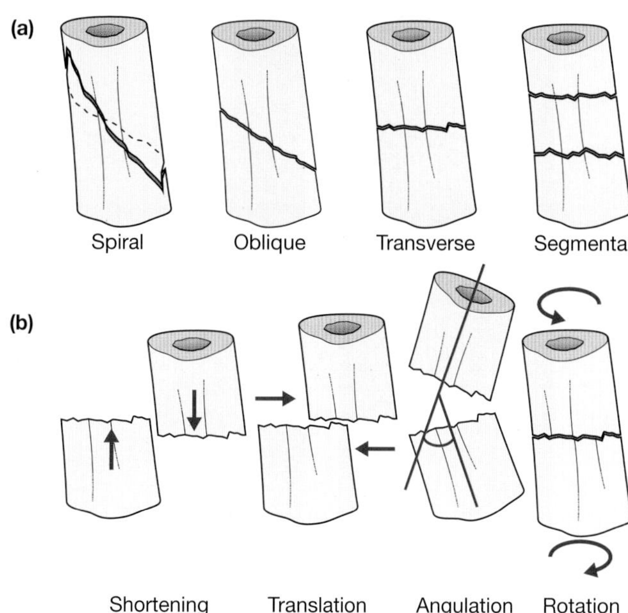

Figure 32.5 Descriptive terms for fractures (a) and type of displacement (b).

Peripheral nerve injury

Seddon classified nerve injuries into neurapraxia, axonotmesis and neurotmesis:

- Neurapraxia – no loss of nerve sheath continuity or peripheral Wallerian degeneration. If the pressure is removed from the nerve, recovery potential is good but may take months.
- Axonotmesis – nerve sheath remains intact, with internal nerve fibre damage and associated Wallerian degeneration. The neural tube (endoneurium) can guide the regenerating nerve fibres to their target. Good potential for recovery; nerve fibre regrowth is at 1 mm per day.
- Neurotmesis – complete division of the nerve, nerve sheath and nerve fibre. Functionally poor outcome without surgical intervention to restore continuity of the nerve sheath.

Although the Seddon classification is useful in understanding the pathoanatomy, the critical discriminator in defining recovery, and need for possible surgical intervention, is the presence or lack of continuity of the enveloping nerve sheath.

Bony injury

Description

Describing the bony injury depends on several characteristics and includes the:

- name of the bone that has been injured;
- region of bone injured (epiphysis, metaphysis, diaphysis);
- pattern of fracture line: transverse, oblique, spiral, segmental or multifragmentary (*Figure 32.5*);
- presence of compression: compression fractures occur when cancellous bone collapses; for example, vertebral wedge compression fracture;
- presence of displacement of the fracture fragments: undisplaced or displaced;
- type and degree of displacement: shortening, translation, angulation, rotation (mnemonic STAR) (*Figure 32.5*); occasionally, the magnitude of rotational displacement can be quite dramatic (*Figure 32.6*) or, indeed, very subtle to assess on a radiograph – hence the need for standardised radiographs assessing the area in question and the joint above and below, but also clinical corroboration;
- presence of pre-existing pathology (e.g. fracture through a tumour or in close proximity to a joint replacement); associated joint pathology: dislocation or subluxation.

In children and adolescents the fracture line may be incomplete because of the plastic, less brittle nature of their bones (*Figure 32.7*). These incomplete fractures are called greenstick (*Figure 32.8*) fractures, where one tension cortex fails. If the compression cortex buckles, they are called torus (*Figure 32.9*) or buckle fractures. Paediatric bone may also simply undergo plastic deformation without a visible fracture line.

Summary box 32.2

Describing an injury

Use plain language to describe:

- Location
- Soft-tissue component
- Bony injury

Sir Herbert J Seddon, trained at St Bartholomew's Hospital, London University and the Royal National Orthopaedic Hospital, Stanmore, UK. He became the second Nuffield Professor of Orthopaedic Surgery in Oxford, UK.

Augustus Volney Waller, 1816–1870, general practitioner of Kensington, London, UK (1842–1851), subsequently worked as a physiologist in Bonn, Germany; Paris, France; Birmingham, UK; and Geneva, Switzerland.

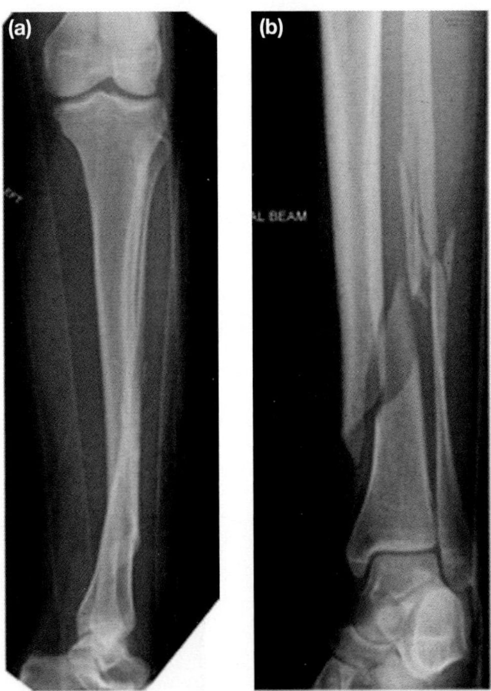

Figure 32.6 Describing fractures: the importance of rotation. (a) Anteroposterior (AP) view of the knee seen at the top of the radiograph and lateral view of the ankle at the bottom, showing a spiral fracture at the junction of the middle and distal thirds of the tibia. (b) AP radiograph of the ankle on the same patient. Note the varied diameter of the fracture fragments; this implies rotational deformity. The distal fragment has translated laterally by 50%. There is no significant angulation on this view.

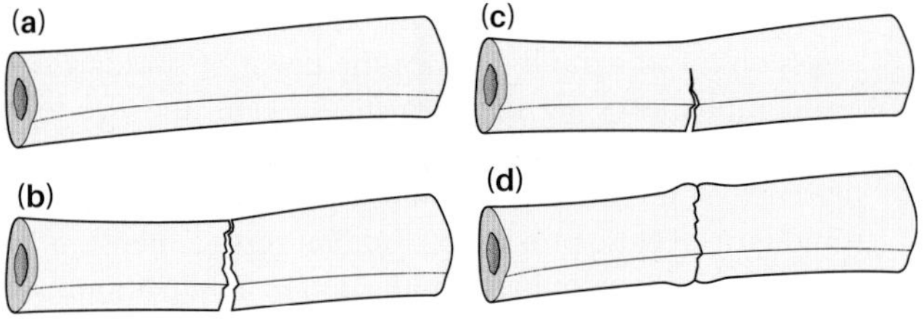

Figure 32.7 Types of bony injury: (a) uninjured bone; (b) adult transverse fracture failure across the whole bone; (c) greenstick fracture; the bone has failed on the tension side; (d) torus or buckle fracture; the bone has failed on the compression side.

Classification

For each specific bony injury there may be several injury-specific classification systems.

AO classification

The AO (Arbeitsgemeinschaft für Osteosynthesefragen) system provides a comprehensive classification of all fractures (*Figure 32.10*). The first number defines the bone injured and the second number the segment of bone injured: proximal metaphysis, diaphysis, distal metaphysis. The letter and number that follows further defines the nature of the injury

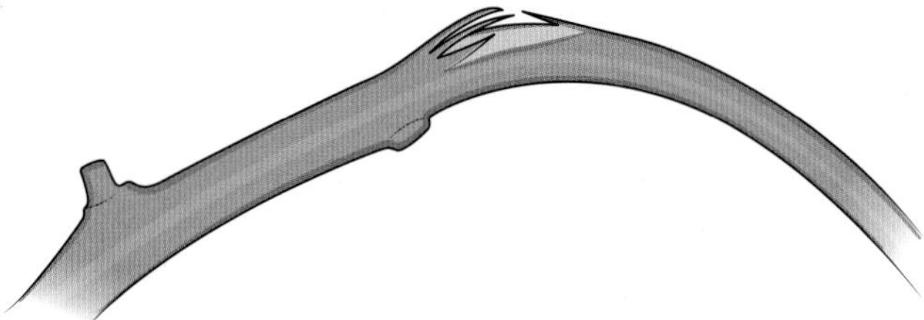

Figure 32.8 Greenstick fractures take their name from the way in which a 'green' stick (one that is alive and has sap flowing through it) breaks.

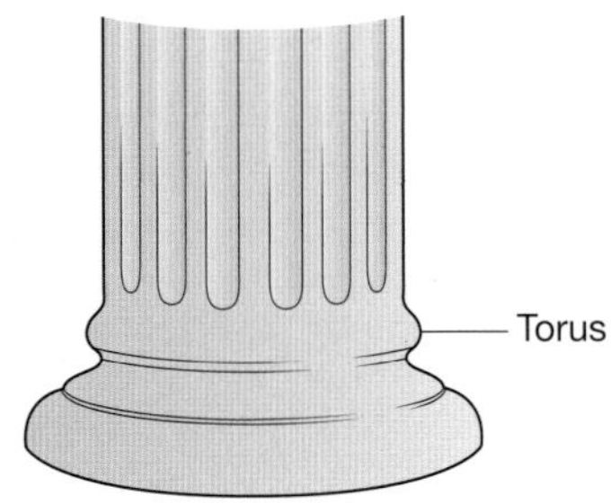

Figure 32.9 Torus fractures take their name from an architectural torus, which is the 'bulge' at the base of a column.

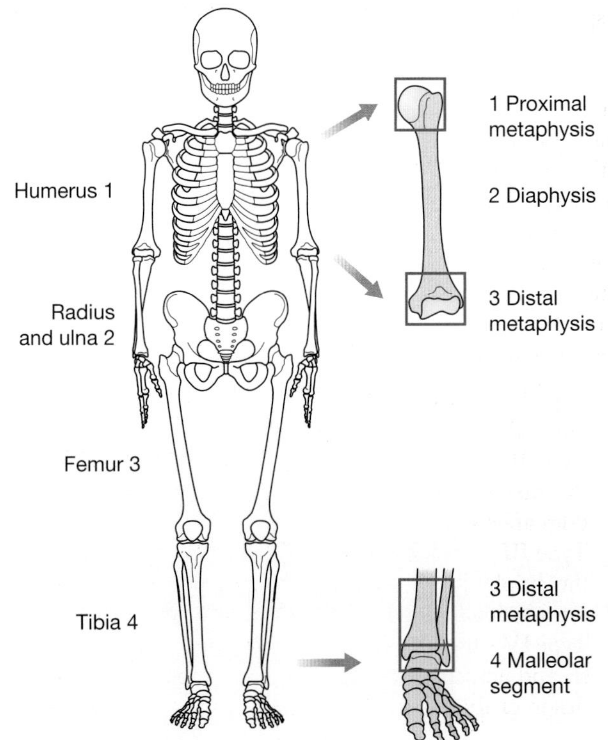

Figure 32.10 The AO classification system: the first two numbers specify the site of the fracture.

AO, Arbeitsgemeinschaft für Osteosynthesefragen, may be translated from the German as 'Working Party on Problems of Bone Repair'.

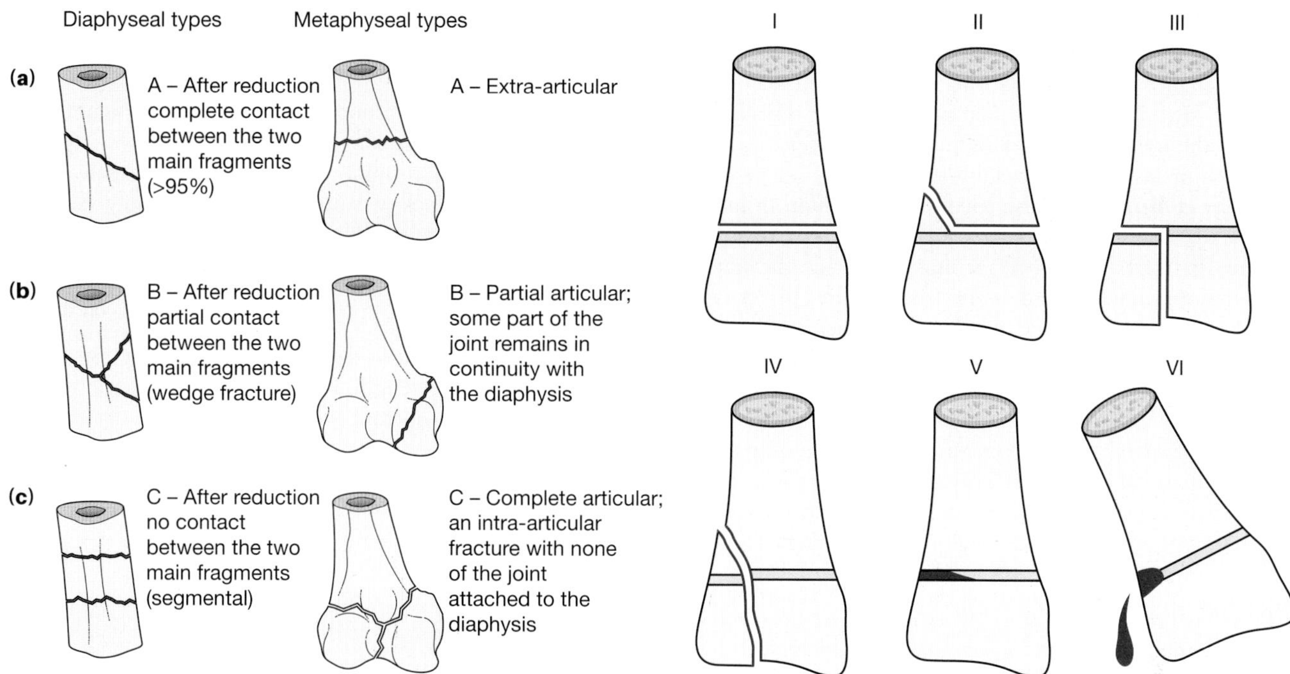

Figure 32.11 The AO classification system: the letter defines the nature of the fracture.

Figure 32.12 The Salter–Harris classification of growth plate injuries.

(*Figure 32.11*). For example, the previously described humeral fracture would be 12-A1 (1 humerus, 2 diaphysis, A simple, 1 spiral). (For more detail see ***Further reading***.)

Growth plate injury classification

In child and adolescent injuries involvement of the growth plate (physis) can lead to abnormal growth or growth arrest, either complete or partial. Complete growth arrest will result in length abnormalities and partial growth arrest might result in angular deformities. The severity of injury to the physis is classified in the Salter–Harris classification, which considers whether the fracture line passes through the epiphysis, physis, metaphysis or combinations of all the above. Salter–Harris described five and Mercer Rang added the sixth (*Figure 32.12*):

- Type I – simple fracture line just involving the physis. Seldom affects growth.
- Type II – fracture line through the physis exiting through the metaphysis, producing a metaphyseal fragment. Seldom affects growth.
- Type III – fracture line through the physis exiting through the epiphysis (intra-articular). Seldom affects growth, but intra-articular affecting joint surface.
- Type IV – fracture line across the epiphysis, across the physis and across the metaphysis. This injury can cause focal fusion of the physis, leading to abnormal growth.
- Type V – a crush injury of the physis. Growth disturbance is common and may be the first radiological sign of an injury.
- Type VI – injury to perichondral structures by direct trauma. Rare injury, high chance of abnormal growth.

FRACTURE HEALING

It is useful to review fracture healing, as it relates to treatment and outcome. Following a fracture, bone can heal in two different ways: direct (primary) bone healing or indirect (secondary) bone healing. One can conceptualise direct bone healing as being akin to a wound that is stitched together whereas indirect bone healing is similar to forming a scab that over time turns to normal tissue. Through intervention, the clinician is able to influence the healing response of the tissue: direct bone healing being more likely if the two bone ends are squeezed together (compression), and indirect healing should there be movement (termed strain) at the fracture site. If there is too much movement, i.e. the fracture is too unstable, healing of the fracture may not occur.

- **Direct bone healing**, as the name implies, heals directly with bone and without callus formation. It happens in an environment of cortical apposition and absolute stability with no movement or gap between the fracture fragments.

Robert Bruce Salter, 1924–2010, Professor of Orthopaedic Surgery, University of Toronto, Ontario, Canada. A pioneer in the field of paediatric orthopaedic surgery, he received international awards for medical science and the Distinguished Achievement for Orthopaedic Research award.
W Robert Harris, 1922–2005, formerly Professor, University of Toronto, President of the Canadian Orthopaedic Foundation (1968) and President of the Canadian Orthopaedic Association (1975 and 1976).
Charles Mercer Rang, 1933–2003, British orthopaedic paediatric surgeon.

The normal osteoclastic-mediated remodelling of bone is directed across the fracture interface. Osteoclastic cutting cones cut across the fracture line, with following osteoblasts laying down lamellar bone across the fracture. This is similar to the normal remodelling process that occurs in bone all the time as part of skeletal homeostasis.

- **Indirect bone healing** involves a transition from one tissue to another with callus formation. It is the most common form of bone healing. Following the injury, haematoma fills the gap at the fracture site. In response to a varying strain and under the influence of bone-stimulating factors, the tissue undergoes differentiation, from haematoma to fibrous tissue and then to soft callus, followed by mineralisation and formation of mature bone. The amount of strain determines the nature of tissue it differentiates into: under 100% leads to fibrous tissue, under 10% soft callus, less than 2% hard callus and progressive mineralisation (Perren's theory of bone healing). Hence a little movement is good, too much movement is bad.

Bone healing requires not only an advantageous mechanical environment but also an advantageous biological environment. Principally this can be described in terms of blood supply and the preservation of blood supply from the surrounding soft tissues, the periosteum and the nutrient arterial supply to bone. Should the inflow be affected through trauma or peripheral vascular disease, or should there be an extensive soft-tissue injury causing poor bone perfusion, bone healing can be affected. Similarly, microscopic inflow issues at the tissue perfusion level, e.g. as a result of diabetes, may also lead to poor bone healing. Infection may also create a biological insult to bone healing; therefore, open fractures with their extensive soft-tissue injury and increased probability of infection are prone to impaired bone healing.

Terminology of bone healing after fracture

Union

The fracture has healed sufficiently from a clinical perspective to withstand physiological loads, with very little pain and minimal tenderness at the fracture site. Radiologically a fracture has united when the callus bridges the fracture site.

Delayed union

This description can be applied to a fracture that is slow to heal and that has not healed in the expected time frame.

Non-union

This description can be applied to a fracture that has not healed and shows no potential to heal without further intervention. A non-union can also be defined as a fracture that fails to demonstrate clinical or radiological improvement over 3 months. In general, you do not describe a fracture as 'non-union' until 6 months after the injury.

There are a number of different types of non-union: atrophic, hypertrophic and infected. It is useful to consider certain factors with regard to the non-union: the biology of the fracture, the mechanical environment and the host (patient factors such as diabetes and smoking).

In an atrophic non-union, the problem is generally a biological one, with a lack of stimulus or blood supply. A hypertrophic non-union generally occurs when there is too much movement at the fracture site.

Consolidation

This follows union and demonstrates that the bone has returned to normal strength. Radiologically it is demonstrated by the return of the normal cortical pattern.

Remodelling

In children, and to a lesser degree in adults, bone remodels based on the forces passing through it.

Summary box 32.3

Fracture healing

- Direct – cortical apposition and absolute stability
- Indirect – secondary bone healing, requires some movement

TREATMENT

The main principle of extremity fracture management builds on the classical concept of reduction and stabilisation of the fracture. Treatment can be considered under the following headings (see ***Apley's system of orthopaedics and fractures [Further reading]***):

- reduce;
- hold;
- heal;
- rehabilitate.

The main objective of any treatment is to return the patient to normal function as soon and as safely as possible. Broadly speaking, treatment may be operative or non-operative, with differing risks and benefits (*Table 32.3*).

Reduce

The first thing to consider is the degree of displacement of the fracture fragments. It is useful to ask the following question: if the bone were to heal in this position, would it be compatible with optimum function in the short and long term?

In general, fractures involving the articular joint surface need to be reduced perfectly back to their original anatomical position, to restore normal joint movement in the short term and avoid degenerative joint disease in the long term – **intra-articular fracture = anatomical reduction**.

Stephan M Perren, 1932–2019, Director, AO Research Institute, Davos, Switzerland, 1967–1996.

TABLE 32.3 Risks and benefits of fracture treatment.

Benefits	Risks
• Pain relief • Prevention of infection • Restoration of anatomy • Early movement of the limb • Early movement of the patient • Improved function • Reduced risk of secondary arthritis • Financial cost (time off work)	• Anaesthesia • Introduction of infection • Damage to soft tissues and neurovascular structures • Devitalising bone • Need for implant removal • Financial cost (cost of treatment)

Fractures that do not involve the joint surface generally require restoration of mechanical alignment of the joints above and below. The fracture fragments do not need to be reduced perfectly. Focus on acceptable alignment, length and rotation – **extra-articular fracture = mechanical alignment**.

In children an extra-articular fracture has the ability to remodel, and therefore an increased degree of displacement can be accepted.

If a fracture requires reduction, it can be reduced open or closed. A closed reduction is where the bones are manipulated and moved without exposing the bone. Often the best way to reduce a fracture is to reverse the sequence of injury, without tearing or further damaging the intact soft tissues and periosteum. On occasion this may mean exaggerating the deformity (*Figure 32.13*).

Open reduction is utilised if an acceptable closed reduction is not achieved or likely to succeed. A combination of closed and open methods can be used to reduce a fracture. Care should be taken during an open reduction not to unduly devitalise the fracture fragments by stripping intact periosteum. A balance between maintaining a blood supply to the fracture fragments (biology) and achieving anatomical reduction needs to be maintained.

Adequacy of reduction is complex and depends on many factors. If intra-articular, the joint surface involved needs to be considered. By way of an example, 2 mm of residual displacement of the articular surface may be acceptable in the patella and tibial plateau and may be acceptable in fractures involving the distal radius, but is not acceptable in the condylar joints of the fingers. In general consider the relative thickness of the articular surface involved.

On occasion consideration of how you intend to subsequently hold the fracture may affect the primary form of reduction.

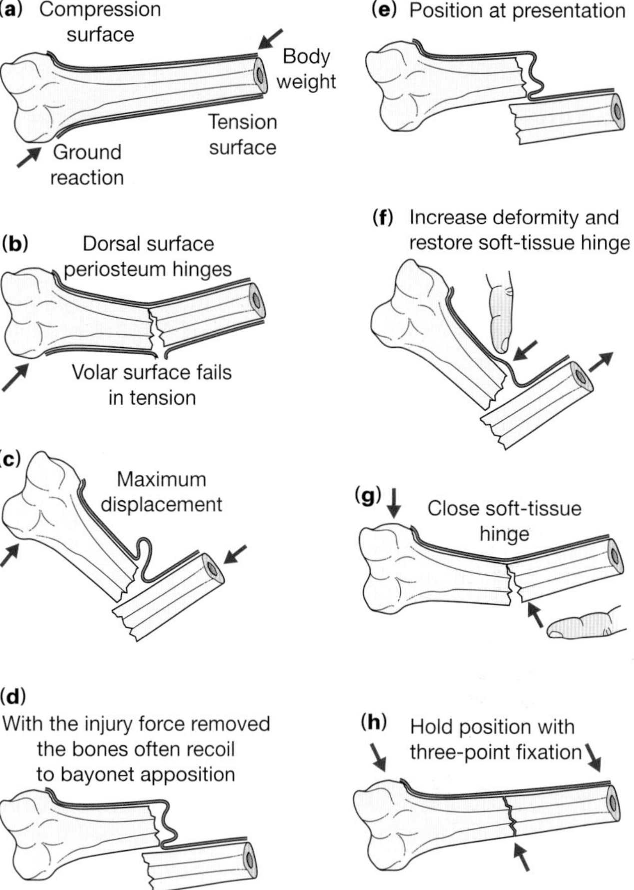

Figure 32.13 (a–d) Representation of how the mechanism of injury causes the bony and soft-tissue injury. (e–h) Representation of how the residual mechanical properties of the tissues may be used to effect and hold a reduction.

Summary box 32.4

Reduction

- Reduction has two components: reducing the fragments and assessing adequacy of reduction
- Reduction can be performed open or closed
- The principle is to reverse the movement that created the fracture
- Over-angulation allows the intact periosteum to guide the fragments into position

Hold

If the fracture fragments are in an acceptable position, or have been reduced into an acceptable position, they then need to be held in that position until they heal. When choosing a method to hold a fracture the aim is to:

- optimise the biological and mechanical environment to create the most favourable conditions possible for fracture healing;
- minimise the period of disability by speeding up the healing process or providing enough stability to return to normal function while the fracture heals.

There are several methods of holding fracture fragments in place:

- plaster cast/splints;
- traction;
- Kirschner (K-) wires;

Martin Kirschner, 1879–1942, Professor of Surgery, Heidelberg, Germany, introduced the use of skeletal traction wires in 1909.

- external fixation;
- plates and screws;
- intramedullary nails.

Note: Arthroplasty may be used where fragments cannot be held together.

On occasion a combination of holding methods may be used; for example, K-wires and a moulded cast in the case of a simple extra-articular distal radial fracture. It is important to consider the way of holding the reduction in terms of outcome and ensure that this is part of the overarching goal to optimise the patient's return to function as safely and as fast as possible.

For example, a displaced clavicle fracture in a 10-year-old has a 99% chance of sound union within a few months if treated non-operatively. In contrast, a displaced multifragmentary middle third clavicle in a 35-year-old woman will carry a 35% chance of going on to a non-union at 6 months. Therefore, even though this fracture may heal with non-operative treatment, with appropriate explanation and shared decision making, a patient may choose to have surgery early in order to get back to normal function as soon as possible.

Stability can be absolute or relative:

- **Absolute stability**. Implies no displacement or movement and is achieved by accurate anatomical reduction with compression across the fracture fragments to optimise the environment for direct bone healing. This is desirable in intra-articular fractures, where callus at the fracture site might inhibit movement. Intra-articular fractures require an anatomical reduction and absolute stability.
- **Relative stability**. Allows a little movement at the fracture site, optimising the environment for callus formation and indirect bone healing.

Selected examples of achieving absolute and relative stability are shown in ***Figure 32.14***.

Plaster cast and splints

Plaster casts and splints are generally used to hold stable fractures or supplement the fixation of unstable fractures (e.g. below-elbow cast applied to a distal radial fracture after K-wire fixation [see ***Kirschner wires***]).

Plaster casts come in two forms: plaster of Paris and synthetic casting materials. Plaster of Paris is the preferred method in acute fractures; where more support is needed, it is easier to mould plaster of Paris than a synthetic cast. In acute injuries, where there is a risk of swelling and compartment syndrome, a backslab will often be applied. A backslab is not always positioned on the dorsal surface as the name suggests, but is a partial cast where a layer of plaster of Paris or synthetic cast is applied along roughly half the circumference. An alternative to a backslab includes a full cast that is split along its full length to allow for swelling. The use of an incomplete cast does not remove the risk of swelling and compartment syndrome and must always be accompanied by close clinical observation.

Moulding of the cast is an art form requiring appropriate skill to achieve the desired effect. Three-point moulding is used to control the position, often using the intact dorsal periosteal hinge to mould against (***Figure 32.13***). Often, a correctly

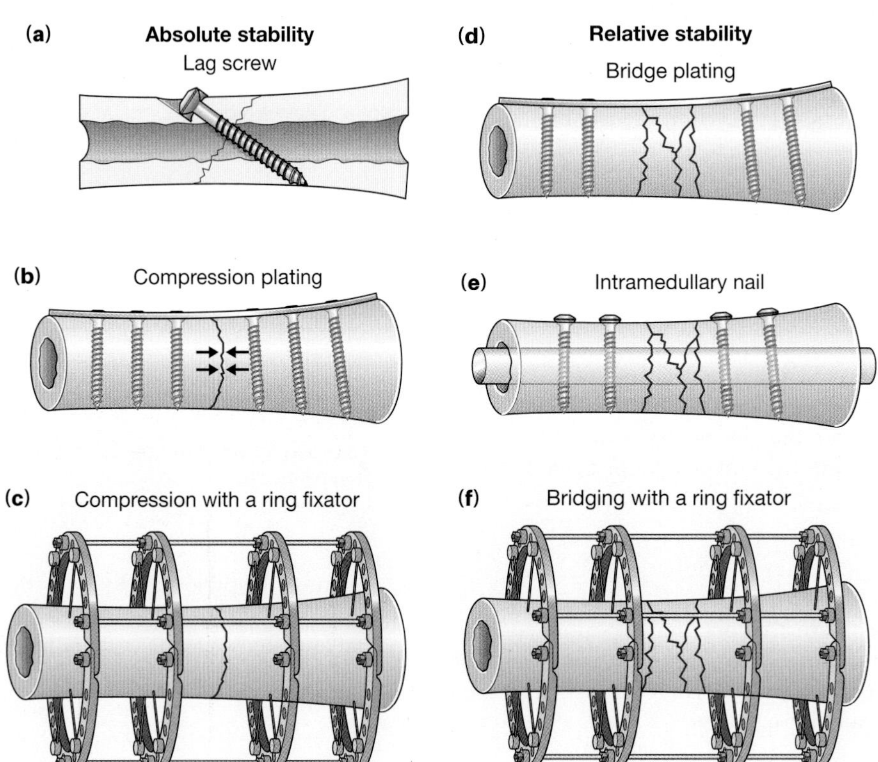

Figure 32.14 (a–f) How absolute and relative stability can be achieved. The same implants may be used to achieve different mechanical effects.

Plaster of Paris is a white crystalline powder, calcium sulphate hemihydrate $CaSO_4{\cdot}0.5H_2O$, which sets hard when water is added to it.

moulded cast will look crooked, leading to the adage 'bent casts make straight bones' (*Figure 32.15*).

Commercially available upper limb and lower limb splints provide comfort, support and social protection to stable fractures. Ease of application and the ability to remove them make them very useful for patients to return to activities of daily living, including bathing and showering.

The advantages and disadvantages of plaster cast and splint usage are described in *Table 32.4*.

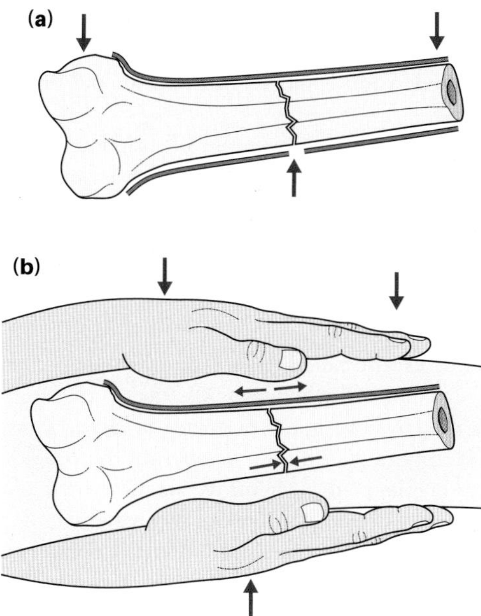

Figure 32.15 (a) The position achieved at the end of the manipulation described in *Figure 32.13*. (b) Demonstration of how, by moulding the cast, the intact periosteum is kept under tension and the bone under compression; thus, the remaining mechanical properties are used to achieve stability.

TABLE 32.4 Advantages and disadvantages of casting and splinting.

Advantages	• No wound • No interference with the fracture site • Cheap • Adjustable • No implants to remove
Disadvantages	• Limited access to the soft tissues • Cumbersome (particularly in the elderly) • Interferes with function • Poor mechanical stability • 'Plaster disease' – joint stiffness and muscle wasting

Traction

Traction is defined as a stretching force on a limb to pull a fracture straight. After appropriate pain control, simply pulling on the limb using manual traction will help realign fracture fragments, returning overall length and alignment. If the fracture is simple and off-ended (displaced so the two bone ends are translated and misaligned), it may require more than simply pulling to reduce it (see reduction in *Figure 32.13*). Once reduced, however, continued longitudinal traction will often hold it reduced.

A traction force can be applied and maintained by a variety of systems and techniques. It is easy to apply traction to any extremity; however, it is cumbersome and requires a fixed point to pull on. This can require the patient to be fixed to one place and limit return to normal function (see *Table 32.5* for advantages and disadvantages of traction).

TABLE 32.5 Advantages and disadvantages of traction.

Advantages	• No wound in zone of injury • No interference with fracture site • Materials cheap • Adjustable
Disadvantages	• Restricts mobility of patient • Expensive in hospital time • Skin pressure complications • Pin site infection • Thromboembolic complication

Traction is often used in the treatment of femoral shaft fractures in adults as a temporary measure for comfort and to allow transfer of the patient, until definitive fixation can be undertaken. A Thomas splint is applied to the limb initially in a static fashion (*Figure 32.16a*) and then, once in bed, balanced traction is applied to help pull the leg out to length and pull the splint off the ischial tuberosity (*Figure 32.16b*).

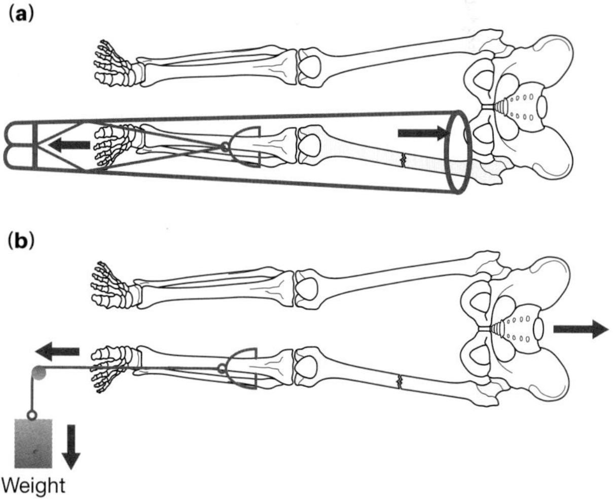

Figure 32.16 (a) Static traction with a Thomas splint. The force and counterforce are contained within a static system. The load is applied to the patient through the tibial traction pin via a cord tightened with a Spanish windlass. The counterforce is applied through pressure by the splint on the ischial tuberosity. (b) A dynamic system in which the load is applied by weights suspended from the tibial pin and the counterforce is the patient's own weight.

Hugh Owen Thomas, 1834–1891, general practitioner of Liverpool, UK, is regarded as the founder of orthopaedic surgery, although never holding a hospital appointment and preferring to treat patients in their own homes. He introduced the Thomas splint in 1875.

The anchor point on the limb may be either skin, by applying an adhesive or non-adhesive bandage, or skeletal traction, where a pin is placed in the proximal tibia or distal femur.

A common everyday example of traction is the use of a collar and cuff in proximal humeral fractures. When the patient is upright, the lower part of the arm, under the action of gravity, provides longitudinal traction, thus aligning the fracture fragments.

Kirschner wires

Kirschner wires (also called K-wires) are smooth, non-threaded, thin flexible wires often between 0.9 and 2.5 mm in diameter. They are used to hold small fragments in place. They may be used in a temporary fashion intraoperatively to hold fracture fragments in place until definitive fixation with plates and screws can be performed. They are inexpensive and simple to use. Moreover, they are extensively used for definitive fixation of injuries around the hand and wrist. The flexible nature of the wires can often require supplementation, as a hybrid construct of K-wires and plaster cast fixation.

In distal radial fractures the wires are placed percutaneously after closed reduction, with the trailing end of the wire left proud of the skin and the end bent to limit wire migration. K-wires around the distal radius can be removed in the clinic setting 4–6 weeks after insertion. Complications of K-wires include pin site infection, wire breakage, loss of fixation and wire migration. Wire migration may be a potentially serious problem in certain locations. It is not advisable to use non-threaded K-wires around the shoulder girdle and clavicle as migration into the thoracic cavity and heart has been reported (*Table 32.6*).

TABLE 32.6 Indications for K-wire insertion.

- Temporary fixation
- Definitive fixation – with small fracture fragments (e.g. wrist fractures and hand injuries)
- Tension band wiring (fractures of the patella and olecranon)
- Temporary immobilisation of a small joint

External fixation

External fixation involves percutaneous placement of metal rods or fine wires into bone to anchor a metal frame on the outside (*Table 32.7*). The frame construct itself may consist of tubular rods with connectors, or a circular ring construct – the 'Ilizarov' frame. Hybrid variations are infinite, with combinations of anchor fixation modalities and frame constructs. The Taylor spatial frame allows for gradual correction of deformity (*Figure 32.17*).

The major drawback of external fixation is that they can be cumbersome to the patient and pin site infection can be a problem (*Table 32.7*).

Specific indications for external fixators include:

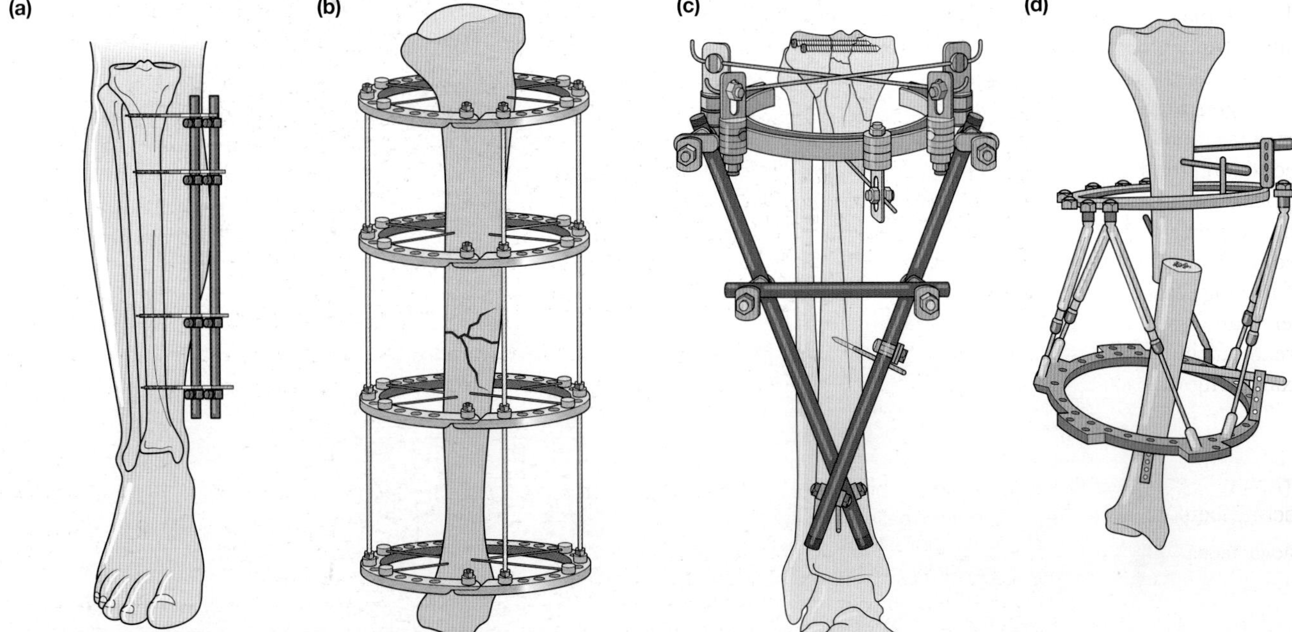

Figure 32.17 (a) Monolateral tubular frame with a metal rod (half pin anchorage to bone). (b) Circular ring fixator with fine wire anchorage to bone. (c) Hybrid circular/tubular rod frame construct with a combination of half pin and fine wire anchorage to bone. (d) Taylor spatial frame; allows for gradual correction of deformity.

Gavriil Abramovich Ilizarov, 1921–1993, orthopaedic surgeon, Kurgan, Western Siberia, Russia. He did not attend school until he was 11 years old as his family was too poor to buy him shoes.
J Charles Taylor, orthopaedic surgeon, Memphis, TN, USA.

TABLE 32.7 Advantages and disadvantages of external fixation.

Advantages	• No interference with fracture site • Adjustable after application: alignment; biomechanics • Soft tissues accessible for plastic surgery • Rapid stabilisation of fracture • Hardware easy to remove
Disadvantages	• Pin site infection • Interferes with plastic surgical procedures • Soft-tissue tethering • Cumbersome for the patient

- emergency stabilisation of a long bone fracture in the polytrauma patient thought too unwell to have other interventions – damage control orthopaedics;
- stabilisation of a dislocated joint after reduction (e.g. a spanning fixator across the knee joint while the vascular surgeons repair an arterial injury with a knee dislocation);
- complex periarticular fractures to provide temporary stabilisation and allow the soft-tissue damage to recover before definitive fixation (e.g. a distal tibial [pilon] fracture);
- fractures associated with infection;
- treating fractures with bone loss.

Plates and screws

Plates and screws can be used in many different ways. A 'lag screw' can be used to generate compression across a fracture site, optimising the environment for direct bone healing. Similarly, compression can be achieved using a dynamic compression plate. A plate might also be used simply to neutralise forces, buttress a fracture or work as an internal–external fixator (*Figure 32.14*).

In general, plates and screws are used where possible in articular and periarticular fractures where an anatomical reduction is required, often via open means, followed by the application of the plate and screws to achieve a rigid construct. In extra-articular fractures, where mechanical alignment is required together with relative stability, one option is the use of locking plate technology. This allows a closed reduction and percutaneous placement of the plate with locking screws to create an internal construct, which behaves like an external fixator. Injury-specific plating systems have revolutionised the ability to treat certain injuries, with plates pre-bent and pre-shaped for specific anatomical regions and specific injury patterns (see *Table 32.8* for the advantages and disadvantages of plate fixation).

TABLE 32.8 Advantages and disadvantages of plate and screw fixation.

Advantages	• Can be used when anatomical reduction is required • Allows early mobilisation • Can provide absolute or relative stability
Disadvantages	• May interfere with the fracture site • Periosteal/soft-tissue damage • Does not normally allow for immediate load-bearing • Potential for infection • Metalwork complications • Possible need for plate removal

Intramedullary nails

Diaphyseal fractures are best suited for intramedullary nailing. Where mechanical alignment is required together with relative stability, they allow for indirect bone healing. After nail insertion, mechanical alignment is checked particularly for length, alignment and rotation. Locking screws are then placed proximally and distally to maintain length and alignment. Intramedullary nailing of metaphyseal and articular fractures is a challenge. However, with improved implant design and the ability to lock the nails very distally and in multiple directions, the indications for intramedullary nailing are expanding.

Intramedullary nails may be placed in an unreamed or reamed fashion. Reaming is the process whereby the intramedullary canal is widened slightly to allow passage of a larger diameter nail, relating to the last reamer size used. *Table 32.9* compares reamed with unreamed nails.

Intramedullary nailing can be a technically demanding procedure. The advantages and disadvantages are summarised in *Table 32.10*.

TABLE 32.9 A comparison of reamed and unreamed nailing (an assumption is that nails used unreamed are usually thinner than those used reamed).

	Reamed IMN	Unreamed IMN
Insertion time	Longer	Quicker
Time to union	Shorter	Longer
Size of implant	Larger	Smaller
Reduction of distal fractures	Easier	More difficult
Strength of construct	More	Less

IMN, intramedullary nail.

TABLE 32.10 Advantages and disadvantages of intramedullary nailing.

Advantages	• Minimally invasive • Early weight-bearing • Less periosteal damage than open reduction and internal fixation • Seldom need removal
Disadvantages	• Increased risk of fat emboli/chest complications • Infection difficult to treat • Difficult to remove if broken

Arthroplasty

Arthroplasty is indicated in certain acute circumstances: articular fractures that are not reconstructible or injuries where the vascularity of the articular segment is compromised (e.g. displaced intracapsular femoral neck fracture in an older patient).

The patient's demographics and functional demands need to be considered in choosing arthroplasty as a treatment option. Implant longevity and level of activities following implant insertion need to be matched. Traditionally, arthroplasty for trauma was limited to hip and shoulder hemiarthroplasty.

Total hip replacement, acute distal femoral replacement, radial head replacement, total and hemielbow arthroplasty and reverse polarity shoulder arthroplasty are current treatment options for older patients with osteoporotic periarticular fractures. The selection of a particular technique will depend on clinical evidence and our previously stated aim to return patients to optimal function as soon as possible. It should be considered in the context that it can be expensive and require considerable other resources to make the procedure safe and long-lasting.

Heal

Time to fracture healing depends on several factors: patient comorbidities, the age of the patient, bone involved (upper limb or lower limb), patient factors (diabetes) and choice of treatment. Well-known factors that slow down bone healing include diabetes mellitus (doubles time to union), diminished blood supply (peripheral vascular disease, vascular injury at the time of injury), smoking, non-steroidal anti-inflammatory drugs and infection at the fracture site.

Several chemical and mechanical methods have been attempted to enhance fracture healing, including bone marrow injections into the fracture site and other orthobiologics such as bone morphogenic proteins. Mechanical methods include controlled axial micromotion (using an external fixator), electromagnetic stimulation and low-intensity pulsed ultrasound. There is good basic scientific evidence to support their theoretical benefit; however, to date there is little clinical evidence for their use in the primary treatment of closed fractures. The surgical strategy is important in determining how bones heal. As surgeons, our technique helps dictate whether the injury heals by primary bone healing, through compression; secondary bone healing, through forming callus that becomes ossified to bone over time; and, indeed, whether the fracture heals at all. Respecting the biological and biomechanical environment of the fracture is an important consideration when planning operative and non-operative management of fractures.

TABLE 32.11 Indications for surgery in limb trauma. The main indication is that operation will produce a better outcome; the principles are given in the text.

- A fracture requiring treatment that is unsuitable for non-operative measures
- Open fractures
- Failed non-operative management
- Multiple injuries
- Pathological or impending pathological fractures
- Displaced intra-articular fractures
- Fractures through the growth plate, where arrest is possible (Salter–Harris types III–V)
- Avulsion fractures that compromise the functional integrity of a ligament/tendon around a joint (e.g. olecranon fracture)
- Established non-unions or malunions

Rehabilitate

The main aim of treatment is to return the patient to a similar level of premorbid function as quickly as possible. Rehabilitation begins as soon as feasible. It is often not necessary to wait until bone union before beginning rehabilitation. It is important to move the affected joints and the joints in close proximity to the fracture (e.g. elbow and shoulder exercise while in a cast for a distal radial fracture), limiting global stiffness and wasting of the muscles on that limb.

TREATMENT BY FRACTURE LOCATION

In general, the principles of treatment described above are dependent on the fracture location: diaphyseal, metaphyseal and intra-articular.

Table 32.11 outlines some indications for operative stabilisation.

Diaphyseal fractures

Extra-articular fractures do not require an anatomical reduction, but rather a mechanical restoration by correction of length, alignment and rotation (*Figure 32.18*).

Angular malunion of a diaphyseal fracture of the weight-bearing long bones will lead to abnormal joint forces on the joint above and below, leading to pain and secondary degenerative joint disease.

Diaphyseal fractures are generally well suited to intramedullary fixation techniques, as previously discussed.

Summary box 32.5

Diaphyseal fractures

- Restore length, alignment and rotation
- Consider whether primary or secondary bone healing is the objective
- Radius and ulna need precise reduction to function

Metaphyseal fractures

In the AO classification metaphyseal fractures are classified into A type – extra-articular, B type – partial articular, and C type – complete articular.

In A-type fractures, joint congruity is not an issue and as such the principles of mechanical alignment, length and rotation need to be considered. Fixation of metaphyseal fractures is less predictable with intramedullary nailing, therefore plate and screw fixation, external fixation or, in the smaller joints, K-wire fixation is used. Metaphyseal fractures are close to the joint and so consideration is given to stable fixation to allow early joint movement and rehabilitation.

Intra-articular fractures

AO type B and type C fractures are intra-articular and as such the principles of treating intra-articular fractures need to be

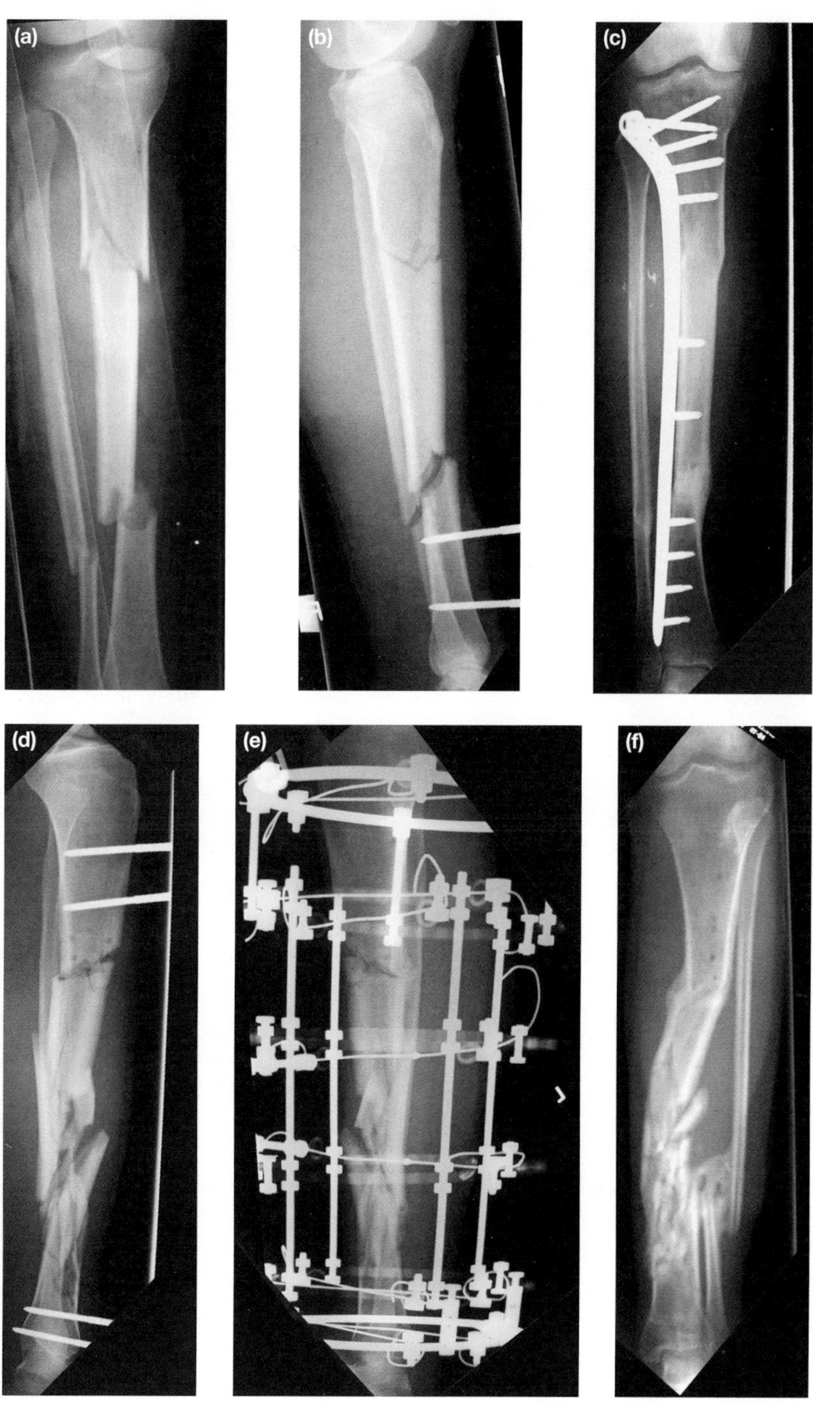

Figure 32.18 (a) and (d) are C-type or segmental tibial fractures. Each was a high-energy injury; (b) and (e) show a temporary spanning external fixator applied in each case; (c) and (f) show definitive relative stability was achieved with different methods of bridging fixation. Healing was by indirect means in both cases. Despite irregularities at the fracture sites the overall alignment in coronal and sagittal planes was satisfactory and function was good.

respected; namely, anatomical reduction of the articular surface and rigid stabilisation to allow early joint movement and avoidance of degenerative joint disease (*Figure 32.19*). However, these principles have to be balanced with the increased wound complications of open surgery and devitalising bone fragments with excessive exposure of the bone.

Osteoporotic intra-articular fractures are a considerable challenge. Although anatomical reduction may be achieved, rigid fixation devices may cut out of soft bone, particularly in the metaphysis of the bone where pull-out strength of the fixation is reduced. Plate design and the introduction of locking plates where the screw secures itself into the plate are design

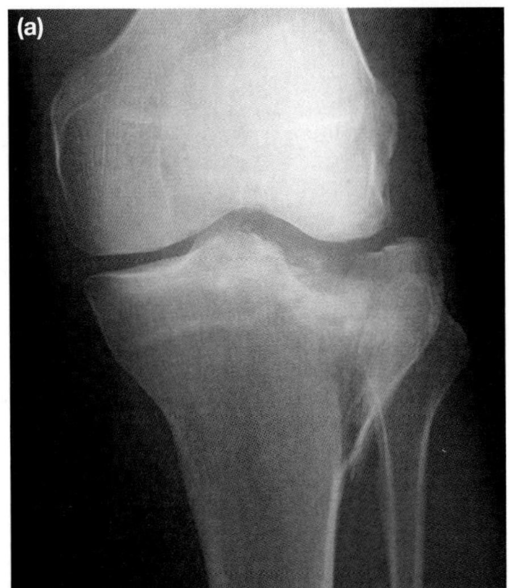

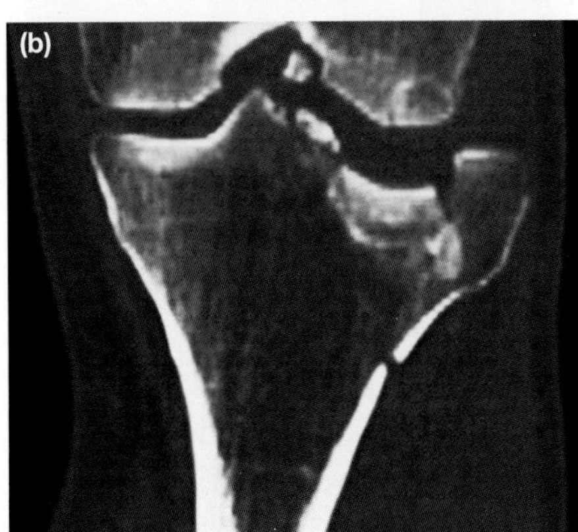

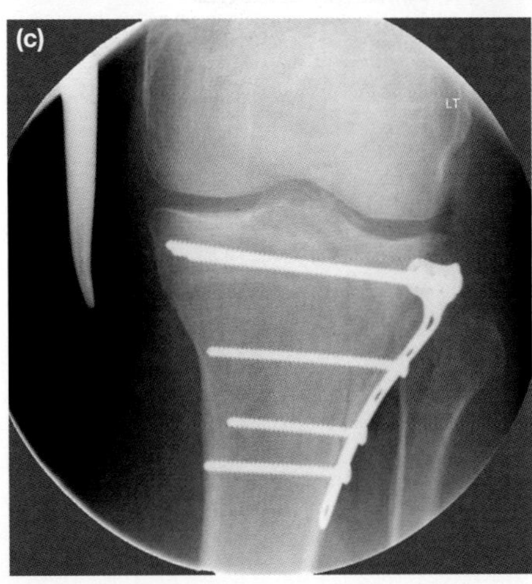

Figure 32.19 A B-type or partial articular fracture. (a) Plain radiograph; (b) computed tomography clarifies the injury; (c) fixation with plate and screws achieving compression across a previously reduced fracture.

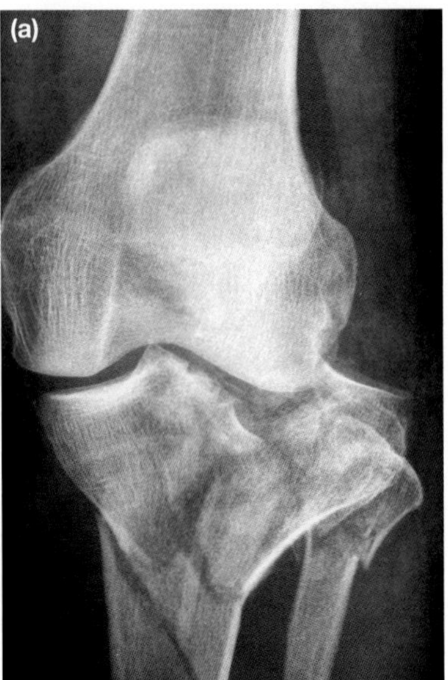

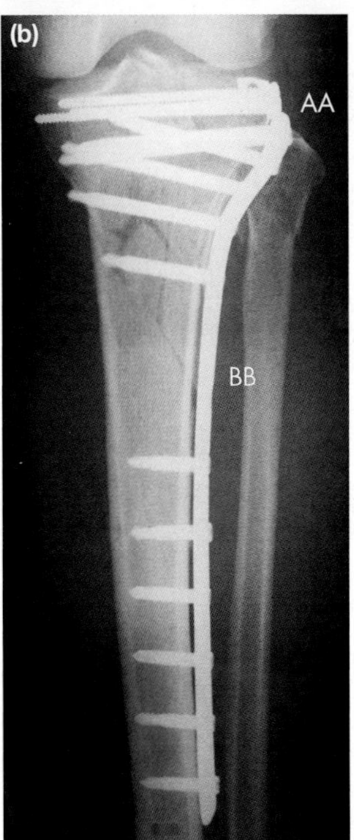

Figure 32.20 (a) A C-type proximal tibial articular fracture (i.e. none of the joint remains attached to the diaphysis). (b) The small plate and screws (AA) are used to compress the joint fragments, aiming for absolute stability. The heavy duty fixed angled device (BB) spans the fracture and provides relative stability. Although the image is historical and techniques vary with time, there has been good restoration of alignment and joint congruity.

features to help improve cut-out strength and may help reduce failure of fixation in osteoporotic bone. Injectable bone substitutes may be used to fill bone voids and augment fixation. If stable fixation is not possible, then consideration might be given to non-operative treatment and delayed joint replacement or, on occasion, primary joint replacement may be undertaken.

In type C fractures where the articular surface has separated from the metaphysis, the articular surface is initially anatomically reduced and held with temporary K-wires or lag screws and then the articular block is reattached to the shaft using methods as described above – plate, nail or frame (***Figure 32.20***).

TREATMENT BY REGION (FROM TOP TO TOE)

Scaphoid fracture

The blood supply to the scaphoid enters distally and supplies the scaphoid in a retrograde fashion. As such, a displaced waist of scaphoid fracture interrupts the blood supply to the proximal pole, leading to avascular necrosis. An undisplaced fracture of the scaphoid may not be visible on the initial radiographs. If a fracture is not evident on the initial radiographs and the patient is tender in the anatomical snuff box following a fall on the outstretched hand, special scaphoid view radiographs should be requested (*Figure 32.21*).

If a fracture is not evident on the initial radiographs and the patient remains tender in the anatomical snuff box, then treat as a suspected scaphoid fracture until a fracture is actively excluded. The standard protocol of a suspected scaphoid fracture is to immobilise the wrist and examine again 10–14 days later. If tenderness remains, repeat the scaphoid views. If facilities and resources allow, an earlier diagnosis may be made with a bone scan, MRI or CT.

Undisplaced fractures can be treated non-operatively in a below-elbow cast. It is not necessary to include the thumb as a routine. In displaced or unstable fractures (>1 mm) consideration should be given to open reduction and rigid fixation with a headless compression screw. Complications of scaphoid fractures include: non-union, avascular necrosis, malunion and carpal instability.

Carpal instability

The most commonly involved carpal bone is the lunate. A lunate dislocation is where the lunate bone dislocates out of the radiocarpal joint. In a perilunate dislocation the lunate remains in the radiocarpal joint and the rest of the carpus dislocates around the lunate. Lunate and perilunate dislocations are easily missed unless careful attention is paid to carpal alignment on the lateral radiograph (*Figure 32.22*). Review of the radiographs should particularly ensure the anatomical location of the lunate in the radiocarpal fossa and that the capitate in the 'cup' of the lunate is maintained.

Acute injuries should be reduced closed initially to remove pressure from the median nerve. Anatomical carpal alignment is difficult to hold and therefore surgical reconstruction of damaged intrinsic ligaments, together with K-wire fixation of the carpal bones, is often undertaken. Ligamentous healing is slow and may be incomplete. K-wires are kept in place for 8 weeks and the wrist casted or splinted for 3 months.

Thumb metacarpophalangeal ulnar collateral ligament

Injury to the thumb metacarpal ulnar collateral ligament is a unique injury often termed 'gamekeeper's thumb' or 'skier's thumb'. Owing to the unique anatomical arrangement of adductor pollicis, if the ligament undergoes complete rupture the aponeurosis may become interposed, inhibiting

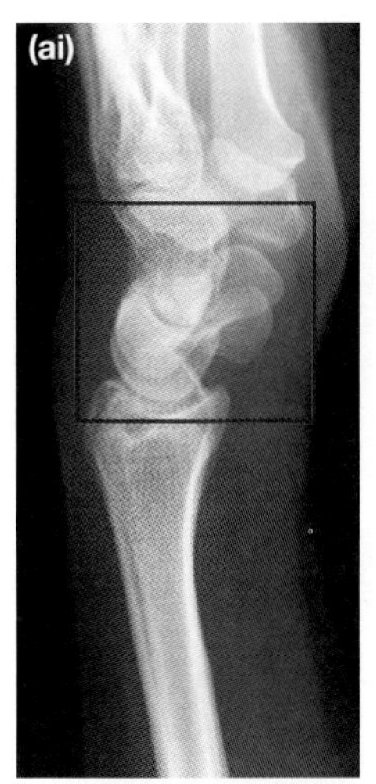

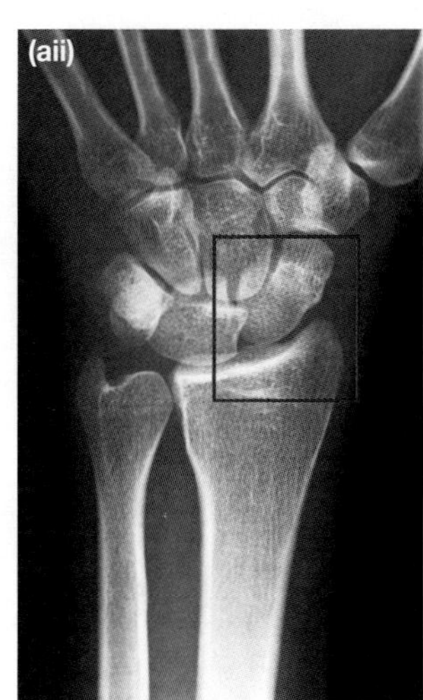

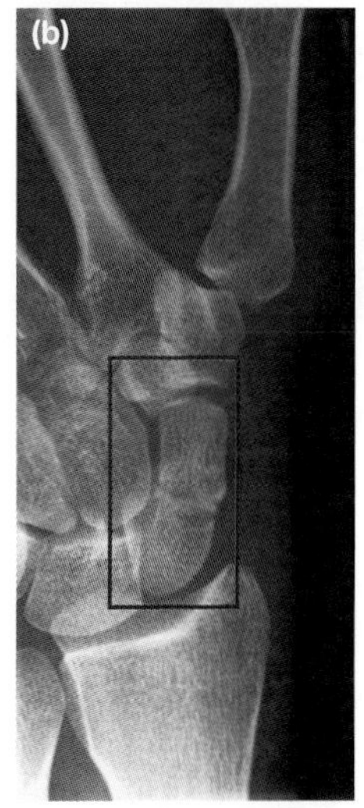

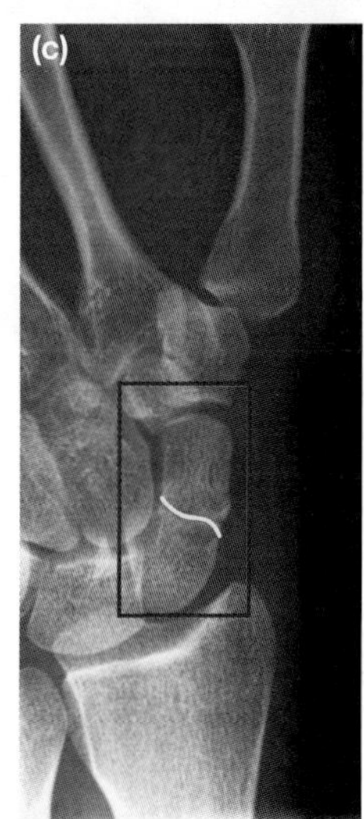

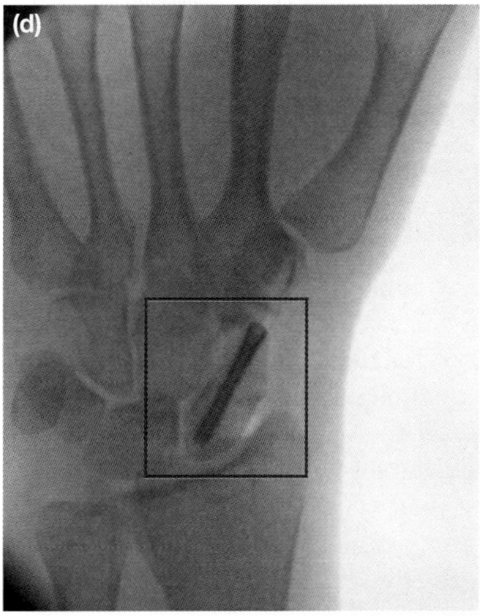

Figure 32.21 Scaphoid fracture. (a) Anteroposterior (i) and lateral (ii) views in which the injury is difficult to see; (b, c) oblique views with the fracture line highlighted; (d) in this case of a young patient, the fracture was treated with early fixation.

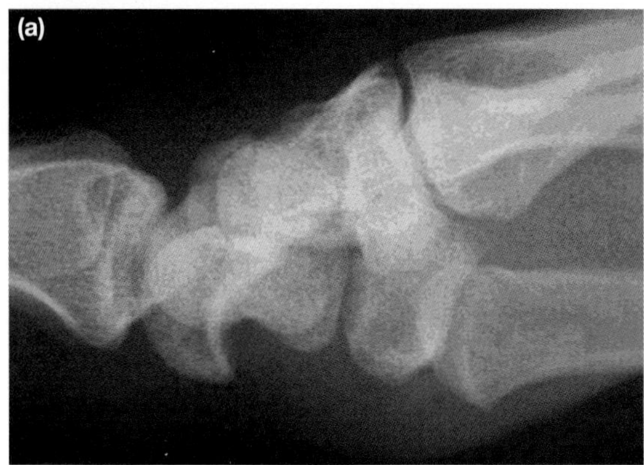

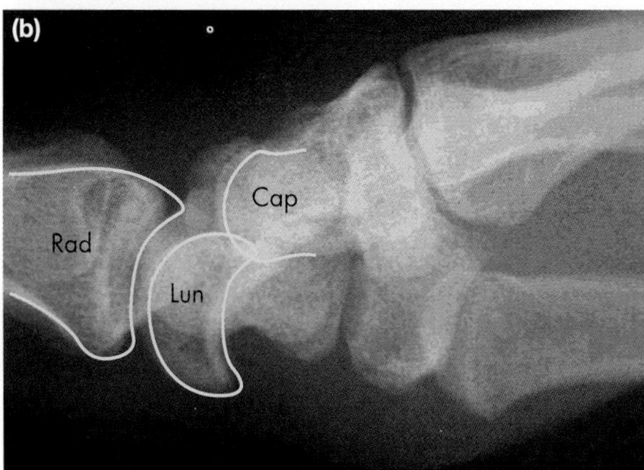

Figure 32.22 Perilunate dislocation. (a) A plain lateral radiograph of the wrist; (b) the outline of the perilunate dislocation is highlighted. Cap, capitate; Lun, lunate; Rad, radius.

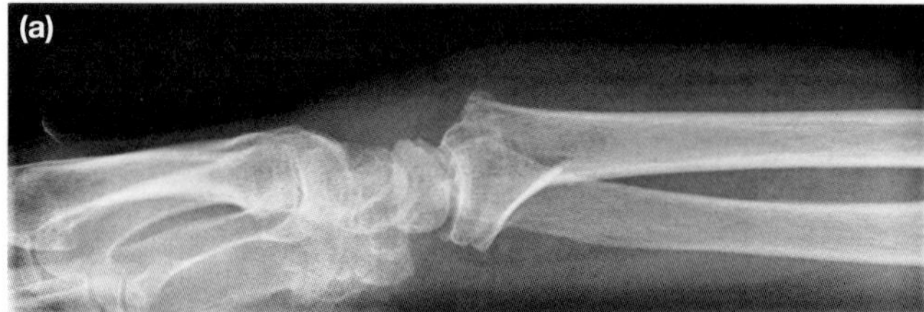

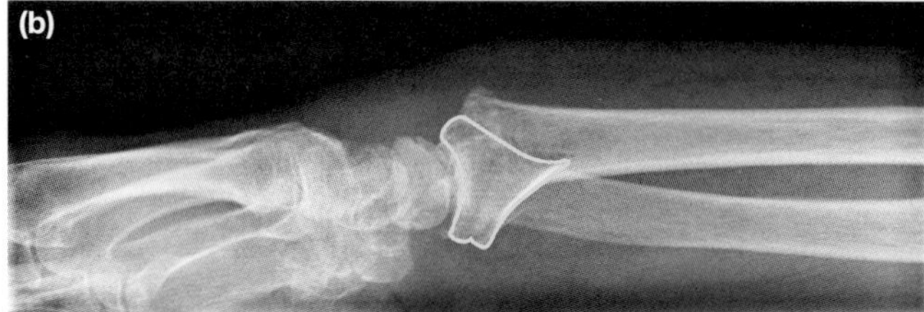

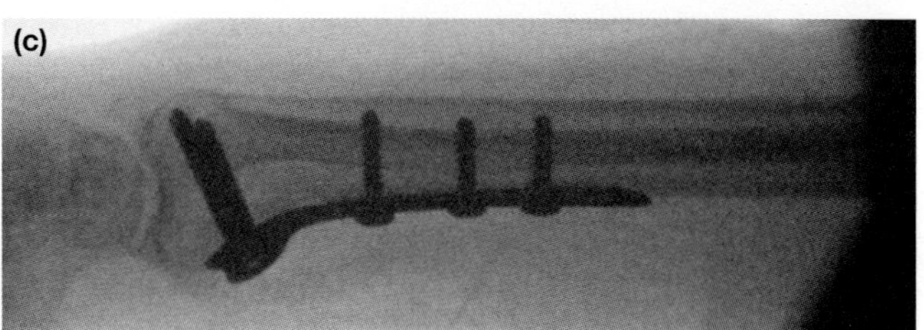

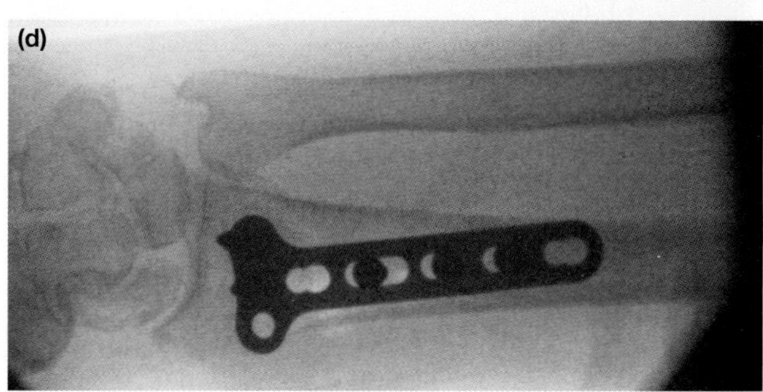

Figure 32.23 An A-type or extra-articular metaphyseal fracture. A plain lateral radiograph of this Smith-type fracture (a, b). Fracture fixed to a plate. There is no interfragmental compression. The plate is pushing against or buttressing the distal fragment (c, d).

ligament-to-bone healing. A rupture of the ulnar collateral ligament should be suspected when an ulna-directed force is directed across the metacarpophalangeal (MCP) joint. A tender swelling on the ulnar side of the MCP joint may signify the Stener lesion. Increased laxity may be clinically evident; if there is uncertainty, stress radiographs can demonstrate the degree of injury. Complete ruptures with a Stener lesion (interposed aponeurosis) require open reduction of the ligament to restore bone contact, with a suture anchor repair of the associated ulnar collateral ligament.

Distal radial fractures

Extra-articular (type A) fractures of the distal radius may displace in a volar or dorsal direction. It is possible to reduce volar displaced fractures (Smith's fracture) of the distal radius with a closed technique. However, they tend to be unstable and displace if held in a cast. Hence most volar displaced extra-articular distal radial fractures are reduced and held with a volar buttress plate (*Figure 32.23*).

Most dorsally displaced fractures (Colles fracture) can be addressed with closed reduction and held in a cast. However, some will slip or collapse with cast treatment, and so close review for the first few weeks is advocated.

Fractures with significant initial displacement and dorsal comminution are at risk of early and late collapse. After thorough counselling the patient may choose to have the fracture reduced and then held surgically with K-wires, plate and screw fixation (volar or dorsal) or external fixation. The K-wires may be placed across the fracture fragments or intrafocally, going through the fracture site. The latter can be used to help reduce the fracture and then used to lock the fracture fragments in place (*Figure 32.24*).

Treatment is individualised based on patient and fracture pattern factors. Intra-articular fractures (types B and C) of the

Bertil Stener, 1920–1999, Swedish orthopaedic surgeon, described the anatomy and treatment of a displaced ulna collateral ligament injury to the thumb in 1962.
Robert William Smith, 1807–1873, Professor of Surgery, Trinity College, Dublin, Ireland, described the reverse Colles fracture in 1847.
Abraham Colles, 1773–1843, President of the Royal College of Surgeons of Ireland (1802), Professor of Anatomy, Physiology and Surgery (1804) and described distal radial fracture in 1814.

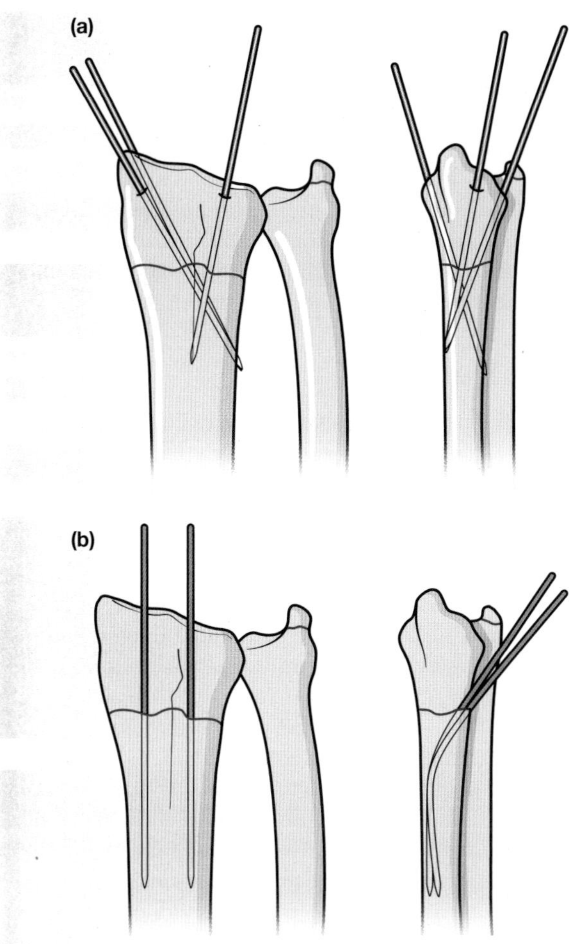

Figure 32.24 (a) K-wires placed across fracture fragments; (b) intrafocal K-wires used to help reduce the fracture.

distal radius require anatomical reduction of the joint surface; a gap or step of less than 2 mm can be accepted in the radius. The distal radius fails fairly predictably with splitting of the lunate fossa fragment in the coronal plane and separation of the radial styloid.

If a closed reduction can be achieved with manipulation, the fracture fragments can subsequently be held with K-wires, plate and screw fixation or external fixation. The most common form of treatment is closed reduction and percutaneous K-wire fixation, supplemented with a plaster cast for 4–6 weeks.

Forearm fractures (radius and ulna)

Fractures of the diaphyseal shaft of the radius and ulna are technically, in the anatomical sense of the word, extra-articular. However, the forearm bones work together, being coupled at the proximal and distal radioulnar joints to allow for forearm pronation and supination. Therefore, when considering treatment the principles that apply to intra-articular fractures need to be considered: anatomical reduction and rigid fixation to allow for early joint motion. Most fractures that involve both radius and ulna in adults require open reduction, anatomical alignment and rigid plate fixation.

Isolated fractures of the ulna, the so-called nightstick fracture, are a little more controversial, as non-operative management is possible but in this location risks delayed union and non-union, hence treatment depends on patient factors. Operative fixation with plate and screw fixation is technically simple and allows early predictable return to function.

Olecranon fractures

Olecranon fractures may be displaced or undisplaced. Undisplaced fractures with <2 mm gap or step at the articular surface can be treated non-operatively. In displaced fractures the extensor mechanism is interrupted and the articular surface requires anatomical reduction and stable fixation to allow early movement. Fixation may comprise K-wire and figure-of-eight tension band wiring or plate fixation. In multifragmentary fractures or fractures associated with an elbow dislocation, increased stability is required with the use of a plate and screws.

Humeral fractures

Fractures of the diaphyseal portion of the humeral shaft are extra-articular fractures and as such require mechanical alignment. Non-operative treatment with functional bracing will achieve union in an acceptable position within 12 weeks in over 80% of cases. Gravity can provide traction on the arm and in conjunction with a humeral brace helps to hold alignment and allow early range of motion of the elbow. Active shoulder abduction is avoided until fracture union to prevent varus deformity.

Shoulder movement must not be absent during treatment and so gravity-assisted pendulum exercises are instituted early on to prevent shoulder stiffness. As the fracture approaches the metaphyseal region of the humerus it becomes more difficult to control with humeral bracing. Distal third extra-articular fractures of the humerus can be treated non-operatively in a humeral brace but have a tendency to go into varus. Articular fractures of the distal humerus require anatomical reduction and stable fixation to allow early joint movement.

Internal fixation is indicated for displaced intra-articular fractures, non-union or delayed union, open fractures, multiple injuries and those fractures not held in an acceptable position with brace treatment. Fixation of diaphyseal fractures can be achieved with intramedullary nailing or plate and screw fixation. Plate fixation is associated with higher union rates and lower rates of reintervention (*Figure 32.25*).

The radial nerve is the most commonly injured nerve in humeral shaft fractures. Treatment of a humeral shaft fracture with a concomitant radial nerve palsy remains topical. Most will recover spontaneously. In general, if the nerve injury occurs at the time of the original injury, non-operative treatment can be considered. If it occurs after the injury, for example at the time of brace application, then it should be explored. When exploring the radial nerve, plate and screw fixation is then undertaken to stabilise the humerus.

Fractures of the proximal humerus

In fractures of the proximal humerus consideration is given to the vascularity of the humeral head. The most common

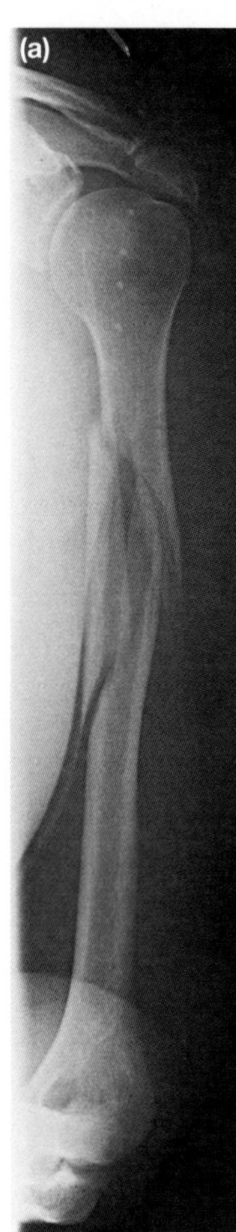

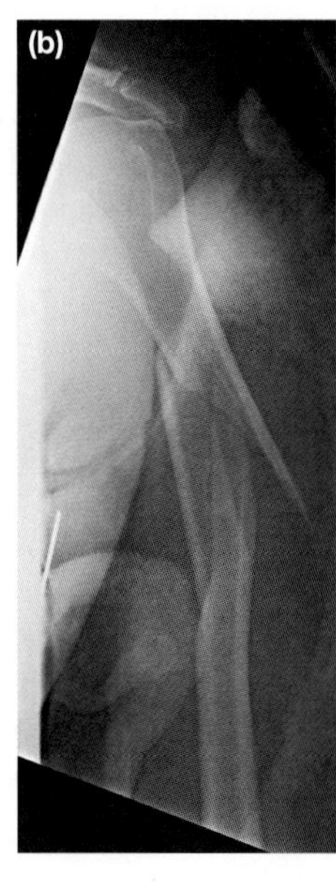

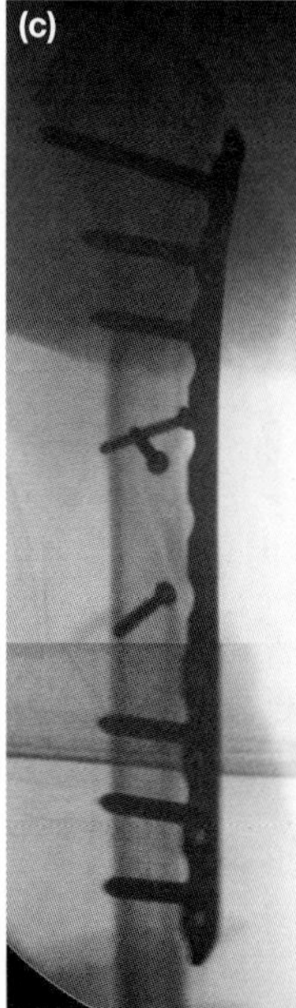

Figure 32.25 (a–c) A B-type humeral shaft fracture. This fracture could not be controlled by non-operative means and was treated with lag screws protected by a plate.

classification of the proximal humerus is the Neer classification, which looks at the four individual pieces of the proximal humerus (articular head fragment, lesser tuberosity, greater tuberosity and the shaft).

If a fragment is displaced by more than 1 cm or angulated by more than 45° in respect of another fragment, it is considered a part. As such, based on the fracture pattern, it may be undisplaced, or in two parts, three parts or four parts. Consideration is then given to potential joint dislocation, anterior or posterior. The greater the number of parts, the higher the chances of interruption of the vascularity to the humeral head and the more complex the injury.

Three factors can be used to predict avascularity of the humeral head:

1 fracture through the anatomical neck;
2 loss of the medial hinge;
3 less than 8 mm of bone along the medial calcar.

In situations where there is a high risk of failure of both fixation and non-operative treatment, owing to avascular necrosis or implant fixation failing from bone loss or loss of function (e.g. with displaced fractures in lower demand patients and those with osteoporosis and other comorbidities), consideration may be given to replacing the humeral head. This may take the form of an anatomical hemiarthroplasty. One of the limitations of trauma hemiarthroplasty for proximal humeral fractures involves reliable healing of the tuberosities and the rotator cuff. Increasingly, a primary reverse polarity shoulder prosthesis is being used. This implant does not rely on tuberosity healing, as it functions under the power of the deltoid muscle.

In younger patients reduction and fixation may be considered. A variety of fixation methods are available: percutaneous fixation, intramedullary nails and plate fixation.

Clavicle fractures

Diaphyseal fractures of the middle third of the clavicle have traditionally been treated non-operatively with a broad arm sling for comfort and social protection, followed by increasing use of the arm.

Most mid-third fractures of the clavicle will unite with non-operative treatment. There is, however, a subset of clavicle fractures that may be slow to heal and that do impact on shoulder girdle function. Displaced, comminuted fractures show a propensity to be slow to heal and increasing age and female gender further negatively impact on fracture healing. It has been shown that 2 cm of shortening of the clavicle impacts on shoulder girdle function, with weakness and fatigability when working above shoulder height.

Internal fixation with an intramedullary device or plate and screw construct can restore length, alignment and rotation. This can improve the speed and amount of functional restoration, but carries all the risks of surgical treatment. Treatment is individualised to patient needs and expectations.

Proximal femoral fractures

The blood supply to the femoral head is a prime consideration in treating femoral neck fractures. The blood supply comes via the hip capsule and although vascular anatomy is variable it is chiefly through the medial and lateral branches of the deep circumflex femoral artery in addition to the occasionally redundant artery of the ligamentum teres (a branch of the obturator artery). The joint capsule anteriorly inserts along the intertrochanteric line and posteriorly half-way along the femoral neck. Fractures proximal to the hip capsule are intracapsular and those distal to the capsule are extracapsular fractures.

Intracapsular femoral neck fractures

Intracapsular fractures are further broken down into whether they are displaced or undisplaced. Undisplaced intracapsular fractures are generally stable and interruption of the blood supply to the femoral head is rare. Therefore, treatment is aimed at ensuring that the head fragment does not displace during rehabilitation. This can be achieved with cannulated screws inserted along the femoral neck into the head.

A displaced intracapsular fracture may cause disruption of the blood supply either through direct injury to the arteries

Charles Sumner Neer II, 1917–2011, American orthopedic surgeon, emeritus professor at Columbia University, developed a widely used shoulder prosthesis and also developed a common classification system for proximal humerus fractures.

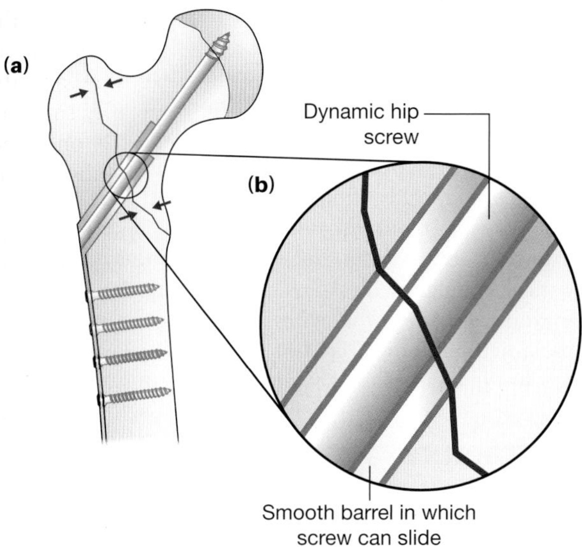

Figure 32.26 (a) A dynamic hip screw for fixing a trochanteric proximal femoral fracture. This allows for compression at the fracture site on load-bearing and protects the femoral head from penetration by the screw when the osteoporotic bone settles; (b) insert to show the sliding screw in the barrel.

or joint capsule intra-articular haematoma can affect the survival of the femoral head, leading to avascular necrosis. If the patient is physiologically young, reduction and internal fixation with cannulated screws or a dynamic hip screw might be attempted to preserve the native head.

If the patient is older and would benefit from a single operation, the head may be sacrificed and replaced with a prosthetic head. Arthroplasty of the proximal femur may take the form of hemiarthroplasty or total hip replacement, depending on the patient's functional demands.

Extracapsular femoral neck fractures

If the fracture is extracapsular, vascularity of the head is not an issue. Extracapsular femoral neck fractures are subdivided into stable or unstable. Unstable fractures include a reverse oblique pattern or where the medial calcar is a comminuted (lesser trochanter) fracture. Stable extracapsular fractures simply require connection of the head to the shaft, often using a dynamic hip screw (***Figure 32.26***).

In unstable fractures a dynamic hip screw can also be used, but, owing to the unfavourable mechanical environment relating to the loss of the medial calcar or a reverse oblique pattern, an intramedullary device might be considered.

Femoral shaft fractures

It is possible to treat diaphyseal fractures of the femoral shaft non-operatively. The fracture can be reduced and held in position until union with traction; however, it takes 3 months. This is a long time to be in hospital and carries all the potential risks of prolonged bed rest. Most femoral shaft fractures are treated with a locked intramedullary nail.

With modern locked intramedullary implants, the patient will be up and out of bed the following day and, if it is an isolated injury, home within a few days. Weight-bearing depends on the fracture pattern and implant used. If there is a simple fracture pattern with cortical apposition, it will be possible to mobilise with crutches, weight-bearing as comfort allows. Although it may still take 3 months or more for the fracture to unite, the implant will be able to carry the load until union, allowing earlier return to function out of the hospital.

Distal femoral fractures

Metaphyseal osteoporotic fractures of the distal femur are amenable to internal fixation with locked intramedullary nails or plate and screw fixation. If the fracture extends into the articular surface, reconstruction may be undertaken with cannulated screws augmented with intramedullary nailing or injury-specific locking plates for the distal femur. More commonly now these injuries are often next to a knee replacement (periprosthetic fracture), which can add technical complexity; surgical decision making is influenced by whether the implant is attached to bone or is loose, the amount of bone to fix into and the health status of the patient. More recently, primary and revision arthroplasty have been considered in these situations to allow early mobilisation.

Patellar fractures

Similar to olecranon fractures, undisplaced fractures in which the extensor mechanism is intact can be treated non-operatively. A simple assessment of this is if the patient can straight leg raise to test the extensor mechanism, but beware of the patient who is able to 'cheat' by using the iliotibial band to internally rotate the leg to compensate for the deficient extensor mechanism. Displaced fractures require anatomical reduction of the articular surface and reconstitution of the integrity of the extensor mechanism. The cartilage on the patella is very thick; as such, increased amounts of displacement compared with other joints may not lead to degeneration.

Surgical treatment of simple displaced fractures can be achieved with two K-wires and figure-of-eight tension band wiring.

Multifragmentary patellar fractures can be very challenging. Patellar excision is an option but significantly reduces the mechanical advantage of the extensor apparatus. A tension band construct may be augmented by using circumferential wiring of the patella.

Tibial plateau fractures

Intra-articular fractures of the tibial plateau are common. Injuries may involve the lateral or medial side or both. The joint articular surface may be split, depressed or a combination of both. A CT scan should be performed to see the full extent of the injury. Undisplaced fractures may be treated non-operatively with a hinged knee brace and progressive protected weight-bearing over 8–12 weeks. The surgical considerations here are to restore alignment and joint congruity.

Displaced fractures require reduction and stabilisation. The articular surface, once reduced, is often held with plate and screw fixation or fine wire external fixation.

Tibial shaft fractures

For an undisplaced non-comminuted fracture of the tibial shaft, closed reduction and an above-knee cast is a safe and inexpensive treatment. At 4–6 weeks this may be converted to a patellar tendon below-knee cast to allow knee movement. Prolonged casting can lead to stiffness of the knee and the subtalar joint. Cast treatment requires close and constant monitoring of the position of the fracture site. To correct minor angular deformities the cast can be wedged.

A patient may choose to have an intramedullary nail to allow free knee and ankle movement. This, however, risks infection of the implant and anterior knee pain. This is another situation in which information and shared decision making can allow the patient to select the most appropriate treatment option.

For comminuted and complex fractures of the tibial shaft, although cast treatment is possible, intramedullary nailing is preferred despite the potential complications of infection and anterior knee pain. Fractures at the diaphyseal–metaphyseal junction at the knee and ankle are difficult to hold with an intramedullary nail and as such may be held with a plate and screws.

Tibial fractures are also very amenable to external fixation with either a monolateral frame or fine wire circular construct, particularly where surgical skills and implants are not available for intramedullary nailing.

Ankle fractures

Ankle fractures are very common. As with all intra-articular fractures one should strive for an anatomical reduction. Because of the biconvex saddle shape of the articular surface, small amounts of talar shift significantly increase joint surface contact pressures.

It is useful to think of the ankle mortise as having three columns: medial, lateral and posterior. Each column has a bony and a soft-tissue component. On the lateral side there are the lateral malleolus, lateral collateral ligament and syndesmotic ligaments. On the medial side there are the medial malleolus and medial collateral ligament (deltoid ligament). The posterior column has the posterior syndesmotic ligaments attached from the lateral part of the posterior malleolus to the posterior lateral malleolus.

If only one column (either the bony or soft-tissue component) has been injured, then it is considered a stable injury and can be treated non-operatively with cast or splint protection for 6–8 weeks.

If both or all three columns are involved or there is evidence of talar shift, it is an unstable injury. Depending on the patient's age and risk factors for wound complications, in general unstable fractures are treated with open reduction and rigid fixation to hold the fracture anatomically.

Non-operative treatment may be used for unstable fractures in elderly patients or patients with poor skin and unfavourable soft tissues, but this approach requires close observation and careful attention to casting technique.

Calcaneal fractures

The os calcis injury is most frequently caused by a fall from a height. It is important to exclude associated injuries to the lumbar spine, which occur in 20% of cases. Most os calcis fractures involve the posterior facet of the subtalar joint. The severity of the injury is often best appreciated with CT scans (***Figure** 32.27*). Treatment depends on the severity of the injury to the subtalar joint and widening of the heel leading to peroneal impingement. An os calcis fracture is a significant injury and outcomes following surgical or non-operative treatment are unpredictable. On occasion in severe injuries, primary fusion of the subtalar joint may be considered.

Talus fracture

The talus consists of a head, neck and body. The most common injury is a talar neck fracture. This is caused by forced dorsiflexion of the forefoot (aviator's astragalus). The blood supply to the body of the talus is interrupted in displaced talar neck fractures. In high-energy injuries the talus can not only be fractured but also dislocated, at either the talonavicular joint, subtalar joint or tibiotalar joint. These are very serious injuries to the foot that can affect the patient's long-term function through the development of either degenerative changes or avascular necrosis. To optimise outcome and reduce the possibility of avascular necrosis, anatomical reduction and stable fixation of the talar neck should be performed. Fixation of the talus to achieve compression can be technically very challenging. An operative issue with talus fractures is that there tends to be comminution that does not allow effective compression of the fracture fragments together, or when compression is achieved the shape of the talus is inadvertently altered, thereby affecting the shape of the foot. In addition, the injury to the blood supply from the initial trauma may result in avascular necrosis of the talus, non-union and later degeneration between it and the adjacent joints (tibiotalar, talocalcaneal and talonavicular).

Tarsometatarsal (Lisfranc) joint injuries

Injuries to the midfoot are associated with significant morbidity ranging from a midfoot sprain to complete rupture of the ligaments connecting the forefoot to the midfoot. Injury classically follows forced plantarflexion of the midfoot. An alternative mechanism of injury are crush injuries where the foot is forced flat by a heavy weight. Lisfranc's ligament connects the second metatarsal to the medial cuneiform. Poorly treated injuries to the midfoot lead to significant morbidity and, if suspected, a CT of the foot should be undertaken. Treatment options range from closed reduction and plaster cast application to open reduction and internal fixation. In severe cases primary tarsometatarsal fusion may be considered.

Achilles tendon rupture

Complete rupture of the Achilles tendon is a common injury; 20% of acute injuries are missed. Active plantarflexion of the

Jacques Lisfranc de St Martin, 1790–1847, Professor of Surgery and Operative Medicine, Paris, France.

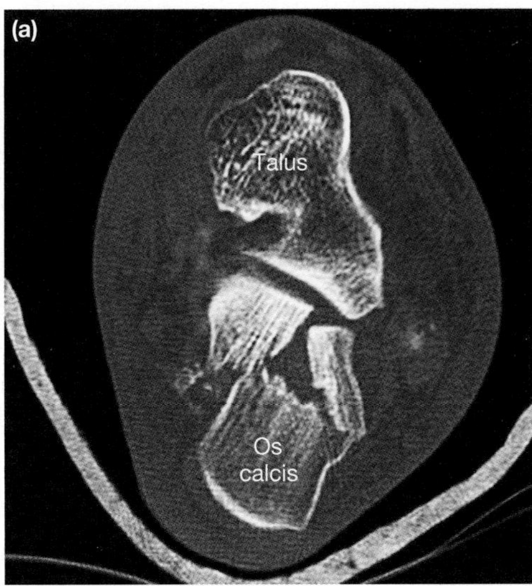

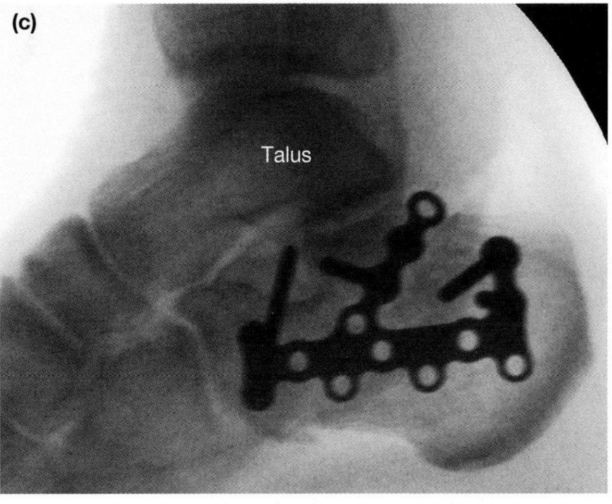

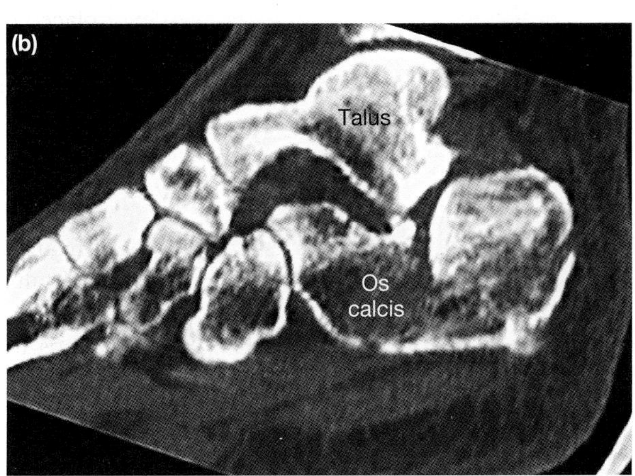

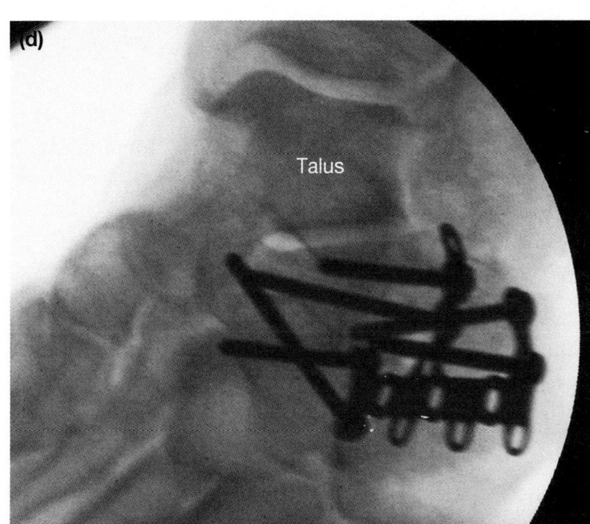

Figure 32.27 Axial (a) and sagittal (b) views of a displaced intra-articular fracture of the os calcis. (c, d) Intraoperative views of the reconstruction. Both the overall shape and the articular surface have been restored.

ankle is still possible, although weak, through the use of the toe plantarflexors.

A classic history is a feeling of being kicked in the heel and feeling something go. The most common activity leading to Achilles tendon rupture is badminton or squash following sudden forced contraction of the calf.

On examination a palpable gap may be felt. The diagnosis is confirmed by placing the patient prone on the examination couch, feet off the edge of the bed; squeezing the calf fails to elicit passive plantarflexion of the foot. If doubt exists, an ultrasound can confirm the diagnosis.

Treatment of acute Achilles tendon rupture involves surgical repair or functional management. There is an increasing trend to functional management as opposed to direct surgical repair.

TREATMENT OF FRACTURES IN THE SKELETALLY IMMATURE

The treatment principles that were described for the adult are equally applicable to the child (i.e. reduce, hold, heal, rehabilitate).

A major difference to consider is that in extra-articular fractures there is a remodelling potential, which means that increased degrees of deformity may be accepted. Remodelling happens best in the plane of the joint and the closer the injury is to the growth plate. Rotational and joint surface remodelling are poor. Fractures occurring near the site of greatest longitudinal growth will remodel the most (e.g. fractures around the distal femur have a greater remodelling potential than the proximal femur). The younger the patient, the greater the remodelling potential. Significant remodelling essentially ceases when the growth plates have closed.

A further difference is that paediatric fractures heal more rapidly and, as such, do not need to be held as long as in the adult counterpart. Similarly, fixation does not need to be as rigid, as fracture union is more rapid.

Growth plate injuries require special mention (*Figure 32.12*). In general, growth plate injuries should be anatomically reduced to minimise the potential for growth disturbance. However, in the process of reducing the fracture, further injury to the growth plate should be avoided.

Repeated manipulation of physeal injuries should be avoided. Injury to the perichondral ring and placing metalwork across the physis (where possible) should similarly be avoided. If fixation necessitates crossing the physis, consider limited damage by using the smallest smooth K-wires with a single pass in the middle of the physis if possible.

The paediatric periosteum is often thick and very strong; this needs to be considered when reducing the fracture, requiring an exaggeration of the deformity and pushing the fracture back into place instead of just applying longitudinal traction. The periosteal hinge should be preserved as it also allows for better holding of the fracture if it remains intact, as previously described (*Figure 32.12*).

Always consider the possibility of non-accidental injury, as discussed in *Chapters 26 and 44*.

SPECIFIC PAEDIATRIC INJURIES

Distal radial fractures

Fractures of the distal radius are very common in children. The bone either fails at the physis, leading to Salter–Harris type 2 fractures of the distal radius, or the metaphysis fails. The treatment principle of physeal fractures is to achieve an anatomical reduction. This can often be achieved with closed manipulation and the fracture held in position until healing with a below-elbow plaster cast. Growth arrest is rare after physeal fractures of the distal radius.

Complete metaphyseal fractures of the distal radius require close attention (*Figure 32.28*). In most cases an acceptable closed reduction can be achieved, but holding the distal fragment in an acceptable position can be challenging with cast immobilisation. Brachioradialis, which is attached to the radial styloid, is a continual deforming force. If non-operative treatment using a cast application is chosen, the position should be checked with radiographs weekly for the first 3 weeks; if re-displacement occurs, repeat manipulation and K-wire fixation may be required.

Distal humerus (supracondylar fracture)

Supracondylar humeral fractures are very common injuries in children. The distal humerus may go into flexion or extension, extension being by far the most common. Treatment depends on the degree of displacement. Undisplaced fractures may be protected in a collar and cuff or backslab for 3 weeks and then progressive mobilisation.

If displaced, the fracture can often be reduced with closed manipulation. If the dorsal periosteal hinge is intact, above-elbow cast immobilisation for 3–4 weeks is often sufficient to hold the fracture until union. If the periosteal hinge is broken, percutaneous K-wires are used to hold the fracture, supplemented with an above-elbow cast.

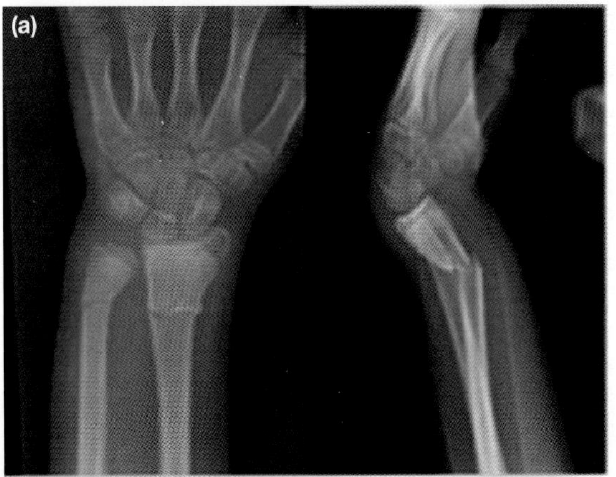

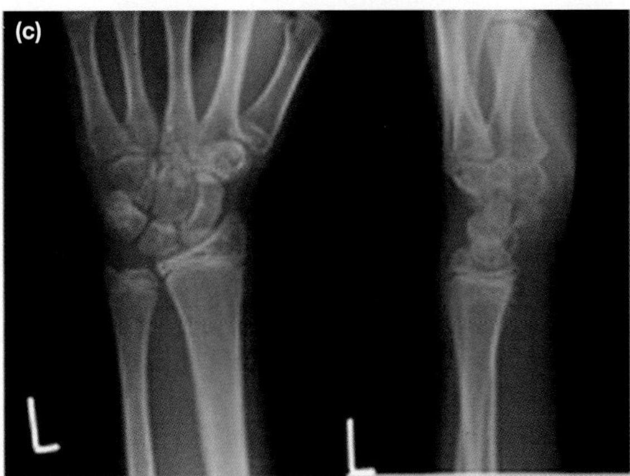

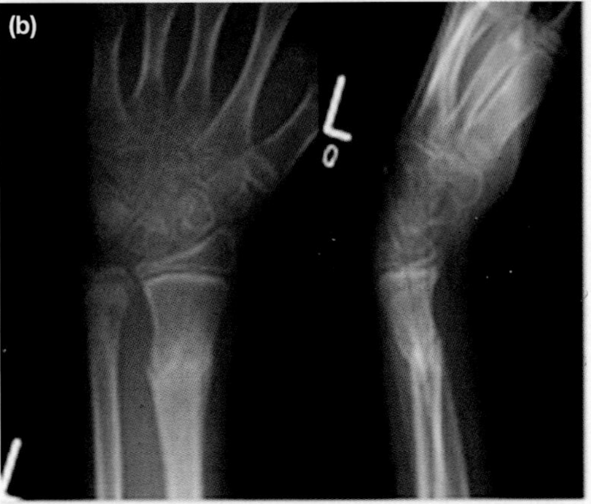

Figure 32.28 (a) Anteroposterior and lateral radiographs of a 10-year-old child showing a dorsally angulated metaphyseal fracture of the radius and undisplaced fracture of the ulna. (b) The injury was treated with closed manipulation and cast application. Eight weeks' postinjury radiograph out of the cast. The fracture is united, with residual 11° dorsal angulation. (c) Radiograph of the wrist following repeat injury 2 years later at age 12, showing complete remodelling. No residual deformity.

A very rare but feared complication of paediatric supracondylar fractures is Volkmann's ischaemic contracture. This is due to excessive swelling and missed compartment syndrome in the forearm. It is particularly important not to put the elbow into deep flexion if there is a lot of swelling. If deep flexion is the only way to hold the fracture, then K-wire fixation should be considered.

Neurovascular injury at the time of a supracondylar fracture is not uncommon. Careful attention should be paid to the neurovascular status of the limb. The white pulseless hand is a surgical emergency and requires immediate attention, assessment and urgent reduction. If the pulse does not return with reduction, then the vessels should be explored by appropriately trained surgeons.

The pink pulseless hand is more controversial and requires early senior decision making. If there is satisfactory perfusion of the limb, no suggestion of compartment syndrome and no neurological injury, then reduction and stabilisation of the fracture is warranted and a more expectant approach to the vascular injury can be taken. Often the pulse will return within 24–48 hours.

Neurological injury is common, most often a neuropraxia. They often resolve on fracture reduction, stabilisation and resolution of the swelling.

Malunion in varus or valgus remains a problem. Often the elbow will remodel the deformity in the anteroposterior flexion–extension plane, but varus and valgus malunion remodels less. Careful attention needs to be paid to the adequacy of the reduction and K-wire placement to hold the fracture to avoid angular malunion.

Lateral condylar mass fracture of the elbow

Lateral condylar mass fractures of the elbow are easily missed and often considered benign as there is often only a small flake of bone visible. This thin sliver of metaphyseal bone on the lateral side of the elbow is very deceptive. Do not underestimate the significance of this injury (*Figure 32.29*).

Treatment depends on the stability of the lateral mass fragment. If stable, non-operative treatment is acceptable. If unstable, anatomical reduction and fixation should be attempted to avoid complications.

Unstable fractures are suggested by significant soft-tissue swelling, by fracture displacement of more than 2 mm or by the fracture being visible on both anteroposterior and lateral views of the elbow.

Unstable fractures require anatomical reduction and rigid fixation with K-wires or screw fixation to avoid displacement and complications. Avascular necrosis of the capitellum and non-union of the lateral condyle lead to the so-called 'fish tail' deformity.

Slipped upper femoral epiphysis

A slipped upper femoral epiphysis classically occurs in a child approaching puberty. It is easily missed as symptoms may be mild and the predominant symptom may be knee pain referred from the hip. A history of trauma may be offered and the child may limp.

Examination of the limb reveals a hip that flexes into external rotation. Radiographs should include a good lateral view of the femoral head and neck (*Figure 32.30*). If the radiographs are normal, consider an MRI, looking for a preslip; if found, consider prophylactic fixation. If treated in the early stages, the prognosis is very good. A severely displaced slipped upper femoral epiphysis might lead to avascular necrosis of the femoral head and chondrolysis. This is a very difficult condition to treat effectively in young patients.

Femoral shaft fractures

Femoral shaft fractures in children are treated based on the age and size of the child:

- infants (0–18 months);
- toddlers and small children (18 months–4 years);
- children (4–12 years);
- older children/adolescents.

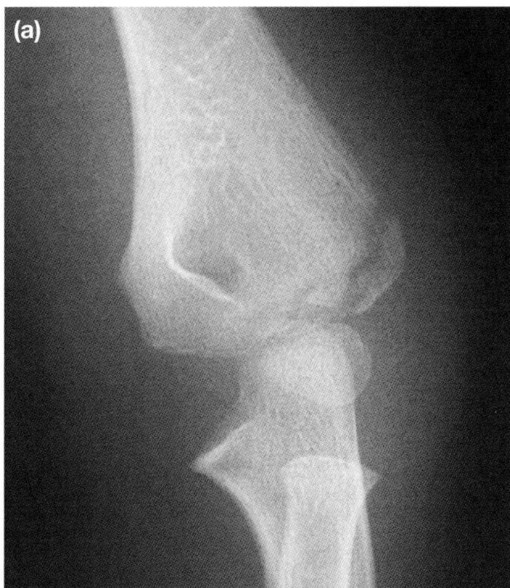

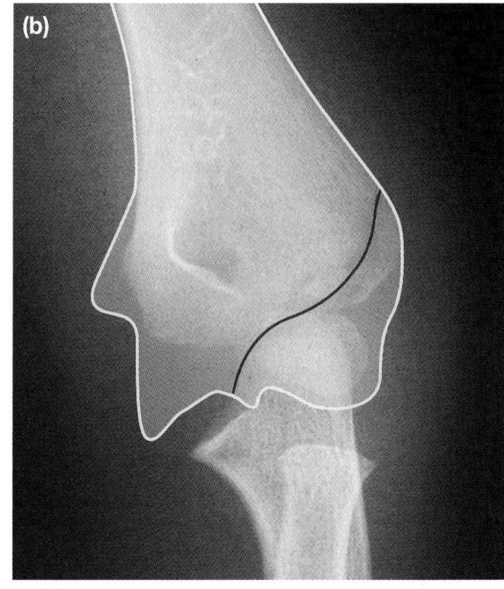

Figure 32.29 Lateral condylar mass fracture. (a) The metaphyseal fracture. (b) The yellow shows the shape of the distal humerus, including the cartilaginous analogue, and the red shows the true extent of the injury (i.e. a significant intra-articular fracture).

Richard von Volkmann, 1830–1889, Professor of Surgery, Halle, Germany.

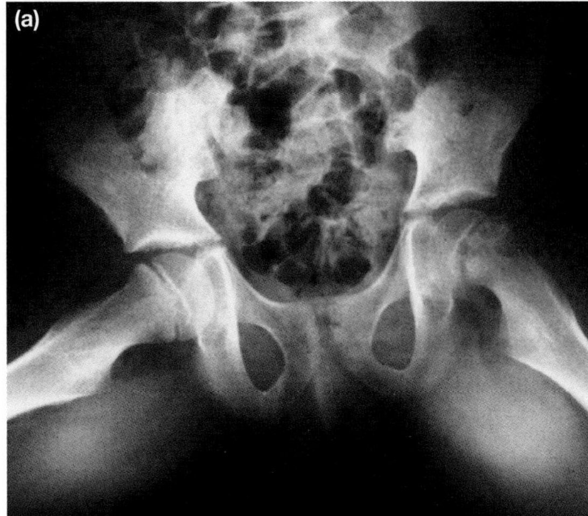

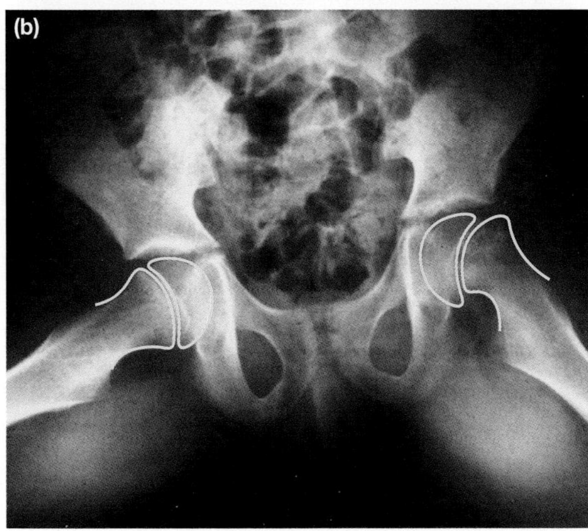

Figure 32.30 Slipped left upper femoral epiphysis. (a) Plain radiograph; (b) the injury highlighted.

In infants (0–18 months), ensure that there is no evidence of non-accidental injury. In infants under 12–15 kg, gallows traction is acceptable. This traction involves suspension of the legs vertically with the buttocks just off the bed. In toddlers and small children treatment is by traction initially followed by hip spica application. Shortening of up to 1 cm and angulation of 15–20° can be accepted depending on the age of the child because of extensive remodelling potential.

As the child gets older and time to union increases, the non-operative measures of traction and hip spica become more cumbersome.

In children from 4 to 12 years several treatment options exist: traction and hip spica, elastic stable intramedullary nailing (ESIN), external fixation or plate fixation. Definitive treatment depends on surgeon skills, facilities and patient and parent needs.

In older children and adolescents, non-operative treatment with traction and hip spica cast application becomes less tolerable. Depending on the size and build of the patient, operative treatment may include ESIN (*Figure 32.31*), external fixation or plate fixation. In larger overweight adolescents, titanium elastic nails may not be strong enough to resist bending forces and locked intramedullary nailing may be considered.

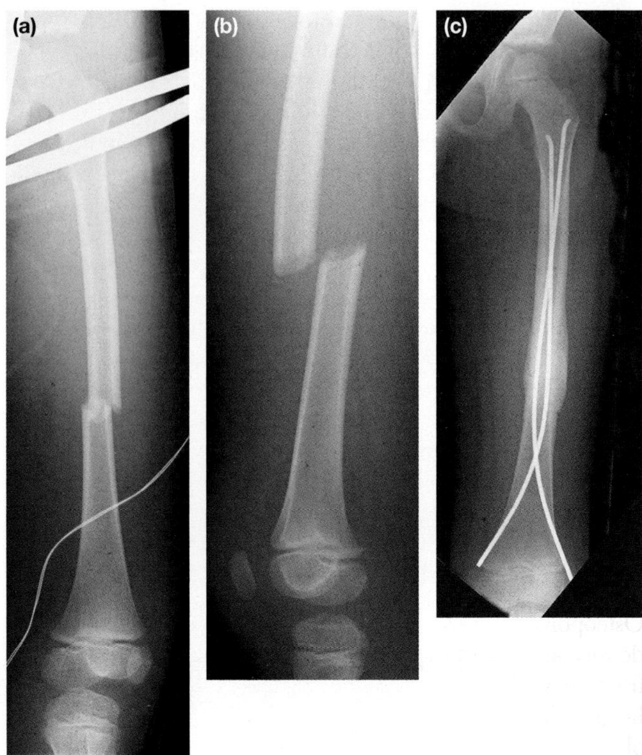

Figure 32.31 (a–c) Femoral shaft fracture in a child that has been stabilised with elastic nails.

Summary box 32.6

Fractures in the skeletally immature

- Do not forget non-accidental injury
- Be reluctant to remanipulate a physeal injury
- Elastic nails are a significant step forward in fracture treatment in children
- Not many fractures require operative intervention in children

It is important, however, to remember that there is a small chance of avascular necrosis of the femoral head if an antegrade intramedullary nail is used prior to or just after physeal closure. This is a rare but devastating complication in this age group. Far lateral entry point nails on the greater trochanter have been developed to limit the effect on the blood supply to the femoral head; however, the risk of avascular necrosis persists.

Tibial shaft fractures

Tibial fractures in children are often very amenable to non-operative treatment, starting with an above-knee cast, followed by conversion to a Sarmiento patellar tendon

Augusto Sarmiento, b. 1927, Colombian orthopaedic surgeon, Professor and Chairman of the Department of Orthopedics, University of Southern California, Los Angeles, CA, USA.

below-knee cast at 4–6 weeks. Remodelling in the tibia is somewhat limited; as such, less angular deformity (only 10–15°) can be accepted and no rotational deformity. Some shortening of the tibia can be accepted as the tibia is expected to overgrow by 0.5 cm in response to injury. If it is not possible to hold the fracture in an acceptable position with a cast, then external fixation, elastic stable intramedullary nailing (ESIN)/titanium elastic nails (TENS; thin flexible nails inserted in the canal of a long bone to splint it) or plating is an option.

SPECIAL CONSIDERATIONS

Special consideration needs to be given to osteoporotic and pathological fractures, for example the ability to hold the fracture until union. Furthermore, open fractures require urgent appropriate treatment to ensure bone healing in the absence of infection.

Osteoporotic fractures

Osteoporosis is a condition characterised by low bone mineral density and reduced strength. Osteoporotic bone is liable to fracture with low-energy injuries (e.g. a fall from standing height). Treatment of lower limb osteoporotic fractures in older patients is challenging. As there may be additional and pre-existing mobility problems, such patients are unable to partially weight-bear and so fixation should be strong enough to allow immediate weight-bearing and to hold the position until union. Locking plate technology improves fixation in osteoporotic bone, and bone void fillers can be utilised (*Figure 32.32*).

Pathological fractures

When abnormal bone fails under normal load this is referred to as a pathological fracture. Depending on the cause of the pathological fracture the bone may not heal and consideration should be given to a load-bearing device not load-sharing. If involving the joint surface or close to the joint surface, the affected area may be excised en bloc and a joint replacement performed.

The bone may be weakened by a primary bone tumour, secondary metastatic deposits, haematological malignancy (myeloma, lymphoma, leukaemia), osteomyelitis and metabolic bone disease (osteomalacia, Paget's disease, osteoporosis).

A pathological fracture should be suspected if the history is not consistent with the severity of the injury. The patient may give a history of low-energy injury that normally would not cause a fracture. If a pathological fracture is suspected, the cause should be actively sought. Where a primary bone tumour is suspected, treatment should be planned to prevent disseminating the disease (see *Chapter 42*).

In patients with metastatic bone disease, the primary source should be sought if multiple metastatic deposits are identified. If life expectancy is poor, then stabilisation with a load-bearing device may be considered. If an isolated metastasis is identified and an overall good prognosis is offered by the oncologists, a more aggressive curative approach may be taken with en bloc excision of the primary and the isolated secondary deposit.

If a metastatic deposit is identified prior to fracture, prophylactic fixation should be considered if impending fracture is likely. Prophylactic stabilisation with a load-bearing device is once again advocated. If life expectancy is good and the deposit periarticular, an en bloc excision and joint arthroplasty may be considered to optimise return to near normal function as soon as possible.

Open fractures

Any fracture with an overlying wound should be considered an open fracture. The term previously used was a compound fracture. Open fractures require particular mention because adequate stabilisation of the bony injury and appropriate management of the soft-tissue injury are paramount to ensure a good outcome with a low complication rate. The treatment of bone and joint infection is expensive, laborious and time-consuming for the professional as well as the patient. An infected femoral shaft fracture following intramedullary nailing will typically take 3 years and five operations to clear the infection and achieve union.

The Gustilo and Anderson classification of open fractures is the most frequently used classification (*Table 32.2*). The definitive grade is determined intraoperatively after thorough debridement. It is not based on size of wound alone but takes into account several factors; for example, a farmyard or heavily contaminated wound of under 1 cm may still be considered a grade III injury.

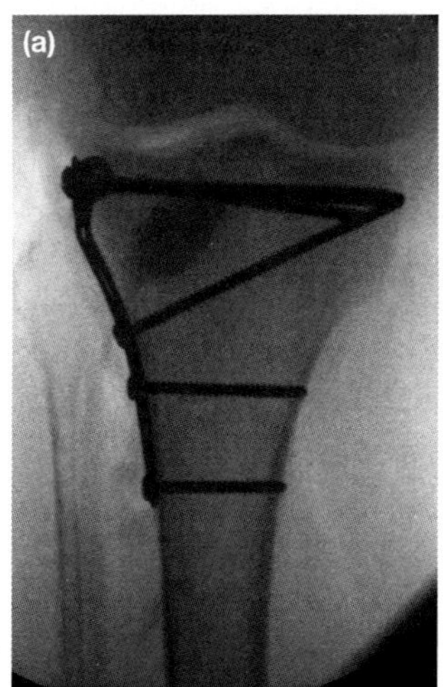

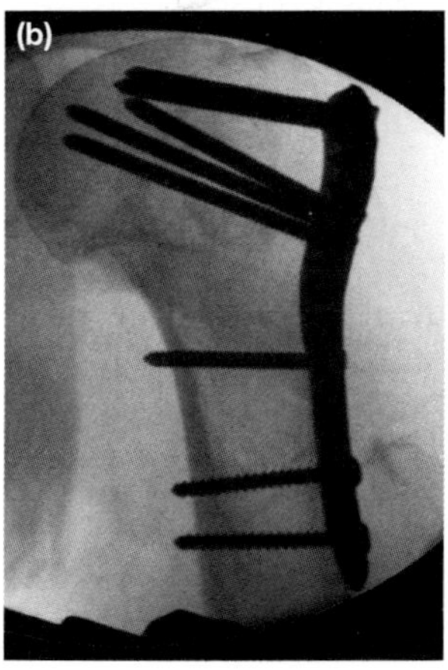

Figure 32.32 Variations in fixation technique suited to osteoporotic bone. (a) Norian bone substitute has been injected to support the lateral tibial plateau in the partial articular fracture. (b) A locking plate in a proximal humerus. The screws are threaded into the plate to make a fixed-angle device.

Sir James Paget, 1814–1899, surgeon, St Bartholomew's Hospital, London, UK.

The aim of open fracture management is to achieve bony union, optimise function and avoid infection. The treatment of open fractures should be considered in two phases: the emergency department presurgical phase and the surgical phase.

Presurgical phase

1 Take a photograph to document the severity of the injury and limit the need for repeated opening of dressings. (Do not delay steps below unduly.)
2 Assess neurovascular status; if compromised and the fracture is displaced, quickly remove any macroscopic dirt and reduce the fracture/dislocation. It is not essential to achieve an anatomical reduction; simply remove the pressure from the soft tissues (make a leg look like a leg and an arm look like an arm). If the bone was out of the skin and is reduced under the skin, then document clearly and inform the surgical team.
3 Once overall alignment is achieved, splint the affected limb; treatment of an open fracture is treatment of the soft tissues.
4 Apply a moist saline dressing to the wound. It is acceptable to irrigate the wound with saline in the emergency department to remove any macroscopic dirt, but definitive debridement and washout of the wound should be undertaken in a theatre environment.
5 Administer intravenous antibiotics according to local protocols. It has been shown that early administration of intravenous antibiotics is one of the most important steps. A broad-spectrum antibiotic should be chosen covering Gram-positive, Gram-negative and, if there is severe contamination, anaerobic organisms.
6 Obtain a tetanus immunisation history and treat accordingly.
7 Inform a senior orthopaedic surgeon of the injury as soon as possible and make preparations for the surgical phase.

Surgical phase

In the past an open fracture was considered a contraindication to internal fixation. It is increasingly evident that stable fixation of the bony injury is very important to prevent deterioration of the soft tissues, allowing recovery and healing.

Fracture stabilisation may come in the form of external fixation or internal fixation with screws/plates/intramedullary nails, depending on the setting.

Summary box 32.7

Special considerations

- Osteoporotic fractures in older patients may require specialised fixation techniques with locking screw/plate technology and injectable bone cement augmentation
- Pathological fractures may not heal and require load-bearing not load-sharing implants
- Arthroplasty in suitable patients bypasses the problems of blood supply and weak bone and allows early full weight-bearing and return to function
- Open fractures require prompt debridement, stabilisation and adequate soft-tissue cover to prevent infection

Management of the soft tissues is critical to prevent the zone of injury spreading. Thorough debridement of any contaminated or non-vital soft tissue is important. Any loose or devitalised bone fragments should be discarded. Bone defects are easier to deal with than an infected non-union.

Soft-tissue reconstruction may involve primary or delayed primary closure of the wound, or more sophisticated soft-tissue reconstruction options including microvascular free tissue transfer.

Continue intravenous antibiotics until 48 hours after definitive wound closure.

COMPARTMENT SYNDROME

Compartment syndrome is raised pressure in a fascial compartment to a level that compromises tissue perfusion. There are several causes of compartment syndrome, fractures being the most common (70%), followed by soft-tissue contusions (23%). Rarer causes include: bleeding disorders, including anticoagulation; burns (particularly circumferential third-degree burns); postischaemic swelling (reperfusion injury); tight casts/dressings; and extravasation of intravenous infusions (contrast under pressure).

The pathophysiology involves increased tissue pressure, which leads to reduced microperfusion, resulting in tissue ischaemia and irreversible muscle damage from cellular anoxia.

Compartment syndrome is a clinical diagnosis characterised by pain out of proportion, increasing pain, and pain on passive stretch, with paraesthesia possible. Paralysis, numbness and pallor are late signs and pulselessness is an extremely late sign.

Compartment pressure monitoring may be useful in cases of diagnostic uncertainty and in patients with altered levels of consciousness (intubated, head injury).

Measure multiple sites near but not in the fracture site, in all the compartments of the affected limb. Generally accepted pressure thresholds include an absolute pressure greater than or equal to 30 mmHg or pressure difference (diastolic pressure – compartment pressure) less than or equal to 30 mmHg.

Emergency treatment involves splitting casts and/or dressings to the skin and elevating the extremity. Senior input should be sought and arrangements put in place to perform definitive treatment with fasciotomies.

There are some common pitfalls to remember. The incidence of compartment syndrome associated with high- and low-energy injuries is nearly equal. Compartment syndrome can occur in open fractures. Have a high index of suspicion and be particularly vigilant in patients with an altered level of consciousness.

CONCLUSION

The correct identification of extremity trauma, combined with timely and appropriate treatment, is essential to return patients to normal function as safely and as quickly as possible. The same injury may be treated in different ways based on patient factors, age, functional demands and comorbidities. Surgeon and resource-based factors also need to be considered.

Summary box 32.8

Summary of extremity trauma

- Realise that an injury exists
- Find the characteristics of the injury, describe it and classify it
- Consider the natural history of the injury
- Treatment is guided by outcome if known or by principle if not
- Beware of injuries that are 'easily missed'

FURTHER READING

Blom A, Warwick D, Whitehouse M. *Apley's system of orthopaedics and fractures*, 10th edn. Boca Raton, FL: CRC Press, 2017.

Bone LR, Johnson KD, Weight J, Scheinberg RJ. Early versus delayed stabilization of femoral fractures. *J Bone Joint Surg* 1989; **71A**: 33640.

British Orthopaedic Association. *BOA standards for trauma and orthopaedics (BOASTs)*. Available from https://www.boa.ac.uk/standards-guidance/boasts.html (accessed 31 March 2022).

Charnley J. *The closed treatment of common fractures*. Edinburgh: E&S Livingstone, 1950.

Gustilo RB, Anderson JT. Prevention of infection in the treatment of 1025 open fractures of long bones. *J Bone Joint Surg* 1976; **8A**: 453–8.

Mast J, Jakob R, Ganz R. *Planning and reduction technique in fracture surgery*. Berlin: Springer-Verlag, 1989.

Medicines and Healthcare products Regulatory Agency. *Guidance: Magnetic resonance imaging equipment in clinical use: safety guidelines*. London: MHRA, 2014. Available from https://www.gov.uk/government/publications/safety-guidelines-for-magnetic-resonance-imaging-equipment-in-clinical-use

Muller ME, Nazarian S, Koch P. *The AO classification of fractures*. Schatzker J (trans). Berlin: Springer-Verlag, 1988.

Rajasekaran S, Sabapathy SR, Dheenadhayalan J *et al.* Ganga hospital open injury score in management of open injuries. *Eur J Trauma Emerg Surg* 2015; **41(1)**: 3-15.

Tornetta P, Ricci W, Court-Brown CM *et al.* (eds). *Rockwood and Green's fractures in adults*, 9th edn. Philadelphia, PA: Wolters Kluwer, 2019.

Tscherne H, Oestern HJ. Die Klassifizierung des Weichteilschadens bei offenen und geschlossenen Frakturen (A new classification of soft-tissue damage in open and closed fractures [author's transl]). *Unfallheilkunde* 1982; **85(3)**: 111–15. German.

CHAPTER 33 Disaster surgery

Learning objectives

To recognise and understand:

- The common features of various disasters
- The principles behind the organisation of the relief effort and of triage in treatment and evacuation
- The role and limitations of field hospitals in disaster
- The features of conditions peculiar to disaster situations and their treatment

INTRODUCTION

Natural disasters provide a constant reminder of the power and capricious nature of our planet. The depletion of the ozone layer and global warming mean that the future may hold in store calamitous events with even greater magnitude than those experienced before. National conflicts and ideological differences have not lessened and the resultant 'unnatural disasters' have the potential to rival the natural ones in enormity (see *Chapter 34*). Disasters by their very nature are unpredictable and no two are alike. Nevertheless, there are numerous common elements and it has been shown that countries that invest in disaster preparedness are better equipped to cope with such catastrophes. Recent wars and disasters have highlighted the increasingly crucial role of surgeons in these scenarios.

COMMON FEATURES OF MAJOR DISASTERS

Any event that results in the loss of human life is disastrous, but most accidents, such as aeroplane and train crashes, are limited in the number of people involved. Conversely, natural disasters, such as earthquakes and tsunamis, leave in their wake massive destruction over large areas that can transcend national boundaries. All the apparatus of a society that responds to such disasters (the civil administration, emergency services, fire brigades and hospitals) may itself be involved and unable to respond (*Figure 33.1*). Large numbers of people may require immediate shelter, clean water and food, in addition to any medical needs.

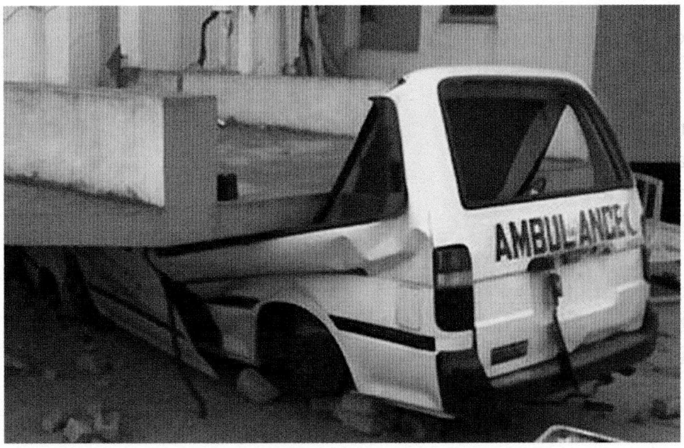

A breakdown of communication is inevitable and can be accompanied by widespread panic and disruption of civil order. Access to the disaster area may be limited because of the destruction of bridges, affecting road and rail links.

Figure 33.1 Damage to emergency medical services.

Summary box 33.1

Common features of major disasters

- Massive casualties
- Damage to infrastructure
- A large number of people requiring shelter
- Panic and uncertainty among the population
- Limited access to the area
- Breakdown of communication

FACTORS INFLUENCING RELIEF EFFORTS AND PROVISION OF MEDICAL AID

Good communication is critical for the authorities to respond quickly to a disaster. Wireless technology and satellite imagery have revolutionised the way in which real-time information can be obtained (*Figure 33.2*). Nonetheless, there is an inevitable lag period between the occurrence of the disaster and the response from the establishment.

The location of the disaster area has a bearing on relief efforts. In large cities emergency and medical services are better developed. However, these areas are densely populated and

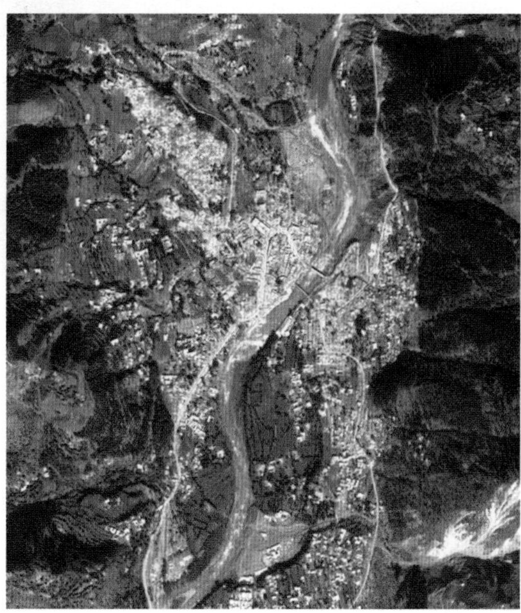

Figure 33.2 Satellite image showing destruction of a bridge as a result of flooding.

may have limited access by road and air. Disasters in remote areas can be particularly difficult to manage because relief efforts are hampered by geographical isolation and the lack of infrastructure.

The time frame in which a disaster occurs also impacts on the relief efforts. Earthquakes can unleash havoc in seconds but floods and hurricanes may continue for several days. Another important factor is the state of resources of the country; disasters in poorer countries can seldom be managed without significant outside assistance

Summary box 33.2

Factors influencing rescue and relief efforts

- Status of communications
- Location, whether rural or urban
- Accessibility of the location
- Time frame in which disaster occurs
- Economic state of development of the area

SEQUENCE OF RELIEF EFFORTS AFTER A DISASTER

Establishing a chain of command

Many countries have dedicated organisations that deal with disasters. In other countries, an administrative hierarchy is established to coordinate the teams participating in relief efforts (*Figure 33.3*).

Damage assessment

The first objective in disaster management is an assessment of the damage and the number of casualties. All sources of information must be employed. The 24-hour news services are frequently the first on the scene and can be an important source of information. Drones are now a quick and inexpensive option for a rapid view of a disaster area.

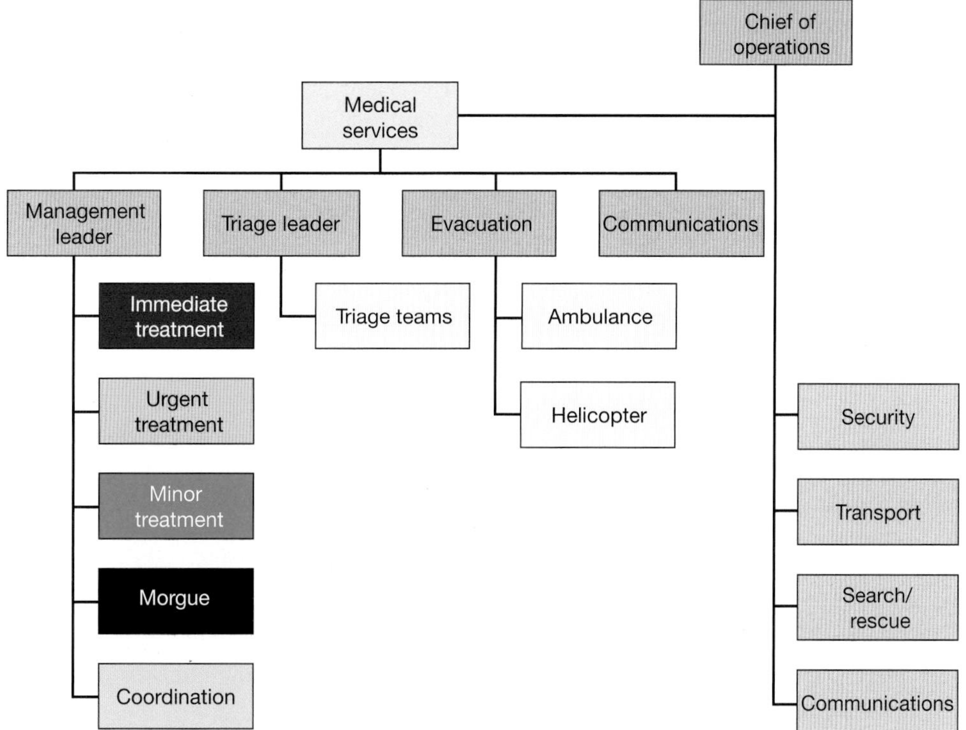

Figure 33.3 Organisation chart for disaster management.

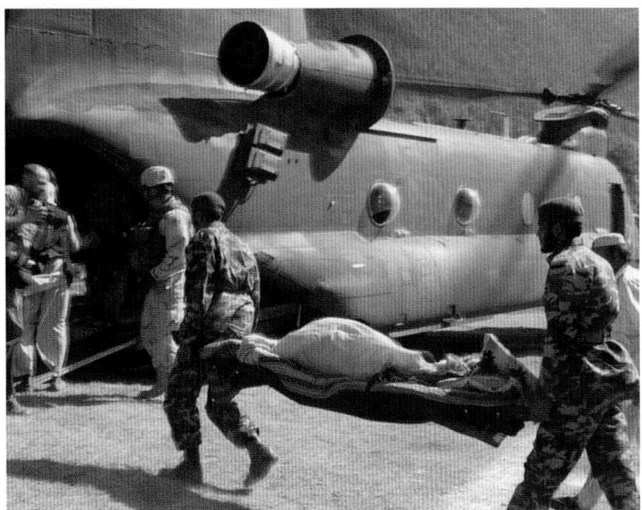

Figure 33.4 Heli-evacuation.

Mobilising resources

The next step is mobilisation of human and material resources appropriate to the extent of the disaster. Although all modes of transport need to be considered, helicopters provide the quickest access for the first responders (*Figure 33.4*). The teams that make up the initial response must include experienced staff who can assess the situation and who have the authority to take immediate decisions.

Rescue operation

Early coordination of the rescue effort allows optimal use of resources. The first priority is to prevent further damage from occurring, both to people and to the infrastructure. The types of injuries encountered by rescue workers depend on the delay between the onset of the disaster and their arrival. Patients with head injuries and abdominal and thoracic trauma will either have been treated or have succumbed to their injuries within 48–72 hours of a disaster. After the first week, the only casualties requiring treatment are those with complex limb trauma and infected wounds (*Figure 33.5*).

Coordination with relief agencies

A laudable aspect of globalisation is the outpouring of help from governments and non-governmental organisations in response to a disaster. Some, such as Rescue And Preparedness In Disasters (RAPID), deal with search and rescue, whereas others, such as the International Committee of the Red Cross and Oxfam, provide general disaster-related relief (*Figure 33.6*). The various United Nations agencies deal with medical care, food provision and refugees. Coordinating the efforts of these organisations is essential for optimal results, as medical aid in isolation is inadequate without the simultaneous provision of safe drinking water, food, clothing and shelter.

Summary box 33.3

Sequence of the relief effort in major disasters

- Establish chain of command
- Set up lines of communication
- Carry out damage assessment
- Mobilise resources
- Initiate rescue operation
- Triage casualties
- Start emergency treatment
- Arrange evacuation
- Start definitive management

Dealing with the media

Disasters act like a magnet for the media. In today's world of 24-hour news coverage, this plays an important part in shaping public opinion. It is essential to establish a working relationship between the media and the rescue teams. With careful handling the media can become a powerful ally and play a constructive role in identifying problems, galvanising aid and keeping the public informed.

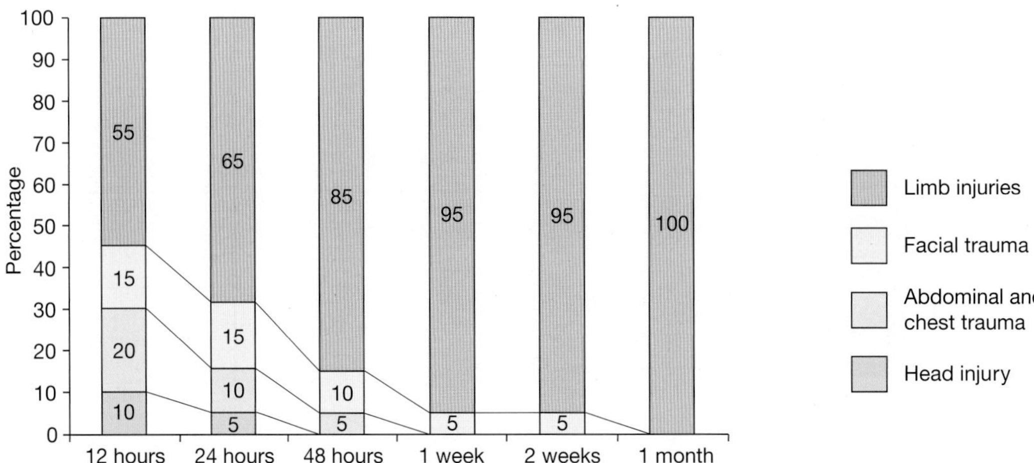

Figure 33.5 Time line showing the type of injuries encountered at different times in a disaster.

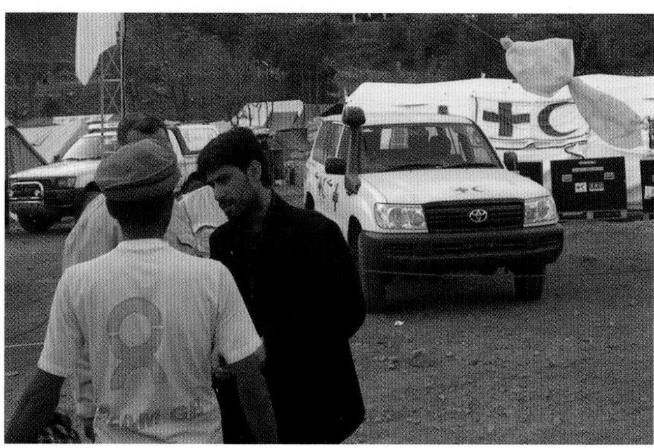

Figure 33.6 Oxfam and the International Committee of the Red Cross provide generalised relief.

Triage

Derived from the French verb *trier*, triage means 'to sort' and is the cornerstone of the management of mass casualties. It aims to identify those patients who will benefit the most by being treated the earliest, ensuring 'the greatest good for the greatest number'. Numerous studies show that only 10–15% of disaster casualties are serious enough to require hospitalisation. By sorting out the minor injuries, triage lessens the immediate burden on medical facilities. Deciding who receives priority when faced with hundreds of seriously injured victims is a daunting prospect. Triage should be undertaken by someone senior, who has the experience and authority to make these critical decisions. To keep pace with the changing clinical picture of an injured person, triage needs to be undertaken in the field, before evacuation and again at the hospital.

Triage areas

For efficient triage the injured need to be brought together into any undamaged structures that can shelter a large number of wounded. A good water supply, good lighting and ease of access are useful. Separate areas should be reserved for patient holding, emergency treatment and decontamination (in the event of discharge of hazardous materials).

Practical triage

Emergency life-saving measures should proceed alongside triage and can actually help the decision-making process. The assessment and restoration of airway, breathing and circulation are critical and are discussed in *Chapter 27*. Vital signs and a general physical examination should be combined with a brief history, taken by a paramedic or by a volunteer worker if one is available.

Documentation for triage

Accurate documentation is an inseparable part of triage and should include basic patient data, vital signs with timing, brief details of injuries (preferably on a diagram) and treatment given. A system of colour-coded tags attached to the patient's wrist or around the neck should be employed by the emergency medical services. The colour denotes the degree of urgency with which a patient requires treatment (*Figure 33.7*).

Triage categories

All methods of triage use simple criteria based on vital signs. A rapid clinical assessment should be made taking into account the patient's ability to walk, their mental status and the presence or absence of ventilation or capillary perfusion. A commonly used four-tier system is presented in *Table 33.1*.

Evacuation of casualties

Decisions regarding the best destination for each patient need to be based on how far it is safe for them to travel and whether the facilities that they need for definitive treatment will be available. A quick retriage is very useful in this situation. The paramedics accompanying the casualties should be committed to preventing a 'second accident' (damage caused inadvertently by transport and treatment). An adequate supply of essentials such as intravenous fluids, dressings, pain medication and oxygen must be arranged (see *Chapter 34*).

TABLE 33.1 Triage categories.

Priority	Colour	Medical need	Clinical status	Examples
First (I)	Red	Immediate	Critical, but likely to survive if treatment given early	Severe facial trauma, tension pneumothorax, profuse external bleeding, haemothorax, flail chest, major intra-abdominal bleed, extradural haematomas
Second (II)	Yellow	Urgent	Critical, likely to survive if treatment given within hours	Compound fractures, degloving injuries, ruptured abdominal viscus, pelvic fractures, spinal injuries
Third (III)	Green	Non-urgent	Stable, likely to survive even if treatment is delayed for hours to days	Simple fractures, sprains, minor lacerations
Last (0)	Black	Unsalvageable	Not breathing, pulseless, so severely injured that no medical care is likely to help	Severe brain damage, very extensive burns, major disruption/loss of chest or abdominal wall structures

Triage is the earliest example of clinical risk management. This is done on the basis of need so that resources can be allocated by good prioritisation. The process was first used in 1792 by Baron Dominique Jean Larrey, Surgeon in Chief to Napoleon's Imperial Guard. The concept of triage emerged from the French Service de Santé des Armées so that resources could be used to the optimum – 'most for the most'.

(a)

FRONT

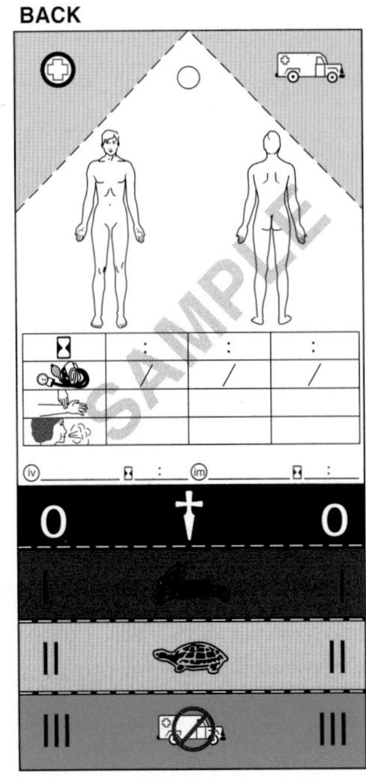

(b)

Figure 33.7 Triage tags ((a) courtesy of TACDA & METTAG products, The American Civil Defense Association; (b) courtesy of Disaster Management Systems).

Field hospitals

The decision to deploy field hospitals depends on the location, the number of casualties and the speed with which evacuation can be organised (*Figure 33.8*). Whether the traditional tented structure or the modular type, housed in containers, is employed, the facility must be equipped with radiograph capability, operating rooms, vital signs monitors, sterilising equipment, a blood bank, ventilators and basic laboratory facilities.

Management in the field

Field hospitals principally function in three main areas (*Table 33.2*).

> **Summary box 33.4**
>
> **Essentials of casualty evacuation**
>
> - Retriage to upgrade priorities among the injured
> - Select appropriate medical facilities for transfer
> - Choose appropriate means of transport
> - Prevent the 'second accident' during transfer
> - Ensure an adequate supply of materials to accompany the patient

First aid

Care for patients with minor injuries involves cleaning and dressing wounds, suturing lacerations and splinting simple fractures. Most of these 'walking wounded' can be sent away with antibiotics and simple pain relief.

Damage control surgery

Damage control surgery (DCS) is the concept that only life- and limb-saving surgery should be performed in field hospitals to allow safe transfer of a patient to a definitive treating facility. This will include ensuring that the airway is secure, haemorrhage is under control and compartments are decompressed in the chest, skull, abdomen and the limbs. Devitalised tissue should be removed and any contamination prevented from developing into infection. DCS is explained in more detail, in the context of early management and other settings, throughout the chapters in Part 4.

Emergency care for immediate life-threatening injuries

There are many patients who may be saved by relatively simple measures, provided that these are taken urgently. Endotracheal intubation and tracheostomy may be needed to provide a secure airway. A needle thoracocentesis will relieve a tension pneumothorax and a chest drain will be needed before a patient with a significant chest injury is transferred by air. An open pneumothorax should be closed. Damaged major vessels

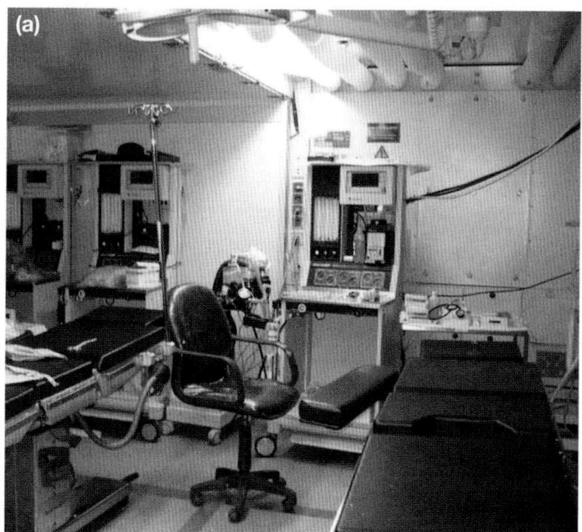
(a)

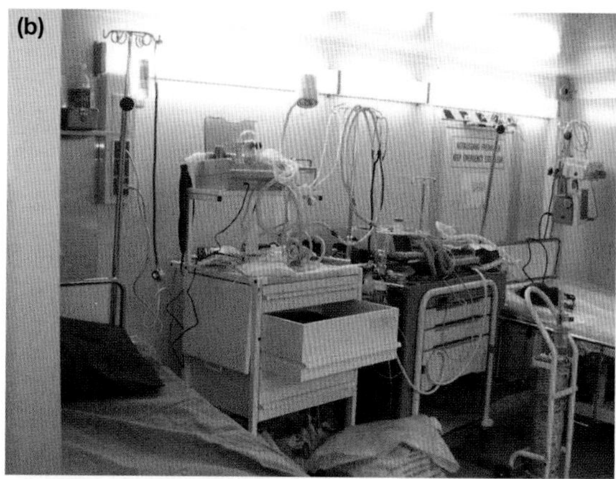
(b)

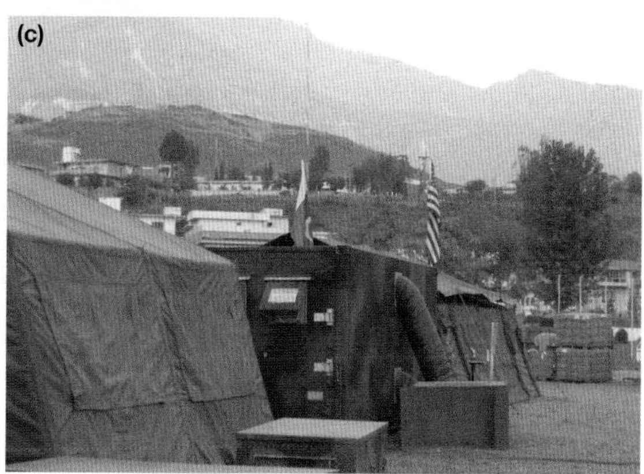
(c)

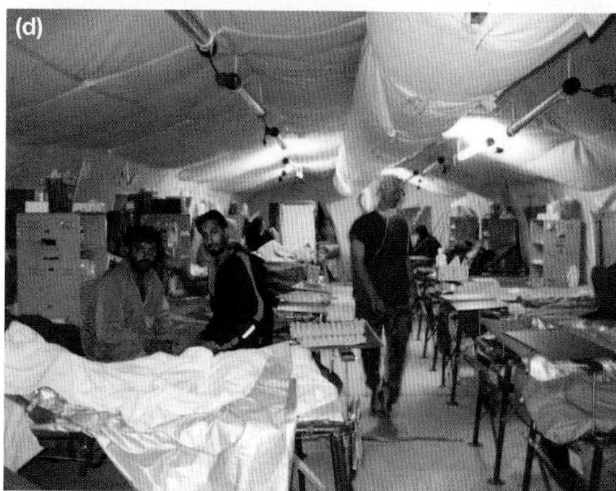
(d)

Figure 33.8 Field hospitals: (a, b) modular type; (c) tented structure; (d) interior of a tented field hospital.

TABLE 33.2 Type of treatment given in field hospitals.

	Examples	Further
First aid	Suturing cuts and lacerations, splinting simple fractures	Review at local hospital
Emergency care for life-threatening injuries	Endotracheal intubation, tracheostomy, relieving tension pneumothorax, stopping external haemorrhage, relieving an extradural haematoma, emergency thoracotomy/laparotomy for internal haemorrhage	After damage control surgery, transfer patients to base hospitals once stable
Initial care for non-life-threatening injuries	Debridement of contaminated wounds, reduction of fractures and dislocations, application of external fixators, vascular repairs	Transfer patients to base hospitals for definitive management

to limbs should be repaired if possible. Fasciotomies will be needed for muscle compartments that are swelling from injury or from reperfusion. Amputation for clearly devitalised limbs and gas gangrene should be undertaken at field hospitals as delay will be fatal. Specific aspects of care are discussed in the relevant chapters elsewhere in this book.

Initial care for non-life-threatening injuries

Many patients sustain serious injuries that require prolonged care. These include compound limb fractures, degloving injuries, dislocations of major joints, major facial injuries and complex hand injuries. These patients will need specialised care requiring transfer to the appropriate facility. Replantations of amputated limbs and other extensive procedures should not

Summary box 33.5

Principles of DCS

- Do the minimum needed to allow safe transfer to a definitive facility
- Take actions that prevent deterioration of that patient during transfer
- Secure the airway – may require tracheostomy
- Control bleeding – may require craniotomy, laparotomy, thoracotomy, repair of major limb vessels
- Prevent pressure build-up – may require burr holes, chest drain, laparotomy, fasciotomy
- Prevent infection by extensile exposure and removing dead and contaminated tissue

be attempted in field hospitals as they are time-consuming and divert resources and personnel to the treatment of a few patients.

Debridement

Taken from the French, meaning to 'unleash or cut open', debridement plays a crucial part in the management of trauma. Wounds sustained in disasters are often heavily contaminated, containing foreign bodies and non-viable tissues (*Figure 33.9*). Debridement reduces the chances of anaerobic and necrotising infections and can prevent systemic sepsis. The following principles of debridement apply to all contaminated wounds:

- After the administration of anaesthesia, the injured area is copiously irrigated with normal saline. Lavage using a pressurised system is controversial, with concerns over tissue trauma and spread of debris (*Figure 33.10*). A water-jet based system that simultaneously clears the debris after debriding is very useful. The wound is palpated and all foreign matter removed. Dirt and debris enmeshed in soft tissues can only be removed by excision of those tissues. Open joints should be thoroughly irrigated and all foreign material removed.
- Wounds with extensive cavitation should be enlarged longitudinally to gain better access and allow full decompression of the underlying muscles. This should be carried out under tourniquet. This helps to visualise the damaged structures and allows the surgeon to gain proximal and distal control of vascular injuries and to identify severed ends of major nerves and tendons.
- The next step is excision of all dead and devitalised tissue. At this stage the tourniquet is let down to check the vascularity of the tissues. Skin excision is kept to a minimum and only the margins of the wound need be trimmed back to healthy bleeding edges. Excision of devitalised muscle should be undertaken generously. Muscle that is pale or dark in colour, that does not contract on pinching and that does not bleed on cutting must be removed. In patients with traumatic amputations, the bone ends are tidied, the skin and muscle edges trimmed to the lowest level possible and the wound left open.
- In patients with associated fractures, skeletal stabilisation should be obtained before embarking on any repairs. External fixators are invaluable for this and make wound management much easier (*Figure 33.11*).
- In the acute setting, only vascular repairs are justified. For lacerated vessels the ends are trimmed and an anastomosis performed. In the case of loss of substance of the vessel wall, a vein patch or reversed vein graft may be employed. Silicone tubing may be used as a temporary bypass (stent) while vascular repair is being carried out in patients with critically compromised distal circulation.
- Nerves and tendons should not be dissected out nor should any attempt be made at definitive repair in wounds with tissue devitalisation, as this leads to poor results. The key

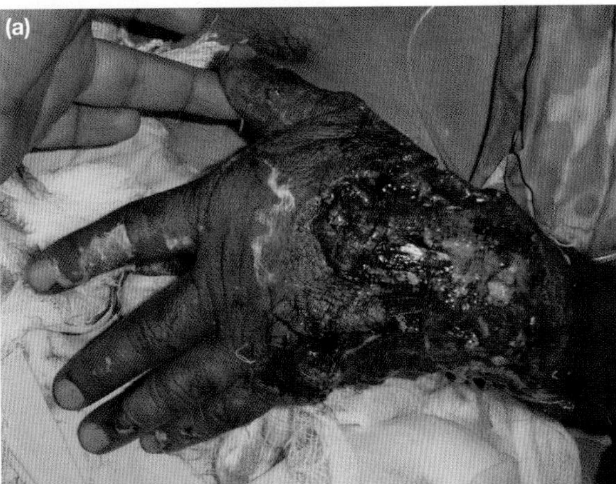

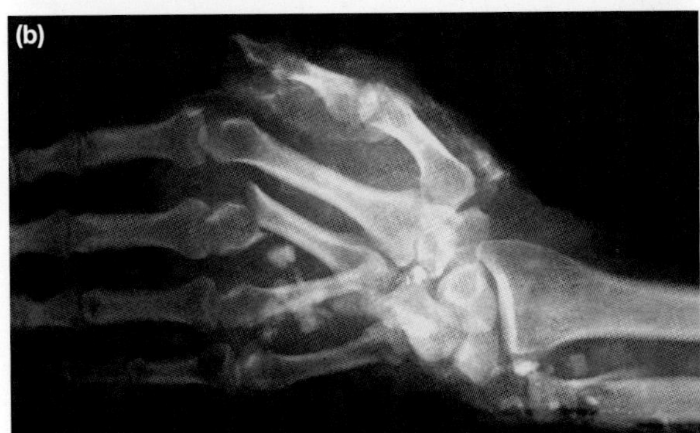

Figure 33.9 (a, b) Gross contamination typically seen in wounds sustained in disasters. The radiograph shows numerous radio-opaque foreign bodies in the soft tissues.

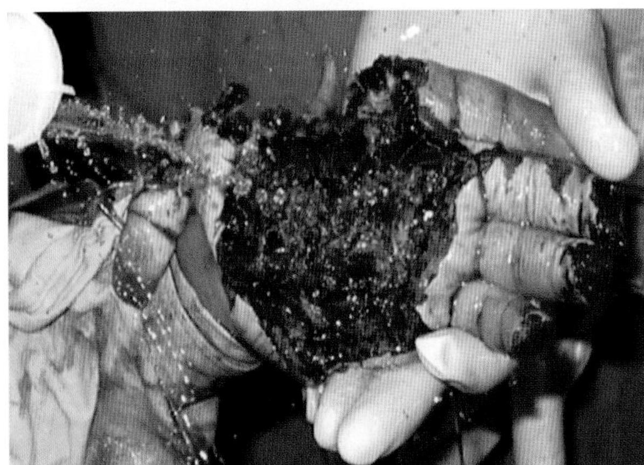

Figure 33.10 Lavage with normal saline to decontaminate a wound.

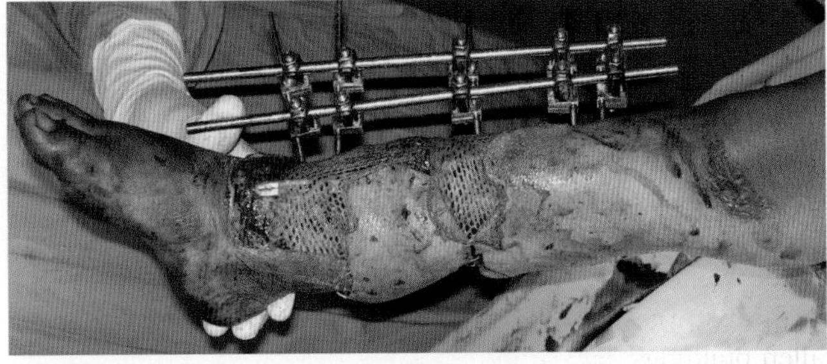

Figure 33.11 External fixators provide skeletal stabilisation and allow easy management of the soft tissues.

structures should be identified and the edges trimmed and tagged with non-absorbable sutures to facilitate repair during subsequent exploration.

- Wounds sustained in disasters are heavily contaminated and are not suitable for primary closure. However, blood vessels and exposed joint surfaces need to be covered. This can be achieved by loosely tacking adjoining muscle over the exposed area. The wound is then covered with fluffed gauze and sterile cotton and the extremity splinted with a plaster of Paris slab. For extremity injuries, elevation is critical to reduce oedema.
- Broad-spectrum antibiotics, such as third-generation cephalosporins, are started prophylactically and continued for 5–7 days.
- The wound is reinspected at 24–48 hours to assess the viability of the tissues. Wounds are closed between the fourth and sixth day if there is no infection. Tension should be avoided and one should not hesitate to use skin grafts to obtain cover.
- In wounds with gross infection no attempt at closure is made until infection is eradicated. These wounds are re-explored to make sure that there are no residual foreign bodies or devitalised tissue. Tissue should be taken for microbiological culture. Vacuum-assisted closure (Vac-Pac) has emerged as a very useful tool for deeply cavitating wounds. It utilises low-pressure suction to evacuate exudate, promote granulation tissue and reduce the size of the wound (*Figure 33.12*). Once the wounds are free from infection secondary closure can be undertaken.

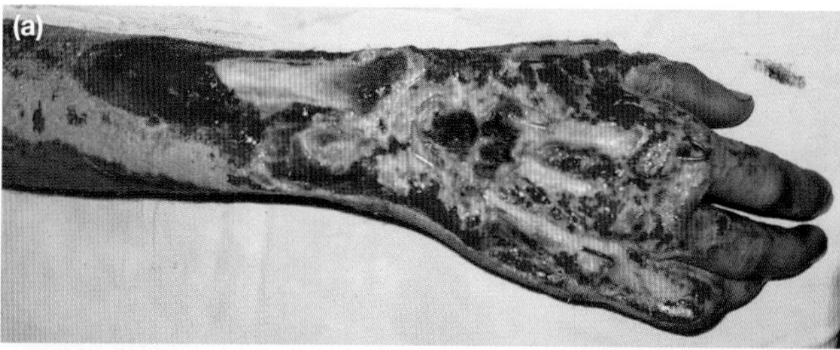

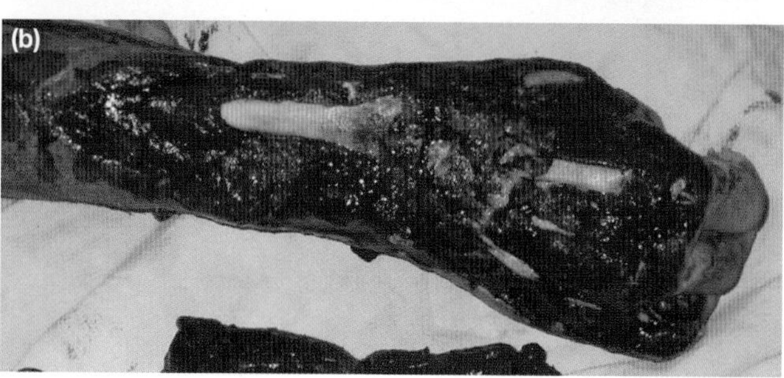

Figure 33.12 (a, b) Use of low-pressure vacuum therapy in preparing a wound for secondary closure.

Summary box 33.6

Principles of debridement and initial wound care

- Obtain generous exposure through skin and fascia
- Identify neurovascular bundles
- Excise devitalised tissue
- Remove foreign bodies
- Repair major vessels
- Obtain skeletal stabilisation with external fixators
- Only tag tendons and nerves that have been cut
- Leave the wound open and delay primary closure
- Avoid tight dressings
- Elevate the injured limb

DEFINITIVE MANAGEMENT

The hospitals designated to undertake definitive management should be selected on the basis of the facilities available and the number of injured that they can handle. The resources required for trauma patients are more than the typical case mix of a hospital. A rule of thumb is that only half the bed strength of a hospital can be utilised to provide optimum trauma care in an emergency situation.

Hospital reorganisation

In hospitals receiving mass casualties some reorganisation of services is unavoidable. This includes transferring patients with non-urgent conditions to other facilities, augmenting surgical services, reorganising the specialist rota and redesignating medical wards as surgical care areas. An appeal for blood donations should be broadcast.

SPECIFIC ISSUES

There is no injury that is peculiar to disasters and the whole spectrum of external injuries from minor cuts and compound fractures to amputations is seen. Internal organ damage is frequent and, unless immediate help is available, this accounts for the majority of early mortality figures. People trapped under fallen buildings may suffer crush injuries and crush syndrome if the duration is prolonged. Crush injuries and missile injuries cause extensive tissue damage and gross contamination, both favourable conditions for anaerobic and microaerophilic infections.

Limb salvage

The Mangled Extremity Severity Score (MESS) and its modifications are useful in deciding about limb salvage. Extensive tissue loss, neurovascular damage and loss of long fragments of bone are traditionally indications for amputation. Currently, wounds of any dimension can be covered with microvascular flaps and distraction osteogenesis and vascularised bone can be used to restore bony continuity. If performed in time, vascular repairs can salvage most acutely ischaemic limbs. Because of these developments the indications for amputation in trauma have undergone a paradigm shift and the majority of patients who reach a tertiary-care facility within 24 hours are candidates for limb salvage (*Figure 33.13*). This assumes

Plaster of Paris is a white crystalline powder, calcium sulphate hemihydrate $CaSO_4 \cdot 0.5H_2O$, which sets hard when water is added to it.

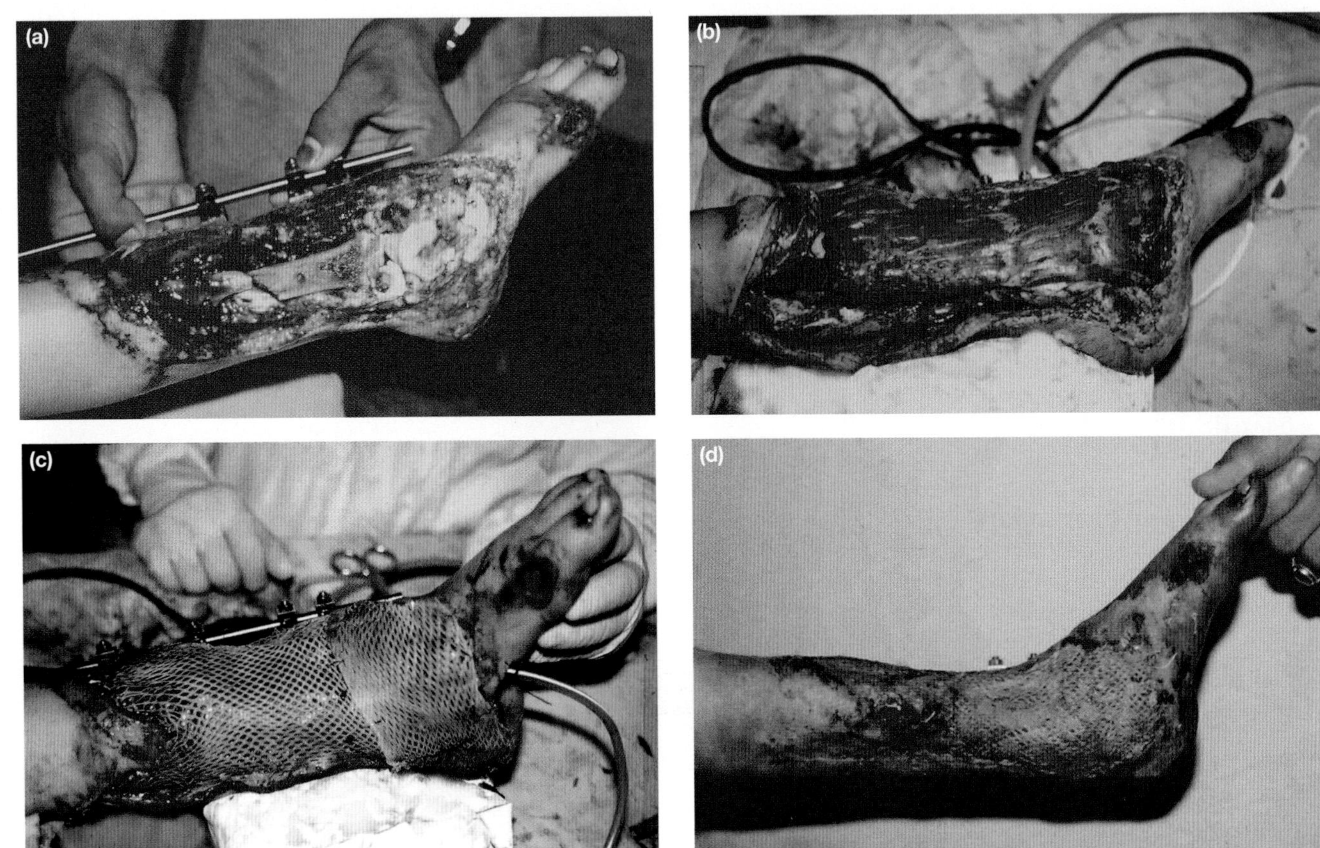

Figure 33.13 (a–d) Badly traumatised lower limb. Reconstruction has been performed using a microvascular rectus abdominis flap covered with a skin graft.

that debridement and, if required, vascular repairs have been performed in a field medical facility. A limb is unlikely to survive if the vascular repair of major limb vessels has been delayed for more than 4–6 hours.

Facial injuries

The management of facial injuries follows the same general principles of debridement and delayed closure as already outlined. Because of the functional and cosmetic importance of facial structures, skin and soft-tissue excisions are kept to a minimum. The face has a robust vascularity and a high ability to counter infection. Even in patients who present late with gross contamination, careful debridement followed by delayed primary closure can lead to good results (***Figure 33.14***).

Tetanus

This potentially fatal condition, also called 'lockjaw', is caused by *Clostridium tetani*, a Gram-positive spore-forming bacillus occurring naturally in the intestines of humans and in the soil. It enters the body through a wound and replicates, thriving on the anaerobic conditions present in devitalised tissues. It produces tetanospasmin, an exotoxin that binds to the neuromuscular junctions of the central nervous system neurones, rendering them incapable of neurotransmitter release. This leads to failure of inhibition of motor reflex responses to sensory stimulation and generalised contractions of agonist and antagonist muscles produce tetanic spasms. The median incubation period is 7 days, ranging from 4 to 14 days.

Early symptoms are painful spasms of the facial muscles, resulting in risus sardonicus (***Figure 33.15***). The spasms spread to involve the respiratory and laryngeal musculature. Spasms of the paravertebral and extensor limb musculature produce opisthotonus, an arching of the whole body. Laryngeal muscle spasm leads to apnoea and, if prolonged, to asphyxia and respiratory arrest. The spasms can be brought on by the slightest of sensory stimulus.

The diagnosis is obvious once it is fully manifest. There are three aspects of management:

- **Prevention**. Wounds contaminated with soil can harbour tetanus spores, and active immunisation is indicated by administering 0.5 mL of tetanus toxoid intramuscularly. Patients with gross contamination of cavitating wounds should also receive 250–500 U of human anti-tetanus globulin (ATG) intramuscularly to provide passive immunisation and to neutralise the circulating toxin. In full-blown

Hans Christian Joachim Gram, 1853–1938, Professor of Pharmacology (1891–1900) and of Medicine (1900–1923), Copenhagen, Denmark, described this method of staining bacteria in 1884.

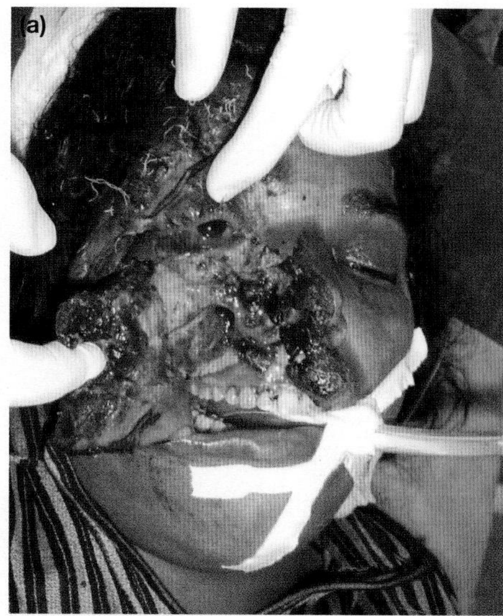

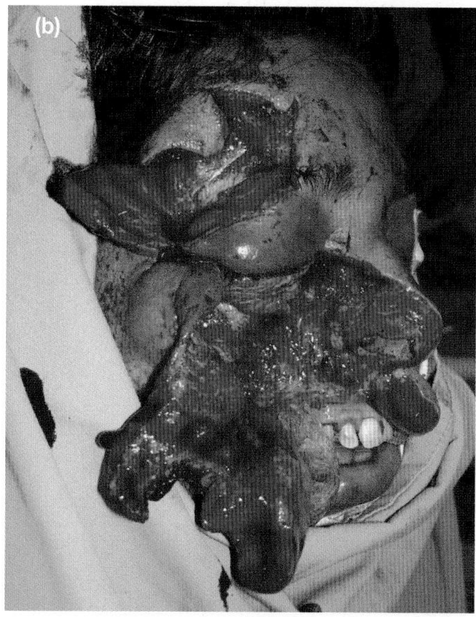

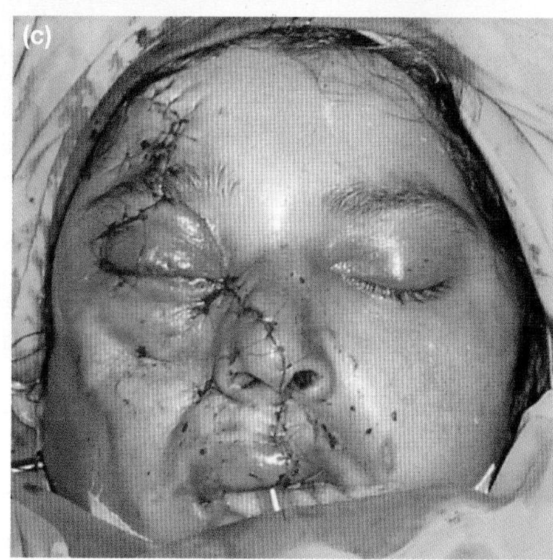

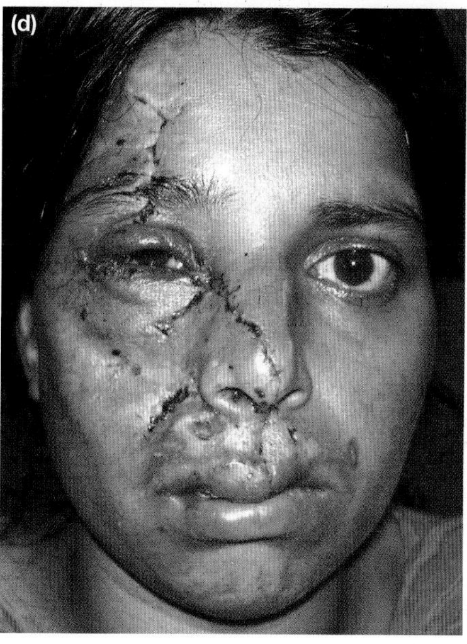

Figure 33.14 (a–d) Late-presenting facial injury with gross contamination. A thorough debridement followed by delayed primary closure has yielded good results.

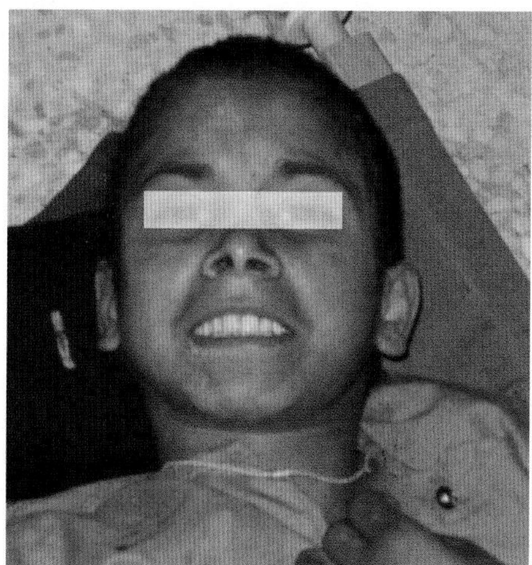

Figure 33.15 Risus sardonicus of 'lockjaw' (courtesy of Dr Samira Ajmal, FRCS).

clinical tetanus, 3000–10 000 U of ATG should be administered. Wound manipulation should be avoided for 2–3 hours after ATG administration to minimise tetanospasmin release.

- **Local wound care**. This includes a thorough wound debridement to eliminate the anaerobic environment. Intravenous administration of $10–24 \times 10^6$ U per day of penicillin G should be continued for 10–14 days. The wound should be closed using the delayed primary or secondary closure techniques.
- **Supportive care for established disease**. These patients are nursed in an intensive care unit (ICU) environment, free from strong sensory stimuli. Diazepam is useful in preventing the onset of spasms but, if these become sustained, the patient is paralysed, intubated and placed on a ventilator. The patient is then gradually weaned off the ventilator under cover of anticonvulsants. The overall mortality rate is around 45%, prognosis being determined

by the incubation period and the time from the first symptom to the first tetanic spasm. In general, shorter intervals indicate a poorer prognosis. Recently, intrathecal antitoxin administration has been used for spasm control to avoid ventilatory support. Nevertheless, without access to mechanical ventilation the mortality remains high and even those who survive may require several weeks of hospitalisation.

Summary box 33.7

Tetanus

- Caused by *C. tetani*
- Spores are present in the soil
- Thrives in dead or contaminated tissue
- Produces tetanospasmin, an exotoxin
- Produces spasm of muscles
- Make sure patients are immunised
- For heavily contaminated wounds give ATG

Necrotising fasciitis

Necrotising fasciitis is a rapidly spreading infection that produces necrosis of the subcutaneous tissues and overlying skin. It is caused by β-haemolytic streptococci and, occasionally, *Staphylococcus aureus*, but may take the form of a polymicrobial infection associated with other aerobic and anaerobic pathogens, including *Bacteroides*, *Clostridium*, *Proteus*, *Pseudomonas* and *Klebsiella*. It is termed Fournier's gangrene when it affects the perineal area and Meleney's gangrene when it involves the abdominal wall. The underlying pathology includes acute inflammatory infiltrate, extensive necrosis, oedema and thrombosis of the microvasculature. The area becomes oedematous, painful and very tender. The skin turns dusky blue and black secondary to the progressive underlying thrombosis and necrosis (*Figure 33.16*). The area may develop bullae and progress to overt cutaneous gangrene. It spreads contiguously but occasionally produces skip lesions that later coalesce. It is accompanied by fever and severe toxicity. Renal failure may occur as a result of hypovolaemia and cardiovascular collapse caused by septic shock. The rate of progression is dramatic and unless aggressively treated it leads to serious consequences with mortality approaching 70%.

The diagnosis is made on clinical grounds. Creatinine kinase levels may show enormous elevation and biopsy of the fascial layers will confirm the diagnosis. Patients should be admitted to the ICU and treated with careful monitoring of volume derangements and cardiac status. Oxygen supplementation is beneficial and endotracheal intubation is required in patients unable to maintain their airway.

High-dose penicillin G along with broad-spectrum antibiotics, such as third-generation cephalosporins and metronidazole, are given intravenously. The cornerstone of management is surgical excision of the necrotic tissue. The devitalised tissue is removed generously, going beyond the area of induration. The wound is lightly packed with gauze and dressed.

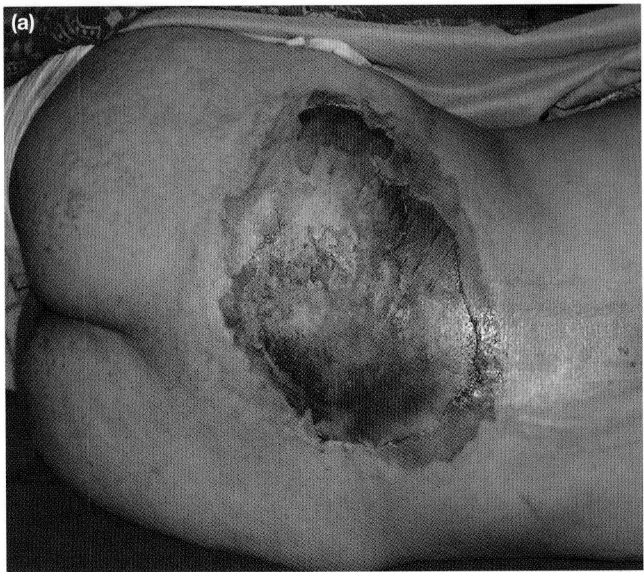

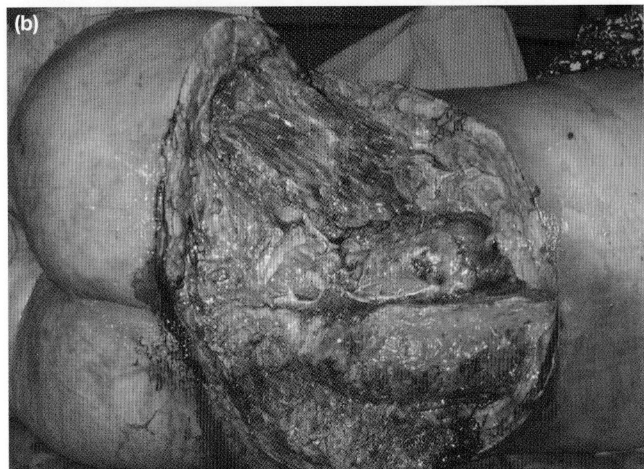

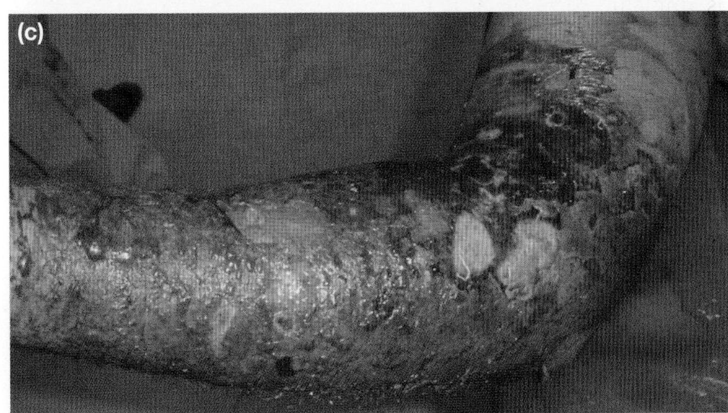

Figure 33.16 (a) Necrotising fasciitis at presentation and (b) rapid progression seen after 24 hours. (c) Typical bullae and induration.

Theodor Albrecht Edwin Klebs, 1834–1913, Professor of Bacteriology, successively at Prague, Czechoslovakia; Zurich, Switzerland; and then the Rush Medical College, Chicago, IL, USA.
Jean Alfred Fournier, 1832–1915, syphilologist, the Founder of the Venereal and Dermatological Clinic, Hôpital St Louis, Paris, France.
Frank Lamont Meleney, 1889–1963, Professor of Clinical Surgery, Columbia University, New York, NY, USA.

This process is repeated daily as the necrosis is prone to spread beyond the edges of the excised wound. In patients who survive, this results in a large wound, which will require skin grafting or flap coverage.

Summary box 33.8

Necrotising fasciitis

- Caused by β-haemolytic *Streptococcus* or is polymicrobial
- Also called Fournier's or Meleney's gangrene
- Progress is rapid and renal failure is an early complication
- Treat with radical surgical excision repeated every 24 hours
- Give oxygen and penicillin

Recently, the role of hyperbaric oxygen (HBO) has become more established with a reduction in mortality in patients treated with HBO (9–20%) compared with patients who did not receive HBO (30–50%).

Gas gangrene (clostridial myonecrosis)

Gas gangrene is a dreaded consequence of late-presenting missile wounds and crushing injuries. It is a rapidly progressive, potentially fatal condition characterised by widespread necrosis of the muscles and soft-tissue destruction. The common causative organism is *Clostridium perfringens*, a spore-forming, Gram-positive saprophyte that flourishes in anaerobic conditions. Other organisms implicated in gas gangrene include *Clostridium bifermentans*, *Clostridium septicum* and *Clostridium sporogenes*. Non-clostridial gas-producing organisms such as coliforms have also been isolated in 60–85% of cases of gas gangrene.

C. perfringens produces many exotoxins but their exact role is unclear. Alpha-toxin, the most important, is a lecithinase that destroys red and white blood cells, platelets, fibroblasts and muscle cells. The phi-toxin produces myocardial suppression while the kappa-toxin is responsible for the destruction of connective tissue and blood vessels.

Devitalised tissue or premature wound closure provides the anaerobic conditions necessary for spore germination. The usual incubation period is <24 hours but ranges from 1 hour to 6 weeks. A vicious cycle of tissue destruction is initiated by rapidly multiplying bacteria and locally and systemically acting exotoxins. This causes spreading necrosis of muscle and thrombosis of blood vessels. The typical feature of this condition is the production of gas that spreads along the muscle planes. Systemically, the exotoxins cause severe haemolysis and, combined with the local effects, this leads to the rapid progression of the disease, hypotension, shock, acute kidney injury and acute respiratory distress syndrome.

Pain that rapidly increases in severity is the earliest symptom. The limb swells up and the wound exudes a serosanguineous discharge. The skin is involved secondary to muscle necrosis, turning brown and progressing to a blue–black colour with haemorrhagic bullae (*Figure 33.17*). The characteristic sickly sweet odour and soft-tissue crepitus appear with established infection but their absence does not exclude the diagnosis.

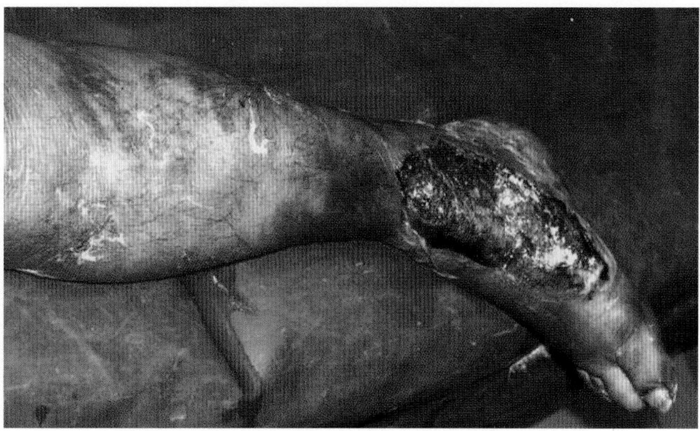

Figure 33.17 Typical picture of spreading gas gangrene caused by a crush injury.

These local signs are accompanied by pyrexia, tachycardia, tachypnoea and altered mental status.

The diagnosis is made on the basis of history and clinical features. A peripheral blood smear may suggest haemolysis and a Gram stain of the exudate reveals large Gram-positive bacilli without neutrophils. The biochemical profile may show metabolic acidosis and renal failure. Radiography can visualise gas in the soft tissues and is particularly useful in patients with chest and abdominal involvement.

Patients should be admitted to the ICU and treated aggressively with careful monitoring. High-dose penicillin G and clindamycin, along with third-generation cephalosporins, should be given intravenously. Surgical treatment is the same as for necrotising fasciitis (see *Necrotising fasciitis*). In established gas gangrene with systemic toxicity, amputation of the involved extremity is life-saving and should not be delayed. No attempt is made at closure; amputation stumps are left open and the wound is lightly packed with saline-soaked gauze and then dressed.

The role of HBO is not as clear as in necrotising fasciitis. However, considering the frequent catastrophic outcomes, it is recommended in severe cases if the facilities are available.

Summary box 33.9

Gas gangrene

- Caused by *C. perfringens*
- Spores are present in the soil
- Thrives in anaerobic conditions and produces many exotoxins
- Treat with radical and regular surgical excision
- Give oxygen and penicillin
- Early amputation may be life-saving

Crush injury and syndrome

A crush injury occurs when a body part is subjected to a high degree of force or pressure, usually after being squeezed between two heavy or immobile objects. Damage related to a crush injury includes lacerations, fractures, bleeding, bruising, compartment syndrome and crush syndrome (*Figure 33.18*).

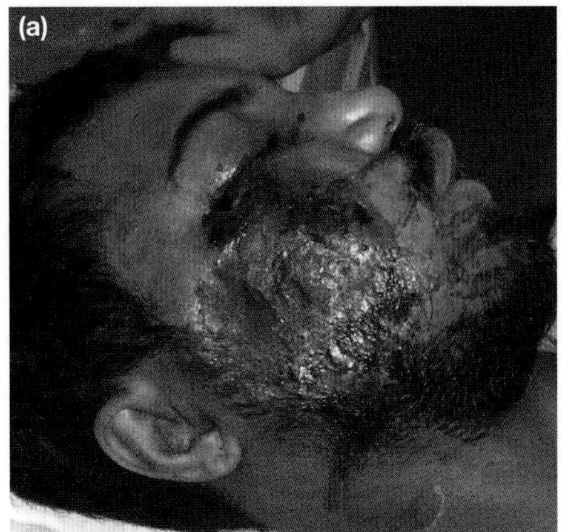

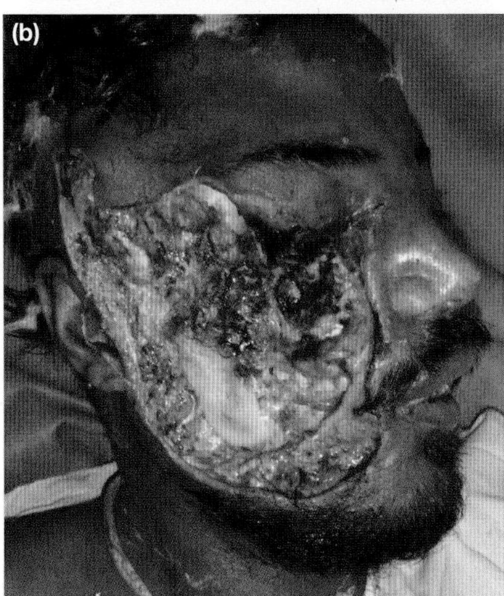

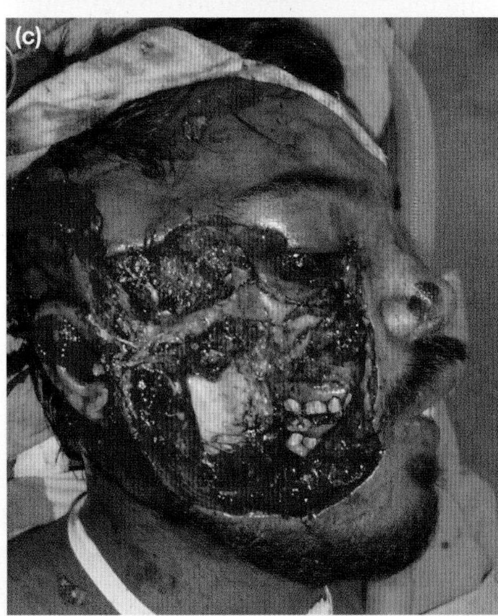

Figure 33.18 (a–c) Extensive crush injury in a man trapped in a fallen house. The depth to which the soft tissues have been devitalised is seen clearly.

Crush syndrome

The association between crush injury, rhabdomyolysis and acute kidney injury was first reported in victims trapped during the 'London Blitz'. It is seen in earthquake and mining accident survivors and in battlefield casualties. Prolonged crushing of muscle leads to a reperfusion injury when the casualty is rescued. This releases myoglobin and vasoactive mediators into the circulation. It also sequesters many litres of fluid, reducing the intravascular volume and resulting in renal vasoconstriction and ischaemia. The myoglobinuria leads to renal failure from tubular obstruction.

The treatment of crushed casualties should begin as soon as they are discovered. Rescuers must be alert to the presence of associated injuries (*Figure 33.19*). Aggressive volume-loading of patients, preferably before extrication, is the best treatment. After provision of first aid and starting intravenous fluids the patient should be catheterised to measure urine output. In adults, a saline infusion of 1000–1500 mL/h should be initiated. This should be continued until myoglobin is no longer detectable in the urine. Mannitol administration can reduce the reperfusion component of this injury. Once a flow of urine is observed, a mannitol–alkaline diuresis of up to 8 litres per day should be maintained, keeping the urinary pH greater than 6.5. An early fasciotomy can decompress muscle compartments and prevent severe loss of limb function. A late fasciotomy, when it is obvious that the muscles of that compartment must be dead, is only likely to cause a massive release of myoglobin, as well as potentially introducing infection into dead tissue. It is therefore best not to perform a fasciotomy in cases where entrapment has been for over 12 hours. Intensive care is required with close attention to fluid balance and renal dialysis if required.

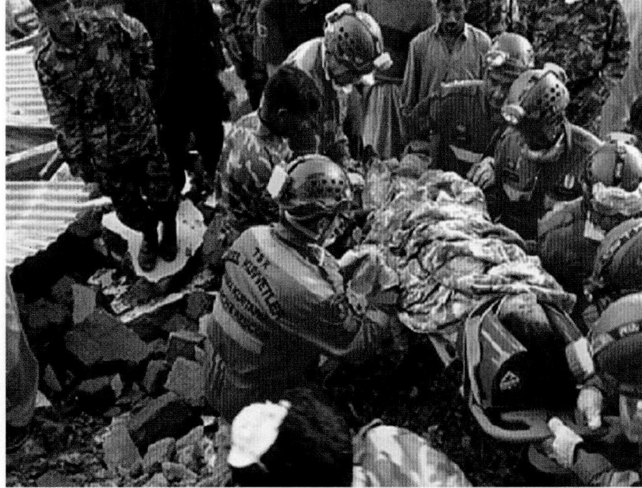

Figure 33.19 Rescuers must be prepared for injuries to the spine. Treatment of crush syndrome should start before extrication.

The **London Blitz** is the name given to the German air raids on London between 7 September 1940 and 17 May 1941, during which it is estimated that more than 15 000 people were killed. Blitz is short for *Blitzkrieg*, which is German for 'lightning war'.

Summary box 33.10

Crush syndrome

- Arises as a result of reperfusion
- Acute kidney injury and renal failure from myoglobinuria is a complication
- A late fasciotomy may make things worse not better

Compartment syndrome

A compartment syndrome develops when the pressure within a muscle compartment starts to rise as a result of trauma (see *Chapter 32*). This occurs in muscles enclosed in a fascia such as the calf and forearm muscles and the intrinsic muscles of the hand and foot. A tight bandage or plaster, haemorrhage from a fracture or severe blunt trauma leads to a rise in pressure in the compartment until it exceeds venous drainage pressure. If the pressure rises further, it will cut off perfusion of the muscle. Passive stretching of the affected muscle will cause extreme pain and this is diagnostic of the condition. If the condition is left unrelieved, then nerves passing through the compartment will cease to function and the muscle will die and then undergo fibrosis and shortening, producing a Volkmann's ischaemic contracture. Removal of any constricting agent and, if necessary, a fasciotomy will relieve the pressure and muscle perfusion will restart. Pressure studies are not reliable; if in doubt, perform a fasciotomy.

Summary box 33.11

Compartment syndrome

- Commonest in a closed fracture or soft-tissue crush injury
- Pain on passive extension of the muscles is diagnostic
- Intracompartmental pressure studies are not reliable
- If there is any suspicion, then fasciotomy must be performed early

Frostbite and immersion injuries (trench foot)

Frostbite occurs when a part of the body freezes. The cells are disrupted and the tissue dies. It is in effect a 'cold' burn and can be categorised according to the depth that it affects in the same way as a conventional burn. Other mechanisms at play include vasoconstriction caused by cold, capillary sludging and reperfusion injury with the release of free radicals, which occurs on rewarming the part. It commonly involves the fingers, toes, cheeks, the tip of the nose and the ears. When frozen the tissue feels hard and cannot be indented. Immersion injury is a cold injury that does not involve actual freezing of the tissue and is commonly caused by prolonged immersion in cold water (hence trench foot). The patient may also be hypothermic. Warming should be gentle as the heat used may actually cause a burn! Rehydration with warm fluids and use of non-steroidal anti-inflammatory drugs such as ibuprofen are beneficial. Demarcation will occur between dead and viable tissue and at this stage no surgery should be undertaken as there is often considerable deep recovery. The injured area should be kept clean and dry and efforts made to prevent further injury, as well as to prevent infection. Definitive surgery to excise dead tissue can be left for many months. Recent developments, such as the use of tissue plasminogen activator and nerve blocks, show promising results in reducing amputations, but have to be started within 24 hours and are seldom possible in the field.

Summary box 33.12

Frostbite

- Can be superficial or deep like a burn
- Rewarm gently
- Allow demarcation to occur naturally
- Protect against further trauma and infection

HANDING OVER

Follow-up and secondary problems

The medical aspect of disaster management does not involve a single short-term effort. It requires a long-term commitment and involvement of various disciplines. Because of the large numbers of casualties, the initial treatment is directed towards the anatomical restoration of damaged structures. There are therefore numerous patients who will need secondary procedures for functional restoration. This second wave of patients is encountered 3–6 months after a major catastrophe and arrangements should be made to deal with this.

Designated centres

Initially, the casualties may be scattered among many hospitals. After the first few weeks most of the acute problems have been dealt with and only those patients who require longer term treatment remain. At this point it is advisable to designate a particular hospital as a centre for these patients. This concentrates resources and expertise and makes follow-up easier.

DISASTER PLANS

Disasters are unforeseen events and planning for them may seem paradoxical. It has, however, been shown that disaster planning not only works but also saves lives. Disaster planning is a wide field but a résumé of the important aspects follows.

Establishment of a national disaster management organisation

This is the first step in the planning for disasters. Most resource-rich countries already have such an agency, which can formulate policy at the national level and has the infrastructure to react quickly when the need arises.

Richard von Volkmann, 1830–1889, Professor of Surgery, Halle, Germany.

Anticipating disasters

Areas near active volcanoes and geological fault lines are at risk from seismic disturbances, whereas regions along major rivers are liable to flooding. The urban centres of all countries are now potential targets for terrorist attacks. It is important to not only carry out threat assessments but also, if possible, set up an early warning system.

Evacuation planning

Evacuation of large population centres as a prelude to, or in the wake of, an impending disaster is a complex exercise. Yet it may be the most prudent course of action to remove as many people as possible from harm's way. Clear identification of exit routes must be determined and communicated to the populations at risk.

Organisation of emergency services

Emergency services such as the fire brigade, police and ambulance service must have defined roles and areas of responsibility to ensure a coordinated response during a crisis. Members of these teams must be included in the planning phase to ensure that the final plan is practicable and reflects the situation on the ground.

Summary box 33.13

Disaster planning

- Disaster can be anticipated and should be prepared for
- Evacuation of a whole population may be the best option
- Coordination between military, police, fire, ambulance and medical services is important

Medical planning

Identification of hospitals able to take large numbers of casualties and the location of areas that can be used for patient holding and triage in case of mass casualties is important. Hospitals that offer specialised services should be identified and their role during a major crisis defined. Suitable hospitals in the surrounding areas must be designated as overflow hospitals in the eventuality of a very large volume of patients.

FURTHER READING

Bartholdson S, von Schreeb J. Natural disasters and injuries: what does a surgeon need to know? *Curr Trauma Rep* 2018; **4**: 103–8.

Ciottone GR, Biddinger PD, Darling RG *et al. Çiottone's disaster medicine*, 2nd edn. Philadelphia, PA: Elsevier, 2016.

Trelles M, Dominguez L, Stewart BT. Surgery in low-income countries during crisis: experience at Médecins Sans Frontières facilities in 20 countries between 2008 and 2014. *Trop Med Int Health* 2015; **20**(8): 968–71.

World Health Organization. *Disaster management guidelines: emergency surgical care in disaster situations*. Geneva: WHO, 2009. Available from https://www.who.int/surgery/publications/EmergencySurgicalCareinDisasterSituations.pdf

World Health Organization. *WHO integrated management on emergency and essential surgical care (IMEESC) tool kit* (CD), 2011. Available from https://www.who.int/publications/i/item/integrated-management-for-emergency-and-surgical-care-(-imeesc)-toolkit/.

CHAPTER 34 Conflict surgery

Learning objectives

To understand and appreciate:

- Fundamental differences of war surgery
- Injury patterns of modern warfare
- Principles of war surgical management
- Blast and ballistic injury

INTRODUCTION

He who wishes to be a surgeon must first go to war.
Hippocrates (*c*.460–377 BCE)

The treatment of war wounds is as ancient as warfare itself. The Edwin Smith papyrus has been dated to 1600 BCE and is the oldest known treatise on trauma surgery and anatomy.[1] The history of battlefield surgery is the history of surgical advancement and the importance of the medical lessons learned from war have long been recognised.

While almost every conflict has served to increase our knowledge of the treatment of war injuries, and many individuals have played significant parts in the development of war surgery, Dominque Jean Larrey is considered by many to be the first modern military surgeon. Larrey, a French battlefield surgeon and favourite of Napoleon, devised some of the first systems of triage and casualty care that still form the fundamentals of modern military medicine. These systems must be in place in order to overcome the difficulties and logistical challenges of providing medical care to a battlefield.

HOW IS WAR SURGERY DIFFERENT?

While civilian trauma surgery bears some of the hallmarks of the battlefield, there are fundamental contrasts in environment and injury pattern that must be appreciated:

- The environment of war is likely to be austere. While recent long-term deployment has led to the establishment of some well-equipped field hospitals, logistical and personnel restrictions mean that sophisticated diagnostic and therapeutic techniques may not be available.
- War is hostile and potentially dangerous. Necessary workforce protection must be considered to ensure the safety of medical personnel and patients alike. Modern fighting forces employ physician-led resuscitation, along with forward surgical teams. Moving medical personnel closer to the fighting may increase their personal risk.
- War injuries are different from civilian trauma. Modern weapons may deliver such amounts of energy that the tissue destruction and patterns of injury seen are unlike all but the most extreme of civilian trauma.
- War is a mass casualty situation. Although casualty numbers vary between treatment facilities, triage is an important aspect of military surgery. The dictum 'do the best for the most, not everything for everyone' is important and may require a change in thinking for many used to civilian practice.
- War surgery is usually delivered in stages. The principles of damage control are often applied to allow transfer of patients between echelons of care. Careful planning, coordination and communication are essential.

ETHICAL AND LEGAL CONSIDERATIONS

International Humanitarian Law (IHL) regulates humanitarian issues during armed conflict. Modern IHL is derived from a variety of sources, notably the Geneva Conventions and their additional protocols, along with further specific regulations from the United Nations and The Hague Conventions. IHL provides medical personnel with rights in times of armed war, but also assigns duties to them surrounding the rights of protected personnel under their care.

Importantly, medical personnel are bound by medical ethics and IHL to treat patients solely based on need and without regard for their nationality, race and class or their religious or political beliefs.

Along with providing medical support to deployed forces, treatment is offered to both home nation and enemy combatants. The treatment of such patients may require a change in the approach to their definitive care. Evacuation of these

The papyrus is named after Edwin Smith, the Egyptologist who discovered it in 1866; it is held at the New York Academy of Medicine, NY, USA.
Dominique Jean Larrey, 1766–1842, French surgeon in Napoleon's Grand Armée.

personnel to certain categories of subsequent facility (see *Medical support roles*) may not be possible and the staged approach to care may need modification. Transfer to host nation medical facilities may be possible but dependent on local capability.

This scenario may require an adaptation to clinical thinking. As an example, consider the ethical and logistical dilemma in performing revascularisation and orthoplastic procedures for a local patient in a country without rehabilitation facilities.

Medical personnel and facilities are protected under IHL and should not be attacked. However, the nature of modern conflict is unconventional; guerrilla warfare and the inability of deployed forces to define the enemy combatant requires the security of facilities and personnel to be of the highest priority.

MEDICAL SUPPORT ROLES

The term 'role' is used to designate the tiers of medical support that integrate into a modern military operation.[2] An appreciation of the capabilities and limitations of these roles is essential to improving the care of casualties at each stage. Different nations and forces will have medical support configured with some variability but, overall, systems are similar in order to ensure that the basic treatment, supply and evacuation needs that are essential for a military operation are available.

- **Role 1** medical support provides for routine primary health care, specialised first aid, triage, resuscitation and stabilisation. It is integrated within a small unit. The capabilities of role 1 care will depend greatly on the size of the unit and the training of the personnel within it.
- **Role 2** provides an intermediate capability for the reception and triage of casualties, as well as being able to perform resuscitation and treatment of shock to a higher technical level than role 1. It is prepared to provide evacuation from role 1 facilities. It has capability for damage control surgery (DCS) and may include a limited holding facility for the short-term holding of casualties until they can return to duty or be evacuated.
- **Role 3** medical support is deployed hospital care and the elements required to support it. This includes a mission-tailored variety of clinical specialties, including primary surgery and diagnostic support. In recent conflicts role 3 facilities grew and evolved into sophisticated hard-built hospitals.

Summary box 34.1

Medical support roles

- R1– unit-level medical care including first aid and primary health care
- R2 – intermediate unit for resuscitation, damage control and stabilisation
- R3 – deployed hospital care with multispecialty capability
- R4 – definitive hospital care within the home or allied nation

- **Role 4** provides the full spectrum of definitive medical care that cannot be deployed to the area of operations or is too time-consuming to be conducted there. It is normally provided in the country of origin or an allied nation depending on the location of deployment and time-lines of transfer.

It is important to appreciate that these roles are highly variable both within and between different nations. The size and scale of the operations as a whole, along with predictions of both civilian and military medical requirements, will dictate the structure of the medical support.

MEDICAL EVACUATION

Medical evacuation refers to the movement and en route care of casualties within a conflict zone. The evacuation may be the initial movement from a battlefield or between other more sophisticated echelons of care, up to and including repatriation to a home nation.

Aeromedical evacuation using either fixed or rotary wing aircraft has had a major impact on evacuation timelines. Certain considerations must be made prior to and during aeromedical evacuation:

- the patient should be sufficiently stabilised for the anticipated mode and duration of travel;
- the patient's airway and breathing are adequate for movement;
- intravenous access, surgical drains, urinary catheters and any other tubes should be firmly secured;
- patients at high risk for thoracic barotrauma should be considered for prophylactic chest tube placement before prolonged aeromedical evacuation;
- blankets and/or warmers should cover the patient securely to mitigate against hypothermia.

The capability of different evacuation platforms may vary from highly sophisticated mobile critical care units to the simple transportation of casualties by non-medical personnel. These capabilities, along with the timelines and distances involved in casualty movement, should be major considerations for the planning of medical support operations.

The 'golden hour' is an oft-quoted principle in trauma medicine and refers to the initial time period following injury during which a life is most likely lost or saved. Although the origins and applicability of the term are disputed,[3] the principle is ubiquitously understood. Within the military setting, death is certainly seen to occur most commonly within the prehospital environment and within a short period after injury, with better outcomes seen after rapid transport to surgical care.[4]

Improvement in outcomes from severe deployed trauma may rely upon either the shortening of time to damage control care or lengthening of the 'golden hour'. Shortening of timelines may be achieved with change in transport systems or deployment of surgical teams further 'forward', or even the use of telemedical technology to utilise remote expertise. Lengthening of the golden hour may perhaps be achieved by the use of novel prehospital haemorrhage control techniques or an increase in the availability of prehospital blood products.[5–8]

PATTERNS OF MODERN WAR SURGERY

Modern warfare has changed over recent decades. The causes of injury are particular to the individual conflict, nation and armed service.[9] Historically, penetrating trauma was predominantly sustained by combat infantry, whereas naval and air personnel sustained more blunt injuries (*Table 34.1*).

Improvements in trauma scoring systems and the development of a concise system for the recording of injuries and casualty care have increased the ability of modern armed services to analyse the injury patterns of their deployed personnel.

TABLE 34.1 Historical causes of injury among US service personnel.

	Service			
Mechanism	Infantry (%)	Armoured (%)	Sea (%)	Air (%)
Ballistic	90	50	25	5
Blunt	2–3	5	10	50
Blast	2–3	5	10	<10
Thermal	2–3	25	30	25
Combined	<5	15	25	10

Adapted from Champion *et al.*[9]

A cohort analysis of combat injuries incurred by US forces[10] showed significant differences in injury patterns sustained in the most recent Afghanistan and Iraq conflicts compared with those sustained in the Second World War and the Korean and Vietnamese Wars. Head and neck injuries were far more common in recent conflict whereas thoracic and extremity injuries were less so. This is probably because of the increased use of body armour and similar personnel protective equipment in more recent conflicts.

The mechanism of injury has also changed. Although ballistic injuries remain an important contributor to battlefield trauma, injuries due to explosions (which include improvised explosive devices [IEDs], landmines, mortars, grenades and rockets) have become increasingly common and are now the predominant mode of wounding and fatality. The relative proportions of injuries caused by explosive and ballistic weapons are shown in *Table 34.2*.

The emergence of explosive patterns of injury is due to the increasing use of IEDs within conflicts. IEDs have been the signature weapon within operations in Afghanistan and Iraq; however, their use has not been limited to these regions. The relative low cost, ease of production and widespread expertise means that IEDs are likely to play significant roles in most contemporary and future conflicts.

TABLE 34.2 Relative proportion of injuries caused by gunshot wounds and explosions among US personnel.

	Gunshot (% of total injuries)	Explosion (% of total injuries)
US Civil War	91	9
First World War	65	35
Second World War	27	73
Korean War	31	69
Vietnamese War	35	65
Iraq/Afghanistan War	19	81

Adapted from Owens *et al.*[10]

PRINCIPLES OF WAR SURGERY

Battlefield death occurs early (or immediately) because of devastating central nervous system injury and haemorrhage, or late because of infection. Some of the injuries causing immediate death (including brain, heart and great vessel injury) are non-survivable[11] and may only be managed with prevention.

Treatment of haemorrhage is therefore the mainstay of military trauma medicine. Bleeding should be recognised and managed from the point of wounding.[12] Tourniquets are indicated for the control of catastrophic extremity bleeding. Non-compressible torso haemorrhage carries a poor prognosis,[13] although it may be amenable to methods of endovascular control not yet commonly used.[14]

A damage control approach to surgery must be employed to stop bleeding, to remove necrotic tissue and foreign material and to reduce contamination. In addition to life-saving surgery, procedures to salvage limbs, including revascularisation (or temporary shunting) and fasciotomy, should be considered early, when physiology allows.

DAMAGE CONTROL SURGERY

DCS was first described by Rotondo *et al.*,[15] although the idea of an abbreviated laparotomy for the unwell patient was not totally novel. The concepts of DCS were initially applied to complex trauma patients with combined vascular and visceral injuries. Improved outcomes were seen following DCS principles compared with conventional definitive surgery.

The DCS approach is to restore physiology over anatomy and is typically divided into several phases:

- **Phase 1**. Recognition of injury severity and the need for damage control principles, both surgical and resuscitative. Features of phase 1 include rapid-sequence induction of anaesthesia and intubation, early rewarming and prompt movement to the operating theatre.
- **Phase 2**. Immediate laparotomy with rapid control of bleeding and contamination, abdominal packing and temporary wound closure.
- **Phase 3**. Movement to the intensive care unit (ICU) for ongoing resuscitation with normalisation of biochemical and physiological parameters.
- **Phase 4**. Re-exploration in the operating theatre to perform definitive repair of all injuries. Multiple procedures on multiple occasions may be required. Even at this stage, non-essential procedures may be truncated or delayed if physiology deteriorates.

The selection of patients for damage control management may not be straightforward. While various physiological and biochemical markers of injury have been suggested, there is no validated threshold. Hypothermia, coagulopathy, acidosis, blood loss and anticipated operative time should all be considered (see *Chapters 26 and 27*).

The benefits of a DCS approach to those patients who need it has been repeatedly shown, but liberal, and perhaps overzealous, use of DCS is unlikely to be beneficial to those who would tolerate definitive repair. DCS puts a heavy toll on theatre and ICU resources. In addition, multiple trips to theatre may increase the likelihood of morbidity, including abdominal wall hernias, fistulae and infection.

Damage control resuscitation (DCR) should be concurrent with DCS. The principles of DCR include permissive hypotension, the avoidance of crystalloid with haemostatic resuscitation and the recognition and management of acute traumatic coagulopathy (ATC). The application of these principles to military patients is uncertain because of longer timelines. Prolonged periods of permissive hypotension are likely to be harmful,[16] whereas haemostatic resuscitation and management of ATC is ineffectual in the absence of haemorrhage control.[17]

MASSIVE TRANSFUSION

While haemorrhage control prior to the need for massive transfusion is ideal, this is often not the case. The degree of injury and associated massive blood loss associated with war injuries may necessitate large-volume transfusion. The use of crystalloids to resuscitate exsanguinating patients is strongly discouraged, but the optimal ratio of blood products has not yet been ascertained. Massive transfusion protocols exist within most deployed units. The use of such a protocol in a UK role 3 facility, along with aggressive resuscitation and use of blood products, has been associated with improved trauma outcomes.[18] The success of such a protocol is highly dependent on a steady stream of blood products and reflects the sophisticated transfusion infrastructure that should be woven into a deployed capability.

Blood transfusion is increasingly administered in a more forward location (within both role 1 and role 2 environments) with limited volumes of blood transported to the point of wounding by aeromedical response teams. Future resuscitative strategies are under much scrutiny. The use of whole blood (and the possibility of 'walking blood banks') may be combined with alternatives to conventional blood components, which can join adequate oxygen carriage with positive or neutral effects on patient coagulation.[19]

DECISION MAKING WITHIN THE DEPLOYED ENVIRONMENT

The damage control approach is vital in a proportion of war injuries, but thought must be given to available resources. Within a well-established role 3 unit, both DCS and definitive procedures are likely to be possible. Blood and blood products are also likely to be available and restocked regularly. In this scenario, patient physiology is the major determinant of the mode of care.

In contrast, decision making becomes more crucial within the austere environment. Theatre space, intensive care beds, equipment and blood products may be limited. Long evacuation times may contraindicate permissive hypotension.

Limited resources, such as blood, may need to be divided among casualties. Within a role 1 or role 2 facility, immediate evacuation may be undertaken in preference to more thorough stabilisation.

Decision making of this nature is complex and difficult and requires practice in the context of simulation, exercises and courses.

WEAPON EFFECTS

Ballistics

The ability to manage conflict injuries relies on an understanding of the underlying mechanism of wounding, which is likely to be different from that in civilian trauma. As stated, while ballistic injuries are no longer the most common cause of battlefield injury, firearms remain a common element in all conflict. Civilian trauma practice, depending on local firearm laws, may well encompass a significant volume of gunshot wounds, although patterns of injury with war wounds may well differ as a result of the weapons used. An understanding of the mechanism of ballistic wounding is required to treat these wounds effectively.

The earliest recorded depiction of a firearm is from 1326, but firearms became ubiquitous on the battlefield during the seventeenth century.[20] Ballistic weapons all work with the same principles – an explosion is used to propel a projectile along and out of a straight tube – but have evolved considerably from rudimentary cannons to sophisticated modern-day firearms. The explosive force within a modern firearm comes from propellant encased within a cartridge. The basic design of a cartridge is shown in *Figure 34.1*.

Internal ballistics describes the characteristics of a projectile while inside the weapon. The hammer mechanism strikes a primer at the base of the cartridge, which ignites the propellant. Hot gas produced by the explosion expands and forces the bullet away from the cartridge and along the barrel. Spiral grooves, or rifling, impart spin on the bullet, which aids accuracy and stabilisation.

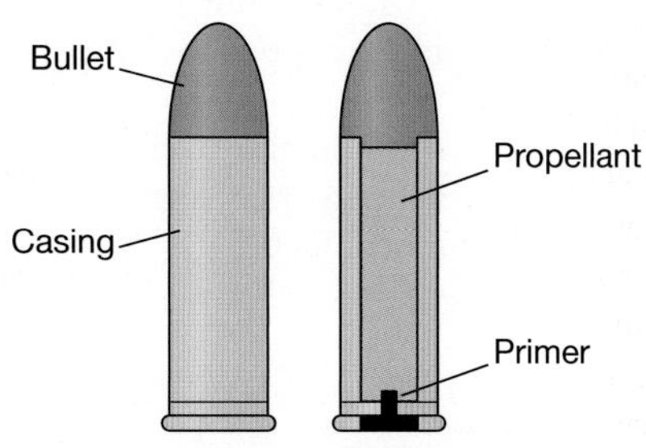

Figure 34.1 Diagram of basic cartridge structure.

While the basic principles apply to nearly all firearms, advances in firearm design have served predominantly to improve accuracy, reliability and rate of fire. Ammunition is normally held within a magazine or belt that loads directly into the chamber of the weapon. The loading mechanism determines the rate of fire. In a semiautomatic or fully automatic system, the recoil forces of the spent cartridge eject the cartridge while resetting the chamber and accepting a new cartridge from the magazine, such that the process may be repeated rapidly.

Shotguns utilise a similar mechanism except that a collection of smaller projectiles – 'shot' – are expelled rather than a single bullet. These smaller projectiles disperse away from one another after leaving the barrel. The degree of dispersal is dependent on the relative length of the barrel.

External ballistics describe the characteristics of a projectile in free flight. It may be influenced by ammunition type and ambient conditions. Ammunition differs widely with the most pronounced difference between pistol and rifle ammunition. Rifles are expected to be accurate at ranges up to and beyond 1000 metres, while pistols are intended for far shorter ranges. Rifle cartridges are longer and typically have a greater proportion of propellant to projectile. The characteristics of ammunition that determine wound effects are the size or calibre (which describes the internal diameter of the weapon barrel) and the material components of the bullet:

- Full metal jacket ammunition has an outer coating of harder metal around a softer core. This reduces breakdown of the bullet along the barrel and improves accuracy, reliability and target penetration.
- Soft tip and hollow point ammunition have a degree of exposed lead that flattens and deforms on impact. These bullets have less penetrating ability but rapidly transfer energy to the impacted tissue and cause large wounds.

Ballistic injuries

Terminal ballistics (or wound ballistics) describes the interaction between projectiles and target tissue. This interaction and subsequent transfer of energy cause injury. The kinetic energy of the bullet is related to the mass and velocity of the impacting projectile. Both the mass and velocity of military firearms may be considerably greater than those commonly seen in civilian trauma, leading to higher energies and more severe wounds. While the weapon and ammunition type may be a determinant in the potential injury caused, many other factors, including range, angle, clothing, armour and anatomical variation, will determine the actual wound pattern. Although an understanding of ballistic science may allow a surgeon to anticipate possible injuries, each should be evaluated and managed individually.

In consideration of the damage done, tissue may be described by the areas of disruption caused by the projectile and the permanent and temporary wound cavity, which are illustrated in *Figure 34.2*.

The permanent cavity is the localised area of definitive tissue injury caused by contact with the projectile. This area of cell necrosis is the result of direct contact, crushing and laceration of tissues in the path of the projectile. The size and

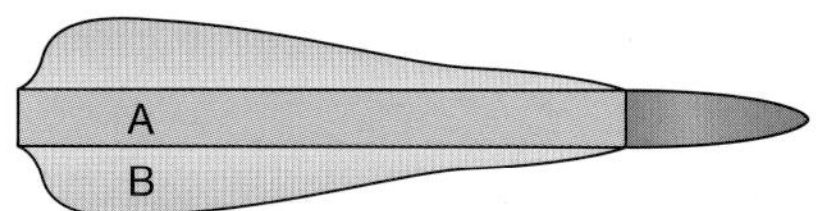

Figure 34.2 Diagram showing the permanent wound cavity (A) and the temporary wound cavity (B). This relatively large temporary cavity is more typical of a higher energy weapon.

trajectory of the projectile determines the cavity size. This type of cavity is the predominant wound effect of pistol bullets, which have relatively low energy. Higher energy projectiles, including military rifle and machine gun bullets, may be subject to greater degrees of deformation and tumbling as they travel through tissue. This increases the effective cross-sectional area of the projectile and may lead to a larger and less regular permanent wound cavity.

In contrast, the temporary wound cavity is created by lateral displacement of tissue that has not been in direct contact with the bullet. The degree of damage in this area is dependent on the amount of energy transferred by the bullet and the material properties of the tissue itself. Individual tissues have an elastic strength that resists the stretching caused by a projectile. As the energy increases, the tissue is no longer able to rebound and, above certain thresholds, contusion, laceration and permanent damage may occur. Skin, muscle, lung and bowel wall tissues have good elastic strength and may rebound well following stretch, with minimal damage within the temporary wound cavity. In contrast, liver, brain and spleen have poor elasticity and are more likely to shatter when stretched. The incompressibility of fluids within hollow organs (bowel and bladder) means that they are vulnerable to stretch despite favourable properties of the tissue wall itself.

Summary box 34.2

Ballistics

- Internal ballistics – characterise the projectile within the weapon during firing
- External ballistics – characterise the projectile in free flight
- Terminal ballistics – characterise the projectile/tissue interaction

MANAGEMENT OF GUNSHOT WOUNDS

The management of gunshot wounds in a conflict setting may differ from that in civilian practice. The typical low-energy wounds caused by pistols are sometimes managed conservatively in civilian trauma centres with adequate wound care, cleaning and antibiotics. Military wounds are associated with higher energies, higher rates of infection and more severe injury. The extent of these injuries, including the size of the wound cavities, may not be adequately assessed without thorough surgical examination (*Figure 34.3*). As such, most penetrating wounds in the military setting are explored under anaesthetic. The extent and capacity for recovery of the temporary wound

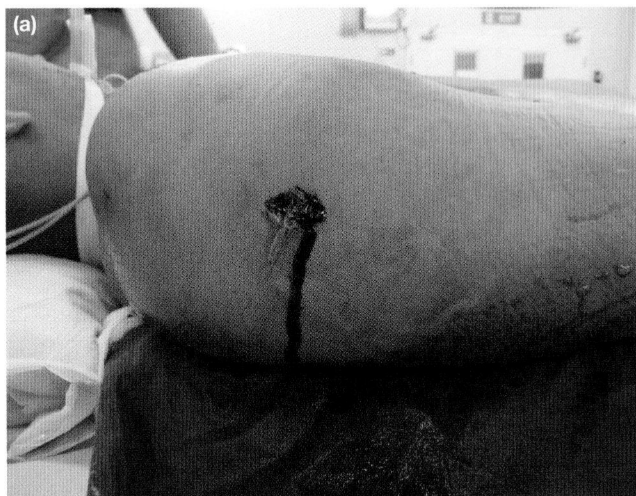

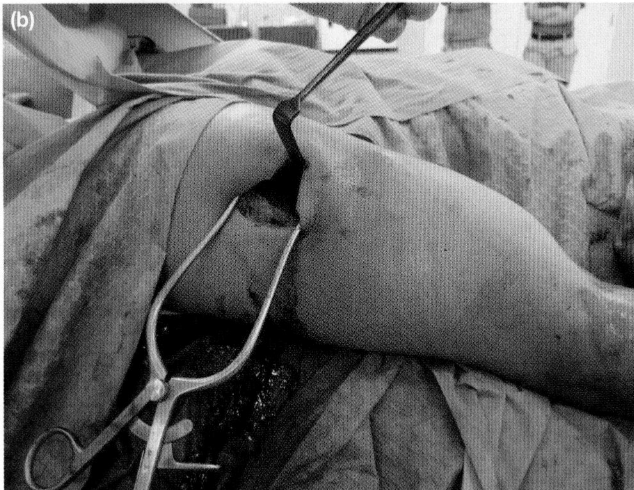

Figure 34.3 Entry wound to the right shoulder (a) with the wound extended in order to assess it adequately (b).

cavity may not be appreciated at the time of the first operation. A damage control approach should be adopted if the physiology of the patient dictates it. An interval period may also allow for adequate appreciation of the permanent wound cavity, along with the response of the surrounding structures and demarcation of non-viable tissue.

BLAST

As already discussed, blast has become the predominant mechanism of injury in recent conflicts. Unfortunately, terrorist attacks within urban centres mean that these injuries are increasingly encountered within civilian practice.

While explosives come in many forms and their effects vary as a result, fundamental principles underlie all blast events.

An explosive may be defined as 'a substance that can be made to undergo a rapid chemical reaction that will transform a liquid or solid into gas, liberating a large amount of energy'.[21] The explosive properties of such a material are determined by the chemical composition of the material and the speed at which energy is expelled. Low explosives react by a process called deflagration, whereby the reaction is propagated by flame passing through the material at a rate significantly slower than the speed of sound. They are made up of a combustible material and an accompanying oxidant. Low explosives include gunpowder, gasoline and pyrotechnics such as fireworks and flares. Low explosives more commonly cause burns than typical blast injuries and will not be discussed further.

In contrast, high explosives degrade via detonation. Shockwaves are passed through the material at supersonic speeds and the resultant energy is expelled at very high rates. High explosives include plastic explosive and trinitrotoluene (TNT). The input of a relatively small amount of energy results in the production of a very large volume of gas, at high speed and pressure. The outward expansion causes a wave of compressed air that moves away from the point of detonation at supersonic speeds and in a uniform sphere (within a free field).

The change in surrounding pressure is described as the blast overpressure. Following detonation within a free field, there is a near instantaneous pressure rise, which falls exponentially. This is classically described by the Friedlander curve (*Figure 34.4*).

This characteristic pressure peak is only seen during a truly free (almost theoretical) scenario. Enclosure of the blast or reflection of blast waves by people, vehicles or buildings is likely to change the overpressure profile such that high pressures may be sustained for longer periods and have a greater propensity to cause injury. For this reason, blasts within enclosed spaces are notable for causing a greater range and severity of injury.

In addition to expanding gases, detonation of explosives may result in the expulsion of fragments. These fragments may be part of a device casing, separate material deliberately added with the intention of fragmentation or environmental material flung by the blast.

Blast winds are generated by the displacement of surrounding air. The direction of these winds may change as the blast

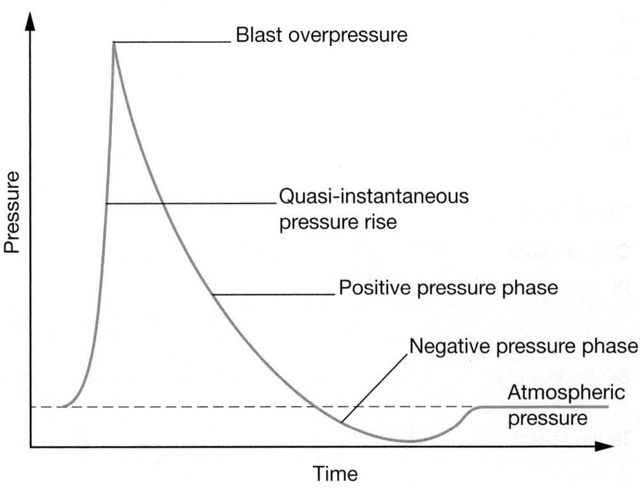

Figure 34.4 Theoretical blast overpressure changes within a free field.

Frederick Gerard Friedlander, 1917–2001, Austrian mathematician, lived and worked in the UK from 1934.

overpressure drops transiently beneath ambient pressure and creates a partial vacuum.

Improvised explosive devices

The characteristic weapon of modern warfare has been the IED, which was the leading cause of death among coalition troops during conflicts in Iraq and Afghanistan.[22] These devices may range from rudimentary homemade explosives to sophisticated devices containing high explosives. Within this broad range of devices are further categories including roadside explosives and blast mines, suicide bombers and explosive formed projectiles (EFPs). EFPs are a particular form of device with a deformable plate on the uppermost surface. The detonation of the device and expansion of the explosive products deforms this plate into a missile shape, while simultaneously accelerating it upwards to very high velocities. Alternatively, copper plates may melt to create a high-speed molten jet (a shaped charge). Upon contact with a target (typically a vehicle), the missile impacts the hull of the vehicle with a degree of penetration dependent on the device and vehicle armour. Huge amounts of kinetic energy are dispersed through the vehicle and occupants. Injuries may be caused by both direct impact of the deforming hull and gross upwards acceleration followed by downwards deceleration of the whole vehicle.

BLAST INJURIES

Blast injuries are classified by the blast mechanism (*Table 34.3*).

Primary blast injury

Primary blast injuries result from the overpressure and are, as such, unique to blast. The effect of blast overpressure is most marked at the interface between air and tissue or liquid.

Tympanic membrane (TM) rupture is the most common primary blast injury. Patients may be asymptomatic or have a degree of transient hearing loss and otorrhoea. Previously, the presence of TM rupture was used as a marker for other occult blast injuries. This has been challenged recently by findings that show TM injury is not ubiquitous in the presence of more severe primary blast injury. The blast environment and orientation of the ear canal to the shockwave are likely to determine the chance of injury.

TABLE 34.3 Classification of blast injuries.

Classification	Injury type	Examples
Primary blast	Overpressure	Tympanic membrane injury, blast lung, intestinal blast injury
Secondary blast	Penetrating/ fragmentation	All penetrating injuries
Tertiary blast	Blunt	Blunt and crush injuries, traumatic amputation
Quaternary blast	Miscellaneous	Burns, inhalation injury
Quinary blast	Effect of device additions	Radiation sickness, infection

Primary blast lung injury, or blast lung, is the most widely researched blast phenomenon. The exact mechanism of blast lung remains contested but it depends on the propagation of energy from the shockwave into the lung tissue, where it causes disruption. Proposed mechanisms of injury include spalling (disruption of tissues at air–liquid interfaces), implosion (compression and re-expansion of air-filled structures) and rapid acceleration of tissues of different densities. Large animal models have demonstrated that the level of injury is related to the rate of chest wall displacement, rather than the maximal depth of deflection.[23] The severity of injury is dependent on the strength of the blast, the range from detonation and the surrounding environment.

Those working closely with explosives may wear personal armour that assists in decoupling the effect of the primary blast. Current examples of such armour tend to be cumbersome. More common varieties of torso body armour provide protection against penetrating injury but probably do little to mitigate the effects of primary blast.

The pathophysiology of blast lung includes both immediate and delayed responses. There is an immediate bradycardia and apnoea of variable length, which is likely to be a vagally mediated reflex.[24] The lung injury itself is typified by alveolar capillary rupture with subsequent intrapulmonary bleeding and oedema. The extent of this injury is proportional to the blast exposure and may range from microscopic petechial injury to areas of frank haemorrhage.

While rarely seen in isolation, primary blast may leave little external evidence of injury since the skin itself is rarely affected. Clinical features of blast lung include progressive hypoxia, which may not be apparent at the time of injury and is related to the inflammatory response to intrapulmonary haemorrhage and worsening oedema.

Other structural lung injuries are associated with primary blast, although the prediction of these injuries by blast conditions is not consistent and is likely to be complicated by tertiary impact. Pneumothoraces may occur as a result of pleural rupture in the absence of penetrating injury. Injury to the larger vessels may lead to haemothoraces and the formation of alveolar–venous or bronchovenous fistulae. Air embolism due to such fistulae may cause acute hypoxia with cardiovascular collapse and is a leading cause of death in those who do not survive until treatment.

The diagnosis of blast lung is clinical with findings of hypoxia following blast exposure. Typical 'bat-wing' pulmonary infiltrates are seen on the chest radiograph and computed tomography may discriminate these injuries from the more peripheral contusions seen in blunt trauma. Imaging may be useful in detecting associated structural lung injuries.

Treatment of blast lung is largely supportive. Mechanical ventilation may be required but consideration should be given to the possibility of air embolism and pneumothorax that may be exacerbated. Some centres advocate the use of prophylactic bilateral pleural decompression, although there is little evidence to suggest an effect on outcomes. Patients with significant blast lung injury are highly likely to have sustained other blast-related injuries and any management plan should consider their overall condition.

The abdomen may also be subject to primary blast. The incidence of abdominal injury due to air blast has not been extensively examined, although a recent review of multiple incidents, including a variety of blast conditions, showed that abdominal injury is not common – seen in around 3% of incidents.[25]

Damage is dependent on coupling of the blast overpressure and the shockwave to a stress wave that travels through the abdomen. The effect of shockwave dispersal is most marked at tissue–air interfaces. As such, the hollow organs are those most commonly injured. The caecum is probably most sensitive to intestinal blast injury. Conversely, the small bowel and its extensive mesentery may be more susceptible to large shear waves causing mesenteric tearing.

The presentation of primary blast injury to the bowel may be delayed relative to the acute onset of blast lung. Abdominal symptoms may be absent initially with progression to pain and frank peritonitis, should perforation and contamination occur. Given the lack of external injury, indications for operative intervention are largely clinical, as with conventional blunt abdominal trauma. The patient should be assessed anaesthetically with particular consideration to the effect of anaesthesia and ventilation on any concomitant blast lung injury.

The most common operative finding of intestinal blast is subserosal haemorrhage.[25] Tearing of the mucosal surface with bleeding into the lumen of the tract may occur following repeated exposure to relatively lower blast overpressures. As in blunt injury, there is a propensity for mural haematomas to progress to perforation as a result of tissue necrosis. Full-thickness injuries to the bowel with immediate perforation can occur with a greater exposure to blast overpressure.

The surgical management of blast bowel injury is that of any penetrating and blunt trauma, with primary repair or resection as indicated. Surgical judgement is essential regarding the findings of non-perforated but contused bowel. A damage control approach to such injuries may allow for repeat assessment later, but in a physiologically well patient, in whom a relook would not be justified, the surgeon must decide to resect a segment or risk future progression of these lesions to perforation.

The solid organs are more resistant to primary blast. Parenchymal disruption due to the shockwave has been described at very high levels of overpressure, although the experimental data for these injuries are sparse. Injury, with subsequent bleeding, may result from rapid distractions of organ attachments and mesenteries. These blast conditions are more likely to be encountered in enclosed conditions and differentiation of primary from tertiary injuries is difficult.

Secondary blast injury

Secondary blast injury refers to the effect of fragments that are accelerated away from the device following detonation. Sources of fragments include:

- the casing of the device;
- purposefully placed fragments within the device; these may include nails, bolts or ball bearings and are embedded within the device or adherent to the exterior;
- nearby objects including glass and stones;

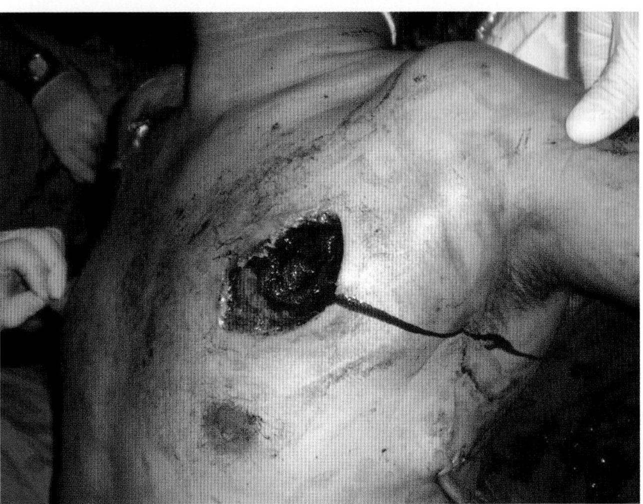

Figure 34.5 Large anterior fragmentation injury.

- biological material including bone may be expelled, particularly following a suicide bomb or antipersonnel mine attack.

Shrapnel is often used to describe explosive fragments, although the term is more strictly applied to a specific form of artillery shell.

The energy of a primary blast wave disperses quickly in proportion to the distance from the blast; it is subject to the inverse cube law. As such, only those within a reasonably small radius of the blast are affected. Conversely, the velocity and wounding potential of an energised fragment are subject to the inverse square law. Secondary blast injuries may occur at long range from the detonation. Fragments may be accelerated up to very high velocities. As with ballistics, injuries are dependent on the range and energy of the fragment.

In contrast to bullet wounds, the variability of fragments produces a wide range of wounds and no two wounds will be the same (*Figure 34.5*). The irregular surfaces of fragments cause complex patterns of yaw and tumble. Both permanent and temporary wound cavities may be unpredictable and irregular.

The management of fragment wounds is similar to ballistic and conventional penetrating trauma. Wounds should be adequately debrided. Fragment wounds should be considered dirty and principles of septic surgery applied. Where possible, serial debridement and delayed primary closure should be attempted.

The fragments should be removed at the time of surgery if easily accessible. Other indications for early removal include fragments within joint spaces or adjacent to structures with danger of erosion and further injuries. Late indications for fragment removal include ongoing sepsis, pain or lack of function.

Tertiary blast injury

Tertiary blast injury is the result of gross movement of personnel, objects or infrastructure by blast wind. Tertiary injury is analogous to conventional blunt trauma and may cause a wide variety of injuries to all organ systems. Traumatic amputation is typically included within this category, although primary blast and the shattering or 'brisance' effect on bone may play a part.

Quaternary and quinary injury

Quaternary blast injury refers to a miscellaneous group of injuries that do not fall within other categories. These include burns, inhalational injuries and late-onset respiratory problems. Quinary injury refers to injury caused by the intentional addition of either biologically or radioactively active material to an explosive device.

Environmental effects

As already alluded to, the shockwave of blast overpressure is modified by an enclosed or partially enclosed space. Environmental variations may make marked differences to injury rates and clinical presentations following blast. Higher rates of blast lung and TM rupture are seen following enclosed blast (in which both the casualty and blast are enclosed). In contrast, secondary blast injuries may be lower in number as more people are protected from energised fragments. Tertiary injury is difficult to predict based on blast characteristics but a higher proportion of blunt injuries have been seen following enclosed blast.

A distinct pattern of injury has been described following underbody blast against military vehicles. Underbody blast casualties have a greater range of injuries and are overall more severely injured.[26] In addition to blunt injury sustained from displacement within the vehicle, the effect of blast is manifested by propagation of the shockwave through a solid, with both upwards deformation of the floor and a rapid upwards acceleration of the whole vehicle and subsequent deceleration following impact with the ground. The solid blast injury burden includes severe foot and ankle[27] and pelvic injuries.[28] Mortality from underbody blast is most commonly caused by head injury and non-compressible torso haemorrhage, including aortic disruption and liver laceration.[29]

Complex dismounted blast injury

In contrast, the dismounted IED casualty may sustain a characteristic pattern of injuries, including lower limb amputation, pelvic fracture and genital, perineal and rectal injuries.[30,31] The most common cause of death in such casualties is from haemorrhage.[26] Initial management is therefore focused upon control of bleeding with tourniquets and swift proximal vascular control. This group may in the future benefit from the judicious use of resuscitative endovascular balloon occlusion of the aorta (REBOA) as a bridge to definitive control.[14,32] The role of REBOA in civilian trauma remains greatly contested and its use in military and austere settings may be complicated by long timelines entailing a prohibitively high burden of ischaemic injury.

Following control of bleeding and DCR, management principles for complex dismounted blast injury include the identification and repair of specific injuries, with serial debridement and delayed reconstruction of soft tissues.

Orthopaedic considerations include external fixation of pelvic injuries and the retention of maximal limb length for rehabilitation. High rates of rectal injuries require careful rectal examination with proctoscopy and early consideration of faecal diversion. Genitourinary injuries should be managed with careful catheterisation if possible (and consideration of suprapubic catheters) with exploration of scrotal wounds.[33]

INFECTION

Battlefield wounds are by their very nature grossly contaminated and the treatment and prevention of infection is one of the basic functions of war surgery. Wounds sustained during warfare are high-energy wounds with large areas of devitalised tissue. This is particularly the case for dismounted blast injuries where there is massive disruption of tissue planes with soil and debris forced into the zones of injury (*Figure 34.6*).

Wounding agents are all non-sterile and highly likely to be contaminated by bacteria. Both large-calibre ballistic wounds and blast wounds may contain dirty clothing or contaminated fragments. Multiple steps in casualty evacuation and substantial delays before treatment may allow progression of contamination to clinically significant infection.

Specific organism patterns will depend on endemic flora, but commonly seen bacteria include:

- Gram-positive cocci, including staphylococci, streptococci and enterococci;
- Gram-negative rods, including *Escherichia coli*, *Proteus* and *Klebsiella*;
- *Pseudomonas*, *Enterobacter*, *Acinetobacter* and *Serratia* are common nosocomial pathogens that are usually expected among casualties following long periods of hospitalisation;
- *Salmonella*, *Shigella* and *Vibrio* should be suspected in cases of bacterial dysentery.

Fungal infection, including *Candida*, should be considered in casualties hospitalised for prolonged periods, those who are malnourished or immunosuppressed or those who have received broad-spectrum antibiotics, adrenocortical steroids or parenteral nutrition.

Techniques to reduce the infectious burden are part of every aspect of war surgery. At the point of wounding, sterile dressings should be applied. Antibiotics, if available, should be administered if evacuation and further treatment are likely to be delayed.

Empirical antibiotic therapy should be commenced or continued following movement to a medical facility. The mainstay of treatment is prompt surgical control of the infectious cause with adequate debridement of non-viable tissue and drainage of infective material. Extensive irrigation should be employed to remove dead tissue and foreign bodies. High-pressure wound lavage has been shown to increase bacterial propagation into soft tissue and is not indicated.

With few exceptions (such as facial wounds), closure of contaminated war wounds should not be performed at the time of first operation. The open wound should be left with clean,

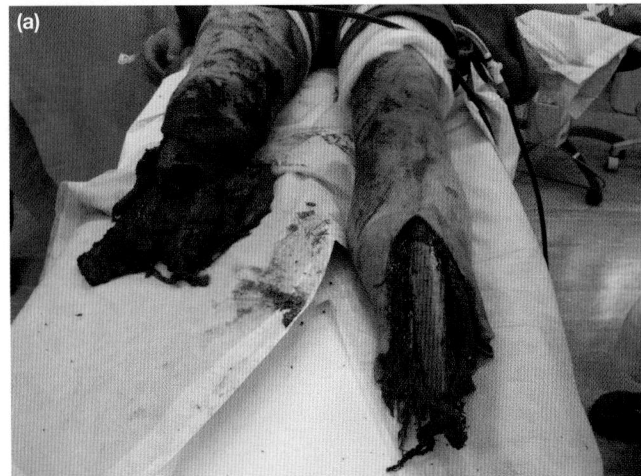

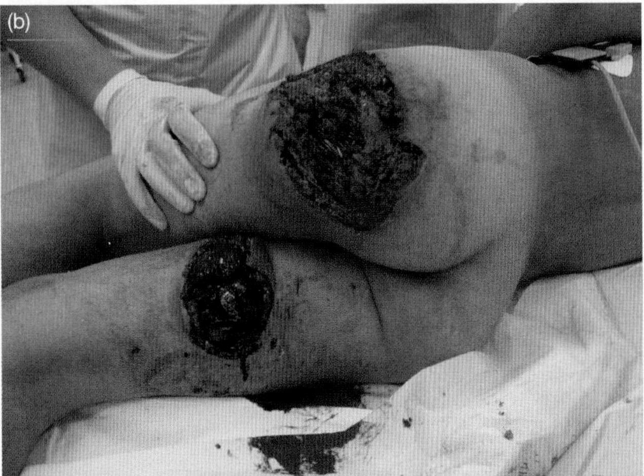

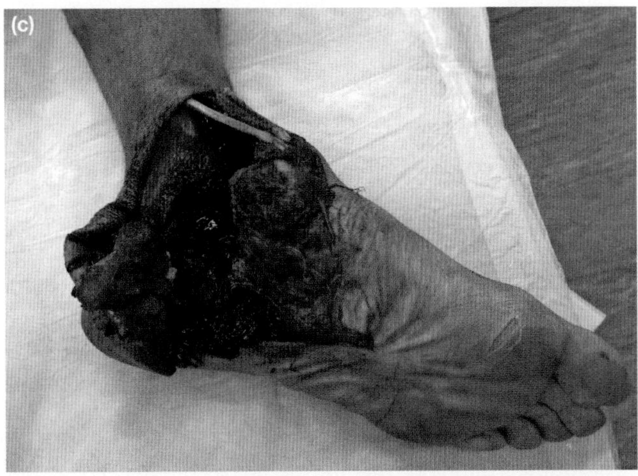

Figure 34.6 Blast injuries including bilateral lower limb amputation (a), buttock and thigh soft tissue injury (b) and complex hind foot injury (c). The need for extensive debridement is evident from the level of wound contamination and non-viable tissue.

moist dressings. Negative pressure wound therapy should be considered for larger wounds.

Antibiotic therapy should be tailored to specific wounds with the empirical antibiotic choice dependent on the injured body region or cavity. Microbial culture will aid the guidance of therapy for more established infection. Contaminated war wounds should be considered tetanus prone and appropriate tetanus prophylaxis administered.

Clinical experience and judgement are essential in the assessment of war wounds. Adequate exposure, often with extension of the wound, is mandated to ensure debridement of all devitalised tissue. Serial operations may be required. Early consideration should be given to soft-tissue coverage. The skin is often remarkably resilient to injury and conservative debridement of it may facilitate more successful reconstruction.

REFERENCES

1 Atta HM. Edwin Smith Surgical Papyrus: the oldest known surgical treatise. *Am Surg* 1999; **65**(12): 1190–2.
2 North Atlantic Treaty Organization. *NATO logistics handbook*. Brussels: NATO Headquarters, 2012. Available from https://www.nato.int/docu/logi-en/logistics_hndbk_2012-en.pdf.
3 Lerner EB, Moscati RM. The golden hour: scientific fact or medical 'urban legend'? *Acad Emerg Med* 2001; **8**(7): 758–60.
4 Howard JT, Kotwal RS, Santos-Lazada AR *et al.* Reexamination of a battlefield trauma golden hour policy. *J Trauma Acute Care Surg* 2018; **84**(1): 11–18.
5 Fisher AD, Teeter WA, Cordova CB *et al.* The role I resuscitation team and resuscitative endovascular balloon occlusion of the aorta. *J Spec Oper Med* 2017; **17**(2): 65–73.
6 Russo RM, Williams TK, Grayson JK *et al.* Extending the golden hour: partial resuscitative endovascular balloon occlusion of the aorta in a highly lethal swine liver injury model. *J Trauma Acute Care Surg* 2016; **80**(3): 372–80.
7 Benavides LC, Smith IM, Benavides JM *et al.* Deployed skills training for whole blood collection by a special operations expeditionary surgical team. *J Trauma Acute Care Surg* 2017; **82**(6S Suppl 1): S96–102.
8 Nettesheim N, Powell D, Vasios W *et al.* Telemedical support for military medicine. *Mil Med* 2018; **183**(11–12): e462–70.
9 Champion HR, Bellamy RF, Roberts CP, Leppaniemi A. A profile of combat injury. *J Trauma* 2003; **54**(5 Suppl): S13–19.
10 Owens BD, Kragh JF, Wenke JC *et al.* Combat wounds in operation Iraqi Freedom and Operation Enduring Freedom. *J Trauma* 2008; **64**(2): 295–9.
11 Eastridge BJ, Hardin M, Cantrell J *et al.* Died of wounds on the battlefield: causation and implications for improving combat casualty care. *J Trauma* 2011; **71**: S4–8.
12 Hodgetts TJ. ABC to <C>ABC: redefining the military trauma paradigm. *Emerg Med J* 2006; **23**(10): 745–6.
13 Morrison JJ, Stannard A, Rasmussen TE *et al.* Injury pattern and mortality of noncompressible torso hemorrhage in UK combat casualties. *J Trauma Acute Care Surg* 2013; **75**(2 Suppl 2): S263–8.
14 Morrison JJ, Ross JD, Rasmussen TE *et al.* Resuscitative endovascular balloon occlusion of the aorta: a gap analysis of severely injured UK combat casualties. *Shock* 2014; **41**(5): 388–93.
15 Rotondo M, Schwab C. 'Damage control': an approach for improved survival in exsanguinating penetrating abdominal injury. *J Trauma* 1993; **35**(3): 375–82.
16 Garner J, Watts S, Parry C *et al.* Prolonged permissive hypotensive resuscitation is associated with poor outcome in primary blast injury with controlled hemorrhage. *Ann Surg* 2010; **251**(6): 1131–9.
17 Khan S, Brohi K, Chana M *et al.* Hemostatic resuscitation is neither hemostatic nor resuscitative in trauma hemorrhage. *J Trauma Acute Care Surg* 2014; **76**(3): 561–7; discussion 567–8.
18 Jansen JO, Morrison JJ, Midwinter MJ, Doughty H. Changes in blood transfusion practices in the UK role 3 medical treatment facility in Afghanistan, 2008-2011. *Transfus Med* 2014; **24**(3): 154–61.
19 Naumann DN, Khan MA, Smith JE *et al.* Future strategies for

remote damage control resuscitation after traumatic hemorrhage. *J Trauma Acute Care Surg* 2019; **86**: 163–6.
20 Breeze J, Penn-Barwell J, Keene D *et al* (eds). *Ballistic trauma: a practical guide*, 4th edn. Cham, Switzerland: Springer, 2017.
21 Stuhmiller J, Phillips Y, Richmond DR. The physics and mechanisms of primary blast injury. In: Bellamy RF, Zajtchuk R (eds). *Conventional warfare: ballistic, blast and burn injuries*. Washington, DC: Department of the Army, Office of the Surgeon General, 1991: 241–70.
22 Ramasamy A, Hill AM, Clasper JC. Improvised explosive devices: pathophysiology, injury profiles and current medical management. *J R Army Med Corps* 2009; **155**(4): 265–72.
23 Cooper GJ, Taylor DE. Biophysics of impact injury to the chest and abdomen. *J R Army Med Corps* 1989; **135**(2): 58–67.
24 Guy RJ, Kirkman E, Watkins PE, Cooper GJ. Physiologic responses to primary blast. *J Trauma* 1998; **45**(6): 983–7.
25 Owers C, Morgan JL, Garner JP. Abdominal trauma in primary blast injury. *Br J Surg* 2011; **98**(2): 168–79.
26 Singleton JA, Gibb IE, Hunt NC *et al.* Identifying future 'unexpected' survivors: a retrospective cohort study of fatal injury patterns in victims of improvised explosive devices. *BMJ Open* 2013; **3**(8): e003130.
27 Ramasamy A, Hill AM, Masouros S *et al.* Blast-related fracture patterns: a forensic biomechanical approach. *J R Soc Interface* 2011; **8**(58): 689–98.
28 Webster C, Masouros S, Gibb I, Clasper JC. Fracture patterns in pelvic blast injury: a retrospective analysis and implications for future preventative strategies. *Bone Joint J* 2015; **97-B**(Suppl 8): 14.
29 Pearce AP, Bull AMJ, Clasper JC. Mediastinal injury is the strongest predictor of mortality in mounted blast amongst UK deployed forces. *Injury* 2017; **48**(9): 1900–5.
30 Cannon JW, Hofmann LJ, Glasgow SC *et al.* Dismounted complex blast injuries: a comprehensive review of the modern combat experience. *J Am Coll Surg* 2016; **223**(4): 652–64.
31 Smith S, Devine M, Taddeo J, McAlister VC. Injury profile suffered by targets of antipersonnel improvised explosive devices: prospective cohort study. *BMJ Open* 2017;**7**(7): e014697.
32 Rees P, Waller B, Buckley AM *et al.* REBOA at Role 2 Afloat: resuscitative endovascular balloon occlusion of the aorta as a bridge to damage control surgery in the military maritime setting. *J R Army Med Corps* 2018; **164**(2): 72–6.
33 Sharma DM, Webster CE, Kirkman-Brown J *et al.* Blast injury to the perineum. *BMJ Mil Health* 2013; **159**: i1-i3.

CHAPTER 35 History taking and clinical examination in musculoskeletal disease

Learning objectives

To understand how to:

- Take a comprehensive musculoskeletal history
- Perform a structured and systematic musculoskeletal examination
- Use and interpret special tests
- Use findings to understand the impact on a patient's pain and function

INTRODUCTION

The components of the musculoskeletal (MSK) system include the bones, joints, ligaments, muscles and tendons as well as the neurological and vascular structures. A simple system allows a concise yet comprehensive history to be taken and a reliable examination to be performed. This will permit diagnosis of the common, the rare and the clinically urgent MSK problems that are likely to be encountered in clinical practice.

HISTORY

Introduction

- Ensure you have followed appropriate hand hygiene guidance.
- Introduce yourself and check the patient's name and date of birth.
- Request presence of a chaperone as appropriate.
- Explain what you are going to do, obtain verbal consent and ensure that the patient is comfortable.

Take a history

- **Presenting complaint**. Start with an open-ended question. Ask the patient to 'explain what the problem is' in their own words and ask the patient what their hopes and expectations are from the interview.
- **History of the presenting complaint ('the three Ws')**. **W**hen did you first notice the problem? **W**hat were you doing when it started? **W**as the onset sudden or did it develop gradually?
- **Associated symptoms**. Ask about the following: pain; swelling; instability – 'giving way'; mechanical symptoms (e.g. locking, clicking, clunking); loss of power; altered sensation.
- **Functional impairment**. Ask whether the patient is having difficulties performing activities of daily living: upper limb, e.g. personal hygiene, feeding; lower limb, e.g. putting on shoes and socks, standing, walking and climbing stairs.
- **Past medical history (PMH)**. Check for comorbid conditions which may contribute to the presenting problem or affect the patient's fitness for an anaesthetic, e.g. diabetes, asthma, previous heart attack or stroke. Check for any previous problems with anaesthesia.
- **Past surgical history**. Ask about relevant surgical procedures.
- **Drug history**. Ask about all medication and the following in particular: anticoagulants, steroids, aspirin, immunosuppressant therapy, oral contraceptive pill and hormone replacement therapy.
- **Social history**. Tailor questions to the patient's condition: patient's age; hand dominance; employment status; dependants; alcohol consumption; smoking; hobbies; home help; accommodation – own house, residential or nursing home; use of walking aids; mental test score assessment.
- **Family history**. This may reveal a history of MSK disease.

Summary box 35.1

Taking a history

- Introduce yourself and put the patient at ease
- Explain what you are doing and ensure that the patient agrees
- Start with an open question to understand the presenting complaint
- Check for history of the presenting complaint and associated symptoms
- Ask about functional impairment
- Check past medical history and relevant surgical and family history
- Check drug and social history

MUSCULOSKELETAL EXAMINATION

General principles

Apley described a useful and systematic approach to clinical examination. This approach is divided into three parts:

1 look;
2 feel;
3 move.

Look

The inspection begins as soon as you enter the examination room. Look for any walking aids. Remember to look at the whole patient and not just at the joint of interest. For example:

- look at the hands for rheumatoid arthritis;
- look at the eyes for Horner's syndrome;
- look for any obvious upper or lower limb or spinal deformity.

Gait

The gait cycle is all of the activity between the initial contact of the foot with the ground and the succeeding initial contact of the same limb. There are two main stages: the stance phase (60%) and the swing phase (40%). Ask the patient to stand, and inspect from the front, side and back. Then, ask the patient to walk using any walking aids. Some of the types of limp that might be present are described in ***Table 35.1***.

Focused inspection

Adequately expose the joint above and below. Expose the opposite limb for comparison. Make sure that the patient is comfortable. It may be easier for you and the patient if they remain standing for the first part of the examination. When a couch is used, make sure that it is in the centre of the room (not against the wall) so that you can work on both sides of the patient. Remember that all joints are covered by an envelope of soft tissues and skin. Look at the skin for:

- surgical scars (arthroscopy scars may be difficult to see);
- bruising (may indicate recent injury or a bleeding disorder);
- erythema (e.g. cellulitis);
- ulcers (e.g. arterial, vascular or neuropathic);
- rashes;
- sinuses (e.g. secondary to osteomyelitis);
- hair loss and the presence or absence of sweating;
- pigmentations or raised lesion (e.g. café-au-lait spots or neurofibromas).

Look at the soft tissues for:

- swelling (e.g. may indicate a joint effusion);
- lumps (consider which tissue layer they are arising from);
- muscle wasting (e.g. may be secondary to disuse atrophy, neuropathy);
- muscle fasciculation (lower motor neurone pathology).

Look at the bones for:

- abnormal limb alignment – comparison with the other side may be helpful;
- deformity.

Feel

Ask the patient if they have any areas of tenderness. Ensure that you do not cause the patient pain – watch their face as you feel. It may be easier (especially with children) to feel the normal side first.

TABLE 35.1 Types of limp.

Cause	Pathogenesis	Presentation
Long	Osteoarthritis (in other leg)	Head dips. Cadence dash/dash
Incoordinated	Cerebral palsy	Head movement lacks coordination. No regular cadence
Muscle weakness	Osteoarthritis hip	Head moves from side to side (windscreen wiper)
Pain	Osteoarthritis hip	Head dips. Cadence dot/dash
Stiff	Arthrodesis hip	Head rocks to and fro
Limp	**Pathology**	
Antalgic	Hip joint arthritis	
Trendelenburg	Weakness of hip abductors	
High-stepping gait	Foot drop secondary to common peroneal nerve palsy	
Spastic	Cerebral palsy	
Ataxic	Cerebellar pathology	

Alan Graham Apley, 1914–1996, Director of Orthopaedic Surgery, St Thomas' Hospital, London, UK. As a consultant also at Rowley Bristow Orthopaedic Hospital, he conducted the most popular orthopaedic postgraduate course for the FRCS examination in Pyrford, UK, which became internationally known as the 'Pyrford Orthopaedic Course'.

Johann Friedrich Horner, 1831–1886, Professor of Ophthalmology, Zurich, Switzerland, described this syndrome in 1869.

Friedrich Trendelenburg, 1844–1924, Professor of Surgery successively at Rostock (1875–1882), Bonn (1882–1895) and Leipzig (1895–1911), Germany. The Trendelenburg position was first described in 1885.

Skin

The aim of sensory testing is to establish a pattern of sensory loss. Look for a dermatomal (may indicate spinal root or peripheral nerve pathology) or glove-and-stocking distribution (may indicate a neuropathy, e.g. diabetes). Perform a screening test by lightly stroking both limbs. Record whether the patient feels a difference. If none is noticed there is no need to spend more time on the neurological examination. If there is a difference, then a full neurological examination should now be performed.

Soft tissues

- **Tenderness**. Try to determine the actual anatomical structure from which the pain arises (e.g. subcutaneous fat, bursae, nerves, arteries).
- **Lumps and effusions**. Determine the characteristics of any lump or effusion using *Table 35.2* as a guide.
- **Pulses**. Palpate the distal pulses (or capillary return) of the limb. Recording distal neurovascular status both before and after surgery is important. Absence of distal pulses is an absolute contraindication to elective surgery in that limb. Acute loss of circulation to a limb is a surgical emergency.

Bone

Palpate the contours of the joint and assess for tenderness. For superficial joints, such as the knee, the joint line can be felt and checked for lumps and tenderness.

TABLE 35.3 Terminology used to describe the direction of movement.

Flexion	Forward or anterior movement of the trunk or limb
Lateral flexion	Bending of the forward-facing head and trunk to either side
Extension	Backward or posterior movement
Abduction	A movement away from the midline of the body
Adduction	A movement towards the midline of the body
Internal rotation	Rotation towards the midline of the body
External rotation	Rotation away from the midline
Supination	Movement of the forearm so that the palm faces anteriorly
Pronation	Movement of the forearm so that the palm faces posteriorly
Circumduction	A combination of flexion, abduction, extension and adduction without rotation
Inversion	Movement of the foot that directs the sole of the foot medially
Eversion	Movement of the foot that directs the sole of the foot laterally
Retraction	Backwards movement of the head, jaw or shoulders

Move

There are three stages to assessing movement. The words used to describe a particular movement are shown in *Table 35.3*.

- **Active**. Ask the patient to move the joint within the limits of their pain.
- **Passive**. Move the limb or joint yourself. Record the range of movement in 'degrees' (a goniometer may be helpful). Comparison of active and passive range allows the three causes of loss of range of movement to be distinguished. In limitation caused by pain or stiffness the ranges are the same but one is painful. In weakness passive range is greater than active.
- **Stability**. Stability has a static and a dynamic component: static tests assess the integrity of the ligaments and joint (bone) surfaces; dynamic tests assess the integrity and functions of the muscles and tendons. Ask the patient to move the joint actively through its range of motion while you try to stop the movement. Record power using the Medical Research Council (MRC) grading system as illustrated in *Table 35.4*. Consider the muscles that drive each movement, the peripheral nerves that supply them and the nerve root values (*Table 35.5*).

In the following sections, in addition to the approach of 'look, feel, move', we have included details of special tests for each joint as well as neurological examination of the limb. The peripheral nerve examination comprises sensory and motor testing, reflexes, tone and coordination and proprioception.

TABLE 35.2 Swelling: an acronym for history and examination of a lump.

Start	Did it appear after trauma or gradually on its own?
Where	Anatomical site and layer (skin, fat, muscle); does it move in relation to these?
External features	Size, surface and definition of margins
Lymph nodes	Are the local ones enlarged?
Liquid	Is it fluctuant? Can it be transilluminated?
Internal features	Is it hard? Is it tender?
Noise	Is there a thrill? Is there a bruit?
General	Examination of the whole patient for general lumps

TABLE 35.4 The Medical Research Council grading system of muscle power.

Grade	Description
0	No movement
1	Flicker of movement
2	Active movement with gravity elimination
3	Active movement against gravity
4	Active movement against resistance but power less than full
5	Normal power

TABLE 35.5 Peripheral nerves.

Root level	Sensation	Motor	Reflex
C5	Lateral upper arm	Deltoid	Biceps
C6	Lateral forearm	Wrist extension	Brachioradialis
C7	Middle finger	Triceps	Triceps
C8	Little finger	Finger flexors	–
T1	Medial forearm	Interossei	–
L1	Anterior thigh	Psoas	–
L2	Anterior thigh/groin	Quadriceps	–
L3	Anterior and lateral thigh	Quadriceps	–
L4	Medial leg and foot	Tibialis anterior	Knee jerk
L5	Lateral leg and first dorsal web space	Extensor hallucis longus	–
S1	Lateral and plantar foot	Gastrocnemius/perineals	Achilles
S2–S4	Perianal	Bladder and foot intrinsics	–

Assessment of joint hypermobility

Increased movement and flexibility of a joint can often cause joint pain and symptoms of instability. A formal assessment of joint mobility can help document the degree of mobility. The Beighton score alone cannot be used to diagnose hypermobility in terms of its underlying causes; however, it acts as a standardised clinical assessment across both upper and lower limbs and the spine.

The Beighton score is calculated as follows (***Figure 35.1***):

- 1 point if, while standing forward bending, the patient can place their palms on the ground with legs straight;
- 1 point for each elbow that bends backwards;
- 1 point for each knee that bends backwards;
- 1 point for each thumb that touches the forearm when bent backwards;
- 1 point for each little finger that bends backwards beyond 90°;
- total score out of 9.

Summary box 35.2

MSK examination

- Hand hygiene and chaperone presence
- Introduce yourself and put the patient at ease
- Assess the gait
- Look
- Feel
- Move
- Special tests
- Neurological examination
- Pulses

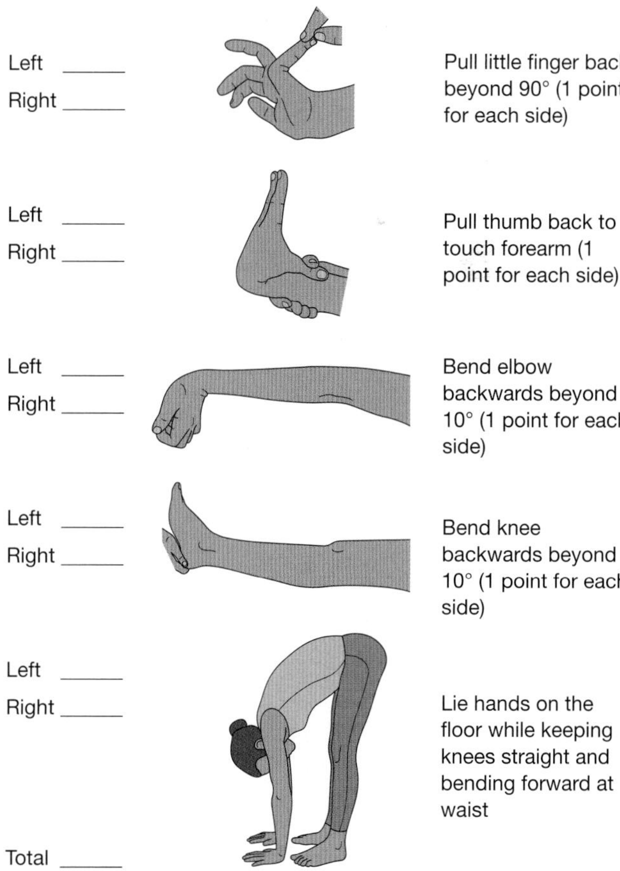

Figure 35.1 Beighton score (a screening technique for hypermobility).

Peter H Beighton, b. 1934, British medical geneticist. With Francis T Horan published 'Orthopedic aspects of the Ehlers-Danlos syndrome' in 1969.

CLINICAL EXAMINATION OF THE SPINE

The spinal column consists of 33 vertebrae with 23 intervertebral discs. This is supported by numerous ligaments and paraspinal muscles.

When observed from the front (coronal plane) with the patient standing and the hips and knees fully extended, the head should be centred over the sacrum. A 'plumb line' dropped from the spinous process of C7 should fall through the gluteal crease (*Figure 35.2*). If it falls to either side of the cleft, lateral tilt of the spine is present. The ear, shoulder and greater trochanter of the hip should lie in the same vertical plane. When the patient is observed from the side, assess the four physiological sagittal plane curves (cervical and lumbar lordosis, and thoracic and sacral kyphosis) (*Figure 35.3*).

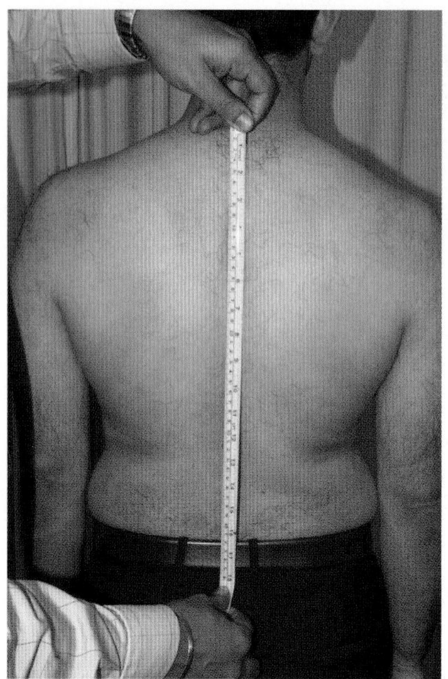

Figure 35.2 Plumb line.

Cervical spine

Look

Ensure that the shoulders, back muscles and scapulae can be seen. Look for muscle wasting and asymmetry of the neck creases and check that the shoulders are level and that there is a normal cervical lordosis (range 20–40°).

Feel

Stand behind the patient and support the patient's chin.

- **Soft tissues**. Feel for spasm of the paraspinal muscles.
- **Bone**. Palpate the spinous processes (tenderness and alignment); the spinous processes of C7 (vertebra prominens) and T1 are usually large and are easily palpable at the base of the neck.

Move

Motion occurs in three planes: flexion/extension, lateral bending and rotation (*Figure 35.4*).

- **Flexion (45°)/extension (55°)**. Ask the patient to bend their neck forwards – place the chin on the chest. Measure the distance from the chin to the sternum. Ask the patient to extend their neck by looking up at the ceiling.

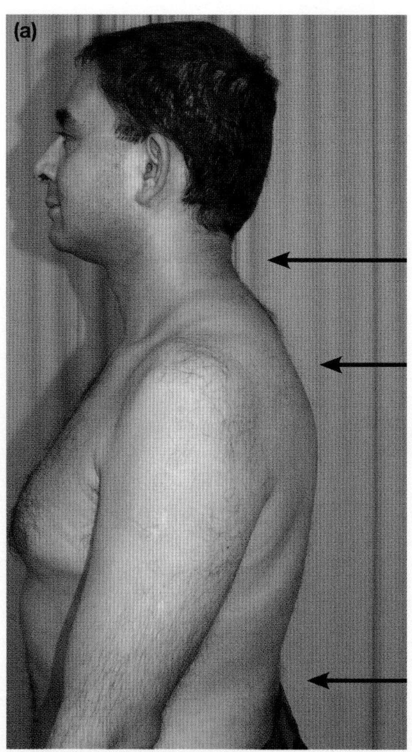

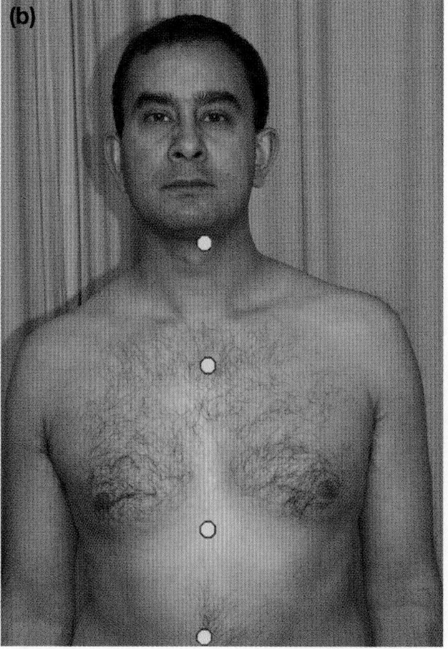

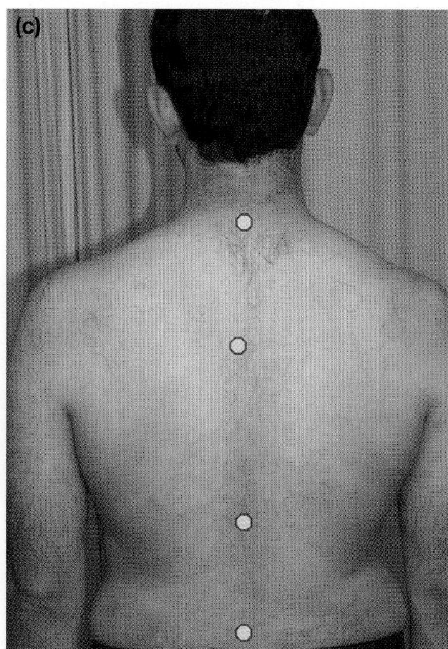

Figure 35.3 (a) Standing sagittal profile showing cervical and lumbar lordosis, with thoracic kyphosis. (b, c) Normal alignment whole spine from front and behind patient.

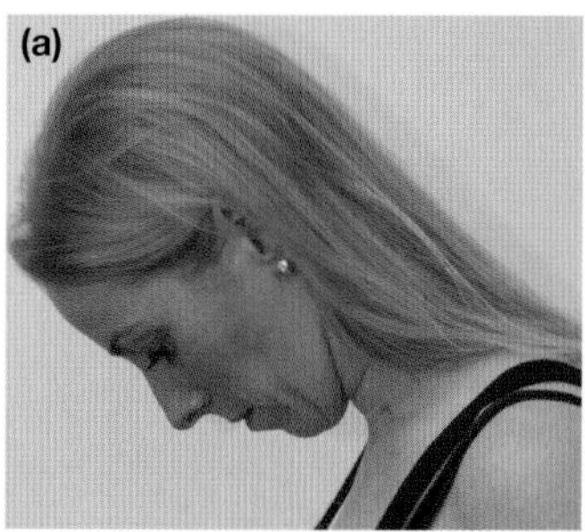

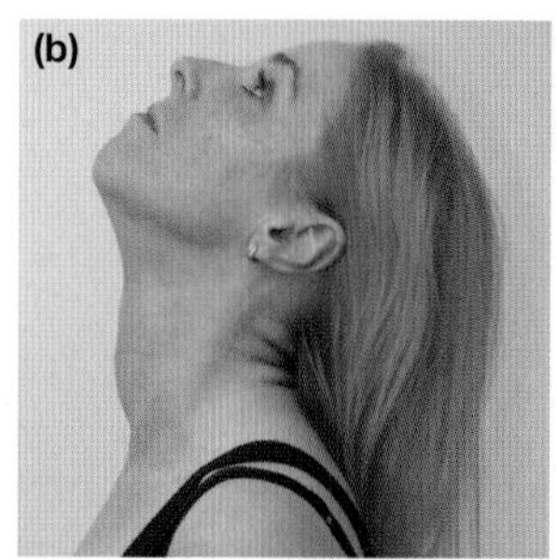

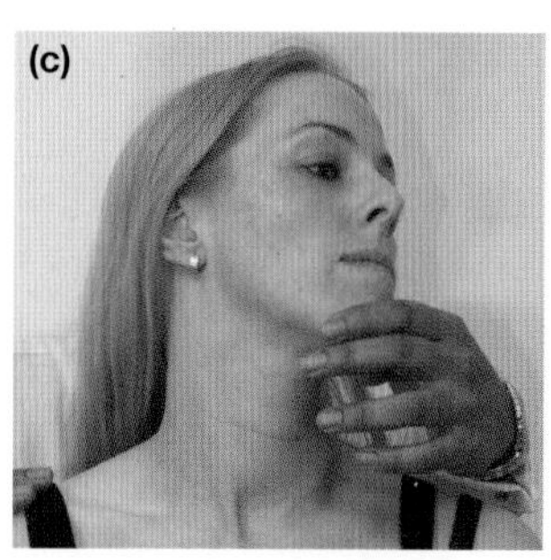

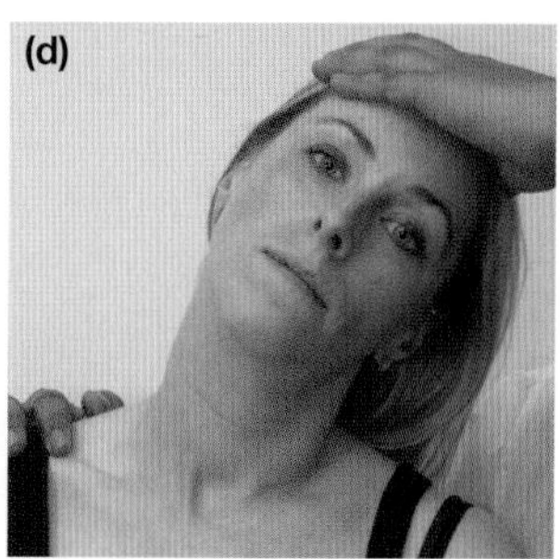

Figure 35.4 Cervical spine flexion/extension (a, b), rotation (c) and bending (d).

- **Right/left rotation (70°)**. Ask the patient to look over each shoulder while not moving the chest wall.
- **Right/left lateral bending (40°)**. Ask the patient to lay their ear on their ipsilateral shoulder.

Neurological

Focus your examination on the C5 to T1 nerve roots. These supply the upper extremities (***Figure 35.5***).

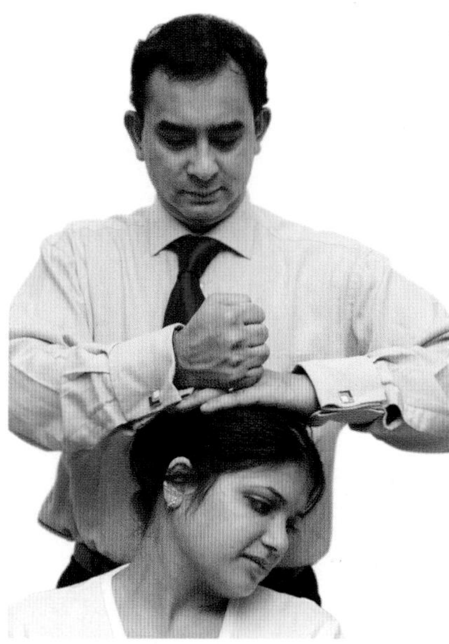

Figure 35.5 Spurling's test for cervical spine nerve root entrapment. The examiner turns the patient's head to the affected side while extending and applying downward pressure to the top of the patient's head.

Thoracic spine

Pathology commonly presents with pain and deformity. The thoracic spine is normally convex with a gentle kyphosis (normal range 20–45°).

Look

Ensure that the front and the back from the neck to the gluteal cleft can be visualised. Note skin markings (e.g. café-au-lait spots, hairy patches). These may suggest occult neurology or bony pathology.

- **Front**. Check for asymmetry of the shoulder and ribcage suggesting scoliosis.
- **Back**. Look for a difference in the height of the iliac crests (pelvic tilt). Assess for coronal plane deformity, such as scoliosis (lateral curvature of the thoracic spine with rotation). A rib hump suggesting a structural scoliosis may be visible.
- **Side**. Assess for sagittal plane deformity, such as an increased kyphosis.

Feel

Palpate, with one hand supporting the patient's pelvis.

Move

Range of motion is limited in the thoracic spine:

- **Forward bending test** (***Figure 35.6***). Ask the patient to bend forwards to touch their toes:
  - *structural scoliosis*: a rib hump will increase in size (bulge posteriorly on the thoracic convex side) as the patient bends forwards; this is diagnostic of idiopathic thoracic scoliosis (rotatory deformity);
  - *functional scoliosis*: the spine straightens as the patient bends forwards and no rib hump is visible; this flexible deformity is secondary to other abnormalities such as abnormal leg lengths and muscle spasm in the lumbar region.
- **Lateral bending**. This can be used to assess the flexibility of a scoliosis. Radiographs can be taken in this position to supplement the assessment.

Lumbar spine

Examination should include the pelvis, hips, lower limbs, gait and peripheral vascular system as well as the lumbar region. Irritation of nerves in the lumbar spine can mimic problems in the lower limb. Always consider referred pain.

Look

- **Back**. Check the skin at the base of the spine for hairy tufts and dimples (underlying spina bifida). Prominence of the spinal muscles on one side may be the result of muscle spasm secondary to pain.
- **Side**. The lumbar spine has a smooth concavity known as the lumbar lordosis (normal range is 40–60°). Muscle spasm is a cause of loss of the normal lordosis.

Roy Glenwood Spurling, 1894–1968, American neurosurgeon, first described the Spurling test with William Beecher Scoville.

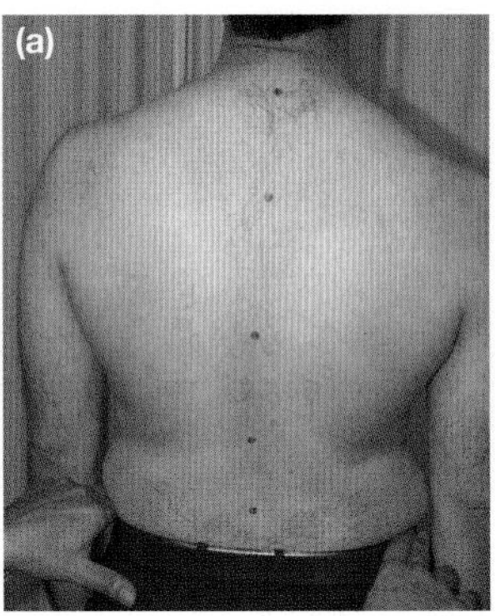

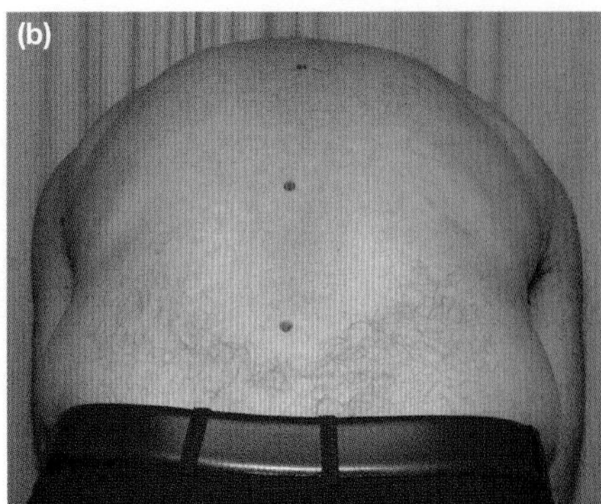

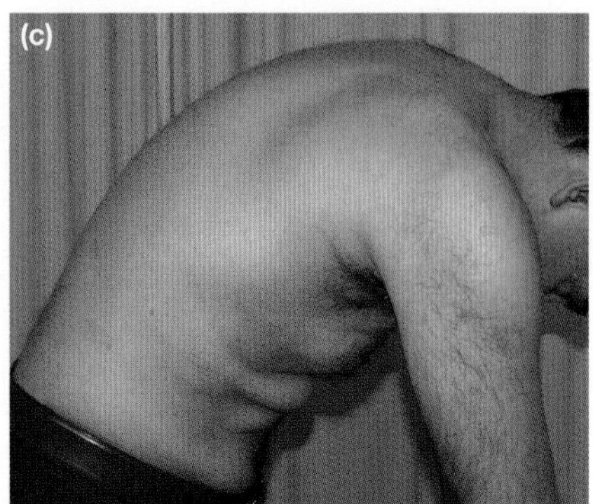

Figure 35.6 (a–c) Forward bending test.

Feel

Feel for any 'step-off' in the spinous processes. This may indicate forward slippage of one of the vertebrae on another.

Move

Movement occurs in flexion, extension, lateral bending and rotation (*Figure 35.7*). Record the motion in each plane in degrees. Remember that a significant portion of lumbar flexion is achieved through the hip joint.

- **Forward flexion**. This is a measure of lumbar flexibility. The skin of the lumbar spine stretches as the patient bends forwards. To measure flexion, place the tip of your thumb over the T12/L1 junction and the tip of your index finger of the same hand over the lumbosacral junction. Ask the patient to bend forwards and touch the toes (normal range 40–60°). Measure the distance by which your thumb and the tip of your index finger separate.
- **Lateral bending**. Ask the patient to slide their right hand down the outside of their right leg and then their left hand down the outside of their left leg. Note the distance that each hand moves down that side of the thigh.
- **Rotation**. Stand behind the patient and hold their pelvis still with both hands. Ask the patient to twist around and look over their shoulder. Note the angle that the shoulder girdle forms with the pelvis (range 3–18°).

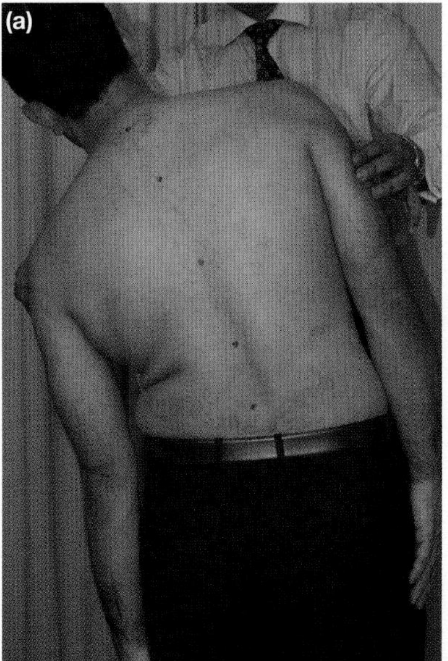

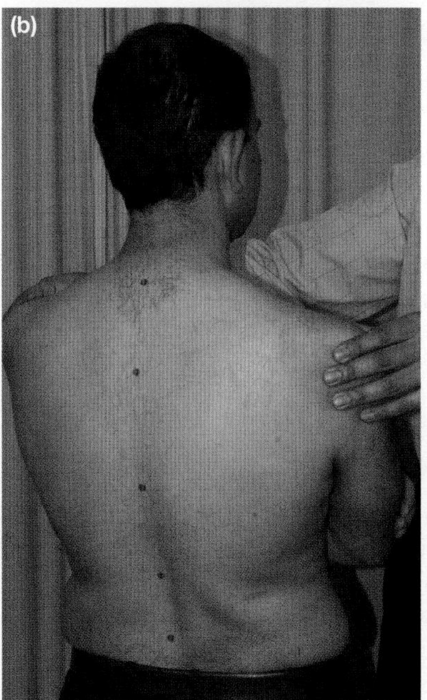

Figure 35.7 Lumbar examination; lateral bending (a) and rotation (b).

Special tests

- **Lasègue's straight leg raise test** (*Figure 35.8*). This test increases tension along the sciatic nerve (L5 and S1 nerve roots). With the patient supine, elevate the leg with the knee bent to check pain-free movement of the hip. Then, straighten the knee and note the angle at which the hamstrings allow the hip to flex. Finally, allow the hip to extend until tension is removed from the hamstring muscles and then the ankle is dorsiflexed firmly (but without excessive force), which in turn pulls on the sciatic nerve. If the patient experiences pain running down the leg, then the test is positive.

Charles Ernest Lasègue, 1816–1863, Professor of Medicine, University of Paris, and Physician, La Salpêtrière, Paris, France. This test was described by Lasègue's student, who named it after his teacher.

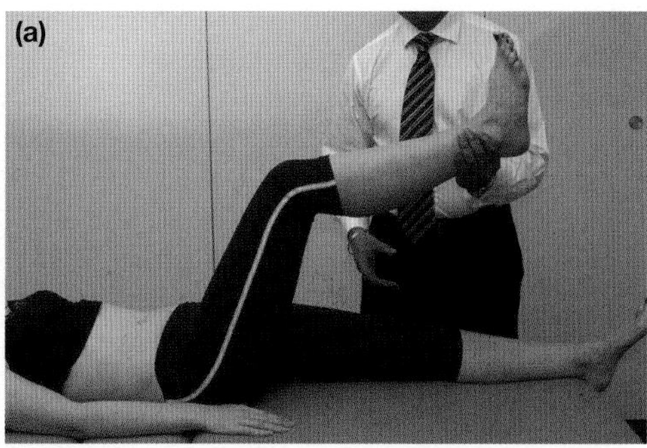

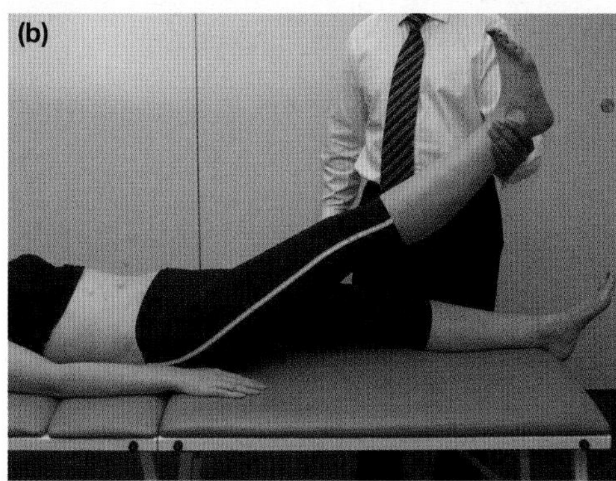

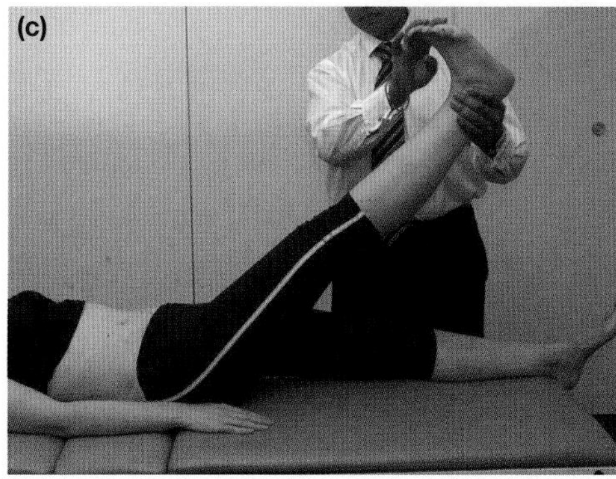

Figure 35.8 (a–c) Lasègue's straight leg test.

- **Contralateral stretch test**. Elevate the asymptomatic leg; if pain is reproduced in the other leg the test is considered positive.

Summary box 35.3

Spine examination

- Inspection of the standing patient
  - From the front and back (coronal plane)
  - From the side (sagittal plane)
- Palpation
  - Palpation of the posterior bony elements and the paraspinal muscles
- Move
  - Assess flexion, extension, lateral rotation and lateral bending
- Neurological
  - Assess sensation, tone, power, reflexes, proprioception and coordination
- Special tests
  - Spurling's test
  - Forward bending test
  - Lasègue's straight leg test
  - Contralateral stretch test

CLINICAL EXAMINATION OF THE HAND AND WRIST

The hand and wrist should be thought of as one functional unit. The muscles may be divided into extrinsic (the muscle bellies in the forearm) and intrinsic (origins and insertions within the hand alone). The 'flexors' (volar side) flex the wrist and fingers and the 'extensors' (dorsal surface) extend the digits and fingers.

Look

Inspect the posture of both hands. A nerve lesion will produce a specific resting position (e.g. an ulnar nerve lesion will produce clawing of the little and ring fingers).

- **Skin**. Assess for scars, discoloration (café-au-lait spots, erythema) and loss of hair. The nails may reveal systemic disease (e.g. psoriatic pitting). Look for tight bands in the palm (Dupuytren's contracture). Loss of sweating is seen in complex regional pain syndrome.
- **Soft tissue**. Centrally located swellings at the wrist may indicate a ganglion arising from the wrist joint itself; de Quervain's tenosynovitis may present with a swelling around the radial styloid.
- **Muscle wasting**. Check for thenar, hypothenar (***Figure 35.9***) and intrinsic muscle wasting. To assess thenar eminence wasting, place the hands side by side with the thumbs upwards and look down and compare the thenar regions. Patterns of muscle wasting are shown in ***Table 35.6***.
- **Bones**. Look for bony deformity (dinner fork deformity, Colles' fracture). Typical bony deformities are described in ***Table 35.7***.

TABLE 35.6 Patterns of muscle wasting in the hand.

Thenar wasting	Median nerve palsy (C8)
Hypothenar wasting	Ulnar nerve palsy (T1)
Intrinsic wasting	Ulnar nerve palsy (T1)

Baron Guillaume Dupuytren, 1777–1835, surgeon, Hôtel Dieu, Paris, France, described the condition in 1831.
Friedrich Joseph de Quervain, 1868–1940, Professor of Surgery, Berne, Switzerland, described this form of tenosynovitis in 1895.
Abraham Colles, 1773–1843, President of the Royal College of Surgeons of Ireland (1802), Professor of Anatomy, Physiology and Surgery (1804) and described distal radial fracture in 1814.

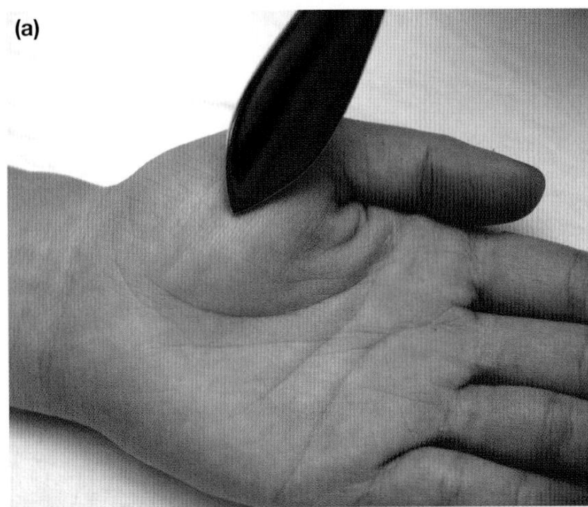

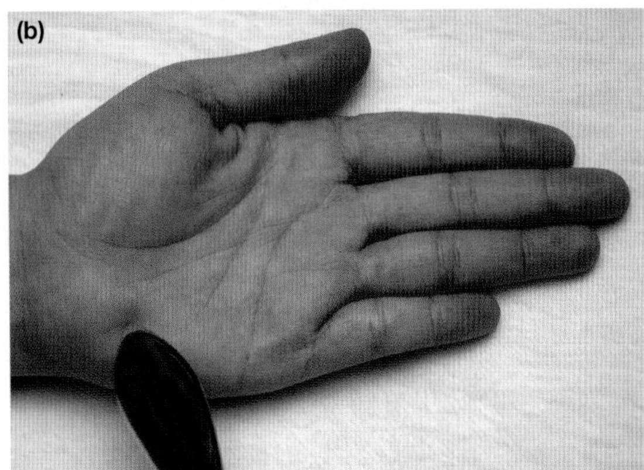

Figure 35.9 Thenar (a) and hypothenar (b) wasting.

Feel

- **Skin**. If there is any question of abnormal sensation on a simple stroke test comparing both sides, proceed to the two-point discrimination test using the sharp ends of a paper clip. Record the minimum distance between the tips of the paper clip at which the patient is able to recognise two points. ***Table 35.8*** describes the anatomical regions supplied by the median, ulnar and radial nerves.
  - *Pen sliding test*. To assess the absence or presence of sweating, slide a pen along the radial border of the index finger. If the pen slides smoothly, this may indicate loss of sweating.
- **Soft tissue**. Feel for muscle bulk and tendon thickening. Feel bony prominences, radial styloid, ulnar styloid and the anatomical snuff box. Feel for sensation using two-point discrimination of the medial nerve (radial aspect of the index finger), radial nerve (in the anatomical snuff box) and ulnar nerve (ulnar aspect of the little finger).

TABLE 35.7 Bony deformities of the hand.

Anatomical site	Name	Association
DIPJ	Heberden's nodes	Osteoarthritis
PIPJ	Bouchard's node	Osteoarthritis
Hyperextension of the MCPJ, flexion of the PIPJ and hyperextension of the DIPJ	Boutonnière deformity	Rheumatoid arthritis
Hyperextension of the MCPJ and PIPJ and flexion of the DIPJ	Swan neck deformity	Rheumatoid arthritis
Flexion of the MCPJ with hyperextension of the interphalangeal joint	Z deformity of the thumb	Rheumatoid arthritis
Subluxation of the MCPJ	Ulnar drift	Rheumatoid arthritis

DIPJ, distal interphalangeal joint; MCPJ, metacarpophalangeal joint; PIPJ, proximal interphalangeal joint.

  - *Blood vessels*: check the radial and ulnar artery pulses; assess the capillary refill time, which is normally less than 2 seconds; Allen's test should also be performed before surgery (***Table 35.9 and Figure 35.10***).
  - *Nerves*: compressive neuropathies are most commonly seen affecting the median nerve (see Tinel's [***Figure 35.11a***] and Phalen's [***Figure 35.11b***] tests in ***Table 35.9***).
  - *Palmar fascia*: feel for palmar thickening and skin pits; long finger-like structures (cords), most commonly affecting the ring and little fingers, are suggestive of Dupuytren's disease.
- **Bones**. Palpate from the radial to the ulnar side of the wrist joint. In the trauma setting, palpate the anatomical snuff box (***Figure 35.12***): a fracture of the scaphoid may cause tenderness (see ***Chapter 32***). The scaphoid tubercle, pisiform and the hook of hamate are all palpable on the volar aspect of the wrist.

TABLE 35.8 Sensory distribution of the nerve supply to the hand.

Nerve	Sensory distribution
Ulnar	Little finger and ulnar half of the ring finger
Median	Thumb, index, middle and radial half of the ring finger
Radial	Base of the thumb on the dorsum of the hand

William Heberden (Senior), 1710–1801, physician, practised first in Cambridge and later in London, UK.
Charles Jacques Bouchard, 1837–1915, physician, Dean of the Faculty of Medicine, Paris, France.
Boutonnière is French for 'buttonhole'.
Edgar van Nuys Allen, 1900–1961, Professor of Medicine, The Mayo Clinic, Rochester, MN, USA.
Jules Tinel, 1879–1952, Physician, Hôpital Beaujon, Paris, France.
George S Phalen, contemporary orthopaedic surgeon and Chief of Hand Surgery, The Cleveland Clinic, Cleveland, OH, USA. He helped to establish the American Society for Surgery of the Hand.

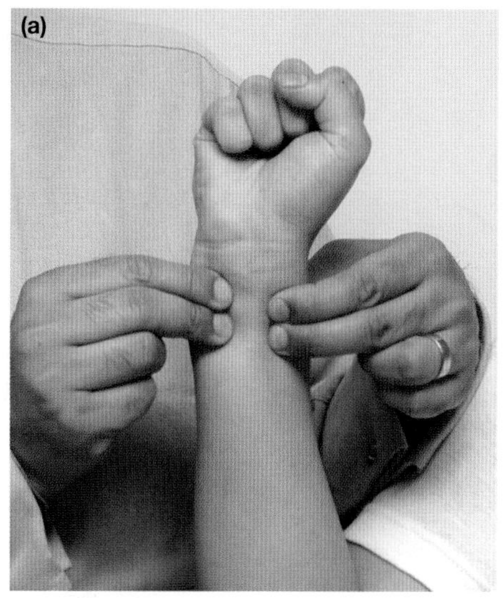
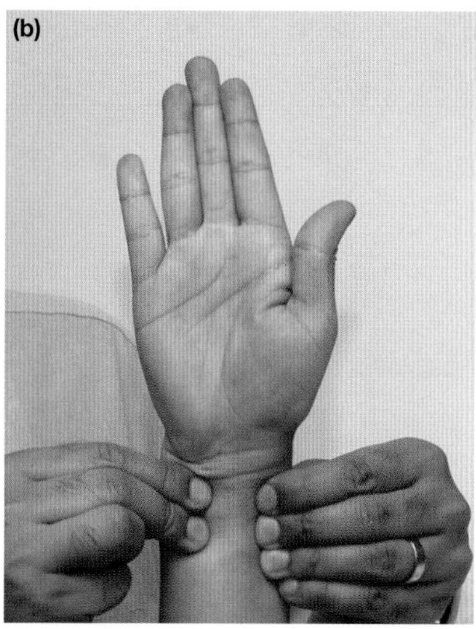
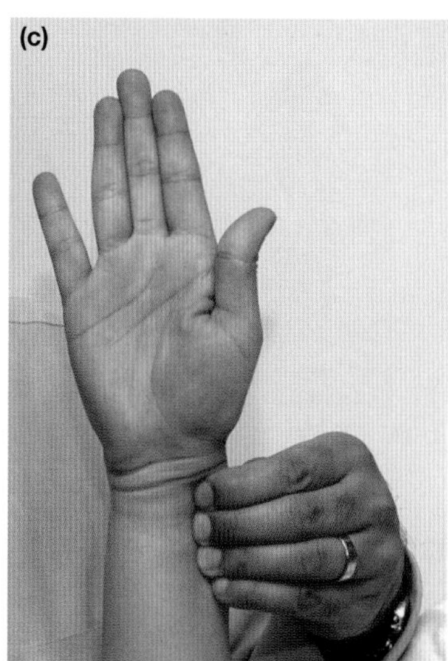

Figure 35.10 (a–c) Performing Allen's test.

TABLE 35.9 Special hand tests.

Test	Technique	Significance
Allen's test	Elevate the hand and apply digital pressure on the radial and ulnar arteries to occlude them. Ask the patient to make a fist several times. The tips of the fingers should go pale. Release each artery in turn and observe the return of colour	Tests the adequacy of the blood supply to the hand from the radial and ulnar arteries and the arcade between them
Tinel's test	Tap over the nerve of interest. Tingling may indicate nerve compression	Identifies compression of a peripheral nerve
Phalen's test	Place the wrist in maximum flexion with the elbows extended	Compression of the medial nerve causes paraesthesia
Froment's sign	Ask the patient to grip a sheet of paper between the index finger and thumb of both hands. Grip the paper yourself similarly. Ask the patient to resist as you attempt to pull the paper away	A positive test indicated by flexion of the thumb interphalangeal joint suggests weakness of the adductor pollicis muscle supplied by the ulnar nerve. Recruitment of the median nerve-innervated flexor pollicis brevis explains the thumb posture

Move

The wrist can be moved into flexion and extension, and ulnar and radial deviation.

- **Wrist**. Extension is tested by asking the patient to push the hands together into a 'prayer' position (***Figure 35.13a***). If there is loss of extension, the palms will not meet and/or one forearm will be dropped. Palmar flexion is tested in a similar fashion but with the hands pointing down and the back of the hands in contact (***Figure 35.13b***). Ulnar and radial deviation are tested by taking the patient's hand in your own and moving the hand into these directions.
- **Hand**. A general screening assessment is to ask the patient to roll up their fingers from full extension to full flexion. This will reveal a trigger finger.

Extensors and flexors

Asking the patient to grip two of your fingers in their fist tests the power of the extensors of the wrist (radial nerve) because they are needed to brace the wrist. It also tests the power of the flexors in the forearm (median nerve). Asking the patient then to extend and spread their fingers apart against resistance tests the intrinsic muscles of the hand (mainly the ulnar nerve).

Finger flexors

- **Superficialis tendon test**. The flexor digitorum profundus (FDP) usually has one muscle belly from which tendons to all of the fingers arise. The FDP can be immobilised by holding all of the fingers (except the one being examined) in extension; this allows the superficialis tendon to be tested in isolation. If the test finger is able to flex, despite profundus being immobilised, then the superficialis tendon to that finger is working. Repeat the test for the other fingers and examine FDP (***Figure 35.14***).

Thumb and thenar eminence

- **Abductor pollicis brevis, opponens pollicis and flexor pollicis brevis** can be tested together by opposing the thumb to the little finger.

Jules Froment, 1878–1946, Professor of Clinical Medicine, Lyons, France.

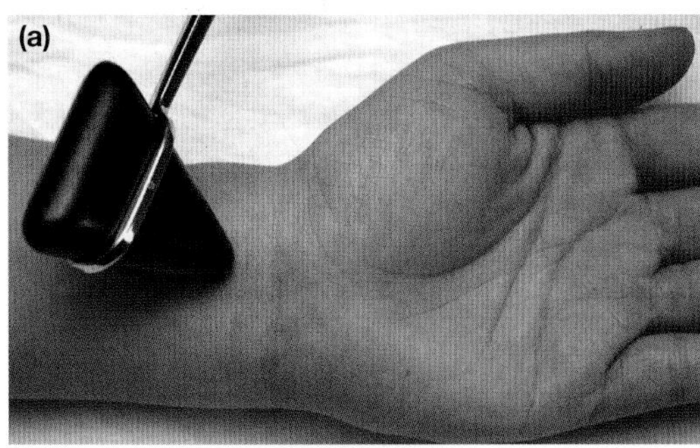

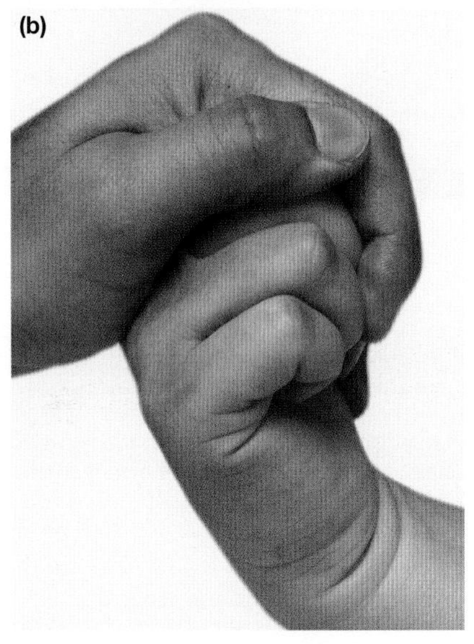

Figure 35.11 (a) Tinel's test; (b) Phalen's test.

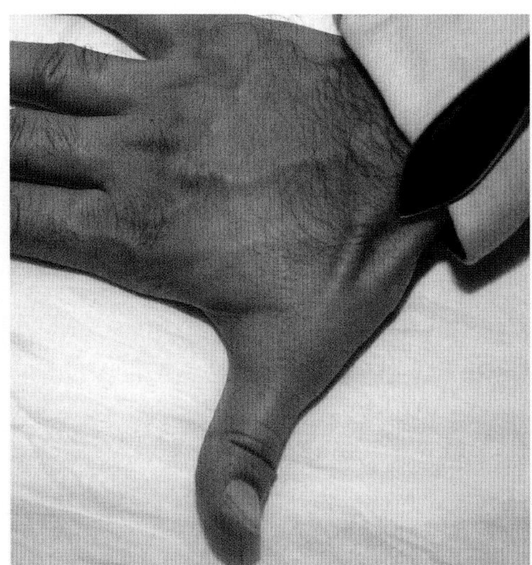

Figure 35.12 Palpating the anatomical snuff box between the tendons of extensor pollicis longus and abductor pollicis brevis.

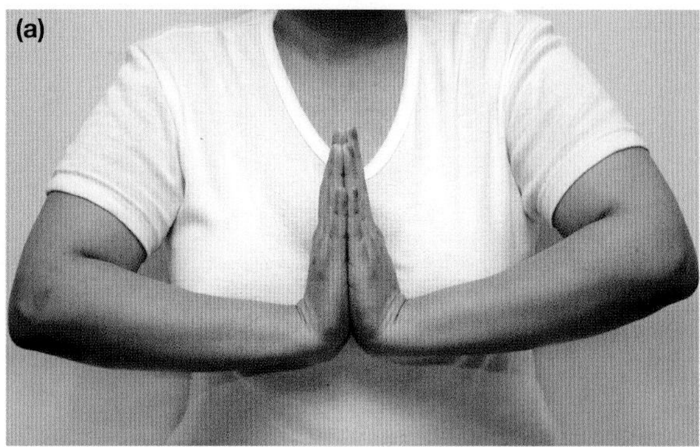

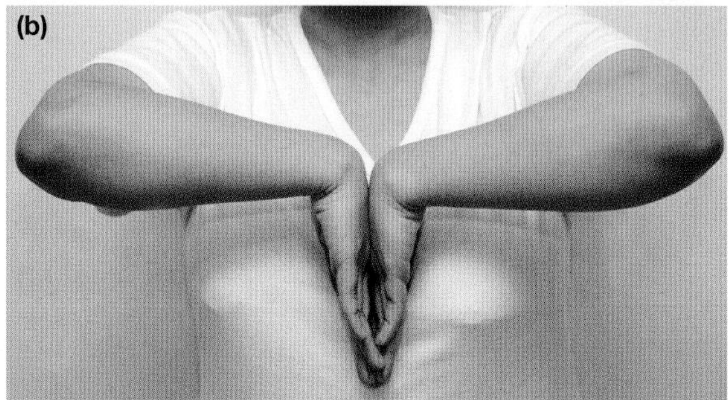

Figure 35.13 Testing the range of (a) wrist extension; (b) wrist flexion.

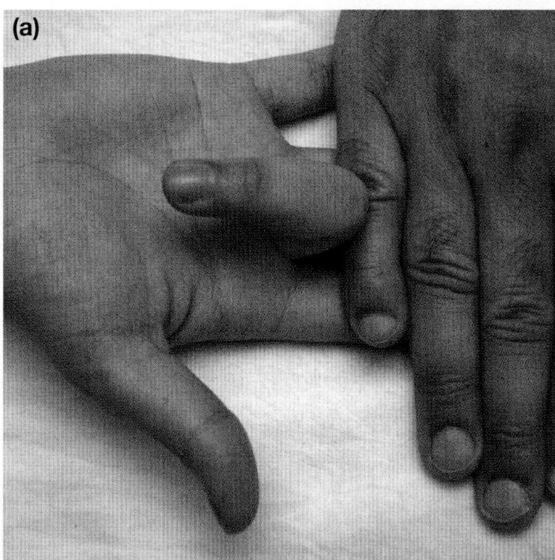

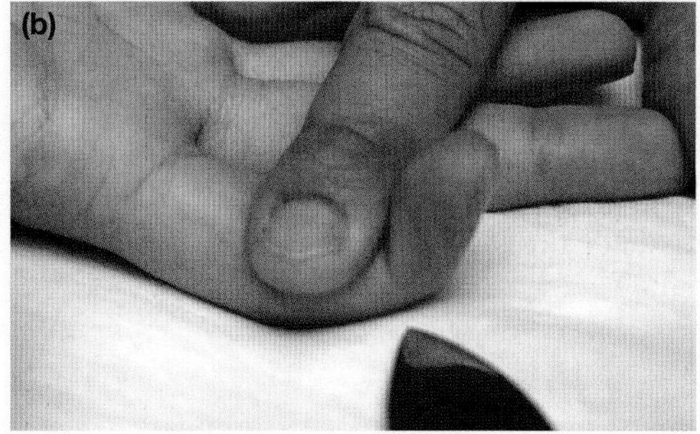

Figure 35.14 Testing the (a) flexor digitorum superficialis; (b) flexor digitorum profundus.

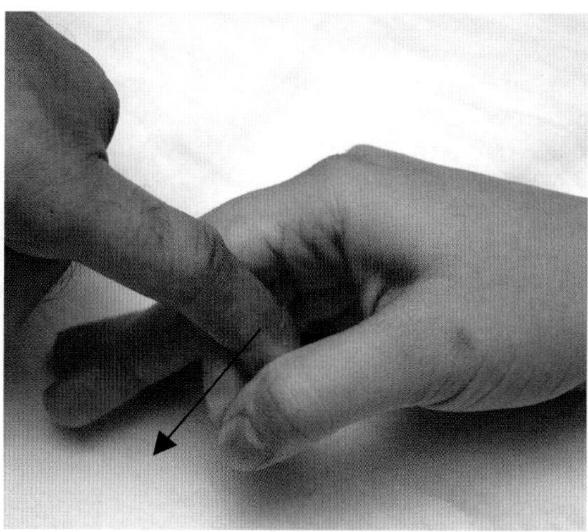

Figure 35.15 Test for flexor pollicis longus supplied by the anterior interosseus nerve.

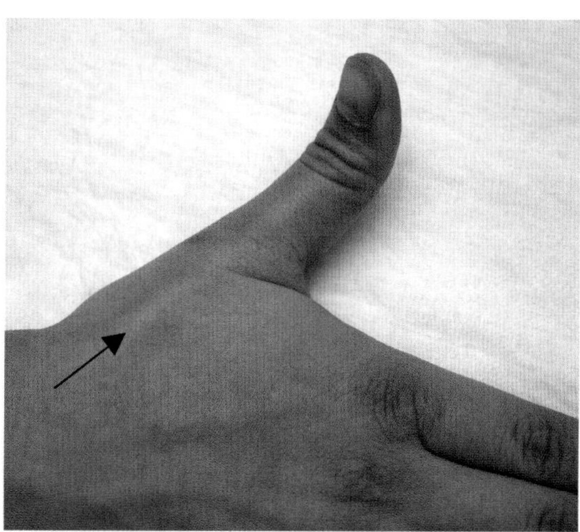

Figure 35.16 Testing the integrity of extensor pollicis longus.

- **Flexor pollicis longus**. The muscle is supplied by the anterior interosseus nerve (branch of the median nerve) and can be tested by asking the patient to bring the tips of the thumb and index finger together (the 'OK' sign; *Figure 35.15*).
- **Extensor pollicis longus**. The integrity of the tendon is tested by asking the patient to lift the thumb off a table with the palm flat on the table (*Figure 35.16*).
- **Adductor pollicis**. Test using Froment's sign (see *Table 35.9 and Figure 35.17*).
- **Abductor pollicis brevis**. This muscle is supplied by the median nerve. With the hand lying flat on a table with the palm facing upwards, ask the patient to raise the thumb towards the ceiling. Ask the patient to resist as you push the thumb back towards the palm (*Figure 35.18*).

Summary box 35.4

Hand and wrist examination

- Inspection of the standing patient
  - Dorsum and palm – asymmetry, deformity, muscle wasting
  - Inspection of the supine patient
  - Skin, scars, soft tissues
  - Palpation of bony structures and joints of the hand
- Movements
  - Wrist – flexion and extension, ulnar and radial deviation
  - Hand – thumb movements, metatarsophalangeal joints and small joints of the hand
- Special tests
  - Allen's test
  - Tinel's and Phalen's tests for the median nerve
  - Froment's sign
  - Finkelstein's test

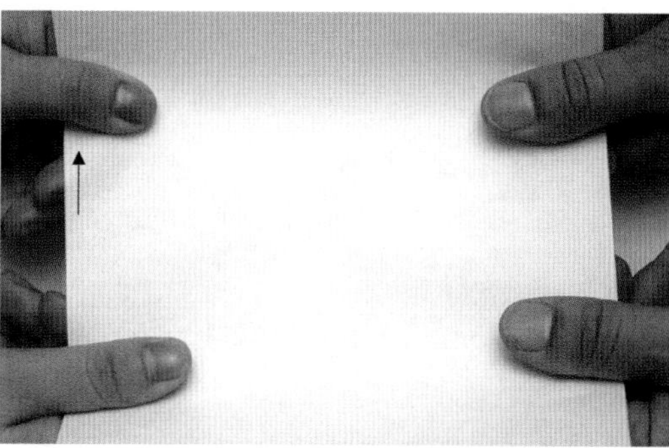

Figure 35.17 Froment's sign; the arrow illustrates the flexed posture of the thumb interphalangeal joint, indicating weakness of the ulnar nerve-innervated adductor pollicis muscle.

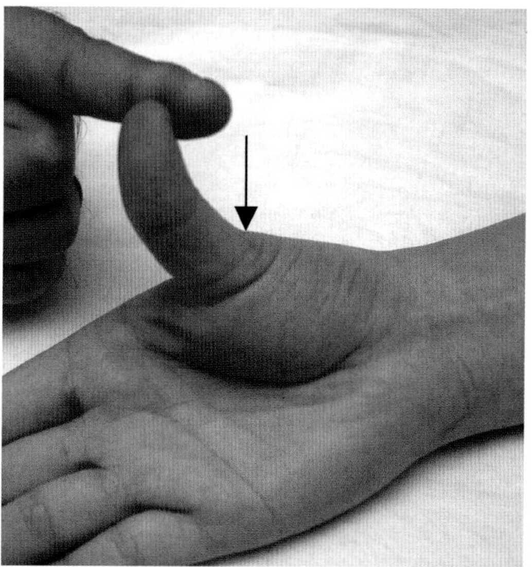

Figure 35.18 Testing the power of the abductor pollicis brevis supplied by the median nerve.

Harry Finkelstein, 1883–1975, American surgeon, one of the cofounders of the Hospital for Joint Diseases, New York, NY, USA. In 1932, along with E J Haboush invented a stabilising apparatus and operative technique for bone lengthening, anticipating by decades the current widely utilised Ilizarov technique.

CLINICAL EXAMINATION OF THE ELBOW

The elbow is a hinge joint formed by the articulation of the ulna and radius with the humerus.

Look

- **Skin**. Check the extensor surface for signs of psoriasis.
- **Soft tissues**. Look for any swellings, e.g. olecranon bursa, rheumatoid nodules, gouty tophi.
- **Muscle wasting**. Examine the biceps and triceps muscle bulk. Note that compression of the ulnar nerve at the elbow leads to wasting distally in the hypothenar eminence and intrinsic muscles of the hand – assess the hand for the presence of clawing and wasting.
- **Bone**. With the elbow in extension, look at the axis between the upper arm and forearm. There is a physiological valgus ('carrying angle') of 9–14° (2–3° greater in women) (***Figure 35.19***). This angle allows the elbow to be tucked into the waist depression above the iliac crest:
  - *cubitus varus* (gun-stock deformity): the carrying angle is reversed, secondary to a malunited supracondylar fracture;
  - *cubitus valgus*: the carrying angle is increased, caused by malunion of a distal humeral fracture;
  - *hyperextension*: there is normally a physiological hyperextension of the elbow (5°).

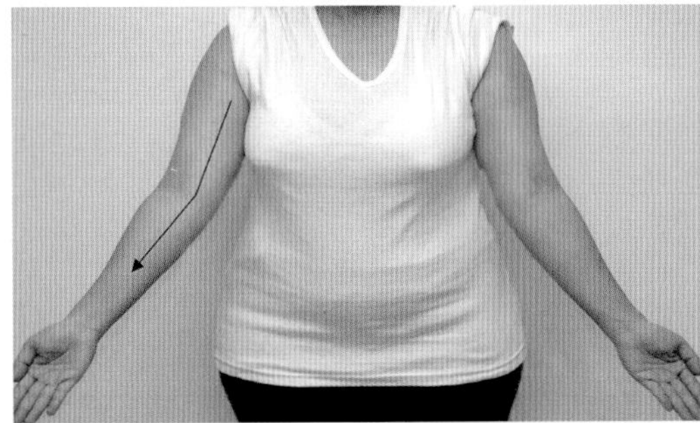

Figure 35.19 Carrying angle of the elbow illustrating the normal cubitus valgus.

Feel

- **Soft tissues**. An effusion may be detected by performing a cross-fluctuation test. The ulnar nerve can be rolled under your fingers placed between the medial epicondyle and the olecranon. Test the distal sensation in the hand (especially in the distribution of the ulnar nerve) and assess the vascular status.
- **Bones**. The three palpation landmarks are the medial and lateral epicondyles and the apex of the olecranon. These form an equilateral triangle when the elbow is flexed to 90°. The radial head is palpated with the examiner's thumb while the other hand pronates and supinates the forearm. On the medial side, palpate the medial epicondyle. Posteriorly, palpate the olecranon fossa.

Move

- **Flexion–extension**. The normal range is from –5° (slight hyperextension) to 150°. Ask the patient to bend the elbow from the fully straight position (***Figure 35.20***).
- **Pronation and supination**. With the elbows at 90° and the palms facing upwards (full supination), ask the patient to turn the forearm so that the dorsum of the hand faces upwards (full pronation) (***Figure 35.21***). The normal values are 70° pronation and 90° supination.

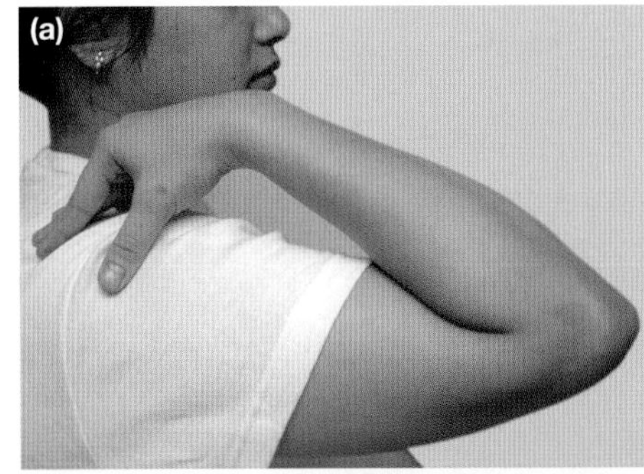

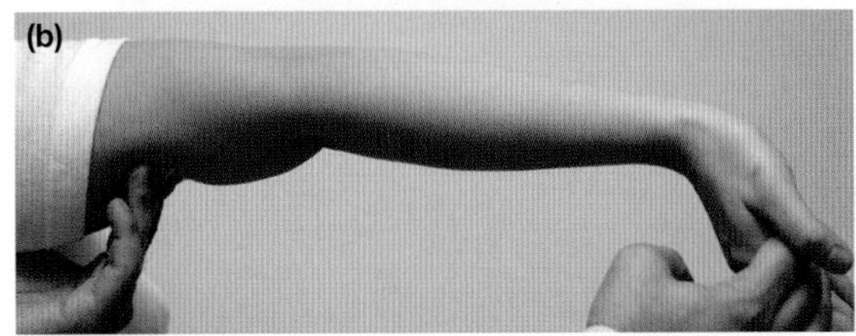

Figure 35.20 (a) Elbow flexion; (b) elbow extension.

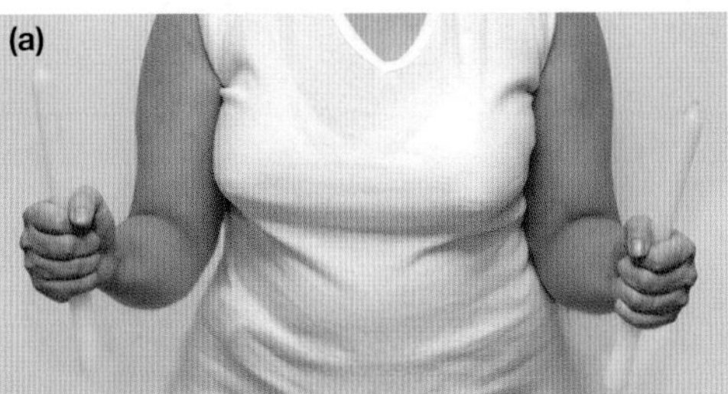

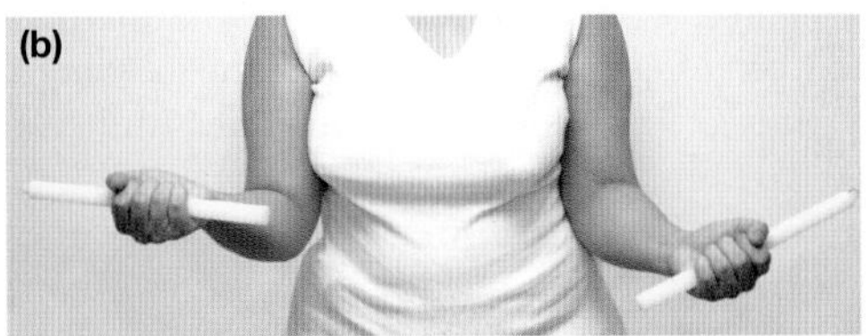

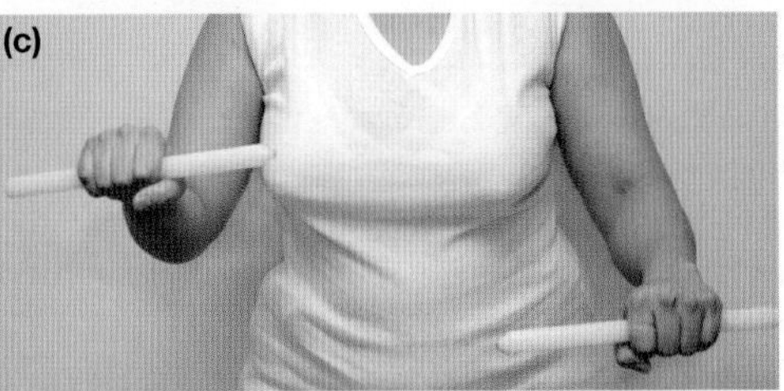

Figure 35.21 Testing forearm rotation: (a) mid-prone position; (b) full supination; (c) full pronation.

Special tests and diagnoses

Tennis elbow and golfer's elbow

Both conditions are inflammatory processes of the tendons that attach the large muscle mass of the forearm to the lateral or medial epicondyle.

- **Medial epicondylitis** (synonym golfer's elbow). The medial epicondyle is the common origin of the forearm flexors and the pronator muscle. Palpate the medial epicondyle for tenderness. The diagnostic test is resisted wrist flexion, which reproduces the pain over the medial epicondyle.
- **Lateral epicondylitis** (synonym tennis elbow). The lateral epicondyle is the common origin of the forearm extensors. Palpate for tenderness – usually just distal (5–10 mm) to the epicondyle near the origin of the extensor carpi radialis brevis muscle. Wrist extension against resistance with the elbow extended should provoke the patient's symptoms.

Summary box 35.5

Elbow examination

- Inspection of the standing patient
  - Front – asymmetry, carrying angle, deformity
  - Back – olecranon fossa
- Inspection of the supine patient
  - Skin, scars, soft tissues, deformity
  - Palpation of bony structures
- Movements
  - Flexion and extension, pronation and supination
- Special tests
  - Tennis and golfer's elbow

CLINICAL EXAMINATION OF THE SHOULDER

Pain arising from the shoulder joint may be felt anterolaterally. Referred pain may present from the cervical spine, heart, mediastinum and the diaphragm.

Look

Assess the attitude of the limb.

- **Skin**. Check for surgical scars. An anterior scar is used for the deltopectoral approach. At the side, the deltoid splitting approach and lateral arthroscopic portals may be seen. Posteriorly, arthroscopic portal sites can be seen.
- **Soft tissues**. Wasting of the deltoid muscle is commonly seen after shoulder dislocation when there is a temporary loss of function of the axillary nerve that supplies it. The rotator cuff comprises four muscles: supraspinatus, infraspinatus, subscapularis and teres minor. Wasting of these muscles may occur following a rotator cuff problem.
- **Bone**. Look for any obvious deformity or prominence. A fracture of the middle third clavicle is the most common cause. A dislocation may be suspected by a loss of normal shoulder contour. The more common anterior dislocation often presents with an anterior bulge and a squared-off shoulder.

Feel

Generalised pain in the shoulder may arise from the neck or the shoulder joint itself. More localised pain is often indicative of acromioclavicular joint pathology.

- **Skin**. Test sensation in the upper part of the lateral aspect of the arm ('regimental badge area') (***Figure 35.22***). Loss may indicate damage to the axillary nerve (following shoulder dislocation).
- **Bones**. Palpate the acromioclavicular and sternoclavicular joints and the clavicle.

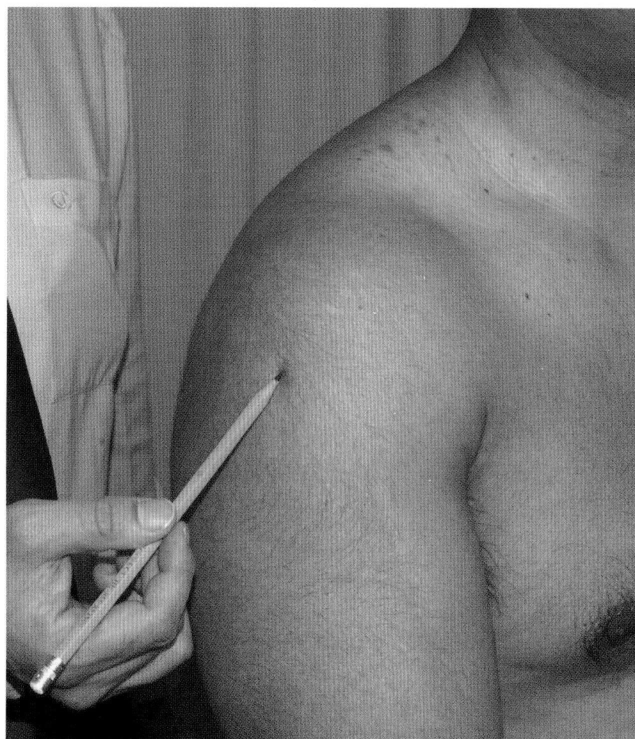

Figure 35.22 The area of skin supplied by the axillary nerve – the 'regimental badge area'.

Move

Differentiate between movements of the shoulder joint and scapulothoracic movement of the scapula on the chest wall. Patients with a painful shoulder will commonly move from the scapulothoracic joint. Stabilise the scapula by placing the thumb over the coracoid process and the fingers of the same hand over the spine of the scapula. Start in the 'neutral position' with the arms by the sides, elbows extended and the palms facing forwards. Note any pain throughout the range of movement (***Figure 35.23***).

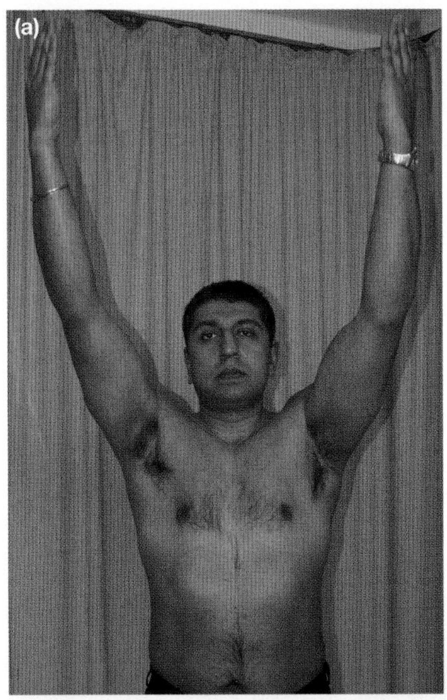
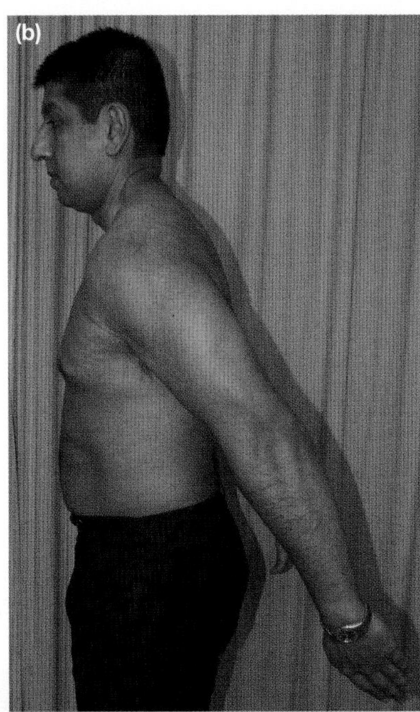
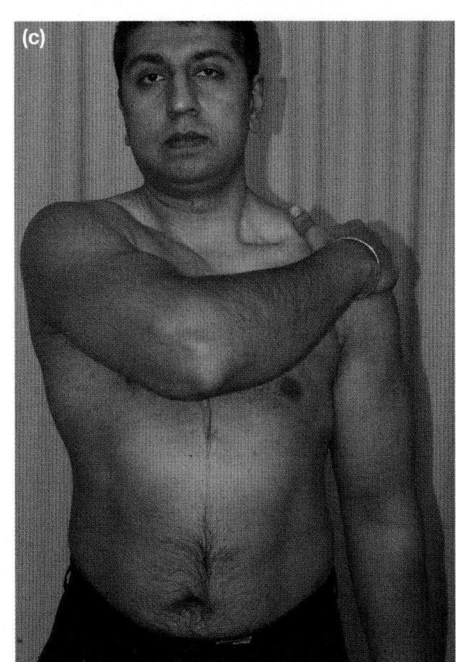
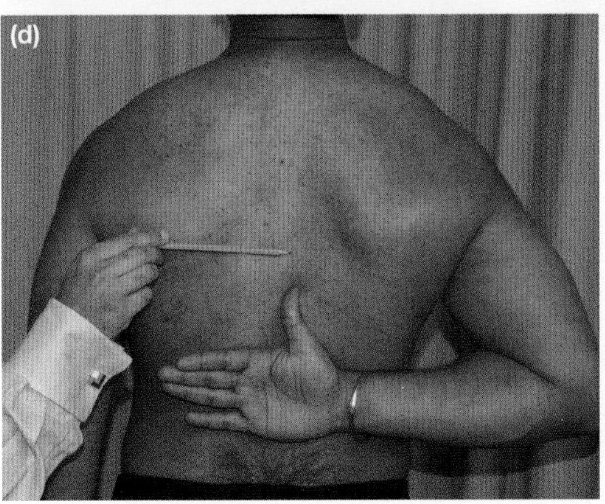
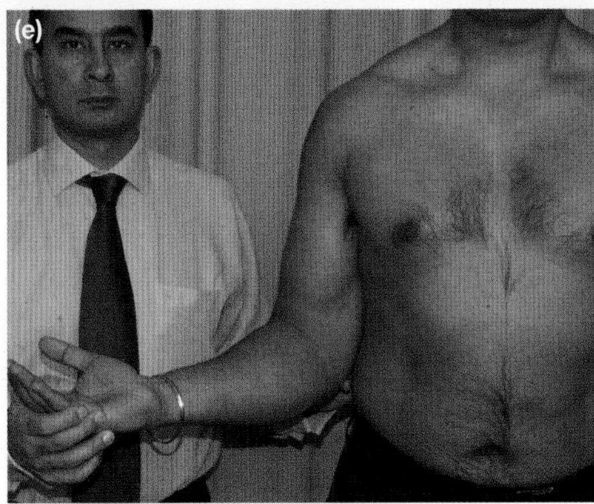

Figure 35.23 Movements of the shoulder: (a) forward flexion; (b) extension; (c) adduction; (d) internal rotation; (e) external rotation.

- **Forward flexion**. Ask the patient to raise their hands in front to touch the ceiling while keeping the elbows extended (0–180°).
- **Extension**. Ask the patient to extend both arms behind (0–30°).
- **Abduction**. Shoulder abduction involves the glenohumeral joint and scapulothoracic movement. The first 60° of movement is mainly at the glenohumeral joint. Beyond this the scapula begins to rotate on the thorax and final movements are almost entirely scapulothoracic. Raise the arms sideways until the fingers point to the ceiling (180°).
- **Adduction**. Ask the patient to touch their other shoulder tip.
- **Internal rotation**. Ask the patient to touch their back with the dorsum of the hand and to raise their hand up the back as high as possible (normal range is thoracic spine level T7–9).
- **External rotation**. With the arms by the sides, bend the elbows to 90° and rotate the forearms to the mid-prone position. Ask the patient to separate their hands as much as possible (0–40°).

Special tests and diagnoses

Impingement syndrome

This is impairment of rotator cuff function within the subacromial bursa. It may lead to inflammation (tendinitis) or a partial- or full-thickness tear. Impingement is characterised by pain and weakness on abduction and internal rotation.

- **Painful arc test** (*Figure 35.24*). Ask the patient to abduct their arms from their sides. The presence of pain from 60° to 120° is positive.
- **Jobe's test (empty can)** (*Figure 35.25*). Ask the patient to abduct the arm to 90° elevation in the scapular plane with full internal rotation (empty can position). Ask the patient to resist downward pressure. The presence of pain is a positive test.

Christopher Jobe, contemporary, American orthopedic surgeon, specialising in shoulder and knee surgery, diagnostic musculoskeletal ultrasound and sports injuries.

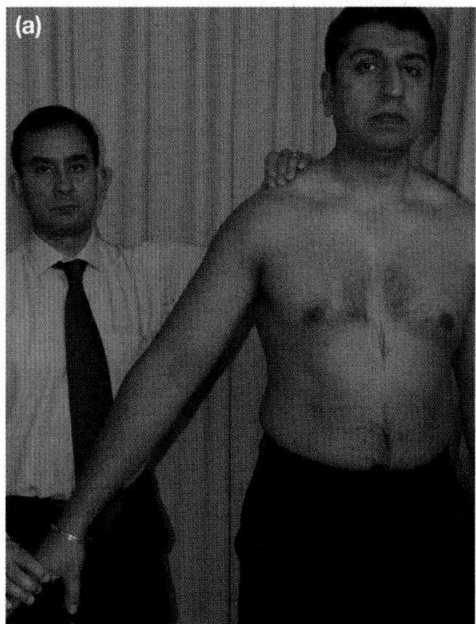

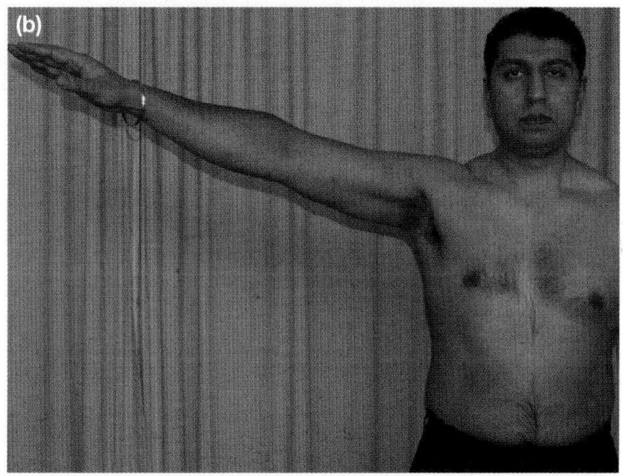

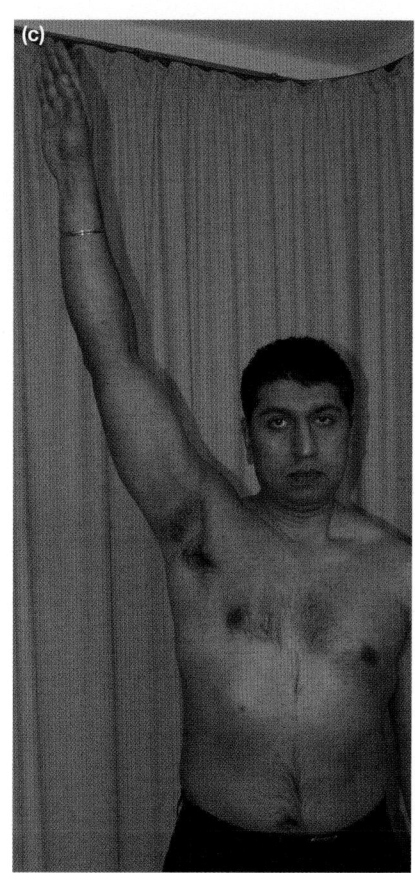

Figure 35.24 (a–c) Painful arc test for rotator cuff impingement.

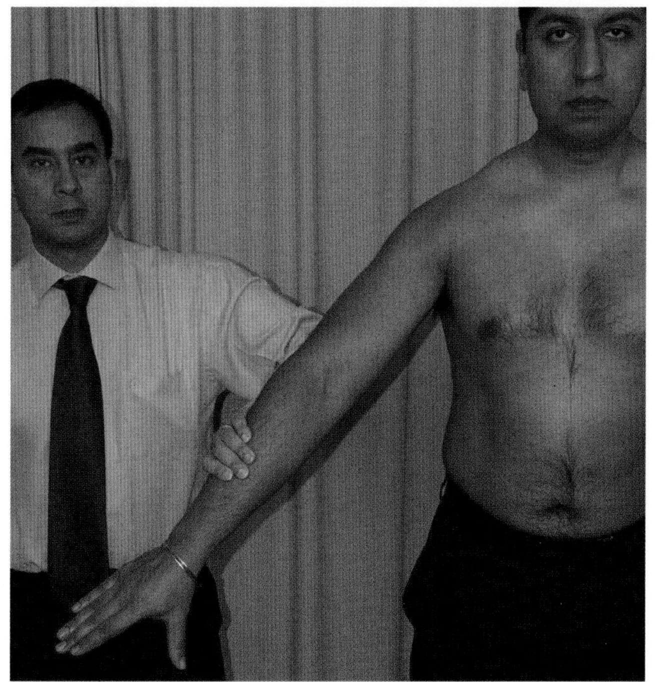

Figure 35.25 Jobe's test for rotator cuff impingement.

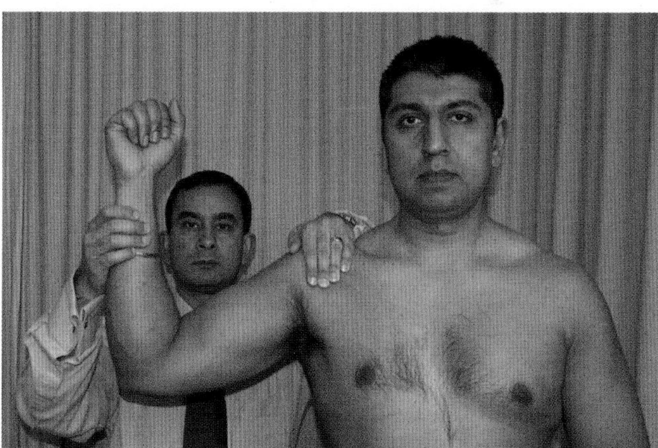

Figure 35.26 Anterior apprehension test for anterior shoulder instability.

Shoulder instability

Instability may be defined as a shoulder that slips in and out of joint (dislocation) more than once or twice, or frequently slips partially out of joint and then returns on its own. Instability can be anterior, posterior, inferior or multidirectional.

- **Apprehension test** (*Figure 35.26*). With the patient supine or standing, flex the elbow to 90° and abduct the shoulder to 90°. Now externally rotate the shoulder. Apprehension indicates anterior instability.

Summary box 35.6

Shoulder examination
- Inspection of the standing patient
  - Front – asymmetry, deformity
  - Side – muscle wasting
  - Back – muscle wasting, scapula
- Inspection of the supine patient
  - Skin, scars, soft tissues, deformity
  - Palpation of shoulder girdle (sternum to scapula)
- Movements
  - Flexion and extension, abduction and adduction, internal and external rotation
- Special tests
  - Impingement syndrome – painful arc, Jobe's test, Hawkins' test (see also *Chapter 38*)
  - Shoulder instability – apprehension, relocation test, sulcus sign
  - Rotator cuff assessment
  - Acromioclavicular joint pathology
  - Frozen shoulder versus glenohumeral osteoarthritis

CLINICAL EXAMINATION OF THE HIP JOINT

The hip is a synovium-lined ball-and-socket joint. Typical clinical diseases of the hip that may be encountered in children and adults are shown in *Table 35.10*. A patient complaining of hip pain should undergo a careful examination of the spine, abdomen, pelvis, groin and thigh. In addition, consider a gynaecological examination in women.

Look

With the patient standing, look at the front, side and back of the hip. Look around the room for walking aids and heel raises in the shoes.

- **Skin**. Look for scars and sinuses.
- **Soft tissues**. Muscle wasting may be present as a consequence of hip arthritis or primary muscle or neurological disease.
- **Bone**. Look at the posture of the limb and assess for adduction deformity; fixed adduction may be present in severe osteoarthritis and cerebral palsy, and makes the leg appear short because the pelvis is tilted (apparent shortening).

TABLE 35.10 Common clinical diseases of the hip in children and adults.

Children	Adults
• Developmental dysplasia of the hip • Transient synovitis of the hip • Perthes' disease • Septic arthritis and osteomyelitis • Slipped capital femoral epiphysis • Juvenile idiopathic arthritis	• Primary osteoarthritis • Secondary osteoarthritis • Inflammatory arthritis • Avascular necrosis • Femoroacetabular impingement • Labral tears • Referred pain

Feel

- **Soft tissues**. Tenderness overlying the greater trochanter may suggest trochanteric bursitis or an abductor enthesopathy.
- **Bone**. Bony landmarks can be palpated; these include the anterior superior iliac spine (ASIS), iliac crest and the greater trochanter of the femur.

Other areas for palpation include the inguinal ligament, which may have a local hernia or lymphadenopathy. The femoral artery can be palpated as it passes under the inguinal ligament at its midpoint halfway between the ASIS and the pubic tubercle.

Move

The hip joint can be moved into flexion, extension, abduction and adduction, and internal and external rotation (*Figure 35.27*). True hip movement ends when the pelvis begins to move. To detect true hip movement, simultaneously place a finger/hand on the ASIS contralateral to the hip being examined. Remember to compare both sides.

Passive movement

Hip flexion (120–0°) when lying supine

The patient is asked to lie on their back and then roll themselves into a ball, flexing the hips and the spine fully. A comparison of the flexion of the two hips can be made in this position. The patient is then asked to hold onto the knee of the 'bad' leg with both hands (thereby fixing the pelvis in flexion) and the other leg is allowed to extend down onto the couch. A note is made of any fixed flexion deformity (inability of the thigh to come down onto the couch). This 'good' hip is then returned to full flexion and the patient grasps that knee while dropping the other, 'bad', hip into extension. This modified Thomas's test is the most comfortable and accurate way of measuring flexion and extension of the hip, minimising movement of the painful hip (*Figure 35.28*).

Richard J Hawkins, contemporary, Canadian orthopaedic surgeon, based in Colorado and a founding member and Past President of the American Shoulder and Elbow Surgeons.

Georg Clemens Perthes, 1869–1927, Professor of Surgery, Tübingen, Germany, described osteochondritis of the femoral capital epiphysis in 1910.

Hugh Owen Thomas, 1834–1891, general practitioner, Liverpool, UK. He is regarded as the founder of orthopaedic surgery although never holding a hospital appointment, preferring to treat patients in their own homes. He introduced the Thomas splint in 1875.

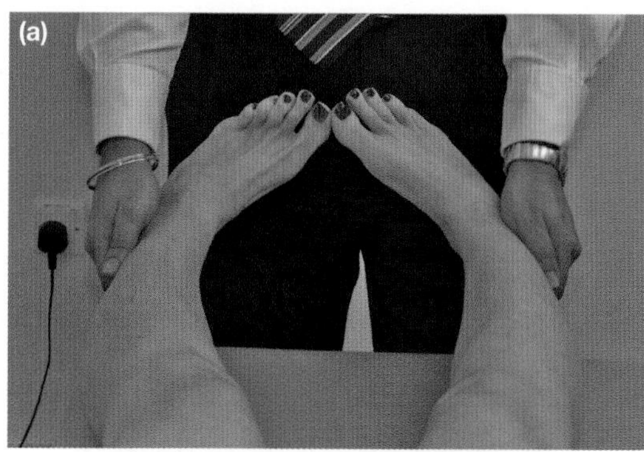

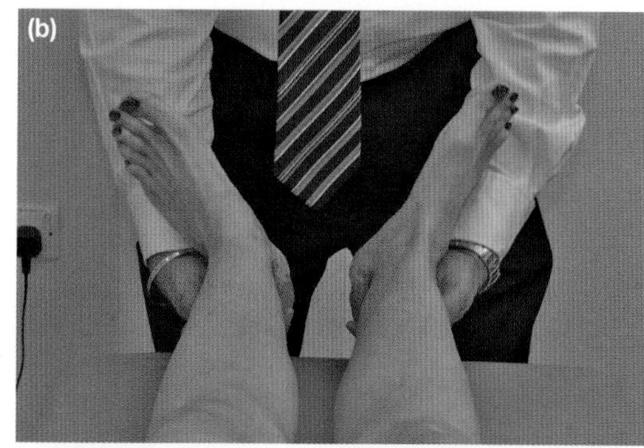

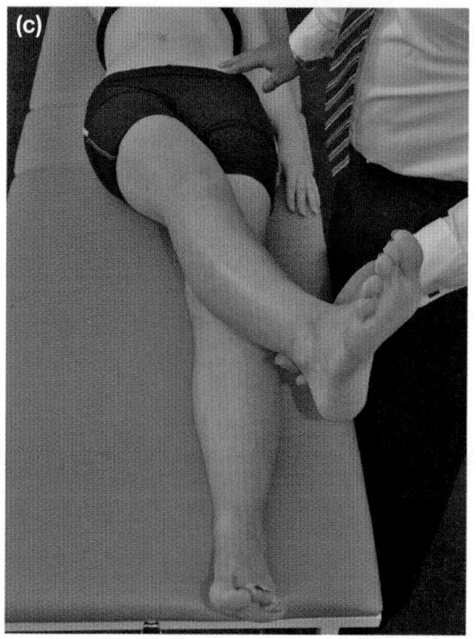

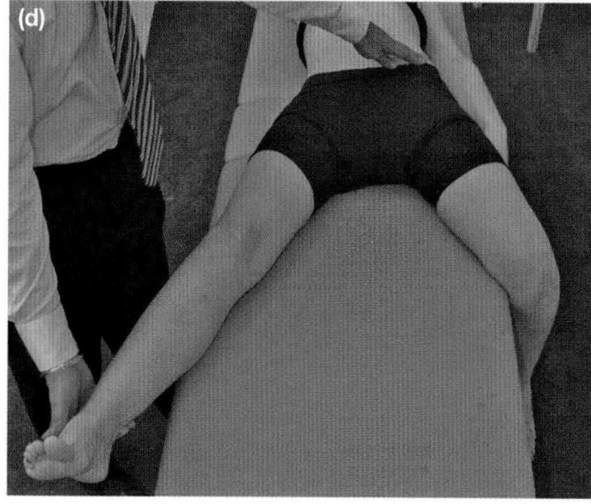

Figure 35.27 Hip movements: (a) internal rotation; (b) external rotation; (c) adduction; (d) abduction.

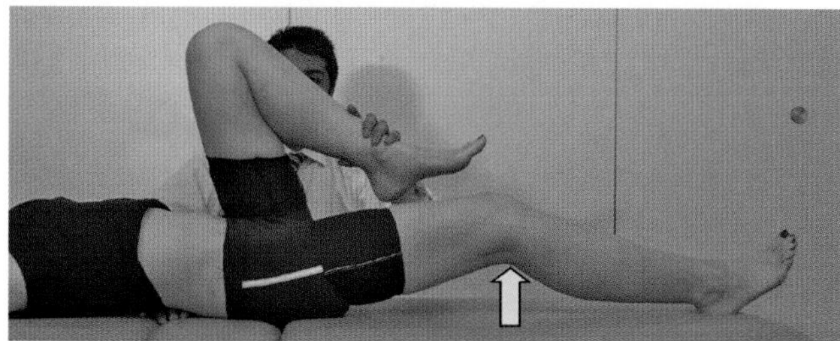

Figure 35.28 Modified Thomas's test for assessing a fixed flexion deformity. A fixed flexion deformity of the right hip is indicated by an inability to fully straighten the right leg (arrow).

Hip extension (0–10°) when lying in a prone position

Hip extension can be measured by asking the patient to roll onto their front and extend the hip.

Rotation

- **Internal rotation (45°)**. With the hip flexed to 90° and the knee in 90° of flexion, hold the front of the knee with one hand and the foot with the other. Internally rotate the hip (the foot goes outwards), then externally rotate the hip (the foot goes in). The angle that the tibia makes with the vertical indicates the range of movement. Pain at the extremes of movement suggests inflammation in the hip.
- **Abduction (40°)**. The hip should be abducted by moving the leg away from the midline with the other hand on the patient's pelvis to detect any tilt in the pelvis.

Special tests

- **Trendelenburg test** (*Figure 35.29*). Face the patient and ask them to place their hands on the palm of your hands for support. Then ask them to stand first on one leg, then the other. Increased pressure from the opposite hand as they take weight through the weak hip indicates a positive Trendelenburg test.
- **Leg length discrepancy (LLD)**. The inequality may be in the hip joint, femur, tibia, ankle or foot or a combination of these. The pathology may be from the bone being too short or too long. When assessing LLD, square the pelvis. If that is not possible then place both legs in the same position. For example, if there is an adduction deformity present in the affected leg, place the good leg in the same degree of adduction. LLD can be caused by a real difference in the leg lengths (the bones are different lengths) or by a deformity that makes the leg appear short because the pelvis must be tilted to get the leg onto the ground. The first is called 'real' LLD, measured ASIS to medial malleolus. The second is called 'apparent' LLD, measured midline, e.g. xiphisternum to medial malleolus. Each differs in cause and therefore treatment. The LLD apparent to the

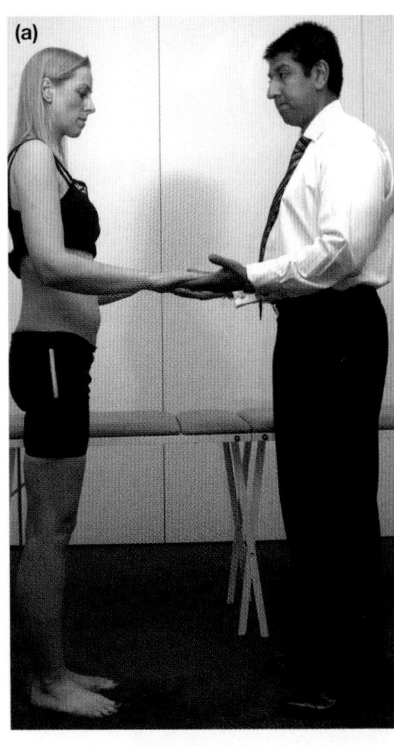

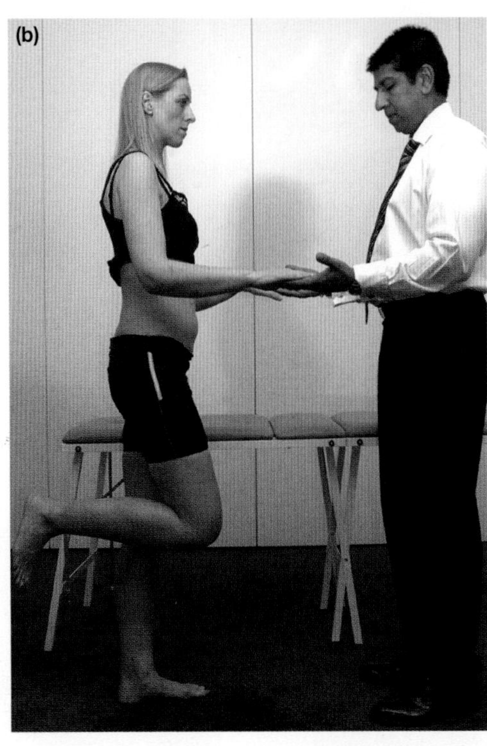

Figure 35.29 (a, b) Trendelenburg test.

patient can also be measured using wooden blocks placed under the patient's 'short' leg until the patient feels level.

- **Gait**. Hip disease can present with an altered gait pattern. The common types of abnormal gait are described in *Table 35.11* (see also *Summary box 35.8*).
- **Impingement**. Two commonly performed tests relate to femoroacetabular impingement. The FADDIR test, performed with hip flexion at 90° and subsequent adduction and internal rotation (F-ADD-IR) can reproduce the hip pain in impingement. The FABER test combines hip flexion, abduction and external rotation (F-AB-ER) and can reproduce hip pain in impingement but also pain from other locations, e.g. sacroiliac.

Snapping hip

Snapping hip is a condition in which the patient feels a snapping sensation or hears a popping sound in their hip when they walk, get up from a chair or swing their leg around. The snapping sensation occurs when a muscle or tendon (the strong tissue that connects muscle to bone) moves over a bony protrusion in the hip region, e.g. psoas and iliotibial band. Although snapping hip is usually painless and harmless, the sensation can be annoying. In some cases, snapping hip leads to bursitis, a painful swelling of the fluid-filled sacs that cushion the hip joint.

Summary box 35.7

Common causes of LLD in the hip

- Osteoarthritis
- Hip fracture
- Hip dislocation
- Hip dysplasia
- Avascular necrosis
- Fixed flexion deformity

TABLE 35.11 Common limps observed in hip disease.

Gait pattern	Description
Weak: Trendelenburg	May lead to pelvic sway or tilt. The patient swings the body over the weak hip to stay in balance when it is weight-bearing
Painful: antalgic	The rhythm is dot–dash, with a short period spent on the painful limb
Unbalanced: broad-based	May be caused by ataxia, e.g. cerebellar pathology. The rhythm also tends to be disordered
Loss of muscle control: high-stepping	May be due to loss of proprioception or a drop foot. This leads to difficulty in clearing the toes during the swing phase: the patient compensates by externally rotating the leg and flexing the hip and knee
Deformity: in-toeing	Can be caused by persistent femoral anteversion. The foot may catch on the back of the calf of the weight-bearing leg, tripping the patient

CLINICAL EXAMINATION OF THE KNEE

The knee is a synovial hinged joint. There are three compartments: medial, lateral and patellofemoral. The quadriceps, quadriceps tendon, patella, patellar tendon and tibial tuberosity constitute the extensor mechanism of the knee.

The anterior cruciate ligament (ACL) provides primary restraint to anterior displacement of the tibia. The posterior cruciate ligament (PCL) provides posterior restraint of the tibia. The medial collateral ligament (MCL) resists valgus and

Summary box 35.8

Hip examination

- Inspection of the standing patient
  - Front – pelvic tilt, rotational deformity
  - Side – lumbar lordosis
  - Back – pelvic tilt, scoliosis, gluteal wasting
  - Gait – Trendelenburg, antalgic
- Inspection of the supine patient
  - Skin, scars, soft tissues, deformity
- Palpation of the anterior joint line, adductor origin, greater trochanter, ischial tuberosity
- Movements
  - Flexion and extension
  - Abduction and adduction
  - Internal and external rotation
- Special tests
  - Thomas's test
  - Trendelenburg test
  - Leg length assessment – real/apparent
  - Impingement tests
  - Snapping hip tests

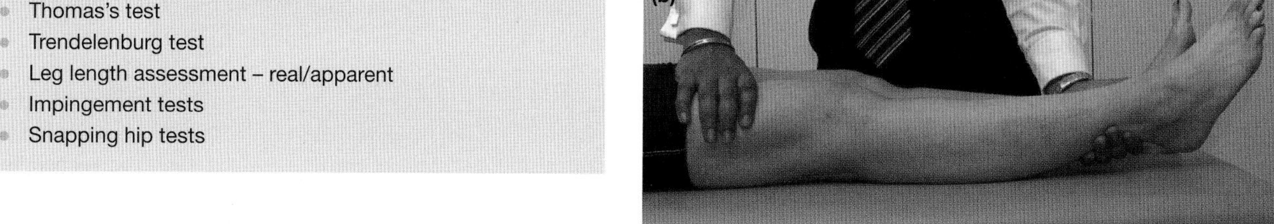

Figure 35.30 (a) Knee flexion; (b) extension.

external rotation forces whereas the lateral collateral ligament (LCL) resists varus forces.

Look

Look at the front, sides and back of both knees and for any walking or mobility aids or external appliances.

- **Skin**. Check for scars.
- **Soft tissues**. Look for wasting of the quadriceps and swelling in front of and behind the knee.
- **Bone**. Look for overall alignment (varus or valgus deformity). Measure the intermalleolar distance if a valgus deformity is present. With varus deformity, measure the distance between the medial aspects of the knees. From the side of the knee, look for fixed flexion or recurvatum (hyperextension).

Gait

Look for antalgic gait (osteoarthritis) and varus thrust (collapse of the knee into more varus as weight is taken on that leg).

Feel

- **Soft tissue**. Feel the tendons for quadriceps and patellar tendon rupture.
- **Fluid displacement or stroke test**. First empty the medial side of the knee by stroking any fluid up from the medial side into the suprapatellar pouch. Then place your hand on the superior aspect of the suprapatellar pouch and move it inferiorly, attempting to displace any fluid into the knee joint. Maintain your hand at the level of the superior pole of the patella. Now look to see whether the normal gutters on either side of the knee are less noticeable because of fluid distension. Stroke the back of your hand over each gutter in turn. Look at the opposite gutter to see if there is cross-filling.
- **Patellar tap test**. This test is used when a large effusion is present. Place one hand on either side of the patella and, with the other hand, push down on the patella. With an effusion, fluctuance is present as the patella moves towards the joint.
- **Bone**. Feel the tibial tuberosity, inferior pole of the patella, patellar facets, origin and insertion of the knee ligaments and joint line (medial and lateral). Remember to palpate for any popliteal swellings. Note the height of the patella.

Move

The knee moves principally in flexion (0–135°) and extension (from 0 to –10°) (***Figure 35.30***). Assess hyperextension by placing one of your hands on the anterior aspect of the distal femur. Now lift the distal tibia with the other hand. Measure the angle or the height that the heel can be lifted off the couch before the knee starts to move.

Perform a lag test to assess the integrity of the extensor mechanism. The patient is asked to lift the whole leg up off the bed (10°) with the knee straight. They are then asked to bend the knee and then try to straighten it again with the leg still held in the air. If they are unable to re-straighten the knee they have a positive lag. This indicates significant weakness of the quadriceps mechanism.

In the presence of an apparent fixed flexion deformity of the knee (seen in osteoarthritis), decide whether this is arising

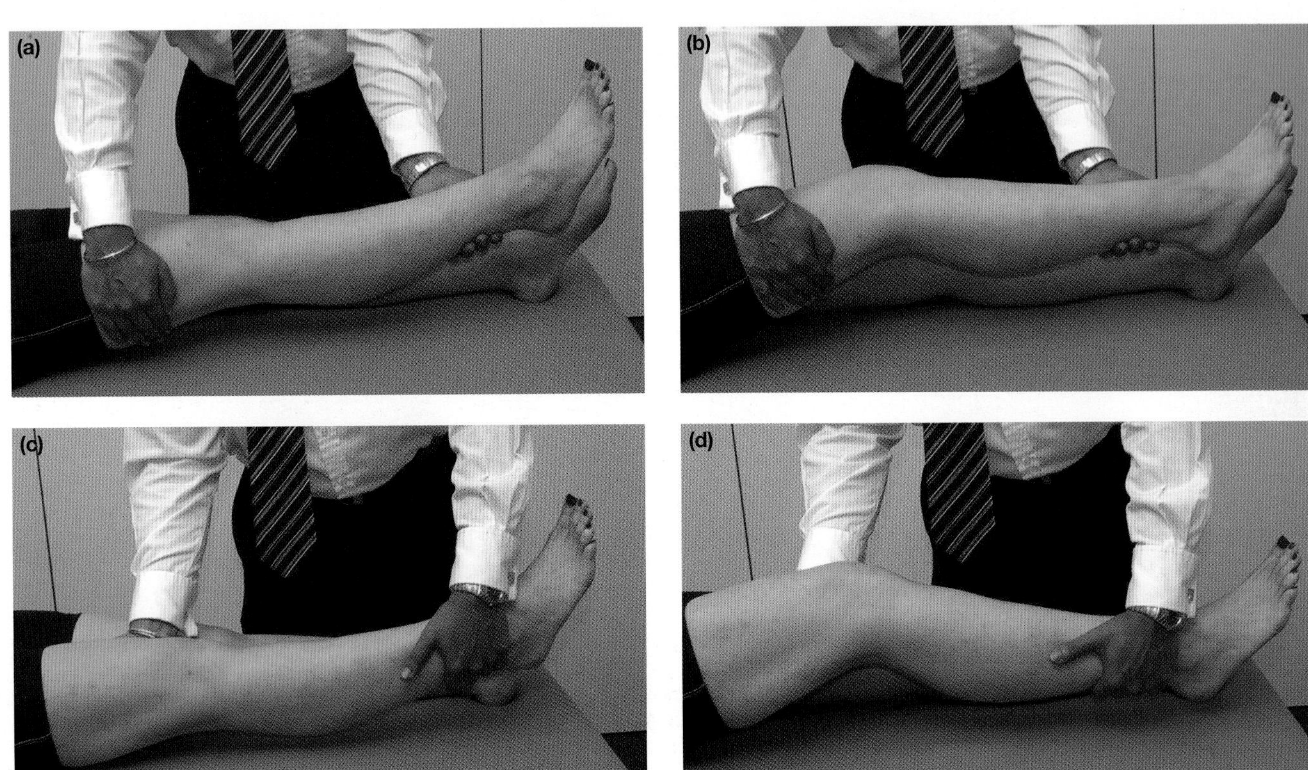

Figure 35.31 Assessing the medial (a, b) and lateral (c, d) collateral ligaments.

from the knee or the hip joint. To differentiate, sit the patient up with the knees hanging over the edge of the couch; this obliterates the effect of any hip flexion deformity. Passively try to extend the knee fully. With a flexion deformity of the knee, this is not possible.

Special tests

Collateral ligaments

To assess the ligaments, place the leg under your arm. Flex the knee to 30° (not more) to relax the posterior capsule (the MCL and LCL are taut in full extension and lax in flexion). Stress each ligament in turn by applying a valgus or varus force. With your index fingers simultaneously palpate over the collateral ligaments. Assess for signs of instability (excessive opening of the joint). The quality of the end point should be noted (is it firm or spongy?). Compare both sides (*Figure 35.31*).

- **Medial collateral ligament**. A lax MCL or deficient lateral compartment may cause knee instability when applying a valgus stress. It is important to note that the valgus stress test should be applied with the knee in 30° of flexion. Valgus instability in full extension (0°) should alert you to a possible posterior structure injury (e.g. posterior capsule, PCL).
- **Lateral collateral ligament**. A lax LCL or deficient medial compartment may cause knee instability when applying a varus stress in 10° of flexion. Instability in full extension (0°) suggests injury to the posterior structures. In a suspected lateral injury, evaluation of the peroneal nerve must be performed.

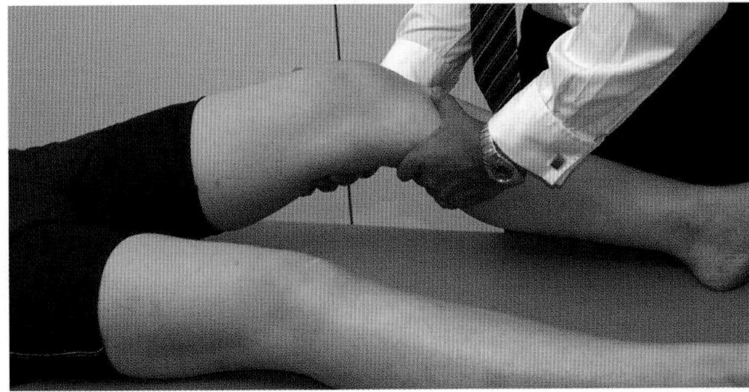

Figure 35.32 Lachman's test: flex the knee to 15–30° and pull the proximal tibia forwards.

Anterior cruciate ligament

The most sensitive test for evaluation of the ACL is the Lachman test.

- **The Lachman test** (*Figure 35.32*). Flex the knee to 15–30° and pull the proximal tibia gently forwards. Excessive laxity may indicate rupture of the ACL. Anterior translation of the tibia associated with a soft or no end point is a positive test. The test may be negative in chronic ruptures because the ACL stump can scar to the PCL.

John W Lachman, 1919–2007, Professor and Chairman of the Orthopedic Department at Temple University in Philadelphia, PA, USA.

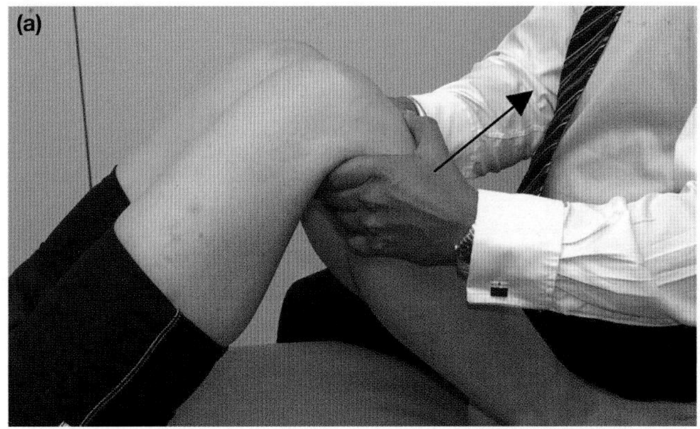

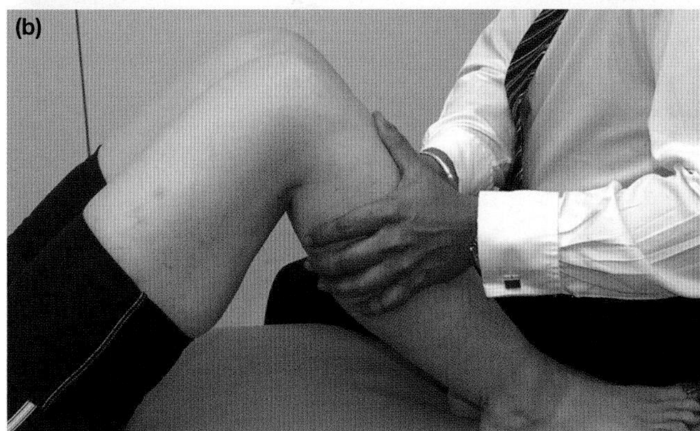

Figure 35.33 (a) Anterior draw test for anterior cruciate ligament stability; (b) posterior draw test for posterior cruciate ligament stability.

- **Anterior draw test** (*Figure 35.33a*). Flex both knees to 90° and look for a posterior sag (compare the height of the tibial tuberosities looking from the side). This may indicate an injury to the PCL. Stabilise the feet by sitting on them. Now place your hands around the proximal and posterior aspect of the tibia. With your index fingers, push up the hamstrings to encourage them to relax. Now draw the tibia gently forwards and measure any laxity, comparing it with the other knee. The degree of laxity can be graded: grade I (0–5 mm), grade II (5–10 mm) and grade III (>10 mm).

Posterior cruciate ligament

The PCL is the primary restraint to posterior tibial translation between 30° and 90° of knee flexion. At 90° knee flexion, the PCL controls the majority of posterior translation of the tibia. Look for a posterior sag with the knees flexed to 90°. The posterior draw test is the most reliable clinical test for a PCL injury.

- **Posterior draw test** (*Figure 35.33b*). Perform the test with the knee flexed to 90°. Push the anterior aspect of the proximal tibia posteriorly and compare any laxity with the other side. If more than 10 mm of posterior tibial translation is noted at 30° and/or 90° of knee flexion, a combined PCL and posterolateral corner injury may be present. An evaluation of the competency of the posterolateral corner is necessary.

Menisci

The presence of palpable joint line tenderness is the most sensitive clinical examination test for a meniscal tear. Flex the knee to 90° and palpate the joint line using your thumb and index finger. Note any areas of tenderness. Tests for meniscal damage are not very reliable but, combined with a history of mechanical symptoms, locking, catching and pain, may be helpful. With posterior medial meniscal tears patients suffer pain on high flexion or squatting. The well-known test for meniscal tears is McMurray's test. The patient lies supine with their knee flexed to 45° and hip flexed to 45°. The examiner braces the lower leg: one hand holds the ankle; the other hand holds the knee. For assessment of the medial meniscus, palpate the medial joint line with the knee flexed. A 'click' may be felt, suggesting meniscus relocation. A valgus stress is applied to the flexed knee. Externally rotate the leg (toes point outward), and slowly extend the knee while it is still in valgus.

Patellofemoral joint

The patella normally enters the trochlea from a lateral position and becomes centralised with increasing knee flexion, travelling in a 'J' pattern.

- **Patellar tracking** (*Figure 35.34*). Sit the patient and ask them to let their legs hang off the end of the couch with the knees flexed to 90°. Ask the patient to extend the knee slowly to full extension. Towards the end of extension, look for lateral subluxation of the patella ('J' sign). This indicates maltracking.
- **Patellar apprehension** (Fairbank's) test (for instability). Attempt to displace the patella laterally with the knee in extension. Patients with instability contract their quadriceps muscle or complain of pain. With the patient supine and the quadriceps relaxed, flex the knee to 30° while trying to push the patella laterally. With instability the patient may react with apprehension. In addition, the quadriceps muscle may contract in an attempt to realign the patella.

Patellar tendon

The patellar tendon serves as the distal limit of the extensor mechanism. Rupture usually occurs at the osseotendinous junction. This results in an inability to actively perform and maintain full knee extension. A rupture presents with diffuse swelling in the anterior knee. A high-riding patella (patella alta) is present secondary to the unopposed pull of the quadriceps muscle. A defect in the tendon is usually palpable. When the rupture extends through the medial and lateral retinacula, active extension is lost.

Thomas Porter McMurray, 1887–1949, Professor of Orthopaedic Surgery, Liverpool University, Liverpool, UK.
Sir Harold Arthur Thomas Fairbank, 1876–1961, orthopaedic surgeon, King's College Hospital, London, UK.

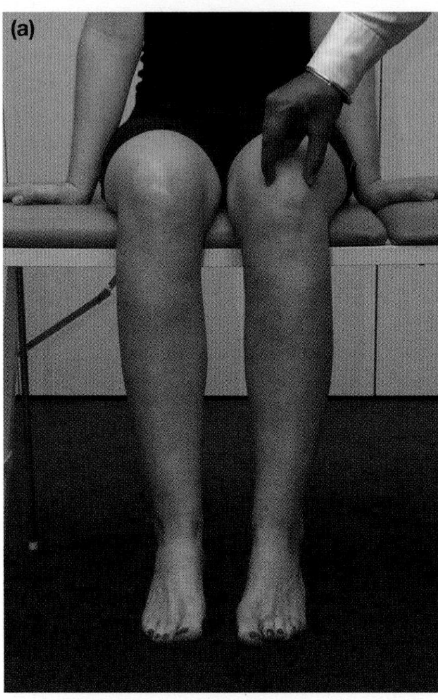

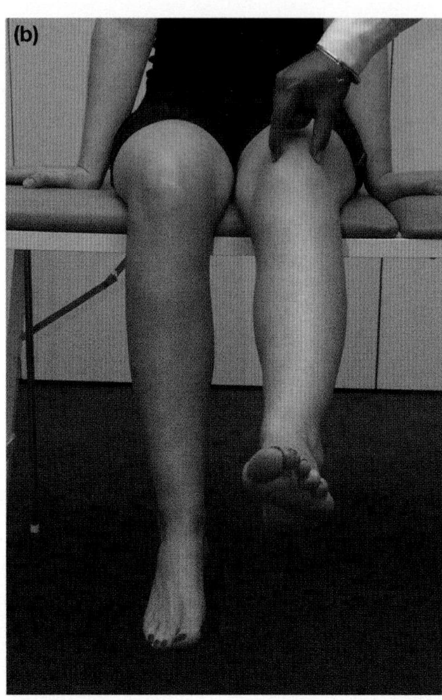

Figure 35.34 (a, b) Patellar tracking.

Summary box 35.9

Knee examination

- Inspection of the standing patient
  - Front – alignment (varus/valgus/rotational deformity), muscle bulk
  - Side – fixed flexion deformity
  - Back – popliteal swellings, hamstrings
  - Gait – antalgic, high-stepping gait (foot drop), varus thrust
- Inspection of the supine patient
  - Skin, scars, soft tissues, deformity
  - Palpation of the extensor mechanism, medial and lateral joint lines and collateral ligaments, hamstrings, tibial tuberosity, fibular head
- Movements
  - Flexion and extension
- Special tests
  - Patellar apprehension test and extensor mechanism
  - Cruciate ligaments
  - Collateral ligaments
  - Menisci

CLINICAL EXAMINATION OF THE FOOT AND ANKLE

The foot can be divided into three parts: the hindfoot (calcaneus, talus), the midfoot (navicular, cuboids, cuneiforms) and the forefoot (metatarsals and phalanges).

Look

Ask the patient to stand and assess the overall limb alignment. Assess pelvic obliquity, LLD (and its level), valgus/varus deformities of the knee and rotational alignment. Check for contractures of the hips and knees. Now focus your attention on the foot itself:

- **Foot shape**. Assess the overall shape of the forefoot from the front. From the side, look for the normal medial arch (***Figure 35.35a***). The hindfoot is best appreciated from behind. Now look at the vertical relationship between the Achilles tendon and the calcaneus (normal heel valgus of 5–7°). Look from behind and count the number of toes that can be seen. The 'too many toes' sign demonstrates increased forefoot abduction (pes planus [flat foot]) and a splayed forefoot. Foot shapes that may be encountered include neutral foot (no overall deformity), skew foot (hindfoot valgus and forefoot adduction), metatarsus adductus (neutral hindfoot and adduction of the metatarsus), pes planus (collapse of the medial arch) and pes cavus or high arch (increased medial arch) (***Figure 35.35b***). The possible causes of pes planus and pes cavus are shown in ***Summary boxes 35.10 and 35.11***, respectively.
- **Skin**. A bunion or red swelling on the medial aspect of the metatarsophalangeal joint (MTPJ) is common. This is an area of inflamed skin with an underlying subcutaneous bursa and a joint osteophyte. Systemic manifestations include gouty tophi and thin fat pads under the metatarsal heads as seen in rheumatoid arthritis. Corns are callosities which form where toes rub against the inside of shoes. Remember to assess the appearance of the nails.
- **Soft tissues**. Swelling may indicate soft-tissue or joint pathology. Muscle wasting is most commonly seen on the dorsum of the foot and in the clefts between the metatarsals. If this is present, a full neurological examination of the upper and lower limbs should be performed, including the spine.
- **Bones**. Look for any bony prominences or exostoses. Common forefoot deformities are shown in ***Table 35.12***.

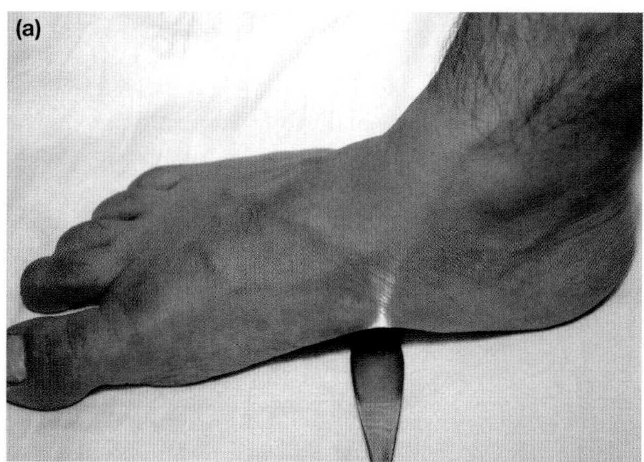

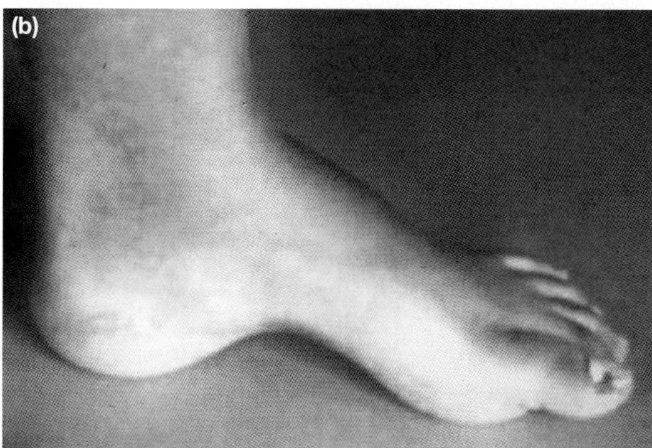

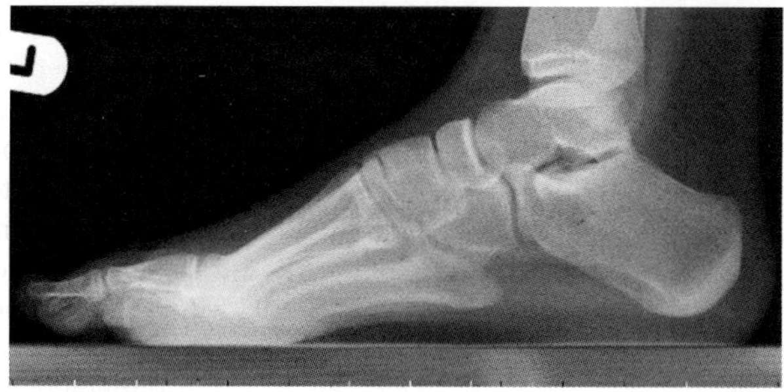

Figure 35.35 (a) Normal medial longitudinal arch of the foot. (b) Clinical and radiological appearance of pes cavus.

Summary box 35.10

Causes of pes planus
- Normal variant
- Hyperlaxity syndrome, e.g. Marfan's syndrome
- Tarsal coalition – rigid and painful flat foot (see *Figure 35.40a*)
- Tibial posterior dysfunction

Summary box 35.11

Causes of pes cavus (*Figure 35.35b*)
- Spinal anomalies, e.g. spina bifida
- Hereditary sensorimotor neuropathies, such as Charcot–Marie–Tooth disease
- Charcot foot (e.g. neuropathic foot)
- Post-compartment syndrome (e.g. Volkmann's ischaemic contracture)

Gait

Look for a high-stepping gait (foot drop), painful (antalgic) gait (ankle and foot joint pain) and a short propulsive phase (forefoot pain).

Footwear

Inspect the footwear. This may reveal areas of abnormal weight-bearing. With normal wear of the sole, a corner is typically worn off the posterolateral aspect of the heel (heel strike). In addition, there may be a circular wear pattern under the ball of the big toe (toe-off phase).

- **External appearance**. Look at the materials used, the metal supports and heel raise, depth and width.
- **Internal appearance**. Look at the insoles, arch supports and heel cups.

Feel

- **Skin**. Reduced sensation in a glove-and-stocking distribution is seen with diabetes.

TABLE 35.12 Common forefoot deformities.

Deformity	Metatarsophalangeal joint	Proximal interphalangeal joint	Distal interphalangeal joint
Claw toe	Hyperextension	Flexion	Flexion
Hammer toe	Normal	Flexion	Flexion
Mallet toe	Normal	Normal	Flexion
Hallux valgus or varus	Valgus or varus position	Normal	–

Antoine Bernard-Jean Marfan, 1858–1942, physician, Hôpital des Infants-Malades, Paris, France, described this syndrome in 1896.
Jean Martin Charcot, 1825–1893, physician, La Salpêtrière, Paris, France.
Pierre Marie, 1853–1940, neurologist, Hospice de Bicêtre, Paris, France, later became Professor of Pathological Anatomy in the Faculty of Medicine, and finally, in 1918, Professor of Neurology.
Howard Henry Tooth, 1856–1925, physician, St Bartholomew's Hospital and the National Hospital for Nervous Diseases, London, UK, described peroneal muscular atrophy in 1886, independently of Charcot and Marie.
Richard von Volkmann, 1830–1889, Professor of Surgery, Halle, Germany.

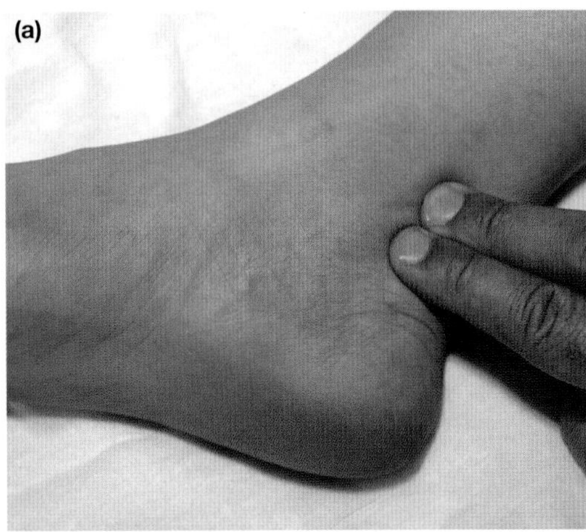

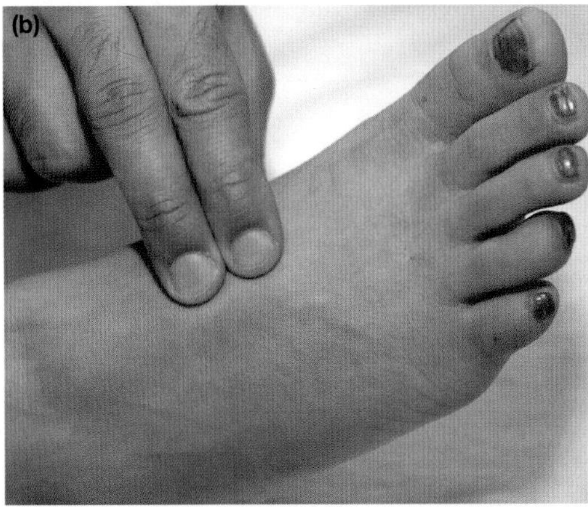

Figure 35.36 (a) Palpation of the posterior tibial pulse. (b) Palpation of the dorsalis pedis pulse.

- **Soft tissues**. The posterior tibial and the dorsal pedis pulses should be identified (***Figure 35.36***). Palpate the tibialis anterior tendon and the long extensor tendons on the dorsum of the foot. From the back, palpate the Achilles tendon. Palpate the peroneal tendons from the lateral side and the tibialis posterior tendon from the medial side. The sinus tarsi can be assessed. This is an anatomical space bounded by the talus and calcaneus and is recognisable as a soft-tissue depression anterior to the lateral malleolus. It is filled with fat and the extensor digitorum brevis muscle. Sinus tarsi syndrome may occur. This may be caused by injury to the interosseous talocalcaneal ligament or the subtalar joint. There is pain and tenderness over the sinus tarsi with subjective hindfoot instability. The pain is characteristically relieved by local anaesthetic injection.
- **Bones**. Feel for deformity, bony prominences and loose bodies:
  - *ankle joint*: the medial and lateral malleoli, anterior and posterior joint line, lateral gutter and ligament complex, the syndesmosis (front of the ankle), medial gutter and medial ligament complex;
  - *subtalar joint*: palpate each facet;
  - *midtarsal joints*: the talonavicular and calcaneocuboid joints;
  - *tarsometatarsal joints* (TMTJ): note that the second TMTJ is several millimetres proximal to the others; movement is minimal in the second ray, limited in the third ray, moderate in the fourth and fifth rays and very variable in the first ray.
- **Specific structures to palpate:**
  - *calcaneus* (heel bone): the most common cause of pain is plantar fasciitis; this may present with numbness, burning and electric shock sensations, which are worse in the morning and improve as the day goes on; identify the exact point of tenderness;
  - *tendons*: examine for contracture of the Achilles tendon insertion and the peroneal or tibialis posterior tendons;
  - *head of talus*: invert and evert the patient's foot;
  - *sustentaculum tali*: palpate one fingerbreadth below the medial malleolus; this important structure serves as an attachment for the spring ligament;
  - *cuneiforms* (medial, middle and lateral), MTPJs, web spaces and all the forefoot bones.

Move

The movements of the foot and ankle are linked via the ankle, subtalar and midfoot joints. Remember the acronyms PAED – pronation, abduction, eversion and dorsiflexion – and SAPI – supination, adduction, plantarflexion and inversion. These are the two common general foot deformities.

Ankle (Figure 35.37)

- **Dorsiflexion**. Test dorsiflexion with the knee both flexed and extended. If restriction is greater with the knee extended than flexed, the contracture is principally in the gastrocnemius. Restriction that is equal in all knee positions is caused by a contracture principally of the soleus.
- **Plantarflexion**. Ask the patient to touch the floor with their foot (15°). Weakness suggests injury to the Achilles tendon or pathology affecting the S1 nerve root.

Subtalar joint (Figures 35.38 and 35.39)

Hold the talar neck and ask the patient to move their heel from side to side. Repeat using a hand on the heel to move the joint and apply a varus and valgus stress while feeling for movements of the talus. Holding the talus as opposed to the tibia isolates the subtalar from ankle motion. (Normal range is 5° in each direction.)

- **Inversion**. Ask the patient to move their foot in towards them.
- **Eversion**. Ask the patient to move their foot out to the side.

Midtarsal joint

Hold the heel with one hand and move the forefoot medially (adduction = 20°) and laterally (abduction = 10°) with the other hand.

Tarsometatarsal joint

Hold the midfoot and manipulate each metatarsal up and down to estimate the passive range of movement.

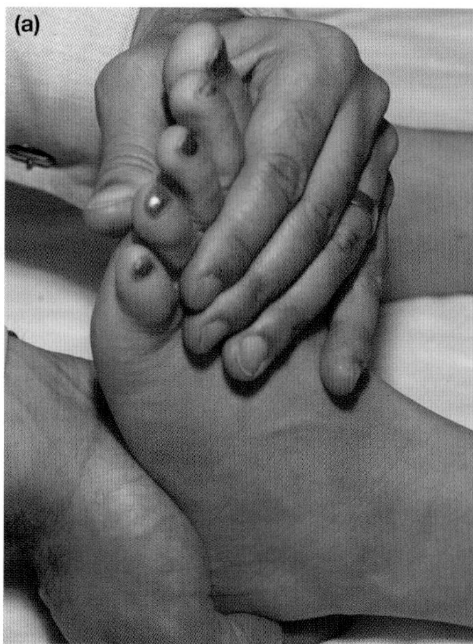

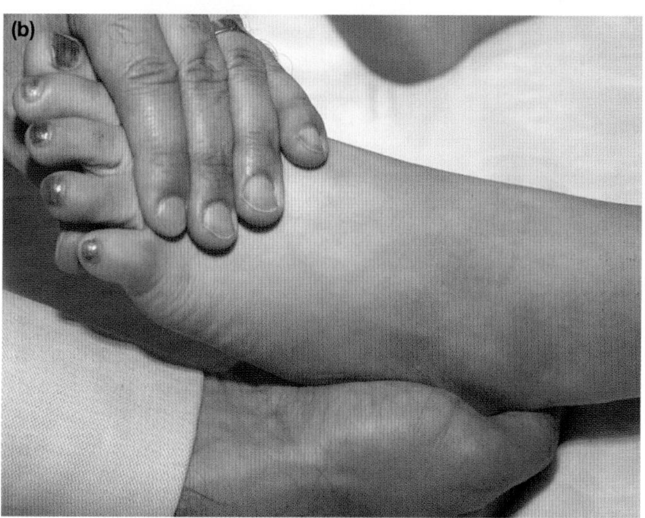

Figure 35.37 (a) Ankle dorsiflexion and (b) ankle plantarflexion.

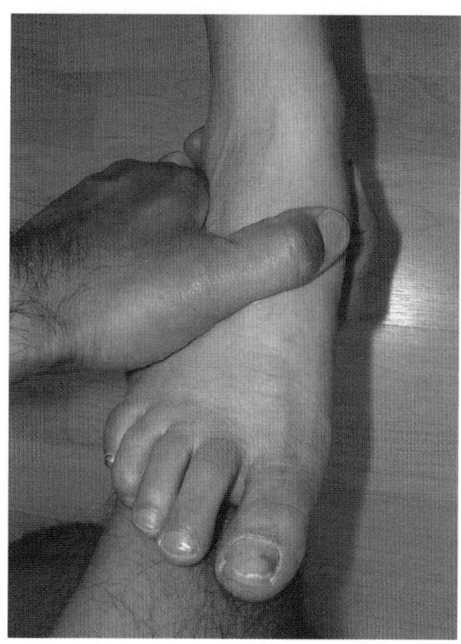

Figure 35.38 Testing subtalar joint motion.

Metatarsophalangeal joint

Test extension (70–90°) by asking the patient to lift the toes to the ceiling and test flexion (45°) by pointing the toes to the floor. Normal toe-off requires 35–40° of dorsiflexion.

Special tests

Achilles tendon

Feel the gastrocnemius and soleus bellies and the whole length of the tendon for gaps (rupture), tenderness or swelling. Also identify the posterolateral (Haglund's) prominence of the calcaneus and palpate the retro-Achilles bursa.

The test for integrity of the tendon is the Thompson or Simmonds test. Do not be misled by the patient's ability to stand on tiptoes – some people can do this using their long toe flexors alone. Lie the patient prone and allow their calves to rest on your forearms. Squeeze each calf in turn and watch for movement at the ankle joint. Lack of movement may indicate a rupture.

Subtalar joint flexibility

Ask the patient to stand on their toes and observe the heel from behind; the heel moves normally from valgus to varus, indicating flexibility. The Coleman block test is used to assess the flexibility of the subtalar joint. Ask the patient to stand on a 2-cm block with the great toe over the medial edge, resting on the floor. Now look from behind. If the hindfoot varus remains, the subtalar joint is fixed. If it corrects to valgus, the joint is mobile (*Figure 35.39*).

Flat foot flexibility

Use the windlass and Jack's tests to distinguish a flexible from a fixed flat foot (*Figure 35.40*).

- **Windlass test**. Ask the patient to stand on their toes and observe the arch of the foot on the medial aspect. As soon as the patient stands on their toes, the arch forms. Failure of this indicates a fixed flat foot.

Patrik Haglund, 1870–1937, Swedish orthopaedic surgeon.
Theodore Campbell Thompson, 1902–1986, American orthopedic surgeon, made many contributions to orthopaedic surgery, especially in the field of post-polio deformities.
Franklin Adin Simmonds, 1911–1983, orthopaedic surgeon, Rowley Bristow Hospital, Pyrford, UK.
Sherman S Coleman, 1922–2004, Chief Surgeon, Intermountain Unit of the Shriners Hospital, and Chairman, Division of Orthopedics, University of Utah, Salt Lake City, UT, USA.
Ewan A Jack, 1909–1953, Scottish orthopaedic surgeon.

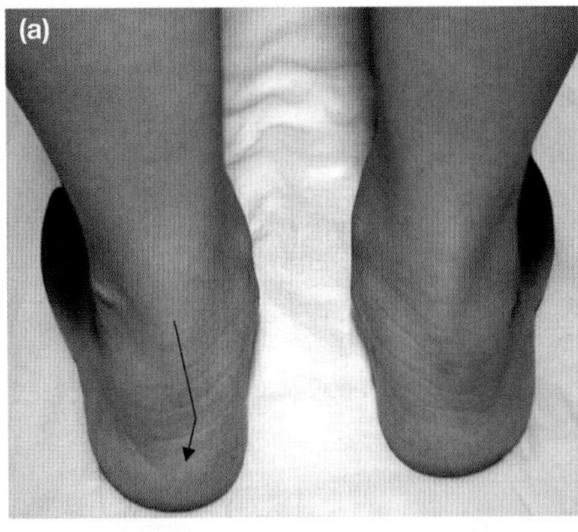

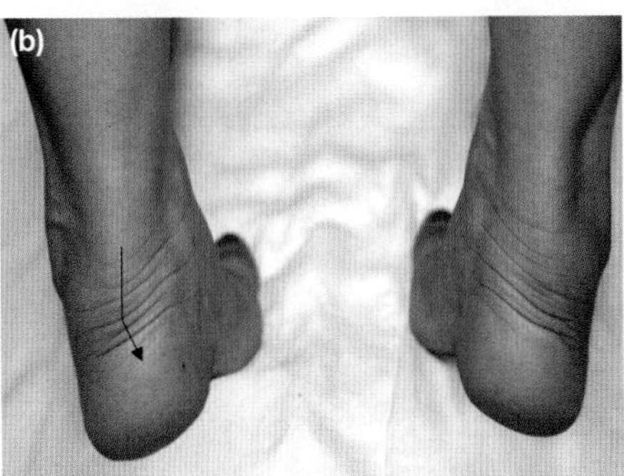

Figure 35.39 (a, b) Testing subtalar joint flexibility.

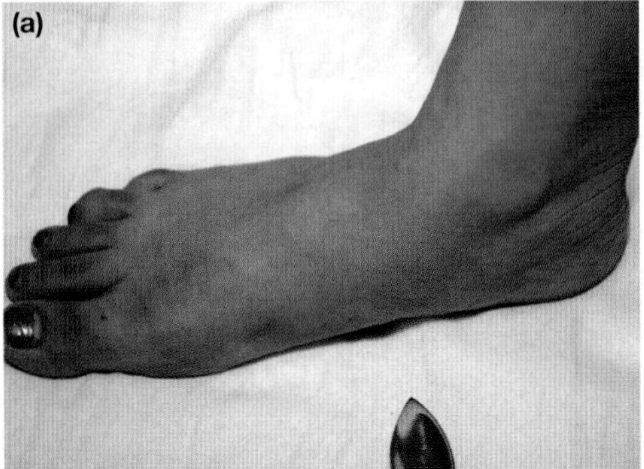

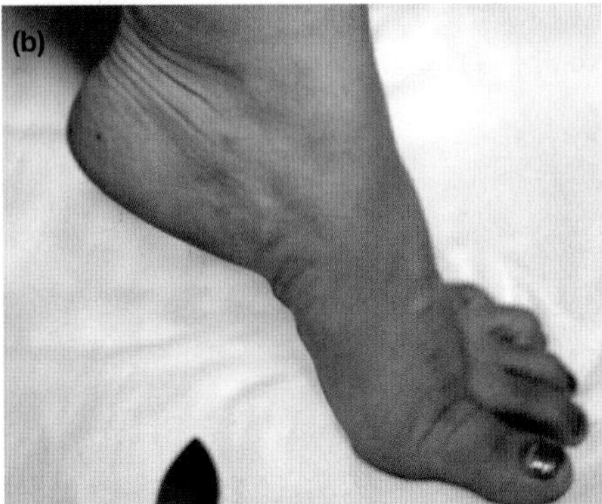

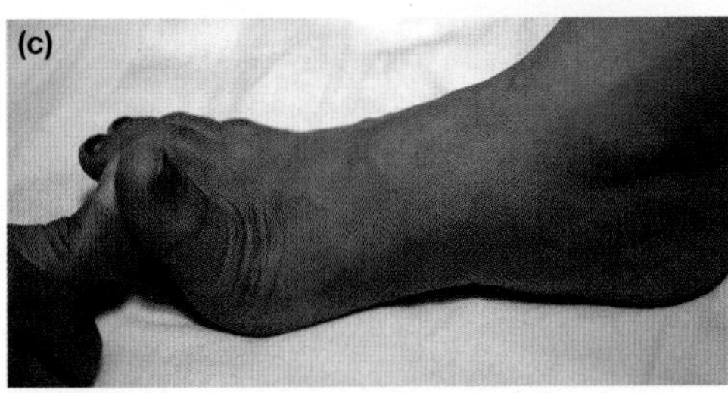

Figure 35.40 (a) Flat foot appearance with a reduced medial longitudinal arch; (b) windlass test; (c) Jack's test.

- **Jack's test**. With the patient standing, lift up the great toe. The arch should form in the flexible flat foot.

Ankle stability

Trauma to the ankle is a common cause of instability. Accurate assessment may be difficult in the acute setting because of pain.

- **Anterior draw test**. With the foot resting over the bed, hold the heel with one hand and the front of the tibia with the other. Move the heel forwards on the fixed tibia. Compare with the other side. Instability of the syndesmosis may be palpable (***Figure 35.41***).
- **Squeeze test for distal tibiofibular stability**. Compress the proximal calf. Pain at the ankle may indicate separation of the distal fibula from the tibia.
- **Tilt test**. Hold the talus at the neck rather than the heel so that you can be sure that any tilt is in the ankle and not the subtalar joint.

Tarsometatarsal joint stability

Stability can be assessed by pushing each joint up and down. Standing lateral radiographs may be used in addition.

Tibialis anterior

Ask the patient to walk on their heels with their feet inverted; the tibialis anterior tendon can be seen. With the patient's feet resting over the edge of the couch, ask the patient to actively dorsiflex and invert their foot to reach your hand. Palpate the tibialis anterior muscle.

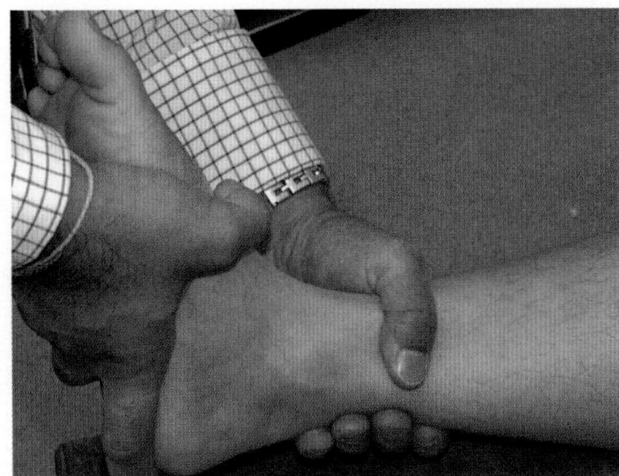

Figure 35.41 Anterior draw test.

Tibialis posterior

Pathology of the tibialis posterior typically presents with posteromedial ankle pain, swelling and gradual onset of a flat foot. When assessing the tendon, look for swelling along its course, a flat foot with heel valgus, the 'too many toes' sign and prominence of the talar head. Palpate for tenderness, swelling or gaps in the tendon.

- **To test integrity**, ask the patient to perform a single-foot tiptoe test on both sides. The inability to lift the affected heel off the ground is suggestive of a tibialis posterior tendon injury or insufficiency.
- **To test strength**, position the foot in the plantarflexed and inverted position. Ask the patient to hold this position while you push against their foot.

Dorsiflexors

Tendinitis of the long toe dorsiflexors usually presents in athletes. Pain affects gait in the early contact phase. Palpate for swelling, gaps or any tenderness. Ask the patient to move the foot into dorsiflexion and to hold this position while you push the foot down.

Inability to dorsiflex the foot is referred to as foot drop. Causes include stroke, spinal injury, spinal stenosis or disc prolapse, peripheral nerve injury (e.g. sciatic, common and deep peroneal) or a peripheral neuropathy.

Peroneal tendons

Peroneal tendon pathology presents with swelling and/or pain of the lateral hindfoot or midfoot. There may be a history of the ankle 'giving way'. Presentations of peroneal tendon pathology include:

- **'peroneal spasm'**: may be seen in tarsal coalition; here, the muscles are usually contracted secondary to the hindfoot valgus;
- **peroneal tendon dislocation**: attempt to dislocate the tendons by dorsiflexing and everting the foot.

The peroneus longus may be palpated just before it crosses under the foot to insert onto the base of the first metatarsal. Ask the patient to plantar flex the first metatarsal. Test strength and integrity by active and resisted eversion while you palpate the tendons for swelling, tenderness or gaps.

Morton's neuroma

This condition represents thickening of the tissue that surrounds the digital nerve leading to the toes as the nerve passes under the ligament connecting the metatarsals in the forefoot. It is most frequent between the third and fourth toes. A neuroma presents with burning pain in the ball of the foot that radiates to the involved toes. The condition is difficult to diagnose and requires a high index of suspicion. Palpate in the web space between the symptomatic toes for a mass. Compression of the metatarsals may elicit a 'click' between the bones (Mulder's click).

Summary box 35.12

Ankle and foot examination

- Inspection of the standing patient
  - Front – alignment, foot shape and deformity
  - Side – medial arch
  - Back – heel position
  - Gait – antalgic, high-stepping gait (foot drop)
- Inspection of the supine patient
  - Skin, scars, soft tissues, bony deformity
  - Palpation of the ankle, subtalar, midfoot and forefoot joints
- Movements
  - Dorsiflexion, plantarflexion, inversion, eversion
- Special tests
  - Flexibility of the subtalar joint and a flat foot
  - Joint stability, Morton's neuroma
  - Tendons – tibialis posterior and anterior, Achilles tendon, peroneals and dorsiflexors

FURTHER READING

Beighton PH, Horan F. Orthopedic aspects of the Ehlers-Danlos syndrome. *J Bone Joint Surg* 1969; **51-B**: 444–53.

Ellenbecker TS, Nirschl R, Renstrom P. Current concepts in examination and treatment of elbow tendon injury. *Sports Health* 2013; **5**(2): 186–94.

Guosheng Y, Chongxi R, Guoqing C *et al.* The diagnostic value of a modified Neer test in identifying subacromial impingement syndrome. *Eur J Orthop Surg Traumatol* 2017; **27**(8): 1063–7.

Martin HD, Palmer IJ. History and physical examination of the hip: the basics. *Curr Rev Musculoskelet Med* 2013; **6**(3): 219–25.

Rossi R, Dettoni F, Bruzzone M *et al.* Clinical examination of the knee: know your tools for diagnosis of knee injuries. *Sports Med Arthrosc Rehabil Ther Technol* 2011; **3**: 25.

Warwick D, Blom A, Whitehouse M. *Apley and Solomon's concise system of orthopaedics and trauma*, 5th edn. Abingdon: CRC Press, 2022.

Thomas George Morton, 1835–1903, surgeon, Pennsylvania Hospital, Philadelphia, PA, USA.
Jacob D Mulder, 1901–1965, Dutch surgeon and podiatrist.

CHAPTER 36 Sports medicine and sports injuries

Learning objectives

- To review some common sports injuries
- To understand the basics of history, physical examination and imaging for common injuries
- To assess the patient and offer treatment and rehabilitation plans

INTRODUCTION

In addition to a clinical assessment, an understanding of the biomechanics of injury associated with sporting activity can facilitate diagnosis, treatment and management of the patient according to their competitive level and recovery goals. This chapter aims to provide a brief clinically directed overview of selected common injuries, with the examples associated with a wide variety of sports.

DIAGNOSIS OF SPORTS INJURIES

Within the history, there are some additional questions that need to be asked when treating a patient with a sports injury:

- How was the injury sustained?
- When was the injury sustained?
- What intervention(s) has the patient tried and what rehabilitation have they had?
- How many hours of training is the patient doing and has this changed recently?
- Has the patient had a previous injury?
- What are the patient's competitive goals?

The examination should follow the general system described in *Chapter 35*.

COMMONLY ENCOUNTERED REGIONAL INJURIES

Shoulder

Shoulder instability and rotator cuff tear

Background

Shoulder injuries affect athletes of all ages; however, the distribution of shoulder injuries varies between young and older participants. In athletes younger than 30 years old, especially those participating in contact sports, anterior shoulder dislocations can occur in instances of traumatic or forced shoulder abduction and external rotation. Unfortunately, such dislocations, even if reduced, lead to some degree of stretching of the anterior capsule and tearing of the anteroinferior labrum, which places the patient at risk for further instability events. In older patients who experience falls and sustain the same anterior shoulder dislocations, additional pathologies, including rotator cuff tears, can occur.

History and physical examination

Patients who sustain a shoulder dislocation often describe a violent injury event such as a fall or tackle with the arm in some degree of abduction. Patients will often describe a sensation of their shoulder feeling out of place, especially if the shoulder does not spontaneously reduce. An important component of the history involves the details of the dislocation(s): self-reduction versus emergency department reduction, length of time dislocated prior to reduction, prior dislocations, extremity numbness, general ligamentous laxity and activity profile – all of these details have implications for management. Examination in the acute period should focus on evaluating anterior apprehension or subjective patient discomfort and fear of re-dislocation in the positions of abduction and external rotation of the shoulder, as well as rotator cuff strength and neurovascular integrity, especially of the axillary nerve (see *Further reading*).[1,2]

Imaging

Radiographs, including at least true anteroposterior (AP) or Grashey, scapular Y, axillary or Velpeau views, should be obtained in all circumstances and evaluated to confirm glenohumeral reduction while ruling out associated fractures, such as Hill–Sachs deformities or glenoid rim fractures.

Rudolph Grashey, 1876–1950, Professor of Roentgenology, University of Cologne, Cologne, Germany.
Alfred-Armand-Louis-Marie Velpeau, 1795–1867, French anatomist and surgeon.
Harold Arthur Hill, 1901–1973, radiologist, San Francisco, CA, USA.
Maurice David Sachs, 1909–1987, radiologist, San Francisco, CA, USA.

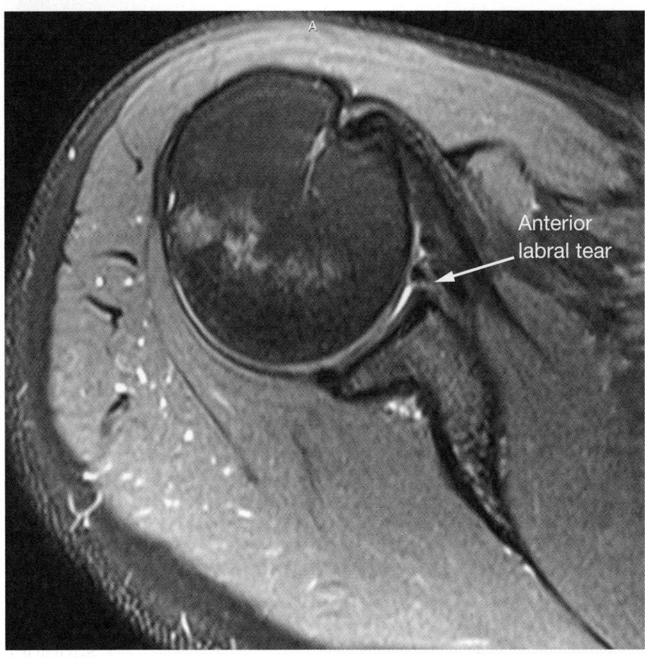

Figure 36.1 Axial fluid-sensitive magnetic resonance image of the shoulder demonstrating an anterior labral tear.

Specific views, including the West Point axillary and the Stryker notch views, can be helpful for evaluating glenoid rim or Bankart fractures or Hill–Sachs lesions, respectively. In cases of recurrent instability where glenoid bone loss is suspected, computed tomography (CT) with or without three-dimensional reconstruction can be helpful in further determining the extent of bone loss. In most instances of anterior instability, magnetic resonance imaging (MRI) is recommended (*Figure 36.1*) to evaluate for concomitant soft-tissue injuries, including rotator cuff tears, humeral avulsions of the glenohumeral ligament (HAGL), glenolabral articular disruptions (GLAD) or anterior labrum periosteal sleeve avulsion (ALPSA).

Treatment

After reduction of an acute anterior glenohumeral dislocation, patients are typically placed in a sling for the first few days.[2] It is important to begin early gentle range of motion of the shoulder through pendulum exercises but also to continue to move the elbow, wrist and digits actively to maintain range of motion in those distal joints. The initial period is then progressed to increased passive and then active and active-assisted range of motion of the shoulder. Once range of motion has returned to near normal, rotator cuff and scapular strengthening is progressed. Surgery is considered for even first-time dislocators based upon stratification of several factors, including younger age, activity profile and pathology present on imaging. Furthermore, depending upon the pathology present, the surgical options exist on a continuum from arthroscopic capsulolabral repair to open capsulolabral repair and capsular shift to glenoid bony augmentation procedures.[3,4] Regardless of the treatment method chosen, athletes are cleared to return to sport once their range of motion and strength have returned to normal levels.

Older athletes who acutely tear their rotator cuff in the setting of shoulder dislocations can be considered for acute rotator cuff repair.[5] The treatment of rotator cuff tears has evolved over several years and current techniques of arthroscopic repair with a knotless, linked, double-row construct (*Figure 36.2*) have demonstrated excellent patient-reported outcomes with low re-tear rates.

Differential diagnosis

- Proximal humerus fracture.
- Greater tuberosity fracture.
- Acromioclavicular joint separation.

> **Summary box 36.1**
>
> **Shoulder instability**
>
> - Dislocations occur in instances of traumatic or forced shoulder abduction and external rotation
> - Details of the reduction, time dislocated, history of prior dislocations, general ligamentous laxity and activity profile have implications for management
> - Radiographs to confirm glenohumeral reduction include true AP or Grashey, scapular Y, axillary or Velpeau views
> - A sling should be used for a few days following an acute anterior glenohumeral dislocation
> - Surgery is considered based upon stratification of several factors, including younger age, activity profile and pathology present on imaging

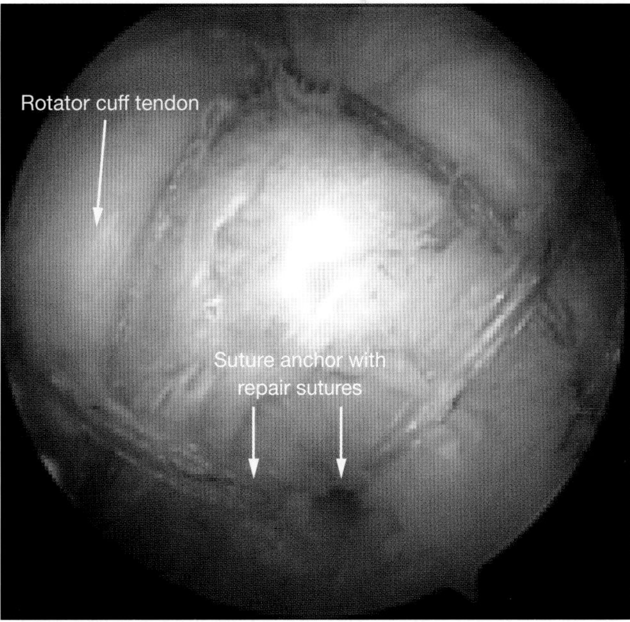

Figure 36.2 Shoulder arthroscopic image of a rotator cuff repair viewed from the subacromial space through a lateral portal with a 30° arthroscope.

William Schamel Stryker, 1916–2015, orthopedic surgeon and Captain in the United States Navy.
Arthur Sydney Blundell Bankart, 1879–1951, orthopaedic surgeon, The Middlesex Hospital, London, UK.

Elbow

Ulnar collateral ligament tear

Background

The anterior band of the ulnar collateral ligament (UCL) is the primary stabiliser to valgus stress at the elbow. Anatomically this ligament courses from the medial epicondyle of the humerus to the sublime tubercle of the ulna. Although it can be injured acutely through mechanisms of elbow dislocations, pathology is most frequently encountered in repetitive throwing athletes, such as baseball pitchers and javelin throwers. In the late cocking and early acceleration phases of throwing the ligament is under its maximum stress and at this stage is at the highest risk of rupture and chronic attenuation.

History and physical examination

Throwers who sustain ruptures of their UCL commonly present with two sets of complaints. Rarely, the thrower will recall an acute episode when they heard a pop in the throwing cycle followed by medial elbow pain and pain worse with throwing. The vast majority of throwers complain of medial elbow pain and tightness coupled with decreased velocity that comes on more insidiously. Examination focuses on provocative manoeuvres that are specific for the UCL, including valgus stress and the moving valgus stress tests or milking manoeuvre (***Figure 36.3***), in which the examiner provides a valgus stress through elbow range of motion.[6] Pain at the medial elbow during these manoeuvres is specific for UCL pathology. The examiner should also focus on both ulnar nerve sensory and motor symptoms in the hand in addition to ulnar nerve subluxation as these pathologies can affect the proposed treatment algorithm.

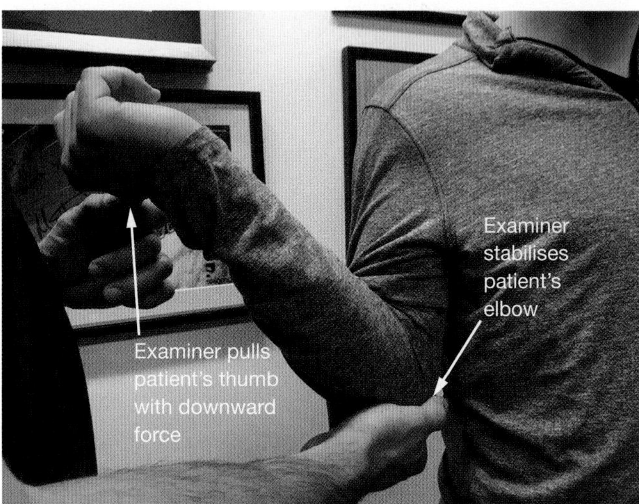

Figure 36.3 Demonstration of the milking manoeuvre. This is considered a positive test when this provocative manoeuvre elicits pain in the medial elbow, indicating ulnar collateral ligament injury.

Imaging

Radiographs of the elbow include a series of AP, lateral, internal and external oblique views. These can help rule out other commonly encountered phenomena seen in overhead throwing athletes, including medial epicondyle fractures, posteromedial impingement and capitellar osteochondral defects. When UCL pathology is suspected, dynamic ultrasound is a helpful imaging modality to help characterise the location of the UCL pathology. Moreover, it permits easy examination of the contralateral elbow, which can help to quantify incongruities in medial elbow joint space gapping, an indirect gauge of tear severity. MRI is commonly obtained to precisely define the location of the UCL tear as well as to better evaluate the articular cartilage and the flexor pronator mass, which can also commonly be affected.

Treatment

Conservative management of UCL injuries is considered first-line treatment and typically entails a period of several months of cessation of throwing followed by structured rehabilitation that includes strengthening of secondary stabilising muscles about the elbow and a gradual return of throwing.[6] The use of biological injections, including platelet-rich plasma, has been proposed for partial-thickness ligament tears in some centres, but more clinical evidence is required. Although ligament repair with an internal brace has recently been demonstrated to have efficacy in certain types of tears, the gold standard for surgical treatment is UCL reconstruction or Tommy John surgery. The surgery involves an autograft tendon harvest, commonly utilising the ipsilateral palmaris longus tendon, and reconstruction of the ligament through bone tunnels in both the humerus and ulna.[6] This surgery can be coupled with *in situ* decompression or transposition of the ulnar nerve, if indicated. Ulnar reconstruction surgery is indicated for the highest level of throwers who wish to continue playing their respective sport, with return to sport taking anywhere from 12 to 18 months.

Differential diagnosis

- Flexor pronator mass sprain.
- Ulnohumeral arthritis.
- Ulnar nerve compression or subluxation.
- Loose body.

Summary box 36.2

UCL tears

- Injury seen among repetitive throwing athletes
- Onset can be acute ('pop') or insidious with medial elbow pain, tightness and decreased throwing velocity
- Dynamic ultrasound or MRI can be used to characterise the location of the UCL pathology
- First-line treatment is conservative management with cessation of throwing followed by structured rehabilitation
- Surgical options include UCL reconstruction (gold standard) or ligament repair with an internal brace

Tommy John surgery, named after Thomas Edward John Jr, the first major league baseball pitcher who received an ulnar collateral ligament reconstruction in 1974.

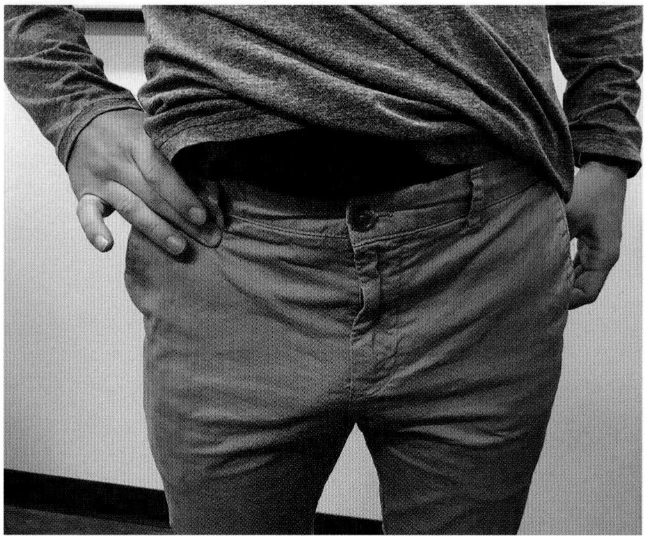

Figure 36.4 Example of the C-sign for intra-articular hip pathology when asking a patient to demonstrate where they feel their pain.

Hip

Femoroacetabular impingement and dysplasia

Background

Intra-articular hip derangements most commonly manifest as anterolateral groin pain in a characteristic distribution, referred to as a 'C-sign' (*Figure 36.4*). In a young patient, two common sources of groin pain with intra-articular origin are femoroacetabular impingement (FAI) and dysplasia. These conditions are considered in some detail in *Chapter 39* but are described here as they can present as a sports-related injury.

History and physical examination

Young patients with a history of groin pain or repetitive 'groin or hip flexor sprains' should be evaluated for dysplasia or FAI. Physical examination focuses on hip range of motion, strength, palpation and provocative manoeuvres. Some important manoeuvres include the FADIR examination, which stands for hip Flexion, ADduction and Internal Rotation, which is specific for impingement pathologies, but the FABER (Flexion, ABduction and External Rotation) manoeuvre as well as resisted hip flexion (Stinchfield testing) can also identify true intra-articular pathologies.[7]

Imaging

Initial imaging includes radiographs of the pelvis and the affected hip. Anteroposterior pelvis and false profile views can help determine lateral or anterior coverage of the acetabulum, respectively, while 45° Dunn lateral radiographs of the hip are the optimal projection for detecting the presence of a cam lesion (*Figure 36.5*). Three-dimensional imaging, including CT and MRI, is helpful for better defining the bony morphology and soft-tissue (i.e. labral) integrity, respectively.

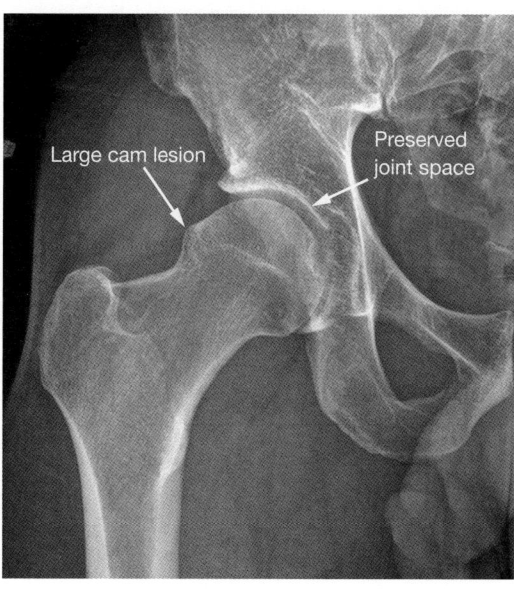

Figure 36.5 Anteroposterior right hip radiograph demonstrating a large cam lesion in the setting of the preserved hip joint space.

Treatment

Once the correct diagnosis is determined both pathologies can initially be treated conservatively using anti-inflammatory drugs, physical therapy and at times intra-articular injection, for example corticosteroid. Should these modalities fail, both FAI and dysplasia have their own specific surgical interventions: arthroscopy (*Figure 36.6*) and osteotomy, respectively (see *Chapter 39*). Importantly, the aforementioned interventions are only a consideration prior to the development of joint space narrowing and osteoarthritis in an effort to preserve the hip joint.[7]

Differential diagnosis

- Adductor strain.
- Hip osteoarthritis.
- Athletic pubalgia.
- Lumbar radiculopathy.

Summary box 36.3

Femoroacetabular impingement and dysplasia

- Intra-articular hip derangements can manifest with anterolateral groin pain in a characteristic distribution ('C-sign')
- Consider pathologies in young patients with a history of groin pain or repetitive 'groin or hip flexor sprains'
- Initial imaging includes radiographs of the pelvis and the affected hip
- Three-dimensional imaging includes CT (bony morphology) and MRI (soft-tissue integrity)
- Conservative treatment involves using anti-inflammatory drugs, physical therapy and/or intra-articular injection
- Surgical interventions are arthroscopy (FAI) and osteotomy (dysplasia) prior to the development of joint space narrowing and osteoarthritis

Frank E Stinchfield, 1910–1992, American orthopaedic surgeon and founder of The Hip Society.
Denis M Dunn, 1916–2001, British orthopaedic surgeon.

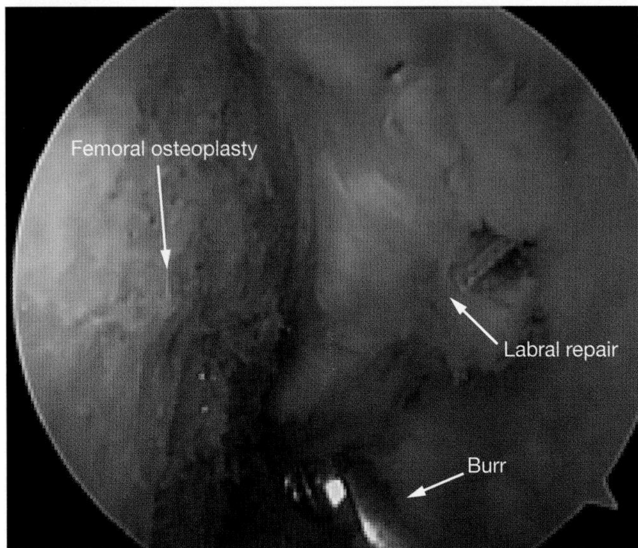

Figure 36.6 Hip arthroscopic image viewed through the mid-anterior portal with a 70° arthroscope.

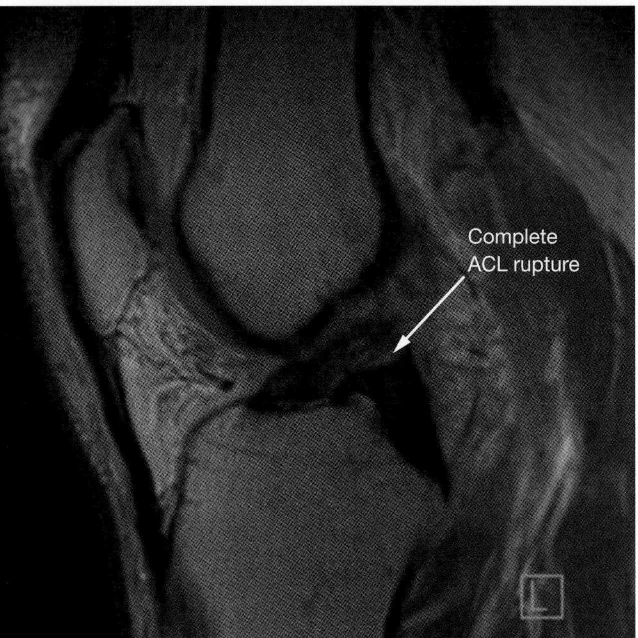

Figure 36.7 Sagittal proton density magnetic resonance image of the knee demonstrating a complete proximal anterior cruciate ligament (ACL) rupture.

Knee anterior cruciate ligament rupture with meniscus tear

Background

Acute knee injuries are extremely common in most sports that require jumping, twisting and contact. Sports with physical impact or tackling, such as rugby or American football, can result in contact knee injuries that often lead to varus or valgus stresses to the knee, resulting in collateral ligament injuries (i.e. lateral collateral ligament or medial collateral ligament) in addition to concomitant cruciate ligament, meniscus or articular cartilage injuries. More frequently, however, acute non-contact injuries of the knee lead to injury to the anterior cruciate ligament (ACL). The most common mechanism of these injuries is a deceleration when the knee falls into valgus and the tibia externally rotates, leading to a subluxation of the knee. These injuries are often associated with either medial or lateral meniscus injuries.

History and physical examination

Patients with an acute ACL injury will often report hearing or feeling a pop in their knee followed by a notable effusion and/or haemarthrosis. Once the effusion resolves, they may report a paucity of knee pain, often leading the patient to believe that the injury has healed itself. However, patients usually present to a physician after attempting subsequent cutting and pivoting activities, which can lead to recurrent instability. Given that the ACL's primary function is to restrict anterior translation of the tibia on the femur, the most commonly utilised tests to evaluate the competency of the ACL are the anterior drawer and Lachman tests (see ***Chapter 35***).

Imaging

The initial evaluation of an acute knee injury with effusion and/or haemarthrosis necessitates radiographic evaluation. AP, lateral and merchant views are the minimum recommended. These radiographs can be useful for identifying any concomitant injuries, including fractures. A Segond fracture located on the anterolateral tibia is pathognomonic for an ACL injury. If an ACL injury is suspected by physical examination, an MRI is performed to better evaluate the intra-articular structures and to aid in surgical planning. A systematic evaluation of the MRI is necessary to ensure that no additional pathology is missed (***Figure 36.7***). 'Kissing lesions' of bony oedema seen on fluid-sensitive sequences on the posterolateral tibia and lateral femoral condyle are also pathognomonic for ACL rupture and represent the pivot shift knee subluxation seen in the setting of ACL rupture.

Treatment

ACL injuries can be managed conservatively through activity modification and bracing. Should these modalities fail, surgery is an excellent option for restoration of knee stability and to decrease the potential for further meniscal or articular cartilage degeneration. ACL repair has recently become a resurging option for proximal-type tears when the ACL can be restored back to its anatomic footprint on the femur. The bridge-enhanced ACL repair (BEAR) technique using a collagen scaffold is currently under clinical trial and may emerge as an option in the future. The gold standard for ACL, however, is reconstruction. In younger patients, large multicentre cohort studies have indicated that autograft reconstruction offers the best durability and lowest chance for re-rupture. Options for autograft reconstruction include bone–patellar tendon–bone, hamstring and quadriceps–tendon autografts. For older and

John W Lachman, 1919–2007, Professor and Chairman of the Orthopedic Department at Temple University in Philadelphia, PA, USA.
Paul Ferdinand Segond, 1851–1912, French surgeon who was a founder of obstetrics and also an expert of the knee, Paris, France.

low-demand patients with symptomatic instability, allograft tendon reconstruction provides an additional graft option.

Meniscal tears are frequently encountered in the setting of ACL rupture.[8] Common tear patterns encountered include radial tears, root tears and bucket-handle tears where the torn portion of the meniscus can flip like a bucket handle into the centre of the joint. Previously, meniscus tears were treated with partial excision to remove any mechanical disruptions and associated pain, but in recent years the joint preservation functions of the menisci as well as their contribution to stability of the knee have been better appreciated, leading to efforts to preserve as much meniscal tissue as possible, especially in younger patients. Various methods of meniscus repair are currently utilised to restore the meniscus anatomy, including all-inside devices, inside-out, outside-in and root repair techniques, the details of which are beyond the scope of this chapter. Biological strategies, to augment the repair, are being evaluated in some centres.

Differential diagnosis

- Patellar dislocation.
- Posterior cruciate ligament rupture.
- Medial collateral ligament knee rupture.
- Posterolateral corner knee ligament injury.
- Patellar tendon rupture.

Summary box 36.4

ACL ruptures

- Mechanism is commonly a non-contact pivoting injury or a direct impact to the lateral knee
- Patients often hear or feel a pop in their knee followed by a notable effusion and may experience instability when returning to cutting and pivoting activities
- Radiographic evaluation includes AP, lateral and merchant views
- MRI is performed to better evaluate the intra-articular structures, aid in surgical planning and ensure that no additional pathology is missed
- ACL injuries can be managed conservatively through activity modification and bracing
- Surgical options include ACL reconstruction (gold standard) and repair in certain select scenarios

Ankle

Low ankle sprains

Background

Ankle sprains are a common injury that can prevent athletes from competing. These injuries are prevalent in sports that involve cutting actions or uneven surfaces while running, such as basketball, rugby, soccer, football and trail running. The ankle primarily resists inversion through the lateral collateral ligament complex, which is composed of the anterior talofibular ligament (ATFL), posterior talofibular ligament (PTFL) and calcaneofibular ligament (CFL). The ATFL is the most frequently injured ligament in the complex; it attaches at the most distal aspect of the fibula and spans anteromedially to the lateral aspect of the talus to prevent inversion during plantarflexion. The CFL is the next most injured ligament; it attaches proximal and posterior to the ATFL origin on the fibula and traverses posteromedially to the lateral aspect of the calcaneus. The position and orientation of the CFL results in resistance against inversion of the ankle while dorsiflexed. The PTFL is the strongest ligament in the complex and is rarely involved in ankle sprains.

History and physical examination

Patients with ankle sprains can often recall the injury and will report the feeling of the ankle inverting. Post injury, many patients will have swelling and bruising on the lateral aspect of their ankle, which can travel to a dependent position on their foot. Examiners should perform all examination manoeuvres on the contralateral and ipsilateral sides to assist in comparisons. The patient may exhibit tenderness to palpation at the lateral collateral ligament complex. The anterior drawer test can be used to evaluate for ATFL injuries. In this test, the ankle is placed into mild plantarflexion while a posterior force is applied to the distal tibia and an anterior translation force is applied to the calcaneus. This test is positive when there is excessive anterior translation of the talus on the tibia compared to the contralateral side. The talar tilt examination evaluates both the CFL and the ATFL. This test is performed with mild plantarflexion of the foot, followed by stabilisation of the distal tibia with one hand while the other hand places varus stress on the talus. Excessive tilt during this manoeuvre is indicative of ATFL injury, whereas CFL injury is indicated by excessive tilt when placing the foot in slight dorsiflexion with varus stress on the talus being applied.

Imaging

Radiographs of the ankle are indicated if the patient fulfils any of the Ottawa ankle rules (***Table 36.1***). Foot radiographs are obtained if the patient has tenderness at the base of the fifth metatarsal or at the navicular bone or if they are unable to bear weight on the foot. Typically, radiographs include weight-bearing AP, mortise and lateral views along with a talar tilt view. These can help rule out other pathologies that may be contributing to ankle pain, such as various types of fractures or osteochondral lesions of the talus. If the examiner is concerned about a high ankle sprain, an external rotation radiograph can be obtained. MRI is not a standard modality utilised in the evaluation of ankle sprains but should be obtained for patients with chronic ankle pain or instability to evaluate for osteochondral lesions of the talus, tendon injury, anterolateral impingement or tibiofibular syndesmosis injury.

TABLE 36.1 Ottawa ankle rules.

- Bone tenderness along the distal 6 cm of the posterior margin or at the tip of the lateral malleolus
- Bone tenderness along the distal 6 cm of the posterior margin or at the tip of the medial malleolus
- Inability to bear weight at the time of the accident or at the time of examination

Treatment

Ankle sprains are often treated conservatively with rest, ice, compression and elevation. Athletes should limit weight-bearing initially, with care being directed towards pain control, reducing swelling and proprioceptive exercises. Strengthening of the peroneal muscles and stretching can occur once the patient is able to tolerate bearing weight on the ankle. Consider supportive braces to further stabilise the ankle from inversion and eversion. Surgery is indicated in patients with persistent pain and recurrent ankle sprains. This can be achieved through anatomical reconstruction by imbrication of the attenuated ATFL with or without reinforcement using the inferior extensor retinaculum.[9] Several non-anatomical lateral ankle ligament reconstruction techniques have also been described for use in chronic ankle instability. The prognosis following an ankle sprain depends on the severity of the injury, but many patients are back participating in sports after a few weeks.

Differential diagnosis

- Anterolateral ankle impingement.
- Peroneal tendon disruption.
- Fracture of the lateral talar process.
- Syndesmotic sprain.
- Osteochondral lesion of the talus.
- Malleolar fracture.
- Lateral process of the calcaneus fracture.

Summary box 36.5

Low ankle sprains

- Common injury among athletes in sports that involve cutting actions or running on uneven surfaces
- Patients may report the feeling of the ankle inverting and present with subsequent swelling and bruising on the lateral aspect of their ankle
- Radiographs of the ankle are indicated if the patient fulfils any of the Ottawa ankle rules
- Foot radiographs are obtained if the patient has tenderness at the base of the fifth metatarsal or at the navicular bone or if they are unable to bear weight on the foot
- Ankle sprains are often treated conservatively with rest, ice, compression and elevation
- Surgery is indicated in patients with persistent pain and recurrent ankle sprains

INJURIES ASSOCIATED WITH INDIVIDUAL SPORTS

Golf

The shoulder and the back are the common sites of overuse injuries. Golfer's elbow or medial epicondylitis is due to a common flexor origin tendinosis that also commonly occurs in weightlifters and rodeo athletes.

Tennis

Tennis elbow or lateral epicondylitis is angiofibrous dysplasia of the common extensor origin. Treatment consists of bracing, activity modification, injection (with some centres using platelet-rich plasma) and surgery if conservative measures fail.

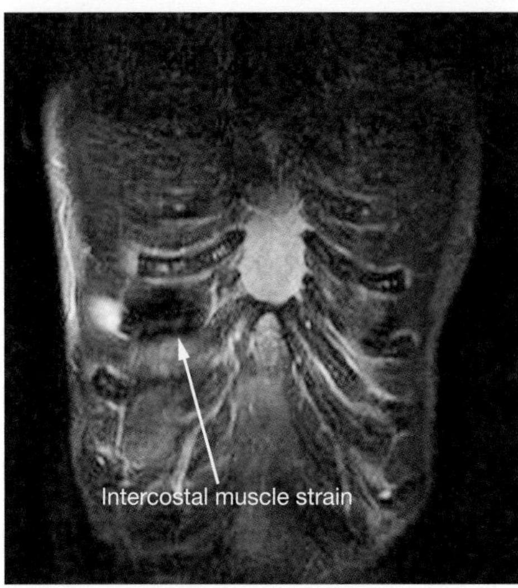

Figure 36.8 Coronal magnetic resonance imaging scan of the chest showing an intercostal muscle injury in a rower.

Partial ruptures of the calf muscles, especially the medial head of the gastrocnemius, are also found in tennis players (called tennis leg), and in patients who take part in other sports requiring sudden extreme acceleration.

Rowing

The common injuries that are encountered in rowing but that are rare in other athletics include rib stress fractures and intercostal muscle tears (***Figure 36.8***), which occur from the repetitive engagement of the latissimus dorsi muscles. Forearm tendon issues such as intersection syndrome (a tendinosis where the first and second extensor tendon compartments of the forearm cross) are also a commonly encountered problem in rowing athletes.

American football

This contact sport produces a variety of unique injuries, the main ones of which are closed head injuries, fractures, hip dislocations, twisting injuries to the knees and ankles leading to ligament tears, and turf toe.

Rugby

This is a high-intensity contact sport. Patients present with neck injuries including fractures of the cervical spine; acromioclavicular joint and finger injuries including dislocation of the phalanges; and tendon injuries such as jersey finger, in which there is injury to the flexor digitorum profundus tendon.

Javelin

Javelin throwers experience various injuries to the kinetic chain given the violent and abrupt throwing approach. Injuries due to abnormal stresses on the elbow are similar to those seen in baseball. This causes abnormalities of the hip, shoulder, UCL and phalanges.

Swimming

Shoulder injuries are more common in swimmers, especially in those performing the crawl or the butterfly stroke because of multidirectional instability, which can provide a competitive advantage for swimming but can become pathological.

Ballet dancing

Ballet dancers have problems with posterior impingement of the ankle and tendinopathy of the flexor hallucis longus tendon when working *en pointe* (tiptoe). Stress fractures are also found in female dancers as a result of repetitive training and can be more frequent in the female athlete triad (osteoporosis, disordered eating and amenorrhoea) (***Figure 36.9***).

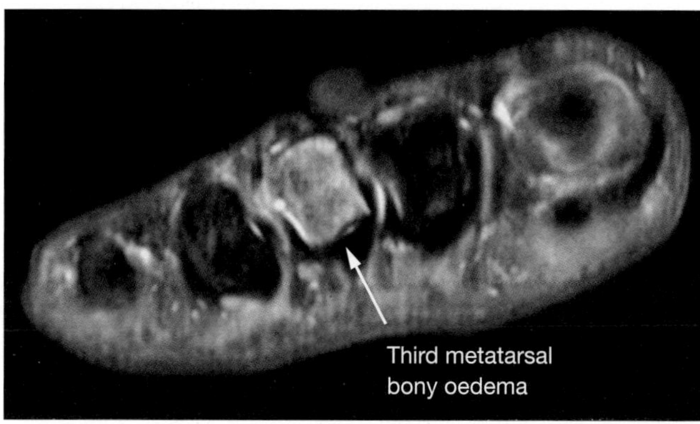

Figure 36.9 Magnetic resonance imaging short T1 inversion recovery axial sequence showing a stress injury to a metatarsal.

Snowboarding and skiing

Participants in both snowboarding and skiing have the full range of injuries associated with these high-speed sports. The rigid high boots used by skiers protect the ankle but increase the loads transmitted up the limb, risking fracture of the tibia and ligament disruption of the knee (especially the anterior cruciate). Novice snowboarders tend to get wrist fractures, while all levels of snowboarder can injure the acromioclavicular joint.

Marathon running

Most common problems include electrolyte abnormalities during events and iliotibial band syndrome and stress fractures in the feet and shins chronically.

SUMMARY

Athletic activities commonly result in a variety of injuries. For providers who take care of athletes, a basic knowledge of both common injuries and treatment algorithms as well as various sport-specific injury patterns is necessary to provide optimal care.

ACKNOWLEDGEMENT

The authors are grateful for and wish to acknowledge the contribution of Dylan Rakowski MD in the preparation of this chapter.

FURTHER READING

1 Goldenberg BT, Lacheta L, Rosenberg SI *et al.* Comprehensive review of the physical exam for glenohumeral instability. *Phys Sportsmed* 2020; **48**(2): 142–50.
2 Norte GE, West A, Gnacinski M *et al.* On-field management of the acute anterior glenohumeral dislocation. *Phys Sportsmed* 2011; **39**(3): 151–62.
3 Godin JA, Altintas B, Horan MP *et al.* Midterm results of the bony Bankart bridge technique for the treatment of bony Bankart lesions. *Am J Sports Med* 2019; **47**(1): 158–64.
4 Martetschläger F, Kraus TM, Hardy P, Millett PJ. Arthroscopic management of anterior shoulder instability with glenoid bone defects. *Knee Surg Sports Traumatol Arthrosc* 2013; **21**(12): 2867-76.
5 Bhatia S, Greenspoon JA, Horan MP *et al.* Two-year outcomes after arthroscopic rotator cuff repair in recreational athletes older than 70 years. *Am J Sports Med* 2015; **43**(7): 1737–42.
6 Jones KJ, Osbahr DC, Schrumpf MA *et al.* Ulnar collateral ligament reconstruction in throwing athletes: a review of current concepts. AAOS exhibit selection. *J Bone Joint Surg Am* 2012; **94**(8): e49.
7 Philippon MJ, Maxwell RB, Johnston TL *et al.* Clinical presentation of femoroacetabular impingement. *Knee Surg Sports Traumatol Arthrosc* 2007; **15**(8): 1041–7.
8 Millett PJ, Willis AA, Warren RF. Associated injuries in pediatric and adolescent anterior cruciate ligament tears: does a delay in treatment increase the risk of meniscal tear? *Arthroscopy* 2002; **18**(9): 955–9.
9 Chen ET, Borg-Stein J, McInnis KC. Ankle sprains: evaluation, rehabilitation, and prevention. *Curr Sports Med Rep* 2019; **18**(6): 217–23.

CHAPTER 37 The spine

Learning objectives

To learn:
- The salient features relating to the history and examination of the spine
- The investigations commonly used in the field of spinal disorders
- The treatment principles for common conditions affecting the spine
- The global issues in spinal surgery

EPIDEMIOLOGY

The lifetime prevalence of low back pain has been reported to be 60–80%. By contrast, the lifetime prevalence of true sciatica is 2–4%. It is generally accepted that 90% of acute low back pain episodes settle, allowing return to work within 6 weeks. However, some 5–7% of the population aged between 45 and 64 years will report back problems as a 'chronic sickness'. Up to 70% of acute episodes of sciatica resolve within 3 months.

Summary box 37.1

Epidemiology
- Low back pain is extremely common
- 90% of acute low back pain episodes settle within 6 weeks
- Sciatica is much less frequent
- 70% of acute sciatic episodes settle within 3 months

CLINICAL ANATOMY

The normal cervical lordosis measures between 35° and 45°. The normal lumbar lordosis is between 40° and 80° (mean 60°) and decreases with age. Most lumbar lordosis occurs between L4 and S1. The normal thoracic kyphosis is between 20° and 50° (mean 35°) and increases with age. When standing, the normal sagittal vertical axis (sagittal plumb line) falls from the odontoid process through the C7/T1 disc space and crosses the spinal column at the T12/L1 disc space, before reaching the posterosuperior corner of the S1 vertebral body. For an energy-efficient posture, cervical and lumbar lordosis will balance thoracic kyphosis.

The spinal canal is formed behind the articulated vertebral body by the posterior elements of the vertebral column and can be divided into a **central** portion and two **lateral** portions. The central portion is occupied by the thecal sac containing the spinal cord, which terminates behind the body of L1. The lateral portions contain the nerve roots.

The spinal nerve roots comprise 8 cervical, 12 thoracic, 5 lumbar, 5 sacral and 1 coccygeal. Dorsal and ventral roots join to form spinal nerves. The ventral root and the dorsal root ganglion lie within the intervertebral foramen. This foramen is bounded superiorly and inferiorly by pedicles, anteriorly by the disc and posteriorly by the facet joint. Degenerative changes in these structures may lead to neural compromise. Laminar overlap within the lumbar spine decreases from L1 to S1 so that, at the L5/S1 level, access to the intervertebral disc requires less bone removal than at a more proximal level.

The blood supply of the spinal cord is derived from the vertebral, deep cervical, intercostal and lumbar arteries. The arteries of the spinal cord include the anterior spinal artery and two posterior spinal arteries, with the anterior spinal artery providing the majority of the vascular supply to the spinal cord. The radicular artery of Adamkiewicz makes a major contribution to the anterior spinal artery, supplying the lower spinal cord. It originates on the left in 80% of people, usually accompanying the ventral root of T9, T10 or T11, but can originate anywhere from T5 to L5. Ligation of this important artery may lead to critical ischaemia of the spinal cord. Ligating segmental vessels over the midpoint of the vertebral body will minimise the risk of injury to this important artery during anterior approaches to the spine.

PATIENT HISTORY

The commonest reasons for referral to a spinal clinic include **pain** and **spinal deformity**. A detailed history of the pain, including site, type, severity, duration, frequency and aggravating factors, should be sought. Has there been any history of

Albert Adamkiewicz, 1850–1921, Professor of Pathology, the University of Kraków (Cracow), Poland, described the arterial supply to the spinal cord in 1882.

trauma? Is the pain present at night? Is there associated pain in the upper limbs (brachialgia) or lower limbs (sciatica)? Is there associated numbness, tingling, weakness or difficulty with gait? Is there a family history of ankylosing spondylitis or rheumatoid arthritis? Are there concurrent medical conditions such as diabetes, peripheral vascular diseases, osteoarthritis of the hip or previous malignancies? Are there systemic symptoms such as unexplained weight loss, chills or fever?

Patients should always be asked about the presence of perineal numbness (saddle area) and difficulties or changes in sensation when passing urine or faeces, as these symptoms may indicate a cauda equina syndrome (CES) (***Table 37.1***).

Patients should be asked whether the pain is interfering with their ability to work. What treatment has the patient already tried and how effective were these treatments (e.g. analgesics, exercise, physiotherapy or spinal injections)? Pending litigation or worker's compensation claims may have a negative prognostic effect on future treatments.

Spinal deformities, e.g. scoliosis and excessive kyphosis (>50°), are generally painless in children but may be symptomatic in adult life. How quickly has the spinal deformity progressed? It is important to assess skeletal maturity and whether the child has gone through a recent growth spurt. Has menstruation commenced in the female or has the voice dropped in the male, indicating the onset of puberty?

TABLE 37.1 Cauda equina syndrome

- Low back pain
- Uni- or bilateral sciatica
- Saddle anaesthesia
- Motor weakness in the lower extremities
- Variable rectal and urinary symptoms

PHYSICAL EXAMINATION

The patient should be undressed and posture should be evaluated in both frontal and sagittal planes. Shoulder or waist asymmetry suggests the presence of scoliosis. The Adams forward bend test will accentuate trunk asymmetry and allow appreciation of rib or loin prominence on the convex side of each curve. The skin should be examined for cutaneous neurofibromata, café-au-lait patches or axillary freckling commonly present in neurofibromatosis. Neurological examination should include abdominal reflexes. Leg lengths should be measured. In the case of kyphosis, the sagittal alignment and forward gaze should be assessed.

Palpation is useful to locate specific areas of tenderness. The normal range of motion in the cervical spine is 45° of flexion, 55° of extension, 70° of rotation and 40° of lateral bend. The normal range of motion in the lumbar spine is 40–60° of flexion, 20–35° of extension, 15–20° of lateral bending and 3–18° of rotation. Schober's test is a simple clinical test to evaluate spinal mobility. A tape measure is used to mark the skin midway between the posterior superior iliac spines and at points 10 cm proximal and 5 cm distal to this mark while the patient is standing. The patient is then asked to bend forwards as far as possible and the distance between the two points is measured with the patient in the flexed position. Normally one would expect to see an increase of at least 5 cm between the two points in the erect and flexed positions. A distance of less than 5 cm between these points may indicate ankylosing spondylitis.

Neurological examination of the upper and lower limbs will focus on tone, power, coordination, reflexes, sensation and gait (***Tables 37.2 and 37.3***). A rectal examination and assessment of perineal sensation should be performed if there is any concern about cauda equina integrity. The superficial abdominal reflex is an upper motor neurone (UMN) reflex. It is performed by stroking one of four abdominal quadrants in succession. The umbilicus should move towards the quadrant that was stroked. The reflex should be symmetrical from side to side. Absent or asymmetrical abdominal reflexes may indicate intraspinal pathology such as syringomyelia or spinal cord injury.

Myelopathy or UMN lesions are reported by spasticity, motor weakness, hyper-reflexia, positive Hoffmann's sign (forced flexion of the distal phalanx of the middle finger results in flexion of the thumb and index finger), upgoing Babinski response and patellar and ankle clonus.

Summary box 37.2

UMN lesions are characterised by:

- Increased tone – spastic
- Hyper-reflexia
- Muscle spasms
- Motor weakness
- Disuse atrophy
- Positive Hoffmann's sign
- Ankle and patellar clonus
- Upgoing plantar response

Typical signs of radiculopathy (lower motor neurone [LMN] lesion) include sensory loss, motor weakness, flaccid paralysis, muscle atrophy, loss of reflexes and muscle fasciculation. The straight leg raise (SLR) test is performed with the patient in the supine position. The leg is elevated with the knee straight to increase tension along the L5 and S1 nerve roots. The test is positive if the leg elevation provokes radicular pain. The crossed SLR test is carried out by elevating the asymptomatic leg; if positive, this produces sciatic symptoms in the opposite leg. A positive test is associated with a herniated disc

William Adams, 1820–1900, described the forward bending test for scoliosis in 1865. His understanding of the nature of the rotational element of scoliosis was given by a postmortem examination he performed on an eminent surgeon and geologist, Gideon Mantell.
Paul Schober, 1865–1943, German physician.
Johann Hoffmann, 1857–1919, Professor of Neurology, Heidelberg, Germany.
Joseph Francis Felix Babinski, 1857–1932, neurologist, Hôpital de la Pitié, Paris, France.

TABLE 37.2 Neurological evaluation of the upper limb.

Neurological level	Motor	Sensation	Reflexes
C5	Deltoid	Lateral arm	Biceps (C5/6)
C6	Wrist extensors	Lateral forearm	Brachioradialis (C5/6)
C7	Triceps	Middle finger	Triceps (C7/8)
C8	Long finger flexors	Medial forearm	No reflex
T1	Interosseus muscles	Medial arm	No reflex

TABLE 37.3 Neurological evaluation of the lower limb.

Neurological level	Motor	Sensation	Reflexes
L2	Hip flexion	Anterior thigh, groin	No reflex
L3	Knee extension	Anterior and lateral thigh	Patellar (L3/4)
L4	Ankle dorsiflexion	Medial leg and foot	Patellar (L3/4)
L5	Extensor hallucis longus	Lateral leg and foot	No reflex
S1	Ankle plantarflexion	Lateral foot and little toe	Achilles (S1/2)

in 97% of patients. Lasègue's sign denotes radicular pain aggravated by ankle dorsiflexion.

The femoral nerve stretch test is performed with the patient in the prone position by extending the hip and flexing the knee. This creates tension on the L2, L3 and L4 nerve roots. The femoral nerve stretch test is considered positive if radicular pain occurs in the anterior thigh region during the test.

The examination should include, where appropriate, examination of the shoulder, hip, knee, sacroiliac joint and vascular system, as dual pathology is common in the ageing community.

In 1979, Waddell and colleagues (see ***Further reading***) developed and validated a series of signs and tests that have proved helpful in identifying individuals who are magnifying or exaggerating symptoms, possibly for secondary gain (***Table 37.4***)

TABLE 37.4 Non-organic physical signs in low back pain.

- **Tenderness:** superficial or non-anatomical
- **Simulation tests***:* axial loading or rotation
- **Distraction tests***:* variable straight leg raises
- **Regional disturbances***:* non-anatomical sensory or motor loss
- **Over-reaction***:* grimacing, muscle tremor, etc.

Summary box 37.3

LMN lesions are characterised by:

- Decreased tone – flaccid
- Hyporeflexia
- Denervation fasciculations
- Motor weakness
- Sensory loss
- Severe atrophy
- Downgoing plantar response

Red flags

After taking a history and examining the patient it is important to consider 'red flags' (***Table 37.5***), which allow diagnostic triage into those with serious pathology of the spine, such as CES, fractures, tumours and infection, and those without.

Non-spinal causes of back pain

Pain may arise from the spine, but non-spinal causes of pain must also be considered (***Table 37.6***).

INVESTIGATIONS

The most common diagnostic imaging tests used to evaluate spinal disorders include plain radiographs, computed tomography (CT), magnetic resonance imaging (MRI), CT myelography and isotope bone scanning. These investigations are extremely sensitive, but relatively non-specific. For example, at least one-third of asymptomatic patients have been noted to have 'abnormalities' on MRI scans. All investigations must therefore be carefully correlated with the clinical findings.

Plain radiographs

It is not appropriate to order spine radiographs for every patient presenting with neck or low back pain. Patients with red flag signs or symptoms and those who have not responded to conservative treatment require imaging, with most units in resource-rich countries utilising MRI (no radiation penalty) in this situation. Standing radiographs of the whole spine are important for the assessment of scoliosis. Radiographs cannot diagnose early-stage tumour or infection, because significant bone destruction (between 40% and 60% of bone mass) must occur before a radiographic abnormality is detected.

Charles Ernest Lasègue, 1816–1863, Professor of Medicine, University of Paris, and physician, La Salpêtrière, Paris, France

TABLE 37.5 'Red flags': serious conditions whose signs and symptoms can cause low back pain.

Condition	Signs and symptoms
Cauda equina syndrome	• Severe or progressive bilateral neurological deficit of the legs, such as major motor weakness with knee extension, ankle eversion or foot dorsiflexion
	• Recent-onset urinary retention (caused by bladder distension because the sensation of fullness is lost) and/or urinary incontinence or alteration of function (caused by loss of sensation when passing urine)
	• Recent-onset faecal incontinence (due to loss of sensation of rectal fullness)
	• Perianal or perineal sensory loss (saddle anaesthesia or paraesthesia)
	• Unexpected laxity of the anal sphincter
Spinal fracture	• Sudden onset of severe central spinal pain that is relieved by lying down
	• A history of major trauma (e.g. road traffic collision or fall from a height), minor trauma or just strenuous lifting in people with osteoporosis who take corticosteroids
	• Structural deformity of the spine such as a step from one vertebra to an adjacent vertebra
	• There may be point tenderness over a vertebral body
Cancer	• The person being 50 years of age or more
	• Gradual onset of symptoms
	• Severe unremitting pain that remains when the person is supine, aching night pain that prevents or disturbs sleep, pain aggravated by straining (for example, at stool or when coughing or sneezing) and thoracic pain
	• Localised spinal tenderness
	• No symptomatic improvement after 4–6 weeks of conservative low back pain therapy
	• Unexplained weight loss
	• Past history of cancer; breast, lung, gastrointestinal, prostate, renal and thyroid cancers are more likely to metastasise to the spine
Infection (such as discitis, vertebral osteomyelitis or spinal epidural abscess)	• Fever
	• Tuberculosis or recent urinary tract infection
	• Diabetes
	• History of intravenous drug use
	• HIV infection, use of immunosuppressants or where the person is otherwise immunocompromised

HIV, human immunodeficiency virus.

TABLE 37.6 Non-spinal causes of low back pain: referred pain.

- Respiratory, e.g. mesothelioma
- Vascular, e.g. abdominal aortic aneurysm
- Renal, e.g. pyelonephritis
- Gastrointestinal, e.g. peptic ulcer, pancreatitis
- Urogenital, e.g. testicular, ovarian or prostatic carcinoma

Computed tomography

This investigation is the best test for assessing bone anatomy. Three-dimensional reconstructions are often useful for the assessment of congenital spinal deformity. However, one should remember that a typical CT of the lumbar spine will expose the patient to an effective dose of 5–10 millisieverts (mSv), which would be equivalent to 2.5–5 years of natural background radiation; those who travel on 7-hour flights (0.05 mSv per 7-hour flight) would need to make 100–200 journeys in their lifetime to be exposed to the same effective dose.

Magnetic resonance imaging

This allows detailed visualisation of the spinal cord, thecal sac, epidural space, intervertebral discs, nerve roots, paraspinal soft tissues and bone marrow. It is contraindicated for patients with certain pacemakers and coronary stents, intracranial metal clips, metallic bodies in the eye, spinal cord stimulators and certain drug pumps.

Bone scintigraphy

Isotope bone scans are highly sensitive, but non-specific, tests that are useful for screening the skeletal system for metastatic disease, discitis or vertebral body osteomyelitis, or to assess the relative activity of bone lesions such as osteoid osteoma, osteoblastoma, defects in the pars interarticularis or a pseudarthrosis (incomplete fusion). In the case of multiple myeloma or purely lytic metastases, the bone scan may not show increased activity as these tumours may not stimulate a significant **osteoblastic** response.

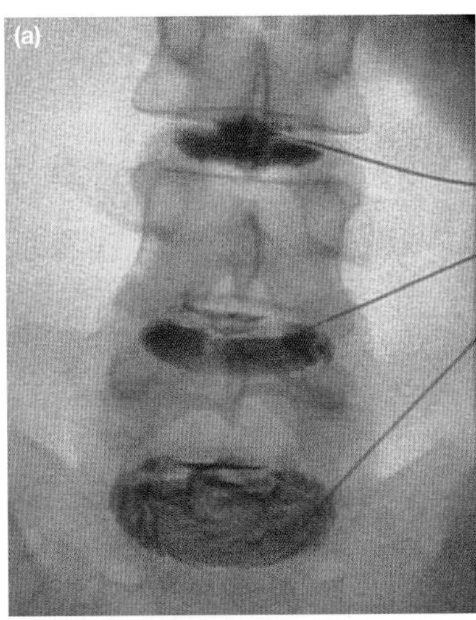

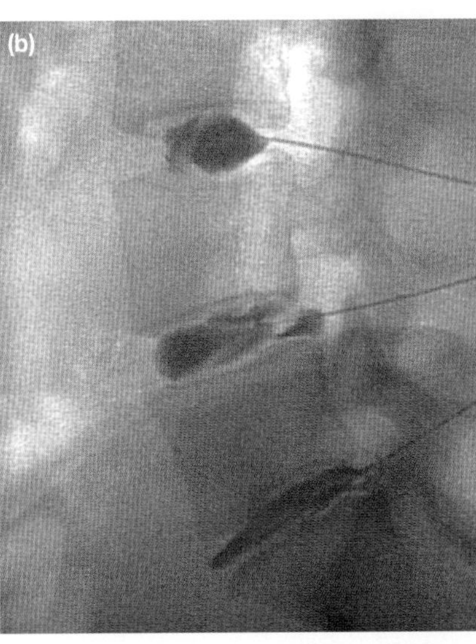

Figure 37.1 Lumbar discography. Anteroposterior (a) and lateral (b) radiographs following injection of contrast medium into the lower three lumbar discs. Morphology: L3/4 cotton ball, L4/5 fissured, L5/S1 ruptured. Concordant low back pain was reproduced when injecting the L4/5 and L5/S1 discs. No pain was experienced when the L3/4 disc was injected. The patient underwent a posterolateral fusion L4 to S1.

Bone densitometry

Bone density and osteoporosis can be measured using dual energy x-ray absorptiometry (DEXA) of the hip, wrist and spine.

Provocative discography

This investigation involves the placement of a 24-gauge needle into the centre of the intervertebral disc in a conscious patient. Radio-opaque contrast agent (1–3.5 mL) is then injected into the disc. The contrast pattern will allow the discrimination of different degrees of disc degeneration; cotton ball or lobular would be considered normal whereas irregular, fissured or ruptured would be considered degenerate (***Figure 37.1***). The patient is asked if they are experiencing their 'usual type of back pain'. To diagnose discogenic low back pain one must document evidence of disc degeneration and concordant pain during the injection. Treatment options may include spinal fusion or disc replacement.

Facet joint injections

For patients with facet joint arthropathy, x-ray-guided local anaesthetic and steroid injections may be both diagnostic and therapeutic for 4–6 weeks. Longer term relief may be obtained by facet joint rhizolysis. This percutaneous procedure denervates the facet joint.

Foraminal epidural steroid injections

For patients with radiculopathy due to a prolapsed intervertebral disc or lateral recess stenosis, a targeted foraminal epidural injection of local anaesthetic and steroid may provide important diagnostic information and have a lasting therapeutic effect.

Spinal biopsy

Either CT-guided or open biopsy is often performed to obtain tissue for diagnostic study in cases of suspected tumour and/or infection.

DEGENERATIVE CONDITIONS OF THE SPINE

Cervical radiculopathy

Patients present with neck and arm pain (brachialgia), paraesthesia and motor weakness in the distribution of the compromised nerve root (radiculopathy). This may be caused by disc herniation or degenerative stenosis. Symptoms often respond to conservative treatment, including physiotherapy and medication for neuropathic pain (amitriptyline, gabapentin or pregabalin), or CT-guided foraminal epidural steroid injections of local anaesthetic and steroid. Intractable pain and/or functional neurological deficit are indications for surgical intervention. Surgical options include anterior cervical discectomy and fusion (using a cage packed with bone graft and plate), cervical total disc replacement (***Figure 37.2***) or posterior procedures to enlarge the canal such as laminoplasty and laminoforaminotomy. Randomised controlled trials have compared anterior cervical discectomy and fusion with cervical disc replacement. Similar clinical outcomes have been observed in both groups. However, cervical disc replacements preserve motion in the operated level and may protect against adjacent segment disease in the longer term.

Cervical myelopathy

Degenerative change in the cervical spine leading to spinal cord compression is the commonest cause of cervical myelopathy in patients over 55 years of age. LMN changes occur **at the level** of the lesion, with atrophy of the upper extremity muscles, particularly the intrinsic muscles of the hands. UMN findings are noted **below** the level of the lesion and may involve both upper and lower extremities. If surgery is considered an anterior or posterior decompression may be required.

Thoracic disc herniation

Thoracic disc herniations that require surgical intervention are rare, accounting for less than 2% of all discectomy procedures.

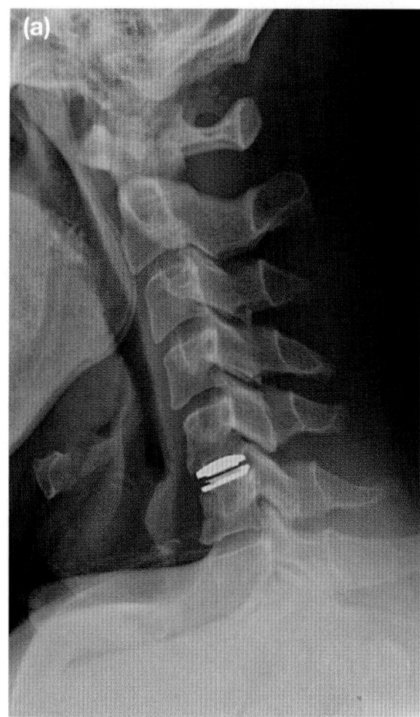

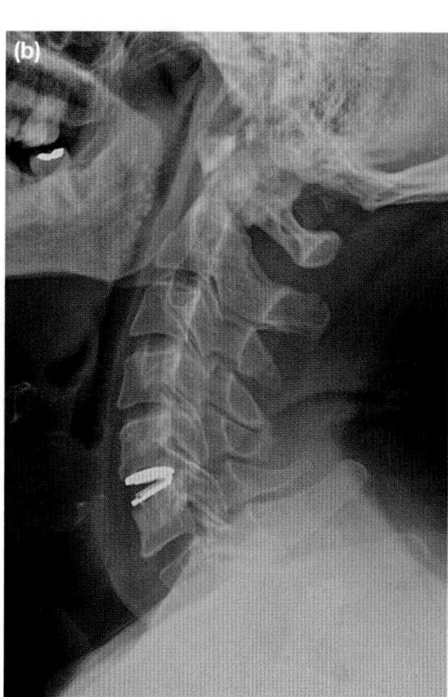

Figure 37.2 Cervical total disc replacement. The patient presented with severe left-sided C6 radiculopathy. Magnetic resonance imaging scan confirmed a left C5/6 disc herniation. The patient underwent a C5/6 discectomy and decompression of the left traversing C6 nerve root, followed by insertion of a cervical disc replacement. Lateral radiographs in flexion (a) and extension (b) show restored motion to the C5/6 level.

Typically, the patient presents with axial pain, radiculopathy or myelopathy. Conservative treatment including non-steroidal anti-inflammatory drugs, physiotherapy and general fitness improvement should be considered initially. If required, thoracic discectomy may be performed via thoracotomy or, for a soft disc prolapse, via a thoracoscopic approach.

Cauda equina syndrome

CES is a very serious and urgent condition that arises from compression of the cauda equina nerve roots, which supply the perineum and genital regions and bladder, bowel and sexual function. The most frequent cause is a massive central lumbar disc protrusion at L4/5 or L5/S1; other causes include lumbar fractures, postoperative epidural haematoma, spinal stenosis and spinal tumours. Occlusion of the lumbar arteries by dissection or aneurysm of the abdominal aorta can lead to similar dysfunction of the cauda equina without compression.

CES is rare, accounting for only 2–6% of all lumbar disc herniations. However, it is important as timely treatment can prevent catastrophic incontinence; delay in treatment is a major cause of litigation in many countries.

CES presents most commonly in the 20- to 45-year age group, with some or all of the following symptoms: low back pain; unilateral or bilateral sciatica; lower limb motor weakness; and sensory abnormalities, including saddle anaesthesia, bladder dysfunction (initially sensory changes, later painless retention and overflow incontinence in later stages) and sexual and bowel dysfunction. CES may result from acute or chronic compression of the cauda equina nerve roots.

TABLE 37.7 Classification of cauda equina syndrome (CES).

Name	Abbreviation	Definition	Investigation after initial diagnosis	Treatment if MRI positive for compression of CES
CES suspected	CES-S	Large disc herniation or bilateral sciatica but normal S2–5 motor and sensory function	MRI within 24 hours	Discuss risks and benefits of surgery versus conservative treatment
CES early	CES-E	Some perineal sensory change but normal bladder and bowel function	MRI immediate	Urgent decompression
CES incomplete	CES-I	Impaired bladder function or sensation but executive/ voluntary control of bladder maintained	MRI immediate	Urgent decompression
CES retention	CES-R	Bladder retention and overflow incontinence	MRI immediate	Urgent decompression on next daytime list if patient presents overnight
CES complete	CES-C	Complete loss of cauda equina function	MRI in working hours	Decompression if improvement considered possible

MRI, magnetic resonance imaging.

Cauda equina nerve roots lack epineurium and perineurium and only have a thin endoneurium root sheath, making them more susceptible to compression forces when compared with peripheral nerves. The syndrome can result in permanent motor deficit and bladder, bowel and sexual dysfunction. It represents a true spinal emergency and requires urgent surgical decompression. The outcome for patients who undergo surgical decompression within 24 hours of the onset of loss of bladder or bowel control is significantly better than that of those who undergo surgery beyond this 24-hour period.

Cauda equina syndrome classification

The key classification of CES (***Table 37.7***) is into cases where there is still executive or voluntary control of the bladder (CES-I) and cases where there is bladder retention and overflow incontinence (CES-R). CES-I cases are considered to be more urgently in need of decompression to prevent deterioration to CES-R. Most surgeons now believe that continued compression causes a continuous deterioration in function and therefore early decompression is of benefit.

Summary box 37.4

Cauda equina syndrome

- Commonest presenting symptoms: perineal numbness, alteration in bladder function and sensation leading to painless urinary retention, overflow incontinence and faecal incontinence
- Urgent investigation with MRI is required for all suspected cases
- Confirmed CES requires surgical decompression within 24 hours to achieve optimum outcomes

Lumbar disc herniation

Symptomatic lumbar disc herniation occurs during the lifetime in approximately 2–4% of the population. Risk factors include family history, male gender, age (30–50 years), heavy lifting or twisting, stressful occupation, lower income and cigarette smoking.

Over 90% of lumbar disc herniations occur at the L4/5 or L5/S1 levels. A posterolateral disc protrusion will affect the **traversing** root, e.g. an L4/5 disc protrusion will affect the L5 nerve root. A far-lateral disc protrusion (extraforaminal) will affect the **exiting** nerve root, e.g. a far-lateral L5/S1 disc protrusion will affect the L5 nerve root. Symptoms typically commence with a period of back pain followed by sciatica. There may be paraesthesia, motor weakness, loss of reflexes and a reduction in SLR.

For simple sciatica, a period of 6–12 weeks of conservative treatment is advised. Up to 70% of patients will settle within this period. A trial of pregabalin (GABA analogue) and/or a transforaminal epidural steroid injection may be helpful. Microdiscectomy is the standard surgical intervention for those in whom conservative treatment has failed. The procedure is carried out in the prone position with radiographic confirmation of the correct level. Loupes with a headlight or use of the operating microscope greatly facilitate the procedure. A 3- to 4-cm incision is made with a unilateral take down of the multifidus. The spinal canal is entered via removal of the ligamentum flavum under the lamina. The thecal sac and traversing nerve root are identified. The dura and nerve root are retracted medially and the offending disc prolapse incised via a transverse annulotomy. The disc fragment is removed and the disc space cleared of any remaining nuclear material with rongeurs and multiple washouts of the disc space. The wound is closed. Patients are generally discharged the next morning.

Spinal stenosis

Spinal stenosis may be defined as any type of narrowing of the spinal canal, nerve root canal or intervertebral foramen. The resultant nerve root compression leads to nerve root ischaemia, presenting with back, buttock or leg pain provoked by exercise. Spinal stenosis may be congenital, as is the case in achondroplasia, or acquired, as is the case for degenerative types (commonly presenting between 50 and 70 years of age). The narrowing is caused by facet joint hypertrophy, disc bulging and ligamentum flavum thickening.

Symptoms of spinal claudication can be distinguished from vascular claudication because they are frequently associated with neurological symptoms, are often worse in extension and pedal pulses are present on clinical examination. Symptoms progress in approximately 20–33% of patients who receive no treatment. The condition may be treated successfully by surgical decompression alone with preservation of the facet joints.

Summary box 37.5

Spinal stenosis

- Extremely common condition in the 50- to 70-year age group
- Classic symptoms: back, buttock, thigh and calf pain
- Provoked by walking and extended posture
- Relieved by flexed posture
- Symptoms progress in up to one-third of untreated patients

Discogenic low back pain

Discogenic low back pain has been defined as a continuum of diagnostic categories (internal disc disruption, degenerative disc disease, segmental instability) reflecting various stages of degenerative pathology affecting the intervertebral disc. Not all degenerate discs are painful. Patients typically present with chronic relapsing episodes of low back pain between the ages of 40 and 60 years.

A recent study has compared rehabilitation with spinal fusion for discogenic pain. Both groups reported reductions in disability, with the authors strongly recommending a course of rehabilitation **before** surgical intervention. For those who fail to improve with conservative measures, provocative lumbar discography (***Figure 37.1***) may help to identify the source of pain, and surgery in the form of a lumbar spinal fusion (***Figure 37.3***) or lumbar disc replacement (***Figure 37.4***) may be considered.

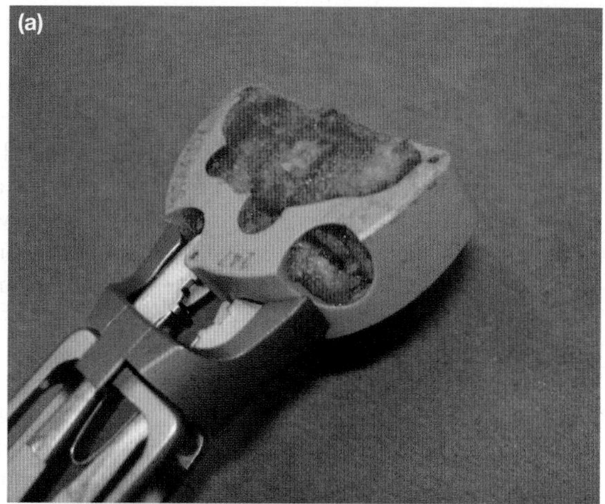

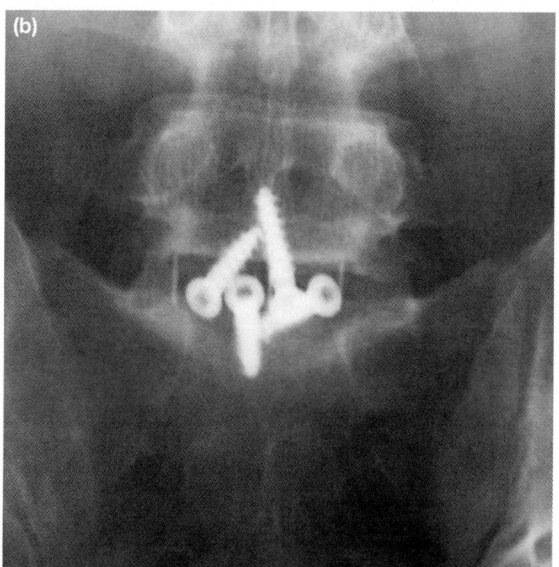

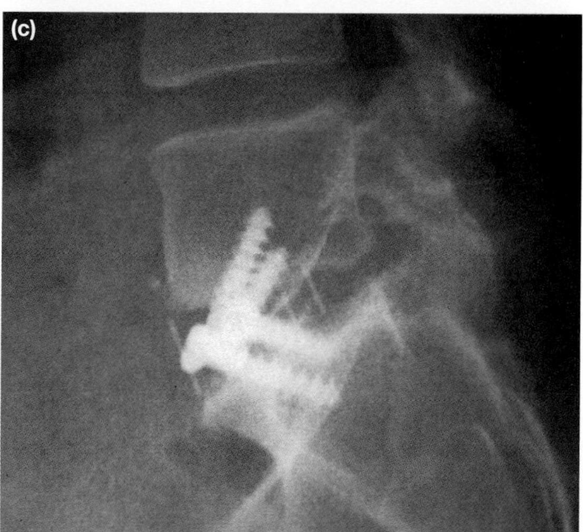

Figure 37.3 Anterior lumbar interbody fusion. (a) The PEEK (poly-ethyl-ethyl-ketone) cage has been packed with bone graft prior to insertion; (b, c) show the anteroposterior and lateral postoperative radiographs, respectively.

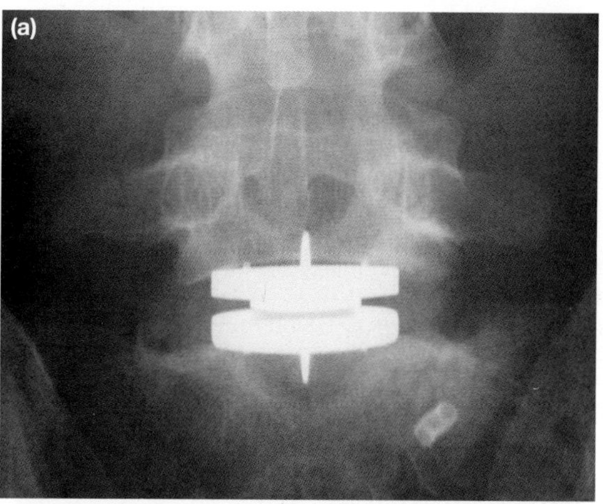

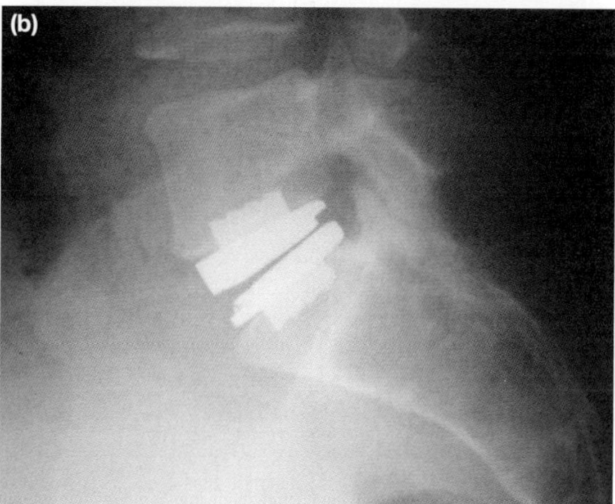

Figure 37.4 Lumbar total disc replacement. (a) Anteroposterior radiograph with 30° of cranial inclination. (b) Lateral radiograph with the implant appropriately positioned.

SPONDYLOLYSIS AND SPONDYLOLISTHESIS

Spondylolysis

This is a unilateral or bilateral defect in the pars interarticularis without vertebral slippage. The incidence is reported in approximately 6% by the age of 14 years, but is much higher in the young athletic population. The diagnosis is difficult to confirm with plain radiographs. Reverse gantry CT, MRI and single photon emission computed tomography (SPECT) are useful investigations for this condition. Treatment involves rest, non-steroidal anti-inflammatory medication, activity modification and a lumbosacral orthosis. For patients who remain symptomatic despite an adequate trial of non-operative care, surgery in the form of a direct repair of the pseudarthrosis by a Buck's fusion may be indicated.

J E Buck, surgeon, Brook General Hospital, London, UK, described the direct repair of the defect in spondylolisthesis in 1970.

Summary box 37.6

Spondylolysis

- Incidence in general population 6% by 14 years
- Incidence in athletic population 15–47%
- May be completely asymptomatic/incidental finding on radiograph
- Difficult to image, but MRI proving more useful
- Conservative treatment: activity modification, anti-lordotic brace
- Surgical treatment: direct repair preserving motion or spinal fusion if associated disc degeneration

Spondylolisthesis

Spondylolisthesis is a forward slippage of the vertebral body engendered by a break in the continuity or elongation of the pars interarticularis and presents in 4% of the adult population. Spondylolisthesis can be classified into six types by causation (*Table 37.8*) or by the degree of slip (*Table 37.9*).

For skeletally immature patients (<18 years old) who have progressive slips in the spine, and in individuals with intractable low back or radicular pain or neurological symptoms, surgery may be indicated. For low-grade slips (Meyerding grades I and II) fusion-*in-situ* is the procedure of choice. If there is **objective** evidence of neural compression (e.g. weakness of extensor hallucis longus), a spinal decompression should be performed at the same time. For high-grade slips (Meyerding grades III or IV) (*Figure 37.5*), opinion is divided on whether to reduce the slip first and then fuse, or simply to fuse *in situ*.

TABLE 37.8 Wiltse classification of spondylolisthesis (see *Further reading*).

Type 1	Dysplastic	• Associated with congenital deficiency of the L5/S1 articulation
Type 2	Isthmic	• Associated with a lesion of the pars interarticularis • Three subtypes: ◦ 2A: lytic defect of the pars ◦ 2B: elongated or attenuated pars ◦ 2C: acute pars fracture
Type 3	Degenerative spondylolisthesis	• Segmental instability due to disc degeneration/facet arthrosis
Type 4	Traumatic	• Acute fracture in the region of the posterior elements, other than the pars interarticularis
Type 5	Pathological	• Generalised bone disease resulting in attenuation of the pars (e.g. metabolic, neoplastic)
Type 6	Post surgical	• After decompression of the lumbar spine

TABLE 37.9 The Meyerding classification for the degree of slip of spondylolisthesis.

Grade I	1–25%
Grade II	26–50%
Grade III	51–75%
Grade IV	76–100%

TUMOURS OF THE SPINE

Metastatic tumours

The commonest malignancies that metastasise to the spine are shown in *Table 37.10*. Red flags picked up on history or examination will alert the clinician to this possible diagnosis.

Over 80% of patients with spinal metastases present with progressive pain, and only 20% present with spinal cord compression. Relevant investigations include full blood count (FBC), urea and electrolytes, liver function tests, calcium, erythrocyte sedimentation rate (ESR), C-reactive protein (CRP), prostate-specific antigen (PSA), serum protein electrophoresis, thyroid function tests (where a thyroid mass has been palpated) and nutritional indices. Plain radiographs may show an absent pedicle ('winking owl' sign), vertebral cortical erosion and/or vertebral collapse. MRI of the whole spine will detect most metastases. Most metastases are **osteoblastic** and will show up on bone scintigraphy; however, **osteolytic** lesions such as multiple myeloma and renal cell carcinoma may not show up on an isotope bone scan. Metastases from the prostate may be sclerotic. Biopsies may be obtained via a percutaneous CT-guided method or open biopsy.

TABLE 37.10 Commonest malignancies that metastasise to the spine and their frequency.

Breast	21%
Lung	14%
Prostate	7.5%
Renal	5%
Gastrointestinal	5%
Thyroid	2.5%

Treatment options include orthotics, steroids (dexamethasone), radiotherapy, chemotherapy, hormonal therapy, surgery or a combination of any of the above. Radiotherapy promotes reossification of the vertebral body and reduces tumour load. It can be very effective for reducing 'bone pain'. Lymphoma, breast, lung and prostate metastases are **highly radiosensitive**. Gastrointestinal adenocarcinoma, metastatic melanoma, thyroid and renal carcinoma are **radioresistant**. Small cell carcinoma of the lung, Ewing's sarcoma, thyroid carcinoma, breast carcinoma and neuroblastoma are usually sensitive to chemotherapy and should have chemotherapeutic agents as the first-line management. Adenocarcinoma of the lung is resistant to chemotherapy. Prostate metastases may respond well to antiandrogenic hormone medication.

Henry W Meyerding, 1884–1969, Professor of Orthopaedic Surgery, Mayo Clinic, Rochester, MN, USA.
James Ewing, 1866–1943, Professor of Pathology, Cornell University Medical College, New York, NY, USA, described this type of sarcoma in 1921.

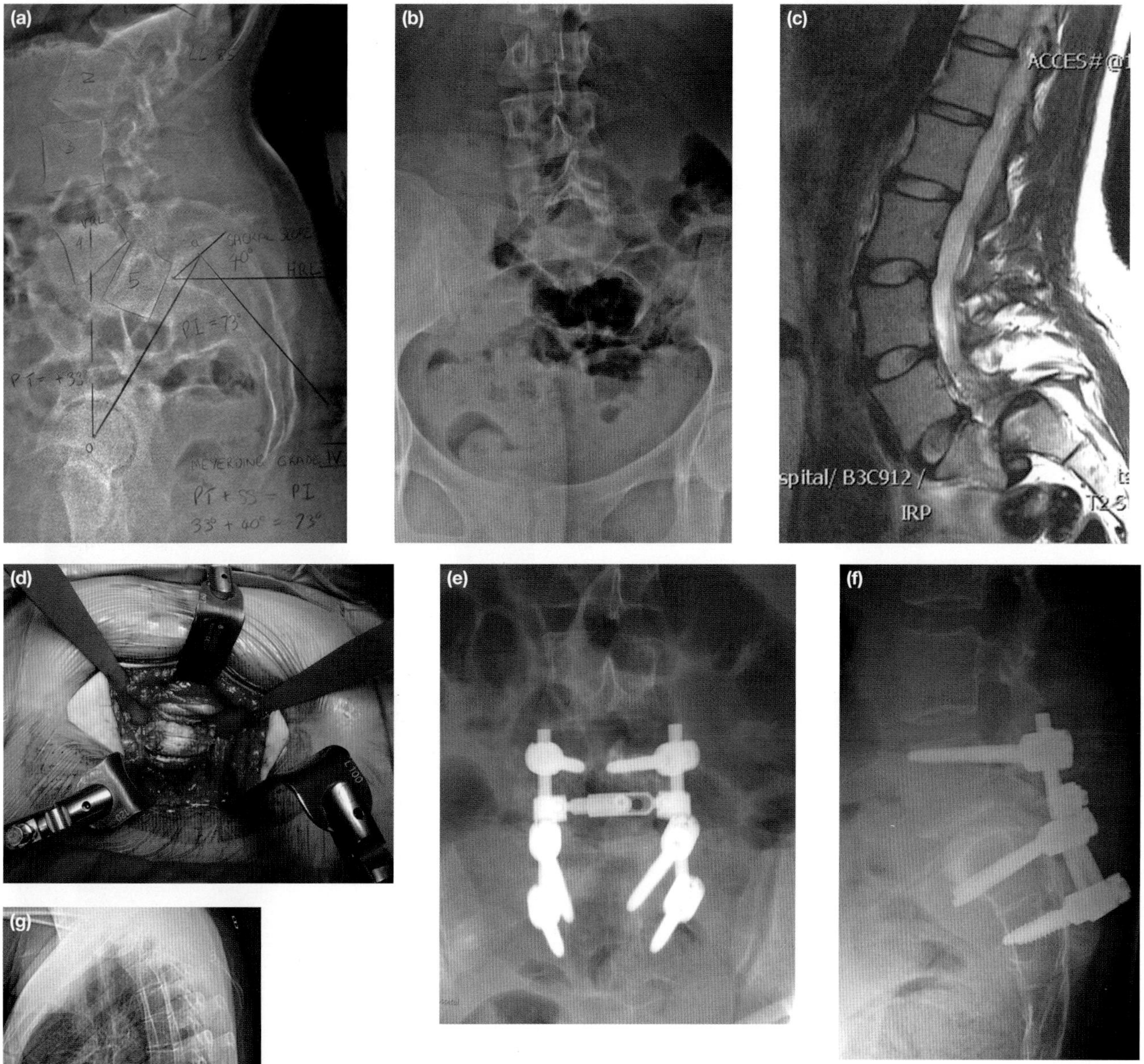

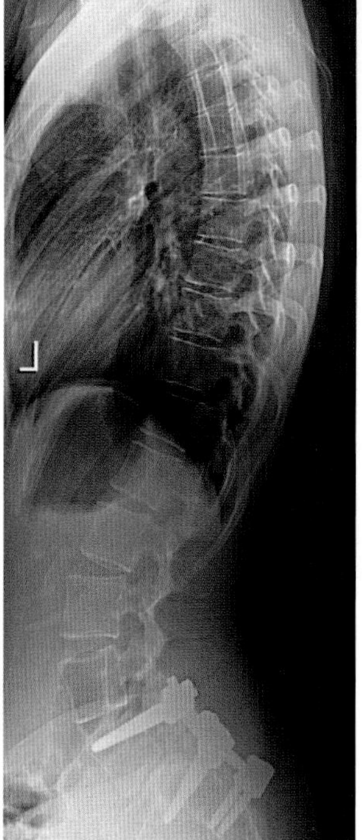

Figure 37.5 High-grade spondylolisthesis. Lateral standing radiograph (a) demonstrates Meyerding grade IV slip associated with high pelvic incidence. Anteroposterior (AP) radiograph (b) demonstrates the inverted Napoleon hat sign. T2-weighted mid-sagittal magnetic resonance imaging scan (c) shows the 'domed sacrum'. The patient underwent a modified Gaines procedure under one anaesthetic (d) with anterior vertebral resection of L5 along with the L4/5 and L5/S1 intervertebral discs, followed by resection of the posterior elements, articular process and L5 pedicles. AP (e) and lateral (f) radiographs demonstrate final reduction of L4 onto the sacrum with pedicle fixation from L4 to S2. (g) Postoperative full-length lateral standing radiograph at 12 months.

Robert W Gaines Jr, contemporary, surgeon, Department of Orthopaedic Surgery, University of Missouri, Columbia, MO, USA.

Extensive reconstructive tumour surgery should be reserved for those patients whose life expectancy exceeds 3–6 months. For patients with malignant spinal cord compression, the combination of decompressive surgery with stabilisation and postoperative radiotherapy has been shown to be superior in outcome when compared with radiotherapy alone. In one randomised trial, surgery and radiotherapy permitted most patients to remain ambulatory for the remainder of their lives, whereas patients treated with radiotherapy alone spent a large portion of their remaining time as paraplegics.

Summary box 37.7

Metastatic tumours of the spine

- Commonest presentation is progressive spinal pain
- Whole-spine MRI will detect most metastases
- Surgery is indicated for instability, pain, progressive deformity or neurological deficit

Primary tumours of the spine

Primary bone tumours of the spine account for only 2% of all spinal tumours. They arise *de novo* in the bone, cartilage, neural or ligamentous structures of the spine. They may be benign, intermediate or malignant. Benign primary spine tumours include osteoid osteoma, osteoblastoma (***Figure 37.6***), chondroma, chondroblastoma, chondromyxoid fibroma, giant cell tumours, haemangioma, lymphangioma and lipoma. Intermediate primary spine tumours include aggressive osteoblastoma, haemangiopericytoma, haemangioendothelioma and chordoma. Malignant primary spinal tumours include osteosarcoma, chondrosarcoma, Ewing's sarcoma, neuroectodermal tumours, malignant lymphoma, myeloma, angiosarcoma, fibrosarcoma and liposarcoma. The reader is

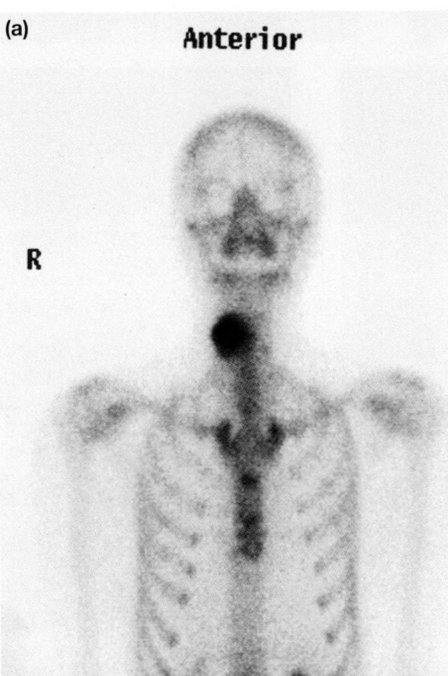

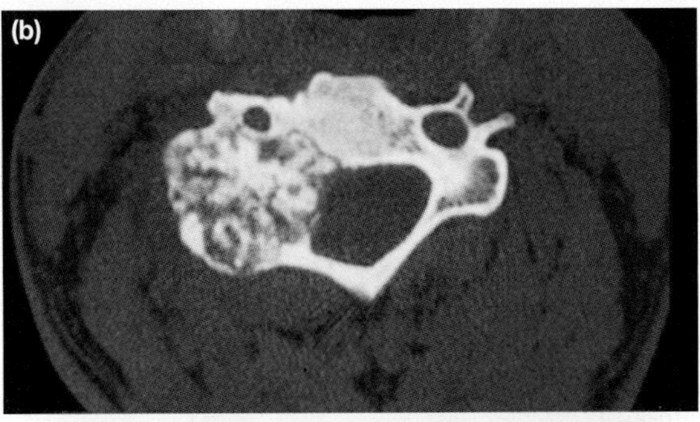

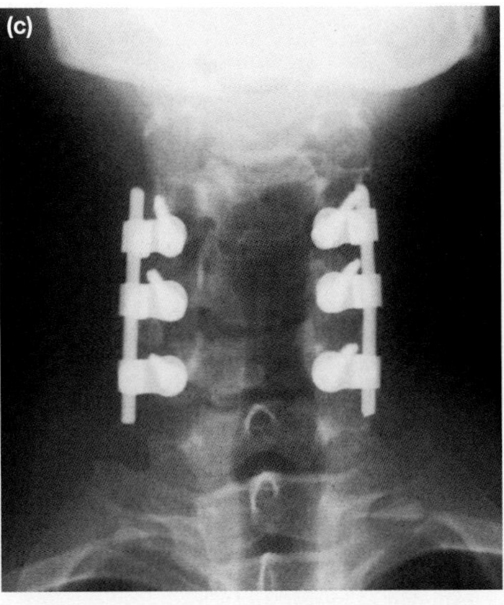

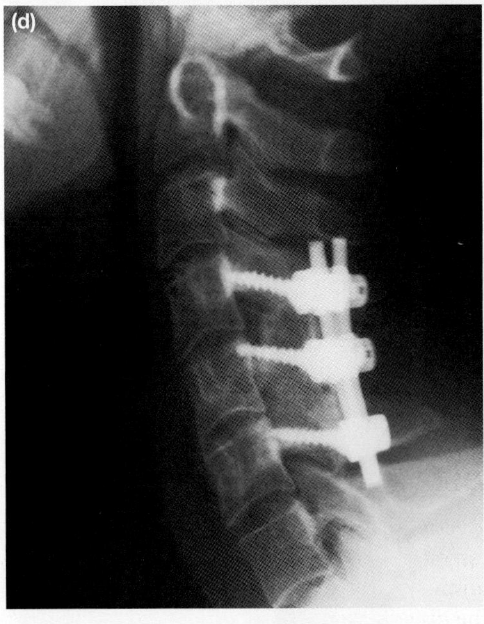

Figure 37.6 Osteoblastoma arising from the posterior elements of C5. This 21-year-old man presented with severe unremitting neck pain. Isotope bone scan (a) demonstrated increased uptake in C5. An axial computed tomography scan (b) further delineated the expansive lesion. The tumour was successfully removed with the aid of an intraoperative gamma probe to confirm complete excision; (c, d) postoperative anteroposterior and lateral radiographs, respectively, following reconstruction with a tricortical bone graft, lateral mass screws and rods.

referred to *Chapter 42* for further information on orthopaedic oncology.

In patients less than 18 years of age, 68% of all tumours are benign. For those patients who present over 18 years of age, more than 80% of tumours are malignant. Benign tumours tend to occur in the posterior elements; malignant tumours tend to involve the vertebral body.

Intradural tumours

These are rare. They may be intramedullary (within the substance of the spinal cord) or extramedullary (outside the cord). Most are extramedullary and benign; the commonest are meningiomas and neurofibromas.

Meningiomas are usually benign and arise from the meninges. They are generally slow growing and often warrant radiological surveillance. If the lesion is large and impinges on the spinal cord or nerve roots, steroids and early surgery may be indicated.

Neurofibromas are benign tumours that arise from the nerve sheath. There are three major types of neurofibroma: cutaneous, spinal and plexiform. In 90% of cases they present as solitary lesions, with the remainder presenting in patients with neurofibromatosis type 1 (NF-1), an autosomal dominant genetically inherited disease. NF-1 occurs in 1 in 3000 births and has been referred to as peripheral neurofibromatosis or von Recklinghausen disease. Diagnosis of NF-1 is confirmed when an individual has two or more of the following: at least six café-au-lait macules >5 mm diameter before puberty or six café-au-lait macules >15 mm after puberty, two or more neurofibromas of any type or one plexiform neurofibroma, multiple freckles in the axillary or inguinal regions, a distinctive bone abnormality involving the eye socket or arm/leg bones, optic glioma in the brain, two or more Lisch nodules in the eye, and a parent, sibling or child with NF-1. Neurofibromatosis type 2 (NF-2) is a genetically determined disorder that affects 1 in 40 000 individuals worldwide. A diagnosis of NF-2 is made when an individual has the following findings: schwannomas on both eighth cranial (vestibular) nerves or a parent, sibling or child with NF-2 plus one vestibular schwannoma in a person less than 30 years of age, or any two of the following: meningioma, glioma, schwannoma, juvenile cataracts.

INFECTIONS OF THE SPINE

Pyogenic infections

Pyogenic vertebral osteomyelitis is primarily a lesion of the disc and its osseous margins. The most common method by which an organism spreads to the spine is via the haematogenous route. The disc is nearly always involved in pyogenic vertebral infection. In contrast, granulomatous infection, such as tuberculosis, typically does not involve the disc space.

Risk factors for pyogenic vertebral osteomyelitis include advancing age, intravenous drug abuse, diabetes, renal failure, recent infections and trauma. *Staphylococcus aureus* accounts for 30–55% of the infections. Gram-negative organisms such as *Escherichia coli*, *Pseudomonas* species and *Proteus* species are associated with recent genitourinary infections and intravenous drug abuse. Anaerobic infections are uncommon, but may be seen in diabetic patients and after penetrating trauma.

If there is a failure of medical management (persistent pain, elevated erythrocyte sedimentation rate, C-reactive protein), operative interventions that should be considered are shown in *Table 37.11*.

TABLE 37.11 Operative interventions in pyogenic infections that should be used from a surgical perspective.

- Open biopsy (when a closed biopsy has failed)
- Drainage of abscesses
- Decompression of spinal cord compression
- Correction of progressive spinal deformity
- Stabilisation of progressive spinal instability

Epidural abscess

This condition is often a surgical emergency. The majority of cases occur within the thoracic spine. Without treatment, neurological deficit, including paralysis, may develop.

Tuberculosis

This is discussed in *Chapters 6 and 43*.

INFLAMMATORY SPONDYLOARTHROPATHY

Rheumatoid arthritis

Disease-modifying anti-rheumatic drugs (DMARDs) are a class of drugs indicated for the treatment of rheumatoid arthritis. Conventional medications have been used such as methotrexate, leflunomide, hydroxychloroquine and sulfasalazine. Newer biological agents are now available, including infliximab, adalimumab and etanercept. These medications have improved the outcomes significantly.

Between 33% and 50% of patients develop atlantoaxial subluxation (AAS) within 5 years of the diagnosis of rheumatoid arthritis. Some 2–10% of patients with AAS develop myelopathy over the next 10 years. Once diagnosed with myelopathy, 50% of patients may die within 1 year. The degree of subluxation may need to be checked by performing flexion and extension radiographs, and the theatre staff (especially the anaesthetist) need to be warned to take special care especially with intubation. The indications for surgery to stabilise the cervical spine are given in *Table 37.12*.

Friedrich Daniel von Recklinghausen, 1833–1910, Professor of Pathology, Strasbourg, France, described generalised neurofibromatosis in 1882.
Karl Lisch, 1907–1999, ophthalmologist, Wörgl, Austria.
Friedrich Theodor Schwann, 1810–1882, Professor of Anatomy successively at Louvain (1839–1848) and Liège, Belgium (1849–1880).
Hans Christian Joachim Gram, 1853–1938, Professor of Pharmacology (1891–1900) and of Medicine (1900–1923), Copenhagen, Denmark, described this method of staining bacteria in 1884.
Theodor Escherich, 1857–1911, Professor of Paediatrics, Vienna, Austria, discovered the *Bacterium coli commune* in 1886.

TABLE 37.12 Recommendations for spinal surgery in rheumatoid arthritis.

- AAS with a PADI of 14 mm or less
- AAS with at least 5 mm of basilar invagination
- Subaxial subluxation with a sagittal canal diameter of 14 mm or less

AAS, atlantoaxial subluxation; PADI, posterior atlantodental interval.

Ankylosing spondylitis

Should a patient with ankylosing spondylitis present following trauma, a high index of suspicion for occult fractures should be present. It is common for patients with ankylosing spondylitis to develop epidural haematomas with subtle neurological deficit.

Patients with a significant fixed flexion deformity at the cervicothoracic junction ('chin-on-chest' deformity), limited forward gaze and eating and swallowing difficulties may be treated with a closing wedge osteotomy at the cervicothoracic junction (*Figure 37.7*). Extension osteotomies can also be performed in the thoracic and lumbar spine.

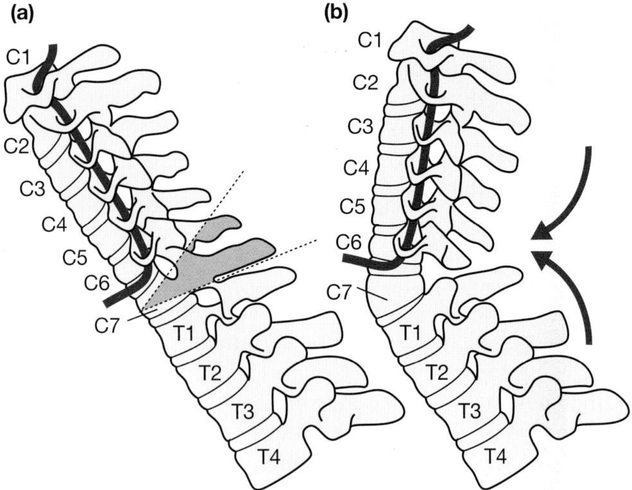

Figure 37.7 C7 closing wedge osteotomy for correction of cervicothoracic kyphosis in patients with ankylosing spondylitis. Planned resection lateral view (a) and lateral view after closure of the osteotomy (b).

SPINAL DEFORMITY

Spinal deformity may be categorised into a coronal plane deformity (scoliosis) or a sagittal plane deformity (kyphosis and lordosis). Further classification may be made on the basis of aetiology into congenital, neuromuscular, idiopathic or syndromic. Appropriate radiographs for the assessment of scoliosis include a full posteroanterior and lateral standing spine. When surgery is contemplated, supine lateral bending radiographs are obtained to assess the flexibility of the curve(s). Curve magnitude is measured in degrees and is known as the Cobb angle. The criterion for diagnosis of scoliosis is a Cobb angle of 10° or more. The causes of scoliosis are given in *Table 37.13*.

TABLE 37.13 Aetiology of scoliosis.

- Idiopathic
- Neuromuscular
- Congenital
- Syndrome-related

Idiopathic scoliosis

Idiopathic scoliosis accounts for 70% of presentations. It can be classified into **early onset** (before 8 years of age) (*Figure 37.8*) and **late onset** (after 8 years of age; typical adolescent idiopathic scoliosis). The distinction is important, as the number of alveoli in the lung does not increase after the age of 8 years. Patients with severe curves in the early-onset group may develop cor pulmonale and right ventricular failure resulting in premature death. Adolescent idiopathic scoliosis is associated with a normal or near-normal life expectancy.

The prevalence of curves with a Cobb angle >10° is between 0.5% and 3%. The prevalence of curves >30° is between 1.5 and 3 per 1000. Risk factors for progression include female gender, remaining skeletal growth, curve location and curve magnitude. Not all curves stabilise when skeletal maturity is reached. In long-term studies, 68% experienced curve progression; the most marked progression of 1° per year was observed in patients with thoracic curves between 50° and 75°.

Idiopathic curves of less than 25° are monitored with clinical and radiographic examination. In growing children (premenarchal) with curves between 20° and 29°, a brace may be indicated. Bracing is used to **prevent** curve progression and generally does not lead to permanent curve correction. Curves beyond 45° are not amenable to brace treatment.

Surgery in the form of corrective instrumentation and spinal fusion is indicated for curve progression beyond 40°, truncal imbalance and unacceptable cosmesis. During surgery, continuous spinal cord monitoring is used in the form of somatosensory evoked potentials (SSEPs), motor-evoked potentials (MEPs) and free-run and stimulated electromyographic (EMG) activity to minimise the risk of neurological damage. The risk of neurological injury is 0.4% (1 in 250).

Neuromuscular scoliosis

This may be due to neuropathic disorders, such as cerebral palsy, spinocerebellar degeneration, syringomyelia, tetraplegia (*Figure 37.9*), spinal muscular atrophy and poliomyelitis, or **myopathic** disorders, such as Duchenne muscular dystrophy and myotonic dystrophy. There is good evidence that stabilisation of the spine in children with Duchenne muscular dystrophy who are able to walk (before respiratory compromise is too severe to preclude a general anaesthetic) may increase their lifespan by several years.

John R Cobb, American surgeon, wrote a paper in 1948 on how to measure the angle on a radiograph in scoliosis.
Guillaume Benjamin Amand Duchenne, 1806–1875, neurologist, worked successively in Boulogne and Paris, France, but never held a hospital appointment.

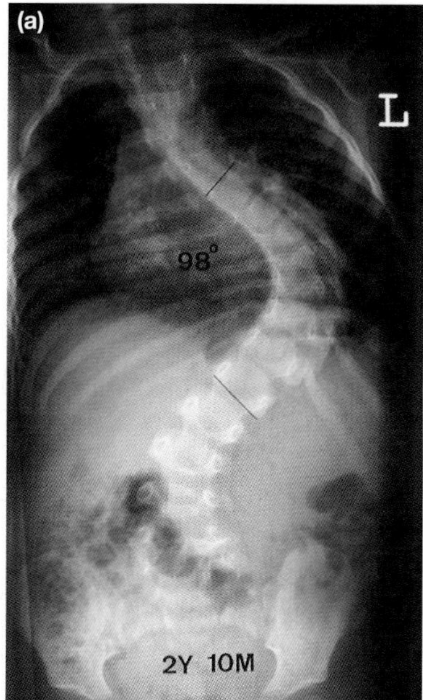

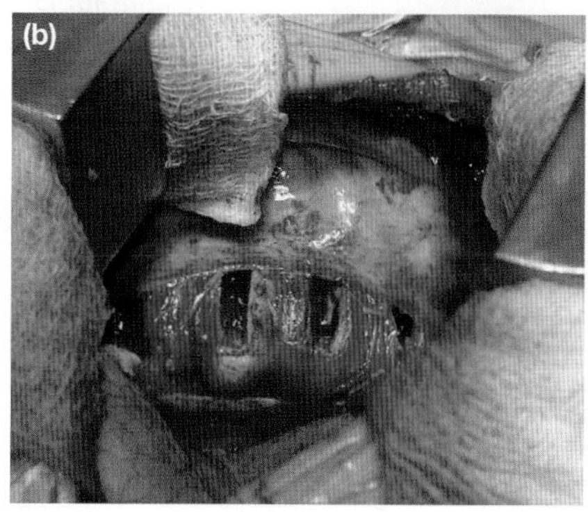

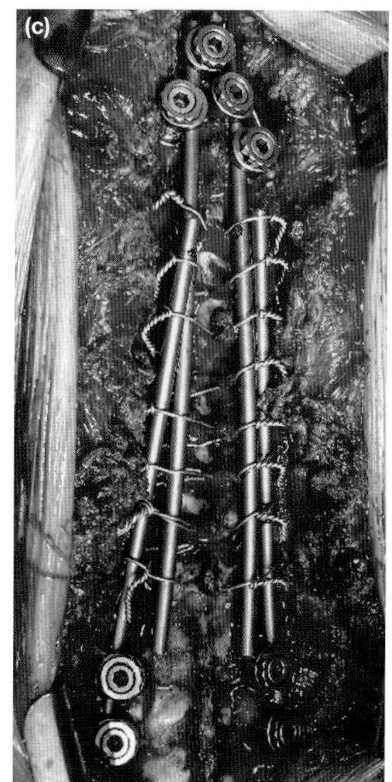

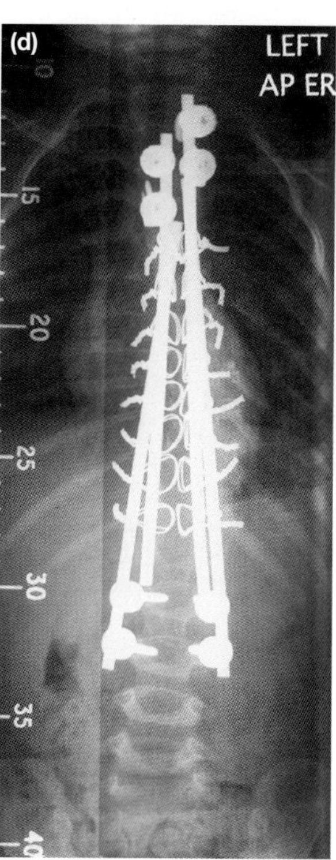

Figure 37.8 Early-onset idiopathic scoliosis. The anteroposterior standing radiograph (a) demonstrates a Cobb angle of 98° and dextrocardia. This 34-month-old boy underwent a convex hemiepiphysiodesis over the apical four discs (b), followed by Luque trolley instrumentation **without** fusion to correct the spinal deformity and allow growth (c, d).

Congenital scoliosis

This is caused by vertebral anomalies that produce a frontal plane growth asymmetry. The anomalies are present at birth, but the curvature may take years to be clinically evident. Close observation of spinal growth is required until skeletal maturity is reached. Brace treatment is ineffective for the primary structural curves, which are often short and rigid, but it may have a role in the control of compensatory curves. For progressive curves, surgical options include growing rod constructs such as magnetically controlled growing rod procedures, hemivertebra excision, correction and fusion or posterior instrumented correction and fusion.

Summary box 37.8

Spinal deformity

- Early-onset idiopathic scoliosis (<8 years old) has the potential to impair lung function
- Neuromuscular scoliosis: timely surgery may prolong life
- Congenital scoliosis: rigid curves do not respond to brace treatment

Scheuermann's kyphosis

Typically, in this condition, there is wedging of the seventh to 10th thoracic vertebrae. The patient presents with both apical pain and low back pain (due to attempts by the lumbar musculature to compensate for the thoracic hyperkyphosis). The incidence has been estimated at 1–8% of the population, and it is more common in males. Physiotherapy may be useful. Bracing for skeletally immature patients with kyphosis up to 65° may be effective in arresting progression. Indications for surgery include pain (apical or low back pain produced by compensatory hyperlordosis), progressive deformity greater than 70°, unacceptable cosmesis and neurological and/or cardiopulmonary compromise. If surgery is contemplated, it may require anterior release followed by posterior correction and fusion. Increasingly, posterior chevron osteotomies carried out at the time of posterior instrumentation may prevent the need for the initial anterior release.

DEVELOPMENTAL ABNORMALITIES

Developmental abnormalities of the spine and spinal cord can be divided into primary bony disorders (e.g. congenital

Eduardo Luque, contemporary, professor, Shriners Hospital for Crippled Children, Mexico City, Mexico.
Holger Werfel Scheuermann, 1877–1960, radiologist, Municipal Hospital, Sundby, Copenhagen, Denmark, described juvenile kyphosis in 1920.

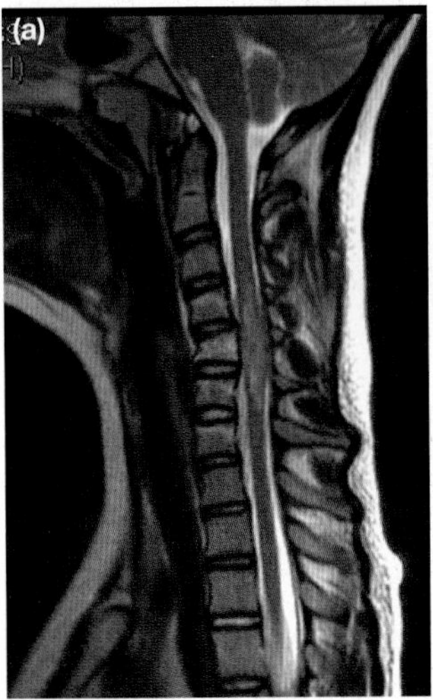

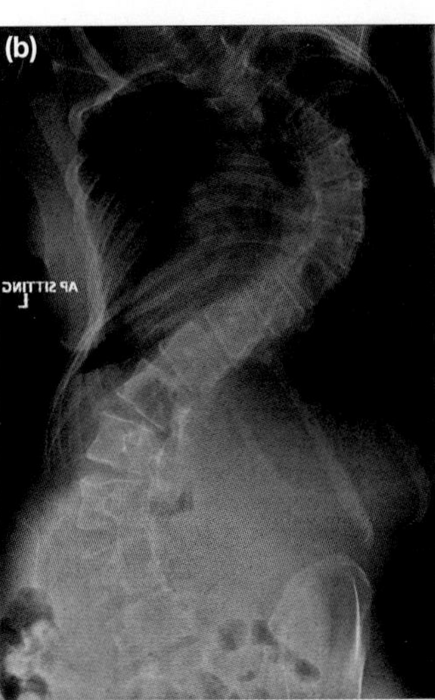

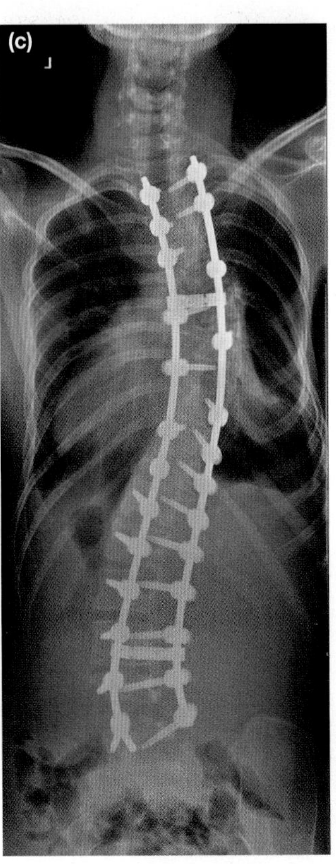

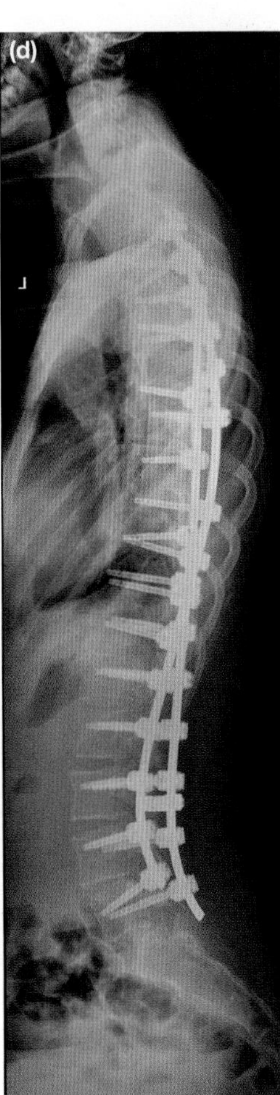

Figure 37.9 This 13-year-old girl sustained a cervical spinal cord injury (SCI) following a dive into a swimming pool. The International Standards for Neurological Classification of Spinal Cord Impairment (ISNCSCI), commonly referred to as the American Spinal Injury Association (ASIA), are based on a standardised sensory and motor assessment. The ASIA Impairment Scale splits these grades into: grade A (complete), grade B (sensory incomplete), grade C (motor incomplete, muscle grade <3), grade D (motor incomplete, muscle >3) and grade E (normal). The patient was diagnosed with a C5 ASIA B SCI. The T2 sagittal magnetic resonance imaging scan (a) demonstrated signal change maximal at the C6 level. The patient developed significant neuromuscular scoliosis. The anteroposterior (AP) sitting radiograph (b) demonstrates a right thoracic curve with a Cobb angle of 104° and a left lumbar curve with a Cobb angle of 82°. Following pedicle screw instrumentation and fusion from T2 to L5, the right thoracic curve corrected to 40° and the left lumbar curve corrected to 38° as noted on the AP radiograph (c) with restoration of sagittal balance (d).

scoliosis, as discussed above) and primary neurological disorders (e.g. spina bifida, Arnold–Chiari malformation and spinal dysraphism).

Spina bifida

Spina bifida is caused by a failure of fusion of the vertebral arches and possibly the underlying neural tube. Spina bifida cystica has an incidence of 1 in 300 live births and is associated with hydrocephalus. It is now decreasing as a consequence of folic acid supplementation, antenatal ultrasound and the measurement of α-fetoprotein (AFP) levels. There are two basic types:

- **Meningocele**: the meninges herniate through the bony defect and are covered by skin.
- **Myelomeningocele**: the roof of the defect is formed by exposed neural tissue, with 75% of patients developing hydrocephalus.

A meningocele with good-quality skin over the defect may be treated conservatively. A meningocele with a more prominent sac can be excised at 3–6 months. The management of myelomeningocele is more controversial. Enthusiasm for closing all defects has been replaced by a more selective approach with the recognition that it was inappropriate to operate on children with severe hydrocephalus, a large open defect and no distal neurological function. The majority of these children die in their first year if closure is not attempted. With antibiotics, early surgical closure and shunts to prevent hydrocephalus, half the children who survive the first 24 hours will reach school age, but long-term problems remain, including skin problems, neuromuscular scoliosis, bone and joint deformity and the complications associated with a neuropathic bladder.

Arnold-Chiari malformation

Arnold–Chiari malformation occurs when the medulla oblongata and the cerebellar tonsils extend through the foramen magnum into the cervical spinal canal, causing pressure on the lower medulla. Hydrocephalus and impaired neurological function are common, and there is a strong association

Julius Arnold, 1835–1915, Professor of Pathological Anatomy, University of Heidelberg, Heidelberg, Germany, described this condition in 1894.
Hans Chiari, 1851–1916, Professor of Pathological Anatomy, Strasbourg, Germany (Strasbourg was returned to France in 1918 after the end of the First World War), gave his account of this condition in 1891.

with spina bifida and syringomyelia. Symptoms may include headache, vomiting, visual disturbances, mental impairment, cerebellar ataxia, sensory disturbances or paralysis. Management consists of decompressing the foramen magnum and, usually, the posterior arch of the atlas to restore normal cerebrospinal fluid flow.

Spinal dysraphism

This is a group of disorders arising from abnormal embryological formation of tissues; all are associated with a progressive neurological deficit as the result of spinal cord tethering and traction or cord compression. There is a strong association with spina bifida.

In diastematomyelia, there is an abnormal bony or cartilaginous spur projecting across the middle of the vertebral canal, dividing the dural tube and spinal cord in two. Between 50% and 70% of patients are seen to have a skin naevus, dimple or hairy patch when the spine is examined. Surgical release of the tethering has variable results.

Syringomyelia

Patients may present with sensory disturbance, weakness of the hands, loss of pain and temperature sensation, asymmetrical abdominal reflexes or progressive kyphoscoliosis. It is associated with Arnold–Chiari malformation and spinal cord tumours. Where syringomyelia is associated with an Arnold–Chiari malformation and scoliosis, a posterior cranial fossa decompression should be carried out first to resolve the syringomyelia. The scoliosis may then be corrected at a later date.

METABOLIC BONE DISEASES AFFECTING THE SPINE

Osteoporosis

Patients with osteoporosis may present with pain following minimal trauma, loss of height and exaggerated thoracic kyphosis. Medications used to prevent and treat osteoporosis include calcium, vitamin D, bisphosphonates (alendronate, risedronate, once-yearly intravenous zoledronic acid), denosumab, strontium ranelate, selective oestrogen receptor modulators (SERMs) such as raloxifene, hormone replacement therapy and teriparatide.

Patients with painful thoracic fractures may be treated with short-term bed rest, analgesics and a spinal orthosis. If the back is still painful 6 weeks after the injury, patients may be considered for vertebroplasty or kyphoplasty. Vertebroplasty involves the injection of polymethylmethacrylate (PMMA) bone cement under pressure into the vertebral body with fluoroscopic guidance. The goals of the procedure are to **stabilise the spine** and **decrease the pain** associated with compression fractures. Kyphoplasty, on the other hand, involves inserting bilateral bone tamps with balloons into the vertebral body. These are inflated under fluoroscopic control with the bone tamp re-expanding the body, and elevating the end plates to reduce the fracture deformity. The balloons are then deflated and removed, and PMMA is placed in the cavity created by the balloons. The goals of kyphoplasty are **spinal stabilisation, pain relief and restoration of vertebral body height**. Significant complications have been reported, including nerve root injury and spinal cord injury resulting from cement extravasation, along with cement embolism, infection and hypotension.

GLOBAL ISSUES IN SPINE SURGERY

It is important that the information presented in this chapter, which is widely used throughout the world for teaching and training, outlines the very best evidence-based treatment that is available for surgical conditions. The text has covered the essentials of spine surgery and has very rightly demonstrated current techniques that involve up-to-date equipment. It is, however, an inescapable fact that the majority of the world's population does not have access to state-of-the-art spinal surgery. There are two main reasons for this: first, the cost of spinal surgery and, second, the lack of trained surgeons.

Cost implications of modern spinal surgery

There have been dramatic advances in spinal surgery owing to modern imaging, modern instruments and implants, and advanced spinal cord monitoring equipment. The widespread availability of MRI in high-income countries such as the USA, the UK and most of Europe has meant that diagnostic accuracy is available to the whole population in these countries. This is not, however, the case for most of the world, where there is no free or state-sponsored MRI service, and a private scan costing US$500 is unaffordable to most. If a family cannot afford a scan, then they also cannot afford the cost of an operation, the spinal implants, spinal cord monitoring and the use of expensive disposable instruments such as high-speed burrs.

The lack of trained spinal surgeons

In the last 25 years high-income countries have seen the rapid development of spinal surgery, and the rapid development of spinal surgery as a complete career. It is now normal in such countries for spinal surgeons to practise only in the field of spinal surgery and no longer to undertake general orthopaedic or neurosurgical operations. This has inevitably led to refinement of skills and increasing subspecialisation. In low-income countries, where there may be a single orthopaedic surgeon for 1 million people, doing 'just spinal surgery' is not an option, and a much more general approach is needed. In the map shown in ***Figure 37.10***, each country in the world is represented with an area proportional to the number of people in the population per active surgeon. This represents surgeons of all types, but it shows that, in many parts of Africa, there are more than half a million people per surgeon. The map showing the population covered by each **spinal** surgeon would be even more striking.

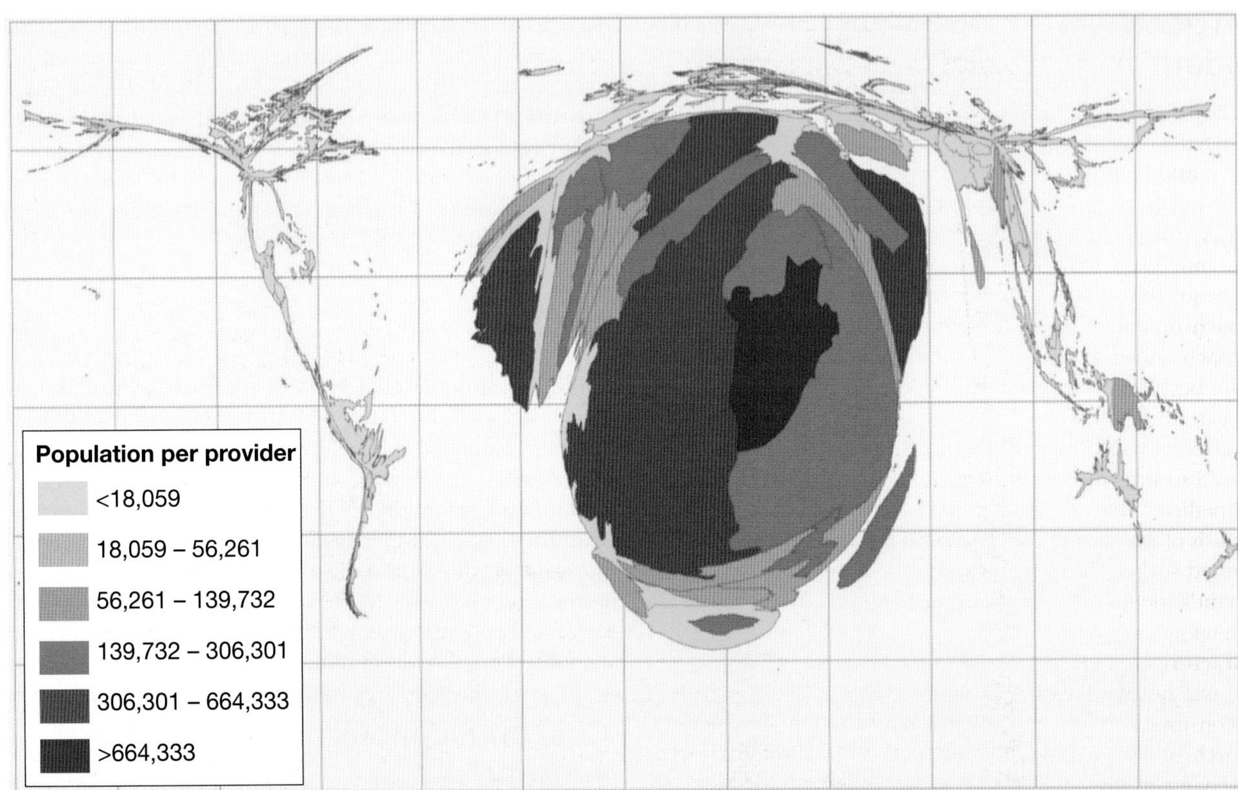

Figure 37.10 Global distribution of surgeons, anaesthetists and obstetricians. Each country in the world is represented with an area proportional to the number of the population per active surgeon. (Reproduced with permission from Holmer H, Lantz A, Kunjumen T *et al*. Global distribution of surgeons, anaesthesiologists, and obstetricians. *Lancet Glob Health* 2015; **3**(Suppl 2): S9–11.)

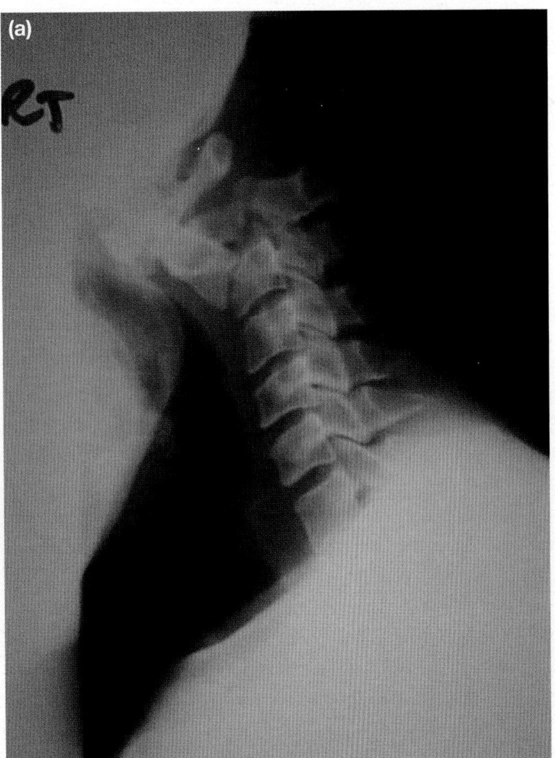

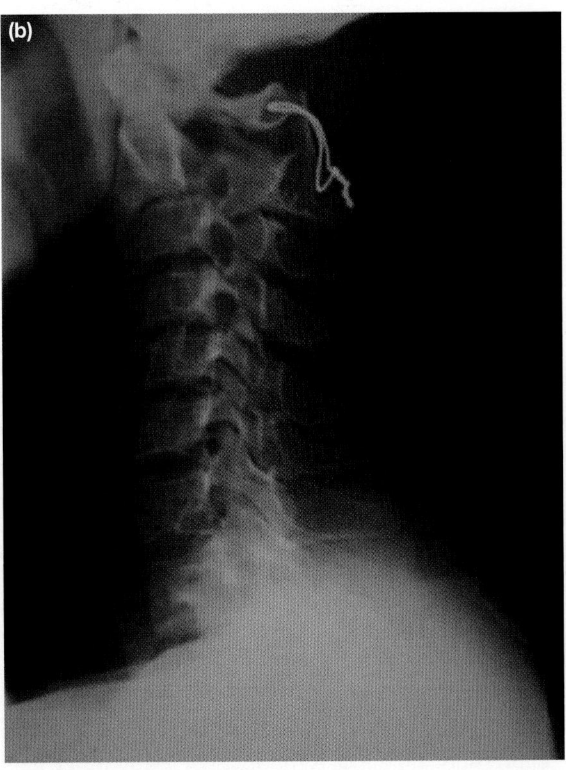

Figure 37.11 (a) Lateral cervical spine radiograph with a fracture/dislocation at C2/3 sustained by a patient living in a low-income country. (b) The surgeon used a low-risk, low-technology technique, wiring the arch of C1 to the spine of C2 with a piece of stainless steel wire, then laying on corticocancellous bone graft.

Can good spine care be given without modern imaging and equipment?

The key to good surgery in all disciplines is a surgeon who is dedicated to the care of his or her patient, who takes a good history and examination and then offers the best treatment that is available under the circumstances. In a high-income country this will often involve MRI scanning, dissection under microscope control and expensive titanium implants. In a resource-poor, low-income country it may involve just as much time and skill, but often a much more conservative approach. When surgery is needed the surgeon may have to do the best that he or she can with the equipment available. The case in ***Figure 37.11*** illustrates this point well. Note the lateral cervical spine radiograph with a fracture/dislocation at C2/3 sustained by a patient living in a low-income country. The pedicles of C2 are fractured, allowing C2 to subluxate forwards on C3 and compress the spinal cord. The patient was admitted several days after a car crash, holding his head with his hands for stability. In a high-income country where there is imaging and fluoroscopic-guided pedicle screw fixation, the fracture could easily be fixed. In the low-income country, there was no cervical spine instrumentation available and the surgeon used a low-risk, low-technology technique of wiring the arch of C1 to the spine of C2 with stainless steel wire, then laying on corticocancellous bone graft. The reduction was stable, the graft incorporated and the patient was thankful. It is not appropriate to say that this was inadequate treatment compared with the best that the world has to offer, because the best that the world has to offer was not available.

FURTHER READING

Debnath UK, Freeman BJ, Gregory P *et al.* Clinical outcome and return to sport after the surgical treatment of spondylolysis in young athletes. *J Bone Joint Surg Br* 2003; **85**(2): 244–9.

Fairbank J, Frost H, Wilson-McDonald J *et al.* Randomised controlled trial to compare surgical stabilisation of the lumbar spine with an intensive rehabilitation programme for patients with chronic low back pain: the MRC spine stabilisation trial. *BMJ* 2005; **330**: 1233–8.

Fritzell P, Hägg O, Wessperg P *et al.* Volvo Award in Clinical Science: lumbar fusion versus non-surgical treatment for chronic low back pain. A multi-centre randomised controlled trial from the Swedish Lumbar Spine Study Group. *Spine* 2001; **26**: 2521–34.

Gardner A, Gardner E, Morley T. Cauda equina syndrome: a review of the current clinical and medico-legal position. *Eur Spine J* 2011; **20**(5): 690–7.

Holmer H, Lantz A, Kunjuman T *et al.* Global distribution of surgeons, anaesthesiologists, and obstetricians. *Lancet Glob Health* 2015; **3**: S9–11.

Janssen ME, Zigler JE, Spivak JE *et al.* ProDisc-C total disc replacement versus anterior cervical discectomy and fusion for single-level symptomatic cervical disc disease. Seven-year follow-up of the prospective randomized U.S. Food and Drug Administration investigational device exemption study. *J Bone Joint Surg Am* 2015; **97**(21): 1738–47.

Meara JG, Leather AJ, Hagander L *et al.* Global Surgery 2030: evidence and solutions for achieving health, welfare, and economic development. *Lancet* 2015; **386**: 569–624.

Patchell RA, Tibb PA, Regine WF *et al.* Direct decompressive surgical resection in the treatment of spinal cord compression caused by metastatic cancer: a randomised trial. *Lancet* 2005; **366**: 643–8.

Srikandarajah N, Noble A, Clark S, *et al.* Cauda Equina Syndrome Core Outcome Set (CESCOS): an international patient and healthcare professional consensus for research studies. *PLoS ONE* 2020; **15**(1): e0225907.

Tokala DP, Lam KS, Freeman BJ *et al.* C7 decancellisation closing wedge osteotomy for the correction of fixed cervico-thoracic kyphosis. *Eur Spine J* 2007; **16**(9): 1471–8.

Waddell G, McCulloch JA, Kummel ED *et al.* Volvo Award in Clinical Science: non organic physical signs in low-back pain. *Spine* 1979; **5**: 117–25.

Wiltse LL, Newman PH, Macnab I. Classification of spondylosis and spondylolisthesis. *Clin Orthop* 1976; **117**: 23–9.

CHAPTER

38 The upper limb

Learning objectives

To understand:
- Anatomy and physiology relevant to upper limb pathology

To be able to explain:
- The diagnosis and treatment of common upper limb conditions

SHOULDER GIRDLE

Anatomy and function

The shoulder girdle (clavicle, scapula and the humerus, which articulates directly with the scapula at the glenohumeral joint) is controlled and supported by muscles crossing between the spine, thorax, scapula and humerus. The sternoclavicular joint is the only synovial joint between the upper limb and the axial skeleton. The glenohumeral joint is most closely controlled by the deltoid and rotator cuff muscles (subscapularis, supraspinatus, infraspinatus and teres minor), although 26 muscles in total act across this articulation, which controls the upper limb with respect to the torso. The scapula is integral to shoulder motion, both gliding and rotating on the posterolateral surface of the thorax. Of the 180° of elevation possible at the shoulder, around 50° is provided by scapular rotation on the chest while the clavicle elevates 30–60° concurrently. The remainder of the range of elevation occurs at the glenohumeral joint. During elevation both the humerus and clavicle rotate significantly: external rotation of the humerus bringing the greater tuberosity and cuff attachments from beneath the acromion, where they would otherwise limit the range (*Figure 38.1*).

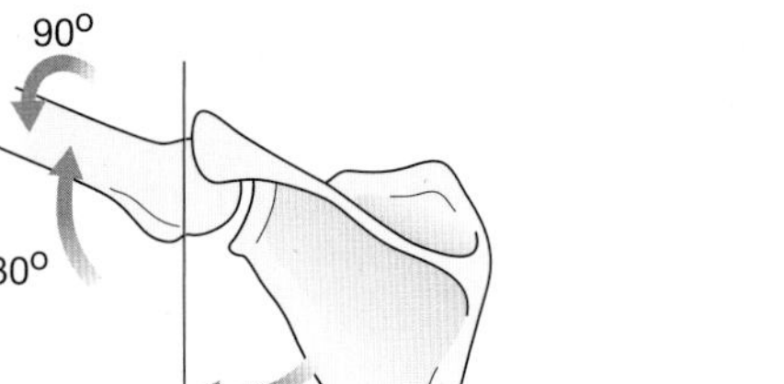

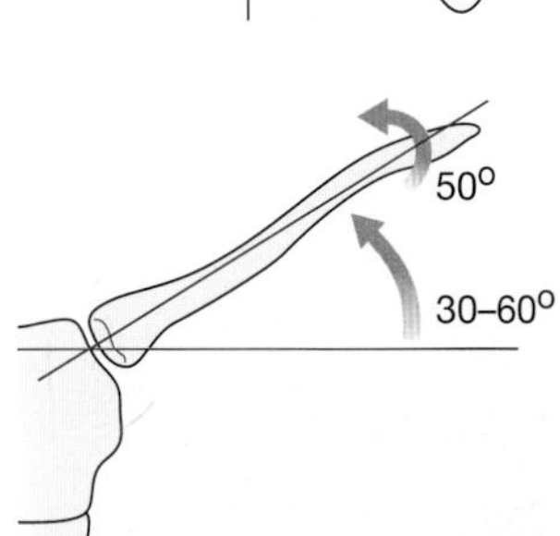

Figure 38.1 Relative motion of the elements of the shoulder girdle.

Congenital abnormalities

Sprengel's shoulder

The commonest congenital abnormality is due to abnormal scapular descent from its embryonic midcervical position. The typical presentation is a high, small, rotated scapula that remains connected to the cervical spine by a bony bar, fibrous band or an omovertebral body (*Figure 38.2*). Other congenital deformities impacting on upper limb function are rib abnormalities and cervical or thoracic abnormalities, including scoliosis and Klippel–Feil syndrome (congenital fusion of cervical vertebrae). Pseudarthrosis of the clavicle is a congenital abnormality that can be mistaken for a birth-related fracture. In later life it can be mistaken for a non-union when radiographs are taken after trauma and attempts to plate and graft the lesion are usually doomed to failure.

Acquired abnormalities

History

Patients usually associate the onset of their symptoms with an unusual event (trauma or excessive activity) even though the

Otto Gerhard Karl Sprengel, 1852–1915, surgeon, Grossherzogliches Krankenhaus (the Grand Ducal Hospital), Brunswick, Germany, described congenital high scapula in 1891.
Maurice Klippel, 1858–1942, neurologist, Hôpital Tenon, Paris, France.
André Feil, 1884–1955, neurologist, Paris, France. Klippel and Feil described this condition in a joint paper in 1912.

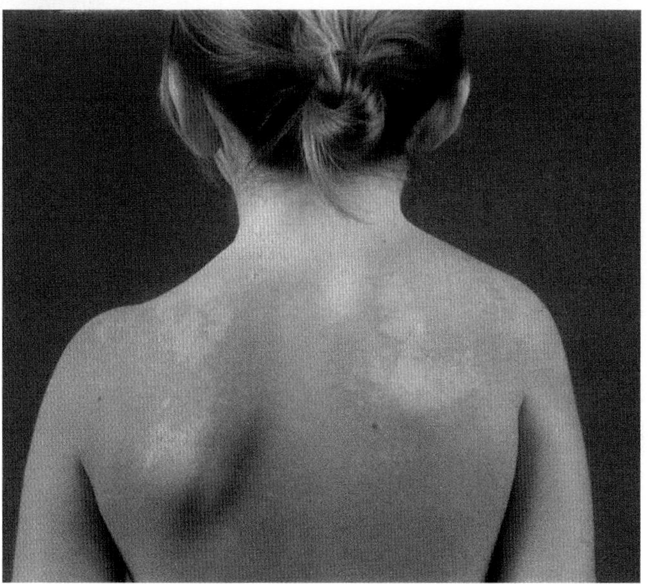

Figure 38.2 Sprengel's shoulder (right) of a 4-year-old girl.

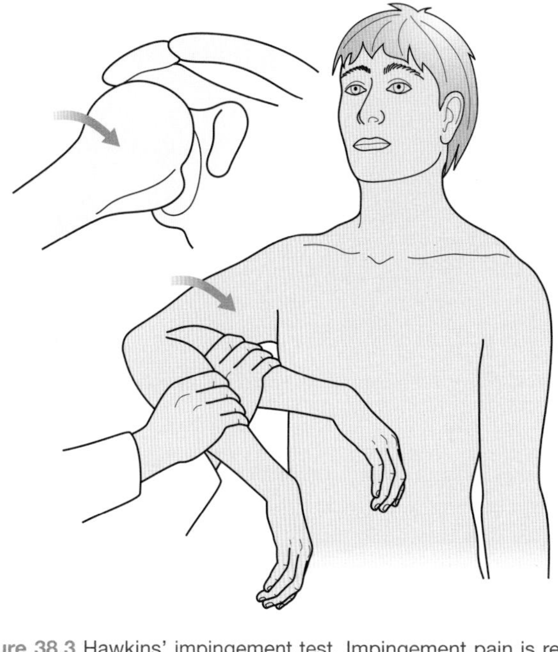

Figure 38.3 Hawkins' impingement test. Impingement pain is reproduced when the shoulder is internally rotated with 90° of forward flexion, thereby locating the greater tuberosity and anterior rotator cuff underneath the acromion and coracoacromial ligament.

causation may not be as clear as the patient thinks. Even so, the onset (sudden or gradual) and duration are important details to establish, as is the age, occupation and hand dominance of the patient. Pain presenting in the shoulder (or anywhere in the upper limb) can arise from the nerves of the neck, so the history should enquire about neck problems.

Examination

If the patient can localise the pain to an exact point around or within the shoulder, then the problem is unlikely to be referred from the neck. Tests for inflammation and impingement involve trying to reproduce the pain by loading the limb in the position that creates the problem (e.g. Hawkins' test for impingement; *Figure 38.3*). Tests for tears in structures such as the rotator cuff look specifically for weakness, while apprehension tests check for instability (such as may predispose to recurrent shoulder dislocation).

Investigations

Radiographs are often of limited value because most shoulder pain arises from soft-tissue structures. However, a reduced subacromial space may be clearly visible in full-thickness rotator cuff tears (*Figure 38.4a*). The appearance of a typical subacromial spur can be seen on the radiograph in *Figure 38.4b* and morphological variants of the acromion are shown in *Figure 38.5*. Patients with impingement pain and rotator cuff tears are much more likely to have a hooked acromion. The appearance of a spur, which produces the hook, is usually due to calcification within the coracoacromial ligament (CAL) insertion and it may be a secondary consequence of degenerative cuff disease rather than a causative lesion.

(a)

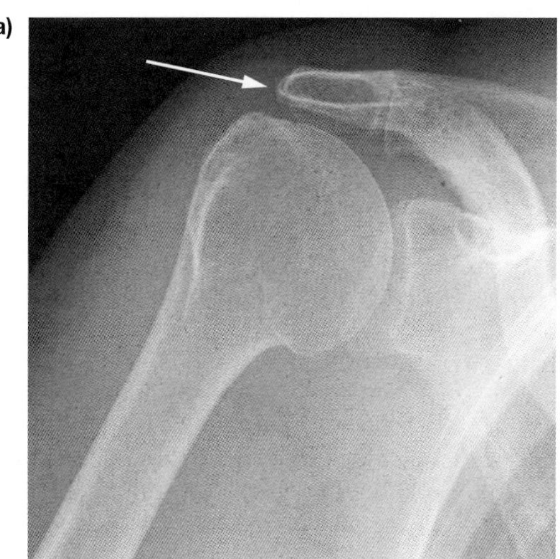

(b)

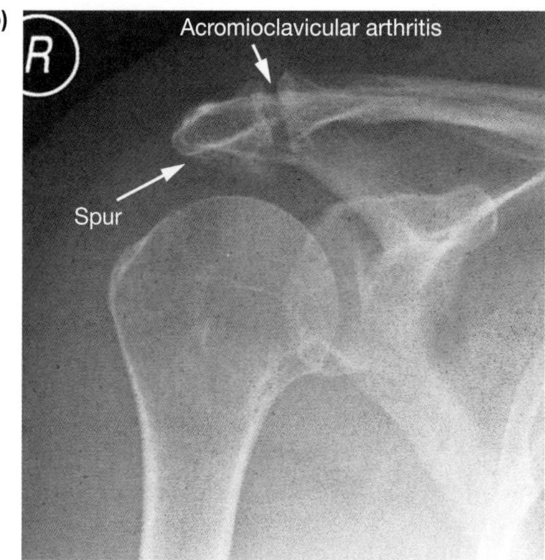

Figure 38.4 (a) Radiograph showing sclerosis on the undersurface of the acromion and the greater tuberosity, with reduced subacromial space. (b) Radiograph showing an acromial spur and arthritis of the acromioclavicular joint.

Richard J Hawkins, contemporary, Canadian orthopaedic surgeon.

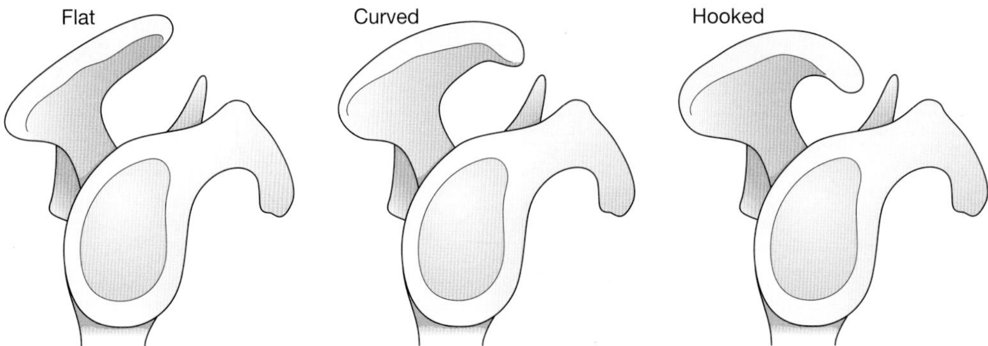

Figure 38.5 The three commonest acromial morphologies seen in adults. Children almost always have the flat morphology.

Both ultrasound and magnetic resonance imaging (MRI) allow the integrity and health of the rotator cuff to be checked whereas magnetic resonance (MR) arthrography also gives information on the integrity of the labrum of the glenohumeral joint (*Figure 38.6*).

Local anaesthetic injections may help to localise the source of pain. For example, a painful arc on forward elevation (Neer's sign) may be completely relieved by injecting local anaesthetic into the subacromial bursa in cases of subacromial impingement (Neer's test positive).

Rotator cuff degeneration and impingement

The rotator cuff moves in a confined space between the humeral head, the acromion and the CAL. Blood vessels cannot cross the glenohumeral joint cavity below the supraspinatus tendon or through the subacromial space above it, and vessels that enter from the insertional and muscle belly ends become constricted when the tendon is tensioned around the curved humeral head when the cuff is active. Blood flow is therefore limited, the tendon is exposed to external forces as it operates in a confined space and its capacity for self-repair is limited. More than any other tendon, therefore, it is prone to age-related degeneration, leading to tendinosis and partial- and full-thickness tearing; the rate of this is at least partly genetically determined. Even a trivial injury can inhibit rotator cuff function, so that it does not glide so easily in its subacromial space, starting a progression of inflammation, swelling and pain in the subacromial region. This subacromial pain may be termed impingement, which is felt to be attributable to abrasion of the cuff and bursa on the undersurface of the acromion. The impingement itself causes further bursal inflammation and pain, which further inhibits rotator cuff function, and a vicious circle is set up. The likelihood of subacromial pain developing is increased in patients with a spur beneath the acromion, which is seen increasingly commonly with age (*Figure 38.5*) and may be an effect rather than a cause of painful subacromial degeneration, as described earlier in this paragraph. The result is a painful arc of movement for the patient, which corresponds to the position where the inflamed segment of the supraspinatus tendon passes under the anterior acromial spur. The examiner may find that, although the patient cannot actively lift their arm through this segment (because of the pain), passively lifting the arm for the patient enables them to continue with pain-free movement once the area of impingement is passed (*Figure 38.7*).

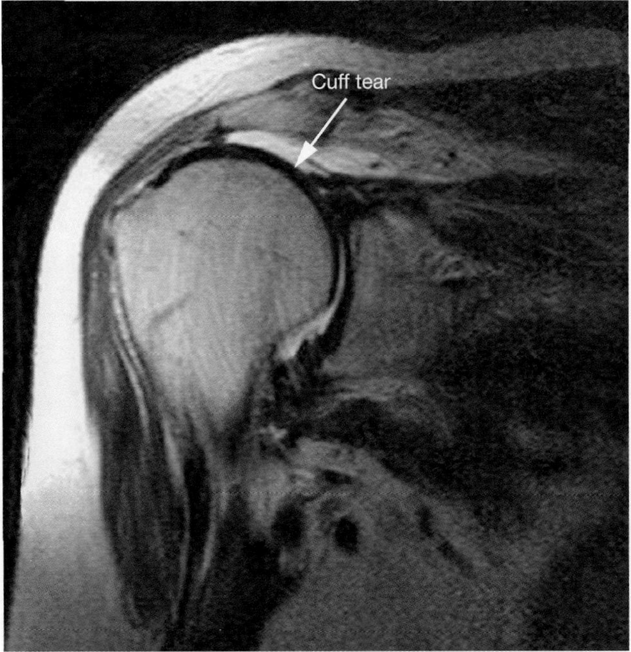

Figure 38.6 Magnetic resonance imaging scan showing a retracted cuff tear.

Treatment

Injection of steroid into the inflamed subacromial bursa may break the cycle of inflammation and impingement (*Figure 38.8*), allowing rotator cuff function to resume without impingement. Physiotherapy promotes normal cuff activity once the pain has been relieved in this way. A commonly performed procedure is arthroscopic removal of the subacromial spur, anteroinferior acromion and the CAL, which has been shown to give good relief of symptoms (*Figure 38.9*), but there is no evidence that it either improves the long-term prognosis or reduces the risk of rotator cuff tears developing.

Charles Sumner Neer II, 1917–2011, orthopedic surgeon, Columbia University, New York, NY, USA, developed the first widely used shoulder arthroplasty.

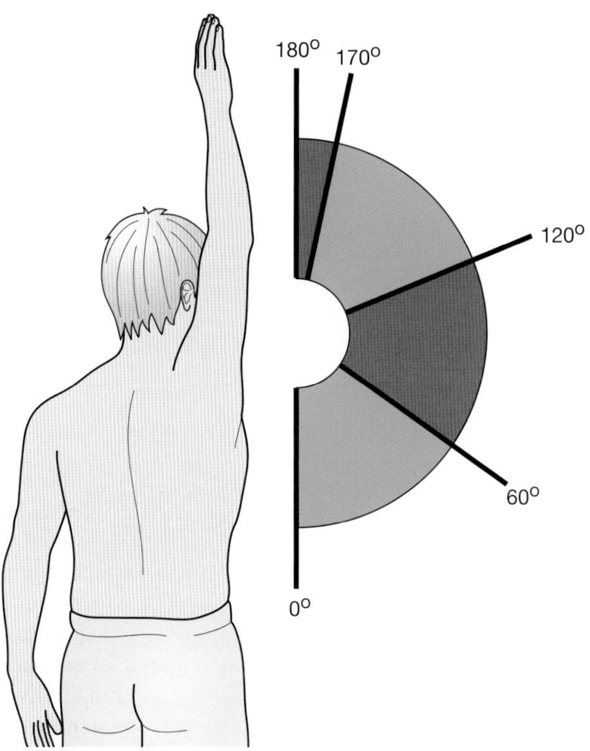

Figure 38.7 Arcs of shoulder girdle motion with subacromial impingement pain between 60° and 120° of abduction, and acromioclavicular joint pain between 170° and 180°.

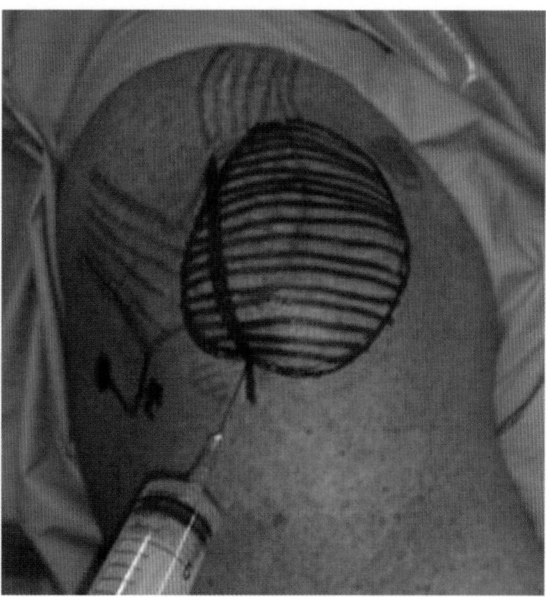

Figure 38.8 Technique of administering an injection into the subacromial bursa.

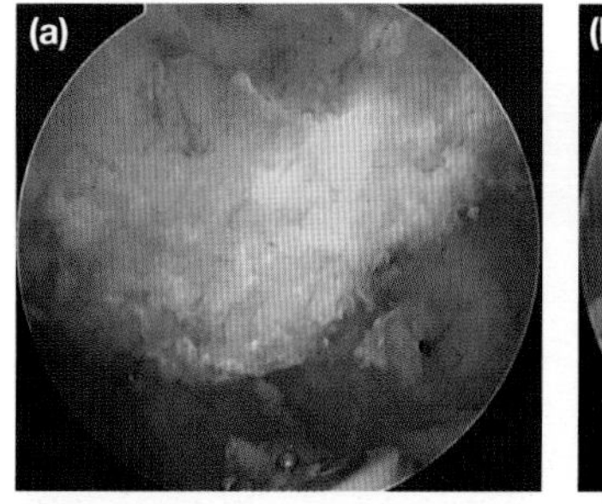

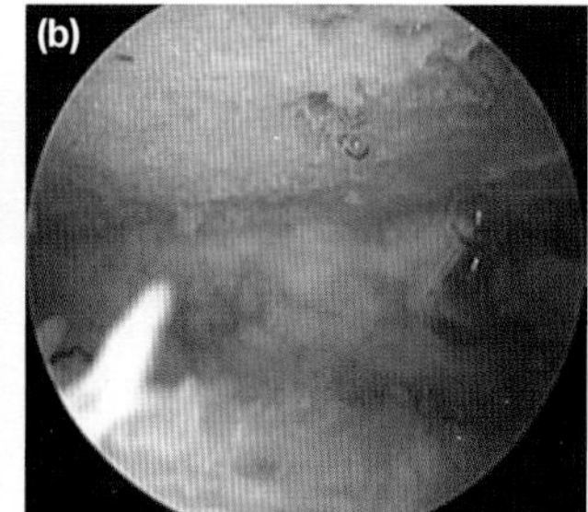

Figure 38.9 (a) Arthroscopic view of an acromial spur. (b) Arthroscopic view after the acromial spur has been removed and the cuff decompressed.

Summary box 38.1

Rotator cuff degeneration and impingement

- Tendinosis and bursitis produce weakness secondary to pain (often a painful arc)
- A tendon tear produces weakness that is only secondarily painful
- Injection of local anaesthetic and retesting can distinguish those who do from those who do not have a tear – weakness persists if there is a significant tear

Summary box 38.2

Treatment of subacromial impingement

- Non-operative treatment includes injections and rotator cuff rehabilitation
- Surgery may be indicated if symptoms persist beyond 3–6 months of non-surgical management
- Surgery restores a flat acromion and makes more room for rotator cuff gliding but there is no evidence that it improves the long-term outlook

Rotator cuff tears

The rotator cuff has a relatively poor blood supply in the segment that glides between the humeral head and acromion, as described in ***Rotator cuff degeneration and impingement***. The cuff thins with age and eventually develops defects that are termed tears, whether or not there has been any trauma involved in their appearance. This means that tears are more common in older adults, and at any age they do not heal spontaneously. Tears usually begin at the anterolateral edge of the supraspinatus, and progress posteriorly to involve the infraspinatus and teres minor tendons. This creates a bare area over the greater tuberosity, as the torn cuff retracts medially (***Figure 38.10***).

History

In the younger patient with a healthier cuff the onset often requires relatively major trauma, e.g. breaking a fall from a motorcycle or significant height with the outstretched hand, but in older adults the onset may follow a simple fall, a painful period of tendinitis or the condition may apparently occur spontaneously.

Examination

The patient may have a mixed picture of subacromial pain and a tear, but if the pain is removed by injection of local anaesthetic the weakness will persist. Symptomatic tears are

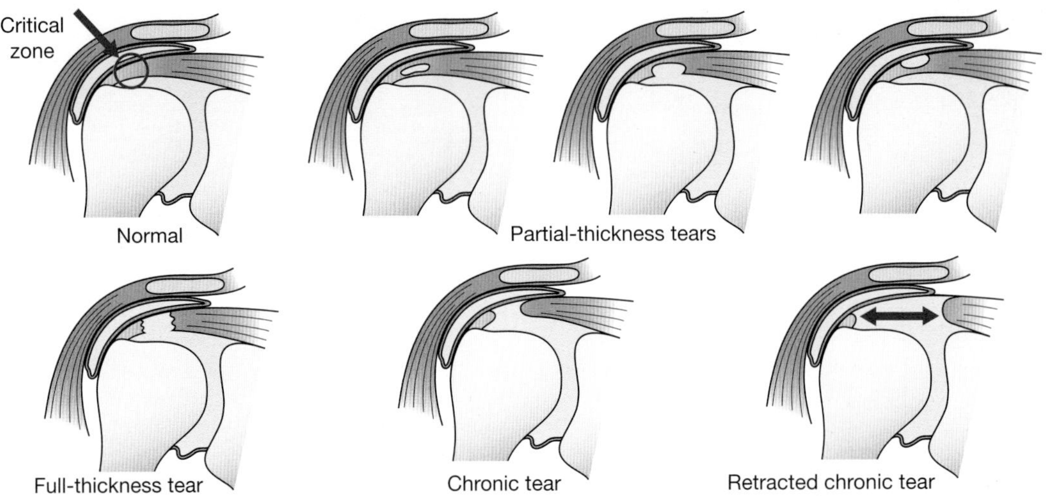

Figure 38.10 Various stages of rotator cuff tear. Initial partial-thickness tears progress to full–thickness and retracted tears but this process may be asymptomatic.

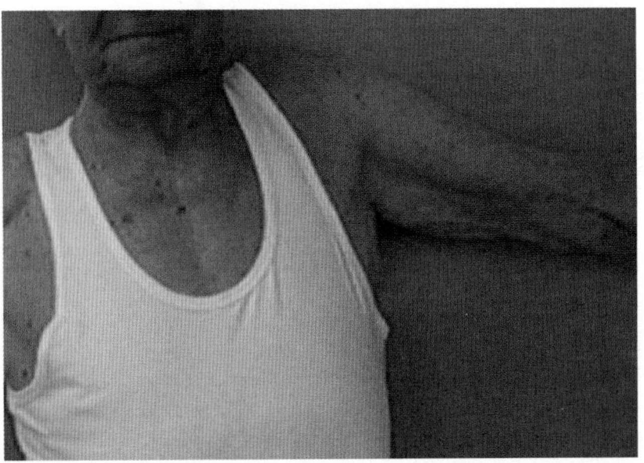

Figure 38.11 A 75-year-old man with a >5 cm retracted cuff tear attempting to abduct his shoulder; the lack of a stable fulcrum provided by the rotator cuff means that the deltoid is less effective and can only abduct to 60°.

associated with pain, weakness, limited active abduction, cuff muscle wasting and hunching of the shoulder when attempting abduction (***Figure 38.11***). Specific tests can localise the tear by identifying which muscles are affected, e.g. the 'empty can test' for supraspinatus.

Investigation

Both ultrasound scanning, in the hands of an experienced operator, and MRI are excellent tools for detecting rotator cuff tears and assessing the tissue quality. Tears are classified as small (less than 1 cm), intermediate (2–4 cm) and large (more than 5 cm).

Treatment

Treatment depends on the patient's age, lifestyle and severity of symptoms. Three to six months of rehabilitation are required after surgical repair before resuming full overhead loading, so this is not an operation to be carried out in those who cannot rest the shoulder, including those who need it for weight-bearing through bilateral crutches. Arthroscopic or mini-open repair with subacromial decompression can be considered for all tears, but is likely to give a better outcome in the young than in the old. It may not be possible to repair large tears owing to their size, or the attempt at repair may be fruitless because of fatty atrophy of the rotator cuff and loss of muscle contractility, in which case complex surgery, e.g. tendon transfers, patch grafts or reverse joint replacement (***Figure 38.12***), will need to be considered.

Summary box 38.3

Rotator cuff tears

- Occur more commonly in older age groups
- 4–20% of 40- to 50-year-olds have asymptomatic rotator cuff tears
- Up to 30% of 70-year-olds have an asymptomatic full-thickness tear
- Acute tears may present with little pain but profound weakness
- Earlier repair after traumatic onset with acute loss of function gives better results

Frozen shoulder (adhesive capsulitis)

This is an idiopathic condition causing stiffness and pain, most commonly affecting females in their fifties. It is also associated with diabetes, heart and thyroid disease.

History and examination

Frozen shoulder is characterised by the onset of severe pain that is often spontaneous, though patients may recall an episode of minor trauma, which is of unknown relevance. It may also complicate surgery or other painful shoulder conditions. The differential diagnosis includes infection, fractures and rotator cuff tear, though if the stiffness is global and there is no redness or temperature then osteoarthritis is the main

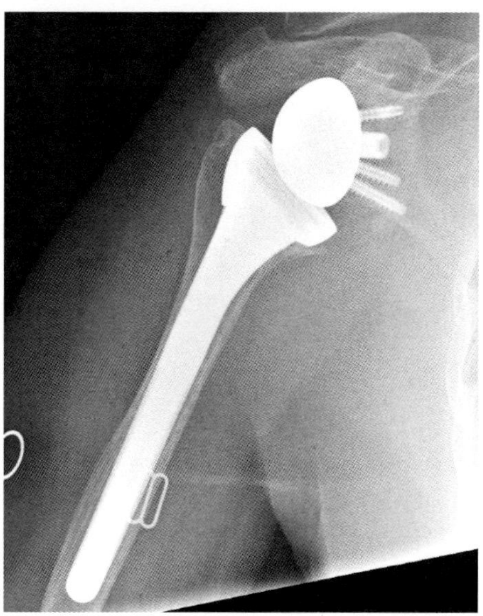

Figure 38.12 Reverse geometry total shoulder replacement.

alternative diagnosis. Initially there is severe pain but this improves with time. However, there is global loss of active and passive movement, limited by pain. The pathognomonic sign is loss of active external rotation. Radiographs are normal and distinguish it from osteoarthritis.

Treatment

The clinical course typically lasts 1–2 years, often considerably longer in individuals with diabetes, and is divided into painful, stiffening (freezing and frozen) and thawing phases. If untreated, frozen shoulder will resolve, and the majority of patients are left with no functional problems. In the first phase of the condition, treatment is pain relief. Corticosteroids can also be injected into the subacromial space or glenohumeral joint, although this is more often considered in the second phase. The latter can also be combined with a large volume (20–30 mL) of local anaesthetic to produce a distension injection. Despite the pain, the patient should be encouraged to perform as much active and passive movement as they can, and distension injections facilitate this. Operative options include manipulation under anaesthesia or arthroscopic release of the tight capsule, which usually produce pain relief and are indicated for prolonged stiffness.

Summary box 38.4

Frozen shoulder (adhesive capsulitis)

- Most commonly occurs in females in their fifties
- Spontaneous onset
- Produces severe pain with reduced glenohumeral motion
- Spontaneous resolution can occur over 1–2 years
- Differential diagnoses: calcific tendinitis and rotator cuff tear
- Injections, distension with saline, manipulation and surgical release may all help

Calcific tendinitis

Calcium salt deposition within the supraspinatus tendon is believed to be part of a degenerative process, possibly linked to the processes producing partial degenerative tears of the tendon. However, large deposits can occur in relatively young individuals with acute calcific tendinitis. Calcific deposits can be found coincidentally on radiographs taken for other purposes, but acute calcific tendinitis is agonisingly painful and associated with florid opaque lesions on radiographs. There is a spectrum of presentations between these two extremes

History and examination

In acute calcific tendinitis there is a rapid onset of severe shoulder pain with painful, restricted motion. However, in contrast to adhesive capsulitis, external rotation is usually possible. Subacromial calcific deposits can be seen on plain radiographs (***Figure 38.13***) and are well delineated on ultrasound scanning, with the calcifications casting acoustic shadows.

Treatment

Subacromial corticosteroid injections may help and can be accompanied by needling, aspiration or flushing of the deposits (barbotage). The condition is often self-limiting, with resorption of the calcium deposits. Surgery for resistant cases includes arthroscopic or open subacromial decompression and release or excision of the calcific deposits if they are prominent.

Arthritis of the shoulder

Rheumatoid arthritis

The glenohumeral joint is commonly involved in rheumatoid arthritis (***Figure 38.14***). As is typical of this condition, there is osteoporosis, destruction of the articular cartilage and synovial proliferation with pannus formation. The rotator cuff is weakened and frequently tears. Arthroscopic synovectomy may slow the progress of the joint destruction and lead to a reduction in pain and improvement in range of movement but has been effectively superseded, in many locations, by the introduction of biological therapies for rheumatoid disease.

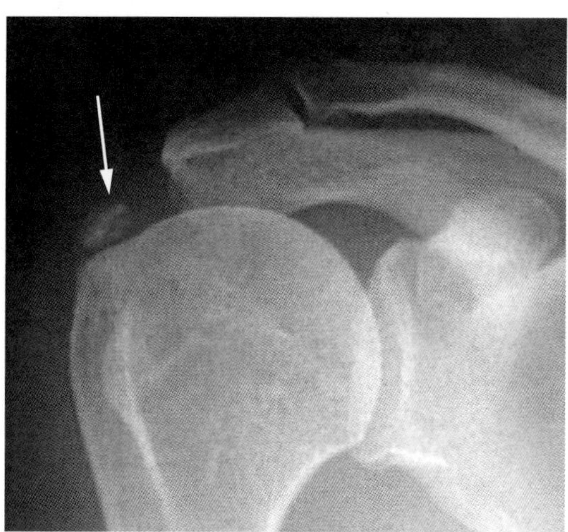

Figure 38.13 Radiograph demonstrating calcific tendinitis.

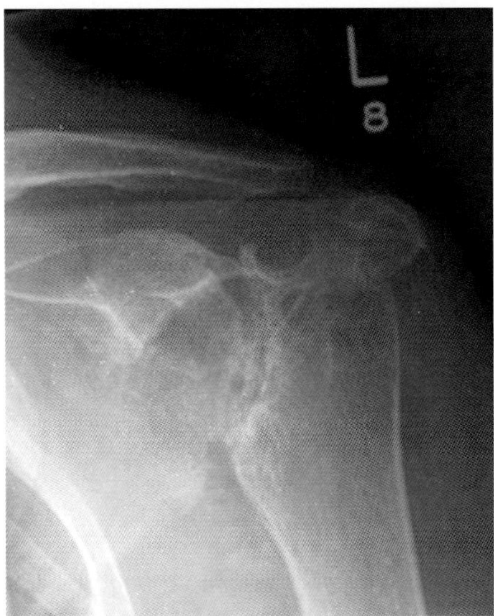

Figure 38.14 Rheumatoid arthritis of the shoulder.

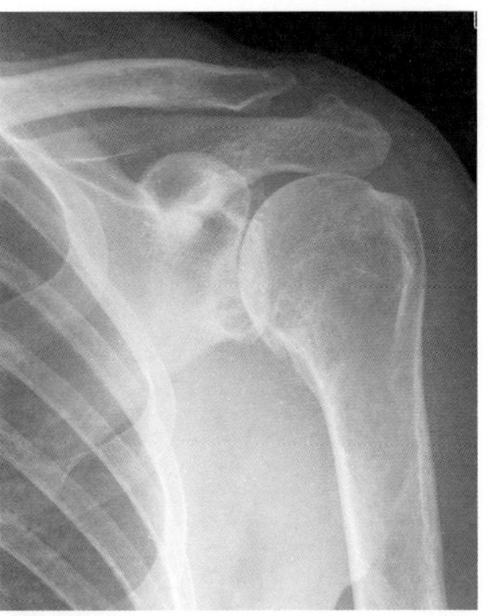

Figure 38.15 Osteoarthritis of the glenohumeral joint.

Intra-articular steroid injections may be helpful. Shoulder replacement is complicated by poor bone stock and anatomical shoulder replacement is further compromised by damage to the stabilising structures around the shoulder, especially the rotator cuff. In these patients reverse shoulder replacement may be an option if bone stock is preserved, although the patient should only expect a reduction in pain. Any increase in range of movement is a bonus, though is more likely with reverse shoulder replacement.

Summary box 38.5

Shoulder problems in rheumatoid arthritis

- Arthroscopic synovectomy may be effective but rarely needed
- Rotator cuff tears are common
- Glenohumeral joint replacement improves pain, but motion depends on rotator cuff involvement

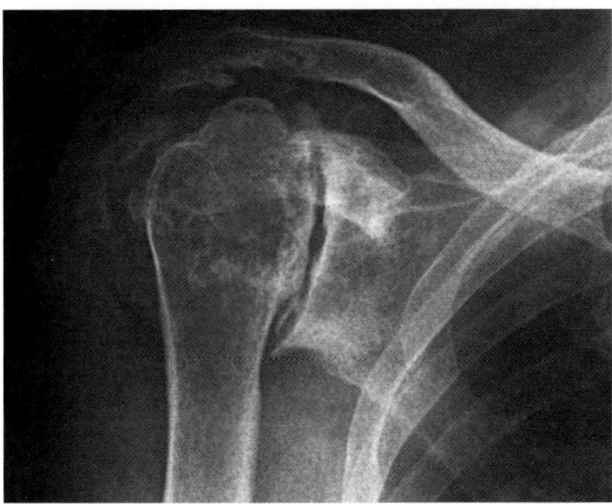

Figure 38.16 Post-traumatic arthritis with malunion of the proximal humerus, collapse of the humeral head, subchondral sclerosis and osteophytes.

Osteoarthritis of the shoulder

Glenohumeral joint osteoarthritis is either primary (***Figure 38.15***), secondary to trauma (***Figure 38.16***) or end-stage rotator cuff disease, i.e. cuff arthropathy (***Figure 38.17***).

Treatment

If medical treatment has failed, the surgical options are arthroscopic debridement or joint arthroplasty. Debridement is not predictable and is often reserved for young, active patients to delay the need for arthroplasty. Both total shoulder replacement (***Figure 38.18***) and hemiarthroplasty (***Figure 38.19***) have good reported results in appropriate patients, although pain relief is better with total arthroplasty, with the rate of hemiarthroplasty falling as the rate of total arthroplasty increases. An anatomical total shoulder arthroplasty can be performed if the rotator cuff is intact. However, in most patients with rheumatoid arthritis, and all patients with cuff tear arthropathy,

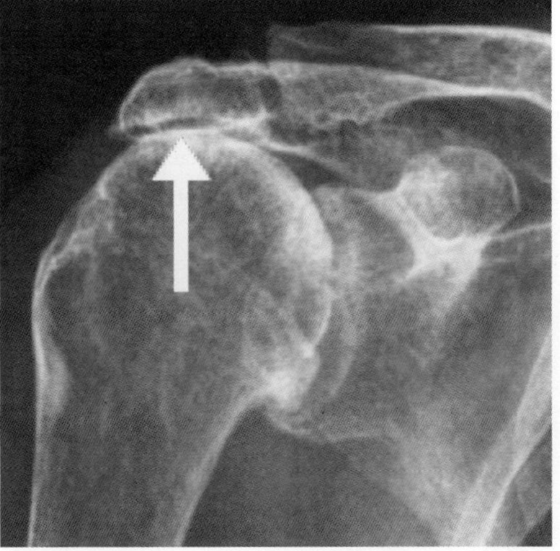

Figure 38.17 A massive cuff tear that has led to superior migration of the humeral head and secondary osteoarthritis of the glenohumeral joint.

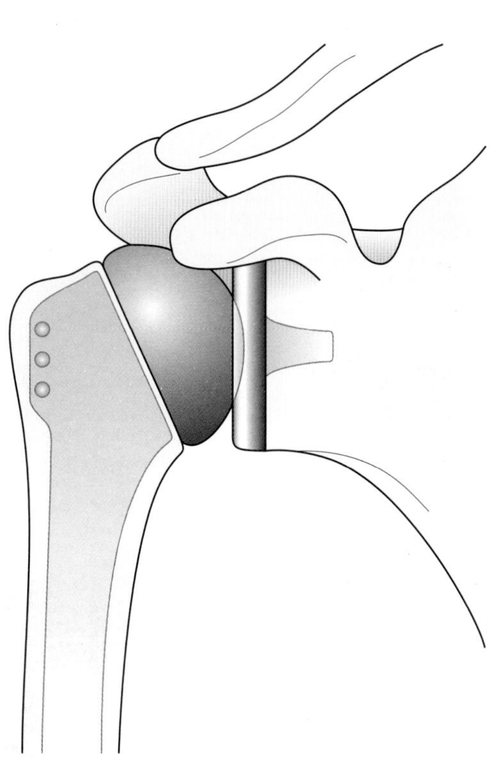

Figure 38.18 Anatomical total shoulder replacement performed for osteoarthritis. An intact rotator cuff is essential.

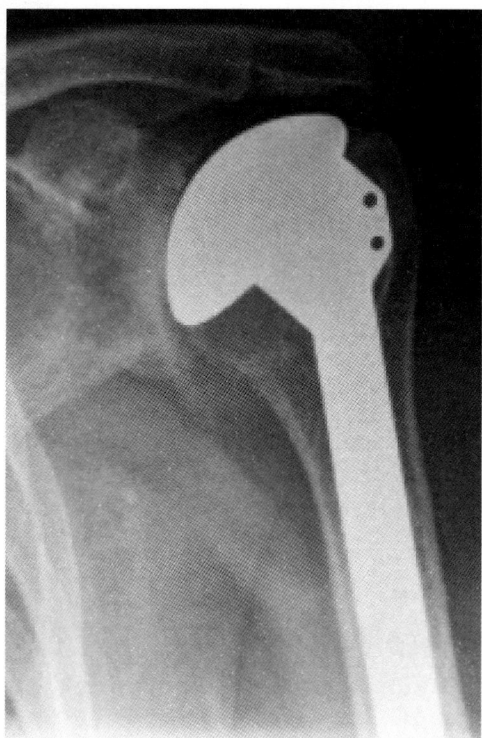

Figure 38.19 Shoulder hemiarthroplasty can be performed for arthritis, particularly if there is a deficient rotator cuff or in very young, active patients with a well-preserved glenoid.

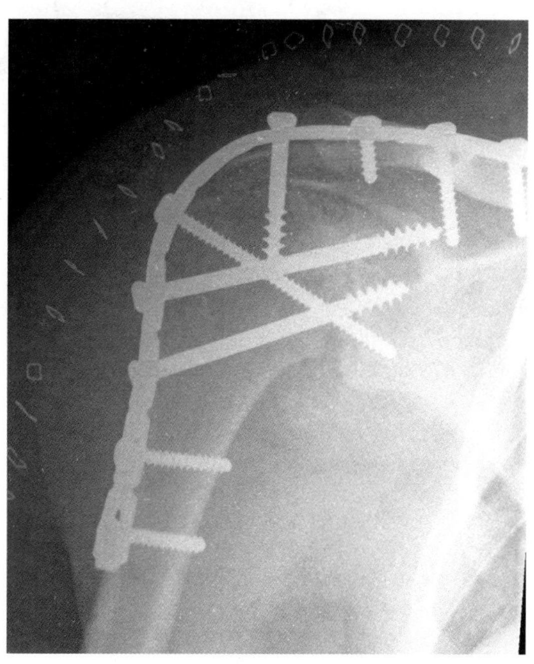

Figure 38.20 Arthrodesis of the shoulder.

the cuff is deficient and either a hemiarthroplasty or a reverse polarity total shoulder arthroplasty (***Figure 38.12***) should be used. Shoulder arthroplasty is an effective pain-relieving procedure, but less predictable in restoring motion, especially above shoulder level.

Arthrodesis of the joint is an alternative in younger patients with a history of sepsis or neurological problems (***Figure 38.20***). It is also used after brachial plexus injury, when nerve repair restores hand and elbow function but the shoulder remains flail because of loss of the C5 supply. Good scapulothoracic control, tested by the ability to shrug the shoulder powerfully, is a prerequisite to successful arthrodesis. Patients retain a moderate range of movement at the shoulder girdle as a result of scapulothoracic motion, which normally makes up approximately one-third of apparent shoulder elevation, the remaining two-thirds being glenohumeral movement, which is lost in arthrodesis.

Summary box 38.6

Arthritis of the shoulder

- Severe cases are treated with hemiarthroplasty or total shoulder arthroplasty
- Anatomical total shoulder replacement should not be performed if the rotator cuff is deficient but reverse shoulder replacement is appropriate
- Pain relief is good following arthroplasty, although improvement in range of motion is less predictable
- Glenohumeral arthrodesis is an option in the young or those with a history of sepsis
- Post arthrodesis, motion is fair but is entirely scapulothoracic

Acromioclavicular joint

Acromioclavicular joint (ACJ) arthritis is common and is often asymptomatic, noted as an incidental finding on radiographs (***Figure 38.4b***). Symptoms typically arise in males aged 20–50 years. Inferior osteophytes can impinge on the underlying rotator cuff.

History and examination

There may be a history of trauma to the ACJ. Pain is activity related and worse when using the arm overhead. There is prominence of the lateral end of the clavicle. The joint line is tender. Flexing and adducting the arm to place the hand around the opposite shoulder reproduces pain. There is a high painful arc, pain being worst for the last 20–30° of elevation. If symptoms are related to inferior osteophytes, impingement symptoms and signs can also be present.

Treatment

An intra-articular corticosteroid injection will usually help; even if the effect is short-lived it localises the problem accurately. Surgery involves arthroscopic or open excision of the lateral 0.5–1 cm of the clavicle (***Figure 38.21***). This gives good pain relief. In patients with symptoms that are predominantly those of impingement, arthroscopic removal of the inferior osteophytes with subacromial decompression should be performed.

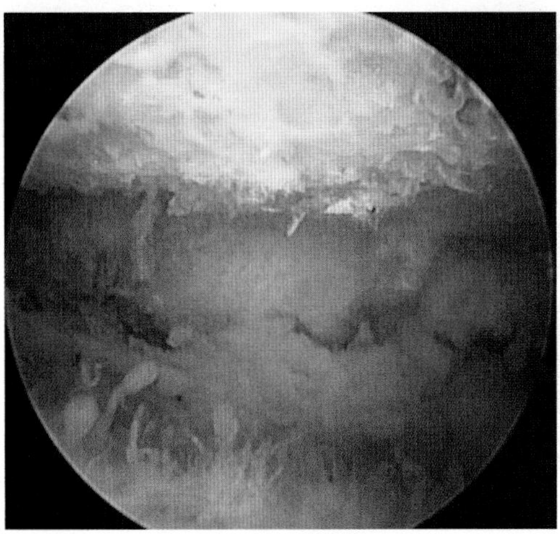

Figure 38.21 Arthroscopic end-on view of the clavicle after excision of its distal end.

Summary box 38.7

ACJ problems

- ACJ arthritis is common and is often asymptomatic
- It may become symptomatic secondary to trauma or repetitive overload
- Intra-articular steroid and local anaesthetic injection may relieve symptoms
- Excision of the lateral end of the clavicle gives good results

Long head of biceps tendon rupture

Rupture of the long head of biceps usually occurs in older adults and is due to constriction and degeneration of the tendon in the bicipital groove, especially at the superior end, beneath the anterior acromion. It is associated with rotator cuff tears. Most patients present with few symptoms, although they often seek advice because of the bulge they notice in their arm.

History and examination

Patients feel a sense of 'something giving way' in front of the shoulder, sometimes with relief of pain if there was any present beforehand due to biceps tendinitis. The upper arm is bruised and elbow flexion produces a swelling in the front and middle of the arm (***Figure 38.22***). The lump will be permanent and is initially tender. Power is slightly diminished in the early stages, when there may also be cramping pains on use of the arm.

Treatment

Reassurance that pain and bruising will resolve is sufficient. Power improves over several months and surgery (biceps tenodesis) is not needed for function, although it may help the cosmetic appearance.

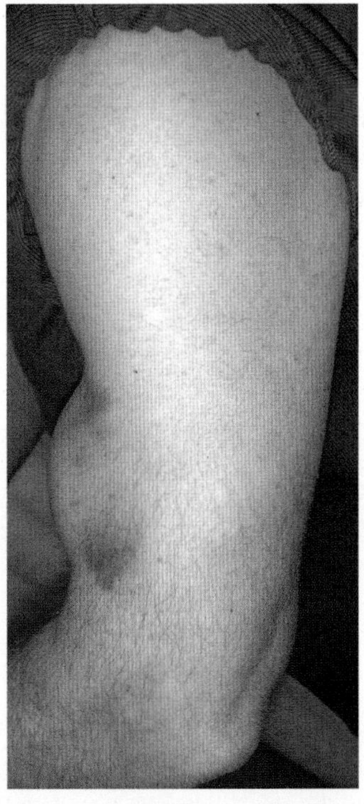

Figure 38.22 Bruising and change in the upper arm shape due to rupture of the long head of biceps.

Dislocation of the shoulder and instability of the glenohumeral joint

Three broad groups of shoulder instability exist.

Classification of glenohumeral instability

- **Traumatic**: unidirectional; involuntary; surgery is usually successful.
- **Atraumatic**: multidirectional, painful; involuntary; responds to surgery.
- **Habitual**: voluntary, with ligament laxity, painless; surgery usually contraindicated.

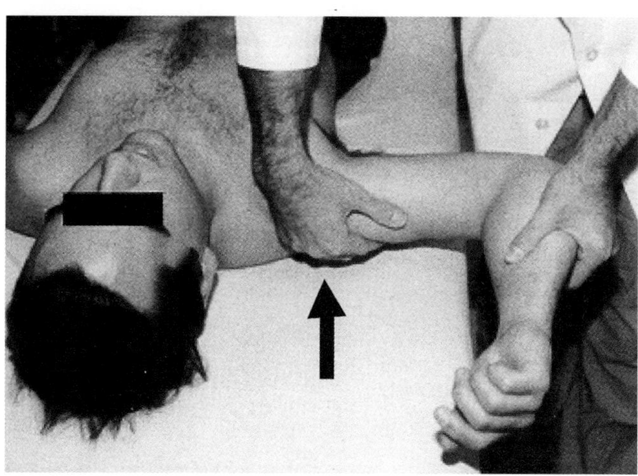

Figure 38.23 Apprehension test for anterior instability.

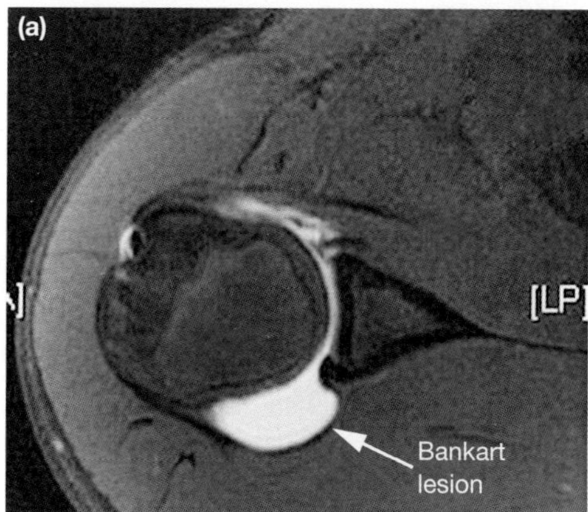

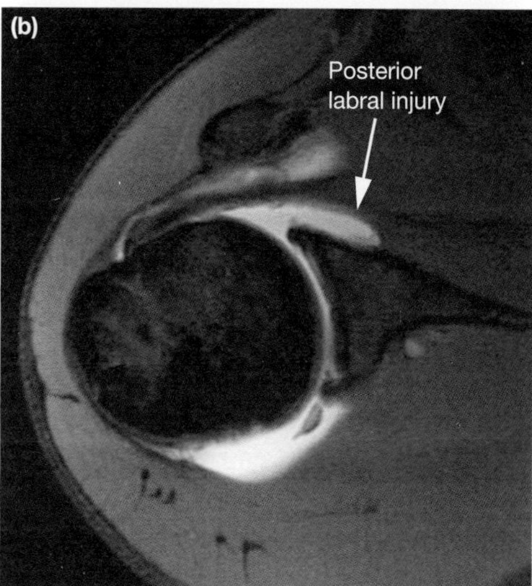

Figure 38.24 (a) Magnetic resonance (MR) arthrogram showing an anterior Bankart lesion. (b) MR arthrogram showing a posterior labral injury.

Recurrent traumatic anterior instability

History

Traumatic shoulder dislocation is the commonest of all dislocations, usually first presenting in patients under 25. The shoulder usually dislocates anteroinferiorly and initially there is a notable traumatic event. Subsequent dislocations usually require less force. The shoulder may sublux and relocate, or actually dislocate (complete separation of the joint surfaces).

Examination

Assuming that the patient presents with a history of instability following a previous anterior dislocation (after which the joint was reduced), examination of the shoulder reveals a full range of motion. However, with forced abduction and external rotation the patient experiences apprehension (a sense of impending doom as the patient feels the shoulder about to re-dislocate!) (***Figure 38.23***).

Investigations

On computed tomography (CT) or MR arthrography (***Figure 38.24***) detachment of the anteroinferior labrum (Bankart's lesion) (***Figures 38.25 and 38.26***) and damage to the humeral head (Hill–Sachs lesion) can often be seen. On CT without arthrography only the bone lesions will be seen, which can also include a marginal fracture of the anteroinferior glenoid margin (bony Bankart).

Treatment

The relative indications for surgery are repeated dislocations, or symptoms of instability that persist after reduction of the first dislocation, that are interfering with the patient's quality of life. Anterior instability can be treated with arthroscopic or open repair of the Bankart lesion with retensioning of the stretched anterior/inferior capsule, which prevents further dislocations in up to 90–95% of patients. Bony defects of the glenoid, and occasionally large Hill–Sachs lesions, may have to

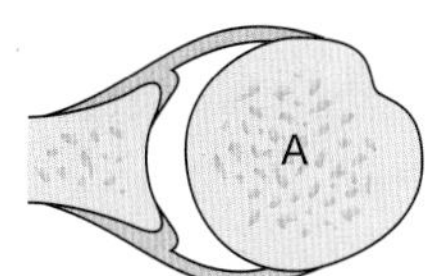

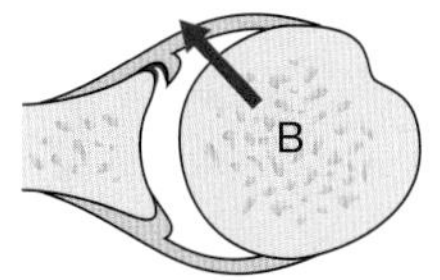

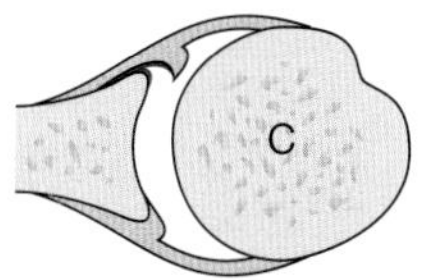

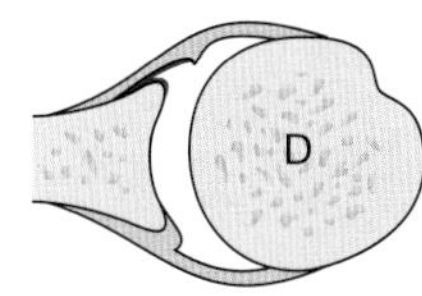

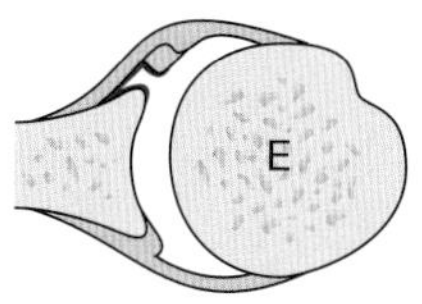

Figure 38.25 Schematic representation of Bankart's lesion, which forms a spectrum of pathology from minor labral detachment (B) to large detachments with glenoid rim fractures (bony Bankart; E).

Arthur Sydney Blundell Bankart, 1879–1951, orthopaedic surgeon, The Middlesex Hospital, London, UK.
Harold Arthur Hill, 1901–1973, radiologist, San Francisco, CA, USA.
Maurice David Sachs, 1909–1987, radiologist, San Francisco, CA, USA.

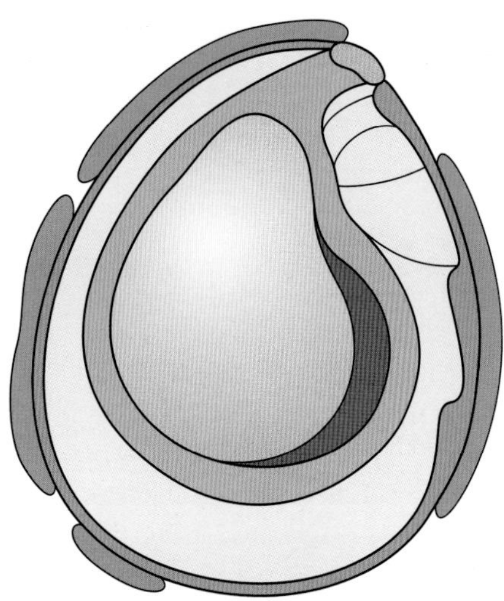

Figure 38.26 An end-on view of the glenoid labrum, demonstrating anteroinferior labral detachment (red) with the rotator cuff muscles (brown), long head of biceps tendon and labrum (grey).

be grafted. For the less common recurrent posterior instability, repair of the damaged labrum and tightening of the posterior capsule is needed.

Posterior dislocation of the shoulder

This is a relatively rare event and is easy to miss. The clue is often in the history, as the patient will often have had either an electric shock or an epileptic fit or been subject to severe restraint when their arm has been forced up their back (a half-Nelson) – all are mechanisms producing forced internal rotation of the glenohumeral joint.

The patient may be in severe pain but can be difficult to examine properly if they are post-ictal or are recovering from an electric shock. For the same reason, the radiographer may only be able to get an anteroposterior view of the shoulder; on this view, the shoulder may look normal to the unwary (*Figure 38.27*). It is the high 'index of suspicion' from the history that gives the best chance of making the diagnosis.

Treatment

This dislocation may be difficult to reduce if the posterior margin of the glenoid is embedded in the humeral head (a 'locked' posterior dislocation), so that open reduction is needed. A number of techniques are available, such as gently abducting the internally rotated arm above shoulder height while maintaining axial traction then externally rotating the arm before returning it down to the side – the reduced shoulder

Summary box 38.8

Recurrent traumatic shoulder instability

- An appreciable force leads to the first dislocation or subluxation
- Subsequent dislocations/subluxations require less force
- The commonest direction of dislocation is anteroinferior
- There is a positive apprehension sign
- Surgical treatment repairs the labral lesion and reverses traumatic laxity of the capsule

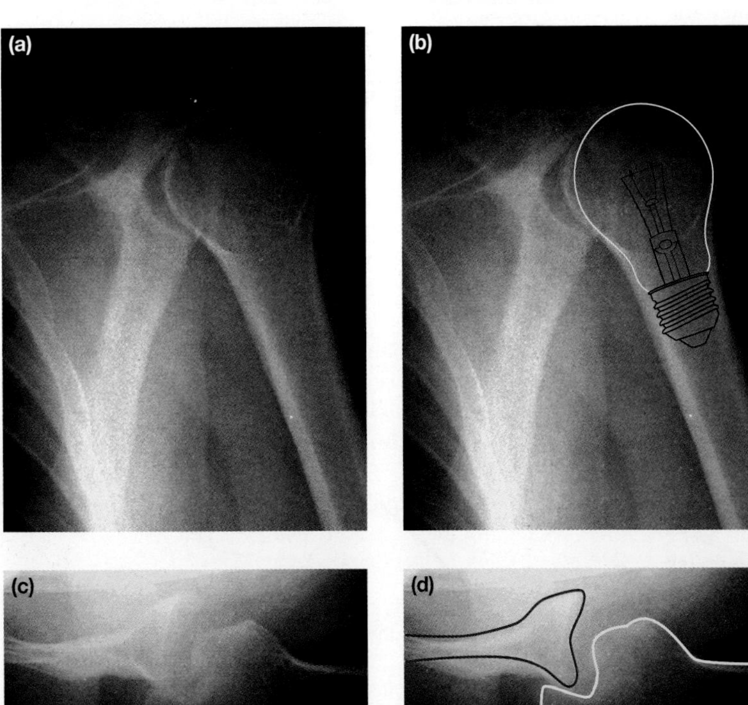

Figure 38.27 Posterior dislocation of the shoulder. (a) Anteroposterior view; (b) origin of the light bulb sign; (c) axial projection demonstrating how much easier it is to visualise the injury on this view; (d) axial projection highlighting this joint and further demonstrating the impacted fracture in the humeral head, or anterior Hill–Sachs lesion.

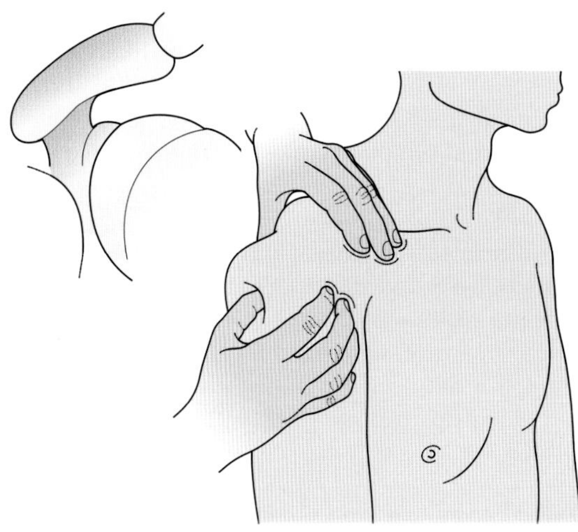

Figure 38.28 Generalised laxity can be appreciated by drawing the humeral head in anterior and posterior directions and feeling it slide up to, and possibly even over, the glenoid rim. A sulcus will be produced under the acromion if the humerus is drawn inferiorly (sulcus sign).

should then be placed in an external rotation brace to allow the stretched and torn posterior structures an opportunity to heal.

Atraumatic instability

History

There is usually no history of an initial injury. Instability may be multidirectional and is usually associated with subluxation rather than dislocation. The patient is often able to reduce the shoulder without assistance.

Examination

Generalised ligament laxity is common (see Beighton score in *Chapter 35*). Apprehension tests are positive, but often in more than one direction. Anterior and posterior drawing of the humeral head allows laxity to be tested in these directions, whereas downward traction on the humerus may produce a 'sulcus sign' as the deltoid is sucked into the space created by inferior subluxation of the humeral head (*Figure 38.28*). Overactivity of muscle groups such as pectoralis major should be sought, as this gives an avenue of treatment through rehabilitation.

Treatment

Specialist physiotherapy should be tried first in these patients, aiming to improve both the proprioception and firing patterns of the muscles around the shoulder (for instance, biofeedback to control an overactive pectoralis major or strengthening of underactive muscle groups). If this fails then surgery may be considered, by way of capsular tightening.

Habitual dislocation

Habitual dislocators are patients who can sublux the shoulder at will, usually either anteroinferiorly or posteriorly. The manoeuvre is painless. Patients have generalised joint laxity and may subluxate the shoulder as a 'party trick'.

Patients should be advised to stop subluxating the shoulder, which may then allow the capsule to tighten naturally with age. They may benefit from assessment and advice from a specialist physiotherapist. Surgery is associated with a high failure rate and should be avoided.

DISORDERS OF THE ELBOW

Anatomy and function

The elbow joint allows flexion and extension through the ulnohumeral articulation as well as rotation of the radial head, which articulates with both the capitellum of the distal humerus (radiocapitellar joint) and the proximal ulna (proximal radioulnar joint [PRUJ]). The rotation of the radius at the PRUJ, in concert with the distal radioulnar joint and interosseous membrane, permits pronation and supination of the forearm. The elbow joint possesses a slim soft-tissue envelope, traversed by multiple neurovascular structures. At the front, from medial to lateral, are found the median nerve, brachial artery and radial nerve. At the back, just behind the medial epicondyle is found the ulnar nerve.

Tennis elbow (lateral epicondylitis) and golfer's elbow (medial epicondylitis)

These are discussed in *Chapters 35 and 36*.

Arthritis of the elbow

Rheumatoid arthritis

Surgery may be required, especially in end-stage disease (*Figure 38.29*). Arthroscopic or open radial head excision and synovectomy are effective for painful, restricted pronation and supination. Elbow arthroplasty is effective for pain relief and functional restoration.

Osteoarthritis

Osteoarthritis of the elbow is usually primary (*Figure 38.30*) or secondary to trauma.

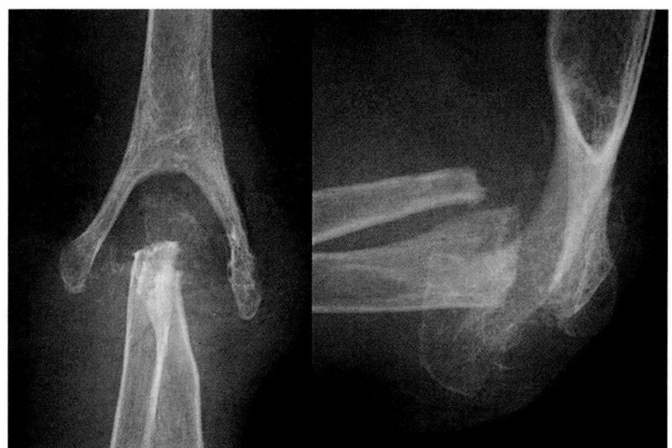

Figure 38.29 Typical end-stage unstable and destroyed rheumatoid elbow.

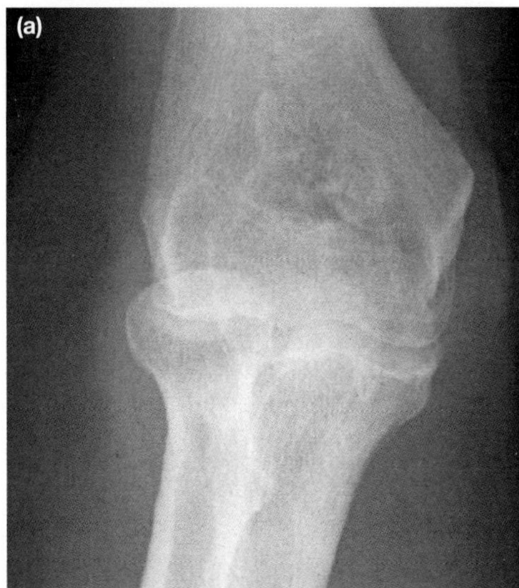

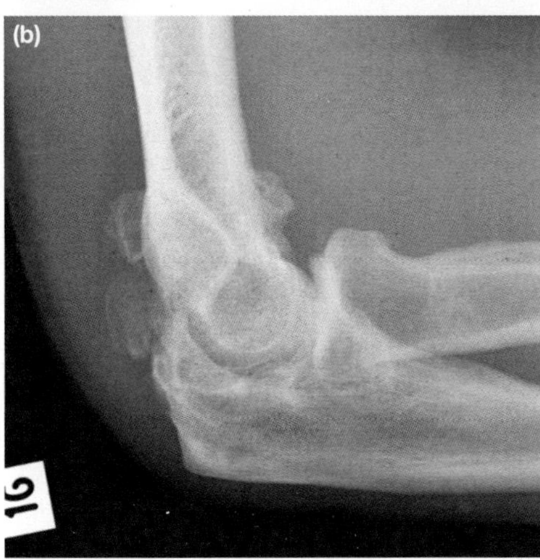

Figure 38.30 (a, b) Radiographs showing osteoarthritis of the elbow joint.

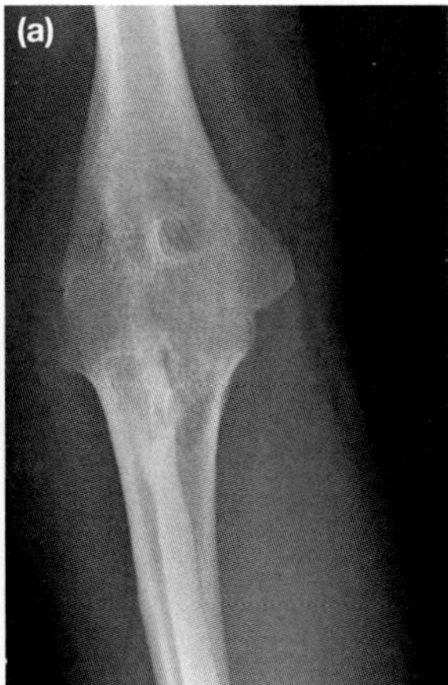

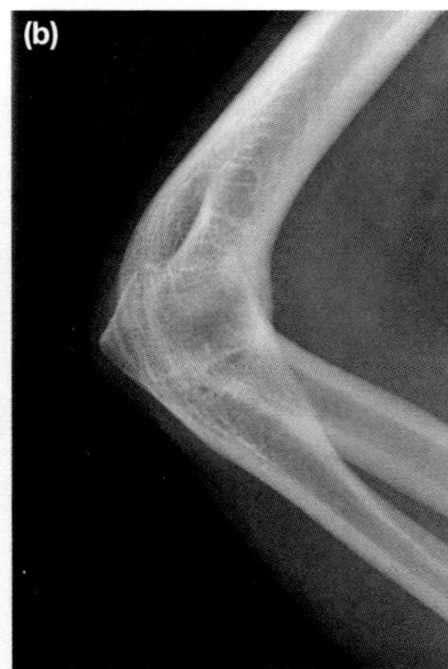

Figure 38.31 (a, b) Ankylosed elbow after tuberculosis. Arthrodesis is a surgical procedure to achieve the same end result, by excising the articular surfaces and compression plating across the joint.

History

Typical patients are middle-aged men in manual occupations. Symptoms can include pain, locking, crepitus and painful motion with loss of terminal flexion and extension. Ulnar nerve entrapment symptoms may be present.

Examination

There is restriction of extension and flexion with impingement pain as osteophytes and soft tissues are pressed together at the end of the available range. Pronation and supination tend to be spared in comparison with rheumatoid arthritis but there may still be crepitus felt over the radiocapitellar joint on rotation and pain when this is done with the fist clenched ('grip and grind' test).

Treatment

Surgery should be considered only if medical treatment fails. Arthrodesis may very rarely be offered for those performing heavy manual work (***Figure 38.31***) but is associated with significant residual functional loss. However, joint replacement will not survive long under heavy loading. Surgical debridement alleviates pain and increases range of motion by removing anterior and posterior osteophytes, the thickened capsule and loose bodies through a lateral approach (lateral column procedure). In earlier stages the olecranon osteophytes can be accessed through the triceps tendon, creating an olecranon foramen by drilling through the olecranon fossa to access the coronoid tip osteophyte and any loose bodies (the so-called 'OK' procedure). Interposition arthroplasty (for example, Achilles tendon allograft) may be considered in younger patients, although it can be associated with significant bone loss with time, possibly restricting future treatments. Prosthetic joint arthroplasty provides more predictable symptomatic relief (***Figure 38.32***) but high activity levels are associated with early loosening.

Summary box 38.9

Arthritis of the elbow

- Excision of the radial head and synovectomy improves pain and pronation–supination in rheumatoid arthritis
- Total elbow replacement gives good results in rheumatoid and low-demand osteoarthritic patients
- Arthrodesis may be the only surgical option in a high-demand manual labourer

Loose bodies in the elbow

The common causes are osteoarthritis, osteochondritis dissecans in the young (***Figure 38.33***) and synovial chondromatosis (***Figure 38.34***). Patients describe sudden pain and locking, and the need to manipulate the elbow for relief. Plain radiographs will usually confirm the diagnosis (***Figure 38.35***) but if there is doubt a CT or MR arthrogram will demonstrate filling defects in the intra-articular contrast. Arthroscopic clearance of the joint produces good results (***Figure 38.36***).

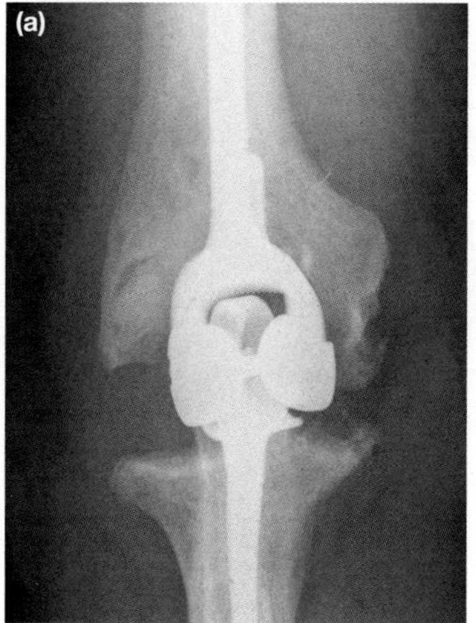

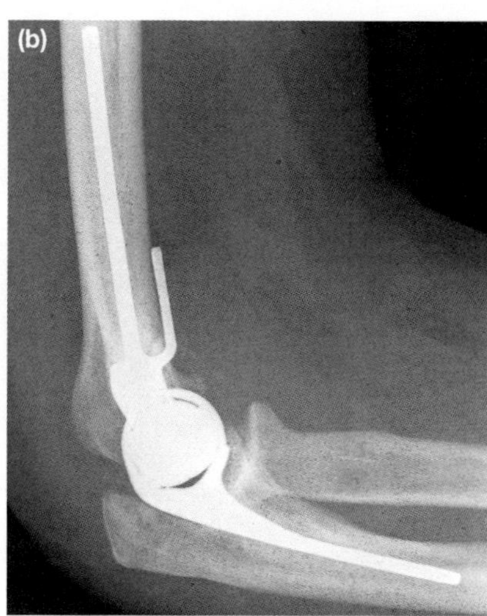

Figure 38.32 (a, b) Linked total elbow replacement.

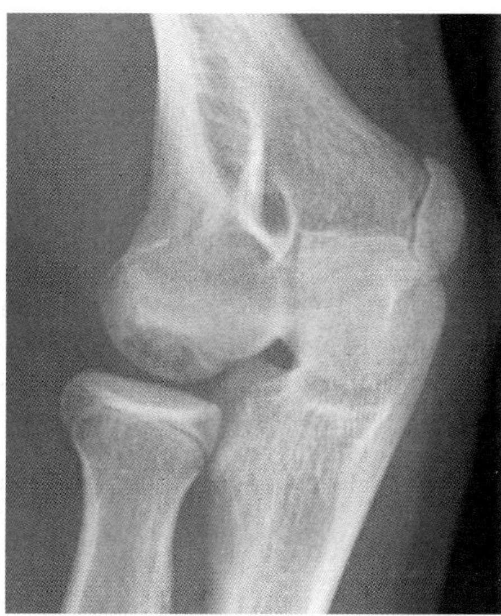

Figure 38.33 Osteochondritis dissecans of the capitellum (Panner's disease).

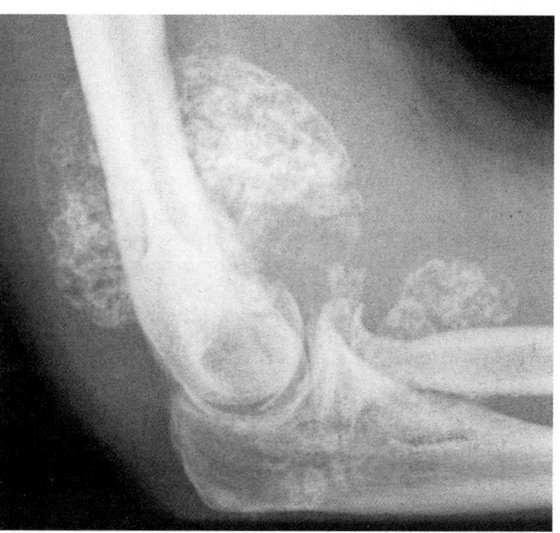

Figure 38.34 Synovial chondromatosis.

Olecranon bursitis

This is a relatively common disorder in which the point of the elbow becomes red, warm, swollen and painful. Initially, septic arthritis may be suspected. However, on examination signs and symptoms are confined to the extensor aspect of the elbow (***Figure 38.37***), over the olecranon, and movement within an arc of 30–130° is almost always possible. Most cases settle with anti-inflammatory drugs. If the patient is pyrexial antibiotics should be given. Formal drainage of the bursa is indicated if purulent material is present.

Chronic olecranon bursitis may be associated with calcific nodules of the bursal lining (***Figure 38.38***). These can be excised if they prove troublesome.

Ulnar nerve compression

Compression of the ulnar nerve most commonly occurs in the cubital tunnel (behind the medial epicondyle) within the arcade of Struthers. It may become compressed by the medial intermuscular septum as the nerve passes into the posterior compartment of the distal humerus. Distally it may also become compressed as the nerve passes between the heads of the flexor carpi ulnaris (***Figure 38.39***).

History and examination

Patients describe tingling/numbness in the little and ring fingers. A positive Tinel's sign is usually present at the compression site, with wasting and weakness of the intrinsic muscles

Hans Jessen Panner, 1871–1930, radiologist, Copenhagen, Denmark, described this condition in 1927.
Sir John Struthers, 1823–1899, Professor of Anatomy, University of Aberdeen, Aberdeen, UK.
Jules Tinel, 1879–1952, physician, Hôpital Beaujon, Paris, France.

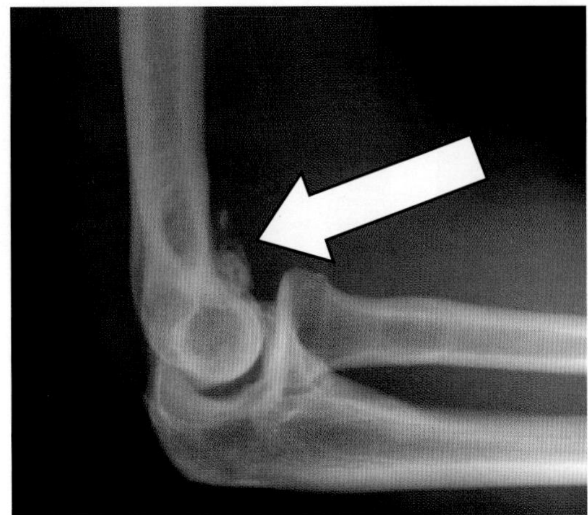

Figure 38.35 Radiographs showing loose bodies in the elbow (arrow).

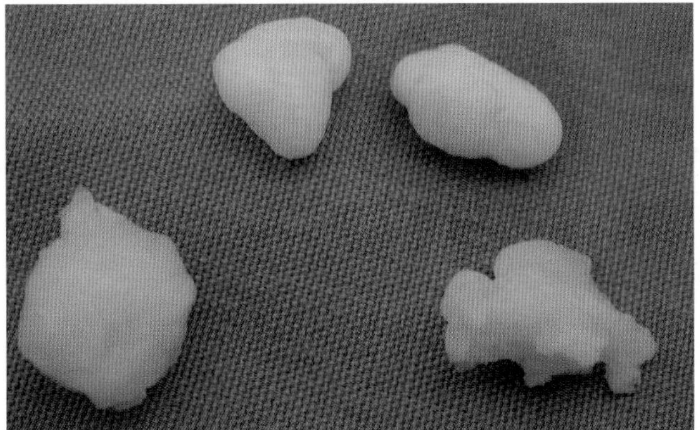

Figure 38.36 Loose bodies removed arthroscopically from the patient in *Figure 38.35*.

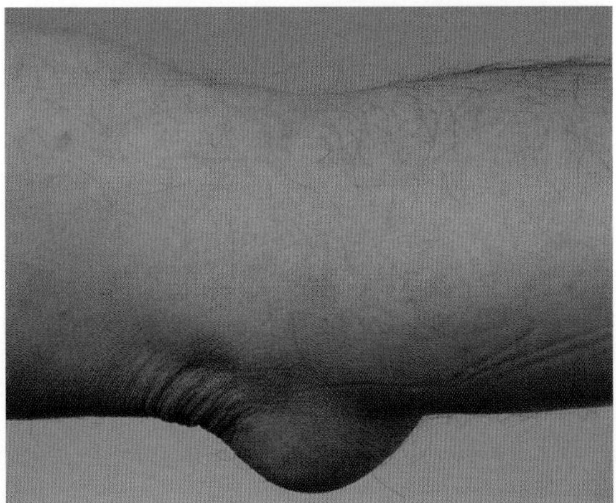

Figure 38.37 Olecranon bursitis.

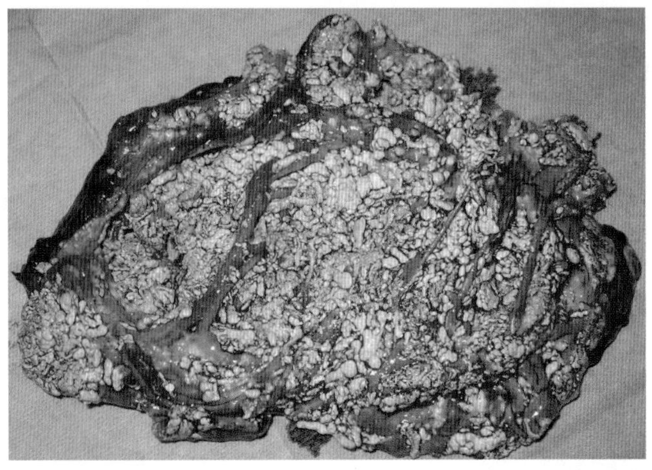

Figure 38.38 Large chronic olecranon bursa with dense calcific deposit.

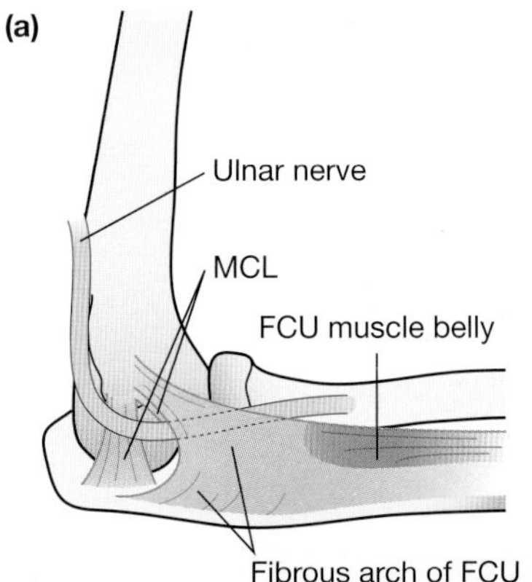

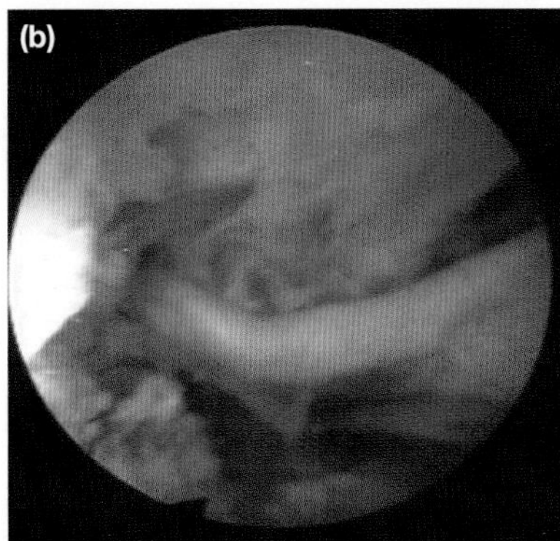

Figure 38.39 (a) Anatomy of the cubital tunnel site for ulnar nerve compression, with (b) a view of arthroscopic ulnar nerve decompression. FCU, flexor carpi ulnaris; MCL, medial collateral ligament.

of the hand (*Figure 38.40*). Froment's sign may be positive if there is weakness of the adductor pollicis (*Figure 38.41*). Nerve conduction studies have an unpredictable diagnostic value in the early stages. Radiographs may confirm medial osteophytes or loose bodies if compression is secondary to arthritis.

Treatment

Splints preventing elbow flexion at night may be useful if only night symptoms are a problem for the patient. If symptoms persist, surgery can be performed; options include simple nerve decompression (most cases), partial medial epicondylectomy and/or anterior transposition of the nerve. Transposition is necessary in cases of valgus deformity or if the nerve is unstable after decompression.

Jules Froment, 1878–1946, Professor of Clinical Medicine, Lyons, France.

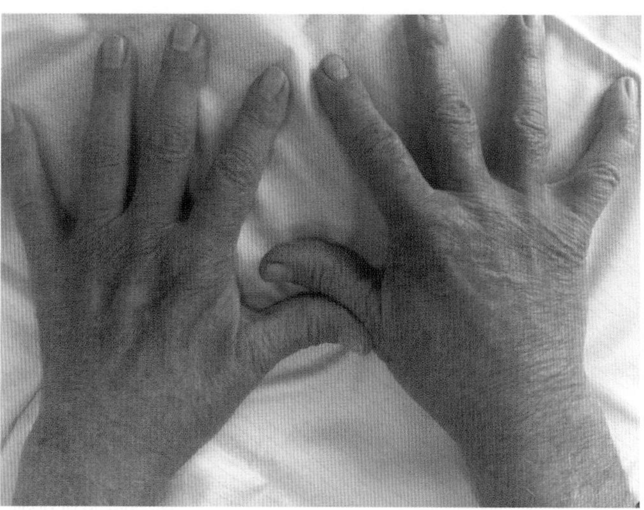

Figure 38.40 Intrinsic muscle wasting on the left due to ulnar neuropathy.

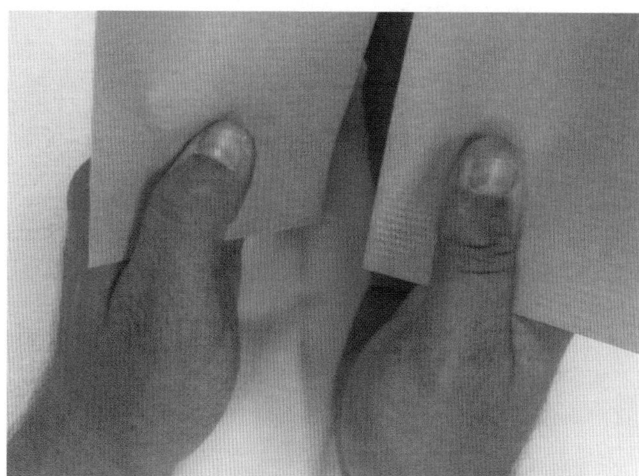

Figure 38.41 Froment's sign tests the adductor pollicis. The patient is asked to hold a piece of paper in a side pinch between the thumb and the index finger. The examiner attempts to pull the paper out. Owing to weakness of the adductor pollicis, the patient will compensate by flexing the flexor pollicis longus, which is supplied by the anterior interosseous nerve (median nerve).

Summary box 38.10

Other common elbow problems

- Loose bodies cause locking and can be removed arthroscopically
- If the ulnar nerve is compressed, weakness and wasting will be seen in the hands
- Simple decompression is usually successful

TUMOURS OF THE UPPER LIMB

Tumours are discussed in ***Chapter 42***.

HAND AND WRIST

The hand and wrist work in concert to interact with the environment in which they are placed. The index finger works against the thumb for pinch grip; the thumb can press against the side of the flexed index finger for a key-pinch grip; the tips of the thumb, index and middle fingers provide a tripod pinch; all fingers curl for hook grip while the little and ring fingers provide the most power when making a fist. A mobile and stable wrist is required to optimise hand function through maximising range of movement and strength.

Clinical history and physical examination

History

Asking about the patient's occupation, hobbies (sport, musical instruments, fine art) and hand dominance are important when taking a history. In considering the problem concerned there are a number of symptoms that patients complain of: pain, swelling, stiffness, instability and pins and needles are commonly encountered in the hand and wrist. Sometimes these present together and sometimes in isolation, but all affect the function of the hand. It is vital to ask which of these issues causes the functional deficit, since there is no value in fusing a painful finger that is stiff if the main concern of the patient is the stiffness rather than the pain. A history of other medical comorbidities is important to glean, since these may well be part of the pathology or alter the management strategies that can be considered, e.g. carpal tunnel syndrome may be the first presentation of diabetes mellitus.

Examination

The examination of the hand should assess sensation, movement, power and clinically relevant special tests for the issues encountered. Perfusion is seen (pink is well perfused) and felt (slightly warm to the touch with palpable radial and ulnar pulses). Sensory innervation of the median (radial 3.5 volar digits), ulnar (ulnar 1.5 volar digits) and radial (first dorsal web space and back of the hand) nerves is required. To test the motor innervation one can assess the abductor pollicis brevis for the median nerve and the first dorsal interosseous muscle for the ulnar nerve. The radial nerve does not supply any muscles in the hand but supplies the muscles that drive wrist extension. In assessing movement and power, one should start by evaluating functional combined movements such as grip, 'thumbs up', flat hand, palm up (supination) and palm down (pronation) as well as wrist movements (flexion, extension, radial and ulnar deviation). After that, a more detailed assessment of each individual muscle/tendon group is required. While assessing movements, obvious side-to-side asymmetry may be encountered, such as rotational malalignment of the digits (***Figure 38.42***). There are also a number of special tests relevant to different pathologies seen.

Investigations

Radiographs can be used to assess for arthritis or bone tumours. Electrophysiological studies may be required to evaluate nerve function, assessing both sensory and motor supply. Ultrasound

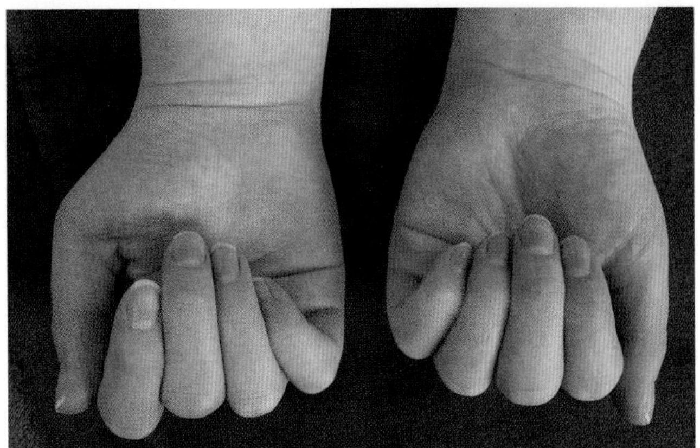

Figure 38.42 Rotational deformity of the little finger.

is a very useful investigation as it can assess soft tissues in a dynamic way while the patient is asked to perform movements, identifying issues such as tendon instability. In addition, since the hand has a thin soft-tissue envelope, many structures can be seen very well with ultrasound that would not normally be evaluated (e.g. erosions within the joints of the fingers as an early sign of inflammatory joint disease). MRI is useful for diagnosing avascular necrosis, ligament injuries or to characterise soft-tissue tumours.

Hand swelling and stiffness

Swelling followed by stiffness is the arch enemy of hand rehabilitation. The hand will swell after injury, surgery or infection. In response, the wrist flexes and then there is compensatory metacarpophalangeal joint (MCPJ) extension and interphalangeal joint (IPJ) flexion. If action is not taken swiftly, this position will become permanent, as collateral ligaments shrink and tissues fibrose. Hand elevation to reduce swelling, splintage in the position of safety to prevent collateral shortening (Edinburgh position: wrist extension, MCPJ flexion, IPJ extension) and early mobilisation prevent permanent stiffness.

Summary box 38.11

General principles of treatment

Avoid swelling and stiffness by:

- Elevation – reduce swelling
- Splintage – avoid contractures
- Movement – pump away swelling and encourage suppleness

Thumb ulnar collateral ligament injury

Chronic thumb overuse or overloading leads to stretching of the ulnar collateral ligament and instability (gamekeeper's thumb). The ligament can also rupture acutely if the thumb is forcibly abducted (skier's thumb). If valgus stress on examination causes significant opening of the joint on the ulnar side then the ligament needs to be repaired surgically, as the adductor aponeurosis interposes between the torn end of the ligament and its insertion (*Figure 38.43*), preventing healing and causing chronic instability.

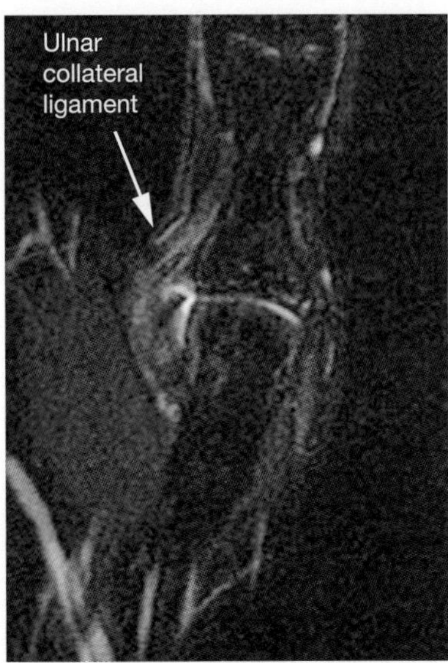

Figure 38.43 Magnetic resonance imaging showing rupture of the ulnar collateral ligament of the thumb (skier's thumb).

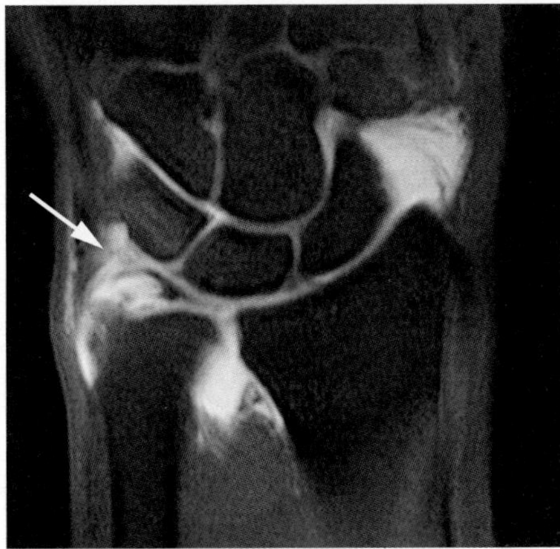

Figure 38.44 Magnetic resonance arthrogram showing peripheral detachment of the triangular fibrocartilage complex.

Triangular fibrocartilage complex

The triangular fibrocartilage complex (TFCC) consists of the ulnocarpal ligaments, extensor carpi ulnaris tendon sheath and a meniscus-like structure between the distal ulna and the carpus. It is continuous with the dorsal and volar wrist capsules and stabilises the distal radioulnar joint. It can undergo traumatic or degenerative tears, presenting with ulna-sided wrist pain and distal radioulnar instability. An MRI arthrogram or wrist arthroscopy aids diagnosis (*Figure 38.44*). Peripheral tears of the TFCC can be repaired open or arthroscopically, while central degenerative tears can be arthroscopically debrided.

Infections

Paronychia

Nail bed infection is the most common hand infection (*Figure 38.45*). After initial inflammation, pus accumulates beside and sometimes under the nail. It is best treated with incision, drainage and appropriate antibiotic therapy. This

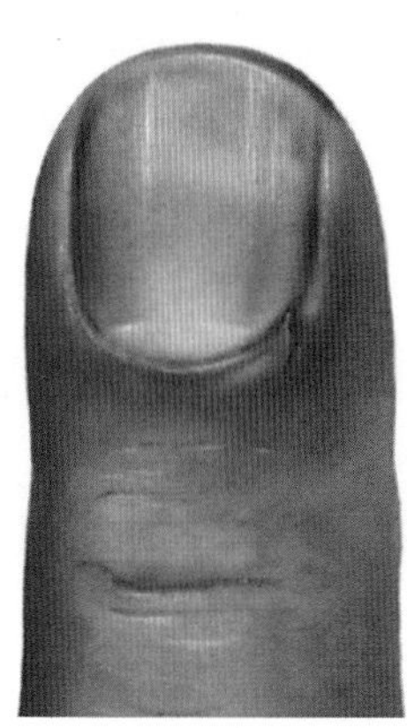

Figure 38.45 Acute paronychia.

is occasionally facilitated by partial nail removal to allow full drainage of the collection.

Felon

A felon is an abscess within the specialised fibrous septae of the fingertip pulp. It causes intense pain and may lead to terminal phalangeal osteomyelitis. Incision and drainage through the midline of the pulp of the finger in the location of maximal swelling, followed by intravenous antibiotics, are recommended.

Flexor tendon sheath infection

Flexor tendon sheath infections present with Kanavel's cardinal signs:

- the affected finger is held in flexion;
- there is uniform swelling over the tendon and digit;
- tender to the touch;
- pain on passive extension of the finger.

Flexor sheath anatomy is important to understand, since infection within flexors 2 (index) to 4 (ring) is usually confined to that finger, whereas infections arising in the sheath of the thumb or little finger may extend via the radial and ulnar bursae, respectively, towards the wrist. Treatment is by open irrigation throughout the tendon sheath course; small incisions are made at the proximal and distal ends of the affected sheath and the sheath is washed out, delivering irrigation via a small nasogastric or feeding tube. The whole finger may require opening if the viability of the digit is threatened. This is followed by what is often an extended course of intravenous antibiotics. If infection is untreated tendon adhesions and necrosis occur. Infection can spread proximally, damaging the whole hand.

Summary box 38.12

Treatment of hand infections

- Elevate and splint in a functional position and give intravenous antibiotics
- Surgical drainage should include tendon sheath irrigation
- Early mobilisation

Mycobacterial infections

Tuberculosis may involve the tenosynovium, joints or bone. The most dramatic form is a compound palmar ganglion, with synovial swelling proximal and distal to the transverse carpal ligament, occasionally causing symptoms of carpal tunnel syndrome. The diagnosis is made by taking a biopsy. Synovectomy should be performed and the patient treated with the appropriate antibiotics.

Deep palmar infections

These infections occur in the palm but may be limited to a web space. The whole hand becomes swollen and tender as pus collects on either side of the septum. Treatment is incision and drainage with thorough washout of the wound. It is important that all deep spaces are opened: incisions on both the dorsal and volar aspects of the hand may be needed. If in doubt, an ultrasound scan or MRI can delineate the extent of the collections within the deep palmar spaces.

Arthritis

Rheumatoid arthritis

Rheumatoid arthritis presents with classic symptoms: morning stiffness, symmetrical arthritis, hand deformities and rheumatoid nodules. Diagnostic criteria include seropositive rheumatoid factor and radiographic changes (*Table 38.1*). The inflamed rheumatoid synovium (pannus) destroys ligaments, tendons and joints, producing pain, deformity and loss of function. Typical rheumatoid deformities in the hand include boutonnière (*Figure 38.46*), swan neck (*Figure 38.47*) and radial drift of the wrist (due to supination of the carpus), with compensatory ulnar deviation of the MCPJs (*Figure 38.48*). Pannus can cause extensor tendon ruptures, classically starting with the little finger and progressing stepwise in a radial direction (Vaughan-Jackson syndrome). With progressive deformity and instability of the wrist and hand, activities such as key pinch and the opening of jars become impossible to perform. The treatment should be dictated by the patient's levels of pain and disability, not purely on the basis of deformity.

TABLE 38.1 Radiographic differences between rheumatoid and osteoarthritis.

Rheumatoid arthritis	Osteoarthritis
Periarticular osteoporosis/ subchondral erosions	Subchondral sclerosis and cysts
Periarticular soft-tissue swelling	Less pronounced swelling
Joint space narrowing	Joint space narrowing
Marginal erosions	Marginal osteophytes
Joint deformity/malalignment	Less pronounced deformities
Ankylosis	Less common ankylosis

Allen B Kanavel, 1874–1938, Professor of Surgery, Northwestern University Medical School and President of the American College of Surgeons (1931–1932).
Boutonnière is French for 'buttonhole'.
Oliver J Vaughan-Jackson, 1907–2003, consultant orthopaedic surgeon, The London Hospital, London, UK, and a specialist in hand surgery.

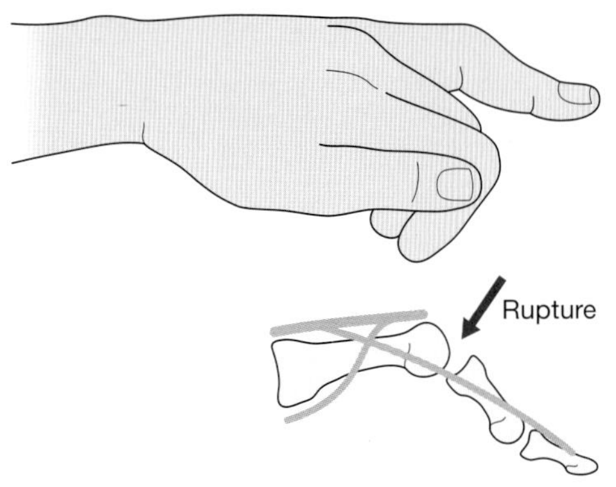

Figure 38.46 Boutonnière deformity.

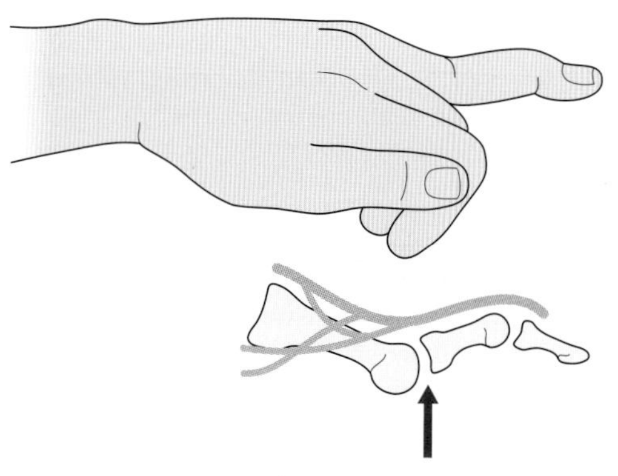

Figure 38.47 Swan neck deformity.

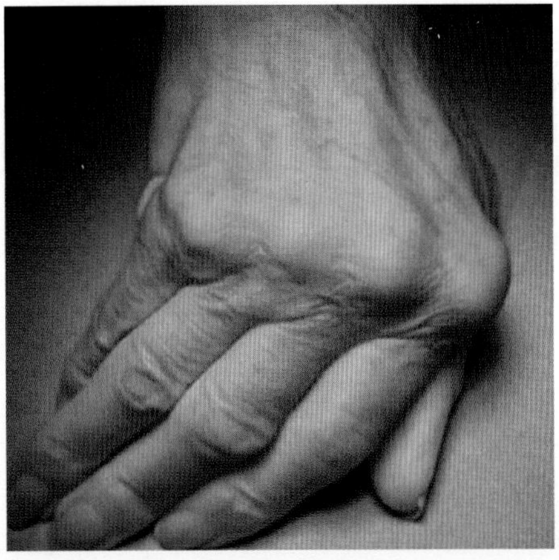

Figure 38.48 Rheumatoid hand showing ulnar drift at the metacarpophalangeal joints, which is seen compensating for radial deviation at the wrist joint.

Summary box 38.13

Manifestations of rheumatoid arthritis in the hand

- Swan neck, boutonnière finger deformities
- Extensor tendon ruptures (Vaughan-Jackson syndrome)
- Flexor tendon synovitis or rupture
- MCPJs: flexion, ulnar deviation, subluxation, dislocation
- Wrist: radial deviation, carpal supination, prominent ulnar head (caput ulnae), extensor tenosynovitis

Management

The primary indications for surgery are: (i) pain relief; (ii) functional improvement; (iii) to prevent disease progression; and (iv) cosmesis. Patients may require many surgical procedures over time and a helpful axiom is to start proximally and work distally, alternating between motion-sacrificing and motion-sparing procedures. The various procedures that can be considered are:

1 Synovectomy: improves pain, increases function and prevents tendon rupture.
2 Trigger finger releases and nerve decompression surgery (carpal tunnel syndrome).
3 Distal ulna excision: reduces pain, prevents extensor tendon rupture or protects repaired extensor tendons. Distal ulna excision leads to instability and so, in the young patient, a constrained ulnar head arthroplasty is preferred.
4 Arthrodesis of the wrist, thumb and some of the smaller joints: gives good pain relief and creates a stable axis against which other parts can function.
5 MCPJ and IPJ replacements: provide pain relief and functional improvement. Total wrist arthroplasty will also provide good pain relief and some motion (***Figure 38.49***).
6 Tendon reconstructions: some ruptured tendons can cause significant morbidity (***Figure 38.50***) and are often treated by either a tendon transfer or a local joint fusion.

Osteoarthritis

Wrist

The radiocarpal joint can develop primary or secondary osteoarthritis (after intra-articular trauma or infection). If conservative measures have failed then operative management includes limited or total wrist arthrodesis and total wrist replacement.

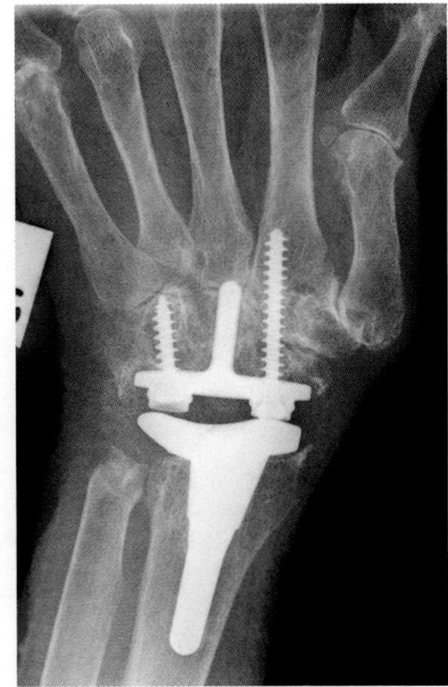

Figure 38.49 Total wrist replacement.

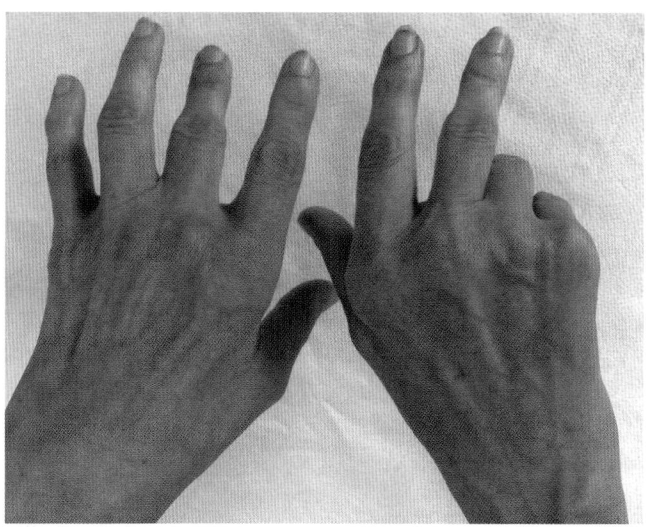

Figure 38.50 Rupture of the extensor tendons to the little and ring fingers.

Hand

Females are more commonly affected than males. The commonly affected joints are the distal interphalangeal (Heberden's nodes), proximal interphalangeal (PIP) (Bouchard's nodes) and the thumb carpometacarpal joints (*Figure 38.51*). Symptoms rarely correlate with the appearance, either clinically or radiographically. Treatment includes splinting, physiotherapy and steroid injections. Surgical options include arthrodesis for distal interphalangeal (DIP) and PIP joints (*Figure 38.52*), joint replacement (PIP and MCPJs) and excision arthroplasty (excision of the trapezium [trapeziectomy] for thumb carpometacarpal joint arthritis). Joint arthrodesis eliminates pain at the expense of motion, but function is often well preserved.

Other forms of arthritis in the hand

Psoriasis particularly affects the IPJs, but is asymmetrical in nature and causes fusiform swelling of the digits along with nail changes. Gout causes pain, joint swelling and redness, as well as occasionally tophi (monosodium urate crystal deposits), and can be difficult to differentiate from septic arthritis. Serum urate is not always raised in acute attacks but finding negatively birefringent sodium urate crystals on microscopy of aspirated joint fluid is diagnostic.

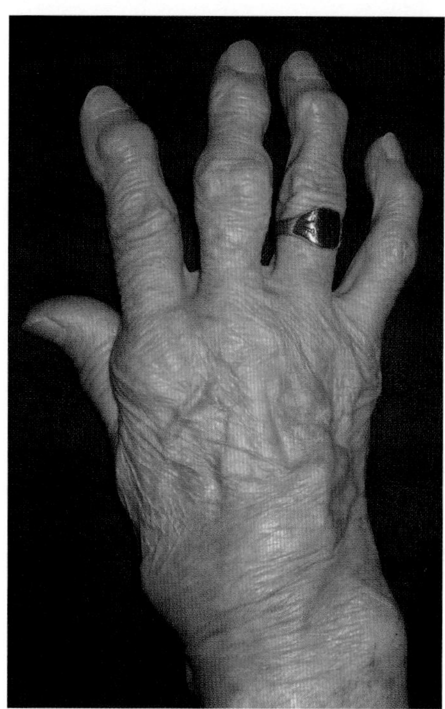

Figure 38.51 Hand deformities secondary to osteoarthritis.

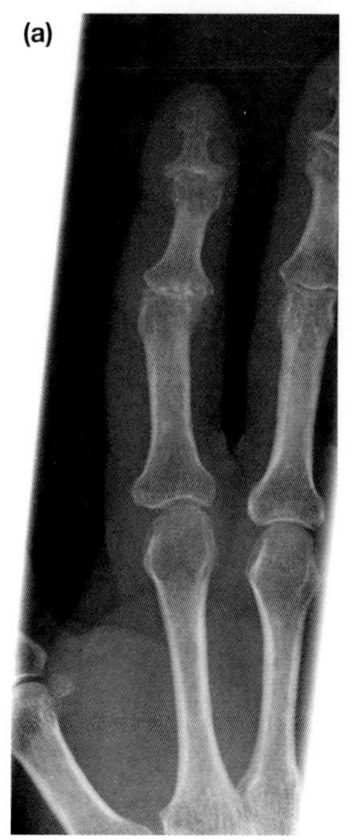

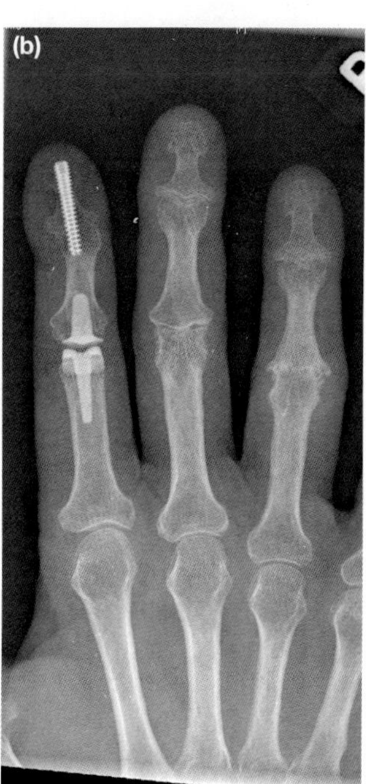

Figure 38.52 Radiographs of the distal interphalangeal (DIPJ) and proximal interphalangeal (PIPJ) joints treated with DIPJ arthrodesis and PIPJ arthroplasty/joint replacement. (a) Preoperative image; (b) after surgery.

Dupuytren's contracture

Dupuytren's contracture is most often characterised as an autosomal dominant condition, common in northern Europe, predominantly in men in the fifth to seventh decades of life. Four out of seven cases occur in those with a family history but there are also many sporadic cases. It is associated with smoking, trauma, epilepsy, hypothyroidism, alcoholic cirrhosis and possibly human immunodeficiency virus (HIV) infection. It also appears very frequently as a clinical case in postgraduate examinations! The characteristic features are palmar nodules, skin puckering, cords of the palm and digits, and flexion

William Heberden (Senior), 1710–1801, physician, who practised first in Cambridge and from 1748 in London, UK, described these nodes in 1802.
Charles Jacques Bouchard, 1837–1915, physician, Dean of the Faculty of Medicine, Paris, France.
Baron Guillaume Dupuytren, 1777–1835, surgeon, Hôtel Dieu, Paris, France, described this condition in 1831.

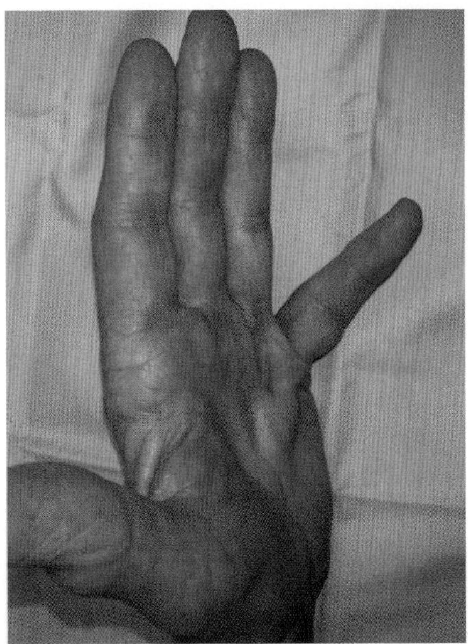

Figure 38.53 Dupuytren's contracture of the little finger metacarpophalangeal joint with a significant palmar cord.

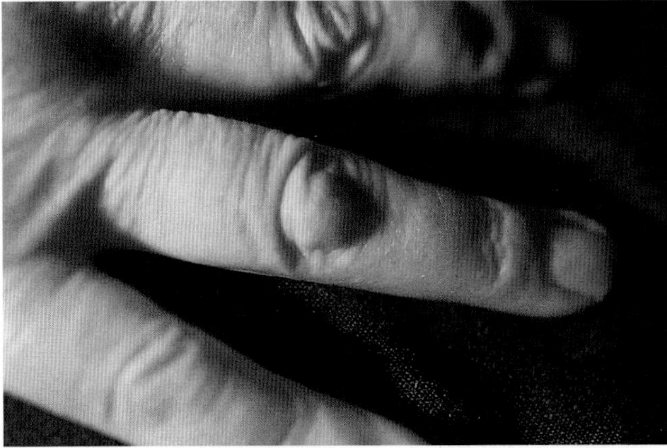

Figure 38.54 Garrod's knuckle pads.

contractures of the digits (*Figure 38.53*). It is commonest on the ulnar side of the hand. Garrod's knuckle pads (thickened skin on the dorsum of the PIP joint) are another feature visible on examination and seen in more severe forms of the disease (*Figure 38.54*). The condition can also produce cords in the penis, causing it to become curved (Peyronie's disease) and may also produce plantar thickening on the sole of the foot (Ledderhose disease). Intervention is indicated when the patient cannot put the affected hand flat on the table owing to fixed deformity ('table-top test') or when any flexion contracture develops in the PIP joint. Milder cases may be treated by needle fasciotomy or collagenase injections, while more severe cases are managed surgically. Great care should be taken during surgery to avoid damage to the digital nerves, which may be trapped in the fibrous tissue. At the end of surgery, it may not be possible to obtain primary closure of the skin, so one should consider performing Z-plasties to lengthen the skin, full-thickness skin grafting taken from the anteromedial proximal forearm (hairless) or occasionally leaving an open wound to heal by secondary intention.

In late-stage disease a fixed contracture of the MCPJs and PIP joints may develop. In these cases excision of the fibrous bands may produce no improvement in the condition; if the contracted finger is preventing useful function of the hand, amputation may have to be considered.

Summary box 38.14

Dupuytren's contracture

- Autosomal dominant inheritance but many sporadic cases
- Fibroblastic hyperplasia with resultant skin nodules, cords and deformities
- Intervention is indicated if hand cannot be placed flat
- Severe disease is signified if hand cannot be placed flat; severe fixed flexion deformities may mean that amputation is the only surgical option

Tendon disorders

Trigger digit

Triggering occurs in the fingers or in the thumb as a result of a size mismatch between the flexor tendon and the sheath (usually at the A1 pulley) in which it glides.

The patient complains of painful locking or snapping of the finger, usually when attempting to straighten a bent finger. Occasionally, it may present as a finger that is too painful to bend, associated with pain and tenderness at the A1 pulley. There is often a palpable nodule in the tendon. Management is a steroid injection into the sheath; if this fails surgical tendon sheath (A1 pulley) release should be performed under local anaesthesia, taking care not to cut too much of the pulley and create bowstringing of the flexor tendon. Trigger digits, especially the thumb, can occur in infants and in such cases usually resolve spontaneously.

De Quervain's disease

De Quervain's disease is caused by tenosynovitis of the abductor pollicis longus (APL) and extensor pollicis brevis (EPB) in the first dorsal wrist extensor compartment (1st EC). It is predominantly seen in middle-aged females and is associated with pregnancy (new mother's wrist) and inflammatory arthritis. The clinical features are radial wrist pain, tenderness, swelling

Sir Archibald Edward Garrod, 1857–1936, Regius Professor of Medicine, University of Oxford, Oxford, UK, described this condition in 1893.
Francois de la Peyronie, 1678–1747, surgeon to King Louis XIV of France and founder of the Royal Academy of Surgery, Paris, France.
Georg Ledderhose, 1855–1925, German surgeon, described this disease in 1894.
Fritz de Quervain, 1868–1940, Professor of Surgery, Berne, Switzerland, described this form of tenosynovitis in 1895

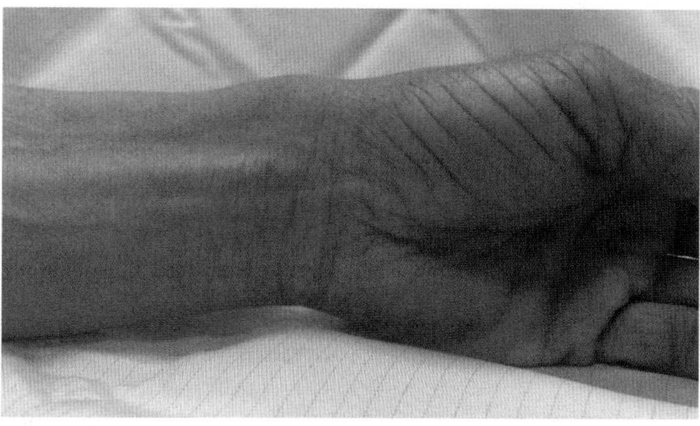

Figure 38.55 De Quervain's disease.

(*Figure 38.55*) and a positive Finkelstein's test (pain over the 1st EC associated with ulnar deviation of the wrist when the thumb is clasped in the palm). The management options are non-steroidal anti-inflammatories, splintage, steroid injections and surgical release of the extensor retinaculum of the first dorsal compartment. If surgery is considered, careful attention should be paid to fully releasing the APL and EPB, which frequently consist of bundles of separate tendon slips that lie in separate sheaths.

Compressive neuropathies

Median nerve (carpal tunnel syndrome)

The majority of cases of carpal tunnel syndrome are idiopathic. It is, however, associated with diabetes, thyroid disorders, alcoholism, amyloidosis, inflammatory arthritis, pregnancy and obesity.

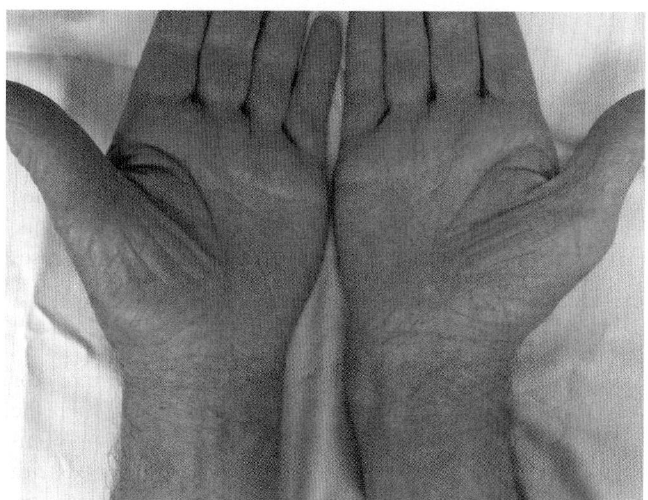

Figure 38.56 Thenar muscle wasting in carpal tunnel syndrome.

History

The patient presents with tingling and infrequently numbness of the volar aspects of the radial three and a half digits. Patients also complain of being woken at night by pain and tingling, and that hanging their hand out of the bed provides relief. They may also complain of clumsiness when picking up small objects or when carrying heavy ones. Symptoms and signs are often bilateral.

Examination

Wasting of the thenar eminence is visible (*Figure 38.56*) in chronic severe cases, and there is sometimes weakness specifically of the abductor pollicis brevis. The tests for carpal tunnel compression are described in *Chapter 35* but the most reliable are: (i) Tinel's – percussion over the carpal tunnel and (ii) Phalen's test – reproduction of paraesthesia with full prolonged wrist flexion. More recently, Durkan's compression test, in which digital pressure over the carpal tunnel reproduces the symptoms, has been shown to be highly sensitive and specific. Electrophysiological studies may confirm the diagnosis, with evidence of slowing of nerve conduction through the carpal tunnel, however they can also be normal. Non-operative treatment includes night splintage of the wrist in extension and steroid injections. If surgery is required the median nerve is surgically decompressed by incising the roof of the tunnel (transverse carpal ligament), as either an open or an endoscopic percutaneous procedure.

Summary box 38.15

Carpal tunnel syndrome

- Night pain is common and relieved by shaking the hand
- Thenar wasting is an advanced sign
- Tinel's, Phalen's and Durkan's tests are useful
- Treatment includes splints and surgical decompression

Ulnar nerve (Guyon's tunnel syndrome)

Ulnar nerve compression in Guyon's canal can lead to tingling and numbness in the ring and little fingers with hypothenar wasting. There is preservation of dorsal sensation over the little and ring fingers, because, although these areas are innervated by the ulnar nerve, the dorsal sensory branches are given off prior to Guyon's canal and are thus unaffected. Compression is usually due to a ganglion, ulnar artery aneurysm or a fracture of the hook of hamate.

Harry Finkelstein, 1883–1975, American surgeon, one of the cofounders of the Hospital for Joint Diseases, New York, NY, USA.
George S Phalen, contemporary, orthopaedic surgeon and Chief of Hand Surgery, The Cleveland Clinic, Cleveland, OH, USA. He helped to establish the American Society for Surgery of the Hand.
John A Durkan, contemporary, American surgeon, specialist in orthopaedic and sports medicine.
Jean Casimir Felix Guyon, 1831–1920, Professor of Genitourinary Surgery, Paris, France.

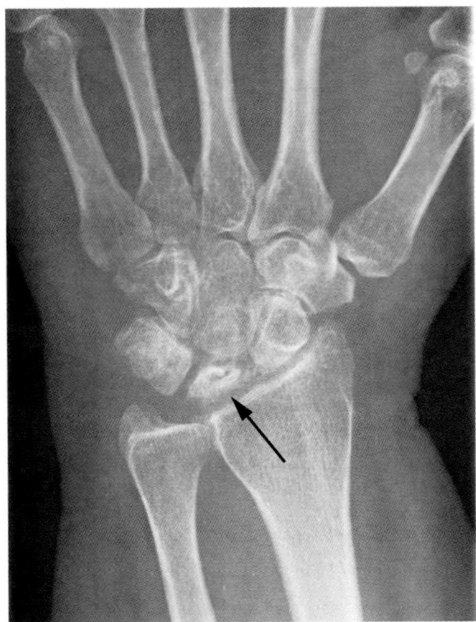

Figure 38.57 Avascular necrosis of the lunate (Kienböck's).

Avascular necrosis of carpal bones

Idiopathic avascular necrosis of the lunate (Kienböck's disease; *Figure 38.57*) or scaphoid (Preiser's disease) can occur. The clinical presentation is of wrist pain and the diagnosis can be confirmed with radiographs and MRI. The natural history of the condition is that it leads to collapse of the avascular carpal bones and subsequent arthritis of the carpus, which may be best treated with a partial or complete fusion of the wrist. This will at least give a strong and painless wrist. The limitation in movement caused by arthrodesis procedures is not as great as might be expected.

Ganglion cysts

Ganglion cysts are the commonest cause of a swelling in the hand and they are found most often on the dorsal (*Figure 38.58*) and volar (*Figure 38.59*) surfaces of the wrist, over the dorsum of the DIP joint (digital mucous cyst) or within the flexor tendon sheath at the base of the finger (seed ganglion). Dorsal and volar wrist ganglions can cause discomfort. The swellings are smooth, fluctuant and transilluminate brightly. Mucous cysts may discharge and can cause nail changes (*Figure 38.60*). Seed ganglions can be painful when gripping. Aspiration or surgical excision can be considered. Patients should be informed regarding possible recurrence.

Congenital malformations

There are many congenital malformations of the upper limb and these are discussed in *Chapter 44*. A classification summarising the main congenital defects and based on aetiology appears as *Table 38.2*.

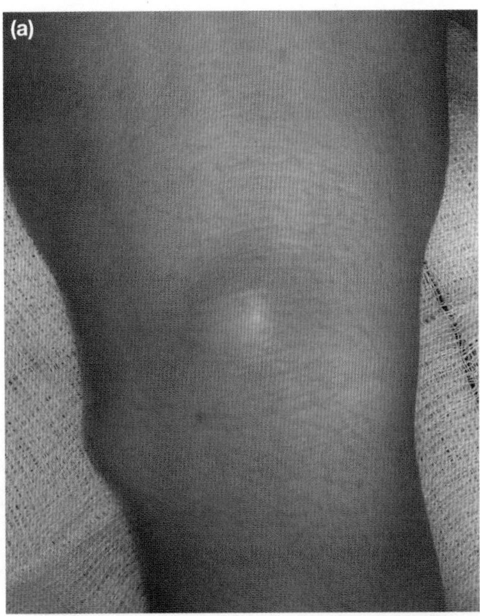

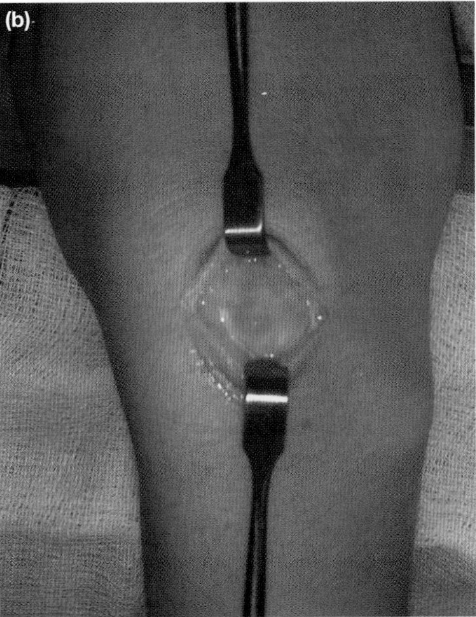

Figure 38.58 (a) Clinical and (b) surgical appearance of a dorsal wrist ganglion.

Robert Kienböck, 1871–1953, Professor of Radiology, Vienna, Austria, described this condition in 1910.
Georg K F Preiser, 1876–1913, German orthopaedic surgeon, published the first study on the vascular supply of the scaphoid bone in 1910.

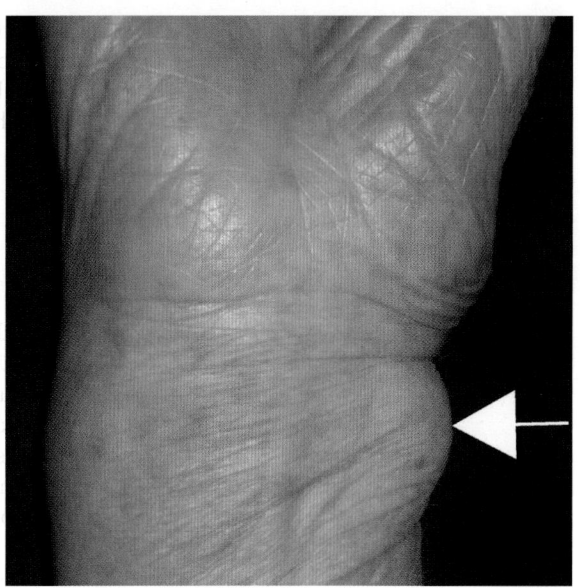

Figure 38.59 Volar wrist ganglion.

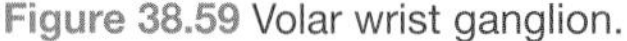

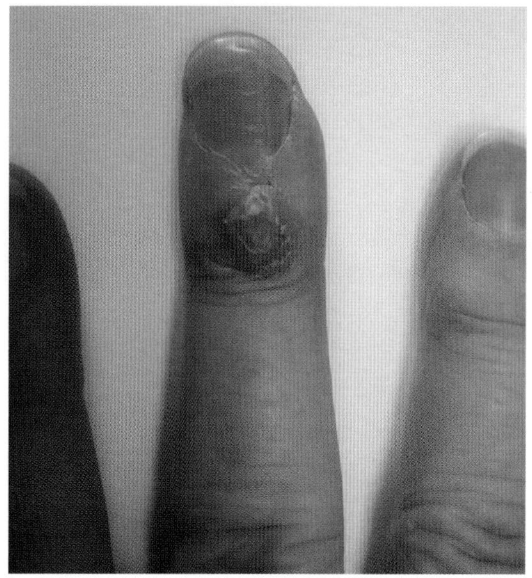

Figure 38.60 Myxoid cyst with changes in the nail.

TABLE 38.2 Congenital malformations (hand and wrist).

A Defects in formation due to arrested development	1 Transverse agenesis 2 Longitudinal agenesis (a) radial ray aplasia; (b) median ray aplasia; (c) ulnar ray aplasia 3 Thumb aplasia/hypoplasia
B Defects in differentiation/separation	1 Syndactyly 2 Camptodactyly 3 Clinodactyly 4 Kirner's deformity 5 Radioulnar synostosis
C Duplications	1 Supernumerary phalanges 2 Supernumerary digits (polydactyly)
D Excess development/hyperplasia	Macrodactyly
E Insufficient development/hypoplasia	Thumb hypoplasia
F Constricting (amniotic) bands	Simple amniotic band syndrome
G Generalised skeletal anomalies	Marfan, Turner and Down syndromes

FURTHER READING

Burden EG, Batten TJ, Smith CD *et al.* Reverse shoulder arthroplasty: a systematic review and meta analysis of complications and patient outcomes dependent on prosthesis design. *Bone Joint J* 2021; **103-B**(5): 813–21.

Carr AJ, Cooper CD, Campbell AK *et al.* Clinical effectiveness and cost-effectiveness of open and arthroscopic rotator cuff repair (the UK Rotator Cuff Surgery [UKUFF] randomised trial). *Health Technol Assess* 2015; **19**(80): 1–218.

Gill DR, Morrey BF. The Coonrad-Morrey total elbow arthroplasty in patients who have rheumatoid arthritis. A ten to fifteen-year follow-up study. *J Bone Joint Surg Am* 1998; **80**: 1327–35.

Mizuno N, Denard PJ, Raiss P *et al.* Long-term results of the Latarjet procedure for anterior instability of the shoulder. *J Shoulder Elbow Surg* 2014; **23**(11): 1691–9.

Neer CS. Anterior acromioplasty for the chronic impingement syndrome in the shoulder: a preliminary report. *J Bone Joint Surg [Am]* 1972; **54-A**: 41–50.

O'Driscoll SW, Bell DF, Morrey BF. Posterolateral rotatory instability of the elbow. *J Bone Joint Surg Am* 1991; **73**: 440–6.

Poppen NK, Walker PS. Normal and abnormal motion of the shoulder. *J Bone Joint Surg [Am]* 1976; **58-A**: 195–201.

Rangan A, Brearley SD, Keding A *et al.* Management of adults with primary frozen shoulder in secondary care (UK FROST): a multicentre, three-arm, superiority randomised clinical trial. *Lancet* 2020; **396**: 977–89.

Rowe CR, Patel D, Southmayd WW. The Bankart procedure: long-term end-result study. *J Bone Joint Surg [Am]* 1978; **60-A**: 1–16.

Singh JA, Sperling JW, Schleck S *et al.* Periprosthetic infections after total shoulder arthroplasty: a 33-year perspective. *J Shoulder Elbow Surg* 2012; **21**(11): 1534–41.

Joseph Kirner, 1888–1964, Chief Physician, Waldshut Hospital, Baden, Germany.

Bernard Jean Antonin Marfan, 1858–1942, physician, L'Hôpital des Enfants-Malades, Paris, France, described this syndrome in 1896.

Henry Hubert Turner, 1892–1970, Professor of Medicine, University of Oklahoma, Oklahoma City, OK, USA.

John Langdon Haydon Down (sometimes given as Langdon-Down), 1828–1896, physician, The London Hospital, London, UK.

CHAPTER

39 The hip

Learning objectives

To understand:

- The anatomy and biomechanics of the hip and their clinical implications
- The clinical presentation, aetiology and management of common hip pathologies
- The principles of joint replacement including important complications
- The advances in surgical practice in this field

ANATOMY AND BIOMECHANICS

Applied anatomy

The hip is a ball-and-socket joint formed by the head of the femur and the cup-shaped acetabulum (Latin: 'little vinegar cup') (***Figure 39.1***). The joint allows a considerable range of movement in different planes and is still inherently stable because of its bony anatomy and the static and dynamic stabilisers. The static stabilisers are composed of the iliofemoral and pubofemoral ligaments anteriorly and the ischiofemoral ligament posteriorly; together with the joint capsule and the labrum (***Figure 39.1***). The muscles running across the joint (short external rotator muscles and gluteus maximus posteriorly, the iliopsoas anteriorly and the hip abductors laterally) constitute the dynamic stabilisers. The acetabular labrum is a fibrocartilaginous structure that is triangular in cross-section and attaches to the rim of the acetabulum, except at its base, where it is replaced by a ligament called the transverse acetabular ligament. The labrum helps in deepening the socket, thereby enhancing stability. It also acts as a fluid seal and thereby helps to improve joint lubrication. The femoral head derives its blood supply mainly from the retinacular branches of the medial circumflex femoral artery and has a small contribution from the artery of the ligamentum teres.

Summary box 39.1

Anatomy

- The hip joint is a ball-and-socket joint, with both static and dynamic stabilisers
- Static stabilisers include the capsule, ligaments and labrum
- Dynamic stabilisers consist of the muscles acting across the joint
- Blood supply to the femoral head is mainly derived from the medial circumflex femoral artery

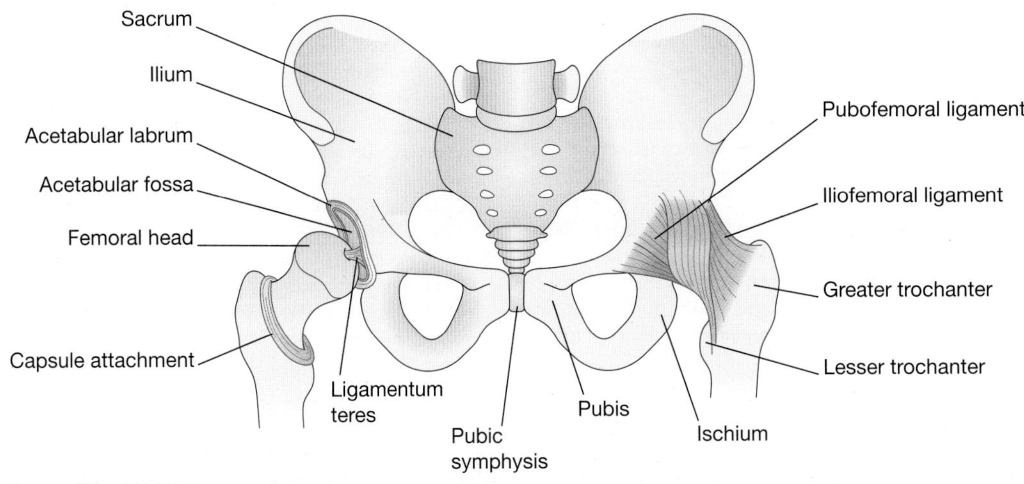

Figure 39.1 Anatomy of the hip joint.

Biomechanics of the hip joint

Kinetic analysis reveals that forces as high as three times body weight can be exerted across the hip joint during activities of daily living, and eight times body weight during physically demanding activities. This is primarily the result of contraction of muscles crossing the hip joint. The abductors, because of their insertion at the greater trochanter, help in supporting the pelvis when the patient stands on the ipsilateral leg and thereby form the basis of the Trendelenburg test (***Figure 39.2***).

> **Summary box 39.2**
>
> Forces going through the hip joint
> - Lifting leg from bed – one and a half times body weight
> - Standing on one leg – three times body weight
> - Running and jumping - ten times body weight

CONDITIONS AFFECTING THE HIP

Common hip pathologies in the paediatric age group and secondary to trauma are covered in ***Chapters 29, 32 and 44***. This chapter focuses on the acquired pathological conditions in the adult.

Avascular necrosis

Avascular necrosis (AVN), or osteonecrosis of the femoral head, occurs because of an interruption in the blood supply to the femoral head, leading to bone death. This results in collapse of the femoral head initially, and eventually secondary osteoarthritis (OA). AVN can be primary (idiopathic) or secondary to other pathology (***Table 39.1***).

TABLE 39.1 Aetiology of avascular necrosis of the femoral head.

- Steroids
- Alcohol excess
- Idiopathic (see Perthes' disease; see ***Chapter 44***)
- Sickle cell disease
- Haemoglobinopathies
- Caisson disease ('the bends' in divers)
- Hyperlipidaemia
- Systemic lupus erythematosus
- Gaucher's disease
- Chronic liver disease
- Antiphospholipid antibody syndrome
- Radiotherapy
- Chemotherapy
- Human immunodeficiency virus
- Hypercoagulable states (protein C and protein S deficiency)

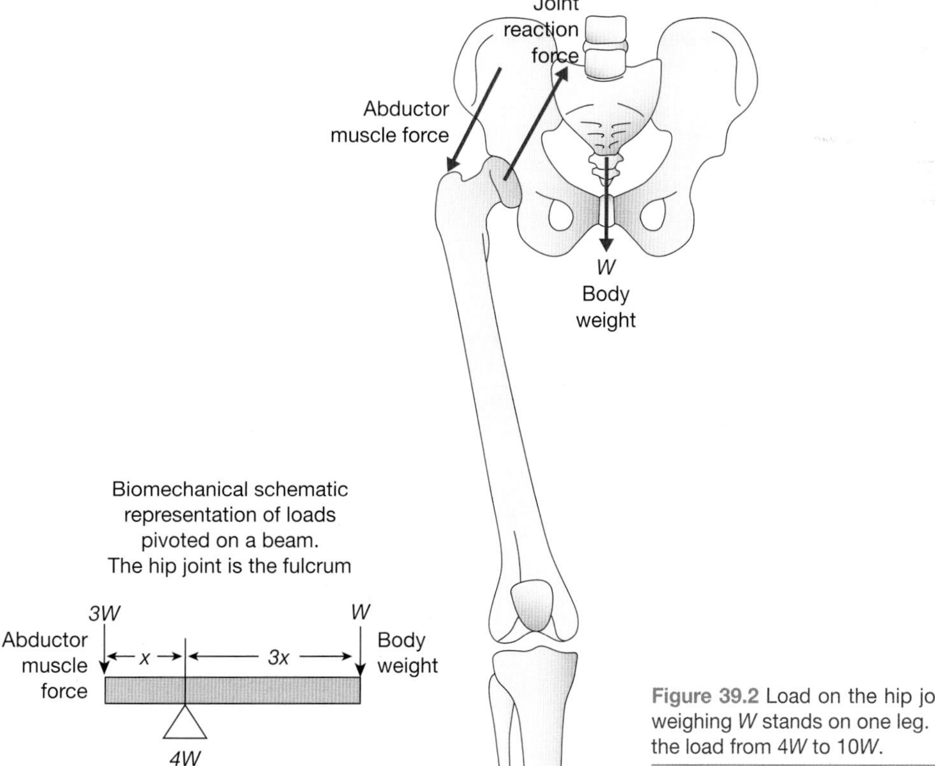

Figure 39.2 Load on the hip joint when a subject weighing W stands on one leg. Hopping increases the load from $4W$ to $10W$.

Friedrich Trendelenburg, 1844–1924, Professor of Surgery successively at Rostock (1875–1882), Bonn (1882–1895) and Leipzig (1895–1911), Germany. The Trendelenburg position was first described in 1885.

A **caisson** is a watertight chamber used to protect construction workers during the building of underwater structures by means of pressurised air introduction.

Philippe Charles Ernest Gaucher, 1854–1918, physician, Hôpital St Louis, Paris, France, described familial splenic anaemia in 1882.

Georg Clemens Perthes, 1869–1927, Professor of Surgery, Tübingen, Germany, described osteochondritis of the femoral capital epiphysis in 1910.

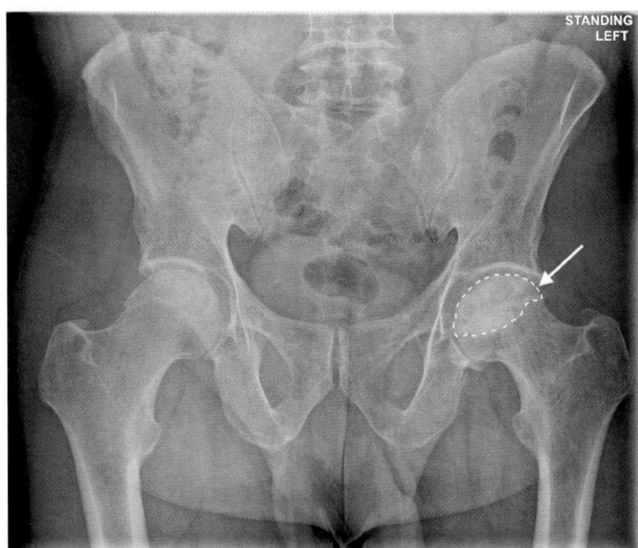

Figure 39.3 Radiological appearance of avascular necrosis of the femoral head of the left hip. There is evidence of femoral head sclerosis (dashed line and arrow) as a consequence of avascular necrosis.

Clinical features

AVN usually affects men aged 35–45 and is bilateral in over 50% of patients. The patient is frequently asymptomatic in the early stages. As the disease progresses the patient may complain of an ache in the groin and walk with a limp. Clinical examination in the early stages is usually normal but may reveal a positive Thomas's test and limitation in the range of movement as the disease progresses.

Investigations

A weight-bearing anteroposterior (AP) radiograph of the pelvis along with a lateral radiograph will show the classical features of AVN, including increased sclerosis in the early stages and the crescent sign indicating subchondral bone resorption. In the late stages there may be femoral head irregularity indicating the onset of arthritis (***Figure 39.3***), and flattening, indicating a segmental head collapse. However, radiographs may be normal in the early stages of the disease and, therefore, the most sensitive and specific way of investigating these patients is with magnetic resonance imaging (MRI). MRI allows accurate assessment of the extent of involvement of the femoral head and can also identify associated bone marrow changes. This helps in early diagnosis and the prediction of prognosis (***Figure 39.4***). In 1985, Ficat classified the disease into five stages. In 1995, Steinberg modified this classification into seven stages (0–VI) based upon both radiograph and MRI appearance (***Table 39.2***). Stages I–IV are further divided according to the extent of femoral head involvement (A; mild, B; moderate and C; severe).

Management

Conservative treatment in well-established cases usually leads to poorer outcomes and is therefore not recommended. The choice of surgical treatment depends upon whether the femoral head has collapsed or not. In the pre-collapse stage the principle is to preserve and preferably encourage revascularisation of the femoral head, whereas in the collapse stage the aim is to bring the undamaged parts of the femoral head into the load-bearing zone of the hip joint.

The surgical treatment for the pre-collapse stage includes core decompression, which is aimed at relieving the intravascular congestion in the femoral head and thereby pain. This can be achieved with or without bone grafting or combined with bone-marrow-derived cell therapies; a vascularised bone graft can also be used to stimulate bone formation and support the femoral head. Once the femoral head has collapsed, either a femoral osteotomy (which aims to transfer the weight-bearing area of the femoral head and thereby protect the collapsed segment) or a joint replacement (if degenerative changes have set in) is the preferred option (see ***Primary total hip replacement***).

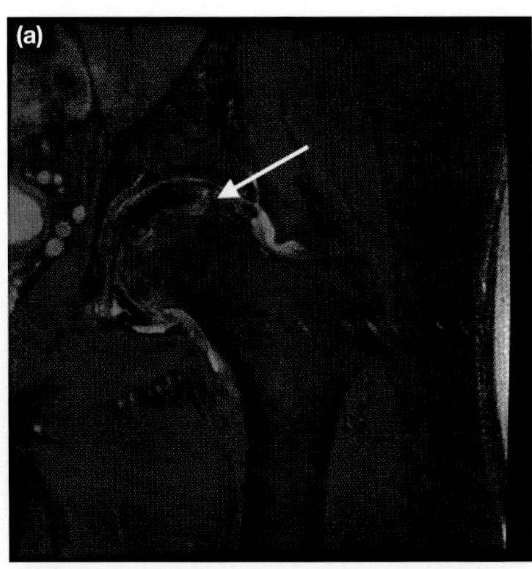

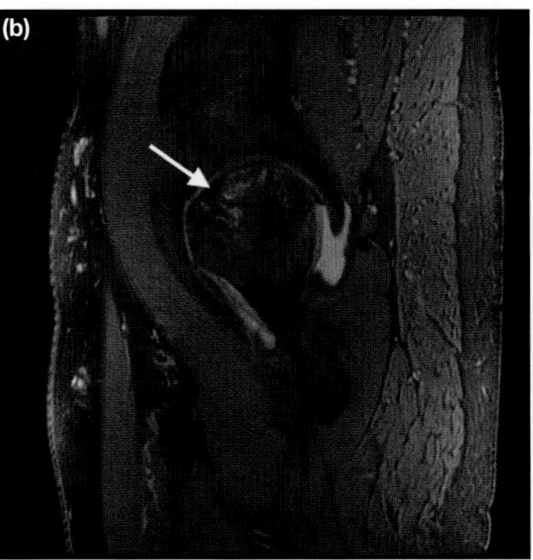

Figure 39.4 Magnetic resonance imaging scan of the hip joint showing avascular necrosis (arrows). (a) Coronal view; (b) sagittal view.

Hugh Owen Thomas, 1834–1891, general practitioner, Liverpool, UK. He is regarded as the founder of orthopaedic surgery although never holding a hospital appointment, preferring to treat patients in their own homes. He introduced the Thomas splint in 1875.
R Paul Ficat, 1917–1986, Professor of Clinical Orthopaedic Surgery and Traumatology, Université Paul Sabatier, Toulouse, France.
Marvin E Steinberg, contemporary, Professor of Orthopedic Surgery, Philadelphia, PA, USA.

TABLE 39.2 Steinberg's classification of avascular necrosis of the femoral head based on the type of radiological change on radiographs and magnetic resonance imaging (MRI).

Stage	Description
0	Normal or non-diagnostic radiograph, bone scan or MRI
I	Normal radiograph, abnormal MRI or bone scan
II	Sclerosis and cysts
III	Subchondral collapse, crescent sign
IV	Flattening of the head, normal acetabulum
V	Acetabular involvement
VI	Obliteration of joint space

Summary box 39.3

AVN of the femoral head

- Patients can be asymptomatic in the early stages and therefore a high index of suspicion is necessary for initial diagnosis
- MRI scan is required for early diagnosis
- Treatment is based on whether the patient presents before or after the femoral head has collapsed
- In the pre-collapse stage treatment focuses on revascularisation of the femoral head
- In the collapsed stage, the aim is to reorient the damaged area of the femoral head or replace the joint if degenerative changes have set in
- Prognosis is dependent upon the extent of femoral head involvement

Femoroacetabular impingement

Femoroacetabular impingement (FAI) has recently been recognised as a cause of hip pain in the young adult and may lead to secondary hip OA. Two distinct types of FAI have been described – cam and pincer – although many patients have a mixed picture with both morphologies occurring simultaneously. Cam FAI is secondary to abnormal morphology of the femoral head and neck junction whereas pincer FAI is a result of anterior overcoverage or retroversion of the acetabulum. The cam deformity is typically described as an abnormal bony bump at the femoral head–neck junction (*Figure 39.5a*), measured as an alpha angle of >55° (*Figure 39.5b,d*). The alpha angle is ideally measured on the Dunn view, which is a 45° lateral view of the hip. This view is useful to identify subtle cam deformities that are not clearly visible on the AP radiograph (*Figure 39.5c,d*, arrow pointing to the cam deformity). The alpha angle can be measured on the AP radiograph if severe but the extent is accurately assessed on the Dunn view. The alpha angle is the angle made by a line along the centre of the femoral neck to the centre of the femoral head and another from the centre of the femoral head to the point on the femoral head outside the imaginary circle, as shown in *Figure 39.5b,d*.

On the other hand, pincer deformity is defined by a lateral centre–edge angle (LCEA) measured on the AP radiograph (*Figure 39.5b*) of over 40° (normal 25–40°). The LCEA is the angle formed between an imaginary vertical line from the centre of the femoral head and another from the centre of the femoral head to the lateral edge of the acetabulum.

The impingement, which occurs during deep hip flexion or earlier with internal rotation as a result of the abnormal morphology, results in damage to the labrochondral junction. Patients typically present with groin pain and limitation of activities related to deep bending and rotation. Plain radiographs are useful in evaluating the bony deformity. Further evaluation with MRI typically reveals acetabular labral and chondral lesions and abnormal femoral head morphology in the case of cam deformity. Computed tomography (CT) scan, especially three-dimensional (3D) CT, is helpful in accurately assessing the proximal femoral morphology, acetabular coverage and posterior joint space and allows for planning management. Treatment options for FAI depend on the patient's symptoms and vary from non-operative treatment to hip preservation procedures that aim to address labral, chondral and bony pathology; this can be achieved with arthroscopy, safe surgical hip dislocation or osteotomy of the femur and/or acetabulum.

Hip dysplasia in young adults

Hip dysplasia is a condition in which there is under-coverage of the femoral head, secondary to a shallow acetabulum. Hip dysplasia is defined as an LCEA of <20° and/or an acetabular index of >10° (*Figure 39.6*). The acetabular index (also called the Tönnis angle) is the angle formed by an imaginary line through the superior weight-bearing portion of the acetabulum and an imaginary horizontal line (*Figure 39.6*).

Thorough screening and timely management of developmental dysplasia of the hip (DDH) as a child is aimed at preventing problems during early adulthood. In mild cases of DDH symptoms are not present until the person is a teenager or an adult. Abnormal biomechanics in hip dysplasia leads to progressive chondral damage and labral tears. Treatment options depend on the severity of dysplasia and the extent of damage in the hip joint, with options being hip arthroscopy, periacetabular osteotomy or total hip replacement (THR) in cases where there is evidence of arthritis.

Extra-articular hip pathology

Hip pain can also occur as a result of impingement of extra-articular structures resulting in restriction of activities. *Table 39.3* shows the common causes of extra-articular hip impingement. Snapping hip syndromes (shown in *Table 39.3*) can also present with hip pain. Imaging modalities such as ultrasound and MRI may aid the diagnosis. Treatment begins with non-operative measures such as physiotherapy with surgical procedures aimed at treating the primary pathology in refractory cases. See *Further reading* for additional information.

Denis M Dunn, 1916–2001, consultant orthopaedic surgeon at the Colchester and District Hospital Group and honorary assistant surgeon at The London Hospital, London, UK.
Dietrich Tönnis, 1927–2010, German paediatric orthopaedic surgeon. He had an interest in the hip joint, especially dysplastic hips.

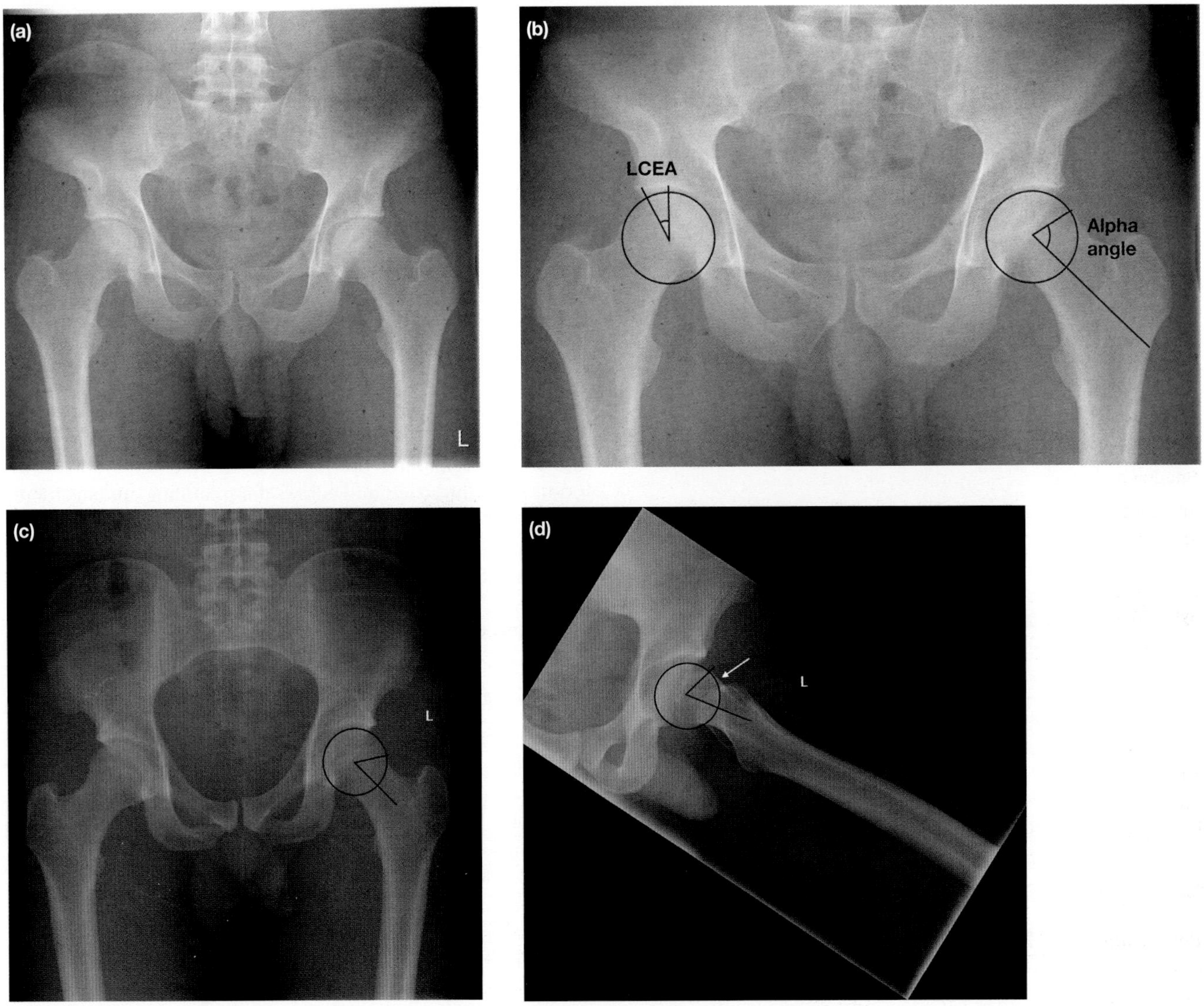

Figure 39.5 Radiograph showing cam femoroacetabular impingement (a), marked over the femoral head (b) with the arrow pointing to the cam deformity. (c) Anteroposterior radiograph and (d) a subtle cam lesion picked up on the lateral view. The alpha angle measurement is used to assess the severity of cam deformity (normal ≤55°). The lateral centre–edge angle (LCEA) is a measure of acetabular coverage (normal = 25–40°).

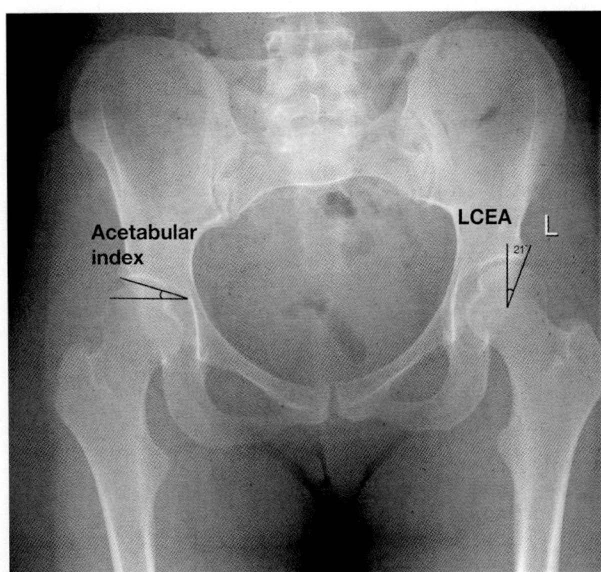

Figure 39.6 Plain radiograph showing bilateral hip dysplasia: uncovering of the femoral head as measured by a centre–edge angle (CEA) of less than 20°. Normal CEA is 25–40°. A CEA of 20–25° is categorised as borderline dysplasia of the hip. An acetabular index of >10° is suggestive of hip dysplasia.

TABLE 39.3 Extra-articular hip impingement and externally snapping hip syndromes.	
Pathology	Description
Extra-articular hip impingement	
Iliopsoas impingement	Impingement between the iliopsoas muscle and the labrum, resulting in distinct anterior labral pathology
Subspine impingement	Impingement between an enlarged or malorientated anterior inferior iliac spine and the distal anterior femoral neck
Ischiofemoral impingement	Compression of the quadratus femoris muscle between the lesser trochanter and the ischial tuberosity
Deep gluteal syndrome	Entrapment of the sciatic nerve in the deep gluteal space resulting in pain in the buttock
Snapping hip syndromes	
Internal snapping hip syndrome	Iliopsoas tendon glides over the hip joint, producing a snapping sensation and eventually leading to labral tear
External snapping hip syndrome	Iliotibial band glides over the greater trochanter and snaps, producing an audible and/or visible snap

HIP PRESERVATION PROCEDURES

For the conditions above, in which degenerative change is not predominant, a variety of surgical procedures are now described with the aim of preserving the hip joint.

Diagnostic hip injection

Identification of the source of symptoms is essential to ensure appropriate management. Since the hip joint is deeply seated, several extra-articular pathologies can present with hip and groin pain and the diagnostic hip injection can help elucidate whether the pain is extra- or intra-articular in origin. This is performed as a day case procedure under image intensifier (portable x-ray machine) guidance under appropriate anaesthesia. Using aseptic precautions, a long spinal needle is inserted into the hip joint. The position of the needle is confirmed by injecting either a small amount of radio-opaque contrast dye or air to provide a contrast arthrogram. Once the intra-articular position is confirmed, a mixture of local anaesthetic and steroid is injected into the hip joint.

The procedure can also be therapeutic and is an essential tool that can help in prognosis as well prior to proceeding with hip preservation procedures (arthroscopy or osteotomy), especially in cases of uncertainty relating to the source of the pain and therefore the diagnosis.

Arthroscopy of the hip

The hip joint presents challenges to arthroscopy in terms of access and instrumentation of the deeply recessed femoral head in the acetabulum and the surrounding thick fibrocapsular and muscular envelope. Technical advances, including an improved ability to manage the capsule and gain exposure, have led to an expanding list of applications, including the treatment of symptomatic labral tears, FAI and the removal of loose bodies, e.g. synovial chondromatosis. Arthroscopy allows a clear view of the femoral and acetabular articular surfaces, the labrum, the ligamentum teres and the head–neck junction, along with the surrounding synovium and its folds, and the peritrochanteric space. Advantages include minimally invasive access to all these structures coupled with rapid recovery, in comparison with open surgery. However, there is a steep learning curve with hip arthroscopic procedures and adequate training of this procedure with a mentored independent practice in the early part of a surgeon's career is an essential part of achieving a successful outcome.

Osteotomies around the hip

The goal of an osteotomy around the hip is to redistribute forces evenly across the joint, thereby eliminating excessive point loading. This can be achieved by performing an osteotomy on the femoral or the acetabular side, depending upon the desired goal, e.g. an excessive valgus neck–shaft angle and an uncovered femoral head on the lateral aspect can be corrected by carrying out a varus femoral osteotomy. Similarly, a redirection osteotomy on the acetabular side can also be performed to improve coverage of the femoral head in cases of hip dysplasia. The common indications for an osteotomy around the hip in the adult age group are shown in ***Table 39.4***. Ideally, an osteotomy should be considered in a young patient who maintains a good range of movement of the hip and whose imaging studies (radiographs and/or CT scan or MRI scan) show a joint devoid of significant degenerative change.

TABLE 39.4 Indications for osteotomy around the hip in the adult age group.	
Femoral osteotomy	Periacetabular osteotomy (PAO)
Perthes' disease Osteoarthritis in a young patient Slipped capital femoral epiphysis Avascular necrosis	Developmental dysplasia of the hip Acetabular retroversion (reverse PAO)

Thorough preoperative planning is essential to assess whether the desired position can be achieved. Increasingly 3D CT scans are used for preoperative planning. In addition, 3D printing has been used to understand the problem and plan surgical correction. Computer navigation and robotics are novel adjuncts that are aimed at obtaining an accurate correction of the concerned deformity.

DEGENERATIVE AND INFLAMMATORY DISORDERS OF THE HIP

Osteoarthritis

OA is referred to as primary when no predisposing cause can be found, and secondary when it develops after an insult to the hip joint. A multitude of factors, including genetic, biochemical and mechanical influences, have been implicated in the development of primary OA. The exact mechanism for the development of primary OA remains unknown and it is therefore termed idiopathic. However, FAI has been proposed as an aetiological factor responsible for the development of OA by a Swiss group in 1999 (see ***Further reading***). Secondary OA develops following trauma, AVN, dysplasia, slipped capital femoral epiphysis, inflammatory arthropathy or other known predisposing causes. The causes of OA of the hip are provided in *Table 39.5*.

TABLE 39.5 Aetiology of osteoarthritis.

Primary	• Cause unknown, termed idiopathic • Associations: for example, genetics, obesity
Secondary	• Trauma • Avascular necrosis • Inflammatory arthropathy (e.g. rheumatoid arthritis) • Perthes' disease • Developmental dysplasia of the hip • Slipped capital femoral epiphysis • Septic arthritis • Femoroacetabular impingement implicated as a possible cause

Clinical features

OA of the hip affects 10–25% of those aged 65 years or older. The most consistent symptoms are groin pain and limitation of movement. The pain may also radiate down to the knee joint; in some cases the only presenting feature may be a painful knee. In the early stages of the disease, pain is activity related but as the disease progresses the patient also complains of pain at rest. The patient frequently complains of night pain and may also find it difficult to get into a comfortable position while sleeping. Functionally, any activity that involves flexion and rotation is difficult to perform, e.g. putting on shoes and socks and getting into and out of a bath or a car. As the pain increases the hip joint gradually loses its movement because of muscle spasm, capsular contracture and osteophyte formation, leading to further limitation of activities.

Clinical examination may reveal gluteal muscle wasting. There may also be a limp, with a positive Trendelenburg's test. Leg length discrepancy, usually shortening, and limitation of movement, particularly internal rotation, are consistent features. Many patients present with a fixed flexion deformity that is best elicited by a modified Thomas's test (see *Chapter 35*).

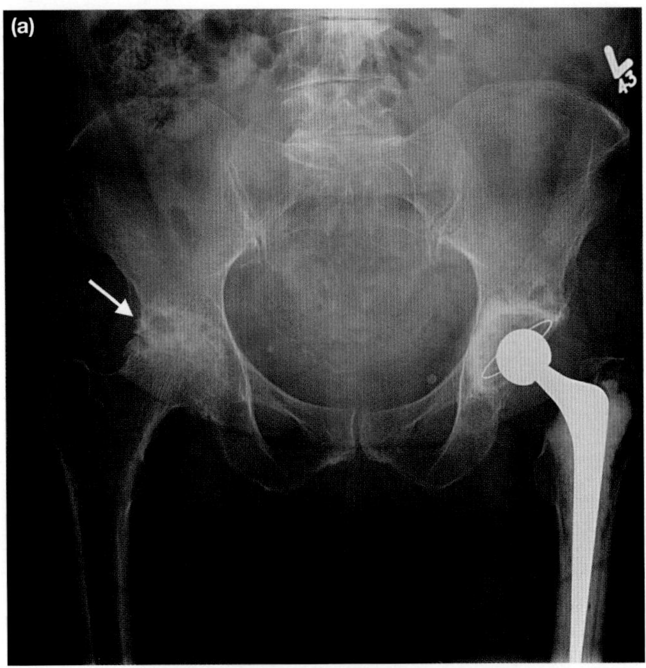

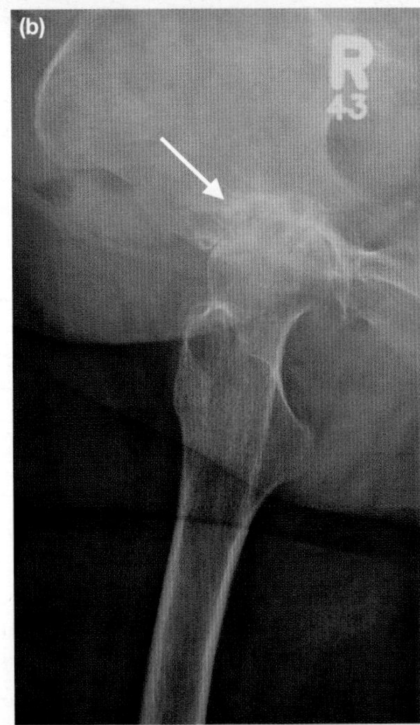

Figure 39.7 (a) Anteroposterior radiograph of the hip joint showing severe osteoarthritis of the right hip (arrow) and a cemented total hip replacement on the left; (b) lateral view of the right hip.

Investigations

The characteristic features on a plain radiograph are (i) a reduction of the joint space, (ii) sclerosis in the subchondral bone, (iii) subchondral cysts, and (iv) osteophyte formation (***Figure 39.7***). Eventually, a collapsed femoral head may also be evident.

Management

There is no specific pharmacological therapy for OA; however, non-operative treatment with non-steroidal anti-inflammatories, regular exercise, physiotherapy and modification of lifestyle with loss of weight does help. Patients should also be encouraged to use walking aids (usually a walking stick in the opposite hand) to offload the affected hip joint and to reduce the workload of the ipsilateral abductors.

The indications for surgery are relentless pain (usually night pain), limitation of lifestyle and activities of daily living and failure of non-operative treatment. The surgical options include an arthrodesis (fusion), an osteotomy (realignment)

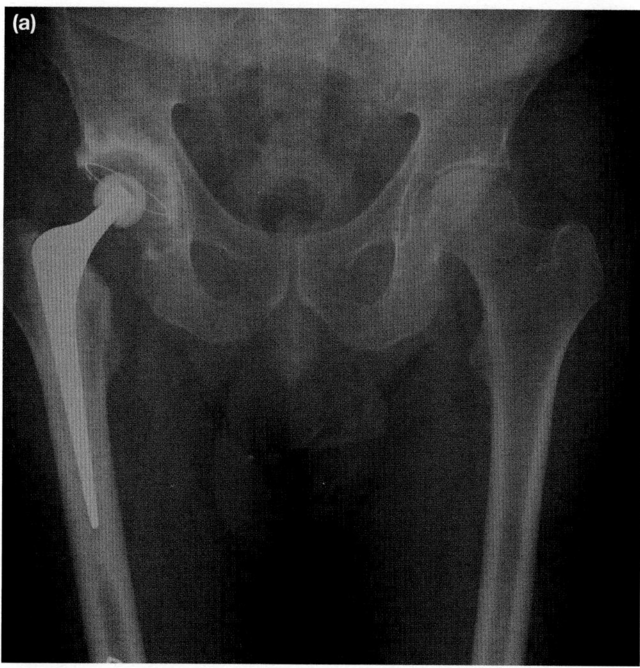

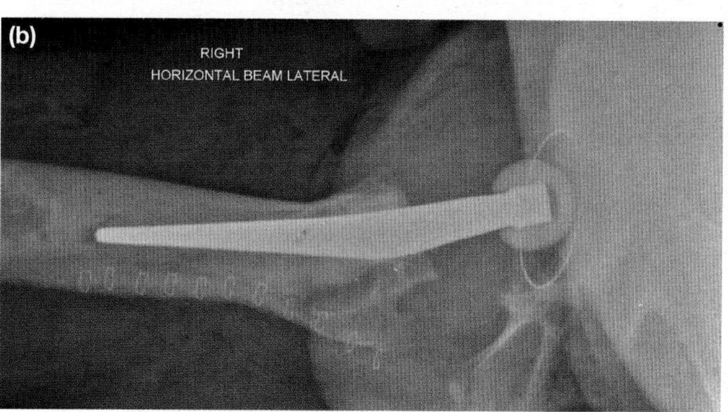

Figure 39.8 Radiographs showing a cemented total hip replacement *in situ*. (a) Anteroposterior view and (b) lateral view.

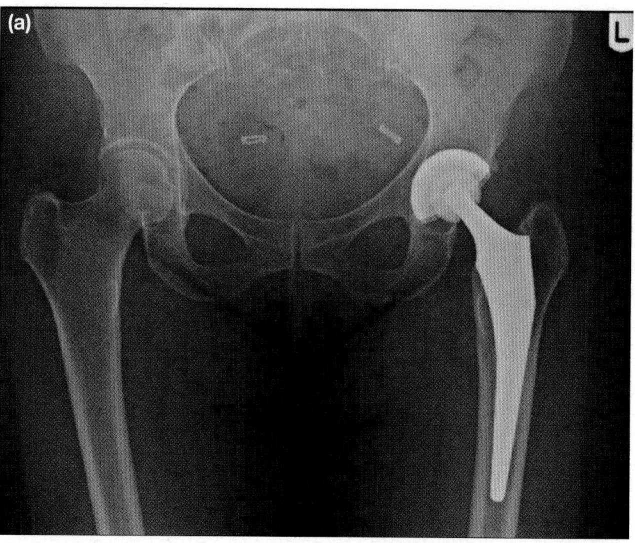

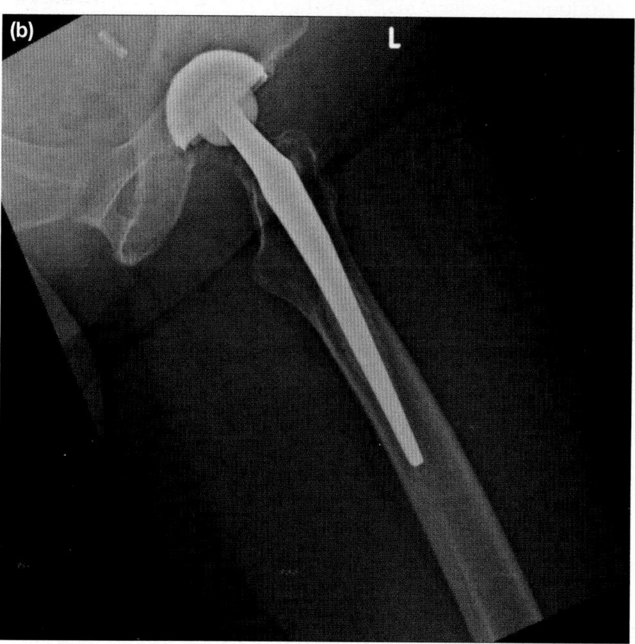

Figure 39.9 Radiographs of an uncemented total hip replacement. (a) Anteroposterior view and (b) lateral view.

or a joint replacement (***Figures 39.7a, 39.8 and 39.9***). The indications are based on limitation of lifestyle and individual needs, thereby making it a truly life-improving and life-changing operation.

Summary box 39.4

OA of the hip

- OA is a degenerative condition leading to progressive damage of the articular cartilage and other joint structures
- The most consistent clinical features are groin pain and limitation of movement
- Characteristic radiological features are reduced joint space, subchondral sclerosis, subchondral cysts and osteophyte formation
- Non-operative treatment includes walking aids, non-steroidal analgesics, physiotherapy and weight loss
- Surgical options include osteotomy, arthrodesis or a joint replacement

Inflammatory arthritis

The hip joint can also be affected by inflammatory arthritides; however, these are not as common as OA. This group includes rheumatoid arthritis, ankylosing spondylitis, gout and chondrocalcinosis, juvenile rheumatoid arthritis and systemic lupus erythematosus.

SURGICAL PROCEDURES FOR DEGENERATIVE HIP CONDITIONS

Arthrodesis of the hip

Arthrodesis or fusion of the hip is an uncommon operation. It is generally reserved for young patients with severe OA who have heavy manual jobs and in whom joint replacements are likely to fail early. The aim is to achieve a painless joint by fusing it in a functional position, which is about 30° of flexion, 15° of external rotation and 5° of abduction. This can be achieved by an intra-articular dynamic hip screw or by an extra-articular plate with screws.

Several problems can occur following an arthrodesis, including altered gait and excessive loading of the ipsilateral knee, the contralateral hip and the spine. Degenerative change in these joints in the long term is the rule rather than the exception.

Summary box 39.5

Features of an ideal joint replacement

- Biocompatible
- Well fixed to the host tissue, stable and allowing a good range of movement
- Bearing surfaces should be designed to minimise friction and have improved wear characteristics
- Material released from the bearings should be non-toxic
- Remove the minimum amount of bone
- Produce mechanical stability
- Should ideally outlive the patient

Primary total hip replacement

Over 95 000 primary THRs are performed annually in the UK (National Joint Registry, UK). The success rate for THR is very high and the evidence supports the results being more than encouraging. In the modern era, with evidence-based technique and selection of prosthesis, over 95% of patients will have a well-functioning THR at 10 years after surgery. In the best series, 85% will still be functioning at 20 years, although some are still in place because the patient may have increasing comorbidities, preventing revision of the THR. Following surgery, pain is reduced and there is improvement in mobility and sleep, as well as social and sexual function. Nevertheless, with the ever-increasing number of patients with joint replacements, the number of patients whose replacement has failed and come to the point of revision, or even re-revision, is rising.

Principles and design of hip replacements

Joint replacement should be biocompatible and made of inert materials. It should be well fixed to the host tissue and the design should incorporate features that allow a good range of movement and stability. The bearing surfaces should produce low friction and minimise the amount of wear particles produced which in turn prevents early loosening. The material released from the bearing surface should be non-toxic. The procedure should remove the minimum amount of the patient's bone so that revision is possible, and it should create a biomechanically stable joint. Finally, any implanted joint should ideally outlive the patient and be cost-effective.

Materials for the femoral component

Implants available currently are made of cobalt chrome alloy, stainless steel or titanium. Metal implants are able to withstand high loads, are relatively inert and can be manufactured easily. However, they do pose problems in terms of ion release if they are used as bearing surfaces. Also, corrosion can be a cause for concern if two dissimilar metals are used.

Bearing surfaces

The design described by Charnley in 1961 revolutionised THR and became a gold standard by using a bearing surface of metal on high-density polyethylene. This is described as a hard-on-soft bearing surface and has a low coefficient of friction, which in turn produces lower wear of the polyethylene component, resulting in longer survival of the prosthesis. Hence the phrase low-friction arthroplasty was given to this implant. High-density polyethylene has good shock-absorbing properties but does wear slowly over the years, producing small particles that can stimulate an inflammatory response in the joint, which then leads to osteolysis and aseptic loosening of the implants. The activated macrophages resorb bone and may also stimulate osteoclasts to do the same. There has therefore been a move towards using bearing surfaces with a lower wear rate, such as ceramic on ceramic. With metal-on-metal bearing surfaces, although the wear rate is lower, the wear particles are smaller (nano rather than micro) and can lead to an adverse reaction, particularly in the soft tissues, resulting in failure. There is increasing evidence that these implants are less forgiving than conventional metal-on-polyethylene THRs, appearing to require more precise implant positioning. Ceramic femoral head bearings on polyethylene cups are low friction, but ceramic femoral heads on ceramic acetabular cups have the lowest friction of all. However, ceramic-on-ceramic bearings are expensive to manufacture, and are another example of hard-on-hard bearings and produce small-sized wear particles. A summary of the advantages and disadvantages of each bearing surface is provided in ***Table 39.6***.

Fixation of implants

Artificial joints must be securely fixed to the bone on each side of the joint so that the implant does not work loose. This can be achieved with the help of cement or biological interdigitation between the prosthesis and bone (***Table 39.7***).

Traditionally, hip replacements were fixed into a bed of polymethylmethacrylate (PMMA) cement (***Figure 39.8***). The cement acts as a grout (spacer) and not as a glue between the implant and the bone. In the majority of cases, it gives an excellent outcome as shown by data in several national joint registries. However, it can cause potential problems: cement pressurisation can result in release of cement and marrow contents into the patient's blood stream. This can cause a drop in blood pressure. Improvements in cementing techniques allow for no gaps in the cement mantle between the femoral component and the bone. In spite of all the measures taken, occasionally there may be small areas in the cement mantle without cement.

Sir John Charnley, 1911–1982, Professor, Wrightington Hospital, UK, pioneer in hip replacement design, particularly the concept of low-friction arthroplasty.

TABLE 39.6 Bearing surfaces for hip replacements.

Type of bearing	Advantages	Disadvantages	Current use
Metal on polyethylene	Proven efficacy; easy to manufacture; cheap	Comparatively high friction; high wear rates; wear particles excite an inflammatory response that leads to osteolysis	Favourable in older age group >70 years
Ceramic on polyethylene	Lower wear rate	Expensive; ceramic fracture can be a problem	Preferrable in younger patients <70 years. Newer polyethylene – UHMWPE – has low wear rate
Metal on metal	Lower wear rate	Problem with metal ion release leading to adverse reaction to metal debris and severe osteolysis. Published examples of failure requiring early revision; implant recalls; expensive	Only a select group of patients – young male. Use head size larger than 48 mm
Ceramic on ceramic	Newer delta ceramics have the lowest wear rate	Very expensive; ceramic can fracture; squeaking	High-functioning young patients

UHMWPE, ultra-high-molecular-weight polyethylene.

TABLE 39.7 Fixation of implants.

Method of fixation	Component	Advantages	Disadvantages
Cemented	Femur	Implant does not need to fit cavity exactly; well-proven results	Cement polymerisation is exothermic with possibility of thermal injury; fragments may cause third-body wear and stimulate aseptic loosening; difficult to remove at revision
	Acetabulum	Cheap, can be used in osteoporotic bone	Higher shear forces leading to failure
Uncemented	Femur	No cement required; fixation more secure; dynamic and biological fixation	Risk of fracture; fit must be perfect; osseous integration may not be established; expensive
	Acetabulum	Good fixation into acetabulum; can be augmented with screws to secure fixation	Improper technique can lead to acetabular fracture

On the other hand, this problem can be obviated by using an uncemented prosthesis in which biological fixation can be achieved by providing a rough surface on the prosthesis for bone to grow into the porous surface of the prosthesis or by coating the surface of the prosthesis with hydroxyapatite, an osteoconductive agent, to encourage bone to bond to the prosthesis (*Figure 39.9*). These uncemented devices have also shown good long-term outcomes, although they can be associated with higher implant costs, increased risk of intraoperative fracture and difficulty in removing them if revision surgery is required in the future.

Surgical approaches to the hip, postoperative course and complications

The operation can be performed via a posterior approach, a trochanteric osteotomy, an anterolateral or Hardinge approach or an anterior approach (*Table 39.8*). Each approach has its own advantages and disadvantages. Minimally invasive surgery has been described that shortens the size of the incision and attempts to lessen soft-tissue damage. As access can be restricted, specialised instruments have been developed to facilitate this. Although the concept is attractive, no long-term benefits have been conclusively shown in minimally invasive hip surgery over the conventional technique. Eventually, whichever approach is used, it is essential to be able to implant a prosthesis so as to reproduce the patient's anatomy such that the implant has the correct offset, is at the correct centre of rotation with the correct component orientation, restores leg length and carries minimal risk of complications.

The postoperative course generally involves a 2- to 3-day stay in hospital but day case hip replacements are being performed in a select group of patients in some centres. The physiotherapist encourages the patient to mobilise safely and independently, avoiding any movements that might lead to a dislocation (*Figure 39.10*). Postoperative plain radiographs are essential to ensure that implants are in correct alignment and orientation, and rule out any iatrogenic fracture. Prior to discharge, the occupational therapist assesses the patient's home circumstances and arranges for any modifications that may be

Kevin Hardinge, b. 1939, orthopaedic surgeon, Wrightington Hospital, UK, described the direct lateral approach to the hip in 1982.

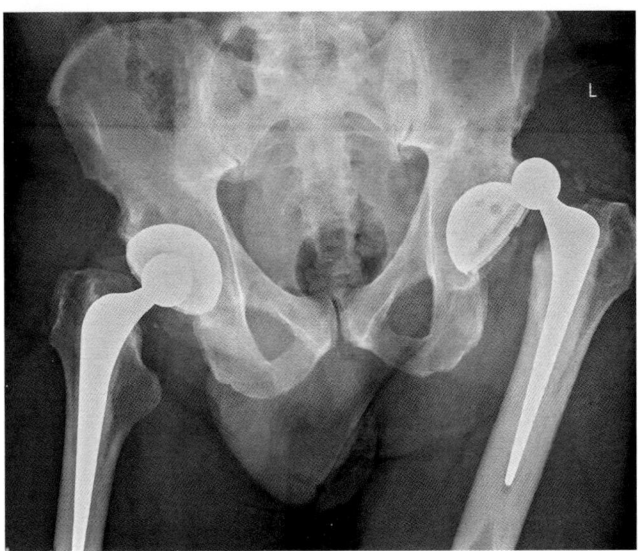

Figure 39.10 Anteroposterior radiograph showing dislocation of a left hybrid total hip replacement (cemented femoral stem and uncemented acetabular component).

required to assist the patient, e.g. a raised toilet seat. For the first 6 weeks patients are advised to avoid movements that make the THR prone to dislocation. Outpatient follow-up visits are arranged at 6 weeks and at 1 year post surgery. Although THR is generally a successful and safe procedure, it does have associated complications. A comprehensive list of complications is provided in ***Table 39.9***. Perioperative administration of antibiotics is a very important part in prevention of infection in addition to adequate aseptic precautions in the operating theatre. Venous thromboembolism is a risk following THR and deep vein thrombosis (DVT) is relatively common if no precautions are taken to reduce this risk. DVT can lead to pulmonary embolism (PE), which can be fatal. Hence steps need to be taken to minimise the risk for both DVT and PE, including adequate hydration, the use of regional anaesthesia and early postoperative mobilisation. In addition, both mechanical device (thromboembolic deterrent [TED] stockings, foot pumps or intermittent pneumatic calf compression devices) and chemical thromboprophylaxis (low-molecular-weight heparin, warfarin or oral anticoagulants) are commonly prescribed for a period of 4–6 weeks after surgery to reduce the risk of DVT (this depends on local and national guidelines).

TABLE 39.8 Surgical approaches to the hip.

Surgical approach	Anatomical interval and muscle
Posterior	Along the fibres of the gluteus maximus, and dividing the short external rotators
Trochanteric	A trochanteric osteotomy is required
Anterolateral/ Hardinge	Parts of the gluteus medius and minimus are reflected off the greater trochanter
Anterior	The interval is developed between the sartorius and tensor fascia lata superficially and rectus femoris and gluteus medius deeply

TABLE 39.9 Complications of total hip replacement.

Intraoperative complications	• Nerve injury – sciatic, femoral and obturator nerves • Vascular injury – femoral vein and artery • Femoral or acetabular fracture • Fragments of cement left in joint
Postoperative complications	• Infection • Deep vein thrombosis and pulmonary embolism • Leg length inequality • Dislocation • Heterotopic ossification • Septic/aseptic loosening • Implant breakage/failure

Revision total hip replacement

Revision of a THR is required if the patient is symptomatic secondary to failure of the implant by loosening (***Figure 39.11***), recurrent dislocations or a periprosthetic fracture. Rarely the femoral prosthesis itself can fracture, leading to pain and disability requiring revision surgery. Loosening of the implant can occur as a result of an infection or aseptic loosening. Aseptic osteolysis is caused by an inflammatory response secondary to particle wear, which can be from either polyethylene or metal.

In the initial stages of loosening the patient complains of pain, which is experienced mainly on weight-bearing. Thorough assessment to rule out infection is essential to plan further treatment. A history of infection (can also be reported as problems with wound healing) in the immediate postoperative period may suggest infection as a cause of premature implant loosening. The infection can be low grade, with *Staphylococcus*

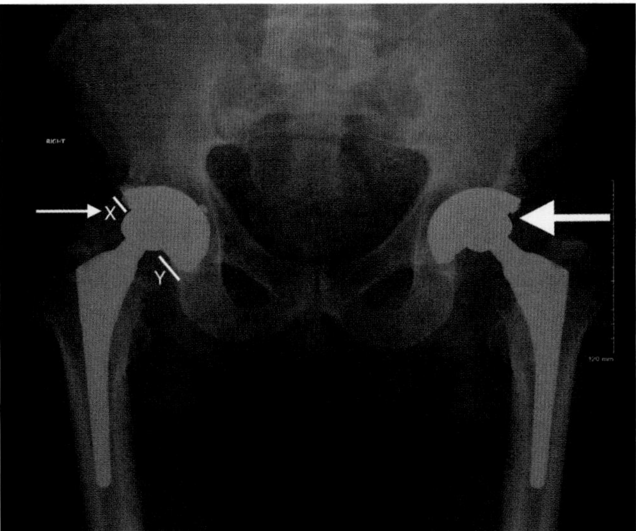

Figure 39.11 Significant acetabular wear, eccentric position of the femoral head (arrow indicating left side wear) and osteolysis behind the acetabular component. Right hip wear is also seen (thin arrow). Distance X should be equal to distance Y. Here, distance X is considerably smaller than distance Y, indicating eccentric wear of the polyethylene (thin arrow).

epidermidis multiplying slowly within a glycocalyx coating, and therefore normal measures of infection such as a raised C-reactive protein (CRP) may be equivocal (see ***Chapter 43***). The Musculoskeletal Infection Society (MSIS) has defined several criteria (major and minor) to help with the diagnosis of prosthetic joint infection. The diagnosis of infection is aided by an elevated CRP and erythrocyte sedimentation rate; a joint aspirate or biopsy is also useful to identify a pathogen. In addition, a labelled white cell scan and single photon emission CT (SPECT) can provide additional information.

Revision THR can be a single-stage or a two-stage procedure depending on the indication. If the loosening is secondary to infection, a two-stage revision is usually preferred. The first stage consists of implant removal, thorough debridement and implantation of an antibiotic-loaded cement spacer. Multiple deep specimens are sent for bacteriology to determine the organism and its antimicrobial sensitivity. The patient is subsequently prescribed an appropriate antibiotic regime (see ***Chapter 43***). At the second stage of the procedure, the cement spacer is removed and a new prosthesis implanted. In the case of aseptic loosening, revision is performed as a single-stage procedure. If there has been a significant amount of bone loss, bone grafting or trabecular metal augments may be required. The results following a revision hip replacement are not as good as those following a primary THR and the rate of complications, especially dislocation, is also higher. Specialised acetabular components such as dual-mobility implants are favoured in a revision setting, especially for recurrent dislocation in those with poor muscle function.

FURTHER READING

Ben-Shlomo Y, Blom A, Boulton C *et al. The National Joint Registry 18th annual report 2021*. London: National Joint Registry; 2021. Available from https://www.ncbi.nlm.nih.gov/books/NBK576858/

Bulstrode C, Wilson-MacDonald J, Eastwood DM *et al. Oxford textbook of trauma and orthopaedics*, 2nd edn. Oxford: Oxford University Press, 2017.

Ganz R, Parvizi J, Beck M *et al.* Femoroacetabular impingement: a cause for osteoarthritis of the hip. *Clin Orthop.* 2003; **417**: 112–20.

Houcke JV, Khanduja V, Pattyn C, Audenaert E. The history of biomechanics in total hip arthroplasty. *Indian J Orthop* 2017; **51**(4): 359–67. Erratum in: *Indian J Orthop* 2017; **51**(5): 629.

Khanduja V, Villar RN. Arthroscopic surgery of the hip: current concepts and recent advances. *J Bone Joint Surg Br* 2006; **88**(12): 1557–66.

Magrill ACL, Nakano N, Khanduja V. Historical review of arthroscopic surgery of the hip. *Int Orthop* 2017; **41**(10): 1983–94.

Matsumoto K, Ganz R, Khanduja V. The history of femoroacetabular impingement. *Bone Joint Res* 2020; **9**(9): 572–7.

Miller M, Thompson SR. *Miller's review of orthopaedics*, 8th edn. Philadelphia: Elsevier, 2019.

Nakano N, Yip G, Khanduja V. Current concepts in the diagnosis and management of extra-articular hip impingement syndromes. *Int Orthop* 2017; **41**(7): 1321–8.

Palmer AJR, Ayyar Gupta V, Fernquest S *et al.* FAIT Study Group. Arthroscopic hip surgery compared with physiotherapy and activity modification for the treatment of symptomatic femoroacetabular impingement: multicentre randomised controlled trial. *BMJ* 2019; **364**: l185. Erratum in: *BMJ* 2021; **372**: m3715.

Parvizi J, Tan TL, Goswami K *et al.* The 2018 definition of periprosthetic hip and knee infection: an evidence-based and validated criteria. *J Arthroplasty* 2018; **33**(5): 1309–14.e2.

Sunil Kumar KH, Rawal J, Nakano N *et al.* Pathogenesis and contemporary diagnoses for lateral hip pain: a scoping review. *Knee Surg Sports Traumatol Arthrosc* 2021; **29**(8): 2408–16.

Warwick D, Blom A, Whitehouse M. *Apley and Solomon's concise system of orthopaedics and trauma*, 5th edn. Abingdon: CRC Press, 2022.

Bailey & Love Bailey & Love Bailey & Love Bailey & Love Bailey & Love

CHAPTER 40 The knee

Learning objectives

To understand:

- The anatomy and biomechanics of the knee and their clinical implications
- The clinical presentation, aetiology and management of common knee pathologies
- The principles of joint replacement, including important complications
- The advances in surgical practice in this field

APPLIED ANATOMY

The knee joint is a synovial hinge joint. It consists of two condyloid tibiofemoral joints and a sellar (or saddle shaped) patellofemoral joint. The shape makes the joint inherently unstable, but stability is achieved by a combination of static (ligaments) and dynamic (muscles) stabilisers acting across the joint.

Interposed between the tibia and femoral condyles are the medial and lateral menisci. These fibrocartilaginous structures aid shock absorption, increase the area over which load is dissipated and have a role in anteroposterior stability (*Figure 40.1*). Loss of the protective function of the meniscus through injury, degeneration or meniscectomy can accelerate degenerative change and progression to arthritis. Medial meniscal tears are three times more common than those in the more mobile lateral meniscus. Tears or meniscectomy that disturb the circumferential fibres and defunction the protective hoop stresses (such as radial tears, disruption of the root attachments or removal or large portions of the meniscus) can cause rapid deterioration of the joint.

The medial and lateral collateral ligaments are the primary restraints to valgus and varus stress, respectively. The medial collateral ligament (MCL) is a broad, flat ligament composed of a superficial and a deep layer. The deep layer is attached to the medial meniscus and to the tibia, close to the joint. The superficial MCL attaches more distally on the tibia. The MCL is commonly injured, but frequently heals with conservative management. The lateral collateral ligament (LCL) is a simple cord-like structure but works in combination with other structures (including the popliteus, biceps, popliteofibular ligament, iliotibial band, joint capsule) to form the lateral/posterolateral ligament complex. Injuries to the LCL are less likely to heal with conservative management and are more likely to require reconstruction.

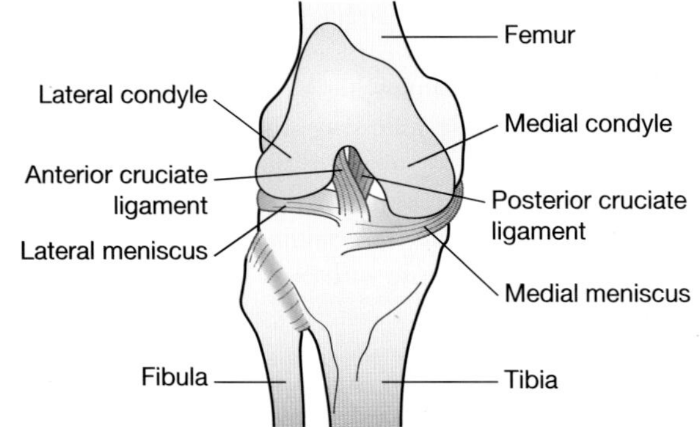

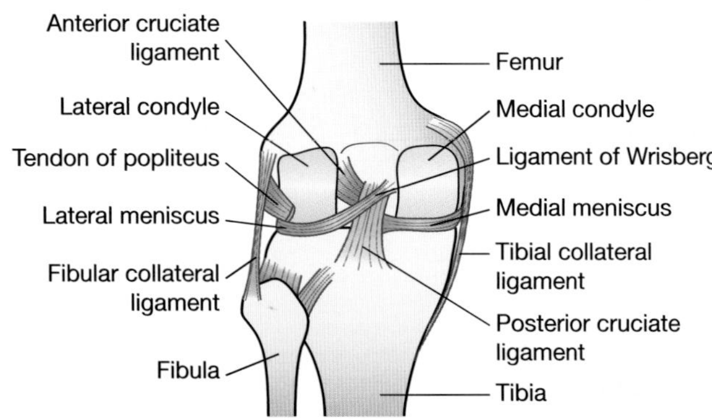

Figure 40.1 Anatomy of the knee joint.

The anterior and posterior cruciate ligaments are each made up of two bundles. The anterior cruciate ligament (ACL) has an anteromedial bundle that is tight in flexion and a posterolateral bundle that is tight in extension. The posterior cruciate ligament (PCL) has an anterolateral bundle (tight in flexion) and a posteromedial portion (tight in extension). The ACL and PCL prevent anterior and posterior translation of

Heinrich A Wrisberg, 1739–1808, German anatomist and gynaecologist.

the tibia on the femur, respectively. Single ligament or meniscal injuries are more likely to occur during sport. Multiple ligament injuries completely disrupt two or more of the four main ligaments and are associated with high-energy trauma such as car crashes. This can result in complete dislocation of the joint and damage to arteries and nerves.

Hyaline articular cartilage is a highly specialised connective tissue that lines the joint surface and has a low coefficient of friction. Hyaline cartilage is devoid of blood vessels, lymphatics and nerves and has a limited capacity for repair. The configuration of cartilage changes with ageing and with disease predisposing to injury.

The knee has bursae surrounding it that can become inflamed and infected.

Summary box 40.1

Anatomy of the knee joint

- Complex synovial hinge joint
- The shape of the joint surfaces makes it inherently unstable
- The static stabilisers are the joint capsule, menisci, cruciate and collateral ligaments
- The dynamic stabilisers are the quadriceps and hamstring muscles

BIOMECHANICS

Axes of the lower limb

The anatomical axes of the femur and tibia are defined by their medullary canal. The mechanical axis of the lower limb runs from the centre of the femoral head, through the intercondylar notch of the knee to the centre of the ankle joint. The angle between the anatomical and mechanical axes of the femur is usually between 5° and 7° (often called the valgus cut angle in arthroplasty) (*Figure 40.2*). A total knee replacement (TKR) is traditionally performed with the goal of lining up the components using cuts perpendicular to the mechanical axis. Knees with malalignment are more prone to injury or degeneration in the loaded compartment. Realignment surgery (tibial or femoral osteotomy) can offload the damaged compartment to reduce symptoms and slow progression to arthritis.

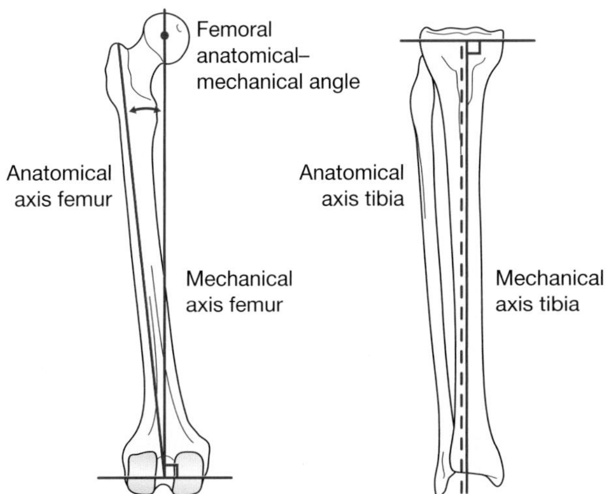

Figure 40.2 Axes of the lower limb. Anatomical and mechanical axes are coincident in the tibia but not the femur. (Adapted from Miller M. *Review of orthopaedics*, 4th edn. Philadelphia: Elsevier, 2004. By kind permission of the publishers.)

Kinematics and kinetics

Knee motion is predominantly in the sagittal plane. A limited degree of rotation also occurs and increases as knee flexion increases. The normal range of motion is between 5° of hyperextension and 135° of flexion. Magnetic resonance imaging (MRI) of cadaveric knees has revealed that, during knee flexion, a combination of rolling and sliding of the femur on the tibia occurs in addition to internal rotation of the tibia. This is because the larger medial femoral condyle rolls back less than the smaller lateral femoral condyle. This motion is facilitated by a more mobile lateral meniscus and lateral ligaments that are more lax in flexion.

The biomechanical role of the patella is to function as a pulley for the quadriceps. It increases the power of the quadriceps by increasing the lever arm. It has the thickest articular cartilage in the body and is designed to withstand loads as high as 20 times body weight when jumping. Abnormal alignment, surface contour, soft-tissue constraints or muscle balance can result in patellar dislocation.

Summary box 40.2

Biomechanics of the knee joint

- The femur has different anatomical and mechanical axes because of the offset of the proximal femur at the hip. These axes are the same in a normal tibia
- Knee motion is mainly in the sagittal plane with some rotation
- The patella acts as a pulley, increasing the lever arm of the quadriceps
- Loads of up to 20 times body weight are transmitted across the patella when jumping

CONDITIONS AFFECTING THE KNEE JOINT

The commonest conditions affecting the knee include injury to the soft-tissue structures and osteoarthritis (OA).

Soft-tissue knee problems

These can present as acute injures or as delayed, more chronic cases with additional degenerative problems. Specific structures commonly involved are the menisci, ligaments and tendons. These can also be associated with chondral or osteochondral injury.

Meniscal tears

The pattern of meniscal injury or degeneration is variable and can affect either the medial and/or the lateral meniscus.

There are several recognised patterns of meniscal tear: circumferential, radial, horizontal, flap and degenerate. MRI scan is the investigation of choice for identifying meniscal tears. Meniscal tears seldom heal. Meniscal tears associated with a specific injury or with mechanical symptoms, e.g. catching, locking and giving way, generally respond well to arthroscopic repair or debridement. Factors making a tear amenable to repair include younger age of patient, early presentation, simple tear configuration, knee stability and a tear in the vascular outer third of the meniscus. Degenerate tears in ageing joints, without an episode of injury and without mechanical symptoms, are primarily treated conservatively with arthroscopy considered after failure of conservative treatment.

Anterior cruciate ligament injury

The ACL rupture is the most common serious ligament injury in the knee. Injury is usually caused by a twisting or landing injury in a pivoting sport. It may be associated with an audible 'pop', immediate swelling and the need to be 'carried off' the field. The injury risk is higher among females; this is thought to be due to smaller ligaments, smaller femoral notches and different landing biomechanics. ACL deficiency can cause instability resulting in further damage to other structures, complex meniscal tears and chondral injury. Examination findings confirming an ACL injury include a positive Lachman test and a positive pivot shift test. MRI scan confirms the ACL rupture and identifies possible injury to secondary structures such as meniscus or cartilage.

Isolated ACL injuries are generally initially managed non-operatively with a knee brace, painkillers, swelling reduction and physiotherapy. Surgical reconstruction is considered in multiligament injuries, in cases of persisting instability after non-operative management, or in young patients or high-demand athletes who tend to fail conservative treatment (see ***Chapter 36***). Surgical reconstruction of the ACL is best undertaken when the knee has recovered from the acute injury and has a good range of knee motion and muscle function.

Extensor mechanism rupture

This includes ruptures of either the quadriceps or patellar tendons. These are usually high-energy injuries but can occur more easily in those on steroids, following steroid injections or following previous open knee surgery that may have compromised the blood supply to these structures. They usually present with significant pain and swelling and the inability to actively extend the knee. Prompt surgical repair or reconstruction is required to avoid a significant long-term loss of knee function.

Articular cartilage injury

These can occur in isolation or in association with ACL injuries or patellar dislocations. Partial-thickness defects do not show any potential to heal. Full-thickness defects in younger patients may mount a healing response with fibrocartilage. In higher energy injury, bone may be included in the surface fragment (osteochondral injury). If picked up acutely the chondral and osteochondral lesions may be surgically fixed back in place. Delayed options for full-thickness defects include: removal of the loose body, microfracture, microfracture covered by a collagen membrane, osteochondral transplant (mosaicplasty) or chondrocyte transplant. Chondrocyte transplant usually involves autologous chondrocyte implantation (ACI) or matrix-assisted ACI (MACI). The age of the patient and the site and size of the defect determine the most appropriate treatment.

Osteoarthritis

OA commonly affects the knee joint. The prevalence of symptomatic knee OA in adults aged 60 years or older is approximately 10% in men and 13% in women. OA can be either primary (idiopathic) or secondary. Patients with primary OA tend to have other joints involved and may have a family history of arthritis. Secondary OA may occur following a previous intra-articular fracture, meniscectomy, ligament injury, osteonecrosis or in a neuropathic joint.

Clinical features

Patients usually describe pain, stiffness and swelling. Pain is usually worse with loading and with activity. Patellofemoral OA pain is worse on stairs and rising from a seated position. The natural history of OA is of a gradual steady deterioration from episodes of short-lived flare-ups progressing to constant pain that often affects sleep. Mobility deteriorates, walking distance reduces and walking aids are frequently required. In severe cases, patients may become dependent on a wheelchair or become housebound.

Examination reveals an antalgic gait in which the patient limps, spending a short time on the painful limb, and moves their centre of gravity to minimise the weight they are taking through this limb. In knee OA the deformity is usually varus, with bone loss on the medial side. Valgus deformity is more common in women, in rheumatoid arthritis and after lateral meniscectomy. The joint appears bulky owing to effusion, synovial thickening and growth of osteophytes. An effusion is frequently present and movement, particularly extension, is restricted. Crepitus can be both palpable and audible.

Investigation

Plain radiographs are the investigation of choice with typical features of joint space narrowing, subchondral sclerosis, osteophytes and subchondral cysts (***Figure 40.3***). These are best performed weight-bearing to show the extent of joint narrowing. MRI scan is not routinely required prior to knee replacement.

Treatment

Non-operative methods are the first line of treatment. Patients should be encouraged to lose weight, undertake regular exercise to prevent joint stiffness and use anti-inflammatory medication. Walking aids, such as a stick, orthotics and off-loader braces, may be beneficial. Intra-articular steroid injections can be used to settle an arthritic flare-up but are no longer recommended as a long-term solution because of concerns about infection and causing further joint cartilage damage.

John W Lachman, 1919–2007, Professor and Chairman of the Orthopedic Department at Temple University in Philadelphia, PA, USA.

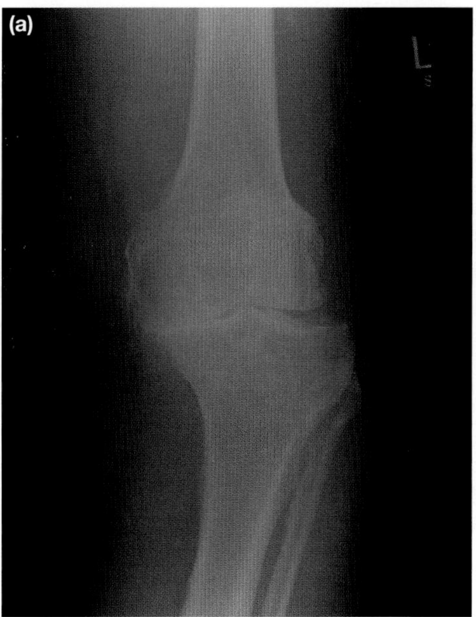

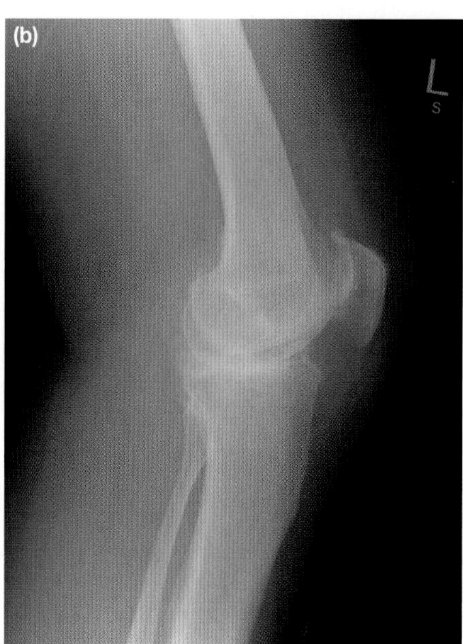

Figure 40.3 Anteroposterior (a) and lateral (b) radiographs of osteoarthritis of the knee.

Surgical options include osteotomy, partial knee replacement, TKR or arthrodesis.

Summary box 40.3

Knee OA

- More common in females
- Can be primary (idiopathic) or secondary (e.g. post traumatic)
- The main symptom is pain made worse by use
- Examination reveals swelling and a reduced range of motion with or without deformity
- The key radiographic features are joint space narrowing, subchondral sclerosis and cysts, and osteophytes
- Treatment is non-operative initially. Knee replacement is reserved for end-stage disease

SURGICAL PROCEDURES

Knee operations can be done either arthroscopically or open. Arthroscopic treatment is possible for most soft-tissue problems, while open surgery is required for osteotomy, replacements and arthrodesis. Procedures amenable to arthroscopic treatment are summarised in ***Table 40.1***.

TABLE 40.1 Indications for knee arthroscopy.

- Torn meniscus resection or repair
- Anterior/posterior cruciate ligament reconstruction
- Loose body removal
- Cartilage regeneration techniques, including microfracture
- Septic arthritis washout
- Inflammatory arthritis and pigmented villonodular synovitis (PVNS) – synovectomy
- Diagnosis of unexplained knee pain
- Tibial plateau fractures – allows intraoperative assessment and reduction of the articular surface

Meniscal surgery

This is performed arthroscopically, commonly using two portals, usually as a day case under general anaesthetic. The meniscus is inspected to define the configuration of the tear and whether it is in a part of the meniscus with sufficient blood supply to allow healing. If the tear is not amenable to repair, a combination of punches and arthroscopic shavers are used to remove any unstable or unhealthy meniscus, back to a healthy stable rim. Attempts should be made to repair meniscal tears in the young, and if the tear is repairable; commonly these will be circumferential or 'bucket-handle' tears. Repair includes freshening the repair site and then fixation with a combination of inside-out, outside-in or all-inside sutures or meniscal repair devices. Postoperative protection of the repair usually includes restriction of weight-bearing and use of a brace for between 6 weeks and 3 months.

Cruciate reconstruction

An isolated ACL injury is most commonly treated with an arthroscopic intra-articular reconstruction. The graft can be a bone–patellar tendon–bone or four-strand hamstring autograft. Screws or fixation devices hold the graft in bone tunnels in the femur and tibia until it has healed. Return to full sport can take up to a year. Postoperative rehabilitation programmes are crucial to a favourable outcome. Complications following ACL surgery are usually a result of incorrect tunnel placement (placing the femoral tunnel too far anteriorly limits knee flexion) and early surgery. The graft re-rupture rate is approximately 1% per year.

Osteotomy

Varus or valgus alignment or deformity of the knee can abnormally load the medial or lateral compartment, resulting in premature degenerative change in that compartment. Osteotomy aims to divide the bone, correct the deformity and alter the load-bearing mechanics of the joint. The most

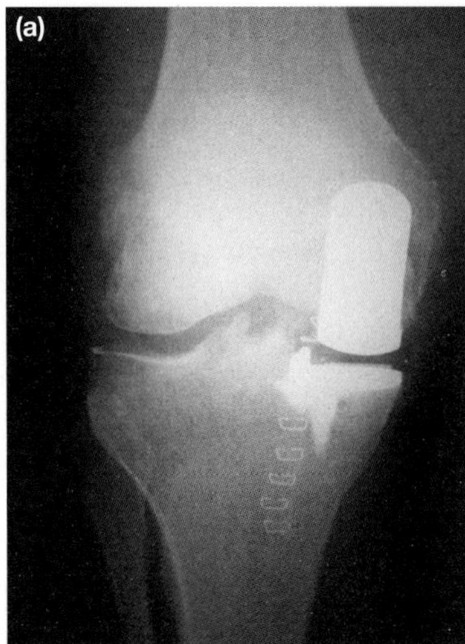

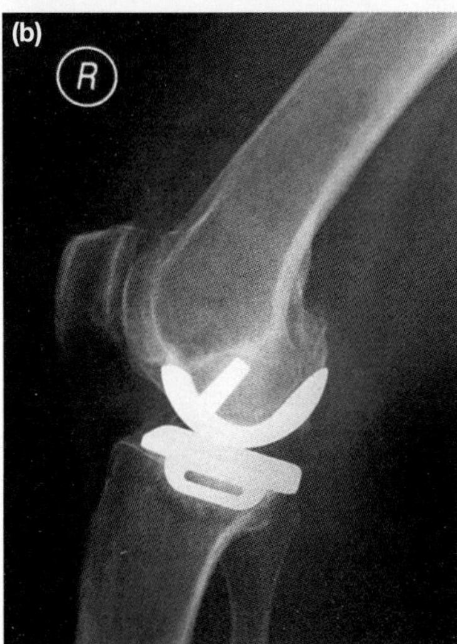

Figure 40.4 Anteroposterior (a) and lateral (b) radiographs of a unicompartmental knee replacement.

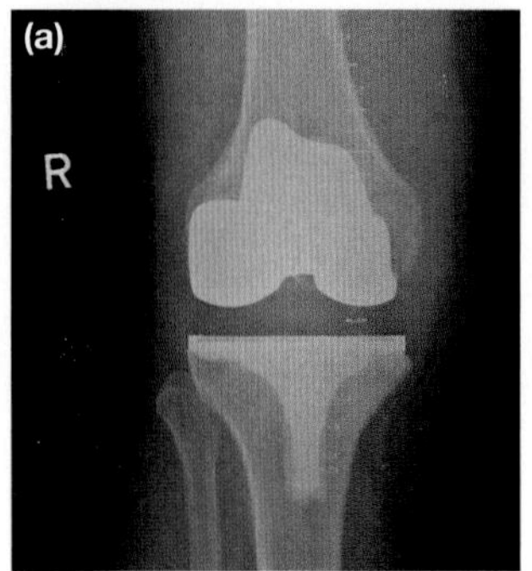

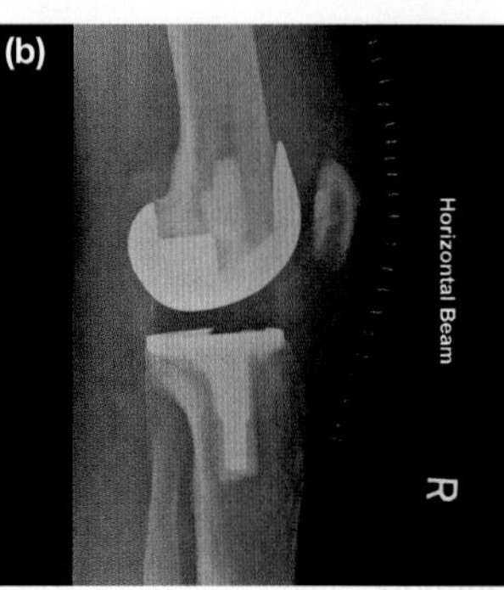

Figure 40.5 Anteroposterior (a) and lateral (b) radiographs of a total knee replacement.

commonly performed operation is a high tibial osteotomy (HTO) for a varus knee. Realignment is achieved with either an opening-wedge medial HTO or a closing-wedge lateral HTO. The amount of angular correction is calculated preoperatively and then created in theatre with jigs under radiographic control. Fixation with modern plates and locking screws allows early weight-bearing and mobilisation. The ideal patient for osteotomy is a young, active and well-motivated individual with disease limited to one compartment.

Knee joint replacement

There are three compartments within the knee: medial and lateral tibiofemoral, and patellofemoral. In 20–50% of cases, OA affects only one compartment and these patients may be suitable for a partial or unicompartmental knee replacement (UKR) (***Figure 40.4***), while in tricompartmental disease a TKR is indicated (***Figure 40.5***).

Patients are suitable for UKR if disease is limited to one compartment, if ligaments are intact and if fixed deformity is less than 15°. UKR has complication rates of one-third to one-half those of TKR with a lower infection rate, lower medical risks and lower risk of death. UKR is associated with a more rapid recovery, shorter hospital stay, preservation of knee kinematics and generally superior function to that of TKR. Revision rates for UKR are significantly influenced by the surgeon's experience and the implant. In optimal conditions the revision rates are similar to TKR, but on national registries UKRs have higher 10-year revision rates (6–12 %) than TKRs (2–6%).

Isolated patellofemoral replacement is also performed but the numbers are low in view of the scarcity of isolated patellofemoral disease. Revision rates are higher than other partial knee replacements, largely because of progression of arthritis in the remaining compartments.

A TKR can be regarded as a resurfacing procedure in which the femoral articular surface is replaced with metal and the tibial articular surface is replaced by a tough polyethylene insert, usually inserted into a metal tibial baseplate. TKR is one of the most successful surgical interventions, with most patients getting significant pain reduction and improvement in mobility. Revision rates are less than 5% at 15 years. Patient satisfaction with TKR is generally lower than that achieved with hip replacement.

TKR implants are generally cemented into the bone using polymethylmethacrylate (PMMA) cement. The design of the articulation can provide varying amounts of stability or constraint. Unconstrained TKRs are the most common and can either retain or sacrifice the PCL; these implants are called cruciate-retaining (CR) or PCL-sacrificing (PS), respectively. The more constrained the implant the greater the force transmitted to the implant–cement–bone interfaces, therefore increasing the risk of loosening. More constrained implants are generally only used in revision cases. If the joint is very unstable or deformed then a hinged knee replacement is used as it does not rely on the ligaments for stability. Modern knee replacements try to reduce wear by using enhanced bearing surfaces such as cross-linked polyethylene, vitamin E-enriched polyethylene or ceramicised surface coatings.

The TKR surgical technique aims to correct the deformity and leave the leg aligned with the mechanical axis and with the joint parallel to the ground. More modern philosophies of TKR try to match the patient's more individual alignment in the hope that this feels more natural to the patient, but it may require additional technology to allow this to be done accurately, e.g. computer navigation or robotics. It is important that the ligaments and soft-tissue envelope are well aligned and balanced to allow good stability, range of motion and patellar tracking. Early weight-bearing and mobilising are now possible, with some patients treated as day cases but most staying in hospital for 2–4 days.

Complications following TKR can be broadly classified into intraoperative and postoperative (***Table 40.2***).

TABLE 40.2 Complications of total knee replacement.

Intraoperative
- Implant malposition and malalignment; with subsequent contribution to instability, stiffness or pain
- Nerve or vessel injury, including tourniquet damage
- Fracture
- Patellar tendon avulsion
- Fat embolism

Postoperative
- Infection
- Deep vein thrombosis/pulmonary embolism
- Pain/stiffness
- Instability
- Osteolysis
- Component loosening
- Dislocation

Summary box 40.4

Aims of TKR
- Correct deformity caused by arthritis
- Align the knee to the mechanical axis or slightly under-corrected
- Joint line perpendicular to the mechanical axis
- Balanced collateral ligaments
- Ensure patellofemoral joint tracks normally

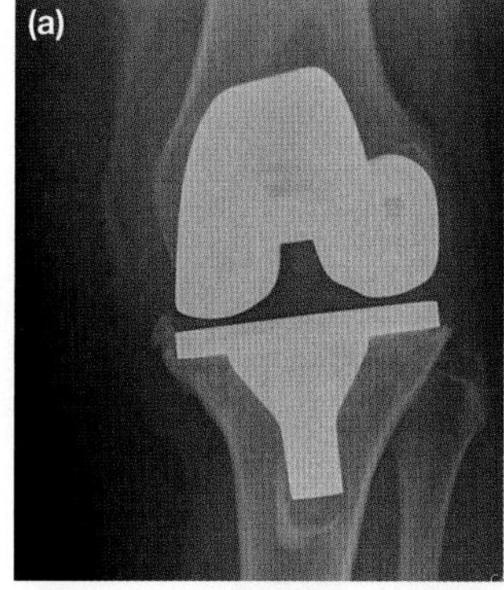

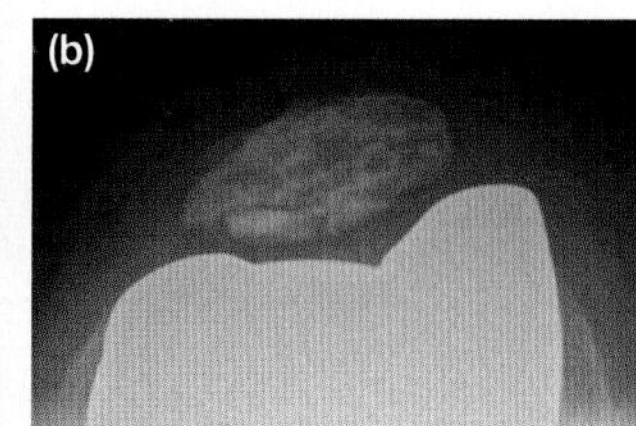

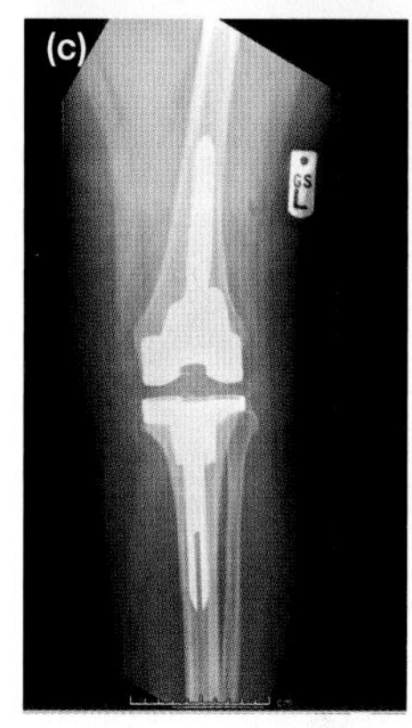

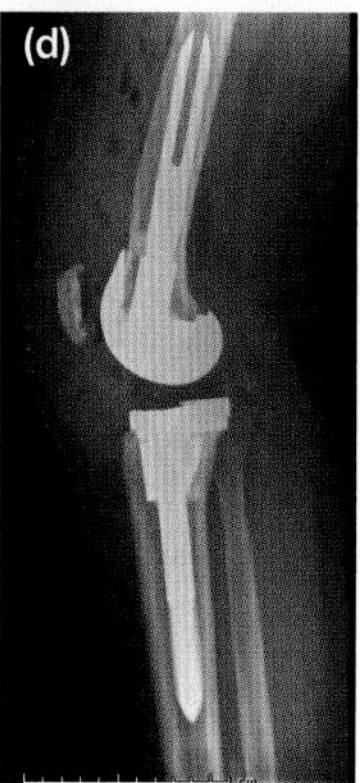

Figure 40.6 Radiographs of a malaligned knee (a, b) and a well-aligned revised knee (c, d).

Knee arthrodesis

Knee arthrodesis is rare and is largely a historic procedure that is seldom acceptable to modern patients. It is therefore used as a salvage option after failure of multiply-revised and infected joint replacements, particularly if there is disruption of the extensor mechanism. It is occasionally considered as a primary intervention in rare cases where neurological abnormality would prevent the patient from having the muscle control necessary to control a knee replacement, e.g. stroke, spina bifida, polio, Charcot arthropathy. The ideal position of fusion is 7° of valgus and 15° of flexion. Arthrodesis can be performed using intramedullary nails, plates or extramedullary fixators.

Revision knee replacement

TKRs have excellent long-term survival, with 82% lasting over 20 years and over 95% lasting 10–15 years. In the first few years, revision surgery is most likely to be due to infection, and non-infective causes, such as instability and malalignment. Beyond 10 years, revision is usually a result of aseptic loosening of components, which is often a result of wear of the plastic insert and polyethylene-induced osteolysis. With any failed joint replacement, infection should be excluded as this can compromise the result of surgery and may require a different surgical strategy, e.g. a two-stage rather than a single-stage procedure. Revision arthroplasty is technically more challenging, requires more complex and expensive implants and has a higher complication rate. When done for the correct indication, results are very good. As with a primary TKR, the goal remains to provide a well-aligned, stable and pain-free knee (***Figure 40.6***).

FURTHER READING

Bulstrode C, Wilson MacDonald J, Eastwood D *et al. Oxford textbook of trauma and orthopaedics*, 2nd edn. Oxford: Oxford University Press, 2017.

Howells NR, Brunton LR, Robinson J *et al.* Acute knee dislocation: an evidence based approach to the management of the multiligament injured knee. *Injury* 2011; **42**(11): 1198–204.

Miller MD, Thompson SR. *Miller's review of orthopaedics*, 8th edn. Philadelphia, PA: Elsevier, 2019.

National Joint Registry for England, Wales, Northern Ireland and the Isle of Man. *16th annual report 2019*. Hemel Hempstead: National Joint Registry, 2019.

Scott WN. *Insall & Scott surgery of the knee*, 6th edn. Philadelphia, PA: Elsevier, 2017.

Warwick D, Blom A, Whitehouse M. *Apley and Solomon's concise system of orthopaedics and trauma*, 5th edn. Abingdon: CRC Press, 2022.

Jean Martin Charcot, 1825–1893, physician, La Salpêtrière, Paris, France.

CHAPTER 41 The foot and ankle

Learning objectives

To understand:

- The basic anatomy and biomechanics of the foot and ankle
- The common problems affecting the foot and ankle in each age group
- The principles behind the treatment of each condition, be it conservative or surgical
- The significance of progressive neurological diseases

ANATOMY

There are 26 (25 with variant) main bones in the foot (seven tarsal bones, five metatarsals and 14 phalanges [13 in the biphalangeal fifth toe variant]) plus the two sesamoids of the hallux and a variable number of other sesamoid and accessory bones.

Movements at the ankle joint are mainly dorsiflexion and plantarflexion, but are more complex than this. The joint is actually a truncated section of a cone, meaning that the motion is not simply a hinge; in addition, movement of the ankle leads to rotation of the fibula at the syndesmosis. This means that the foot externally rotates with dorsiflexion and internally rotates with plantarflexion.

Stability is conferred upon the ankle by the congruence of the mortice and the integrity of principally the medial, lateral and inferior tibiofibular ligaments.

The subtalar joint is divided into anterior, middle and posterior facets and, along with the talonavicular and calcaneocuboid joints, makes up the triple joint complex. These joints are responsible for inversion and eversion of the hind- and midfoot. The joints are co-dependent such that limitation of one affects movement at the others. Fusion of the triple complex slightly affects movement at the ankle and vice versa.

The second tarsometatarsal (TMT) joint is recessed relative to the first and third and acts as a 'keystone'. Disruption of this joint (Lisfranc's injury) leads to loss of the transverse arch and an acquired flat foot.

The lower leg is divided into four compartments:

- the superficial posterior – gastrocnemius, soleus and plantaris;
- the deep posterior – tibialis posterior, flexor digitorum longus and flexor hallucis longus (FHL);
- the lateral – peroneus brevis and peroneus longus;
- the anterior – tibialis anterior, extensor hallucis longus, extensor digitorum longus and peroneus tertius.

There is only one muscle on the dorsum of the foot, the extensor digitorum brevis. The muscles on the plantar aspect of the foot are divided into four layers, the first being the most superficial, and the course of the neurovascular structures is a favourite examination topic. The plantar fascia is a very important structure that takes its origin from the heel and inserts into the bases of the proximal phalanges of the toes. At toe-off, the fascia tightens and accentuates the medial plantar arch and helps provide a rigid lever arm, the so-called 'windlass mechanism'. This is essential in the preservation of the integrity of the arch of the foot and function of the toes.

The blood supply of the foot is from the anterior tibial, the posterior tibial and the peroneal arteries. The following nerves supply sensation to the foot: posterior tibial, saphenous, sural, superficial and deep peroneal (***Figure 41.1***).

Summary box 41.1

Anatomy of the foot

- There are 26 major bones in the foot
- There are four layers of muscles in the sole of the foot
- The blood supply of the foot is from the anterior and posterior tibial arteries plus the peroneal artery

Jacques Lisfranc, 1790–1847, Professor of Surgery and Operative Medicine, Paris, France.

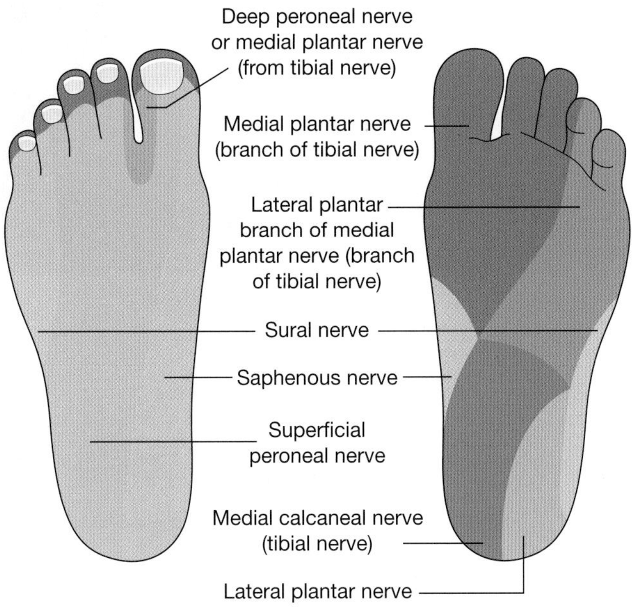

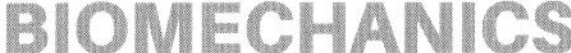

Figure 41.1 Cutaneous nerve supply of the foot (courtesy of Bartleby.com).

BIOMECHANICS

The walking cycle is divided into the stance (60%) and swing (40%) phases. The stance phase is divided into three intervals: (i) heel strike to foot flat; (ii) foot flat until the body passes over the ankle; and (iii) ankle joint plantarflexion to toe-off. During walking up to 12% of the gait cycle is spent with both feet in the stance phase, but with running there is a period when neither foot is in contact with the ground – the 'float' phase. During running the cycle time is shortened but the forces generated are very much increased.

Summary box 41.2

Biomechanics

- The gait cycle is divided into swing and stance phases
- Running generates increased forces, shortens the gait cycle and has a float phase when neither foot touches the ground

Examination

The examination of the foot is described in *Chapter 35*. The patient should be watched walking, and both the foot and the footwear of the patient need examining when looking for abnormal load and wear.

PAEDIATRIC CONDITIONS

These are discussed in *Chapter 44*.

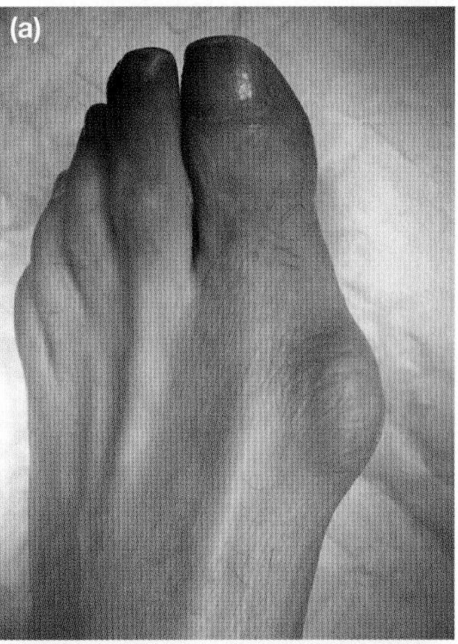

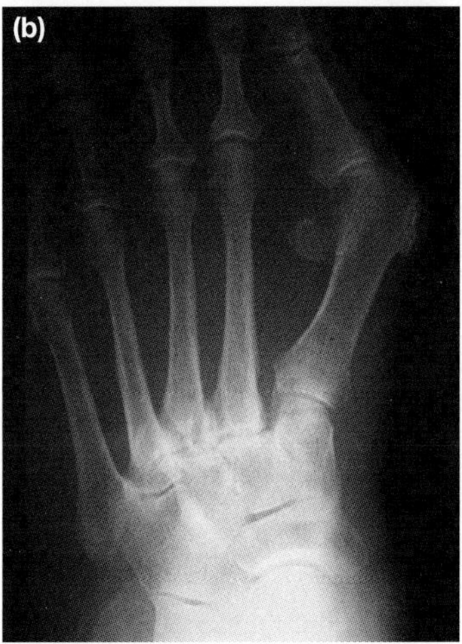

Figure 41.2 (a, b) Hallux valgus and bunion.

PATHOLOGY IN THE ADULT

The forefoot

Hallux valgus

Hallux valgus is deviation of the big toe away from the midline, i.e. towards the lesser toes, and is usually associated with a bunion, a swelling made up of both bone and bursa on the medial aspect of the first metatarsal head (*Figure 41.2*). It is a common condition that affects women more than men, and that is often bilateral. It is believed that the tendency to hallux valgus is inherited and that fully enclosed shoes accelerate the development of the condition, although not all agree.

With increasing deformity the first ray becomes defunctioned and elevated, and overload of the second metatarsophalangeal (MTP) joint often results in pain, swelling and eventually plantar plate disruption and dislocation. This can present with a prominent callosity beneath the second MTP joint and eventually hammering of the second toe.

Non-operative treatment of hallux valgus includes a wider toe box and pressure relief. Surgical intervention is commonly offered, but has a 10% rate of dissatisfaction.

For mild deformities a distal osteotomy (e.g. chevron) is usually adequate. For moderate deformities the surgeon is

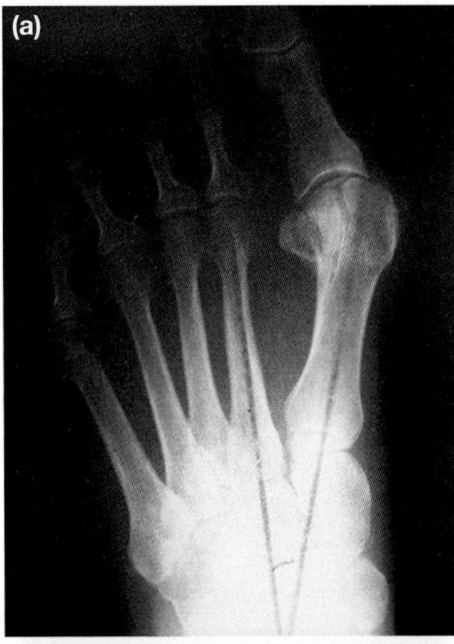

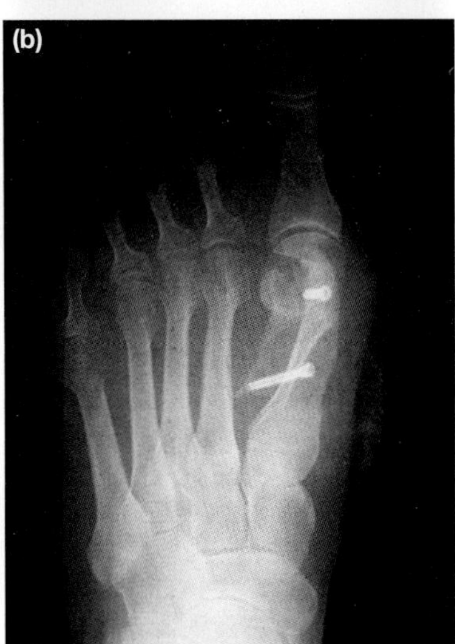

Figure 41.3 Pre- (a) and postoperative (b) radiographs of a scarf osteotomy.

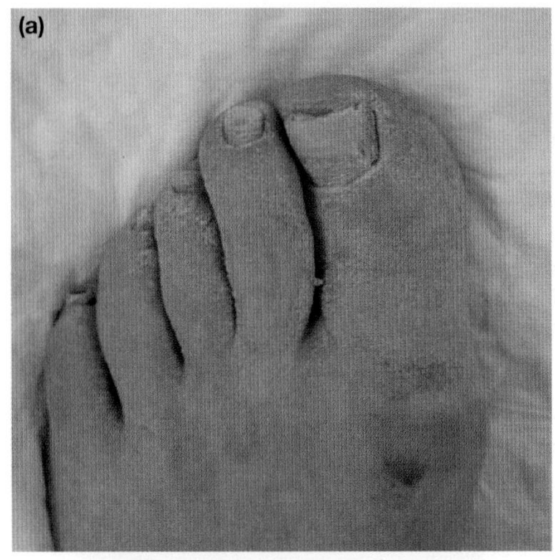

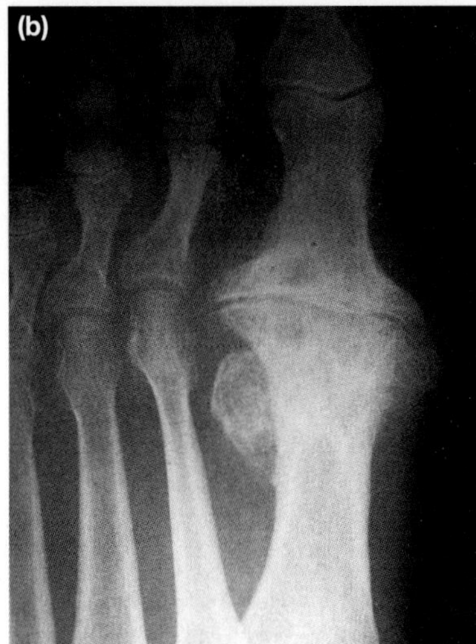

Figure 41.4 Clinical (a) and radiographic (b) appearance of hallux rigidus.

more likely to use a shaft, e.g. scarf (*Figure 41.3*) or Ludloff, or a basal (proximal chevron or crescentic) osteotomy. Severe deformities can be corrected by shaft and basal osteotomies but sometimes a fusion of the first TMT joint (modified Lapidus) or a first MTP joint fusion can be effective and is the preferred option for hypermobile or unstable TMT1 joint deformities. Minimally invasive techniques are developing and are widespread, especially in Europe, but there are few peer-reviewed series of outcomes from the UK and it has not become mainstream.

Basal osteotomies and fusions have a higher risk of abnormal elevation or depression of the rays, resulting in overload of the rest of the forefoot. However, they do allow a massive correction. They are best stabilised using plates.

Operations such as a Keller's excision arthroplasty, where the proximal third of the proximal phalanx is excised, serve to defunction the toe and sesamoids and are reserved for low-demand, high-risk patients in whom there is a high risk that healing of an osteotomy might fail.

The complications of bunion surgery are infection, cutaneous nerve damage, recurrence or overcorrection of deformity, stiffness and overload of the second MTP joint (transfer lesion); 10% of patients have significant reservations and 20% mild reservations about their outcome. Occasionally patients develop early arthritis following surgery and require revision to fusion.

Hallux rigidus

Hallux rigidus is a painful condition of the hallux MTP joint characterised by loss of motion, especially in dorsiflexion, and osteophyte formation on the dorsum and sides of the joint (*Figure 41.4*).

A **scarf** osteotomy is named after a carpentry term; it is an elongated Z-shaped osteotomy along the metatarsal.

Karl Ludloff, 1864–1945, German orthopaedic surgeon.

Paul W Lapidus, 1893–1981, Russian-born orthopaedic surgeon, Chief of the first Orthopedic Foot Clinic and Service, Hospital for Joint Diseases, New York, NY, USA.

William Lordan Keller, 1874–1959, Head of the Department of Surgery, Walter Reed Hospital, Washington, DC, USA, described this operation in 1904.

Summary box 41.3

Hallux valgus

- Bunions affect women more often than men
- Patients with hallux valgus have inherited a tendency to develop the condition
- Not all patients need surgery
- The choice of operation is determined by the severity of the deformity and presence or absence of any arthritis, instability of the joints or hypermobility

In adults there is often a history of trauma or repetitive microtrauma (sport) but, occasionally, there is a strong family history of the condition. Gout and rheumatological conditions may present in this way. Patients complain of stiffness and pain on weight-bearing.

The most effective non-operative treatment is provision of a stiff-soled shoe with a deep toe box or a rocker-soled shoe, which are now available on the high street.

The mainstays of surgical management are injection/manipulation, cheilectomy (a radical debridement and excision of the part of the joint blocking movement), fusion and interposition arthroplasty (Keller-type procedure or silicone interposition). Prosthetic arthroplasty, with hemi-, total, interposition or spacer arthroplasty, is available but many prostheses have been withdrawn because of high failure rates and few series extend beyond 9 years. Newer prosthetic inserts with claimed joint-preserving capabilities similarly fail to show advantages with regards to pain and have a high revision/reoperation rate but are still preferred by some who wish to retain mobility at MTP1 in the short to medium term.

Fusion is for the severely affected and is an effective means of abolishing pain, but affects the biomechanics and some patients are left with intractable pain beneath the sesamoids. A fusion will still usually allow sports participation.

Summary box 41.4

Hallux rigidus

- Hallux rigidus can affect adolescents as well as adults
- Stiff-soled shoes with a deep toe box are the most comfortable type of shoe
- Cheilectomy and fusion are the mainstays of surgical treatment

Sesamoid/sesamoid complex problems

Turf toe

Acute injuries (turf toe) can be managed non-operatively or surgically depending on the grade of the injury and the occupation of the patient. Grade 4 acute rupture may require surgery.

Turf toe is a plantar plate disruption usually from hyperextension injuries at MTP1 and may involve sesamoid fractures. Low-grade injuries can be treated non-operatively but high-grade injuries require reconstruction, especially in athletes (see ***Chapter 36***).

Chronic conditions range from stress fracture to avascular necrosis (AVN) and sesamoiditis but are probably all the same phenomenon. Management includes offloading with orthotics, injections of steroids and, rarely, shaving/excision. Excision surgery carries a high risk.

Lesser toe deformities

Hammer, mallet and claw toes are frequent and are usually nonindicative but may be secondary to other deformities in the foot or to underlying neurological disease. Nonoperative treatment involves appropriate padding and footwear modification. For symptomatic flexible deformities soft-tissue surgery such as flexor/extensor tenotomies with/without capsulotomy is usually adequate, but for fixed deformities bony procedures are required such as interposition arthroplasty, fusion or excision arthroplasty.

Isolated lesser toe MTP extension/subluxation may result from a ruptured plantar plate at MTP joints and repair techniques have evolved recently, but the results are moderate at best and the trend is back to non-operative management where possible. Ultrasound and magnetic resonance imaging (MRI) are now well established for these injuries.

Freiberg's disease

Freiberg's disease (***Figure 41.5***) is an ischaemic necrosis of the epiphysis, resulting in pain and swelling of the joint. It will often settle with rest. Reshaping osteotomies are described, or excision of the proximal phalangeal head for severe adult cases with joint destruction. Excision of the whole metatarsal head should never be performed.

Morton's neuroma and metatarsalgia

Metatarsalgia usually occurs secondary to joint problems, overload or irritation of a nerve. Morton's neuroma is a painful

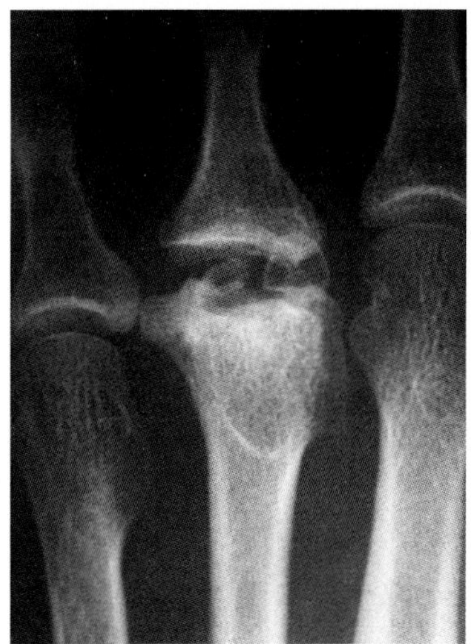

Figure 41.5 Freiberg's disease.

Albert Henry Freiberg, Professor of Orthopaedic Surgery, University of Cincinnati, Cincinnati, OH, USA, gave his account of this condition in 1926.
Thomas George Morton, 1835–1903, surgeon, Pennsylvania Hospital, Philadelphia, PA, USA, described this condition in 1876.

condition that, in most cases, arises from compression of the common digital nerve, most commonly between the third and fourth metatarsal heads and the second/third and is usually secondary to other forefoot pathology.

The diagnosis is confirmed by ultrasound or MRI. Non-operative treatments include advice about footwear, an orthosis (premetatarsal dome) to splay the metatarsal heads or an injection of steroids. Cryotherapy and even alcohol injections have been reported.

Surgery involves resection (the affected toes will be permanently partly hemi-numb if the nerve is removed) but this is not without risk of patient dissatisfaction, pain and recurrence, with around 5% reporting bad outcomes, often permanent. European colleagues often simply transect the intermetatarsal ligament instead.

Summary box 41.5

Morton's neuroma

- Morton's neuroma most commonly affects the second or third web space
- Surgical excision of neuroma is often successful but has a risk of pain syndrome
- Guided injections form the mainstay of treatment for most

Stress fracture

This may occur following sport or may be incipient. It usually presents in the forefoot and may mimic Morton's neuroma or metatarsalgia. An unexplained aetiology might require biochemical or biomechanical evaluation. Forefoot fractures can usually be managed non-operatively.

Stress fractures may occur in any bone. Those of the navicular, talus and tibial sesamoid often present with vague symptomatology but early diagnosis with MRI and management are essential with immediate offloading and protection with early fixation – if required, urgently – if a full fracture is seen developing. Vague, poorly defined midfoot pain in an athlete or military recruit mandates urgent scanning and offloading.

Follow-up investigation of bone metabolism/density and exclusion of myeloma may be required.

The midfoot

The midfoot comprises the cuneiforms and the cuboid and related joints.

Midfoot arthritis

The aetiology is usually not known but the risk factors include microtrauma, rheumatological causes, flat foot, Lisfranc or similar injuries (which may have been missed), Charcot and cavus foot. Patients are best managed non-operatively with orthotics, shoes, analgesia and modifications of their lifestyle.

Pain, often with palpable dorsal osteophytes, is the commonest finding. Injections and orthotics are the mainstay of treatment, with surgery high risk and having moderate outcomes. Fusion or interposition arthroplasty of the lateral two TMT joints has a universally poor outcome.

Charcot

An acute hot, red, swollen foot (which may or may not be painful) may be indicative of Charcot (often secondary to diabetes, which may as yet be undiagnosed) or other neuropathy. Immediate offloading in plaster and urgent management are indicated; National Institute for Health and Care Excellence (NICE) guidelines are available in the UK.

The presence of any unexplained swelling, heat, ulcer or deformity in a diabetic foot mandates an emergency and referral along NICE guidelines; failure to follow such guidelines can lead to significant sums being paid out by indemnity organsiations.

Tendinopathy

Rarely, dorsal pain may be due to tibialis anterior tendinosis at its insertion; management is usually non-operative. Injection carries a slight risk of rupture, which is ameliorated by a surgical boot with deep vein thrombosis (DVT) prophylaxis.

Ganglions

Midfoot ganglions are common and may cause neuralgia over dorsal bosses. Injection/aspiration should be attempted. Surgery may be required but recurrence is high and secondary neuralgia not infrequent.

The hindfoot and ankle

Ankle arthritis

The definitive operative treatment for arthritis of the ankle will usually be in the form of total ankle replacement (TAR) or more commonly arthrodesis (fusion); the latter is often carried out via an open approach but arthroscopic techniques have better outcomes, more rapid recovery and fewer complications and almost all surgical units in the UK now offer such techniques. Such techniques are mandatory in the presence of a poor soft-tissue envelope or in the presence of a clotting diathesis.

A UK national trial is currently under way to evaluate the relative outcomes of TAR versus arthrodesis (the TARVA trial), which are as yet undefined; the trial has been complicated further by the withdrawal/failure of the two leading implants.

The advantage of fusion is that it has a known track record, good outcomes (over 90% of patients do well) and minimal morbidity, especially with modern arthroscopic techniques, but not all do well with fusion. Function following isolated fusion is virtually normal for most patients and this is probably due to increased mobility at other joints. However, this may precipitate arthralgia elsewhere.

TARs were until recently three-component devices (except in the USA) but a two-component device is now the market leader in the UK by far. It is not yet known if this is relevant but allows an easier regulatory pathway in the USA. Outcomes

Jean Martin Charcot, 1825–1893, physician, La Salpêtrière, Paris, France.

seem to be related to accuracy of placement and modern instrumentation may be a key factor; custom implants based on preoperative computed tomography (CT) scans are becoming mainstream. TARs allow preservation of joint mobility but at the expense of larger incisions and possible eventual failure. Revision rates of <1% to 7% per annum are reported, with most showing an approximately 3% failure rate per year. Survivorship analysis does not record patients who are doing badly but who do not have further surgery and a recent paper showed revisions are under-reported. The changes in the regulatory pathways in the UK/European Union relating to the development of new implants may limit the development of TARs in these regions to the same levels of efficacy seen by total hip replacements and total knee replacements.

Hindfoot (excluding ankle) arthritis

The triple complex refers to the subtalar (talocalcaneal), calcaneocuboid and talonavicular joints. These joints are often affected by arthritis. Treatment options are limited and, if simple measures have failed, a fusion should be performed. Smokers and patients with diabetes have a massively increased non-union rate for all foot fusion procedures and should be warned of this when they give consent. Late presentation of coalitions usually requires fusion.

Ankle combined with other hindfoot arthritis

If surgical input is required, one option is to treat one set of joints and then see how the patient fares. For example, offer the patient an ankle fusion or replacement and then assess the outcome. Secondary surgery to the other joints can then be performed if required. The alternative is to treat all joints at once. The non-union rates of the ankle following a subtalar fusion or vice versa are high (up to 75%). For this reason, some clinicians advise TAR, not ankle fusion, following a previous subtalar/triple fusion.

Modern techniques now use third-generation hindfoot fusion nails that fuse both the ankle and subtalar joints. These are inserted with an open or arthroscopic fusion technique.

A pantalar fusion is quite disabling but may be necessary in patients with rheumatoid arthritis or with deformities/stress fractures and in those with a failed arthroplasty with subtalar joint involvement, pantalar arthritis or AVN with collapse of the talus.

Summary box 41.6

Midfoot and hindfoot

- Joint disorders are degenerative or inflammatory
- The mainstay of surgical treatment remains fusion, although ankle replacements are becoming more successful
- Rheumatoid arthritis must be medically controlled as well as possible before surgery
- Knee deformities should be corrected before tackling foot problems

Rheumatological presentations in the foot

The early presentations of rheumatological disease may include synovitis of the lesser MTP joints and widespread small joint disease, often in association with enthesopathy such as plantar fasciitis or Achilles tendinosis. However, the classic deformity is of hallux valgus with or without hallux rigidus deformity and subluxation or even dislocation of the lesser MTP joints in the forefoot and arthritis and deformity in the mid/hindfoot.

The patient may present with a bunion and prominent lesser metatarsal heads, which can often be felt to be dislocated on clinical examination and are painful to palpation. Joint-sparing surgery is preferred, with preservation of the metatarsal heads if possible, often shortening and relocating the MTP joints. Destruction of the joints can be treated with proximal phalangeal partial excisions. Fusion of the first MTP joint is the usual requirement. Late recurrence can be managed with excision arthroplasty.

Excision of the metatarsal heads produces an almost instantaneous and gratifying relief of pain. If a plantar approach is used an ellipse of skin can be excised to move the metatarsal padding back over the end of the metatarsal. While most surgeons avoid scars on the plantar aspect of the foot wherever possible, this is one procedure where the results are good. However, such surgery leaves no room for revision in later years.

The requirement for rheumatoid forefoot correction has fallen dramatically in the last 20 years with the advent of disease-modifying drugs; most trainee surgeons will now have never seen a Fowler's procedure (or similar), which was once a mainstream and common procedure.

Midfoot

Rheumatological disease may also affect the midfoot and here the outcome is usually just pain and stiffness. Options are limited to injections and fusion surgery if non-operative measures have failed.

Hindfoot and ankle

Rheumatological disease also affects the hindfoot and ankle. Many patients require surgical hindfoot fusions and the options for the ankle are discussed in ***Ankle arthritis***. Outcomes of TAR are favourable in patients with rheumatoid arthritis, although increased deformities may make the outcomes less predictable.

The rheumatological diseases also affect soft tissues. Patients are more prone to developing enthesopathy, tendinitis and tendinosis, and even tendon rupture. The Achilles tendon should never be injected with steroid for fear of rupture; similarly, the tibialis anterior and tibialis posterior tendons are risky for injection.

Tendon disorders

Tenosynovitis/tendinitis is probably a misnomer as the histological data support neither pathology in many cases. It often occurs as a result of injury or overuse or is secondary to inflammatory disease. Rest, anti-inflammatory medication

Alan W Fowler, 1920–2013, orthopaedic surgeon, Bridgend Hospital, UK.

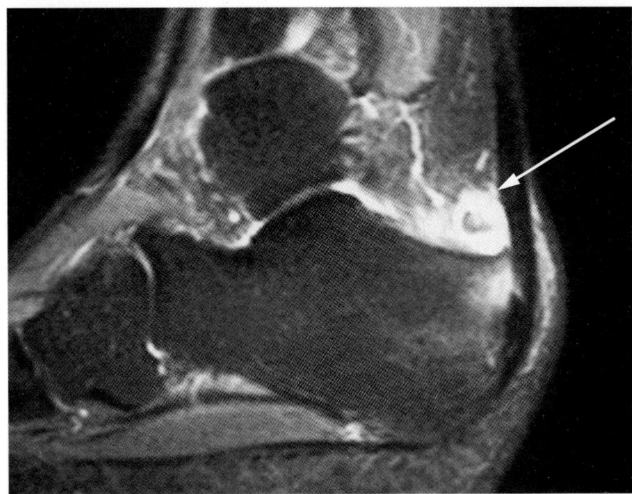

Figure 41.6 Insertional Achilles tendinitis (arrow).

and physiotherapy are often helpful but, in inflammatory conditions, tenosynovectomy may be required.

The tendons most commonly affected by degeneration are the Achilles (***Figure 41.6***), tibialis posterior and the peronei (brevis more than longus).

Ruptured Achilles tendon

The Achilles tendon rupture is relatively frequent in the 40- to 50-year-old age group who are undertaking vigorous sport after a long period away from such activities, but can occur in any age and with little provocation. One-quarter are missed in primary care or in the accident and emergency department and the recording of the Simmonds test is mandatory. The test is non-reliable after 1 week. Management of acute rupture is more frequently non-operative nowadays, provided ultrasound has shown closure of the gap in plantarflexion (although the importance of this even is now debated), and many protocols are described for non-operative management. Surgical fixation is an alternative but large meta-analyses have shown little if any advantage of surgical fixation with an increased complication rate.

Many patients do not suffer the acute rupture classically described in all textbooks and many seem to have a series of micro-tears that gradually lead to total rupture. Studies have shown that older adult patients with Achilles rupture regained 70–90% of the normal power with no treatment whatsoever when reviewed at 1 year; for many patients, this is enough to allow some of them to return to normal function.

Non-operative options for a missed rupture include a sprung ankle–foot orthotic ankle brace, while operative options involve reconstructive surgery with or without FHL tendon augmentation or synthetic ligament replacement.

Achilles tendinosis

Non-insertional tendinosis is frequent, often related to overuse and is usually managed non-operatively. Multiple tendon problems should alert the clinician to the presence of seronegative arthritides. Shockwave therapy is a recent addition to the armoury. Steroid injections may rupture the Achilles tendon and are discouraged; high-volume saline, dry-needling and sclerosant injections have all been described but are used less frequently with the advent of shockwave. Surgery for non-insertional tendinosis has moderate success.

Insertional tendinosis is usually associated with a Haglund's bony deformity or the presence of intratendinous bony spurs/shelves seen on lateral radiograph. Significant intratendinous bony spurs rarely get better without surgical input in the author's experience. Minimally invasive or mini-open excision of the prominent posterolateral corner of the calcaneum in Haglund's deformity, detachment, debridement and reattachment or reshaping osteotomy form the mainstay of modern surgical techniques for insertional problems, but both conditions have a relatively high rate of failure and complication with surgery.

Peroneal tendon problems

The peroneal tendons may develop tendinosis, may subluxate or may become involved in an inflammatory process with or without bony overgrowth at the inferior retinaculum (***Figure 41.7***). An associated varus heel will amplify the problem and will need addressing with an appropriate reconstruction/osteotomy or fusion. Investigation as to whether the varus heel caused the peroneal problem or vice versa should be established or recurrence is guaranteed.

Peroneal tendon subluxation can occur spontaneously or after injury. It may be associated with the groove at the back of the fibula being too shallow to contain the peroneal tendons, but may just be secondary to a superior retinaculum tear. The patient may be able to demonstrate a tendon subluxation over the fibula. Surgical repair is usually required and involves deepening of the groove.

Tendinosis/tendinitis can be managed non-operatively, although injections have occasionally caused rupture. Surgical debridement or repair of splits/tears/ruptures is well described but has only moderate success.

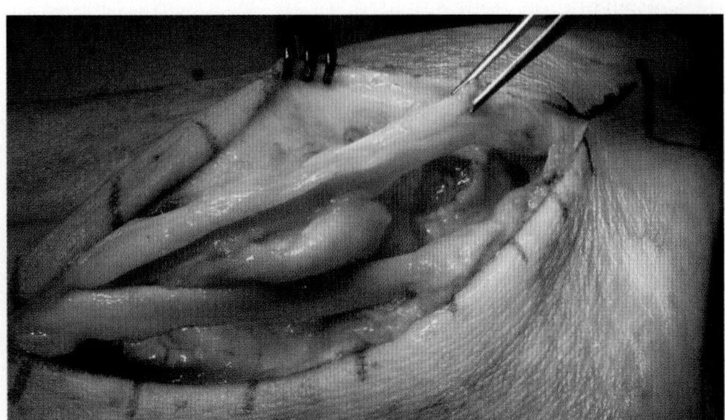

Figure 41.7 Split and degenerate peroneus brevis.

Franklin Adin Simmonds, 1911–1983, orthopaedic surgeon, The Rowley Bristow Hospital, Pyrford, Surrey, UK.
Patrik Haglund, 1870–1937, Swedish orthopaedic surgeon.

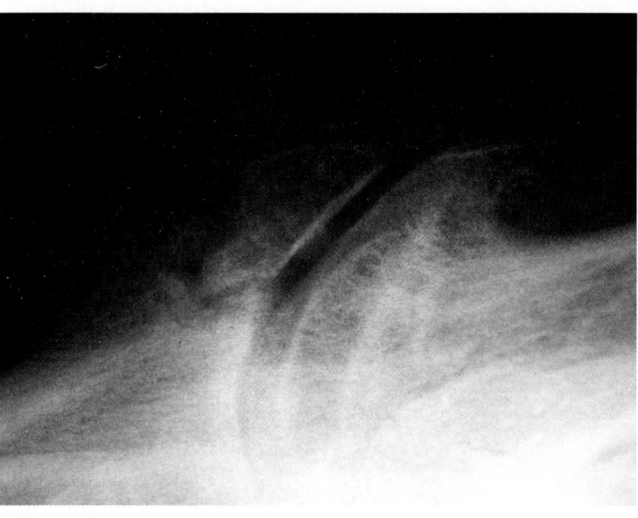

Figure 41.8 Tarsometatarsal arthritis.

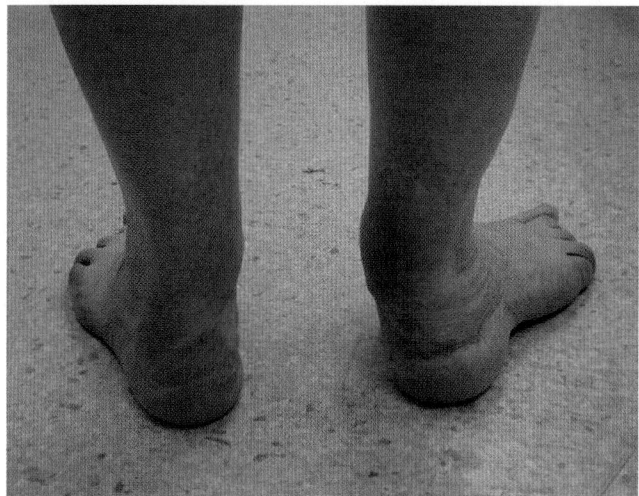

Figure 41.9 A tibialis posterior tendon-deficient foot.

Acquired flat foot

There is a wide range of normal appearance of adult feet. Pathological causes of a flat foot include:

- tibialis posterior tendon dysfunction;
- tarsometatarsal arthritis/injury (***Figure 41.8***);
- Charcot neuroarthropathy, e.g. diabetes (see ***Diabetes***);
- inflammatory/degenerative arthritis of the subtalar/talonavicular/naviculocuneiform joints;
- spring ligament rupture;
- tarsal coalition.

Summary box 41.7

Acquired flat foot

- Tibialis posterior tendon dysfunction and tarsometatarsal osteoarthritis are common causes of an acquired flat foot
- Orthoses, rest and non-steroidal anti-inflammatory drugs (NSAIDs) can help with symptomatic relief
- Surgery is a major undertaking but is often highly successful at achieving symptomatic relief

The tibialis posterior tendon tends to fail in overweight individuals and those who have flat feet. Often, after unaccustomed exercise, the tendon swells and is painful. The condition occurs mainly in women; the key test, which is that the patient cannot stand on tiptoe on that leg alone, indicates a significant advanced stage tendon problem. Many individuals will require surgical treatment in the form of a medial displacement calcaneal osteotomy, flexor digitorum longus or FHL tendon transfer and spring ligament repair. Failure to treat this condition can lead to spectacular deformity (***Figure 41.9***).

An acute traumatic flat foot may develop in young athletes and military recruits after traumatic injury. Examination shows a new-onset flat foot but with a functioning tibialis posterior tendon with single-leg tiptoe preserved; here the injury is an isolated spring ligament tear and early surgery prevents late-onset secondary deformity.

Ankle instability

Most people who sustain an ankle sprain will recover, particularly if they receive prompt physiotherapy. However, some individuals develop significant instability. On examination an unstable ankle due to ligament disruption will show a marked 'anterior drawer' sign.

If physiotherapy is unsuccessful at resolving the problem, a reconstruction may be needed with ligament augmentation. Anatomical techniques such as the Broström procedure are favoured and may be supplemented with synthetic augments for early mobilisation. Peroneal tendon harvesting for reconstruction is now obsolete with the new reconstruction techniques and implants.

Other aetiologies of instability include osteochondritis dissecans (OCD) lesions, syndesmosis instability and peroneal tendon pathology.

Osteochondral lesion of the talus

Patients with persistent pain (and sometimes instability) in the ankle following an injury should be suspected of having an osteochondral lesion, with MRI or CT usually required for diagnosis.

Repair of cartilage is not yet possible and large meta-analyses of experimental techniques such as grafting, cell culture, implants and stem cells have not yet shown any statistical benefit. Debridement and microabrasion/microfracture form the mainstay of treatment. Large fragments seen early might benefit from early fixation. Juveniles seem to have a high spontaneous recovery rate and surgery should not be necessary.

L Broström, described the surgical treatment of chronic ligament ruptures in 1966.

Synovitis

Many patients have ongoing pain following ankle injury that is simply due to synovitis within the ankle joint, prominence of the syndesmotic ligament into the joint, impaction injury or undiagnosed fracture or OCD lesion. MRI is mandatory for these cases but usually misses the synovitis. Synovitis may be treated non-operatively, with an injection of steroid. Persistent symptoms may require arthroscopic debridement.

Neurological foot conditions

Pes cavus

The development of unilateral pes cavus is likely to be due to an upper motor neurone lesion, so an appropriate neurological examination should be performed and spinal imaging is mandated.

Pes cavus is usually bilateral and most cases will be associated with an underlying neurological condition, the most common being Charcot–Marie–Tooth disease. These patients may present with characteristic progressive small muscle wasting, thin calf musculature, hand symptoms, aches and pains, and cavovarus feet. Examination may show early loss of vibration sense. Precise diagnosis is confirmed with nerve conduction studies and genetic testing.

The key deforming force is always relative preservation of the tibialis posterior tendon. Surgical correction of the deformity is often required. The principal goal of treatment is to obtain a foot that can be placed flat on the ground, and with the power of the muscles around the ankle in balance. It will always be necessary to transfer the tibialis posterior tendon. The most commonly performed procedure is to transfer the tibialis posterior tendon to the dorsolateral side of the foot, with a lateralising heel osteotomy and dorsiflexion osteotomy of the first ray with or without a Jones procedure to the great toe and Hibbs procedure to the lesser toes. Older textbooks all universally relay the mistaken belief that it is peroneal overactivity that is the deforming force … it isn't!

Summary box 41.8

Pes cavus

- Pes cavus needs neurological investigation
- About 80% of cases of pes cavus are associated with a neurological disease
- The commonest cause is Charcot–Marie–Tooth disease
- Unilateral pes cavus – think diastematomyelia/tumour

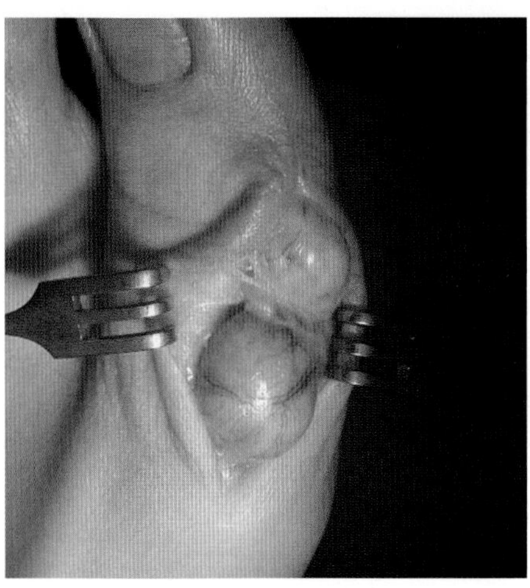

Figure 41.10 Angioleiomyoma of the hallux.

Tumours

The most common benign tumours of the foot are ganglia, giant cell tumour and angioleiomyomas (***Figure 41.10***); these tumours may need surgical excision.

Pigmented villonodular synovitis is a locally aggressive condition found in the ankle and is diagnosed by MRI or at histology. Imatinib medical therapy and en bloc resection are becoming more mainstream for cure rather than repeated arthroscopic suppression. Surveillance for recurrence is mandatory.

The most common 'tumour' seen in the foot is the plantar fibroma or Ledderhose's disease, which presents as a painful, often growing, lump in the sole along the plantar fascia. The condition is linked to Dupuytren's contracture and Peyronie's disease. Surgery should be avoided. Ultrasound or MRI will confirm the multifocal nature of the disease and exclude other pathology.

Any large or growing lump in the foot needs formal work-up along tumour guidelines, especially in the presence of night pain.

Infection

Septic arthritis in the foot or ankle is rare except in patients with diabetes and constitutes a surgical emergency; when it occurs it usually follows a surgical procedure but it can also arise as a result of haematogenous spread. Treatment is immediate surgical drainage and administration of appropriate high-dosage antibiotics once cultures are obtained.

Pierre Marie, 1853–1940, neurologist, Hospice de Bicêtre, Paris, France, later becoming Professor of Pathological Anatomy in the Faculty of Medicine, and finally, in 1918, Professor of Neurology.
Howard Henry Tooth, 1856–1925, physician, St Bartholomew's Hospital and the National Hospital for Nervous Diseases, London, UK, described peroneal muscular atrophy in 1886 independently of Charcot and Marie.
Sir Robert Jones, 1857–1933, British orthopaedic surgeon.
Russell A Hibbs, 1869–1932, Professor of Orthopedic Surgery, Columbia University, New York, NY, USA, described an operation for 'claw foot' in 1919.
Georg Ledderhose, 1855–1925, German surgeon, described this disease in 1894.
Baron Guillaume Dupuytren, 1777–1835, surgeon, Hôtel Dieu, Paris, France, described this condition in 1831.
François de la Peyronie, 1678–1747, surgeon to King Louis XIV of France and founder of the Royal Academy of Surgery, Paris, France.

The most common causative organism is *Staphylococcus aureus* with methicillin-resistant *S. aureus* (MRSA) becoming more common. Even with prompt treatment chondrolysis often occurs and subsequent degenerative changes develop rapidly.

In immunocompromised patients, opportunistic infections can arise and, in those with diabetes, failure to treat with debridement can lead to amputation. It is important to realise that radiographs in the early stages of infection are usually normal and that diagnosis is made on clinical suspicion and with blood tests and more sophisticated imaging such as MRI or bone scanning.

Tuberculosis can affect the foot and is associated with major bony damage; it responds surprisingly well to debridement and appropriate antituberculous therapy (***Figure 41.11***).

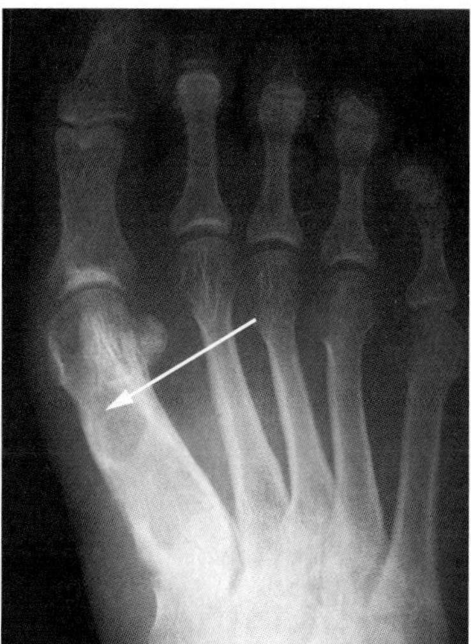

Figure 41.11 Tuberculosis of the foot (arrow).

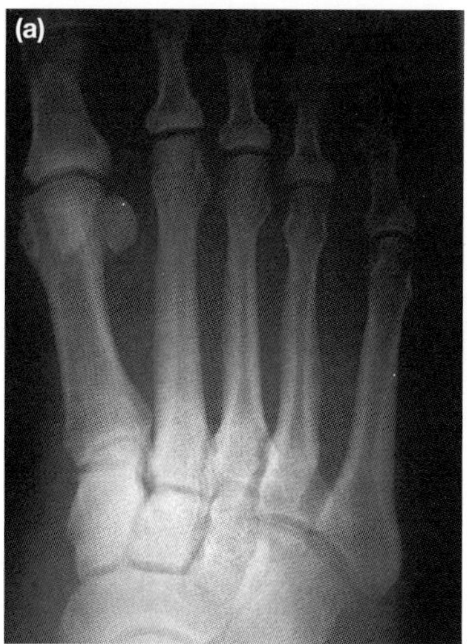

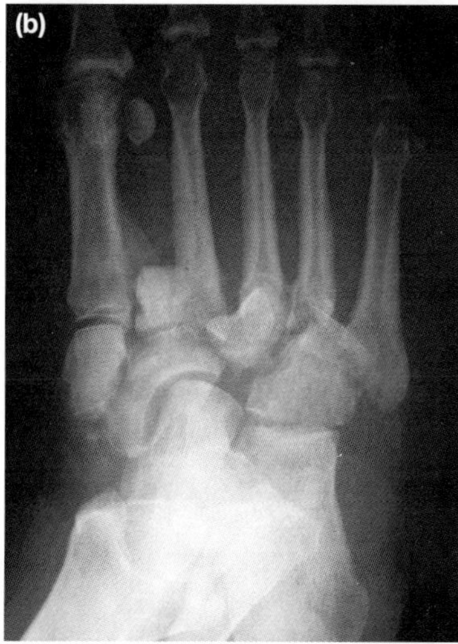

Figure 41.12 Charcot foot: radiographs taken at the time of a trivial injury (a) and 6 weeks later (b).

Diabetes

Patients with diabetes have foot problems secondary to neuropathy and microvascular changes. They are at increased risk of infection and ulceration, and trauma (sometimes trivial) can lead to collapse of the foot, also known as Charcot neuroarthropathy (***Figure 41.12***).

Ulceration and amputation

Ulceration can lead to major morbidity and amputation (***Figure 41.13***). Ulcers need to be treated urgently, and when ulcer healing has occurred the aim should be to keep the foot ulcer free. NICE guidelines detail optimal management pathways with urgent admission and radiological and clinical assessment in a multidisciplinary team setting, followed by debridement, antibiotics if required and formal offloading. Ulceration is a surgical emergency and mandates immediate referral along NICE guidelines in the UK. Most amputations are preceded by ulceration.

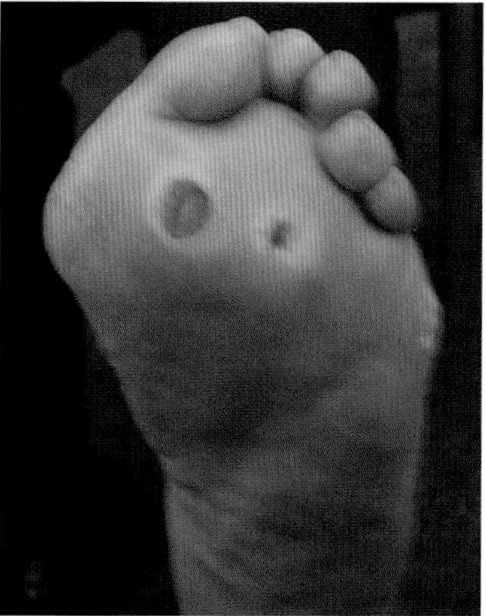

Figure 41.13 Diabetic foot ulcer.

Charcot

Charcot is a condition in which patients develop a neuropathic destruction of the joints. It is often described as painless but actually the majority of patients have some pain. In the western world diabetes is the biggest cause but in the rest of the world leprosy is also important. However, any other neurological condition can cause this disease.

Charcot often presents with a hot, swollen, red extremity. It is often misdiagnosed as cellulitis, gout, fracture or DVT, and many present late because of the difficulty in diagnosis.

If there is no history of skin damage, infection is unlikely, but MRI and even biopsy can help differentiate between infection and Charcot. From initiation through to bone consolidation may take up to 18 months. The principle of treatment throughout is to maintain a foot-shaped foot to prevent late pressure ulcers. The acute Charcot foot requires appropriate splintage in a Charcot retaining orthotic walker (CROW) or a total contact cast (TCC), but many surgeons offer an aggressive early surgical approach if bony prominence/ulceration is thought to be inevitable. Surgical excision of a bony prominence dramatically reduces ulceration and amputation risk and reconstruction in the early phases of Charcot is now becoming more mainstream, but surgical risks are high. Long-segment fixation with implants and intramedullary nailing is now regularly undertaken. Failure of non-operative or operative treatment results in ulceration and amputation.

Summary box 41.9

Diabetes

- Patients with diabetes are prone to infection because of:
  - Peripheral neuropathy
  - Peripheral vascular disease
  - Impaired resistance to infection
- A Charcot foot is often misdiagnosed but is a surgical emergency and requires urgent admission and management
- An ulcer in a diabetic foot is a surgical emergency and requires urgent admission and management

Entrapment neuropathies

Any nerve supplying the foot can become entrapped and result in pain, and treatment often requires surgical decompression. Tarsal tunnel syndrome is much rarer than carpal tunnel syndrome and is confirmed with nerve conduction. A high proportion of patients retain neurology and pain despite release.

Heel pain

The commonest cause of heel pain is plantar fasciitis. Pain is located inferomedially within the heel and is worst first thing in the morning and after periods of rest. The majority of cases settle within 18 months and surgery is rarely required or successful. Ultrasound-guided injection or shockwave forms the mainstay of treatment for the non-resolving cases. The differential diagnosis list includes calcaneal stress fracture, tarsal tunnel syndrome, seronegative arthropathy and Ledderhose's disease.

FURTHER READING

Bulstrode C, Wilson MacDonald J *et al. Oxford textbook of trauma and orthopaedics*, 2nd edn. Oxford: Oxford University Press, 2017.

Miller MD, Thompson SR. *Miller's review of orthopaedics*, 8th edn. Philadelphia, PA: Elsevier, 2019.

Warwick D, Blom A, Whitehouse M. *Apley and Solomon's concise system of orthopaedics and trauma*, 5th edn. Abingdon: CRC Press, 2022.

CHAPTER 42 Musculoskeletal tumours

Learning objectives

- List the symptoms and signs associated with a musculoskeletal tumour
- Understand why a patient with a suspected musculoskeletal tumour should be referred to a specialist centre for staging, biopsy and multidisciplinary management
- Understand why staging should be completed before biopsy
- Explain why a diagnosis is required before treatment
- Understand the principles of biopsy
- Describe the principles of surgical treatment of musculoskeletal tumours
- List the aims of surgical treatment for metastatic bone disease
- Understand how to manage patients with an impending or completed pathological fracture
- Evaluate the risk of pathological fracture

INTRODUCTION

Musculoskeletal tumours include primary and secondary benign and malignant tumours of bone and soft tissue. The most common malignant tumours in bone are metastatic carcinomas (*Figure 42.1*). Advances in oncological treatment mean that the number of patients living with metastatic bone disease is increasing. The most common carcinomas that metastasise to bone originate in the breast, prostate, lung, kidney, thyroid and colon (*Figure 42.2*).

Haematopoietic tumours may also arise in bone: multiple myeloma (*Figure 42.3*) is a malignant neoplasm arising from plasma cells in the bone marrow, leading to multiple lesions in the skeleton. When solitary, this type of tumour is called a plasmacytoma.

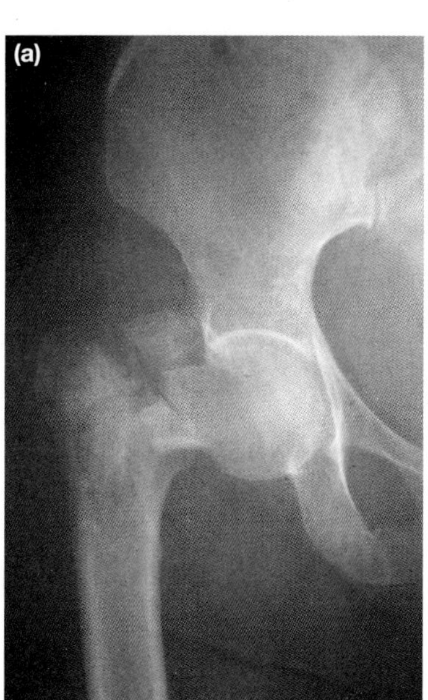

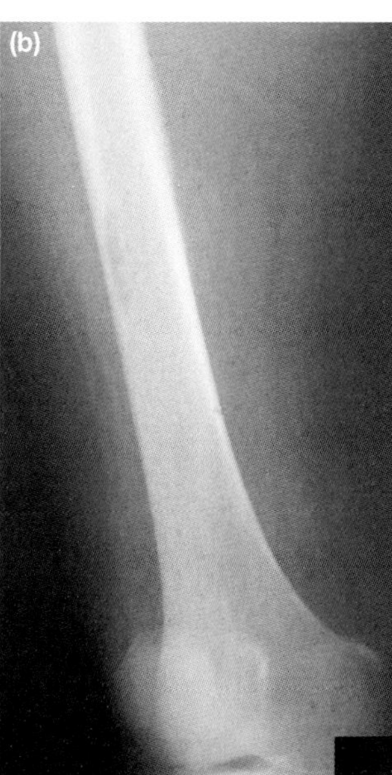

Figure 42.1 (a) Pathological fracture of the proximal femur through metastatic breast carcinoma. **(b)** Radiographs of the whole femur show a further, more distal metastatic deposit.

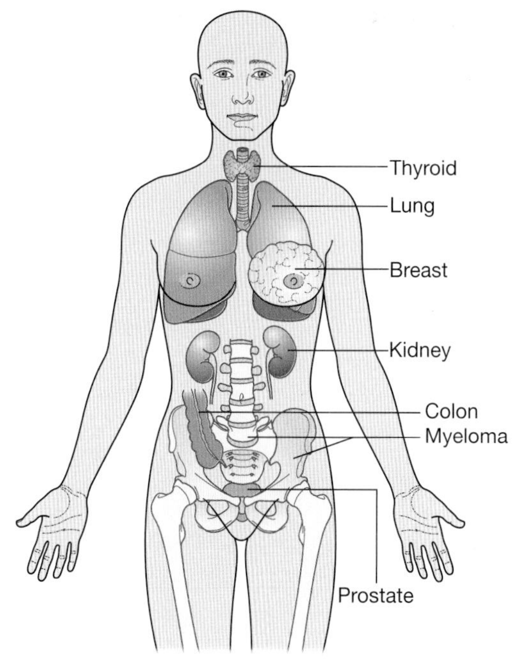

Figure 42.2 Common malignant tumours involving bone (courtesy of Mr Andy Biggs, The Robert Jones and Agnes Hunt Orthopaedic Hospital NHS Foundation Trust).

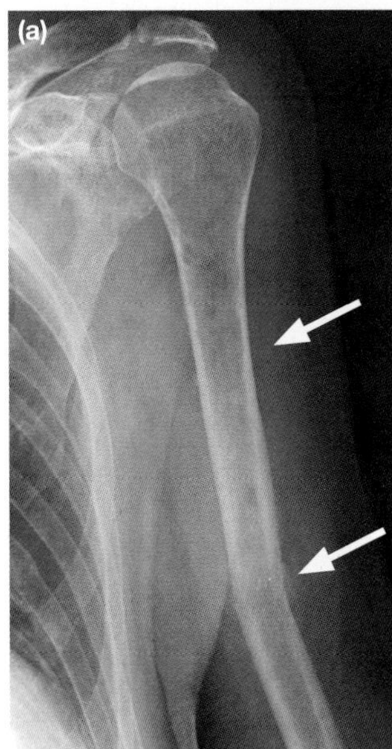

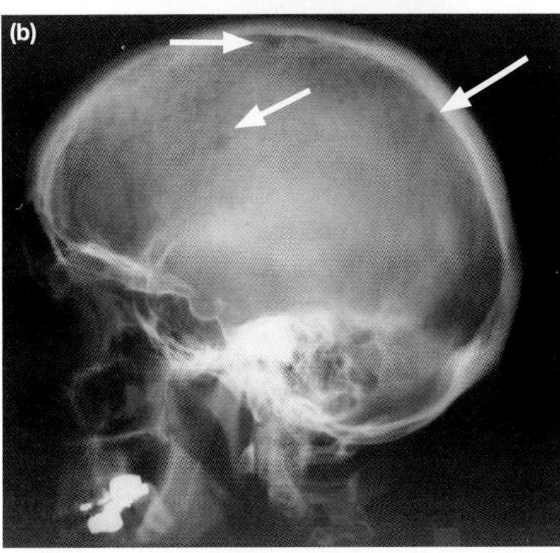

Figure 42.3 (a) Multiple myeloma affecting the left humerus with a pathological fracture (arrows). (b) Multiple myeloma with multiple deposits in the skull (arrows).

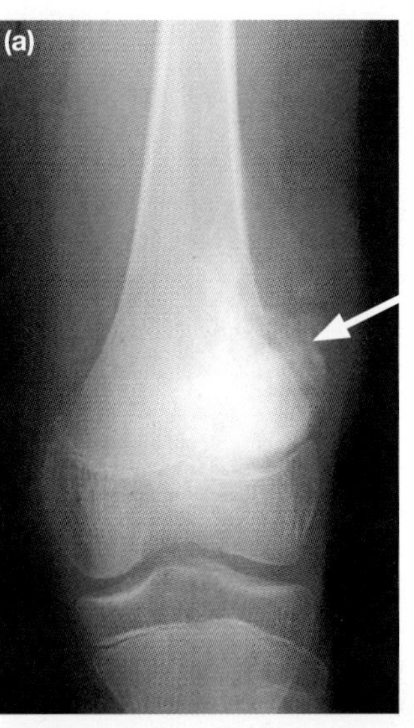

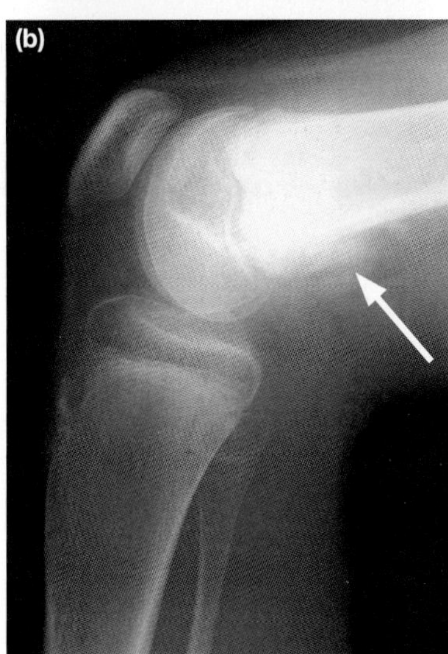

Figure 42.4 (a, b) Sclerotic osteosarcoma of the distal femur in a child (arrows).

Malignant primary bone tumours (sarcomas) are very rare, but notably can occur in children and young adults. The most common malignant primary bone tumours are osteosarcoma (***Figure 42.4***), chondrosarcoma (***Figures 42.5, 42.6 and 42.7***) and Ewing's sarcoma (***Figure 42.8***).

Soft-tissue tumours are common. However, only one in a 100 is malignant (***Figure 42.9***).

BONE TUMOURS

Tumours found in bone are classified according to their morphological appearances. These include:

- metastatic carcinomas; may show histological features of their tissue of origin;
- haematopoietic tumours; e.g. myeloma;
- osteogenic tumours; e.g. osteosarcoma;
- chondrogenic tumours; e.g. chondrosarcoma;
- others; e.g. Ewing's sarcoma.

Osteosarcoma has two age incidence peaks: one in adolescence and the other later in life. Osteosarcomas in older patients usually arise in association with Paget's disease, osteonecrosis or after radiotherapy treatment. Ewing's sarcoma occurs in adolescence, whereas the incidence of chondrosarcoma increases from middle age onwards.

Some conditions are associated with an increased likelihood of developing malignant tumours in bone and/or cartilage (***Table 42.1***).

James Ewing, 1866–1943, Professor of Pathology, Cornell University Medical College, New York, NY, USA, described this type of sarcoma in 1921.
Sir James Paget, 1814–1899, surgeon, St Bartholomew's Hospital, London, UK, described osteitis deformans in 1877.

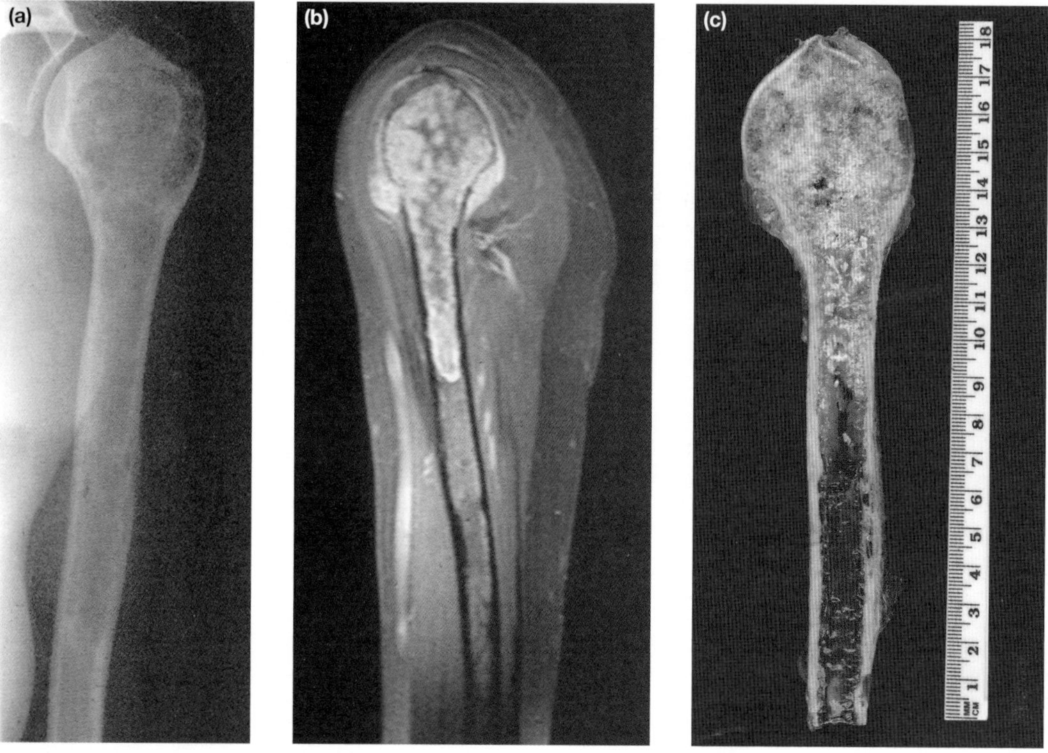

Figure 42.5 (a) Chondrosarcoma of the proximal humerus with multiple calcifications. (b) Magnetic resonance imaging scan showing extensive involvement. (c) Excised chondrosarcoma of the proximal humerus.

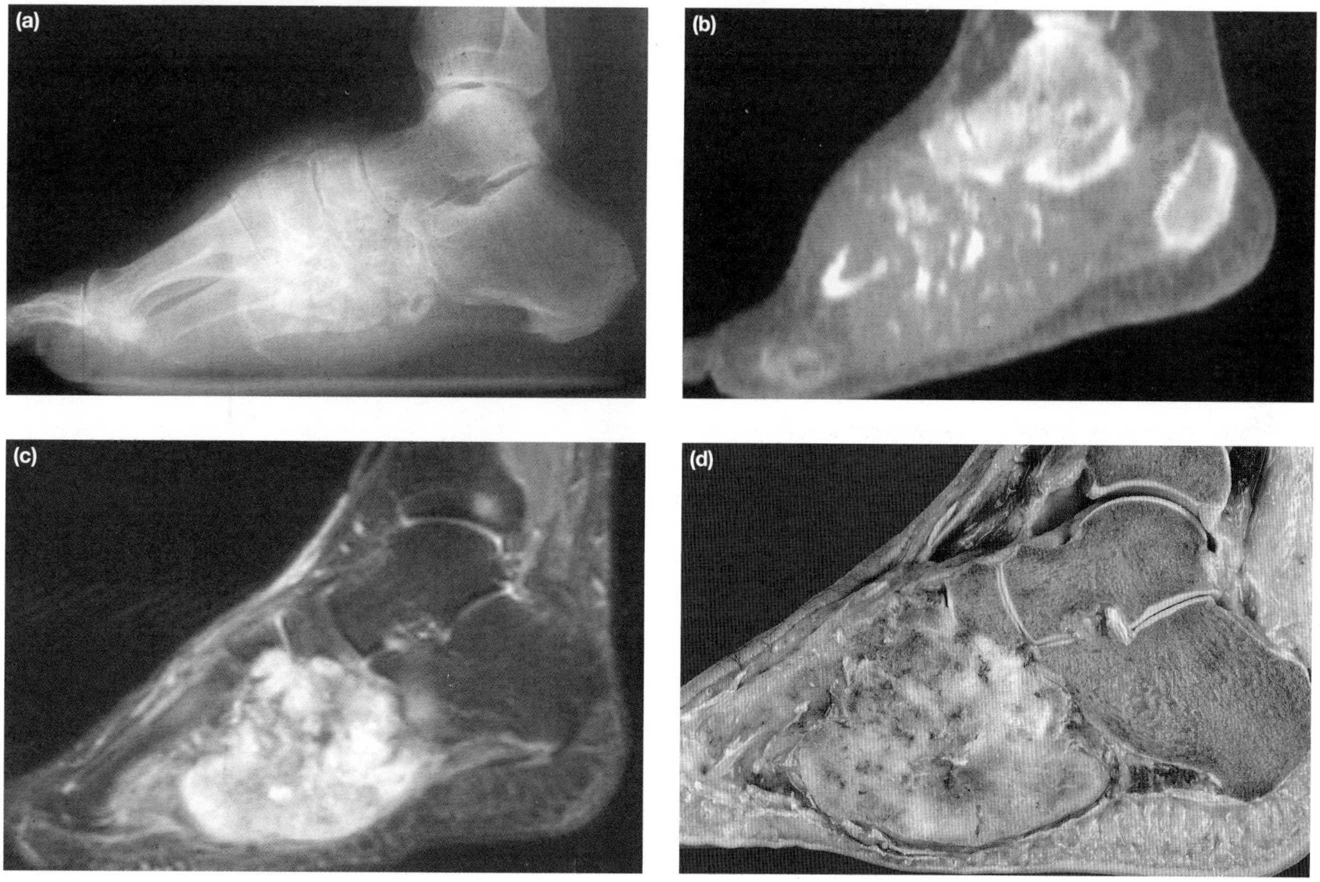

Figure 42.6 (a) Chondrosarcoma of the foot. (b) Computed tomography scan reconstruction showing multiple calcifications. (c) T2-weighted magnetic resonance imaging scan shows high signal in the chondrosarcoma. (d) Excised chondrosarcoma of the foot.

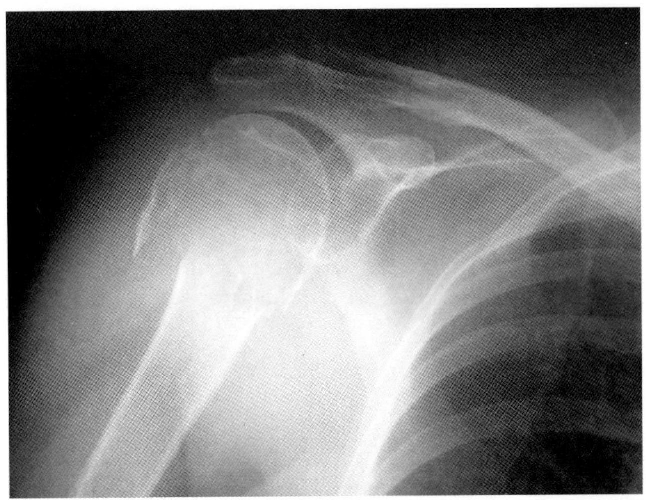

Figure 42.7 Pathological fracture through a primary chondrosarcoma of the proximal humerus.

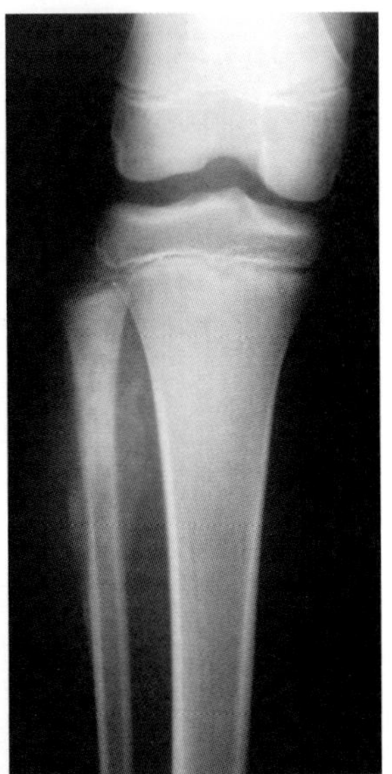

Figure 42.8 Ewing's sarcoma of the proximal fibula. The tumour is metadiaphyseal in location with a periosteal reaction and subtle onion-skinning.

TABLE 42.1 Conditions associated with an increased risk of malignant disease in bone and cartilage.

High risk	Moderate risk	Low risk
Maffucci syndrome (enchondromatosis and angiomas of soft tissue)	Hereditary multiple exostoses	Chronic osteomyelitis
Ollier's disease (enchondromatosis)	Polyostotic Paget's disease	Osteonecrosis
Familial retinoblastoma syndrome	Radiation osteitis	Fibrous dysplasia, osteogenesis imperfecta, osteoblastoma and chondroblastoma

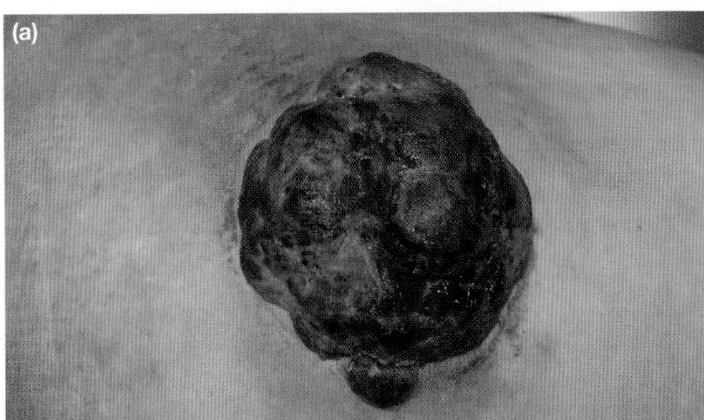

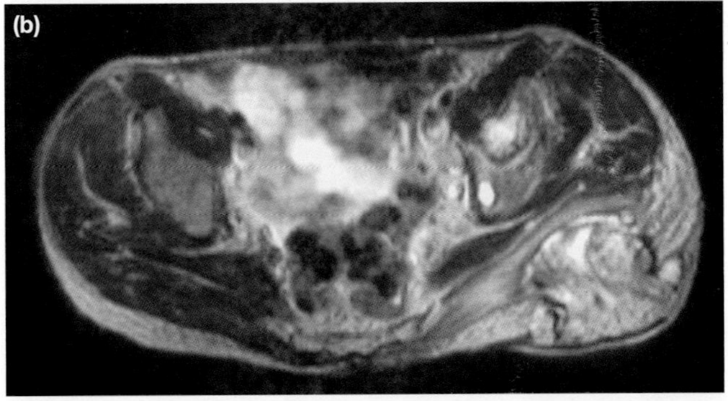

Figure 42.9 (a) Large fungating soft-tissue sarcoma of the buttock. (b) Magnetic resonance imaging scan from the same patient showing a large fungating sarcoma of the buttock.

Metastatic bone disease

Most tumours that metastasise to bone are carcinomas. Sometimes, despite further investigations, the primary tumour is never found: these patients are described as having 'carcinoma of unknown primary'. However, with advanced diagnostics and laboratory investigations the origin of most bone metastases can be identified.

Carcinomas usually spread to bone by the haematogenous route: the spine is the third most common site for metastases, after the lung and liver. Although most patients with metastatic cancer will have bone metastases in the spine before they die, only 10% are symptomatic.

Tumour cells metastasise to the spine via Batson's venous plexus. These retroperitoneal veins have no valves and allow retrograde embolic spread to the spine and proximal long bones (***Figure 42.10***).

Bone metastases can be lytic, sclerotic or mixed. Lytic metastases are usually highly vascular or locally aggressive such that there is no healing response from the bone. Metastases from prostate cancer may appear sclerotic.

Metastases are rare in children, but bone metastases can occur from neuroblastoma, rhabdomyosarcoma and clear cell carcinoma of the kidney.

Angelo Maffucci, 1847–1903, Professor of Pathological Anatomy, Pisa, Italy, described enchondromatosis in association with soft tissue haemangiomas in 1881.
Louis Xavier Edouard Léopold Ollier, 1830–1900, Professor of Surgery, Lyons, France, described enchondromatosis in 1899.
Oscar V Batson, 1894–1979, American otolaryngologist.

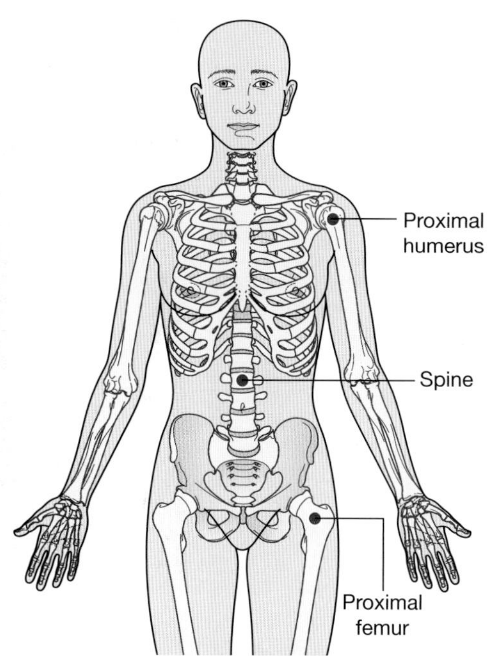

Figure 42.10 Common sites of metastatic bone disease (courtesy of Mr Andy Biggs, The Robert Jones and Agnes Hunt Orthopaedic Hospital NHS Foundation Trust).

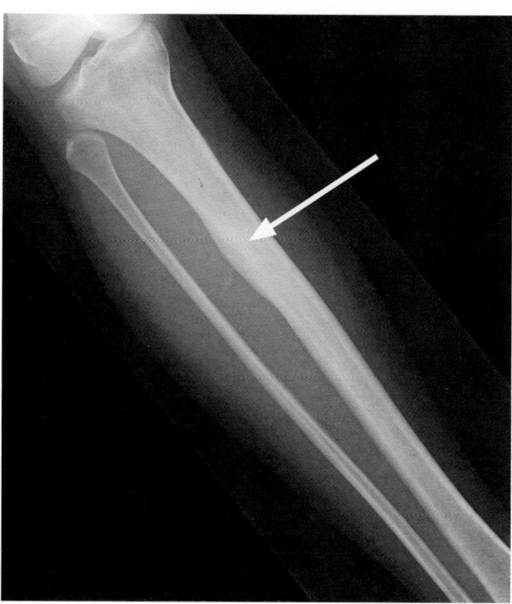

Figure 42.11 Radiograph showing an osteoid osteoma of the tibial diaphysis with reactive bone formation (arrow).

Summary box 42.1

Most common tumours metastasising to bone (93%)

- Breast
- Prostate
- Lung
- Renal
- Thyroid
- Colon

Summary box 42.2

Most common sites of bone metastases

- Spine
- Proximal femur and pelvis
- Proximal humerus

Haematopoietic tumours

Malignant haematopoietic tumours that commonly present in orthopaedic clinics are either solitary plasmacytoma/multiple myeloma (arising from plasma cells; *Figure 42.2*) or lymphomas (arising from lymphoid cells).

Osteogenic tumours

These tumours characteristically produce osteoid or bony matrix, which may be seen on imaging studies or on histological examination.

Osteoid osteoma (*Figures 42.11 and 42.12*) is a benign bone-forming lesion that is small but very painful. Usually, pain occurs at night and is typically relieved by non-steroidal anti-inflammatory medication. Osteoid osteomas usually occur in children and adolescents. They can arise in any bone, particularly the proximal femur, and cause a dense cortical reaction in the centre of which is a nidus (*Figure 42.12*).

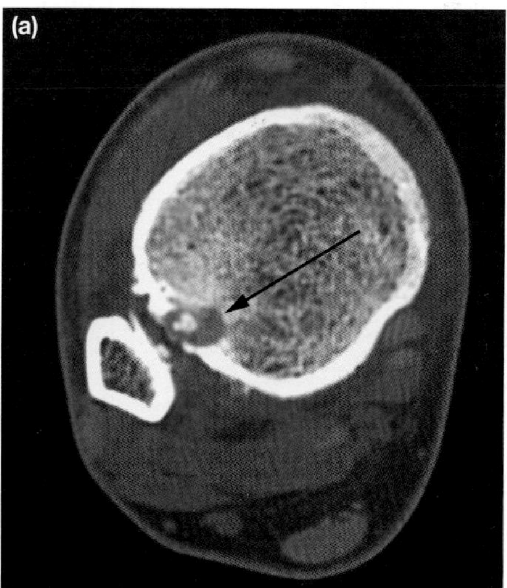

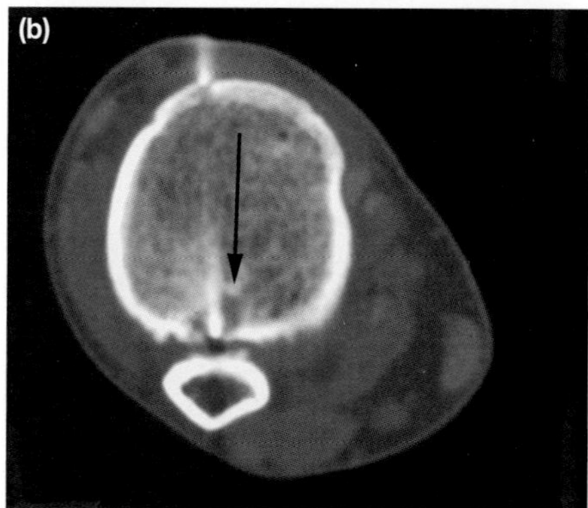

Figure 42.12 (a) Axial computed tomography (CT) scan showing an osteoid osteoma nidus in the distal tibia (arrow). (b) CT-guided radiofrequency thermocoagulation of an osteoid osteoma of the distal tibia. The scan shows the electrode *in situ* (arrow).

Summary box 42.3

Malignant bone tumours
- Plasmacytoma – solitary form of multiple myeloma
- Osteosarcoma – usually secondary to Paget's disease and radiotherapy in older patients
- Chondrosarcoma
- Ewing's sarcoma

Osteoid osteomas can cause irritation and effusions if they occur close to a joint.

Osteoblastoma is the larger (>2 cm), more aggressive counterpart of osteoid osteoma and more typically occurs in the spine.

Osteosarcoma (*Figure 42.4*) is a malignant bone-forming tumour, most common in the distal femur, followed by the proximal tibia, proximal humerus and distal tibia. The radiological and histological classification of osteosarcomas includes sclerotic (*Figure 42.4*), chondroblastic, telangiectatic and other more unusual forms. Usually, osteosarcomas are intraosseous, but they can also arise from the surface of bones. Parosteal osteosarcoma (*Figure 42.13*) is a low-grade osteosarcoma that arises from the surface of the bone, typically of the distal femur or proximal tibia. Symptoms are often mild and longstanding.

Summary box 42.4

Tumours producing bone
- Osteoid osteoma – small, painful; produce dense cortical reaction
- Osteoblastoma – larger and more aggressive than osteoid osteoma
- Osteosarcoma – malignant; commonest in lower femur and upper tibia

Chondrogenic tumours

These tumours produce chondroid matrix and include a wide range of benign and malignant tumours.

Osteochondroma (*Figures 42.14 and 42.15*) is a benign cartilage-capped bony projection, thought to originate from the physis. The bony projection always grows away from the joint towards the diaphyseal region of the bone. It has no structures attached to it. Osteochondromas can be pedunculated (with a stalk) or sessile (without a stalk). The stalk or base is always continuous with the intramedullary cavity of the bone, and the continuity of the cortex of the bone into an osteochondroma is a characteristic radiological feature. They are usually solitary, but some patients have multiple osteochondromas (hereditary multiple exostoses, autosomal dominant inheritance) (*Figure 42.16*). Osteochondromas can cause local irritation and complications include mechanical symptoms, nerve impingement, vascular pseudoaneurysm, fracture and infarction. Increasing size or pain, particularly after skeletal maturity, is concerning and may indicate malignant transformation. The incidence of malignant transformation is less than 1% in solitary osteochondromas and 1–3% in patients with multiple osteochondromas.

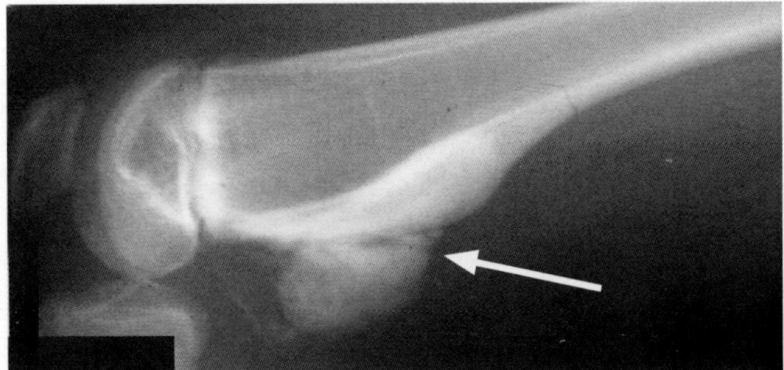

Figure 42.13 Parosteal osteosarcoma of the distal femur in an unusually young patient. There is no continuity between the tumour and the intramedullary cavity of the femur (arrow).

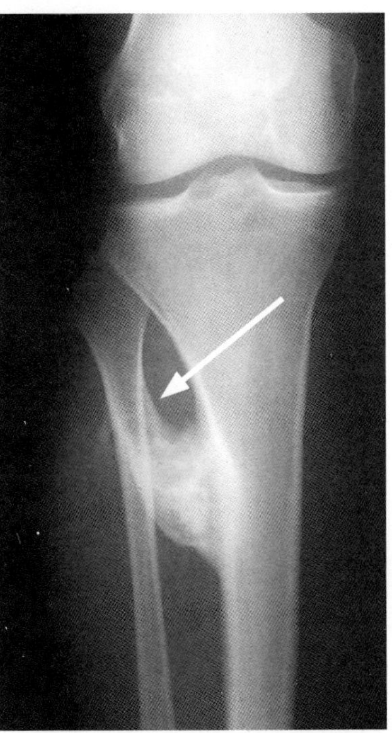

Figure 42.14 Pedunculated osteochondromas (arrow) of the proximal fibula with pseudarthrosis. Osteochondromas always grow away from the physis and are in continuity with the intramedullary cavity of the bone they arise from.

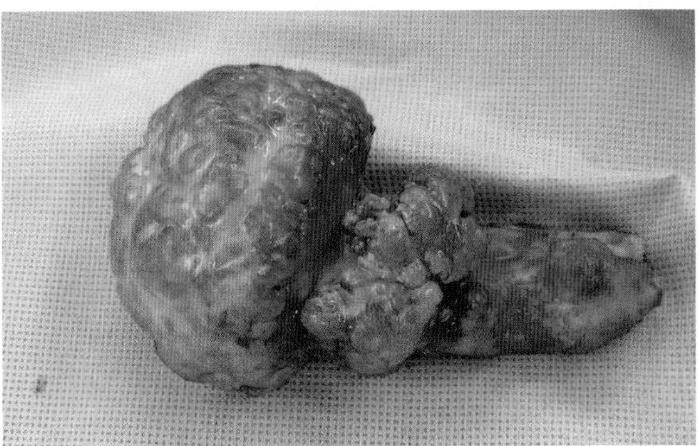

Figure 42.15 Excised pedunculated osteochondroma showing a cartilage cap.

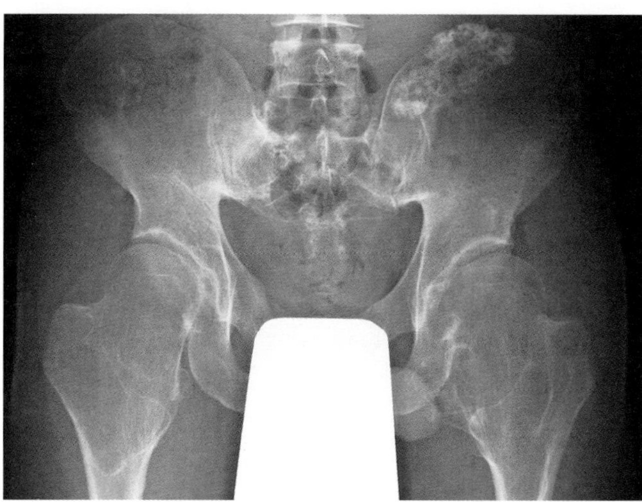

Figure 42.16 Multiple osteochondromas in hereditary multiple exostoses. Note the multiple bone involvement and the flask-shaped femoral metaphyses.

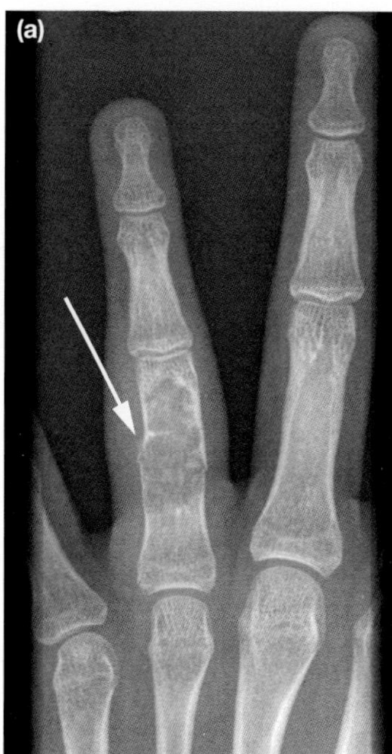

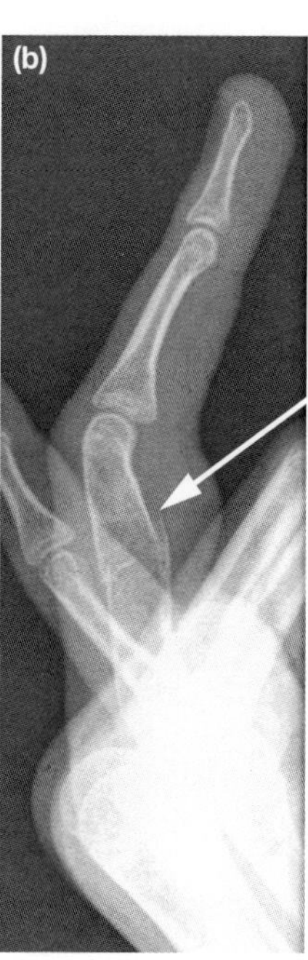

Figure 42.17 (a, b) Calcification and pathological fracture in a benign enchondroma of the proximal phalanx of the ring finger (arrows).

Enchondroma (*Figure 42.17*) is a benign cartilaginous neoplasm within the intramedullary cavity of bone. Approximately 50% are in the hands and feet: enchondromas are the most common bone tumours in the hand. Although they can present with pain, swelling or pathological fracture, many are entirely asymptomatic and are detected incidentally. Patchy calcification, expansion and scalloping can be visible on radiographs, but some are only diagnosed on magnetic resonance imaging (MRI) scan.

Ollier's disease is a developmental condition characterised by multiple enchondromas. In Maffucci syndrome, multiple enchondromas are associated with multiple angiomas. Malignant transformation to chondrosarcoma can occur in approximately 20% of patients with Ollier's disease and is almost inevitable in patients with Maffucci syndrome.

Chondroblastoma (*Figure 42.18*) is a benign cartilage-producing tumour that occurs in the epiphyses of bones in children. It is most common around the knee. Pain is often severe, with associated inflammation and possibly joint effusion. On plain radiographs, there is an often barely visible lytic lesion in the centre of the epiphysis. Previously, the diagnosis was often missed, but this has become less frequent with MRI scanning, which usually identifies the lesion with an intense inflammatory response.

Chondrosarcoma (*Figures 42.5, 42.6 and 42.7*) is a malignant tumour with cartilage differentiation. The biological behaviour ranges from very low-grade lesions to highly aggressive dedifferentiated tumours. Patients usually present with pain and/or swelling and symptoms may be longstanding. Many chondrosarcomas arise in pre-existing lesions such as osteochondromas or enchondromas. Diagnosis of a chondrosarcoma requires clinical, radiological and pathological correlation. Clear cell chondrosarcoma is a rare form of chondrosarcoma that occurs in the epiphysis (*Figure 42.19*).

Summary box 42.5

Tumours producing cartilage

- Osteochondroma – cartilage capped; grows away from physis
- Enchondroma – inside bone; commonest in hands and feet
- Chondroblastoma – in epiphyses of adolescents
- Chondrosarcoma – of varying malignancy

Others

Simple (unicameral) bone cyst (*Figure 42.20*) is a membrane-lined cavity filled with serous fluid within a bone. It usually occurs in the proximal long bones of children. Associated thinning of the cortex of the bone can lead to fracture. Such fractures usually heal with conservative treatment, but the cyst may only partially resolve.

Aneurysmal bone cyst (*Figure 42.21*) is a benign cystic lesion of bone consisting of blood-filled spaces separated by fibrous septa. The lesion is more aggressive than a simple bone cyst and often presents with pain and swelling. Plain radiographs commonly show aggressive features with eccentric expansion of the cortex and an open physis. Scans often show multiple fluid levels (*Figure 42.21b*).

Giant cell tumour of bone (*Figure 42.22*) is a locally aggressive tumour with large osteoclast-like giant cells. It usually occurs between the ages of 20 and 45, after the physes have closed. Giant cell tumour of bone typically extends into the epiphysis of long bones and erodes bone under the articular cartilage, especially around the knee, proximal humerus and distal radius. 'Benign' metastases are rare.

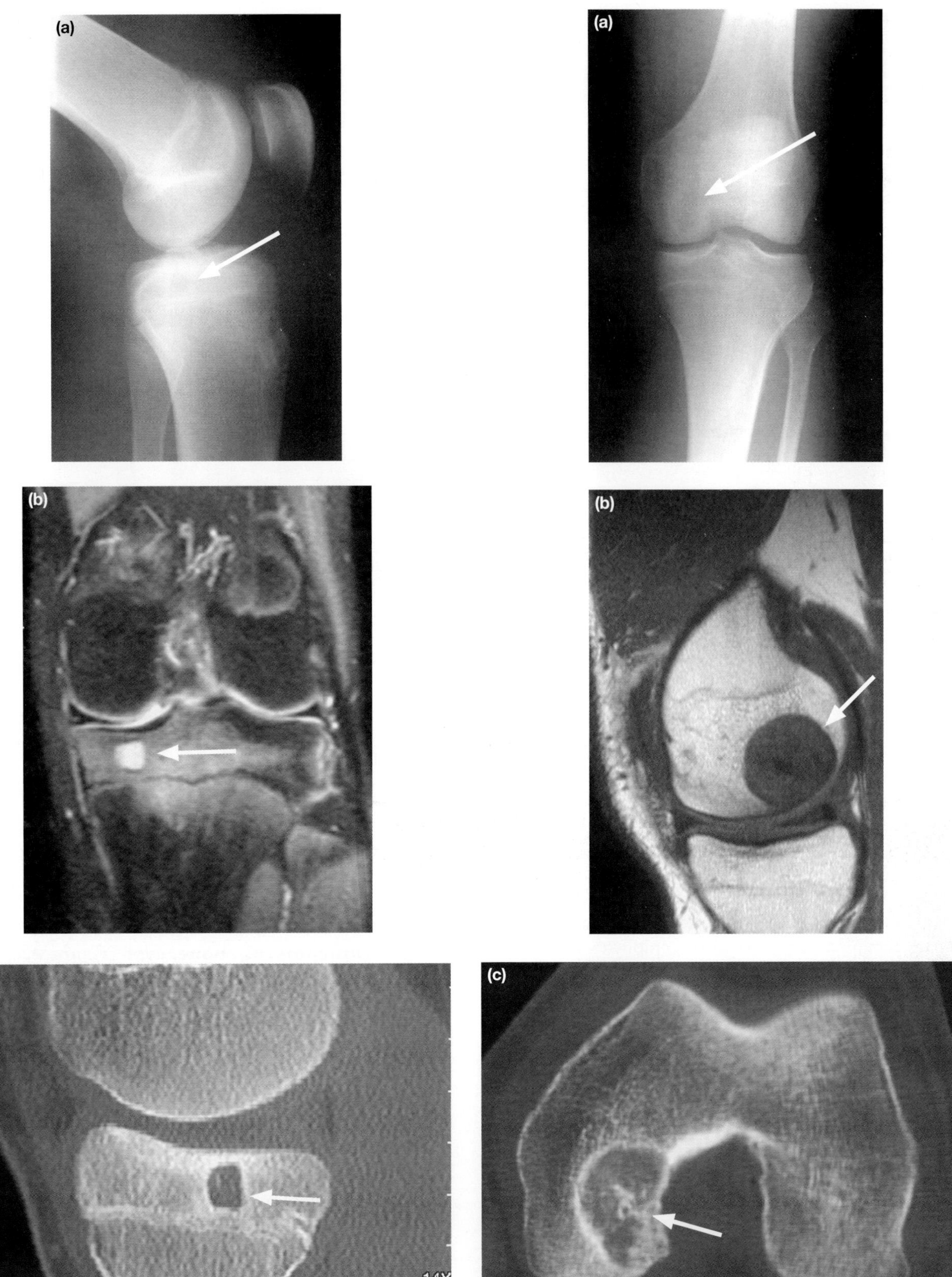

Figure 42.18 (a) Lateral radiograph with a barely visible chondroblastoma in the epiphysis of the proximal tibia (arrow). (b) Coronal T2-weighted magnetic resonance imaging scan showing a chondroblastoma (arrow) in the epiphysis of the proximal tibia with surrounding oedema. (c) Sagittal computed tomography reconstruction showing calcification within a chondroblastoma (arrow) of the proximal tibial epiphysis.

Figure 42.19 (a) Clear cell chondrosarcoma of the medial femoral condyle (arrow). (b) Sagittal T1-weighted magnetic resonance imaging scan showing a clear cell chondrosarcoma (arrow) in the medial femoral condyle. (c) Computed tomography scan reconstruction shows calcification (arrow) within the lesion.

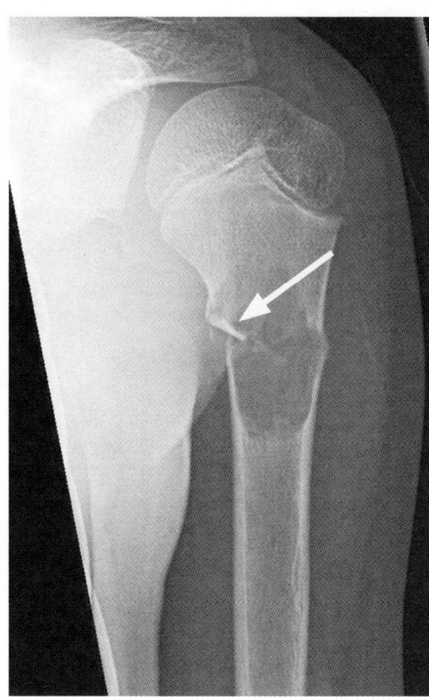

Figure 42.20 Pathological fracture through a simple bone cyst (arrow) with the pathognomonic fallen leaf sign. The fracture healed and the cyst consolidated without operative intervention.

Eosinophilic granuloma is a rare neoplasm of Langerhans cells (*Figure 42.23*). It can be unifocal (eosinophilic granuloma), multifocal (Hand–Schüller–Christian disease) or disseminated (Letterer–Siwe disease). There is a predilection for the skull and the diaphyses of long bones. In the spine it can present with collapse, known as vertebra plana. The radiographic appearance can be aggressive and similar to Ewing's sarcoma.

Fibrous dysplasia (*Figure 42.24*) is a benign, developmental, fibro-osseous lesion that can be mono- or polyostotic. It usually affects the long bones, ribs and skull. Patients can present with pain, swelling and/or fracture, but many lesions are detected incidentally. Hip fractures can produce a 'shepherd's crook' deformity of the proximal femur. Radiologically there is often expansion and a ground-glass appearance, sometimes with cystic change.

Ewing's sarcoma (*Figure 42.8*) is a malignant round cell sarcoma of bone in which cells usually have a characteristic 11:22 translocation. However, other mutations have been described. It tends to arise in the diaphysis of a long bone, pelvis or scapula. Patients usually present with a painful mass and may have systemic symptoms, including fever, anaemia and increased erythrocyte sedimentation rate (ESR). Radiologically the bone appears moth-eaten and may show an 'onion skin' periosteal reaction. MRI may show a large extraosseous soft-tissue mass as well as significant inflammation with oedema.

Bone tumours usually occur in characteristic anatomical locations (*Table 42.2*), and epiphyseal tumours are likely to be benign (*Table 42.3*).

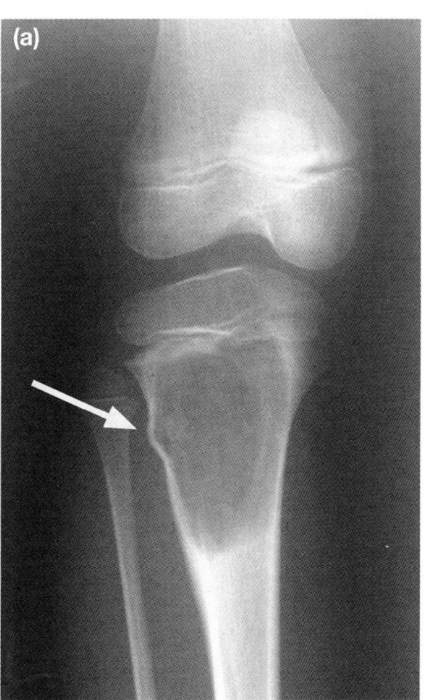

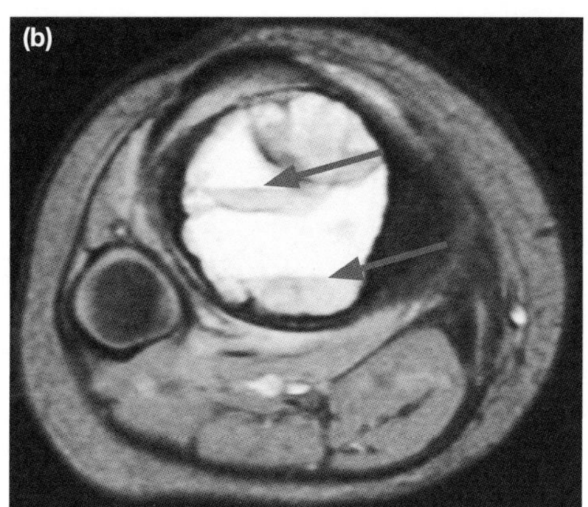

Figure 42.21 (a) Aneurysmal bone cyst with pathological fracture (arrow) of the proximal tibia. (b) Magnetic resonance imaging scan shows multiple fluid levels (arrows).

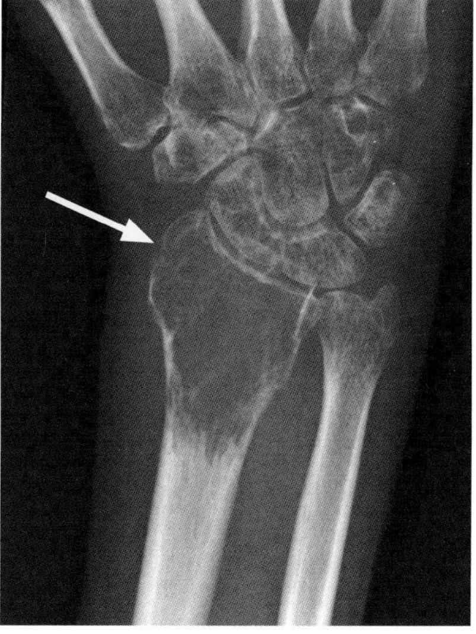

Figure 42.22 Giant cell tumour of the distal radius (arrow). Note the classic epiphyseal/metaphyseal location with subarticular involvement, as well as a permeative margin proximally in the radius indicating locally aggressive behaviour.

Paul Langerhans, 1847–1888, Professor of Pathological Anatomy, Freiberg, Germany.
Alfred Hand Jr, 1868–1949, American pediatrician, described the eponymous disease in 1893.
Artur Schüller, 1874–1957, Austrian neuroradiologist, described the eponymous disease in 1915.
Henry A Christian, 1876–1951, American physician, described the eponymous disease in 1919.
Erich Letterer, 1895–1982, German pathologist.
Sture A Siwe, 1897–1966, Swedish paediatrician.

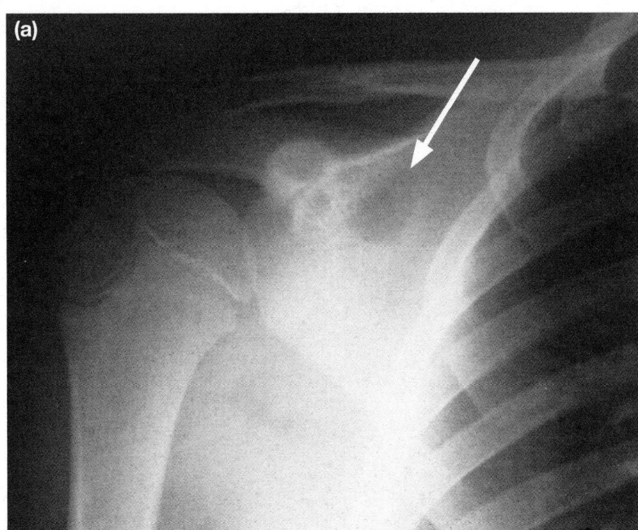

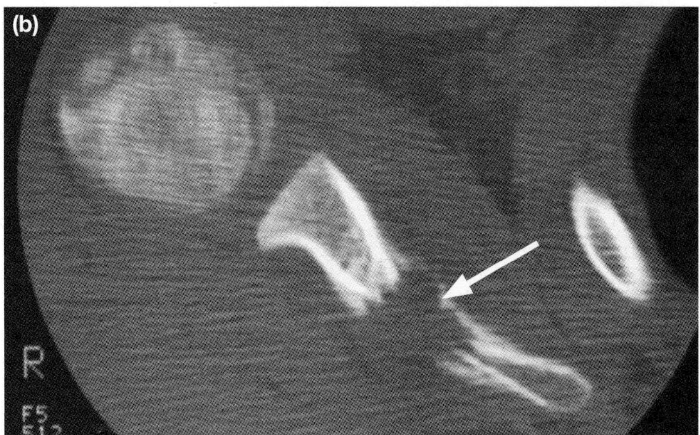

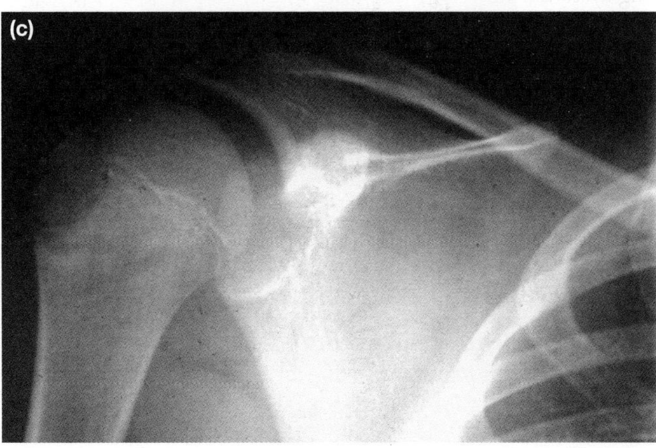

Figure 42.23 (a) Eosinophilic granuloma of the scapula (arrow). (b) Computed tomography scan shows a 'punched-out' lesion (arrow). (c) Spontaneous resolution.

TABLE 42.2 Classification of bone tumours by site.

Site	Tumour
Diaphyseal	• Eosinophilic granuloma • Osteoid osteoma • Fibrous dysplasia • Adamantinoma • Ewing's sarcoma
Metaphyseal	• Most
Epiphyseal	• Chondroblastoma • Intra-articular osteoid osteoma • Giant cell tumour (physis closed) • Clear cell chondrosarcoma

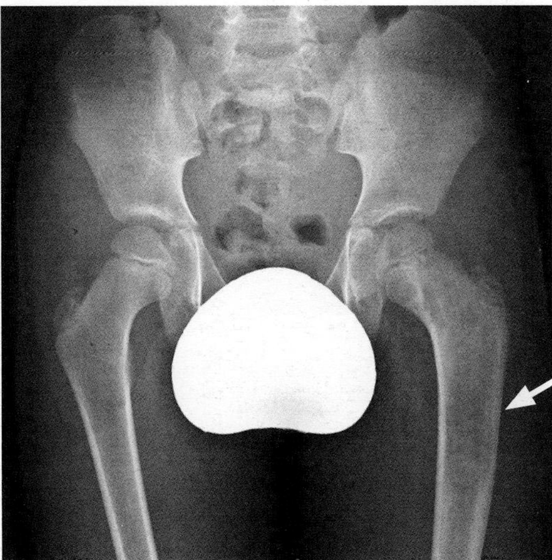

Figure 42.24 Fibrous dysplasia affecting the left proximal femur (arrow). There is expansion of the bone with a ground-glass appearance.

TABLE 42.3 Common diaphyseal bone tumours according to age.

Age	Most common diaphyseal tumour
<10 years	Eosinophilic granuloma
Teenage	Ewing's sarcoma
Adult	Lymphoma
>60 years	Metastasis/myeloma

Summary box 42.6

Other bone tumours

- Simple bone cyst – proximal long bones of children
- Aneurysmal bone cyst – more aggressive, expanding
- Giant cell tumour – found in epiphyses around the knee
- Fibrous dysplasia – may be multiple; long bones, ribs and skull
- Ewing's – round cell sarcoma; patients may have fever and anaemia

Staging of primary bone tumours

In the Enneking system, benign tumours are staged as:

- latent (e.g. osteochondroma);
- active (e.g. osteoid osteoma);
- aggressive (e.g. giant cell tumour).

William F Enneking, 1926–2014, American orthopedic oncologist.

Latent lesions are usually asymptomatic and often discovered incidentally. Active lesions, such as osteoid osteoma, present with mild symptoms and continue to grow. Aggressive lesions tend to grow rapidly and destroy bone.

The Enneking staging system for malignant tumours combines the local extent of the tumour and the histological grade (***Table 42.4***). The compartment is the bone in which the tumour arises. A tumour is extracompartmental when it has breached the cortex of the bone. Most primary malignant bone tumours are Enneking stage 2B at diagnosis, meaning they have extended outside the bone of origin but metastases are not detectable. The American Joint Committee on Cancer (AJCC)/Union for International Cancer Control (UICC) staging system is also widely used.

TABLE 42.4 The Enneking staging system for bone tumours.

Low grade	Intracompartmental	1A
	Extracompartmental	1B
High grade	Intracompartmental	2A
	Extracompartmental	2B
Any grade	Metastases	3

Summary box 42.7

Warning signs - bone tumour

- Non-mechanical bone pain
- Especially around the knee in young adolescents
- Concerning radiographs

SOFT-TISSUE TUMOURS

Soft-tissue tumours have also historically been classified according to their morphological appearance and presumed cell of origin. The range of biological behaviour is wide and most morphological types have a benign and malignant counterpart, for example lipoma (***Figure 42.25***) and liposarcoma. Other more frequent types include undifferentiated pleomorphic sarcoma and synovial sarcoma. Patients with suspected or confirmed soft-tissue sarcomas should be assessed and managed in a specialist centre.

Summary box 42.8

Warning signs - soft-tissue tumour

- Larger than 5 cm
- Increasing in size
- Painful
- Deep to the fascia
- Recurrence after previous excision

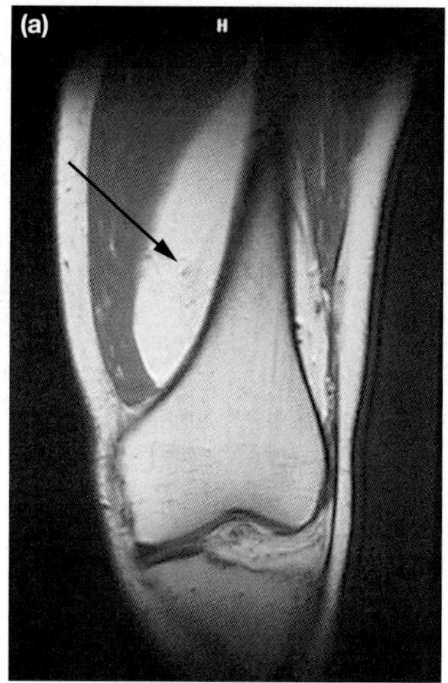

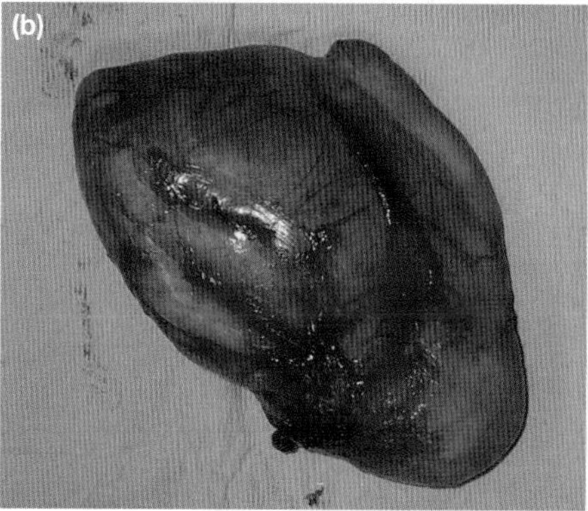

Figure 42.25 (a) Coronal T1-weighted magnetic resonance imaging scan showing a benign lipoma deep to the quadriceps muscle (arrow). (b) Excised benign lipoma.

The Trojani system, based on tumour differentiation, mitotic count and tumour necrosis, is the standard for grading malignant soft tissue tumours. The AJCC / UICC system is used to stage malignant soft tissue tumours.

EVALUATION AND INVESTIGATION OF THE PATIENT WITH A SUSPECTED BONE OR SOFT-TISSUE TUMOUR

The diagnosis and treatment of patients with primary bone and/or soft-tissue tumours requires a high index of suspicion, appropriate and prompt investigation, and early referral to a specialist multidisciplinary team for diagnosis, biopsy and appropriate treatment. When a musculoskeletal tumour is suspected, clinicians should:

- stop;
- think;
- investigate.

Monique Trojani, contemporary, described the histopathological grading system in 1984.

The assessment and investigation of any patient with a bone or soft-tissue tumour can be divided into three phases. The first two phases can be performed at the referring hospital, but the third phase may be best done in a specialist centre (*Table 42.5*).

TABLE 42.5 The three phases of assessment of lesions.

Phase 1 (within 24 hours)	Phase 2 (within first week)	Phase 3 (at specialist centre)
• History and examination • Blood tests • Radiograph whole bone • Chest radiograph	• Bone scan • Ultrasound scan abdomen • CT scan chest	• CT scan lesion • MRI scan lesion • Biopsy

CT, computed tomography; MRI, magnetic resonance imaging.

History and examination

It is important to take a thorough history, including a pain history. Non-mechanical and/or night pain, particularly in the young adolescent, is a concerning symptom and a primary bone tumour should be suspected. Relief with non-steroidal anti-inflammatory drugs may suggest an osteoid osteoma.

Patients with a history of malignancy who present with back pain should be considered to have metastatic bone disease until proven otherwise. Plain radiographs of the spine and routine blood tests are the minimum that is required. An MRI of the spine is a more sensitive test for the detection of a malignant tumour and may demonstrate soft-tissue extension into the spinal canal. Multiple myeloma (*Figure 42.3*) is the most common primary malignancy of bone in adults and should be considered in all patients over 65 years of age with back pain. Back pain associated with an ESR >100 mm/h indicates multiple myeloma until proven otherwise. Monoclonal gammopathy or elevated urinary and serum Bence Jones proteins are diagnostic. All patients with suspected cancer in the spine should be examined for signs of spinal cord compression, a potential surgical emergency.

Great care should be taken when managing a patient with an apparently 'solitary' bone metastasis. This could be a primary bone tumour, and further investigation including biopsy is required.

Soft-tissue tumours are common and the vast majority are benign. However, a soft-tissue mass meeting any of the following criteria may be malignant and the patient should be referred to a specialist centre:

- painful;
- increasing in size;
- more than 5 cm in diameter.

In addition, tumours that have recurred after previous excision and tumours located deep to the fascia are more likely to be malignant. It is important to note that tumours that appear mostly superficial but involve the deep fascia are classified as deep tumours.

Investigation

The investigation of a patient with a suspected primary bone or soft-tissue tumour should include the following.

- Local investigations:
  - ultrasound scan (for soft-tissue tumours);
  - plain radiographs of the whole affected bone or soft-tissue lesion (*Figure 42.1*);
  - MRI of the whole affected bone or soft-tissue mass;
  - computed tomography (CT) scan may be helpful in addition to an MRI scan.
- Distant:
  - blood tests, including full blood count, ESR, urea and electrolytes, bone profile and protein electrophoresis;
  - plain radiographs or CT scan of the chest (more sensitive);
  - whole-body isotope bone scan (for suspected primary or metastatic bone tumours);
  - ultrasound or CT scan of the abdomen (if renal metastasis is a possibility).

Plain radiographs are usually the most useful imaging investigations in determining the diagnosis of a primary bone tumour, but further appropriate scans are usually required for confirmation and staging. Imaging should always include the whole of the affected bone to look for satellite lesions and skip metastases. Satellite lesions occur within, whereas skip lesions occur beyond, the reactive zone of the tumour, which is the layer of compressed tissues, inflammatory cells and tumour infiltration that surrounds the tumour.

Both primary bone and soft-tissue sarcomas metastasise to the lungs, and a CT scan of the chest is an essential part of staging.

Patients who present with a lytic bone lesion could have a primary renal carcinoma and an ultrasound or CT scan of the abdomen is advised. Surgery to a renal metastasis can lead to significant blood loss.

Summary box 42.9

Staging

- Plain radiography is most informative for bone tumours
- Always image the whole bone in the case of skip lesions
- CT of the lung detects lung metastases
- Lytic lesions require imaging of the abdomen to check for a primary renal carcinoma

Biopsy

A biopsy is performed only when local staging investigations have been completed. Because removal of the biopsy track is an important principle in the treatment of sarcomas, and specialist pathology is required, biopsies should be performed either in, or after consultation with, the specialist centre where the definitive surgical procedure will be performed.

Henry Bence Jones, 1813–1873, physician, St George's Hospital, London, UK.

Image-guided biopsies (usually ultrasound- or CT-guided) have a higher diagnostic accuracy because areas of radiological concern can be targeted. If image-guided biopsy is performed, close discussion between radiologist and surgeon is required to ensure an appropriate biopsy route is used (***Figures 42.26 and 42.27***).

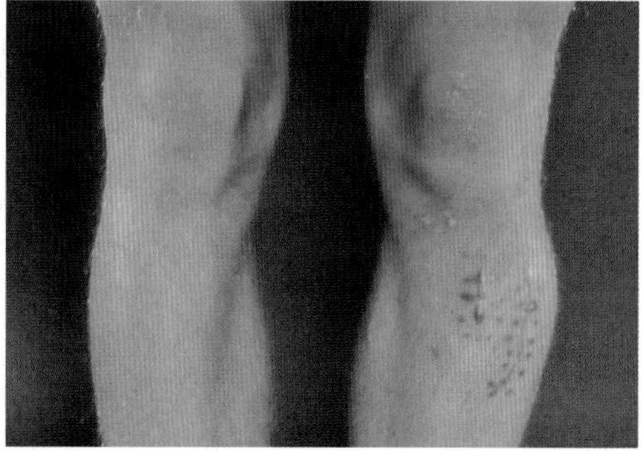

Figure 42.26 Poorly placed biopsies can make subsequent surgical excision of the track difficult or not possible.

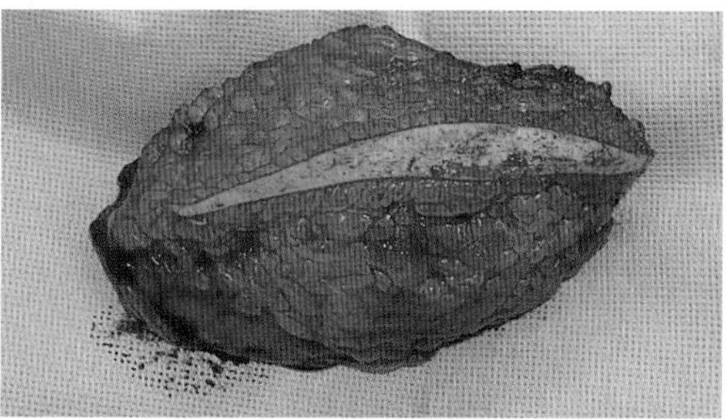

Figure 42.27 *En bloc* excised tumour and biopsy track.

Summary box 42.10

Biopsy

- Only biopsy once local staging is completed
- Biopsy should be performed at, or after discussion with, the specialist centre
- Image-guided biopsy is more reliable
- The biopsy track should be excised at definitive surgery
- Jamshidi needles for bone; Trucut needles for soft tissues

Biopsies for bone tumours are usually taken using a Jamshidi or other hollow needle (***Figure 42.28***), while Trucut needles are preferred for soft-tissue tumours.

Although most biopsies are performed with a needle, sometimes an open biopsy is required, which should be performed according to the following principles.

- A tourniquet can be used; but exsanguination by compression should be avoided as this may disseminate the tumour.

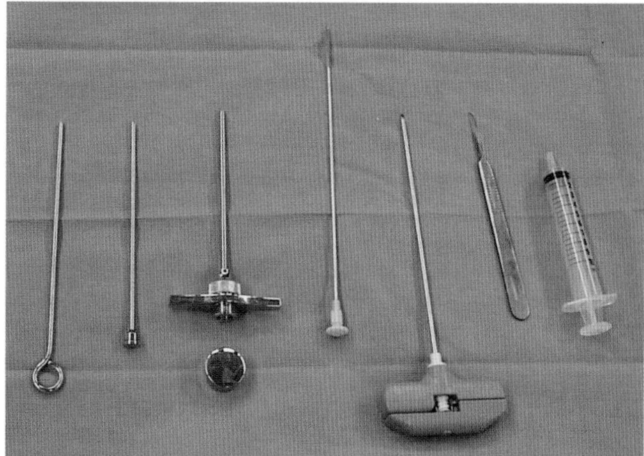

Figure 42.28 Bone biopsy instruments.

- Use longitudinal incisions that are part of an extensile approach.
- Do not cross anatomical compartments or contaminate critical anatomical structures (e.g. nerves or blood vessels).
- Use a biopsy track that can be excised at the time of definitive surgery.
- Ensure specimens are sent for microbiology as well as histopathology.
- Some specimens should be sent fresh to the laboratory for genetic studies.

PRINCIPLES OF TREATMENT

Primary bone tumours

Benign

Most latent and active benign bone tumours that need treatment are treated by intralesional curettage. Packing of the cavity with a graft or bone substitutes is usually not required.

Simple bone cysts can heal following pathological fracture and an initial conservative approach following fracture is best. If the cyst persists following union of the fracture, and the risk of further fracture is deemed to be high, then a variety of treatments, including injection with steroid or bone marrow and surgical curettage, have been described.

Osteoid osteomas can resolve spontaneously. However, symptoms are often pronounced, and most patients are treated by CT-guided thermocoagulation. Surgical removal (which usually requires burring down onto the surface of the nidus and removing it) is seldom required.

Large or more rapidly growing benign bone tumours may require more extensive surgical excision and reconstruction. Giant cell tumours of bone are associated with a high local recurrence rate and are usually treated with thorough curettage or, when very extensive, surgical resection of the affected bone. The RANK-ligand (receptor activator of nuclear factor ligand) antibody denosumab has an evolving role in treating these tumours.

En bloc is French for 'in a block'.
Khosrow Jamshidi, contemporary, Iranian haematologist.

Malignant tumours

Malignant primary bone tumours require a multidisciplinary approach that may include chemotherapy and radiotherapy as well as surgery. Osteosarcoma and Ewing's sarcoma are treated with neoadjuvant (before surgery) chemotherapy and surgery. Chondrosarcomas are not sensitive to chemotherapy or radiotherapy and treatment is surgical excision where possible.

The aim of surgery for a primary malignant bone tumour is to remove it completely (usually with a layer of normal tissue around it that includes the biopsy track) and then to reconstruct the limb to maximise physical function.

Following excision the surgical margins can be classified as shown in ***Table 42.6***.

TABLE 42.6 Classification of surgical resection margins.

Intralesional	Resection through the tumour
Marginal	Resection through the reactive zone of the tumour
Wide	Resection outside the reactive zone of the tumour
Radical	Resection of the whole anatomical compartment

In most cases, limb salvage with excision and reconstruction is possible (***Figure 42.29***). Only a minority of patients (10–15%) require primary amputation, either because of neurovascular invasion or because the reconstructed limb may be less functional than an amputation (e.g. for some tumours in the foot and ankle). Limb salvage is associated with a slightly higher rate of local recurrence than amputation. However, no difference in overall survival has been demonstrated. The surgical options for malignant primary bone tumours include:

- amputation or van Nes rotationplasty;
- excision alone (for dispensable bones, e.g. the fibula, or areas where reconstruction is difficult, e.g. in parts of the pelvis);
- excision and reconstruction with a structural graft or massive endoprosthesis.

The complications of massive endoprosthetic reconstruction of a limb include infection, instability and wear or loosening of the prosthesis.

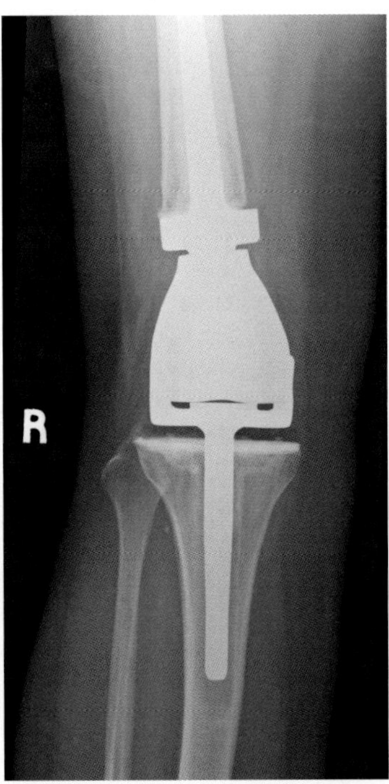

Figure 42.29 Endoprosthetic replacement of the distal femur.

Summary box 42.11

Treatment of benign bone tumours
- Benign lesions can usually be simply curetted
- CT-guided thermocoagulation is used for osteoid osteoma
- Large benign tumours may require reconstruction

Summary box 42.12

Treatment of malignant bone tumours
- Osteosarcomas and Ewing's sarcoma require neoadjuvant chemotherapy
- Chondrosarcomas are insensitive to radiotherapy or chemotherapy
- Most malignant tumours can be treated with limb salvage
- There is no difference in survival between amputation and limb salvage

Metastatic bone disease

Patients with confirmed metastatic bone disease may require resuscitation for electrolyte imbalance, anaemia, cardiorespiratory problems or hypercalcaemia before surgical treatment can be considered. Hypercalcaemia can be treated effectively with fluid resuscitation and bisphosphonate infusion.

Surgical treatment in patients with metastatic bone disease is usually palliative; although complete resection of solitary metastases in selected patients may confer some survival benefit, the evidence for this is not strong.

Surgery of the spine may be required for stabilisation and/or decompression when tumour extension puts the spinal cord at risk. Surgery in the peripheral skeleton is mainly for treatment of pain and (impending) pathological fracture.

Renal metastases tend to be very vascular and massive blood loss can be encountered during surgery. Therefore, preoperative embolisation should be considered just before surgery to prevent blood loss (***Figure 42.30***).

Treatment of myeloma is mainly haematological. Nonsurgical treatments including radiotherapy can lead to healing

Cornelis Pieter van Nes, 1897–1972, Dutch orthopaedic surgeon, who practised in Leiden and described rotationplasty in 1950.

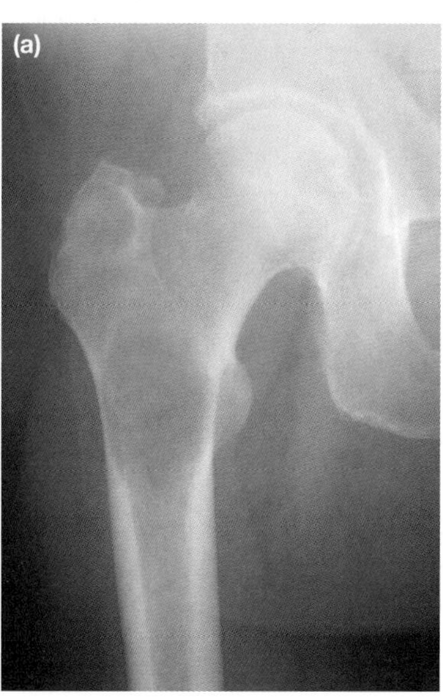

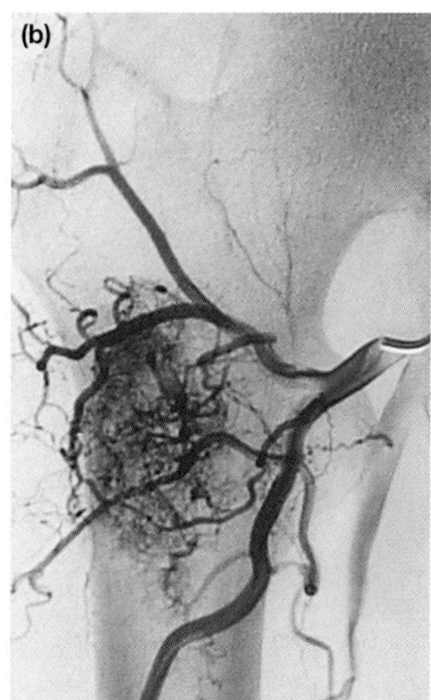

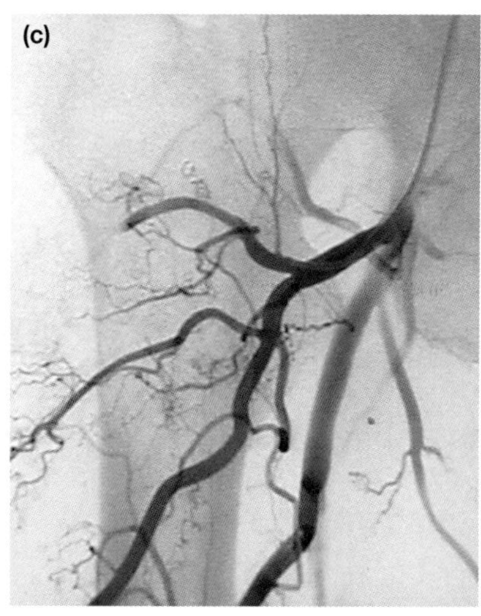

Figure 42.30 **(a)** Lytic metastasis of renal cell carcinoma. **(b)** Angiogram shows increased vascularity. **(c)** Following embolisation.

of bone lesions in some cases. Surgical treatment is often required for complications such as fracture and spinal cord compression.

The following factors should be considered when contemplating surgical treatment for patients with metastatic bone disease:

- likely survival (***Figure 42.31***) – consider the primary diagnosis and performance status;
- quality of life;
- fitness for anaesthesia and surgery;
- fracture risk;
- single or multiple bone lesions;
- response to adjuvant treatment such as radiotherapy and hormonal treatment;
- radiotherapy can be administered pre- or postoperatively.

The risk of pathological fracture can be assessed using the Mirels score (***Table 42.7***). However, this scoring system is prone to inter- and intraobserver variation.

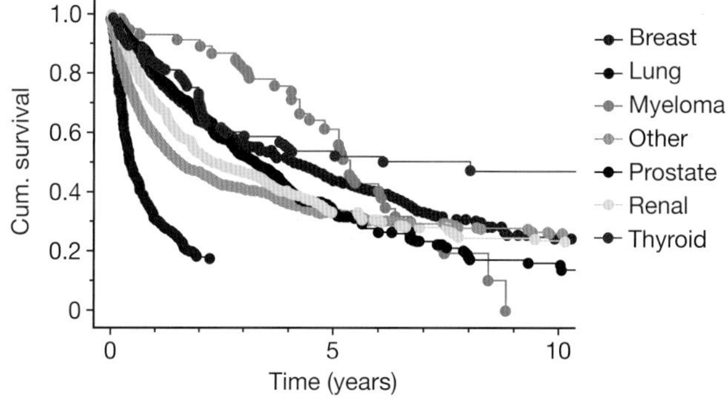

Figure 42.31 Cumulative survival curves of patients who present with bony metastasis.

TABLE 42.7 The Mirels scoring system for risk of pathological fracture.

	Score		
	1	2	3
Site	Upper limb	Lower limb	Peritrochanteric
Pain	Mild	Moderate	Functional
Size	<1/3	1/3–2/3	>2/3
Lesion	Blastic	Mixed	Lytic

Score >8, high risk of fracture – urgent prophylactic fixation should be considered; score <8, low risk of fracture – orthopaedic intervention may not be required.

Bone healing following a fracture through a metastasis is unpredictable and there can be local recurrence of the tumour after treatment. The approach is therefore different from the treatment of other fractures. The aim of surgery should be to improve pain and maintain mobility. Approaches that require prolonged protected weight-bearing to allow healing are not appropriate in this group of patients with reduced life expectancy. Therefore, as a general rule, prosthetic replacement of bones is preferred, particularly for epiphyseal and metaphyseal lesions. Metastases in the diaphysis may be most appropriately treated with an intramedullary nail. In the shoulder, prosthetic replacements have a poor function and internal fixation may give better physical functioning. However, for hip lesions, the best treatment is often replacement surgery.

Patients with solitary breast and renal metastases can have prolonged disease-free survival, so excision and replacement rather than fixation should be considered.

Hilton Mirels, contemporary, South African orthopaedic surgeon who now practises in the USA.

Summary box 42.13

Treatment of bone metastases

- Surgery cannot lengthen life but may shorten it
- The spine may need to be stabilised and nerves or the cord decompressing
- Long bones will need to be stabilised if a pathological fracture is imminent
- Patients who have a possibility of long-term survival may need excision and prosthetic reconstruction
- Radiotherapy often relieves pain

Soft-tissue tumours

The treatment of soft-tissue tumours should take account of tumour type and the response to other treatments including radiotherapy. Large low-grade or benign lipomatous tumours may be excised in a deliberately marginal or close but complete fashion. Soft-tissue sarcomas should however be excised with a margin of normal tissue around them, which includes the biopsy track, wherever possible (***Figure 42.27***). Skin involvement may require resection of the skin and reconstruction with a split-skin graft or skin flap.

Following surgical excision of high-grade soft-tissue sarcomas, adjuvant radiotherapy should be considered. Preoperative radiotherapy can also have good results, but there is a risk of wound-healing problems following surgery. Chemotherapy has a limited role in the treatment of soft-tissue sarcomas.

FURTHER READING

British Orthopaedic Oncology Society and British Orthopaedic Association. *Metastatic bone disease. A guide to good practice.* Oxford: BOOS; London: BOA, 2015.

Cool P, Grimer R. Pathological fractures of the extremities. *Trauma* 2000; **2**: 101–11.

Cool P, Grimer R, Rees R. Surveillance in patients with sarcoma of the extremities. *Eur J Surg Oncol* 2005; **31**(9): 1020–4.

Dangoor A, Seddon B, Gerrand C *et al.* UK guidelines for the management of soft tissue sarcomas. *Clin Sarcoma Res* 2016; **6**: 20.

Enneking WF, Spanier SS, Goodman MA. A system for the surgical staging of musculoskeletal sarcoma. *Clin Orthop Relat Res* 1980; **153**: 106–20.

Gerrand C, Athanasou N, Brennan B *et al.* on behalf of the British Sarcoma Group. UK guidelines for the management of bone sarcomas. *Clin Sarcoma Res* 2016; **6**: 7.

Mankin HJ, Lange TA, Spanier SS. The hazards of biopsy in patients with malignant primary bone and soft tissue tumors. *J Bone Joint Surg* 1982; **64-A**: 1121–7.

Mirels H. Metastatic disease in long bones. *Clin Orthop* 1989; **249**: 256–64.

Wedin R, Bauer HC. Surgical treatment of skeletal metastatic lesions of the proximal femur: endoprosthesis or reconstruction nail? *J Bone Joint Surg Br* 2005; **87**(12): 1653–7.

World Health Organization, International Agency for Research on Cancer. *WHO classification of tumours.* Vol. 3. *Soft tissue and bone tumours*, 5th edn. Lyon: IARC Press, 2019.

Union for International Cancer Control. *TNM classification of malignant tumours*, 8th edn. Oxford/Hoboken, NJ: John Wiley & Sons, 2017.

CHAPTER 43 Infection of the bones and joints

Learning objectives

To understand:

- Characteristic features of septic arthritis, acute and chronic osteomyelitis and implant infections
- Diagnostic principles in bone and joint infection
- Treatment of infection of native bones and joints
- Treatment of fracture-related and prosthetic joint infections

INTRODUCTION

Osteomyelitis is an old disease, identified in dinosaur bones, early hominids and skeletons from ancient civilisations. It is named from the components of the disease (*osteo*, bone; *myelos*, marrow; *itis*, inflammation; Greek) and is caused by bacterial invasion of the bone. Worldwide, acute infection of bones and joints remains common in children. In adults, open fractures and orthopaedic implant surgery produce a large number of severe infections each year.

Orthopaedic infection can present acutely, with major systemic upset, local inflammation and purulence, or insidiously, with gradual bone destruction leading to loss of function and slowly evolving local symptoms, with or without systemic features.

Bone and joint infections cause a substantial burden of complex morbidity. Acute infections can be life- or limb-threatening, while chronic disease may produce prolonged disability, pain and ill-health. This has major implications for patient mental health and social interactions.

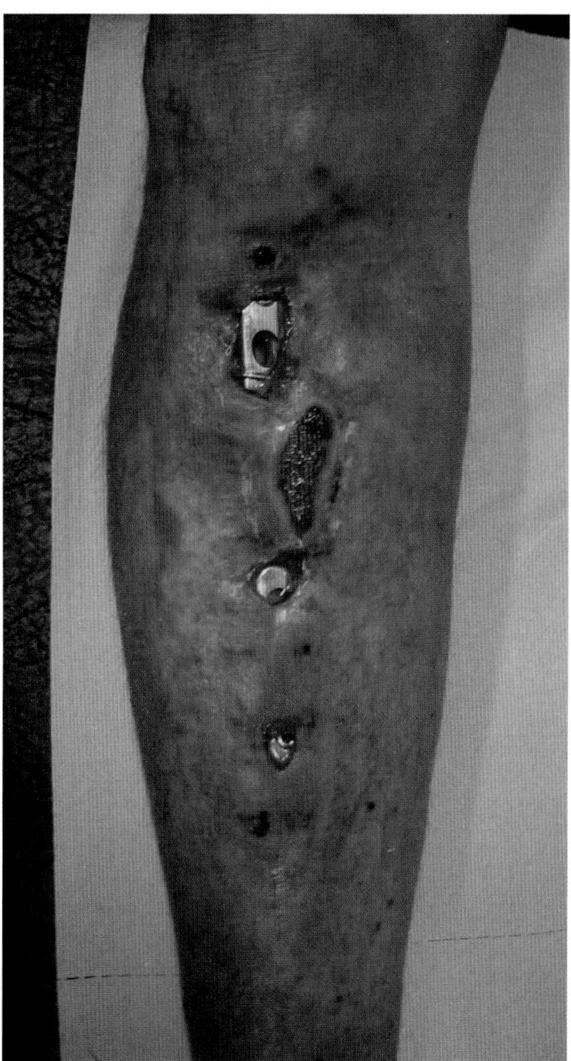

Figure 43.1 This open fracture of the tibia was treated with internal fixation using a plate. An early fracture-related infection developed, with skin breakdown and exposure of the metalwork.

EPIDEMIOLOGY

The pattern of bone infection is changing, and the incidence is increasing. Bone and joint infection affects around 1 per 10 000 children across the world. Inadequate initial treatment generates chronic infections in up to one-third of cases. In the developed world, bone infection is frequently seen after injury or surgery (contiguous focus osteomyelitis) and is often implant related (***Figure 43.1***). Increasing life expectancy, obesity, medical comorbidities (diabetes, peripheral vascular disease, immunocompromise) and increased rates of bone surgery contribute to a group of patients with increased susceptibility to infection. Prosthetic joint replacement is a highly successful therapy for joint disease but is complicated by infection in at least 1% of cases. It was estimated that joint replacement generated more than 70 000 new cases of prosthetic joint infection (PJI) in the USA in 2020. These are difficult and expensive to treat, costing over US$1.5 billion. The incidence of infection after fracture has decreased but increased use of internal fixation has increased the prevalence of post-traumatic bone infection overall. This will produce a significant economic burden for healthcare providers in the future.

Summary box 43.1

Epidemiology of bone infection

- Bone and joint infections from haematogenous spread remain common worldwide
- The increased use of implants for joint replacement and fracture fixation are an important source of new infections
- Immunocompromised patients are another increasing source (e.g. diabetes, cancer treatment)

GENERAL PRINCIPLES OF ORTHOPAEDIC INFECTION

Pathology

Bone infection has all the elements of any inflammatory condition but bone produces some specific pathological features. Acute osteomyelitis occurs when pathogenic organisms cause infection, leading to inflammation in the bone and surrounding tissues. The medullary bone may form abscesses and pus may track through the cortex to form periosteal elevation and soft-tissue extension. This process will devascularise the cortical bone, causing bone death – the characteristic feature of chronic osteomyelitis.

Bacteria can adhere to dead bone or implant surfaces, forming a complex community enveloped in a polysaccharide matrix, known as a biofilm. These bacteria alter their metabolic state, making them more resistant both to the host immune system and to antibiotics. Toxins and lytic enzymes from bacteria cause early damage to articular cartilage.

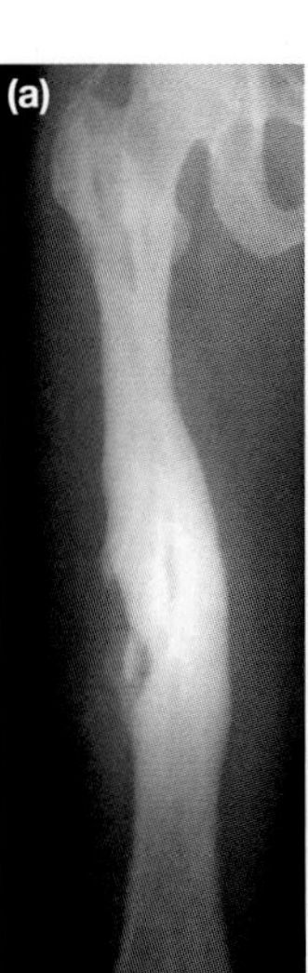

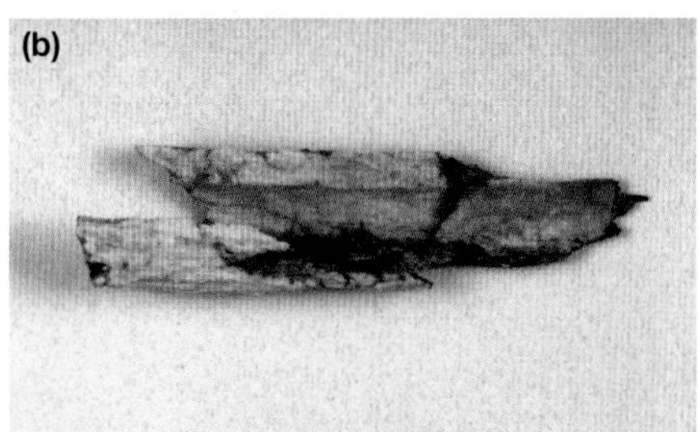

Figure 43.2 (a) Radiograph of chronic infection of the femur with a large central sequestrum and well-developed involucrum. (b) The sequestrum that was removed from the mid-femur at surgery.

The infected bone reacts to the infection by separating dead fragments of bone (sequestration) and forming sinuses to drain pus and discharge small bone fragments. New bone is laid down around the infection from the periosteum (involucrum) (***Figure 43.2***).

In septic arthritis, infection may follow direct ingress of bacteria after injury or surgery, or may result from discharge of an adjacent acute osteomyelitis into the joint. Particularly in neonates or the elderly, bacteraemia may infect a previously normal joint.

Summary box 43.2

Pathology of bone infection

- Bacteria infecting bone form a resistant biofilm on dead bone and implant surfaces
- Infected bone dies and forms a sequestrum
- The periosteum around lays down new bone – an involucrum

Microbiology

Virulent Gram-positive organisms, particularly *Staphylococcus aureus*, are the most common cause of bone or joint infection in native tissue. However, once prosthetic material is implanted, a wide range of organisms can be involved. This includes organisms with low virulence that are usually considered skin commensals, such as coagulase-negative staphylococci, α-haemolytic streptococci and *Cutibacterium acnes* (***Table 43.1***).

Diagnosis

Clinical

Diagnosis is predominantly clinical with confirmation using other tests, as outlined below.

Biomarkers

Raised inflammatory markers (erythrocyte sedimentation rate [ESR], C-reactive protein [CRP] and white cell count [WCC]) are characteristic of acute infection, but they are neither sufficiently sensitive nor sufficiently specific to rule infection in or out. Recently, new synovial fluid markers (α-defensin and calprotectin) have shown high accuracy in diagnosis of PJI.

Imaging

Plain radiographs can demonstrate dead bone, periosteal reaction, involucrum formation and loosening of implants. However, they are often normal in the first few days of infection. A normal radiograph does not exclude infection. Over time, radiographs will show progressive implant loosening, bone lysis or sequestration in chronic osteomyelitis.

Ultrasonography is ideal for identifying soft-tissue collections and joint effusions and can be used to guide bone biopsy and aspiration.

Computed tomography (CT) scans are helpful in assessing bone union of infected fractures. Small sequestra and cortical

Hans Christian Joachim Gram, 1853–1938, Professor of Medicine, Copenhagen, Denmark.

TABLE 43.1 Organisms most commonly involved in bone and joint infection.

Classification of infection	Group(s) of organisms	Examples of specific organisms and context in which infection occurs
Gram positive	Staphylococci	*Staphylococcus aureus* (commonest across all settings) Coagulase-negative staphylococci (common in implant-associated infection)
	Streptococci	α-Haemolytic streptococci, including *Streptococcus pneumoniae, Streptococcus milleri* group and *Streptococcus viridans* (in implant-associated infection)
		β-Haemolytic streptococci (e.g. *Streptococcus pyogenes, Streptococcus agalactiae*)
	Cutibacteria	Increasingly recognised in implant-associated infection and septic arthritis of the shoulder
	Enterococci	Common in diabetic foot infection and chronic osteomyelitis
Gram negative	Enterobacteriaceae	*Escherichia coli* (especially at extremes of age)
		Klebsiella spp.
		Salmonella spp. (particularly associated with sickle cell disease)
	Pseudomonas spp.	Associated with diabetic foot infections, osteomyelitis underlying chronic wounds/ulcers, patients heavily exposed to a hospital environment and/or prior antibiotics
	Kingella kingae	Common cause of septic arthritis in children under 4 years
	Haemophilus spp.	*Haemophilus influenzae* (consider in non-immunised children)
	Neisseria spp.	*Neisseria meningitidis*
		Neisseria gonorrhoeae (consider risk factors for sexually transmitted infection)
Others	Fungi, especially *Candida* spp.	Cause infection in immunocompromised and/or heavily antibiotic-exposed hosts. Common after prolonged use of negative-pressure wound therapy
	Mycobacterium tuberculosis	Present without pulmonary disease Geographical distribution Common with HIV
	Atypical mycobacteria (*Mycobacterium marinum, Mycobacterium ulcerans*)	May be a component of disseminated infection in HIV-infected patients; also cause post-surgical infection in immunocompetent hosts
Mixed	Any combination of the above organisms	More common after trauma, recurrent surgery and with poor wound healing and sinuses, or resulting from contiguous spread from an infected source (e.g. skin, GI tract)
'Culture negative'	No growth from cultures, but diagnosis of infection made on clinical/radiological/ histopathological grounds	Most common in patients who have had recent antimicrobial exposure prior to surgical sampling

GI, gastrointestinal; HIV, human immunodeficiency virus.

erosions are best seen with CT and these scans can be used to plan surgery for excision of dead bone (***Figure 43.3a***).

Isotope bone scans are of very limited value as they are non-specific and give no information that may guide diagnosis or treatment. The combination of ^{18}F-fluorodeoxyglucose positron emission tomography (^{18}FDG-PET) with a CT scan allows localisation of active infection in chronic osteomyelitis and may facilitate planning of surgery. ^{18}FDG-PET/CT is not specific to infection and so cannot reliably distinguish infective from aseptic loosening around implants.

Magnetic resonance imaging (MRI) scanning is the investigation of choice, in the absence of metal implants. It is highly sensitive and specific, showing all components of the disease (***Figure 43.3b***). However, it can overestimate the extent of infection when there is widespread reactive oedema.

Microbiological diagnosis

Good treatment starts with a reliable microbiological diagnosis. Superficial swabs from wounds or spontaneously draining pus are unreliable. Cultures from these do not reflect the pathogens in the bone. Microbiological samples may be falsely negative if antibiotics are given first. Synovial tissue samples are particularly important in producing a higher diagnostic yield for infection with mycobacteria or fungi.

In chronic infections, particularly those involving prosthetic material, multiple biopsy samples are needed. It is recommended to take at least five tissue samples; each one with a separate, sterile instrument. Samples should be promptly transferred to the laboratory with clinical details of the infection. Culture should be maintained for at least 10 days in musculoskeletal infections to allow identification of slow-growing

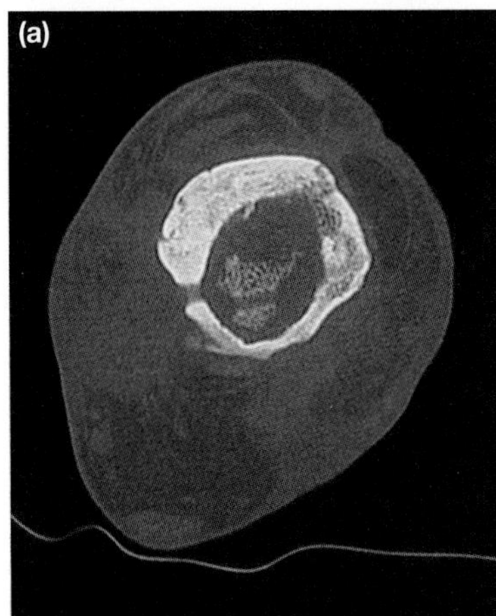

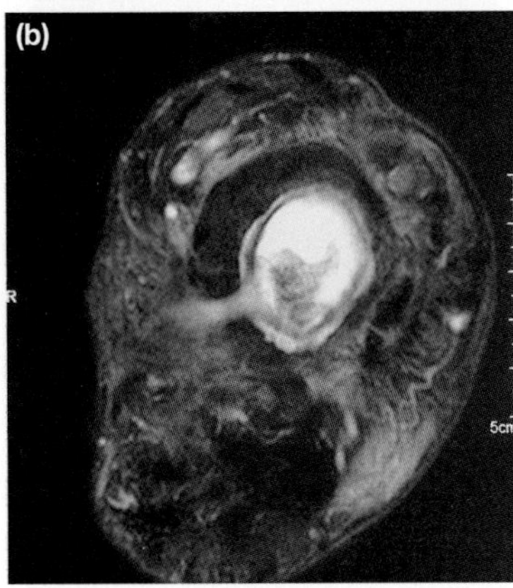

Figure 43.3 (a) Transverse computed tomography scan of the femur with a central sequestrum, sinus and cortical bone erosion. (b) Magnetic resonance imaging scan of the same femur with better resolution of the medullary infection and soft-tissue involvement.

organisms such as *C. acnes*. A positive tissue diagnosis is confirmed when phenotypically identical organisms are cultured from at least two of the five tissue samples. A single positive culture may suggest infection.

It is also possible to culture organisms from removed implants that have been subjected to ultrasonic vibration to disrupt biofilm (sonication).

Summary box 43.3

Principles of diagnosis

- ESR and CRP are neither sensitive nor specific in making a diagnosis of bone infection
- Plain radiographs may be normal in the early phase
- Ultrasonography is valuable for identifying fluid/pus collections
- MRI is usually the investigation of choice
- Superficial swabs are of no value in identifying the organism causing deep infection
- If the patient is on antibiotics, cultures may be falsely negative
- Multiple biopsy specimens should be obtained to optimise microbiological diagnosis
- A neutrophil infiltrate on histology can confirm infection

Histopathology

The histological diagnosis of infection (rather than other sources of inflammation) depends on identifying organisms on a Gram stain or the presence of a neutrophilic infiltrate. Histology can directly diagnose tuberculosis and atypical mycobacterial osteomyelitis (caseating and non-caseating granulomas), actinomycosis and fungal hyphae. The presence of five or more polymorphonuclear neutrophils per high-powered field is diagnostic in fracture-related joint infections and PJIs. Histology is valuable in confirming the presence of infection in culture-negative cases.

Management

Successful treatment requires accurate diagnosis and a multidisciplinary approach to deliver a package of care, summarised as follows:

- Preoperative:
  - patient assessment and clinical staging of disease;
  - full discussion of all treatment options with potential complications;
  - diagnostic tests for general health;
  - optimisation of patients and treatment of comorbidities.
- Operative:
  - exposure for multiple, deep bone sampling;
  - excision of all affected tissue;
  - intravenous antibiotics after sampling;
  - bone stabilisation, if necessary;
  - dead-space management;
  - soft-tissue cover, which may include plastic surgery.
- Postoperative:
  - functional rehabilitation;
  - continued antimicrobial therapy guided by culture results, with regular clinical monitoring.

The principles listed above dictate that a range of surgical and medical specialists will be needed to treat patients with bone and joint infections. If the patient is systemically well, there is often time to complete investigations, optimise patient health and plan interventions. Complex infections should be referred early to centres that specialise in these cases. Attention to diabetes control, peripheral vascular disease, nutrition and smoking cessation is essential. Many patients will benefit from psychological support or at least good counselling around the difficulties of eradicating infection and the components of treatment.

Antibiotic therapy

Patients with septic shock, or with rapidly advancing local or systemic signs of infection, should receive prompt empiric antibiotic therapy. When delay in antibiotics would be unsafe, blood cultures, local aspiration of pus or radiologically guided biopsy may give valuable culture material immediately prior to starting antibiotics.

In most cases, it is safe to delay antibiotics until definitive operative microbiological samples have been taken, particularly in chronic or implant-related infections. For patients who have already been started on antibiotics, a clinical assessment should be made; if safe to do so, antibiotics should be stopped at least 2 weeks before biopsy or surgery.

Local guidelines should be followed, but most hospitals recommend a 'community-acquired' level of cover using an agent such as co-amoxiclav. Additional antibiotics to cover resistant Gram-positive organisms (e.g. vancomycin for methicillin-resistant *S. aureus* [MRSA]) are considered if there has been significant prior hospital exposure or if the patient is known to be colonised with these organisms. Cover for resistant Gram-negative organisms (e.g. meropenem for *Pseudomonas*) is considered in certain settings, including severe diabetic foot infection.

In the past, prolonged intravenous antibiotic courses (i.e. 4–6 weeks of treatment) were often recommended. The recent OVIVA trial has shown that oral therapy is equally effective, providing that the organism(s) is susceptible and the patient can tolerate the chosen antibiotic.

Summary box 43.4

Antibiotics for osteomyelitis

- Septic shock needs treatment without delay, with antibiotics chosen empirically based on local guidelines
- In clinically stable patients, antibiotics should be delayed until specimens have been taken
- In elective surgery for osteomyelitis, antibiotics should be stopped at least 2 weeks in advance
- Agents such as co-amoxiclav or ceftriaxone are appropriate for most community-acquired infection
- Vancomycin or meropenem may be indicated for resistant species
- Oral therapy is effective if susceptible organisms are cultured

NATIVE JOINT SEPTIC ARTHRITIS

Epidemiology

Bacterial infection of native joints occurs with an estimated incidence of 4–10 per 100 000 population per year in western Europe, with higher rates associated with socioeconomic deprivation and in developing countries. The condition most characteristically affects patients at extremes of age, usually with pre-existing arthropathy or immunocompromise (*Table 43.2*).

Joint infection may arise as a result of haematogenous dissemination of bacteria from another focus (e.g. endocarditis) or may occur as a result of direct inoculation or local extension from an infected source (e.g. traumatic wound or adjacent osteomyelitis).

TABLE 43.2 Risk factors for native joint septic arthritis.

- Extremes of age
- Underlying joint abnormality, especially rheumatoid arthritis
- Immunocompromise (e.g. diabetes mellitus, HIV infection, immunosuppressive therapy)
- Joint instrumentation (e.g. steroid injection, arthroscopy)
- Intravenous drug abuse
- Indwelling central venous catheter
- Bacteraemia (especially *Staphylococcus aureus*)

HIV, human immunodeficiency virus.

Clinical features

Most patients present after an acute or subacute history with a single hot, swollen, painful joint. In children, there is often a history of recent minor trauma. The joint is held immobile in the 'position of comfort', with 'pseudoparalysis' in neonates. There is severe pain if any attempt is made to move the affected joint actively or passively. In children and adults, the knee joint is most frequently affected, whereas in neonates it is the hip. Fever and other systemic signs are usually present, but their absence does not rule out the diagnosis. Fever is absent in about one-third of cases.

Diagnosis

Aspiration and/or biopsy of intra-articular fluid or tissue will allow a Gram stain to be performed (although this is positive in only about one-third of infected cases). Culture of a causative organism from synovial fluid is diagnostic (positive in 80–90%) but results are delayed by the time taken to grow and identify the organism in the laboratory. A high WCC in joint fluid (e.g. 50–150 000 cells/mm^3), with a neutrophil predominance (>90%), is characteristic of infection. However, other inflammatory conditions can also cause a raised cell count, and crystals may be seen in infected joints as well as in gout or pseudogout. The limited sensitivity of direct microscopy and Gram stain and the time taken to obtain a positive culture should not delay early treatment for the infection. The decision to perform a surgical washout and give antibiotics should be based on the clinical picture.

Summary box 43.5

Presentation of septic arthritis

- Children may be toxic and febrile but adults may have only a low-grade fever
- Usually symptoms affect only one joint, often with pre-existing arthropathy
- The joint is swollen and held in a characteristic 'position of comfort'
- **Any** movement causes extreme pain

Management

Surgical management

Medical treatment alone is rarely indicated in joint sepsis. Prompt surgical drainage is a priority to avoid further damage to the cartilage. Arthroscopic washout is commonly performed but it may be difficult to remove loculated areas of infection. Washout should be with Ringer's solution or

Sidney Ringer, 1835–1910, Professor of Clinical Medicine, University College Hospital, London, UK.

0.9% sodium chloride. Antiseptics should be avoided because of the risk of chondrolysis. There should be a low threshold for open arthrotomy, particularly if a joint is not settling. A synovectomy is recommended if there is major synovial thickening, aggressive synovitis or subchondral erosions seen on radiology (Gächter stages 3 and 4). Inadequate clearance may lead to chronic infection with destruction of the joint (***Figure 43.4***). Treatment may then require joint excision, joint fusion or staged joint replacement.

Medical management

Antibiotics are usually given for 3–6 weeks (beginning with intravenous therapy). There are sparse data to guide duration. Longer courses should be considered if the infection is slow to resolve, if more than one washout is required, if the patient is bacteraemic and/or if the infection is caused by *S. aureus*. The choice of antibiotics is as given in ***Summary box 43.4***.

> **Summary box 43.6**
>
> Native joint septic arthritis
> - Most common at extremes of age, in patients with rheumatoid arthritis and in association with immunocompromise
> - Most commonly affects hips in neonates and knees in adults and children
> - The commonest pathogen is *S. aureus*
> - Joints should be aspirated for microbiology before starting antibiotics, if safe to do so
> - Management is prompt surgical joint washout, followed by 3–6 weeks of antibiotics

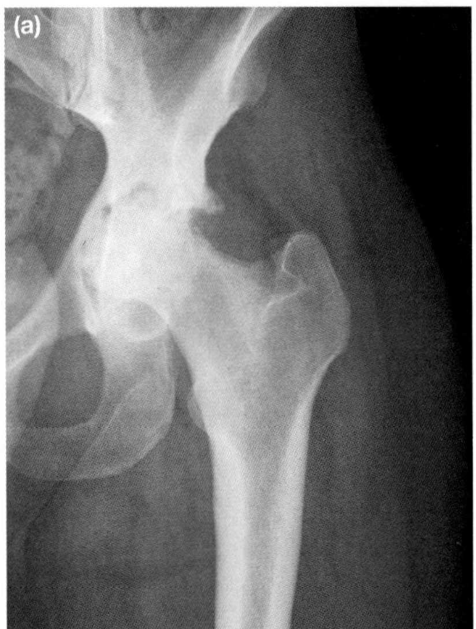

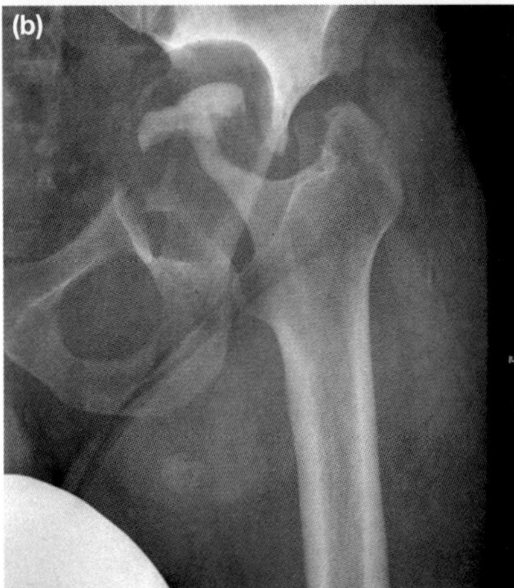

Figure 43.4 (a) Septic arthritis of the hip in a person who injects drugs. This was untreated for several weeks, resulting in destruction of the joint surface. (b) The same hip after 9 months without treatment. The proximal femur and acetabulum have been grossly eroded by infection.

PROSTHETIC JOINT INFECTION

Epidemiology

The incidence of PJI is around 1% per joint per year, with upper limb joints at a higher risk. Infection can be minimised with improved operative practice, prophylactic systemic antibiotics, local antibiotics in cement and the use of surgical 'care bundles'. Risk factors include obesity, skin disease, diabetes, malignancy, inflammatory arthritis, prolonged or complicated surgery, revision surgery, fracture and postoperative wound infection or haematoma.

Clinical features

PJIs may present early (within 3 months of surgery), in a delayed manner (3–24 months from surgery) or late (after 2 years).

- **Early infections** are acquired at surgery and are usually caused by virulent organisms (e.g. *S. aureus*). They present with a discharging wound, cellulitis, pain, inflammation and swelling.
- **Delayed infections** are more characteristically due to low-virulence organisms (e.g. coagulase-negative staphylococci or cutibacteria).
- **Late infections** are more likely to present with an indolent clinical syndrome of joint discomfort or mechanical dysfunction ('start-up' symptoms are particularly characteristic), with or without a discharging sinus. Late presentations are usually due to haematogenous infection of a previously uninfected joint, from bacteraemia. The source may indicate the microbiology (e.g. pneumococci from respiratory origin, *Salmonella* spp. from the gut, *Escherichia coli* from the urinary tract).

Diagnosis

Infection should be suspected in any patient with a leaking wound over an implant, unresolved pain or new pain around a previously pain-free implant. Routine blood tests may be helpful in acute infection but are often falsely reassuring.

André Gächter, contemporary, Swiss orthopaedic surgeon.

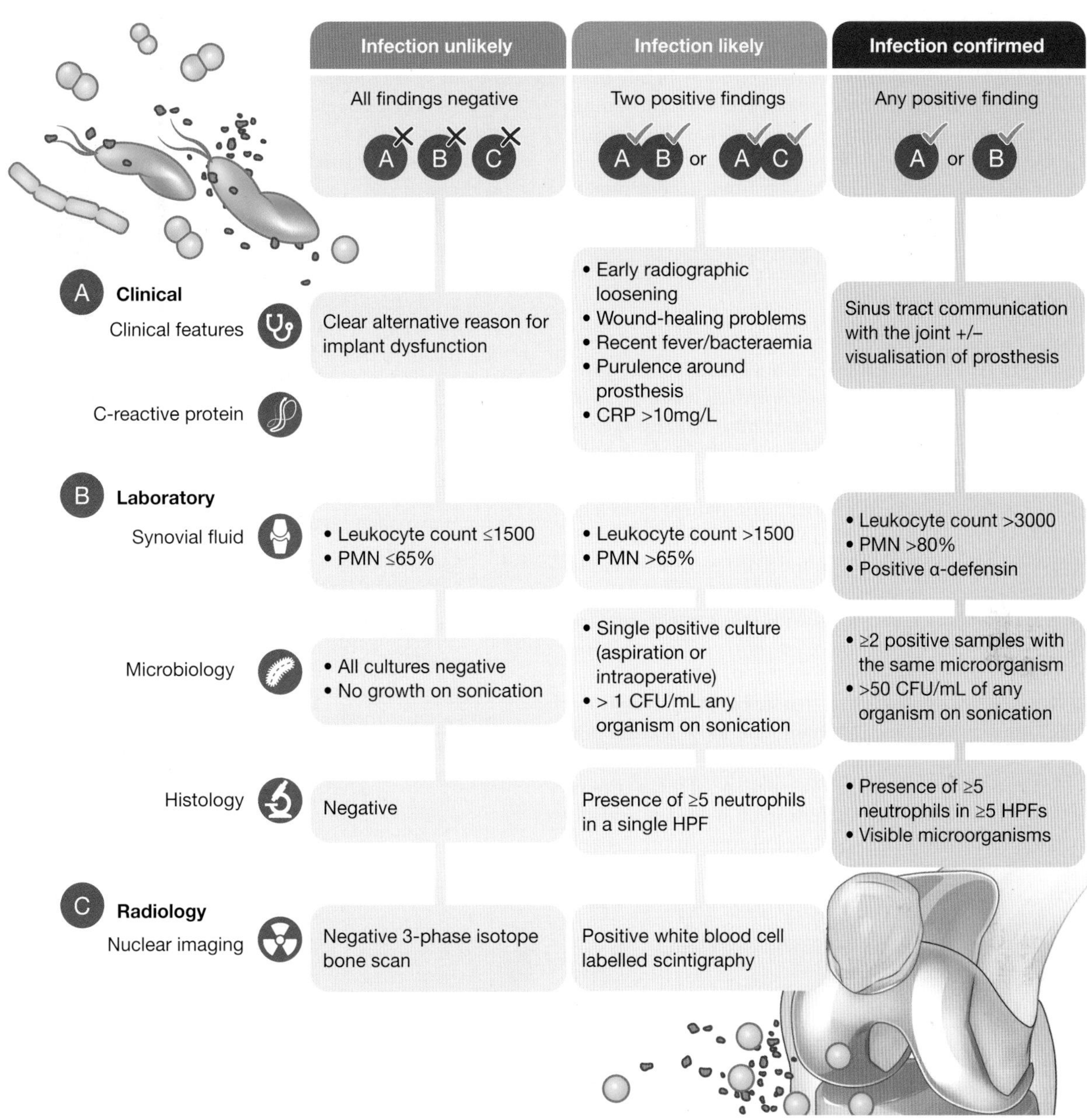

Figure 43.5 The European Bone and Joint Infection Society definition of prosthetic joint infection. CFU, colony-forming unit; CRP, C-reactive protein; HPF, high-power field; PMN, polymorphonuclear cells. (Reproduced with permission from McNally MA, Sousa R, Wouthuyzen-Bakker M *et al*. Infographic: The EBJIS definition of prosthetic joint infection: a practical guide for clinicians. *Bone Joint J* 2021; **103-B**(1): 16–17.)

The European Bone and Joint Infection Society (EBJIS) has produced diagnostic criteria for PJI. Infection is confirmed if there is a sinus communicating with the joint or there is a high synovial fluid WCC (>3000/μL), a positive microbiological culture or positive histology (more than five polymorphs per high-power field) (***Figure 43.5***) Plain radiographs may show features of loosening of a chronically infected prosthesis, and ultrasound may identify associated collections. Nuclear scans cannot reliably distinguish aseptic loosening from PJI.

Management

A multidisciplinary approach is required, including orthopaedics, plastic surgery, infectious diseases/microbiology, pharmacy, nursing, occupational therapy and physiotherapy, centred on the patient's understanding and wishes regarding their condition. Many patients have other medical comorbidities that should also be addressed and optimised. PJI can be associated with a range of emotional, psychological and mental health issues, ranging from anger about surgical complications to depression arising from chronic symptoms, lack of function and prolonged hospitalisation.

The choice of surgical strategy for prosthetic joints can be categorised as:

- salvage of an infected implant;
- removal of the infected implant with or without reimplantation.

Some groups have used the timing of presentation to determine this (i.e. salvage for early infection versus removal and revision for late infection). Others regard any firmly fixed implant as potentially salvageable, irrespective of the timing (and there are now several studies showing that this is feasible). However, it is agreed that loose infected implants should always be removed (***Figure 43.6***). Furthermore, it is essential to achieve soft-tissue cover of bone and prosthetic material. This may be difficult around the knee, requiring local muscle flaps.

Management options can be divided into the following broad approaches.

- **Debridement, antibiotics and implant retention - 'DAIR'**. This can only be undertaken if the prosthesis is well fixed. DAIR is not a form of washout as all infected soft tissue and necrotic bone must be fully excised and modular components exchanged. This cannot be achieved by arthroscopic surgery. Good soft-tissue cover is essential. Following debridement, the patient is treated with long-term antibiotics (frequently 6 weeks of intravenous therapy followed by 6 months or more of oral antibiotics). Prolonged infection-free intervals can be achieved in 80% of patients but success with this strategy may be lower in infections caused by *S. aureus* or with multiresistant organisms.
- **Two-stage joint revision surgery**. A thorough excision is undertaken and all cement and loose foreign material is removed. An antibiotic-impregnated spacer may be implanted (which may be articulating). This is a temporary measure and cannot withstand full weight-bearing. The patient is treated with oral or intravenous antibiotics, most commonly for 6 weeks. A new prosthesis is implanted after the course of antibiotics has been completed. In recent years there has been a trend towards shorter intervals between stages, often within the 6-week antimicrobial therapy.
- **Single-stage joint revision surgery**. The procedure is the same as above, but removal and reimplantation are undertaken in the same operating session. Healthy soft tissues around the new implant are essential to prevent reinfection. Some centres consider single-stage revisions when less florid signs of infection are present (i.e. absence of collections or sinus tracts), or for frail patients for whom the risk of a second operation is higher. There are no adequate trial data comparing outcomes with the two-stage approach.
- **Joint removal or fusion**. When reconstruction options are not technically possible or are ruled out by comorbid conditions, removal of the prosthesis without reimplantation may palliate symptoms. An example is the Girdlestone excision arthroplasty of the hip. In prosthetic infections of the knee, ankle or wrist, it may be possible to create a joint fusion after prosthesis removal. This is complex surgery, which may involve major bone reconstruction. Amputation may be necessary for knee or ankle implants.
- **Suppressive therapy with antibiotics**. In patients who are not medically fit for any operative intervention, or who choose to decline all surgical options, long-term treatment with antibiotics may help to suppress the symptoms of infection. There are limited data, but anecdotally the success rate of this approach is low.

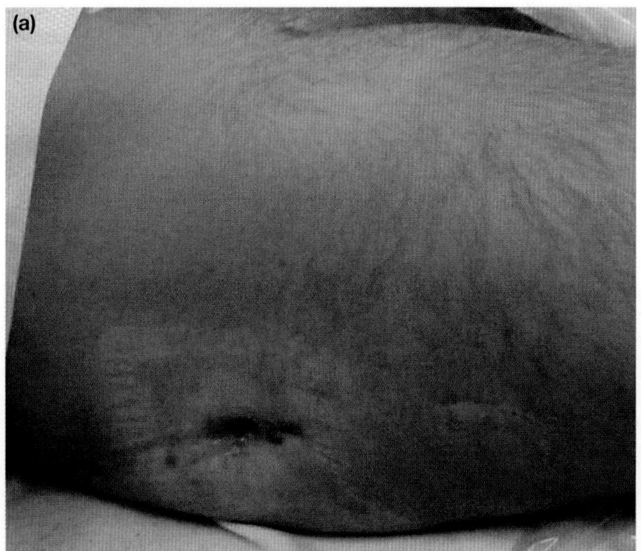

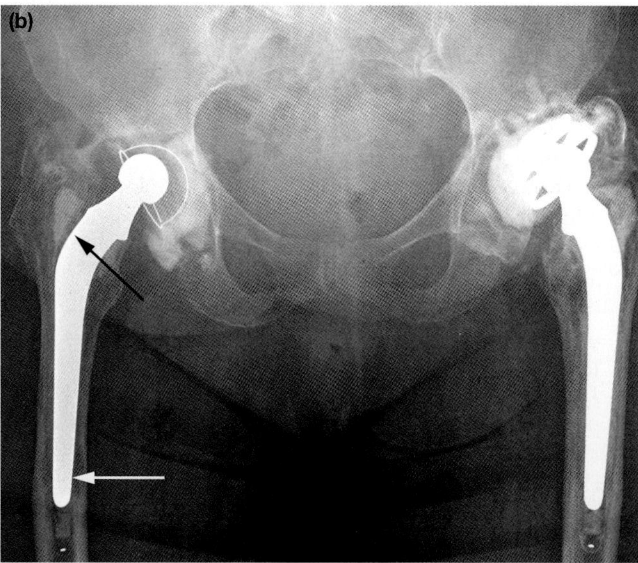

Figure 43.6 (a) Sinus draining from the scar over the lateral side of the hip. This patient had a total hip replacement 14 years before that had been complicated by a wound haematoma and infection. (b) Radiograph of both hips of same patient. Both hips are loose but only the right side has definite infection (arrows).

Gathorne Robert Girdlestone, 1881–1950, Nuffield Professor of Orthopaedics, University of Oxford, UK, described excision arthroplasty of the hip for septic arthritis.

Summary box 43.7

Prosthetic joint infection

- Well-fixed prostheses may be Debrided, treated with Antibiotics and the Implant Retained ('DAIR' approach)
- Loose prostheses must be removed
- Replacement can be made at the initial surgery (one stage) or after a delay to allow infection to be eradicated with antibiotics (two stage)
- Multiple surgical samples are crucial for identifying a pathogen
- Thorough excision of infected tissue is a key determinant of outcome
- Long-term antibiotics may be used for patients who are not suitable for major revision surgery

FRACTURE-RELATED INFECTION

Infection complicates around 3–5% of all fracture fixations. Open tibia fractures are a high-risk group with up to 25% becoming infected after fixation. Calcaneal fractures and ankle fracture fixation in the elderly also have high infection rates.

Many of the principles outlined above for PJI can be applied to infections associated with metalwork used to fix fractures.

There are several clinical scenarios which must be addressed:

- **Unhealed fracture with *stable* fixation**. This is usually seen early after fixation and can be managed with deep sampling, debridement of infected tissues and management of dead spaces (often with local antibiotic carriers) ('DAIR' approach). It is extremely important to provide good soft-tissue cover over the fracture. In the tibia, this will most often require a plastic surgical reconstruction. After debridement, systemic antibiotics must be given to suppress infection until bone union.
- **Healed fracture with infected implant**. In these cases, the implant can be removed, but there should still be a careful debridement, deep sampling, dead space management and soft-tissue cover.
- **Unhealed fracture with *unstable* fixation**. Stability is essential for bone healing and eradication of infection. If the implant is not stable, it should be removed and replaced by an external fixator. Radical excision of the infected fracture is needed and the resulting defect may present a major reconstructive challenge (***Figure 43.7***). Recently, antibiotic-coated locking nails have been used to restabilise infected fractures with some success.

ANTIMICROBIAL THERAPY FOR PROSTHETIC JOINT INFECTION AND FRACTURE-RELATED INFECTION

Following surgical sampling, empiric broad-spectrum intravenous antibiotic therapy (e.g. vancomycin and meropenem) should be given. This can be rationalised when culture results are available. In culture-negative cases, ongoing therapy to cover the most likely pathogens should be instituted.

The duration of therapy is determined according to the surgical approach, with 6 weeks for those in whom prosthetic material is completely removed versus 6 months for patients undergoing a 'DAIR' strategy, and prolonged (occasionally lifelong) treatment for patients in whom all other options are contraindicated or intolerable. In a few patients, the best therapy is no intervention, when chronic low-grade symptoms are well controlled and preferable to the risks of either surgery or long-term antibiotic therapy.

The antibiotic regimen should be planned with the advice of a microbiologist and supervised carefully to promote compliance and to detect and manage side effects. Monitoring of the joint is largely on clinical grounds; biomarkers including CRP are not predictive of treatment failure. Serial radiographs are helpful to detect progressive bone loss, which may be an indicator of recurrent active infection and can predispose to periprosthetic fracture and implant loosening.

ACUTE OSTEOMYELITIS

This presents like septic arthritis with a short history of pain, swelling, loss of function and systemic upset. In adults, the vertebral column is the commonest site; in children, long bones are most frequently affected. In young children, a fever and refusal to weight-bear may be the only clues.

Diagnosis

In the early phase (2–3 days) radiographs may be normal but MRI will show bone oedema and periosteal elevation. After 5–7 days, plain radiographs may show subtle abnormality with osteopenia and periosteal new bone formation. WCC and CRP are often elevated in the early phase. Treatment should not be delayed pending investigations.

Management

Acute osteomyelitis can be treated with antibiotics alone, when the diagnosis is made within 2–3 days of onset of symptoms, there is no dead bone on imaging and there is no adjacent septic arthritis. Culture results help to guide therapy, so blood cultures should be taken, and radiologically guided sampling should be considered. Empirical intravenous therapy against Gram-positive organisms is given (cephalosporins or flucloxacillin), adding gentamicin to cover Gram-negative organisms in children under 1 year.

The limb should be splinted and good analgesia given. Intravenous antibiotics should be converted to oral therapy, depending on clinical progress and the results of cultures, and therapy is continued for a total of 2–3 weeks. If the patient does not respond rapidly, if the limb deteriorates or if there is imaging evidence of progression of disease, surgery is indicated to prevent bone destruction and the onset of chronic osteomyelitis.

With prompt treatment, acute bone infection has a good prognosis with a 90% cure rate. Failure to treat adequately produces chronicity, with recurrent infection over many years. In children, the adjacent growth plates and joints may be affected with subsequent deformity and joint destruction.

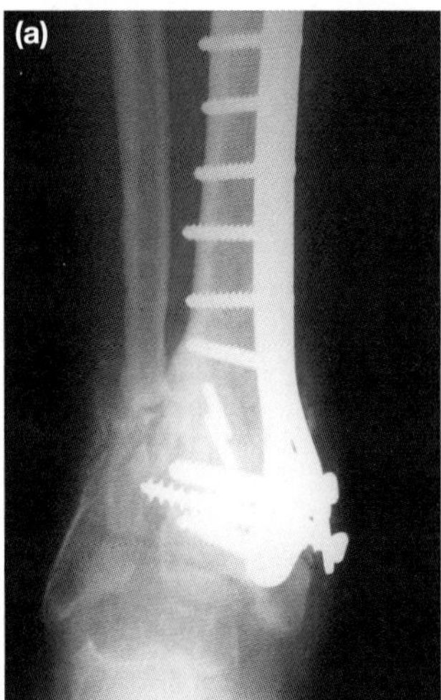

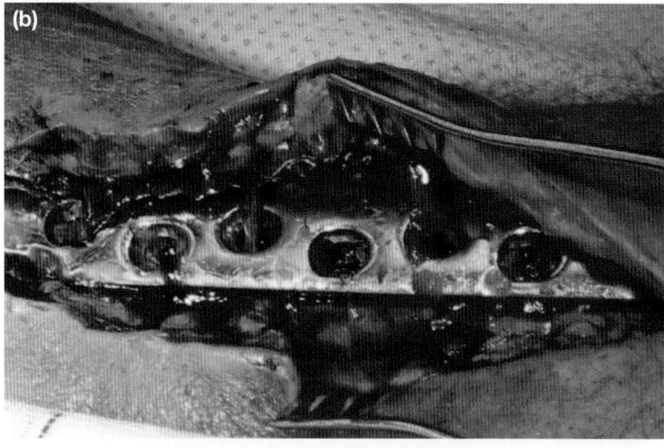

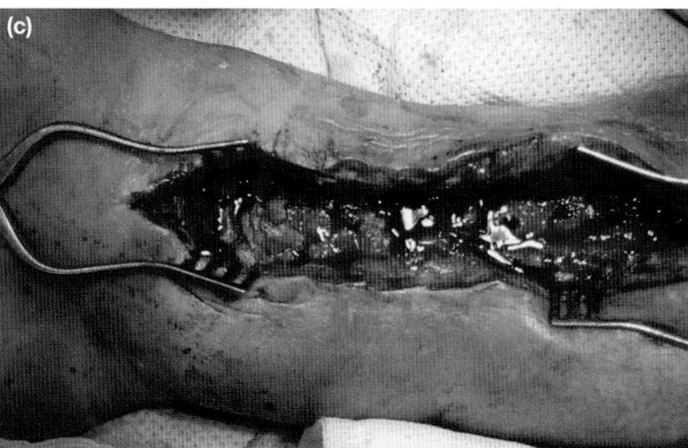

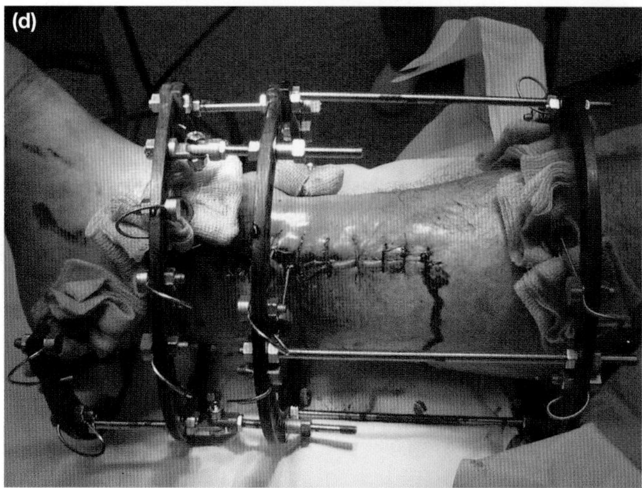

Figure 43.7 (a) Radiograph of a complex distal tibia fracture that was internally fixed but complicated by deep infection. (b) At operation, the plate was loose and grossly infected. (c) The plate and all infected tissue was excised. Deep samples were sent for microbiology and histology. The defect at the lower end was filled with an absorbable antibiotic carrier. (d) The bone was stabilised with an Ilizarov circular external fixator and the skin primarily closed.

Summary box 43.8

Acute osteomyelitis

- Presents in children with toxaemia, fever and unwillingness to move the limb
- May affect the vertebral column in adults, where back pain may be the only symptom
- Radiographs may be normal for up to 1 week so are of limited value in early diagnosis
- MRI is the investigation of choice
- WCC and CRP are usually raised
- Early diagnosis is treated with high dose intravenous antibiotics, started empirically and modified with culture results
- Late diagnosis and/or failure of medical treatment requires surgical debridement

CHRONIC OSTEOMYELITIS

This is a serious condition that may affect the patient for decades. Chronic bone infection is best treated within a dedicated multidisciplinary team that has the skills to deal with all aspects of the condition, the associated comorbidities and the range of surgical reconstructive options.

Diagnosis

Plain radiographs can delineate soft-tissue swelling, subperiosteal reaction, bone destruction and sequestra. CT scans are good for cortical bone imaging (***Figure 43.8***). MRI is the imaging test of choice (see ***General principles of orthopaedic infection***). Blood tests are often normal in chronic osteomyelitis. Confirmation of the diagnosis is with culture from deep surgical samples and histology. [18]FDG-PET CT scanning can be helpful for surgical planning.

Gavriil Abramovich Ilizarov, 1921–1992, orthopaedic surgeon, Kurgan, Western Siberia, Russia, pioneered this eponymous approach to bone reconstruction in the 1960s for the management of osteomyelitis, fractures and limb deformities.

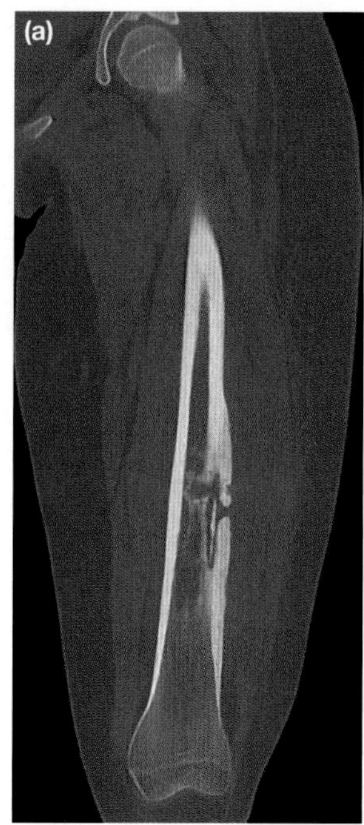

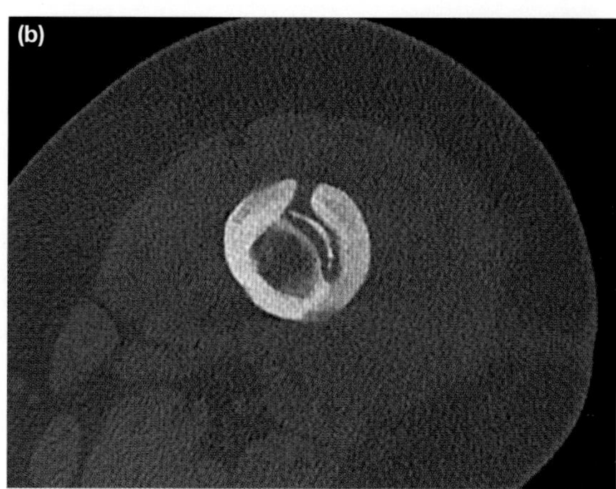

Figure 43.8 (a) Coronal computed tomography scan of the femur showing diaphyseal chronic osteomyelitis. (b) A transverse section clearly shows the sequestration of the lateral cortex and overlying new bone formation (involucrum).

Management

The BACH classification divides patients into 'uncomplicated', 'complex' and 'limited options available' based on the four important features of the infection (***Figure 43.9***). These are: the anatomical location in the bone (B), the antimicrobial profile (A), the need for soft-tissue cover (C) and the health of the host (H). Treatment must always address all four parts of the classification to achieve good outcomes. All infected unhealed fractures and infected non-unions are complex.

As with PJI, comorbidities should be optimised before surgery. The interaction between the patient's health status and the extent of the bone infection greatly affects the outcome after surgery. In chronic infection, it is essential to address medical conditions that may impair wound healing (e.g. smoking, peripheral vascular disease, diabetes, steroid use) prior to surgery. This approach has been shown to improve cure rates. A joint assessment by an orthopaedic surgeon, plastic surgeon and infectious disease physician will allow good preoperative planning.

	Bone involvement	**A**ntimicrobial options	**C**overage of soft tissue	**H**ost status
Uncomplicated	B1 Cavitary involvement (including medullary, cortical and non-segmental corticomedullary)	Ax Unknown/culture negative A1 <4 resistant tests ≥80% susceptibility tests sensitive	C1 Direct closure possible Plastic surgery expertise *not required*	H1 Patient fit and well or has well-controlled disease
Complex	B2 Segmental involvement Any infection with joint involvement	A2 >4 resistant tests <80% susceptibility tests sensitive	C1 Direct closure not possible Plastic surgery expertise *required*	H2 Patient with either poorly controlled disease, severe disease or recurrent osteomyelitis
Limited options	B3 Whole bone involvement	A3 Sensitivity to either 0 or 1 susceptibility test		H3 Unfit for anaesthetic Patient declines surgery Surgery not indicated

Figure 43.9 The BACH classification of osteomyelitis.

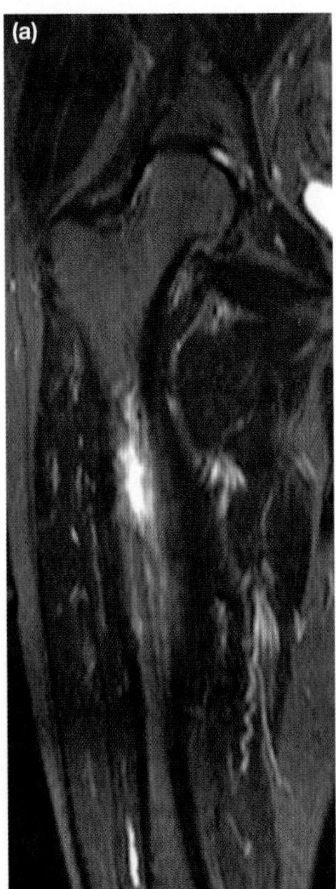

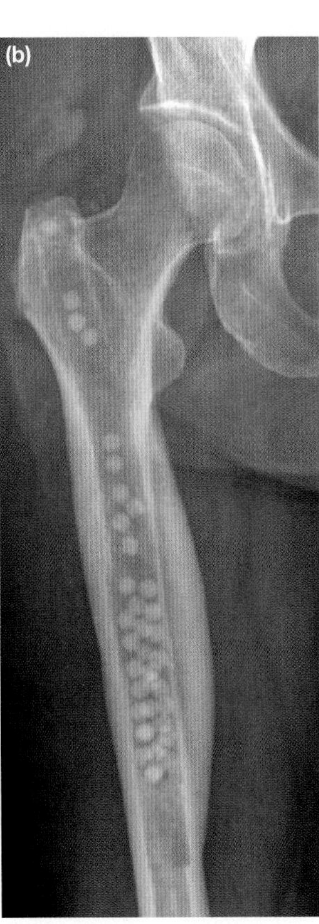

Figure 43.10 (a) This magnetic resonance imaging scan shows a BACH uncomplicated medullary osteomyelitis of the femur. (b) The infected bone has been removed by reaming and the central defect filled with absorbable calcium sulphate pellets with gentamicin.

In uncomplicated disease, excision of the dead bone, with local and systemic antibiotics and direct wound closure, is highly effective (*Figure 43.10*). If more than one-third of the cortical circumference is excised, splintage is essential, often with external fixation to prevent fracture. Secondary bone grafting may be needed.

When the infection is segmental (BACH complex), or when the soft-tissue envelope cannot be closed directly, major reconstruction will be required. Curative resection must be segmental and bone stabilisation will always be required. The Ilizarov method, which uses distraction osteogenesis to fill bone defects, is a powerful and successful technique in these cases. It can be combined with free tissue transfer. This allows reconstruction to proceed in parallel with rehabilitation.

After surgery, patients should be given antibiotics. In total segmental excision of infection a short course may be indicated, but in most chronic infections 6–12 weeks is often advised. If there is any doubt about the adequacy of removal of the dead bone, a long antibiotic course will be needed and recurrence will be more likely. In chronic fracture-related infection, antibiotics should continue until fracture union.

There is now increasing interest in the use of local antibiotic absorbable carriers. These can deliver high doses of antibiotics into the bone, without systemic effects. Some ceramic materials (with hydroxyapatite) can form new bone in the defect, avoiding the need for secondary bone grafting.

Summary box 43.9

Chronic osteomyelitis

- Chronic disease requires specialist surgery with excision, stabilisation and reconstruction
- Host status should be optimised before surgery
- Following surgery, antibiotic therapy is typically continued for at least 6 weeks

DIABETIC FOOT INFECTION

The global prevalence of diabetes has increased exponentially in recent years. Foot infections are a leading cause of hospital admissions in this group, with an annual incidence of foot complications of 1–2% per year owing to the combined influence of macro- and microvascular insufficiency, mechanical disruption, peripheral and autonomic neuropathy, immune defects and impaired tissue healing. Ulceration of the calcaneum and bones of the forefoot is common (*Figure 43.11*) and will result in amputation in up to one-fifth of cases.

Infection begins as invasion of bacteria into the compromised tissues and will rapidly spread to deep structures. Diagnosis is made on the clinical signs and symptoms of local inflammation and systemic upset. The presence of a wound/ulcer, spreading cellulitis, fevers or critical ischaemia indicate a more severe infection and the need for urgent treatment.

Blood tests are frequently unhelpful, as inflammatory markers may be normal or only mildly raised. Plain radiographs may show evidence of osteomyelitis but can be normal (particularly early in infection). MRI is the most sensitive imaging modality for diagnosis of bone involvement. Superficial swabs

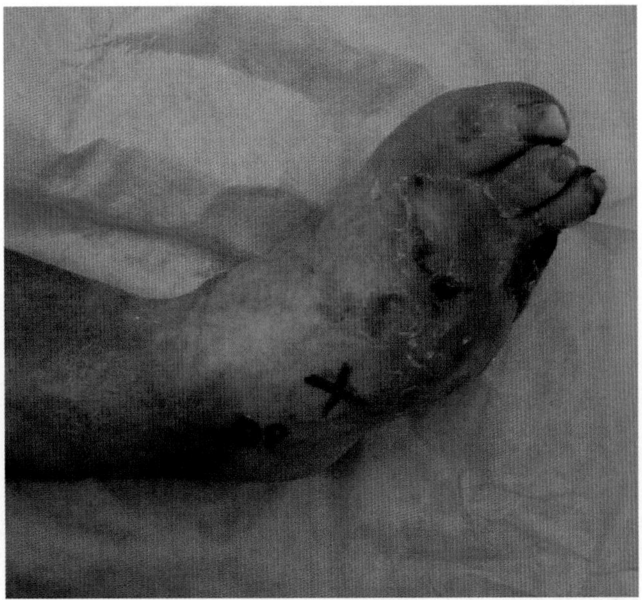

Figure 43.11 A severe diabetic foot infection, with marked infection, necrosis and tissue loss. The patient was neuropathic and had ankle and hindfoot deformity. The foot was salvaged with a corrective triple fusion of the hindfoot, excision of the infected ulcer, antibiotic therapy and primary closure of the lateral soft tissues.

or cultures from ulcers or sinus tracts are not reliable in determining the organisms responsible for underlying deep-seated infection. A combination of the 'probe-to-bone' test with elevated inflammatory markers and abnormal plain radiographs confirms the diagnosis.

The aetiological agents of diabetic foot infection are the same as for bone infection in non-diabetic individuals, namely *S. aureus*, β-haemolytic streptococci and aerobic Gram-negative bacilli. *Pseudomonas* is over-represented, and empirical therapy for severe infections should include cover for this organism. Anaerobes may also be present and addition of metronidazole (particularly for abscesses and/or devitalised tissue) should be considered.

Surgical debridement is required for collections, necrotic areas or more extensive osteomyelitis. Thought should be given to distinguishing superficial osteitis, resulting from loss of soft-tissue cover (often in association with vascular compromise), from more extensive bone involvement. In the former, biopsy and antibiotic therapy may be of limited importance and optimising glycaemic control, improving vascular supply and relieving pressure, with appropriate footwear, much more important. This approach may avoid more extensive tissue loss or later amputation.

Many patients with diabetes with foot infection have significant vascular compromise and neuropathy, which makes healing after surgery unreliable. A full vascular assessment is mandatory in those with poor peripheral pulses. Proximal angioplasty or bypass surgery may improve distal vascularity to a level where infection surgery in the foot may be more successful.

Amputation is not an easy option in diabetic foot disease and wound healing can be problematic. In general, excision should be adequate to remove all infected material and excess bone may need to be resected to allow tension-free skin closure. If there is extensive peripheral neuropathy, a below-knee amputation in an area with better sensation may be more appropriate.

Summary box 43.10

Diabetic foot infection

- The most important risk factor for osteomyelitis is the presence of a foot ulcer
- Ulcer swabs are not reliable in determining the pathogens responsible for osteomyelitis
- Bone biopsy for culture should be considered in extensive/complex infection but may not be necessary in mild disease
- In severe disease, surgical debridement of collections and/or necrotic tissue is required, followed by antibiotics tailored according to culture results

MUSCULOSKELETAL INFECTION CAUSED BY MYCOBACTERIA

Tuberculous arthritis/osteomyelitis remains prevalent in low- and middle-income countries. There is now a resurgence across the world as a consequence of migration and immunocompromise (including human immunodeficiency virus [HIV]). The most common organism is *Mycobacterium tuberculosis*. Around half of all cases affect the spine, typically manifesting as para-discal infection but also causing discitis and vertebral osteomyelitis. Native joint infection typically presents with monoarticular pain in a weight-bearing joint.

For optimal management of tuberculosis, the patient must be referred to a specialist multidisciplinary team for input that includes the following components.

- Baseline screening for HIV and other blood-borne viruses.
- Assessment for other sites of mycobacterial infection.
- Measurement of baseline renal and liver function, to be repeated at intervals throughout treatment. Drug-induced hepatitis is the commonest serious side effect that may require temporary withdrawal or alteration of therapy.
- Baseline and follow-up testing of hearing (if injectable agents to be used) and colour vision (if ethambutol to be used).
- Consideration of any potential drug interactions (rifampicin is a potent inducer of the cytochrome P450 system; it can interact with many classes of drug, including anticonvulsants, antiretroviral therapy, anticoagulants, antibiotics and antifungals).
- Institution of appropriate infection control precautions and contact tracing.
- Appropriate education and support to optimise adherence to therapy.
- Prescription of an appropriate combination of drug therapy.
    - For fully sensitive *M. tuberculosis*, the preferred regimen is oral rifampicin, isoniazid, pyrazinamide and ethambutol for 2 months, followed by rifampicin and isoniazid for a further 4 months.
    - Worldwide, there is an increase in the prevalence of drug-resistant tuberculosis, classified as multidrug resistant (MDR) and extensively drug resistant (XDR). Infection with these organisms requires a treatment regimen that includes an injectable agent (typically amikacin, kanamycin or capreomycin) together with oral agents selected according to the susceptibility profile of the isolate (these may include cycloserine, ethionamide, para-aminosalicylic acid [PAS], fluoroquinolones and linezolid). Prolongation of therapy is required, and side effects/toxicity are common.
- Surgery is only recommended to decompress or stabilise the spine and occasionally to confirm the diagnosis by tissue biopsy.

Non-tuberculous mycobacteria are ubiquitous environmental organisms. They are best recognised as agents of disease in patients with underlying immunocompromise (including HIV, diabetes and organ transplantation) or other risk factors for introduction of infection (such as penetrating trauma or the presence of a prosthesis). However, they may occasionally also cause infection in hosts without obvious risk factors.

Treatment can be difficult; these organisms are resistant to the standard agents used for first line antituberculous therapy; surgery to debride and drain sites of infection can therefore be particularly important to reduce the bacterial burden. There is no single standardised drug regimen or duration, so choice of therapy depends on the *in vitro* susceptibility of the organism and length of treatment depends on the location of disease; extent of surgical debridement; the identification and phenotypic characteristics of the organism; and the patient's underlying condition, presence of immunocompromise and response to therapy. As for treatment of *M. tuberculosis*, expert medical oversight is crucial throughout treatment.

ACKNOWLEDGEMENTS

Dr Philip Bejon and Dr Philipa Matthews contributed to earlier versions of this chapter, and I remain grateful for their input.

FURTHER READING

Coakley G, Mathews C, Field M *et al.* BSR & BHPR, BOA, RCGP and BSAC guidelines for management of the hot swollen joint. *Rheumatology* 2006; **54**: 1039–41.

Dudareva M, Hotchen AJ, Ferguson J *et al.* The microbiology of osteomyelitis: changes over ten years. *J Infection* 2019; **79**: 189–98.

Ferguson J, Athanasou N, Diefenbeck M, McNally MA. Radiographic and histological analysis of a synthetic bone graft substitute eluting gentamicin in the treatment of chronic osteomyelitis. *J Bone Joint Infect* 2019; **4**(2): 76–84.

Hotchen AJ, Dudareva M, Corrigan RA *et al.* Can we predict outcome after treatment of long bone osteomyelitis? A study of patient-reported quality of life, stratified with the BACH classification. *Bone Joint J* 2020; **102-B**(11): 1587–96.

Iliadis AD, Ramachandran M. Paediatric bone and joint infection. *EFORT Open Rev* 2017; **2**(1): 7–12.

Li H-K, Rombach I, Zambellas R *et al.* Oral versus intravenous antibiotics for bone and joint infection. *N Engl J Med* 2019; **380**: 425–36.

Lipsky BA, Senneville E, Abbas ZG *et al.* Guidelines on the diagnosis and treatment of foot infection in persons with diabetes (IWGDF 2019 update). *Diabetes Metab Res Rev* 2020; **36**(S1): e3280.

McNally MA. Osteomyelitis. In: Chen AF (ed.). *Management of orthopaedic infections: a practical guide.* New York, NY: Thieme, 2021: ch. 5, 61–87.

McNally MA, Ferguson JY, Lau ACK *et al.* Single-stage treatment of chronic osteomyelitis with a new absorbable, gentamicin-loaded, calcium sulphate/hydroxyapatite biocomposite. *Bone Joint J* 2016; **98-B**: 1289–96.

McNally M, Govaert G, Dudareva M *et al.* Definition and diagnosis of fracture-related infection. *EFORT Open Rev* 2020; **5**: 614–19.

McNally MA, Sousa R, Wouthuyzen-Bakker M *et al.* The EBJIS definition of prosthetic joint infection: a practical guide for clinicians. *Bone Joint J* 2021; **103-B**(1): 18–25.

Metsemakers W-J, Morgenstern, M, Senneville E *et al.* General treatment principles for fracture-related infection: recommendations from an international expert group. *Arch Orthop Trauma Surg* 2020; **140**(8): 1013–27.

Middleton R, Khan T, Alvand A. Update on the diagnosis and management of prosthetic joint infection in hip and knee arthroplasty. *Bone Joint 360* 2019; **8**(4): 5–13.

Mifsud M, Ferguson JY, Stubbs DA *et al.* Simultaneous debridement, Ilizarov reconstruction and free muscle flaps in the management of complex tibial infection. *J Bone Joint Infect* 2020; **6**: 63–72.

CHAPTER 44 Paediatric orthopaedics

Learning objectives

To be familiar with:
- Physiological versus pathological development of the musculoskeletal system
- Diagnosis and treatment of developmental dysplasia of the hip
- Presentation and management of other childhood hip conditions
- Management of club foot
- Problems associated with musculoskeletal infection in childhood

INTRODUCTION

Immature skeletons heal rapidly and can remodel with growth but physeal injury or muscle imbalance may lead to progressive deformity. The conservative treatment of common conditions, such as developmental dysplasia of the hip (DDH), considers remodelling ability with an understanding of the Hueter–Volkmann principle and Wolff's law (*Table 44.1*): improving the biomechanical environment may reverse abnormal growth. In contrast, in conditions such as Blount's disease, a poorly functioning growth plate leads to asymmetrical growth and deformity. Advances in genetics and molecular science have improved our understanding of certain conditions and may lead to new treatments.

TABLE 44.1 Laws governing the remodelling of bone.

Hueter–Volkmann principle
• Compressive forces inhibit growth
• Tensile forces stimulate growth
Wolff's law
• Bone deposition and resorption depend on the stresses applied

DEVELOPMENT OF THE MUSCULOSKELETAL SYSTEM

The upper limb bud forms on the lateral wall of the 4-week embryo, followed promptly by the lower limb bud. By 2 months, differentiation of the limb elements is complete. Most congenital limb anomalies arise during this period.

Three coordinated signalling centres control limb development. The **apical ectodermal ridge** (AER) guides mesodermal differentiation in a proximal-to-distal direction, controlling digit formation via the production of fibroblast growth factors (FGFs). The mesodermal **zone of polarising activity** (ZPA) directs anteroposterior development via the sonic hedgehog protein, which is itself sustained by FGFs. The ectodermal driven **wingless-type** (Wnt) signalling centre develops dorsoventral axis configuration and limb alignment.

Certain limb anomalies are directly related to alterations in these centres. Experimentally, removal of the AER leads to a truncated limb, similar to a congenital amputation, and prevents interdigital necrosis resulting in syndactyly. An additional ZPA results in a mirror duplication of the distal limb.

Factors causing fetal limb anomalies may also influence other organ formation, resulting in potentially life-threatening disorders.

Summary box 44.1

Development of the musculoskeletal system
- Occurs 4–8 weeks after fertilisation
- AER controls proximal-to-distal differentiation and interdigital necrosis
- ZPA directs posterior-to-anterior differentiation
- Wnt influences dorsal-to-ventral differentiation

NORMAL VARIANTS

Many normal variants of growth and development cause parental concern. The common problems relate to tripping and falling, an intoeing gait, bowlegs, knock knees and flat feet. In general, if they are symmetrical, symptom-free and in an otherwise normal child, they require no intervention. If the

Carl Hueter, 1838–1882, Professor of Surgery, University of Greifswald, Germany.
Richard von Volkmann, 1830–1889, Professor of Surgery, Halle, Germany.
Julius Wolff, 1836–1902, Professor of Orthopaedic Surgery, Berlin, Germany.

child fails to achieve their developmental milestones or there are functional problems, further investigation may be required.

Intoeing gait

Intoeing is defined as a negative foot progression angle and results from one or more lower limb torsional anomalies (*Figure 44.1 and Table 44.2*).

Persistent femoral neck anteversion presents clinically with excessive internal rotation at the hip joint, which is best assessed with the patient prone (*Figure 44.2a*). All femurs are anteverted at birth but as the femur lengthens it rotates with spontaneous improvement in the anteversion. If, by 10–12 years, a persistent deformity is associated with functional difficulties, corrective osteotomy may be justified. In such cases, the child has no ability to externally rotate the extended hip. In others, compensatory external tibial torsion may develop, in which case the foot progression angle will be normal but the child may have symptoms of the miserable malalignment syndrome, including knee pain and feelings of instability.

TABLE 44.2 Common sites and causes of intoeing gait in childhood.

Site	Cause
Femur/hip	Persistent femoral neck anteversion
Tibia	Internal tibial torsion
Foot	Metatarsus adductus

Internal tibial torsion is assessed by the thigh–foot angle and is commonly associated with physiological tibia vara in infants (*Figure 44.2b*). Spontaneous correction occurs by age 4, as the tibia rotates with growth.

Metatarsus adductus (*Figure 44.2c*) is usually flexible and corrects by age 2–4 years. For the more rigid foot, stretching, with or without plaster casts or straight-last shoes, may help. Surgical release is rarely indicated.

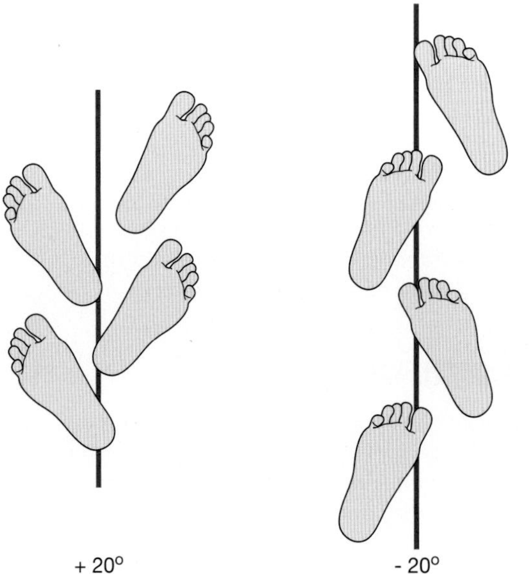

Figure 44.1 Foot progression angle: a positive angle represents an extoeing gait; a negative angle, an intoeing gait.

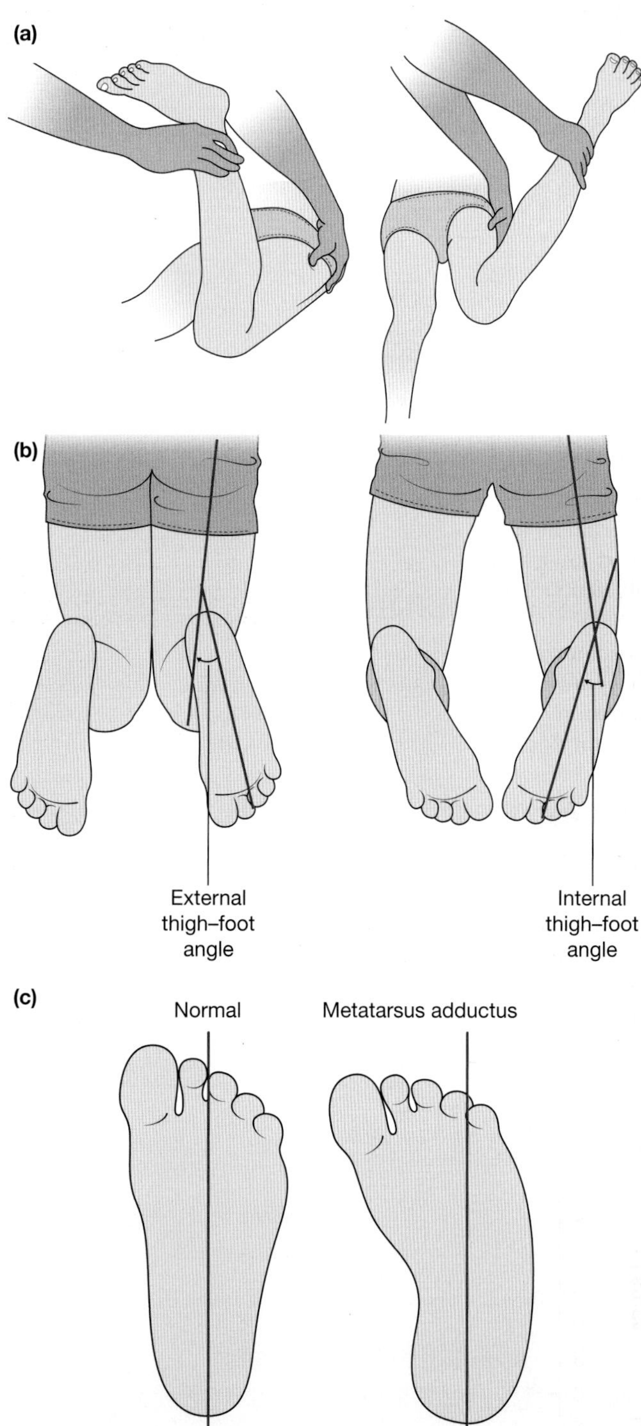

Figure 44.2 Assessment of the torsional profile: all assessments are done with the child prone. (a) Femoral neck anteversion measured as the range of internal hip rotation with the hip extended and the knee flexed. Craig's test measures the degree of internal rotation present when the greater trochanter is at its most prominent (also called the trochanteric prominence test). (b) The thigh–foot angle measures the angle between the relaxed hindfoot and the thigh. (c) The bean-shaped foot of metatarsus adductus viewed from above: a curved lateral border with/without a medial crease.

Other abnormalities of gait

Extoeing is less common but results from relative femoral retroversion, external tibial torsion or flexible flat feet. The child may walk late because of poor balance associated with the foot posture and overall alignment. Gait improves with growth/time.

Toe walking is a phase in normal gait development. If the gait does not mature to a heel–toe pattern by 3 years, physiotherapy may help, and older children benefit from surgical lengthening of a contracted gastrocsoleus complex, if it is present. If toe walking starts after walking age, a spinal or neuromuscular aetiology such as a tethered cord or a muscular dystrophy must be considered; in the unilateral case, an orthopaedic cause for a short leg, such as a dislocated hip, must be excluded.

Knock knees and bowlegs

All children start life with bowlegs, often accompanied by internal tibial torsion. By the age of 2–3 years they have developed knock knees, which regress towards the normal adult tibiofemoral angle of 7° valgus by age 7 (*Figure 44.3*).

The intercondylar or intermalleolar distance is often used to quantify the deformity but radiographs are needed when the deformity is severe, asymmetrical or symptomatic. The most common pathological causes are previous trauma, rickets or a skeletal dysplasia.

Flat foot

All children (<3 years) have flat feet with a fat pad obscuring the arch. Over time, the longitudinal arch develops but 15% of adults have flat feet influenced by familial and racial factors.

All flat feet have a flattened medial arch with a valgus heel but two types are distinguishable (*Table 44.3*). The painless, flexible flat foot needs no treatment. Orthoses **do not** alter the natural history but can alleviate symptoms **if** they are present.

The symptomatic, rigid flat foot is due to inflammation or a tarsal coalition and requires investigation and medical or surgical management (*Figure 44.4*).

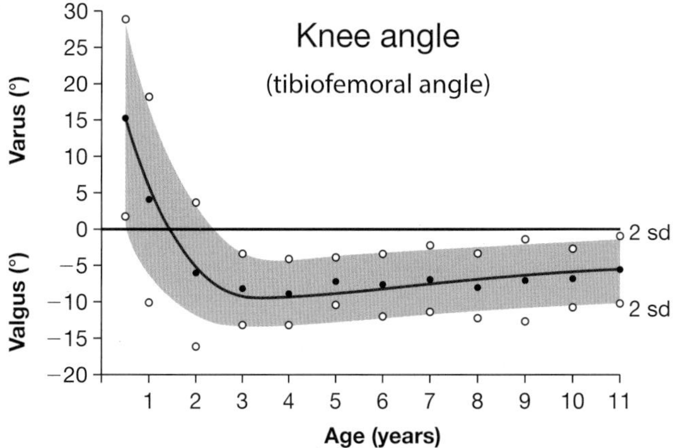

Figure 44.3 Graph to show the normal tendency of limb alignment to change from varus to valgus with growth; normal is slight valgus after the age of 7–8 years.

TABLE 44.3 Flat feet.

Type	Characteristics
Flexible	• On tiptoe the arch returns and the heel corrects into varus • Subtalar joint movements are full and pain free
Rigid	• On tiptoe the arch fails to return and the heel remains in valgus • Subtalar joint movements are restricted and often painful

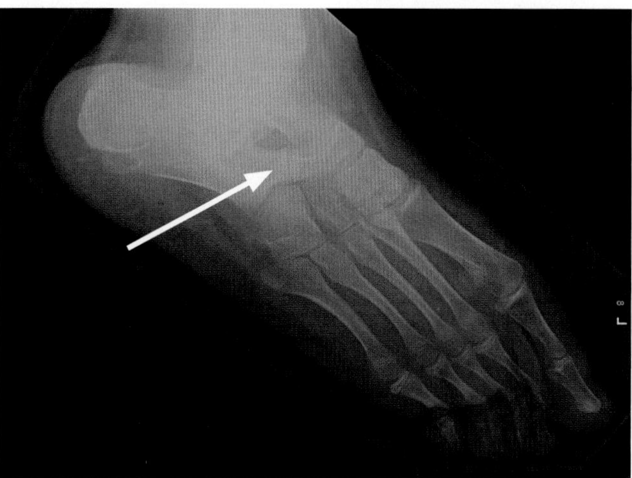

Figure 44.4 Oblique radiograph of the foot that shows the most common form of tarsal coalition: an incomplete calcaneonavicular bar (arrow).

Summary box 44.2

Normal variants

- Legs are often bowed until age 2 years and then knock-kneed until age 6–7 years
- Neuromuscular pathology must be excluded in toe walkers, particularly when the onset is late
- Intoeing or extoeing is associated with excessive femoral or tibial torsion or foot deformity
- Flexible, pain-free flat feet require no treatment

Postural abnormalities

Many babies are subjected to moulding pressures *in utero*. At birth they exhibit 'postural abnormalities', such as torticollis, calcaneovalgus feet and plagiocephaly, which improve with time and/or stretching exercises.

CONGENITAL AND DEVELOPMENTAL ABNORMALITIES OF THE SKELETON

Although many skeletal abnormalities are identified antenatally or at birth, others become apparent with growth. Skeletal disorders are often linked to focal or generalised soft-tissue abnormalities; the presence of a skin dimple or a vascular malformation should be a 'red flag', as should the 'featureless' limbs of a child with arthrogryposis multiplex congenita (AMC) (*Table 44.4 and Figure 44.5*).

TABLE 44.4 Classification of congenital limb malformations.

Category	Example
Failure of formation of parts	
• Transverse	• Congenital amputation of the forearm/lower limb
• Longitudinal	• Fibula hemimelia
Failure of differentiation	Radioulnar synostosis; vertebral body fusion
Duplication	Extra digits
Overgrowth	Gigantism; macrodactyly
Undergrowth	
Congenital constriction band syndrome	Often affects hands/feet with poor formation of the digits distally
Generalised skeletal abnormalities	Skeletal dysplasia, e.g. achondroplasia

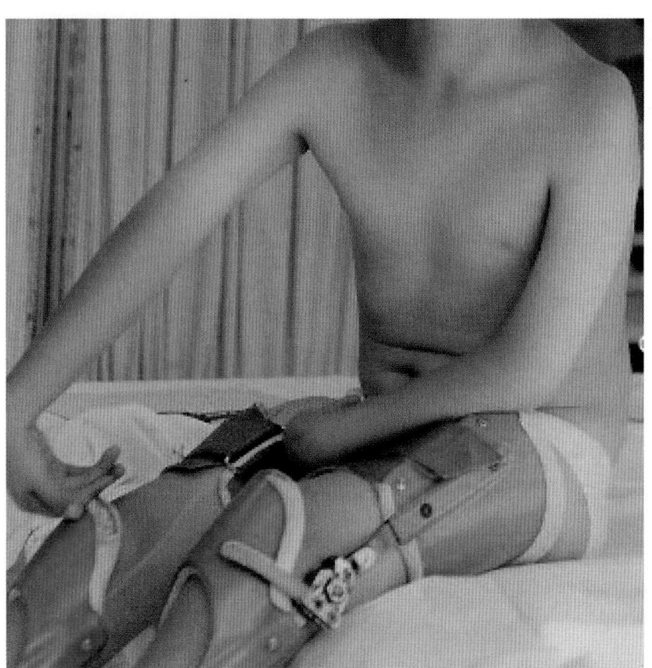

Figure 44.5 A child with arthrogryposis multiplex congenita and featureless upper limbs (no skin creases or muscle definition). He mobilises with the help of knee–ankle–foot orthoses.

Many anomalies require little treatment and cause minimal functional disability whereas others, such as proximal femoral focal deficiency (PFFD), pose considerable challenges to both the patient and their doctors. In these cases the functional and cosmetic needs of the child and family must be balanced against available resources and expertise (*Figure 44.6*). Despite advances in limb reconstruction techniques there are few high-quality data from skeletally mature patients to support their widespread use. Concurrently, significant advances are occurring with amputation prosthetics, which may result in better patient-reported outcome scores (PROMSs), particularly in certain regions.

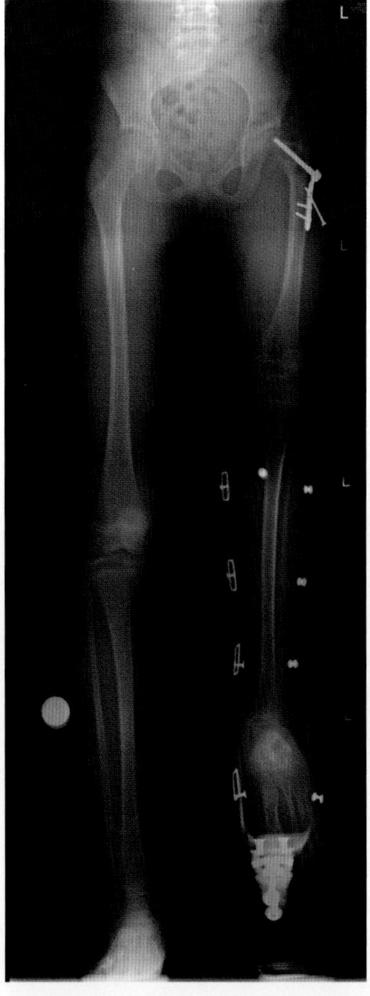

Figure 44.6 Radiograph of a child born with proximal femoral focal deficiency. A proximal femoral osteotomy improved her hip mechanics and stability (a screw has come loose from the plate). She opted to keep her foot and not to undergo leg lengthening. She functions well with an extension prosthesis.

Generalised skeletal dysplasias

Achondroplasia

Achondroplasia is caused by a gain-in-function mutation in the FGFR3 (fibroblast growth factor receptor 3) gene, located on the short arm of chromosome (Chr) 4, which affects enchondral bone formation. It is autosomal dominant. Patients present with disproportionate short stature where the limbs are shorter than the trunk, together with classical clinical and radiographic features (*Figure 44.7*).

Underdevelopment of the foramen magnum and spinal stenosis can cause neurological difficulties. Correction of limb alignment may be necessary and limb-lengthening techniques are used in some countries.

Hereditary multiple exostoses

An autosomal dominant condition related to a loss-of-function mutation in either the *EXT1* (Chr 8q) or *EXT2* gene (Chr 11p), leads to dysregulated growth and exostosis formation. Exostoses consisting of a cartilaginous cap on a bony stalk may be sessile or pedunculated. They grow as the child grows and may cause cosmetic or functional difficulties, justifying excision. Differential growth between the paired bones of the forearm and lower leg can lead to joint deformity and dislocation of the radial head, exacerbated by the effects of altered mechanical forces on growth. Treatment aims to prevent deformity (*Figure 44.8*). Continued growth after skeletal maturity may represent malignant transformation of a benign osteochondroma: a rare occurrence (see ***Chapter 42***).

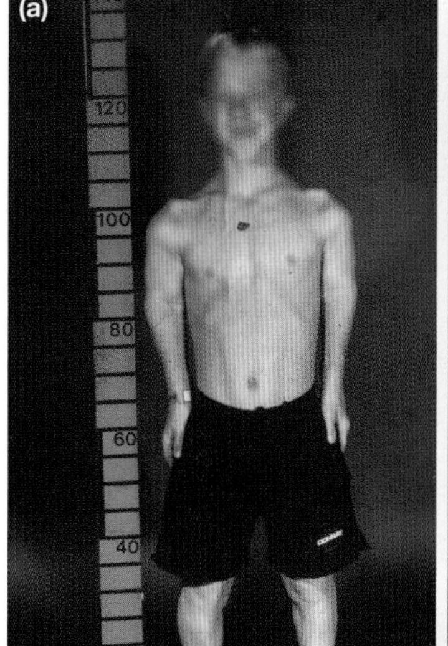

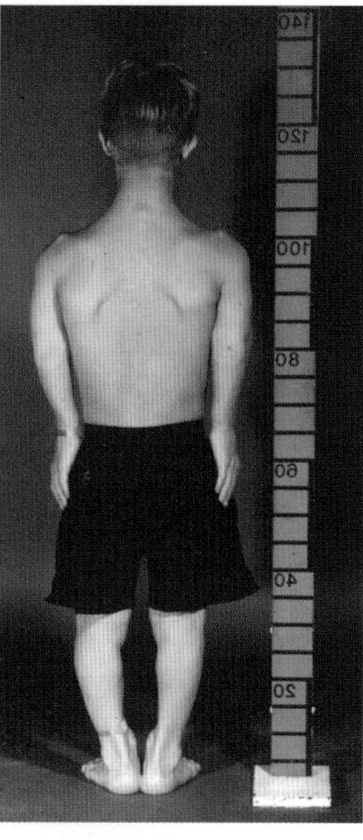

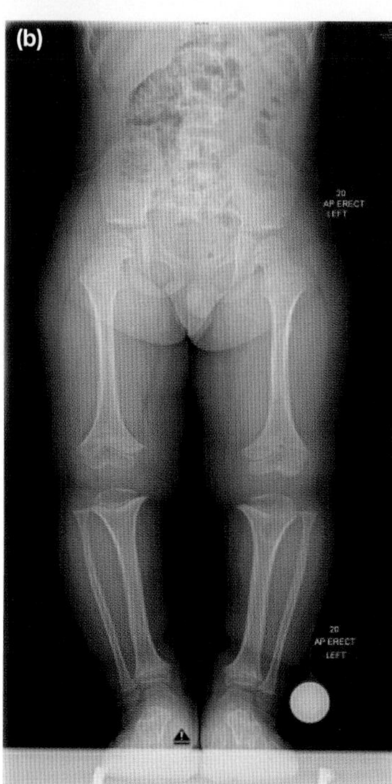

Figure 44.7 Achondroplasia. (a) A child with achondroplasia: his upper limbs are short and his hands do not reach midthigh. (b) Standing leg length/alignment radiograph of a different child demonstrating short limbs, widened metaphysis, an overlong fibula and slight bowing. The acetabulum is horizontal and the pelvic wings seem square: classical features of achondroplasia.

Enchondromatosis (Ollier's disease)

Enchondromas arise from chondrocyte rests within the medullary canal of tubular bones: they consist of mature hyaline cartilage (*Figure 44.9*). Larger lesions may show calcification on radiographs and vertical lucent streaks (representing cartilage columns) in the metaphysis. Pathological fractures are common. In Maffucci's syndrome there are also soft-tissue haemangiomas and lymphangiomas (see ***Chapter 42***).

Fibrous dysplasia

This common disorder is often a chance radiographic finding, particularly in its monostotic form. It is a localised defect in osteoblastic differentiation and maturation in which normal bone is replaced by fibrous stroma. With polyostotic fibrous dysplasia, limb deformity and pathological fractures are common. In patients with precocious puberty and Coast of Maine café-au-lait spots, the diagnosis is McCune–Albright syndrome (*Figure 44.10*).

Summary box 44.3

Congenital and developmental abnormalities of the skeleton

- Achondroplasia affects enchondral ossification and presents with disproportionate short stature
- Exostoses may cause functional and/or cosmetic problems
- Patients with Ollier's disease (multiple enchondromatosis) often have lesions in the hands and feet

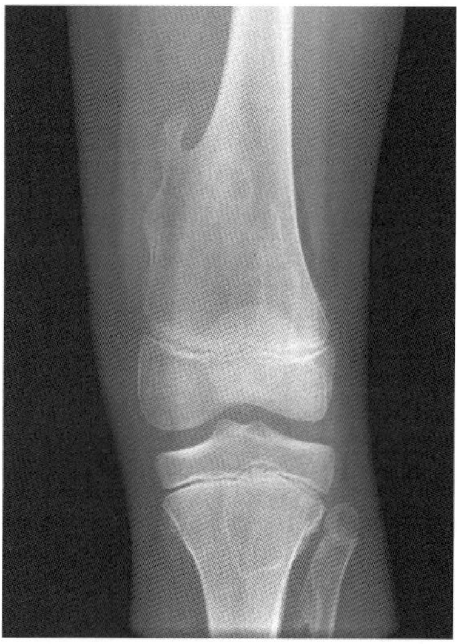

Figure 44.8 Radiograph of the knee showing multiple broad-based osteochondromas.

Louis Xavier Edouard Léopold Ollier, 1830–1900, Professor of Surgery, Lyons, France, described enchondromatosis in 1899.
Angelo Maffucci, 1845–1903, Professor of Pathological Anatomy, Pisa, Italy, described enchondromatosis in association with soft-tissue haemangiomas in 1881.
Donovan James McCune, 1902–1976, American paediatrician.
Fuller Albright, 1900–1969, physician, Massachusetts General Hospital, Boston, MA, USA.

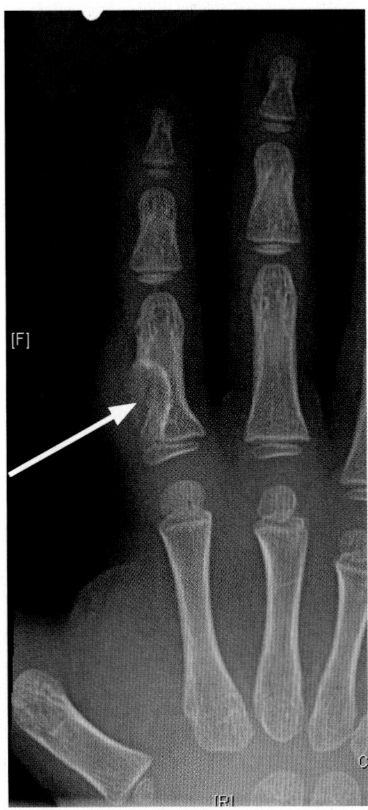

Figure 44.9 Anteroposterior radiograph of the index finger of a child showing a solitary enchondroma (arrow): note the opacity in the soft tissues, which represents the extent of the cartilaginous lesion.

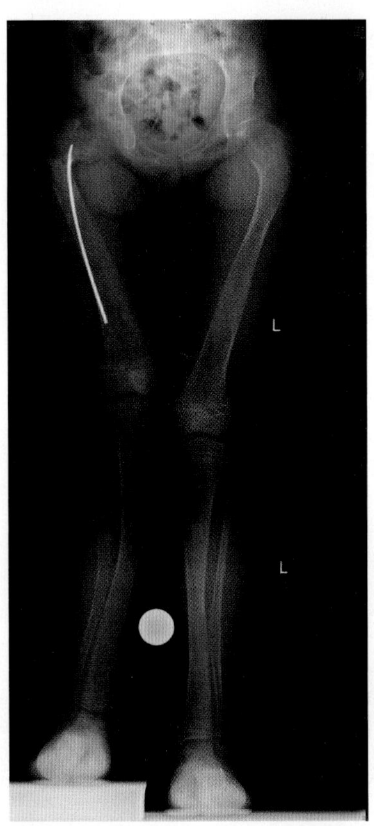

Figure 44.10 Standing leg length/alignment radiograph of a child with polyostotic fibrous dysplasia. The diaphyseal lesions have a 'ground-glass' appearance. The bones are often deformed and the limb may be short, as seen on the right. The femur has fractured previously and one intramedullary nail remains in place.

METABOLIC BONE DISEASE

Rickets

In rickets, the primary problem is inadequate mineralisation of growing bone (***Table 44.5***). In severe cases the classic radiographic features are seen at all physes with significant deformity (***Figure 44.11***). Medical treatment improves mineralisation and deformity corrects with growth. Once the medical condition has stabilised, surgery may be indicated to treat residual limb deformity. Guided growth techniques are often used in preference to osteotomies.

TABLE 44.5 Common causes of rickets.

Nutritional	Reduced intake of vitamin D and calcium
Environmental	Inadequate exposure to sunlight
Gastrointestinal disease	Crohn's disease, gluten-sensitive enteropathy
Genetic	X-linked hypophosphataemia (excess FGF23 production)
Renal disease	End-stage renal failure, renal tubular anomalies Secondary hyperparathyroidism may be present

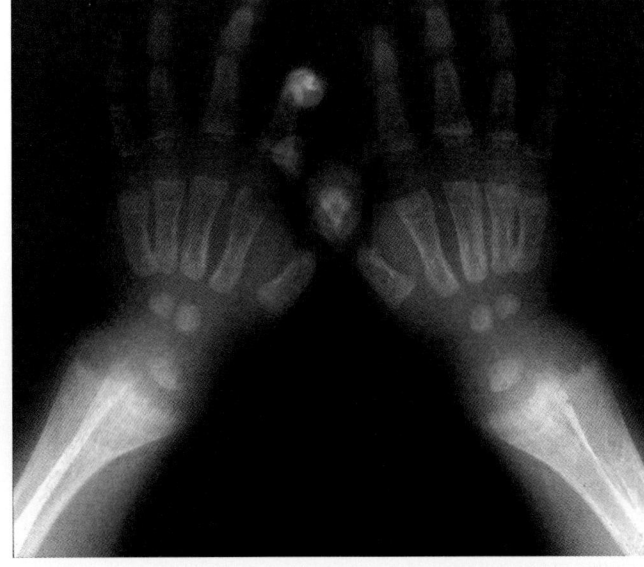

Figure 44.11 Radiographs in cases of rickets demonstrate widened physes with cupped, flared metaphyses.

Burrill Bernard Crohn, 1884–1983, gastroenterologist, Mount Sinai Hospital, New York, NY, USA, described regional ileitis in 1932.

Osteogenesis imperfecta (brittle bone disease)

Osteogenesis imperfecta (OI) represents a spectrum of conditions linked by a qualitative and/or quantitative abnormality of collagen production. Most identified mutations affect the collagen genes. The bone may break easily but it heals promptly and well. All structures containing collagen may be affected, accounting for the ligamentous laxity, blue sclerae and poor teeth in some phenotypes.

Cyclical bisphosphonate treatment decreases bone resorption and turnover. This reduces bone pain and the fracture rate, promoting weight-bearing mobility and bone strength (*Figure 44.12*).

Following fracture, treatment options range from simple casting techniques to more specialised surgical procedures to correct/maintain bony alignment while allowing growth. Intramedullary techniques for stabilisation of fractures or osteotomies are preferred to plate fixation. Rehabilitation should start promptly.

Summary box 44.4

Metabolic bone disease

- Rickets, from nutritional or other causes, is characterised by a failure of bone mineralisation
  - X-linked hypophosphataemic rickets is a dominant condition, affecting boys and girls; in some countries, treatment is with monoclonal FGF23 antibodies
- In OI:
  - There is defective type I collagen production
  - In severe forms frequent fractures lead to progressive deformity, which in turn increases fracture risk
  - Systemic treatment with bisphosphonates reduces the fracture rate

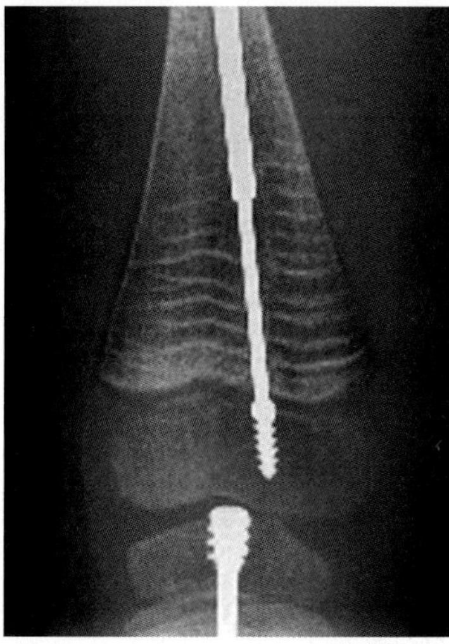

Figure 44.12 Radiograph of a child with osteogenesis imperfecta who has been treated with cyclical bisphosphonates. Multiple growth lines are visible in addition to intramedullary devices in both the femur and tibia.

ABNORMALITIES OF THE HIP

Developmental dysplasia of the hip

DDH defines the spectrum of hip instability, ranging from the hip that is in joint but has a shallow (dysplastic) acetabulum and may be 'pushed out' (Barlow positive) to the dislocated hip that is irreducible (Ortolani negative). The clinical picture varies with the pathology and the age at presentation: neonatal hips may be unstable, a toddler may limp, adolescents may experience exercise-induced pain and an adult may have pain secondary to degenerative arthritis.

Incidence

The incidence of neonatal instability is approximately 20 per 1000 live births, whereas that of true dislocation is approximately 2 per 1000 live births; many hips stabilise spontaneously.

Aetiology of developmental dysplasia of the hip

- **Gender**. Four to five times more common in girls, possibly related to hormonal factors causing temporary joint laxity in the peripartum period.
- **Breech presentation**. More common in breech babies, particularly with the extended breech position.
- **Birth order**. More common in firstborns and in the left hip because of the common fetal position (left occipito-anterior) in a tight primigravid uterus where movement is restricted.
- **Oligohydramnios**. Restricts fetal movement. The presence of other postural deformities (torticollis and metatarsus adductus) raises the possibility of DDH.
- **Family history**. A positive family history significantly increases the risk of DDH.
- **Regional and racial variation**. More common in certain regions and in certain races because of a combination of genetic, environmental and cultural factors.
  - Swaddling the legs together exacerbates hip instability, whereas carrying the baby astride the carer's hip or back encourages hip flexion and abduction that improve stability.

Hip dislocation is often found in association with generalised syndromes or neuromuscular conditions. These teratological hips are often resistant to the simpler treatments and a holistic approach to the child's overall condition and prognosis must be taken.

Diagnosis

Neonate

- **Clinical assessment and screening**. In many countries, neonates are screened for limitation of hip abduction and hip joint instability. In the UK, as part of the newborn and infant physical examination (NIPE) guidelines, the hips are examined again at 6 weeks. The knees and hips are flexed and the thigh held by the examiner with the thumb

Thomas Geoffrey Barlow, 1915–1975, orthopaedic surgeon, Salford Royal Hospital, Salford, UK.
Marius Ortolani, 1904–1987, orthopaedic surgeon, Instituto Provinciale Per L'Infanzia di Ferrara, Italy, described this test in 1937.

along the medial aspect and a finger behind the greater trochanter. The hips are abducted gently: if abduction is limited, the hip may be dislocated. The examiner's finger then lifts the greater trochanter upwards; a soft clunk – the **Ortolani test** – with improved hip abduction signifies hip reduction (***Figure 44.13a***). If the hip does abduct fully, then the flexed hip is brought back to neutral and then adducted while downward pressure is applied to the knee with the examiner's thumb and palm: an unstable hip may dislocate or sublux – the **Barlow test** (***Figure 44.13b***). With an irreducible hip there is no clunk of reduction but there will be limitation of abduction. Bilateral dislocation may be missed because abduction is symmetrical and abduction may be normal when there is low muscle tone and joint laxity. In a dislocated hip, the femoral head may be palpable in the buttock.
- **Ultrasonographic assessment**. Ultrasonography defines the anatomy and the stability of the hip joint. It is used as a screening tool (universally or selectively for 'at-risk' patients) (***Figure 44.14***). Screening scans should be performed between 4 and 6 weeks of age and treatment, when necessary, started by 6 weeks. The sonographic appearance of most hips improves (in terms of both hip stability and acetabular dysplasia) spontaneously as the baby grows.
- **Radiography**. Plain radiographs are used from 4–5 months of age, when the relationship of the femoral ossific nucleus to the acetabulum can be assessed; late ossification of the nucleus is common in DDH (***Figure 44.15***).

Infant

Hip checks, looking for limitation of abduction in more than 90° of flexion and limb shortening, are part of developmental monitoring.

Child

Children present with a Trendelenburg gait and/or unilateral tiptoeing, as the affected leg is short. Abduction in flexion is limited and there may be an extra thigh crease. The signs may be subtle and easily missed in an unsteady toddler. If both hips are affected there will be a waddling gait and a lumbar lordosis.

Adolescent

Discomfort after exercise is common but the pain may be in the knee.

In all age groups, radiographs may show dysplasia, subluxation or dislocation.

Summary box 44.5

The neonatal clinical examination must ask and answer the following questions:

- Is the hip dislocated?
  - If so, is it reducible (Ortolani positive) or not (Ortolani negative)?
- If the hip is not dislocated, is it dislocatable (or subluxable)?
  - If so, it is Barlow positive
- If the hip is not dislocated or dislocatable, is it clinically normal?
  - If so, do the risk factors in the history still demand further assessment with an ultrasound scan or plain radiograph?

Summary box 44.6

Diagnosis of DDH

- Based on the history and clinical examination and confirmed by appropriate investigations
- All neonates are screened clinically (Barlow and Ortolani tests) at birth and at 6 weeks
- Ultrasound is used as a selective screening test in 'at-risk' babies
- Radiography is useful from 4 months onwards
- Older children present with a limp and/or tiptoeing and a lumbar lordosis in bilateral cases

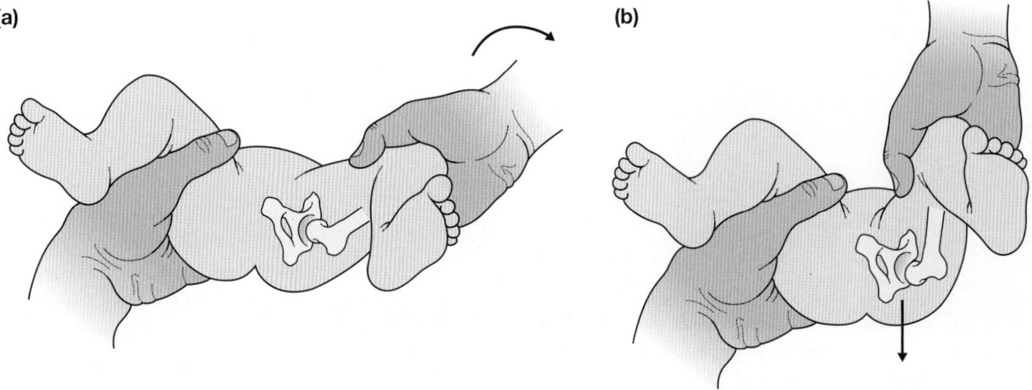

Figure 44.13 Line diagram illustrating the **(a)** Ortolani and **(b)** Barlow tests for developmental dysplasia of the hip. For the Barlow test the femur must be at 90° to the bed.

Friedrich Trendelenburg, 1844–1924, successively Professor of Surgery at Rostock (1875–1882), Bonn (1822–1895) and Leipzig (1895–1911), Germany.

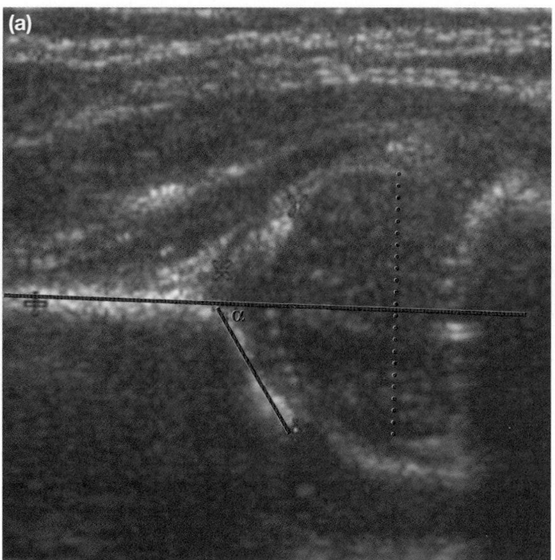

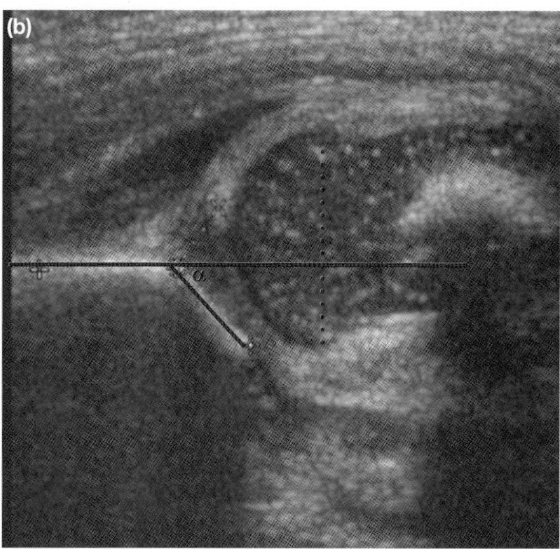

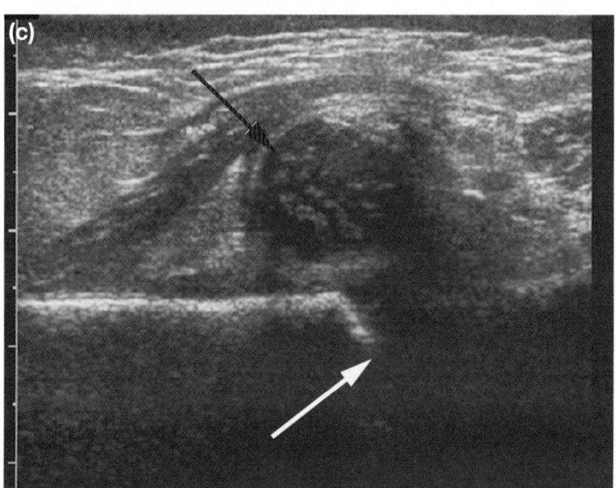

Figure 44.14 Ultrasound images of an infant hip. (a) Normal hip with a high α angle and a Morin index of 50% (defined as the percentage of the femoral head covered by the acetabulum, i.e. the portion lying below the horizontal red line). (b) Grossly dysplastic hip with a low α angle and a Morin index of <50%. This hip is likely to be unstable on dynamic ultrasound scanning, i.e. Barlow positive. (c) A dislocated hip joint (dislocated femoral head, red arrow; 'empty' acetabulum, white arrow).

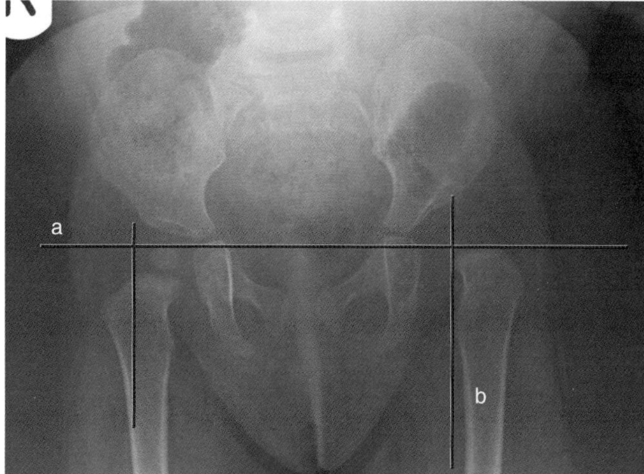

Figure 44.15 Anteroposterior pelvic radiograph showing Hilgenreiner's line (a) and Perkins' line (b). The femoral head (ossific nucleus) of a normal hip lies in the inner lower quadrant. The right hip is normal; the left hip has developmental dysplasia of the hip.

Management

The objective is to obtain a stable, congruous reduction of the femoral head within the acetabulum while avoiding damage to the capital epiphysis (avascular necrosis [AVN]), which causes stiffness and proximal femoral deformity.

Neonate

Owing to the peripartum hormonal effects many neonatal hips are unstable. Most stabilise spontaneously by 6 weeks.

Hips that remain unstable or that are dislocated at rest are treated with harnesses or splints that obtain and maintain reduction with the hip abducted and flexed. Joint stability is monitored with ultrasound scanning. Most harnesses (***Figure 44.16***) allow controlled movement while splints hold the hips more rigidly and may carry a greater risk of AVN and femoral nerve palsy. If the hips fail to relocate or stabilise, treatment should be discontinued.

Infant

Successful harness treatment is unusual after the age of 4–6 months. For the late-presenting hip or one that fails conservative treatment, an examination under anaesthetic may achieve a closed reduction. A psoas/adductor release can

Christian Morin, contemporary, French paediatric orthopaedic surgeon.
Heinrich Hilgenreiner, 1870–1954, German surgeon and orthopaedist.
George Perkins, 1892–1980, Professor of Surgery, St Thomas' Hospital, London, UK, described signs by which to diagnose congenital dislocation of the hip in 1928.

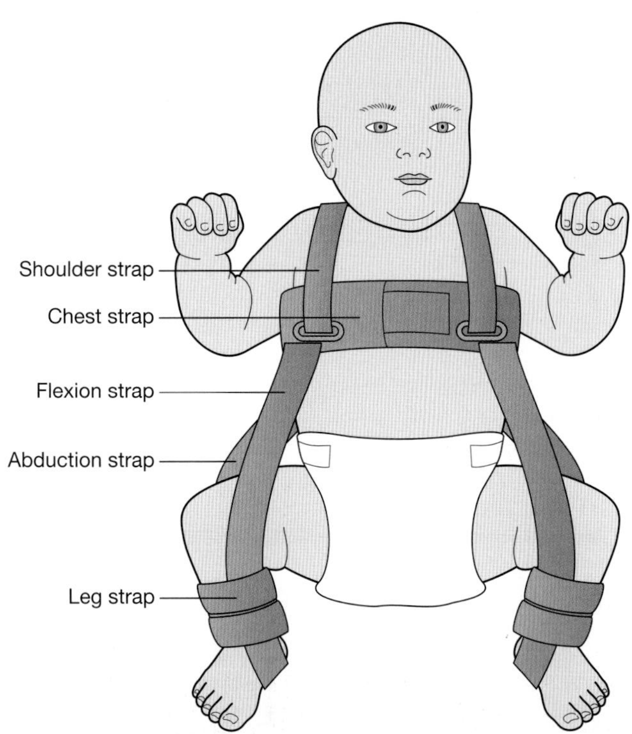

Figure 44.16 The anterior strap of the Pavlik harness controls hip flexion, whereas the posterior strap limits adduction and encourages abduction.

be performed if the arthrogram suggests they are blocking reduction or limiting stability. Postoperatively, a spica cast maintains hip reduction.

If the hip is irreducible or can only be held reduced in an extreme position then treatment should be abandoned and an open reduction considered via a medial or anterior approach.

Summary box 44.7

Management of early DDH

- Many hips that are unstable in the first 2–3 weeks of life require no treatment as they improve spontaneously
- Up to age 4–6 months, a harness or splint is effective treatment
- In older babies, closed reduction is often possible
- For failed closed treatment, open surgical reduction is required

Child

A medial approach open reduction can be performed between 6 and 24 months of age. An anterior approach to the hip (from 9–12 months of age) allows for a simultaneous capsulorrhaphy. In the older child, a pelvic osteotomy may be required to reorientate the acetabulum, and femoral shortening or derotation osteotomies will improve stability (*Figure 44.17*).

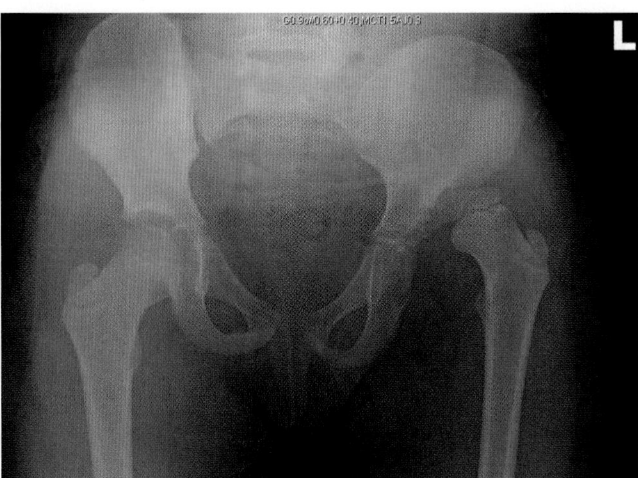

Figure 44.17 Anteroposterior pelvic radiograph showing acetabular dysplasia with subluxation (developmental dysplasia of the hip) of the left hip. This child presented at age 7 years.

Surgery is contraindicated in children over the age of 6–8 years in bilateral cases and the age of 8–10 years in unilateral cases (*Figure 44.18*).

Adolescent

Hips are often dysplastic and subluxated. If the hip is reducible, the joint can be reconstructed with a combination of pelvic and femoral osteotomies. For the irreducible hip, acetabular augmentation may reduce symptoms and delay the onset of degenerative change.

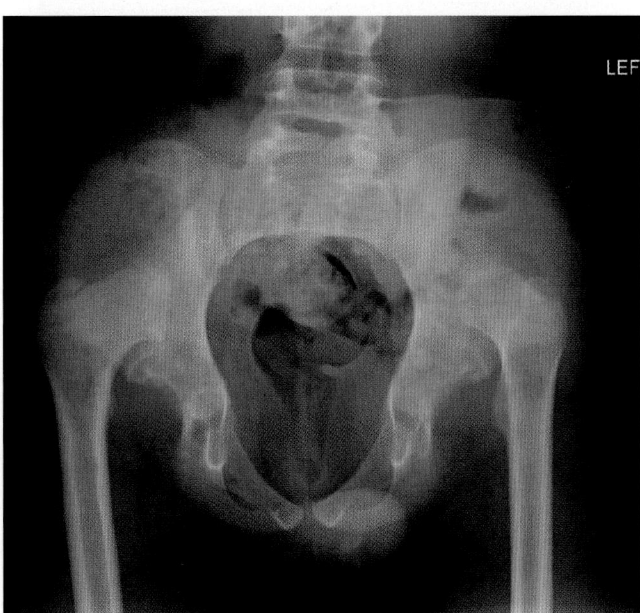

Figure 44.18 Anteroposterior pelvic radiograph showing bilateral true dislocations in a 9-year-old child; the decision was made not to offer an operation. The pathology in these hips is different from that shown in *Figure 44.17*.

Arnold Pavlik, 1902–1962, Czech orthopaedic surgeon, became famous mainly for the development of a functional, active method of treating developmental dysplasia of the hip.

Summary box 44.8

Management of late-presenting DDH

- The older the child, the more likely it is that they will require surgery
- Femoral osteotomy improves hip stability
- Pelvic osteotomy redirects or reshapes the acetabulum
- The potential for acetabular remodelling decreases after the age of 3–4 years
- Avascular necrosis is a risk with all DDH treatment

Secondary procedures and complications

At follow-up, acetabular remodelling is assessed with the acetabular index or the centre–edge angle (***Figure 44.19***). Surgery may be required for residual dysplasia or subluxation. AVN with trochanteric overgrowth causes a Trendelenburg limp: the outcome is poor (***Figure 44.20***). Occasionally, a leg length difference needs treatment. There is an increased risk of osteoarthritis and hip arthroplasty later in life.

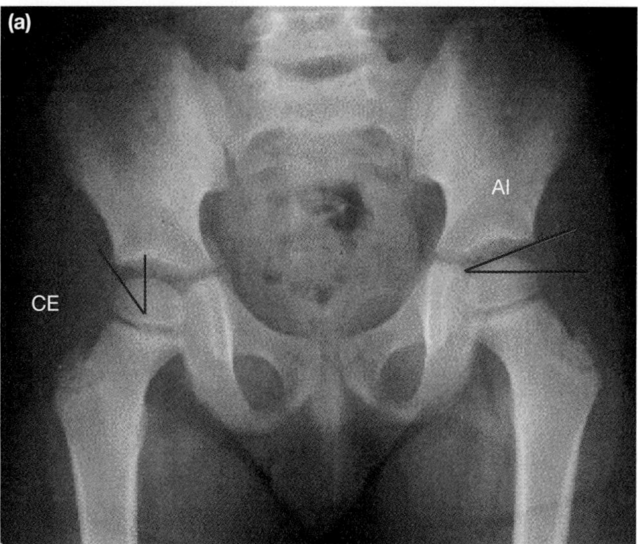

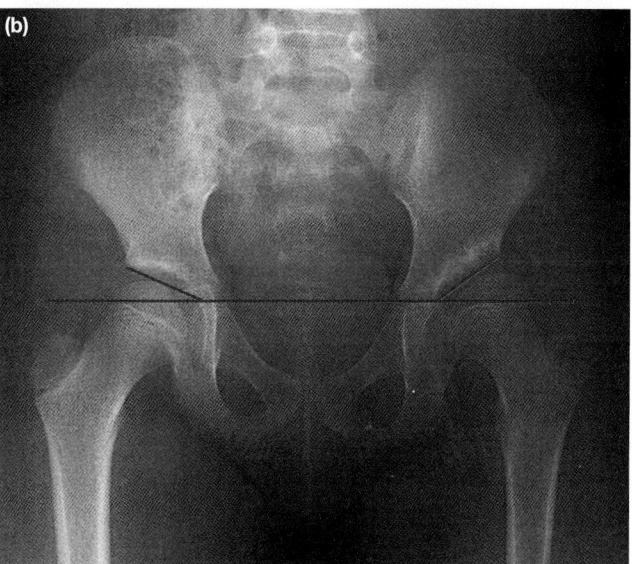

Figure 44.19 Anteroposterior pelvic radiographs demonstrating the acetabular index (AI) and the centre–edge (CE) angle: (a) normal hips; (b) the left hip shows residual dysplasia. The AI is increased when compared with the normal right hip. The left CE angle would be smaller too, but it has not been measured on this radiograph.

Legg-Calvé-Perthes disease

Incidence and aetiology

This rare condition, characterised by the development of AVN of the proximal femoral epiphysis, predominantly affects boys aged 4–7 years; 10% develop bilateral disease. Although the aetiology is unclear, factors such as socioeconomic deprivation and passive smoking have been implicated. Other causes of femoral head AVN must be considered, particularly in bilateral cases (***Table 44.6***).

TABLE 44.6 Causes of avascular necrosis of the femoral head.

- Steroids
- Infection/surgery/previous injury
- Perthes' disease
- Sickle cell disease
- Hypothyroidism
- Multiple epiphyseal dysplasia will show AVN-like appearances in both femoral heads

Pathology

Once established the process follows a well-described course. The avascular change may affect all or part of the femoral epiphysis. If the avascular bone collapses, this is followed by revascularisation, resorption and fragmentation of the dead ossific nucleus within the cartilaginous femoral head, and finally by reossification and regeneration ('healing') of the bony epiphysis. In this respect, Perthes' disease is a self-limiting condition but, during the collapse and fragmentation phases, femoral head deformity occurs as the cartilage 'follows' the shape of the reossifying epiphysis. This change in shape is irreversible and has a permanent effect on hip function.

Diagnosis

The history, clinical examination and anteroposterior and 'frog' lateral pelvic radiographs make the diagnosis. An intermittently painful hip (or knee) with a limp and irritability or restriction of hip movements requires investigation. The radiographic features vary with the disease stage and may not correlate with the clinical condition (***Figure 44.21***).

Legg, Calvé and Perthes all described osteochondritis of the head of the femur independently in 1910.
Arthur Thornton Legg, 1874–1939, orthopaedic surgeon, The Children's Hospital, Boston, MA, USA.
Jacques Calvé, 1875–1927, orthopaedic surgeon, La Fondation Franco-Americaine, Berck Plage, Pas-de-Calais, France.
Georg Clemens Perthes, 1869–1927, Professor of Surgery, Tübingen, Germany.

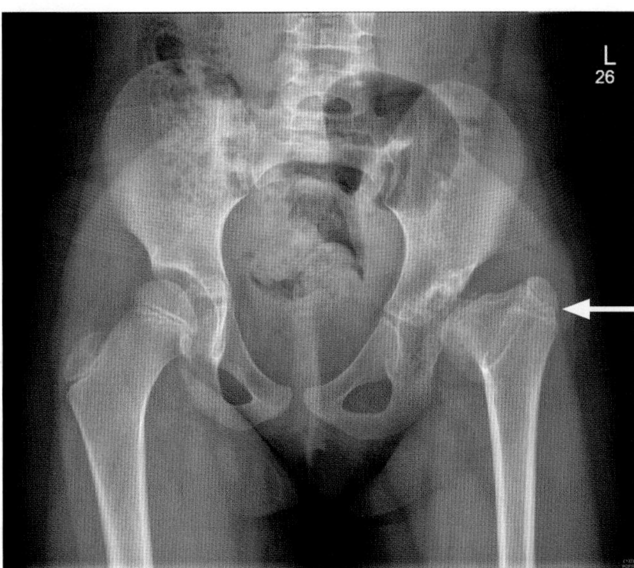

Figure 44.20 Anteroposterior pelvic radiograph of a 7-year-old girl who developed avascular necrosis secondary to a postoperative wound infection following a closed reduction of her dislocated left hip. Note the destruction of the femoral head and the proximal femoral physis, so that the femoral neck is short and the greater trochanter relatively high (arrow).

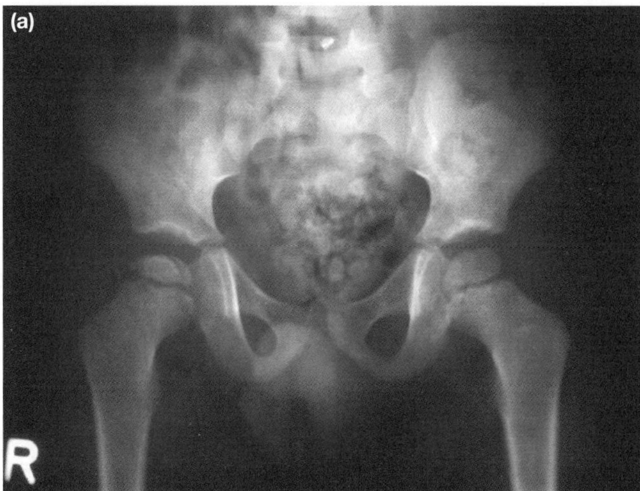

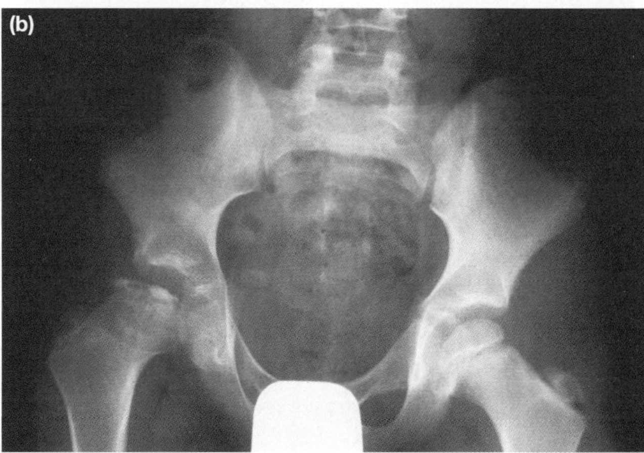

Figure 44.21 Anteroposterior pelvic radiographs of Perthes' disease demonstrating whole head involvement: (a) right-sided disease; the process is in an early phase and the area of dense necrotic bone is visible; (b) there has been collapse and fragmentation. The Herring classification relates to the height of the lateral pillar (lateral portion of the epiphysis) in the fragmentation phase of the disease.

Management

The prognosis, and hence the management, is influenced by the extent of AVN and the degree of collapse. The Herring classification is popular but can only be applied when the head is in the fragmentation phase. If the anterolateral portion of the head is preserved, the prognosis is good.

Treatment aims to minimise femoral head deformity and the risk of secondary acetabular dysplasia by maintaining a good range of joint movement with analgesia and physiotherapy. The use of crutches and/or wheelchairs is discouraged because they promote a flexion/adduction posture. Brace management does not alter the natural history.

The role of operative treatment is controversial. Surgery can be performed early to prevent deformity secondary to femoral head collapse or late to 'salvage' a poor mechanical situation when deformity is limiting movement (***Table 44.7***).

Summary box 44.9

Legg-Calvé-Perthes disease

- Most common in boys aged 4–7 years
- AVN leads to femoral head collapse; the return of the blood supply heralds the resorption and reossification phases that allow the femoral head to 'heal'
- The prognosis is better in younger children (and in boys), who have more remodelling potential before skeletal maturity
- Management aims to maintain femoral head sphericity
- Treatment may be non-surgical (to maximise range of movement) or surgical (early for containment or late for 'salvage')

Not all hips with deformity require 'salvage' surgery: young children, with more time to remodel, have a better prognosis as the acetabular changes (in response to the altered femoral head shape) result in an aspherical but congruent joint. Degenerative change may occur in adult life.

Slip of the capital (upper) femoral epiphysis (SCFE/SUFE)

The physis connects the proximal femoral epiphysis (the femoral head) to the metaphysis (femoral neck). In certain physiological or pathological conditions a 'stress fracture' through the physis allows the epiphysis to displace as it would with an intracapsular femoral neck fracture, so the leg lies short and externally

John A Herring, contemporary, pediatric orthopedic surgeon, chief of staff emeritus, Texas Scottish Rite Hospital for Children, and professor, UT Southwestern Medical Center, Dallas, TX, USA.

TABLE 44.7 A guide to some of the surgical options available for the management of Perthes' disease.

Timing	Type of procedure	Comments	Aim
Early	Femoral osteotomy	• Varus and derotation • Consider an opening wedge osteotomy to maintain length	To cover ('contain') the vulnerable femoral head
	Innominate osteotomy		
	Shelf acetabuloplasty		
Intermediate	Arthrodiastasis	Hinged distraction to allow movement, primarily flexion/extension	To reduce deforming pressures on the femoral head
Late	Femoral osteotomy	• Valgus • With extension to undo a fixed flexion deformity or flexion to remove the anterior bump from impinging on the acetabulum	To improve joint congruity and hence function; to improve joint mechanics
	Arthrotomy	To remove osteochondral fragments	
	Head–neck osteoplasty	After physeal closure	To improve head shape by reducing femoroacetabular impingement and increasing head/neck offset
	Trochanteric epiphysiodesis or distal transfer	Epiphysiodesis not effective after age 7–8 years	To improve lever arm function
Contralateral limb	Distal femoral epiphysiodesis		To reduce leg length discrepancy and effects on hip joint mechanics

rotated. There is painful limitation of hip movement. Hilton's law, which states that a joint is supplied by the same nerves as the muscles that move the joint, explains why many children present with knee pain although the pathology is in the hip.

Incidence and aetiology

SCFE is rare, with an incidence of approximately 5 per 100 000 population. Boys are affected most commonly. The peak incidence is related to the start of puberty and hence is earlier in girls. As a result of hormonally stimulated growth, the strength of the physis, its resistance to shear and its orientation are reduced. The hip is therefore 'at risk' and normal forces, exacerbated by obesity and repetitive minor trauma, precipitate a slip. Other conditions such as hypothyroidism, renal failure and previous radiotherapy treatment (local or to the pituitary) also increase the risk.

Diagnosis

The diagnosis is suggested by the history and examination and confirmed on plain radiographs (***Figure 44.22***). Displacement is often more obvious on a lateral view and the diagnosis can be missed if only the anteroposterior radiograph is checked.

Classification

A SCFE can be classified according to three parameters: timing, severity and stability. The onset of symptoms divides slips into those that are acute, chronic or acute on chronic. Slip severity is assessed on the lateral radiograph in terms of percentage uncovering of the metaphysis (***Table 44.8***) or by measuring the slip angle of Southwick (***Figure 44.23***). An unstable slip is defined by Loder as one in which the patient cannot bear weight on the limb.

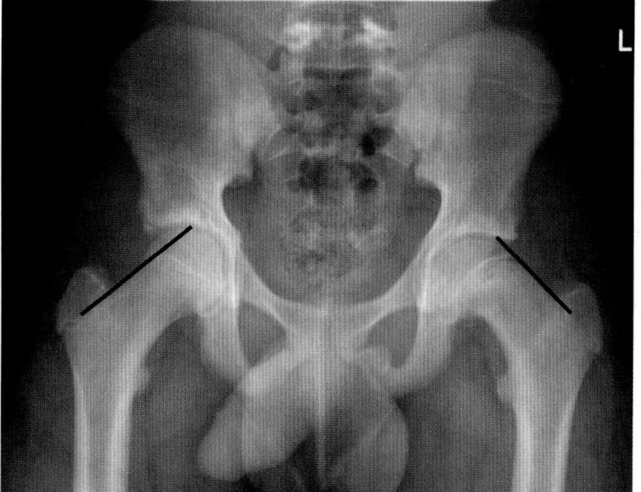

Figure 44.22 Anteroposterior pelvic radiograph demonstrating a mild slip of the upper (capital) femoral epiphysis on the left side. A line drawn along the upper margin of the femoral neck should transect the femoral head (right side); if it does not do so (left side) a slip is present. There are many other radiographic features that help to confirm the diagnosis but the changes are often subtle and may be seen first on the frog lateral view.

John Hilton, 1805–1878, surgeon, Guy's Hospital, London, UK.
Wayne O Southwick, 1923–2016, American surgeon and academic, first chairman of the Department of Orthopaedics and Rehabilitation, Yale University, New Haven, CT, USA, from 1958 to 1979.
Randall Loder, contemporary, Professor of Orthopaedic Surgery, Philadelphia, PA, USA.

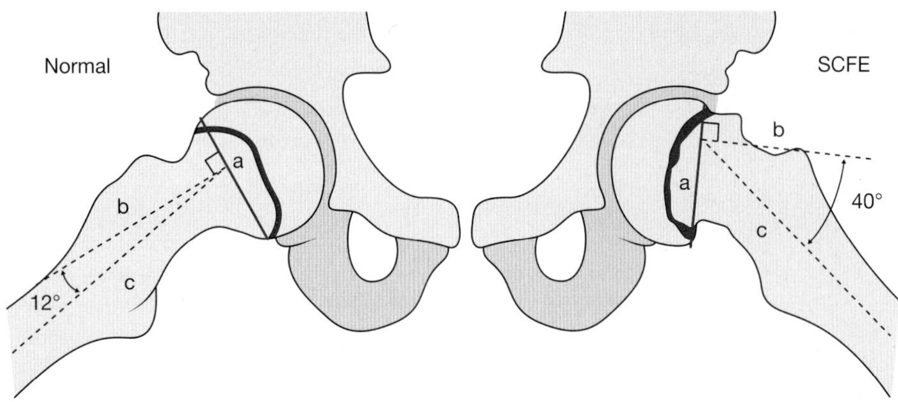

Figure 44.23 The Southwick slip angle is measured on a lateral radiograph and denotes how far the epiphysis has slipped off the metaphysis. The value on the normal side must be subtracted from the value on the abnormal side to get the true value. SCFE, slip of the capital femoral epiphysis.

Management

Following an acute episode the patient is often unable to weight bear and the slip is considered to be **unstable**.

TABLE 44.8 Grading of the severity of slip of the capital femoral epiphysis.

Slip severity	Metaphysis uncovered (%)
Mild	<33
Moderate	33–66
Severe	>66

Displacement is often moderate or severe. This situation is equivalent to a displaced intracapsular femoral neck fracture. This means that an acute unstable SCFE is an emergency. The AVN risk is considerable (***Figure 44.24***).

With the reduction in muscle spasm that accompanies a general anaesthetic, a gentle repositioning of the femoral epiphysis occurs as the externally rotated limb is lifted into the neutral position using no force. A capsulotomy reduces the tamponade effect on the epiphyseal vessels. To be effective such treatment should take place within 24 hours of injury. If delayed, the AVN rate may increase.

With **chronic** slips the patient is able to weight bear, albeit with pain, and the slip is stable. Screw or pin fixation *in situ* relieves pain and movement improves but there will be permanent reduction in abduction, flexion and internal rotation (***Figure 44.25***). The leg will be slightly short.

In the **chronic severe** slip it may be impossible to place a screw in a satisfactory position centrally within the epiphysis. Once healed, there may be significant, persistent deformity leading to restriction of joint movement. In these cases a realignment osteotomy may be considered. As with all osteotomies, the closer the correction is to the site of deformity, the better the outcome. However, in this situation the centre of rotation of angulation (CORA) for the deformity is at the level of the physis; the risk of AVN or chondrolysis may be unacceptably high with an osteotomy at this level, and so an intertrochanteric osteotomy could be considered. The slipped epiphysis is associated with a 'cam' type of femoroacetabular impingement and this may require treatment with a head–neck osteoplasty to restore the offset between the head and neck.

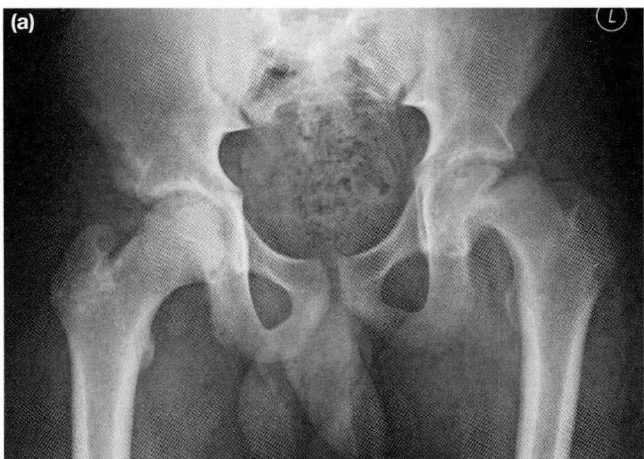

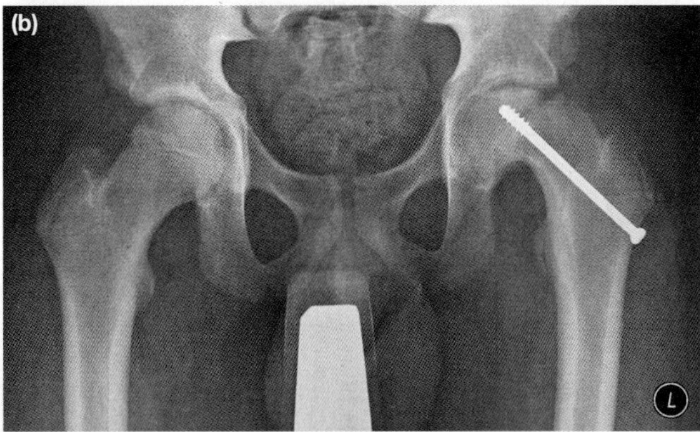

Figure 44.24 Anteroposterior pelvic radiograph showing a left-sided acute severe unstable slip of the capital femoral epiphysis: (a) at presentation; (b) following partial repositioning and fixation with a cannulated screw. When this heals, because of the incomplete reduction it is likely that the metaphysis will impinge on the acetabulum (femoroacetabular impingement) during movement, causing pain and leading to degenerative change.

Bilateral slips do occur and prophylactic pinning of the normal but 'at-risk' hip may be indicated.

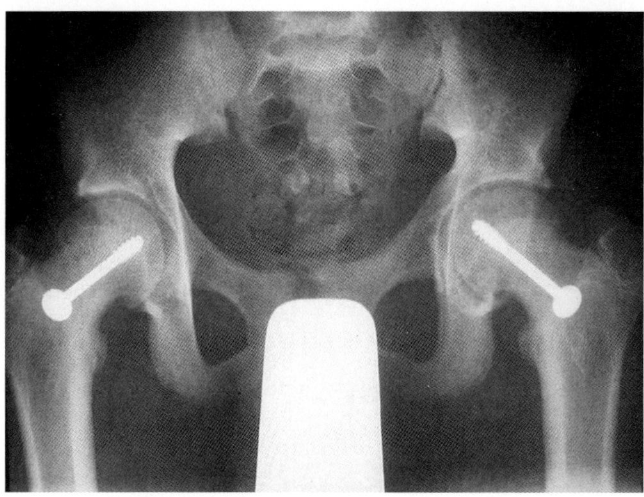

Figure 44.25 Anteroposterior radiograph showing screw fixation in situ of a case of bilateral chronic slip of the capital femoral epiphysis. Note the position of the screw: the more severe the slip, the more proximal and more anterior the screw entry point must be on the femoral neck.

Summary box 44.10

Slip of the upper (capital) femoral epiphysis

- Occurs in prepubertal children, boys more commonly than girls
- Often presents with knee pain, and a short and externally rotated leg
- Classification systems relate to timing, severity and stability – all affect the prognosis
- Most slips are pinned *in situ* with a single screw into the centre of the epiphysis
- AVN is a feared complication of both the condition and its treatment

ABNORMALITIES OF THE KNEE AND LOWER LEG

Many knee problems in children or adolescents are self-limiting. Others require surgical consideration to reduce the risk of later degenerative change.

Osteochondritis dissecans

Osteochondritis dissecans (OCD) affects the lateral aspect of the medial femoral condyle of the distal femur (but also the talus and the humerus). An osteochondral fragment becomes partially or completely separated from the joint surface. Magnetic resonance imaging (MRI) is the best method for demonstrating the site, extent and stability of the lesion. In mild cases, the osteochondral fragment remains attached and heals, particularly if treated early with activity modification. If it detaches, partially or completely, mechanical symptoms necessitate treatment either to encourage bone healing via fixation of the fragment or to remove a loose body. Younger children have a better prognosis.

Discoid meniscus

This invariably affects the lateral meniscus, which is abnormally thick and covers most of the tibial plateau. The child presents with a painful clunk on knee extension. MRI is usually diagnostic. Surgery is indicated for relief of pain or mechanical symptoms.

Anterior knee pain

In adolescents the extensor mechanism of the knee is a common site of knee pain.

Osgood–Schlatter disease is a traction apophysitis of the patellar tendon insertion. Pain, tenderness and swelling at the tibial tubercle, exacerbated by exercise, are diagnostic and radiographs are unnecessary (although, in unilateral cases, it may be important to exclude other diagnoses such as a malignancy). Treatment is relative rest and analgesia, and the condition resolves once the apophysis has fused.

Patellofemoral pain is common and often attributed to an adolescent growth spurt: symptoms are exacerbated either by activity or by resting with the knee flexed. Alterations to activity levels and sitting position and physiotherapy to stretch and strengthen both the hamstrings and the quadriceps muscles usually result in a return to normal within a few months.

Patellofemoral pain may be associated with patellar maltracking and/or instability. Physiotherapy develops the quadriceps muscles, particularly the vastus medialis oblique (VMO), and counteracts wasting secondary to the pain. Many operations improve patellar tracking and these include options for realignment of the extensor mechanism both proximally and distally.

Fibular hemimelia

In fibular hemimelia there is a congenital failure of formation of the lateral 'column' of the lower leg (***Figure 44.26*** and ***Table 44.9***).

TABLE 44.9 Classical radiographic features of fibular hemimelia.

Foot and ankle	Absent lateral rays; tarsal coalition; ball-and-socket ankle joint
Lower leg	Absent or deficient fibula; short, bowed tibia
Knee	Absent tibial spine (no cruciate ligament); deficient lateral femoral condyle
Femur	Relative hypoplasia
Limb length and alignment	Short; external rotation with/without valgus

Robert Bailey Osgood, 1873–1956, Professor of Orthopaedic Surgery, Harvard University Medical School, Boston, MA, USA.
Carl Schlatter, 1864–1934, Professor of Surgery, Zurich, Switzerland. Osgood and Schlatter described osteochondritis of the tibial tubercle independently in 1903.

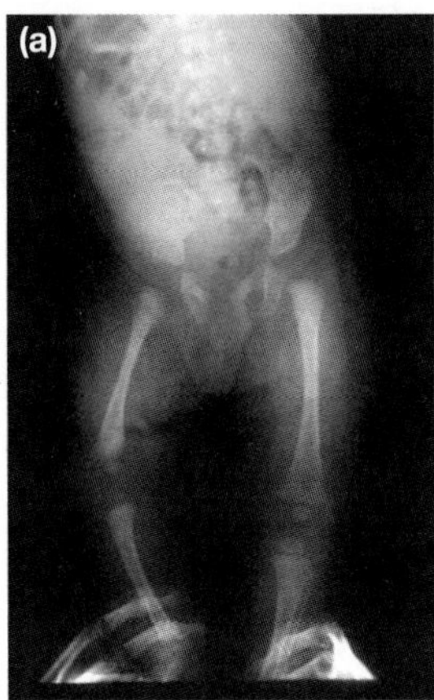

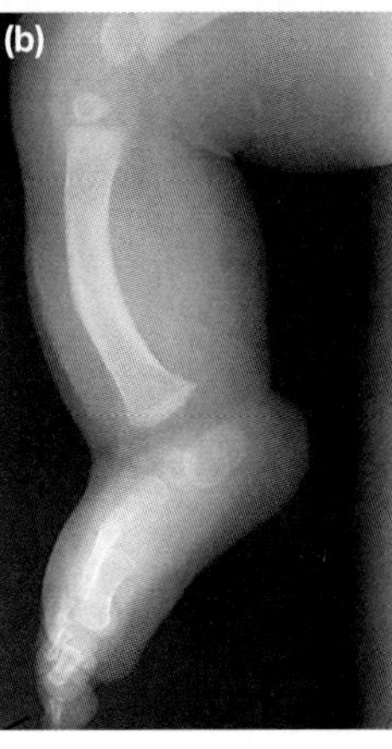

Figure 44.26 Anteroposterior (a) and lateral (b) radiographs of two lower limbs showing some of the features of a fibular hemimelia: absent fifth ray in the foot, absent fibula and deformed tibia.

Management is tailored to the severity of the deficiency. Treatment options range from a shoe raise, through multiple episodes of limb equalisation surgery to amputation for the worst cases. An early prediction of the leg length discrepancy at maturity allows a realistic treatment plan to be devised for the patient, which should include consideration of a contralateral epiphysiodesis.

Blount's disease

The aetiology of the disordered growth in the posteromedial proximal tibial physis is unknown. The infantile form is more common in Afro-Caribbean children but adolescent-onset disease affects all ethnic groups. The child presents with progressive and often severe tibia vara with significant intoeing. The radiographic features are diagnostic (***Figure 44.27***).

Treatment is surgical: following correction of limb alignment via an osteotomy, an epiphysiodesis of the remaining physis prevents recurrence. In unilateral cases, the limb – once straightened – is short and concomitant tibial lengthening with an external fixator is often an attractive option.

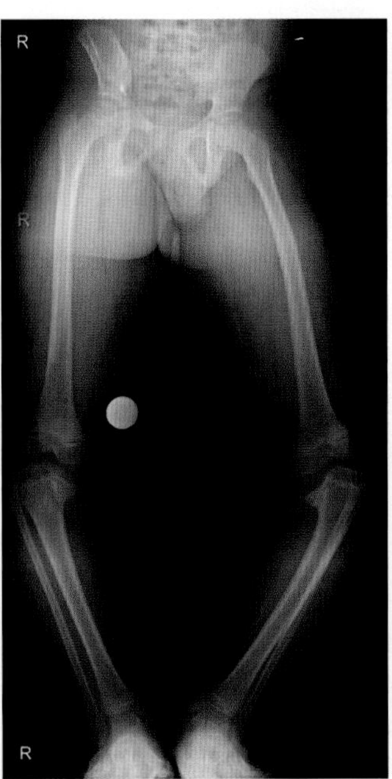

Figure 44.27 Standing leg length and alignment radiograph of a child with bilateral asymmetrical bow legs. Both proximal medial tibial physes/epiphyses are abnormal: this is bilateral Blount's disease.

Congenital pseudarthrosis of the tibia

This rare condition presents with an anterolateral bow of the tibia with or without a fracture. Classic radiographic changes are noted and 50% are associated with neurofibromatosis. Once fractured the tibia is reluctant to heal. Long-term orthotic treatment may be necessary, with subsequent surgical procedures designed to obtain bony union and restore leg length (***Figure 44.28***).

Summary box 44.11

Abnormalities of the knee and lower leg

- OCD – better prognosis in children than in adults
- Discoid meniscus – usually lateral, may require surgery
- Anterior knee pain – treatment usually conservative
- Fibular hemimelia – associated with abnormalities from the foot proximally (foot worse than hip); the tibial bow has an anteromedial apex
- Blount's disease – clinically, a sharp proximal tibial angulation
- Congenital pseudarthrosis of the tibia – the tibial bow has an anterolateral apex
- Apex posteromedial tibial bow – the bow improves with time but the limb may be short

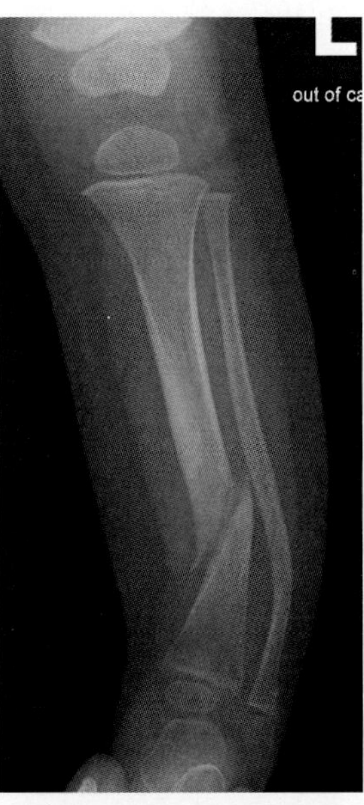

Figure 44.28 Anteroposterior radiograph of a child showing a congenital tibial pseudarthrosis and abnormal fibula. She was born with a bowed lower leg that subsequently fractured. She has a family history of neurofibromatosis.

Walter Putnam Blount, 1900–1992, Professor of Orthopaedic Surgery, Marquette University, Milwaukee, WI, USA, described this condition in 1937.

ABNORMALITIES OF THE FOOT AND ANKLE

Parents are often concerned that minor abnormalities will limit function but this is rarely the case.

Congenital talipes equinovarus (the 'club foot')

In true congenital talipes equinovarus (CTEV) the three-dimensional deformity is fixed (***Figure 44.29***). Intrauterine moulding can cause an identical pattern that is postural and therefore correctable.

Incidence and aetiology

The incidence varies from 1 to 6 per 1000 live births, depending on ethnic differences. It is more common in boys and is bilateral in 50% of cases. A family history is common but inheritance is multifactorial. The diagnosis may be made during an antenatal ultrasound: the sensitivity is higher in bilateral cases, which are more likely to have a syndromic association. In some countries, the detection of CTEV may be grounds for a termination of the pregnancy but the parents should be reassured that, with treatment, their child will function as well as his/her peers.

Most cases are idiopathic but because the outcome varies with the aetiology it is important to consider the cause when planning treatment (***Table 44.10***). Many idiopathic cases will have some weakness of the evertor muscles.

Pathology

The talonavicular joint is subluxed, with the navicular displaced medially with respect to the talar head. Ligaments, particularly the calcaneofibular ligament, and tendon sheaths, such as the posterior tibial tendon sheath, are shortened and thickened and contain contractile myofibroblasts. The gastrocsoleus and posterior tibial muscles are smaller than normal, with reduced myofibrils and increased connective tissue, possibly because of a local neuromuscular abnormality. The vascular supply via the dorsalis pedis may be diminished. It remains unclear which abnormalities are primary and which occur as the deformity develops.

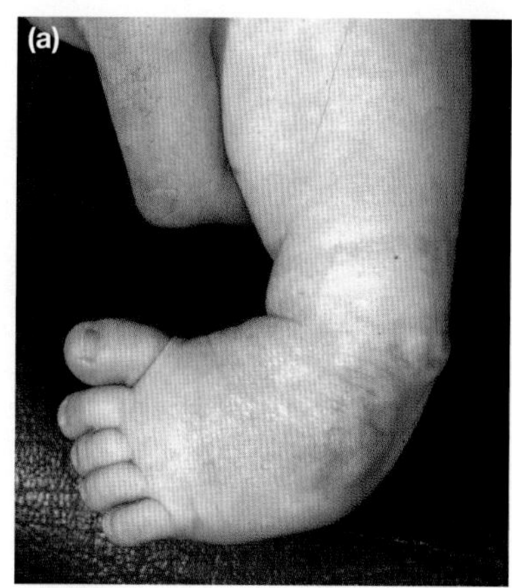

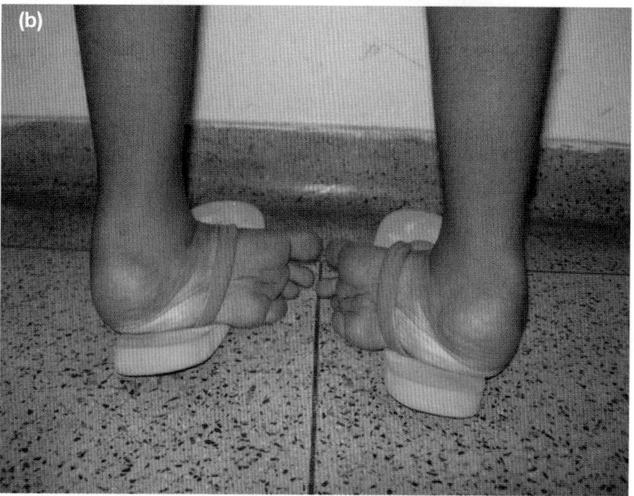

Figure 44.29 (a) Anteroposterior photograph of a foot showing the classic deformities associated with a club foot. The hindfoot (not seen) is in equinus and varus, there is midfoot cavus and the forefoot lies adducted and apparently supinated, although it is actually pronated relative to the hindfoot. (b) Untreated congenital talipes equinovarus in a child aged 7 years. Shoe wear is difficult although some independent mobility is possible.

Clinical assessment

The postural club foot may benefit from physiotherapy stretches but, by definition, it must be normal by 3 months of age.

TABLE 44.10 Several different types of club foot are recognised.

Type	Example
Postural	
Idiopathic	
Neuromuscular	Spina bifida; arthrogryposis
Syndromic	Trisomy 15 or Disastrophic Dysplasia or Amniotic Band Syndrome

In contrast, the structural idiopathic club foot has fixed deformity with elements of hindfoot equinus and varus, midfoot adductus and pronation of the first ray, giving the appearance of forefoot cavus. The heel feels 'empty' as the calcaneus is pulled up by the shortened tendo-Achilles. There is a deep medial and a single posterior crease.

All children with structural club-foot deformity will have a small calf and foot. Tibial shortening may become apparent with growth. Children should be examined carefully for signs of intraspinal pathology.

Both the Pirani and Diméglio classification systems are based on the appearance of the foot in its position of maximal correction. They predict treatment response and hence outcome.

Shafique Pirani, contemporary, Clinical Professor, Department of Orthopaedic Surgery, University of British Columbia, Vancouver, Canada.
Alain Diméglio, contemporary, orthopaedic surgeon, Montpellier, France.

Summary box 44.12

Club foot

- Multiplanar deformity: hindfoot equinus and varus, midfoot adductus and forefoot cavus
- Incidence is 1–6 per 1000 live births, more common in boys and with a familial tendency
- Most cases are idiopathic but neuromuscular causes include spina bifida and arthrogryposis
- Scoring systems (Pirani/Diméglio), are used to assess severity

Treatment

Ponseti method

The Ponseti method corrects foot deformity in 95% of idiopathic cases without the need for a formal surgical release and is the treatment of choice for all feet. Treatment commences within a few weeks of birth. A specific set of manoeuvres, followed by a series of well-moulded above-knee plaster casts, results in gradual correction of the deformity (***Figure 44.30***). The head of the talus is the fulcrum around which the rest of the foot rotates. After the forefoot has been corrected, most feet lack 15° of dorsiflexion and require a percutaneous Achilles tenotomy (performed under local anaesthetic in the clinic setting).

Once corrected the foot position is maintained by a foot abduction orthosis (FAO) that holds the foot in external rotation and slight dorsiflexion. The FAO is worn full time for 3 months and at 'night and nap time' for up to 4 years. Poor compliance with the FAO is associated with a higher relapse rate. Recurrent deformity can be treated with further plasters, but a tibialis anterior tendon transfer (TATT) may be required around the age of 2.5–4 years for persisting dynamic supination.

Feet treated with the Ponseti method are less stiff, less likely to be painful and less subject to overcorrection than those treated surgically. The Ponseti method also works reasonably well in non-idiopathic feet but both the failure and relapse rates are higher.

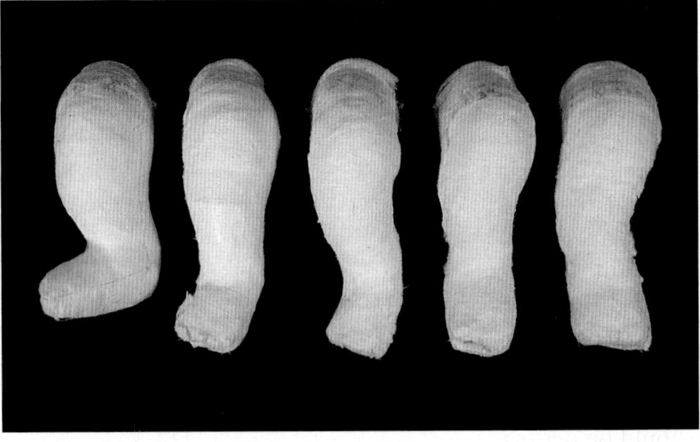

Figure 44.30 A series of casts documenting the stepwise correction of the foot deformity with the Ponseti method of serial manipulation and casting.

Surgical treatment

If conservative treatment fails, surgical intervention is required, ideally before walking age; this is more likely in non-idiopathic deformities.

Surgical release is generally performed 'à la carte', with sequential release of the pathologically tight structures via either Turco or Cincinnati incisions to reduce the subluxated joints. Stabilisation may include temporary Kirschner wire fixation. Following correction, wound closure can be difficult but the Cincinnati incision heals well by secondary intention during the postoperative casting period.

Good or excellent results can be achieved but stiffness and over- or undercorrection are common complications.

Surgery for recurrent deformity requires a careful assessment of the forefoot, hindfoot and tibial torsion. The foot becomes progressively stiffer with each surgical intervention.

Summary box 44.13

Treatment of club foot

- The Ponseti method of serial casting is successful in 95% of feet when defined as avoiding formal surgical release

  The standard sequence of manipulations is:

  C – correction of the apparent forefoot **cavus** by elevation of the first ray

  A – gradual forefoot abduction to 60°, and simultaneous

  V – correction of the hindfoot **varus**

  E – correction of hindfoot **equinus** usually follows a percutaneous Achilles tenotomy, which is an integral part of treatment
- TATT is used to correct dynamic supination in older children

If the Ponseti method fails:

- Surgical release addresses posterior, medial, plantar and lateral structures, and results in a stiffer foot than one treated conservatively

Other foot and ankle conditions

Most postural deformities such as metatarsus adductus and calcaneovalgus feet improve spontaneously.

Congenital vertical talus (CVT) is rare and frequently associated with neuromuscular conditions such as

Ignacio Ponseti, 1914–2009, faculty member of the University of Iowa, USA. Born in Menorca, fled Spain during the Civil War because of the political situation, worked as a general practitioner in Mexico and then went to Iowa to train in orthopaedics. The technique that bears his name only became popular years after he retired – but it brought him back to work for another 20 years.

Vincent J Turco, 1916–1999, Chief of Orthopedic Surgery, St. Francis Hospital, Hartford, CT, and Assistant Clinical Professor, Yale University Medical School, New Haven, and the University of Connecticut Medical School, Farmington, CT, USA.

Martin Kirschner, 1879–1942, Professor of Surgery, Heidelberg, Germany, introduced the use of skeletal traction wires in 1909.

arthrogryposis and spinal dysraphism. Clinically, there is a stiff 'rocker-bottom' foot with dorsal dislocation of the navicular on the talus (*Figure 44.31*). A 'reverse' Ponseti method with a limited surgical approach to reduce and Kirschner (K)-wire the talonavicular joint and a percutaneous Achilles tenotomy may be preferable to more extensive surgical releases.

In **tarsal coalition** there is failure of segmentation of adjacent tarsal bones. School-aged children present with hindfoot pain and recurrent ankle sprains. The most common coalitions are talocalcaneal and calcaneonavicular (*Figure 44.4*). Radiographs, computed tomography (CT) or MRI are used to confirm the diagnosis. Treatment is initially conservative, but if the coalition requires surgical excision this should be performed before degenerative changes develop.

Other causes of foot pain in children include the osteochondroses, in which the radiographic changes are similar to AVN. These 'heal' but the change in shape of the affected bone may lead to secondary joint stiffness and loss of function. (Similar 'diseases' affect the lunate [Kienböck's] and the capitellum of the humerus [Panner's].)

- **Freiberg's osteochondrosis** presents with forefoot pain and avascular change in the second metatarsal head. Symptomatic bony spurs and osteochondral fragments may need excision but often it is asymptomatic and seen as an incidental finding on a radiograph.
- **Köhler's disease** presents with dorsal forefoot pain and swelling in young children. The navicular becomes avascular with alteration in the ossification process.
- **Sever's disease** (enthesopathy of the calcaneal apophysis) presents with heel pain related to activity. Tightness in the calf muscle complex may be a contributing factor. The 'features' on a radiograph are, in fact, part of normal growth and development.

Flexed, medially curved 'curly toes' are common and rarely need treatment. Strapping is ineffective. Flexor tenotomy is used when there are symptoms or cosmetic concerns.

Summary box 44.14

Other foot and ankle conditions

- CVT – presents as 'rocker-bottom' foot
- Tarsal coalition – presents as a stiff, painful flat foot
- Osteochondroses – almost always self-limiting
- Curly toes are common – most do not need treatment

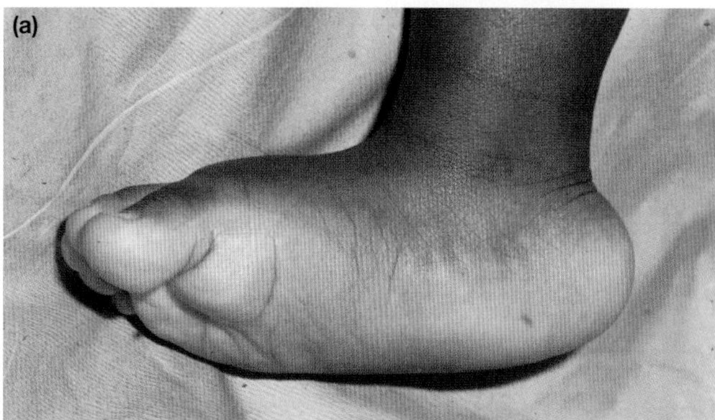

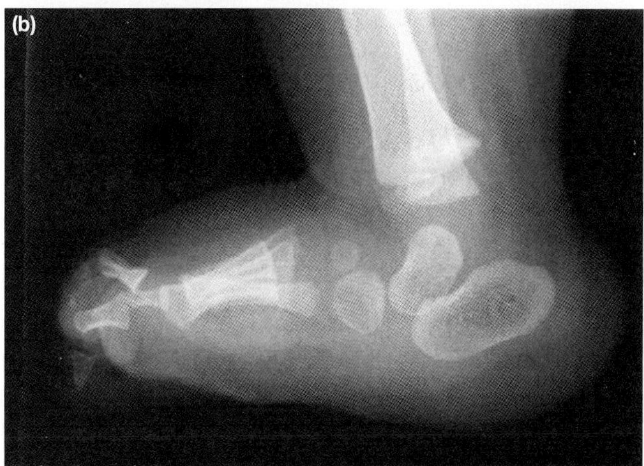

Figure 44.31 Congenital vertical talus: (a) lateral photograph demonstrating a 'rocker-bottom foot'; (b) lateral radiograph showing hindfoot equinus and suggesting dorsal subluxation of the non-ossified navicular and forefoot with respect to the head of the talus.

ABNORMALITIES OF THE UPPER LIMB

Minor finger abnormalities are common (*Table 44.11*) but not all require surgical intervention. Comfort and function are more important than appearance.

Function is also the most important consideration when managing more extensive upper limb abnormalities. Treatment is often delayed until hand dominance is established and it is clear what problems a specific deformity is causing any given child. Children are very adaptable and cope with disabilities much more readily than their parents/doctors expect.

Radial club hand

This longitudinal failure of formation is commonly associated with other malformations, for example as part of the VACTERL (abnormal vertebrae, anus, cardiovascular system, trachea, oesophagus, renal system and limb buds) syndrome. The clinical problem depends on whether the thumb is present and functional (*Figure 44.32*). Treatment is a balance of conservative measures, including physiotherapy and splinting, and judicious surgery to centralise and stabilise the hand and wrist on the single bone forearm. Thumb reconstruction may be technically challenging. In later childhood, forearm lengthening may be considered.

Robert Kienböck, 1871–1953, Professor of Radiology, Vienna, Austria, described this condition in 1910.
Hans Jessen Panner, 1871–1930, radiologist, Copenhagen, Denmark, described this condition in 1927.
Albert Henry Freiberg, 1869–1940, Professor of Orthopaedic Surgery, The University of Cincinnati, Cincinnati, OH, USA, described this disease in 1926.
Alban Köhler, 1874–1947, radiologist, of Wiesbaden, Germany, described this disease in 1908.
James Warren Sever, 1878–1964, orthopaedic surgeon, The Children's Hospital, Boston, MA, USA, described apophysitis of the os calcis in 1912.

TABLE 44.11 Common minor congenital anomalies affecting the hand.

Anomaly	Definition	Treatment
Extra/accessory digits		Excise/amputate when necessary
Syndactyly	Failure of separation of digits	Separation with/ without skin grafting for functional or cosmetic reasons
Trigger thumb (digit)		Release of the A1 pulley of the flexor tendon sheath
Clinodactyly (usually the fifth digit)	Abnormal angulation of the digit in the radioulnar plane	Surgical treatment of the delta phalanx if deformity is progressive or interfering with hand function
Camptodactyly (usually the fifth digit)	Fixed flexion deformity of the proximal interphalangeal joint	Splinting/ physiotherapy; surgery rarely indicated

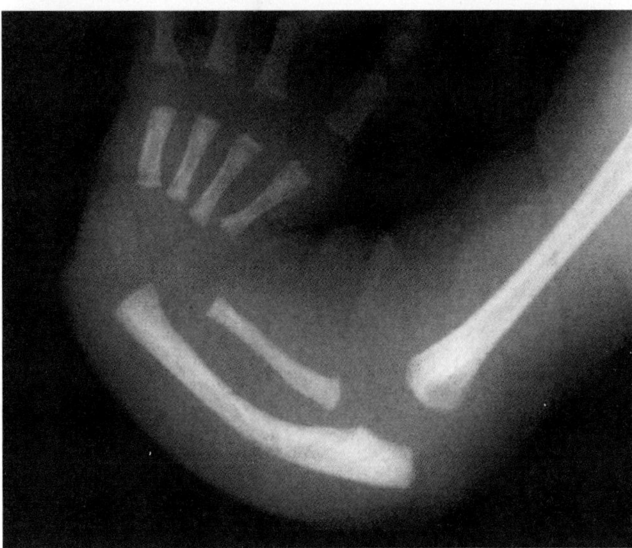

Figure 44.32 Anteroposterior radiograph of a radial club hand demonstrating a short radius, a deformed ulna and an absent thumb.

Radioulnar synostosis

Failure of proximal separation of the embryonic radius and ulna means that the forearm has no ability to pronate/supinate. The hand, on the end of the forearm, is therefore in a fixed position along the arc from full pronation–neutral–full supination. The child presents if this fixed position results in functional difficulties. Osteotomy of the forearm bones changes the fixed position (for example, from pronation to neutral) but does not restore movement. The choice of the postoperative position depends on hand dominance, cultural considerations and functional demands. Undoing the synostosis is not successful.

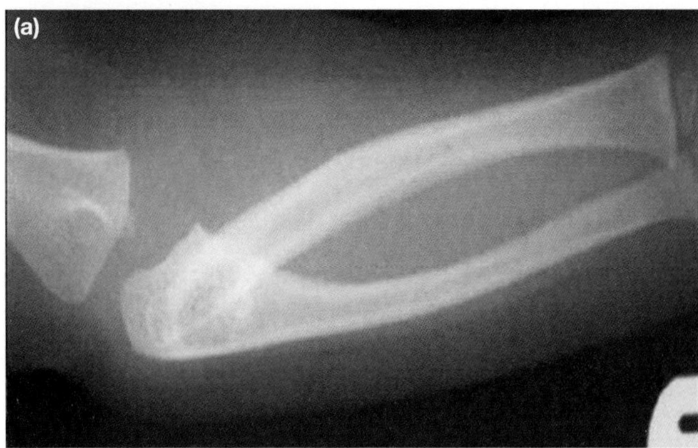

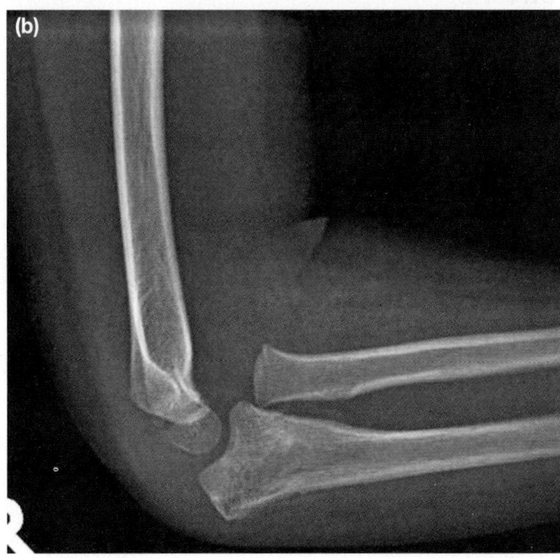

Figure 44.33 Radial head dislocation: (a) lateral radiograph of a forearm showing a proximal radioulnar synostosis with a congenital posterolateral dislocation of the radial head. Note the underdeveloped radial head and neck and compare with (b), a lateral radiograph of a traumatic anterior dislocation of the radial head with a normal appearance to the head and neck and a deformity in the proximal ulna.

Congenital radial head dislocation

The dislocation is usually posterolateral, compared with the classic traumatic anterior dislocation (*Figure 44.33*). Some restriction of elbow joint movement and forearm rotation is noted along with discomfort on activity. Surgical treatment should be avoided in children.

Summary box 44.15

Upper limb abnormalities

- Radial club hand is frequently associated with other congenital anomalies, for example the VACTERL or Holt–Oram syndromes
- Radioulnar synostosis presents with a fixed forearm position
- Congenital radial head dislocation is usually posterolateral

Mary Clayton Holt, 1924–1993, cardiologist, The London Hospital for Women and Children, London, UK.
Samuel Oram, 1913–1991, cardiologist, King's College Hospital, London, UK. Holt and Oram described this syndrome in a joint paper in 1960.

SPINAL DEFORMITIES AND BACK PAIN

Congenital deformities

Congenital vertebral deformities are failures either of formation (a hemivertebra) or of segmentation (unilateral or bilateral fusions or bars). The clinical result is usually a scoliosis (*Figure 44.34*). Treatment should be based on the potential for curve progression. When a kyphosis develops, progressive neurological deficit is common. Bracing is ineffective for congenital vertebral deformities.

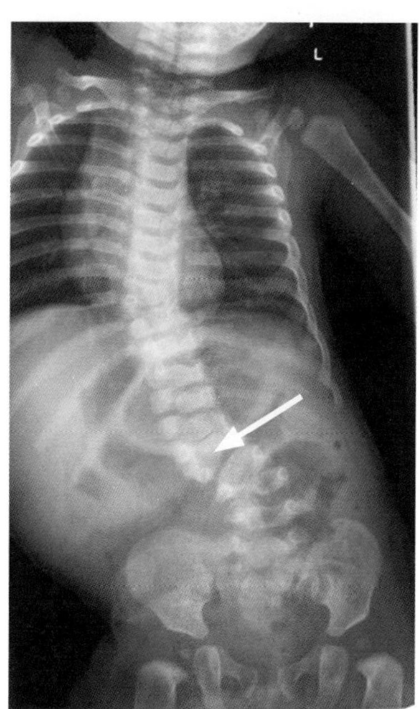

Figure 44.34 Anteroposterior radiograph of the spine demonstrating multiple congenital vertebral anomalies including hemivertebrae. The arrow points to one of the congenital vertebral anomalies.

Scoliosis

The term 'scoliosis' describes spinal deformity in three planes: lateral curvature is the most obvious deformity while the rotational component is most apparent in forward flexion when the rib asymmetry creates a 'rib hump' (*Figure 44.35*). The cause may be idiopathic, neuromuscular, related to a syndrome or congenital. Both the aetiology and the age of onset affect the natural history (*Table 44.12*). In general, the earlier the onset, the more likely the deformity is to be progressive. As most lung development occurs in early childhood, the management of early-onset scoliosis must preserve growth: casting techniques or the use of 'growing rods' may be appropriate.

The adolescent idiopathic curve is the most common, affecting girls more than boys. Idiopathic scoliosis is generally not painful and, therefore, in the presence of significant pain tumour and infection must be excluded. The Cobb angle is a radiological measurement that defines severity and guides treatment (*Figure 44.36*). Curves <20° do not need treatment, progressive curves of 25–40° may be braced and those >40° are considered for surgery, which involves instrumenting and fusing the spine (see also *Chapter 37*).

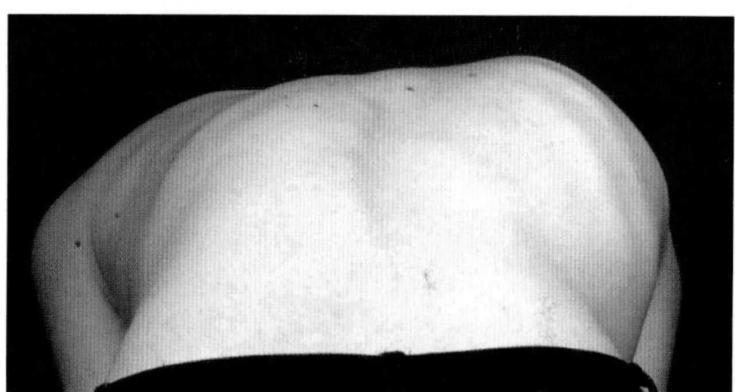

Figure 44.35 Clinical photograph of the Adams forward bend test that demonstrates the presence of a rib hump on the right and a prominence of the lumbar paravertebral muscles on the left.

TABLE 44.12 Classification of idiopathic scoliosis.

Type	Age at onset
Early onset	<10 years
Adolescent	11–18 years
Adult	Onset at maturity

Summary box 44.16

Scoliosis

- Multiplanar deformity includes a rotational component
- Aetiology may be congenital (underlying bony malformation), neuromuscular, syndromic or idiopathic
- A leg length discrepancy causes a postural scoliosis
- Adolescent idiopathic scoliosis is the most common structural scoliosis
- Back pain associated with scoliosis may be due to infection or tumour
- Treatment depends on the severity and likelihood of curve progression – it varies from observation, through bracing to surgery

Kyphosis

When a kyphosis exceeds the normal 20–50° the cause may be postural or structural. Scheuermann's disease presents as a progressive structural adolescent kyphosis characterised radiologically by >5° vertebral wedging at three adjacent levels with end-plate changes. The aetiology is unknown. Treatment ranges from physiotherapy and bracing to surgery.

William Adams, 1820–1900, described the forward bending test for scoliosis in 1865.
John R Cobb, American surgeon, wrote a paper in 1948 on how to measure the angle on a radiograph in scoliosis.
Holger Werfel Scheuermann, 1877–1960, radiologist, The Municipal Hospital, Sundby, Copenhagen, Denmark, described juvenile kyphosis in 1920.

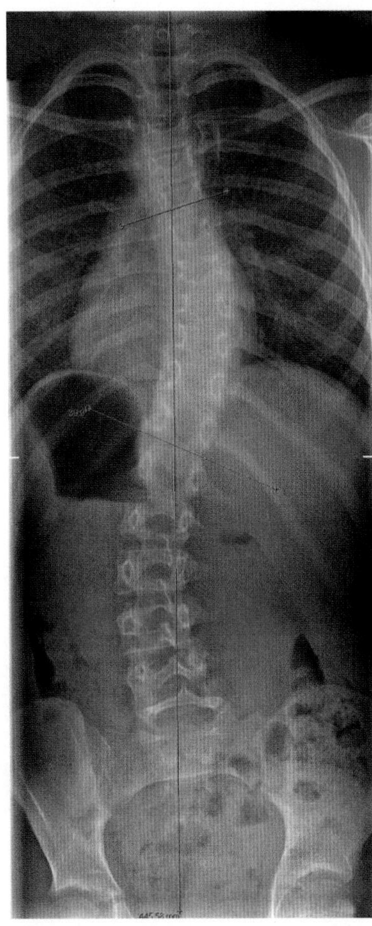

Figure 44.36 Posteroanterior radiograph of a spine with a scoliosis (right thoracic), with a Cobb angle of 40°.

Spondylolisthesis

Spondylolysis defines a defect in the pars interarticularis of the vertebra. There are six types including congenital and traumatic. Spondylolisthesis occurs when the upper vertebra slips forward on the lower; it is graded according to the percentage slip, measured by relating the slipped vertebra to the one below (*Table 44.13*).

Mild slips are often asymptomatic and require no treatment. Treatment (physiotherapy, bracing and surgery) depends on the degree of slip and symptoms; mechanical back pain may respond to conservative methods, but neurological involvement usually requires surgical intervention.

TABLE 44.13 Classification of spondylolisthesis according to severity of the slip.

Grade	Percentage slip
0	No slip
1	<25
2	26–50
3	51–75
4	>75
Spondyloptosis	>100 – complete translation

Torticollis

In torticollis the head is tilted towards and rotated away from the tight sternocleidomastoid muscle.

Congenital torticollis is usually secondary to intrauterine moulding but may present with a fixed sternocleidomastoid contracture or a palpable 'tumour' within the muscle. Most cases resolve with stretching but persistent cases develop facial asymmetry requiring release of the origin and/or insertion of the sternocleidomastoid muscle.

Acquired torticollis is rare and may be caused by inflammation/infection, ocular problems, atlantoaxial rotatory subluxation or a posterior fossa tumour.

Back pain

Children report back pain less frequently than adults, although >50% will have had one episode by late adolescence. Back pain in a child is a 'red flag' for serious spinal pathology; however, if it is mild, intermittent or occurring only on strenuous activity, it is usually self-limiting. Many adolescents do suffer posture-related discomfort. Physiotherapy to improve core strength and stability reduces symptoms if exercises are performed regularly.

Summary box 44.17

'Red flag' symptoms and signs for spinal pathology

- Systemic illness, fever or weight loss
- Progressive neurological deficit
- Unrelenting or night pain
- Spinal deformity

All 'red flag' signs require urgent investigation with a full blood count (FBC), erythrocyte sedimentation rate (ESR), C-reactive protein (CRP), plain radiograph and MRI or other imaging. Other causes of back pain include intra-abdominal, renal and systemic pathology.

Summary box 44.18

Other spinal conditions

- Excessive kyphosis may be due to Scheuermann's disease
- Spondylolisthesis is a forward slip of one vertebra on another; it may cause mechanical and, rarely, neurological symptoms
- Torticollis may be congenital and usually responds to stretching of the sternocleidomastoid muscle
- Acquired torticollis may be due to one of several significant pathologies
- Back pain with red flag symptoms and signs requires urgent investigation

NEUROMUSCULAR CONDITIONS

Joint stability and limb function rely on the complex integration of the musculoskeletal and neurological systems. Damage to either leads to one of several conditions linked only by the fact that they are incurable and often progressive, particularly during the period of skeletal growth. Management is directed at helping the child cope with their disability, minimising further deterioration and maximising function. It is important to have an understanding of what the damage is and what the future holds (***Table 44.14***).

Spina bifida and polio are classic lower motor neurone lesions, whereas cerebral palsy and head injuries affect upper motor neurones and the higher centres. There are often other disabilities such as blindness, epilepsy and intellectual difficulties to consider.

TABLE 44.14 Factors to be considered in the assessment of a neuromuscular disability.

- Is the insult to the neurological system progressive or non-progressive?
- Is it located centrally or peripherally?
- Is it general or focal?
- Is it associated with other abnormalities or not?
- If the insult is not neurological, is it myopathic?

In children, even if the initial insult to the neuromuscular system is non-progressive, the effects of the insult change with growth. Damage at any level of the neuromuscular system leads to an alteration in tone and muscle imbalance associated with decreased control of movement. Abnormal muscle pull, particularly in combination with the effects of gravity, alters bone growth, leading to deformity and joint contracture. Muscles are relatively weak and, with body growth and a weight increase, they are no longer strong enough to control a heavier limb, particularly when deformity means they are working at a mechanical disadvantage.

A multidisciplinary approach to management is essential. Physiotherapy and orthotic management may reduce the need for surgical intervention and postoperatively they ensure that the surgical benefits are maximised. In conditions such as Duchenne muscular dystrophy there is substantial evidence for the benefits of certain surgical procedures; however, in other conditions (cerebral palsy) there are fewer such long-term validated studies.

In general, it is important to maintain good joint movement, muscle length and tendon excursion. This is easier to achieve in patients with a flaccid paralysis or low tone. The maintenance of muscle strength is also important. The use of splints, positioning techniques and seating and sleeping systems is common with the aim of preventing fixed contractures.

Surgery has a valuable role in the management of selected patients (***Table 44.15***).

The surgeon must understand that altering ankle posture may affect knee and hip posture/function and vice versa. The patient must have the intellectual ability and motivation to recover from the surgical procedure. Some of the factors mentioned previously (***Table 44.14***) must be considered in any holistic approach to the patient.

Summary box 44.19

Principles of treatment of neuromuscular conditions

- A neurological defect, whether progressive or not, may cause progressive deformity with skeletal growth
- A multidisciplinary approach is essential
- Primary therapy aims to maintain range of movement and prevent fixed contractures with an emphasis on managing tone and position
- Surgery has a limited role in the management of neuromuscular conditions

Cerebral palsy

Cerebral palsy (CP) is caused by a non-progressive insult to the developing brain in the perinatal period; in most cases only risk factors, such as prematurity, rather than specific causes, such as hypoxia (hypoxic ischaemic encephalopathy [HIE]), can be identified. The effects of CP may only become apparent as the child grows and fails to reach developmental milestones. Investigations may identify the aetiology and predict the pattern of the CP: premature babies may show evidence of periventricular leukomalacia (PVL) on MRI, associated with a spastic diplegia and relative preservation of intellectual function.

TABLE 44.15 General types of surgical procedure that may be considered in the management of a patient with a neuromuscular condition.

Surgical procedure	Aim of treatment
Lengthening of the muscle–tendon unit	Restores joint range (but results in relative muscle weakness)
Tendon transfer	Improves functional movement; rebalances muscle forces, after correction of fixed deformity
Release of joint contracture; correction of bony deformity	Restores mechanical alignment and allows muscles to work in a more efficient manner
Fuse/stabilise/relocate joints	Improves posture/function; reduces pain
Neurological procedures: • selective dorsal rhizotomy (SDR) • intrathecal baclofen pumps (ITB)	Reduce spasticity – ***not*** useful in dystonia
Leg equalisation procedures	Improve lower limb mechanics

Guillaume Benjamin Amand Duchenne (Duchenne de Boulogne), 1806–1875, neurologist, worked successively in Boulogne and Paris, France, but never held a hospital appointment.

TABLE 44.16 Classification of cerebral palsy with respect to muscle tone and site of involvement.

	Characteristics
Tone	
Spastic ('high')	• Commonest type of abnormality; due to pyramidal system damage • Velocity-dependent increased muscle tone and brisk reflexes
Dyskinetic • Dystonic • Choreoathetoid	 • Increased tone but reduced activity – stiff movements • Low tone but increased activity – uncoordinated jerky movements • Due to damage in the extrapyramidal system
Ataxia	• Generalised low tone, loss of muscle coordination • Due to cerebellar damage
Mixed	• No one tone/movement disorder predominatesw • Combination of spasticity and dystonia is common
Hypotonia	Usually a phase (which may last years) before the features of spasticity develop
Site	
Unilateral • Hemiplegia	 Arm more affected than leg
Bilateral • Diplegia • Total body involvement	 Legs more affected than arms Often significant intellectual impairment and associated difficulties

In general, the pattern of involvement can be classified according to the anatomical site involved and the effect on muscle tone (***Table 44.16***). The prognosis for walking can be predicted by identifying evidence of neurological development, i.e. gaining motor skills and losing primitive reflexes. The age-related Gross Motor Function Classification System (GMFCS) has five categories that relate to mobility and prognosis (GMFCS I – near-normal versus GMFCS V – wheelchair based). Many children with GMFCS V CP have multiple associated problems and a short life expectancy.

An important aspect of management is the control of high tone. Tone can be reduced with drugs (e.g. diazepam and baclofen). Alternatively, neuromuscular blockers such as botulinum toxin allow a focal reduction in tone by preventing acetylcholine release at the neuromuscular junction. The effect is temporary, giving a 'window' during which the physiotherapists can stretch agonists and strengthen antagonists. It is important to differentiate between dynamic and fixed contractures; the latter will not respond to tone management or splinting.

The classic CP gait patterns demonstrate flexor spasticity. The child with spastic diplegia has problems at all levels of the lower limb. Single-event multilevel surgery (SEMLS) is popular, and gait analysis (both observational and computerised) contributes to the selection of an appropriate management plan for an individual patient. Computerised analysis provides objective evidence of joint movement and mechanics in multiple planes (***Figure 44.37***). Appropriate bone and soft-tissue procedures can then be planned. Botulinum toxin helps with postoperative pain and spasm.

In the child with total body involvement (TBI) and high muscle tone, hip subluxation leading to dislocation is common (***Figure 44.38***). Current thinking is that symmetry and pelvic position are important so the hips should be kept in joint with early surgical intervention if necessary. Aggressive management of a spinal deformity initially concentrates on seating position and subsequently emphasises spinal bracing or surgery.

Overall, it is important to remember that, in adulthood, independent mobility, even if in a wheelchair, and effective communication are the most important requirements.

Summary box 44.20

Cerebral palsy

- Brain injury is non-progressive
- Classified as unilateral or bilateral involvement: hemiplegia, diplegia or TBI
- Tone may be high, low or variable but there is always a generalised, relative muscle weakness
- In ambulant children, gait analysis may be used to plan management
- In TBI, primary concerns are hip subluxation and spinal deformity

Polio

Despite an effective polio vaccine, this disease still occurs. About 1–2% of patients develop neurological problems when the virus affects the anterior horn cells. Muscle weakness is proportionate to the number of motor units destroyed. Patients develop trick movements to adjust to their muscle weakness and minor joint contractures may improve function (for example, ankle equinus in the presence of weak quadriceps muscles). Careful preoperative assessment is required and both the surgeon and the patient must understand the goals of treatment.

Spina bifida

The extent of the disability varies with the level of the lesion: upper motor neurone involvement will produce spasticity while the more classic lower motor neurone lesion produces a flaccid paralysis. Muscle imbalance leads to secondary joint deformity but the accompanying sensory disturbance may affect the choice of surgical and non-surgical options. Many children require a ventriculoperitoneal (VP) shunt to drain the hydrocephalus that develops following closure of the myelocele. With growth, a tethered cord or a blocked VP shunt may develop with a deterioration in the neurological picture.

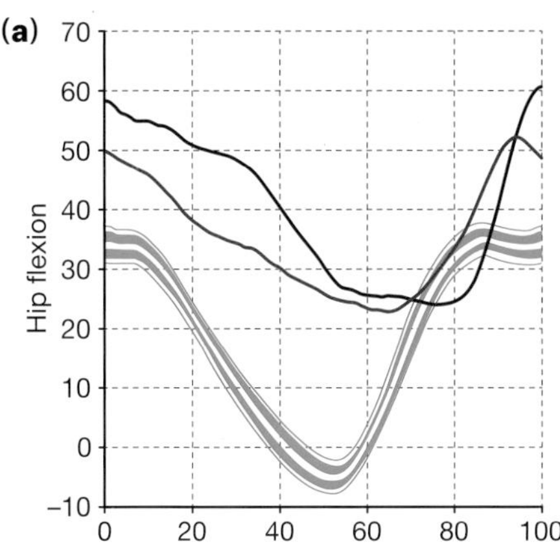

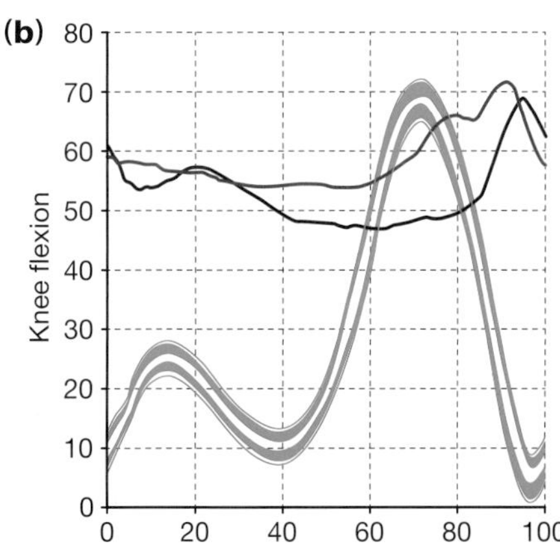

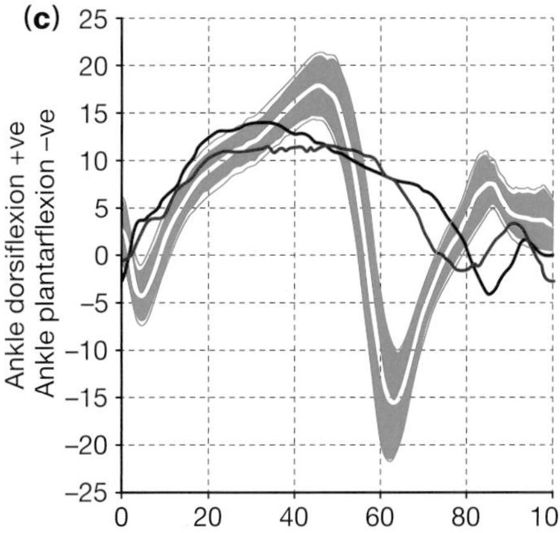

Figure 44.37 Gait analysis graphs such as these demonstrate the normal range of joint movements (green band) at the hip (a), knee (b) and ankle (c) during the stance and swing phases of the gait. The abnormal joint ranges are shown in red (right leg) and blue (left leg) and demonstrate the excessive hip flexion, lack of knee extension and abnormal ankle mechanics associated with the 'crouch' gait of a child with cerebral palsy.

Muscular dystrophy

Many types of muscular dystrophy exist that vary in severity and distribution of involvement. Surgical intervention aims to improve quality of life. This is best achieved by operating early to release joint contractures and maintain the ability to walk with a good spinal posture.

Brachial plexopathy

Neonatal brachial plexus injury is still common, with a devastating effect on upper limb function, particularly if antigravity motor activity has not recovered by 6 months. Physiotherapy is the mainstay of early treatment to maintain muscle length and joint range of movement and thus reduce the risk of glenohumeral dislocation. Neural repair may be necessary in the infant. Later surgical interventions aim to release joint/muscle contractures and improve function, perhaps with tendon transfers.

INFECTION

Worldwide, osteoarticular infection remains a frequent cause of significant morbidity.

Septic arthritis

Joint infection is usually secondary to haematogenous spread but direct inoculation can occur, for example during a neonatal venepuncture. Diagnosis can be difficult in the very young and in those presenting with overwhelming sepsis. Neonates, children with immunocompromise and those with sickle cell

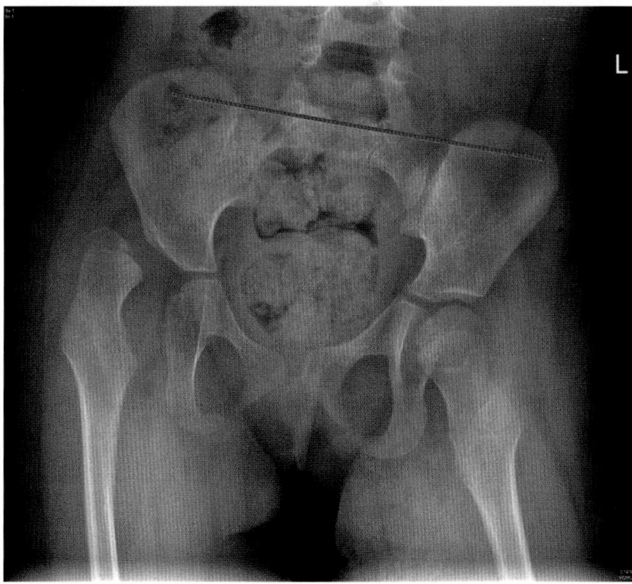

Figure 44.38 Anteroposterior pelvic radiograph of a child with spastic cerebral palsy. The right hip is dislocated: none of the head lies medial to the vertical Perkins line. The acetabulum is dysplastic. The left hip is in abduction. There is often a 'windswept' appearance with one leg stiff in abduction and the other stiff in adduction. The red line demonstrates the pelvic obliquity; many children also have a scoliosis. Note the significant constipation; this can cause significant pain, which will increase spasm and increase the pain still further.

disease are at increased risk. At the other end of the spectrum the differentiation between joint sepsis and transient synovitis of the hip can also be difficult.

Classically, the child presents with pain, fever and a reluctance to move the joint; in the lower limb, this implies a reluctance to weight bear. On examination, local tenderness and painful restriction of movement are apparent and in superficial joints inflammation may be obvious, with a hot, swollen joint.

Investigations include FBC, ESR, CRP and blood cultures. Plain radiographs help exclude other diagnoses and may identify osteomyelitis. Ultrasound scans of deep joints, such as the hip, will identify joint effusions (***Figure 44.39***). MRI is considered the investigation of choice but this resource is not available to all (in a timely manner) and, in young children, it requires a general anaesthetic. Good clinical skills, regular patient review and a high index of suspicion are still the most valuable tools. Four clinical predictors can differentiate between septic arthritis and transient synovitis (***Table 44.17***).

Pus in a joint is destructive: the proteases produced by leukocytes destroy both the bacteria and the collagen matrix of the articular cartilage. AVN may occur secondary to pressure effects or ischaemic infarction. The treatment of a presumed septic arthritis therefore requires the prompt removal of pus from the joint and appropriate adequate antibiotic therapy. Pain relief and rest are also important, as are the general health and nutrition of the patient. The joint is aspirated and, if pus is confirmed, a formal washout is mandatory; standard teaching states that the joint must be opened, irrigated and free drainage encouraged via the capsulotomy. Recent literature supports repeated aspiration/irrigation via a large-bore cannula or a small arthroscope for all joints except the hip. Antibiotic usage is guided by local hospital policy, the source of the infection, the Gram stain and, in due course, the culture and sensitivity of the organism identified. Joint instability, particularly in the hip joint (***Figure 44.40***), may require the reduced joint to be splinted while the inflammatory process settles.

TABLE 44.17 Septic arthritis.

(a) The clinical predictors of Kocher *et al.* (2004) for the diagnosis of septic arthritis:
- History of fever >38.5°C
- Non-weight-bearing
- Erythrocyte sedimentation rate >40 mm/h
- White cell count >12 × 10^9/L

(b) The value of the clinical predictors of Kocher *et al.* in determining the likelihood of a joint being septic:

Number of positive predictors	Predicted probability of joint sepsis
0	2.0%
1	9.5%
2	35.0%
3	72.8%
4	93.0%

The most frequently identified organism is *Staphylococcus aureus*. Streptococcal infection is also common and other organisms are more prevalent in certain age groups, e.g. the neonate, in certain conditions, e.g. sickle cell disease, or in certain countries. The *Haemophilus influenzae* type B (Hib) vaccine has essentially eliminated *H. influenzae* as a cause of infection, but in some countries *Kingella kingae* has taken its place.

Improvement is judged clinically and by monitoring the inflammatory markers. Reaccumulation of pus does occur and must be suspected and treated promptly if the child fails to improve.

Summary box 44.21

Septic arthritis
- Diagnosis is difficult in neonates and the immunocompromised
- Typical presentation is pain, fever and a reluctance to move the joint or weight bear
- Investigations should include FBC, ESR, CRP, blood cultures and appropriate imaging studies, combined with astute clinical skills
- Pus in a joint destroys articular cartilage and causes avascular necrosis of intra-articular epiphyses
- Treatment is prompt removal of pus, appropriate antibiotic therapy, pain relief and splintage

Osteomyelitis

As with septic arthritis, bone infection is usually caused by haematogenous spread. Infection starts in the metaphyses of long bones, where the slow flow through the looped vessels combined with microtrauma encourages seeding of infection during a bacteraemia (***Figure 44.41a***). Inflammation follows

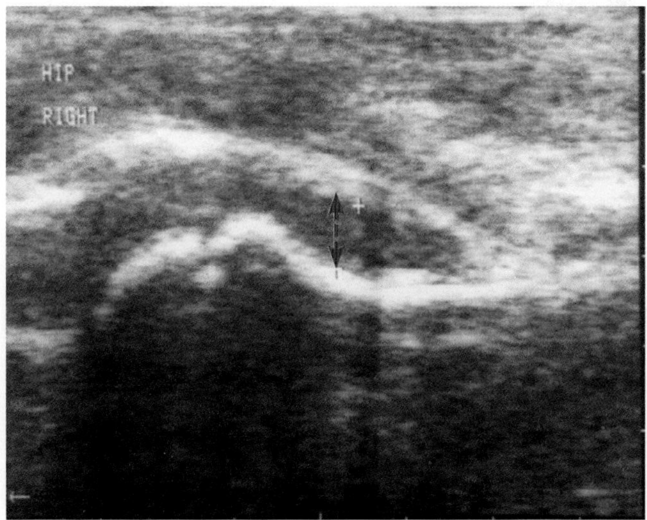

Figure 44.39 Ultrasound scan of a hip joint. A large effusion is distending the joint capsule. The dotted line represents the distance between the femoral neck and the joint capsule.

Hans Christian Joachim Gram, 1853–1938, Professor of Pharmacology (1891–1900) and of Medicine (1900–1923), Copenhagen, Denmark, described this method of staining bacteria in 1884.

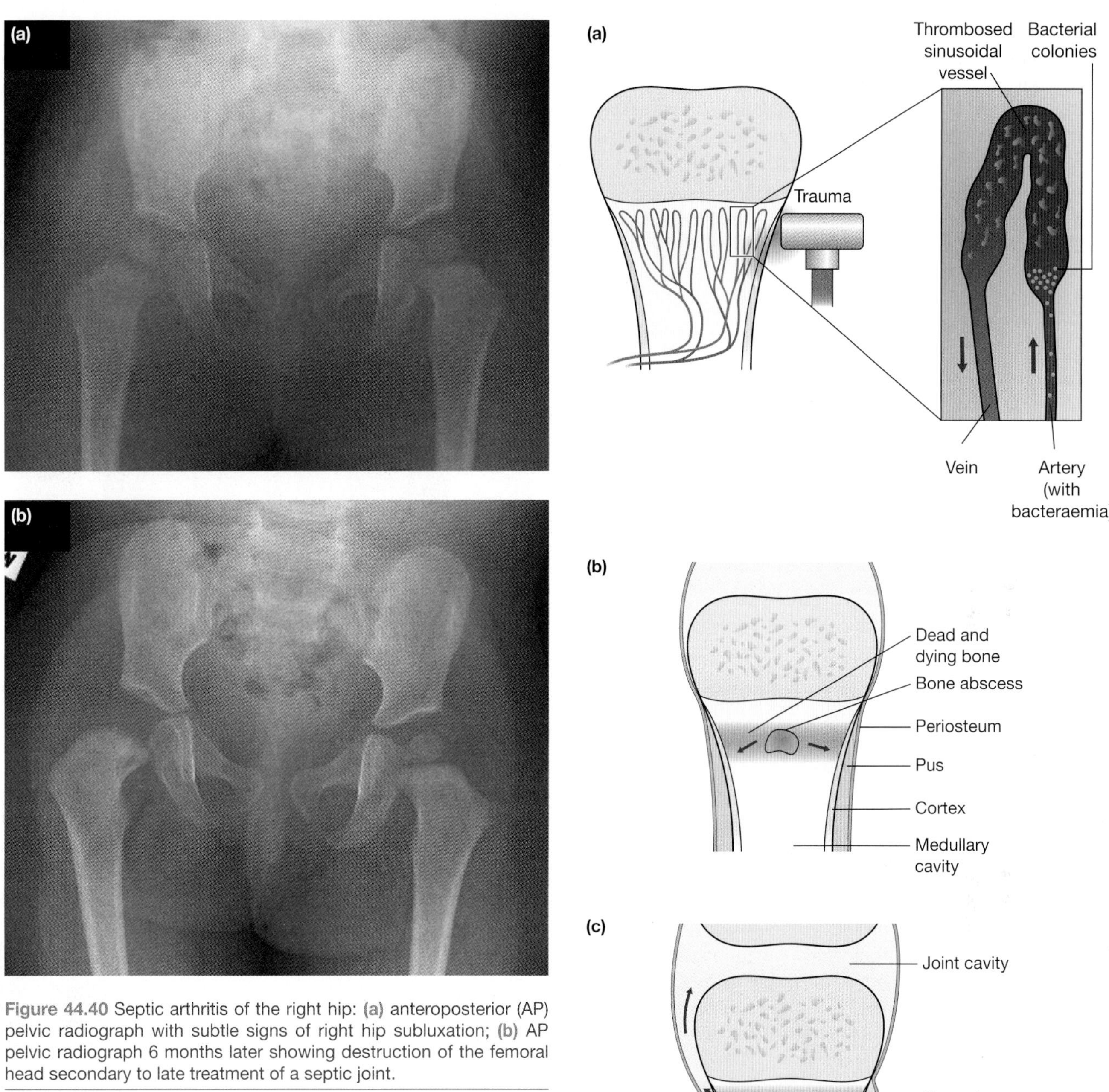

Figure 44.40 Septic arthritis of the right hip: (a) anteroposterior (AP) pelvic radiograph with subtle signs of right hip subluxation; (b) AP pelvic radiograph 6 months later showing destruction of the femoral head secondary to late treatment of a septic joint.

Figure 44.41 (a–c) Diagrams illustrating the pathology underlying the development of osteomyelitis. The longer the infection goes untreated the greater the destruction, with the possibility of sequestrum formation and secondary joint infection.

and, if purulent material forms, the pressure effects secondary to the abscess formation lead to bony destruction. Pus passes through cortical bone and when it does so it elevates the strong periosteum, which may render the cortical bone avascular. As in cases of trauma or tumour, the periosteal elevation is a potent stimulus for new bone formation. In cases of untreated or chronic infection this new bone or involucrum may surround the dead bone, the sequestrum, leading to a 'bone-within-a-bone' appearance (*Figure 44.41b*).

The presentation and investigation of osteomyelitis can be similar to those for joint sepsis. The differentiation between the two may be difficult and a sympathetic joint effusion may occur with metaphyseal osteomyelitis. Thus, if there are no organisms seen on microscopy of a joint aspirate, the possibility of a coexisting osteomyelitis must be considered. The metaphysis of a long bone may be intracapsular and infection may spread easily into the joint once the periosteum is breached. In the neonate, proximal femoral osteomyelitis and septic arthritis are essentially the same condition (*Figure 44.41c*).

General principles for the management of infection should be followed. Pus needs to be drained but otherwise the treatment is medical. Debate continues over the duration of treatment and indeed whether antibiotics should be parenteral or oral: management varies from region to region and relates to the local bacteriological prevalences. Methicillin-resistant *S. aureus* (MRSA) is common in some areas and the presence of the Panton–Valentine leukocidin gene increases morbidity.

The shortened intravenous and oral treatment regimes are for **uncomplicated** cases of osteomyelitis and septic arthritis only, and only for patients who are improving clinically and haematologically.

Summary box 44.22

Bone and joint infection

- Occurs by haematogenous spread, enhanced by microtrauma
- In untreated and/or chronic osteomyelitis, new involucrum envelops dead sequestrum
- In addition to antibiotics, treatment consists of:
  - Rest/splintage of affected limb
  - Analgesia
- A joint effusion may be sympathetic, a primary septic arthritis or caused by direct spread from the adjacent metaphyseal infection
- Treatment involves:
  - Drainage of pus when present
  - Appropriate and often prolonged antibiotic therapy: parenteral and then oral
  - Treatment of the underlying condition, e.g. nutritional deficiency, sickle cell disease

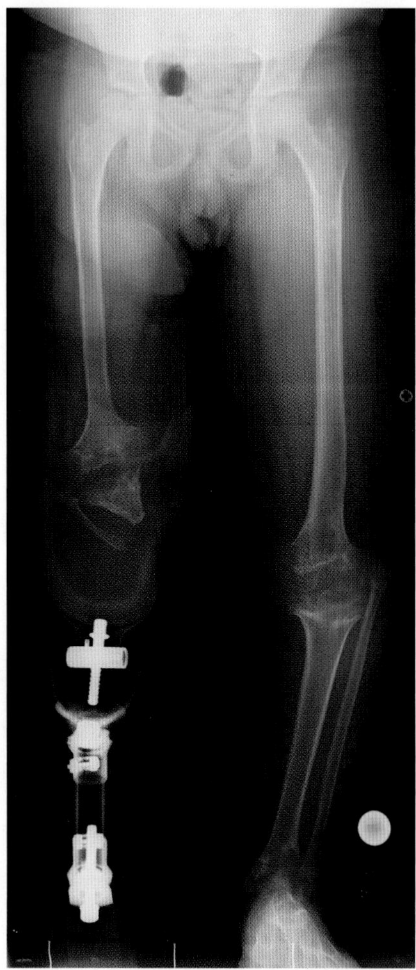

Figure 44.42 Anteroposterior leg length and alignment radiograph of an adolescent who had meningococcal septicaemia as a child. He has a right below-knee amputation. Many of his lower limb physes are not growing well so he has deformity of his remaining right proximal tibia, a short left tibia and an overgrown fibula. His right femur is also short.

Complications of bone and joint sepsis

Treated appropriately, most cases of sepsis resolve with no sequelae. However, significant complications can occur, particularly in terms of chronic infection and where there has been damage to the joint and/or the physis and the epiphyseal growth centres. In the neonate, vascular channels pass through the physis, connecting the metaphysis with the epiphysis, and a poorer outcome may ensue (***Figure 44.40b***). Orthopaedic follow-up should be continued until normal growth patterns are documented.

Meningococcal sepsis

The often debilitating, late orthopaedic sequelae of meningococcal septicaemia are secondary to endotoxin-induced microvascular injury and ischaemic physeal damage (***Figure 44.42***).

Tuberculosis

Globally, tuberculosis is common. The clinical presentation is often insidious, with malaise and weight loss combined with a boggy joint swelling, muscle wasting and joint contractures. Spinal deformity and neurological symptoms are particular problems.

Chronic relapsing/recurrent multifocal osteomyelitis

The radiographic features suggest subacute or chronic osteomyelitis (or tumour) but laboratory and histopathological findings are non-specific and cultures negative. This is an inflammatory (**not** infective) condition.

Discitis

Children who refuse to weight bear and complain of back pain may have discitis. The aetiology of this condition may be infective or inflammatory but if vertebral bodies are involved, infection is assumed.

Sir Philip Noel Panton, 1877–1950, Consultant Adviser in Pathology, Ministry of Health, UK.
Francis Valentine, 1897–1957, described Panton–Valentine leukocidin as a dermo-necrotic and leukocidal toxin while working with Philip Panton at the Hale Clinical Laboratory, London, UK, in 1932.

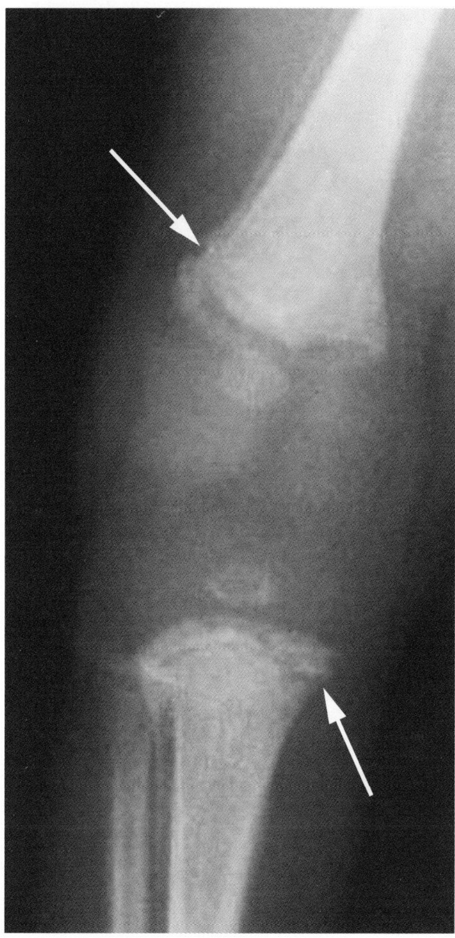

Figure 44.43 Anteroposterior radiograph of a knee showing metaphyseal corner fractures that are considered to be pathognomonic of non-accidental injury.

Brodie's abscess

Chronic infections may present with radiographic features of a sclerotic walled cyst.

CLINICAL DILEMMAS

The limping child

Children may limp because of pain, weakness, deformity or to gain attention; the causes vary from sepsis to a spinal tumour and from a leg length discrepancy to a simple blister. Serious causes must be excluded and the 'surgical sieve' helps identify the most likely diagnoses (*Table 44.18*).

TABLE 44.18 A guide to the clinical assessment of the limping child.

- Symptom onset: sudden or gradual?
- Symptom duration
- Concurrent events: recent viral infection, trauma, new sport?
- General health: is the child well?

The examination must include all joints and soft tissues and, in addition, a brief neurological examination, measurement of leg length and an assessment of pain at rest or on weight-bearing.

Many conditions, such as sepsis and juvenile arthritis, can present at any age but certain hip conditions are more likely in particular age groups (*Table 44.19*).

Plain radiographs should include both anteroposterior and 'frog' lateral views of the pelvis. Always bear in mind the possibility of a tumour; further imaging such as MRI may be required.

TABLE 44.19 Age at presentation of certain hip conditions.

Age (years)	Diagnosis
1–3	• Sepsis • Late presenting developmental dysplasia of the hip
3–10	• Transient synovitis • Perthes' disease
11–15	• Slipped upper femoral epiphysis

Non-accidental injury

No child is exempt but some children are at particular risk, including those under 3 years of age, those with disabilities and those in families suffering socioeconomic deprivation. A careful clinical assessment is required (*Figure 44.43* and *Table 44.20*). Characteristic patterns should alert the clinician to the possibility of non-accidental injury (NAI) (*Table 44.21*).

NAI occurs in different forms: emotional, physical, sexual and neglect. When suspected it should be discussed with child safeguarding teams. All injuries should be documented carefully. It may be prudent to admit the child until further checks have been made.

TABLE 44.20 Factors that raise concern in the clinical assessment of suspected non-accidental injury.

History
- Delay in seeking medical advice
- Variable story
- Mechanism inconsistent with injury pattern

Examination
- Unexpected bruising to the buttocks/back of legs
- 'Finger-mark' bruises
- Bruises of various ages
- Burns, deep scratches, etc.

TABLE 44.21 Fracture patterns with a high specificity for non-accidental injury.

- Multiple fractures at different stages of healing/old fractures
- Posterior rib fractures
- Corner or bucket-handle metaphyseal fractures
- Scapular fractures
- Any fracture in a child below walking age

Sir Benjamin Collins Brodie, 1783–1862, surgeon, St George's Hospital, London, UK, described 'Brodie's abscess' in 1828.

FURTHER READING

Bulstrode CJK, Wilson-MacDonald J, Eastwood DM *et al.* (eds). *Oxford textbook of trauma and orthopaedics*, 2nd edn. Oxford: Oxford University Press, 2017.

Flynn JM, Weinstein SL (eds). *Lovell and Winters pediatric orthopaedics*, vols 1 and 2, 8th edn. Philadelphia, PA: Lippincott, Williams & Wilkins, 2020.

Global Help. *Paediatric orthopaedics*. Available from https://global-help.org/pediatric-orthopaedics (accessed 25 March 2021).

Kocher MS, Mandiga R, Zurakowski D *et al.* Validation of a clinical prediction rule for the differentiation between septic arthritis and transient synovitis of the hip in children. *J Bone Joint Surg Am* 2004; **86**(8): 1629-35.

CHAPTER 45 Skin and subcutaneous tissue

Learning objectives

To understand:

- The structure and functional properties of skin
- The classification of vascular skin lesions
- The cutaneous manifestations of generalised disease as related to surgery
- The classification of benign skin tumours
- The management of malignant skin tumours

FUNCTIONAL ANATOMY AND PHYSIOLOGY OF SKIN

Skin can be divided into two layers: the outer epidermis and the inner dermis. Deep to the dermis lies subcutaneous fat and any remnants of the panniculus carnosus.

Epidermis

The epidermis constitutes 5% of the skin and is composed of five layers of keratinised, stratified squamous epithelium – the strata: basalis (deep), spinosum, granulosum, lucidum and corneum (superficial).

Most epidermal cells are keratinocytes arranged in layers. The basal epidermis (stratum basalis) also contains melanocytes. Keratinocytes are classified according to their depth in the epidermis and their degree of differentiation. Keratinocytes grow and are replaced via mitosis in the cells of the stratum granulosum as they progress from deep to superficial, losing their nuclei and organelles as they ascend, before forming the stratum corneum. The other keratinocyte layers in the skin (strata lucidum, granulosum and spinosum) are variably thick according to body site; for instance, all three are thick in the glabrous skin of the palms and soles of the feet and almost absent in eyelid skin.

Melanocytes are dendritic cells of neural crest origin, usually located in the basal epidermis. Each melanocyte synthesises melanin, a brown-black pigment, which is transferred via membrane processes to the keratinocytes in the strata granulosum and spinosum. Melanin provides protection against ultraviolet radiation (UVR). Ethnic differences in skin colour are determined by variations in the amount, combination and distribution of melanin within the keratinocytes, not by differences in the number of melanocytes.

The surface of the epidermis is coated with a mixture of secreted molecules and microorganisms and generally has an acid pH, which is protective against harmful flora.

Dermis

The dermis constitutes 95% of the skin and is structurally divided into a superficial papillary layer, which is composed of delicate collagen and elastin fibres in ground substance, into which a capillary and lymphatic network ramifies, and a deeper reticular layer, which is composed of coarse branching collagen, layered parallel to the skin surface (***Figure 45.1***).

The epidermis and dermis meet at the dermoepidermal junction in a three-dimensional wave-like arrangement in which epidermal rete ridges project down, interdigitating with upward-pointing, dermal papillae containing vascular and lymphatic plexi.

The skin also contains specialised cells such as Langerhans cells, whose role is to engulf antigens and present them to T cells. Merkel cells, and Meissner's and Pacinian corpuscles have roles in mechanosensation.

Skin adnexa

Adnexal structures such as hair follicles, sebaceous glands and sweat glands span both the epidermal and dermal layers and contain some keratinocytes in their ducts. In injuries where epidermis is lost, re-epithelialisation occurs from these structures as well as from the wound margins.

Paul Langerhans, 1847–1888, Professor of Pathological Anatomy, Freiberg, Germany.
Friedrich Sigmund Merkel, 1845–1919, Professor of Anatomy, successively at Rostock, Königsberg (now Kaliningrad in Russia) and Göttingen, Germany.
George Meissner, 1829–1905, Professor of Physiology, Göttingen, Germany.
Filippo Pacini, 1812–1883, Professor of Anatomy and Physiology, Florence, Italy.

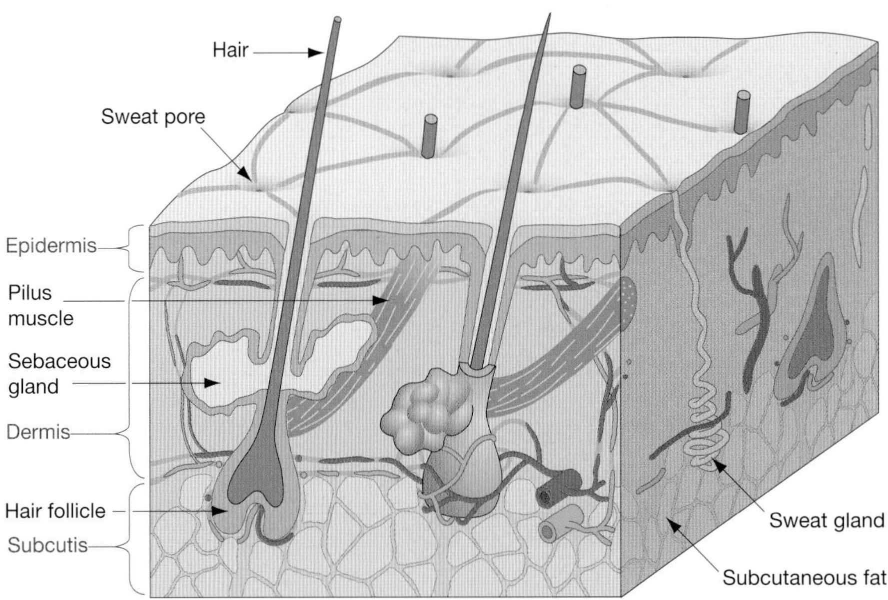

Figure 45.1 Three-dimensional diagram of the structural layers of the skin and its adnexal structures. (Reproduced from Simonsen T, Aarbakke J, Kay I *et al. Illustrated pharmacology for nurses*. London: Hodder Arnold, 2006 with kind permission of the illustrator, Roy Lysaa.)

Hair follicles are tubular invaginations of the epidermis, from which grow hair shafts (dead keratinised tissue). Strips of smooth muscle (arrector pili) are inserted into the wall of the hair follicle and elevate it in response to stress and cold.

Sebaceous glands are hair follicle appendages situated between the follicle and arrector pili muscle such that muscle contraction compresses the gland and sebum is released (holocrine secretion) along the elevated hair.

Simple eccrine and apocrine sweat glands open into pores in hair follicles. Eccrine glands are distributed throughout the entire body surface, except the lips. They secrete sweat in response to emotion or during thermoregulation. Apocrine glands are found in the axillae and groins and become active at puberty. Their secretion, characteristically malodorous after bacterial degradation, is in response to emotion and hormone secretion.

Skin dimensions

The skin is a large organ. In an adult it may have an area of 1–2 m^2 and weigh 15–20 kg. Skin thickness varies with age, location and sun damage, but in any given region it is thinner in children than in adults. The dermis is between 15 and 40 times thicker than the epidermis, but starts to thin during the fourth decade. The epidermis is thickest on the palms, soles, back and buttocks and thinnest on eyelids (0.5–1 mm on the sole of the foot; 0.05–0.09 mm on the eyelid).

Blood supply of the skin

The body can be envisaged as three-dimensional segments of tissue called angiosomes, each with an arterial supply and a venous drainage. Blood equilibrates and flows between neighbouring angiosomes via 'choke' vessels, which tend to be situated within muscles. Cutaneous arteries, direct branches of segmental arteries (concentrated at the dorsoventral axes and intermuscular septae), perforate the underlying muscles or run directly within fascial layers to the skin from the deep tissues (***Figure 45.2***).

The blood supply to the skin anastomoses in subfascial, fascial, subdermal, dermal and subepidermal plexi. The epidermis contains no blood vessels so cells there derive nourishment by diffusion.

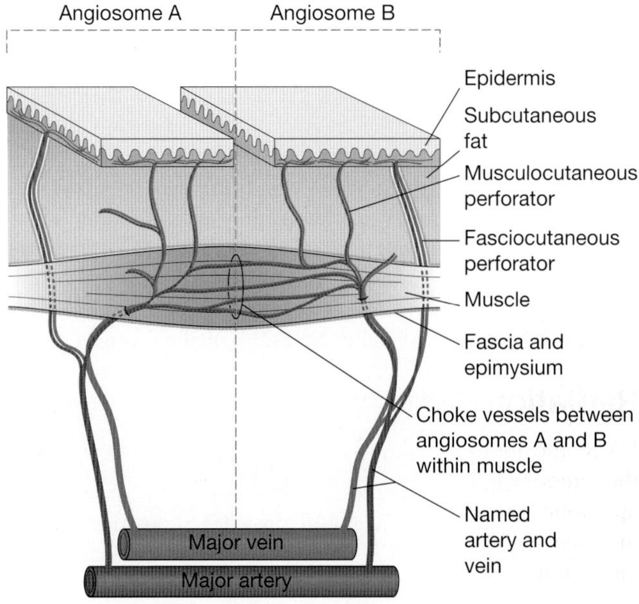

Figure 45.2 Schematic showing two neighbouring angiosomes. Note the choke vessels within the muscle spanning the two cutaneous territories of angiosomes A and B; two common examples of myocutaneous flaps that utilise this physiology include the rectus abdominis and the latissimus dorsi flaps.

The venous drainage of the skin is via both valved and unvalved veins. Unvalved veins allow oscillating flow in the subdermal plexus between cutaneous territories, equilibrating flow and pressure. The valved cutaneous veins drain via plexi to the deep veins.

Anomalies of skin metabolism

Skin has the potential for a blood supply 20–100 times greater than its metabolic and thermoregulatory requirements. This apparent excess enables restitution of mechanical integrity after the myriad of trivial injuries (scratching, stretching, compressing, thermal) to which skin is subjected; however, blood supply is inadequate to support full-thickness wound healing, which requires primary closure or granulation tissue.

Skin functions optimally at temperatures below body core temperature and can tolerate long periods of ischaemia, allowing it to be both grafted and/or expanded for use in reconstruction.

FUNCTION OF THE SKIN

Skin and subcutaneous tissue have several important functions:

- Barrier to the environment enveloping the body and protecting against trauma, radiation and pathogens. Secreted sebum and sweat mix to form a microscopic acidic film across the epidermis – 'the acid mantle' – which is protective against microorganisms and toxic substances.
- Regulates temperature and water homeostasis.
- Organ of excretion for urea, sodium chloride, potassium and water, as well as sulphur-containing metabolites from drugs (e.g. dimethyl sulphoxide) or food (garlic, cumin).
- The skin has significant endocrine and metabolic functions and interactions. Skin cells contain receptors for and respond to peptides, steroid sex hormones, thyroid hormones and neurotransmitters and they both produce (cholecalciferol) and metabolise (androgens) hormones and precursors to activate, potentiate and inactivate their functions.
- Sensory organ with multiple receptors for pain, pressure and movement.

PATHOPHYSIOLOGY OF THE SKIN AND SUBCUTANEOUS TISSUES

Radiation damage

UVR and ionising radiation (IR) damage cellular DNA via the tumour suppressor gene *p53*, inhibiting cellular repair and apoptotic mechanisms. There is also evidence that efferent immune responses are impaired after skin exposure to UVR, facilitating neoplasia.

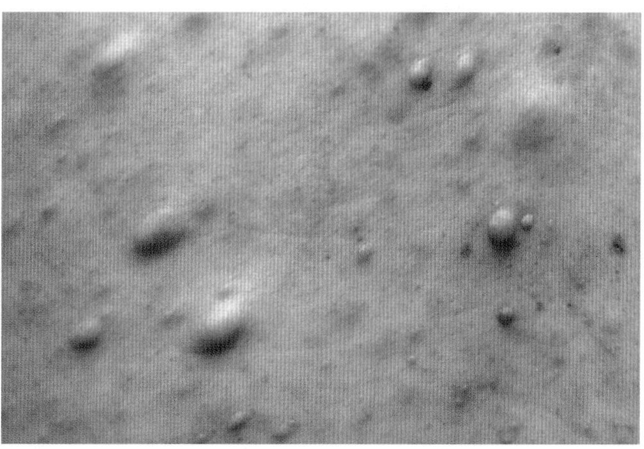

Figure 45.3 Neurofibromatosis (courtesy of St John's Institute for Dermatology, London, UK).

Ultraviolet radiation

UVR is divisible into A, B and C according to wavelength. UVR, inducing oxidative damage, is the principal cause of skin cancer in all skin types as well as sunburn and skin ageing. UVA and UVB are the principal natural causes of ultraviolet (UV)-induced damage (UVC is absorbed by the atmosphere, but can be emitted by artificial sources). UVA has a longer wavelength than and less energy per photon than UVB, but penetrates more deeply. The effects of UVR are attenuated by melanin and there is an inverse relationship between melanin content and skin susceptibility to UV-induced neoplasia. Some protection is afforded by the stratum corneum, which reflects and refracts UVR, and by clothing, protective creams, cloud cover, particulate air pollution and buildings.

Ionising radiation

The effects of IR are dose, wavelength and time dependent. The skin, with its rapid cellular turnover, shows signs soon after exposure. High-frequency rays cause electron coupling at the molecular level, damaging proteins, polysaccharides and lipids.

Infrared radiation

Infrared radiation generates heat; cumulative exposure can cause thermal burns.

Congenital/genetic disorders

Neurofibromatosis

There are two distinct neurofibromatosis (NF) syndromes, in which Schwann cells form tumours (***Figure 45.3***). Each is caused by different genes on different chromosomes: 70% are autosomal dominant and 30% arise from sporadic mutations. NF-1 (Von Recklinghausen's disease) is the commoner variant,

---

Friedrich Theodor Schwann, 1810–1882, Professor of Anatomy, successively at Louvain (1839–1848) and Liege, Belgium (1849–1880). Original research before the age of 27 laid the foundation of the physiology of nerve and muscle. The first to deal with problems related to living matter on a purely physical and chemical basis and to recognise the cell as the unit of living matter. Discovered pepsin and the role of living organisms in fermentation.

Friedrich Von Recklinghausen, 1833–1910, German Professor of Pathology, also described haemochromatosis.

affecting approximately 1:4000 births. It arises from a gene mutation on chromosome 17. Skin manifestations appear in early life, with the development of more than five smooth-surfaced café-au-lait spots, subcutaneous neurofibromata, armpit or groin freckling and Lisch nodules. NF-2 produces multiple central nervous system tumours.

Naevoid basal cell carcinoma (Gorlin's) syndrome

This is an autosomal dominant inherited condition caused by an abnormal tumour suppressor gene on chromosome 9q 22–31 coding the 'patched' protein; 90% of patients develop multiple basal cell carcinomas (BCCs). Patients may exhibit specific phenotypical characteristics, including overdeveloped supraorbital ridges; broad nasal roots; hypertelorism; bifid ribs; scoliosis; brachymetacarpalism; palmar pits; and molar odontogenic cysts; patients are also prone to other tumours.

Xeroderma pigmentosum

This syndrome is caused by an abnormality on the 'patched' gene of chromosome 9q, resulting in aberrant nucleotide repair during cellular DNA maintenance. It confers a >2000-fold increase in skin cancer risk and has autosomal recessive inheritance. Sufferers are intolerant of UVR, leading to premature skin ageing and development of multiple neoplasms. Most affected individuals die in early adulthood from metastatic disease (60% mortality by 20 years of age).

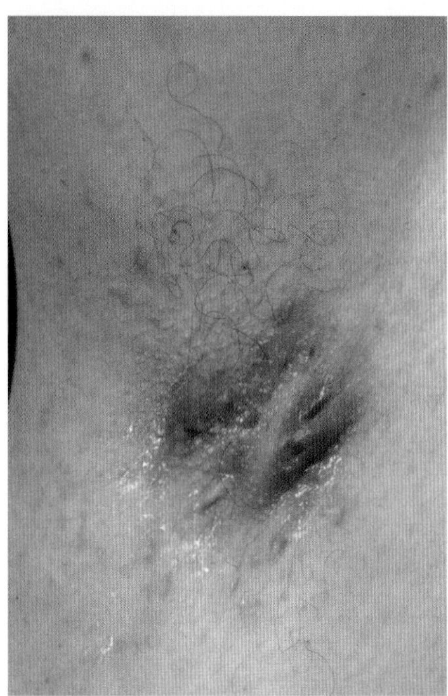

Figure 45.4 Hidradenitis suppurativa affecting the axilla (courtesy of St John's Institute for Dermatology, London, UK).

Gardner's syndrome

This syndrome is an autosomal dominant disease variant of familial adenomatous polyposis (FAP), which is caused by *APC* gene mutations on chromosome 5q 22. Gardner's syndrome can cause the development of cutaneous pathology, such as multiple epidermoid cysts and lipomata.

Ferguson-Smith syndrome

A rare autosomal dominant inherited abnormality on chromosome 9q in which affected individuals develop multiple self-healing squamous cell carcinomas (SCCs) without relation to sun exposure.

Cutaneous manifestations of generalised disease

Many diseases have cutaneous manifestations that present in surgical practice. These include: necrobiosis lipoidica, granuloma annulare in diabetes mellitus and pyoderma gangrenosum in inflammatory bowel disease. Their management should be sought in appropriate texts.

Hyperhidrosis

This involves excessive eccrine sweating of the palms, soles of the feet, axillae and groins, causing functional and social problems. It can be treated with antiperspirants or periodic local injections with botulinum toxin A. More resistant cases are treated by transthoracic endoscopic sympathectomy.

Lipodystrophy

Lipodystrophy (lipoatrophy) is a localised or generalised loss of fatty tissue, which can be primary or secondary. It can be a complication of long-term administration of insulin, following treatment of human immunodeficiency virus (HIV) with protease inhibitors or in transplant recipients.

It can be treated in selected cases by autologous fat grafting, injections of poly-l-lactic acid and free tissue transfer.

Inflammatory conditions

Hidradenitis suppurativa

Characterised by follicular occlusion, folliculitis and secondary infection (usually with *Staphylococcus aureus* and *Propionibacterium acnes*), hidradenitis suppurativa culminates in chronic suppurative, painful skin abscesses, sinus tracts and scarring. It affects apocrine gland-bearing skin in the axillae, groins and, less often, scalp, breast, chest and perineum (***Figure 45.4***). Affecting four women for every man, it has a genetic predisposition, but variable penetrance, and is strongly associated with obesity, smoking and sex hormones (it starts at puberty and often resolves at menopause).

Karl Lisch, 1907–1999, ophthalmologist, Wörgl, Austria.
Robert J Gorlin, 1923–2006, American dentist and Professor of Oral Pathology, published over 400 articles on craniofacial syndromes.
Eldon John Gardner, 1909–1989, geneticist, The University of Utah, Salt Lake City, UT, USA, described this syndrome in 1950.
John Ferguson-Smith, 1888–1978, Glaswegian dermatologist.

Management. Patients should stop smoking and lose excess weight. Symptoms can be reduced by the use of antiseptic soaps, tea tree oil and wearing non-compressive and aerated underwear. Medical treatments include topical and oral antibiotics and antiandrogen drugs. In selected cases, patients require radical excision of the affected skin and subcutaneous tissue. Reconstruction after excision avoids contracture and functional impairment.

Pyoderma gangrenosum

Characterised by rapid onset and painful cutaneous ulceration with purple undermined edges, pyoderma gangrenosum is secondary to heightened immunological reactivity, usually from another disease process, such as inflammatory bowel disease, rheumatoid arthritis, non-Hodgkin's lymphoma or granulomatosis with polyangiitis (***Figure 45.5***). Ulcers generally respond to steroids; surgery is rarely indicated and may exacerbate the condition.

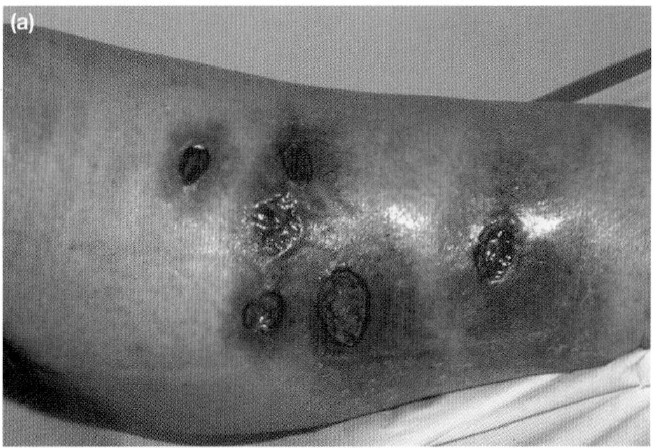

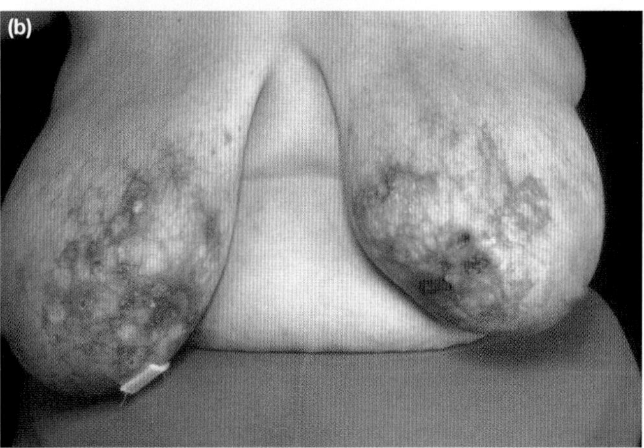

Figure 45.5 Pyoderma gangrenosum affecting the legs **(a)** and the breasts **(b)** (courtesy of St John's Institute for Dermatology, London, UK).

Infections

Skin and soft-tissue infections can be localised or spreading, necrotising or non-necrotising. Localised or spreading non-necrotising infections usually respond to broad-spectrum antibiotics. Localised necrotising infections need surgical debridement as well as antibiotic therapy. Spreading necrotising soft-tissue infection constitutes a life-threatening surgical emergency, requiring immediate resuscitation, intravenous antibiotic therapy and urgent surgical intervention with radical debridement.

Impetigo

Impetigo is a superficial infection of skin with staphylococci, streptococci or both (***Figure 45.6***). It is highly infectious and is characterised by blisters that rupture and coalesce to form a honey-coloured crust; it usually affects children. Treatment is directed at washing the affected areas and applying topical antistaphylococcal treatments; broad-spectrum oral antibiotics are required if streptococcal infection is also implicated.

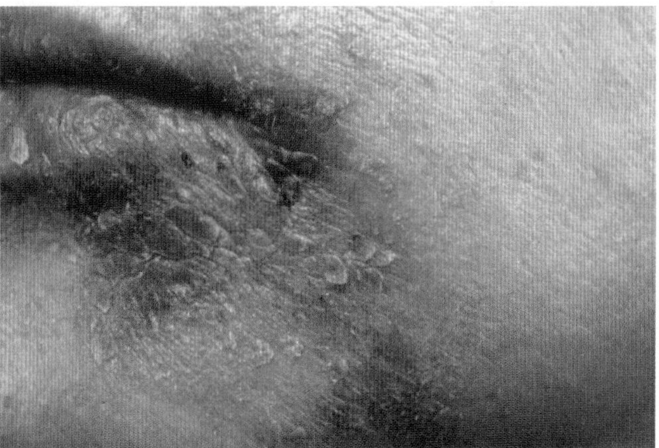

Figure 45.6 Impetigo. Note the honey-coloured crust (courtesy of St John's Institute for Dermatology, London, UK).

Erysipelas

Erysipelas is a sharply demarcated streptococcal infection of the superficial lymphatics, usually associated with broken skin on the face (***Figure 45.7***). The area affected is erythematous and oedematous. The patient may be febrile and have a leukocytosis. Prompt administration of broad-spectrum antibiotics after swabbing the area for culture and sensitivity is usually all that is necessary.

Cellulitis/lymphangitis

This is a bacterial infection of the skin and subcutaneous tissue that is more generalised than erysipelas. It is usually associated with broken skin or pre-existing ulceration. It is characterised by an expanding area of erythematous, oedematous tissue that is painful, in association with fever, malaise and leukocytosis. Erythema tracking along lymphatics may be visible (lymphangitis) (***Figure 45.8***). The commonest causative organisms are *Streptococcus pyogenes* and *S. aureus*. Blood and skin cultures for sensitivity should be taken before prompt administration of broad-spectrum intravenous antibiotics and elevation of the affected extremity.

Thomas Hodgkin, 1798–1866, curator of the museum and demonstrator of morbid anatomy, Guy's Hospital, London, UK.

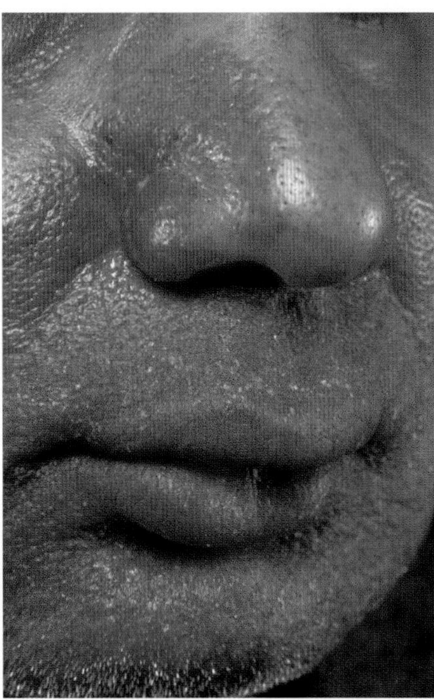

Figure 45.7 Erysipelas (courtesy of St John's Institute for Dermatology, London, UK).

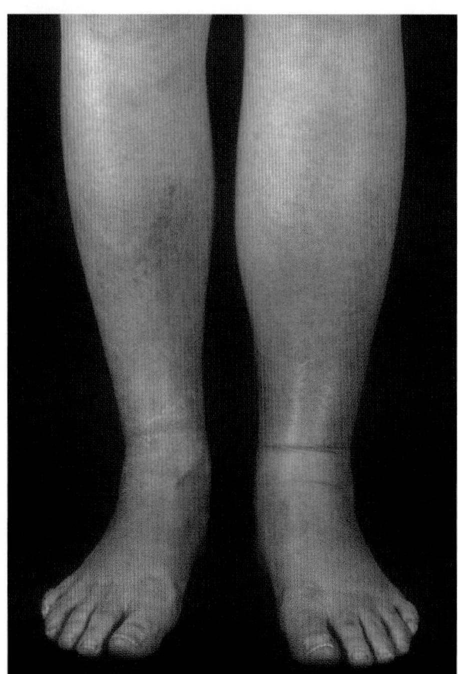

Figure 45.8 Cellulitis affecting the left leg (courtesy of St John's Institute for Dermatology, London, UK).

Necrotising fasciitis

Meleney's synergistic gangrene and Fournier's gangrene are variants of a similar disease process.

Necrotising fasciitis results from synergistic polymicrobial infection, most commonly a group A β-haemolytic *Streptococcus* in combination with *Staphylococcus*, *Escherichia coli*, *Pseudomonas*, *Proteus*, *Bacteroides* or *Clostridium*; 80% of patients have a history of previous trauma/infection and over 60% of cases commence in the lower extremities. Predisposing conditions include diabetes mellitus, smoking, penetrating trauma, pressure sores, immunosuppression, intravenous drug abuse, perineal infection (perianal abscess, Bartholin's cysts) and skin damage/infection (abrasions, bites, boils).

Summary box 45.1

Necrotising fasciitis

- Surgical emergency
- Polymicrobial synergistic infection
- 80% have a history of previous trauma or infection
- Rapid progression to septic shock
- Urgent resuscitation, antibiotics and surgical debridement
- Mortality 30–50%

Classical clinical signs include oedema stretching beyond visible skin erythema; a woody-hard texture to the subcutaneous tissues; an inability to distinguish fascial planes and muscle groups on palpation; disproportionate pain in relation to the affected area, with associated skin vesicles and soft-tissue crepitus (***Figure 45.9***). Lymphangitis tends to be absent. Early on, patients may be febrile and tachycardic, with a very rapid progression to septic shock. Radiographs, which should not have delayed urgent treatment, may demonstrate air in the tissues.

Management should commence with urgent fluid resuscitation, monitoring of haemodynamic status and administration of high-dose intravenous broad-spectrum antibiotics. This is a surgical emergency and the diseased area should be debrided as soon as possible until viable, healthy, bleeding tissue is reached. Early surgical review and further debridement is advisable, together with the use of vacuum-assisted dressings. Early skin grafting in selected cases may minimise protein and fluid losses. Where available, hyperbaric oxygen therapy after debridement may be helpful. Mortality of between 30% and 50% can be expected, even with prompt operative intervention.

Purpura fulminans

This is a relatively rare condition in which intravascular thrombosis produces rapid skin necrosis and haemorrhagic infarction, which progresses rapidly to septic shock and disseminated intravascular coagulation. Usually seen in children, it can occur in adults and may be subdivided into three types based on the aetiological mechanism: 'acute infectious', 'neonatal' and 'idiopathic' purpura fulminans.

Acute infectious is the commonest form. It is associated with a mortality rate of 40–50%, usually from multiorgan

Frank Meleney, 1889–1963, American surgeon in the First World War, then became a Professor at Columbia Medical School in New York, NY, USA.
Jean Fournier, 1832–1914, French dermatologist, also described tertiary syphilis.
Caspar Bartholin (Secundus), 1655–1709, Professor of Medicine, Anatomy and Physics, Copenhagen, Denmark, described these glands in 1677.

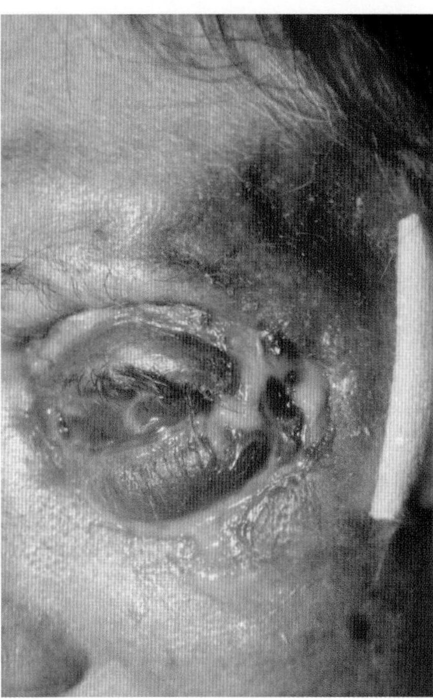

Figure 45.9 Necrotising fasciitis affecting the left orbit and facial skin (courtesy of St John's Institute for Dermatology, London, UK).

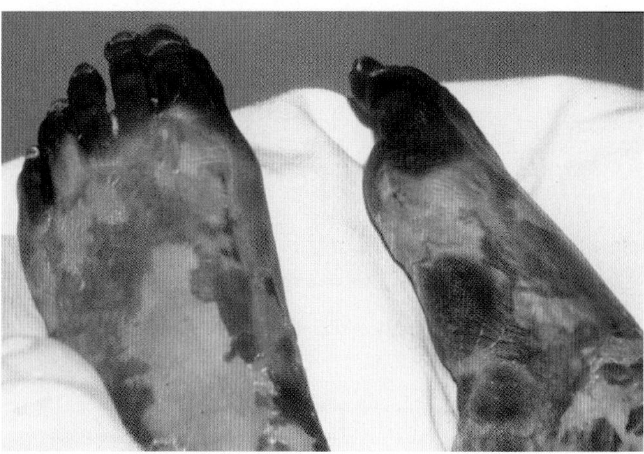

Figure 45.10 Acute infectious purpura fulminans caused by meningococcal septicaemia. Note the sharply demarcated necrotic areas distal to the affected end or perforating arteries with surrounding normal skin (courtesy of St John's Institute for Dermatology, London, UK).

failure, and is secondary to either an acute bacterial (*Neisseria meningitidis*) or viral infection (varicella). It is most common in children under 7 years, following an upper respiratory tract infection or in asplenia. Endotoxins produce an imbalance in procoagulant and anticoagulant endothelial activity, producing protein C deficiency; this gives the clinical picture of an initial petechial rash developing into confluent ecchymoses and haemorrhagic bullae, which necrose to form well-demarcated lesions that form hard eschars. Extensive tissue loss is common, which often culminates in limb amputation (***Figure 45.10***).

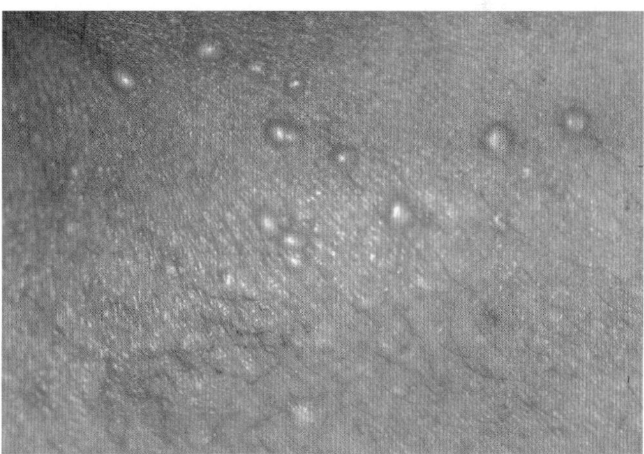

Figure 45.11 Milia (courtesy of St John's Institute for Dermatology, London, UK).

Skin and soft-tissue cysts

Milia

Small, hard, keratin retention cysts (***Figure 45.11***) seen both in babies and, after chronic sun exposure, in the elderly as part of Favre–Racouchot syndrome (solar comedones, pseudocysts and leathery, furrowed sun-damaged skin – heightened by smoking).

Epidermal cysts

These cysts are lined with true stratified squamous epithelium, derived from hair follicle infundibuli or traumatic inclusion. Commonly known as sebaceous cysts, they can occur anywhere. They are fixed to the skin and usually have a central punctum (***Figure 45.12***).

Treatment depends on the clinical state of the cyst. When inflamed or infected, they should be incised and drained initially; they should be removed later once the inflammation and induration has subsided. It is important to excise the cyst in its entirety as failure to do so usually results in recurrence.

Meibomian cysts are epidermal cysts found on the free edge of the eyelid. Trichilemmal (pilar/pilosebaceous) cysts are derived from the epidermis of the external root sheath of the hair follicle; 90% are found in the scalp and 70% are multiple. They are usually distinguished from epidermal cysts by pathologists, rather than clinically.

Albert Ludwig Siegmund Neisser, 1855–1916, Director of the Dermatological Institute, Breslau, Germany (now Wrocław, Poland).
Maurice Favre, 1876–1954, French dermatologist.
Jean Racouchot, 1908–1994, French dermatologist.
Heinrich Meibom (Meibomius), 1638–1700, Professor of Medicine, History and Poetry, Helmstadt, Germany, described these glands in 1666.

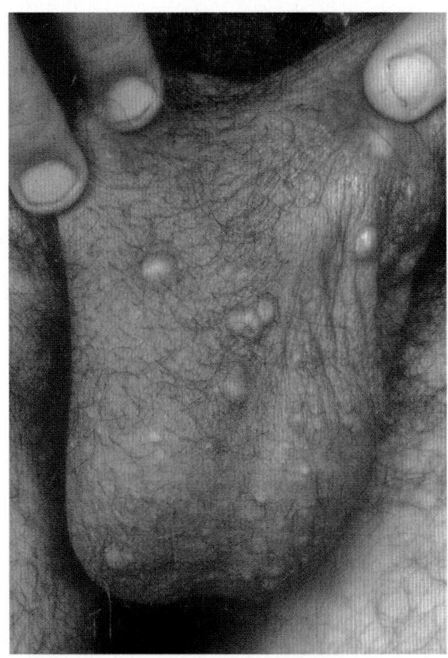

Figure 45.12 Multiple scrotal epidermal cysts (courtesy of St John's Institute for Dermatology, London, UK).

SKIN TUMOURS

Benign lesions

Basal cell papilloma (seborrhoeic keratosis, senile keratosis, verruca senilis)

Their appearance varies from macular to soft, excrescent, warty lesions – often pigmented and hyperkeratotic – but may be flesh-coloured or pink. They are formed from the basal layer of epidermal cells and contain melanocytes.

Papillary wart (verruca vulgaris)

This is a benign skin tumour arising from infection with the human papillomavirus (HPV), which is also responsible for plantar warts and condylomata acuminata.

Freckle (ephelis)

A freckle is an area of skin that contains a normal number of melanocytes, producing an abnormally large number of melanin granules.

Lentigo

These are small, circumscribed pigmented macules that stem from sun damage and some systemic syndromes. Solar lentigos are commoner in fairer skins.

Moles/naevi

Melanocytes migrate from the neural crest to the basal epidermis during embryogenesis. When melanocytes aggregate in the dermis or at the dermoepidermal junction, they are called naevus cells.

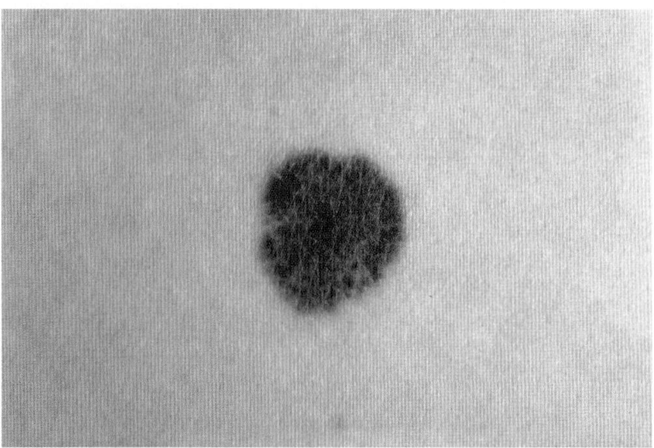

Figure 45.13 Junctional naevus (courtesy of St John's Institute for Dermatology, London, UK).

Junctional naevus

A junctional naevus is a dermoepidermal proliferation of naevus cells, visible as deeply pigmented macules or papules that occur commonly in childhood or adolescence, usually progressing to form compound or intradermal naevi with advancing age. Benign mucosal lesions tend to be junctional naevi (***Figure 45.13***).

Compound naevus

This is a maculopapular, pigmented lesion that becomes most prominent during adolescence (***Figure 45.14***). It represents a junctional proliferation of naevus cells, with nests and columns in the dermis.

Intradermal naevus

Intradermal naevi are faintly pigmented papules in adults that show no junctional proliferation; however, they do show a cluster of dermal melanocytes (***Figure 45.15***).

Spitz naevus

These are reddish brown (occasionally deeply pigmented) nodules, previously termed 'juvenile melanoma' (***Figure 45.16***). They most commonly occur on the face and legs, growing rapidly initially then remaining static or regressing. The differential diagnosis is melanoma and excision biopsy is warranted if there is doubt as to the diagnosis.

Spindle cell naevus

Spindle cell naevi are dense black lesions that contain spindle cells and atypical melanocytes at the dermoepidermal junction. They are commonly seen on the thighs and affect women more frequently. They may have malignant potential.

Halo naevus

The halo of depigmentation around any benign naevus represents an antibody response to melanocytes. Depigmentation may also be a feature of a malignant melanoma. Halo naevi are associated with vitiligo (***Figure 45.17***).

Sophie Spitz, 1910–1956, American dermatopathologist at the Memorial Sloan Kettering Cancer Center, published the first case series of 'juvenile melanoma' in 1948.

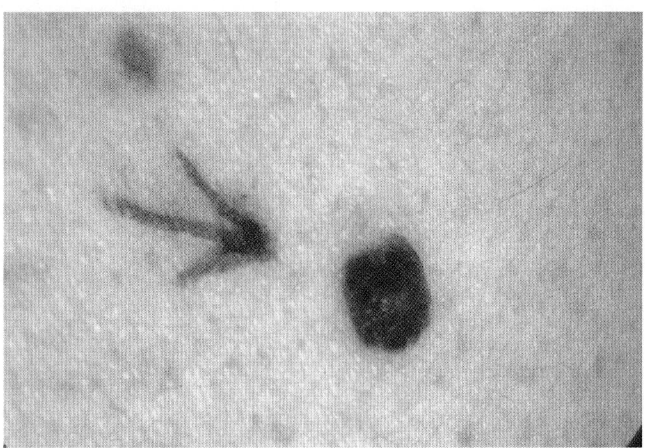

Figure 45.14 Compound naevus (courtesy of St John's Institute for Dermatology, London, UK).

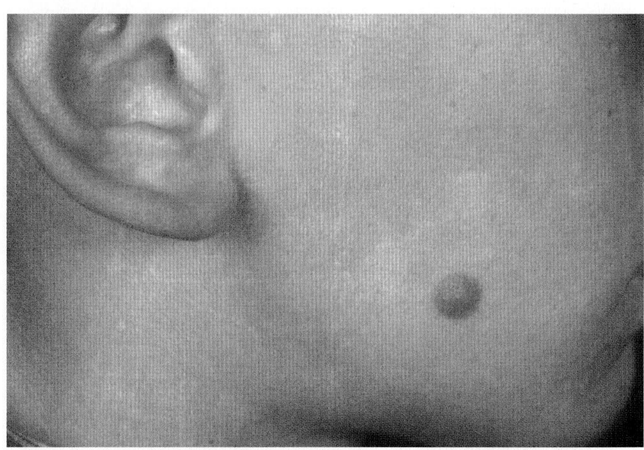

Figure 45.16 Spitz naevus (courtesy of St John's Institute for Dermatology, London, UK).

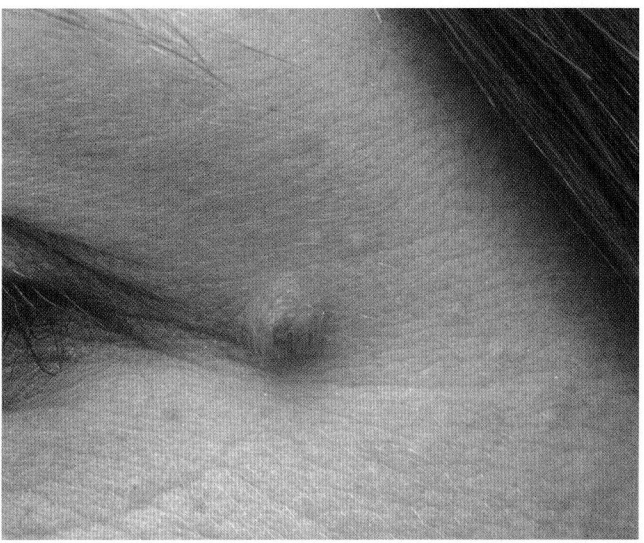

Figure 45.15 Intradermal naevus (courtesy of St John's Institute for Dermatology, London, UK).

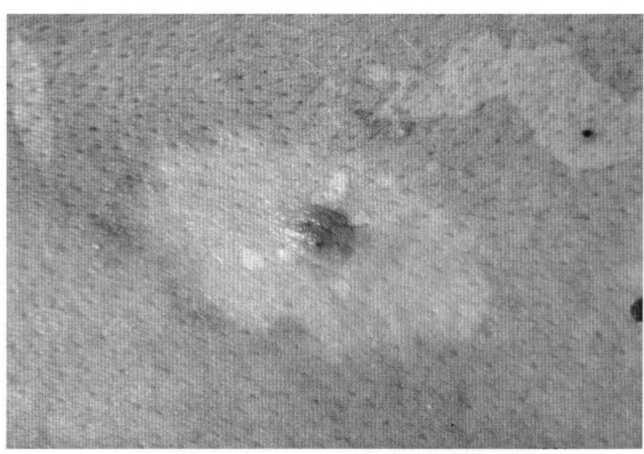

Figure 45.17 Halo naevus (courtesy of St John's Institute for Dermatology, London, UK).

Café-au-lait spots

These are coffee-coloured macules of variable size (from a few millimetres to 10 cm) (***Figure 45.18***). Multiple lesions are associated with NF-1 and McCune–Albright syndromes. They are more common in dark-skinned people.

Naevus spilus (speckled lentiginous naevus)

These are similar in appearance to café-au-lait spots but with hyperpigmented speckles throughout (***Figure 45.19***). They are benign lesions that are associated with various cutaneous diseases, but whose speckled appearance can be confused with malignant change. The mainstay of management is observation and serial photography as malignant transformation is rare.

Mongolian spot

A Mongolian spot is a congenital blue-grey macule found on the sacral skin (***Figure 45.20***). Pigmentation initially deepens and then regresses completely by age 7 years.

Blue naevus

This is a benign skin lesion that is four times more common in children, typically affecting the extremities and face (***Figure 45.21***).

Naevi of Ota and Ito

A naevus of Ota is a dermal melanocytic hamartoma visible as a blue or grey macule in the trigeminal V1 and V2 dermatomes. It is four times more common in women and most frequently seen in Asian and African people (***Figure 45.22***).

A naevus of Ito is characterised by dermal melanocytosis in the shoulder region and can occur simultaneously in patients with naevus of Ota (***Figure 45.23***).

Donovan James McCune, 1902–1976, American pediatrician.
Fuller Albright, 1900–1969, physician, Massachusetts General Hospital, Boston, MA, USA.
Masao Ota, 1885–1945, Japanese dermatologist.
Minoru Ito, 1892–1986, Professor of Dermatology, Tohoku University, Sendai, Honshu, Japan.

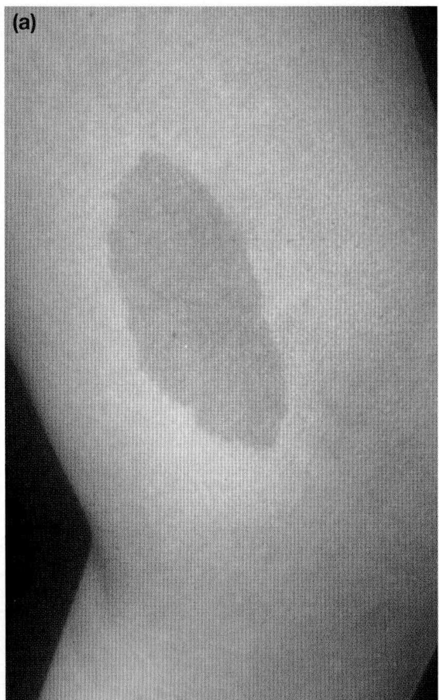

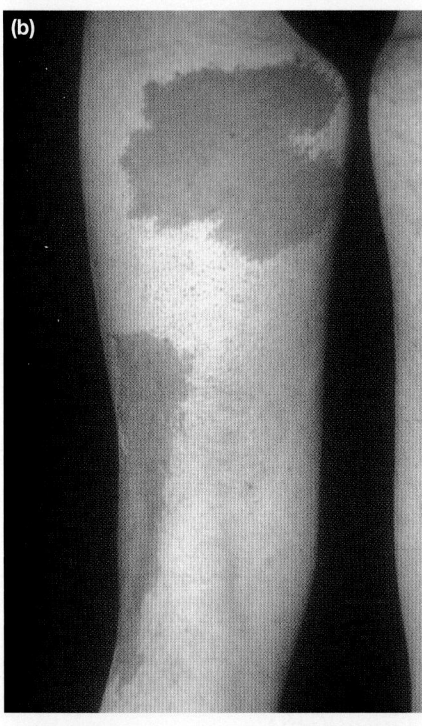

Figure 45.18 Café-au-lait spots. Note the two topographical variants: in (a) the spot has a smooth 'coast of California' border, whereas the upper spot in (b) has an irregular 'coast of Maine' border. Multiple smooth-bordered lesions are commonly associated with syndromes (courtesy of St John's Institute for Dermatology, London, UK).

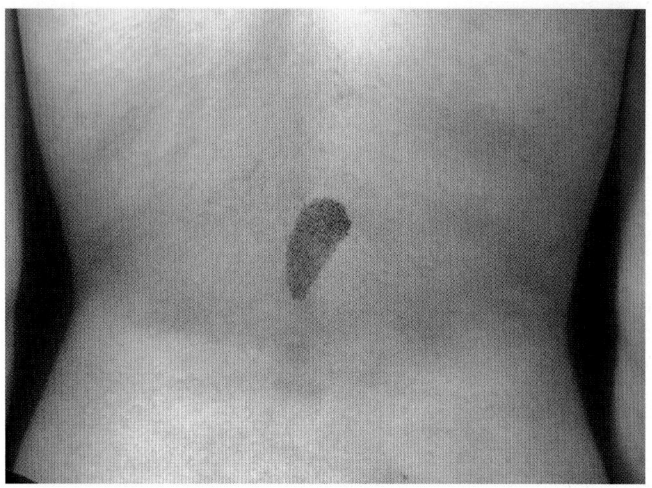

Figure 45.19 Naevus spilus (courtesy of St John's Institute for Dermatology, London, UK).

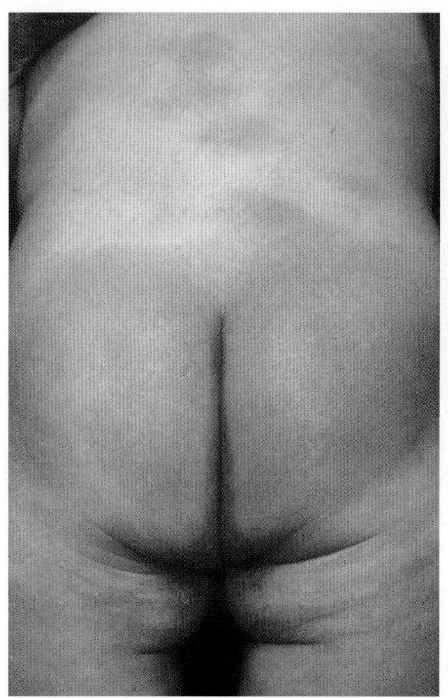

Figure 45.20 Mongolian spot (courtesy of St John's Institute for Dermatology, London, UK).

Hair follicles

Trichoepithelioma

These are small skin-coloured nodules found most often in the nasolabial folds. Trichoepithelioma is clinically and histologically similar to a BCC.

Pilomatrixoma (calcifying epithelioma of Malherbe)

These are benign hair matrix cell tumours that often calcify; 40% are found in the under-10 age group.

Albert Hippolyte Malherbe, 1845–1945, Professor of Histology, Anatomy and Surgery, Nantes, France.

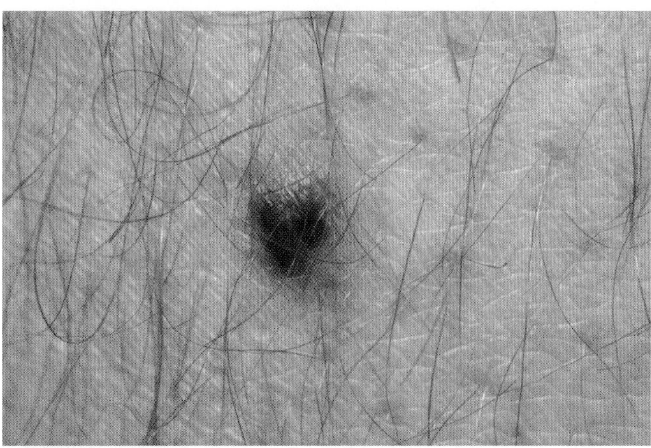

Figure 45.21 Blue naevus (courtesy of St John's Institute for Dermatology, London, UK).

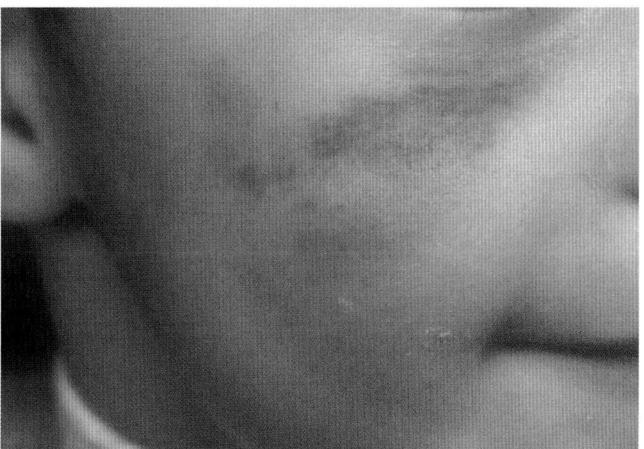

Figure 45.22 Naevus of Ota (courtesy of St John's Institute for Dermatology, London, UK).

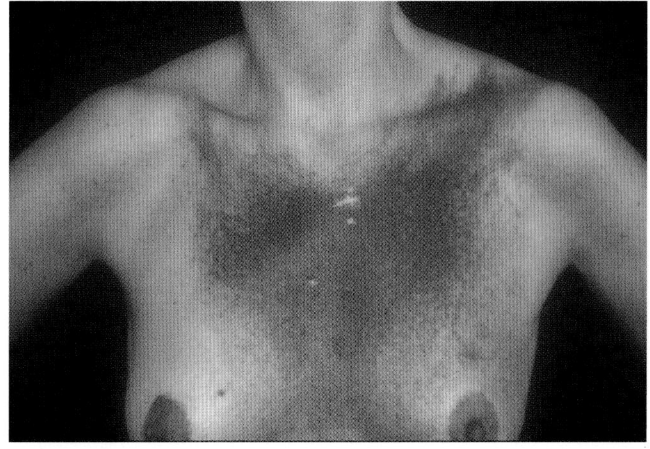

Figure 45.23 Naevus of Ito (courtesy of St John's Institute for Dermatology, London, UK).

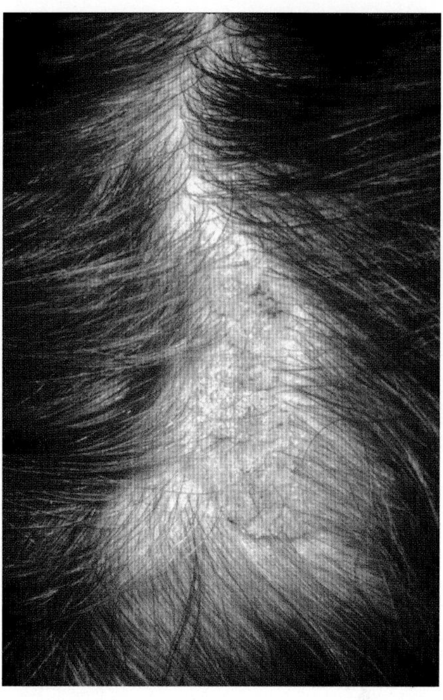

Figure 45.24 Naevus sebaceous of Jadassohn (courtesy of St John's Institute for Dermatology, London, UK).

Trichilemmoma (naevus sebaceous of Jadassohn)

Trichilemmoma is a congenital hamartoma with the appearance of a linear verrucous naevus; 10% lifetime risk of forming a BCC (*Figure 45.24*).

Adenoma sebaceum (tuberous sclerosis, Bourneville disease)

These are facial papules (angiofibromata) that are red-brown depending on skin colour and usually appear on the nasolabial folds, cheek and chin. They usually appear in children before 10 years of age and increase in size and number until adolescence. Cosmetic removal by argon or pulsed-dye lasers or scalpel is indicated (*Figure 45.25*).

Rhinophyma

Rhinophyma is the end-stage sequela of nasal acne rosacea (*Figure 45.26*). It is nasal sebaceous gland hypertrophy and hyperplasia and tends to affect elderly men (male-to-female ration 12:1). Occult BCCs exist in 3%. Treatment by dermabrasion or laser resurfacing produces good results.

Sweat glands

Cystadenoma (hydrocystadenomas, hidradenomas)

These are 1- to 3-cm translucent blue cystic nodules.

Josef Jadassohn, 1863–1936, dermatologist, Breslau, Germany (now Wrocław, Poland).
Desire M Bourneville, 1840–1909, physician, Le Bicêtre, Paris, France.

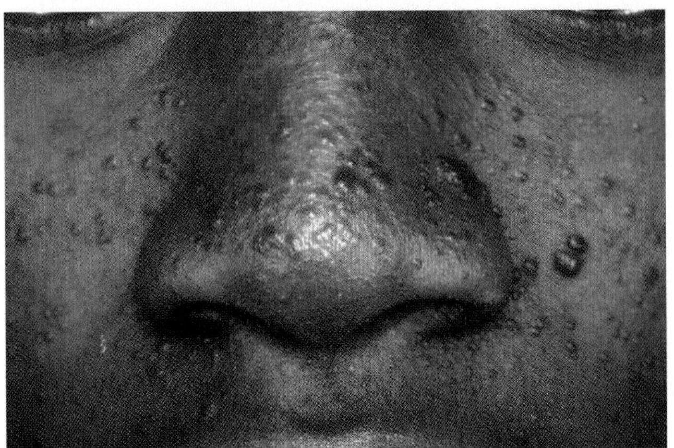

Figure 45.25 Adenoma sebaceum (courtesy of St John's Institute for Dermatology, London, UK).

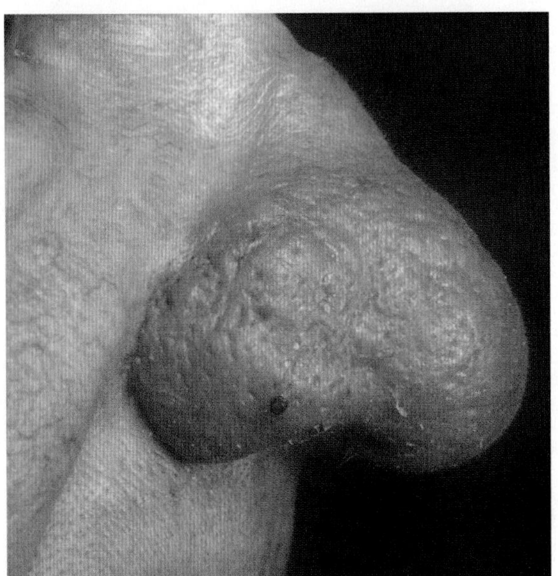

Figure 45.26 Rhinophyma (courtesy of St John's Institute for Dermatology, London, UK).

Eccrine poroma (papillary syringoma)

These are single raised or pedicled lesions found most often on the palm or sole.

Cylindroma (turban tumour)

A variant of eccrine spiradenoma that coalesce when multiple on the scalp, forming a 'turban tumour'.

Premalignant lesions

Extramammary Paget's disease (intraepidermal adenocarcinoma)

This occurs in cutaneous sites that are rich in apocrine glands such as the axillae and the genital and perianal regions. Approximately 25% are associated with an underlying *in situ* or invasive adenocarcinoma. Early skin changes are subtle and may present as an eczematous lesion or intertrigo. Surgical excision forms the basis of treatment, with up to 20% demonstrating invasive disease after pathology assessment (***Figure 45.27***).

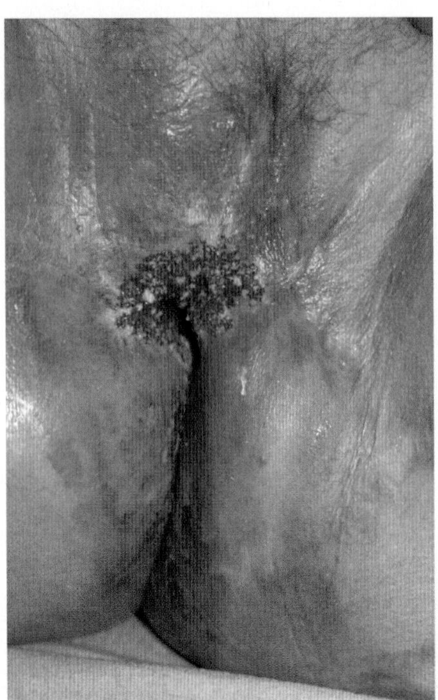

Figure 45.27 Extramammary Paget's disease involving the perineum (courtesy of St John's Institute for Dermatology, London, UK).

Giant congenital pigmented naevus or giant hairy naevus

This hamartoma of naevo-melanocytes causes confusion because its definition and management are contentious. It has a similar histology to compound naevi, but with naevus cells distributed variably throughout all skin layers and into the subdermal fat and muscle and with a tendency to dermatomal distribution (***Figure 45.28***). Giant congenital pigmented naevi (GCPNs) are precursors of melanoma but the magnitude of this risk is unclear, largely because of the lack of well-conducted studies and variable classification of the naevus. A 3–5% lifetime risk of melanoma is quoted. One in three childhood malignant melanomas arise in patients with GCPN, but the risk decreases with age: 15% of malignant melanomas present at birth, 62% present by puberty and 99% by 45 years of age.

A multidisciplinary management approach is advocated, with initial investigations examining for neurocutaneous melanosis as there may be leptomeningeal involvement. Removal of GCPN should be considered for both aesthetic and oncological reasons.

Atypical (dysplastic) naevus

To be 'atypical naevi', lesions must have three of the following characteristics: variegated pigmentation; ill-defined borders;

Sir James Paget, 1814–1899, surgeon, St Bartholomew's Hospital, London, UK.

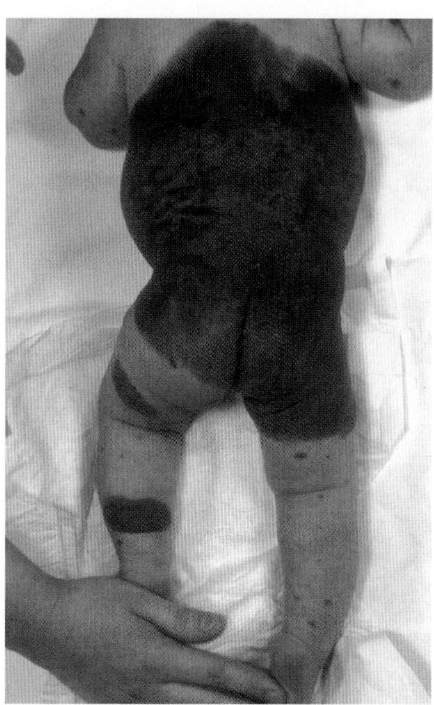

Figure 45.28 Giant congenital pigmented naevus (courtesy of St John's Institute for Dermatology, London, UK).

undulating irregular surfaces; or size >5 mm. Terminology is confused because, although the terms 'dysplastic' and 'atypical' are often used interchangeably, dysplasia is a histological diagnosis with findings of irregular proliferations of melanocytes at the basal layer of the epidermis. In fact, a small proportion of clinically 'atypical naevi' are actually dysplastic when examined microscopically.

Atypical naevi can be sporadic or familial (familial atypical multiple mole–melanoma [FAMMM] syndrome). Possession of more than five lesions confers a relative risk of melanoma six times greater than usual; within FAMMM syndrome, they confer a 100% risk of malignant melanoma and patients with FAMMM syndrome should be screened for melanoma 6-monthly, lifelong (***Figure 45.29***).

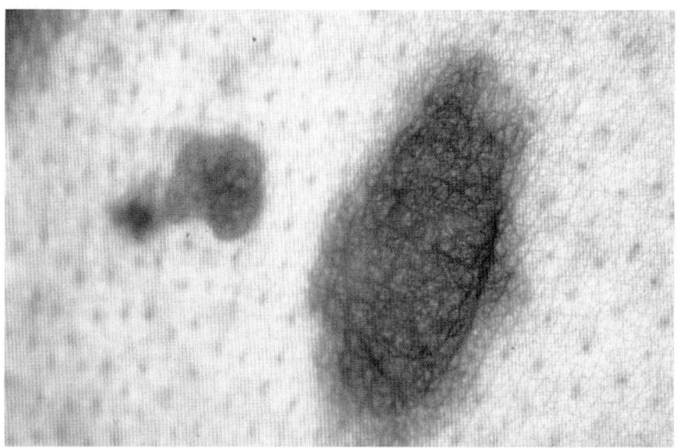

Figure 45.29 Dysplastic naevus (courtesy of St John's Institute for Dermatology, London, UK).

Malignant lesions

Data from the World Health Organization suggest that both non-melanoma and melanoma skin cancers continue to increase in incidence, despite educational programmes and wide-ranging changes in uptake of sun protective measures and improvements in sunscreens. Skin cancer is the commonest malignancy in white-skinned people, constituting 33% of all recorded malignancies annually, with 2–3 million new non-melanoma skin cancers and 132 000 new malignant melanomas (4.5% of all new cancers are melanomas) diagnosed each year.

Basal cell carcinoma

This is usually a slow-growing, locally invasive, malignant tumour of pluripotential epithelial cells arising from basal epidermis and hair follicles; hence, it affects the pilosebaceous skin.

Summary box 45.2

Basal cell carcinoma

- Slow growing
- Risk factor – UVR
- 90% nodular/nodular cystic
- High- and low-risk BCC

Epidemiology

The strongest predisposing factor to BCC is UVR. It occurs in the elderly or the middle-aged after excessive sun exposure, with 95% occurring between the ages of 40 and 80 years. The incidence of BCC rises with proximity to the equator, although 33% arise in parts of the body not usually exposed to the sun. Other predisposing factors include exposure to arsenical compounds, coal tar, aromatic hydrocarbons and IR and genetic skin cancer syndromes. White-skinned people are almost exclusively affected. BCC is more common in men than in women.

Pathogenesis

BCCs have no apparent precursor lesions and their development is proportional to the initial dose of the carcinogen, but not duration of exposure. The most likely model of pathogenesis for BCCs involves mesodermal factors as intrinsic promoters coupled with an initiation step. BCCs metastasise extremely rarely.

Macroscopic

BCCs can be divided into localised (nodular, nodulocystic, cystic, pigmented and naevoid) and generalised (superficial: multifocal and superficial spreading; or infiltrative: morphoeic, ice pick and cicatrising). Nodular and nodulocystic variants account for 90% of BCCs.

Microscopic

Twenty-six histological subtypes have been described. The characteristic finding is of ovoid cells in nests with a single 'palisading' layer. It is only the outer layer of cells that actively divide, explaining why tumour growth rates are slower than their cell cycle speed would suggest and why incompletely excised lesions are more aggressive. Morphoeic BCCs synthesise type 4 collagenase and so spread rapidly (***Figure 45.30***).

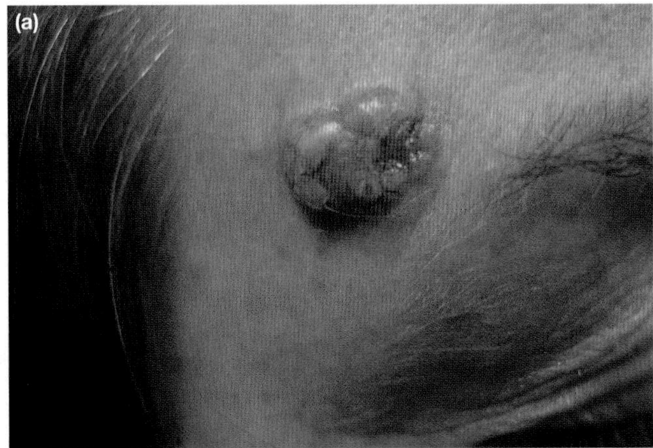

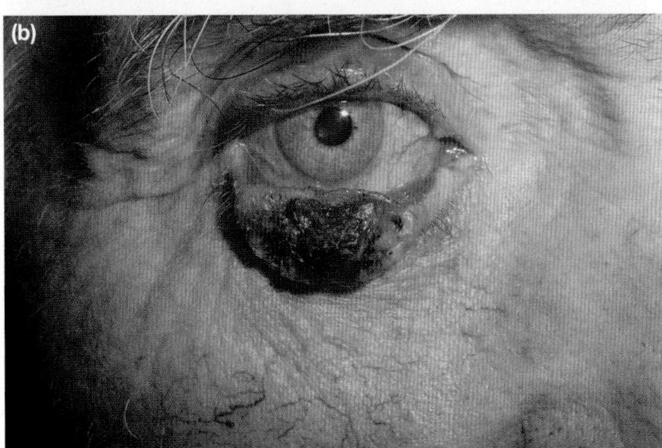

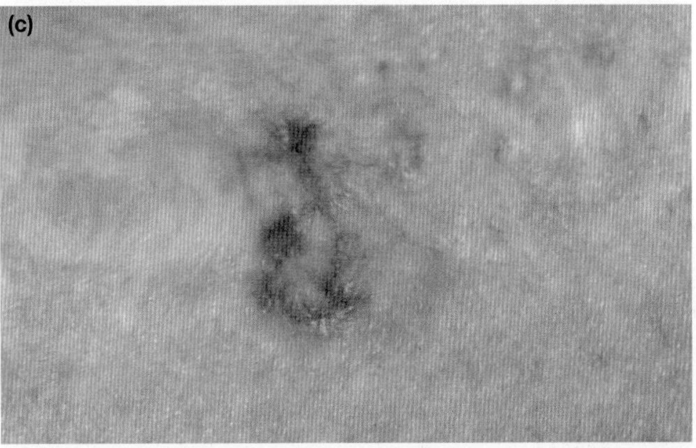

Figure 45.30 (a) A nodulocystic basal carcinoma (BCC). Note the characteristic pearly surface with telangiectasia. **(b)** An ulcerating BCC on the lower eyelid. **(c)** A recurrent morphoeic BCC. (**(a, b)** courtesy of Mr AR Greenbaum; **(c)** courtesy of St John's Institute for Dermatology, London, UK.)

Prognosis

There are 'high-risk' and 'low-risk' BCCs. High-risk BCCs: are large (>2 cm); are located at sites where direct invasion gives access to the cranium (near the eye, nose and ear); are recurrent tumours; are tumours forming in the presence of immunosuppression; or have micronodular or infiltrating histological subtypes.

Management

Treatment can be surgical or non-surgical. Tumour and surrounding surgical margins should always be assessed and marked under loupe magnification, the latter varying between 2 and 15 mm depending on the macroscopic variant. Where margins are ill-defined or tissue is at a premium (nose, eyes), either a two-stage surgical approach with subsequent reconstruction after confirmation of clear margins or Mohs' micrographic surgery is advisable. The histological sample must be orientated and marked for pathological examination.

Mohs' micrographic surgery is a method used by dermatological surgeons (dermatologists who have undergone extra training in techniques of cutaneous surgery and histopathology) to excise skin cancer under microscopic control.

In elderly or infirm patients, radiotherapy produces similar recurrence rates to surgery, but with the risk of generating further malignancy after one to two decades. Biopsy-proven, superficial tumours can be treated with topical treatments (5-fluorouracil, imiquimod).

Unless excision of a BCC is complete, there is a 67% recurrence rate if margins are grossly involved and a 33% recurrence rate within 2 years with microscopic involvement or when reported 'close'.

Patients with uncomplicated, completely excised lesions can be discharged. Follow-up is reserved for patients with tumours in high-risk areas; for those with globally sun-damaged skin; for those with syndromes; and for those who decline further surgery after incomplete excisions.

Cutaneous squamous cell carcinoma

SCC is a malignant tumour of keratinising cells of the epidermis or its appendages. It arises from the stratum basalis of the epidermis and expresses cytokeratins 1 and 10.

Epidemiology

Four BCCs occur for every SCC, which is the second most common form of skin cancer. It is strongly related to cumulative sun exposure and damage, especially in white-skinned individuals living nearer the equator. In the northern hemisphere it affects the elderly, whereas it is not uncommon in sun-damaged, middle-aged white people in the southern hemisphere. Everywhere, it is more common in men than in women. SCC is also associated with chronic inflammation (chronic sinus tracts, pre-existing scars, osteomyelitis, burns, vaccination points) and immunosuppression. When a SCC appears in a scar it is known as a Marjolin's ulcer.

Frederic E Mohs, 1910–2002, American physician and general surgeon, University of Wisconsin, Madison, WI, USA, developed Mohs' micrographic surgical technique in 1938 for cutaneous malignant lesions.

Jean-Nicolas Marjolin, 1780–1850, surgeon, Paris, France, described the development of carcinomatous ulcers in scars in 1828.

Summary box 45.3

Squamous cell carcinoma

- Associated with UVR, chronic inflammation, immunosuppression and chemical carcinogens
- High- and low-risk SCC
- Metastasis in 2% of low-risk and up to 30% of high-risk cases

IR causes SCC, as do chemical carcinogens (arsenicals, tar) and infection with HPV subtypes 5 and 16. There is also evidence that current and previous tobacco use doubles the relative risk of SCC.

In the past, actinic (solar) keratoses (AKs), i.e. cutaneous horns and keratoacanthomas, were considered to be premalignant lesions leading to SCC. Current thinking is to classify these lesions on a continuum of lesions, some of which can improve, as with other squamous cell tumours such as cervical intraepithelial neoplasia.

AKs are areas of permanent sun damage in which there is dyskeratosis, partial-thickness cellular atypia and subepidermal inflammation, but an intact basement membrane (***Figure 45.31***). They 'wax and wane' macroscopically between macular and papular, with and without keratinous surfaces. Most improve after moisturisation and remain as erythematous macules; however, up to 20% form SCC.

When an AK has a keratinous surface with a height greater than its base diameter, it is termed a keratin horn; 10% will have an underlying SCC (***Figure 45.32***).

Keratoacanthomas are rapidly growing, nodular tumours exhibiting symmetry around a central keratin-filled crater.

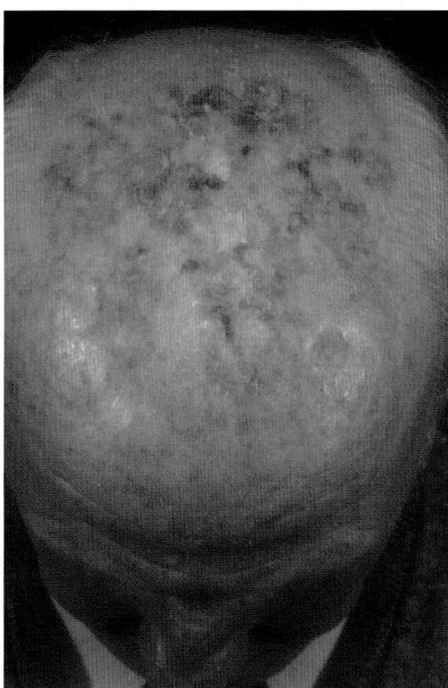

Figure 45.31 Actinic keratosis (courtesy of St John's Institute for Dermatology, London, UK).

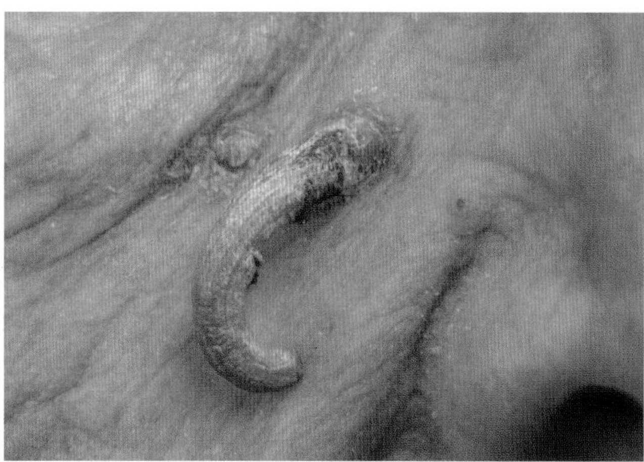

Figure 45.32 Cutaneous horn (courtesy of St John's Institute for Dermatology, London, UK).

Current thinking is that, rather than being separate premalignant entities, they are better considered as self-healing SCCs and, as such, are often reported by pathologists as 'keratoacanthoma-like SCCs' (***Figure 45.33***). Keratoacanthomas are twice as common in men as in women and are usually found on the face or limbs of chronically sun-damaged 50- to 70-year-old white-skinned individuals. They may be caused by HPV in a hair follicle during the growth phase and are also associated with smoking and chemical carcinogen exposure. Excision is recommended, rather than observation, as the differential diagnosis includes anaplastic SCC and the excision scar is often better than that which remains after resolution.

Bowen's disease is SCC *in situ* and often develops as full-thickness dysplasia in hypertrophic AKs (***Figure 45.34***). SCC *in situ* usually presents as a slowly enlarging erythematous scaly plaque and may occur anywhere on the mucocutaneous surface of the body. On the glans penis, it is called erythroplasia of Queyrat (***Figure 45.35***). Topical therapy with 5-fluorouracil or imiquimod is an effective treatment. Alternatives include surgical excision with a 4-mm margin or Mohs' micrographic surgery for larger or recurrent lesions.

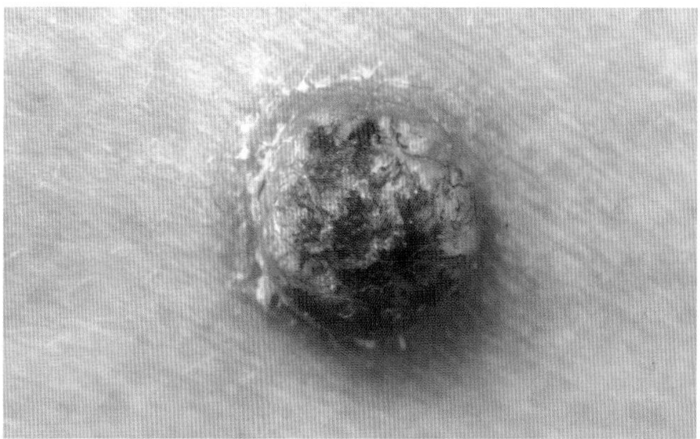

Figure 45.33 Keratoacanthoma (courtesy of St John's Institute for Dermatology, London, UK).

John T Bowen, 1857–1941, Professor of Dermatology, Harvard University Medical School, Boston, MA, USA, described this condition in 1912.
August Queyrat, 1856–1933, dermatologist, Paris, France, described this condition in 1911.

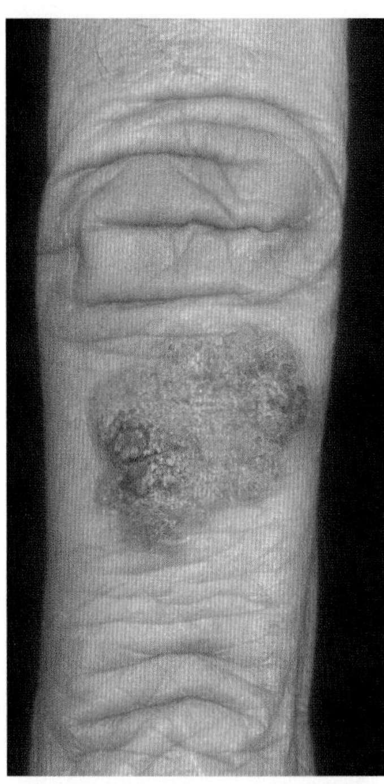

Figure 45.34 Bowen's disease – squamous cell carcinoma *in situ* (courtesy of St John's Institute for Dermatology, London, UK).

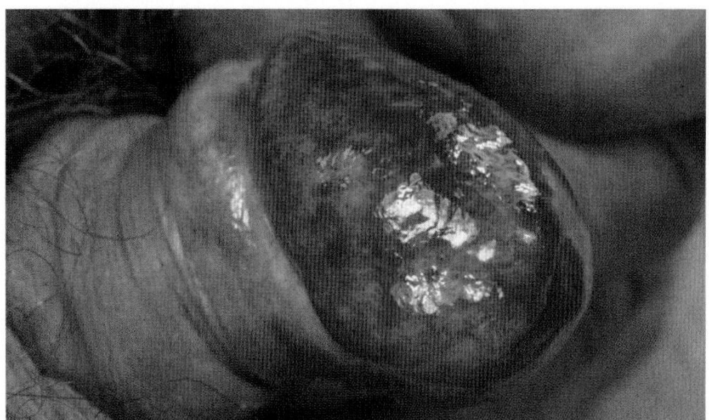

Figure 45.35 Erythroplasia of Queyrat – squamous cell carcinoma *in situ* on the glans penis; also called Paget's disease of the penis (courtesy of St John's Institute for Dermatology, London, UK).

Macroscopic

The appearance of SCC may vary from smooth nodular, verrucous, papillomatous to ulcerating lesions. All ulcerate eventually as they grow. The ulcers have a characteristic everted edge and are surrounded by inflamed, indurated skin. Differential diagnoses of SCC include: AK; BCC; pyoderma gangrenosum; warts; and lichen simplex chronicus (***Figure 45.36***).

Microscopic

Characteristic irregular masses of squamous epithelium are noted to proliferate and invade the dermis from the basal layer. The tumour stains positive for cytokeratins 1 and 10. SCC can be graded histologically according to Broders' grading, which describes the proportion of dedifferentiated cells in the tumour. ***Table 45.1*** presents tumour classification and staging.

Prognosis

There are several independent prognostic variables for SCC:

- Depth: the deeper the lesion, the worse the prognosis. For SCC <2 mm, metastasis is highly unlikely; if SCC >6 mm, 15% will have metastasised.

TABLE 45.1 Tumour–node–metastasis (TNM) classification and staging of squamous cell carcinoma.

Size	Nodes	Metastases	Stages
TX Primary tumour cannot be assessed	NX Nodal involvement cannot be assessed	M0 No metastatic disease	Stage 0 Tis, N0, M0
T0 No evidence of primary tumour	N0 No regional nodes	M1 Metastatic disease present	Stage I T1, N0, M0
Tis *In situ* (confined to full-thickness epidermal) disease	N1 Spread to 1 ipsilateral nearby node that is <3 cm in diameter		Stage II T2, N0, M0
T1 Primary <2 cm	N2a Spread to 1 ipsilateral nearby node that is 3–6 cm in diameter		Stage III T3, N0, M0 or T1–T3, N1, M0
T2 Primary >2 cm	N2b Spread to >1 ipsilateral nearby nodes but none >6 cm in diameter		Stage IV T1–T3, N2, M0 or any disease that is N3, or T4 or M1
T3 Primary invasion of a facial bone	N2c Spread to contralateral node(s) but none are >6 cm in diameter		
T4 Invasion of muscle, base of skull or other bones	N3 Spread to any node >6 cm in diameter		

Albert Compton Broders, 1885–1964, American pathologist, MN, USA, and Chairman of the Department of Surgical Pathology, Mayo Clinic, Rochester, MN, USA; for 1 year in 1935 Professor of Surgical Pathology and Director of Cancer Research, University of Virginia, Charlottesville, VA, USA. Broders also graded rectal cancer in the USA in a similar manner to the one that Cuthbert Dukes used to classify it in the UK. A combination of Broders' grading and Dukes' classification gave a more accurate prognosis for rectal carcinoma than either method alone.

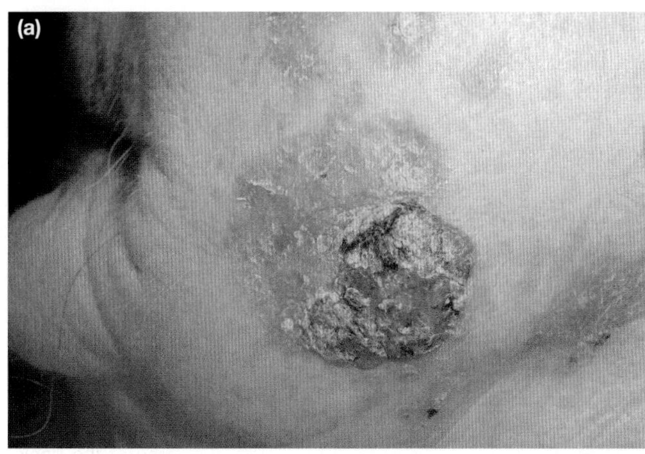
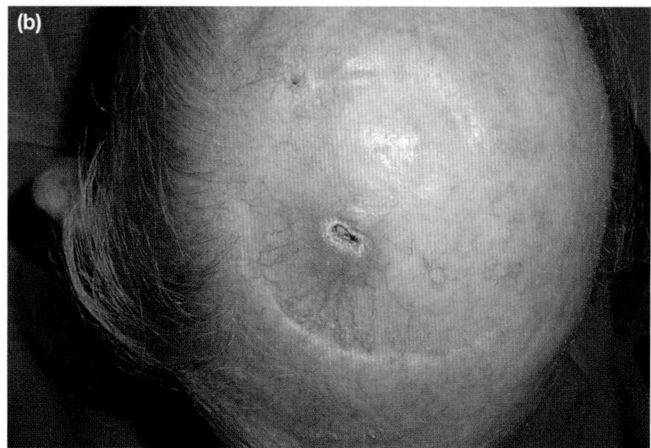
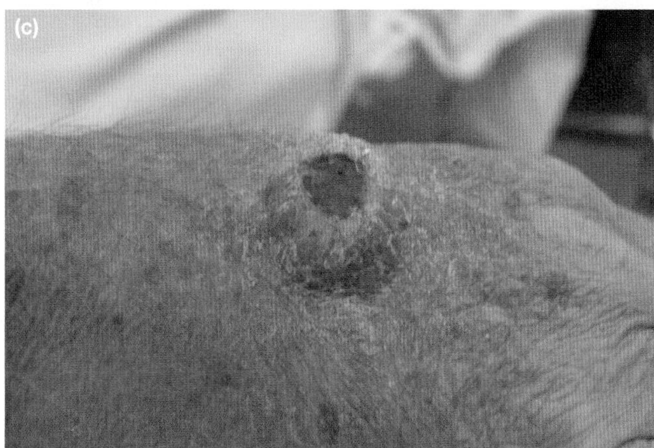
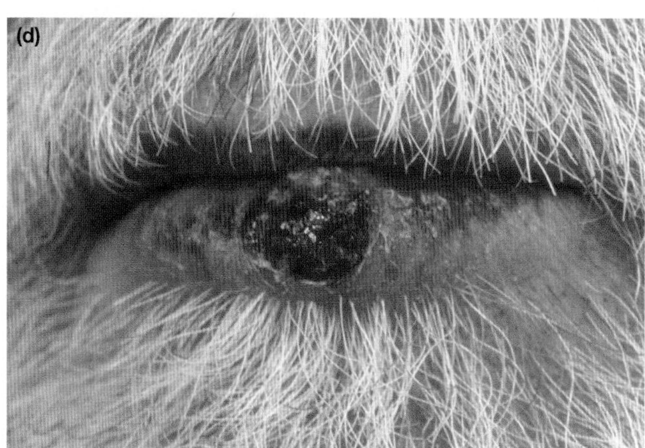

Figure 45.36 **(a)** A squamous cell carcinoma (SCC) on the face. **(b)** A recurrent SCC arising in a previously skin-grafted area of the scalp. **(c)** SCC arising on the dorsum of the hand in a renal transplant recipient on immunosuppressive therapy. **(d)** SCC arising on the lip of a smoker who worked outside on a farm. (**(a–c)** courtesy of Mr AR Greenbaum; **(d)** courtesy of St John's Institute for Dermatology, London, UK.)

- Surface size: lesions >2 cm have a worse prognosis than smaller ones.
- Histological grade: the higher the Broders' grade, the worse the prognosis.
- Microscopic invasion of lymphovascular spaces or nerve tissue carries a high risk of metastatic disease.

Therefore, as well as information on pathological pattern, cellular morphology and Broders' grade, any histopathology report for SCC should include the depth of invasion, the presence of perineural or lymphovascular invasion and the deep and peripheral margin clearance.

- Site: SCCs on the lips and ears have higher local recurrence rates than lesions elsewhere, and tumours at the extremities fare worse than those on the trunk.
- Aetiology: SCCs that arise in burn scars, osteomyelitis skin sinuses, chronic ulcers and areas of skin that have been irradiated have a higher metastatic potential.
- Immunosuppression: SCCs will invade further in those with impaired immune response.

The overall rate of metastasis varies between 2% and 30% for SCC (usually to regional nodes) with a local recurrence rate of 20%.

Management

SCC is a heterogeneous tumour with a malignant potential that varies between subtypes. Management must address the tumour's tendency for lymphatic metastasis and the possibility of in-transit metastasis.

Surgical excision is the only means of providing accurate information on histology and clearance. The margins for primary excision should be tailored to surface size in the first instance. This should ideally be assessed using surgical loupe magnification. A 4-mm clearance margin should be achieved if the SCC measures <2 cm across, and a 1-cm clearance margin if the SCC measures >2 cm; 95% of local recurrence and regional metastases occur within 5 years, thus follow-up beyond this period is not indicated.

Cutaneous malignant melanoma

Melanoma is a cancer of melanocytes and can, therefore, arise in skin, mucosa, retina and the leptomeninges.

Epidemiology

Observational data suggest that cutaneous melanoma is caused by exposure to UVR, but this general observation, which is a generally reliable fact, may hide some of the nuanced variables that contribute to melanoma formation.

Generally speaking, its rise in incidence reflects increased recreational activity in the sun and emigration among white-skinned people not suited to sun exposure. Although it accounts for less than 5% of skin malignancy (and 1.6% of all malignancy worldwide), it is responsible for over 75% of skin malignancy-related deaths.

It is the commonest cancer in young adults (20–39 years) and the most likely cause of cancer-related death.

Distribution between the sexes varies around the world and reflects occupational and recreational exposure to sunlight. Likewise, geographical distribution reflects exposure of white-skinned individuals to sunlight: Australia and New Zealand, countries with a predominantly white-skinned, immigrant population, have an incidence of 33.6 per 100 000. Five per cent of all patients with malignant melanoma will develop a second primary melanoma; 7% of malignant melanomas present as occult metastasis from an unknown primary.

What is less clear within data on cutaneous melanoma is the contribution by variables such as serum vitamin D levels and vitamin receptor genotypes, because thinner melanomas and lower recurrence rates have been linked to higher serum vitamin D levels, and why some forms of melanoma seem more attributable to cumulative sun exposure (superficial spreading) than others (nodular). Studies exploring whether there may be benefit from a degree of sun exposure that avoids 'sunbathing' and burning and whether sun-related vitamin D production in skin, rather than supplemental vitamin D, is beneficial are ongoing, but our best information still bases sun avoidance at the centre of melanoma prevention.

Pathophysiology

Cumulative UV exposure favours the development of lentigo maligna melanoma (LMM) and later onset of disease, whereas 'flash fry' exposure, typical of rapidly acquired holiday tans, favours the other morphological variants and early onset of disease.

A small proportion of malignant melanoma is genetically mediated and develops at an earlier age. People at most risk of developing malignant melanoma include: those with genetic syndromes; those with a past history of malignant melanoma or with a first-degree relative who has malignant melanoma; those who have more than 30 sun-acquired naevi or a history of five significant sunburns before the age of 16; fair-skinned/red-haired people living close to the equator; anyone with excessive UVR exposure (environmental or salon-delivered); or anyone with immunosuppression (which increases malignant melanoma incidence 20- to 30-fold). Male gender and solitary living are both associated with thicker melanomas at diagnosis. In women, higher socioeconomic status is positively correlated with developing melanoma.

> **Summary box 45.4**
>
> **Malignant melanoma**
> - Rising incidence
> - Genetic and acquired risk factors
> - Superficial spreading form the most common
> - Breslow thickness is the most important prognostic indicator
> - Sentinel node biopsy (SNB) is useful for staging

Macroscopic

Only 10–20% of malignant melanomas form in pre-existing naevi, with the remainder arising *de novo* in previously normally pigmented skin. The most likely naevi to form malignant melanoma are atypical naevi, atypical junctional lentiginous naevi (usually facial) and giant pigmented congenital naevi.

Macroscopic features in a pre-existing naevus that suggest malignant change are listed in ***Summary box 45.5***.

There are four common macroscopic variants of malignant melanoma and several other notable, but rarer, forms, as follows.

Superficial spreading melanoma (SSM). This is the most common presentation (70%); usually arises in a pre-existing naevus after several years of slow change, followed by rapid growth in the months before presentation (***Figure 45.37***). Nodularity within SSM heralds the onset of the vertical growth phase.

Nodular melanoma (NM). NM accounts for 15% of all malignant melanoma and tends to be more aggressive than SSM, with a shorter clinical onset. These lesions often arise *de novo* in skin and are more common in men than in women, often presenting in middle age and usually on the trunk, head or neck (***Figure 45.38***). They typically appear as blue/black papules, 1–2 cm in diameter, and because they lack the horizontal growth phase they tend to be sharply demarcated. Up to 5% are amelanotic.

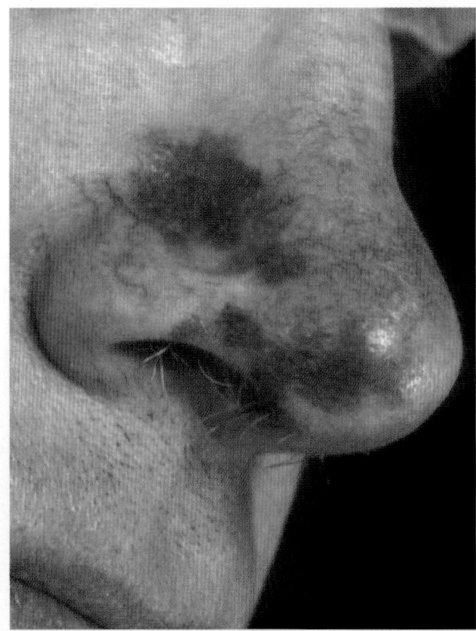

Figure 45.37 Superficial spreading melanoma (courtesy of St John's Institute for Dermatology, London, UK).

Alexander Breslow, 1928–1980, pathologist, George Washington University, Washington, DC, USA, first reported in 1970 that the prognosis depends upon the thickness of the tumour.

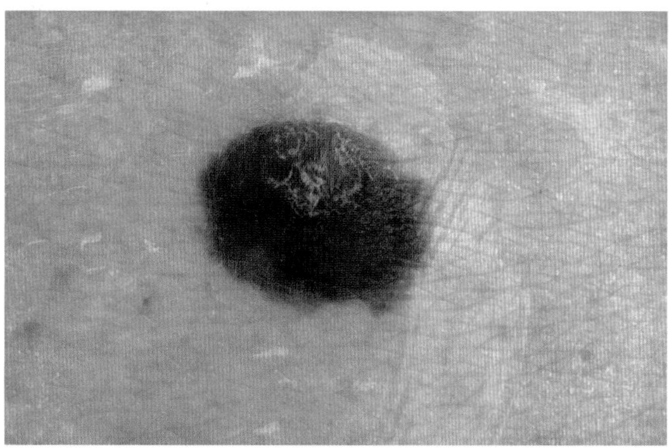

Figure 45.38 Nodular melanoma (courtesy of St John's Institute for Dermatology, London, UK).

Lentigo maligna melanoma. LMM was previously also known as Hutchinson's melanotic freckle. This variant presents as a slow-growing, variegated brown macule on the face, neck or hands of the elderly (***Figure 45.39***). They are positively correlated with prolonged, intense sun exposure and affect women more than men. They account for between 5% and 10% of malignant melanomas.

LMMs are thought to have less metastatic potential than other variants as they take longer to enter a vertical growth phase. Nonetheless, when they have entered the vertical growth phase their metastatic potential is the same as any other melanoma.

Acral lentiginous melanoma (ALM). ALM affects the soles and palms. It is rare in white-skinned individuals (2–8% of malignant melanoma) but more common in Afro-Caribbean, Hispanic and Asian populations (35–60%). It usually presents as a flat, irregular macule in later life; 25% are amelanotic and may mimic a fungal infection or pyogenic granuloma.

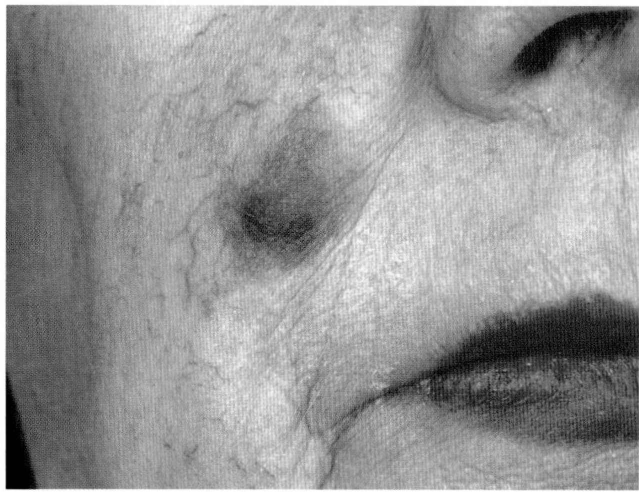

Figure 45.39 Lentigo maligna melanoma (courtesy of St John's Institute for Dermatology, London, UK).

Malignant melanomas under the fingernail are usually SSM rather than ALM. For finger- or toenail lesions it is vital to biopsy the nail matrix rather than just the pigment on the nail plate. A classical feature of a subungual melanoma is Hutchinson's sign: nail fold pigmentation that widens progressively to produce a triangular pigmented macule with associated nail dystrophy. The differential diagnosis is 'benign racial melanonychia', which produces a linear dark streak under a nail in a dark-skinned individual. Malignancy is unlikely if the nail fold is uninvolved (***Figure 45.40***).

Miscellaneous

- Amelanotic melanoma may present as a flesh-coloured skin lesion; as a metastasis from an unknown skin primary; or in the gastrointestinal tract, with obstruction or intussusception.

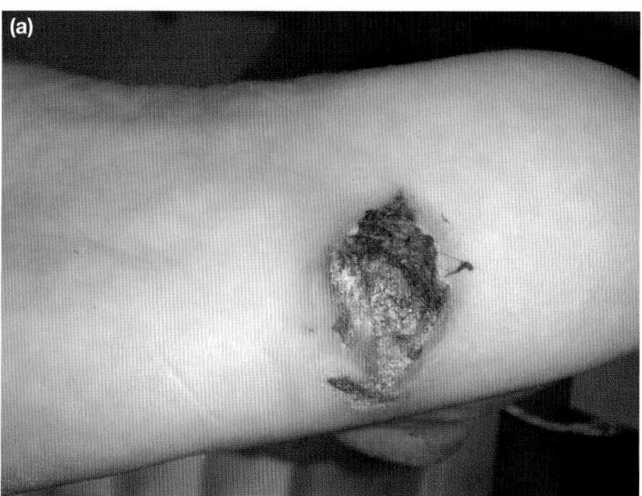

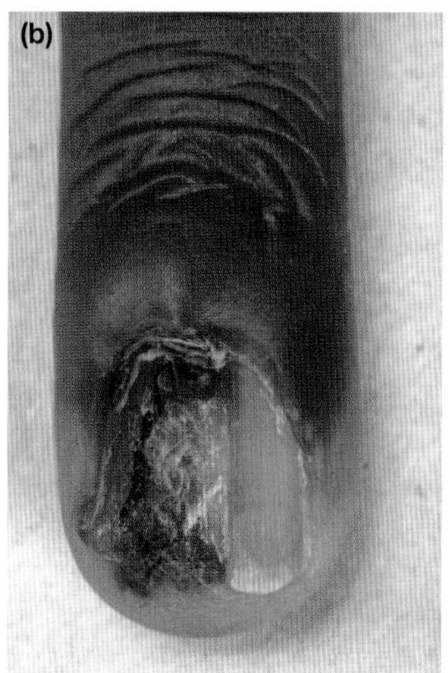

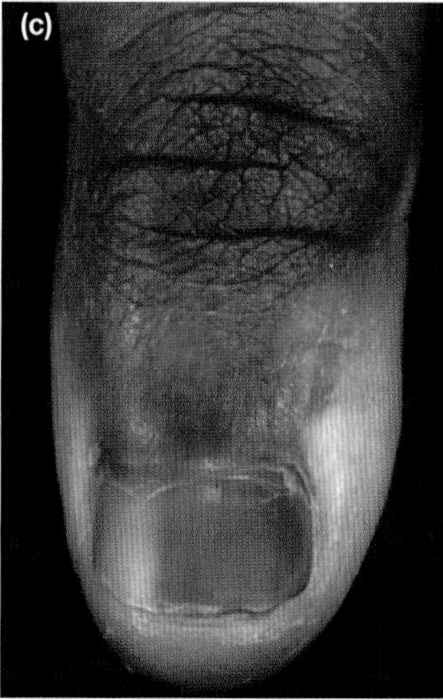

Figure 45.40 (a) Acral lentiginous melanoma on the sole of the foot. **(b)** Subungual melanoma – probably a superficial spreading melanoma. Note the swelling proximal to the nailfold. **(c)** Benign racial melanonychia. (**(a)** courtesy of Mr AR Greenbaum; **(b, c)** courtesy of St John's Institute for Dermatology, London, UK.)

Sir Jonathan Hutchinson, 1828–1913, surgeon, St Bartholomew's Hospital, London, UK.

- Desmoplastic melanoma is mostly found on the head and neck region. It has a propensity for perineural infiltration and often recurs locally if not widely excised. It may be amelanotic clinically.

Summary box 45.5

Macroscopic features in naevi suggestive of malignant melanoma

- Change in size
- Shape
- Colour
- Thickness (elevation/nodularity or ulceration)
- Satellite lesions (pigment spreading into surrounding area)
- Tingling/itching/serosanguineous discharge (usually late signs)

Microscopic

Malignant change occurs in the melanocytes in the basal epidermis, while *in situ* atypical melanocytes are limited to the dermoepidermal junction and show no evidence of dermal involvement. During the horizontal growth phase, cells spread along the dermoepidermal junction; although they may breach the dermis, their migration is predominantly radial. During the vertical growth phase, the dermis may be invaded. The greater the depth of invasion, the greater the metastatic potential of the tumour.

Management

History and clinical examination should be directed at discovering the primary lesion and identification of local, regional or distant spread.

An excision biopsy with a 2- to 3-mm margin of skin and a cuff of subdermal fat is acceptable. Incision biopsy is occasionally indicated: for instance, in large lesions on the face where an excision biopsy of the whole lesion would be disfiguring.

In experienced hands, observation and review every 2 months may avoid biopsies in equivocal cases, but serial clinical and dermoscopic photography by a clinician with expertise in dermoscopy is mandatory when observation is chosen, rather than excision biopsy for definitive histopathological diagnosis. Dermoscopy coupled to computers with learning capability may soon outperform clinicians in melanoma diagnosis to the point where screening becomes much easier.

Biopsy and pathological examination provide the first step towards staging melanoma. The Breslow thickness of a melanoma (measured to the nearest 0.1 mm from the granular layer to the base of the tumour) is the most important prognostic indicator in the absence of lymph node metastases. The American Joint Committee on Cancer (AJCC) staging system takes lymph node involvement, distant metastases and evidence-based prognostic factors into account; these can then be used to guide optimum care and inclusion in research studies for adjuvant or other treatments where applicable.

The detail of the AJCC melanoma staging system has become too specialised for the ambit of this text; most specialists look up its detail as they assign a stage to a patient (***Table 45.2***).

Investigations

Guidelines for staging are controversial. The author suggests that investigations should be directed towards detecting occult disease, so as to upstage patients and treat them accurately and appropriately, the only cure for malignant melanoma currently being appropriate surgery. Thus, offering SNB to patients with T2a disease and greater is critical and investigations for T3a disease and greater should be directed to individual clinical presentation.

Local treatment

The treatment for melanoma is surgery. Lentigo maligna (melanoma *in situ*) should be excised completely in most clinical situations because of the risk of it entering the vertical growth phase to become LMM. A complete excision requires no further treatment.

For melanoma *in situ* a wide excision of 5 mm is sufficient; for melanoma <1 mm deep, a 1-cm margin is sufficient; and for deeper lesions, a 2-cm only margin is recommended, as there is no evidence that wider margins make a difference.

Regional lymph nodes

The likelihood of metastatic spread to regional lymph nodes is proportional to the Breslow thickness of the melanoma. Management of regional lymph nodes has been a contentious topic for well over a century. Some advocated simultaneous elective lymph node clearance at the time of wide excision of the primary melanoma. Others favoured a therapeutic lymphadenectomy if regional metastases became clinically evident. Ideally, one would like to be able to select for treatment those patients with the highest risk of metastatic spread. SNB, an investigation based on the fact that lymphatic metastases proceed in an orderly fashion and can be predicted by mapping the lymphatic drainage from a primary tumour to the first or 'sentinel' node in the regional lymphatic basin, offered that potential, but prospective controlled studies have shown no survival benefit from lymphadenectomy after positive SNB involving micrometastasis <0.2 mm in a single node. This may be because most patients have been treated by removing the sentinel node, which was the only node involved at that stage.

However, completion lymphadenectomy after positive SNB remains, on current evidence, the optimum method for regional control, if patients accept the morbidity associated with regional lymphadenectomy.

Adjuvant therapy

When mutation locks BRAF protein signalling to 'on', it affects the mitogen-activated protein kinase (MAPK) cellular pathway, promoting initiation, malignant transformation, tumour progression and metastasis in the 50% of malignant melanomas with BRAF V600 mutations. Targeted therapy in stage IV melanoma using dabrafenib or vemurafenib, which block BRAF action, has shown promising results with metastatic melanoma. Trametinib has a different action on the MAPK pathway: stopping cell growth and promoting apoptosis. Combined use with dabrafenib to counter acquired tumour resistance via MAPK pathway reactivation shows promising results in stage IV disease. Also, the selective immune

TABLE 45.2 Summary of the American Joint Committee on Cancer melanoma staging, 8th edition.

Primary tumour		Regional nodes		Distant metastases
TX Primary tumour cannot be assessed (has been curettage or has severely regressed)		NX Patients in whom nodes cannot be assessed (e.g. previous excision)		
T0 No evidence of primary tumour		N0 No node involvement		M0 No detected distant metastases
Tis Melanoma *in situ*				
T1 <1.0 mm	a: <0.8 mm, no ulceration b: 0.8–1.0 mm, no ulceration; or <1.0 mm with ulceration	N1 1 node	a: Micrometastasis (no MSI) b: Macrometastasis (no MSI) c: MSI present	M1a Skin, subcutaneous or distant lymph node metastases (normal serum LDH levels)
T2 1.01–2.0 mm	a: No ulceration b: With ulceration	N2 2 or 3 nodes	a: Micrometastasis (no MSI) b: Macrometastasis (no MSI) c: MSI present	M1b Lung metastases (normal serum LDH levels)
T3 2.01–4.0 mm	a: No ulceration b: With ulceration	N3	a: Micrometastasis, >3 nodes (no MSI) b: Micrometastasis, >3 nodes or matted or 1 clinical node (no MSI) c: >1 clinical or occult node with MSI present	M1c All other visceral metastases or any distant metastases with elevated serum LDH levels
T4 >4 mm	a: No ulceration b: With ulceration			M1d Brain metastases
Clinical staging of melanoma				
Stage 0: Tis, N0, M0 Stage Ia: T1a, N0, M0 Stage Ib: T1b or T2a, N0, M0		Stage IIa: T2b or T3a, N0, M0 Stage IIb: T3b or T4a, N0, M0 Stage IIc: T4b, N0, M0		Stage III: any T, >N1, M0 Stage IV: any T, any N1, M1

LDH, lactate dehydrogenase; MSI denotes the presence of satellite lesions, in-transit lesions or local recurrence.

checkpoint inhibitors ipilimumab and nivolumab demonstrate benefit in metastatic or unresectable melanoma.

Over the last 5 years, five randomised prospective trials of adjuvant therapy have reported findings in the treatment of patients with stage II to IV disease. While all five trials showed a significant improvement in relapse-free survival, only two of the trials were mature enough to report on overall survival.

Prognosis

The Breslow thickness of the primary tumour offers the best correlation with survival in stage I disease. The higher the mitotic index, the poorer the prognosis of the primary tumour. This has greater significance than the presence or absence of ulceration.

The presence of lymph node metastases is the single most important prognostic index in melanoma, outweighing both tumour and host factors. The number of affected nodes and the presence of extranodal extension are also significant outcome predictors. Once regional nodes are clinically involved, 70–85% of patients will have occult distant metastases.

Merkel cell (dermal mechanoreceptor) tumour

This is an aggressive malignant tumour of Merkel cells and usually affects the elderly. It is four times more common in women than in men (***Figure 45.41***). Treatment is with wide local excision, aiming for a 25- to 30-mm margin, followed by radiotherapy.

VASCULAR LESIONS

Congenital: haemangiomata and vascular malformations

These can be subclassified biologically into vascular tumours or vascular malformations based on their endothelial characteristics, or radiologically into haemangiomata, vascular and lymphatic malformations based on their vascular dynamics.

Haemangiomata

These are benign endothelial tumours that affect three girls for every boy. Thirty per cent have a herald patch at birth, which then grows rapidly in the first year of life and slowly involutes over several years, with 70% having resolved by 7 years of age. Large haemangiomata can trap platelets, leading to thrombocytopenia (Kasabach–Merritt syndrome).

Vascular malformations

Vascular malformations affect boys and girls equally and are associated with numerous syndromes. They are invariably

Haig H Kasabach, 1898–1943, radiologist, Presbyterian Hospital, New York, NY, USA.

Katharine K Merritt, 1886–1986, pediatrician, Babies Hospital, Columbia University College of Physicians and Surgeons, New York, NY, USA. Kasabach and Merritt described the condition as a joint paper in 1940.

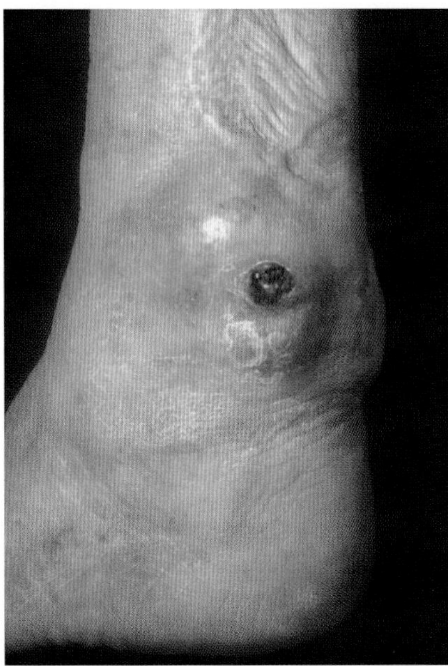

Figure 45.41 Merkel cell tumour (courtesy of St John's Institute for Dermatology, London, UK).

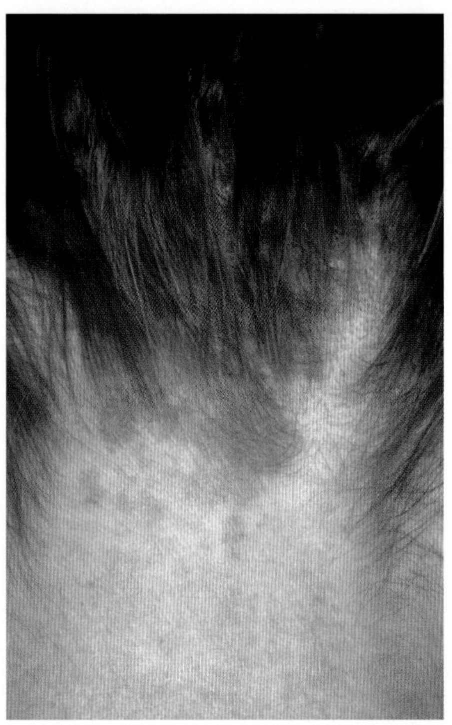

Figure 45.42 Salmon patch (courtesy of St John's Institute for Dermatology, London, UK).

present at birth but may be missed if deep to the skin. Vascular malformations subsequently grow in proportion to the child's growth (rather than in response to sepsis or hormonal stimulation). Stasis can lead to a localised, consumptive coagulopathy in large venous malformations. Low-flow malformations may cause skeletal hypoplasia, while high-flow malformations can cause hypertrophy.

Common vascular birthmarks

Salmon patch

A salmon patch is a vascular malformation that presents as a pinkish macule, usually at the nape of neck (***Figure 45.42***). It is caused by an area of persistent fetal dermal circulation that usually disappears at 1 year.

Capillary haemangioma (strawberry naevus)

This is the commonest 'birthmark', occurring most frequently on the head and neck (***Figure 45.43***). Ninety per cent are present at birth; as a consequence of intravascular thrombosis, fibrosis and mast cell infiltration, 10% resolve each subsequent year, with 70% resolved by 7 years old.

White skin is affected most commonly and girls are affected three times more than boys.

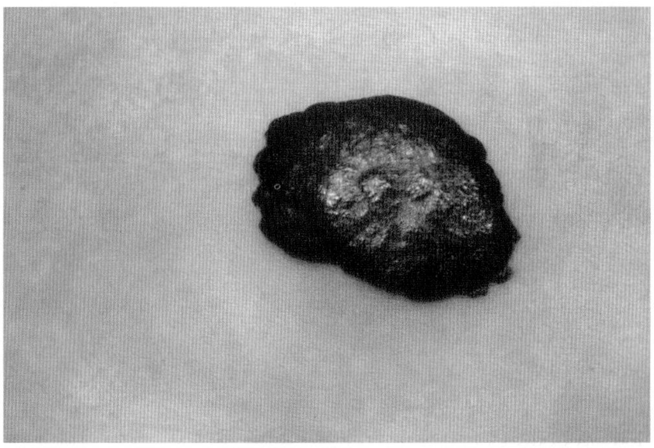

Figure 45.43 Capillary haemangioma (courtesy of St John's Institute for Dermatology, London, UK).

Capillary vascular malformations ('port-wine' stains)

Capillary vascular malformations ('port-wine stains' [PWSs]) are 20 times less common than capillary haemangiomata and result from defective maturation of the cutaneous sympathetic innervation during embryogenesis, leading to localised intradermal capillary vasodilatation (***Figure 45.44***). They appear at birth as flat, smooth, intensely purple-stained areas, most frequently on the head and neck, often within the maxillary and mandibular dermatomes of the trigeminal nerve.

Treatment with intense pulsed light and pulsed-dye laser is successful. PWSs may be associated with various syndromes.

Acquired

Campbell de Morgan spots

These are arteriovenous fistulae at the dermal capillary level in sun-exposed skin of older patients (***Figure 45.45***).

Campbell Greig de Morgan, 1811–1876, surgeon, Middlesex Hospital, London, UK. First to propose that cancer started locally and then spread first to lymph nodes and beyond.

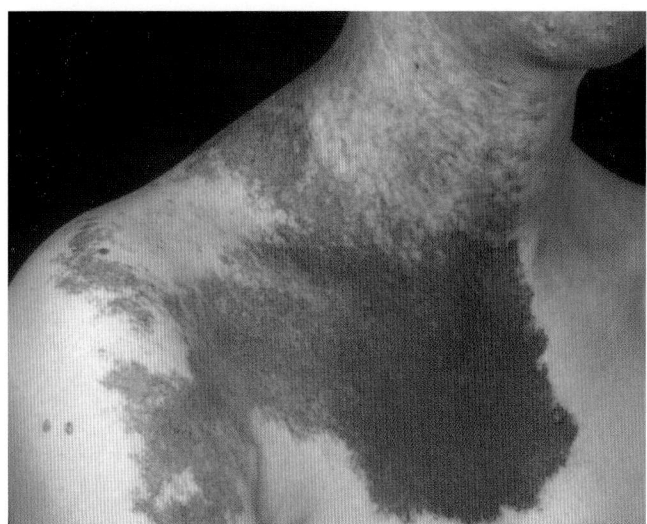

Figure 45.44 'Port-wine' stain (courtesy of St John's Institute for Dermatology, London, UK).

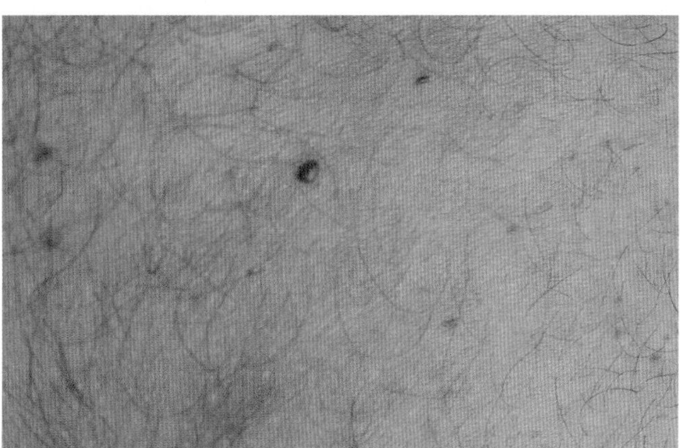

Figure 45.45 Campbell de Morgan spot (courtesy of Mr AR Greenbaum).

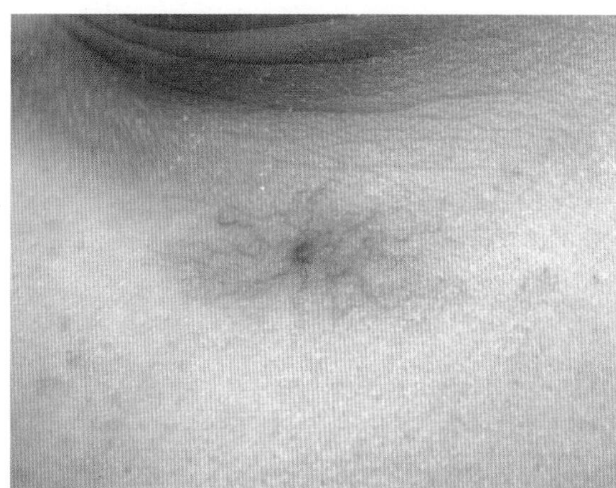

Figure 45.46 Spider naevus (courtesy of St John's Institute for Dermatology, London, UK).

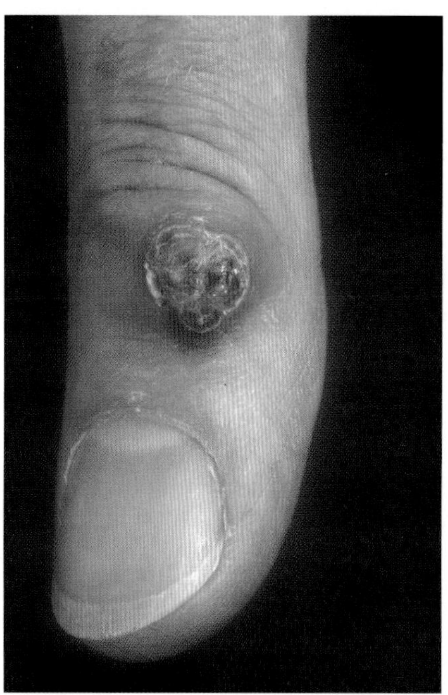

Figure 45.47 Pyogenic granuloma (courtesy of St John's Institute for Dermatology, London, UK).

Spider naevi

These are angiomata that appear (and may disappear) spontaneously at puberty or in two-thirds of pregnant women, usually disappearing in the puerperium (***Figure 45.46***). Spider naevi are also associated with chronic liver disease. They can be treated with intense pulsed light or pulsed-dye laser.

Pyogenic granuloma

These share many histological characteristics of haemangiomata and are probably a subtype thereof (***Figure 45.47***). Most are small (0.5–1.5 cm), raised, pedunculated, soft, red nodular lesions showing superficial ulceration and a tendency to bleed after trivial trauma. They should be excised with a minimal margin.

Glomus tumour

This arises from a subcutaneous arteriovenous shunt (Sucquet–Hoyer canals), especially in the corium of the nail bed. Typically, it is a small, purple nodule measuring a few millimetres in size, which is disproportionately painful in response to insignificant stimuli, including cold exposure (***Figure 45.48***). Subungual varieties may be invisible causes of paroxysmal digital pain.

Angiosarcoma ('malignant angioendothelioma')

A rare, highly malignant tumour arising from the endothelial cells (***Figure 45.49***). The lymphangiosarcoma variant arises from lymphatic endothelium and can develop in lymphoedematous tissue, particularly an extremity. Proliferation is rapid with early systemic spread.

JP Sucquet, 1840–1870, anatomist, Paris, France.
Heinrich Hoyer, 1834–1907, Professor of Histology, Embryology and Anatomy, Central Medical School, The Polish University, Warsaw, Poland.

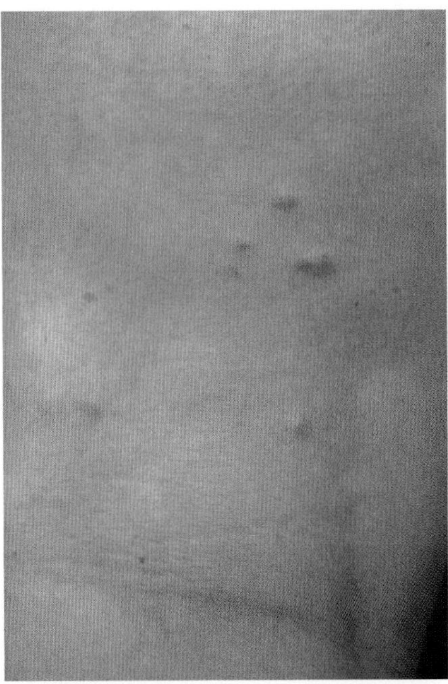

Figure 45.48 Glomus tumour (courtesy of St John's Institute for Dermatology, London, UK).

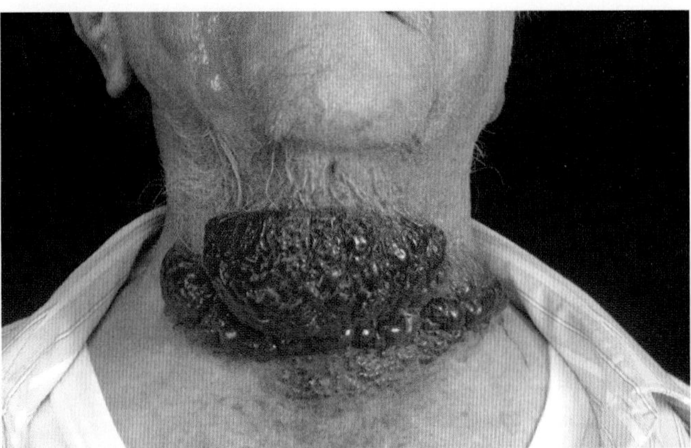

Figure 45.49 Angiosarcoma (courtesy of St John's Institute for Dermatology, London, UK).

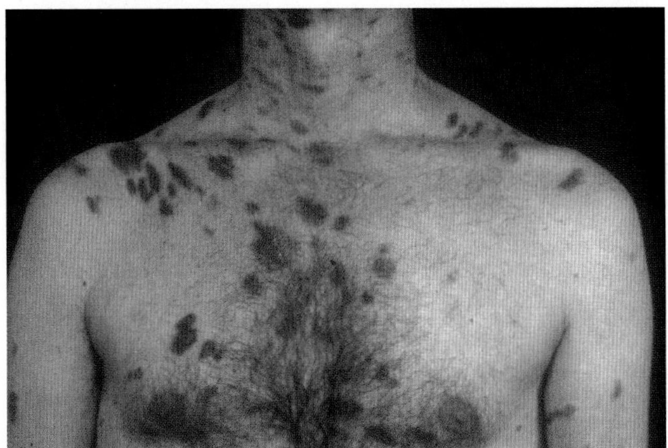

Figure 45.50 Kaposi's sarcoma (courtesy of St John's Institute for Dermatology, London, UK).

Kaposi's sarcoma

Kaposi's sarcoma is a malignant, proliferative tumour of vascular endothelial cells, which was first described in elderly Jewish men but is now most commonly associated with immune compromise after transplantation or HIV infection (***Figure 45.50***). There appears to be a causal link with infection by human herpesvirus 8. Kaposi's sarcoma usually starts as a red-brown, indurated, plaque-like skin lesion that becomes nodular and then ulcerates. Treatment is with radiotherapy.

WOUNDS

Congenital

Cutis aplasia congenita

This is a rare condition characterised by the congenital absence of epidermis, dermis and, in some cases, subcutaneous tissues, with underlying bony defects in 20%. Treatment depends on the severity of the presentation, but usually involves plastic surgery.

Parry-Romberg disease (linear morphoea)

A rare variant of scleroderma affecting up to 3:100 000 children. It is linked to certain HLA subtypes and to a family history of autoimmune disease. It is three times more common in females and often develops after an external physical trigger, such as friction or trauma.

Parry–Romberg disease is a progressive, hemifacial atrophy of skin, soft tissue and bone. The disease commonly starts in the late twenties but can present in childhood, when the resulting deformity is worse because it is magnified by differential growth elsewhere. The condition is self-limiting, usually by 5–10 years after onset. Once stable, plastic surgery techniques can be employed alone or in combination to reconstruct an aesthetic contour. Coup de sabre is a variant that affects the cranium and scalp and resembles a 'blow from a sabre'.

Spina bifida

Failure of closure of the caudal neuropore during the fourth week *in utero* results in incomplete development of some or all of the structural elements posterior to the spinal cord. This can occur anywhere, but is commonest in lumbar vertebrae and presents as gross variants: spina bifida occulta, in which there is a bony defect without neural protrusion, and spina bifida cystica, in which there is herniation of the meninges (meningocele), spinal cord (myelocele) or, most commonly,

Moritz Kaposi, 1837–1902, Austrian dermatologist, described xeroderma pigmentosum in 1874. He also described a rare cutaneous sarcoma in Ashkenazi Jews, now more often an AIDS-defining condition.
Caleb Hillier Parry, 1755–1822, physician, The General Hospital, Bath, UK.
Moritz Heinrich Romberg, 1795–1873, neurologist, Director of the University Hospital, Berlin, Germany.

both (meningomyelocele). Management ideally involves a multidisciplinary approach and is directed towards protecting the spinal cord and preventing cerebrospinal fluid contamination, secondary hydrocephalus and meningitis.

Acquired

Pressure sores

These begin with tissue necrosis at a pressure point and develop into a cone-shaped volume of necrotic loss. As many as 10% of acute hospital inpatients will have some degree of pressure sore. The majority affect the elderly and patients with spinal injury or decreased sensibility; 80% of paraplegics will get a pressure sore and 8% die as a result.

The pathogenesis of pressure sores revolves around unrelieved pressure: an increase in local tissue pressure above that of perfusion pressure produces ischaemic necrosis that is directly proportional to the duration and degree of pressure and inversely proportional to the area over which it is applied. Muscle and fat are more susceptible to pressure than skin.

In a patient who has no predisposing factors management is aimed at debridement and repair of the defect, on the assumption that recurrence will not occur once normal function and sensibility returns. In the paraplegic patient, recurrence is likely, so management should involve a multidisciplinary approach. Primary treatment involves relieving pressure (special mattress, nursing care, relief of muscle spasm and contractures), optimising nutrition, correcting anaemia and preventing infection. Surgery involves thorough debridement to promote healing and plastic surgery to reconstruct the defect.

Ulcers

An ulcer is a discontinuity of an epithelial surface. It is characterised by destruction of the surface epithelium and a granulating base. Ulcers can be classified as non-specific, specific and malignant (***Figure 45.51***).

Sinus

A sinus is a blind-ending tract connecting a cavity lined with granulation tissue (often an abscess cavity) to an epithelial surface (***Figure 45.52a***). Sinuses may be congenital or acquired. Congenital sinuses arise from the remnants of persistent embryonic ducts. Acquired sinuses can result from: a retained foreign body (ingrown hair or suture material); chronic infection (tuberculosis, osteomyelitis or actinomycosis); chronic inflammation (Crohn's disease); malignancy; or inadequate surgical drainage of a cavity.

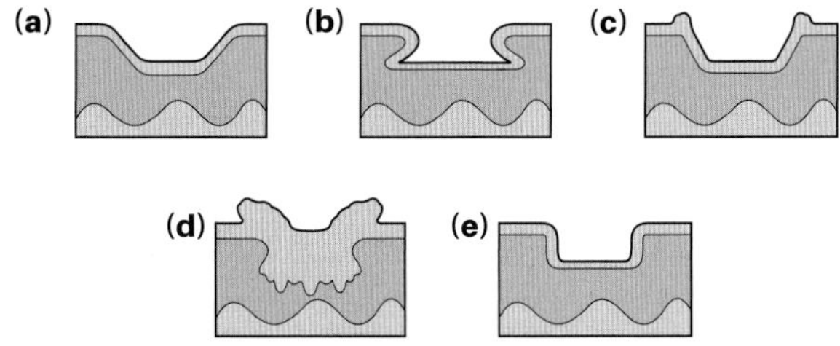

Figure 45.51 Some characteristic shapes of the edges of ulcers. **(a)** Non-specific ulcer: note the shelving edge. **(b)** Tuberculous ulcer: note the undermined edge. **(c)** Basal cell carcinoma (rodent ulcer): note the rolled edge, which may exhibit small blood vessels. **(d)** Epithelioma: note the heaped-up, everted edge and irregular thickened base. **(e)** Syphilis: note the punched-out edge and thin base, which may be covered with a 'wash-leather' slough.

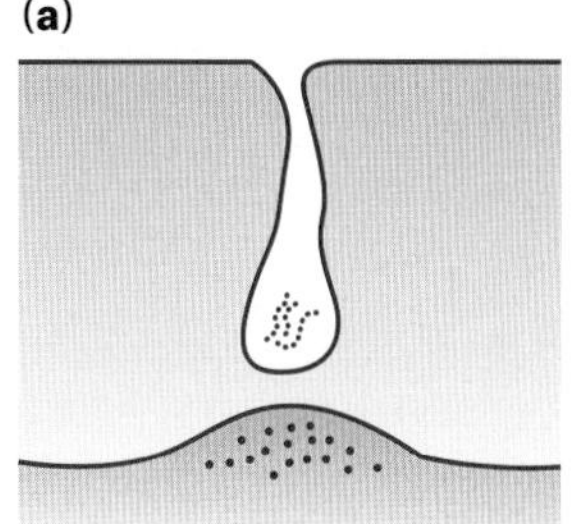

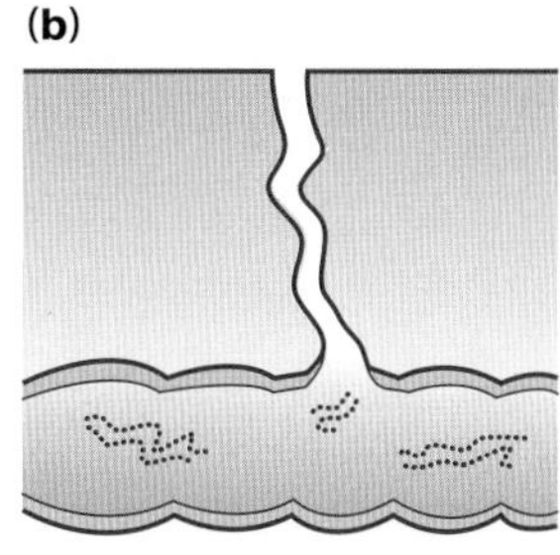

Figure 45.52 A sinus **(a)** and a fistula **(b)**; both usually arise from a preceding abscess. **(a)** This is a blind track, in this case a pilonidal abscess. **(b)** This is a track connecting two epithelium-lined surfaces, in this case a colocutaneous fistula from colon to skin.

Treatment of a sinus is directed at removing the underlying cause. Biopsies should always be taken from the wall of a sinus to exclude malignancy or specific infection. For specific management of the disease conditions, please refer to the appropriate chapter.

Fistula

A fistula is an abnormal communication between two epithelium-lined surfaces (***Figure 45.52b***). This communication or tract is usually lined by granulation tissue, but may become epithelialised in chronic cases. Fistulae may be congenital (e.g. tracheo-oesophageal and branchial fistulae) or acquired (e.g. enterocutaneous complicating Crohn's disease or surgery, or arteriovenous). Management of a fistula is directed at the underlying aetiology (see the appropriate chapters).

FURTHER READING

Calonje JE, Brenn T, Lazar A, Billings S. *McKee's pathology of the skin*, 5th edn. Amsterdam: Elsevier, 2019.
Soyer HP, Argenziano G, Hoffmann-Wellenhof R, Zalaudek I. *Dermoscopy: the essentials*, 3rd edn. Philadelphia, PA: Mosby Wolfe, 2020.

WEBSITE ADDRESSES

American Joint Committee on Cancer for TNM classifications of tumours and up-to-date staging: https://cancerstaging.org/.
Dermnet New Zealand – a reliable online educational resource run by a community of dermatologists and other health specialists: https://www.dermnetnz.org/.
International Dermoscopy Society – free to join, this society is run by dermatologists to promote clinical research and education in dermoscopy: https://dermoscopy-ids.org/.

Burrill Bernard Crohn, 1884–1983, gastroenterologist, Mount Sinai Hospital, New York, NY, USA, described regional ileitis in 1932.

CHAPTER 46 Burns

Learning objectives

To assess:
- The area and depth of burns in adults and children
- The requirement for transfer to a specialist burn unit

To understand:
- The pathophysiology of burn injury and the systemic effects
- Methods for calculating the rate and quantity of fluids required
- Principal techniques for treating burns and the patient
- The pathophysiology of electrical and chemical burns

INTRODUCTION

The last 50 years have seen great strides made to reduce both morbidity and mortality from burn injuries. The coming years will see a better understanding of the control of physiology along with improvements in reconstruction and rehabilitation and utilising new technology.

A large burn injury will have a significant effect on the patient's family and friends and the patient's future. The importance of multidisciplinary care needs to be stressed for the adequate and effective care of the burn patient.

Incidence and mechanism of burn injury

The incidence of burn injury varies greatly among countries and cultures. In the UK (with its population of 67 million), each year around 175 000 people visit accident and emergency departments with burns; of these, about 13 000 need to be admitted. About 1000 have severe burns requiring fluid resuscitation, and half of the victims are under 16 years of age.

The mechanism of burn injury varies according to age, with the extremes of age being particularly vulnerable. The majority of burns in children are scalds caused by accidents with kettles, pans, hot drinks and bath water. It is important in this age group to screen for non-accidental injury as this may become a safeguarding issue. Delay in presentation, inconsistent history from care givers or an unexpected burn pattern/depth should trigger a concern and further investigation; alerting senior staff is essential. Among adolescent patients, burns are usually caused by experimentation with matches and flammable liquids. In adults flame burns are more frequent, and scald burns and contact burns (such as a fall against a radiator and an inability to extract) become more common with age. Often a burn injury in the elderly is the trigger point at which increasing frailty and inability to self-care are recognised. Again, non-accidental injuries should be screened for in this vulnerable age group. The majority of electrical and chemical injuries occur in adults and are frequently associated with occupation. Cold and radiation are rarer thermal injuries. Associated conditions in adults, such as mental disease (attempted suicide or assault), epilepsy and alcohol or drug abuse, are underlying factors in as many as 80% of patients with burns admitted to hospital in some populations.

Summary box 46.1

Screening for non-accidental burn injury
- Delay in presentation, perceived lack of concern by the care giver
- Inconsistency with the history of the burn and the burn pattern/depth
- Other unexplained injuries such as bruises/fractures
- Frequent hospital attendances

Burn prevention

Legislation, health promotion and appliance design have reduced the incidence of burns: regulations regarding flame-retardant clothes and furniture; the promotion of smoke alarms; the design of cookers and gas fires; the almost universal use of cordless kettles; and the education of parents to set their hot water thermostat to 60°C all play their part. Recent campaigns have included highlighting the dangers of leaving hot hair straighteners near children and the slogan 'hot water burns like fire' in relation to the danger of scald injuries.

Summary box 46.2

Prevention of burns

A significant proportion of burns can be prevented by:
- Implementing good health and safety regulations
- Educating the public
- Introducing effective legislation

THE PATHOPHYSIOLOGY OF BURN INJURY TO THE SKIN

Burns cause a multisystem injury, but by far the most common organ affected is the skin. An understanding of the function and the structure of the skin is essential when assessing and treating a burn injury (see *Chapter 45*).

Summary box 46.3

Functions of the skin

- Waterproofing and protection from ultraviolet light
- Immune response
- Thermoregulation
- Vitamin D production
- Facilitates movement, sensation and cosmesis

INJURY TO THE AIRWAY AND LUNGS

Burns can also damage the airway and lungs, with life-threatening consequences. Inhalation injury of hot, smoked-filled air has three components, each of which can present alone or in any combination. They are: upper airway injury, lower airway injury (true smoke inhalation) and metabolic poisoning. Airway injuries occur when the face and neck are burned; the significance of being trapped in an enclosed space (burning room or car) cannot be underestimated.

Summary box 46.4

Warning signs of burns to the respiratory system

- Burns around the face and neck, blistering inside the mouth
- A history of being trapped in an enclosed space
- Change to/hoarseness of voice
- Stridor
- Singeing of facial and nasal hair

Metabolic poisoning

Incomplete combustion of carbonaceous materials may produce carbon monoxide, and burning of nitrogen-containing polymers releases hydrogen cyanide. Carbon monoxide poisoning is the most common immediate cause of death from fire. It is an odourless, colourless gas that binds with erythrocyte haemoglobin approximately 250 times more avidly than oxygen. Carboxyhaemoglobin is inactive in oxygen transport and impairs oxygen delivery at the tissue level. Additionally, it competes with, and inhibits, oxygen binding to cytochrome oxidase. This disrupts aerobic metabolism and decreases the capacity for cellular respiration. The treatment for carbon monoxide poisoning is early recognition and therapy with high-flow, high-concentration oxygen. Cyanide combines with trivalent iron in the mitochondrial cytochrome A3 complex, inhibiting electron transport and cellular respiration.

Mechanical block on rib movement

Full-thickness burned skin loses its elasticity, becoming stiff and leathery in appearance. This, combined with subcutaneous oedema, can physically stop rib expansion when the burn extends across the chest, compromising respiratory function.

Summary box 46.5

Dangers of smoke, hot gas or steam inhalation

- Inhaled hot gases can cause supraglottic airway burns and laryngeal oedema
- Inhaled steam can cause subglottic burns and loss of respiratory epithelium
- Inhaled smoke particles can cause chemical pneumonitis and respiratory failure
- Inhaled poisons, such as carbon monoxide, can cause metabolic poisoning
- Full-thickness burns to the chest can cause mechanical blockage to rib movement

INFLAMMATION AND CIRCULATORY CHANGES

The circulatory changes initiated by a burn injury are complex and multifactorial, originating from both the actual injury of burned skin (eschar) and the inflammatory cascade. It is governed by a complex series of events. The release of neuropeptides and the activation of complement are initiated by the stimulation of pain fibres and the alteration of proteins by heat. The activation of Hageman factor initiates a number of protease-driven cascades, altering the arachidonic acid, thrombin and kallikrein pathways. Fluid is lost from capillaries and oedema formation occurs.

Summary box 46.6

The shock reaction after burns

- Burns produce an inflammatory reaction
- This leads to vastly increased vascular permeability
- Water, solutes and proteins move from the intra- to the extravascular space
- The volume of fluid lost is directly proportional to the area of the burn
- Above 15% of surface area, the loss of fluid produces shock requiring resuscitation

OTHER LIFE-THREATENING EVENTS WITH MAJOR BURNS

The immune system and infection

The inflammatory changes caused by the burn have an effect on the patient's immune system. Cell-mediated immunity is significantly reduced in large burns, leaving them more

John Hageman was a 37-year-old railroad brakeman, in whom this factor deficiency was discovered by Dr Oscar Ratnoff in 1955.

susceptible to bacterial and fungal infections. There are many potential sources of infection, primarily from the burn wound and from the lung if this is injured, but also from any central venous lines, tracheostomies or urinary catheters present.

Changes to the intestine

The inflammatory stimulus and shock can cause microvascular damage and ischaemia to the gut mucosa. This reduces gut motility and can prevent the absorption of food. Failure of enteral feeding in a patient with a large burn is a life-threatening complication. This process also increases the translocation of gut bacteria, which can become an important source of infection in large burns. Gut mucosal swelling, gastric stasis and peritoneal oedema can also cause abdominal compartment syndrome, which splints the diaphragm and increases the airway pressures needed for respiration.

Danger to peripheral circulation

In full-thickness burns, the collagen fibres are coagulated. The normal elasticity of the skin is lost. A circumferential full-thickness burn to a limb acts as a tourniquet as the limb swells. If untreated, this will progress to limb-threatening ischaemia.

Summary box 46.7

Other complications of burns

- Infection from the burn site, lungs, gut, lines and catheters
- Malabsorption from the gut
- Circumferential burns may compromise circulation to a limb

IMMEDIATE CARE OF THE BURN PATIENT

Prehospital care

Good prehospital care is essential in ensuring rapid assessment and transfer. The key principles are:

- **Ensure rescuer safety**. This is particularly important in the case of electrical and chemical injuries and building fires.
- **Stop the burning process**. Stop, drop and roll is a good method of extinguishing fire burning on a person.
- **Check for other injuries**. A standard ABC (airway–breathing–circulation) check followed by a rapid secondary survey will ensure that no other significant injuries are missed. Patients burned in explosions or even escaping from fires can have coexisting fractures or blast pattern injuries.
- **Cool the burn wound**. This provides analgesia and slows the delayed microvascular damage that can occur after a burn injury. Cooling should occur for a minimum of 20 minutes and is effective up to 1 hour after the burn injury. It is a particularly important first aid step in partial-thickness burns, especially scalds. In temperate climates, cooling should be at about 15°C – tepid water – and hypothermia must be avoided, particularly in the extremes of age.
- **Give oxygen**. Anyone involved in a fire in an enclosed space should receive oxygen, especially if there is an altered consciousness level.
- **Elevate**. Sitting a patient up with a burned airway may prove life-saving in the event of a delay in transfer to hospital care. Elevation of burned limbs will reduce swelling and discomfort.
- **Analgesia**. Administration of analgesia prior to or during transfer will alleviate pain.

Hospital care

The principles of managing an acute burn injury follow the advanced trauma life support (ATLS) principles as per any major trauma:

- A, airway control;
- B, breathing and ventilation;
- C, circulation;
- D, disability – neurological status;
- E, exposure with environmental control;
- F, fluid resuscitation.

The possibility of injury additional to the burn must be sought both clinically and from the history, and treated appropriately. The major determinants of severity of any burn injury are the percentage of total body surface area (TBSA) that is burned, the presence of an inhalation injury, the depth of the burn and the age/comorbidities of the patient.

Not all burned patients will need to be admitted to a burns unit, but the main criteria are given in ***Table 46.1***.

Summary box 46.8

Major determinants of the outcome of a burn

- Percentage surface area involved
- Depth of burns
- Presence of an inhalational injury
- Age and comorbidities of the patient

TABLE 46.1 The criteria for acute admission to a burns unit.

- Suspected airway or inhalational injury
- Any burn likely to require fluid resuscitation
- Any burn likely to require surgery
- Patients with burns of any significance to the hands, face, feet or perineum
- Patients whose psychiatric or social background makes it inadvisable to send them home
- Any suspicion of non-accidental injury
- Any burn in a patient at the extremes of age
- Any burn with associated potentially serious sequelae, including high-tension electrical burns and concentrated hydrofluoric acid burns

Airway

Summary box 46.9

Recognition of the potentially burned airway
- A history of being trapped in the presence of smoke or hot gases
- Burns on the palate or nasal mucosa, or loss of all the hairs in the nose
- Deep burns around the mouth and neck
- Hoarseness/change in voice

The burned airway creates problems for the patient by swelling and, if not managed proactively, can completely occlude the upper airway. The treatment is to secure the airway with an endotracheal tube until the swelling has subsided, which is usually after about 48 hours (***Figure 46.1***). The indications of laryngeal oedema, such as a change in voice, stridor, anxiety and respiratory difficulty, are very late symptoms. Intubation at this point is often difficult or impossible owing to swelling, so acute cricothyroidotomy equipment must be at hand when intubating patients with a delayed diagnosis of airway burn. Because of this, early intubation of suspected airway burn is the treatment of choice in such patients. The time frame from burn to airway occlusion is usually between 4 and 24 hours, so there is time to make a sensible decision with senior staff and allow an experienced anaesthetist to intubate the patient. Although antidotes exist to some specific components of smoke (carbon monoxide and cyanide), the treatment of smoke inhalation usually involves endotracheal intubation and ventilatory support (sometimes for several weeks).

Summary box 46.10

Initial management of the burned airway
- Early elective intubation is safest
- Delay can make intubation very difficult owing to swelling
- Be ready to perform an emergency cricothyroidotomy if intubation is delayed

Breathing

Inhalational injury

Time is a major factor; anyone trapped in a fire for more than a couple of minutes must be observed for signs of smoke inhalation. Other signs that raise suspicion are the presence of soot in the nose and the oropharynx and a chest radiograph showing patchy consolidation.

The clinical features are a progressive increase in respiratory effort and rate, rising pulse, anxiety and confusion and decreasing oxygen saturation. These symptoms may not be apparent immediately and can take 24 hours to 5 days to develop.

Treatment starts as soon as this injury is suspected and the airway is secure. Physiotherapy, nebulisers and warm humidified oxygen are all useful. The patient's progress should be monitored using the respiratory rate, together with blood gas measurements. If the situation deteriorates, continuous or intermittent positive pressure may be used with a mask or T-piece. In the severest cases, intubation and management in an intensive care unit will be needed. Nebulised heparin can be useful in preventing the formation of the fibrin casts, although heparin requires antithrombin for its efficacy (which is deficient after burn injury) and some providers suggest additional antithrombin administration. The efficacy of inhaled heparin therapy may be enhanced by the simultaneous administration of the mucolytic agent *N*-acetylcysteine. Bronchodilators, such as albuterol, may also be of value, additionally stimulating mucosal repair, demonstrating anti-inflammatory properties and decreasing inflammatory mediators such as histamine, leukotrienes and tumour necrosis factor.

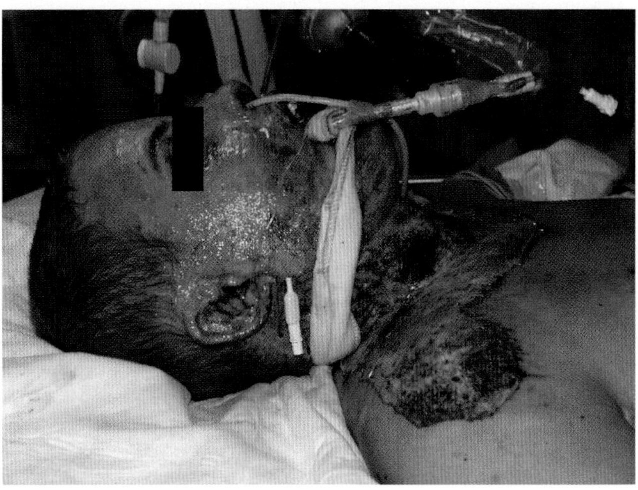

Figure 46.1 Burns to the face and neck with inhalation injury requiring intubation.

The key, therefore, in the management of inhalational injury is to suspect it from the history, institute early management and observe carefully for deterioration.

Thermal burn injury to the lower airway

These rare injuries can occur with steam injuries. The management is supportive and the same as that for an inhalational injury.

Metabolic poisoning

Any history of a fire within an enclosed space and any history of altered consciousness are important clues to metabolic poisoning. Blood gases must be measured immediately if poisoning is a possibility. Carboxyhaemoglobin levels raised above 10% must be treated with high inspired oxygen for 24 hours to speed its displacement from haemoglobin. Metabolic acidosis is a feature of many forms of poisoning. Modern treatment of cyanide poisoning involves the intravenous administration of vitamin B12 (hydroxycobalamin), which interacts with cyanide to form cyanocobalamin, which is water soluble and excreted in the urine. Once again the key to diagnosis is the history and blood gas measurement will confirm the diagnosis.

Mechanical block to breathing

Any mechanical block to breathing from the eschar of a significant full-thickness burn on the chest wall is obvious from the examination. There will also be carbon dioxide retention and high inspiratory pressures if the patient is ventilated. The treatment is to make some scoring cuts through the burned skin to allow the chest to expand (escharotomy).

ASSESSMENT OF THE BURN WOUND

Assessing size

The defining feature of any burn referral and usually the first question to seek clarification is 'What is the size of the burn?'

From this simple question the burn team can establish the correct method of transfer and the resources needed to appropriately manage the patient with burn on arrival.

The standard method of estimating burn size is to use percentage body surface area. As per the Emergency Management of Severe Burns (EMSB) the distal wrist crease to fingertips of an adult patient's hand is approximately 1% TBSA (1.25%), due to the inherent error in measurement this is useful for small burns of up to 10% TBSA. An estimation of burn size (greater than 15% in an adult; 10% in extremes of age) will also determine whether fluid resuscitation is required.

A useful aide-memoire in the prehospital and emergency setting is the Wallace rule of nines. In this schematic each body part is assigned a burn percentage: each upper limb is 9%, head is 9%, lower limbs are 18% each, posterior torso and buttocks is 18% and the anterior torso 18% (chest 9% and abdomen 9%). The remaining 1% is assigned to the genitalia. The rule of nines has been in established clinical practice for 70 years but it is not without drawbacks. In terms of accuracy there is a tendency to overestimate burn size, and in the obese patient the proportion of surface area of the arms and head decreases as the surface area of the torso and legs increase. A modification of 5% for the arms, 20% for the legs and 50% for the torso has been suggested but is not widely used. However, the rule of nines is an excellent means to quickly and reliably assess the size of a burn in an emergency setting, providing the clinician is aware of the limitations; it is not suitable for children under 10 years of age.

On arrival at a burns unit, the standard formatting for assessment and documentation is the Lund and Browder chart (***Figure 46.2***). Developed in 1942 following a mass casualty burn event at a nightclub in Boston, MA, USA, the chart is a schematic representation of the anterior and posterior body. It further subdivides body areas and allows for differentiation of burn depth by shading.

The Lund and Browder chart can be completed at multiple points during a burn admission to document changes in burn size/depth and can also be used as an adjunct to surgical notes, when skin graft donor sites and grafted areas can be shaded.

In an increasingly digital era, it is worth noting the easy availability of burn management apps that are readily compatible with smart phones. These invariably involve shading

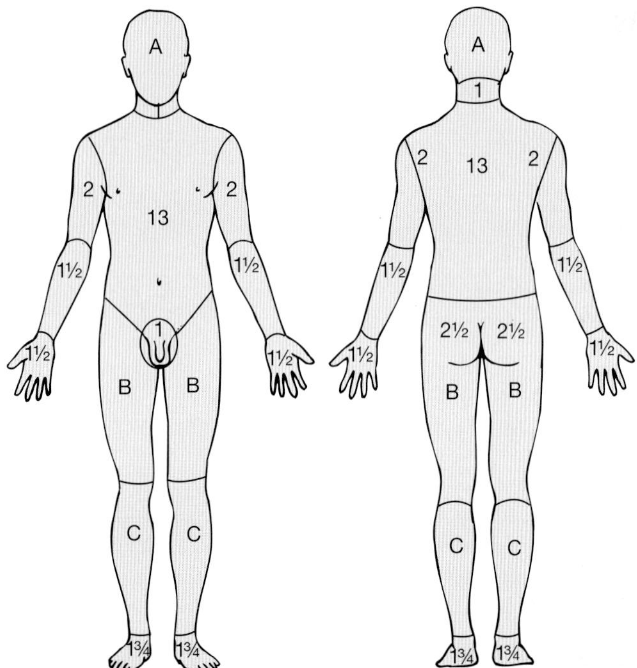

Relative percentage of area affected by growth

Age in years	0	1	5	10	15	Adult
A Head	9	8	6	5	4	3
B Thigh	2	3	4	4	4	4
C Leg	2	2	3	3	3	3

Figure 46.2 Modified Lund and Browder table and diagram.

a pictorial representation of the body, which then calculates a burn size. Additional features include adding age and weight to allow automatic estimation of fluid resuscitation requirements.

Burn size calculation: children

The body proportions of children necessitate adjustment of the above-mentioned scales. An infant's head is proportionally larger than an adult's and this adjustment is represented on the modified Lund and Browder chart for children, where at birth the head represents 18% and the lower limbs 13.5% each. For each year 1% is subtracted from the head, with 0.5% being added to each lower limb until the age of 10, when the body proportions are roughly equivalent to those of an adult.

Summary box 46.11

Assessing the area of a burn

- The patient's hand is 1% TBSA, and is a useful guide in small burns
- The Lund and Browder chart is useful in larger burns
- The 'rule of nines' is adequate for a first approximation only

Alexander Burns Wallace, 1906–1974, Scottish plastic surgeon and founding member of the British Association of Plastic Surgeons.
Charles C Lund, 1895–1972, American surgeon, Boston City Hospital, Boston, MA, USA.
Newton C Browder, 1893–1969, American surgeon, Boston City Hospital, Boston, MA, USA. Lund and Browder developed the chart based on their experiences in treating over 300 burn patients injured in a fire in Boston in 1942.

Assessing depth from the history

The first indication of burn depth comes from the history (*Table 46.2*). The burning of human skin is temperature and time dependent. It takes 6 hours for skin maintained at 44°C to suffer irreversible changes, but a surface temperature of 70°C for 1 second is all that is needed to produce epidermal destruction. Taking an example of hot water at 65°C: exposure for 45 seconds will produce a full-thickness burn; for 15 seconds a deep partial-thickness burn; and for 7 seconds a superficial partial-thickness burn (*Figure 46.3*).

TABLE 46.2 Causes of burns and their likely depth.

Cause of burn	Probable depth of burn
Scald	Superficial, but with deep dermal patches in the absence of good first aid. Will be deep in a young infant or the elderly
Fat burns	Deep dermal to full thickness
Flame burns	Mixed deep dermal and full thickness
Alkali burns, including cement	Often deep dermal or full thickness
Acid burns	Weak concentrations superficial; strong concentrations deep dermal
Electrical contact burn	Full thickness

Summary box 46.12

Assessing the depth of a burn

- The history is important: temperature, time and burning material
- Superficial burns have capillary filling
- Deep partial-thickness burns do not blanch, but have some sensation
- Full-thickness burns feel leathery and have no sensation

Superficial partial-thickness burns

The damage in these burns goes no deeper than the papillary dermis. The clinical features are blistering and/or loss of the epidermis. The underlying dermis is pink and moist and will exudate fluid for up to 36 hours post burn injury. The capillary return is clearly visible when blanched. There is little or no fixed capillary staining. Pinprick sensation is normal. Superficial partial-thickness burns heal without residual scarring in 2 weeks (*Figure 46.4*). The treatment is supportive.

Deep partial-thickness burn

These burns involve damage to the deeper parts of the reticular dermis. Clinically, the epidermis is usually lost. The exposed dermis is not as moist as that in a superficial burn. There is often abundant fixed capillary staining, especially if examined after 48 hours. The colour does not blanch with pressure under the examiner's finger. Sensation is reduced, and the patient is unable to distinguish sharp from blunt pressure when examined with a needle. Deep dermal burns take 3 weeks or more to heal without surgery and usually lead to hypertrophic scarring.

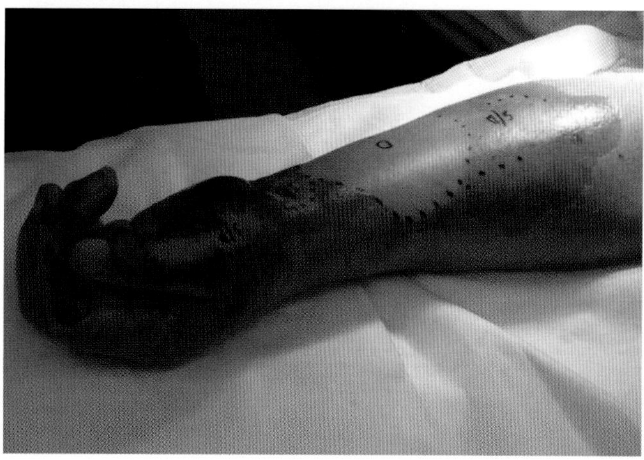

Figure 46.3 Photograph showing the difference between superficial dermal (S/D) and deep dermal (D). The burn wound is less than 24 hours old and has been meticulously cleaned in theatre.

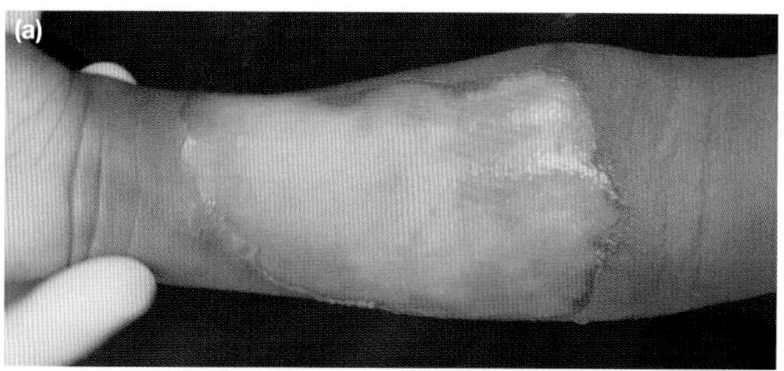

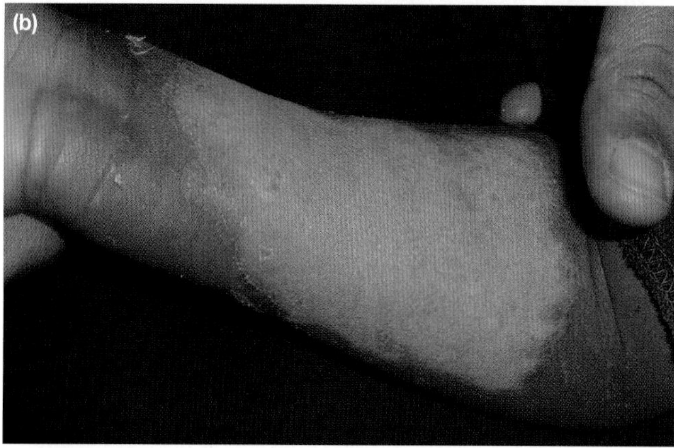

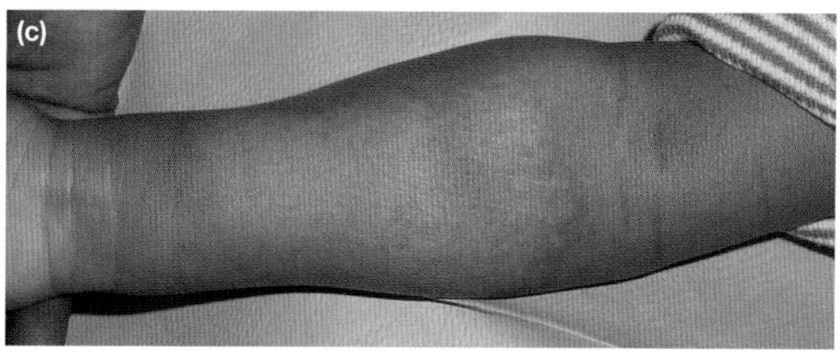

Figure 46.4 (a) A superficial partial-thickness scald 24 hours after injury. The dermis is pink and blanches to pressure. **(b)** At 2 weeks, the wound is healed but lacks pigment. **(c)** At 3 months, the pigment is returning.

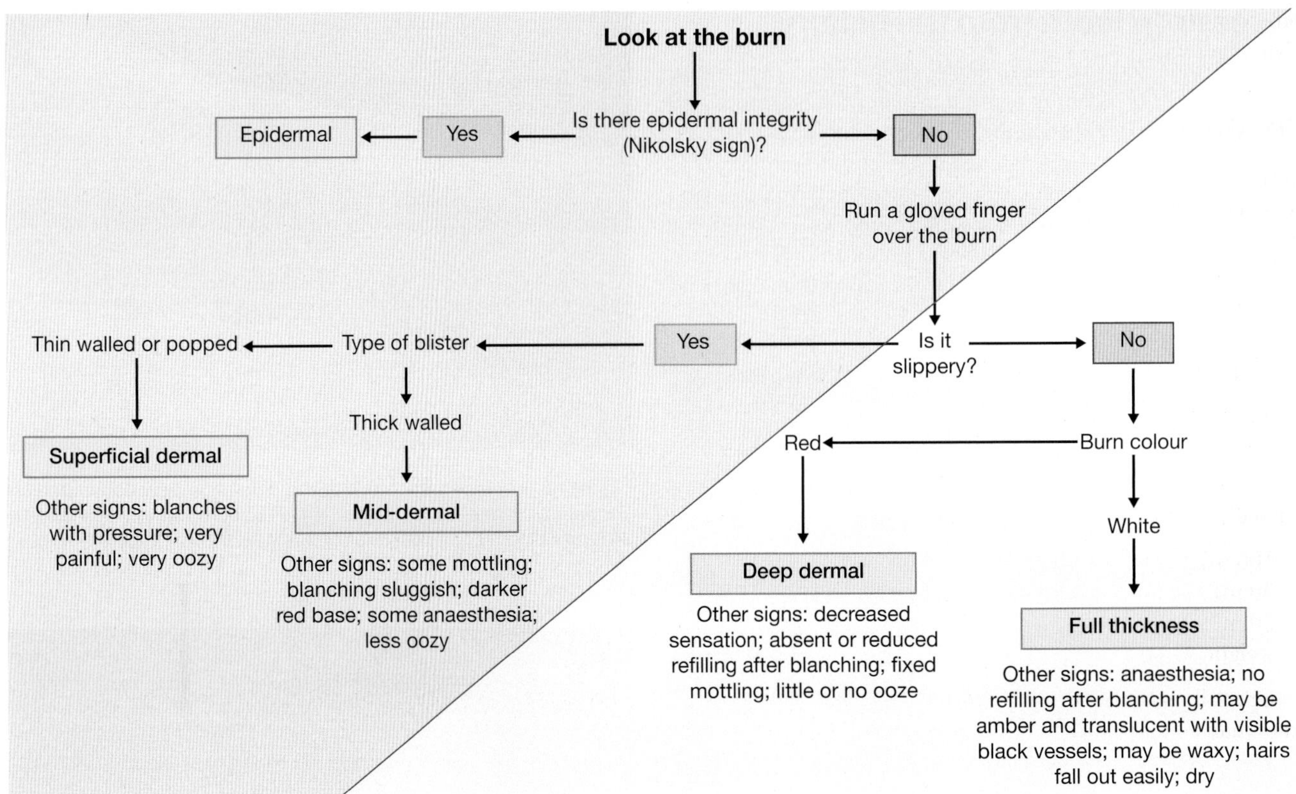

Figure 46.5 Protocol for assessing depth of burn. The Nikolsky sign refers to detachment of the epidermis from the dermis when lateral pressure is applied to the skin.

Full-thickness burns

The whole of the dermis is destroyed in these burns. Clinically, they have a hard, leathery feel. The appearance can vary from that similar to the patient's normal skin to charred black, depending upon the intensity of the heat. There is no capillary return. Often, thrombosed vessels can be seen under the skin. These burns are completely anaesthetic – a needle can be stuck deep into the dermis without any pain or bleeding.

Concept of two burn depths

In treatment terms, there are two burn depths. There are those burns which, with optimal support and good wound management, are superficial enough to heal spontaneously and quickly (within 14 days), leaving an excellent functional and cosmetic result, defined in this chapter as group A. Group B includes those burns that are sufficiently deep to undergo prolonged healing by secondary intention. This process takes weeks or months and involves the degradation and separation of the eschar (burned tissue), the formation of granulation tissue and the process of wound contraction. The course of healing by secondary intention *must* be aborted and replaced as closely as possible by a process of primary intention healing with direct closure, skin graft and skin substitutes.

Figure 46.5 is a pictorial representation of this with burns in the pink section to the left of the line belonging to group A and burns in the blue section to the right to group B.

FLUID RESUSCITATION

As the understanding of 'fluid shifts' developed, the introduction of fluid resuscitation guidelines greatly improved the survival rates for patients with large burns. Standard guidelines and formulae are taught to emergency department and first-responder personnel. Resuscitation fluid should commence from time of burn injury and any delay in commencement must be caught up.

Intravenous resuscitation is appropriate for any adult with a burn greater than 15% TBSA and any child with a burn greater than 10% TBSA. Extremes of age require extra care: for children, additional maintenance fluid is required; in the elderly, judicious monitoring is necessary owing to concurrent comorbidities and the inherent physiology of ageing.

Depending on resources available, the commencement of intravenous fluid resuscitation approaches 30% TBSA in some countries. If oral resuscitation is necessary then additional salt solutions (such as Dioralyte) are required as hyponatraemia and water intoxication can be fatal.

There are three variables in the calculation of fluid requirements: the percentage of TBSA burned, the weight of the patient and the rate/type of fluid. Fluid loss is maximum in the first 8 hours and slows by 24–36 hours, by which stage normal fluid replacement is required.

There are three main fluids used in the resuscitation stage: crystalloid (by far the most common), colloid and, in

Pyotr Nikolsky, 1858–1940, Russian dermatologist.

some centres, hypertonic saline. Each resuscitation fluid has advantages and disadvantages.

Crystalloid resuscitation

Hartmann's solution or Ringer's lactate is the most commonly used crystalloid as it most closely replicates the osmolality of plasma. It is considerably less expensive than colloid and can maintain intravascular volume.

The modified Parkland formula is the most commonly used:

$$\text{TBSA\% burn} \times \text{weight (kg)} \times 4 = \text{volume in mL}$$

The first half is given in 8 hours and the second over 16 hours to complete the 24-hour resuscitation time frame.

In children maintenance fluid must also be given. This is normally dextrose–saline given as follows:

- 100 mL/kg for 24 hours for the first 10 kg;
- 50 mL/kg for the next 10 kg;
- 20 mL/kg for 24 hours for each kilogram over 20 kg body weight.

Crystalloid resuscitation requires eight-fold greater volumes than colloid which can result in increased tissue oedema.

Hypertonic saline

Hypertonic saline is used in some centres; it produces hyperosmolality and hypernatraemia, resulting in a reduction in the shift of intracellular water to the extracellular space. Proponents of this resuscitation fluid cite advantages that include less tissue oedema and a resultant decrease in escharotomies and intubations. However, prolonged hypernatraemia without careful monitoring can be problematic and lead to renal dysfunction.

Colloid resuscitation

The most commonly used colloid is human albumin solution. Plasma proteins are responsible for inward oncotic pressure that counteracts the outward capillary hydrostatic pressure. Albumin should be preferably administered after the first 12 hours post burn as the massive fluid shifts drive proteins out of the cells.

The most common colloid-based formula is the Muir and Barclay formula, which estimates the amount of fluid that needs to be infused during the first 36 hours post burn:

- the basic formula is: TBSA% × weight (kg) × 0.5 = one portion;
- six portions are given in total over 36 hours:
  - give one infusion 4 hourly for 12 hours (three portions in total);
  - then one infusion 6 hourly for 12 hours (two portions in total);
  - the final infusion to be given over 12 hours.

The original Muir and Barclay formula utilised fresh-frozen plasma as the colloid of choice. Both albumin and fresh-frozen plasma are maintained in the blood bank and are more expensive; excessive use can cause additional pressure on the renal system.

Monitoring of resuscitation

Although fluid resuscitation has defined guidelines it is critical to understand that the process is dynamic and rigid adherence to protocols should be avoided. The key to monitoring of resuscitation is urine output. Urine output should be between 0.5 and 1.0 mL/kg body weight per hour. If the urine output drops and the patient is showing signs of hypoperfusion (tachycardia, cool peripheries and a high lactate/metabolic acidosis), then a bolus of 10 mL/kg body weight should be given. It is important that patients are not over-resuscitated; urine output in excess of 2 mL/kg body weight per hour should warrant a decrease in infusion.

Other measures of tissue perfusion such as lactate levels can be useful, particularly in larger burns. A persistent raised lactate/metabolic acidosis can indicate a missed systemic toxicity from cyanide or carbon monoxide. Patients with underlying comorbidities, particularly cardiac or renal, will require further intensive monitoring such as central venous pressure measurement in an intensive care setting.

Summary box 46.13

Fluids for resuscitation

- In children with burns over 10% TBSA and adults with burns over 15% TBSA, consider the need for intravenous fluid resuscitation
- If oral fluids are to be used, salt must be added
- Fluids needed can be calculated from a standard formula and start from time of burn
- The key is to monitor urine output

Temperature management

When undergoing burn assessment and fluid resuscitation it is vital that the patient maintains an adequate core temperature. A key function of skin is thermoregulation and in large burns this is severely impacted. Hypothermia is a component of the 'lethal triad of trauma', which includes acidosis and coagulopathy; the combination of all three significantly increases mortality. Measures to counteract hypothermia include infusing warmed fluids, external warmers such as the 'Bair Hugger' and increasing the ambient room temperature in the emergency department/assessment room.

Alexis Frank Hartmann, 1898–1964, pediatrician, St Louis, MO, USA, described the solution; should not be confused with the name of Henri Albert Charles Antoine Hartmann, French surgeon, who described the operation that goes by his name.
Sidney Ringer, 1835–1910, Professor of Clinical Medicine, University College Hospital, London, UK.
Parkland Memorial Hospital, Dallas, TX, USA.
Ian Fraser Kerr Muir, 1921–2008, plastic surgeon, Aberdeen Royal Infirmary, Aberdeen, UK, referred to as 'a gentle giant of plastic surgery'.
Thomas Laird Barclay, 1925–2007, plastic surgeon, Royal Infirmary, Bradford, UK.

TREATING THE BURN WOUND

Group A burns: superficial dermal partial-thickness burns

There are two key concepts for managing partial-thickness burns:

- prevent any factor that may result in the burn 'changing group', predominantly infection;
- control pain, particularly during dressing changes and therapy.

An array of treatment options are used worldwide for the treatment of these wounds, ranging from honey and simple dressings to synthetic biological dressings with porcine collagen or live cultured keratinocytes.

The ideal dressing should be easy to apply, non-painful, pain-reducing, simple to manage and locally available. The crucial factor is to prevent the borderline mid-dermal burns from progressing to deep dermal. Here, the choice of dressing can make the difference between scar and no scar and/or operation and no operation.

If the wound is heavily contaminated as a result of the accident, then it is prudent to clean the wound formally under a general anaesthetic. With more chronic contamination, silver sulphadiazine cream dressing for 2 or 3 days is very effective and can be changed to a dressing that is more efficient at promoting healing after this period.

The simplest method of treating a superficial burn wound is by exposure, but this is usually only suitable for small burns on the face as this method is painful and requires an intensive amount of nursing support. A variation on this theme is to cover the wound with a permeable wound dressing, such as Mefix® or Fixomull®. This allows the wounds to dry but, because it is a covering, it avoids the problems of the wound adhering to sheets and clothes. A similar method of managing these types of burn is to place a Vaseline-impregnated gauze (with or without an antiseptic, such as chlorhexidine) over the wound. An alternative is a fenestrated silicone sheet (e.g. Mepitel®). To provide antibacterial cover Acticoat dressings with silver nanocrystals are also used. They can be left in place for up to 7 days.

More interactive dressings include hydrocolloids and biological dressings. Hydrocolloid dressings need to be changed every 3–5 days. They are particularly useful in mixed-depth burns as the high protease levels under the occlusive dressing aids debridement of the deeper areas of burn. They also provide a moist environment, which is good for epithelialisation. Duoderm® is a hydrocolloid dressing. There is good evidence for its role in burns.

Biosynthetic (e.g. Biobrane®) and natural (e.g. amniotic membranes) dressings also provide good healing environments and do not need to be changed. They are ideal for one-stop management of superficial burns, being easy to apply and comfortable (***Figure 46.6***). However, they will become detached if applied to deep dermal wounds as the eschar needs to separate. They are therefore not as useful in mixed-depth wounds.

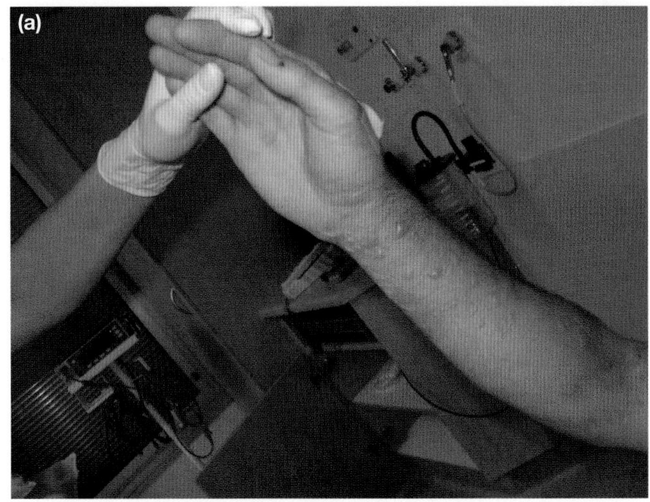

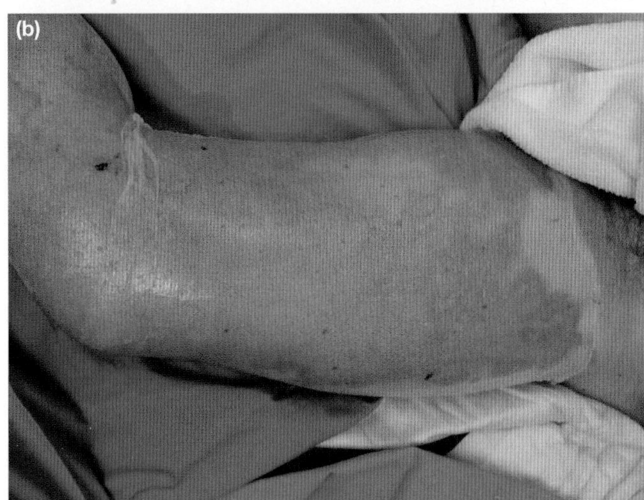

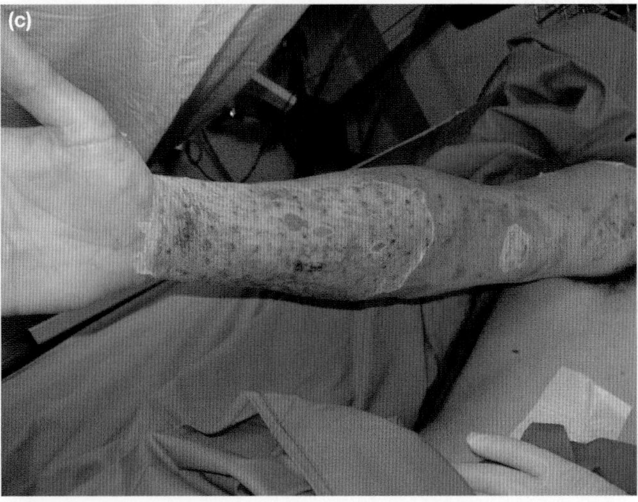

Figure 46.6 Treatment of partial-thickness burns with Biobrane. **(a)** Prior to surgical scrubbing and shaving. **(b)** Following surgical debridement and application of Biobrane; note that the Biobrane is adherent to the wound. **(c)** As the burn wound re-epithelialises the Biobrane lifts and can be trimmed at each dressing change. Normally the Biobrane is fully removed by 3 weeks.

Summary box 46.14

Treatment goals for group A burns

- Prevent burn becoming infected
- Use of appropriate dressings
- Manage pain
- Prevent progression to deeper burn (group B burns)

Group B burns: full-thickness and deep dermal burns

The management of the burn wound remains the same, irrespective of the size of the injury. The burn needs to be cleaned, and the size and depth need to be assessed. For full-thickness burns and deep partial-thickness burns an escharotomy may be required. All but the very smallest of full-thickness burns are likely to involve excision. Smaller deep dermal burns of intermittent depth may require 48 hours to declare but will require appropriate dressing management.

Escharotomy

Circumferential full-thickness burns to the limbs and torso require emergency surgery. The burn has a tourniquet-like effect compromising respiration (torso) and peripheral circulation (limbs). The tourniquet effect of this injury is treated by incising the whole length of full-thickness burns (***Table 46.3***).

For the chest this comprises two longitudinal and two horizontal incisions. Performance of chest escharotomy should show evidence of immediate improvement of respiration and, if intubated, the ventilation pressures. For the limbs the escharotomy incision is performed in the midaxial line, avoiding major nerves (***Figure 46.7***). An escharotomy can cause significant blood loss; therefore consider use of cutting diathermy and have appropriate dressings and blood available.

TABLE 46.3 Key features of escharotomy placement.

Upper limb	Midaxial. Anterior to the elbow medially to avoid the ulnar nerve
Hand	Midline in the digits Release muscle compartments if tight Best done in theatre
Lower limb	Midaxial. Posterior to the ankle medially to avoid the long saphenous vein and anterior to the head of the fibula to avoid the common peroneal nerve
Chest	Down the chest lateral to the nipples, across the chest below the clavicle and across the chest at the level of the xiphisternum
General rules	Extend the wound beyond the deep burn Diathermy any significant bleeding vessels Apply haemostatic dressing and elevate the limb postoperatively

Surgical treatment

Early versus staged full-thickness burn excision

Opinion varies on the timing of burn eschar excision. Early total burn excision refers to excision of the entire burn on arrival at the burns unit or as soon as logistically possible. Once the patient is cleared of trauma in the emergency department, the airway is secure and intravenous access and monitoring achieved, then the decision is whether to take the patient straight to theatre for burn wound debridement/escharectomy or to transfer the patient to the intensive care unit.

The advantage of early burn excision is to exploit the time period or 'window' before the overwhelming systemic response to the burn reaches a crescendo.

The 'anaesthetic' window refers to the effect of the burn on the airway – an upper airway burn can be bypassed by endotracheal intubation but a lower airway burn inhalational injury can cause chemical pneumonitis that may progress to acute respiratory distress syndrome. This usually becomes problematic after 48 hours; therefore, it is prudent to exploit this window and perform the burn excision during the time prior to lung injury decompensation.

The 'haemodynamic' window refers to the progressive inflammatory vasodilation and potential coagulopathy. This leads to an increasing resistance to vasoconstrictor agents in tumescence fluids with the potential for blood loss and need for blood transfusion which can drive further immunocompromise. Excising a full-thickness burn early, prior to these changes, can result in less blood loss. Additionally removing the eschar, which plays a role in driving the fluid shifts, will result in less oedema and lower fluid requirements.

Finally the 'bacterial' window is also important. Excising a full-thickness burn, which is essentially necrotic material, can help to reduce the bacterial load, thereby reducing the risk of infection.

Summary box 46.15

Early burn excision

- Removal of eschar reduces bacterial load
- Majority of surgery is performed prior to substantial lung injury
- Allows effective use of vasoconstrictive fluids
- Requires adequate theatre, staff and facilities

Early burn excision is dependent on the appropriate staff, resources, equipment and time. When these are not readily available a staged approach is also utilised. This involves serial debridement of the burn over several operating sessions in the first week of the burn. Proponents of this approach advocate shorter operating times and reducing the requirements for blood transfusions.

This technique also relies on managing the remaining burn eschar until excision to prevent bacterial colonisation and to prepare for surgery. This is achieved by using silver-based dressing/creams containing antibacterial properties including *Pseudomonas aeruginosa* and methicillin-resistant *Staphylococcus aureus*.

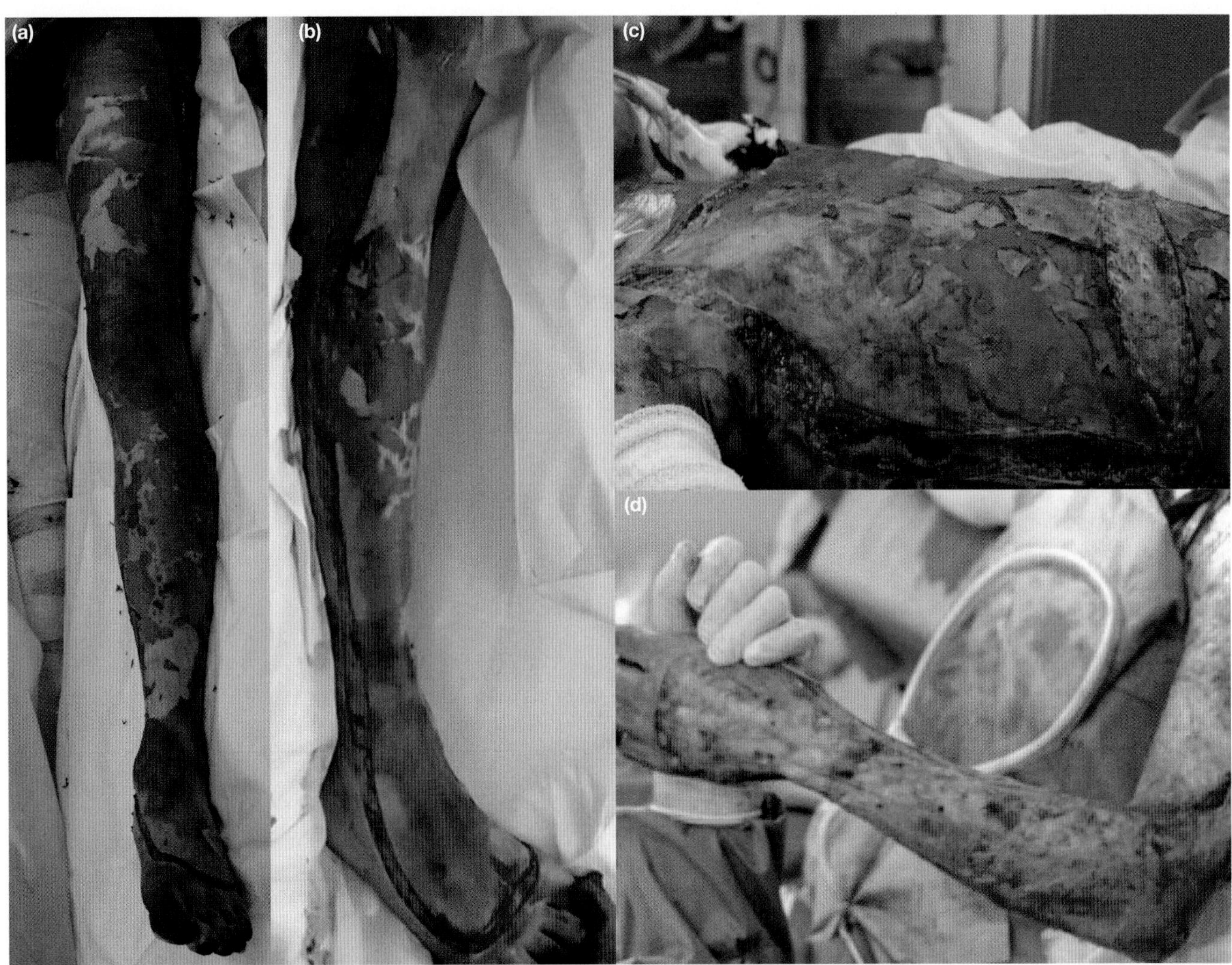

Figure 46.7 (a-d) Extensive full-thickness burns at first operation. Note the placement of the escharotomies on the chest and the lower limb. The leg had an escharectomy followed by escharotomy.

Dressings with silver that are commonly used include:

- **Silver sulphadiazine cream (1%)**. This gives broad-spectrum prophylaxis against bacterial colonisation.
- **Mafenide acetate cream**. This is popular, especially in the USA, but is painful to apply and has been associated with metabolic acidosis. It is usually used as a 5% topical solution.
- **Silver sulphadiazine and cerium nitrate**. This induces a sterile eschar on the burned skin and has been shown in certain instances, especially in elderly patients, to reduce some of the cell-mediated immunosuppression that occurs in burns. It is especially useful in treating burns when a conservative treatment option has been chosen. Cerium nitrate has also been shown to boost cell-mediated immunity in these patients.
- **Acticoat**. This is a nanocrystalline silver barrier dressing and is an effective antimicrobial against a broad spectrum of bacteria.

The keystone of burns surgery is control, regardless of whether early or staged excision is the plan. A wide-bore cannula should be used and the patient's blood pressure must be monitored adequately. If a large excision is considered, then an arterial line (to monitor blood pressure) and central venous access are needed. The anaesthetist also needs measurements and control of the acid–base balance, clotting time and haemoglobin levels. The core temperature of the patient must not drop below 36°C, otherwise clotting irregularities will be compounded.

For most burn excisions, subcutaneous injection of a dilute solution of adrenaline (epinephrine) 1:1 000 000 or 1:500 000 and tourniquet control are important for controlling blood loss. The tumescence fluid is injected into both the burn eschar and the donor sites.

Summary box 46.16

Staged burn excision

- Shorter but more frequent surgical theatre trips
- Will require managing/binding of remaining eschar

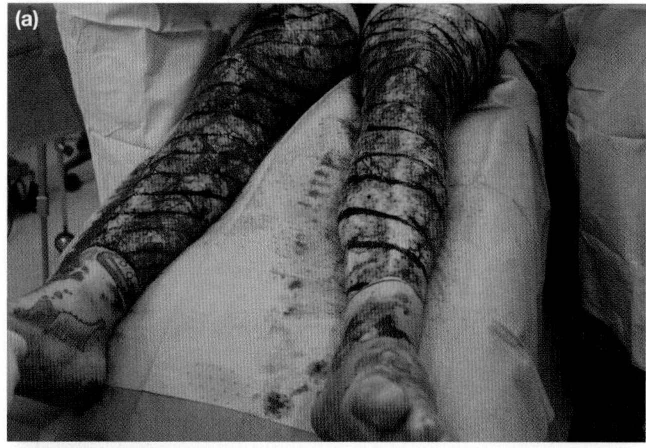

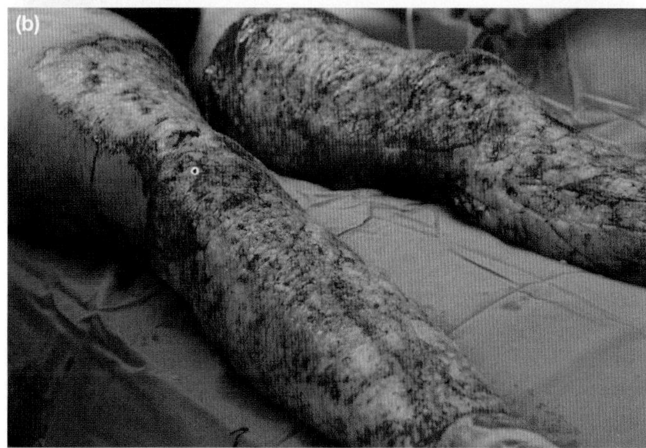

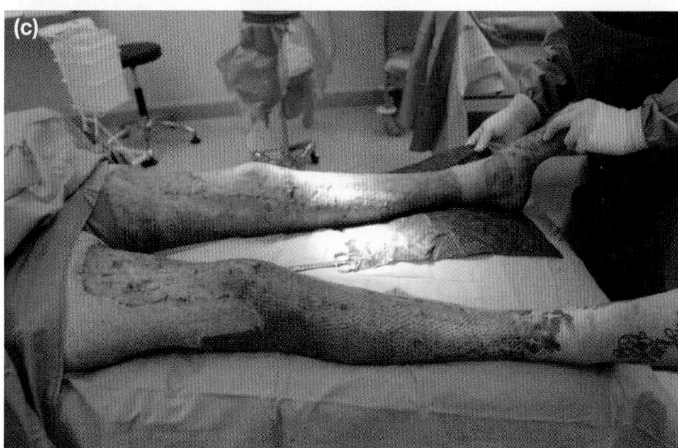

Figure 46.8 Full-thickness leg burns. **(a)** Marked for excision; **(b)** excised to healthy tissue fat/fascia; **(c)** skin graft at first dressing change.

In deep dermal burns, tangential excision is performed until punctate bleeding is observed and the dermis can be seen to be free of any small, thrombosed vessels. A topical solution of 1:500 000 adrenaline also helps to reduce bleeding, as does the application of the skin graft/substitute.

Full-thickness burns require full-thickness excision of the skin. In certain circumstances, it is appropriate to go down to the fascia but, in most cases, the burn excision is down to viable fat. Wherever possible, a skin graft/substitute should be applied immediately (***Figure 46.8***).

Graft application results in primary intention healing in the plane deep to the graft and at the horizontal margins where it meets unburned skin. Split-skin grafts can be left as intact sheets where function (over major joints, hands and fingers, anterior neck), cosmesis (face, dorsum of hands) and future growth (developing breasts) are particularly important; however, skin grafts can never result in 'normal' skin. Because we rely on spontaneous healing of the site from which they are harvested (the donor site), they are thin, consisting of the epidermis and a variable proportion of the superficial dermis.

They are often harvested as between 0.30 and 0.38 mm and thus their application into the burn wound creates a donor defect. Because the dermal component of the graft is thin, graft contraction post application occurs. The thinner the harvested graft, the greater the degree of contraction and the greater the degree of functional disability and dysaesthesia. The donor site is painful; as a result techniques must be employed to reduce the size of the donor site in an effort to minimise the pain. These include meshing the graft by putting it through a series of blades mounted on rollers that create offset incisions in the skin graft in horizontal lines. Post meshing, these cuts can be pulled open, extending the graft and resulting in diamond-shaped defects. This has the advantage of reducing the likelihood of graft haematoma/seroma. Meshing can be performed at different ratios. As the ratio increases, the size of the diamond defect increases.

Since the burn bed after excision of deep burn does not contain tissue capable of healing without modification of the bed structure, a small bleb of granulation tissue forms in these diamonds between the graft struts. This results in a characteristic mesh pattern scarring. The wider the mesh, the worse the appearance.

Although the epidermis can regenerate, the dermis removed from the donor site during skin graft harvesting can only repair and a layer of scar forms under the new epidermis at the donor site, which is 'thinner' than it was pre-harvest. The donor site is thus not an infinite resource. With serial graft harvesting, the donor site can become so deep a wound that adnexal structures are no longer present and the donor site has to heal by secondary intention, or receive a skin graft itself. In very extensive burns, where the burn size exceeds donor site availability, the surgeon tends to rely on higher ratios (1:3, up to 1:9) and harvests the skin grafts more thinly. This allows the donor site to heal more rapidly, facilitating earlier reharvest when serial grafting is required.

Postoperative management of these patients requires careful evaluation of fluid balance and levels of haemoglobin. The outer dressings will require attention and regular changing because of expected fluid leaks.

Physiotherapy and splints are important in maintaining range of movement and reducing joint contracture. Elevation of the appropriate limbs is important. The hand must be splinted in a position of function after grafting, although the graft needs to be applied in the position of maximal stretch. Knees are best splinted in extension; axillae in abduction. Supervised movement by the physiotherapists, usually under direct vision of any affected joints, should begin after about 5 days.

Summary box 46.17

Burn excision surgery

- Deep dermal burns need tangential shaving and split-skin grafting or dermal substitutes
- All but the smallest full-thickness burns need surgery
- The anaesthetist needs to be ready for significant blood loss
- Tumescence fluid and topical adrenaline reduces bleeding
- All burnt tissue needs to be excised
- Stable cover, permanent or temporary, should be applied

The use of skin grafts and skin substitutes

Until very recently, the early definitive closure of wounds proved problematic when full-thickness burns exceeded 50% of the TBSA. The mainstay of burn wound repair has been the split-skin autograft and, at >50% TBSA, the burn area exceeds the donor site area. A number of manoeuvres have been established to facilitate coverage of these wounds by grafting, all of which are utilised in patients with the most extensive burn wounds. Techniques include serial episodes of grafting surgery, harvesting very thin autografts (to allow more rapid re-epithelialisation of the donor sites, facilitating earlier reharvest and allowing a greater number of harvests from the same donor site), widely meshing the grafts or using a Meek–Wall technique (Meek, Humeca, Enschede, the Netherlands). This latter technique involves using small pieces of graft, placed in a specialised holder on a cork board and run through a series of blades perpendicular to each other, to create small squares of graft each 3 mm × 3 mm. Once cut, the holding platform can be pulled apart (to differing distances – the 'mesh ratio'), separating the tiny grafts. Although 'fiddly' and laborious, this technique minimises graft wastage, since even small pieces of graft can be meshed in this way.

The use of cadaver skin to cover the non-grafted wounds pending donor site re-epithelialisation and 'reharvestability' gained popularity in the late twentieth century as issues of consent and techniques for harvest and storage (banking) were refined. The use of cadaver skin has a number of limitations. Skin banks are frequently short, or devoid, of stock. Its presence 'passively' temporises the wound, 'buying time' but not improving the wound bed, merely allowing undirected granulation. It cannot be used unless the patient is pathologically immune suppressed.

The dermal matrix strategy, pioneered by Jack Burke, sought to redress some of these issues. In producing a 'scaffold' to allow autologous tissue in-growth and establish a 'neodermis' ('active' temporisation), he improved the outcome of the thin, meshed skin graft. A completely synthetic, biodegradable polymer version has also been developed (***Figures 46.9 and 46.10***).

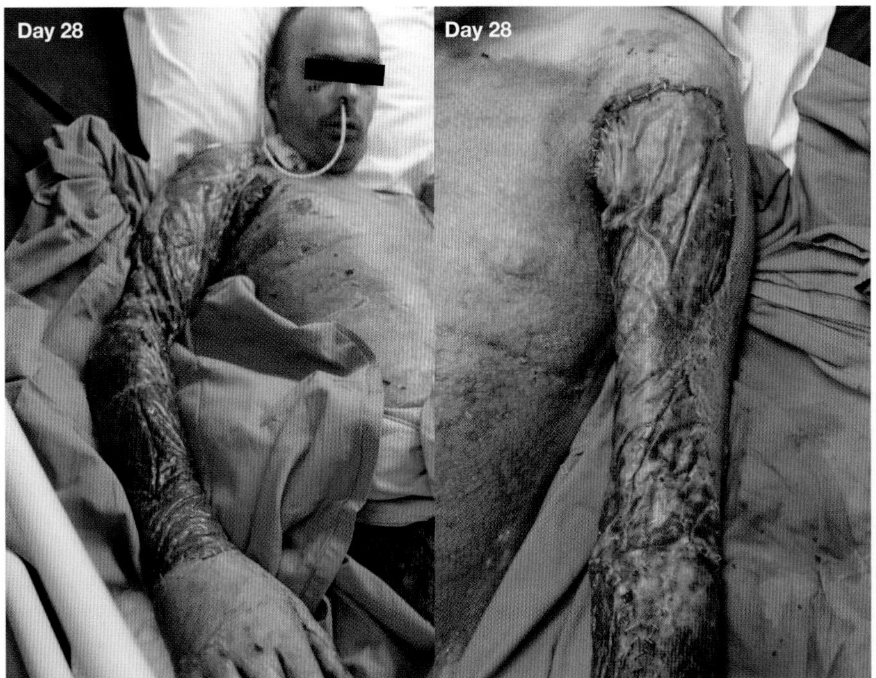

Figure 46.9 Day 28 post-full-thickness burns treated with early skin grafting using the Biodegradable Temporising Matrix (BTM) (a synthetic, biodegradable polyurethane dermal matrix) on the arms and immediate skin graft to chest.

Cicero Parker Meek, 1914–1979, general practitioner with a special interest in the treatment of burn patients, Aiken County Hospital, SC, USA.
SP Wall Jr, engineer, developed the Meek–Wall microdermatome with CP Meek in 1963.
John F Burke, 1922–2011, medical researcher, Harvard University, Boston, MA, USA, widely known for his co-invention of synthetic skin substitute in 1981 with Ioannis V Yannas.

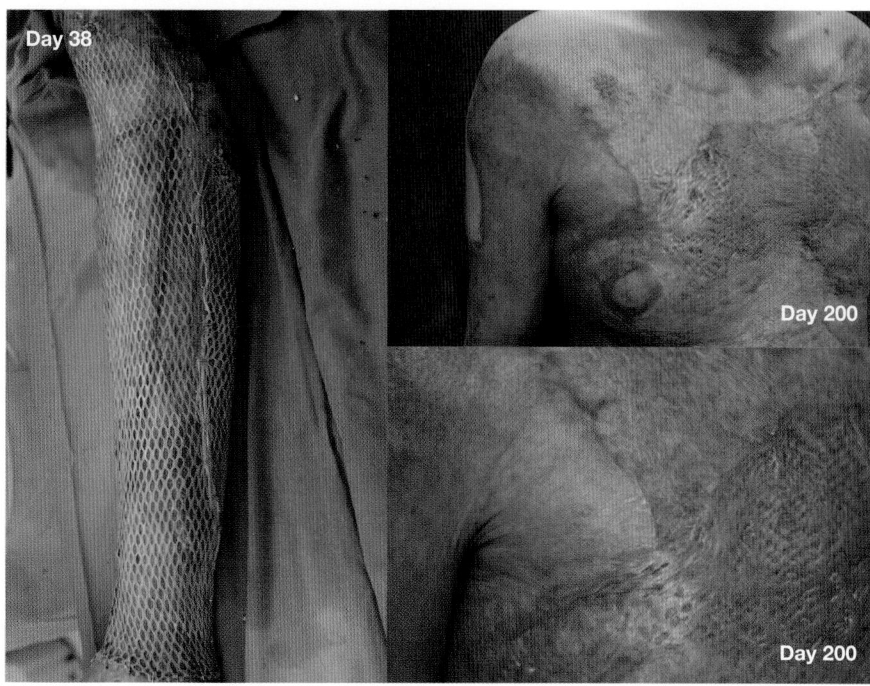

Figure 46.10 Day 38 picture shows a mesh graft on the arm after the dermal substitute has been removed. The day 200 pictures show the difference in scar outcome between the immediate skin graft to the chest and a Biodegradable Temporising Matrix (BTM) and skin graft to the arm and axilla. Both skin grafts had the same mesh ratio.

ADDITIONAL ASPECTS OF TREATING THE BURNED PATIENT

Analgesia

Acute

Analgesia is a vital part of burns management. Small burns, especially superficial burns, respond well to simple oral analgesia, paracetamol and non-steroidal anti-inflammatory drugs. Topical cooling is especially soothing. Large burns require intravenous opiates for the initial management; intramuscular administration should be avoided as uptake is variable.

Subacute

In patients with large burns, continuous analgesia is required, beginning with infusions and continuing with oral tablets. Powerful, short-acting analgesia should be administered before dressing changes. Administration is guided by anaesthetists, as in the case of general anaesthesia or midazolam and ketamine, or less intensive supervision, as in the case of morphine and nitrous oxide. Early support by colleagues from the pain team is beneficial in controlling pain.

Energy balance and nutrition

Any adult with a burn greater than 15% (10% in children) of TBSA has an increased nutritional requirement. All patients with burns of 20% of TBSA or greater should receive a nasogastric or nasojejunal tube and feeding should start within 6 hours of the injury to reduce gut mucosal damage. The advantage of the nasojejunal tube is that fasting is not necessary for trips to theatre. A number of different formulae are available to calculate the energy requirements of patients. This should be managed by a specialist dietician as part of the multidisciplinary team.

Burn injuries are catabolic in the acute episode. Successful management of the patient's energy balance involves a number of strategies. The catabolic drive continues while the wound remains unhealed and, therefore, rapid excision of the burn and stable coverage of the wound are the most significant factors in reversing this. Obligatory energy utilisation must be reduced to a minimum by keeping the patient warm with good environmental control. The excess energy requirements must be provided for and the nutritional balance monitored by measuring weight and nitrogen balance.

Monitoring and control of infection

Patients with major burns steadily become immunocompromised, having large portals of entry to pathogenic and opportunistic bacteria and fungi via the burn wound. They have compromised local defences in the lungs and gut owing to oedema, and usually have monitoring lines and catheters, which themselves represent portals for infection. Control of infection begins with policies on handwashing and other cross-contamination prevention measures. Bacteriological surveillance of the wound, catheter tips and sputum helps to build a picture of the patient's flora. If there are signs of infection, then further cultures need to be taken and antibiotics started. This is often initially on a best guess basis, hence the usefulness of prior surveillance; close liaison with a microbiologist is essential. In patients with large burns who remain

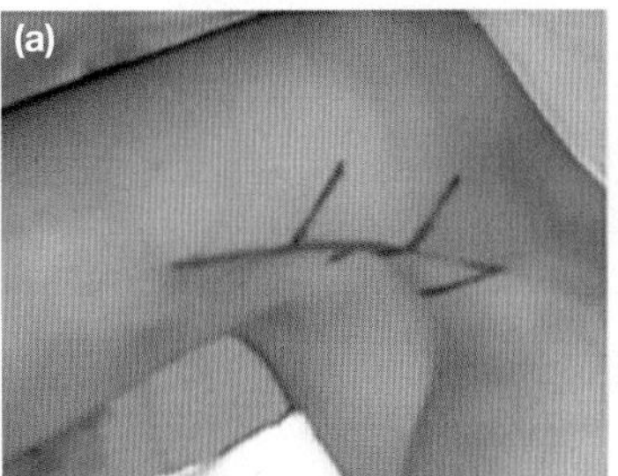

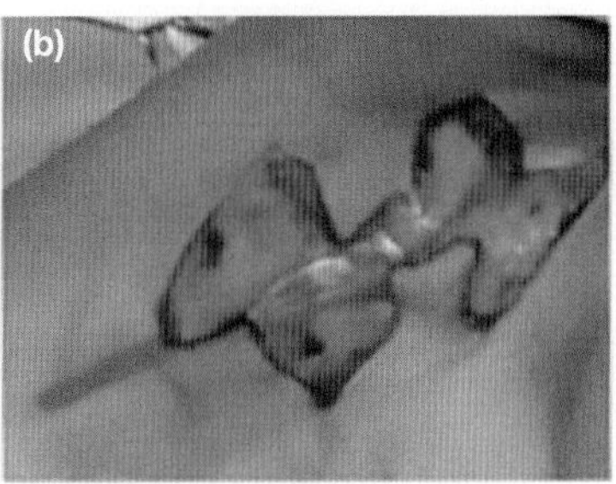

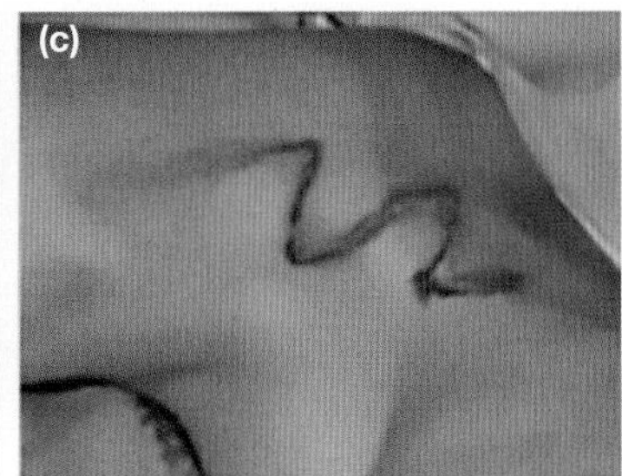

Figure 46.11 **(a)** Scar band contracture marked with multiple Z-plasties. **(b)** Release of the scar intraoperatively. **(c)** Reorientation of the scar when the Z-plasties are sutured.

catabolic, the core temperature is usually reset by the hypothalamus above 37°C. Significant temperatures are those above 38.5°C, but often other signs of infection are more useful to the clinician. These include significant rise or fall in the white cell count, thrombocytosis, increasing signs of catabolism and decreasing clinical status of the patient.

Nursing care

Burns patients require particularly intensive nursing care. Nurses are the primary effectors of many decisions that directly affect healing. Bandaged hands and joints that are stiff and painful need careful coaxing. Personal hygiene, baths and showers all become time-consuming and painful, but are vital parts of the patient's physiotherapy. Their success or failure has a powerful psychological impact on the patient and his or her family.

Physiotherapy and occupational therapy

All burns cause swelling, especially burns to the hands. Elevation, splintage and exercise reduce swelling and improve the final outcome. The physiotherapy needs to be started on day 1, so that the message can be reinforced on a daily basis. As the burn wounds heal scar management and rehabilitation to previous activities of daily living become increasingly important.

Psychological

A major burn is an overwhelming event, outside the normal experience, which stretches the patient's coping ability, suspends the patient's sense of safety and causes post-traumatic reactions. These are normal and usually self-limiting, receding as the patient heals. The features of this intensity of experience are of intrusive reactions, arousal reactions and avoidance reactions. Early intervention with psychology and development of coping strategies is of vital importance.

Delayed reconstruction and scar management

Delayed reconstruction of burn injuries is common for large full-thickness burns. These techniques were pioneered by McIndoe and Gillies. In the early healing period, acute contractures around the eye need particular attention. Eyelids must be grafted at the first sign of difficulty in closing the eyelids, and this must be done before the patient has any symptoms of exposure keratitis. Other areas that require early intervention are any contracture causing significant loss of range of movement of a joint. This is particularly important in the hand and axilla.

An established contracture can be treated in a number of ways. Burn alopecia is best treated with tissue expansion of the unburned hair-bearing skin. Tissue expansion is also a useful technique for isolated burns and other areas with adjacent normal skin. Z-plasty is useful where there is a single band and a transposition flap is useful in wider bands of scarring (***Figure 46.11***). In areas of circumferential or very broad areas of scarring, the only real treatment is incision and replacement with tissue. By far the best tissue for replacement is from either a full-thickness graft, dermal substitute with split-skin graft or vascularised tissue as in a free flap.

Summary box 46.18

Delayed reconstruction of burns

- Eyelids must be treated before exposure keratitis arises
- Transposition flaps and Z-plasties with or without tissue expansion are useful
- Full-thickness grafts and free flaps may be needed for large or difficult areas
- Hypertrophy is treated with pressure garments
- Pharmacological treatment of itch is important

The Guinea Pig Club. Sir Archibald McIndoe, 1900–1960, born in New Zealand, was appointed in 1938 as Consultant Plastic Surgeon to the Royal Air Force. He trained with his cousin, **Sir Harold Delf Gillies**, another internationally reputed plastic surgeon. McIndoe became world famous for his pioneering work on Battle of Britain pilots who were badly burnt. His work on these airmen, who needed several operations, and using his innovative technical and psychological methods, was the start of a lifelong service. The young fighter pilots were therefore referred to as 'guinea pigs' – thus was formed The Guinea Pig Club. McIndoe referred to his patients as 'the boys', who in turn called him 'the boss' or 'the maestro'. To this day, some of the members of the Guinea Pig Club from all over the world still meet on an annual basis in Sussex. McIndoe founded the British Association of Plastic Surgeons (BAPS).

Hypertrophy of many scars will respond to pressure garments. These need to be worn for a period of 6–18 months. Where it is difficult to apply pressure with pressure garments, or with smaller areas of hypertrophy, silicone patches will speed scar maturation, as will intralesional injection of steroid. Itching and dermatitis in burn scar areas are common. Pharmacological treatment of itch is an essential adjunct to therapy.

NON-THERMAL BURN INJURY

Electrical injuries

Electrical injuries are usually divided into low- and high-voltage injuries, the threshold being 1000 V.

Summary box 46.19

Electrical burns

- Low-voltage injuries cause small, localised, deep burns
- They can cause cardiac arrest through pacing interruption without significant direct myocardial damage
- High-voltage injuries damage by flash (external burn) and conduction (internal burn)
- Myocardium may be directly damaged without pacing interruption
- Limbs may need fasciotomies or amputation
- Look for and treat acidosis and myoglobinuria

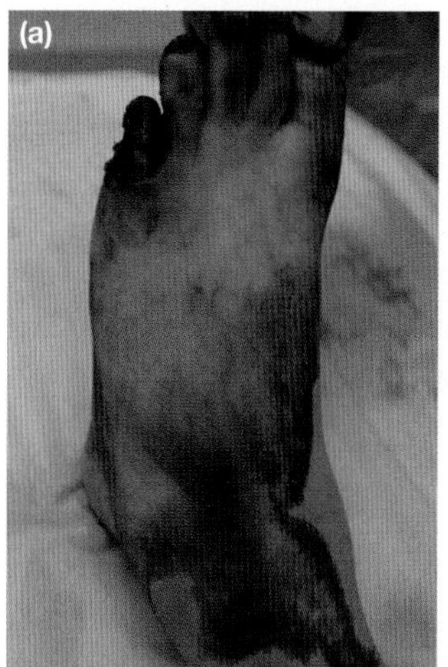

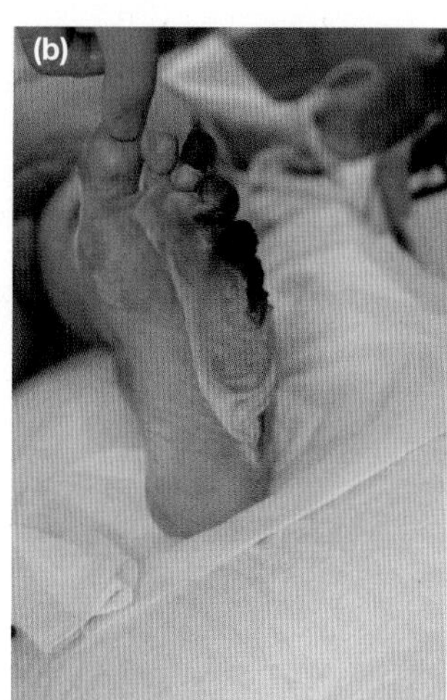

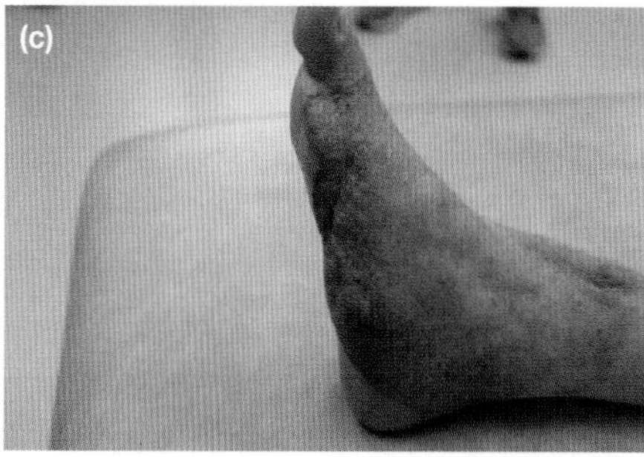

Figure 46.12 (a, b) High-voltage electrical injury resulting in amputation of the lateral three toes and the lateral foot. **(c)** One year post injury after treatment with a dermal substitute (Biodegradable Temporising Matrix [BTM]) and skin grafting.

Low-tension injuries

Low-tension or domestic appliance injuries do not have enough energy to cause destruction to significant amounts of subcutaneous tissues when the current passes through the body. The resistance is too great. The contact point, normally in the fingers, suffers small deep burns; these may cause underlying tendon and nerve damage, but there will be little damage between. The alternating current creates a tetany within the muscles, and thus patients often describe how they were unable to release the device until the power was turned off. The main danger with these injuries is from the alternating current interfering with normal cardiac pacing. This can cause cardiac arrest. The electricity itself does not usually cause significant underlying myocardial damage, so resuscitation, if successful, should be lasting.

High-tension injuries

High-tension electrical injuries (***Figure 46.12***) can be caused by one of three sources of damage: the flash, the flame and the current itself.

When a high-tension line is earthed, enormous energy is released as the current travels from the line to the earth. As the current travels through the air, the air is heated and expands in an explosive manner, which can propel the victim. A flash burn is the contact of superheated air with the skin for a short duration. The flash, however, can go on to ignite the patient's clothes and so cause a normal flame burn.

In accidents with overhead lines, the patient often acts as the conduction rod to earth. In these injuries, there is enough current to cause damage to the subcutaneous tissues and muscles. The entry and exit points are damaged but, importantly, the current can cause huge amounts of subcutaneous damage between these two points. These can be extremely serious injuries.

The damage to the underlying muscles in the affected limb can cause the rapid onset of compartment syndrome requiring urgent fasciotomies. The release of the myoglobin will cause myoglobinuria and subsequent renal dysfunction. Therefore, during the resuscitation of these patients, efforts must be made to maintain a high urine output of up to 2 mL/kg body weight per hour. Severe acidosis is common in large electrical burns and may require fluid and bicarbonate boluses. These patients are also at risk of myocardial damage as a result of direct muscle damage, rather than by interference with cardiac pacing. This gives rise to significant electrocardiogram changes, with raised cardiac enzymes. If there is significant damage, there is rapid onset of heart failure. In the case of a severe injury through a limb, primary amputation is sometimes the most effective management.

Chemical injuries

There are over 70 000 different chemicals in regular use within industry. Occasionally, these cause burns. Ultimately, there are two aspects to a chemical injury. The first is the physical destruction of the skin and the second is any poisoning caused by systemic absorption.

The initial management of chemical burns is to ascertain whether it is in a solid powder or liquid state. Water irrigation should not be used for solid powders as this will result in further reaction, these substances require removal with forceps. Examples include phosphorous, a component of military devices and elemental sodium, which is occasionally present in laboratory explosions. It is rare that a medical practitioner will encounter these burns. The more common injuries are caused by either acids or alkalis. Alkalis are usually the more destructive and are especially dangerous if they have come into contact with the eyes. After copious lavage, the next step in the management of any chemical injury is to identify the chemical and its concentration and to elucidate whether there is any underlying threat to the patient's life if absorbed systemically.

Summary box 46.20

Chemical burns

- Damage is from corrosion and poisoning
- Copious lavage with water helps in most cases
- Then identify the chemical and assess the risks of absorption

One acid that is a common cause of acid burns is hydrofluoric acid, although generally a weak acid, it chelates calcium and magnesium in tissues. Burns affecting the fingers and caused by dilute acid are relatively common. The initial management is with calcium gluconate gel topically; however, severe burns or burns to large areas of the hand can be subsequently treated with Bier's blocks containing calcium gluconate 10% gel. If the patient has been burnt with a concentration greater than 50%, the threat of hypocalcaemia and subsequent arrhythmias then becomes high, and this is an indication for acute early excision. It is best not to split-skin graft these hydrofluoric acid wounds initially, but to do this at a delayed stage.

Ionising radiation injury

These injuries can be divided into groups depending on whether radiation exposure was to the whole body or localised. The management of localised radiation damage is usually conservative until the true extent of the tissue injury is apparent. Should this damage have caused an ulcer, then excision and coverage with vascularised tissue is required.

Whole-body radiation causes a large number of symptoms and may be fatal. A patient who has suffered whole-body irradiation and has acute desquamation of the skin has received a lethal dose of radiation, which can cause a particularly slow and unpleasant death. Non-lethal radiation has a number of systemic effects related to the gut mucosa and immune system dysfunction. Other than giving iodine tablets, the management of these injuries is supportive.

Summary box 46.21

Radiation burns

- Local burns causing ulceration need excision and vascularised flap cover, usually with free flaps
- Systemic overdose needs supportive treatment

Cold injuries

Cold injuries are principally divided into two types: acute cold injuries from industrial accidents and frostbite.

Exposure to liquid petroleum gas (LPG), liquid nitrogen and other such liquids will cause epidermal and dermal destruction. The tissue is more resistant to cold injury than to heat injury, and the inflammatory reaction is not as marked. The assessment of depth of injury is more difficult, so it is rare to make the decision for surgery early.

Frostbite injuries affect the peripheries in cold climates. The initial treatment is with rapid rewarming in a bath at 42°C. The cold injury produces delayed microvascular damage similar to that of ischaemia–reperfusion injury. The level of damage is difficult to assess, and surgery usually does not play a role in its management, which is conservative, until there is absolute demarcation of the level of injury.

RECENT ADVANCES

Advanced technology, newer drugs and skin substitutes are the major advances in burn care. The next steps will focus on cultured autologous skin incorporating the patient's own keratinocytes and fibroblasts. An intelligent use of these modalities is essential to make an effective case for cost–benefit ratios.

FURTHER READING

Australian and New Zealand Burn Association. *Emergency management of severe burns (EMSB) Course manual*, 19th edn, pre-course reading. Australian and New Zealand Burn Association, 2021.

Herndon D (ed.). *Total burn care*, 5th edn. Philadelphia, PA: Saunders and Elsevier, 2017.

August Karl Gustav Bier, 1861–1949, Professor of Surgery, Berlin, Germany.

CHAPTER 47 Plastic and reconstructive surgery

Learning objectives

To be aware of:
- A variety of plastic surgical techniques used to restore bodily form and function

To know:
- The relevant anatomy and physiology of skin

To understand:
- The different types of skin grafts
- The principles and use of flaps
- The concept of microsurgical reconstructive surgery

WHAT IS RECONSTRUCTIVE PLASTIC SURGERY?

Reconstructive plastic surgery is a surgical specialty that aims to restore form and function. The word *plastic* derives from the ancient Greek *plassein* – to mould or shape. Unlike all other specialties, plastic surgery is not bound by anatomical or functional region. Instead, it involves the use of a wide array of surgical techniques to reconstruct tissues that have been damaged by congenital loss, infection, trauma, cancer or even the process of ageing. Hence the reconstructive plastic surgeon often works in collaboration with other specialists wherever necessary, including head and neck surgeons, oral surgeons, orthopaedic surgeons, ophthalmologists, urologists, paediatric surgeons, gynaecologists, general surgeons and dermatologists. Modern plastic surgery techniques enable clinicians to perform complex surgical procedures that would not have been previously possible, such as major oncological head and neck resections or skeletal fixation of open limb fractures with significant soft-tissue defects.

Since plastic surgery involves the restoration of form, it is necessarily closely related to aesthetic (or cosmetic) surgery, which has gained much attention in the media in recent decades. Many of the surgical techniques, including liposuction, fat grafting, scar management, tissue expansion and flap contouring, are shared between the two specialties. However, plastic surgery also aims to achieve restoration of function. An example would be the use of a free neurotised gracilis muscle transfer from the thigh to the face to restore a smile in facial palsy, or the use of a jejunal free flap to restore swallowing following a pharyngolaryngectomy for squamous cell carcinoma. Indeed, the microsurgical techniques developed to enable tissue transplantation within the same individual and the replantation of severed body parts (i.e. autografts) have, together with the discovery of immunosuppressive agents, heralded the field of composite tissue allotransplantation in the latter half of the twentieth century – including face, hand and abdominal wall transplants (i.e. homografts).

HISTORY

Although the evolution of plastic surgery as a surgical specialty is comparatively recent, with the 'masters' of the First World War years, including Sir Harold Gillies, a New Zealand otolaryngologist working in London, considered to be the founding fathers, its origins hark back to ancient times and were driven by the need to treat burns, congenital deformity and acquired injuries (whether judicial, vindictive or sustained in battle). The 'pre-scientific period' included a description by the pioneering Indian surgeon Sushruta in 600 BCE of numerous facial flaps (including a method to repair the split earlobe), which predated the forehead flap being used for nasal reconstruction by some 400 years. Anatomical understanding improved markedly from the mid-fifteenth century – the 'scientific period' – as human dissection became widely practised and the development of printing allowed anatomical drawings to be reproduced and disseminated. During this period the 'Italian rhinoplasty', which utilised a two-stage brachial flap technique, was popularised by Tagliacozzi. The 'modern period' – from the nineteenth century to the present day – witnessed a detailed appreciation of the anatomy of the cutaneous circulation, although the significance of the early research undertaken by Manchot took almost a century to be fully recognised, such that the random-pattern 'waltzed' tubed

Sir Harold Delf Gillies, 1882–1960, the 'father of plastic surgery', became the first President of the British Association of Plastic Surgeons in 1946.
Sushruta, *c.* 600 BCE, Indian surgeon; his eponymous Samhitá ('compendium') was translated into English in 1907.
Gaspare Tagliacozzi, 1545–1599, Professor of Surgery, University of Bologna, Bologna, Italy.
Carl Herman Manchot, 1866–1932, was born in Switzerland and studied medicine at the University of Strasbourg, Strasbourg, France.

pedicle flap was superseded by axial pattern flaps, including the musculocutaneous latissimus dorsi flap by Tansini (1896). This era of surgical discovery was greatly facilitated by the advent of antisepsis by Semmelweis (1847) and Lister (1883), the discovery of anaesthesia by Morton (1846), antibiotics by Fleming (1928) and immunosuppression by Hench (1949) and Calne (1962).

The past 50 years have seen an explosion in the complexity of microsurgical reconstructive techniques, culminating in vascularised composite tissue transplantation becoming part of routine clinical practice. A timeline of some of the key advances in the history of plastic surgical innovation is given in *Table 47.1*.

SURGICAL ANATOMY OF THE SKIN

Skin is the largest end organ, covering the body's entire external surface. Together with its derivatives, including hair, nails and sweat glands, it forms the integumentary system. The skin serves a number of functions that are critical for survival. It provides a protective barrier against mechanical, thermal and irradiation (ultraviolet) injury and infection. It also plays a role in homeostasis by preventing fluid loss and regulating temperature. As the primary interface with the external environment, it acts as a sensory organ and also produces vitamin D. Hence restoration of the skin is essential even if the underlying structures await delayed reconstruction.

TABLE 47.1 A selection of key advances in the history of plastic surgery innovation.

Year	Surgeon	Nationality	Innovation
c. 1800 BCE	–	Ancient Egypt	Wound care techniques
c. 600 BCE	Sushruta	India	Local flaps for nasal reconstruction
c. 25 CE	Celsus	Rome	Local flaps for lip reconstruction
c. 1000 CE	Al-Zahrawi	Spain	Introduced catgut sutures and developed numerous surgical instruments
c. 1400 CE	Branca	Sicily	Distant (arm) flap for nasal reconstruction
1789	Desault	France	Recognition of the importance of definitive wound debridement
1854	Hamilton	USA	Concept of flap 'delay' with the distant cross-leg flap
1862	Wood	UK	Concept of axial pattern flaps with the pedicled groin flap (*Figure 47.1*)
1889	Manchot	Germany	Cutaneous arterial supply using cadaveric arterial injection studies
1894	Dauriac	France	First description of a pedicled muscle (rectus abdominis) flap
1896	Tansini	Italy	Breast reconstruction using a pedicled musculocutaneous latissimus dorsi flap
1912	Carrel	France	Nobel Prize for the development of vascular anastomosis and its application to organ transplantation
1916–1917	Filatov and Gillies	Russian Empire and UK	Tubed pedicled flaps and concept of 'waltzing'
1954	Murray	USA	Nobel Prize for the first renal transplant between identical twins
1968	Cobbett	UK	Free toe-to-hand transfer
1973	Daniel and Taylor	Australia	Free groin flap to foot
1978	Taylor	Australia	Concept of the 'angiosome'
1979	Yang	China	Free radial forearm ('Chinese') flap
1989	Koshima	Japan	Perforator flaps (*Figure 47.2*)
1998	Dubernard	France	Hand transplant
2004	Chen	Taiwan	Vascularised lymph node transfer
2005	Devauchelle	France	Partial face transplant
2006	Barret	Spain	Full face transplant

Iginio Tansini, 1855–1943, Professor of Surgery, University of Pavia, Pavia, Italy.
Ignaz Philipp Semmelweis, 1818–1865, Professor of Obstetrics, University of Pest, Pest, Hungary.
Joseph Lister, Baron Lister of Lyme Regis, 1827–1912, Professor of Surgery, University of Glasgow, Glasgow, UK.
William Thomas Green Morton, 1819–1868, an American dentist.
Sir Alexander Fleming, 1881–1955, a Scottish microbiologist who discovered penicillin at St Mary's Hospital, London, UK, for which he was jointly awarded the Nobel Prize in 1945.
Philip Showalter Hench, 1986–1965, Professor of Medicine, Mayo Clinic, Rochester, USA, was jointly awarded the Nobel Prize in 1950 for his pioneering work on cortisone.
Sir Roy Yorke Calne, b. 1930, Emeritus Professor of Surgery, University of Cambridge, Cambridge, UK.

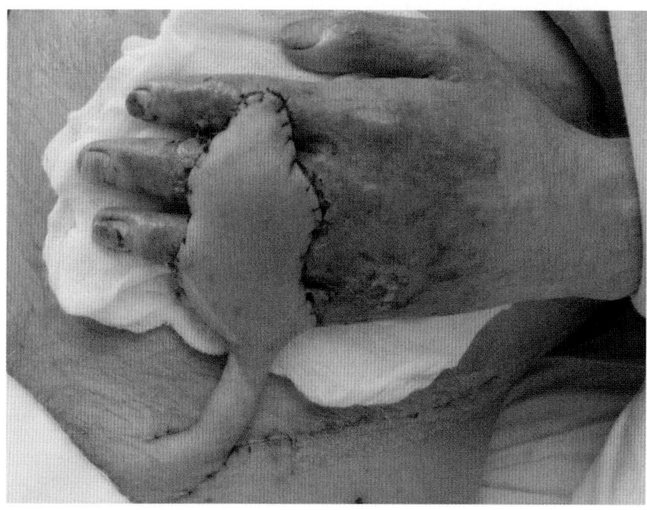

Figure 47.1 Pedicled groin flap. Full-thickness burn wounds over the dorsum of multiple digits. The exposed extensor tendons were covered by a pedicled groin flap. The pedicle was divided at 3 weeks and the digits were subsequently separated in stages.

The skin's structure consists of the outer epidermis (ectodermal in origin), the dermis and the inner hypodermis (of mesodermal origin). The deepest layer of the epidermis is the *stratum basale,* where stem cells differentiate into keratinocytes and migrate upwards towards the outermost *stratum corneum,* an acellular layer made of dead keratinocytes acting as a barrier to fluid loss and protection against invasion by microorganisms. The epidermis regenerates from deeper follicular elements such as hair follicles and sweat glands.

The dermis is connected to the epidermis via the basement membrane and consists of the upper papillary layer, composed of loose connective tissue, and a deeper reticular layer, which is thicker and consists of dense connective tissue and collagen fibres. The dermis houses the hair follicles, sweat glands, sensory receptors and blood vessels.

The hypodermis contains the subcutaneous fat as well as skin appendages, including hair follicles, sensory receptors, neurones and blood vessels.

The relative composition of these layers varies depending on the functional requirements of the region concerned. Specialised areas such as hair-bearing scalp skin or glabrous heel skin can be challenging to reconstruct as there are limited donor sites. However, for non-specialised skin, the abdomen and groin make ideal donor sites as they are elastic and thin and, thus, amenable to primary closure.

Blood vessels are found in the dermis and hypodermis and are arranged in a number of plexuses between each anatomical layer (***Figure 47.3***). Ultimately, they all originate from a main feeding or source vessel, via fine perforating vessels ('perforators') either directly or indirectly by traversing through fascia, muscle or bone. This observation gave rise to Taylor's 'angiosome' concept, in which angiosomes refer to three-dimensional blocks of tissue including skin and deeper tissue layers that are supplied by specific source arteries. Thus, any skin or other tissue types can be detached as a 'flap' provided the vessel course from the source vessel to the end organ that is to be transferred is kept intact.

Cutaneous nerves tend to run axially out of the major nerve trunks but are less defined than most perforating blood vessels. It is possible to coapt nerve ends between a cutaneous nerve within a flap and one at the recipient site, so-called 'neurotisation', to regain some sensation in the flap.

WOUND HEALING

There are various ways in which a wound can heal (see ***Chapter 3***). Plastic surgeons can affect the way in which wounds heal. Primary healing, or 'healing by primary intention', occurs when the wound is closed soon after the injury by reapproximating the wound edges. This is typically achieved with sutures, although glue, tape and staples can also be used. Incisions are designed so that they lie along the lines of relaxed

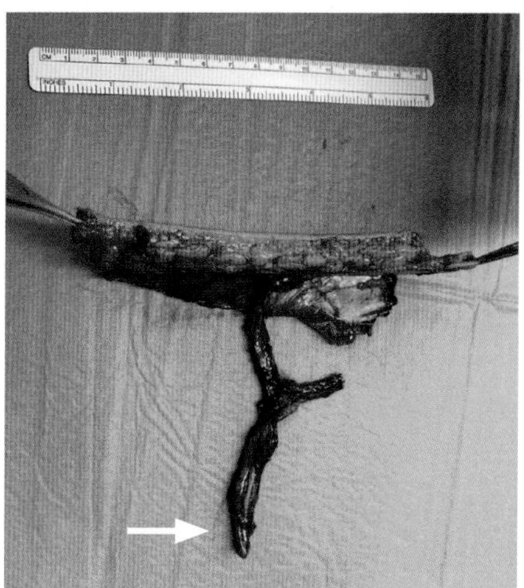

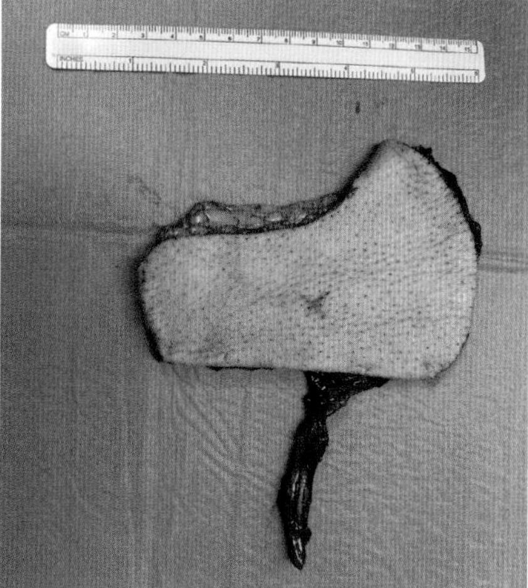

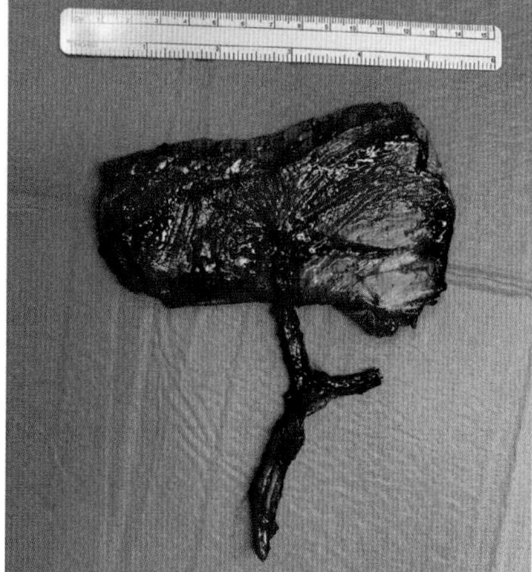

Figure 47.2 Three views of an anterolateral thigh flap on detachment from the donor site prior to anastomosis at the recipient site. Pedicle (arrow) consisting of one perforator artery and two vena comitans.

Geoffrey Ian Taylor, contemporary, Professor of Plastic Surgery, University of Melbourne, Melbourne, Australia.

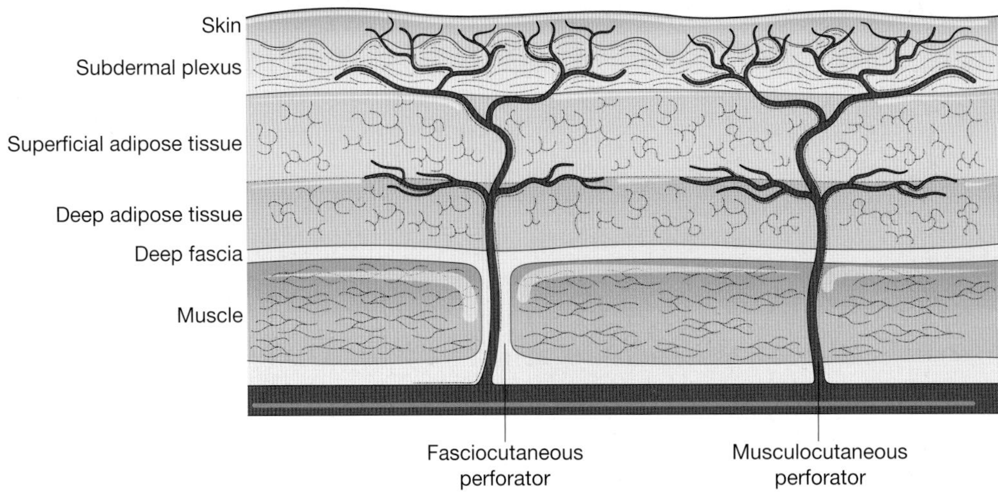

Figure 47.3 Diagram of skin anatomy with vascular plexus.

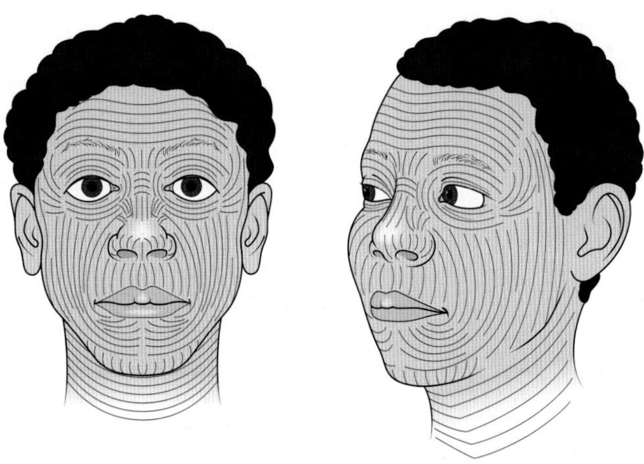

Figure 47.4 Lines of relaxed skin tension.

skin tension to reduce the appearance of the scar, particularly on the face and in areas of tension (***Figure 47.4***). Secondary healing, or 'healing by secondary intention', occurs when the wound is left to heal from its base. The wound is typically kept clean with sterile non-adherent dressings. Over the course of days and weeks, the wound contracts and skin cells migrate across the wound through a process called epithelialisation. Secondary healing is typically employed for wounds that have poor healing potential, such as leg and pressure ulcers, in which surgery risks exacerbating the wound-healing burden.

Every reconstructive procedure depends on the potential for wound healing. Furthermore, much of reconstructive plastic surgery involves the creation of wounds to heal other wounds – hence the aphorism 'rob Peter to pay Paul'. Therefore, the plastic surgeon must consider how to maximise the chances of success and adopt their approach accordingly. For example, in genetic conditions such as Ehlers–Danlos syndrome and epidermolysis bullosa (for which there is currently no cure), the surgeon is required to be less aggressive in their approach as surgical intervention risks creating additional iatrogenic wounds that may fail to optimally heal, thus potentially worsening the patient's situation (Hippocrates: *primum non nocere*; first, do no harm). Systemic comorbidities including diabetes, peripheral vascular disease, renal failure, corticosteroid use and immunodeficiency are significant causes of delayed wound healing and must be addressed preoperatively. For example, diabetic control may be optimised with the help of an endocrinologist, and preoperative angioplasty may augment blood flow in a chronically ischaemic lower limb. Nutrition is essential for wound healing; vitamin and protein deficiencies should be addressed preoperatively with the guidance of a dietician. Smoking is particularly detrimental as it causes vasoconstriction and decreases local oxygen delivery to tissues, thus impairing healing; patients are therefore advised to cease smoking at least 6 weeks prior to elective surgery if possible.

Furthermore, it is crucial to optimise a wound bed to promote healing. For example, the wound may require formal debridement and washout to minimise bacterial colonisation and hence the risk of surgical site infection. Perioperative antibiotics may also be necessary.

ABERRANT HEALING

Scarring can be aberrant owing to a combination of genetic predisposition and environmental factors. The two main types of abnormal scarring are hypertrophic and keloid scars.

Hypertrophic scars are elevated within the borders of the original scar and affect up to 15% of wounds. They tend to occur soon after injury, subsiding over time, and arise in areas of tension, particularly flexor surfaces. They may be successfully

Edward Ehlers, 1863–1937, Professor of Clinical Dermatology, Copenhagen, Denmark.
Henri Alexandre Danlos, 1844–1912, dermatologist, Hôpital St Louis, Paris, France, gave his account of this condition in 1908.
Hippocrates of Kos, *c*. 460–375 BCE, was a physician in Ancient Greece and considered to be the 'father of medicine'.

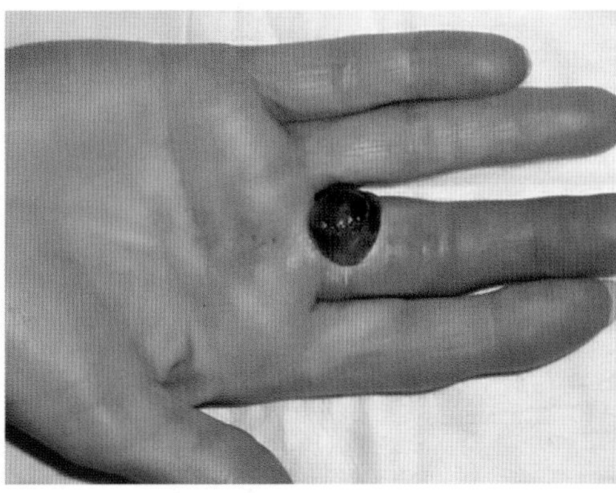

Figure 47.5 Pyogenic granuloma following a glass laceration to the base of the right middle finger.

treated with topical silicone, intralesional corticosteroid injection, compression therapy or surgical excision.

Keloid scars, by contrast, extend beyond the original wound borders and can be locally destructive; in extreme cases, they are debilitating. They occur more commonly in darker skin types and may arise some months after the injury, most commonly affecting the face, earlobes, deltoid area and presternal region. They are more resistant to treatment and may require repeated excision with adjuvant radiotherapy.

Scars may also be widened, thin and depressed owing to excess tension across the wound. Scars may also be unstable and prone to recurrent ulceration and breakdown; this is most frequently seen at mobile sites (such as overlying major joints or the neck) when healing has been achieved secondarily. These scars can be excised (serially if necessary) or resurfaced with a flap in order to provide more robust coverage.

Wounds that fail to heal properly may become populated with unstable and highly vascular granulation tissue ('over-granulated') that is fragile and prone to intermittent bleeding. These may be treated with topical silver nitrate or corticosteroid or may require formal excision and reconstruction.

A traumatic wound can lead to the development of a pyogenic granuloma. This is a benign proliferation of capillary blood vessels of the skin and presents as a painless red fleshy nodule that grows rapidly over several weeks and bleeds intermittently (***Figure 47.5***). It may be treated topically as per over-granulation tissue but frequently requires surgical excision.

In chronic wounds, such as in pressure sores, burns or osteomyelitis, the chronicity of the inflammatory environment can lead to the development of a Marjolin ulcer. This is a rare but aggressive form of squamous cell carcinoma that has a high propensity for distant metastasis. A low index of suspicion must be observed in chronic wounds that undergo sudden phenotypic change, so early biopsy is advocated.

WOUND DRESSINGS

These are a vital part of wound care and are used to optimise healing. The most suitable dressing is selected based on the type of wound being treated. The 'ideal dressing' should provide a moist environment to facilitate epidermal migration, enable gas exchange between the wound and environment, provide protection against bacterial infection and be non-adherent (to avoid trauma on removal). Furthermore, the dressing should be sterile, non-toxic, non-allergenic and readily available at minimal expense.

One of the most traditional dressings in regular use is gauze (tulle) impregnated with petroleum jelly (e.g. Jelonet®); it is ideal for clean wounds with minimal exudate. Semipermeable foam dressings (e.g. Allevyn®) are suitable for moderately to highly exudating wounds such as leg ulcers. Hydrocolloid dressings (e.g. Duoderm®) contain an inner colloidal layer with an impermeable outer layer and are ideal for moderately exudating wounds such as minor burns. Alginate dressings (e.g. Kaltostat®) are derived from seaweed and contain calcium salts that facilitate haemostasis; they can be used on moderate to heavily exudating wounds such as split-thickness skin graft donor sites. Mepitel® is a non-adherent dressing comprising a perforated silicone sheet that is designed for prolonged applications of up to 2 weeks; it is therefore popular in paediatric wounds. Some dressings contain antimicrobial agents such as ionic silver (e.g. Aquacel Ag®) or povidone iodine (e.g. Inadine®) that may have additional functionality in contaminated wounds.

Negative-pressure wound therapy (e.g. vacuum-assisted closure; VAC®) uses intermittent or continuous topical negative pressure (up to −125 mmHg) through a sealed foam dressing in order to stimulate the formation of granulation tissue, reduce local oedema and tissue exudate and reduce bacterial load. The technique has numerous applications, including as a dressing to secure a skin graft to its recipient bed, temporary coverage of a complex acute wound (e.g. an open abdomen; ***Figure 47.6***) until definitive cover can be achieved or to manage chronic wounds such as pressure ulcers.

RECONSTRUCTIVE TECHNIQUES

These range from the simple, including healing by secondary intention or skin grafting, to the complex, including free tissue transfer or vascularised composite allotransplantation. They also include the use of autologous tissue, allograft material, biocompatible materials such as skin substitutes, internal and external fixators and tissue expanders. Improved understanding of the blood supply to different tissue types including skin has vastly expanded the number of flap options (see below) available to reconstruct different parts of the body. The introduction of the operating microscope has ushered in the era of microsurgical reconstruction that has enabled free tissue transfer and replantation, procedures whereby the blood supply to a flap is detached from the donor site and re-established through vessel anastomosis to local source vessels at the recipient site.

Reconstructive plastic surgery is almost always undertaken to improve healing. Without it, wounds may heal poorly with unacceptable consequences, including chronic or non-healing wounds, unsightly and debilitating scars or the risk of deep infection. A common scenario is a skin defect that is too large

Jean-Nicolas Marjolin, 1780–1850, Professor of External Pathology, Hôtel-Dieu de Paris, Paris, France.

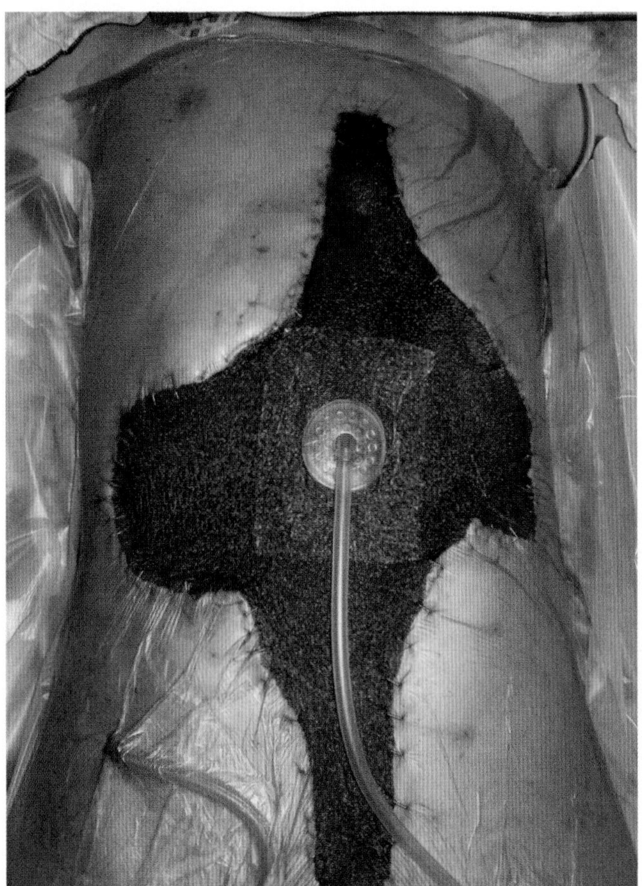

Figure 47.6 Negative-pressure wound therapy to promote wound healing in an open abdomen. The system consists of a non-adherent dressing overlaid by a sponge that is sealed with an airtight membrane and connected to a suction device.

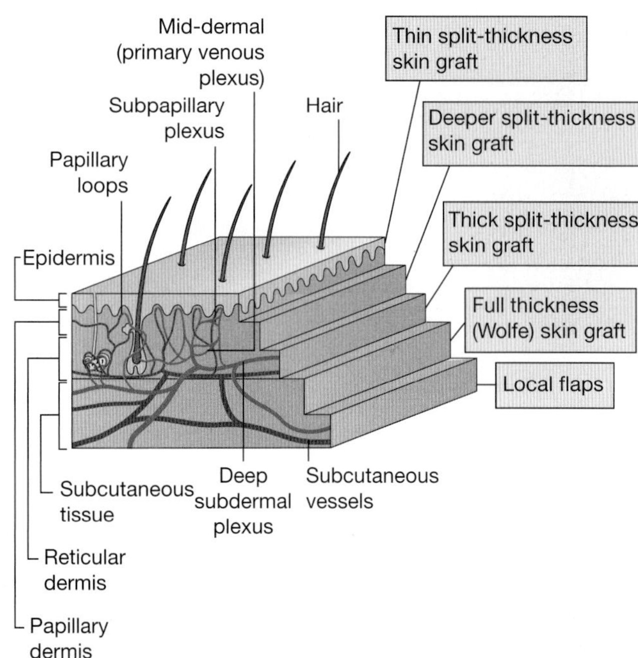

Figure 47.7 Schematic anatomy of the skin and its relationship to harvesting skin grafts (of varying thicknesses) and raising local flaps.

to be closed primarily, thus requiring surgical techniques or adjuncts to achieve wound closure. Several conceptual frameworks exist for the appropriate selection of techniques, including the now obsolete reconstructive ladder which advocates using the simplest methods first, and the patient-centred 'reconstructive elevator'. In essence, the modern patient-centred reconstructive technique employed must be considered in the context of each individual case, including patient factors, available skills, resources and the consequences of success and failure to achieve the best long-term outcome.

In acute burns, for example, split-thickness skin grafting is almost always used to restore skin as soon as possible in order to preserve life. Following facial tumour excision, a local flap is often superior to a skin graft in terms of contour and aesthetics such as skin quality and colour match. For pressure sore reconstruction, a local flap comprising both skin and muscle (for dead-space obliteration) would be more durable than a skin graft or primary closure, both of which would place the scar at the site of greatest pressure. For open lower limb fractures, free tissue transfer is often required as there is a lack of local tissue availability; this option provides healthy vascularised tissues to cover the fracture site (including any orthopaedic metalwork), thus significantly reducing the risk of limb-threatening deep infection or osteomyelitis.

Grafts

Grafts are tissues that are transferred without their blood supply and therefore need to be revascularised through the recipient wound bed. To maximise the success of this procedure, the wound bed must be healthy with a good blood supply such that angiogenesis into the graft tissue can occur. Graft failure occurs most commonly as a result of shear forces disrupting the graft from the wound bed, infection (particularly with group A β-haemolytic *Streptococcus* spp.) and haematoma or seroma formation (which can lift the graft away from the underlying wound bed).

Skin grafts are used to achieve wound closure in situations where the skin defects are too large for primary closure and healing by secondary intention may be inappropriate or lead to an unreasonable delay in complete healing. There are two types of skin grafts, depending on the depth at which they are taken (***Figure 47.7***):

- **Split-thickness skin grafts** consist of epidermis and a variable amount of dermis and are sometimes referred to as Thiersch grafts. They are commonly harvested from the thigh using a dermatome or graft knife to achieve a consistent depth (***Figure 47.8***). It is relatively simple to harvest large areas of skin to reconstruct sizeable defects such as those following a significant burn injury (see ***Chapter 46***). The grafted skin can then be meshed or fenestrated to

Karl Thiersch, 1822–1895, Professor of Surgery, Leipzig University, Leipzig, Germany.

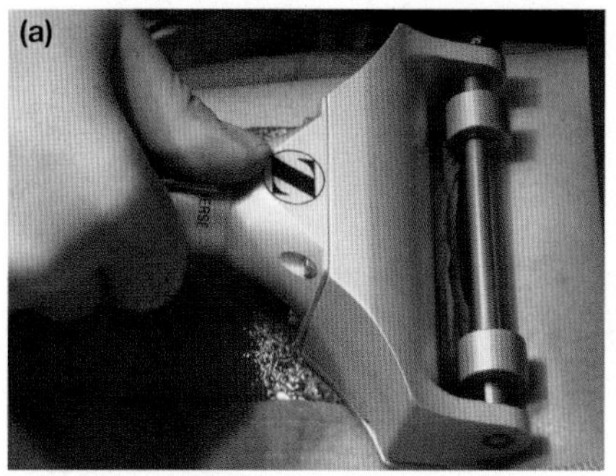
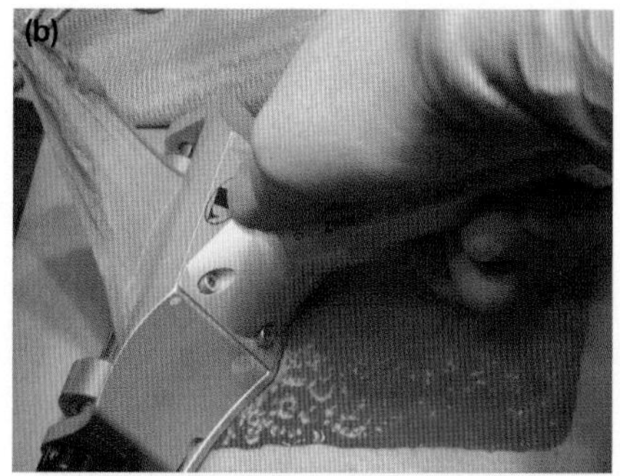
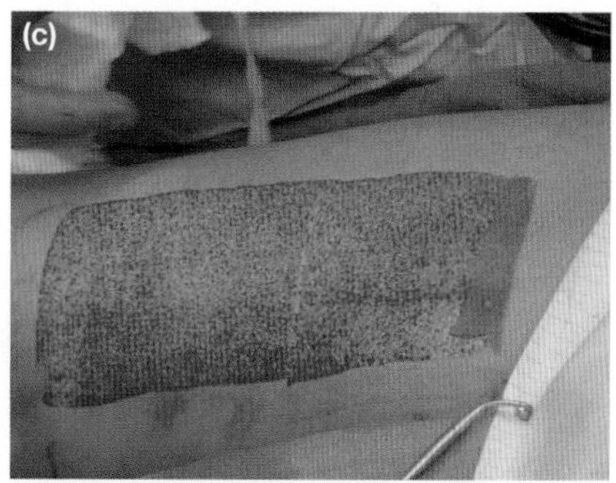
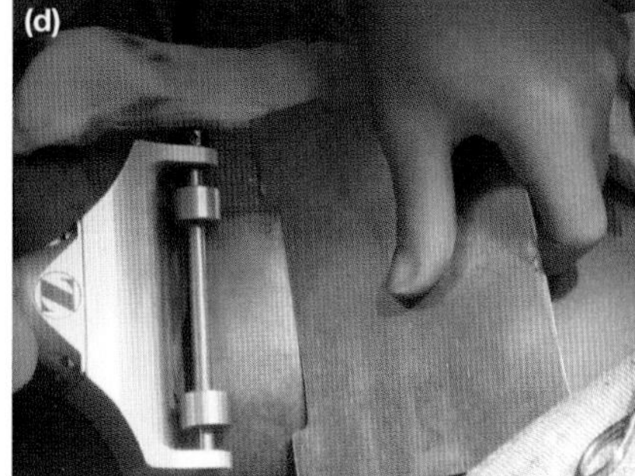
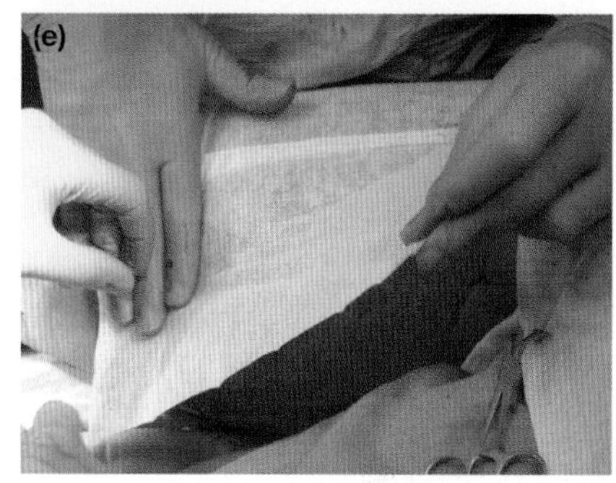

Figure 47.8 Power dermatome harvest of a split-thickness skin graft, with the correct method of providing skin tension **(a–d)** and applying a sterile dressing **(e)**.

expand and cover a wider surface area as well as avoid the accumulation of an underlying haematoma. The graft is typically sutured, glued or stapled to the recipient site. However, grafts are not entirely robust, for example they can shear off, and may contract significantly over time. The donor area usually heals by secondary intention within 2 weeks by means of simple dressings (***Figure 47.9***).

- **Full-thickness skin grafts** consist of epidermis and dermis. As they include the entire thickness of the dermis, they retain their elasticity and are less prone to secondary scar contracture. However, this also means that the area harvested is limited by the ability to primarily close the donor site. The common sites for harvest include the supraclavicular skin, groin crease and posterior auricular region (known as a Wolfe graft), where there is adequate skin laxity. Full-thickness grafts are commonly used for syndactyly release in the hand, reconstruction of facial defects following skin cancer excision or contracture releases following burns (***Figure 47.10***).
- **Composite skin grafts** are a combination of skin and another tissue type, such as fat or cartilage. A commonly used composite skin graft is to harvest a skin/cartilage graft from the helical root of the ear to reconstruct the alar of the nose following skin cancer excision. A hair-bearing composite scalp graft can be used to reconstruct an eyebrow.

Nerve grafts are used to reconstruct peripheral nerves (including the brachial plexus) and in the surgical management of facial palsy (by utilising a cross-facial nerve graft) and corneal paraesthesia. Common donor nerves include the sural nerve, medial antebrachial cutaneous nerve and the sensory branch of the posterior interosseous nerve (ideal for digital nerve grafts). Whereas vessels are 'anastomosed', nerves are 'coapted' – typically using epineurial sutures with or without fibrin glue in a tension-free manner.

Tendon grafts are utilised for the reconstruction of tendons in the upper and lower extremities as a result of trauma, infection (e.g. leprosy) or neurological injury (peripheral nerve or spinal transection). Commonly used donor tendons include palmaris longus, extensor digitorum longus and plantaris.

Autologous cartilage grafts can be used for support and augmentation (such as the cartilaginous framework of a staged reconstruction for microtia, a congenital deformity of the outer ear), to correct contour irregularities (such as the nasal dorsum) or to repair or resurface damaged joints (such as the temporomandibular joint or small joints of the hand).

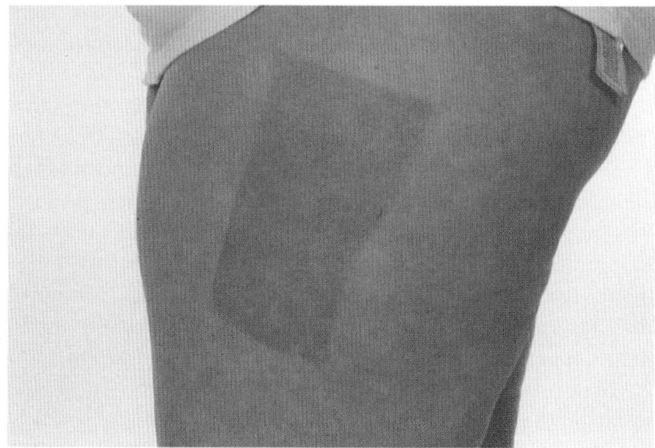

Figure 47.9 Typical appearance of a split-thickness skin graft donor site on the left lateral thigh 6 months after harvest. The mild hyperpigmentation is expected to fade over time.

John Reissberg Wolfe, 1824–1904, Professor of Ophthalmology, University of Glasgow, UK.

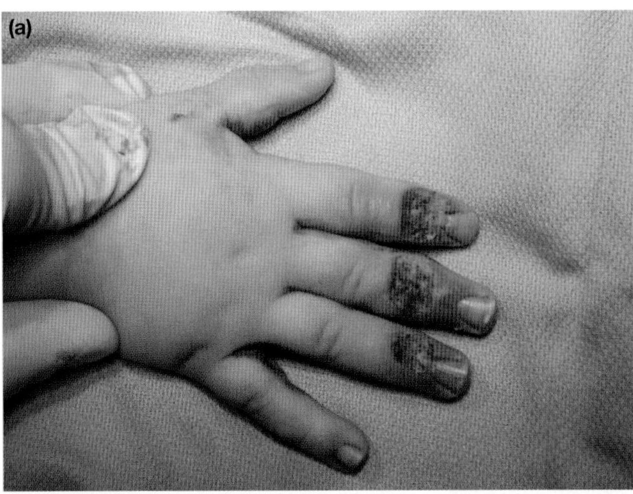
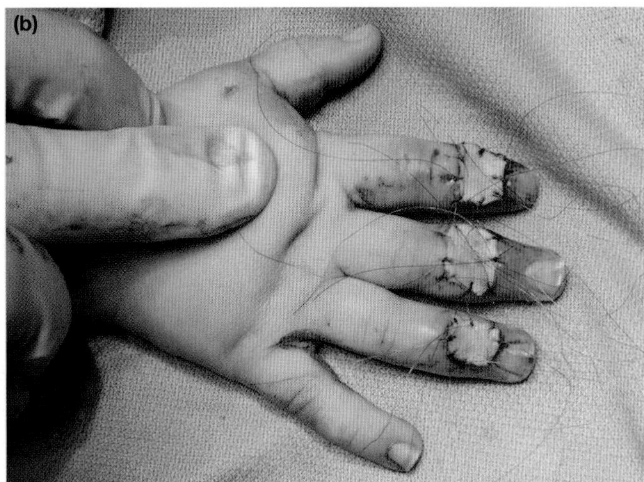
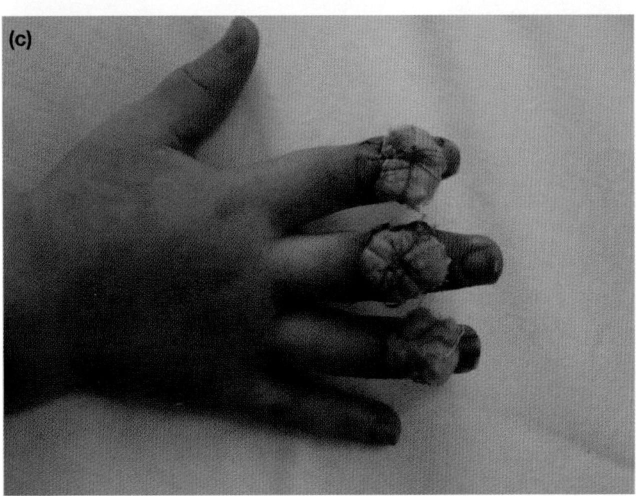
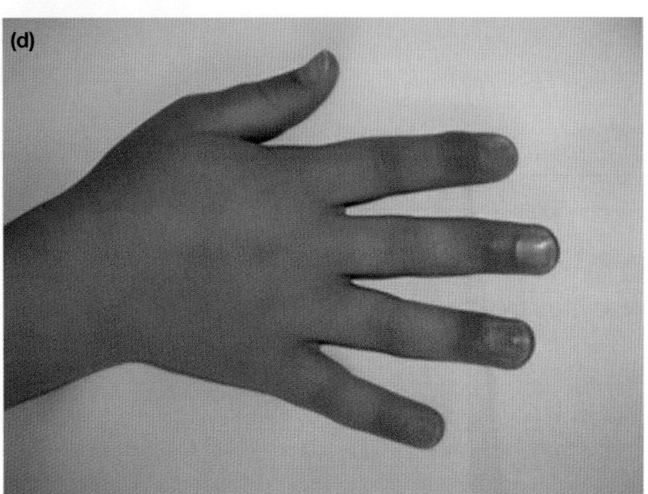

Figure 47.10 Full-thickness skin graft reconstruction of a contact burn to the dorsum of the digits. **(a)** Post excision of burn wounds. **(b)** Full-thickness skin grafts from the groin sutured to the wounds. **(c)** Tie-over dressings applied to avoid shearing of the graft off the wound bed. **(d)** Postoperative appearance at 1 year.

Common donor sites include the conchal bowl of the ear (elastic cartilage), the nasal septum (which provides rigid hyaline cartilage) and costal cartilage (a plentiful source of hyaline cartilage).

Whereas autograft (i.e. graft harvested from the same individual) is considered the 'gold standard' for most elective surgical indications, there are certain circumstances when allografting (i.e. from another individual of the same species) or xenografting (i.e. from another species) might be necessary to minimise donor site morbidity or because of a lack of donor tissue. For example, cadaveric allograft or porcine xenograft may be used as a temporising 'dressing' following the initial debridement of an extensive burn or necrotising fasciitis.

Skin substitutes are engineered dressings that are designed to facilitate wound healing by replicating as many of the key functions as possible. They can either replace the epidermal or dermal components (or both) and can have either a cellular or acellular dermal matrix. Dermal substitutes include Alloderm® (human dermal matrix) or Integra® (bovine collagen with chondroitin and a silastic membrane) whereas Epicel® is an example of an epidermal substitute derived from autologous keratinocytes. Apligraf® is a double-layered bioengineered skin substitute derived from human fibroblasts and keratinocytes and is licensed for the treatment of diabetic and venous ulcers. Their advantage is one of ready availability (in large quantities if required) without the creation of a donor site defect; however, they are expensive and must be employed using a meticulous surgical technique to avoid failure.

Tissue expansion is the creation of extra skin and soft tissue by using a subcutaneous silicone balloon in order to reconstruct locoregional defects. The tissue expander is placed within a subcutaneous pocket and then inflated with saline solution at regular (e.g. weekly) intervals via a filling port (which can be buried or externalised). The overlying skin and soft tissue have viscoelastic properties; in response to the underlying mechanical force, they permanently elongate through the processes of 'creep' and stress relaxation. Angiogenesis leads to increased vascularity within the expanded skin flap and the local response to a 'foreign body' creates a fibrous capsule. Thus large flaps can be created that have similar physical and mechanical properties to the skin that is to be replaced. Common indications include scalp reconstruction following skin cancer excision

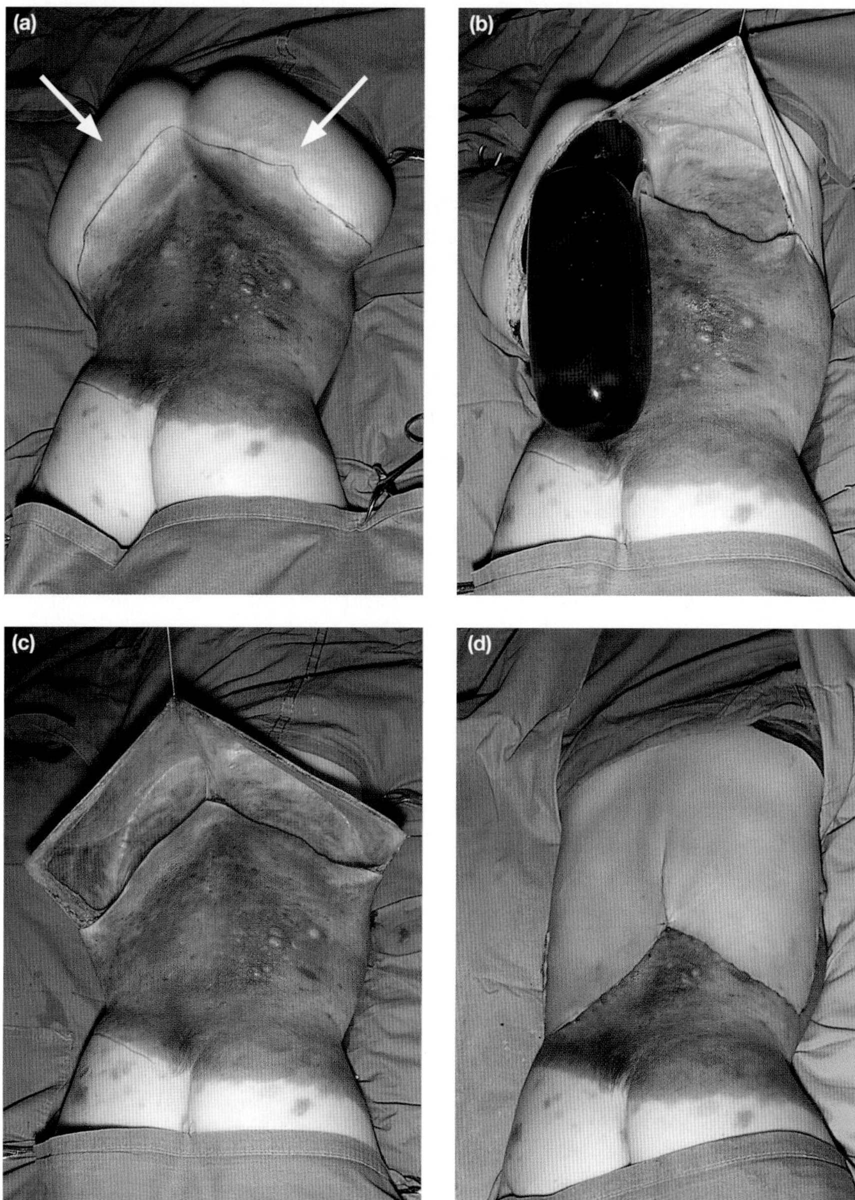

Figure 47.11 Tissue expansion provides local autologous tissue for reconstruction of large defects. **(a)** Extensive congenital melanocytic naevus of the back with tissue expanders *in situ* (arrows). **(b)** Explantation of inflated tissue expanders. **(c)** Advancement of expanded skin flaps to determine the extent of naevus excision. **(d)** Immediate postoperative appearance after partial excision of the naevus and skin flap closure. The flaps were subsequently re-expanded to facilitate excision of the residual naevus.

(ideal for reconstructing hair-bearing skin), breast reconstruction following mastectomy and auricular reconstruction. Occasionally, more than one expander is used to reconstruct complex or large defects, such as giant congenital melanocytic naevi (***Figure 47.11***). Caution must be exercised when considering expansion of irradiated tissue or in patients with comorbidities including diabetes or connective tissue disorders as wound healing is impaired in these scenarios.

Prosthetics are widely used in plastic surgery – ranging from ocular, nasal and auricular to hand prostheses. Alloplastic implants are routinely employed in reconstructive plastic surgery, including titanium plates for cranioplasties (replacing lost calvarial bone), porous polyethylene (Medpor®) onlay implants to augment the facial skeleton (e.g. cheek bones or chin tip) and breast implants. Breast implants comprise an outer shell (typically a silicone elastomer that may be smooth or textured) and a filling material (saline or silicone gel) and come in a variety of shapes (round or anatomical) and a vast array of volumes. Implants are prone to capsular contracture, may interfere with mammographic cancer surveillance and are associated with the development of anaplastic large-cell lymphoma in a small percentage of cases.

Lipotransfer

Lipotransfer, or autologous fat grafting, is a useful reconstructive technique to achieve soft-tissue augmentation, i.e. increase the volume in a specific region, hence it is sometimes referred to as 'lipomodelling'. Common indications include facial defects in progressive hemifacial atrophy (Parry–Romberg syndrome)

Caleb Hillier Parry, 1755–1822, physician, Bath General Hospital, Bath, UK.
Moritz Heinrich Romberg, 1795–1873, German neurologist, Director of the University Hospital, Berlin, Germany.

and breast reconstruction, although the greatest demand comes from the aesthetic industry for facial rejuvenation and buttock/breast augmentation. Lipotransfer is also used to improve scar remodelling, particularly after radiotherapy, the rationale being that adipose tissue contains adipose-derived stromal cells, which can modulate the healing process.

Autologous fat is an ideal filler material for soft-tissue reconstruction as it is biocompatible, non-immunogenic, inexpensive and can be easily and repeatedly harvested. This technique was systematised and popularised by Coleman in the late twentieth century. The stages of lipotransfer include: (i) harvesting or 'liposuction', whereby adipose tissue is suctioned from a body part, usually the abdomen , thigh or buttock, using local anaesthetic and a cannula; (ii) fat preparation, including centrifugation of the fat aspirate; and (iii) injection, using a specialised cannula, at the recipient site. One disadvantage is that the grafted fat undergoes an unpredictable amount of fat resorption (typically approximately 20% but may reach 80%). Current research is focused on how to improve the survival of the grafted fat, including through enrichment with a freshly isolated stromal vascular fraction. Although generally safe, there is a small risk of fat embolism, which can have serious complications (including blindness and stroke) and can be fatal.

Flaps

A flap is a block of tissue that contains an innate blood supply that may be transferred from a donor site to reconstruct a secondary defect; the pedicle is the 'base' of the flap that contains the blood supply. Unlike a graft, a flap can therefore be used to reconstruct a defect that does not have a vascularised wound bed, such as exposed tendon, cortical bone or a prosthesis. There are numerous methods of classifying flaps: according to their blood supply, their proximity to the defect, the method by which they are transferred and the tissue that they contain.

The five Cs methodology is a useful flap classification system based on their circulation, composition, contiguity, contour and conditioning (***Figure 47.12***).

1 **Circulation**: random pattern flaps have no dominant blood supply whereas axial flaps have a dominant feeding vessel.
2 **Composition**: cutaneous, fasciocutaneous, fascial, musculocutaneous, muscle, osseocutaneous, osseous, omentum/bowel.
3 **Contiguity**: local (where the flap shares a side with the defect) (***Figure 47.13***), regional (where the flap is near but not immediately adjacent to the defect) (***Figures 47.14 and 47.15***) and distant (where the flap is far from the defect and can be either pedicled or free) (***Figures 47.16 and 47.17***).
4 **Contour**: the method by which the flap is transferred into the defect – advancement (***Figures 47.18 and 47.19***), transposition (***Figure 47.20***), rotation (***Figure 47.21***), interpolation, waltzing, crane principle and free.
5 **Conditioning**: whether the flap is delayed by partially elevating and resetting the flap prior to definitive elevation and transfer. Delay enables a larger flap to be harvested by improving its blood supply.

Fasciocutaneous flaps comprise a fascial component that augments the flap blood supply owing to a network of subfascial, fascial and suprafascial vessels. Fasciocutaneous flaps may be classified according to Cormack and Lamberty (1984) (***Figure 47.22***):

- Type A: multiple perforators that can be direct or indirect (e.g. Pontén flap).
- Type B: single perforator that is usually direct and runs along the axis of the flap (e.g. the scapular or parascapular flaps).
- Type C: segmental perforators that arise from the same source vessel (e.g. the radial forearm and lateral arm flaps) (***Figure 47.23***).
- Type D: similar to type C; however, the flap is raised as an osteomyofasciocutaneous flap (e.g. the free fibular flap).

In muscle and musculocutaneous flaps the motor nerve is always accompanied by a vascular pedicle, which is often the major source of the flap circulation. A dominant pedicle can sustain an entire muscle whereas a minor pedicle can normally only sustain a portion of the flap. The skin in a musculocutaneous flap is supplied by perforators. Muscle flaps are classified by Mathes and Nahai (1981) (***Figure 47.24***):

- Type I: single vascular pedicle (e.g. tensor fascia lata and gastrocnemius).
- Type II: one dominant pedicle with one or more minor pedicles (e.g. gracilis, biceps femoris, sternocleidomastoid, soleus and trapezius); the flap cannot survive on the minor pedicle(s) alone.
- Type III: dual dominant pedicles (e.g. gluteus maximus, pectoralis minor, rectus abdominis, serratus anterior and temporalis).
- Type IV: segmental pedicles (e.g. flexor hallucis longus, sartorius and tibialis anterior).
- Type V: dominant pedicle with several smaller segmental pedicles (e.g. latissimus dorsi and pectoralis major) (***Figures 47.25 and 47.26***); the flap can survive on the minor pedicles alone.

A chimeric flap consists of multiple otherwise spatially independent flaps, each of which has an independent vascular supply, with all pedicles linked to a common source vessel. For example, the descending branch of the lateral femoral

Sydney Reese Coleman, contemporary, plastic surgeon, New York, NY, USA.
George Carl Cormack, contemporary, plastic surgeon, Cambridge, UK.
Byrom George Harker Lamberty, contemporary, plastic surgeon, Cambridge, UK.
Bengt Pontén, 1923–2007, Associate Professor of Plastic Surgery, Uppsala University, Uppsala , Sweden.
Stephen John Mathes, 1943–2007, Professor of Surgery, University of California, San Francisco, CA, USA.
Foad Nahai, contemporary, Professor of Surgery, Emory University, Atlanta, GA, USA.

(a)

TRANSPOSITION FLAP

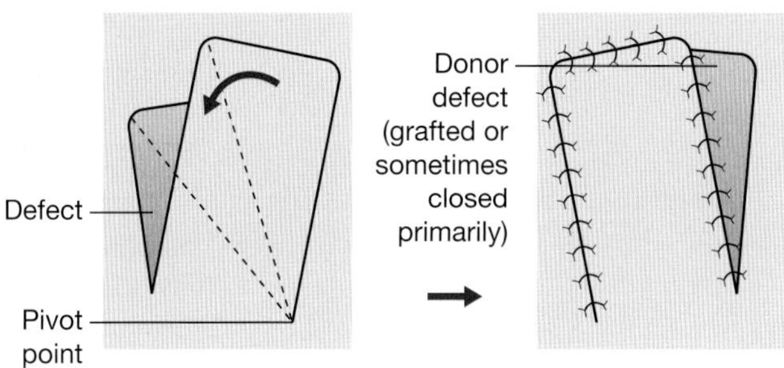

Z-PLASTY

Two triangular transposition flaps interposed

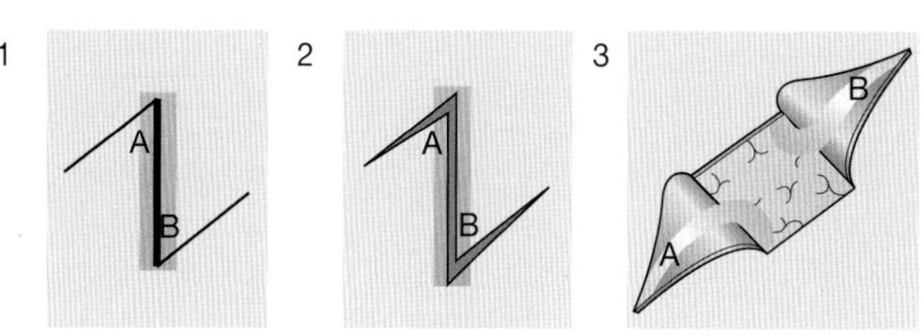

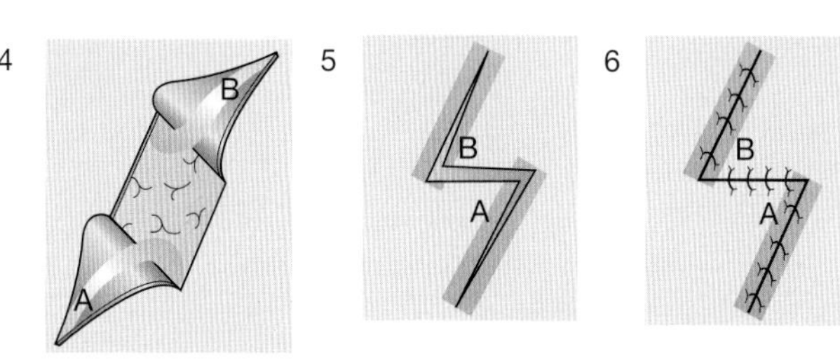

(b)

BILOBED FLAP

Uses a flap to close a convex defect, and a second smaller flap to close the donor site

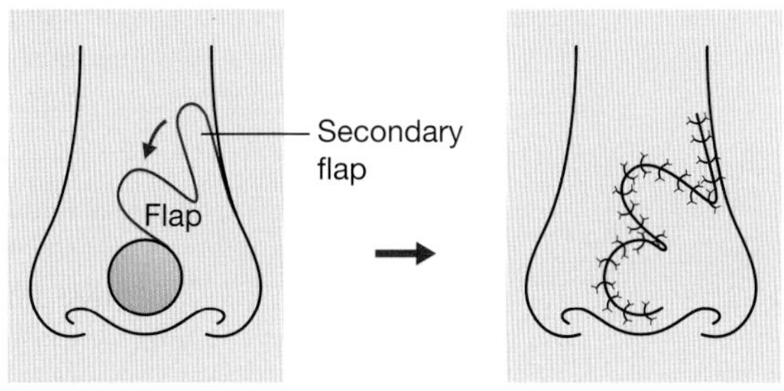

BIPEDICLE FLAP

A 'bucket-handle' flap supplied from both ends. Useful to rebuild the lower eyelid

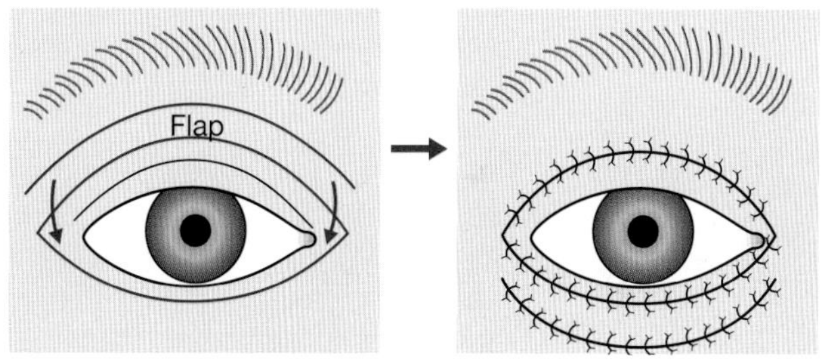

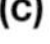

RHOMBOID FLAP

A parallelogram-shaped transposition flap

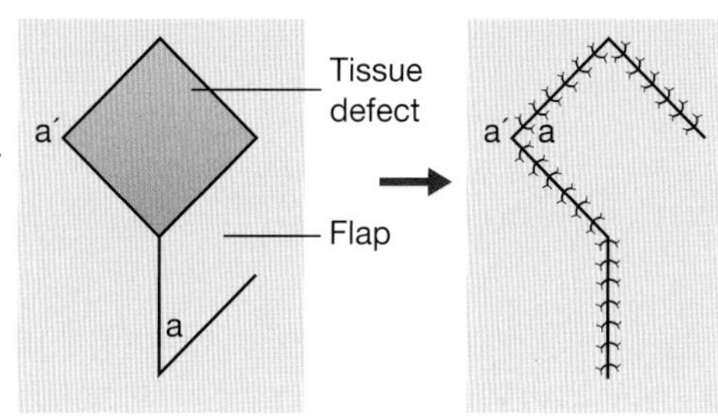

ROTATION FLAP

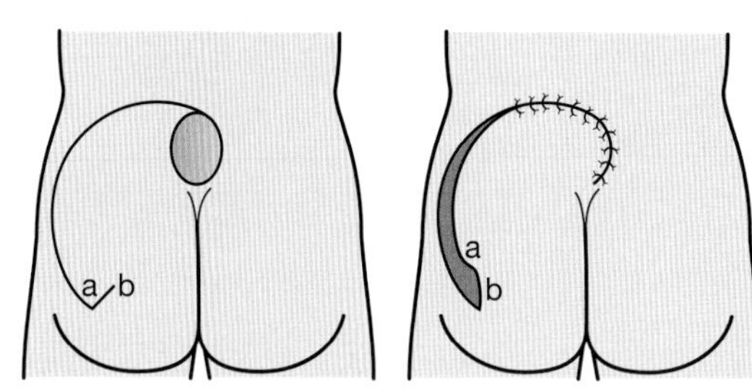

Figure 47.12 Local flap diagrams. **(a)** Transposition and Z-plasty flaps. **(b)** Bilobed and bipedicled flaps. **(c)** Rhomboid and rotation flaps. *(continued overleaf)*

(d)

ADVANCEMENT FLAP

Simple rectangular
(with or without Burow's triangle excision at base)

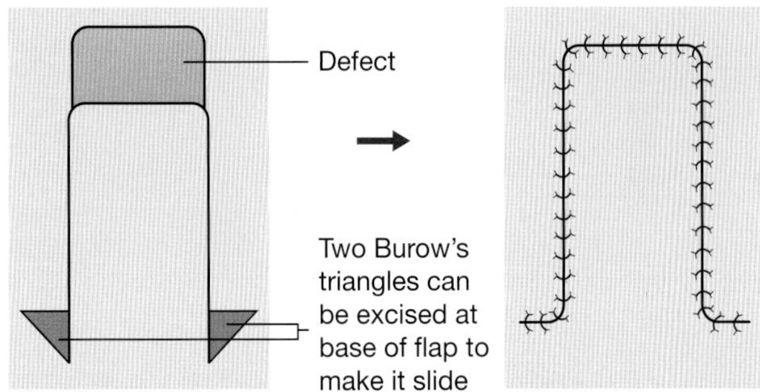

V to Y

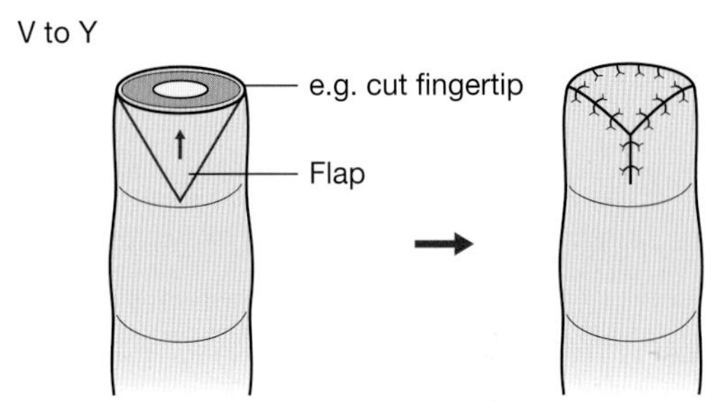

Y to V

Usually multiple to release band scars over joints

This is one of the most effective means of releasing moderate isolated band burn scars over flexion creases

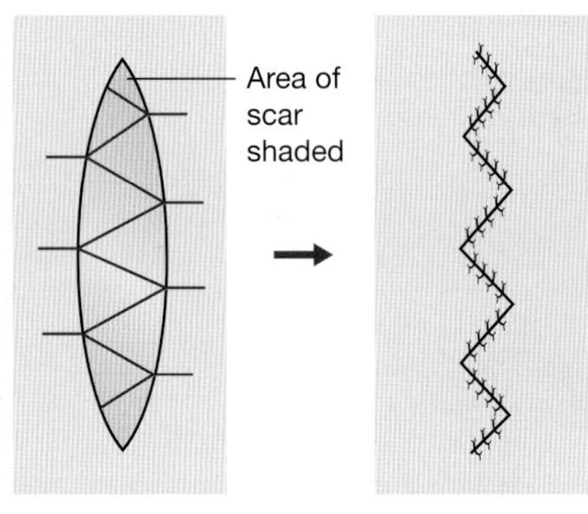

(e)

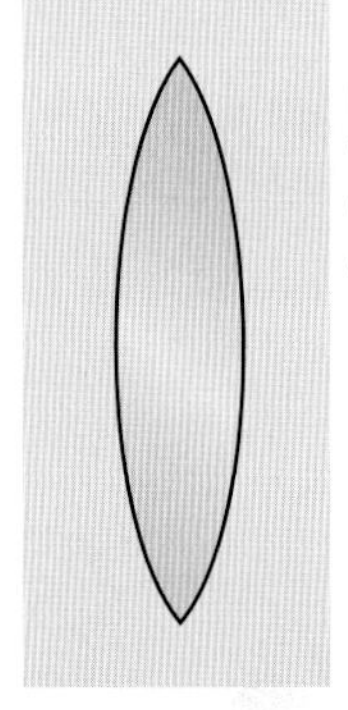

1
Burn scar with long ellipse around it

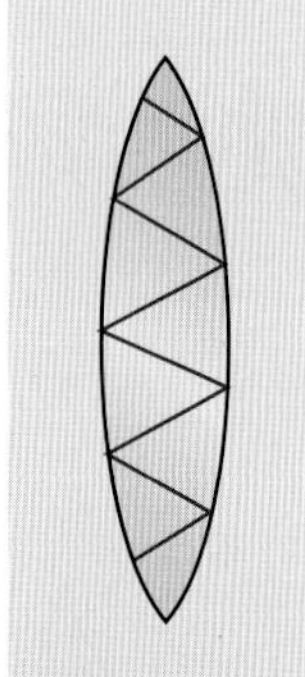

2
Mark a long zig-zag along the scar

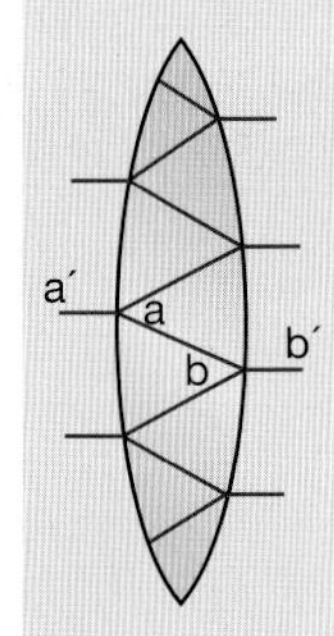

3
Add in the horizontal lines to the zig-zag; each becomes a 'Y'

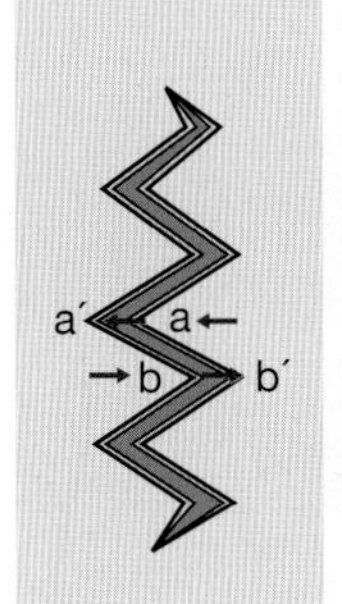

4
The cut lines will look something like this

Advance the tips of the zig-zags into the spaces

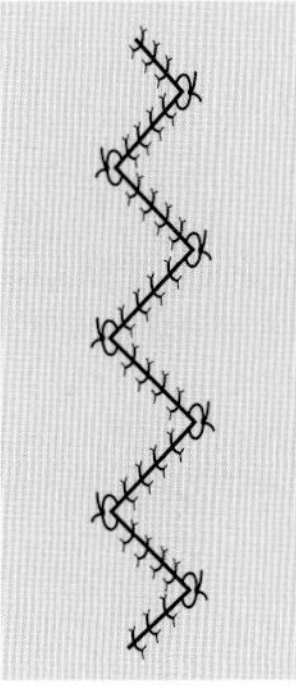

5
The finished wound will look something like this

Pad it well, and be sure to splint open when not exercising

Figure 47.12 (*continued*) Local flap diagrams. **(d)** Advancement flaps. **(e)** Multiple Y-to-V plasty for burn scar.

Karl August von Burow, 1809–1874, surgeon, Königsberg, Germany.

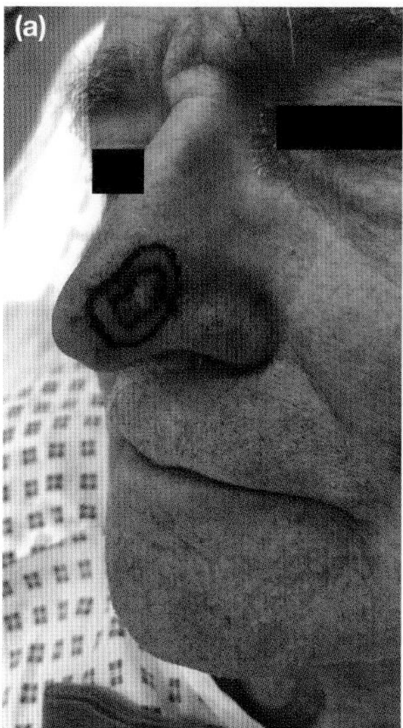
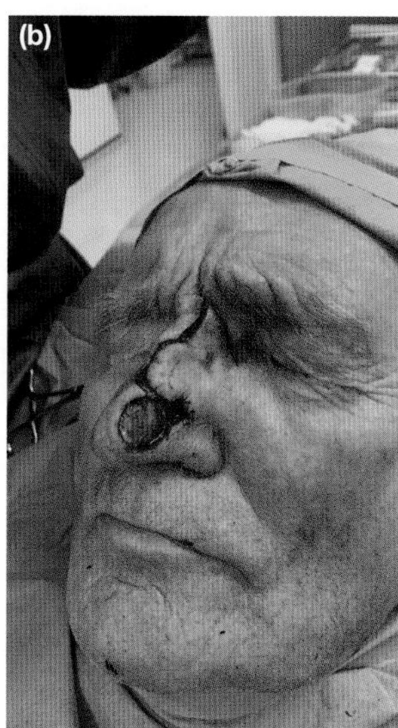
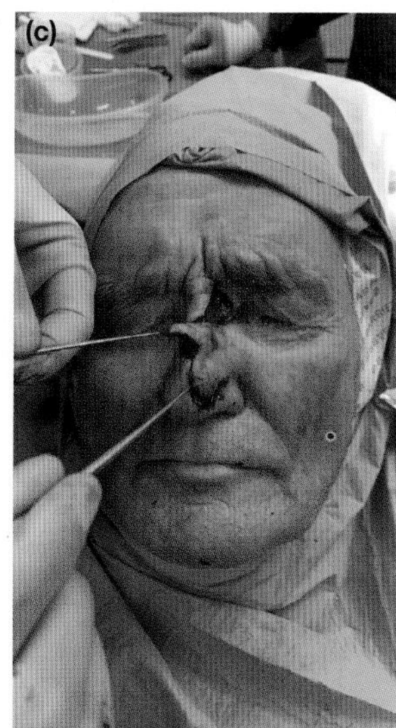
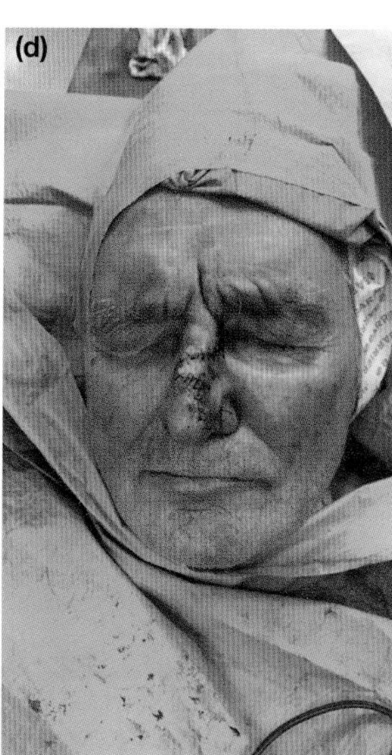

Figure 47.13 Bilobed flap reconstruction of a nasal defect following excision of a basal cell carcinoma. **(a)** Excision markings. **(b)** Bilobed flap raised. **(c)** Transposition of bilobed flap. **(d)** Immediate postoperative appearance.

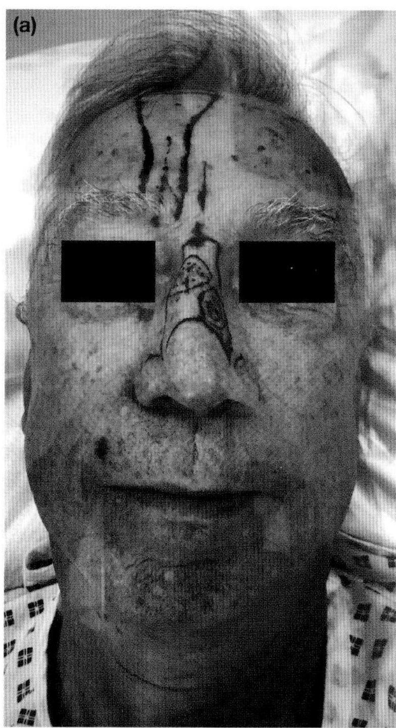
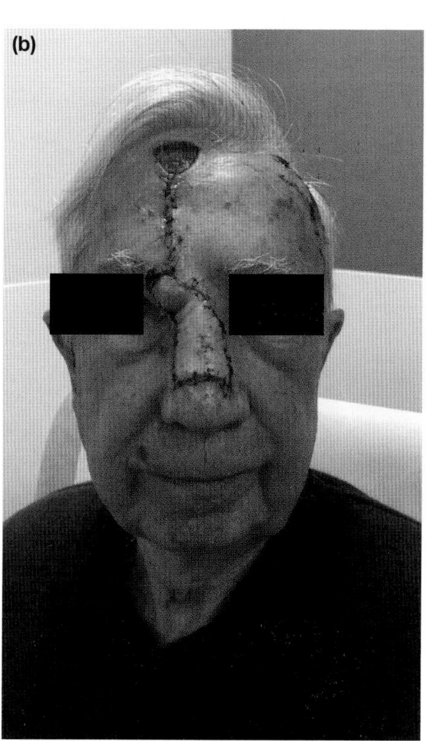
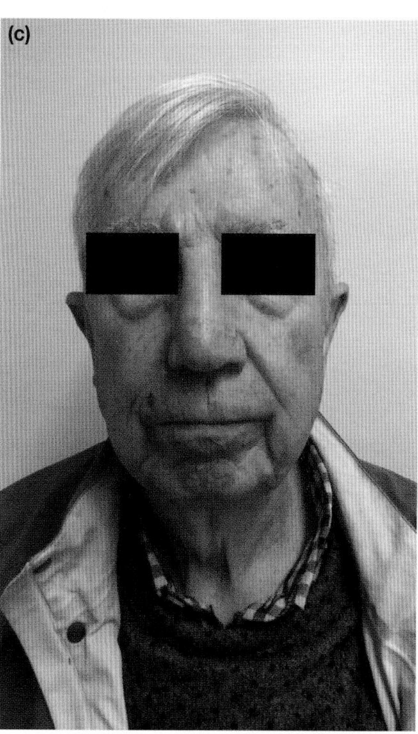

Figure 47.14 Forehead flap reconstruction of nasal defect following excision of multiple basal cell carcinomas. **(a)** Preoperative markings demonstrating the forehead flap based on the right supratrochlear artery. The pedicle position is confirmed using a hand-held Doppler probe. **(b)** Flap inset to nose – note the bulky pedicle at the right medial eyebrow; donor site closed primarily except at the widest point, where it is allowed to heal by secondary intention. **(c)** The flap pedicle was divided at a second stage, allowing contouring of the flap. Appearance at 6 months.

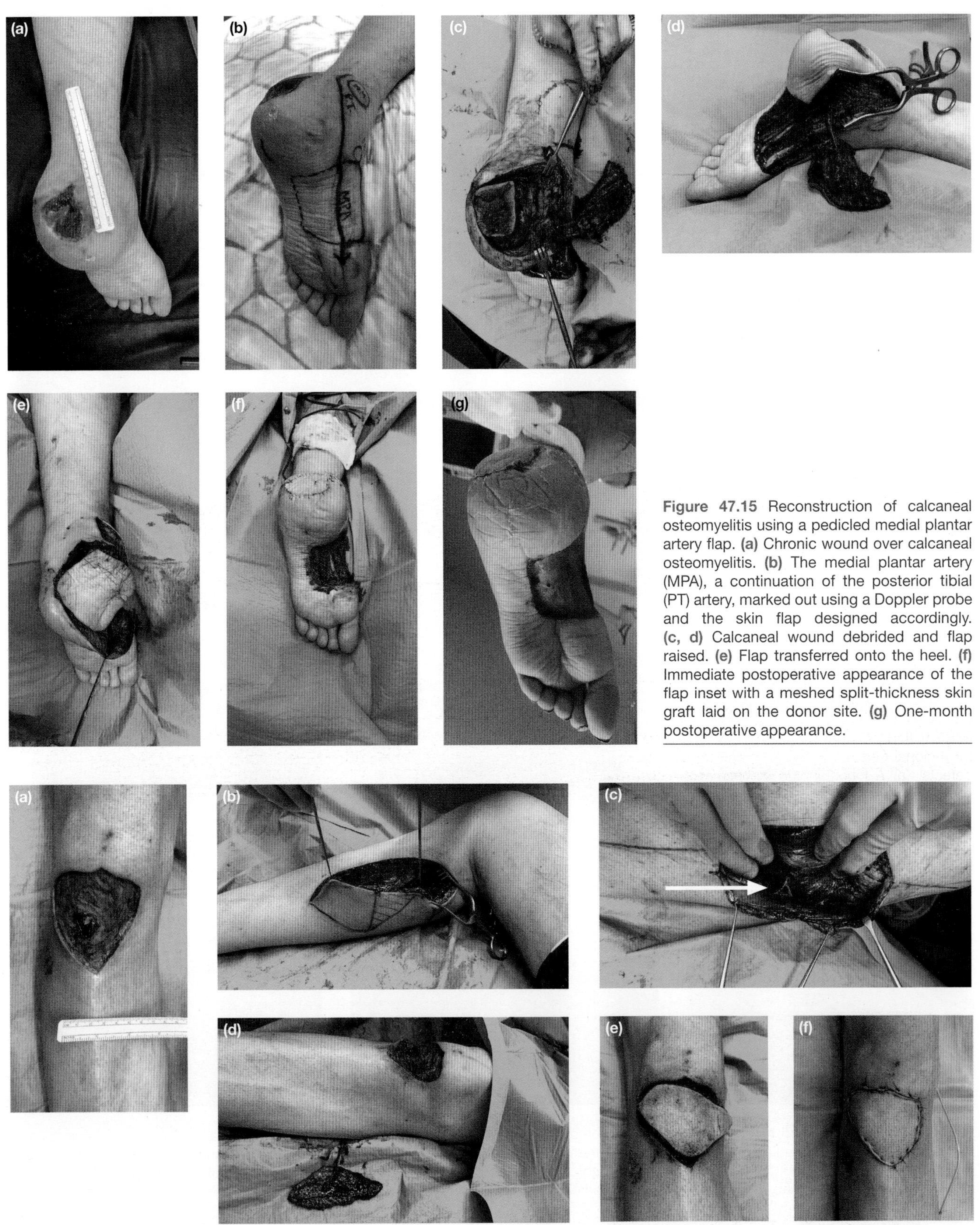

Figure 47.15 Reconstruction of calcaneal osteomyelitis using a pedicled medial plantar artery flap. **(a)** Chronic wound over calcaneal osteomyelitis. **(b)** The medial plantar artery (MPA), a continuation of the posterior tibial (PT) artery, marked out using a Doppler probe and the skin flap designed accordingly. **(c, d)** Calcaneal wound debrided and flap raised. **(e)** Flap transferred onto the heel. **(f)** Immediate postoperative appearance of the flap inset with a meshed split-thickness skin graft laid on the donor site. **(g)** One-month postoperative appearance.

Figure 47.16 The medial sural artery perforator (MSAP) flap can be used as a pedicled flap for regional defects or as a free flap for distant defects. **(a)** Traumatic defect of the anterior knee with a partially transected patellar ligament and cortical loss of the tibial tuberosity following wound debridement. **(b, c)** The MSAP flap is harvested – the perforator (arrow) is identified arising from the substance of the gastrocnemius muscle belly. **(d, e)** The flap remains attached to a pedicle and is transferred through a subcutaneous tunnel to the anterior knee defect. **(f)** Appearance after inset of the flap.

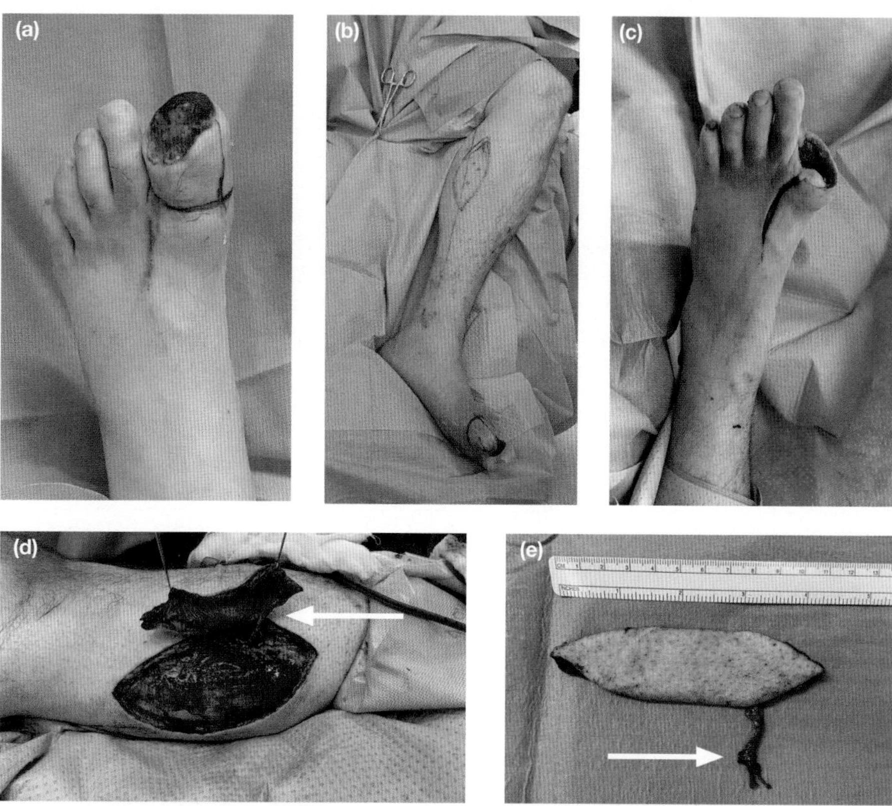

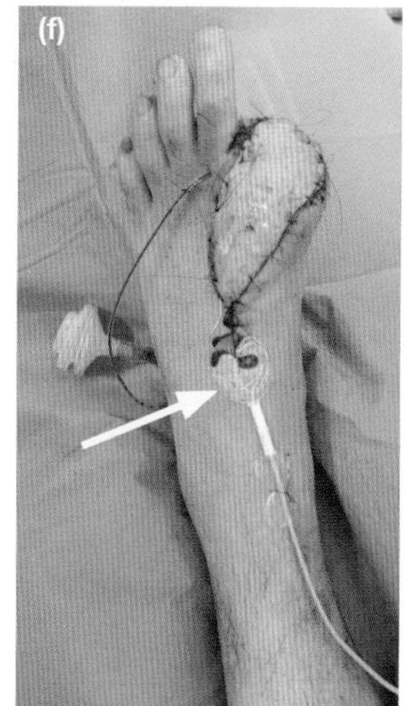

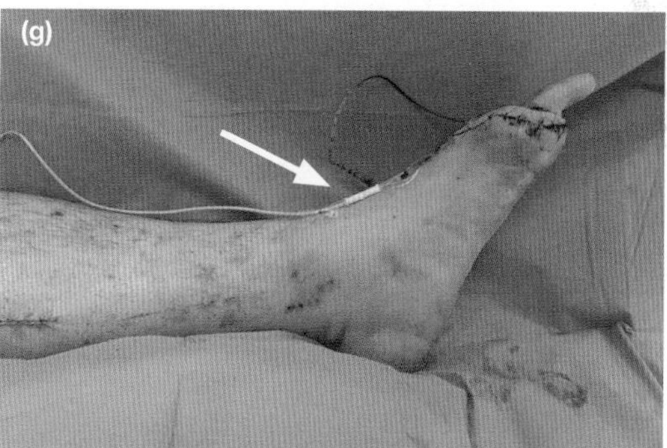

Figure 47.17 The medial sural artery perforator (MSAP) flap can be used as a pedicled flap for regional defects or as a free flap for distant defects. **(a)** A longstanding diabetic foot ulcer of the left hallux with underlying osteomyelitis. **(b)** Marking of the MSAP flap. **(c)** Amputation of the hallux – direct closure would have necessitated proximal excision of the first metatarsal bone, thereby compromising weightbearing. **(d)** The MSAP pedicle (arrow) dissected. **(e)** The detached MSAP flap with the pedicle (arrow). **(f, g)** Immediate postoperative appearance of the flap, with indwelling Doppler monitoring (arrows) for venous anastomosis patency.

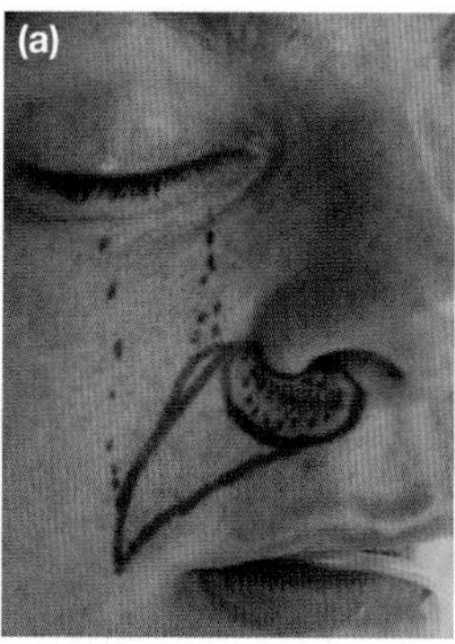

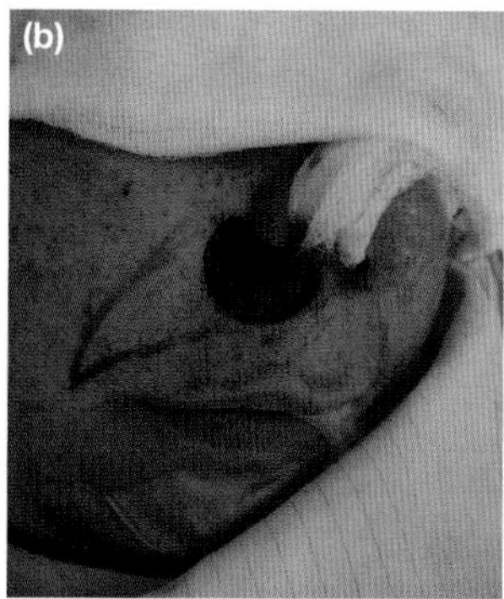

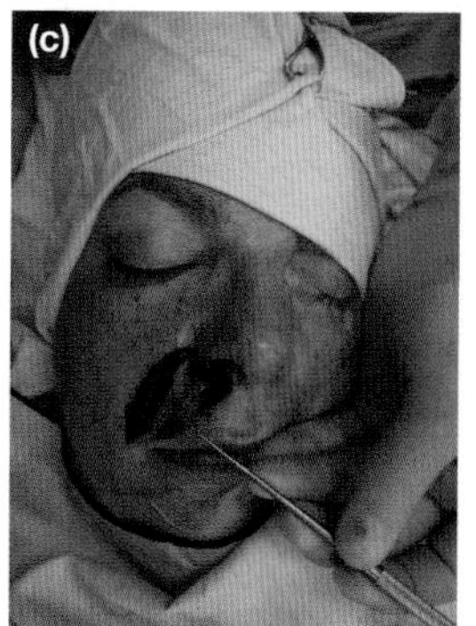

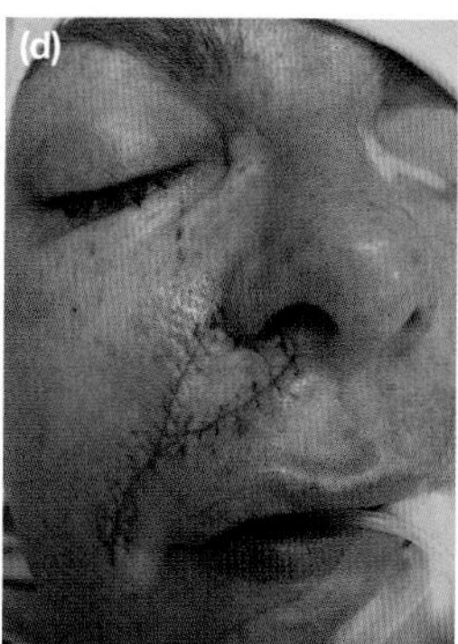

Figure 47.18 Excision of a basal cell carcinoma of the right alar groove and reconstruction with a V-to-Y nasolabial advancement flap. **(a)** Tumour excision margins and flap design markings. **(b)** The defect following excision of the basal cell carcinoma. **(c)** Raising the nasolabial flap. **(d)** Advancement and inset of the flap.

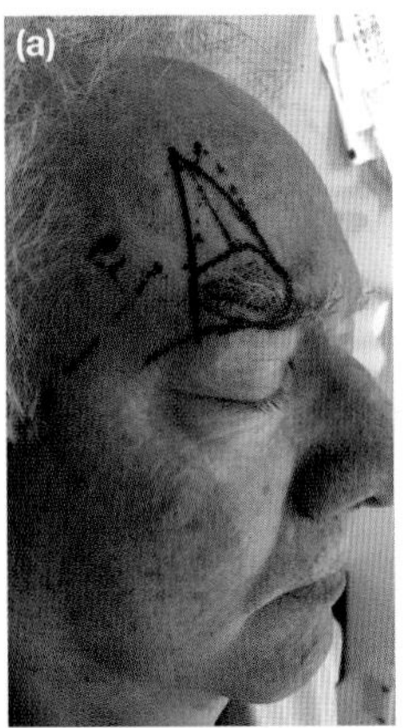

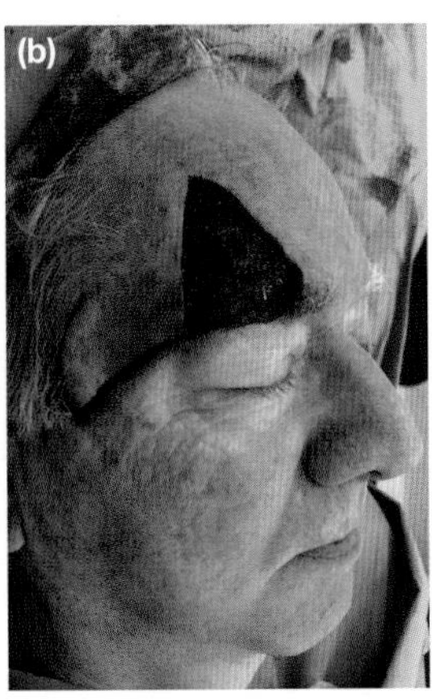

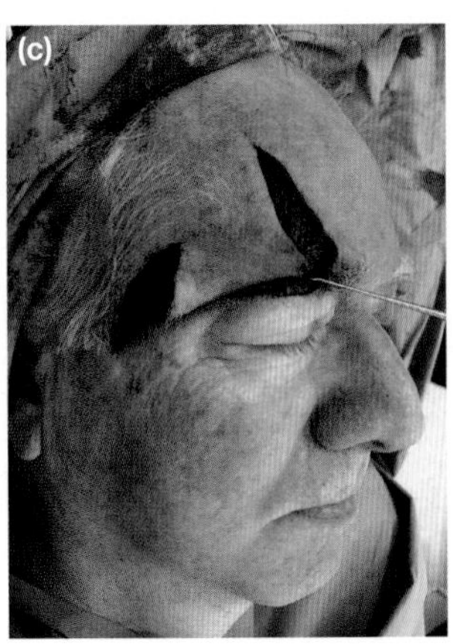

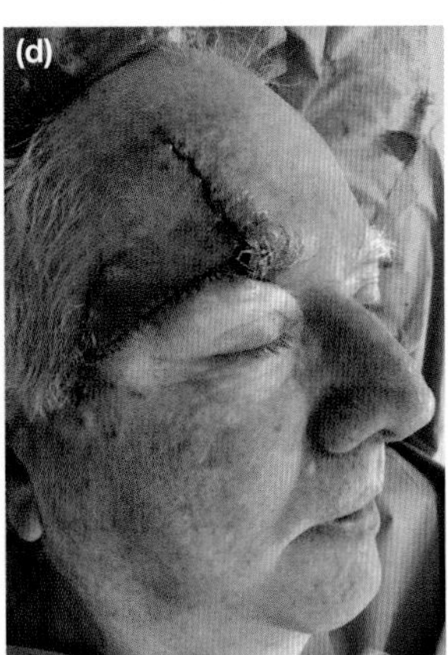

Figure 47.19 Hatchet flap reconstruction following excision of a skin cancer of the right eyebrow. **(a)** Preoperative planning. **(b)** Post excision of the tumour with a back cut to enable flap advancement. **(c)** Insetting of the flap. **(d)** Immediate postoperative appearance.

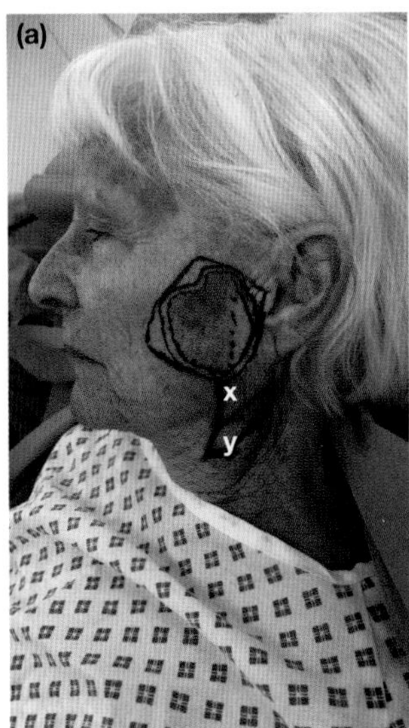

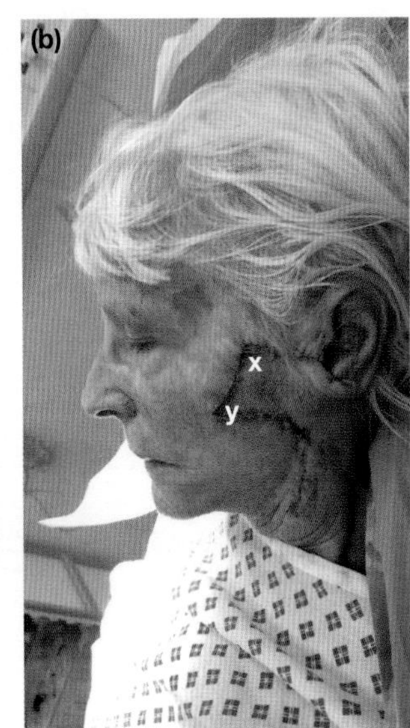

Figure 47.20 Reconstruction of a melanocytic lesion of the left pre-auricular region using a rhomboid (transposition) flap. **(a)** Preoperative markings. **(b)** Immediate postoperative appearance.

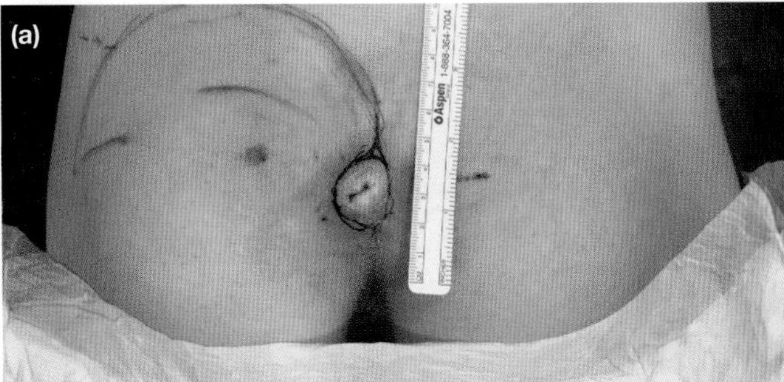

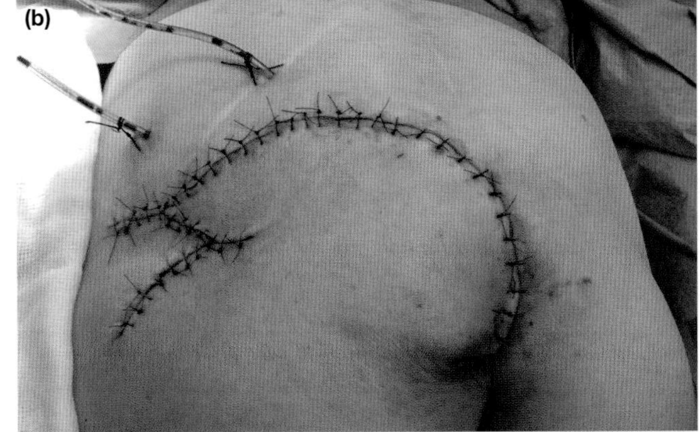

Figure 47.21 Rotation flap reconstruction following excision of a pilonidal sinus. **(a)** Preoperative marking of the rotational flap with a back cut. **(b)** Immediate postoperative appearance.

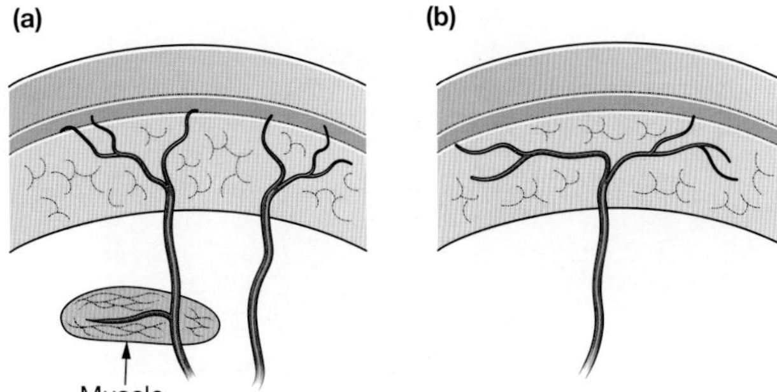

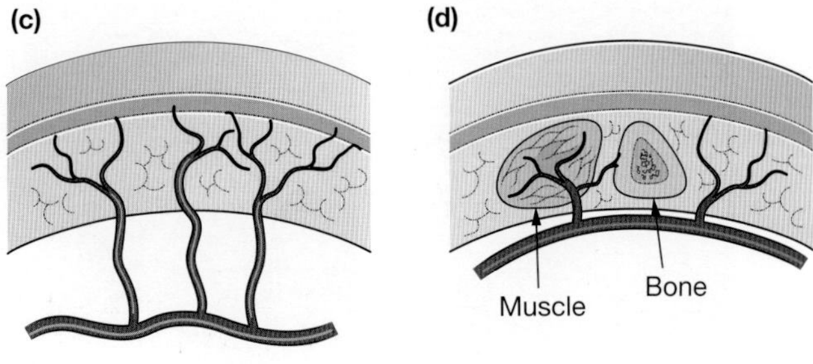

Figure 47.22 Cormack and Lamberty classification of fasciocutaneous flaps. **(a)** Multiple large perforators. **(b)** Single large perforator. **(c)** Multiple, small, segmental perforators. **(d)** Osteomyofascial perforators.

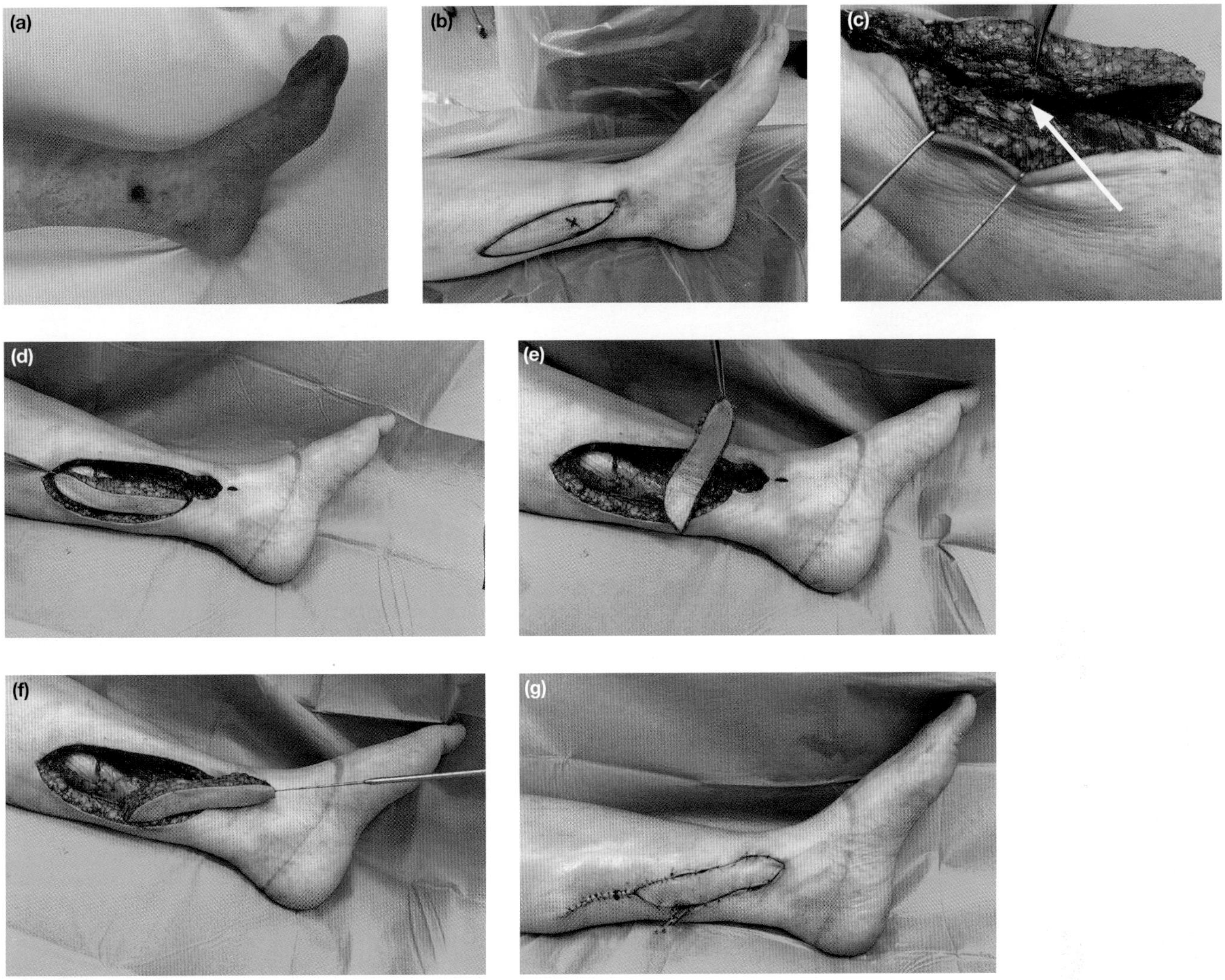

Figure 47.23 Wound debridement and reconstruction with a pedicled flap based on a perforator arising from the posterior tibial artery. **(a)** Chronic sinus overlying internal fixation of a medial malleolar fracture. **(b)** The perforator has been identified using a Doppler probe and marked on the skin (X). **(c)** The perforator (arrow) and a pair of vena comitans were dissected and the fasciocutaneous flap islanded. **(d–f)** The flap is propellered 180° clockwise to reconstruct the defect. **(g)** The donor site was able to be closed primarily owing to local skin laxity.

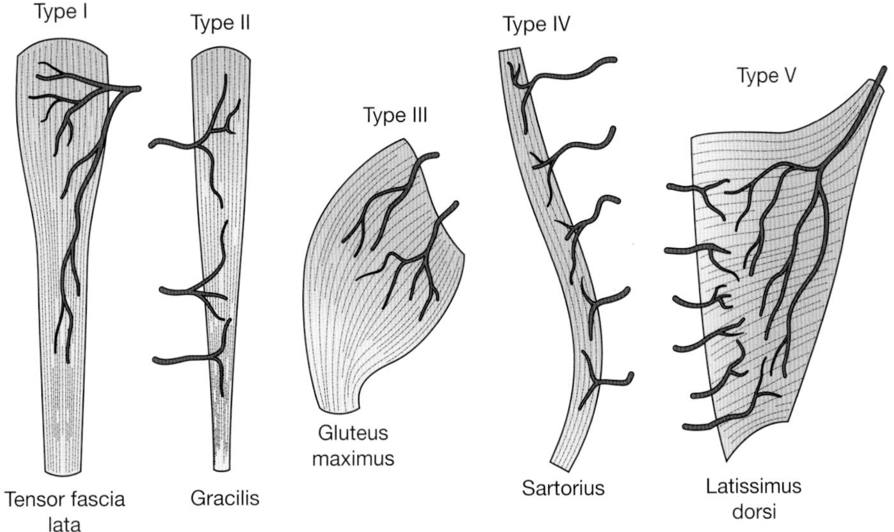

Figure 47.24 The Mathes and Nahai classification of muscle flaps.

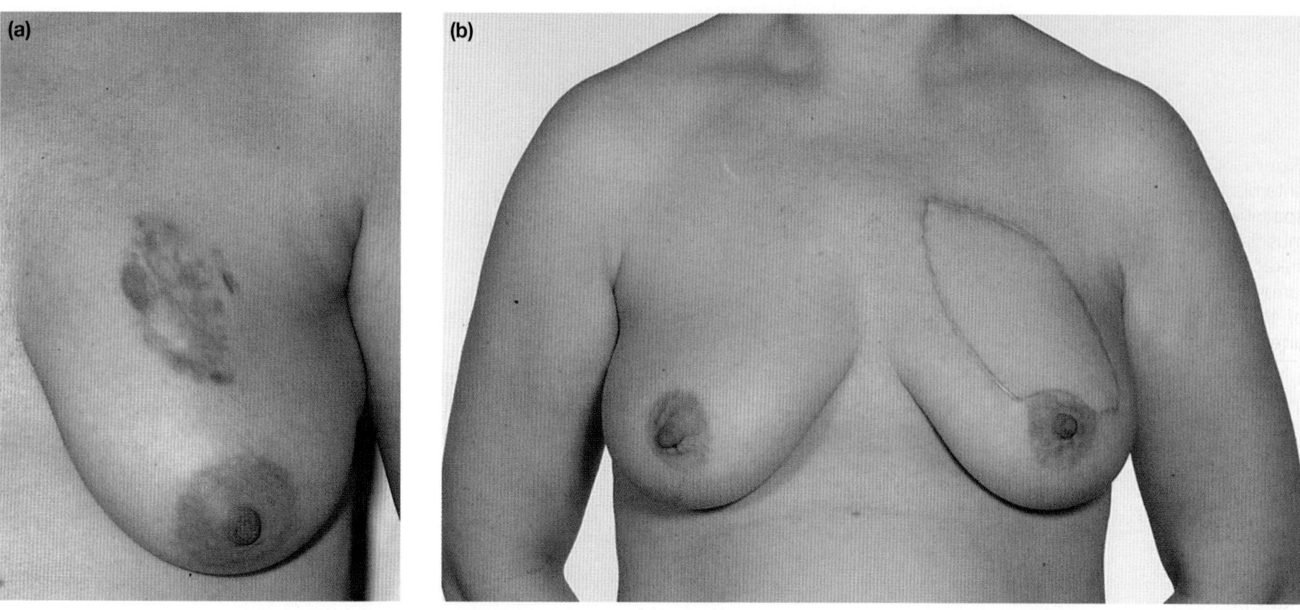

Figure 47.25 The latissimus dorsi flap can be used as a pedicled flap to reconstruct regional defects or as a free flap to reconstruct distant defects. **(a)** Dermatofibrosarcoma protuberans of the left breast. **(b)** Reconstruction using a pedicled musculocutaneous latissimus dorsi flap.

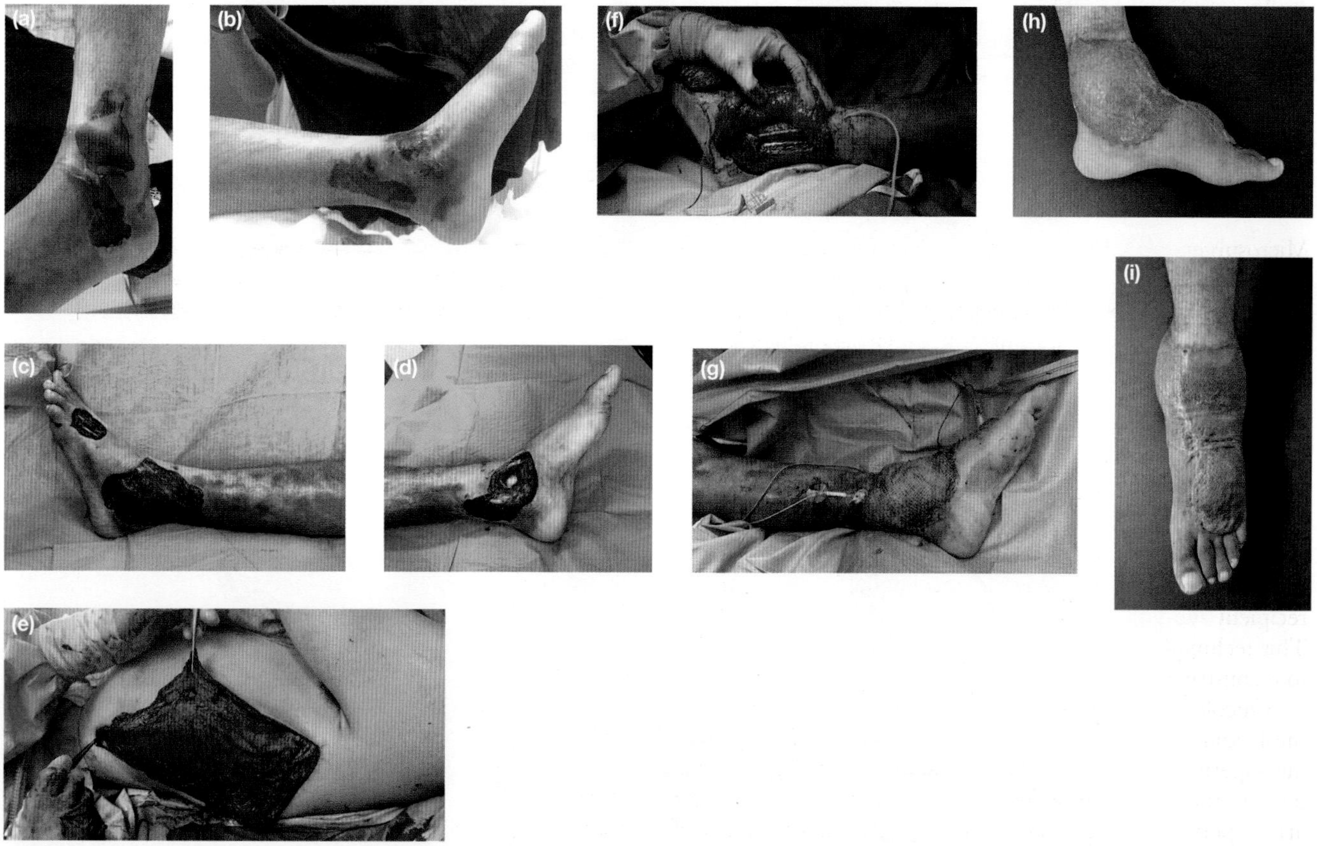

Figure 47.26 (a, b) Limb-threatening, multiplanar degloving injury of the left foot and ankle from a road traffic accident. **(c, d)** Following wound debridement, multiple skin defects with exposed extensor tendons and tibiotalar joint. **(e)** Harvest of left latissimus dorsi and serratus anterior flaps as two separate free flaps. **(f, g)** Immediate postoperative appearance with meshed split-thickness skin grafts laid over the muscle flaps. **(h, i)** Postoperative appearance at 6 months with normal ambulation.

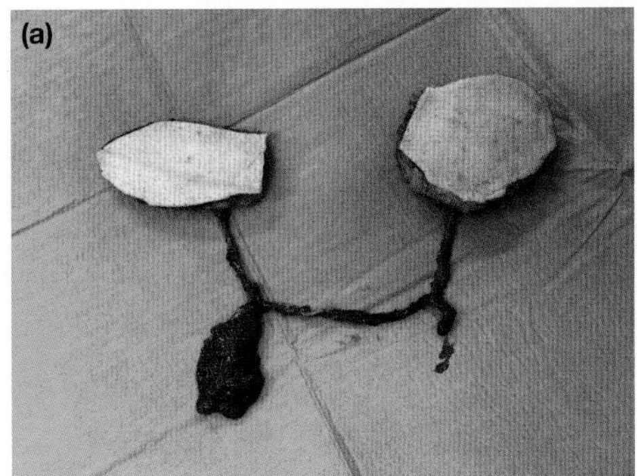

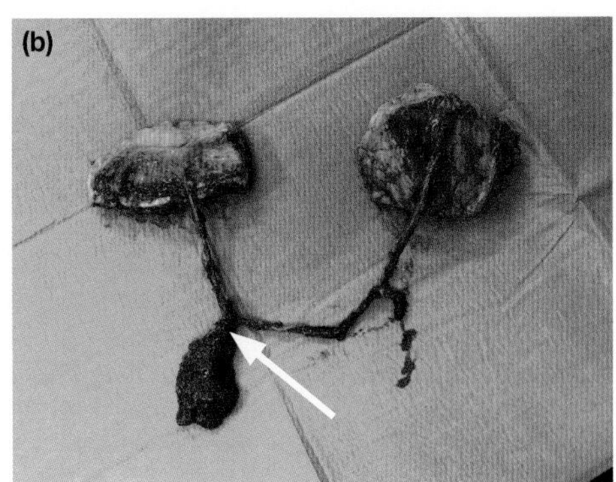

Figure 47.27 (a, b) Chimeric anterolateral thigh flap comprising spatially independent skin and muscle flaps with all pedicles linked to a common source vessel (arrow), the descending branch of the lateral femoral circumflex artery.

circumflex artery pedicle can support multiple skin and muscle flaps (***Figure 47.27***) or the subscapular vascular pedicle can support a scapular flap, a parascapular flap, a latissimus dorsi flap and a serratus anterior flap. This enables the reconstruction of complex composite defects involving different tissues. For example, following resection of a maxillary sinus tumour, a chimeric scapular flap can be used to reconstruct both the bony and skin defects.

Venous flow-through flaps are based on a venous rather than arterial pedicle so that the vein delivers both inflow and outflow of blood. These flaps are thin and pliable but prone to venous congestion and partial necrosis as there is no arterial input and the flap survives on deoxygenated blood. There is minimal donor site morbidity. Examples include the saphenous flap and those based on the superficial veins of the forearm.

MICROSURGERY

Microsurgery is a surgical subspecialty that makes use of magnification, precision tools and surgical techniques to enable the anastomosis of small blood vessels and coaptation of nerves. The diameter of a typical suture is between 0.01 and 0.03 mm. The advent of microvascular anastomotic techniques renders it feasible to transplant tissue to every region of the body, thus vastly expanding the reconstructive armamentarium as it is no longer necessary to rely on grafts that must revascularise from an underlying wound bed or on pedicled flaps that are limited by size, length or the distance they can 'travel'. Provided the course from the source vessel to the end organ is preserved, it is possible to transfer flaps from any region of the body to any recipient site provided an appropriate recipient vessel exists. This technique offers a highly versatile and flexible approach to reconstructive surgery.

Oncological reconstruction for head and neck cancer or mastectomy defects often requires the use of free flaps, providing superior functional and aesthetic outcomes. Typical flaps include the anterolateral thigh and deep inferior epigastric artery perforator flaps, based on the descending branch of the lateral circumflex femoral artery and the deep inferior epigastric artery, respectively. For complex limb injuries or osteomyelitis, microsurgical reconstruction has meant that limb salvage is now possible rather than amputation (***Figure 47.26***). Common flaps used in this context include the gracilis or latissimus dorsi muscle flaps.

Microsurgical flaps are not always used to reconstruct skin defects. Free functional muscle flaps are used to reanimate the face or the upper limb in facial and brachial plexus palsies, respectively. Free bone flaps such as the free fibular flap may also be used to reconstruct the mandible following oncological resection or to provide a strut following excision of an osteomyelitic segment of tibia.

Microsurgery has also made it possible to replant amputated digits and limbs, or reconstruct missing fingers with free vascularised functioning and sensate toes (***Figure 47.28***). Furthermore, the technique has also made vascularised composite allotransplantation possible, including of the hand and face.

Anastomoses are usually hand sewn (using specialist microinstruments with the aid of an operating microscope), although the adoption of mechanical coupler devices for venous anastomoses is becoming increasingly popular as they are often technically less demanding and faster than a hand-sewn approach.

Supermicrosurgery involving microneurovascular anastomosis of vessels and coaptation of single nerve fascicles of the order of 0.3–0.8 mm has further expanded the field. It has enabled the reconstruction of fingertip injuries, which traditionally would have been treated with amputation, and the creation of lymphaticovenous anastomosis for the treatment of chronic lymphoedema.

FLAP MONITORING

Following microvascular free-flap reconstruction, patients may be monitored in a high-dependency unit setting as it is crucial to keep the patient physiologically optimised in order that the flap remains well perfused at all times. The traditional adage is that the patient should be kept 'wet, warm and comfortable'. Strict fluid balance is monitored with the aim of keeping the circulation hyperdynamic; the flap is kept warm with a Bair Hugger® device and analgesia is carefully controlled to minimise excessive catecholamine production as a result of pain. The flap is monitored regularly by specialist nurses who assess the colour, warmth and turgor of the flap. Pressure applied to the skin of a musculocutaneous flap enables the capillary refill time to be assessed; if necessary the flap can be pricked with a

Christian Andreas Doppler, 1803-1853, Director of the Institute of Physics, University of Vienna, Vienna, Austria.

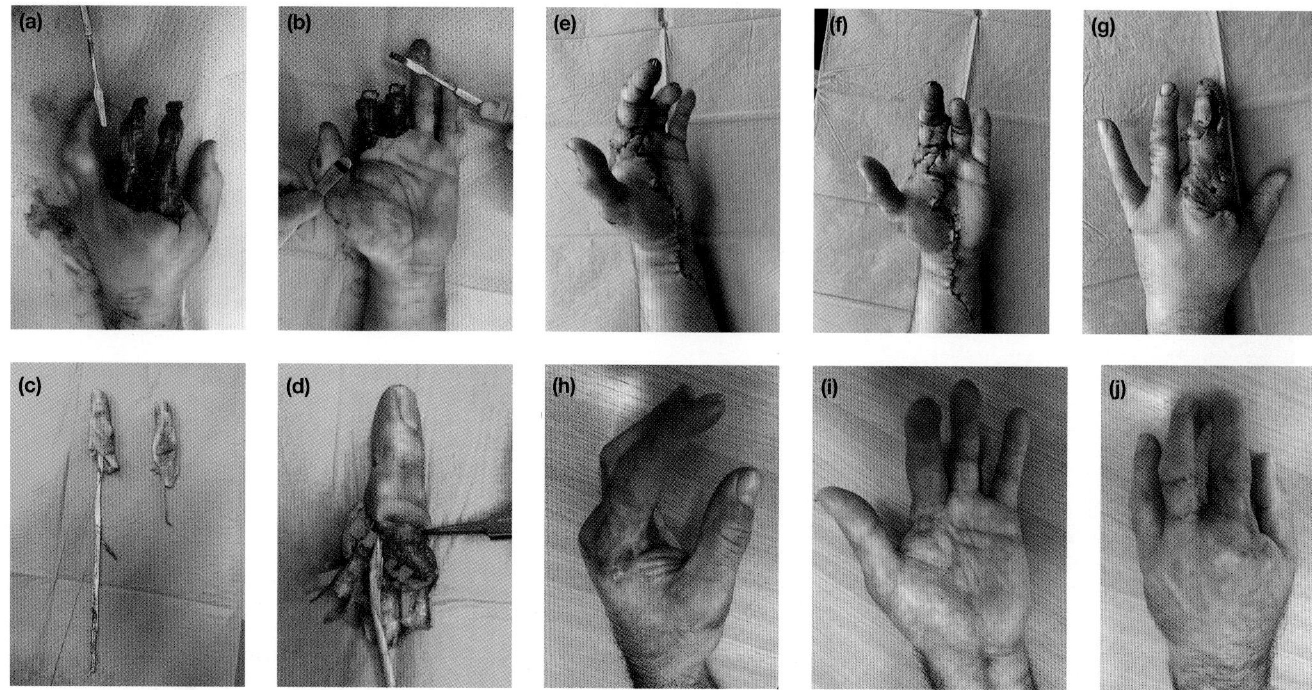

Figure 47.28 Replantation of digit. **(a–c)** Complete avulsions of the index and middle fingers at the distal interphalangeal joints. The avulsed middle finger was not salvageable. **(d)** The avulsed index finger was dissected and the digital arteries, veins and nerves were identified. Heterotopic replantation of the avulsed index finger to the middle. **(e–g)** Immediate postoperative appearance. **(h–j)** One-year postoperative appearance with the range of motion demonstrated.

hypodermic needle to assess bleeding. The arterial and venous flow to a flap can often be monitored with a hand-help Doppler device, whereas some surgeons use an implantable Doppler (attached to the venous outflow of the flap), which is especially useful for muscle flaps (without the benefit of a skin paddle to monitor) or those flaps that are buried and thus not accessible for direct visual monitoring.

The survival of a free flap is usually threatened by an interruption to arterial inflow or venous drainage; rapid identification of a problem is essential as an immediate return to theatre is required to salvage the flap. Approximately 5% of free flaps will require exploration in theatre for vascular compromise; of these, more than 60% can be salvaged. The earlier a flap is explored the greater the likelihood of salvage success. Approximately two-thirds of cases of vascular compromise are venous in aetiology, with one-third being arterial; combined inflow and outflow issues are sometimes seen, and in some situations the vessels may be patent but compromised by external pressure (such as a haematoma or an excessively tight dressing). Thus, when assessing a compromised flap at the bedside, the surgeon must ensure that the dressings are loosened and any overly tensioned sutures released. Close flap monitoring is of most value in the first 48 hours with rapid detection of vascular compromise facilitating early salvage and improved flap survival.

A free-flap survival rate in excess 95% is typical in routine elective reconstructive cases such as breast reconstruction using a transverse rectus abdominis (TRAM) or deep inferior epigastric perforator (DIEP) flap. Flap survival rates are slightly lower in, for example, cases of complex polytrauma or head and neck reconstruction.

LEECH THERAPY

The European medicinal leech (*Hirudo medicinalis*) is an invertebrate annelid; its saliva contains hirudin (an anticoagulant), hyaluronidase (which facilitates anticoagulant penetration into the wound) and histamine (to maintain vasodilatation). The primary indication for leech therapy is to improve drainage from flaps that are venously congested, i.e. those that are dusky blue with a brisk capillary refill and a rapid, dark pinprick. Such congestion may result from a particular vein being too small or not present or a venous anastomosis not being technically possible (e.g. a distal digital replant where an artery is reconstructed but not the vein). Leeches are not normally used in cases of suspected venous obstruction of a free flap as immediate surgical exploration is required; likewise they are of no benefit in an arterially compromised flap as, again, immediate surgical exploration is mandated.

As leeching is used for venous (as opposed to arterial) insufficiency, a typical course of treatment may last for up to 2 weeks – until new vein formation occurs at the margins of the flap (***Figure 47.29***). The anticoagulant effect persists once the leech has detached from the patient, with bleeding occurring for some hours; each leech will imbibe up to 5 mL of blood and up to 150 mL of blood may be lost in the subsequent ooze; thus, all patients must have their haemoglobin level monitored regularly and blood transfusion may be necessary.

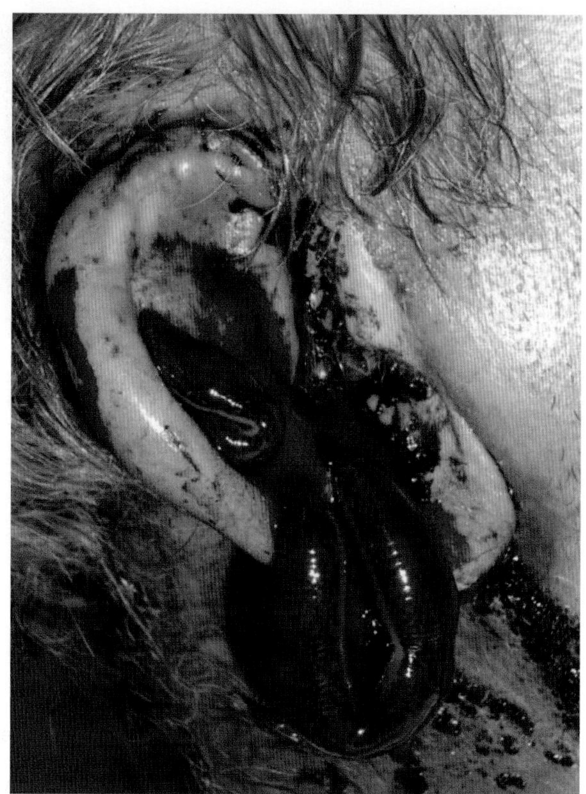

Figure 47.29 Leeching used for a venously congested replanted right external ear.

Leeches contain *Aeromonas hydrophila*, so patients require prophylactic antibiotics (typically a quinolone) until wound closure is complete.

FUTURE DIRECTIONS

Anatomical discoveries, such as a detailed understanding of the blood supply to the skin as well as technical and engineering innovations that brought about microsurgery, have enabled the field of reconstructive plastic surgery to blossom. As populations age and life expectancies continue to improve, the demand for reconstructive surgery, particularly among the elderly population for chronic degenerative and neoplastic conditions, will continue apace. The key to the next phase of reconstructive plastic surgery advances will likely be a combined approach across multiple scientific and surgical disciplines.

The scientific areas that will lead to significant breakthroughs include wound healing, bioengineering, cancer treatment and immunotolerance for vascularised allotransplantation. Recent discoveries of the genetic, epigenetic and molecular mechanisms that underlie conditions such as craniosynostosis, cleft lip and palate, Dupuytren's disease and delayed wound healing now provide a rational basis for the development of therapeutic interventions. Bioengineering and tissue engineering will certainly play a major role in modern reconstruction; for example, smart tissue expansion for cleft palate reconstruction and biocompatible scaffolds that simultaneously promote *in situ* tissue regeneration as well as deliver treatment by eluting antibiotics or chemotherapeutic agents for musculoskeletal and cancer reconstruction. Furthermore, as the cultural and political landscapes evolve, new areas of reconstructive surgery have emerged, including gender-affirming surgery. One of the most exciting areas of reconstructive plastic surgery has been the increasing success of vascularised composite allotransplantation, including of the face and upper limb. Outcomes are expected to continue to improve with better understanding of immunological tolerance and increasing social acceptance of the donation of body parts.

The field of robotic surgery continues to expand. It is particularly useful to assist in surgical approaches where access is limited, such as cleft surgery. The latest devices are able to eliminate hand tremor, increase dexterity and range of motion, provide haptic feedback and three-dimensional views that assist greatly in challenging dissections, and have been successfully adopted in oncological head and neck reconstruction.

Reconstructive plastic surgery is unique in its creativity, breadth and variety of reconstructive techniques. While this affords the specialty powerful means to serve the patient, it does also mean the practice of evidence-based surgery is challenging. There are often numerous techniques to treat the same conditions with a lack of high-quality evidence. Moreover, there are often situations where surgery may be technically feasible but not in the best interest of the patient. For example, patients with complex multifragmentary open tibiofibular fractures and neurovascular compromise may have a better quality of life with a below-knee amputation than with a salvage reconstruction with free tissue transfer. Hence, well-designed pragmatic clinical trials and the development of rigorous tools to capture the most relevant data, such as patient-reported outcome measures, together with the building of large-scale clinical research networks at both national and international levels will be crucial to drive complex shared decision making between surgeon and patient.

FURTHER READING

MacGregor AD, MacGregor IA. *Fundamental techniques in plastic surgery*, 10th edn. Edinburgh: Churchill Livingstone, 2000.
Neligan PC (ed.). *Plastic surgery*. Philadelphia, PA: Saunders, 2012.
Santoni-Rugiu P, Sykes PJ. *A history of plastic surgery*. London: Springer, 2007.
Taylor GI, Palmer HK. The vascular territories (angiosomes) of the body: experimental study and clinical applications. *Br J Plast Surg* **40**(2), 113–41.
Wei F-C, Mardini S. *Flaps and reconstructive surgery*, 2nd edn. Philadelphia, PA: Saunders, 2016.

Baron Guillaume Dupuytren, 1777–1835, Surgeon in Chief, Hôtel-Dieu, Paris, France.

CHAPTER 48 Cranial neurosurgery

Learning objectives

- To understand the physiology of raised intracranial pressure, cerebrospinal fluid circulation and intracranial blood flow
- To recognise central nervous system infection, and understand the acute management
- To be familiar with causes of spontaneous intracranial haemorrhage and the principles of management of subarachnoid haemorrhage
- To recognise common intracranial tumours, their presentation, investigation and treatment
- To be aware of common developmental and other pathologies encountered in paediatric neurosurgical practice and emergency paediatric care
- To understand the indications and approaches available for the management of epilepsy, pain syndromes and movement disorders
- To note key practical and ethical issues relating to consent and risks, Creutzfeldt–Jakob precautions and the diagnosis of brainstem death

RAISED INTRACRANIAL PRESSURE

The importance of intracranial pressure (ICP) management in the context of head injury has been discussed elsewhere (see ***Chapter 28***). Likewise ICP is key to presentation and management across the spectrum of cranial neurosurgery.

Clinical features of raised intracranial pressure

Symptoms of raised ICP include a 'high-pressure headache' that is worse on coughing or bending forward. By contrast, low-pressure headaches, typically associated with excessive cerebrospinal fluid (CSF) drainage, are worse on standing. High-pressure headaches may be accompanied by nausea and vomiting, blurred vision and double vision: cranial nerve compression can result in eye movement and pupil abnormalities. Fundoscopy can detect papilloedema (***Figure 48.1***), but this takes time to develop so may be absent in the acute phase.

Before closure of the skull sutures in infancy, raised ICP presents differently with an increase in head circumference, prominent scalp veins and a tense bulging fontanelle. In infants and older children, raised CSF pressure results in dorsal midbrain compression with a loss of upgaze known as sunsetting, a feature of Parinaud's syndrome (***Figure 48.2***).

Raised ICP requires urgent evaluation and management: delay risks progression to cerebral herniation resulting in cardiovascular instability, neurological deficit and death. Vision may also deteriorate rapidly and irreversibly. Where there are pupil changes or a deterioration in conscious level, anaesthetic and

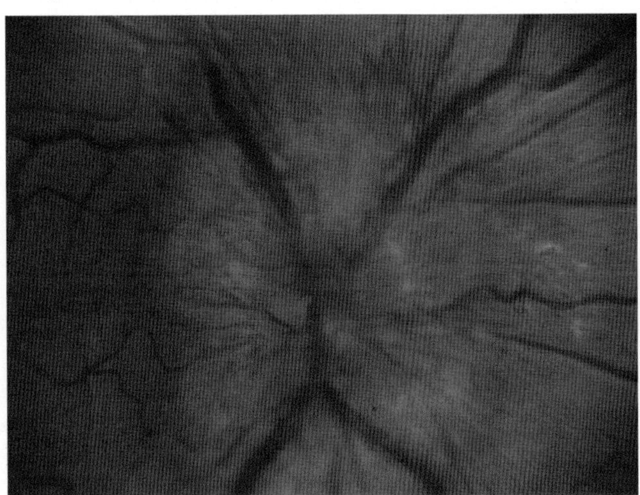

Figure 48.1 Papilloedema. The optic disc is swollen with blurred margins.

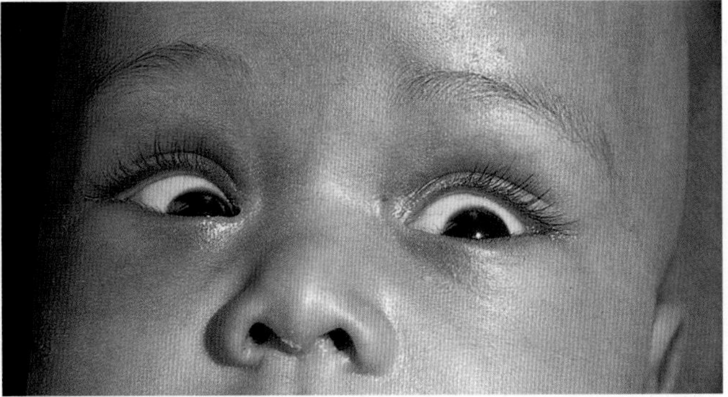

Figure 48.2 Parinaud's syndrome with sunsetting.

Henri Parinaud, 1844–1905, French ophthalmologist and pioneer in neuro-ophthalmology.

neurosurgical help may be needed: raise the head of the bed, administer hypertonic saline or mannitol and arrange urgent computed tomography (CT) imaging.

Investigation of raised intracranial pressure

CT is a first-line investigation to identify causes of raised ICP, including mass lesions, bleeds, cerebral oedema and hydrocephalus, and to guide treatment. Outside the emergency setting many pathologies, as well as the anatomy relating to potential treatments such as third ventriculostomy, may be better visualised on magnetic resonance imaging (MRI). The gold standard for quantifying ICP and monitoring in real time is by transducing CSF pressure through an external ventricular drain or insertion of a pressure monitor into the brain substance (***Figure 48.3***).

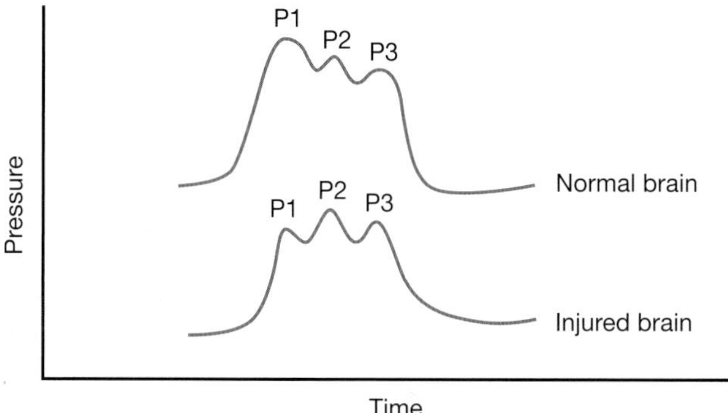

Figure 48.3 The intracranial pressure waveform. The P1 percussion wave corresponds to arterial pulsation. Reduced brain compliance in the setting of traumatic brain injury among others is associated with a prominent P2 tidal wave. The P3 dicrotic wave represents venous pulsation.

Summary box 48.1

Raised ICP

Acutely raised ICP is a neurosurgical emergency. Clinical features include:

- Headache
- Nausea and vomiting
- Diplopia and blurred vision
- Drowsiness then coma

HYDROCEPHALUS

The total volume of CSF is normally about 150 mL. Production from the walls of the ventricles and the choroid plexus is about 20 mL/h. Hydrocephalus refers to an increase in CSF volume with ventricular enlargement, often presenting symptoms of raised ICP.

Physiology of cerebrospinal fluid flow

CSF flows from the lateral ventricles through the foramen of Monro to the third ventricle, then down the cerebral aqueduct to the fourth ventricle, where it exits to the subarachnoid space via the midline foramen of Magendie and the lateral foramina of Luschka (***Figure 48.4***). CSF is reabsorbed into the arachnoid villi along the superior sagittal sinus.

Obstructive and communicating hydrocephalus

Hydrocephalus (***Figure 48.5***) almost always reflects obstruction to circulation (an obstructive hydrocephalus; ***Figure 48.6***) or failure of reabsorption (a communicating hydrocephalus; ***Figure 48.7***) (***Table 48.1***). The distinction is important since obstructive hydrocephalus especially can cause very sudden

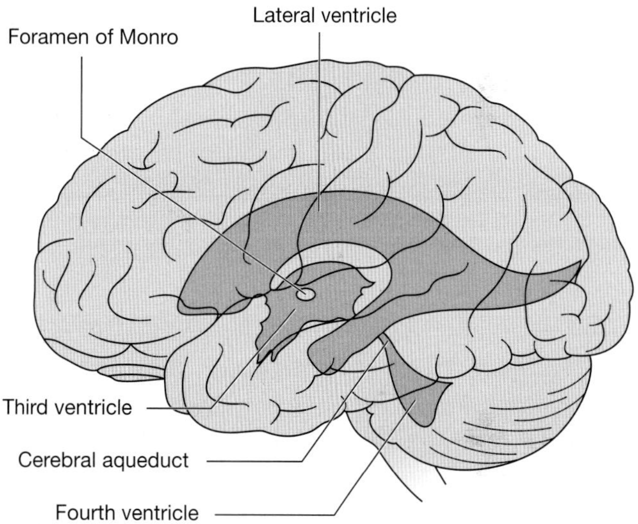

Figure 48.4 'CSF pathways'. Cerebrospinal fluid (CSF) is produced by the choroid plexus of the lateral ventricles and flows through the ventricular system to exit into the subarachnoid space through the foramina of Magendie and Luschka in the fourth ventricle.

TABLE 48.1 Aetiology of hydrocephalus.

Obstructive hydrocephalus	• Lesions within the ventricle • Lesions in the ventricular wall • Lesions distant from the ventricle but with a mass effect
Communicating hydrocephalus	• Post haemorrhagic • CSF infection • Raised CSF protein
Excessive CSF production (rare)	Choroid plexus papilloma/carcinoma

CSF, cerebrospinal fluid.

Alexander Monro, 1733–1817, Professor of Anatomy, The University of Edinburgh, Edinburgh, UK, a post also held by his father, Alexander Monro (primus), and son, Alexander Monro (tertius).

Francois Magendie, 1783–1855, Physician and Professor of Pathology and Physiology, Paris, France. Also described the Magendie sign, a downward and inward rotation of the eye due to a cerebellar lesion.

Hubert von Luschka, 1820–1875, anatomist, University of Tübingen, Tübingen, Germany.

deterioration with coma and death, and because lumbar puncture in this context carries a risk of herniation of the brainstem and cerebellar tonsils owing to the resulting differential pressure changes (sometimes termed 'coning'). For communicating hydrocephalus, lumbar puncture is of diagnostic value, deriving an opening pressure and assessment of the CSF contents. It is also therapeutic: drainage of typically between 10 and 30 mL of CSF can relieve hydrocephalus temporarily.

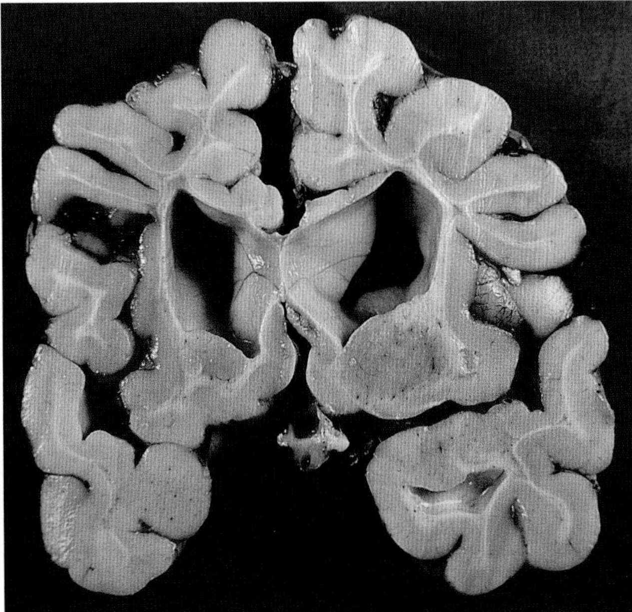

Figure 48.5 Pathological specimen of a hydrocephalic brain.

Treatment of hydrocephalus in the emergency setting usually involves CSF diversion, for example using an external ventricular drain. Disorders of CSF flow with poorly understood mechanisms manifest in two syndromes: normal pressure hydrocephalus and idiopathic intracranial hypertension (IIH).

Normal pressure hydrocephalus

Normal pressure hydrocephalus is an important cause of dementia since it is readily reversible. It may be idiopathic or develop in the context of previous brain insults, including subarachnoid haemorrhage (SAH), head injury, meningitis and tumour. The CSF pressure at lumbar puncture is typically normal, but it is believed that reduced brain compliance in this condition results in transient spikes of ICP that contribute to clinical deterioration. Patients typically present with the triad of gait disturbance, incontinence and cognitive decline. Ventriculomegaly is evident on imaging, but this can also be the result of cortical atrophy due to other dementia pathologies. Diagnosis typically depends on lumbar infusion and/or drainage studies to demonstrate altered compliance and/or clinical improvement associated with CSF drainage. Treatment is typically by insertion of a ventriculoperitoneal shunt.

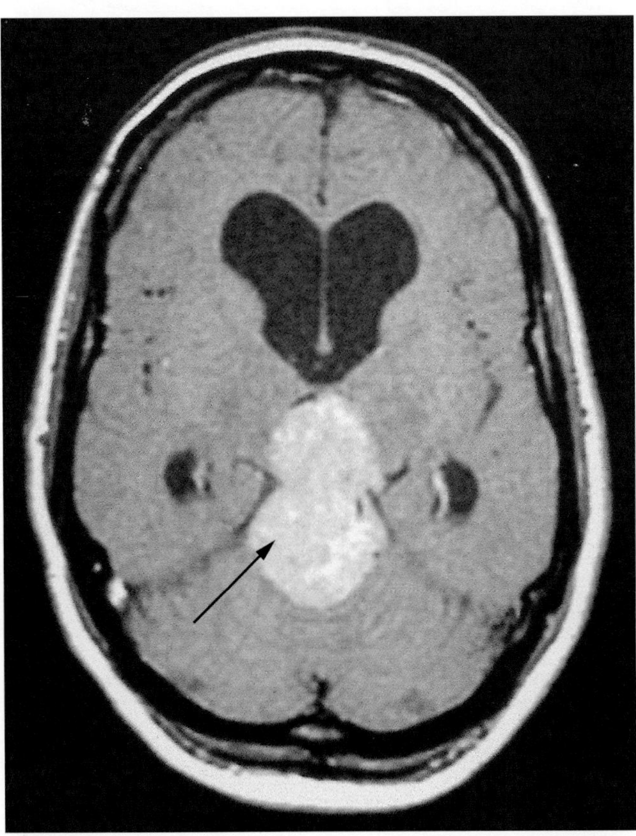

Figure 48.6 Pineal region tumour (arrow) causing obstructive hydrocephalus.

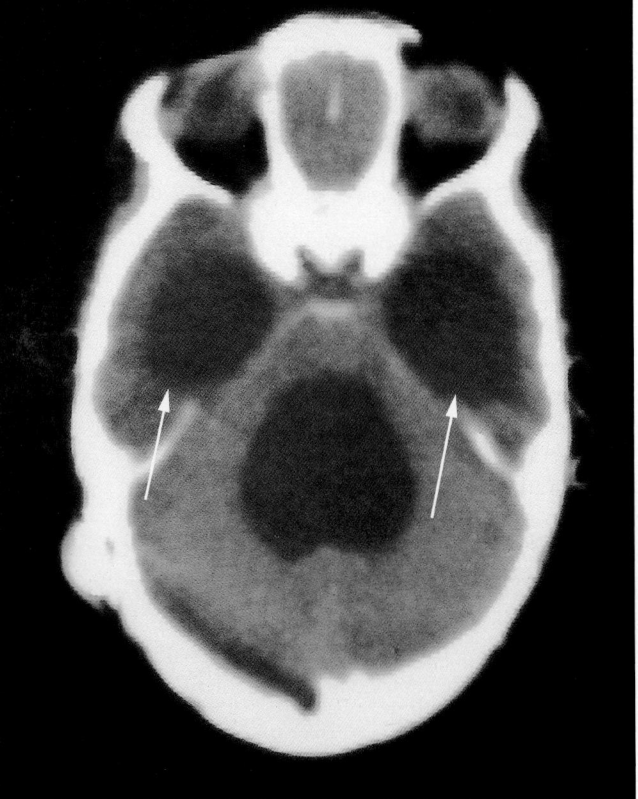

Figure 48.7 Gross hydrocephalus in a neonate with very prominent temporal horns (arrows) and fourth ventricle.

Idiopathic intracranial hypertension

Patients with IIH develop raised ICP without an underlying mass lesion. Patients are classically young overweight women with high-pressure headaches and visual deterioration. Examination may reveal papilloedema, and occasionally cranial nerve palsies. Imaging is unremarkable, but lumbar puncture demonstrates a raised opening pressure >25 mmHg. The diagnosis is one of exclusion, and the aetiology is not well understood. Impaired CSF resorption may reflect raised venous pressure, either as a result of sinus thrombosis or secondary to raised intra-abdominal pressure in obese patients. Weight loss and cessation of certain medications, including the oral contraceptive pill, is often effective. This is combined with medical therapy using acetazolamide to reduce CSF production. For patients with visual field loss or visual failure despite medication, lumboperitoneal or ventriculoperitoneal shunting is offered. There may be a role for optic nerve sheath fenestration or venous sinus stenting in select cases.

Summary box 48.2

Hydrocephalus and disorders of CSF flow

- Obstructive or communicating hydrocephalus may occur as a result of neurosurgical pathology or its treatment
- CT is the first line of investigation. Lumbar puncture can confirm raised CSF pressure in communicating hydrocephalus and relieve it temporarily, but is dangerous in obstructive hydrocephalus
- Normal pressure hydrocephalus is a potentially reversible cause of dementia, presenting with gait disturbance, incontinence and cognitive decline
- IIH causes headaches and even visual loss in young people; it can be managed with weight loss, acetazolamide, serial lumbar puncture and CSF diversion as a last resort

Treatment of hydrocephalus

Acute obstructive hydrocephalus is an emergency because of the risk of rapid progression to coma and death, sometimes with very sudden deterioration, a 'hydrocephalic attack'. It may be relieved by addressing the underlying pathology, for instance by excision of a tumour responsible for an obstructive hydrocephalus. Most often, however, temporary ventricular drainage is required as a precaution in the preoperative and perioperative period or as an emergency in an obtunded or deteriorating patient.

External ventricular drain

External ventricular drains (EVDs) are an effective temporary measure to relieve hydrocephalus. Most commonly they are inserted through a burr hole at Kocher's point (right of midline, anterior to the coronal suture), perpendicular to the brain surface, so that the catheter tip rests adjacent to the foramen of Monro in the lateral ventricle. Intrathecal antibiotics may also be delivered through the EVD. Lumbar drains are an alternative means of temporary CSF diversion.

Ventriculoperitoneal shunts

Ventriculoperitoneal shunting comprises the insertion of a proximal or ventricular catheter into the lateral ventricle, while a distal catheter is tunnelled subcutaneously to the abdomen. Ventriculoatrial, ventriculopleural and lumboperitoneal shunting are also occasionally employed. A shunt valve inserted between the proximal and distal catheters regulates flow through the system by opening at a predetermined pressure (*Figure 48.8*); the shunt valve typically incorporates a CSF reservoir, which allows for percutaneous sampling. An anti-siphon system may also be incorporated to prevent excessive drainage in the standing position. Programmable valves offer variable opening pressures, adjusted magnetically using a device applied externally over the valve.

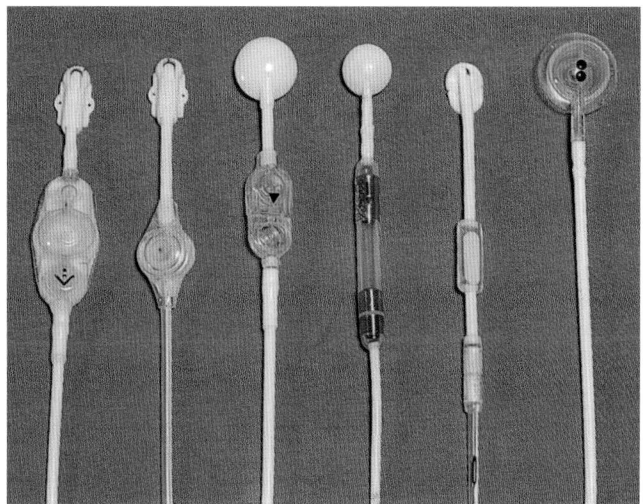

Figure 48.8 Examples of ventriculoperitoneal shunt valves.

Shunt complications

Shunts are vulnerable to disconnection, infection, blockage and overdrainage, so that 15–20% require replacement within 3 years.

Features of shunt infection typically include fever, headache and meningism; 75% of infections present within 1 month, reflecting introduction at the time of insertion. The diagnosis can be confirmed by CSF tap from the shunt reservoir or lumbar puncture if safe to do so. The shunt is removed and external ventricular drainage or serial lumbar punctures instituted to cover a course of antibiotic therapy. Once CSF sampling confirms resolution of the infection and a normal protein concentration, a shunt can be inserted at a new site.

Patients with blocked shunts present clinical features of hydrocephalus, which can be confirmed on CT, and the shunt reservoir may be difficult to compress or refill only slowly. The majority of blockages are attributable to cellular and proteinaceous debris, especially due to infection, but choroid plexus adhesion, blood clot or failure of the valve mechanism may also be responsible. In the context of obstructive and congenital

Emil Theodor Kocher, 1841–1917, Professor of Surgery, Berne, Switzerland. In 1909, he was awarded the Nobel Prize in Physiology or Medicine for his work on the thyroid.

hydrocephalus especially, shunt blockage is an emergency because of the potential for rapid deterioration owing to uncontrolled rises in ICP.

Overdrainage can result in low-pressure headaches, which are typically worse on standing. Collapse of the ventricles can cause accumulation of fluid or blood in the subdural space, resulting in subdural hygroma or subdural haematoma. The slit ventricle syndrome describes the situation in children treated with shunts, whose ventricles and subarachnoid spaces are underdeveloped, resulting in poor brain compliance. In these patients normal fluctuations in ICP are exaggerated so that coughing and straining may cause symptoms of raised ICP. Any shunt blockage may not be evident on scan as the ventricles fail to enlarge.

Endoscopic third ventriculostomy

This procedure is especially useful in obstructive hydrocephalus due to aqueduct stenosis. A neuroendoscope is inserted into the frontal horn of the lateral ventricle and then into the third ventricle via the foramen of Monro. The floor of the ventricle is then opened between the mamillary bodies and the pituitary recess. Free drainage between the third ventricle and the adjacent subarachnoid cisterns is then possible, without the infection risk posed by implanted tubing. Reblockage of this route is common, however, and many patients will subsequently require a shunt. Rare but serious complications include damage to the basilar artery or forniceal damage, resulting in permanent memory impairment.

Summary box 48.3

Treating hydrocephalus

- Temporary CSF diversion can be achieved with an EVD
- In the long term a shunt, usually connecting the lateral ventricles with the peritoneal cavity in the abdomen (ventriculoperitoneal shunt), is the mainstay of management
- Shunt blockage and infection are common complications
- In certain cases, obstructive hydrocephalus can be managed by endoscopic third ventriculostomy

INTRACRANIAL INFECTION

Meningitis

Meningitis describes inflammation of the meninges of the brain and spinal cord, most commonly and most seriously due to bacterial infection. The clinical features of meningeal irritation or meningism are fever, headache, neck stiffness and photophobia. Community-acquired bacterial meningitis can progress rapidly without antibiotic treatment to subpial encephalopathy, venous thrombosis, cerebral oedema and death. Meningitis as a complication of head injury or surgery typically follows a more insidious course, but nonetheless remains a feared complication requiring prompt intervention.

TABLE 48.2 Principles of central nervous system antibiotic therapy.

- Treatment should be initiated as soon as feasible, allowing for sampling of collections or CSF first if the patient's clinical condition allows
- High-dose empirical intravenous antibiotics are administered according to local protocol, broad spectrum initially and then according to sensitivities of the organisms responsible once identified
- Extended treatment over 6 weeks or more is typically required, but a switch to oral therapy may be appropriate after an interval and in consultation with the microbiology team

Typical organisms are *Staphylococcus aureus*, Enterobacteriaceae, *Pseudomonas* and pneumococci.

Meningitis after head injury is common, affecting 25% of patients with base of skull fracture and CSF leak. Repair of the CSF leak may be required, and empirical antibiotics (***Table 48.2***) should have activity against commensal nasal organisms, including Gram-positive cocci and Gram-negative bacilli in the presence of symptoms/signs of clinical meningitis.

Summary box 48.4

Meningitis

- A feared complication of neurosurgery and of head injury
- CT head allows exclusion of raised ICP prior to lumbar puncture
- CSF should be sent for microscopy and culture, and for assay of protein and glucose levels
- Treatment, pending identification of an organism, is with broad -spectrum antibiotics, including anaerobic cover

Brain abscess and empyema

Abscesses arise when the brain is exposed directly, for example as a result of fracture or infection of an air sinus, or at surgery. They also result from haematogenous spread, typically in association with respiratory and dental infections or endocarditis. In 25% of cases, no underlying primary infection is found. The organisms involved are normally bacteria, but immunocompromised hosts in particular are vulnerable to a broad range of pathogens (***Table 48.3***).

Typical presenting features include low-grade fever, confusion, seizures and focal deficit, often with equivocal blood markers of inflammation; blood cultures should be obtained at an early stage. CT scan with contrast is the initial imaging modality of choice. Hypodense oedematous brain representing early cerebritis is visible in the first few days (***Figure 48.9***). The classic appearances of a smooth-walled, well-defined, ring-enhancing mass develop as the abscess matures (***Figure 48.10***). The distinction between abscess and tumour can be difficult and has important management implications since abscesses generally require urgent drainage. Restricted diffusion evident

Hans Christian Joachim Gram, 1853–1938, Professor of Pharmacology (1891–1900) and of Medicine (1900–1923), Copenhagen, Denmark, described this method of staining bacteria in 1884.

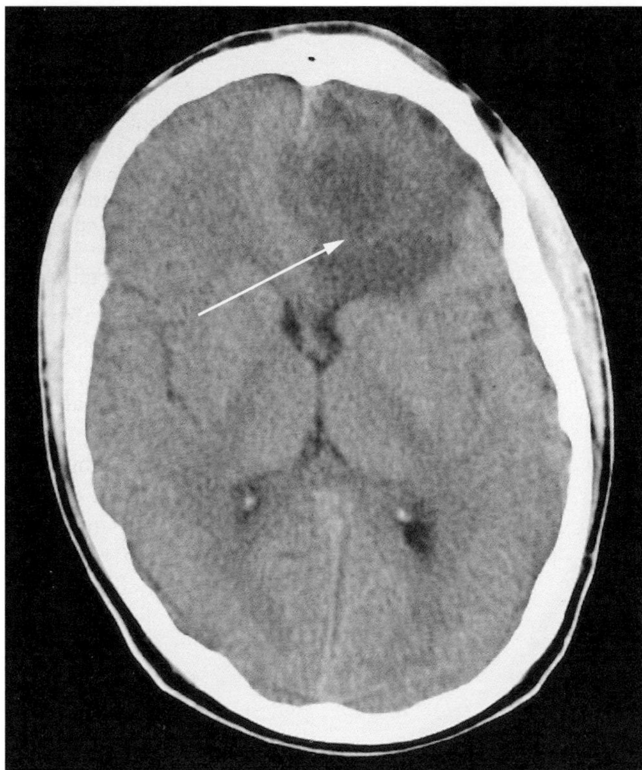

Figure 48.9 Axial computed tomography scan with contrast of a patient with frontal sinusitis presenting with seizures. Early cerebritis is evident in the left frontal region (arrow).

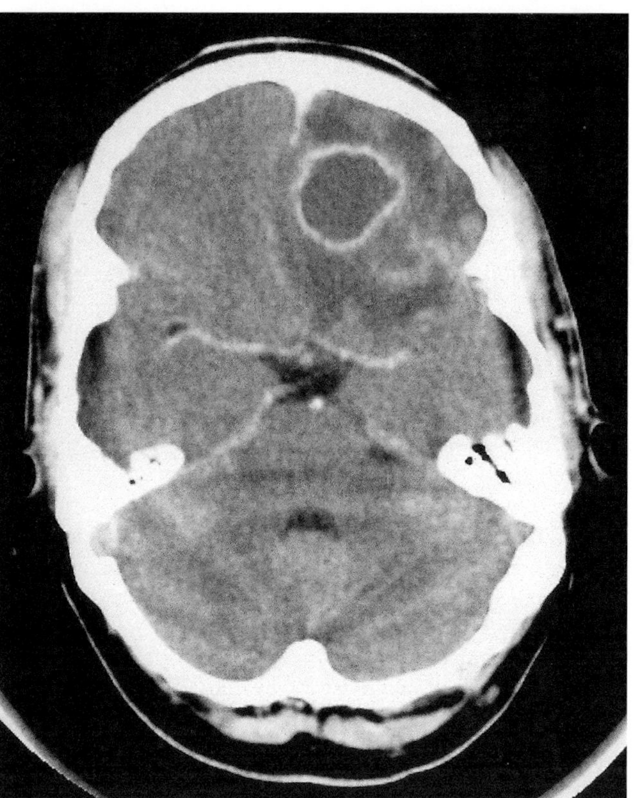

Figure 48.10 Axial computed tomography scan with contrast in the same patient as in Figure 48.9 2 weeks later. A ring-enhancing, smooth-walled lesion is evident; this is an abscess suitable for image-guided drainage.

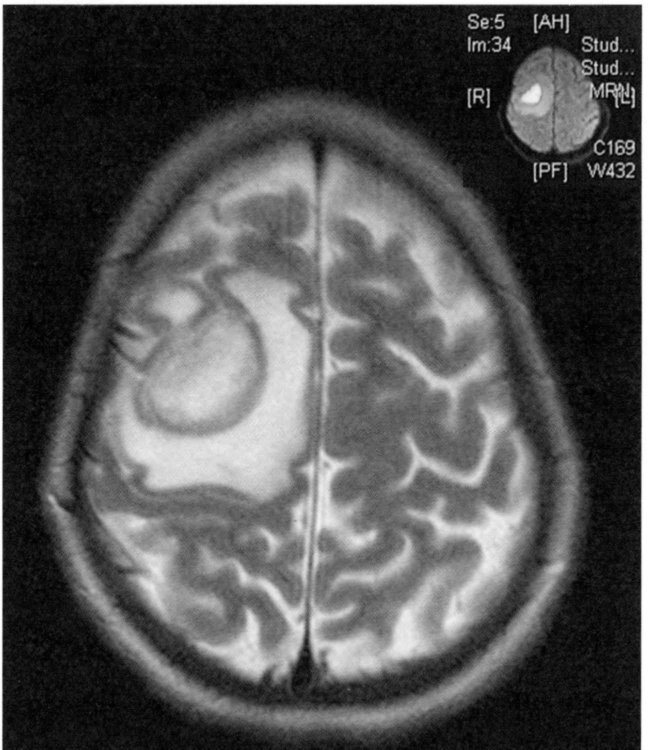

Figure 48.11 The right frontal lesion evident on T2-weighted magnetic resonance imaging (MRI) (main image) exhibits high signal on diffusion-weighted MRI sequences (top right inset) indicative of brain abscess.

on diffusion-weighted MRI sequences is a valuable indicator of infective pathology (*Figure 48.11*).

The mainstay of abscess management is early surgical drainage: mortality for patients treated in this way is about 4%, whereas it is greater than 80% in cases of ventriculitis due to rupture of an abscess into the ventricles. Up to 50% of patients with brain abscess will develop seizures at some stage, so that prophylactic anticonvulsants should be considered.

TABLE 48.3 Common causative organisms.

Condition	Organisms
Sinus/mastoid infection	Streptococci; *Bacteroides*; enterobacteria; staphylococci; *Pseudomonas*
Haematogenous spread	*Bacteroides*; streptococci
Penetrating trauma	*Staphylococcus aureus*; *Clostridium*; *Bacillus*; enterobacteria
Food contamination	*Toxoplasma*; pork tapeworm (neurocysticercosis)
Immunocompromise	HIV; *Toxoplasma* (protozoal); *Cryptococcus* (fungal); JC virus

HIV, human immunodeficiency virus; JC, John Cunningham.

Summary box 48.5

Brain abscesses

- Presenting features are those of infection and intracranial mass lesion
- Imaging reveals a 'ring-enhancing lesion', with tumour usually the main differential
- Early diagnosis, usually followed by drainage, is key for good outcome

Subdural empyema

Subdural empyema refers to an infected fluid collection in the subdural space. This may develop as a result of sinusitis, mastoiditis or meningitis, and can complicate trauma or surgery. ***Figure 48.12*** shows a subdural empyema associated with osteomyelitis of the frontal bone and associated scalp swelling – Pott's puffy tumour. In empyema, pus will generally collect in the parafalcine region and over the convexity, triggering inflammation and thrombosis in the cortical veins, which helps to explain the high mortality of 8–12%. Presentation mimics that of meningitis and cerebral abscess; typical CT appearances are of hypodense or isodense subdural collection, with contrast enhancement at the margins and often swelling and midline shift.

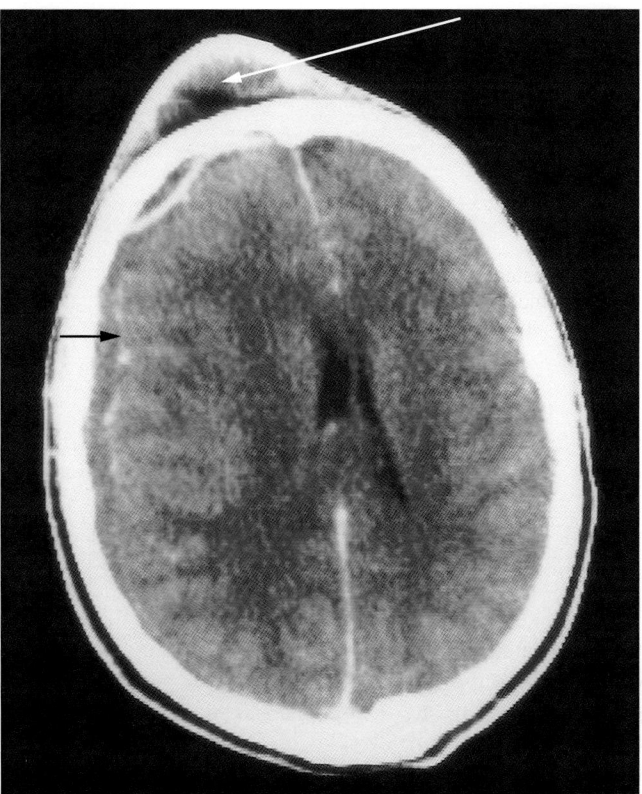

Figure 48.12 Axial computed tomography scan with contrast showing a right hemisphere subdural empyema (short arrow) and a right frontal Pott's puffy tumour (long arrow) (osteomyelitis of the frontal bone).

Summary box 48.6

Subdural empyema

- Presenting features are similar to those of meningitis or cerebral abscess
- Typically a crescentic collection with a contrast-enhancing rim is evident on CT
- Drainage is the mainstay of treatment

Tuberculosis

Tuberculosis (TB) infection of the central nervous system (CNS) represents haematogenous spread from primary pulmonary foci. A high index of suspicion is required, especially when population or individual risk factors are present. TB can result in a diverse but overlapping spectrum of pathology, including in the head:

- tuberculous meningitis – this commonly affects young children; CT demonstrates intense meningeal enhancement and hydrocephalus is a common complication;
- tuberculoma – discrete tumour-like granulomas at the base of the cerebral hemispheres, presenting with mass effect;
- tuberculous abscess – seen predominantly in immunocompromised hosts, this represents progression of a tuberculoma with prominent central caseating necrosis;
- miliary tuberculosis – describes a diffuse distribution of multiple small tuberculomas throughout the brain substance.

Where the meninges are involved, lymphocytes can be expected to predominate in the CSF, rather than the polymorphs seen with other bacterial meningitides. The increase in protein content and reduction in glucose concentration are also less marked. Ziehl–Neelsen staining for mycobacteria is frequently negative, and polymerase chain reaction (PCR) testing offers relatively rapid diagnosis compared with culture for acid-fast bacilli, which may take weeks. A 20- to 30-mL CSF sample allows spinning to increase the culture yield. Management is with antituberculous therapy; hydrocephalus may require shunt insertion.

VASCULAR NEUROSURGERY

Subarachnoid haemorrhage

'Spontaneous' SAH is usually the result of bleeding from a ruptured aneurysm (approximately 80% of SAH) or an arteriovenous malformation (AVM). Most ruptured aneurysms are located in the circle of Willis, at branch points in the arterial

Percival Pott, 1714–1788, surgeon, St Bartholomew's Hospital, London, UK. Besides the 'puffy tumour', described in 1760, Pott established the first association between a cancer and an environmental carcinogen, when he noted the high incidence of (squamous cell) scrotal cancers in chimney sweeps.
Franz Ziehl, 1857–1926, German bacteriologist and professor in Lübeck, Germany.
Friedrich Carl Adolf Neelsen, 1854–1894, German pathologist and professor at the Institute of Pathology, University of Rostock, Germany.

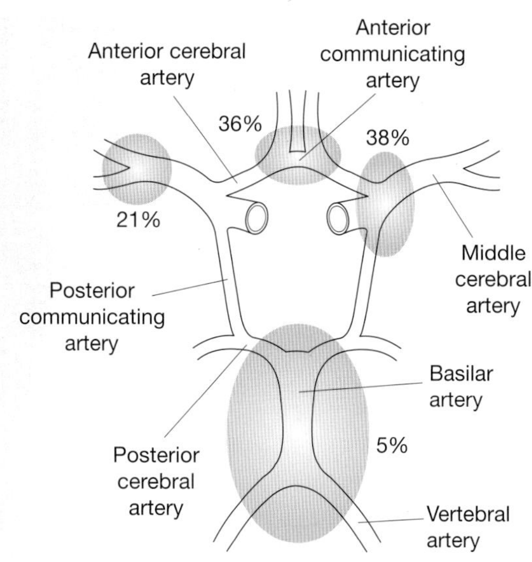

Figure 48.13 Common sites of aneurysm in the circle of Willis.

tree associated with turbulent blood flow (*Figure 48.13*). A distinct subgroup of patients with SAH suffer bleeds confined to the basal cisterns anterior to the midbrain and pons, without an underlying lesion evident on angiogram. This is termed perimesencephalic SAH, is believed to represent venous bleeding and has an excellent prognosis. Aneurysms may also develop as a result of infective infiltration of arterial walls in the context of bacteraemia (mycotic aneurysm), often in the setting of intravenous drug use or infective endocarditis. Pseudoaneurysms may also develop after trauma or after surgery.

Aneurysmal bleeding has an incidence of 10–15 per 100 000 population per year. Risk factors include age, female sex, hypertension, smoking, cocaine abuse and a family history with two first-degree relatives affected. A range of genetic disorders, in particular adult polycystic kidney disease, fibromuscular dysplasia, neurofibromatosis type 1, Ehlers–Danlos and Marfan syndrome, are known to predispose patients to this condition.

History and examination

The typical presentation of an SAH includes a 'thunderclap' headache, which is both sudden and severe and is outside the patient's normal experience. Some patients describe prodromal headaches preceding the event, potentially representing aneurysm growth or subclinical bleeds. The sudden onset occurs commonly but not exclusively during exertion, and may be associated with seizure (10%), unresponsiveness (50%) and vomiting (70%). Sometimes it is difficult to establish whether SAH has caused a fall or a fall with head injury is responsible for the SAH. Approximately one-third of SAHs are incorrectly diagnosed at initial presentation. Patients are then at high risk of succumbing to early complications, especially a rebleed.

Neurological examination may be normal ('good clinical grade') or the patient may have focal deficits and an impaired conscious level ('poor grade'). The World Federation of Neurosurgical Societies (WFNS) grading of SAH is measured against the condition of the patient after resuscitation rather than at the time of ictus (*Table 48.4*). A painful third nerve palsy is typically the result of compression from a posterior communicating artery aneurysm. Meningitic features of neck stiffness and photophobia often develop over hours. Intraocular haemorrhages, classically subhyaloid, may be visible on fundoscopy. The combination of SAH and vitreous haemorrhage is known as Terson's syndrome and occurs in 15–20% of patients. Papilloedema should be sought, but may not be evident early in the course of a developing hydrocephalus.

Investigation

CT scan is the imaging of first choice; when performed within 12 hours of ictus, it will confirm bleeding in more than 98% of cases. This makes a diagnostic lumbar puncture unnecessary (*Figure 48.14*).

TABLE 48.4 World Federation of Neurosurgical Societies (WFNS) grading of subarachnoid haemorrhage.

Grade	Glasgow Coma Scale	Focal deficits[a]
I	15	–
II	13–14	–
III	13–14	+
IV	7–12	±
V	3–9	±

[a]Focal deficit = dysphasia or limb weakness.

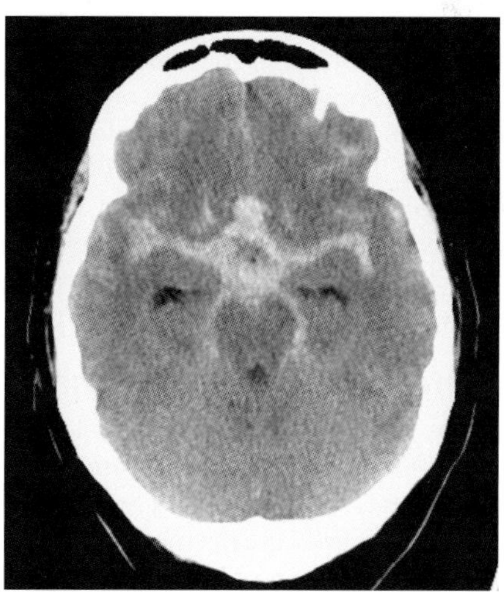

Figure 48.14 Diffuse subarachnoid bleeding from a ruptured anterior communicating artery aneurysm extends to the prepontine and ambient cisterns around the brainstem and into both Sylvian fissures.

Thomas Willis, 1621–1675, Sedleian Professor of Natural Philosophy at Oxford. Also the first anatomist to number the cranial nerves in the order used today.
Edward Ehlers, 1863–1937, Professor of Clinical Dermatology, Copenhagen, Denmark.
Henri Alexandre Danlos, 1844–1912, dermatologist, Hôpital St Louis, Paris, France, gave his account of this condition in 1908.
Bernard Jean Antonin Marfan, 1858–1942, physician L'Hôpital des Enfants-Malades, Paris, France, described this syndrome in 1896.
Albert Terson, 1867–1935, French ophthalmologist.
Franciscus Sylvius, 1614–1672, a Dutch physician, chemist, physiologist and anatomist.

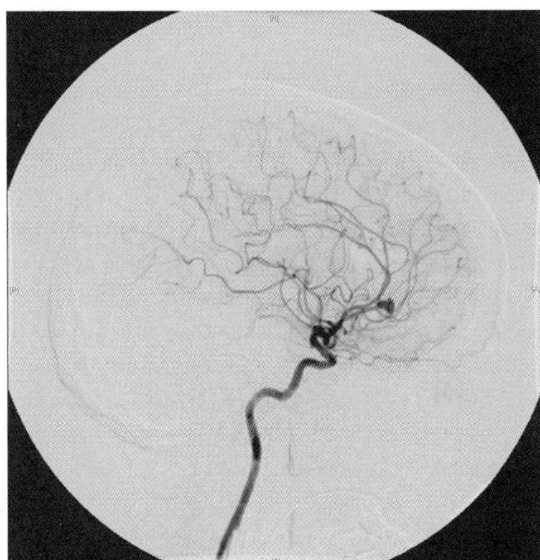

Figure 48.15 There is a small saccular aneurysm of the pericallosal branch of the anterior cerebral artery.

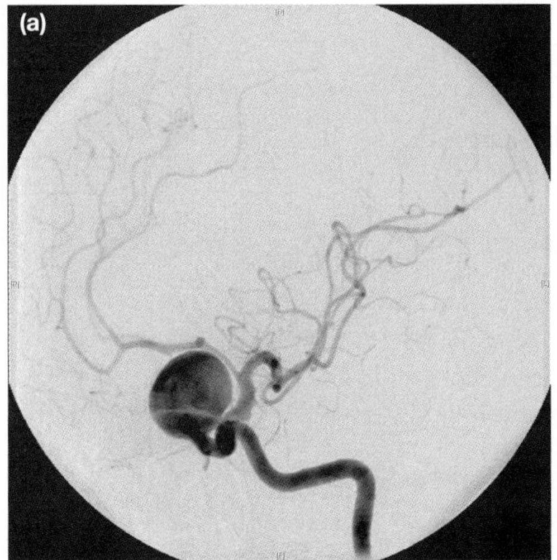

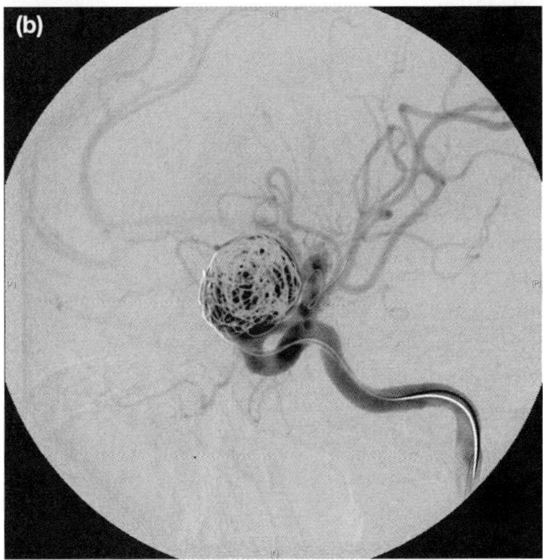

Figure 48.16 (a) A giant aneurysm of the internal carotid artery. (b) Angiographic embolisation (coiling) of the giant aneurysm. Note the single displaced coil passing into the distal internal carotid artery and then the middle cerebral artery.

The sensitivity of CT scan, however, deteriorates to less than 50% at 1 week after a bleed. In light of this, patients with a suggestive history and negative CT scan will require lumbar puncture, especially where presentation is delayed. The CSF supernatant should be analysed by spectrophotometry (visual inspection is not reliable) for the spectra of haemoglobin breakdown products oxyhaemoglobin and bilirubin. These are present in samples taken at least 6 and preferably 12 hours after SAH, but not in CSF mixed with fresh blood due to traumatic puncture and analysed immediately. Failure to exclude SAH with an adequate lumbar puncture sample can result in diagnostic confusion and overtreatment.

Aneurysms can be visualised by CT and magnetic resonance angiography, but the gold standard remains digital subtraction angiography (DSA), which involves access to both vertebral and carotid arteries through the femoral artery under local anaesthetic. This allows visualisation of the vascular anatomy by injection of contrast medium with simultaneous radiographic screening (***Figure 48.15***). The serious potential risks include ischaemic stroke or arterial dissection (1–2%), and renal failure or allergic reactions attributable to contrast.

Surgical/interventional management

Aneurysms may be removed from the circulation surgically by craniotomy and 'clipping' or by endovascular embolisation, also known as 'coiling' (***Figure 48.16***). Sometimes mesh stents may also be used to help secure the metal coils within the aneurysm sac as part of this procedure. Class 1 evidence suggests that coiling has slightly better outcomes where feasible, but clipping remains necessary or preferable in many cases; these decisions are shared between surgeons, radiologists and the patient. A rebleed risk of 4% in the first 24 hours then 1.5% per day thereafter is quoted for untreated aneurysms; 80% of patients who rebleed have an eventual poor outcome. For this reason, and to permit optimal management of vasospasm, the current consensus favours early intervention, despite the surgical challenges presented by brain swelling and blood load.

Unruptured aneurysms represent a thorny management problem: incidentally detected small anterior circulation aneurysms represent a minimal bleeding risk. Screening, even in high-risk groups, is therefore of questionable benefit.

Medical management

Patients should be placed on bed rest with hourly neuro-observations. They require strict input–output monitoring and intravenous fluid replacement with normal saline initially. Oral nimodipine at a dose of 60 mg every 4 hours is administered to reduce the incidence of vasospasm and delayed ischaemic neurological deficit. Analgesics, laxatives, antiemetics, gastric protection and compression stockings are also likely to be necessary. After resuscitation, the priorities in SAH are to:

1 prevent rebleeding by identifying and controlling any underlying lesion;
2 recognise and manage:
   - neurological complications, especially vasospasm, delayed ischaemic neurological deficit and hydrocephalus;

- systemic complications, including electrolyte imbalance, severe hypertension, cardiac infarct and arrhythmia, and neurogenic pulmonary oedema.

These goals are best served by early transfer of the patient to a neurosurgical centre. In elderly patients with a poor WFNS grade, a decision to offer only supportive management may be appropriate.

Neurological deterioration should prompt a repeat scan to exclude evidence of rebleeding and of hydrocephalus. This is typically the communicating type, which is a common complication of haemorrhage. Where these complications are not demonstrated, deterioration may reflect delayed ischaemic neurological deficit (DNID), which commonly develops 3–10 days after aneurysmal haemorrhage and can progress rapidly to infarction. The process is attributed to cerebral vasospasm in response to, and correlating with, the blood load. This process can be visualised angiographically or by perfusion CT, and the velocity of blood flow in the cerebral vasculature measured using transcranial Doppler ultrasound can also provide an indirect assessment of the degree of stenosis. Outcomes are optimised by the prophylactic administration of nimodipine and maintenance of fluid volume, typically with 2.5–3 L/day of normal saline. In established vasospasm, the goal is to maintain cerebral perfusion by administration of fluid and inotropes.

Hyponatraemia is a frequent complication of SAH, attributed to cerebral salt wasting in the context of fluid depletion and to the syndrome of inappropriate antidiuretic hormone secretion otherwise. This is associated with a higher incidence of DNID; practical management, irrespective of the underlying pathology, is based on sodium replacement with hypertonic infusions if necessary. Fluid restriction is not appropriate in these patients since this risks further compromising perfusion.

Summary box 48.7

Subarachnoid haemorrhage

- Most result from rupture of an aneurysm in the circle of Willis
- Plain CT and lumbar puncture are first-line investigations
- Even 'good grade' patients treated promptly have a significant morbidity owing to vasospasm, cardiac arrhythmias, neurogenic pulmonary oedema, etc.

Intracerebral haemorrhage

Intracerebral haemorrhage (ICH) typically presents with sudden focal deficit and a reduced conscious level. Following initial resuscitation, these patients will require CT scan to establish the diagnosis and the size and position of the bleed (***Figure 48.17***). They require reversal of anticoagulation, ongoing hourly neuro-observations and blood pressure monitoring. High blood pressure may be longstanding and associated with adaptations to autoregulation, so attempts at lowering it acutely with intravenous antihypertensives should be made only if the values are very high (e.g. mean arterial pressure >130 mmHg).

Spontaneous ICH accounts for 10–15% of strokes and has a mortality of 40% at 1 year. The majority occur in the context of hypertension or amyloid angiopathy, or as a complication of ischaemic stroke. Coagulation disorders, especially patients being treated with warfarin, are a major risk factor. In younger patients and where the pattern of bleeding is atypical, dedicated imaging to rule out an underlying vascular anomaly or tumour is required. For example it is critically important to identify ICH due to aneurysm rupture or AVM before considering surgical intervention.

Craniotomy and evacuation may be used to alleviate raised ICP. Importantly this surgery may be life-saving by relieving raised ICP but cannot reverse deficits resulting from the haematoma directly. Surgical evacuation would typically be a good option for younger, fitter patients with signs of raised ICP and haematomas close to the cortical surface or in the posterior fossa.

Summary box 48.8

Intracerebral haemorrhage

- These account for 10–15% of strokes
- Presentation is with headache, focal deficits and signs of raised ICP
- High blood pressure may be chronic so should only be reduced with care
- Anticoagulants should be reversed
- In fit patients, clot evacuation is an option to relieve raised ICP but not reverse deficits
- Further imaging may be required to exclude an underlying vascular or neoplastic lesion

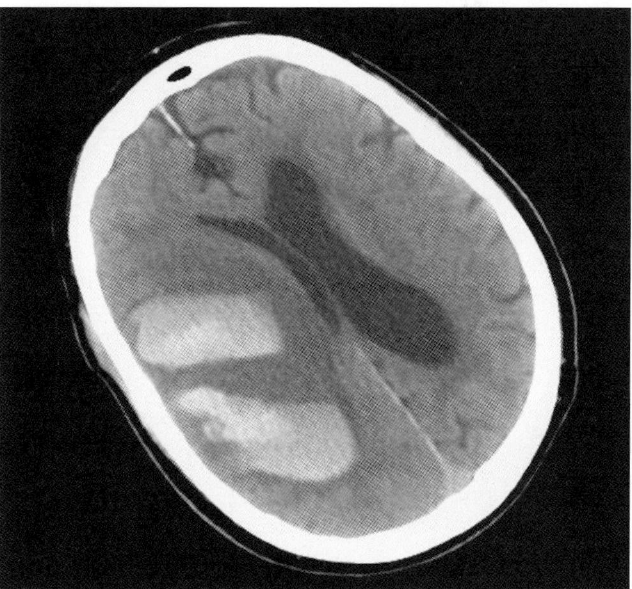

Figure 48.17 Large acute intracerebral haemorrhages in the right frontal and parietal lobes are evident, with surrounding oedema and midline shift.

Christian Johann Doppler, 1803–1853, Professor of Experimental Physics, Vienna, Austria, enunciated the 'Doppler principle' in 1842.

Vascular malformations

Vascular malformations are usually congenital in origin, with certain key exceptions discussed below. They may present with headaches, pulsatile tinnitus, seizures or focal deficit, or else acutely with rupture and haemorrhage.

AVMs are responsible for a small proportion of SAHs and ICHs. Vessels and calcification may be apparent on CT or MRI and the lesion is confirmed on angiography (***Figure 48.18***).

Depending on the size, location and venous drainage patterns, surgery or radiosurgery are usually preferred treatment options. In some cases endovascular embolisation with tissue glue may have a role, and for many AVMs there is no treatment with a satisfactory risk–benefit ratio.

Vein of Galen malformations are AVMs feeding into an embryological venous remnant dorsal to the brainstem, presenting in childhood. High-flow malformations may cause cardiac failure. They may be treated by embolisation.

Dural arteriovenous fistulae (DAVFs) are shunts between dural arteries and veins or sinuses. They are proposed to arise as a result of vessel remodelling in response to dural sinus thrombosis and subsequent recanalisation. They may present with subarachnoid, intracerebral or subdural bleeding, or with headache and pulsatile tinnitus. A carotid cavernous fistula is a spontaneous or traumatic DAVF between the internal carotid artery and surrounding cavernous sinus, typically producing eye pain, ocular muscle palsies and exophthalmos. Angiography is diagnostic.

Cavernomas (***Figure 48.19***) are discrete venous anomalies within brain tissue, visible on MRI but not angiography, that can bleed repeatedly, causing progressive deficit. They can be removed surgically if required.

Related lesions, usually clinically silent, include developmental venous anomalies and capillary telangiectasia.

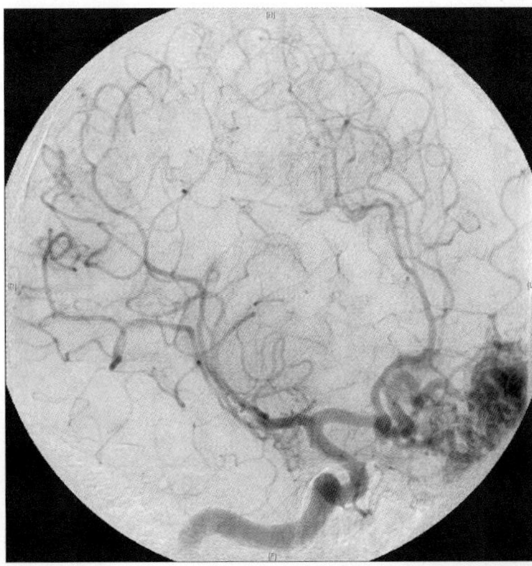

Figure 48.18 An arteriovenous malformation supplied by the anterior cerebral, middle cerebral and middle meningeal arteries is demonstrated at the 4 o'clock position in this angiogram.

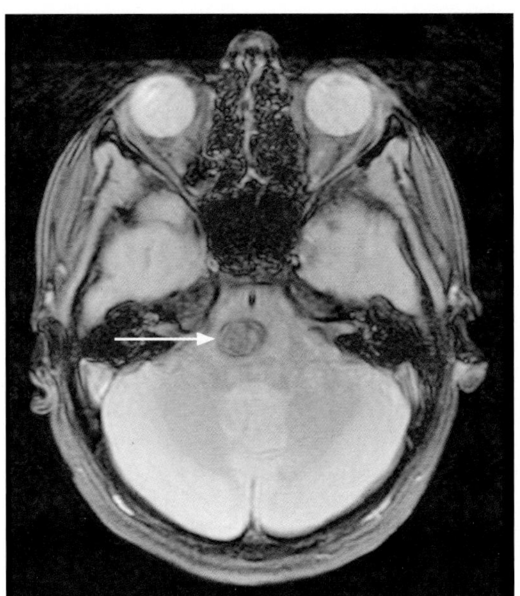

Figure 48.19 A brainstem cavernoma (arrow).

Neurosurgery in occlusive vascular disease

In a subgroup of patients with completed ischaemic strokes, generally in the middle cerebral artery territory or posterior fossa, there is a role for decompressive craniectomy in the 2–3 days after ictus to manage brain swelling and raised ICP associated with the infarct.

There is class 1 evidence for the role of carotid endarterectomy in reducing the risk of stroke in patients with symptomatic carotid stenosis, and a debatable role for the procedure in patients with no previous transient ischaemic episodes.

Moyamoya disease entails the progressive obliteration of one or both internal carotid arteries, thought to represent an autoimmune process. The development of external carotid circulation collaterals produces the angiographic 'puff of smoke' appearance from which the term derives. It presents in youth or early middle age with ischaemia or haemorrhage. Untreated, the majority of patients suffer major deficit or die within 2 years. Ischaemia may be addressed by a variety of bypass techniques, for example by anastomosing the superficial temporal artery (arising from the external carotid) to the middle cerebral artery.

BRAIN TUMOURS

The term 'brain tumour' applies to more than 100 distinct pathologies detailed in the World Health Organization (WHO) classification. Many are malignant, but even histologically benign tumours may carry a grave prognosis when they encroach on key structures that also limit surgical access. The commonest brain tumour is a metastasis. Primary brain

Galen, 130–200, Roman physician, commenced practice as Surgeon to the Gladiators at Pergamum (now Bergama in Turkey) and later became personal physician to the Emperor Marcus Aurelius and to two of his successors. He was a prolific writer on many subjects, among them anatomy, medicine, pathology and philosophy. His work affected medical thinking for 15 centuries after his death. (Gladiator is Latin for 'swordsman'.)

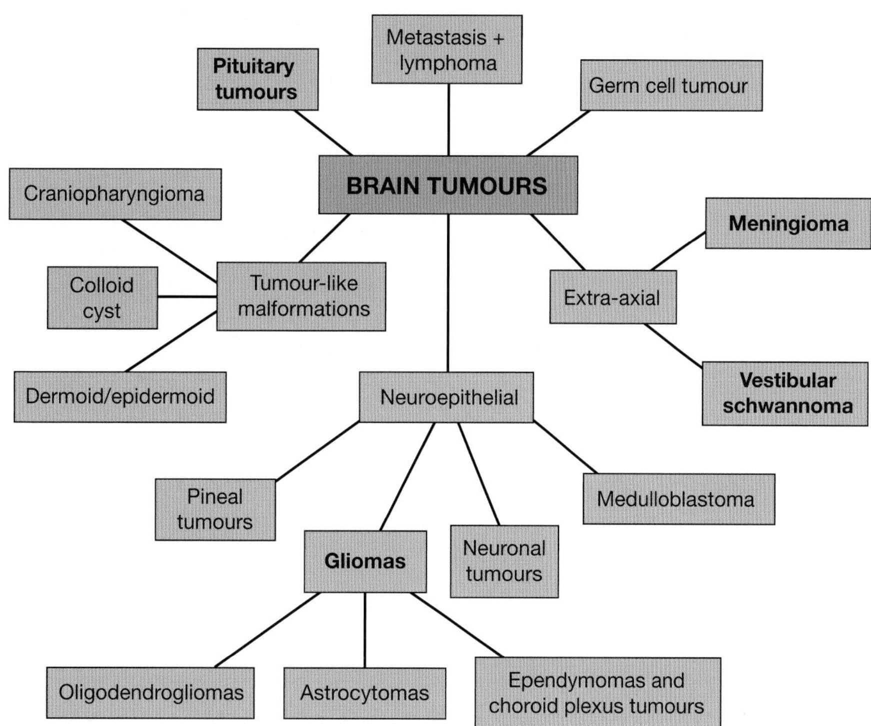

Figure 48.20 Brain tumour classification. A simplified schema encompassing some of the key brain tumour categories. Highlighted in bold are the pathologies discussed in more detail in this chapter.

tumours represent 1.5% of all cancers, with an incidence of 19 per 100 000 person-years. Nevertheless many, especially glial, tumours present commonly in younger age groups and are incurable, so that they are a leading cause of life-years lost to cancer.

Classification

WHO classifies primary brain tumours on the basis of cell of origin and histological grade (***Figure 48.20***), with the 2016 edition including a number of additional molecular classifications assigned in parallel to constitute an 'integrated' diagnosis.

Common adult primary brain tumours include gliomas, meningiomas (15–20% of total), pituitary adenomas (10–15% of total) and vestibular schwannomas.

Grade I is applied to 'benign' lesions, while grade IV implies high-grade malignancy.

Aetiology

The common primary brain tumours mentioned above mostly occur sporadically. There is no proven risk due to environmental factors, except for radiation exposure, but germline genetic syndromes may also predispose (***Table 48.5***).

TABLE 48.5 Chromosomal abnormalities associated with brain tumours.

Syndrome	Gene defect	Tumour
Neurofibromatosis type 1	*Neurofibromin* (chromosome 17)	Astrocytomas; neurofibromas
Neurofibromatosis type 2	*Schwannomin* (chromosome 22)	Acoustic neuromas (bilateral); meningiomas
Cowden's disease	*PTEN* (chromosome 10)	Astrocytomas
Hereditary non-polyposis colorectal cancer	Multiple	Astrocytomas
Li–Fraumeni syndrome	*p53* (chromosome 17)	Astrocytomas

PTEN, phosphatase and tensin homologue.

Presentation

Most tumours present with one or more features belonging to three cardinal categories: these are seizure, raised ICP and focal neurological deficit. Pituitary adenomas may also present with endocrine disturbance.

Theodor Schwann, 1810–1882, Professor of Anatomy, Louvain and Liège, Belgium. German physiologist who established the cellular basis of differentiated tissues including feathers.

One of the few clinical syndromes named for the patient rather than the clinician. **Rachel Cowden** was, in 1963, the first patient described with the syndrome. She died from breast cancer at the age of 20.

Frederick Pei Li, 1940–2015, Professor of Medicine, Harvard University Medical School, Boston, MA, USA.

Joseph F Fraumeni, b. 1933, Director of Cancer Epidemiology and Genetics, The National Cancer Institute, Bethesda, MD, USA.

Seizures

Seizures are a common presenting feature, especially of low-grade gliomas arising in the cortical hemispheres. Simple partial seizures, involving focal twitching or similar with preserved consciousness, are the rule, but temporal location will commonly produce complex partial seizures, and any seizure may progress to a secondary generalised tonic–clonic fit.

Patients who have had a seizure should be started on an antiepileptic drug, typically levetiracetam. Routine prophylaxis in patients with tumours who have no history of seizures is not recommended, although a short course at the time of craniotomy for tumour excision may be warranted.

Raised intracranial pressure

Headache is a presenting feature in only about 50% of patients. It is classically worse in the morning and on straining (high-pressure features) and is accompanied by nausea and vomiting. Pressure effects develop as a result of the tumour mass effect and surrounding oedema, especially in fast-growing metastases and high-grade gliomas (see main section on ***Raised intracranial pressure***). After excluding the possibility of brain abscess (see ***Brain abscess and empyema***), the mass effect is controlled initially using high-dose glucocorticoids (e.g. dexamethasone) and, especially in the case of posterior fossa tumours, early external ventricular drainage may be required to treat obstructive hydrocephalus.

Focal neurological deficit

A focal deficit that is progressive over time, as opposed to the sudden onset of a vascular accident, is suspicious of tumour. Lesions in specific locations can produce characteristic patterns of deficit due to compression of local structures (***Table 48.6***).

TABLE 48.6 Patterns of deficit generally associated with certain tumours.

Tumour location	Expected deficit
Pituitary (e.g. pituitary adenoma)	Bitemporal hemianopia; gaze palsies
Cerebellopontine angle (e.g. vestibular schwannoma)	Hearing loss; balance disturbance; tinnitus
Anterior skull base (e.g. olfactory groove meningioma)	Anosmia; ipsilateral optic atrophy; contralateral papilloedema (Foster Kennedy syndrome)
Occipital (e.g. glioma, metastasis)	Homonymous hemianopia with central sparing
Parietal (dominant hemisphere)	Acalculia; agraphia; left–right disorientation; finger agnosia (Gerstmann's syndrome)
Parietal (e.g. glioma)	Sensory inattention; dressing apraxia; astereognosis
Temporal (e.g. glioma)	Memory disturbance; contralateral superior quadrantanopia; dysphasia (dominant hemisphere)
Frontal (e.g. glioma)	Personality change; gait disturbance; urinary incontinence
Brainstem (e.g. brainstem glioma)	Multiple cranial nerve deficits; long tract signs; nystagmus
Posterior fossa (e.g. medulloblastoma)	Ataxia; hydrocephalus

Summary box 48.9

Brain tumours

Most brain tumours will present with one or more features related to the following triad:

- Raised ICP
- Seizures
- Focal deficit

Common brain tumours

Cerebral metastases

Cerebral metastases (***Figure 48.21***) are the most common intracranial tumours and are diagnosed in 25% of patients with cancer, a proportion that is increasing with extended survival associated with more effective treatment of primary cancers. The tumours of origin and their contribution to the burden of cerebral metastases are detailed in ***Table 48.7***. Traditionally

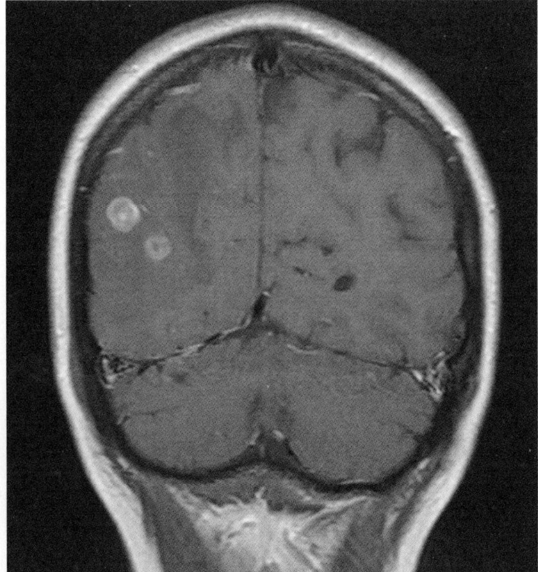

Figure 48.21 T1-weighted magnetic resonance imaging with contrast. Two right occipital lung metastases are demonstrated. They are well demarcated and enhance with gadolinium contrast.

Robert Foster Kennedy, 1884–1952, British Neurologist, awarded the Chevalier de la Légion d'honneur in recognition of his service in French front-line field hospitals in the First World War.

Josef Gerstmann, 1887–1969, Austrian neurologist who fled to America in 1938 to escape the Nazis.

patients with multiple cerebral metastases were deemed unsuitable for surgery. In patients with good functional status and well-controlled systemic disease, craniotomy for resection of a single focus, and in selected cases multiple lesions, may confer symptomatic and survival benefits. New molecular therapies can control systemic disease in many cancers; in these cases craniotomy and resection of one or more lesions responsible for the mass effect or hydrocephalus with medical treatment of the remaining lesions may be well warranted. Occasionally diagnostic biopsy may be warranted where the primary is unknown.

TABLE 48.7 Tissue of origin for brain metastases (approximate).

Origin	Percentage
Lung	40
Breast	15
Melanoma	10
Renal/genitourinary	10
Other/unknown	25

Glioma

These are intrinsic tumours with glial histology, with subtypes including astrocytomas, oligodendrogliomas, ependymomas and mixed tumours. This is a tissue diagnosis, but imaging often predicts both a glial origin and the grade of tumour (***Figure 48.22***). Low-grade glioma (WHO grade II) has a peak incidence in the fourth decade of life, and commonly presents with seizures initially. High-grade gliomas include anaplastic astrocytoma (WHO grade III) and glioblastoma (WHO grade IV), the commonest glial tumour (***Figure 48.23***). They typically present *de novo* with the peak incidence in the fifth and sixth decades of life, respectively, or arise by transformation of low-grade tumours.

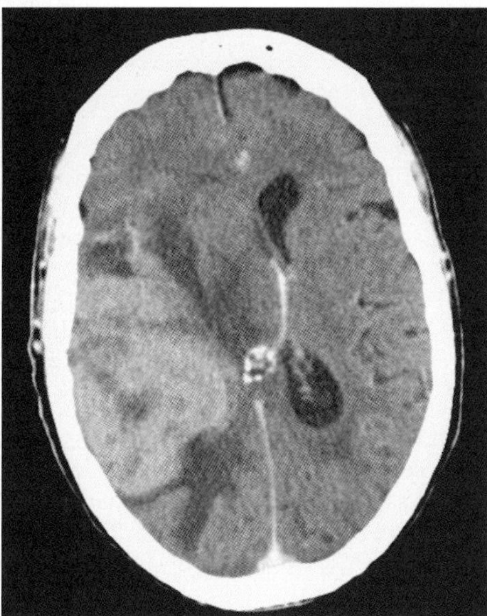

Figure 48.22 Computed tomography with contrast demonstrates a heterogeneous right frontoparietal lesion with mass effect and midline shift, almost certainly a glioblastoma multiforme. A magnetic resonance imaging scan with and without contrast will aid evaluation.

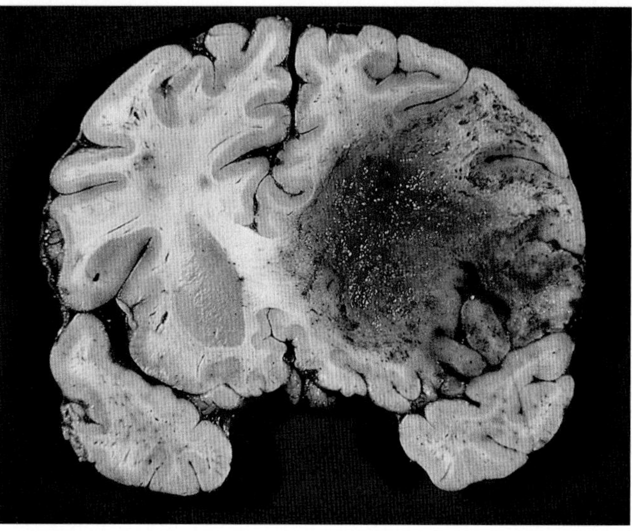

Figure 48.23 Pathological specimen of glioblastoma multiforme.

MRI of the head with and without contrast is the preferred modality, generally combined with CT of the chest, abdomen and pelvis to exclude an extracranial primary, since metastasis is usually the main differential diagnosis. Diffusion-weighted MRI sequences are valuable in excluding another key differential diagnosis – brain abscess, which is associated with prominent restricted diffusion in these images.

Initial management of these tumours should generally include high-dose steroids to alleviate any mass effect. Antiepileptics are administered when seizures are a presenting feature or are anticipated in view of the temporal location. Surgical resection is usually the primary treatment, with the aim of reducing disease burden and obtaining tissue for diagnosis. When tumours encroach on the eloquent cortex, especially the speech areas of the dominant hemisphere which are not consistently anatomically localised, awake craniotomy allows for mapping of speech function. Except for grade I pilocytic astrocytomas typically found in children, gliomas are notable for diffuse infiltration into the surrounding brain, so that recurrence after even macroscopically complete resection is the rule.

The classification of gliomas has been significantly updated with the recent addition of integrated molecular diagnostic categories to the WHO 2016 classification (***Figure 48.24***). Gliomas with low-grade histology often carry characteristic mutations; for example, point mutations in isocitrate dehydrogenase (*IDH*) enzymes and 1p/19q chromosomal co-deletion, the latter specific to oligodendrogliomas. Glioblastomas are WHO grade IV tumours and include *IDH* wild-type 'primary' glioblastoma and occasional *IDH* mutant 'secondary' glioblastomas. These are thought to arise from transformation of previously diagnosed, or clinically silent, low-grade gliomas. *IDH* wild-type status is a strong predictor of aggressive malignant behaviour, even in the absence of high-grade histological features. Active treatment consists of maximal surgical resection, typically with the assistance of intraoperative neuronavigation systems to accurately localise the tumour.

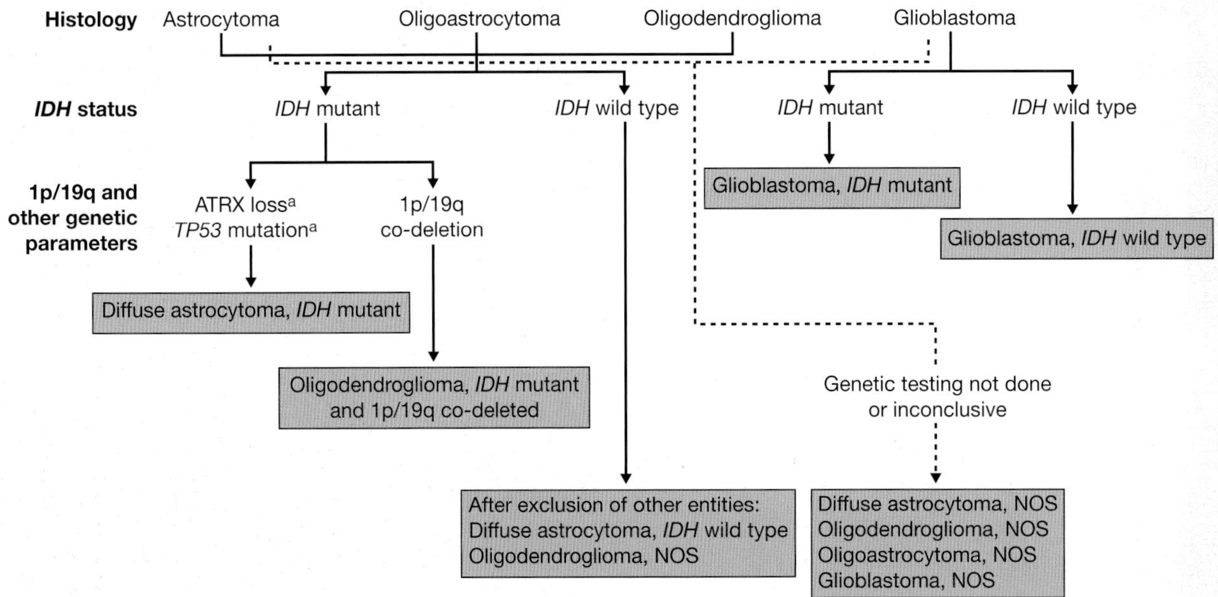

Figure 48.24 World Health Organization 2016 classification of gliomas. ATRX, α-thalassaemia/mental retardation syndrome X-linked; IDH, isocitrate dehydrogenase; NOS, not otherwise specified. [a]Characteristic but not required for diagnosis. (Reproduced from Louis DN, Perry A, Reifenberger G *et al*. The 2016 World Health Organization classification of tumors of the central nervous system: a summary. *Acta Neuropathol* 2016; **131**(6): 803–20, with permission from Springer.)

Patients can also be dosed with 5-aminolevulinic acid (5-ALA) preoperatively. Protoporphyrin IX, a fluorescent metabolite of this drug, accumulates selectively in glioma cells, causing them to glow pink under ultraviolet light, so providing a real-time assessment of tumour infiltration at the resection boundaries.

First-line adjuvant treatment in malignant glioma includes high-dose focused radiation therapy and alkylating chemotherapy with oral temozolomide. Median survival for glioblastoma remains just over 12 months.

Meningioma

Meningiomas are usually benign lesions, although anaplastic variants do occur. They arise from the meninges and typically present as a result of the mass effect from the tumour, compounded by vasogenic oedema in the adjacent brain and obstructive hydrocephalus where CSF drainage is impaired. Imaging will demonstrate a contrast-enhancing mass distinct from the brain with a dural base (***Figure 48.25***).

These are generally slow-growing lesions: smaller lesions, perhaps detected incidentally in an elderly patient, may well warrant a 'watch-and-wait' approach. If the lesion is large or positioned so as to impinge on key structures, the patient may require steroids and early surgery. The degree of resection predicts recurrence, with rates of 10% at 10 years for total excision with a clear dural margin and 30% at 10 years for subtotal excision. Lesions that are difficult to approach surgically may be managed with radiotherapy or stereotactic radiosurgery.

Summary box 48.10

Common supratentorial brain tumours

- Metastases and gliomas are common tumours arising within brain substance, appearing as 'ring-enhancing' lesions on contrast CT. Surgery is usually life-extending rather than curative
- Meningiomas arise from the meninges around the brain and typically enhance uniformly on contrast CT. Most are benign and amenable to curative resection
- MRI is usually the best modality for evaluating brain tumours. Diffusion-weighted sequences help to exclude abscess when glioma or metastasis is suspected
- Metastasis is the main differential diagnosis, and CT of the body is useful in identifying extracranial primary tumours
- Steroids, along with proton pump inhibitor treatment for gastric protection, are administered to control swelling and the mass effect in the short term

Pituitary tumours

Most tumours in the sellar region are benign pituitary adenomas, but pathology in this region can also include malignant variants as well as craniopharyngiomas, meningiomas, aneurysms and Rathke's cleft cysts (***Figure 48.26***).

Microadenomas are less than 10 mm in size and usually present incidentally or with endocrine effects. Macroadenomas are larger than 10 mm and often present with visual

Martin Heinrich Rathke, 1793–1860, German anatomist.

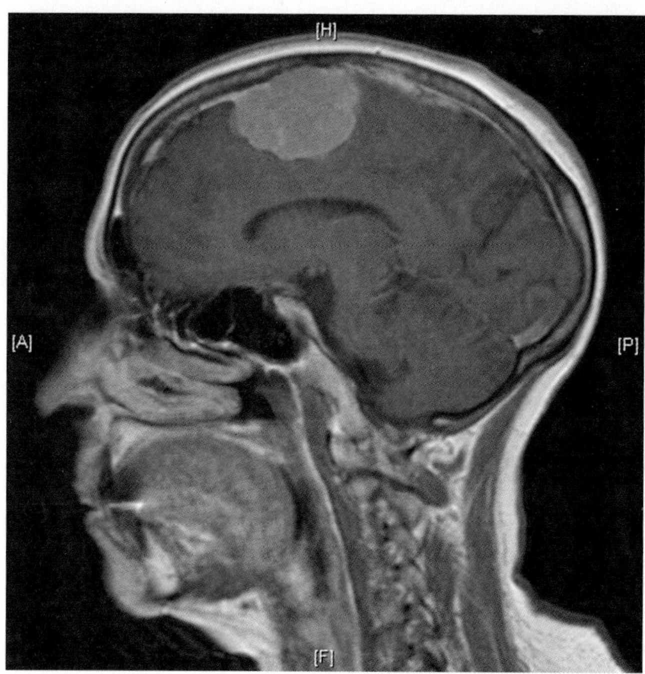

Figure 48.25 On T1-weighted magnetic resonance imaging an extra-axial, durally based lesion is seen to arise in the region of the falx. This is a meningioma.

field deficits. Thirty per cent of adenomas are prolactinomas, 20% are non-functioning, 15% secrete growth hormone and 10% secrete adrenocorticotropic hormone (ACTH).

Features of note in the initial assessment include any history of galactorrhoea (suggestive of prolactinoma) and Cushingoid or acromegalic features pointing to ACTH- or growth hormone-secreting tumours, respectively. Baseline assessment of pituitary function should include serum prolactin, follicle-stimulating hormone and luteinising hormone together with testosterone in males or oestradiol in females, thyroid function tests and fasting serum growth hormone and cortisol. Preoperative prolactin levels are crucial since prolactinomas may be managed with dopamine agonists such as bromocriptine and cabergoline rather than surgery. Growth hormone-secreting tumours may also respond to dopamine agonists or to somatostatin analogues such as octreotide. The cortisol level is also important since deficiency must be corrected, especially in the perioperative period. Diagnosis of ACTH-secreting tumours can be difficult and may require the use of specialised tests such as petrosal sinus sampling and the dexamethasone suppression test.

Effective treatment requires close cooperation between the neurosurgical team and an endocrinologist. Compression of the chiasm with any evidence of visual compromise is the main indication for urgent surgical intervention.

Surgical resection is usually performed by a transsphenoidal approach through the nose, using a microscope or endoscope. Sometimes large tumours also require a craniotomy. After operation patients are at risk of CSF leak and pituitary insufficiency. Diabetes insipidus resulting from manipulation

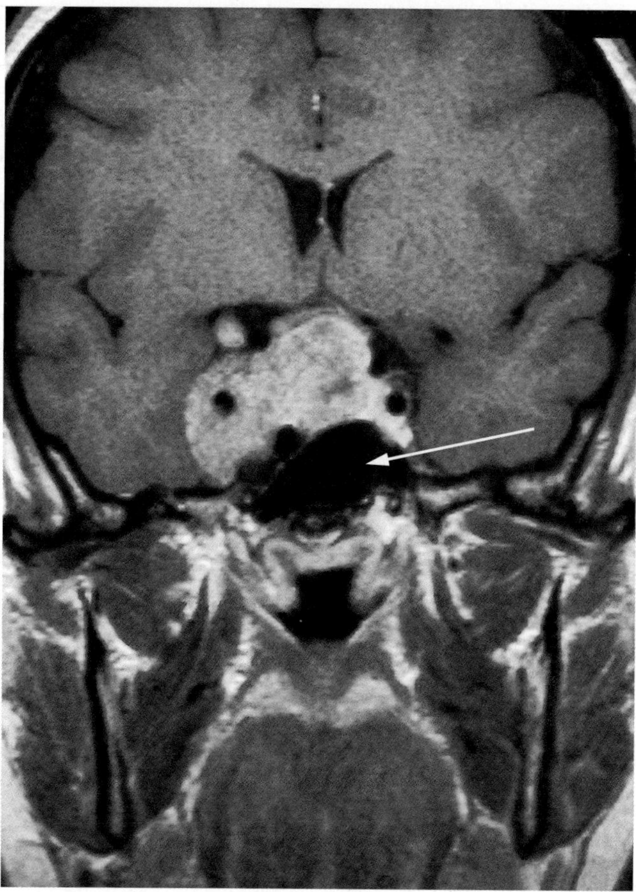

Figure 48.26 Non-functioning pituitary macroadenoma (arrow) compressing the optic chiasm superiorly, extending into the right cavernous sinus and encasing the right carotid artery.

of the pituitary stalk is possible in the immediate postoperative period and usually resolves spontaneously. Where it is suspected, the patient will require hourly measurement of urine output and blood and urine samples for calculation of sodium concentration and osmolality. If confirmed, the condition can be managed with desmopressin in consultation with endocrinology.

Pituitary apoplexy is a syndrome associated with haemorrhage or infarction in a pituitary tumour. It presents with sudden headache, visual loss and ophthalmoplegia with or without impaired conscious level. Endocrine resuscitation with intravenous steroids is the priority and surgical decompression may be required.

Vestibular schwannoma

These are nerve sheath tumours arising in the cerebellopontine angle (***Figure 48.27***) that present with hearing loss, tinnitus and balance problems. Facial numbness and weakness are less common, while large tumours may present with features of brainstem compression or hydrocephalus. The differential

Harvey Williams Cushing, 1869–1939, Professor of Surgery, Harvard University Medical School, Boston, MA, USA; credited as the father of modern neurosurgery; described the eponymous disease but also pioneered new techniques in bacteriology, blood pressure measurement and electrocautery.

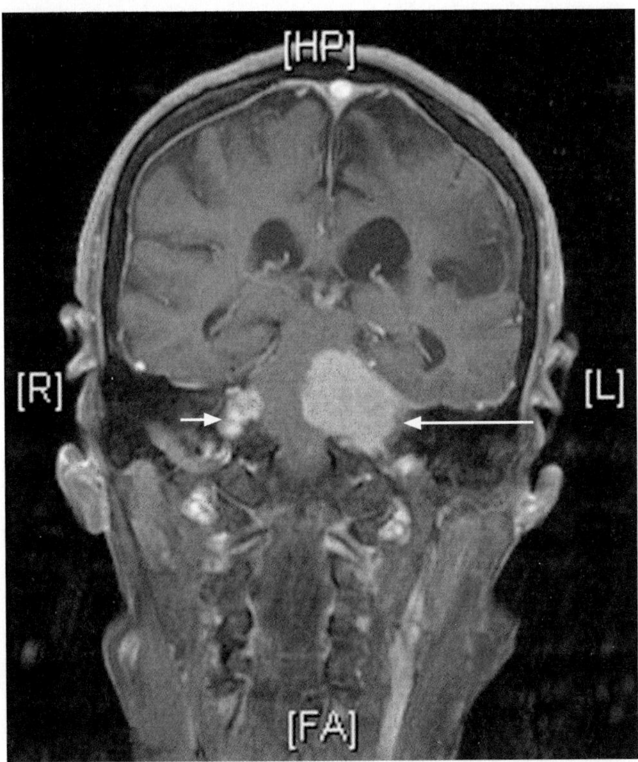

Figure 48.27 The appearances of a meningioma in the left cerebellopontine angle (CPA) (long arrow), with a coexisting vestibular schwannoma in the right CPA (short arrow).

diagnosis includes meningioma, metastasis and epidermoid cyst.

Small intracanalicular tumours (within the internal auditory canal) may be managed with surveillance. For intermediate size tumours, radiosurgery is an alternative to operation. Large lesions (>4 cm), especially with brainstem compression, will require excision and consideration of ventriculoperitoneal shunt to relieve hydrocephalus. Translabyrinthine, retrosigmoid and middle fossa approaches are possible, the latter options offering potential preservation of hearing in smaller tumours with some intact function at presentation. Patients with larger tumours will typically have no serviceable hearing in the affected ear and the focus is then on preserving facial nerve function.

Summary box 48.11

Skull base and paediatric tumours

- Pituitary tumours typically present with endocrinological disturbance (microadenomas) or visual deficits due to compression (macroadenomas). Some of these tumours are managed surgically, in close cooperation with endocrinologists
- Vestibular schwannomas (acoustic neuromas) are benign nerve sheath tumours, usually presenting with hearing loss, tinnitus and balance problems. Their proximity to the brainstem allows them to cause significant morbidity and mortality and can present a major surgical challenge

PAEDIATRIC NEUROSURGERY

Paediatric neurosurgery incorporates the management of tumours and developmental abnormalities, for example cysts, neural tube defects and posterior fossa malformations. In general these present with combinations of developmental delay, seizures and macrocephaly or hydrocephalus. Early fusion of one or more cranial sutures, craniosynostosis, is also a common neonatal presentation.

Brain tumours in children

Brain tumours are the most common solid tumours in children but are nonetheless seen only infrequently outside specialist units. They typically present with developmental regression and enlarging head circumference in the youngest, with headache, seizure and focal deficits prominent in older children.

Posterior fossa tumours are relatively more common in children, in particular:

- medulloblastoma;
- ependymoma;
- pilocytic astrocytoma.

Treatment will typically combine surgical resection or biopsy, CSF diversion, chemotherapy and/or radiotherapy.

Cysts

These benign fluid-filled intracranial lesions typically present incidentally or with mass effect or hydrocephalus. Treatment of symptomatic or enlarging lesions is usually surgical, involving excision, endoscopic fenestration into a cistern or ventricle or shunting for hydrocephalus. Cyst types include:

- arachnoid cyst: typically middle fossa, CSF enclosed in an envelope of arachnoid mater;
- colloid cyst: occur in the roof of the third ventricle, believed to represent embryonic endoderm remnants;
- dermoid and epidermoid cysts: epithelium-lined structures arising from displaced ectodermal remnants, typically in the posterior fossa (midline) and cerebellopontine angle, respectively;
- porencephalic cysts: brain cavities lined with gliotic white matter, containing CSF in communication with the ventricles or subarachnoid space.

Neural tube defects

Failure of closure of the neural tube is associated with folate deficiency, family history and some anticonvulsants. Prenatal screening, using serum α-fetoprotein levels and ultrasound, and diagnostic testing, using amniocentesis, are possible. The spectrum of conditions associated with failed closure of the posterior neuropore includes the conditions described below.

Spina bifida occulta

A congenital absence of a spinous process, without exposure of meninges or neural tissue, but presenting a characteristic shallow hair-covered hollow at the base of the spine. This is common and rarely clinically significant.

Sometimes it may be associated with tethered cord syndrome, which involves thickening of the filum terminale, resulting in traction on the cord. Presentation is with progressive deficits, spasticity, bladder dysfunction or scoliosis, and treatment involves surgical exploration and untethering of the cord.

Meningocele

A sac of meninges, covered by skin and containing CSF alone, herniates through an anterior or posterior bony defect.

Myelomeningocele

A herniating sac of meninges without covering skin contains spinal cord, nerves or both. This is always associated with Chiari II malformation (see ***Posterior fossa malformations***). Open myelomeningocele presents a high infection risk and requires early surgical repair.

Lipomyelomeningocele

Adipose tissue adherent to the spinal cord herniates through a bony defect to the sacrolumbar soft tissue. This may be associated with bladder dysfunction and require surgical relief of the resultant cord tethering.

Failure of closure of the anterior neuropore produces anencephaly, which is uniformly fatal; the spectrum of spinal dysraphisms, however, is replicated in the skull. Cranium bifidum is a failure of fusion, often in the occipital region. This may be associated with herniation of meninges and CSF (meningocele) and potentially also brain substance (encephalocele) (***Figure 48.28***).

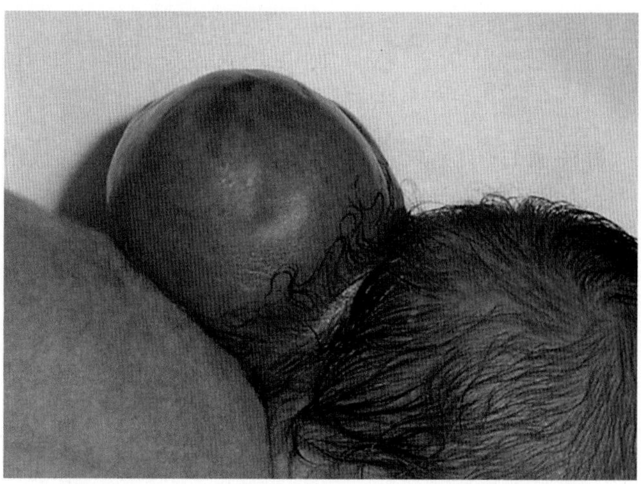

Figure 48.28 An occipital encephalocele.

Posterior fossa malformations

Chiari malformations involve cerebellar herniation through the foramen magnum:

- Normal: up to 5 mm of cerebellar tonsillar descent through the foramen magnum.
- Chiari I: >5 mm of tonsillar descent; presents typically in young adults with cough headaches and neurological disturbance reflecting brainstem/cerebellar compression and/or formation of a fluid-filled syrinx in the spinal cord as a result of disordered CSF flow. Shunting and foramen magnum decompression are the mainstay of treatment.
- Chiari II: descent of the tonsils and vermis associated with myelomeningocele and hydrocephalus, so clinically apparent in infancy.

Dandy–Walker malformations present in infancy with macrocephaly, developmental delay and hydrocephalus; most patients have associated abnormalities in the CNS and other organ systems. Imaging demonstrates a hypoplastic cerebellar vermis, with the posterior fossa occupied by a large thin-walled cyst. Treatment usually involves shunt placement.

Craniosynostosis

Normal fusion of the coronal, lambdoidal, squamosal and sagittal sutures occurs between 6 and 12 months of age; others such as the frontal suture fuse later. Craniosynostosis is the premature fusion of one (simple craniosynostosis) or more (complex craniosynostosis) cranial sutures, preventing growth perpendicular to the suture. This results in a range of skull deformities (***Table 48.8*** and ***Figures 48.29 and 48.30***) and hydrocephalus. Syndromic craniosynostosis, often associated with abnormalities of the fibroblast growth factor receptor genes, is accompanied by developmental delay and other abnormalities. The surgical treatment aims to correct deformity and prevent development of raised ICP.

TABLE 48.8 Types of craniosynostosis.

Type	Suture involved	Clinical features
Scaphocephaly	Sagittal suture	Narrow boat-shaped head
Brachycephaly	Coronal suture	Shortened/broad forehead
Microcephaly	All sutures involved	Small head
Plagiocephaly	Unilateral coronal/ lambdoid suture	Asymmetric skull
Trigonocephaly	Metopic suture	Pointed narrow forehead

FUNCTIONAL NEUROSURGERY

Functional neurosurgery aims to relieve epilepsy, movement disorders or pain by ablation or stimulation of brain tissue and nerves.

Hans Chiari, 1851–1916, Professor of Pathological Anatomy, Strasbourg, Germany (Strasbourg was returned to France in 1918 after the end of the First World War), gave his account of this condition in 1891.
Walter Edward Dandy, 1886–1946, American neurosurgeon and scientist, considered one of the founding fathers of neurosurgery.
Arthur Earl Walker, 1907–1995, Canadian-born neurosurgeon, neuroscientist and epileptologist.

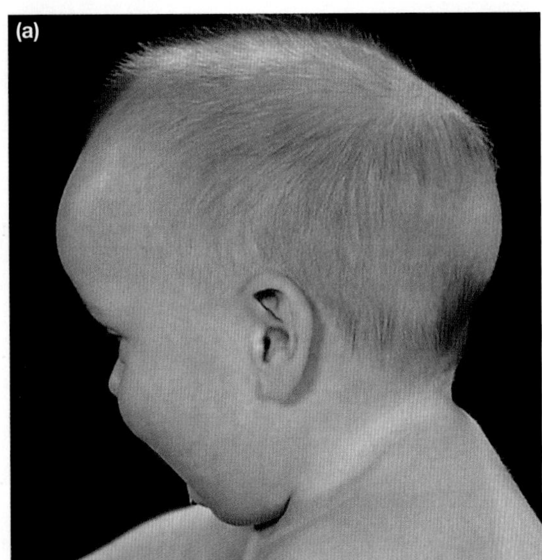

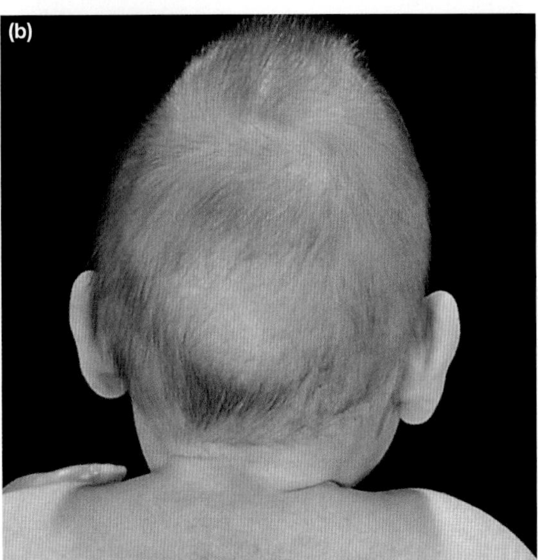

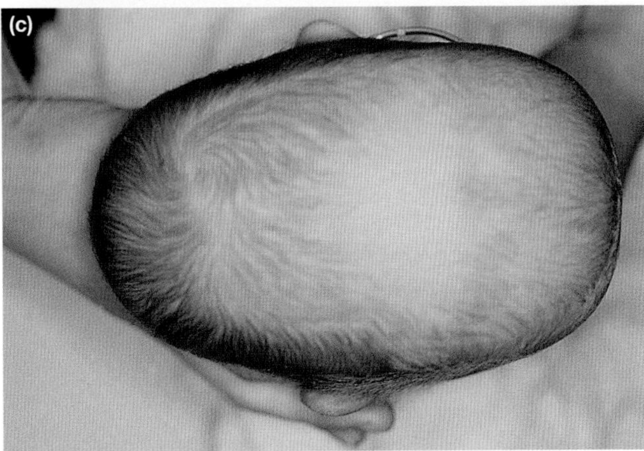

Figure 48.29 (a–c) Characteristic appearance of scaphocephaly due to sagittal suture synostosis.

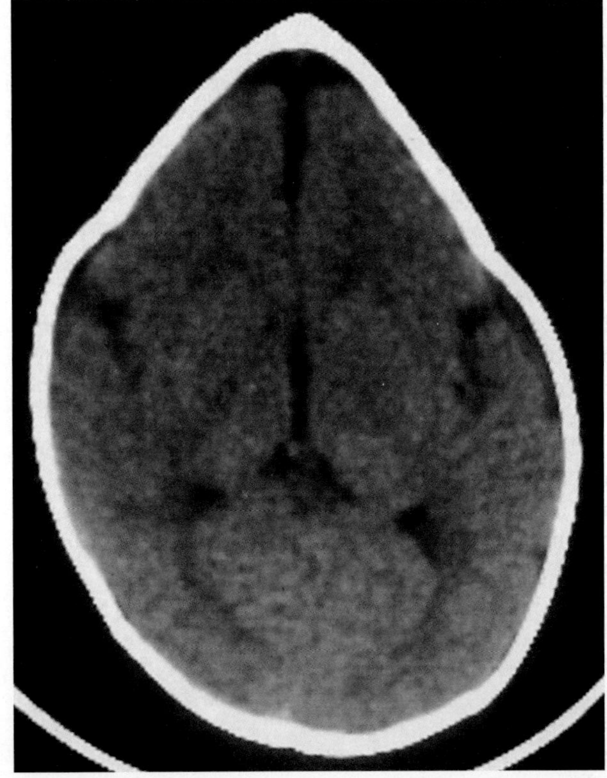

Figure 48.30 Axial computed tomography scan showing severe trigonocephaly due to premature fusion of the metopic suture.

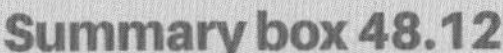

Summary box 48.12

Paediatric neurosurgery

- A large variety of mostly neuroectodermal brain tumours represent the most common solid organ tumours in children
- Children manifest a range of developmental pathologies requiring neurosurgical management, including:
  - Cysts
  - Neural tube defects
  - Posterior fossa abnormalities
  - Craniosynostosis
- Generic features of intracranial pathology include developmental delay, seizures, macrocephaly and hydrocephalus

Epilepsy

Up to 10% of the population will suffer a seizure at some point in their lives, and epilepsy, a syndrome of recurrent unprovoked seizures, represents the most common neurological disorder. About 20–30% of patients fail to achieve adequate seizure control with drugs, and many of these focal epilepsies may benefit from surgery. Where a primary lesion such as a tumour, AVM or cavernoma is present, lesionectomy alone may be appropriate. Over time, however, repeated seizures can trigger hippocampal atrophy, which can then present a second seizure focus. This dual pathology is clinically important because seizure control may require removal of the atrophic hippocampus as well as the primary pathology.

Investigation

MRI is a mainstay, demonstrating, for example, reduced hippocampal volume and distorted architecture in mesial temporal sclerosis. Nuclear medicine modalities, including single-photon emission CT (SPECT) and positron emission tomography (PET), are sometimes used to demonstrate ictal and interictal metabolic abnormalities.

Electroencephalography (EEG) entails recording from an array of scalp electrodes and comparison between ictal and interictal recordings. This is especially helpful in lateralising the focus of complex partial seizures in temporal lobe epilepsy and is combined with video monitoring of the seizure in a videotelemetry suite. A more detailed localisation may be achieved invasively by the preoperative placement of subdural or depth electrodes, preoperatively or by intraoperative electrocorticography (ECoG).

Neuropsychological evaluation is used to evaluate the patient's preoperative function, looking for concordant focal impairments and, using the Wada test (***Table 48.9***), assessing the risk of postoperative language and memory deficits in temporal lobe epilepsy surgery.

TABLE 48.9 Wada test.

- Sodium amytal is injected into each internal carotid artery in turn, with simultaneous speech and memory testing to localise function
- The aim is to confirm language laterality, and hence that resection on the side of the lesion will not significantly impair verbal memory functions

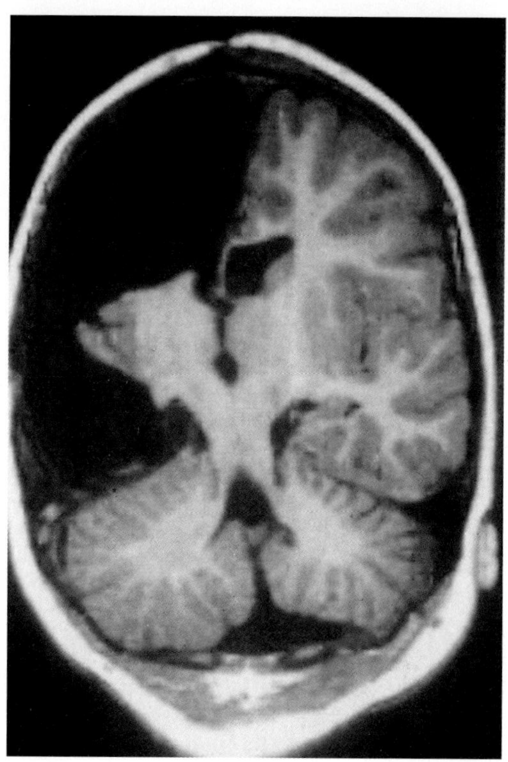

Figure 48.31 Coronal T2-weighted magnetic resonance image following anatomical hemispherectomy.

Surgical management

The seizure focus may be resected, generally where it is in non-eloquent brain, or otherwise a disconnection can be performed. Awake craniotomy, allowing mapping particularly of speech centres, is increasingly employed.

Mesial temporal epilepsy is commonly medically refractory and can be addressed surgically by amygdalohippocampectomy or resection of the temporal lobe including the mesial structures. With careful patient selection, cure rates of up to 70% or greater can be achieved.

Functional, or rarely anatomical, hemispherectomy (***Figure 48.31***) may be performed for specific epilepsy syndromes associated with hemiplegia, such as infantile hemiplegia syndrome. This is usually considered in the early years of life when plasticity and potential for functional recovery is greatest.

Disconnection procedures include corpus callosotomy, which is used for patients suffering drop attacks, and subpial transections to isolate a seizure focus in eloquent brain from the surrounding cortex.

Vagal nerve stimulators can be implanted in severe drug-refractory epilepsy, with electrodes applied to the vagus nerve in the carotid sheath in the neck. This option can achieve significant reductions in seizure frequency, especially in children, although the mechanism is not clear.

Movement disorders

Prior to the development of levodopa drug therapy, surgical ablation of the subthalamic nucleus (STN) or globus pallidus interna (GPi) was a mainstay of management for Parkinson's disease. Inhibition of the action of these centres remains a valuable tool later in the course of the disease as the therapeutic window using levodopa narrows, but this is now achieved using deep brain stimulation with electrodes. This offers the advantage of an adjustable and reversible effect and can be performed bilaterally where equivalent lesioning surgery would probably result in deficits.

Deep brain stimulation is also an option for other movement disorders where less invasive approaches are ineffective. These include dystonias, which may be amenable to bilateral GPi stimulation, and essential tremor, where the ventralis intermediate nucleus (Vim) of the thalamus is a preferred target.

Pain syndromes

Neurosurgical approaches to the relief of pain may address the underlying aetiology directly or may seek to interrupt or modulate the transmission responsible for the pain. The contrasting

Juhn Atsushi Wada, b. 1924, Japanese–Canadian neurologist known for research into epilepsy and human brain asymmetry, including his description of the Wada test for cerebral hemispheric dominance of language function.
James Parkinson, 1755–1824, general practitioner of Shoreditch, London, UK, published *An essay on the shaking palsy* in 1817.

approaches are demonstrated in the management of trigeminal neuralgia. This manifests, generally in middle age or later, with paroxysmal lancinating pain in the distribution of one or more divisions of the trigeminal nerve. The pain occurs without other neurological disturbance and may be triggered by trivial stimuli such as eating or brushing the teeth. The pain is often attributable to impingement on the nerve by the superior cerebellar artery or other vessels, as first postulated by Walter Dandy. Occasionally another primary lesion is responsible; for example demyelination due to multiple sclerosis can result in nerve impulses 'jumping' from adjacent sensory nerves to pain fibres, a process termed ephaptic transmission. When medications such as gabapentin and carbamazepine cannot achieve control, surgical options include the following.

- **Craniotomy and microvascular decompression** (MVD): this is designed to address the proposed origin of the neuropathic pain by applying material between the nerve and adjacent vessel to prevent direct contact and stimulation. It achieves long-lasting relief of symptoms in over 90% of patients with evidence of neurovascular compression on MRI. In other patients success rates are lower, and for older patients the risks associated with craniotomy may be hard to justify.
- **Stereotactic radiosurgery** is non-invasive but symptom improvement can take weeks or months; overall efficacy is lower than for MVD.
- **Percutaneous Gasserian rhizolysis** involves needle placement under radiographic guidance at the Gasserian ganglion in Meckel's cave. This permits lesioning of the ganglion by glycerol injection, radiofrequency thermocoagulation or balloon compression, with the aim of disrupting aberrant pain transmission. Facial numbness and recurrence of pain within 2 years are common after these procedures, and overall efficacy is lower than for MVD.

Treatment of pain elsewhere may also be based on lesioning of nerve tracts. For example pain related to brachial plexus infiltration or injury may be treated by sectioning the spinothalamic tract (cordotomy) or the dorsal root entry zone (DREZ operation). These approaches are limited by the potential for producing deficits, and especially by the occurrence of deafferentation ('phantom limb') pain syndromes, which are particularly unpleasant and difficult to treat.

Electrical stimulation is used to modulate pain transmission: for example, spinal cord stimulators can be applied to a range of pain syndromes, especially those associated with failed spinal surgery. Deep brain stimulation targeting the periaqueductal grey and sensory thalamic nuclei has a role in chronic pain arising in the context of thalamic stroke. Implanted devices may also be used for intrathecal delivery of opiates for pain control or baclofen to alleviate spasticity.

Summary box 48.13

Functional neurosurgery

- Intractable epilepsy can be treated surgically by implantation of a vagal nerve stimulator or by resection of one or more seizure foci
- Deep brain stimulation using implanted electrodes has largely replaced lesioning of these structures for management of drug-refractory Parkinson's disease
- Microvascular decompression is offered for trigeminal neuralgia, and other neuropathic pain syndromes may respond to lesioning of nerve tracts

PRACTICAL AND ETHICAL ISSUES

Creutzfeldt-Jakob disease

Creutzfeldt–Jakob disease (CJD) is a rare transmissible spongiform encephalopathy producing a rapidly progressive dementia; it is uniformly fatal. The causative agent seems to be a misfolded protein – a prion – that is not destroyed by conventional sterilisation techniques. UK practice involves undertaking preoperative checks to exclude any risk factors for CJD infection. These include family history, receipt of pituitary-derived human growth hormone, receipt of cadaveric dura mater grafts and previous brain or spinal surgery prior to 1997. Where risk factors are present, instruments must be quarantined or destroyed postoperatively.

Risks of craniotomy

The risks associated with craniotomy are important to appreciate in discussing operations with patients and family, and in evaluating patients who deteriorate postoperatively. Specific risks depend on the anatomy of each approach. The following figures quoted in brackets will vary significantly between individual procedures and even between centres:

- infection (5%) and wound breakdown;
- intracerebral haemorrhage;
- seizures;
- CSF leak;
- permanent neurological deficit;
- death (1%).

Brainstem death

This is defined as the irreversible loss of cerebral and brainstem function. Brainstem death is legally equivalent to death, and is a precondition for the harvesting of organs for transplant from heart-beating donors.

Johann Lorenz Gasser, 1723–1765, Professor of Anatomy, Vienna, Austria.
Johann Friedrich Meckel (the elder), 1724–1774, German anatomist, has 'the elder' appended to his name to avoid confusion with his famous grandson, Johann Friedrich Meckel (1781–1833), who was also an anatomist.
Hans Gerhard Creutzfeldt, 1885–1946, neurologist, Kiel, Germany.
Alfons Maria Jakob, 1884–1931, neurologist, Hamburg, Germany.

Diagnosis requires:

- identification of the cause of irreversible coma;
- exclusion of reversible causes of coma;
- clinical demonstration of the absence of brainstem function.

In the UK, this entails testing twice, by two clinicians, to demonstrate the absence of:

- response to pain;
- respiratory drive (apnoea despite a PCO_2 >6.7 kPa);
- pupillary light reflex;
- corneal reflex;
- vestibulo-ocular reflex;
- oculocephalic reflex;
- gag reflex.

FURTHER READING

Greenberg MS. *Handbook of neurosurgery,* 9th edn. New York, NY: Thieme, 2019.

Patton J. *Neurological differential diagnosis,* 2nd edn. New York, NY: Springer, 1998.

Samandouras G. *The neurosurgeon's handbook.* Oxford: Oxford Publishing, 2010.

CHAPTER 49 The eye and orbit

Learning objectives

To understand and appreciate:

- The anatomy of the eye and orbit
- The common ocular disorders and their symptoms and specific signs
- The value of special investigations
- When specialist referral is appropriate
- Recent advances in ocular surgery

OCULAR ANATOMY

Adnexae

The lids comprise skin, connective tissue, the orbicularis oculi (cranial nerve VII) and the tarsal plate, with multiple meibomian glands opening posterior to the lashes and lined with conjunctiva, which is reflected onto the sclera. The upper lid is elevated by the levator muscle (cranial nerve III) and has a horizontal strip of sympathetically innervated Müller's muscle, giving rise to 2 mm of ptosis in Horner's syndrome. The frontalis muscle may also contribute to eyelid elevation, particularly when the levator muscle is weak. Both lids are attached to the orbital rim by the medial and lateral canthal tendons. Both have a rich vascular supply and are innervated by the V1 division of the trigeminal nerve (cranial nerve V) above and the V2 division below.

Lacrimal system

The almond-shaped lacrimal gland lies under the upper outer orbital rim and opens into the upper conjunctival fornix through 10–15 ducts. Tears are swept across the globe by the lids and evaporate or pass into the upper and lower lid puncta, and then into the canaliculi to join the common canaliculus, which passes into the lacrimal sac under the medial canthal tendon. The sac is drained by the nasolacrimal duct into the nose, opening in the inferior meatus under the inferior turbinate.

The globe

The cornea is the 12-mm-diameter window of the eye, 550 μm thick centrally on average; its clarity is due to the regular arrangement of collagen bundles and relative dehydration. It merges into the sclera at the corneoscleral junction (the limbus), the insertion of the bulbar conjunctiva. The sclera, which is 1 mm thick, constitutes four-fifths of the wall of the eye and gives attachment to the extraocular muscles (***Figure 49.1***). It is perforated by the long and short posterior ciliary arteries and the vortex veins and is contiguous with the optic nerve sheath.

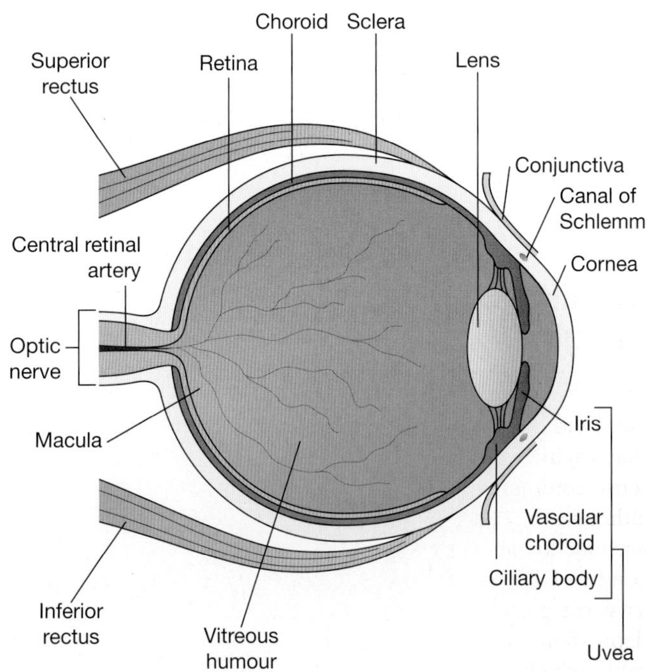

Figure 49.1 Anatomy of the eye.

Heinrich Meibom (Meibomius), 1638–1700, Professor of Medicine, History and Poetry, Helmstadt, Germany, described these glands in 1666.
Johannes Peter Müller, 1801–1858, Professor of Anatomy and Physiology, Berlin, Germany.
Johan Friedrich Horner, 1831–1886, Professor of Ophthalmology, Zurich, Switzerland, described this syndrome in 1869.

The uvea comprises the iris, ciliary body and vascular choroid. Photoreceptor cells in the outer retina sense light and send impulses to retinal ganglion cells in the inner retina via bipolar cells. The retinal pigment epithelium underlies the photoreceptors and is responsible for reprocessing of photopigments. The optic nerve conveys the axons of retinal ganglion cells from the eye to the brain. The most high-resolution part of the retina – the macula – lies at the posterior pole within the vascular arcade. The biconvex lens and capsule are suspended by the lens zonules, over 300 tiny fibres attached to the ciliary muscle. Aqueous humour arises from the ciliary processes, hydrates the vitreous gel, passes through the pupil into the anterior chamber between the iris and the cornea and then drains out through the trabecular meshwork into Schlemm's canal in the drainage angle and from there to the episcleral venous circulation. The balance between production and drainage of aqueous humour determines the intraocular pressure, which in most normal eyes is regulated at a level of 10–21 mmHg. The inner retina is supplied by the central retinal artery and drained by the central retinal vein.

Orbit

The orbit is four-sided and pyramidal in structure, housing the globe, optic nerve, the four rectus and two oblique muscles, the lacrimal gland, orbital fat, the cranial nerves III–VI, the ophthalmic artery with its tributaries and the ophthalmic veins, which anastomose anteriorly with the face and posteriorly with the cranial cavity. Above is the frontal lobe of the brain, temporally the temporal fossa, inferiorly the maxillary sinus and nasally the lacrimal sac and ethmoidal and sphenoidal air sinuses. The optic nerve passes through the optic canal to the chiasm, with other nerves and vessels passing through the superior ophthalmic fissure.

PERIORBITAL AND ORBITAL SWELLINGS

Swellings related to the supraorbital margin

Dermoid cysts

Dermoid cysts are benign congenital choristomas of the orbit that originate from fetal bone suture lines during development, most commonly the frontozygomatic suture (***Figure 49.2***), although they may also occur more medially. Dermoid cysts account for about half of childhood orbital neoplasms and consist of keratinised epithelium and adnexal structures such as sweat glands and hair follicles. They often cause a bony depression and they may have a dumbbell extension into the orbit, which is of particular importance should they need to be excised. Dermoid cysts can also erode the orbital plate of the frontal bone to become attached to dura; for this reason it is important to image the area by computed tomography (CT) before excision.

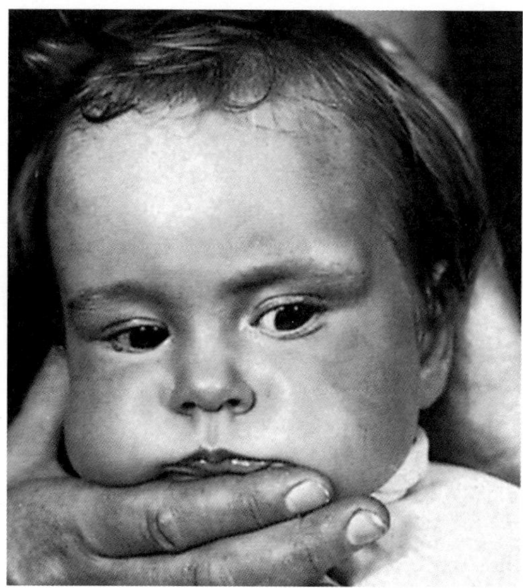

Figure 49.2 External angular dermoid.

Neurofibromatosis

Neurofibromatosis may also produce swellings above the eye. The diagnosis can usually be confirmed by an examination of the whole body, as there are often multiple lesions. Proptosis can also result (***Figure 49.3***). Other ophthalmic features may be present.

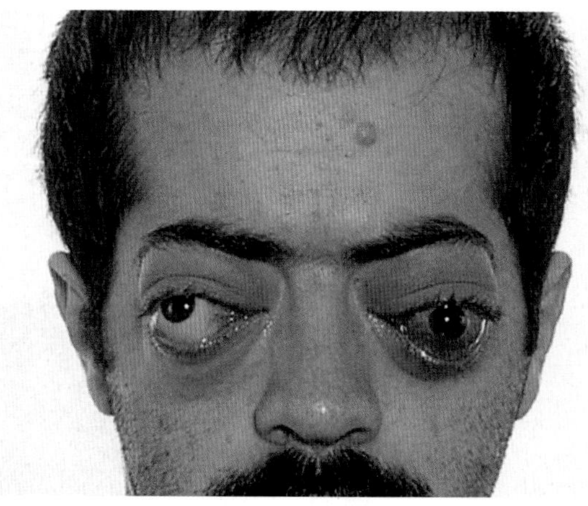

Figure 49.3 Neurofibroma in the orbit with proptosis, and also similar lesions in the forehead.

Swellings of the lids

Meibomian cysts (chalazion)

These are the most common lid swellings (***Figure 49.4***). A meibomian cyst is a chronic granulomatous inflammation of a meibomian gland. It may occur on either upper or lower lids and presents as a smooth, painless swelling. It can be felt by rolling the cyst on the tarsal plate. It can be distinguished from

Friedrich Schlemm, 1795–1858, Professor of Anatomy, Berlin, Germany.

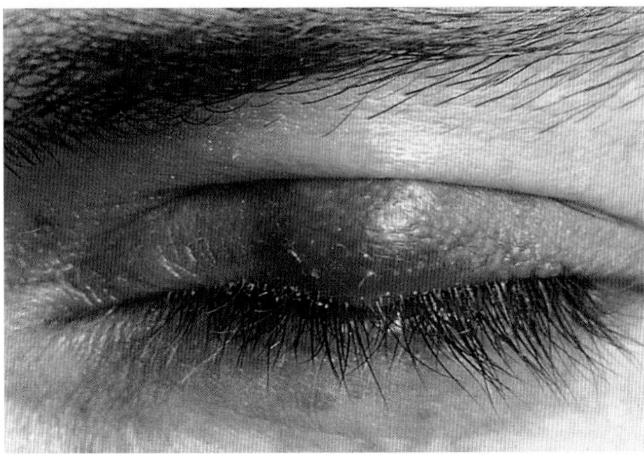

Figure 49.4 Meibomian cyst (courtesy of Mr D Spalton, FRCS).

a stye (hordeolum), which is an infection of a hair follicle and is usually painful. Persistent meibomian cysts that do not resolve with conservative treatment (hot compresses) are treated by incision and curettage from the conjunctival surface. Styes are treated by antibiotics and local heat.

Basal cell carcinoma (rodent ulcer)

This is the most common malignant tumour of the eyelids (***Figure 49.5***). Basal cell carcinomas may be locally invasive but do not tend to metastasise. They are more common on the lower lids, often start as a small pimple that ulcerates and has raised edges ('rodent ulcer') and are usually easily excised in the early stages. Histological confirmation that the excision is complete is required. More extensive lesions may require specialist techniques such as Mohs' micrographic surgical excision controlled by frozen section. Local radiotherapy or cryotherapy can be carried out; however, recurrence is more common, more aggressive and more difficult to detect.

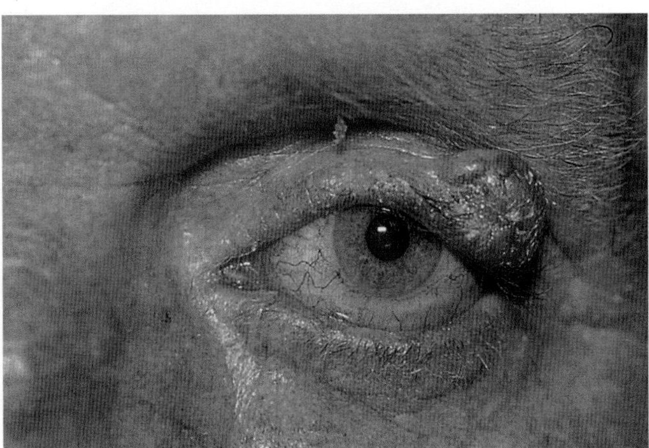

Figure 49.5 Rodent ulcers (courtesy of Mr J Beare, FRCS).

Summary box 49.1

Basal cell carcinomas

- Basal cell carcinomas are the most common malignant eyelid tumour
- Treatment is by wide local excision with careful histopathological margin control
- All unusual eyelid lesions (especially in the elderly) should be biopsied

Other lid swellings

Other types of lid swelling are less common. They include squamous cell carcinoma and malignant melanoma, sebaceous cyst, papilloma, keratoacanthoma, cyst of Moll (sweat glands) (***Figure 49.6***) or Zeis (sebaceous glands) and molluscum contagiosum. When molluscum contagiosum occurs on the lid margin, it can give rise to a mild viral chronic keratoconjunctivitis and should be curetted or excised.

Carcinoma of the meibomian glands and rhabdomyosarcomas are rare lesions; they need to be treated by radical excision. Atypical or meibomian cysts that recur should be biopsied to exclude sebaceous gland carcinoma.

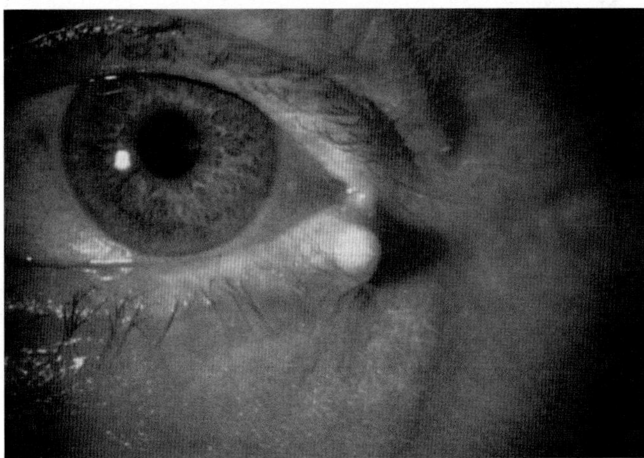

Figure 49.6 Cyst of Moll.

Swellings of the lacrimal system

Lacrimal sac mucocele

This occurs from obstruction of the lacrimal duct beyond the sac and results in a fluctuant swelling that bulges out just below the medial canthus. It can become infected to give rise to a painful tense swelling (acute dacryocystitis). If untreated, it may give rise to a fistula. Treatment is by performing a bypass operation between the lacrimal sac and the nose (a dacryocystorhinostomy). Watering of the eye can also occur as a result of eversion of the lower lid (ectropion), which causes loss of contact between the lower punctum and the tear film, or from

Frederic E Mohs, 1910–2002, developed the technique of micrographic surgical excision while a medical student at University of Wisconsin, USA.
Jacob Antonius Moll, 1832–1913, ophthalmologist of The Hague, The Netherlands.
Eduard Zeis, 1807–1868, Professor of Surgery, Marburg (1844–1850), who later worked at Dresden, Germany, described these glands in 1835.

reflex hypersecretion as a result of irritation, for example by inturning lashes in entropion, and these must be distinguished from a mucocele.

Lacrimal gland tumours

These are swellings of the lacrimal glands, which lie in the upper lateral aspect of the orbit. Eventually they lead to impairment of ocular movements and displacement of the globe forwards, downwards and inwards. Pathologically the tumours resemble parotid tumours and they can be pleomorphic adenomas with or without malignant change, carcinomas or mucoepidermoid tumours.

Orbital swellings

Orbital swellings result in displacement of the globe and limitation of movement. A full description of orbital swellings is outside the realm of this text, but some of the most common causes include the following.

- **Pseudoproptosis**. This results from a large eyeball, as seen in congenital glaucoma or high myopia.
- **Orbital inflammatory conditions** that result in orbital cellulitis (*Figure 49.7*).
- **Haemorrhage** after trauma or retrobulbar injection.
- **Neoplasia** affecting the lacrimal gland, the optic nerve, the orbital walls or the nasal sinuses (e.g. glioma [neurofibromatosis, *Figure 49.3*], meningioma and osteoma [*Figure 49.8*]).
- **Thyroid eye disease** (*Figures 49.9–49.11*). This is the most common cause of unilateral and bilateral proptosis in adults and may occur in the absence of active thyroid disease or after thyroidectomy. Management of severe thyroid eye disease may require large doses of systemic steroids, radiotherapy or even orbital lateral wall decompression if the eyeball is threatened by exposure or optic nerve compression. The disease is often more severe in smokers and those with poorly controlled thyroid function. CT and

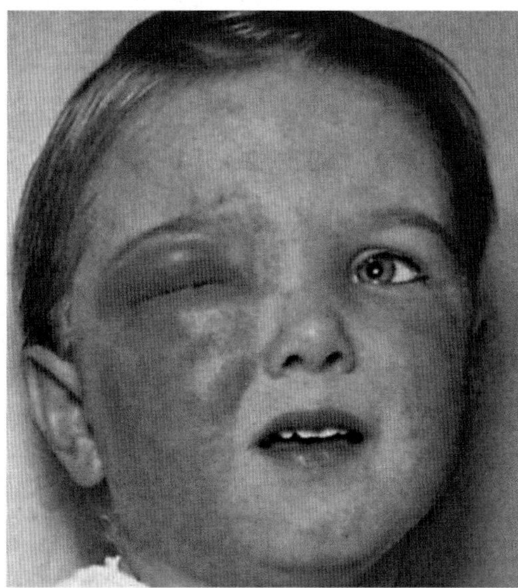

Figure 49.7 Orbital cellulitis.

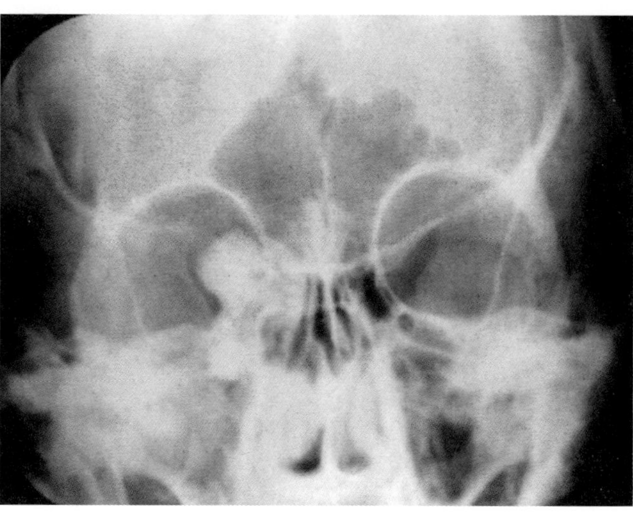

Figure 49.8 Radiograph showing an osteoma on the nasal side of the orbit giving rise to proptosis.

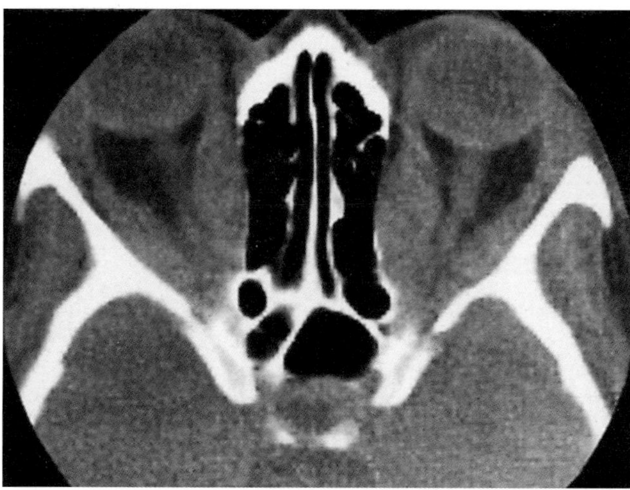

Figure 49.9 Computed tomogram of the orbit in dysthyroid exophthalmos, showing swollen muscles (courtesy of Dr Glyn Lloyd).

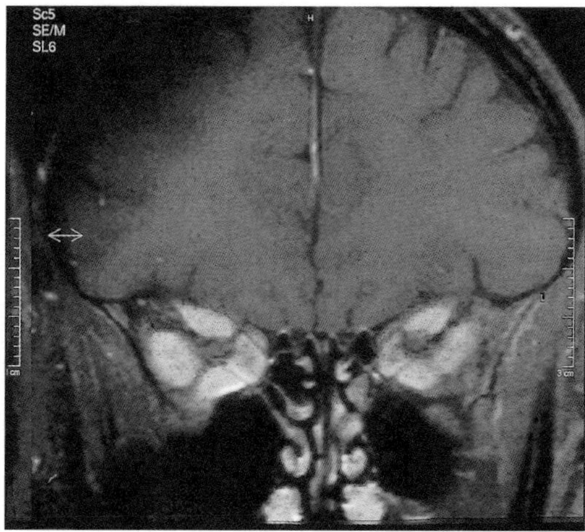

Figure 49.10 Magnetic resonance imaging scan of a coronal view of the orbit, showing enlarged muscles in thyroid disease (courtesy of Dr Juliette Britton).

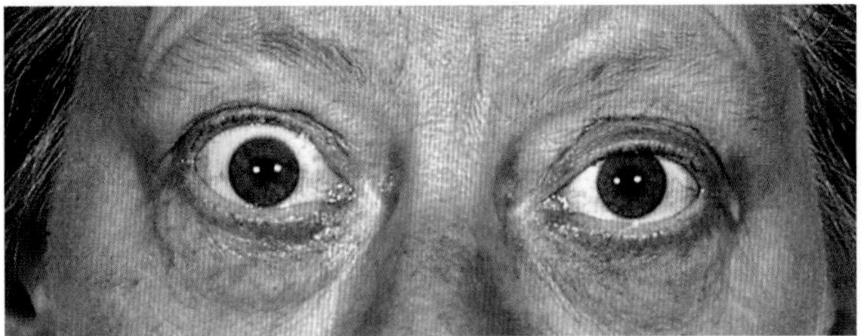

Figure 49.11 Exophthalmos in dysthyroid eye disease.

magnetic resonance imaging (MRI) scans are useful in diagnosis. MRI with short tau inversion recovery (STIR) sequences is particularly useful for identification of active inflammation within the orbital tissues.

- **Pseudotumour**, or malignant lymphoma.
- **Haemangiomas** of the orbit (***Figure 49.12***).
- **Tumour metastases**. These are rare. In children they usually arise from neuroblastomas of the adrenal gland, whereas in adults the oesophagus, stomach, breast and prostate can be sites of primary lesions.

Diagnostic aids

Diagnostic aids include radiography, CT, MRI, ultrasonography and, less commonly, tomography and orbital venography.

Treatment

Treatment is directed to the cause of the lesion, taking care to prevent exposure of the eye, diplopia or visual impairment from optic nerve compression.

INTRAOCULAR TUMOURS

Children

Retinoblastoma, the most common ocular malignancy of childhood, is a malignant tumour of the retina that can be bilateral in around one-third of cases. Half of cases are hereditary (autosomal dominant) and are due to mutation of the *RB1* gene on chromosome 13; children with a family history should be carefully monitored from birth. Remaining cases occur sporadically. Inherited retinoblastoma is more likely to be bilateral. Retinoblastoma is often not spotted until the tumour fills the globe and presents as a white reflex in the pupil or as a squint (***Figure 49.13***). The differential diagnosis includes retinopathy of prematurity, persistent fetal vasculature (PFV) and intraocular infections. If the tumour is large, enucleation may be required, but radiotherapy, cryotherapy, chemotherapy or laser treatment can cure small lesions. Liaison with a paediatric oncologist is essential.

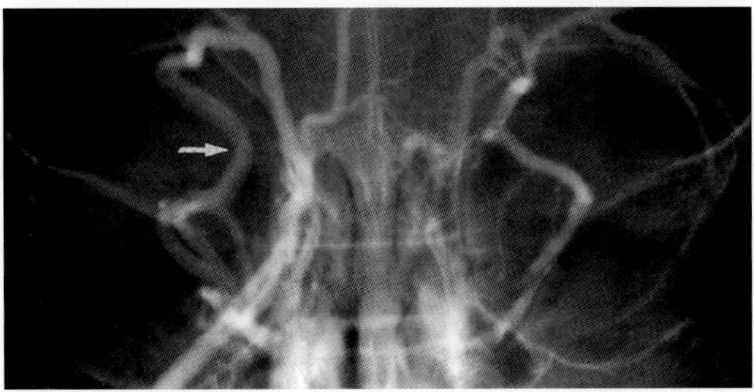

Figure 49.12 Capillary haemangioma in a child. An orbital venogram demonstrates displacement of the second part of the superior ophthalmic vein (arrow) (courtesy of Dr Glyn Lloyd).

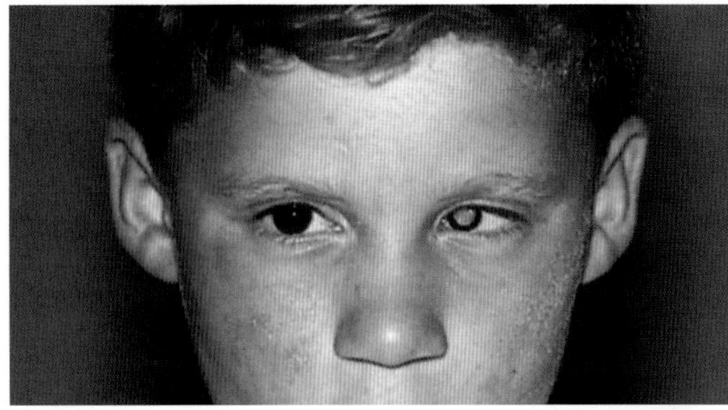

Figure 49.13 Retinoblastoma giving rise to a white pupillary reflex. This child was first seen with a convergent squint and discharged without a fundus examination. He was next seen many years later with a 'white reflex' and died soon after diagnosis (courtesy of MA Bedford, FRCS).

Summary box 49.2

Intraocular tumours

- Any child with a white pupil (leukokoria) should be referred to an ophthalmologist to exclude retinoblastoma, although congenital cataracts may also cause this sign
- A blind painful eye may hide a melanoma or other ocular tumour

Adults

Malignant melanoma is the most common primary malignant tumour of the eye and originates in the pigmented cells of the choroid (***Figure 49.14***), ciliary body or iris. It can present with a reduction in vision, a vitreous haemorrhage or by the chance finding of an elevated pigmented lesion in the eye. Tumour growth is variable but, as a general rule, the more posterior the lesion, the more rapidly progressive it is likely to be. Spread may be delayed for many years; however, the liver is frequently involved, hence the advice 'beware of the patient with a glass eye and an enlarged liver'. Treatment options vary by size and location of the tumour but include laser photocoagulation, radioactive plaque, radiotherapy/proton beam therapy, enucleation and, in selected cases, local excision. Diagnosis is made by direct observation and/or ultrasonography, which shows a solid tumour, often with low internal reflectivity on ultrasound (***Figure 49.15***).

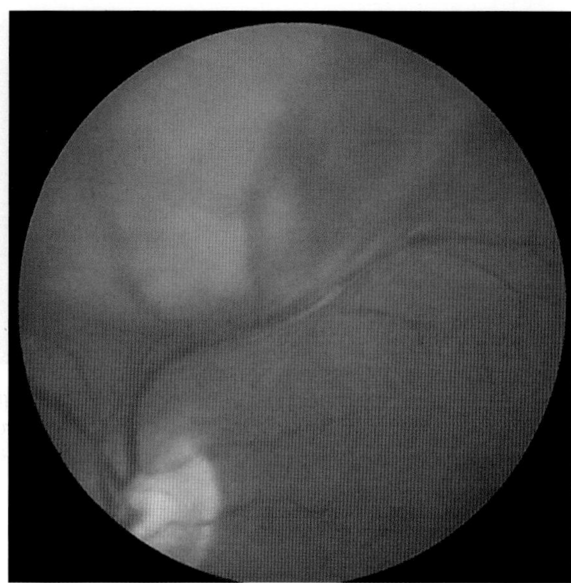

Figure 49.14 Choroidal melanoma.

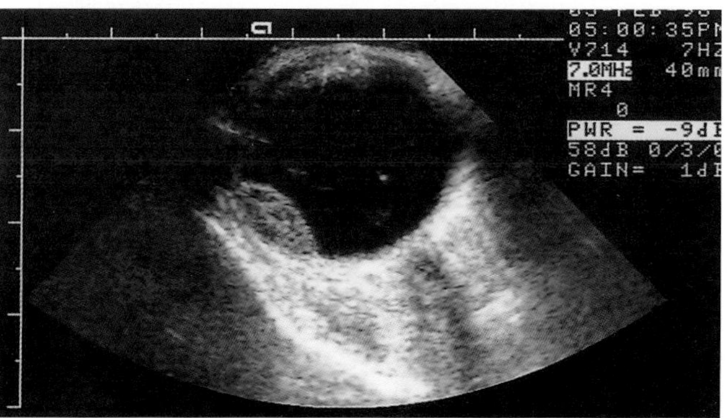

Figure 49.15 B-scan showing choroidal melanoma (courtesy of Dr Marie Reston).

INJURIES INVOLVING THE EYE AND ADJACENT STRUCTURES

Corneal abrasions and ulceration

The cornea is frequently damaged by direct trauma or by foreign bodies (*Figure 49.16*). Ulceration can occur with infection, exposure (for example in severely ill patients with incomplete eye closure) or after damage to the facial nerve. Postherpetic ulceration is common and serious if not treated. Fluorescein instillation illuminated by blue light shows up corneal ulceration at an early stage, with areas of epithelial loss fluorescing green.

Treatment of sterile corneal abrasions or exposure is by topical lubrication or padding of the eye. If bacterial infection is suspected, a swab or scrape may be performed for microbiological diagnosis and topical antibiotics such as 0.5% chloramphenicol or ofloxacin eye drops are commonly used.

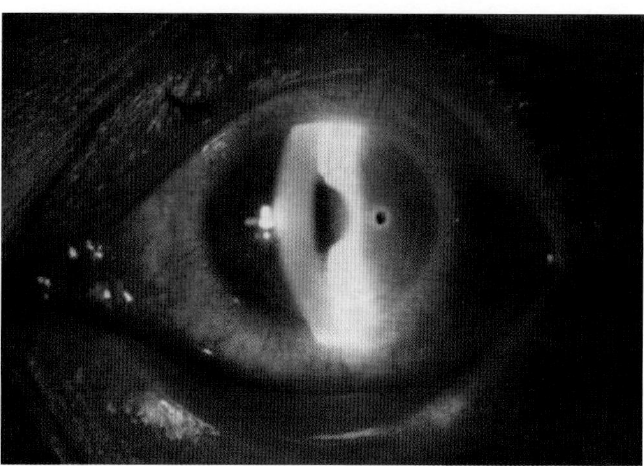

Figure 49.16 Corneal foreign body.

The eye is made more comfortable by the use of mydriatics such as cyclopentolate to reduce photophobia. Herpes simplex dendritic ulcers are treated with aciclovir ointment. In countries in the Far and Middle East, chronic infection with trachoma can cause corneal opacification and blindness, although the worldwide incidence of this condition is falling. Corneal grafting is the only cure for an opaque cornea. Until recently, full-thickness penetrating keratoplasty was the only corneal graft technique. For some conditions this has largely been replaced by lamellar or partial-thickness graft surgery, in a technique termed DSEK or 'Descemet's stripping endothelial keratoplasty'. However, penetrating keratoplasty remains the treatment of choice for severe corneal damage due to infection or injury. Rarely, osteo-odonto-keratoprosthesis can be attempted in very severe cases of opaque corneas that are not suitable for grafting. Artificial corneal prostheses have also been developed. Acanthamoeba is a rare serious cause of corneal infection. This infection usually follows the use of contact lenses. Specialist management and treatment is recommended.

Summary box 49.3

Corneal abrasions

- A drop of fluorescein dye illuminated by a blue light reveals even the smallest corneal abrasion
- Corneal ulcers are often more serious in contact lens wearers and require prompt assessment and treatment
- Development of white infiltrate in/around a corneal abrasion is a sign of infection

Blunt injuries to the eye and orbit

The floor of the orbit is its weakest wall and in blunt trauma, such as a blow from a fist, it is often fractured without fractures of the other walls. This is called a blow-out fracture. Clinical signs are enophthalmos, bruising around the orbit, maxillary hypoaesthesia and limitation of upward gaze owing to entrapment of the inferior rectus muscle leading to vertical diplopia.

Jean Descemet, 1732–1810, French physician and botanist.

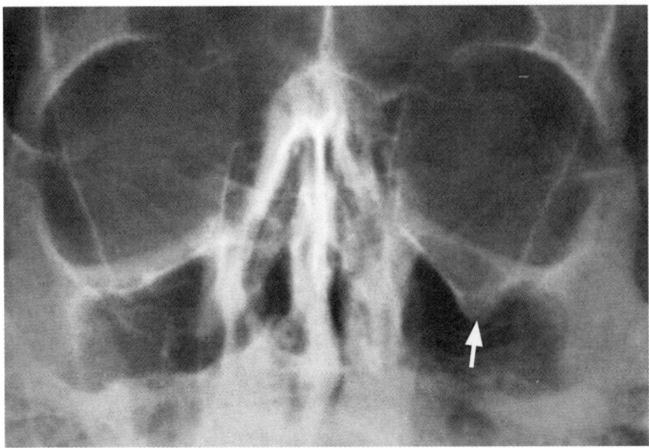

Figure 49.17 Radiograph showing a blow-out fracture of the orbit (left) with soft tissue in the antrum (arrow) (courtesy of Dr Glyn Lloyd).

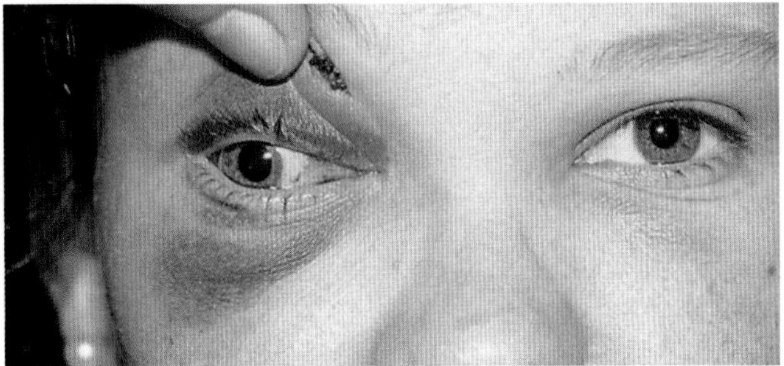

Figure 49.18 Injury from a ski pole into the right brow. Vision reduced to 'no perception of light' (courtesy of J Beare, FRCS).

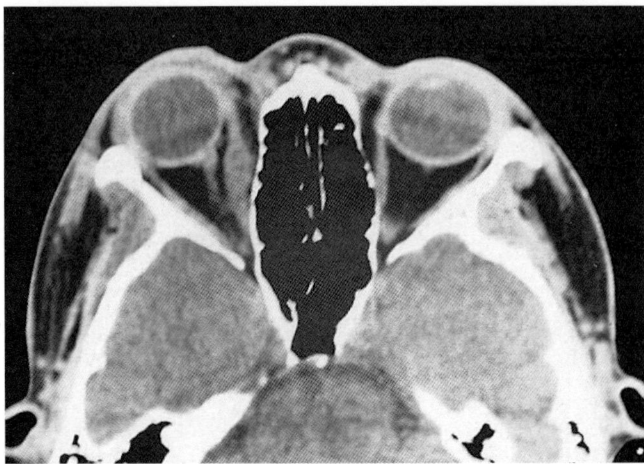

Figure 49.19 Scan of orbit from *Figure 49.18* showing a massive swelling of the medial rectus (courtesy of J Beare, FRCS).

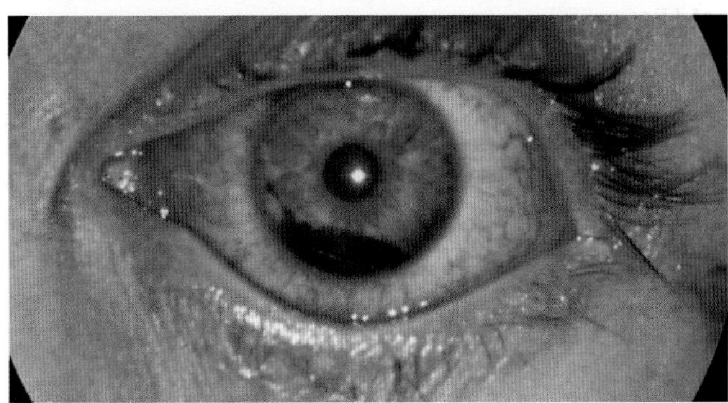

Figure 49.20 Hyphaema. Blood in the vitreous chamber after a concussional injury.

This occurs when the extraocular muscles or orbital septa become trapped in the fracture and can be identified as a soft-tissue mass in the antrum on a radiograph (*Figure 49.17*), although CT scans or tomograms may be necessary. Surgical repair of the orbital floor with freeing of the trapped contents may be necessary if troublesome diplopia persists or enophthalmos is marked. A child with an orbital floor fracture requires urgent assessment, particularly if upgaze is restricted, as trapping of the inferior rectus muscle may cause ischaemia and require urgent surgery. If an orbital haemorrhage is too extensive to examine the eye, it may be necessary to examine the eye under anaesthesia because there may be a hidden perforation of the globe. Injuries to the lids and lid margins must be repaired; if the lacrimal canaliculi are damaged, they should be repaired if possible, especially the lower canaliculus, as 75% of tear drainage goes through it.

Blunt injuries can also cause damage to the optic nerve, which can result in blindness and a total afferent nerve defect (*Figures 49.18 and 49.19*).

Blunt ocular injuries

Blunt injuries to the eye can give rise to several problems, which include the following:

- **Iritis**. Inflammation; treated with topical steroids.
- **Hyphaema** (blood in the anterior chamber) (*Figure 49.20*). Rest and sedation, particularly in children, are advised because the main danger in this condition is secondary bleeding, resulting in an acute rise in intraocular pressure and blood staining of the cornea. The use of antifibrinolytic agents (ε-aminocaproic acid) has been advocated; if the pressure rises, surgery to wash out the blood may be necessary.
- **Subluxation of the lens**. This is suspected if the iris, or part of the iris, 'wobbles' on movement (iridodonesis).
- **Secondary glaucoma**. This is often associated with recession of the iridocorneal drainage angle.
- **Retinal and macular haemorrhages and choroidal tears** (*Figure 49.21*).
- **Retinal dialysis**. This may lead to a retinal detachment and permanent damage to vision (*Figure 49.22*).

Penetrating eye injuries

These occur when the globe is penetrated, often in road traffic and other major accidents (*Figure 49.23*) and also in injuries from sharp instruments. The compulsory wearing of seat belts in motor vehicles has substantially reduced the incidence of this type of eye injury, by up to 73% in the UK. The presence of an irregular pupil suggests prolapse of the iris and should arouse suspicion of a penetrating injury. Treatment is prompt primary repair to restore the integrity of the globe.

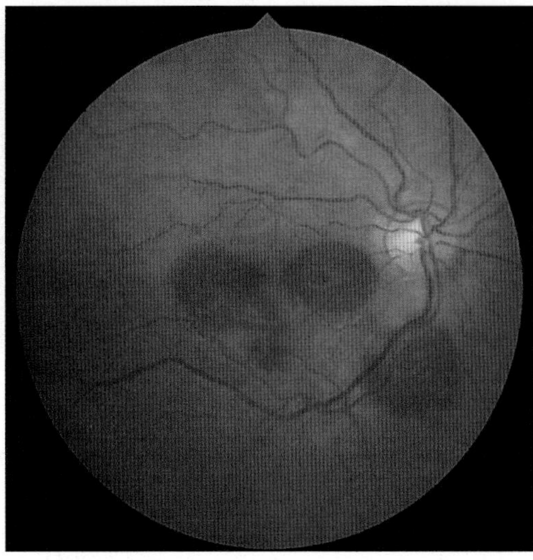

Figure 49.21 Retinal haemorrhage from a cricket bat injury (courtesy of J Beare, FRCS).

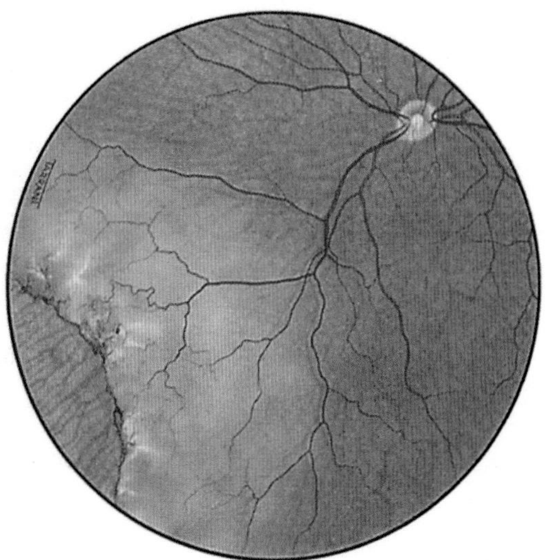

Figure 49.22 Retinal dialysis after blunt ocular injury.

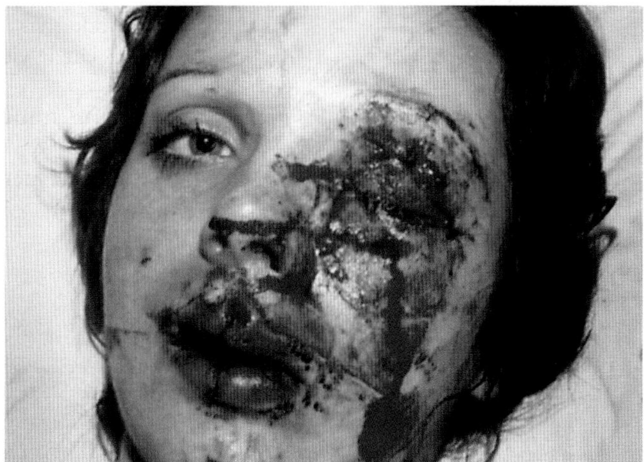

Figure 49.23 Facial lacerations from a windscreen injury. Beware of a perforating eye injury.

If a perforation is suspected, extensive eye examination should not be attempted before anaesthesia because this may lead to further extrusion of the intraocular contents. If the fundal view is poor, ultrasonography and orbital imaging are indicated. Secondary corneal grafting, lensectomy and vitrectomy have considerably improved the visual prognosis; these must be done by an experienced eye surgeon. Injuries to the optic nerves must also be excluded in severe accidents.

Intraocular foreign bodies

Intraocular foreign bodies must always be excluded when patients attend the accident and emergency department with an eye injury and a history of working with a hammer and chisel or a history of a potentially high-velocity injury. Radiography of the orbits must be performed. Ferrous and copper foreign bodies should always be removed, sometimes requiring the use of a magnet. B-scan ultrasonography can also assist in localising foreign bodies when a vitreous haemorrhage or cataract is present. CT can be used, but MRI is contraindicated if a ferrous intraocular foreign body is suspected.

Summary box 49.4

Penetrating eye injuries

- A distorted and irregular pupil warrants the careful exclusion of a penetrating eye injury
- Avoid extensive eye examination if globe rupture is suspected to avoid worsening the injury prior to surgical repair

Burns

Radiation burns

Corneal injury may occur after exposure to ultraviolet radiation, for example after arc welding or excessive sunlight (snow blindness) and sun lamps. Such burns cause intense gritty burning pain and photophobia as a result of keratitis (corneal inflammation), which starts some hours after exposure. Mydriatic and local steroids with antibiotic drops ease the condition, and healing usually occurs after 24 hours.

Thermal burns

If these involve the full thickness of the lids, corneal scarring may occur from exposure and immediate corneal protection is necessary. A splash of molten metal may cause marked local necrosis and may lead to permanent corneal scarring. Treatment is to remove any debris by irrigation and to instil local atropine, antibiotics and steroids to prevent superadded infection and scarring. Lid reconstruction may be necessary.

Chemical burns

Chemical burns, and especially alkali burns, can be serious because ocular penetration occurs quickly and ischaemic necrosis can result (***Figure 49.24***). Immediate copious irrigation until the pH is neutral will ensure that the chemical is diluted as much as possible, and all particles should be removed from the fornices. Treatment can then be continued as with thermal burns. Well-fitting goggles should prevent such injuries.

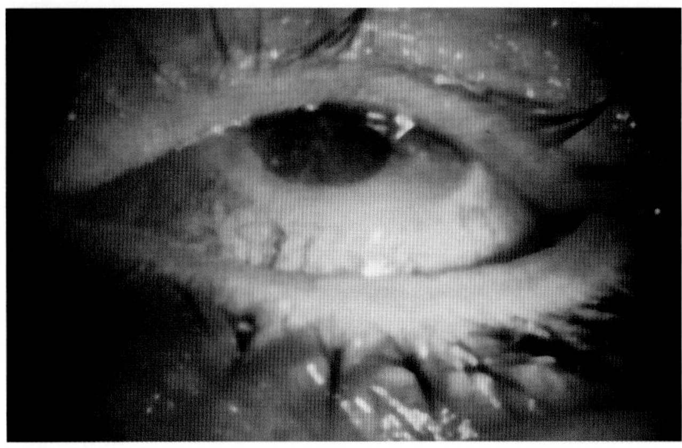

Figure 49.24 Chemical burn showing conjunctival necrosis.

DIFFERENTIAL DIAGNOSIS OF THE ACUTE RED EYE

This is important in the management of minor ocular complaints and the recognition of conditions that require expert attention. Possible causes of the acute red eye include:

- subconjunctival haemorrhage;
- conjunctivitis;
- keratitis;
- uveitis;
- episcleritis and scleritis;
- acute glaucoma.

Any condition with pain, visual impairment or a pupil abnormality suggests a more serious diagnosis.

Subconjunctival haemorrhage

This presents as a bright red eye, often noticed incidentally with only minimal discomfort and normal vision. Causes include coughing, sneezing, minor trauma, hypertension and, rarely, a bleeding disorder. Subconjunctival haemorrhages are more common in those receiving antiplatelet or anticoagulation therapy. Reassurance and treatment of the underlying cause are required. Most settle within a week, but can recur.

Conjunctivitis

Symptoms are grittiness, redness and discharge. Causes are infective, chemical, allergic or traumatic. In the newborn it can be serious; gonococcal and chlamydial infection must be excluded. Bacterial conjunctivitis is purulent, usually self-limiting and treated with topical broad-spectrum antibiotics. Chlamydial and adenovirus infections must be considered. Adenoviral infections are common and usually affect one eye much more in severity and onset, tending to be more watery than sticky, and are often associated with a palpable preauricular gland.

Vernal conjunctivitis (*Figure 49.25*) is a form of allergic conjunctivitis that is characterised by itchy eyes, usually worse in the spring and early summer and often associated with other allergic problems such as hay fever. Clinically, most signs are under the upper lid, which may have a cobblestone appearance instead of a smooth surface.

Giant papillary conjunctivitis with large papillae under the upper lid may be seen in soft contact lens wearers. This is usually caused by an allergy to the sterilising solutions and lens protein and may be helped by either using a preservative-free solution or using daily-wear disposable lenses.

Kaposi's sarcoma, often associated with human immunodeficiency virus (HIV) infection, can rarely present like a subconjunctival haemorrhage (*Figure 49.26*).

Considerable conjunctival and corneal irritation can be caused by the lids turning in (entropion) (*Figure 49.27*) or turning out (ectropion) (*Figures 49.28 and 49.29*), and by ingrowing lashes. The lids should be repaired surgically to their normal position.

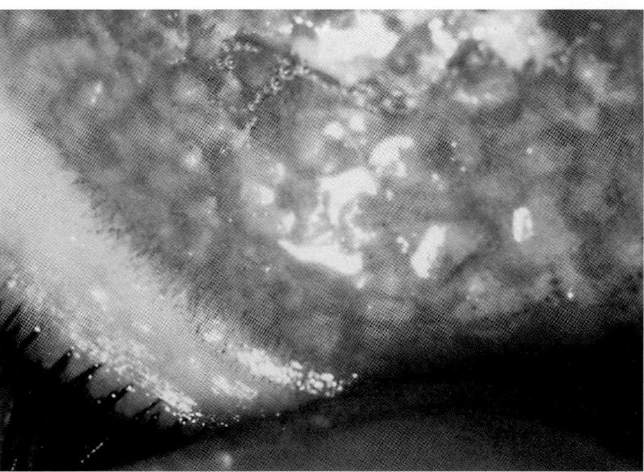

Figure 49.25 Vernal conjunctivitis (spring catarrh) showing cobblestone appearance under the upper lid.

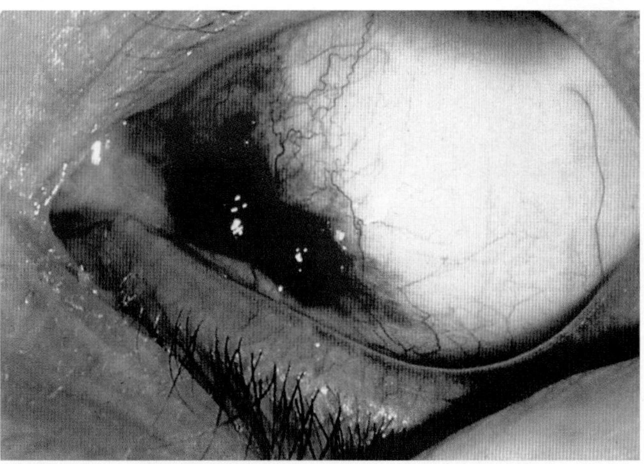

Figure 49.26 Kaposi's sarcoma of conjunctiva.

Moritz Kaposi, 1837–1902, Professor of Dermatology, Vienna, Austria, described pigmented sarcoma of the skin in 1872.

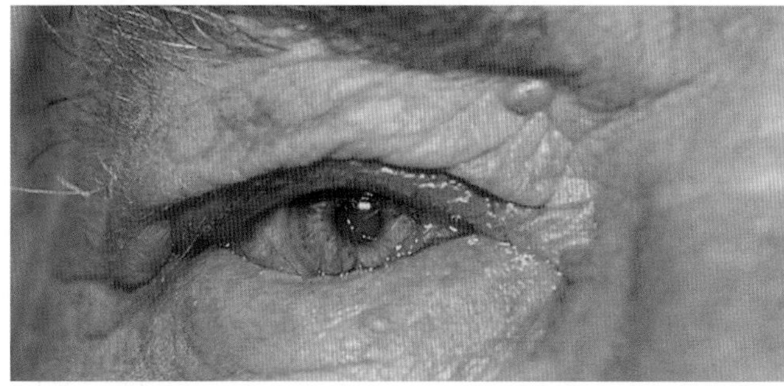

Figure 49.27 Entropion (courtesy of J Beare, FRCS).

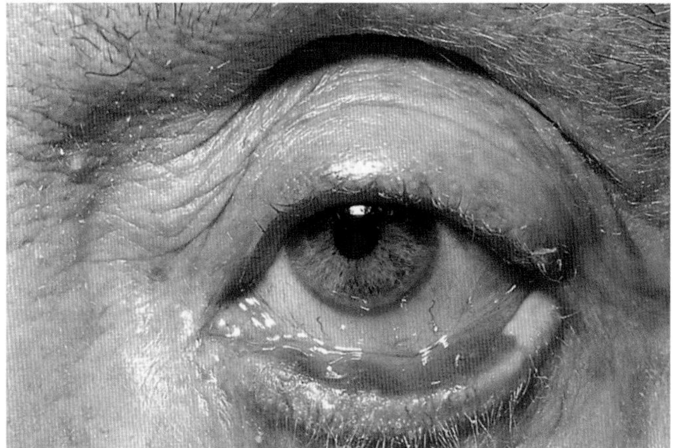

Figure 49.28 Ectropion, lower lid (courtesy of J Beare, FRCS).

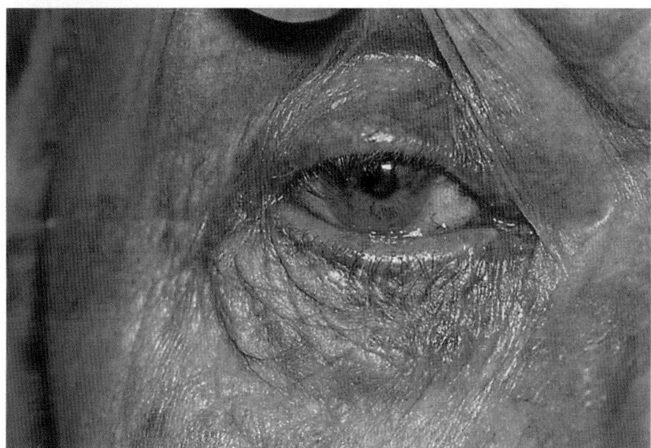

Figure 49.29 Ectropion, upper lid – chronic staphylococcal infection (courtesy of J Beare, FRCS).

Vision is not commonly affected in conjunctivitis but, with some viral infections, a keratitis may be present and result in visual impairment and pain. All of the other conditions below are painful and usually affect vision.

Keratitis (inflammation of the cornea)

Herpes simplex infection presents as a dendritic (branching) ulcer, shown easily by staining with fluorescein or Rose Bengal. It is treated with aciclovir ointment five times per day. The use of steroid drops must be avoided as this can make the condition much worse (***Figure 49.30***).

Corneal ulceration may occur as a result of ingrowing lashes or corneal foreign bodies, marginal ulceration and infected abrasions. Infected ulcers can occur in patients wearing soft contact lenses or elderly immunocompromised individuals. Herpes zoster (shingles) may affect the ophthalmic division of cranial nerve V and can give rise to a keratitis and uveitis. It is important to avoid the use of steroid drops until a diagnosis has been made. Local anaesthetic drops should also not be given on a regular basis.

Uveitis

This can be anterior (iritis) or, more rarely, posterior. In anterior uveitis, the pupil is sometimes small and/or irregular owing to formation of posterior synechiae (adhesions between the iris and the lens). There is often circumcorneal injection and there may be keratic precipitates present on the posterior surface of the cornea. Pain, photophobia and some visual loss are usually present. Posterior uveitis can present with a white eye and blurred vision. It usually takes a chronic course. Granulomatous diseases, Behçet's disease, Reiter's syndrome, toxoplasmosis and cytomegalovirus infection should be excluded. Topical systemic steroids and, sometimes, immunosuppressive drugs are useful in treating these conditions; management should be under the care of an ophthalmologist.

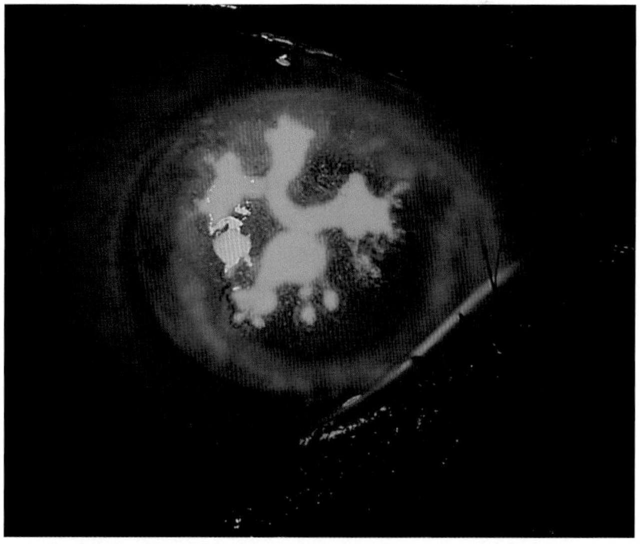

Figure 49.30 Dendritic staining caused by herpes keratitis.

Rose Bengal (or Bengal Rose) is dichlorotetraiodofluorescein.
Hulusi Behçet, 1889–1948, Professor of Dermatology, Istanbul, Turkey, described this disease in 1937.
Hans Conrad Julius Reiter, 1881–1968, President of the Health Service and Honorary Professor of Hygiene at the University of Berlin, Germany, described this disease in 1916.

Episcleritis and scleritis

Episcleritis or inflammation of the episcleral tissue often occurs as an idiopathic condition (*Figure 49.31*). Scleritis is a less common, more serious, condition in which the deeper sclera is involved. There is often an associated uveitis and severe pain. Thinning of the sclera may result. Systemic non-steroidal anti-inflammatory drugs or steroids/other immunomodulatory agents may be required to treat the condition adequately. Approximately half of patients with scleritis have an underlying systemic disorder.

Scleritis is often associated with severe rheumatoid conditions. The presence of scleritis suggests that there is active systemic disease and this requires systemic work-up, including renal function tests.

Acute angle closure

This usually occurs in older, often hypermetropic, patients. The prevalence is much higher in some Asian populations. The cornea becomes hazy, the pupil oval, dilated and non-reacting, the vision poor and the eye feels hard. In severe cases pain may be accompanied by vomiting and the condition can be mistaken for an acute abdominal problem. Tonometry (intraocular measurement) and examination of the iridocorneal angle by gonioscopy (using a prism placed on the cornea) is diagnostic. Urgent treatment to reduce the pressure with pilocarpine eyedrops, oral acetazolamide and, if refractory, mannitol should be started, followed by yttrium aluminium garnet (YAG) laser iridotomy, laser iridoplasty, anterior chamber paracentesis or surgical iridectomy. The condition is usually bilateral and the second eye usually needs a prophylactic iridotomy at the same time.

Except for a simple conjunctivitis and subconjunctival haemorrhage, which are self-limiting, the management of an acute red eye requires expert treatment and a specialist opinion should be sought. A painful eye with a cranial nerve III palsy (ptosis, dilated pupil, globe down and out) often signifies an intracranial aneurysm and should be investigated immediately.

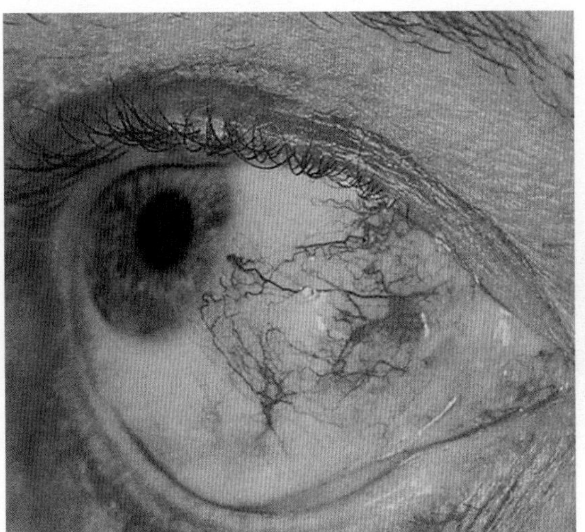

Figure 49.31 Episcleritis.

PAINLESS LOSS OF VISION

This may occur in one or both eyes, and the visual loss may be transient or permanent. Possible causes are:

- **Acute**:
  - obstruction of the central retinal artery (*Figure 49.32*);
  - obstruction of the central retinal vein (*Figure 49.33*);
  - ischaemic optic neuropathy;
  - migraine and other vascular causes;
  - vitreous and retinal haemorrhages;
  - retinal detachment (*Figure 49.34*);
  - macular hole, cyst or haemorrhage;
  - cystoid macular oedema, often after surgery;
  - hysterical blindness.
- **Chronic**:
  - cataract;
  - glaucoma;
  - macular degeneration.
  - diabetic retinopathy.

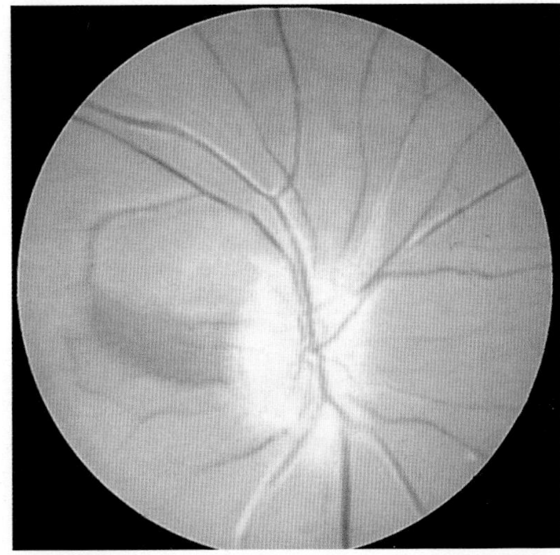

Figure 49.32 Retinal artery occlusion.

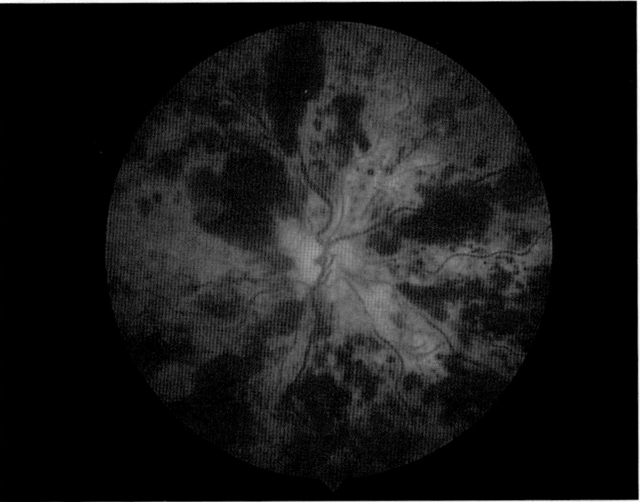

Figure 49.33 Central retinal vein occlusion.

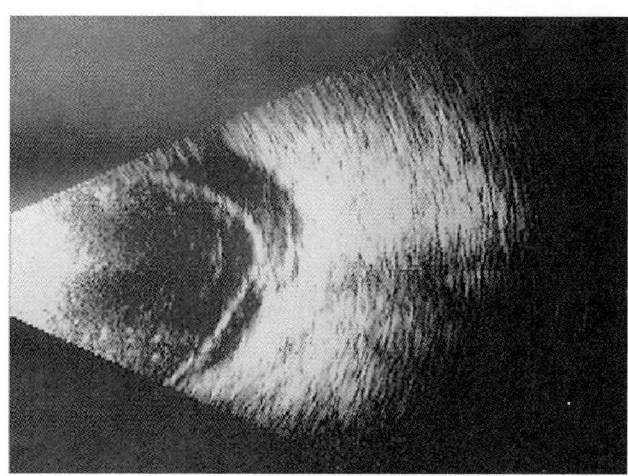

Figure 49.34 B-scan of a retinal detachment.

Specialist help should be sought in any case of loss of vision. The possibility of temporal arteritis should always be considered in the differential diagnosis of sudden visual loss, as prompt treatment of this condition is extremely important. Elderly patients with sudden visual loss should be specifically asked for symptoms of scalp tenderness and jaw claudication and temporal arteries should be palpated for pulsation and tenderness. The erythrocyte sedimentation rate and C-reactive protein should be measured immediately if temporal arteritis is suspected, and the carotid system should be examined for bruits and other signs of arteriosclerosis in cases of ischaemic optic neuropathy and central retinal artery occlusion. Glaucoma, hypertension, hyperviscosity syndromes and diabetes should be looked for in cases of central vein thrombosis.

RECENT DEVELOPMENTS IN EYE SURGERY

In the last three decades, eye surgery has become a microsurgical specialty. Cataract surgery has been transformed by changes in local anaesthesia, implants, phacoemulsification and small-incision surgery, which allows compressible/foldable silicone or acrylic implants to be inserted through a 2-mm incision. The implant power can be more accurately measured by new formulae and the use of A-scan ultrasonography or laser wavefront biometry, and multifocal and accommodative lenses are now available. An even more recent advance in cataract surgery is the development of femtosecond laser technology, which allows extremely controlled corneal incisions, lens capsule opening and lens fragmentation to be achieved automatically together with the facility to adjust the shape of the cornea at the time of surgery to improve visual outcome for some patients. The extent to which this technology improves long-term visual outcomes remains to be seen.

There are new treatments for eye disorders that involve abnormal growth of blood vessels in the back of the eye, such as the wet form of age-related macular degeneration. Anti-vascular endothelial growth factor (VEGF) antibodies, such as the drug ranibizumab, may be injected directly into the vitreous cavity to reduce new vessel proliferation. Intravitreal steroid injections or anti-VEGF agents are now also being used to treat patients with macular oedema caused, for example, by diabetic retinopathy or retinal vein occlusion.

Developments in vitreous surgery have enabled membranes to be peeled off the retina and macular holes to be repaired, and have also increased success rates in retinal detachment surgery with the additional use of gases and silicone oil or heavy liquid inserted into the vitreous cavity to tamponade the retina. Advances in technology have also led to the development of photosensitive chips and camera systems that can be implanted into the eye to restore some vision in patients with severe and otherwise untreatable macular diseases.

Some paralytic squints can be helped by the use of adjustable sutures or injections of botulinum toxin into the overacting muscles.

Refractive errors can be treated by the excimer laser. These can be combined with *laser in situ* keratomileusis (LASIK) surgery, which involves cutting a corneal flap (by femtosecond laser or surgery) and performing the laser surgery at a deeper level. There have been some concerns about defective contrast sensitivity and problems with night vision after laser correction of myopia. Phakic implants have also been used to correct high refractive errors. Corneal topography aids the accuracy of corneal and refractive surgery and the increased use and quality of CT and MRI scans has revolutionised the diagnosis of orbital and intracranial lesions involving the optic pathways (***Figures 49.35–49.37***).

Fluorescein angiography and ocular coherence tomography (OCT) are invaluable in the diagnosis and treatment of macular conditions. OCT angiography has recently been developed; this allows assessment of the retinal microvasculature without the need for systemically administered agents. This technology may reduce the need for fluorescein angiography in the future. OCT as well as scanning laser polarimetry of the retinal nerve fibre layer and Heidelberg retinal tomography (HRT) are widely used in the diagnosis and management of glaucoma. Surgical glaucoma management is also developing rapidly. Trabeculectomy surgery, where eye pressure is reduced by creating a fistula between the anterior chamber

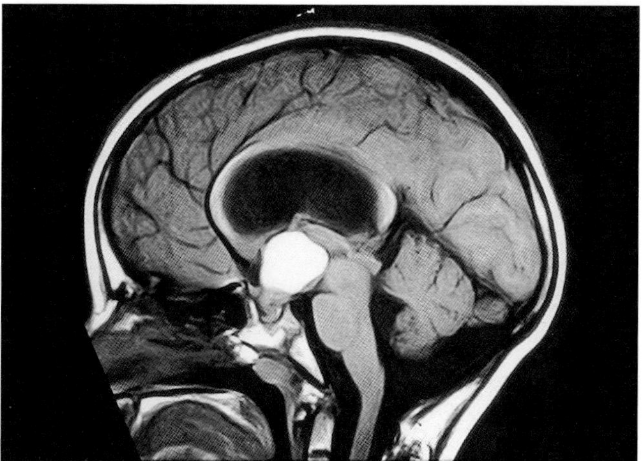

Figure 49.35 Magnetic resonance imaging scan, sagittal view. Craniopharyngioma. The mass in the suprasellar cistern is of high signal intensity because of the proteinaceous fluid that the cyst contains (courtesy of Dr Juliette Britton).

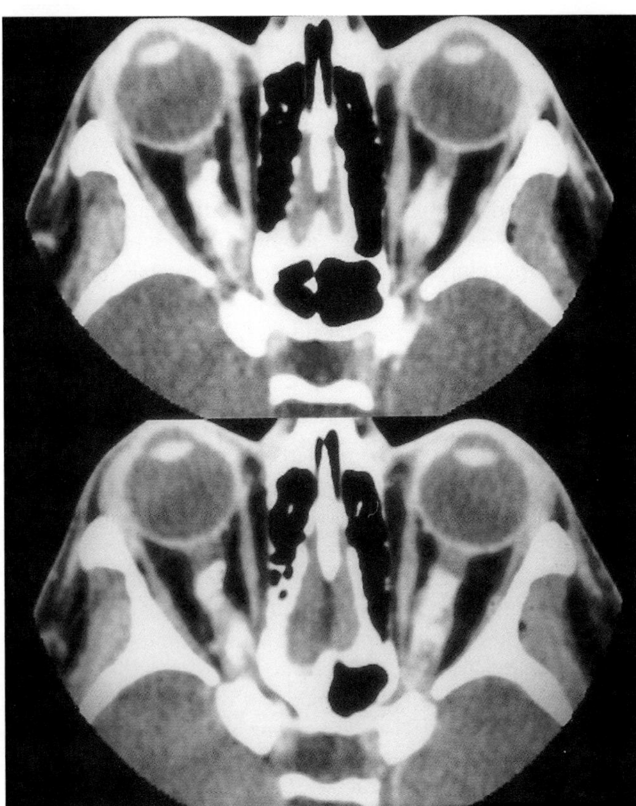

Figure 49.36 High-resolution computed tomography through the orbits showing dense calcification of the optic nerve sheaths typical of optic nerve meningioma (courtesy of Dr Juliette Britton).

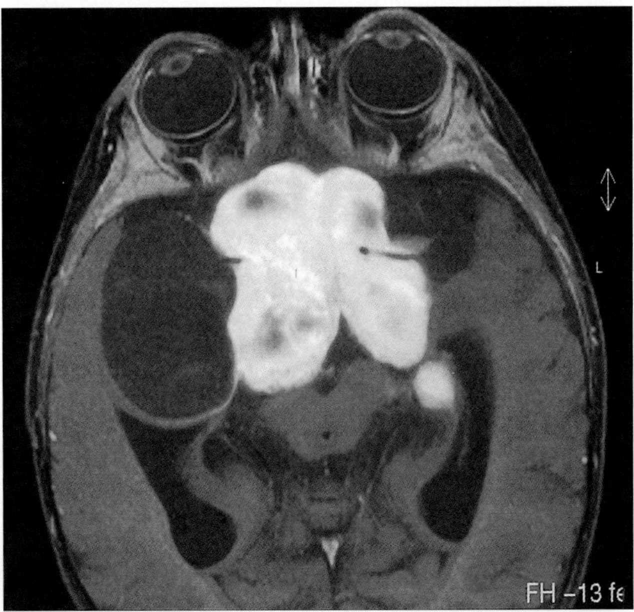

Figure 49.37 Axial enhanced magnetic resonance imaging scan showing a mass involving the optic chiasma and extending down the optic nerves and tracts.

and the subconjunctival space, remains widely used and has become more refined in recent years, with better control of wound healing using topical application of antiscarring drugs such as mitomycin C. Alternatives to trabeculectomy have been developed using devices such as Baerveldt and Ahmed shunts that drain aqueous from the eye to lower the pressure. A new revolution is also under way using minimally invasive glaucoma surgical techniques, with a variety of tiny devices now available to shunt aqueous and reduce eye pressure.

LASERS IN OPHTHALMOLOGY

Blue-green lasers (argon or frequency-doubled YAG) or diode lasers are used to treat the retina in diabetic retinopathy (pan-retinal photocoagulation for proliferative disease or focal treatment for leaky microaneurysms) and may also be used to close retinal tears or breaks that might lead to retinal detachment.

Argon laser or selective laser trabeculoplasty can be used to open the drainage angle to control elevated intraocular pressure in open angle glaucoma. Trans-scleral diode photocoagulation of the ciliary body is used to treat refractory secondary glaucoma with uncontrolled ocular pressure.

Laser iridotomy with the neodymium-doped YAG (Nd:YAG) laser is used to treat both the affected and fellow eye in acute angle closure glaucoma. The Nd:YAG laser is also used to photodisrupt and clean an opaque posterior capsule, which occurs in 5–10% of cases following cataract surgery.

SURGICAL PROCEDURES

Excision of an eyeball/enucleation

Indications include a blind, painful eye, a blind, cosmetically poor eye/intraocular neoplasm and, in cadavers, for use in corneal grafting.

The operation

The speculum is introduced between the lids and opened. The conjunctiva is picked up with toothed forceps and divided completely all round as near as possible to the cornea. Tenon's capsule is entered and each of the four rectus and two oblique muscle tendons is hooked up on a strabismus hook and divided close to the sclera. The speculum is now pressed backwards and the eyeball projects forwards. Blunt scissors, curved on the flat, are insinuated on the inner side of the globe, and these are used to sever the optic nerve. The eyeball can now be drawn forwards with the forceps, and the oblique muscles, together with any other strands of tissue that are still attaching the globe to the orbit, are divided. A swab, moistened with hot water and pressed into the orbit, will control the haemorrhage. If an orbital implant is inserted to give better eye movement, the muscles are sutured to the implant at the appropriate sites. The subconjunctival tissues and conjunctiva are closed in layers.

George G Baerveldt, 1945–2021, ophthalmologist, Emeritus Professor of Ophthalmology, UC Irvine, CA, USA.
A Mateen Ahmed, contemporary, Nigerian ophthalmologist, based in California, USA, developed the shunt that was approved by the US Food and Drug Administration in 1993.
Jacques Rene Tenon, 1724–1816, surgeon, La Salpêtrière, Paris, France.

Evisceration of an eyeball

Evisceration is preferred to excision in endo-ophthalmitis, minimising the risk of orbital and intracranial spread with meningitis. The sclera is transfixed with a pointed knife a little behind the corneosclerotic junction, and the cornea is removed entirely by completing the encircling incision in the sclera. The contents of the globe are then removed with a curette, care being exercised to remove all of the uveal tract. At the end of the operation the interior must appear perfectly white. A ball orbital implant made of acrylic or hydroxyapatite may be placed within the orbit behind the sclera to improve the appearance when the artificial eye is fitted.

Incision and curettage of chalazion (meibomian cyst)

The lid margin is everted to allow the application of a meibomian clamp. The ring of the clamp is placed on the palpebral conjunctiva with the granuloma in the centre. An incision is made with a small blade in the axis of the gland. The herniating granulomatous tissue is removed with a curette and the cavity is scraped clean. Recurrent cysts may have to have the cyst wall dissected away with scissors. A biopsy may be necessary in atypical or recurrent cysts to exclude malignant change.

FURTHER READING

Denniston A, Murray P. *Oxford handbook of ophthalmology*, 4th edn. Oxford: Oxford University Press, 2018.

Friedman NJ, Kaiser PJ, Trattler WB. *Review of ophthalmology*, 3rd edn. Edinburgh: Elsevier, 2017.

Jackson TL. *Moorfields manual of ophthalmology*, 3rd edn. London: JP Medical Ltd, 2019.

Salmon J. *Kanski's clinical ophthalmology: a systematic approach*, 9th edn. Edinburgh: Elsevier, 2019.

Wills Eye Hospital. *The Wills eye manual: office and emergency room diagnosis and treatment of eye disease*, 8th edn. Philadelphia, PA: Walters Kluwer, 2021.

CHAPTER 50 Developmental abnormalities of the face, mouth and jaws: cleft lip and palate

Learning objectives

To understand:

- The range and complexity of craniofacial anomalies
- The principles driving interventions for the developing child with a craniofacial anomaly
- In more depth the epidemiology, pathogenesis and management of cleft lip and palate

INTRODUCTION

Congenital abnormalities of the head and neck are complex and often confusing. For these reasons it is helpful to have a classification system that helps to understand the variety of conditions. For any classification system to be useful it should ideally help to explain the aetiology and pathogenesis of the abnormality and to determine treatment. For these multi-faceted and multifactorial conditions an ideal classification system is not available. Consequently, there are a number of different systems available: some are purely descriptive (e.g. Tessier's classification of clefts), while others apply only to single conditions, such as the OMENS (O, orbital abnormalities; M, mandibular deformity; E, ear deformity; N, nerve involvement; and S, soft-tissue abnormalities) classification of hemifacial (craniofacial) microsomia, which has utility in instituting treatment protocols.

CLASSIFICATION OF CRANIOFACIAL ABNORMALITIES

van der Meulen and his colleagues proposed a classification system that has significant utility in helping to understand the variety and complexity of craniofacial malformations. This classification considers the embryological development of the craniofacial region. First, in terms of the formation and fusion of the processes (branchial arches): the failure of the fusion

TABLE 50.1 Types of developmental abnormalities of the face, mouth and jaws.

Type	Examples
Cerebrocranial dysplasias	Anencephaly, microcephaly
Cerebrofacial dysplasias	Rhinencephalic and oculo-orbital dysplasias
Craniofacial dysplasias with clefting	Lateronasomaxillary, medionasomaxillary, intermaxillary, maxillomandibular clefting
Craniofacial dysplasias with dysostosis	Sphenoidal, sphenoidal frontal, frontal, frontofrontal, frontonasoethmoidal, internasal, nasal, premaxillomaxillary, nasomaxillary, maxillozygomatic, zygomatic, zygoauromandibular, temporoauromandibular, mandibular, intermandibular
Craniofacial dysplasias with synostosis	• Craniosynostosis: lambdoid and sagittal • Craniofaciosynostosis: metopic, coronal, bicoronal • Faciosynostosis: vomeropremaxillary (Binder syndrome)
Craniofacial dysplasias with dysostosis and synostosis	Crouzon, Apert and Pfeiffer syndromes
Craniofacial dysplasias with dyschondrosis	Achondroplasia

After van der Meulen JC, Mazzola R, Vermey-Keers C *et al.* A morphogenetic classification of craniofacial malformations. *Plast Reconstr Surg* 1983; **71**(4): 560–72.

Paul Tessier, 1917–2008, French maxillofacial surgeon, considered the 'father of modern craniofacial surgery'.
Jacques C H van der Meulen, 1929–2017, Professor in Plastic and Reconstructive Surgery, Erasmus University, Rotterdam, The Netherlands.
Karl Heinz Binder, 1923–2016, German dentist, documented the facial features of three children with the condition that now bears his name.
Louis Edouard Octave Crouzon, 1874–1938, neurologist, Paris, France, described this syndrome in 1912.
Eugene Apert, 1868–1940, physician, L'Hôpital des Infants Malades, Paris, France, described this syndrome in 1906.
Rudolf Arthur Pfeiffer, 1931–2012, geneticist, Münster, Germany, described this syndrome in 1964.

of these processes leads to clefting disorders, for example the failure of fusion between the frontonasal process and the maxillary process results in a cleft lip, either unilaterally or bilaterally. Second, in the formation of bone and cartilage; if this is abnormal it is termed dysostosis or dyschondrosis. Third, the formation and growth at the sutures between the various bones of the craniofacial skeleton: premature fusion leads to synostosis. Superimposed on this concept is the consideration of the development of the central nervous system; this leads to a number of types of abnormality, as outlined in ***Table 50.1***.

In addition, and in common with all classification systems, there is another large group of conditions that do not sit within the system outlined above and also listed in ***Table 50.1***.

EPIDEMIOLOGY

The incidence of congenital craniofacial anomalies varies in different parts of the world and is often not easy to quantify. ***Table 50.2*** outlines the various incidences of the more common craniofacial abnormalities.

TABLE 50.2 Approximate incidence data from multiple sources.

Condition	Incidence
Apert syndrome	1 in 100 000
Pfeiffer syndrome	1 in 100 000
Crouzon syndrome	1 in 62 500
Treacher Collins syndrome	1 in 50 000
Unicoronal synostosis	1 in 10 000
Metopic synostosis	1 in 7000
Sagittal synostosis	1 in 5000
Hemifacial microsomia	1 in 3500
Neurofibromatosis	1 in 2600
Cleft lip and palate	1 in 600

DIAGNOSIS

The diagnosis of the craniofacial anomalies has, in recent years, undergone a massive change on two fronts: first, advances in ultrasonography have increased the rate of prenatal diagnosis and impacted management significantly; second, the rapid expansion in genetic understanding has led to many more mutations being linked to particular phenotypes. Despite these advances the diagnosis of the majority of these conditions remains clinical.

MANAGEMENT

In considering the management of this vast range of heterogeneous congenital abnormalities it is very difficult to generalise about management protocols. The vast majority of management is delivered by multidisciplinary teams (MDTs) within specialist centres.

Prenatal management

There have been a few reported cases of prenatal surgery when a diagnosis was made or suspected prenatally. However, these procedures remain at present experimental; in general, the options open are for termination or best supportive care in preparation for the birth. This can often provide the parents with a period of time to adjust to the impending birth of a child with additional demands and needs. The opportunity to meet parents, adults and children who have experienced the same condition is often very valuable. Termination and its therapeutic uses is obviously a contentious and very personal issue. However, some parents may request this for very treatable conditions (e.g. isolated cleft lip); in these circumstances, the local ethics board must be involved and ultimately on occasions the advice of the courts must also be sought.

Neonatal management

In the neonatal period management is aimed at addressing the urgent issues relating to the airway, breathing, eye protection and establishing feeding.

In many of the craniofacial conditions the airway can be affected and may be fully or partially obstructed. This may be because of a retropositioned hypoplastic maxilla – the tongue falling back to close off the upper airway; this is often compounded by a hypoplastic mandible. The trachea itself may also be abnormal and tracheomalacia can lead to respiratory problems. Neonates are obligate nasal breathers and some forms of nasal obstruction can precipitate airway symptoms. In the most severe cases intubation is not possible as a result of the abnormal anatomy and a tracheostomy may be necessary. In emergency situations it may be helpful to nurse the baby prone, allowing the tongue to fall forwards.

In some cases, particularly the syndromic craniosynostoses such as Apert syndrome, Pfeiffer syndrome or Crouzon syndrome, the combination of midface retrusion and brachycephalic forehead shape can lead to severe exorbitism. In the worst cases this can cause ocular dislocation with the eyelids closing behind the globe. In severe exorbitism the eyelids do not close adequately to moisturise and protect the cornea; without intervention this may lead to irreversible corneal damage.

In neonates with airway embarrassment, even without anatomical abnormalities, the effort of breathing can be exhausting and this can significantly compromise the ability to feed. Structural anomalies can also affect the ability to feed; expert input from a specialist feeding nurse is often helpful. The use of specialised teats may be helpful but in some cases naso- or orogastric feeding may be necessary.

Management in infancy (0–12 months)

At this age treatment falls into two categories: that directed at major functional issues as for neonatal care and that directed at skull surgery in cases of craniosynostosis.

Edward Treacher Collins, 1862–1932, ophthalmic surgeon, Royal London Ophthalmic Hospital and Charing Cross Hospital, London, UK, described this syndrome in 1900.

In the older child the indications for surgery remain the same; however, there is the possibility of surgery to advance the mandible in the severely retrognathic patient. This can be used to obviate the need for a tracheostomy or to allow for early decannulation. The most effective technique is distraction osteogenesis (or distraction histogenesis), which utilises the same basic principles as in limb lengthening. The bone is cut and a device placed across the osteotomy site; after a short latent period the bone ends are gradually separated, distracting the callus. In the mandible, unlike the long bones, it is not necessary to limit the bone cut to the cortex (corticotomy) and a complete osteotomy is used. The technique allows for a lengthening of approximately 1 mm/day, after which there is a retention period to allow for consolidation of the callus.

Craniosynostosis results in premature fusion of one or more of the skull sutures. The conditions may be isolated or part of a syndrome. This can result in abnormalities of both the skull and, particularly in syndromic cases, the facial skeleton. In 10–20% of single-suture cases and a higher proportion of syndromic multisuture cases the infants develop raised intracranial pressure, which presents as episodes of distress, listlessness and disturbed sleep. This may be associated with papilloedema and, untreated, can lead to visual failure. The diagnosis is confirmed with intracranial pressure monitoring.

Some congenital lesions may obstruct the vision of one or both eyes and this type of problem needs to be addressed to minimise the chances of amblyopia developing. An example of this would be the development of a large true haemangioma of the eyelids threatening to obscure the child's vision out of one eye.

Management in early childhood (1-12 years)

In early childhood management should be aimed at dealing with functional problems – airway obstruction, speech and feeding issues – but there is an increasing imperative for surgery to address the appearance of the child. There is no doubt that visible differences can affect a child's development, both socially and emotionally; however, there is a significant role for psychological and emotional support for the whole family and in some cases for the school community to help the child, family and school understand and deal with the additional pressures that visible difference makes. Surgery can make a significant difference for some patients, but for many surgery should be delayed as long as possible for an optimal outcome in the long term.

In the older child airway issues can become a problem and their identification is more difficult. The usual presentation is of sleep apnoea, which often has an insidious onset; the history should be actively sought as parents may be accustomed to noisy snoring and daytime tiredness in the child and may not consider it abnormal. Initial investigation is with a home overnight oxygen saturation monitor, which, if abnormal, should trigger a comprehensive sleep study. The management of obstructive sleep apnoea includes the use of tonsillectomy/adenoidectomy, midface advancement and mandibular distraction as well as a variety of ventilator support devices.

Management in late childhood to maturity

Airway and other functional issues are usually stabilised by this time and interventions are aimed at optimising the overall appearance. The transition from primary school to secondary school is often a period of distress for patients with visible differences and their families. If there are pressing psychological reasons corrective surgery can be offered, although this is usually best postponed until growth is complete. In general, a comprehensive integrated corrective plan should be developed within the MDT. This would usually address the skeletal and dental abnormalities first and then address the soft tissues. The majority of the major craniofacial abnormalities should be managed by a formal MDT.

CLEFT LIP AND PALATE

Introduction

Cleft lip and/or palate is the most common congenital abnormality affecting the orofacial region. These conditions most commonly occur as isolated deformities but can also be associated with other medical conditions, e.g. congenital heart disease. They are also an associated feature in over 300 recognised syndromes. All children born with a cleft are screened for other congenital abnormalities. Where the cleft is thought to be associated with a syndrome any appropriate further investigations, including genetic counselling, will be organised.

Incidence

The incidence of cleft lip and/or palate is around 1:600 live births. There are geographical and ethnic variations, with a higher incidence among the South East Asian and Native American populations than elsewhere in the world. The accuracy of these figures may be questionable owing to a variance in reporting and healthcare infrastructure.

The typical distribution of cleft types is:

- cleft lip alone: 15% (***Figure 50.1a,b***);
- cleft lip and palate: 45%;
- isolated cleft palate: 40% (***Figure 50.1c***).

Classification of cleft

Cleft lip and/or palate presents in a heterogeneous manner. In simple terms these conditions can be divided into two clinical types (phenotypes):

1 isolated cleft palate;
2 cleft lip with or without involvement of the alveolus (tooth-bearing portion of the jaw) or palate.

Within these broad classifications a variety of combinations of cleft type can exist. These all aim to define the extent and laterality of the cleft (left/right/bilateral) (***Figure 50.2***). This information is both diagnostic and, increasingly, of prognostic value. Many have argued for a single classification system to be

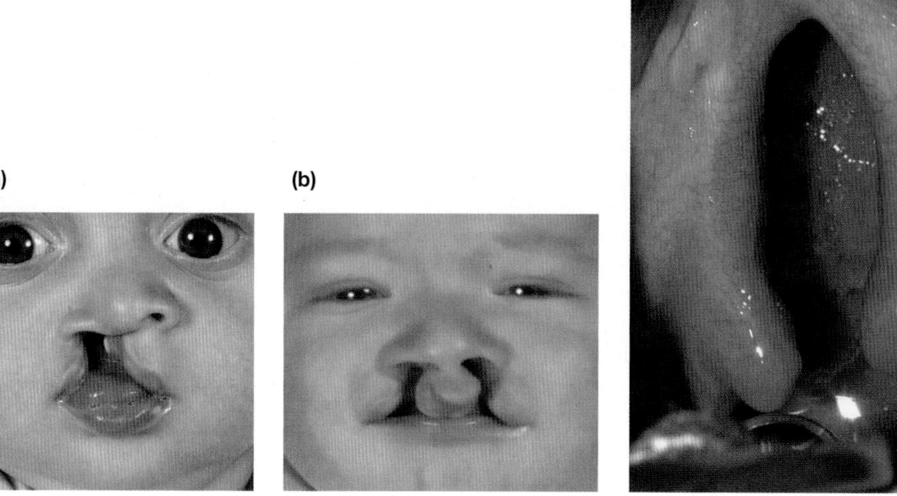

Figure 50.1 (a) Unilateral cleft lip. (b) Bilateral cleft lip. (c) Isolated cleft palate.

(a)

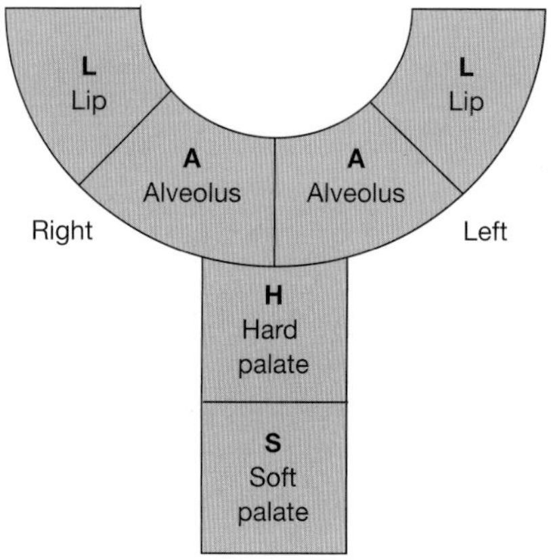

(b)

Class	Description
I	Soft palate only
II	Hard and soft palate to the incisive foramen
III	Complete unilateral of soft, hard, lip and alveolar ridge
IV	Complete bilateral of soft, hard and/or lip and alveolar ridge

Figure 50.2 (a) The LAHSHAL code. (b) The Veau classification system.

adopted: even when the same system is being used, clinicians may interpret the findings inconsistently.

In the UK, national audit data are collected for outcomes in unilateral cleft lip and palate (UCLP), thus allowing intercentre comparison. Cleft lip and/or palate is more common in males, whereas isolated cleft palate is more common in females. In UCLP the condition affects the left side in 60% of cases.

Summary box 50.1

Overview of cleft lip and palate

- Cleft lip and/or palate has two main phenotypes
- Cleft palate is more common in females and cleft lip and/or palate is more common in males
- The incidence/prevalence demonstrates geographical variation
- There are simple classification systems that describe phenotype

Aetiology

Non-syndromic cleft lip and/or palate may present as new diagnosis within a family or with a clear family history. A family history of cleft lip and palate in which a first-degree relative is affected increases the risk of subsequent cleft cases in the family, supporting the theory that there are underlying genetic mutations contributing to the aetiology. Isolated cleft palate is more commonly associated with a syndrome than cleft lip and palate and isolated cleft lip. Over 150 named syndromes are associated with cleft lip and palate, although Stickler (ophthalmic and musculoskeletal abnormalities), DiGeorge (cardiac/thymic anomalies), Down, Apert and Treacher Collins syndromes are most frequently encountered.

Victor Veau, 1871–1949, French surgeon and author of several books on cleft lip and cleft palate surgery.
Gunnar B Stickler, 1925–2010, born in Germany, Chair of Section of Paediatrics and later Paediatric Cardiology, The Mayo Clinic, Rochester, MN, USA.
Angelo Mario DiGeorge, 1921–2009, Italian American physician and pediatric endocrinologist.
John Langdon Haydon Down (sometimes given as Haydon-Down), 1828–1896, physician, The London Hospital, London, and Superintendent, Earlswood Asylum for Idiots, Surrey, UK, described this syndrome in 1866.

Various environmental factors have been implicated in the aetiology of cleft lip and/or palate, including maternal epilepsy (and associated medication) and drugs (e.g. steroids, diazepam, sodium valproate and phenytoin). The role of antenatal folic acid supplements in preventing cleft lip and/or palate remains equivocal.

Pierre Robin sequence is a condition worth considering in specific terms. This sequence comprises isolated cleft palate, retrognathia and a posteriorly displaced tongue (glossoptosis), which is associated with early airway and feeding difficulties.

Although airway obstruction does not commonly occur in babies with a non-syndromic cleft lip and/or palate, in babies with an airway obstruction, e.g. Pierre Robin sequence, hypoxic episodes during sleep and feeding can be life-threatening. Intermittent airway obstruction is more frequent and is managed conservatively. In more severe cases the children will often require adjunctive support for their airway compromise such as supplemental oxygen, nasopharyngeal airway and even tracheostomy. More controversially, surgical adhesion of the tongue to the lower lip (labioglossopexy) in the first few days after birth is an alternative but less commonly practised method of management. Mandibular distraction surgery has advocates but numerous attempts at developing a consensus view in support of this procedure for airway compromise in cleft have been unsuccessful.

> **Summary box 50.2**
>
> Aetiology of cleft lip and palate
>
> - The cause of cleft lip and/or palate is multifactorial
> - Most cases occur without a clear family history or known risk factors
> - Clefts can be associated with many craniofacial/medical syndromes

Cleft lip and/or palate: embryology and pathogenesis

Embryologically, the lip and palate are derived from facial prominences/processes.

1. The lip/nose complex is derived from a mixture of the median nasal process and the maxillary processes.
2. The primary palate is derived from the median nasal process and consists of all anatomical structures anterior to the incisive foramen, namely the alveolus and philtral portion of the upper lip. The remainder of the lip is derived from the maxillary processes.
3. The secondary palate is derived from the maxillary processes and is defined as the remainder of the palate behind the incisive foramen, which is divided into the hard palate and, more posteriorly, the soft palate. Cleft palate results in failure of fusion or descent of the two palatal shelves. This failure to descend, fuse or remain fused can result in a cleft affecting any part of the palate.

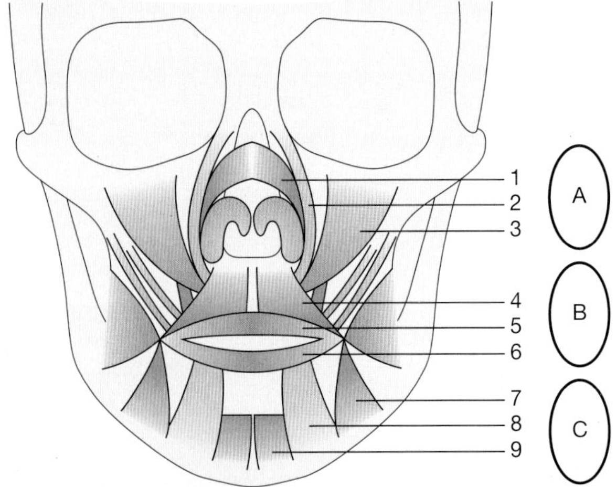

Figure 50.3 The muscle chains of the face: frontal view. The nasal cartilages are represented in blue. A, nasolabial (muscles 1–3); B, bilabial (muscles 4–6); C, labiomental (muscles 7–9); 1, transverse nasalis; 2, levator labii superioris alaeque nasi; 3, levator labii superioris; 4, orbicularis oris (oblique head) – upper lip; 5, orbicularis oris (horizontal head) – upper lip; 6, orbicularis oris – lower lip; 7, depressor anguli oris; 8, depressor labii inferioris; 9, mentalis.

Clinical anatomy

The muscle chains of the face are shown in ***Figure 50.3***. Their disruption in unilateral cleft lip is shown in ***Figure 50.4***.

> **Summary box 50.3**
>
> Embryology and pathogenesis of cleft lip and/or palate
>
> - Clefts occur at the points of fusion of facial processes
> - Normal anatomical structures are displaced and disrupted
> - Abnormal muscle insertion results in aesthetic and functional sequelae

Cleft lip

The abnormalities in cleft lip are the direct consequence of disruption of the muscles of the upper lip and nasolabial region. The muscle continuity is disrupted, leading to the cleft lip and also abnormal insertions of the muscle at the cleft edge. The effect of this can be seen on the nasal septum and the nose itself.

Unilateral cleft lip

In the unilateral cleft lip, the muscle rings are disrupted on one side, resulting in an asymmetric upper lip and/or nose. This involves the external nasal cartilages, nasal septum and anterior maxilla (premaxilla). This influences the mucocutaneous tissues, causing a displacement of nasal skin onto the lip and a retraction of labial skin, as well as changes to the vermilion and lip mucosa. All these changes need to be considered in planning the surgical repair of the unilateral cleft lip.

Pierre Robin, 1867–1950, Professor, The French School of Dentistry, Paris, France, described this syndrome in 1929.

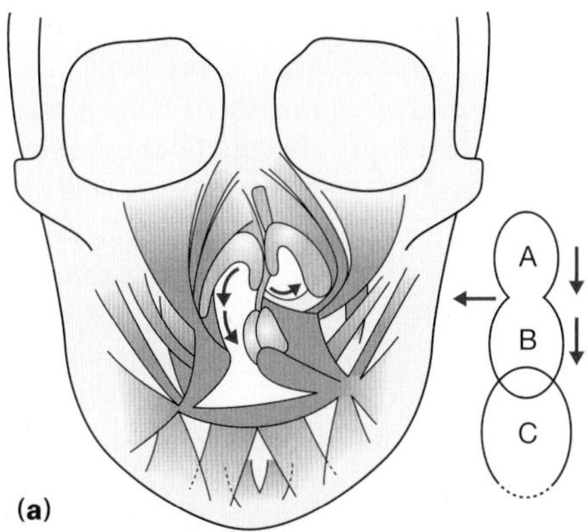

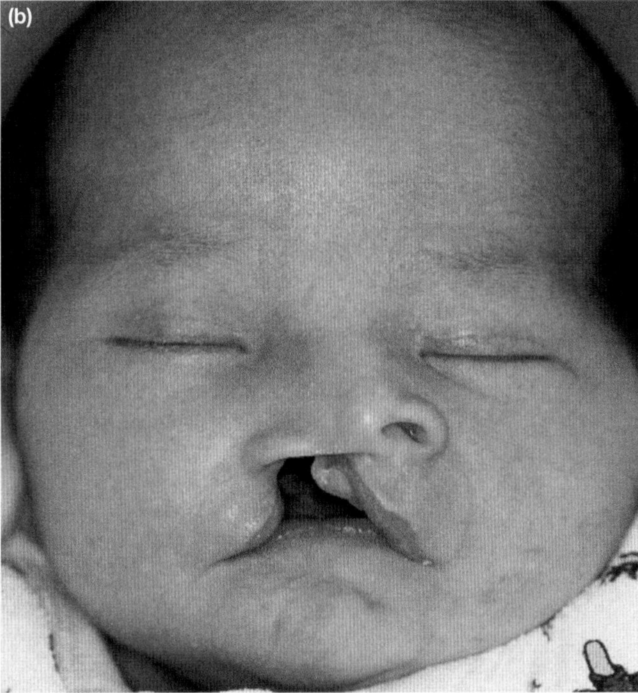

Figure 50.4 (a) Schematic representation of disruption of the nasolabial and bilabial muscle chains in unilateral (right) cleft lip. A, nasolabial; B, bilabial; C, labiomental. (b) Unilateral cleft lip before muscular reconstruction (courtesy of William P Smith).

Bilateral cleft lip

In the bilateral cleft lip the disruption is greater but often symmetrical. Muscular continuity is disrupted bilaterally, producing a flaring of the nose (caused by a lack of nasolabial muscle continuity), a protrusive premaxilla and an area of skin in front of the premaxilla devoid of muscle, known as the prolabium. As in the unilateral cleft lip, the muscular, cartilaginous and skeletal deformities influence the mucocutaneous tissues, which must be respected in planning the repair of the bilateral cleft lip.

Cleft palate

Embryologically, the primary palate consists of all anatomical structures anterior to the incisive foramen, namely the alveolus and upper lip. The secondary palate is defined as the remainder of the palate behind the incisive foramen, divided into the hard palate and, more posteriorly, the soft palate.

Cleft palate results in failure of fusion of the two palatine shelves. This failure may be confined to the soft palate alone or involve both hard and soft palate. When the cleft of the hard palate remains attached to the nasal septum and vomer, the cleft is termed incomplete. When the nasal septum and vomer are completely separated from the palatine processes, the cleft palate is termed complete.

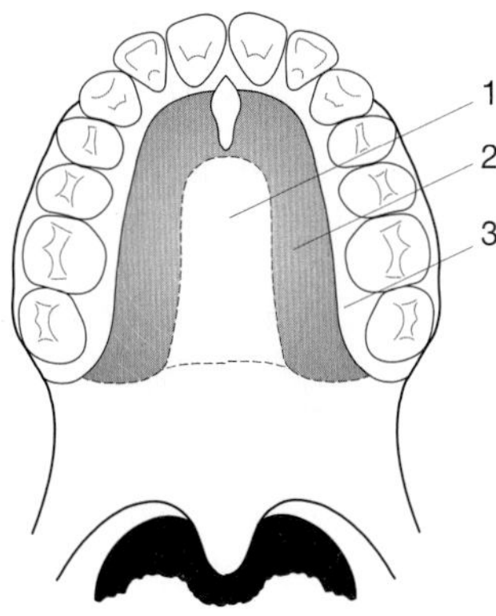

Figure 50.5 The three mucosal zones of the hard palate. 1, palatal fibromucosa; 2, maxillary fibromucosa; 3, gingival fibromucosa.

Soft palate

In the non-cleft soft palate, closure of the velopharynx, which is essential for normal speech development, is achieved by elevation of the soft palate. Although this is achieved by coordinated muscular activity, it is the levator veli palatini that is the key muscle in achieving this. In general, the muscle fibres of the soft palate are orientated transversely with no significant attachment to the hard palate. In a cleft palate the muscle fibres are orientated in an anteroposterior direction, inserting into the posterior edge of the hard palate.

Hard palate

The hard palate can be divided into three anatomical and physiological zones (***Figure 50.5***). The central palatal fibromucosa is very thin and lies directly below the floor of nose. The maxillary fibromucosa is thick and contains the greater palatine neurovascular bundle. The gingival fibromucosa lies more lateral and adjacent to the teeth.

In performing surgical closure of a cleft palate, the changes associated with the cleft must be understood to obtain an anatomical and functional repair. In complete cleft palate the median part of the palatal vault is absent and the palatal fibromucosa is reduced in size. The maxillary and gingival fibromucosa are not modified in thickness, width or position.

The cleft multidisciplinary team and primary management

The cleft team

Modern cleft services rely on well-coordinated patient pathways. The pathways and protocols may vary from country to country but the aims of treatment are consistent. Care is provided from diagnosis onwards to ensure that every patient with cleft lip and/or palate has appropriate access to the correct clinician and care at the optimal time. In the UK, most children with a cleft involving the lip are diagnosed antenatally. Scanning protocols now include an 'anomaly scan' at around 20 weeks. Isolated cleft palate cannot be diagnosed antenatally using routine scanning techniques. Some researchers have suggested that Doppler studies may help in diagnosing isolated cleft palate. When an antenatal diagnosis is confirmed, referral to a cleft team is appropriate. Clinical nurse specialist involvement would commence from this point onwards.

The cleft MDT therefore has a range of clinical expertise and specialisms within it. These are:

- **Cleft coordinator/administrator**. This is vital to ensure that patients and families have clinical episodes organised as per the protocol of the service. Responsive administrative support is vital for patients, families and clinicians.
- **Clinical nurse specialist** (CNS). The role of the CNS is central to the safe and effective delivery of cleft care. These clinicians will, in most cases, be the first clinical contact with the team. The CNS will assess the child and provide initial support to the family. Assessment of feeding, airway and general well-being is carried out. The role of the CNS is vital in ensuring that each child is optimally prepared for surgery.
- **Paediatrician**. Most children who have a cleft will be otherwise well. In some cases there may be associated or coexisting medical problems, e.g. cardiac or respiratory. These will require appropriate specialist input and perhaps coordination of care by a paediatrician.
- **Speech and language therapist** (SLT). The input of an SLT is vital where palatal involvement exists in the cleft type. Assessment and therapy are provided where required. Outcome measurements and diagnosis of palatal dysfunction are key elements of the SLT's role in cleft care.
- **Ear–nose–throat (ENT)/audiology**. Regular hearing tests and effective intervention for hearing loss are vital in ensuring speech development. This is a key part of early cleft care.
- **Paediatric dentist**. Traditionally dental/oral health has been poor for this patient group. A greater emphasis on disease prevention has resulted in much improved dental outcomes. A key part of early health care would involve a paediatric dentist.
- **Orthodontist**. The role of the orthodontist varies in different services. Some services will have early orthodontic intervention to mould the anterior cleft presurgically. This is not undertaken in many countries, e.g. the UK. The orthodontist, therefore, becomes a key figure at around 7 years of age as the child enters the early 'mixed dentition' phase. Assessment and preparation for alveolar bone grafting (ABG) as well as definitive orthodontic alignment are undertaken where required. The orthodontist is a key member of the team delivering orthognathic (jaw alignment) surgery at the point of skeletal maturity if required.
- **Clinical psychologist**. These clinicians are involved throughout the clinical pathway, providing support to patients, families and team members. Key outcomes in relation to quality of life are assessed by these clinicians.
- **Cleft surgeon**. The cleft surgeon's role is to provide assessment and intervention to patients. The main aim of cleft surgery is to correct the underlying anatomical abnormalities that can lead to issues with appearance and function. Optimal clinical outcomes can be achieved for most patients with limited surgical intervention. One to three operative interventions (depending on the type of cleft) in childhood are all that would be planned as part of a cleft pathway/protocol. Outcomes of surgery/cleft care are audited annually in most countries.

Immediate/neonatal care

Feeding

Babies born with a cleft involving the palate will feed well and thrive, provided that they receive the appropriate CNS input. The feeding aids for a child with a cleft palate aim to improve the efficiency of delivery of milk, reducing the effort of feeding. Expressed breast milk is best. A range of modified bottles and teats are available. Soft bottles allow the parents to do much of the work of milk delivery for the child by synchronising their 'squeeze' to the baby's 'suck'. Feeding plates, constructed from a dental impression of the upper jaw, were used in the past in the UK and may still be used in other parts of the world.

In some units, babies are provided with an active plate that aims not only to improve feeding but also to reduce the width of the cleft and improve the shape of the nose prior to surgery – nasoalveolar moulding (NAM). The evidence in the literature of long-term benefit using such a regime is conflicting.

Summary box 50.4

Immediate/neonatal care for a patient with a cleft and/or palate

- Babies born with a cleft may have issues with feeding and airway
- A team of clinicians is required to meet all the needs of a child with a cleft
- Most of the care delivered to a child with a cleft lip and/or palate is non-surgical in the initial phase

PRINCIPLES OF CLEFT SURGERY

The ultimate aim in cleft lip and palate management is to facilitate normal development and well-being. In seeking this, surgical repair is aimed at producing normal anatomy in the lip, nose and palate. Essentially, oral and dental health should also be optimised in the management. Key outcomes measured include speech, facial growth, general well-being and dental health.

With the exception of rare conditions such as holoprosencephaly, there is no true hypoplasia of the tissues involved

Christian Johann Doppler, 1803–1853, Professor of Experimental Physics, Vienna, Austria, enunciated the 'Doppler principle' in 1842.

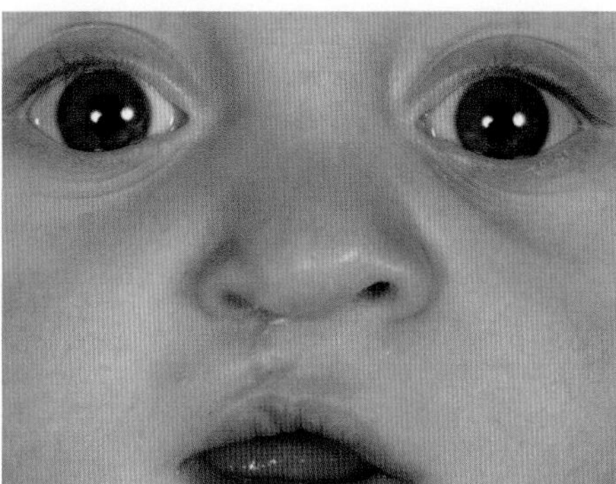

Figure 50.6 Postoperative unilateral cleft lip repair.

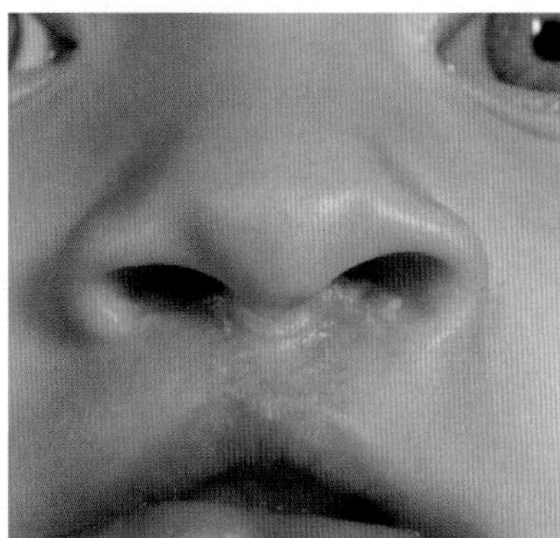

Figure 50.7 Postoperative bilateral cleft lip repair.

on either side of the cleft. There is, however, displacement, deformation and underdevelopment of the muscles and facial skeleton. Emphasis is placed on muscular reconstruction of the lip, nose and face as well as muscles of the soft palate.

Normal or near-normal anatomy promotes normal function, thereby encouraging normal growth and development of lip, nose, palate and facial skeleton. An in-depth understanding of the anatomy of the cleft is invaluable if the surgeon is to achieve normal, or near-normal, anatomical reconstruction.

Surgical techniques

Much debate and variation exist across the world in the timing and techniques employed in cleft repair. All have the common aims stated above. Restoration of form and function can be achieved using many of these protocols, but the following protocol is that which is used in the UK and was popularised in Norway.

- Cleft lip/nose and anterior palate repair is performed between 3 and 6 months of age (***Figures 50.6 and 50.7***).
- The anterior palate closure is achieved by using a single-layer mucosal flap from the vomer. The lip is closed using a variety of described techniques but most surgeons believe that the muscle repair is more important than the skin incision, hence the variation.

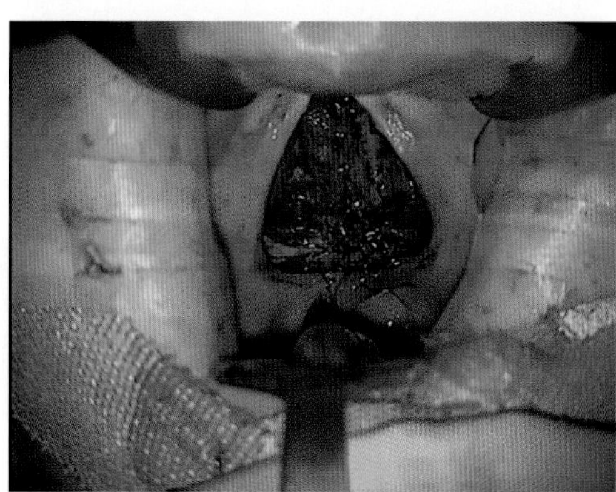

Figure 50.8 Dissection of the levator muscles.

- Definitive cleft palate repair is carried out between 6 and 12 months. There is conflicting evidence within the published literature relating to optimal timing of palate repair. The principle applied in the UK is that of closure during the early stages of speech development.
- The most common surgical approach in cleft palate repair is the intravelar veloplasty (IVVP), in which incisions along the cleft edge provide access to the soft palate muscle. The levator muscles are dissected free (***Figure 50.8***) and sutured together in the midline to recreate a muscular sling.

Summary box 50.5

Primary surgery for cleft lip and/or palate

- Treatment staged from anterior (lip) to posterior (soft palate) in the UK
- Multiple eponymous skin incisions for lip repair but muscle reconstruction is key
- Management of the levator sling is key in cleft palate repair

Age 1–7 years: early years care/follow-up

Following primary surgery, regular review by an MDT is essential. Many aspects of cleft care require review during the early years of childhood:

- hearing;
- speech;
- dental development;
- wound healing and aesthetics.

Hearing

Eustachian tube dysfunction plays a central role in the pathogenesis of otitis media with effusion (OME) in babies and children born with a cleft palate. Children with a cleft lip alone exhibit the same frequency of otitis media as their age-matched counterparts, whereas those children with palatal involvement may have an increased incidence of OME. Regardless of the

Bartolomeu Eustachio (Eustachius), 1513–1574, Professor of Anatomy, appointed physician to the Pope in 1547.

incidence it is important for normal speech development that hearing is within normal limits.

All children are screened at birth, but those who have a cleft palate are monitored regularly with audiological screening.

Speech

In the UK, specialist SLTs involved in cleft care engage at an early stage with families and children. Some teams will run group sessions to encourage speech development. Speech is constantly monitored during development and early intervention is advisable if speech pathology is suspected or diagnosed.

The problems that may present can be considered in two broad groups:

1. **Velopharyngeal incompetence** (VPI). Where the soft palate fails to achieve adequate velopharyngeal closure, which is required for certain sounds in speech, air escape occurs, leading to the resonance issue of hypernasality. This can lead to unintelligible speech because of either the hypernasality itself or the adaptations made by the child in an attempt to achieve velopharyngeal closure.
2. **Articulation errors**. These either arise as a compensatory mechanism, as stated above to overcome VPI, or, less commonly, are caused by jaw/dental and occlusal abnormalities.

To investigate these problems, the cleft team relies upon the specialist SLT assessment and investigations such as lateral videofluoroscopy and nasendoscopy. These investigations are used to visualise the palate as it moves in real time during speech.

Secondary speech surgery may be offered when there are structural issues to overcome such as VPI. Cleft palate repair is carried out when the palatal function is assessed to be suboptimal but other procedures that alter the dynamics of airflow during speech to reduce nasal escape may also be employed. These interventions are broadly termed pharyngoplasty procedures.

Dental

Dental anomalies are common findings in children with cleft lip and/or palate. Various phenomena, including delayed tooth development, delayed eruption of teeth and morphological abnormalities, are well documented. The number of teeth may be reduced (hypodontia) or increased (hyperdontia), occurring most commonly in the region of the cleft alveolus and involving the maxillary lateral incisor tooth. These abnormalities can occur in both primary and secondary dentition. All children with cleft lip and palate should undergo regular dental examination. Dental management should also include preventive measures such as dietary advice, fluoride supplements and fissure sealants. A well-maintained and disease-free dentition in childhood provides the optimal situation for successful orthodontic treatment.

Wound healing/aesthetics

Wound infections are rare but if they occur may lead to revision surgery. If this is a lip wound infection then revision can be timed to be pre-school or, if the problem is subtle, the lip can be revised opportunistically at the time of, for example, ABG.

Palatal dysfunction may require cleft palate repair or pharyngoplasty as described earlier in *Speech*.

Age 7-12 years: late childhood care/follow-up

Alveolar bone grafting

ABG is a key surgical intervention for patients with alveolar involvement. The procedure can be carried out at the same time as primary cleft lip surgery and is defined as primary bone grafting. More commonly the procedure is a separate surgical intervention later in development. In this case the term secondary bone grafting is used. Secondary bone grafting is timed in relation to the development of the underlying adult dentition in the region of the cleft. Dental development can be assessed radiographically and the optimal window for bone grafting is thus easily defined. The lateral incisor tooth is commonly absent or diminutive but, if present and of normal morphology, the bone graft can be timed around the root development of this tooth (often described as early secondary grafting at age 5–7 years).

The canine tooth is most commonly used in assessment and timing. The optimal timing for intervention is at the point when the canine root is one-half to two-thirds formed (often described as late secondary grafting at age 8–11 years). As there is wide variation in the rate of dental development it is better to assess each patient and their dentition on an individual basis and tailor the treatment to this.

Patients may undergo a short period of orthodontic treatment prior to bone grafting. Less than 50% of patients with UCLP will require this. When carried out, the aim is to expand the alveolar cleft to improve surgical access. Occasionally the adjacent teeth may be aligned in advance of surgery if they are interfering with access. It is vital in a bilateral cleft to be able to stabilise the mobile anterior (premaxillary) segment to facilitate bone healing. Adjunctive secondary procedures can be carried out simultaneously, e.g. cleft lip revision.

The success rate of ABG is high. There are a variety of scoring systems used to measure outcome. Close teamwork between the cleft surgeon and the orthodontist is vital. In the situation where there is significant hypodontia in the region of the cleft a decision may be taken **not** to perform ABG. In this case the missing teeth can be replaced with a variety of restorative options, including a denture, an adhesive bridge or an implant-retained prosthesis. Bone grafting will be required for implant placement but this is better carried out when the patient is skeletally mature.

The primary objectives when performing ABG are to:

- provide adequate bony support for the adult teeth to enable subsequent orthodontic alignment;
- enable the eruption of adult teeth into the line of the dental arch;
- stabilise the premaxilla in bilateral clefts;
- definitively close the residual alveolar cleft.

The secondary objectives or associated benefits may include aesthetic improvements to the nasolabial region.

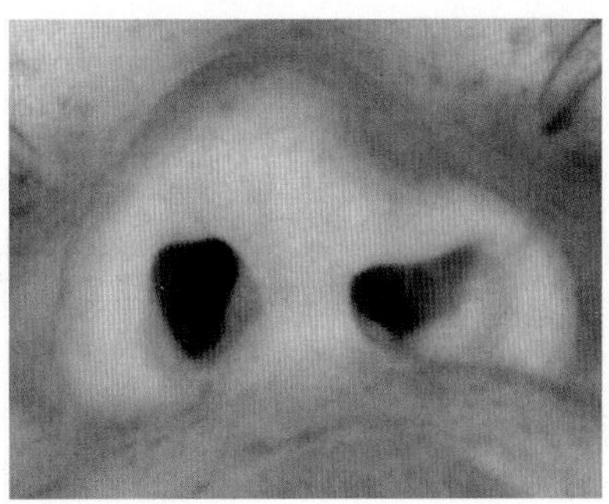

Figure 50.9 Nasal asymmetry.

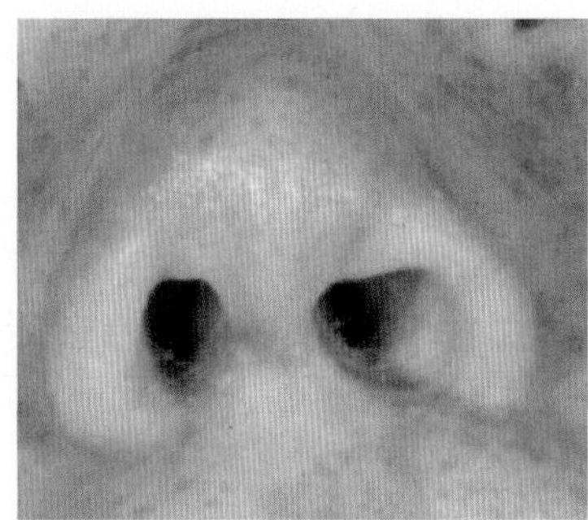

Figure 50.10 Nasal asymmetry addressed by open surgical revision.

Orthodontic treatment

Children with cleft lip and alveolar involvement will often benefit from orthodontic treatment. Orthodontic treatment is commonly carried out in two phases:

1. Mixed dentition (8–10 years): to prepare the alveolar cleft for ABG (see ***Alveolar bone grafting***).
2. Permanent dentition (12–18 years): to definitively align the dental arches, aiming for a normal functioning occlusion. This phase of treatment may be linked to preparation for orthognathic surgery (jaw alignment surgery).

SECONDARY/REVISION SURGERY

These procedures are undertaken to improve aesthetics and/or function. They may be considered as procedures that were unplanned at the time of primary surgery. Specific examples are as follows.

Cleft lip/nose revision

Indications for revisional surgery to a previously repaired cleft lip are dependent on the site and severity of the residual deformity.

Relative indications for lip revision include:

- misaligned vermilion;
- lip asymmetry.

Relative indications for residual nasal deformity include:

- incorrect alar base position;
- poor nasal tip projection;
- deviation of cartilaginous nasal septum into the non-cleft nostril.

Residual nasal deformity is an external manifestation of incomplete reconstruction of the nasolabial muscle ring (see ***Clinical anatomy***). It is thought less than ideal to surgically interfere with the nasal septum in the growing child. Minor adjustments are possible before the age of 14–15 years (***Figures 50.9 and 50.10***), but more major nasal surgery is usually delayed until after this age.

Open septorhinoplasty may be considered for definitive surgical nasal correction. In patients with cleft lip and palate, open surgery is preferred to gain access to the external cartilaginous framework, which is frequently affected by the primary issues of muscle attachment related to the cleft. One common feature is collapse of the lower lateral cartilage on the cleft side together with a dislocation of the cartilaginous septum into the non-cleft nostril. The open method ensures adequate access and repositioning of the cartilaginous framework as a tertiary procedure to improve nasal tip projection, correct septal deformity and relocate alar cartilages. Grafting techniques are often employed using harvested septal (nasal) cartilage or conchal (ear) cartilage.

Orthognathic surgery

Impaired growth of the midface (maxilla) is a consequence of a number of factors, which are poorly understood. Genetic factors as well as local factors following primary surgery may be involved. Elective maxillary advancement or bimaxillary surgery may be indicated to restore aesthetics and dental occlusal harmony. Orthognathic surgery is usually performed when facial growth is complete (16–17 years in female patients, 17–19 years in male patients).

The principal dentofacial deformity associated with cleft lip and palate is underdevelopment in both the horizontal and vertical direction of the maxilla. This jaw size discrepancy can be corrected with orthognathic surgery (***Figure 50.11***).

SUMMARY

Cleft care has been the subject of significant reorganisation in recent years. Coordinated care is provided in most countries by MDTs. Specific training pathways exist in many countries for cleft surgery. Better collection and collation of outcome data will drive evidence-based improvements in care and service development.

Summary box 50.6

Summary of care for patients with cleft lip and/or palate

- Cleft surgery in infants is time sensitive
- Aesthetic and functional outcomes are important and are measured
- Surgery involves restoration of muscle position to as close to normal as possible
- Planned surgery includes bone grafting in children with alveolar involvement
- Revision/secondary surgery optimises aesthetic and functional outcomes

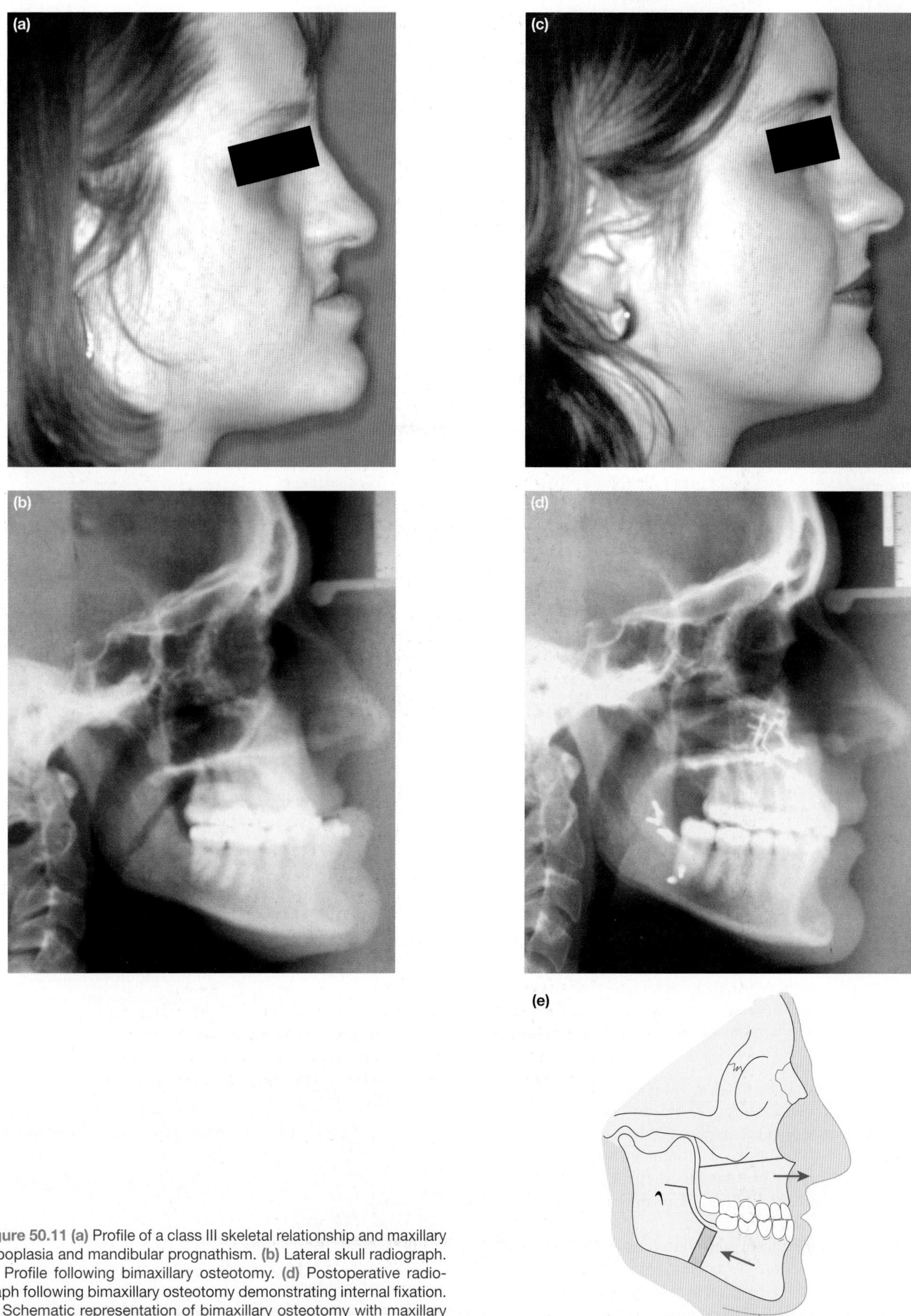

Figure 50.11 (a) Profile of a class III skeletal relationship and maxillary hypoplasia and mandibular prognathism. (b) Lateral skull radiograph. (c) Profile following bimaxillary osteotomy. (d) Postoperative radiograph following bimaxillary osteotomy demonstrating internal fixation. (e) Schematic representation of bimaxillary osteotomy with maxillary advancement and mandibular retrusion (courtesy of William P Smith).

FURTHER READING

Bearn D, Mildinhall S, Murphy T *et al.* Cleft lip and palate care in the United Kingdom – the Clinical Standards Advisory Group (CSAG) study. Part 4: outcome comparisons, training, and conclusions. *Cleft Palate Craniofac J* 2001; **38**(1): 38–43.

Bongaarts CA, Prahl-Andersen B, Bronkhorst EM *et al.* Infant orthopedics and facial growth in complete unilateral cleft lip and palate until six years of age (Dutchcleft). *Cleft Palate Craniofac J* 2009; **46**(6): 654–63.

Boorman JG, Sommerlad BC. Levator palati and palatal dimples: their anatomy, relationship and clinical significance. *Br J Plast Surg* 1985; **38**(3): 326–32.

Boorman JG, Sommerlad BC. Musculus uvulae and levator palati: their anatomical and functional relationship in velopharyngeal closure. *Br J Plast Surg* 1985; **38**(3): 333–8.

Boyne PJ, Sands NR. Secondary bone grafting of residual alveolar and palatal clefts. *J Oral Surg* 1972; **30**(2): 87–92.

Boyne PJ, Sands NR. Combined orthodontic-surgical management of residual palato-alveolar cleft defects. *Am J Orthod* 1976; **70**(1): 20–37.

Fudalej PS, Wegrodzka E, Semb G, Hortis-Dzierzbicka M. One-stage (Warsaw) and two-stage (Oslo) repair of unilateral cleft lip and palate: craniofacial outcomes. *J Craniomaxillofac Surg* 2015; **43**(7): 1224–31.

Furlow Jr LT. Cleft palate repair by double opposing Z-plasty. *Plast Reconstr Surg* 1986; **78**(6): 724–38.

Harville EW, Wilcox AJ, Lie RT *et al.* Cleft lip and palate versus cleft lip only: are they distinct defects? *Am J Epidemiol* 2005; **162**(5): 448–53.

Harville EW, Wilcox AJ, Lie RT *et al.* Epidemiology of cleft palate alone and cleft palate with accompanying defects. *Eur J Epidemiol* 2007; **22**(6): 389–95.

McBride WA, McIntyre GT, Carroll K, Mossey PA. Subphenotyping and classification of orofacial clefts: need for orofacial cleft subphenotyping calls for revised classification. *Cleft Palate Craniofac J* 2016; **53**(5): 539–49.

Naran S, Kirschner RE, Schuster L *et al.* Simonart's band: its effect on cleft classification and recommendations for standardized nomenclature. *Cleft Palate Craniofac J* 2017; **54**(6): 726–33.

Noverraz RL, Disse MA, Ongkosuwito EM *et al.* Transverse dental arch relationship at 9 and 12 years in children with unilateral cleft lip and palate treated with infant orthopedics: a randomized clinical trial (DUTCHCLEFT). *Clin Oral Investig* 2015; **19**(9): 2255–65.

Sandy J, Williams A, Mildinhall S *et al.* The Clinical Standards Advisory Group (CSAG) cleft lip and palate study. *Br J Orthod* 1998; **25**(1): 21–30.

Sandy JR, Williams AC, Bearn D *et al.* Cleft lip and palate care in the United Kingdom – the Clinical Standards Advisory Group (CSAG) study. Part 1: background and methodology. *Cleft Palate Craniofac J* 2001; **38**(1): 20–3.

Sell D, Grunwell P, Mildinhall S *et al.* Cleft lip and palate care in the United Kingdom – the Clinical Standards Advisory Group (CSAG) study. Part 3: speech outcomes. *Cleft Palate Craniofac J* 2001; **38**(1): 30–7.

Sitzman TJ, Mara CA, Long Jr RE *et al.* The Americleft Project: burden of care from secondary surgery. *Plast Reconstr Surg Glob Open* 2015; **3**(7): e442.

Sommerlad BC. Surgical management of cleft palate: a review. *J R Soc Med* 1989; **82**(11): 677–8.

Sommerlad BC. The use of the operating microscope for cleft palate repair and pharyngoplasty. *Plast Reconstr Surg* 2003; **112**(6): 1540–1.

Sommerlad BC. A technique for cleft palate repair. *Plast Reconstr Surg* 2003; **112**(6): 1542–8.

Sommerlad BC, Fenn C, Harland K *et al.* Submucous cleft palate: a grading system and review of 40 consecutive submucous cleft palate repairs. *Cleft Palate Craniofac J* 2004; **41**(2): 114–23.

Wilcox AJ, Lie RT, Solvoll K *et al.* Folic acid supplements and risk of facial clefts: national population based case-control study. *BMJ* 2007; **334**(7591): 464.

Williams AC, Bearn D, Mildinhall S *et al.* Cleft lip and palate care in the United Kingdom – the Clinical Standards Advisory Group (CSAG) study. Part 2: dentofacial outcomes and patient satisfaction. *Cleft Palate Craniofac J* 2001; **38**(1): 24–9.

CHAPTER

51 The ear, nose and sinuses

Learning objectives

To be familiar with:
- The anatomy of the ear
- The conditions of the outer, middle and inner ear
- The examination of the ear, including hearing tests
- The basic anatomy of the nose and paranasal sinuses
- The principles of managing post-traumatic nasal and septal deformity
- The causes and management of epistaxis

To understand:
- The outer layer of the tympanic membrane migrates outwards
- The facial nerve can be damaged by trauma and ear disease
- Chronic ear disease can lead to intracranial sepsis
- There are two types of hearing loss: conductive and sensorineural
- The clinical features of sinus infection, its treatment and potential complications
- The diagnosis and management of chronic rhinosinusitis with and without nasal polyposis
- The common sinonasal tumours, their presentation, investigation and principles of treatment

INTRODUCTION

Disorders affecting the ear, nose and sinus are common reasons for primary care attendance; however, few surgeons will encounter such diseases in day-to-day practice. Nonetheless, traumatic, infective and neoplastic processes can impact on these organs and their anatomical proximity to critical anatomical structures demands a basic understanding in order to efficiently diagnose, refer and treat conditions. A full and detailed review of the management of ear and nose conditions is beyond the scope of this text. Instead, the aim of this chapter is to familiarise the reader with the basic anatomy and pathology relevant to patients who present with conditions affecting the ear, nose and sinuses.

THE EAR

The mammalian ear is an evolutionary masterpiece. Its highly complex 'three-dimensional anatomy' is best learnt by dissecting cadaver temporal bones.

The external ear

The external and middle ear develop from the first two branchial arches. The external ear canal is 3 cm in length; the outer two-thirds is cartilage and the inner third is bony. The skin on the lateral surface of the tympanic membrane is highly specialised and migrates outwards along the ear canal. As a result of this migration most people's ears are self-cleaning. The external canal is richly innervated and the skin is tightly bound down to the perichondrium so that swelling in this region results in severe pain.

The lymphatics of the external ear drain to the retroauricular, parotid, retropharyngeal and deep upper cervical lymph nodes.

The tympanic membrane and middle ear

The anatomy of the tympanic membrane and ossicles is shown in ***Figure 51.1***. The relations of the middle ear are important (***Figure 51.2***). The tympanic membrane and ossicles act as a transformer of vibrations in the air to vibrations within the fluid-filled inner ear.

The inner ear

The inner ear comprises the cochlea and vestibular labyrinth (saccule, utricle and semicircular canals). These structures are embedded in dense bone called the otic capsule.

The cochlea is a coiled shell of two and three-quarter turns. Within the cochlea is a spiral structure called the cochlear duct (***Figure 51.3***), which contains endolymph that is partitioned by Reissner's membrane from the perilymph of the scala vestibuli and the basilar membrane from the perilymph of the scala tympani. The perilymph sits uninterrupted from the oval window and stapes footplate at the start of the scala vestibuli in continuity with the round window membrane at the end of the scala tympani (***Figure 51.4***). The endolymph has a high concentration of potassium, similar to intracellular fluid, and

Ernst Reissner, 1824–1878, Professor of Anatomy at Dorpat and later at Breslau, Germany (now Wrocław, Poland), described the vestibular membrane of the cochlea in 1851.

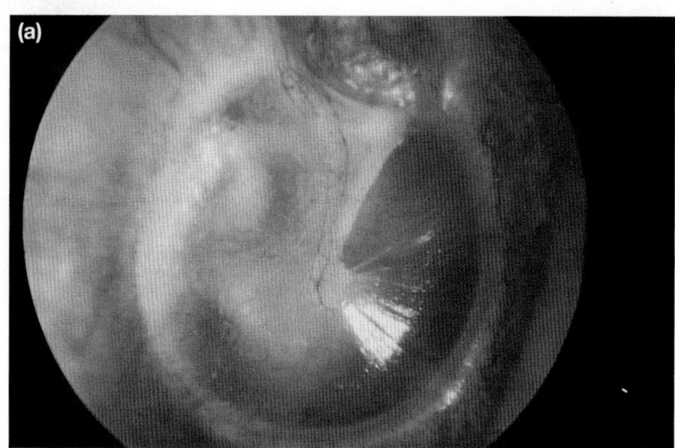

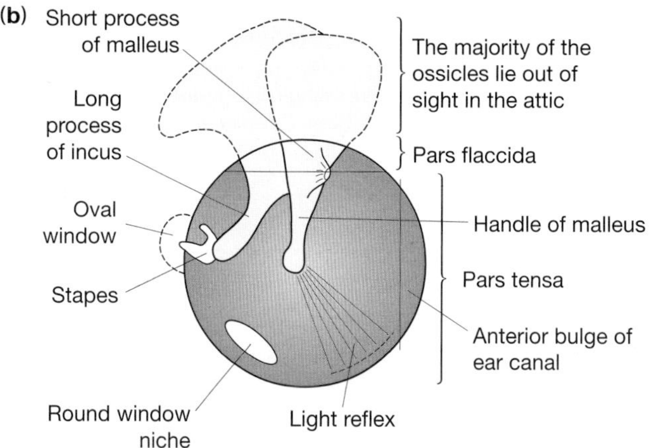

Figure 51.1 (a) Right tympanic membrane and (b) diagram to illustrate the anatomy of the tympanic membrane and ossicles (courtesy of Dr Christian Deguine).

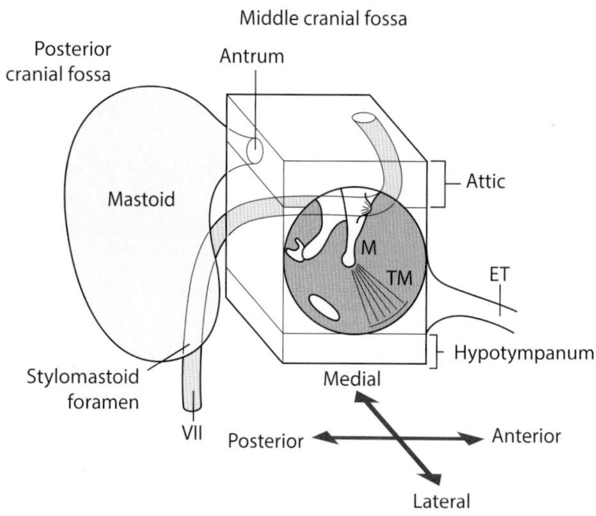

Figure 51.2 Diagram of the right ear to show the relationships of the middle ear. ET, Eustachian tube; M, malleus; TM, tympanic membrane; VII, facial nerve (courtesy of Dr Christian Deguine).

the perilymph has a high sodium concentration and communicates with the cerebrospinal fluid (CSF). Maintenance of the ionic gradients is an active process and is essential for neuronal activity.

There are approximately 15 500 hair cells in the human cochlea. They are arranged in rows of 3500 inner and 12 000 outer hair cells. Movement of the stapes footplate causes a pressure wave through the perilymph, resulting in vibration of the basilar membrane and a shearing motion between the tops of the hair cells and the tectorial membrane. The inner hair cells act as mechanicoelectric transducers, converting the acoustic signal into an electric impulse. The outer hair cells contain contractile proteins and serve to tune the basilar membrane on which they are positioned. Each inner hair cell responds to a particular frequency of vibration. When stimulated, it depolarises and passes an impulse to the cochlear nuclei in the brainstem.

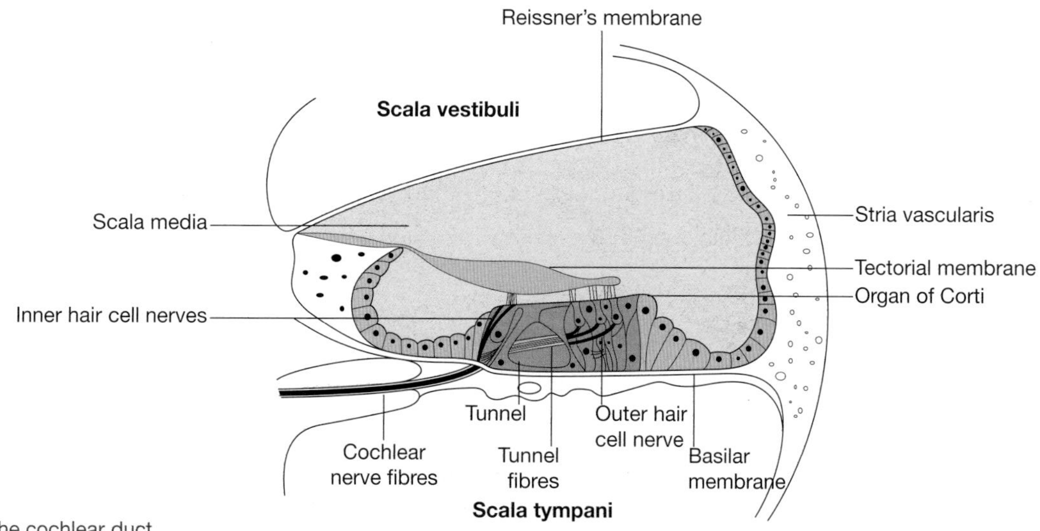

Figure 51.3 The cochlear duct.

Bartolomeu Eustachio (Eustachius), 1513–1574, Professor of Anatomy, appointed physician to the Pope in 1547.
Alfonso Giacomo Gaspare Corti, 1822–1876, Italian anatomist.

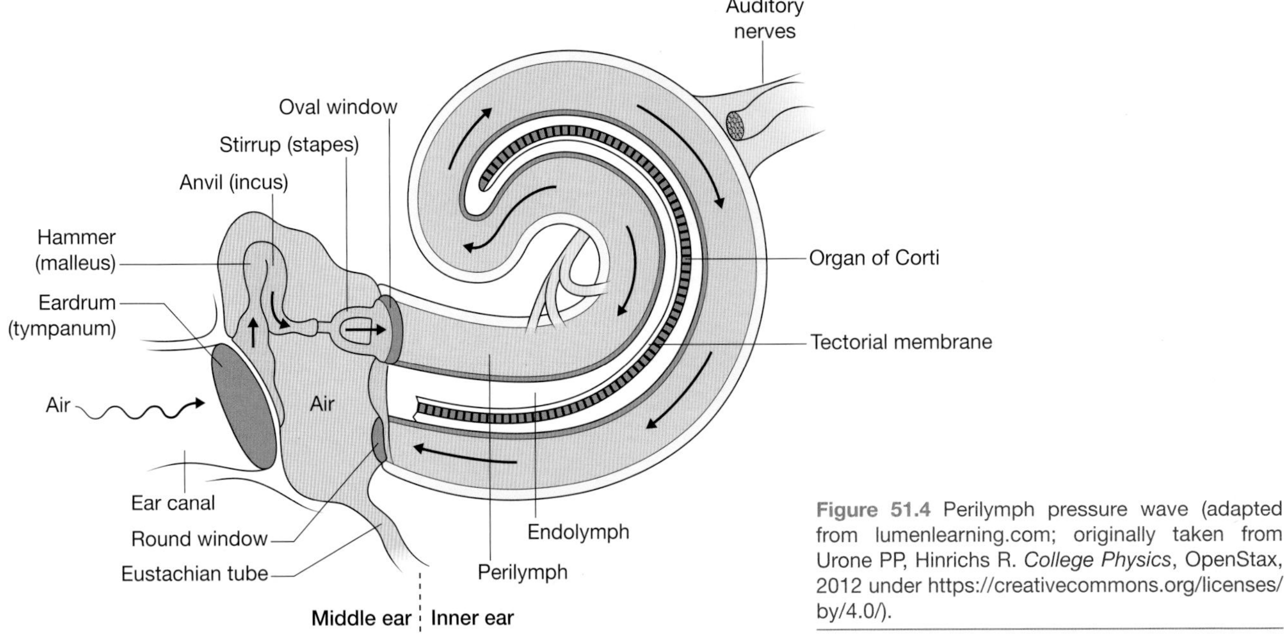

Figure 51.4 Perilymph pressure wave (adapted from lumenlearning.com; originally taken from Urone PP, Hinrichs R. *College Physics*, OpenStax, 2012 under https://creativecommons.org/licenses/by/4.0/).

The vestibular labyrinth consists of the semicircular canals, utricle and saccule and their central connections. The three semicircular canals are arranged in the three planes of space at right angles to each other. Like the auditory system, hair cells are present. In the lateral canals, the hair cells are embedded in a gelatinous cupula. Shearing forces, caused by angular movements of the head, produce hair cell movements and generate action potentials. In the utricle and saccule the hair cells are embedded in an otoconial membrane, which contains particles of calcium carbonate. These respond to changes in linear acceleration and the pull of gravity.

Impulses are carried centrally by the vestibular nerve and connections are made to the spinal cord, cerebellum and external ocular muscles. Its function is to record the position and movements of the head.

The sensory nerve supply

The external ear is supplied by the auriculotemporal branch of the trigeminal nerve (cranial nerve [CN] V) and the greater auricular nerve (C2/3), together with branches of the lesser occipital nerve (C2). CNs VII, IX and X also supply small sensory branches to the external ear. The middle ear is supplied by the glossopharyngeal nerve (CN IX).

This complicated and rich sensory innervation means that referred otalgia is common and may originate from the normal area of distribution of any of the above nerves. A classic example is the referred otalgia caused by cancer of the larynx or hypopharynx.

Taking a thorough history is the most important part of the assessment; the symptoms that need to be enquired after are listed in *Table 51.1*.

Summary box 51.1

Applied anatomy

- The skin on the outer surface of the eardrum migrates outwards so that the ear canal is 'self-cleaning'
- Infection of the middle ear and mastoid can easily spread to the cranial cavity
- The facial nerve pursues a tortuous course through the middle ear
- The ear has a rich sensory innervation so that 'referred otalgia' is common
- Cancer of the larynx or lower pharynx can present with otalgia

TABLE 51.1 History taking.

Ask about:
- Earache, pain and itch
- Hearing loss
- Discharge: type, quantity and smell
- Tinnitus
- Vertigo
- Facial weakness
- Speech and development (in children)
- Past history: head injury, baro- or noise trauma, ototoxics, family history and previous ear surgery

EXAMINATION OF THE EAR

The instruments required for examination are shown in *Figure 51.5*. Examination of the ear is part of the general ear, nose and throat (ENT) examination. Rinne and Weber tuning fork tests are used to distinguish between a conductive

Friedrich Heinrich Adolf Rinne, 1819–1868, otologist, Göttingen, Germany, described this test in 1855.
Friedrich Eugen Weber-Liel, 1832–1891, otologist, University of Berlin and Jena, Germany, described the operation of tenotomy of the tensor tympani used for certain forms of partial deafness.

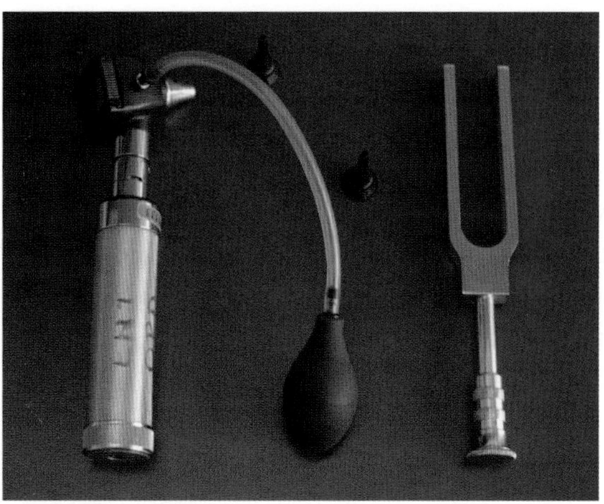

Figure 51.5 Tools of the trade: a fibreoptic otoscope, with pneumatic attachment and a selection of specula. Also a 512-Hz tuning fork.

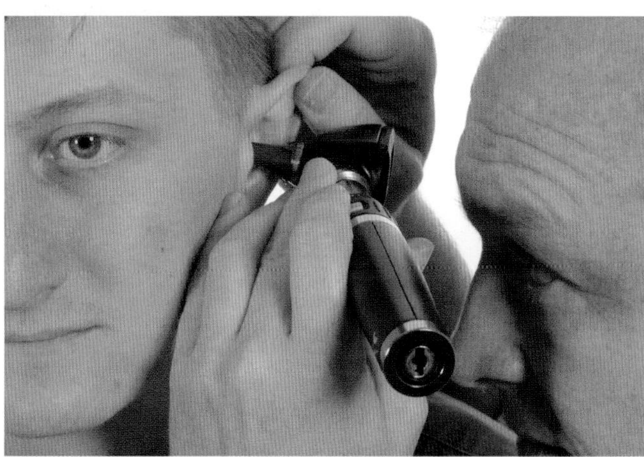

Figure 51.6 The correct method of holding the otoscope. Note the pinna is retracted to straighten the ear canal. Hold the barrel of the otoscope so that the examiner's little finger is balanced on the patient's cheek; this prevents the speculum impinging on the tympanic membrane in case of sudden movement.

and a sensorineural hearing loss. The correct way to hold an otoscope is shown in ***Figure 51.6***.

The CNs and especially the function of the facial nerve should be examined. Although conversational testing can give a useful guide to the level of hearing, pure tone audiometry in a soundproof booth is the best way of establishing the air and bone hearing levels (***Figure 51.7***). Other common audiological tests include speech audiometry, tympanometry, stapedial reflexes, electric response audiometry, otoacoustic emissions, caloric testing and electronystagmography (see ***Further reading***).

Radiological investigation

Computed tomography (CT) scanning of the temporal bones is commonly performed before mastoid surgery to show detailed individual anatomy, as well as alerting the surgeon to anatomical variants. Pus, bone and air are shown well on high-resolution CT (***Figure 51.8***).

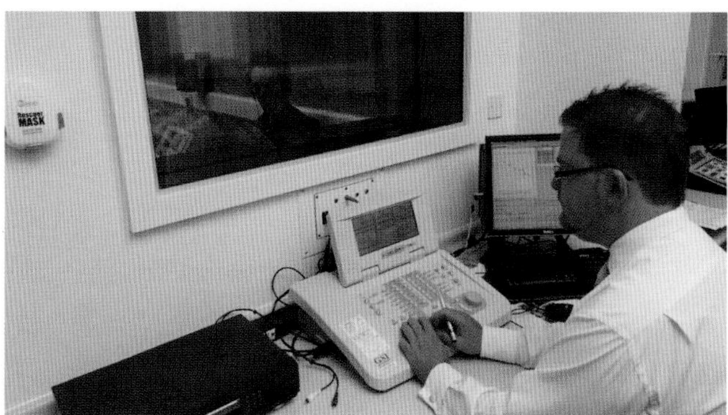

Figure 51.7 Audiometry. The patient sits in a soundproof room and the audiologist presents sounds at different thresholds and records the responses.

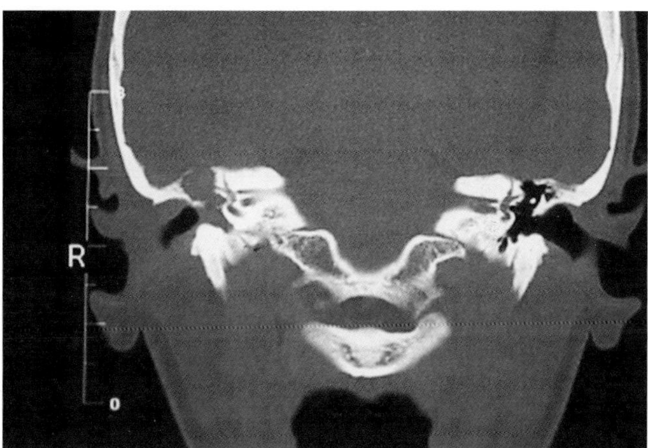

Figure 51.8 Computed tomography scan showing a normal left ear. The air-filled middle ear and the incus and stapes, the semicircular canals and internal acoustic meatus can be seen. In the right ear the entire middle ear and mastoid are opaque and filled with soft tissue. This is the typical appearance of a cholesteatoma.

Magnetic resonance imaging (MRI) is better than CT at imaging soft tissue (e.g. facial and auditory nerve) and is the best method for imaging tumours of the acoustic nerves (***Figure 51.9***). Diffusion-weighted MRI is also commonly used to detect recurrent cholesteatoma.

CONDITIONS OF THE EXTERNAL EAR

Congenital anomalies

The external and middle ear originate from the first and second branchial arches, but the cochlea is neuroectodermal in origin. An individual can have a congenital abnormality of the pinna and middle ear with a normal cochlea and therefore the potential for normal hearing.

Trauma

A haematoma of the pinna occurs when blood collects under the perichondrium. The cartilage receives its blood supply

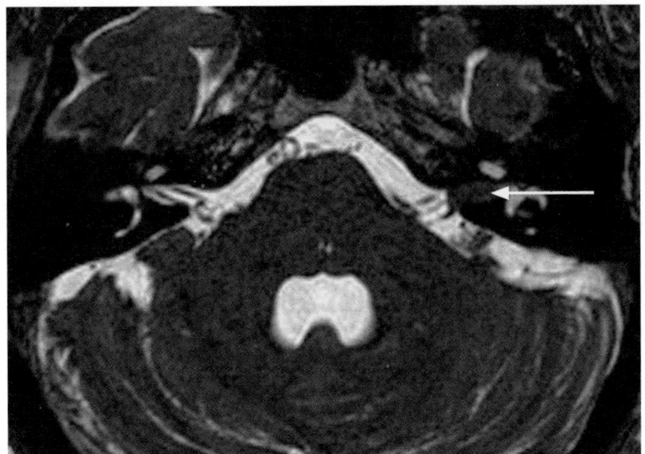

Figure 51.9 Computed tomography scan showing a vestibular schwannoma occluding the left internal acoustic meatus (arrow).

from the perichondrial layer and will die if the haematoma is not evacuated, resulting in a so-called cauliflower ear. A generous incision under anaesthetic, with a pressure dressing or compressive sutures and antibiotic cover, is recommended (***Figure 51.10***).

Foreign bodies in the ear canal are most easily removed at the first attempt by an experienced practitioner with the aid of a microscope. General anaesthesia may be required in children and those with learning difficulties. Batteries need to be removed within the hour (***Figure 51.11***).

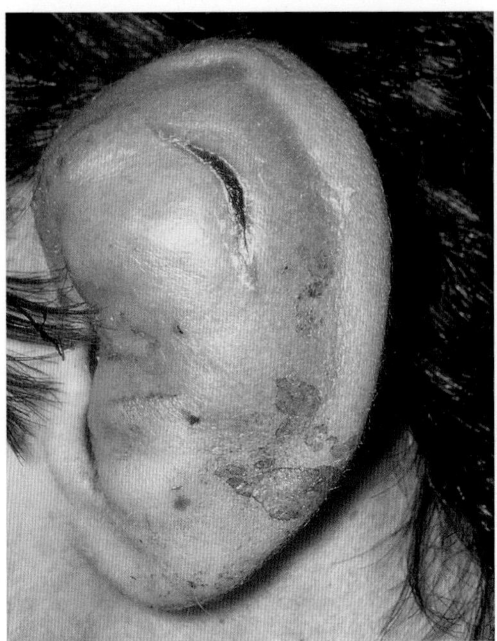

Figure 51.10 Haematoma of the pinna.

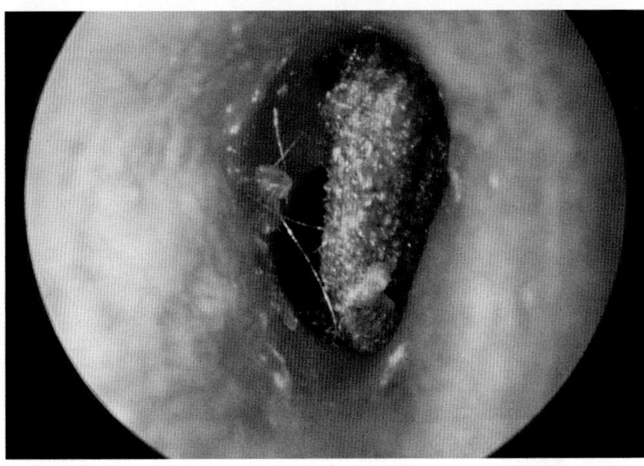

Figure 51.11 Removal of a foreign body from the ear canal can be a challenge (courtesy of Dr Christian Deguine).

Summary box 51.2

Trauma of the external ear

- A haematoma of the pinna requires thorough drainage, antibiotics and a compressive dressing or sutures
- Foreign bodies in the ear canal are most easily removed at the first attempt with the aid of a microscope
- Batteries need to be removed urgently

Inflammation and infection

Otitis externa is very common and consists of generalised inflammation of the skin of the external auditory meatus. The cause is often cotton bud use, a moist environment, immunocompromise, allergies or skin disorders, such as psoriasis and eczema. Common pathogens are *Pseudomonas* and *Staphylococcus* bacteria, *Candida* and *Aspergillus*. Once the skin of the ear canal becomes oedematous, skin migration stops and debris collects in the ear canal. This acts as a substrate for the pathogens. Movement of the pinna elicits pain, which distinguishes it from otitis media.

The initial treatment is with a topical antibiotic and steroid ear drops together with analgesia. If this fails, meticulous removal of the debris with the aid of an operating microscope is required. Fungal infection can be recognised by the presence of hyphae within the canal (***Figure 51.12***). Fungal infection causes irritation and itch. The treatment is meticulous removal of the fungus and any debris, as well as stopping any concurrent antibiotics. Systemic antibiotics are rarely required for otitis externa but should be used if cellulitis of the pinna occurs (***Figure 51.13***).

Necrotising otitis externa is a rare but important condition because, if left untreated, it has a high mortality. It presents as a severe, persistent, unilateral otitis externa possibly with facial weakness in an immunocompromised individual (e.g. elderly patient with diabetes). Usually the infecting organism is *Pseudomonas aeruginosa*. Osteomyelitis of the skull base may result in lower CN palsy (VII–XII). A multidisciplinary approach

Friedrich Theodor Schwann, 1810–1882, Professor of Anatomy and Physiology, successively at Louvain (1839–1848) and Liège (1848–1880), Belgium, described the neurilemma in 1839.

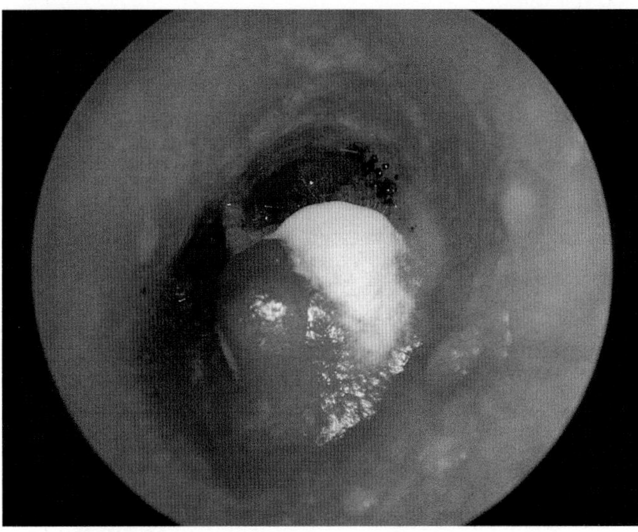

Figure 51.12 Fungal otitis externa. Note the spores.

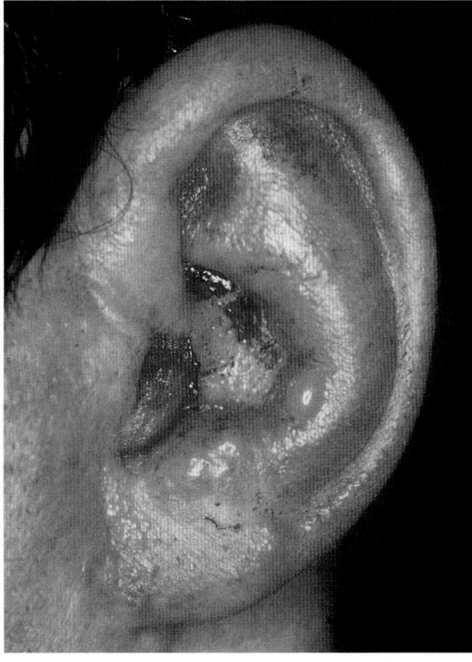

Figure 51.13 Cellulitis of the pinna.

involving microbiology and radiology is required with long-term systemic antibiotic treatment.

Neoplasms

Exostosis is an area of hyperostosis rather than a neoplasm that arises from the bone of the ear canal in individuals who swim in cold water (synonym 'surfer's ear') (***Figure 51.14***). No treatment is required unless the exostosis obstructs the canal. Osteomas are true neoplasms, often singular and more lateral than exostosis. Other benign tumours include papillomas and adenomas.

Malignant primary tumours of the external ear are either basal cell or squamous cell carcinomas (***Figure 51.15***).

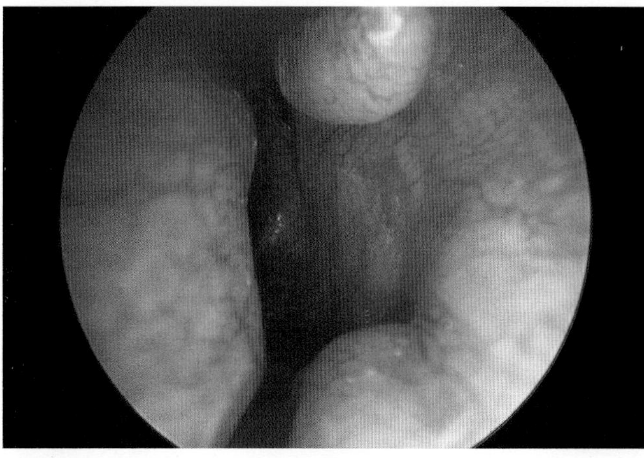

Figure 51.14 Exostoses grow from the bony part of the ear canal in response to cold and so are found in swimmers, surfers and divers. Treatment is only required if the exostoses occlude the ear canal.

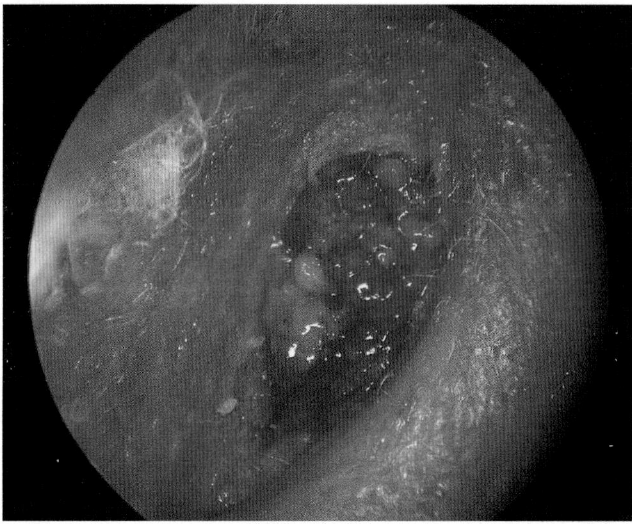

Figure 51.15 Squamous cell carcinomas of the external ear usually originate from the pinna. In this case the tumour is growing from the canal (courtesy of Mr P Beasley).

Summary box 51.3

Types of otitis externa

- Acute bacterial otitis externa is very common and painful; treat with topical steroid and antibiotic drops
- Systemic antibiotics should be reserved for cellulitis of the pinna
- Chronic otitis externa needs the underlying dermatitis to be treated
- Fungal otitis externa itches and can be diagnosed by the presence of hyphae and spores; treat with meticulous cleaning and stop antibiotics
- Necrotising otitis externa is a progressive skull base infection that occurs in immunocompromised individuals and can be life-threatening; intensive long-term antibiotic treatment is required

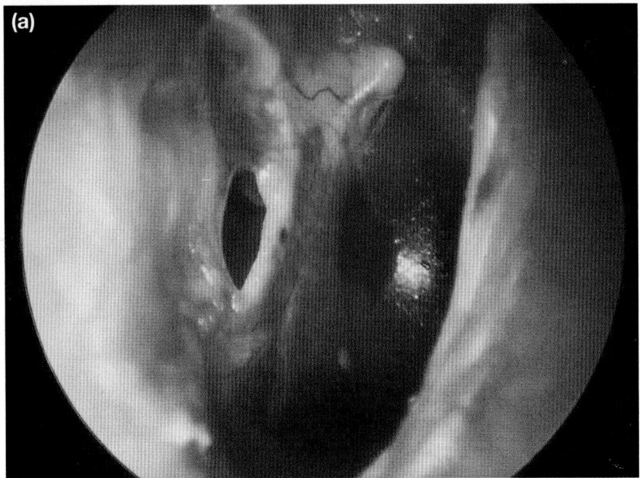

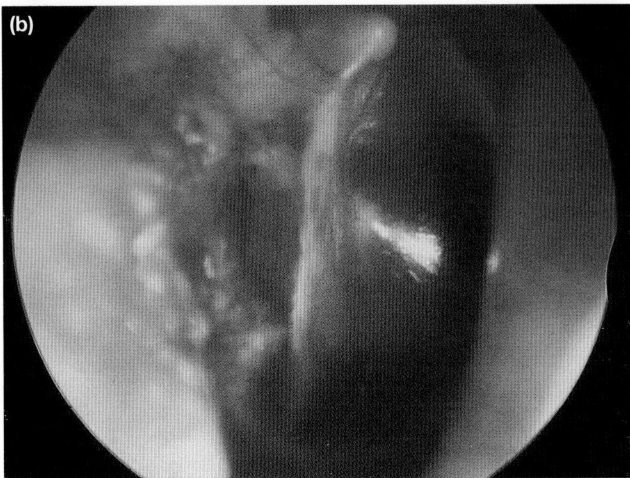

Figure 51.16 (a) Traumatically perforated tympanic membrane. (b) The same tympanic membrane 2 days later (courtesy of Dr Christian Deguine). (Reproduced with permission from O'Donoghue GM, Bates GJ, Narula A. *Clinical ENT*: an illustrated textbook. Oxford: Oxford University Press, 1991.)

Both may present as ulcerating or crusting lesions that grow slowly and may be ignored by elderly patients. Squamous cell carcinomas metastasise to the parotid and/or neck nodes. The ear canal may be invaded by tumours from the parotid gland and postnasal space carcinomas, which 'creep' up the Eustachian tube. All resectable malignant tumours of the ear are treated primarily with surgery, with or without the addition of radiation therapy.

CONDITIONS OF THE MIDDLE EAR

Congenital anomalies

Aural atresia and congenital anomalies of the middle ear occur in 1/10 000 to 1/20 000 births and are typically unilateral and non-syndromal but may be associated with other branchial arch syndromes (e.g. Pierre Robin, craniofacial dysostosis, Down and Treacher Collins syndromes).

Trauma

Trauma to the middle ear can result in a perforated tympanic membrane (***Figure 51.16a***); 90% of such perforations heal spontaneously within 6 weeks (***Figure 51.16b***). Trauma can also result in ossicular discontinuity and it is usually the incus that is displaced. A damaged ossicular chain and tympanic membrane are repaired by ossiculoplasty or tympanoplasty, respectively.

> **Summary box 51.4**
>
> **Congenital anomalies and trauma of the middle ear**
>
> - Congenital anomalies may be isolated or associated with general congenital deformities
> - Traumatic perforations of the tympanic membrane usually heal spontaneously but explosive and welding injuries do not
> - A myringoplasty is an operation that repairs the tympanic membrane
> - With severe head trauma the incus can be displaced, which leads to a conductive hearing loss

Acute otitis media

Acute otitis media (AOM) is one of the most common childhood illnesses with a peak incidence between 6 and 18 months of age. It has occurred in 70% of children by the age of 2 and in 90% by the age of 6. It is characterised by purulent fluid in the middle ear. The tympanic membrane bulges because of pressure from the pus in the middle ear (***Figure 51.17***). The child suffers pain, fever and lethargy. The most common infecting organisms are *Streptococcus pneumoniae* and *Haemophilus influenzae*. Treatment is with analgesics and antipyretics. Systemic antibiotics should be reserved for children under 2 years with bilateral disease or those with other risk factors for complications.The most common complication is mastoiditis because the mastoid air cells connect freely with the middle ear space. Mastoiditis (***Figure 51.18***) requires hospital admission for intravenous antibiotics, for consideration of CT scanning and to monitor for complications such as facial nerve palsy, lateral sinus thrombosis and meningitis. If infection does not resolve quickly abscess aspiration and myringotomy (with/without grommet insertion) is performed. A cortical mastoidectomy is carried out if complications arise.

Otitis media with effusion (glue ear)

Otitis media with effusion (OME) is a middle ear effusion with no evidence of infection. It has a bimodal incidence affecting

Pierre Robin, 1867–1950, Professor, The French School of Dentistry, Paris, France, described this syndrome in 1929.

John Langdon Haydon Down (sometimes given as Langdon-Brown), 1828–1896, physician, The London Hospital, London, UK, published the classification of ailments in 1866.

Edward Treacher Collins, 1862–1932, ophthalmic surgeon, The Royal London Ophthalmic Hospital and Charing Cross Hospital, London, UK, described this syndrome in 1900.

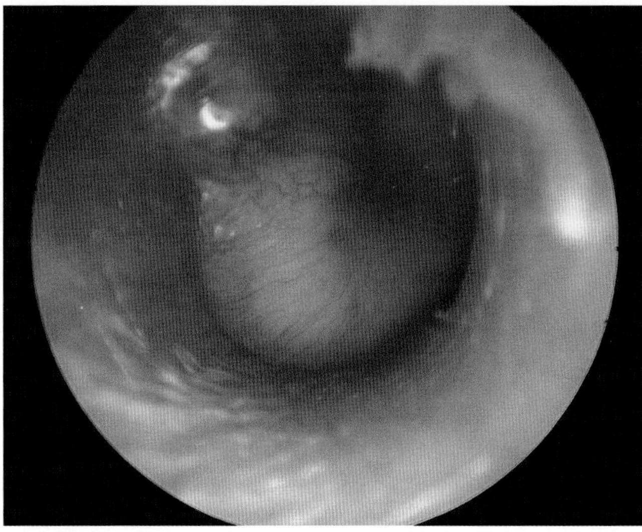

Figure 51.17 Acute otitis media of the left ear. Note the bulging tympanic membrane.

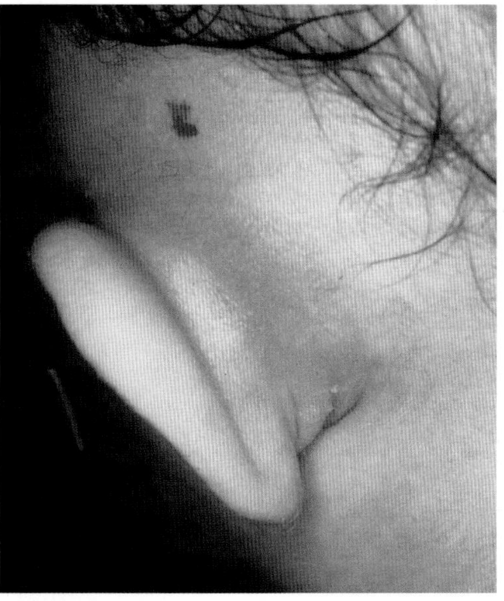

Figure 51.18 Child with acute mastoiditis whose tympanic membrane is shown in *Figure 51.16*.

40% of 2-year-olds (age of starting nursery) and 20% of 5-year-olds (age of starting school). It arises mainly in the winter months, suggesting an infective aetiology. Infection and inflammation of the immature Eustachian tube results in poor middle ear ventilation, negative pressure and the transudation of fluid.

The following symptoms may be associated with glue ear:

- hearing impairment, which often fluctuates;
- delayed speech;
- behavioural problems;
- recurrent ear infections (the exudate is an ideal culture medium for microorganisms);
- reading and learning difficulties at school.

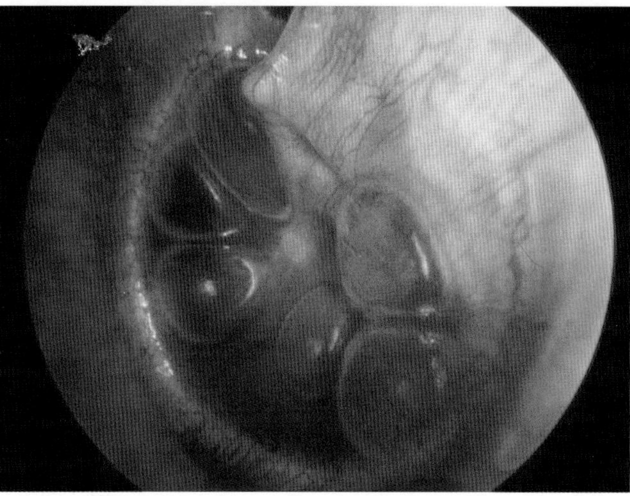

Figure 51.19 The initial serous transudate of glue ear, left ear (courtesy of Dr Christian Deguine). (Reproduced with permission from O'Donoghue GM, Bates GJ, Narula A. *Clinical ENT: an illustrated textbook*. Oxford: Oxford University Press, 1991.)

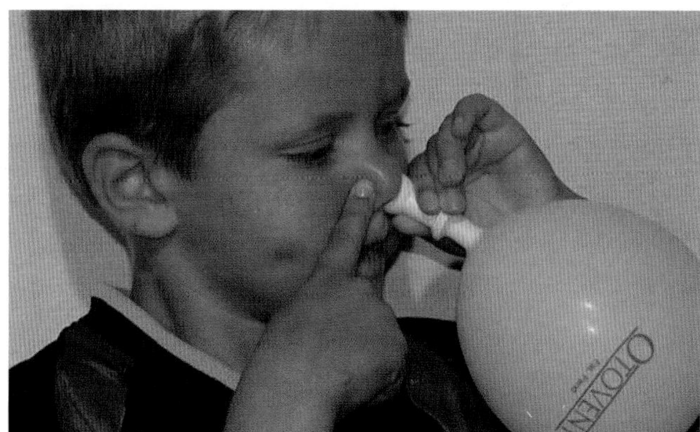

Figure 51.20 Otovent® device.

Otoscopic findings with glue ear

The otoscopic findings of exudative glue ear are of a dull drum that is immobile on pneumatic otoscopy. The tympanic membrane is retracted and radial blood vessels may be present (*Figure 51.19*).

In children first presenting with bilateral glue ear, 50% will be better within 12 weeks, therefore a 'wait and watch' policy is appropriate. If a bilateral conductive hearing loss persists, there is some evidence of reduced IQ and behaviour changes. However, speech delays are reversed by age 8.

Medical treatment is of limited value. Valsalva manoeuvres and the Otovent® device (*Figure 51.20*) are worth trying for patients old enough to comply in an attempt to improve Eustachian tube function. Surgical insertion of ventilation tubes (grommets) (*Figure 51.21*) and adenoidectomy are effective and should be discussed if there is no resolution after a period of watchful waiting. A middle ear effusion in adults is often associated with an upper respiratory tract infection.

Antonio Maria Valsalva, 1666–1723, Italian physician and anatomist.

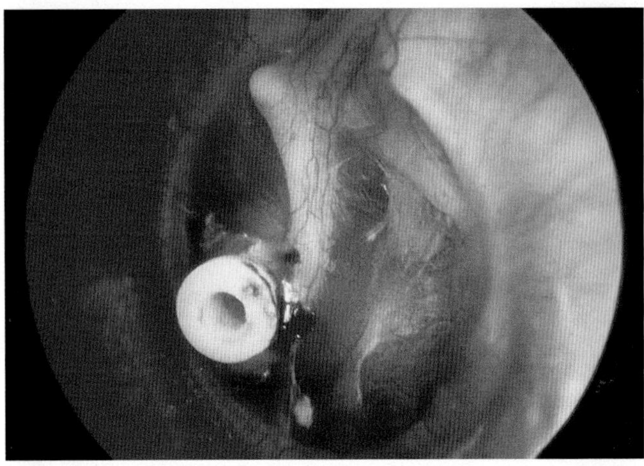

Figure 51.21 Ventilation tube in the tympanic membrane, left ear (courtesy of Dr Christian Deguine).

A persistent unilateral effusion in an adult requires examination of the postnasal space to exclude obstructive nasopharyngeal carcinoma, which is the most common carcinoma in men in southern China.

Summary box 51.5

AOM and OME

- AOM is very common but rarely associated with severe complications such as mastoiditis
- OME is very common in children and usually resolves without treatment
- Persistent OME and/or recurrent AOM are best treated with grommets and/or adenoidectomy
- A persistent middle ear effusion in an adult may be caused by a nasopharyngeal carcinoma; this is commonest in people from southern China

Chronic otitis media

Chronic otitis media (COM) is a persisting (at least 2 weeks to 3 months) abnormality of the tympanic membrane from previous recurrent AOM and/or OME. It is classified as active (i.e. inflammation and pus present), inactive (potential to become active) or healed (no potential to become active). Active and passive are then further subclassified as mucosal or squamous (*Figure 51.22*).

Active mucosal COM implies a perforation with otorrhoea (ear discharge) due to inflamed middle ear mucosa with or without granulation tissue. Inactive mucosal COM implies a dry perforation without inflammation. Surgery in the form of tympanoplasty (repair of the perforation) is indicated in patients with recurrent infection (to reduce symptoms of otorrhoea and prevent further deterioration of the hearing due to the ototoxic effects of infection) and where there is a likelihood that it will restore hearing in the operated ear to 30 dB or better or to within 15 dB of the contralateral ear (this is known as the Belfast rule of thumb).

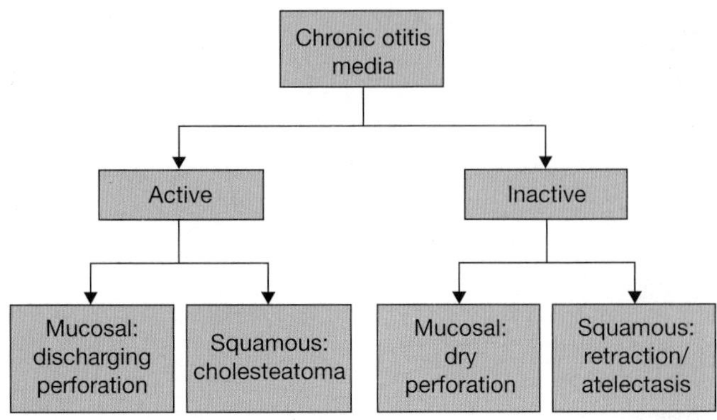

Figure 51.22 Classification of chronic otitis media.

Active squamous COM is otherwise known as acquired cholesteatoma. This represents a quarter of all active COM with an incidence of 1/10 000. It usually presents with persistent otorrhoea and hearing loss as a result of keratinising squamous epithelium within the middle ear. The cholesteatoma matrix destroys the structures in its path through the release of lytic enzymes, inflammatory mediators and pressure necrosis. If left, there is a risk of all the complications attributable to AOM. The lifetime risk of intracerebral abscess is 1/200 in a 30-year-old patient. The recommended treatment is mastoid surgery using a drill under microscopic or endoscopic guidance to access and remove the cholesteatoma. Often the ossicles are involved or eroded so an ossiculoplasty (to restore hearing by reconstructing the ossicular chain) may be performed at the same time.

Otosclerosis

This is an autosomal dominant condition of variable penetrance in which excess bone is laid down around the footplate of the stapes, impeding mobility of the stapes and resulting in a conductive hearing loss (*Figure 51.23*). A diagnosis should be suspected in any patient with a conductive hearing loss and a normal tympanic membrane.

The treatment options are simple reassurance, a conventional hearing aid, a stapedotomy operation or bone conduction hearing aid (*Figure 51.24*).

Neoplasms

Middle ear tumours are rare, with the most common being a glomus tumour (*Figure 51.25*). Glomus tumours are paragangliomas arising from non-chromaffin paraganglionic tissue (the carotid body tumour arising in the neck is an example of this type of tumour). In the temporal bone, two types of glomus tumour are recognised and classification depends on the location: glomus tympanicum (arising in the middle ear) and glomus jugulare (arising next to the jugular bulb).

Symptoms include pulse synchronous tinnitus and conductive and sensorineural hearing loss. Palsies of CNs VII, IX, X, XI and/or XII may occur. The classic sign is a cherry-red mass lying behind the tympanic membrane. The treatment of

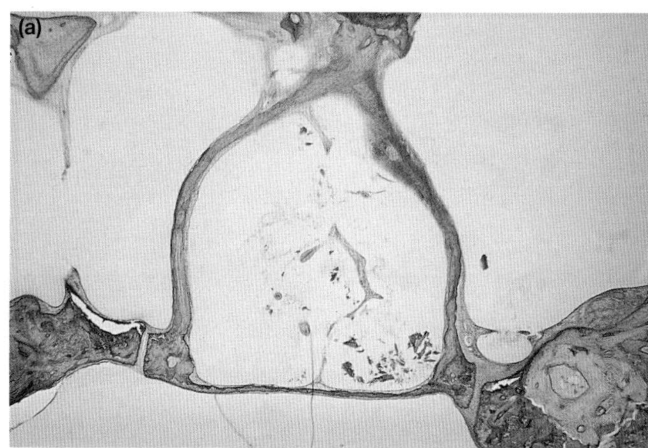

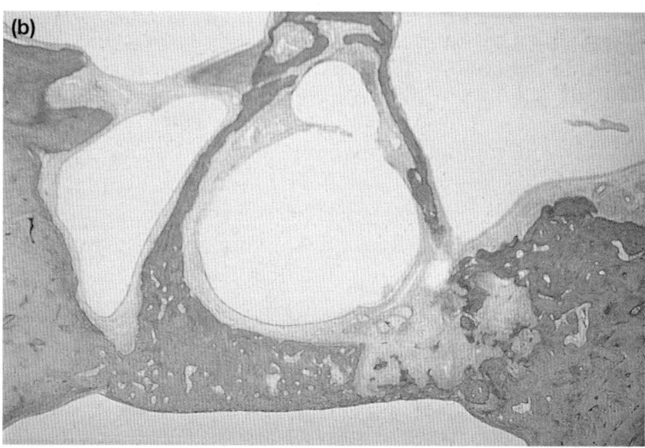

Figure 51.23 Section of normal stapes **(a)** and section of stapes affected by otosclerosis **(b)**.

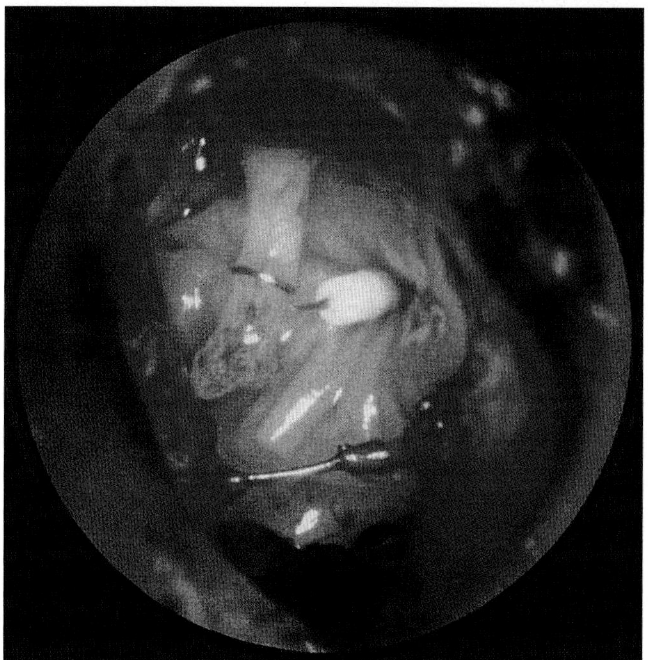

Figure 51.24 The stapedotomy operation showing the piston linking the incus to the vein graft, left ear.

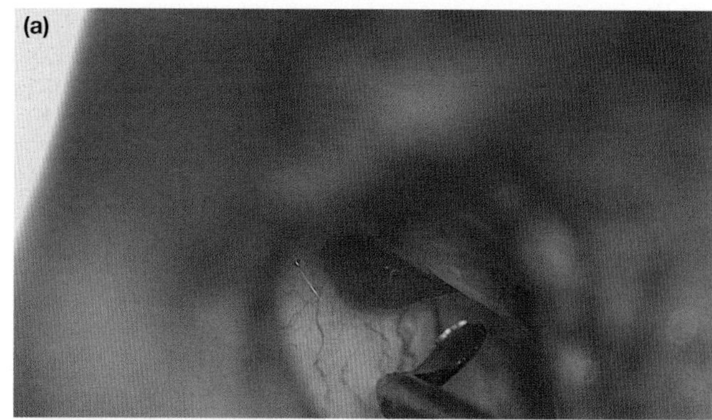

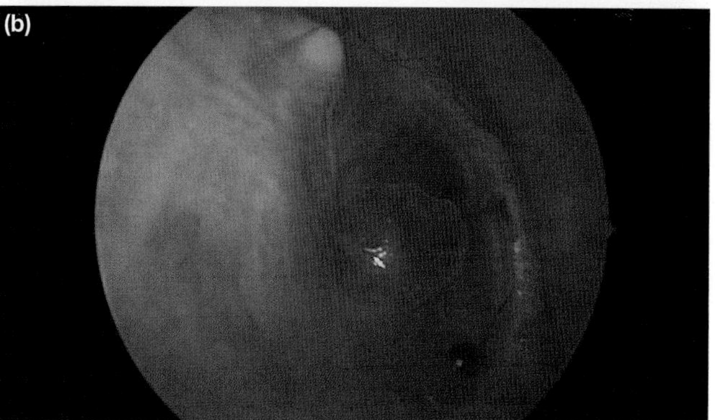

Figure 51.25 (a, b) Glomus tumour in the middle ear, left ear (courtesy of Professor Peter Rea, Leicester).

choice is preoperative embolisation followed by surgical excision. Radiotherapy is also effective.

Squamous cell carcinoma may also occur within the middle ear. It usually presents with deep-seated pain and a blood-stained discharge. Facial paralysis often occurs. Squamous carcinomas usually arise in a chronically discharging ear and can arise in a chronically infected mastoid cavity. Radical surgical excision with or without radiotherapy provides the only chance of cure.

Summary box 51.6

Neoplasms of the middle ear

- Highly vascular glomus tumours are rare and may present with pulsatile tinnitus
- Squamous cell cancer usually presents with pain and facial paralysis

CONDITIONS OF THE INNER EAR

Congenital sensorineural hearing loss

Half of congenital sensorineural hearing loss is genetic and half is acquired. Of the genetic hearing loss 75% is non-syndromic, of which the most common is a connexin 26

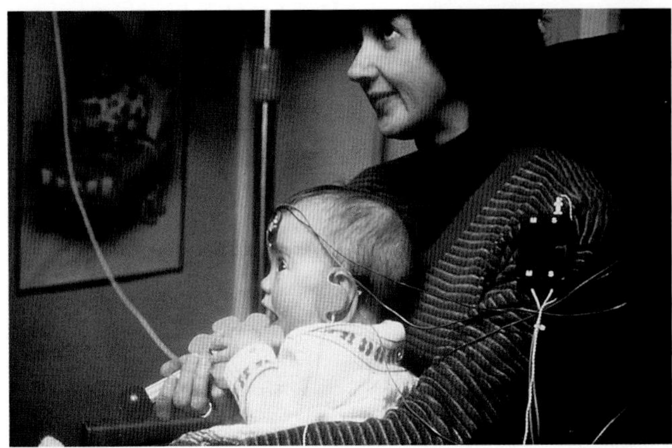

Figure 51.26 Evoked-response audiometry. A simple non-invasive objective test of hearing thresholds. (Reproduced with permission from O'Donoghue GM, Bates GJ, Narula A. *Clinical ENT: an illustrated textbook*. Oxford: Oxford University Press, 1991.)

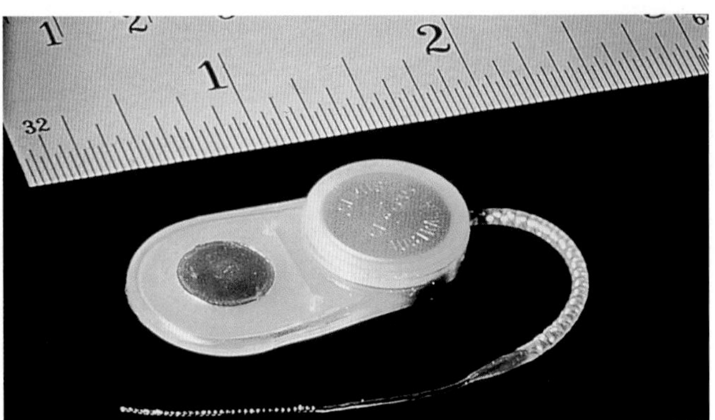

Figure 51.27 Multichannel cochlear implant (Cochlear Corporation).

gene mutation. Syndromic causes include Usher, Pendred, Jervell and Lange-Nielsen, Waardenburg, Treacher Collins, Alport, Stickler, neurofibromatosis type 2 and branchio-oto-renal syndromes.

Acquired causes are intrauterine infections, including rubella, toxoplasmosis and cytomegalovirus infection; perinatal hypoxia, jaundice and prematurity; and postnatal meningitis.

All newborn babies in the UK are now screened at birth for deafness by measuring otoacoustic emissions in response to 'clicks' in the ear. Children failing this are referred for auditory brainstem response to establish hearing thresholds (***Figure 51.26***). If some hearing is present, the early fitment of hearing aids can maximise the neural plasticity that is present in the developing brain. If a child has a profound hearing loss, early intervention with a cochlear implant is essential for the development of the auditory cortex (***Figure 51.27***). Most cases of profound sensorineural hearing loss are due to loss of cochlear hair cells, so an implant inserted through the round window can selectively stimulate the cochlear neurones, which usually remain intact.

Presbycusis

Presbycusis is characterised by a gradual loss of hearing in both ears, with or without tinnitus. The hearing loss usually affects the higher frequencies and a classical audiogram is shown in ***Figure 51.28***. The consonants of speech lie within the high-frequency range, which makes speech discrimination difficult.

Many patients with presbycusis are concerned that they may lose their hearing completely and need reassurance. Hearing aid technology has improved dramatically over recent years and most patients can derive benefit (***Figure 51.29***).

Tinnitus

Tinnitus is the perception of sound when no external sound source is present. It may have an extrinsic cause; for example, the pulsatile tinnitus of a glomus tumour. Usually, however, the tinnitus is generated within the internal auditory pathway. Thirty per cent of people will experience tinnitus at some time in their lives. Tinnitus frequently accompanies presbycusis, as well as any other condition that affects hearing. Most individuals habituate to the presence of tinnitus but in some patients it proves intrusive. Treatment is with reassurance, masking and hearing aids (for patients with hearing loss).

Sudden sensorineural hearing loss

Defined as >30 dB sensorineural hearing loss at three frequencies within 3 days. History and examination should focus on a cause, which may be infective, neoplastic, traumatic, ototoxic, neurological or autoimmune. Investigations such as MRI are important (1% of acoustic neuromas present as sudden sensorineural hearing loss) but screening blood tests are of low yield where there is nothing in the history to suggest a cause. The majority are idiopathic and the recommended treatment is oral steroids with/without intratympanic steroids with salvage intratympanic steroids for those who do not recover after 2 weeks.

Trauma

Noise exposure

Hair cells within the cochlea are damaged by sudden acoustic trauma (blast injury or gunfire) or prolonged exposure to excessive noise. The sensorineural hearing loss that results is greatest between 3 and 6 kHz and is often accompanied by tinnitus (***Figure 51.30***). The law in the UK requires that workers are protected from noise.

Charles Howard Usher, 1865–1942, ophthalmologist, Aberdeen Royal Infirmary, Aberdeen, UK.
Vaughan Pendred, 1869–1946, general practitioner, Durham, UK.
Anton Jervell, 1901–1987, physician, University of Oslo, Oslo, Norway.
Fred Lange-Nielsen, 1919–1989, physician and jazz musician, Oslo, Norway.
Petrus Johannes Waardenburg, 1886–1979, ophthalmologist, Utrecht, The Netherlands.
Arthur Cecil Alport, 1880–1959, Professor of Medicine, King Fuad I Hospital, University of Cairo, Egypt.
Gunnar B Stickler, 1925–2010, pediatrician, Mayo Clinic, USA.

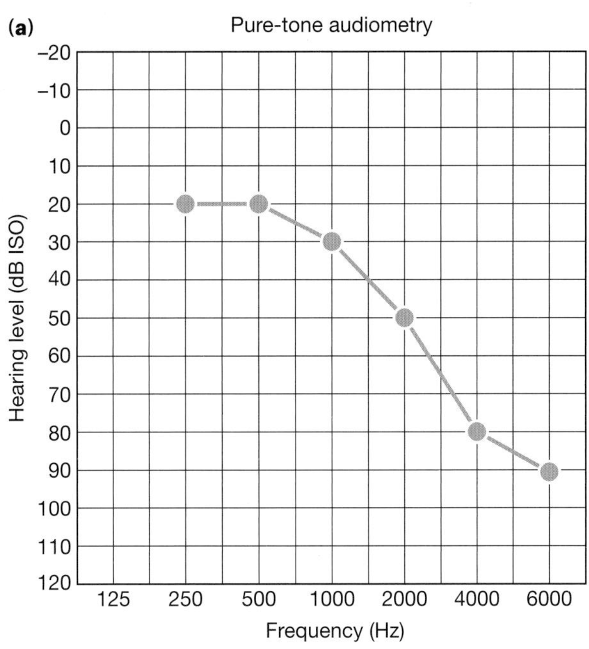

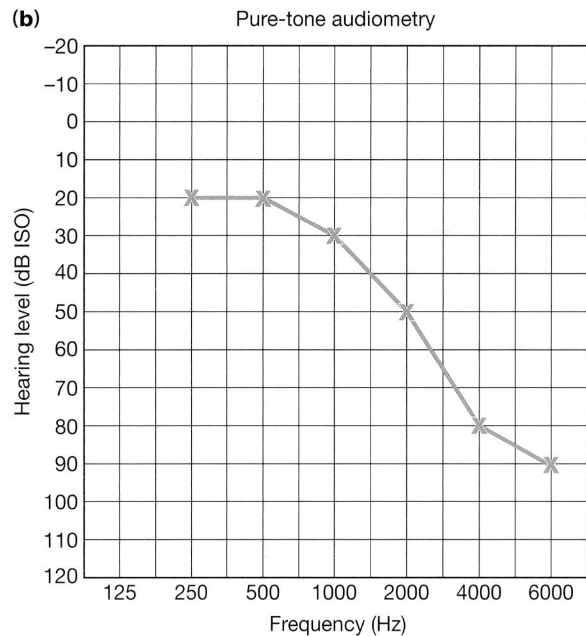

Figure 51.28 Typical audiogram of presbycusis: **(a)** right ear; **(b)** left ear.

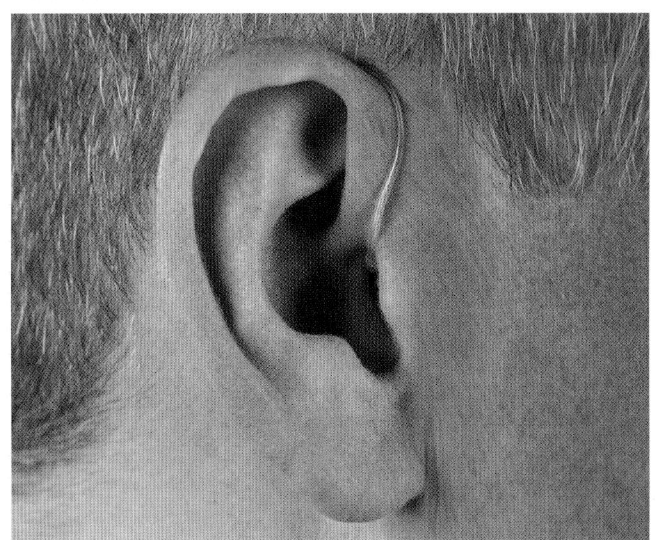

Figure 51.29 Modern hearing aid.

Head injury

The otic capsule is the hardest bone in the body but, if trauma to the head is severe, temporal bone fractures may occur. These are traditionally described as either longitudinal (80%) or transverse (20%); however, the majority have longitudinal and transverse components. Longitudinal fractures may lead to fracture of the external auditory canal, conductive hearing loss and CSF otorrhoea. Transverse fractures may involve the facial nerve, leading to palsy, and labyrinth, leading to a sensorineural hearing loss that is permanent. Profound vertigo occurs initially, followed by gradual compensation.

Drug ototoxicity

Antibiotics such as aminoglycosides, vancomycin and erythromycin, loop diuretics such as frusemide, chemotherapy agents such as cisplatin and carboplatin, and salicylates such as aspirin and quinine are all ototoxic. Recognition of risk factors, such as poor renal function in patients being treated with aminoglycosides, is therefore important. Although many topical ear drops contain aminoglycosides, there is little evidence that short periods of topical treatment cause sensorineural hearing loss.

Balance disorders

Vertigo is the hallucination of movement.

Benign paroxysmal positional vertigo

Benign paroxysmal positional vertigo (BPPV) is the most common form of vertigo. It is caused by otoliths (calcium carbonate crystals) most commonly within the posterior semicircular canal abnormally triggering the ampullary hair cells. Typically, the vertigo is triggered by turning, only lasts for a few seconds and is not associated with other otological symptoms. A positive Hallpike test confirms the diagnosis. The condition is usually self-limiting but recovery may be expediated by an Epley manoeuvre.

Charles Skinner Hallpike, 1900–1979, aural surgeon, National Hospital for Neurology and Neurosurgery, London, UK.
John W Epley, contemporary, Director, Portland Otology Clinic, Portland, OR, USA, established his clinic in 1975; he developed the Epley manoeuvre for treating benign paroxysmal positional vertigo (BPPV).

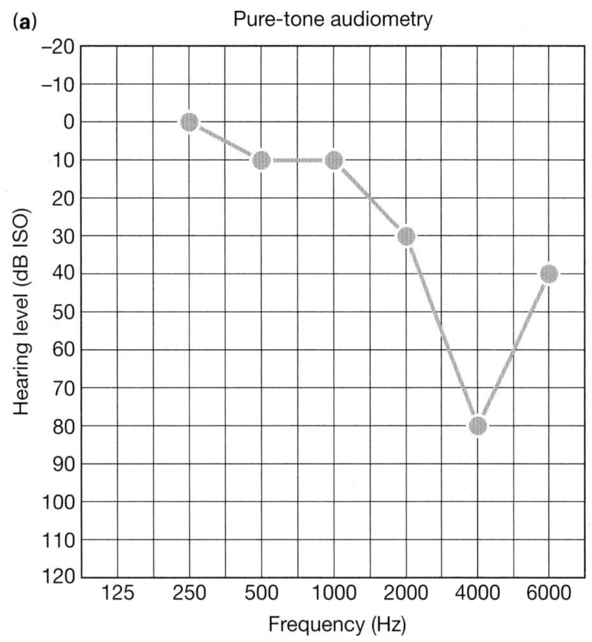

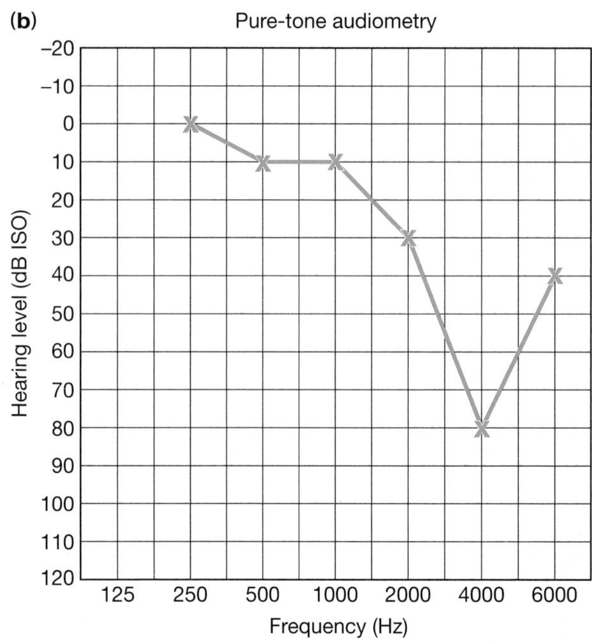

Figure 51.30 A typical audiogram of noise damage: (a) right ear; (b) left ear.

Vestibular neuronitis

Infection or inflammation of the superior vestibular nerve results in persistent vertigo lasting a few days. If the hearing is also affected, this is known as labyrinthitis. Treatment is supportive with vestibular sedatives, such as prochlorperazine, in the first few days, early mobilisation and consideration of systemic steroids.

Menière's disease

It has been said that clinicians not only disagree on the cause of Menière's disease, but they also disagree on the spelling. There is certainly evidence of endolymphatic hydrops (longstanding high-pressure changes within the inner ear) in pathological specimens of patients who have had the condition. The condition is characterised by a triad of symptoms: intermittent attacks of vertigo, a unilateral fluctuating sensorineural hearing loss and tinnitus. The patient often has a sensation of pressure in the affected ear before an attack. The hearing loss typically affects the lower frequencies. The vertigo characteristically lasts between 30 minutes and 6 hours and is often accompanied by nausea and vomiting. The investigations include pure tone audiometry and an MRI scan (to exclude an acoustic neuroma). The only evidence-based medical treatment is intratympanic injections of dexamethasone or gentamicin into the middle ear.

Vestibular migraine

Often confused with Menière's disease, this condition is five times more prevalent, presenting with similar symptoms but without the hearing loss or tinnitus. The migrainous process affects the labyrinth in up to 40% of migraineurs. Treatment includes addressing the risk factors, such as lifestyle and dietary triggers, with prophylactic medication such as propranolol, tricyclic antidepressants and antiepileptic medication for those with ongoing symptoms.

Facial paralysis

Seventy-five per cent of all facial palsies are due to Bell's palsy. This probably results from a herpes simplex viral infection of the facial nerve. The nerve swells and is compressed within the temporal bone. Early treatment with high-dose steroids and eye protection is mandatory. Not all facial nerve palsies are due to viral infection and a thorough otoneurological examination is required. The facial nerve can be damaged at the cerebellopontine angle, within the internal auditory meatus, within the middle ear, at the skull base and within the parotid gland. It is essential to consider these potential sites of facial nerve damage in any patient with CN VII paralysis and perform an MRI scan if appropriate.

Summary box 51.7

Facial paralysis

- The facial nerve passes through the middle ear and mastoid
- When considering a paralysis, think 'complete' or 'partial'
- Protect the eye: carry out a full otoneurological examination to find the cause
- If acute, consider steroids

Prosper Menière, 1799–1862, physician, The Institute of Deaf Mutes, Paris, France, described this condition in 1861.
Sir Charles Bell, 1774–1842, surgeon, The Middlesex Hospital, London UK, and from 1835 until his death, Professor of Surgery, The University of Edinburgh, Edinburgh, UK.

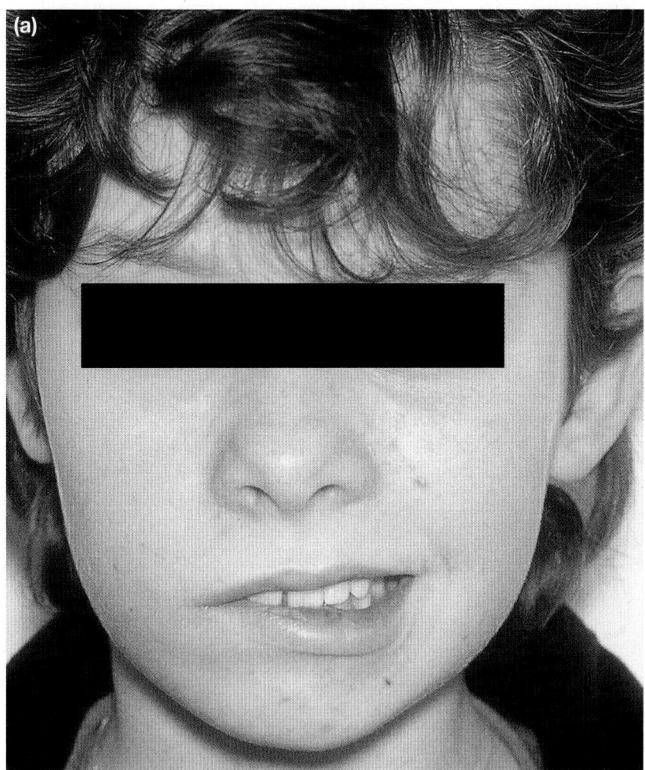

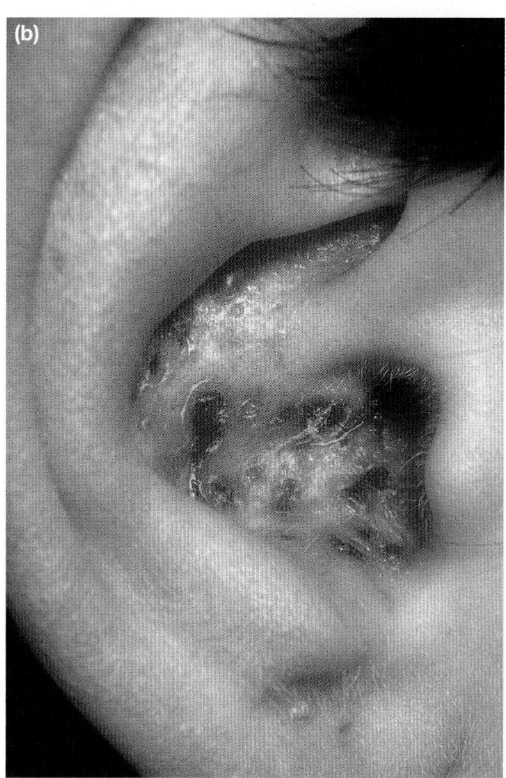

Figure 51.31 Herpes zoster infection of right cranial nerve (CN) VII (a) and right CN VIII (b) with vesicles on the pinna.

Ramsay Hunt syndrome

This is caused by herpes zoster virus and is characterised by facial paralysis, pain and the appearance of vesicles on the tympanic membrane, ear canal, pinna or inside of the cheek (*Figure 51.31*). It may be accompanied by vertigo and sensorineural hearing loss (CN VIII). Treatment with aciclovir is effective if given early.

Neoplasms

These are uncommon but can present with sensorineural hearing loss, tinnitus and vertigo. Acoustic neuromas, which are actually schwannomas of the vestibular division of CN VIII, are the most common, followed by meningiomas. Acoustic neuromas grow slowly and somewhat unpredictably and as they expand can cause CN palsies, brainstem compression and raised intracranial pressure. The early symptoms are a unilateral sensorineural hearing loss or unilateral tinnitus, or both. Therefore, it is essential to perform MRI on all patients with persistent unilateral sensorineural hearing loss or tinnitus. Relatively asymptomatic acoustic neuromas that are less than 2 cm in diameter and growing less than 2 mm/year (70%) are generally treated with a 'watch, wait and rescan' policy or occasionally stereotactic radiotherapy. Tumour volumes greater than 2 cm in diameter are often best treated by skull base surgery in the form of a translabyrinthine, retrolabyrinthine or middle fossa approach.

Summary box 51.8

Conditions of the inner ear

- Presbycusis is the bilateral high-frequency loss associated with ageing
- Unilateral tinnitus or sensorineural hearing loss needs to be investigated to exclude acoustic neuroma
- Sudden sensorineural hearing loss needs immediate treatment with steroids and routine MRI to exclude acoustic neuroma
- Menière's disease presents with the triad of sensorineural hearing loss, tinnitus and vertigo

THE NOSE AND SINUSES

BASIC ANATOMY OF THE NOSE AND PARANASAL SINUSES

The supporting structures of the nose are shown in *Figure 51.32*. The septum consists of the anterior quadrilateral cartilage, the perpendicular plate of the ethmoid and the vomer (*Figure 51.33*). The lateral wall of the nasal cavity contains the superior, middle and inferior turbinates, which warm and moisten nasal airflow (*Figure 51.34*). There are paired frontal, sphenoid, maxillary and anterior and posterior ethmoid sinuses. The anterior nasal sinuses (frontal, maxillary and anterior ethmoid) drain into the middle meatus (between

James Ramsay Hunt, 1874–1937, Professor of Neurology, Columbia College of Physicians and Surgeons, New York, USA.

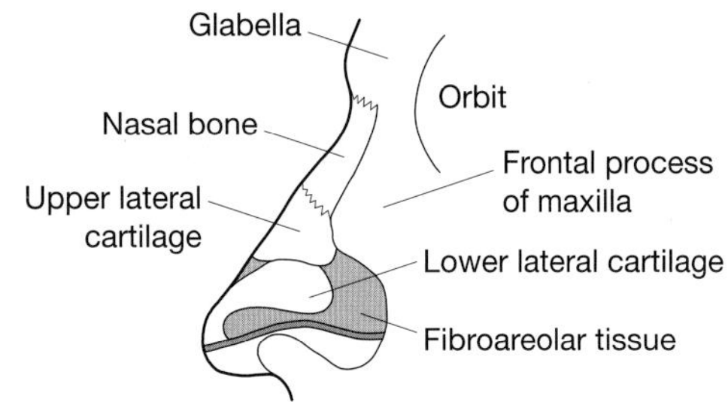

Figure 51.32 The nasal skeleton.

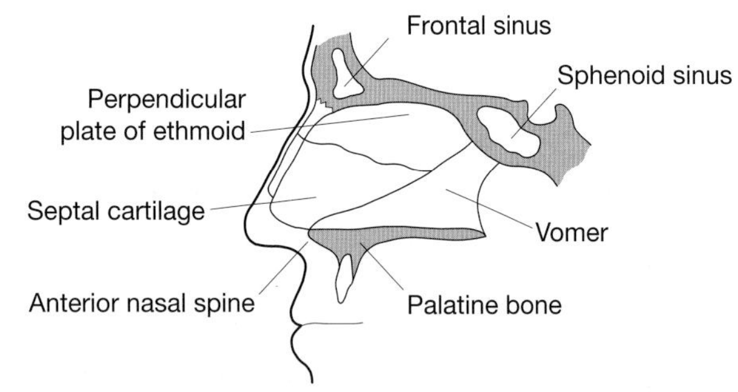

Figure 51.33 The left side of the nasal septum.

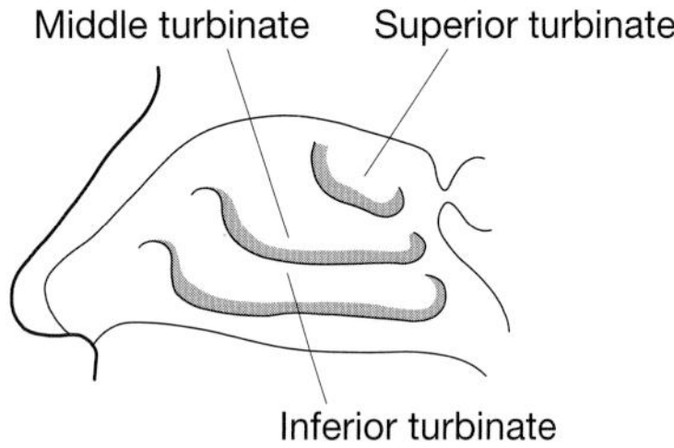

Figure 51.34 The right lateral nasal wall.

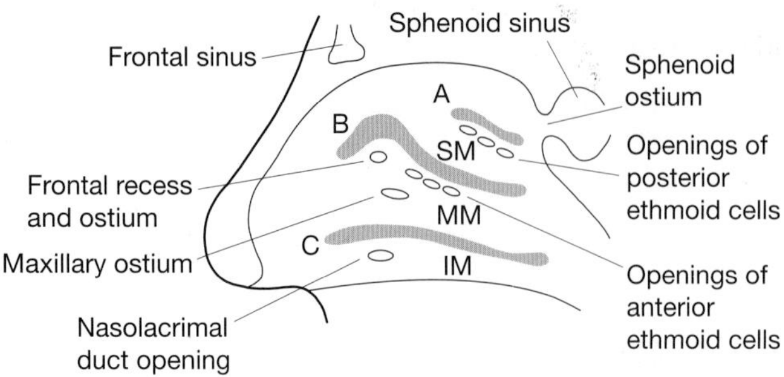

Figure 51.35 The right lateral nasal wall with turbinates removed to show the sinus ostia. A, insertion of superior turbinate; B, insertion of middle turbinate; C, insertion of inferior turbinate; IM, inferior meatus; MM, middle meatus; SM, superior meatus.

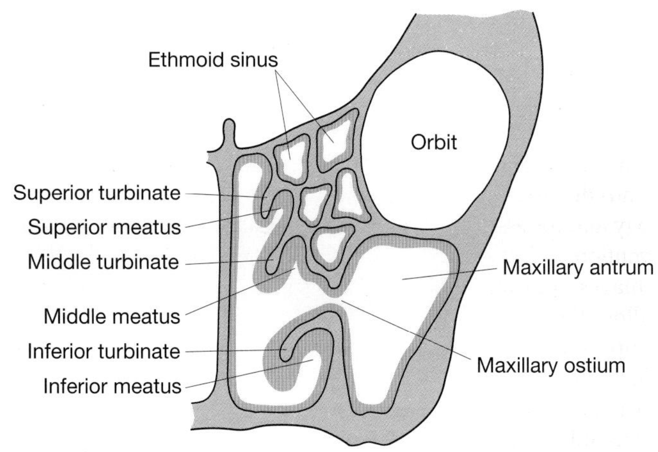

Figure 51.36 Coronal section through the left maxillary and ethmoid sinuses.

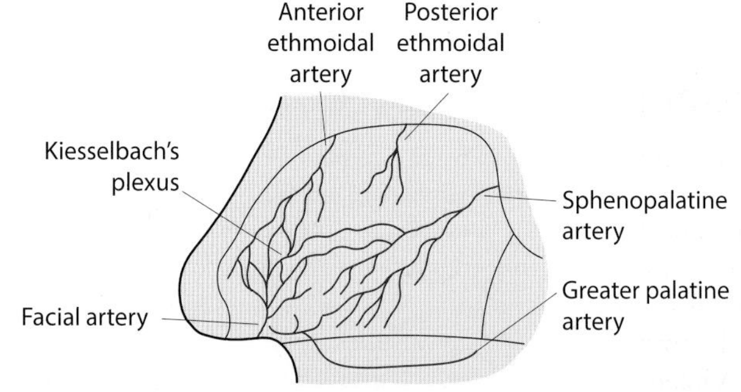

Figure 51.37 Arterial blood supply to the left side of the nasal septum.

the middle turbinate and lateral wall of the nose). The posterior ethmoid and sphenoid sinuses drain into the superior meatus and sphenoethmoidal recess (between the superior turbinate and nasal septum), respectively (***Figures 51.35 and 51.36***).

The nasal fossae and sinuses receive their blood supply via the external and internal carotid arteries. The external carotid artery supplies the interior of the nose via the maxillary and sphenopalatine arteries. The greater palatine artery supplies the anteroinferior septum via the incisive canal. The contribution from the internal carotid artery is via the anterior and posterior ethmoidal arteries, which are branches of the ophthalmic artery (***Figure 51.37***). All these arteries anastomose to form a plexus of vessels (Kiesselbach's plexus) on the anterior part of the nasal septum. Venous drainage is via the ophthalmic and facial veins and the pterygoid and pharyngeal plexuses. Intracranial drainage into the cavernous sinus via the ophthalmic vein is of particular clinical importance because of the potential for intracranial spread of nasal sepsis.

EXAMINATION OF THE NOSE AND PARANASAL SINUSES

Internal inspection of the nasal fossae can be achieved to a limited extent with the use of a Thudichum speculum. The anterior nasal septum, nasal vestibule and anterior inferior turbinate can be assessed. A more detailed examination of the nose is possible with the use of either rigid or flexible endoscopes

Wilhelm Kiesselbach, 1839–1902, Professor of Otology, Erlangen, Germany.
Johann Ludwig Wilhelm Thudichum, 1829–1901, biochemist and general practitioner, London, UK.

(*Figure 51.38*). The endoscopes are attached to a light source and camera and the image is displayed on a monitor.

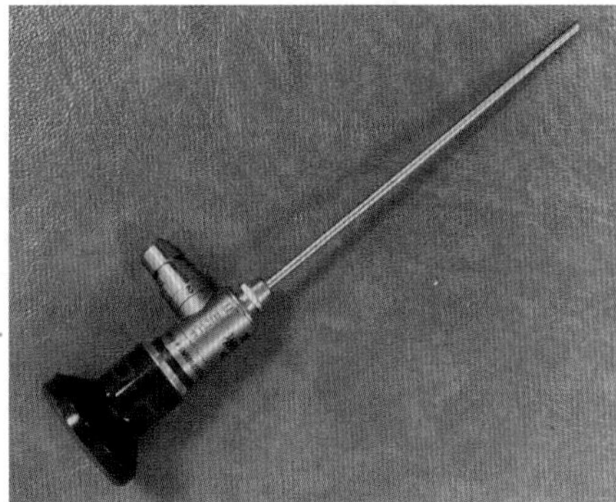

Figure 51.38 Rigid nasendoscope.

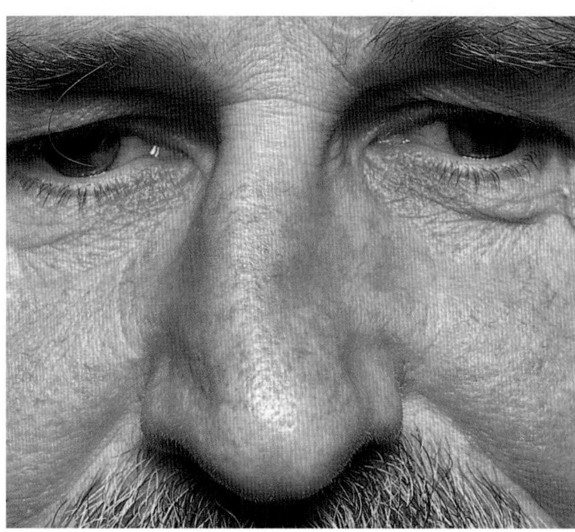

Figure 51.39 Fracture of the nasal bones with displacement of the bony nasal complex to the right side.

IMAGING OF PARANASAL SINUSES

Plain radiographs are of limited value in the assessment of sinus disease. CT is far superior in demonstrating sinus pathology and for assessing bony anatomy to plan any surgical intervention. CT scans are acquired and reconstructed to produce images in axial, coronal and sagittal planes. The three planes allow the drainage of the frontal sinus to be identified and important surgical landmarks can be reviewed preoperatively, including the cribriform plate, anterior skull base, lamina papyracea and location of the anterior ethmoid artery. MRI is useful in sinus pathology to assess any intracranial or orbital extension of disease.

TRAUMA TO THE NOSE AND PARANASAL SINUSES

Fracture of the nasal bones

Blunt injury to the nose may fracture the nasal bones (*Figure 51.39*). The fracture line can extend into the lacrimal bone and tear the anterior ethmoidal artery, producing catastrophic haemorrhage. This may be delayed, occurring only as the soft-tissue swelling subsides, reducing the tamponade effect on the torn vessel.

Violent trauma to the frontal area of the nose can result in a fracture of the frontal and ethmoid sinuses with potential extension into the anterior cranial fossa. Dural tears and brain injuries, either open or closed, are then at risk from sinonasal ascending infection, which may progress to meningitis or brain abscess. CSF rhinorrhoea is a certain sign of a dural tear. CSF rhinorrhoea can be confirmed by collecting a sample of the fluid and sending for β_2-transferrin assay. A bony defect in the anterior skull base following trauma can be identified on high-resolution CT. The CSF leak will often settle with conservative management but, if persistent, it can be repaired endoscopically.

Management of fractured nasal bones

Fractured nasal bones are normally accompanied by extensive overlying soft-tissue swelling and bruising, which may hinder the assessment of any underlying bony deformity. Reviewing after 4–5 days when the soft-tissue swelling has diminished will allow a better assessment of any deformity. If there is a significant degree of nasal deformity, this can be corrected by manipulation of the nasal bones under local or general anaesthesia. This should be carried out within 3 weeks of the injury while the bony fragments are still mobile. After this period, if there is significant cosmetic or functional issues, a septorhinoplasty can be performed at least 6 months following the injury.

Septal injury

A blunt injury of moderate force may lead to lateral displacement or deformity of the septal cartilage, restricting the nasal airway. Unlike the nasal bones the nasal septum cannot be manipulated back into position and requires a formal septoplasty procedure to restore the anatomy and the patency of the nasal airways.

Bleeding under the mucoperichondrium of the septum will cause a septal haematoma and nasal obstruction. Untreated, a septal haematoma will progress to abscess formation and ultimately result in necrosis of the septal cartilage, septal perforation and nasal collapse. A septal haematoma should be treated by incision and drainage of the blood clot, insertion of a small silicone drain and packing of the nasal fossa. A broad-spectrum prophylactic antibiotic should be prescribed.

Summary box 51.9

Nasal trauma

- Do not overlook a septal haematoma
- Displaced nasal bone fractures should be reduced within 3 weeks of injury
- Severe persistent epistaxis after trauma suggests lacrimal bone fracture and injury to the anterior ethmoid artery
- CSF rhinorrhoea indicates a fracture involving the anterior skull base with a dural tear

THE NASAL SEPTUM

Septal deformity

Deviation of the nasal septum may occur naturally or arise as a result of nasal trauma and is readily apparent on anterior rhinoscopy (***Figure 51.40***). Surgical correction can be achieved by a submucous resection (SMR) of the septum where the deformed septal cartilage is excised while preserving a caudal and dorsal strut for support (***Figure 51.41***). The alternative is a septoplasty procedure during which the septal cartilage is preserved but the anatomical abnormalities giving rise to its deformity, such as a twisted maxillary crest or inclination of the bony septum posteriorly, are corrected.

Complications of septal surgery include septal perforation. If too much cartilage is excised in the SMR procedure, loss of support to the dorsum of the nose may result in a supra-tip depression or drooping of the tip of the nose.

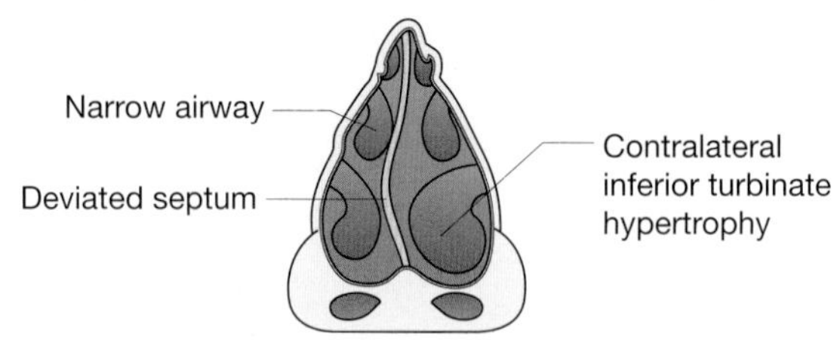

Figure 51.40 Coronal section through the anterior nasal fossae with deviated nasal septum to the right side.

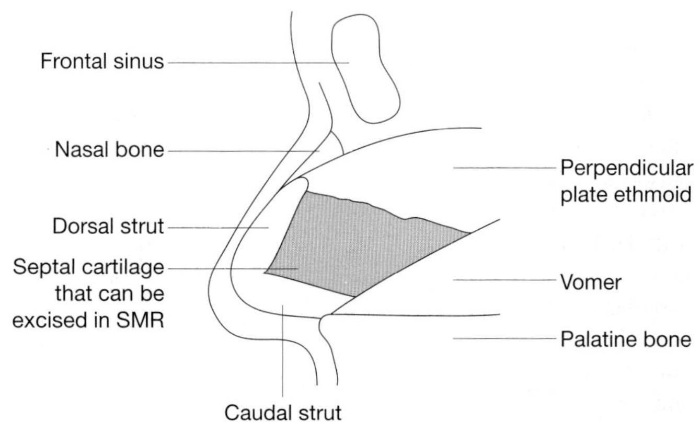

Figure 51.41 Area of cartilage that can be removed in submucous resection (SMR) leaving dorsal and caudal strut for support.

Septal perforation

A hole in the nasal septum causes turbulent airflow through the nose and a resulting sensation of nasal blockage, extensive nasal crusting, bleeding and whistling. The causes of septal perforation are listed in ***Summary box 51.10***.

Septal perforations seldom heal spontaneously. A great variety of operations have been described to close septal perforations but none has met with universal success. These have included closing the perforation using cartilage or synthetic material and covering with local flaps. Alternatively, the perforation may be occluded by inserting a Silastic biflanged prosthesis or 'septal button' (***Figures 51.42 and 51.43***). In some cases, particularly those patients with significant whistling and bleeding from the posterior edge, the perforation can be enlarged and mucosa folded around the posterior edge to stabilise it.

Granulomatosis with polyangiitis is a systemic idiopathic autoimmune disease affecting the nose, lungs and kidneys. Mucosal granulations on the nasal septum destroy cartilage, producing a septal perforation with saddle deformity of the nose. Laboratory findings include a high erythrocyte sedimentation rate, impaired creatinine clearance and antineutrophil cytoplasmic antibodies (c-ANCA) in most cases.

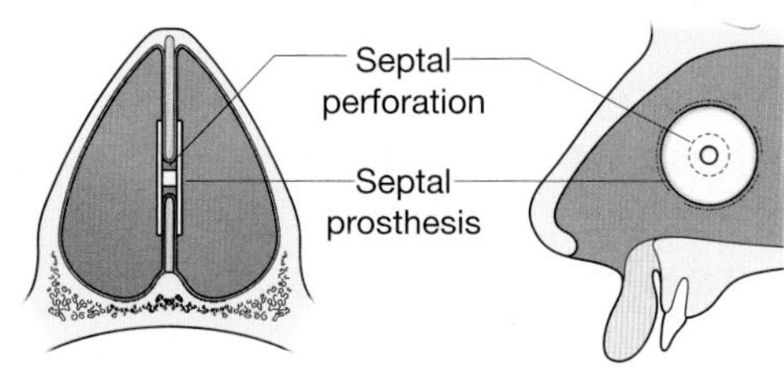

Figure 51.42 Anterior and lateral views of septal perforation occluded with a prosthesis.

Summary box 51.10

Causes of septal perforations

- Trauma
  - Iatrogenic following septal surgery
  - Nose picking
  - Following a septal haematoma from nasal injury
- Infection
  - Syphilis
  - Tuberculosis
- Vasculitis
  - Granulomatosis with polyangiitis
- Tumours
- Toxins
  - Chrome salts
  - Cocaine
- Idiopathic

EPISTAXIS

The causes of epistaxis are listed in ***Table 51.2***. The most common site of bleeding is from Kiesselbach's plexus in Little's area of the anterior portion of the septum (***Figure 51.37***). Anterior bleeding is common in children and young adults owing to nose blowing or picking. In the elderly, anticoagulants and hypertension are the underlying causes of arterial bleeding from the posterior part of the nose.

James Laurence Little, 1836–1885, Professor of Surgery, The University of Vermont, Montpelier, VT, USA.

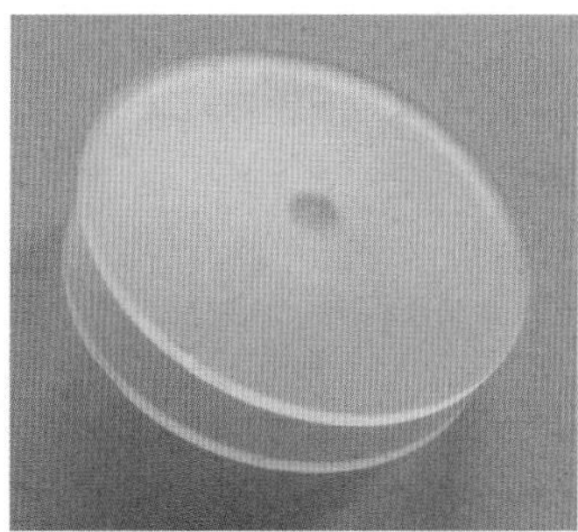

Figure 51.43 Silastic prosthesis for septal perforation.

Hereditary haemorrhagic telangiectasia (HHT) (Osler's disease) gives rise to recurrent multifocal bleeding from thin-walled vessels deficient in muscle and elastic tissue (*Figure 51.44*).

Juvenile angiofibroma is an uncommon condition that affects adolescent boys and may lead to massive life-threatening episodes of bleeding. Diagnosis is made with contrast CT or MRI. Anterior bowing or indentation of the posterior antral wall (Holman–Miller or antral sign) is the classical finding but may be seen in other expansive lesions in this area. It is a very vascular tumour, which should not be biopsied because of the risk of uncontrollable haemorrhage. Excision is best carried out by an experienced surgeon and is usually performed endoscopically, often using image guidance (*Figure 51.45*). Preoperative embolisation of the feeding blood vessels may help to reduce blood loss during surgery.

TABLE 51.2 Causes of epistaxis.

Local	• Nose picking • Nasal trauma • Nasal foreign bodies • Tumours • Infection • Granulomatous disorders • Juvenile angiofibroma
Systemic	• Hypertension • Warfarin therapy • New anticoagulants (rivaroxaban) • Aspirin, clopidogrel therapy • Haemophilia • von Willebrand's disease • Leukaemia • Hereditary haemorrhagic telangiectasia (Osler's disease)

Management of epistaxis

Anterior bleeding from Kiesselbach's plexus may be controlled by silver nitrate cautery under local anaesthesia. Even in more posterior epistaxis, the bleeding point can often be identified using rigid nasendoscopy and controlled with the use of a topical vasoconstrictor, and then dealt with directly using electrocautery. However, posterior bleeding, as seen in the elderly, may require anterior nasal packing either with Vaseline-impregnated ribbon gauze or a non-absorbable sponge. There are also many haemostatic, absorbable materials that can be used to pack the nose to help control bleeding. An alternative to anterior packing is the use of an inflatable epistaxis balloon catheter (*Figure 51.46*). The catheter is passed into the nose and the distal balloon is inflated in the nasopharynx to secure it. The proximal balloon, which is sausage shaped, is then inflated within the nasal fossa to compress the bleeding point. Although usually effective, they can be uncomfortable.

Postnasal packing may be required in refractory cases whereby a gauze pack is positioned in the nasopharynx under general anaesthesia. Endoscopic sphenopalatine artery clipping is an effective treatment for significant epistaxis not responding to direct cautery or nasal packing.

For uncontrolled life-threatening epistaxis in which the above methods have proved ineffective, haemostasis is secured by vascular ligation. Depending on the origin of bleeding it may be necessary to ligate the internal maxillary artery in the pterygopalatine fossa (which can be accessed endoscopically) and the anterior and posterior ethmoidal arteries. An alternative measure is external carotid artery ligation above the origin of the lingual artery. Another option is to involve the interventional radiologist for possible embolisation. It is also important to recognise, and treat, any factors contributing to the epistaxis, such as clotting or platelet abnormalities.

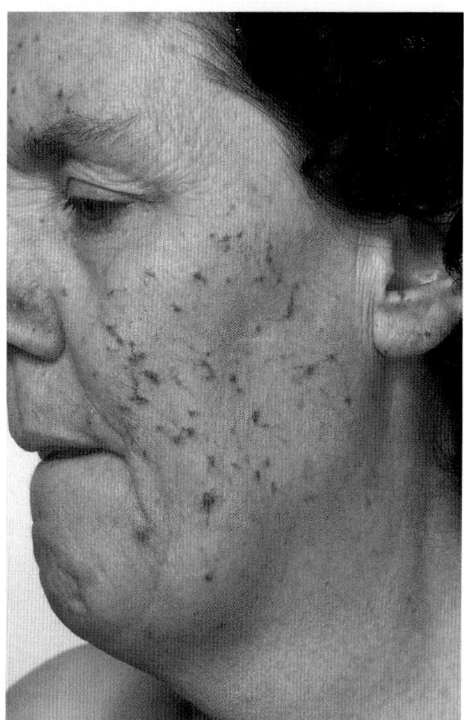

Figure 51.44 Hereditary haemorrhagic telangiectasia (Osler's disease) showing multiple telangiectasia.

Sir William Osler, 1849–1919, Professor of Medicine, successively at McGill University, Montreal, Canada, University of Pennsylvania, Philadelphia, PA, and Johns Hopkins University, Baltimore, MD, USA, finally becoming Regius Professor of Medicine at Oxford University, Oxford, UK, in 1904.
Colin B Holman, 1917–2008, American radiologist, Mayo Clinic.
W Eugene Miller, American radiologist, Mayo Clinic, with Colin Holman described the eponymous sign on plain radiographs in 1965.
Erik Adolf von Willebrand, 1870–1949, physician, Diakonissanstaltens Hospital, Helsinki, (Helsingfors), Finland, described hereditary pseudohaemophilia in 1926.

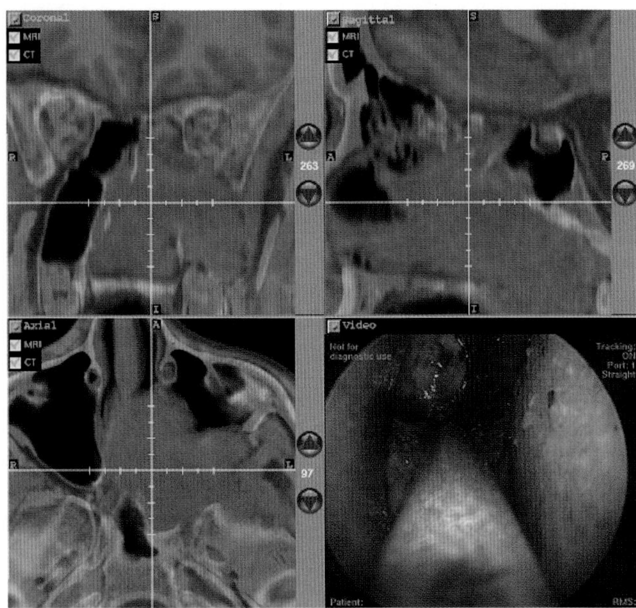

Figure 51.45 Endoscopic resection of juvenile angiofibroma using image guidance (merged computed tomography and magnetic resonance imaging scans).

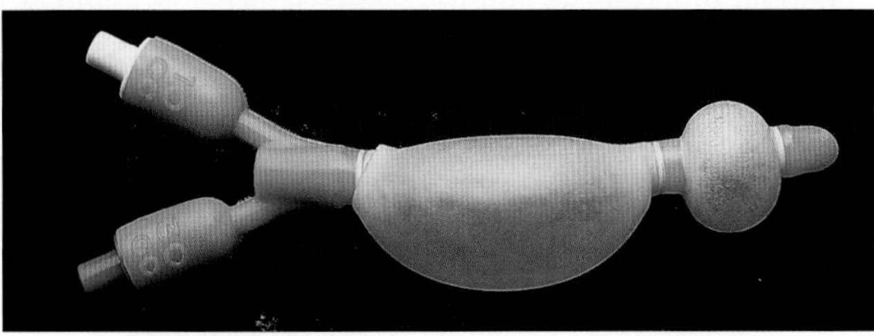

Figure 51.46 Epistaxis balloon catheter.

In HHT, anterior nasal packing is best avoided if at all possible because it is most likely to lead to further mucosal trauma and bleeding. High-dose oestrogen induces squamous metaplasia of the nasal mucosa and has been used effectively in treating this condition. Medications that block vessel growth, such as bevacizumab, and those that slow the disintegration of clots, such as tranexamic acid, help reduce the bleeding associated with HHT. There are also surgical options, including cautery/ablation of the telangiectasia, septodermoplasty or surgical closure of the nostril (Young's procedure).

RHINOSINUSITIS

Rhinosinusitis is inflammation of the sinonasal mucosa and is defined as the presence of nasal congestion or nasal discharge and at least one of facial pain or hyposmia with endoscopic and/or CT changes to confirm the diagnosis. It can be divided into acute rhinosinusitis (ARS) and chronic rhinosinusitis (CRS) depending on the timing of symptoms. Symptoms are present for less than 12 weeks in ARS and more than 12 weeks in CRS.

Summary box 51.11

Epistaxis

- The most common causes are nose picking, hypertension and anticoagulant therapy
- Young people bleed from the anterior septum – Kiesselbach's plexus
- Elderly people bleed from the posterior part of the nose
- Epistaxis is ideally treated with direct cautery to the bleeding point under endoscopic guidance
- Silver nitrate cautery can be used to control anterior bleeding
- Moderate bleeding may require anterior nasal packing
- Severe bleeding may require anterior and posterior nasal packing
- Persistent bleeding may require endoscopic sphenopalatine artery ligation

Acute rhinosinusitis

ARS is thought to result from bacterial superinfection of virally damaged mucosa. The commonest bacteria involved are *S. pneumoniae*, *H. influenzae* and *Moraxella catarrhalis*. Upper dental sepsis may also predispose to acute maxillary sinusitis. Patients with maxillary sinusitis have a mucopurulent discharge, facial pain and nasal obstruction. Irritation of the superior alveolar nerve may give rise to referred upper toothache. In ARS nasendoscopy reveals inflamed and swollen nasal mucosa with mucopurulent secretions in the middle meatus. Dental sepsis from anaerobic organisms causes around 10% of cases of maxillary sinusitis. The resultant mucopurulent nasal secretion has a foul taste and smell. Plain sinus radiographs may show a fluid level in the antrum or complete opacity (***Figure 51.47***). However, plain radiographs are now seldom used and have been superseded by CT scans to investigate ARS. CT scans confirm opacification and mucosal thickening of the maxillary sinus as well as providing anatomical detail prior to endoscopic surgical intervention (***Figure 51.48***).

Acute frontoethmoidal sinusitis can also occur and presents with mucopurulent discharge, facial pain (including frontal headache), nasal congestion and hyposmia. Again, mucopus is seen on endoscopy in the middle meatus and is investigated with CT.

Treatment

Penetration of antibiotics into chronically inflamed sinus mucosa is reduced and, therefore, treatment may need to be prolonged. Topical nasal decongestants, such as ephedrine nasal drops, will often encourage the sinus to drain and topical corticosteroids are used to reduce inflammation. Saline douches can also be beneficial.

Antral lavage under local or general anaesthesia was previously used to confirm the diagnosis and provided the opportunity to obtain samples for bacteriology. Nowadays, pus in the middle meatus can simply be sampled endoscopically in clinic and antral lavage is rarely performed. Endoscopic sinus surgery allows a more functional approach to diseases of the paranasal sinuses and enables the drainage pathways of the paranasal

Austen Young, 1914–2005, ENT surgeon, Sheffield, UK, first described surgical closure of the nostril for the management of atrophic rhinitis.

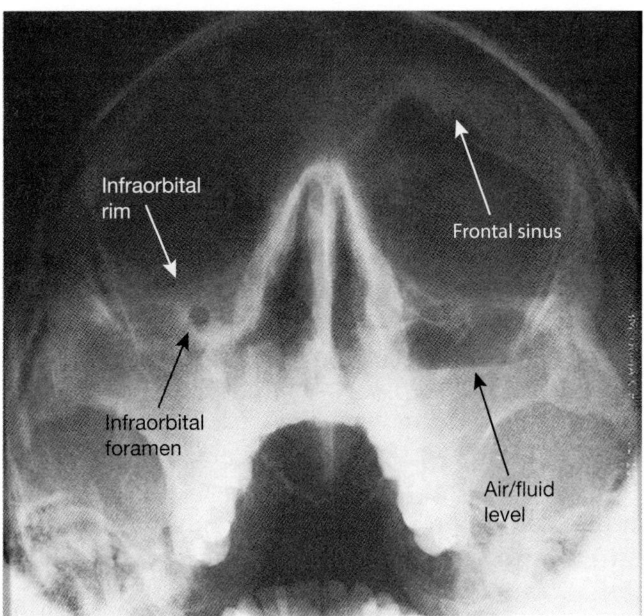

Figure 51.47 Plain radiograph showing the fluid level in the left maxillary antrum and total opacity of the right antrum.

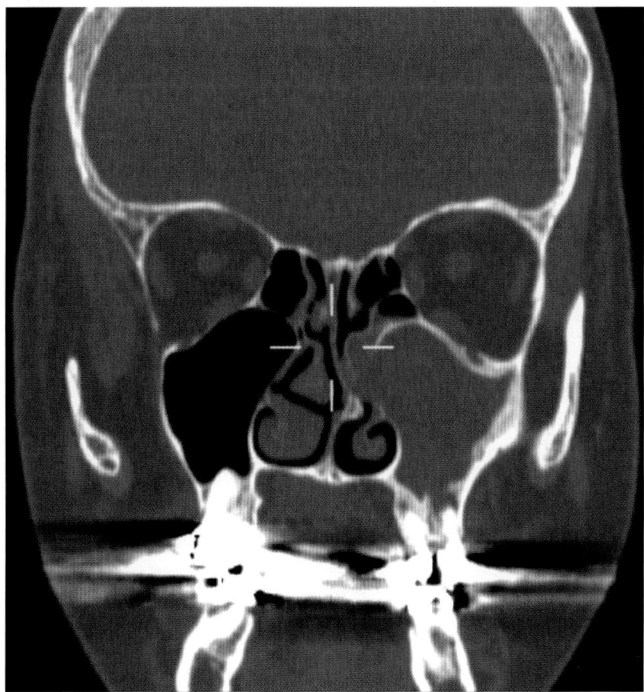

Figure 51.48 Coronal computed tomography scan showing left-sided maxillary sinus opacification due to maxillary sinusitis.

sinuses to be opened. Most cases of ARS can be treated conservatively with antibiotics and topical treatment. Surgery is used for those patients unresponsive to medical management or with complications. The majority of patients with ARS who require surgery are treated endoscopically. However, in some cases an open surgical approach may be necessary.

Summary box 51.12

Acute rhinosinusitis

- The most common causative organisms are *S. pneumoniae, H. influenzae, M. catarrhalis*
- Anaerobic infection of the maxillary sinus may result from dental sepsis
- Acute infection should be treated with antibiotics, topical decongestants and corticosteroids
- Endoscopic sinus surgery may be required

Complications

Complications of ARS include orbital and intracranial problems. The spread of infection from the sinuses occurs either through diploic veins or directly through bone erosion. This can result in epidural, subdural or cerebral abscesses or in meningitis/encephalitis. Cavernous sinus thrombosis may also result and can present with bilateral ptosis, proptosis, retro-ocular pain, ophthalmoplegia, papilloedema and spiking fevers.

Orbital complications of ARS are more common. Most often this is related to ethmoid sinus infection (***Figure 51.49***). An ophthalmology review is essential because of the threat to vision and intravenous antibiotics covering aerobic and anaerobic organisms are used. If there are any concerns regarding the eye, including proptosis, chemosis, ophthalmoplegia or reduced visual acuity, then CT with contrast is required (***Figure 51.50***). If an abscess is identified, this should be drained (endoscopically or open).

Summary box 51.13

Complications of acute rhinosinusitis

- Orbital – cellulitis, abscess
- Orbital infections may threaten sight
- Intracranial spread may cause meningitis, cerebral abscess or cavernous sinus thrombosis
- Osteomyelitis of the bones, particularly frontal, may occur

Summary box 51.14

Chandler classification of orbital complications of sinusitis

- I – preseptal cellulitis
- II – orbital cellulitis
- III – subperiosteal abscess
- IV – orbital abscess
- V – cavernous sinus thrombosis

Osteomyelitis of the frontal bones can also occur as a complication of ARS. If the anterior table of the frontal sinus is involved and becomes dehiscent, it can present with significant swelling of the skin of the forehead and a mass – Pott's puffy tumour (***Figure 51.51***).

Percivall Pott, 1714–1788, surgeon, London, UK.

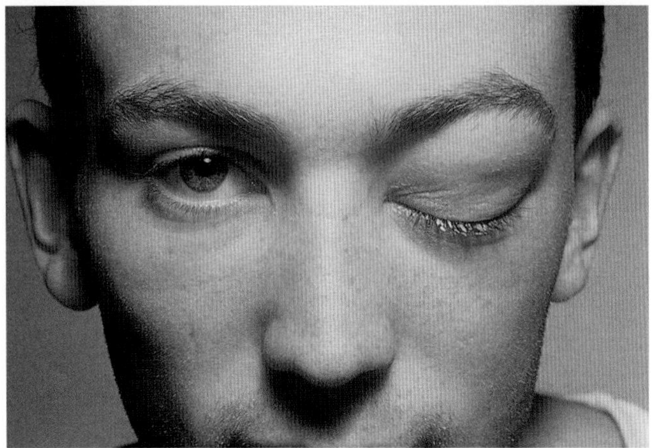

Figure 51.49 Left periorbital cellulitis complicating acute left ethmoiditis.

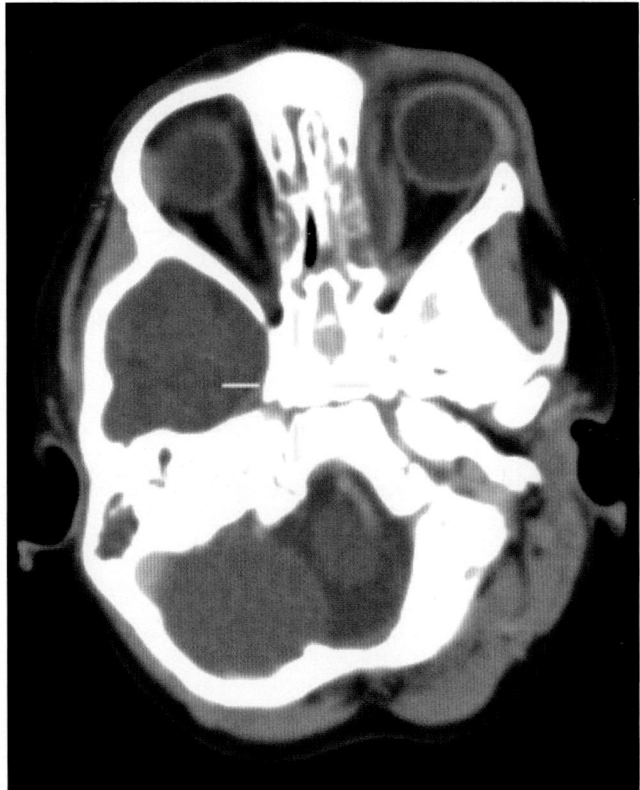

Figure 51.50 Axial computed tomography scan showing a subperiosteal abscess in the left orbit.

Chronic rhinosinusitis

CRS is common, affecting around 11% of the population. The aetiology is multifactorial and a number of factors have been linked to CRS, including ciliary dyskinesia, allergy, asthma, bacteria (*Staphylococcus aureus*), fungi and a number of host factors, including anatomical variations (deviated septum, concha bullosa of the middle turbinates). CRS has traditionally been divided into CRS with nasal polyps (CRSwNPs) and without (CRSsNPs). More recently CRS has been classified into primary or secondary, and local or diffuse disease.

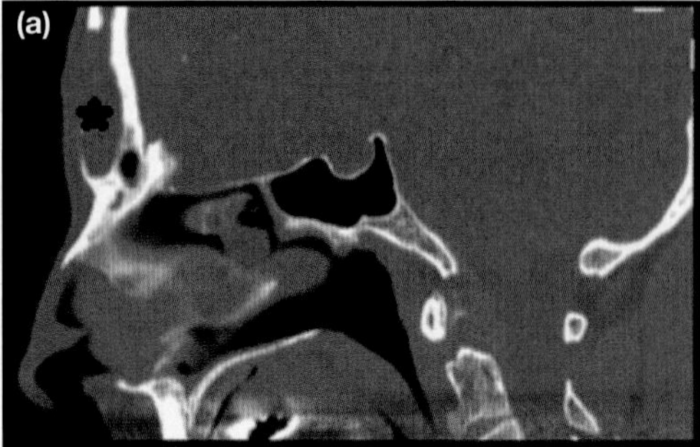

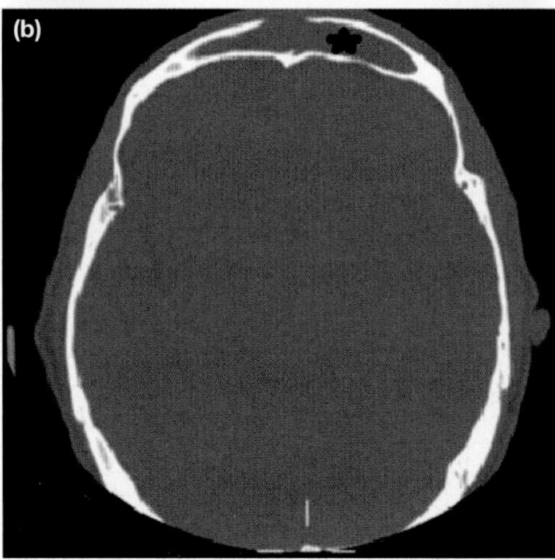

Figure 51.51 Sagittal (a) and axial (b) computed tomography scans showing complete opacification of the frontal sinus (marked with an asterisk) due to frontal sinusitis. The anterior wall of the frontal sinus is absent owing to infection.

Pathology

Nasal polyps are benign swellings of the sinus mucosa of unknown origin. Histologically, the polyps contain an oedematous stroma infiltrated with inflammatory cells and eosinophils. Inflammatory polyps tend to be bilateral and extend into the middle meatus. A single large polyp arising from the maxillary antrum is referred to as an antrochoanal polyp (***Figure 51.52***). This usually fills the nose and eventually prolapses posteriorly down into the nasopharynx.

Clinical features

Patients with CRSwNPs present with nasal obstruction, watery rhinorrhoea, postnasal drip and often hyposmia/anosmia. Pain does not tend to be a significant feature. Polyps are easily identifiable within the nose as pale semitransparent grey masses, which are mobile and insensitive when palpated with a fine probe (***Figure 51.53***). This allows them to be distinguished from hypertrophied turbinates. In CRSsNPs the middle meatus is often congested, with mucopus present.

Malignancy should be considered in adults with unilateral nasal polyps whereas in children such polyps must be distinguished from a meningocele or encephalocele by high-resolution CT scanning of the anterior cranial fossa. Nasal polyps are unusual in children; however, they do occur in conjunction with cystic fibrosis in 10% of cases.

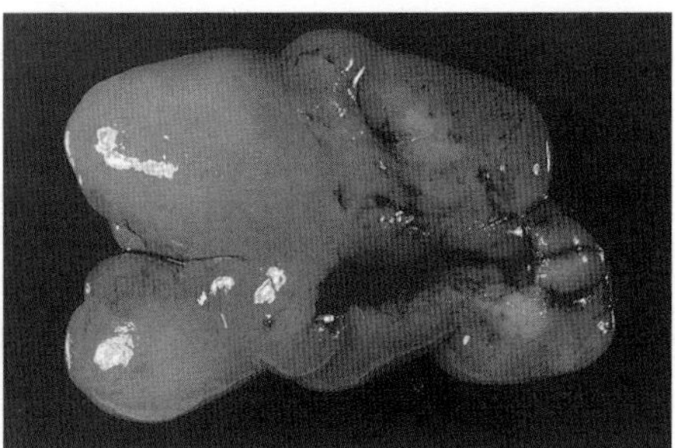

Figure 51.52 Antrochoanal polyp.

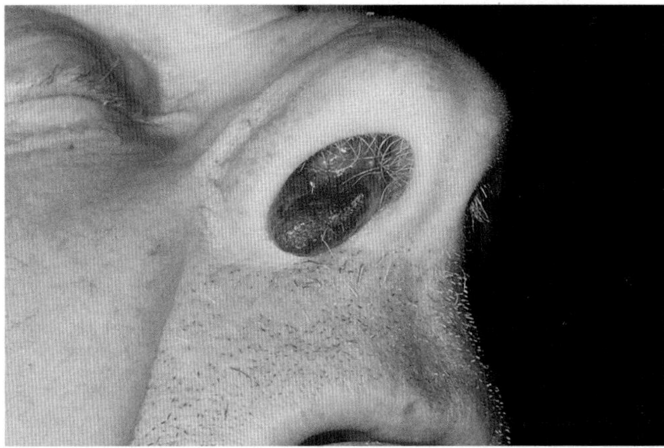

Figure 51.53 Nasal polyp in the right nasal vestibule.

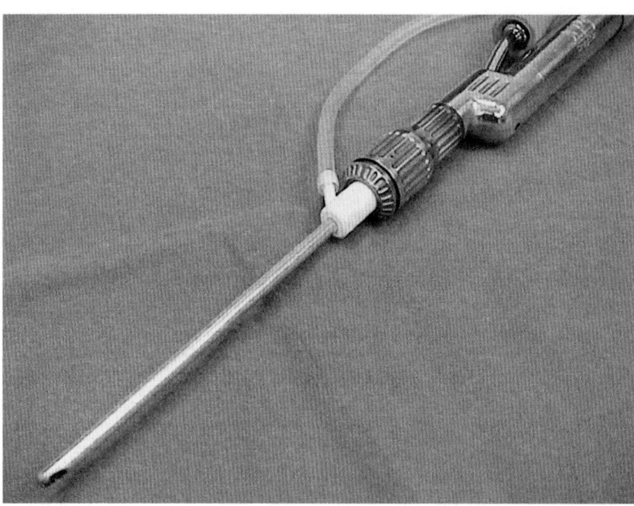

Figure 51.54 Powered nasal microdebrider.

Summary box 51.15

Nasal polyps

- Polyps are insensitive to touch and are mobile
- Inflammatory polyps are usually bilateral
- Unilateral nasal polyps should be removed for histology
- Bleeding polyps may indicate malignancy
- Meningocele and encephalocele must be excluded in children with polyps
- Polyps are removed using a powered microdebrider

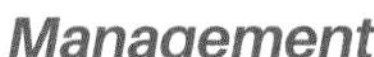

Management

Medical treatment of CRSwNPs with systemic steroids will often reduce the size of the nasal polyps and give short-term relief of nasal blockage. Unfortunately, the polyps tend to recur when the treatment stops. Topical corticosteroid drops and sprays are also used along with saline douching. Biological treatments using monoclonal antibodies are a potential new therapy for CRSwNPs. In CRSsNPs, in addition to topical treatments, a long course of low-dose antibiotics (macrolides) can be used in those patients with a normal level of immunoglobulin E. Surgical treatment is indicated in patients who do not respond to medical treatment. Endoscopic nasal polypectomy and functional endoscopic sinus surgery (FESS) is performed following a CT scan that confirms the extent of disease and shows the important bony anatomy preoperatively. Serious complications following FESS include CSF leak and orbital problems, including orbital haematoma, and so it is important to review the level and symmetry of the anterior skull base and the integrity of the lamina papyracea on the CT scan prior to surgery. Endoscopic polypectomy is performed using a powered nasal microdebrider (***Figure 51.54***).

Image guidance can be used in endoscopic sinus surgery and extended endoscopic procedures such as pituitary and anterior skull base surgery to provide real-time feedback of instrument position in the nose based on preoperative CT or MRI scans.

TUMOURS OF THE NOSE AND SINUSES

Tumours arising in the nose or paranasal sinuses may present with unilateral nasal obstruction, persistent unilateral anterior rhinorrhoea, postnasal drip, epistaxis, unilateral bloodstained rhinorrhoea, facial swelling or proptosis.

Benign tumours

Simple papillomas or viral warts can grow inside the nasal vestibule. They can be confused with carcinomas and are best excised for histological diagnosis.

Osteomas of the nasal skeleton are not uncommon and are often detected on radiology as an incidental finding (***Figure 51.55***). In symptomatic individuals the osteoma can be removed endoscopically or via an open procedure.

Inverted (transitional cell) papillomas can occur in both the nasal cavity and the nasal sinuses. They are inverted papillomas because histologically the hyperplastic epithelium inverts into the underlying stroma. The papillomas are covered with transitional epithelium. Calcification within the tumour may be seen on CT along with sclerosis of the bone at the margins of the growth (***Figure 51.56***). Inverted papillomas can undergo malignant change. Full surgical resection is required, and this can usually be performed endoscopically.

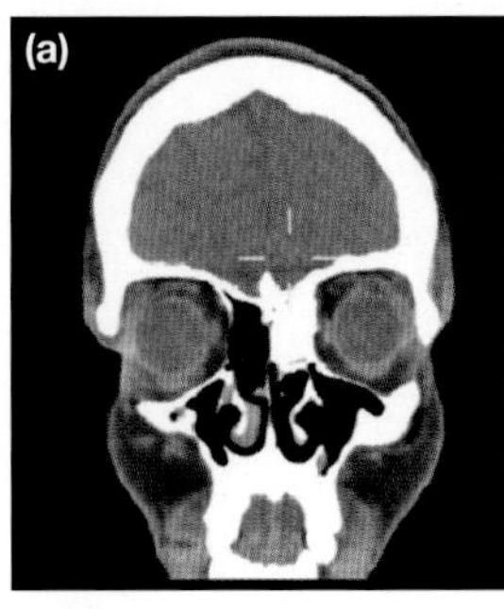

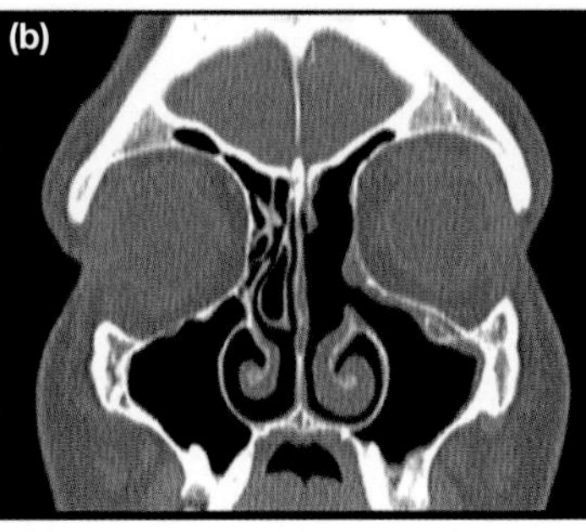

Figure 51.55 Coronal computed tomography (CT) scan showing an osteoma in the left anterior ethmoid sinus adjacent to the orbit (a). The second coronal CT scan is following endoscopic excision of the osteoma (b).

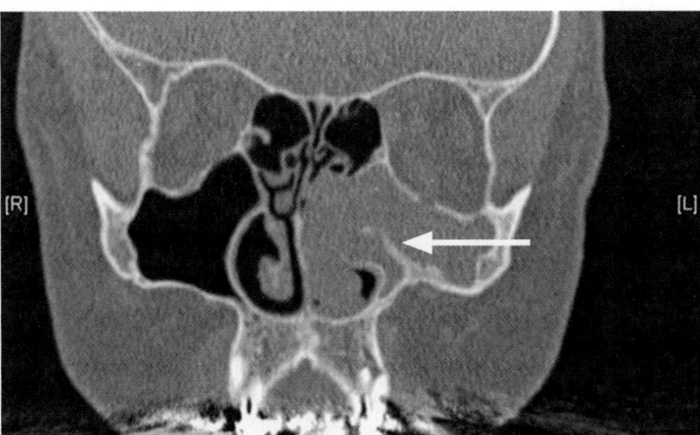

Figure 51.56 Coronal computed tomography scan showing an extensive inverted papilloma involving the left maxillary sinus; arrow indicates calcification within the tumour.

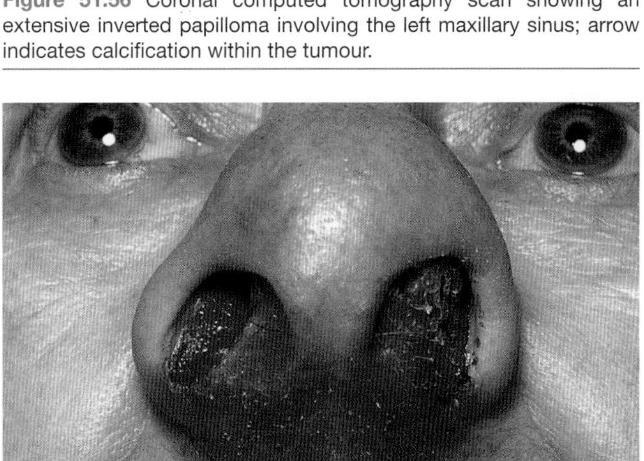
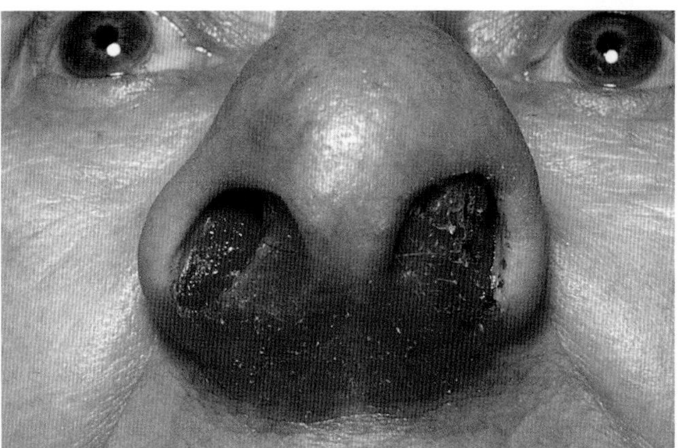

Figure 51.57 Squamous cell carcinoma of the nasal septum.

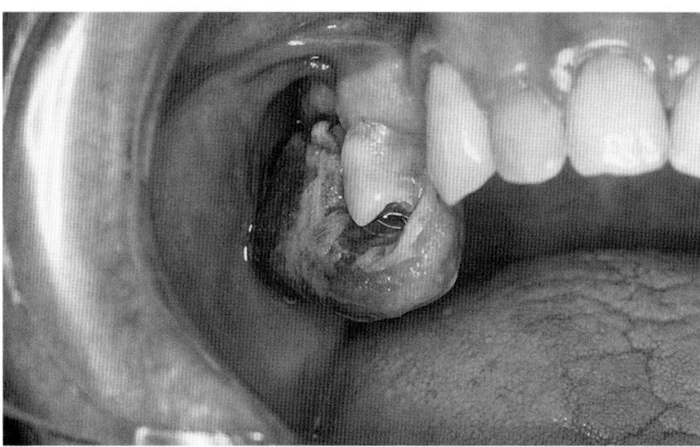

Figure 51.58 Maxillary antral carcinoma presenting through an oro-antral fistula.

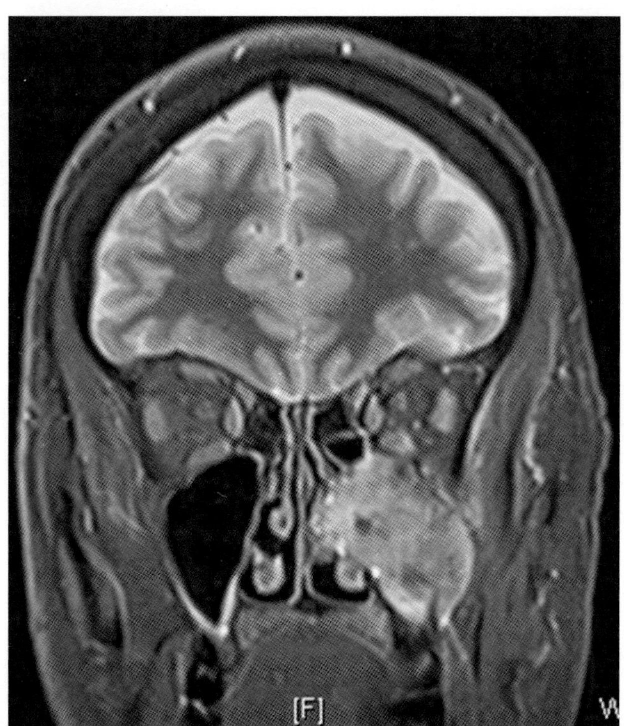

Figure 51.59 Coronal magnetic resonance imaging scan of the paranasal sinuses showing extensive left maxillary antral carcinoma invading adjacent structures.

Malignant tumours

The most common malignant tumours to occur within the nasal cavity and paranasal sinuses are squamous cell carcinomas (*Figure 51.57*), adenoid cystic carcinomas and adenocarcinomas. Adenocarcinoma has been linked to exposure to hard wood dust in the furniture industry. Adenoid cystic carcinomas arise from minor salivary glands, which can be found in the nose. Suspicious signs of invasion of neighbouring tissues include diplopia, proptosis, loosening of the teeth (*Figure 51.58*), trismus, CN palsies and regional lymphadenopathy. *Figure 51.59* shows invasion of a left maxillary antral carcinoma into adjacent structures, including the orbit, on an MRI scan.

Patients with sinus or intranasal malignancy are best managed in a combined clinic where the expertise of ENT surgeons, maxillofacial surgeons and oncologists can be employed.

Summary box 51.16

Tumours of the nose and sinuses

- Unilateral nasal blockage, discharge and bleeding are often presenting symptoms in nasal or sinus tumours
- Osteomas are often asymptomatic
- Inverted papilloma is a benign tumour, which presents as a unilateral polyp that can undergo malignant change
- Squamous cell carcinoma is the most common malignant tumour
- Almost 50% of sinonasal cancers arise on the lateral nasal wall and 33% in the maxillary antrum
- Multidisciplinary management of malignant sinonasal tumours requires input from ENT surgeons, maxillofacial surgeons and oncologists

FURTHER READING

Fokkens WJ, Lund VJ, Hopkins C *et al.* European position paper on rhinosinusitis and nasal polyps. *Rhinology* 2020; **58**(Suppl S29): 1–464.

Watkinson JC, Clarke RW (eds). *Scott-Brown's otorhinolaryngology and head and neck surgery*, 8th edn. Boca Raton, FL: CRC Press, 2018.

CHAPTER 52 The pharynx, larynx and neck

Learning objectives

To understand:

- The relevant anatomy, physiology, disease processes and investigations of the pharynx, the larynx and the neck
- The diagnosis and emergency treatment of airway obstruction
- The aetiology, natural history and management of squamous cell carcinoma of the upper aerodigestive tract

CLINICAL ANATOMY AND PHYSIOLOGY

The pharynx

The pharynx is a fibromuscular tube forming the upper part of the respiratory and digestive passages. It extends from the base of the skull to the level of the sixth cervical vertebra at the lower border of the cricoid cartilage, where it becomes continuous with the oesophagus. It is divided into three parts: the nasopharynx, oropharynx and hypopharynx (*Figure 52.1*).

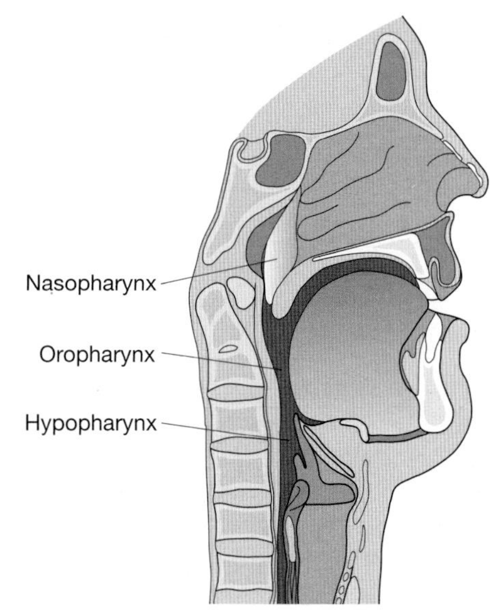

Figure 52.1 The component parts of the pharynx.

Nasopharynx

The nasopharynx lies anterior to the first cervical vertebra. The adenoids, which constitute the superior component of Waldeyer's ring, are situated at the junction of the roof and posterior wall of the nasopharynx. Waldeyer's ring is a ring of lymphoid tissue comprising, in addition to the adenoids, the palatine and lingual tonsils of the oropharynx. It is situated at the entry to the air and food passages and is constantly exposed to new inspired or ingested antigenic stimuli. Accordingly, it is an important part of the mucosa-associated lymphoid tissue (MALT), which processes antigens and presents them to T-helper cells and B cells (*Figure 52.2*), thereby facilitating a first-line immune response mechanism, which is particularly important in childhood. The tissue of Waldeyer's ring undergoes physiological hypertrophy during early childhood as the child is exposed to increasing amounts of antigenic stimuli, and there is often a similar hypertrophy of the cervical lymph nodes.

The Eustachian tubes, leading from the middle ear cleft, open into the posterosuperior aspect of the lateral wall. Dorsal and superior to the openings, bounded anteriorly by a ridge formed by the salpingopharyngeus muscle, are the fossae of Rosenmüller, a common site for the development of nasopharyngeal carcinoma (*Figure 52.3*).

Oropharynx

This is bounded superiorly by the soft palate, inferiorly by the lingual surface of the epiglottis and anteriorly by the anterior faucial pillars and the circumvallate papillae of the tongue. The palatine tonsils are situated in the lateral wall between the anterior and posterior pillars of the fauces. The lateral wall, and in particular the tonsil, takes its blood supply from the facial artery, which may be closely related to the lower pole,

Heinrich Wilhelm Gottfried Waldeyer-Hartz, 1836–1921, Professor of Pathological Anatomy, Berlin, Germany.
Bartolomeo Eustachio (Eustachius), 1513–1574, appointed physician to the Pope in 1547, and Professor of Anatomy, Rome, Italy, in 1549.
Johann Christian Rosenmüller, 1771–1820, Professor of Anatomy and Surgery, Leipzig, Germany.

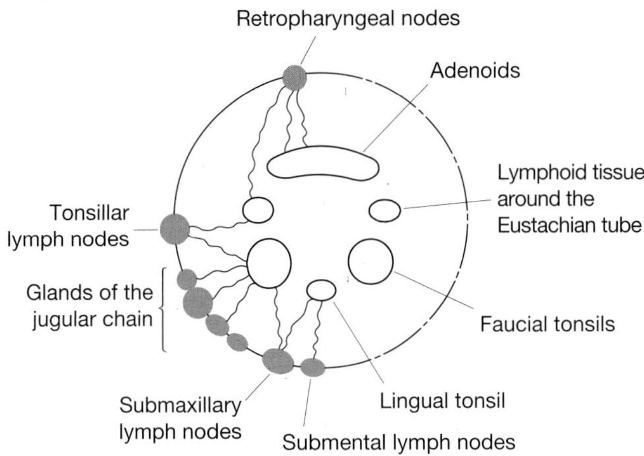

Figure 52.2 Waldeyer's ring.

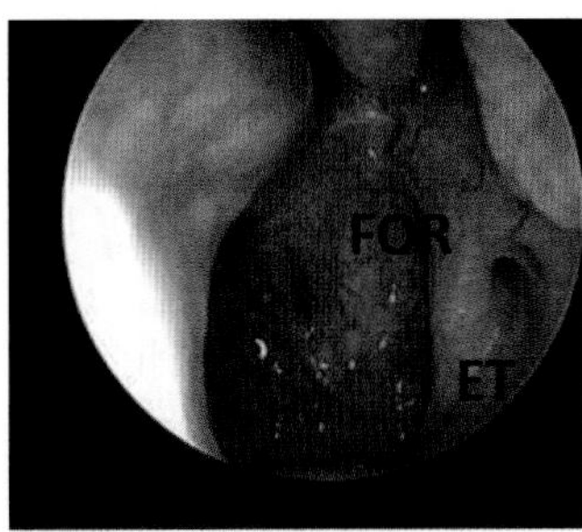

Figure 52.3 Endoscopic view of the left nasopharynx. ET, Eustachian tube; FOR, fossa of Rosenmüller.

and laterally a plexus of paratonsillar veins, which may be the source of significant venous bleeding following tonsillectomy.

Hypopharynx

The superior border of the hypopharynx is at the level of the laryngeal inlet. Its inferior border is the lower border of the cricoid cartilage where it continues into the oesophagus. The hypopharynx is commonly divided into three areas: the right and left piriform fossae, the posterior pharyngeal wall and the postcricoid region. The mucosa of these areas is, however, continuous so disease processes, such as squamous cell carcinomas, often involve more than one area as a result of overt or submucosal spread.

The multifaceted complex process of swallowing, which consists of the oral, pharyngeal and oesophageal phases (*Figure 52.4*), is mediated via afferent fibres passing to the medulla oblongata through the second division of the trigeminal nerve (V), glossopharyngeal nerve (IX) and vagus nerve (X). The efferent pathway is from the nucleus ambiguus and is mediated via the glossopharyngeal (IX), vagus (X) and hypoglossal (XII) nerves. Damage to these major cranial nerves at any point along their pathway, by trauma or disease, may cause dysphagia and/or aspiration.

Videofluoroscopy, in which the passage of a bolus of radio-opaque food of different textures from the point at which it enters the oral cavity down to its passage within the stomach is examined radiologically, is the investigation of choice when investigating swallowing (dys)function.

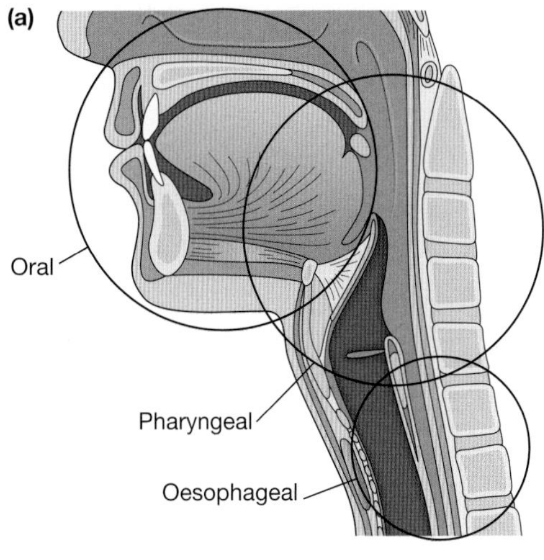

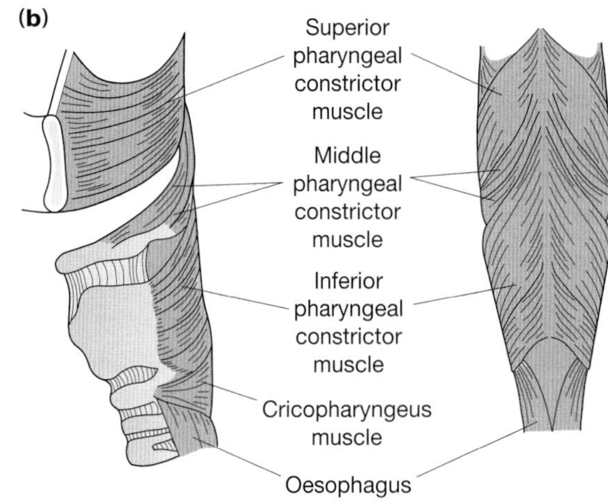

Figure 52.4 The three phases of swallowing (a) and the muscles (b).

Anatomical relationships of the pharynx

Some of these are illustrated in *Figure 52.5*.

Parapharyngeal space

This potential space lies lateral to the pharynx and is shaped like an inverted pyramid with its base at the base of the skull and its apex at the level of hyoid. It is divided into a prestyloid space, which contains the deep lobe of the parotid gland, blood vessels, lymph nodes and fat tissue, and a poststyloid space (also known as carotid space), which contains cranial nerves IX–XII, the carotid artery, internal jugular vein, deep cervical lymph nodes and cervical sympathetic trunk.

Infection and necrosis of the cervical lymph nodes in the parapharyngeal space most commonly occur from infections of the tonsils or teeth (particularly the third lower molar tooth). As the parapharyngeal space is not anatomically divided, infection may therefore spread from the skull base cranially to the superior mediastinum caudally and consequently often presents a surgical challenge.

Retropharyngeal space

This potential space lies posterior to the pharynx, bounded anteriorly by the constrictor muscles and the covering

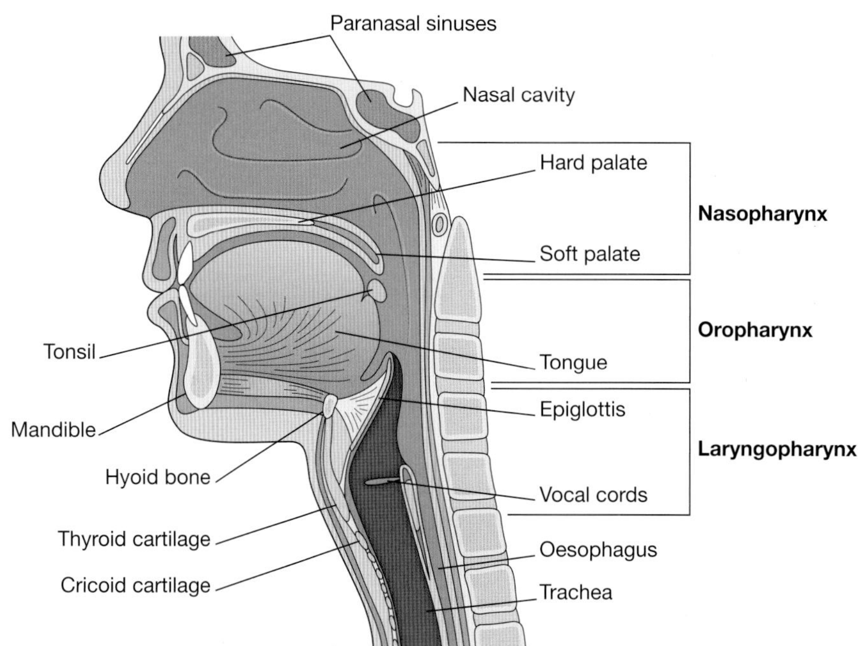

Figure 52.5 Sagittal diagram of the upper aerodigestive tract.

buccopharyngeal fascia and posteriorly by the prevertebral musculature and its overlying prevertebral fascia. It contains the retropharyngeal lymph nodes, which are usually paired lateral nodes but which are separated by a tough midline fibrous condensation that connects the prevertebral and buccopharyngeal fascia.

As with the lymphoid tissue of Waldeyer's ring, these nodes are more active in infancy and young children, and it is at this age that they are most likely to be involved in inflammatory processes, which, if severe, may affect swallowing and respiration as a consequence of gross swelling and suppuration of the retropharyngeal space.

Larynx

It is important to appreciate that the main function of the larynx is not the production of voice but the protection of the tracheobronchial airway and lungs. In order to achieve this, the larynx, together with the base of the tongue, forms the protective sphincter that closes off the airway during swallowing. It is only an evolutionary by-product that, in humans and some other mammals, the larynx is responsible for the production of sound.

The larynx comprises a cartilaginous framework (that may ossify in later life), which consists of the hyoid bone above, the thyroid and cricoid cartilages and the intricate arytenoid cartilages posteriorly.

The cricoid cartilage is the only complete ring in the entire airway and bounds the subglottis, which is the narrowest point of the airway in children. This is the most common site for damage from an endotracheal tube used for intensive care unit ventilation in seriously ill patients.

A purely anatomical description of the larynx divides it into the supraglottis, glottis and subglottis (*Figure 52.6*). The true

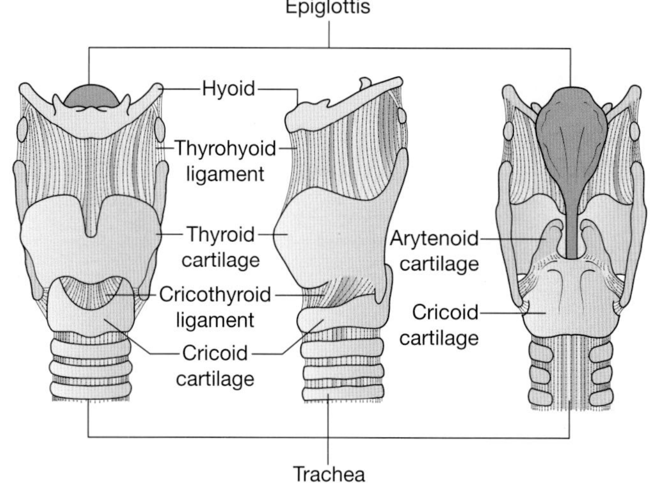

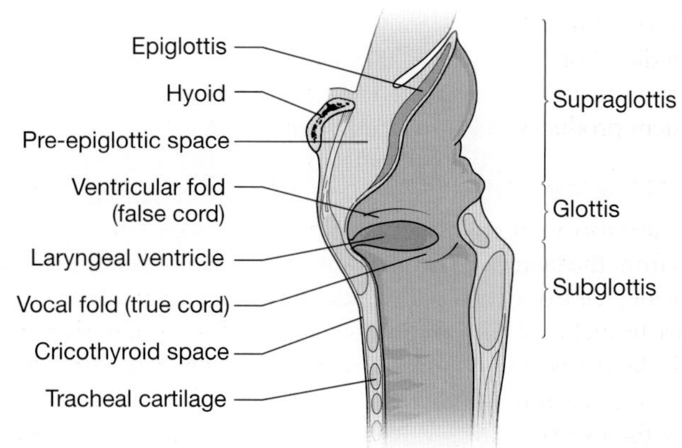

Figure 52.6 Anatomy of the larynx.

(a)

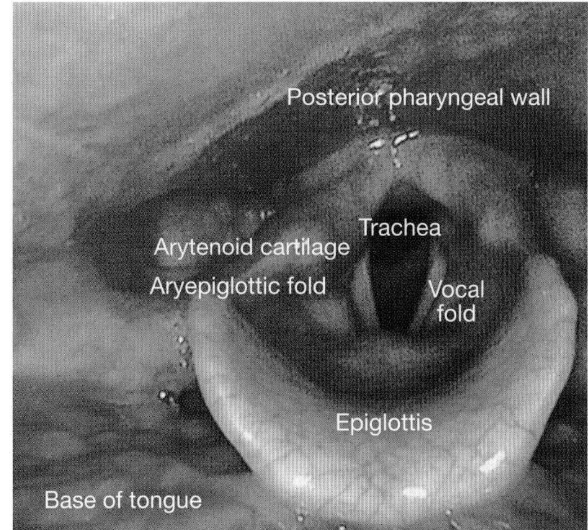

(b)

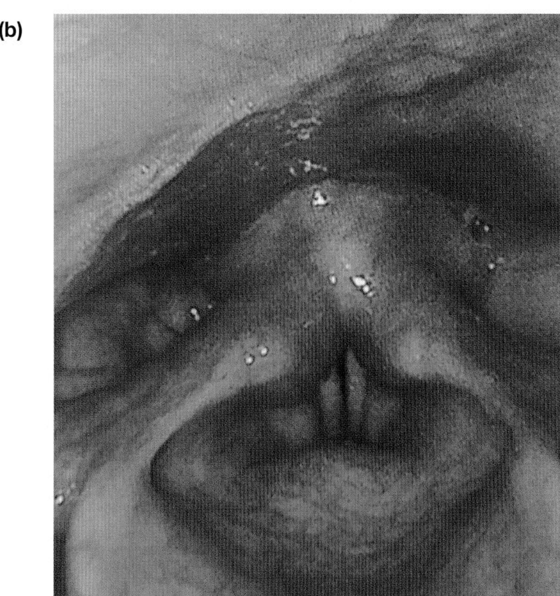

Figure 52.7 (a) Flexible nasendoscopy view of the larynx with the vocal folds abducted. (b) Flexible nasendoscopy view of the larynx with the vocal folds adducted.

vocal folds (often incorrectly called the vocal cords) are normally white, in contrast to the pink mucosa of the rest of the larynx and airway. The true vocal folds meet anteriorly at the midlevel of the thyroid cartilage, whereas posteriorly they are separate and attached to an arytenoid cartilage. This arrangement produces the 'V' shape of the glottis (***Figure 52.7***).

Nerve supply

The sensory nerve supply to the larynx above the true vocal folds is from the internal branch of the superior laryngeal nerve and, below, it is from the recurrent laryngeal nerve. Both these nerves are branches of the vagus nerve (X). The motor nerve supply to the larynx is from the recurrent laryngeal nerve, which supplies all intrinsic muscles except the cricothyroid, which is supplied by the external branch of the superior laryngeal nerve. Only one of these intrinsic muscles, the posterior cricoarytenoid, abducts the vocal folds during respiration. All other intrinsic muscles adduct the cords. Damage to the recurrent laryngeal or vagus nerve above the recurrent laryngeal nerve branch will cause paralysis of the vocal fold on the side of the damage. Additionally, cadaver studies have described the 'human communicating nerve', which is an anastomosis between the external branch of the superior laryngeal nerve and the recurrent laryngeal nerve, seen in 70% of human larynges. This nerve provides the sensory supply to the subglottis and motor innervation to the thyroarytenoid muscle.

Phonation/speech

The larynx functions by closing the vocal fold against the air being exhaled from the lungs, but the rise in subglottic pressure forces the vocal folds apart slightly for an instant of time, resulting in an accompanying sinusoidal wave-like vibration of the vocal fold epithelium. The human vocal folds have a specialised tissue morphology with resultant biomechanical properties that allow phonation. The opening and closing occurs in rapid sequence to produce a vibrating column of air, which is the source of sound that can be articulated by the structure of the oral cavity to produce speech.

Paralysis or disease of the vocal folds or closely associated laryngeal structures will give rise to disturbance of the sound, producing hoarseness.

The functions of the larynx are given in ***Summary box 52.1***.

Summary box 52.1

Functions of the larynx

- Protection of the lower respiratory tract by:
  - Closure of the laryngeal inlet
  - Closure of the false cords
  - Closure of the glottis
  - Cessation of respiration
  - Cough reflex
- Phonation
  - Vocal folds produce sound by quasiperiodic vibration
- Respiration
  - Control of pressure
- Fixation of chest
  - Aids lifting, straining and climbing

Neck

The neck is divided into anterior and posterior triangles by the sternocleidomastoid muscle. The anterior triangle extends from the inferior border of the mandible to the sternum below and is bounded by the midline and the posterior border of the sternocleidomastoid muscle. The posterior triangle extends backwards to the anterior border of the trapezius muscle and inferiorly to the clavicle. The upper part of the anterior triangle, above the hyoid bone, is commonly subdivided into the submandibular triangle above the digastric muscle bellies, and the submental triangle anteriorly, between the anterior digastric bellies of each side. The lymphatic drainage of the head and neck is of considerable clinical importance (***Figure 52.8***).

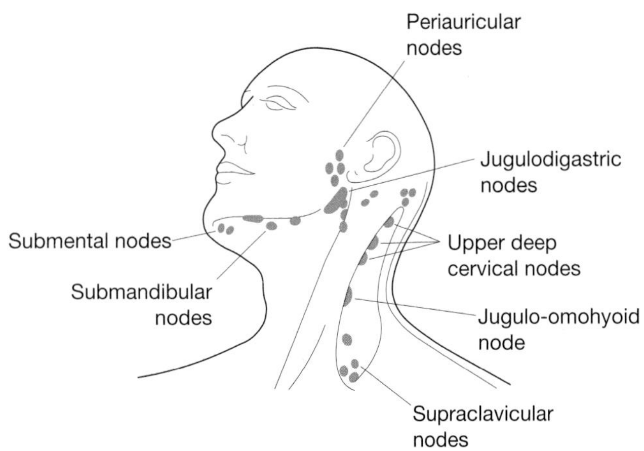

Figure 52.8 Distribution of cervical lymph nodes.

The most important chain of nodes are the jugular nodes, which run adjacent to the internal jugular vein. The other main groups are the submental, submandibular, pre- and postauricular, occipital and posterior triangle nodes.

A system of levels is used to describe the location of these neck nodes (***Figure 52.9***). Of particular note are the jugular nodal levels, which include levels II, III and IV; these relate to the upper, middle and inferior third of the carotid sheath, respectively. The level II nodes, which contain the large jugulodigastric node, drain the naso- and oropharynx, including the tonsils, posterolateral aspects of the oral cavity and the superior aspects of the larynx and piriform fossae. They are the most common sites of enlargement and may be palpated along the anterior border of the sternocleidomastoid muscle.

Metastatic spread of squamous cell carcinoma (80% of head and neck cancers) most commonly occurs from tumours arising in the upper aerodigestive tract mucosa, which comprises the following sites: oral cavity, nasopharynx, oropharynx, larynx and hypopharynx. When an enlarged neck node is detected and malignant disease is suspected, these sites must be carefully examined.

CLINICAL EXAMINATION

Pharynx and larynx

Before examination of the pharynx, the oral cavity should be examined with the aid of a good light and tongue depressors. Historically, a reflecting mirror on the head was used as a source of examination light. However, a headband-mounted fibreoptic light source is widely available and more commonly used. Either option permits the use of both hands to hold instruments. Inspection should include the buccal mucosa and lips, the palate, the tongue and floor of the mouth, all surfaces of the teeth and gums, the salivary ductal orifices, opening and closing of the mouth and dental occlusion. Patients should be asked to elevate the tongue to the roof of the mouth and protrude the tongue towards both the right and the left. Grasping the protruded tongue with a gauze aids the examination. Intraoral palpation may be required gently using one

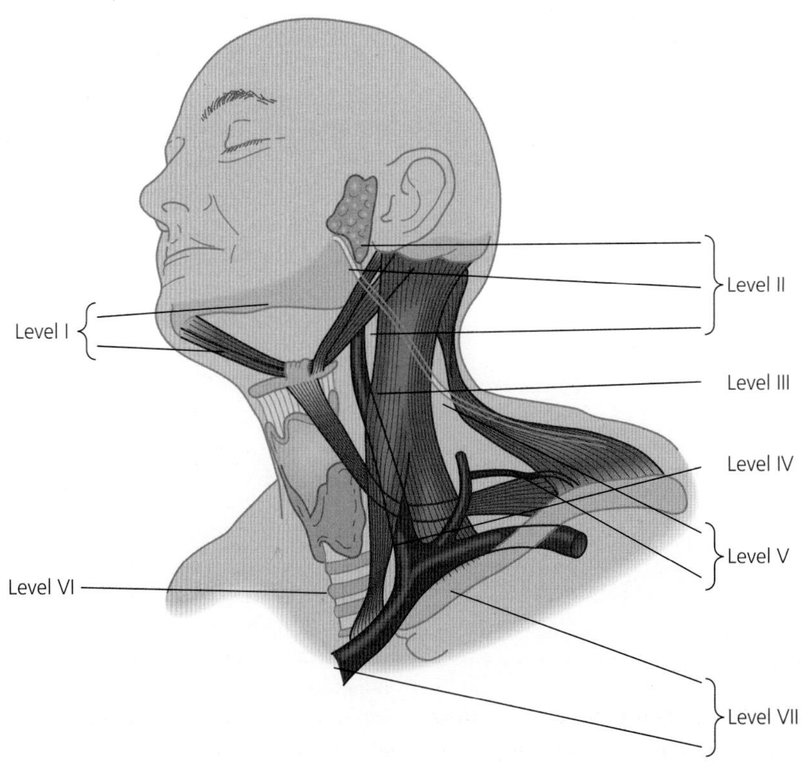

Figure 52.9 The level system for describing the location of lymph nodes in the neck. Level I, submental and submandibular group; level II, upper jugular group; level III, middle jugular group; level IV, lower jugular group; level V, posterior triangle group; level VI, anterior compartment group; level VII, superior mediastinal nodes. (Reproduced with permission from Watkinson JC, Gilbert RW. *Stell & Maran's textbook of head and neck surgery and oncology*, 5th edn. Boca Raton, FL: Hodder Arnold/CRC Press, 2012.)

or two fingers to feel any swellings. Intraoral palpation may be combined with extraoral bimanual palpation of the submental and submandibular lymph nodes and salivary glands to aid the characterisation and/or localisation of any swelling detected.

Following examination of the oral cavity, the oropharynx is then inspected with the tongue depressor placed firmly onto the tongue base to depress it inferiorly. Care must be taken to, if possible, avoid provoking a gag reflex. The anterior and posterior faucial pillars, the tonsil, retromolar trigone and posterior pharyngeal wall should all be inspected for colour changes, ulceration, mass lesions, mucopus, foreign bodies and swellings. Pain and trismus as a consequence of pharyngolaryngeal or neck pathology may add to the difficulty of the examination but are significant clinical findings in their own right.

While angled mirrors and a headlight may be used in expert hands, modern flexible fibreoptic endoscopes passed through the nose, with or without topical anaesthesia, allow high-quality examination of the entire nasopharynx, oropharynx, larynx and often the hypopharynx in almost every patient. Moreover, a camera attached to the endoscope permits the taking of high-quality photographs to record and present pertinent clinical findings. A rigid 0° fibreoptic endoscope (Hopkins' rod) is often used in preference to inspect the nasal cavities and nasopharynx.

Neck

The patient should be examined in the sitting position with the whole neck exposed so that both clavicles are clearly seen. The neck is inspected from the front and the patient asked to swallow, preferably with the aid of a sip of water. Movements of the larynx and any swellings in the neck are noted. The patient should be asked to protrude the tongue if there is a midline neck swelling, as a thyroglossal duct cyst will move upwards with the tongue protrusion. The neck is then examined from behind, one side at a time, with the chin flexed slightly downwards and the neck tilted to the same side being palpated to remove any undue tension in the strap muscles, platysma and sternocleidomastoids.

On examining for a lump in the neck, it is often helpful to ask the patient to point to the lump first. Ask if the lump is tender. All five palpable neck node levels (I–V) should be examined systematically.

If malignancy is suspected (hard, irregular or fixed to overlying skin or to deep structures), inspection of the upper aerodigestive tract mucosa, as described above, is mandatory.

Summary box 52.2

Key points of history and examination

Mouth

- Adequate light source and two spatulas to examine the mouth
- Examine
  - Lips
  - Teeth, gums, gingival sulci
  - Buccal mucosa, opening of parotid ducts
  - Floor of mouth and opening of submandibular salivary ducts
  - Hard and soft palate
  - Retromolar trigone region
  - Anterior and posterior faucial pillars, tonsils
  - Posterior pharyngeal wall
  - Tongue (observe full movements)
- Palpate
  - Salivary glands/ducts
  - Any mass lesions or ulcers in the mouth

Larynx, oropharynx and hypopharynx

- Indirect laryngoscopy
  - Mirror and headlight
- Flexible fibreoptic pharyngolaryngoscopy

Nasopharynx

- Rigid Hopkins' rod endoscopy
- Flexible fibreoptic nasendoscopy

Neck

- Inspection
  - Tongue protrusion
  - Observe swallowing
- Palpation
  - If a mass is palpable, evaluate for size, site, shape, consistency, superficial and deep fixation, fluctuation, transillumination, auscultation

INVESTIGATION OF THE PHARYNX, LARYNX AND NECK

Plain lateral radiographs

Plain lateral radiographs of the neck and cervical spine may show soft-tissue abnormalities, although their sensitivity and specificity is low; of particular importance is the depth and outline of the prevertebral soft-tissue shadow on sagittal section as an indication of retropharyngeal pathology. The outline of the laryngotracheal airway may be a useful guide to the presence of disease in the pharynx and larynx. There should be no air within the upper oesophagus. If air is seen, endoscopy is advised. Radio-opaque foreign bodies may be seen impacted in the pharynx, larynx or upper oesophagus on these radiographs (***Figures 52.10 and 52.11***).

Barium swallow and videofluoroscopy

Barium (or water-soluble contrast if a pharyngeal or oesophageal perforation is suspected) is used to perform dynamic videofluoroscopic studies, which record the movement of a small quantity of radio-opaque food of various textures and allow detailed evaluation of the oral and pharyngeal phases of swallowing (***Figure 52.12***).

Harold Horace Hopkins, 1918–1994, Professor of Applied Optics, University of Reading, Reading, UK, invented the rigid rod endoscope (Hopkins' rod, 1954) and contributed to the development of the fibres for flexible endoscopes.

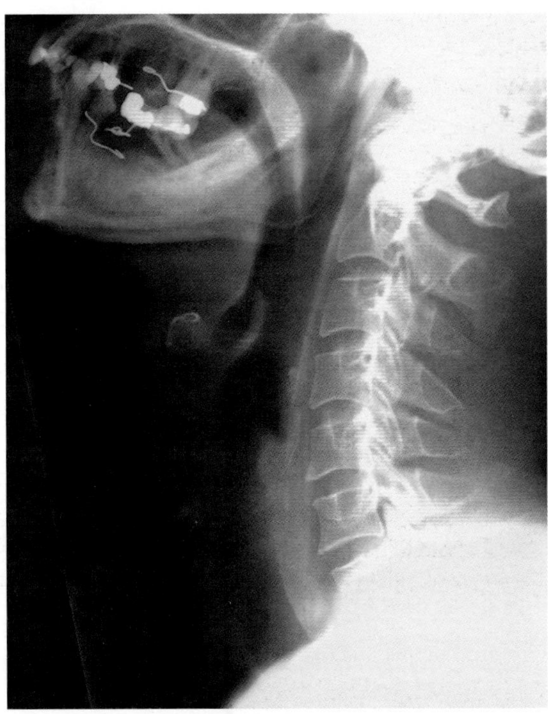

Figure 52.10 Plain lateral radiograph showing normal anatomy.

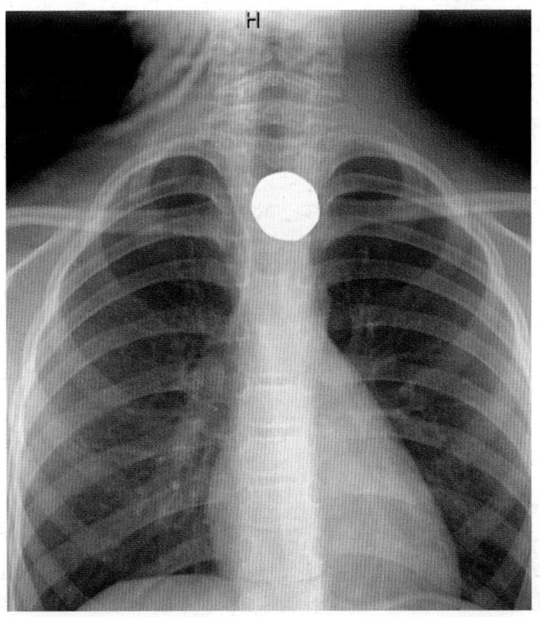

Figure 52.11 Plain radiograph demonstrating a coin in the oesophagus.

Computed tomography scanning

Computed tomography (CT) scanning provides high-resolution imaging of disease in the pharynx, larynx and neck. Intravenous contrast given at the same time as the CT scan (dynamic scanning) further improves the demonstration of disease in these areas (***Figure 52.13***).

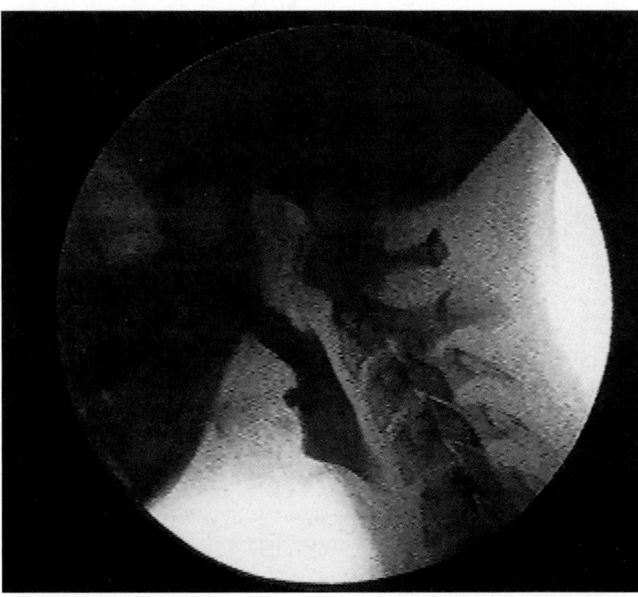

Figure 52.12 Static image grab from a videofluoroscopy sequence showing liquid barium in the upper pharynx in a normal swallow.

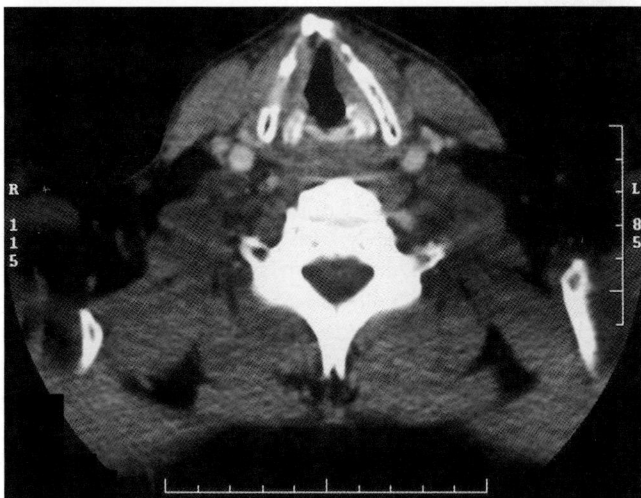

Figure 52.13 Axial computed tomography scan through the neck and larynx at the level of the glottis.

Other imaging

Magnetic resonance imaging (MRI) gives better soft-tissue definition and is preferred for primary tumour staging except for paranasal sinus cancers. Drawbacks of this approach include a reduction in image quality as a result of movement artefact, poorer definition of bony and cartilaginous structures and upstaging of tumours as a result of oversensitivity (***Figure 52.14***). Ultrasound scanning can be useful in differentiating solid lesions (e.g. malignant lymph nodes) from cystic lesions such as a branchial cyst and is particularly helpful when fine-needle aspiration is needed to establish the diagnosis; this modality is also invaluable for salivary gland pathology.

If a head and neck malignancy is suspected, then CT imaging of the thorax should also be performed to detect distant

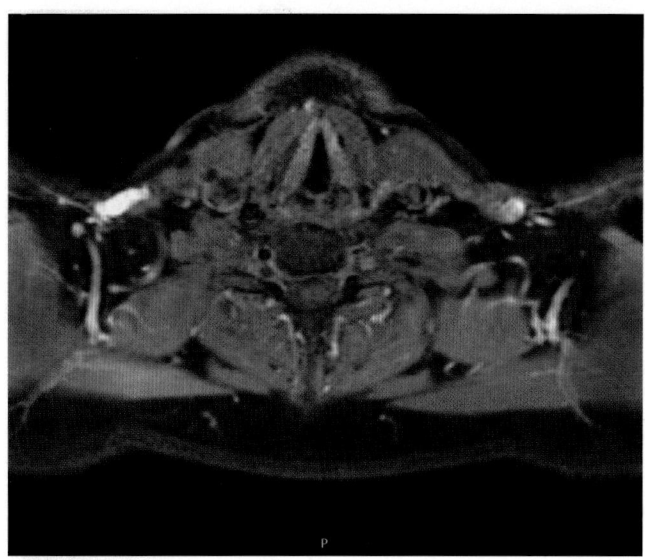

Figure 52.14 An axial magnetic resonance imaging scan at the same level as *Figure 52.13*.

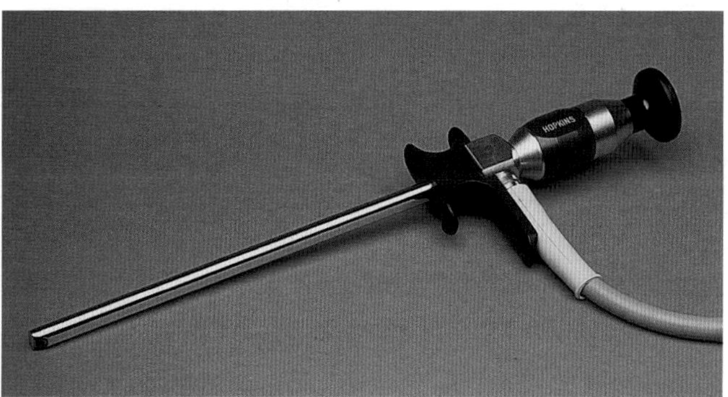

Figure 52.15 A rigid Hopkins' rod or endoscope.

metastases and synchronous primary bronchogenic tumours (approximately 5%), as the presence of these diagnoses will change treatment options.

Positron emission tomography (PET)-CT scans are performed during a single examination, in which the cross-sectional anatomical detail of a CT is fused with the metabolic information available from using a radiotracer. 18-Fluorodeoxyglucose (FDG) is the most commonly used radiotracer, with molecules similar to glucose; it accumulates in areas of high metabolic activity, which may represent tumour or inflammation. PET-CT is particularly used in patients being investigated for carcinoma of unknown primary to help identify the primary site of tumour, to look for distant metastases and to assess response to cancer treatment.

Fine-needle aspiration cytology and core biopsy

This is the investigation of choice when attempting to determine the nature of a neck or thyroid mass. Fine-needle aspiration cytology (FNAC) is aided by ultrasound (CT guided for deep-seated lesions) to the extent that ultrasound-guided FNAC or core biopsy is now the standard of care in many units around the world. Core biopsy is the preferred technique in investigating a neck node as immunohistochemistry tests can be performed on the tissue samples to determine positivity to human papillomavirus (HPV) or Epstein–Barr virus (EBV) in current-day practice. The technique is safe and well tolerated and has high diagnostic sensitivity and specificity, especially when diagnosing cervical lymph node enlargement.

Angiography or digital subtraction vascular imaging

These techniques may be indicated if a vascular lesion such as a carotid body tumour is suspected. Angiography may have a therapeutic role to play by facilitating embolisation of vascular tumours prior to planned surgical procedures. Magnetic resonance angiography (MRA) offers excellent resolution of vascular anatomy and is less invasive.

Direct pharyngoscopy and laryngoscopy

Examination of the pharynx, larynx and neck under general anaesthesia may be required to assess the stage and resectability of the primary site, or in instances where comprehensive examination has not been possible; such scenarios include an inadequate clinical examination caused by trismus from pain, poor patient compliance or large obstructive pharyngeal or laryngeal pathology. These examinations may be further aided by the use of an operating microscope or rigid straight and angled (30° and 70°) endoscopes (Hopkins' rods) (***Figure 52.15***).

The advantages and disadvantages of laryngeal examination techniques are given in ***Summary box 52.3***.

Summary box 52.3

Advantages and disadvantages of larynx and pharynx examination techniques

- Flexible nasolaryngoscopy
  - Well-tolerated examination
  - Can also examine nasal passages and postnasal space
  - Need fibreoptic light source
- Rigid endoscopy
  - Can be used with stroboscope for evaluation of voice
  - High-definition view
  - Needs fibreoptic light source
  - Bulky and difficult if prominent gag reflex present
- Laryngeal mirror
  - Does not need fibreoptic light source
  - No record of examination
  - Low-resolution image
  - Difficult if prominent gag reflex present

Michael Anthony Epstein, b. 1921, formerly Professor of Pathology, University of Bristol, Bristol, UK.
Yvonne Barr, 1931–2016, virologist who emigrated to Australia. Epstein and Barr discovered this virus in 1964.

DISEASES OF THE PHARYNX

NASOPHARYNX

Enlarged adenoid

The most common cause of an enlarged adenoid (there is only one nasopharyngeal adenoid, despite the common use of the term 'adenoids') is physiological hypertrophy in childhood. The size of the adenoid alone is not an indication for removal. Of more importance is the consequence of hypertrophy (e.g. nasal obstruction). Adenoid hypertrophy (***Figure 52.16***) is often associated with hypertrophy of the other lymphoid tissues of Waldeyer's ring. Of particular note, if excessive adenoidal hypertrophy causes blockage of the nasopharynx in association with tonsil hypertrophy, the upper airway may become compromised during sleep causing, obstructive sleep apnoea (OSA).

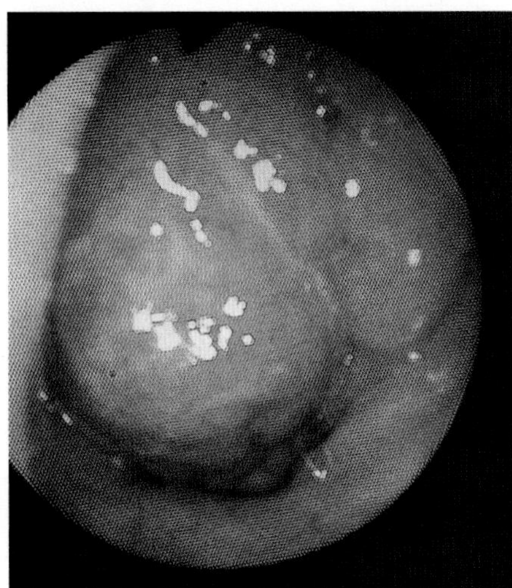

Figure 52.16 Adenoid hypertrophy.

Obstructive sleep apnoea

This condition is becoming increasingly diagnosed in children and is important because it can cause sleep deprivation and secondary cardiac complications. It has been implicated in some cases of sudden infant death syndrome. The most common symptom is snoring, which is typically irregular, with the child ceasing respiration (apnoea) and then restarting with a loud inspiratory snort. The child is often restless and may take up strange sleep positions as he or she tries to improve the pharyngeal airway. Surgical removal of the tonsils and adenoid is curative, but it is important to avoid sedative premedications and opiate analgesics postoperatively because they may further depress the child's respiratory drive.

OSA may also occur in adults, where the obstruction may result from nasal deformity, a hypertrophic soft palate associated with an altered nasopharyngeal isthmus, obesity and general narrowing of the pharyngeal airway, or supraglottic laryngeal pathology. The initial investigation may include a sleep study, during which measurements of the patient's sleep pattern and arterial oxygenation are undertaken. Continuous positive airway pressure devices may ameliorate OSA by splinting the obstruction open. Surgery may also be indicated, depending on the level(s) of the obstruction.

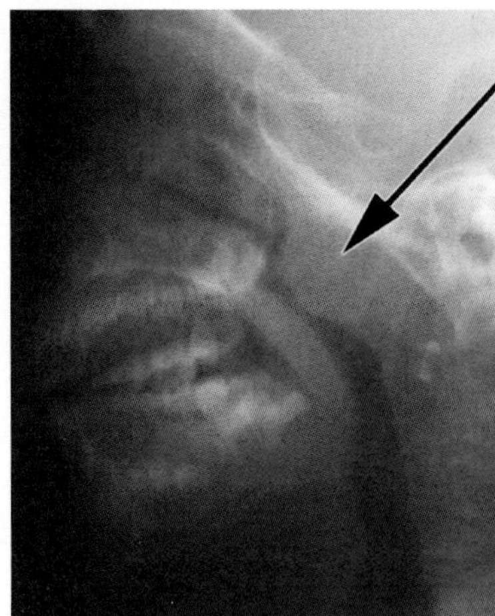

Figure 52.17 Plain lateral radiograph showing a large pad of adenoid tissue (arrow) in the postnasal space.

Hypertrophy of adenoid tissue most commonly occurs between the ages of 4 and 10, but the adenoid tissue usually undergoes spontaneous atrophy during puberty, although some remnants may persist into adult life (***Figure 52.17***). The relationship of adenoid enlargement to recurrent secretory otitis media or recurrent acute otitis media is not entirely clear.

Adenoidectomy

Adenoid tissue can be removed alone or in conjunction with a tonsillectomy. The indications for adenoidectomy are:

- OSA associated with postnasal obstruction;
- recurrent acute otitis media or prolonged serous otitis media, usually longer than 3 months' duration;
- recurrent rhinosinusitis*;
- postnasal discharge*.

*Relative indications

Operative technique

With the patient placed in a supine position with the neck in a neutral position, the adenoid tissue is removed with a guarded curette pressed against the roof of the nasopharynx before sweeping downwards to deliver the excised adenoid into the oropharynx (***Figures 52.18 and 52.19***). A postnasal swab is placed into the nasopharynx until all haemorrhage has ceased. A mirror can be used to guide the direction of the adenoid curette. Alternatively, suction monopolar diathermy or a coblator may be used to remove adenoid tissue.

Reactionary or secondary haemorrhage during the recovery period may require a nasopharyngeal pack under a further anaesthetic. This can occasionally cause respiratory depression in children and adults, and strict observation is required while the pack is in place.

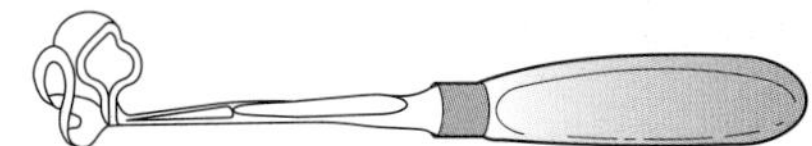

Figure 52.18 St Clair Thomson adenoid curette.

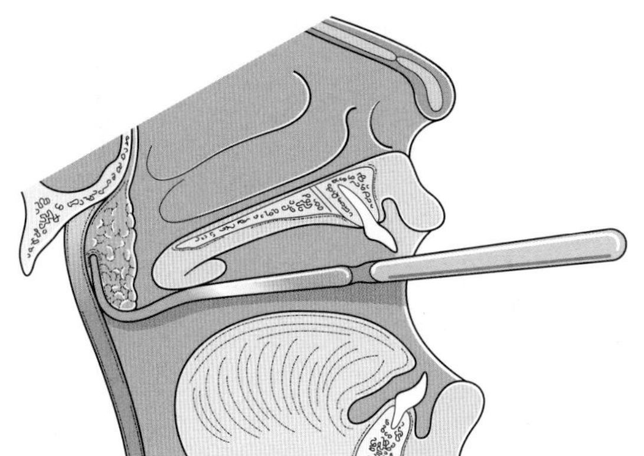

Figure 52.19 Curettage of the adenoid.

Tumours of the nasopharynx

Benign

There are two main types of benign tumours of the nasopharynx: the angiofibroma and the antrochoanal polyp. Both are rare.

Angiofibroma

This tumour is confined to young male patients most commonly between the ages of 8 and 20 years. It usually causes progressive nasal obstruction, recurrent severe epistaxis, purulent rhinorrhoea and occasionally loss of vision because of compression of the optic nerve by superior extension of the tumour through the skull base. Although the tumour is rare, these symptoms in a young male patient should always arouse suspicion. The tumour is more common in northern India, although the reasons for this are unknown. Clinical examination typically shows a mass in the nasal cavity or nasopharynx, but CT scanning best demonstrates the extent of the tumour and any associated bony erosion. MRI scanning defines the soft-tissue extent and, with these two modalities, combined with the history and clinical examination, a diagnosis can safely be arrived at. Angiography and embolisation are usually performed 24–48 hours prior to surgery to minimise intra-operative bleeding. Biopsy should be avoided unless clinical and radiological examinations are not diagnostic because of the risk of bleeding.

Surgical resection requires adequate exposure through either a midfacial degloving approach or lateral rhinotomy (***Figures 52.20 and 52.21***). Both allow ligation of the feeding maxillary artery. More recently, endoscopic resection has been used for smaller lesions.

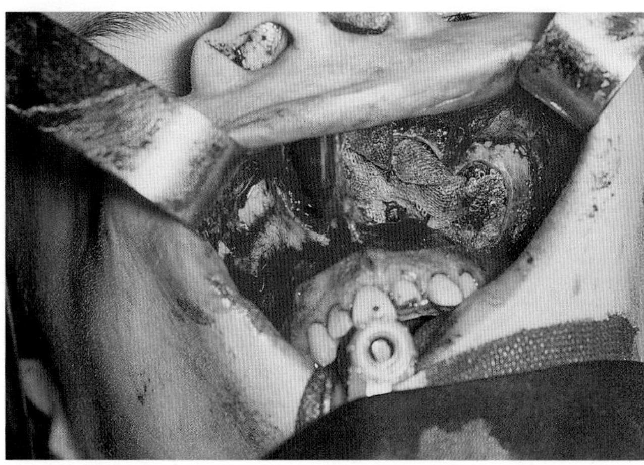

Figure 52.20 Intraoperative photograph showing exposure during a midfacial degloving approach.

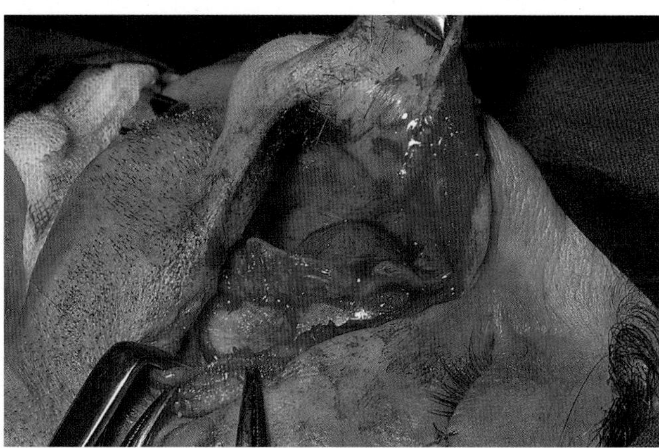

Figure 52.21 Intraoperative photograph showing an incision in lateral rhinotomy.

Antrochoanal polyp

This relatively uncommon lesion is a benign mucosal polyp that arises in the maxillary antrum and prolapses into the nasal cavity, where it expands backwards into the nasopharynx and occasionally into the oropharynx (***Figures 52.22 and 52.23***). It may mimic an angiofibroma, from which it is distinguished by its avascularity and pale colour, as well as its site of origin, which is determined on endoscopic examination and imaging. It requires complete removal via an endoscopic approach through the middle meatus of the maxillary sinus or, rarely, via an open Caldwell–Luc approach.

Malignant

Nasopharyngeal carcinoma

Nasopharyngeal carcinoma has a marked geographically variable incidence. There is classically a tumour involving the nasopharynx that may extend into the nasal cavity, oral

Sir St Clair Thomson, 1859–1943, British surgeon and professor of laryngology.

George Walter Caldwell, 1834–1918, otolaryngologist, who practised successively in New York, San Francisco and Los Angeles, USA, devised this operation for treating suppuration in the maxillary antrum in 1893.

Henri Luc, 1855–1925, otolaryngologist, Paris, France, described his operation in 1889.

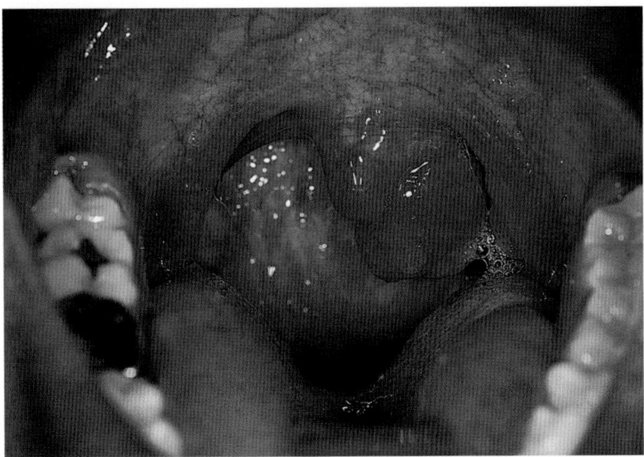

Figure 52.22 Intraoral view showing a fleshy polyp hanging in the oropharynx.

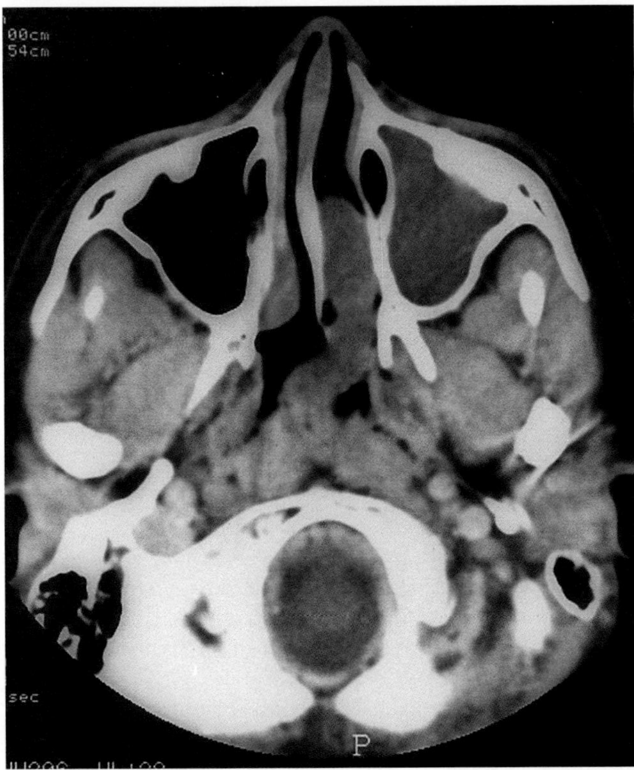

Figure 52.23 Axial computed tomogram of an antrochoanal polyp (as seen in *Figure 52.22*), with an opaque maxillary antrum and a mass in the nasal cavity and nasopharynx.

cavity, parapharyngeal space, bones and sinuses or brain. It has a male-to-female ratio of 3:1. In most parts of the world, it is rare with an annual incidence of 1 case per 100 000 population; however, among southern Chinese populations the rate is 30–50 cases per 100 000 population. The aetiology of nasopharyngeal carcinoma is multifactorial. Genetic susceptibility, tobacco smoking, early infection by EBV and consumption of traditional diets, particularly salted fish, are known to contribute.

Summary box 52.4

Aetiological factors in nasopharyngeal carcinoma

- Genetic (e.g. Cantonese population)
- Infective (e.g. EBV)
- Environmental (e.g. salted fish)
- Tobacco smoking

The majority of nasopharyngeal tumours are undifferentiated with a characteristic morphology, constituting over 90% of nasopharyngeal malignancy in endemic areas. Rare epithelial tumours are adenocarcinoma and adenoid cystic carcinoma, which arise from minor salivary glands. B- and T-cell lymphomas also occur in the nasopharynx and should not be confused with the more common undifferentiated carcinoma. Nasopharyngeal carcinoma has a bimodal distribution with an increased incidence in teenagers and young adults and then again in the 50- to 60-year-old age group.

Clinical features. Symptoms are closely related to the position of the tumour in the nasopharynx and the degree of regional and/or distant spread. Early symptoms are often minimal and may be ignored by both patient and doctor. Approximately 50% of patients will present with a malignant node or nodes in the neck, indicating an advanced tumour. While investigation of the lymph node will involve fine-needle aspiration or a biopsy, such a clinical presentation mandates an immediate thorough examination of the nasopharynx. In about 5% of patients, the nasopharynx may look normal or minimally asymmetrical but contains submucosal nasopharyngeal carcinoma. MRI or CT of the head and neck should be performed as part of the diagnostic work-up; even if a nasopharyngeal mass is not identified clinically or radiologically, a biopsy of the nasopharynx, targeting the fossa of Rosenmüller, will reveal the site of the primary tumour in patients with a malignant neck lump that shows EBV positivity. In contrast, nasal complaints (obstruction with/without rhinorrhoea) occur in one-third of patients and aural symptoms of unilateral deafness as a consequence of Eustachian tube obstruction and secretory otitis media occur in approximately 20% of patients. Neurological complications with cranial nerve palsies as a result of disease in the skull base occur relatively late in the disease, but are a poor prognostic sign, as is trismus resulting from tumour involvement of the pterygoid musculature.

Summary box 52.5

Nasopharyngeal carcinoma: main presenting complaints

- Regional
  - Cervical lymphadenopathy
- Local
  - Hearing loss (unilateral serous otitis media), otalgia
  - Nasal obstruction, bloody discharge, epistaxis
  - Cranial nerve palsies, especially III–VI then IX–XII
  - Trismus

Investigation. This is by direct inspection with a flexible or rigid nasendoscope and biopsy under topical or general anaesthesia. Serological investigation for EBV-associated antigenic markers in combination with the clinical and histological examination is valuable for the early detection of disease. Highly sensitive assays for antiviral antibodies together with virus-associated serological markers are useful in early detection and in post-treatment surveillance. Immunoglobulin (Ig) A antiviral capsid antigen antibody and early antigen antibody have been evaluated in mass surveys in southern China and have been found to be an excellent screening method for early detection of nasopharyngeal carcinoma in high-risk groups.

Imaging. This is essential for staging and to determine the extent of disease. The imaging of choice is MRI, which allows for assessment of brain parenchyma, cavernous sinus and the closely associated cranial foramina and for treatment planning. CT or PET-CT of the head, neck and chest has a major role in planning radiotherapy and assessing the response to treatment, diagnosing recurrence and detecting complications.

Treatment. The primary treatment of nasopharyngeal carcinoma is non-surgical as it is highly radiosensitive and depends on the stage of the disease. Intensity-modulated radiotherapy is the treatment of choice for early stages I and II and cisplatin-based chemotherapy with concurrent radiation therapy for stages III and IV. Surgery is reserved for local recurrence that would require a nasopharyngectomy, which can be performed either transorally with a robot, transnasally with a rigid telescope or via an open approach; regional recurrence in the neck is managed by a neck dissection. Given the complexity of the anatomy and proximity of vital neurovascular structures, ongoing trials with proton beam therapy at selected centres around the world have demonstrated promising results with lesser adverse effects. For early disease, 5-year disease-free survival rates of more than 75% are common; however, in advanced disease the results are less good, with 5-year disease-free survival rates of 30–50%.

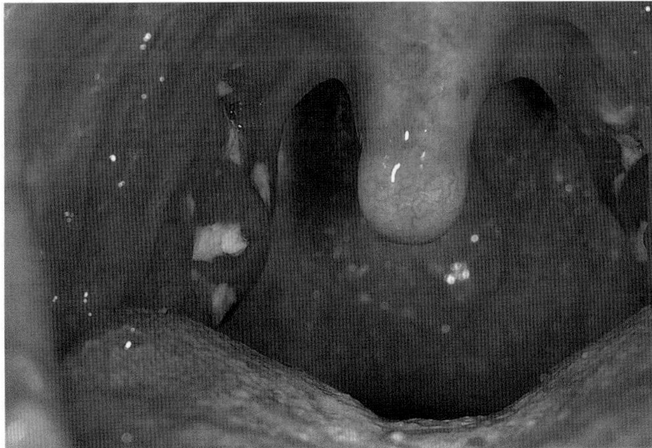

Figure 52.24 Acute follicular tonsillitis.

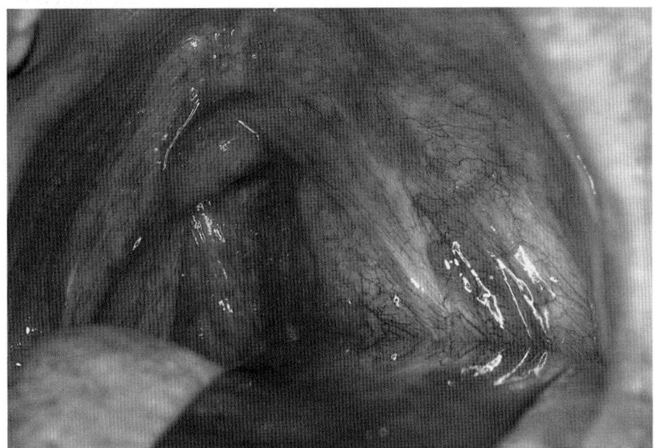

Figure 52.25 Quinsy (peritonsillar abscess).

OROPHARYNX

Acute tonsillitis

This common condition is characterised by a sore throat, fever, general malaise, dysphagia, enlarged upper cervical nodes and sometimes referred otalgia. Approximately half the cases are bacterial, the most common cause being a pyogenic group A *Streptococcus*. The remainder are viral and a wide variety of viruses have been implicated, in particular infectious mononucleosis (glandular fever), which may be mistaken for bacterial tonsillitis.

On examination, the tonsils are swollen and erythematous, and yellow or white pustules may be seen on the palatine tonsils, hence the name 'follicular tonsillitis' (***Figure 52.24***). A throat swab should be taken at the time of examination as well as blood for EBV testing to confirm or refute the diagnosis of glandular fever.

Treatment

Paracetamol and/or other analgesia may be administered to relieve pain and saline gargles are soothing. The condition is frequently sensitive to benzyl- or phenoxymethylpenicillin (penicillin V) and these are given until antibiotic sensitivities are established. Ampicillin is avoided as it may precipitate a rash in patients with infectious mononucleosis. Most cases resolve in a few days.

Quinsy

This is an abscess in the peritonsillar region that causes severe pain and trismus (***Figure 52.25***). The trismus, which is caused by spasm induced in the pterygoid muscles, may make examination difficult but may be overcome by instillation of local anaesthesia into the posterior nasal cavity (anaesthetising the sphenopalatine ganglion) and the oropharynx. Inspection reveals a diffuse swelling of the soft palate just superior or lateral to the involved tonsil, displacing the uvula medially. In more advanced cases, pus may be seen pointing underneath the thin mucosa.

Treatment

In the early stages, intravenous broad-spectrum antibiotics may produce resolution. However, if there is frank abscess

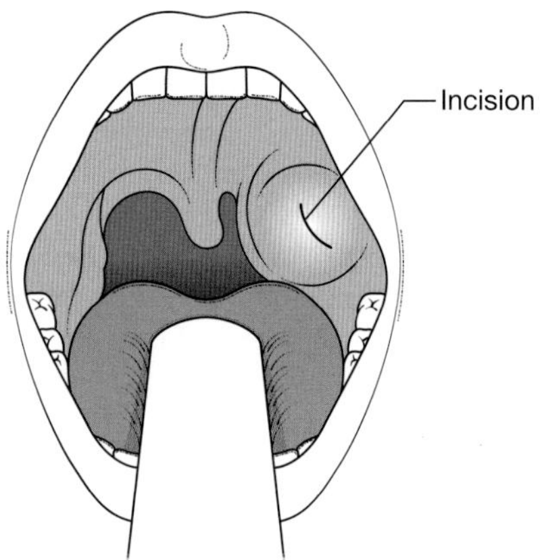

Figure 52.26 Site of incision in a peritonsillar abscess.

TABLE 52.1 Indications for tonsillectomy.	
Absolute	• Sleep apnoea, chronic respiratory tract obstruction, cor pulmonale • Suspected tonsillar malignancy
Relative	• Documented recurrent acute tonsillitis • Chronic tonsillitis • Peritonsillar abscess (quinsy) • Tonsillar asymmetry • Tonsillitis resulting in febrile convulsions • Diphtheria carriers • Systemic disease caused by β-haemolytic *Streptococcus* (nephritis, rheumatic fever)

formation, incision and drainage of the pus can be carried out under local anaesthesia. A small scalpel is best modified by winding a strip of adhesive tape around the blade so that only 1 cm of the blade projects. In teenagers and young adults, the patient sits upright and an incision is made approximately midway between the base of the uvula and the third upper molar tooth (***Figure** 52.26*). This may produce immediate release of pus, but, if not, a dressing forceps is pushed firmly through the incision and, on opening, pus may then be encountered. Needle aspiration of the pus, with or without ultrasound guidance, is an alternative treatment. In small children, general anaesthesia is required.

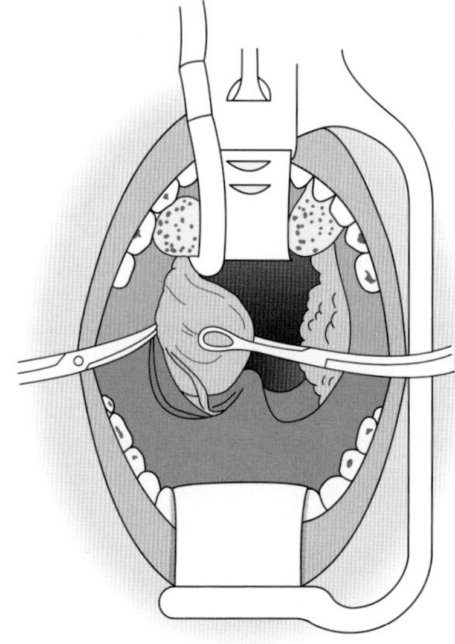

Figure 52.27 Removal of the tonsils.

Chronic tonsillitis

Chronic tonsillitis usually results from repeated attacks of acute tonsillitis in which the tonsils become progressively damaged by inflammatory processes and provide a reservoir for infective organisms.

Tonsillectomy

The indications for a tonsillectomy are either diagnostic, therapeutic or for surgical access. Recurrent acute tonsillitis is the most common relative indication for tonsillectomy in children and adolescents, although it is important that these attacks are well documented, frequent and do not simply constitute a minor viral sore throat. Chronic tonsillitis more frequently affects young adults, in whom it is important to establish that chronic mouth breathing secondary to nasal obstruction is not the main problem rather than the tonsils themselves. Tonsillectomies are occasionally performed as a means to gain surgical access to the parapharyngeal space laterally in the oropharynx or to access an elongated styloid process. Absolute indications for tonsillectomy are when the size of the tonsils is contributing to airway obstruction or a malignancy of the tonsils is suspected (***Table** 52.1*).

Ideally, the procedure should be undertaken when the tonsils are not acutely infected, and it is important to discuss factors that may increase the tendency to bleed. Blood transfusion is rarely required, but it is normal practice to type and screen blood for cross-match in children under 15 kg in weight.

Dissection tonsillectomy is carried out under general anaesthesia. The mucosa of the anterior faucial pillar is incised and the tonsil capsule identified. Using blunt dissection, the tonsil is separated from its bed until only a small inferior pedicle is left (***Figure** 52.27*). It is then separated from the lingual tonsil. A tonsil swab is placed in the tonsillar bed and pressure applied for some minutes, following which bleeding points may be controlled by ligature or by bipolar diathermy. (Coblation and laser dissection is commonly used in the resource-rich world in an attempt to reduce postoperative pain and bleeding.)

Following surgery, the patient is kept under close observation for any systemic or local evidence of bleeding, with regular pulse and blood pressure measurements and observation to monitor whether the patient is swallowing excessively (***Figure** 52.28*). Postoperatively, patients are encouraged to eat normally and take regular oral analgesics. Patients are allowed home on the same or following day and are warned that they may experience otalgia as a result of referred pain from the glossopharyngeal nerve and that secondary haemorrhage may occur up to 10 days following the surgery.

Haemorrhage is the most common complication in the immediate postoperative period. Local pressure may help in mild cases, but reactionary haemorrhage usually requires return to theatre for definitive treatment, particularly in

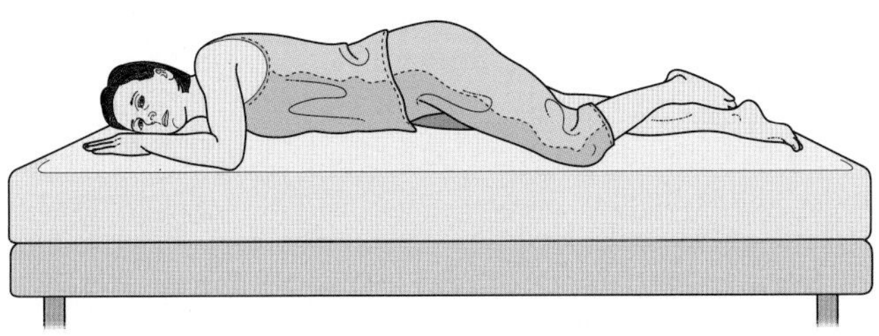

Figure 52.28 Positioning of the patient after tonsillectomy.

younger patients. Under general anaesthesia, it may be possible to identify a bleeding spot, but often a more generalised ooze is observed and suturing of the tonsil bed combined with the application of haemostatic gauze and bipolar diathermy is often more successful than attempted placement of ligatures.

Late haemorrhage is sometimes secondary to infection and patients are usually started on broad-spectrum intravenous antibiotics. Any residual clot in the tonsil fossa should be removed and regular gargling with a dilute solution of hydrogen peroxide may be beneficial. Significant or persistent bleeding may require a further general anaesthetic and haemostasis, which may require diathermy and/or undersewing of the granulating, sloughy tonsil fossa. Postoperative tonsillar haemorrhage is still a serious and life-threatening complication and should not be underestimated, particularly in the younger patient.

Summary box 52.6

Complications of tonsillectomy

- Haemorrhage (immediate or late)
- Infection
- Pain/otalgia
- Postoperative airway obstruction
- Velopharyngeal insufficiency
- Injury to oral cavity and oropharyngeal structures

Parapharyngeal abscess

Parapharyngeal abscess may be confused with a peritonsillar abscess, but the maximal swelling is behind the posterior faucial pillar and there may be little or no oedema of the soft palate. The patient is usually a young child and there may be a severe general malaise and obvious neck swelling. A large parapharyngeal abscess may compromise both the airway and swallowing. MRI or CT scanning of the head and neck is often an invaluable aid to diagnosis and management as it allows assessment of the extent of the abscess and facilitates planning of the optimal surgical approach. In early cases, admission to hospital and the institution of fluid replacements coupled with intravenous antibiotics may produce resolution. However, when a collection is evident, transcervical drainage is required under general anaesthesia, which usually requires the expertise of a senior anaesthetist. In instances where an obvious abscess points into the oropharynx, drainage may be carried out with a blunt instrument (***Figure 52.29***).

Acute retropharyngeal abscess

This is the result of suppuration of the retropharyngeal lymph nodes and, again, is most commonly seen in children, with most cases occurring under the age of 1 year. It is associated with infection of the upper aerodigestive tract and is frequently accompanied by severe general malaise, neck rigidity, dysphagia, drooling, a croupy cough, an altered cry and marked dyspnoea.

Dyspnoea may be the prominent symptom and may also be accompanied by febrile convulsions and vomiting. These children should always be carefully examined by the most senior clinicians available. Inspection of the posterior wall of the pharynx may show gross swelling and an abscess pointing beneath the thinned mucosa.

In countries where diphtheria still occurs, an acute retropharyngeal abscess may be confused with this, but the presence of the greyish-green membrane aids differentiation. Occasionally, a foreign body, most commonly a fish bone that has perforated the posterior pharyngeal mucosa, will give rise to a retropharyngeal abscess in older children and young adults. Intravenous antibiotics are commenced immediately but surgical drainage of the abscess is often necessary. It requires an experienced anaesthetist because, on induction, care must be taken to avoid rupturing the abscess. The airway is protected by placing the child in a head-down position while a pair of dressing forceps, guided by the finger, may be thrust into an obvious abscess in the posterior wall and the contents evacuated. On other occasions, an approach anterior and medial to the carotid sheath via a cervical incision may be preferable.

Chronic retropharyngeal abscess

This condition is now rare and is most commonly the result of an extension of tuberculosis (TB) of the cervical spine, which has spread through the anterior longitudinal ligament to reach the prevertebral space. In addition to the pharyngeal

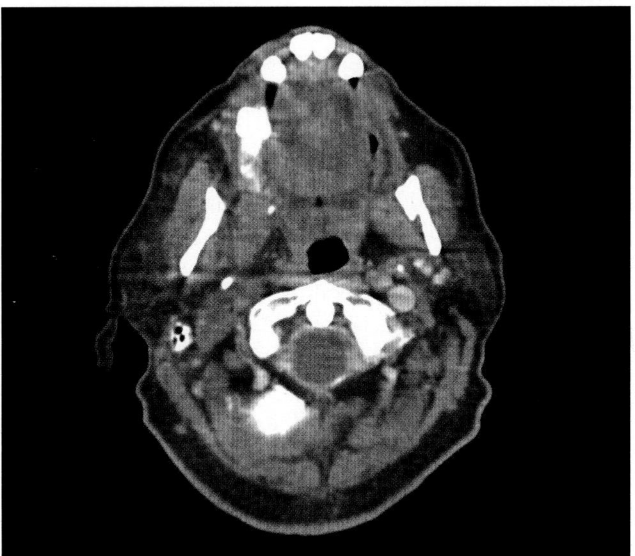

Figure 52.29 Axial computed tomography scan of the neck demonstrating right parapharyngeal abscess.

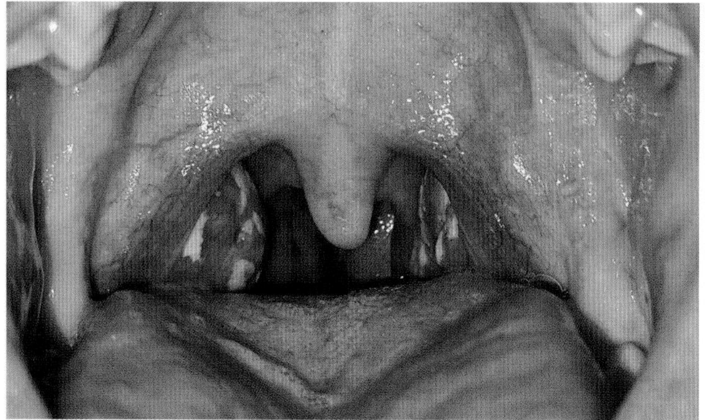

Figure 52.30 Infectious mononucleosis.

swelling seen intraorally, there may be fullness behind the sternocleidomastoid muscle on one side. In contrast to an acute retropharyngeal abscess, this condition occurs almost solely in adults. Radiology usually shows evidence of bone destruction and loss of the normal curvature of the cervical spine. The spine may be quite unstable and undue manipulation may precipitate a neurological event.

In contrast to an acute abscess, a chronic retropharyngeal abscess must not be opened into the mouth, as such a procedure may lead to secondary infection. Drainage of the abscess may not be necessary if suitable treatment of the underlying TB disease is instituted. If it is necessary, drainage should be carried out through a cervical incision anterior to the sternocleidomastoid muscle with an approach anterior and medial to the carotid sheath to enter the retropharyngeal space. The cavity is opened and suctioned dry after taking biopsy material. Occasionally, surgery is required to decompress or stabilise the spinal cord if there is a progressive neurological deficit.

Glandular fever (infectious mononucleosis)

This systemic condition is usually caused by EBV, but similar features can be caused by cytomegalovirus or toxoplasmosis. The tonsils are typically erythematous with a creamy grey exudate and appear almost confluent, usually symmetrical (***Figure 52.30***). In addition to the discomfort and dysphagia, patients may drool saliva and have respiratory difficulty, particularly on inspiration. They commonly have a high temperature and gross general malaise with marked cervical or generalised lymphadenopathy. Occasionally, an enlarged spleen or liver may be detected. The condition is most frequent in teenagers and young adults. The diagnosis can be confirmed by serological testing for EBV, which has now commonly replaced Paul–Bunnell testing, an absolute and relative lymphocytosis, and the presence of atypical monocytes in the peripheral blood.

Treatment

Analgesia and maintenance of fluid intake are important. A small number of patients require admission to hospital if the airway is compromised or if oral intake of fluids is not possible, and a short course of steroids may be helpful. Antibiotics are of little value and ampicillin is contraindicated because of the frequent appearance of a widespread skin rash. Rarely, if the airway is severely compromised, an elective tracheostomy under local anaesthesia is safer and less traumatic than an emergency intubation. Emergency tonsillectomy is contraindicated because of the generalised pharyngeal oedema and compromised airway.

Human immunodeficiency virus (HIV)

Acquired immunodeficiency syndrome (AIDS) can affect the ear, nose and throat (ENT) system at any point during the disease. The initial seroconversion may present with the symptoms of glandular fever; this is followed by an asymptomatic period of variable length. In the pre-AIDS period, before the full-blown symptoms of the AIDS-related complex, many patients have minor upper respiratory tract symptoms that are often overlooked, such as otitis externa, rhinosinusitis and a non-specific pharyngitis. As the patient moves into the full-blown AIDS-related complex, a persistent, generalised lymphadenopathy is frequently found affecting the cervical nodes, which is usually due to follicular hyperplasia. However, patients may also develop tumours such as Kaposi's sarcoma, sometimes seen in the oral cavity, and high-grade malignant B-cell lymphoma affecting the cervical lymph nodes and nasopharynx. In addition, multiple ulcers may be found in the oral cavity or pharynx associated with herpesvirus infection. Severe *Candida* may affect the oral cavity, pharynx, oesophagus or even larynx, and a hairy leukoplakia may affect the tongue (***Figure 52.31***).

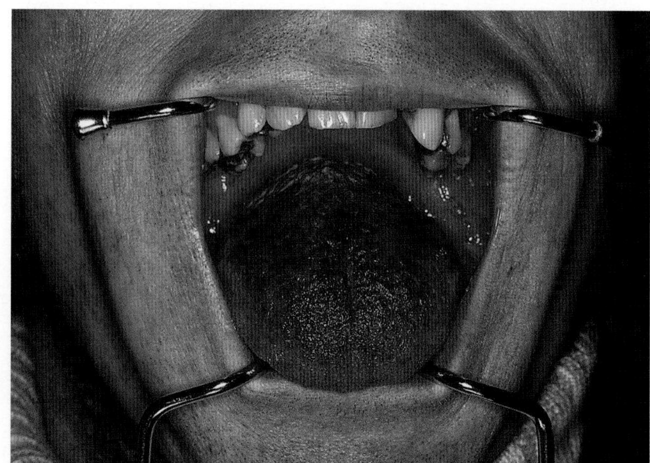

Figure 52.31 Intraoral view showing a hairy tongue in a human immunodeficiency virus-positive patient.

John Rodman Paul, 1893–1971, Professor of Preventative Medicine, Yale University, New Haven, CT, USA.
Walls Willard Bunnell, 1902–1966, American physician. Paul and Bunnell described this test in 1932.
Moritz Kaposi, 1837–1902, Professor of Dermatology, Vienna, Austria, described pigmented sarcoma of the skin in 1872.

The globus syndrome

A wide variety of patients experience the feeling of a lump in the throat (from the Latin *globus* = lump). The symptom most commonly affects adults between 30 and 60 years of age. This feeling is not true dysphagia as there is no difficulty in swallowing. Most patients notice the symptom more if they swallow their own saliva (i.e. a forced, dry swallow) rather than when they eat or drink.

The aetiology of this common symptom is unknown, but some patients may have gastro-oesophageal reflux or spasm of their cricopharyngeus muscle. Radiological and endoscopic investigation may be necessary to exclude an underlying cause and/or for patient reassurance.

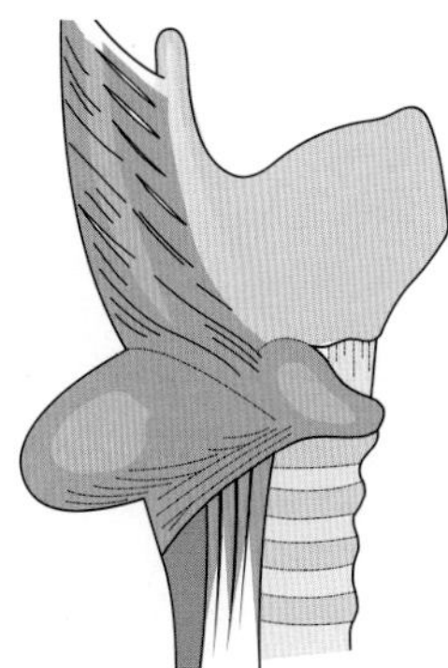

Figure 52.32 A pharyngeal pouch.

Pharyngeal pouch

A pharyngeal pouch is a protrusion of mucosa though Killian's dehiscence, a weak area of the posterior pharyngeal wall between the oblique fibres of the thyropharyngeus and the transverse fibres of cricopharyngeus at the lower end of the inferior constrictor muscle (***Figure 52.32***). These fibres, along with the circular fibres of the upper oesophagus, form the physiological upper oesophageal sphincter mechanism. Videofluoroscopic and manometric studies have been unable to elucidate the cause of the pouch. Many patients with pharyngeal pouches have been demonstrated to have normal relaxation of the upper oesophageal sphincter mechanism in relation to swallowing, but others have been shown to have incomplete pharyngeal relaxation, early cricopharyngeal contraction and abnormalities of the pharyngeal contraction wave. When enlarged, the pouch almost invariably deviates to the left side of the neck.

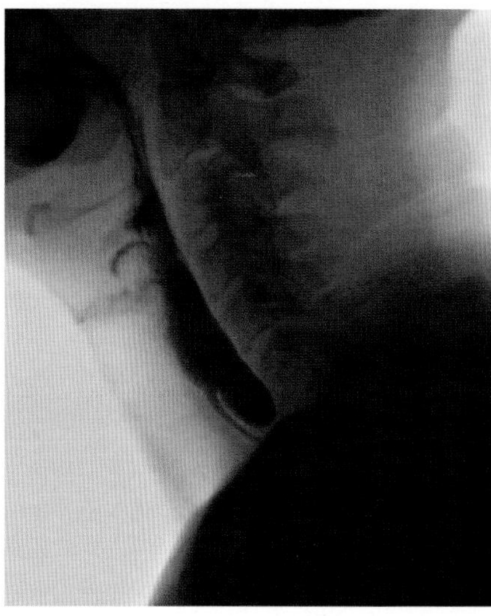

Figure 52.33 Pharyngeal pouch on barium swallow.

Clinical features

Patients with this condition are commonly more than 60 years of age and it is more common in men than in women. As the diverticulum enlarges, patients may experience regurgitation of undigested food, sometimes hours after a meal, particularly if they are bending down or turning over in bed at night. They sometimes wake at night with a feeling of tightness in the throat and a fit of coughing. Occasionally, they may present with recurrent, unexplained chest infections as a result of aspiration of the contents of the pouch. As the pouch increases in size, patients may notice gurgling noises from the neck on swallowing and the pouch may become large enough to form a visible swelling in the neck. Dysphagia may also be a presenting symptom.

Radiological examination

A thin emulsion of barium is given to the patient as a barium swallow (***Figure 52.33***) or ideally as part of a videofluoroscopic swallowing study. Care should be exercised in patients who cough on swallowing, indicating they may have aspiration. A small volume of barium is sufficient to outline the pharynx, pouch and upper oesophagus. The videofluoroscopic study gives additional information about the pharyngeal contraction waves and the performance of the upper oesophageal sphincter.

Treatment

Surgery is indicated when the pouch is associated with progressive symptoms and particularly when a prominent cricopharyngeal bar of muscle is associated with abnormality of the upper oesophageal sphincter mechanism and causes considerable dysphagia. In elderly patients, a decision to operate may be influenced by their general condition. However, surgical intervention is mandated in all but the most poorly patients as, in most cases, it is the pouch that is contributing significantly to the underlying debilitation. Of particular importance is the risk of recurrent pneumonia from aspiration and overspill of pouch contents, as well as increasing dysphagia as the pouch opening becomes larger than the oesophageal opening and the enlarged pouch exerts extramural pressure on the oesophagus. Accordingly, preoperative chest physiotherapy and attention to the respiratory, cardiovascular and nutritional aspects of the patient are important.

Gustav Killian, 1860–1921, Professor of Laryngology at Freiburg, and later at Berlin, Germany.

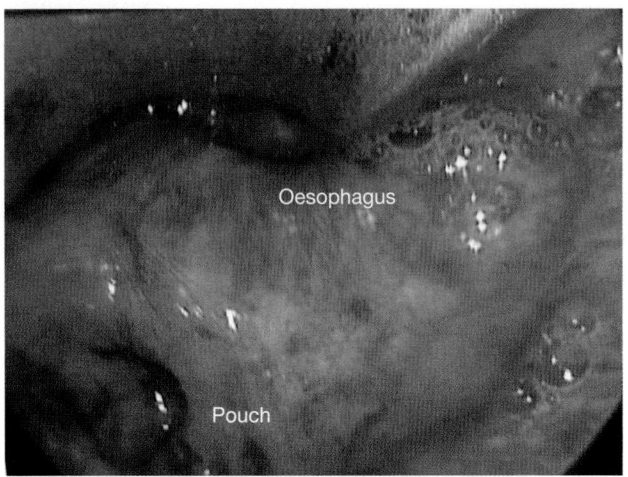

Figure 52.34 Endoscopic view of a pharyngeal pouch.

The surgical technique typically used is endoscopic stapling of the diverticular wall. A double-bladed rigid endoscope (diverticuloscope) is passed, with one blade in the diverticulum and one blade positioned in the oesophagus (***Figure 52.34***). Opening of the bivalve scope reveals the pathognomonic 'bar' formed by the cricopharyngeus muscle and overlying mucosa, which forms the boundary between the posterior wall of the oesophagus and the anterior wall of the pouch. At this stage the pouch should be emptied of food content and the mucosa should be inspected for the rare occurrence of carcinoma in the pouch. An endoscopic linear stapler is then introduced to sit astride the 'bar'. One jaw of the stapler is placed in the oesophagus, the other in the pouch. The stapler is fired, dividing the wall separating the two. The process should be repeated until the bottom of the pouch is reached. This has the effect of opening the pouch, incorporating it as part of the oesophageal wall and dividing the cricopharyngeus muscle. If the patient is symptom free after the procedure, they may start graded oral intake and be discharged early. Division of the 'bar' using a carbon dioxide laser, as an alternative to stapling, is gaining popularity in some centres. Flexible endoscopic division of the cricopharyngeal bar is a new technique popularised over the last decade, with equally good results, and can be used in patients who have poor access with rigid endoscopes.

In instances where endoscopic access is difficult or for very large pouches, an open excision of the pouch becomes necessary. In the classic external operation, the opening to the pouch is first identified using a pharyngoscope and a nasogastric tube placed into the oesophageal lumen for postoperative nutrition. This initial endoscopy is often difficult because the normal oesophageal opening is small compared with the lumen of the pouch, but it may be better visualised using a Dohlman's rigid endoscope. The pouch may be packed with ribbon gauze to further aid identification of its neck.

A lower neck incision along the anterior border of the left sternocleidomastoid muscle, or a transverse crease incision, is used and the muscle and carotid sheath are retracted laterally and the trachea and larynx medially. The pouch is found medially behind the lower pharynx and is carefully isolated and dissected back to its origin at Killian's dehiscence. It is then excised and the pharynx closed in two layers or, if it is small, the pouch may be invaginated into the pharyngeal lumen before closing the muscle layers. Care must be taken to protect the recurrent laryngeal nerve during the procedure. In all cases, a myotomy dividing the fibres of the cricopharyngeus muscle and the upper oesophageal circular muscle fibres must be performed. The wound is usually closed with drainage and the patient fed through a nasogastric tube for 3–7 days. A water-based swallow test is performed on day 5 to ascertain that there is no leak prior to commencing oral feeds.

The average operating time with an endoscopic procedure is 20–30 minutes compared with 60–90 minutes with an external procedure. Inpatient stay is also decreased for patients undergoing an endoscopic procedure. The endoscopic technique is associated with a high symptomatic success rate and a low morbidity, which is particularly important in the elderly.

Complications

The classic operation has been associated with wound infection, mediastinitis, pharyngeal fistula formation, recurrent laryngeal nerve palsy and stenosis of the upper oesophagus. Endoscopic division is associated with the same risks but at much lower rates. The recurrence rates between the two procedures appears to be equal; longer term follow-up will establish this. Endoscopic stapling will also allow for safe reoperation if necessary. It must be noted that contrast swallows will demonstrate the pouch in patients who have undergone stapling and are an inappropriate modality to evaluate recurrences.

Sideropenic dysphagia

Prolonged iron deficiency anaemia may lead to dysphagia, particularly in middle-aged women. In addition, they may have koilonychia, cheilosis and angular stomatitis together with lassitude and poor exercise tolerance. The dysphagia is caused by a postcricoid or upper oesophageal web and these patients have a higher incidence of postcricoid malignancy. The syndrome is associated with the names of Plummer and Vinson, Paterson and Brown Kelly.

Tumours of the oropharynx

Benign

Benign tumours of the oropharynx are rare, papillomas being the most common. These are usually incidental findings and are rarely of any importance.

Gösta Dohlman, 1890–1983, Swedish physician and professor.
Henry Stanley Plummer, 1874–1937, physician, The Mayo Clinic, Rochester, MN, USA, described this syndrome in 1912.
Porter Paisley Vinson, 1890–1959, physician, The Mayo Clinic, Rochester, MN, who later practised in Richmond, VA, USA.
Donald Rose Paterson, 1863–1939, surgeon, The Ear, Nose and Throat Department, The Royal Infirmary, Cardiff, UK.
Adam Brown Kelly, 1865–1941, surgeon, The Ear, Nose and Throat Department, The Royal Victoria Infirmary, Glasgow, UK. Vinson, Paterson and Kelly all described this syndrome independently in 1919.

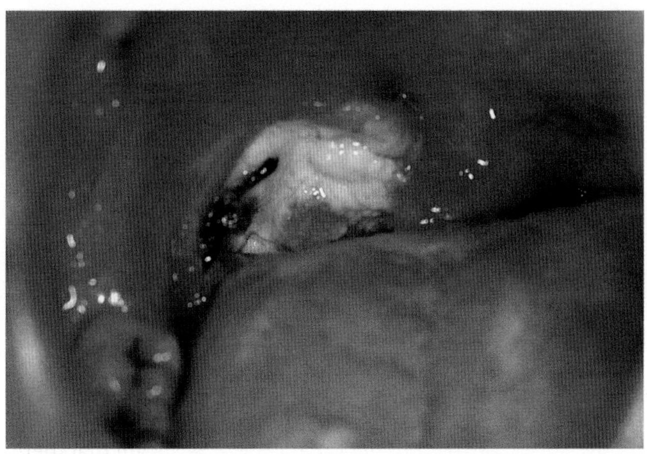

Figure 52.35 Squamous cell carcinoma of the right tonsil.

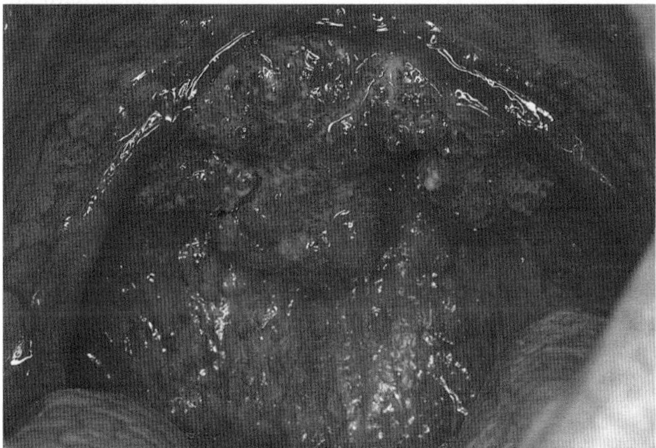

Figure 52.36 Squamous cell carcinoma of the soft palate.

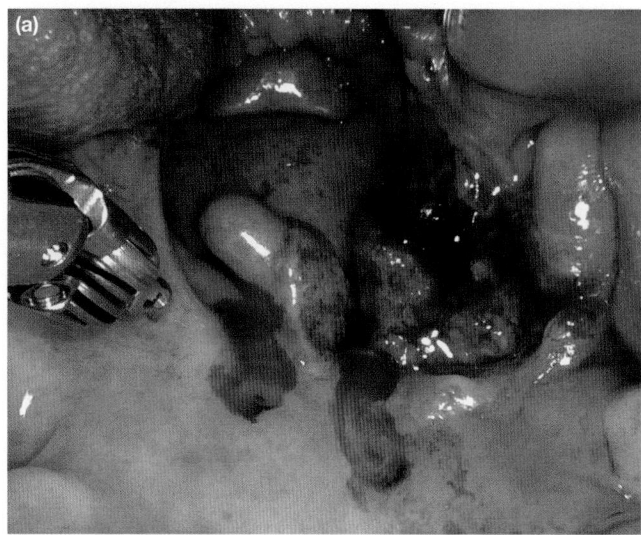

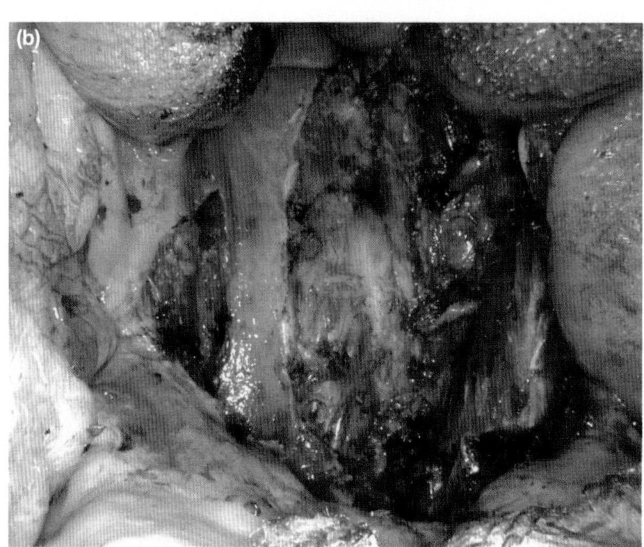

Figure 52.37 (a) Recurrent cancer of the soft palate and tonsil set up for transoral robotic resection. (b) Completed resection of the cancer. Note prevertebral fascia that is now continuous with the parapharyngeal fat.

Malignant

The most important epithelial tumour is squamous cell carcinoma, which constitutes approximately 90% of all epithelial tumours in the upper aerodigestive tract (***Figures 52.35 and 52.36***). In the oropharynx, the proportion is less (70%) because of the higher incidence of lymphoma (25%) and salivary gland tumours (5%). Because of the rich lymphatic drainage of the oropharynx, cervical node metastases are common. They may be the only presenting feature with a primary pharyngeal tumour often being unsuspected and missed in the tonsil or tongue base.

Aetiology

While it has been long established that oropharyngeal squamous cell carcinoma (OPSCC) is strongly associated with cigarette smoking and consumption of alcohol, over recent decades there has been a near epidemic increase in HPV-associated OPSCC (HPV+OPSCC) in the resource-rich world, with prevalences of up to 70% being commonly reported in the USA, UK and northern Europe. That HPV+OPSCC constitutes a separate disease entity is undoubted, as these patients are typically younger with less or no history of alcohol and tobacco use. The presenting features of HPV+OPSCC include multiple large cystic cervical lymph nodes with a small primary; these are usually associated with better outcomes after treatment.

Treatment

Treatment varies with facilities around the world, but early-stage tumours may be cured by transoral laser surgery, transoral robotic surgery or radiotherapy. Intermediate- or late-stage disease is usually managed with concurrent chemoradiotherapy or based on institutional choices, with open surgery and reconstruction using myocutaneous pedicles or free flaps. Recurrent disease following radiotherapy with/without chemotherapy is a surgical challenge; smaller tumours can be treated by transoral robotic surgery (***Figure 52.37***), but larger recurrences require open surgery and reconstruction. Neck dissection is required in most cases where surgery is the primary treatment modality and is also required for patients who have only partially responded following chemoradiotherapy. Postoperative dysphagia with aspiration as a result of interference in the complex neuromuscular control of the second phase of swallowing is a particular problem in these patients. The advent of HPV+OPSCC has created a clinical need to define novel de-intensified treatments that maintain current advantageous survival rates while reducing the late morbidity of treatment. Management of such tumours should be multidisciplinary and is best carried out at tertiary centres undertaking this work on a regular basis.

Lymphoma of the head and neck

Lymphomas of the head and neck may arise in nodal or extranodal sites and both Hodgkin's disease and non-Hodgkin's lymphoma commonly present as lymph node enlargement in the neck. Hodgkin's disease is rare in the oropharynx, but non-Hodgkin's lymphoma accounts for 15–20% of tumours at this site in some countries. Most are of the B-cell type and have features in common with other MALT tumours. Further evaluation with CT scanning of the thorax and abdomen and bone marrow evaluation are essential. Core biopsy, or, often, excision biopsy to improve tissue yield, is frequently required to establish a firm diagnosis and aid in the classification of lymphomas.

Radiotherapy is the treatment of choice for localised non-Hodgkin's lymphoma; for widespread non-Hodgkin's lymphoma, systemic treatment is needed.

HYPOPHARYNX

Tumours of the hypopharynx

Benign

Benign tumours of the hypopharynx are very rare, the most common being the fibroma and the leiomyoma. They show a smooth, submucosal mass lying in the lumen of the hypopharynx or oesophagus.

Malignant

Malignant tumours of the hypopharynx are almost exclusively squamous cell carcinomas and typically behave aggressively. The tumours are usually classified according to their probable anatomical site of origin from the piriform fossa, postcricoid region or posterior pharyngeal wall. Marked differences in the incidence of these tumours occur globally because of factors such as iron deficiency anaemia (see ***Sideropenic dysphagia***). They may be associated with marked submucosal spread, which further complicates evaluation. Tumours arising from the piriform fossa and posterior pharyngeal wall may spread to upper or lower cervical nodes. Tumours arising in the postcricoid area typically metastasise to paratracheal and paraoesophageal nodes, which may not be palpable. As with other non-HPV head and neck cancers, alcohol and tobacco are two principal carcinogens. Postcricoid carcinoma, though rare, is more common in women than in men.

The diagnosis of hypopharyngeal carcinoma should be considered in all patients presenting with dysphagia, hoarseness or referred otalgia, particularly if they have a history of smoking or significant alcohol consumption.

Fibreoptic endoscopic examination in the clinic may show only subtle signs such as oedema or pooling of saliva unilaterally in the piriform fossa. Note should also be made that this region is not well seen on flexible gastroscopy. The preferred investigation is with direct rigid pharyngoscopy and oesophagoscopy with biopsy under a general anaesthetic. All regions of the neck must be assessed in a systematic manner. Fine-needle aspiration is advocated for suspicious nodes.

Radiological examination

As for other head and neck cancers, a suspected primary tumour requires an MRI or CT scan of the neck together with a CT scan of the thorax and upper abdomen.

Treatment

Squamous cell carcinoma of the hypopharynx commonly presents late and carries a poor prognosis. Early lesions may be treated with radiotherapy or transoral robotic or transoral laser microsurgical resection and a neck dissection plus postoperative radiotherapy. Non-surgical strategies, designed to preserve function, rely on chemoradiotherapy. Major open excisional surgery is generally used for recurrence after radiotherapy or as primary excision in advanced disease. Total laryngectomy and either partial or total pharyngectomy followed by pharyngeal reconstruction involving myocutaneous or free flap reconstruction (e.g. jejunum or anterolateral thigh) or gastric transposition is commonly required (***Figure 52.38***). Swallowing and voice

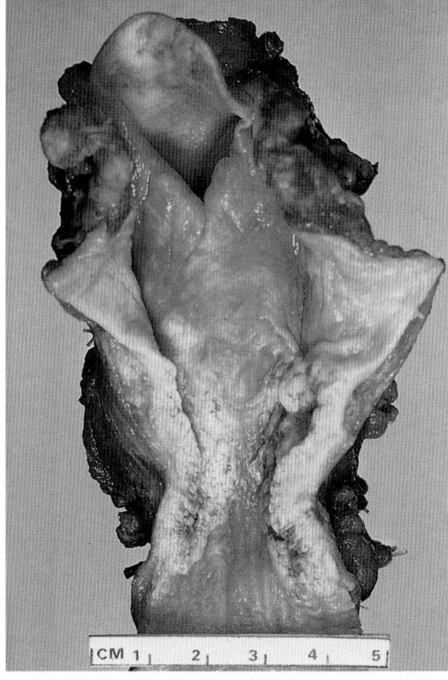

Figure 52.38 Total pharyngolaryngectomy specimen showing hypopharyngeal carcinoma (hypopharynx opened from the posterior aspect of the resection).

Thomas Hodgkin, 1798–1866, Curator of the Museum and Demonstrator of Morbid Anatomy, Guy's Hospital, London, UK, described lymphadenoma in 1832.

rehabilitation are necessary to support patients after this major surgery if they are to adjust and maintain some quality of life.

Summary box 52.7

Tumours of the hypopharynx

- Variable symptoms – discomfort, pain, dysphagia, hoarseness
- Incidence increased by history of smoking and alcohol
- Expert examination with nasendoscopy
- Late presentation
- Referral to multidisciplinary team for detailed assessment and treatment – radiotherapy with/without chemotherapy, transoral or open surgery

DISEASES OF THE LARYNX

EMERGENCIES

Stridor

Stridor means noisy breathing. It may be inspiratory or expiratory or occur in both phases of respiration. Inspiratory stridor is usually due to an obstruction at or above the vocal folds and is most commonly the result of an inhaled foreign body or acute infections such as epiglottitis. Expiratory stridor is usually from the lower respiratory tract and gives rise to a prolonged expiratory wheeze. It is most commonly associated with acute asthma or acute infective tracheobronchitis. Biphasic stridor is usually due to obstruction or disease of the tracheobronchial airway and distal lungs.

Summary box 52.8

Stridor

- Inspiratory
  - Foreign body or epiglottitis
- Expiratory
  - Acute asthma or infective tracheobronchitis
- Biphasic
  - Obstruction, disease of tracheobronchial airway or distal lungs

Stridor in children

Infants and children presenting with stridor need careful assessment with a full history and examination as appropriate. If, on presentation, a child is cyanosed and severely unwell, the airway must be secured as soon as possible, but a brief history with important pointers can often be obtained from the parents.

History

In infants in the first year of life, it is important to establish if the stridor is associated with particular activities such as swallowing, crying or movement. These may suggest congenital laryngomalacia or subglottic stenosis. If the stridor is exacerbated by feeding, particularly in the first 4 weeks of life, this suggests a vascular ring compressing the oesophagus or tracheo-oesophageal fistula. If the cry is weak or abnormal, this suggests a vocal fold palsy. If the problem only occurs in association with an upper respiratory tract infection and, in particular, is biphasic, this suggests congenital subglottic stenosis. In a young child, inspiratory stridor and drooling suggest acute epiglottitis, whereas biphasic stridor without drooling suggests laryngotracheobronchitis or croup.

Examination

It is important, when possible, to observe the child carefully at rest. Once a baby starts to cry, it may be impossible to study its resting respiratory pattern for some time. Ask the mother, not a nurse or a colleague, to move a baby or young child into different positions, such as face down and supine, and watch for changes in respiratory pattern and level of distress. Observe any drooling and, with neonates and infants, always try to watch the child being fed, listening to the trachea and chest with a stethoscope if possible. Always examine the whole child, looking for any evidence of congenital abnormalities before attempting any examination of the throat.

Summary box 52.9

Acute paediatric stridor

Congenital

- Laryngomalacia
- Laryngeal web
- Subglottic stenosis

Acquired

- Inflammatory
  - Angioneurotic oedema
- Traumatic
  - Impacted foreign body, laryngeal fracture
- Infective
  - Epiglottitis, laryngotracheobronchitis
- Neurological
  - Vocal fold palsy
- Neoplasia
  - Benign laryngeal papillomatosis

If a child is stridulous and drooling, do not attempt to lay them down and do not attempt to look inside the mouth. These manoeuvres are potentially life-threatening as the child may aspirate a large quantity of thick saliva contained within the oral cavity. It is particularly important in acute epiglottitis as the aspiration of thick saliva may be associated with further laryngeal spasm and a respiratory arrest. Restlessness, increasing tachycardia and cyanosis are important signs of hypoxia. If the child is not distressed and drooling, and not markedly stridulous, they may be cooperative enough that it is possible to look inside the mouth and check the palate, tongue and oropharynx. In stridulous children, particularly neonates and infants, a transcutaneous oximeter is invaluable. A resuscitation trolley with the necessary equipment for emergency intubation or tracheostomy should be close at hand before commencing examination.

Investigation

Plain lateral radiographs of the neck and a chest radiograph can be obtained but only if the child's condition permits. If a child is severely stridulous, they should not be sent to a radiography department without access to medical staff or resuscitation equipment.

Examination under anaesthesia is essential in all children whose diagnosis remains in doubt. This requires a high level of anaesthetic and surgical skill, with appropriate selection of rigid laryngoscopes, bronchoscopes and telescopes. Equipment for an urgent tracheostomy should also be readily available at all times.

Acute epiglottitis

In children acute epiglottitis is of rapid onset. It tends to occur in children of 2 years of age and over. Stridor is usually associated with drooling of saliva. The condition is caused by *Haemophilus influenzae* infection, which initially causes a severe pharyngitis that extends to involve the laryngeal inlet, causing inflammation and oedema. Further progression involves the whole of the supraglottic larynx, with severe oedema of the aryepiglottic folds and epiglottis being the most notable component, hence the commonly used term 'acute epiglottitis'.

These children frequently require intensive management with emergency intubation or tracheostomy followed by oxygenation, humidification, continuous oximetry and antibiotics. There may be associated septicaemia, so blood cultures should be obtained. Attempted examination with a spatula into the mouth may precipitate a respiratory arrest and should be avoided. The incidence of acute epiglottitis has plummeted where *H. influenzae* vaccination programmes are in place.

Laryngotracheobronchitis (croup)

Croup is usually of slower onset than acute epiglottitis and occurs most commonly in children under 2 years of age. It is usually viral in origin and the cases often occur in clusters. The children have biphasic stridor and are often hoarse with a typical barking cough. Airway intervention is required less often, but admission to hospital with oxygenation and humidification, coupled with antibiotics, may be necessary if there are signs of secondary infection.

Foreign bodies

Both children and adults may inhale foreign bodies. Young children will attempt to swallow a wide variety of objects, but coins, beads and parts of toys are particularly common. In adults, the aspiration is usually food, particularly inadequately chewed bones and meat. This is more common in elderly edentulous adults. Occasionally, portions of dentures may be inhaled, particularly in association with road traffic accidents.

Clinical features

The history is paramount and a history of foreign body ingestion or inhalation in a child, even though the pain, dysphagia, coughing, etc. may have settled, should always be taken seriously.

Adults usually have a clear recall, which facilitates diagnosis. Fish bones may lodge in the tonsils or base of tongue with minimal symptoms, but small fish bones may give rise to delayed para- and retropharyngeal abscess formation.

Examination

Examination may be prevented by trismus, pain and anxiety, but the presence of a foreign body may be suspected by salivary pooling within the piriform fossa or adjacent oedema and erythema of the pharyngolaryngeal mucosa.

Radiology

Radiology may be helpful but is not critical. Fish bones are often invisible on plain radiographs and a normal plain radiograph does not exclude a foreign body within the pharynx, larynx, oesophagus or lungs.

Specialised studies may help in cases of doubt, using a CT scan or a contrast swallow in the case of a suspected oesophageal foreign body.

Treatment

In the case of an inhaled foreign body causing severe stridor in a neonate or infant, it may be removed either by hooking it from the pharynx with a finger or by inverting the child carefully by the ankles and slapping their back. In a larger child, it may be more appropriate to bend the child over your knee with the child's head hanging down and again strike the child firmly between the shoulders. In the case of adults, an impacted laryngeal foreign body may be coughed out using abdominal thrusts (often referred to as a Heimlich manoeuvre). This involves standing behind the patient, clasping the arms around the lower thorax, such that the knuckles of the clasped hands come into contact with the patient's xiphisternum, and then a brief, firm compression of the lower thorax may aid instant expiration of the foreign body. If none of these immediate emergency measures removes the foreign body and the patient is cyanosed and severely stridulous, an immediate cricothyroidotomy or tracheostomy may be necessary. In less urgent cases, and when a foreign body is strongly suspected, endoscopy under general anaesthesia may be indicated.

Other causes of acute pharyngolaryngeal oedema

Angioneurotic oedema, radiotherapy and laryngeal trauma associated with road traffic accidents, corrosives, scalds and smoke ingestion may all cause significant pharyngolaryngeal oedema, in addition to the acute infective conditions

Henry Jay Heimlich, 1920–2016, thoracic surgeon, Xavier University, Cincinnati, OH, USA.

mentioned above. Hoarseness is the predominant symptom along with dysphagia prior to the increase in dyspnoea. If flexible laryngoscopic examination is possible, marked oedema of the supraglottis and pharynx can be seen. Humidified oxygen, adrenaline (epinephrine) nebulisers, systemic antihistamines and steroids may be valuable. Opioids should not be given as they may cause respiratory depression and respiratory arrest. If the dyspnoea progresses, intubation or tracheostomy will be necessary.

TRACHEOSTOMY AND OTHER EMERGENCY AIRWAY MEASURES

This procedure relieves airway obstruction or protects the airway by fashioning a direct entrance into the trachea through the skin of the neck. Tracheostomy may be carried out as an emergency for acute airway obstruction when the larynx cannot be intubated, but it is not always an easy procedure, particularly in an obese patient. An easier alternative for the inexperienced is insertion of a large intravenous cannula or a small tube into the cricothyroid membrane, which lies in the midline immediately below the thyroid cartilage. The time to do a tracheostomy is when you first think it may be necessary.

If time allows, the following should be undertaken:

- inspection and palpation of the neck to assess the laryngotracheal anatomy in the individual patient;
- indirect or direct laryngoscopy;
- assessment of pulmonary function by auscultation.

Whenever possible, the procedure should be adequately explained to the patient beforehand, with particular emphasis on the inability to speak immediately following the operation. Ample reassurance is required that they will not have 'lost' their voice permanently. The indications for tracheostomy are shown in ***Summary box 52.10***.

Within the theatre or intensive care setting, the 'can't intubate, can't oxygenate' situation occurs after attempts to secure the airway by a facemask, a supraglottic airway device and an endotracheal tube have failed. Only a narrow window exists to avoid profound hypoxia and its consequences and local protocols should be agreed upon to manage these situations beforehand using appropriate emergency front of neck access options (cricothyroidotomy or tracheostomy).

Emergency tracheostomy

If a skilled anaesthetist is unavailable, local anaesthesia is employed, but in desperate cases when the patient is unconscious, none is required. In patients who have suffered severe head and neck trauma and who may have an unstable cervical spine fracture, cricothyroidotomy may be more suitable. If it is possible, the patient should be laid supine with padding placed under the shoulders and the extended neck kept as steady as possible in the midline. This aids palpation of the thyroid and cricoid cartilage between the thumb and index finger of the free hand. The movements of the fingers of the free hand are important in this technique. The operation is more difficult in small children and thick-necked adults as the landmarks are difficult to palpate (***Figures 52.39 and 52.40***).

Summary box 52.10

Indications for tracheostomy

- Acute upper airway obstruction
  - For example, an inhaled foreign body, a large pharyngolaryngeal tumour or acute pharyngolaryngeal infections in children
- Potential upper airway obstruction
  - For example, after or prior to major surgery involving the oral cavity, pharynx, larynx or neck
- Protection of the lower airway
  - For example, protection against aspiration of saliva in unconscious patients as a consequence of head injuries, maxillofacial injuries, comas, bulbar poliomyelitis or tetanus
- Patients requiring prolonged artificial respiration
  - Best performed within 10 days of ventilation

A vertical midline incision is made from the inferior aspect of the thyroid cartilage to the suprasternal notch and continued down between the infrahyoid muscles. There may be heavy bleeding from the wound at this point, particularly if the neck is congested as a result of the patient's efforts to breathe around an acute upper airway obstruction. No steps should be taken to control this haemorrhage, although an assistant and suction are valuable. The operator should feel carefully for the cricoid cartilage using the index finger of the free hand while retracting the skin edges by pressure applied by the thumb and middle finger. If the situation is one of extreme urgency, a further vertical incision straight into the trachea at the level of the second, third and fourth rings should be made immediately without regard to the presence of the thyroid isthmus. The knife blade is rotated through 90°, thus opening the trachea. At this point the patient may cough violently as blood enters the airway. The operator should be aware of this possibility and avoid losing the position of the scalpel in the open trachea. Any form of available tube should be inserted into the trachea as soon as possible and blood and secretion sucked out. Once an airway has been established, haemostasis is then secured. With the emergency under control, the tracheostomy should be refashioned as soon as possible.

Should additional equipment and more time be available once the cricoid cartilage has been identified, blunt finger dissection inferiorly can be used to mobilise the thyroid isthmus, which should be clipped and divided, clearing the trachea before making a vertical incision through the second to the fourth rings. A tracheal dilator is inserted through the tracheal incision and the edges of the tracheal wound are separated gently. This is likely to induce coughing and so, particularly in cases where there is a suspected infection risk, as far as possible care should be taken to minimise the risk of contaminating the operator(s). A tracheostomy tube is inserted into the trachea and the dilator removed. It is important that the surgeon/assistant keeps a finger on the tube while it is secured with sutures to the neck skin. Additional securing of the tube is achieved by means of tapes attached to the flange of the device passed behind the neck and secured to the opposite side with the neck in a neutral position.

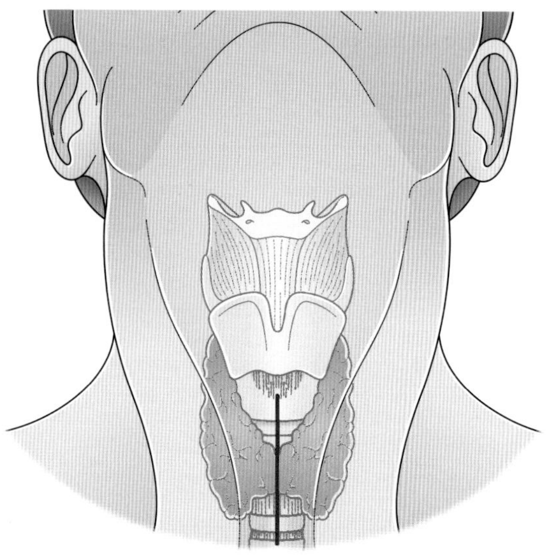

Figure 52.39 Position of the skin incision in an emergency tracheostomy.

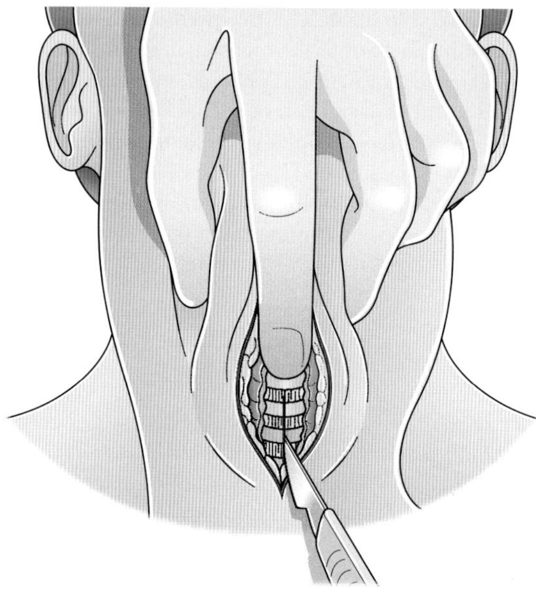

Figure 52.40 An incision in the trachea in an emergency tracheostomy.

Elective tracheostomy

The advantage of an elective surgical procedure is that there is complete airway control at all times, unhurried dissection and careful placement of an appropriate tube. Close cooperation between the surgeon, anaesthetist and scrub nurse is essential, and attention to detail will markedly reduce possible complications and morbidity from the procedure.

Following induction of general anaesthesia and endotracheal intubation, the patient is positioned with a combination of head extension and placement of an appropriate sandbag under the shoulders (***Figure 52.41***). There should be no rotation of the head. Children's heads should not be overextended, as it is possible to enter the trachea in the fifth and sixth rings in these circumstances. A transverse incision may be used in the elective situation (***Figure 52.42***). The thyroid isthmus is divided carefully and oversewn and tension sutures placed either side of the tracheal fenestration in children (***Figure 52.43***). A Bjork flap may be used in adults (***Figures 52.44 and 52.45***).

The advantages of a Bjork flap outweigh the potential disadvantages, as performed correctly it is safe and allows reintroduction of a displaced tube with the minimum of difficulty, reducing the risk of replacing the displaced tube in a false track anterior to the trachea into the superior mediastinum. Although not routinely used, this is described here for completion.

The inferiorly based flap is created by starting with an incision into the trachea between the first and second or second and third tracheal rings. In order to reduce the risk of subglottic stenosis, damage to the first tracheal ring should be avoided at all costs. A stay suture is inserted around the cartilage at the free edge of the flap. Lateral incisions are made in a caudal direction extending through two tracheal rings to create the flap. One option is to leave the stay suture attached and taped to the chest wall to allow retraction of the flap to obliterate the pretracheal space when replacing a displaced tube. An alternative is to suture the free edge of the flap to the edge of the inferior transverse skin incision.

In a paediatric patient a vertical incision is made between the second and third tracheal rings. No tracheal tissue is removed. A cuff of anterior neck subcutaneous fat pad may be removed in children for adequate access. Prior to incision of the trachea, vertical stay sutures are placed lateral to the midline through the tracheal rings and left in place. These can provide traction for the trachea and allow for rapid tracheostomy tube reinsertion if accidental decannulation occurs prior to the establishment of the tract. Some surgeons will suture skin flaps to the trachea for additional safety (maturation sutures). It is essential to stick to the midline during dissection as more lateral dissection risks a pneumothorax, as the cupula of the cervical pleura extends into the neck on either side of the trachea.

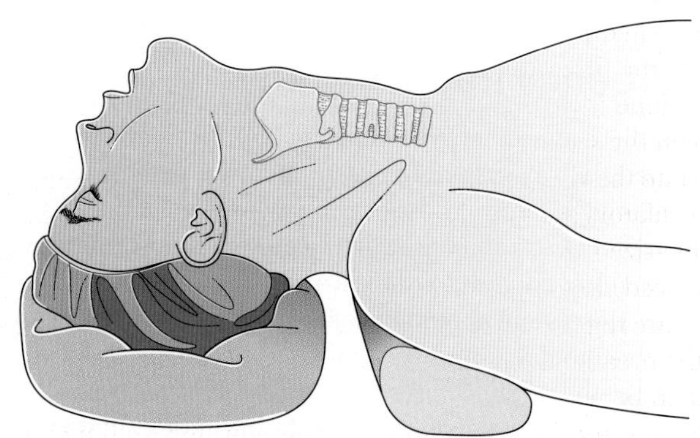

Figure 52.41 Position of the patient for elective tracheostomy.

Viking Olaf Bjork, 1918–2009, cardiac surgeon, Karolinska Sjukset, Stockholm, Sweden.

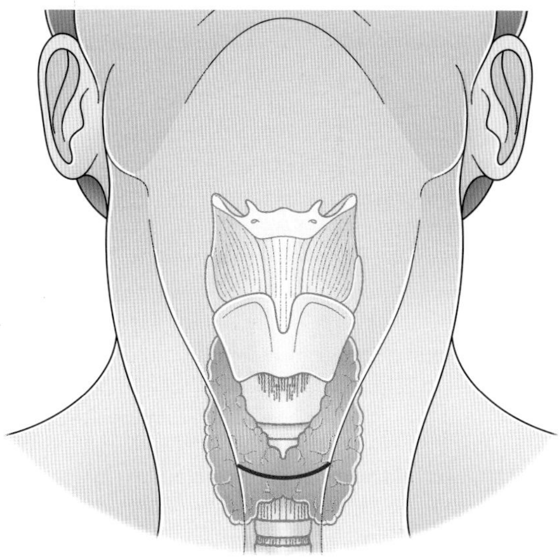

Figure 52.42 Position of the skin incision in an elective tracheostomy.

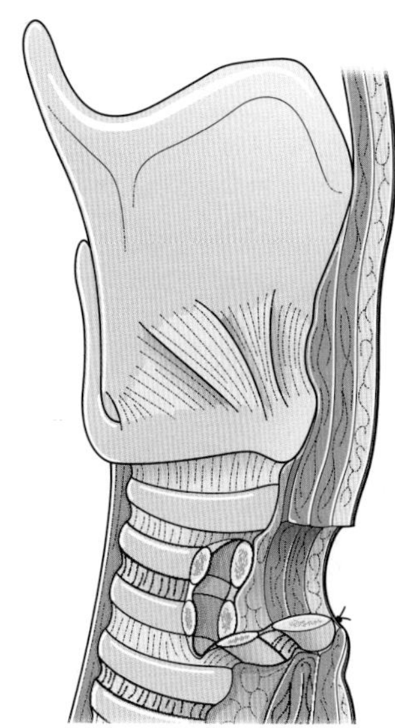

Figure 52.44 Bjork flap.

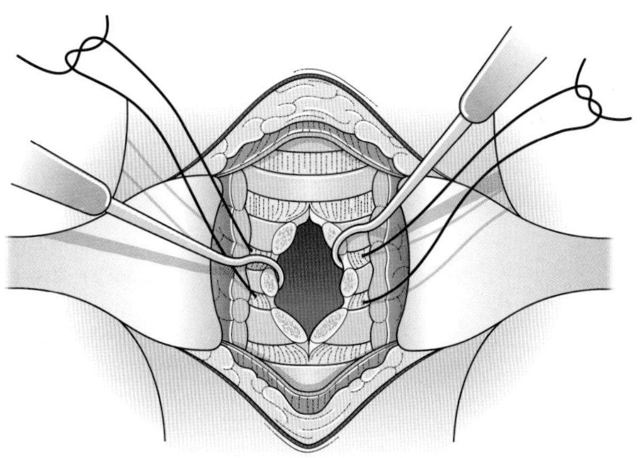

Figure 52.43 Tracheal fenestration in an elective tracheostomy.

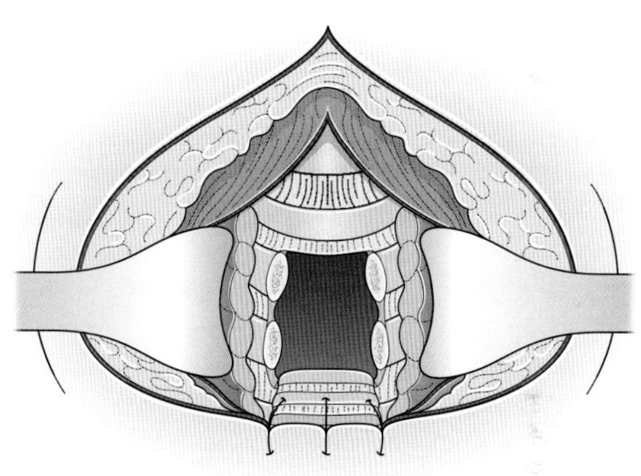

Figure 52.45 Fenestration in a Bjork flap.

Percutaneous tracheostomy

As an alternative to open tracheostomy, a percutaneous tracheostomy is commonly performed in the critical care setting in an intubated patient. A transverse skin incision is made at the level of the first and second tracheal rings; blunt dissection of the midline is then performed. A 22-gauge needle is inserted between the second and third tracheal rings. When air is aspirated into the syringe, the guidewire is introduced. Sequentially larger dilators are then inserted over the guidewire to create a suitable-sized tracheostome. Finally, the tracheotomy tube is introduced along the guidewire and dilator. The guidewire and dilator are removed, the cuff of the tracheotomy tube is inflated and the breathing circuit is connected. The endotracheal tube can then be removed.

Patients must have appropriate anatomy and no limitation of neck movement. If any doubt arises as to the suitability of a patient for percutaneous tracheostomy, a surgical approach should be adopted. Percutaneous tracheostomy is rarely performed in children.

Tracheostomy tubes

Most modern tracheostomy tubes are made of plastic (***Figure 52.46***). Tubes of various sizes with varying curves, angles, cuffs, inner tubes and speaking valves are available. After a newly fashioned tracheostomy is created, a cuffed tube is used initially to protect the airway from secretions or bleeding. This may be changed after 3–4 days to a non-cuffed tube. The pressure within the tube cuff should be carefully monitored and should be low enough so as not to occlude circulation in the mucosal capillaries, which promotes scar tissue formation and subglottic stenosis. When in position, the tube should be retained by double tapes threaded through the flanges and passed around the patient's neck. It is important that the patient's head is flexed when the tapes are tied, otherwise they may become slack when the patient is moved from the position of extension, thereby resulting in a possible displacement of the tube if the patient coughs. Alternatively, the flanges of the plastic tube may be stitched directly to the underlying neck skin. A removable inner tube, which is easily cleaned, should

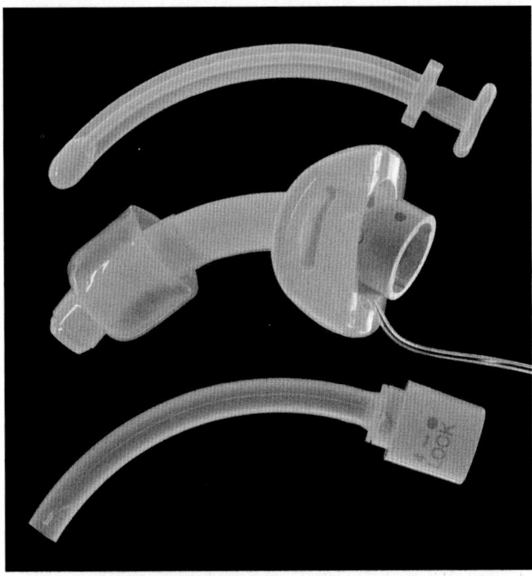

Figure 52.46 Modern plastic tracheostomy tube with the introducer, low-pressure cuff and inner cannula.

always be used to prevent lumen occlusion by thickened, dried secretions from the trachea.

All forms of tracheostomy and cricothyroidotomy bypass the upper airway and have the following advantages:

- the anatomical dead space is reduced by approximately 50%;
- the work of breathing is reduced;
- alveolar ventilation is increased;
- the level of sedation needed for patient comfort is decreased and, unlike endotracheal intubation, the patient may be able to talk and eat with a tube in place.

However, there are several disadvantages:

- loss of heat and moisture exchange in the upper respiratory tract;
- desiccation of tracheal epithelium, loss of ciliated cells and metaplasia;
- the presence of a foreign body in the trachea stimulates production of mucus; where no cilia are present, the mucociliary stream is therefore impeded;
- the increased mucus is more viscid and thick crusts may form and block the tube;
- although many patients with a tracheostomy can feed satisfactorily, there is some splinting of the larynx, which may prevent normal swallowing and lead to aspiration; this aspiration may be silent.

Postoperative treatment is designed to counteract these effects and frequent suction and humidification are most important. A trolley must be placed by the bed containing a tracheal dilator, duplicate tubes and introducers, retractors and dressings. Oxygen is at hand and, in the initial period, a nurse must be in constant attendance. Humidification will render the secretions less viscid and a sucker with a catheter attached should be on hand to keep the tracheobronchial tree free from secretions.

Summary box 52.11

Tracheostomy: postoperative management

- Suction – efficient, sterile and as often as required
- Humidification (with or without oxygen)
- A warm, well-ventilated room
- Position of the tube and patient
- Spare tube, introducer, tapes, tracheal dilator
- Change of tube, inner tube, possible speaking valve
- Physiotherapy
- Initiation of local decannulation protocols where indicated

Complications of tracheostomy

The intraoperative, early and late postoperative complications of tracheostomy are listed in ***Table 52.2***.

TABLE 52.2 Tracheostomy: complications.

Intraoperative complications	• Haemorrhage • Injury to paratracheal structures, particularly the carotid artery, recurrent laryngeal nerve and oesophagus • Damage to the trachea
Early postoperative complications	• Apnoea caused by a fall in the PCO_2 • Haemorrhage • Subcutaneous emphysema, pneumomediastinum and pneumothorax • Accidental extubation, anterior displacement of the tube, obstruction of the tube lumen and tip occlusion against the tracheal wall • Infection • Swallowing dysfunction
Late postoperative complications	• Difficult decannulation • Tracheocutaneous fistula • Tracheo-oesophageal fistula, tracheoinnominate artery fistula with severe haemorrhage • Tracheal stenosis

PCO_2, partial pressure of carbon dioxide.

OTHER EMERGENCY AIRWAY PROCEDURES

Fibreoptic endotracheal intubation

In most emergency situations, endotracheal intubation is the most direct and satisfactory method of securing the airway. Nasotracheal 'awake' intubation in expert hands is also a well-established technique and is particularly useful if the patient has trismus, severe mandibular injuries, cervical spine rigidity or an obstructing mass within the oral cavity or lower down in the upper aerodigestive tract. This is facilitated by passing a fibreoptic endoscope through the centre of an endotracheal tube, hence guiding it into the larynx and trachea under direct vision.

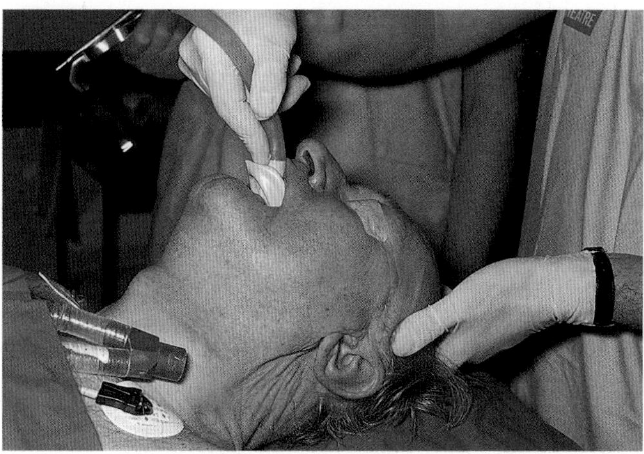

Figure 52.47 A laryngeal mask airway being inserted.

Laryngeal mask airway

The laryngeal mask airway (LMA) is a wide-bore airway with an inflatable cuff at the distal end, which forms a seal in the pharynx around the laryngeal inlet. Provided the laryngotracheal airway is clear, the LMA provides a clear and secure airway. The technique can easily be learnt by non-anaesthetists and secures an airway in most cases. It comes in a range of sizes covering infants to large adults. It is particularly useful in cases of difficult intubation where mouth opening is unimpeded (***Figure 52.47***). A newer variation of this is the i-gel® device, which replaces the inflatable cuff with a rim that conforms to the anatomical shape around the laryngeal inlet.

Transtracheal ventilation

This technique is simple and effective and allows ventilation for periods in excess of 1 hour, providing time to allow for more elective intubation. The cricothyroid membrane is located as discussed above, and a 14- or 16-gauge plastic sheathed intravascular needle attached to a 10-mL syringe containing a few millilitres of lidocaine is introduced in the midline and directed downwards and backwards into the tracheal lumen. The needle is advanced steadily and negative pressure is placed on the syringe until bubbles of air are clearly seen (***Figure 52.48***). The tissues of the neck may be infiltrated with the anaesthetic if desired and the tracheal mucosa likewise partly anaesthetised by the introduction of 1–2 mL of lidocaine after gaining the lumen. The needle is removed and the plastic sheath cannula left in the tracheal lumen; it must be carefully held and fixed in place by the operator so that it does not come out of the lumen into the soft tissues of the neck. It is attached by means of a Luer connection to the high-pressure oxygen supply. Ventilation may be undertaken in a controlled manner with a jetting device, with the chest being observed for appropriate movements.

If there is severe obstruction of the laryngopharynx by the foreign body or tumour, the exhaled outflow of gases can be aided by the placement of one or two further cannulae as exhalation ports. This procedure gains extremely rapid control of ventilation and requires a minimum of technical expertise. Its only notable complication is surgical emphysema of the neck tissues if the cannula dislodges from the tracheal lumen.

Cricothyroidotomy

Cricothyroidotomy has the advantages of speed and ease, requiring minimal equipment and surgical expertise, and has great value in the emergency setting when conditions are not optimal to perform a tracheostomy.

Cricothyroidotomy is performed through the cricothyroid membrane, which is a fibroelastic condensation connecting the thyroid cartilage to the cricoid cartilage. The cricothyroid artery and vein, the pyramidal lobe of the thyroid gland and lymph nodes may overlie the membrane. The membrane should be identified precisely before undertaking the procedure to avoid injury to adjacent structures; the patient's neck is extended and the area between the prominence of the thyroid cartilage and the cricoid cartilage below is palpated with the index finger of the free hand and, if necessary, the 'laryngeal handshake technique' can be used to define the membrane (***Figure 52.49***).

Cricothyroidotomy can be performed using the scalpel or cannulae. The scalpel–bougie tube technique is the fastest and most reliable method of securing the airway; a number 10 blade, a bougie and a 6-mm cuffed endotracheal tube are needed to perform this, with the patient receiving 100% oxygen and full neuromuscular blockade. A vertical skin incision is recommended with dissection rapidly carried down to the cricothyroid membrane. A 1-cm transverse incision is made through the membrane immediately above the cricoid cartilage and the scalpel twisted through a right angle to gain access to the airway. If available, an artery forceps, bougie, dilator or tracheal hook will improve the aperture and insertion of an

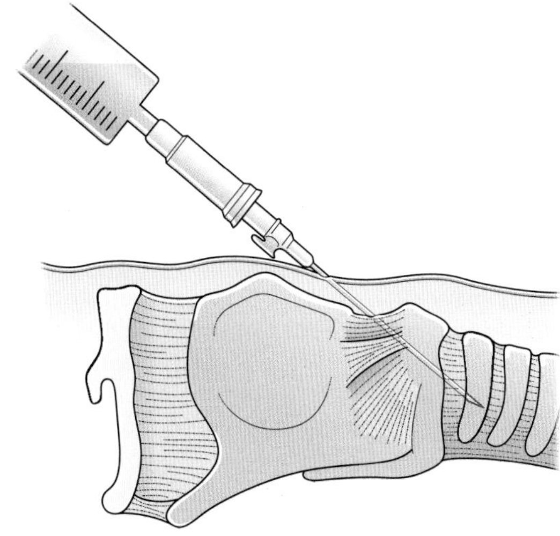

Figure 52.48 Transtracheal needle introduction.

Hermann Adolph Wülfing-Lüer, 1836–1909, German instrument maker who was working in Paris, France, at the end of the nineteenth century.

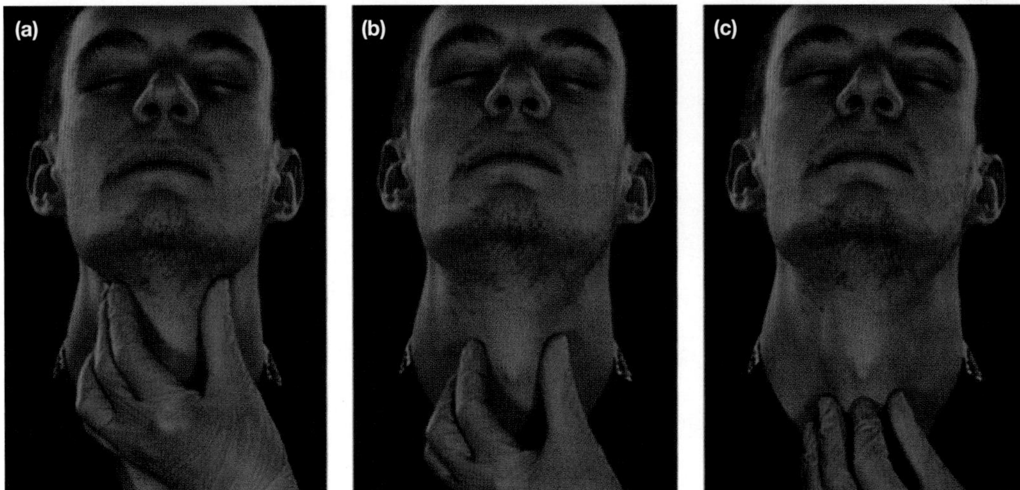

Figure 52.49 Laryngeal handshake technique as described in the Difficult Airway Society (DAS) 2015 guidelines. (a) The index finger and thumb grasp the top of the larynx (the greater cornu of the hyoid bone) and roll it from side to side. The bony and cartilaginous cage of the larynx is a cone, which connects to the trachea. (b) The fingers and thumb slide down over the thyroid laminae. (c) The middle finger and thumb rest on the cricoid cartilage, with the index finger palpating the cricothyroid membrane. (Reproduced with permission from Drew T, McCaul CL. Laryngeal handshake technique in locating the cricothyroid membrane: a non-randomised comparative study. *Br J Anaesth* 2018; **121**(5): P1173–8.)

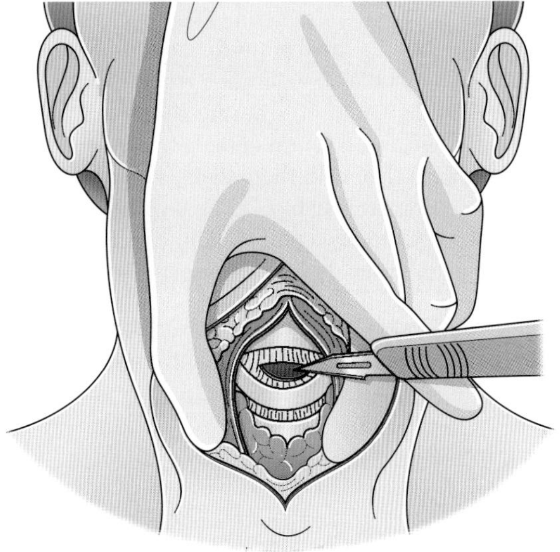

Figure 52.50 Incision in a cricothyroidotomy.

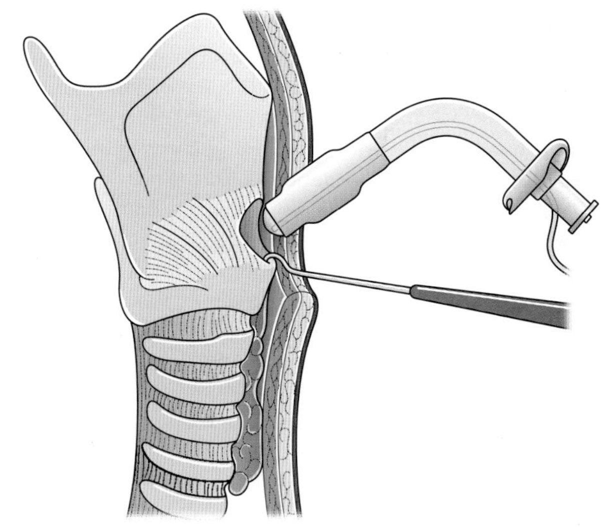

Figure 52.51 Insertion of a tube after cricothyroidotomy.

available tube (***Figures 52.50 and 52.51***). The endotracheal tube allows ventilation using conventional low-pressure equipment. Cannula cricothyroidotomy can be performed with a narrow-bore (internal diameter ≤2 mm) or wide-bore (internal diameter ≥4 mm) cannula to facilitate oxygenation. Specialist equipment is available for this, but both techniques are associated with kinking of the cannula and complications, such as device displacement and barotrauma.

As soon as practicably possible, the cricothyroidotomy should be converted to a tracheostomy. Although there is debate about the frequency of subglottic stenosis following this procedure, there is general agreement that it is much increased if any long-term ventilation is undertaken via even a modestly size tracheostomy tube through the cricothyroid membrane.

LARYNGEAL DISEASE CAUSING VOICE DISORDERS

Vocal nodules

These are fibrous thickenings of the vocal folds at the junction of the middle and anterior thirds (***Figure 52.52***) and result from vocal abuse; they are known as singers' nodules in adults and screamers' nodules in children. Speech therapy is therefore the preferred treatment and the lesions will resolve spontaneously in most cases. Occasionally, the nodules will need to be surgically removed using modern microlaryngoscopic dissection or laser techniques, but speech therapy will still be required for postoperative voice rehabilitation.

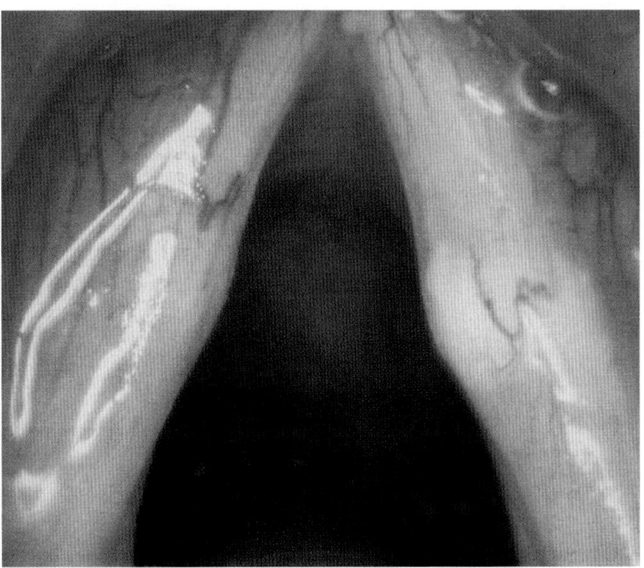

Figure 52.52 Vocal fold nodules.

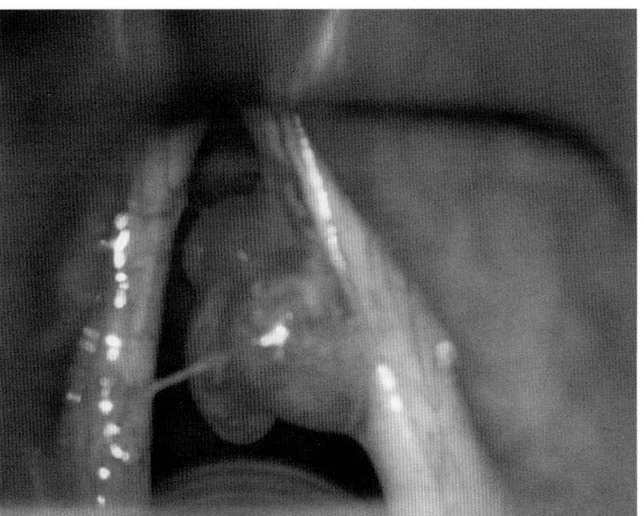

Figure 52.53 A vocal fold polyp.

Vocal fold polyps

These are usually unilateral and may be associated with an acute infective episode, cigarette smoking or vocal abuse (*Figure 52.53*). Speech therapy is again indicated, but they do usually require removal by microdissection or laser surgery.

Summary box 52.12

Causes of hoarseness

- Mucosal disease (e.g. vocal nodule, polyps or laryngeal papillomatosis, acute or chronic laryngitis)
- Neurological disease (e.g. vocal fold palsy)
- Neoplasia (e.g. laryngeal tumours)
- Non-specific voice disorders, functional dysphonia

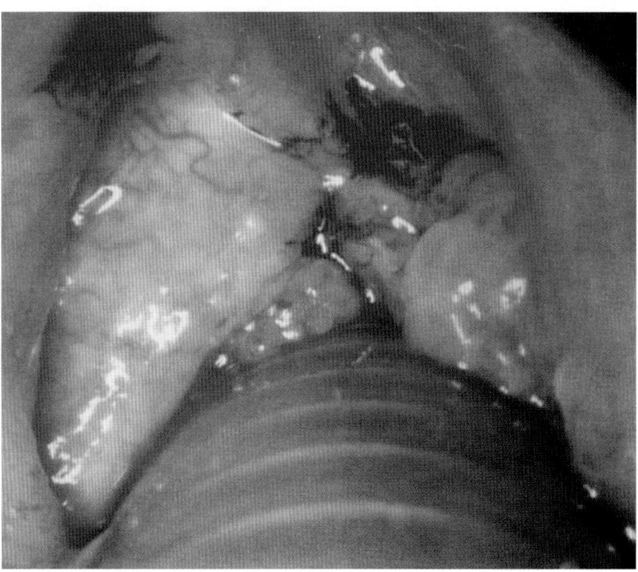

Figure 52.54 Laryngeal papillomas.

Laryngeal papillomata

These are rare benign tumours occurring mainly in children but can also present in adults. They are most commonly found on the vocal folds but may spread throughout the larynx and tracheobronchial airway (although this is less likely in adults) (*Figure 52.54*). They are caused by papillomaviruses (most frequently HPV 6 and 11) and need repeated removal usually by laser microsurgery or microdebrider to maintain a reasonable voice and airway. These patients are best managed in specialist centres, with the appropriate expertise. The evidence to date is mixed with regard to antiviral use, and existing data are insufficient to support the regular use of antiviral agents such as cidofovir in the management of laryngeal papillomatosis. Vaccination against papilloma has shown some therapeutic benefit in reducing the recurrence of the disease. There is a greater appreciation of the role that gastro-oesophageal reflux may play in this setting and many centres opt to place patients on proton pump inhibitors or H_2 blockers.

Acute laryngitis

This often occurs as part of an upper respiratory tract infection in association with a cough and pharyngitis. Usually viral, it may be localised to the larynx and it settles quickly if the voice is rested during the acute inflammation. Steam inhalations are soothing along with mild analgesia, but antibiotics are unnecessary.

Summary box 52.13

Warning

- Hoarseness lasting for 3–4 weeks should always be referred for an ENT opinion

Chronic laryngitis

Chronic laryngitis may be specific and can be caused by mycobacteria, syphilis and fungi. Treatment is directed towards the causative organism. Non-specific laryngitis is common, the main predisposing factors being smoking, chronic upper and lower respiratory sepsis and voice abuse. Gastro-oesophageal reflux has been implicated as a factor in laryngitis, vocal fold nodules and polyps, but the evidence is controversial. However, antireflux medication and proton pump inhibitors are commonly prescribed. Diagnosis of chronic laryngitis should not be made unless the larynx has been fully evaluated by a laryngologist.

Vocal fold palsy

This may be unilateral or bilateral (***Figure 52.55***). Unilateral cord palsy is most commonly idiopathic. In non-idiopathic cases, left vocal fold palsy is most common because of the long intrathoracic course of the left recurrent laryngeal nerve, which arches around the aorta and may be commonly involved in inflammatory and neoplastic conditions involving the left hilum or lung apex. Lung cancer should be considered the cause of a left vocal fold palsy until proved otherwise.

Tumours of the nasopharynx, larynx, thyroid gland or oesophagus may also cause vocal fold palsy. Bilateral vocal fold paralysis is uncommon and tends to occur after thyroid surgery or head injuries.

> **Summary box 52.14**
>
> Causes of vocal fold palsy
>
> **Congenital (infants)**
>
> **Acquired**
> - Traumatic
>   - Direct to neck
>   - Post surgery (e.g. thyroidectomy)
> - Infective
>   - Viral (rare)
> - Neoplastic
>   - Carcinoma of the lung involving the left hilum
>   - Carcinoma of the nasopharynx, larynx, thyroid and oesophagus
> - Vascular
>   - Aortic aneurysm
> - Neurological
>   - Lower motor neurone disease

Clinical features

Unilateral recurrent laryngeal nerve palsy of sudden onset produces hoarseness, difficulty in swallowing liquids and a weakened cough. These symptoms may be short-lived and the voice may return to normal within a few weeks as the muscles in the opposite vocal fold compensate and move it across the midline to meet the paralysed vocal fold, which usually lies in the paramedian position. Bilateral recurrent laryngeal nerve palsy is an occasional and serious complication of total thyroidectomy. On anaesthetic reversal, acute dyspnoea occurs as a result of the paramedian position of both vocal folds, which reduce the airway to 2–3 mm and which tend to get sucked together on inspiration. This can be temporarily relieved by positive pressure mask ventilation, but, in severe cases, tracheostomy or intubation is necessary immediately, otherwise death occurs from asphyxia.

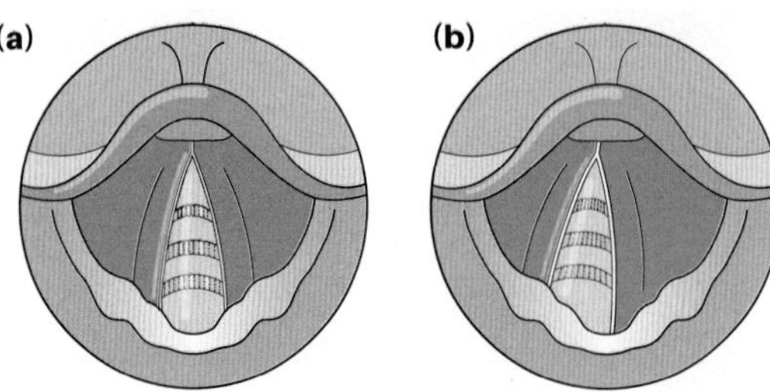

Figure 52.55 Vocal fold positions: (a) normal; (b) unilateral vocal fold palsy.

Investigation of vocal fold paralysis is by a CT scan from the skull base (including posterior fossa) to the diaphragm. Approximately 20–25% of vocal fold paralysis occurs without known pathology and spontaneous recovery may occur. When compensation does not occur, a unilateral paralysed fold may be medialised by injection or external thyroplasty.

In bilateral vocal fold palsy, surgery may be carried out to divide the posterior aspect of one vocal fold (cordotomy) or a portion of one arytenoid cartilage (arytenoidectomy). These procedures are most easily performed endoscopically with a carbon dioxide laser. They increase the size of the posterior glottic airway, allowing the patient to be decannulated or even avoid an initial tracheostomy.

Tumours of the larynx

Benign tumours of the larynx are extremely rare. Squamous cell carcinoma is the most common malignant tumour, being responsible for more than 90% of tumours within the larynx. It is the second most common head and neck cancer (oral cavity is more common) and previously usually occurred in elderly male smokers. However, over the past decades, the incidence among women has risen because of increased smoking. The incidence of laryngeal cancer in the three subsites – supraglottis, glottis and subglottis – varies around the world.

Clinical features

Patients typically present with voice change. Other symptoms include dysphagia, odynophagia and neck lumps. Advanced tumours can present with airway compromise, usually as inspiratory stridor (***Figure 52.56***).

Investigations

Direct laryngoscopy, followed by a general anaesthetic assessment, together with angled (30° and 70°) Hopkins' rod examination, allows precise determination of the extent of the tumour and biopsy confirms the histology. CT and MRI give further details of the extent of larger tumours, demonstrating

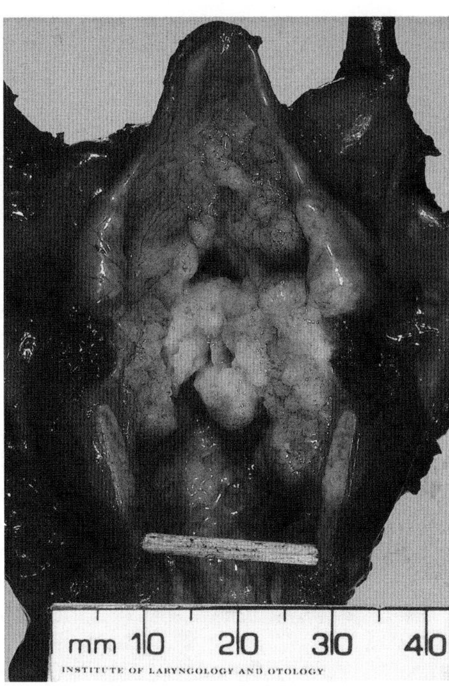

Figure 52.56 A total laryngectomy specimen with a transglottic tumour.

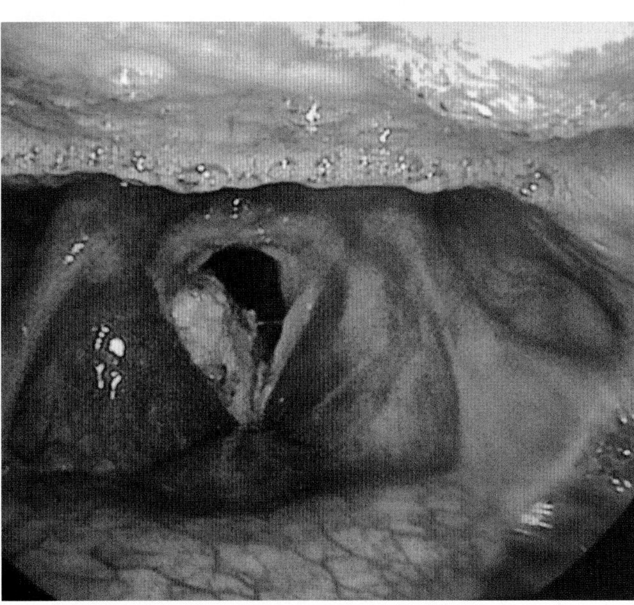

Figure 52.57 Flexible nasendoscopy demonstrating a laryngeal tumour seen involving the entire length of the right vocal fold.

spread outside the larynx and suspicious nodal involvement within the neck, which may not be obvious clinically.

Treatment

Early laryngeal cancer (T1 and T2)

Early-stage supraglottic and glottic tumours can be treated with a single modality: radiotherapy or endoscopic surgical resection, with the aim of preservation of function. Although both modalities are associated with similar survival rates (approximately 95% local control), transoral laser resection is commonly used as it usually involves day case surgery and more therapeutic options are available for the small number of patients who have local recurrence (***Figure 52.57***).

Advanced laryngeal cancer (T3 and T4)

Organ preservation should be a priority when treating locally advanced cancer without extralaryngeal spread and/or laryngeal dysfunction. The non-surgical standard of care is concurrent chemoradiotherapy; while a variety of open partial laryngectomy procedures are also available, these are best undertaken in specialist centres.

Laryngeal cancer with gross extralaryngeal extension is usually best treated with total laryngectomy and adjuvant postoperative radiotherapy or chemoradiotherapy (***Figure 52.56***).

After the larynx has been removed, the remaining trachea is brought out onto the lower neck as a permanent tracheal stoma and the hypopharynx, which is opened at the time of the operation, is closed to restore continuity for swallowing (***Figure 52.58***). Thus, the upper aero- and digestive tracts are permanently disconnected. Part or all of the thyroid gland and associated parathyroid glands may also be removed, depending on the extent of the disease.

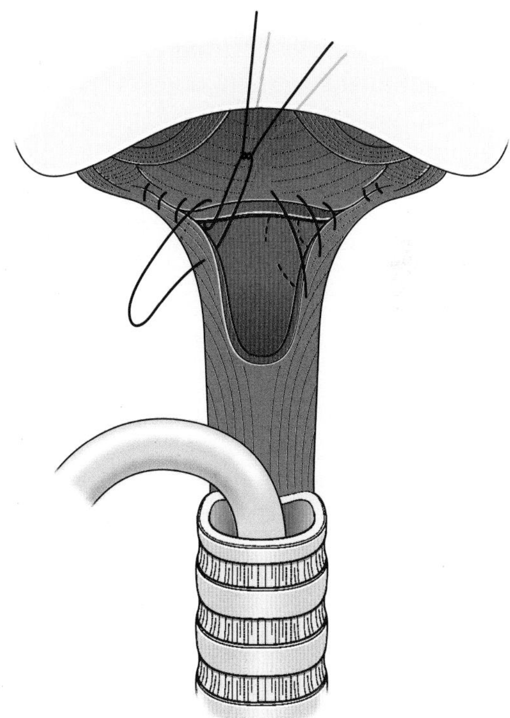

Figure 52.58 Transverse closure of the pharynx with an endotracheal tube in the end tracheostome.

Voice rehabilitation

The loss of the larynx as a generator of sound does not prevent patients speaking as long as an alternative source of sound can be created by vibration in the pharynx. This can be achieved in one of three ways:

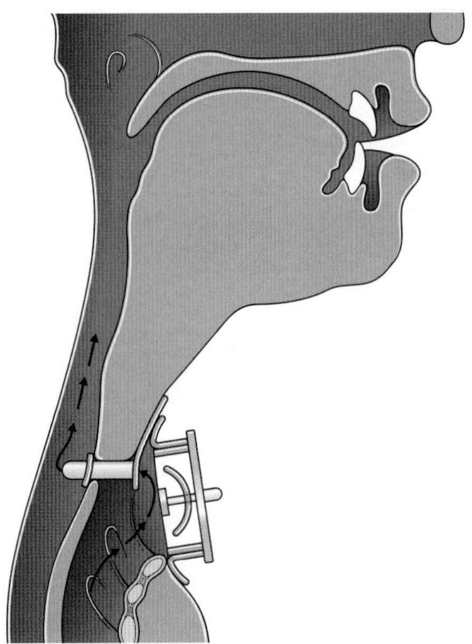

Figure 52.59 A Blom–Singer valve within a surgically fashioned tracheo-oesophageal fistula and an outer stoma valve.

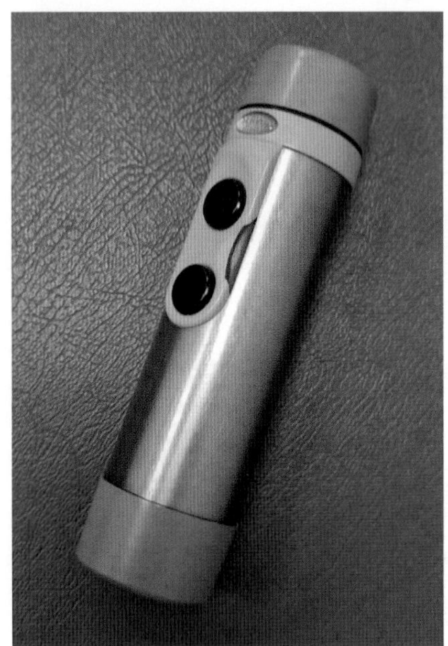

Figure 52.61 Electrolarynx.

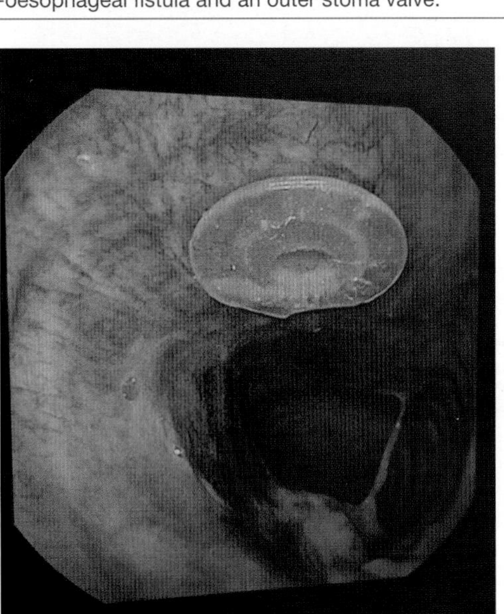

Figure 52.60 Provox voice valve prosthesis viewed in rear wall of trachea.

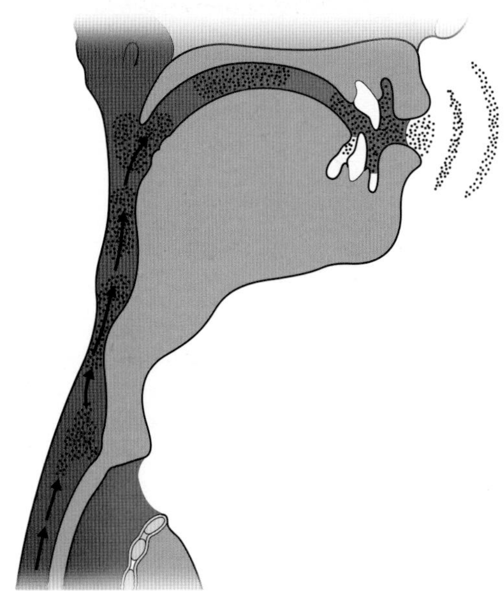

Figure 52.62 Production of oesophageal speech.

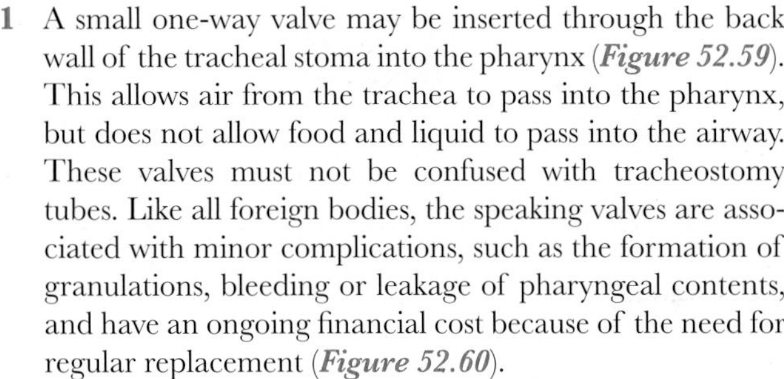

1 A small one-way valve may be inserted through the back wall of the tracheal stoma into the pharynx (*Figure 52.59*). This allows air from the trachea to pass into the pharynx, but does not allow food and liquid to pass into the airway. These valves must not be confused with tracheostomy tubes. Like all foreign bodies, the speaking valves are associated with minor complications, such as the formation of granulations, bleeding or leakage of pharyngeal contents, and have an ongoing financial cost because of the need for regular replacement (*Figure 52.60*).

2 An external battery-powered vibrating device that when applied to the soft tissues of the neck produces sound, which is turned into speech by the vocal tract comprising the tongue, pharynx, oral cavity, lips, teeth and nasal sinuses (*Figure 52.61*).

3 Oesophageal speech, when air is swallowed into the pharynx and upper oesophagus. On regurgitating the air, a segment of the pharyngo-oesophageal mucosa vibrates to produce sound, which is modified by the vocal tract into speech (*Figure 52.62*).

Mark I Singer, contemporary, head and neck surgeon, San Francisco, CA, USA.
Eric D Blom, contemporary, speech pathologist and medical device inventor, Carmel, IN, USA.

DISEASES OF THE NECK

LUMP IN THE NECK

On presentation, a careful history and examination are essential. The clinical signs of size, site, shape, consistency, fixation to skin or deep structures, pulsation, compressibility, transillumination or the presence of a bruit must be established and recorded.

Branchial cyst

A branchial cyst (*Figure 52.63*) develops from the vestigial remnants of the second branchial cleft, is lined by squamous epithelium and contains thick, turbid fluid. The cyst usually presents in the upper neck in early or middle adulthood and is found at the junction of the upper third and middle third of the sternomastoid muscle at its anterior border. It is a fluctuant swelling that may transilluminate and is often soft in its early stages so that it may be difficult to palpate.

Summary box 52.15

Diagnosis of a lump in the neck

- History
- Physical signs
  - Size
  - Site
  - Shape
  - Surface
  - Consistency
  - Fixation: deep/superficial
  - Pulsatility
  - Compressibility
  - Transillumination
  - Bruit

If the cyst becomes infected, it becomes erythematous and tender and the differential diagnosis is broadened. Ultrasound and fine-needle aspiration both aid diagnosis and treatment is by complete excision, which is best undertaken when the lesion is quiescent. It passes superficial to the hypoglossal and glossopharyngeal nerves, but deep to the posterior belly of the digastric. These structures and the spinal accessory nerve must be positively identified to avoid damage. In patients over 35 years of age, a high index of suspicion for a necrotic metastatic lymph node should exist and malignancy should be excluded before excision.

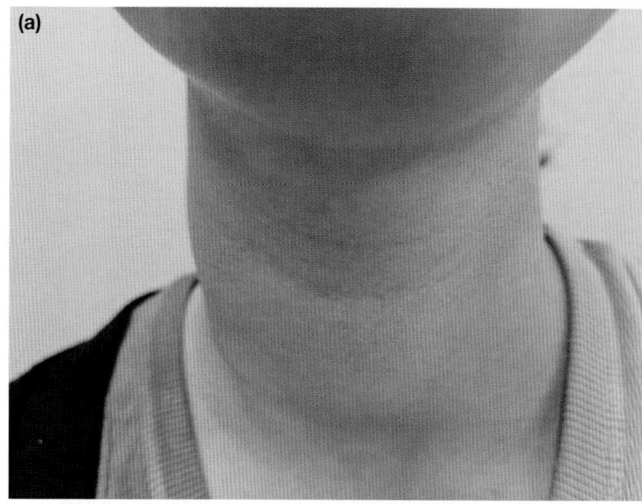

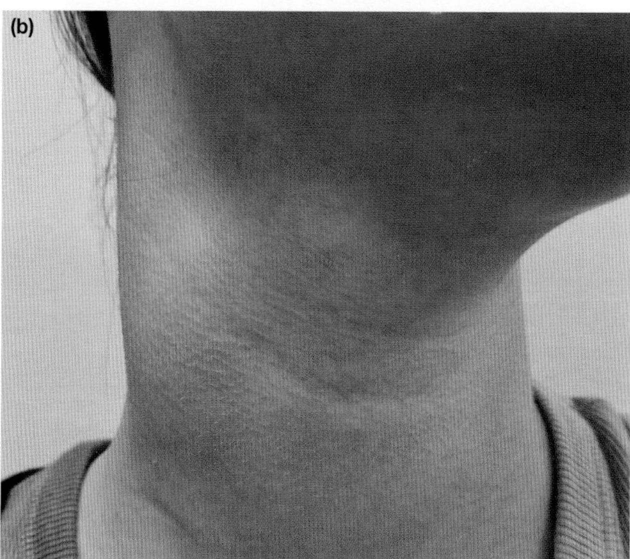

Figure 52.63 Right branchial cyst: anterior **(a)** and oblique **(b)** views.

Branchial fistula

A branchial fistula (*Figure 52.64*) may be unilateral or bilateral and is thought to represent a persistent second branchial cleft. The external orifice is nearly always situated in the lower third of the neck near the anterior border of the sternocleidomastoid muscle, while the internal orifice is located on the anterior aspect of the posterior faucial pillar just behind the tonsil. Although the anterior aspect of the tract is easy to dissect, it may pass backwards and upwards through the bifurcation of the common carotid artery as far as the pharyngeal constrictors. The internal aspect of the tract may, however, end blindly at or close to the lateral pharyngeal wall, constituting a sinus rather than a fistula. The tract is lined by ciliated columnar epithelium and, as such, there may be a small amount of recurrent mucopurulent discharge onto the neck. The tract follows the same path as a branchial cyst and requires complete excision to avoid recurrence.

Cystic hygroma

Cystic hygromas (*Figure 52.65*) usually present in the neonate or in early infancy, and occasionally may present at birth and be so large as to obstruct labour. The cysts are filled with clear lymph and lined by a single layer of epithelium with a mosaic appearance. Swelling usually occurs in the neck and may involve the face, submandibular region, tongue and floor of the mouth. The swelling may be bilateral and is soft and partially compressible, visibly increasing in size when the child coughs or cries. The characteristic that distinguishes it from all other neck swellings is that it is brilliantly transilluminant. The cheek, axilla, groin and mediastinum are other less frequent sites for a cystic hygroma.

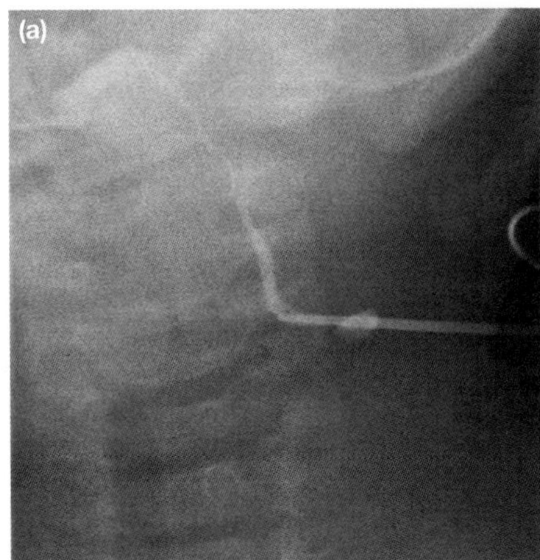

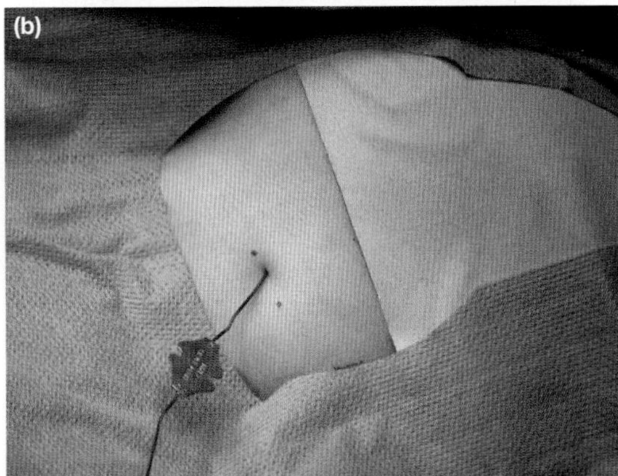

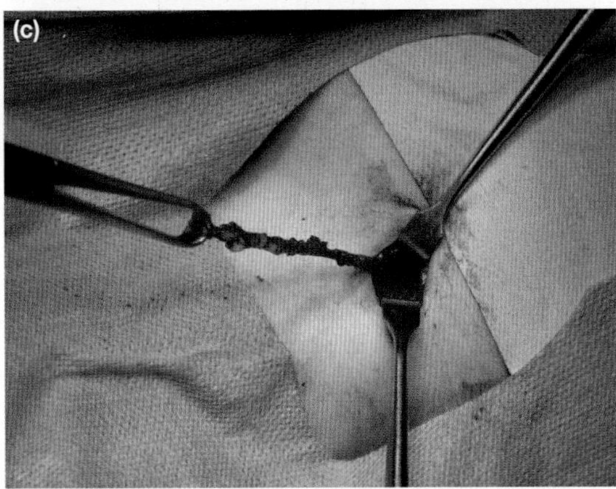

Figure 52.64 (a) Plain radiograph with radio-opaque dye in the fistula tract. (b) Probing of the fistula tract. (c) Excision of the fistula tract.

The behaviour of cystic hygromas during infancy is unpredictable. Sometimes the cyst expands rapidly and occasionally respiratory difficulty ensues, requiring immediate aspiration and even occasionally a tracheostomy. The cyst may become infected.

Definitive treatment involving complete excision of the cyst at an early stage is best if possible. Injection of a sclerosing agent is an alternative strategy and may reduce the size of the cyst; however, they are commonly multicystic and therefore complete resolution is a challenge.

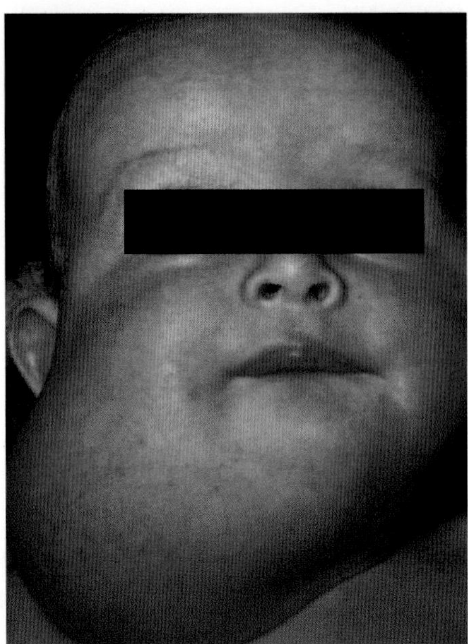

Figure 52.65 Cystic hygroma.

Thyroglossal duct cysts

Embryology

The thyroid gland descends early in fetal life from the base of the tongue towards its position in the lower neck with the isthmus lying over the second and third tracheal rings. At the time of its descent, the hyoid bone has not been formed and the track of the descent of the thyroid gland is variable, passing in front, through or behind the eventual position of the hyoid body. Thyroglossal duct cysts represent a persistence of this track and may therefore be found anywhere in or adjacent to the midline from the tongue base to the thyroid isthmus. Rarely, what appears to be a thyroglossal cyst is an incompletely migrated thyroid gland that contains the only functioning thyroid tissue in the body. Ultrasound neck imaging is used to confirm a cyst and the presence of a thyroid gland in the normal location.

Clinical features

The cysts almost always arise in the midline but, when they are adjacent to the thyroid cartilage, they may lie slightly to one side of the midline. Classically, the cyst moves upwards on swallowing and with tongue protrusion, but this can also occur with other midline cysts such as dermoid cysts, as it merely indicates attachment to the hyoid bone.

Thyroglossal cysts may become infected and rupture onto the skin of the neck, presenting as a discharging sinus. Although they often occur in children, they may also present in adults, even as late as the sixth or seventh decade of life (***Figure 52.66***).

Treatment

Treatment must include excision of the whole thyroglossal tract, which involves removal of the body of the hyoid bone and

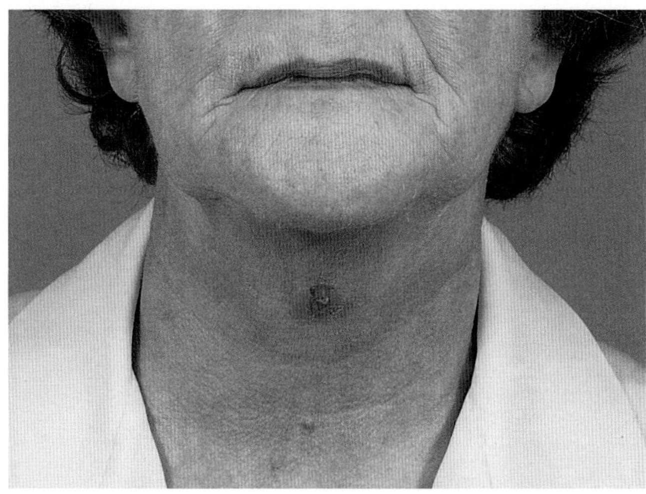

Figure 52.66 A patient with a thyroglossal fistula from a cyst in the midline of the neck.

the suprahyoid tract through the tongue base to the vallecula at the site of the primitive foramen caecum, together with a core of tissue on either side. This operation is known as Sistrunk's operation and minimises recurrence, most notably from small side branches of the thyroglossal tract.

TRAUMA TO THE NECK

The management of penetrating neck trauma depends on the structures that have been injured. The neck is classified into three zones for this purpose (***Table 52.3***). (Note: this is different from the levels used to describe cervical lymphadenopathy.) The majority of injuries occur commonly in zone 2. Critical clinical assessment coupled with appropriate imaging such as a CT scan or CT angiogram is crucial in managing these patients.

TABLE 52.3 The zones of the neck and structures contained within.

Zone	Boundary	Structures within
1	From clavicle/ sternal notch to cricoid cartilage	Trachea, oesophagus, innominate artery, arch of aorta, brachial plexus, thoracic duct, carotid artery
2	From cricoid cartilage to angle of mandible	Larynx, hypopharynx, carotid artery (common/internal/external), internal jugular vein, sympathetic plexus, recurrent laryngeal nerve
3	From angle of mandible to skull base	Facial nerve, carotid artery (internal/branches of external), jugular vein

Wounds above the hyoid bone

The cavity of the mouth or pharynx may have been entered and the epiglottis may be transected. These wounds require repair with absorbable sutures under a general anaesthetic. If there is any degree of associated oedema or bleeding, particularly in relation to the tongue base or laryngeal inlet, it is advisable to perform a tracheostomy to avoid any subsequent airway compromise.

Wounds of the thyroid and cricoid cartilage

Blunt crushing injuries or severe laceration injuries to the laryngeal skeleton can cause marked haematoma formation or swelling and rapid loss of the airway. There may be significant disruption of the laryngeal skeleton. These patients should not have an endotracheal intubation for any length of time, even if this is the initial emergency way of protecting the airway. The larynx is a delicate three-tiered sphincter and the presence of a foreign body in its lumen after severe disruption gives rise to major fibrosis and loss of laryngeal function. These injuries frequently require a low tracheostomy, following which the larynx can be carefully explored, damaged cartilages repositioned and sutured or plated and the paraglottic space drained.

An indwelling stent of soft sponge shaped to fit the laryngeal lumen and held by a nylon retaining suture through the neck may be left in place for 5–10 days to minimise webbing. This stent can be removed endoscopically after cutting the retaining suture and, as the laryngeal damage heals, the patient may then be decannulated.

Division of the trachea

Wounds of the trachea are rare. They should all be formally explored and, to obtain adequate exposure, it is usually necessary to divide and ligate the thyroid isthmus. A small tracheostomy below the wound followed by repair of the trachea with a limited number of submucosal sutures is appropriate. In self-inflicted wounds, the recurrent laryngeal nerves, which lie protected in the tracheo-oesophageal grooves, are rarely injured. Primary repair of the nerve is rarely possible but may be undertaken at the time of formal exploration of a major neck wound.

Neurovascular injury

Penetrating wounds of the neck may involve the common carotid or the external or internal carotid arteries. Major haemorrhagic shock may occur. Venous air embolism may occur because of damage to one of the major veins, most commonly the internal jugular. Compression, resuscitation and exploration under general anaesthetic, with control of vessels above and below the injury and primary repair, should be undertaken. All cervical nerves are vulnerable to injury, particularly the vagus and recurrent laryngeal nerves and cervical sympathetic chain.

Thoracic duct injury

Wounds to the thoracic duct are usually iatrogenic and usually left sided, occurring when lymph node level IV is dissected during a neck dissection. When damage to the duct is not

Walter Ellis Sistrunk Jr, 1880–1933, Professor of Clinical Surgery, Baylor University College of Medicine, Dallas, TX, USA.

recognised at the time of operation, chyle may subsequently leak from the wound in amounts up to 2 L/day with profound effects on nutrition.

Should the damage be recognised during an operation, the proximal end of the duct must be ligated. Ligation of the duct is not harmful because there are a number of anastomotic channels between the lymphatic and venous systems in the lower neck. If undetected, chyle usually starts to discharge from the neck wound within 24 hours of the operation. Low-flow chyle leaks (less than 500 mL/day) can be managed conservatively with a low-fat diet and systemic octreotide. The patient's fluid and electrolyte balance must be closely monitored. Total parenteral nutrition and surgical re-exploration may be warranted in high-output leaks.

INFLAMMATORY CONDITIONS OF THE NECK

Ludwig's angina

Ludwig described a clinical entity characterised by a brawny swelling of the submandibular region combined with inflammatory oedema of the mouth. These clinical features, as well as accompanying putrid halitosis, define the condition.

The infection is often caused by a virulent streptococcal infection associated with anaerobic organisms. There may also be an underlying oral cavity cancer. The infection tracks deep to the mylohyoid muscle, causing oedema and inflammation such that the tongue is displaced upwards and backwards, giving rise to dysphagia and subsequently to painful obstruction of the airway. Unless treated, cellulitis may extend beneath the deep fascial layers of the neck to involve the larynx, causing glottic oedema and further airway compromise.

Antibiotic therapy should be instituted as soon as possible using intravenous broad-spectrum antibiotics, with anaerobic cover. If the swelling does not subside rapidly with such treatment, or in advanced cases where pus is evident, a curved submental incision may be used to drain both submandibular triangles. The mylohyoid muscle may be incised to decompress the floor of the mouth and corrugated drains placed in the wound, which is then lightly sutured. Although this operation may be conducted under local anaesthetic, a general anaesthetic approach is preferred as it provides a more controlled setting, allowing for optimal exposure and drainage without undue stress to the patient. Rarely, a tracheostomy may be necessary.

Cervical lymphadenitis

Cervical lymphadenitis is common owing to infection or inflammation in the oral and nasal cavities, pharynx, larynx, ear, scalp and face.

Acute lymphadenitis

The affected lymph nodes are enlarged and tender, and there may be varying degrees of general constitutional disturbance such as pyrexia, anorexia and general malaise. The treatment in the first instance is directed to the primary focus of infection, for example tonsillitis or a dental abscess.

Chronic lymphadenitis

Chronic, painless lymphadenopathy may be caused by TB in young children or adults or be secondary to malignant disease, most commonly from a squamous cell carcinoma in older individuals. Lymphoma and/or HIV infection may also be present in the cervical nodes.

Summary box 52.16

Causes of cervical lymphadenopathy

Inflammatory
- Reactive hyperplasia

Infective
- Viral
  - For example, infectious mononucleosis, HIV
- Bacterial
  - *Streptococcus, Staphylococcus*
  - Actinomycosis
  - TB
  - Brucellosis
- Protozoan
  - Toxoplasmosis

Neoplastic
- Malignant
  - Primary (e.g. lymphoma)
  - Secondary (e.g. squamous cell carcinoma)
    - Known primary
    - Occult primary

Tuberculous adenitis

This condition most commonly affects children or young adults but can occur at any age. The deep upper cervical nodes are most commonly affected, but there may be a widespread cervical lymphadenitis with matted nodes. In most cases, the tubercular bacilli gain entrance through the ipsilateral tonsil. In approximately 80% of patients, the tuberculous process is limited to the clinically affected group of lymph nodes, but a primary focus in the lungs must always be suspected.

Rarely, the patient may develop a natural resistance to the infection and the nodes may be detected at a later date, as evidenced by calcification on radiography. This can also be seen after appropriate general treatment of TB adenitis. If treatment is not instituted, the caseated node may liquefy and break down with the formation of a cold abscess in the neck. The pus is initially confined by the deep cervical fascia, but after weeks or months this may become eroded at one point and the pus flows through the small opening into the space beneath the superficial fascia. The process has now reached the well-known stage of a 'collar-stud' abscess. The superficial abscess enlarges steadily and, unless suitably treated, a discharging sinus results.

Wilhelm Friedrich von Ludwig, 1790–1865, Professor of Surgery and Midwifery, Tübingen, Germany.

Investigation

Fine-needle aspirate taken from neck nodes with a suspicion of TB should be tested for the presence of acid-fast bacilli. Systemic investigation should not be neglected, with a chest radiograph and tuberculin skin test (Mantoux) useful as first-line investigations. The drawback of the Mantoux test is the poor sensitivity in immunocompromised patients and low specificity in patients with prior bacille Calmette–Guérin (BCG) vaccination.

The interferon-γ release assay (QuantiFERON®-TB Gold In-Tube; QFT-GIT; Cellestis, Carnegie, Australia) with T-SPOT®.*TB* (Oxford Immunotec, Abingdon, UK), in contrast, is more specific than a Mantoux test as the results are not confounded by previous BCG vaccination. This blood test measures the cellular immune response to antigens derived from *Mycobacterium tuberculosis*. Although active or latent infection cannot be specifically differentiated with this test, a positive test in a patient with negative clinical and radiological evidence of TB indicates latent TB infection. Depending on the country of origin, where TB is diagnosed or suspected, the coexistence of other infectious diseases such as HIV and malaria should not be overlooked.

Treatment

The patient should be treated using appropriate chemotherapy, dependent on the sensitivities derived from the abscess contents. If an abscess fails to resolve despite appropriate chemotherapy and general measures, occasionally excision of the abscess and its surrounding fibrous capsule is necessary, together with the relevant lymph nodes. If there is active TB of another system, for example pulmonary TB, then removal of tuberculous lymph nodes in the neck is inappropriate. The matted nodes are associated with significant fibrosis, making surgery difficult to the extent that the sacrifice of adjacent structures such as the internal jugular vein or sternocleidomastoid muscle may be necessary. The resected nodes should be sent for both histology and microbiology.

PRIMARY TUMOURS OF THE NECK

Neurogenic tumours

Paraganglioma (carotid body tumour)

This is a rare tumour that has a higher incidence in areas where people live at high altitudes because of chronic hypoxia leading to carotid body hyperplasia. The tumours most commonly present in the fifth decade. Approximately 10% of patients have a family history, with familial cases caused by mutations in the genes for succinate dehydrogenase (SDH) enzyme. There is an association with phaeochromocytoma in familial cases, and thus appropriate tests should be undertaken to rule out synchronous catecholamine-secreting tumours during the work-up. The tumours arise from the chemoreceptor cells on the medial side of the carotid bulb and, at this point, the tumour is adherent to the carotid wall. These tumours are usually benign with only a small number of cases producing proven metastases (***Figures 52.67 and 52.68***).

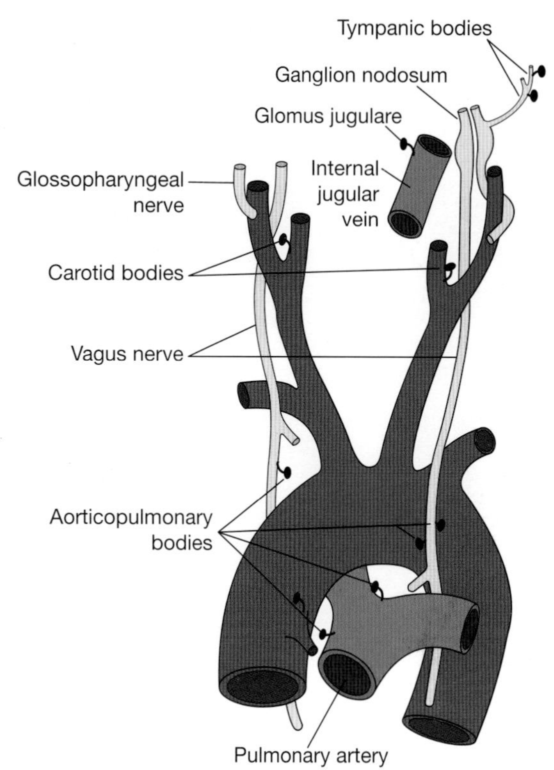

Figure 52.67 Sites for chemodectomas.

Clinical features

There is often a long history of a slowly enlarging, painless lump at the carotid bifurcation. About one-third of patients present with a pharyngeal mass that pushes the tonsil medially and anteriorly. The mass is firm, rubbery, pulsatile, mobile from side to side but not up and down and can sometimes be emptied by firm pressure, after which it slowly refills in a pulsatile manner. A bruit may also be present. Swellings in the parapharyngeal space, which often displace the tonsil medially, should not be biopsied from within the mouth.

Investigations

When a paraganglioma is suspected, a carotid angiogram can be carried out to demonstrate the carotid bifurcation, which is usually splayed, and a blush, which outlines the tumour vessels. MRI scanning also provides excellent detail in most cases. This tumour must not be biopsied and fine-needle aspiration is also contraindicated.

Charles Mantoux, 1877–1947, physician, Le Cannet, Alpes Maritimes, France, described the intradermal tuberculin skin test in 1908.
Albert Leon Charles Calmette, 1863–1933, and **Jean-Marie Camille Guérin**, 1872–1961, microbiologists at the Institute Pasteur, Lille, France, introduced the bacille Calmette–Guérin in 1908.

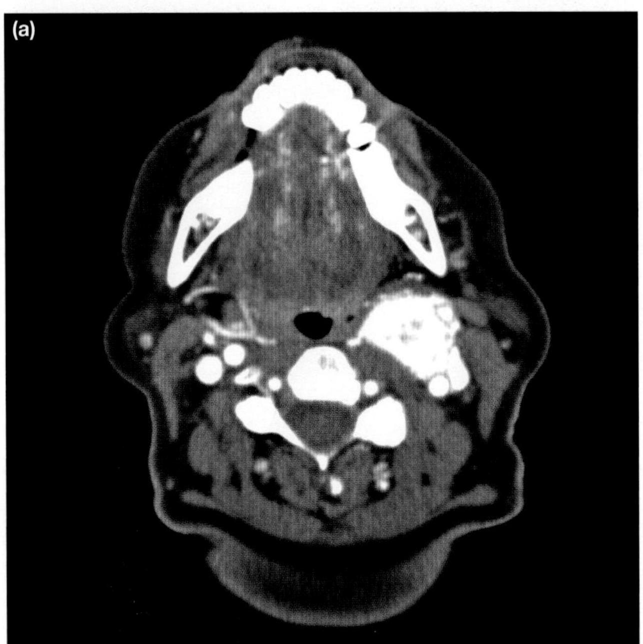

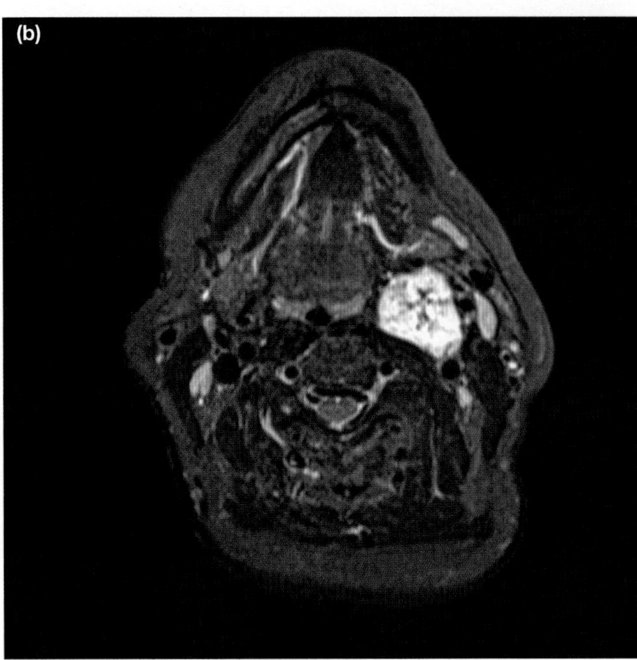

Figure 52.68 Axial view computed tomography angiogram (a) and magnetic resonance imaging (b) demonstrating a left carotid body tumour.

Treatment

The Shamblin classification is used to determine the surgical resectability of these tumours. Type I tumours are localised and do not involve more than 180° of the carotid vessels; type II tumours surround the vessel by over 180°; and type III tumours completely encase the vessels and are more challenging to resect with higher complications and a possible need for vessel reconstruction.

Because these tumours rarely metastasise and their overall rate of growth is slow, the need for surgical removal must be considered carefully as complications of surgery are potentially serious. The operation is best avoided in elderly patients. Radiotherapy will not cure the tumour but can prevent further growth. In some cases it may be possible to dissect the tumour away from the carotid bifurcation but, at times, when the tumour is large, it may not be separable from the vessels and resection will be necessary, such that all appropriate facilities should be available to establish a bypass while a vein autograft is inserted to restore arterial continuity in the carotid system.

Vagal body tumours

Vagal paragangliomas arise from nests of paraganglionic tissue of the vagus nerve just below the base of the skull near the jugular foramen. They may also be found at various sites along the nerve down to the level of the carotid artery bifurcation. They also present as slowly growing and painless masses in the anterolateral aspect of the neck, and may also have a long history, commonly of 2–3 years, before diagnosis. They may spread into the cranial cavity. Diagnosis is confirmed by CT and MRI scanning and additional MRA or arteriography if necessary. Treatment is surgical excision following appropriate consent of resulting hoarseness.

Peripheral nerve tumours

Schwannomas are solitary and encapsulated tumours attached to or surrounded by nerve, although paralysis of the associated nerve is unusual. The vagus nerve is the most common site. Neurofibromas also arise from the Schwann cell and may be part of von Recklinghausen's syndrome of multiple neurofibromatosis. Multiple neurofibromatosis is an autosomal dominant, hereditary disease; the neurofibromas may be present at birth and are often multiple.

Diagnosis requires CT or MRI scanning to differentiate them from other parapharyngeal tumours but, on occasions, the diagnosis must wait until excision (***Figure 52.69***).

Secondary carcinoma

Metastatic spread of squamous cell carcinoma to the cervical lymph nodes is a common occurrence from head and neck primary cancers; occasionally, this may be the sole presenting feature of the disease (***Figure 52.70***). The upper aerodigestive tract mucosa must be carefully examined for a primary site before considering surgery to the neck nodes. When a primary site is not seen on clinical examination, they are most often found in the oropharynx. Appropriate radiological

William R Shamblin, Mayo Graduate School of Medicine (University of Minnesota), Rochester, MN, USA, described this classification in 1971.
Friedrich Theodor Schwann, 1810–1882, Professor of Anatomy and Physiology, successively at Louvain (1839–1848) and Liège (1848–1880), Belgium, described the neurilemma in 1839.
Friedrich Daniel von Recklinghausen, 1833–1910, Professor of Pathology, Strasbourg, France, described generalised neurofibromatosis in 1882.

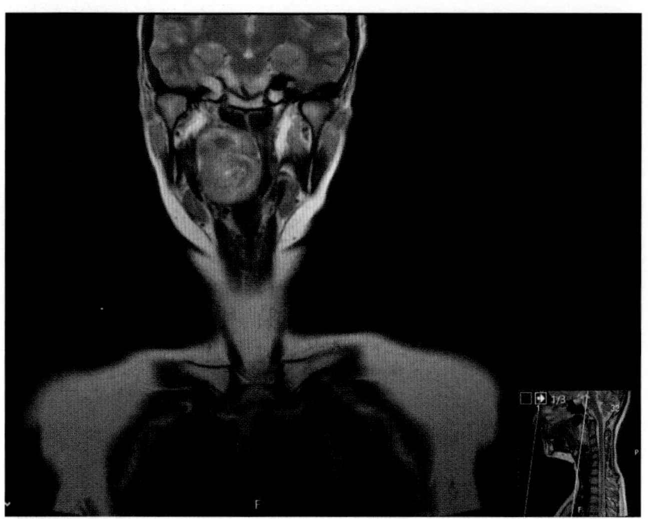

Figure 52.69 Magnetic resonance imaging scan demonstrating a large parapharyngeal tumour. The imaging characteristics of the tumour suggested a paraganglioma or a schwannoma. Resection confirmed the latter.

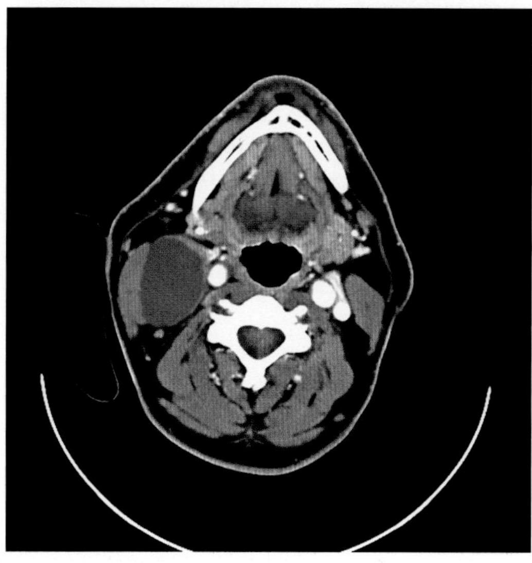

Figure 52.70 Axial computed tomography scan demonstrating a large cystic metastatic node from an unknown primary. Core biopsy confirmed a squamous cell cancer.

investigations (MRI, PET-CT) must be undertaken to define subclinical primaries, as management will be dictated by this. If radiological assessment shows no primaries, tonsillectomy and robot-assisted tongue base mucosectomy are performed as a diagnostic procedure because the oropharynx is the most common site for a clinically and radiologically unknown primary cancer.

Management

The management of malignant cervical lymph nodes depends on the overall treatment regime:

- if surgery is being used to treat the primary disease and the cervical nodes are palpable and <3 cm, they may be excised with the primary lesion as part of a neck dissection;
- if radiotherapy or chemoradiotherapy is used initially with resolution of the primary tumour, but there is subsequent residual or recurrent nodal disease, then this situation will require cervical lymph node dissection.

Type of neck dissection

Classical radical neck dissection (Crile)

The classic operation involves resection of the cervical lymph nodes (levels I–V) and those structures closely associated: the internal jugular vein, the accessory nerve, the submandibular gland and the sternocleidomastoid muscle. These structures are all removed en bloc and in continuity with the primary disease if possible. The main disability that follows the operation is weakness and drooping of the shoulder due to paralysis of the trapezius muscle as a consequence of excision of the accessory nerve. Bulky nodal disease may dictate the need for a radical neck dissection, but this operation is less commonly performed owing to a better understanding of the lymphatic drainage of the primary sites and as most patients with advanced disease need adjuvant radiation.

Modified radical neck dissection

This term denotes a procedure in which one or more of the non-lymphatic structures are preserved (the accessory nerve, the sternocleidomastoid muscle or the internal jugular vein) with clearance of all nodal levels (I–V).

Selective neck dissection

In this type of dissection, one or more of the major lymph node groups is preserved along with the sternocleidomastoid muscle, accessory nerve and internal jugular vein. In these circumstances, the exact groups of nodes excised must be documented.

It must be noted that, when neck dissections are performed for residual disease after (chemo)radiation therapy, the neck is often fibrotic and scarred and the operation may not fall into any of the above categories. For instance, lymph nodes in levels II and III may be removed, along with the sternomastoid muscle for access; thus, meticulous annotation of the procedure is more important than ascribing a name to the operation.

SUMMARY

The anatomical and physiological performance of the pharyngolarynx is involved in the important mechanisms of breathing, coughing, voice production and swallowing. A variety of congenital, traumatic, infectious and neoplastic conditions disturb these functions, giving rise to the common symptoms of pain, swelling, hoarseness, dyspnoea and dysphagia.

Squamous cell carcinomas are the most common malignancies, accounting for approximately 80% of all head and

George Washington Crile, 1864–1943, Professor of Surgery, The Western Reserve University, and one of the founders of the Cleveland Clinic, Cleveland, OH, USA.

neck tumours. Their incidence and anatomical site vary around the world, but they are mainly caused by the preventable aetiological agents of smoking and alcohol, although nasopharyngeal and oropharyngeal squamous cell carcinomas have additional genetic and environmental factors. All head and neck cancers have a high morbidity and mortality and require expert treatment.

FURTHER READING

Bull P, Clarke R. *Diseases of the ear, nose and throat.* Oxford: Blackwell, 2007.

Dhillon R, East C. *Nose and throat, head and neck surgery*, 4th edn. Amsterdam: Elsevier, 2013.

Lau A, Jacques T, Tandon S, Lesser T. *Evidence-based emergency ENT care.* Scotts Valley, CA: Createspace, 2015.

Paleri V, Roland NJ (eds). Head and neck cancer: United Kingdom national multidisciplinary guidelines. *J Laryngol Otol* 2016; **130**(S2): S3–224.

Paleri V, Jones TM, Woolford T, White N (eds). Volume 3: Head and neck surgery. In Watkinson JC, Clarke RW (eds). *Scott-Brown's otorhinolaryngology and head and neck surgery*, 8th edn. Boca Raton, FL: CRC Press, 2018.

Probst R, Grevers G, Iro H. *Basic otorhinolaryngology.* Stuttgart: Georg Thieme, 2006.

Wackym PA, Snow JB (eds). *Ballenger's otorhinolaryngology head and neck surgery*, 18th edn. Raleigh, NC: PMPH, 2016.

Watkinson JC, Clarke RW (eds). *Scott-Brown's otorhinolaryngology and head and neck surgery*, 8th edn. Boca Raton, FL: CRC Press, 2018.

Watkinson J, Gilbert RW (eds). *Stell & Marans textbook of head and neck surgery and oncology*, 5th edn. London: Hodder & Arnold, 2012.

CHAPTER 53 Oral cavity cancer

Learning objectives

To understand:

- The epidemiology and aetiology of oral cancer
- The cardinal features of malignant lesions of the oral cavity (signs and symptoms)
- Broad steps necessary for investigation and management of oral cavity cancers

INTRODUCTION

The oral cavity (***Figure 53.1***) extends from the mucosal surface of the lips to the junction of the hard and soft palate. It does not include the soft palate, uvula or tonsils, which form part of the oropharynx. Oral cavity cancer is the eighth most common cancer worldwide, with an estimated 350 000 cases arising annually. While there have been significant advances in the understanding and management of oral cavity cancer, the morbidity and prognosis associated with it have remained largely unchanged. In this chapter, we will outline the aetiology and epidemiology of oral cavity cancer, as well as risk factors for this disease, and highlight important geographical variations. Additionally, we will explore the investigation and management of oral cavity cancer. Lastly, we will outline emerging techniques and technologies utilised in oral cavity cancer treatment.

EPIDEMIOLOGY

There is considerable geographical variation in the incidence of oral cancers worldwide, reflecting differing lifestyles and risk factor exposure.

For clarity, and in keeping with the 11th revision of the *International Classification of Diseases* (ICD-11), we will include cancers of the lip, gum, tongue, palate and floor of the mouth as well as the rest of the mouth in oral cavity cancer. Cancers of the nasopharynx, hypopharynx and major salivary glands are excluded. The oropharynx includes the base of the tongue, the soft palate/uvula, the pharyngeal walls and the tonsils. Cancers arising in the oropharynx are discussed separately in ***Chapter 52***.

Incidence

There are approximately 350 000 new cases of oral cavity cancer per year worldwide. The vast majority of these are squamous cell carcinomas (SCCs). In 2015, the estimated age-standardised ratio of oral cavity cancer was 5.8 in men and 2.3 in women per 100 000. This 2:1 ratio has narrowed recently but still probably reflects the higher consumption of alcohol and tobacco by men worldwide. Two-thirds of all oral cancers occur in low-income countries, with half of those in South Asia. India, for example, has 100 000 new cases per annum.

Rates of oral cancer vary significantly worldwide. High-incidence areas include South East Asia, Papua New Guinea, parts of western Europe (e.g. Portugal and France), parts of eastern Europe (e.g. Slovakia and Hungary), as well as areas in Latin America (e.g. Brazil).

The incidence of oral cancer increases with age, with most cases occurring in those over 50 years. The mean age at presentation is 62 years, with a strong correlation between lower socioeconomic class and disease incidence. However, there is an increasing trend for cases affecting younger patients (45 years or younger), many of whom lack exposure to traditional risk factors.

The 5-year survival rate for early-stage cancers is 80%. Despite recent advances, the overall 5-year survival for oral cancer has not markedly improved and remains at 50%. In South Asia, this figure is often below 50%, with a reported 5-year survival of 35% in India.

Regional variations

Oral cancer is one of the most common cancers in India, with an age-adjusted incidence rate of 20 per 100 000.[1] The disease accounts for over one-third of all cancers in India. In contrast to western populations, cancers of the buccogingival/retromolar area account for over 40% of cancers in India and South East Asia, reflecting the commonplace use of the known carcinogens betel quid/gutka, along with smokeless tobacco.

In Europe, there is significant variation reflecting the varying cultures and lifestyles, especially between eastern and western Europe. Eastern Europe has one of the highest age-standardised incidence rates of oral cancer worldwide, with Hungary recording the highest rates. In these populations,

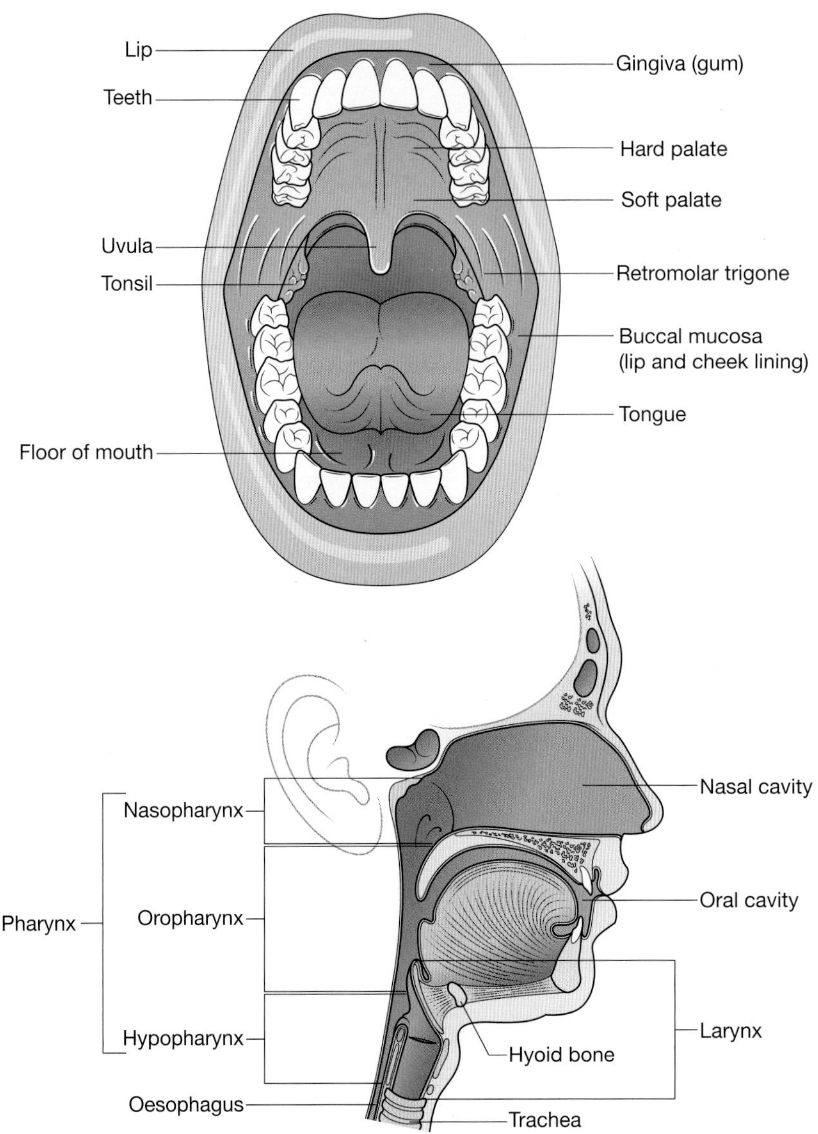

Figure 53.1 The oral cavity.

the lateral border of the tongue and the floor of the mouth constitute particularly high-risk sites.

In the USA, Surveillance, Epidemiology, and End Results (SEER) Program statistics indicate that the age-adjusted rate for oral cancer is 11.2 per 100 000 per year, while the number of deaths is 2.5 per 100 000 per year.

Risk factors

Tobacco, alcohol and betel quid (areca nut, catechu, slaked lime wrapped in a piper betel leaf) are long-established risk factors for oral cavity squamous cell carcinoma (OCSCC). There is a dose–response relationship between the use of tobacco, alcohol and betel quid and the development of oral cancer.

Transcriptionally active human papillomavirus (HPV) accounts for only a small percentage (approximately 5%) of OCSCCs, which is in stark contrast to oropharyngeal squamous cell cancers (OPSCCs), where 50–70% are caused by HPV. Although HPV-positive SCC has prognostic significance in the oropharynx (see ***Chapter 52***), this survival advantage does not appear to be conferred within the oral cavity.

Other risk factors include previous exposure to radiation, chronic infection, immunosuppression and hereditary conditions such as Fanconi anaemia and Li–Fraumeni syndrome.

Guido Fanconi, 1892–1979, Swiss paediatrician, named several conditions, including Fanconi anaemia, a rare genetic disorder of DNA repair leading to bone marrow failure and the development of haematological and solid malignancies typically within early life.

Frederick Pei Li, 1940–2015, Boston, MA, USA, and **Joseph F Fraumeni Jr**, b. 1933, National Institutes of Health, Bethesda, MD, USA, described a familial syndrome of soft-tissue sarcomas, breast cancer and other malignancies in 1969.

Summary box 53.1

Risk factors for oral cavity malignancy

- Smoking
- Alcohol
- Betel quid
- HPV
- Hereditary conditions
- Immunosuppression
- Chronic infection
- Potentially/premalignant lesions

Premalignant lesions

The majority of oral cancers do not originate from a pre-existing lesion. However, there are a group of oral premalignant lesions, or more accurately described potentially malignant lesions, that are mucosal abnormalities from which oral cancer can arise. These lesions include leukoplakia, erythroplakia, erythroleukoplakia, proliferative verrucous leukoplakia (PVL), oral submucous fibrosis, oral lichen planus and lupus erythematosus, as well as inherited conditions such as epidermolysis bullosa and dyskeratosis congenita. A leukoplakia is a white patch or plaque that cannot be rubbed off, while an erythroplakia is a bright red velvety plaque, neither of which can be characterised clinically or pathologically as any other recognisable condition. A speckled leukoplakia or erythroleukoplakia is essentially a combination of both; it carries the greatest risk for malignant change.

The management of premalignant lesions is challenging, not least because of an inconsistency with nomenclature internationally but also because the natural history of these lesions remains unclear.

The reported rates of malignant transformation vary widely between studies and countries. A systematic review of observational studies in 2016 reported that malignant transformation in oral leukoplakia could vary from 0.13% to 34.0%.[2]

Risk assessment forms the cornerstone of the management of these lesions. Among these lesions, erythroleukoplakia, PVL and dyskeratosis congenita carry the highest risk for malignant transformation. Clinical factors to be considered include size, location and lifestyle exposure to known carcinogens. Biopsy of lesions is advocated for accurate pathological diagnosis as well as to ascertain the degree of dysplasia (mild, moderate, severe), or indeed the presence of malignancy in a lesion.

Summary box 53.2

Factors associated with increased risk for malignant change in pre-existing (dysplastic) lesions

- Female sex
- Size >200 mm^2
- Non-homogeneous lesion
- Non-smoker
- Presence of multiple lesions
- Location (e.g. lateral border of tongue/floor of mouth)

It should be pointed out that surgical removal of a premalignant or dysplastic lesion does not completely remove the risk of transformation and as such appropriate surveillance regimes are necessary.

Molecular biology

According to The Cancer Genome Atlas (TCGA), alterations in *p53* (83%) and *CDKN2A* (57%) are the two most frequent genomic mutations noted in HPV-negative cancers of the head and neck (of which oral cancer is an example). This contrasts with HPV-positive tumours, found most frequently in the oropharynx, which have a considerably lower mutational burden and consistently retain *p53* 'wild-type' status. It is, however, important to note that, as yet, the current standard of care in head and neck squamous cell carcinoma (HNSCC), including oral cavity cancers, is not based on or influenced by genetic profiling or molecular biology.

STAGING

Staging is required to document tumour size, location and disease extent, as well as to formulate a treatment plan and facilitate discussion of prognosis with the patient. Additionally, it is an important tool for comparative outcome reporting. The eighth edition of the Union for International Cancer Control (UICC)/American Joint Committee on Cancer (AJCC) tumour–node–metastasis (TNM) staging manual (***Table 53.1***) has introduced changes in how oral cavity cancers are staged. The most significant updates for oral cancer are: (i) the inclusion of depth of invasion (DOI) as an element for determining the T stage of primary tumours and (ii) recognition of extranodal extension (ENE) as a feature necessitating upstaging of nodal disease. This recognition of additional negative prognostic factors in the eighth edition should allow improved stratification of outcomes for patients.

T stage

The size and extent of tumours are typically determined by thorough clinical examination (supported by examination under anaesthesia [EUA] where necessary) and by radiographic assessment with cross-sectional imaging (e.g. computed tomography [CT], magnetic resonance imaging [MRI]). While the DOI can be estimated radiologically, it remains a pathologically determined feature from a surgically resected specimen. ***Figure 53.2*** illustrates the influence that T stage, and therefore depth of invasion, has on overall survival.

N stage

The system for describing the anatomy of regional lymph node metastases has been well described previously and is outlined in ***Figure 53.3***. It divides the lateral neck nodes into five separate levels, based on their relationship to certain anatomical structures.

SCC in the oral cavity and lips tends to metastasise to lymph nodes at levels I, II and III. However, with SCC of the

TABLE 53.1 Outline of the T category from the American Joint Committee on Cancer (AJCC) tumour–node–metastasis (TNM) staging manual, 8th edition.

T category	T criteria
TX	Primary tumour cannot be assessed
Tis	Carcinoma *in situ*
T1	Tumour ≤2 cm, ≤5 mm DOI
T2	Tumour ≤2 cm, DOI >5 mm and ≤10 mm *or* tumour >2 cm but ≤4 cm, and ≤10 mm DOI
T3	Tumour >4 cm *or* any tumour >10 mm DOI
T4	Moderately advanced or very advanced local disease
T4a	Moderately advanced local disease: (lip) tumour invades through cortical bone or involves the inferior alveolar nerve, floor of mouth or skin of face (i.e. chin or nose); (oral cavity) tumour invades adjacent structures only (e.g. through cortical bone of the mandible or maxilla, or involves the maxillary sinus or skin of the face); note that superficial erosion of bone/tooth socket (alone) by a gingival primary is not sufficient to classify a tumour as T4
T4b	Very advanced local disease; tumour invades masticator space, pterygoid plates or skull base and/or encases the internal carotid artery

DOI, depth of invasion (not tumour thickness).

Reproduced with permission from AJCC, Chicago, IL, USA. The original source for this material is the *AJCC Cancer Staging Manual*, 8th edition (2017) published by Springer Science+Business Media LLC (springer.com) (Amin MB, Edge SB, Greene FL *et al*. (eds). AJCC *cancer staging manual*, 8th edn. New York, NY: Springer International Publishing: American Joint Commission on Cancer, 2017).

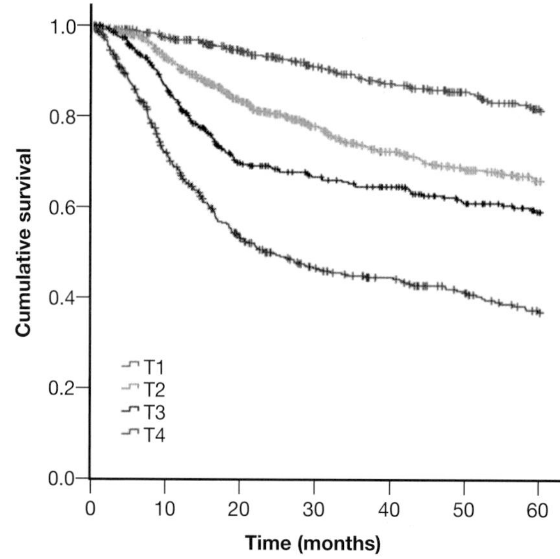

No. of patients	0	12	24	36	48	60
T1	429	376	313	262	222	179
T2	564	460	345	276	233	191
T3	377	286	206	180	151	121
T4	422	256	166	133	108	83

Figure 53.2 The influence that T stage, and therefore depth of invasion, has on overall survival. (Reproduced with permission from AJCC, Chicago, IL, USA. The original source for this material is the *AJCC Cancer Staging Manual*, 8th edition (2017) published by Springer Science+Business Media LLC (springer.com) (Amin MB, Edge SB, Greene FL *et al*. (eds). AJCC *cancer staging manual*, 8th edn. New York, NY: Springer International Publishing: American Joint Commission on Cancer, 2017).)

oral tongue there is a risk of skip metastasis directly to lymph node levels III or IV, without the involvement of higher level lymph node groups. By contrast, tumours arising in the oropharynx commonly metastasise to lymph node levels II–IV, as well as retropharyngeal and contralateral nodal groups. In addition to the number, size and location of involved nodes, ENE has now been included as a contributor to nodal staging (*Table 53.2*). ENE has been reliably shown to be an adverse prognosticator in all oral cavity tumours.

M stage

Routine assessment of the chest (as a minimum) for evidence of distant metastasis and/or synchronous lung primary tumours is the norm as part of staging prior to treatment. M0 denotes no distant metastases, whereas M1 signifies distant metastases present. The presence of any distant metastases automatically places a patient in the stage 4C group, currently without curative therapeutic options.

Prognostic stage groupings

The eighth edition AJCC stage groupings are outlined in *Table 53.3*.

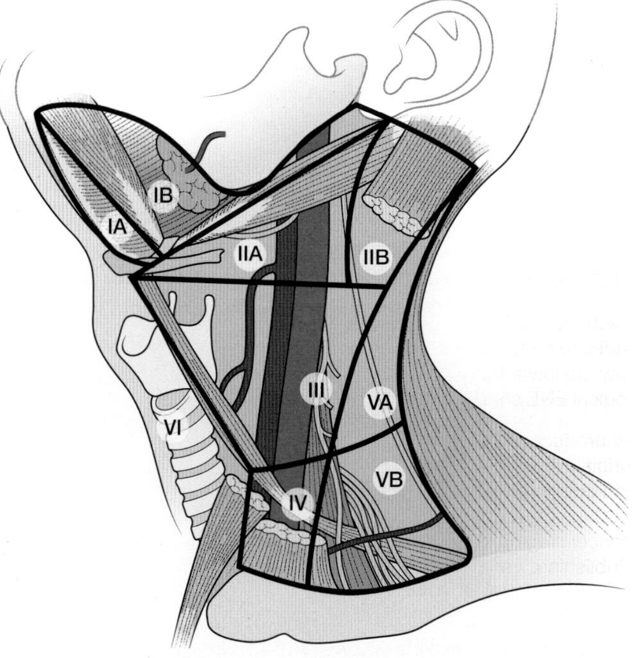

Figure 53.3 Cervical lymph node levels.

TABLE 53.2 Outline of the pathological N category from the American Joint Committee on Cancer (AJCC) tumour–node–metastasis (TNM) staging manual, 8th edition.

N category	N criteria[a]
NX	Regional lymph nodes cannot be assessed
N0	No regional lymph node metastasis
N1	Metastasis in a single ipsilateral lymph node, 3 cm or less in greatest dimension and ENE-negative
N2	Metastasis in a single ipsilateral lymph node, 3 cm or less in greatest dimension and ENE-positive; *or* more than 3 cm but not more than 6 cm in greatest dimension and ENE-negative; *or* metastases in multiple ipsilateral lymph nodes, none more than 6 cm in greatest dimension and ENE-negative; *or* metastases in bilateral or contralateral lymph nodes, none more than 6 cm in greatest dimension and ENE-negative
N2a	Metastasis in a single ipsilateral or contralateral lymph node 3 cm or less in greatest dimension and ENE-positive; *or* metastasis in a single ipsilateral lymph node more than 3 cm but not more than 6 cm in greatest dimension and ENE-negative
N2b	Metastasis in multiple ipsilateral lymph nodes, none more than 6 cm in greatest dimension and ENE-negative
N2c	Metastasis in bilateral or contralateral lymph nodes, none more than 6 cm in greatest dimension and ENE-negative
N3	Metastasis in a lymph node more than 6 cm in greatest dimension and ENE-negative; *or* metastasis in a single ipsilateral lymph node more than 3 cm in greatest dimension and ENE-positive; *or* metastasis in multiple ipsilateral, contralateral or bilateral lymph nodes, with any ENE-positive
N3a	Metastasis in a lymph node more than 6 cm in greatest dimension and ENE-negative
N3b	Metastasis in a single ipsilateral lymph node more than 3 cm in greatest dimension and ENE-positive; *or* metastasis in multiple ipsilateral, contralateral or bilateral lymph nodes, with any ENE-positive

ENE, extranodal extension.

[a]Note that a designation of 'U' or 'L' may be used for any N stage to indicate metastasis above the lower border of the cricoid ('U') or below the lower border of the cricoid ('L'). Similarly, clinical and pathological ENE should be recorded as ENE-negative or ENE-positive.

Reproduced with permission from AJCC, Chicago, IL, USA. The original source for this material is the *AJCC Cancer Staging Manual*, 8th edition (2017) published by Springer Science+Business Media LLC (springer.com) (Amin MB, Edge SB, Greene FL *et al*. (eds). *AJCC cancer staging manual*, 8th edn. New York, NY: Springer International Publishing: American Joint Commission on Cancer, 2017).

TABLE 53.3 Prognostic stage groupings from the American Joint Committee on Cancer (AJCC) tumour–node–metastasis (TNM) staging manual, 8th edition.

Stage	T category	N category	M category
0	Tis	N0	M0
I	T1	N0	M0
II	T2	N0	M0
III	T3 T1, T2, T3	N0 N1	M0 M0
IVA	T4a T1, T2, T3, T4a	N0, N1 N2	M0 M0
IVB	Any T T4b	N3 Any N	M0 M0
IVC	Any T	Any N	M1

Reproduced with permission from AJCC, Chicago, IL, USA. The original source for this material is the *AJCC Cancer Staging Manual*, 8th edition (2017) published by Springer Science+Business Media LLC (springer.com) (Amin MB, Edge SB, Greene FL *et al*. (eds). *AJCC cancer staging manual*, 8th edn. New York, NY: Springer International Publishing: American Joint Commission on Cancer, 2017).

PATHOLOGY OF ORAL CANCERS

The vast majority (>95%) of oral cavity cancers are squamous cell carcinomas (OCSCCs). The World Health Organization (WHO) tumour grading system, based on cellular differentiation, is routinely used in pathological analysis and diagnosis of OCSCC. The histological parameters routinely described in OCSCC include:

- histological type;
- tumour grade/differentiation;
- pattern of invasion;
- tumour thickness and DOI;
- perineural invasion (PNI);
- lymphovascular invasion (LVI);
- bone involvement;
- nodal metastases.

Histological type

The vast majority of OCSCCs are conventional squamous-type carcinomas, reflecting their cell of origin. Other less commonly encountered variants include papillary, adenosquamous, acantholytic, basaloid, spindle cell and verrucous carcinomas, along with carcinoma cuniculatum.

Tumour grade (differentiation)

Often cited as an important prognosticator, the 'WHO grade' is based on Broders' original classification and includes well (G1), moderate (G2) or poorly differentiated (G3) grading. The grade is essentially based on how similar the tumour tissue appears relative to the normal tissue from which it originated.

In general, well-differentiated OCSCCs are less aggressive than their poorly differentiated counterparts, which infiltrate

Albert Compton Broders, 1885–1964, American pathologist, Minnesota, USA, and Chairman of the Department of Surgical Pathology, The Mayo Clinic, Rochester, MN, USA; for 1 year in 1935 Professor of Surgical Pathology and Director of Cancer Research, University of Virginia, VA, USA.

and metastasise more readily. Poorly differentiated tumours carry a worse prognosis.

Pattern of invasion

The pattern of invasion refers to the shape of the advancing front or border of the tumour. Like tumour grade/differentiation, it is of important prognostic value. The UK Royal College of Pathologists recommends the grading of pattern of invasion into two broad categories: cohesive and non-cohesive.

Tumour thickness and depth of invasion

Tumour thickness is measured as the maximum vertical dimension between the tumour surface and the deepest point of invasion. Although frequently used interchangeably with DOI, it is the latter that carries greater importance from a prognostic viewpoint as well as the propensity for metastases. DOI is the distance from the level of the basement membrane of the closest adjacent normal mucosa to the deepest point of the tumour invasion.

Perineural invasion

While there is no clear consensus on the criteria for diagnosing PNI, it is generally described as being present if at least one-third of the circumference of a nerve is surrounded by tumour cells and/or if deposits of tumour are found in any of the three layers of the nerve sheath.

PNI is a marker for the biological aggressiveness of a tumour and an independent risk factor for cervical metastases, local recurrence and therefore poorer prognosis.

Lymphovascular invasion

LVI represents the presence of tumour cells within an endothelium-lined space, irrespective of whether it is a vein or lymph channel.

Bone invasion

Three patterns of bone invasion, namely infiltrative, erosive or mixed, have been described. There is strong evidence that most tumours enter the bone at the point of contact in an erosive fashion, and not via foramina or the periodontal membrane. It is important to point out that cortical erosion as opposed to medullary invasion does not equate to a T4 tumour.

Metastases

As outlined previously, HPV-negative cervical node metastases are associated with decreased overall and disease-specific survival. While skip metastases have been described, most OCSCC metastases occur in levels I and II of the neck. ENE occurs when the capsule is breached and this is now accounted for in the UICC/AJCC eighth edition TNM staging system.

Distant metastases are rare in OCSCCs, with reported rates of 2–9%, and are associated most commonly with ENE and bilateral neck disease.

EXAMINATION, INVESTIGATION, DIAGNOSIS AND WORK-UP

These can be summarised as follows:

- history and examination;
- biopsy;
- clinical and radiographic staging investigations;
- comorbidity and functional status;
- multidisciplinary team (MDT)/tumour board discussion and treatment plan formulation;
- pathological staging;
- adjunctive treatments if appropriate.

When a lesion is suspicious for malignancy, a histopathological diagnosis is essential. Prior to this a thorough history and examination of the oral cavity, oropharynx and neck should be completed.

Radiographic assessment, in the form of a CT and MRI, is also mandatory. In some centres sentinel lymph node biopsy (SLNB) has become an established technique used for investigation and staging of early oral cancers that have no clinical or radiographic evidence for cervical metastases. A positive SLNB necessitates subsequent management of the neck (typically with completion neck dissection).

EUA is often used to further assess a tumour, especially in cases where a biopsy is not possible in the outpatient setting or where the extent of the tumour cannot be properly assessed via clinical examination in an awake patient. An EUA can support treatment planning and decision making with regards to access, extent of resection and reconstructive plans.

Oral cavity

All sites in the oral cavity are examined under direct visualisation. ***Table 53.4*** details the signs and symptoms that are suggestive of a neoplastic process. ***Figure 53.4*** demonstrates the wide clinical presentation of OCSCCs, which range from small areas of (erythro)leukoplakia to larger erosive and cavitated lesions that invade surrounding tissues. Reduced tongue movement, sensory nerve deficit, trismus, otalgia and dysphagia are all in keeping with late-stage disease. Fibreoptic examination is not routinely performed in oral cavity assessment but may support assessment of the posterior extent of the tumour. The incidence of synchronous primary tumours of the upper digestive tract is 2.4–4.5%.

TABLE 53.4 Signs and symptoms of oral cavity neoplasm.

Signs	Symptoms
• Non-healing ulcer (>2 weeks) • Persistent neck mass/ lymphadenopathy • Lesion, pigmentation with progressive increase in size • Lesion with associated induration • Persistent red or white lesion • Non-resolving 'inflammatory' lesion • Soft-tissue lesion with associated radiographic changes • Unexplained tooth mobility	• Sensory nerve deficit • Chronic otalgia • Trismus of unknown aetiology • Dysphagia

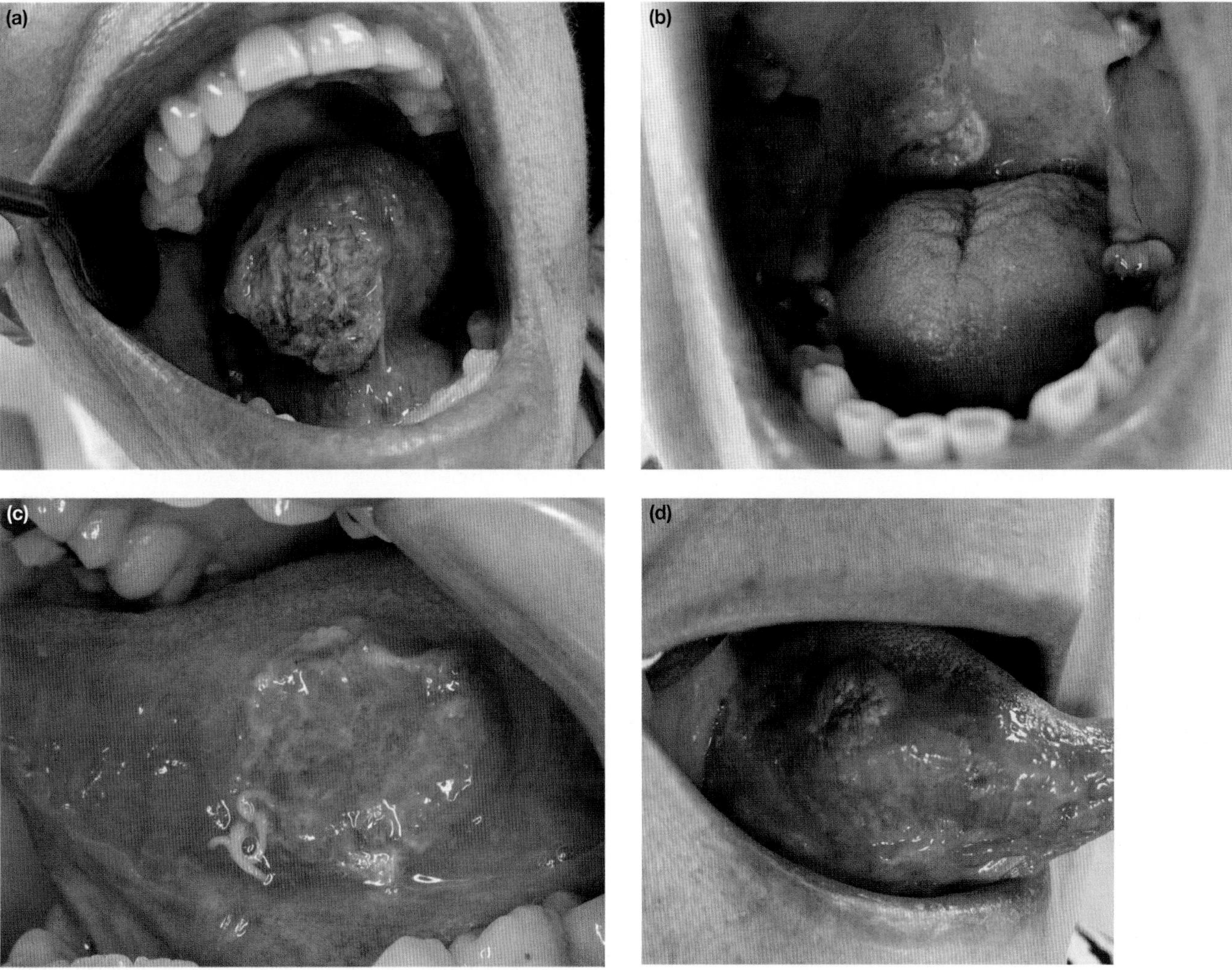

Figure 53.4 Clinical presentations of oral cavity squamous cell carcinoma (SCC). Note the cardinal features consistent with malignancy; namely speckled appearance, raised rolled edges, contact bleeding and variable ulceration. (a) Right ventral tongue SCC. (b) Right soft palate SCC. (c) Left posterolateral tongue SCC. (d) Right lateral tongue SCC.

The neck

All levels of the neck must be palpated thoroughly, to assess for lymphadenopathy. However, it is important to note that, along with clinical examination, cross-sectional imaging of the neck is also required. Clinical examination without imaging has a 74% sensitivity for detecting lymphadenopathy. The presence of a neck metastasis decreases a patient's prognosis by approximately 50%.

Biopsy

Primary tumour

Histopathological diagnosis via a formal biopsy is the gold standard prior to further investigation and treatment. An incisional biopsy is preferred. It is important to avoid necrotic areas, and a narrow deep biopsy is more useful than a shallow broad one. Other biopsy techniques such as exfoliative cytology and brush biopsy lack sensitivity and are therefore not commonly employed.

Neck lump

Fine-needle aspiration cytology (FNAC) is the first-line biopsy for the investigation of neck lymphadenopathy. This technique carries a sensitivity of 89–98%. It will help in differentiating between thyroid malignancy, oropharyngeal and oral cavity lesions (utilising HPV diagnostic tests) and lymphoma.

Imaging

Contemporary cross-sectional imaging techniques are essential in the management of head and neck cancer. They inform treatment decisions and prognosis. CT and/or MRI are the gold standard imaging modalities to stage a tumour of the oral cavity. Plain film radiography and ultrasonography, along with positron emission tomography–computed tomography (PET-CT) are useful adjuncts. The aims of imaging are as follows:

- outline the anatomical extent of the primary tumour (T stage), as well as the 'resectability' of the tumour based on its relationship to vital structures;

- detection of locoregional metastases;
- detection of metastatic disease precluding cure;
- detection of synchronous primary tumours of the lung and upper aerodigestive tract;
- monitoring of disease response following non-surgical treatment and for detection of disease recurrence.

Computed tomography

Contrast-enhanced CT (CECT), typically modern multi-detector slice computed tomography (MDCT), is a commonly available staging tool. This offers the advantage of rapidly acquired spatially accurate cross-sectional images. Hard-tissue detail is a particular advantage of CT, relative to MRI; this is particularly important when assessing bony involvement (mandible/maxilla) in oral SCC. CT is also the usual imaging modality for thoracic staging.

Magnetic resonance imaging

By comparison with CT, MRI has improved soft-tissue contrast resolution and, depending upon specialist radiologist preference, it is frequently the imaging modality of choice for defining the primary extent of oral cavity cancers. Additionally, it offers more information on perineural spread and bone marrow invasion. T1-weighted 'anatomical' images have good spatial resolution, while T2-weighted images preferentially highlight oedema and therefore pathology.

MRI has a sensitivity of 82% and specificity of 66.7% for the detection of bone/bone marrow invasion in the mandible. The ability of MRI to detect neck metastases is comparable to that of CT.

Positron emission tomography combined with computed tomography

PET-CT is not a first-line imaging investigation for head and neck cancer and its use is usually restricted to detection of distant metastases or synchronous tumours, investigation of tumours of unknown primary and post-treatment surveillance.

Plain film and panoramic radiographs

Plain film or panoramic radiographs can be helpful in defining gross bony involvement during tumour staging; however, their main utility is for evaluation of the dentition to plan essential prophylactic dental treatment and highlight infection or inflammation.

Ultrasound

Ultrasonography is a non-invasive, chair-side investigation that is now most commonly used to guide FNAC sampling of suspicious lymph nodes. It is operator dependent but in experienced hands is very useful in the detection of lymphadenopathy. It is of limited value in investigation of oral cavity tumours. It has 85% sensitivity and 78.9% specificity for cervical lymphadenopathy.

Sentinel lymph node biopsy

Sentinel lymph node biopsy (SLNB) has become a recognised technique to support staging of the neck in patients who do not have clinical or radiological evidence of lymph node metastases (cN0). The sentinel node is the first node to which cancer cells are most likely to spread. SLNB seeks to determine the presence of nodal metastasis within the first draining node(s) and guides the necessity (or otherwise) for further treatment of the neck.

There is robust evidence that, in patients with a T1/2 oral cavity SCC, performing a prophylactic elective neck dissection as opposed to adopting a 'watch and wait' policy leads to superior overall and disease-free survival.[3] However, not all patients will have nodal metastases and as such provision of a neck dissection for all will inevitably result in overtreatment of a significant proportion. SLNB can be utilised to highlight those patients with occult metastases and who can then proceed to formal neck dissection. Additionally, SLNB may demonstrate unexpected contralateral lymph node drainage that would not otherwise have been identified or treated. Despite its potential benefits, the SLNB technique has a false-negative rate of 14%.[4] To date, evidence providing a comparative analysis of elective neck dissection versus SLNB (where survival is the primary end point) is still lacking.

SURGICAL MANAGEMENT

Surgery, with adjuvant radiotherapy (or chemoradiotherapy) if indicated, remains the mainstay for management of oral cavity cancer. Over time, surgical techniques have evolved to become more refined with a greater emphasis on function-sparing techniques and a move away from more radical procedures. Reconstruction of postablative defects with an associated improvement in quality of life is a cornerstone of the surgical management of oral cavity cancer. This evolution in surgical management has been influenced by an improved understanding of tumour biology, more accurate staging investigations and microvascular free tissue transfer reconstruction. Overall and disease-specific survival is largely dictated by tumour biology, with features such as nodal metastases with ENE of greatest importance. Notwithstanding this, surgeons can optimise the outcome for patients by considering the following principles:

- patient selection;
- key surgical decisions;
- reconstruction;
- multidisciplinary care.

Patient selection

As outlined previously, patients' comorbidities and functional status as well as their social circumstances play a significant role in their ability to tolerate surgery and rehabilitation. The early involvement of an MDT including physicians, anaesthetists, physiotherapists and dieticians is important particularly in high-risk patients in order to optimise their performance status preoperatively.

The 'operability' of a tumour is determined largely by its size and relationship to important anatomical structures of the head and neck. In the AJCC eighth edition TNM staging system T4b tumours are those that may be unresectable owing to involvement of or proximity to the skull base, masticator space, pterygoid plates and/or the internal carotid artery.

Key surgical decisions

Once the decision has been made that surgery is appropriate, a few key decisions are to be made. These are as follows:

- airway management;
- access to the tumour;
- tumour resection;
- management of the neck;
- reconstruction.

Airway management

Airway management in patients undergoing surgery for OCSCC is largely centred on protecting the airway against acute embarrassment in the perioperative period. The available options are immediate postoperative extubation, overnight intubation/delayed extubation, submental intubation and tracheostomy. The choice of airway is a joint decision made between the anaesthetist and surgeon, and is influenced heavily by the ability to re-establish a patient's airway quickly should a life-threatening event occur. Immediate postoperative extubation is generally reserved for smaller well-lateralised tumours in uncomplicated patients who may not require reconstruction. In selected patients, overnight intubation is considered when tracheostomy is unlikely yet can still be sited on postoperative day 1 if warranted; this approach is burdensome on resources given the higher level of care for the first night, but it reduces length of stay via a quicker restoration of speech and swallow.

A low threshold for placing a tracheostomy is appropriate in patients having a bilateral neck dissection or previous neck dissection; large resection with reconstruction; and in patients with a difficult airway. Consideration should also be given to placing a tracheostomy in patients having a segmental mandibular resection; lateralised resections involving the floor of mouth and reconstruction; as well as previously irradiated patients.

Access surgery

The goal in surgical management of OCSCC is to remove the tumour with an adequate margin circumferentially. While most tumours can be removed via a transoral approach, some cannot be resected safely without an access procedure. These might include large maxillary tumours, posteriorly located tumours and tongue base tumours, or patients who have previously had surgery and/or radiotherapy. The most commonly used access procedures include the lip-split mandibulotomy (LSM) (***Figure 53.5***), the mandibular lingual release, the visor flap and the Weber–Fergusson approach (***Figure 53.6***), which provides excellent access to the maxilla and, if extended infraorbitally, to the periorbital area.

Lip-split mandibulotomy

This is the most commonly used access procedure and provides excellent access to the posterior oral cavity, tongue base and oropharynx. It involves making an osteotomy in the mandible in order to 'swing' it laterally, thereby facilitating access. Care must be taken to ensure that the lingual mucosa does not tear in an uncontrolled fashion towards the tumour resection margin.

Tumour resection

The gold standard in OCSCC is resection with a 1-cm clinical margin circumferentially, vital structures permitting.

Mandibular resection

Decisions regarding management of the mandible when tumour lies close to, abuts or invades the bone are critical. If there is evidence of infiltrative bone invasion, either segmental or rim resection of the involved mandible is required.

Segmental resection involves removing the full height of the invaded section of the mandible such that there is loss of continuity of the lower border. Rim resection or 'marginal mandibulectomy' involves removing a partial thickness of mandible such that continuity of the lower border remains. A rim resection is sometimes performed when a tumour lies close to but does not definitively invade the mandible, in order to achieve a satisfactory soft-tissue margin.

Maxillary resection

Owing to anatomical differences such as thinner bone, the presence of sinuses, tightly adherent palatal mucosa and proximity to the orbit and skull base, maxillary resection considerations differ from those in the mandible. Small tumours of the maxillary alveolus can be managed by transoral partial maxillectomy. More extensive tumours involving the floor of the maxillary sinus require wider access by a Weber–Fergusson incision (***Figure 53.6***). If the preoperative investigations demonstrate extension of the disease into the pterygoid space or the infratemporal fossa, the prognosis is poor as surgical clearance is difficult or not possible. Tumour extending into the orbit requires simultaneous orbital exenteration or, in some instances, a combined neurosurgical resection. The various methods of maxillary reconstruction can be guided by the extent of resection and tissues involved. Reconstruction seeks to provide an oral seal and restore facial profile and tissue loss, while facilitating a means to achieve dental rehabilitation.

Management of the neck

In surgical terms, 'management of the neck' refers to a neck dissection – elective or therapeutic. In patients with clinical and/or radiographic evidence of cervical metastases, treatment of the neck in the form of a therapeutic neck dissection is indicated (primary radiotherapy is less common). In patients with early-stage disease and in whom there is no clinical or radiographic evidence for cervical metastases, there is now strong evidence showing that patients who have an up-front or elective neck dissection have better overall and disease-specific survival relative to patients who have a 'watch-and-wait' policy and a therapeutic neck dissection only when a metastasis becomes apparent.[5] SLNB can be utilised as a staging investigation to better guide the indications for a neck dissection in the setting of a small tumour where occult metastases may still be present.

Over the last 100 years, neck dissections have evolved to achieve a less radical extent as evidence emerged for the oncological safety of more selective or nuanced procedures.[6] For elective neck dissections, a selective neck dissection involving

Sir William Fergusson, 1808–1877, Scottish surgeon, described and published a modification of the original Weber incision to access the midface.

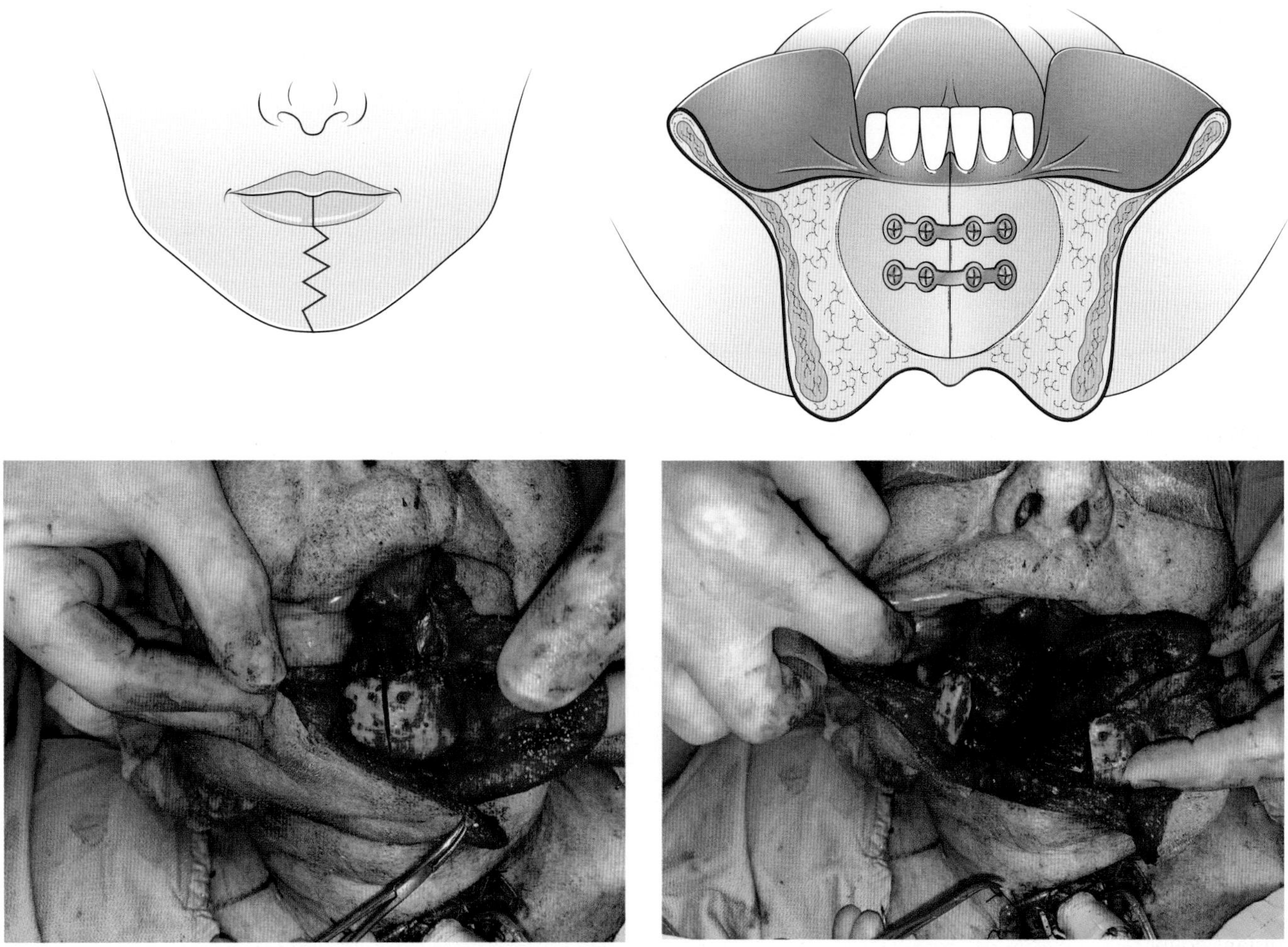

Figure 53.5 Lip-split mandibulotomy.

levels I–III of the neck is indicated for the management of OCSCC.[7]

A neck dissection is performed not only to stage a disease and aid prognosis, but also for therapeutic purposes as well as informing the need for adjuvant therapy. Additionally, it provides access to recipient vessels within the neck, which may be used in microvascular free tissue reconstruction.

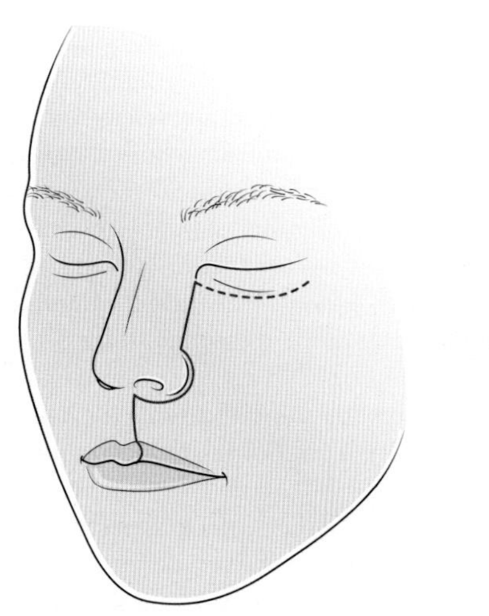

Figure 53.6 Weber–Fergusson approach.

Reconstruction

Reconstruction following tumour ablation is a key component in the management of OCSCC. Decision making with regards to reconstruction should not influence the ablative procedure. Notwithstanding the importance of facial aesthetics, preservation or restoration of speech, chewing, swallow and oral continence are of paramount importance. The oral cavity is a unique site. It contains hard and soft tissues, including the dentition, is bathed in saliva and is anatomically complex. It is the opening to the aerodigestive tract and has a multitude of motor and sensory nerves. Like any defect, reconstruction of the oral cavity should aim to replace resected tissue with similar tissue. The reconstruction ladder (***Figure 53.7***) is a useful algorithm and can be applied to the oral cavity.

Additionally, general reconstruction principles apply: namely, use the simplest method that will meet reconstruction aims, replace lost tissue with similar tissue, consider vascularised tissue in a previously irradiated recipient site and always have an alternative should your primary reconstruction fail.

- Healing by secondary intention
- Primary closure
- Skin grafting
- Local flaps
- Regional flaps
- Microvascular free tissue transfer

Figure 53.7 The reconstruction ladder.

While free tissue transfer ('free flaps') has revolutionised reconstruction following ablation of an OCSCC, there are instances, for example owing to patient comorbidities, where a local or regional flap is appropriate.

Owing to the extensive and consistent blood supply in the head and neck, local flaps in this region are safe and predictable. Smaller defects not requiring substantial soft tissue or bone for reconstruction can be reliably reconstructed with flaps such as, but not limited to, the facial artery myomucosal (FAMM), nasolabial, buccal fat pad, tongue and palatal flaps. Regional and pedicled flaps include tissue(s) from other parts of the head and neck, such as the temporalis and platysma flaps, as well as those from more distant sites such as the latissimus dorsi, deltopectoral and pectoralis major flaps.

Free flaps

A free flap is a portion of vascularised tissue harvested from a distant donor site and transferred to an area requiring reconstruction where its artery and vein are anastomosed locally, thereby providing an independent blood supply. Most tissue types, including skin, fascia, muscle, tendon and bone, can be harvested. Therefore, within the oral cavity both bone and soft tissue can be replaced with similar tissue(s).

Soft-tissue reconstruction

In oral cavity reconstruction, common soft-tissue flaps used include the radial forearm free flap (RFFF; ***Figure 53.8***) and anterolateral thigh (ALT) flap. Alternative soft-tissue free flaps include rectus abdominis, latissimus dorsi, medial sural artery perforator and lateral arm flaps. The relative merits of these flaps are outlined in ***Table 53.5***.

Composite reconstruction

The fibula is the most commonly used bone-containing (composite) flap globally, while the iliac crest (DCIA), scapula (including tip of scapula) and composite RFFFs are also used, each carrying specific pros and cons. Chimeric flaps, where osseous and soft-tissue components are independently mobile (e.g. the thoracodorsal system of free flaps), are advocated for certain complex reconstructions. The relative merits of the more common composite flap donor sites are outlined in ***Table 53.6***.

Reconstruction by anatomical subsite

Soft-tissue reconstruction

Intraorally this includes the tongue, floor of the mouth, buccal and retromolar mucosa as well as the soft palate. As outlined previously the most commonly used soft-tissue flaps are the RFFF and ALT. The RFFF provides a thin, non-hirsute and pliable flap with a long vascular pedicle and so can be useful where significant bulk is not required. The ALT (***Figure 53.9***), however, owing to its increased bulk, is far more suited to tongue reconstruction where bulkiness is crucial in creating a seal between the oral cavity and soft palate during speech and swallowing. The ALT also facilitates multiple skin paddles and/or muscle components, where necessary.

TABLE 53.5 Relative merits of common soft-tissue flaps.

Donor site	RFFF	ALT	MSAP	TDAP	Lateral arm	Rectus	LD
Donor site morbidity	+++	++	++	++	++	+++	++
Pedicle length	++++ 18 cm	+++ 12 cm	++ 10 cm	++++ 15 cm	+ 6 cm; increased with ELAF	+ 7 cm	++ 8.5 cm
Quality of vessels	++++	+++	+++	++++	++	++++	++++
Diameter	Artery: 3 mm Vein: 1.5 (3 mm if cephalic) No atherosclerosis	Artery: 2.1 mm Vein: 2.3 mm	Artery: 1.25 mm Vein: 2 mm	Artery: 2.7 mm Vein: 3.4 mm No atherosclerosis	Artery: 1.5 mm Vein: 2.5 mm	Artery: 3.5 mm Vein: 4 mm	Artery: 2.7 mm Vein: 3.4 mm No atherosclerosis
Soft-tissue paddle	++ 12 × 5 cm	++++ 16 × 8 cm	++ 10 × 5 cm	++++ 25 × 10 cm	++ 12 × 5 cm	+++ Muscle: 6 × 25 cm Skin: 13 × 25 cm	++++ Muscle: 35 × 20 cm Skin: 18 × 7 cm
Two-team operating	+++	++++	++++	+	++	+++	+

ALT, anterolateral thigh; ELAF, extended lateral arm flap; LD, latissimus dorsi; MSAP, medial sural artery perforator; RFFF, radial forearm free flap; TDAP, thoracodorsal artery perforator.

TABLE 53.6 Relative merits of composite flap donor sites.

Donor site	Fibula	DCIA	Scapula	Thoracodorsal/tip of scapula	Composite RFFF
Donor site morbidity	++	+++	+++	+++	+
Pedicle length	+++	+	+	+++	++++
Quality of vessels	+++/+ (may be affected by atherosclerosis)	++ (potentially small diameter)	++++ (large, spared from atherosclerosis)	++++ (large, spared from atherosclerosis)	+++ (spared from atherosclerosis)
Volume of bone	++	++++	+++	++	+
Length of bone	++++ (14 cm)	+++ (12 cm)	++ (10 cm)	++ (6 cm)	+++ (12 cm)
Suitability for implants	+++	++++	+++	+	Not suitable
Soft-tissue paddle	+++ (occasionally unreliable)	+ (internal oblique or DCIA perforator)	++++ (two soft-tissue flaps and/or chimera with LD or TAP)	++++ (allows chimeric flap with two independently mobile skin paddles with/without LD muscle)	+++ (reliable skin flap, but lacks bulk)
Two-team operating	++++	+++	+	+	+++

DCIA, deep circumflex iliac artery; LD, latissimus dorsi; RFFF, radial forearm free flap; TAP, thoracodorsal artery perforator.

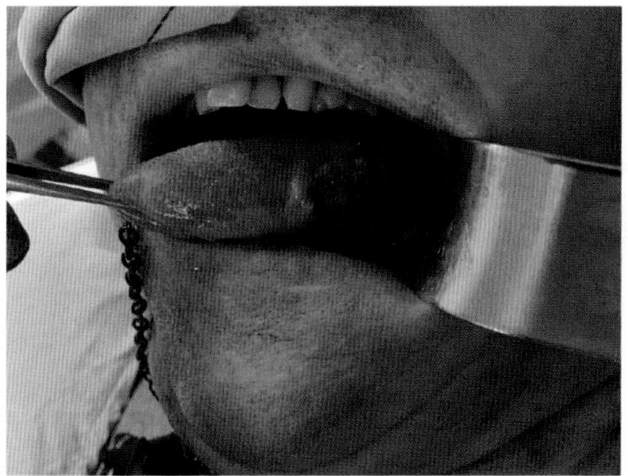

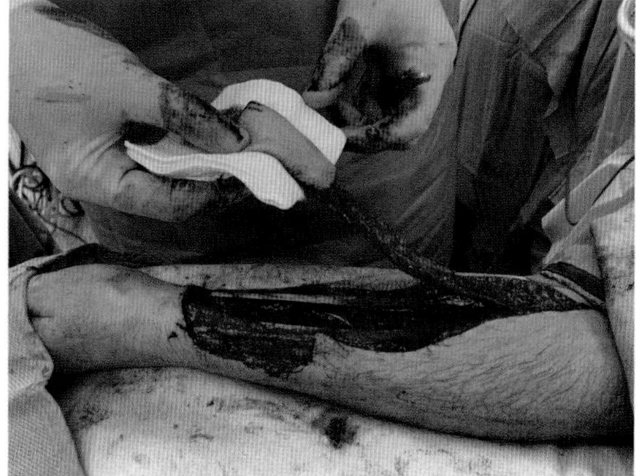

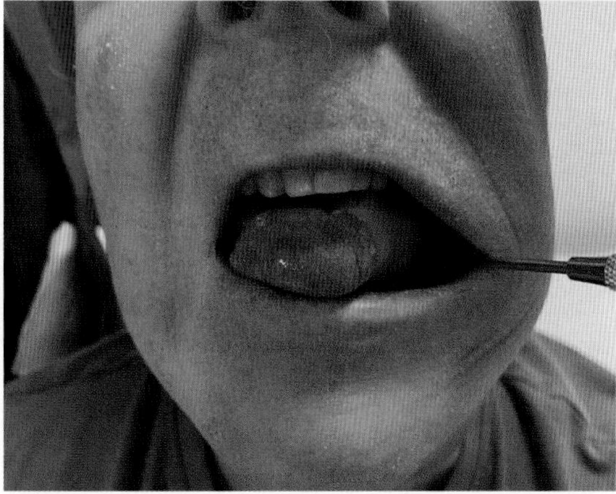

Figure 53.8 Radial forearm free flap used to reconstruct a left lateral tongue defect. Note the suitable bulk/composition of the thin and pliable radial forearm tissue for a modest soft-tissue defect.

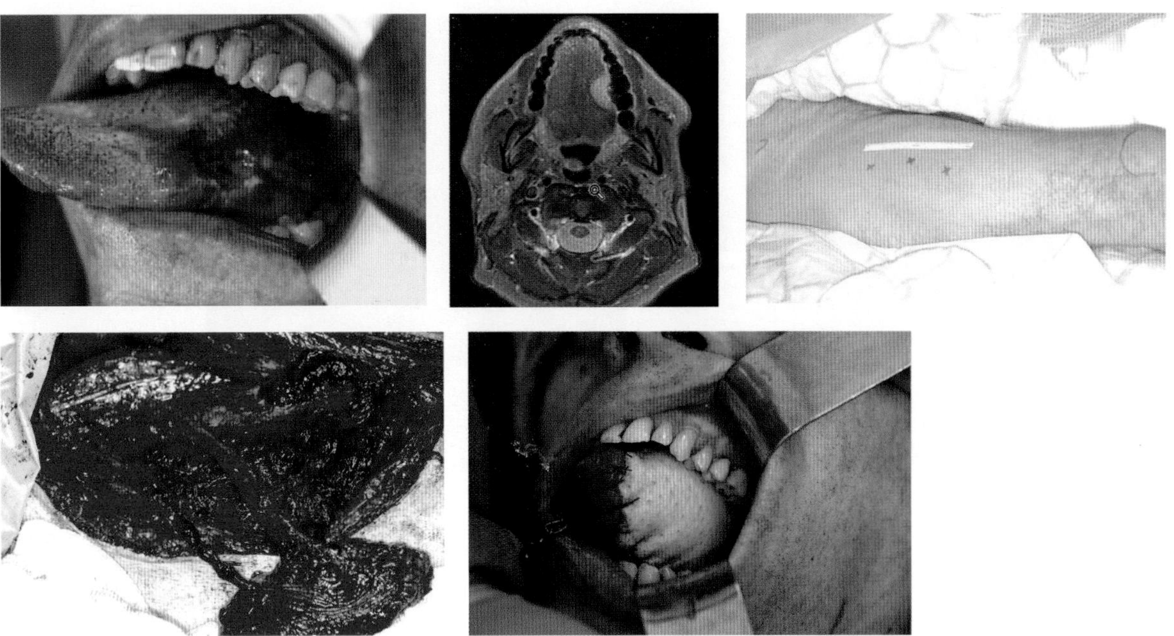

Figure 53.9 The use of an anterolateral thigh flap to reconstruct a left partial glossectomy/floor of the mouth ablative defect.

Mandible reconstruction

Reconstruction with composite free flaps is now the gold standard for segmental mandibular defects (***Figures 53.10 and 53.11***). The choice of flap is varied and depends on factors including the site, size and complexity of the defect, patient comorbidities and indeed surgeon training and preference.

While it is possible to leave small posterior sites unreconstructed, reconstruction of an anterior defect is particularly important, and challenging, in order to achieve satisfactory function for the patient.

The following general principles may help to plan mandibular reconstruction:

- reconstruction of the anterior mandible is always more challenging;
- although the lengths of the bone and pedicle are often cited as factors in choosing the donor site, the average defect is 6–10 cm and usually immediately adjacent vessels for microvascular anastomosis mean that these are not usually an impediment;
- use the curvature of the chosen bony flap to follow the natural shape of the mandible, thereby reducing the number of potential osteotomies;
- in an edentulous case, it may be helpful to slightly reduce the span of the mandibular segment to avoid a resultant class III appearance, where the mandible protrudes beyond the opposing maxilla, giving a very prominent chin position;
- free bone can become a nidus for persistent infection, particularly following radiotherapy.

Maxillary reconstruction

The main aims of maxillary reconstruction are as follows:

- restore facial contours and aesthetics;
- separate sinonasal cavities from the mouth;
- restore soft palate competence to facilitate speech and swallowing;
- restore/provide for replacement of dentition.

A classification system for maxillary defects is useful for both treatment planning and discussion with colleagues. The most widely adopted classification is that proposed by Brown and Shaw; this classification considers both the vertical and horizontal extent of the defect. Classes I–VI (***Figure 53.12***) describe the increasing size in a vertical dimension, while the horizontal extent is described by the letters a–c. Although not absolute, one of the advantages of this classification system is that it implies management.

Class I defects are easy to repair with the only reconstructive requirement being to separate the oral and nasal/antral cavities. Local flaps are often satisfactory, and the RFFF is the most commonly used free flap. Class II defects can be restored in a similar fashion to class I, especially when more posteriorly located. However, composite (bone-containing) free flaps are usually required for anterior defects, and class IIc defects, as well as situations where the existing dentition is not adequate to retain a prosthesis.

In classes III and IV, support for the contents of the orbit is lost, as well as support for the anterior cheek and alveolus. A prosthesis alone will provide a suboptimal result. The reconstructive goals are to support the orbital contents and facial skin, ensure bony continuity between the remaining alveolus and zygomatic buttress (ideally sufficient to facilitate endo-osseous implant placement), as well as seal the oral and nasal cavities. Therefore, a composite free flap (e.g. the thoracodorsal free flap) is suitable for fulfilling these requirements.

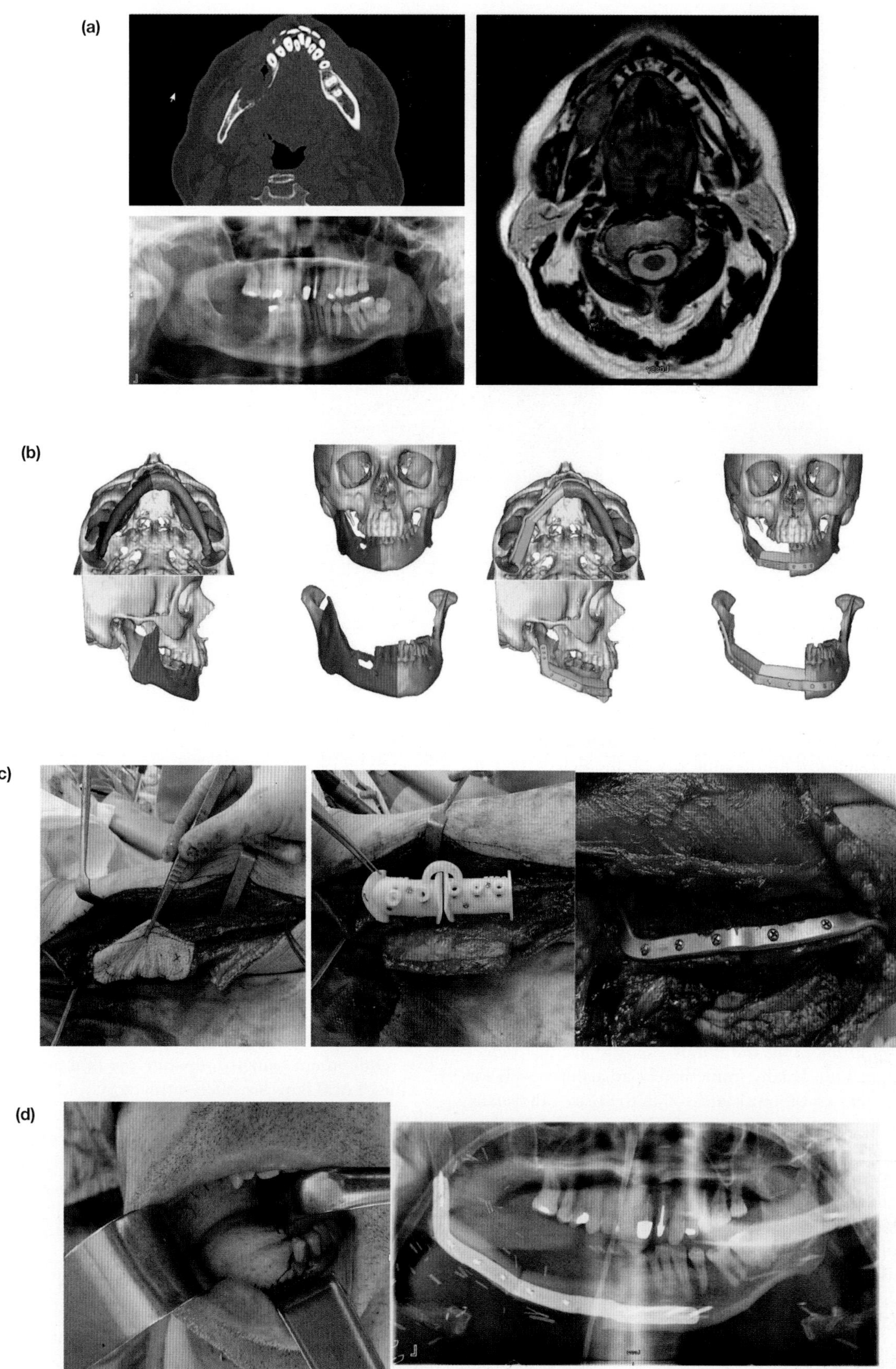

Figure 53.10 Management of a right mandibular squamous cell carcinoma utilising virtual surgical planning (VSP) and a fibula free flap. (a) Radiographic images demonstrating tumour in the right mandible. (b) VSP highlighting both resection and reconstruction. (c) The fibula free flap with the cutting guide *in situ*. (d) Final reconstruction clinically and radiographically.

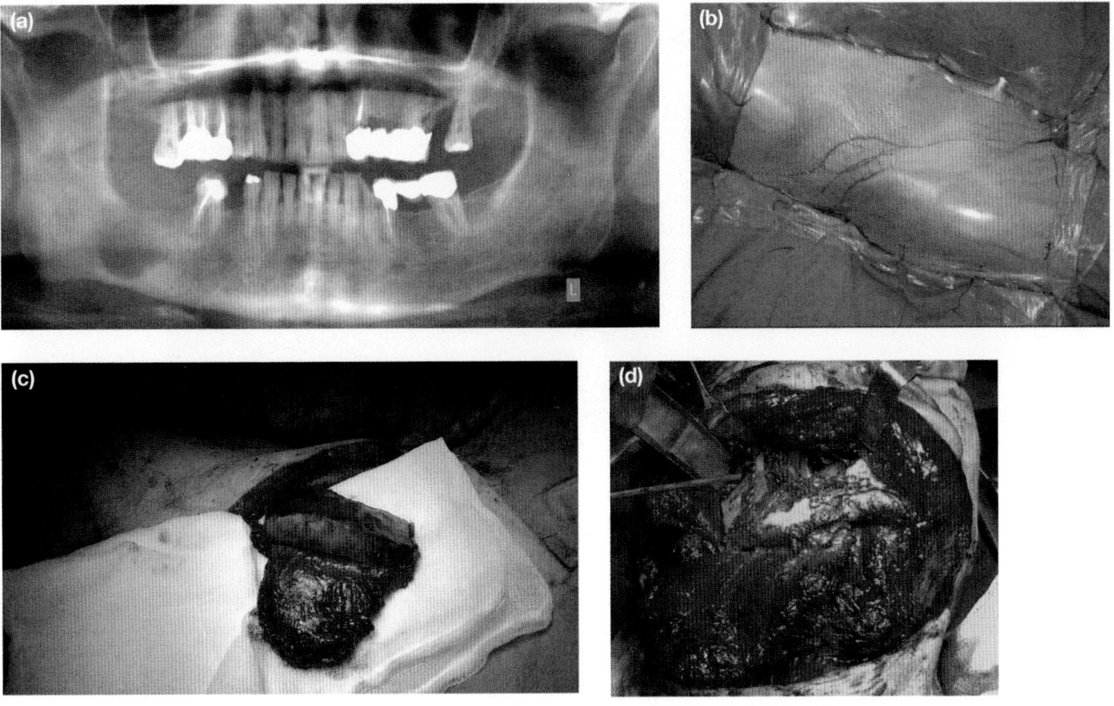

Figure 53.11 Right mandibular squamous cell carcinoma ablative defect. Orthopantomogram showing the bony defect in the right body/angle (a). This was reconstructed with a deep circumflex iliac artery (DCIA)/iliac crest free flap. The surface anatomical markings for a right DCIA free flap are demonstrated with a typical incision (b). Note the virtual surgical planning cutting guide on the iliac crest bone component and the associated well-vascularised muscle paddle (internal oblique muscle) (c) subsequently inset for the mandibular and intraoral defect reconstruction (d).

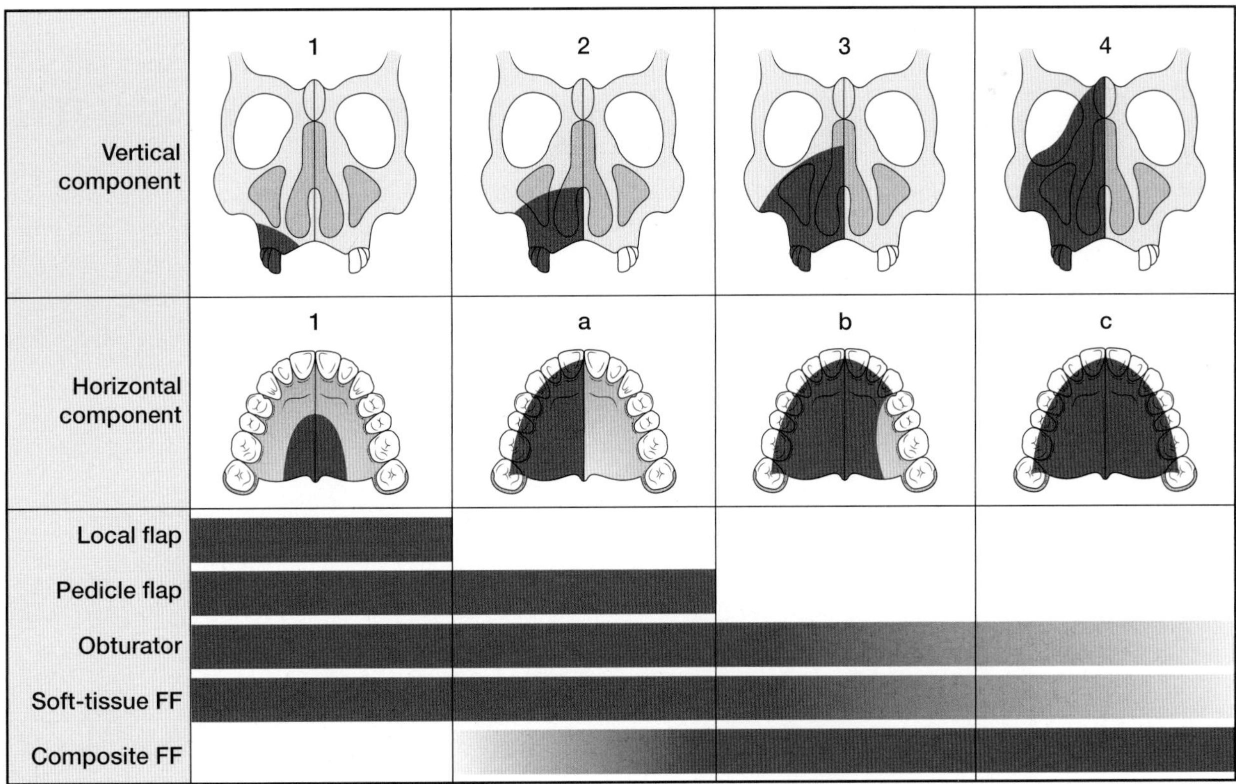

Figure 53.12 Maxillectomy defect classification and proposed reconstructions. Note that an updated version was published in 2010, but this diagram provides a useful visual representation of proposed reconstruction according to the class of defect. (Reproduced with permission from Brown JS, Rogers SN, McNally DN, Boyle M. A modified classification for the maxillectomy defect. *Head Neck* 2000; **22**(1): 17–26.)

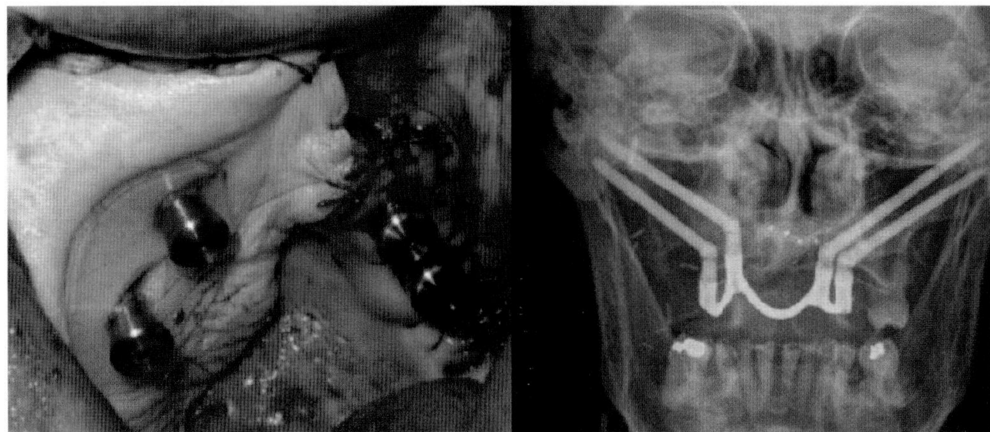

Figure 53.13 A zygomatic implant perforator used to reconstruct a left hemi-maxillectomy defect (courtesy of Prof. C Butterworth).

Evolution in zygomatic implant technology can support prosthetic rehabilitation and restoration of low-level maxillectomy defects in combination with soft-tissue flaps. In select cases, this can remove the necessity for composite free flaps.

It should be pointed out that prosthetic reconstruction, using an obturator denture, of a maxillary defect remains a reasonable and sometimes appropriate alternative to free tissue reconstruction. However, studies have shown that free flap reconstruction results in improved functional and aesthetic outcomes when compared with prosthetic obturation.

Zygomatic implants and zygomatic implant perforator (ZIP) flaps

Zygomatic as well as oncological or co-axis implants, used in conjunction with a fixed or removable prosthesis, or indeed with a free flap, have improved our ability to quickly restore dentition post maxillectomy. Recently, the use of zygomatic implants that perforate a soft-tissue free flap (used to close an oroantral/oronasal communication) and placed immediately after tumour ablation has been described (***Figure 53.13***).

Virtual surgical planning

The use of virtual surgical planning (VSP) in oral cavity reconstruction is increasing. Potential benefits include reduced operating time, greater accuracy and improved aesthetic/functional outcomes.

Patient-specific surgical stents and cutting guides for both the tumour and donor sites are made preoperatively, based on CT scans and software (***Figure 53.14***). The surgeon performs the surgery virtually; based on the resection and therefore the size and shape of reconstruction required, cutting guides are provided for both the oral resection and donor site harvesting (***Figure 53.15***). Prefabricated reconstruction plates can also be made.

ADJUVANT THERAPY FOR THE MANAGEMENT OF ORAL CAVITY CANCER

While primary chemoradiotherapy can be offered to patients who are unsuitable for or refuse surgery, primary surgery, with/without adjuvant (chemo)radiotherapy, is the standard

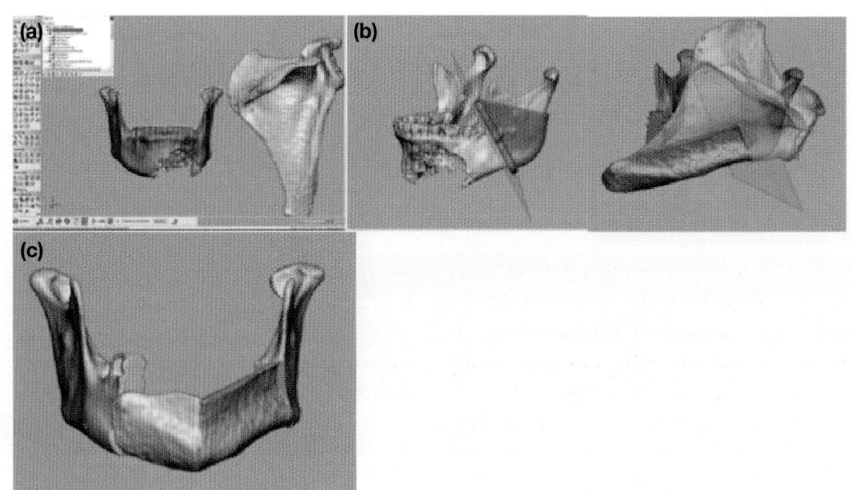

Figure 53.14 Virtual surgical planning. (a) A virtual mandible (green) with an obvious bony defect. (b) The resection cutting plane with the scapula overlaid. (c) The final reconstruction plan with a two-part (osteotomised) scapula osseous component.

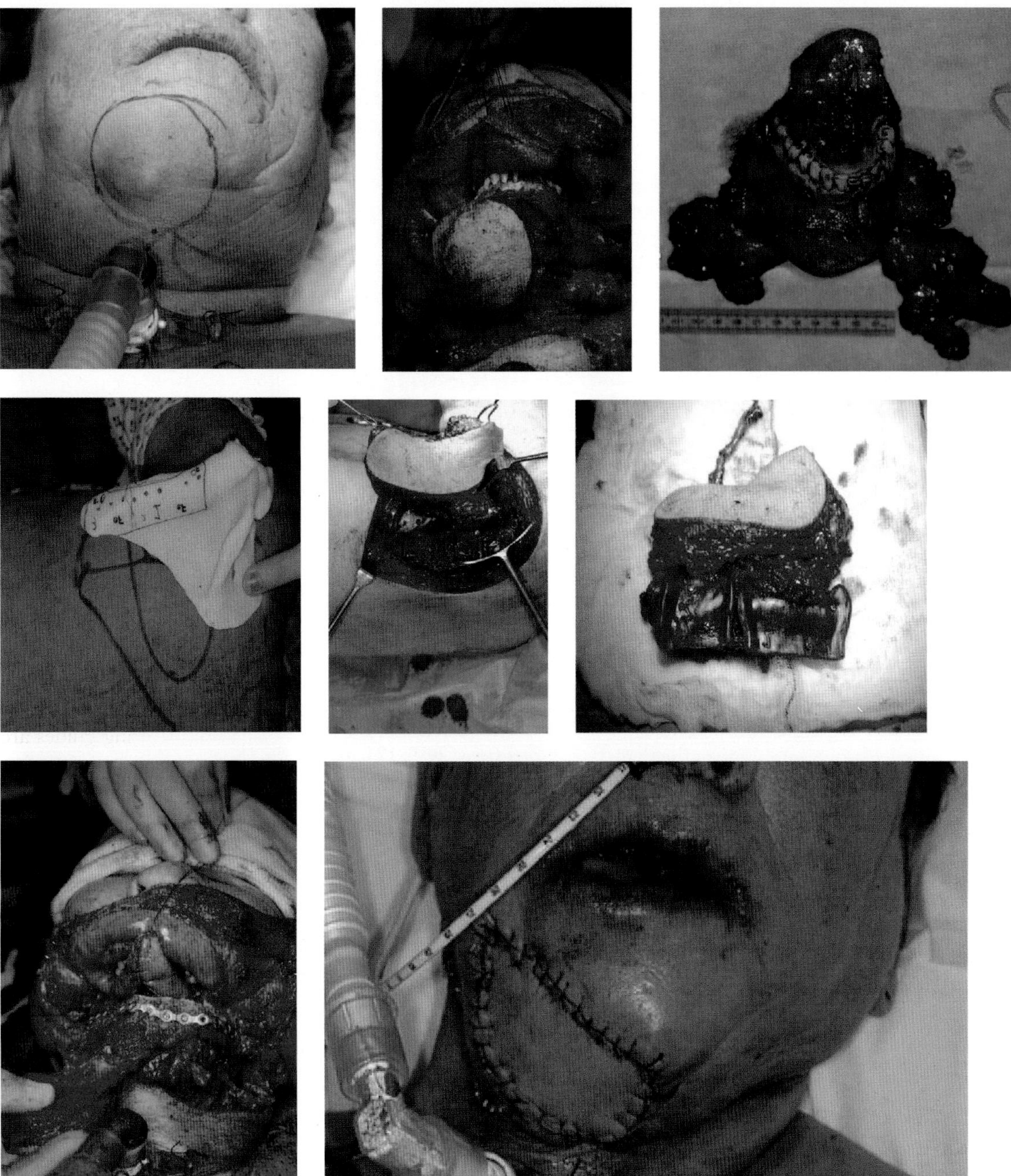

Figure 53.15 Series demonstrating the management of a T4 squamous cell carcinoma involving the right anterior floor of the mouth, mandible and overlying skin. Virtual surgical planning and cutting guides were used to harvest and inset the scapula free flap.

treatment for oral cavity cancer. Adjuvant therapy is given based on pathological features of the tumour. Radiotherapy is administered typically via external beam radiotherapy. In high-risk cases, chemotherapy (usually cisplatin-based) is included as a radiosensitiser within the adjuvant regime for suitably fit patients.

As outlined in previous sections, the adverse pathological features associated with locoregional recurrence and decreased overall and disease-specific survival include ENE, close/involved margins, LVI and PNI. It is these, among other, adverse features that inform the decision to administer adjuvant therapy.

While there is no absolute international agreement regarding the criteria for radiotherapy, the current consensus is that one major criterion (ENE and/or involved margin [<1 mm]) or two minor criteria (close margin [1–4.9 mm], multiple involved nodes, largest node >3 cm, LVI/PNI, T3/4) would indicate the need for adjuvant radiotherapy.[8]

Adjuvant chemoradiotherapy

The landmark RTOG 9501 and EORTC 22931 randomised trials form the basis for the contemporary role of adjuvant chemotherapy (CRT) in high-risk OCSCC (although only 25%

of recruited patients had OCSCC). These studies looked at the benefit conferred by adding high-dose cisplatin to conventional postoperative radiotherapy (RT), with primary end points of locoregional control and progression-free survival, respectively. Positive surgical margins and extracapsular extension (ECE; now ENE) were used to classify patients as high risk in both studies, while several other criteria unique to each were also investigated. Ultimately, and following several associated long-term, subgroup and pooled analyses, these trials provided strong evidence for the use of concurrent cisplatin-based CRT in high-risk patients.

Immunotherapy

Antitumour immunotherapy is based on the principle that tumours can sometimes escape immune response/checkpoints owing to adaptations in immune surveillance and the tumour microenvironment. Immunotherapy represents a change in the treatment paradigm.

The pathway of the programmed death receptor-1 (PD-1) and its ligand (PD-L1) has become an increasingly important target for immunotherapy in HNSCC. The receptor–ligand interaction is a major mechanism used by tumours to evade the immune system. Multiple randomised phase III trials have demonstrated that exposure to a PD-1 inhibitor prolongs survival in recurrent or metastatic HNSCC.

These results, among others, highlight the potential for research assessing the role of checkpoint inhibition in the management of HNSCC.

MANAGEMENT OF RECURRENT AND/OR METASTATIC DISEASE

Patients with a low burden of disease or oligometastatic deposit(s) and a satisfactory performance status can be offered salvage surgery and/or radiotherapy with curative intent. Patients with a recurrence not amenable to surgery and/or radiotherapy are eligible for systemic treatment. Current standard of care options depend on previous exposure to platinum-containing chemotherapy, but include both immunotherapy and palliative chemotherapy regimens. Nonetheless, the poor prognosis for these patients remains.

ACKNOWLEDGEMENTS

The authors acknowledge Professor RJ Shaw, Professor JS Brown and Professor C Butterworth for clinical photographs utilised in this chapter.

REFERENCES

1 Coelho KR. Challenges of the oral cancer burden in India. *J Cancer Epidemiol* 2012; **2012**: 701932.
2 Warnakulasuriya S, Ariyawardana A. Malignant transformation of oral leukoplakia: a systematic review of observational studies. *J Oral Pathol Med* 2016; **45**(3): 155–66.
3 D'Cruz AK, Vaish R, Kapre N *et al.* Elective versus therapeutic neck dissection in node-negative oral cancer. *N Engl J Med* 2015; **373**(6): 521–9.
4 Schilling C, Stoeckli SJ, Haerle SK *et al.* Sentinel European Node Trial (SENT): 3-year results of sentinel node biopsy in oral cancer. *Eur J Cancer* 2015; **51**(18): 2777–84.
5 Hutchison IL, Ridout F, Cheung SMY *et al.* Nationwide randomised trial evaluating elective neck dissection for early stage oral cancer (SEND study) with meta-analysis and concurrent real-world cohort. *Br J Cancer* 2019; **121**(10): 827–36.
6 Lindberg R. Distribution of cervical lymph node metastases from squamous cell carcinoma of the upper respiratory and digestive tracts. *Cancer* 1972; **29**(6): 1446–9.
7 Shah JP. Patterns of cervical lymph node metastasis from squamous carcinomas of the upper aerodigestive tract. *Am J Surg* 1990; **160**(4): 405–9.
8 Expert Panel on Radiation Oncology–Head and Neck; Salama JK, Saba N, Quon H *et al.* ACR appropriateness criteria® adjuvant therapy for resected squamous cell carcinoma of the head and neck. *Oral Oncol* 2011; **47**(7): 554–9.

CHAPTER 54 Disorders of the salivary glands

Learning objectives

To understand:

- The surgical anatomy of the salivary glands
- The presentation, pathology and investigation of salivary gland disease
- The medical and surgical treatment of various pathologies affecting the salivary glands

INTRODUCTION

The parotid, submandibular and sublingual glands are the three paired major salivary glands; the minor salivary glands are multiple and situated mainly in the lips, buccal mucosa, tongue and palate, but they can be present anywhere along the aerodigestive tract. Obstructive and inflammatory conditions, tumours and autoimmune-mediated conditions affect these glands.

Saliva is an important secretion that performs a number of essential functions, such as clearing substances from the mouth, maintaining pH and tooth mineralisation and influencing the oral microbiome, which protects the body and helps with wound healing. Moreover, saliva not only neutralises some harmful dietary components but also lubricates and hydrates oral mucosal surfaces. This has been the topic of study for centuries, with the oldest reference to salivary glands, and more specifically to saliva, found in clay tablets at the Akka Library, which was created by the Assyrian King Assurbanipal from old Mesopotamia around 2500 BCE. It even referred to the use of the plant belladonna for curing excessive salivary flow.

CLINICAL ANATOMY AND EMBRYOLOGY

The parotid, submandibular and sublingual glands are three paired glands whereas there are innumerable minor salivary glands (***Figure 54.1***). The glandular architecture is essentially a series of ducts that open into the oral cavity and are surrounded by acini, which produce the saliva. The extracellular matrix includes the myoepithelial cells, myofibroblasts, immune cells, endothelial cells, stromal cells and nerve fibres. The parotid is ectodermal in origin, while the submandibular and sublingual glands are endodermal. The parotid represents the largest of the salivary glands and is situated in front of the external acoustic meatus between the ramus of the mandible and the sternocleidomastoid muscle. Each gland is encapsulated and is composed of fat and cells that secrete mainly serous fluids. The major duct of the parotid gland is called Stensen's duct, which opens into the vestibule of the mouth opposite the crown of the upper second molar tooth, while the submandibular duct is Wharton's duct, which opens into the floor of the mouth paramedian to the frenulum. The parotid gland, being primarily serous, secretes watery saliva while the rest are mixed serous and mucinous glands.

> **Summary box 54.1**
>
> **Surgical anatomy of the salivary glands**
>
> - Three pairs of major salivary glands – parotid, submandibular and sublingual
> - Approximately 800 minor salivary glands

Parotid gland

Understanding a gland's development gives us insight into the pathophysiology of the various disorders afflicting it. The parotid gland is ectodermal in origin and develops in the sixth week of gestation, when the epithelial buds invaginate from the oral mucosa into the surrounding mesenchyme. A tunnel develops from this groove and the gland is formed at its blind end by proliferation, budding and extensive branching. The secretory acini develop from the epithelial tissue, whereas the capsule of the gland and the connective tissue develop from the mesenchyme. The parotid, unlike other glands in the body, does not become encapsulated early to form a regular gland. The other structures in the vicinity, including the vessels, nerves and lymphatics, develop before encapsulation. The gland goes on to

Niels Stensen, 1638–1686, Danish anatomist, natural scientist and theologist.
Thomas Wharton, 1616–1673, physician, St Thomas' Hospital, London, UK, described the submandibular duct in 1656.

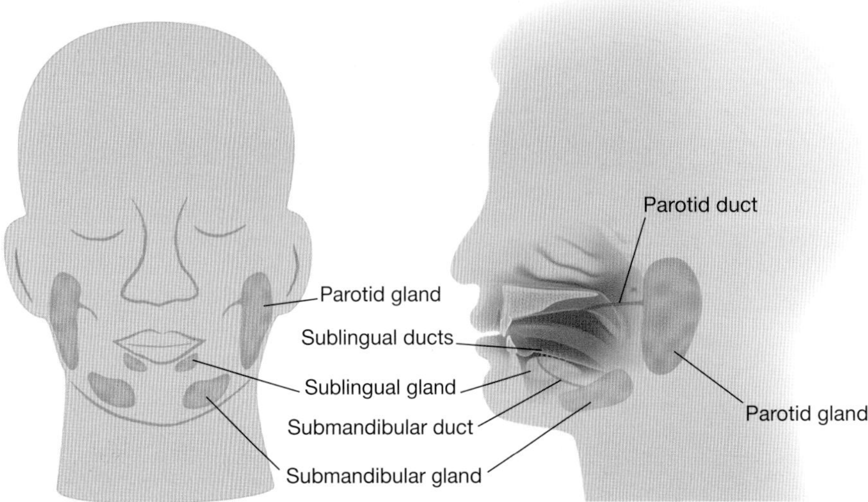

Figure 54.1 Anatomical position of the three major salivary glands.

envelop the facial nerve, the terminal branches of the external carotid artery, the retromandibular and superficial temporal vein and the lymph nodes. The capsule thus merges with the investing fascia from the zygoma, over the temporomandibular joint and the masseter and reaches the styloid base, posterior digastric belly and the sternocleidomastoid muscle. The superficial musculoaponeurotic system is closely approximated to this capsule. The parotid gland is, thus, irregular in shape and wedged in a recess between the ramus of the mandible, the base of the skull and the mastoid process.

The parotid (Stensen's) duct passes over the masseter muscle and enters the buccal mucosa through the buccinator muscle at the level of the upper second molar tooth. In some cases, an accessory gland is found along the course of the duct. Salivary tissue that is separated from the main parotid gland is referred to as an accessory parotid gland. These lie on the masseter muscle in front of Stensen's duct and have a secondary duct joining Stensen's duct. According to autopsy studies, the incidence of an accessory parotid gland is 21–61%. Embryologically, the growing, budding salivary glands originate from the oral cavity epithelium outwards into the mesenchyme as it differentiates into the various facial structures. The late completion of parotid gland encapsulation needs to be considered when planning surgery for accessory gland pathology that might also require removal of a superficial parotid gland. Following superficial parotid gland removal, the remnant unencapsulated acinar system in the glandular structure may also account for sialocele formation (a localised cavity or cyst containing saliva). Also after parotid gland surgery the acinar system with its ductules can be exposed to the wound, resulting in breakdown and leakage of saliva with fistula formation.

The facial nerve gets enveloped within the substance of the gland as it grows laterally, dividing the parotid gland into the superficial and deep lobes. Generally, the major functional component (80%) is superficial whereas the deep lobe is usually the retromandibular component with minimal functional gland tissue.

The lymphatic system develops within the parotid glandular tissue after encapsulation of the submandibular and sublingual glands. This results in the majority of the lymphatic structures, including the lymph nodes, being embedded within the parotid. The retromandibular vein, which drains these lymphatics, generally lies deep to the facial nerve and is a constant landmark that is useful during the retrograde method of identification of the main trunk of the facial nerve. Most of the lymph nodes lie in the superficial (preauricular) lobe of the parotid gland lateral to the masseter while very few lie in the deep (retromandibular) lobe of the parotid.

Summary box 54.2

Parotid gland

- Parotid gland and minor salivary glands are ectodermal in origin whereas the submandibular and sublingual glands are endodermal
- Parotid gland develops in the sixth week but has delayed encapsulation
- Facial vessels, facial nerve and lymphatic tissue are embedded in the substance of the parotid gland before the capsule fuses

Parotid innervation and Frey's syndrome

The glossopharyngeal nerve (cranial nerve IX) carries preganglionic parasympathetic fibres from the inferior salivatory nucleus. The Jacobson nerve, a branch of cranial

Lucja Frey, 1896–1944, physician, The Neurological Clinic, Warsaw, Poland.
Ludwig Levin Jacobson, 1783–1843, Danish anatomist.

nerve IX, enters via the inferior tympanic canaliculus to form the tympanic plexus in the middle ear. The lesser petrosal nerve carrying the preganglionic fibres from here exits via the foramen ovale, where it synapses with the postganglionic secretomotor parasympathetic fibres in the otic ganglion. These fibres exit the otic ganglion and join the auriculotemporal nerve in the infratemporal fossa, which innervates the parotid gland for the secretion of saliva.

Within the gland, acetylcholine (ACh) stimulates both acinar activity and ductal transport, leading to vasodilatation of the glands and contraction of the myoepithelial cells. Atropine decreases salivation by competing with ACh for the salivary receptor site and is useful in reducing salivary secretion. Regeneration of parasympathetic fibres to the sweat glands leads to abnormal autonomic reinnervation. ACh can act as a neurotransmitter for both postganglionic sympathetic and parasympathetic fibres; this might contribute to 'gustatory sweating' (Frey syndrome), which involves sweating and flushing of the skin overlying the parotid region while eating in some patients following parotidectomy.

Submandibular gland

The submandibular glands originate from the junctional tissue between ectoderm and endoderm from the floor of the mouth. They grow from the 18th to the 25th embryonic week and acquire connective capsules.

They lie in the submandibular space between the digastric muscles and extend upwards deep to the mandible. They consist of a larger superficial and a smaller deep lobe that is continuous around the posterior border of the mylohyoid muscle. The deep part of the gland lies on the hyoglossus muscle in close relation to the lingual nerve. The submandibular ganglion innervates the submandibular gland by the postganglionic parasympathetic fibres from the superior salivatory nucleus of the pons, through the chorda tympani and lingual nerve. The ganglion connections are required to be separated to free the gland and preserve the lingual nerve during excision.

The gland is surrounded by a well-defined capsule derived from the deep cervical fascia, which splits to enclose it. Wharton's (submandibular) duct lies between the hyoglossus and mylohyoid muscle after arising from the deep part of the gland. It drains at the sublingual papilla into the anterior floor of the mouth. The facial vein lies superficial to the gland to reach the anterior border of the mandible. The facial artery enters deep to the posterior belly of the digastric and stylohyoid muscles and passes through or superficial to the gland to reach the anterior border of the mandible. The glandular branches need to be ligated when preserving the facial artery during submandibular gland removal. The facial artery is commonly used as the recipient artery in microvascular anastomosis in free tissue transfer in head and neck reconstruction. The marginal mandibular branch of the facial nerve lies in the superficial fascia, traversing over the facial vessels. Martin described the technique of ligating these vessels and flipping them above in order to preserve the mandibular division of the facial nerve during neck dissection.

Sublingual gland

The sublingual glands contribute around 5% of saliva production and are the smallest of the major salivary glands. They lie above the mylohyoid muscle and below the floor of mouth mucosa and are bordered by the mandible laterally and by the genioglossus muscle medially. Their secretions are drained by small ducts (Rivinus's ducts) that exit along the sublingual fold at the floor of the mouth. A few anterior ducts may join together to form a common duct called Bartholin's duct, which empties close to or into Wharton's duct near the sublingual caruncle.

The pathology of the sublingual glands mainly involves the formation of a mucous retention cyst (ranula). Tumours of sublingual glands are very rare.

Summary box 54.3

Sublingual gland

- Problems are rare
- Minor mucous retention cysts may need surgery
- A plunging ranula is a retention cyst that tunnels deep
- Nearly all tumours are malignant

Minor salivary glands

Minor salivary glands appear at about the 12th week of gestation, forming directly from upper respiratory ectoderm. They develop as individual units with simple tubuloacinar systems.

The minor salivary glands lack a distinct capsule and merge with the surrounding connective tissue in the submucosal region. They are widely distributed in the head and neck region and are mainly located (70–90%) in the oral cavity and oropharynx, including the palate, the tongue, the lips, the buccal mucosa and the retromolar trigone. The other sites are the nose, paranasal sinuses, pharynx and the larynx. They contribute 8–10% of the saliva and play a major role in saliva production during sleep.

COMMON DISORDERS

Mucoceles

Extravasation mucoceles and retention cysts are formed by mucous extravasation. Both have similar clinical features but variable distinct pathogenesis (*Figure 54.2*).

Hayes Martin, 1892–1977 Attending Surgeon, Memorial Hospital; Chief, Head and Neck Surgery, Memorial Sloan Kettering Cancer Centre; Professor of Surgery, Cornell University Medical College, New York, NY, USA.

Augustus Quirinus Rivinus, 1652–1723, German physician and botanist, studied the anatomy of salivary glands and also developed ways of classifying plants.

Thomas Bartholin, 1616–1680, Professor of Anatomy, Copenhagen University, Copenhagen, Denmark.

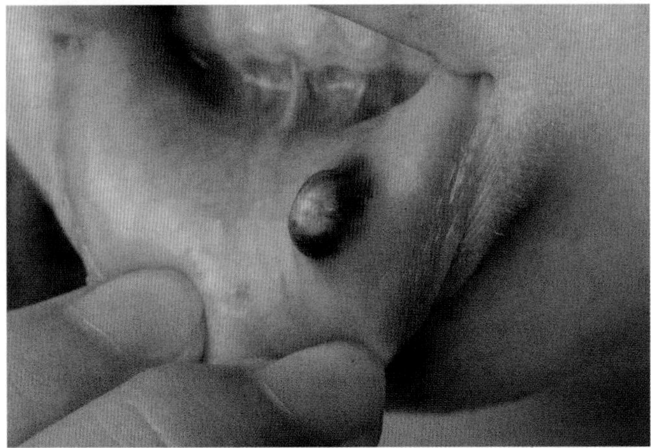

Figure 54.2 Mucous retention cyst. A translucent swelling on the lower lip is typical.

Extravasation mucocele

Trauma to the minor salivary gland duct causes accumulation of saliva in the surrounding connective tissue, followed by an inflammatory reaction. They occur commonly in children and adolescents and are mainly found on the lower lip. A ranula is a type of extravasation mucocele.

Ranula (little frog)

Ranulas, first described by Banister in his surgical compilation of 1585, are caused either by the rupture of the main duct or by the rupture of obstructed acini of the sublingual gland. They appear as a characteristic bluish swelling in the anterior floor of the mouth and resemble the belly or air sac of a frog. They can remain localised or insinuate through the mylohyoid muscle to present as a submental swelling called a 'plunging ranula'. They are usually soft, fluctuant and painless unless infected. Imaging corroborates the clinical diagnosis and aspiration yields the thick sticky saliva that distinguishes them from a lymphangioma (***Figures 54.3 and 54.4***).

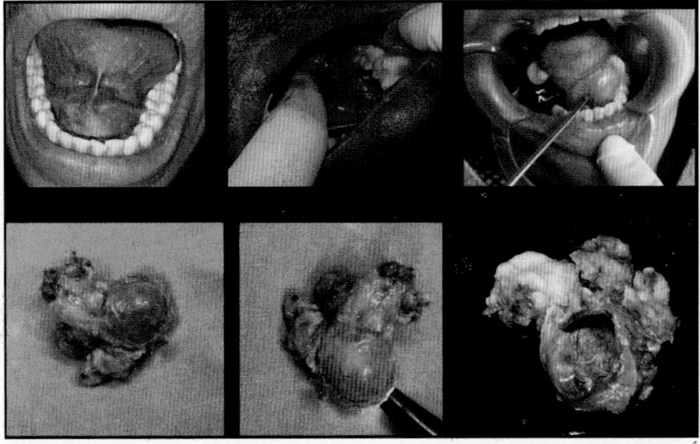

Figure 54.3 Ranulas in the floor of mouth, transillumination and specimen (courtesy of Dr Shirish Ghan, Nasik, India).

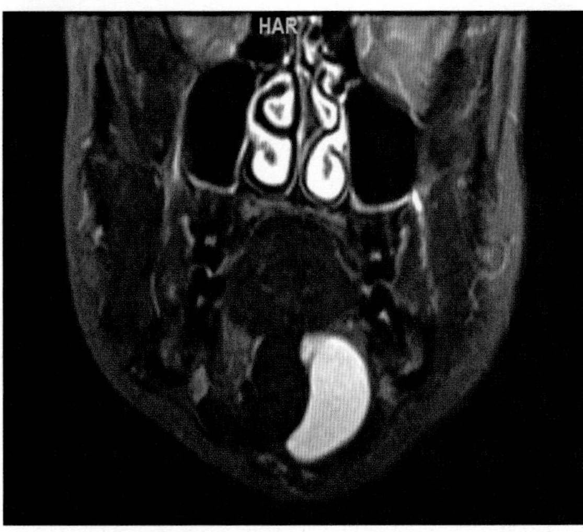

Figure 54.4 Magnetic resonance imaging scan showing a ranula in the floor of mouth.

Treatment should include removal of the sublingual gland as this gland has multiple ducts and ranulas can recur if the gland is left behind. Incision, drainage and marsupialisation have low success rates. Injecting OK-432 at the local site produces inflammation and fibrosis. Injection of botulinum toxin has shown a good success rate but needs further evaluation.

Retention cyst

These result from obstruction of the duct by periductal scars, sialolithiasis (salivary gland stone formation) or pressure from surrounding tissue. These cysts are mainly found in the ductal system of a minor salivary gland. The cyst cavity may contain fragments of a sialolith or mucous material. Some may regress spontaneously but are best treated by surgical excision.

Acute necrotising sialometaplasia

This usually occurs on the palate and primarily affects the minor salivary glands. It initially presents as a swelling that goes on to develop a central crater with rolled out margins, mimicking a malignant ulcer. Clinically it can be mistaken for a malignancy and the biopsy also raises doubt because of the presence of necrosis and hyperplasia. However, the lobular architecture of the glands is generally preserved and the lack of cellular atypia might help the pathologist to reach the right diagnosis. Ultimately, the lesion heals in a few weeks. The exact aetiology is unknown but is suspected to follow trauma or be caused by an injection to that area or by excessive vomiting.

Immunological conditions

Sjögren's syndrome

Sjögren's syndrome (SjS) is a chronic autoimmune disease with lymphocytic infiltration and autoimmune injury to the salivary and lacrimal glands, leading to dryness of the mouth

John Banister, 1533–1610, English anatomist, surgeon and teacher.
Henrik Samuel Conrad Sjögren, 1899–1986, Professor of Ophthalmology, Gothenburg, Sweden, described this condition in 1933.

(xerostomia) and eyes. The understanding of the pathophysiology of the disease is evolving and is a complex interaction among genetic elements, environmental factors and abnormal host immunity. It mainly affects women in the fourth to fifth decades, who present with enlargement of the salivary glands, especially the parotid. Typically there is a delay in the time taken to diagnosis of the disease. Studies have shown a delay of 2–6 months between the first consultation and diagnosis. SjS can be considered to have four stages: initiation stage, preclinical stage, asymptomatic SjS stage and overt SjS stage.

Primary SjS is not associated with any illness or disease, whereas secondary SjS is associated with other autoimmune disorders, including systemic lupus erythematosus, rheumatoid arthritis and scleroderma (***Table 54.1***).

With no diagnostic markers, the diagnosis is based on a set of five criteria proposed by the European Alliance of Associations for Rheumatology (EULAR). One of them is a biopsy of the sublabial salivary glands, which shows histological features of focal lymphocytic sialadenitis. The criteria required for diagnosis of SjS involve at least one focus score of more than 50 lymphocytes per 4 mm^2 of parenchymal tissue. Other tests for early diagnosis are evolving; these include testing for increasing levels of biomarkers such as complement C3 and neutrophil elastase in saliva and tears. In addition, identification of traditional antibodies such as anti-nuclear antibodies (anti-SSA/Ro or anti-SSB/La) and rheumatoid factor can also be used. However, a significant proportion of patients with SjS may be seronegative.

Treatment depends on disease activity and the organs involved. Tear substitutes can be used and xerostomia is treated by dental and oral surgeons. Randomised controlled trials have not shown any benefit with hydroxychloroquine or disease-modifying antirheumatic drugs (DMARDs). Treatment with glucocorticoids and/or immunosuppressant drugs should be considered in severe systemic manifestations.

TABLE 54.1 Degenerative disorders of the salivary glands.

Primary Sjögren's syndrome	• More severe xerostomia • Widespread exocrine gland dysfunction • No connective tissue disorder
Secondary Sjögren's syndrome	• Male-to-female ratio 1:10 • Middle age • Underlying connective tissue disorder
Benign lymphoepithelial lesion	• Diffuse parotid swelling 20% bilateral • 5% develop lymphoma

Scleroderma

This is an immunologically mediated disease with complex interactions between the vascular network, inflammatory markers and collagen tissue. It mainly affects adults with a female preponderance. Multiple organs may be affected by excessive deposition of collagen in various organs. While skin is more commonly affected, it can also involve the heart, lungs, kidneys and gastrointestinal tract. Salivary gland parenchyma may be replaced by collagen tissue, leading to clinical xerostomia. Biopsy of a minor salivary gland may be useful for diagnosis.

Sarcoidosis

This is an inflammatory disorder characterised by multiple non-caseating granulomas in multiple systems. A dry cough, fatigue and shortness of breath are its main symptoms. The chest radiograph typically shows bilateral hilar lymphadenopathy and reticular opacities in the lungs. Skin, heart, kidney, eyes, joints, exocrine glands and the central nervous system may be involved. The aetiology is unclear but one proposed mechanism is where an individual with a susceptible genotype is exposed to one or more potential antigens, resulting in a sustained inflammatory response. The disease most commonly occurs in those aged 20–60, in people of African or northern European descent and in those with a family history of the disease. Triggers are thought to include infection (mycobacteria, propionic bacteria and viruses) or exposure to certain chemicals or dust. The function of an organ can begin to be affected as granulomas form and enlarge.

For the salivary glands, the patient can present with a localised tumour-like swelling, usually in the parotid – the so-called sarcoid pseudotumour along with xerostomia. In the absence of other disease, the diagnosis is usually made following surgical excision for a presumed neoplasm. Heerfordt's syndrome is a rare manifestation of sarcoidosis that involves parotid swelling, anterior uveitis, facial palsy and fever.

Ectopic/aberrant salivary gland tissue

The presence of ectopic salivary tissue in the mandible can manifest as circumscribed unilocular osteolytic radiolucency of the jaw, known as a Stafne bone cyst. They are possibly caused by either congenital entrapment of salivary tissue during mandibular development or pressure resorption from the adjacent ectopic salivary gland and facial artery. On orthopantomogram, the size ranges from 0.5 to 2 cm, with a median of 1.2 cm. They are mainly located in the posterior region of the mandible, especially between the first molar and the angle of the mandible. The other sites of ectopic salivary tissue include the cervical lymph nodes, middle ear, parathyroid glands, thyroid gland, pituitary gland, cerebellopontine angle and soft tissue medial to the sternocleidomastoid muscle.

Sialadenitis

Inflammation of a salivary gland can be acute or chronic (***Table 54.2***). Acute causes include viral and bacterial infection. It mainly affects the young adolescent population. Parotid glands are more commonly involved than submandibular glands.

Christian Frederick Heerfordt, 1871–1953, Danish ophthalmologist, described this syndrome in 1909.
Edward C Stafne, 1894–1981, dental surgeon, The Mayo Clinic, Rochester, MN, USA, described these cysts in 1942.

TABLE 54.2 Various causes of acute and chronic sialadenitis.

Acute sialadenitis	Chronic sialadenitis
• Viral: ◦ Mumps ◦ Coxsackie ◦ Cytomegalovirus ◦ Paramyxovirus • Bacterial: ◦ *Staphylococcus aureus* (acute suppurative parotitis)	• Granulomatous: ◦ TB ◦ Cat scratch disease ◦ Actinomycosis ◦ Sarcoidosis • HIV • Abscess (parotid and submandibular) • Recurrent subacute parotitis • Radiation sialadenitis

HIV, human immunodeficiency virus; TB, tuberculosis.

Viral infections are more common than bacterial infections. The causative organisms are most commonly paramyxovirus (mumps), followed by cytomegalovirus, coxsackie virus, human immunodeficiency virus (HIV), parainfluenza virus types I and II, influenza virus A and herpesvirus.

Among bacteria, *Staphylococcus aureus* is the most common organism and usually results in a retrograde spread of infection through the duct. Duct obstruction and xerostomia in the elderly population are predisposing factors. The patient will present with a painful red swelling over the gland region.

Viral sialadenitis is self-limiting in most cases, requiring symptomatic supportive care, while bacterial infection will require antibiotics.

Human immunodeficiency virus sialadenitis

This is mainly characterised by bilateral enlargement of the parotid glands. This may mimic SjS. HIV sialadenitis is usually seen in young individuals with an absence of any serological antibodies, whereas SjS is mainly seen in middle-aged women. The prevalence is between 5% and 10% and it has been postulated that it is more common in women on highly active antiretroviral therapy (HAART) (mainly protease inhibitors).

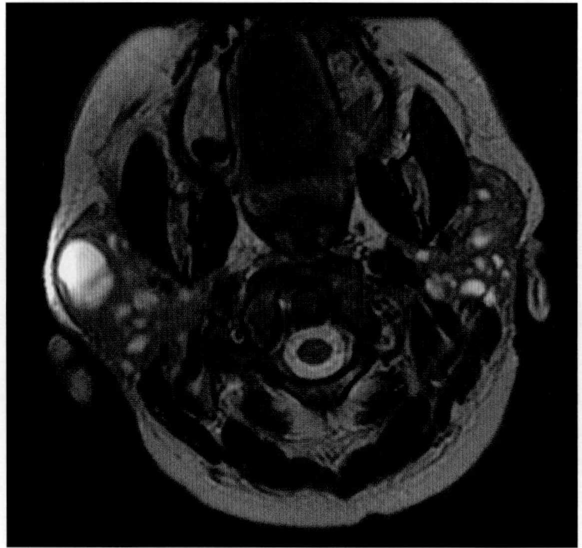

Figure 54.5 Lymphoepithelial cysts in a human immunodeficiency virus-infected patient.

Patients also complain of xerostomia, which may be due to HAART or parenchymal disease of the salivary gland as a result of HIV (***Figure 54.5***).

Biopsy reveals perivascular, periductal and periacinar areas predominantly infiltrated with CD8 cells. Abnormal deposition of fat seen in the parotid gland (parotid lipomatosis) as well as in the abdomen and dorsal cervical areas may be associated with the use of protease inhibitors.

Benign lymphoepithelial cysts are HIV-related reactive lymphoproliferation, which may occur in the intraparotid lymph nodes (***Table 54.1***). The parotid glandular epithelium may get trapped within the normal intraparotid lymph nodes, resulting in cystic enlargement or migration of HIV-infected cells into the parotid gland, which could trigger lymphoid proliferation, salivary duct dysplasia, ductal obstruction and cyst formation. Ultrasonography is usually diagnostic. There may be a rare conversion into lymphoma. Diffuse infiltrative lymphocytosis syndrome manifests with bilateral enlargement caused by constant infiltration of CD8 in the parotid glands.

Summary box 54.4

HIV sialadenitis

- Incidence 5–10%
- More common in women on HAART
- Mimic SjS, but absent antibody
- Infiltration of CD8 in the parotid glands

Recurrent parotitis of childhood

This is characterised by rapid swelling of one or both parotid glands that is aggravated by chewing and eating. Systemic upset with fever and malaise is variable. The symptoms usually last about a week and are followed by a quiescent period for weeks to several months. It is mainly seen between the ages of 3 and 6 years. It is postulated to be caused by an incompetent parotid duct punctum, leading to ductal contamination with oral fluids. The diagnosis is based on the characteristic history. In addition, sialography shows a characteristic punctate sialectasis (snowstorm). The condition is difficult to manage if it becomes established and the initial treatment is important. The treatment consists of long courses of antibiotics and endoscopic washouts.

Sialadenosis

This is a non-inflammatory bilateral enlargement of the parotid glands. The swelling is generally painless with reduced saliva and is associated with chronic malnutrition, obesity, alcoholism, liver disease, diabetes and drugs such as guanethidine, thioridazine or isoprenaline. It requires differentiation from any neoplastic disorder. Treatment mainly consists of management of the underlying systemic disorder.

Sialolithiasis

Salivary gland stones can form in the gland ducts. Patients between the ages of 30 and 60 with sialolithiasis typically present with cyclical postprandial swelling of the major salivary

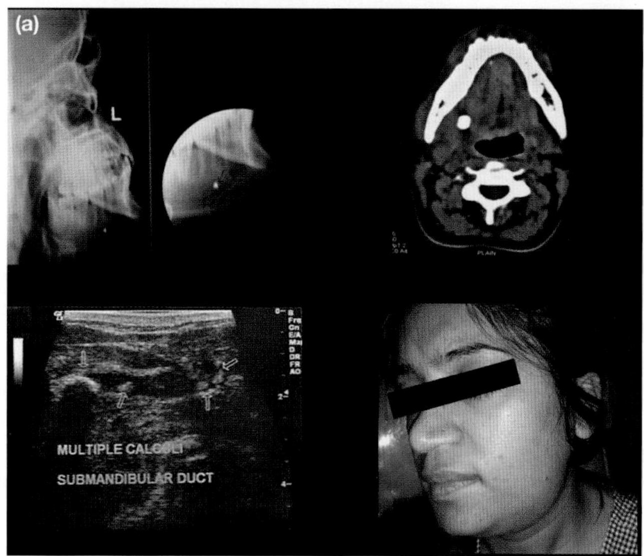

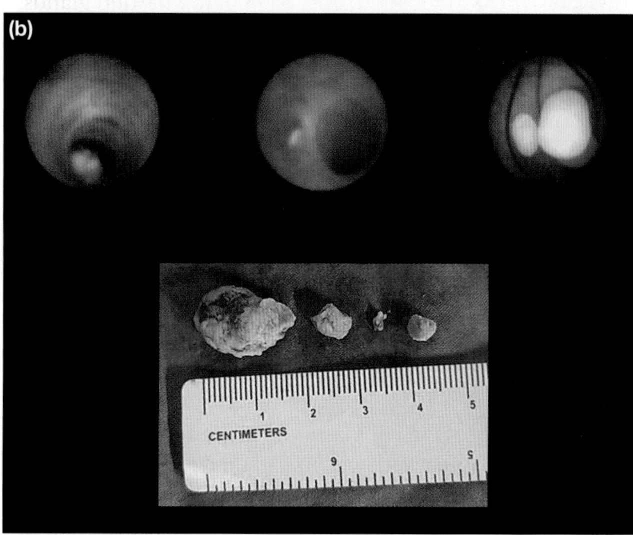

Figure 54.6 (a) A submandibular gland sialolithiasis. (b) Sialo-endoscopy with submandibular gland calculus removal (courtesy of Dr Shirish Ghan, Nasik, India).

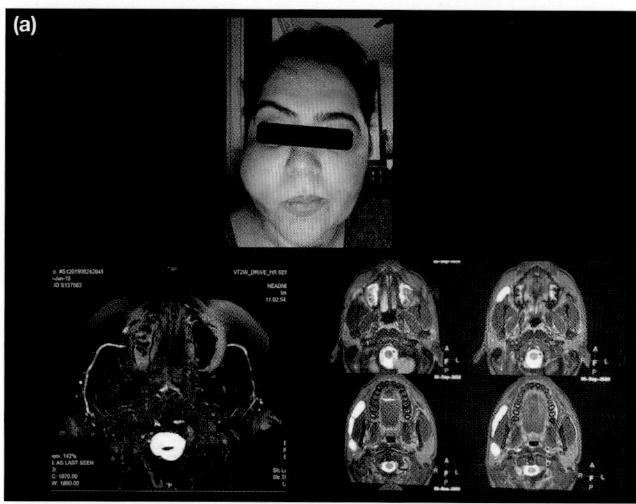

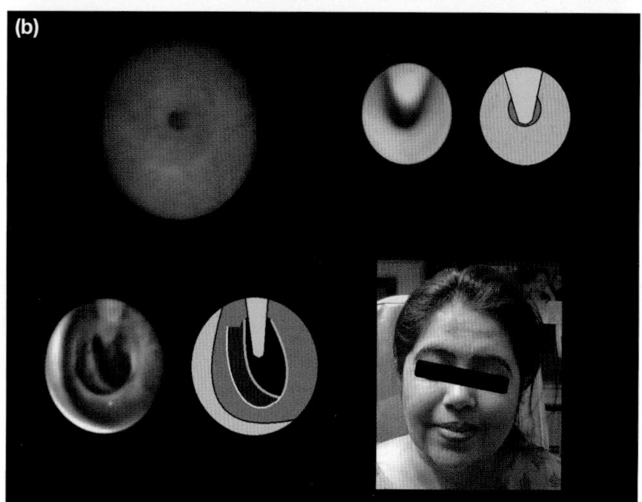

Figure 54.7 (a) Parotid gland swelling due to lithiasis and secondary stricture. (b) Sialendoscopic stricture dilatation (courtesy of Dr Shirish Ghan, Nasik, India).

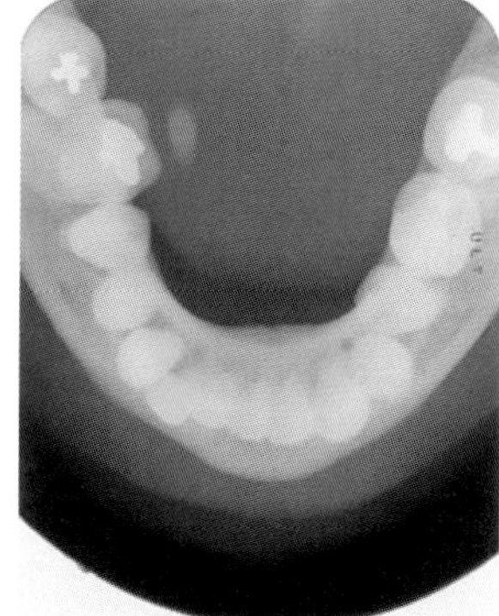

Figure 54.8 Occlusal view showing a stone in the submandibular gland.

glands and dryness possibly due to decreased salivary flow. Duct abnormality, inflammation and increased calcium content of the saliva may contribute to an increased risk of sialolithiasis. Chronic dehydration and pharmacological causes of decreased salivary flow are often implicated. The submandibular gland is most commonly affected (85%) owing to the ascending course of its duct, predisposing it to stagnation of the mucinous as well as the more viscous saliva it produces (***Figure 54.6***). The alkaline saliva precipitates calcium and phosphate and predisposes to stone formation. On examination, there is an asymmetrical enlargement of the gland and a large proximal stone may be palpated in certain cases. Submandibular gland duct stones are mainly proximal and parotid gland duct stones are mainly distal (***Figure 54.7***). Sialolithiasis complicated by a secondary bacterial infection may present with an abscess.

Conventional radiographs are considered as an initial diagnostic test (***Figure 54.8***). However, small stones may be missed and only 80% of stones are radio-opaque. In such cases, computed tomography (CT) scanning, ultrasonography and a magnetic resonance sialogram will be more sensitive for diagnosis and localisation. Sialography is the gold standard for diagnosis and involves injecting a dye into the duct of the salivary gland. It not only helps in diagnosis of sialolithiasis but also identifies any pathology in the duct. In addition, it may be therapeutic in certain cases. Sialendoscopy provides direct visualisation of the duct and can be used for removal of stones. It is a safe procedure that can be performed under local anaesthesia with better outcomes than open surgery. The smaller (<5 mm) distal stones can be removed with endoscopy while the larger (>5 mm) distal stones may require duct slitting. For an impacted stone, the transoral route is used. Intraparenchymal stones between 5 and 7 mm can be extracted endoscopically while larger stones require transoral slitting. Stones that are not palpable and not visualised endoscopically can be removed using external shock wave lithotripsy (ESWL). However, ESWL is not suitable for stones larger than 7–10 mm. Hilar stones are removed using an endoscope. Excision of the submandibular gland should be considered as a last resort. Parotid stones (<7 mm) can be removed endoscopically and difficult cases might need a combined transcutaneous approach. ESWL can be considered for impacted stones. Again gland removal should be considered only as a final remedy.

Xerostomia

Normal salivary flow decreases with age. Typical complaints are of a dry mouth, difficulty swallowing and speaking, intolerance to spicy, acidic and crunchy food, a loss of taste and denture-wearing issues. Xerostomia is more common among postmenopausal women, who complain of a burning tongue or mouth. Common causes of xerostomia are chronic anxiety states and depression; dehydration; anticholinergic drugs, especially antidepressants; salivary gland disorders (e.g. SjS); and radiotherapy to the head and neck region. Xerostomia and salivary gland hypofunction diagnosis requires a thorough history and examination as well as documentation with one of the several questionnaires available. Treatments include proper hydration, humidification at night, avoiding harmful dentifrices and crunchy/hard foods and the use of sugar-free chewing gums and lozenges. Medications include lubricants, saliva substitutes or stimulants.

Sialorrhoea

Excess salivation is rarely symptomatic in healthy individuals as it is swallowed spontaneously. Certain drugs and oral infection produce a transient increase in salivary flow; however, uncontrolled drooling is usually seen in the presence of normal salivary production in children with mental and physical disability, most notably cerebral palsy. Sialorrhoea can be managed with antisialogogues or with intraparenchymal injection of botulinum toxin injection. Most resting salivary flow arises from the submandibular glands and surgery should focus on either bilateral excision or repositioning of the salivary duct to control sialorrhoea.

Trauma

Trauma to the salivary glands or ducts is uncommon and is usually associated with polytrauma due to penetrating injuries, blasts or vehicular accidents. This can result in injury to the salivary glandular tissue, the duct and the surrounding nerves, such as the facial and hypoglossal nerves. Often these injuries go unnoticed and manifest later with a salivary fistula, nerve palsy and/or sialoceles.

The basic principles of all wound care management apply to salivary gland injuries, including removal of foreign bodies, wound washout, debridement and tension-free closure of the wound. Besides this, the glandular tissue, the duct and the nerves in the vicinity require utmost attention to prevent late complications. These are often overlooked and missed.

Facial nerve

A cranial nerve examination guides the clinician towards the possibility of nerve injuries. The wound is examined for nerve injuries. If the branches are severed anteriorly to an imaginary line dropped vertically down from the lateral canthus of the eye, they are not repaired. If the injury is posterior to this line, a direct nerve repair or grafting is carried out depending on the wound status. If not feasible at that time the nerve endings are tagged for later.

Salivary duct

Within the first 72 hours a duct injury should be repaired with a direct end-to-end anastomosis over a cannula. If there is a loss of duct tissue of over 1 cm, the proximal portion is either cannulated for subsequent marsupialisation into the oral cavity or a duct rerouting is considered. In cases with significant parenchyma and duct injury a ductal ligation along with gland excision should be considered.

NEOPLASMS OF THE SALIVARY GLAND

Primary salivary gland neoplasms are extremely rare and form less than 3% of head and neck malignancies. The incidence is 0.4–13.5 cases per 100 000 for benign neoplasms and 0.4–2.6 per 100 000 for malignant tumours. These neoplasms present after the fourth decade and affect both sexes equally. Warthin's tumours are more common in older men, while pleomorphic adenomas are slightly more common in women.

With a varied spectrum of pathologies, salivary gland neoplasms present a diagnostic and therapeutic challenge. The World Health Organization (WHO) first classified these in 1972, and its last update was in 2017 (***Table 54.3***). Most salivary gland tumours (>80%) occur in the major salivary glands and the majority of them are benign. Minor salivary gland tumours, in contrast, are more likely to be malignant (>50%) (***Figure 54.9***). The commonest benign neoplasm is the pleomorphic adenoma (mostly seen in the parotid glands), while the commonest malignant tumour is the mucoepidermoid carcinoma.

Radiation exposure has been implicated in the development of both benign and malignant salivary gland tumours, while there is a strong association of smoking with Warthin's tumour. Viral infections, environmental factors and industrial exposure, such as rubber manufacturing, nickel compounds and hair dyes, have been reported to be associated with the development of salivary gland tumours.

Aldred Scott Warthin, 1866–1931, Professor of Pathology, University of Michigan, Ann Arbor, MI, USA.

TABLE 54.3 World Health Organization classification of salivary gland neoplasms (2017).

Malignant epithelial tumours	Benign epithelial tumours

• Acinic cell carcinoma
• Mucoepidermoid carcinoma
• Adenoid cystic carcinoma
• Polymorphous low-grade adenocarcinoma
• Epithelial–myoepithelial carcinoma
• Clear cell carcinoma, not otherwise specified
• Basal cell adenocarcinoma
• Sebaceous carcinoma
• Sebaceous lymphadenocarcinoma
• Cystadenocarcinoma
• Low-grade cribriform cystadenocarcinoma
• Mucinous adenocarcinoma
• Oncocytic carcinoma
• Salivary duct carcinoma
• Adenocarcinoma, not otherwise specified
• Myoepithelial carcinoma
• Carcinoma ex pleomorphic adenoma
• Carcinosarcoma
• Metastasising pleomorphic adenoma
• Squamous cell carcinoma
• Small cell carcinoma
• Large cell carcinoma
• Lymphoepithelial carcinoma
• Sialoblastoma
	• Pleomorphic adenoma
	• Myoepithelioma
	• Basal cell adenoma
	• Warthin's tumour
	• Oncocytoma
	• Canalicular adenoma
	• Sebaceous adenoma
	• Lymphadenoma
	  ◦ Sebaceous
	  ◦ Non-sebaceous
	• Ductal papillomas
	  ◦ Inverted ductal papilloma
	  ◦ Intraductal papilloma
	  ◦ Sialadenoma papilliferum
	• Cystadenoma
	
	Soft-tissue tumours
	• Haemangioma
	
	Haematolymphoid tumours
	• Hodgkin's lymphoma
	• Diffuse large B-cell lymphoma
	• Extranodal marginal zone B-cell lymphoma
	
	Secondary tumours

Histological grades of salivary gland cancers	
High grade	**Low to intermediate grade**
• High-grade mucoepidermoid carcinoma • Salivary duct carcinoma • Adenoid cystic carcinoma • Carcinoma ex pleomorphic adenoma • Squamous cell carcinoma • Anaplastic or undifferentiated carcinoma • Malignant mixed carcinoma	• Low-grade mucoepidermoid carcinoma • Acinic cell carcinoma • Polymorphous low-grade adenocarcinoma • Epithelial–myoepithelial carcinoma

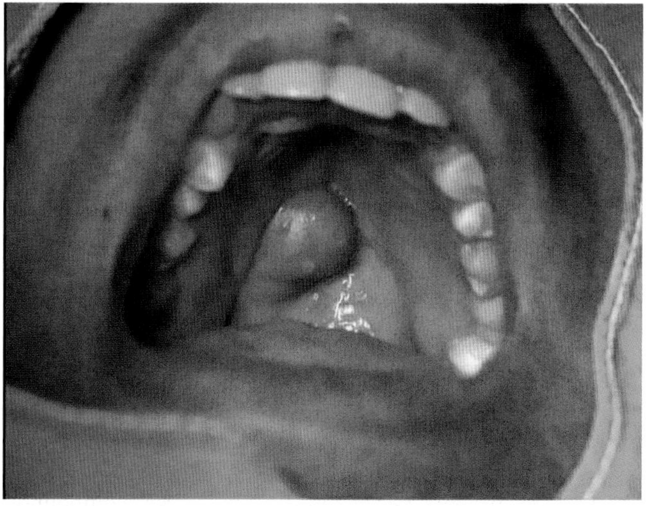

Figure 54.9 Mucoepidermoid carcinoma of the palate.

Benign tumours

Pleomorphic adenoma

These are the most common benign salivary gland tumours. They can occur at all ages, but are most commonly seen between the third and sixth decade. The average age of presentation is 45 years and they are more frequently seen in women. They occur most frequently in the parotid glands (>80%), but are also seen in the submandibular gland and hard palate. Pleomorphic adenoma presents as a painless, well-defined solitary mobile mass with gradual progression over many years and can reach enormous proportions (***Figure 54.10***). Occasionally they can present as metachronous and synchronous tumours. When they arise from the deep lobe of the parotid they may present as a paratonsillar bulge. A sudden increase in size or facial nerve palsy is associated with malignant transformation, which is rare. Treatment involves surgical excision with a cuff of surrounding normal tissue, where possible, to include the

Thomas Hodgkin, 1798–1866, curator of the museum and demonstrator of Morbid Anatomy, Guy's Hospital, London, UK, described lymphadenoma in 1832.

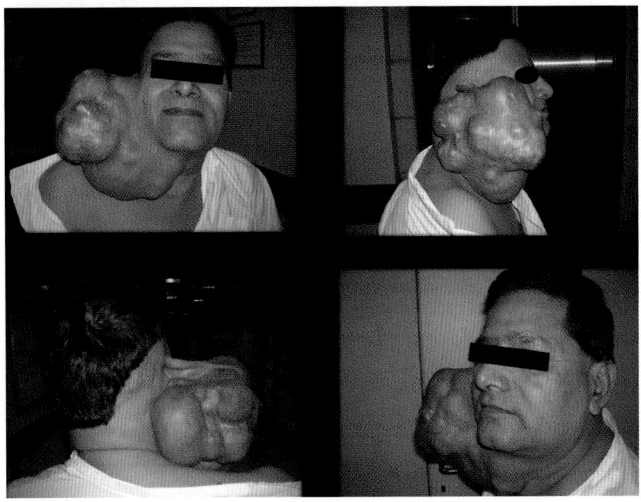

Figure 54.10 Double head: large pleomorphic adenoma grown over 15 years.

pseudopods from the tumour capsule. Enucleation may result in capsular breach and tumour spillage, increasing the possibility of local recurrence; it should be avoided.

Histopathology

On gross examination, pleomorphic adenoma presents as a well-circumscribed, nodular, firm mass with a white to tan cut surface, sometimes showing cartilaginous areas. Large tumours may show areas of degeneration and cystic changes. On microscopy, the tumour comprises mixed epithelial, myoepithelial and stromal components. A spectrum of architectural and cellular features is seen, including oval, epithelioid, spindle shaped, plasmacytoid and clear cells, in variable amounts of myxoid to chondroid and hyalinised stroma. The presence of ductal atypia, diffuse fibrosis and necrosis should be evaluated further to rule out malignancy. In immunohistochemistry, luminal cells express CK7 (strong and diffuse) and myoepithelial cells express p63, S-100, SOX10 and SMA.

Warthin's tumour

Warthin's tumour, also known as adenolymphoma or cystadenoma lymphomatosum, is a benign tumour composed of oncocytic epithelial cells lining ductal, papillary and cystic spaces in a reactive lymphoid tissue. They are the second most common benign salivary gland tumours (5–15%) and are mainly seen in older men, after the sixth decade of life. They have been associated with cigarette smoking as well as radiation exposure. They are almost exclusively seen in the parotid gland, especially in the inferior pole, and are rarely seen in the periparotid nodes. They can occur synchronously or metachronously in the same or bilateral glands. They are also known to occur with other salivary gland neoplasms such as pleomorphic adenoma and salivary duct carcinoma. Clinically, they present as painless, slow-growing swellings. Facial palsy is rare. Malignant transformation is extremely rare (<1%) and can occur in both the epithelial (Warthin's adenocarcinoma) and lymphoid (lymphoma) components. Complete surgical excision with an adequate margin is the treatment of choice. Recurrences are very rare and may be due to multifocal tumours.

Histopathology

On gross examination, they are well circumscribed and ovoid to spherical with a cut surface showing solid and cystic areas containing mucoid to brownish fluid and papillary projections. On microscopy, the tumours have papillary and cystic structures lined by bilayered oncocytic epithelial cells in a lymphoid stroma with germinal centres. The epithelium may show metaplastic changes, including squamous, sebaceous, ciliated and mucous cells.

Malignant tumours

Mucoepidermoid carcinoma

Mucoepidermoid carcinomas are malignancies consisting of mucinous, intermediate and squamoid tumour cells in variable proportions. They are the most common salivary gland malignancies in children and young adults, with a peak incidence in the second decade of life. They are known to occur following radiation or chemotherapy in childhood. They occur in both major and minor salivary glands, with the parotid being the most common site involved. They generally present as soft to firm, painless masses with a gradual increase in size. The tumours are classified as low, intermediate or high grade based on histology. High-grade mucoepidermoid carcinomas tend to be locally aggressive with bone and/or skin involvement and nodal metastases. Distant metastases are seen mainly to the lungs. Complete surgical excision with wide margins is advocated for mucoepidermoid carcinoma. Appropriate adjuvant radiotherapy is the treatment of choice for intermediate- to high-grade mucoepidermoid carcinomas.

On gross examination, the tumours are circumscribed or infiltrative and partially cystic. On histopathology, mucoepidermoid carcinomas have squamoid, mucin-producing and intermediate cells in variable proportions. There can be a cystic and solid growth pattern. Low-grade mucoepidermoid carcinomas are generally cystic, well circumscribed and rich in mucous cells. Intermediate-grade tumours are less circumscribed and more solid, usually with a predominant intermediate cell component. High-grade mucoepidermoid carcinomas are usually solid, infiltrative and show nuclear atypia, mitosis, necrosis, perineural invasion and lymphovascular emboli. Demonstration of at least focal intracellular mucin is essential for the diagnosis of high-grade mucoepidermoid carcinoma.

Summary box 54.5

Mucoepidermoid carcinoma

- Most common salivary gland malignancy
- Can occur in minor and major salivary glands
- Most common site: parotid

Adenoid cystic carcinoma

Adenoid cystic carcinoma is a slow-growing malignancy composed of both epithelial and myoepithelial cells and characterised by a high predilection for perineural invasion. It has varying outcomes with good 5-year control but poor 10-year survival owing to the higher incidence of delayed distant metastases. They occur mainly in the fifth to sixth decades, with a slight female preponderance (1.5:1). Most of these malignancies occur in the major salivary glands, but they can also be seen in minor glands in the oral cavity, paranasal sinuses, tracheobronchial tree, etc. Most patients will present with slow-growing masses, with the presence of numbness, paraesthesia or pain. Facial and other neural palsies may be present depending on the site of the tumour. Nodal metastases are seen with high-grade lesions and asymptomatic distant metastases, especially lung metastases, are a frequent presentation. In addition, bone, liver and brain metastases are also seen. Radical surgical excision with or without adjuvant radiotherapy is the treatment of choice. Single-modality radiotherapy is associated with inferior control outcomes. There is an emerging role of proton ion and carbon ion therapy, especially in unresectable/metastatic disease. Factors influencing survival include the tumour site, stage, nodal disease, presence of perineural spread and grade of tumour.

Grossly, adenoid cystic carcinoma presents as a poorly circumscribed, firm, grey-white and solid mass. On histopathology, it is an unencapsulated, infiltrative biphasic neoplasm with variable proportions of epithelial and myoepithelial cells and shows cribriform tubular and solid patterns. The cells show small, angulated, hyperchromatic nuclei with scant cytoplasm. The cribriform pattern is characterised by neoplastic cells arranged around small, sharply punched out cylindromatous spaces containing basophilic matrix. The tubular pattern shows bilayered tubules with a true lumen. The solid pattern is less common and shows sheets and nests of tumour cells without lumen formation. Perineural invasion is widely seen in adenoid cystic carcinoma. High-grade transformation can occur. Immunohistochemically, the ductal cells are positive for c-KIT, and myoepithelial cells are positive for p63 and SMA.

Acinic cell carcinoma

Acinic cell carcinoma is composed of neoplastic acinar cells. It is a low- to intermediate-grade tumour occurring mostly (90%) in the parotid gland. They typically present in the fifth decade and have a slight female predilection (1.5:1). They are generally slow-growing, painless, mobile, solitary tumours and rarely present with facial palsy. A small proportion may be high grade and may metastasise to cervical nodes and lung. Complete excision with an adequate margin is the recommended treatment. Recurrences can occur in cases of incomplete resection, deep lobe involvement and larger size tumours. On histopathology, the tumours show characteristic serous acinar cells and variable proportions of other cell types, including clear, vacuolated, intercalated duct-type oncocytic and hobnail features. They can have solid (most common), follicular or microcystic patterns with a prominent lymphoid infiltrate. Mitoses, necroses and nuclear pleomorphism are rare. Immunohistochemically, the neoplastic cells are positive for DOG1 and SOX10, whereas they are immunonegative for mammaglobin, differentiating them from secretory carcinoma.

Carcinoma ex pleomorphic adenoma

Carcinoma ex pleomorphic adenoma (epithelial and/or myoepithelial) arises in association with primary or recurrent pleomorphic adenoma. The carcinoma component can be either purely epithelial or myoepithelial in presentation, with infiltration into the surrounding glandular and extraglandular tissue. It occurs mainly in the parotid gland, is more common in women and presents a decade later than pleomorphic adenoma (sixth decade). It often presents as a rapidly growing mass (within a longstanding swelling) associated with pain and facial palsy. Radical surgical excision with or without adjuvant radiotherapy is the treatment of choice. Local and distant metastases occur in 70% of cases with poor 5-year survival outcomes of 25–65%.

On histopathology, the tumour shows variable proportions of both pleomorphic adenoma and high-grade adenocarcinoma such as salivary duct carcinoma or myoepithelial carcinoma. It is subclassified as non-invasive or intracapsular (tumour is confined within pleomorphic adenoma), minimally invasive (tumour breaching the pleomorphic adenoma capsule) and widely invasive into adjacent salivary gland and soft tissue. TP53 mutations and amplification of HER2 (in salivary duct carcinoma) with a high degree of genetic instability and copy-number alterations are seen.

Salivary duct carcinoma

Also known as high-grade ductal carcinoma, salivary duct carcinoma is a high-grade adenocarcinoma, resembling high-grade mammary ductal carcinoma. The tumour may arise *de novo* or as a malignant component of carcinoma ex pleomorphic adenoma. It is relatively less common and mostly arises in the parotid. It is commonly seen in elderly men in their sixth or seventh decade. Salivary duct carcinoma is an aggressive tumour presenting as a rapidly growing mass, often with facial palsy, pain and cervical lymphadenopathy. Complete excision with wide margins (total parotidectomy) with neck dissection is the treatment of choice. On histopathology, it resembles high-grade invasive ductal breast cancer with a large duct-like configuration with comedo necrosis and cribriform and Roman bridge-like features. Vascular and perineural invasion is seen. Salivary duct carcinoma also shows androgen receptor and HER2 receptor positivity in a significant percentage of cases, making it a target for treatment, especially in the recurrent/metastatic setting. It has a high predilection for local recurrence and regional and distant metastases and a poor overall survival.

INVESTIGATIONS

Imaging

Various modalities, from plain radiography to ultrasonography, CT, MRI and sialography are available to clinicians. In most cases, CT scans are considered superior for differentiating neoplasms from inflammatory conditions, while MRI scans give better differentiation between benign and malignant neoplasms.

High-resolution ultrasonography

Ultrasonography is a very useful diagnostic tool, especially for lesions of major salivary glands. Acute inflammatory conditions may be picked up by enlarged glands with increased blood flow, compared with chronic inflammation, in which the glands may be smaller in size and hypoechoic. Sialolithiasis will present with distinct acoustic shadowing. Benign tumours such as pleomorphic adenoma are generally visualised as well-lobulated, hypoechoic lesions with some calcifications. Malignant tumours will have irregular shapes and a hypoechoic, inhomogeneous appearance with blurred margins. However, ultrasonography cannot adequately characterise lesions of the deep lobe of the parotid gland and when there is suspected involvement of the skull base; in these cases, cross-sectional imaging such as CT/MRI is preferred.

Computed tomography/magnetic resonance imaging scans

These are the best tools for almost complete imaging of the salivary glands. They detect both cystic and solid masses with good accuracy as well as help in diagnosing and localising sialolithiasis. CT scans are especially useful in determining the extent of the tumour, erosion of surrounding osseous structures, extraglandular involvement and the presence of metastatic nodes. MRI scans, especially diffusion-weighted (DW) and gadolinium-enhanced dynamic MRI, can differentiate benign and malignant neoplasms based on the apparent diffusion coefficient (ADC) values, peak enhancement and washout ratios.

Positron emission tomography with computed tomography (PET-CT) scans

These scans are used mainly in the detection of distant metastases in high-grade malignancies or if the salivary glands are involved as the site of metastasis with an unknown primary.

Cytology

Fine-needle aspiration cytology

Fine-needle aspiration cytology (FNAC) is a widely available, simple and relatively safe diagnostic tool. It is used in the clinical setting of mass-forming lesions, often performed under ultrasound guidance. It can differentiate between inflammatory conditions and neoplasms with a high sensitivity (96%) and specificity (98%). Systematic reviews have reported FNAC to have a high sensitivity (80%) and specificity (97%) in differentiating benign from malignant lesions. The Milan system (***Table 54.4***) for reporting salivary gland cytopathology is an effective tool to assess the adequacy of the cytopathology specimen and quantify the risk of malignancy.

TABLE 54.4 The Milan system for reporting salivary gland cytopathology.

Diagnostic criteria	Risk of malignancy	Usual management
I Non-diagnostic	25%	Clinical and radiological correlation/repeat FNAC
II Non-neoplastic	10%	Clinical follow-up and radiological correlation
III AUS	20%	Repeat FNAC or surgery
IV Neoplasm		
IVA Benign	<5%	Conservative surgery or clinical follow-up
IVB SUMP	35%	Conservative surgery[a]
V Suspicious for malignancy	60%	Surgery[a]
VI Malignant	>90%	Surgery[a] (extent depends on type and grade of malignancy)

AUS, atypia of undetermined significance; FNAC, fine-needle aspiration cytology; SUMP, salivary gland neoplasm of uncertain malignant potential.

[a]Intraoperative frozen section may be helpful to determine the extent of surgery.

Adapted from Pusztaszeri M, Rossi ED, Baloch ZW, Faquin WC. Salivary gland fine needle aspiration and introduction of the Milan reporting system. *Adv Anat Pathol* 2019; **26**(2): 84–92.

Core needle biopsy

FNAC has a high specificity but a lower sensitivity in diagnosing malignancies. Being operator dependent, there is a high variability in practice. In addition, in lymphoma or high-grade malignancies, ancillary studies such as flow cytometry and immunohistochemistry are required to confirm the diagnosis. In these settings, core needle biopsy has greater diagnostic accuracy than FNAC. It provides more tissue for diagnosis and preserves the cellular architecture for further classification of malignancies. However, as it is a more invasive procedure, it is often reserved as a supplement to FNAC for problem solving.

STAGING OF SALIVARY GLAND MALIGNANCIES

Major salivary gland malignancies are staged using the eighth edition of the American Joint Committee on Cancer (AJCC) staging. However, minor salivary gland malignancies are staged as per their site of origin. The primary tumour (T) staging is as given in ***Table 54.5***. The nodal (N) and distant metastasis (M) staging is similar to that for head and neck squamous cell carcinomas.

TREATMENT OF SALIVARY GLAND MALIGNANCIES

The treatment guidelines are based on retrospective studies, with very little randomised evidence to guide treatment decisions. Surgery forms the mainstay of treatment with a goal to extirpate the tumour with microscopic margins of at least 0.5 cm. The extent of resection is determined not only by the size and stage of the malignancy but also by the grade of differentiation. The preservation of the facial nerve should be planned, but not at the cost of residual disease. Elective neck dissection should be offered for T3/T4 and high-grade tumours. In node-positive disease, comprehensive neck dissection is mandatory. Adjuvant radiotherapy is advocated for stage III and IV tumours, high grade of differentiation as

TABLE 54.5 T staging of salivary gland tumours as per the American Joint Committee on Cancer system.

T category	T criteria
TX	Primary tumour cannot be assessed
T0	No evidence of primary tumour
Tis	Carcinoma *in situ*
T1	Tumour 2 cm or smaller in greatest dimension without extraparenchymal extension[a]
T2	Tumour larger than 2 cm but not larger than 4 cm in greatest dimension without extraparenchymal extension[a]
T3	Tumour larger than 4 cm and/or tumour having extraparenchymal extension[a]
T4a	Moderately advanced disease Tumour invades skin, mandible, ear canal and/or facial nerve
T4b	Very advanced disease Tumour invades skull base and/or pterygoid plates and/or encases carotid artery

[a]Extraparenchymal extension is clinical or macroscopic evidence of invasion of soft tissues. Microscopic evidence alone does not constitute extraparenchymal extension for classification purposes.

well as the presence of high-risk features such as close/positive surgical margins, the presence of perineural or lymphovascular invasion and nodal metastases with extranodal extension. The role of chemoradiation in the adjuvant setting is still under investigation. In unresectable or metastatic tumours, palliative chemotherapy and/or targeted therapy is being explored.

SURGERY AND COMPLICATIONS

Submandibular gland resection

The submandibular gland is surrounded by important structures and its removal is fairly straightforward if planned well. The approaches to the submandibular gland are transcutaneous (such as lateral transcervical, submental and retroauricular) or transoral. Visualisation during the various approaches can be improved with endoscopic or robotic assistance, potentially reducing complications.

Summary box 54.6

Important anatomical relations to the submandibular gland

- Lingual nerve
- Hypoglossal nerve
- Marginal mandibular branch of the facial nerve
- Anterior facial vein
- Facial artery

Planning the surgery

Decision making is determined by the nature of the disease. In benign lesions only the gland is removed, preserving surrounding nerves. In malignant lesions, depending on the stage and histology, there may be a consideration for a supraomohyoid neck dissection involving levels I–III.

Anaesthesia

General anaesthesia is usually preferred unless there is any contraindication, in which case local anaesthesia may be considered.

Incision

The incision planned should ensure complete access to the tumour, be extendable to encompass intraoperative surprises and be safe and cosmetically acceptable. The standard incision is placed in a neck crease at least two finger breadths below the mandible. The horizontal incision is along the lines of relaxation, which results in a cosmetic scar (***Figure 54.11a***).

Flap elevation

After incising the skin the platysma is exposed and divided in the same plane. The skin is retracted with skin hooks and the flap is elevated in the avascular subplatysmal plane, taking care that the veins remain in the investing fascia. The flap is elevated up to the attachment of the platysma on the mandible, which helps in identification of the marginal mandibular nerve (***Figure 54.11b***).

Marginal mandibular nerve preservation

The fascia above the facial vessels is palpated in the midportion of the body of the mandible. The nerve is usually identified in the fascia above the vessels and is dissected along its path horizontally to expose it as it exits the parotid and traverses onto the muscles anteriorly.

Gland mobilisation

The facial vein and artery are ligated below the marginal nerve, exposing the lower edge of the body of the mandible. The submandibular gland is now retracted downwards and outwards to expose the mylohyoid muscle (***Figure 54.11c***); the fascia overlying the submandibular gland is dissected, exposing the submental artery and vein, which are secured and ligated. The lateral edge of the mylohyoid is delineated and retracted with a curved retractor. This exposes the deeper portion of the submandibular gland as well as Wharton's duct. The submandibular gland is then retracted downwards to expose the lingual nerve (***Figure 54.11d***) and the connecting submandibular ganglion, which is divided. The gland is then retracted superiorly and posteriorly, exposing the deep fascia alongside the ranine veins above the hypoglossal nerve (***Figure 54.11e***). Wharton's duct is then clamped, divided and ligated close to the floor of the mouth to prevent retention of debris or stones, reducing the chance of infection. The gland is retracted downwards and laterally, exposing the facial artery above the common tendon of the digastric muscle. The facial artery is clamped, divided and ligated, completing the gland excision.

Malignant submandibular tumours

Treatment for low-grade tumours that are less than 4 cm without extraparenchymal spread is submandibular gland removal with clearance of the perivascular group of lymph nodes around

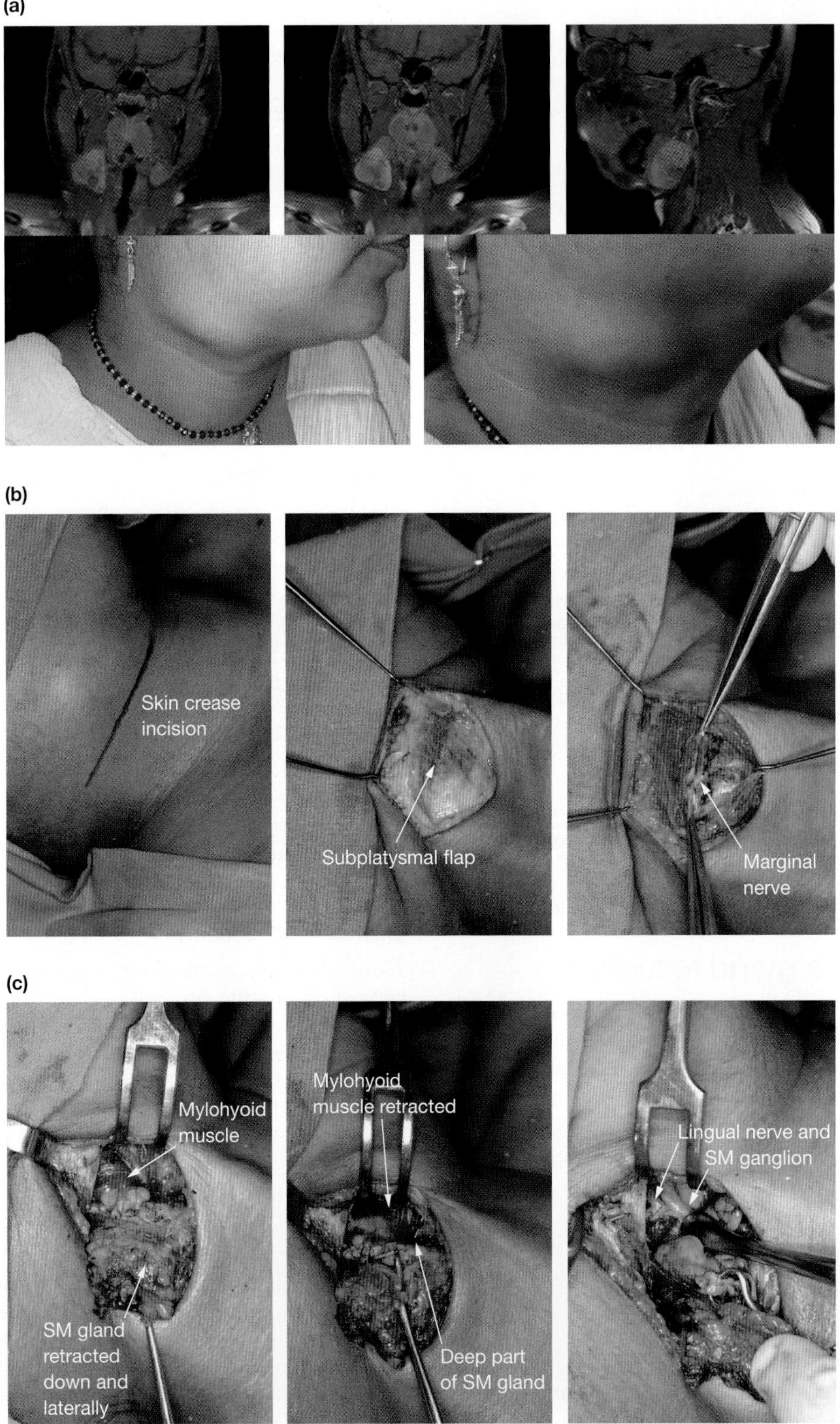

Figure 54.11 (a) Submandibular (SM) pleomorphic adenoma: clinical presentation and T1-weighted magnetic resonance imaging with contrast view showing the tumour. (b) A horizontal skin crease incision, subplatysmal flap elevation and identification of the marginal mandibular nerve. (c) The gland is retracted downwards and outwards to identify and retract the mylohyoid muscle to locate the lingual nerve.

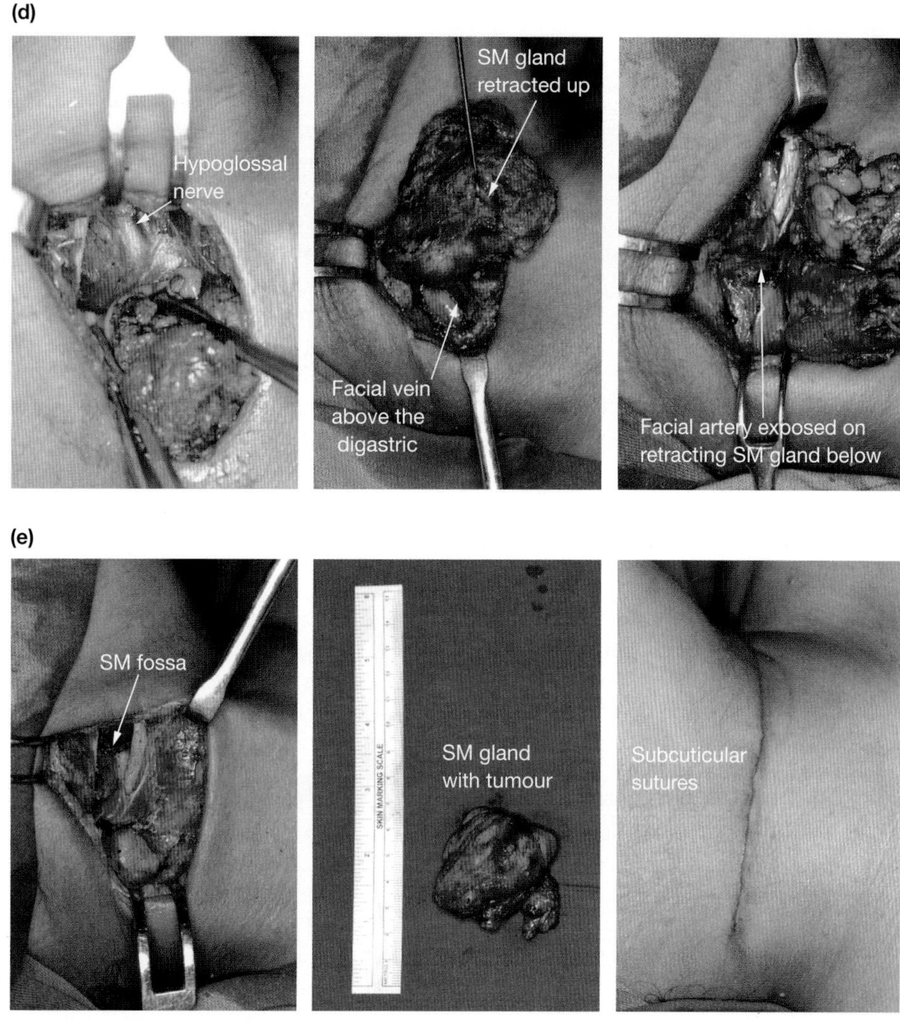

Figure 54.11 (d) The gland is retracted downwards and outwards to identify the hypoglossal nerve and the facial vein and artery before removing the gland. (e) The submandibular fossa after tumour-laden gland removal and closure with subcuticular sutures.

the facial vein. In high-grade tumours, supraomohyoid neck dissection (levels I–III) is recommended, whereas node-positive tumours require a comprehensive neck dissection (levels I–V).

For tumours with extraparenchymal spread, radical clearance of the involved structures along with a formal comprehensive neck dissection is required.

Closure

Haemostasis is achieved and an antiseptic wash is given. Intraoral communication is ruled out before placing a suction drain over the mylohyoid with the tip pointing laterally to prevent migration into the oral cavity. The wound is closed by approximating the platysma with absorbable sutures and the skin with absorbable or non-absorbable sutures.

Complications

Nerve palsy

The proximity of the three nerves (marginal division of the facial, lingual and hypoglossal) to the submandibular gland makes them susceptible to injury. Care should be taken, especially in recurrent sialadenitis, which causes dense adhesions, increasing the possibility of nerve injury.

Haemorrhage

The facial artery and the ranine veins along the hypoglossal are notorious for postoperative haemorrhage and should be double-checked prior to closure.

Parotidectomy

In parotidectomy, the tumour is removed with a cuff of normal surrounding tissue where possible. The embryological development of the parotid with its late encapsulation not only embeds vessels, nerves and lymph nodes within the capsule but also fuses widely with the investing fascia from the temporalis above to the digastric below and from the buccinator anteriorly to the mastoid posteriorly. The facial nerve traverses the parotid, making the removal of this gland difficult.

Summary box 54.7

Types of parotid surgery as per the extent of resection (conservative to radical)

- Extracapsular dissection
- Adequate parotidectomy
- Superficial parotidectomy
- Total conservative parotidectomy
- Radical parotidectomy

Planning the surgery

Decision making should take into consideration:

1. presumed tumour histology;
2. relation to the facial nerve plane (Patey's faciovenous plane);
3. location of the tumour (deep lobe of the parotid);
4. facial nerve function.

Traditionally, the type of parotidectomy is based on the location of the tumour either lateral to the plane of the facial nerve, necessitating a superficial parotidectomy, or deep to it, requiring a total parotidectomy. A total conservative parotidectomy usually preserves the facial nerve whereas a radical parotidectomy involves its sacrifice.

Today, with a focus towards reducing morbidity and preserving gland function, variations of parotidectomy have evolved in the management of benign tumours:

- Extracapsular tumour dissection does not require a formal facial nerve dissection; this reduces the incidence of temporary facial nerve palsy.
- Adequate parotidectomy involves removal of the tumour with a cuff of normal tissue in tail of parotid lesions, preserving function. It may not be possible to excise the tumour with a cuff of normal tissue in all the cases, especially when the lump is abutting the facial nerve.
- Deep lobe parotid tumours can be removed, preserving the entire superficial parotid gland, which is functional as well as cosmetic.

Anaesthesia

General anaesthesia is usually preferred unless there is any contraindication, in which case local anaesthesia may rarely be considered.

Incision

The planned incision should ensure complete access to the tumour, be extendable to encompass intraoperative surprises and be safe and cosmetically acceptable. The Blair incision is a straight preauricular incision curving slightly below the ear lobule. Bailey modified the inferior segment towards the mastoid and along the anterior border of the sternocleidomastoid.

The modern 'lazy S' incision gently curves downwards along the natural skin crease of the neck (***Figure 54.12a***) and has three components: (i) the horizontal part along the skin crease two finger breadths from the angle of the mandible, (ii) the vertical part close to the tragus in a skin crease if present, and (iii) the communicating part connecting the horizontal and vertical components in a gentle curve.

The facelift incision has two components: the anterior preauricular component is similar to the modified Blair incision while the posterior limb curves at right angles, reaching the hairline and avoiding any neck incision.

Flap elevation

The horizontal component of the modified Blair incision is incised first to identify the platysma, the external jugular vein and the greater auricular nerve. The vertical component is then incised and connected inferiorly. The platysma is divided and the subplatysmal flap is raised until the parotid gland is visualised and continued above, remaining below the superficial musculoaponeurotic fascia, which connects the temporalis fascia and the platysma. This allows a suitable flap to be raised with the entire subcutaneous fat lifted off the parotid gland. The flap is developed anteriorly with elevation over the parotid gland but not onto the masseteric fascia to prevent damage to the nerve branches as they exit the gland (***Figure 54.12b***).

Parotid gland mobilisation

The fascia between the sternocleidomastoid and the parotid is dissected in the avascular plane. The greater auricular nerve is dissected up to the ear lobule and its anterior branches are divided (***Figure 54.12c***). The gland is then dissected off the sternomastoid muscle and fibrofatty tissue overlying the internal jugular vein to identify the posterior belly of the digastric muscle, which is then traced to the mastoid process. The external jugular vein is preserved as it provides a good landmark for the facial nerve plane. The parotid is then mobilised from the tragal cartilage and the bony external auditory meatus, exposing its tip – the 'tragal pointer'. The two avascular planes are then connected by blunt and sharp dissection, identifying the tympanomastoid suture.

Facial nerve localisation

The facial nerve is usually identified by the antegrade technique using anatomical landmarks, which are fairly constant, and is delineated from the trunk to the peripheral branches (***Figure 54.12d***):

- tragal (Conley's) pointer: the facial nerve lies 1 cm deep and inferior to the tip of the tragal cartilage;
- digastric muscle: the facial nerve can be identified above the upper border of the posterior belly of the digastric muscle;
- tympanomastoid suture: the facial nerve lies inferior to this suture line as it overlies the stylomastoid foramen.

David Howard Patey, 1899–1976, surgeon, The Middlesex Hospital, London, UK.
Vilray Papin Blair, 1871–1955, described the incision that bears his name in 1912.
Henry Hamilton Bailey, 1894–1961, surgeon, The Royal Northern Hospital, London, UK.
John J Conley, 1912–1999, otolaryngologist, St. Vincent's Hospital and Medical Center, USA, made important contributions in the treatment of head and neck cancer.

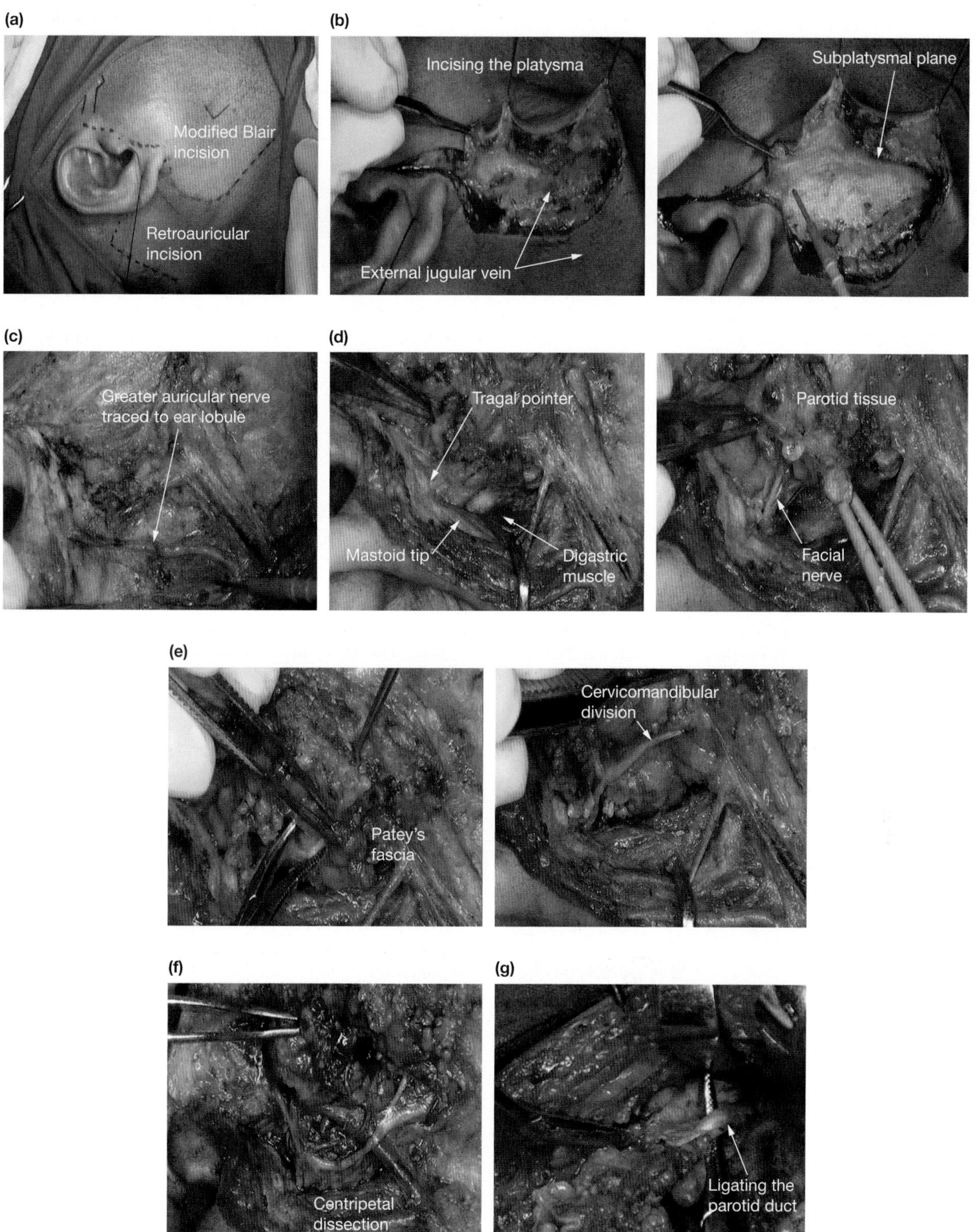

Figure 54.12 (a) Incision planning showing the modified Blair incision and the retroauricular incision. (b) Subplatysmal flap elevation to identify the superficial musculoaponeurotic system layer, preserving the external jugular vein. (c) Greater auricular nerve traced as far as the ear lobule, dividing the branches going on to the parotid gland. (d) Tragal pointer and the digastric muscle used in combination to identify the facial nerve exiting the stylomastoid foramen in the centre. (e) Dissection of the nerve in Patey's fascia: dissecting the nerves of the main trunk from the periphery to the centre. (f) Centripetal dissection of the parotid gland towards the parotid duct in the centre. (g) Ligation of the parotid duct.

At the stylomastoid foramen, the facial nerve is encircled by the parotid gland, fibrofatty tissue and the stylomastoid branch of the posterior auricular artery. Dissection of the glandular tissue and artery exposes the nerve. Bleeding can be brisk; this can be controlled with pressure, adrenaline (epinephrine) neuropatties and bipolar electrocautery.

Identification of the facial trunk by a retrograde dissection technique is useful in revision cases with altered anatomy and fibrosis. It relies on the identification of one of the main branches of the nerve (usually the buccal branch in relation to the parotid duct), which is then traced proximally to the main trunk.

Centripetal dissection

Once the main trunk is identified, a curved fine artery forceps is used to dissect in Patey's plane above the nerve, taking care to avoid stretching the nerve (***Figure 54.12e***). The glandular tissue is dissected off the nerve and divided laterally. Starting with the lower cervicomandibular division and its further divisions into the cervical, marginal mandibular and lower buccal branches, the entire course of each branch is identified until it exits the gland. Each of the branches is dissected in a sequential manner in a centripetal dissection working towards the parotid duct (***Figure 54.12f***). Thereafter, the upper temporozygomatic division is traced onto its temporal, zygomatic and upper buccal branches, similarly reaching the duct. Thus at the end of the dissection the entire superficial part of the gland remains attached to the parotid duct, which can be clamped and ligated to deliver the specimen (***Figure 54.12g***).

Total conservative parotidectomy

In a tumour straddling the superficial and deep lobes across Patey's plane, following removal of the superficial lobe, the deep lobe is dissected off the temporal veins and terminal branches of the external carotid artery. This results in complete removal of the suprafacial and subfacial parotid gland with preservation of the facial nerves – a total conservative parotidectomy.

Radical parotidectomy

In malignant tumours with extraparenchymal spread and facial nerve invasion, it is imperative to remove the involved structures. Radical parotidectomy involves removal of all parotid gland tissue and elective division of the involved facial nerve branches as well as the structures involved, most commonly the masseter muscle. It is imperative to repair the facial nerves when a segment has been removed. The branches supplying the orbicularis oculi and oris are prioritised in the reconstruction using cable grafts from either the greater auricular nerve or the sural nerve.

Extracapsular dissection

Extracapsular dissection for select benign parotid tumours is practised to avoid facial nerve dissection. It is reported to be as safe as parotidectomy. With a similar incision the subcutaneous flap is elevated above the platysma. At the site of the tumour the fascia is incised in a cruciate or curvilinear manner to expose the tumour. The tumour is dissected carefully in an extracapsular plane, visualising the facial nerve branches. Use of intraoperative nerve monitoring makes this safer. However, in the absence of monitoring, careful dissection and a high level of suspicion before cutting any tissue is critical for uneventful surgery. After excision the fascia is sutured with absorbable sutures, followed by skin closure.

Drain placement and closure

Sternomastoid muscle flaps or acellular dermal sheets may be used to cover the parotid bed. This attempts to prevent cross-innervation of the subcutaneous gland and overlying skin by the auriculotemporal nerve to avoid Frey's syndrome. A suction drain tube is placed and anchored beneath the posterior belly of the digastric muscle. The drain is brought out posterior to the suture line. The skin is sutured in layers.

Complications

Temporary facial palsy is commonly seen in the lower branches, especially the marginal mandibular nerve. Most patients tend to recover over time. When the zygomaticotemporal division is affected, eye care is essential to protect the cornea.

Parotidectomy is a clean operation and hence infection is rare. Postoperative management of the drains following aseptic precautions and timely removal decreases the risk of infection.

Haematoma is uncommon and is usually preventable with appropriate intraoperative haemostasis. Small haematomas usually resolve without intervention. Extreme collection causing discoloration suggests a possible bleeding diathesis that requires appropriate management and evacuation of the haematoma.

Sialocele is preventable by underrunning the capsule, where possible, to avoid exposure of the main acinar ductal system. Treatment includes the use of anticholinergics to reduce salivary secretion, aspiration and pressure dressings. Longstanding salivary fistulae may require low-dose radiation.

Hollowing of the retromandibular area can be reduced with autologous fat grafts, which can be placed at the time of primary surgery.

Frey's syndrome (gustatory sweating) results from cross-innervation of the dermal sweat glands by the regenerating postganglionic parasympathetic nerve fibres of the auriculotemporal nerve. It occurs in most patients but is often not significant; patients rarely mention it unless it is excessive. Common presentations are sweating and flushing in the preauricular region during meals. Minor's starch iodine test identifies the region affected. In it iodine is painted in the preauricular region, dried and covered with starch. Salivary stimulation causes sweating, which turns the starch blue. Frey's syndrome can be reduced either by raising a thick flap with all subcutaneous fat over the parotid or by interposition of tissue, such as a sternocleidomastoid flap, temporalis fascia, allodermal tissue or autologous fat between the skin and the surgical bed. Its incidence can be reduced by extracapsular

Victor Minor, Russian neurologist, described the starch iodine test in 1928.

dissection and careful closure of the superficial musculo-aponeurotic system. Treatment includes use of antiperspirants in mild cases; in more severe cases, tympanic neurectomy or botulinum toxin injection at the site of perspiration is used, which is very effective.

Summary box 54.8

Complications of parotid gland surgery

- Haematoma formation
- Infection
- Deformity: unsightly scar and retromandibular hollowing
- Temporary facial nerve weakness
- Transection of the facial nerve and permanent facial weakness
- Sialocele
- Facial numbness
- Permanent numbness of the ear lobe associated with great auricular nerve transection
- Frey's syndrome

Summary box 54.9

Management of established Frey's syndrome

- Antiperspirants, usually containing aluminium chlorohydrate
- Denervation by tympanic neurectomy
- The injection of botulinum toxin into the affected skin

FURTHER READING

El-Naggar AK, Chan JKC, Grandis JR *et al.* (eds). *Tumours of the salivary glands*, 4th edn. Lyon: IARC Press, 2017.

Pusztaszeri M, Rossi ED, Baloch ZW, Faquin WC. Salivary gland fine needle aspiration and introduction of the Milan reporting system. *Adv Anat Pathol* 2019; **26**(2): 84–92.

Schmidt RL, Hall BJ, Wilson AR, Layfield LJ. A systematic review and meta-analysis of the diagnostic accuracy of fine-needle aspiration cytology for parotid gland lesions. *Am J Clin Pathol* 2011; **136**: 45–59.

Speight PM, Barrett AW. Salivary gland tumours. *Oral Dis* 2002; **8**(5): 229–40.

Valstar MH, de Ridder M, van den Broek EC *et al.* Salivary gland pleomorphic adenoma in the Netherlands: a nationwide observational study of primary tumor incidence, malignant transformation, recurrence, and risk factors for recurrence. *Oral Oncol* 2017; **66**: 93–9.

PART 8 | Endocrine and breast

CHAPTER 55 The thyroid gland

Learning objectives

- To understand the development and anatomy of the thyroid gland
- To know the physiology and investigation of thyroid function
- To be able to select appropriate investigations for thyroid swellings
- To know when to operate on a thyroid swelling
- To describe thyroidectomy
- To know the risks and complications of thyroid surgery

EMBRYOLOGY

The embryology of the thyroid and parathyroid glands underlies the anatomical position, anatomical variations and congenital conditions of these structures; it is therefore vital for surgery (*Figure 55.1*). The thyroglossal duct develops from the median bud of the pharynx. The foramen caecum at the junction of the anterior two-thirds and posterior one-third of the tongue is the vestigial remnant of the duct. This initially hollow structure migrates caudally and passes in close continuity with, and sometimes through, the developing hyoid cartilage. The parathyroid glands develop from the third and fourth pharyngeal pouches. The thymus also develops from the third pouch. As it descends, the thymus takes the associated parathyroid gland with it, which explains why the inferior parathyroid, which arises from the third pharyngeal pouch, normally lies inferior to the superior gland. However, the inferior parathyroid may be found anywhere along this line of descent (see also *Chapter 56*). The developing thyroid lobes amalgamate with the structures that arise in the fourth pharyngeal pouch, i.e. the superior parathyroid gland and the ultimobranchial body. Parafollicular cells (C cells) from the neural crest reach the thyroid via the ultimobranchial body.

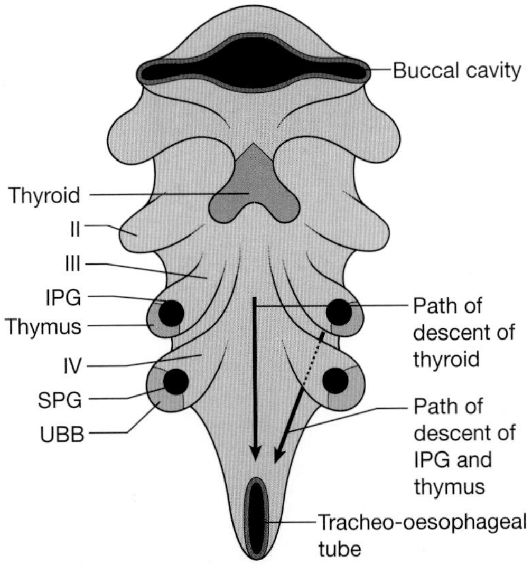

Figure 55.1 Embryology of the thyroid and parathyroid. Diagram of an anterior view of the pharynx in a 4-week embryo showing the relationship of the third and fourth pharyngeal pouches to the final position of the thyroid and parathyroid glands. IPG, inferior parathyroid; SPG, superior parathyroid; UBB, ultimobranchial body.

SURGICAL ANATOMY

The normal thyroid gland weighs 20–25 g. The functioning unit is the lobule supplied by a single arteriole and consists of 24–40 follicles lined with cuboidal epithelium. The follicle contains colloid in which thyroglobulin is stored (*Figure 55.2*). The arterial supply is rich, and extensive anastomoses occur between the main thyroid arteries and the branches of the tracheal and oesophageal arteries (*Figure 55.3*). There is an extensive lymphatic network within and around the gland. Although some lymph channels pass directly to the deep cervical nodes, the subcapsular plexus drains principally to the central compartment juxtathyroid – 'Delphian' and paratracheal nodes and nodes on the superior and inferior thyroid veins (level VI) – and from there to the deep cervical (levels II, III, IV and V) and mediastinal groups of nodes (level VII) (*Figure 55.4*).

The relationship between the recurrent laryngeal nerve (RLN) and the thyroid is of supreme importance to the

Delphi, a sacred site near the Gulf of Corinth in Greece, is the place where Pythia, the snake-woman oracle, resided. She sat on a tripod clutching the ribbons of the monolithic 'omphalos' of the world and, after inhaling sulphurous fumes, would utter meaningless jargon, which was interpreted equivocally by the attendant priests for those who came to consult her. Formerly the purpose of these lymph nodes was uncertain, and they were therefore called 'Delphic'.

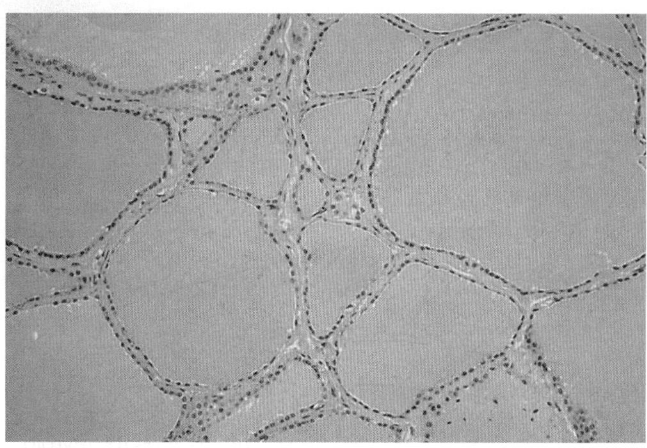

Figure 55.2 Histology of the normal thyroid.

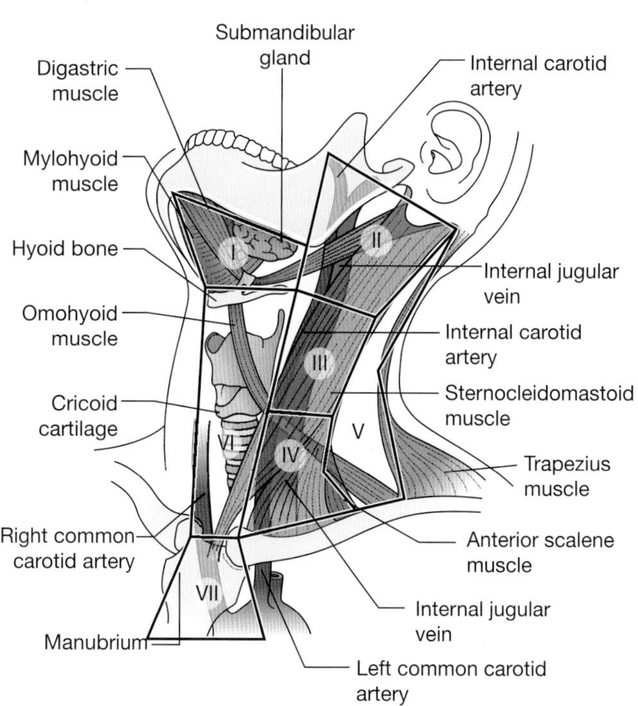

Figure 55.4 Cervical lymph node levels.

operating surgeon. A branch of the vagus, the nerve recurs round the arch of the aorta on the left and the subclavian artery on the right. The clinical significance of this is that on the left the nerve has more distance in which to reach the tracheo-oesophageal groove and therefore runs in a medial plane. On the right, there is less distance and the nerve runs more obliquely to reach the tracheo-oesophageal groove. Approximately 2% of nerves on the right are non-recurrent and will enter the larynx from above.

The nerve runs posterior to the thyroid and enters the larynx at the cricothyroid joint. This entry point is at the level

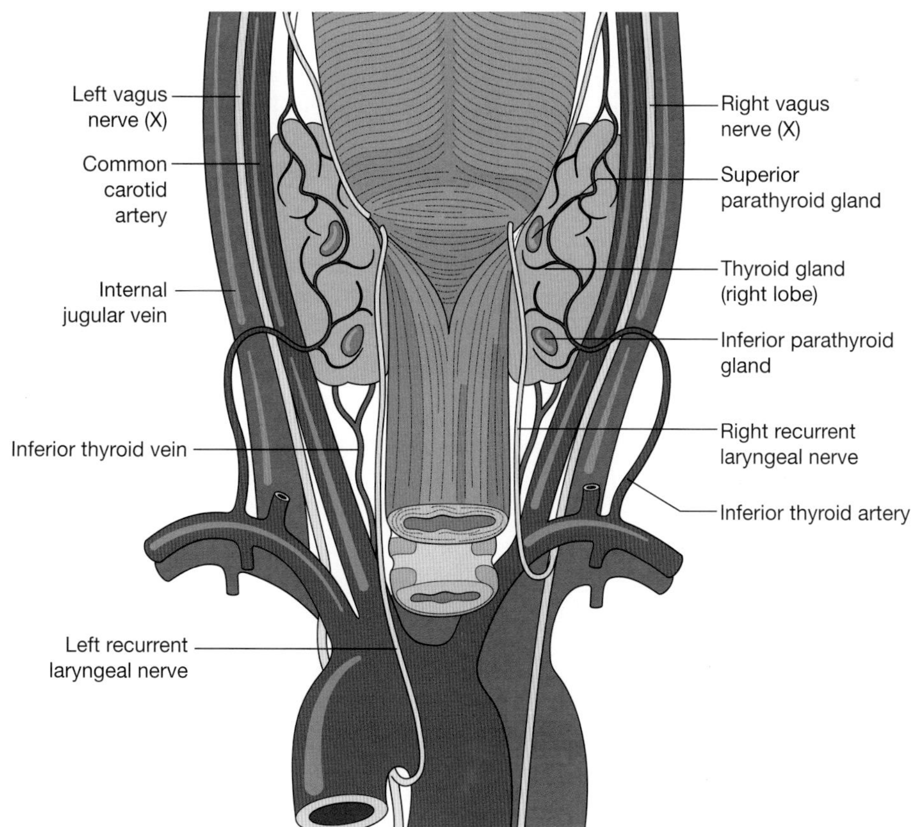

Figure 55.3 The thyroid gland from behind.

of Berry's ligament, a condensation of pretracheal fascia that binds the thyroid to the trachea. This is the point at which the nerve is at most risk of injury during surgery. In terms of surgical anatomy, the nerve can be located in the tracheo-oesophageal groove, where it forms one side of Beahrs' triangle (the other two sides are the carotid artery and the inferior thyroid artery) or at the cricothyroid joint. The nerve will normally be found as the thyroid lobe is mobilised laterally, lying under the most posterolateral portion of the gland called the tubercle of Zuckerkandl.

PHYSIOLOGY

Thyroxine

The hormones tri-iodothyronine (T_3) and L-thyroxine (T_4) are bound to thyroglobulin within the colloid. Synthesis within the thyroglobulin complex is controlled by several enzymes, in distinct steps:

- trapping of inorganic iodide from the blood;
- oxidation of iodide to iodine;
- binding of iodine with tyrosine to form iodotyrosine;
- coupling of monoiodotyrosines and di-iodotyrosines to form T_3 and T_4.

When hormones are required, the complex is resorbed into the cell and thyroglobulin is broken down. T_3 and T_4 are liberated and enter the blood, where they are bound to serum proteins: albumin, thyroxine-binding globulin (TBG) and thyroxine-binding prealbumin (TBPA). The small amount of hormone that remains free in the serum is biologically active.

The metabolic effects of the thyroid hormones are due to unbound free T_3 and T_4 (0.3% and 0.03% of the total circulating hormones, respectively). T_3 is the more important physiological hormone and is also produced in the periphery by conversion from T_4. T_3 is quick acting (within a few hours), whereas T_4 acts more slowly (4–14 days).

Calcitonin

The parafollicular C cells of the thyroid are of neuroendocrine origin and arrive in the thyroid via the ultimobranchial body (*Figure 55.1*). They produce calcitonin.

The pituitary-thyroid axis

Synthesis and release of thyroid hormones from the thyroid is controlled by thyroid-stimulating hormone (TSH) from the anterior pituitary. Secretion of TSH depends upon the level of circulating thyroid hormones and is modified in a negative feedback manner. In hyperthyroidism TSH production is suppressed, whereas in hypothyroidism it is stimulated. Regulation of TSH secretion also results from the action of thyrotrophin-releasing hormone (TRH) produced in the hypothalamus.

Thyroid-stimulating antibodies

A family of IgG immunoglobulins bind with TSH receptor sites (TRAbs) and activate TSH receptors on the follicular cell membrane. They have a more protracted action than TSH (16–24 versus 1.5–3 hours) and are responsible for virtually all cases of thyrotoxicosis not due to autonomous toxic nodules. Serum concentrations are very low but their measurement is not essential to make the diagnosis.

Serum thyroid hormones

Serum thyroid-stimulating hormone

TSH levels can be measured accurately down to very low serum concentrations with an immunochemiluminometric assay. Interpretation of deranged TSH levels depends on knowledge of the T_3 and T_4 values. In the euthyroid state, T_3, T_4 and TSH levels will all be within the normal range. Florid thyroid failure results in depressed T_3 and T_4 levels, with gross elevation of TSH. Incipient or developing thyroid failure is characterised by low normal values of T_3 and T_4 and elevation of TSH. In toxic states, the TSH level is suppressed (*Table 55.1*).

Thyroid autoantibodies

Serum levels of antibodies against thyroid peroxidase (TPO) and thyroglobulin are useful in determining the cause of thyroid dysfunction and swellings. Autoimmune thyroiditis may be associated with thyroid toxicity, failure or euthyroid goitre. Levels above 25 units/mL for TPO antibody and titres of greater than 1:100 for antithyroglobulin are considered significant,

TABLE 55.1 Results of thyroid function tests in normal and pathological states.

Thyroid functional state	TSH (0.3–3.3 mU/L)	Free T_4 (10–30 nmol/L)	Free T_3 (3.5–7.5 μmol/L)
Euthyroid	Normal	Normal	Normal
Thyrotoxic	Undetectable	High	High
Myxoedema	High	Low	Low
Suppressive T_4 therapy	Undetectable	High	High (often normal)
T_3 toxicity	Low/undetectable	Normal	High

T_3, tri-iodothyronine; T_4, L-thyroxine; TSH, thyroid-stimulating hormone.

Sir James Berry, 1860–1946, surgeon, Royal Free Hospital, London, UK.
Oliver H Beahrs, 1914–2006, surgeon, Mayo Clinic, Rochester, MN, USA.
Emil Zuckerkandl, 1849–1901, Austro-Hungarian anatomist, brother of urologist Otto Zuckerkandl.
Myxoedema was first described in 1873 by Sir William Withey Gull, 1816–1890, physician, Guy's Hospital, London, UK.

although a proportion of patients with histological evidence of lymphocytic (autoimmune) thyroiditis are seronegative. The presence of antithyroglobulin antibody interferes with assays of serum thyroglobulin, with implications for follow-up of thyroid cancers. TSH receptor antibodies (TSH-RAb or TRAB) are often present in Graves' disease. They are largely produced within the thyroid itself.

Summary box 55.1

Thyroid investigations

Essential

- Serum: TSH (T_3 and T_4 if abnormal); thyroid autoantibodies
- Fine-needle aspiration cytology (FNAC) of palpable discrete swellings

Optional

- Corrected serum calcium
- Serum calcitonin (carcinoembryonic antigen may be used as an alternative screening test for medullary cancer)
- Imaging: chest radiograph and thoracic inlet if tracheal deviation/retrosternal goitre; ultrasonography, computed tomography (CT) and magnetic resonance imaging (MRI) scan for known cancer, some reoperations and some retrosternal goitres; isotope scan if discrete swelling and toxicity coexist

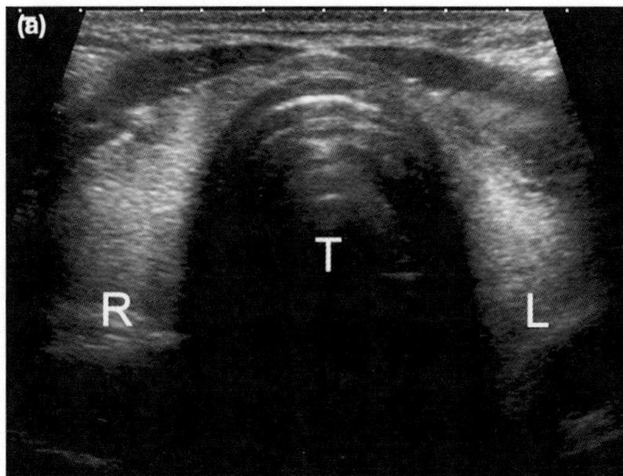

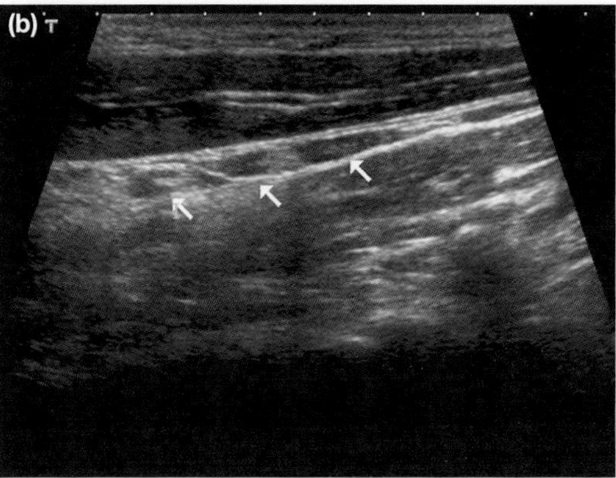

Figure 55.5 Ultrasonography. (a) Transverse scan of a normal thyroid. R, right lobe; L, left lobe; T, trachea. (b) Longitudinal scan of normal jugular lymph nodes (white arrows).

Thyroid imaging

The workhorse investigation in thyroid disease for the surgeon is ultrasonography. This modality allows assessment of the gland and the regional lymphatics. Not only can the characteristics of the gland substance be quantified, but critically the presence and features of thyroid nodules can be described. Number, size, shape, margins, vascularity and specific features such as the presence of microcalcifications can be used to predict the risk of malignancy within a specific nodule. Regional lymphatics, particularly in the lateral neck, can be assessed accurately for the presence of metastatic deposits. During ultrasonography, fine-needle aspiration (FNA) can be performed more accurately than free-hand techniques allow.

Ultrasonography has the advantages that it is not associated with ionising radiation and is non-invasive and cheap (*Figure 55.5*). Visualisation of the central neck nodes, in particular those behind the sternum, is however limited. For this reason, when metastatic disease is detected cross-sectional imaging is required to fully stage the disease. Retrosternal extension, which can often be predicted on a plain chest radiograph (*Figure 55.6*), also requires more advanced techniques to determine the extent adequately prior to considering management. For most of these indications, the imaging modality of choice is CT. Rapid acquisition times minimise artefacts secondary to breathing and the lung fields can be accurately assessed simultaneously.

In the setting of an invasive primary thyroid cancer, both CT and MRI may have a role. Contrast-enhanced CT is useful

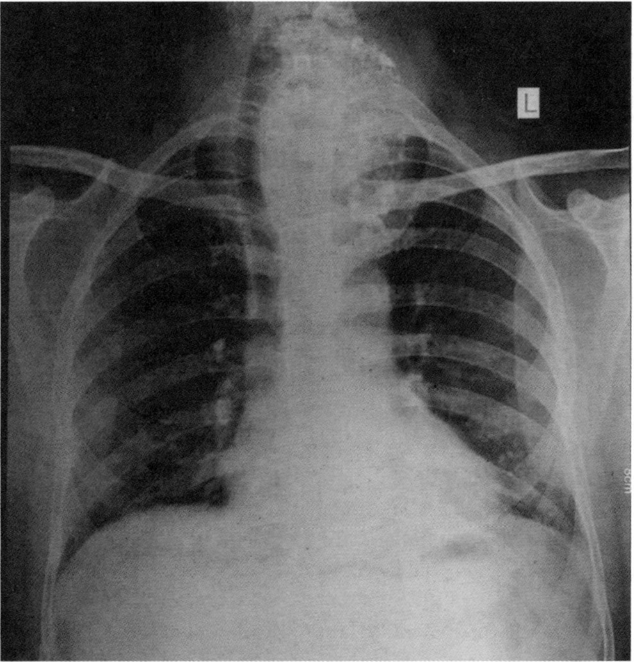

Figure 55.6 Chest radiograph showing a retrosternal goitre with calcification and tracheal displacement (courtesy of Dr Achleshwar Dayal, Hoshangabad, MP, India).

Robert James Graves, 1796–1853, physician, Meath Hospital, Dublin, Ireland, published an account of exophthalmic goitre in 1835. He was President of the Royal College of Physicians of Ireland and elected Fellow of the Royal Society (London, UK) in 1849.

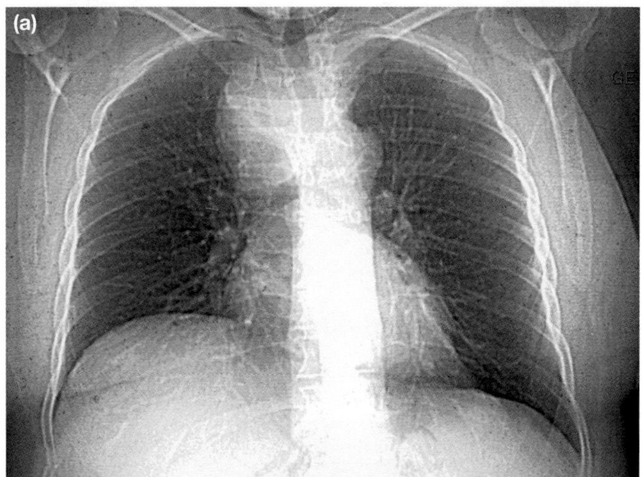

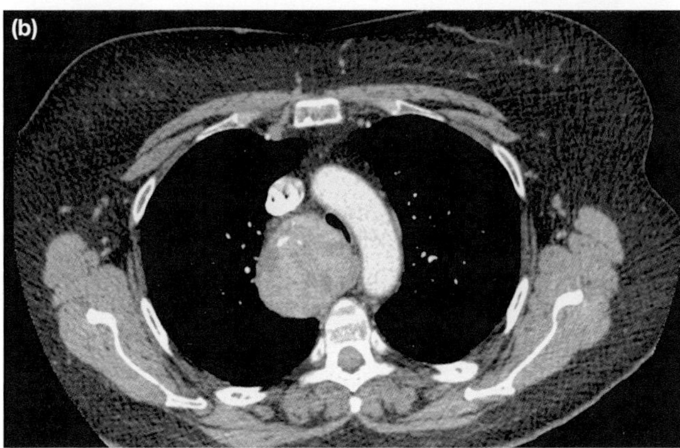

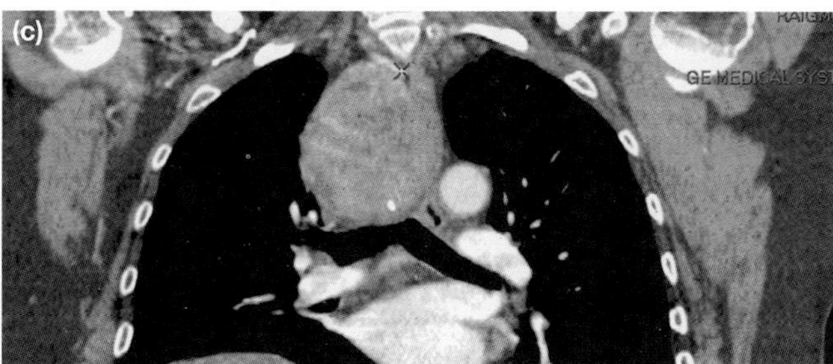

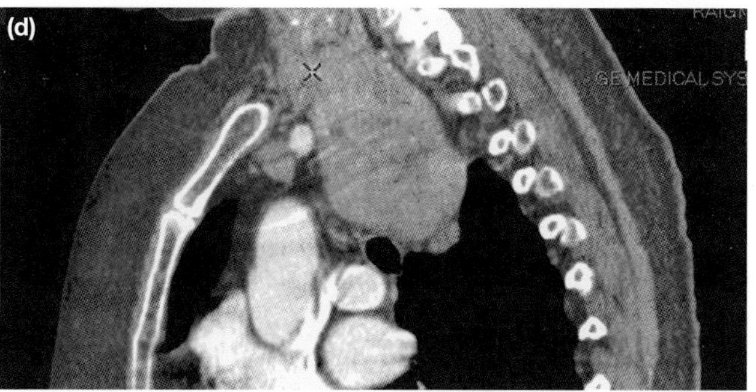

Figure 55.7 (a) Scout film showing retrosternal goitre. (b) Axial computed tomography (CT) section showing goitre extending to below the aortic arch with tracheal compression. (c) Coronal CT section showing goitre extending to the tracheal bifurcation. (d) Sagittal CT section showing goitre filling the posterior mediastinum.

for determining the extent of airway invasion (*Figure 55.7*) and MRI is superior at determining the presence of prevertebral fascia invasion.

Positron emission tomography (PET) scans have limited application in thyroid disease. They may be considered in the setting of recurrent thyroid cancer. This is particularly useful when the disease does not concentrate iodine, at which point fluorodeoxyglucose (FDG) uptake increases and lesions become positive on PET scans.

Isotope scanning

The uptake by the thyroid of a low dose of either radiolabelled iodine (^{123}I) or the cheaper technetium (^{99m}Tc) will demonstrate the distribution of activity in the whole gland. Routine isotope scanning is unnecessary and inappropriate for distinguishing benign from malignant lesions because the majority (80%) of 'cold' swellings are benign and some (5%) functioning or 'warm' swellings will be malignant. Its principal value is in the toxic patient with a nodule or nodularity of the thyroid. Localisation of overactivity in the gland will differentiate between a toxic nodule with suppression of the remainder of the gland and toxic multinodular goitre with several areas of increased uptake with important implications for therapy (*Figure 55.8*).

Whole-body scanning is used to demonstrate metastases. However, the patient must have all normally functioning thyroid tissue ablated by either surgery or radioiodine before the scan is performed because metastatic thyroid cancer tissue cannot compete with normal thyroid tissue in the uptake of iodine.

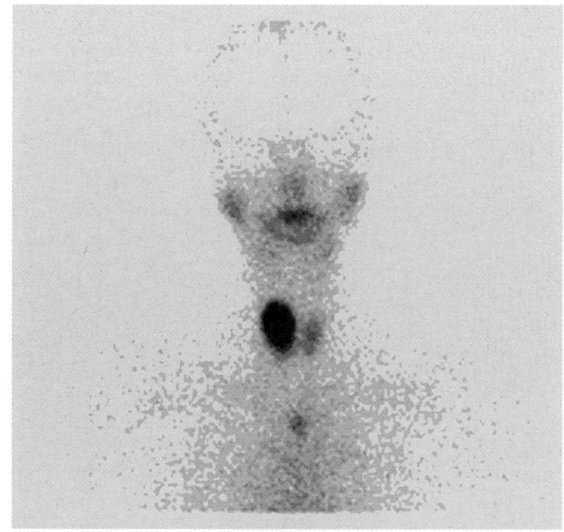

Figure 55.8 Technetium thyroid scan showing the appearance of a 1-cm 'toxic' adenoma in the right thyroid lobe with suppression of uptake in the left lobe. The intense uptake gives a false impression of the size of the swelling.

Fine-needle aspiration cytology

FNAC is the investigation of choice in discrete thyroid swellings. FNAC has excellent patient compliance, is simple and quick to perform in the outpatient department and is readily repeated. This technique, developed in Scandinavia 40 years ago, is now routine throughout the world. FNAC results should be reported using standard terminology (*Table 55.2*). Ultrasound guidance allows more accurate sampling and reduces the rate of unsatisfactory aspirates.

TABLE 55.2 Classification of fine-needle aspiration cytology reports.

Thy1	Non-diagnostic
Thy1c	Non-diagnostic cystic
Thy2	Non-neoplastic
Thy3	Follicular
Thy4	Suspicious of malignancy
Thy5	Malignant

TABLE 55.3 Classification of thyroid swellings.

Simple goitre (euthyroid)	Diffuse hyperplastic	• Physiological • Pubertal • Pregnancy
	Multinodular goitre	
Toxic	Diffuse (Graves' disease)	
	Multinodular	
	Toxic adenoma	
Neoplastic	Benign	
	Malignant	
Inflammatory	Autoimmune	Chronic lymphocytic thyroiditis
		Hashimoto's disease
	Granulomatous	de Quervain's thyroiditis
	Fibrosing	Riedel's thyroiditis
	Infective	Acute (bacterial thyroiditis, viral thyroiditis, 'subacute thyroiditis')
		Chronic (tuberculous, syphilitic)
	Other	Amyloid

THYROID ENLARGEMENT

The normal thyroid gland is impalpable. The term goitre (from the Latin guttur = the throat) is used to describe generalised enlargement of the thyroid gland. A discrete swelling (nodule) in one lobe with no palpable abnormality elsewhere is termed an isolated (or solitary) swelling. Discrete swellings with evidence of abnormality elsewhere in the gland are termed dominant.

A scheme for classifying thyroid enlargement is given in *Table 55.3*.

Simple goitre

Aetiology

Simple goitre may develop as a result of stimulation of the thyroid gland by TSH, either as a result of inappropriate secretion from a microadenoma in the anterior pituitary (which is rare) or in response to a chronically low level of circulating thyroid hormones. The most important factor in endemic goitre is dietary deficiency of iodine (see ***Iodine deficiency***), but defective hormone synthesis probably accounts for many sporadic goitres (see ***Dyshormonogenesis***).

TSH is not the only stimulus to thyroid follicular cell proliferation as other growth factors, including immunoglobulins, exert an influence. The heterogeneous structural and functional response in the thyroid resulting in characteristic nodularity may be due to the presence of clones of cells particularly sensitive to growth stimulation.

Iodine deficiency

The daily requirement of iodine is about 0.1–0.15 mg. In nearly all districts where simple goitre is endemic, there is a very low iodide content in the water and food. Endemic areas are in the mountainous ranges, such as the Rocky Mountains, the Alps, the Andes and the Himalayas, and in the UK areas of Derbyshire and Yorkshire. Endemic goitre is also found in lowland areas where the soil lacks iodide or the water supply comes from far away mountain ranges, e.g. the Great Lakes of North America, the plains of Lombardy, the Struma Valley, the Nile Valley and the Congo. Calcium is also goitrogenic and goitre is common in low-iodine areas on chalk or limestone, for example Derbyshire and southern Ireland. Although iodides in food and water may be adequate, failure of intestinal absorption may produce iodine deficiency.

Dyshormonogenesis

Enzyme deficiencies of varying severity may be responsible for many sporadic goitres, i.e. in non-endemic areas (*Figure 55.9*). There is often a family history, suggesting a genetic defect. Environmental factors may compensate in areas of high iodine intake; for example, goitre is almost unknown in Iceland where the fish diet is rich in iodine. Similarly, a low intake of iodine encourages goitre formation in those with a metabolic predisposition.

Hakaru Hashimoto, 1881–1934, Director, The Hashimoto Hospital, Mie, Japan, described chronic lymphocytic thyroiditis in 1912.
Friedrich Joseph de Quervain, 1868–1940, Professor of Surgery, Berne, Switzerland, described this form of thyroiditis in 1902.
Bernhard Riedel, 1846–1916, Surgeon, University of Jena, Thuringia, Germany
Struma. The River Struma arises in the mountains of Bulgaria and flows into the Aegean Sea. Along its banks and those of its tributaries dwell peoples of several nationalities, among whom endemic goitre has long been prevalent. Struma is a European continental term for goitre.

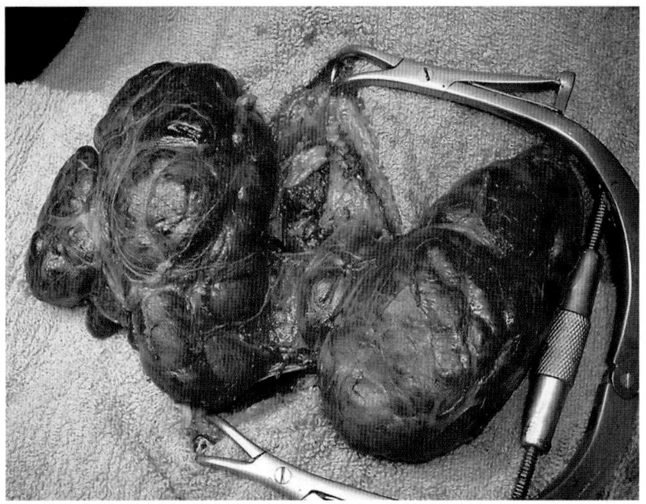

Figure 55.9 Total thyroidectomy for dyshormonogenetic goitre in a 14-year-old girl.

Goitrogens

Well-known goitrogens are the vegetables of the brassica family (cabbage, kale and rape), which contain thiocyanate, drugs such as para-aminosalicylic acid (PAS) and the antithyroid drugs. Thiocyanates and perchlorates interfere with iodide trapping; carbimazole and thiouracil compounds interfere with the oxidation of iodide and the binding of iodine to tyrosine.

Surprisingly, iodides in large quantities are goitrogenic because they inhibit the organic binding of iodine and produce an iodide goitre. Excessive iodine intake may be associated with an increased incidence of autoimmune thyroid disease.

The natural history of simple goitre

Stages in goitre formation are:

- Persistent growth stimulation causes diffuse hyperplasia; all lobules are composed of active follicles and iodine uptake is uniform. This is a diffuse hyperplastic goitre, which may persist but is reversible if stimulation ceases.
- Later, as a result of fluctuating stimulation, a mixed pattern develops with areas of active lobules and areas of inactive lobules.
- Active lobules become more vascular and hyperplastic until haemorrhage occurs, causing central necrosis and leaving only a surrounding rind of active follicles.
- Necrotic lobules coalesce to form nodules filled either with iodine-free colloid or a mass of new but inactive follicles.
- Continual repetition of this process results in a nodular goitre. Most nodules are inactive, and active follicles are present only in the internodular tissue.

Diffuse hyperplastic goitre

Diffuse hyperplasia corresponds to the first stages of the natural history. The goitre appears in childhood in endemic areas; in sporadic cases, it usually occurs at puberty, when metabolic demands are high. If TSH stimulation ceases the goitre may regress, but tends to recur later at times of stress such as pregnancy. The goitre is soft, diffuse and may become large enough to cause discomfort. A colloid goitre is a late stage of diffuse hyperplasia, when TSH stimulation has fallen off and when many follicles are inactive and full of colloid (*Figure 55.10*).

Nodular goitre

Nodules are usually multiple, forming a multinodular goitre (*Figure 55.11*). Occasionally, only one macroscopic nodule is found, but microscopic changes will be present throughout the gland; this is one form of a clinically solitary nodule. Nodules may be colloid or cellular, and cystic degeneration and haemorrhage are common, as is subsequent calcification. Nodules appear early in endemic goitre and later (between 20 and 30 years) in sporadic goitre, although the patient may be unaware of the goitre until his or her late forties or fifties. All types of simple goitre are more common in the female than in the male owing to the presence of oestrogen receptors in thyroid tissue.

Diagnosis

Diagnosis is usually straightforward. The patient is euthyroid and the nodules are palpable and often visible; they are smooth, usually firm and not hard and the goitre is painless and moves

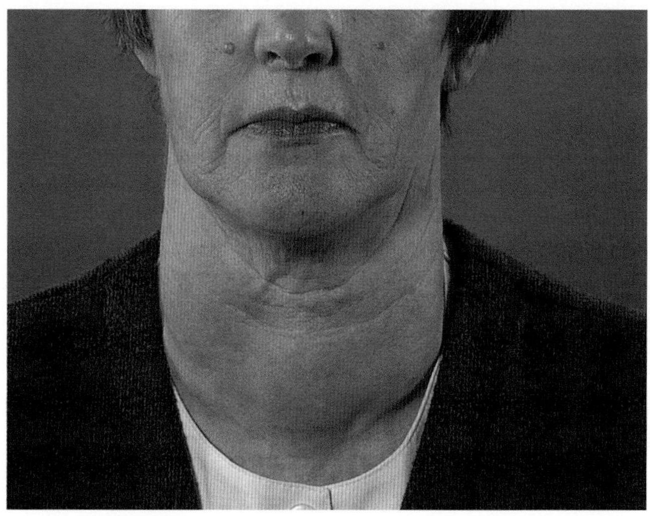

Figure 55.10 Colloid goitre.

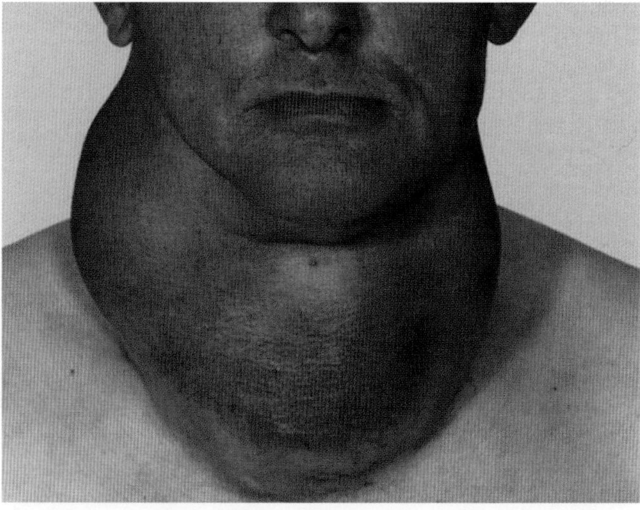

Figure 55.11 Large multinodular goitre.

freely on swallowing. Hardness and irregularity, due to calcification, may simulate carcinoma. A painful nodule, sudden appearance or rapid enlargement of a nodule raises suspicion of carcinoma but is usually due to haemorrhage into a simple nodule. Differential diagnosis from autoimmune thyroiditis may be difficult and the two conditions frequently coexist.

Investigations

Thyroid function should be assessed to exclude hyperthyroidism, and the presence of circulating thyroid antibodies tested to differentiate from autoimmune thyroiditis. Ultrasonography is the gold standard assessment when undertaken by a suitably trained and experienced operator. FNAC is only required for a nodule within the goitre that demonstrates ultrasonographic features of concern. This may or may not be the largest 'dominant' nodule. The biopsy should be performed under ultrasound guidance to ensure that the correct nodule is sampled. If there are swallowing or breathing symptoms then a CT scan of the chest and neck is the best modality to assess tracheal or oesophageal deviation or compression.

Complications

Tracheal obstruction may be due to gross lateral displacement or compression in a lateral or anteroposterior plane by retrosternal extension of the goitre (*Figure 55.7*). Acute respiratory obstruction may follow haemorrhage into a nodule impacted in the thoracic inlet.

Secondary thyrotoxicosis

Transient episodes of mild hyperthyroidism are common, occurring in up to 30% of patients.

Carcinoma

An increased incidence of cancer (usually follicular) has been reported from endemic areas. Dominant or rapidly growing nodules in longstanding goitres should always be subjected to aspiration cytology.

Prevention and treatment of simple goitre

In endemic areas the incidence of goitre has been strikingly reduced by the introduction of iodised salt. In the early stages, a hyperplastic goitre may regress if thyroxine is given in a dose of 0.15–0.2 mg daily for a few months.

Although the nodular stage of simple goitre is irreversible, more than half of benign nodules will regress in size over 10 years. Most patients with multinodular goitre are asymptomatic and do not require operation. Surgery is indicated for nodular goitres with features of underlying malignancy, for pressure symptoms if other causes have been excluded or for cosmetic reasons if the patient finds the goitre unsightly. If the goitre is causing tracheal compression then surgery should be considered. Many such patients are found incidentally and are asymptomatic and often very elderly. As these goitres often grow very slowly the risks and benefits of surgery should be considered carefully, particularly if a sternal split may be required for access.

There is a choice of surgical treatment in multinodular goitre: total thyroidectomy with immediate and lifelong replacement of thyroxine or some form of partial resection to conserve sufficient functioning thyroid tissue to subserve normal function while reducing the risk of hypoparathyroidism that accompanies total thyroidectomy. Historically subtotal thyroidectomy involves partial resection of each lobe, removing the bulk of the gland and leaving up to 8 g of relatively normal tissue in each remnant. The technique is essentially the same as described for toxic goitre, as are the postoperative complications. A significant problem with this approach is the propensity for regrowth. Therefore, unless there is a local shortage of thyroxine, most surgeons now favour total thyroidectomy in the setting of bilateral disease. More often, however, the multinodular change is asymmetrical, with one lobe more significantly involved than the other. In these circumstances, particularly in older patients, total lobectomy on the more affected side is the appropriate management. Although this can be used in combination with subtotal resection of the contralateral lobe (Dunhill procedure), most surgeons now prefer no intervention on the less affected side because of the potential for regrowth and the increased rate of complications associated with reoperation. In many cases, the causative factors persist and recurrence is likely.

Reoperation for recurrent nodular goitre is more difficult and hazardous and, for this reason, an increasing number of thyroid surgeons favour total thyroidectomy in younger patients. However, when the first operation comprised unilateral lobectomy alone for asymmetric goitre, reoperation and completion total thyroidectomy is straightforward if required for progression of nodularity in the remaining lobe. Total lobectomy and total thyroidectomy have the additional advantage of being therapeutic for incidental carcinomas.

Clinically discrete swellings

Discrete thyroid swellings (thyroid nodules) are common and are palpable in 3–4% of the adult population in the UK and USA. They are three to four times more frequent in women than in men.

Diagnosis

A discrete swelling in an otherwise impalpable gland is termed isolated or solitary, whereas the preferred term is dominant for a similar swelling in a gland with clinical evidence of generalised abnormality in the form of a palpable contralateral lobe or generalised mild nodularity. About 70% of discrete thyroid swellings are clinically isolated and about 30% are dominant. The true incidence of isolated swellings is somewhat less than the clinical estimate. Clinical classification is inevitably subjective and overestimates the frequency of truly isolated swellings. When such a gland is exposed at operation or examined by ultrasonography, CT or MRI, clinically impalpable nodules are often detected. The true frequency of thyroid nodularity compared with the clinical detection rate by palpation is shown in *Figure 55.12*.

Sir Thomas Peel Dunhill, 1876–1957, surgeon, St Bartholomew's Hospital, London, UK.

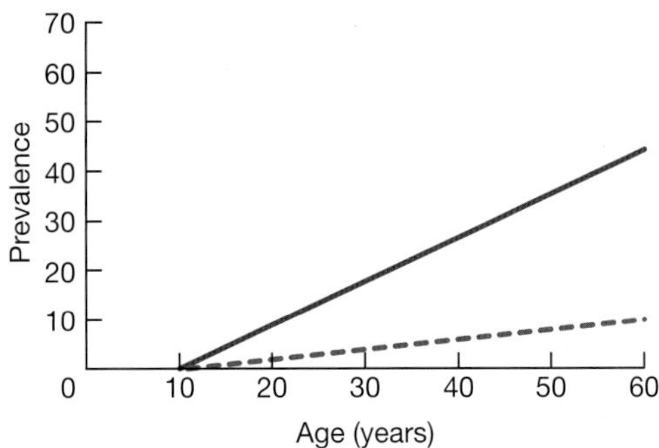

Figure 55.12 The prevalence of thyroid nodules detected on palpation (dashed line) or by ultrasonography or postmortem examination (solid line) (after Mazzaferri).

Demonstrating the presence of impalpable nodules does not change the management of palpable discrete swellings and begs the question of the necessity of investigating incidentally found nodules. The importance of discrete swellings lies in the risk of neoplasia compared with other thyroid swellings. Some 15% of isolated swellings prove to be malignant and an additional 30–40% are follicular adenomas. The remainder are non-neoplastic, largely consisting of areas of colloid degeneration, thyroiditis or cysts. Although the incidence of malignancy or follicular adenoma in clinically dominant swellings is approximately half of that of truly isolated swellings, it is substantial and cannot be ignored (*Figure 55.13*).

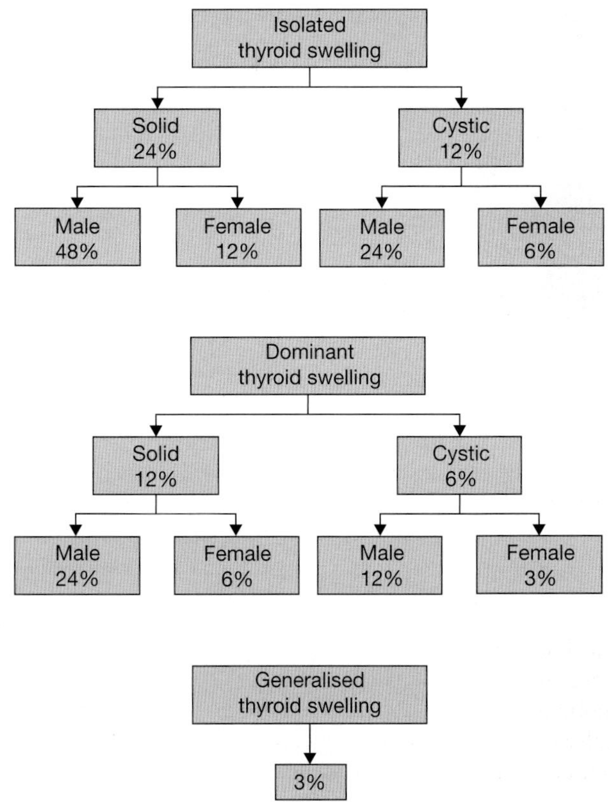

Figure 55.13 The risk of malignancy in thyroid swellings ('rule of 12'). The risk of cancer in a thyroid swelling can be expressed as a factor of 12. The risk is greater in isolated versus dominant swellings, solid versus cystic swellings and in men versus women.

Investigation

Thyroid function

Serum TSH and thyroid hormone levels should be measured. If hyperthyroidism associated with a discrete swelling is confirmed biochemically, it indicates either a 'toxic adenoma' or a manifestation of toxic multinodular goitre. The combination of toxicity and nodularity is important and is an indication for isotope scanning to localise the area(s) of hyperfunction.

Autoantibody titres

The autoantibody status may determine whether a swelling is a manifestation of chronic lymphocytic thyroiditis. The presence of circulating antibodies increases the risk of thyroid failure after lobectomy.

Isotope scan

Isotope scanning used to be the mainstay of investigation of discrete thyroid swellings but has been abandoned except when toxicity is associated with nodularity.

Ultrasonography

This is used to determine the physical characteristics of thyroid swellings. There are a number of ultrasonographic features in a thyroid swelling associated with thyroid neoplasia, including microcalcification and increased vascularity, but only macroscopic capsular breach and nodal involvement are diagnostic of malignancy. Ultrasonography should be used as the primary investigation of any thyroid nodule as a reassuring appearance mitigates the need for FNAC (see ***Fine-needle aspiration cytology***).

Fine-needle aspiration cytology

FNAC should be used, ideally under ultrasound guidance, on all nodules that do not fulfil a fully benign (U2) classification on ultrasonography. FNAC is reliable in identifying papillary thyroid carcinoma (PTC) but cannot distinguish between a benign follicular adenoma (*Figure 55.14*) and follicular carcinoma, as this distinction is dependent not on cytology but on histological criteria, which include capsular and vascular invasion.

FNAC is both highly specific and sensitive. Using ultrasonography improves this further, particularly in part cystic, part solid nodules in which ultrasonography allows targeting of the solid element for biopsy.

Radiology

Plain films have previously been used to assess tracheal compression and deviation, but the modality of choice now is CT scanning. CT scanning is also useful if ultrasonography has identified metastatic disease in the neck as it can assist surgical planning and also assess the superior mediastinum and lungs.

Ernest L Mazzaferri, 1936–2013, endocrinologist, Ohio State University School of Medicine, Columbus, OH, USA.

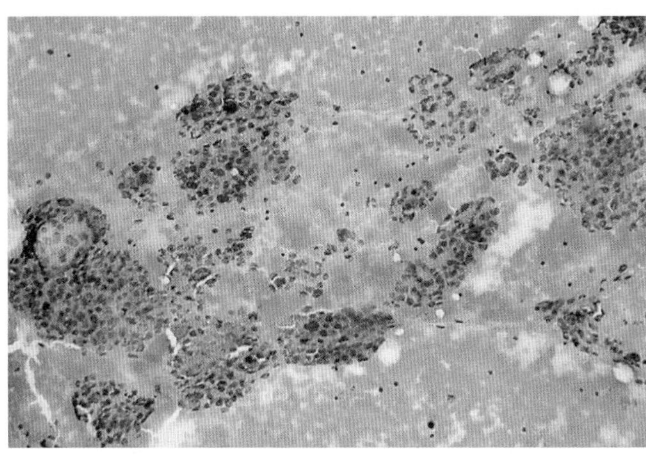

Figure 55.14 Thy3 aspiration cytology (*Table 55.2*). Follicular neoplasm showing increased cellularity with a follicular pattern.

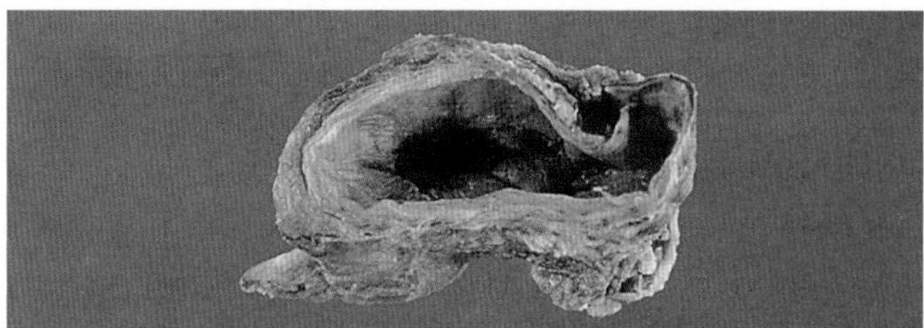

Figure 55.15 Apparently simple cystic thyroid swelling, the wall of which comprised follicular neoplastic tissue.

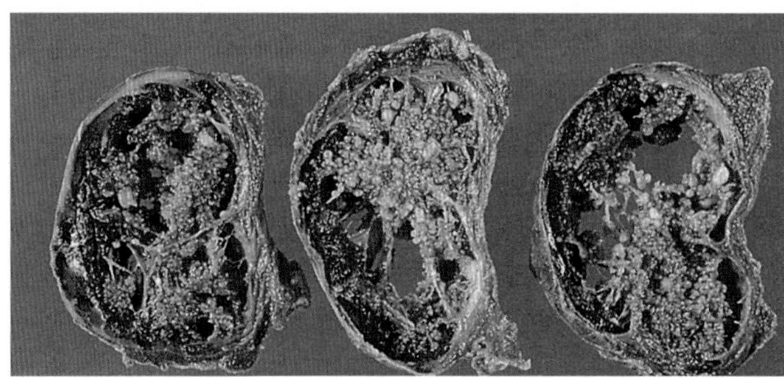

Figure 55.16 Cyst formation in a papillary carcinoma.

Laryngoscopy

Flexible laryngoscopy has rendered indirect laryngoscopy obsolete and is widely used preoperatively to determine the mobility of the vocal cords. The presence of a unilateral cord palsy coexisting with an ipsilateral thyroid nodule of concern is usually diagnostic of malignant disease.

Core biopsy

Core biopsy is rarely indicated in thyroid masses owing to the vascularity of the thyroid gland and the risk of postprocedure haemorrhage. It can be useful in the rapid diagnosis of widely invasive malignant disease, for example anaplastic carcinoma, or in the diagnosis of lymphadenopathy.

Indication for surgery

The main indication for operation is the risk of neoplasia, which includes follicular adenoma as well as malignant swellings. The reason for advocating the removal of all follicular neoplasms is that it is seldom possible to distinguish between a follicular adenoma and carcinoma cytologically. Even when the cytology is negative, the age and sex of the patient and the size of the swelling may be relative indications for surgery, especially when a large swelling is responsible for symptoms.

There are useful clinical criteria to assist in selection for operation according to the risk of neoplasia and malignancy. Hard texture alone is not reliable as tense cystic swellings may be suspiciously hard but a hard, irregular swelling with any apparent fixity, which is unusual, is highly suspicious. Evidence of RLN paralysis, suggested by hoarseness and a non-occlusive cough and confirmed by laryngoscopy, is almost pathognomonic. Cervical lymphadenopathy along the internal jugular vein in association with a clinically suspicious swelling is almost diagnostic of PTC. In most patients, however, such features are absent. The incidence of thyroid carcinoma in women is about three times that in men, but a discrete swelling in a male is much more likely to be malignant than in a female. The risk of carcinoma is increased at either end of the age range and a discrete swelling in a teenager of either sex must be provisionally diagnosed as carcinoma.

Thyroid cysts

Routine FNAC (or ultrasonography) shows that over 30% of clinically isolated swellings contain fluid and are cystic or partly cystic. Tense cysts may be hard and mimic carcinoma. Bleeding into a cyst often presents with a history of sudden painful swelling, which resolves to a variable extent over a period of weeks if untreated. Aspiration yields altered blood but reaccumulation is frequent. About 55% of cystic swellings are the result of colloid degeneration or are of uncertain aetiology because of an absence of epithelial cells in the lining. Although most of the remainder are the result of involution in follicular adenomas (*Figure 55.15*), some 10–15% of cystic follicular swellings are histologically malignant (30% in men and 10% in women). PTC is often associated with cyst formation (*Figure 55.16*).

Most patients with discrete swellings, however, are women, aged 20–40 years, in whom the risk of malignancy, although significant, is low and the indications for operation are not clear-cut.

Ultrasonography is the most useful tool for assessing cysts. If there is no discernible solid element, the cyst is almost certainly benign and does not need to be further investigated. As stated above, simple aspiration is associated with high rates of reaccumulation. However, ablation using either ethanol or thermal probes (radiofrequency, microwave, laser or high-frequency ultrasound) achieves cyst resolution in up to 90% of cases and should be considered for recurrent, symptomatic cysts. If there is an associated solid element, then consideration should be given to targeting that area with ultrasound-guided FNAC.

The indications for operation in isolated or dominant thyroid swellings are listed in *Table 55.4*.

TABLE 55.4 Indications for operation in thyroid swellings.

Neoplasia	FNAC positive Thy3–5	
	Clinical suspicion	• Age • Male sex • Hard texture • Fixity • Recurrent laryngeal nerve palsy • Lymphadenopathy • Recurrent cyst
Toxic adenoma		
Pressure symptoms		
Cosmesis		
Patient's wishes		

FNAC, fine-needle aspiration cytology; Thy3–5, see *Table 55.2*.

Selection of thyroid procedure

The choice of thyroid operation depends on:

- diagnosis (if known preoperatively);
- risk of thyroid failure;
- risk of RLN injury;
- risk of recurrence;
- Graves' disease;
- multinodular goitre;
- differentiated thyroid cancer;
- risk of hypoparathyroidism.

Total and near-total thyroidectomy do not conserve sufficient thyroid tissue for normal thyroid function and thyroid replacement therapy is necessary. In two-thirds of patients with negative antithyroid antibodies, one thyroid lobe will maintain normal function.

Subtotal resections for colloid goitre or Graves' disease run the risk of later growth of the remnant and, if a second operation is required years later, this greatly increases the risk to the RLN and parathyroid glands. In young patients, total thyroidectomy should be considered. It may be preferable to leave the least affected lobe untouched to permit a straightforward lobectomy in the future if required, rather than carry out subtotal resections.

In Graves' disease, preserving large remnants increases the risk of recurrence of the toxicity and, in these cases, it is better to err on the side of removing too much thyroid tissue rather than too little (*Table 55.5*). Thyroid failure should not be regarded as a failure of treatment, but recurrent toxicity is.

The relative merits of routine total versus selective total thyroidectomy in differentiated thyroid cancer are discussed below.

Summary box 55.2

Thyroid operations

All thyroid operations can be assembled from three basic elements:

1. Total lobectomy
2. Isthmusectomy
3. Subtotal lobectomy

Total thyroidectomy = 2 × total lobectomy + isthmusectomy

Subtotal thyroidectomy = 2 × subtotal lobectomy + isthmusectomy

Near-total thyroidectomy = total lobectomy + isthmusectomy + subtotal lobectomy (Dunhill procedure)

Lobectomy = total lobectomy + isthmusectomy

Retrosternal goitre

Retrosternal goitre tends to arise from the slow growth of a multinodular gland down into the mediastinum. As the gland enlarges within the thoracic inlet, pressure may lead to dysphagia, tracheal compression and eventually airway symptoms. The vast majority of patients have minimal symptoms. Patients should be considered for surgery if there is significant airway compression, if symptoms are present or in young patients in whom symptoms are likely to develop. In elderly patients with incidentally discovered retrosternal goitres, most surgeons would observe rather than treat prophylactically. Clearly a balance between risk and benefit must be made.

If a decision is made to proceed to surgery, assessment of the extent of disease is critical. The vast majority (>95%) of retrosternal goitres can be removed transcervically. Patients most at risk of requiring conversion to an open sternotomy approach include those with malignant disease or who are undergoing revision, those whose goitres that extend into the posterior mediastinum and those in whom the diameter of the goitre exceeds that of the thoracic inlet. In such cases a joint case with thoracic surgery should be planned.

All patients should have cross-sectional imaging. Ideally this is performed in the surgical position and, when interpreting CT chest scans, the surgeon should pay attention to the arm position. If the arms are up (as for standard CT chest)

TABLE 55.5 Comparison of surgical options for Graves' disease.

	Total thyroidectomy	Subtotal thyroidectomy
Control of toxicity	Immediate	Immediate
Return to euthyroid state	Immediate	Variable – up to 12 months
Risk of recurrence	None	Lifelong – up to 5%[a]
Risk of thyroid failure	100%	Lifelong – up to 100% at 30 years[a]
Risk of permanent hypoparathyroidism	5%	1%
Need for follow-up	Minimal	Lifelong

[a]The risks of recurrence and late failure are a function of the size of the remnant as a proportion of the total gland weight. Large remnants in small glands have a higher risk of recurrence and a low risk of failure, and small remnants in large glands have a higher risk of thyroid failure but a low risk of recurrence.

there will be a great deal of difference in thyroid position compared with when the arms are down and the neck extended.

The approach to surgery is as described in ***Surgical technique of thyroidectomy***. A longer incision is required. The surgeon may mobilise the sternomastoid muscle from the strap muscles to improve access. The ligamentous tissue between the sternal heads of the clavicles may be gently divided to increase the opening for gland delivery. Blunt dissection on the capsule of the gland allows mobilisation. Gentle traction is applied to deliver the gland into the neck. If the goitre has developed from a posteriorly positioned nodule there is a risk that the RLN may be displaced anteriorly, so great care must be taken in dividing apparent fascial bands that overlie the gland. The blood supply is from the neck, reducing the risk of catastrophic bleeding from the great vessels. Nonetheless, care should be taken in the region of the major blood vessels in the neck and chest.

If the gland is fixed and immobile or too large to deliver through a cervical approach, a midline sternotomy is performed and the gland can be dissected from below to achieve a safe total thyroidectomy.

HYPERTHYROIDISM

Thyrotoxicosis

The term thyrotoxicosis is retained because hyperthyroidism, i.e. symptoms due to a raised level of circulating thyroid hormones, is not responsible for all manifestations of the disease. Clinical types are:

- diffuse toxic goitre (Graves' disease);
- toxic nodular goitre;
- toxic nodule;
- hyperthyroidism due to rarer causes.

Diffuse toxic goitre

Graves' disease, a diffuse vascular goitre appearing at the same time as hyperthyroidism, usually occurs in younger women and is frequently associated with eye signs (***Figure 55.17***). The syndrome is that of primary thyrotoxicosis; 55% of patients have a family history of autoimmune endocrine diseases. The whole of the functioning thyroid tissue is involved, and the hypertrophy and hyperplasia are due to abnormal TSH-RAb that bind to TSH receptor sites and produce a disproportionate and prolonged effect.

Toxic nodular goitre

A simple nodular goitre is present for a long time before the hyperthyroidism, usually in the middle-aged or elderly, and very infrequently is associated with eye signs. The syndrome is that of secondary thyrotoxicosis.

In many cases of toxic nodular goitre, the nodules are inactive, and it is the internodular thyroid tissue that is overactive. However, in some toxic nodular goitres, one or more nodules are overactive and here the hyperthyroidism is due to autonomous thyroid tissue as in a toxic adenoma.

Toxic nodule

A toxic nodule is a solitary overactive nodule, which may be part of a generalised nodularity or a true toxic adenoma. It is autonomous and its hypertrophy and hyperplasia are not due to TSH-RAb. TSH secretion is suppressed by the high level of circulating thyroid hormones and the normal thyroid tissue surrounding the nodule is itself suppressed and inactive.

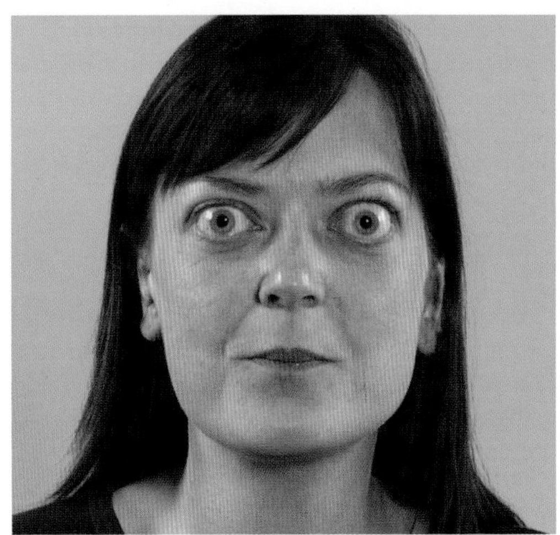

Figure 55.17 Graves' disease.

Histology

The normal thyroid gland consists of acini lined with flattened cuboidal epithelium and filled with homogeneous colloid (***Figure 55.2***). In hyperthyroidism (***Figure 55.18***), there is hyperplasia of acini, which are lined by high columnar epithelium. Many of them are empty, and others contain vacuolated colloid with a characteristic 'scalloped' pattern adjacent to the thyrocytes.

Principles of treatment of thyrotoxicosis

Non-specific measures are rest and sedation and in established thyrotoxicosis should be used only in conjunction with specific measures, i.e. the use of antithyroid drugs, surgery and radioiodine.

Antithyroid drugs

Those in common use are carbimazole and propylthiouracil. Antithyroid drugs are used to restore the patient to a euthyroid

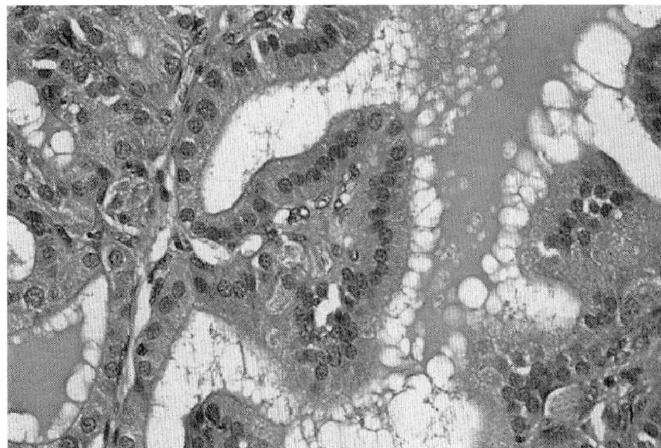

Figure 55.18 Histology of thyrotoxicosis.

state and to maintain this for a prolonged period in the hope that a permanent remission will occur, i.e. that production of TSH-RAb will diminish or cease. Antithyroid drugs cannot cure a toxic nodule. The overactive thyroid tissue is autonomous and recurrence of the hyperthyroidism is certain when the drug is discontinued.

- **Advantages**. No surgery and no use of radioactive materials.
- **Disadvantages**. Treatment is prolonged and the failure rate is at least 55%. The duration of treatment may be tailored to the severity of the toxicity, with milder cases being treated for only 6 months and severe cases for 2 years before stopping therapy.

Surgery

In diffuse toxic goitre and toxic nodular goitre with overactive internodular tissue, surgery cures by reducing the mass of overactive tissue by reducing the thyroid below a critical mass. After subtotal thyroidectomy the patient should return to a euthyroid state, albeit after a variable period of hypothyroidism. There are, however, long-term risks of recurrence and eventual thyroid failure. In contrast total/near-total thyroidectomy accepts immediate thyroid failure and lifelong thyroxine replacement to eliminate the risk of recurrence and simplify follow-up. Operation may result in a reduction in TSH-RAb. In the autonomous toxic nodule, and in toxic nodular goitre with overactive autonomous toxic nodules, surgery cures by removing all the overactive thyroid tissue; this allows the suppressed normal tissue to function again.

- **Advantages**. The goitre is removed, the cure is rapid and the cure rate is high if surgery has been adequate.
- **Disadvantages**. Recurrence of thyrotoxicosis occurs in at least 5% of cases when subtotal thyroidectomy is carried out. There is a risk of permanent hypoparathyroidism and nerve injury. Young women tend to have a poorer cosmetic result from the scar.

Every operation carries a risk, but with suitable preparation and an experienced surgeon the mortality is negligible and the morbidity low.

Radioiodine

Radioiodine destroys thyroid cells and, as in thyroidectomy, reduces the mass of functioning thyroid tissue to below a critical level.

- **Advantages**. No surgery and no prolonged drug therapy.
- **Disadvantages**. Isotope facilities must be available. The patient must be quarantined while radiation levels are high and avoid pregnancy and close physical contact, particularly with children. Eye signs may be aggravated.

Choice of therapy

Each case must be considered individually. Below are listed guiding principles on the most satisfactory treatment for a particular toxic goitre at a particular age; these must, however, be modified according to the facilities available and the personality and wishes of the individual patient and any other coexistent medical or surgical condition. Access to post-treatment care and availability of replacement thyroxine can be important considerations in some areas.

Diffuse toxic goitre

Most patients have an initial course of antithyroid drugs with radioiodine for relapse. Exceptions are those who refuse radiation, those who have large goitres or progressive eye signs and those who are pregnant.

Toxic nodular goitre

Toxic nodular goitre is often large and uncomfortable and enlarges still further with antithyroid drugs. Large goitres should be treated surgically because they do not respond as well or as rapidly to radioiodine or antithyroid drugs as does a diffuse toxic goitre.

Toxic nodule

Surgery or radioiodine treatment is appropriate. Resection is easy, certain and has limited morbidity. Radioiodine is a good alternative for patients over the age of 45 years because the suppressed thyroid tissue does not take up iodine and thus there is minimal risk of delayed thyroid insufficiency.

Failure of previous treatment with antithyroid drugs or radioiodine

In this case, surgery or thyroid ablation with ^{123}I is appropriate.

Surgery for thyrotoxicosis

Preoperative preparation

Traditional preparation aims to make the patient biochemically euthyroid at operation. Preparation is as an outpatient and only rarely is admission to hospital necessary on account of severe symptoms at presentation, failure to control the hyperthyroidism or non-compliance with medication. Care should be coordinated with endocrinology input.

Carbimazole 30–40 mg/day is the drug of choice for preparation. When euthyroid (after 8–12 weeks), the dose may be reduced to 5 mg 8-hourly or a 'block and replace' regime used. In this case, the high dose of carbimazole is continued to inhibit T_3 and T_4 production and a maintenance dose of 0.1–0.15 mg thyroxine is given daily. The last dose of carbimazole may be given on the evening before surgery. Iodides are not used alone because, if the patient needs preoperative treatment, a more effective drug should be given.

An alternative method of preparation is to abolish the clinical manifestations of the toxic state, using β-adrenergic blocking drugs. These act on the target organs and not on the gland itself. Propranolol also inhibits the peripheral conversion of T_4 to T_3. The appropriate dosages are propranolol 40 mg three times daily. Clinical response to β-blockade is rapid and the patient may be rendered clinically euthyroid and operation arranged in a few days rather than weeks. The dose of β-adrenergic blocking drug is increased to achieve the required clinical response and quite often larger doses (propranolol 80 mg three times daily or nadolol 320 mg once daily) are necessary.

β-Adrenergic blocking drugs do not interfere with synthesis of thyroid hormones, and hormone levels remain high during treatment and for some days after thyroidectomy. It is, therefore, important to continue treatment for 7 days postoperatively.

Iodine may be given with carbimazole or a β-adrenergic blocking drug for 10 days before operation. Iodide alone produces a transient remission and may reduce vascularity, thereby marginally improving safety. The use of iodine preparations is not universal because of more effective alternatives. Iodine gives an additional measure of safety in case the early morning dose of β-adrenergic blocking drug is mistakenly omitted on the day of operation.

The extent of the resection depends on the size of the gland, the age of the patient, the experience of the surgeon, the need to minimise the risk of recurrent toxicity and the wish to avoid postoperative thyroid replacement (***Table 55.5***).

Surgical technique of thyroidectomy

The aim of thyroidectomy is to remove the entire thyroid lobe (bilaterally if total thyroidectomy), encompassing all disease and preserving the cervical strap muscles, external branches of the superior laryngeal nerve, the RLN, parathyroid glands and their blood supply in each case while minimising cosmetic impact.

Set-up. With the patient under general anaesthesia, supine, arms at their side, with their head on a ring and neck extended with a shoulder roll or the head of the table extended with the head of the bed raised (reverse Trendelenburg), the operative field is prepared from lower lip to upper chest.

A nerve monitor endotracheal tube or electrode wrap can be used (see ***New technology in thyroidectomy***). The position of the tube should be checked after positioning the patient as extending the neck can withdraw the tube and compromise the contact of the electrodes in the larynx.

Either use a head drape or square off the surgical site. If head draping, include the nerve monitor leads in the head drape. Alternatively, squaring off the surgical site can give easier access to the endotracheal tube if required.

Exposure. The skin incision is placed in a skin crease as close as possible to the cricoid at the superior edge of the thyroid isthmus, which is usually palpable. The length of the incision is determined by the size of the thyroid; however, there is little benefit in extending the incision much beyond the medial edge of the sternocleidomastoid muscle. Mark the incision before prepping and infiltrate with local anaesthetic and adrenaline (epinephrine).

A scalpel is used for the skin incision. Incise through the dermis, making sure to use the full extent of the incision.

Monopolar diathermy can be used to expose and divide the platysma. This plane is then used to raise a subplatysmal flap to the thyroid notch of the thyroid cartilage superiorly and to the suprasternal notch inferiorly.

The midline is identified between the strap muscles superiorly as, often, the sternohyoid muscles separate around the thyroid eminence. The sternohyoid muscles are raised with toothed forceps and monopolar diathermy is used to divide the fascia, avoiding injury to the anterior jugular veins. A Langenbeck retractor helps dissect superior and inferior limits.

The plane is developed to dissect between the muscle layers, elevating sternohyoid laterally until the ansa cervicalis is visualised. The sternothyroid muscle is then mobilised from the gland, taking great care with the delicate vasculature. If required, the strap muscles may be divided superiorly to afford greater exposure. There is usually an artery and a vein travelling between the two strap muscles superiolaterally; these can be injured if overly enthusiastic blunt dissection is used. Once the internal jugular vein is identified dissection medial and deep to this will allow identification of the common carotid artery, and between the vessels the vagus nerve. This should be stimulated to prove that the nerve monitor is functioning properly. If the latency reading on the nerve monitor is unexpectedly short on the right side then consider a non-recurrent right laryngeal nerve.

At this point the gland is exposed and ready for dissection. Minimal blood loss should have been encountered.

Upper pole. The assistant now places Langenbeck retractors under sternohyoid, one lateral to the upper pole and one medial. This displays the superior thyroid vascular pedicle, which is controlled with ties or a bipolar energy device. This not only mobilises the superior pole but also preserves the blood supply to the superior parathyroid gland. In addition, it minimises risk to the superior laryngeal nerve, which can often be seen passing medially towards the cricothyroid muscle. Gradually the superior pole is mobilised, taking care not to dissect below the cricoid cartilage, at which point the RLN is at risk (***Figure 55.19***).

Mobilising the rest of the gland. Gentle traction on the fascia over the gland, immediately next to the superior plane, will show a plane to follow over the main thyroid. This is followed inferiorly, avoiding excessive lateral dissection to prevent inadvertent damage to the RLN. Blunt dissection will allow much of this fascia to be mobilised. Occasional vessels require bipolar cautery.

Next, the trachea is identified in the midline below the isthmus, staying on the cartilage and close to the gland in order to prevent damage to vessels that may contribute to arcades supplying the inferior parathyroid gland.

At this point, the RLN is superior and lateral to the trachea and inferior to the plane developed superiorly. Depending on just how compliant the fascia is and how large the lobe is, much of the dissection may now be complete. A pledget may be used to brush fascia laterally.

Identification of the recurrent laryngeal nerve. It is not uncommon that the RLN can be seen at this point. Assuming

---

Friedrich Trendelenburg, 1844–1924, successively Professor of Surgery at Rostock (1875–1882), Bonn (1822–1895) and Leipzig (1895–1911), Germany. The Trendelenburg position was first described in 1885.

Bernhard Rudolf Konrad von Langenbeck, 1810–1887, Professor of Surgery, successively at Kiel and Berlin, Germany.

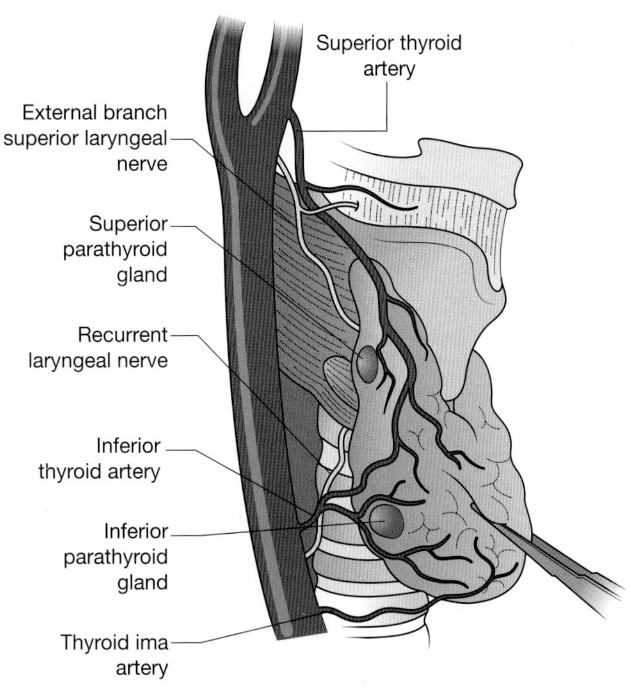

Figure 55.19 General anatomy of a thyroidectomy.

it is not, dissection proceeds by gently mobilising the fascia around the gland, staying directly on the gland and not dividing anything that could be neural. The RLN will be close, often but not always behind the inferior thyroid artery (approximately 70%). By remaining vigilant, never dividing any structure that could remotely be neural and slowly dissecting fascia, the lobe can be delivered from above and below, mobilising in the direction of Berry's ligament. Using this approach, the RLN will be identified and can be confirmed with the nerve stimulator.

Once the nerve has been identified a number of approaches are possible. Ideally the nerve is largely lateral to the gland. This allows dissection to progress until only Berry's ligament remains. However, if the nerve lies medially, it may actually lie on the thyroid and require gentle dissection to free it from the thyroid surface. If this is the case, stay directly on the nerve and slowly dissect the nerve free of the surrounding tissue, endeavouring not to injure the nerve by direct pressure.

The nerve should be traced towards the cricothyroid joint as it enters the larynx. The pretracheal fascia condenses into Berry's ligament at this point. Small vessels within the ligament retract if not controlled with bipolar cautery or ties, and the resulting bleeding can disorientate the surgeon, placing the nerve at risk. In order to avoid this, pre-emptive diathermy to the ligament and careful layer-by-layer dissection allows final mobilisation of the thyroid lobe. Some surgeons prefer to isolate the ligament and apply a careful tie to achieve haemostasis. Whichever method is preferred, great care must be taken at this point.

Management of Berry's ligament. The exact anatomy here will depend on how extensive the condensation of fascia (Berry's ligament) is and how it relates to the RLN. This is variable and this relationship dictates how easy the next steps are. In some the ligament is distant from the nerve. In others the nerve runs up to and even through the ligament. Keeping the nerve in direct vision, minimal division of the ligament allows the RLN to move back and expose more of the ligament, allowing the process to continue, layer by layer, until the nerve is well lateral and the ligament has been divided.

If, during this process, bleeding is encountered the use of targeted pressure and occasionally fine-tip suction to identify the specific bleeding point and careful use of bipolar cautery will achieve haemostasis. This must be meticulous as re-exploration of this area for bleeding puts the RLN at significant risk.

Delivery of the gland. Loose pretrachea fascia can now be opened with monopolar diathermy over the trachea to the midline and beyond to remove the isthmus, which is divided, encompassing any pyramidal lobe tissue. The residual isthmus is either oversewn or sealed with bipolar cautery. If a total thyroidectomy is required, the procedure is repeated on the other side.

Closure. The operative field should be inspected. Irrigation with saline helps identification of small bleeding points. The anatomy should be confirmed, ideally with confirmation of neural integrity by stimulating the vagus (if previously located). Bipolar cautery is used carefully to avoid nerve or parathyroid injury.

Most surgeons do not place a drain. Interrupted sutures are placed through the sternohyoid muscle to prevent adhesion between the trachea and skin. The aim is not to perform a watertight closure of the muscle in case this promotes pressure in the event of a haematoma.

The platysma closure is followed by subcuticular skin closure with an absorbable suture.

New technology in thyroidectomy

The major immediate risk following thyroidectomy is haemorrhage; conventionally, artery forceps, ligatures and sutures have been used to secure the meticulous haemostasis necessary to minimise the risk of this potentially life-threatening complication. Ultrasonic shears, enhanced bipolar diathermy and harmonic vessel sealing devices are increasingly used in thyroid surgery and may be advantageous in complex procedures.

Monitoring of the RLN and vagus nerve has become available over the last few years. By placing electrodes on the endotracheal tube between the vocal cords, movements can be detected when the nerve is stimulated. Such intermittent nerve monitoring is gaining in popularity. Advocates consider the monitor particularly useful in recurrent operations where scar tissue makes the nerve difficult to identify. In addition, some find that operative time is reduced and that this is a valuable tool for training. There is also some support for the use of nerve monitoring during bilateral thyroid surgery, as the information provided can aid in the identification of a unilateral palsy to prevent bilateral palsy that can require tracheostomy. Those who do not support the use of the nerve monitor highlight the lack of evidence that there is any real difference in outcome associated with this practice. In addition, there is the expense of the base machine and the electrodes.

In contrast to intermittent nerve monitoring that allows identification of a damaged nerve, continuous nerve monitoring has now been developed. In theory, this provides the opportunity to identify a nerve when function is threatened (by excessive traction, for example). This technique, although theoretically advantageous, requires an electrode to be placed on the vagus nerve and has not gained widespread acceptance (*Figure 55.20*).

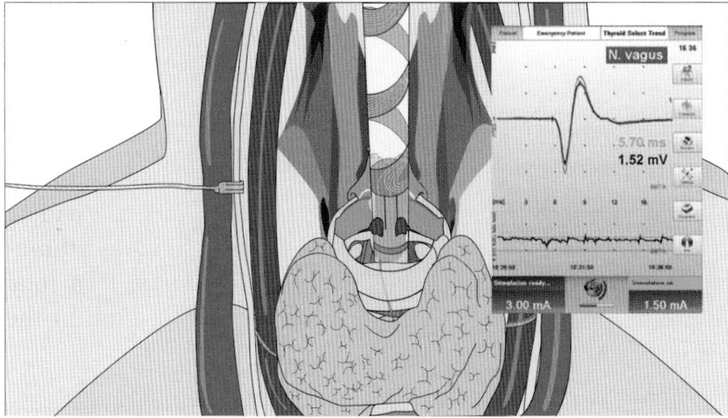

Figure 55.20 Continuous monitoring of the vagus nerve (adapted from an image provided by Inomed UK Ltd).

Alternative surgical techniques

Over the past two decades, increasing experience has been gained in alternative approaches to thyroid surgery. Minimally invasive video-assisted techniques have been developed that allow surgeons to operate through an incision <2 cm in length. With appropriately modified dissectors, experienced operators and advanced haemostatic electrosurgical devices, such procedures offer reduced scar length. However, they are only appropriate for small-volume disease and as such are not suitable for many thyroid cases.

Remote access thyroid surgery is of increasing interest. A number of approaches have been developed via axillary or breast incisions and also through the oral cavity. These approaches can be used with laparoscopic or robotic techniques to allow a magnified view of the operative site. Such 'maximally invasive' techniques require extended dissection over the chest wall or neck and again are most suitable for small-volume disease. Experienced centres continue to expand the indications for these techniques. However, they are associated with increased and significant time, which currently limits their application to most thyroid surgical practice.

Postoperative complications

Haemorrhage is the most frequent life-threatening complication of thyroidectomy. Around 1 in 50 patients will develop a haematoma, and in almost all cases this will develop in the first 24 hours. If an arterial bleed occurs, the tension in the central compartment pressure can rise until it exceeds venous pressure. Venous oedema of the larynx can then develop and cause airway obstruction, leading to death. Although improvements in understanding of the blood supply to the larynx and technical developments in terms of haemostatic technologies have been made, this complication has not been eliminated. Although many surgeons worldwide practise day case thyroidectomy, bleeding is the reason that, in the UK, thyroidectomy remains an inpatient procedure.

Intraoperative attention to detail in terms of haemostasis is critical. When closing the wound, avoiding a watertight closure of the strap muscles may allow a haematoma to escape into the subcutaneous tissues. Wound drains have not been shown to have a protective effect. Close monitoring of the wound is advised postoperatively. If a haematoma develops, clinical staff should know to remove skin sutures in order to release some pressure and seek senior advice immediately. Endotracheal intubation should be used to secure the airway while the haematoma is evacuated and the bleeding point controlled.

RLN paralysis and voice change RLN injury may be unilateral or bilateral, transient or permanent. Early routine postoperative laryngoscopy reveals a much higher incidence of transient cord paralysis than is detectable by simple assessment of the integrity of the voice and cough. Such temporary dysfunction is not clinically important, however, but voice and cord function should be assessed at first follow-up 4 weeks postoperatively. A British Association of Endocrine and Thyroid Surgeons audit revealed an RLN palsy rate of 1.8% at 1 month, declining to 0.5% at 3 months for first-time operations. Permanent paralysis is rare if the nerve has been identified at operation.

If an RLN is injured during surgery and the transected ends are identified, they should be reanastomosed. In the event that a length of nerve is excised (owing to invasion by malignancy, for example), anastomosis of the ansa cervicalis may be considered. This does not return mobility of the vocal cord but maintains neurological input to the muscles of the larynx. By avoiding denervation and related muscle atrophy, the vocal quality is improved. Permanent vocal cord paralysis should be treated conservatively with speech therapy. If voice quality is unacceptable, medialisation procedures can be performed. Nerve grafting has shown promise but experience is limited.

Injury to the external branch of the superior laryngeal nerve is more common because of its proximity to the superior thyroid artery. This leads to loss of tension in the vocal cord with diminished power and range in the voice. Patients, particularly those who use their voice professionally, must be advised that any thyroid operation will result in change to the voice even in the absence of nerve trauma. Fortunately, for most patients the changes are subtle and only demonstrable on formal voice assessment.

Thyroid insufficiency. Thyroxine replacement will be required following total thyroidectomy. Around one in three patients who has a lobectomy will require supplementation; rates are higher in those with thyroid autoantibodies. Subtotal thyroidectomy was at one time performed with the aim of leaving sufficient tissue to maintain thyroid function. However, this is difficult to judge and, over the years, the benign process that necessitated primary surgery may recur, requiring difficult revision procedures. For this reason, the practice of subtotal thyroidectomy has been more or less abandoned outside environments where exogenous thyroxine is not available.

Parathyroid insufficiency. This is due to removal of the parathyroid glands or infarction through damage to the parathyroid end arteries; often both factors occur together. Vascular injury is probably far more important than inadvertent removal. The incidence of permanent hypoparathyroidism should be less than 1% and most cases present dramatically 2–5 days after operation; very rarely, the onset is delayed for 2–3 weeks or a patient with marked hypocalcaemia may be asymptomatic. The complication is limited to total thyroidectomy, as when lobectomy is performed the contralateral parathyroid glands are sufficient to maintain calcium levels. In particular, total thyroidectomy with central neck dissection places the parathyroid glands and their vascular supply at great risk and should only be performed when there is evidence of metastatic disease or high risk of occult disease in the regional lymph nodes.

Thyrotoxic crisis (storm). This is an acute exacerbation of hyperthyroidism. It occurs if a thyrotoxic patient has been inadequately prepared for thyroidectomy and is now extremely rare. Very rarely, a thyrotoxic patient presents in a crisis and this may follow an unrelated operation. Symptomatic and supportive treatment is for dehydration, hyperpyrexia and restlessness. This requires the administration of intravenous fluids, cooling the patient with ice packs, administration of oxygen, diuretics for cardiac failure, digoxin for uncontrolled atrial fibrillation, sedation and intravenous hydrocortisone. Specific treatment is by carbimazole 10–20 mg 6-hourly, Lugol's iodine 10 drops 8-hourly by mouth or sodium iodide 1 g intravenously. Propranolol intravenously (1–2 mg) or orally (40 g 6-hourly) will block β-adrenergic effects.

Wound infection. Cellulitis requiring prescription of antibiotics, often by the general practitioner, is more common than most surgeons appreciate. A significant subcutaneous or deep cervical abscess is exceptionally rare and should be drained.

Hypertrophic or keloid scar. This is more likely to form if the incision overlies the sternum and in dark-skinned individuals. Intradermal injections of corticosteroid should be given at once and repeated monthly if necessary. Scar revision rarely results in significant long-term improvement.

Stitch granuloma. This may occur with or without sinus formation and is seen after the use of non-absorbable, particularly silk, suture material. Absorbable ligatures and sutures should be used throughout thyroid surgery.

Postoperative care

Following surgery, the patient should be returned to the recovery room and nursed overnight on the ward. Wound care should include vigilance for signs of a haematoma. Following total thyroidectomy, calcium levels should be checked postoperatively. Not all patients develop immediate hypocalcaemia and they should be educated about the signs (paraesthesia of the fingers and toes or around the mouth). Serial calcium monitoring should be recommended for those at highest risk.

Those patients who had a total thyroidectomy require thyroxine replacement, which should start on day 1 postoperatively. On clinic review, in addition to checking the histology report, the wound should be inspected and the larynx examined for vocal cord function. Biochemical assessment of thyroid function and calcium, if required, should be arranged.

NEOPLASMS OF THE THYROID

Classification of thyroid neoplasms is presented in *Table 55.6* and the relative incidence of malignancies in *Table 55.7*.

TABLE 55.6 Classification of thyroid neoplasms.

Benign	Follicular adenoma		
Malignant	Primary	Follicular epithelium – differentiated	Follicular Papillary
		Follicular epithelium – poorly differentiated	Anaplastic
		Parafollicular cells	Medullar
		Lymphoid cells	
	Secondary	Metastatic	
		Local infiltration	

TABLE 55.7 Relative incidence of primary malignant tumours of the thyroid gland.

Malignancy	Relative incidence (%)
Papillary carcinoma	80
Follicular carcinoma	10
Poorly differentiated/anaplastic carcinoma	5
Medullary carcinoma	2.5
Lymphoma	2.5

Benign tumours

Follicular adenomas present as clinically solitary nodules (*Figure 55.21*) and the distinction between a follicular carcinoma and an adenoma can only be made by histological examination; in the adenoma there is no invasion of the capsule or of pericapsular blood vessels. For this reason, FNA, which provides cytological detail but not tissue architecture, cannot differentiate between benign and malignant follicular lesions. Diagnosis and treatment is, therefore, by wide excision, i.e. total lobectomy. The remaining thyroid tissue is normal so that prolonged follow-up is unnecessary.

Malignant tumours

The vast majority of primary malignancies are carcinomas derived from the follicular cells (*Table 55.6*). Such tumours

Jean Guillaume Auguste Lugol, 1786–1851, Physician, Hôpital Saint-Louis, Paris, France.

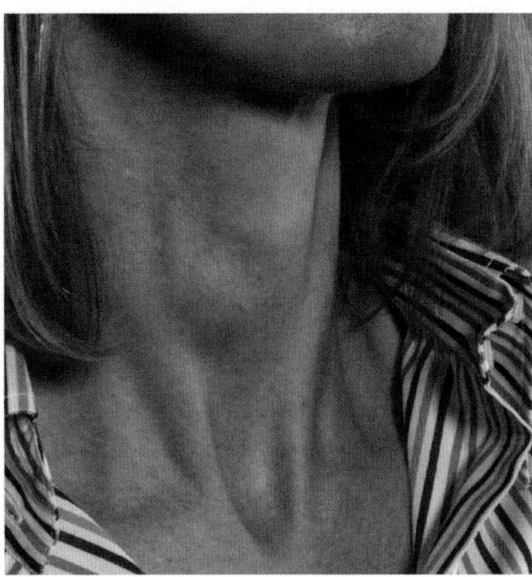

Figure 55.21 Isolated swelling in the upper pole of the right thyroid lobe.

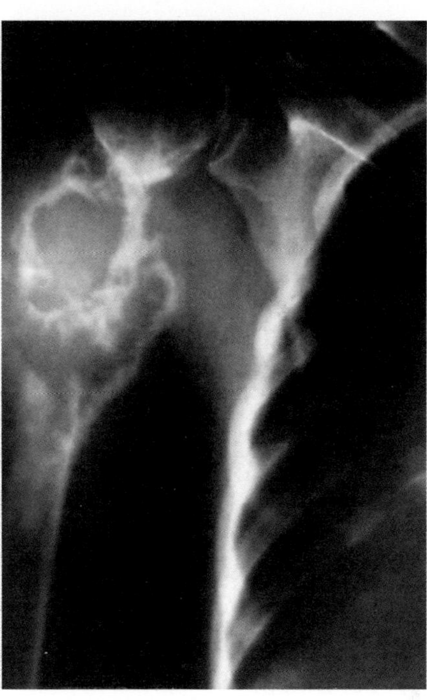

Figure 55.22 Metastasis in the humerus from thyroid carcinoma (courtesy of DS Devadatta, Vellore, India).

were thought of as differentiated (papillary, follicular and Hürthle cell) and undifferentiated (anaplastic). However, now an intermediate class of 'poorly differentiated carcinoma' is recognised, which is likely to represent a state of dedifferentiated – between classic differentiated and undifferentiated diseases. The parafollicular C cells can undergo malignant transformation into medullary carcinoma, and thyroid lymphoma is another primary thyroid malignancy. In addition, the thyroid can be involved by direct spread from surrounding structures (larynx and oesophagus) or metastases (most commonly from renal cell carcinoma). Lymph node and blood-borne metastases of thyroid cancer occur primarily to bone and lung and may be the mode of presentation (*Figure 55.22*).

Aetiology of malignant thyroid tumours

The great majority of thyroid cancers have no known aetiological factor. The most important identifiable aetiological factor in differentiated thyroid carcinoma (particularly papillary) is irradiation of the thyroid under 5 years of age. In the town of Gomel, Ukraine, the incidence of childhood thyroid cancer rose from <1 per million to 96 per million following the Chernobyl nuclear disaster.

Short latency aggressive PTC is associated with the *ret/PTC3* oncogene and later developing, possibly less aggressive, cancers with *ret/PTC1*. The incidence of follicular carcinoma is high in endemic goitrous areas, possibly because of TSH stimulation. Malignant lymphomas sometimes develop in autoimmune thyroiditis, and the lymphocytic infiltration in the autoimmune process may be an aetiological factor.

Clinical features of thyroid cancers

The annual incidence is about 0.8 per million of the population and the sex ratio is three females to one male. However, the incidence of PTC is increasing rapidly across the world. This is mostly due to increased rates of imaging detecting previously occult disease. For that reason, although the incidence is increasing, the mortality rates remain static at over 80% 5-year survival for all groups. In particular, anaplastic carcinoma predicts poor outcome with differentiated carcinomas generally having excellent outcomes. The most common presenting symptom is a thyroid swelling (*Figures 55.21 and 55.23*). Enlarged cervical lymph nodes may be the presentation of PTC. RLN paralysis is very suggestive of locally advanced disease.

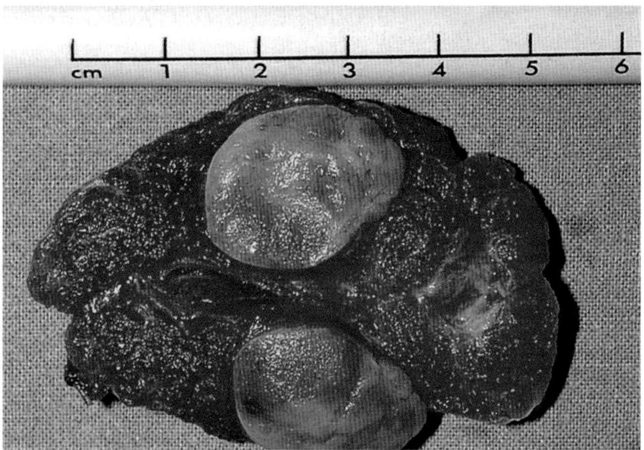

Figure 55.23 Follicular neoplasm of the thyroid presenting as an isolated swelling.

Karl Hürthle, 1866–1945, histopathologist, Breslau, Germany (now Wrocław, Poland).

Anaplastic cancers are usually hard, irregular and infiltrating. A differentiated carcinoma may be suspiciously firm and irregular, but is often indistinguishable from a benign swelling. Small papillary tumours may be impalpable, even when lymphatic metastases are present. Pain, often referred to the ear, is suggestive of nerve involvement from infiltrating tumours.

Diagnosis of thyroid neoplasms

Clinical history and examination continue to be the cornerstone of diagnosis of thyroid neoplasms. As previously mentioned, radiation exposure and family history should be discussed. Examination of the central neck and regional lymphatics should be combined with assessment of vocal cord function. Biochemical assessment of thyroid function should also be considered in this first encounter, if not already performed.

Following initial assessment, the next step is ultrasonography. This non-invasive investigation is most accurate at assessing thyroid swellings. Not only can a judgement be made on the presence, size and number of thyroid nodules present, but an estimate of risk of malignancy can be made depending on these findings.

Following ultrasonography, lesions can be categorised as benign, indeterminate or malignant. Benign lesions require no further assessment unless surgery is considered for compressive symptoms. Indeterminate or malignant lesions should be investigated with FNAC.

Occasionally, the surgeon will encounter a thyrotoxic patient. Such cases are one of the few indications for a radioiodine uptake scan. This allows assessment of the function of a nodule. Hot nodules are very rarely malignant. Cold nodules will require assessment as for all other thyroid neoplasms.

Following clinical, ultrasonographic and cytological assessment, the vast majority of lesions will be characterised as benign, malignant or indeterminate. Further treatment will be planned accordingly.

Certain situations require specific consideration. For patients with widespread nodal disease or suspicion of locally invasive disease affecting the airway, contrast-enhanced imaging should be considered. This should cover the neck and chest. This not only allows accurate assessment of any visceral invasion, but is superior to ultrasonography at defining disease in the mediastinum and thorax. Concerns over the impact of iodine-containing contrast on delays to radioactive iodine therapy have been overplayed, and it is more critical that the surgeon has an accurate assessment of disease extent prior to surgery.

Patients with a rapidly growing thyroid mass, particularly if solid and fixed, should be considered at risk of anaplastic carcinoma. However, this diagnosis can be difficult to differentiate from thyroid lymphoma or occasionally thyroiditis. Despite the difficulty, an accurate diagnosis is critical as anaplastic carcinoma is rapidly fatal and palliative measures are generally recommended, whereas confounding disease processes may respond to therapy. In this setting, core or even open biopsy may be required to make a confident diagnosis.

Papillary thyroid carcinoma

PTC is the most common thyroid malignancy. Interestingly, up to 30% of patients who die of non-thyroid disease have deposits of PTC in autopsy studies, suggesting that many patients live with this disease undetected. Nonetheless, when PTC is diagnosed most patients will be offered treatment. The disease is known for its propensity for lymph node metastases. These are more common in younger patients, in whom they do not affect the otherwise excellent survival. This finding is in contrast to most malignancies, where the finding of metastatic disease confers a poor outcome. One contentious finding in patients with PTC is a high rate of occult micrometastases (as high as 40% of N0 patients in the central neck). Despite the presence of metastases, few patients progress to have clinically meaningful disease and the role of elective nodal surgery is in question. Distant metastases are uncommon in PTC.

Recently, increasing interest has focused on 'papillary microcarcinoma'. This term is used to describe PTC that is <10 mm in size. These lesions are common (detected in about 10% of benign thyroid resections) and not associated with adverse outcomes, including recurrence or non-survival. As such, management and follow-up of patients with these lesions of doubtful clinical significance is controversial. In Korea, for example, national screening has led to a significant increase in these cases. In Japan groups are opting for an observational approach without surgery. These studies have shown that at least two-thirds never progress. In the USA some groups are attempting non-surgical management with ablation techniques using ethanol or radiofrequency. In most of the world, however, groups try to avoid diagnosing these small, insignificant lesions by limiting biopsies to >10 mm lesions and being conservative in the management of lesions following their diagnosis.

Follicular carcinoma

Follicular carcinoma can normally only be differentiated from follicular adenoma by the architecture on histology. For this reason, follicular lesions on FNA are unable to be diagnosed as malignant in the absence of clinical features such as metastases (***Figure 55.24***). Multiple foci of follicular carcinoma are seldom seen and lymph node involvement is much less common than in PTC. Blood-borne metastases are more common and the eventual mortality rate, although still low, is twice that of PTC (***Figure 55.25***).

Hürthle cell tumours are a rare variant of follicular neoplasm in which oxyphil (Hürthle, Askanazy) cells predominate histologically. Hürthle cell cancers are associated with a poor prognosis.

Prognosis in differentiated thyroid carcinoma

The prognosis in differentiated thyroid cancers is generally excellent. In terms of survival, older patients, those with large tumours or those with extrathyroid extension or distant metastases have worse outcomes. A system of risk stratification can

Max Askanazy, 1865–1940, Professor of Pathology, Geneva, Switzerland

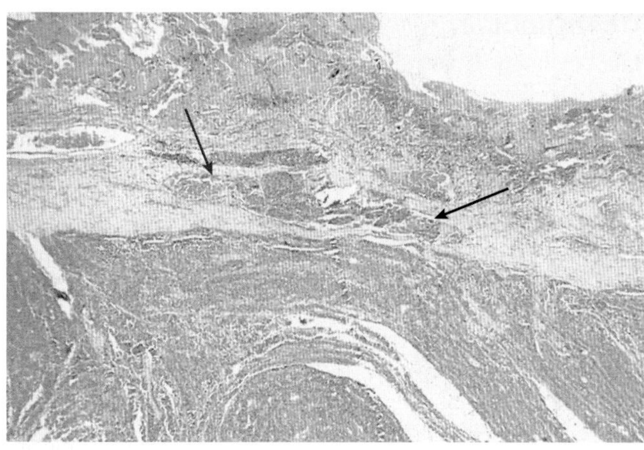

Figure 55.24 Histology of follicular thyroid carcinoma showing vascular (red arrow) and capsular (black arrow) invasion (courtesy of Dr SWB Ewen, Aberdeen, UK).

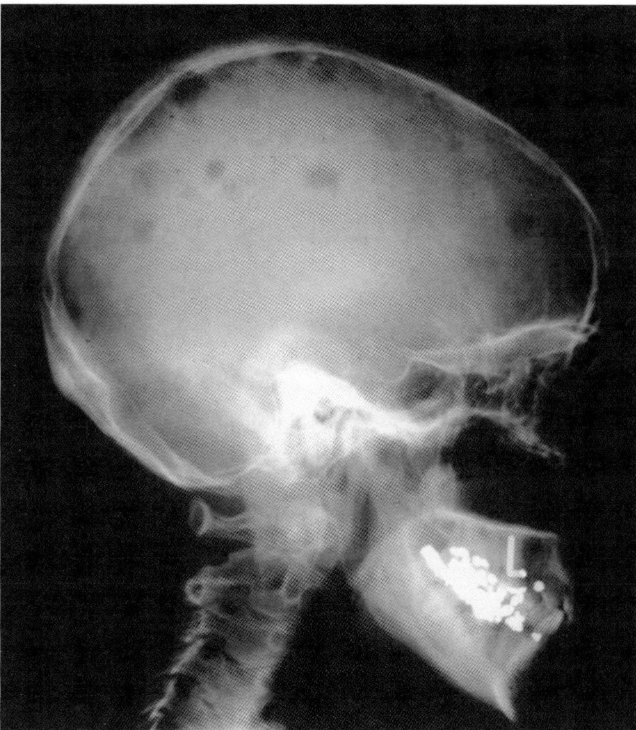

Figure 55.25 Follicular carcinoma of the thyroid with skull secondaries.

be used to predict the risk on an individual basis. In a young patient with a low-risk tumour, the risk of death following appropriate treatment is almost zero. In an older patient with a high-risk tumour (extrathyroid extension or distant metastases), the risk is as high as 55% at 5 years. Older patients with low-risk tumours and younger patients with high-risk tumours are an intermediate-risk group. Nodal metastases deserve special mention. In younger patients they predict for recurrence but not for death. This is because recurrent neck disease in young patients can almost always be successfully salvaged. In contrast, for older patients neck metastases (particularly in the lateral neck) are a marker of distant metastases in some, and therefore carry a negative prognostic implication for both recurrence and death.

The American Joint Committee on Cancer system stages all patients <55 years as stage I unless they have distant metastases, when they are stage II. Older T1N0M0 patients are stage I and T2N0M0 patients are stage II. The presence of nodal disease upstages older patients to stage II, as does T3 disease. All older patients with locally invasive primary disease (T4) or distant metastases are stage IV.

Surgical treatment for differentiated thyroid cancer

This subject has many contentious aspects. For the vast majority of patients, outcome is excellent irrespective of the extent of surgery. The low number of recurrences and deaths has made prospective trials difficult; as such, very few exist.

The aim of surgery is to rid the patient of macroscopic disease, reduce the chance of recurrence and minimise surgical morbidity. Achieving a balance between these aims is critical. In addition, the surgeon must consider whether radioactive iodine is to be recommended. In low-risk cases this is rarely indicated, whereas in high-risk patients it is used almost universally. Risk stratification is therefore critical.

In high-risk patients with nodal or distant metastases, total thyroidectomy will be performed to eradicate disease in the thyroid and prepare the patient for radioactive iodine. For low-risk patients with a single focus of disease limited to the thyroid, a thyroid lobectomy can be offered. This has the significant advantage of protecting the contralateral RLN and parathyroid glands. This approach is now considered appropriate unless there are high-risk features of disease.

In terms of the neck, when metastatic disease is present, a therapeutic compartment-orientated neck dissection should be performed to remove disease from the central or lateral neck, depending on the site of involvement.

The role of elective neck surgery when no disease in the nodes is detected preoperatively is far more controversial. Lateral neck dissection carries significant morbidity and, despite high rates of occult metastases in PTC, has been abandoned. The reason for this is that, even in patients who are thought to have occult metastases, very few progress to clinically meaningful disease. In contrast, the morbidity of central neck dissection is lower, and the compartment has to be opened during a thyroidectomy. In addition, salvage surgery in the central neck carries a high risk to the RLN and parathyroid glands. For these reasons elective central neck dissection has been popular in the last few decades. However, increased recognition that performing such surgery in all patients with PTC leads to high rates of morbidity and the lack of evidence that outcomes improve as a result of more aggressive surgery have led to a move away from this practice. At this point, patients who are considered at highest risk of having occult metastases in the central neck (those with extrathyroid extension, for example) are considered most likely to benefit from elective surgery. It is not recommended routinely in low-risk patients.

Many patients will only be diagnosed with their thyroid cancer following a diagnostic lobectomy. In this setting, risk assessment is again critical. If the patient is considered low risk, further surgery is unlikely to be beneficial and active surveillance should be considered. This approach, pioneered in Japan, has been adopted in a number of centres for PTCs <1 cm as only 30% of patients develop tumour growth that requires intervention. Larger tumours and younger patients are at higher risk and radioactive iodine may be recommended, in which case completion thyroidectomy may be required.

Given the complexity of decision making in thyroid cancer and the different groups involved (surgeons, endocrinologists, radiologists, cytologists, pathologists and nuclear medicine physicians), all cases should be discussed in a multidisciplinary setting.

Thyroxine

Following surgery, thyroid cells (both normal and malignant) can be suppressed using high doses of thyroxine. This was once considered routine for all differentiated thyroid cancers during follow-up. Again, risk stratification has modified the approach to these patients. Following surgery, patients can be considered high or low risk. For those patients at high risk from disease, thyroxine will be prescribed at levels that suppress TSH without making the patient biochemically hyperthyroid. In contrast, low-risk patients may be considered for thyroxine replacement at physiological levels. In this patient group, a balance of benefit (remember these patients have extremely low rates of recurrence or death) versus risk must be made. In particular, long-term TSH suppression can result in cardiac arrhythmia and osteoporosis. As such the multidisciplinary team should consider all risks during follow-up to strike this balance.

Radioiodine

^{131}I can be given to deliver tumoricidal doses of radioactivity directly to thyroid tissue, both benign and malignant. In the setting of thyroid cancer, all normal tissue should be removed (total thyroidectomy) along with any gross neck disease (neck dissection) in order for any residual microscopic disease or distant metastases to receive an optimal dose. Radioiodine treatment is not an alternative to surgical resection for resectable disease.

In order to effectively drive the radioiodine into cells, high levels of TSH are required. This can be achieved by rendering the patient hypothyroid (off thyroxine) or by using recombinant TSH, which is injected prior to radioiodine administration.

Following radioiodine administration, an uptake scan is performed. This demonstrates areas of iodine uptake in the whole body and can be used to identify any metastatic disease not recognised on initial imaging. This information is useful for risk stratification following initial therapy.

Outside the setting of primary treatment, radioiodine treatment may be considered in cases of recurrence. Multiple doses can be used to treat unresectable disease or distant metastases.

Most differentiated thyroid cancers will concentrate iodine. However, with advancing patient age and particularly if disease is multiply recurrent the tumour will lose iodine avidity. This is called radioiodine refractory disease. Such cases may be considered for external beam radiotherapy, although this is uncommon.

Thyroglobulin

Thyroglobulin is a tumour marker produced by normal thyroid cells and most differentiated thyroid cancers and offers an extremely accurate method of following patients postoperatively. If a lobectomy has been performed the level will not be undetectable, but trends can be used to monitor for recurrence. Following total thyroidectomy, the aim is to have an undetectable thyroglobulin. Patients who achieve this point are at extremely low risk of recurrence. Serial thyroglobulin measurement (6- to 12-monthly) combined with ultrasonographic assessment of the neck can then be used to monitor patients during follow-up.

If an undetectable level is not achieved, the thyroglobulin can be followed. If it increases, imaging should be performed to look for gross recurrent disease. Resectable disease should be addressed surgically, and normally further radioactive iodine would be indicated. The role of radioactive iodine in a rising thyroglobulin without structural disease is controversial.

Undifferentiated (anaplastic) carcinoma

This is one of the most aggressive malignancies in humans. Thankfully it is rare. It may develop *de novo* or present as dedifferentiation of a papillary or poorly differentiated carcinoma. The disease is characterised by rapid growth, visceral invasion and distant metastases. The surgeon's role in this disease is crucial. Thyroid lymphoma can be incorrectly diagnosed as anaplastic cancer and so biopsy is critical. This can be done using a core or open technique.

Management is controversial because of the extremely poor prognosis. Occasional patients may present with disease limited to the neck, which appears resectable on imaging. Such patients seem to have a slightly better outcome if treated with aggressive surgery and postoperative adjuvant therapy (radiotherapy with/without chemotherapy). However, in the majority, treatment is palliative. Those who develop airway symptoms are generally better managed without tracheostomy, despite the potentially distressing mode of death.

Medullary carcinoma

These are tumours of the parafollicular (C cells) derived from the neural crest that are not unlike those of a carcinoid tumour (***Figure 55.26***). High levels of serum calcitonin and carcinoembryonic antigen are produced. Calcitonin levels fall after resection and rise again with recurrence, making it a valuable tumour marker in the follow-up of patients with this disease. Diarrhoea is a feature in 30% of cases and this may be due to 5-hydroxytryptamine or prostaglandins produced by the tumour cells.

Medullary carcinoma may occur in combination with adrenal phaeochromocytoma and hyperparathyroidism (usually due to hyperplasia) in the syndrome known as multiple endocrine neoplasia type 2A (MEN-2A). The familial form of the disease frequently affects children and young adults, whereas the sporadic cases occur at any age with no sex predominance. When the familial form is associated with prominent mucosal

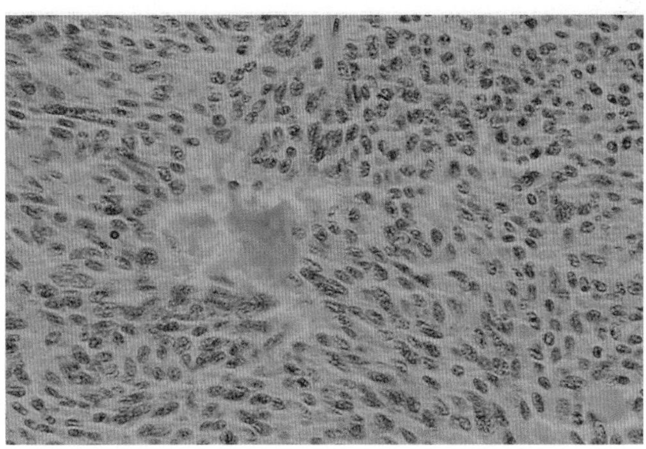

Figure 55.26 Histology of medullary carcinoma showing characteristic 'cell balls' and amyloid (courtesy of Dr SWB Ewen, Aberdeen, UK).

neuromas involving the lips, tongue and inner aspect of the eyelids, with a Marfanoid habitus, the syndrome is referred to as MEN type 2B (see *Chapter 57*).

Involvement of lymph nodes occurs in 55–60% of cases and blood-borne metastases are common. Tumours are not TSH dependent and do not take up radioactive iodine. The prognosis is variable and depends on the stage at diagnosis. Any nodal involvement virtually eliminates the prospect of cure and, unfortunately, even small tumours confined to the thyroid gland may have spread by the time of diagnosis, particularly in familial cancers. In common with many endocrine tumours the progression of disease may be very slow, with a characteristically indolent course and long survival, even in the absence of cure.

In familial cases of medullary thyroid cancer, genetic screening of relatives should be recommended and the information used to make recommendations concerning prophylactic thyroidectomy. Some relatives may be monitored into adulthood with serial calcitonin monitoring. In contrast, the highest risk mutations are associated with early-onset disease and total thyroidectomy is recommended during infancy.

Treatment

When medullary carcinoma is diagnosed, staging of the neck and chest should be performed. For patients with disease confined to the thyroid, total thyroidectomy is recommended to remove all C cells with elective dissection of the central neck nodes. If there is evidence of nodal metastases, gross disease should be excised but the surgeon should be mindful of morbidity. Such patients are highly likely to develop recurrent disease, hence a pragmatic approach should be adopted (see *Chapter 56*).

Malignant lymphoma

In the past, many malignant lymphomas were diagnosed as small round-cell anaplastic carcinomas. Response to irradiation is dramatic (*Figure 55.27*) and radical surgery is unnecessary once the diagnosis is established by biopsy. In patients with tracheal compression, isthmusectomy is the most appropriate form of biopsy, although the response to therapy is so rapid that this should rarely be necessary unless there has been difficulty in making a histological diagnosis. The prognosis is good, particularly if there is no involvement of cervical lymph nodes. Rarely, the tumour is part of widespread malignant lymphoma disease and the prognosis in these cases is worse. Most lymphomas occur against a background of lymphocytic thyroiditis.

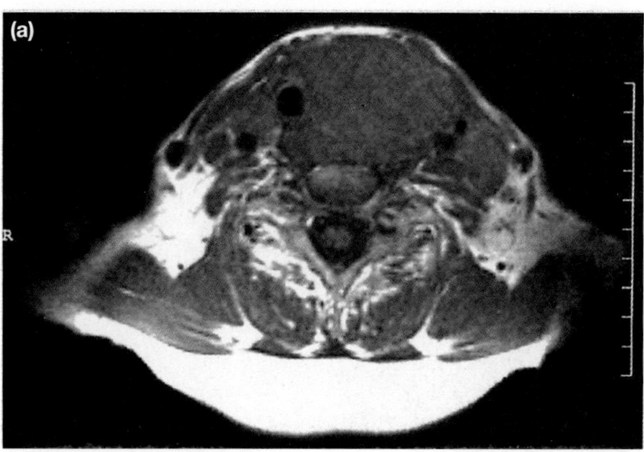

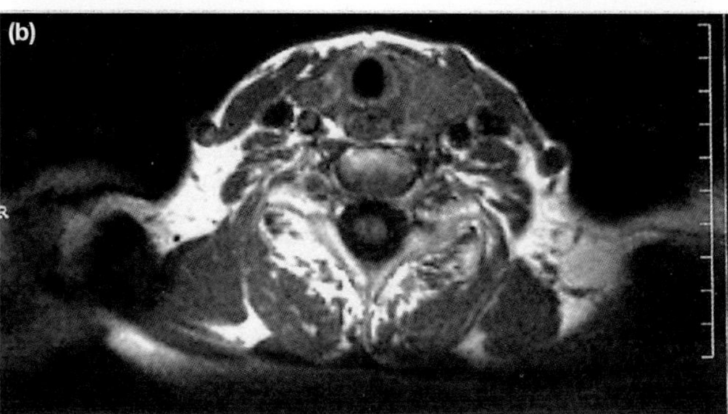

Figure 55.27 Magnetic resonance imaging scans of extensive malignant lymphoma (a) before and (b) after 7 days of external beam radiotherapy (courtesy of Dr FW Smith, Aberdeen, UK).

THYROIDITIS

Chronic lymphocytic (autoimmune) thyroiditis (Hashimoto's disease)

This common condition is usually associated with raised titres of thyroid antibodies. It commonly presents as a goitre, which may be diffuse or nodular with a characteristic 'bosselated' feel or with established or subclinical thyroid failure. The diagnosis often follows investigation of a discrete swelling. Features of chronic lymphocytic (focal) thyroiditis are commonly present on histological examination in association with other thyroid disease, notably toxic goitre (*Figure 55.28*). Primary

Antoine Marfan, 1858–1942, paediatrician, University of Paris, France.
Bosselated: covered in multiple bosses (small protuberences).

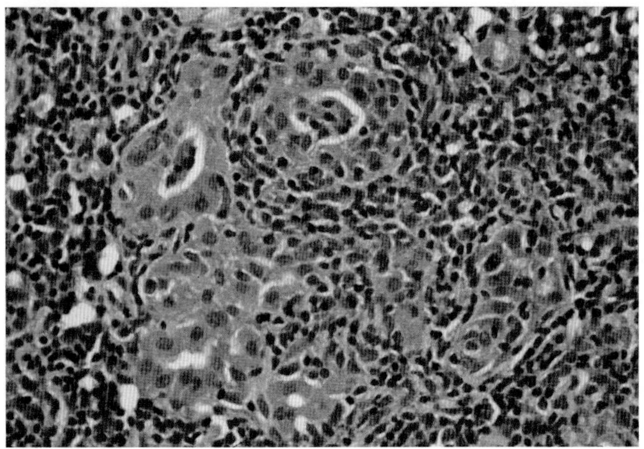

Figure 55.28 Autoimmune thyroiditis (Hashimoto's disease; struma lymphomatosa). Intense lymphocytic–plasma cell infiltration, acinar destruction and fibrosis.

myxoedema without detectable thyroid enlargement represents the end stage of the pathological process.

Granulomatous thyroiditis (subacute thyroiditis, de Quervain's thyroiditis)

This may follow a viral infection. In a typical subacute presentation, there is pain in the neck, fever, malaise and a firm, irregular enlargement of one or both thyroid lobes. There are raised inflammatory markers, absent thyroid antibodies, the serum T_4 is high normal or slightly raised and the ^{123}I uptake of the gland is low. The condition is self-limiting and, in a few months, the goitre subsides and there may be a period of months of hypothyroidism before eventual recovery.

In 10% of cases the onset is acute, the goitre is very painful and tender and there may be symptoms of hyperthyroidism. One-third of cases are asymptomatic but for the presence of the goitre. If diagnosis is in doubt, it may be confirmed by FNAC, radioactive iodine uptake and a rapid symptomatic response to prednisone. The specific treatment for the acute patient with severe pain is to give prednisone 10–20 mg daily for 7 days and the dose is then gradually reduced over the next month. If thyroid failure is prominent, treatment with thyroxine may be required until function recovers.

Riedel's thyroiditis

This is very rare, accounting for 0.5% of goitres. Thyroid tissue is replaced by cellular fibrous tissue, which infiltrates through the capsule into muscles and adjacent structures, including parathyroids, recurrent nerves and the carotid sheath. It may occur in association with retroperitoneal and mediastinal fibrosis and is most probably a collagen disease. The goitre may be unilateral or bilateral and is very hard and fixed. The differential diagnosis from anaplastic carcinoma can be made with certainty only by biopsy, when a wedge of the isthmus should also be removed to free the trachea. If unilateral, the other lobe is usually involved later and subsequent hypothyroidism is common. Treatment is with high-dose steroids, tamoxifen and thyroxine replacement. Reduction in the size of the goitre and long-term improvement in symptoms are to be expected if treatment is commenced early.

FURTHER READING

Bible KC, Kebebew E, Brierly J *et al.* 2021 American Thyroid Association guidelines for management of patients with anaplastic thyroid cancer. *Thyroid* 2021; **31**: 337–86.

Chadwick D, Kinsman R, Walton P. *The British Association of Endocrine and Thyroid Surgeons fifth national audit report.* Henley-on-Thames: Dendrite Clinical Systems Ltd, 2017.

Chen A, Bernet V, Carty SE *et al.* American Thyroid Association statement on optimal surgical management of goiter. *Thyroid* 2014; **24**: 181–9.

Gharib H, Papini E, Valcavi R *et al.* American Association of Clinical Endocrinologists and Associazione Medici Endocrinologi medical guidelines for clinical practice for the diagnosis and management of thyroid nodules. *Endocr Pract* 2006; **12**: 63–102.

Haugen BRM, Alexander EK, Bible KC *et al.* American Thyroid Association management guidelines for adult patients with thyroid nodules and differentiated thyroid cancer. *Thyroid* 2016; **26**: 1–133.

Perros P, Boelaert K, Colley S *et al.* Guidelines for the management of thyroid cancer. *Clin Endocrinol* 2014; **81**(Suppl 1): 1–122.

Wells Jr SA, Asa SL, Dralle H *et al.* Revised American Thyroid Association guidelines for the management of medullary thyroid carcinoma. *Thyroid* 2015; **25**: 567–610.

Yeh MW, Bauer AJ, Bernet VA *et al.* American Thyroid Association statement on preoperative imaging for thyroid cancer surgery. *Thyroid* 2015; **25**: 3–14.

CHAPTER 56 The parathyroid glands

Learning objectives

To understand:

- The anatomy of the parathyroid glands
- The physiology of calcium regulation
- The underlying causes of hypercalcaemia and appropriate emergency management
- The aetiology, presentation, investigation and management of primary hyperparathyroidism and associated special cases
- The aetiology, presentation, investigation and management of secondary and tertiary hyperparathyroidism
- The aetiology and management of parathyroid carcinoma

INTRODUCTION

The parathyroid glands were first described by Sir Richard Owen in a neck dissection of an Indian rhinoceros at the London Zoological Gardens in 1850. Credit for recognition of the 'glandulae parathyreoidae' goes, however, to Sandström, who published a monograph in 1887 on dissection of the parathyroid glands and their blood supply in animals and human cadavers. Unfortunately, Sandström committed suicide at the age of 37 and it was not until the 1890s that his work was rediscovered by Gley, who associated tetany following thyroid surgery with removal of the parathyroid glands. In 1905, MacCallum found that he could relieve postoperative tetany by the injection of parathyroid extract. While the association between parathyroid enlargement and bone disease was reported in 1907, it was not until 1925 that the first parathyroidectomy was performed by Mandl in Vienna on Albert Gahne, a tram conductor with severe primary hyperparathyroidism (PHPT) and osteitis fibrosa cystica.

ANATOMY OF THE PARATHYROID GLANDS

The developmental embryology and surgical anatomy of the parathyroid glands are intimately linked, and knowledge of both is essential for successful surgical treatment of parathyroid disease.

The parathyroid glands, of which there are four, develop from the third and fourth pharyngeal pouches between the fifth and 12th weeks of gestation. They are typically described as 'Portland brick' (yellow/brown) in colour and weigh approximately 30 mg. Approximately 13% of the population have abnormal parathyroid tissue, with 5% having a true supernumerary gland. The blood supply of both the superior and inferior parathyroid glands arises from the inferior thyroidal artery. While the location of the individual glands may vary significantly, there appears to be a degree of symmetry between opposite sides that can be helpful during surgical dissection.

The inferior parathyroid gland and the thymus arise from the third pharyngeal pouch. As a result of the longer normal embryological descent, there is correspondingly more variation in their anatomical position. However, in more than 50% of cases they are located at the inferior pole of the thyroid gland, on the anterior, lateral or posterior surface. The gland itself is freely mobile within a globule of fat adjacent to the lower pole (*Figure 56.1a*).

The superior parathyroid glands arise from the dorsal portion of the fourth pharyngeal pouch. As a result of their more limited embryological descent they are more constant in position. In more than 80% of patients, the superior parathyroid glands are located at the posterior aspect of the thyroid lobe in an area 2 cm in diameter, centred 1 cm around the junction of the inferior thyroid artery and the recurrent laryngeal nerve in strict proximity to the cricothyroid junction (*Figure 56.1b*). The parathyroid glands are closely associated with, but contained within, a halo of fat that is freely mobile over the thyroid capsule.

Sir Richard Owen, 1804–1892, English comparative anatomist and palaeontologist. First director of the Natural History Museum, London, UK, and Hunterian Professor at the Royal College of Surgeons of England.
Ivar Viktor Sandström, 1852–1889, medical student, Uppsala, Sweden.
Marcel Eugene Gley, 1857–1930, French pathologist.
William J MacCallum, 1874–1944, Professor of Pathology, Johns Hopkins Hospital, Baltimore, MD, USA.
Felix Mandl, 1892–1957, Professor of Surgery, Vienna, Austria.

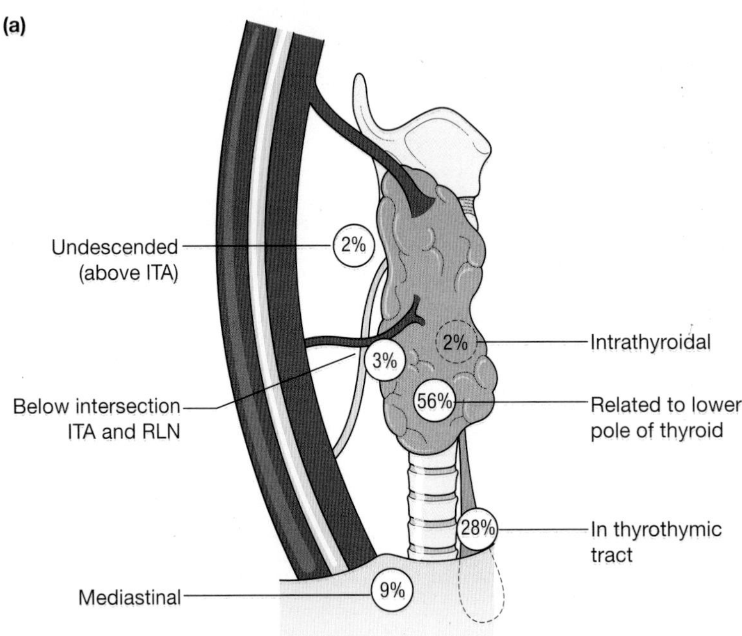

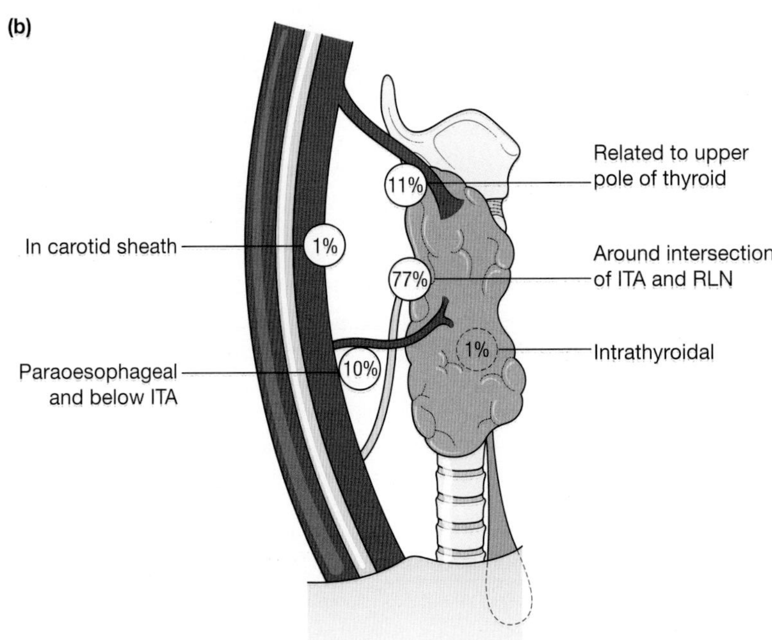

Figure 56.1 Potential locations of the inferior (a) and superior (b) parathyroid glands. ITA, inferior thyroid artery; RLN, recurrent laryngeal nerve.

CALCIUM AND PARATHYROID HORMONE REGULATION

The parathyroid glands play a central role in the regulation of serum calcium levels through the production of the active 84-amino-acid peptide, parathyroid hormone (PTH). PTH is secreted in response to low serum calcium or high serum magnesium levels. It is initially cleaved in the liver, yielding an inactive C-terminal that is cleared by the kidneys. The N-terminal fragment is responsible for the biological activity of PTH on peripheral tissues. The active circulating molecule has a half-life of approximately 3–5 minutes in patients with normal renal function.

PTH acts directly on the kidneys, bone and the gastrointestinal tract to activate intracellular second messengers, including cyclic AMP and calcium. In the kidneys, PTH increases serum calcium levels by increasing resorption of calcium from the renal tubules and increasing the hydroxylation of 25-hydroxyvitamin D to the biologically active 1,25-dihydroxyvitamin D. Active vitamin D increases both the resorption of phosphorus in the kidneys and the absorption of calcium from the gastrointestinal tract. In bone, PTH acts on osteoblasts and osteoclasts to increase bone turnover, thereby increasing the amount of calcium in the extracellular space (*Figure 56.2*).

Calcitonin, which is synthesised by the parafollicular C cells of the thyroid gland, acts as the physiological antagonist to PTH. Calcitonin decreases serum calcium by decreasing bone turnover.

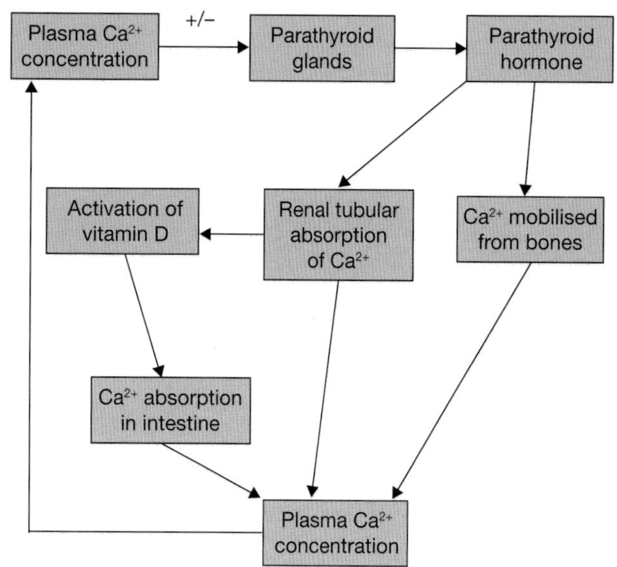

Figure 56.2 The actions of parathyroid hormone.

PRIMARY HYPERPARATHYROIDISM

The early descriptions of patients with PHPT were dominated by those with osteitis fibrosa cystica. Brown tumours of the long bones and associated subperiosteal bone reabsorption, distal tapering of the clavicles and the classical 'salt and pepper' erosions of the skull were typical findings. Over 80% of patients had associated renal stones, significant neuromuscular dysfunction and muscle weakness. This led to the traditional mnemonic that patients with PHPT presented with 'bones, stones, abdominal groans and psychiatric overtones'. The introduction of the automated serum chemical autoanalyser in the 1970s as well as the radioimmune assay to accurately measure circulating PTH levels radically improved early diagnosis of PHPT, such that the majority of patients are now identified incidentally on routine biochemical investigations and are asymptomatic. The current controversies, therefore, centre on the indications for intervention, either surgically or medically.

Presentation

PHPT is defined as hypercalcaemia in the presence of an unsuppressed and therefore relatively, or absolutely, elevated PTH level. Prevalence of the disease is reported to be 0.2–0.5%, with approximately 100 000 new cases per year in the USA. The majority of PHPT is sporadic in nature. Familial disease can occur in multiple endocrine neoplasia (MEN) type 1 or type 2A or as a familial cluster. Patients usually present in the fifth or sixth decades and there is a female predominance with a ratio of 3:1.

Patients are typically identified incidentally with an elevated total calcium or following routine assessment of bone densitometry (DEXA scan). Most patients will, however, have some vague constitutional symptoms, such as fatigue, muscle weakness, depression or some mild memory impairment on questioning. The presence of kidney stones remains the most common clinical manifestation of symptomatic PHPT. Between 15% and 20% of patients will have nephrolithiasis and over 40% of patients will have hypercalciuria. Increasingly, postmenopausal women present with significant osteopenia or osteoporosis in the distal one-third of the radius with a minimal reduction in the lumbar spine, which prompts further investigation. This distribution arises as PTH appears to be catabolic at cortical sites (distal one-third of the radius) and anabolic at cancellous sites (lumbar spine).

PHPT may present with pancreatitis, although it is rarely seen in patients with milder forms of the disease. Common epidemiologically linked disorders, such as hypertension and peptic ulcer disease, are often encountered. Clinical examination is usually normal. Band keratopathy, pathognomonic of the disease and due to deposition of calcium phosphate crystals in the cornea, is now rarely identified.

The differential diagnosis of PHPT includes other causes of hypercalcaemia, which are usually readily distinguishable (*Table 56.1*). It is important to exclude the presence of a widespread malignancy, in which patients will typically have other symptoms. The exception to this rule is multiple myeloma, in which hypercalcaemia can be the presenting

TABLE 56.1 Causes of hypercalcaemia.

Endocrine	• Primary hyperparathyroidism • Thyrotoxicosis • Phaeochromocytoma
Renal failure	• Secondary hyperparathyroidism • Tertiary hyperparathyroidism
Malignant disease	• Skeletal metastatic disease • Multiple myeloma, lymphoma, leukaemia • Solid tumours (PTH-related peptide mediated): lung, renal, squamous cell carcinoma of the head and neck, oesophagus, genital tract
Nutritional	• Excessive vitamin D ingestion • Vitamin A intoxication • Milk-alkali syndrome • Aluminium intoxication
Granulomatous	• Sarcoidosis • Tuberculosis
Inherited disease	• Hypercalciuric hypercalcaemia
Immobilisation	
Paget's disease	
Drug related	• Lithium

PTH, parathyroid hormone.

Sir James Paget, 1814–1899, surgical pathologist, Royal College of Surgeons of England.

complaint. Improvements in the immunoradiometric and immunochemiluminometric assays for PTH can help to distinguish these conditions, as in malignancy PTH levels are typically suppressed.

Hypercalcaemic crisis: presentation and management

Hypercalcaemia is documented in 0.5% of the general population and in up to 5% of hospitalised patients. The vast majority are asymptomatic with a mild to moderate elevation of serum calcium (<3 mmol/L and 3–3.5 mmol/L, respectively) and respond to treatment of the underlying aetiology with associated dietary modification. A small proportion of patients will present symptomatically with a total calcium of >3.5 mmol/L. This is referred to as a hypercalcaemic crisis and requires aggressive medical management.

Although symptoms can be varied, the typical presentation is of acute confusion, abdominal pain, vomiting, dehydration and anuria. Prolongation of the PR interval with a shortened QT interval can be identified on an electrocardiogram (ECG) prior to potentially lethal cardiac arrhythmias. Where the calcium is >4.5 mmol/L, coma and cardiac arrest can occur.

Treatment revolves around increasing renal excretion of calcium, reducing skeletal release of calcium and treatment of the underlying cause. Aggressive rehydration plays a pivotal role. Typically, 200–500 mL/h of normal saline is given to maintain a urine output >100 mL/h, with the caveat that this may be modified to account for associated patient comorbidities. Once intravascular volume has been adequately restored, loop diuretics, such as furosemide, can be used to enhance the renal excretion of calcium. The majority of patients will have normalisation of their calcium with these simple measures.

In patients with advanced malignancy and a serum calcium level >3 mmol/L, agents that blunt the release of calcium from skeletal stores may be required. First-line treatment includes administration of bisphosphonates. These are pyrophosphate analogues that inhibit osteoclast activity in areas of high bone turnover. In the acute setting, these are given intravenously owing to poor absorption in the gastrointestinal tract. Calcitonin can be used to both decrease osteoclastic activity and increase renal excretion of calcium. It has a short duration of action and is usually used as a bridge to reduce calcium until the sustained action of the bisphosphonates is seen. Finally, glucocorticoids (prednisolone) can be used to enhance the action of calcitonin. They increase calciuresis and decrease intestinal absorption of calcium. As a result, they may also play a role in diseases associated with vitamin D excess.

Pathology

The underlying aetiology of PHPT is usually a solitary parathyroid adenoma; however, in a small number of patients (2–4%) there are double adenomas. It may occur in a sporadic fashion or it can be familial (approximately 10%) (MEN type 1, type 4, type 2A or hyperparathyroidism–jaw tumour syndrome [HPT-JT]) in nature.

The only known risk factor for the development of PHPT is a history of prior neck irradiation. The underlying genetic pathogenesis of PHPT remains unclear. However, genes regulating the cell cycle, such as *MEN1* and *CCND1*, have been recognised as playing an important role owing to the clonal nature of adenomas. Somatic mutations in *MEN1*, which encodes menin, occur in 12–35% of sporadic cases and rearrangements or overexpression of *CCND1*, which encodes cyclin D1, have been demonstrated in 20–40% of patients. Upregulation of cyclin D may lead to a clonal proliferation within the parathyroid glands. This does not alter the set point of calcium but the hyperplasic nature of the parathyroid cells themselves causes excessive secretion of PTH.

Multigland disease is less common, occurring in approximately 15% of patients. No clinical features differentiate single from multigland disease, although multigland disease is more commonly associated with familial syndromes such as MEN types 1 and 2A, as well as the chronic ingestion of lithium.

Diagnosis

PHPT is a biochemical diagnosis. Only when the disease has been confirmed biochemically should localisation studies be undertaken. Positive imaging does not confirm the diagnosis and negative findings cannot rule it out.

PHPT is defined as an elevated total, or more specifically ionised, calcium in the presence of an inappropriately elevated or unsuppressed PTH. It is associated with a low serum phosphate in the setting of normal creatinine and vitamin D levels; 24-hour urinary excretion of calcium may be normal or elevated. It is important to perform a 24-hour urinary collection to rule out the presence of the rare familial hypocalciuric hypercalcaemia (FHH). Alkaline phosphatase may be elevated in patients in whom there is concomitant bone disease. This is important to recognise preoperatively as the surgeon should anticipate significant postoperative hypocalcaemia due to the development of hungry bone syndrome.

Localisation studies

> In my opinion, the only localising study required in a patient with untreated primary hyperparathyroidism is to localise an experienced parathyroid surgeon.
>
> John Doppman, 1986

Historically, preoperative localisation studies for PHPT were considered less important than identifying an experienced surgeon. However, with a shift away from the traditional four-gland (cervical neck) exploration to more minimally invasive procedures, accurate preoperative identification is critically important to guide surgical strategy.

There are a variety of both non-invasive and invasive studies commonly in use. Non-invasive radiology includes nuclear medicine-based studies, ultrasonography and four-dimensional (4D) computed tomography (CT) scanning. Invasive imaging is largely reserved for reoperative surgery and includes ultrasound or CT-guided fine-needle aspiration with

John L Doppman, 1928–2000, radiologist, National Institutes of Health, USA, developed the technique of selective venous sampling for parathyroid localisation.

concomitant PTH assays, parathyroid angiography or selective venous sampling for the PTH gradient.

Nuclear medicine-based studies (sestamibi scanning)

The use of sestamibi (2-methoxy-2-methylpropylisonitrile [MIBI]) for parathyroid localisation was first described in 1989 and is now regarded as the most accurate and reliable method for imaging the parathyroid glands. It is safe and reproducible and, while it has a sensitivity and specificity similar to ultrasonography, it may image glands in ectopic positions better (*Figure 56.3a*).

Sestamibi accumulates in mitochondria and therefore washes out at differential rates depending on the number of mitochondria within individual tissues. Parathyroid adenomas often have a high concentration of oxyphilic cells with high mitochondrial content. These retain tracer, and adenomas are therefore associated with a slow washout when compared with the thyroid gland. There are three different protocols for sestamibi scanning: single-isotope dual-phase scan, dual-isotope subtraction imaging and single-photon emission computed tomography (SPECT). The sensitivity and specificity of sestamibi, regardless of the protocol used, are 79% and 90%, respectively. False positives are rare but may arise from some solid thyroid nodules, such as Hürthle cell nodules, that are associated with high oxyphilic content. These can be reduced by the addition of a thyroid-specific radioactive tracer, such as ^{99}Tc-pertechnetate and subsequent subtraction images.

Ultrasonography

Ultrasonography is a non-invasive, inexpensive method of imaging the parathyroid glands (*Figure 56.3b*). Parathyroid adenomas are typically oval or elongated, bi- or multilobed hypoechoic structures. Rarely, adenomas may be cystic or heterogeneous in nature. Giant adenomas are described as those over 3 cm in size. Ultrasonography is not associated with any radiation exposure and has the advantage of being able to identify and facilitate biopsy of any concomitant thyroid pathology. However, ultrasonography is operator, lesion size and location dependent. Critically, ultrasonography may

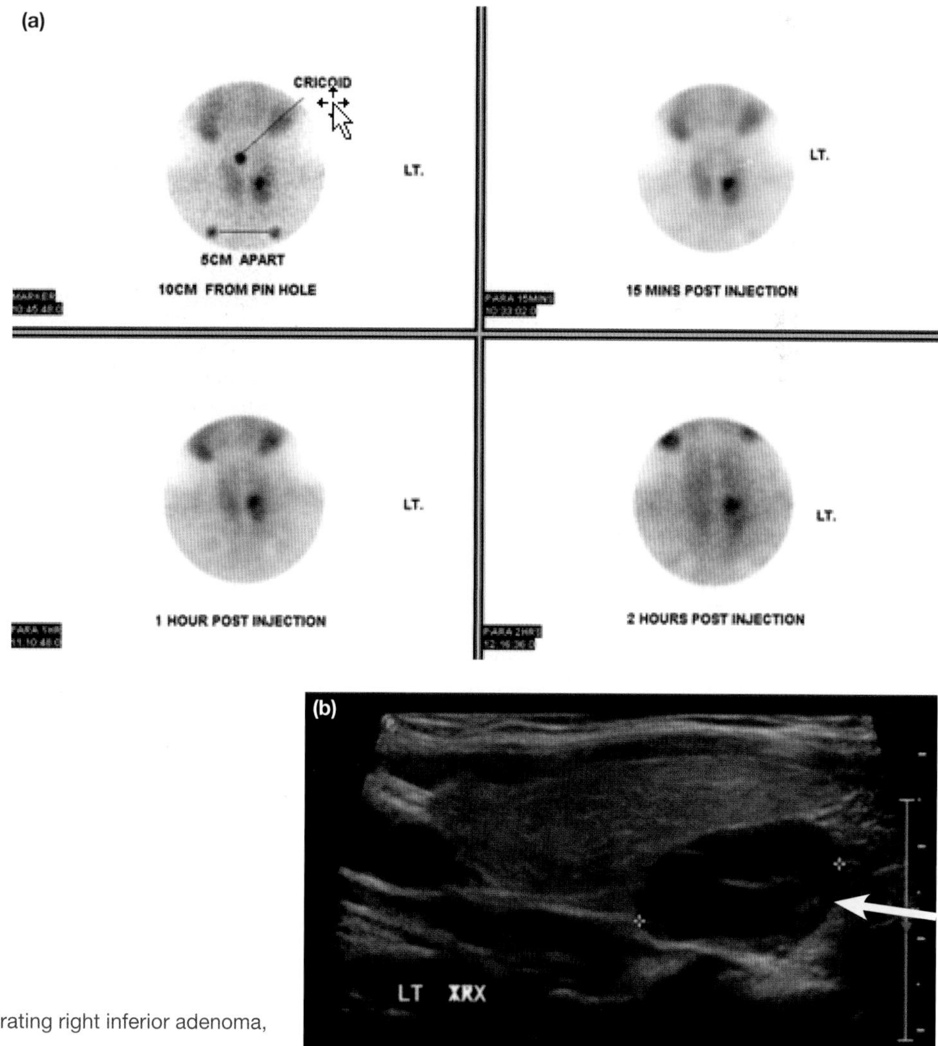

Figure 56.3 Sestamibi scan (a) demonstrating right inferior adenoma, with concordant ultrasonography (b).

Karl Hürthle, 1866–1945, histopathologist, Breslau, Germany (now Wrocław, Poland).

miss adenomas located in retro-oesophageal, retrosternal or retrotracheal areas. It can also be difficult to differentiate between a small parathyroid gland and a normal-appearing lymph node. A meta-analysis of preoperative localisation techniques in PHPT demonstrated that ultrasonography and sestamibi-SPECT have comparable accuracy, with pooled sensitivities of 76.1% and 78.9%, respectively, and positive predictive values (PPVs) of 93.2% and 90.7%, respectively (Krakauer *et al.*, 2016).

Four-dimensional computed tomography scanning/positron emission tomography-computed tomography

Multiphase CT imaging (4D-CT) has become widely utilised to localise disease (***Figure 56.4***). It gives both anatomical and functional information about the parathyroid glands. Using precontrast, postcontrast and delayed images, it demonstrates not only detailed anatomical localisation but, combined with rapid uptake and washout, allows hyperfunctioning glands to be differentiated from lymph nodes that demonstrate a progressive enhancement pattern. The potential disadvantage of 4D-CT scanning is the higher radiation dose when compared with traditional imaging modalities. Modification of the protocol now allows fewer phases to be obtained without compromising outcomes. The initial study in 2006 reported a sensitivity of 88% for lateralisation and 70% for localisation of parathyroid adenomas (Rodgers *et al.*, 2006). A more recent meta-analysis, although limited by the small number of studies, demonstrated a sensitivity and PPV of 89.4% and 93.5%, respectively, when 4D-CT was used as the primary imaging modality. This was reduced to 71.8% and 74.9%, respectively, in cases of negative or inconclusive prior imaging (Cheung *et al.*, 2012).

Positron emission tomography (PET) scanning remains expensive and is not widely available. However, recent data suggest that there may be an incremental value to ^{18}F-fluorocholine PET with the addition of CT scanning for localisation of ectopic adenomas.

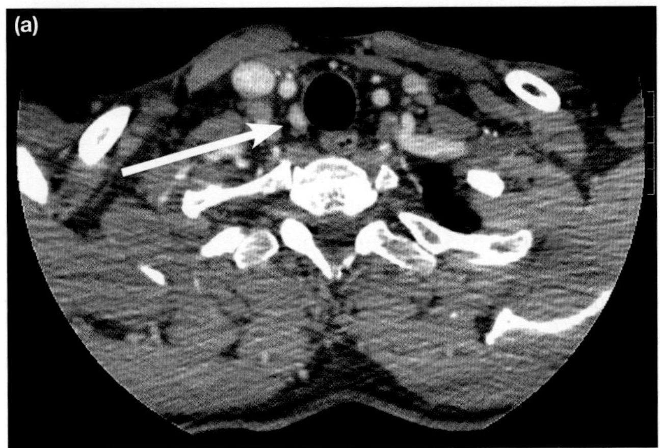

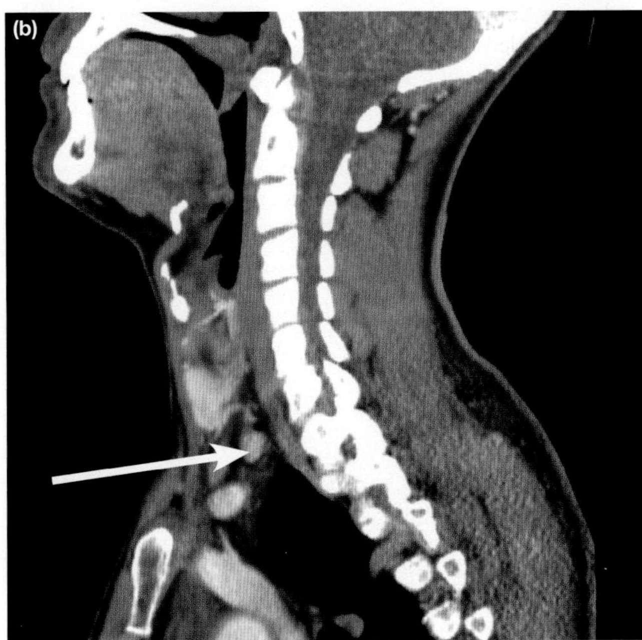

Figure 56.4 (a, b) Four-dimensional computed tomography scanning demonstrating a right inferior parathyroid adenoma (arrows).

Magnetic resonance imaging

Magnetic resonance imaging (MRI) is not commonly used to image the parathyroid glands. However, on T2-weighted images, enlarged parathyroid glands demonstrate significantly increased intensity. In reoperative cases or where the adenoma is located in the mediastinum, MRI may be beneficial, with higher reported sensitivities (50–88%). While the sensitivity of MRI is slightly better than that for CT (64–88%) in primary disease, it has significant limitations. It is expensive, patients can be poorly compliant owing to claustrophobia and the resolution for normal glands or adenomas <5 mm is poor. Similarly, it can be difficult to localise superior glands because of their posterior location, which allows them to be obscured by the thyroid gland.

Parathyroid angiography and venous sampling for parathyroid hormone

Parathyroid angiography is reserved for reoperative cases and is now rarely required owing to improvements in non-invasive imaging modalities. It involves examination of both thyrocervical trunks, both internal mammary arteries and both carotids, with occasional selective superior thyroid artery catheterisation. Vascular parathyroid adenomas appear as a persistent oval or round 'stain' on angiography. Serious complications such as contrast-induced renal failure, embolisation and neurological damage have limited its utility.

Selective venous sampling for PTH can allow accurate localisation of adenomas but an experienced interventional radiologist is vital for success. The venous drainage of the lesion is established when there is a twofold drop in the PTH between the sampled blood and the serum PTH. The sensitivity is reported to be 80% and is equally effective in localising cervical and mediastinal adenomas. However, the false-positive rate of between 6% and 18% limits its utility to reoperative cases.

Management strategies

Surgical management

The mainstay of treatment for PHPT is surgery, addressing the underlying aetiology and allowing not only resolution of biochemical abnormalities but also sustained improvements in end-organ damage. Traditionally a bilateral cervical exploration was performed with reported cure rates of 95–98%. With improvements in preoperative radiological localisation, a more minimally invasive approach has been developed and widely adopted (*Figure 56.5*).

All symptomatic patients should be offered surgery. An expert panel published recommendations on which asymptomatic patients should be considered for surgical intervention (*Table 56.2*). Guidelines from the American Association of Endocrine Surgeons have more liberal indications for surgery. These included patients with cognitive or psychiatric symptoms attributable to PHPT, cardiovascular disease (excluding hypertension) and more non-specific symptoms, such as muscle weakness, impaired functional capacity and abnormal sleep patterns. When criteria have been met and where a single adenoma has been confidently identified by radiological means, a minimally invasive parathyroidectomy may be offered. Conversely, where there is discordant imaging or where imaging fails to identify any parathyroid abnormalities, then a bilateral neck exploration and a three-and-a-half-gland parathyroidectomy or a four-gland parathyroidectomy and autotransplantation should be performed.

Consent for a parathyroidectomy must include the possibility of recurrent laryngeal nerve damage (risk <1%), permanent hypoparathyroidism (requiring lifelong calcium and vitamin D supplementation; risk 0.5%) and persistent (5%) or recurrent hyperparathyroidism. Persistent disease is defined as an elevated serum calcium within 6 weeks of surgical intervention and recurrent disease is defined as an increase in calcium levels after 6 months but with an intervening period of normocalcaemia.

TABLE 56.2 Consensus guidelines for surgical intervention in asymptomatic primary hyperparathyroidism.

Measurement of serum calcium	0.25 mmol/L (1.0 mg/dL) above the upper limit of normal
Skeletal	• BMD by DEXA; T score –2.5 at lumbar spine, total hip, femoral neck or distal one-third of radius • Vertebral fracture
Renal	• Creatinine clearance <60 mL/min • 24-hour urinary calcium >10 mmol/dL (>400 mL/day) or increased risk of stone formation by risk analysis
Age	<50 years

BMD, bone mineral density; DEXA, bone densitometry.
Adapted from Bilezikian *et al*. (2014).

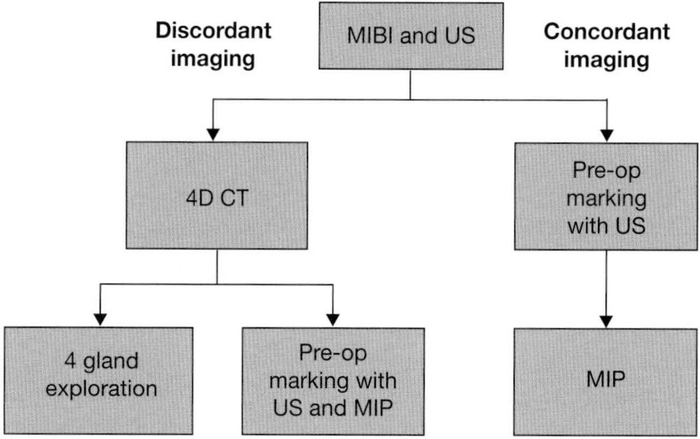

Figure 56.5 Localisation paradigm and management strategies. 4D CT, four-dimensional computed tomography; MIBI, 2-methoxy-2-methylpropylisonitrile; MIP, minimally invasive parathyroidectomy; US, ultrasonography.

Minimally invasive (focused) parathyroidectomy

Minimally invasive approaches are based on the principle that over 80% of individuals with PHPT have a single adenoma. Although there is no strict definition of the procedure, it commonly refers to the removal of a localised abnormal parathyroid gland through an incision less than 3 cm in length (*Figure 56.6*). The term encompasses open approaches (central and lateral incisions) and video-assisted and radio-guided parathyroidectomies. A number of randomised studies have shown that the focused approach has similar cure rates to

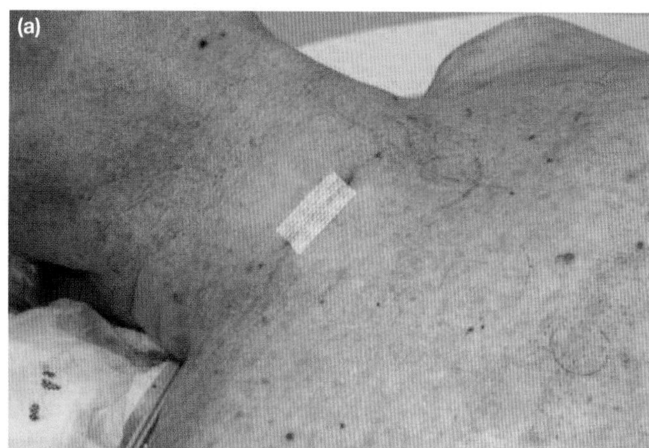

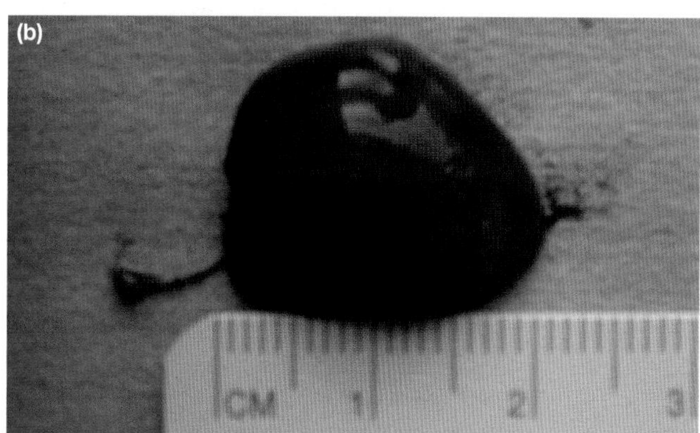

Figure 56.6 **(a)** Minimally invasive parathyroidectomy through a lateral approach; **(b)** the excised parathyroid adenoma.

a cervical exploration but with reduced rates of postoperative hypocalcaemia, shorter operating times, potentially less pain and better cosmesis.

The need to convert from a focused to a cervical exploration may be guided by the use of intraoperative PTH measurements. Routine use is, however, controversial owing to high false-positive and false-negative rates. The basic concept is that the half-life of circulating PTH is 3–5 minutes and there should therefore be a significant drop detected in the plasma PTH following resection of a single adenoma. If no such drop is detected, then multigland disease may be suspected and conversion to a bilateral neck exploration should be considered. The Miami criteria were developed to determine the extent of resection. A drop in the PTH into the normal range and to less than half the maximum preoperative PTH at 10 minutes appears to accurately predict single-gland disease (*Figure 56.7*).

Bilateral neck exploration

A traditional cervical neck exploration is required where imaging is negative or discordant, in MEN (type 1 or type 2A) or in lithium-induced PHPT. A transverse collar (Kocher's) incision is made and the subplatysmal plane developed. The deep cervical fascia is divided between the strap muscles and these are retracted. The thyroid lobes are mobilised and the middle thyroid vein may be divided when present.

Identification of the recurrent laryngeal nerve and the middle thyroid artery allows a starting point for a systematic exploration (see *Chapter 55*). All four glands are identified. Three and a half glands are resected, with half of a vascularised parathyroid left *in situ*. The other half of the gland should be sent for frozen section to confirm the presence of parathyroid tissue (*Figure 56.8*). Ideally the most normal-appearing parathyroid is left *in situ*. With this caveat in mind, where possible an inferior gland should be left. It is marked with a non-absorbable suture to aid identification in the presence of recurrent disease, where resection can be achieved without increasing the risk of damage to the recurrent laryngeal nerve. Alternatively, all four glands can be resected and a forearm autotransplant created. Small pieces of parathyroid are sutured into pockets created in the brachioradialis muscle. Cure rates and rates of persistent and recurrent disease appear to be similar, regardless of the type of procedure used. However, in recurrent disease it can be difficult to identify the location of the recurrent tissue when an autotransplant is performed.

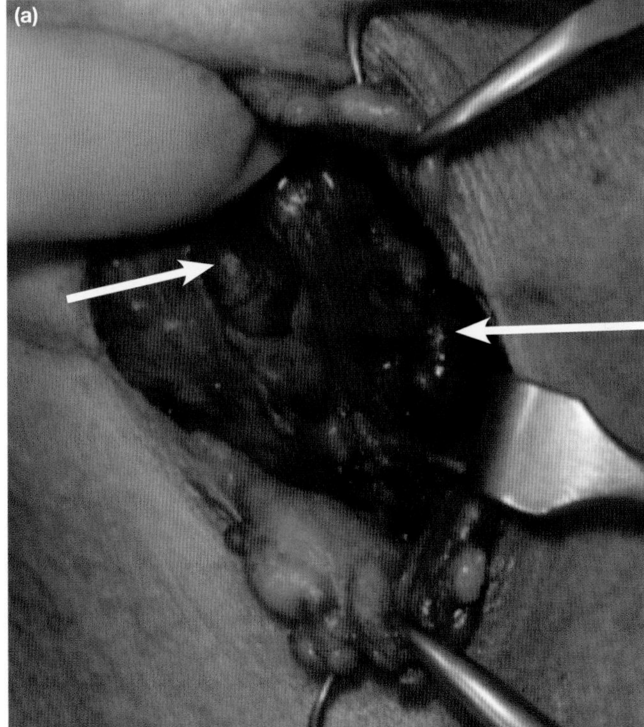

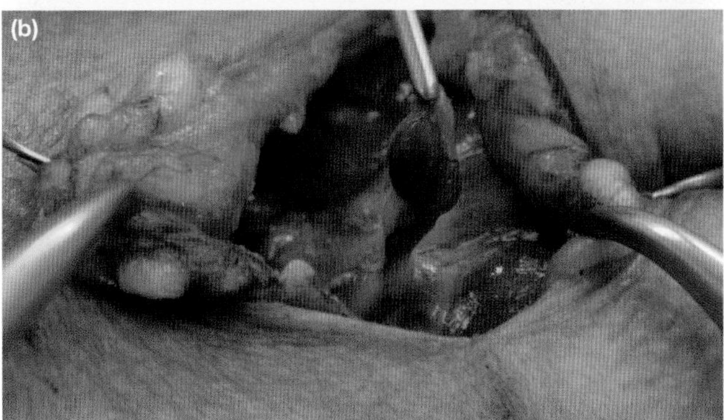

Figure 56.8 Parathyroidectomy with exposure of the left superior and inferior parathyroid glands (white arrows) *in situ* (a) and left superior gland mobilised on its vascular pedicle (b).

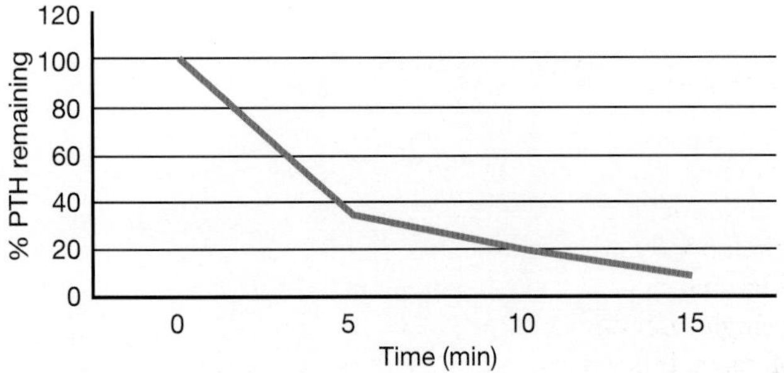

Figure 56.7 Miami criteria for intraoperative parathyroid hormone (PTH) measurement. Drop of PTH into the normal range and less than half the maximum value at 10 minutes postresection.

Thymectomy and resection of mediastinal adenomas

The incidence of clinically significant supernumerary glands is increased in patients with multigland disease or those with hereditary syndromes. A thymectomy should be routinely undertaken for patients with *MEN1*-associated PHPT or in secondary hyperparathyroidism. A cervical thymectomy is performed by dissecting close to the thymic capsule, exploring the cervical part of the gland. The mediastinal part of the gland can be removed by gentle upwards traction, with ligation of the veins draining into the innominate vein. The end of the

Emil Theodor Kocher, 1841–1917, surgeon, Berne, Switzerland, awarded the Nobel Prize in Physiology or Medicine in 1909 for his research on the thyroid.

gland is tapered and rarely requires formal ligation. A median sternotomy is not required where a prophylactic thymectomy is being performed.

Mediastinal adenomas are rare, accounting for less than 1% of all parathyroid adenomas. They will be typically identified on preoperative imaging. Resection can be achieved either by an open sternotomy or increasingly by a thoracoscopic approach. A minimally invasive approach can be particularly effective where the abnormal gland lies immediately deep to the mediastinal pleura. It can confer significant advantages in length of hospital stay and complication rates.

Permanent hypoparathyroidism

Permanent hypoparathyroidism is defined as the continuing need for calcium and/or vitamin D replacement at 1 year postoperatively. It is a rare complication when surgery is undertaken for PHPT (0.5%), but in secondary hyperparathyroidism it can range from 4% to 12%. Symptoms and signs relate to serum calcium levels. Symptoms include mild circumoral or digital numbness and paraesthesia, carpopedal or laryngeal spasms and cardiac arrhythmias. Chvostek's and Trousseau's signs may be elicited. Chvostek's sign refers to contraction of the ipsilateral facial muscles on percussion of the facial nerve below the zygoma. Trousseau's sign refers to the development of carpopedal spasm secondary to occlusion of the arm (usually with a blood pressure cuff).

Biochemical investigations include total and ionised calcium levels as well as serum magnesium levels. An ECG may demonstrate a prolonged QT interval or QRS complex changes. Mild hypocalcaemia can be treated with oral calcium and vitamin D supplementation. Acute symptomatic hypocalcaemia is an emergency and should be corrected with intravenous as well as oral calcium and vitamin D replacement. Traditionally, 10 mL of 10% calcium gluconate is administered slowly intravenously. Supplemental magnesium may also be required, owing to the synergistic action of transporters for calcium and magnesium.

Medical management

Medical management is warranted in patients who are deemed unfit or who have contraindications to surgical intervention, in patients with failed surgical intervention or in the long-term management of parathyroid carcinoma. The aims are to prevent skeletal complications (improve bone mineral density and reduce fracture risk) and to stabilise biochemical parameters. There are only limited data on the long-term efficacy of such an approach as surgery is known to provide durable responses.

Bisphosphonates/denosumab

Bisphosphonates are pyrophosphate analogues that are concentrated in areas of high bone turnover. They inhibit osteoclast activity and apoptosis, thereby increasing bone mineralisation and reducing bone turnover. Studies looking at the management of PHTP utilising bisphosphonates are limited by small numbers and short follow-up. However, use does appear to stabilise bone mineral density without markedly altering the underlying serum biochemistry. Denosumab is a monoclonal antibody that works as a receptor activator of nuclear factor- κB (RANK) ligand inhibitor. Data from the DENOCINA trial suggest that it may be a valid treatment option for patients in whom surgery is undesirable.

Hormone replacement therapy and selective oestrogen receptor antagonists

Hormone replacement therapy (HRT) has been shown to improve bone mineral density and reduce the associated fracture risk in postmenopausal women by reducing bone turnover. Two non-randomised controlled trials have shown a durable and similar response to surgery for PHTP at 4 years, with improvements in bone mineral density but without any improvement in the underlying serum biochemistry. The rationale for the use of selective oestrogen receptor antagonists (SERMs) is that they should confer the benefits of HRT but without the potential adverse vascular and breast effects. The effect on the bone mineral, however, appears to be less significant than that of HRT.

Calcimimetics

The extracellular calcium-sensing receptor on the parathyroid cell surface negatively regulates secretion of PTH. Activation of the receptor decreases secretion of PTH, thereby decreasing bone turnover. Calcimimetics, such as cinacalcet, amplify the sensitivity of the calcium-sensing receptor to extracellular calcium, altering the set point and thereby decreasing PTH production. Cinacalcet was approved for use in PHPT by the European Medicines Agency in 2008 and subsequently by the US Food and Drug Administration in 2011 for the treatment of severe hypercalcaemia in patients with PHPT who were unfit for parathyroidectomy. Normalisation of serum calcium levels can be achieved with a similar reduction in the level of PTH, although not to within the normal range. Despite this, neither the urinary calcium nor the bone mineral density appear to change even after 3 years of treatment. Drug tolerance, especially gastrointestinal side effects, can be problematic and may limit the duration of usage.

SPECIAL CASES

Lithium-induced hyperparathyroidism

Lithium-induced hyperparathyroidism occurs in 10–15% of patients treated with long-term lithium. It is generally associated with a mild elevation in calcium with failure to suppress PTH. The underlying aetiology can be either gland hyperplasia, with lithium originally thought to stimulate all parathyroid tissue, or a single adenoma, which has been shown to occur in 33–49% of cases. It has recently been suggested that the hyperparathyroidism may be caused by interference with the parathyroid kinase C signal transduction system and the Wnt pathway. Biochemical abnormalities may resolve with discontinuation

Frantisek Chvostek, 1835–1884, physician, The Jasefsacademie, Vienna, Austria.
Armand Trousseau, 1801–1867, physician, Hôtel Dieu, Paris, France.

of lithium. Surgery is indicated where ongoing treatment with lithium is required or where abnormalities persist following withdrawal of lithium. Minimally invasive surgery is relatively contraindicated in these patients because of the high incidence of multigland disease. Excision, however, should be limited to those glands that are obviously enlarged at exploration rather than a formal three-and-a-half-gland excision.

Familial syndromes

Familial hyperparathyroidism can be part of a well-recognised endocrine disorder, but it may also occur in isolation in a non-syndromic form. PHPT occurs as a central facet in multiple MEN type 1, type 4, type 2A, HPT-JT, autosomal dominant mild hyperparathyroidism and FHH.

Familial isolated hyperparathyroidism

Familial isolated hyperparathyroidism occurs when patients have PHPT without any other associated endocrinopathies. The underlying genetic abnormality has yet to be fully elucidated, but the syndrome has been linked to known mutations in the *MEN1* gene, the *HRPT2* gene as well as the calcium-sensing receptor gene. A significant proportion of patients will belong to the MEN 1 family, with documented recognised mutations but without expression of other endocrinopathies. Hyperparathyroidism should be treated with a formal bilateral neck exploration and management as per patients with MEN.

MEN type 1-associated hyperparathyroidism

MEN type 1 is a rare autosomal dominant syndrome consisting of tumours of the parathyroids, endocrine pancreas–duodenum and the pituitary (the three Ps). It occurs in approximately 1 per 30 000 individuals. It can also be associated with adrenal adenomas or carcinoma, foregut carcinoids and lipomas. Mutations, of which there are over 1000 identified in different families, occur in the *MEN1* gene, which encodes the protein menin. Menin acts as a tumour suppressor. Patients typically present with young onset (20–30 years of age) of symptomatic hyperparathyroidism and over 95% of patients will have PHPT before the age of 40 years.

Surgical intervention in MEN type 1 aims to obtain and maintain normocalcaemia for the longest time possible. In general, it is associated with the presence of multigland parathyroid disease and as such has mandated a bilateral cervical exploration with at least a subtotal parathyroidectomy and cervical thymectomy. A subtotal parathyroidectomy removes three and a half glands with half of the most normal-appearing parathyroid left *in situ* with a marking stitch to facilitate reoperative intervention. A total parathyroidectomy and forearm autotransplantation is an acceptable alternative. Detailed intraoperative notes, including diagrams, should be kept. Despite meticulous and extensive surgery, the rates of both persistent and recurrent disease remain high in this group of patients (up to 62%) regardless of the type of surgery performed. Unfortunately, the rates of postoperative permanent hypocalcaemia are also high, with published rates up to 47%.

MEN type 4-associated hyperparathyroidism

MEN type 4 is an autosomal dominant syndrome that comprises the same combination of tumours as MEN type 1 but is a rarer cause of hereditary PHPT. It arises as a result of an inactivating pathogenic variant in the cyclin-dependent kinase inhibitor *CDKN1B* gene. It should be managed in the same fashion as MEN type 1.

MEN type 2A-associated hyperparathyroidism

MEN type 2A consists of medullary thyroid carcinoma (MTC), unilateral or bilateral phaeochromocytomas and PHPT. PHPT occurs in approximately 20% of patients and is associated with mutations in codon 634 in the RET proto-oncogene. The majority of patients will be asymptomatic, with a mild elevation in calcium and asymmetrically enlarged parathyroid glands. It is extremely important that the presence of a phaeochromocytoma is excluded prior to surgical intervention. Surgery is usually performed for MTC, with the parathyroid enlargement often being a coincidental intraoperative finding (see *Chapter 55*). In this setting, with extensive surgery for MTC, the primary aim of treatment is to avoid hypoparathyroidism. A conservative stance is adopted with resection of grossly enlarged glands, but with preservation of parathyroid tissue where possible and identification with a marking stitch in the neck.

Hyperparathyroidism-jaw tumour syndrome

HPT-JT is a rare cause of PHPT. It arises as a result of inactivating mutations in the *HRPT2/CDC73* gene on chromosome 1q21–q31, encoding parafibromin. It classically presents with early-onset PHPT (mean age of 32 years), the aetiology of which can be either single- or multigland disease but is predominantly cystic in nature. It presents with severe hypercalcaemia and is associated with an increased risk of an underlying parathyroid carcinoma. Approximately 40% of patients will have the pathognomonic ossifying jaw fibromas of the maxilla or mandible. Other associated abnormalities include renal pathology (hamartomas, polycystic kidney disease and adult Wilms' tumours) and female patients may have uterine malignancies. Surgical intervention involves removal of all enlarged parathyroid glands.

Where there is concern for a parathyroid carcinoma, great care must be taken to avoid tumour spillage. Whether or not an en bloc resection of the enlarged suspicious parathyroid and the adjacent thyroid lobectomy is required remains controversial.

Autosomal dominant mild hyperparathyroidism

This is a rare autosomal dominant syndrome presenting with hypercalcaemia and hypercalciuria. It is associated with a mutation in the calcium-sensing receptor gene. It typically presents in patients who are over 40 years of age and all patients have PHPT. Surgical intervention requires a bilateral neck exploration as it is associated with multigland disease.

Max Wilms, 1867–1918, Professor of Surgery, University of Heidelberg, Germany.

Familial hypocalciuric hypercalcaemia

FHH is not a surgical disease and therefore preoperative diagnosis is imperative for the surgeon. FHH arises as a result of heterozygous mutations in the calcium-sensing receptor gene on chromosome 3. Benign FHH typically presents with mild hypercalcaemia in young (<10 years of age) asymptomatic patients. Patients with FHH have a normal or slightly elevated PTH level, increased serum magnesium levels and hypocalciuria. A low urinary calcium–creatinine clearance ratio is used to discriminate between FHH and mild PHPT. Patients rarely require intervention and surgical intervention is not indicated.

Criteria for genetic testing

In clinical practice, specific criteria can be employed to determine which patients are at the highest risk of hereditary PHPT. The current NHS England National Genomic Test Directory testing criteria from March 2019 for familial hyperparathyroidism state that testing should be considered for patients with PHPT and a creatinine clearance ratio >0.02 who meet **one** of the following criteria:

1. presenting before the age of 35 years **or**
2. presenting before the age of 45 years with **one** of:
   a. proven multigland involvement **or**
   b. hyperplasia on histology **or**
   c. ossifying fibroma(s) of the maxilla or mandible **or**
   d. at least one first-degree relative with unexplained hyperparathyroidism.

The testing criterion for FHH is a creatinine clearance ratio <0.02.

Summary box 56.1

Primary hyperparathyroidism

- Presentation is now typically asymptomatic rather than the classical 'bones, stones, abdominal groans and psychiatric overtones'
- The diagnosis of PHPT is a biochemical one
- Presence of an elevated ionised calcium with an inappropriately elevated/not suppressed PTH level confirms the diagnosis
- Sestamibi and focused neck ultrasonography are the first-line radiological investigations
- 85% of cases are due to a single adenoma
- Minimally invasive parathyroidectomy is a safe and acceptable alternative to a four-gland exploration in the presence of localised disease
- Familial syndromes and disease that is not localised require a formal four-gland exploration and three-and-a-half-gland parathyroidectomy

SECONDARY HYPERPARATHYROIDISM

Secondary hyperparathyroidism is defined as a derangement in calcium homeostasis, which leads to a compensatory increase in PTH secretion. It occurs primarily as a result of chronic kidney disease and is therefore sometimes referred to as renal hyperparathyroidism. Other underlying causes include gastrointestinal malabsorption, vitamin D deficiency, liver disease or chronic lithium usage.

The pathogenesis of secondary hyperparathyroidism is related to renal dysfunction. Abnormalities in the renal tubular absorption of phosphate lead to hyperphosphataemia. This acts directly on the parathyroid cells and stimulates PTH secretion. More recent translational research has identified a novel phosphaturia hormone, fibroblast growth factor 23 (FGF23). This is progressively secreted from osteocytes to compensate for chronic phosphate retention that in turn leads to a reduction in 1,25-dihydroxyvitamin D, which by reducing the intestinal absorption of calcium also acts to increase secretion of PTH. Previous studies in patients with chronic renal disease have shown that there is a reduction in the expression of the vitamin D receptor and the calcium-sensing receptor, with associated skeletal resistance to PTH. These factors interact to form the complex pattern leading to progressive secondary hyperparathyroidism in the setting of chronic renal disease.

The pathological characteristics associated with secondary hyperparathyroidism include hyperplasia, asymmetrical glandular enlargement or nodularity. This differentiation is important as, when the parathyroid gland becomes nodular, it loses expression of the vitamin D receptor and the calcium-sensing receptor gene. It has been proposed that nodular parathyroid glands may be resistant to calcimimetics and therefore refractory to medical management.

Diagnosis

The classical symptoms associated with secondary hyperparathyroidism are seen less commonly now, with greater awareness of the disease and the resultant earlier medical intervention. However, progressive bone disease, especially bone pain, can occur with associated soft-tissue calcium deposits (***Figure 56.9***).

The diagnosis of secondary hyperparathyroidism is characterised by hypocalcaemia or normocalcaemia with an elevated PTH. Patients have a high serum phosphate and a low vitamin D. Traditional plain radiographs now rarely demonstrate the pathognomonic osteitis fibrosa cystica. However, bone densitometry (DEXA scan) typically demonstrates osteopenia or osteoporosis.

The diagnosis of secondary hyperparathyroidism is a biochemical one. In general, localisation studies are not undertaken as minimally invasive surgery is not indicated. However, neck ultrasonography can be performed to identify patients with nodular hyperplasia who may be refractory to medical management. Localisation studies are helpful in patients with recurrent disease in order to identify ectopic parathyroid tissue, especially in the mediastinum. In cases of recurrent disease, when there is no evidence of active disease in the neck and a previous allograft has been used to the forearm, selective venous sampling for PTH in the neck and the brachial vein on the side of the graft can be useful. This is known as the Casanova test and to prove that the recurrent disease is located in the grafted arm (graft hyperplasia) the ratio must be greater than 20:1.

Daniel Casanova, contemporary, University of Cantabria, Santander, Spain.

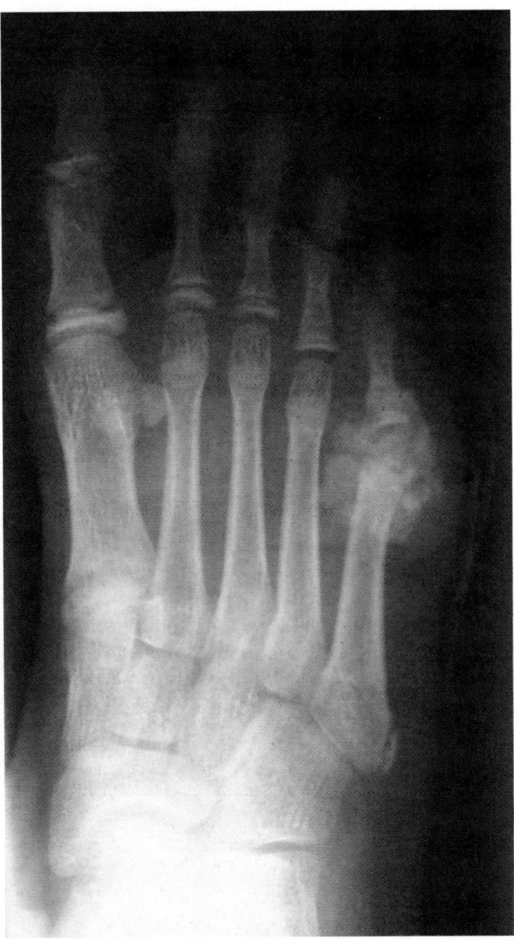

Figure 56.9 Secondary hyperparathyroidism. Radiograph showing ectopic calcification.

Calciphylaxis

Calciphylaxis (calcific uraemic arteriolopathy) is a syndrome of disseminated calcification resulting in both vascular calcification and skin necrosis. It accounts for approximately 4% of patients undergoing surgical intervention for secondary hyperparathyroidism. It presents with expanding painful cutaneous purpuric lesions, predominantly on the extremities, although they can also be seen on the lower abdomen. The underlying tissue calcification within the arteriolar and small vascular walls leads to ischaemic necrosis and the development of gangrene, which in turn leads to overwhelming sepsis and death. The majority of these patients will have an elevated calcium × phosphate product but it is not usually associated with an extremely high PTH level. The underlying aetiology remains unclear but a number of potential factors have been postulated. A reduction in the serum levels of a calcification inhibitory protein, α_2-Heremans–Schmid glycoprotein, and abnormalities in smooth muscle cell biology in uraemic patients may play a role in the development of the syndrome. Prognosis for these patients is extremely poor, with a mortality of up to 87%. An urgent parathyroidectomy has been shown to decrease pain, improve wound healing and reduce the risk of amputation in these patients. It has also been associated with an increase in median survival.

Management

Renal transplantation remains the only definite treatment for secondary hyperparathyroidism. Other therapies are a bridge to this or aim to provide symptom relief. Standard management includes replacement of calcium and vitamin D and the reduction of phosphate levels by the use of phosphate binders. Treatment of this disease changed radically with the introduction of calcimimetic drugs, such as cinacalcet. Calcimimetics alter the set point of the calcium-sensing receptor, thereby reducing the constant stimulation of the parathyroid glands and lowering the PTH level. This obviously does not address the underlying renal disease. It remains controversial as to which patients may benefit from the use of calcimimetics and which patients may benefit from earlier surgical intervention. Indications for pursuing medical management include those patients who are deemed non-surgical candidates by reason of medical comorbidities. Similarly, where there is persistent or recurrent disease, the origin of which cannot be clearly elucidated, surgical management should be avoided. However, there are definite indications for surgical intervention in secondary hyperparathyroidism (*Table 56.3*), although these have been modified to reflect the current use, where available, of calcimimetics (*Table 56.4*).

There are a wide variety of operations that can be utilised for the management of secondary hyperparathyroidism, none of which appears significantly superior in terms of clinical outcomes (persistent or recurrent disease). These include a subtotal parathyroidectomy, a total parathyroidectomy with autograft or a total parathyroidectomy without autograft. Cryopreservation of resected tissue, where available, should be

TABLE 56.3 Indications for surgical intervention in secondary hyperparathyroidism.

Essential components
1. Persistently high serum level of intact PTH >500 pg/mL 2. Hyperphosphataemia (serum PO_4 >6 mg/dL) or hypercalcaemia (serum Ca >2.5 mmol/L or 10 mg/dL) which is refractory to medical management 3. Estimated volume of the largest gland >300–500 mm^3 or long axis >1 cm
Clinical findings
If patients have one of these symptoms, parathyroidectomy should be recommended: • Severe osteitis fibrosa with associated high bone turnover • Subjective symptoms (bone and joint pain, arthralgia, muscle weakness, irritability, pruritus, depression) • Progressive ectopic calcification • Calciphylaxis • Progressive reduction in bone mineral content • Anaemia resistant to ESA • Dilated cardiomyopathy/cardiac failure

ESA, erythropoietin-stimulating agent; PTH, parathyroid hormone.

J F Heremans, 1927–1975, Professor of Medicine, Catholic University of Louvain, Belgium.
Karl Schmid, 1920–2009, Biochemist, Boston Medical Center, Boston, MA, USA.

TABLE 56.4 Proposed indications for surgical management of secondary hyperparathyroidism (SHPT) in the era of calcimimetics.

- When SHPT is refractory to vitamin D replacement or vitamin D analogues and prolonged survival is anticipated
- Severely impaired quality of life owing to either SHPT or intolerance to calcimimetics
- When sufficient reduction in parathyroid hormone cannot be achieved with use of calcimimetics
- Thyroid surgery is also required (thyroid carcinoma)

performed in cases of significant postoperative hypocalcaemia. The first two procedures are most widely accepted and the type of operation performed depends upon the surgeon.

A subtotal parathyroidectomy is where three and a half parathyroid glands are excised, with the remnant being marked with a non-absorbable stitch to facilitate identification in the event of recurrent disease. A biopsy of the final gland that is to be left *in situ* is mandatory to confirm the presence of residual parathyroid tissue. Ideally an inferior gland is left *in situ* to facilitate reoperative surgery and minimise potential damage to the recurrent laryngeal nerve in that setting (***Figure 56.10***). A total parathyroidectomy with a forearm autograft involves removal of all parathyroid tissue in the neck, with reimplantation of a small amount of morcellated tissue within a pocket formed in the brachioradialis muscle. Overall, regardless of the operative approach utilised the cure rate ranges between 90% and 96%, with similar complication rates. A randomised study looking at 40 patients who underwent either a subtotal or total parathyroidectomy with autotransplant demonstrated no significant difference between the two operations in terms of efficacy and recurrence rate (Rothmund *et al.*, 1991).

The response to surgical intervention is often dramatic. The biochemical parameters may resolve almost immediately and appear to be sustained for up to 3 years postoperatively. Patients subjectively report improvements in the symptoms of secondary hyperparathyroidism, including bone pain, pruritus, fatigue and depression. Finally, bone metabolism is improved with an approximate 10% increase in trabecular bone, with almost immediate suppression of bone resorption and acceleration of new bone formation.

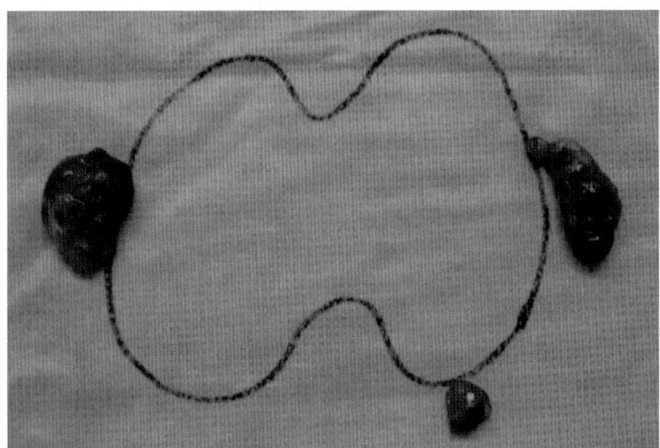

Figure 56.10 Subtotal parathyroidectomy for parathyroid hyperplasia. Right inferior gland biopsied and half left *in situ*.

Summary box 56.2

Secondary hyperparathyroidism

- Primarily due to underlying chronic kidney disease
- Associated with parathyroid hyperplasia
- Diagnosis is made biochemically with a low or normal calcium and an elevated PTH. High phosphate levels and low vitamin D levels are seen
- No localisation studies are required
- Mainstay of treatment is renal transplantation. Medical management with calcium and vitamin D replacements and phosphate binders is a bridge to transplantation
- Use of calcimimetics has reduced the requirement for surgical intervention
- Subtotal parathyroidectomy remains the surgical intervention of choice when indicated

TERTIARY HYPERPARATHYROIDISM

Tertiary hyperparathyroidism is a persistent autonomous hypercalcaemic hyperparathyroidism occurring after kidney transplantation. A number of proposed factors may prevent involution of the hyperplastic parathyroid glands following resolution of the underlying renal impairment. These include impaired graft function, non-suppressible PTH secretion, slow involution of enlarged glands or insufficient calcitriol conversion by the transplanted kidney.

The biochemical diagnosis is confirmed by an elevated total or ionised calcium, with an associated elevated or unsuppressed PTH and a reduced phosphate occurring at least 1 year post renal transplantation. Differentiation from PHPT can be difficult. Fewer than 1% of patients with tertiary hyperparathyroidism will require surgical intervention (***Table 56.5***). The only new evidence for intervention is the presence of nodular hyperplasia of the glands themselves. Traditionally, localisation studies or imaging of the neck was not indicated in tertiary hyperparathyroidism. However, increasing knowledge of the clonal nature of gland hyperplasia suggests that where there is a nodule within the parathyroid with a volume of tissue greater than 500 mm^3, then resolution of electrolyte abnormalities is unlikely.

TABLE 56.5 Indications for surgical intervention in tertiary hyperparathyroidism.

- Subacute severe hypercalcaemia (>3 mmol/L)
- Impaired graft function
- Nodular hyperplasia of the parathyroid gland(s)
- Progressive symptoms (>2 years following transplantation)
  - Worsening bone disease (pain, fracture, bone loss)
  - Renal stones/nephrocalcinosis
  - Soft-tissue or vascular calcifications

The use of calcimimetics in tertiary hyperparathyroidism remains controversial and has not been approved for this indication. However, isolated reports have documented control of hypercalcaemia with minimal side effects in individual patients. Surgical intervention remains the definitive management strategy. Subtotal parathyroidectomy or total parathyroidectomy with autotransplantation are acceptable surgical options. The majority of endocrine surgeons will opt for a subtotal parathyroidectomy in this setting, leaving a gland approximately four times normal in volume to minimise postoperative complications. Total parathyroidectomy without an autograft is not a treatment option because of the postoperative and persistent difficulties in managing the associated hypocalcaemia.

Summary box 56.3

Tertiary hyperparathyroidism

- Persistent autonomous hypercalcaemic hyperparathyroidism occurring after kidney transplantation
- Diagnosis is made by demonstrating an elevated total or ionised calcium with an associated elevated or unsuppressed PTH and a reduced phosphate occurring at least 1 year post renal transplantation
- Localisation studies are not required but a focused neck ultrasonography may confirm the presence of nodular enlargement
- Surgical intervention remains the mainstay of treatment and involves a subtotal parathyroidectomy

PARATHYROID CARCINOMA

Parathyroid carcinoma is a rare malignancy occurring in approximately 1% of cases of PHPT, with an estimated prevalence of 0.005% of all cancers. While the aetiology remains unclear, recent advances in molecular biology suggest that there may be an underlying genetic basis. Currently, a history of previous neck irradiation remains the only known environmental risk factor. However, given that it can arise in patients with end-stage renal disease as well as in those with MEN type 1, malignant transformation in hyperplastic glands may also occur.

A significant proportion of patients (>10%) with a parathyroid carcinoma will have HPT-JT. The underlying mutation is in the *HRPT2/CDC73* gene at chromosome 1q21–q31, a tumour suppressor gene that encodes the protein parafibromin. Parafibromin is involved in the regulation of cellular transcription and histone modification. *HRPT2* mutations, leading to inactivation of parafibromin, are therefore an important contributor to the pathogenesis of parathyroid carcinoma. Similarly, up to 18% of patients with a parathyroid carcinoma will have an inactivating mutation of the *PRUNE2* gene, located on chromosome 9q21.2. This is a tumour suppressor gene that encodes the RAS homologue family member A, leading to suppression of oncogenic cellular transformation.

Parathyroid carcinoma remains difficult to diagnose preoperatively as it biochemically resembles PHPT. There are, however, a number of suggestive features. First, the diagnosis is typically made a decade earlier, with an equal gender preponderance when compared with PHPT. Second, a greater proportion of these patients will be symptomatic at presentation. A palpable neck mass is found in 36–52% of patients with parathyroid carcinomas but rarely (<5%) in cases of PHPT. Finally, the biochemical abnormalities tend to be exaggerated with an average total calcium of between 3.75 and 3.97 mmol/L and a PTH level 5–10 times the normal range.

The leading cause of morbidity and mortality from parathyroid carcinoma is hypercalcaemia due to inappropriate PTH secretion. Treatment is focused on controlling hypercalcaemia and removal of the carcinoma where possible. Surgery remains the mainstay of treatment for primary presentations and locally recurrent disease. Complete resection of the tumour, avoiding spillage, is vital in preventing seeding and thus recurrent disease. En bloc resection of the tumour, associated thyroid lobectomy and central neck dissection remain controversial.

Complete R0 resection was thought to provide the only means of a cure. However, a number of recent studies have failed to demonstrate an improvement in local recurrence rates with such comprehensive resection. Adjuvant chemotherapy has not been shown to confer a disease-free or overall survival benefit. Use of external beam radiotherapy should be considered on an individual basis. Traditionally, it has not been deemed effective, but more recent single-institution case series challenge this assumption. It may be considered where it is difficult to achieve a complete surgical resection or in patients with multifocal recurrent soft-tissue deposits.

Histological confirmation of a parathyroid carcinoma remains difficult. The World Health Organization criteria (2017) for the diagnosis of a parathyroid carcinoma emphasise the need for definite invasion of the surrounding soft tissue and/or metastatic disease. The classical description that included trabecular architecture, mitotic figures, thick fibrous bands and capsular and vascular invasion is largely non-specific. New molecular markers may aid the diagnosis and stratify patients for more intensive follow-up (*Figure 56.11*). Immunohistochemical evidence of downregulation of parafibromin has a sensitivity of 67% and a specificity of 100% for detecting parathyroid carcinoma and the protein gene product 9.5 (PGP 9.5). Parafibromin immunohistochemistry may be used with immunohistochemistry for PGP 9.5. This is a protein encoded by ubiquitin carboxyl-terminal esterase LI. It is upregulated in parathyroid carcinoma and has a sensitivity of 78% and a specificity of 100%. All parafibromin-negative and PGP 9.5-positive tumours should be considered for genetic screening.

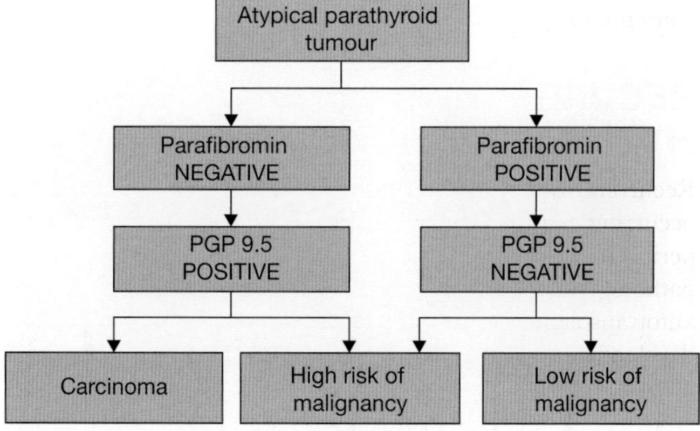

Figure 56.11 Proposed decision tree for atypical parathyroid tumours using parafibromin and PGP 9.5 immunohistochemistry.

Parathyroid carcinoma is an indolent but progressive disease. Metastatic spread can occur to the lungs, liver and bones. Recurrence rates range from 33% to 80% and it typically occurs in the first 3 years. Overall survival is reported to be 85–90% at 5 years and 49–77% at 10 years.

Summary box 56.4

Parathyroid carcinoma

- Accounts for approximately 1% of all cases of PHPT
- A history of previous neck irradiation remains the only known environmental risk factor
- The tumours remain difficult to diagnose preoperatively as they biochemically resemble PHPT
- Treatment is focused on controlling hypercalcaemia and removal of the carcinoma where possible
- Surgery remains the mainstay of treatment for primary presentations and locally recurrent disease. Complete resection of the tumour avoiding spillage is vital in preventing seeding and thus recurrent disease

PERSISTENT HYPERPARATHYROIDISM

Persistent hyperparathyroidism is defined as an elevated calcium within 6 weeks of surgical intervention. For all parathyroid operations (minimally invasive parathyroidectomy [MIP] and bilateral exploration) the rate of persistent hypercalcaemia is approximately 6% in sporadic disease and between 16% and 20% in hereditary disease. It usually arises as a result of a technical error during the first operation because of either a missed adenoma or asymmetrical disease. When this occurs all preoperative biochemistry, radiological imaging, intraoperative findings and pathology must be carefully reviewed. If reoperation is appropriate, repeat imaging of the neck and mediastinum is required (sestamibi, ultrasonography and 4D-CT scanning). Surgical intervention can be straightforward where there are intact tissue planes, such as following a minimally invasive parathyroidectomy. Complications, including recurrent laryngeal nerve damage and permanent hypocalcaemia, are increased when extensive previous dissection has occurred and the patient must be consented appropriately.

RECURRENT HYPERPARATHYROIDISM

Recurrent hyperparathyroidism is defined as hypercalcaemia occurring 6 months after surgery but with an intervening period of normocalcaemia. Common causes include missed pathology at the first operation; hyperplasia in remaining or autotransplanted tissue; parathyromatosis; or, very rarely, the development of a second parathyroid adenoma. Parathyromatosis refers to disseminated parathyroid tissue within the soft tissues of the neck and superior mediastinum owing to rupture of the parathyroid gland during the primary surgery. A definitive indication for surgical intervention must be present prior to embarking on localisation studies. Surgical intervention will be guided by the radiological imaging. Complication rates of recurrent laryngeal nerve damage and permanent hypocalcaemia are higher in reoperative surgery.

FURTHER READING

Agarwal A, Mishra AK, Lombardi CP, Raffaelli M. Applied embryology of the thyroid and parathyroid glands. In: *G.W. Randolph surgery of the thyroid and parathyroid glands*. Philadelphia, PA: Saunders, 2013: 15–24.

Barczyński M, Bränström R, Dionigi G, Mihai R. Sporadic multiple parathyroid gland disease – a consensus report of the European Society of Endocrine Surgeons. *Langenbecks Arch Surg* 2015; **400**(8): 887–905.

Bilezikian JP, Brandi ML, Eastell R *et al.* Guidelines for the management of asymptomatic primary hyperparathyroidism: summary statement from the Fourth International Workshop. *J Clin Endocrinol Metab* 2014; **99**: 3561–9.

Carneiro-Pla D, Pellitteri PK. Intraoperative PTH monitoring during parathyroid surgery. In: *G.W. Randolph surgery of the thyroid and parathyroid glands*. Philadelphia, PA: Saunders, 2013: 605–12.

Certani F, Pardi E, Marcocci C. Update on parathyroid carcinoma. *J Endocrinol Invest* 2016; **39**(6): 595–606.

Cheung K, Wang TS, Farrokhyar F *et al.* A metaanalysis of preoperative localisation techniques for patients with primary hyperparathyroidism. *Ann Surg Oncol* 2012; **19**(2): 577–83.

Howell VM, Gill A, Clarkson A *et al.* Accuracy of combined protein gene product 9.5 and parafibromin markers for immunohistochemical diagnosis of parathyroid carcinoma. *J Clin Endocrinol Metab* 2009; **94**(2): 434–41.

Iacobone M, Carnaille B, Palazzo FF, Vriens M. Hereditary hyperparathyroidism – a consensus report of the European Society of Endocrine Surgeons. *Langenbecks Arch Surg* 2015; **400**(8): 867–86.

Jeong HS, Dominguez AR. Calciphylaxis: controversies in pathogenesis, diagnosis and treatment. *Am J Med Sci* 2016; **356**(1): 217–27.

Krakauer M, Wieslander B, Myschetzky PS *et al.* A prospective comparative study of parathyroid dual-phase scintigraphy, dual-isotope subtraction scintigraphy, 4D-CT, and ultrasonography in primary hyperparathyroidism. *Clin Nucl Med* 2016; **41**(2): 93–100.

Mihai R, Simon D, Hellman P. Imaging for primary hyperparathyroidism – an evidence-based analysis. *Langenbecks Arch Surg* 2009; **394**(5): 765–84.

Pitt SC, Sipple RS, Chen H. Secondary and tertiary hyperparathyroidism: state of the art surgical management. *Surg Clin North Am* 2009; **89**(5): 1227–39.

Rodgers SE, Hunter GJ, Hamberg LM *et al.* Improved pre-operative planning for directed parathyroidectomy with 4-dimensional computed tomography. *Surgery* 2006; **140**(6): 932–40.

Rothmund M, Wagner PK, Schark C. Subtotal parathyroidectomy versus total parathyroidectomy and autotransplantation in secondary hyperparathyroidism: a randomized trial. *World J Surg* 1991; **15**(6): 745–50.

Silverberg SJ, Clarke BL, Peacock M *et al.* 2014. Current issues in the presentation of asymptomatic primary hyperparathyroidism. *Proc Fourth Int Workshop* 2014; **99**: 3580–94.

Walker DM, Silverberg SJ. Primary hyperparathyroidism. *Nat Rev Endocrinol* 2018; **14**(2): 115–125.

CHAPTER 57 The adrenal glands and other abdominal endocrine disorders

Learning objectives

Adrenal gland

- To understand the investigation and diagnosis of disorders of the adrenal gland
- To know of the principles and postoperative management of adrenalectomy

Pancreatic endocrine disorders and gastrointestinal neuroendocrine tumours (GI-NETs)

- To understand the investigation and diagnosis of pancreatic endocrine tumours/GI-NETs
- To know the principles of management of pancreatic endocrine tumours/GI-NETs, including surgery
- To understand the immediate and long-term care after surgery

Multiple endocrine neoplasia (MEN syndromes)

- To understand the genetics and various presentations of patients with MEN
- To be able to manage patients with MEN disorders and familial medullary thyroid cancer
- To understand the principles of surgery and postoperative management of patients with MEN

INTRODUCTION

Two major systems are held responsible for the regulation of homeostasis of the human body: the endocrine and neuroendocrine systems. Both interact with their target organs or target tissues via secretion of ubiquitous messenger molecules, which can be peptides, amines or steroids.

The **endocrine system** consists of various specialist cells in a variety of richly vascularised ductless glands that synthesise and release hormones into the bloodstream.

The **neuroendocrine system** involves neuroendocrine cells that receive nerve impulses to release neurohormones into the bloodstream. Neuroendocrine glands are found in almost every organ of the body. They are mainly found scattered in the gastrointestinal tract, pancreas (islet cells) and thyroid (C cells). For this reason they are known as the diffuse neuroendocrine system. A shared characteristic in the adrenal medulla, gut and pancreatic endocrine tissues are the amine precursor uptake and decarboxylation (APUD) cells, now known as neuroendocrine cells. For many years they were believed to have a common embryological derivation in the neural crest, from which cells migrated to tissues throughout the body. It is now believed that, along with neurones, they share a common neuroendocrine programming influence during their differentiation (see *Further reading*). Finally, somatostatin receptors (SSTRs) are present on the cell surface of neuroendocrine cells, providing a unique and specific molecular target for imaging and therapy. Nuclear imaging physicians and specialists in radiopharmaceutical therapy are important additional members of the endocrine surgery multidisciplinary team.

Throughout the chapter, the diagnosis and management of various conditions are considered. For each and every disease the principles of endocrine surgery are followed in a stepwise manner:

- confirm the diagnosis with biochemical tests;
- render the patient safe (e.g. treat hypertension, hypoglycaemia, hypokalaemia);
- consider whether localisation studies are necessary;
- decide if surgery is indicated;
- if so, what operative approach is best?

ANATOMY

Adrenal glands

The weight of a normal adrenal gland is approximately 4 g. The adrenal glands are paired and situated in the retroperitoneum, near the upper poles of the kidneys, within Gerota's capsule. They are not symmetrical. The right adrenal gland is located between the right liver lobe and the diaphragm, close to and partly behind the inferior vena cava (IVC). The left adrenal gland lies superior–medial to the upper pole of the left kidney and the renal pedicle. It is covered by the pancreatic tail and the spleen (*Figure 57.1*). Each adrenal gland is supplied by multiple small arterial branches from three main vessels: the aorta, the inferior phrenic artery and the renal artery. A usually single large adrenal vein drains into the IVC on the right side and into the renal vein on the left side.

Dumitru Gerota, 1867–1939, Professor of Surgery, Bucharest, Romania.

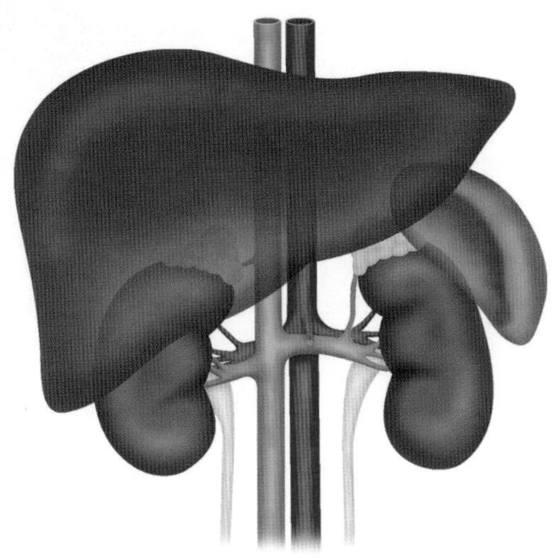

Figure 57.1 Anatomy of the adrenal glands.

Extra-adrenal paraganglia

Paraganglia are neuroendocrine cells associated with the autonomic nervous system. They can be adrenal (medulla) or extra-adrenal. Extra-adrenal paraganglia occur throughout the sympathetic nervous system and along some branches of the parasympathetic glossopharyngeal and vagus nerves. There are four subgroups:

1. **Sympathetic**: the largest cluster is the organ of Zuckerkandl, which is located at the aortic bifurcation or close to the origin of the inferior mesenteric artery.
2. **Chemoreceptor**: including aortic and carotid bodies that assist in the regulation of respiration.
3. **Visceral–autonomic**: in the urinary bladder and peripheral blood vessels.
4. **Intravagal**: situated within or adjacent to the vagal trunk.

Neoplasms of extra-adrenal paraganglia are called paragangliomas (PGLs). Tumours of chemoreceptors are usually referred to as chemodectomas (see *Chapter 52*) and those from parasympathetic ganglia are termed glomus tumours.

EMBRYOLOGY

There are two distinct functional units in the adrenal gland: cortex and medulla. The cortex is derived from the mesoderm. At about the fifth week of life the fetal cortex develops; this is subsequently surrounded by a second wave of mesothelial cells that will eventually form the definitive cortex. After birth the fetal cortex regresses except for its outermost layer, which differentiates into the reticular zone. The adrenal medulla is derived from ectodermal chromaffin cells that are believed to have migrated from the neural crest.

The adrenal cortex represents 90% of the gland and is arranged in a zonal configuration. The outer **zona glomerulosa** contains small, compact cells loosely arranged in cords. The central **zona fasciculata** can be identified by larger, lipoid-rich cells, which are arranged in radial columns. This is the largest layer (70%). Compact and pigmented cells characterise the inner **zona reticularis**.

The adrenal medulla is the inner core that consists of a thin layer of large chromaffin cells (stain yellow with chromium), which synthesise, store and secrete catecholamines.

PHYSIOLOGY

The outer **zona glomerulosa** secretes the C21 steroid aldosterone. The **zona fasciculata** secretes (C21 steroid) cortisol and the inner **zona reticularis** secretes (C19 steroid) androgens.

Aldosterone regulates sodium–potassium homeostasis; it promotes sodium retention and potassium excretion. The target organs of aldosterone are the kidneys, the sweat and salivary glands and the intestinal mucosa. The most important regulators of aldosterone secretion are the renin–angiotensin system and serum potassium concentration.

Renin, produced by the juxtaglomerular cells in the kidneys, acts on its substrate angiotensinogen to generate angiotensin I. Angiotensin I is converted by angiotensin-converting enzyme (ACE) to the octapeptide angiotensin II, which is modified to angiotensin III. Both stimulate secretion of aldosterone from the adrenal cortex. A decrease in renal blood flow (haemorrhage, dehydration, salt depletion, orthostasis, renal artery stenosis) or hyponatraemia increases renin secretion, resulting in sodium retention, potassium excretion and an increased plasma volume.

Cortisol secretion by the cells of the **zona fasciculata** is regulated by adrenocorticotropic hormone (ACTH), which is produced by the anterior pituitary gland. The hypothalamus controls ACTH secretion by secreting corticotropin-releasing hormone (CRH). The serum cortisol level inhibits the release of CRH and ACTH via a closed-loop system (negative feedback loop).

Cortisol has numerous metabolic and immunological effects. It increases gluconeogenesis and lipolysis, decreases peripheral glucose utilisation, inhibits immunological response and, in time, reduces muscular mass. It affects fat distribution, wound healing and bone mineralisation; it also alters mood (causing euphoria or, rarely, depression) and brain cortical activity and alertness. Cells in the zona reticularis synthesise adrenal androgen dehydroepiandrosterone (DHEA) and its sulphate, DHEAS. Adrenal androgen accounts for about 20% of total male activity and is under the control of ACTH.

Cells of the adrenal medulla synthesise mainly adrenaline (epinephrine; 80%) but also noradrenaline (norepinephrine; 20%) and dopamine. Unlike other adrenergic neurones, those of the medulla express phenylethanolamine-*N*-methyltransferase (PNMT), which catalyses the conversion of noradrenaline to adrenaline. These catecholamines act as hormones as they are secreted directly into the circulation. Their effects, which are mediated through α and β receptors on target organs, include the cardiovascular system, resulting in an increase in blood pressure, heart rate and cardiac contractility; vasoconstriction of vessels in the splanchnic system and vasodilatation of vessels

Emil Zuckerkandl, 1849–1910, Professor of Anatomy, Vienna, Austria

in the muscles; bronchodilatation; and increased glycogenolysis in liver and muscles, all of which are necessary for the flight/fight response.

INCIDENTALOMA

Definition

An asymptomatic adrenal mass detected on imaging not performed for suspected adrenal disease is termed an incidentaloma. The aetiology includes benign and malignant tumours of the cortex and medulla or of extra-adrenal origin. These tumours can be either non-functioning (silent) or functioning (secreting excess hormones).

Incidence

Autopsy studies suggest a prevalence of clinically inapparent adrenal masses of the order of 2%, which increases with age. Radiological incidentalomas are seen in about 3% of scans at the age of 50, rising to 10% in the elderly.

Investigation

Incidentaloma embraces all adrenal pathology and so the steps to management are described here and the detail for each pathology will follow in the individual sections of the chapter.

A clear evidence-based algorithm for assessing patients with adrenal incidentaloma has been derived (*Figure 57.2*). The following should be assessed in parallel:

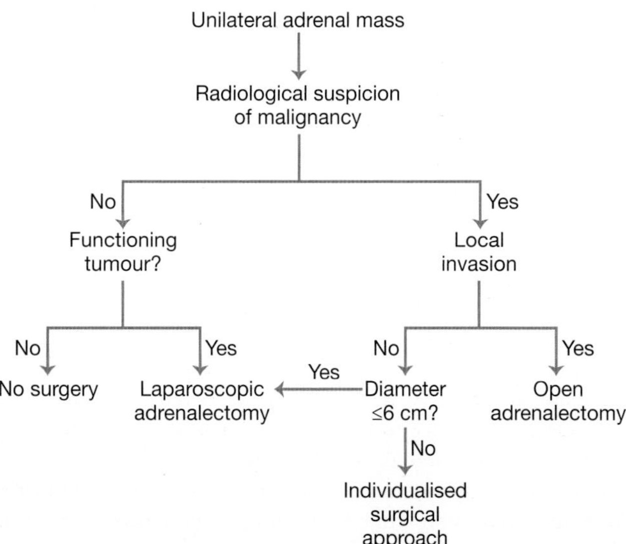

Figure 57.2 Algorithm for the investigation of adrenal incidentaloma. (After Fassnacht M, Arlt W, Bancos I *et al*. Management of adrenal incidentalomas: European Society of Endocrinology Clinical Practice Guideline in collaboration with the European Network for the Study of Adrenal Tumors. *Eur J Endocrinol* 2016; **175**(2): G1–G34.)

- **Is the tumour benign or malignant?** Clinically, Cushing's syndrome and virilising tumours are associated with higher rates of malignancy (50% and 30%, respectively). The optimal way to determine malignancy is by means of a non-contrast computed tomography (CT) scan and measurement of the density of the lesion by Hounsfield units (HU). Benign tumours are low density (≤10 HU). In cases of uncertainty, consideration is given to fluorodeoxyglucose (FDG)–positron emission tomography (PET) scanning, magnetic resonance imaging (MRI) with chemical shift or contrast CT and measurement of washout. Radiological findings suspicious of malignancy are shown in *Summary box 57.1*.
- **Is the tumour functionally active?** This is determined by:
  - Clinical assessment
  - 1 mg overnight dexamethasone suppression test (DST)
  - Measurement of plasma or urinary metanephrines
  - Plasma aldosterone–renin ratio (ARR)
  - Sex hormones and steroid precursors

Summary box 57.1

Radiological features suspicious of adrenal malignancy

- Diameter >40 mm and >10 HU density
- Contrast-enhanced washout CT
  - Relative <40%
  - Absolute <60%
- MRI chemical shift: no change in signal intensity on out-of-phase imaging
- FDG-PET: positive uptake

Management

All patients should be discussed in a multidisciplinary setting. Small (<40 mm), benign non-functioning tumours do not require surgery, but patients should undergo a follow-up CT/MRI at 6 months. There is no consensus about follow-up beyond that period. However, there is evidence that a tumour >30 mm has an increased risk of developing hyperfunction over time.

Adrenalectomy is the standard of care for patients with unilateral tumours causing hormone excess. Adrenalectomy is recommended for all tumours >40 mm in diameter, tumours showing imaging characteristics of malignancy and tumours showing significant growth.

Laparoscopic adrenalectomy is recommended for unilateral adrenal masses with radiological findings suspicious of malignancy and a diameter <60 mm, but without evidence of local invasion. Open adrenalectomy is recommended for unilateral adrenal masses with radiological findings suspicious of malignancy. An individualised approach is required for patients whose tumours fall outside the above categories.

Harvey Williams Cushing, 1869–1939, Professor of Surgery, Harvard University Medical School, Boston, MA, USA.
Sir Godfrey Newbold Hounsfield, 1919–2004, British electrical engineer, won the 1979 Nobel Prize in Physiology or Medicine for helping to develop the diagnostic imaging technique known as X-ray computed tomography.

DISORDERS OF CORTEX

Conn's syndrome (primary hyperaldosteronism)

Definition

First described in 1957 in a patient with hypertension and low serum potassium, primary hyperaldosteronism (PA) now comprises a heterogeneous group of disorders characterised by hypertension and inappropriately raised plasma aldosterone concentrations. It is of importance not only because, if left untreated, it can lead to cardiovascular and renal complications, but also because a significant proportion of patients can be improved or cured with surgery.

Incidence

PA is the most common cause of endocrine hypertension and may be present in up to one-fifth of patients investigated for hypertension. It is twice as common in females as in males and its prevalence increases significantly in those with drug-resistant hypertension. About 30–40% of cases are due to an aldosterone-producing adenoma (APA) of the cortex and just over one-third of patients will have hypokalaemia at presentation.

Pathology

Although Conn originally described a patient with an APA, PA may also be due to bilateral adrenal hyperplasia, adrenocortical carcinoma (ACC), unilateral hyperplasia and familial hyperaldosteronism (FH). Determining the underlying cause is key because this will determine the most appropriate treatment modality (surgery versus medical therapy). In all its forms, PA is characterised by volume expansion secondary to sodium retention and the variable occurrence of hypokalaemia due to increased potassium excretion into the renal tubule. Resultant hypertension leads to an increased risk of cardiovascular morbidity (stroke, myocardial infarction and atrial fibrillation) and mortality compared with matched controls. Furthermore, glucose intolerance, type 2 diabetes and the metabolic syndrome are also more common in those with PA.

Aldosterone-producing adenoma

Arising in the zona glomerulosa, these tumours are typically between 10 and 20 mm in maximal diameter at presentation, well circumscribed and macroscopically golden yellow on slicing (the 'canary tumour'). Ninety per cent contain somatic mutations; although these may be associated with certain clinical features, their presence does not yet affect clinical management. The most common mutations are those of the potassium channel encoded by the *KCNJ5* gene; these are present in approximately 40% of patients with APA. Mutations are thought to trigger calcium influx into glomerulosa cells, resulting in aldosterone secretion and cellular proliferation. Phenotypically, they are more prevalent in females and are associated with larger tumours and higher aldosterone levels, but are not associated with adrenal hyperplasia. In contrast, less common variants, including somatic mutations in the *ATP1A1*, *ATP2B3*, *CACNA1D* and *CTNNB1* genes, exhibit a stronger male preponderance.

Bilateral adrenal hyperplasia (idiopathic hyperplasia)

Traditionally thought to result from diffuse hyperplasia of the zona glomerulosa, the pathophysiology of bilateral adrenal hyperplasia and its drivers remain poorly understood. More recently, aldosterone-producing cell clusters with a high prevalence of somatic mutations in the *CACNA1D* l-type calcium channel gene have been identified in the adrenal cortex of patients with bilateral hyperplasia and these 'micro-APAs' have been cited as the putative cause.

Familial hyperaldosteronism types I–IV

These rare genetic variants of PA are all inherited in an autosomal dominant fashion (50:50 chance that offspring of an affected individual will inherit the disorder).

FH type I or glucocorticoid-remediable aldosteronism (GRA) arises as a result of a *CYP11B1/CYP11B2* chimeric gene and presents with (typically normokalaemic) hypertension when the patient is in their early twenties. The chimeric gene leads to ACTH-dependent aldosterone secretion and is treated by administering physiological doses of glucocorticoids, which suppress ACTH release. Thus treatment is always medical.

FH types II–IV (caused by germline *CLCN2* pathogenic variants, *KCNJ5* pathogenic variants and *CACNA1H* pathogenic variants, respectively) all result in early-onset PA within affected kindreds. Type II FH may lead to APAs or bilateral adrenal hyperplasia; type III massive bilateral adrenal hyperplasia; and type IV developmental disorder with bilateral adrenal hyperplasia. Genetic testing for these disorders is in evolution and, currently, it is recommended that treatment should be as for patients with sporadic PA.

Clinical presentation

Aside from hypertension, patients may be asymptomatic unless they are hypokalaemic, in which case muscle weakness, cramps and fatigue may be present. Hypokalaemia-induced palpitations after initiation of diuretic therapy or polyuria and polydipsia from nephrogenic diabetes insipidus are also described. Physical signs include hypertension, associated bruits and retinopathy. It is worth noting that the following presentations might also warrant screening for PA: drug-resistant hypertension, hypertension and obstructive sleep apnoea, hypertension with incidentaloma, patients with first-degree relatives with PA, and a family history of early-onset hypertension or stroke.

Diagnosis

Biochemical

Although routine tests may reveal hypokalaemia and/or metabolic alkalosis, the diagnosis depends on the presence of non-suppressed plasma aldosterone (pmol/L) and a suppressed plasma renin activity (nmol/L/h). The two are combined to give a plasma ARR: if >850 this is suggestive of PA; if >1700 it is very likely to be PA. Because most, if not all, patients will be prescribed antihypertensives, it is important to stop agents that might interfere with interpretation of the ARR. Although

Jerome William Conn, 1907–1981, Professor of Internal Medicine, University of Michigan, Ann Arbor, MI, USA.

most can be continued, predictably, those that interfere with the renin–angiotensin system, i.e. ACE inhibitors, angiotensin receptor blockers, direct renin inhibitors and aldosterone antagonists (spironolactone and eplerenone), should be stopped for 2 weeks beforehand. More severe biochemical disease is more likely to be due to an APA.

Radiological

Once a biochemical diagnosis is secure, the primary objective is to determine whether it is due to a unilateral APA (or, rarely, carcinoma) or bilateral hyperplasia. High-resolution (2- to 3-mm slices) adrenal CT is the initial investigation of choice and APAs typically appear as a hypodense (<10 HU) unilateral 1- to 2-cm adrenal nodule; carcinomas are heterogenous and >60 mm; and bilateral hyperplasia presents as bilateral bulky adrenal enlargement.

Diagnosis of a unilateral APA on CT alone is controversial: tumours are often small and this, combined with the increasing preponderance for adrenal nodules with advancing age, means that a missed contralateral nodule could be the underlying cause. For this reason, adrenal vein sampling (AVS) is considered the gold standard for confirming unilateral secretion. Surgery based on biochemistry and a unilateral adrenal lesion on imaging alone is effective in those younger than 35 years, leaving AVS for patients older than 35 years or with negative imaging or bilateral nodules. PET scanning with ^{11}C-metomidate, an 11β–hydroxylase (CYP11B1) and aldosterone synthase (CYP11B2) inhibitor, has been compared with AVS and found to be 86% specific and 76% sensitive for lateralising PA; it is therefore a useful adjunct in patients with failed or equivocal AVS results (***Figure 57.3***) (see ***Further reading***).

Treatment

Medical

Prior to surgery, hypertension and hypokalaemia should be adequately corrected. The preoperative response to aldosterone receptor antagonist (spironolactone/eplerenone) therapy is a useful surrogate for predicting likely success. In general, the shorter the time to diagnosis, the better the likely outcome from surgery.

Surgical

Unilateral APA should be managed by minimally invasive adrenalectomy, which results in resolution of hypertension and hypokalaemia or a reduction in antihypertensive requirement in the vast majority of patients.

Bilateral disease

Unless hyperplasia is marked, with dominant nodules >40 mm that are indeterminate, patients with bilateral disease should be managed medically with aldosterone antagonists and other antihypertensives. If this is unsuccessful, lateralising investigations may be used to determine if one side is dominant, in which case excision of that side may improve medical control.

Familial hyperaldosteronism

These disorders are extremely rare and are best managed in a multidisciplinary fashion in conjunction with tertiary

(a)

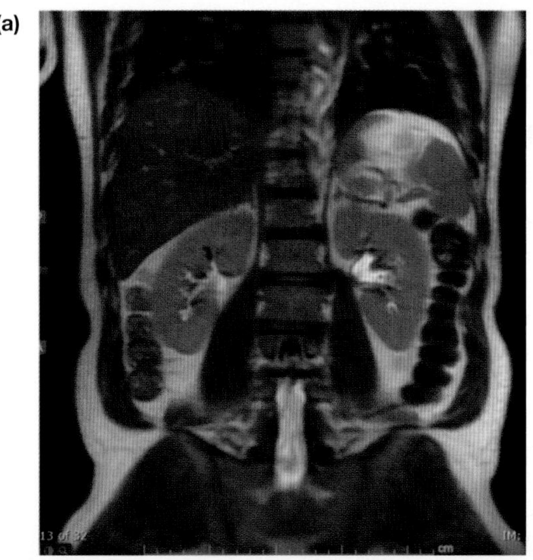

(b)

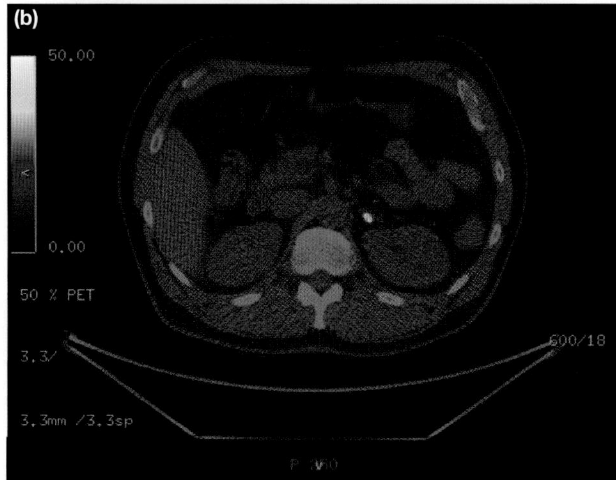

(c)

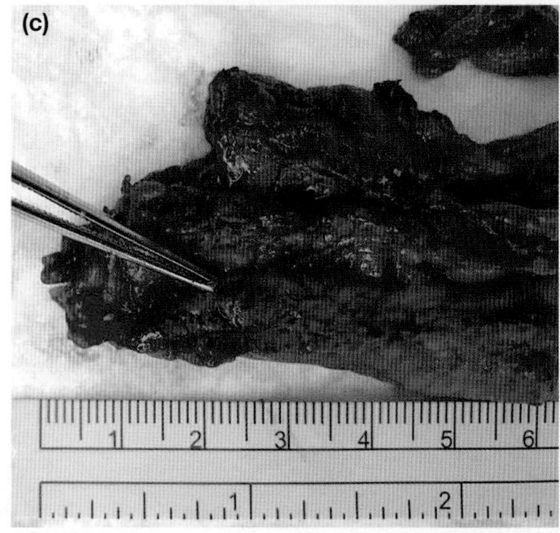

Figure 57.3 A patient with confirmed Conn's syndrome. Magnetic resonance imaging (a) failed to demonstrate a lesion but a 30-SUVmax lesion was demonstrated on a ^{11}C-metomidate positron emission tomography (PET)–computed tomography (CT) scan (b). (c) Surgical specimen sliced to reveal a 6-mm aldosterone-producing adenoma in the medial limb. The patient's hypertension resolved with laparoscopic left adrenalectomy (PET-CT image courtesy of Mark Gurnell, Addenbrooke's Hospital, Cambridge). SUVmax, maximum standard unit value.

endocrinology input. However, surgery should be considered if a unilateral secreting lesion is found to be the cause.

Cushing's syndrome

Definition

Hypercortisolism may arise as a result of excess ACTH secretion (termed pituitary dependent; Cushing's disease), ectopic ACTH secretion from a non-pituitary tumour, exogenous corticosteroid therapy or autonomous secretion of endogenous glucocorticoids from cortical tumours of the adrenal glands (pituitary independent; Cushing's syndrome). ACTH-secreting pituitary tumours account for 70–80% of cases, whereas ectopic ACTH production from foregut neuroendocrine tumours and small cell lung tumours are the cause in 10%. In the remaining 10–15%, Cushing's syndrome arises from unilateral cortisol-secreting adenomas and occasionally ACCs or bilateral nodular adrenal hyperplasia. Left untreated, hypercortisolism leads to a fivefold increase in the risk of death from cardiovascular disease. The principal aim therefore is to determine and treat the underlying cause, while avoiding, if possible, long-term hormonal deficiency or dependence on medication.

Incidence

Iatrogenic Cushing's syndrome is likely to be most prevalent as a result of the widespread use of corticosteroids for other diseases but this is poorly documented. The incidence of pituitary-dependent disease is around six or seven per million per year, whereas the incidence of ectopic ACTH syndrome is around one per million per year. Although adrenal tumours are extremely common, 99% do not present with endocrine disease and so adrenal Cushing's syndrome is also quite uncommon (one or two per million per year). Both ACTH-dependent and -independent Cushing's have a strong female preponderance (four to six times), whereas ectopic ACTH syndrome is twice as common in men. The incidence increases significantly from age 50.

Pathology

Similar to PA, the most common cause of adrenal Cushing's (syndrome) is an adrenocortical adenoma, although it can arise in the setting of bilateral nodular hyperplasia or less commonly ACC (see *Adrenocortical carcinoma*).

Adrenal adenoma

Tumours are well circumscribed, nodular in appearance and composed of polygonal eosinophilic and lipidised cells in a nested pattern. The resulting hypercortisolism leads to suppressed ACTH, which causes atrophy of fasciculata and reticularis, not glomerulosa, in the residual or opposite adrenal gland.

Primary bilateral macronodular adrenal hyperplasia

Primary bilateral macronodular adrenal hyperplasia (BMAH) is a relatively uncommon cause of Cushing's syndrome. It may present as bilateral adrenal incidentalomas and is characterised by the presence of bilateral non-pigmented adrenal nodules ranging from 10 to 40 mm in size. It may also present with subclinical Cushing's.

Clinical presentation

Because of the pleiotropic actions of cortisol, the clinical features of Cushing's syndrome are broad and multisystem (*Summary box 57.2*). The typical patient is characterised by a facial plethora, a buffalo hump and a moon face in combination with hypertension, diabetes, central obesity and proximal muscle-wasting, traditionally referred to as the 'lemon on sticks' appearance (*Figures 57.4 and 57.5*). Clinical signs can be minimal or absent in patients with subclinical Cushing's syndrome.

Summary box 57.2

Clinical features of Cushing's syndrome

Clinical feature	Incidence (%)
Obesity	90
Hypertension	85
Facial plethora	70
Hirsutism	75
Glucose intolerance/diabetes	75
Hyperlipidaemia	70
Abdominal striae	50
Acne	35
Easy bruising	35
Osteoporosis	80
Proximal myopathy	65
Depression/mania/psychosis	85
Menstrual disorders	70
Decrease libido/impotence	85
Renal stones	50

Adapted from Raff H, Sharma ST, Nieman LK. Physiological basis for the etiology, diagnosis, and treatment of adrenal disorders: Cushing's syndrome, adrenal insufficiency, and congenital adrenal hyperplasia. *Compr Physiol* 2014; **4**: 739–69.

Diagnosis

Biochemical

It is important to exclude iatrogenic Cushing's due to ingested steroid therapy, including potent inhaled corticosteroids. Investigations should then determine **if** hypercortisolism is present **and** whether it is ACTH dependent or independent. Imaging should not be pursued until the diagnosis is secure. Endocrine Society 2008 guidance states that two of the following tests should be abnormal for diagnosis:

- late-night salivary cortisol (two measurements): raised levels signify a loss of diurnal rhythm;
- 24-hour urinary free cortisol (UFC) excretion (two measurements): more than three times the upper limit signifies overspill into the urine;

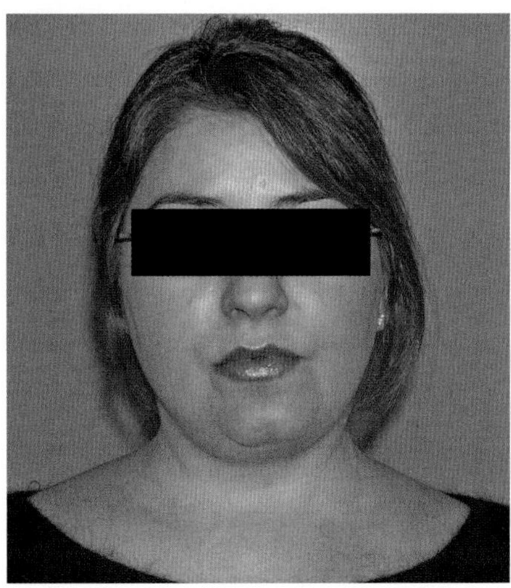

Figure 57.4 A 34-year-old patient with Cushing's syndrome whose symptoms included thickening of the face, weight gain and acne. Today patients with Cushing's syndrome rarely have the full-blown appearance shown in older textbooks.

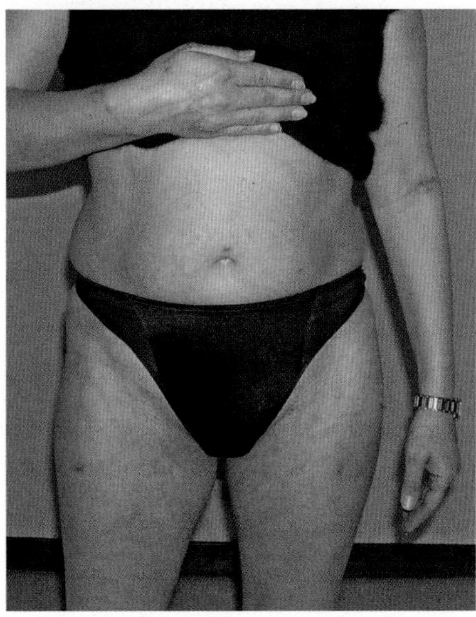

Figure 57.5 Discrete central obesity, ecchymosis and fragile skin in a patient with Cushing's syndrome.

- overnight 1-mg DST (dexamethasone suppression test): non-suppressed morning cortisol >50 nmol/L;
- raised serum ACTH signifies pituitary-dependent disease; if it is adrenal in origin, the ACTH is suppressed (<5 pg/mL).

Radiological

These tests should determine the causative lesion. The ACTH result will determine which diagnostic pathway is taken.

- **ACTH raised**: pituitary MRI and inferior petrosal sinus sampling to exclude pituitary microadenoma. If both are negative, this suggests ectopic ACTH syndrome, which warrants CT imaging of the thorax, abdomen and pelvis. Functional imaging with ^{68}Ga-SSTR PET-CT is a useful adjunct and is 75–80% sensitive in confirming the source of ectopic ACTH.
- **ACTH suppressed**: dedicated adrenal CT or MRI to determine if unilateral adenoma or bilateral nodular hyperplasia (or rarely adrenocortical cancer) are present. Benign lesions are typically hypodense and <10 HU on non-contrast CT.

Treatment

Medical

Metyrapone or ketoconazole therapy reduces steroid synthesis and secretion by CYP11B1 inhibition and can be used to prepare patients with severe hypercortisolism preoperatively or as primary therapy if surgery is not possible. In patients who are critically ill with Cushing's syndrome, intravenous etomidate infusion (even at non-hypnotic doses) can reduce serum cortisol levels to normal within 24 hours, providing a suitable window for surgery. This requires monitoring in an intensive care unit setting.

Surgical

ACTH-producing pituitary tumours are treated by transsphenoidal resection and/or radiotherapy. Resection of ectopic ACTH-secreting tumours will also correct hypercortisolism. Patients who have undergone failed pituitary surgery or those with an unresectable or unlocalised ectopic ACTH-secreting tumour may require bilateral adrenalectomy to control hormone excess. This will render them steroid dependent. Unilateral adenoma should be treated by minimally invasive adrenalectomy provided adrenocortical cancer is not suspected. In cases of bilateral ACTH-independent disease (***Figure 57.6***), the extent of adrenalectomy is contentious; bilateral adrenalectomy should be employed in severe Cushing's and equally enlarged adrenals. In asymmetric disease, excision

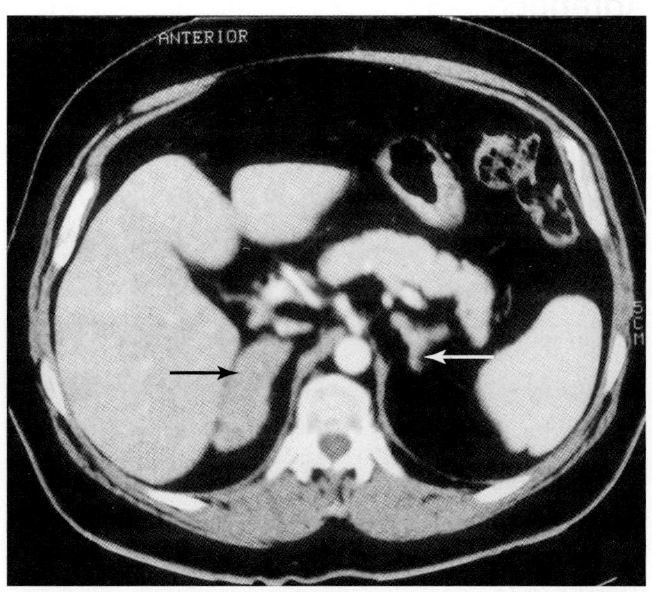

Figure 57.6 Bilateral asymmetrical hyperplasia of the adrenal glands (arrows) in a patient with Cushing's syndrome.

of the larger gland may be curative with a low risk of recurrence. In cases of subclinical Cushing's syndrome and a unilateral adenoma, unilateral adrenalectomy is indicated if the tumour is >4 cm or <4 cm with features of the metabolic syndrome.

Preoperative management. Cushing's syndrome predisposes patients to increased risk of venous thromboembolism, cardiac events, infection and poor wound healing. Patients should therefore receive chemical and mechanical thromboprophylaxis as well as perioperative broad-spectrum antibiotics. Accompanying diabetes should also be adequately controlled. As unilateral or bilateral adrenalectomy in the setting of Cushing's syndrome will result in steroid deficiency in the postoperative period, patients should receive intraoperative corticosteroids (50–100 mg intravenous hydrocortisone) and close liaison with the endocrinology team is strongly advised to guide postoperative management.

Postoperative management. After unilateral adrenalectomy the contralateral gland will be suppressed and so all patients should be commenced on 15–25 mg daily of hydrocortisone. In total, 15 mg/h is required parenterally for the first 12 hours followed by a daily dose of 100 mg for 3 days, which is gradually reduced thereafter. After unilateral adrenalectomy, the contralateral suppressed gland may need up to a year to recover adequate function. A synacthen test is used to confirm adequate adrenal function prior to stopping hydrocortisone supplementation. In 10% of patients with Cushing's disease who undergo a bilateral adrenalectomy after failed pituitary surgery, the pituitary adenoma causes Nelson's syndrome owing to continued ACTH secretion at high levels, resulting in hyperpigmentation due to uncontrolled secretion of pro-opiomelanocortin (POMC). POMC is cleaved to produce ACTH and melanocyte-stimulating hormone, excess of the latter resulting in hyperpigmentation.

Adrenocortical carcinoma

Definition

ACC is a rare aggressive malignancy that arises from the adrenal cortex. The prognosis is variable but is generally poor, in part owing to its tendency to present at a late stage. Although most ACCs are sporadic, a minority occur as part of genetic tumour syndromes such as multiple endocrine neoplasia type 1 (MEN 1), familial adenomatous polyposis and the Li–Fraumeni and Lynch syndromes. Optimal surgery remains the best way of curing the patient and so preoperative diagnosis and planning are key in ensuring this outcome.

Incidence

Estimated incidence is one or two cases per 1 000 000 population per year and, in keeping with benign adrenocortical tumours, a female predominance is observed (1.5:1). ACCs can occur at any age but the peak incidence is in the fourth and fifth decades.

Pathology

Tumours are often large (>10 cm) with a cut surface that ranges from orange to brown (*Figure 57.7*). Necrosis is usually present. Distinguishing between benign and malignant adrenocortical tumours may be difficult, with the presence of local invasion or distant metastasis being the only definitive criteria. If neither are present, the modified Weiss histopathological system may be used to guide management. It comprises five criteria: >6 mitoses/50 high-power fields, ≤25% clear tumour cells in cytoplasm, abnormal mitoses, necrosis and capsular invasion. If a criterion is absent, it is scored 0; if present, it scores 2 for the first two criteria and 1 each for the last three. A total score ≥3 is suggestive of malignant behaviour. More recently the use of the Ki-67 proliferation index has been advocated, with increasing count suggesting poorer prognosis.

Clinical presentation

Patients may present with hormonal excess (50–60%) or symptoms of an abdominal mass such as abdominal or back pain (30–40%). Around one in six ACCs present as adrenal incidentalomas. Those that are hormonally active usually cause Cushing's syndrome or a mixed picture of Cushing's and virilisation in women. Mineralocorticoid excess is rare, as is feminisation in male patients.

Diagnosis

Although radiological investigations are critical in diagnosis, the presence of autonomous secretion of glucocorticoids, sex hormones and steroid precursors should also be carefully evaluated. Phaeochromocytoma (PCC) must also be excluded.

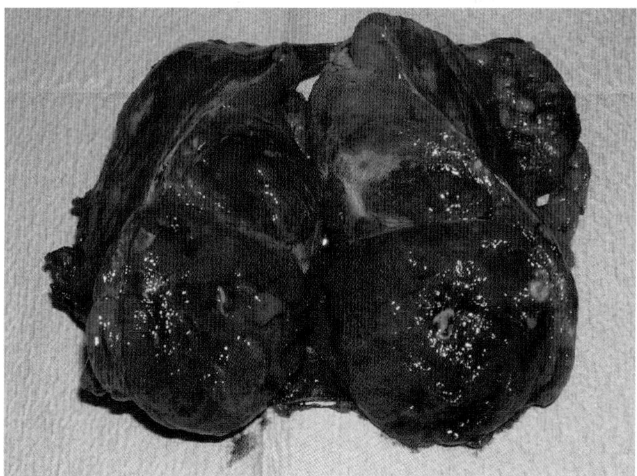

Figure 57.7 Adrenocortical carcinoma that caused Cushing's syndrome and virilisation in a female patient.

Don H Nelson, 1925–2010, Professor of Medicine, University of Utah, Salt Lake City, UT, USA
Frederick Pei Li, 1940–2015, Professor of Clinical Cancer Epidemiology, Harvard, USA
Joseph F Fraumeni Jr, b. 1933, Director of the National Cancer Institute, MD, USA.
Henry T Lynch, 1928–2019, Professor of Cancer Research, Creighton University School of Medicine, Omaha, NE, USA.
Lawrence M Weiss, contemporary, pathologist, Aliso Viejo, Ca, USA.

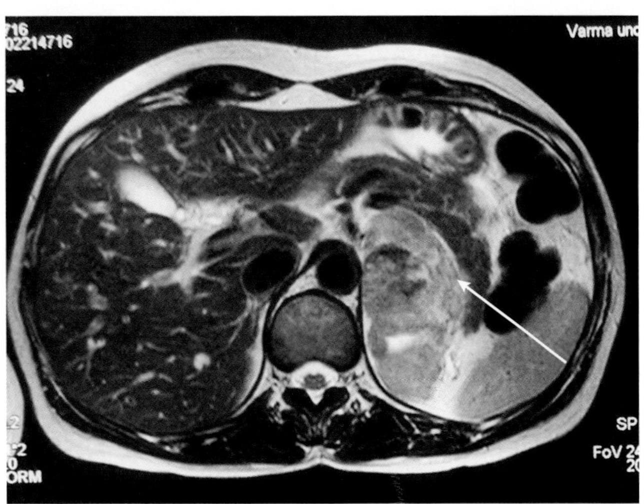

Figure 57.8 Magnetic resonance imaging of adrenocortical carcinoma (arrow) in a patient with cortisol and testosterone excess.

Radiology

ACC is often readily diagnosed on CT or MRI (*Figure 57.8*), where size (>6 cm), heterogeneous appearance and presence of necrosis are suggestive and local invasion and metastatic disease are diagnostic. Common sites of metastases are the lungs and liver, so staging should include the thorax. FDG-PET scanning is complementary and is advised to exclude occult metastatic disease in suspicious lesions. A maximum standard unit value (SUVmax) >40 or 1.5 times higher than the liver both suggest malignant tumours. The use of ^{11}C-metomidate PET may improve diagnostic accuracy but is not widely available. In terms of tissue diagnosis, adrenal biopsy is discouraged and fine-needle aspiration cannot distinguish benign from malignant tumours. Biopsy may have a role in patients with widespread metastatic disease at presentation to guide palliative systemic treatment.

Biochemistry

Glucocorticoid excess should be excluded by careful history and examination, followed by low-dose overnight DST. Serum levels of adrenal androgens (DHEAS, androstenedione, testosterone, 17-hydroxyprogesterone) and serum oestradiol in men and postmenopausal women should also be measured. In patients who are hypertensive, the aldosterone–renin ratio should be measured along with the serum potassium. Steroid precursors can be measured in 24-hour urine collections and may demonstrate a particular pattern on mass spectrometry although use is not widespread at present. Lastly, 24-hour urine or plasma metanephrines should be measured in all patients to exclude PCC.

Treatment

Surgery

Successful R0 resection of the tumour should be the aim of surgery and offers the best chance of cure for the patient. Preoperative assessment should therefore focus on determining whether any adrenal tumour is potentially malignant as this will guide the operative strategy. Treatment should take place in a multidisciplinary setting in a unit with experience of treating this rare disease. Patients with cortisol excess should be given perioperative hydrocortisone. At presentation, there are three common scenarios:

- **Indeterminate or probably malignant tumour <6 cm**: laparoscopic adrenalectomy may be feasible in this situation, but if there is evidence of local invasion on imaging or suspicion of it at laparoscopy open surgery is mandated.
- **Indeterminate or probably malignant tumour >6 cm**: laparoscopic surgery is not advised. In this scenario open radical resection must be undertaken, if necessary *en bloc* with involved adjacent organs (see ***Surgery of the adrenal glands***).
- **Indeterminate or probably malignant tumour <6 cm with synchronous metastatic disease**.

For **limited metastatic disease**, open resection of the tumour and intra-abdominal metastases is advised. For distant disease, resection of the primary followed by adjuvant systemic or surgical treatment of metastases is appropriate.

For **widespread metastatic disease**, initial surgery is no longer routinely advised. Instead, palliative treatment with mitotane with or without chemotherapy should be pursued. If there is significant disease regression after 3–6 months, surgery may then become an option.

More rarely, patients present with locally advanced disease with tumour extension into the great vessels. In this situation, it is recommended that such patients are referred to centres with experience of treating these cases.

Oncological treatment

Patients at high risk of recurrence (size >5 cm, Ki-67 >10%, tumour rupture at surgery, tumour thrombus) and those with metastatic disease should commence mitotane therapy as soon as possible (for up to 5 years) as this has been shown to improve disease-free and overall survival. Palliative EDP (etoposide–doxorubicin–cisplatin) chemotherapy may also be an option if there is disease progression despite mitotane therapy. Unless there is ongoing steroid excess, all patients treated with mitotane should receive oral hydrocortisone replacement therapy.

According to the European Network for the Study of Adrenal Tumours (ENSAT) classification, the 5-year, disease-specific survival rates for ACC are: 82% in stage I (tumour <5 cm; T1N0M0), 61% in stage II (tumour size >5 cm; T2N0M0), 50% for stage III (tumour of any size with at least one of the following factors: tumour infiltration in surrounding tissues [T3], tumour invasion into tumour thrombus in the vena cava or renal vein [T4], positive lymph nodes [N1] but no distant metastases) and 13% for stage IV (distant metastases) (see ***Further reading***).

Metastases

Definition

Adrenal metastases are not uncommon and often portend disseminated incurable disease. Primary tumours that commonly spread to the adrenals include lung, renal, gastric, breast and colorectal cancers.

Diagnosis

The decision regarding surgical intervention must be multidisciplinary and in conjunction with the patient, following careful diagnostic work-up to determine whether it is an isolated adrenal metastasis (seen most often with renal, lung and colorectal primaries) or a more widespread metastatic picture. Patients should therefore undergo CT thorax, abdomen and pelvis and PET-CT to exclude disease at other sites. They should also be screened for catecholamine and cortisol excess to exclude a coincident hormonally active tumour.

Treatment

If disease is widespread, metastasectomy will not usually be appropriate and systemic or palliative treatment should be the norm. Adrenal metastasis diagnosed at presentation (synchronous disease) should be removed if ipsilateral to a renal cell cancer (radical nephrectomy). In the case of other primary tumours, it should be observed with interval scanning at 3–6 months; if the lesion remains stable and isolated, resection should be considered. If adrenal metastasis arises more than 6 months after initial treatment (metachronous), PET-CT should be performed to exclude widespread disease; if the lesion is solitary, excision can be considered.

Surgery

Laparoscopic adrenalectomy is the preferred surgical option. Metastases often induce a significant desmoplastic reaction that can make excision more difficult, particularly when lesions are >4 cm. If there is evidence of local invasion, but the surgery is likely to improve survival, open surgery and *en bloc* excision may be appropriate. Note that, in the setting of previous nephrectomy with adrenalectomy, excision of an affected contralateral adrenal gland will render the patient steroid dependent.

Congenital adrenal hyperplasia (adrenogenital syndrome)

Virilisation and adrenal insufficiency in children are pathognomonic of congenital adrenal hyperplasia (CAH). This is an autosomal recessive disorder caused by a variety of enzymatic defects in the synthetic pathway of cortisol and other steroids from cholesterol. The most frequent defect (95%) is the 21-hydroxylase deficiency, which has an incidence of 1 in 5000 live births. Excessive ACTH secretion secondary to the loss of cortisol leads to an increase in androgenic cortisol precursors and to CAH. CAH may present in girls at birth with ambiguous genitalia or as late-onset disease at puberty. Hypertension and short stature, caused by the premature epiphyseal plate closure, are common signs. Affected patients are treated by replacement of hydrocortisone and fludrocortisone. Large hyperplastic adrenals may need to be removed if symptomatic.

ADRENAL INSUFFICIENCY

Adrenal insufficiency may be primary, secondary or tertiary. Primary insufficiency (Addison's disease) is due to adrenocortical disease, whereas secondary and tertiary insufficiency arise from pituitary and hypothalamic pathology, respectively. Addison's disease most commonly occurs when there is autoimmune (70–90%) or tuberculous destruction of the adrenal cortex and results in glucocorticoid and mineralocorticoid insufficiency. This is in contrast to secondary disease (lack of ACTH) and tertiary disease (lack of CRH secretion), where

TABLE 57.1 Causes and classification of adrenal insufficiency.

Cause of adrenal insufficiency	Pathophysiology	Type of AI
Autoimmune adrenalitis (polyglandular autoimmune syndromes)	Serum antibodies against the steroidogenic enzymes	Primary AI
Infective tuberculous disease	Caseating granulomatous destruction	
Bilateral adrenal infarction	Severe bacterial sepsis in children, e.g. meningococcal septicaemia[a]	
Bilateral adrenal haemorrhage	Traumatic obstetric delivery	
Malignancy	Infiltration by secondary cancers	
Congenital adrenal hyperplasia (adrenogenital syndrome)	Genetic disorders of steroidogenesis	
Pituitary destruction	Infarction, trauma, haemorrhage or infiltration, e.g. craniopharyngioma	Secondary AI
Cessation of chronic glucocorticoid therapy	Zona fasciculata and reticularis atrophy owing to long-term CRH suppression by exogenous corticosteroids	Tertiary AI
Treatment of Cushing's syndrome and Cushing's disease	CRH suppression following removal of ACTH-secreting or cortisol-secreting tumours	
Hypothalamic disorders	Trauma, stroke, tumour infiltration, radiation, infection	

ACTH, adrenocorticotropic hormone; AI, adrenal insufficiency; CRH, corticotropin-releasing hormone.
[a]Waterhouse–Friderichsen syndrome.

Thomas Addison, 1795–1860, physician, Guy's Hospital, London, UK, described the effects of disease of the suprarenal capsules in 1852.
Rupert Waterhouse, 1873–1958, physician, Royal United Hospital, Bath, UK, described this syndrome in 1911.
Carl Friderichsen, 1886–1979, Medical Superintendent, Sundby Hospital, Copenhagen, Denmark, gave his account of the syndrome in 1918.

only glucocorticoid deficiency ensues and aldosterone secretion (under control of the renin–angiotensin system) is spared. The causes are summarised in *Table 57.1*.

Acute adrenal insufficiency (adrenal or Addisonian crisis)

This is a medical emergency. Owing to its non-specific features (shock with some or all of the following: fever, nausea, vomiting, abdominal pain, hypoglycaemia and electrolyte imbalance), it can be difficult to diagnose. It is also rapidly fatal unless prompt and appropriate treatment is instituted early in its course. Typically there is a precipitating illness that may unmask longstanding adrenal insufficiency or a history of trauma or severe sepsis that result in adrenal haemorrhage or infarction (Waterhouse–Friderichsen syndrome), respectively. Because intestinal symptoms and fever are frequent, Addisonian crisis may often be misdiagnosed as an acute abdominal emergency.

Chronic adrenal insufficiency

Patients with chronic adrenal insufficiency may also be difficult to diagnose because symptoms appear insidiously over time. They may experience anorexia, weakness and nausea and, in the case of primary adrenal insufficiency, hyperpigmentation of the skin and oral mucosa because of the loss of negative feedback on secretion of ACTH and POMC. Hypotension, hyponatraemia, hyperkalaemia and hypoglycaemia are commonly observed due to the deficiency of mineralocorticoids.

Diagnosis

The diagnosis of adrenal insufficiency relies on demonstrating cortisol deficiency and then determining whether this is ACTH dependent or independent by performing an ACTH stimulation test (synacthen test). Blood is drawn for basal ACTH and cortisol. If both are low, the diagnosis is secondary or tertiary adrenal insufficiency. If the ACTH is high and the cortisol is low, the cause is adrenal disease (primary adrenal insufficiency). Synacthen testing is used because it is the quickest way to determine if there is any adrenal function; adrenal function is present for some after the onset of pituitary or hypothalamic disease, whereas there will be no response when the adrenal glands are diseased.

Treatment

If acute adrenal insufficiency is suspected, treatment must be commenced immediately while the results of confirmatory testing are awaited. Blood should be drawn for plasma ACTH, serum cortisol, plasma renin activity and aldosterone and therapy with intravenous saline and hydrocortisone should be commenced. A typical regime would consist of a 100-mg bolus of intravenous hydrocortisone followed by 50 mg intravenous hydrocortisone 6-hourly and 2–3 litres of 0.9% saline in 6 hours, with careful cardiovascular monitoring to prevent fluid overload. Concomitant infections, which are frequently present, should also be treated. Fluids and steroids are then tapered as the patient stabilises.

Chronic adrenal insufficiency is treated by replacement therapy with daily oral hydrocortisone (15–25 mg orally in two or three divided doses) and fludrocortisone (0.05–0.2 mg each morning orally). Patients must be advised about the need to take lifelong glucocorticoid and mineralocorticoid replacement therapy. To prevent an Addisonian crisis, patients must be aware of the need to double the dose in cases of illness or stress ('sickness day rules'). If patients with adrenal insufficiency are scheduled for surgery, appropriate steroid cover must be administered.

ADRENAL HAEMORRHAGE

Definition

Adrenal haemorrhage is a serious condition that can result in adrenal insufficiency, shock, acute adrenal crisis and mortality if not managed with adequate treatment. The adrenal glands are, per weight of tissue, one of the most vascular tissues in the body. A number of factors predispose to haemorrhage, including infection (sepsis), myocardial infarction, anticoagulants, trauma, surgery and antiphospholipid syndrome. Clinical presentation can vary from non-specific abdominal pain to adrenal insufficiency or hypovolaemic shock.

Investigation

CT scanning is the most common way to diagnose the condition (*Figure 57.9a*).

Management

Most adrenal bleeds are successfully managed conservatively. Anticoagulation therapy should be stopped temporarily. Rarely, interventional radiology may be necessary to staunch the bleed (*Figure 57.9b*). In cases of bilateral haemorrhage, the possibility of adrenal insufficiency should be considered.

DISORDERS OF THE ADRENAL MEDULLA AND DIFFUSE NEUROENDOCRINE SYSTEM

Phaeochromocytoma and paraganglioma

Definition

Tumours that arise from the neuroectodermal tissue of the adrenal medulla are termed phaeochromocytomas (PCCs) and those arising from the extra-adrenal parasympathetic and sympathetic ganglia are termed paragangliomas (PGLs). PCCs and PGLs are collectively abbreviated to PPGL.

PGLs are either parasympathetic or sympathetic. Parasympathetic PGLs are sited mainly in the head and neck (HNPGLs) and 95% do not secrete catecholamines or other hormones. The common types of HNPGL are carotid body, vagal and jugulotympanic. Sympathetic PGLs usually secrete catecholamines.

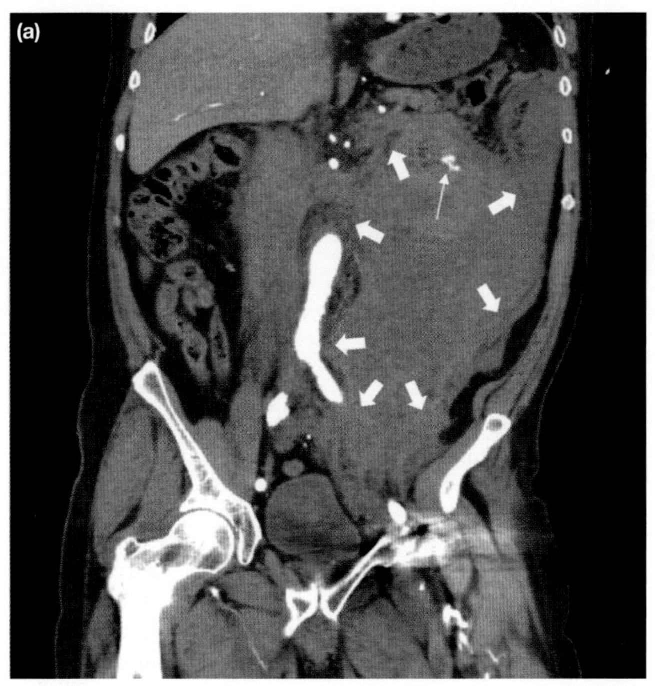

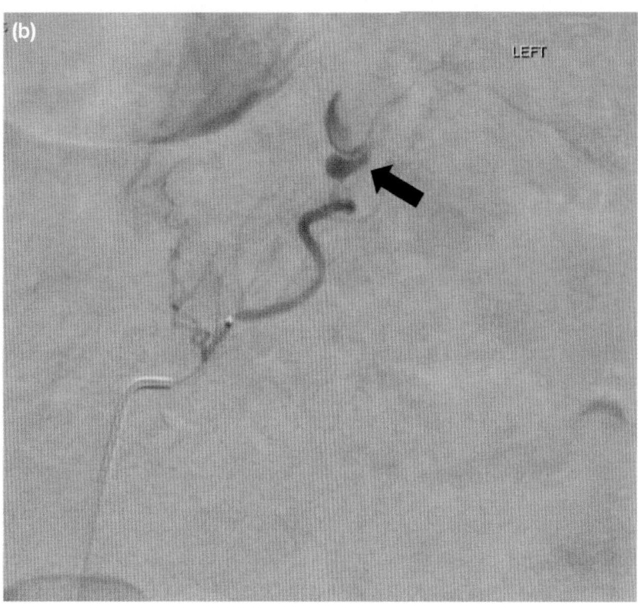

Figure 57.9 (a) Massive left retroperitoneal haematoma (edges outlined by wide white arrows) secondary to left adrenal haemorrhage (contrast extravasation marked by thin white arrow). (b) Selective catheterisation of the left middle adrenal artery demonstrating extravasation (seen in (a)). The bleeding was arrested with injection of gel foam and coils.

Incidence

The incidence of PCC is about 0.6 in 100 000 and 75% are thought to be sporadic. The incidence of sporadic PGL is not known, but is less common than PCC, and the association with hereditary conditions is more common. Overall, about 70% of PPGLs are sporadic and the rest occur as part of inherited endocrine tumour syndromes, which include:

- hereditary PPGL syndromes
- MEN 2
- von Hippel–Lindau disease (VHL)
- neurofibromatosis type 1 (NF1)

Hereditary PPGL syndromes

These are associated with germline mutations in genes, including succinate dehydrogenase (SDH) subunits, Myc-associated protein X (MAX) and transmembrane protein 127 (TMEM127) (*Table 57.2*). Loss-of-function mutations in SDH lead to accumulation of Krebs cycle precursors, which act as oncometabolites. Loss-of-function TMEM127 and MAX mutations result in PPGL development through cell death escape and enhanced survival. *SDHB* gene variants account for the majority of secreting PGLs whereas *SDHD* mutations account for the majority of non-secreting HNPGLs. Affected individuals are regularly surveilled with annual blood tests and 3-yearly MRI (neck and or abdomen).

von Hippel–Lindau disease

An autosomal dominant disease characterised by central nervous system and retinal haemangiomas (60–80%), renal cysts (50–70%), clear cell renal cell carcinoma (30%), pancreatic neuroendocrine tumours (P-NETs) (8–17%), PPGL (20%), endolymphatic sac tumours (6–15%) and epididymal/broad ligament cyst adenoma (50%). VHL is defined by its genotype as type I (deletions) without PPGL and type II (missense mutations), which is associated with PPGL. Patients develop PCC much more frequently than PGL. VHL tumours overproduce only noradrenaline.

Neurofibromatosis type 1

This is a syndrome characterised by the development of café-au-lait spots (100%), axillary freckling (90%), neurofibromas (84%), Lisch nodules of the iris (70%), typical osseous lesions (14%) and optic glioma (4%). PPGL (PCC 96%) are found in 7% of affected patients. *NF-1* is a tumour-suppressor gene and loss-of-function mutations lead to cell proliferation and cancer development.

Pathology

PCCs are greyish-pink on the cut surface and are usually highly vascularised. Areas of haemorrhage or necrosis are often observed. Microscopically, tumour cells are polygonal but the configuration varies considerably. Approximately 10% of

Eugen von Hippel, 1867–1939, Professor of Ophthalmology, Göttingen, Germany.
Arvid Lindau, 1892–1958, Professor of Pathology, Lund, Sweden.
Sir Hans Adolf Krebs, 1900–1981, German-born British biologist, physician and biochemist, his discovery of the citric acid (Krebs) cycle earned him the Nobel Prize in Physiology or Medicine in 1953.
Karl Lisch, 1907–1999, Ophthalmologist, Wörgl, Austria.

TABLE 57.2 Hereditary PPGL syndromes.

Gene	Distinguishing clinical features				
	PGL versus PCC	Bilateral PCC or multiple PGL	Biochemical phenotype	Malignancy risk	Mode of inheritance
MAX	PCC	• 60% bilateral	Mixed	25%	Possibly paternal
SDHA	PGL, PCC	Single	Mixed	Low	AD
SDHAF2	HNPGL	• 90% multiple	Unclear	Low	Paternal[a]
SDHB	PGL	• 20% multiple	Noradrenaline/ normetanephrine	34–97%	AD
SDHC	PGL	• 20% multiple	Noradrenaline/ normetanephrine	Low	AD
SDHD	HNPGL and PGL	• 50% multiple	Noradrenaline/ normetanephrine, often silent	<5%	Paternal[a]

AD, autosomal dominant; HNPGL, head and neck paraganglioma; PCC, phaeochromocytoma; PGL, paraganglioma; PPGL, collective term for PCCs and PGLs.
[a]Only mutations inherited from the father will result in the development of tumours.

PCCs are malignant. The differentiation between malignant and benign tumours is difficult, except when metastases are present. An increased PASS (phaeochromocytoma of the adrenal gland scale score), a high number of Ki-67-positive cells, vascular invasion or a breached capsule all lean more towards malignant rather than benign.

PCCs may also produce calcitonin, ACTH, vasoactive intestinal polypeptide (VIP) and parathyroid hormone-related protein (PTHrP). In patients with MEN 2, the onset of PCC is preceded by adrenomedullary hyperplasia, sometimes bilateral. PCC is rarely malignant in MEN 2 (3–5%) but often malignant with *SDHB* mutations (50%).

Clinical presentation

Functioning PPGLs typically present with symptoms and signs of catecholamine excess, and these are typically intermittent (***Table 57.3***). In total, 90% of patients with the combination of headache, palpitations and sweating in the presence of an adrenal tumour have a PCC. Paroxysms may be precipitated by physical training, induction of general anaesthesia and numerous drugs and agents (contrast medium, tricyclic antidepressant drugs, metoclopramide and opiates). Hypertension may occur continuously, be intermittent or absent.

HNPGLs present with the side effects arising from their local mass effect (e.g. neck mass, dysphonia or tinnitus).

TABLE 57.3 Range and incidence of symptoms from PPGL.

Symptoms	Prevalence (%)
Hypertension	80–90
Paroxysmal	50–60
Continuous	30
Headache	60–90
Sweating	50–70
Palpitation	50–70
Pallor	40–45
Weight loss	20–40
Hyperglycaemia	40
Nausea	20–40
Psychological effects	20–40

PPGL, collective term for phaeochromocytomas and paragangliomas.

Diagnosis

Biochemical

The diagnosis of PPGL is confirmed by elevated catecholamine metabolites (metanephrines) in plasma and/or raised 24-hour urinary excretion of fractionated metanephrines. Metanephrines are produced as a result of intratumour conversion of catecholamines by the enzyme catecholamine-*O*-methyltransferase. Measurement of plasma and urinary metanephrines is more sensitive (99% and 97%, respectively) than plasma and urinary catecholamine measurement (86% and 84%, respectively). Measurements of one or more of these substances that are four times greater than the upper limit of the reference range are 100% diagnostic. Plasma dopamine can be regarded as a marker of tumour burden in malignant PPGL.

Radiological

Once a biochemical diagnosis is established, imaging by CT or MRI is undertaken to determine tumour location and assess its size and risk of malignancy. Size is not a predictor of malignancy for PCC. Malignant PPGLs are diagnosed by the presence of local invasion or metastatic disease. Tumours appear vascular and frequently possess cystic areas or central necrosis (***Figure 57.10***). If initial imaging is negative or reveals extra-adrenal disease, functional investigation with ^{123}I-MIBG (meta-iodobenzylguanidine; 80–90% sensitive) or ^{111}In-octretide scanning (50–70% sensitive) is undertaken

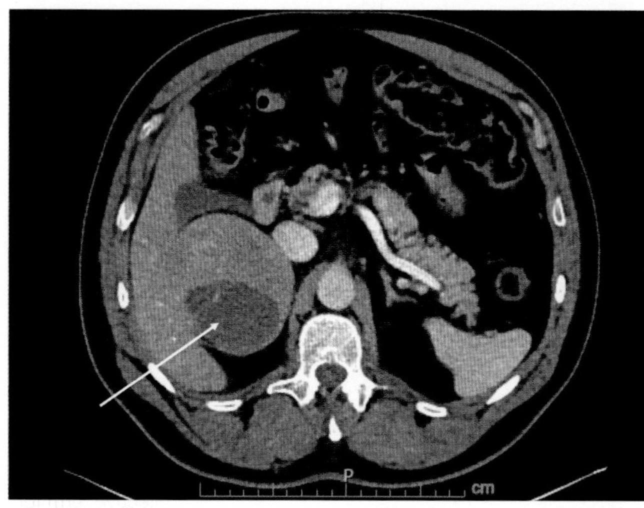

Figure 57.10 A cross-section computed tomography scan of a large phaeochromocytoma showing characteristic central necrosis (arrow).

(*Figure 57.11*). Routine use is not advocated in well-localised adrenal lesions. More recently, 6-[^{18}F]fluorodopamine PET scanning has shown promise, particularly in the setting of PGLs, where conventional imaging and MIBG scanning are negative.

Medical management

Biochemical diagnosis and localisation of PPGLs should be followed by medical preparation to control blood pressure and prompt surgical excision.

Preoperative control of blood pressure

Once a PCC has been diagnosed, an α-adrenoceptor blocker (phenoxybenzamine) is used to block the effects of catecholamine excess and its consequences during surgery. With adequate medical pretreatment, the perioperative mortality rate has decreased from 20–45% to less than 3%. A dose of 20 mg of phenoxybenzamine initially should be increased daily by 10 mg until a daily dose of 100–160 mg is achieved and the

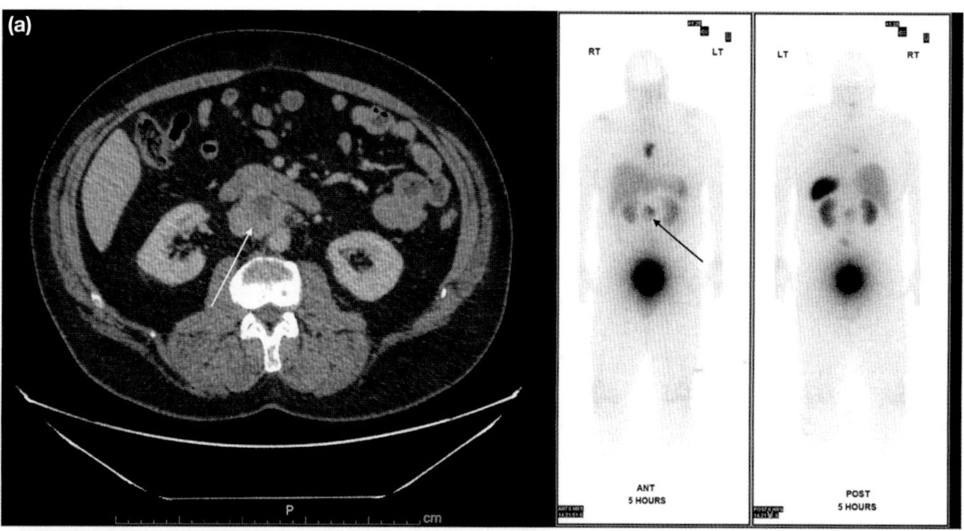

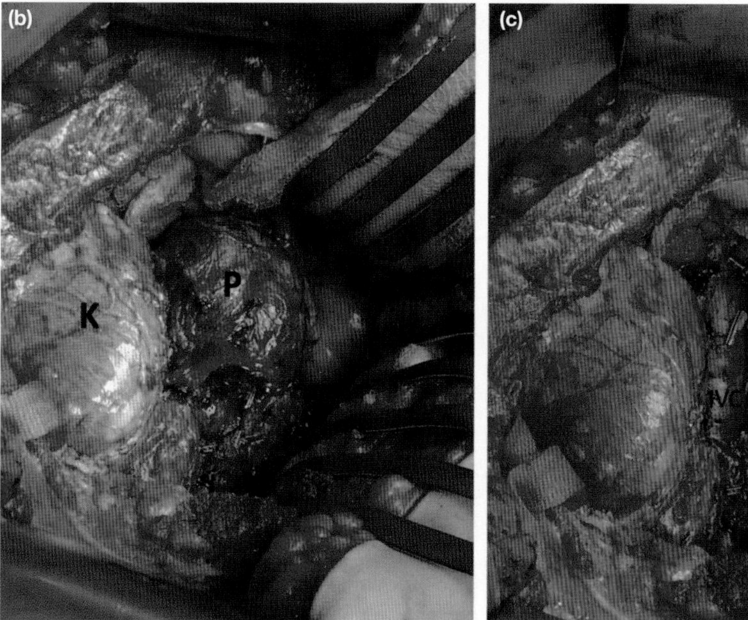

Figure 57.11 (a) A cross-section computed tomography scan showing a paraganglioma anterior to the abdominal aorta (white arrow) and an ^{111}In-octretide scan demonstrating uptake by the tumour (black arrow). Operative photographs before (b) and after (c) extraction of the tumour. AA, abdominal aorta; IVC, inferior vena cava; K, right kidney; P, paraganglioma.

patient reports symptomatic postural hypotension. Additional β-blockade is required if tachycardia or arrhythmias develop; this should not be introduced until the patient is α-blocked. Other regimens have been described, e.g. α-blockade with doxazosin or prazosin, with and without β-blockade, using calcium channel blockers alone and using the catecholamine synthesis blocker metyrosine in the setting of cardiac failure. However, familiarity and experience with a particular pharmacological regime are probably more important than the regime itself. At this point surgery is safe to proceed.

With adequate α-blockade preoperatively, anaesthesia should not be more hazardous than in patients with a non-functioning adrenal tumour; however, in some patients, dramatic changes in heart rate and blood pressure may occur and require sudden administration of pressor or vasodilator agents. A central venous catheter and invasive arterial monitoring are used. Special attention is required when the adrenal vein is ligated as a sudden drop in blood pressure may occur. The infusion of large volumes of fluid or administration of noradrenaline can be necessary to correct postoperative hypotension in the presence of unopposed α-blockade.

Postoperative care

Patients should be observed for 24 hours as hypovolaemia and hypoglycaemia may occur. Lifelong yearly biochemical tests should be performed to identify recurrent, metastatic or metachronous PCC.

Surgical treatment

PPGLs are excised by either laparoscopic or open surgery.

Adrenalectomy for phaeochromocytoma

Laparoscopic resection is now routine in the treatment of PCC. If the tumour is larger than 10 cm or radiological signs of malignancy are detected, an open approach should be considered.

Surgery for paraganglioma

Tumours along the sympathetic chain can be technically challenging owing to their posterior relationship to the great vessels and visceral arterial branches, which may hide smaller lesions. Furthermore, hereditary PGLs are associated with increased risk of local recurrence. For this reason, minimally invasive surgery may not be feasible; open surgery is the preferred option.

Special circumstances

Malignant phaeochromocytoma. Surgical excision is the only chance for cure. If there is direct invasion, laparotomy and *en bloc* excision of involved adjacent organs offers the best chance of cure. In the presence of metastases, excision of the primary tumour is still recommended to improve symptom control and improve the efficacy of adjuvant radiolabelled MIBG and octreotide therapy. The natural history is highly variable with a 5-year survival rate of less than 50%.

Phaeochromocytoma in pregnancy. PCC in pregnancy may be silent and present as a hypertensive emergency or it may mimic an amnion infection syndrome or pre-eclampsia. Without adequate α-blockade, mother and unborn child are threatened by a hypertensive crisis during delivery. In the first and second trimesters the mother should be scheduled for laparoscopic adrenalectomy after adequate α-blockade; the risk of a miscarriage during surgery is high. In the third trimester, elective caesarean with delayed consecutive adrenalectomy 6 weeks later should be performed. The maternal mortality rate is 50% when a PCC remains undiagnosed.

Neuroblastoma

Definition

Neuroblastoma (NB) is the most common and deadliest solid extracranial malignancy in children. It is derived from the primitive nerve cells (neuroblasts) of the sympathetic nervous system, derived from the neural crest. It is often termed the 'clinical enigma' as the prognosis ranges from spontaneous regression to treatment resistance, metastasis and death.

Incidence

NB accounts for 7% of all childhood cancers, with an incidence of 10 per million children under the age of 15 years.

Pathology

The tumour arises from neuroblasts populating the adrenal medulla and sympathetic ganglia in other sites. Forty per cent of NBs are adrenal in origin. The histopathological diagnosis is established from immunohistochemistry (neurofilaments, synaptophysin and neurone-specific enolase). Biopsy tissue is also analysed for genetic alterations. Genomic amplification of *MYCN* is reported in 25% of tumours and is the strongest predictor of poor prognosis. There are many other chromosome arm-level alterations, notably deletion of 1p and 11q and gain of 17q. There is current interest in the analysis of circulating analytes (so-called 'liquid biopsy'), which is less invasive and can be repeated over the therapeutic course.

Clinical presentation

Most (40%) present under the age of 1 year, 35% between ages 1 and 2 years and 25% older than 2 years. Many present with signs and symptoms related to tumour growth or they may be incidental ultrasonographic findings. Presenting symptoms include malaise and/or pain or obstruction of veins or lymphatics or hydronephrosis. Acute or subacute paraplegia can develop from spinal cord or nerve root involvement. Many children (70%) have metastases at the time of presentation. Rarely the tumour secretes VIP, which results in diarrhoea, dehydration and hypokalaemia.

Diagnosis

NBs may secrete catecholamines, leading to elevated 24-hour urinary metanephrines. Serum lactate dehydrogenase is a useful tumour marker. An unequivocal diagnosis is from histology of either the tumour or bone marrow aspirate. Imaging is undertaken to stage the disease using CT or MRI and MIBG (*Figure 57.12*). In children with regional or metastatic disease, biopsy is necessary for diagnosis and prognostication.

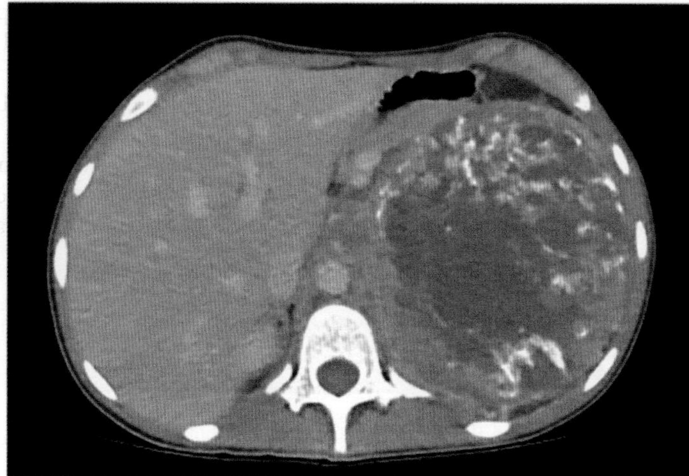

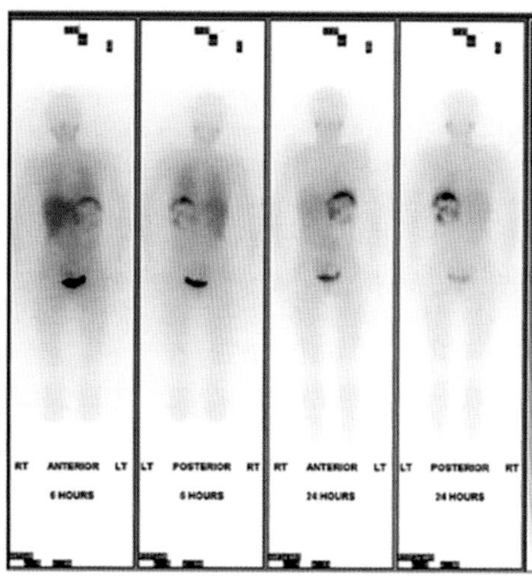

Figure 57.12 Huge left-sided neuroblastoma with central necrosis on computed tomography scan and MIBG (meta-iodobenzylguanidine) scan.

Treatment

Prognosis can be predicted by the tumour stage and the age at diagnosis. Patients are classified as low, intermediate or high risk. Low-risk patients are treated by surgery alone whereas intermediate-risk patients are treated by surgery with adjuvant multiagent chemotherapy. For those patients with localised disease, surgical resection is curative. Postchemotherapy surgery may be performed for complete resection. Patients assigned to the low-risk, intermediate-risk and high-risk groups have overall 3-year survival rates of 90%, 70–90% and 30%, respectively.

Ganglioneuroma

Definition

Ganglioneuromas (GNs) are benign differentiated tumours of neural crest-derived cells in the autonomic nerves.

Incidence

GNs are rare, affecting one per million of the population. Most are sporadic but they can be associated with neurofibromatosis type II and MEN 2B.

Pathology

GNs are benign and are most often located in the mediastinum (20%), retroperitoneum (10%) and adrenal gland (30%). However, GNs can arise anywhere sympathetic nervous tissue is found, such as tongue, bladder, uterus, bone and skin. They are composed of an admixture of ganglion cells and Schwannian stroma/cells.

Clinical presentation

GNs develop in childhood but typically present later as they are non-secreting and slow growing. Two-thirds of patients are under the age of 20 years. They are usually asymptomatic and are identified incidentally. When large, GNs may cause local pressure symptoms such as abdominal pain or bloating. Occasional reports of elevated metanephrines exist and the differential diagnosis is PCC.

Diagnosis

Once a mass is discovered CT and MRI are usually performed to characterise the lesion. They are well defined with a capsule and calcification may be present. GN has a low T1- and a high T2-weighted signal on MRI. Radiology cannot definitively diagnose a GN; histology is required and so preoperative diagnosis can be challenging.

Treatment

Excision is the treatment of choice. A laparoscopic approach is preferred. The prognosis is excellent as recurrences are rare.

SURGERY OF THE ADRENAL GLANDS

Since its description in the 1990s by Gagner, laparoscopic adrenalectomy has become the gold standard in the resection of adrenal tumours, except for tumours with signs of malignancy. Since then, the retroperitoneoscopic modification of the posterior open approach described by Walz has gained popularity. The transperitoneal laparoscopic approach offers a better view of the adrenal region than open surgery and, because the anatomy is more familiar, it is more commonly employed. However, the retroperitoneoscopic approach requires less dissection because it is extraperitoneal; it is most advantageous in patients with small and/or bilateral tumours, e.g. inherited disease. For adrenal surgery as a whole, the mortality rate is less than 0.5% but is higher in the setting of malignant adrenal tumours. The open anterior approach should be undertaken if there are radiological signs of invasion, limited metastases,

Theodore Schwann, 1810–1882, Professor of Anatomy, Leuven, Belgium.
Michel Gagner, b. 1960, Professor of Surgery, Montreal, Canada.
Martin K Walz, contemporary, Professor of Surgery, Essen, Germany.

large tumours (>8–10 cm) or a distinct hormonal pattern to suggest malignancy. To avoid steroid dependence, subtotal adrenalectomy is an option in patients with bilateral tumours provided they are small (<3 cm). It is important to emphasise that these excellent outcomes depend on an experienced surgical team and close liaison with endocrinology colleagues to ensure that any hormonal excess is identified preoperatively, controlled to render surgery safe then supplemented if needed in the postoperative period.

Minimally invasive adrenalectomy

Transperitoneal laparoscopic adrenalectomy

Familiarity with the anatomy of the adrenal region is essential and it should be noted that the approaches for the right and left sides are distinct. Careful haemostasis is essential as small amounts of blood impair the view; direct grasping of the adrenal tissue/tumour should be avoided to reduce the risk of capsular rupture.

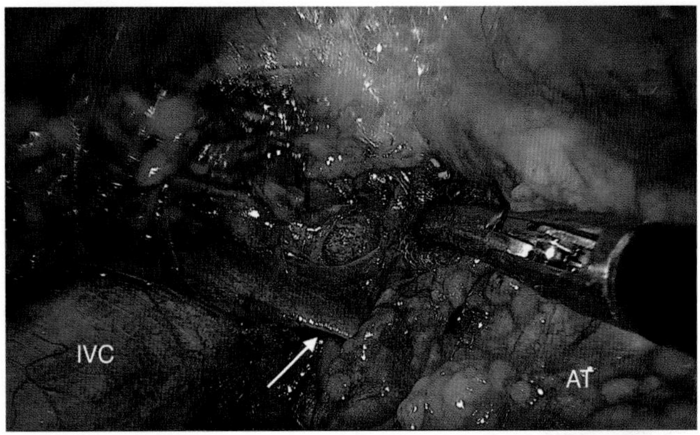

Figure 57.13 View of the right adrenal vein draining (arrow) into the inferior vena cava (IVC) during posterior retroperitoneoscopic adrenalectomy (courtesy of Fausto Palazzo, Hammersmith Hospital, London, UK). AT, adrenal tumour.

Right transperitoneal laparoscopic adrenalectomy

The patient is positioned right side up, with table break. Four ports are used. The liver is retracted cranially and the peritoneal fold between the liver and the tumour is divided from the lateral border of the IVC to the right triangular ligament with the preferred energy device. The peritoneum is then opened caudally along the lateral border of the IVC to the upper renal pole. This allows the tumour to be retracted laterally; the space between it and the IVC is developed, in the process exposing the short right adrenal vein. At this point the posterior abdominal wall (quadratus lumborum) is visible. The vein is clipped and divided and the inferior and lateral attachments are divided and the tumour is removed in a tissue retrieval bag.

Left transperitoneal laparoscopic adrenalectomy

The patient is positioned left side up, with table break. Three ports are used. In the initial phase, the aim is to perform a limited medial visceral rotation of the splenic flexure of the colon, spleen and pancreatic tail. This is achieved by dividing the lateral peritoneal attachments of the colon and the anterior layer of the lienorenal ligament cranially, a distance of 1 cm from the spleen, until the gastric fundus is visible. Further dissection and gravity allow the spleen and pancreatic tail to 'fall' medially to expose the kidney/perinephric fat, covered in Gerota's fascia. The fascia is opened to allow identification of the adrenal vein as it drains into the left renal vein. Once the vein has been clipped and divided, the tumour is retracted away from the renal hilum and resection is completed by mobilising the adrenal gland along its superior, inferior and lateral borders. The inferior phrenic tributary of the adrenal vein may be encountered and is dealt with by clipping. The tumour is then placed in a tissue retrieval bag for removal.

Posterior retroperitoneoscopic adrenalectomy

This technique may be favoured when there has been extensive upper abdominal surgery or for reoperative adrenalectomy (being outside the abdominal cavity affords a better view) as well as for bilateral adrenalectomy. It may not be feasible with larger tumours (>5–6 cm) and in the very obese patient (body mass index >40). The patient is placed prone with the hips and knees flexed to abolish the lumbar lordosis. The first port is placed at the distal end of the 12th rib with a combination of scissor and digital dissection into the retroperitoneum. Gerota's fascia is swept off the posterior abdominal wall and space is made for insertion of the medial (10 mm) and lateral (5 mm) ports, which are inserted with finger guidance. A balloon port is then inserted into the initial port and CO_2 insufflated to 20–25 mmHg; a 30° endoscope is used. Gerota's fascia is opened, avoiding a peritoneal rent laterally. Dissection continues through the perirenal fat to the superior renal pole. The tumour is then mobilised along its lateral and medial borders. The medial border of a right-sided tumour is dissected off the IVC to expose the right adrenal vein, which can then be ligated and divided (*Figure 57.13*). On the left side, the adrenal vein is located at the medial inferior pole of the adrenal gland. After venous ligation, the superior attachments are divided to excise the tumour. The inflation pressure is then reduced to check for haemostasis before tumour extraction with a tissue retrieval bag.

Open adrenalectomy

This operation should be performed when a malignant adrenal tumour is suspected, or for very large tumours (>8–10 cm). In the case of adrenocortical cancer, the aim is to remove the tumour in continuity with any invaded adjacent organs *en bloc* and obtain negative resection margins (R0). Consequently, if there is a risk or intention to perform nephrectomy, splenectomy, distal pancreatectomy or limited right hemihepatectomy, the patient should be consented (and, in the case of splenectomy, vaccinated) accordingly. Similarly, a multidisciplinary approach should be employed for tumours that are invading the liver or IVC. Surgical access is via a rooftop incision extending to the appropriate flank, with Mercedes-Benz extension if necessary. On the right, the hepatic flexure of the colon is mobilised, the

The **Mercedes-Benz** sign takes its name from the insignia displayed on the bonnet of a Mercedes-Benz car.

TABLE 57.4 Characteristics of pancreatic neuroendocrine tumours.

Tumour (syndrome)	Incidence (%)	Presentation	Malignancy (%)
Insulinoma	70–80	Weakness, sweating, tremor, tachycardia, anxiety, fatigue, dizziness, disorientation, seizures	<10
Gastrinoma	20–25	Intractable or recurrent peptic ulcer disease (haemorrhage, perforation), complications of peptic ulcer, diarrhoea	60–90
Non-functional tumours	30–50	Obstructive jaundice, pancreatitis, epigastric pain, duodenal obstruction, weight loss, fatigue	60–90
VIPoma	4	Profuse watery diarrhoea, hypotension, abdominal pain	40–70
Glucagonoma	4	Migratory necrolytic skin rash, glossitis, stomatitis, angular cheilitis, diabetes, severe weight loss, diarrhoea	50–80
Somatostatinoma	<5	Cholelithiasis, diarrhoea, neurofibromatosis	>70
Carcinoid	<1	Flushing, sweating, diarrhoea, oedema	60–90
ACTHoma	<1	Cushing's syndrome	>95
GRFoma	<1	Acromegaly	Unknown

ACTH, adrenocorticotropic hormone; GRH, growth hormone-releasing factor; VIP, vasoactive intestinal polypeptide.

duodenum Kocherised and, if the tumour extends cranially, the right liver lobe is mobilised to achieve optimal exposure of the IVC and tumour. Dissection is from lateral to medial and then along the lateral border of the IVC, inferior to and including the kidney if that is involved. On the left side the adrenal gland can be exposed after mobilisation of the splenic flexure of the colon. If invasion of the pancreas is suspected, distal pancreatectomy is performed with or without splenectomy. If not, they are medially rotated as for the transperitoneal laparoscopic operation. The retroperitoneum is then dissected lateral to medial, including the kidney if necessary, and then along the lateral border of the left crura and cranially towards the diaphragm. If pancreatectomy is performed, a drain should be left to manage a potential pancreatic fistula.

PANCREATIC NEUROENDOCRINE TUMOURS

Introduction

As with neuroendocrine cells in the intestine, pancreatic neuroendocrine cells are believed to be derived from pluripotent stem cells that differentiate into endocrine cells. From these, tumours may arise that are known as P-NETs. They are a heterogeneous group of tumours with diverse morphologies and behaviour. Non-functioning tumours constitute a substantial proportion of all P-NETs (25–100%). The subtypes of P-NET are listed in *Table 57.4*. This section focuses on insulinoma, gastrinoma and non-functioning tumours because they represent 90% of all P-NETs.

Physiology of the endocrine pancreas

The endocrine cells of the pancreas are grouped in the islets of Langerhans, which constitute approximately 1–2% of the mass of the pancreas (*Figure 57.14*). There are about 1 million islets in a healthy adult human pancreas and their combined weight is 1–1.5 g. There are four main types of cell in the islets of Langerhans, which can be classified according to their secretions:

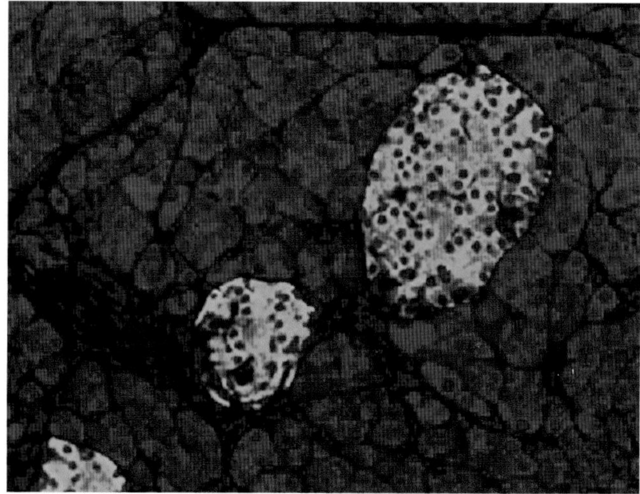

Figure 57.14 Immunofluorescent labelling of endocrine (insulin [green]) and exocrine (amylase [red]) pancreatic cells and the nuclear marker DAPI (4′,6-diamidino-2-phenylindole; blue) (courtesy of Dr Esni, Department of Surgery, University of Pittsburgh, USA).

1. β cells producing insulin (65–80% of the islet cells);
2. α cells producing glucagon (15–20%);
3. δ cells producing somatostatin (3–10%);
4. pancreatic polypeptide (PP) cells containing polypeptide (1%).

Theodor Kocher, 1841–1917, Professor of Surgery, Berne, Switzerland, awarded the Nobel Prize in Physiology or Medicine in 1909.
Paul Langerhans, 1847–1888, Professor of Pathological Anatomy, Freiberg, Germany.

Insulinoma

Definition

This is an insulin-producing tumour of the pancreas.

Incidence

These are rare tumours with an incidence of four (1–32) per million. Insulinomas have been diagnosed in all age groups, with the highest incidence found in the fourth to the sixth decades. Women seem to be slightly more frequently affected.

Pathology (including prognosis)

The aetiology of insulinomas is unknown. They are equally scattered throughout the pancreas. Tumours are graded according to World Health Organization (WHO) NET criteria (*Table 57.5*). Tumours <2 cm in diameter without signs of invasion are considered benign. More than 90% are both benign and solitary. Approximately 10% are associated with MEN 1.

TABLE 57.5 World Health Organization neuroendocrine tumour (NET) classification of tumour grades.

Grade	Mitoses/10 HPFs	Ki-67 index
Grade 1 NET	<2	<3
Grade 2 NET	2–20	3–20
Grade 3 NET (well differentiated with high proliferative index)	>20	>20
NEC (poorly differentiated NEC)	>20	>20

HPF, high-power field; NEC, neuroendocrine carcinoma.

Clinical presentation

Patients typically develop sporadic symptoms of neuroglycopenia. Classically these manifest while fasting or during exercise, but some (18%) may develop symptoms postprandially and these may be the only symptoms. Some patients develop loss of consciousness and coma. The release of catecholamines produces symptoms such as sweating, weakness, hunger, tremor, nausea, anxiety and palpitations. The diagnosis can be elusive owing to its rarity and it is not uncommon for patients to have been investigated for epilepsy (fitting, loss of consciousness) or drug abuse (altered mental state) before the correct diagnosis is established. It is typical that patients will have put on weight prior to presentation (learning to eat to survive).

Diagnosis (with differential)

The cornerstone of diagnosis remains Whipple's triad:

- symptoms induced by fasting;
- hypoglycaemia at the time of symptoms;
- symptoms relieved by administration of glucose.

The key test is a 72-hour fast looking for documented endogenous hyperinsulinism in association with symptoms and signs of low plasma glucose (<3.0 mmol/L), elevated insulin and high C-peptide. If the test is negative and the suspicion of insulinoma is high, a prolonged oral glucose tolerance test is done.

Differential diagnoses include postprandial syndrome after gastrointestinal surgery, dumping syndrome, factitious hypoglycaemia, ethanol ingestion and pancreatic transplantation. Nesidioblastosis is a rare disorder, mainly encountered in children, that is characterised by replacement of normal pancreatic islets by diffuse hyperplasia of islet cells.

After a positive fast test, a CT or MRI is performed. In only a small percentage (<5–10%) insulinomas are elusive on cross-sectional imaging. In such a situation endoscopic ultrasonography (EUS) is undertaken with a positive detection rate in excess of 90%. Visceral angiography with arterial stimulation venous sampling is reserved for negative EUS studies or when more than one lesion has been identified. Another promising method is scintigraphy with radiolabelled glucagon-like peptide 1, which is often overexpressed by insulinomas. However, this is not universally available. MEN 1 should be considered in younger patients and those with multiple lesions. Chromogranin A is not a useful test for this tumour.

Treatment (medical and surgical)

Patients require treatment because of their symptoms.

Surgery

Most insulinomas are small, sporadic and solitary. In most cases enucleation is possible. Contraindications to enucleation are close proximity to the main pancreatic duct and larger tumours. In most cases a laparoscopic approach is recommended for localised tumours and this achieves a high success rate (98–100%). Postoperatively, blood sugar levels begin to rise in most patients within the first few hours after removal of the tumour. To preserve pancreatic function and reduce the risk of iatrogenic diabetes mellitus, patients in whom tumour localisation is not successful at operation should not undergo blind resection.

For patients with MEN 1, tumours may be multifocal. The classical approach was to enucleate tumours in the 'right' pancreas (dictated by the portal vein) and perform a distal pancreatectomy owing to the high number of non-functioning NETs associated with the mutation. Laparoscopic enucleation of localised tumours has become the procedure of choice.

Medical

All patients undergoing surgery should be treated with diazoxide, which suppresses insulin secretion by direct action on the β cells, and receive frequent small meals to avoid hypoglycaemia. Somatostatin analogue (SSA) therapy may also be useful.

For patients with unresectable or metastatic disease, SSAs and everolimus are effective in controlling hypoglycaemia. Other options include chemotherapy, peptide receptor radionuclide therapy (PRRT) and chemoembolisation.

George Hoyt Whipple, 1878–1976, Professor of Pathology, University of Rochester, Rochester, NY, USA, described this disease in 1907. He shared the 1934 Nobel Prize in Physiology or Medicine with George Richards Minot and William Parry Murphy 'for their discoveries concerning liver therapy against anaemias'.

Gastrinoma

Definition

Zollinger–Ellison syndrome (ZES) is a condition that includes: (i) fulminating ulcer diathesis in the stomach, duodenum or atypical sites; (ii) recurrent ulceration despite 'adequate' therapy; and (iii) non-β islet cell tumours of the pancreas (gastrinoma).

Incidence

This is a rare disease affecting between 0.5 and 4 in a million. Approximately 0.1% of patients with duodenal ulcers have evidence of ZES. Up to 20–25% of ZES is associated with MEN.

Pathology

In sporadic disease the tumours are mostly located in the duodenum (60–80%) and are small (<5 mm) and multiple. In MEN 1, all tumours are in the duodenum. The vast majority (approximately 90%) occur within the 'gastrinoma triangle', an area bounded by the junction of the neck and body of the pancreas medially, the junction of the second and third parts of the duodenum inferiorly and the junction of the cystic and common bile ducts superiorly (***Figure 57.15***). Tumours are graded according to WHO NET criteria (***Table 57.5***). In general, the progression of gastrinomas is relatively slow with a 5-year survival rate of 65% and a 10-year survival rate of 51%. Patients with complete tumour resection have excellent 5- and 10-year survival rates (90–100%). Patients with pancreatic tumours have a worse prognosis than those with primary tumours in the duodenum. There is no established marker to predict the biological behaviour of gastrinoma.

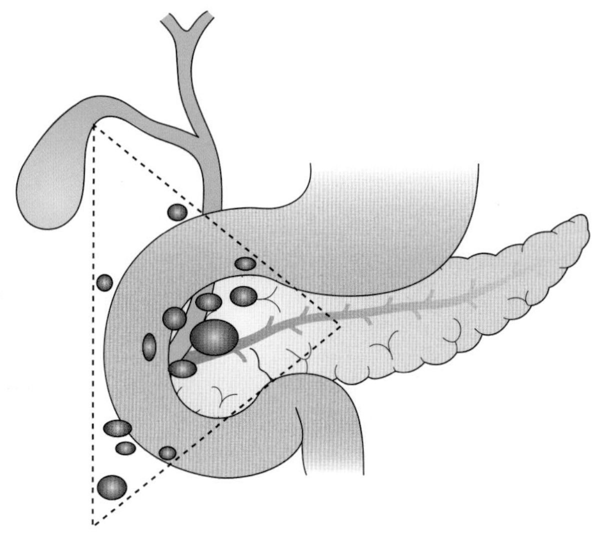

Figure 57.15 The gastrinoma triangle.

Clinical presentation

Over 90% of patients with gastrinomas have peptic ulcer disease, often multiple or in unusual sites. Diarrhoea is another common symptom, caused by the large volume of gastric acid secretion. Abdominal pain from either peptic ulcer disease or gastro-oesophageal reflux disease remains the most common symptom, occurring in more than 75% of patients. Around 60–95% have a history of high alcohol use, which may be a risk factor. The majority of tumours have metastasised by the time of presentation.

Diagnosis (with differential)

The cornerstone of diagnosing ZES is an elevated fasting serum gastrin (FSG). If elevated, the gastric pH is measured. If the pH is <2 and the FSG is more than 10-fold elevated, the diagnosis is confirmed. If the FSG is less than 10-fold higher, a secretin provocation test should be performed. The diagnosis is becoming more difficult because of unreliability of some commercial gastrin assays and the widespread use of proton pump inhibitors (PPIs), which not only increases the pH of the stomach but also leads to inappropriate elevation of FSG in the presence of hypergastrinaemia when gastric acid secretion is present.

Hypergastrinaemia is seen in atrophic gastritis, PPI therapy and *Helicobacter pylori* infections and so all conditions feature in the differential diagnosis. Once a diagnosis is confirmed all patients are screened for MEN 1 (biochemical and genetic).

Localisation studies are then indicated as the tumours are often small and multiple. The majority of gastrinomas have a high density of somatotropin receptors. ^{68}Ga-labelled SSAs with PET-CT have been found to be sensitive and specific. If not available, somatostatin scintigraphy (SRS) and EUS should be done. Chromogranin A is an unreliable test for gastrinoma.

Treatment

Surgery

All patients with sporadic gastrinoma without metastases should have a surgical operation by an experienced surgeon. At the time, the peritumoral lymph nodes should be sampled for histological assessment.

In MEN 1/gastrinoma, surgery is not recommended for patients with tumours <2 cm. Tumours >2 cm are enucleated. Parathyroidectomy reduces gastric acid secretion.

Medical

PPI therapy is the management of choice. Even when patients undergo a surgical cure, most (60%) require continued medical treatment. For patients with advanced locoregional disease or metastases, PPI remains the first-line treatment supplemented with SSA therapy. In refractory cases, locoregional ablative therapy (radiofrequency ablation or chemoembolisation) or PRRT may be effective.

Robert Milton Zollinger, 1903–1992, Professor of Surgery, The Ohio State University, Columbus, OH, USA.
Edwin Homer Ellison, 1918–1970, Professor of Surgery, Marquette University, Milwaukee, WI, USA. Zollinger and Ellison described this condition in a joint paper in 1957 when they were both working at The Ohio State University.

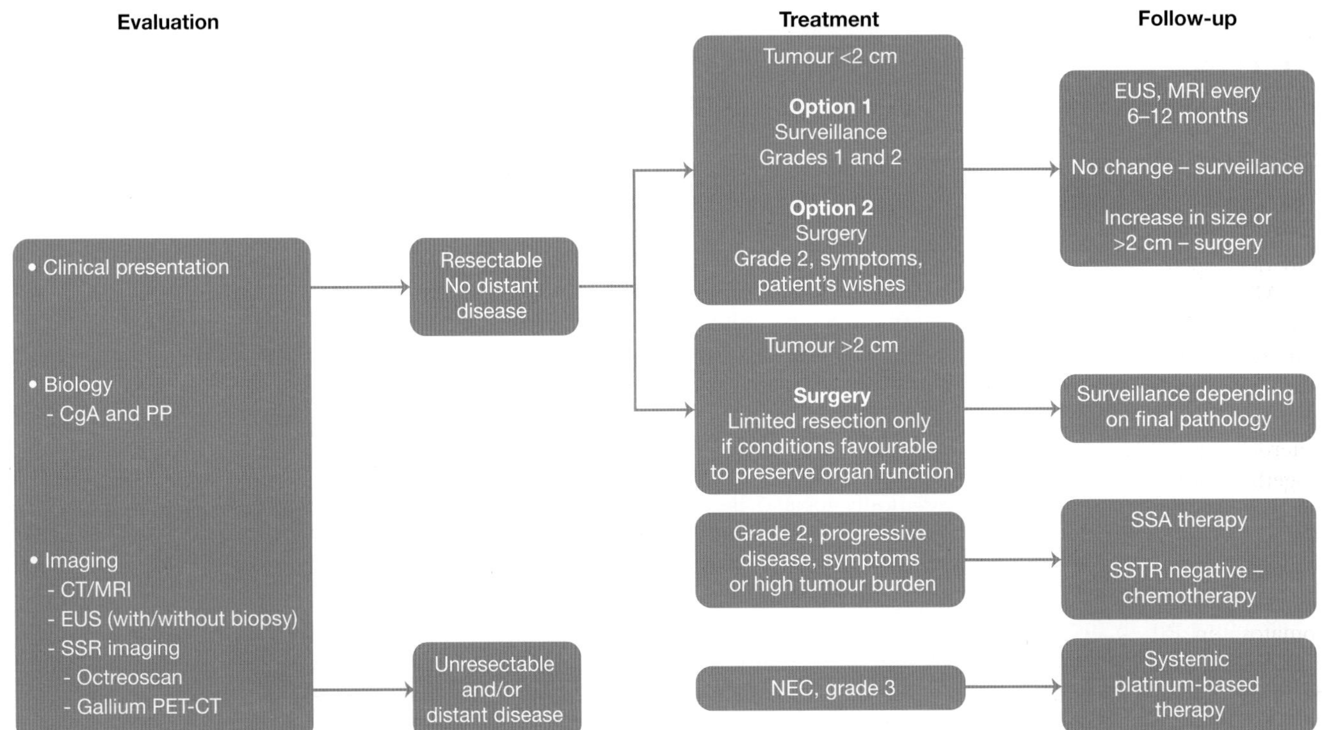

Figure 57.16 Algorithm for the investigation and management of non-functioning pancreatic neuroendocrine tumours. CgA, chromogranin A; CT, computed tomography; EUS, endoscopic ultrasonography; MRI, magnetic resonance imaging; NEC, neuroendocrine carcinoma; PET, positron emission tomography; PP, pancreatic polypeptide; SSA, somatostatin analogue; SSR, somatostatin scintigraphy; SSTR, somatostatin receptor.

Non-functioning pancreatic neuroendocrine tumours

Definition

P-NETs are clinically classified as non-functioning (NF-P-NET) when they do not cause a clinical syndrome.

Incidence

NF-P-NETs account for 60–90% of all P-NETS.

Pathology

NF-P-NETs cannot be distinguished from functional tumours by immunocytochemistry because they may also express hormones such as gastrin and insulin. They usually stain positively for chromogranin A and synaptophysin. The tumours are usually large (>5 cm) and unifocal except in MEN 1 syndrome. They are distributed throughout the pancreas with a head to body to tail ratio of 7:1:1.5.

Clinical presentation

They are generally diagnosed at a more advanced stage owing to their indolent nature, slow growth and lack of functional secretion causing a delay in the onset of symptoms. Therefore, in contrast to functioning PETs, patients with NF-PETs present with various non-specific symptoms, including jaundice, abdominal pain, weight loss and pancreatitis. In some cases liver metastases are the first presentation.

Diagnosis

Increased levels of chromogranin A and PP are usual. The majority of these tumours are large and are easily identified by transabdominal ultrasonography or CT scanning. Differentiation from the more aggressive pancreatic adenocarcinoma is extremely important (see *Chapter 72*). Recognition of NF-P-NETs is imperative because of their resectability and excellent long-term survival compared with their exocrine counterparts.

Treatment (medical and surgical)

For grade 1 and 2 unresectable tumours, SSAs may be effective because of their antiproliferative properties. Alternatively novel targeted drugs (everolimus and sunitinib) could be considered. Platinum-based chemotherapy is the treatment of choice for grade 3 and NEC tumours. The algorithm for the management is summarised in *Figure 57.16*.

NEUROENDOCRINE TUMOURS OF THE STOMACH AND SMALL INTESTINE

Embryology and physiology

The embryology of the intestine is developed from the foregut, midgut and hindgut. The bronchus and lungs are also developed from the foregut. Throughout these tissues are APUD neuroendocrine cells. In the stomach they were described by Kulchitsky and are recognised as neuromodulating cells with serotonin (5-hydroxytryptamine [5-HT]) as their main neurotransmitter. These cells play a crucial role in intestinal motility and secretion. Within the gastric pits are enterochromaffin-like (ECL) cells that secrete histamine. Together with gastrin, these cells are critical in the regulation of gastric acid secretion. All cells of the system secrete different neuroendocrine markers, such as synaptophysin, chromogranin A and neurone-specific enolase, and produce peptide hormones that are stored in granules, e.g. serotonin, somatostatin, PP (pancreatic polypeptide) or gastrin. In clinical practice chromogranin A is utilised as a tumour marker. The main functional test for NETs of the jejunum and ileum (the NETs that are most often encountered) is measurement of the serotonin metabolite 5-hydroxyindoleacetic acid (5-HIAA) in urine.

Gastrointestinal neuroendocrine tumours (GI-NETs) were formerly divided into foregut (stomach, duodenum and pancreas), midgut (small intestine, appendix and caecum) and hindgut carcinoids (large bowel except caecum and rectum). Nowadays, the definition of NET does not consider the organ of origin; instead, a common definition is used that is based on the tissue of origin and histological factors such as the Ki-67 index or mitotic index and size according to the WHO criteria (*Table 57.5*).

Pathogenesis

Historically, tumours arising from the neuroendocrine cells were referred to as 'karzinoide' (carcinoma-like) tumours by Oberndorfer. Now they are termed neuroendocrine tumours (NETs). NETs can be either benign or malignant.

In the gastrointestinal tract, especially the small intestine, they secrete excess 5-HT, which is rapidly metabolised by the liver. In the presence of liver metastases, NET metastases secrete 5-HT into the IVC, avoiding hepatic first-pass metabolism and leading to symptoms of 5-HT excess, known as **carcinoid syndrome**. The cardinal features are sweating, flushing, bronchospasm and restrictive cardiomyopathy secondary to fibrotic right heart valvular disease (Hedinger syndrome).

The overall incidence of GI-NETs is 2.5–5.0 per 100 000 people per year, with a much higher prevalence of 35 per 100 000. Their relative distribution in the gastrointestinal tract is shown in *Table 57.6*.

TABLE 57.6 Relative distribution of neuroendocrine tumours in different organs.

Site	Distribution (%)
Lung	10
Stomach	5
Duodenum	2
Small bowel	25
Appendix	40
Colon	6
Rectum	15

Stomach

Incidence

These are rare with an incidence of 0.2 per 100 000 population per year.

Pathology

There are three types:

1. Type I polyps: associated with atrophic gastritis with high pH and gastrin levels.
2. Type II polyps/small tumours (<1 cm): arise secondary to small gastrinoma with low gastric pH and high gastrin levels (ZES).
3. Type III: these are larger tumours (>1–2 cm), associated with low gastrin.

Types I and II are derived from ECL cells. Type III are almost always malignant and are treated like gastric adenocarcinoma, although liver metastases are common at the time of presentation.

Clinical presentation

Type I (70–80%) are usually found at gastroscopy in the investigation of vague dyspeptic symptoms. Type II (5%), ZES (see ***Pancreatic neuroendocrine tumours***), presents with multiple and complicated peptic ulcers. Type III (15–25%) typically present with bleeding or discomfort.

Diagnosis

Upper intestinal endoscopy is the gold standard with biopsy of identified lesions. EUS is pivotal in measuring tumour depth. Staging is done with CT, SRS or ^{68}Ga-DOTATOC PET.

Treatment

Medical

Type I is managed with vitamin B12 and type II with PPIs with or without endoscopic resection of all visible tumours. Patients are then subjected to annual endoscopic surveillance.

Surgical

Absolute indications for surgery include:

Nikolai Kulchitsky, 1856–1925, Professor of Histology, Kharkov Imperial University, Ukraine.
Siegfried Oberndorfer, 1876–1944, Professor of Pathology, Munich, Germany.
Christoph Hedinger, 1917–1999, pathologist, Zurich, Germany.

- local excision of type I polyps >10 mm;
- a visualised gastrinoma;
- type III gastric NET.

Duodenum

Incidence

These are exceptionally rare tumours, accounting for 1–3% of all GI-NETs.

Pathology

They are usually small (<20 mm) and submucosal. They can be functional (gastrin, somatostatin) or non-secreting. Gastrinoma is often associated with MEN 1.

Clinical presentation

Gastrinoma presents as per type II gastric NETs or as part of MEN 1. Somatostatinoma is associated with NF-1 and gallstones.

Diagnosis (including staging)

Gastrin will be elevated in gastrinoma and low in other cases. Chromogranin A is often elevated for all NETs. Identification and staging is achieved using a combination of endoscopy, EUS, CT and SRS. Patients must be screened for genetic disease.

Treatment (medical and surgical)

PPI therapy successfully manages gastrinoma. In the presence of MEN 1, parathyroidectomy reduces gastric acidity. Duodenal gastrinomas are often elusive and can be successfully managed with PPIs. However, when localised and in the absence of lymph node metastases, resection is the treatment of choice, either endoscopically or by open surgery (see *Further reading*).

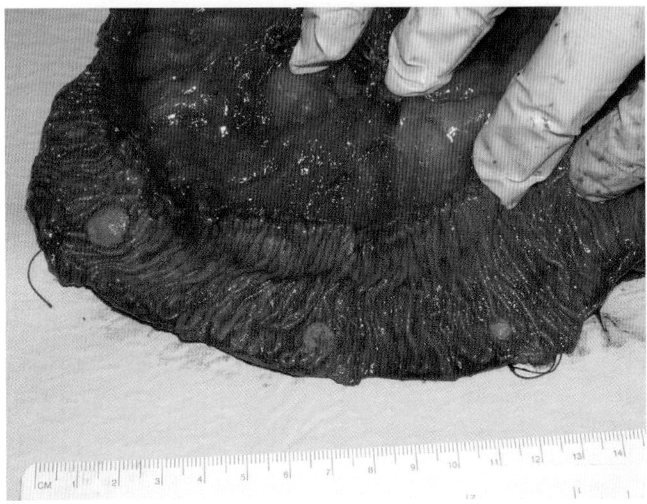

Figure 57.17 Multiple neuroendocrine tumours in the small bowel.

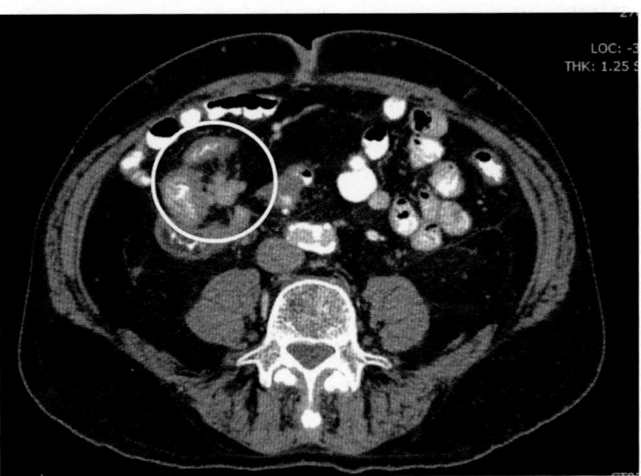

Figure 57.18 Contrast-enhanced (bowel) cross-sectional computed tomography scan with mesenteric lymph node metastasis drawing in the adjacent mesenteric vessels in the desmoplastic reaction (white circle).

Small intestine

Incidence

Midgut carcinoids are the most common NETs with a peak age of diagnosis at 60–70 years. They are the second most common small bowel malignancy.

Pathology

They arise from the enterochromaffin cells and secrete serotonin and substance P. They are either solitary or multiple (30%) (*Figure 57.17*) and the primary tumour can be small (5–20 mm). They are often indolent but often discovered at an advanced stage when regional (lymph nodes; 36%) and distant (liver; 48%) disease is present. From the latter, the patient may develop carcinoid syndrome.

Clinical presentation

Chronic abdominal pain is the most frequent initial symptom. The carcinoid syndrome is seen in 20–30% of patients with liver metastases. Small bowel ischaemia producing pain and diarrhoea arises from involved lymph node metastases, which constrict the mesenteric vessels. However, up to 20% of patients are diagnosed during the investigation of liver metastases or they may be incidentally found during surgery for another reason (laparotomy or appendicectomy).

Diagnosis

Chromogranin A is often elevated (non-specific) and elevated 24-hour urinary 5-HIAA is specific. Cross-sectional CT or MRI often shows the mesenteric lymph nodes with a characteristic spiralling of vessels trapped in the desmoplastic reaction (*Figure 57.18*) and will demonstrate if liver metastases are present. Biopsy is diagnostic and Ki-67 grading is an important prognostic factor and is mandatory for reporting. This is often via an ultrasound-guided liver biopsy. In the search for a primary tumour, CT and/or MRI is followed by ^{68}Ga-DOTATOC PET, fused with CT.

Patients must be evaluated for the presence of Hedinger syndrome (right heart valve fibrosis). A referral is made to the cardiology department, where transthoracic echocardiography will be carried out.

Summary box 57.3

Stratified treatment of NETs based on stage

Disease status	Localised	Regional	Distant		
Stage	I/II	III (N1)	IV (M1)		
Surgical approach	Radical resection		Radical – curative intent	Palliative resection	No resection
	Resection of • primary • nodes (along mesentery)		Resection of • primary • nodes (along mesentery) • liver metastases	Resection of • primary • nodes (along mesentery) • liver metastases	Due to • irresectable • comorbidities
Aim	R0		R0	To avoid obstructive complications (R1)	

Treatment

ENETS (European Neuroendocrine Tumor Society) has developed an algorithm for the treatment of small intestine NETs (*Summary box 57.3*).

Surgical

Patients without distant metastases (stages I–III) are all potential candidates for curative surgery of the primary tumour and regional nodal metastases. All patients should be discussed in a multidisciplinary team meeting. Surgery is only undertaken if it is thought that an R0 resection can be achieved. The limiting factor is often lymph node involvement around the superior mesenteric artery, especially in the presence of severe desmoplastic reaction. Concomitant cholecystectomy should be considered owing to the risk of gallstone formation secondary to SSAs.

In the presence of stage IV (metastatic disease) surgery is contemplated when the patient has obstructive symptoms (palliative) or if an R0 resection (curative) can be achieved with concomitant liver metastasectomy(ies). In this setting, patients should have peroperative protection with intravenous SSAs to avoid a carcinoid crisis.

When curative intent is not possible, there are a number of locoregional therapies to the liver. Patients are always treated with SSAs to prevent a crisis. Therapeutic options include radiofrequency ablation, embolisation and chemoembolisation. Liver transplantation is only considered in a highly selected population (see also *Chapters 69 and 74*).

Medical

SSAs are an effective treatment for syndrome control for functional NETs. SSAs may also be used for antiproliferative purposes in stable or progressive disease in tumours up to a Ki-67 index of 10% (grades I and II). Loperamide or other similar agents may be useful in the control of diarrhoea. When SSA treatment fails, a second-line option is PRRT. Currently yttrium- or lutetium-labelled SSAs are most frequently used. For grade III tumours (NEC), cisplatin-based systemic chemotherapy is the treatment of choice.

Appendiceal carcinoid

Incidence

Appendiceal NETs are the commonest neoplasm in the appendix (30–80%). They are diagnosed in 3–5 in 1000 appendicectomies for acute appendicitis.

Pathology

They are classified in the same way as other NETs. Staging is determined by tumour size and involvement of either the subserosa or mesoappendix (T) as well as nodal (N) and distant metastases (M).

Treatment

Tumours <10 mm in size have an excellent prognosis and appendicectomy achieves cure. A right hemicolectomy should be considered in the rare situations of positive or unclear margins or deep mesoappendiceal invasion (>3 mm). An oncological right hemicolectomy should be performed for tumours >20 mm. Low-risk tumours do not require any follow-up (see also *Chapter 76*).

MULTIPLE ENDOCRINE NEOPLASIA

MEN is a group of heterogeneous disorders characterised by a predisposition of benign and malignant tumours involving two or more endocrine glands. There are four varieties, the most common being MEN 1 and MEN 2.

Multiple endocrine neoplasia type 1

Epidemiology and genetics

MEN 1 is an autosomal dominant inherited disorder. It was originally called Wermer's syndrome. It is rare (1 in 30 000) in the general population but accounts for 10% of primary hyperparathyroidism (PHPT) in patients under 30 years and 30–40% of all cases of gastrinoma. The tumour-suppressor gene *MEN1* encodes for menin, a protein that regulates transcription, cell division and proliferation. The pathophysiology

Paul Wermer, 1898–1975, physician, The Presbyterian Hospital, New York, NY, USA, described this condition in 1954.

consists of a two-hit methodology: a germline mutation followed by a second-hit somatic mutation in the specific tissues. There are many hundreds of germline mutations of *MEN1* on chromosome 11, but there is no genotype/phenotype association.

Clinical presentation

The manifestations of MEN 1 are listed in *Table 57.7*. Virtually all patients develop PHPT (see *Chapter 56*). In screening programmes, non-functioning P-NETs are seen in up to 70% of patients. The most common functioning P-NET is gastrinoma, followed by insulinoma. The remainder are extremely rare. Most pituitary tumours are microadenomas and are either non-functioning or secrete prolactin. The latter can be treated medically.

TABLE 57.7 Clinical manifestations of multiple endocrine neoplasia type 1 (MEN 1).

Tumour site	Frequency (%)
PHPT (four-gland disease)	95
Pancreatic islet cell tumours • Gastrinoma • NF-P-NET • Insulinoma • Glucagonoma • VIPoma • Somatostatinoma	30–80
Pituitary tumours • Prolactin (60%) • Growth hormone (25%) • ACTH (5%) • Non-functioning	15–50
Adrenocortical tumours – mainly non-functioning	40–50
NET lung, thymus, stomach	3–10
Lipomas	5–10
MEN 1 is also associated with meningiomas and facial angiofibromas	

ACTH, adrenocorticotropic hormone; NET, neuroendocrine tumour; NF-P-NET, non-functioning pancreatic neuroendocrine tumour; PHPT, primary hyperparathyroidism; VIP, vasoactive intestinal polypeptide.

Surgery

MEN 1 PHPT treatment differs from sporadic disease because it is secondary to four-gland hyperplasia and so the surgical approach is always bilateral neck exploration. Whether to perform subtotal or total parathyroidectomy with autotransplantation is debatable. All patients should receive counselling about the inevitability of recurrent hyperparathyroidism. At the time of cervical surgery, a prophylactic thymectomy is also performed (see also *Chapter 56*).

Gastrinoma is typically managed medically for tumours <2 cm in diameter. Functioning P-NETs are excised as previously described, but the treatment of NF-P-NET is challenging owing to the widespread distribution of multiple tumours in the pancreas. A balance is sought between tumour resection and the preservation of endocrine function. Functional adrenal tumours in MEN 1 are rare and have to be operated on. Non-functioning tumours should be resected if they reach a size of 4 cm.

Multiple endocrine neoplasia type 2A

Epidemiology and genetics

MEN 2A has a prevalence of 1 in 25 000 people. It is an autosomal dominant condition caused by germline mutations in *RET*, which encodes a transmembrane tyrosine kinase receptor (TKR) that activates pathways involved in proliferation, survival, migration and angiogenesis. Gain-of-function *RET* mutations lead to activation of the TKR and cancer initiation through deregulated proliferation and increased cell survival. The mutation is sited in chromosome 10. There is a strong genotype–phenotype correlation, not seen in MEN 1.

Clinical presentation

The patterns of disease in MEN 2 are shown in *Table 57.8*. Nearly all patients develop medullary thyroid carcinoma (MTC), which is the determinant of survival in this syndrome. PCCs are more likely to be bilateral, but are rarely malignant. PHPT is usually mild and asymptomatic and may not need surgery. A subtype of MEN 2, known as familial MTC (FMTC), is a variant of MEN 2 in which MTC occurs in isolation. MTC combined with PCC alone is known as Sipple's syndrome.

TABLE 57.8 Genotype–phenotype associations for disorders arising from RET gene mutations.

Syndrome	Frequently affected *RET* gene codons	MTC (%)	PHPT (%)	PCC (%)
MEN 2A	609, 634, 790, 804	90–100	20–30	10–70
FMTC	533, 630, 768, 844	90–100	–	–
MEN 2B	883, 918	100	–	10–60

FMTC, familial medullary thyroid carcinoma; MEN, multiple endocrine neoplasia; MTC, medullary thyroid carcinoma; PCC, phaeochromocytoma; PHPT, primary hyperparathyroidism.

Multiple endocrine neoplasia type 2B

Epidemiology and genetics

This has a prevalence of 0.2 in 100 000. MEN 2B is also caused by *RET* mutations, half of which are *de novo*.

Clinical presentation

A variant of MEN 2 characterised by an aggressive and early-onset form of MTC (100%), PPGL (59%), marfanoid habitus and ganglioneuromatosis of the oral mucosa and gut (*Figure 57.19*). MTC is associated with rapid growth and a poor prognosis.

John H Sipple, b. 1930, physician, The State University of New York, Syracuse, NY, USA.

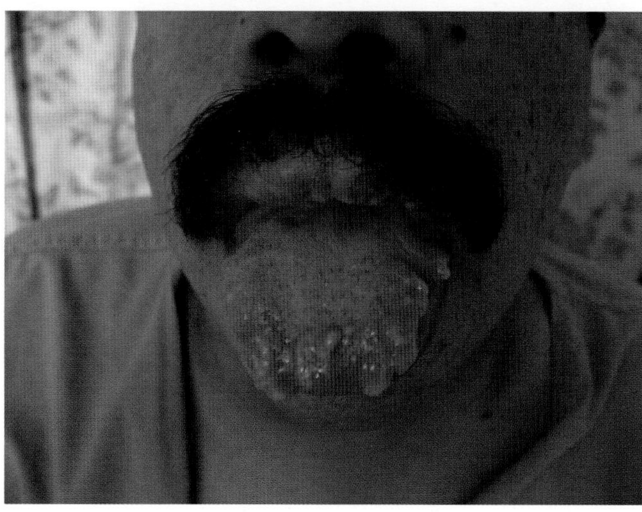

Figure 57.19 Ganglioneuromatosis of the oral mucosa in multiple endocrine neoplasia type 2B.

Surgery for MEN types 2A and 2B

Kindred of known MEN 2 patients are tested for the presence of a mutation. MEN 2B infants should undergo a thyroidectomy in the first year of life. Children who carry *MEN2* mutations are screened for calcitonin, which can detect the presence of the precursor to MTC – C-cell hyperplasia. This allows a thyroidectomy to be undertaken before invasive MTC has developed (so-called prophylactic thyroidectomy) (see also *Chapter 55*). Owing to the strong genotype–phenotype relationship, the specific mutations guide clinicians with regard to the timing of prophylactic surgery (*Table 57.9*).

TABLE 57.9 Risk of medullary thyroid carcinoma and genetic mutations in multiple endocrine neoplasia syndromes.

Risk level, codon	Age of *RET* testing	Age of required first calcitonin	Age of prophylactic surgery
D, 918; 804	As soon as possible, within first year of life	6 months if not already done	As soon as possible, within first year of life
C, 634	<3–5years	>3–5years	Before 5 years
B, 609, 611, 618, 620	<3–5years	>3–5years	Consider before 5 years, may delay
A, 833, 819, 891, 912	<3–5years	>3–5years	Between 10 and 15 years

Multiple endocrine neoplasia type 4

Described in 2006, this is an exceptionally rare autosomal dominant syndrome consisting of *MEN1*-associated tumours (parathyroid and pituitary) in association with tumours of the kidney, adrenal glands and reproductive organs. P-NETs have also been described. The disease is thought to be due to mutations in *CDNK1B*. Treatment is the same as for MEN 1.

FURTHER READING

Alesina PF, Hommeltenberg S, Meier B *et al.* Posterior retroperitoneoscopic adrenalectomy for clinical and subclinical Cushing's syndrome. *World J Surg* 2010; **34**: 1391–7.

American Thyroid Association Guidelines Task Force, Wells SA, Asa SL, Dralle H et al. Revised American Thyroid Association guidelines for the management of medullary thyroid carcinoma. *Thyroid* 2015; **25**: 567–610.

Andrew A, Kramer B, Rawdon BB. The origin of gut and pancreatic neuroendocrine (APUD) cells—the last word? *J Pathol* 1998; **186**: 117–18.

Bornstein SR, Allolio B, Arlt W *et al.* Diagnosis and treatment of primary adrenal insufficiency: an Endocrine Society clinical practice guideline. *J Clin Endocrinol Metab* 2016; **101**: 364–89.

Burton TJ, Mackenzie IS, Balan K *et al.* Evaluation of the sensitivity and specificity of (11)C-metomidate positron emission tomography (PET)-CT for lateralizing aldosterone secretion by Conn's adenomas. *J Clin Endocrinol Metab* 2012; **97**: 100–9.

Dekkers T, Prejbisz A, Kool LJS *et al.* Adrenal vein sampling versus CT scan to determine treatment in primary aldosteronism: an outcome-based randomised diagnostic trial. *Lancet Diabetes Endocrinol* 2016; **4**: 739–46.

Fassnacht M, Arlt W, Bancos I *et al.* Management of adrenal incidentalomas: European Society of Endocrinology clinical practice guideline in collaboration with the European Network for the Study of Adrenal Tumors. *Eur J Endocrinol* 2016; **175**: G1–34.

Fassnacht M, Dekkers O, Else T *et al.* European Society of Endocrinology clinical practice guidelines on the management of adrenocortical carcinoma in adults, in collaboration with the European Network for the Study of Adrenal Tumors. *Eur J Endocrinol* 2018; **179**: G1–46.

Fave GD, Delle Fave G, O'Toole D *et al.* ENETS consensus guidelines update for gastroduodenal neuroendocrine neoplasms. *Neuroendocrinology* 2016; **103**: 119–24.

Gagner M, Lacroix A, Bolté E. Laparoscopic adrenalectomy in Cushing's syndrome and pheochromocytoma. *N Engl J Med* 1992; **327**: 1033.

Nanba K, Omata K, Else T *et al.* Targeted molecular characterization of aldosterone-producing adenomas in white Americans. *J Clin Endocrinol Metab* 2018; **103**: 3869–76.

Omata K, Satoh F, Morimoto R *et al.* Cellular and genetic causes of idiopathic hyperaldosteronism. *Hypertension* 2018; **72**: 874–80.

Osswald A, Quinkler M, Di Dalmazi G *et al.* Long-term outcome of primary bilateral macronodular adrenocortical hyperplasia after unilateral adrenalectomy. *J Clin Endocrinol Metab* 2019; **104**: 2985–93.

O'Toole D, Kianmanesh R, Caplin M. ENETS 2016 consensus guidelines for the management of patients with digestive neuroendocrine tumors: an update. *Neuroendocrinology* 2016; **103**: 117–18.

Patel N, Egan R, Scott-Coombes D, Stechman M. Adrenalectomy in the UK: results from the British Association Endocrine and thyroid surgeons UKRETS database. *Eur J Surg Oncol* 2017; **43**: 2398.

Raff H, Sharma ST, Nieman LK. Physiological basis for the etiology, diagnosis, and treatment of adrenal disorders: Cushing's syndrome, adrenal insufficiency, and congenital adrenal hyperplasia. *Compr Physiol* 2014; **4**: 739–69.

Thiesmeyer JW, Ullmann TM, Stamatiou AT *et al.* Association of adrenal venous sampling with outcomes in primary aldosteronism for unilateral adenomas. *JAMA Surg* 2021; **156**: 165–71.

CHAPTER 58 The breast

Learning objectives

To understand:
- Appropriate investigation of breast disease
- Aberrations of Normal Development and Involution (ANDI) concept and management of benign breast disease
- Types and management of mastitis
- Modern management of breast cancer

COMPARATIVE AND SURGICAL ANATOMY

The breast in adult females overlies the pectoral region, extending from the second rib above to the sixth rib or inframammary crease below. Medially it extends to the lateral border of the sternum and laterally it reaches the anterior axillary line or the mid-axillary line. In adult males the breast tissue is rudimentary and about 2 cm in diameter; it lies deep to the areola and extends up to the areolar edge. The anatomy of the breast is illustrated in *Figure 58.1 and* ▶ *58.1*.

The axillary tail of the breast is palpable in some women and can be seen in the premenstrual period or during lactation. A well-developed axillary tail is sometimes mistaken for a mass of enlarged lymph nodes, a breast mass or a lipoma.

The **breast parenchyma** consists of ductolobular and supportive tissue. The terminal ductule together with the lobule constitute the **t**erminal **d**uctal **l**obular **u**nit, which is referred to by the acronym TDLU. The TDLU is the most active part of the breast tissue and responds to a number of hormones: namely, oestrogen, progesterone, prolactin and growth hormone. There are five to nine major lactiferous (milk) ducts carrying milk from the lobes. Approximately 10–100 lobules empty via ductules into a lactiferous duct. Each lactiferous duct is lined with a spiral arrangement of contractile myoepithelial cells.

Most diseases of the breast arise from the TDLU. About 50% of the ductolobular tissue is located in the upper outer quadrant and about 20% in the central region. Hence, during breast examination particular attention must be paid to the upper outer quadrant, retroareolar region and the nipple–areola complex.

The **supportive tissue** of the breast comprises fibrous tissue in the form of suspensory ligaments of Cooper, adipose

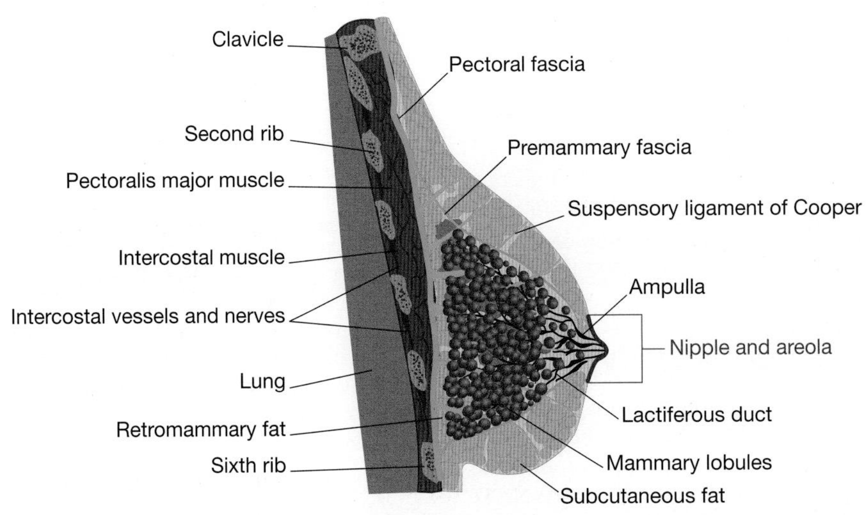

Figure 58.1 Cross-sectional anatomy of the breast.

tissue, blood vessels, nerves and lymphatics. The **ligaments of Cooper** are attached to the undersurface of the dermis superficially and to the pectoral fascia deeply.

The **areola and nipple** contain involuntary muscle arranged in concentric rings as well as radially in the subcutaneous tissue. The circular muscle fibres constitute Sappey's muscle (causes erection of the nipple), whereas longitudinal fibres form the Myerholtz muscle (causes retraction of the nipple). The areolar epithelium contains numerous sweat glands and sebaceous glands; the latter enlarge during pregnancy and serve to lubricate the nipple during lactation (Montgomery's tubercles).

The nipple is covered by thick skin with corrugations. Near its apex lie the orifices of the lactiferous ducts.

The lymphatics of the breast drain predominantly into the axillary and internal mammary lymph nodes. The axillary nodes receive approximately 85% of the lymph from the breast and are arranged in the following groups:

- lateral nodes along the lower border of the axillary vein lying lateral to the thoracodorsal vascular pedicle;
- anterior or pectoral nodes between the lateral borders of pectoralis major and pectoralis minor and the lateral thoracic vessels; these are the sentinel lymph nodes in most patients;
- posterior along the subscapular and thoracodorsal vessels just anterior to the latissimus dorsi muscle;
- a central or medial group of nodes embedded in fat in the centre of the axilla;
- interpectoral or Rotter's nodes – a few nodes lying between the pectoralis major and minor muscles;
- apical nodes that lie above and medial to the pectoralis minor tendon and lateral to the first rib; the apical nodes receive the efferent lymphatic channels from all the axillary nodes.

The apical nodes are in continuity with the supraclavicular nodes and drain into the subclavian lymph trunk, which enters the great veins directly or via the thoracic duct or jugular trunk. Surgically the axillary lymph nodes are classified into three levels:

- **level I**, below and lateral to the lateral border of the pectoralis minor muscle (the majority);
- **level II**, in front of and behind the pectoralis minor muscle (including Rotter's nodes);
- **level III**, above and medial to the medial border of pectoralis minor.

The internal mammary nodes lie along the internal mammary vessels deep to the plane of the costal cartilages and just superficial to the parietal pleura. These drain the medial half of the breast.

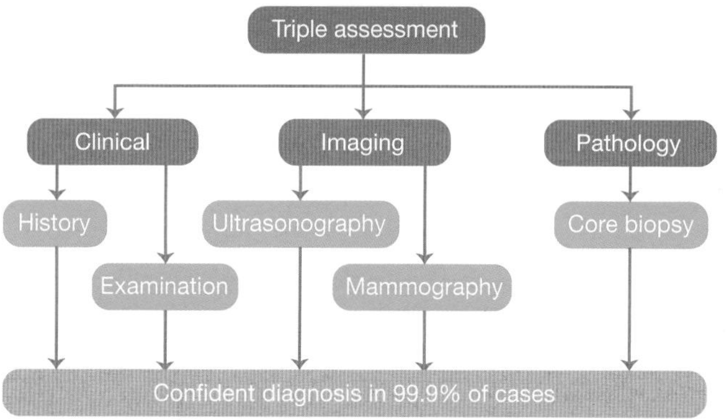

Figure 58.2 Triple assessment.

INVESTIGATIONS FOR BREAST SYMPTOMS

The assessment of women presenting with symptomatic breast disease is carried out in a systematic manner.

Triple assessment

Patients presenting with a breast lump, nipple discharge or other symptoms are assessed by a combination of clinical examination, radiological imaging and tissue sampling taken for either cytological or histological analysis. This combined approach is called 'triple assessment' (*Figure 58.2*). The positive predictive value and diagnostic accuracy of this combination approach 100%.

The clinical assessment should involve a thorough history and clinical breast examination that includes inspection and palpation (*Figure 58.3 and* ■ *58.2*).

Ultrasonography

Ultrasonography is the primary imaging modality in young women with dense breast tissue in whom mammograms are difficult to interpret. Ultrasonography can distinguish cystic from solid lesions. Simple cysts do not require further work-up and follow-up can be avoided. Therapeutic aspiration may be performed for cysts causing pain (*Figure 58.4*). A well-circumscribed, mobile, solid mass in a young woman is suggestive of a fibroadenoma and has an extremely low likelihood of malignancy. Such a finding requires reassurance and imaging follow-up (*Figure 58.5*). Solid masses with an irregular shape and ill-defined margins (indistinct, angular or spiculated) are suspicious for malignancy and require biopsy (*Figure 58.6*). Ultrasonography of the axilla is performed when cancer is diagnosed, with guided percutaneous biopsy of any suspicious lymph glands.

Sir Astley Paston Cooper, 1768–1841, surgeon, Guy's Hospital, London, UK, described these ligaments in 1845.
Marie Philibert Constant Sappey, 1810–1896, French anatomist who published his comprehensive atlas in 1874.
William Fetherston Montgomery, 1797–1859, obstetrician, Dublin, Ireland, described these tubercles in 1837.
Josef Rotter, 1857–1924, German surgeon, described these nodes in the early nineteenth century.

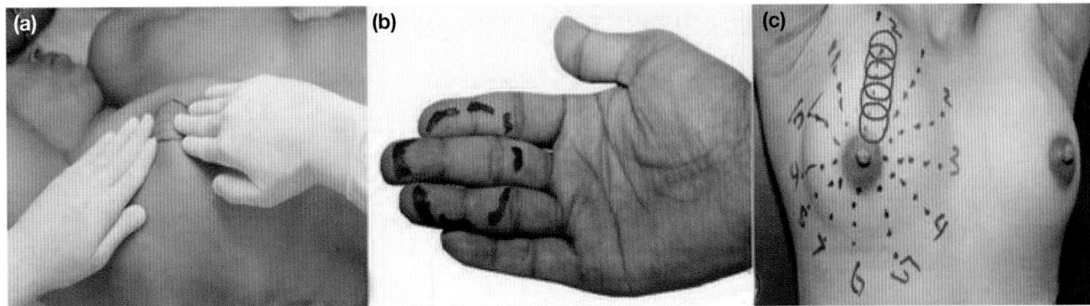

Figure 58.3 Clinical breast examination. (a) Patient lying supine for palpation. (b) Use the pad of three fingers and (c) the dial of a clock method for a comprehensive examination.

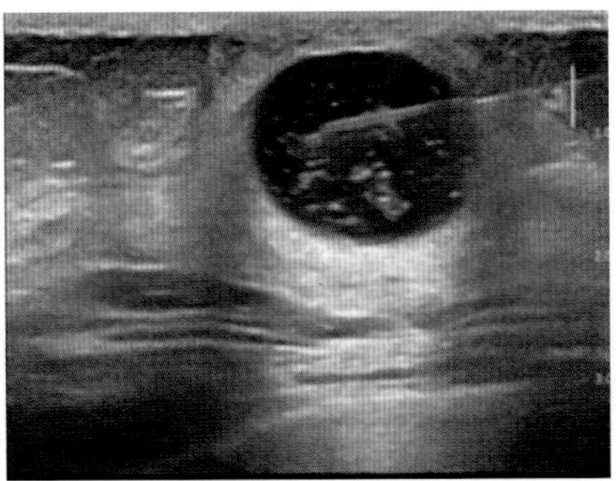

Figure 58.4 Therapeutic aspiration of a complicated cyst. Ultrasonography shows needle aspiration of a sharply defined, anechoic cyst with internal echoes – the floating debris. Breast Imaging Reporting and Data System (BI-RADS) score 2 (*Table 58.1*).

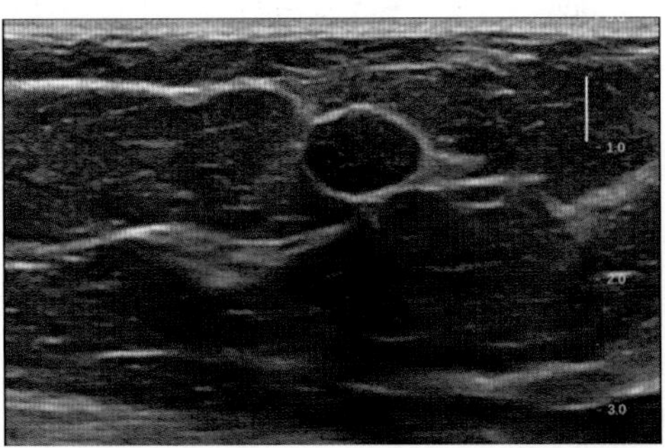

Figure 58.5 Fibroadenoma. Ultrasonography shows a well-circumscribed, solid mass suggestive of fibroadenoma in a young woman. Breast Imaging Reporting and Data System (BI-RADS) score 3 (*Table 58.1*).

Mammography

Mammography in two planes and ultrasonography are the first-line investigations for imaging the breast. Magnetic resonance imaging (MRI) is a valuable adjunctive diagnostic tool because of its high sensitivity for breast pathology. Mammography is also used as an initial screening tool for asymptomatic women in population-based programmes. Radiographs are taken by placing the breast in direct contact with ultrasensitive film and exposing it to low-voltage, high-amperage x-rays. The dose of radiation is approximately 1 mGy per film (*Figure 58.7*). Mammography should be the first investigation in older women who present with breast symptoms. Mammographic features of cancer are shown in *Figure 58.8*. Ancillary signs of malignancy such as lymphadenopathy, breast oedema and skin or areolar thickening or retraction may be seen in advanced cases. The mammographic and ultrasonographic features are not diagnostic of cancer; biopsy is required for definitive diagnosis in lesions with a Breast Imaging Reporting and Data System (BI-RADS) score of 4 or 5 (*Table 58.1*).

Mammography reporting

The American College of Radiology has developed guidelines – BI-RADS – to achieve uniformity and objectivity in the interpretation and reporting of mammograms and ultrasound. The mammographic assessments are categorised from BI-RADS 0 to BI-RADS 6 (*Table 58.1*).

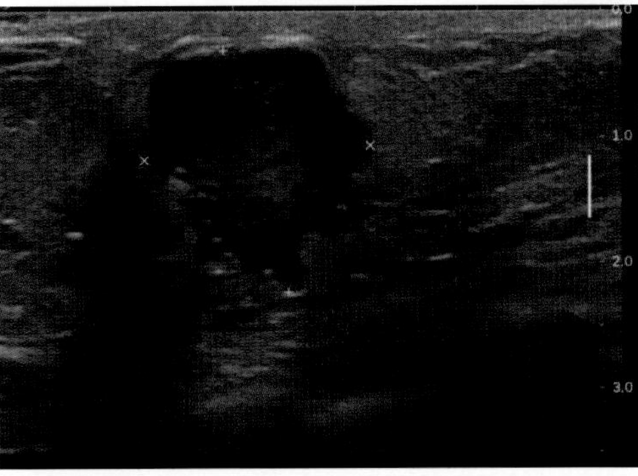

Figure 58.6 Imaging features of breast carcinoma on ultrasonography. This shows a solid, irregular-shaped mass, taller than wider, with angular irregular margins. Breast Imaging Reporting and Data System (BI-RADS) score 5 (*Table 58.1*).

Magnetic resonance imaging

MRI of the breast (*Figure 58.9*) is useful in a number of settings:

- women with dense breasts or discordant or equivocal findings on mammogram/ultrasonography;
- to distinguish scar from recurrence in women who have had previous breast conservation therapy for cancer;

Gy is short for Gray, the SI unit for the absorbed dose of ionising radiation.
Louis Harold Gray, 1905–1965, Director, British Empire Cancer Campaign Research Unit in Radiobiology, Mount Vernon Hospital, Northwood, UK.

TABLE 58.1 Breast Imaging Reporting and Database System (BI-RADS).

Category	Assessment	Probability of malignancy	Follow-up recommendation
0	Assessment is incomplete	Not applicable	Need for additional imaging evaluation and/or prior mammograms for comparison
1	Negative	Essentially 0%	Routine annual screening mammography (for women over age 40)
2	Benign finding(s)	Essentially 0%	Routine annual screening mammography (for women over age 40)
3	Probably benign finding	>0% but ≤2%	Initial short-term follow-up (usually 6 months) examination
4	Suspicious abnormality:		Biopsy should be considered
	4a: Findings needing intervention with a low suspicion for malignancy	>2 to ≤10%	
	4b: Intermediate suspicion of malignancy	>10% to ≤50%	
	4c: Findings of moderate concern, with high suspicion for malignancy	>50% to <95%	
5	Highly suggestive of malignancy	≥95%	Requires biopsy or surgical treatment
6	Known biopsy-proven malignancy	Not applicable	Category reserved for lesions identified on imaging study with biopsy proof of malignancy prior to definitive therapy

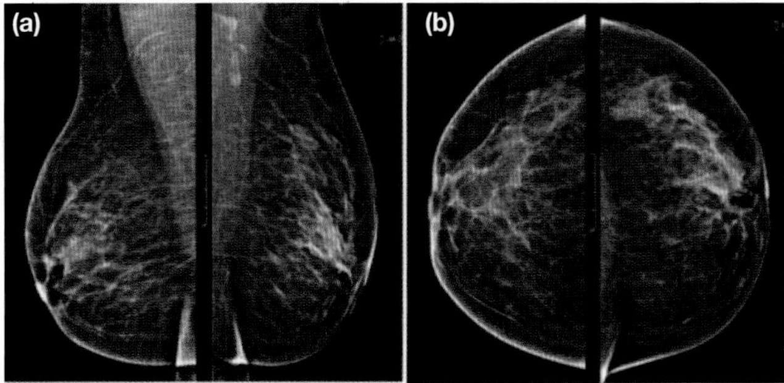

Figure 58.7 Features of a normal mammogram. (a) Mediolateral oblique view; (b) craniocaudal view.

- to assess multifocality and multicentricity and, in lobular cancer, high-grade ductal carcinoma *in situ* (DCIS);
- women with breast cancer (*BRCA*) gene or other genetic mutations or a strong family history;
- women with breast implants.

MRI-guided biopsy may be performed for lesions not visible on ultrasonography or mammogram.

Positron emission tomography

Positron emission tomography (PET) scans are used as a staging investigation in patients with T3, T4, N2, N3 breast cancer and in patients with T1, T2, N0, N1 breast cancer in the presence of symptoms/signs suggestive of metastasis (*Figure 58.10*). Inflammatory lesions (namely, mediastinal lymphadenopathy and pleuropulmonary lesions due to pulmonary tuberculosis [TB]) may give false-positive results, especially in Asian patients. Moreover, PET is very expensive and insurance policies may not cover its cost.

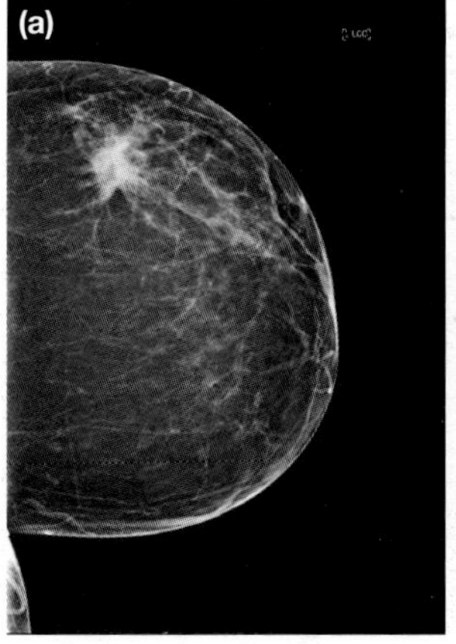

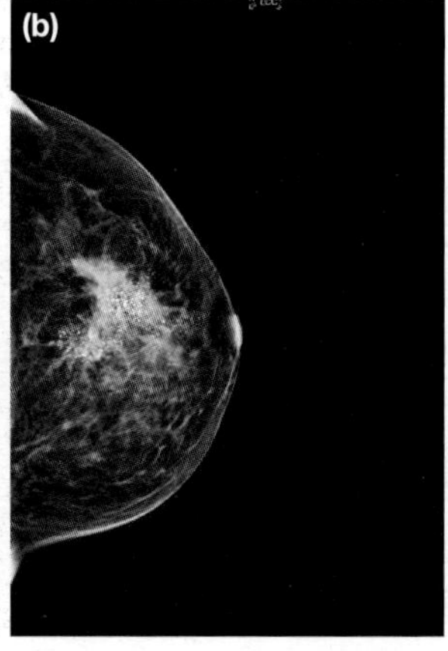

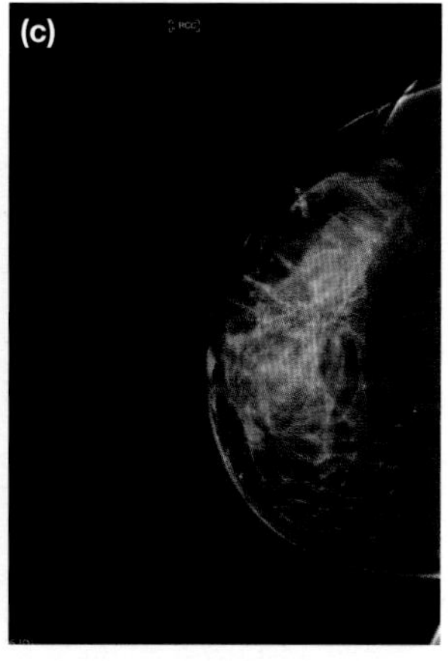

Figure 58.8 Imaging features of breast cancer on mammography (Category BI-RADS 5). (a) Irregular, spiculated mass; (b) fine pleomorphic microcalcifications; (c) architectural distortion.

Otto Heinrich Warburg, 1883–1970, German physiologist, awarded a Nobel prize in 1931 for describing the metabolic dependence of tumour cells on glucose (the Warburg effect). Most primary tumours and metastatic deposits exhibit high uptake of a radiopharmaceutical (^{18}F-fluorodeoxyglucose [^{18}F-FDG]) that may be detected by positron emission tomography.

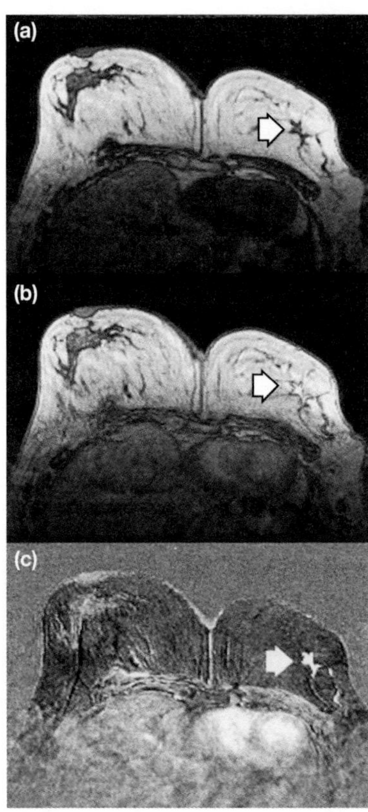

Figure 58.9 Magnetic resonance imaging showing carcinoma of the left breast (arrows). (a) Precontrast; (b) post gadolinium contrast; (c) subtraction image.

Needle biopsy

Tissue for histological examination can be obtained under local anaesthesia using a large-diameter core needle biopsy device (14G for breast tissue and 18G for axillary nodes) (*Figure 58.11*). The core needle biopsy should always be taken under image guidance. The passage of the biopsy needle can be guided by ultrasonography, mammogram or sometimes MRI; the needle tip should be used to take a sample from only the solid part of the mass, avoiding areas of cystic degeneration and blood vessels in and around the lesion.

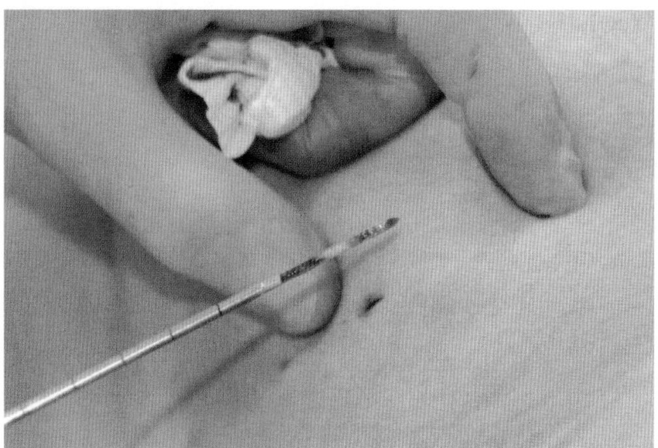

Figure 58.11 Large-diameter core needle biopsy of the breast.

Vacuum-assisted biopsy

The sampling error decreases as the biopsy volume increases and using 8G or 11G needles allows more extensive biopsies to be taken. This is useful in the management of microcalcifications and removal of benign lumps such as fibroadenoma.

BENIGN BREAST DISEASE

Nomenclature

The nomenclature of benign breast disease in the past has been confusing owing to the use of a variety of terms – namely, fibrosis, adenosis, epitheliosis, fibroadenosis and fibrocystic disease – for clinical patterns of pain, nodularity, benign lumps and nipple discharge. However, such terms do not relate to clinical or histological features. Most benign disorders are derived from minor aberrations of the normal process of development, cyclical hormone-related change and involution. To address this confusion, the concept of Aberrations of Normal Development and Involution (ANDI), developed and described by the Cardiff Breast Clinic in the UK, helps in better understanding and treatment of benign breast disease.

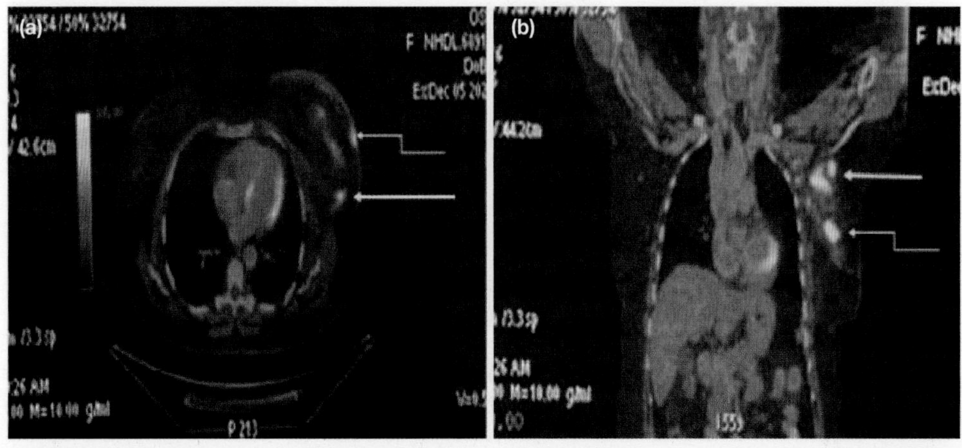

Figure 58.10 Positron emission tomography showing hot spots in the left breast and in axillary lymph nodes in (a) transverse and (b) coronal view.

Aetiology

The breast is a dynamic structure that undergoes alterations due to the cyclical changes in oestrogen and progesterone in every menstrual cycle. These hormones act as growth factors on the epithelial and stromal cells of the TDLU (*58.1*). The pathogenesis of ANDI involves disturbances in the breast physiology extending from a perturbation of normality to well-defined disease processes.

Pathology

This can be considered in three phases: lobule development at 15–25 years, cyclical changes at 15–50 years and involution at 35–55 years of age. It is believed that lobular proliferation leads to the formation of fibroadenoma and involution leads to cyst formation. Aberration in the above phases may lead to a number of benign conditions.

- **Hyperplasia of the epithelium** is defined as the presence of more than two layers of cells in the lining of the ducts and acini. It may occur with or without atypia. If atypia of epithelial cells is seen, the terms **atypical ductal hyperplasia** (ADH) and **atypical lobular hyperplasia** (ALH) are used. If features of ADH are seen to involve more than two ducts or lesions measure >2 mm in diameter, the term **ductal carcinoma *in situ*** (DCIS) is used.
- **Papilloma**. Localised hyperplasia of the ductal epithelium may produce a papilloma within the ducts. It is composed of a central fibrovascular core and papillary projections of the epithelium and myoepithelial cells. The papillary lesions in a duct are of three types:
  - solitary papilloma (relative risk [RR] for cancer 1.5–2);
  - papillomatosis: five or more papillomas in many ducts with peripheral and often bilateral distribution (RR for cancer 3);
  - juvenile papillomatosis, also called **Swiss cheese disease**, affects young women, who present with multiple firm palpable nodules; microscopically, there are multiple papillomas with/without atypia, apocrine cysts, ductal hyperplasia and sclerosing adenosis. A positive family history of breast cancer increases the lifetime cancer risk.
- **Cyst formation**. Kinking or narrowing of ductules is usually due to involution of the stroma and may result in accumulation of secretions in the lobules, forming a microcyst. Many microcysts may join together to form a macrocyst.

Clinical features

The most common manifestations of ANDI are breast pain and benign nodularity. The breast pain usually follows the menstrual cycle, appearing around day 14 and increasing in severity until day 28, when it becomes severe (cyclical pronounced mastalgia with premenstrual exacerbation). Nodularity or lumpiness may be either localised or spread diffusely throughout the breast; it is often bilateral and is most conspicuous in the upper outer quadrant. The nodularity may be cyclical, appearing 1–2 weeks prior to menstruation and regressing with the onset of the menses. A discrete lump in the breast is commonly a fibroadenoma in the young and a cyst in the middle-aged.

Mastalgia

Approximately 50–70% of women attending any breast clinic present with mastalgia (synonym: mastodynia or mazodynia). True mastalgia (arising from breast tissue) is classified into cyclical and non-cyclical types.

Cyclical mastalgia

The pain usually starts around the middle of the cycle on day 14 and gradually increases in severity (measured on a visual analogue scale [VAS] as 0–10) until day 27 or 28. Usually both breasts are involved. The pain is usually relieved with the onset of menses. Severe forms may lead to loss of sleep and impaired sexual and other activities of daily life. The pain may radiate to the upper arm and may be mistaken for angina pectoris.

The cause is unclear and considerations of hormone imbalance, high caffeine intake, low dietary essential fatty acids, water retention or psychoneurosis are not supported by research. In most patients the basal levels of oestrogen, progesterone and prolactin are in the normal range. However, most patients do respond to treatment with antioestrogen drugs, such as tamoxifen, ormeloxifene, luteinising hormone analogues or danazol, suggesting excessive responsiveness of breast tissue to circulating oestrogen.

Non-cyclical mastalgia

The pain presents at any time of the menstrual cycle, at any location of the breast and may occur both before and after menopause. It is often well localised. Some patients may have duct ectasia or periductal mastitis. Breast palpation may reveal a very tender spot confined to a point called the trigger spot or trigger point. Other causes are musculoskeletal, in the form of Tietze's syndrome: a painful costochondral junction with no radiological anomaly and lateral chest wall pain in the anterior axillary line and over serratus anterior. Trauma, cancer or sclerosing adenosis may also result in breast pain. True breast pain must be distinguished from angina, biliary colic, reflex oesophagitis and cervical spondylosis. In low-/middle-income countries, vitamin D and calcium deficiencies are rampant, leading to bony aches and pains that may present as non-cyclical mastalgia. About 5% of breast cancers exhibit pain at presentation, but this is rarely the sole presenting feature.

Treatment

Treatment begins with assessment, including breast examination and imaging. If normal, reassurance that the symptoms are not due to cancer helps the majority of women. The type of pain, cyclical or non-cyclical, should be identified by recording a pain chart for 1 month (*Figure 58.12*). The principles of treatment are outlined in *Table 58.2 and 58.1*. In patients

Alexander Tietze, 1864–1927, Professor of Surgery, Breslau, Germany (now Wrocław, Poland), described this condition in 1921.

DAILY BREAST PAIN CHART

Patient name: Age: Reg. number:

Date:

Month of visit: 0/1/2/3/4/5/6:

Duration of complaint (first visit only): Right Breast___________ Left Breast_________________

Out of ten what was the maximum breast pain score in the last month? Please encircle the number.

(Note: 10 is the maximum pain you ever experienced and 0 is no pain)

On monthly period chart, insert the letter M below the date on days you have menses.

0 1 2 3 4 5 6 7 8 9 10

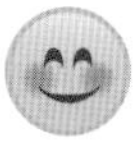

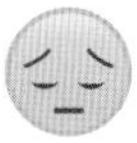

How many days in the last month were painful?

Right breast pain score

Month	1	2	3	4	5	6	7	8	9	10	11	12	13	14	15	16	17	18	19	20	21	22	23	24	25	26	27	28	29	30	31
माह	1	2	3	4	5	6	7	8	9	10	11	12	13	14	15	16	17	18	19	20	21	22	23	24	25	26	27	28	29	30	31

Left breast pain score

Month	1	2	3	4	5	6	7	8	9	10	11	12	13	14	15	16	17	18	19	20	21	22	23	24	25	26	27	28	29	30	31
माह	1	2	3	4	5	6	7	8	9	10	11	12	13	14	15	16	17	18	19	20	21	22	23	24	25	26	27	28	29	30	31

Monthly period

Month	1	2	3	4	5	6	7	8	9	10	11	12	13	14	15	16	17	18	19	20	21	22	23	24	25	26	27	28	29	30	31
माह	1	2	3	4	5	6	7	8	9	10	11	12	13	14	15	16	17	18	19	20	21	22	23	24	25	26	27	28	29	30	31

Note: Please bring this card with you on each visit

Figure 58.12 Breast pain chart. All India Institute of Medical Sciences modification of the Cardiff Breast Pain Chart.

with non-cyclical pain, musculoskeletal pain and other referred causes should be excluded. Trigger point pain may be relieved by local injection of a long-acting corticosteroid such as triamcinolone in combination with lidocaine at the point of maximum tenderness. This may be repeated at intervals until the pain is controlled.

TABLE 58.2 Treatment of breast pain.

Exclude cancer	
Reassure	Use a VAS breast pain chart to record severity
Adequate support	Tight sports brassiere during the day
Consider medication	
Flax seed 30 g daily or oil of evening primrose	Rich sources of omega 3 fatty acids and γ-linolenic acid, respectively
Topical non-steroidal anti-inflammatory cream (diclofenac or piroxicam) four times a day	Useful in mild to moderate mastalgia
Consider systemic medication if pain score >3 on a VAS of 0-10	
Tamoxifen 10 mg daily	For 3–6 months
Danazol 50–300 mg daily	For 3–6 months
Ormeloxifene 30 mg twice a week	For 3–6 months used in both cyclical and non-cyclical mastalgia and for treating nodularity
LHRH agonist alone or with antioestrogen: tamoxifen or ormeloxifene	Short duration: use for 3 months for recalcitrant pain not relieved by the above medications

LHRH, luteinising hormone-releasing hormone; VAS, visual analogue scale.

Nodular or lumpy breasts

Patients who present with painful tender nodularity with mastalgia should be treated for breast pain, as outlined in *Table 58.2*.

Patients with breast nodularity without pain should undergo triple assessment (*Figure 58.2*). The Cardiff–Lucknow nodularity scale – a five-point ordinal scale that grades the nodularity on a scale of 0 to 4, providing an objective measurement of nodularity – has been developed and validated (*Figure 58.13*). In the absence of a discrete lesion on breast imaging, reassurance may be given. If necessary, treatment with an antioestrogen such as tamoxifen or ormeloxifene (Centchroman) has been found to control nodularity within a few weeks.

Discrete lumps in the breast

The main causes of discrete lumps in the breast are listed in *Summary box 58.1*. Sometimes a lump appears in the breast and within a few days regresses on its own. This is called an **evanescent lump**. It is caused by an inflammatory mass of periductal mastitis; the lump, pain and tenderness all disappear together. Sometimes, a cyst or a galactocele may rupture; the lump disappears but pain and tenderness appear. The cyst fluid or milk leaking in the stroma may induce inflammation, causing pain and tenderness.

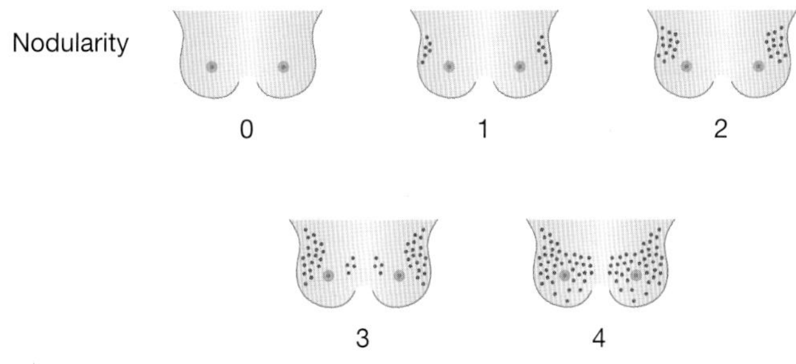

Figure 58.13 The Lucknow–Cardiff breast nodularity scale. A visual analogue scale for nodularity: an ordinal scale. 0, normal or non-nodular; 1, minimal; 2, mild; 3, moderate; 4, severe.

Summary box 58.1

Causes of discrete breast lumps

Benign		Malignant
Non-inflammatory	Fibroadenoma	Carcinoma of the breast (invasive, DCIS)
	Ductal papilloma	Malignant phyllodes
	Phyllodes	
	Hamartoma	
	Galactocele	
	Breast cyst	
	Haematoma	
	Traumatic fat necrosis	
Inflammatory	Breast abscess (acute inflammatory, tubercular)	
	Antibioma	
	Periductal mastitis (evanescent mass)	
	• Granulomatous mastitis • Parasitic: hydatid, filariasis • Fungal: aspergillosis, blastomycosis, *Cryptococcus*, *Histoplasma*	

Breast cysts

Breast cysts are common in the 35- to 55-year-old age group and usually present as a painless lump. Several causative factors contribute as part of ANDI, including lobular involution, increased secretion, ductile obstruction, loss of stroma, hyperoestrogenaemia and hormone replacement therapy. Cysts are often multiple, may be bilateral and can mimic malignancy. They typically present suddenly and cause great alarm; prompt diagnosis by ultrasonography and aspiration under ultrasound guidance provides immediate relief. A smooth-walled cyst without any solid component in its wall is classified as BI-RADS 2 and requires only observation without biopsy. The presence of a solid component in the cyst wall is classified as a **complex cyst** and necessitates a core biopsy to rule out cystadenocarcinoma. This should be distinguished from a **complicated cyst**, which is defined as a cyst containing intracystic floating debris that moves within the cyst with change of posture.

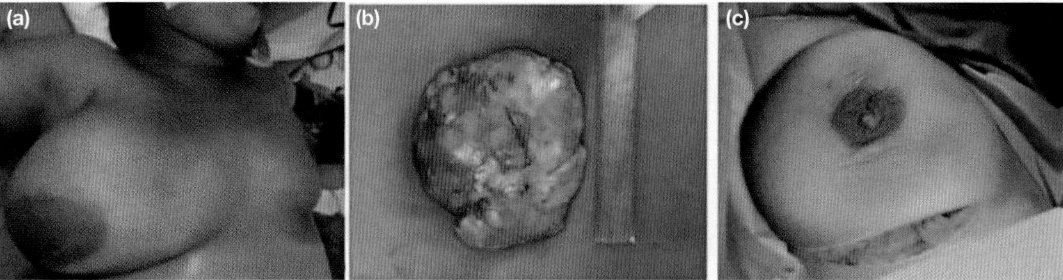

Figure 58.14 Giant fibroadenoma. (a) Clinical picture; (b) excised specimen; (c) submammary (Gaillard Thomas) incision.

Treatment

A solitary cyst or small collection of cysts may be aspirated if associated with pain or inflammation. If the cyst(s) resolve(s) completely, and if the fluid is not bloodstained, no further treatment is required. Cytological examination of cyst fluid is not useful. If there is a residual lump or if the aspirate is bloodstained, a core biopsy or excision for histological diagnosis is advisable. A complicated cyst with associated infection may be treated with a short course of antibiotics.

Galactocele

Galactocele is rare and usually presents as a solitary subareolar milk-filled cyst seen during or just after lactation. It disappears completely and is usually cured by a single aspiration. If it recurs, it may be reaspirated or a nylon strand (2/0) may be passed to clear the blocked duct. Complications of galactocele are non-resolution because of inspissated material and calcification. Surgical excision is rarely indicated. Lactating mothers should be encouraged to continue breastfeeding.

Fibroadenoma

A fibroadenoma is the most common cause of a breast lump in women aged 15–25 years. It arises from hyperplasia of a lobule and usually grows to 2–3 cm in size. It is surrounded by a well-defined capsule. A clinically typical fibroadenoma, confirmed on ultrasonography, may be observed without a biopsy. A biopsy should be obtained if the patient is over 25 or if there are atypical features on ultrasonography. Regression with antioestrogen drugs has been observed with tamoxifen and ormeloxifene (*58.3*).

Giant fibroadenomas occasionally occur during puberty. They are over 5 cm in diameter, often rapidly growing and can be enucleated through a submammary incision (***Figure 58.14***).

The RR of cancer with fibroadenoma ranges from 1.5–1.7 if simple to 3.4–3.7 in the presence of epithelial hyperplasia. Complex fibroadenoma with a family history has an RR for cancer of 3.0–4.0, particularly lobular carcinoma.

Indications for surgical excision are: age over 30 years; suspicious features on imaging, such as microlobulation; atypia on histology; size >5 cm; family history of breast cancer; and the patient's preference. Excision of fibroadenoma in the elderly should include a rim of normal tissue as it may contain malignancy or a phyllodes tumour.

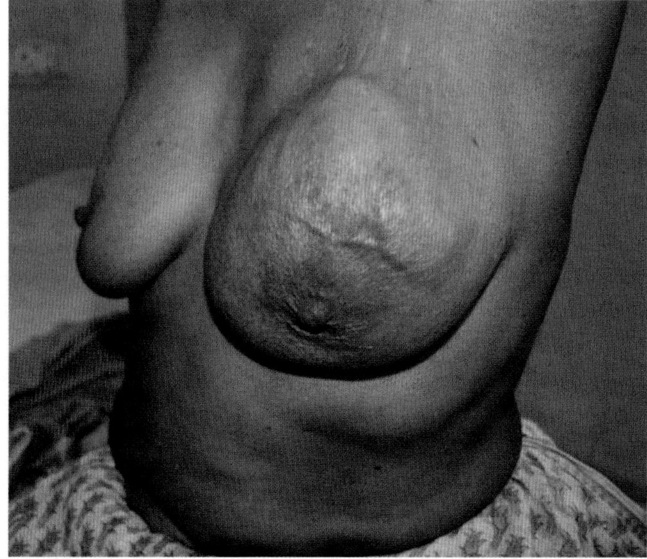

Figure 58.15 Phyllodes tumour of the left breast.

Phyllodes tumour

Previously known as cystosarcoma phyllodes, these benign tumours usually occur in women over the age of 30 years but can appear in younger women and present as a large, sometimes massive, tumour with an unevenly bosselated surface (***Figure 58.15***). Occasionally, the overlying skin is ulcerated owing to pressure necrosis. Despite their size, phyllodes tumours remain mobile on the chest wall and rarely infiltrate the skin until late. It is a true mixed neoplasm comprising both epithelial and mesenchymal elements and resembling a fibroadenoma. Some have a higher mitotic index with infiltrating borders and may rarely metastasise via the bloodstream. Phyllodes tumours are classified according to histological behaviour into benign (mitotic rate <4 per 10 high-power fields [HPF]), borderline (mitotic rate 4–9 per 10 HPF) and malignant (mitotic rate >10 per 10 HPF) tumours.

Treatment

Treatment is by wide local excision (WLE) with a 2-cm margin along with the overlying skin and underlying pectoralis major muscle because of a high incidence of local recurrence.

Theodore Gaillard Thomas, 1831–1903, American gynaecologist, Columbia University College of Physicians and Surgeons, New York, NY, USA.

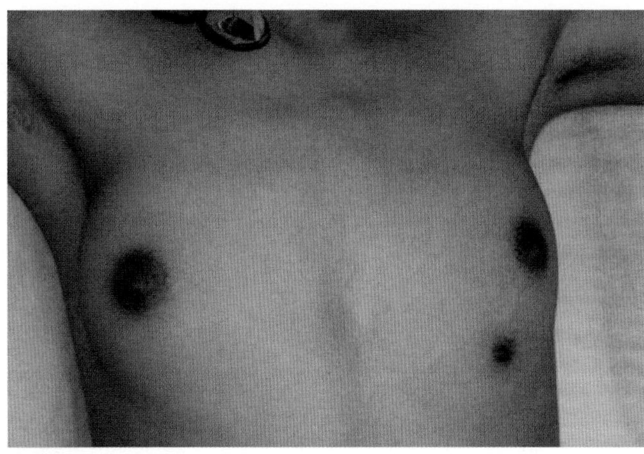

Figure 58.16 Accessory nipple with congenital inversion of the normal nipple.

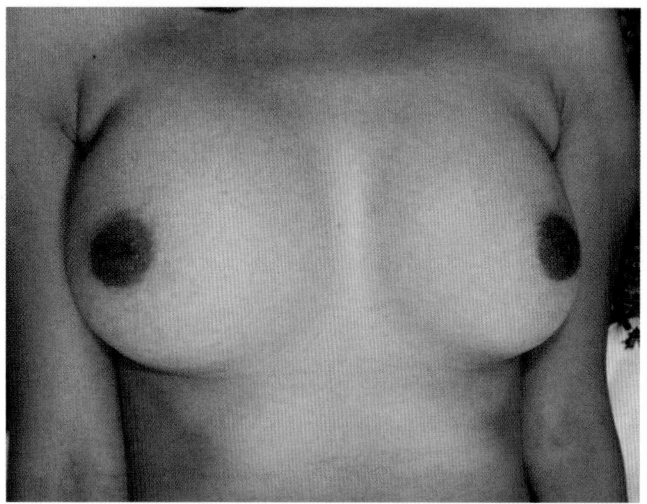

Figure 58.17 Congenital nipple inversion.

Massive tumours, recurrent tumours and those of the malignant type require mastectomy. Postoperative radiotherapy may be offered to women with recurrent or malignant phyllodes tumours. Systemic chemotherapy may be offered for malignant phyllodes.

THE NIPPLE

Absence of the nipple is rare and is usually associated with amazia (congenital absence of the breast). Supernumerary nipples are not uncommon and occur along a line extending from the anterior fold of the axilla to the upper chest (*Figure 58.16*). In the human embryo the milk ridge extends from the axilla to the upper chest only and not to the groin. Rarely, there is duplication of the nipple on a normal areola.

Nipple inversion and retraction

At birth the mammary glands in boys and girls are similar. At around 11–12 years of age, in girls the breast begins to grow. The onset of its growth is called 'the telarche' (1 year before menarche). Initially uniform growth of cells leads to a rounded breast mound. Later elongation of the major milk ducts at age 14–16 years leads to projection of the nipple. Lack of elongation of the major milk ducts leads to failure of the nipple to protrude, called nipple inversion (*Figure 58.17*). An inverted nipple interferes with feeding and may become a source of infection by deposition of debris. It does not predispose to breast cancer.

Nipple retraction is an acquired phenomenon owing to fibrosis in and around the major milk ducts. Retraction of recent onset is always worrisome and may point towards an underlying carcinoma; however, the most common cause of longstanding retraction is periductal mastitis (*Figure 58.18*).

Both nipple inversion and retraction may cause problems with breastfeeding and infection can occur because of retention of secretions. A transverse slit-like or fish mouth-like retraction of the nipple is classically seen in periductal mastitis (*Figure 58.18a*), but circumferential retraction may indicate a carcinoma (*Figure 58.18b*).

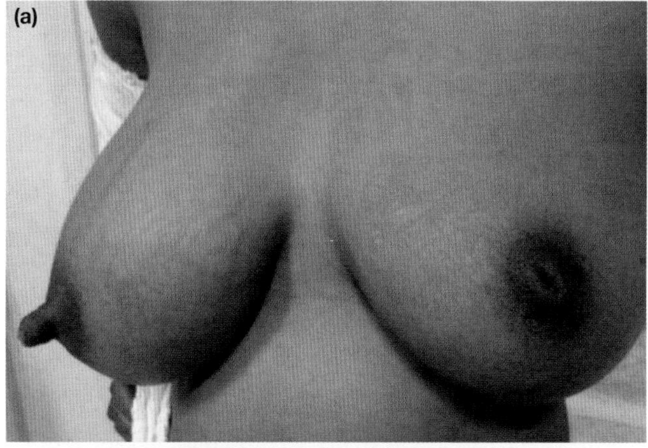

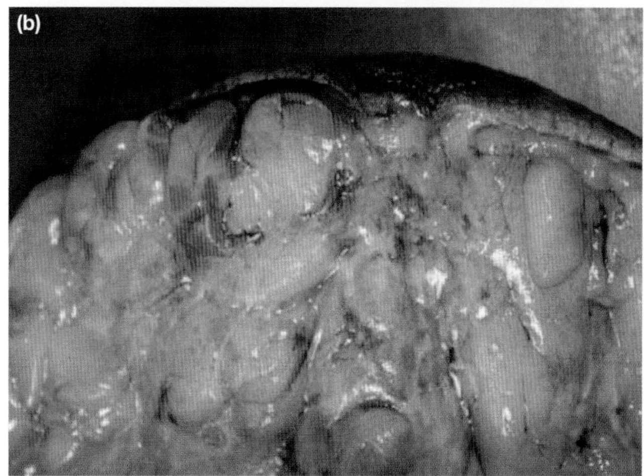

Figure 58.18 Two common causes of retraction of the nipple. (a) Slit-like retraction due to periductal mastitis. (b) Breast cancer with fibrosis around the major milk ducts.

Treatment

Minor degrees of inversion can be corrected by gently pulling the nipple forward. Surgical correction is fraught with division of milk ducts and loss of nipple sensation and the patient should be fully informed of this risk. Mechanical suction devices have been used to evert the nipple, with some benefit.

Cracked nipple

This is observed in about 10% of nursing mothers and is thought to arise from the strong negative force created by suckling. It initiates as a small blister on the nipple that soon ruptures to give rise to a small ulcer. The crack thus formed is often colonised by bacteria or fungi. The microbes from the crack may enter the milk ducts and may progress to lactational mastitis.

If the nipple becomes cracked during lactation, it should be rested for 48 hours and the breast should be emptied with a breast pump. The sore nipple should be gently washed with warm water and moisturising soap followed by application of an antimicrobial cream (mupirocin).

Papilloma of the nipple

Papilloma of the nipple has the same features as any cutaneous papilloma and should be excised with a tiny disc of skin. Alternatively, the base may be tied with a ligature and the papilloma will spontaneously fall off.

Retention cyst of a gland of Montgomery

These glands, situated in the areola, secrete sebum. If they become blocked a sebaceous cyst forms. Rarely they may become infected and need excision.

Eczema

Eczema of the nipple and areola is a rare condition and is often bilateral; it is usually associated with eczema elsewhere on the body. It is treated with 0.1% betamethasone skin cream by local application and by using moisturising soaps. If the nipple fails to heal, Paget's disease must be excluded by taking a wedge biopsy of the lesion.

Paget's disease

Paget's disease is a unique type of DCIS arising in the nipple. It presents as erosion of the nipple that slowly destroys the nipple and encroaches on the areola (*Figure 58.19*). It may become invasive with metastasis to the axillary lymph nodes. Triple assessment is needed to exclude underlying malignancy. Paget's disease without associated underlying malignancy is treated by central core excision, removing a cone of major milk ducts along with the nipple and areola down to the pectoralis major muscle, followed by radiotherapy. Paget's disease with underlying malignancy is treated by mastectomy and evaluation of the axillary nodal status.

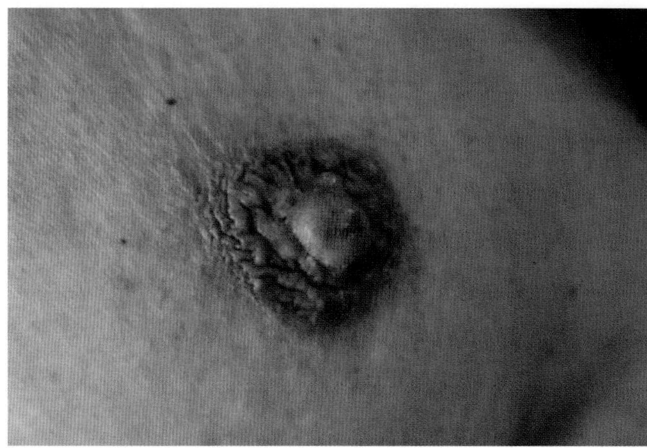

Figure 58.19 Nipple erosion in early Paget's disease.

Discharges from the nipple

Most nipple discharges are caused by physiological aberrations as part of ANDI, may emanate from a single or many milk ducts and may involve one or both sides. The presence of a **s**ingle, **s**erous, **s**anguineous and **s**pontaneous discharge ('**four S**') should be considered pathological and triple assessment should be carried out. Both serous and sanguineous discharges are caused by excessive proliferation of the ductal epithelium, which can be either diffuse or localised or may result from a ductal carcinoma. During pregnancy, the increase in blood flow to the ductolobular tissue may lead to serous or bloody nipple discharge. Hence, a bloody discharge during pregnancy is considered physiological and usually abates spontaneously after childbirth; however, ultrasonography should be performed to rule out malignancy. The clinical significance of the specific colour of the nipple discharge is as follows:

- A clear, serous discharge is commonly caused by ductal papilloma. It is potentially serious and should not be ignored. Multiduct, multicoloured discharge is physiological and the patient may be reassured (*Figure 58.20*).
- A bloodstained discharge may be caused by a duct papilloma, carcinoma or duct ectasia. A duct papilloma is usually single and situated in a major milk duct usually within 5 cm from the nipple.
- A black, green or muddy-coloured discharge is usually the result of duct ectasia.

Galactorrhoea is defined as spontaneous milk discharge from several ducts of both nipples unassociated with childbirth or breastfeeding. It may be associated with a prolactin-secreting adenoma of the pituitary gland. Many drugs can also lead to increased prolactin secretion and galactorrhoea, including haloperidol, chlorpromazine, amitriptyline, metoclopramide and H_2 receptor antagonists (cimetidine).

Sir James Paget, 1814–1899, surgeon, St Bartholomew's Hospital, London, UK, described this disease of the nipple in 1874.

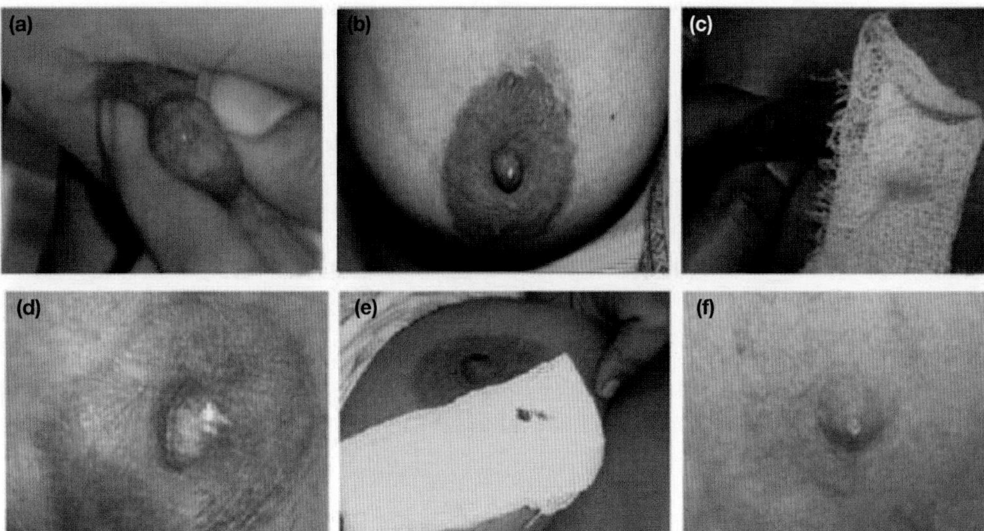

Figure 58.20 Different types of nipple discharge. (a) serous; (b) pus; (c) bloody; (d) cheesy; (e) greenish; (f) watery.

Summary box 58.2

Discharges from the nipple

Discharge from a single duct

- Bloodstained
  - Intraduct papilloma
  - Intraduct carcinoma
  - Duct ectasia
- Serous (sticky translucent fluid)
  - Duct papilloma
  - Ductal hyperplasia
  - Duct ectasia
  - Ductal carcinoma (*in situ* and invasive)

Discharge from more than one duct

- Bloodstained
  - Carcinoma
  - Duct ectasia
- Black, green or muddy
  - Duct ectasia
- Purulent
  - Periductal mastitis

Milk

- Lactation
  - Galactorrhoea
  - Rare causes: hypothyroidism, pituitary tumour
- Discharge from the surface (not from within nipple)
  - Paget's disease
  - Skin diseases (eczema, psoriasis)
  - Rare causes (e.g. chancre)

Management

Triple assessment to exclude carcinoma should be carried out. Ultrasonography may reveal dilated subareolar ducts and a filling defect indicating a duct papilloma with a diagnostic accuracy of 85%.

Ductoscopy (inspection of the internal structure of the duct system) using microendoscopes is technically feasible. Ductography is currently not practised in most centres because of the poor diagnostic yield. Most breast clinics have abandoned the cytological examination of nipple discharge as it has a poor yield for cancer.

Non-bloody discharge

Simple reassurance may be sufficient. However, if the discharge is profuse (wetting of the clothes causing social embarrassment) an operation to remove a 1.5- to 2-cm length of the affected major milk duct (microdochectomy) or ducts (major duct excision) can be performed.

Blood or serous discharge

The risk of cancer is related to the patient's age. Patients below 40 years with a bloody discharge and normal triple assessment may be reassured and followed up with annual imaging. Patients over the age of 40 years should be offered microdochectomy for single-duct discharge or Hadfield's major mammary duct excision for multiduct discharge. A segment of major milk ducts 5 cm in length from the nipple is usually removed as most duct papillomas are located up to a distance of 5 cm from the nipple (*58.4*).

Congenital abnormalities

Amazia

Congenital absence of the breast may occur on one or both sides. It is sometimes associated with Poland's syndrome, which is characterised by the absence of the sternal portion of the pectoralis major and short webbed fingers (symbrachydactyly) on the side of the involved breast (*Figure 58.21*). The breast may be reconstructed with a latissimus dorsi muscle flap and a silicone breast implant.

Geoffrey John Hadfield, 1923–2006, surgeon, Stoke Mandeville Hospital, Aylesbury, UK.
Alfred Poland, 1822–1872, surgeon, Guy's Hospital, London, UK, described this condition in 1841.

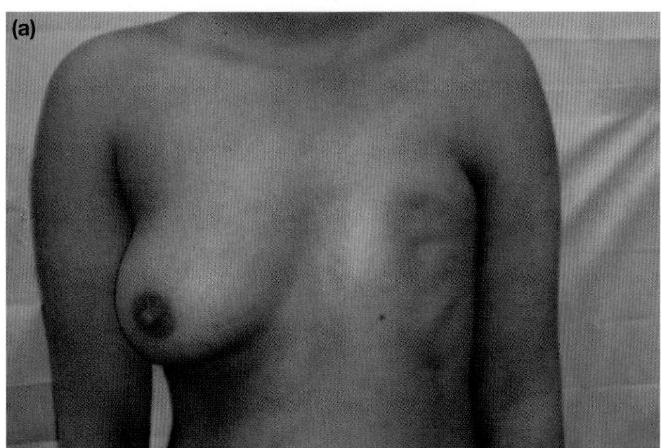

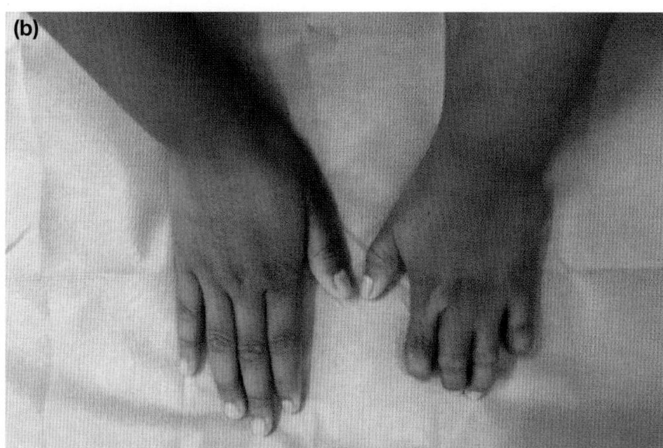

Figure 58.21 Poland's syndrome with congenital absence of the left breast and pectoralis major muscle (a) and symbrachydactyly of the ipsilateral hand (b).

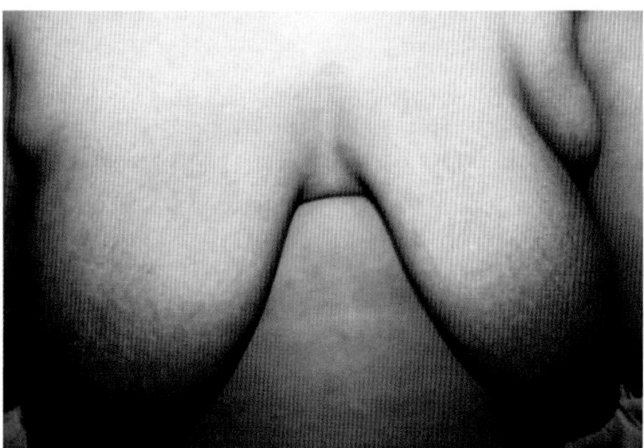

Figure 58.22 Polymazia left side.

Polymazia

Accessory breasts (*Figure 58.22*) have been recorded in the axilla (the most frequent site), groin, buttock and thigh. They have been known to fluctuate in response to hormones in a physiological manner, such as pubertal enlargement and lactation. They may also show the same spectrum of pathological diseases observed in normal breasts. Polymazia may be associated with other congenital diseases, such as vertebral anomalies, cardiac arrhythmias or renal anomalies.

Mastitis of infants

Mastitis of infants may occur in both boys and girls. It is uncommon and is predominantly caused by *Staphylococcus aureus*.

Macromastia

Macromastia is a benign disorder characterised by massive enlargement of one or both breasts disproportionate to the body habitus. The aetiology of this condition is multifactorial: it is usually idiopathic or associated with obesity, the presence of excessive endogenous or exogenous hormones or increased sensitivity of the breast tissues to the hormones. The treatment is reduction mammoplasty (*Figure 58.23*) or a subcutaneous mastectomy along with breast reconstruction.

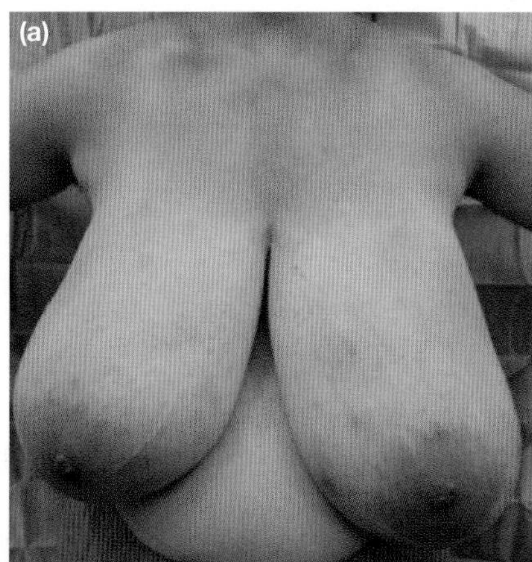

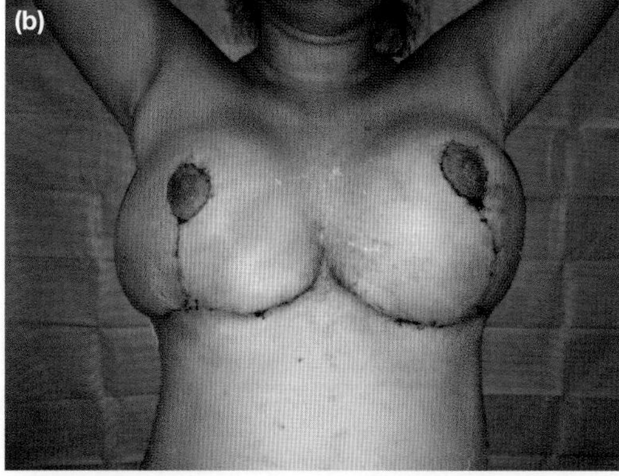

Figure 58.23 Patient with macromastia (a) who underwent inferior pedicle reduction mammoplasty (b) with removal of 1600 g of tissue from the right breast and 1800 g from the left.

Injuries of the breast

Haematoma

Haematoma, particularly a resolving haematoma, gives rise to a lump that, in the absence of overlying bruising, is difficult to diagnose correctly unless it is biopsied.

Traumatic fat necrosis

Traumatic fat necrosis may be acute or chronic and usually occurs in stout, middle-aged women. Following a blow, a lump, which is often painless, appears. This may mimic a carcinoma, even displaying skin tethering and nipple retraction; biopsy is required for diagnosis. A history of trauma is not diagnostic as this may merely have drawn the patient's attention to a pre-existing lump. In a road traffic accident, a seatbelt may transect or avulse the breast off the underlying pectoral muscles owing to a sudden deceleration injury.

Acute inflammation of the breast

Mastitis refers to inflammation of the breast tissue that may or may not be accompanied by infection. Acute mastitis can occur in lactating as well as non-lactating women, with the former being more common.

Lactational (puerperal) mastitis

The incidence of acute mastitis in lactating mothers varies from 3% to 20%. Most cases are caused by *S. aureus* and, if hospital acquired, may be to be due to methicillin-resistant *S. aureus*.

Aetiology

Mastitis may be bacterial or non-bacterial. Bacteria may enter the nipple through a cracked or retracted nipple. In many cases the lactiferous ducts get blocked by epithelial debris, leading to stasis, which is followed by infection. Once within the ampulla of the duct, staphylococci cause clotting of the milk and then multiply within the clot. Abscess formation is most commonly seen at two stages during lactation: in the first month after the first childbirth owing to inexperience or inappropriate and inadequate breastfeeding; and at weaning owing to engorgement and trauma to the nipple by the baby's teeth.

Clinical features

Initially there is generalised cellulitis, which if left untreated progresses to suppuration and abscess formation. An abscess presents as a fluctuant lump (in a deep-seated abscess fluctuation may be absent) with pain, signs of inflammation, fever, malaise and difficulty in feeding. It may also be associated with enlarged tender axillary nodes. Ultrasonography reveals cellulitis (seen as an area of increased echogenicity) and liquefaction necrosis (pus is seen as a hypoechoic collection with floating debris that changes with posture).

Management

During the cellulitic stage, the patient should be treated with anti-staphylococcal antibiotics such as cloxacillin, flucloxacillin or erythromycin. Breastfeeding from both the breasts should be encouraged 2-hourly, followed by emptying the breast. A breast support garment, cold compression on the breast and analgesia aid in symptomatic relief. Any pus seen on ultrasonography should be aspirated and sent for culture and sensitivity. Contrary to the practice of incision and drainage, in a breast abscess ultrasound-guided drainage gives an excellent cosmetic result, does not hamper breastfeeding and can be done as a day-care procedure with a high rate of success. Furthermore, incision and drainage may result in a non-healing milk fistula.

In abscesses >3 cm in diameter or those containing more than 30 mL of pus (assessed on ultrasonography), a vacuum suction catheter is inserted under ultrasound guidance to drain the pus (*Figure 58.24 and* 58.5). The patient should be reviewed on alternate days by clinical examination and ultrasonography. Any residual collection should be aspirated. The antibiotics are modified according to the microbiological culture report. In patients with a suction drain, the catheter is irrigated with cold normal saline (cold to reduce pain) on each visit until complete resolution. Antibiotics should be continued for 14 days.

Subacute and chronic inflammation of the breast

Non-lactational mastitis

Non-lactational mastitis may be defined as inflammation of the breast tissue in a nulliparous woman or occurring after a minimum of 6 months after cessation of lactation. Various forms of non-lactational mastitis include periductal mastitis, idiopathic granulomatous mastitis (IGM) and tubercular mastitis.

Periductal mastitis

This is a chronic non-lactational inflammation around the major milk ducts. The pathogenesis is obscure and thought to be autoimmune in nature. The condition is much more common in smokers.

It may progress to a subareolar inflammatory mass that may suppurate, forming a subareolar abscess. Thick areolar muscles do not allow the abscess to perforate through the areola so the pus follows the path of least resistance, rupturing the skin at the areolar edge and forming a mammary or milk duct fistula (*Figure 58.25*). In some cases, a chronic indurated mass forms beneath the areola, which mimics a carcinoma. Fibrosis in and around major milk ducts causes nipple retraction.

The patient presents with central non-cyclical pain, pus discharge from the nipple and a subareolar tender mass/abscess or mammary duct fistula. The examination reveals a tender, firm subareolar lump or abscess, purulent nipple discharge, thickened tender major milk ducts and a transverse slit-like nipple retraction looking like a fish's mouth (58.6).

Ultrasonography shows thickened major milk ducts with surrounding inflammation or abscess. A lump should be biopsied under ultrasound guidance to confirm the diagnosis. Any pus discharge should be sent for culture sensitivity and GeneXpert® *Mycobacterium tuberculosis* complex and resistance to rifampicin (MTB/RIF) testing to rule out TB. The most common organisms isolated are staphylococci, enterococci, anaerobic streptococci and sometimes *Bacteroides* and mycobacteria.

Many cases of periductal mastitis resolve with a course of antibiotics, combined with needle aspiration of an abscess. However, surgical treatment by major milk duct excision is needed in patients with a subareolar abscess or sepsis and a mammary duct fistula. A 1.5- to 2-cm length of the ductal cone

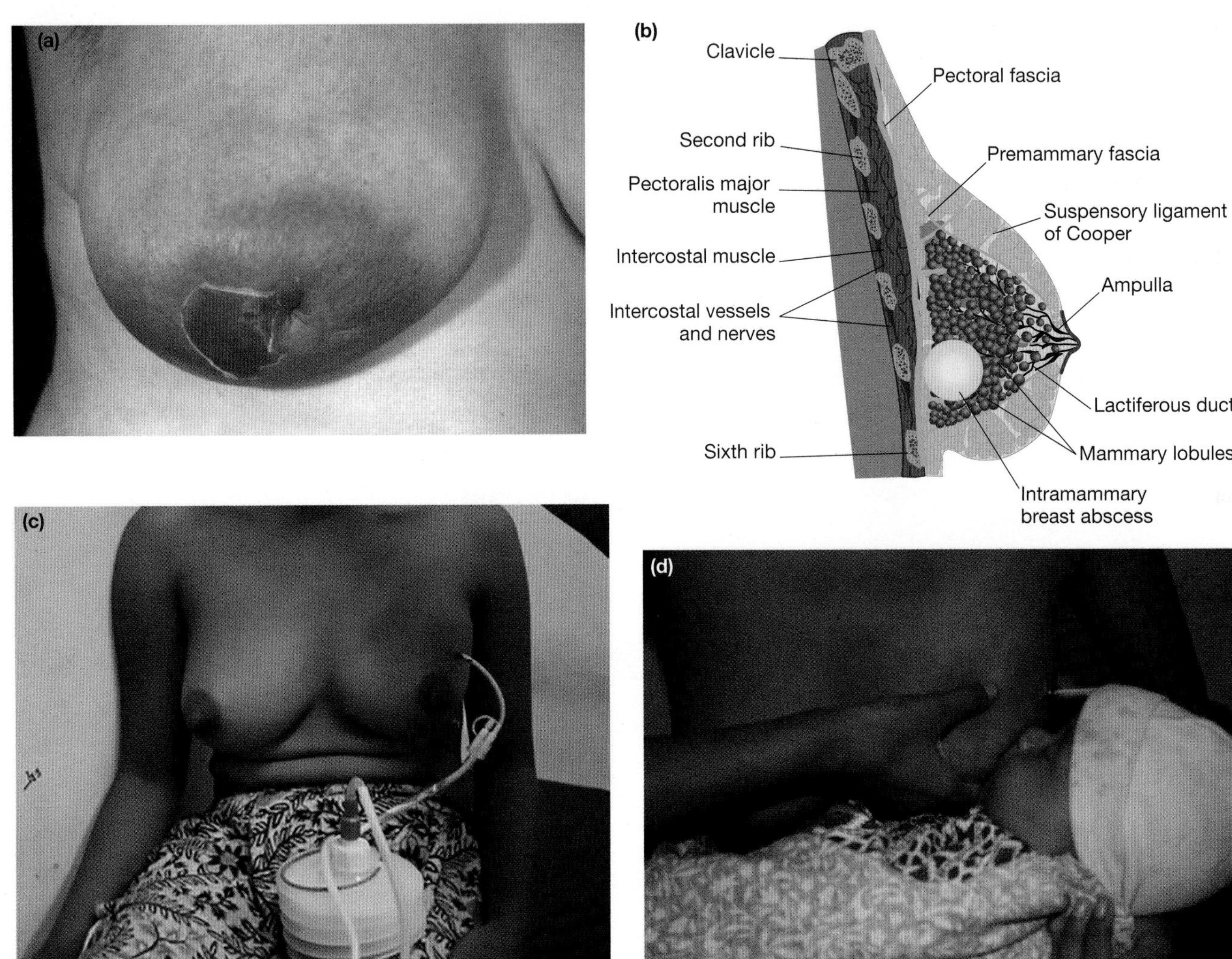

Figure 58.24 (a) Breast abscess; (b) diagrammatic representation; (c) closed suction drainage; (d) breastfeeding while a drainage catheter is in place.

should be excised. Smoking cessation must be encouraged to prevent recurrence.

Idiopathic granulomatous mastitis

This is a benign, self-limiting, inflammatory breast disease of unknown aetiology. It occurs most commonly in young parous women within the first few years after pregnancy. An association between IGM and *Corynebacterium kroppenstedtii* infection has been postulated. IGM may present as single or multiple central or peripheral inflammatory breast masses, with or without abscess formation. IGM may be associated with skin ulceration, nipple retraction, sinus formation, peau d'orange and axillary lymphadenopathy. These findings may mimic cancer.

A needle biopsy of a solid mass establishes the diagnosis of IGM. The tissue/aspirate should also be sent for Gram stain and culture, acid-fast bacilli (AFB) stain and culture and fungal stain and culture. Histologically IGM shows a non-caseating granuloma with chronic inflammation. The differential diagnoses include TB, foreign body reaction and sarcoidosis.

In symptomatic patients and in those with infection, treatment with non-steroidal anti-inflammatory drugs and antibiotics with or without drainage is indicated. In countries where TB is endemic, care should be taken to avoid administering anti-tuberculous therapy as a blanket treatment to all patients with granulomatous mastitis. Anti-tuberculous treatment should only be given to patients with evidence of TB on imaging, histopathology or microbiological analysis and GeneXpert® MTB/RIF. In cases of persistent symptoms or progression, treatment with prednisolone (oral or topical) with or without methotrexate has helped in regression of IGM. A major milk duct excision is indicated in patients with a mammary duct fistula. Excision of chronic abscess cavities is performed in patients with recurrence.

Hans Christian Joachim Gram, 1853–1938, Professor of Pharmacology (1891–1900) and of Medicine (1900–1923), Copenhagen, Denmark, described this method of staining bacteria in 1884.

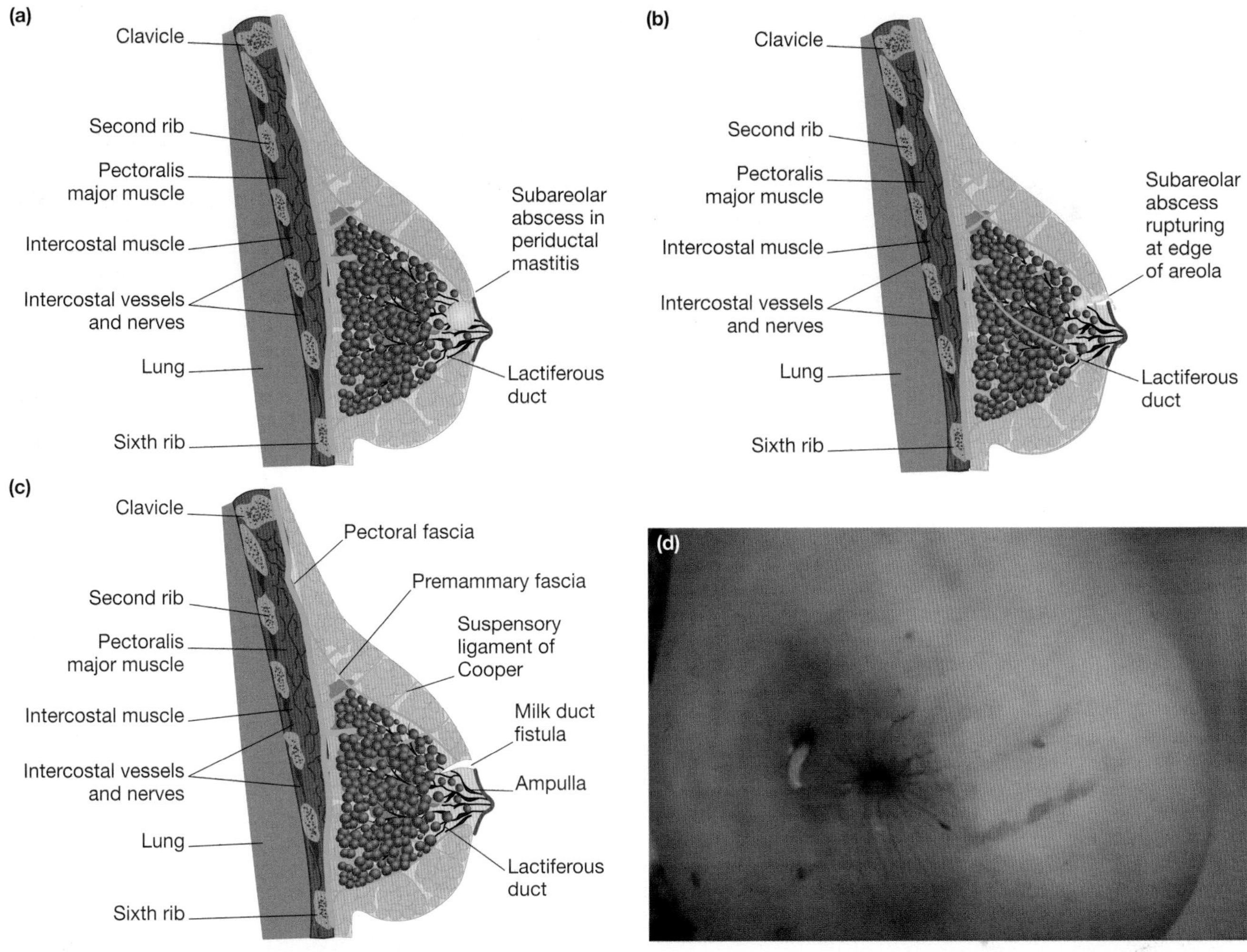

Figure 58.25 Periductal mastitis. (a) Subareoalar abscess due to blockage of a milk duct. (b) Subareolar abscess ruptured at the edge of the areola. (c) Diagrammatic representation of a milk (mammary) duct fistula connecting the mammary duct epithelium to the skin epithelium. (d) Clinical photograph showing a retracted nipple and a milk duct fistula at the areolar edge discharging pus.

Tuberculosis of the breast

TB of the breast is uncommon. It is caused by spread from the axillary or internal mammary lymph nodes or osteitis of the rib or sternum. Sometimes infection may reach the breast from the pleural cavity. Uncommon sources of infection can be entry from a cracked nipple or a haematogenous route. It presents with multiple chronic abscesses and sinuses with a typical bluish discoloration of the surrounding skin. The diagnosis rests on bacteriological and histological examination. Tubercular mastitis results in epithelioid cell granuloma with caseating necrosis. AFB can be seen occasionally in the pus/aspirate from caseation necrosis. Any pus or tissue should be sent for Ziehl–Neelsen staining, GeneXpert® MTB/RIF testing and mycobacterial culture. A computed tomography (CT) scan of the chest and abdomen aids in diagnosis by detecting other foci of present or past TB. A Mantoux test may be done; however, it is of little value in countries where TB is endemic. Treatment consists of anti-tuberculous chemotherapy for 6–9 months. Healing is usual, although often delayed with puckered scars (*Figure 58.26*).

Duct ectasia

Duct ectasia is defined as dilated major milk ducts. It is considered a disorder of involution as part of ANDI. Abnormally dilated ducts are filled with debris. This acts as an irritant and can lead to periductal inflammation and subsequent fibrosis, leading to nipple retraction. Patients usually present with toothpaste-like or coloured (such as brown, green or mud coloured) nipple discharge. The clinical findings of duct ectasia can mimic malignancy as well as benign conditions such as mastitis. Ultrasonography reveals dilated major milk ducts >3 mm in diameter.

Treatment

Triple assessment should be followed by antibiotic therapy if inflammation/infection is present. Co-amoxiclav, flucloxacillin,

Franz Ziehl, 1859–1926, German bacteriologist and a professor in Lubeck, Germany.
Friedrich Carl Adolf Neelsen, 1854–1898, German pathologist and professor at the Institute of Pathology, University of Rostock, Germany.
Charles Mantoux, 1877–1947, physician, Le Cannet, Alpes Maritimes, France, described the intradermal tuberculin skin test in 1908.

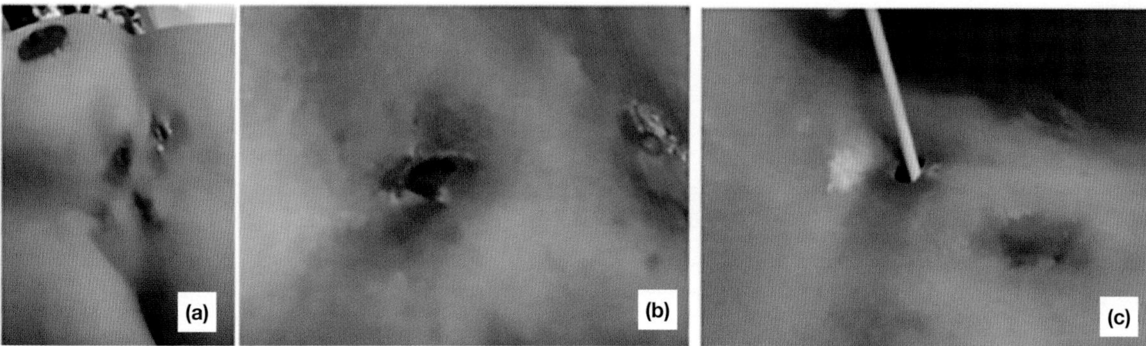

Figure 58.26 Tuberculosis of the breast. (a) Multiple pus-discharging sinuses from the lower part of the breast and lower chest wall. (b) Bluish discoloration of the skin around the tubercular sinus. (c) Undermined edge of a tubercular ulcer.

ciprofloxacin or cefixime along with anti-anaerobic cover with metronidazole or tinidazole for 2–3 weeks is recommended. In patients with profuse nipple discharge or subareolar abscess, major mammary duct excision is performed.

Actinomycosis

Actinomycosis of the breast is very rare. It is caused by anaerobic *Actinomyces* bacteria. The lesions present with multiple chronic, pus-discharging, non-healing sinuses over the breast. The pus demonstrates typical black granules and the specific pathogen on microbiology. The condition requires long-term penicillin injections along with curettage of necrotic granulomas and sinuses.

Mondor's disease

Mondor's disease is thrombophlebitis of the superficial veins of the breast and anterior chest wall.

In the absence of injury or infection, the cause of thrombophlebitis is obscure. The pathognomonic feature is a tender thrombosed subcutaneous cord, usually attached to the skin. When the skin over the breast is stretched by raising the arm, a narrow, shallow, subcutaneous groove alongside the cord becomes apparent (*Figure 58.27*). The differential diagnosis is lymphatic permeation from an occult carcinoma of the breast. The only treatment required is to restrict arm movements. The condition usually subsides within a few months without recurrence, complications or deformity.

CARCINOMA OF THE BREAST

Breast cancer is the most frequent cancer among women, with an estimated 2.3 million new cases diagnosed worldwide in 2020, representing about 25% of all cancers in women. Incidence rates vary widely across the world, from 27 per 100 000 in Middle Africa and East Asia to 92 per 100 000 in North America. In western Europe approximately one in nine women will develop breast cancer, accounting for 3–5% of all deaths in women. In resource-poor countries 1 in 28 women will develop breast cancer in her lifetime and for every 2 women diagnosed with breast cancer 1 dies of cancer.

Risk factors

There are several factors known to increase the RR for developing breast cancer. These are called the risk factors and can be divided into modifiable (those that can be modified by adopting a healthy diet and lifestyle) and non-modifiable risk factors. The events increasing the oestrogenic exposure of the breast are said to be risk factors for breast cancer, such as early menarche, late menopause, nulliparity, late first pregnancy and hormone replacement with high oestrogen therapy. These are listed in *Table 58.3*.

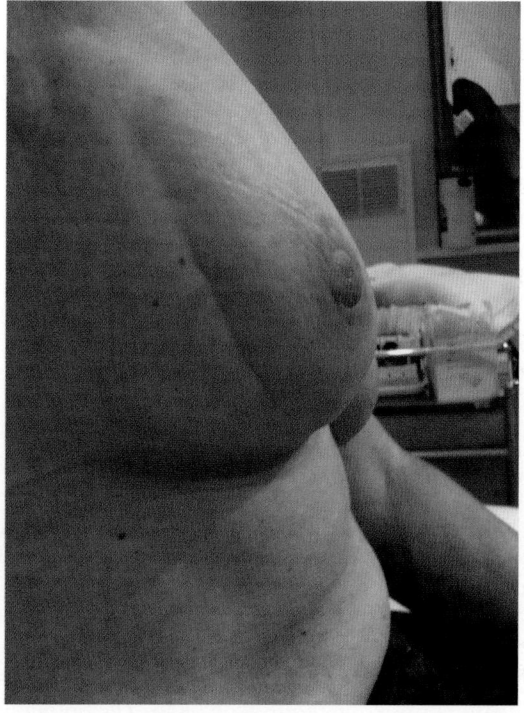

Figure 58.27 Mondor's disease in the lateral aspect of the right breast.

Henri Mondor, 1885–1962, Professor of Surgery, Paris, France.

TABLE 58.3 Risk factors for breast cancer.

	Remarks
Modifiable risk factors	
Obesity: BMI >30	Increased risk in postmenopausal women: RR = 1.29
Parity	Increased risk in nulliparous women or first pregnancy after 35 years of age
Breastfeeding	It is protective for breast cancer and >12 months of breastfeeding by women has a greater protective effect than shorter duration
Age at first childbirth	Early: less risk, <20 years Late: high risk, >35 years
Use of HRT	Use for >10 years increased risk: RR = 1.2
Tobacco use	RR = 1.14 for smoking 25 or more cigarettes/day; RR = 1.07 for smoking for 20 years or more
Alcohol consumption	RR = 1.05 for light drinking (<1 drink/day); RR = 1.32 for moderate drinking (3 or 4 drinks/day); RR = 1.46 for heavy drinking (>4 drinks/day)
Radiation exposure	RR = 6
Non-modifiable risk factors	
Age	Increasing age is a risk factor. While the median age at presentation is around 60 years in the West (UK, USA), it is around 48 years in low-/middle-income nations such as India
Sex	Female sex is a risk factor as only 0.5–1% of all breast cancers occur in males
Ethnicity	American white, African American (age <45 years), Ashkenazi Jew, Parsi in India
Family history of breast cancer	One first-degree relative (mother, sister or daughter) with breast cancer: RR = 2; two first-degree relatives with breast cancer: RR = 3
Genetic predisposition	5–10% of all breast cancers are hereditary; *BRCA1* and *BRCA2* mutations account for up to 70% of hereditary breast cancers
Early menarche (<12 years)	Breast cancer risk increases by around 5% for each year earlier menstruation begins: RR = 1.19 for age <11 years
Late menopause (>55 years)	Breast cancer risk increases by about 3% for each year later menopause begins: RR = 1.12 for menopause at 55 years versus menopause at 45 years
High-risk breast lesions	Proliferative conditions without atypia: RR = 1.8–2 Complex fibroadenoma: RR = 3 Papillomatosis: RR = 3 Proliferative diseases with atypia: atypical ductal and lobular hyperplasia: RR = 4–5 Lobular carcinoma *in situ*: RR = 8–10

BMI, body mass index; *BRCA*, breast cancer; HRT, hormone replacement therapy; RR, relative risk.

Pathology of breast cancer

Breast carcinoma arises from the milk ducts in 90% (ductal carcinoma) or from the lobule in 10% (lobular carcinoma) of patients. The disease may remain confined to the epithelium of the duct or lobule with no breach in the basement membrane; this is called ***in situ* disease**. Infiltration of the surrounding tissue through a breach in the basement membrane leads to 'invasive or infiltrative' ductal or lobular carcinoma. The tumour may be well differentiated, moderately differentiated or poorly differentiated. The modified Bloom–Richardson scoring system for tumour grade includes the sum of individual scores for three variables (percentage of tumour cells with tubule formation, nuclear pleomorphism and the size and number of mitoses/HPF), each of which is assigned from 1 to 3 points according to the degree of deviation from normal breast epithelium. A total score of 3–5 defines grade I; 6 or 7 grade II; and 8 or 9 grade III.

Invasive carcinoma is usually of **no special type** (NST), which represents the most common variety of breast cancer. Rare histological variants, usually carrying a better prognosis, include colloid or mucinous carcinoma, whose cells produce abundant mucin; medullary carcinoma, with solid sheets of large cells often associated with a marked lymphocytic reaction; and tubular carcinoma. The papillary type of carcinoma (both *in situ* and invasive) is a rare type of breast cancer accounting for 0.5–1% of all neoplasms. The lesion is characterised by papillomas with a fibrovascular core and surface covered by epithelial and myoepithelial cells. It usually carries a better prognosis and rarely spreads to lymph nodes and the bloodstream. The tumour cells may overexpress oestrogen receptors (ER positive), progesterone receptors (PR positive), human epidermal growth factor receptor 2/neu (HER2/neu positive) and androgen receptors (AR positive). The degree of mitosis can be detected by the Ki-67 mitotic index.

Gene array analysis has identified five major subtypes: luminal A, luminal B, basal, HER2/neu receptor enriched and a normal-like group (***Table 58.4***). In the absence of gene array testing such as prediction analysis of microarray-50 (PAM-50), immune histochemical receptor staining serves as a surrogate marker of molecular subtypes.

TABLE 58.4 Molecular classification of breast cancer.

Classification	Hormone receptor	HER2/neu	Others
Luminal A	Positive (either or both ER/PR)	Negative	Ki-67 low
Luminal B	Positive (either or both ER/PR)	Negative	Ki-67 high
Basal type (triple negative)	Negative	Negative	Ki-67 usually high
HER2/neu enriched	Negative	Positive	Ki-67 high
Claudin low	Negative	Negative	Claudin low

ER, oestrogen receptor; HER2/neu, human epidermal growth factor receptor 2/neu; PR, progesterone receptor.

Harris JG Bloom, 1923–1988, radiation oncologist, Royal Marsden Hospital, London, UK.
William W Richardson, 1915–2005, pathologist, Middlesex Hospital, London, UK, published a paper with Bloom on the natural history of breast cancer in 1957.

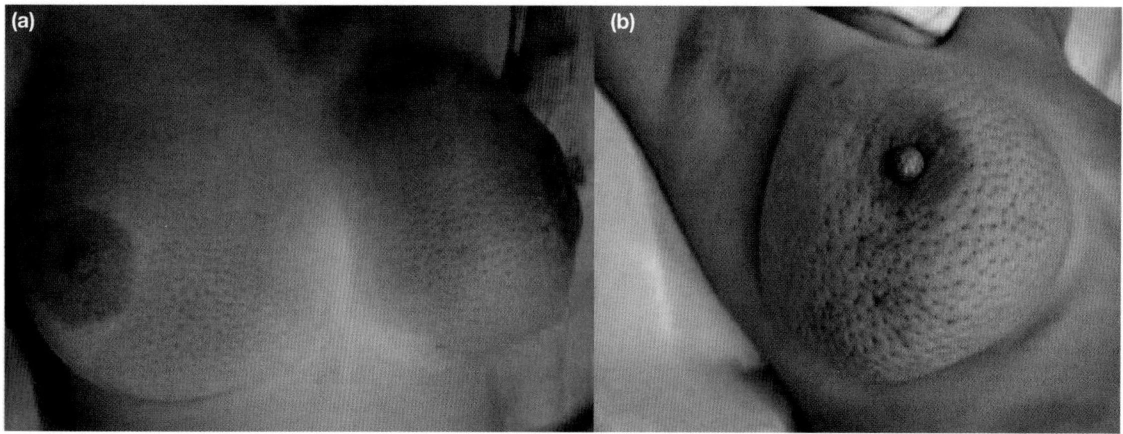

Figure 58.28 (a) Diffuse redness (erythema) and skin oedema involving more than one-third of the breast, with an enlarged left breast – features of inflammatory carcinoma. (b) Peau d'orange refers to the orange peel appearance of the skin of the breast and is a sign of locally advanced disease. Note that in people with darker skins the erythema takes on a brownish hue.

Spread of cancer

Local spread

The tumour increases in size and invades adjacent breast parenchyma. It may involve the skin, leading to ulceration and satellite nodules, and/or involve pectoralis major, serratus anterior and even the chest wall. The tumour cells release a number of growth factors; namely, fibroblast growth factor (FGF), transforming growth factor (TGFα and TGFβ) and vascular endothelial growth factor (VEGF). FGF induces mitosis of adjacent fibrocytes, which convert to fibroblasts and lay down collagen (desmoplastic reaction). Contraction of collagen leads to shortening of Cooper's ligament, pulling the skin inwards and giving rise to the telltale signs of dimpling (shortened single Cooper's ligament), puckering or tethering (many Cooper's ligaments shrunken) or nipple retraction.

Lymphatic metastasis

This occurs mainly to axillary lymph nodes. Tumours from the inner half of the breast may also spread to the internal mammary nodes. Involvement of the contralateral lymph nodes in the absence of a contralateral primary represents metastatic disease (***Table 58.5***).

TABLE 58.5 Causes of contralateral axillary lymph node involvement in breast cancer.

- Haematogenous spread from the contralateral primary
- Spread of cancer from one breast to another via subdermal lymphatics in front of the sternum
- Spread of cancer from one breast to the other via the ipsilateral internal mammary nodes → interconnecting lymphatics behind the sternum → the contralateral internal mammary nodes → the other breast → the opposite axillary nodes
- Tumour developing in an epithelial embryonic cell rest trapped in a lymph node during embryonic development of a node (rare)
- Primary tumour of the opposite breast

Haematogenous spread

At a tumour size of 1–2 mm (10^5 cells) neoangiogenesis occurs. The onset of angiogenesis ushers in rapid growth, invasion and metastatic potential. Haematogenous metastasis occurs to the skeletal system (in order of frequency: lumbar vertebrae, neck of femur, thoracic vertebrae, rib and skull). The bony metastasis is generally osteolytic, although osteosclerotic and mixed types may be seen. Haematogenous metastasis may also occur to the liver, lungs and brain and, occasionally, the adrenal glands and ovaries. In limbs these deposits occur above the elbow and above the knee (haematopoietic vascular bone marrow is confined to the axial skeleton and in limbs above the elbows and the knees). Extensive bone marrow replacement by tumour cells may result in release of immature blast cells in the peripheral blood, giving rise to 'leukoerythroblastic anaemia'. Peripheral blood samples for circulating cell-free tumour deoxyribonucleic acid (cf-DNA) and circulating tumour cells are being studied as potential prognostic markers to predict disease recurrence.

Clinical presentation

A discrete lump in the breast is the most common presentation, and the most common tumour site is the upper outer quadrant of the breast (50% of TDLUs lie there). Other symptoms include nipple retraction, nipple discharge (blood or serous), skin changes such as ulceration, peau d'orange (***Figure 58.28***), satellite nodules or dimpling/tethering. Peau d'orange is a sign of locally advanced disease due to obstruction of cutaneous lymphatic drainage of the breast, by infiltration of either subdermal lymphatics or axillary lymph nodes by tumour cells. **Cancer en cuirasse** (***Figure 58.29***) is due to extensive tumour infiltration of the skin of the breast, chest (in cases of postmastectomy recurrence), upper limb and abdomen.

Few breast cancers in high-income countries present with either locally advanced disease or symptoms of metastatic

Alfred Armand Velpeau, 1795–1867, anatomist and surgeon, Tours, France, described cancer en cuirasse in 1838.

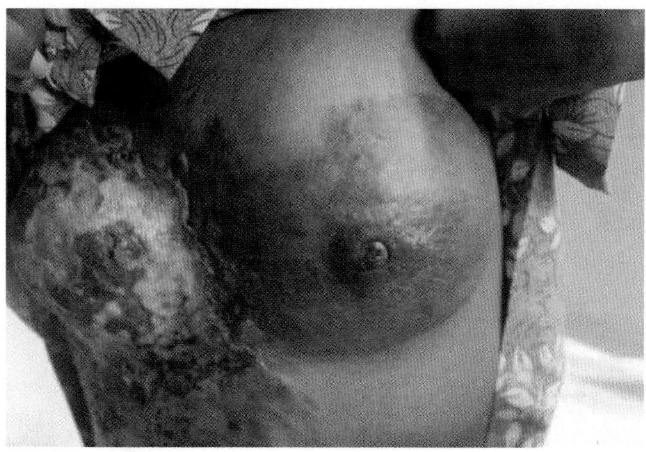

Figure 58.29 Cancer en cuirasse: advanced breast cancer with extensive tumour infiltration of the skin of the breast, upper limb and abdomen.

disease; however, the incidence is much greater in resource-poor countries, where up to 60% of women still present late. Enquiry should be made for the presence of any swelling in the neck or armpit and for the presence of any symptoms due to distant metastasis (bony pain, cough, breathlessness, haemoptysis, headache, visual disturbances, neurological deficit, epileptic fits, abdominal distension, jaundice, anorexia, weakness, weight loss, hypercalcaemia, etc).

Staging of breast cancer

Staging refers to the process of finding out the extent of tumour. The eighth edition of the Union for International Cancer Control (UICC)–American Joint Committee on Cancer (AJCC) TNM staging system is currently used (*Table 58.6*).

In addition to anatomical staging, the eighth edition of the AJCC TNM staging system includes the histological grade, the ER, PR, HER2/neu and Ki-67 assessment, multigene testing with Oncotype DX® and the response to neoadjuvant chemotherapy to refine the prognostic information. The key points in the eighth edition of the AJCC TNM staging system are listed in *Summary box 58.3*.

Summary box 58.3

Key points of the eighth edition of the AJCC TNM staging system

- Lobular carcinoma *in situ* (LCIS) is a high-risk benign lesion not a cancer
- The T categorisation of multiple synchronous tumours is documented using the (m) modifier
- The prefix (y) is used to denote the post-neoadjuvant therapy status
- Satellite nodules in the skin must be separate from the primary tumour for it to be categorised as T4b
- Pathological complete response (pCR) denotes the absence of tumour cells in the breast and axillary nodes in surgical specimens
- Inflammatory carcinoma remains classified as inflammatory carcinoma after NACT, even after complete remission
- Microinvasive (T1mi) carcinomas are defined as invasive tumour foci ≤1.0 mm
- Tumours >1 mm and <2 mm should be reported as rounded to 2 mm
- Tumour size should be measured to the nearest millimetre

Work-up for metastatic breast cancer

Contrast-enhanced CT of the chest, abdomen and pelvis and an isotope bone scan are needed for patients with locally advanced breast cancer (T3, T4 or N2, N3 disease). Patients with early breast carcinoma (T1, T2 and N0, N1 disease) need metastatic evaluation only if they present with symptoms to suggest metastatic disease or raised serum alkaline phosphatase. A PET-CT scan with ^{18}F-fluorodeoxyglucose (^{18}F-FDG) tracer may be used for metastatic work-up.

Treatment of breast cancer

The treatment of breast cancer is multimodal (includes surgery, systemic treatment [chemotherapy, targeted therapy, hormonal therapy] and radiotherapy); hence, specialist breast centres employ a **multidisciplinary team** (MDT) that should include the surgeon, radiologist, pathologist, radiation oncologist, medical oncologist, plastic surgeon and allied health professionals, such as a breast care nurse, psychological counsellor and preferably a genetic counsellor (*58.7*).

While some patients with low disease burden and low biological aggressiveness can be treated with surgery followed by adjuvant therapy, others require downsizing of disease with neoadjuvant systemic therapy or primary systemic therapy.

Neoadjuvant systemic therapy (NAST) consists of **neoadjuvant chemotherapy** (NACT), targeted therapy or hormonal therapy prior to surgery. It aims to downsize the disease and enable clinicians to know the *in vivo* response of the tumour to therapy. The indications for NACT are as follows:

1. Locally advanced breast cancer T3, T4/N2, N3 disease: to downsize the tumour.
2. Select cases of early breast cancer:
   - a to downsize the tumour to facilitate breast conservation surgery (BCS);
   - b HER2/neu-positive tumours;
   - c triple-negative breast cancer (TNBC);
   - d premenopausal women (age <50 years);
   - e patients with axillary node metastasis.

- **Neoadjuvant targeted therapy** (trastuzumab, pertuzumab) is administered for HER2/neu-positive tumours >5 mm in diameter.
- **Neoadjuvant hormonal therapy** is offered to elderly or frail women (with ER and/or -, PR-positive advanced tumours) who are deemed unfit to receive systemic chemotherapy. Neoadjuvant hormonal treatment takes longer (around 3–6 months) for the response to become clinically evident.
- **Response assessment and timing of surgery**: the patient is examined 3 weeks after administration of

TABLE 58.6 Union for International Cancer Control–American Joint Committee on Cancer TNM staging system (eighth edition) for breast cancer.

T category	T criteria
Tx	Primary tumour cannot be assessed
T0	No evidence of primary tumour
Tis(DCIS)	Ductal carcinoma *in situ* (DCIS)
Tis(Paget's)	Paget's disease of the nipple **not** associated with (Paget's) invasive carcinoma and/or carcinoma *in situ* (DCIS) in the underlying breast parenchyma. Carcinomas in the breast parenchyma associated with Paget's disease are categorised based on the size and characteristics of the parenchymal disease, although the presence of Paget's disease should still be noted
T1	Tumour ≤20 mm in greatest dimension
T1mi	Tumour ≤1 mm in greatest dimension
T1a	Tumour >1 mm but ≤5 mm in greatest dimension (round any measurement >1.0–1.9 mm to 2 mm)
T1b	Tumour >5 mm but ≤10 mm in greatest dimension
T1c	Tumour >10 mm but ≤20 mm in greatest dimension
T2	Tumour >20 mm but ≤50 mm in greatest dimension
T3	Tumour >50 mm in greatest dimension
T4	Tumour of any size with direct extension to the chest wall and/or to the skin (ulceration or macroscopic nodules); invasion of the dermis alone does not qualify as T4
T4a	Extension to the chest wall; invasion or adherence to pectoralis muscle in the absence of invasion of chest wall structures does not qualify as T4a
T4b	Ulceration and/or ipsilateral macroscopic satellite nodules and/or oedema (including peau d'orange) of the skin that does not meet the criteria for inflammatory carcinoma
T4c	Both T4a and T4b are present T4a + T4b = T4c
T4d	Inflammatory carcinoma; peau d'orange and redness involving >1/3rd of the surface of the breast with or without a breast lump
cN category	**cN criteria**
cNx	Regional lymph nodes cannot be assessed (e.g. previously removed)
cN0	No regional lymph node metastases (by imaging or clinical examination)
cN1	Metastases to movable ipsilateral level I, II axillary lymph node(s)
cN1mi	Micrometastases (approximately 200 cells, >0.2 mm, but none >2.0 mm)
cN2	Metastases in ipsilateral level I, II axillary lymph nodes that are clinically fixed or matted; **or** in ipsilateral internal mammary nodes in the absence of axillary lymph node metastases
cN2a	Metastases in ipsilateral level I, II axillary lymph nodes fixed to one another (matted) or to other structures
cN2b	Metastases only in ipsilateral internal mammary nodes in the absence of axillary lymph node metastases
cN3	Metastases in ipsilateral infraclavicular (level III axillary) lymph node(s) with or without level I, II axillary lymph node involvement; **or** in ipsilateral internal mammary lymph node(s) with level I, II axillary lymph node metastases; **or** metastases in ipsilateral supraclavicular lymph node(s) with or without axillary or internal mammary lymph node involvement
cN3a	Metastases in ipsilateral infraclavicular lymph node(s)
cN3b	Metastases in ipsilateral internal mammary lymph node(s) and axillary lymph node(s)
cN3c	Metastases in ipsilateral supraclavicular lymph node(s)
M category	**M criteria**
M0	No clinical or radiographic evidence of distant metastases
cM0(i+)	No clinical or radiographic evidence of distant metastases in the presence of tumour cells or deposits <0.2 mm detected microscopically or by molecular techniques in circulating blood, bone marrow or other non-regional nodal tissue in a patient without symptoms or signs of metastases
cM1	Distant metastases detected by clinical and radiographic means

c, clinical.

the second cycle of NACT. Response evaluation criteria in solid tumours (RECIST) are used for reporting the response to NAST. The four RECIST categories are:

- complete response (CR) (lesion not detectable on clinical palpation and imaging);
- partial response (PR) (≥30% reduction in the maximal diameter);
- stable disease (SD) (<30% reduction in maximal diameter);
- progressive disease (PD) (≥20% increase in the maximal diameter).

For patients with CR and PR, the entire chemotherapy regimen may be delivered prior to surgery. If the patient is being planned for BCS, a radio-opaque clip or magnetic marker such as Magseed® is placed under image guidance in the epicentre of the tumour to allow identification at the time of surgery should there be a complete response to NACT. If the facility for clip placement is unavailable, in place of the metal clip a 0.5-cm piece of silicone or a polyvinylchloride (PVC) catheter tip may be inserted through a small skin incision just anterior to the tumour. This catheter tip remains palpable even after complete regression of the tumour and helps the surgeon in performing removal of the index area for BCS, excising 2 cm of tissue all around this catheter. For patients showing stable or progressive disease, after the initial two cycles of chemotherapy, the patient should undergo surgery and be given second-line chemotherapy after surgery.

Surgical management

Surgery plays a central role in the management of breast cancer. There has been a general de-escalation towards more conservative techniques, backed up by clinical trials and meta-analyses showing equal efficacy in locoregional cancer control and survival between mastectomy and WLE/BCS followed by radiotherapy.

The aim of surgery is to remove all disease in the breast and axilla with negative margins. The pathologist reports the distance of the tumour to the nearest excision margin in the breast specimen. Indelible India ink is applied on the specimen surfaces. There should be no tumour cells on the cut edge or 'inked margins' of the tumour for invasive cancer. However, in patients with DCIS a minimum of 2 mm is considered a safe margin.

Early breast cancer (stages 0, I ,II)

The surgical options for the primary tumour include mastectomy or BCS.

Mastectomy is indicated for large tumours (in relation to the size of the breast), multicentric disease, diffuse microcalcification on a mammogram indicative of DCIS, *BRCA*-positive cancers, local recurrence following BCS or the patient's preference. It entails removal of the entire breast tissue, including the skin over the tumour, the nipple–areola complex and the axillary tail. The breast tissue usually extends to a point where the anterior premammary fascia fuses with the posterior pectoral fascia. Therefore, the surgeon should remove the breast to the point of fusion between these two fasciae, which usually extends to the level of the second rib above, to the parasternal edge medially, to the inframammary crease below and to the anterior border of latissimus dorsi laterally. This is different from the traditional view of raising flaps up to the inferior border of the clavicle superiorly and 2–3 cm below the inframammary crease (or up to the upper fibres of the external oblique muscle/rectus abdominis) inferiorly. The radical mastectomy (Halsted) included excision of the breast, all the axillary lymph nodes and both the pectoralis major and minor muscles. It is rarely indicated as it causes excessive morbidity owing to the limitation in movement at the shoulder joint, extensive upper limb lymphoedema, pain and chest wall deformity with no survival benefit compared with less radical surgery. The modified radical mastectomy (MRM) entails mastectomy along with removal of the level I, II and III axillary lymph nodes.

Skin- and nipple-sparing mastectomy is an option in DCIS and early breast cancers where a mastectomy is indicated and the tumour is >1 cm away from the skin and >2 cm away from the nipple. The breast may then be reconstructed using autologous tissue flaps/fat or a silicone breast implant.

Breast conservation surgery (BCS) is aimed at removing the tumour along with a 1-cm margin of normal breast tissue. It is important to orient the surgical specimen with sutures: long lateral ('L' for 'lateral') and short superior ('S' for 'superior'). This is important if one or more margins is positive on histological examination. Patients with involved margins should have a revision of margins called a 'cavity shave'. All patients with BCS receive radiotherapy. BCS together with radiotherapy is called **breast conservation therapy** (BCT): BCS + RT = BCT. BCS is, however, best avoided in patients with a multicentric tumour, diffuse microcalcifications on a mammogram, a large tumour-to-breast ratio, two times positive surgical margins after re-excision, a history of previous breast or chest wall radiation, systemic lupus erythematosus or other collagen vascular disease (these patients have a high risk of a radiation reaction), or ankylosing spondylitis; it is also best avoided in those with severe orthopnoea (as the patient cannot lie on the radiation table).

Wide local excision (WLE) of up to 20% of the breast volume can be achieved by excision of the tumour with adequate margins and closure of the defect by approximation of the breast tissue with absorbable sutures. Volume loss greater than 20% or an unfavourable breast-to-tumour ratio requires an **oncoplastic procedure** to fill the defect so created by mobilising the breast tissue.

Oncoplasty is defined as tumour excision with wide margins followed by repair of the defect by local rearrangement/replacement of the breast tissue and the nipple–areola complex to maintain shape and symmetry. This may be achieved by **volume displacement** (level 1) (***Figures 58.30 and 58.31***) or by **volume replacement** using a distant or local flap (level 2) (***Figure 58.32***) (***Summary box 58.4***).

William Stewart Halsted, 1852–1922, Professor of Surgery, Johns Hopkins Medical School, Baltimore, MD, USA

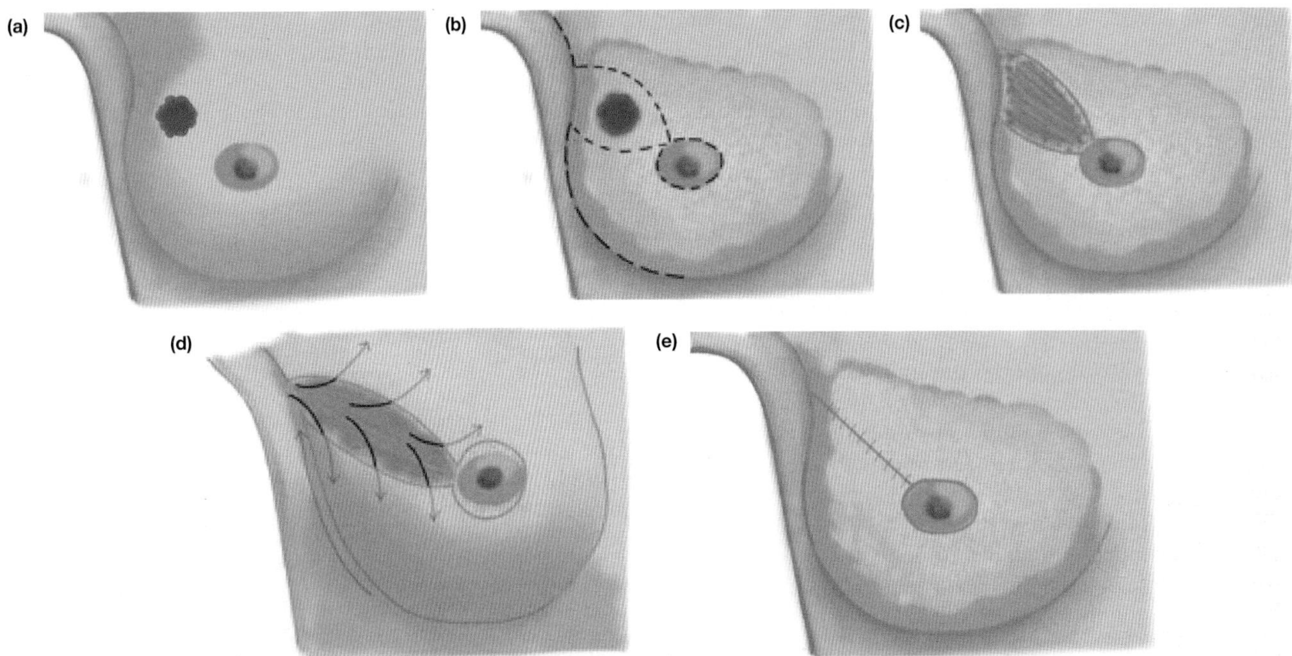

Figure 58.30 Volume displacement oncoplasty for an upper outer quadrant tumour (a). Skin incision markings extending to the periareolar and the lateral mammary crease (b). Full-thickness excision of the tumour with 1-cm margins (c). Dermoglandular pillar mobilisation from the lower outer quadrant of the breast to fill the defect cavity (d). Final sutured wound (e).

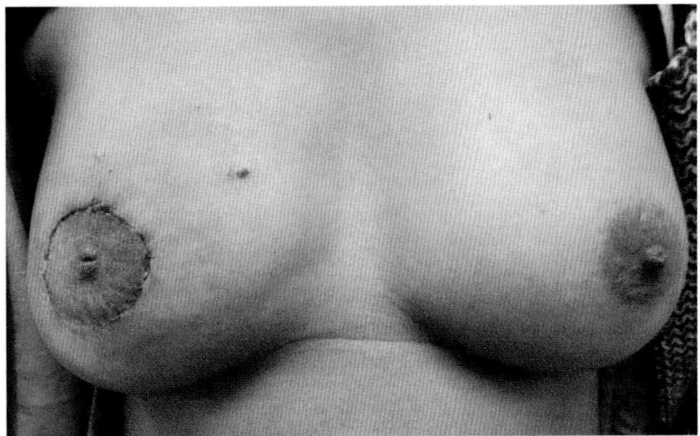

Figure 58.31 A patient with volume displacement with round-block oncoplasty for a right breast tumour.

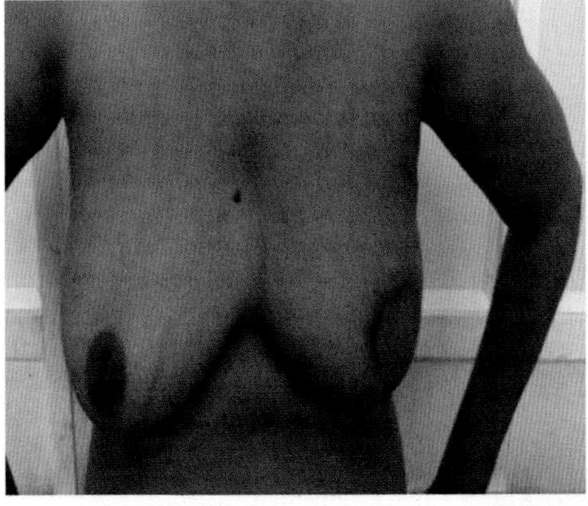

Figure 58.32 A patient with volume replacement oncoplasty with a muscle-sparing latissimus dorsi muscle flap reconstruction for a left breast tumour.

Surgery for the axilla

The role of axillary surgery is to stage the patient (sentinel lymph node biopsy [SLNB]) and to treat disease by axillary lymph node dissection (ALND) for patients with positive axillary nodes (*58.8*).

Sentinel lymph node biopsy. Sentinel means 'a guard'. Like a guard, the first echelon/level of axillary lymph nodes is located at the gateway of the axilla and provides information about the status of axillary node metastasis. The sentinel lymph node refers to the first echelon lymph node in the axilla draining the breast. The sentinel lymph node is identified by the injection of a blue dye (patent blue or methylene blue) and radioisotope technetium-99m-labelled albumin/sulphur colloid/antimony in the breast. The fluorescent dyes fluorescein or indocyanine green can be used if radioisotope is not available. The combination of fluorescein and methylene blue can detect sentinel nodes with >90% identification. Indocyanine green can detect sentinel nodes with 95–100% identification. The dye may be injected into the peritumoral tissue or the periareolar, subareolar or intradermal plane. The tracer(s) passes through lymphatics to the sentinel node and is detected visually as a blue-coloured node and/or a hot node (radioactive) with a handheld gamma ray detection probe or as a fluorescent node with blue light (480 nm for fluorescein) or infrared light (780 nm for indocyanine green) (***Figure 58.33***). The *ex vivo* count of the hot lymph node(s) is noted. All lymph nodes with >10% of the *ex vivo* count of the hottest node and blue lymph nodes are removed and sent for histological confirmation of nodal metastasis. This may be done with

Summary box 58.4

Surgical techniques used to treat breast cancer

Modified radical mastectomy	Mastectomy + level I, II, III axillary lymph node dissection: pectoralis minor muscle is removed in Patey/Madden, retracted in Auchincloss and is divided but not removed in Scanlon modifications
Simple or total mastectomy	Mastectomy including axillary tail without axillary surgery
Skin-sparing mastectomy	Mastectomy: breast skin envelope is preserved, nipple–areola complex removed
Skin + nipple/ areola-sparing mastectomy	Mastectomy: breast skin envelope and nipple–areola complex are preserved
WLE (synonyms lumpectomy; breast conservation surgery, BCS)	Removal of tumour with a three-dimensional clearance of a 1-cm margin of normal tissue
Quadrantectomy	Removal of the tumour-containing quadrant of the breast
Level I oncoplasty	Volume displacement technique involves dual-plane mobilisation of the breast parenchyma (i.e. the dermoglandular plane and the plane between breast parenchyma and pectoralis muscle) to close the defect created after WLE
Level II oncoplasty	More complex procedures that involve skin excision and glandular mobilisation to allow major volume resection, usually more than 20% of breast volume

frozen-section analysis, touch imprint cytology or by molecular methods (GeneSearch Breast Lymph Node Assay™). These methods involve homogenising the node and detecting a gene expression of cytokeratin 19 or mammaglobin by RT-PCR.

Frozen-section evaluation of sentinel nodes has a false-negative rate of 10–12%. Wherever the facility for frozen section is not available, the sentinel node should be sent for formalin-preserved paraffin section processing and haematoxylin and eosin staining.

SLNB is contraindicated in patients with inflammatory breast cancer and in those with T4 disease or a history of previous breast or chest wall surgery, breast scarring (burns) or radiotherapy.

Axillary lymph node dissection. This is indicated for staging and local disease control in patients with axillary lymph node-positive tumours that are clinically and/or biopsy-proven non-palpable nodes and those with three or more sentinel lymph nodes that are positive for macrometastasis.

ALND requires careful anatomical dissection to protect the axillary vein, thoracodorsal vessels, medial and lateral pectoral nerves, intercostobrachial nerves and the long thoracic and thoracodorsal nerves. The intercostobrachial nerve may be divided in the presence of heavy nodal burden to achieve oncological clearance. Level I and II nodes are routinely removed (***Figure 58.34***). Level III axillary dissection is reserved for patients who have enlarged level I and II lymph nodes.

Breast reconstruction

Immediate breast reconstruction offers the advantage of women waking up after surgery with a breast mound. Some women may prefer to undergo delayed reconstruction 6–12 months after completion of their adjuvant treatment.

Immediate reconstruction can be performed using silicone gel breast implants or autologous tissue. Silicone gel implants can be placed superficial to (prepectoral) or underneath

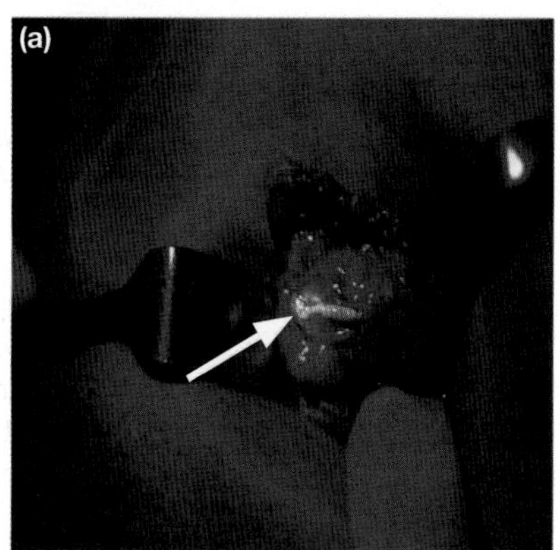

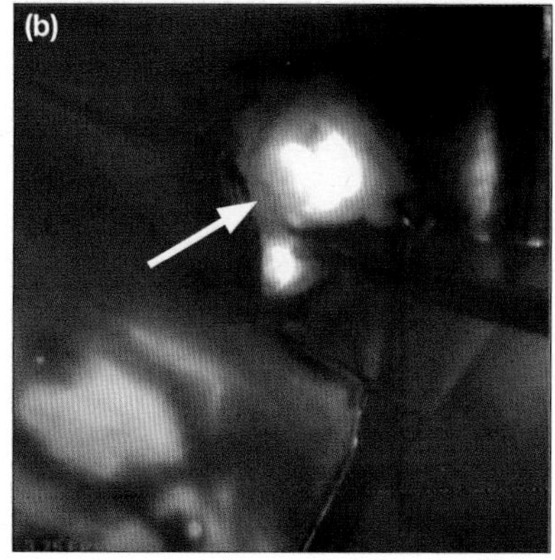

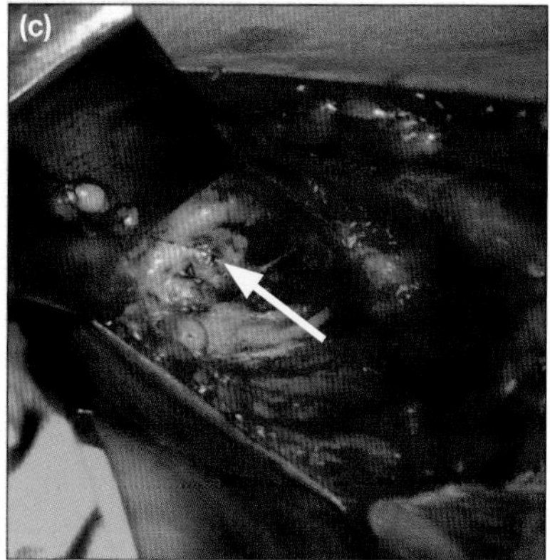

Figure 58.33 Sentinel lymph node biopsy done using (a) fluorescein dye – the fluorescent sentinel lymph node is seen with blue light; (b) indocyanine green – the fluorescent sentinel lymph node is seen using infrared imaging with a 'spy camera'; (c) blue dye (methylene blue) – blue sentinel lymph nodes and lymphatics are seen in the axilla. Sentinel lymph nodes are marked with an arrow.

David Howard Patey, 1899–1976, surgeon, Middlesex Hospital, London, UK.
John L Madden, 1913–1999, surgeon, St Claire Hospital, New York, NY, USA.
Hugh Auchincloss, 1915–1998, surgeon, Columbia College of Physicians and Surgeons, New York, NY, USA.
Edward F Scanlon, 1919–2008, surgeon, Evanston, IL USA.

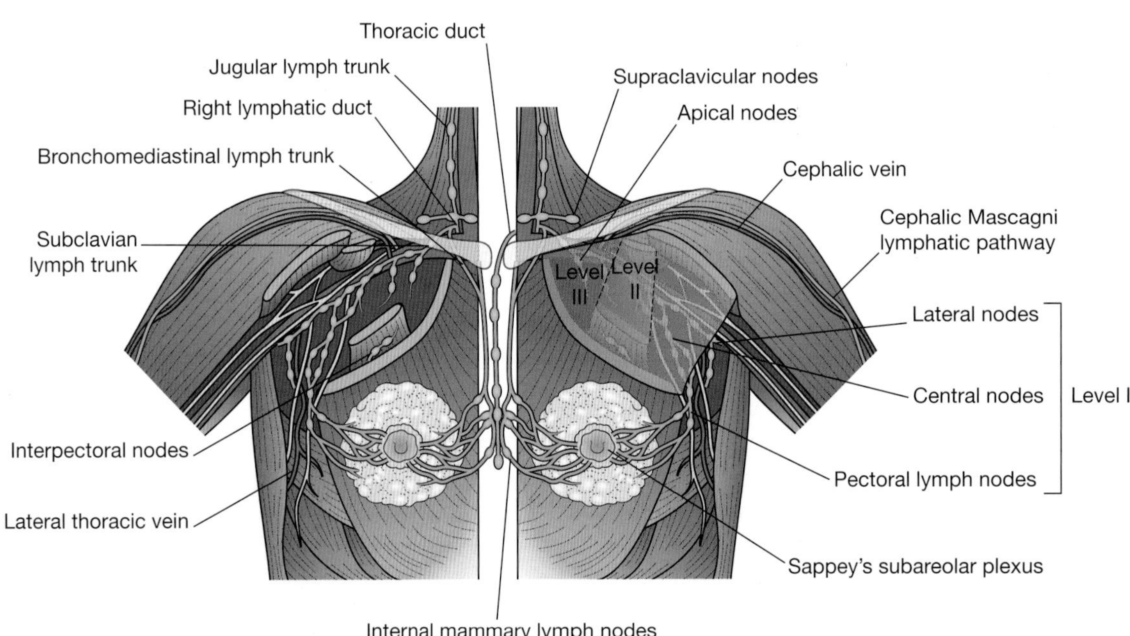

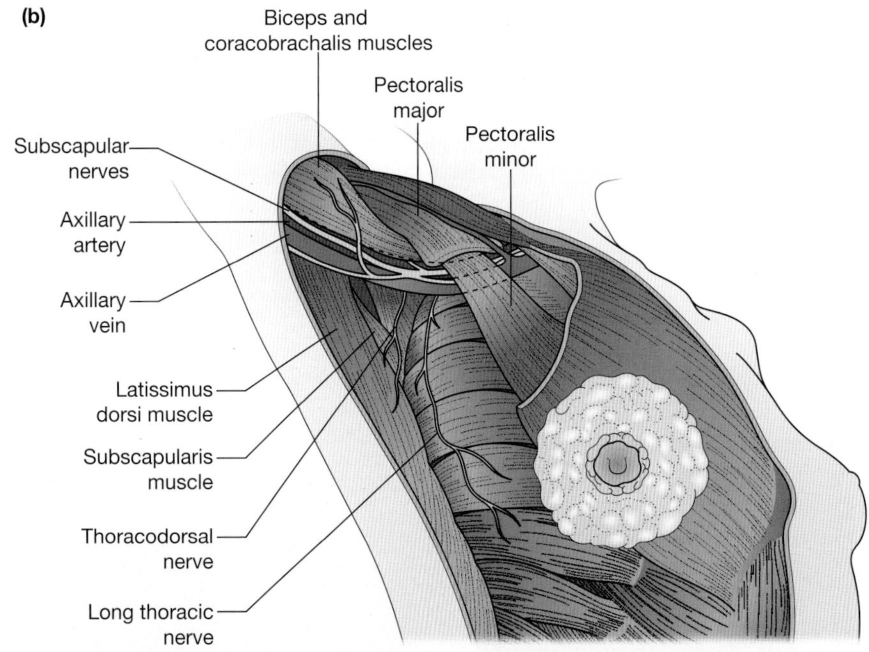

Figure 58.34 (a, b) Lymphatic drainage of the breast depicting level I, II and III lymph nodes.

(subpectoral) the pectoralis major muscle. The tissue flaps commonly used include the latissimus dorsi (*Figure 58.35*), the transverse rectus abdominis myocutaneous (TRAM) (*Figure 58.36*), the anterolateral thigh and the deep inferior epigastric perforator (DIEP) free tissue transfers (*Figure 58.37*). The DIEP flap is commonly used in the UK. It requires microvascular surgical skills and an operative time of about 4 hours. The treatment algorithm for breast reconstruction is set out in *Figure 58.38*.

Radiotherapy after insertion of a silicone prosthesis often leads to a high incidence of capsular contracture and unacceptable results.

To achieve symmetry after breast reconstruction or BCS, the opposite breast may require a cosmetic procedure such as

Paolo Mascagni, 1755–1815, Italian physician and anatomist, published the first complete description of the lymphatic system.

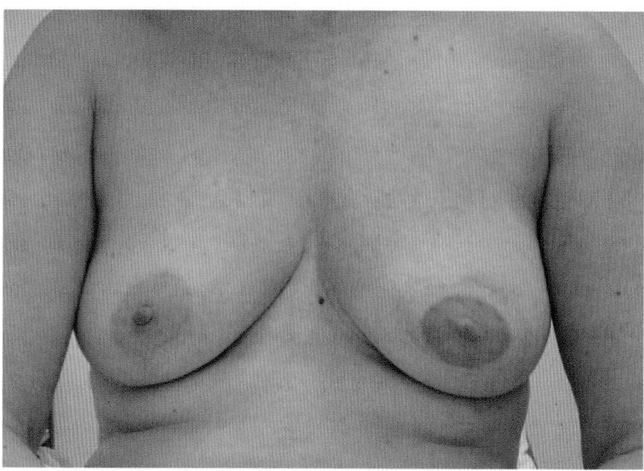

Figure 58.35 Reconstruction with latissimus dorsi flap.

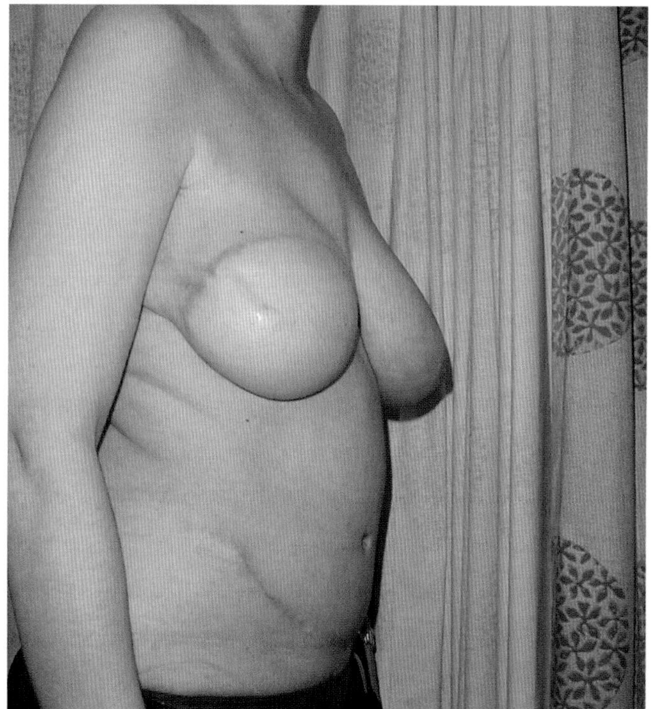

Figure 58.36 Transversus abdominus muscle flap.

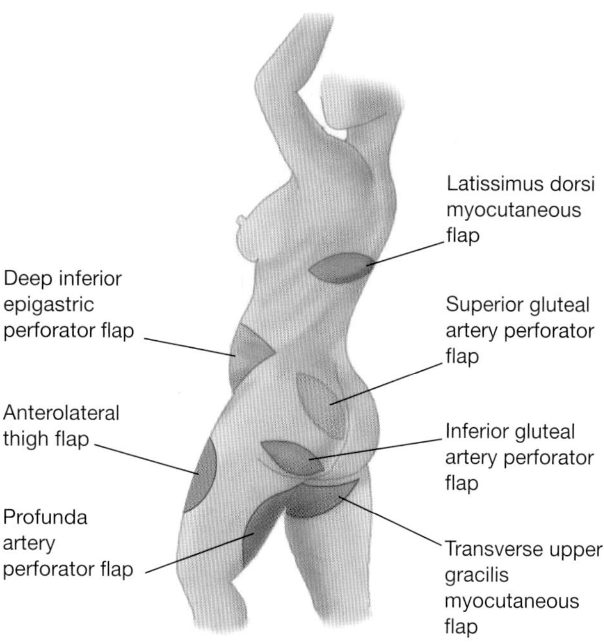

Figure 58.37 Autologous tissue options for breast reconstruction.

reduction or augmentation mammoplasty or mastopexy. The patient needs to be informed that she may require more than one procedure for **symmetrisation**.

Surgical options for locally advanced breast cancers (stages IIIA, IIIB)

Following NACT patients should be offered the option of mastectomy or BCS, if suitable (*Figure 58.38*). Patients with initial skin or chest wall involvement and those with inflammatory carcinoma should undergo MRM (*58.9*).

The role of SLNB in patients with cT3N0 disease and those who become N0 after NACT is currently being studied in a number of trials. A high false-negative rate (>10%) has been reported; this can be reduced if at least three sentinel nodes are removed using dual tracers or using 'targeted SLNB'. In the targeted technique, a metal clip or permanent India ink is applied to a positive node prior to NAST. During surgery after NAST, the node containing the clip or India ink is removed along with SLNB.

Adjuvant treatment

Radiotherapy

Radiotherapy is shown to decrease the risk of locoregional and systemic recurrence and improve survival. The indications include the following:

- patients with locally advanced breast cancers T3, T4, N1, N2, N3 disease;
- following BCS;
- after mastectomy if:
  - tumour size ≥5 cm; skin or chest wall involvement; lymphovascular invasion (LVI), grade 3;
  - axillary lymph node positive for metastasis.

In pathologically lymph node-negative tumours, radiotherapy after BCS is given to the breast only as a dose of 45–50.4 Gy (with or without a boost) delivered in 25 fractions or of 40–42.5 Gy delivered in 15 or 16 fractions (hypofractionation). In patients after mastectomy (T3N0M0), chest wall radiotherapy is given if the sentinel lymph nodes are negative. In patients with lymph node-positive disease locoregional radiotherapy is given covering the chest wall, supraclavicular region, internal mammary nodes and the axilla. The axilla should not be irradiated after axillary node dissection as this increases the risk of lymphoedema.

Accelerated partial breast irradiation (APBI) is a modality of radiotherapy for selected patients meeting the following

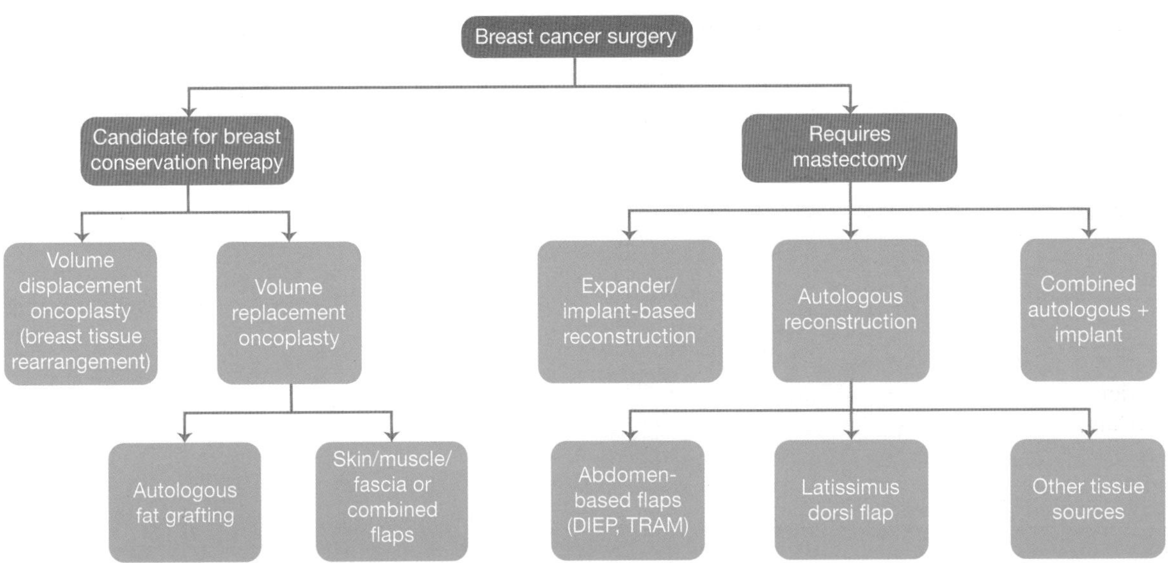

Figure 58.38 Surgical options in women undergoing breast-conserving surgery and reconstructive options for women requiring mastectomy. DIEP, deep inferior epigastric perforator; TRAM, transverse rectus abdominis myocutaneous.

criteria (American Society for Radiation Oncology ABPI guidelines, 2016):

- women 50 years or older with T1 disease and negative resected margins with a margin width of ≥2 mm, invasive ductal carcinoma, no LVI, ER positive, *BRCA* negative and sentinel node negative;
- women 50 years or older with low-risk DCIS (screen detected, low/intermediate nuclear grade, tumour size ≤2.5 cm, negative resected margin widths ≥3 mm).

The tumour bed is irradiated along with a narrow rim of surrounding tissue so as to avoid the potentially harmful effects of irradiation on healthy tissue. It is delivered twice daily for 5 days.

Adjuvant systemic therapy

The purpose of adjuvant systemic therapy is to control putative micrometastases, delay relapse and prolong survival. The results of many international clinical trials, including National Surgical Adjuvant Breast and Bowel Project (NSABP) trials and the Oxford overview meta-analyses by the Early Breast Cancer Trialist Collaborative Group (EBCTCG), demonstrate the benefit of chemotherapy in improving relapse-free survival by approximately 30% and overall survival by 10% at 15 years.

Chemotherapy. This is the most common systemic treatment for breast cancer. The following regimens are used:

- cyclophosphamide (C), methotrexate (M) and 5-fluorouracil (F) (CMF);
- anthracycline-based regimens: CAF (A, Adriamycin [doxorubicin]), CEF (E, epirubicin);
- taxane (docetaxel, paclitaxel)-based regimens.

Adjuvant chemotherapy is indicated for all invasive carcinomas >1 cm in diameter, tumours >0.5 cm with poor prognostic factors (presence of LVI, high grade, HER2/neu positive, TNBC) and node-positive tumours. Currently, decisions to administer chemotherapy as well as to choose a particular regimen are based on tumour stage, tumour biology and discussion with the patient and/or care giver in an MDT.

Gene signature panels help in assessing the benefit of chemotherapy in low-risk tumours, i.e. ER-positive, HER2/neu-negative and node-negative tumours. The risk of recurrence (ROR) scores include Oncotype Dx® (21-gene recurrence score), Prosigna® PAM-50 (breast cancer prognostic gene signature) and MammaPrint® (70-gene breast cancer recurrence assay). Oncotype Dx® is the most widely used ROR score and measures the expression of 16 cancer-related genes and five reference genes on paraffin-embedded tumour tissue. The assay classifies the ROR score as low (<18), moderate (19–30) or high (>30). In patients with a low ROR score, chemotherapy can be avoided.

In patients with endocrine-responsive breast cancer, those with **luminal A tumours** may avoid chemotherapy if they have a low-risk score on Oncotype Dx® and/or clinical risk assessment online tools (e.g. https://breast.predict.nhs.uk/tool); however, patients with a high clinical and genomic risk should be considered for chemotherapy with an anthracycline (epirubicin) or taxane-based therapy. Patients with **luminal B tumours** should receive an anthracycline and/or taxane-based therapy because of the greater risk of relapse. Those with **HER2/neu-positive tumours** should receive trastuzumab+pertuzumab along with chemotherapy (taxane + anthracycline), while those with **triple negative tumours** should receive chemotherapy (taxane + anthracycline). Carboplatin-based regimens may be beneficial for tumours with aggressive biology.

Targeted therapy. The monoclonal antibody trastuzumab (Herceptin®) is effective against the HER2/neu receptor. It is used along with pertuzumab to treat HER2/neu-positive tumours along with chemotherapy. The cytotoxic agent T-DM1 is used in HER2/neu-positive disease: a chemotherapy agent, emtansine, is conjugated to trastuzumab to allow targeted delivery of the chemotherapy to HER2-positive cells.

Hormone therapy. The selective oestrogen receptor modulator tamoxifen and aromatase inhibitors (anastrozole, letrozole, exemestane) are used for hormonal therapy in breast cancer. In premenopausal patients only tamoxifen is used for 5 years in low-risk patients and for 10 years in patients with a high risk of relapse (node positive, tumour >5 cm, LVI).

Aromatase inhibitors are used in postmenopausal women; in an adjuvant setting they have shown beneficial effect compared with tamoxifen in terms of relapse-free survival and overall survival. They are more expensive than tamoxifen and their use is associated with bone density loss and risk of fracture. A bone density scan is advised prior to commencement of treatment with aromatase inhibitors. Bisphosphonates with vitamin D and calcium are used to restore bone loss and may also reduce the risk of recurrence.

Follow-up of operable breast cancer

Follow-up after initial therapy routinely includes clinical examination every 3 months for 2 years, followed by every 6 months for the next 3 years. Thereafter the follow-up is scheduled yearly. A mammogram is also scheduled yearly. Patients with an implant and those with *BRCA* or other genetic mutations need contrast breast MRI annually. Development of any new symptom or sign during follow-up merits detailed clinical evaluation and relevant investigation. Patients presenting with metastatic disease and those with a local/systemic recurrence are seen more frequently depending on the clinical condition.

Metastatic carcinoma of the breast (stage IV)

Treatment of metastatic cancer is aimed at palliating symptoms, improving quality of life, preventing potential disabling complications and attempting to prolong life.

Endocrine therapy for hormone receptor-positive disease is preferred for patients with bony metastasis and limited visceral metastasis. Systemic chemotherapy is preferred for patients with hormone receptor-negative cancers, hormone-refractory metastases and patients with visceral crisis. Oral low-dose metronomic chemotherapy has cytostatic and antiangiogenic effects and may help in improving quality of life.

Patients with bony metastasis should receive palliative radiotherapy to lesions in weight-bearing areas (e.g. vertebra, femur) and to painful bony deposits, along with bisphosphonates. Symptomatic pleural effusions are palliated by intercostal chest drainage and pleurodesis. Surgical resection of metastatic lesions may be indicated in solitary visceral metastasis in patients with good performance status and favourable tumour biology.

Management of local recurrence

The local recurrence should be biopsied as a change in receptor status may occur and influence further therapy. Whole-body MRI or PET-CT scan should be performed to detect metastasis. Systemic chemotherapy should be followed by surgical excision. Most surgeons perform a mastectomy for recurrence; however, second BCS and re-radiotherapy may be considered.

Hereditary and familial breast cancer

Hereditary breast cancer (HBC) runs in families, affecting several close relatives, and is associated with an identifiable genetic mutation. **Familial breast cancer** (FBC) affects several members of a family but is not attributable to any known genetic mutation. HBC accounts for 5–10% and FBC for 20–30% of all breast cancers. HBCs are more aggressive, present at an earlier age and are more often multicentric and bilateral. High-penetrance mutations are found in *BRCA1*, *BRCA2*, Li–Fraumeni syndrome, Cowden syndrome, Peutz–Jeghers syndrome and hereditary gastric cancer syndrome.

BRCA1 (17q21) is associated with a 50–85% lifetime risk of developing breast cancer and up to a 40% risk of ovarian cancer. The breast cancers in *BRCA1* are mostly TNBC. ***BRCA2*** (13q12.3) is associated with an up to 50–60% lifetime risk of breast cancer and a 20% risk of ovarian cancer. It is also associated with cancer of the prostate, colon, gallbladder, bile duct, stomach and pancreas. *BRCA* mutation is more common in males with breast cancer. Genetic risk evaluation should be considered in high-risk individuals (***Summary box 58.5***).

Women with a *BRCA* mutation may be offered a bilateral risk-reducing mastectomy with immediate breast reconstruction. This reduces the risk of breast cancer by 90%. Chemoprophylaxis with tamoxifen or anastrozole may reduce the risk to 50%. Premenopausal women may be offered bilateral salpingo-oophorectomy after they have completed their family at around 35–40 years of age.

Breast cancer in pregnancy

Pregnancy is associated with aggressive tumour biology such as TNBC. Ultrasonography of the breast, mammogram and chest radiograph with abdominal shielding of the fetus may be considered. In cases where bone or brain metastasis is suspected or other investigations are inconclusive, MRI without gadolinium contrast should be used. CT and PET-CT should be avoided (high radiation dose). Genetic counselling should be offered. Surgery can be performed in any trimester.

Frederick Pei Li, 1940–2015, Dana–Farber Cancer Institute, Boston, MA, USA, and **Joseph F Fraumeni Jr**, b. 1933, National Institutes of Health, Washington, DC, USA, in 1969 identified four families with increased susceptibility to cancer. This led to the discovery of mutation in the tumour suppressor gene *p53*.

Cowden syndrome was named after Rachel Cowden, in whom the features were first recognised.

Jan Peutz, 1886–1957, Dutch physician, documented the eponymous condition.

Harold Joseph Jeghers, 1904–1990, Boston, MA, USA, recognised the eponymous syndrome.

Summary box 58.5

Indications for genetic risk evaluation

- An individual at any age with a known pathogenic/likely pathogenic variant in a cancer susceptibility gene within the family
- Breast cancer diagnosed age ≤50 years
- TNBC diagnosed age ≤60 years
- Two breast cancer primaries
- Breast cancer at any age with one or more relative with breast cancer diagnosed ≤50 years, invasive ovarian cancer, male breast cancer, pancreatic cancer, high-grade or metastatic prostate cancer
- Breast cancer at any age with two or more affected relatives
- Male breast cancer
- An individual with a personal or family history of three or more of the following:
  - Breast cancer, sarcoma, adrenocortical carcinoma, brain tumour, leukaemia
  - Colon cancer, endometrial cancer, thyroid cancer, kidney cancer, dermatological manifestations, macrocephaly or hamartomatous polyps of the gastrointestinal tract
  - Lobular breast cancer, diffuse gastric cancer
  - Breast cancer, gastrointestinal cancer or hamartomatous polyps, ovarian sex chord tumours, pancreatic cancer, testicular Sertoli cell tumours or childhood skin pigmentation

Mastectomy is preferred during the first and second trimester as the delay in administering radiotherapy until delivery may be associated with a higher risk of recurrence in the breast. SLNB with low-dose technetium-tagged sulphur colloid is considered safe for the fetus. Chemotherapy should not be administered during the first trimester (period of organogenesis) but can be safely administered during the second and third trimesters (until 34 weeks to allow haematological recovery at the time of delivery). Anthracyclines and taxanes remain the preferred agents. 5-Fluorouracil should be avoided. Anti-HER2/neu and endocrine therapy should be given after delivery, as indicated.

Carcinoma of the male breast

Carcinoma of the male breast (*Figure 58.39*) accounts for less than 0.5% of cases of breast cancer. The most common symptom at presentation is a painless subareolar lump. Involvement of the nipple–areolar complex and underlying pectoral muscles occurs early. Treatment comprises mastectomy with a 2-cm margin along with a portion of underlying pectoralis major muscle followed by radiotherapy. SLNB should be performed in node-negative patients. Tamoxifen 20 mg daily for 5 years is recommended for those with ER-positive tumours.

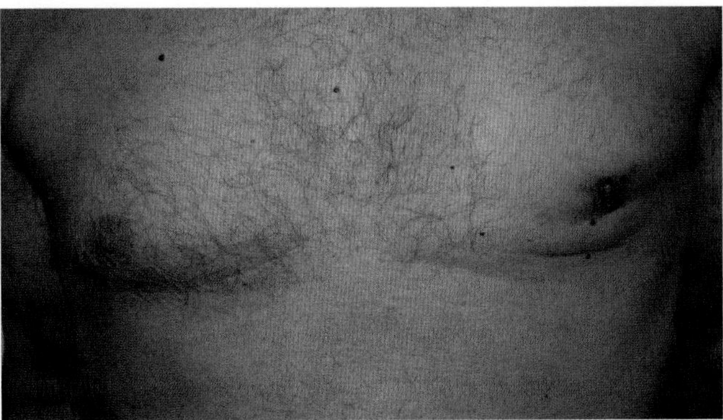

Figure 58.39 Carcinoma of the male left breast (courtesy of Professor Mike Dixon).

Summary box 58.6

Prognosis

Disease factors	Patient factors

• Size of tumour[a]
• Stage of disease
• Axillary lymph node involvement[a]
• Grade of tumour[a]
• Histopathological variant (metaplastic carcinoma is aggressive):
  ◦ Her2/neu positive and triple negative
  ◦ Presence of lymphovascular invasion
  ◦ Extensive DCIS component
  ◦ High Ki-67 index
	• Younger age
	• Premenopausal women
	• *BRCA*-associated tumour
	• Family history of breast cancer
	• Prior history of breast cancer
	• Obesity, sedentary lifestyle
	• Failure to complete intended treatment

DCIS, ductal carcinoma *in situ*.
[a]The Nottingham prognostic index (NPI) is used to determine prognosis following surgery. It is calculated using tumour size (S), number of involved lymph nodes (N) and tumour grade (G). NPI = (0.2 × S) + N + G. Patients are grouped into four categories according to the NPI score: I (excellent) ≤2.4; II (good) >2.4 but ≤3.4; III (moderate) >3.4 but ≤5.4; and IV (poor) >5.4.

Sarcoma

Sarcomas, most commonly fibrosarcoma and angiosarcoma, may arise *de novo* from the mesenchymal tissues of the breast. Some genetic conditions (Li–Fraumeni, neurofibromatosis type 1), exposure to alkylating agents, vinyl chloride or arsenic, prior radiotherapy (e.g. for Hodgkin's lymphoma) and chronic lymphoedema are associated with the development of sarcoma.

Angiosarcoma (*Figure 58.40*) is the most aggressive of all breast tumours and arises from the endothelial cell lining of vascular or lymphatic channels. Angiosarcoma is associated with prior radiotherapy and carries a very poor prognosis.

Screening for breast cancer

Screening for breast cancer involves a highly sensitive diagnostic test to detect the disease in either the preclinical detectable phase or a high-risk precancerous lesion. In most

Enrico Sertoli, 1842–1910, Italian physiologist, discovered the Sertoli cells of the testis in 1865.
Thomas Hodgkin, 1798–1866, lecturer in morbid anatomy and curator of the museum, Guy's Hospital, London, UK, described Hodgkin's lymphoma in 1832.

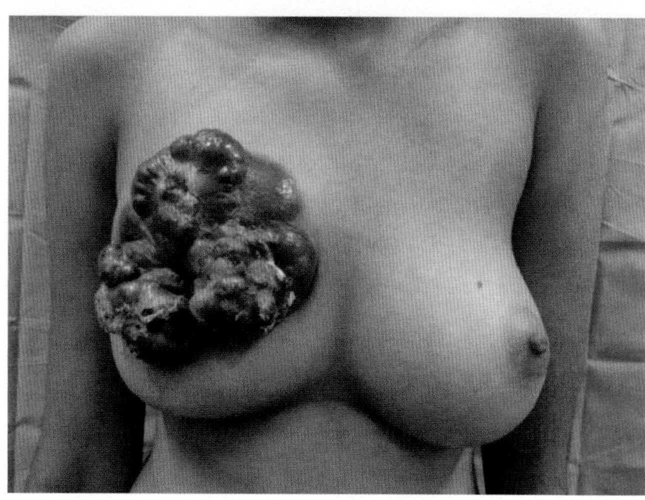

Figure 58.40 Angiosarcoma of the breast in a young woman.

high-income countries population-based mammographic screening achieves very high (90–95%) long-term survival in patients with screen-detected tumours. In the UK, all women aged between 50 and 70 years are invited for mammographic screening every 3 years. In low- and middle-income countries, population-based mammographic screening is not available. In some Asian countries clinical breast examination by a trained healthcare professional along with increasing breast health awareness by breast self-examination is being encouraged as a mode of screening. In India, national screening involves multidisease screening for cancer of the mouth, breast and cervix for all women aged 30–65 years. Clinical breast examination can detect the disease in the early stages while breast self-examination can help women become aware of breast health, detect breast changes and report to the healthcare facility early.

Patients with a suspicious lesion on mammogram are invited for biopsy under image guidance. In small or impalpable lesions a metal clip may be inserted at the site of the lesion. If a carcinoma is found on histology, the metal clip facilitates insertion of a hook wire with its tip near the centre of the lesion to facilitate wire-guided excision. Further therapy is based on histology of the excised specimen after discussion in the MDT.

ACKNOWLEDGEMENTS

The authors are grateful to Professors Smriti Hari and Maneesh Singhal from the All India Institute of Medical Sciences (AIIMS), New Delhi, India, for their assistance in providing illustrations used in the chapter, and to Dr Shivangi Saha of AIIMS, New Delhi, for her contribution to the breast reconstruction section and illustrations. Professor V Seenu of AIIMS critically reappraised the section on sentinel node biopsy. Professor Sandeep Kumar provided insight and critical reappraisal of the section on ANDI and benign breast disease. Dr Deepti Singh helped in the section on mastitis. Professor Manoj Kumar Singh and the team of artists at Virtual Skills Laboratory, AIIMS, designed most of the illustrations and videos for this chapter.

FURTHER READING

Amin MB, Edge S, Greene F *et al.* (eds). *AJCC cancer staging manual*, 8th edn. Cham, Switzerland: Springer, 2017.

Correa C, Harris EE, Leonardi MC *et al.* Accelerated partial breast irradiation: update of an ASTRO evidence-based consensus statement. *Pract Radiat Oncol* 2017; **7**: 73–9.

Early Breast Cancer Trialists Collaborative Group. Long-term outcomes for neoadjuvant versus adjuvant chemotherapy in early breast cancer: meta-analysis of individual patient data from ten randomised trials. *Lancet Oncol* 2018; **19**: 27–39.

Fisher B, Anderson S, Bryant J *et al.* Twenty-year follow-up of a randomized trial comparing total mastectomy, lumpectomy, and lumpectomy plus irradiation for the treatment of invasive breast cancer. *N Engl J Med* 2002; **347**: 1233–41.

Hughes LE, Mansel RE, Webster DJT, Sweetland HM. *Hughes, Mansel & Webster's benign disorders and diseases of the breast*, 3rd edn. Philadelphia, PA: Saunders, 2009.

Kumar S, Rai R, Das V *et al.* Visual analogue scale for assessing breast nodularity in non-discrete lumpy breasts: the Lucknow–Cardiff breast nodularity scale. *Breast* 2010; **19**: 238–42.

Mansel RE, Fallowfield L, Kissin M *et al.* Randomized multicenter trial of sentinel node biopsy versus standard axillary treatment in operable breast cancer: the ALMANAC trial. *J Natl Cancer Inst* 2006; **98**: 599–609.

National Comprehensive Cancer Network. *NCCN guidelines: breast cancer*, v.2.2022. See www.nccn.org/.

Srivastava A, Mansel RE, Arvind N *et al.* Evidence-based management of mastalgia: a meta-analysis of randomised trials. *Breast* 2007; **16**: 503–12.

Srivastava A, Agarwal G, Jatoi I *et al.* Asian Society of Mastology (ASOMA)–proposed standards for care of breast cancer patients. *Indian J Surg* 2021; **83**: 311–15.

CHAPTER 59 Cardiac surgery

Learning objectives

To provide an overall view of:

- The principles of cardiopulmonary bypass
- Incisions, conduits and valve options in cardiac surgery
- The role of investigation and preoperative assessment in planning surgery
- The management of coronary heart disease
- The role of surgery in valvular heart disease
- The role of surgery in congenital heart disease
- The management of aortic pathology
- The management of pericardial disease
- The principles of cardiopulmonary resuscitation after cardiac surgery

INTRODUCTION

Cardiac surgery has developed at a rapid pace since the first procedures in the 1920s. Driven by trauma innovations during the post-war period, the specialty has seen a massive expansion in the range and complexity of conditions treated.

Initially thought to be inoperable, surgery for both acquired and congenital heart disease is now commonplace. There are a variety of techniques to address both ischaemic heart disease (IHD) and valvular disease. These are often performed in conjunction with cardiology colleagues, and minimally invasive approaches are now complementary to surgical techniques.

Surgical correction of congenital defects has given rise to a specialty in its own right, and many patients who would previously have succumbed to heart disease in infancy now have normal life expectancy.

In addition, there are a range of allied technologies that are improving the survival of both adult and paediatric patients undergoing cardiac surgery. Transplantation, mechanical assistance devices and extracorporeal circuits are continuing to have improved outcomes and ensure that cardiac surgery is becoming accessible to more patients than ever.

HISTORICAL PERSPECTIVE

Prior to 1925, when Sir Henry Souttar reported the first mitral commissurotomy in the British Medical Journal, *heart surgery was thought to be impossible*. Souttar wrote that the heart should be as amenable to surgery as any other organ, and the main problem was maintenance of blood flow, particularly to the brain, during surgery.

The first real advances occurred in the late 1940s and early 1950s, driven by surgeons who gained confidence and experience under the pressures and opportunities provided by war. This was followed by the development of cardiopulmonary bypass (CPB) in the mid-1950s, which permitted longer, more complex surgery. Recently, the outlook of patients with congenital, valvular and degenerative heart disease has improved drastically because of advances in the range, complexity and technical expertise in cardiac surgery.

CARDIOPULMONARY BYPASS

CPB was first used successfully in 1953 by Gibbon and has since revolutionised cardiac surgery. It can be used in any procedure in which the heart and lungs need to be stopped temporarily and their function replaced artificially. Before Gibbon's work, heart surgery was mostly confined to epicardial procedures or crude trauma repair. However, valve surgery under direct vision was not possible, nor were the precise reconstructions needed to treat extensive coronary artery disease (CAD). Much of the success of modern CPB is attributable to the development of new biomaterials and sophisticated oxygenating devices, as well as a greater understanding of the pathophysiological consequences of CPB.

Surgical approach to the heart

Median sternotomy is the main approach during cardiac surgery. An incision is made from the suprasternal notch to the xiphisternum. The sternum is divided in the midline and retracted, exposing the thymus superiorly and pericardium inferiorly. The atrophic thymus remains relatively vascular. The thymus and pleurae are dissected from the pericardium, which is opened. Before cannulation for CPB, the patient is fully heparinised. Other incisions can be used, including limited upper or lower sternotomy and left or right anterolateral thoracotomy (in minimally invasive operations or descending aortic surgery).

Sir Henry Sessions Souttar, 1875–1964, surgeon, The London Hospital, London, UK.
John Heysham Gibbon, 1903–1973, worked at Jefferson University, Philadelphia, PA, USA.

Summary box 59.1

Alternative uses of CPB

- Rewarming in hypothermia
- Resuscitation in severe respiratory failure
- As an adjunct in pulmonary embolectomy
- Single- and double-lung transplantation
- In cardiopulmonary trauma
- Certain non-cardiac surgical procedures (e.g. resection of highly vascular tumours or those invading large blood vessels; e.g. the inferior vena cava in renal tumours)

Initiating cardiopulmonary bypass

Arterial cannulation

Conventionally, a perfusion cannula is inserted into the ascending aorta. Two purse-string sutures are usually placed in the selected area for cannulation after manual or epiaortic scan inspection to ensure that it is clear from severe calcification or atherosclerotic lesions that can prevent safe cannulation or lead to increased risk of postoperative complications such as stroke. The aortic cannula is checked for size and inserted into the aorta between the purse-string sutures and secured by tightening them. Air is excluded and the cannula connected to the bypass circuit. Alternatively, when it is either inadvisable (aortic dissection), impractical (aortic root surgery) or impossible (severe adhesions or porcelain [calcified] aorta) to cannulate the aorta, alternative cannulation sites can be used, such as the femoral or the axillary artery. The axillary approach has recently been gaining more popularity as it provides more physiological blood flow in the aorta (antegrade) than femoral cannulation, in which blood flow is opposite to normal physiological conditions (retrograde), and can be utilised to provide selective cerebral perfusion in complex aortic operations. Axillary cannulation has the theoretical advantage of reducing thromboembolic events compared with femoral cannulation. This is related to the differences in the direction of blood flow as flow in femoral cannulation is from the descending aorta to the heart, which means increasing the chances of mobilising calcified plaques from the aorta to the head and neck vessels.

Venous cannulation

A single purse-string suture is placed around the right atrial appendage and a single 'two-stage' venous cannula is placed to establish venous drainage. The venous pipe has end holes that sit in the inferior vena cava and side holes that sit in the right atrium (to drain from the superior vena cava). Alternatively, the superior and inferior venae cavae may be cannulated separately to gain better control over the venous return and facilitate operating on structures in the right ventricle or atrium ('bicaval' cannulation). Venous drainage from the femoral vein can offer an alternative, particularly during thoracic aortic or minimally invasive procedures.

Cardiopulmonary bypass circuit

Once the circuit is connected (***Figure 59.1***) the CPB machine ('pump') gradually takes over circulation and ventilation. Once full flow is established (the required cardiac output depends on many factors, including the patient's body surface area and temperature), the ventilator is stopped and the heart can be isolated from the rest of the circulation and stopped. Blood is drained from the heart to the venous reservoir using a siphon effect (gravity) as it is usually placed 50–70 cm below the level of the heart and oxygenated using an oxygenator that allows gas exchange across its membrane. Oxygenated blood is then pumped back to the patient by the bypass machine via the aortic cannula.

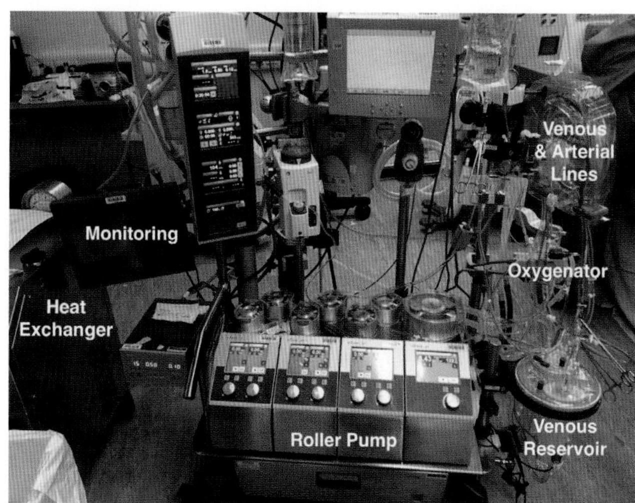

Figure 59.1 The cardiopulmonary bypass circuit shown here in use during 'on-pump' cardiac surgery.

The patient's core temperature can be lowered if needed by passing the returning blood through a heat exchanger, reducing the metabolic demands of the tissues. The degree of cooling is managed according to the severity and complexity of the surgical procedure as well as the surgeon's preference. Suction pumps can be used to keep the operative field clear. Vents, which are small cannulae that are inserted during surgery and connected to the CPB circuit, are used to keep the heart empty by draining any blood that accumulates inside the heart during surgery.

Myocardial protection

Once CPB has been established, the ascending aorta is usually cross-clamped to obtain a bloodless operative field. The heart ceases ejecting and becomes anoxic owing to inhibition of coronary blood flow. Permanent myocardial damage can develop within 15–20 minutes, therefore most cardiac operations require some form of myocardial protection. Techniques of myocardial protection and the operative management of the myocardium have had a significant impact on the complexity of cardiac surgery. Methods of myocardial protection include intracoronary infusion of a cardioplegic solution (antegrade), infusion via the coronary sinus (retrograde), intermittent cross-clamp fibrillation and total circulatory arrest.

Cardioplegia solutions vary in temperature, pH, osmolality and the presence of red cells. Potassium is the most commonly used arresting agent, stopping the heart in diastole by depolarisation of the cardiac myocyte cellular membrane. Cold (4–10°C) isotonic crystalloid or blood solutions aid myocardial protection by reducing metabolic requirements through local hypothermia. Warm cardioplegic solutions, on the other hand, may facilitate better myocardial recovery postoperatively by aiding activation of intramyocardial enzymes. Cardioplegia solutions will need to be given repeatedly every 15–20 minutes during surgery. Other cardioplegia solutions that can be given as a single dose are usually reserved for more complex and longer operations.

Intermittent cross-clamp fibrillation is a technique in which intermittent ventricular fibrillation (VF) is induced by a small electrical charge. The heart does not eject and is relatively still but not bloodless. The aorta is cross-clamped to render the heart ischaemic. The heart can tolerate short periods (10–20 minutes) of ischaemia, providing it is reperfused when the cross-clamp is released and allowed to beat following cardioversion for short periods.

Total circulatory arrest is necessary when visibility and clarity of the operative field is crucial, as in paediatric surgery or in surgery of the ascending arch of the aorta. CPB is established and the core body temperature reduced to 15–18°C (profound hypothermia). The metabolic rate of all body organs is reduced by 50% with every 7°C drop in temperature. Using this technique, circulatory arrest (in which the CPB machine is switched off) can be tolerated for up to 20–30 minutes. Additional cerebral protection can be provided with ice packs placed around the head, pharmacological agents such as thiopental or steroids and cerebral perfusion techniques that allow for longer arrest times.

Discontinuing cardiopulmonary bypass

At the end of the procedure, air must be meticulously excluded from the cardiac chambers (de-airing). Once perfusion is restored to the coronary arteries (by removing the cross-clamp) the heart may beat spontaneously. If VF is present, cardioversion may be required. Epicardial pacing wires are usually placed to treat postoperative bradycardia or heart block. The patient is rewarmed, acidosis and hypokalaemia are corrected and ventilation is restarted. The heart gradually takes over the circulation while the arterial flow from the CPB machine is reduced ('weaning from bypass'). When the blood pressure is acceptable and the surgeon is confident that the heart function is adequate, CPB is discontinued and anticoagulation is reversed by administering protamine and the cannulae are removed.

Complications of CPB

CPB is a complex technique requiring careful interaction and communication between surgeon, anaesthetist and perfusionist to ensure patient safety. Difficulties can occur during cannulation (aortic dissection or atrial injury), at the start of CPB (oxygenator failure) and at the end of CPB (coagulopathy). Other complications can occur following blood exposure to the non-physiological surface of the CPB circuit. This leads to the activation of inflammatory and coagulation cascades, giving rise to a post-CPB systemic inflammatory response syndrome (SIRS) that can lead to multiorgan failure.

Recent improved understanding of the impact of CPB on coagulation and the inflammatory response (SIRS) has resulted in the development of smaller 'mini' CPB circuits, which have demonstrated some advantages in terms of reduced post-CPB inflammatory responses and blood transfusion requirements. Alternative methods include surgery 'off-pump' on a beating heart without the use of CPB; this has some advantages but its use remains restricted to coronary artery bypass grafting (CABG).

CORONARY ARTERY BYPASS SURGERY

Introduction

Before the 1950s, surgical attempts to treat CAD through grafting of non-coronary flow to the myocardium was via pericardial or omental adhesions, with limited success. From the 1960s onwards, the importance of aortocoronary saphenous vein grafts and the value of the internal mammary (internal thoracic) artery were increasingly recognised. Outcomes of CABG surgery were carefully scrutinised and, by the 1970s, multiple large, prospectively randomised, multicentre trials were conducted. All trials showed that a subset of patients had improved survival after surgery, compared with other treatments. With the advent of percutaneous coronary intervention (PCI) in the 1980s, the patient population undergoing CABG has changed, becoming progressively sicker but often with the most to gain. Over the last decade, there have been major advances in PCI, including the use of several generations of drug-eluting stents, as well as biodegradable stents, in an attempt to reduce restenosis. Although the role of CABG in the treatment of IHD has been questioned, several multicentre randomised trials carried out comparing CABG with PCI with drug-eluting stents have clearly shown that CABG remains the gold standard operation in certain groups of patients, such as those with left main stem disease, three-vessel coronary disease, diabetes or those at high risk.

Summary box 59.2

Potential complications of CPB

- Coagulopathy
- Infection
- Air embolism
- Gastrointestinal complications (bowel and liver ischaemia/pancreatitis)
- Microembolisation (eyes, brain)
- Myocardial depression
- Neurological dysfunction
- Postcardiotomy syndrome (similar to Dressler's)
- Pulmonary injury
- Systemic organ dysfunction
- Vascular injury

William Dressler, 1890–1969, cardiologist and Director of Cardiology at Maimonides Medical Center, Brooklyn, NY, USA.

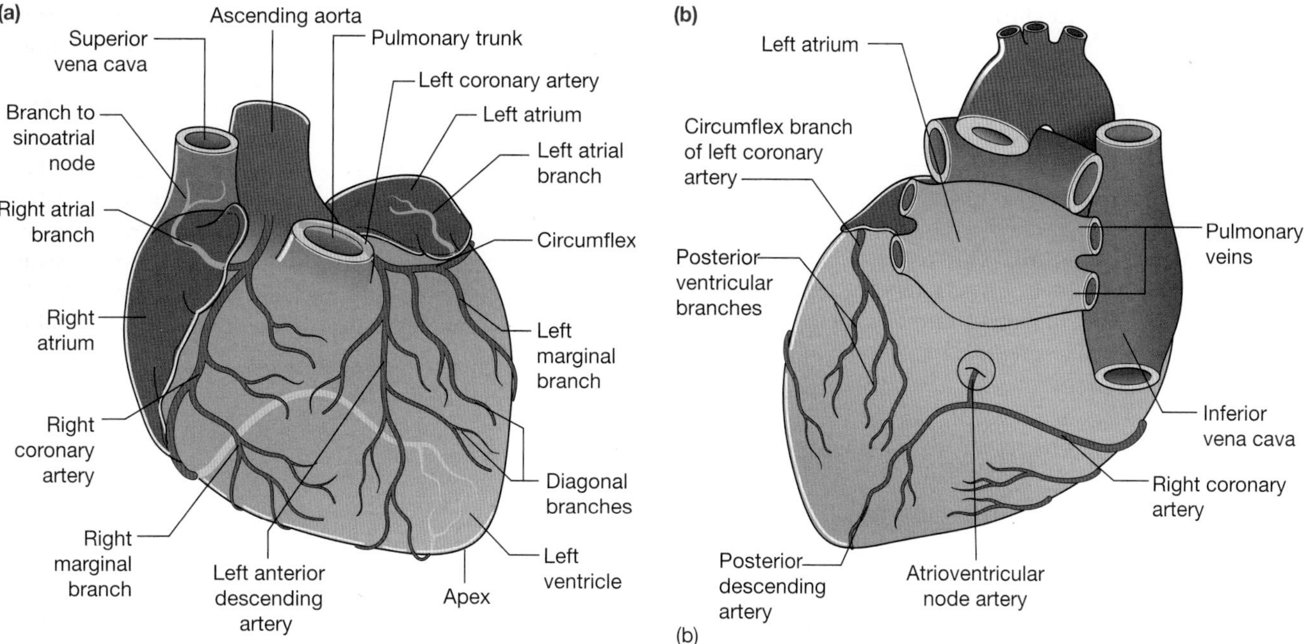

Figure 59.2 The heart, showing the distribution of the left and right coronary arteries. (a) Anterior surface of the heart; (b) base and diaphragmatic surface of the heart.

Coronary artery anatomy

The coronary arteries are branches of the ascending aorta, arising from ostia in the aortic sinuses above the aortic valve, the right from the anterior sinus and the left from the left posterior sinus (***Figure 59.2***).

Summary box 59.3

Coronary artery bypass surgery

- Randomised controlled trials have confirmed improvement in survival following CABG for certain groups of patients
- Randomised controlled trials have confirmed symptomatic benefits (relief of angina) following CABG

Left coronary artery

The left main coronary artery, which arises from the aortic root, can be the site of significant stenosis ('left main stem disease') and carries the worst prognosis in terms of survival without surgery. The artery is inaccessible at its origin and therefore grafts are anastomosed to its branches, the left anterior descending (LAD) artery or anterior interventricular artery and obtuse/marginal (OM) branches of the circumflex artery. The LAD artery is the most frequently diseased coronary artery and most often bypassed during CABG surgery.

Right coronary artery

The right coronary artery (RCA) passes from its origin anteriorly between the right atrial appendage and the pulmonary trunk and courses in the atrioventricular groove around the margin of the right ventricle. It usually forms an anastomosis with the circumflex artery at the junction of the right and left atria and the interventricular septum (the crux) on the back of the heart. It continues as the posterior descending artery or interventricular artery. Common sites of stenosis of the RCA are in its proximal portion or at the bifurcation or crux. In the presence of disease at the bifurcation, a graft can be anastomosed distally to the posterior descending artery.

Anatomical dominance is determined by the artery that supplies the posterior descending artery. In approximately 90% of cases the posterior descending artery arises from the RCA, a pattern referred to as right dominance. The posterior descending artery can also arise from the circumflex artery, a pattern referred to as left dominance, which occurs in approximately 10% of cases. Co-dominance describes the situation in which there are two posterior descending arteries, one each arising from the right coronary and circumflex arteries; the incidence is around 5%.

Ischaemic heart disease

IHD is a major cause of morbidity and mortality in resource-rich countries. The underlying pathology is usually atherosclerosis of the coronary arteries.

Pathophysiology

Atherosclerosis is the process underlying the formation of focal obstructions or plaques in large- and medium-sized arteries. It is a chronic inflammatory process resulting from interactions between plasma lipoproteins, leukocytes (monocyte/macrophages, T lymphocytes), vascular endothelial cells and smooth muscle cells. Different progressive stages of atherosclerosis exist; namely

- **The fatty streak**. The first evidence of atherosclerosis can be found in children aged 10–14 years. This appears as a yellow streak running along the major arteries. The streak consists of smooth muscle cells, which are filled with cholesterol, and foam cells (lipid-laden macrophages).

- **Fibrous plaque**. A fibrous plaque consists of large numbers of smooth muscle cells, foam cells and leukocytes. As the fibrous plaque grows, it projects into the vessel lumen, causing narrowing that, in turn, can lead to ischaemia or infarction.
- **Complicated lesion**. This occurs when the fibrous plaque ruptures, provoking activation of the coagulation cascade and the formation of thrombus. The end result is often a calcified ulcerated plaque with areas of haemorrhage and thrombus.

Clinical manifestations

The principal symptoms of IHD are chest pain or angina, breathlessness, fatigue, peripheral oedema, palpitations and syncope. The severity of symptoms and the extent to which the symptoms interfere with everyday activities and quality of life are important aspects of the clinical history. An assessment of risk factors should be included. Clinical examination follows and, although often normal, any evidence of myocardial ischaemia such as new murmurs or heart sounds associated with heart failure or stigmata of associated disease, such as diabetes or peripheral vascular disease, should be noted.

Summary box 59.4

Risk factors for IHD

- Smoking
- Diabetes mellitus
- Advancing age
- Male gender
- Hyperlipidaemia
- Hypertension
- Family history of IHD
- Obesity
- Reduced physical activity

Investigations

Non-invasive methods of diagnosis

Resting electrocardiography

As a baseline test, a 12-lead resting electrocardiogram (ECG) often provides the first indication of ischaemic cardiac disease and is essential in the acute clinical setting. However, it may be normal even in the presence of severe multivessel coronary disease. Evidence of previous myocardial infarction (MI) is indicated by Q waves and/or non-specific ST- and T-wave changes and angina by ST depression.

Troponin and cardiac isoenzymes

These are useful in assessing patients with an acute coronary syndrome (ACS), which is the umbrella term for STEMI (ST elevated myocardial infarction), non-STEMI and unstable angina, especially when the diagnosis is in doubt. Standard enzyme measurement such as troponin, creatine kinase myocardial band and lactate dehydrogenase can also aid both diagnosis and prognosis.

Exercise tolerance testing

Exercise tolerance testing (ETT) is a valuable technique for assessing myocardial ischaemia, both for diagnostic purposes and as a prognostic tool. However, an abnormal exercise test must be interpreted in the light of the probability of CAD and the physiological response to exercise as measured by the percentage of the maximum predicted heart rate achieved. A positive test with evidence of ischaemia on the ECG (ST depression of ≤2 mm) does not always indicate IHD, and a negative test does not always exclude its presence. ETT should be avoided in patients with cardiac disorders such as aortic stenosis.

Echocardiography

Performed through either a transthoracic or transoesophageal approach, echocardiography is valuable for the evaluation of ventricular function and regional wall motion, as well as valvular lesions. Transoesophageal echocardiography provides essential real-time information intraoperatively.

Stress echocardiography can detect regional wall motion abnormalities brought on by exercise or the use of dobutamine or dipyridamole. It is reliable in identifying viable myocardium. Impaired but recoverable myocardium possesses a functional reserve that allows it to be temporarily recruited into action, whereas scar tissue does not. The development of real-time three-dimensional echocardiography (RT3DE) with the ability to carry out valve reconstruction from different aspects has recently revolutionised preoperative surgical planning in patients with complex valvular lesions.

Radionuclide studies and cardiac magnetic resonance imaging

The main type of radionuclide study used is myocardial perfusion scanning using specific radioisotopes (such as thallium-201) to assess the significance of coronary disease and viability of the myocardium.

Cardiac magnetic resonance imaging (MRI) can be performed to evaluate the ischaemic burden of coronary disease (using pharmacological agents to stress the heart) and to provide details of tissue viability when using gadolinium as a contrast agent. Close gap MRI is also very useful in assessing cardiac tumours, pericarditis and other structural heart diseases.

Positron emission tomography

Positron emission tomography (PET) provides information on myocardial perfusion, metabolism and cell membrane function. Positron-emitting isotopes are used to label physiological substances, which can measure the regional distribution of these substances. PET is valuable in the diagnosis of CAD, particularly when the more widely available imaging modalities are inconclusive. It can identify injured but viable myocardium that is potentially salvageable by revascularisation.

Computed tomography

With the development of ECG-gated computed tomography (CT) scanners, multislice high-resolution CT imaging may become an alternative to coronary angiography. It allows assessment of coronary disease, particularly proximal CAD, and gives some information about the degree of coronary

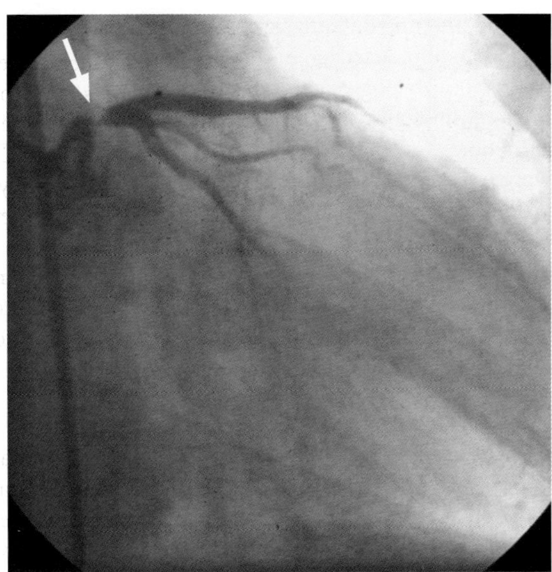

Figure 59.3 Coronary angiogram demonstrating severe stenosis in the left main stem prior to bifurcation of the left anterior descending and circumflex arteries. The arrow indicates the area of severe stenosis.

artery calcification (calcium score) that is very helpful when stratifying patients to determine which ones will benefit from more invasive coronary angiography. It is also useful in patients in whom angiography is challenging (e.g. difficult anatomy).

Invasive methods of diagnosis

Coronary angiography

Selective coronary angiography remains the gold standard diagnostic technique for accurate diagnosis of the presence and extent of CAD (*Figure 59.3*). In spite of the availability of newer imaging techniques such as cardiac MRI, selective coronary angiography provides high image quality, demonstrating the extent, severity and location of coronary artery stenoses and the quality and size of the distal coronary arteries. Different categories of coronary disease are shown in *Table 59.1*. In addition, angiography can assess ventricular function and provide the cardiac surgeon with information to determine operability, operative risk and probability of success.

Coronary angiography only outlines the coronary anatomy; it does not demonstrate ischaemia and it carries an overall complication rate of less than 1%. However, flow measurement across a stenotic area, using techniques such as fractional flow reserve, has been effective in predicting those patients who are likely to benefit from revascularisation. Moreover, intravascular ultrasound can provide more detailed information regarding the degree of stenosis, especially in left main stem disease. A reduction in the luminal diameter of ≥70% usually means an inability to increase coronary flow above resting values.

Summary box 59.5

Coronary angiography

- Gold standard for imaging coronary anatomy
- Demonstrates extent, severity and location of stenosis
- Demonstrates quality and size of distal arterial tree
- Aids diagnosis of ischaemia
- Evaluates suitability for surgery
- Aids in prognostic assessment

Indications for surgery

The decision to offer CABG is based on the balance between expected benefit and potential risks to the patient. Two issues need to be addressed when determining surgical suitability: the appropriateness of revascularisation and the relative merits of CABG versus the alternative PCI. Current best evidence shows that revascularisation can be readily justified on symptomatic grounds in patients with persistent limiting symptoms (angina or angina equivalent) despite optimal medical therapy and/or on prognostic grounds in certain anatomical patterns of disease.

The myocardial revascularisation guidelines of the European Society of Cardiology and the European Association for Cardio-Thoracic Surgery (EACTS) can be useful for identifying patients with certain angiographic features who can benefit from surgery, such as patients with complex coronary anatomy or left main stem disease.

Summary box 59.6

Indications for surgery

- >50% stenosis of the left main stem ('critical left main stem disease')
- >50% stenosis of the proximal left anterior interventricular artery
- Three main coronary arteries diseased ('triple-vessel disease')
- Two-vessel disease including the proximal LAD

Acute coronary syndromes

Substantial benefit is gained with an early invasive revascularisation strategy with PCI or surgery or both. After defining the anatomy with angiography, a decision about the type and extent of intervention can be made. Angiography in combination with ECG changes often identifies the culprit lesion and PCI may be used to treat it. In patients who become stable after an episode of ACS, the indications for CABG are similar to those for patients with stable chronic disease (see *Summary box 59.6*).

TABLE 59.1 Luminal stenosis of coronary arteries and angiographic findings.

	Minimal	Mild	Moderate/significant	Severe	Occluded
Angiographic degree of stenosis	0%	20–49%	50–69%	>70% reduction	Complete occlusion
Luminal cross-sectional stenosis	0%	40–60%	75%	>90%	100%

Optimal timing of revascularisation differs between PCI and CABG. The benefits of PCI in patients with non-ST segment elevation occur with early intervention whereas the benefits of CABG are greatest when patients undergo surgery after several days of medical stabilisation. However, emergency CABG may be indicated for unstable patients with left main stem, multivessel disease and failed PCI.

Surgery for the complications of myocardial infarction

MI leads to myocyte necrosis that usually heals by formation of scar tissue but may lead to rupture of the ventricular wall. Free rupture of the ventricle is usually fatal.

Ventricular septal rupture typically presents 3–7 days after infarction with pulmonary oedema, a pansystolic murmur and haemodynamic instability. Advances in reperfusion therapy such as early access to angiography/PCI services have reduced the incidence to <1%. Diagnosis is usually confirmed with echocardiography, and repair can be performed with a pericardial or artificial Dacron patch in addition to CABG for diseased vessels supplying viable myocardium. Such surgery is usually associated with significant mortality owing to the associated impairment of the ventricular function. Mitral valve papillary muscle necrosis causes acute mitral regurgitation. Diagnosis is made by echocardiography, and right heart catheterisation may be required in the presence of poor right ventricular function and high pulmonary pressure. Mitral valve intervention in addition to CABG is usually necessary, but the mortality rate is higher than in valve intervention for non-ischaemic disease. Ventricular aneurysm may occur following partial-thickness necrosis of the ventricular wall if the free wall is replaced with non-contractile fibrous tissue. Left ventricular function is affected because the fibrous wall balloons out during systole and reduces stroke volume. Repair is undertaken using CPB, and CABG and mitral valve replacement may also be necessary.

Acute failure of percutaneous coronary angioplasty

Since the advent of intracoronary stents, the need for emergency CABG following complications of PCI is low at <1%. The mortality rate of CABG in this group is significantly higher than in the elective setting.

Preparation for surgery

Clinical assessment

Before CABG, the severity and stability of the patient's IHD, the presence of significant valvular disease and the status of left ventricular function should be properly evaluated. Any comorbid risk factors for IHD should be documented and, in particular, the state of coexisting diseases assessed. Attention is paid to the presence of carotid artery disease, peripheral vascular disease, respiratory status, preoperative diabetic control and presence of associated diabetic complications, significant renal dysfunction or coagulopathy. All medications taken by the patient are noted, and some routinely stopped before surgery (e.g. antiplatelet agents, including aspirin; anticoagulants; and oral hypoglycaemics). Others, including diuretics and angiotensin-converting enzyme inhibitors, are stopped at the discretion of the surgeon. Cardiac and antihypertensive medications should be taken preoperatively.

Risk assessment

Myocardial revascularisation by CABG is appropriate when the expected benefits (i.e. survival or health outcomes) exceed the expected negative consequences of the procedure. Therefore, objective methods for risk assessment are essential to determine the patient's suitability for surgery and to provide patients with adequate information for informed consent. Various scoring systems have been developed for risk stratification in cardiac surgery, including the EuroSCORE II and the Society of Thoracic Surgeons (STS) score. EuroSCORE II is the system most commonly used in the UK and takes into account different factors such as age and gender, coexisting conditions such as diabetes and peripheral vascular disease and the proposed operation.

Selection of conduit

Venous grafts

The long saphenous vein is the most commonly used venous conduit as it is straightforward to harvest, provides good length and is easy to handle. Historical studies showed a limited long-term patency rate for long saphenous vein grafts (50–60% at 10 years). However, recent studies suggest that early postoperative use of lipid-lowering agents and antiplatelet agents such as low-dose aspirin can improve vein graft long-term patency. In assessing the patient preoperatively, the legs should be checked for varicose veins. Alternative vein conduits include the short saphenous vein or upper limb veins such as the cephalic vein; however, these grafts are associated with poorer long-term patency rates.

Arterial grafts

The left internal mammary artery (LIMA), or internal thoracic artery, has become the conduit of choice for LAD grafting. Evidence from the mid-1980s to the present day suggests a 10-year patency rate of >95%, with a lower reoperation rate. As this arterial conduit avoids the late complication of vein graft atherosclerosis, interest has focused on the use of bilateral internal mammary artery grafts although there is currently no supporting evidence for this.

The use of the radial artery as an alternative arterial bypass graft has undergone a recent revival. This has been driven by the belief that total arterial revascularisation (avoiding venous conduits) might improve long-term results of coronary surgery. Different studies have demonstrated excellent patency rates at 1 and 5 years with this strategy. When assessing a patient in whom a radial artery harvest is planned, an Allen's test should be performed. The alternative would be vascular assessment of the radial and ulnar arteries with ultrasound.

Edgar Van Nuys Allen, 1900–1961, Professor of Medicine, Mayo Clinic, Rochester, MN, USA.

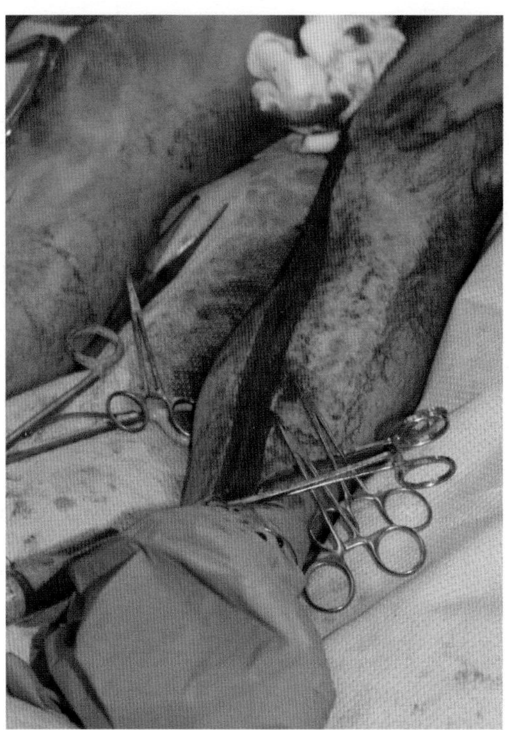

Figure 59.4 Open long saphenous vein harvesting is performed through an incision starting anteriorly to the medial malleolus of the ankle, extending to the groin if necessary.

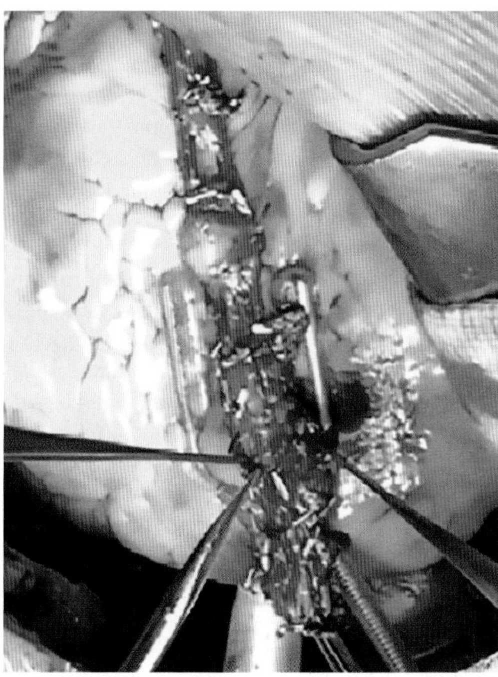

Figure 59.5 A pedicled left internal mammary artery is dissected off the chest wall and divided distally after systemic heparinisation. It is left attached to the subclavian artery proximally.

Summary box 59.7

Allen's test

- The patient repeatedly clenches and unclenches the fist while the surgeon compresses both radial and ulnar arteries digitally at the wrist; this empties blood from the hand
- The hand is then relaxed and compression of the ulnar artery is released; the speed of returning colour to the hand is assessed
- If colour returns in 5–7 seconds, patency and collateral flow from the ulnar artery are confirmed and it is safe to harvest the radial artery

The operation

Intraoperative monitoring includes continuous central venous pressure and blood pressure recording (via a central line in the internal jugular or subclavian vein and radial artery line, respectively), urine output via a urinary catheter, temperature using a nasopharyngeal probe and continuous ECG monitoring.

The operation commences with harvesting of the conduits (long saphenous vein from the leg [*Figure 59.4*] and/or radial artery) while the chest is opened via a median sternotomy and the LIMA is dissected from the chest wall (*Figure 59.5*). The patient is placed on CPB after heparinisation, the aorta is cross-clamped and the heart arrested with cardioplegia. The grafts are anastomosed to coronary arteries distal to the stenoses (*Figure 59.6*).

The aortic cross-clamp is removed and the heart is reperfused with oxygenated blood. A side-biting clamp is applied to the ascending aorta and the proximal anastomoses are completed. Occasionally, the surgeon may opt to carry out the whole operation while the cross-clamp is applied to reduce

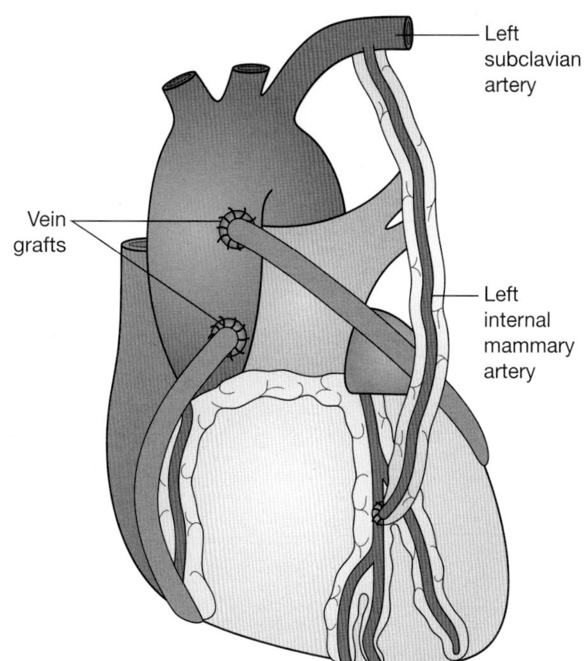

Figure 59.6 Completed coronary artery bypass grafts.

the risks associated with aortic manipulation. The patient is warmed and weaned from CPB. The heparin is reversed and the patient is transferred to the intensive care unit (ICU).

Postoperative recovery

The majority of patients are extubated a few hours postoperatively and remain in the ICU for 24 hours. In some centres, 'fast tracking' appropriate patients allows earlier transfer to a recovery area or high-dependency unit. Discharge is routinely 4–8 days after surgery.

Postoperative complications

Bleeding

Significant bleeding occurs in approximately 2–3% of patients. Rarely, acute cardiac tamponade or profound hypotension may occur in the early postoperative period and requires emergency resternotomy.

Arrhythmias

The most common postoperative arrhythmia is sinus tachycardia, closely followed by atrial fibrillation (AF). AF occurs in around 30–60% of patients undergoing CABG and often spontaneously reverts to sinus rhythm. Treatment includes correction of potassium (>4.5 mmol/L), the use of β-blockers, amiodarone or digoxin and, if necessary, cardioversion.

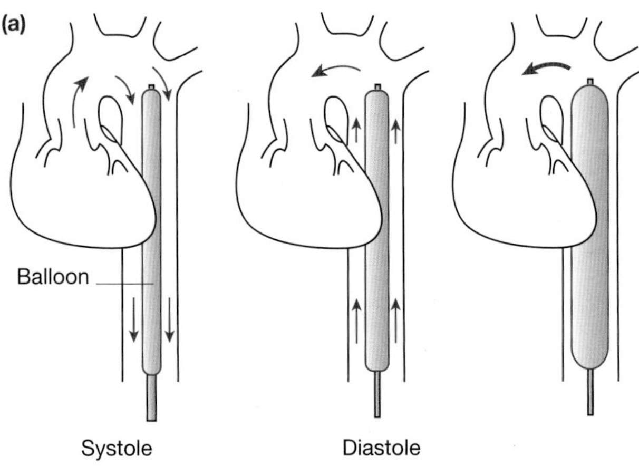

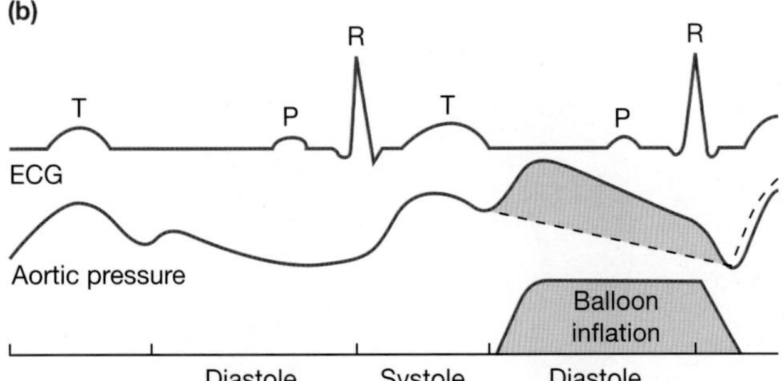

Figure 59.7 Intra-aortic balloon pump counterpulsation. (a) The balloon deflates during systole and thereby lowers systemic resistance. It inflates during diastole and increases coronary perfusion in addition to augmenting the systemic blood pressure. (b) The pressure changes and phases of the electrocardiogram (ECG) are shown.

Bradycardia is rare, but temporary pacing via epicardial pacing wires inserted intraoperatively may be required in the postoperative period.

Poor cardiac output state

Myocardial function typically declines in the first few hours following cardiac surgery, presumably in response to ischaemia/reperfusion-type injury. Inotropic agents are often required at this time to support heart function and maintain the circulation. Occasionally, the patient develops a persistent low cardiac output state. The clinical manifestations include poor peripheral perfusion, low urine output, a developing metabolic acidosis and low blood pressure.

There are several mechanisms that may cause this complication in the early postoperative period, including depressed myocardial contractility, reduced preload, increased afterload and a disturbance in heart rate or rhythm.

Treatment is aimed at the underlying cause but generally includes oxygenation, optimising preload, reducing afterload, managing any rhythm disturbances and improving contractility. If the low cardiac output state persists, the heart may require pharmacological or mechanical support.

Pharmacological support

Different agents can be used to support patients after surgery by altering the systemic vascular resistance, increasing the heart rate and increasing the force of myocardial contractility. Commonly used pharmacological agents include dopamine, dobutamine, adrenaline (epinephrine) and noradrenaline (norepinephrine).

Mechanical support

If low cardiac output persists despite inotropic support, the heart may require mechanical support while it recovers its function. Mechanical support can be achieved using an intra-aortic balloon pump (IABP), ventricular assist device (VAD) or extracorporeal membrane oxygenation (ECMO).

An IABP is a device that is inserted, either percutaneously or under direct vision, into the common femoral artery. It is advanced into the aorta until its tip lies just distal to the aortic arch vessels (***Figure 59.7***). Balloon filling and emptying is triggered by the ECG, deflating during ventricular systole (reducing afterload) and inflating in diastole (displacing blood into the coronary arteries retrogradely).

A VAD is a mechanical circulatory supporting device used to replace the function of a failing heart. It can be used as a short-term measure typically for patients recovering from heart attacks or heart surgery (bridge) or as a long-term support for patients with congestive heart failure (destination). Current VAD devices are all continuous flow and have been shown to be superior to pulsatile flow devices. Blood is exposed in these devices to a non-biological surface that can activate proinflammatory and coagulation cascades, leading to strokes and bleeding. Another important complication associated with VAD is infection.

ECMO is another circulatory support device that is similar to CPB; it can be established using venous access only (VV-ECMO) or venous and arterial access (VA-ECMO). Indications for ECMO include neonates and adults with potentially reversible respiratory failure, postcardiac surgery support or as a temporary stabilisation method for patients who may need a VAD (bridge therapy).

Neurological dysfunction

Stroke leading to a focal neurological deficit occurs in approximately 2% of patients following CABG. Embolisation, probably originating from the aortic arch or heart chambers, is the most common mechanism for territorial infarcts, with hypoperfusion leading to watershed infarcts. Diffuse neurological injury may also occur, leading to subtle cognitive abnormalities in memory, concentration and attention.

Wound infection

Significant deep wound infection resulting in sternal dehiscence and mediastinitis occurs in around 0.5–2% of patients. This is associated with significant morbidity, with a prolonged hospital stay and further surgical interventions for debridement and/or rewiring of the sternum. It has a significant mortality rate of up to 40%. Wound infections are more common in those with diabetes, dialysis patients, smokers, patients with high transfusion requirements and the obese.

Mortality

In the UK, the mortality rate for patients undergoing CABG is 1–3%. Multiple factors have been demonstrated to affect mortality after CABG, including age, gender, existing morbidities, left ventricular function and the use of LIMA.

Surgical outcome

Relief of symptoms

If revascularisation is complete, CABG alleviates or improves anginal symptoms in more than 90% of patients at 1 year; this falls to 80% at 5 years and 60% at 10 years. This symptomatic deterioration usually reflects progression of atherosclerotic disease in vein grafts and native coronary arteries.

Survival

Studies have reported survival rates to be >95% at 1 year, 90% at 5 years, 75% at 10 years and 60% at 15 years. These results may improve in the future because of increased use of arterial conduits and widespread use of dual antiplatelet therapy, β-blockers and lipid-lowering agents.

Summary box 59.8

Coronary artery bypass surgery outcome

Mortality
- 1–3%

Perioperative infarct
- 2–3%

Angina
- Improved in >90% at 1 year
- 80% at 5 years
- 60% at 10 years

Survival
- >95% at 1 year
- 90% at 5 years
- 75% at 10 years
- 60% at 15 years

Off-pump coronary artery surgery

CABG without the use of CPB is gaining popularity and may be combined with a minimally invasive approach or carried out through a conventional sternotomy. It avoids the potential physiological stress associated with CPB and, to some extent, the aortic manipulation that can lead to neurological injury through atherosclerotic embolisation. Since the introduction of cardiac stabilising devices such as the Octopus® (**Figure 59.8**), off-pump coronary artery bypass (OPCAB) grafting has become widespread in the UK and around the world.

The advantages of off-pump surgery over on-pump have recently been questioned, especially with the development of mini-bypass pumps, which offer a closed circuit and minimal non-physiological surface area. This reduces proinflammatory activation but at the same time allows the surgeon to operate on a still, bloodless heart. The disadvantages of OPCAB are mainly related to the quality and number of anastomoses. There is still no evidence to support the superiority of any of the above-mentioned techniques and the final decision is usually based on the surgeon's skills and the required operation.

Minimal access surgery

Minimally invasive direct coronary artery bypass (MIDCAB) grafting is performed through a small incision and avoids the invasive aspects of conventional CABG. Through an anterior submammary incision the LIMA can be dissected using a thoracoscope and grafted to the LAD. More lateral incisions allow access to other coronary vessels, including branches of the circumflex artery. Although not yet evidence based, one approach is to combine MIDCAB (typically LIMA to LAD) with PCI to other less accessible coronary arteries ('hybrid' coronary revascularisation).

VALVULAR HEART DISEASE

Introduction

Early surgical management of valvular heart disease concentrated on valve repair. The heroic early procedures for valve stenosis were closed and therefore 'blind' commissurotomies

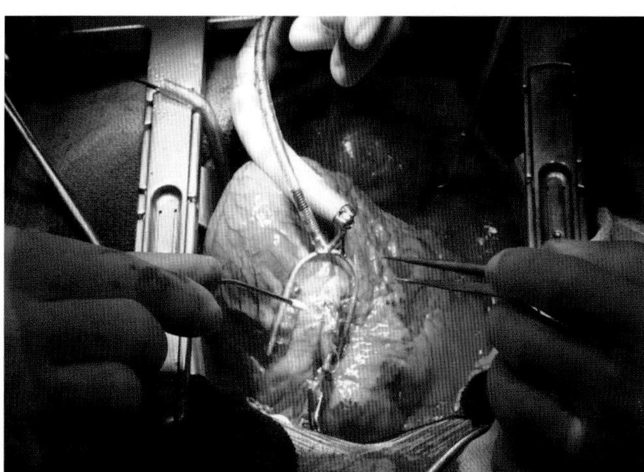

Figure 59.8 Off-pump coronary artery bypass using an Octopus® stabiliser to perform the distal anastomosis.

on a beating heart without CPB. They were replaced by open procedures with full visualisation, allowing precise repair and replacement. The first prosthetic valve replacement was performed by Dwight Harken, who replaced an aortic valve, followed by a mitral valve replacement by Starr a year later. Continued improvements in perioperative care, myocardial protection and, in particular, the development of prosthetic heart valves have improved long-term haemodynamic results, provided symptom relief and prolonged survival. The majority of valvular operations involve surgery on the aortic or mitral valve; tricuspid and pulmonary valve surgery is rarely undertaken in isolation unless it is part of staged congenital surgery.

Surgical anatomy

Heart valves serve to maintain pressure gradients between cardiac chambers, thus ensuring a unidirectional flow of blood through the heart. The aortic valve is tricuspid, with semilunar leaflets attached to the aortic wall at the annulus, the aortic sinuses being above the base of each leaflet, two of which form the origin or ostium of the coronary arteries. The intrinsic shape of the aortic semilunar valve allows blood to leave the ventricle during systole and prevents regurgitation during diastole. If disease leads to disruption of the leaflets or the annulus, valve function will be affected.

The mitral valve is bicuspid; the anterior cusp is larger in area and lies between the orifices of the mitral and aortic valves. The leaflets, like those of the aortic valve, are attached to an annulus. The leaflets join at two commissures and are supported by a subvalvular apparatus, consisting of chordae tendinae and papillary muscles. The papillary muscles contract in ventricular systole, pulling the cusps towards the atrioventricular orifice and holding blood within the ventricle. The proper functioning of the mitral valve depends on the integrity of the annulus, leaflets, chordae and papillary muscles. If surgical repair is required, these structures should be preserved whenever possible (***Figure 59.9***).

Surgical options for heart valve disease

The decision to either repair or replace a valve depends on the underlying pathology, severity of disease and quality and/or involvement of the supporting structures. Generally, repair is favoured when possible in mitral valve disease, particularly in degenerative mitral regurgitation, where it has been shown to have good long-term outcomes. Repair is the operation of choice in tricuspid valve disease, but aortic valve surgery generally involves replacing the diseased valve (***Table 59.2***).

Important factors in selecting the procedure and prosthesis include patient choice, age, existing comorbidities and the need for anticoagulation. Because of uncertainties about its longevity, most surgeons use a bioprosthetic (biological) valve in patients over 60 years. The need for anticoagulation with warfarin may have an impact on choice of valve, particularly in women of childbearing age, the elderly, the presence of congenital or acquired bleeding diathesis and when there is the need for further major surgery.

Types of prosthetic valves

Mechanical valves

Mechanical valves can be used in any age group to replace any valve (***Figure 59.10***). They are extremely durable but thrombogenic and patients require systemic anticoagulation, usually with warfarin. The patient should be warned about the risk of haemorrhagic (intracerebral, epistaxis, gastrointestinal bleed) or thrombotic (cerebral infarction) complications.

Bioprosthetic (biological) valves

Bioprosthetic valves include cadaveric **homograft** (or **allograft**) valves; **autografts**, a patient's own valve; and, most commonly, **heterografts** (or **xenografts**) prepared from animal tissues. All have three semilunar leaflets with central flow, so decreasing pressure gradients and minimising turbulence (***Figure 59.11***). Heterograft 'tissue' valves are the

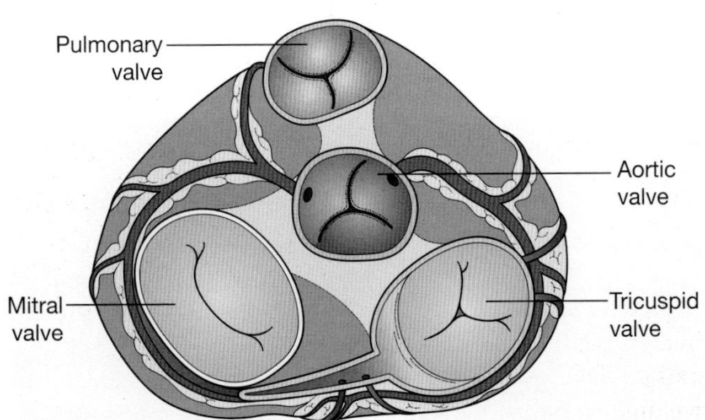

Figure 59.9 Four valves of the heart.

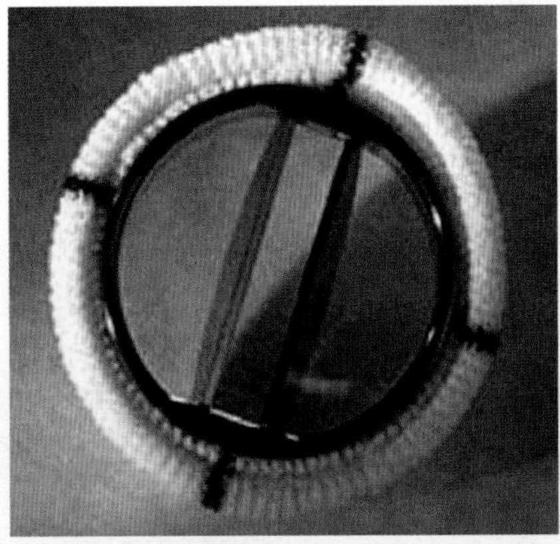

Figure 59.10 Bileaflet mechanical valve.

Dwight Harken, 1910–1993, American surgeon. In June 1948, in Boston, MA, USA, Harken successfully introduced a cardiovalvulotome through the left atrial appendage and into the heart of a 27-year-old with severe mitral stenosis. In 1950, he developed and implanted the first stainless steel cage prosthesis in the aortic position.

Albert Starr, b. 1926, formerly Professor of Surgery, The University of Oregon, OR, USA. Inventor of the world's first durable artificial mitral valve; winner of Lasker award in 2007 – an award given by the Lasker Foundation in the USA to a person (or persons) who has made major contributions to medical science or who has performed public service on behalf of medicine.

TABLE 59.2 Comparing options for heart valve surgery.

Valve repair	Mechanical replacement	Biological valves		
		Stented	Stentless	Homograft
Advantages				
No need for long-term anticoagulation Mimics 'natural' haemodynamics	Can be used in younger patients Good history of evidence	No need for long-term anticoagulation Good evidence base		Does not require anticoagulation Long-term results unknown
Disadvantages				
Technically challenging	Nidus of infection (endocarditis), can be disastrous Requires anticoagulation		Technically more challenging to insert	Requires specialist expertise Increased complexity of surgery
Lifespan				
Variable among techniques and valve involved	Excellent long-term durability (patient lifetime)	Lifespan limited (traditionally 10–15 years, although constantly improving) More suited to older patient		Little evidence, although may be limited
Comments				
Mostly performed for mitral valve disease Evidence for other valves is limited	Many different types and sizes for a range of scenarios	Mostly made of bovine or porcine pericardium Growing evidence for the use of antiplatelet agents postoperatively		Usually taken from deceased donors

most commonly used valves and can be stented with a limited durability of 10–15 years, whereas stentless (or frameless) valves are expected to have less late calcific degeneration but are more technically difficult to insert.

Sutureless and rapid deployment valves

In recent years, there has been an increase in the number of available valves using rapid deployment and sutureless technology. These valves are quicker to implant as they do not require extensive numbers of sutures (usually three in the case of rapid deployment and none in the case of sutureless). These valves are anchored in position with a balloon inflatable stent. This is advantageous in elderly or high-risk patients and in minimally invasive aortic surgery.

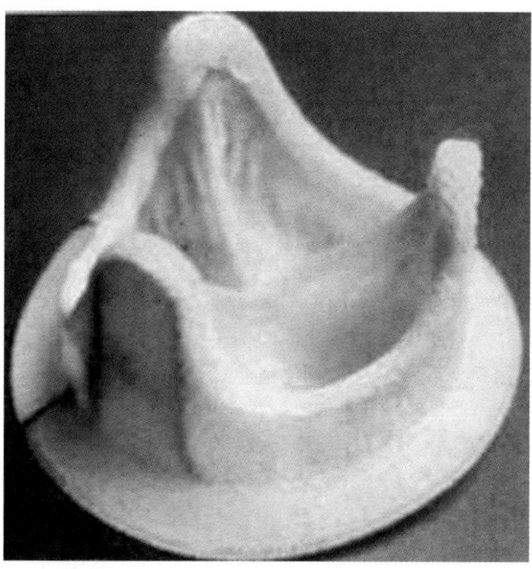

Figure 59.11 Porcine heterograft stented valve.

Prosthetic valve dysfunction and complications

Structural valve failure

Structural failure rates for the currently used bioprosthetic valves, although rare in those over 70 years of age, can reach 60% after 15 years. Structural failure of a mechanical valve is generally uncommon. Recently, a new generation of bioprosthetic valves has been introduced with a novel leaflet preparation method. These valves are associated in theory with more durability and can be used for the younger cohort of patients requiring prosthetic valve replacement.

The increased utilisation of transcatheter aortic valve insertion (TAVI) means that many patients with degenerative prosthetic valve disease can have a new valve inserted inside the old valve without the need for reoperation. This has encouraged many young patients to select a bioprosthetic valve as the preferred choice for replacement.

Paravalvular leak

Early-onset paravalvular leaks usually result from technical difficulties at insertion. Late-onset leaks can occur and may be precipitated by an episode of endocarditis or by leaflet degeneration. The leak can cause haemolytic anaemia or haemodynamic compromise and the valve may need replacement. Recent improvements in catheter techniques have resulted in the ability to close small areas of paravalvular leak with special occlusion devices, thus reducing the need for reoperation.

Thrombosis and thromboembolism

Thrombus formation is the most common complication of a mechanical valve (*Figure 59.12*). The risk of thromboembolism is greater with a mitral valve (mechanical or biological)

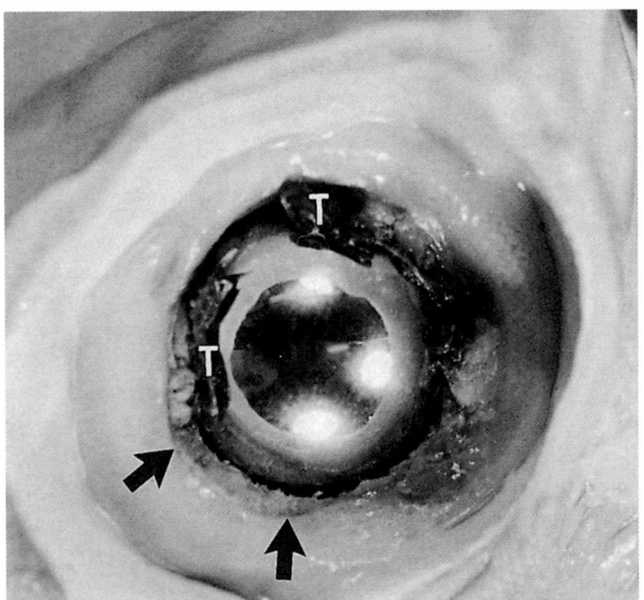

Figure 59.12 Thrombus (marked T and indicated with arrows) on the moving components of a ball-and-cage valve.

than with one in the aortic position. The incidence of thromboembolism in current mechanical valves is 0.5–3% per patient-year. Management depends on the extent of the thrombosis and valve dysfunction and can include either thrombolysis or surgery.

Prosthetic valve endocarditis

The incidence of prosthetic valve endocarditis (PVE) is 2–4%. The risk is lifelong and is at its greatest in the first 3 months after surgery. The incidence of PVE is higher with mechanical and bioprosthetic valves and lowest with homograft and autograft valves. The diagnosis is suspected following symptoms of septicaemia, development of a new murmur or a septic embolus. It is confirmed with echocardiography, which may show vegetations and even abscess formation. A high index of suspicion is required and early multiple blood cultures are needed to confirm the diagnosis, identify the infective organism and choose appropriate antibiotic therapy. The most common organisms in prosthetic and native valve endocarditis are shown in ***Table 59.3***.

The treatment of choice is early aggressive intravenous antibiotic therapy. Serial echocardiography to assess extent of infection and involvement of surrounding myocardial tissue, as well as functional assessment of the infected valve, may help in optimising decisions on timing of surgical intervention. Multidisciplinary team discussion is essential. The principle of surgical treatment is radical debridement of all infective tissue followed by reconstruction of any defects in the annulus and replacement. The prognosis of PVE remains poor, with an overall mortality rate of over 20%.

Postoperative management

Antibiotic prophylaxis

Currently the National Institute for Health and Care Excellence recommends that prophylactic antibiotics are not required for patients with prosthetic valves undergoing dental procedures. Other leading European bodies have recently supported the above recommendation.

Antithrombotic therapy

All patients with mechanical valves require anticoagulation, usually started on the first or second postoperative day. Use of anticoagulants with biological valves is based largely on the manufacturer's guidance.

Direct oral anticoagulants such as apixaban and rivaroxaban are not currently licensed for use with mechanical prosthetic valves. Warfarin is currently the drug of choice and the target international normalised ratio (INR) should be adapted to patient risk factors and thrombogenicity of the prosthesis with evidence supporting a lower INR target for aortic valves; however, the range of INR can vary between 2.5 and 4.

Mitral valve disease

Mitral regurgitation

Any pathological process affecting the mitral valve apparatus may lead to mitral regurgitation. As such, there are many causes of regurgitation and they can be broadly classified into four headings. They are shown in ***Table 59.4***.

Pathophysiology

There is an important distinction between acute and chronic mitral regurgitation. The former is usually the result of

TABLE 59.3 Common organisms in infective endocarditis.

Classification of organism	Native valve	Prosthetic valve
Gram-negative bacteria	*Streptococcus viridans/milleri* HACEK (*Haemophilus* spp., *Aggregatibacter* spp., *Cardio bacterium*, *Eikenella*, *Kingella* spp.)	*Streptococcus* spp.
Gram-positive bacteria	*Staphylococcus aureus/epidermidis* *Streptococcus faecalis*	Coagulase-negative *Staphylococcus* spp. *Staphylococcus aureus* Enterococci
Other	*Candida* *Histoplasma* *Aspergillus*	*Candida* Non-tuberculous mycobacteria

TABLE 59.4 Causes of mitral regurgitation.

Degenerative causes	Ventricular causes	Autoimmune and infective causes	Other causes
Barlow's disease (myxomatous degeneration)	Transient ischaemia and dynamic regurgitation	Infective endocarditis	Trauma (rarely)
Calcification of the leaflets or annulus	Myocardial infarction resulting in papillary muscle rupture	Rheumatic fever (post-streptococcal throat infection)	Congenital defects such as isolated mitral cleft
Marfan/Ehlers–Danlos syndromes and other connective tissue disorders	Cardiomyopathy and annular dilatation		Associated with certain medications (those containing ergotamine)
			Radiotherapy

ischaemic papillary muscle rupture or following infective endocarditis, whereas the latter is the result of longstanding myxomatous degeneration or fibroelastic changes in the leaflets.

In acute mitral regurgitation, the left ventricle ejects blood back into a small, poorly compliant left atrium, imposing a sudden volume load on the left atrium during ventricular systole. This leads to an abrupt rise in left atrial pressure followed by a rise in pulmonary venous pressure and pulmonary oedema.

Chronic mitral regurgitation progresses slowly, allowing compensatory left ventricular dilatation and hypertrophy, and atrial dilatation without significant increase in pressure, protecting the pulmonary circulation. As the disease advances left atrial pressure begins to rise, leading to a rise in pulmonary venous pressure and progressive pulmonary congestion, with eventual congestive cardiac failure.

Clinical features

In acute mitral regurgitation, the patient is usually unwell, presenting with clinical and radiological evidence of acute pulmonary oedema and a loud apical pansystolic murmur. Patients with mild chronic mitral regurgitation are usually asymptomatic. With progressive pulmonary congestion and left ventricular failure, the patient develops fatigue, exertional dyspnoea and orthopnoea. The development of AF with left atrial dilatation is common. The enlarged left ventricle leads to a heaving apical impulse and a pansystolic murmur.

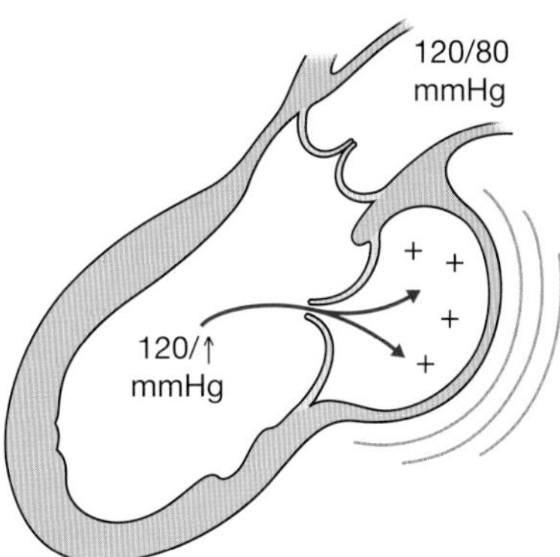

Figure 59.13 Features and pathophysiology of mitral regurgitation. There is a loud parasystolic murmur and the left atrium enlarges. The left ventricle enlarges as a consequence of volume overload.

Investigations

- **ECG**: may show left atrial hypertrophy (bifid P waves, known as 'P mitrale'), left ventricular hypertrophy and AF.
- **Chest radiography**: there may be cardiomegaly with prominent pulmonary vasculature.
- **Echocardiography**: this is often combined with colour flow Doppler imaging, which shows the severity of the regurgitant jet of mitral regurgitation.
- **Coronary angiography**: in patients >40 years of age to investigate the coronary arteries.
- **Cardiac MRI**: increasingly popular as it can give detailed information on structure and function.

Indications for surgery

Indications for surgery in patients with primary mitral regurgitation include severe symptoms or associated changes in left ventricular function or dimension (e.g. left ventricular end-systolic diameter). Evidence suggests that changes in this setting are usually associated with significant mortality if not corrected (***Figure 59.13***). It is also recommended to treat severe mitral disease if a patient is undergoing cardiac surgery for a different reason.

Surgical treatment of primary mitral regurgitation usually involves valve repair. When repair is not feasible, valve replacement with attempts to preserve the subvalvular apparatus should be considered.

The treatment of ischaemic mitral regurgitation remains controversial and current evidence suggests that patients with

John Brereton Barlow, 1924–2008, South African cardiologist.
Bernard Jean Antonin Marfan, 1858–1942, physician, L'Hôpital des Enfants-Malades, Paris, France, described this syndrome in 1896.
Edward Ehlers, 1863–1937, Professor of Clinical Dermatology, Copenhagen, Denmark.
Henri Alexandre Danlos, 1844–1912, dermatologist, Hôpital St Louis, Paris, France.
Christian Johann Doppler, 1803–1853, Professor of Experimental Physics, Vienna, Austria, enunciated the 'Doppler principle' in 1842.

severe ischaemic regurgitation may benefit from mitral valve replacement, while patients with moderate regurgitation should usually undergo repair along with CABG if indicated.

Mitral stenosis

The most common cause of mitral stenosis worldwide remains rheumatic fever, despite the fact that the incidence of overt rheumatic fever in resource-rich countries has decreased. During the healing phase of acute rheumatic fever, the valve leaflets become adherent to each other at their free border so that the commissures become obliterated, narrowing the valve orifice. Symptoms of mitral stenosis usually develop more than 10 years after the acute attack.

Pathophysiology

Mitral stenosis slows diastolic ventricular filling and left atrial pressure rises to maintain cardiac output. This leads to atrial hypertrophy and dilatation. Pulmonary congestion results from the rise in left atrial pressure with time. Although the lungs are protected against pulmonary oedema by constriction of the pulmonary vessels, this adaptive response, along with the passive 'back pressure' generated by the rise in left atrial pressure, leads to pulmonary hypertension (>25 mmHg). This leads to an increased demand on the right ventricle with eventual right heart failure and tricuspid regurgitation. The development of AF is common and can lead to a significant reduction in cardiac output. AF predisposes to thrombi forming in the left atrium, which may embolise to the systemic circulation.

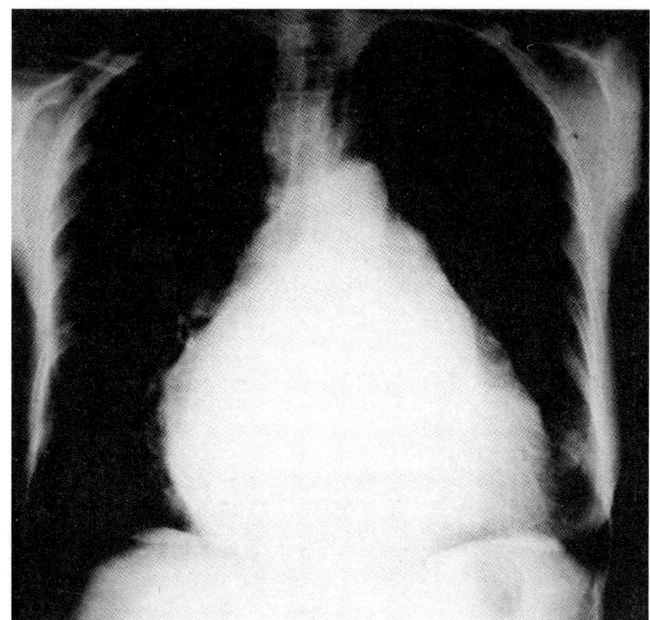

Figure 59.14 Chest radiograph of longstanding mitral stenosis, showing a massive left atrium.

Summary box 59.9

Causes of mitral valve disease

Stenosis
- Rheumatic heart disease (common)
- Calcification of valve or chordae tendinae
- Congenital (rare)

Regurgitation
- Rheumatic heart disease
- Valve prolapse
- Left ventricular dilatation or hypertrophy
- Ischaemia
- Bacterial endocarditis

Clinical features

Some patients may remain asymptomatic for years and then present with symptoms when the heart is stressed by events such as pregnancy, fever, chest infection or with the onset of AF. The common symptoms are fatigue and dyspnoea on exertion, which result from the combination of reduced forward flow and increased back pressure. The resulting pulmonary congestion adds to breathlessness and may produce a cough or haemoptysis.

In severe mitral stenosis, there may also be a right ventricular heave due to right ventricular hypertrophy in response to pulmonary hypertension. Auscultation may reveal an opening snap soon after the second heart sound, as the diseased valve is opened forcibly by the high pressure in the left atrium. The reverse happens when the valve closes and there is a loud 'tapping' first heart sound. In addition, a rumbling mid-diastolic murmur can be heard. The duration of the murmur is related to the severity of the mitral stenosis, increasing in length as the stenosis becomes more severe.

Investigations

- **ECG** may show left atrial enlargement or AF, right axis deviation or other signs of right ventricular hypertrophy (tall QRS complexes in the right ventricular leads V1–3).
- **Chest radiography**: there is a small aortic outline and a prominent pulmonary artery. The left atrium is enlarged (sometimes to an enormous degree) along with upper lobe diversion as a result of the raised pulmonary venous pressure. The right ventricle also appears enlarged (*Figure 59.14*).
- **Echocardiography**, in combination with colour flow Doppler imaging, allows assessment of the flow across the valve and, therefore, the degree of stenosis. Transoesophageal echocardiography (TOE) may be better at assessing valve morphology and excluding the presence of an atrial thrombus.
- **Coronary angiography**: to investigate the coronary arteries.
- **Cardiac MRI**.
- **Right heart catheterisation**.

Indications for surgery

Medical management includes anticoagulation in patients with AF or left atrial enlargement. Tachyarrhythmias should

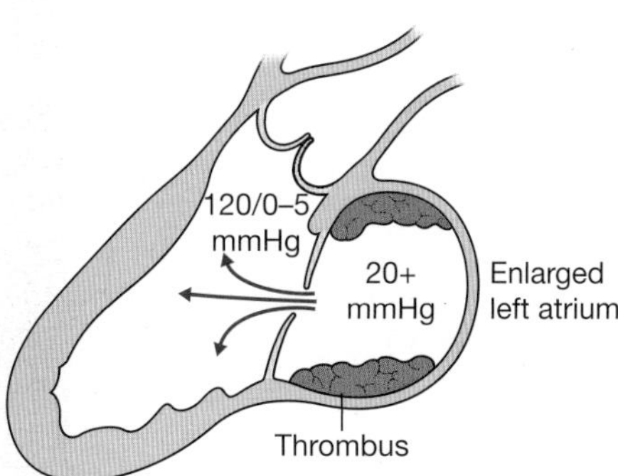

Figure 59.15 Pathophysiology of mitral stenosis. The aorta and left ventricle are relatively small because of chronically reduced cardiac output. The atrium is enlarged and may fibrillate, become stagnant and contain a thrombus. The ventricle fills with a turbulent jet that may be detected as a diastolic murmur or a thrill at the apex.

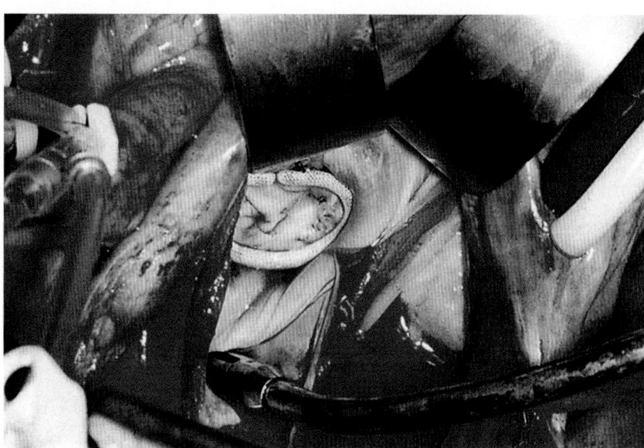

Figure 59.16 Operative view of the mitral valve repair using a Carpentier–Edwards annuloplasty ring (courtesy of A Murday, FRCS).

be treated using pharmacological agents such as digoxin to avoid decompensation and cardiac failure. Diuretics may also provide some benefit. The first-line invasive intervention is balloon valvuloplasty (PMBV); surgery is indicated for severely symptomatic patients who are unsuitable for PMBV or in whom PMBV failed. The prognosis is determined by the severity of the stenosis, the size of the atrium, the presence of AF and rising pulmonary artery pressure (***Figure 59.15***). Surgical options include mitral valve repair or mitral valve replacement. Formerly common surgical procedures such as closed or open commissurotomy are now rarely performed.

Mitral valve operations

Approaches to the mitral valve vary; commonly a median sternotomy or, occasionally, right thoracotomy is performed ('mini'-mitral surgery). The valve can be approached directly through the left atrium in the interatrial groove, through the right atrium and then the interatrial septum or through the left atrial appendage.

Mitral valve repair

Restoration of normal valve function and preservation of the mitral apparatus is preferable to replacement in specific groups of patients, as it can be associated with improved long-term ventricular remodelling and function. This approach reduces the bleeding complications associated with anticoagulants. The functional classification system developed by Carpentier serves as a guideline in valve reconstruction. It classifies mitral insufficiency into one of three groups according to the amplitude of the leaflet motion and provides a useful framework for the mechanisms of failure of the mitral valve. As a rule, several valvular lesions or abnormalities are involved in a functional abnormality, with specific techniques developed to correct each lesion.

At surgery, the anatomy of the valvular apparatus and subvalvular structures is carefully inspected. The extent of annular dilatation, leaflet prolapse and chordal dysfunction is assessed. Repair should respect rather than resect tissues, restoring a good coaptation surface between the two leaflets. The mitral valve repair can employ various techniques, including insertion of a prosthetic ring annuloplasty (***Figure 59.16***); triangular or quadrangular resection of the leaflet; use of a sliding plasty; chordal shortening; chordal transposition; and neochordea implantation.

Many techniques exist, indicating that no one technique addresses all possible findings in mitral regurgitation. Valve repair offers better preservation of ventricular function and avoids prolonged anticoagulation, and valve-related complications such as PVE or structural dysfunction. Recent advances in surgical techniques and the development of different types of rings has led to increased use of mitral valve repair with excellent results, making it the standard operation. The operative mortality is 1–3%. One of the major issues related to mitral repair is the incidence of regurgitation recurrence, which varies between series but can be up to 30% at 5 years. This is related to which leaflet is repaired and the amount of foreign material used in the repair (patch).

Mitral valve replacement

When valve repair is not feasible, mitral valve replacement is necessary. This usually involves a median sternotomy and access to the left atrium on CPB. The diseased valve is excised and a suitably sized mechanical or bioprosthetic valve is implanted. The atriotomy is closed following de-airing of the left heart. Intraoperative TOE can be used to assess adequate valve function.

The mortality rate for elective mitral valve replacement may be up to 5%, depending largely on the state of the myocardium and the general condition of the patient. Common serious in-hospital complications include stroke (<3%) and renal failure (3%). The longer term prognosis for patients following mitral valve replacement is generally good in comparison with the natural history of mitral valve disease. Indeed, more recent evidence suggests that patients with ischaemic severe mitral regurgitation can benefit more from valve replacement than from repair.

Alain Carpentier, b. 1933, cardiothoracic surgeon, Hôpital European Georges Pompidou, Paris, France.

Transcatheter mitral valve repair

The MitraClip® is a device used to reduce mitral valve regurgitation. The method involves suturing of the leaflets of the mitral valve together so that regurgitation into the left atrium is prevented. The valve continues to open through the sides of the suture and therefore blood continues to flow into the left ventricle. Access is usually from the groin where a catheter is inserted in the femoral vein to the right atrium. The left atrium is accessed by making a septal puncture. Although this method is less invasive and associated with rapid recovery and reduced in-hospital stay, it is however technically demanding and long-term durability of the results of the device is unknown.

Data suggest that the MitraClip® may be suitable for a small subset of high-risk patients (e.g. chronic heart failure), but the vast majority are better served by surgery that leaves them with substantially less mitral regurgitation.

Aortic valve disease

Approximately two-thirds of all valve surgery performed in the UK is for aortic valve disease, which remains common despite a reduction in the incidence of rheumatic fever in resource-rich countries.

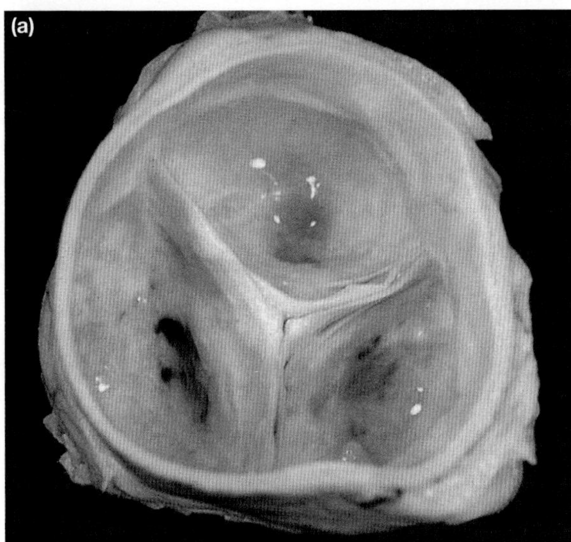

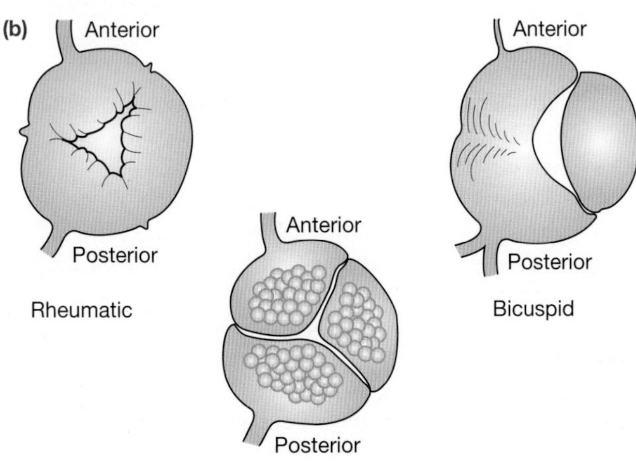

Figure 59.17 (a) Formaldehyde-treated aortic valve (normal tricuspid configuration). (b) Aortic stenosis, different pathologies.

Aortic stenosis

The commonest cause of aortic stenosis in adults is an acquired, degenerative, calcific process that results in immobile aortic valve cusps. Progressive fibrosis and calcification of a congenitally abnormal valve can mimic this degenerative process. The usual congenital abnormality is commissural fusion, leading to a bicuspid aortic valve, which occurs in approximately 1% of the population (***Figure 59.17***).

Pathophysiology

A pressure gradient develops between the left ventricle and the aorta, with the ventricle adapting to this systolic pressure overload by an increase in wall thickness or hypertrophy. This adaptive response is an attempt to normalise left ventricular wall stress in the face of increased left ventricular systolic pressure and may maintain a normal cardiac output, prevent left ventricular dilatation and avoid significant symptoms for a number of years. Eventually, myocardial function is affected and, together with insufficient left ventricular hypertrophy to normalise wall stress (load mismatch), ventricular contractility is reduced.

As aortic stenosis worsens, cardiac output cannot increase with exertion and eventually becomes insufficient at rest. The reduction in ventricular contractility leads to an irreversible decline in left ventricular function, with dilatation and a rise in left ventricular end-diastolic pressure, to the point of overt left heart failure. The severity of aortic stenosis is shown in ***Table 59.5***.

TABLE 59.5 Classification of the severity of aortic stenosis.

	Mild	Moderate	Severe
Valve area (cm^2)	>1.5	1.0–1.5	<1.0
Mean gradient (mmHg)	<20	20–40	>40
Velocity (m/s)	2.6–2.9 (<2.5 found in aortic sclerosis)	3.0–4.0	>4.0
Velocity ratio	>0.50	0.25–0.50	<0.25

Clinical features

Patients are often asymptomatic until decompensation occurs, typically presenting with dyspnoea and angina due to the increased oxygen needs of the hypertrophied left ventricle, reduced coronary filling and inadequate exertional cardiac output. Patients often describe feeling light-headed or 'near' syncope on effort. Arrhythmias can also occur. Auscultation demonstrates an ejection systolic murmur that is typically harsh and best heard over the aortic area with radiation to the carotids. The murmur may become quieter with reduced cardiac output in critical stenosis. The apex beat may be displaced in late disease along with signs of cardiac congestion (***Figure 59.18***).

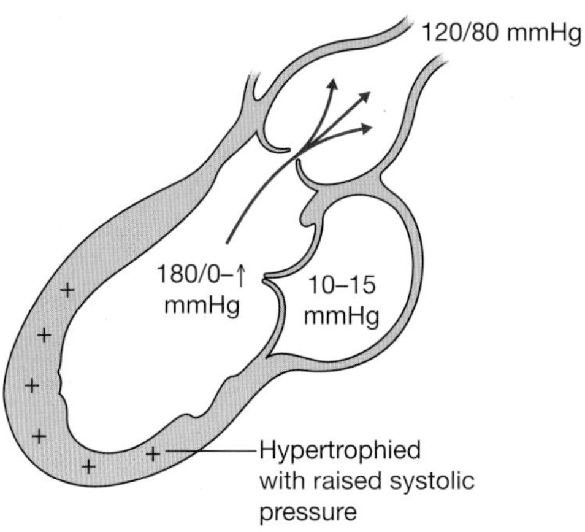

Figure 59.18 Features and pathophysiology of aortic stenosis. Haemodynamic changes in aortic stenosis. Aorta with poststenotic dilatation.

Investigations

- **ECG**: there is left ventricular hypertrophy with tall R waves in the lateral leads and ST depression with inverted T waves – ('strain pattern').
- **Chest radiography** may be normal. Cardiomegaly and pulmonary congestion may be seen with left ventricular failure. Poststenotic dilatation of the aorta is occasionally seen (***Figure 59.19***).
- **Echocardiography** confirms the diagnosis and colour flow Doppler imaging allows assessment of the aortic valve gradient, valve area and evaluation of left ventricular dimensions.
- **Coronary angiography**: to investigate the coronary arteries in patients >40 years of age.

Indications for surgery

Medical management focuses on the avoidance of systemic hypotension and arterial vasodilatation, which may reduce myocardial perfusion pressure and provoke ischaemia.

The natural history of symptomatic patients with aortic stenosis is dismal, with 10-year mortality around 80–90%. The risk of sudden death is related to the severity of stenosis.

Surgery is indicated in asymptomatic patients with severe stenosis and impaired left ventricular function or when the patient is undergoing concomitant procedures such as CABG. An abnormal blood pressure response to exercise (low blood pressure) is also a sign that there is limited reserve in asymptomatic patients.

Aortic regurgitation

The causes of aortic regurgitation can be classified according to the speed of development of the regurgitant jet (acute or chronic) or according to the anatomical location of pathology (valve leaflet or aortic wall). The causes of acute aortic regurgitation include infective endocarditis, aortic dissection and trauma. The common causes of chronic aortic regurgitation include degeneration leading to aortic root and/or annular dilatation, congenital bicuspid valve and previous rheumatic fever or endocarditis. Causes are shown in ***Table 59.6***.

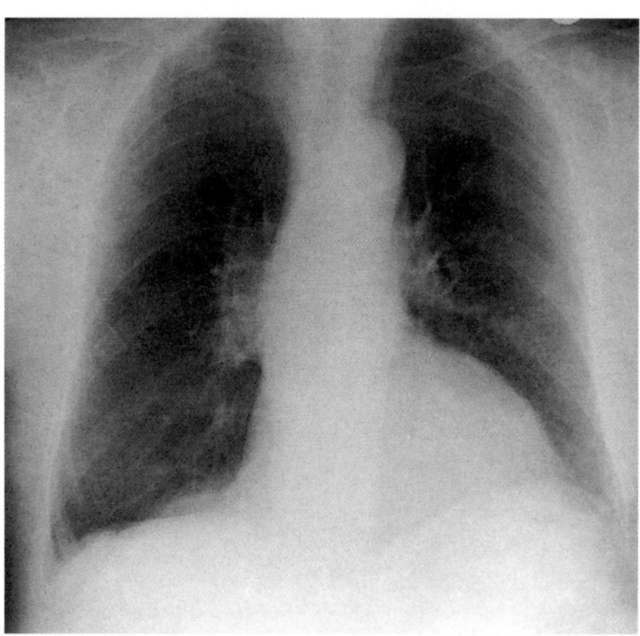

Figure 59.19 Chest radiograph in aortic stenosis.

Pathophysiology

In acute aortic regurgitation, backflow of blood increases ventricular load. It causes a sharp rise in left ventricular end-diastolic pressure, premature closure of the mitral valve and inadequate forward left ventricular filling. The result is sudden haemodynamic deterioration and acute respiratory compromise.

In chronic aortic regurgitation, the left ventricle dilates as a result of volume load, and eccentric hypertrophy is a compensatory mechanism to maintain cardiac output. Systolic and diastolic function is abnormal, and sudden deterioration can occur.

Clinical features

Longstanding aortic regurgitation is usually asymptomatic until left ventricular failure develops, when exertional dyspnoea (predominantly) or angina may develop. A wide pulse pressure due to a reduction in diastolic pressure and a collapsing pulse (water hammer pulse) are commonly seen.

TABLE 59.6 Causes of aortic regurgitation.

Acute aortic regurgitation	Chronic aortic regurgitation
Leaflet abnormalities	
Infective endocarditis Prosthetic valve dysfunction Traumatic leaflet rupture	Bicuspid aortic valve Calcific degeneration Fenfluramine usage (appetite suppressant)
Aortic wall abnormalities	
Aortic wall dissection Aortic trauma	Calcific degeneration Marfan syndrome, Ehlers–Danlos Aortic root dilatation Rheumatoid arthritis, systemic lupus erythematosus, ankylosing spondylitis

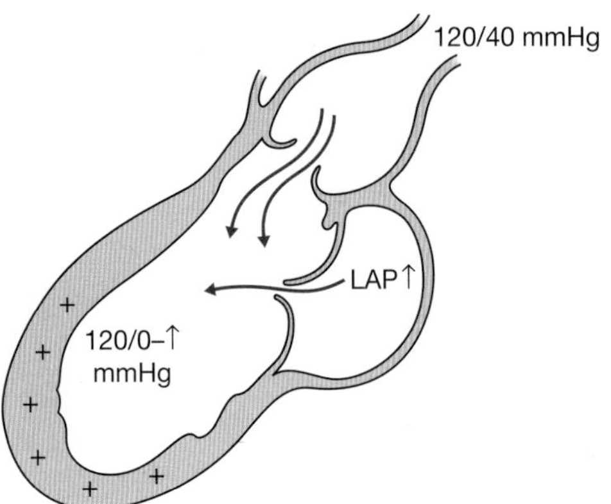

Figure 59.20 Haemodynamic consequences of aortic regurgitation. The left ventricle dilates and hypertrophies and there is a diastolic murmur. LAP, left atrial pressure.

Other manifestations of the wide pulse pressure include visible capillary pulsation of the nail bed (Quincke's sign), pulsatile head bobbing (de Musset's sign), visible arterial pulsation in the neck (Corrigan's sign), a 'pistol shot' sound on auscultating over the femoral artery (Traube's sign) and uvular pulsation (Müller's sign). The apex is displaced laterally and is often visible and hyperdynamic or 'thrusting' in nature because of the left ventricular hypertrophy. Auscultation reveals a high-pitched early diastolic murmur best heard at the left sternal edge (*Figure 59.20*).

Investigations

- **ECG**: there is left ventricular hypertrophy and sometimes a 'strain pattern'.
- **Chest radiography**: cardiomegaly can be seen if the left ventricle is dilating; sometimes, the aortic shadow may also indicate dilatation.
- **Echocardiography**: this allows assessment of the underlying cause and severity of aortic regurgitation and enables the diameter of the aortic root as well as left ventricular dimensions to be determined. Colour flow Doppler imaging quantifies the size of the regurgitant jet.
- **Coronary angiography**: to investigate the coronary arteries in patients >40 years of age.

Indications for surgery

Medical therapy with vasodilator drugs for relief of dyspnoea or angina improves forward stroke volume and reduces regurgitant volume. It is important to note that symptomatic relief does not alter the need for valve surgery.

The indications for surgery include severe regurgitation in symptomatic patients. Asymptomatic patients with severe aortic regurgitation and left ventricular dysfunction should also be offered surgery. Valve replacement should also be considered in asymptomatic patients with severe regurgitation if they are undergoing cardiac surgery for any other reason, or when there is evidence of progressive left ventricular dilatation (left ventricular end-systolic diameter >50 mm). Aortic valve replacement is recommended if there is a decrease in systolic function.

Summary box 59.10

Causes of aortic valve disease

Stenosis
- Congenital
- Rheumatic heart disease
- Acquired calcification and fibrosis of valve

Regurgitation
- Rheumatic heart disease
- Infective endocarditis
- Congenital
- Inflammatory:
  - Systemic lupus erythematosus
  - Rheumatic ankylosing spondylitis
- Dilatation of aortic root:
  - Marfan syndrome
  - Dissection
- Systemic disease:
  - Syphilis
  - Ulcerative colitis

Aortic valve surgery

Unlike mitral valve surgery, there are few occasions when the aortic valve can be repaired and usually the valve requires replacement. However, in neonates and children, aortic valve repair or valvotomy is well established. Percutaneous aortic balloon valvotomy also has a role in children, but appears to only result in temporary benefit in adult aortic valve disease.

Aortic valve replacement

Aortic valve replacement is performed through a median sternotomy or mini-sternotomy on CPB. The aorta is cross-clamped and opened proximally to reveal the diseased valve. Cardioplegic solution is infused into the coronary arteries to arrest the heart in diastole. The valve is excised, leaving the annulus *in situ* but removing as much calcific debris as possible. The annulus is sized and the mechanical or biological valve is then placed into position at the level of the native annulus and the aortotomy is closed.

The operative mortality rate for elective aortic valve surgery is 2–3%. It is higher in emergency surgery, surgery for endocarditis and in older patients.

Heinrich Irenaeus Quincke, 1842–1922, Professor of Medicine, Kiel, Germany.
Louis Charles Alfred de Musset, 1810–1857, French poet and playwright in whom the sign, traditionally, was first noticed.
Sir Dominic John Corrigan, 1802–1880, physician, Jervis Street Hospital, Dublin, Ireland.
Ludwig Traube, 1818–1876, physician, The Charité, Berlin, Germany.
Friedrich von Müller, 1858–1941, physician, Munich, Germany.

Major complications include stroke (2%), perioperative MI (2%) and heart block requiring a permanent pacemaker (<1%). The major determinant of late survival after aortic valve surgery is preoperative left ventricular function. The 5-year survival rate is approximately 75–85%, with the majority of late deaths related to myocardial factors.

Transcatheter aortic valve implantation

Although aortic valve replacement is still the gold standard treatment, a significant number of patients affected by severe aortic stenosis do not undergo surgery because they are high risk (owing to age, frailty or heart failure) or because they are affected by concomitant comorbidities that noticeably increase the operative risk. In such patients TAVI is an attractive alternative to standard aortic valve replacement. Other indications include heavily calcified ('porcelain') ascending aorta and the presence of severe congenital thoracic wall distortion. The advances in TAVI techniques and the currently available evidence suggests that TAVI can be an option in intermediate-risk patients.

There are different approaches for valve implantation; the most commonly used are transapical (retrograde) and transluminal (antegrade).

- **Transapical approach**. In transapical TAVI, the cardiac apex is prepared through a small left anterolateral mini-thoracotomy using a purse-string or a crossing suture reinforced by pledgets. The device is advanced in the left ventricle between the purse-string sutures. This approach reduces the risk of calcium dislodgement due to the passage of a stiff transluminal device into a diseased aortic arch.
- **Transluminal approach**. This can be carried out via direct access to the aorta, or femoral or subclavian arteries. This is a useful technique for patients with previous cardiac surgery; however, the presence of poor access because of peripheral vascular disease, small vessel diameters, tortuous vessels, aortic disease or previous aortic surgery contraindicates this approach.

Whichever approach is used, a balloon catheter is advanced into the left ventricle over a guidewire and positioned at the aortic valve orifice. The existing aortic valve is dilated in order to make room for the prosthetic valve. Rapid right ventricular pacing is used to interrupt cardiac output through the existing aortic valve and to reduce movement during implantation. The new valve, mounted on a metal stent, is manipulated into position and is either self-expanding or deployed using balloon inflation. Deployment leads to obliteration of the existing aortic valve.

Complications associated with TAVI include mortality (5–18% at 30 days), mild-to-moderate aortic regurgitation (30–50%), stroke (3–9%), perioperative open conversion (9–12%), vascular complications (10–15%), atrioventricular block (4–8%) and access artery problems such as bleeding or thrombosis. A recent MI (<3 months), severe pulmonary dysfunction and the presence of an apical thrombus are contraindications for transapical TAVI. Interestingly, recent multicentre trials have demonstrated that the role of TAVI may be offered to intermediate-risk patients, with satisfactory mid-term outcomes.

CONGENITAL HEART DISEASE

Introduction

Congenital heart diseases are abnormalities of cardiac structure that are present from birth. Such developmental abnormalities of the heart typically arise in the third to eighth week of gestation. The first operation for congenital heart disease was patent ductus arteriosus (PDA) ligation by Gross in 1938. With the development of neonatal CPB, improved myocardial protection and microsurgical techniques, an increasing number of corrective and palliative operations are possible.

Development of the heart and fetal circulation and circulatory changes at birth

By 12 weeks of fetal life the primitive vascular tube is fully developed. Fetal circulation differs from that of the adult in that the right and left ventricles pump blood in parallel rather than in series. This arrangement allows the heart and head to receive more highly oxygenated blood. This is possible because of the presence of three structural shunts: the ductus venosus, foramen ovale and ductus arteriosus (***Figure 59.21***).

Soon after birth, pulmonary vascular resistance falls because of the action of breathing and resulting pulmonary vasodilatation. Within 30 minutes of delivery, the ductus arteriosus constricts in response to increasing blood oxygen levels. The result is a reversal of the pulmonary–systemic pressure gradient and termination of blood flow from the pulmonary artery into the aorta.

After birth, cutting and tying of the umbilical cord stops venous blood flow from the placenta. This lowers inferior vena cava pressure and, with falling pulmonary vascular resistance, right atrial pressure falls. The result is closure of the foramen ovale. The abolition of venous return from the placenta also causes the ductus venosus to close.

Closure of the fetal circulatory shunts in the few hours following birth is functional, with complete structural closure typically taking several months. In 20% of adults the structural closure of the foramen ovale remains incomplete, but is of no cardiovascular significance.

Abnormalities of cardiac structure may arise from the persistence of normal fetal channels (PDA, patent foramen ovale), failure of septation (atrial septal defect [ASD], VSD, tetralogy of Fallot), stenosis (intracardiac, supravalvular, valvular, infravalvular or extracardiac coarctation of the aorta), atresia or abnormal connections (transposition of the great vessels

---

Robert E Gross, 1905–1988, Surgeon-in-Chief, Cardiovascular Surgery, Children's Hospital, Boston, MA, USA.
Etienne Arthur Louis Fallot, 1850–1911, Professor of Medicine, Marseilles, France.

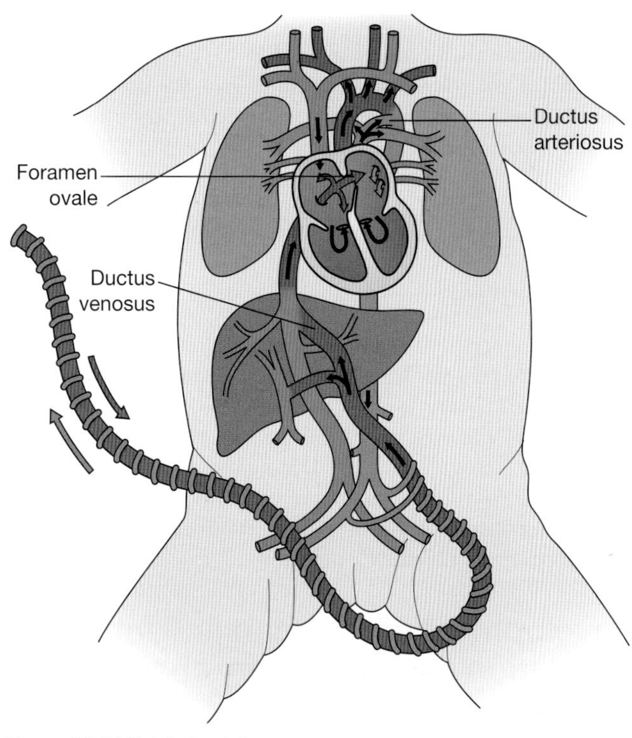

Figure 59.21 Fetal circulation.

(TGV), total anomalous venous drainage). Fetal echocardiography is now sufficiently sensitive to detect intracardiac lesions in the second trimester.

Incidence

Cardiac defects are the most common congenital abnormalities in the UK; the incidence of significant cardiac abnormalities is 8 per 1000 live births. Many spontaneous abortions or stillbirths have cardiac malformations or chromosomal abnormalities associated with structural heart defects. In neonates and children with congenital heart disease, 15% will have more than one cardiac abnormality and 15% will have another extracardiac abnormality.

Aetiology

There is often no obvious aetiology; most abnormalities appear to be multifactorial with both genetic and environmental influences. There are well-recognised associations.

Summary box 59.11

Recognised associations with congenital heart disease

Maternal (environmental) factors

- Infection: rubella
- Disease: systemic lupus erythematosus, diabetes mellitus, maternal phenylketonuria
- Drugs/medications: alcohol abuse, warfarin, phenytoin, lithium, thalidomide

Genetic factors

- Single gene defects: Marfan, Noonan and Holt–Oram syndromes; numerous single-gene disorders
- Chromosomal defects: trisomy 21 (Down syndrome), trisomy 18 (Edwards syndrome), trisomy 13 (Patau syndrome), Turner syndrome, Klinefelter syndrome
- Deletions: DiGeorge and Williams syndromes

Diagnosis

Antenatal diagnosis is occasionally possible, with severe defects detected *in utero* at 16–18 weeks. If an infant has suspected congenital heart disease, a diagnostic evaluation begins with an accurate history from the parents and specific questions about maternal health and drug use. A detailed family history is important because some defects are familial. Clinical examination may reveal a murmur, evidence of heart failure, failure to thrive and cyanosis. In addition, congenital heart disease can present with hypertension, an arrhythmia, evidence of polycythaemia or a thromboembolic event. Investigation is much the same as for the adult patient and, with fetal echocardiography available, cardiac catheterisation is now avoided whenever possible.

Classification

Congenital heart disease can be broadly classified according to the presence or absence of cyanosis, although the distinction is not always clear-cut. Central cyanosis – blueness of the trunk and mucous membranes – results from levels of deoxygenated haemoglobin of >3–5 g/dL in the arterial circulation.

Cyanotic congenital heart diseases make up 25% of cases (8 or 9/1000 live births) and are usually more complex, although they do include simple defects. Cyanotic congenital cardiac lesions can involve:

Jacqueline Anne Noonan, 1928–2020, pediatric cardiologist, the University of Kentucky College of Medicine, Lexington, KY, USA, described this condition in 1963.
Mary Clayton Holt, 1924–1993, cardiologist, The London Hospital for Women and Children, London, UK.
Samuel Oram, 1913–1991, cardiologist, King's College Hospital, London, UK. Holt and Oram described this syndrome in a joint paper in 1960.
John Langdon Haydon Down, 1828–1896, physician, The London Hospital, London, UK.
John Hilton Edwards, 1928–2007, Professor of Genetics, University of Oxford, Oxford, UK.
Klaus Patau, 1908–1975, German-born American geneticist, University of Wisconsin–Madison, Madison, WI, USA.
Henry Hubert Turner, 1892–1970, Professor of Medicine, The University of Oklahoma, Oklahoma City, OK, USA.
Harry Klinefelter, 1912–1990, American rheumatologist and endocrinologist, first described the syndrome in 1942.
Angelo M DiGeorge, 1921–2009, Professor of Pediatrics, Temple University, Philadelphia, PA, USA.
John CP Williams, b. 1922, New Zealand born cardiologist, described the condition in 1961.

- Right–left shunting of blood resulting in decreased pulmonary blood flow. Many lesions consist of septal defects in conjunction with a right-sided obstructive lesion, producing obligatory right-to-left shunts. The most common cause of this is the tetralogy of Fallot.
- Parallel systemic and pulmonary blood flow. If there is no mixing this is incompatible with life; neonates have a patent foramen ovale or VSD that allows some mixing of the two circulations at this level. The most common example of this is TGV.
- Defects in the connections of the heart in which there is mixing of the systemic and pulmonary flows. An example of such a complex lesion is total anomalous pulmonary venous drainage (TAPVD).

Acyanotic congenital heart diseases represent 75% of cases and are usually less complex. They result in an increase in the work imposed on the heart because of either:

- A left-to-right shunt with increased pulmonary blood flow, causing an increase in volume work of the heart. Examples include PDA, ASD and VSD.
- Obstruction of blood flow across a left-sided heart valve, such as aortic stenosis, or in the aorta itself, as occurs with coarctation of the aorta, leading to an increase in pressure and work of the heart.

Typically, acyanotic congenital heart disease presents as heart failure in infancy because of pulmonary congestion caused by increased pulmonary blood flow or increased pulmonary venous blood pressure resulting from an obstructive lesion. The common acyanotic cardiac defects can also present as a murmur in infancy or later.

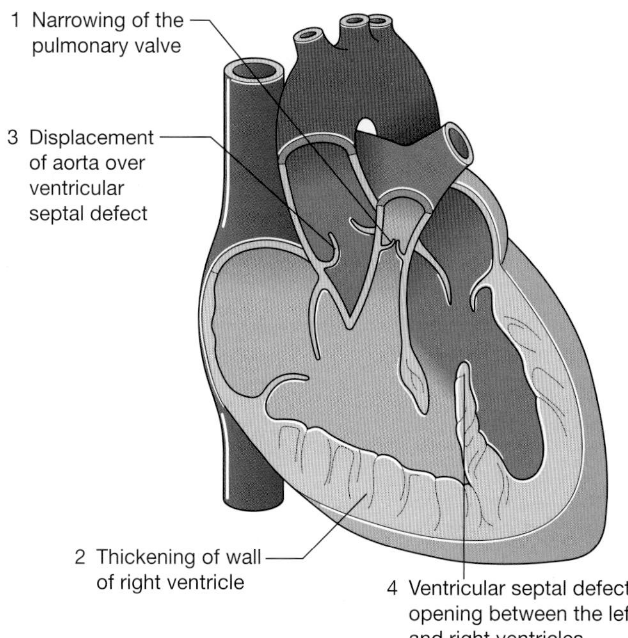

Figure 59.22 Fallot's tetralogy. Four abnormalities that result in insufficiently oxygenated blood being pumped to the body.

Cyanotic congenital heart disease

Tetralogy of Fallot

This is the most common cyanotic congenital heart disease in children surviving to 1 year and accounts for about 4–6% of all congenital heart diseases. The four intracardiac lesions originally described (***Figure 59.22***) were:

- VSD;
- overriding aorta;
- pulmonary (infundibular or subpulmonary) stenosis;
- right ventricular hypertrophy.

There may be no initial clinical signs, but, as pulmonary stenosis progresses, cyanosis typically develops within the first year of life. Squatting is an adaptation by the child to hypoxic spells, increasing systemic vascular resistance and the venous return to the heart. Consequently blood is diverted into the pulmonary circulation, increasing oxygenation. Lethargy and tiredness are also common. Plain radiography classically demonstrates a 'boot-shaped' heart with poorly developed lung vasculature. The diagnosis is confirmed with echocardiography. Surgical correction is the mainstay of treatment and is usually carried out at 4–6 months of age, when possible. Repair is achieved using a patch to close the VSD and resection of the obstructing infundibular septum. Surgical results are good, with a late survival rate of 95% at 5–10 years following correction of tetralogy, an operative mortality rate for a repair of between 5% and 10% and an incidence of reoperation following tetralogy repair of 5–10%.

Transposition of the great vessels

This is the second most common cyanotic congenital heart disease and most common cause of cyanosis from a congenital cardiac defect discovered in the newborn period. TGV results from abnormal development, with the aorta arising from the right ventricle and the pulmonary artery from the left ventricle (***Figure 59.23***). The resulting transposition causes pulmonary and systemic circulations to run in parallel rather than in series; oxygenated pulmonary venous blood returns to the lungs and desaturated systemic venous blood is pumped around the body. The situation is incompatible with life and mixing of the

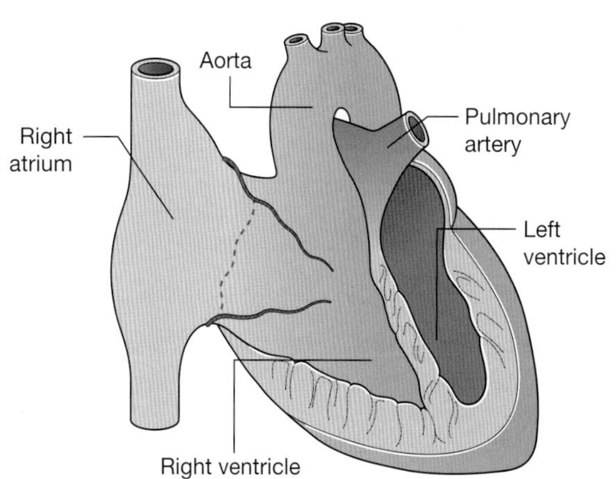

Figure 59.23 Transposition of the great vessels.

blood must occur through associated shunts, such as a patent foramen ovale or VSD.

Patients often present with severe central cyanosis occurring within 48 hours of birth. However, if there is a large ASD or VSD there may be minimal cyanosis initially. Typically, progress is poor and, as pulmonary vascular resistance declines in the neonatal period, high pulmonary flow develops, with cardiac enlargement and left ventricular failure.

The chest radiograph shows pulmonary plethora, with the heart having an 'egg on its side' appearance, with a small pedicle (aorta in front of pulmonary artery). Cardiac echocardiography is sufficient to confirm the diagnosis and delineate the anatomy.

Many infants will die without treatment within 1 month of birth. Initial stabilisation can be achieved by performing percutaneous balloon septostomy to increase the systemic arterial oxygen saturation. Alternatively, intravenous prostaglandins can be administered to keep the PDA open and increase systemic–pulmonary shunting. Arterial switch repair is currently the standard operation and is typically carried out within the first few weeks of life. Long-term outcomes of the operation are excellent and many patients achieve good exercise tolerance; however, some patients will require reoperation for neopulmonary stenosis.

Total anomalous pulmonary venous drainage

TAPVD accounts for 1–2% of congenital heart disease. In TAPVD, the pulmonary venous drainage has disconnected from the left atrium and drains into the systemic venous circulation at some other point (inferior vena cava, superior vena cava, coronary sinus or right atrium). TAPVD presents after the first week of life with cyanosis that is mild to moderate depending on pulmonary flow. Infants with high pulmonary flow develop cardiac failure, recurrent chest infections, failure to thrive and feeding difficulties. If high pulmonary flow is associated with a large ASD, cyanosis is often minimal and the lesion is tolerated well. If there is additional venous obstruction, cyanosis presents at birth with dyspnoea and pulmonary oedema. Echocardiography and cardiac (pulmonary) angiography are necessary to confirm the diagnosis and delineate the anomalous drainage.

The surgical principle is to re-establish the pulmonary venous drainage into the left atrium. The exact operative technique depends on the anatomy and type of TAPVD. The long-term results for survivors of the operation are generally good. Late death following repair is uncommon but, when it occurs, it is often caused by intimal fibroplasia of the pulmonary veins away from the anastomosis.

Eisenmenger syndrome

Eisenmenger syndrome is becoming less common due to development of corrective techniques for congenital heart disease with fewer patients developing a fixed increase in their pulmonary vascular resistance. It follows reversal of a left-to-right shunt, that occurs with, for example, a ASD or VSD, such that de-oxygenated blood now flows from right to left causing cyanosis. These congenital anomalies (ASD, VSD) cause an increase in flow and higher right-sided pressures, which lead to compensatory right ventricular hypertrophy and a subsequent rise in pulmonary artery pressure. Increasing pulmonary hypertension leads to equalisation of pressures either side of the shunt but, at some point, the right-sided pressures will exceed those on the left side, resulting in shunt reversal and desaturated blood entering the left side of the circulation. Cyanosis and dyspnoea are the most common clinical features. Closure of the shunt is contraindicated if pulmonary hypertension is irreversible because the right-to-left shunt now serves to decompress the pulmonary circulation.

Acyanotic congenital heart disease

Patent ductus arteriosus

The ductus arteriosus, a normal fetal communication, facilitates the shunting of oxygenated blood from the pulmonary artery to the aorta, away from the lungs. Normally, functional closure of the ductus occurs within a few hours of birth; it is abnormal if it persists beyond the neonatal period. The ductus closes in response to an increase in peripheral oxygen saturation and a drop in the resistance of the pulmonary circulation as the lungs expand; this causes the ductal tissue to contract through a prostaglandin inhibition mechanism. A cyclo-oxygenase inhibitor (e.g. indomethacin) may be used therapeutically to close the ductus in the first few weeks of life. In premature babies the ductus is more likely to remain patent for longer or permanently. In the isolated case of PDA, there is a left-to-right shunt of blood, resulting in a high pulmonary blood flow. Small shunts usually cause few symptoms and signs apart from the continuous machinery murmur in the left second intercostal space. Larger ducts cause cardiac failure and can uncommonly lead to shunt reversal with cyanosis and clubbing. The diagnosis is best confirmed by echocardiography with colour flow Doppler imaging.

After 6 months of age, PDA closure is rare. Most should be closed by preschool age, regardless of symptoms, if the risks of infective endocarditis, left ventricular failure or, rarely, Eisenmenger syndrome are to be avoided. In the adult, surgical treatment is indicated if there is a persistent left-to-right shunt, even in the presence of reversible pulmonary hypertension. In the premature infant, if medical treatment to close the ductus is unsuccessful, the PDA may be treated by percutaneous interventional cardiology techniques using an umbrella or coil duct occlusion device. If the PDA is very large or the patient very small, surgical closure via a left thoracotomy is preferred. This can be accomplished by either ligation or division of the PDA. The operative mortality rate is low and outcome generally very good.

Coarctation of the aorta

This accounts for 6–7% of congenital heart disease and is defined as a haemodynamically significant narrowing of the

Victor Eisenmenger, 1864–1932, Austrian physician who described this condition in 1897, but the term 'Eisenmenger syndrome' was introduced in 1958 by an Australian cardiologist, **Paul Hamilton Wood** (1907–1962).

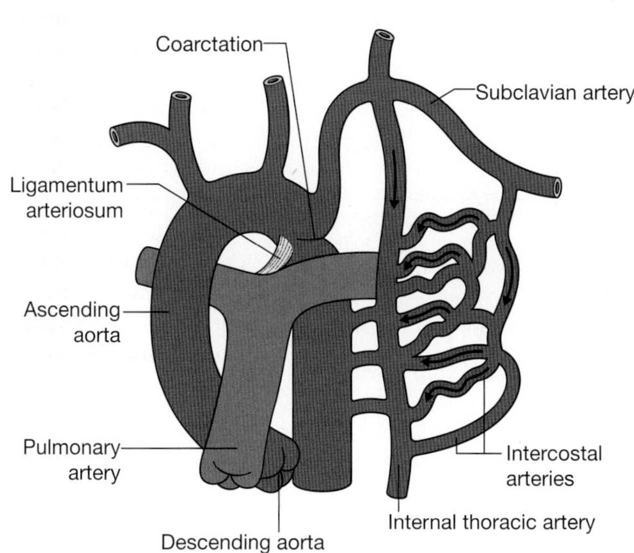

Figure 59.24 Coarctation of the aorta. Coarctation causes severe obstruction of blood flow in the descending thoracic aorta. The descending aorta and its branches are perfused by collateral channels from the axillary and internal thoracic arteries through the intercostal arteries (arrows).

aorta, usually in the descending aorta just distal to the left subclavian artery, around the area of the ductus arteriosus (***Figure 59.24***). The coarctation typically puts a pressure load on the left ventricle, which can ultimately fail. The upper body is well perfused but the lower body, including the kidneys, is poorly perfused, leading to fluid overload, excess renin secretion and acidosis. Coarctation usually affects boys and, if it occurs in girls, is suggestive of Turner syndrome.

In the neonatal period, coarctation ('infantile' or preductal coarctation) presents with symptoms of heart failure. The child may appear well in the first few days of life because the coarctation is bypassed by the ductus arteriosus and oxygenated blood reaches the systemic circulation. As the ductus closes, the child becomes progressively more unwell. In adult-type coarctation (juxtaductal or slightly postductal) obstruction is gradual with complications developing in adolescence or early adulthood. Hypertension is a common presenting problem in older children – often upper body hypertension only with development of enormous collateral vessels that may cause rib-notching and flow murmurs over the scapula. Other symptoms include prominent pulsation in the neck, tired legs or intermittent claudication on exercise. Clinical examination of the pulses may demonstrate a radio-femoral delay and a murmur that is continuous and heard best over the thoracic spine or below the left clavicle.

The chest radiograph classically demonstrates rib-notching because of dilated posterior intercostal vessels. The heart is usually of normal size in the older child and shows a classical 'three sign' replacing the typical aortic knuckle. The upper part of the three sign is the dilated left subclavian, the middle part is the narrowing at the coarctation site and the lower part is the poststenotic dilatation of the descending aorta. Echocardiography is diagnostic. Infant coarctation typically presents with cardiac failure, often requiring vigorous medical treatment, including the administration of prostaglandin to reopen the ductus and general resuscitation before corrective surgery. Definitive treatment is usually surgical repair via a left thoracotomy. Coarctation presenting in the child or later typically requires surgical repair, as most patients die before the age of 40 years because of the associated complications. Percutaneous stenting is currently the standard treatment for adults with isolated coarctation. Without correction, the majority of deaths are caused by heart failure, infective endocarditis, rupture of the aorta or haemorrhagic stroke. The preoperative hypertension may not resolve despite surgical repair.

Atrial septal defects

An ASD is a defect in the septum between the left and right atria leading to a left-to-right shunt, the significance of which is determined by the size of the defect and the relative compliance of the ventricles. The development of the atrial septum is complex and abnormalities of development lead to three commonly recognised ASDs (***Figure 59.25***).

The most common type is an ostium secundum ASD. The anomaly is caused by failure of the septum primum to develop, leading to incomplete coverage of the ostium secundum. These defects are usually asymptomatic in childhood, with symptoms developing insidiously, typically presenting in middle age with congestive cardiac failure secondary to pulmonary hypertension or with atrial arrhythmias.

In ostium primum ASD, the anomaly is a form of partial atrioventricular canal defect or endocardial cushion defect. The abnormalities are confined to the atrial septum and are caused by the endocardial cushions failing to develop and so close the ostium primum part of the interatrial septum. The defect is associated with abnormalities of the mitral valve, leading to mitral regurgitation. There is a relatively high incidence of this abnormality in trisomy 21 (Down syndrome). Typically,

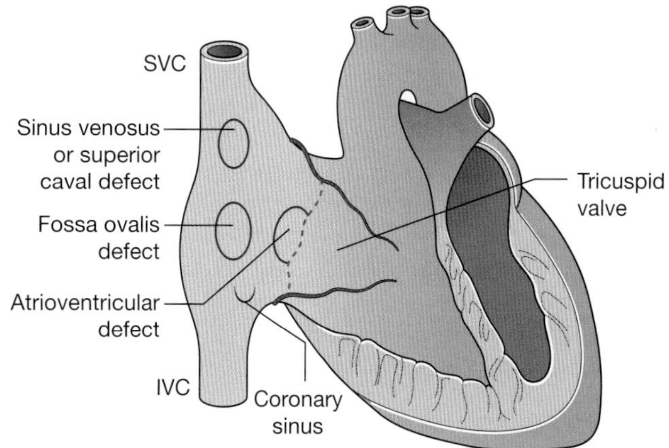

Figure 59.25 Atrial septum viewed from the right. The fossa ovalis is a useful reference point; the most common defect is in this area and is called a fossa ovalis (or ostium secundum) defect. A defect near the atrioventricular junction may be part of the spectrum of atrioventricular septal defects; defects near the entry of the superior vena cava (SVC) are commonly associated with anomalies of venous drainage into the atria. IVC, inferior vena cava.

primum defects present earlier than ostium secundum in childhood, with dyspnoea, recurrent chest infections and, if pulmonary hypertension develops, cyanosis.

A sinus venosus ASD is a rare defect and is the result of failure of partition of the pulmonary and systemic venous circulations. These defects are most commonly located high in the atrial septum at the junction of the superior vena cava and the right atrium. They are frequently associated with anomalous pulmonary venous drainage, with right superior pulmonary veins draining into the superior vena cava or right atrium directly.

Summary box 59.12

Atrial septal defects (ASDs)

Common defects

- Ostium secundum: fossa ovalis defect (approximately 70% of ASDs)
- Ostium primum: atrioventricular septal defect (approximately 20% of ASDs)
- Sinus venosus defect: often associated with anomalous pulmonary venous drainage (approximately 10% of ASDs)
- Patent foramen ovale: common in isolation, usually no left-to-right shunt (not strictly an ASD)

Rarer defects

- Inferior vena cava defects: a low sinus venosus defect and may allow shunting of blood into the left atrium
- Coronary sinus septal defect: also known as unroofed coronary sinus, with the left superior vena cava draining to the left atrium as part of a more complex lesion

Closure is performed during the first decade of life, even in the absence of symptoms, to avoid late-onset right ventricular failure, endocarditis and paradoxical emboli. In adults, closure is still appropriate for symptomatic improvement and avoidance of complications. The traditional method of closure involves open-heart surgery with CPB and closure of the defect, either directly with sutures, as with most secundum defects, or, if the defect is large, using a pericardial or synthetic patch. Closure of small to moderate ASDs using percutaneous catheter-delivered devices in the cardiology catheter laboratory is increasingly common. Primum atrioventricular defect repairs may require additional mitral valve repair. The operative mortality rate for isolated atrioventricular defect repairs is <1%, with an excellent prognosis. Surgical correction of complete atrioventricular canal defects, with closure of the ASD and ventricular septal components and mitral valve repair, is possible, but with a higher surgical mortality rate.

Ventricular septal defects

A VSD is a defect in the interventricular septum that allows left-to-right shunting of blood. VSDs account for 20–30% of congenital heart disease and affect approximately 2 in 1000 live births. They may occur in isolation or as part of a more complex set of cardiac abnormalities (e.g. tetralogy of Fallot,

Summary box 59.13

Types of ventricular septal defects (VSD)

Perimembranous (conoventricular) defect

- The most common defect (70–80%), usually located within the membranous septum and may extend to the tricuspid valve annulus or the base of the aortic valve

Muscular (trabecular) defect

- Occurs in 10% of cases and is located within the membranous septum and can be multiple

Atrioventricular (inlet) defect

- Also called an atrioventricular canal-type defect; occurs in 5% of cases and is located in the atrioventricular canal beneath the tricuspid valve

Subarterial (outlet) defect

- Occurs in 5–10% of cases and lies within the conal septum immediately beneath the pulmonary valve annulus

complete atrioventricular canal defect). Four major anatomical types of VSD are described, based on the anatomical subsections of the interventricular septum (***Figure 59.26***).

The VSD permits a ventricular left-to-right shunt, with subsequent right ventricular volume overload and increased pulmonary blood flow. This may lead to progressive pulmonary oedema and congestive cardiac failure. Persistently elevated pulmonary blood flow and pulmonary vascular resistance also lead to irreversible pulmonary hypertension. They may eventually result in reversal of flow across the defect and Eisenmenger syndrome. The clinical presentation reflects the magnitude of the left-to-right shunt, which, in turn, depends on the size of the VSD and the pulmonary and systemic vascular resistances. Small defects may close or cause little systemic disturbance (maladie de Roger); infants are asymptomatic with normal development. In the first 5 years, up to 50% of VSDs close spontaneously. Clinically, a loud pansystolic murmur can

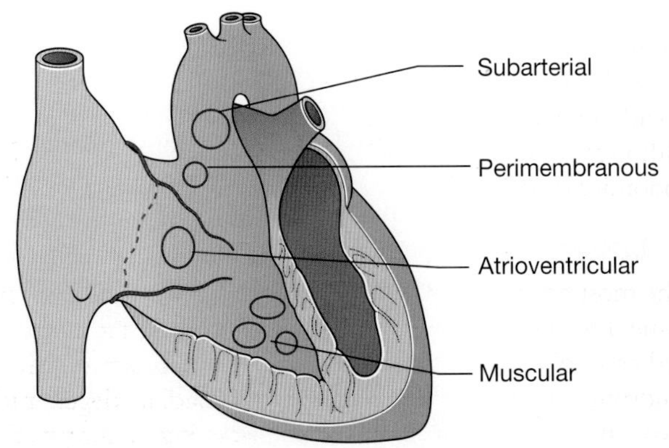

Figure 59.26 Ventricular septum viewed from the right, showing the characteristic sites of ventricular septal defects.

Henri Louis Roger, 1809–1891, physician, Hôpital Sainte-Eugene, Paris, France.

be detected at the left sternal border because of high-pressure flow between the ventricles. Large defects typically present with congestive cardiac failure in the first 2 months of life. Because of the size of the VSD, ventricular pressures are equalised and often only a soft systolic murmur is detected. If left untreated, pulmonary hypertensive changes start from about 1 year of age. Eisenmenger syndrome, secondary to shunt reversal in such cases, may become evident in the second decade of life.

Echocardiography confirms the diagnosis and can estimate the degree of shunting across the defect. Cardiac catheterisation can quantify right and left cardiac pressures and the degree of pulmonary hypertension, as well as demonstrate a step-up in oxygen saturation between left and right ventricles. Generally, surgical closure is indicated for large defects; when there is failure to respond to medical therapy; for left-to-right shunts of >2:1; when there are signs of increasing pulmonary vascular resistance; and in the presence of complications of VSD. These include: (i) aortic regurgitation, which occurs in about 5% of defects; (ii) infundibular stenosis, which tends to be progressive and leads to shunt reversal; and (iii) infective endocarditis, often presenting with pneumonia or pleurisy as the infected 'emboli' in a VSD with a typical left-to-right shunt flows into the pulmonary circulation.

THE THORACIC AORTA

The most common pathologies affecting the thoracic aorta are aneurysm formation and aortic dissection.

Thoracic aortic aneurysms

A true aneurysm is a localised dilatation of a blood vessel involving all three layers of the vessel wall, whereas a false aneurysm has compressed supporting tissue as its wall and is usually the result of a defect in the vessel intima (from trauma, dissection or previous surgery). Aneurysms are described as fusiform when the whole circumference is affected or saccular when only part of the circumference is involved. When the whole length of a vessel is affected, the clinical and anatomical situation is referred to as ectasia.

Aortic aneurysms can develop anywhere along its length, but thoracic aortic aneurysms, including those that extend into the upper abdomen (thoracoabdominal aneurysms), account for 25%, typically occurring in men in the fifth to seventh decade or younger in those with connective tissue disorders. Although a national UK screening programme exists for abdominal aortic aneurysm, this is not true for thoracic disease.

Aetiology

The most common aetiology is atherosclerosis, but connective tissue disorders account for many aneurysms in the aortic root and ascending aorta now that tertiary syphilis is rare. Marfan syndrome is associated with cystic medial degeneration involving the vessel wall and causes widening of the proximal aorta and aortic root, leading to aortic valve insufficiency. It is caused by a mutation in the fibrillin gene. Other disorders associated with aneurysm formation and dissection include Ehlers–Danlos syndrome, which is associated with a range of complications including aortic dissection, joint dislocations, scoliosis and osteogenesis imperfecta.

Many aneurysms are asymptomatic and are discovered incidentally on routine chest radiographs. Others present as a space-occupying lesion in the thorax with pain caused by pressure on adjacent structures (vertebra), hoarseness (left recurrent laryngeal nerve), dysphagia (oesophagus) and respiratory symptoms (left main bronchus). Aortic root aneurysms may lead to dilatation of the aortic root annulus and aortic regurgitation.

Rupture can lead to cardiac tamponade or haemorrhage into the left pleural space, leading to dyspnoea and, if the tracheobronchial airway or oesophagus is involved, haemoptysis or haematemesis.

Investigations

The diagnosis is confirmed by CT or MRI. Arteriography is not necessary for diagnosis but is often required to demonstrate the relation of the arch vessels to the aneurysm.

Indications for surgery

Without treatment the aneurysm is likely to expand and ultimately rupture. Important factors to consider when planning treatment are age, comorbidity and coexisting coronary disease.

In ascending aneurysms, the presence of progressive aortic valve insufficiency is an important indication for surgery. Other indications in this group, including Marfan-related aneurysms, are a diameter of 4.5–5 cm and the presence of symptoms. In descending aneurysms, indications for surgery include symptoms, acute enlargement and a diameter of approximately 6 cm.

Surgical options

The approach adopted for surgical treatment depends on the location of the aneurysm, but typically involves a median sternotomy, CPB and occasionally cooling the patient to 18°C before cross-clamping the aorta above the aneurysm at the distal ascending aorta just before the innominate artery (***Figure 59.27***). If the aortic root is involved, the aorta, together with its annulus and valve, is resected and a composite graft is sutured to the aortic root. The circulation is arrested and, after removal of the aortic cross-clamp, the distal anastomosis is completed. The coronary ostia require reimplantation into the graft (Bentall's operation). More recently there has been increased interest in valve-sparing root surgery or valve repair and root replacement, which is based on two original techniques, namely the remodelling technique described by Magdi Yacoub and the reimplantation technique described by Tirone David. These techniques are associated with reduced thromboembolic complications, but are usually demanding with a small increased risk of requiring reoperation at a later stage.

Hugh Henry Bentall, 1920–2012, Professor of Cardiac Surgery, The Royal Postgraduate Hospital, Hammersmith, London, UK.
Sir Magdi Yacoub, b. 1935, Professor of cardiac surgery, Imperial College, UK.
Tirone David, b. 1944, Professor of Surgery, Toronto, Canada.

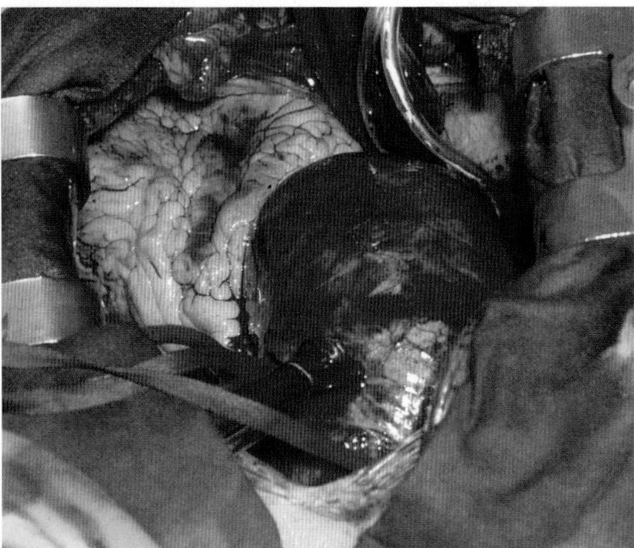

Figure 59.27 A large thoracic aortic aneurysm.

If the ascending aorta is involved, it is resected and replaced with a tube graft. For aortic arch aneurysms, surgery on this section of the aorta is a formidable undertaking because the cerebral and subclavian vessels have to be anastomosed to the graft, either separately or en bloc. Typically, it involves a period of circulatory arrest and some form of cerebral protection. Excision of a descending aortic aneurysm is with graft replacement under CPB, with exposure via a left thoracotomy or with a heparin-bonded shunt. Increasingly, thoracic aneurysms at the aortic arch or more distal are repaired using a percutaneous approach via the femoral artery, with insertion of an endovascular stent graft under radiological guidance.

Surgical outcome

The operative mortality rate is variable depending on the location and type of repair required, but electively is between 5% and 15% and is considerably higher in emergency repairs. Long-term survival depends on underlying pathology but, for ascending aneurysm repairs, the 5-year survival rate is approximately 65%. The major complications of descending aneurysm repairs include paraplegia, renal failure and ventricular dysfunction.

Aortic dissection

This occurs when a defect or flap occurs in the intima of the aorta, resulting in blood tracking into the aortic tissues, splitting the medial layer and creating a false lumen. It most commonly occurs in the ascending aorta or, less often, just distal to the left subclavian artery. It is also more common in men, typically those aged 50–70 years, and in Afro-Caribbean patients.

Aetiology

It usually occurs as a spontaneous or sporadic event, often in a patient with a history of hypertension. Other important associations include Marfan syndrome and pregnancy.

Summary box 59.14

Predisposing factors for aortic dissection

- Age
- Hypertension
- Marfan syndrome
- Pregnancy
- Other connective tissue disorders, e.g. Ehlers–Danlos syndrome, giant cell arteritis, systemic lupus erythematosus
- Coarctation of the aorta
- Turner or Noonan syndromes
- Aortic cannulation site following previous cardiac surgery (iatrogenic)

Clinical features

The presentation is often with tearing interscapular pain not unlike the pain of myocardial ischaemia, and it may be difficult to distinguish between the two. The extent of arterial dissection may produce widespread symptoms and signs.

The dissection can extend distally down the aorta and spiral to involve:

- the renal arteries (renal pain and renal failure);
- the mesenteric arteries (abdominal pain and bowel ischaemia);
- the spinal arteries (paraplegia);
- the iliac arteries (leg pain, pallor, loss of or reduced pulses and acute limb ischaemia).

The dissection may track proximally to involve:

- the head and neck vessels (symptoms and signs of a stroke or transient ischaemic attack);
- the coronary vessels (MI);
- the aortic root (aortic regurgitation).

The dissection may also result in aortic wall rupture into the pericardium (cardiac tamponade) or mediastinum (left haemothorax).

Classification

There are two classifications, both of which are limited in their application but widely used. The DeBakey classification is based on the pattern of dissection, whereas the Stanford classification is based on whether the ascending aorta is involved (***Figure 59.28***).

Investigations

The diagnosis is suspected based on the clinical presentation and careful history taking. Diagnosis is confirmed by CT, which is the standard method for diagnosis. Other imaging modalities such as TOE or MRI can be utilised in cases where the CT is equivocal (***Figure 59.29***).

Management

Initial management of all types of aortic dissection includes blood pressure control (which is usually high at presentation)

Michael Ellis DeBakey, 1908–2008, American cardiac surgeon, Baylor College of Medicine, Houston, TX, USA.

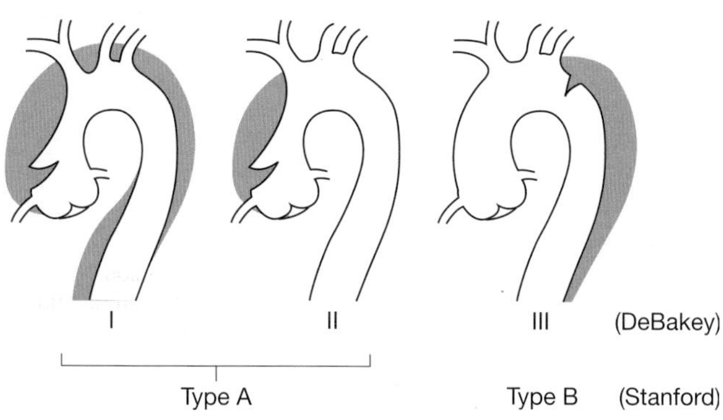

Figure 59.28 Stanford classification of aortic dissections according to whether the ascending aorta is involved (type A) or not (type B). This is simpler than the DeBakey classification (types I, II and III).

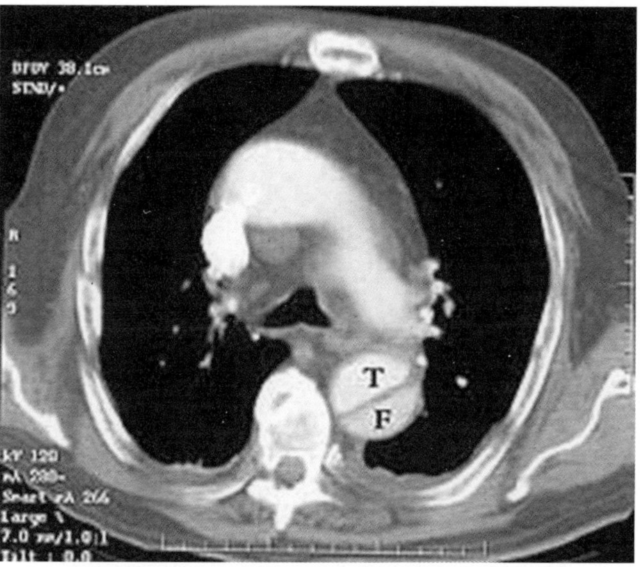

Figure 59.29 Computed tomography scan showing acute dissection of the descending thoracic aorta. F, false lumen; T, true lumen.

and strict pain management, followed by prompt referral for specialist management. The advent of specialist regional centres and regional referral pathways has been shown to improve outcomes in these patients.

Surgical options

Type A (or type I and II) dissections

Those involving the ascending aorta usually require surgical intervention. The chest is opened through a median sternotomy and CPB is commenced, often with core cooling down to 18°C based on the technique used. The aorta is cross-clamped as high up the ascending aorta as possible and opened. Cardioplegic solution is infused into the coronary ostia to arrest the heart in diastole. If the intimal tear is present and localised, the ascending aorta is excised with the tear and replaced with a synthetic graft. The distal anastomosis is performed with circulatory arrest. Recently there have been attempts to carry out endovascular stenting of type A dissections with variable degrees of success. The extent of replacement of the aorta in the setting of acute type I dissection is debatable and is based on the clinical picture and surgical experience.

Type B (or type III) dissections

Initially, these are best managed medically with antihypertensive drugs and monitoring on an acute care unit. Intervention is indicated in complicated cases if the pain increases (signalling impending rupture) or fails to resolve; or when the dissection is associated with evidence of malperfusion (organ, limb or neurological symptoms). The use of percutaneously placed endovascular stents is currently the standard intervention of choice in patients with complicated type B dissection, and surgery is reserved for the rare case that is not suitable for stenting.

Outcomes

If type A dissection is untreated, the mortality rate is 50% within 48 hours and 75% within 1–2 weeks, whereas patients with type B dissections have a better prognosis. Surgical mortality is variable but is around 20–25% for proximal aortic dissection. The overall survival rate for patients leaving hospital, regardless of the type of dissection, is around 80% at 5 years and 40% at 10 years.

PERICARDIAL DISEASES

There is a fibrous envelope covering the heart and separating it from the mediastinal structures. This includes a parietal layer and allows the heart to move with each beat. It can be left wide open after cardiac surgery without any ill effects; however, there are a number of conditions affecting the pericardium that may present to the surgeon.

Pericardial effusion

There is continuous production and resorption of pericardial fluid; if this balance is disturbed, a pericardial effusion may develop. If the pressure exceeds the pressure in the atria, compression will result in reduced venous return and compromised circulation. This state of affairs is called tamponade. A gradual build-up of fluid (e.g. malignant infiltration) may be well tolerated for a long period before tamponade occurs, and the pericardial cavity may contain up to 2 litres of fluid. Acute tamponade (from penetrating trauma, coronary angiography or postoperatively) may occur in minutes with small volumes of blood. The clinical features are low blood pressure with a raised jugular venous pressure and paradoxical pulse. Kussmaul's sign is a characteristic pattern that is seen when the jugular venous pressure rises with inspiration as a result of the impaired venous return to the heart.

Emergency treatment of pericardial tamponade is aspiration of the pericardial space. A wide-bore needle is inserted under local anaesthesia to the left of the xiphisternum, between the angle of the xiphisternum and the ribcage (***Figure 59.30***). The needle is advanced towards the tip of the scapula into the pericardial space. An ECG electrode attached to the needle

Adolf Kussmaul, 1822–1902, Professor of Medicine at, successively, Heidelberg, Erlangen, Freiburg and Strasbourg, Germany.

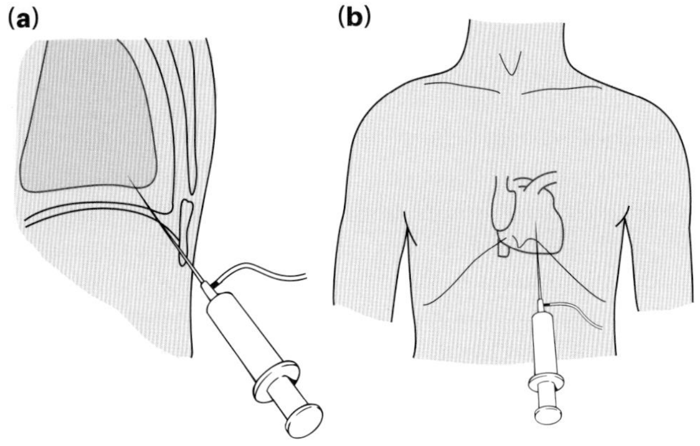

Figure 59.30 (a) Pericardial aspiration through the subxiphoid region. (b) Site of needle insertion for pericardial aspiration.

will indicate when the heart has been touched. This will relieve the situation temporarily until the cause of the tamponade is established. Penetrating wounds of the heart usually require exploration through a median sternotomy. Emergency room thoracotomy is rarely required. Chronic tamponade is usually a result of malignant infiltration of the pericardium (usually secondary carcinoma from breast or bronchus) or, very occasionally, uraemia or connective tissue disease. Treatment sometimes requires a pericardial window between the pericardial space and the pleural or peritoneal space.

Pericarditis

Infection and inflammation may also affect the pericardium. Acute pericarditis usually occurs following a viral illness. Treatment is with non-steroidal anti-inflammatory drugs and bed rest (in case there is an underlying myocarditis). Acute purulent pericarditis is uncommon but requires urgent drainage and intravenous antibiotics, with attention to the underlying cause.

Chronic pericarditis is an uncommon condition in which the pericardium becomes thickened and non-compliant. The heart cannot move freely and the stroke volume is reduced by the constrictive process. The central venous pressure is raised and the liver becomes congested. Peripheral oedema and ascites are also a feature. Treatment is surgical and is aimed at relieving the constriction.

CARDIAC MASSES

Cardiac masses can be either thrombus (blood clots) or tumours. Thrombus can be found in patients with poor left ventricular function or longstanding AF, as well as in patients with proximal pulmonary embolus, in either the ventricles or the left atrium.

Cardiac tumours can be either benign or malignant, which in turn can be secondary (from lung, oesophagus, breast, etc.) or primary.

Atrial myxoma

This is the most common benign cardiac mass in adults. Myxomas are neoplasms of endocardial origin, often appearing as pedunculated masses most commonly seen in the left (75%) or the right (20%) atria. They are rarely found in the ventricles (***Figure 59.31***). Myxomas are associated with a congenital disorder (Carney complex) in 5% of cases. They usually present with symptoms related to blood flow obstruction through heart valves or systemic embolisation. Treatment is by surgical excision and recurrence rates are usually <5%.

Rhabdomyoma

Cardiac tumours in children are incredibly rare (<0.2% of the population), although this is the most common benign cardiac tumour. It usually presents with symptoms related to valve dysfunction or arrhythmias. There are usually multicentric pedunculated masses in either or both ventricles. Rhabdomyoma is associated with tuberous sclerosis in >50% of the cases. Treatment is usually by surgical excision.

Primary malignant cardiac tumours

These are extremely rare and less common than secondary malignancies. They include angiosarcoma, rhabdomyosarcoma and leiomyosarcoma. Patients usually have advanced disease when they are discovered, and they are associated with poor outcomes even with multimodality treatment (surgery and chemoradiation).

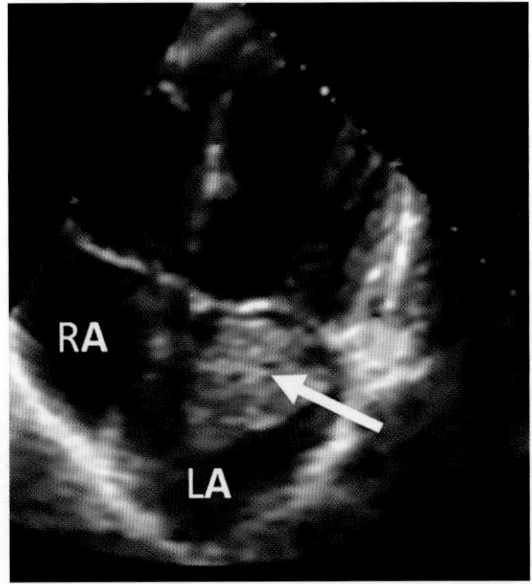

Figure 59.31 Transthoracic echocardiography view of a left atrial (LA) myoma (arrow). RA, right atrium.

J Aidan Carney, b. 1934, County Roscommon, Ireland, pathologist at the Mayo Clinic, described a syndrome of myxomas, spotty pigmentation and endocrine overactivity in 1985.

MANAGEMENT OF CARDIAC ARREST AFTER CARDIAC SURGERY

Introduction

The incidence of cardiac arrest after cardiac surgery is around 0.7–8.0%, with 17–79% survival rates. VF accounts for up to 50% of arrests; tamponade and major bleeding account for most others. Multiple variables may dictate differences in the management of cardiac arrest after cardiac surgery when compared with other situations. Therefore, EACTS published guidelines for resuscitation of cardiac arrest after cardiac surgery, which are summarised below.

Cardiac arrest with 'non-shockable' rhythm

Cardiac surgical patients with a non-VF/ventricular tachycardia (VT) arrest commonly have tamponade, tension pneumothorax or severe hypovolaemia. Prompt treatment is associated with an excellent outcome. Resternotomy should be performed promptly if connecting the pacemaker and atropine fail to resolve the arrest, especially if a prolonged period of CPR is needed, which will be better performed by internal massage.

Emergency resternotomy for ventricular fibrillation or pulseless ventricular tachycardia

A precordial thump may be successful if performed within 10 seconds of the onset of VF or pulseless VT; however, this should not delay cardioversion by defibrillation. In VF or pulseless VT, emergency resternotomy should be performed after three failed attempts at defibrillation.

Emergency resternotomy

After the identification of cardiac arrest, basic life support according to the Advanced Life Support guidelines should be initiated while preparing for emergency resternotomy. Emergency resternotomy may be required in 0.8–2.7% of all patients undergoing cardiac surgery. Emergency resternotomy is a multipractitioner procedure, which should be rapidly performed with a full aseptic technique.

Preparation for emergency resternotomy

- A gown and gloves should be donned in a sterile fashion, but opening should not be delayed in the arrest situation.
- The drape is applied, ensuring that the whole bed is covered (if an all-in-one sterile drape is used then there is no need to prepare the skin with antiseptic).
- The scalpel is used to cut the sternotomy incision, including all sutures, deeply down to the sternal wires.
- All sternal wires are cut with the wire cutters. The sternal edges will separate a little, which may relieve tamponade.
- Suction is used to clear excessive blood or clot.
- The retractor is placed between the sternal edges and the sternum opened.
- If cardiac output is restored expert assistance should then be summoned. If there is no cardiac output, the position of any grafts should be carefully identified and internal cardiac massage and internal defibrillation performed, if required.

Internal cardiac massage

This is a potentially dangerous procedure. Risks include avulsion of a bypass graft, with the LIMA being at particular risk, and right ventricular rupture, especially if it is thin or distended. Therefore, it is important to carefully remove any clot and identify structures at risk such as grafts before placing hands around the heart. There are several methods of internal massage; however, the two-hand technique is the safest.

Two-hand technique

The heart should be inspected to locate the internal mammary and other grafts if present, followed by removal of any blood clots. The right hand is passed over the apex of the heart and then advanced round the apex to the back of the heart, palm up and hand flat. The left hand is then placed flat onto the anterior surface of the heart and the two hands squeezed together at a rate of 100 per minute. Flat palms and straight fingers are important to avoid an unequal distribution of pressure onto the heart, thereby minimising the chance of trauma. If there is a mitral valve replacement or repair, care should be taken not to lift the apex by the right hand, as this can cause a posterior ventricular rupture.

ACKNOWLEDGEMENTS

The author and editors wish to acknowledge the help of Mr Nathan Tyson in the preparation of this chapter.

FURTHER READING

Bojar RM. *Manual of perioperative care in cardiac surgery*, 5th edn. Oxford: Wiley-Blackwell, 2010.

Cohn LH. *Cardiac surgery in the adult*, 5th edn. New York: McGraw Hill Professional, 2017.

Dunning J, Fabbri A, Kolh PH *et al.* Guideline for resuscitation in cardiac arrest after cardiac surgery. *Eur J Cardiothorac Surg* 2009; **36**: 3–28.

Kirklin J, Barratt-Boyes B. *Cardiac surgery*, 4th edn. Philadelphia: Elsevier Saunders, 2013.

Moorjani N, Viola N, Ohri S. *Key questions in cardiac surgery*. Shrewsbury: TFM publishing, 2011.

Nishimura RA, Otto CM, Bonow RO *et al.* AHA/ACC guideline for the management of patients with valvular heart disease. *J Am Coll Cardiol* 2014; **63**(22): e57–e185.

CHAPTER 60 The thorax

Learning objectives

To understand:
- The anatomy and physiology of the thorax
- Investigation of chest pathology
- The role of surgery in pleural disease
- The assessment of patients requiring lung surgery
- Surgical oncology as applied to chest surgery
- Chest wall disorders

INTRODUCTION

Anatomical development of the lungs

The lungs are derived from an outpouching of the primitive foregut during the fourth week of intrauterine life. This bud becomes a two-lobed structure, the ends of which ultimately become the lungs. The lobar arrangement is defined early and is fairly constant but anomalies of fissures and segments leading to anatomical variation in the adult are common.

The primitive lungs drain into the cardinal veins, which ultimately become the pulmonary veins draining into the left atrium. Variability in venous drainage is very common and is usually of little functional significance. At the most severe end of the spectrum is total anomalous drainage, which presents in early infant life because oxygenated blood is all directed back to the right heart.

Anatomy of the lungs

The left lung is divided by the oblique fissure, which lies nearer to the vertical than horizontal, so the upper and lower lobes could also be called anterior and posterior. On the right, the equivalent of the left upper lobe is further divided to give the middle lobe. Each lobe is composed of segments, with anatomically defined and named bronchial, pulmonary arterial and venous connections (***Figure 60.1***).

The right main bronchus (RMB) is shorter, wider and nearly vertical compared with the left main bronchus (LMB). As a consequence, inhaled foreign bodies are more likely to enter the RMB than the left (***Figure 60.2***). The trachea and bronchi have a systemic arterial blood supply delivered by the bronchial arteries, which arise directly from the nearby thoracic aorta.

Lymphatic drainage tends to follow the bronchi. Lymph nodes are both named and identified by numbered 'stations' and more recently into zones, which are of importance in staging of lung cancer (***Figure 60.3***).

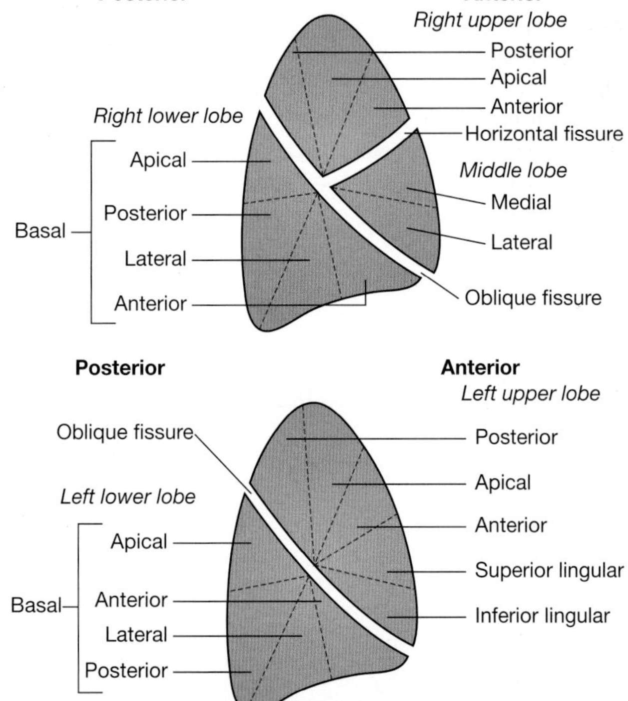

Figure 60.1 The lobar and segmental divisions of the lungs, right lung above and left lung below as if viewed from the side.

Mechanics of breathing

The intercostal muscles contract, causing the ribs to move upwards and outwards, thereby increasing the transverse and anteroposterior dimensions of the chest wall. Along with the diaphragm, which contracts simultaneously and flattens, increasing the vertical dimension of the chest cavity, these muscles are the muscles of respiration. In addition, the accessory muscles of respiration – the neck and spinal muscles such as sternocleidomastoid – may be used particularly during heavy breathing, such as when exercising or during periods of illness

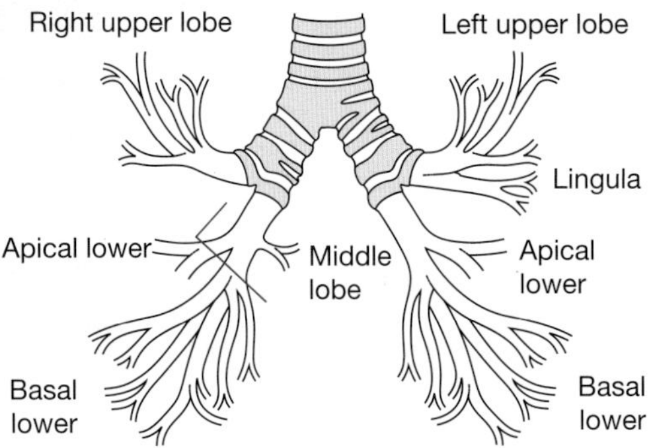

Figure 60.2 Surgical anatomy of the bronchial tree. To surgically remove the right lower lobe and conserve the middle lobe, the surgeon must be prepared to dissect and separately divide the apical bronchial segment (red line).

such as a pneumonia (lung infection). As the volume increases, the intrathoracic pressure falls and air flows in until the alveolar pressure is the same as the atmospheric pressure. The only force used in normal expiration is the elastic recoil of the lung.

Ability to cough comfortably to clear retained secretions is an essential part of recovery from surgery. In a vigorous cough, probably the only muscle in the body that is relaxed is the diaphragm; as the abdomen and chest wall and accessory muscles contract, the limbs are braced and the sphincters are tightened. When the intrathoracic and abdominal pressure is built up, the glottis is opened and the diaphragm is forced up as a piston, or like the plunger of a syringe, to expel air at high velocity.

ASSESSMENT OF FITNESS FOR MAJOR THORACIC SURGERY

The British Thoracic Society (BTS) recommends a tripartite risk assessment model for patients undergoing lung resection, considering the risk of operative mortality, risk of perioperative myocardial events and risk of postoperative dyspnoea (*Figure 60.4*).

Risk of operative mortality

The Thoracic Surgery Scoring System (Thoracoscore) is the most widely used model to assess the risk of operative mortality in thoracic patients. Risk is calculated based on nine variables – age, sex, American Society of Anesthesiologists score, performance status, dyspnoea score, priority of surgery, extent of surgery, malignant diagnosis and composite comorbidity score. It is currently the most robust model available to estimate the risk of death when considering patients for thoracic surgery.

Risk of perioperative myocardial event

History, physical examination and resting electrocardiogram (ECG) form the basics of assessing perioperative cardiovascular risk. Patients who are found to have an active cardiac condition should be evaluated by a cardiologist and optimised (medical, revascularisation or cardiac surgery) before thoracic surgery. Surgery should be avoided within 30 days of myocardial infarction.

Supraclavicular zone
Station 1: low cervical, supraclavicular sternal notch

Upper zone
Station 2: upper paratracheal
Station 3: prevascular/retrotracheal
Station 4: lower paratracheal

Subcarinal zone
Station 7: subcarinal

Hilar/interlobular zone
Station 10: hilar
Station 11: interlobar

Lower zone
Station 8: paraoesophageal
Station 9: pulmonary ligament

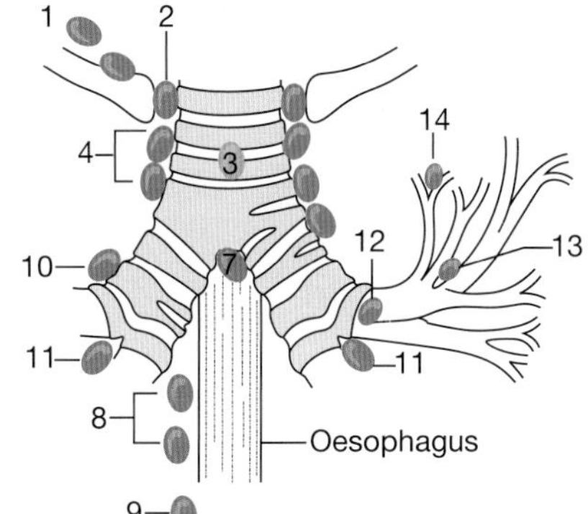

Peripheral zone
Station 12: lobar
Station 13: segmental
Station 14: subsegmental

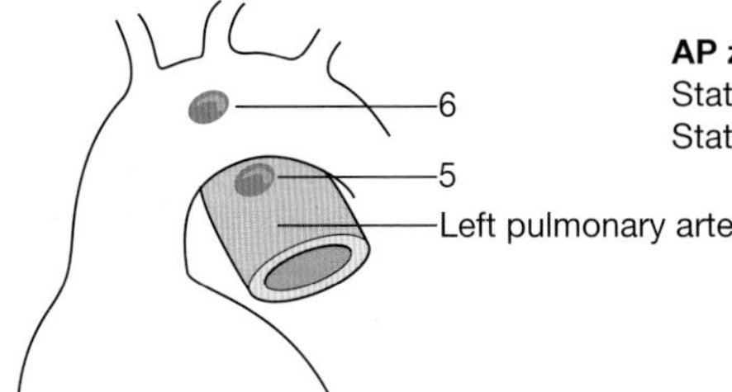

AP zone
Station 5: subaortic
Station 6: para-aortic

Figure 60.3 Lymph node stations related to the bronchial tree are particularly important in the staging of lung cancer, with N1 nodes (10–14) and N2 nodes (2–9) shown. AP, anteroposterior.

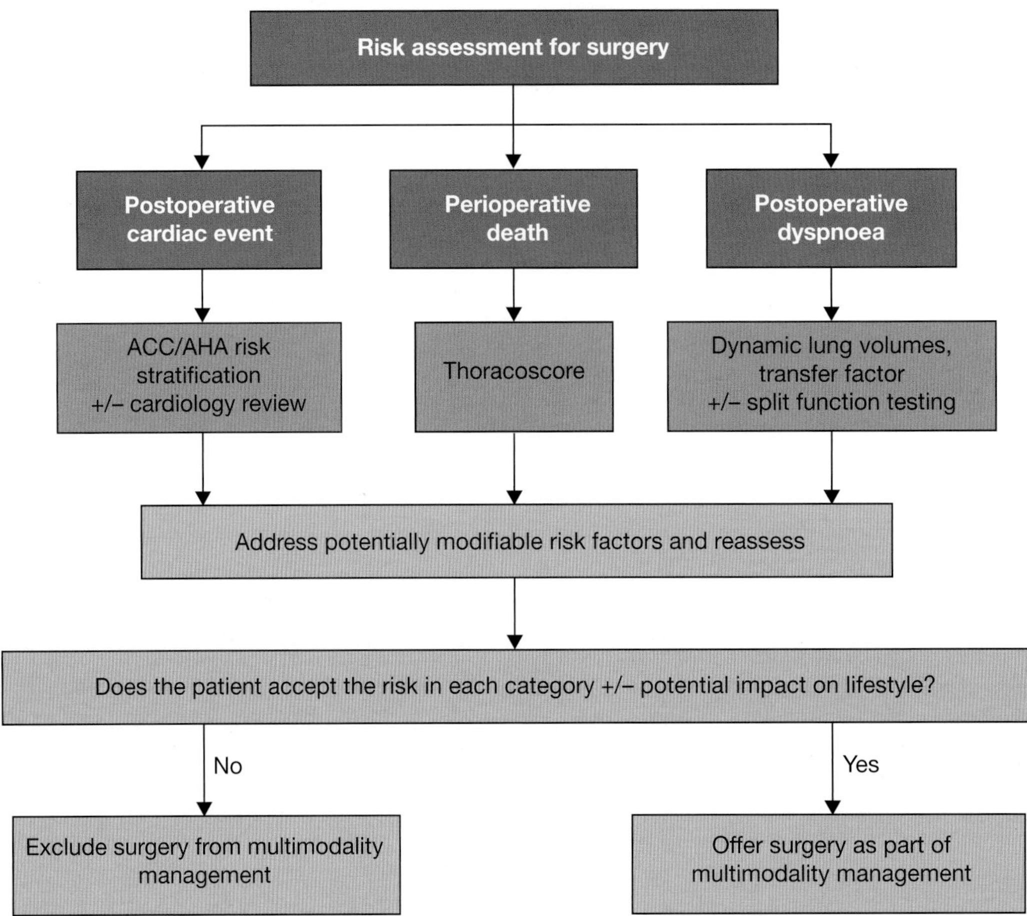

Figure 60.4 Tripartite risk assessment. ACC, American College of Cardiology; AHA, American Heart Association.

Risk of postoperative dyspnoea

Any patient undergoing general anaesthesia requires some assessment of respiratory function. This may be a clinical appraisal of fitness, but more detail is necessary for patients who are undergoing lung resection.

Investigation of the respiratory system

Pulmonary function tests (PFTs) are useful in determining the functional capacity of the patient and the severity of pulmonary disease, and in predicting the response to various treatments. The tests range from simple clinic or bedside measurements to those only available in specialist centres. Spirometry is the most commonly performed PFT and measures specifically the amount (volume) and/or speed (flow rate) of air that can be inhaled or exhaled. It is reported in both absolute values and as a predicted percentage of normal. Normal values vary, depending on gender, race, age and height. The most common parameters measured in spirometry are defined below and illustrated in ***Figure 60.5***.

Peak expiratory flow rate

Peak expiratory flow rate (PEFR) is measured by a Wright peak flow meter or a peak flow gauge. This is the maximum airflow velocity achieved during an expiration delivered with maximal force from the total lung capacity. It is a reliable and reproducible test but has the disadvantage of being effort dependent, and it may therefore be affected by abdominal or thoracic wound pain. PEFR measurements are often used in managing asthma, but there are many other causes of low PEFR such as a problem with large airway patency.

Forced expiratory volume in 1 second

The forced expiratory volume in 1 second (FEV_1) is the amount of air forcibly expired in 1 second. It is low in obstructive lung disease and may be normal in patients with poor gas exchange.

Forced vital capacity

The forced vital capacity (FVC) is the volume of air forcibly displaced following maximal inspiration to maximal expiration. The FEV_1 and the FVC can be measured using a Vitalograph,

Basil Martin Wright, 1912–2001, member of the scientific staff of the Medical Research Council Research Centre, Northwick Park Hospital, Harrow, UK.

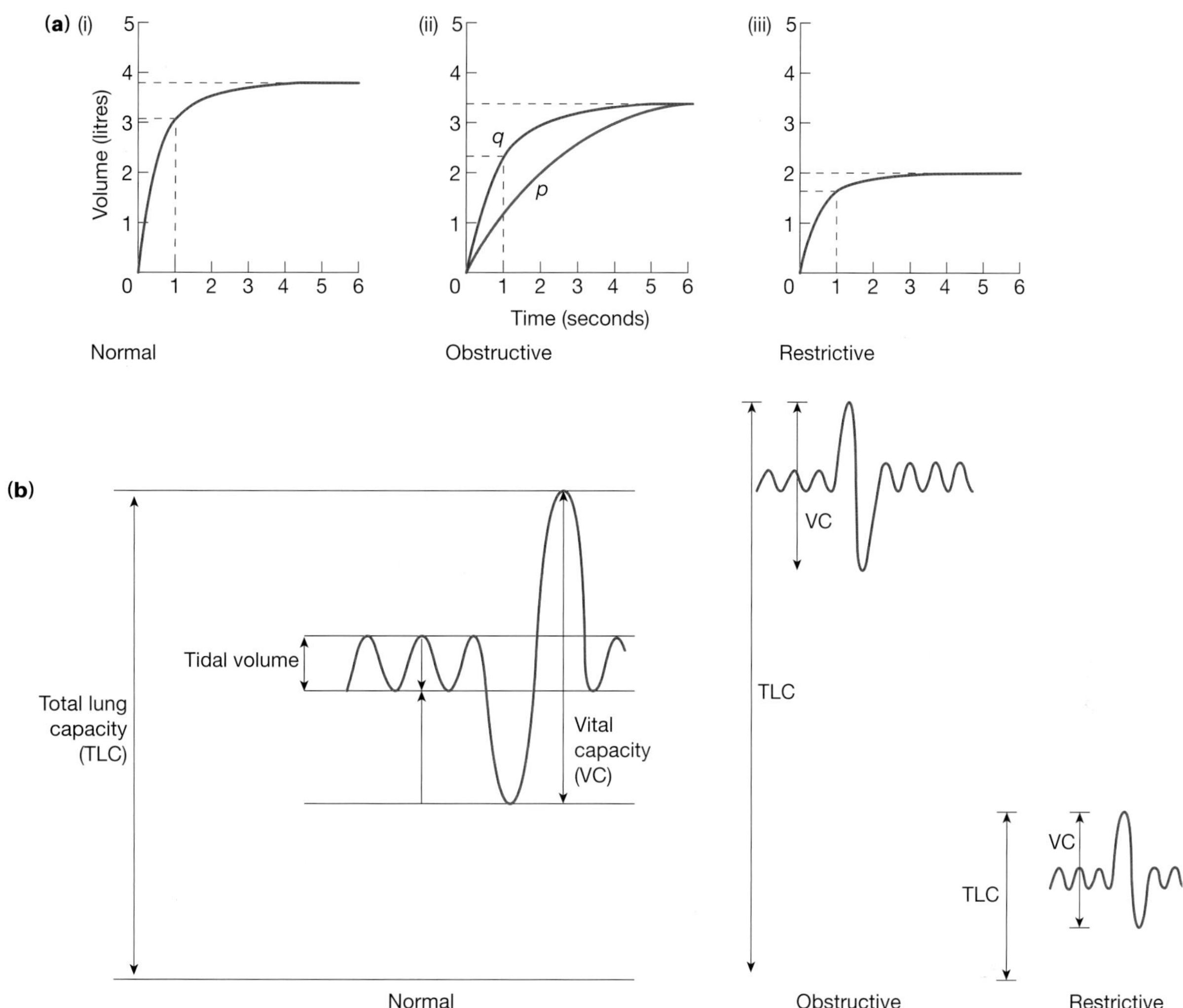

Figure 60.5 Spirometry. (a) Spirogram tracings obtained from a Vitalograph: **(i)** normal forced expiratory volume in 1 s (FEV_1) 3.1 litres, forced vital capacity (FVC) 3.8 litres, FEV_1/FVC 82%; **(ii)** obstructive defect, reversible asthma, *p* before a bronchodilator, FEV_1 1.4 litres, FVC 3.5 litres, FEV_1/FVC 40%; q after a bronchodilator, FEV_1 2.5 litres, FVC 3.5 litres, FEV_1/FVC 71%; **(iii)** restrictive defect, fibrosing alveolitis, FEV_1 1.8 litres, FVC 2.0 litres, FEV_1/FVC 90%. No change with bronchodilators. (b) Changes in lung volume in obstructive and restrictive lung disease. (Reproduced from Gray HH. Pulmonary embolism. *Medicine International* 1993; **21**: 477, by kind permission of the Medicine Group (Journals) Ltd.)

and a ratio (FEV_1/FVC) can be calculated (***Figure 60.5***). A low ratio indicates obstruction and the test should be repeated after bronchodilators. A normal ratio (FVC and FEV_1 reduced to the same extent) indicates a restrictive pathology.

There are two physiological categories of lung disease: obstructive and restrictive (***Table 60.1***). In obstructive conditions such as asthma or emphysema, the flow of air in and out of the lungs is impaired. In restrictive disease, such as lung fibrosis, the lungs have lost size or elasticity, becoming 'stiff' so that they do not fill or expand properly.

TABLE 60.1 Spirometry values in obstructive and restrictive lung diseases.

	Obstructive pattern	Restrictive pattern
PEFR	↓↓	Normal or ↓
FEV_1	↓↓	Normal or ↓
FVC	Normal or ↓	↓↓
FEV_1/FVC	<70	>80

FEV_1, forced expiratory volume in 1 second; FVC, forced vital capacity; PEFR, peak expiratory flow rate.

Diffusion capacity

The diffusion capacity (DLCO) is a measurement of the lung's ability to transfer gases and is often referred to as the 'transfer factor'. It cannot be performed at the bedside, requires the patient's current haemoglobin level and is a test of the integrity of the lung's alveolar–capillary surface area for gas exchange. In lung diseases that damage the alveolar walls, such as emphysema, or that thicken the alveolar membrane, such as lung fibrosis, it may be reduced. In patients who require surgery to remove part of their lung, for example for lung cancer, measurement of DLCO is an important determinant of 'fitness' for surgery and it should be measured formally as part of a lung function test.

Oxygen saturation

Oxygen saturation (S_pO_2) refers to the degree of oxygen molecules (O_2) carried in the blood attached to haemoglobin molecules (Hb). It is a measure of how much oxygen the blood is carrying as a percentage of the maximum it could carry. The common method of monitoring the oxygenation of a patient's haemoglobin is through a pulse oximeter.

Blood gases

The S_pO_2 measured non-invasively with a pulse oximeter measures only oxygenation, not ventilation, and provides no information regarding a patient's carbon dioxide or bicarbonate levels, blood pH or base deficit. This requires arterial blood sampling or 'blood gases' (***Table 60.2***).

TABLE 60.2 Arterial blood gases: 'normal values'.
pH 7.35–7.45
$PaCO_2$ 4.5–6 kPa (35–50 mmHg)
PaO_2 11–14 kPa (83–105 mmHg)
Standard bicarbonate 22–28 mmol/L
Anion gap 10–16 mmol/L
Chloride 98–107 mmol/L

The FEV_1 and DLCO are often used to predict the risk of postoperative dyspnoea after lung resection. The predicted postoperative values can be calculated by considering the volume of lung, more specifically the number of bronchopulmonary segments, expected to be removed at surgery. For example if five segments of the left upper lobe are to be removed, the postoperative predicted FEV_1 in a patient with a preoperative FEV_1 of 2.5 litres (85% predicted) is $((19 - 5)/19) \times 2.5 = 1.84$ litres and $((19 - 5)/19) \times 85\% = 62.6\%$ predicted. This assumes that all bronchopulmonary segments are functioning (e.g. not collapsed) and contribute equally to lung function. Although an optimum cut-off of postoperative predicted FEV_1 of 40% is widely cited, there are currently limited data to provide guidance on this figure to help predict an acceptable degree of postoperative dyspnoea and quality of life. Patients should still be offered surgical resection if the predicted risk of postoperative dyspnoea is moderate or high, as long as they are aware of and accept the risks of dyspnoea and associated complications.

Exercise testing

Other functional assessments, including the shuttle walk test, 6-minute walk test, stair climbing coupled with other tests such as oxygen saturations, as well as cardiopulmonary exercise testing (CPET), could be considered for patients at moderate or high risk of postoperative dyspnoea and may help predict surgical outcome after lung resection. In patients with moderate to high risk of postoperative dyspnoea, using a shuttle walk test distance of >400 m and CPET of >15 mL/kg/min are cut-off values for good function.

The pleura

The key to many aspects of practical chest surgery is an understanding of the pleura and of the mechanics of breathing. Management of the essentially healthy pleural space is logical and simple and needs minimal technology. On the other hand, when pleural disease is advanced, for example when there is gross pleural sepsis surrounding a leaking and trapped lung, management is difficult and the patient may require prolonged care with repeated interventions.

The physiology of pleural fluid

The turnover of fluid in the human pleural space is about 1–2 litres in 24 hours, with only 5–10 mL of fluid present at any one time as a film, about 20 μm thick, between the visceral and parietal pleura.

The mechanisms and equations given are simplifications but serve to explain the clinical conditions encountered. The fluid is produced from the capillaries of the parietal pleura as a transudate, according to the Starling capillary loop pressures. However, there is a further negative force in the pleura. The elastic content of the lung causes it to recoil and collapse if not held open by the negative pressure in the pleura. This elastic recoil exerts about 4 mmHg of negative pressure and favours accumulation of fluid. The secreting forces add up to about 11 mmHg in health. Pleural fluid is mainly reabsorbed (about 90%) by the visceral pleura, whose capillaries are part of the pulmonary circulation. The principal force in absorption of pleural fluid is oncotic pressure (approximately 25 mmHg) minus the difference in mean capillary hydrostatic pressure of the pulmonary capillary (8 mmHg). Thus, the overall absorbing pressure is $25 - 8 = 17$ mmHg, producing a net drying effect $(17 - 11)$ of about 6 mmHg (***Figure 60.6***).

Gas in the pleural space

There is normally no free gas in the pleural space because the same physiological mechanism that absorbs air from a pneumothorax prevents any gas accumulating.

The partial pressures (water as saturated vapour pressure) of the gases in venous/end-capillary blood are:

- PO_2 40 mmHg 5.3 kPa
- PCO_2 46 mmHg 6.1 kPa
- PN_2 573 mmHg 76.4 kPa
- PH_2O 47 mmHg 6.3 kPa

These partial pressures add up to less than atmospheric pressure (760 mmHg). Free gas is therefore absorbed into the blood and lost to the atmosphere through the lungs, with the gases moving in relation to their solubility (carbon dioxide quickest and nitrogen slowest) and relative concentrations in the pleural space and the blood. This does not favour nitrogen, which constitutes about 80% of atmospheric air. Breathing oxygen accelerates nitrogen removal by reducing the content of nitrogen in the blood and increasing the gradient for its absorption. Nitrous oxide anaesthesia is dangerous in the presence of a pneumothorax; nitrous oxide is very soluble and, although not normally present in the pleural space, it will be

Ernest Henry Starling, 1866–1927, Professor of Physiology, University College, London, UK.

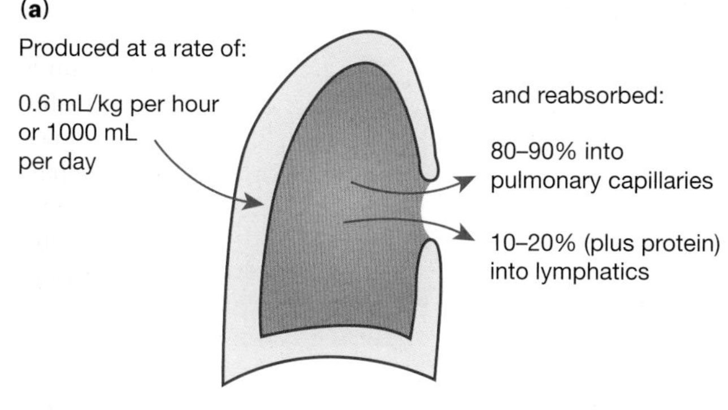

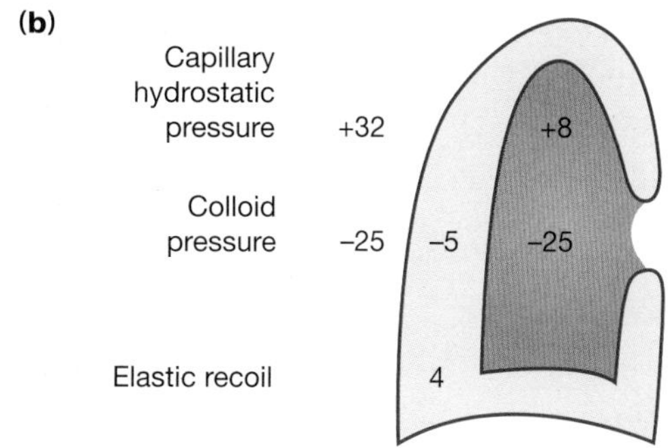

Figure 60.6 (a) Production and absorption of pleural fluid. (b) Normal pleural physiology. (See the text for an explanation of this simplistic physiological model.)

rapidly transported into the space if the patient is given nitrous oxide to breathe.

DISORDERS OF THE PLEURA

Pneumothorax

Pneumothorax is the presence of air outside the lung, within the pleural space. It must be distinguished from bullae or air cysts within the lung. Bullae can be the cause of an air leak from the lung and can therefore coexist with pneumothorax.

Spontaneous pneumothorax occurs when the visceral pleura ruptures without an external traumatic or iatrogenic cause. Cases are divided into primary spontaneous pneumothorax (PSP) and secondary spontaneous pneumothorax (SSP). Pneumothorax can also occur following trauma or iatrogenic injury such as insertion of a central line. Tension pneumothorax is when (independent of aetiology) there is a build-up of positive pressure within the hemithorax, to the extent that the lung is completely collapsed, the diaphragm is flattened, the mediastinum is distorted and, eventually, the venous return to the heart is compromised.

Surgical emphysema is the presence of air in the tissues. It requires a breach of an air-containing viscus in communication with soft tissues, and the generation of positive pressure to push the air along tissue planes. The most serious cause is a ruptured oesophagus. Mediastinal surgical emphysema can also occur with asthma or barotrauma from positive-pressure ventilation. A poorly managed chest drain, with intermittent build-up of pressure, allows air to track into the chest wall through the point where the drain breaches the parietal pleura.

Primary spontaneous pneumothorax

This is a common condition characteristically seen in young people from their mid-teens to late twenties. About 75% of cases are in young men, who tend to be tall and have a family history of the condition. It is due to leaks from small blebs, vesicles or bullae, which may become pedunculated, typically at the apex of the upper lobe or on the upper border of the lower or middle lobes.

Secondary spontaneous pneumothorax

This occurs when the visceral pleura leaks as part of an underlying lung disease; any disease that involves the pleura may cause pneumothorax, including tuberculosis, any cavitating lung disease and necrosing tumours. As such it tends to occur in older patients, often with a history of underlying lung disease such as emphysema. The pneumothorax may be less well tolerated.

The risk of recurrent pneumothorax is increased after the first episode. The best estimates of recurrence rates are:

- of patients who experience a first event, only about one-third experience recurrence;
- of those who have a second episode, about one-half go on to experience a third episode;
- those who have had three episodes will probably go on to have repeated recurrences.

Current recommendations from the BTS are that, in cases of persistent air leak following drain insertion or failure of the lung to re-expand, an early (3–5 days) thoracic surgical opinion should be sought.

Summary box 60.1

Indications for surgical intervention for pneumothorax include:

- Second ipsilateral pneumothorax
- First contralateral pneumothorax
- Bilateral spontaneous pneumothorax
- Pneumothorax fails to settle despite chest drainage
- Spontaneous haemothorax: professions at risk (e.g. pilots, divers)
- Pregnancy

Current recommendations (***Figure 60.7***) focus on the use of small bore (10–14 Fr) chest drains, usually of a Seldinger type, inserted ideally under ultrasound guidance. However, knowledge of the role of the 'surgical' chest drain and how to insert it safely is still required.

Sven Ivar Seldinger, 1921–1998, Swedish radiologist, introduced the Seldinger technique to obtain safe access to blood vessels and other hollow organs.

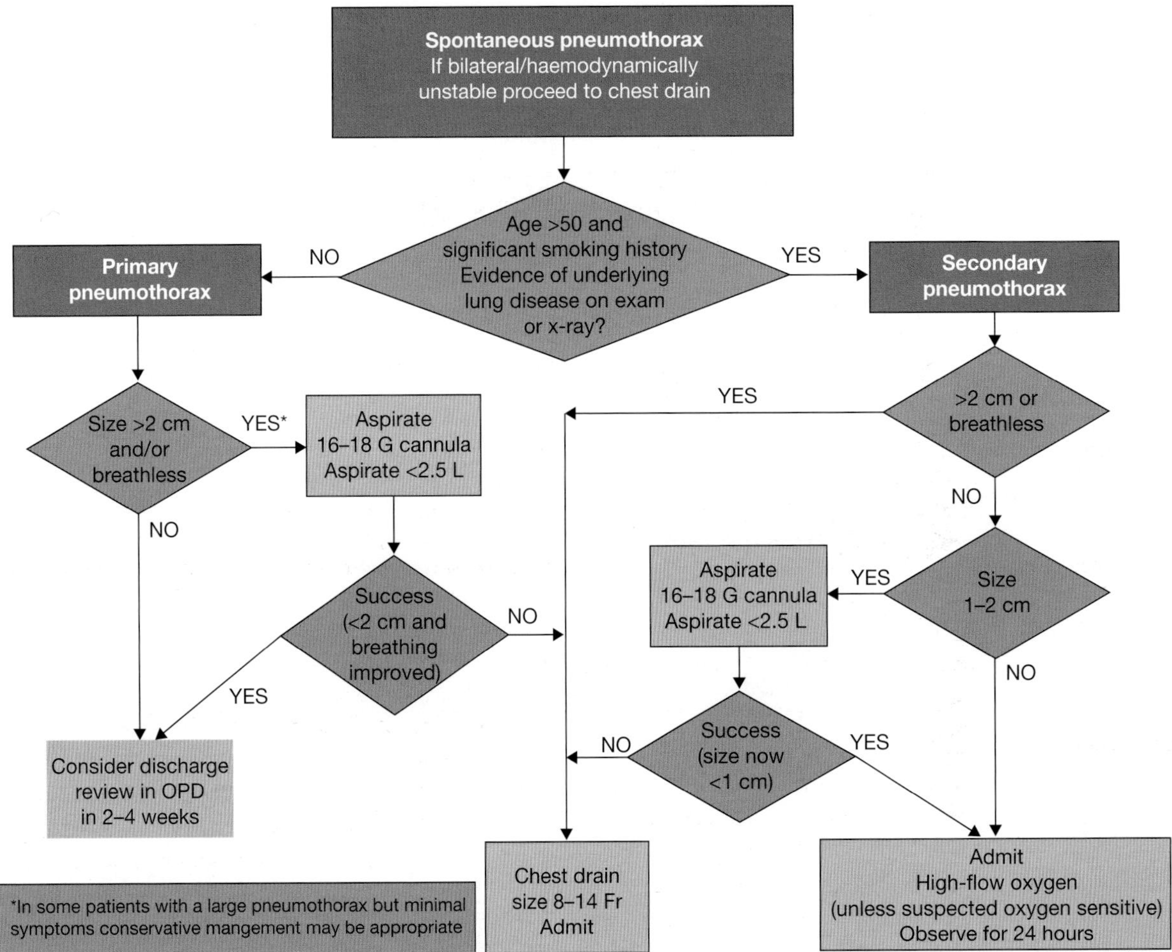

Figure 60.7 British Thoracic Society guidelines on the management of spontaneous pneumothorax (2010) (adapted from www.bts.org.uk). OPD, outpatient department.

Inserting and managing a chest drain

An intercostal tube connected to an underwater seal is central to the management of chest disease; however, the management of the pleura and of chest drains can be troublesome, even in experienced hands.

The safest site for insertion of a drain (***Figure 60.8***) is in the triangle that lies:

- anterior to the mid-axillary line;
- above the level of the nipple;
- below and lateral to the pectoralis major muscle.

This will ideally find the fifth space. The technique includes the following.

- Meticulous attention to sterility throughout.
- Adequate local anaesthesia to include the pleura.
- Sharp dissection to cut only the skin.
- Blunt dissection with artery forceps down through the muscle layers; these should only be the serratus anterior and the intercostals.
- An oblique tract, so that the skin incision and the hole in the parietal pleura do not overlie each other and the drain is in a short tunnel, which reduces the chance of entraining air.
- A drain for pneumothorax and haemothorax should aim towards the apex of the lung. A drain for pleural effusion or empyema should be nearer the base. The drain should pass over the upper edge of the rib to avoid the neurovascular bundle that lies beneath the rib.
- The retaining stitch should be secure but should not obliterate the drain.
- A vertical mattress suture is inserted for later wound closure. This is vital for pneumothorax management but should be omitted if the drain is for empyema (provided there is adherence of the pleura) because that tract should lie open.
- Connect the drain to an underwater seal device which functions as a one-way valve.
- After completion, check that the drain has achieved its objective by taking a chest radiograph.

It is preferable not to apply suction to the drain or clamp it. The danger is that the clamp may be applied for transport and forgotten. Dangers of disconnection and siphoning are small or best averted in other ways apart from clamping.

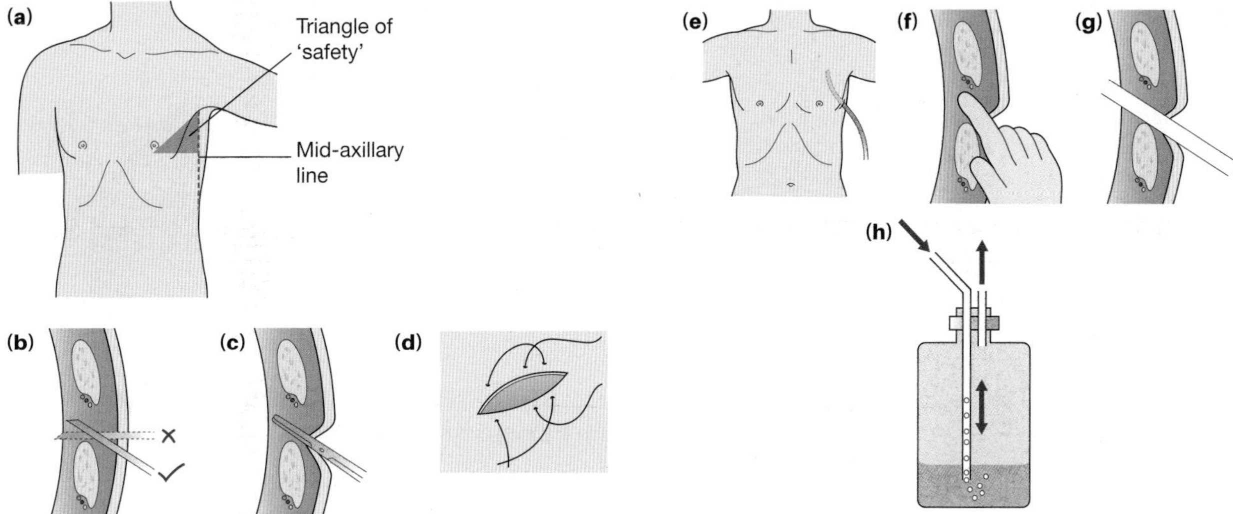

Figure 60.8 Insertion of chest drain: (a) triangle of safety; (b) penetration of the skin, muscle and pleura; (c) blunt dissection of the parietal pleura; (d) suture placement; (e) gauging the distance of insertion; (f) digital examination along the tract into the pleural space; (g) withdrawal of central trochar and positioning of drain; (h) underwater seal chest drain bottle.

A bubbling drain should (almost) never be clamped. Remove the drain when it no longer has a function.

Summary box 60.2

Suction on a pleural tube

- Be aware! Inserting the drain, and not the suction, is the life-saving manoeuvre
- If the lung is reluctant to expand, the suction deviates the mediastinum
- If the lung is fragile, it may worsen an air leak

Surgical management of pneumothorax

Pleurectomy and pleurodesis

Surgery for pneumothorax can be performed by video-assisted thoracoscopic surgery (VATS) or as an open procedure (thoracotomy). The object of the exercise is threefold:

- to deal with any leaks from the lung;
- to search for and obliterate any blebs and bullae;
- to make the visceral pleura adherent to the parietal pleura so that any subsequent leaks are contained and the lung cannot completely collapse.

Pleural adhesion is achieved in one of three ways:

1. **pleurectomy**: systematically stripping the parietal pleura from the chest wall;
2. **pleural abrasion**: a scourer is used to scrape off the slick surface of the parietal pleura;
3. **chemical pleurodesis**: usually talc is used and is insufflated into the chest cavity.

Pleural effusion

Pleural effusion can be readily understood with reference to the physiological mechanisms governing the flux of pleural fluid given above. Pleural effusions are divided into exudates and transudates, depending on protein content (more [exudates] or less [transudates] than 30 g/L), and characterised further according to glucose content, pH and lactate dehydrogenase content. The following are the most common ways in which the pleural fluid balance is disturbed.

Malignant pleural effusion

Pleural effusion is a common complication of cancer. This may be due to:

- lung cancer;
- pleural involvement with primary or secondary malignancy;
- mediastinal lymphatic involvement.

Lung cancer

There may be direct involvement of the parietal and/or visceral pleura, collapse of the lung parenchyma and spread to the mediastinal lymphatics, or a combination of these, causing pleural fluid accumulation. It is usually regarded as a feature that puts lung cancer beyond surgical cure.

Pleural malignancy

The only primary malignancy of the pleura seen with any regularity is malignant mesothelioma. This is a consequence of asbestos exposure, with few exceptions. The peak of asbestos importation into the UK was from 1960 to 1975, with the incidence initially rising but more recently stabilising (2015–2017), with a fall in incidence projected in the future. Mesothelioma commonly presents with breathlessness because of pleural effusions, pain and systemic features of malignancy. Diffuse seeding of the parietal and visceral pleura is a common pattern of dissemination of cancers, particularly adenocarcinoma of any origin.

Mediastinal lymphatic involvement

In many instances, particularly in breast cancer, there is no evident disease in the pleura. The disease is in the mediastinal lymphatics, which are obstructed, and this upsets the balance of physiological forces that control pleural fluid.

Surgery for patients with malignant pleural effusion

The surgeon has two roles: to make the diagnosis and to achieve effective palliation by draining the fluid and pleurodesis.

Diagnosis

Pleural biopsy can be obtained by a range of techniques, with VATS being the most common. An unequivocally positive biopsy is useful, but a negative biopsy may be a sampling error.

Summary box 60.3

Biopsy of the pleura

- Cytological examination of the pleural fluid (low yield)
- Abrams' needle (low yield in malignancy)
- Computed tomography (CT)-guided needle biopsy of a suspicious area
- VATS biopsy
- Open surgical biopsy

Pleural infection and empyema

Empyema is the end stage of pleural infection from any cause. It most commonly results from infection of the underlying lung, involving pneumonia or a lung abscess, but can occur as a complication of any thoracic operation. It is seen if a traumatic haemothorax becomes infected or in the course of management of pneumothorax or pleural effusions. It may be associated with pus under the diaphragm (***Table 60.3***). The pathological diagnosis requires the presence of thick pus with a thick cortex of fibrin and coagulum over the lung.

When empyema presents *de novo* it usually follows pneumonia, and three phases are described:

1 In the exudative phase, there is a protein-rich (>30 g/L) effusion. If this becomes infected with the organisms from the lung (typically *Streptococcus milleri* and *Haemophilus influenzae* in children), the scene is set for empyema. At this stage antibiotics may be all that is required. Aspiration or drainage to dryness in addition is preferred.
2 Over subsequent days, the fluid thickens to what is known as the fibrinopurulent phase. Drainage at this stage is prudent as antibiotics on their own are unlikely to be curative.
3 The organising phase causes the lung to be trapped by a thick peel or 'cortex' for which surgical management may be required.

TABLE 60.3 Conditions that predispose to empyema formation.

Pulmonary infection	Unresolved pneumonia, bronchiectasis, tuberculosis, fungal infections, lung abscess
Aspiration of pleural effusion	Any aetiology
Trauma	Penetrating injury, surgery, oesophageal perforation
Extrapulmonary sources	Subphrenic abscess
Bone infections	Osteomyelitis of ribs or vertebrae

Surgical management of pleural effusions and infections

Thoracoscopy or video-assisted thoracoscopic surgery (VATS)

The direct-vision thoracoscope has been used for many years, but its use was limited mainly to performing biopsies. Since the advent of video-assisted thoracoscopy (***Figure 60.9***) the surgeon's hands are now free because the camera is attached to the thoracoscope, which can be operated by an assistant with the image displayed on a screen. The surgeon is able to manipulate instruments with both hands to perform a variety of procedures. The number of ports required depends on the type and complexity of the surgery. The patient is usually positioned with the diseased side uppermost, having had a double-lumen endotracheobronchial tube (ETT) placed by the anaesthetist to allow for single-lung ventilation. The principal

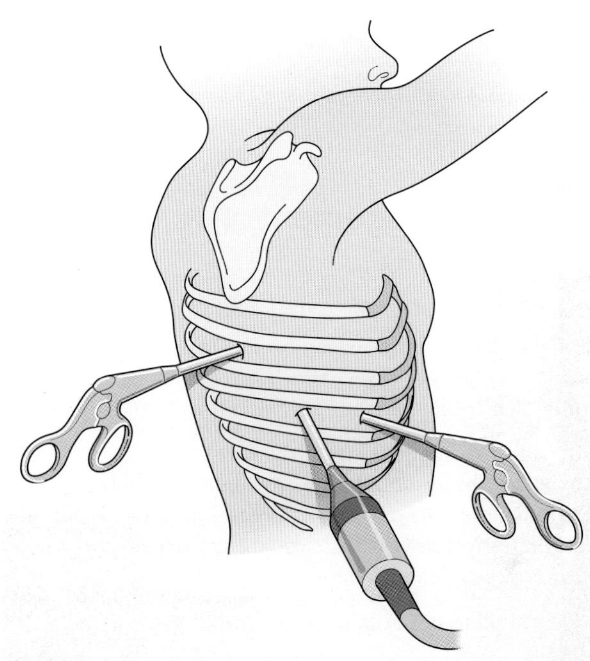

Figure 60.9 Video-assisted thoracoscopic surgery (VATS) utilises modern thoracoscopic instruments and digital technology and avoids large incisions.

Leon David Abrams, 1923–2012, cardiothoracic surgeon, the United Birmingham Hospitals, Birmingham, UK.

advantage is that a large incision is avoided, resulting in less postoperative pain and a more rapid recovery.

VATS drainage, pleural biopsy and talc pleurodesis

VATS drainage, pleural biopsy and talc pleurodesis is increasingly performed for the management of patients with an undiagnosed or malignant pleural effusion. It can be performed using a single port and allows direct visualisation of the pleural cavity for complete drainage, multiple pleural biopsies and excellent talc insufflation to achieve pleurodesis.

VATS debridement of empyema

Pleural infection, particularly early in its evolution, requires drainage, but once the fluid component becomes fibrinopurulent and loculated it requires surgical debridement, which can often be achieved through a VATS approach. The lung is isolated through the use of a double-lumen tube, the patient is positioned disease side up and the pleural cavity is entered. The fluid and debris are vigorously debrided, freeing the lung and allowing for re-expansion. At the end of the case, carefully positioned chest drains are placed to allow for dependent drainage.

Following the procedure, the patient requires good analgesic control, typically using patient-controlled analgesia (PCA), and physiotherapy to help fully re-expand the lung prior to final removal of chest drains.

Decortication

If the lung fails to re-expand after drainage of the empyema, the more radical operation of decortication may be required (*Figure 60.10*). The fibrous cortex or peel from the entrapped underlying lung is removed so that the lung can expand to obliterate the pleural space. This is usually performed through a posterolateral thoracotomy, though in selected cases it can be performed as a VATS procedure. It requires careful dissection to remove the parietal and visceral cortex, taking care not to damage the visceral pleura, so allowing the lung to re-expand fully.

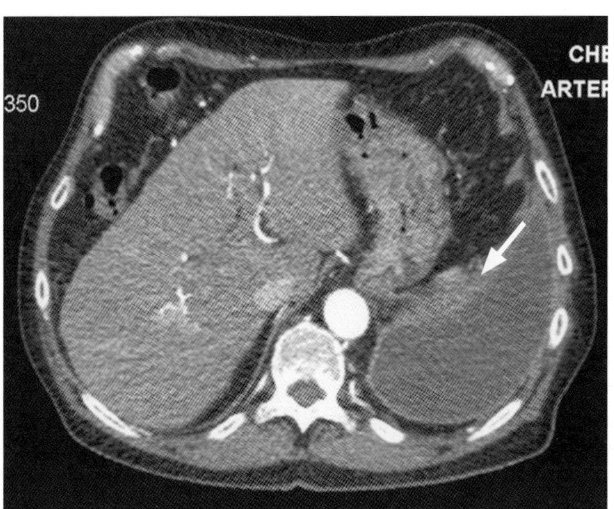

Figure 60.10 Chest computed tomography scan showing an empyema with a grossly thickened pleura (arrow).

DISORDERS OF THE AIRWAY

Haemoptysis

Diseases causing repeated haemoptysis include carcinoma, bronchiectasis, carcinoid tumours and some infections. Severe mitral stenosis is now a rare cause. Patients with repeated haemoptysis should be investigated, at the very least by chest radiography and bronchoscopy. Haemoptysis following trauma may be from a lung contusion or injury to a major airway. Treatment depends on the underlying cause.

Common associated chest symptoms include cough with or without sputum, pain, breathlessness, hoarseness and more general symptoms of systemic upset, including fatigue and loss of weight. Occasionally, chest disease may cause palpitations owing to atrial fibrillation. Any of these symptoms in association with haemoptysis requires urgent investigation.

Investigation

Bronchoscopy

Flexible bronchoscopy (*Table 60.4*) may be performed with the patient awake and the oropharynx anaesthetised with topical lignocaine (*Figure 60.11*). The bronchoscope is passed into the nose or mouth and through the vocal folds under direct vision. As the scope is flexible, its tip can be directed into the segmental bronchi with ease. Tissue and sputum samples may be obtained for diagnostic purposes. There is a greater range of movement with this instrument, but the biopsies are relatively small and suction limited.

TABLE 60.4 Uses of bronchoscopy.

Diagnostic	Confirmation of disease: carcinoma of the bronchus; inflammatory or infective processes
Investigative	Tissue biopsy
Preoperative assessment	Before lung resection Before oesophageal resection Persistent haemoptysis
Therapeutic	Removal of secretions Removal of foreign bodies Stent placement, endobronchial resection, etc.

Rigid bronchoscopy requires general anaesthesia in most instances. It is ideal for therapeutic manoeuvres, such as removal of foreign bodies, aspiration of blood and thick secretions, and intraluminal surgery (laser resection or stent placement). The surgeon and the anaesthetist share control of the airway. The bronchoscope is passed under direct vision into the oropharynx, behind the epiglottis, until the vocal folds are seen and introduced into the trachea.

The tracheal rings and the carina should be easily seen. Advancing the bronchoscope into the RMB or LMB reveals the orifices of the more peripheral bronchi. Operability of an endobronchial tumour may be assessed in terms of its location (e.g. the proximity of a lesion to the carina). Complications are rare but include bleeding, pneumothorax, laryngospasm and arrhythmia.

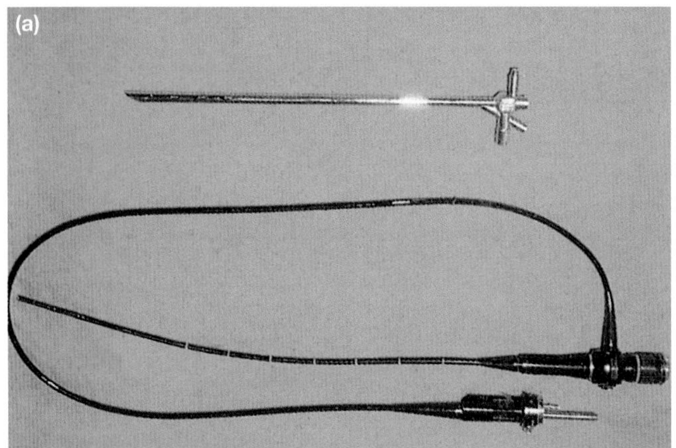

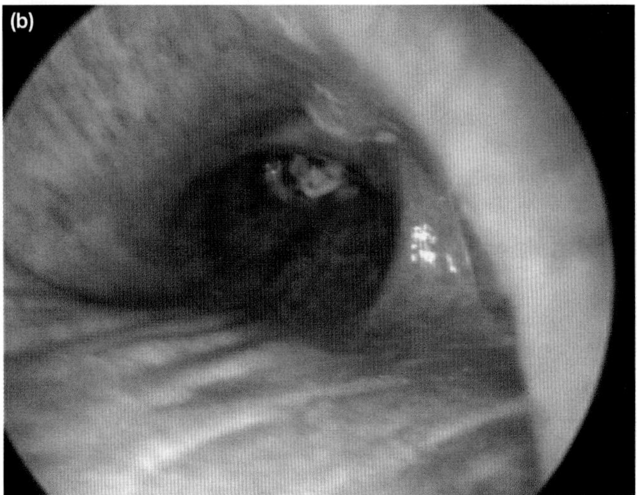

Figure 60.11 (a) Rigid and flexible bronchoscopes. (b) View past the carina into the left main bronchus with a tumour seen in the bronchial lumen.

Rigid bronchoscopy can be combined with endobronchial interventions to tackle airway tumours; these techniques include use of laser or cryotherapy, with heat or cold respectively, to excise potentially obstructing endobronchial tumours and improve airway patency and breathing.

Other techniques of biopsy of intrathoracic lesions are often necessary to confirm diagnosis, stage disease and plan treatment. The options range from percutaneous needle biopsy under radiological control (typically CT scan) to open (VATS) lung biopsy.

Endobronchial ultrasound (EBUS) and navigational bronchoscopy are alternative airway techniques used to obtain intrathoracic biopsies.

Summary box 60.4

Biopsy hazards

- Bleeding disorders
- Systemic anticoagulation
- Pulmonary hypertension

Airway obstruction

Tracheal obstruction may present acutely as a life-threatening emergency or insidiously with little in the way of symptoms until critical narrowing and stridor occur. The more common causes of airway narrowing are outlined in ***Table 60.5***.

Treatment depends on the underlying cause. Tracheostomy may be required to overcome the obstruction, but there are few indications to do this as an emergency. Tracheal replacement resection of up to 6 cm of trachea is possible. Sleeve resections of the major bronchi are also possible.

TABLE 60.5 Causes of airway narrowing.

Intraluminal	Inhaled foreign body Neoplasm
Intramural	Congenital stenosis Fibrous stricture (post intubation or tuberculosis)
Extramural	Neoplasm (thyroid cancer, secondary deposits) Aortic arch aneurysm

Inhaled foreign bodies

This is a fairly common occurrence in small children and is often marked by a choking incident that then apparently passes. Surprisingly large objects can be inhaled and become lodged in the wider calibre and more vertically placed RMB. There are three possible presentations:

1. asymptomatic;
2. wheezing (from airway narrowing) with a persistent cough and signs of obstructive emphysema;
3. pyrexia with a productive cough from pulmonary suppuration.

Either flexible or more often rigid bronchoscopy is required to remove the foreign body.

NEOPLASMS OF THE LUNG

Primary lung cancer

Lung cancer is one of the most common cancers throughout the world. In the UK, there are approximately 45 000 new cases a year. From the time of diagnosis, 60% of patients are dead within 1 year and only 15% survive 5 years, making lung cancer the most common cause of cancer death. Survival is dependent on the stage that the patient presents with lung cancer.

The number of lung cancer operations performed in the UK has significantly increased over the last 10 years. The proportion of lung cancers in which resection is attempted varies but, in most resource-rich countries, is over 30%. Most patients offered lung cancer surgery are in the early stages. The thoracic surgeon working in a cancer team has a role in diagnosis, staging and palliation, in addition to curative resection in appropriate cases. Cigarette smoking is undoubtedly the major risk factor for developing bronchial carcinoma and accounts for 85–95% of all cases. To a lesser extent, atmospheric pollution and certain occupations (mining of radioactive ore and chromium) contribute.

Pathological types

For practical purposes, lung cancers are divided into small cell lung cancer and non-small cell lung cancer (NSCLC), which are seen in a ratio of about 1:4.

- The pattern of disease, the prognosis and the results of treatment for small cell (also known as oat cell) carcinoma differ from all other types sufficiently for these to be managed differently from the outset on the basis of the histological classification.
- Subdivisions of NSCLC according to histological characteristics are much less important, but pathological staging is critical to treatment and outcome.

Histological classification of lung cancer

Small cell lung cancers were known as oat cell cancers because of the packed nature of small dense cells. They are a type of neuroendocrine tumour (NET) and represent about 20% of all lung cancers. They tend to metastasise early to lymph nodes and by blood-borne spread. The median survival is measured in months. The tumours are very responsive to chemotherapy such that median survival may be doubled (although it is still short) but they are rarely, if ever, cured. Surgery is rarely offered unless in very limited stage disease.

Non-small cell lung cancers: adenocarcinoma is now the most common of the NSCLC types, having overtaken squamous cancer. The increasing incidence is partly due to an increasing incidence in women and may be the result, in part, of a move towards lower tar cigarettes that are inhaled more deeply to get the same effect. Squamous carcinoma typically appears as a cavitating tumour.

Large cell undifferentiated is a discrete histological type of NSCLC and is included within NETs. NETs of the lung are a group of lung cancers that include small cell cancer and large cell undifferentiated lung cancer, but also include other less aggressive tumour types, including typical carcinoid and atypical carcinoid tumours. These occur in the major (central) bronchi and 20% are found peripherally. They are characteristically slow growing and highly vascular. Most behave in a benign way; however, approximately 15% metastasise. The patient often presents with a history of recurrent pneumonia or haemoptysis, but carcinoid syndrome is rare unless there are extensive pulmonary or hepatic metastases. Surgical excision is preferred because the prognosis following complete resection is excellent (>90% 10-year survival).

Accurate diagnosis and staging of the tumour are vital if surgery is to be considered.

Clinical features

Clinical features of lung carcinoma depend on:

- the site of the lesion;
- the invasion of neighbouring structures;
- the extent of metastases.

Common symptoms include a persistent cough, weight loss, dyspnoea and non-specific chest pain.

- Haemoptysis occurs in fewer than 50% of patients presenting for the first time.
- Cough, or a changed cough, is a common presentation but non-specific in this population.
- Severe localised pain suggests chest wall invasion with the infiltration of an intercostal nerve. Invasion of the apical area may involve the brachial plexus, leading to Pancoast's syndrome.
- Dyspnoea or breathlessness may come from loss of functioning lung tissue, lymphatic invasion or the development of a large pleural effusion.
- Pleural fluid is an ominous feature and the presence of blood in a pleural effusion suggests that the pleura has been directly invaded.
- Clubbing and hypertrophic pulmonary osteoarthropathy occasionally accompany some lung cancers and may resolve with excision of the primary lesion.
- Invasion of the mediastinum may result in hoarseness (because of recurrent laryngeal nerve involvement), dysphagia (because of the involvement of, or extrinsic pressure on, the oesophagus) and superior vena caval obstruction.
- Small cell carcinoma is associated with the development of myopathies, including the Eaton–Lambert syndrome, which is similar to myasthenia gravis.

Treatment of lung cancer

Careful investigation is required to determine which tumours are operable and will benefit from a major thoracic resection. The internationally agreed tumour–node–metastasis (TNM) staging system gives prognostic information on the natural history of the disease. Tumours graded up to T3, N1, M0 can be encompassed within an anatomical surgical resection and have a much improved prognosis when treated surgically so the tumour must be staged accurately before resection. Increasingly, for higher stage tumours a multi- or trimodality approach is being offered where patients have chemotherapy, with or followed by radiotherapy followed by surgery. A number of non-tumour-related factors, including the general fitness of the patient and the results of lung function tests, help to determine the appropriate treatment. In patients with incurable disease, treatment is palliative to maximise quality of life.

Survival

Carcinoma of the bronchus generally has a low survival rate after diagnosis. Important factors in determining prognosis are the size of the tumour (T status), the spread or stage of the cancer as determined by the TNM classification, the histological type of the tumour and the general condition of the patient. Early detection and surgical resection offer the best hope for cure.

Henry Khunrath Pancoast, 1875–1939, Professor of Radiology, University of Pennsylvania, Philadelphia, PA, USA, described this condition in 1932.
Lee M Eaton, 1905–1958, neurologist who was a professor at the Mayo Clinic, Rochester, MN, USA.
Edward H Lambert, 1915–2003, Professor of Physiology, University of Minnesota, MN, USA. Eaton and Lambert described this condition in a joint paper in 1956.

Diagnosis and staging

Increasing emphasis in recent years has been on the early detection of lung cancer, with guidance on symptoms and signs of potential lung cancer that require urgent chest radiograph and referral to a lung cancer team.

Non-invasive investigations

Chest radiography

A chest radiograph will detect most lung cancers but some, particularly early curable tumours, are hidden by other structures. Secondary effects such as pleural effusion, distal collapse and raised hemidiaphragm may be evident (***Figure 60.12***).

Computed tomography

CT is the first investigation in suspected lung cancer. The surgeon needs to know whether the primary is resectable (T stage) and which, if any, lymph nodes are involved (N stage). Lymph nodes more than 2 cm in diameter are likely to be involved in the disease (70%) (***Figure 60.13***) and those less than 10 mm in the shorter axis are unlikely to be involved. Remote metastases to the liver, adrenal glands or elsewhere may be detected.

Positron emission tomography

The patient is given radiolabelled fluorodeoxyglucose (FDG), which is taken up by all metabolising cells but more avidly by cancer cells. The FDG enters the Krebs cycle but cannot complete it and accumulates in proportion to the glucose avidity of the cells. High accumulation is associated with lung cancers and secondaries. Infection or other inflammation, and lymphadenopathy secondary to it, are also FDG avid.

Sputum cytology

Sputum cytology may reveal malignant cells but the false-negative rate is high.

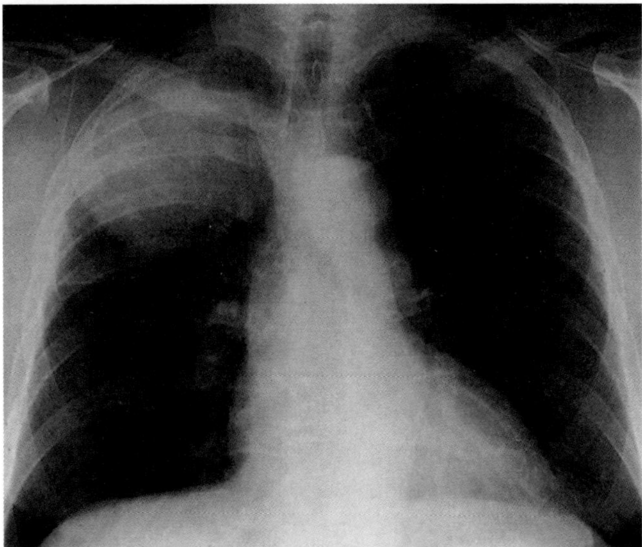

Figure 60.12 Chest radiograph of carcinoma of the lung. This patient has a large mass in the right upper lobe, causing Horner's syndrome, a Pancoast tumour.

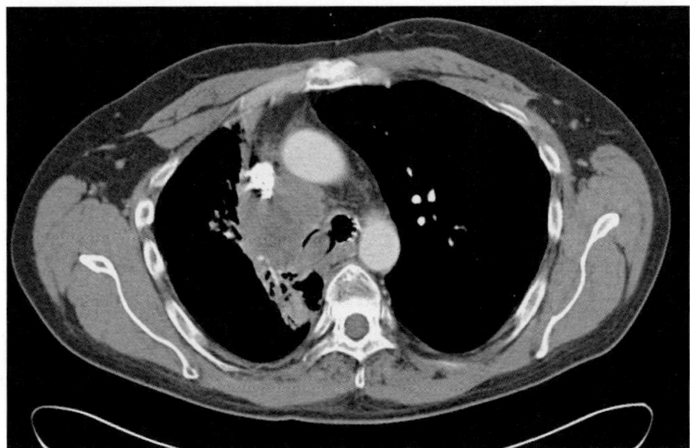

Figure 60.13 Paratracheal lymphadenopathy shown on a computed tomography scan.

Invasive investigations

Once lung cancer is suspected, diagnosis and further staging are sought. The choice of investigation depends on the position of the primary tumour in the lung (peripheral or central) and the clinical stage of the cancer (presence of enlarged lymph nodes or metastasis).

Bronchoscopy

Flexible bronchoscopy is usually performed under sedation, particularly in patients with more centrally placed lung cancers. It allows assessment of the segmental airway, cytological testing through brushing and washing of the concerned segmental bronchi and transbronchial needle aspiration (TBNA).

Endobronchial ultrasound

EBUS allows bronchoscopic assessment of suspicious mediastinal lymph nodes with an ultrasound probe incorporated into the tip of the bronchoscope to aid TBNA (***Figure 60.14***).

Endoscopic ultrasound (EUS) is a similar technique that, by passing the probe down the oesophagus, allows fine-needle aspiration (FNA) of less approachable mediastinal lymph nodes.

Navigational bronchoscopy

Navigational bronchoscopy provides a virtual three-dimensional map of the lung using radiological guidance during a flexible bronchoscopy, which can guide the physician to target, locate and perform an anatomically precise lung biopsy, place markers for radiation therapy and/or facilitate surgical removal of a small peripheral lung lesion or use thermal ablative techniques for peripheral lung lesions.

Johann Friedrich Horner, 1831–1886, Professor of Ophthalmology, Zurich, Switzerland, described this syndrome in 1869.
Sir Hans Adolf Krebs, 1900–1981, Professor of Biochemistry, University of Oxford, Oxford, UK.

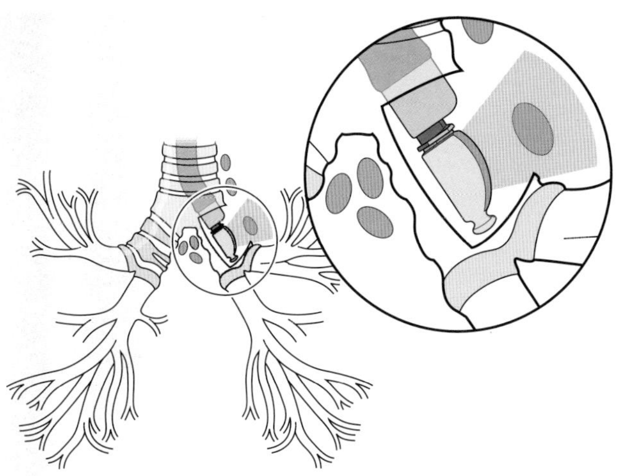

Figure 60.14 Endobronchial ultrasound allows accurate detection of enlarged mediastinal lymph nodes for diagnosis and staging of lung cancer.

Computed tomography-guided biopsy

Percutaneous CT-guided FNA may give a good yield of cells for cytological examination. Alternatively, a core of tissue can be obtained for formal histology. These techniques are best for larger and more peripheral lesions. Pneumothorax is common (10%) but rarely requires intercostal tube drainage. The contraindications include poor respiratory reserve, when even a small pneumothorax would be hazardous.

Surgical diagnosis and staging

Mediastinoscopy, mediastinotomy, VATS or thoracotomy lymph node/lung biopsy are aimed at establishing a tissue diagnosis and assessing the degree of spread (staging), which determines resectability. Histological proof of the status of mediastinal nodes may be important to avoid unnecessary thoracotomy for incurable cancers and, conversely, to avoid denying surgery to patients whose lymph nodes are enlarged but benign.

Mediastinoscopy

Following an incision in the neck and careful blunt dissection in front of the trachea, access to the paratracheal and subcarinal nodes via mediastinoscopy is achieved and biopsies taken (*Figure 60.15*).

These techniques may also be used in the diagnosis of other mediastinal conditions, including:

- lymphoma;
- anterior mediastinal tumours;
- thymoma;
- sarcoid, tuberculosis or any other cause of lymphadenopathy.

VATS mediastinal lymph node and lung biopsy

For inaccessible mediastinal lymph nodes, or when diagnosis of the lung tumour has not been possible through radiological or bronchoscopic techniques, VATS allows diagnosis of the tumour and staging of the mediastinum and gives the opportunity to assess the likely operability of the lung cancer.

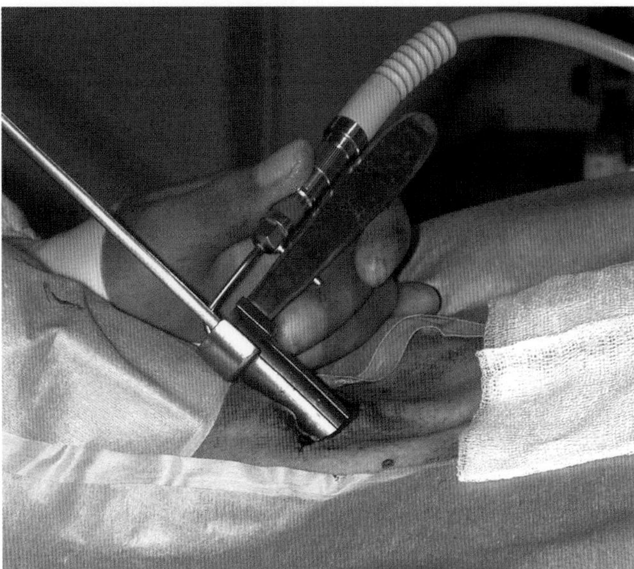

Figure 60.15 Mediastinoscopy. The mediastinoscope slides down immediately in front of the trachea, behind the aortic arch, and behind and between the great vessels of the head and neck.

Surgical approach to lung cancer resection

Thoracotomy

Although the most frequent indication for thoracotomy is lung cancer, all surgeons dealing with trauma should be able to perform a thoracotomy if required. The standard route into the thoracic cavity is through a posterolateral thoracotomy. The incision is used for access to the:

- lung and major bronchi;
- pleura;
- thoracic aorta;
- oesophagus;
- posterior mediastinum.

A double-lumen endotracheal tube is used to allow ventilation of one lung while the other is collapsed, to facilitate surgery and to protect the non-operated lung and retain control of ventilation (*Figure 60.16*). The patient is turned to the

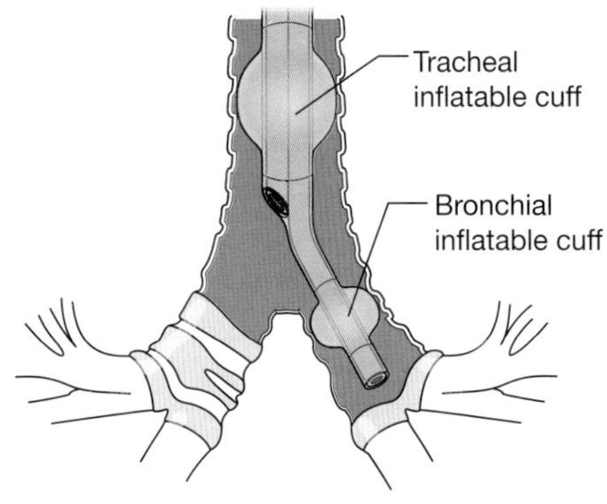

Figure 60.16 The double-lumen tube permits separate ventilation of the right and left lungs.

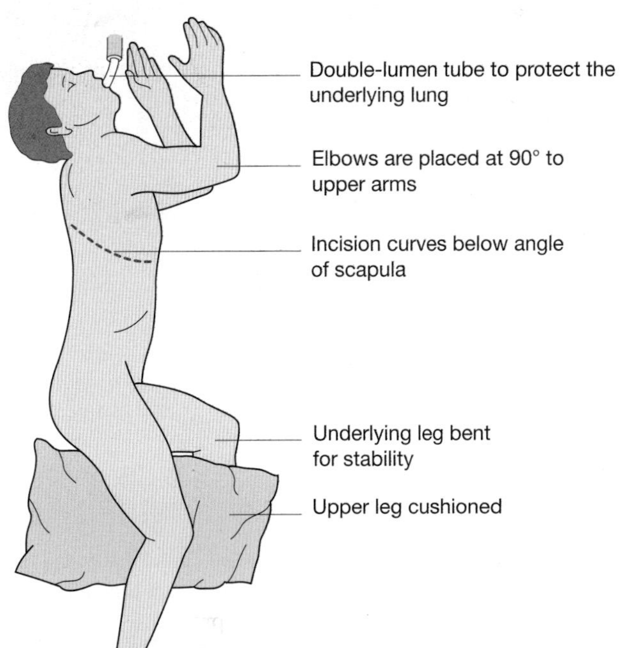

Figure 60.17 Correct positioning for thoracotomy.

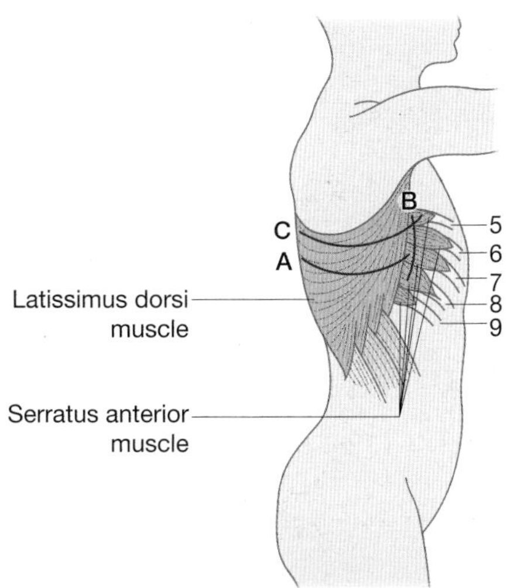

Figure 60.18 Incision and layers encountered during posterolateral thoracotomy. A, The latissimus dorsi is divided in line with the skin incision. B, If the serratus anterior is divided, it should be close to its attachment to ribs 6, 7 and 8. It can be left intact and mobilised along its inferior border. C, The intercostal muscles are stripped off the upper border of the rib.

lateral position with the affected side up (*Figure 60.17*). The incision passes 1–2 cm below the tip of the scapula and extends posteriorly and superiorly between the medial border of the scapula and the spine.

- The incision is deepened through the subcutaneous tissues to the latissimus dorsi. This muscle is divided with coagulating diathermy, taking care over haemostasis.
- A plane of dissection is developed manually, deep to the scapula and serratus anterior. The ribs can be counted down from the highest palpable rib (which is usually the second) and the sixth rib periosteum is scored with the diathermy near its upper border. A periosteal elevator is used to lift the periosteum off the superior border of the rib or, alternatively, the intercostal muscle is cut with diathermy just above the rib (*Figure 60.18*).
- This reveals the pleura, which may be entered by blunt dissection. A rib spreader is inserted between the ribs and opened gently to prevent fracture.

In an emergency thoracotomy for penetrating wounds of the heart, a more anterior approach is used and no specialised supporting equipment is required (*Figure 60.19*). The incision is taken down to the fourth or fifth rib with a scalpel, and the pleural cavity is opened using scissors. This gives rapid access to the left pleural cavity in cases of massive left haemothorax and the pericardium if cardiac tamponade is suspected. A left anterior thoracotomy can be quickly converted to a clamshell or bilateral thoracotomy if necessary.

Analgesia is an important aspect of postoperative care, and the process may be started prior to thoracotomy with an epidural catheter placed by the anaesthetist or intraoperatively by infiltrating the intercostal nerves in the region of the incision with a long-acting local anaesthetic or increasingly via a surgically sited paravertebral catheter. Various strategies have been developed to deliver analgesics postoperatively to facilitate a normal breathing pattern.

Video-assisted thoracoscopic surgery (VATS)

Various approaches utilising thoracoscopic techniques can be used to gain access to the chest cavity and facilitate lung

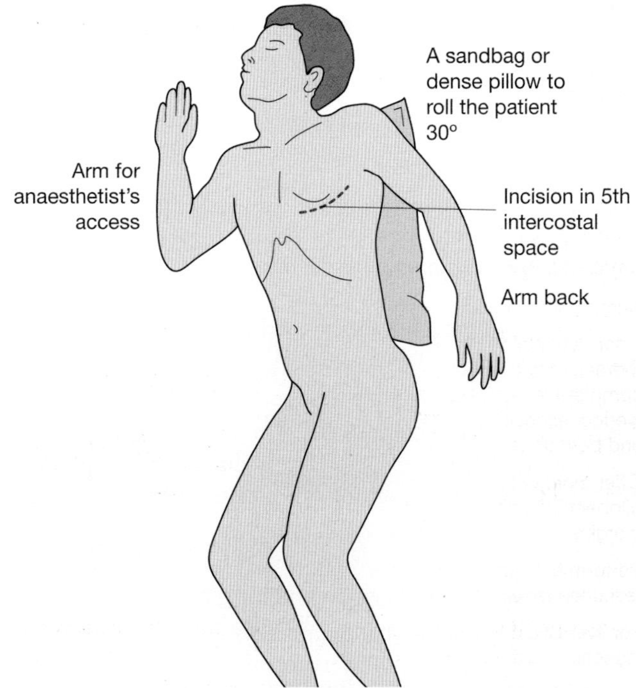

Figure 60.19 Emergency left anterior thoracotomy for access to the heart. This requires no special supports or devices.

resection. VATS is now the approach of choice in early stage lung resections with dissection of the hilar structures and full lymph node staging commonly performed through one- (uniportal), two- or three-port VATS incisions. The technique avoids rib-spreading and appears to reduce postoperative pain and length of stay and aids a speedier recovery, particularly in frail patients.

Robotically assisted thoracic surgery (RATS)

In this approach, the thoracoscopy is done using a robotic system with three-dimensional vision. The surgeon sits at a control panel in the operating room and moves robotic arms to operate through several small incisions in the patient's chest. RATS is similar to VATS in terms of less pain, less blood loss and a shorter recovery time (***Figure 60.20***).

For the surgeon, the robotic system may provide more manoeuvrability and more precision when moving the instruments than standard VATS. It may have advantages when performing more complex lung resections such as segmentectomies or mediastinal tumours (thymectomy).

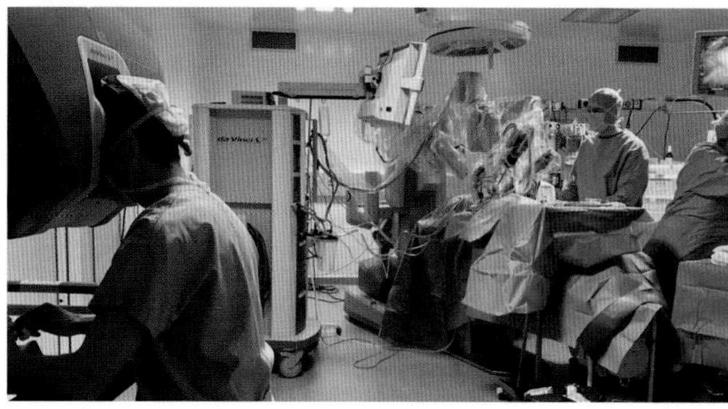

Figure 60.20 A thoracic surgeon performing robotically assisted thoracic (RATS) lung resection remotely from an operating console.

Surgical management of lung cancer

The principle of surgery is to remove all cancer (the primary and the regional lymph nodes) but to conserve as much lung as possible. The selection of patients in terms of the stage of the lung cancer and fitness to undergo such surgery is paramount. Surgery with curative intent is offered to patients with early stage lung cancer (T1–3, N0–1) (***Table 60.6***). Assessment of a patient's fitness to undergo lung cancer resection involves considering premorbid conditions, which can be aided using risk scores such as Thoracoscore, cardiovascular function and lung function; see BTS guidelines in ***Assessment of fitness for major thoracic surgery*** and UK National Institute for Health and Care Excellence (NICE) guidelines in ***Table 60.7***. Lung function, in particular, will aid the surgeon in selecting the type of procedure offered and the likelihood of breathlessness or dyspnoea following lung resection.

TABLE 60.6 UK National Institute for Health and Care Excellence (NICE) recommendations for surgery for non-small cell lung cancer (NSCLC).

Surgery with curative intent for NSCLC
Offer patients with NSCLC who are fit for surgery open or thoracoscopic lobectomy as the treatment of first choice. If complete resection is possible, consider segmentectomy or wedge resection for patients with smaller tumours (T1a–b, N0, M0) and borderline fitness
Offer more extensive surgery (bronchoangioplastic surgery, bilobectomy, pneumonectomy) only when needed to obtain clear margins
Perform hilar and mediastinal lymph node sampling or *en bloc* resection for all patients undergoing surgery with curative intent
For T3 NSCLC with chest wall involvement, aim for complete resection by extrapleural or *en bloc* chest wall resection
For people with operable stage IIIA–N2 NSCLC who can have surgery and are well enough for multimodality therapy, consider chemoradiotherapy with surgery

Choice of lung resection

Segmentectomy and wedge resection

Segmentectomy and wedge resections are performed in patients with small tumours (1–2 cm) that are predominantly ground glass, not solid (lepidic) and with borderline fitness, through thoracotomy or increasingly by VATS or RATS. Each lobe of the lung has segments, which allows anatomical dissection and ligation of the segmental pulmonary artery, vein and bronchus (segmentectomy) (***Figure 60.2***) or non-anatomical excision can be performed (wedge resection) combined with removal of regional lymph nodes.

Lobectomy

Lobectomy remains the treatment of choice for patients with early-stage lung cancer. The surgery can be performed via thoracotomy or VATS. Following dissection of the fissure and hilar structures, the branches of the pulmonary artery and veins to the lobe are isolated and ligated. The bronchus is usually stapled but can be sewn.

The patient does not routinely need intensive care and postoperative ventilation is best avoided. The 30-day mortality rate is 1–2%, with morbidity such as chest infection or cardiac arrhythmia at around 10%. The average length of stay is around 5–7 days.

Pneumonectomy

Pneumonectomy is removal of a whole lung and has a higher mortality rate (5–8%). As such the number of pneumonectomies performed in the UK has fallen and now makes up less than 5% of lung cancer surgery. The surgeon must be satisfied that the patient is fit to tolerate this procedure from the preoperative work-up. This procedure is reserved for either centrally placed tumours involving the main bronchus or those that straddle the fissure.

Bronchoplastic lung resections

Increasingly, owing to the associated complications and higher mortality of a pneumonectomy, preservation of lung tissue is being considered but without compromise of the surgical resection margins. Sleeve lung resections involve removing a central tumour that is invading a major bronchus, such as the LMB or RMB, together with the lobe of the lung involved,

TABLE 60.7 UK National Institute for Health and Care Excellence (NICE) recommendations for assessing fitness for treatment with curative intent (including surgery).

Perioperative mortality	Consider global risk score, such as Thoracoscore	Ensure patient is aware of risk before consenting
Cardiovascular function	Assess risk factors and cardiac functional capacity	Avoid surgery within 30 days of MI
		Optimise primary cardiac treatment and begin secondary cardiac prophylaxis as soon as possible
		Offer surgery if two or fewer risk factors and good cardiac functional capacity
		Seek cardiology review if active cardiac condition, three or more risk factors or poor cardiac functional capacity
		Consider revascularisation before surgery in stable angina
		Continue anti-ischaemic treatment in perioperative period. Discuss perioperative platelet treatment if patient has a coronary stent
Lung function	Perform spirometry, measure TLCO if disproportionate breathlessness or other lung pathology, perform segment count and assess exercise tolerance	Offer surgery if normal FEV_1 and good exercise tolerance or FEV_1 or TLCO below 30% and patient accepts the risks of dyspnoea
	Consider shuttle walk testing (cut-off 400 m) and cardiopulmonary exercise testing (cut-off 15 mL/kg/minute) if moderate to high risk of postoperative dyspnoea	Offer radiotherapy with curative intent if lung function poor but patient is otherwise suitable for radiotherapy with curative intent and volume of irradiated lung is small

FEV_1, forced expiratory volume in 1 s; MI, myocardial infarction; TLCO, transfer factor for carbon monoxide.
From NICE Clinical Guideline 122, available from: www.nice.org.uk/guidance/ng122.

with reanastomosis of the cut major bronchus to the remaining lobar bronchus.

Complications of lung resection

- **Bleeding**. Bleeding should be avoidable by the use of a careful surgical technique but may be severe in the presence of dense adhesions.
- **Respiratory infection**. Many of these patients are ex-smokers and therefore basal collapse and hypoxaemia are common postoperatively.
- **Persistent air leak**. Chest drains are placed at the time of surgery to deal with the air leak. Rarely, the air leak persists and the remaining lung does not expand. Re-thoracotomy may then be necessary to seal the leak.
- **Bronchopleural fistula**. This is a serious complication. Following pneumonectomy, the space left behind is initially filled with air. This is slowly reabsorbed and the space fills with tissue fluid. The fluid level rises until the air is finally reabsorbed (***Figure 60.21***). Dehiscence of the bronchial stump leads to the development of a bronchopleural fistula and the fluid in the space (which is almost inevitably infected) is expectorated in large quantities. This complication has a high morbidity and mortality rate. The patient is nursed sitting up and turned so that the affected space is dependent; this is to prevent infected fluid from entering the remaining lung while arrangements are made to site a pleural drain. This should be connected to an underwater seal but not suction. Bronchopleural fistulae are unlikely to resolve spontaneously and management is highly specialised.

Postoperative care

Enhanced recovery after surgery (ERAS) is a strategy that seeks to reduce patients' perioperative stress response, thereby reducing potential complications, decreasing hospital length of stay and enabling patients to return more quickly to their baseline functional status. These principles have been applied to patients having lung cancer surgery. Postoperatively, patients have limited respiratory reserve following lung resection, so infection and fluid overload are to be avoided. Once air leaks have settled, the drains are removed. Mobilisation, breathing exercises and regular physiotherapy are begun as soon as the patient's condition permits.

Postoperative pain

It is important to deal with postsurgical pain effectively so that a normal breathing pattern and gas exchange are achieved in the early postoperative period. Four strategies are routinely used in combination:

1. paravertebral/extrapleural or epidural catheter-delivered local anaesthetic;
2. intercostal nerve blocks;
3. PCA with intravenous boluses of opiates;
4. background oral analgesia with paracetamol and/or non-steroidal anti-inflammatory drugs.

Long-term postsurgical pain can be reduced by careful attention to detail during the operation. Sources of avoidable chronic pain include rib fracture and the entrapment of intercostal nerves during wound closure.

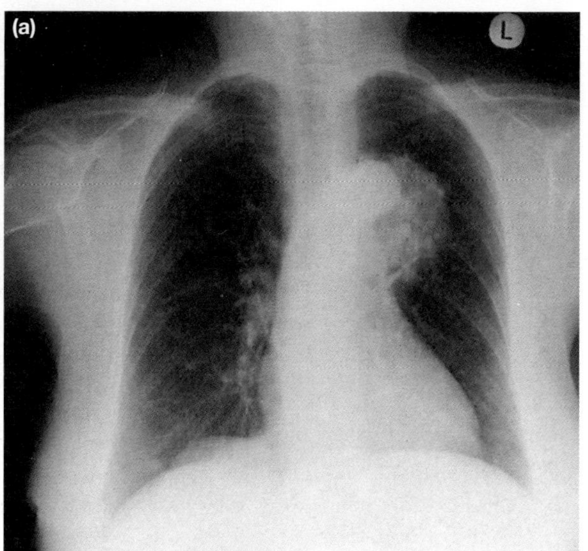

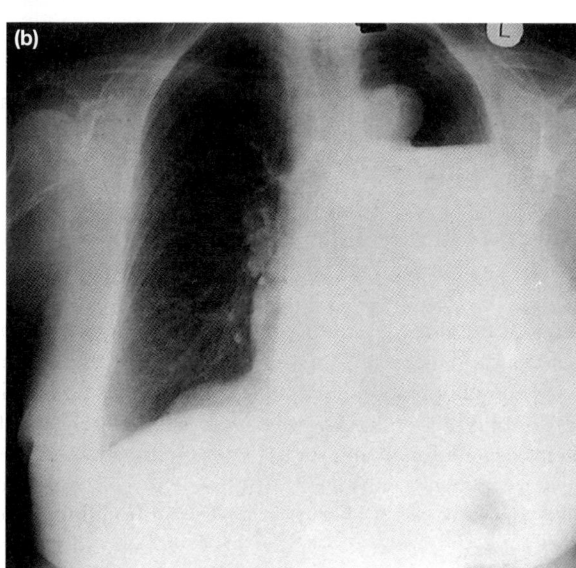

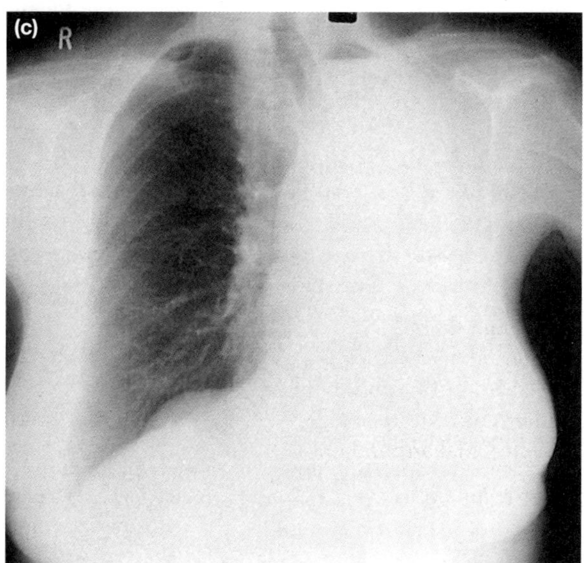

Figure 60.21 Chest radiographs (a) pre- and (b) post-pneumonectomy, with rising fluid level (c) in the left haemothorax.

LUNG METASTASES

For all malignancies, the lung is the most common site of metastases that often develop through haematogenous spread. The presence of metastases is regarded as a sign of advanced disease and few curative treatment options exist; however, surgical resection of lung metastases may result in a survival advantage, particularly with metastases from solid tumours such as colorectal cancer, though the evidence still remains uncertain. The selection criteria often used when considering lung metastasectomy include control of primary tumour; no evidence of metastases outside the lung; possibility of complete resection utilising lung-sparing techniques; and acceptable operative risks with adequate pulmonary function.

Various approaches can be considered, though VATS is increasingly favoured over thoracotomy owing to reduced postoperative pain and length of stay, and therefore speedier recovery. The disadvantage of VATS is the inability to palpate and evaluate the lung in its entirety to locate other nodules deeper within the lung parenchyma, particularly those not identified on prior CT imaging. The main principle when resecting lung metastases is to utilise lung-sparing techniques as much as possible, e.g. wedge resections rather than lobectomy, because it is likely that later reoperations to resect new metastases may be necessary.

Long-term outcome depends on the primary tumour type, with germ cell tumours having the best outcome. Patients with epithelial tumours (carcinomas) generally have a 30–40% 5-year survival, as reported in several retrospective series.

BENIGN LUNG TUMOURS

Benign tumours of the lung are uncommon and account for fewer than 15% of solitary lesions seen on chest radiographs. A peripheral tumour usually causes no symptoms until it is large; a central tumour may present with haemoptysis and signs of bronchial obstruction while still small. A tumour is likely to be benign if it has not increased in size on chest radiographs for more than 2 years or it has some degree of calcification; however, a tissue diagnosis is usually pursued.

Most benign nodules are granulomas (tuberculosis or histoplasmosis). The most common benign tumour is a hamartoma, a developmental abnormality containing mesothelial and endothelial elements. Diagnosis (and definitive treatment) is achieved by excision of the lesion. Any of the mesodermal elements of the lung may form a mesodermal tumour (chondroma, lipoma, leiomyoma). Deposits of amyloid may have a similar radiographic appearance to a nodule (pseudotumour).

THE MEDIASTINUM

The mediastinum refers to the central area in the chest between the thoracic inlet and the diaphragm, between the right and left pleural surfaces, and which extends from the inner aspect of the sternum to the vertebral column. It contains the heart, great vessels, trachea and oesophagus and is arbitrarily subdivided into compartments (superior, inferior, anterior, middle and posterior). Many of the regional lymph node chains draining the chest and its organs are also found

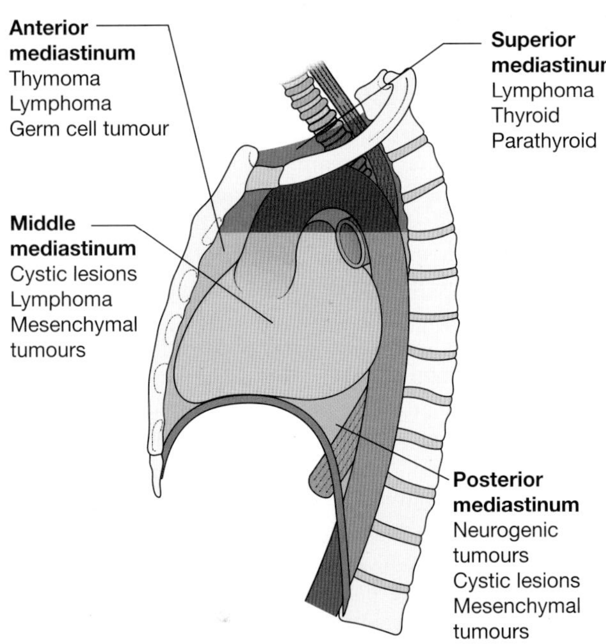

Figure 60.22 Mediastinal pathology. Subdivisions of the mediastinum with the most common mediastinal masses.

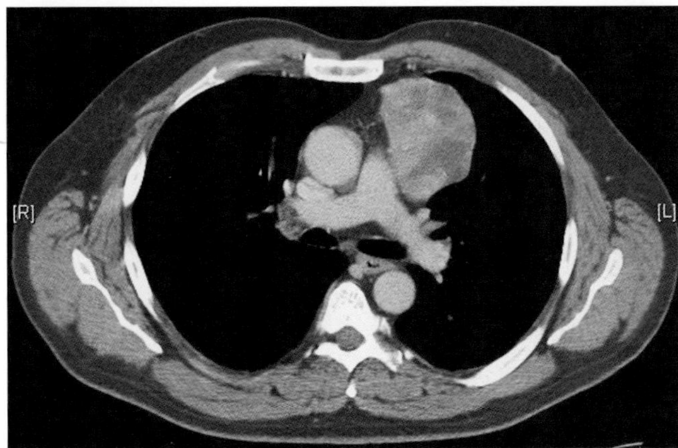

Figure 60.23 Computed tomography scan showing a thymoma presenting as a mediastinal mass.

in the mediastinum. Various surgical procedures to approach structures, and particularly lymph nodes, in the mediastinum are performed, usually as diagnostic procedures. The surgical approach when mediastinal tumours require resection depends on the anatomical location of the tumour (*Figure 60.22*) and includes median sternotomy for anterior mediastinal pathology, thoracotomy or VATS for posterior mediastinal pathology and transcervical (neck incisions) for superior mediastinal pathology. The middle mediastinum can usually be approached through thoracotomy or VATS. Increasingly, a robotic or RATS approach is used, particularly for anterior mediastinal tumours such as thymomas.

Primary tumours of the mediastinum

Thymoma, neurogenic tumours, germ cell tumours and lymphoma are the usual primary tumours of the mediastinum.

- **Thymoma**. This is the most common mediastinal tumour, accounting for 25% of the total, and is derived from the thymus gland (*Figure 60.23*). Thymomas vary in behaviour from benign to aggressively invasive, as reflected in the Masoaka classification system used to stage thymomas and more recently the TNM classification. They are often related to myasthenia gravis, a neuromuscular condition that can have a high associated incidence of thymomas, and interestingly may respond to excision of the thymus gland even when the gland has no associated thymoma present. The only reliable indicator of malignancy is capsular invasion. Diagnosis and treatment are best achieved by complete thymectomy, which for large tumours (>5 cm) or if tumour invasion is suspected a median sternotomy is performed. If the thymoma is small or when the patient has myasthenia gravis and the thymus is being excised as a treatment, various less invasive approaches can be considered, including a VATS approach or a transcervical approach with or without an additional VATS procedure.
- **Germ cell tumour**. The anterior mediastinum is the most common site of extragonadal germ cell tumours. They account for 13% of all mediastinal masses and cysts and contain elements from all three cell types (mesoderm, endoderm and ectoderm). They tend to present in young adults and 75% are benign and cystic, although they may cause compression of neighbouring structures; hence, dermoid cysts are best excised. Malignancy is suspected if elevated levels of serum alpha-fetoprotein, human chorionic gonadotropin and carcinoembryonic antigen are detected. After initial treatment with chemotherapy, a patient with tumour marker normalisation and a persistent mass on CT may be considered for surgical resection. If tumour markers fail to normalise, further chemotherapy is usually offered.
- **Lymphoma**. Lymphoma is a common cause of a mediastinal mass lesion, particularly in the anterior mediastinum, and can lead to superior vena cava obstruction or other symptoms of local compression. The main treatment is chemotherapy, and surgery is rarely required apart from obtaining tissue for diagnosis.
- **Mesenchymal tumours**. Lipomas are common in the anterior mediastinum. Other mesenchymal tumours are very rare.
- **Thyroid**. Ectopic thyroid (and parathyroid) tissue may be found in the anterior mediastinum but usually the mass is an extension of a thyroid lesion (retrosternal goitre). Excision of retrosternal thyroids may be required if there is local airway compression and stridor and can be performed via a transcervical incision, but occasionally median sternotomy may be required.

Akira Masoaka, 1930–2014, Professor of Surgery, Nagoya, Japan.

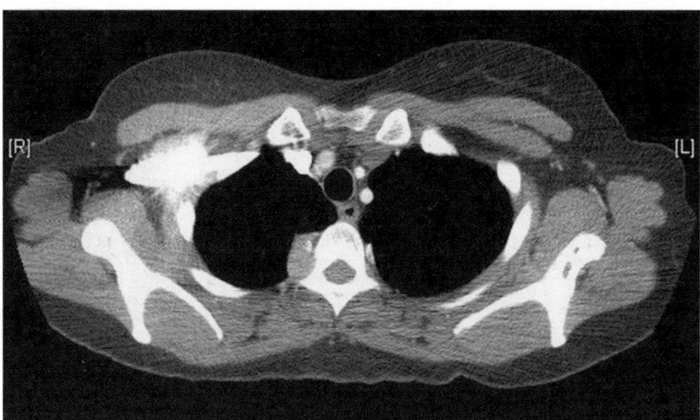

Figure 60.24 Computed tomography scan showing a right-sided paravertebral neurogenic tumour.

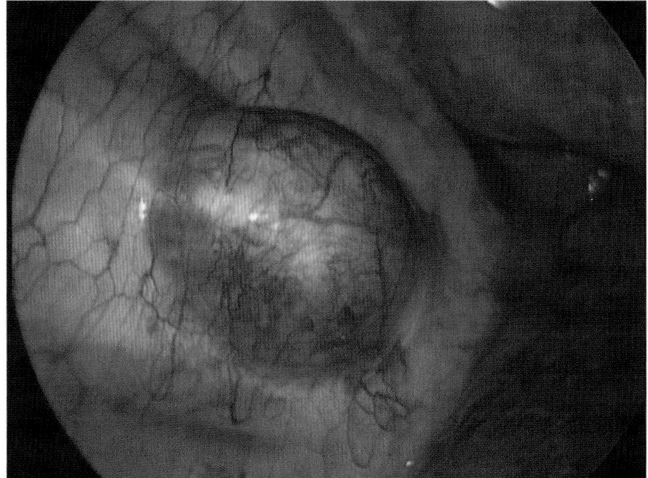
Figure 60.25 Video-assisted thoracoscopic surgery (VATS) image of a neurogenic tumour attached to the posterolateral chest wall prior to excision.

- **Neurogenic tumours**. These may derive from the sympathetic nervous system or the peripheral nerves and are more prevalent in the posterior mediastinum. They may be painful but are more often discovered accidentally on routine chest radiography and can be quite large (***Figure 60.24***). They include neuroblastoma in childhood, and Schwannomas and neurofibromas in adults, which are usually benign. Phaeochromocytoma arises from the sympathetic chain and produces the characteristic endocrine syndrome. Excision of neurogenic tumours is generally recommended, particularly if the patient is developing symptoms. This can be performed through a thoracotomy, though for smaller tumours a VATS approach can be used (***Figure 60.25***).
- Enlarged mediastinal lymph nodes are commonly involved by metastatic tumour, mimicking a primary mediastinal lesion. Symptoms are generally secondary to compression or invasion of a structure within the mediastinum. Surgery such as mediastinoscopy is reserved for diagnosis only.

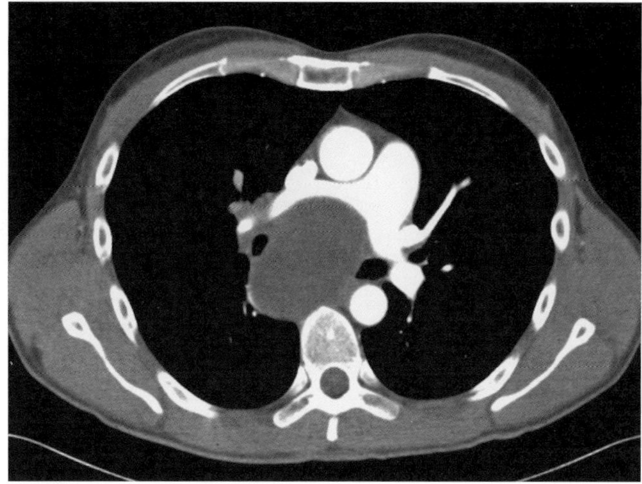
Figure 60.26 Computed tomography scan of the chest showing a bronchogenic cyst splaying the carina.

Other conditions of the mediastinum

Many of the primary tumours such as neurogenic tumours and germ cell tumours can present as cysts or have a cystic quality. In addition, the mediastinum can contain other cysts, often with an embryological aetiology. Thymic, pericardial, bronchogenic and foregut cysts can all present asymptomatically or with local compression (***Figure 60.26***). Surgical excision is recommended if the diagnosis is unclear or the patient has symptoms.

MEDICAL CONDITIONS FOR WHICH SURGERY MAY BE REQUIRED

Bronchiectasis

Bronchiectasis is chronic irreversible dilatation of the medium-sized bronchi, which may occur following a suppurative pneumonia or bronchial obstruction. It is the pathological end stage of a range of conditions. If generalised it is almost never considered for surgical resection. Cases caused by whooping cough and measles are decreasing in frequency in resource-rich countries.

Treatment

Removal of the bronchiectatic part of the lung for bleeding, recurrent infection or copious symptoms can be very effective when the disease is localised.

Lung abscess

The causes of lung abscess are shown in ***Table 60.8***. The chest radiograph shows a cavity with a fluid level or in mycetoma a fungal ball. Most acute abscesses resolve with appropriate antibiotic therapy and postural drainage. Surgery is avoided. Small radiologically sited drains are used sometimes in the intensive care unit.

Theodor Schwann, 1810–1882, Professor of Anatomy and Physiology, successively at Louvain (1839–1848) and Liège, Belgium (1849–1888).

TABLE 60.8 Causes of lung abscess.

Specific pneumonia	Streptococcal Staphylococcal Pneumococcal *Klebsiella* spp. Anaerobic
Bronchial obstruction	Carcinoma Carcinoid Foreign body Postoperative atelectasis
Chronic respiratory sepsis	Sinusitis Tonsillitis Dental infection
Septicaemia	
Penetrating lung injury	

Tuberculosis

Surgery is rarely indicated for tuberculosis in resource-rich countries but, when it is, it must be combined with adequate antitubercular chemotherapy or the benefit of surgery will be lost.

Summary box 60.5

Tuberculosis: indications for surgery

- Suspicious lesion on chest radiograph in which neoplasia cannot be excluded
- Chronic tuberculous abscess, resistant to chemotherapy
- Aspergilloma within a tuberculous cavity
- Life-threatening haemoptysis

Diagnosis

Surgical procedures may be necessary to establish the diagnosis if suspected clinically but sputum or pus cultures are persistently negative.

Complications such as an aspergilloma in a chronic cavity causing life-threatening haemoptysis may require lobectomy.

Pulmonary sequestration

This describes a section of non-functional lung separated from the normal bronchial connection with other abnormalities of development, which often include a direct systemic arterial supply from the aorta. Venous return is to the pulmonary veins in the majority of cases. The segment becomes cystic and infected, resulting in the common appearance of a solid lung mass that may be homogeneous or heterogeneous, occasionally with cystic changes on CT scan. Interlobar sequestration occurs within the lung substance. It may present with recurrent chest infections and/or haemoptysis. Patients with extralobar sequestration are usually asymptomatic because air spaces are not present, and therefore it usually presents as an incidental finding.

Lung cysts

Developmental lung cysts have a tendency to become infected. Acquired lung cysts may contain air or fluid and may be single or multiple. Pulmonary hydatid disease is a cause in endemic areas. Air cysts (bullae) may be spontaneous but may be secondary to emphysematous degeneration (***Figure 60.27***).

LUNG TRANSPLANTATION (see *Chapter 92*)

Lung transplantation is an established therapy for those with end-stage parenchymal or pulmonary vascular disease; it is limited by the number of donor lungs available.

CHEST TRAUMA

The approach to trauma must be methodical and exact because the signs, particularly in the presence of other injury,

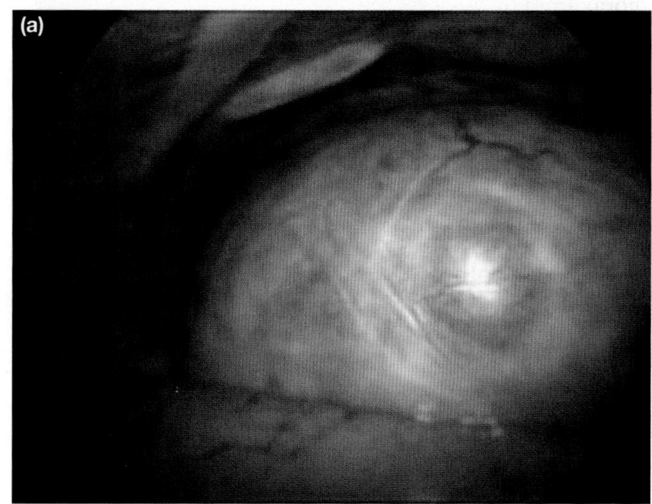

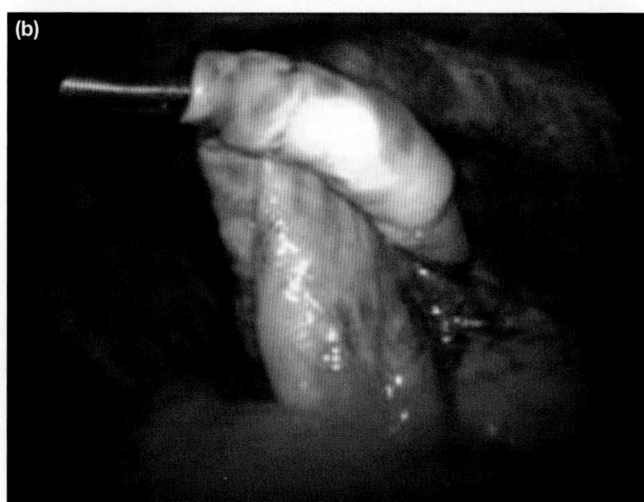

Figure 60.27 (a) A large solitary bulla seen on videothoracoscopy. (b) The bulla deflated and rolled in preparation for staple resection.

Theodor Albrecht Edwin Klebs, 1834–1913, Professor of Bacteriology, successively at Prague, Czech Republic; Zurich, Switzerland; and The Rush Medical College, Chicago, IL, USA.

may easily be missed. The general principles of resuscitation and ATLS (Advanced Trauma Life Support) must be followed.

Thoracic trauma is responsible for over 70% of all deaths following road traffic accidents. Blunt trauma to the chest in isolation is fatal in 10% of cases, rising to 30% if other injuries are present. The indications for emergency room thoracotomy in blunt chest trauma include massive haemothorax, suspected cardiac tamponade and witnessed cardiac arrest in the resuscitation area. Success rates are low. Penetrating thoracic wounds vary according to the prevalence of civil violence, with a mortality rate of 3% for simple stabbing to 15% for gunshot wounds. The indications for emergency room thoracotomy are similar to those for blunt chest trauma. The standard approach is a left anterior thoracotomy, unless the penetrating injury is in the right chest; however, it may be necessary to extend the incision to bilateral thoracotomies or a clam-shell incision.

THE DIAPHRAGM

The diaphragm is the fibromuscular structure separating the thorax from the abdomen.

Disorders of the diaphragm

Disorders of the diaphragm can be broadly classified as disorders of innervation, leading to paralysis of the diaphragm, with elevation and reduction of thoracic volume leading to breathlessness, and disorders of anatomy, which are further categorised into congenital diaphragmatic hernias or acquired hernias, usually secondary to trauma. There are two well-recognised congenital sites where abdominal viscera can herniate into the chest (***Figure 60.28***).

- The foramen of Morgagni: a hernia in the anterior part of the diaphragm with a defect between the sternal and costal attachments. The most commonly involved viscus is the transverse colon.
- The foramen of Bochdalek: through the dome of the diaphragm posteriorly.

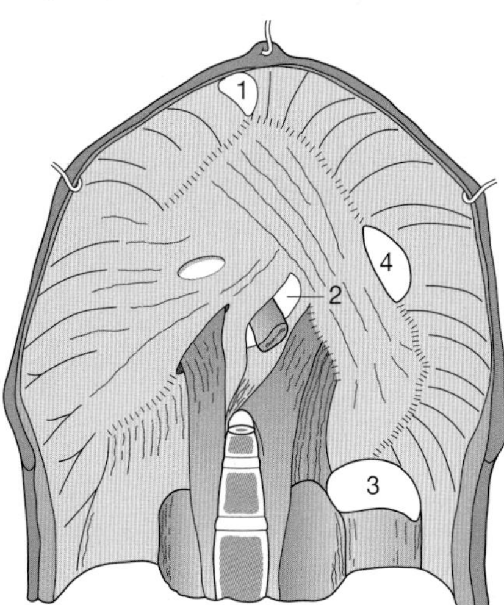

Figure 60.28 Diagram of sites of hernias. The usual sites of congenital diaphragmatic hernia: 1, foramen of Morgagni; 2, oesophageal hiatus; 3, foramen of Bochdalek (pleuroperitoneal hernia); 4, dome.

Traumatic rupture of the diaphragm may occur with blunt trauma. Unless there is severe bleeding or strangulation of the viscera it is best managed after an interval. In a severely injured patient being ventilated it can wait until other injuries are dealt with and weaning from the ventilator is being considered.

When the diaphragm is breached, as in anatomical disorders, repair either with primary closure or with a mesh is usually possible via a thoracotomy. Diaphragmatic paralysis, particularly idiopathic unilateral paralysis, can be treated by plication, returning the diaphragm to a lower position and improving thoracic volume.

DISORDERS OF THE CHEST WALL

Tumours of the chest wall

These can be tumours of any component of the chest wall, i.e. bone, cartilage and soft tissue. They are treated similarly to those that occur at other sites and require specialist surgical input only if major resection and chest wall reconstruction are contemplated.

Other diseases of the chest wall

Congenital abnormalities are often incidental findings on chest radiography (e.g. bifid rib), but there are some important exceptions.

Cervical rib and thoracic outlet syndrome

This rib is usually represented by a fibrous band originating from the seventh cervical vertebra and inserting onto the first thoracic rib. It may be asymptomatic, but because the subclavian artery and brachial plexus course over it a variety of symptoms may occur. The lower trunk of the plexus (mainly T1) is compressed, leading to wasting of the interossei and altered sensation in the T1 distribution. Compression of the subclavian artery may result in a poststenotic dilatation with thrombus and embolus formation. The diagnosis, assessment and surgery are fraught with uncertainties and are best left to those with a well-developed interest in this problem.

Pectus excavatum

The sternum is depressed, with a dish-shaped deformity of the anterior portions of the ribs on one or both sides. Whether it causes cardiopulmonary issues through compression remains unclear but certainly the disfigurement can lead to significant psychological concerns. It can be repaired either as an open procedure (modified Ravitch procedure), which involves resecting the affected costal cartilages and mobilising the sternum, or

Giovanni Battista Morgagni, 1682–1771, Professor of Anatomy, Padua, Italy, for 59 years, regarded as 'the founder of morbid anatomy'.
Victor Alexander Bochdalek, 1801–1883, Professor of Anatomy, Prague, Czech Republic.
Mark M Ravitch, 1910–1989, paediatric surgeon, University of Pittsburgh, PA, USA.
Donald Nuss, contemporary, paediatric surgeon, Norfolk, VA, USA, described this technique in 1987.

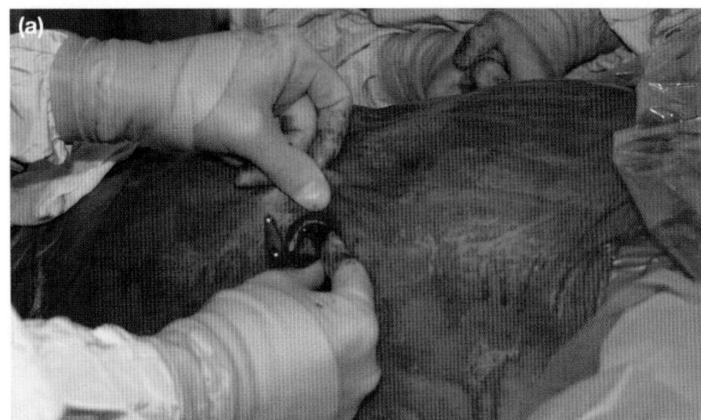

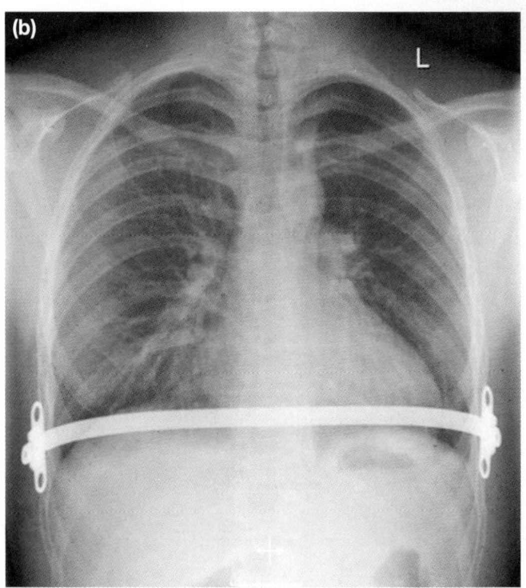

Figure 60.29 (a) Insertion of a preformed bar placed thoracoscopically beneath the pectus excavatum. (b) Chest radiograph following insertion of a metal bar bracing the sternum forward (the Nuss procedure).

as a minimally invasive technique, the Nuss procedure. A metal bar is placed behind the sternum to hold this central panel in its new position; the bar has to be removed after a period of time (***Figure 60.29***).

Pectus carinatum (pigeon chest)

In this condition the sternum is elevated above the level of the ribs and treatment is offered for aesthetic reasons. It often comes to light during the growth spurt at adolescence when, of course, the teenager is particularly sensitive about appearance. Most patients are asymptomatic and the only justification for treatment is on cosmetic grounds. Some surgeons make a very good case for this but the risk of morbidity and of a less than perfect result must be clearly spelt out to the patient and his/her parents. Surgery (modified Ravitch) involves mobilising the sternum with the costal cartilages so that the sternum can be flattened to a more anatomical position. Surgery is best left until the late teens, when further growth of the chest wall is unlikely. Alternatively, an external orthotic brace can be worn in young patients with a pliable chest wall to remodel the chest shape over time.

FURTHER READING

Baas P, Fennell D, Kerr KM *et al.* Malignant pleural mesothelioma: ESMO Clinical Practice Guidelines for diagnosis, treatment and follow-up. *Ann Oncol* 2015; **26**(Suppl 5): v31–9.

Batchelor TJP, Rasburn NJ, Abdelnour-Berchtold E *et al.* Guidelines for enhanced recovery after lung surgery: recommendations of the Enhanced Recovery After Surgery (ERAS®) Society and the European Society of Thoracic Surgeons (ESTS). *Eur J Cardiothorac Surg* 2019; **55**(1): 91–115.

Brierley J, Gospodarowicz MK, Wittekind C. *TNM classification of malignant tumours*, 8th edn. Oxford: Wiley-Blackwell, 2017.

BTS Pleural Disease Guideline Group. British Thoracic Society Pleural Disease Guideline 2010. *Thorax* 2010; **65**(Suppl 2): 1–76.

Lim E, Baldwin D, Beckles M *et al.* Guidelines on the radical management of patients with lung cancer. *Thorax* 2010; **65**(Suppl 3): iii1–27.

National Institute for Health and Care Excellence. *Lung cancer diagnosis and management.* NICE Clinical Guideline 122. London: NICE, 2019. Available from https://www.nice.org.uk/guidance/ng122.

CHAPTER

61 Arterial disorders

Learning objectives

To understand:

- The nature and associated features of occlusive peripheral arterial disease
- The investigation and treatment options for occlusive peripheral arterial disease
- The principles of management of the severely ischaemic limb
- The nature and presentation of aneurysmal disease, including the abdominal aorta and popliteal artery
- The investigation and treatment options for aneurysmal disease
- The arteritides and vasospastic disorders

INTRODUCTION

Arterial disorders represent the most common cause of morbidity and early death in western societies. Much of this is as a result of atheromatous plaque build-up causing stenoses (atherosclerosis) within the arteries that supply the heart muscle (coronary thrombosis and myocardial infarction) and brain (stroke) and the peripheral arterial system. This chapter addresses diseases that are typically the domain of the vascular surgeon, namely those affecting the peripheral arterial system: vascular disease that alters the normal structure and function of the aorta, its visceral branches and the arteries of the lower extremity.

ARTERIAL STENOSIS AND OCCLUSION

Cause and effect

Peripheral arterial stenosis or occlusion is predominantly caused by atherosclerosis and/or thromboembolic disease, but may also occur as a result of trauma. Stenosis or occlusion produces symptoms and signs that relate to the organ supplied by the artery: e.g. lower limb – claudication, rest pain and gangrene; brain – transient ischaemic attacks (TIAs) and stroke; myocardium – angina and myocardial infarction; intestine – abdominal pain and infarction (***Figure 61.1***). The severity of the symptoms relates to the size of the vessel occluded and whether the stenosis or occlusion occurs suddenly (acute) in a previously normal artery or gradually (chronic) with progressive narrowing of the artery over time. In chronic stenosis symptoms may be abated despite being affected by significant steno-occlusive disease as a result of the development of a collateral circulation that provides an alternative, albeit less effective, route for blood to reach the target tissue/organ (***Figure 61.2***).

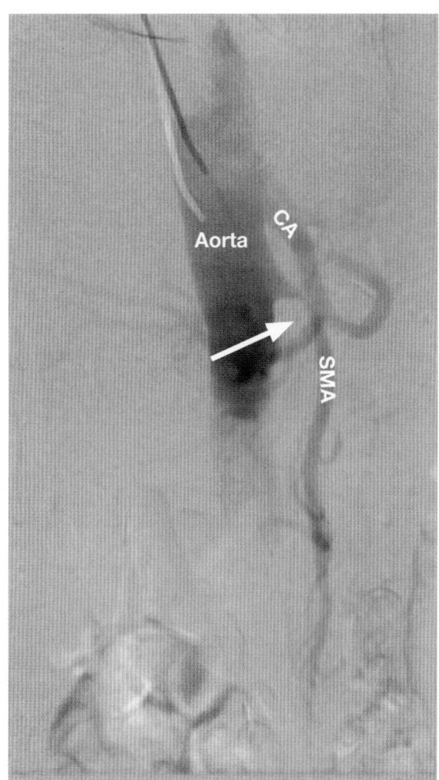

Figure 61.1 Antegrade aortogram via retrograde brachial artery access demonstrating superior mesenteric artery stenosis (arrow). CA, coeliac artery; SMA, superior mesenteric artery.

Claudication from the Latin 'claudicare' – to limp. The Roman emperor Claudius (10 BCE to 54 CE) walked with a limp, which was possibly due to poliomyelitis.

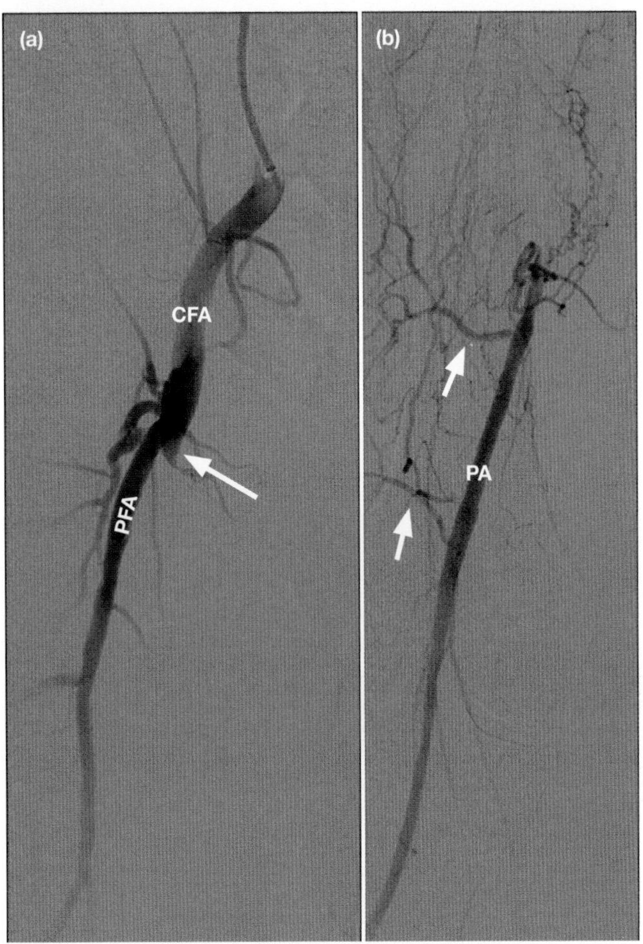

Figure 61.2 (a) Digital subtraction angiogram from the common femoral artery (CFA) demonstrating a flush right superficial femoral artery occlusion (arrow). (b) Reconstitution of the popliteal artery (PA) at the adductor hiatus via collateral flow from the profunda femoris artery (PFA) via the geniculate arteries (arrows).

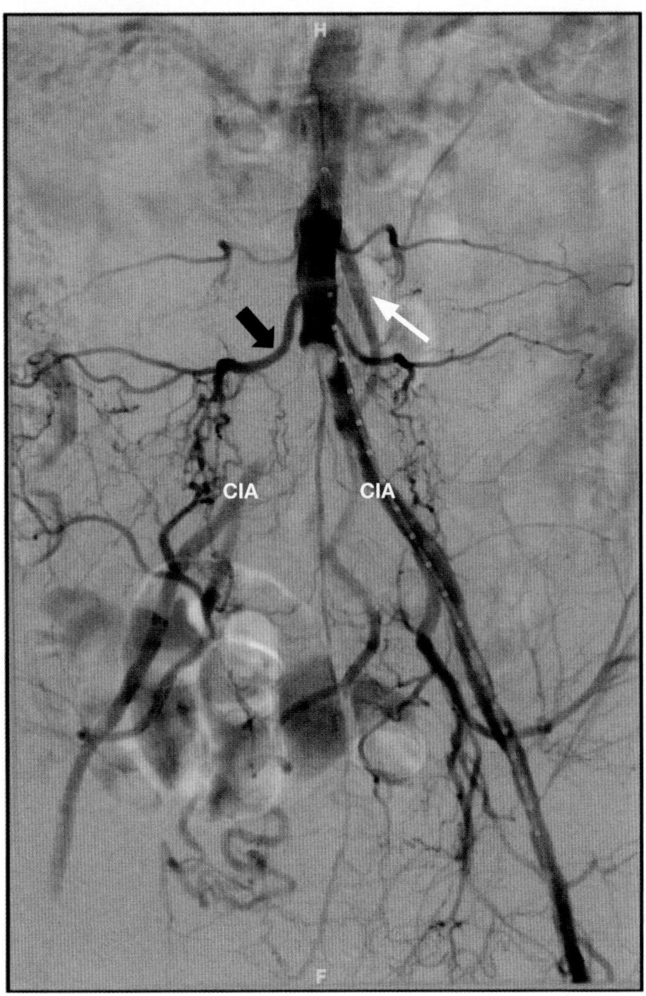

Figure 61.3 Aortoiliac bifurcation disease with an occluded right common iliac artery (CIA) and critically stenosed left CIA. Collateralisation has occurred via the lumbar arteries (black arrow) and the inferior mesenteric artery (white arrow).

Features of chronic arterial stenosis or occlusion in the leg

Intermittent claudication

Intermittent claudication occurs as a result of anaerobic muscle metabolism and is classically described as debilitating cramp-like pain felt in the muscles that is:

- brought on by walking;
- not present on taking the first step (unlike osteoarthritis);
- relieved by rest in both the standing and sitting positions, usually within 5 minutes (unlike nerve compression from a lumbar intervertebral disc prolapse or osteoarthritis of the spine or spinal stenosis, which are typically relieved only when resting in the sitting position for longer than 5 minutes).

The distance that a patient is able to walk without stopping varies (claudication distance) only slightly from day to day. It is decreased, first, by increasing the work demands and hence oxygen requirements of the muscles affected, e.g. walking up hill, increasing the speed of walking and/or carrying heavy weights, and, second, by general health conditions that reduce the oxygen delivery capacity of the arterial system, e.g. anaemia or cardiorespiratory disease.

The muscle group affected by claudication is classically one anatomical level below the level of arterial disease and is usually felt in the posterior calf as the superficial femoral artery is the most commonly affected artery (70% of cases). Aortoiliac disease (30% of cases) may cause thigh or buttock claudication; Leriche's syndrome is buttock claudication combined with sexual impotence, which is secondary to arterial insufficiency (***Figure 61.3***).

Rest pain

As disease progression occurs the claudication distance decreases and perfusion to the leg may be so severely

René Leriche, 1879–1955, Professor of Surgery, Strasbourg, France, described this syndrome.

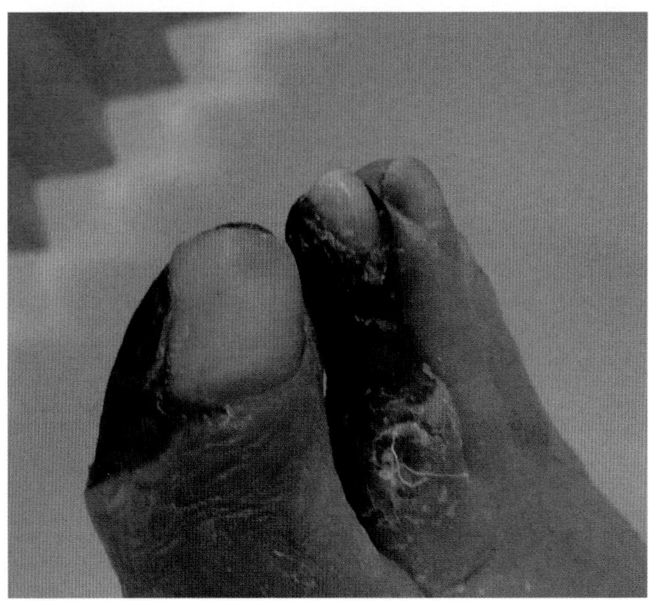

Figure 61.4 Chronic limb-threatening ischaemia with dry gangrene.

compromised that anaerobic respiration occurs even at rest, typically affecting the foot and/or calf. The pain is exacerbated by lying down or elevation of the foot because of the loss of gravitational effects on the perfusion pressure in the foot. The patient characteristically describes pain that is worse at night and may be lessened by hanging the foot out of bed or by sleeping in a chair (effects of gravity restored). Even the pressure of bedclothes on the foot may exacerbate the pain.

Ulceration and gangrene

Ulceration occurs with severe arterial insufficiency and may present as painful erosions between the toes or as shallow, non-healing ulcers on the dorsum of the feet, on the shins and especially around the malleoli. The blackened mummified tissues of frank gangrene are unmistakable (***Figure 61.4***), and superadded infection often makes the gangrene wet. Patients with ischaemic rest pain with or without ulceration/gangrene (tissue loss) are termed to have chronic limb-threatening ischaemia (CLTI). These patients should be considered to have an imminently threatened leg and require urgent vascular assessment/revascularisation to prevent major amputation.

Colour, temperature, sensation and movement

Unlike an acutely ischaemic foot that is often cold, white, paralysed and insensate, a chronically ischaemic limb tends to equilibrate with the temperature of its surroundings and may feel quite warm under the bedclothes. Chronic ischaemia does not produce paralysis and sensation is usually intact. Patients with CLTI who have been waiting for a consultation with their leg in dependence may have a red swollen foot that may be mistaken for cellulitis by the unwary clinician. However, elevation of the limb reveals the severity of the ischaemia with venous guttering and foot pallor that changes to a red/purple colour when the limb is allowed to hang down again (dependent rubor or the sunset foot sign) (***Figure 61.5***). The capillary refill time may be elicited by pressing the skin of the heel or toe pulp, causing blanching (press for 5 seconds), and then releasing to allow colour to return; normally this takes 2–3 seconds but may be prolonged to 10 seconds in severe ischaemia.

Arterial pulses

It is standard practice to examine the femoral, popliteal, posterior tibial and dorsalis pedis arteries together with the abdomen for an aortic aneurysm, which may coexist with lower limb occlusive disease. Diminution of a femoral and/

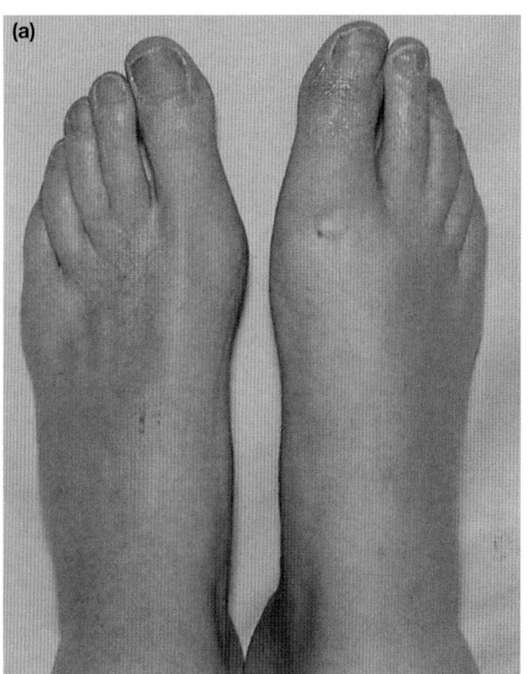

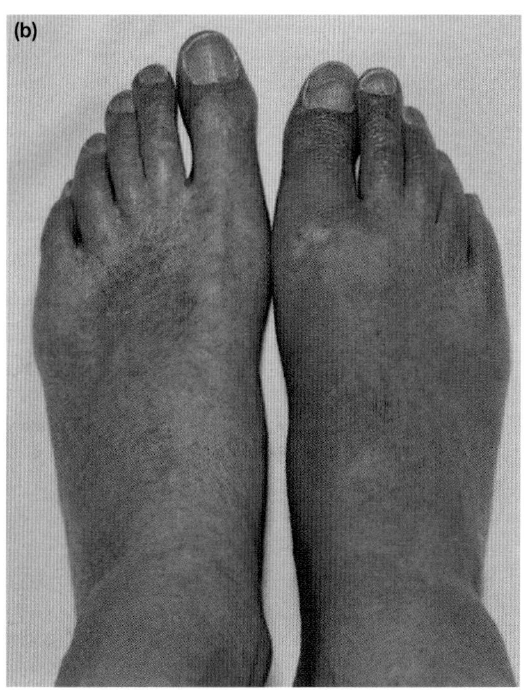

Figure 61.5 Colour changes with elevation **(a)** and dependency **(b)**.

or popliteal pulse can often be appreciated by comparing it with its opposite number; however, pedal pulses are either clinically palpable or absent. Popliteal pulses may be difficult to appreciate; a popliteal artery aneurysm should be suspected if the popliteal pulse is prominent with concomitant loss of the natural concavity of the popliteal fossa. Pulsation distal to an arterial occlusion is usually absent, although the presence of a highly developed collateral circulation may allow distal pulses to be palpable – this is most likely to occur with an iliac stenosis. In this case, exercise (walking until claudication develops) usually causes the pulse to disappear as vasodilation occurs below the obstruction, thereby reducing the pulse pressure. An arterial bruit, heard on auscultation over the pulse, indicates turbulent flow and suggests a stenosis. However, it is an unreliable clinical sign as tight stenoses often do not have bruits. A continuous 'machinery' murmur over an artery usually indicates an arteriovenous fistula.

Summary box 61.1

Features of chronic lower limb arterial stenosis or occlusion

- Intermittent claudication
- Rest pain
- Ulceration
- Gangrene
- Dependent rubor or sunset foot
- Arterial pulsation diminished or absent
- Slow capillary refilling
- Arterial bruit

Relationship of clinical findings to the site of disease

In most cases the anatomical level of arterial stenosis can be determined from accurate assessment of the symptoms and signs (***Table 61.1***). Limb-threatening ischaemia is predominantly caused by multilevel disease, e.g. iliac and femoropopliteal disease.

TABLE 61.1 Relationship of clinical findings to the site of disease.

Aortoiliac obstruction	Claudication in the buttocks, thighs and calves
	Femoral and distal pulses absent in both limbs
	Bruit over the aortoiliac region
	Impotence (Leriche)
Iliac obstruction	Unilateral claudication in the thigh and calf and sometimes the buttock
	Bruit over the iliac region
	Unilateral absence of femoral and distal pulses
Femoropopliteal obstruction	Unilateral claudication in the calf
	Femoral pulse palpable with absent unilateral distal pulses
Distal obstruction	Femoral and popliteal pulses palpable
	Ankle pulses absent
	Claudication in the calf and foot

Investigation of arterial occlusive disease

Most patients with symptomatic lower limb ischaemia present with mild symptomatology and do not require invasive treatment, such as angioplasty or surgical reconstruction, and the decision of whether or not to intervene can often be made without recourse to special investigations. When further investigation is indicated the purpose is to confirm the presence and severity of peripheral arterial disease (PAD), identify the anatomical location of disease and assess the suitability of the patient for intervention.

General investigation

Patients with arterial disease tend to be elderly and atherosclerosis is often a multisystem disease process; the presence of arterial disease in the leg is suggestive of disease in other arterial trees, including the coronary (50%) and cerebral (25–50%) trees. Many patients have other age-related diseases, such as chronic obstructive pulmonary disease and malignancy, that may impact on both their symptoms and suitability for intervention. Blood tests to exclude anaemia, diabetes, renal disease and lipid abnormalities should include a full blood count, blood glucose, lipid profile and serum urea and electrolytes. High blood viscosity (polycythaemia and thrombocythaemia) may be caused by smoking, but may also be associated with cancer; renal impairment (raised serum creatinine and low estimated glomerular filtration rate) may be caused by drugs and may be exacerbated by intravenous contrast agents used during angiography.

An electrocardiogram (ECG) may show coronary ischaemia, left ventricular hypertrophy or a cardiac dysrhythmia, although a normal ECG does not exclude these conditions. More information may be gained by an echocardiogram or exercise testing. Arterial blood gases and a pulmonary function test may be appropriate in patients with severe lung disease.

Doppler ultrasound blood flow detection

A hand-held Doppler ultrasound probe is very useful in the assessment of steno-occlusive arterial disease (***Figures 61.6 and 61.7***). A continuous-wave ultrasound signal is transmitted from the probe at an artery and a receiver within the probe itself picks up the reflected beam. The change in frequency in the reflected beam compared with that of the transmitted beam is due to the Doppler shift, which results from the reflection of the beam by moving blood cells. The frequency change may be converted into an audio signal that is typically pulsatile. Doppler ultrasound equipment can be used in conjunction with a sphygmomanometer to assess systolic pressure in small vessels. This is possible even when the arterial pulse cannot be palpated. Both the pressure and signal quality are important;

Christian Johann Doppler, 1803–1856, Professor of Experimental Physics, Vienna, Austria, enunciated the 'Doppler principle' in 1842.

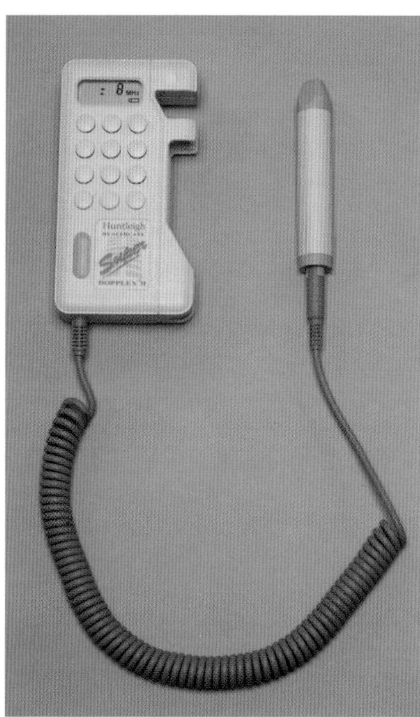

Figure 61.6 A simple hand-held Doppler ultrasound probe.

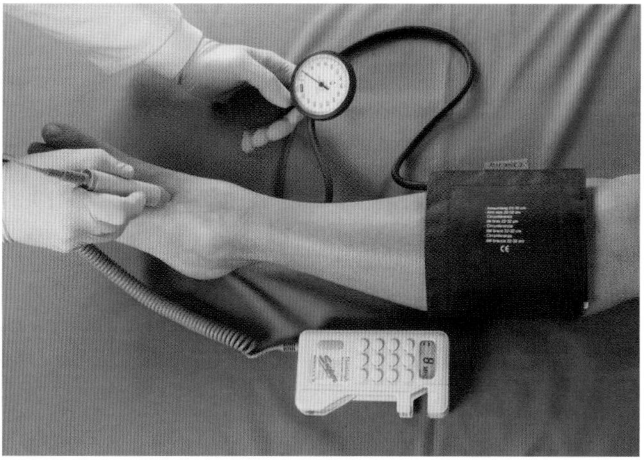

Figure 61.7 A hand-held Doppler probe and sphygmomanometer used to determine systolic pressure in the dorsalis pedis artery, as part of assessing the ankle–brachial pressure index.

a normal artery has a triphasic signal whereas a diseased artery may have a biphasic or monophasic signal depending on the extent of disease. However, although the presence of a Doppler signal indicates moving blood, it does not necessarily indicate that the blood flow is sufficient to maintain limb viability and prevent limb loss.

Quantitative assessment can be carried out at the bedside by performing an ankle–brachial pressure index (ABI), which is the ratio of the systolic pressure at the ankle to that in the ipsilateral arm. The highest pressure in the dorsalis pedis, posterior tibial or peroneal artery serves as the numerator, with the highest brachial systolic pressure being the denominator. The normal resting ABI is 0.9–1.4; values below 0.9 indicate

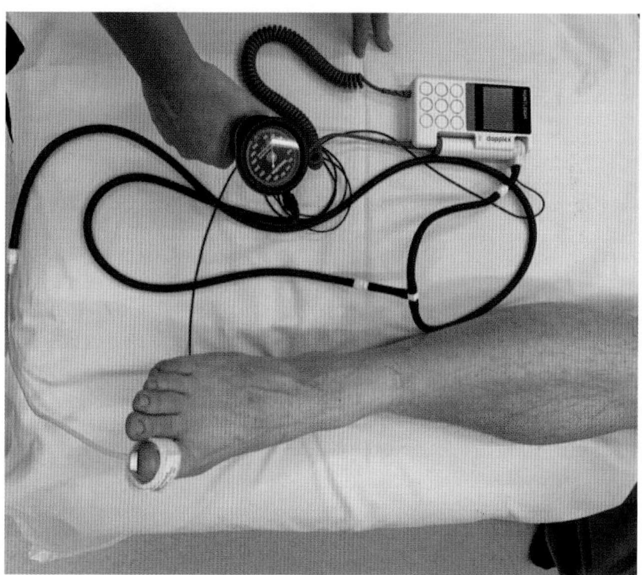

Figure 61.8 Toe pressures being performed from the hallux. An absolute pressure from the hallux of <50 mmHg indicates severe ischaemia that is likely to prevent healing of ulceration.

a haemodynamically significant arterial lesion; a value less than 0.4 suggests CLTI. Values are merely a guide and normal values may be present with intermittent claudication. Retesting after exercise to the onset of pain can be useful; a drop in the resting ABI of >20% after exercise is indicative of flow-limiting arterial disease. Artificially high ABI readings (>1.4) can be caused by media sclerosis and calcification of the arterial wall, causing vessel incompressibility and a falsely elevated ABI; this pattern of disease typically occurs in patients with diabetes mellitus (DM).

Toe (digital) arteries are rarely affected by sclerosis and a toe–brachial pressure index (TBI) in combination with ABI is advocated as a more reliable diagnostic tool for the detection of significant large-vessel steno-occlusive disease in patients with DM. A TBI less than 0.6 suggests a significant arterial lesion that may have been overlooked if ABI was used in isolation (***Figure 61.8***). However, there are limitations to the usage of TBI in the DM population: one in six patients with DM presenting with CLTI will have gangrene or will have undergone an amputation of the hallux.

Duplex Doppler ultrasound

This major non-invasive technique uses B-mode ultrasound to provide an image of vessels (***Figures 61.9 and 61.10***). The image is created because of the varying ability of different tissues to reflect the ultrasound beam. A second ultrasound beam is then used to insonate the imaged vessel and the Doppler shift obtained is analysed by a computer. Most scanners now have colour coding, which allows detailed visualisation of blood flow, turbulence, etc. Different colours indicate changes in direction and velocity of flow with areas of high flow usually indicating a stenosis. In experienced hands, duplex Doppler ultrasound (DUS) is as accurate as angiography and has the advantages of cost-effectiveness and safety. However, there are limitations: the aortoiliac segment can be difficult to visualise because of

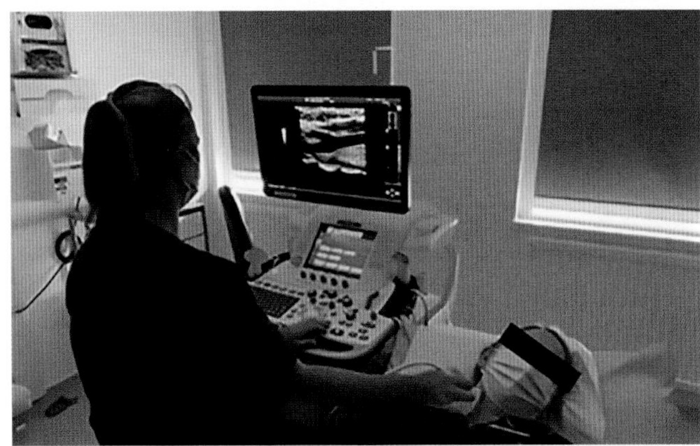

Figure 61.9 Duplex Doppler ultrasound scan being performed of the right carotid bifurcation.

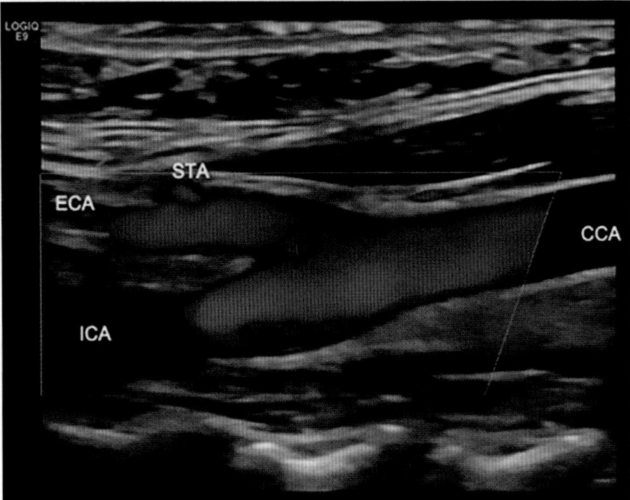

Figure 61.10 Normal duplex Doppler ultrasound of the carotid vessels in the neck. CCA, common carotid artery; ECA, external carotid artery; ICA, internal carotid artery; STA, superior thyroid artery.

bowel gas or obesity; vessels that are heavily calcified may limit the ability of DUS to accurately assess the severity of steno-occlusive disease; the overall accuracy of DUS is determined by operator experience. When DUS inadequately visualises or quantifies the level of disease within an arterial segment an alternative imaging modality, e.g. digital subtraction percutaneous angiography (DSA) or computed tomography angiography (CTA), may be undertaken to delineate the anatomy and extent of disease.

Digital subtraction percutaneous angiography

DSA involves injection of a radio-opaque dye into the arterial tree. Access to the vessel, typically the common femoral artery (CFA), is achieved using the Seldinger technique and is usually done percutaneously (***Figures 61.11 and 61.12***). The images obtained are digitalised by computer and the extraneous background (bone, soft tissues, etc.) is removed to provide clearer images. The benefits of DSA are that it provides dynamic arterial flow information and can be combined with a definitive endovascular intervention when indicated. However, it is associated with potential complications, including bleeding, haematoma, false aneurysm formation, thrombosis, arterial dissection, distal embolisation, renal dysfunction and allergic reaction, which may occur in up to 5% of procedures. Furthermore, it is relatively expensive compared with other investigation modalities and its usage should be limited to patients in whom a concomitant intervention is predicted.

Computed tomography angiography and magnetic resonance angiography

The use of CTA as a minimally invasive alternative to DSA has increased as availability has improved. When used as an adjunct to DSA, CTA is beneficial where DUS is not possible (intrathoracic arteries) or produces poor images (aortoiliac segment). With increased ease of access, better image quality and modern three-dimensional image reconstruction software, CTA has become an invaluable tool when planning revascularisation procedures, enabling the surgeon to visualise and measure diseased arterial segments prior to intervention.

The major concern with CTA, in addition to the exposure to ionising radiation, is the use of iodinated contrast. A substantial proportion of patients presenting with PAD have concomitant renal dysfunction, which may be acutely exacerbated by iodinated contrast, causing contrast-induced nephropathy.

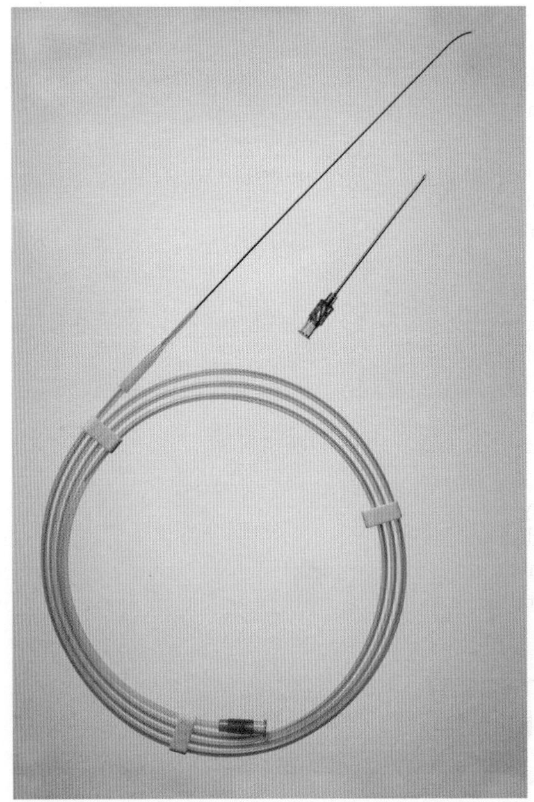

Figure 61.11 A Seldinger needle and guidewire for introducing an arterial catheter.

Sven Ivar Seldinger, 1921–1998, radiologist, Karolinska Institutet, Stockholm, Sweden, introduced percutaneous arterial catheterisation in 1956.

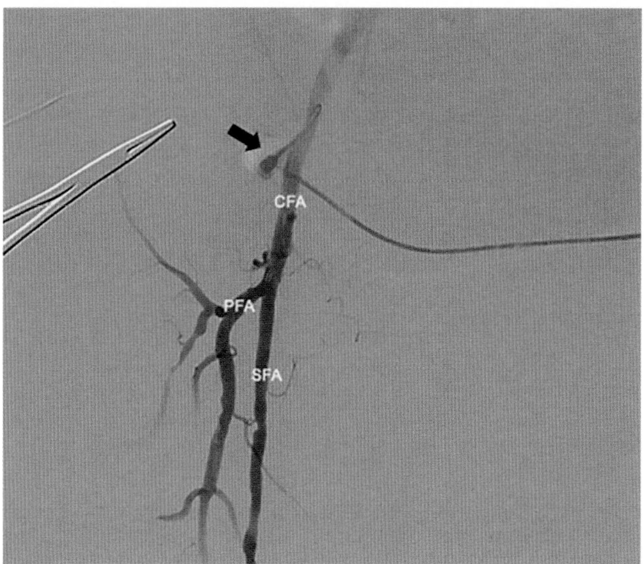

Figure 61.12 Digital subtraction angiogram of the femoral artery complex performed through a sheath (arrow) positioned percutaneously in the common femoral artery (CFA) using the Seldinger technique. PFA, profunda femoris artery; SFA, superficial femoral artery.

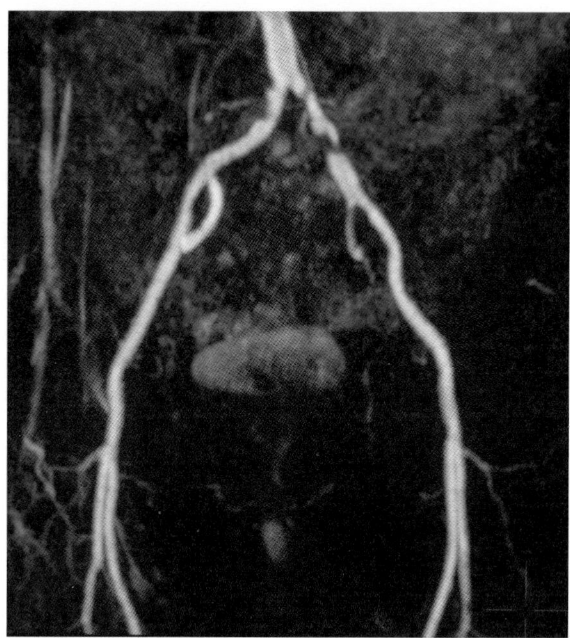

Figure 61.13 Magnetic resonance angiogram showing a tight stenosis at the midpoint of the left common iliac artery.

This is particularly pertinent to the patient with diabetes, in whom one also needs to be mindful of the interactions between contrast and certain pharmacotherapies, e.g. metformin, as their periprocedural usage may cause dangerous metabolic injury.

Magnetic resonance angiography (MRA) is a non-invasive test that avoids the need for ionising radiation and iodinated contrast, thereby having advantages over DSA and CTA. It is becoming more widely utilised, particularly as the proportion of patients with diabetes increases; this patient population typically has calcified crural vessel disease, which is difficult to assess using DUS or CTA.

MRA has the ability to separate out contrast from vessel wall calcification and has become the preferred imaging modality in many institutions.

MRA has a number of limitations and may be contraindicated in patients with claustrophobia or certain metallic implants, e.g. pacemakers. The majority of peripheral arterial stents are now compatible with MRA, although the image quality will often be downgraded, making interpretation of flow difficult. MRA uses gadolinium as a contrast agent and patients with renal dysfunction are at risk of gadolinium-induced nephrogenic systemic fibrosis (***Figure 61.13***).

Management of arterial stenosis or occlusion

General

Only one-quarter of patients presenting with intermittent claudication will experience symptomatic deterioration during their lifetime and the overall risk of progression to CLTI and amputation is small, with <5% of patients requiring amputation over a 5-year period. Patients with an ABI of <0.50 are twice as likely to deteriorate as patients with an ABI of >0.50, and a deteriorating ABI is predictive of future limb loss. For patients with rest pain or tissue necrosis, intervention is usually required to prevent major amputation.

Claudication is often a marker of silent coronary arterial disease whose extent correlates with the ABI: a decrease of 0.1 in ABI below 0.9 is associated with a 10% increase in the relative risk of a major cardiovascular event. Similarly, one-quarter of patients with claudication have significant atherosclerotic disease affecting their carotid and renal arterial systems. It is thus not surprising that the risk of having a major cardiovascular event per year in patients with claudication is >5%, and that 50% of claudicants will die within 10 years from myocardial infarction or stroke. The common modifiable risk factors for PAD mirror those for coronary artery disease: smoking, DM, hypertension and hyperlipidaemia. Therefore, the two main aims when treating claudication are (i) prevention of major cardiovascular morbidity through risk factor modification and (ii) symptom relief/improvement.

Non-surgical management

For many patients with claudication a structured exercise programme of at least 2 hours of exercise per week for 3 months in combination with smoking cessation will lead to sustained improvement in claudication distance and a reduction in cardiovascular risk. DM increases the risk and severity of claudication proportional to the duration of affliction. Strict control in combination with weight loss in obese patients is vital to reduce cardiovascular risk and prevent symptom deterioration.

Drugs

Medication may be required for diseases associated with arterial disorders, such as hypertension and diabetes; some antihypertensives (particularly β-blockers) may exacerbate claudication. Raised blood lipids require active drug treatment, but even when the lipid profile is normal a statin (3-hydroxy-3-methylglutaryl coenzyme A [HMG-CoA] reductase inhibitor) should be prescribed as it may stabilise atherosclerotic plaques and protect against cardiac death independently of baseline serum lipid levels. An antiplatelet agent is also necessary: global guidelines recommend 75 mg per day of clopidogrel or 75 mg per day of aspirin as an alternative. Other agents, such as vasodilators, are unlikely to provide either significant or sustained benefit. Drugs are now available to help with smoking cessation.

Transluminal angioplasty and stenting

Arterial occlusive disease may be treated by inserting a balloon catheter into an artery and inflating it within a stenosed or occluded segment (***Figures 61.14 and 61.15***). This technique is suitable for patients with claudication, rest pain or tissue necrosis (***Figures 61.16 and 61.17***). Following percutaneous femoral artery puncture under local anaesthetic a guidewire is inserted and negotiated through the stenosis or occlusion under fluoroscopic control. A balloon catheter is positioned within the lesion over the guidewire and inflated at high pressure for approximately 30 seconds. Satisfactory dilatation of the lesion is confirmed by performing an angiogram. Percutaneous transluminal angioplasty (PTA) has proved very successful in dilating the iliac and femoropopliteal segments; the results below the knee are less successful but improving. Long occlusions may be treated by the technique of subintimal angioplasty, in which the guidewire crosses the lesion in the subintimal space (in the arterial wall) and a new lumen is created by inflation of the balloon. Complications occur in about 5% of cases and include failure, haematoma, bleeding, thrombosis and distal embolisation; these may impact on the surgeon's ability to perform a subsequent open surgical revascularisation procedure.

If the vessel fails to stay adequately dilated (often caused by elastic recoil of the artery), it may be possible to hold the lumen open using a metallic stent (***Figures 61.18 and 61.19***). This may be introduced on a balloon catheter and expanded

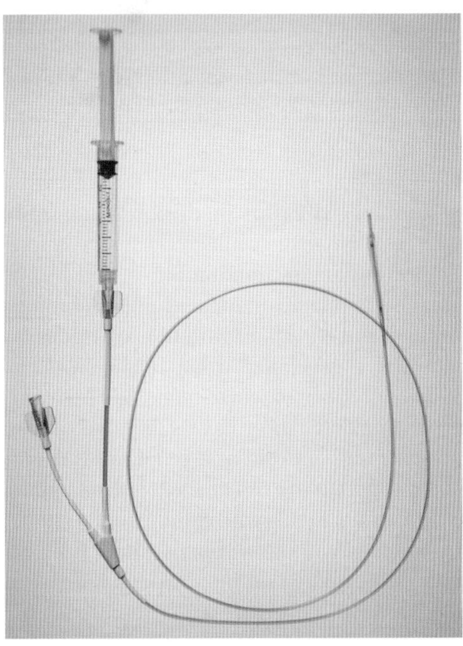

Figure 61.14 Balloon catheter for percutaneous transluminal angioplasty.

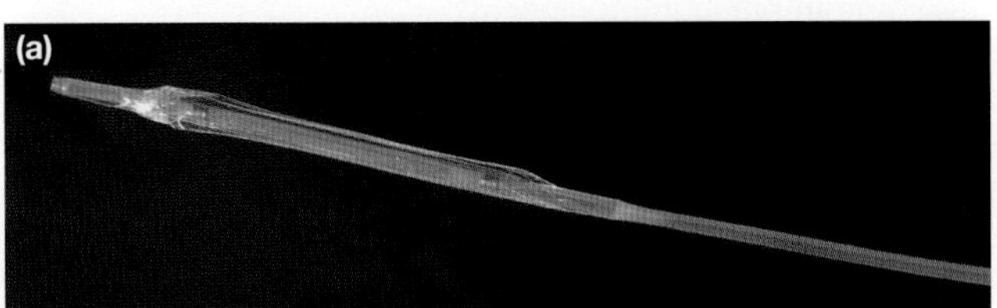

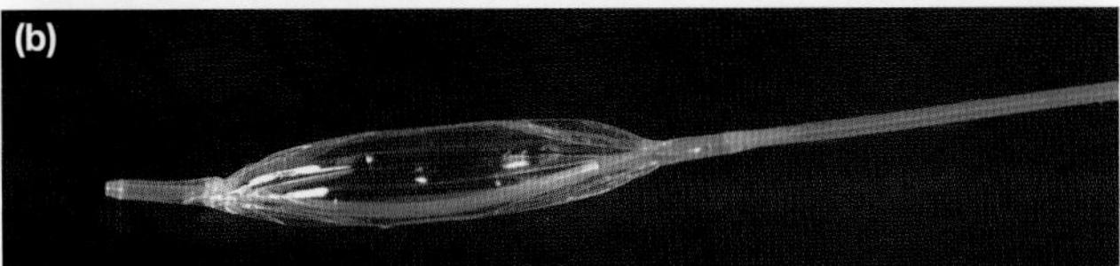

Figure 61.15 (a) Catheter balloon deflated; **(b)** balloon inflated.

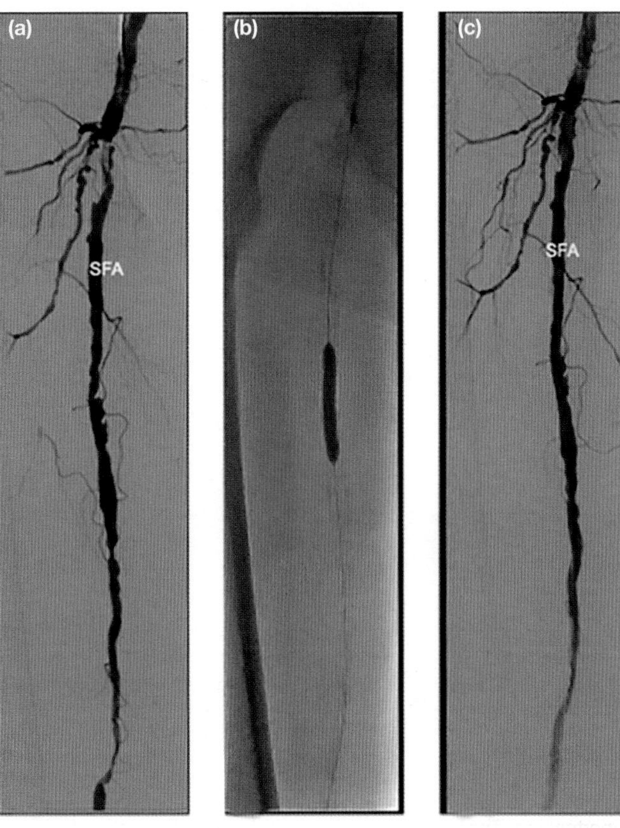

Figure 61.16 (a) Digital subtraction angiogram (DSA) demonstrating multiple stenoses within the superficial femoral artery (SFA). **(b)** Balloon angioplasty of the SFA. **(c)** Postangioplasty DSA of the SFA demonstrating improvement in the previously stenotic regions. This technique can be carried out under local anaesthesia using the Seldinger technique of percutaneous arterial puncture. It is therefore especially useful in the treatment of patients who are medically unfit for major bypass surgery.

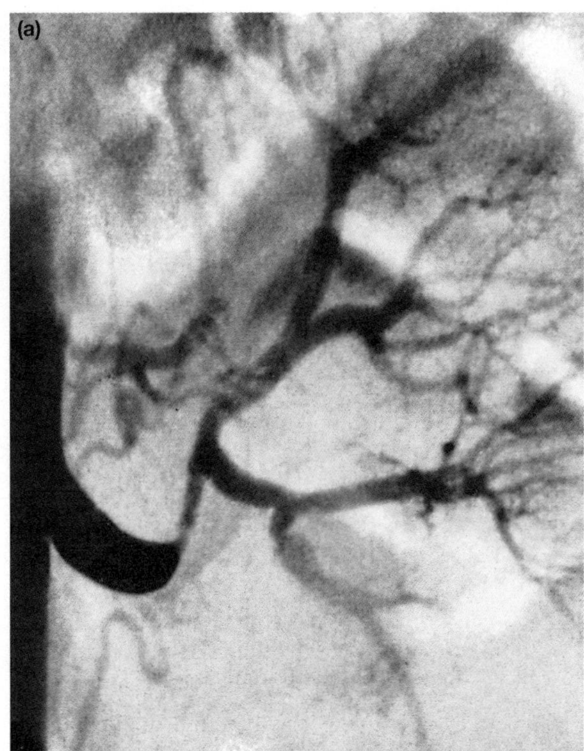

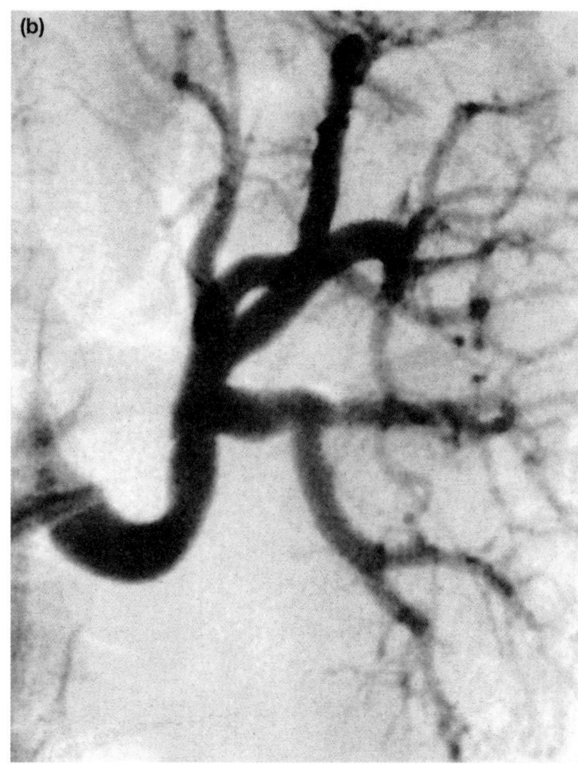

Figure 61.17 Before **(a)** and after **(b)** balloon dilatation of a severely stenosed left renal artery in a 20-year-old woman with uncontrollable hypertension. The patient's blood pressure fell to normal after the procedure. The stenosis was probably due to fibromuscular hyperplasia, but no tissue was available for histological diagnosis.

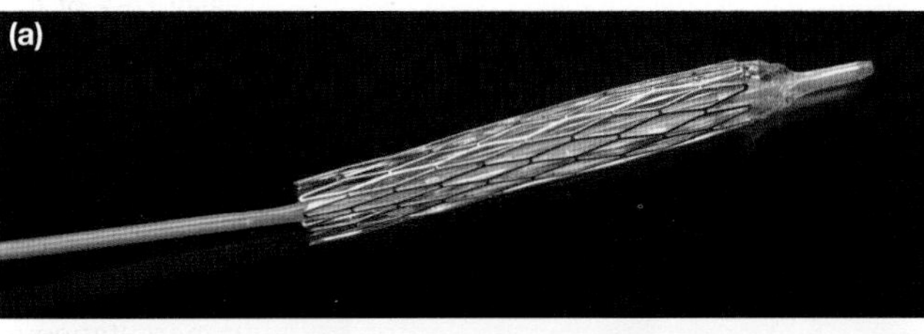

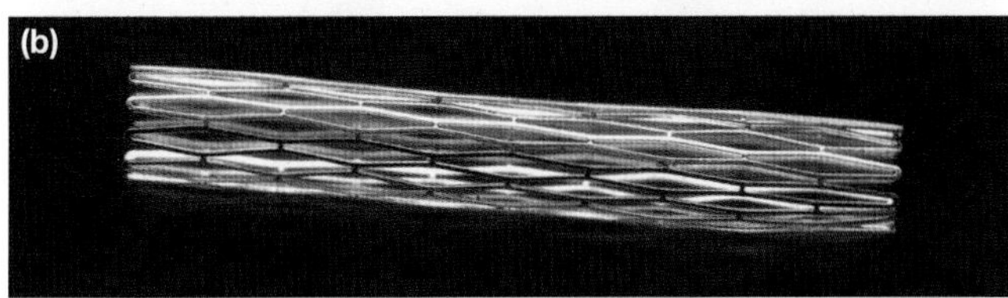

Figure 61.18 (a) A balloon catheter carrying a stent; **(b)** the expanded stent.

by balloon inflation. Alternatively, a self-expanding (typically nitinol) stent may be used; this is contained inside a plastic sheath and deployed by withdrawal of the sheath.

Operations for arterial stenosis or occlusion

Site of disease and type of operation

Surgical operations are usually reserved for patients with severe symptoms (CLTI or lifestyle-limiting claudication) where angioplasty has failed or is not possible. Aortoiliac occlusion responds well to aortobifemoral bypass (***Figure 61.20a***) using a Dacron graft (***Figure 61.21a***), although the operation carries a perioperative mortality and systemic morbidity (stroke, cardiorespiratory failure, renal injury) rate of about 5% and 15%, respectively. In unfit patients, an axillobifemoral bypass is an alternative, although patency rates are less. If only one iliac system is occluded, an iliofemoral or femorofemoral crossover graft may be performed.

Superficial femoral artery disease can be treated by femoropopliteal bypass (***Figure 61.20b***); long-term graft patency is determined by the quality of inflow and outflow, graft length (whether the distal anastomosis is above or below the knee) and the conduit used for the bypass. Autologous great saphenous vein (GSV) gives the best results and can be used reversed or *in situ* after valve disruption. If the GSV is not available from either leg, the lesser saphenous or arm veins may be used. If no vein is available, a prosthetic polytetrafluoroethylene (PTFE) graft may be employed (***Figure 61.21b***), although patency rates are less; many surgeons construct the lower anastomosis using a small collar of vein (Miller cuff or St Mary's boot) between the PTFE and the recipient artery, which may improve patency. Isolated CFA or profunda disease can be treated with endarterectomy and patch (vein or prosthetic) or a short bypass in the groin.

Frequently, in patients with CLTI, particularly those with diabetes, the occlusion extends beyond the popliteal artery into the tibial (crural) vessels. Limb salvage can be attempted with a

Justin H Miller, 1924–1994, vascular surgeon, Royal Adelaide Hospital, Adelaide, Australia.

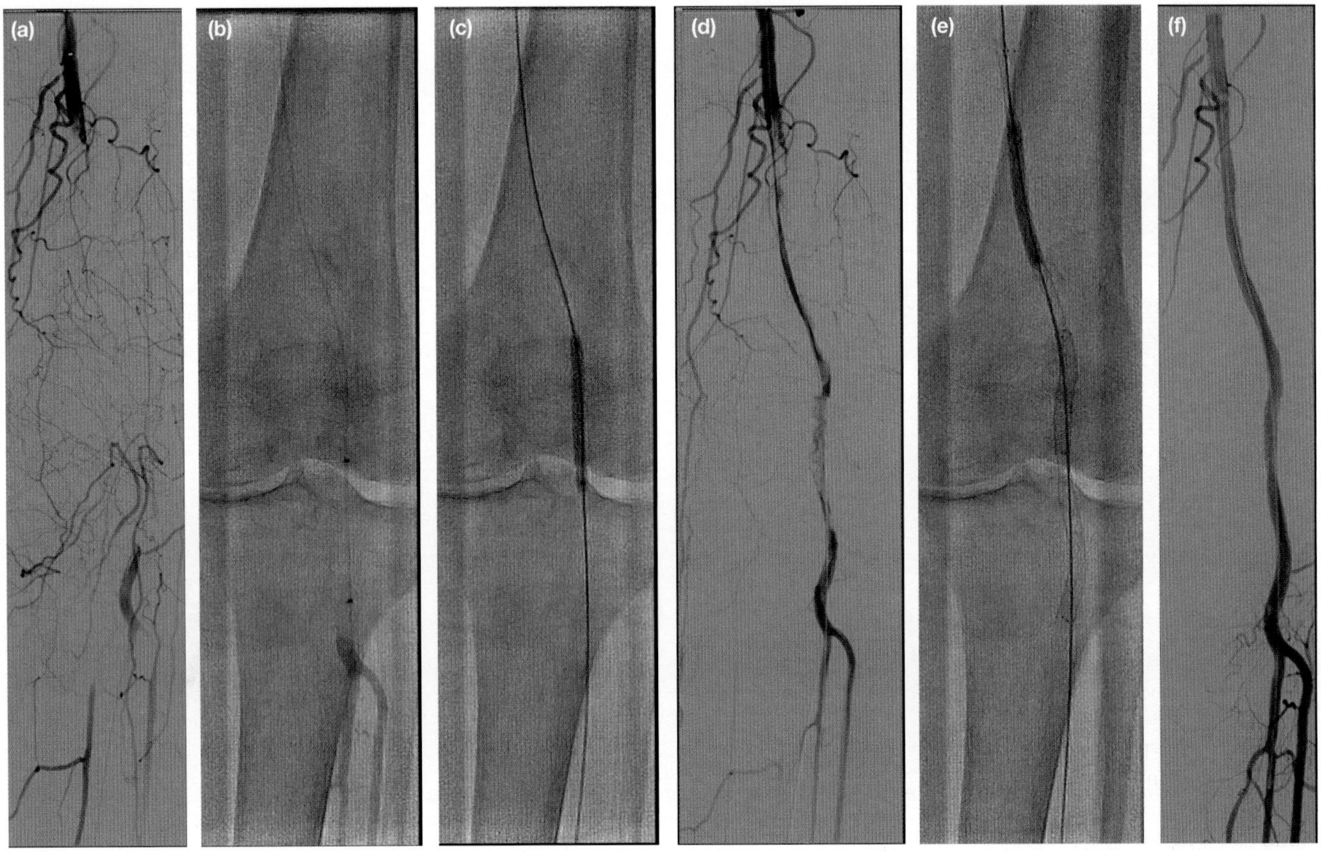

Figure 61.19 (a) Occlusion of the popliteal artery extending into the tibioperoneal trunk. **(b)** A lesion crossed with a catheter angiogram confirming intraluminal positioning beyond the occlusion. **(c)** Balloon angioplasty. **(d)** Angiogram demonstrating vessel recoil. **(e)** Stents inserted to maintain the lumen and balloon moulded. **(f)** Completion angiogram.

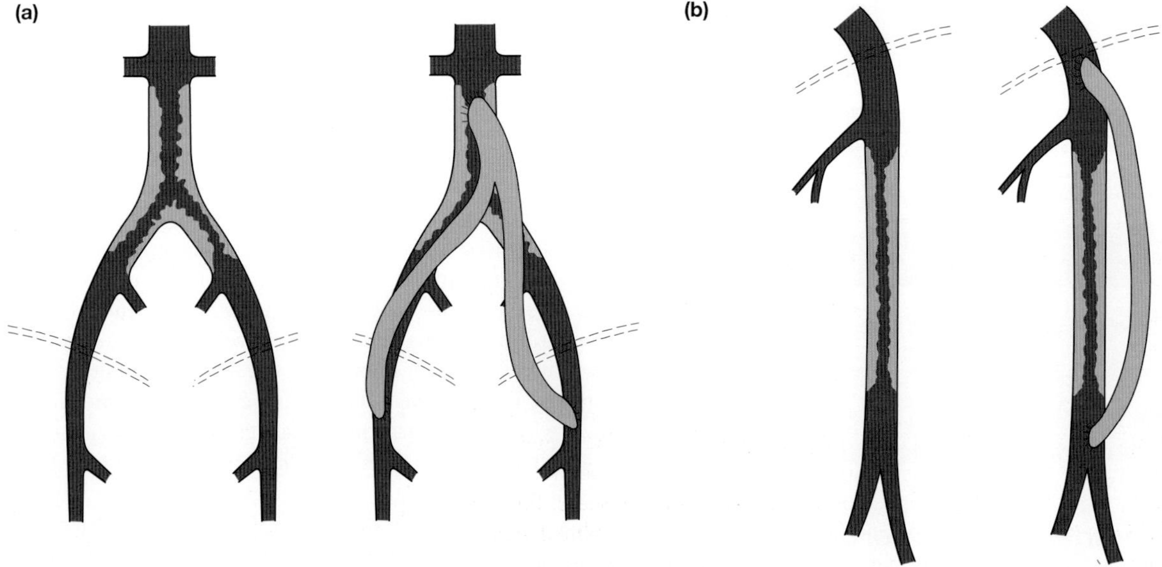

Figure 61.20 (a) Atherosclerotic narrowing of the aortic bifurcation. Aortobifemoral graft to bypass the stenosis. **(b)** Long superficial femoral artery stenosis providing poor collateral circulation. A femoropopliteal graft is used to bypass the occluded area into good 'run-off' below.

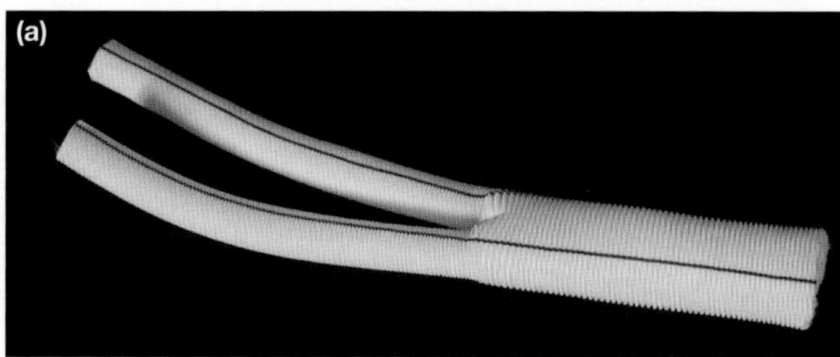

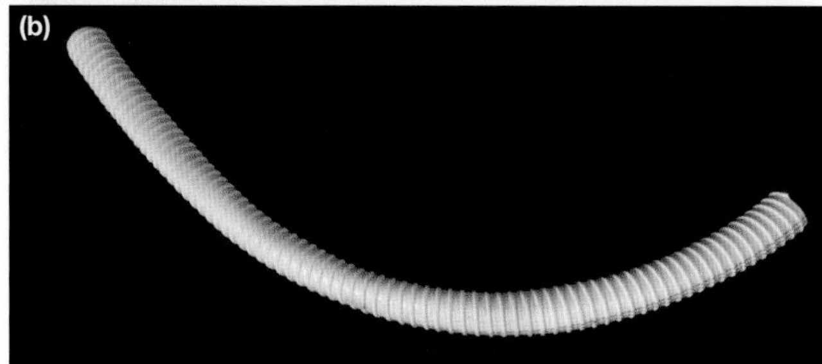

Figure 61.21 (a) A Dacron® bifurcation graft; **(b)** a polytetrafluoroethylene graft.

femorodistal bypass, with success even more dependent on the state of the run-off vessel and the quality of the vein conduit (minimum diameter 3 mm). The risk of early graft failure with limb loss is high (approximately 30% at 30 days) and these long bypasses are only appropriate for limb salvage.

Technical details

For aortobifemoral bypass, the aorta should be approached through a midline abdominal incision; a transverse abdominal incision divides the inferior epigastric vessels (important collateral vessels in patients with an occluded aorta) and should be avoided. The common femoral arteries and their branches are exposed through vertical groin incisions; an oblique or transverse groin incision may be preferred for patients with obesity. The small bowel is retracted to the right and the posterior peritoneum opened. Retroperitoneal tunnels are made from the aorta to the groins. Heparin (5000 U) is given intravenously and the vessels clamped. A vertical incision is made in the anterior aspect of the aorta, to which an obliquely cut, bifurcated Dacron graft is sutured end-to-side with a non-absorbable suture (polypropylene). The graft limbs are then fed down to the groins, where they are anastomosed end-to-side to the common femoral arteries or, if there is evidence of profunda stenosis, to an arteriotomy running from the common femoral vessel down into the profunda. The posterior peritoneum is closed over the Dacron graft to prevent adhesion of the graft to the bowel, and the abdomen and groin wounds are closed.

For femoropopliteal bypass the popliteal artery above or below the knee is exposed through a medial incision. The CFA is exposed at groin level. The GSV may be used in two different ways. First, it may be excised, its tributaries tied and the vein used in a reversed fashion so the valves do not obstruct the flow of blood. Alternatively, it may be left in place (*in situ*) and the valves disrupted with a valvulotome. The graft is sutured to the

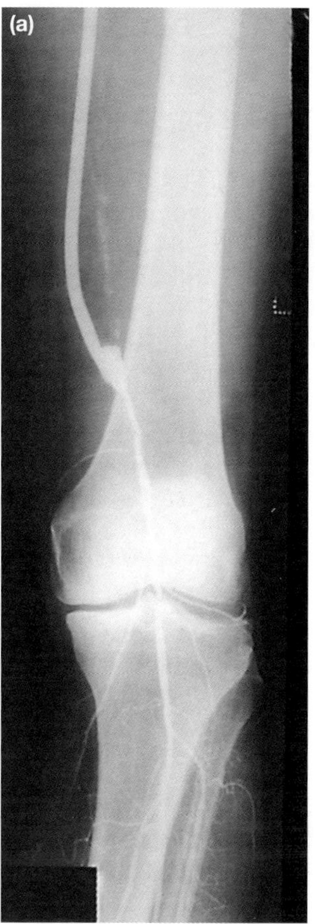

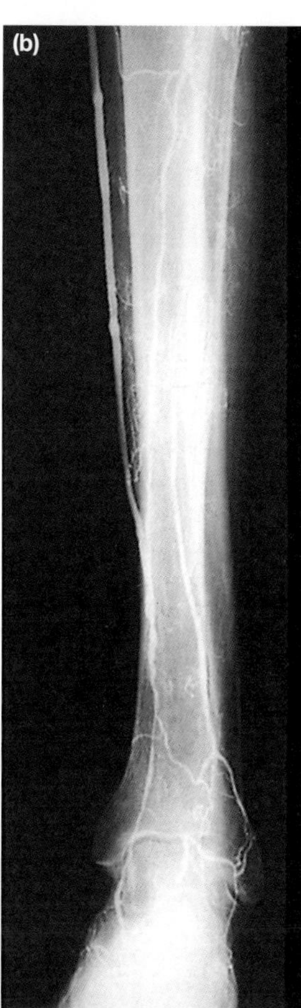

Figure 61.22 (a) Completion angiogram of a femoropopliteal bypass graft (with a Miller cuff). **(b)** Completion angiogram of a femorodistal bypass graft *in situ*.

femoral artery proximally and to the popliteal artery distally. Femorodistal bypass involves fashioning the distal anastomosis to a tibial vessel. If no suitable vein is available, prosthetic material (usually PTFE) may be used, with or without a small vein collar (Miller cuff or St Mary's boot) at its distal end (***Figure 61.22***).

A femorofemoral crossover graft involves tunnelling a prosthetic graft subcutaneously above the pubis between the groins. An axillofemoral graft is tunnelled subcutaneously between the axillary artery proximally to reach one or both of the femoral arteries; the patency rates of an axillobifemoral bypass are better than those for an axillo(uni)femoral bypass.

Results of operation

The long-term results of aortoiliac reconstructive surgery are good and are usually marred only by progressive infrainguinal disease; 90% remain patent at 5 years post surgery. Femoropopliteal surgery is less successful. Immediate postoperative success for vein bypass exceeds 90% but the 5-year patency is around 60%. PTFE bypass yields poorer results than vein bypass, with 5-year success rates of less than 50%. Although the results of femorodistal bypass are even less satisfactory, such surgery can ensure limb salvage in patients who are generally debilitated and whose expected lifespan is limited; long-term patency is less important.

Other sites of atheromatous occlusive disease

The principles of arterial surgery outlined above can be applied at other arterial sites. Carotid stenosis (at the carotid bifurcation in the neck) may cause TIAs. These short-lived mini-strokes are often recurrent and cause unilateral motor or sensory loss in the arm, leg or face, transient blindness (amaurosis fugax) or speech impairment (dysphasia). They are caused by distal embolisation of platelet thrombi that form on the atheromatous plaque into the cerebral circulation. They are a warning of impending major stroke. Patients should be assessed with a duplex scan. If a tight stenosis (>50%) is detected, carotid endarterectomy should be offered (***Figure 61.23***). This involves clamping the vessels, an arteriotomy in the common carotid artery continued up into the internal carotid artery through the diseased segment, removal of the occlusive disease (endarterectomy) and closure of the arteriotomy, often with a patch. Many surgeons also use a temporary shunt to maintain cerebral blood flow while the carotid system is clamped.

Subclavian artery stenosis may cause claudication in the arm or digital ischaemia from distal embolisation. It may be treated by angioplasty or surgical bypass. Sometimes subclavian artery lesions are associated with neck pathology, such as a cervical rib, which should be removed during arterial repair (***Figure 61.24***). Subclavian steal syndrome may occur if the first part of the subclavian artery is occluded. Arm exercise causes syncope because of reversed flow in the vertebral artery, leading to cerebral ischaemia. It can be treated by angioplasty or surgery and is rare.

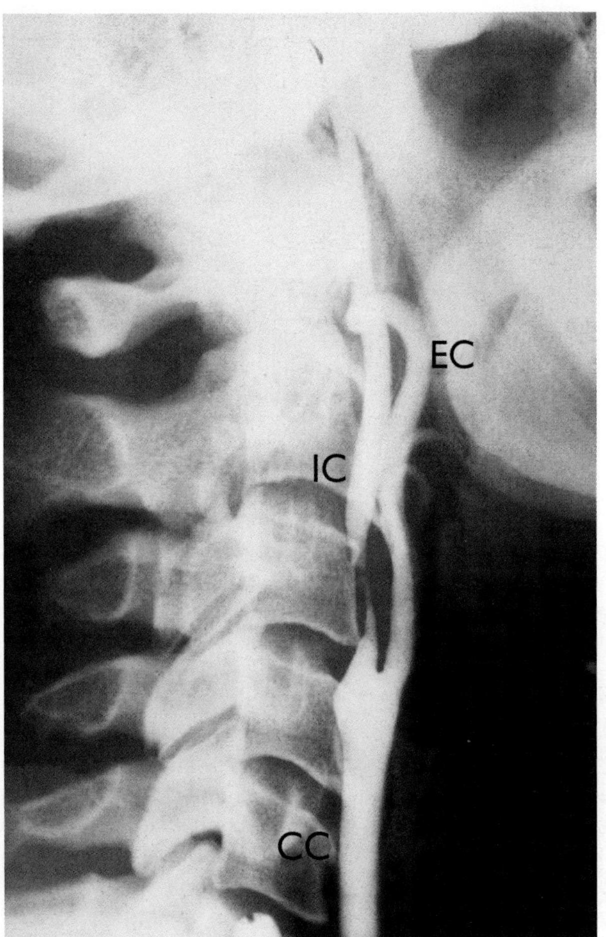

Figure 61.23 Carotid stenosis. A unilateral localised stenosis suitable for operation. CC, common carotid; EC, external carotid; IC, internal carotid.

> **Summary box 61.2**
>
> **Indications for carotid endarterectomy in symptomatic patients**
>
> 50% or greater carotid stenosis and:
> - Ipsilateral amaurosis fugax or monocular blindness
> - Contralateral facial paralysis or paraesthesia
> - Arm/leg paralysis or paraesthesia
> - Hemianopia
> - Dysphasia (if dominant hemisphere)
> - Sensory or visual inattention/neglect

Mesenteric artery occlusive disease may cause pain after eating (intestinal angina) and weight loss. In general, two of the three enteric vessels (coeliac axis, superior mesenteric artery, inferior mesenteric artery) must be occluded to produce symptoms and other intestinal disorders must be excluded before treatment with PTA, endarterectomy or bypass (***Figure 61.25***).

Renal artery stenosis may cause hypertension and eventual renal failure. Although it is possible to improve renal blood flow with PTA or surgery, the mainstays of treatment are drugs to control hypertension, diabetes, etc.

GANGRENE

Gangrene refers to the death of macroscopic portions of tissue, which turns black because of the breakdown of haemoglobin and the formation of iron sulphide. It usually affects the most distal part of a limb because of arterial obstruction (from thrombosis, embolus or arteritis). Dry gangrene occurs when the tissues are desiccated by gradual slowing of the bloodstream; it is typically the result of atheromatous occlusion of arteries. Wet gangrene occurs when superadded infection and putrefaction are present. Crepitus may be palpated as a result of infection by gas-forming organisms, commonly in diabetic foot problems, and should be considered a surgical emergency with urgent tissue debridement or amputation required.

Separation of gangrene

A zone of demarcation between the truly viable and the dead or dying tissue will eventually appear. Separation is achieved by the development of a layer of granulation tissue, which forms between the dead and the living parts. In dry gangrene, if the blood supply of the proximal tissues is adequate, the final line of demarcation appears in a matter of days and separation occurs neatly and with the minimum of infection. If bone is involved, complete separation takes longer than when soft tissues alone are affected, and the stump tends to be conical as the bone has a better blood supply than its coverings. In moist gangrene

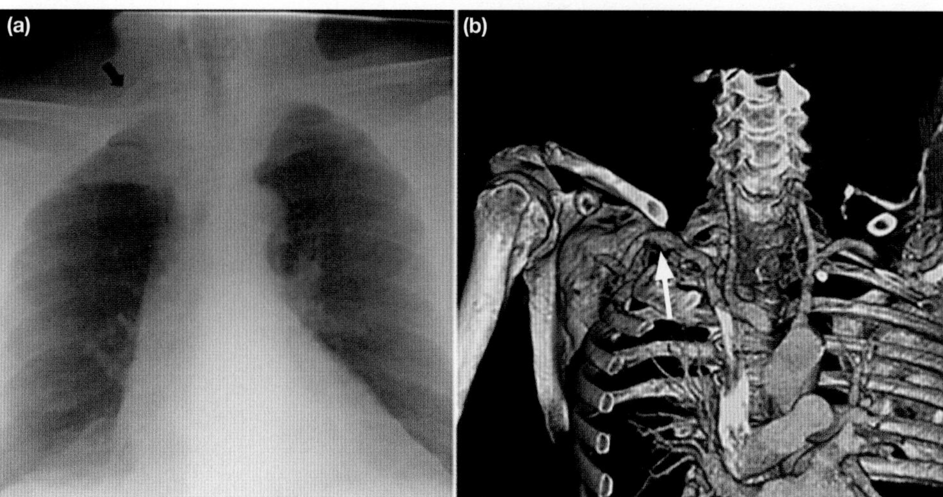

Figure 61.24 This patient presented with an ischaemic right hand. **(a)** A chest radiograph demonstrated a right cervical rib (black arrow). **(b)** A computed tomography angiogram showed stenosis of the subclavian artery (SCA) with poststenotic dilatation (lined with thrombus) (white arrow) caused by the cervical rib. The patient had been embolising from the SCA into the hand. The patient was successfully treated with cervical rib resection, repair of the SCA and distal thromboembolectomy.

the infection and suppuration extend into the neighbouring living tissue, causing the final line of demarcation to be more proximal than in dry gangrene.

If the arterial supply to the proximal living tissue is poor, the line of final demarcation is very slow to form or does not develop at all. Unless the arterial supply can be improved, the gangrene will spread to adjacent tissues or will suddenly appear as 'skip' areas further up the limb. These skip lesions may occur on the other side of the foot, on the heel, on the dorsum of the foot or even in the calf. Infection may also cause gangrene to spread proximally into areas of extensive inflammation. Local amputation in the presence of poor circulation will fail and gangrene will reappear in the wound or skin edges.

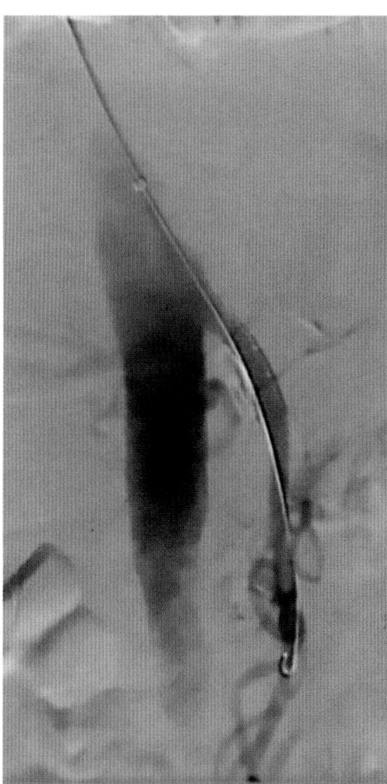

Figure 61.25 The superior mesenteric artery lesion shown in ***Figure 61.1***. It was successfully treated with angioplasty and primary stent insertion.

Treatment of gangrene

How much of a limb or digit can be salvaged depends on the blood supply proximal to the gangrene. Poor circulation should be improved by surgical revascularisation, enabling a more conservative debridement or distal amputation. However, major limb amputation may be required in the presence of life-threatening sepsis, when the blood supply cannot be improved or in patients whose limb is non-functional because of contractures, stroke, etc.

Specific varieties of gangrene

Diabetic gangrene

Diabetic gangrene is usually caused by a combination of three factors: ischaemia secondary to macrovascular disease and microvascular dysfunction; peripheral sensorimotor neuropathy (PSN), which leads to trophic skin changes; and immunosuppression caused by an excess of sugar in the tissues, which predisposes to infection (***Figure 61.26***). Macrovascular

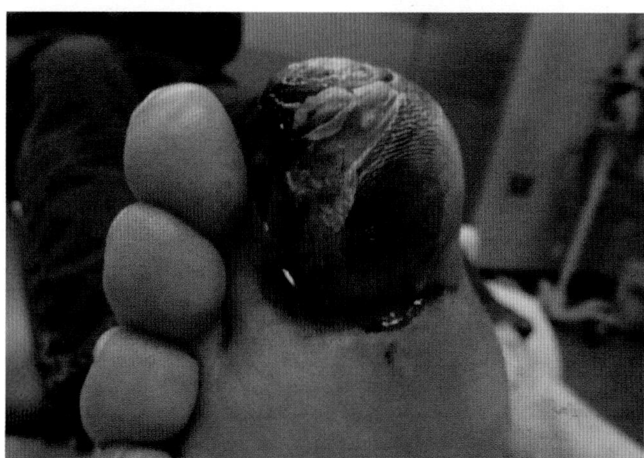

Figure 61.26 Diabetic gangrene.

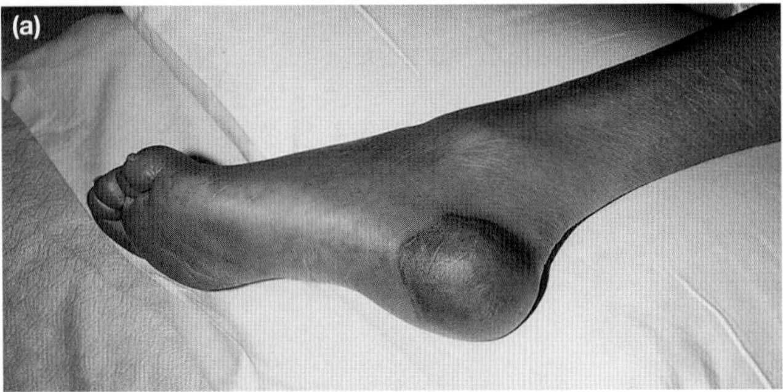

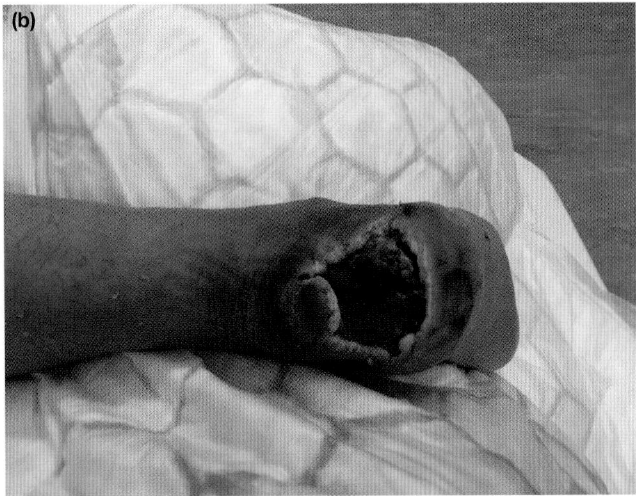

Figure 61.27 Bedsores typically appear over areas exposed to pressure, such as the sacrum and (as in this case) the heel. They can quickly deteriorate from an area of discoloration **(a)** to gross ulceration extending to the calcaneum **(b)**.

disease is atherosclerotic and typically affects the crural vessels with relative sparing of the pedal vessels, whereas increased microcirculatory shunting causes microvascular dysfunction. The PSN is usually sensory in the early phase – classically in a stocking distribution – and renders the patients at high risk of soft-tissue injury and its subsequent neglect. The PSN may extend to the joints of the foot and ankle, resulting in loss of nociceptive and proprioceptive protective reflexes and a repeated cycle of joint injury and bony destruction. Motor involvement causes an imbalance between flexors and extensor muscle groups of the foot, promoting altered foot biomechanics and abnormal pressure loading, which result in thick callosities developing on the sole of the foot.

Ischaemia and PSN act synergistically to increase the risk of diabetic foot ulceration and reduce its subsequent healing potential. Superadded infection due to poor wound care can spread rapidly and proximally in subfascial planes, leading to fulminant foot sepsis, gangrene and death.

Treatment depends on the degree of arterial involvement, which should be investigated and treated rapidly with angioplasty or surgery. The gangrene is treated by drainage of pus, liberal debridement of dead tissue and antibiotics. Unfortunately, a number of patients present with life-threatening systemic upset and should be considered for primary amputation.

Miscellaneous

Other types of gangrene commonly encountered include bedsores and frostbite. Bedsores are gangrene caused by local pressure (***Figure 61.27***), whereas frostbite is caused by exposure to cold (***Figure 61.28***). Both are preventable with adequate protective measures.

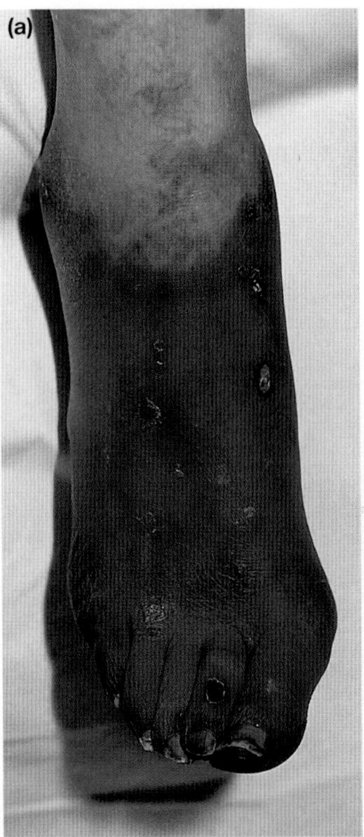

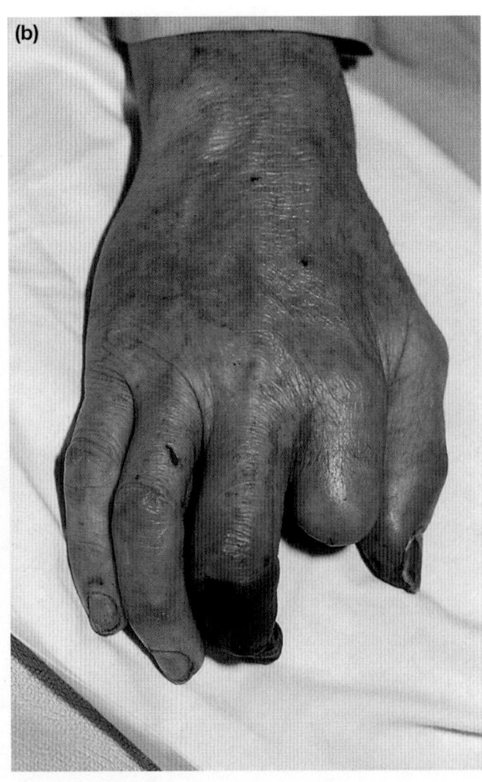

Figure 61.28 (a) Frostbite of the foot. Note the clear demarcation. **(b)** Frostbite of the middle finger in the same patient. The index finger was lost 2 years before, also from frostbite.

ACUTE ARTERIAL OCCLUSION

Sudden occlusion of an artery is usually caused by an embolus. It may also happen when thrombosis occurs on an atherosclerotic plaque, although the outcome is usually less dramatic because collaterals are likely to have developed in chronic arterial stenosis.

Embolic occlusion

An embolus is an object that has become lodged in a vessel and causes obstruction, having been carried in the bloodstream from another site. It is often a thrombus that has become detached from the heart or a more proximal vessel. Sources include the left atrium in atrial fibrillation; a left ventricular mural thrombus following myocardial infarction; vegetations on heart valves in infective endocarditis; and thrombi in aneurysms and on atherosclerotic plaques. Emboli may lodge in any organ and cause ischaemic symptoms.

- **Arm and leg** – pain, pallor, paraesthesia, paralysis and pulselessness (the five Ps of acute limb ischaemia [ALI]) (see ***Acute limb ischaemia***) (***Figure 61.29***). Acute arterial occlusion due to an embolus differs from occlusion due to thrombosis on pre-existing atheroma; in the latter case a collateral circulation has often built up over time (***Figures 61.30 and 61.31***). It is essential to differentiate between the two as they require different management.
- **Brain** – the middle cerebral artery (or its branches) is most commonly affected, resulting in TIA or stroke.
- **Retina** – amaurosis fugax is fleeting blindness caused by a minute thrombus emanating from an atheromatous plaque in the carotid artery passing into the central retinal artery. Lasting obstruction causes permanent blindness.
- **Mesenteric vessels** – possible gangrene and perforation of the corresponding loop of intestine.

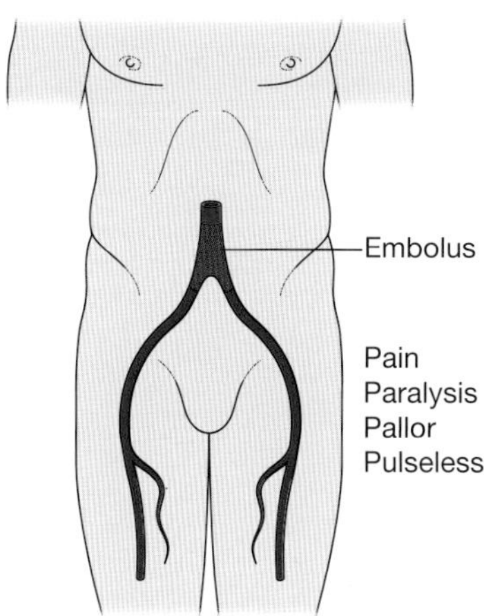

Figure 61.29 The symptoms and signs of embolism (four Ps). The fifth feature, anaesthesia, is often stated to be paraesthesia (the fifth P), but, in truth, complete loss of sensation in the toes and feet is characteristic.

Acute limb ischaemia

ALI is an emergency that requires rapid, accurate clinical assessment and emergency surgical treatment. ALI typically occurs as a result of embolic arterial occlusion or trauma, but less common causes, including thrombosed popliteal artery aneurysm and popliteal artery entrapment, should be kept in mind during patient assessment. Clinicians reviewing a patient with sudden onset leg pain should have a high index of suspicion for ALI as an incorrect diagnosis can be catastrophic for the patient; ischaemia beyond 6 hours is usually irreversible and results in limb loss.

Clinical features

Patients presenting with ALI secondary to embolism typically give no history of prior claudication and complain of the sudden development of severe pain or numbness of the limb. Bedside clinical assessment should be aimed at (i) confirming the diagnosis of ALI, (ii) assessing the severity of the limb ischaemia, and (iii) identifying the underlying cause, including an embolic source.

The skin is initially cold and pale, but as time progresses it slowly becomes mottled; first, non-fixed (blanching to pressure) and then fixed (non-blanching), indicating skin death. Neurological function deteriorates with time, progressing from paraesthesia to eventual complete loss of sensory and motor function, causing an insensate and paralysed limb (a poor prognostic sign). Muscle groups are weakened and painful; manual compression of affected muscle groups may cause pain owing to ischaemia-induced injury – rhabdomyolysis.

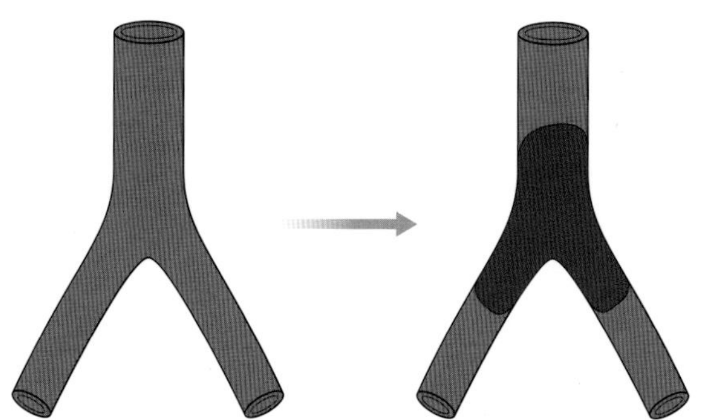

Figure 61.30 Aortic bifurcation embolus. The source of the embolus is a recent myocardial infarct or atrial fibrillation. This causes severe, dramatic symptoms.

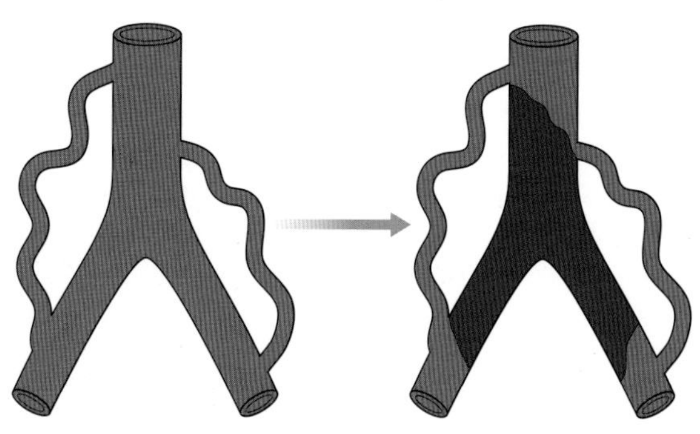

Figure 61.31 Aortic bifurcation thrombosis: claudication is worse but there is no dramatic event owing to the network of collaterals formed as a result of the insidious nature of the stenosis; acute on chronic disease.

TABLE 61.2 Rutherford's classification of acute limb ischaemia.

Grade	Category	Sensory loss	Motor deficit	Doppler signals		Prognosis
				Arterial	Venous	
I	Viable	None	None	Audible	Audible	No immediate threat
IIA	Marginally threatened	None or minimal (toes)	None	Inaudible	Audible	Salvageable if promptly treated
IIB	Immediately threatened	More than toes	Mild/moderate	Inaudible	Audible	Salvageable with immediate revascularisation
III	Irreversible	Profound or insensate	Paralysed	Inaudible	Inaudible	Limb irreversibly damaged, major tissue loss, amputation

Pulses are absent distally but the femoral pulse may be palpable, even thrusting, as distal occlusion results in forceful expansion of the artery with each pressure wave despite the lack of flow. Insonation of the pedal vessels with a hand-held Doppler may elicit faint monophasic signals or no signals at all. Assessment of flow in the limb veins, including the GSV and popliteal vein, can be useful as concurrent venous thrombosis is a very poor prognostic indicator.

Following thorough clinical examination, the limb should be classified according to the Rutherford categories of ALI: class I, viable; class IIa, marginally threatened; class IIb, immediately threatened; and class III, irreversible. The management options and urgency of treatment depend on the appropriate categorisation of the limb (*Table 61.2*).

Investigations should be undertaken as clinically indicated and may include:

- ECG to assess for myocardial infarction and/or atrial fibrillation;
- creatinine kinase to assess for rhabdomyolysis;
- renal function as rhabdomyolysis may lead to myoglobinuria and acute kidney injury;
- imaging assessment of the affected limb's arterial tree, e.g. DUS or CTA, if readily available and not likely to unnecessarily delay emergency treatment when indicated, e.g. Rutherford class IIb

A similar picture will occur in the arm with a brachial embolus.

Treatment

Because of the ensuing stasis, a thrombus can extend distally and proximally to the embolus. The immediate administration of 5000 U of heparin intravenously can reduce this extension and maintain patency of the surrounding (particularly the distal) vessels until the embolus can be treated. The relief of pain is essential because it is severe and constant. Embolectomy and thrombolysis are the treatments available for patients with limb emboli.

Embolectomy

Local or general anaesthesia may be used. The artery (usually the femoral), bulging with clot, is exposed and held in silastic vessel loops. Through a transverse incision the clot begins to extrude and is removed, together with the embolus (*Figure 61.32*), with the help of a Fogarty balloon catheter. The catheter, with its balloon tip, is introduced both proximally and distally until it is deemed to have passed the limit of the clot. The balloon is inflated and the catheter withdrawn slowly, together with any obstructing material (*Figure 61.33*). The procedure is repeated until bleeding occurs. An angiogram

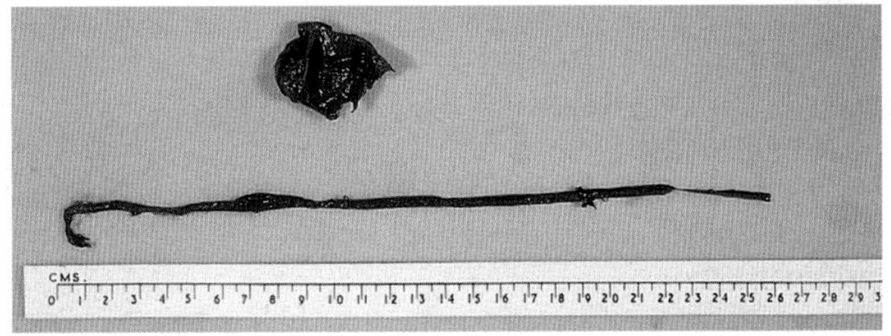

Figure 61.32 Embolic material removed from the common femoral artery, along with a long distal extension thrombus.

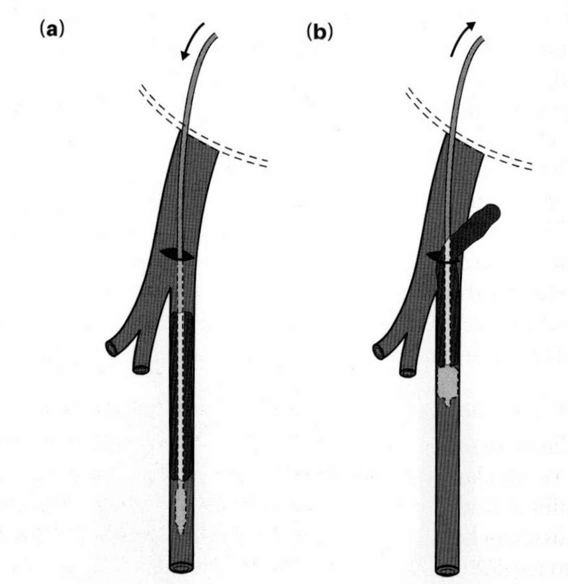

Figure 61.33 **(a)** A Fogarty catheter is inserted through an arteriotomy in the common femoral artery and fed distally down the superficial femoral artery and through the embolus. **(b)** The balloon is inflated and the catheter withdrawn, removing the embolus; the deep femoral and iliac arteries are similarly treated.

Robert Rutherford, 1931–2013, Professor of Surgery, Colorado, USA.
Thomas J Fogarty, b. 1934, surgeon, University of Oregon Medical School, Portland, OR, USA.

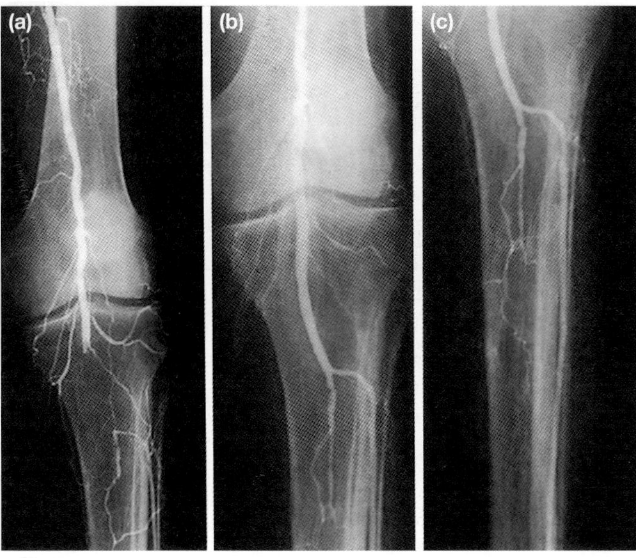

Figure 61.34 Angiogram of an occluded popliteal artery before thrombolysis **(a)**, during successful lysis **(b)** and after completion of lysis **(c)**.

may be performed in the operating theatre at the end of the procedure to ensure that flow to the distal leg has been restored. Postoperatively, heparin therapy is continued until long-term anticoagulation with warfarin is established to reduce the chance of further embolism.

Thrombolysis

If ischaemia is not so severe that immediate operation is essential, it may be possible to treat either embolus or thrombosis by intra-arterial thrombolysis (***Figure 61.34***). At arteriography of the ischaemic limb (usually via the CFA) a narrow catheter is passed into the occluded vessel and left embedded within the clot. Tissue plasminogen activator is infused through the catheter and regular arteriograms are carried out to check on the extent of lysis, which, in successful cases, is achieved within 24 hours. The method should be abandoned if there is no progression of dissolution of clot with time. There are several contraindications to thrombolysis, the most important of which are recent stroke, bleeding diathesis and pregnancy, and results in those over 80 years old are poor.

Compartment syndrome

In limbs that have been subject to sudden ischaemia followed by revascularisation, oedema is likely. Muscles swell within confined fascial compartments and this can itself be a cause of tissue ischaemia, with both local muscle necrosis and nerve damage due to pressure and systemic effects such as renal failure secondary to the liberation of muscle breakdown products.

The classical clinical picture is that of severe pain out of proportion with clinical findings that worsens with time despite appropriate analgesia. The patient often complains of numbness/paraesthesia in the distribution of nerves running within the compartment (non-myelinated type C sensory fibres are most sensitive to hypoxia). Examination of the limb reveals a tense compartment with passive flexion and extension of

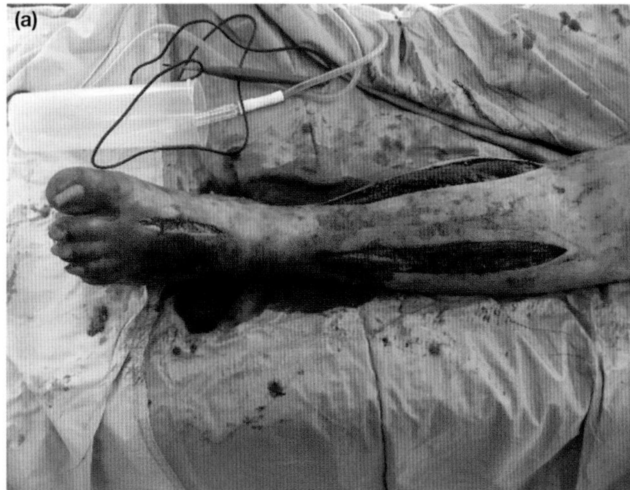

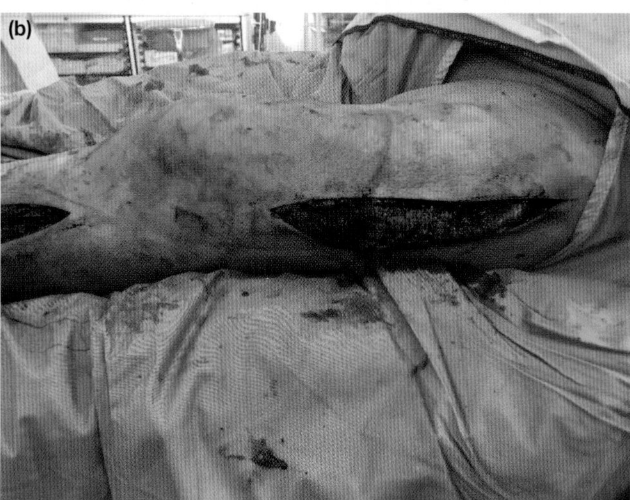

Figure 61.35 (a) Foot and calf fasciotomies; (b) thigh fasciotomy: the medial compartment rarely requires decompression

muscles causing pain. The presence of palpable pulses does not rule out compartment syndrome.

The treatment is urgent compartment fasciotomy to release the compression. The usual site for fasciotomy is the calf (especially the anterior tibial compartment), but compartment syndrome may occasionally affect the thigh, arm and foot. Liberal concomitant usage of calf with/without thigh fasciotomies following revascularisation of a prolonged ischaemic limb is advisable (***Figure 61.35***).

Acute mesenteric ischaemia

Acute mesenteric occlusion may be either thrombotic (following atheromatous narrowing) or embolic. Embolic occlusion results in sudden, severe abdominal pain, with bowel emptying (vomiting and diarrhoea) and a source of emboli present (usually cardiac). Unfortunately, the diagnosis is often only made at laparotomy with widespread infarction of the small and large bowel present; in this situation it is often fatal. Occasionally, the degree of bowel infarction is more limited; resection of the dead bowel and embolectomy of the superior mesenteric artery, or bypass surgery, can reduce the otherwise high mortality rate in these patients. A 'second look' laparotomy 24 hours later to check the viability of the bowel may be indicated.

Other forms of embolism

Infective emboli of bacteria or an infected clot may cause mycotic aneurysms, septicaemia or infected infarcts. Parasitic emboli, caused by the ova of *Taenia echinococcus* and *Filaria sanguinis hominis*, may occur in some countries. Tumour cells (e.g. hypernephroma and cardiac myxoma) are rare causes of emboli. Fat embolism may follow major bony fractures. However, it usually causes venous emboli that travel to the lungs and cause acute respiratory distress syndrome.

Air embolism

Air may be accidentally injected into the venous circulation or sucked into an open vein during head and neck surgery or a cut throat. It may also occur following Fallopian tube insufflation or illegal abortion. If a large volume of air reaches the right side of the heart it may form an airlock within the pulmonary artery and cause acute right heart failure.

The treatment of air embolism is to put the patient in a head-down (Trendelenburg) position to encourage the air to enter the veins in the lower part of the body. The patient should also be placed on the left side to help the air to float to the ventricular apex, away from the ostium of the pulmonary artery. In extreme cases air may be aspirated from the heart through a needle introduced below the left costal margin.

Therapeutic embolisation

This is used to arrest haemorrhage from the gastrointestinal, urinary, gynaecological and respiratory tracts, to treat arteriovenous malformations by blocking their arterial supply and to control the growth of unresectable tumours. Arterial embolisation requires accurate selective catheterisation using the Seldinger technique. A variety of materials may be used, including Gelfoam sponge, plastic microspheres, balloons, ethyl alcohol, quick-setting plastics and metal coils.

AMPUTATION

General

Amputation should be considered when part of a limb is dead, deadly or a dead loss. A limb is dead when arterial occlusive disease is severe enough to cause infarction of macroscopic portions of tissue, i.e. gangrene. The occlusion may be in major vessels (atherosclerotic or embolic occlusions) or in small peripheral vessels (diabetes, Buerger's disease, Raynaud's disease, inadvertent intra-arterial injection). If the obstruction cannot be reversed and the symptoms are severe, amputation is required.

A limb is deadly when the putrefaction and infection of moist gangrene spreads to surrounding viable tissues. Cellulitis and severe toxaemia are the result. Amputation is required as a lifesaving operation. Antibiotic cover should be broad and massive. Other life-threatening situations for which amputation may be required include gas gangrene (as opposed to simple infection), neoplasm (such as osteogenic sarcoma) and arteriovenous fistula.

A limb may be deemed a dead loss in the following circumstances: first, when there is relentless severe rest pain without gangrene and reconstruction is not possible – amputation will improve quality of life; second, when a contracture or paralysis makes the limb impossible to use and renders it a hindrance; and third, when there is major unrecoverable traumatic damage.

Summary box 61.3

Indications for amputation

Dead limb
- Gangrene

Deadly limb
- Wet gangrene
- Spreading cellulitis
- Arteriovenous fistula
- Other (e.g. malignancy)

'Dead loss' limb
- Severe rest pain with unreconstructable critical leg ischaemia
- Paralysis
- Other (e.g. contracture, trauma)

Distal and transmetatarsal amputation

In patients with small-vessel disease, typically caused by DM, gangrene of the toes may occur with relatively good blood supply to the surrounding tissues. In such circumstances local amputation of the digits can result in healing. However, if the metatarsophalangeal joint region is involved, a ray excision is required, taking part of the corresponding metatarsal bone and cutting tendons back. Most surgeons leave the wound open. Early mobility aids drainage, provided that cellulitis is not present. For less extensive gangrene, if amputation is taken through a joint, healing is improved by removing the cartilage from the joint surface. A transmetatarsal amputation may be required when several toes are affected but the proximal circulation is adequate. The wound may be closed with a viable long plantar flap or left open (***Figure 61.36***).

Gabrielle Falloppio (Fallopius), 1523–1563, Professor of Anatomy, Surgery and Botany, Padua, Italy.
Friedrich Trendelenburg, 1844–1924, Professor of Surgery, successively at Rostock, Bonn and Leipzig, Germany.
Leo Buerger, 1879–1943, Professor of Urologic Surgery, New York Polyclinic Medical School, New York, NY, USA, described thromboangiitis obliterans in 1908.
Maurice Raynaud, 1834–1881, physician, Hôpital Lariboisière, Paris, France, described this condition in 1862.

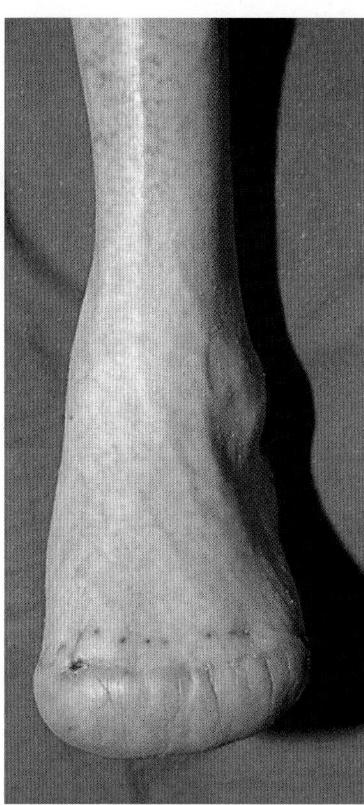

Figure 61.36 Transmetatarsal amputation for diabetic gangrene of the toes.

Major amputation

Choice of operation

The major choice is between an above- and below-knee operation. A below-knee amputation preserves the knee joint and gives the best chance of walking again with a prosthesis (***Figure 61.37***). However, an above-knee amputation is more likely to heal and may be appropriate if the patient has no prospect of walking again. If the femoral pulse is absent, the amputation should be above the knee. Unfortunately, the presence of a femoral pulse does not guarantee healing of a below-knee amputation and sometimes a failed below-knee amputation may require revision to an above-knee procedure.

For above- or below-knee amputations with a good stump shape, it is possible to hold a prosthesis in place simply by suction, without any cumbersome and unsightly straps. The stump should be of sufficient length to give the required leverage, i.e. not less than 8 cm below the knee (preferably 10–12 cm) and not less than 20 cm above the knee.

Through-knee or knee disarticulation has regained popularity as an alternative to above-knee amputation if soft-tissue viability permits. This amputation preserves the full length of the femur and patella and provides a long mechanical lever that is controlled by stronger muscles as the line of muscle transection is distal and occurs through fascial tissue as opposed to thick muscular bellies, as is the case with an above-knee amputation. The bulbous nature of the amputation end, initially thought a hindrance for subsequent prosthetic fitting, is now seen as beneficial as it allows for a self-suspending prosthetic that is less likely to rotate than an above-knee amputation prosthetic. For patients unlikely to mobilise with a prosthetic, e.g. elderly patients or patients with bilateral amputations, the increased length of the stump provides better counterweight to the torso, enabling better core stability.

Postoperative care of an amputee

Opiate pain relief should be given regularly. Care of the good limb must not be forgotten – a pressure ulcer on the remaining foot will delay mobilisation despite satisfactory healing of the stump. Exercise and mobilisation are of the greatest importance. After surgery, flexion deformity must be prevented and exercises started to build up muscle power and coordination. Mobility is progressively increased with walking between bars and the use of an inflatable artificial limb, which allows weight bearing to be started before a pylon or temporary artificial limb is ready (***Figure 61.38***). Early assessment of the home is part of the programme; this allows time for minor alterations, such as the addition of stair rails, movement of furniture to give support near doors and provision of clearance in confined passages.

Complications

Early complications include haemorrhage, which requires return to the operating room for haemostasis; haematoma, which requires evacuation; and infection, usually in association with a haematoma. Any abscess must be drained and appropriate antibiotics given. Gas gangrene can occur in a mid-thigh stump from faecal contamination. Wound dehiscence and gangrene of the flaps are caused by ischaemia; a higher amputation may be necessary. Amputees are at risk of deep vein thrombosis and pulmonary embolism in the early postoperative period and prophylaxis with subcutaneous heparin is essential.

Later complications include pain resulting from unresolved infection (sinus, osteitis, sequestrum), a bone spur, a scar adherent to bone and an amputation neuroma. Patients frequently remark that they can feel the amputated limb (phantom limb) and sometimes remark that it is painful (phantom pain). The surgeon's attitude should be one of firm reassurance that this sensation will almost certainly disappear with time; gabapentin or amitriptyline may help. Other late complications include ulceration of the stump because of pressure effects of the prosthesis or increased ischaemia.

ANEURYSM

General

Dilatations of localised segments of the arterial system are called aneurysms when there is a ≥50% increase in the diameter of the vessel; below 50% they are termed ectatic. They can either be true aneurysms, containing the three layers of the arterial wall (intima, media, adventitia) in the aneurysm sac, or false aneurysms, having a single layer of fibrous tissue as the wall of the sac, e.g. aneurysm following trauma. Aneurysms can also be grouped according to their shape (fusiform,

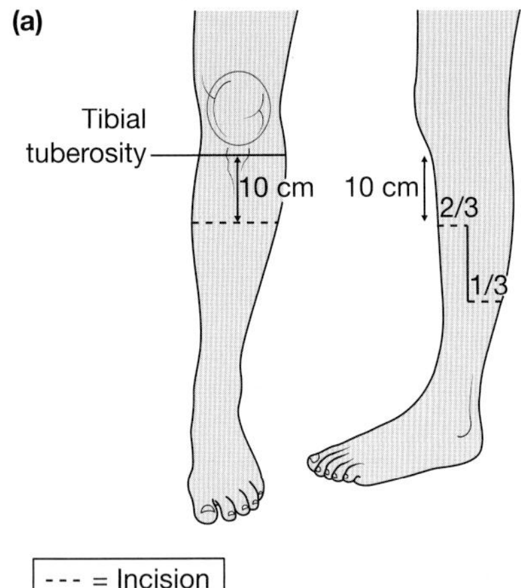

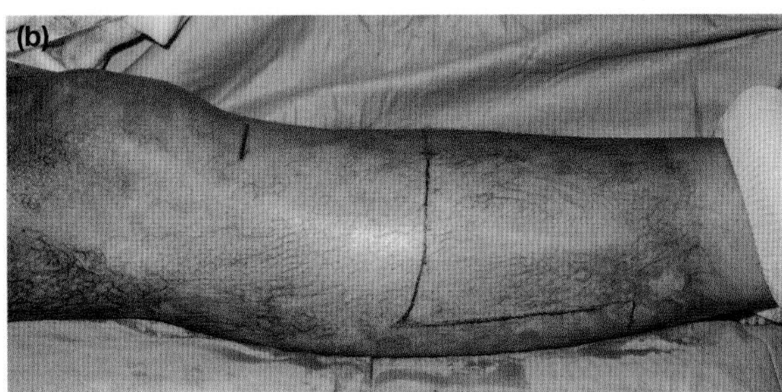

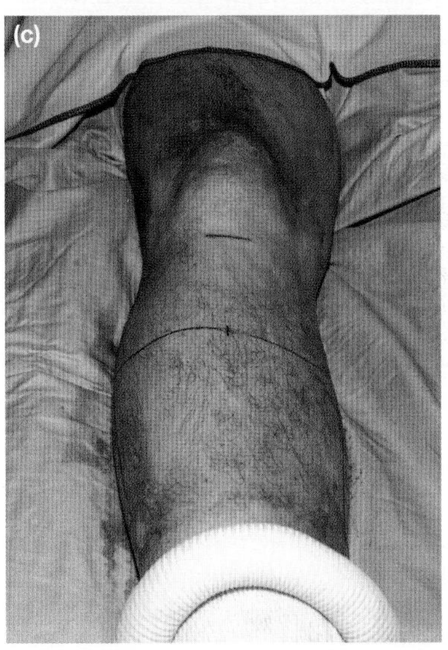

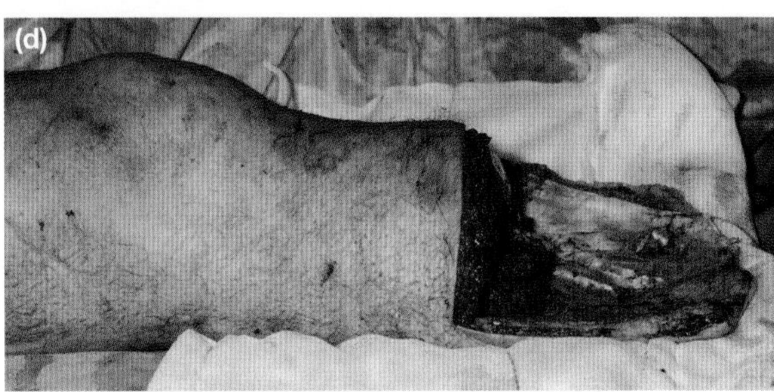

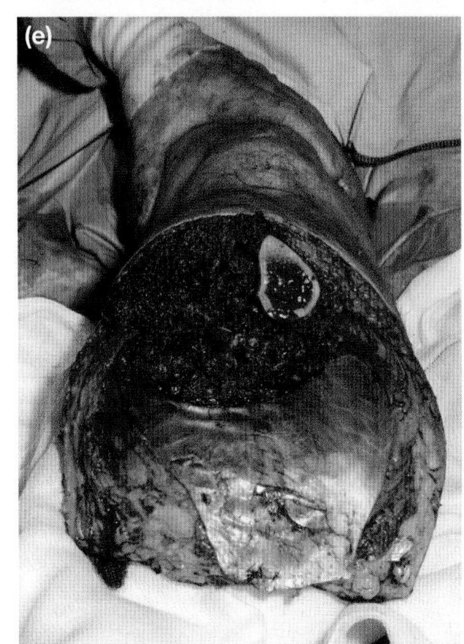

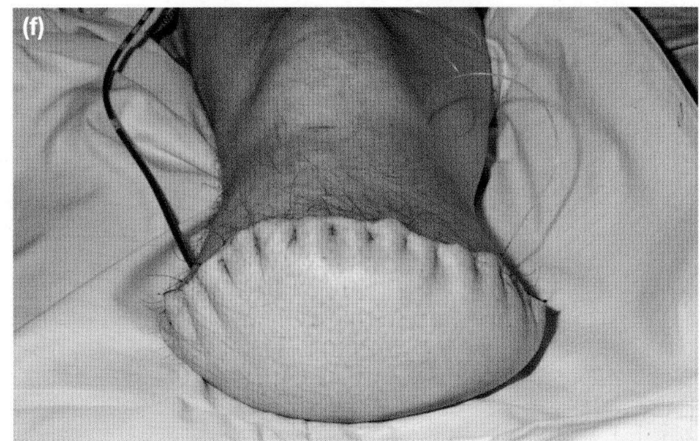

Figure 61.37 **(a)** Schematic representation of operative markings for a long posterior flap below-knee amputation. **(b)** Lateral view of operative markings. **(c)** Anterior view of operative markings. **(d)** Lateral view following removal of the leg. **(e)** Anterior view following removal of the leg. **(f)** Wound closure with a suction drain and local anaesthetic infusion 'stump' catheter.

saccular) or their aetiology (atheromatous, traumatic, mycotic, etc.). The term mycotic is a misnomer because, although it indicates infection as the cause of the aneurysm, it is due to bacteria, not fungi. Aneurysms may occur in the aorta or in the iliac, femoral, popliteal, subclavian, axillary, carotid, cerebral, mesenteric, splenic and renal arteries and their branches. The majority are true fusiform atherosclerotic aneurysms.

Clinical features

The majority of arterial aneurysms are asymptomatic at the time of identification and are often identified during routine health checks or investigations for other pathologies. Aneurysms measuring twice the size of the corresponding normal vessel are at increased risk of becoming symptomatic. The symptoms relate to the vessel affected and the tissues it supplies and occur as a result of compression of surrounding structures, thrombosis, rupture or the release of emboli. Many aneurysms of clinical significance can be palpated and, typically, an expansile pulsation is felt. Transmitted pulsation through a mass lesion, cyst or abscess lying adjacent to a large artery may be mistaken for aneurysmal pulsation. Before incising a swelling believed to be an abscess it is essential to make sure that it does not pulsate. Finally, a tortuous (and often

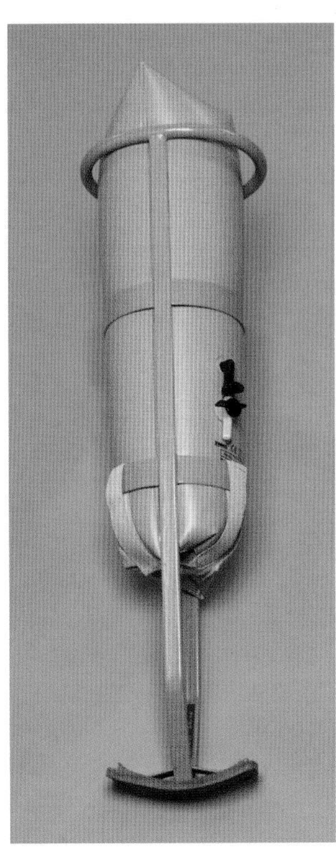

Figure 61.38 Inflatable artificial limb.

Summary box 61.4

Classification of aneurysms

Wall
- True (three layers: intima, media, adventitia)
- False (single layer of fibrous tissue)

Morphology
- Fusiform
- Saccular

Aetiology
- Atheromatous
- Mycotic (bacterial rather than fungal)
- Collagen disease
- Traumatic

ectatic) artery, usually the innominate or carotid, may seem like an aneurysm to the inexperienced clinician.

Abdominal aortic aneurysm

Abdominal aortic aneurysm is by far the most common type of large-vessel aneurysm and is found in 2% of the population at autopsy; 95% have associated atheromatous degeneration and 95% occur below the renal arteries. Most remain asymptomatic until rupture occurs; the risk of rupture increases with increasing size (diameter) of the aneurysm. Asymptomatic aneurysms are found incidentally on physical examination, radiography or ultrasonography investigation. A UK national screening programme for abdominal aortic aneurysm commenced in 2009 offering an ultrasonography scan to men in their 65th year. Symptomatic aneurysms may cause minor symptoms, such as back and abdominal discomfort, before sudden, severe back and/or abdominal pain develops from expansion and rupture. Rarely, symptoms may occur as a result of erosion or compression of surrounding structures, e.g. aortoenteric fistula or ureteric obstruction.

Asymptomatic abdominal aortic aneurysm

An asymptomatic abdominal aortic aneurysm (***Figure 61.39***) in an otherwise fit patient should be considered for repair if >55 mm in diameter, measured by ultrasonography in the anteroposterior plane. The annual incidence of rupture rises exponentially as the aneurysm size passes 55 mm: ≤1% are in aneurysms that are <55 mm in diameter, 5–10% are in those that are 55–60 mm in diameter and ~25% are in those that are ≥70 mm in diameter. Assuming that open elective surgery (transabdominal) carries a 5% mortality rate, the balance is in favour of elective operation once the maximum diameter is >55 mm, provided there is no major comorbidity. Regular ultrasonography surveillance is indicated for asymptomatic aneurysms <55 mm in diameter.

Investigations

Full blood count, electrolytes, liver function tests, coagulation tests and blood lipid estimation should be performed. Blood should be cross-matched a few days prior to surgery. Many

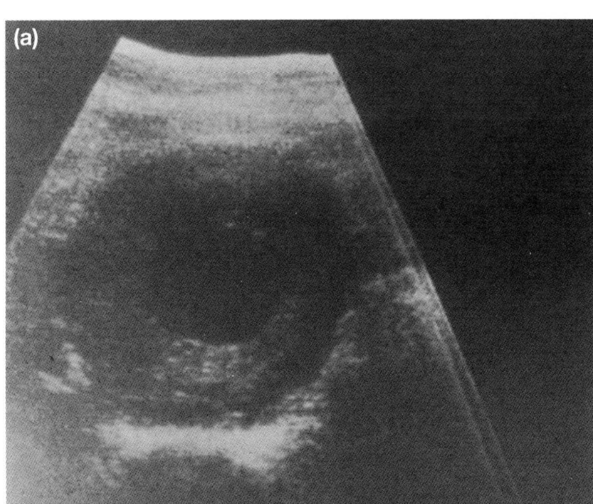

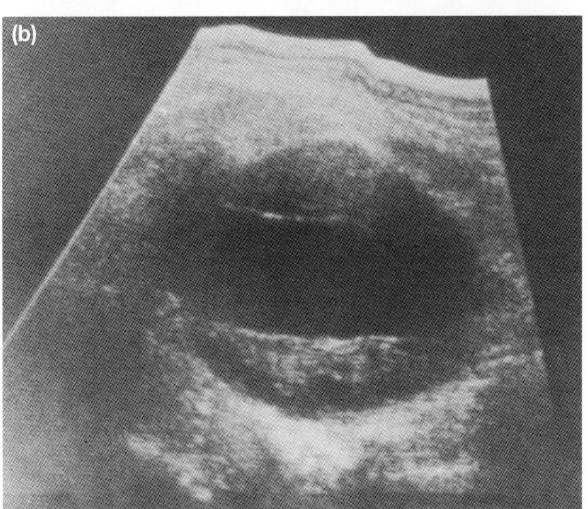

Figure 61.39 Ultrasonogram of an aortic aneurysm showing the large clot-filled sac with a small central lumen (transverse and longitudinal scans).

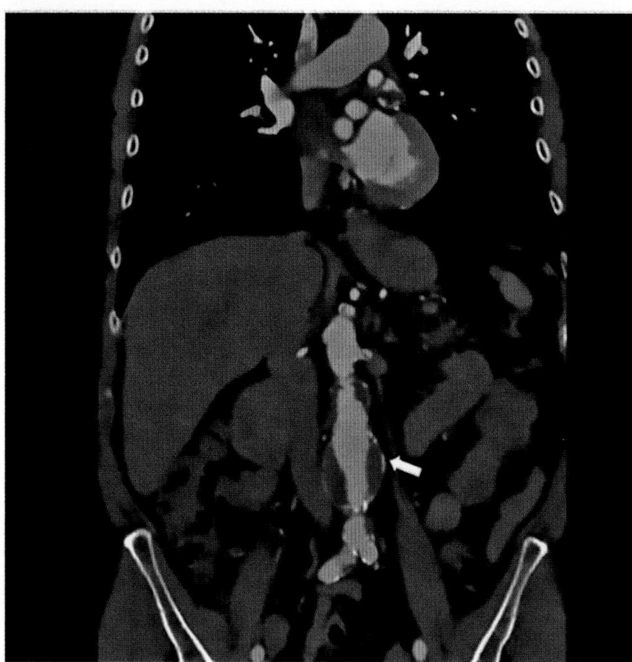

Figure 61.40 Computed tomography of the abdomen showing an infrarenal aortic aneurysm in the coronal plane (arrow). Blood flowing through the thrombus-containing sac is enhanced with contrast agent and appears white.

patients now have an anaesthetic assessment and the need for cardiac and respiratory function tests is decided at this time. ECG and chest radiographs are essential; further assessment may include echocardiograph, cardiopulmonary exercise testing and spirometry.

The morphology of the aneurysm is best assessed by computed tomography (CT) scan; this can be reconstructed on imaging software to create a three-dimensional model of the aneurysm (***Figures 61.40 and 61.41***). Seventy-five per cent of aneurysms are suitable for endovascular (minimally invasive) repair, usually via the femoral arteries in the groin. If lower limb pulses are absent, there may be associated arterial occlusive disease that should be assessed by DUS initially. Further assessment with CT, MRA or digital subtraction angiography may be required and angioplasty may be appropriate. The aneurysm is often filled with circumferential clot (***Figure 61.42a***) that produces a falsely narrowed appearance on DSA (***Figure 61.42b***); this method should not therefore be used to assess aneurysm size.

Choice of operation: open or endovascular repair

In recent years there has been much discussion regarding the optimal way to treat an abdominal aortic aneurysm with both open surgical repair and endovascular aneurysm repair (EVAR) having vocal advocates in the scientific literature. The National Institute for Health and Care Excellence (NICE) in the UK published guidelines in 2020 recommending open surgical repair unless contraindicated, reserving EVAR for high-risk patients or those with a hostile abdomen. This compares to the European Society for Vascular Surgery 2019 guidelines, which recommend EVAR as the first-line treatment option with open surgical repair to be considered for patients with long life expectancy. Pragmatically, the clinician should be prepared to undertake what they and the patient (after a detailed conversation) agree to be the best option, taking into account the skillset and resource availability and often, unfortunately, the financial constraints of the patient or healthcare system.

Open aneurysm repair

Under general anaesthesia, with the patient lying supine, a full-length midline or supraumbilical transverse incision is made. The small bowel is lifted to the patient's right and the aorta identified. The posterior peritoneum overlying the aorta is opened and the upper limit of the aneurysm identified. The aorta immediately above the dilatation is exposed; this is generally just inferior to the left renal vein and renal arteries (***Figure 61.43***). The common iliac arteries are then exposed and clamps applied above and below the lesion.

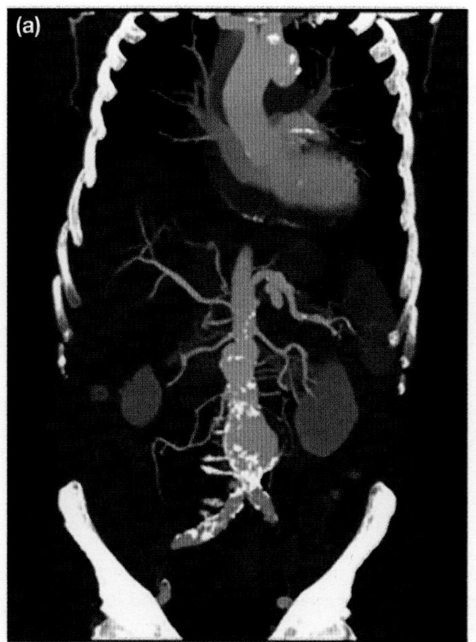

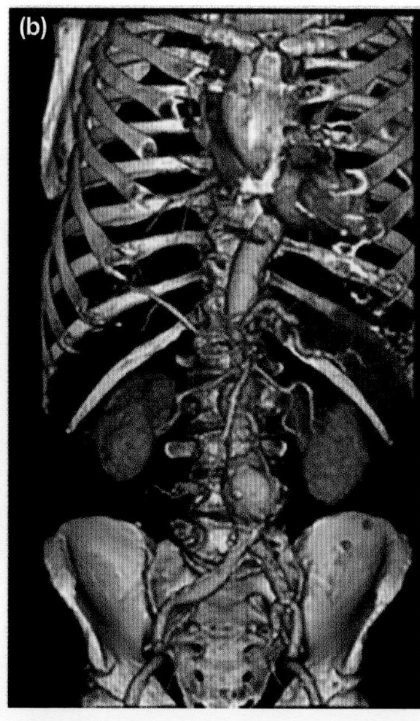

Figure 61.41 (a) Maximum intensity projection reconstruction of an aortic aneurysm from a spiral computed tomogram. **(b)** Three-dimensional reconstruction of an abdominal aortic aneurysm.

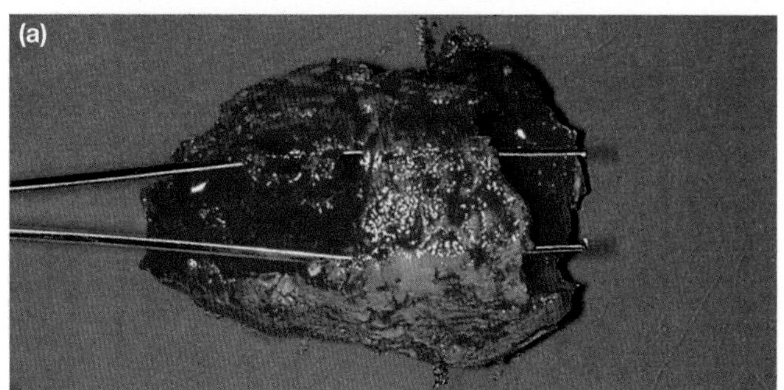

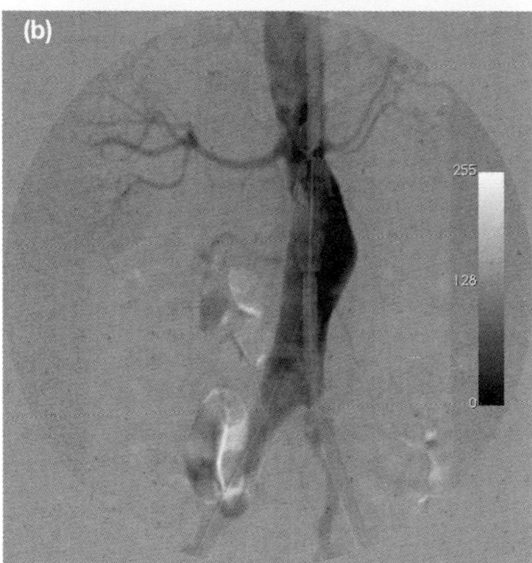

Figure 61.42 (a) Thrombus removed from an abdominal aortic aneurysm; this thrombus is the reason an angiogram may give a false impression of aneurysm diameter on digital subtraction angiography (b).

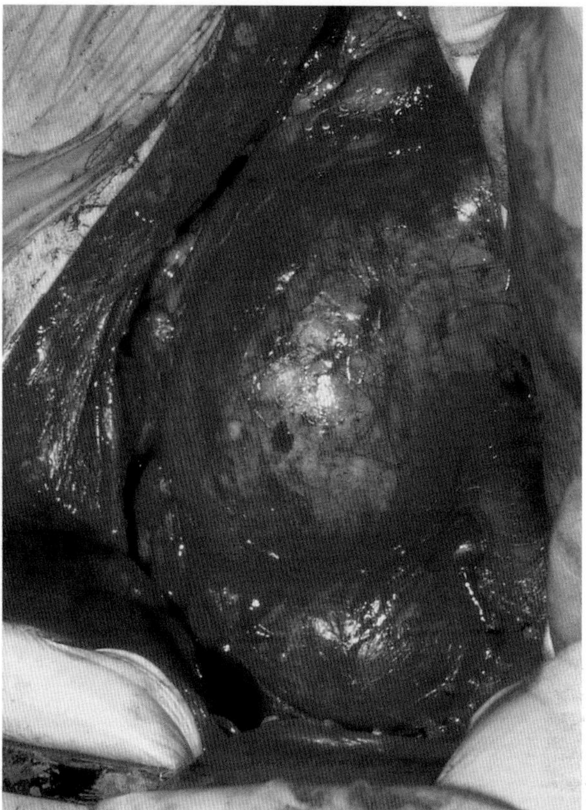

Figure 61.43 Operative appearance of a large, non-ruptured infrarenal abdominal aortic aneurysm.

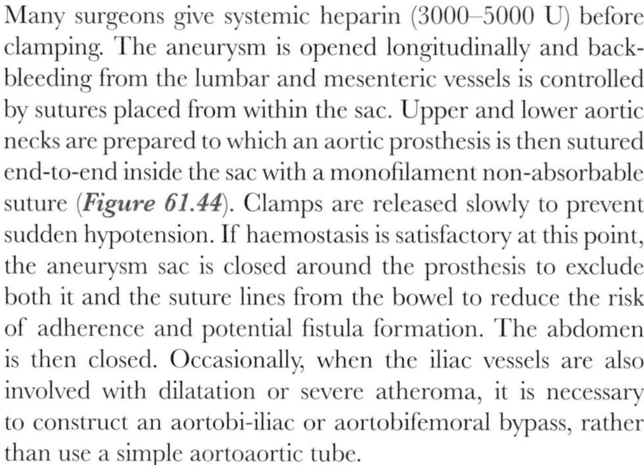

Many surgeons give systemic heparin (3000–5000 U) before clamping. The aneurysm is opened longitudinally and back-bleeding from the lumbar and mesenteric vessels is controlled by sutures placed from within the sac. Upper and lower aortic necks are prepared to which an aortic prosthesis is then sutured end-to-end inside the sac with a monofilament non-absorbable suture (***Figure 61.44***). Clamps are released slowly to prevent sudden hypotension. If haemostasis is satisfactory at this point, the aneurysm sac is closed around the prosthesis to exclude both it and the suture lines from the bowel to reduce the risk of adherence and potential fistula formation. The abdomen is then closed. Occasionally, when the iliac vessels are also involved with dilatation or severe atheroma, it is necessary to construct an aortobi-iliac or aortobifemoral bypass, rather than use a simple aortoaortic tube.

Endovascular aneurysm repair

EVAR is now established in clinical practice and has been shown to reduce mortality compared with open repair over the first 6 years but there are concerns about long-term durability. Currently about 75% of infrarenal aneurysms are suitable for EVAR, depending on the morphology of the aneurysm as assessed by CT scan. Common causes of unsuitability include a short, flared or angulated neck and difficult iliac artery access because of narrowing or tortuosity. The usual technique is to expose both femoral arteries (under general or local anaesthetic), which allows access to the aorta. Then, under radiological control, guidewires and catheters are used to cross the aneurysm and an angiogram performed to mark the level of the renal arteries.

The endovascular prosthesis (often termed a 'stent graft') is usually made up of three separate parts: a main body (***Figure 61.45a***) and two limbs that are enclosed in separate delivery catheters (***Figure 61.45b***). Some types have only two pieces: a main body with an ipsilateral limb attached and a separate contralateral limb. The prosthesis is made from Dacron or PTFE with integral metallic stents for support. The delivery catheter is inserted into the aneurysm sac and the stent–graft deployed by withdrawal of the delivery system. Most systems now have hooks or barbs to anchor the prosthesis in the aortic wall, and some surgeons inflate a moulding balloon catheter in the stent–graft to ensure that the hooks and barbs are engaged and a good seal is obtained (***Figure 61.46***). Although the top edge of the fabric of the stent–graft has to be deployed below the renal arteries (infrarenal fixation), some systems have additional bare metal stents at the proximal end of the main body that lie across the renal arteries to give better support and fixation (suprarenal fixation). Blood flows between the metal struts of the stent into the renal arteries. Success is dependent on a good seal between the stent–graft and the proximal and distal 'landing zones' in the aorta and iliac arteries. Failure to achieve a good seal results in an endoleak, which means that the aneurysm is not excluded from the circulation and may still expand and rupture. Patients who undergo EVAR require lifelong follow-up and surveillance with duplex (***Figure 61.47***) or CT scans to detect endoleak, disconnection

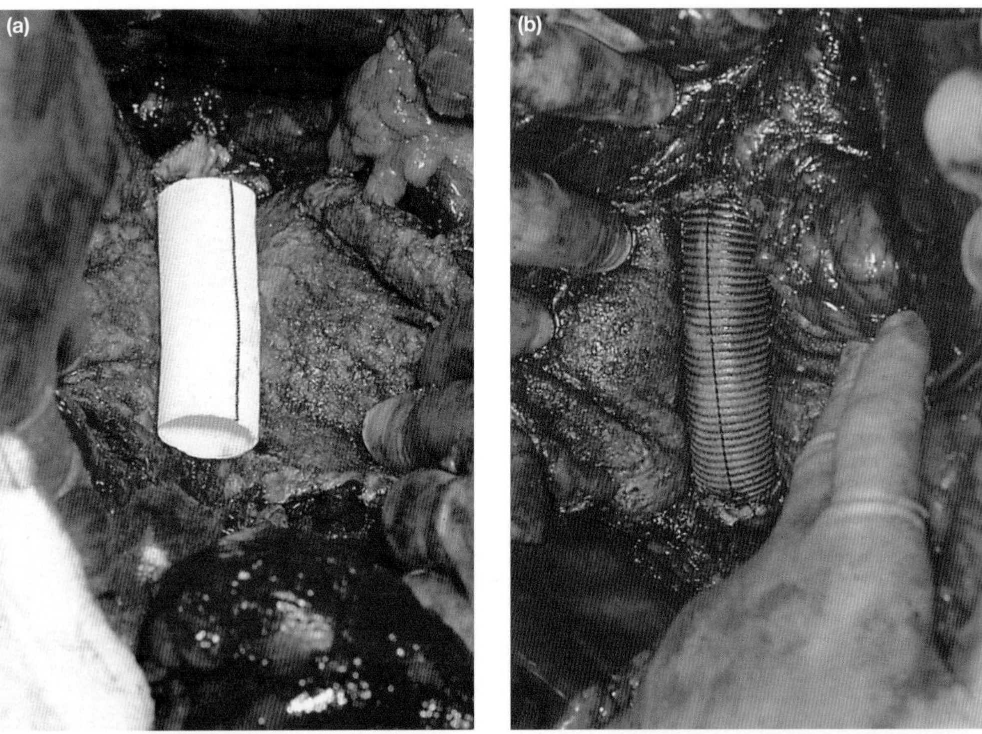

Figure 61.44 (a) Aneurysm sac opened. Note that the posterior wall of the aorta immediately above and below the sac is not divided. A Dacron tube graft is laid in place within the sac ready for suture. (b) The graft is sutured in place and the vascular clamps removed.

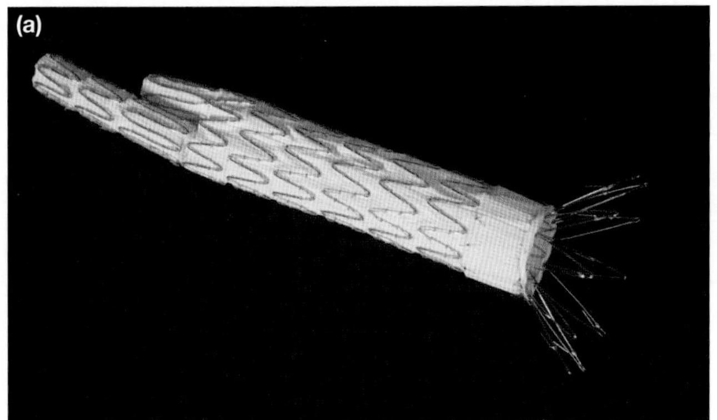

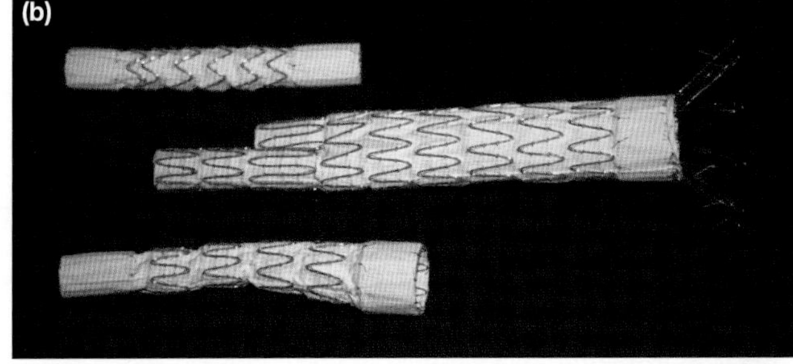

Figure 61.45 (a) Endovascular prosthesis main body; with separate limbs (b).

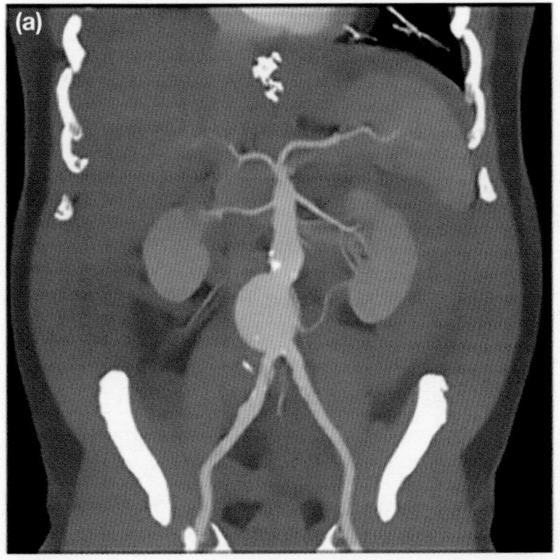

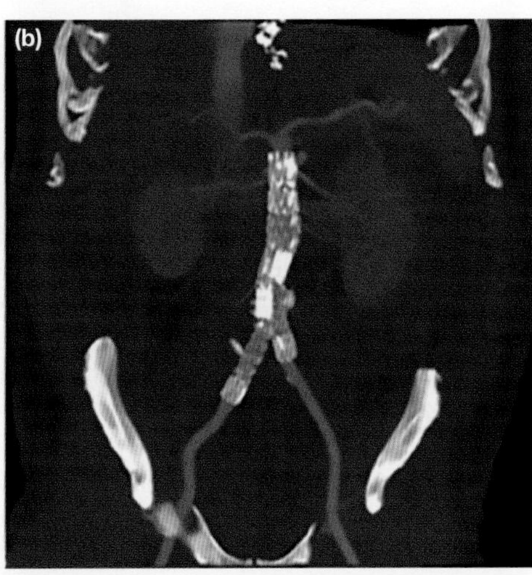

Figure 61.46 Infrarenal aortic aneurysm before (a) and after (b) endovascular aneurysm repair.

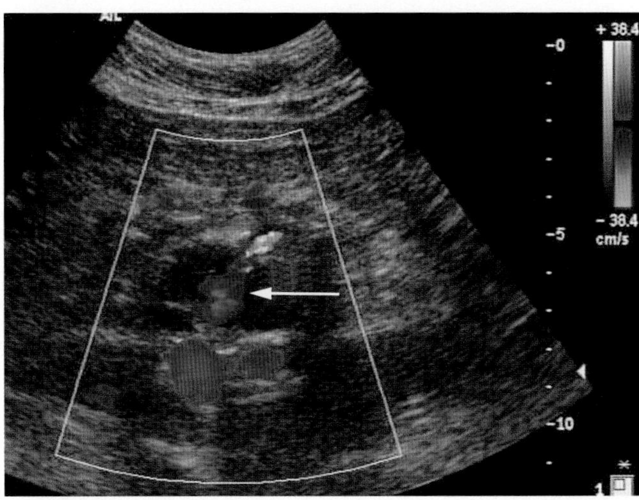

Figure 61.47 Duplex ultrasonography scan post endovascular aneurysm repair (EVAR), showing the aortic sac in cross-section and two limbs of EVAR (red ovals). There is a type II endoleak from the inferior mesenteric artery, with blood flowing retrogradely into the aneurysm sac (arrow).

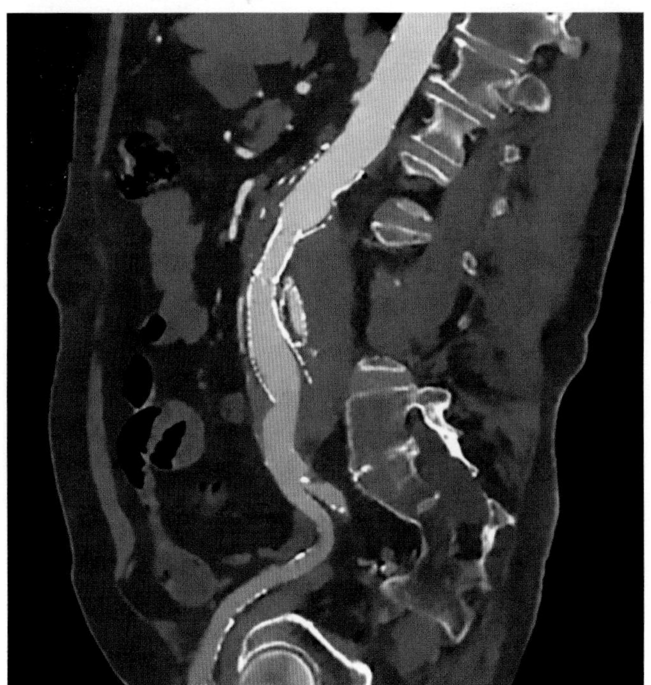

Figure 61.48 A stent–graft retracted into the aneurysm sac, creating a type Ib endoleak.

of the components and migration of the stent–graft, all of which predispose to late rupture (*Figure 61.48*).

Ruptured abdominal aortic aneurysm

Abdominal aortic aneurysms can rupture anteriorly into the peritoneal cavity (20%) or posterolaterally into the retroperitoneal space (80%). Less than 50% of patients with rupture survive to reach hospital. Anterior rupture results in free bleeding into the peritoneal cavity; very few patients reach hospital alive. Posterior rupture on the other hand produces a retroperitoneal haematoma (*Figure 61.49*). Often a brief period ensues when a combination of moderate hypotension and the resistance of the retroperitoneal tissues arrests further haemorrhage and may allow transport to hospital. The patient may remain conscious but in severe pain. If no operation is performed, death is virtually inevitable. Operative mortality is around 50% and the overall combined mortality (community and hospital) is around 80–90%.

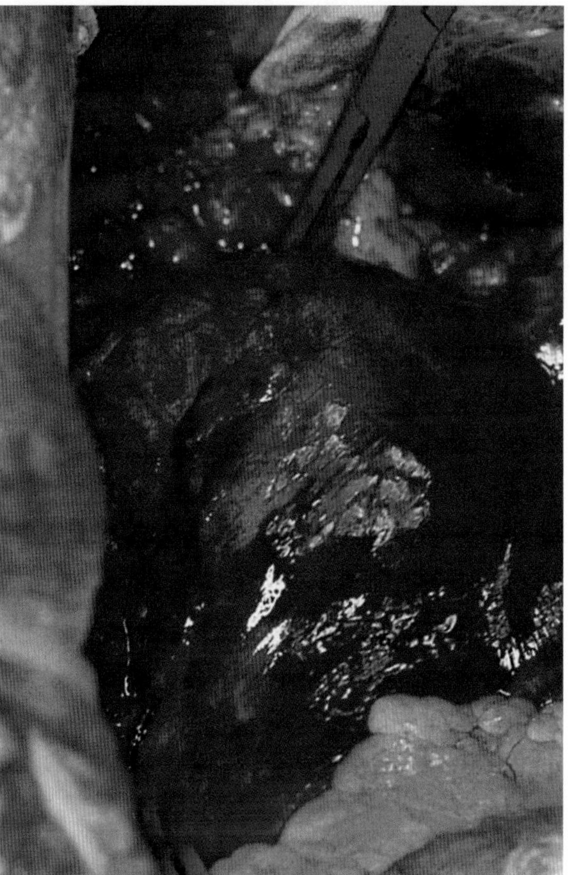

Figure 61.49 The retroperitoneal haematoma of a ruptured aortic aneurysm. The aortic pulsation is palpated through the haematoma at its upper limit and fingers are insinuated on each side of the aorta. With finger control, the upper clamp is positioned and closed on the aorta. The procedure is then as for a planned case. Here, the clamp is at the proximal end of the aneurysm; the haematoma has spread from the left paracolic gutter to encircle the aneurysm and the aortic bifurcation.

Ruptured abdominal aortic aneurysm is a surgical emergency; it should be suspected in a patient with the triad of severe abdominal and/or back pain, hypotension and a pulsatile abdominal mass. If there is doubt about the presence of an aneurysm an ultrasonography scan may help but this cannot diagnose rupture. CT scanning should be used to establish the diagnosis and to confirm a rupture and whether an EVAR is possible: EVAR should be considered as the first-line option for all anatomically suitable ruptured aortic aneurysms.

Good venous access is needed for infusion of saline or volume-expanding fluids, but the systolic blood pressure should not be raised any more than is necessary to maintain consciousness and permit cardiac perfusion (<100 mmHg). After CT scanning, the patient should be transferred immediately to an operating theatre where a urinary catheter and arterial line are usually inserted. If the patient appears stable, surgery may be delayed until cross-matched blood is available but surgery should commence immediately if haemodynamic instability develops. For open surgical repair the abdomen is usually prepared and draped with the patient awake, minimising potential delays in cross-clamping the aorta as general anaesthesia is often accompanied by haemodynamic deterioration. Endovascular repair can often be performed under local anaesthetic and, if indicated, an aortic occlusion balloon catheter can be inserted to gain control in a patient with significant haemodynamic compromise. Always remember that the treatment of ruptured aneurysm is an operation, not monitoring and resuscitation.

Summary box 61.5

Management of ruptured abdominal aortic aneurysm

- Early diagnosis (abdominal/back pain, pulsatile mass, shock)
- Immediate resuscitation (oxygen, intravenous replacement therapy, central line)
- Maintain systolic pressure, but not >100 mmHg
- Urinary catheter
- Cross-match blood
- Rapid transfer to the operating room

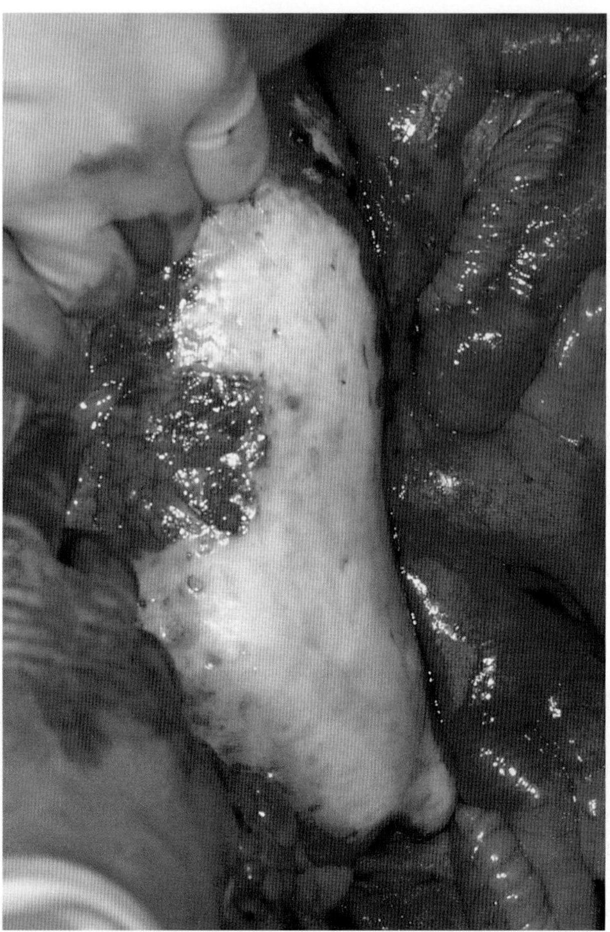

Figure 61.50 An inflammatory abdominal aortic aneurysm. Note the white 'icing' effect. Such lesions can be technically difficult to manage.

Symptomatic abdominal aortic aneurysm

These patients most commonly present with abdominal and/or back pain but the aneurysm is not ruptured on CT scan. Pain may also occur in the thigh and groin because of nerve compression. Gastrointestinal, urinary and venous symptoms can also be caused by pressure from an abdominal aneurysm. About 3% of all aneurysms cause pain as a result of inflammation of the aneurysm itself (***Figure 61.50***). Finally, a few cause symptoms from distal embolisation of intraluminal thrombus. An operation is usually indicated in patients who are otherwise reasonably fit. Pain may be a warning sign of stretching of the aneurysm sac and imminent rupture; surgery should be performed as soon as possible (usually on the next available operating list). The operative mortality of symptomatic aneurysms is usually higher than that for elective cases.

Postoperative complications

The most common complications after open repair are cardiac (ischaemia and infarction) and respiratory (atelectasis and lower lobe consolidation). A degree of colonic ischaemia because of a lack of a collateral blood supply occurs in about 10% of patients, but this usually resolves spontaneously. Acute kidney injury is an uncommon event after elective procedures but may complicate procedures undertaken for rupture. Acute kidney injury is more likely if there is preoperative renal impairment or considerable intraoperative blood loss. Neurological complications include sexual dysfunction and spinal cord ischaemia. An aortoduodenal fistula is an uncommon but treatable complication of abdominal aortic replacement surgery. It should be suspected whenever haematemesis or melaena occurs in the months or years after operation. Prosthetic graft infection is also uncommon; it may require explantation of the original graft and replacement with an autologous deep vein (superficial femoral vein) graft or removal of the original graft with oversewing of the aortic stump and limb revascularisation by insertion of an axillobifemoral bypass. Both techniques are associated with significant risk of perioperative morbidity and mortality.

Cardiac, respiratory, renal and neurological complications are less common after endovascular repair. However, there are complications that are unique to EVAR, such as endoleak (***Table 61.3***), graft migration, metal strut fracture and graft limb occlusion. Lifelong surveillance with duplex or CT scans (together with plain abdominal radiographs for strut fracture) is required to detect endoleak and migration. High-pressure endoleaks may require repeat ballooning or a proximal cuff or distal limb extension to reseal the endograft. Migration may also require extension of the graft. Overall, 10–20% of patients with EVAR will require secondary interventions to treat complications at some future date, although many of the interventions can be performed with a percutaneous approach via the femoral artery in the angiography suite.

TABLE 61.3 Classification of endoleaks following endovascular aneurysm repair.

Type of endoleak	Definition
Type I	Persistent filling of the aneurysm sac owing to an ineffective seal at the proximal (Ia) or distal (Ib) end of the stent–graft
Type II	Persistent filling of the aneurysm sac owing to retrograde flow of blood from aortic collaterals, e.g. IMA, lumbar arteries
Type III	Persistent filling of the aneurysm sac owing to structural failure of the stent–graft as a result of component disconnection (IIIa) or stent fabric tear (IIIb)
Type IV	Persistent filling of the aneurysm sac owing to stent–graft fabric porosity
Type V (endotension)	Persistent filling of the aneurysm sac without evidence of types I–IV endoleak

IMA, inferior mesenteric artery.

PERIPHERAL ANEURYSM

Popliteal aneurysm

Popliteal artery aneurysm accounts for 70% of all peripheral aneurysms classically diagnosed in men in their seventh decade of life; 50% are bilateral. Examination of the abdominal aorta is indicated if a popliteal aneurysm is found because one-third are accompanied by aortic dilatation. Popliteal aneurysms present as a swelling behind the knee or with symptoms caused by complications, such as severe ischaemia following thrombosis or distal ischaemia as a result of emboli. The diagnosis is usually confirmed with DUS but assessment of the distal vessels (with CT, MRA or DSA) is important prior to repair if the foot pulses are diminished or absent. An asymptomatic aneurysm greater than 20 mm in diameter should be considered for elective repair to prevent future complications. Some surgeons would also offer elective repair for smaller diameters if the sac contains thrombus because of a perceived increased risk of distal embolisation. All symptomatic popliteal aneurysms, including those in which single crural vessel embolisation has occurred, should be considered for repair.

Two techniques for surgical repair may be used: exclusion bypass and inlay repair. An exclusion bypass involves a medial approach to the above- and below-knee popliteal arteries, ligation of the aneurysm and restoration of flow to the foot with a bypass graft using saphenous vein. Many surgeons favour this approach because the anatomy is similar to that for a femoropopliteal bypass and therefore familiar. An inlay graft repair is performed through a posterior approach and has the benefits of allowing free ligation of feeding geniculate branches as well as aneurysmectomy in patients with neurovascular compression. However, the posterior approach limits exposure of the superficial femoral and crural arteries and should only be used when the popliteal aneurysm is confined to the popliteal fossa.

In the acute situation, the presentation is usually with a thrombosed aneurysm and an ischaemic foot; popliteal aneurysms very rarely rupture. Aneurysm thrombosis tends to occur following a period of chronic embolisation to the run-off vessels. As successive run-off vessels occlude over time the outflow to the popliteal artery diminishes, resulting in reduced flow rates in the aneurysm sac and eventual thrombosis. In such cases surgery is often unsuccessful because the outflow for the graft reconstruction is chronically diseased. Attempts to re-establish a patent run-off vessel with embolectomy and intra-arterial thrombolysis may be successful, but the limb loss rate is high (50%).

Femoral aneurysm

True aneurysm of the femoral artery is uncommon. Complications occur in less than 3% so conservative treatment is generally indicated, but it is important to look for aneurysms elsewhere as over half are associated with abdominal or popliteal aneurysms. Large aneurysms should be repaired. False aneurysm of the femoral artery occurs in 2% of patients after arterial surgery at this site. Local repair may involve reanastomosis of the bypass in the groin under suitable antibiotic cover. However, if infection is the cause, the treatment may involve excision of the infected graft and insertion of a further bypass routed around the infected area. In the latter case, the failure rate is high, and limb loss may be unavoidable. For false aneurysms caused by femoral artery puncture measuring ≤3 cm, thrombin injection under ultrasonography guidance may be successful and avoids surgery. False aneurysms measuring >3 cm usually require open surgical repair with suturing of the puncture site.

Iliac aneurysm

This usually occurs in conjunction with aortic aneurysm and only rarely on its own. When occurring in isolation it is difficult to diagnose clinically so about half present already ruptured. Open surgery usually involves an inlay graft but some iliac aneurysms may be suitable for endovascular repair.

ARTERIOVENOUS FISTULA

Communication between an artery and a vein may be either a congenital malformation or the result of trauma. Arteriovenous fistulae for haemodialysis access are also created surgically. All arteriovenous communications have a structural and a physiological effect. The structural effect of arterial blood flow on the veins is characteristic; they become dilated, tortuous and thick walled (arterialised). The physiological effect, if the fistula is large, is an increase in cardiac output that may lead to cardiac failure.

A pulsatile swelling may be present if the lesion is superficial. A thrill is detected on palpation and auscultation reveals a buzzing continuous bruit ('machinery murmur'). Dilated veins may be seen and pressure on the artery proximal to the fistula reduces the swelling and the thrill and bruit cease.

Duplex scan and/or angiography confirms the lesion that shows rapid venous filling.

Management

Treatment is often complex and usually involves embolisation. Excision surgery is sometimes used for severe deformity or recurrent haemorrhage; the assistance of a plastic surgeon is wise. Ligation of a 'feeding' artery usually fails and may preclude treatment by embolisation.

ARTERITIS AND VASOSPASTIC CONDITIONS

Thromboangiitis obliterans (Buerger's disease)

This is characterised by occlusive disease of small and medium-sized limb arteries, thrombophlebitis of superficial or deep veins and Raynaud's syndrome; it usually occurs in young male smokers. Histologically, there are inflammatory changes in the walls of arteries and veins, leading to thrombosis. Treatment is total abstinence from smoking, which arrests, but does not reverse, the disease. Established arterial occlusions are treated as for atheromatous disease, but amputations may eventually be required.

Other forms of arteritis

Arteritis occurs in association with many connective tissue disorders, e.g. rheumatoid arthritis, systemic lupus erythematosus and polyarteritis nodosa.

Temporal arteritis is a disease in which localised infiltration with inflammatory and giant cells leads to arterial occlusion, ischaemic headache and tender, palpable, pulseless (thrombosed) arteries in the scalp. Irreversible blindness occurs if the ophthalmic artery becomes occluded. The surgeon may be required to perform a temporal artery biopsy, but this should not delay immediate steroid therapy to arrest and reverse the process before the ophthalmic artery is involved. Takayasu's disease is an arteritis that obstructs major arteries, particularly the large vessels coming off the aortic arch. It usually pursues a relentless course.

Cystic myxomatous degeneration

This is typified by an accumulation of clear jelly (like a synovial ganglion) in the outer layers of a main artery, especially the popliteal artery. The lesion may narrow the vessel, causing claudication. Duplex scan is the investigation of choice. Decompression, by removal of the myxomatous material, may be successful but in some cases excision of the diseased artery with interposition vein graft repair is required.

Raynaud's disease

This idiopathic condition usually occurs in young women and affects the hands more than the feet. There is abnormal sensitivity in the arteriolar response to cold. These vessels constrict and the digits (usually the fingers) turn white and become incapable of fine movements. The capillaries then dilate and fill with slowly flowing deoxygenated blood, resulting in the digits becoming swollen and dusky. As the attack passes off, the arterioles relax, oxygenated blood returns into the dilated capillaries and the digits become red. Thus, the condition is recognised by the characteristic sequence of blanching, dusky cyanosis and red engorgement, often accompanied by pain. Superficial necrosis is very uncommon. This condition must be distinguished from Raynaud's syndrome, which has similar features (see ***Raynaud's syndrome***). Treatment of Raynaud's disease consists of protection from cold and avoidance of pulp and nail bed infection. Calcium antagonists, such as nifedipine, may also have a role to play and electrically heated gloves can be useful in winter. Sympathectomy has been used in the past but it is either ineffective or its effects are short-lived.

Raynaud's syndrome

Raynaud's syndrome is the peripheral arterial manifestation of a collagen disease such as systemic lupus erythematosus or rheumatoid arthritis. The clinical features are as for Raynaud's disease but they may be much more aggressive. Raynaud's syndrome may also follow the use of vibrating tools. In this context it is a recognised industrial disease and is known as 'vibration white finger'.

Treatment is directed primarily at the underlying condition, although the conservative measures outlined above are often helpful. The syndrome when secondary to collagen disease leads frequently to necrosis of digits and multiple amputations. Sympathectomy yields disappointing results and is not recommended. Nifedipine, steroids and vasospastic antagonists may all have a role in treatment. Patients with vibration white finger should avoid vibrating tools.

Acrocyanosis

Acrocyanosis may be confused with Raynaud's disease but it is painless and not episodic. It tends to affect young women and the mottled cyanosis of the fingers and/or toes may be accompanied by paraesthesia and chilblains.

Sympathectomy

Endoscopic transthoracic sympathectomy is now reserved as a minimally invasive treatment of palmar and axillary hyperhidrosis. Open cervical sympathectomy was used in the past as a treatment of vasospastic disorders but was usually unsuccessful. Lumbar sympathectomy was used to treat lower limb ischaemia in the past but has also become obsolete.

FURTHER READING

Bhattacharya V, Stansby G (eds). *Postgraduate vascular surgery: a candidate's guide to the FRCS and Board Exams*. Singapore: World Scientific Europe Ltd, 2018.

Moore WS (ed.). *Vascular and endovascular surgery: a comprehensive review*, 9th edn. Amsterdam: Elsevier, 2018.

Sidway AN, Perler BA (eds). *Rutherford's vascular surgery*, 9th edn. Amsterdam: Elsevier, 2019.

Wind GG, Valentin RJ (eds). *Anatomic exposures in vascular surgery*, 3rd edn. Philadelphia, PA: Lippincott Williams & Wilkins, 2013.

Mikito Takayasu, 1860–1938, Japanese ophthalmologist, described this disease in 1908.

CHAPTER

62 Venous disorders

Learning objectives

To understand:
- Venous anatomy and physiology
- The pathophysiology of venous hypertension
- The clinical significance and management of superficial venous reflux
- The management of venous ulceration
- Venous thromboembolism

INTRODUCTION

Up to 40% of the adult population in resource-rich countries have diseases of the veins of the leg. This extraordinary prevalence along with the associated impairment in health-related quality of life make it a very important area of surgical practice. Surgical intervention has been revolutionised by the development of endovenous techniques, and level 1 evidence has demonstrated that treatment can be associated with very high clinical- and cost-effectiveness. Despite the considerable importance placed on lower limb function during the management of orthopaedic and arterial diseases, venous diseases are often forgotten or dismissed as cosmetic practice. An understanding of the nature and management of venous disease is critical to address this imbalance and improve the quality of patients' lives.

THE ANATOMY OF THE VENOUS SYSTEM OF THE LOWER LIMB

The venous system of the lower limb can be divided anatomically into the **superficial venous system**, which is located within the superficial tissues, and the **deep venous system**, beneath the deep fascia of the leg, accompanying the arterial tree. The superficial veins drain into the deep system, either at junctions or via fascial perforating veins, and the deep veins then return blood to the right atrium of the heart. Venous anatomy is characteristically variable. The terminology used below is consistent with international consensus.

The deep veins of the lower limb (***Figure 62.1a***) include three pairs of venae comitantes, which accompany the three crural arteries (anterior and posterior tibial and peroneal arteries). These six veins intercommunicate and come together in the popliteal fossa to form the popliteal vein, which also receives the soleal and gastrocnemius veins. The popliteal vein passes up through the adductor hiatus to enter the subsartorial canal as the femoral vein, which receives the deep (profunda) femoral vein (or veins) in the femoral triangle before passing behind the inguinal ligament to become the external iliac vein. The internal iliac vein combines with the external iliac vein in the pelvis to form the common iliac vein. The left common iliac vein passes behind the right common iliac artery to join the right common iliac vein on the right side of the abdominal aorta to form the inferior vena cava, which goes on to the right atrium.

Far more anatomical variations exist within the superficial veins of the lower limb, but there are almost always two trunks or axes – the great and small saphenous veins (***Figure 62.1b,c***). These lie superficial to the fascia lata (deep fascia) but deep to the saphenous fascia, in the saphenous 'envelope'.

As the sole of the foot is often placed under significant pressure, the majority of the venous drainage of the foot is into the dorsal venous arch, running in the subcutaneous tissues over the metatarsal heads. The medial end of this arch drains into the first axis: the great saphenous vein (GSV). This is the longest vein in the body and is the most frequently affected by superficial incompetence. The GSV passes anterior to the medial malleolus and ascends the leg accompanied by the saphenous nerve in the superficial tissues medial to the tibia, looping posteriorly at the level of the medial condyle of the femur and continuing in the medial thigh. In the groin, it unites with tributaries corresponding to the arterial branches of the common femoral artery, before piercing the cribriform fascia covering the saphenous opening (approximately 2.5 cm below and lateral to the pubic tubercle, but often somewhat higher) and terminates by draining into the common femoral vein (CFV) at the saphenofemoral junction (SFJ). Throughout its course the GSV unites variably with other superficial tributaries. The anterior accessory of the great saphenous vein (AAGSV) is one of the most common. This is often seen originating around the lateral border of the knee, although it sometimes originates as low as the lateral end of the dorsal venous arch. Occasionally, this vein may also course up the medial aspect of the thigh, anterolateral to the GSV and

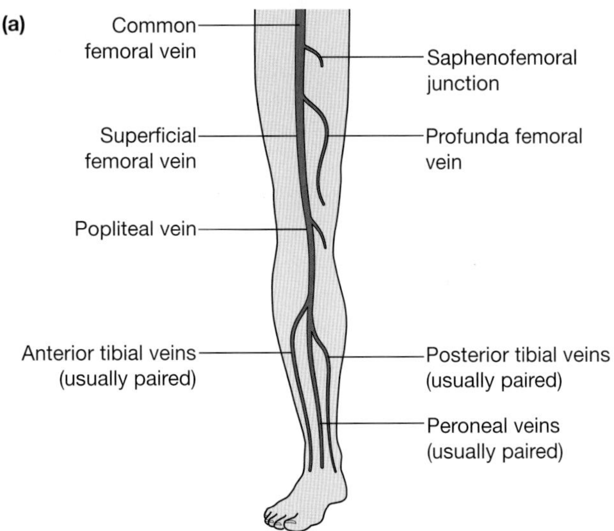

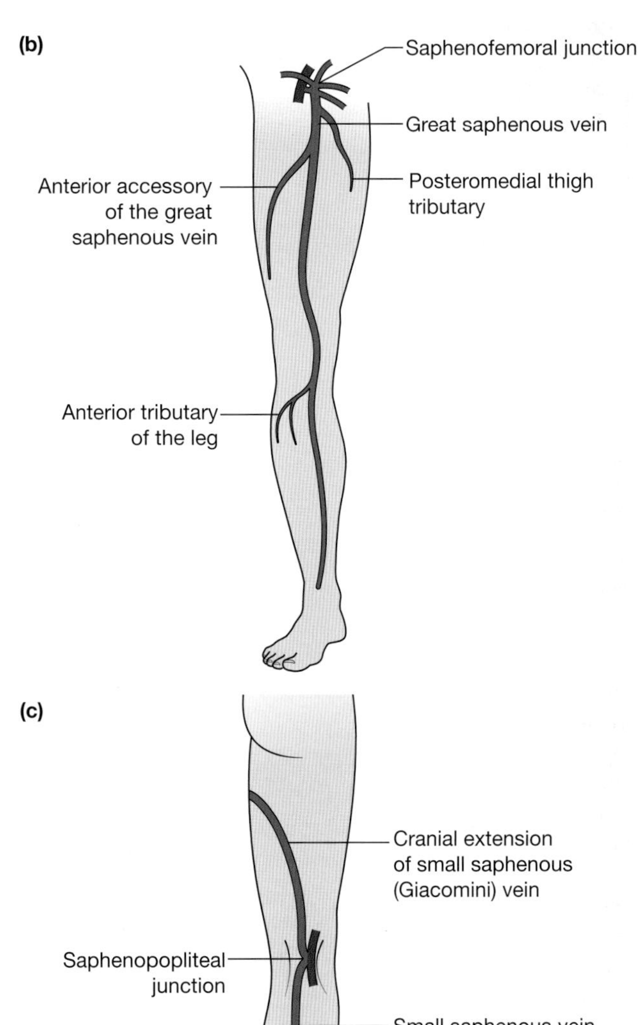

Figure 62.1 (a) Anatomy of the deep veins of the lower limb; **(b)** anatomy of the superficial veins of the lower limb (great saphenous axis); **(c)** anatomy of the superficial veins of the lower limb (small saphenous axis).

following its course. In this instance, its origin is typically a confluence of small tributaries around the knee. There is usually an in-line GSV axis passing uninterrupted from the foot (in some cases this may be hypoplastic), but this pattern of AAGSV is commonly mistaken for the GSV itself (some surgeons will call this a duplex GSV; a true duplex GSV is rare). The AAGSV may drain into the GSV in the thigh, but is typically at or near the junction itself.

The small saphenous vein (SSV) originates from the lateral side of the dorsal venous arch and accompanies the sural nerve as it passes posterior to the lateral malleolus, then upwards in the posterior midline of the leg. In the proximal calf it is usually found sitting in the groove between the two muscular heads of gastrocnemius. Its termination commonly occurs by piercing the fascia of the popliteal fossa to drain into the popliteal vein at the saphenopopliteal junction (SPJ). However, this junction is highly variable and the vein may terminate as low as the mid-calf. The SSV may extend cranially beyond the SPJ, in which case it is known as either a cranial extension of the SSV, which terminates by piercing the fascia in the posterior thigh to drain into the deep system, or the Giacomini vein, which communicates with the GSV system occasionally joining the GSV at or about the SFJ. In some cases, the SSV does not terminate at or below the popliteal fossa at all, but continues on as described above.

In the calf and thigh there are a number of valved perforating (communicating) veins that join the superficial to the deep veins at inconstant sites and which allow blood to flow from the superficial to the deep venous system. The most important of these are the direct perforating veins of the medial and lateral calf and the communicating veins around the knee and in the mid-thigh.

VENOUS PATHOPHYSIOLOGY

The purpose of the venous system is primarily to return blood back to the heart so that it can be delivered into the pulmonary circulation. The venous system contains approximately 60% of the total blood volume, with an average pressure of around 5–10 mmHg. Mechanical factors, alongside the autonomic nervous and endocrine systems, control the rate at which blood is delivered to the right atrium. Through its effects upon myocardial contractility via the Starling mechanism, venous return is one of the factors responsible for determining cardiac output.

Blood enters the lower limb through the femoral arteries before passing through arterioles into the capillaries, which

Carlo Giacomini, 1840–1898, anatomist, Turin, Italy. On his death he left his skeleton to the Anatomical Museum in Turin.
Ernest Henry Starling, 1866–1927, physiologist, University College, London, UK.

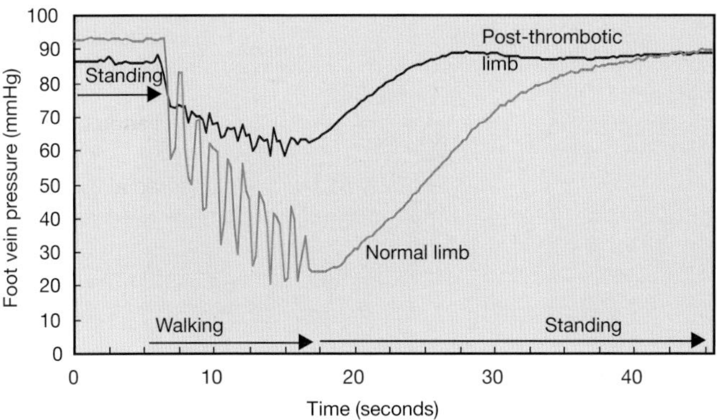

Figure 62.2 Effect of exercise on the superficial venous pressure in health and disease. The light blue line demonstrates the reduction in pressure primarily related to the action of the calf muscle pump. The dark blue line demonstrates how venous dysfunction is associated with reduced net antegrade flow during exercise, resulting in a relative increase in venous pressure when compared with normal (venous hypertension).

have a pressure of about 32 mmHg at their arterial ends. This pressure is reduced along the course of the capillaries and is approximately 12 mmHg at the venular end of the capillary. The pressure continues to fall in the main veins, and is as low as 5 mmHg at the upper end of the vena cava where it enters the right atrium.

The venous pressure in a foot vein on standing is equivalent to the height of a column of blood extending from the heart to the foot, e.g. approximately 100 mmHg. To enable blood to be returned against gravity in the standing position a pressure gradient must exist between the veins in the leg and those in the chest. This gradient is created in two ways. First, the increase in thoracic volume during inspiration decreases intrathoracic pressure. Second, the pressure in the veins of the leg is increased by compression by the surrounding muscles (the 'calf muscle pump') and to a lesser extent the tone of the venous wall. The deep veins of the calf are capacious and are joined by blind-ending sacks called the soleal sinusoids, which force blood into the popliteal and crural veins during calf muscle pump contraction, e.g. walking. The foot pump also ejects blood from the plantar veins during walking. As the calf muscles contract, the veins are compressed and the valves only allow blood to pass in the direction of the heart. The pressure within the calf compartment rises to 200–300 mmHg during muscle contraction. Rapid blood flow in the deep veins at junctions and perforators draws blood from the superficial veins, driving this up the deep veins also. During muscle relaxation, the pressure falls and further blood from the superficial veins enters the deep vein. Each time this occurs the pressure falls in the superficial venous compartment until a threshold is reached, when the venous inflow keeps pace with ejection from the deep veins. This is normally around 30 mmHg, a fall of approximately two-thirds of the resting venous pressure. The net reduction in the pressure of the superficial system is dependent on the presence of a pressure gradient between the leg and the thorax and a patent and compliant venous system containing competent valves (***Figure 62.2***). An absence of one or more of these results in venous hypertension, which leads to further vein wall damage, including loss of compliance, thickening, dilatation and valvular dysfunction. This venous damage goes on to reduce the function of the affected veins, worsening the venous hypertension in a vicious cycle. When exposed to high venous and capillary pressures chronically, the soft tissues of the leg will be damaged, causing a spectrum of damage that becomes irreversible. The causes of venous hypertension are listed in ***Table 62.1***.

TABLE 62.1 Factors causing venous hypertension.

Pressure gradient dysfunction

• Increased abdominal or thoracic pressure
  • COPD
  • Pregnancy
  • Obesity
  • Large tumour
  • Constipation
• Decreased calf muscle pump function
  • Immobility
  • Ankle joint fusion
  • Paralysis

Dysfunction of the venous system

• Venous structural deficit
  • Valvular agenesis
  • Valvular incompetence
  • Venous dilatation
  • Venous tortuosity
  • Loss of vein wall compliance
  • Loss of venous tone
  • Arteriovenous fistula
• Venous occlusion
  • Agenesis
  • Thrombosis
  • Iatrogenic/trauma
• Venous compression
  • May–Thurner syndrome
  • Pelvic/abdominal tumour
  • Pelvic/abdominal radiotherapy

COPD, chronic obstructive pulmonary disease.

The majority of patients with venous disease have a problem primarily with the vein wall structure and in most this is confined to the superficial veins. Little is known about the mechanism of initiation of the changes in the vein wall. These changes are complex, but are typified by valvular failure allowing retrograde flow within the vein with gravity (venous incompetence). It is no longer thought that venous incompetence is caused by a primary mechanical valvular failure.

The vein wall changes include inflammatory cell infiltration and activation, dysfunctional smooth muscle cell proliferation, collagen deposition, decreased elastin content and increased matrix metalloproteinases. These effects typically lead to loss

Rudolf Virchow, 1821–1902, pathologist, Charité Hospital, Berlin, Germany, was the first to be credited with describing iliac vein compression. It was not until 1957 that **May** and **Thurner** (Innsbruck, Austria) clearly described compression of the left common iliac vein by the right common iliac artery.

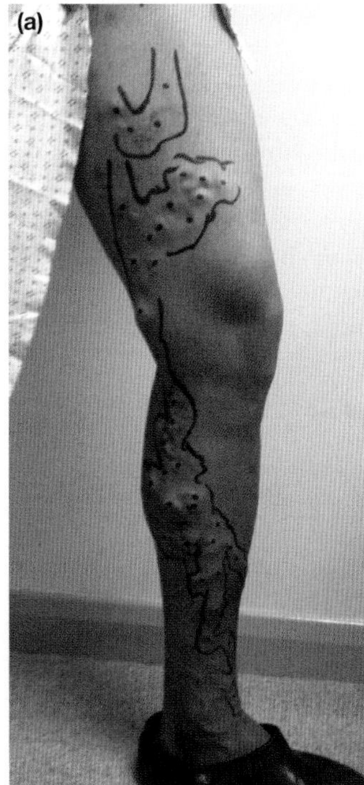

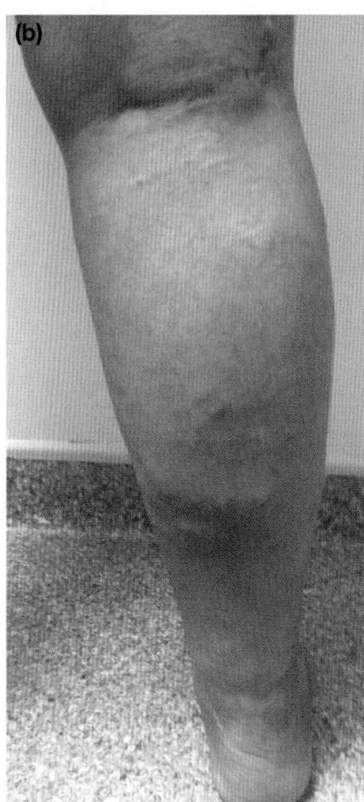

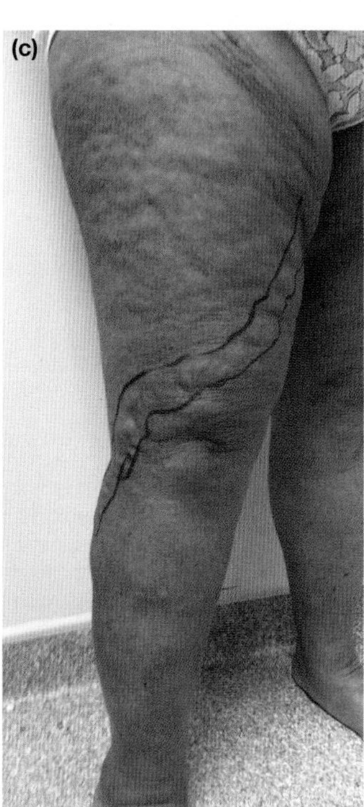

Figure 62.3 Varicose veins: **(a)** left leg varicose veins in the distribution of an incompetent great saphenous vein (marked for intervention); **(b)** right leg varicose veins in the distribution of the small saphenous system with a recent episode of phlebitis; **(c)** varicose veins in the distribution of an isolated incompetent anterior accessory of the great saphenous vein with associated gaiter area skin changes.

of compliance, dilatation, elongation (causing tortuosity) and secondary valvular dysfunction. This process can be initiated anywhere in the venous tree. Secondary varicose veins may develop in patients with post-thrombotic limbs and in patients with congenital abnormalities such as the Klippel–Trénaunay syndrome or multiple arteriovenous fistulae.

The extent and number of incompetent veins governs the extent of the venous hypertension and correlates with the severity of the soft-tissue complications seen. Importantly, however, neither the reflux burden nor the presence of skin changes, short of ulceration, correlate with the presence or degree of symptoms.

CLINICAL FEATURES OF VENOUS HYPERTENSION OF THE LEG

The following clinical features are commonly seen:

- Varicose vein: subcutaneous dilated vein 3 mm in diameter or larger. They are frequently elongated and tortuous, with intermittent 'blowouts', but are defined by the presence of reflux and may be straight and uniform tubes morphologically (***Figure 62.3***).
- Telangiectasia (thread veins, spider veins and hyphen webs): represent tiny intradermal venules less than 1 mm in diameter (***Figure 62.4***).
- Reticular vein: small dilated 'bluish' subdermal vein 1–2.9 mm in diameter, usually tortuous, can be difficult to distinguish this from a normal subdermal vein in someone with white thin transparent skin.
- Saphena varix (***Figure 62.5***) is a (usually painless) groin swelling apparent on standing.
- Corona phlebectatica (malleolar flare): a fan-shaped pattern of telangiectasia on the ankle or foot. This is an early sign of advanced venous disease.
- Oedema: increased volume of fluid in the skin and soft tissues of the leg. Commonly starts distally and moves more proximally with increasing venous dysfunction. Classically this is 'pitting oedema', with firm digital pressure leaving an indentation in the soft tissues.
- Eczema: an erythematous dermatitis, often appears minor, although it may be associated with significant itching and discomfort. In extreme cases it may progress to blistering and weeping (***Figures 62.6–62.8***).
- Pigmentation (haemosiderosis): a brownish discoloration of the skin, usually permanent. It is usually seen around the ankle, but is also seen in proximity to varicose veins and incompetent perforators (***Figures 62.7 and 62.9***).
- Lipodermatosclerosis (LDS): chronic inflammation and fibrosis of the skin and subcutaneous tissues, resulting in a tight, contracted, 'woody' leg on examination. It occasionally results in significant contractures of the Achilles

Maurice Klippel, 1858–1942, neurologist, La Salpêtrière, Paris, France.
Paul Trénaunay, 1875–1938, French neurologist. Klippel and Trénaunay described this condition in a joint paper in 1900.
A **gaiter** is a leather or cloth covering for the lower leg and ankle. The name is derived from the French 'guetre' for the same piece of clothing.

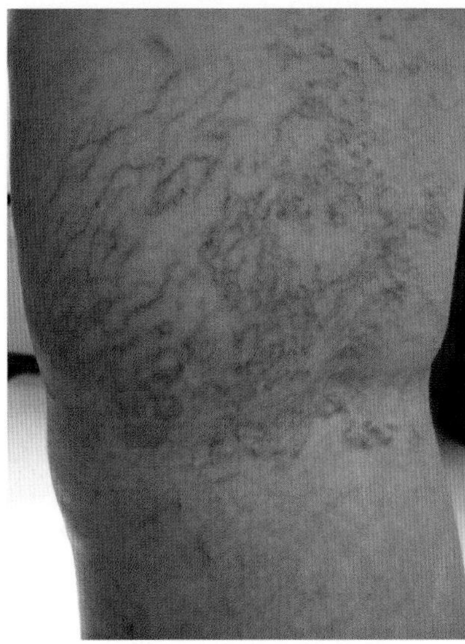

Figure 62.4 Telangiectasia and reticular veins.

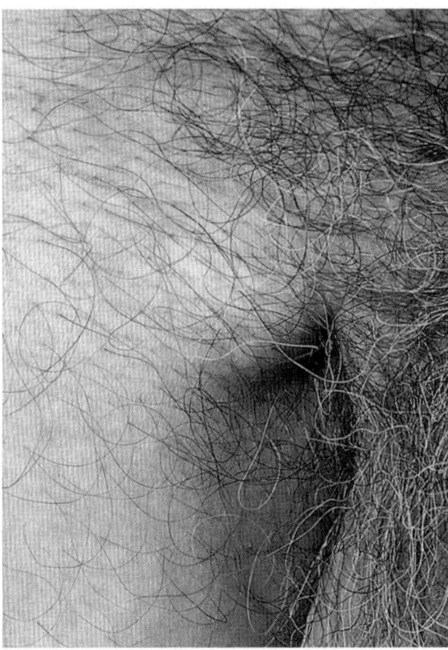

Figure 62.5 A saphena varix.

tendon. This is a sign of severe chronic venous disease (*Figures 62.6 and 62.9*).

- Atrophie blanche: localised areas of atrophic, white skin, often surrounded by telangiectasia and pigmentation. Some authors distinguish this from the white scarring left by ulceration; others do not. Either way, this is a sign of severe chronic venous disease (*Figure 62.6*).
- Venous ulcer: full-thickness skin loss, usually around the ankle, which fails to heal spontaneously and is propagated by continuing venous hypertension and the changes associated with chronic venous disease (*Figure 62.10*).

Classification system

The descriptive CEAP (Clinical–aEtiology–Anatomy–Pathophysiology) classification for chronic venous disorders is widely utilised.

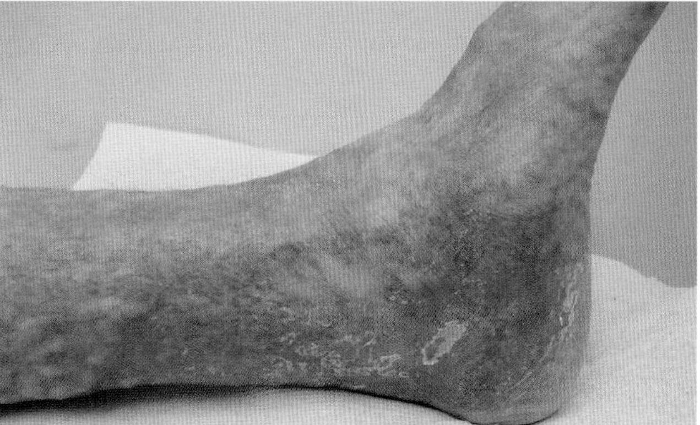

Figure 62.6 Advanced skin changes: lipodermatosclerosis, eczema and atrophie blanche.

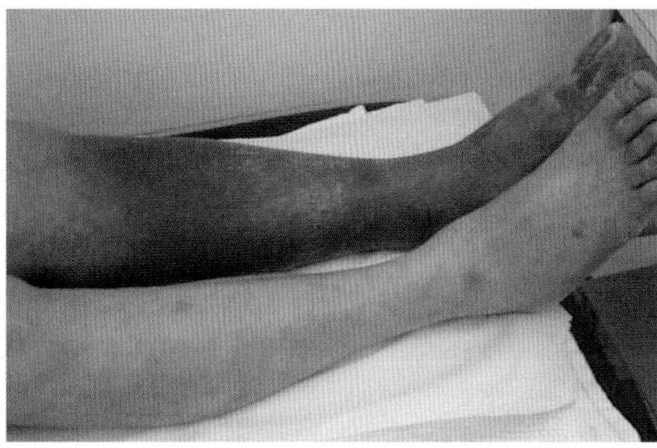

Figure 62.7 Pigmentation (haemosiderosis) and mild eczema.

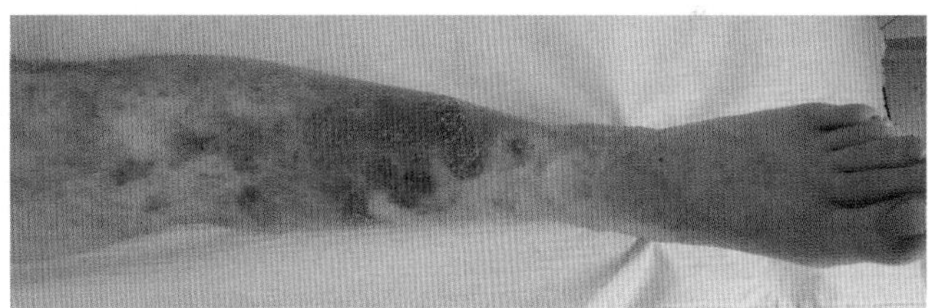

Figure 62.8 Severe eczema.

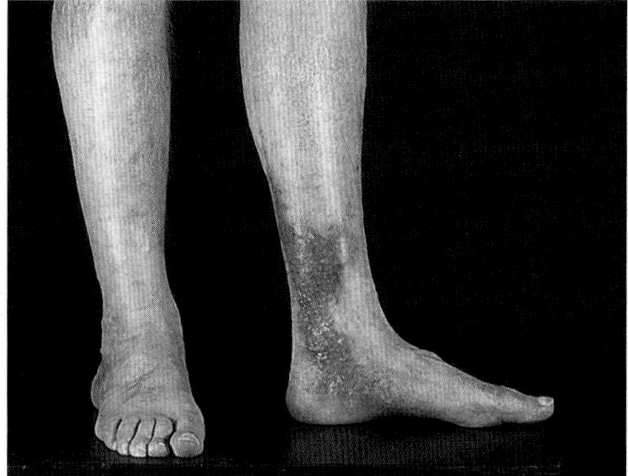

Figure 62.9 Haemosiderosis and mild lipodermatosclerosis of the calf skin.

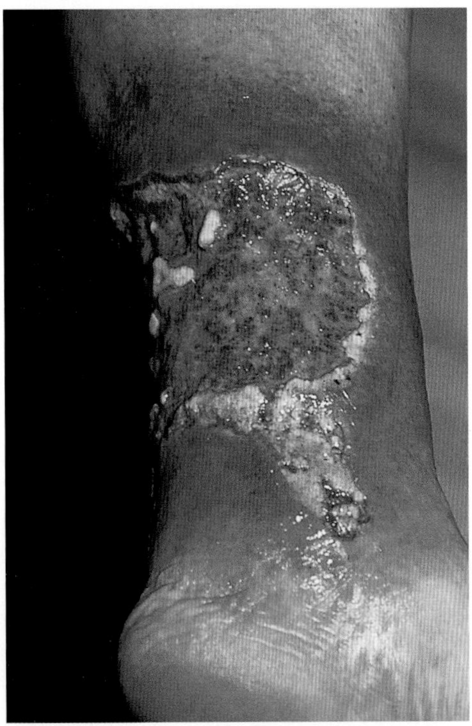

Figure 62.10 Venous ulcer.

For clinical classification:

- C0: no signs of venous disease;
- C1: telangiectasia or reticular veins;
- C2: varicose veins;
- C3: oedema;
- C4a: pigmentation or eczema;
- C4b: LDS or atrophie blanche;
- C4c Corona phlebectatica
- C5: healed venous ulcer;
- C6: active venous ulcer.

Clinical class can be further characterised as symptomatic (s), asymptomatic (a) or recurrent following previous successful treatment or healing (r), e.g. C2a, C2s, C6r.

For aetiological classification:

- Ec: congenital;
- Ep: primary;
- Es: secondary (post-thrombotic);
- En: no venous cause identified.

For anatomical classification:

- As: superficial veins;
- Ap: perforator veins;
- Ad: deep veins;
- An: no venous location identified.

For pathophysiological classification:

- Pr: reflux;
- Po: obstruction;
- Pr,o: reflux and obstruction;
- Pn: no venous pathophysiology identifiable.

VARICOSE VEINS

In clinical practice, patients are normally categorised as having 'varicose veins' or 'venous ulcers'. Cases of varicose veins may be uncomplicated or complicated. Complications may be chronic (as discussed above) or acute, including superficial vein thrombosis (thrombophlebitis) and bleeding. Uncomplicated varicose veins may be asymptomatic or symptomatic.

Epidemiology

The adult prevalence of visible varicose veins is between 30% and 50%. Factors affecting prevalence include:

- Gender: the vast majority of studies report a higher prevalence in women than in men, though community prevalence may differ.
- Age: the prevalence of varicose veins increases with age. In the Edinburgh Vein Study, the prevalence of trunk varicosities in the age groups 18–24 years, 25–34 years, 35–44 years, 45–57 years and 55–64 years was 11.5%, 14.6%, 28.8%, 41.9% and 55.7%, respectively.
- Ethnicity: does seem to influence the prevalence of varicose veins.
- Body mass and height: increasing body mass index and height may be associated with a higher prevalence of varicose veins.
- Pregnancy: increases the risk of varicose veins.
- Family history: evidence supports familial susceptibility to varicose veins.
- Occupation and lifestyle factors: there is inconclusive evidence regarding increased prevalence of varicose veins in smokers, in patients who suffer constipation and in those with occupations that involve prolonged standing.

Symptoms

Varicose veins frequently cause symptoms. Patients describe aching, heaviness, throbbing, burning or bursting over affected areas and sometimes the whole limb. Such symptoms typically increase throughout the day or with prolonged standing, and are relieved by elevation or compression hosiery. Itching is also commonly described, though this is more frequent in the presence of complications, as is swelling of the ankle. Venous symptoms in the absence of complications can be vague and it may be difficult to ascertain from history alone whether they are truly venous in origin and, therefore, whether treatment will help. A trial of compression hosiery can help as venous symptoms should show some beneficial improvement.

Symptoms can be very severe and interfere with a patient's daily activities such as work, recreation and caring for children and adults. Such symptoms are independent of the degree of venous incompetence or the presence of complications, including skin changes short of ulceration. Studies have also shown that symptoms are associated with a significant deficit in health-related quality of life, and significant improvements are seen with treatment to remove or ablate the refluxing veins. The maximal benefit is seen in those with uncomplicated symptomatic varicose veins, as skin changes and a proportion of the associated morbidity are frequently irreversible.

Telangiectasia (not associated with malleolar flare) and reticular veins occur very commonly in the absence of significant reflux or obstruction and in the vast majority do not cause any physical symptoms, though cosmetic treatment is commonly sought.

Signs

The presence of tortuous dilated subcutaneous veins is usually clinically obvious. These are confined to the GSV and SSV systems in approximately 60% and 20% of cases, respectively. The distribution of varicosities may indicate which superficial axis is defective; medial thigh and calf varicosities suggest GSV incompetence (***Figure 62.3a***), posterolateral calf varicosities are suggestive of SSV incompetence (***Figure 62.3b***), whereas anterolateral thigh and calf varicosities may indicate isolated incompetence of the AAGSV (***Figure 62.3c***). Any of the clinical features above may be present. Large, dilated veins around the SFJ may present as a (usually painless) lump, emergent when standing and disappearing when recumbent. This is a saphena varix (***Figure 62.5***). Gentle palpation over the varix during coughing may elicit an impulse and it may be mistaken for a groin hernia.

Investigation

Tourniquet tests and the use of hand-held Doppler have now been abandoned. There is good evidence to support the policy of duplex ultrasound scanning for all patients with varicose veins prior to any intervention. The best clinical results come from clinicians who are personally very skilled in the use of duplex ultrasound and use it to design a bespoke treatment for each individual patient, based upon their unique anatomy.

A high-frequency linear array transducer of 7.5–13 MHz is appropriate for the majority of lower limbs in order to obtain good quality images. The B-mode settings (depth, focal zone, overall gain and dynamic gain) should be optimised to ensure that the area of interest is in the centre and occupies the majority of the image, and that the lumen of the vein appears as a dark void in the subcutaneous and deep tissues. The pulsed wave spectral or colour Doppler settings should be optimised for the low-flow velocities encountered within veins. It is conventional to use blue to represent antegrade venous flow towards the heart and red for the reverse. Visible venous flow can be augmented by a calf squeeze.

The aim of the duplex scan in a patient with varicose veins is to establish:

- the presence of reflux in the deep and superficial venous system;
- the exact distribution and extent of reflux in the superficial venous system, including affected junctions and perforators;
- the presence of obstruction in the deep venous system;
- the suitability of the incompetent superficial veins for the different treatments available (based upon diameter, extent, tortuosity, saphena varix);
- the presence of thrombus within the superficial veins;
- an indication of a pelvic source of reflux or obstruction.

In order to standardise measurements of venous diameter and reflux, it is recommended that examination of the superficial veins is performed with the patient standing. Superficial or crural vein reflux is defined as retrograde flow in the reverse direction to physiological flow lasting for 0.5 seconds or more. The proximal deep veins require a duration of 1 second or more to be classified as incompetent. Reflux may be elicited by release of a calf or foot squeeze for proximal or calf varicosities, respectively, manual compression over varicosity clusters, pneumatic calf cuff deflation, active foot dorsiflexion and relaxation or the Valsalva manoeuvre.

The patient should stand facing towards the examiner with the leg rotated outwards, heel on the ground and weight on the opposite limb (***Figure 62.11***). The use of a platform, ideally with a handle or support bar for the patient and a stool that can drop to a low height, will improve the ergonomic comfort of both the sonographer and the patient. The scan should commence in the groin, using a transverse view to identify the GSV and CFV lying medial to the common femoral artery (the 'Mickey Mouse' sign; ***Figure 62.12***). SFJ competence is assessed in the transverse view and potential destinations for reflux, including the GSV, the AAGSV and other major thigh tributaries superficial to the saphenous fascia, are noted. Any indication of a pelvic source of reflux suggests the need for more proximal imaging. The full length of the GSV within its fascial compartment should be examined (***Figure 62.13***), and its diameter measured if required. The groin is next examined

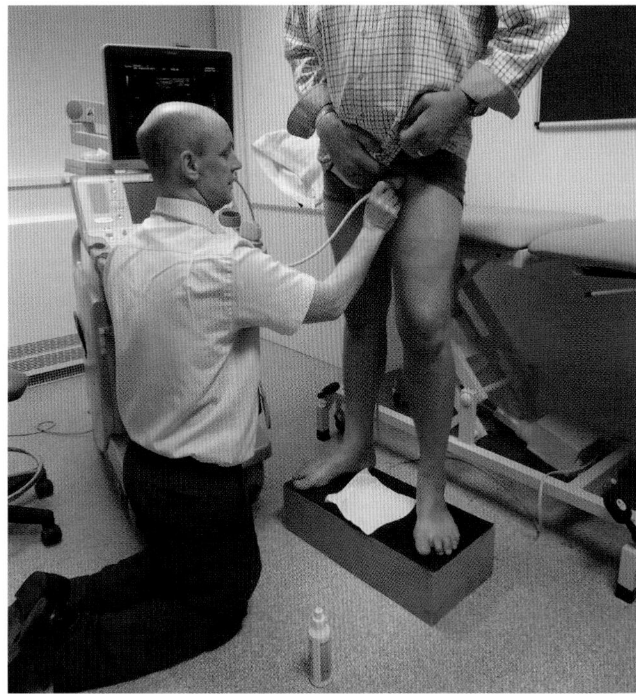

Figure 62.11 Patient position for venous duplex examination of the great saphenous system.

Christian Johann Doppler, 1803–1853, Professor of Experimental Physics, Vienna, Austria, enunciated the 'Doppler principle' in 1842.
Antonio Valsalva, 1666–1723, anatomist, Bologna, Italy. Also described the Eustachian tube and aortic sinuses.

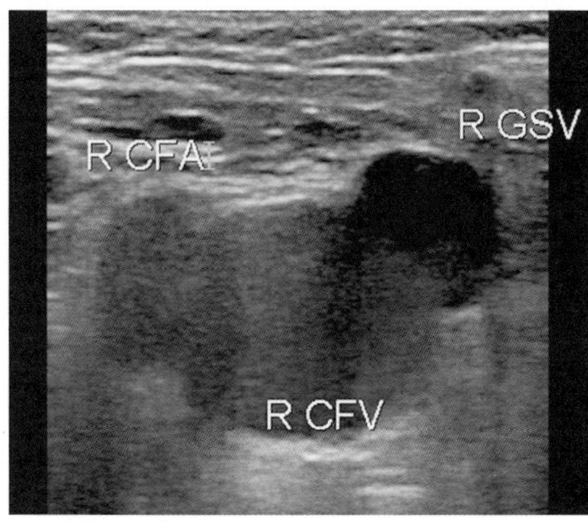

Figure 62.12 'Mickey Mouse' transverse B-mode image of the right (R) common femoral vein (CFV) and artery (CFA), great saphenous vein (GSV) and saphenofemoral junction.

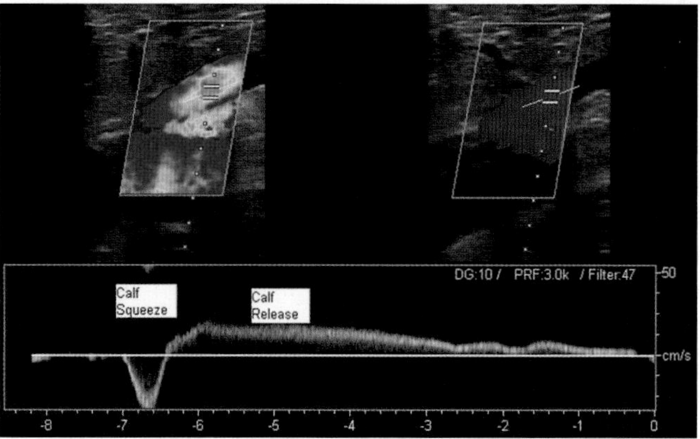

Figure 62.14 Spectral Doppler trace of the saphenofemoral junction showing antegrade and retrograde flow. The downward spike on the trace is the antegrade augmented flow and this is followed by approximately 4 seconds of retrograde flow.

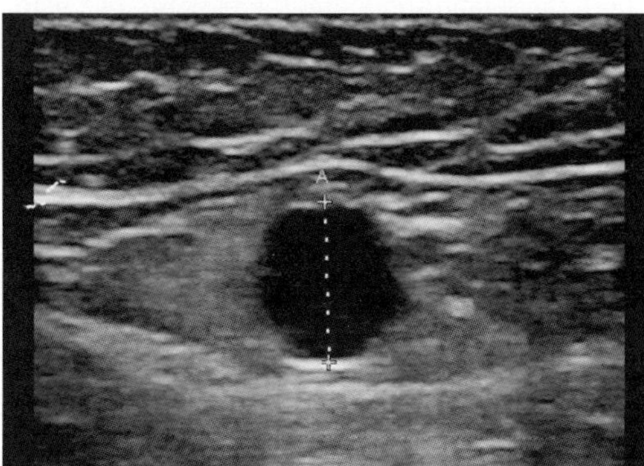

Figure 62.13 'Saphenous eye' transverse B-mode view of the great saphenous vein in fascial compartments of the thigh. The fascial line above the vein is the saphenous fascia. A true great or small saphenous vein will not cross this line, although the fascia may become discontinuous around the knee. The line deep to the vein is the fascia lata, with the muscle beneath.

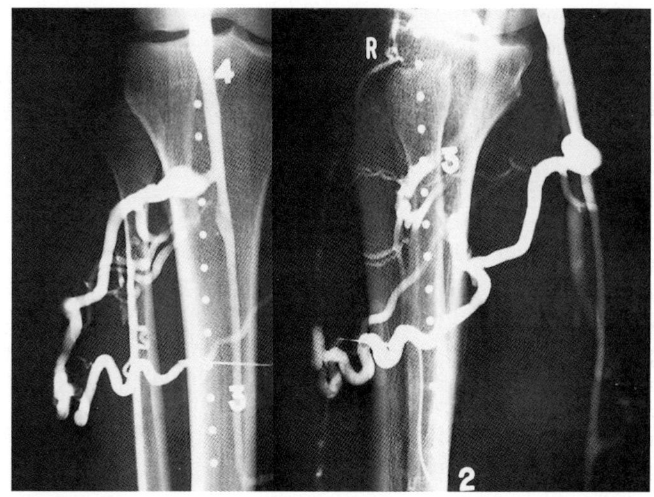

Figure 62.15 Varicogram. (This is now a historical investigation.)

for reflux or obstruction in the CFV, superficial femoral vein and SFJ using spectral and/or colour Doppler (***Figure 62.14***).

A loss of phasic flow with respiration in the CFV suggests upstream obstruction and the need for proximal imaging. The presence and competence of thigh and calf perforators should be noted and the crural veins examined for reflux or obstruction. For examination of the SSV and posterior thigh extension of the SSV (Giacomini vein), the patient is positioned facing away, knee slightly flexed, heel on the ground and the weight taken on the opposite leg. If the SPJ is incompetent, the level of the SPJ in relation to the knee crease and whether the SSV joins the popliteal vein posteriorly, medially or laterally is noted if open surgical ligation is to be entertained. In the transverse view, the SSV vein is followed distally, checking its competence and diameter in the proximal, mid- and distal calf. Finally, the patency and competence of the popliteal vein is assessed.

Pelvic and iliac veins may be investigated using transabdominal or transvaginal duplex. Very occasionally investigations other than duplex are required, and these may be non-invasive, such as magnetic resonance (MR) venography, or invasive, such as contrast venography or intravenous ultrasound (IVUS). The use of varicography has become historical (***Figure 62.15***).

Management

Many patients with asymptomatic varicose veins do not progress to develop complications, although a significant proportion do, and there is no clear confirmatory evidence that treating such patients prevents the development of future complications. There is clear evidence, however, that those with symptoms and/or complications see a significant quality-of-life benefit from treatment to remove or ablate refluxing superficial veins.

When interventional treatment is planned there are considerable variations in practice and treatment strategies. A detailed description of the nuances, merits and criticisms of the various options is beyond the scope of this chapter; however, a description of the basic treatment modalities available is presented below. An experienced surgeon will have his/her own preferred methods, but will frequently employ several or all methods in chosen circumstances, not infrequently in the same patient.

Compression

Compression hosiery relies on graduated external pressure to improve deep venous return and reduce venous pressures. It may be knee length or thigh length; there is no evidence which length of stocking is more effective and hence below-knee stockings are usually prescribed as they are easier to don and have much better patient acceptance. Compression hosiery is classified according to the pressure it exerts: the British classification class 1 stockings exert pressure of 14–17 mmHg, class 2 exert 18–24 mmHg and class 3 exert 25–35 mmHg.

Compression hosiery significantly improves varicose vein symptoms but is not popular with patients, with compliance rates and long-term tolerance being universally poor. There is no evidence to suggest that compression hosiery prevents the occurrence or progression of varicose veins. Furthermore, incorrect application of compression hosiery can have serious consequences (pressure necrosis, tourniquet effects); thus assessment, prescription and application of compression hosiery should be limited to those with the appropriate skills and training. There are level 1 trial data to demonstrate that interventional treatment offers superior improvements in quality of life and is cost-effective. Compression is therefore to be regarded as an adjunct to assessment or treatment, unless by patient choice.

Endothermal ablation

Endothermal ablation technologies replaced surgical ligation and stripping as the gold standard treatment once randomised trials demonstrated that they were marginally safer, have extremely high technical efficacy, offer superior quality of life post procedure (with a rapid recovery) and equivalent improvements in quality of life in the longer term. The techniques are cost-effective as they can be performed as an outpatient under local anaesthetic. The basic concept is that a treatment device is inserted into the incompetent axial vein percutaneously. The vein is surrounded by tumescent local anaesthetic solution. This compresses the vein onto the treatment device, emptying it of blood. It also hydro-dissects tissues such as nerves away from the zone of injury. Finally, it acts as a heat sink, mopping up excess thermal energy to prevent remote damage. The treatment device then produces thermal energy that destroys the structure of the vein, resulting in permanent occlusion. Two broad technologies exist: laser ablation and radiofrequency ablation (RFA).

Laser ablation

Endovenous laser ablation (EVLA) utilises a small flexible glass fibre that is inserted into the vein. Laser energy (typically at a wavelength of 1470 nm) is transmitted down the fibre and is absorbed at the point of treatment at the end of the fibre. Absorption of this radiation results in a vigorous generation of thermal energy. The tip of the fibre may be bare, focusing the energy in a very small area; divergent forward firing, spreading the energy over a larger area; or divergent side or radial firing. It is postulated that the last two designs allow a more even distribution of energy, reducing vein wall perforations that are thought to be associated with postprocedural pain and bruising. There is no clear evidence to support one design over another. This procedure is very good for treatment of any vein that will allow the passage of a guidewire. No technique has reported a higher technical efficacy rate.

The procedure begins with ultrasound-guided marking of the truncal vein to be treated and the site of proposed cannulation. The varicosities are also marked at this stage if concomitant treatment (phlebectomy or foam sclerotherapy) is to be undertaken. The patient is then positioned on the procedure couch in the reverse Trendelenburg position. For the GSV, the patient is supine with the hip of the leg to be treated externally rotated and slightly flexed. A pillow under the contralateral hip/lower back may improve patient comfort. For the SSV the patient is positioned in the prone position. The vein is then cannulated percutaneously under ultrasound guidance, at the lowest point of reflux. Some devices allow passage of the fibre directly through a short sheath, while others use a wire first, allowing passage of a catheter that then carries the laser fibre. The former is slightly faster with fewer steps; the latter allows greater success with more tortuous veins. Accurate positioning of the fibre tip with ultrasound is crucial (***Figure 62.16***), but the exact location is controversial, with some surgeons positioning the tip several centimetres distal to the junction and others aiming for a flush occlusion. Proponents of the former cite that this strategy protects the deep vein from inadvertent damage and/or thrombosis. Proponents of the latter argue that neoreflux in junctional tributaries is a common pattern of recurrence and that in expert hands the rate of deep vein injury is no different and the thrombosis rate may be lower (presumably as there is minimal patent stump in which to form thrombus). Following the administration of perivenous tumescent anaesthesia (***Figure 62.17***), the ablation can be performed. Practice varies as to the power of the laser and the withdrawal speed, but commonly an energy delivery

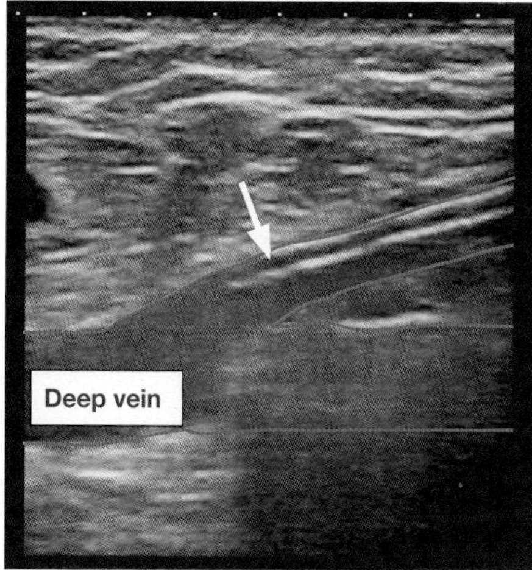

Figure 62.16 Endovenous laser ablation; B-mode longitudinal imaging during catheter tip positioning at the saphenofemoral junction. The saphenofemoral junction is highlighted (in blue) with an arrow pointing to the catheter.

Friedrich Trendelenburg, 1844–1924, Professor of Surgery successively at Rostock (1875–1882), Bonn (1882–1895) and Leipzig (1895–1911), Germany. The Trendelenburg position was first described in 1885.

of around 60–80 J/cm is used to achieve a durable closure. There is no clear evidence to guide the optimal power and pullback speed. Compression is usually applied following treatment, but there is no consensus over the method, degree or duration, and this is true of postprocedural compression with all techniques.

Radiofrequency ablation

RFA uses the same treatment principles, but an electromagnetic current is used to create the thermal energy. A range of different devices have been created but the most popular, which has the most supportive evidence, is the ClosureFast™ device (Medtronic) (***Figure 62.18***). This device has a wire coil on the end of a treatment catheter. The generator passes an electrical current through the coil until the surrounding temperature reaches 120°C. This is then maintained for a treatment cycle of 20 seconds. The coil is then withdrawn for a set length and another treatment cycle is commenced. Coils of 3 cm and 7 cm are produced, with the latter increasing the speed of treatment, while still being suitable for most anatomies.

There have been a range of studies comparing EVLA and RFA. The evidence is generally equivocal, with both treatments having relative advantages and disadvantages; choice often comes down to personal preference. Both are excellent treatment options and can be applied successfully to the majority of patients.

There have been a range of studies comparing EVLA and RFA. The evidence is generally equivocal, with both treatments having relative advantages and disadvantages; choice often comes down to personal preference. Both are excellent treatment options and can be applied successfully to the majority of patients.

Some summary points:

- Both treatments have a very high efficacy (>95% closure rate) and are suitable for treatment of the vast majority of patients presenting with superficial vein reflux in association with superficial axial incompetence.
- Veins that are very tortuous may still be suitable for endothermal ablation but require a guidewire and in the case of EVLA, a catheter-based, rather than direct fibre system. Both techniques offer this.

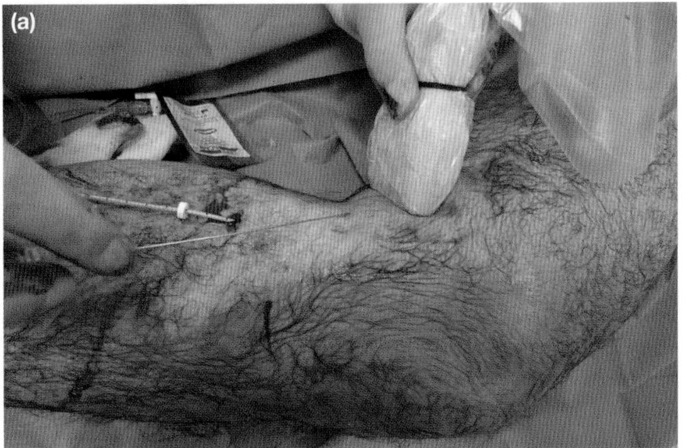

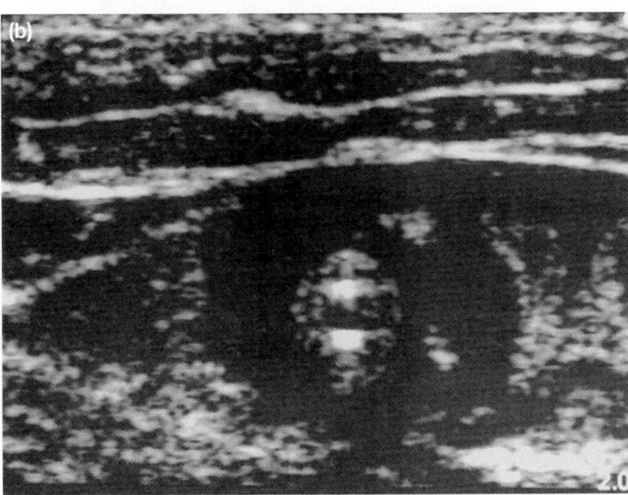

Figure 62.17 (a) Ultrasound-guided infiltration of perivenous tumescent anaesthetic via a long spinal needle. The anaesthetic solution is infiltrated using an electronic foot-operated pump; **(b)** ultrasound image of a perivenous 'halo' of anaesthetic solution around the vein and catheter in transverse section.

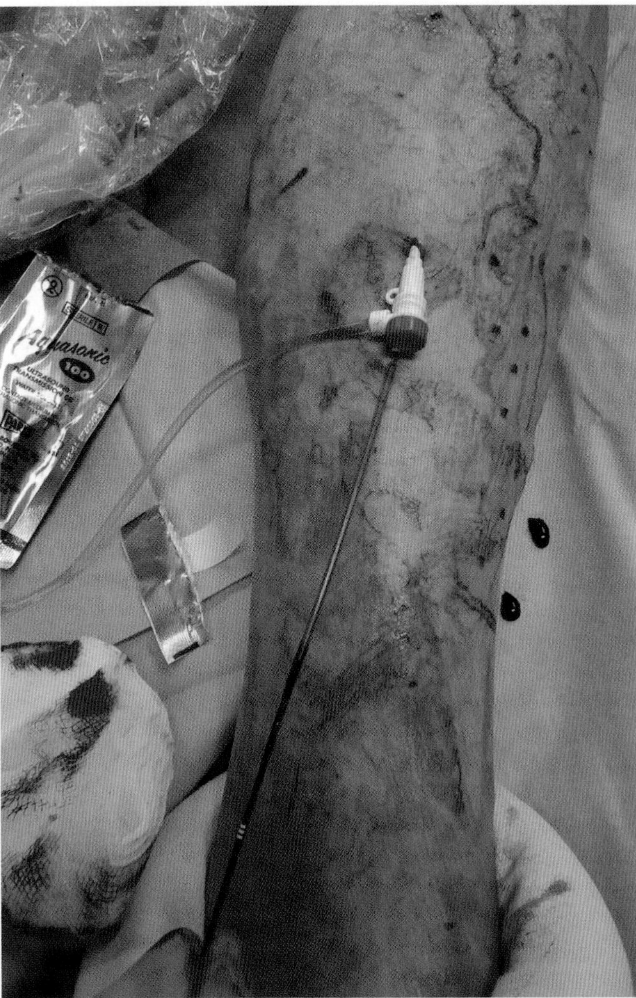

Figure 62.18 Radiofrequency ablation with ClosureFast™ introducing the treatment catheter through a sheath. The distal 7 cm of this device comprises a metal coil.

- Catheter-based systems have the additional advantage of allowing direct and targeted delivery of adjuvant foam sclerotherapy, e.g. to ablate areas of neovascularisation. This is more difficult with radiofrequency catheters due to a smaller lumen (0.018 versus 0.035 in), but it is still possible.

Advantages in favour of RFA over EVLA include:

- The core skill set to plan and perform these procedures is the same; however, EVLA requires an understanding of power settings and pullback speeds, whereas a radiofrequency device typically has a set treatment cycle on a single button press. This reduces the device-specific learning curve and the possibility of a novice making a mistake with the energy delivery.
- The automatic treatment cycle also frees the surgeon's focus, allowing better communication with the patient and with care, concurrent treatment, e.g. infiltrating local anaesthetic into the tributaries and performing phlebectomy, reducing procedural times.
- EVLA requires specific laser safety protocols including the design and function of the room as well as specific training for the operator and theatre team. This can have an impact on the set-up and flexibility of the service.
- RFA may be associated with a marginal reduction in pain and bruising, although this has not been shown to impact on periprocedural quality of life or recovery.

Advantages in favour of EVLA over RFA include:

- When it comes to veins that are very large in diameter (>15 mm) EVLA can be a better option, allowing an increase in energy delivery and higher efficacy rates.
- EVLA consumables are typically much less expensive; however, costs vary by device and market and the price difference has reduced over time.
- A standard EVLA fibre may be used to treat perforators, whereas a specific additional device is typically required for RFA, increasing costs. The clinical utility and indications for perforator management remain uncertain.

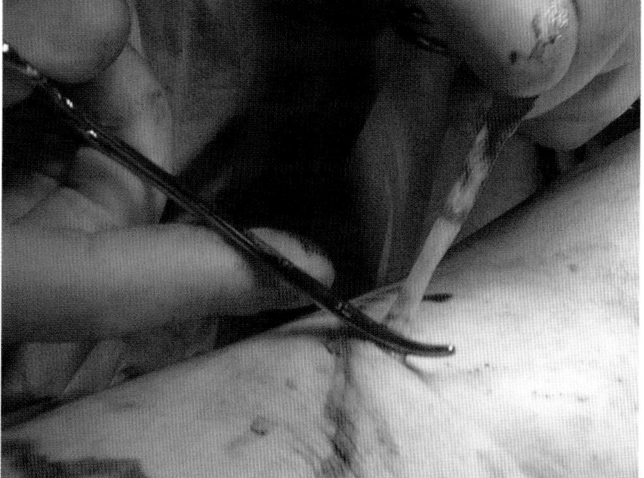

Figure 62.19 Phlebectomy performed under tumescent anaesthesia following endothermal ablation.

As endothermal ablation treats only junctional and truncal incompetence, debate exists regarding the management of varicosities. These can be managed concomitantly or sequentially by either phlebectomy or sclerotherapy. Concomitant phlebectomy (***Figure 62.19***) results in a more rapid improvement in disease-specific quality of life, and allows the vast majority of patients to complete treatment in a single visit.

Non-endothermal, non-tumescent ablation

Endothermal ablation was a large step forwards in the management of superficial incompetence; however, all techniques require the injection of tumescent local anaesthetic solution and this can be uncomfortable for the patient. Other techniques that avoid injection are being developed.

Ultrasound-guided foam sclerotherapy

Sclerotherapy is the original non-endothermal, non-tumescent technique and has been performed for over 100 years. It involves the injection of a sclerosing agent directly into the superficial veins. The most commonly used is sodium tetradecyl sulphate. The direct contact with detergent causes cellular death and initiates an inflammatory response, aiming to result in thrombosis, fibrosis and obliteration (sclerosis). Blood deactivates the action of the sclerosing agent and the doses administered need to be limited to avoid adverse effects, causing a trade-off between poor efficacy and safety. This led to the development of ultrasound-guided foam sclerotherapy (UGFS). The use of foam increases the effective volume of the agent, maximising endothelial contact and displacing any blood that deactivates it.

The procedure commences with the patient standing, and the sites of venous cannulation are selected and marked using ultrasound. With the patient supine, the major venous trunks and superficial varicosities to be treated are then all cannulated using ultrasound guidance prior to any injection (***Figure 62.20***). Once all injection sites are cannulated the foam can be prepared. The most widely used method is that of Tessari; this utilises two syringes connected using a three-way

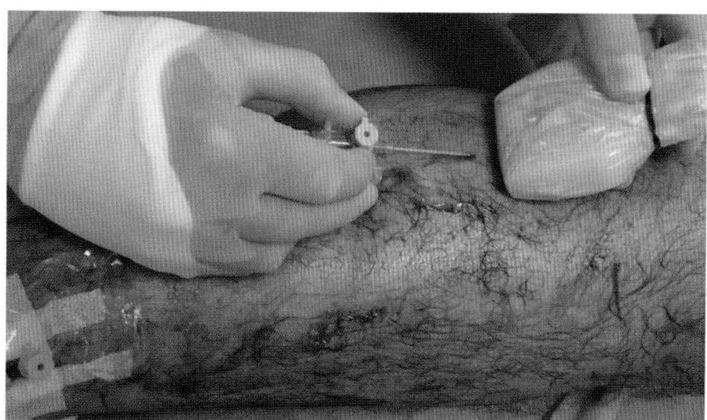

Figure 62.20 Foam sclerotherapy; cannulation of veins during ultrasound-guided foam sclerotherapy.

Lorenzo Tessari, b. 1949, physician, Trieste, Italy.

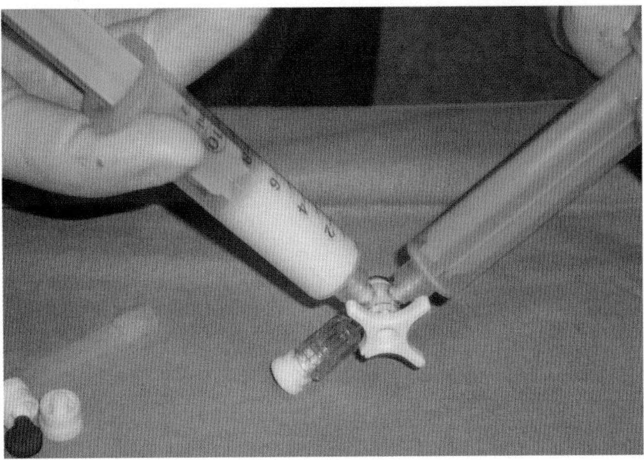

Figure 62.21 Foam sclerotherapy; Tessari method of foam sclerosant preparation.

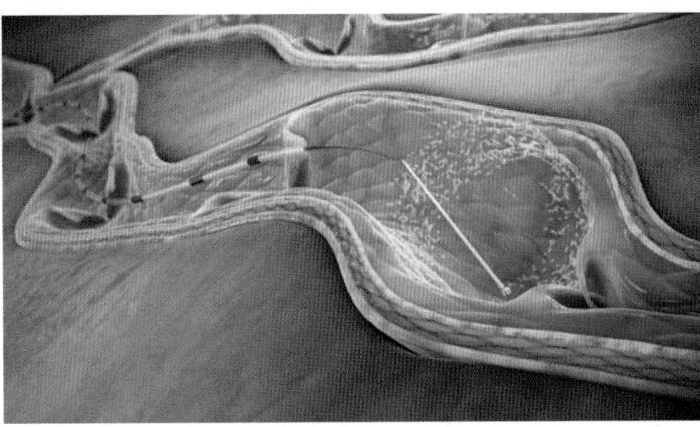

Figure 62.22 Mechanochemical ablation device (reproduced with permission from Vascular Insights).

tap. A 1:3 or 1:4 ratio mixture of sclerosant and air is drawn into one syringe, and is then oscillated vigorously between the two syringes about 10 or 20 times (***Figure 62.21***). The foam produced in this way is stable for about 2 minutes so it should be injected as soon as it has been made. The leg is then elevated to empty the veins of blood, and injection of foam commences first with superficial varicosities and ends with injection of the GSV or SSV. Only 1–2 mL of foam should be injected at a time and the distribution of the foam should be monitored and massaged with the ultrasound probe. When the foam is visualised at the site of junctional incompetence no further foam should be injected. The maximum volume of foam that should be injected at a single session should not exceed 10–12 mL as the incidence of complications is directly related to the volume of foam injected. Compression is then applied as following endothermal ablation. While it is postulated that compression may have a larger effect upon efficacy for this treatment, practice is not informed by evidence and a wide variation exists.

Outside of a small number of centres, the efficacy of UGFS is significantly worse than for endothermal ablation, leading to high reintervention rates, and the rates of complications such as phlebitis and pigmentation can be high. UGFS does however carry some significant advantages:

- It avoids tumescent anaesthetic and is therefore a less painful procedure (although postoperative pain is probably similar).
- No axial or tributary veins are too tortuous.
- It also allows the treatment of calf veins with overlying skin damage or ulceration without the need to pierce through damaged skin.
- Consumable treatment costs are very low.

These factors mean that many surgeons using endothermal techniques also use foam sclerotherapy as an adjunct in specific circumstances.

Catheter-directed sclerotherapy and mechanochemical ablation

The efficacy of sclerotherapy relies on endothelial contact with fresh, undiluted sclerosant. Some have therefore experimented with catheter-delivered sclerotherapy rather than trying to milk the sclerosant down the vein lumen. There is no good evidence to date that this increases efficacy and the technique is not in widespread use.

A related technology that has shown more promise is mechanochemical ablation (***Figure 62.22***). This involves a treatment device that deploys an angled wire from the end. This attaches to a motorised handle. The catheter is placed within the vein lumen as for endothermal ablation. The trigger on the handle is depressed, spinning the wire around and liquid sclerosant is infiltrated via the catheter simultaneously during catheter withdrawal. It is thought that the spinning wire causes physical damage to the endothelium and allows a deeper penetration of the sclerosant into the vein wall. The technique is possible in most cases without tumescent anaesthesia, although a small number of patients find the procedure uncomfortable and the device can 'snag' on the vein, tearing it or rarely stripping it altogether. Comparative studies with endothermal ablation suggest similar early efficacy rates but increased medium-/long-term recanalisation rates. The axial ablation is usually less painful than endothermal ablation, but this advantage is lost when it is combined with phlebectomy of the tributaries; therefore, it is uncertain whether it can replace endothermal ablation, unless axial ablation is to be performed in isolation. Treating longer veins can also be challenging owing to limitations in catheter length and the safe dose of sclerosant. It is a good choice for a patient with needle phobia who is happy to forgo treatment of varicose tributaries.

Endovenous glue

The final non-tumescent technique is the endoluminal application of cyanoacrylate adhesive (***Figure 62.23***). Again, this involves a treatment catheter placed within the vein lumen. A handle is used to infiltrate the adhesive in 0.1-mL applications via the catheter. The vein is then compressed, sealing the lumen closed. Early efficacy results are similarly promising and patients experience minimal intraprocedural pain. Long-term results and the optimal management of tributaries are unknown (similar to mechanochemical ablation). The consumable costs are currently the highest for any venous ablative technique.

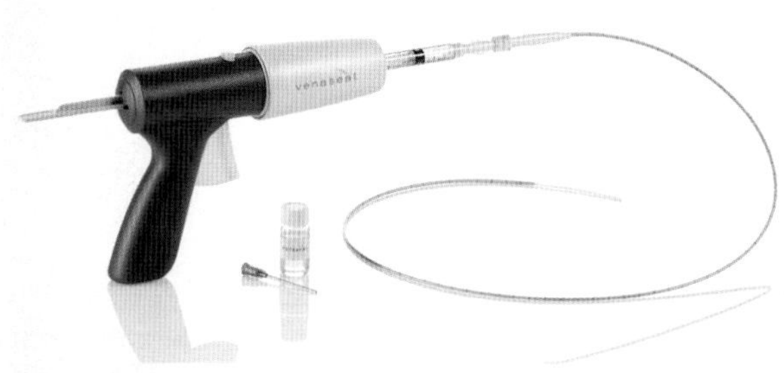

Figure 62.23 Endovenous glue device (reproduced with permission from Medtronic Inc.).

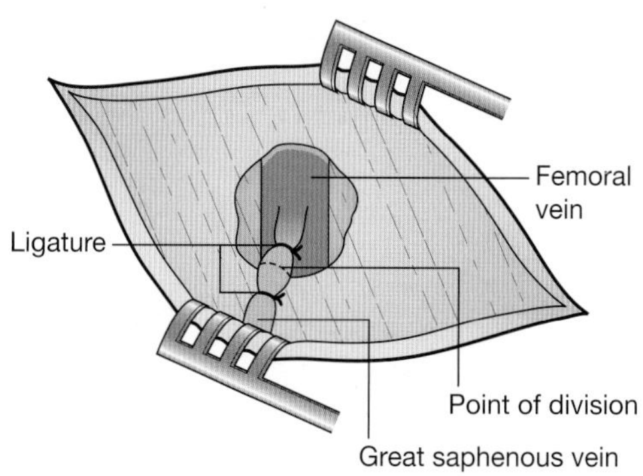

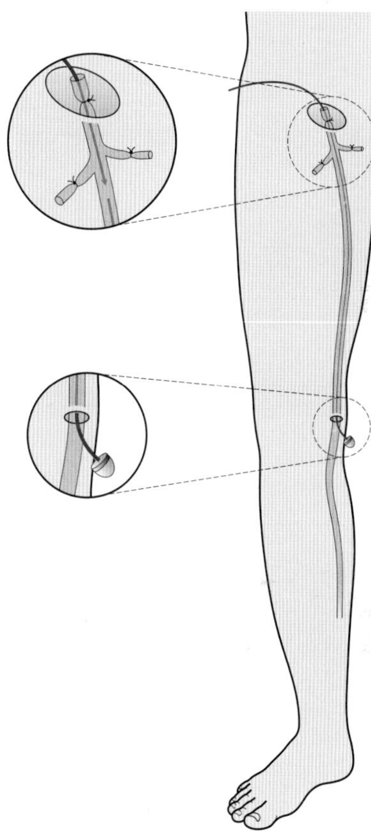

Figure 62.24 Saphenofemoral junction ligation and great saphenous vein stripping.

Open surgery

The principles of traditional ligation and stripping are to fully dissect the point of junctional incompetence and to remove the refluxing axial vein and dilated tributaries. The operation is usually performed under general anaesthesia but locoregional anaesthesia is used by some; the infiltration of tumescent local anaesthesia around the axial vein prior to stripping may have some advantages, but is not widely used.

The role of open surgery as a primary treatment of a refluxing superficial axis has been considerably reduced with the development of the minimally invasive techniques described above, the long-term results of which are at least comparable to open surgery but with significantly less morbidity and faster recovery. Experienced endovenous surgeons do still use open surgery in some circumstances and a venous surgeon needs to be trained and experienced in this area.

Surgical adjuncts including phlebectomy and, occasionally, perforator ligation are much more commonly used, and the former has been shown to have a significant impact upon outcome.

Saphenofemoral ligation and great saphenous stripping

An oblique groin incision is made at the level of, and lateral to, the pubic tubercle, ideally above the groin crease. The GSV is identified and dissected to the SFJ, which should be clearly established before the vein is divided to avoid disastrous inadvertent transection of the superficial femoral vein. The anatomy is often variable but six GSV tributaries may be encountered close to the SFJ:

- Laterally:
  - superficial inferior epigastric vein;
  - superficial circumflex iliac vein.
- Medially:
  - superficial external pudendal vein;
  - deep external pudendal vein.
- Distally:
  - anterior accessory of the great saphenous vein;
  - posteromedial thigh vein.

Classically, these are ligated distal to their divisions. A flush SFJ ligation is then performed and the GSV retrogradely stripped to around the knee (***Figure 62.24***). Phlebectomy is performed as discussed above.

Closure of the cribriform fascia, with sutures or synthetic patches over the ligated SFJ, does not reduce groin recurrence. Stripping to the lowest point of reflux may improve results, but at a cost of increased saphenous nerve complications and is not widely performed. More recently, some surgeons have argued that surgical trauma and subsequent inflammation in the groin are associated with neovascularisation, which in turn may lead to recurrence. Furthermore, others hypothesise that it is the loss of the normal groin tributaries that may be responsible for driving the process of neovascularisation. These concepts have led some to believe that ligation of the refluxing vein should be distal to the tributaries and that the junction itself should be left untouched. There is no clear clinical evidence to support these hypotheses.

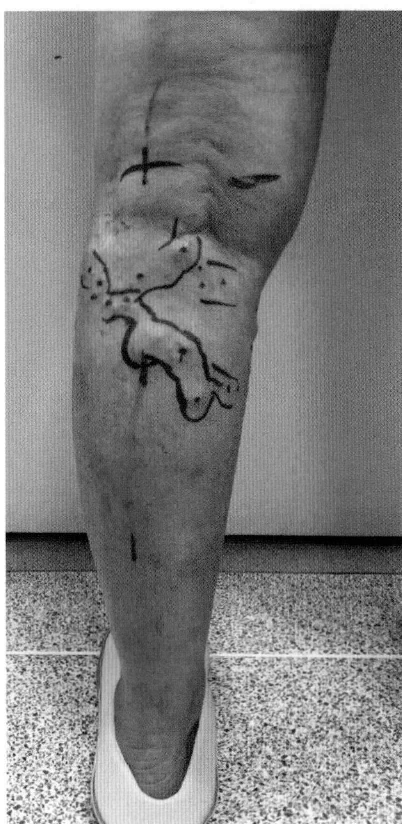

Figure 62.25 Preoperative marking of the saphenopopliteal junction and small saphenous vein mapped using duplex scanning.

Saphenopopliteal junction ligation and small saphenous stripping

Preoperative duplex to mark the position of the SPJ is highly recommended (***Figure 62.25***). The patient is positioned in the prone position, a transverse incision is made over the premarked SPJ, the fascia is divided and the SSV is exposed. The SPJ can then be formally dissected with a flush ligation or the SSV can be gently retracted and ligated as proximally as possible. No good evidence exists to favour one technique over the other; proponents of the flush ligation would argue that it avoids leaving a stump of SSV, a common source of recurrence, while proponents of the simple SSV ligation technique argue that it reduces the incidence of the most common serious complications – nerve injury and popliteal vein injury.

The SSV can then either be stripped or the proximal section of the vein can be resected. Those who strip argue that it reduces the incidence of recurrence, while opponents feel it increases the incidence of sural nerve injury. There are no randomised trials comparing these techniques. Once again, phlebectomy is then performed.

Adjunctive surgical techniques

Phlebectomy

This may be performed following treatment of junctional incompetence and axial vein reflux, or as a sole treatment under local anaesthetic in patients with isolated tributary incompetence, or possibly in very early axial reflux, which reverts to normal upon occlusion of the refluxing tributary on duplex ultrasound. Phlebectomy is usually performed through small stab incisions using small mosquito forceps and/or phlebectomy hooks that have been demonstrated to be superior – in terms of bruising, pain and generic quality of life – to transilluminated-powered phlebectomy (***Figure 62.19***).

Perforator ligation

The majority of studies assessing the role of perforator ligation have been in patients with venous ulcers, analysing the effects on ulcer healing; even in this situation randomised data are lacking. The role of perforator ligation in patients with uncomplicated varicose veins is even less clear. In uncomplicated varicose veins perforators may be ligated through a small, duplex-guided incision, while in patients with skin changes subfascial endoscopic perforator ligation may be preferred, although the benefits are unproven. Perforators can also be ablated with endovenous techniques.

Complications of standard varicose vein surgery

Complications (minor and major) are reported in up to 20% of patients who undergo traditional varicose vein surgery. Wound infections, the most common complication, are reduced by prophylactic antibiotics. Nerve injury is the most common serious complication. The incidence of saphenous nerve neuralgia is up to 7% following GSV stripping to the knee (the incidence is higher with stripping to the ankle). The incidence of sural nerve neuropraxia and common peroneal nerve injury may be as high as 20% and 4%, respectively, following SSV surgery. The incidence of venous thromboembolic complications is approximately 0.5% following varicose vein surgery; however, patient risk factors must be individually assessed and appropriate prophylaxis administered according to guidelines.

Recurrent varicose veins

Approximately 10–20% of patients who present to hospital with varicose veins have had previous intervention. Prospective data on long-term results following intervention for recurrent varicose veins are sparse and the criteria for defining recurrence are variable.

Significant clinical recurrence 5–10 years following varicose vein surgery occurs in 10–35% of patients, but minor/duplex-detected recurrence is much more common, being of the order of 70%. Causes of recurrence include: neovascularisation, reflux in the residual axial vein, inadequate initial surgery and new junctional reflux. Neovascularisation is the development of new veins within postsurgical tissue. These veins lack valves and over time can span the tissue between a ligated junction and nearby tributary veins. If significant in size and/or number, these may contribute to recurrent venous hypertension.

Recurrence is more common following SSV surgery than following GSV surgery, and in patients with high body mass index, while stripping of the incompetent axial vein reduces recurrence rates. Limited data suggest that recurrence rates following endovenous thermal ablation may be lower than following surgery. Recurrent varicose veins often have an atypical distribution and duplex assessment is mandatory (***Figures 62.26 and 62.27***). Open surgery for recurrent varicose veins is associated with a high (40%) complication rate, the most common being lymph leak and wound infection, thus endovenous interventions would seem to offer an attractive alternative, where feasible.

Summary box 62.1

Varicose veins

- Are one of the most common conditions causing a physical impairment in quality of life
- Interventional treatment improves quality of life and is highly cost-effective
- Anatomical and physiological assessment using duplex ultrasound is invaluable in the diagnosis and planning of treatment
- Ultrasound-guided endovenous ablation has revolutionised treatment, minimising procedural morbidity while being highly effective

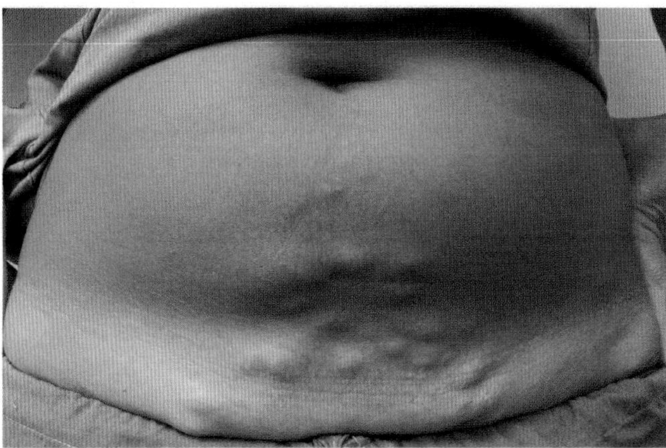

Figure 62.26 Recurrent anterior abdominal wall varicose veins following saphenofemoral junction ligation complicated by iliac deep vein thrombosis.

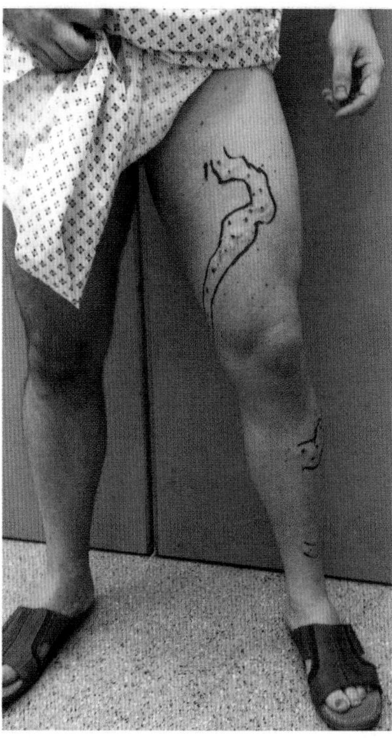

Figure 62.27 Recurrent varicose veins secondary to an incompetent thigh perforator.

VENOUS LEG ULCER

Venous disease is responsible for around 85% of all chronic lower limb ulcers in resource-rich countries. Community-based prevalence is 0.1–0.3% in adults (2–4% in the elderly). Venous leg ulcer has a disproportionate cost to society, with profound impairment in health-related quality of life for both patients and their carers; the dressings alone account for 1–3% of western healthcare expenditure. Furthermore, 15–30% of patients with 'venous' leg ulcers have concomitant arterial occlusive disease. This is termed a 'mixed' ulcer. There are many other causes of leg ulcers and these must be excluded in any patient presenting with ulceration. Causes of leg ulceration include:

- venous disease: superficial incompetence, deep incompetence or obstruction;
- arterial ischaemic ulcers;
- vasculitic ulcers;
- traumatic ulcers;
- neuropathic ulcers;
- neoplastic ulcers;
- infections, especially in low and middle income countries.

Pathophysiology of ulceration

The exact pathophysiology of ulcer development has not been established. Originally, it was thought that static blood within the superficial veins led to hypoxia, which caused tissue death (stasis ulcers). This was not confirmed by investigation of venous oxygen saturation, which was found to be higher in ulcerated limbs. This led to the concept of arteriovenous fistulae, which were thought to develop in response to the high venous pressure; however, this could not be confirmed. High venous pressure was found to be associated with a pericapillary infiltrate. This includes fibrin and other proteins, which are known to lead to fibrosis. It was hypothesised that these 'cuffs' could act as an impediment to diffusion of oxygen and nutrients.

Leukocytes were found to be reduced in the blood returning from legs with venous hypertension. This decrease in leukocyte passage was shown to increase if short-term venous hypertension was induced by application of a tourniquet. This led to the concept of white cell 'trapping', which, however, has not been confirmed by further investigation. Polymorphonuclear leukocytes were not found within the tissues, but increased numbers of mast cells, monocytes and lymphocytes have been found in periulcer tissues.

Reactive oxygen species are increased in the ulcer environment and these may generate free radicals, leading to tissue damage. Proteolytic enzymes are also increased in ulcers and the fibroblasts in the ulcer surrounds are also abnormal, being in a 'senescent' state. Growth factors may be inhibited, leading to poor repair, and their absence may also lead to ulceration. It is debated whether these factors are the cause or effect of an ulcer.

At present, ambulatory venous hypertension is the only accepted underlying cause of venous ulceration. This also explains why venous ulcers are never seen in the upper limb. It is important to try to define the exact mechanism of ulcer development. Venous hypertension may be the result of primary valve incompetence of the saphenous veins, incompetence of the perforating veins or incompetence or obstruction of the deep veins.

Clinical features

The ulcer must be carefully examined. A venous ulcer usually has a gently sloping edge and the floor contains granulation tissue covered by a variable amount of slough and exudate. Any significant elevation of the ulcer edge should indicate the need for a biopsy to exclude a carcinoma (usually a squamous cell).

Venous leg ulcers characteristically develop in the skin of the gaiter region, the area between the muscles of the calf and the ankle. This is the region where many of the Cockett perforators join the posterior tibial vein to the surface vein, known as the posterior arch vein. The majority of ulcers develop on the medial side of the calf, but may develop anywhere in the gaiter area. Extension onto the foot or into the upper calf is uncommon and, if there is ulceration at these sites, other diagnoses should be seriously considered. Ulcers often develop in response to minor trauma; many patients notice some itching, perhaps associated with mast cell degranulation, before the ulcers develop. Almost all venous ulcers have surrounding haemosiderosis (seen as pigmentation) and the more chronic ulcers develop LDS with associated fibrosis of the subcutaneous tissue (***Figure 62.10***). This is manifest as thickening, pigmentation, inflammation and induration of the calf skin. The pigmentation comes from haemosiderin and melanin and the haemosiderin itself may be an important factor in ulcer development.

A full examination of the front and back of the limbs with the patient standing should be carried out to assess the presence of varicosities and truncal incompetence of the saphenous systems (note that venous ulcers are not always accompanied by varicose veins). All patients should have their pulses palpated and, if there is any doubt, their arterial Doppler pressures should be measured. Sensation and proprioception should be assessed to exclude neuropathy, especially in patients with diabetes. A careful examination of the hand and other joints may confirm the presence of rheumatoid arthritis or osteoarthritis.

Investigation

Most vascular surgeons will carry out a duplex scan when the patient with an ulcer is first seen to assess the status of the deep and superficial veins. The presence of reflux in these veins does not confirm a venous ulcer, but supports the diagnosis in the absence of another cause and helps direct treatment.

Venous ulcers are characteristically difficult to heal; however, persistence may indicate that there is another or coexisting cause (e.g. malignancy, rheumatoid arthritis or arterial ischaemia). Biopsies are indicated if malignancy is suspected and it is important to remember that a Marjolin's type of ulcer (a squamous cell or basal cell carcinoma) can develop in a chronic longstanding venous ulcer (***Figure 62.28***).

Patients with atypical or with ulcers not responding to treatment should have a full blood count, blood glucose, erythrocyte sedimentation rate (ESR) or C-reactive protein (CRP) assessment as well as a sickle cell test if they have an appropriate ethnic background. Anaemia can both cause ulcers (e.g. sickle cell disease and pernicious anaemia) and be a result of ulceration (e.g. iron deficiency anaemia and the anaemia of chronic disease). Polycythaemia is a rare cause of ulceration. An antibody screen should be obtained if the ulcer appears 'atypical' or if there is any suggestion of joint disease (e.g. rheumatoid arthritis). All patients presenting with a new ulcer should have their Doppler pressures measured unless the foot pulses are easily palpable and have been confirmed as such by a vascular specialist.

Management

The very best results are seen in specialist multidisciplinary ulcer services. The cause of a venous leg ulcer is venous hypertension and the keystone of management is to decrease this hypertension using venous ablation and compression therapy.

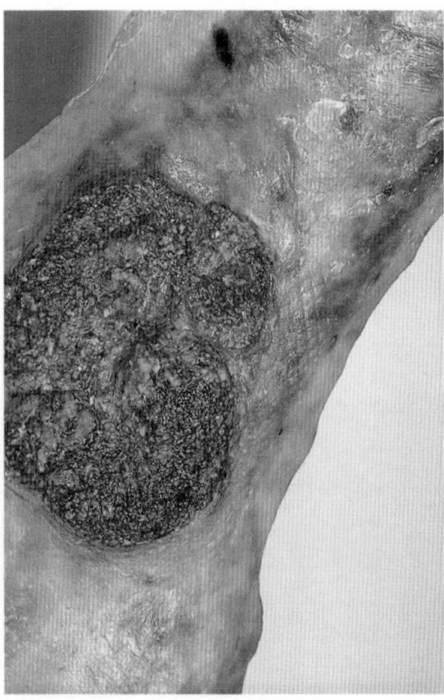

Figure 62.28 A Marjolin's ulcer (a squamous cell cancer arising in a chronic venous ulcer).

Frank Bernard Cockett, 1916–2014, surgeon, St Thomas's Hospital, London, UK.
Jean-Nicholas Marjolin, 1780–1850, surgeon, Paris, France, described the development of malignant ulcers in scars in 1828.

Superficial venous ablation or surgery

In patients with venous leg ulcers, treatment of superficial venous incompetence has been demonstrated to accelerate healing and reduce recurrence; therefore, expeditious referral to a vascular service for assessment is recommended.

Compression

The most clinical and cost-effective compression regimes are two-layer compression hosiery or four-layer compression bandaging. The latter includes:

- Orthopaedic wool: distributes the pressure and reduces undue pressure on sensitive areas susceptible to pressure damage. Also helps to absorb excess exudate that escapes the primary dressing.
- Cotton crepe: smooths the wool and holds it in place.
- Elastic bandage: first compressive layer, contributes about one-third of the interface pressure.
- Cohesive bandage: second compressive layer, increases stiffness and adds approximately two-thirds of the interface pressure.

The ideal interface pressure in pure venous ulceration is 35–40 mmHg. Skilled application of these dressings is essential for both safety and efficacy, and the best results come from specialist nursing teams based either in secondary care or in the community.

Compression in mixed ulcers is controversial, but emerging evidence suggests that it is both safe and effective when performed and monitored appropriately. With an ankle–brachial pressure index (ABPI) of 0.5–0.8 modified compression with an interface pressure of 30 mmHg is safe and effective and pressures of up to 40 mmHg have been described in studies using inelastic bandages without ill effect. Contrary to conventional thinking, studies have shown an increase in perfusion in patients treated in this way, presumably by a reduction in capillary back pressure. Patients do see respectable healing rates in this group, but they remain lower than in those patients with an ABPI >0.8. It is not clear whether revascularisation followed by full compression yields better results, but this is common practice. Patients with an ABPI <0.5 or an ankle pressure <60 mmHg must undergo revascularisation prior to any compression treatment.

Other treatments

Pentoxifylline, which increases microvascular perfusion by decreasing plasma cellular viscosity and cytokine inhibition, has been demonstrated to be a useful adjunct to compression by augmenting ulcer healing.

Horse chestnut seed extract has been shown to be a safe and efficacious treatment for chronic venous hypertension, improving symptoms and reducing leg volume.

A number of biological dressings have been developed, including fetal keratinocytes and collagen meshes, which have been shown to improve healing; however, they are not cost-effective for the majority of ulcers. Pinch grafts and ulcer excision with mesh grafting have been shown to provide good early healing with moderate long-term results (50% healed at 5 years).

Antibiotics do not speed ulcer healing in the absence of cellulitis and all other specific ulcer-healing drugs are of dubious validity. A large range of topical therapies and primary dressings have similarly failed to have an impact.

Prevention of recurrence

Once an ulcer has healed the patient must be re-evaluated in an attempt to prevent recurrence. If not already performed, patients should undergo treatment for their superficial venous incompetence. Class 2 below-knee graduated compression stockings should be prescribed for all patients with residual reflux or deep venous occlusion, or those with recurrent ulceration despite not being in this group. These should be worn for life.

Prognosis

Nearly all venous ulcers can be healed, but, even in those who have successful ablation or wear their stockings religiously, there is a 20–30% incidence of reulceration by 5 years. The greatest risk of reulceration is in the post-thrombotic leg.

Summary box 62.2

Venous leg ulcer

- Is associated with a profound impairment in quality of life
- Ulcers are not infrequently difficult to heal and prone to recurrence
- The treatment of these chronic wounds is associated with high costs to healthcare systems and patients
- The mainstay of treatment is the reduction in venous hypertension, with ablation of superficial venous incompetence and compression
- Early endovenous ablation of superficial reflux almost halves the time to healing of venous leg ulcers, reduces ulcer recurrence rates and is cost-effective

PELVIC CONGESTION SYNDROME

Pelvic congestion syndrome (PCS) is among the differential diagnoses to be considered in female patients presenting with chronic pelvic pain and may be significantly underdiagnosed. PCS sufferers are typically premenopausal, multiparous women aged 20–45 years, who present with severe dull aching pelvic pain thought to be the direct result of ovarian and pelvic varicosities. The pain is usually non-cyclical, and may be precipitated by prolonged standing. Other symptoms include dysmenorrhoea, menorrhagia, rectal discomfort or urinary frequency. Signs may include tenderness over the uterus/ovaries, vulval varicosities and haemorrhoids. There may be vulval and atypically distributed thigh varicosities. The road to a diagnosis of PCS is often a long and laborious one, usually only made following extensive investigations to exclude other more common causes of pelvic pain. Abdominal, pelvic and transvaginal duplex examination allows dynamic visualisation of pelvic blood flow and should be the initial investigation of choice, as these are rapid, readily accessible outpatient procedures that are also valuable in excluding

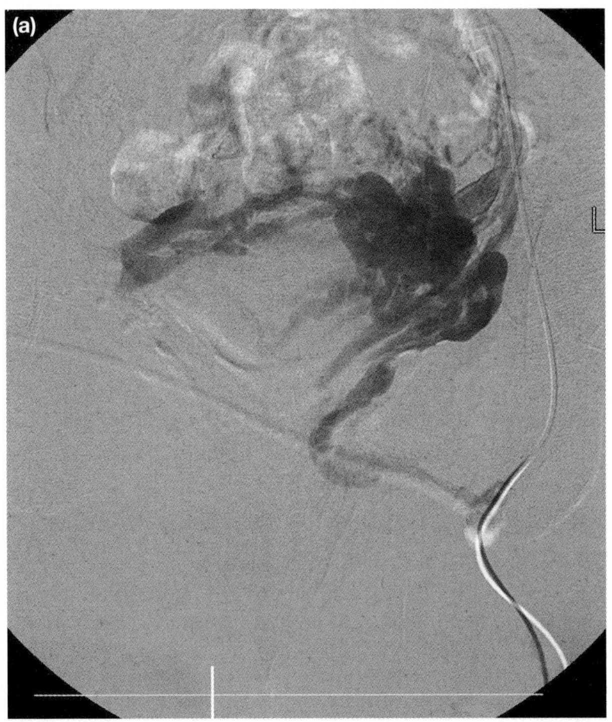

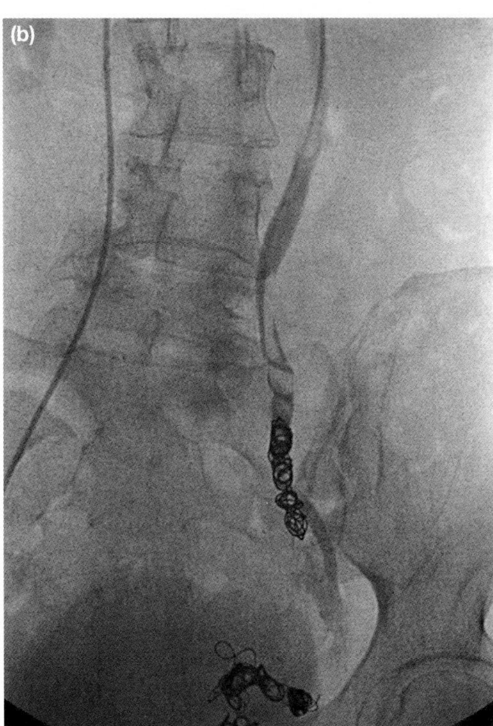

Figure 62.29 (a, b) Left ovarian vein incompetence supplying the pelvic and pudendal varicosities: **(a)** diagnostic venogram; **(b)** therapeutic embolisation.

other pathologies. Alternatives include MR venography and diagnostic venography.

Medical treatments for PCS include psychotherapy, progestins, danazol, gonadotropin receptor agonists (GnRH) with hormone replacement therapy, and non-steroidal anti-inflammatory drugs (NSAIDs). Historical open surgical procedures (extraperitoneal resection of ovarian veins) have now largely been superseded by percutaneous pelvic vein embolisation (***Figure 62.29***), reducing peri- and post-procedural morbidity while maintaining high success rates.

VENOUS THROMBOEMBOLISM

Venous thromboembolism (VTE) is an important condition within surgery, and autopsy studies suggest that it is the most common direct cause of death in surgical patients. Venous thrombosis is the formation of a semisolid coagulum within the venous system and may occur in the superficial system (superficial vein thrombosis [SVT] or 'thrombophlebitis') or the deep system (deep vein thrombosis [DVT]). Venous thrombosis of the deep veins of the leg may be complicated by the immediate risk of pulmonary embolus and sudden death. Subsequently, patients are at risk of developing PTS (***Figure 62.30***) and venous ulceration. While DVT may occur in the upper limb, it is the leg that gives rise to the vast majority of the morbidity and subsequent complications of this condition.

Aetiology

The three factors described by Virchow over a century ago are still relevant in the development of venous thrombosis. These are:

- contact of blood with an abnormal surface (e.g. endothelial damage);
- abnormal flow (e.g. stasis);
- abnormal blood (e.g. thrombophilia).

There are many predisposing causes for VTE. These are listed in ***Table 62.2***. The most important factor is a hospital admission for treatment of a medical or surgical condition. Injury, especially fractures of the lower limb and pelvis, pregnancy and the oral contraceptive pill are other well-recognised predisposing factors. Endothelial damage is now known to be critically important. The interaction of the endothelium with inflammatory cells, or previous deep vein damage, renders the endothelial surface hypercoagulable and less fibrinolytic. Stasis is a predisposing factor seen in many of the conditions described in ***Table 62.2***, especially in the postoperative period, in patients with heart failure and in those with arterial ischaemia.

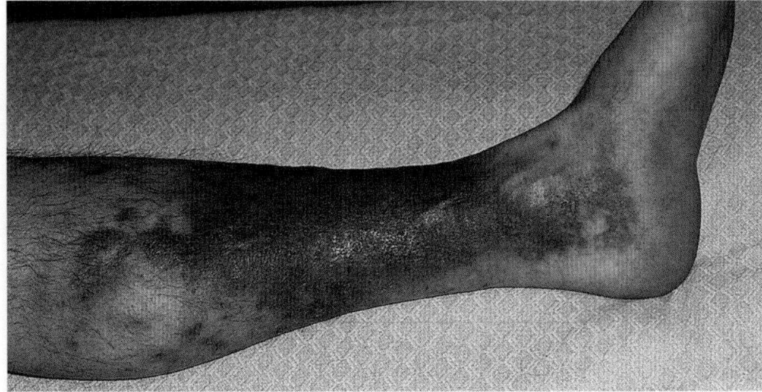

Figure 62.30 Post-thrombotic leg demonstrating features of eczema, pigmentation and mild lipodermatosclerosis.

TABLE 62.2 Risk factors for venous thromboembolism.
Patient factors
• Age
• Obesity
• Varicose veins
• Immobility
• Pregnancy
• Puerperium
• High-dose oestrogen therapy
• Previous deep vein thrombosis or pulmonary embolism
• Thrombophilia (see *Table 62.3*)
Disease or surgical procedure
• Trauma or surgery, especially of pelvis, hip and lower limb
• Malignancy, especially pelvic, and abdominal metastatic
• Heart failure
• Recent myocardial infarction
• Paralysis of lower limb(s)
• Infection
• Inflammatory bowel disease
• Nephrotic syndrome
• Polycythaemia
• Paraproteinaemia
• Paroxysmal nocturnal haemoglobinuria antibody or lupus anticoagulant
• Behçet's disease
• Homocystinaemia

A number of conditions are associated with increased coagulability of the blood (thrombophilia) (***Table 62.3***). Deficiencies of antithrombin, activated protein C and protein S have all been shown to predispose to venous thrombosis in young patients. Activated protein C deficiency is associated with inheritance of the factor V Leiden gene and may account for the higher incidence of venous thrombosis in white populations (being present in 6–7%). It results in a small increase in the risk of VTE, although it may act in concert with some of the other predisposing factors. A thrombophilia should be excluded in any patient presenting with an episode of VTE who gives a family history of VTE or in whom there is no other predisposing factor.

Although the development of DVT is probably multifactorial, immobility (and hence stasis) remains one of the most important factors. DVT is recognised as a complication of long-haul flights and other forms of travel.

Pathology

The thrombus commences as a platelet aggregate. Subsequently, fibrin and red cells form a mesh until the lumen of the vein wall occludes. The coralline thrombus then progresses

TABLE 62.3 Abnormalities of thrombosis and fibrinolysis (thrombophilia) that lead to an increased risk of venous thrombosis.
Congenital
• Deficiency of antithrombin III, protein C or protein S
• Antiphospholipid antibody or lupus anticoagulant
• Factor V Leiden gene defect or activated protein C resistance
• Dysfibrinogenaemias
Acquired
• Antiphospholipid antibody or lupus anticoagulant

as a propagated loose red fibrin clot containing many red cells (***Figure 62.31***). This is likely to extend up to the next large venous branch and it is possible for the clot to break off and embolise to the lung as a pulmonary embolus. In this situation the embolus arising from the lower leg veins becomes detached, passes through the large veins of the limb and vena cava, through the right heart and lodges in the pulmonary arteries. This may totally occlude perfusion to all or part of one or both lungs. This results in a clinical spectrum from tachycardia and pain, through respiratory failure (despite adequate ventilation) to cardiovascular collapse and death. Moderate-sized emboli can cause pyramidal-shaped infarcts on imaging.

Diagnosis

The most common presentation of a DVT is pain and swelling, especially in the calf, usually in one leg; however, bilateral DVTs are common, occurring in up to 30%. When the swelling

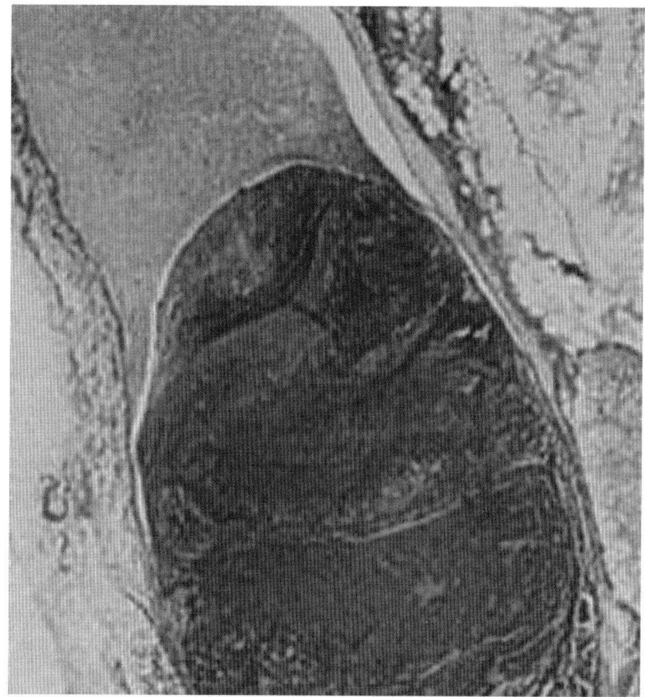

Figure 62.31 An organised thrombus.

Hulusi Behçet, 1889–1948, Turkish dermatologist, described a disease of inflamed blood vessels in 1937.

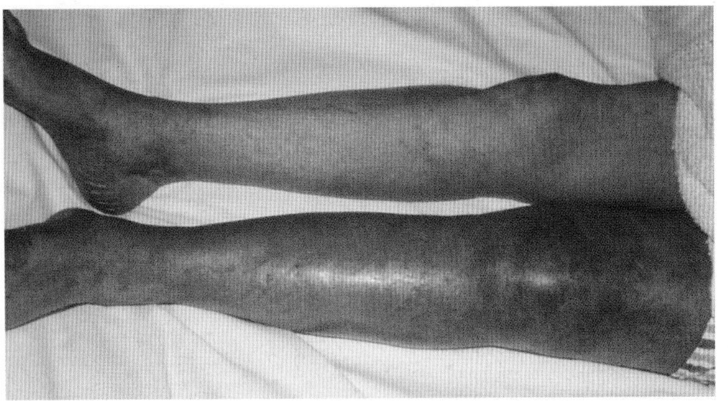

Figure 62.32 Phlegmasia cerulea dolens.

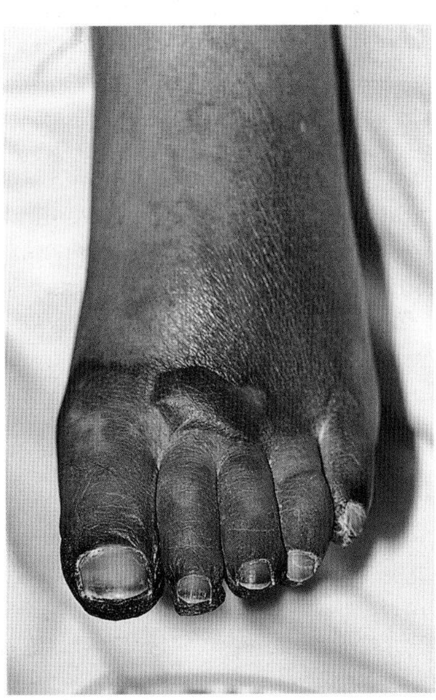

Figure 62.33 A foot with venous gangrene. The gangrene is symmetrical, involving all of the toes. There is no clear-cut edge and there is marked oedema of the foot.

is bilateral, DVT must be differentiated from other causes of systemic oedema, such as hypoproteinaemia, renal failure and heart failure. Some patients have no symptoms of thrombosis and may first present with signs of a pulmonary embolus, e.g. pleuritic chest pain, haemoptysis and shortness of breath. Patients may also develop shortness of breath from chronic pulmonary hypertension. Sometimes the leg appears cellulitic and very occasionally it may be white or cyanosed: phlegmasia alba dolens and phlegmasia cerulea dolens (***Figure 62.32***). This indicates venous pressures that are so high they are impeding tissue perfusion. Patients who present with venous gangrene (***Figure 62.33***) often have an underlying neoplasm.

Clinical examination for DVT is unreliable. Physical signs may also be absent. Mild pitting oedema of the ankle, dilated surface veins, a stiff calf and tenderness over the course of the deep veins should be sought. Leg pain occurs in about 50% of patients with DVT but is non-specific. Homans' sign – resistance (not pain) of the calf muscles to forcible dorsiflexion – is not specific and should not be elicited. Tenderness occurs in 75% of patients but is also found in 50% of patients without objectively confirmed DVT. The pain and tenderness associated with DVT does not usually correlate with the size, location or extent of the thrombus. Clinical signs and symptoms of pulmonary embolus occur in about 10% of patients with confirmed DVT.

A low-grade pyrexia may be present, especially in a patient who is having repeated pulmonary embolus. Patients may have signs of cyanosis, dyspnoea, raised neck veins, a fixed split second heart sound and a pleural rub if they have pulmonary emboli causing right heart strain, although these signs may be subtle or absent.

Investigation

The diagnosis of DVT and pulmonary embolus should be established by special investigations as the symptoms and signs are non-specific and may be absent. In addition, treatment with anticoagulation is not without risk and the diagnosis must be made with reasonable certainty.

Many centres direct investigations based upon the modified Wells score (***Table 62.4***), with further imaging dictated by these results. These scores can be unreliable though, especially in hospital inpatients, and should only be considered a guide.

Venous duplex ultrasound is commonly performed to look for evidence of thrombosis throughout the deep or superficial venous system. Ideally, this should be performed by an experienced vascular sonographer, but the volume of cases is such that compression ultrasound is frequently being performed by non-specialists. Compression ultrasound involves applying pressure with the ultrasound probe over the common femoral

TABLE 62.4 Modified Wells criteria for predicting deep vein thrombosis (DVT).

Variable	Score
Lower limb trauma or surgery or immobilisation in a plaster cast	1
Bedridden for >3 days or surgery in last 4 weeks	1
Tenderness along the line of femoral or popliteal veins	1
Entire limb swollen	1
Calf >3 cm larger circumference than other side 10 cm below tibial tuberosity	1
Pitting oedema	1
Dilated collateral superficial veins (not varicose veins)	1
Previous DVT	1
Malignancy (including treatment up to 6 months ago)	1
Intravenous drug abuse	3
Alternative diagnosis more likely than DVT	–2

Low probability (5%) of DVT (score –2 to 0); moderate probability (17%) of DVT (score 1 or 2); high probability (17–53%) of DVT (score >2).

John Homans, 1877–1957, Professor of Clinical Surgery, Harvard University Medical School, Boston, MA, USA, a founding member of the Society for Vascular Surgery.

Philip Wells, contemporary, physician, University of Ottawa, Ottawa, ON, Canada.

and popliteal veins. Under normal circumstances these veins will compress tightly shut. In the presence of DVT they will not fully compress. It is rapid to both learn and perform, but not ideal and most importantly misses calf vein thrombosis. Calf vein thromboses may propagate to form a more extensive thrombus, which may in turn embolise. The optimal management of calf vein thrombosis when detected is not clear; some units use surveillance, with others anticoagulating such patients upon detection.

Ascending venography, which shows a thrombus as a filling defect, is now rarely required unless thrombolysis is being considered (***Figure 62.34***). MR venography may also be used. Pulmonary embolus is diagnosed definitively by computed tomography (CT) pulmonary angiogram, which will demonstrate the presence of filling defects in the pulmonary arteries (***Figure 62.35***). Pulmonary angiography is rarely required unless thrombolysis is being considered.

The differential diagnosis of a DVT includes a ruptured Baker's cyst, a calf muscle haematoma, a ruptured plantaris muscle, a thrombosed popliteal aneurysm and arterial ischaemia. Duplex scanning will detect many of these conditions but often patients present with non-specific pain in the calf that resolves with no firm diagnosis being made. The differential diagnosis of a pulmonary embolism includes myocardial infarction, pleurisy, pneumonia and aortic dissection.

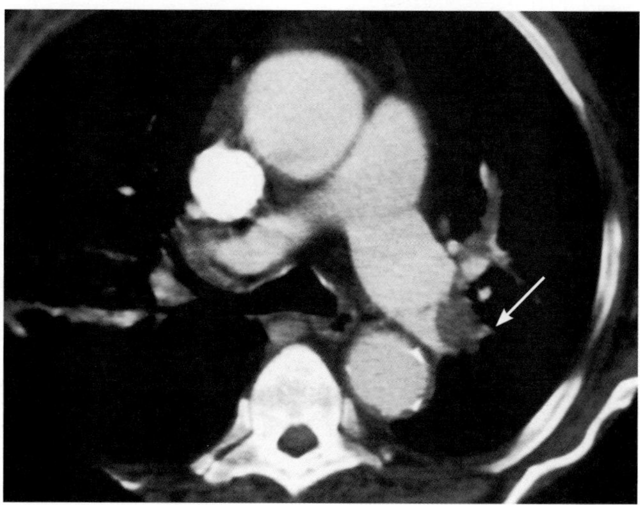

Figure 62.35 A computed tomography pulmonary angiogram showing pulmonary emboli as filling defects (arrow) in the pulmonary artery.

Prophylaxis

Prophylactic methods can be divided into mechanical and pharmacological. A variety of mechanical methods have been tried, but only the use of graduated elastic compression stockings and external pneumatic compression have been shown to be worthwhile by reducing the incidence of thrombosis. Newer devices, such as electronic nerve stimulators, lack evidence of efficacy to date. More recent emerging evidence is casting some doubt on the benefit of mechanical prophylaxis in surgical patients and there are further studies underway. Compression-based prophylactic measures should be avoided in patients with peripheral vascular disease.

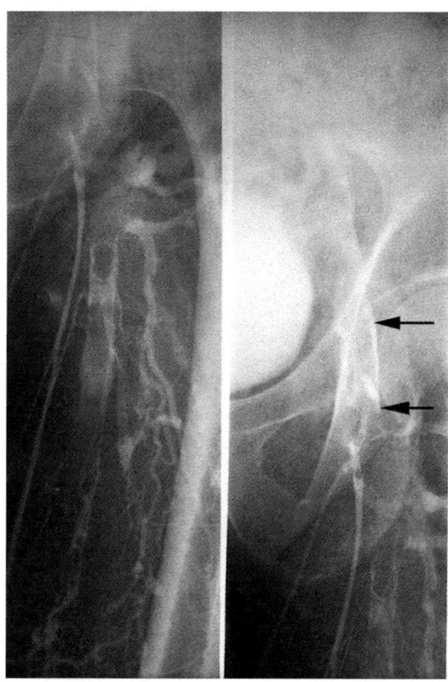

Figure 62.34 An ascending venogram of a deep vein thrombosis seen as filling defects (arrows) with contrast passing around the thrombus.

Pharmacological methods are more effective than mechanical methods at risk reduction, although they carry an increased risk of bleeding. In the past, low-dose unfractionated heparin was used both intravenously and subcutaneously. In the absence of renal impairment, most centres currently use low-molecular-weight heparin (LMWH) given subcutaneously. This is given once daily, does not require monitoring and has a lower risk of bleeding complications.

Patients who are being admitted for surgery may be graded as low, moderate or high risk for pulmonary embolism and VTE (***Tables 62.5 and 62.6***). Patients in the medium- or high-risk groups should be considered for pharmacological

TABLE 62.5 Modified Wells criteria for predicting pulmonary embolism (PE).

Variable	Score
Clinical signs and symptoms of DVT (minimum of leg swelling and pain on palpation of deep veins)	3
Alternative diagnosis less likely than PE	3
Heart rate >100 bpm	1.5
Immobilisation >3 days or surgery within past 4 weeks	1.5
Previous DVT or PE	1.5
Haemoptysis	1
Malignancy (treatment or palliation within past 6 months)	1

A score of <4 means PE is unlikely (12.4%); >4 is suggestive of PE (37.1%).

bpm, beats per minute; DVT, deep vein thrombosis.

William Morrant Baker, 1839–1896, surgeon, St Bartholomew's Hospital, London, UK, described these cysts in 1877.

TABLE 62.6 Low-, medium- and high-risk patient groups for venous thromboembolism.

Low
• Minor surgery <30 minutes; any age; no risk factors
• Major surgery >30 minutes; age <40; no other risk factors
• Minor trauma or medical illness
Medium
• Major surgery; age 40+ or other risk factors
• Major medical illness: heart/lung disease, cancer, inflammatory bowel disease
• Major trauma/burns
• Minor surgery, trauma, medical illness in patient with previous DVT, PE or thrombophilia
High
• Major orthopaedic surgery or fracture of pelvis, hip, lower limb. Major abdominal/pelvic surgery for cancer
• Major surgery, trauma, medical illness in patient with DVT, PE or thrombophilia
• Lower limb paralysis (e.g. stroke, paraplegia)
• Major lower limb amputation

DVT, deep vein thrombosis; PE, pulmonary embolus.

prophylaxis with an anticoagulant medication. Recent level 1 evidence suggests that the addition of mechanical prophylaxis in such patients affords no additional benefit.

Treatment

Deep vein thrombosis

The management of DVT has in the past been focused upon reducing the risk of pulmonary embolus. Patients who are confirmed to have a DVT on duplex imaging should be rapidly anticoagulated with a 'treatment dose' of subcutaneous LMWH. Patients with significant renal impairment should be commenced on intravenous unfractionated heparin. Patients who have a sensitivity towards heparinoids, such as those with heparin-induced thrombocytopenia, should commence on another anticoagulant, such as fondaparinux (an indirect factor Xa inhibitor) or bivalirudin (a direct thrombin inhibitor). This will achieve rapid anticoagulation and reduce the risk of embolisation. Typically, patients will then commence on oral anticoagulation for at least 3 months (or longer depending upon the persistence of risk factors or in recurrent cases). Oral anticoagulation using new or 'novel' anticoagulants (NOACs), which directly inhibit either factor Xa (rivaroxaban and apixaban) or thrombin (dabigatran), is recommended as they are equally effective as vitamin K antagonists (warfarin) in preventing recurrent symptomatic VTE but are associated with less major bleeding complications.

Patients who cannot be safely anticoagulated (usually because of bleeding risks) should be considered for a temporary inferior vena cava filter, until either they are safe to be anticoagulated or the risk of embolisation has subsided and the filter may be retrieved.

Endovascular surgery aiming to restore patency, including thrombus removal, lysis and stenting techniques, are increasingly used in patients with acute DVT aiming to reduce the risk of chronic post-thrombotic syndrome. Research suggests this may be beneficial in selected patients, for example those with iliofemoral thrombosis.

Pulmonary embolus

Most pulmonary emboli can be treated by anticoagulation and observation, but severe right heart strain and shortness of breath indicate the need for thrombolysis or radiologically guided catheter embolectomy.

Superficial vein thrombosis

This condition was previously known as thrombophlebitis. An abnormal endothelium is a much more common precipitating factor than in most DVTs. Common causes include external trauma (especially to varicose veins), venepunctures and infusions of hyperosmolar solutions and drugs. The presence of an intravenous cannula for longer than 24–48 hours often leads to local thrombosis. Some systemic diseases such as thromboangiitis obliterans (Buerger's disease) and malignancy, especially of the pancreas, can lead to a flitting thrombophlebitis (thrombophlebitis migrans), affecting different veins at different times. Finally, coagulation disorders such as polycythaemia, thrombocytosis and sickle cell disease are often associated, as is a concomitant DVT.

The surface vein feels solid and is tender on palpation. The overlying skin may be attached to the vein and in the early stages may be erythematous before gradually turning brown. A linear segment of vein of variable length can be easily palpated once the inflammation has died down.

A full blood count, coagulation screen and duplex scan of the deep veins should usually be obtained. Any suggestion of an associated malignancy should be investigated using

Summary box 62.3

Venous thromboembolism

- May be unprovoked, in which case an association with an inherited thrombophilia should be considered
- Is much more commonly seen as a complication of illness or surgery
- Is associated with both quality-of-life impairment and a risk of mortality
- All healthcare professionals should actively assess the risk and consider preventative measures where this risk is increased
- Management should involve measures to reduce the risk of extension and/or embolisation, typically with systemic anticoagulation
- Early thrombus removal is increasingly being used aiming to prevent chronic post-thrombotic syndrome, and rarely for limb salvage

Leo Buerger, 1879–1943, Professor of Urologic Surgery, The New York Polyclinic Medical School, New York, NY, USA, described thromboangiitis obliterans in 1908.

appropriate endoscopy and imaging studies, such as an abdominal CT scan.

Most patients are treated with NSAIDs and topical heparinoid preparations and the condition resolves spontaneously. Proximity to a deep venous junction or long affected length are indications for short-term anticoagulation and interval duplex assessment. Rarely, infected thrombi require incision or excision. Ligation to prevent propagation into the deep veins is almost never required. Associated DVT or thrombophilia is treated with anticoagulation.

CONGENITAL VENOUS ANOMALIES

There are four main types of anomaly:

- aplasia;
- hypoplasia;
- duplication;
- persistence of vestigial vessels.

Aplasia is most commonly seen in the inferior vena cava and has a similar presentation to the post-thrombotic limb. Membranous occlusion of the left common iliac vein (May–Thurner syndrome) often develops where the vein passes behind the right common iliac artery (iliac vein compression syndrome). This leads to an iliac vein thrombosis, which most commonly affects the left common and external iliac veins. Membranes may also narrow the hepatic veins, which can become totally occluded, leading to a Budd–Chiari syndrome.

Hypoplasia results in a narrow vein, which frequently offers little significant venous function and amounts to a functional venous occlusion, being circumvented by enlarged collateral venous tributaries. Duplications are quite common, with double vena cava, femoral and renal veins; they often present as an incidental finding.

Klippel-Trénaunay syndrome

This is a combined anomaly of a cutaneous naevus, persistent vestigial veins with varicose veins and soft-tissue and bone hypertrophy. The condition is a mesodermal abnormality that is not familial (***Figure 62.36***).

Segments of the deep veins are hypoplastic or aplastic and there may be an associated obstruction of the lymphatics. The condition must be distinguished from the Parkes-Weber syndrome, in which there are multiple arteriovenous fistulae causing venous hypertension, ulceration and high-output cardiac failure.

Virtually all patients with Klippel–Trénaunay syndrome should be treated conservatively with compression hosiery; however, some will benefit from laser ablation of the naevus, stapling of the bones to avoid leg length discrepancy and occasional removal of large superficial varicose veins, provided the deep veins are patent. LMWH should be given to all patients having surgery as this syndrome is associated with an increased risk of VTE.

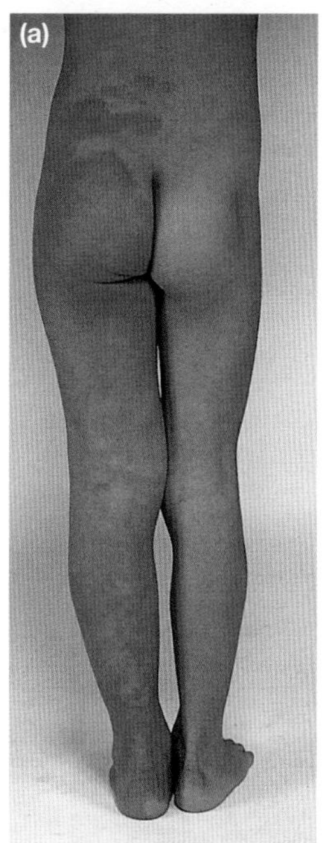

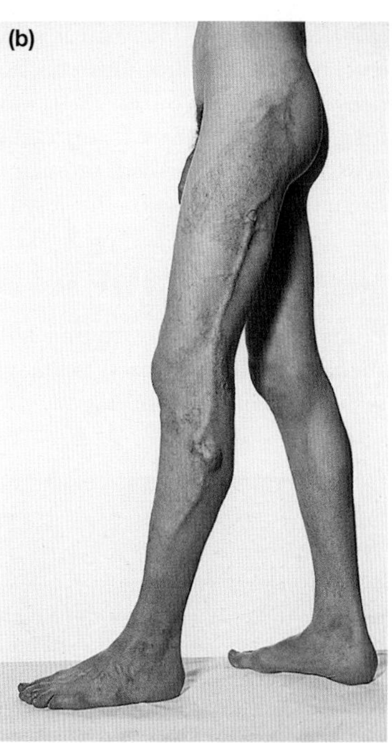

Figure 62.36 Two patients with Klippel–Trénaunay syndrome. **(a)** This patient has a longer leg and a capillary naevus; **(b)** this patient has a large lateral anomalous axial vein.

VENOUS ENTRAPMENT SYNDROMES

The axillary vein and the popliteal vein are the two veins that are most commonly compressed. The former is compressed at the thoracic outlet between the first rib and the clavicle, where it usually presents as an axillary vein thrombosis (see ***Axillary vein thrombosis***) (***Figure 62.37a***). The latter is compressed by an abnormal insertion of the gastrocnemius muscles. Entrapment may cause discomfort and swelling of the limb during exercise before thrombosis develops. Treatment is by surgical decompression, excising the first rib or dividing the abnormal musculature of the gastrocnemius insertion.

AXILLARY VEIN THROMBOSIS

Thrombosis of the axillary vein (Paget–Schrotter disease) may occur following excessive exercise in a patient with an anatomically abnormal thoracic outlet, but is also associated with excessive muscle bulk as found in weight lifters. The vein may be compressed by a cervical rib if this is present

George Budd, 1808–1882, Professor of Medicine, King's College Hospital, London, UK, described this syndrome in 1845.
Hans Chiari, 1851–1916, Professor of Pathological Anatomy, Strasbourg, Germany (Strasbourg was returned to France after the end of the First World War, in 1918), gave his account of this condition in 1898.
Frederick Parkes-Weber, 1863–1962, physician, The German Hospital, Dalston, London, UK.
Sir James Paget, 1814–1899, English surgeon and pathologist, best known for his description of Paget's disease of the bone.
Leopold von Schrotter, 1837–1908, Austrian physician and laryngologist, Chair of Laryngology, University of Vienna, Vienna, Austria.

(*Figure 62.37b*). The arm is swollen and painful and, at an early stage, the thrombus can be disrupted by thrombolysis delivered through one of the arm veins. The vein must then be imaged to see if there is any compression on elevation of the arm. If this is confirmed, thoracic outlet decompression can be carried out by resecting the cervical rib or first rib.

VENOUS INJURY

Blunt or penetrating trauma almost always damages some small and medium-sized veins, which can be safely ignored or ligated without causing any problems. Larger axial venous channels have in the past been ligated when injured, but it is now recognised that these axial veins should be repaired whenever possible to reduce subsequent morbidity (pain and swelling in the tissues being drained) and limb loss when associated with a concomitant arterial injury. Many venous injuries remain undiagnosed at the time of injury (e.g. crural vein damage associated with a fractured tibia) and only present many years later when post-thrombotic changes become apparent. Venous injuries occur from both civilian and military trauma but the incidence of venous military injuries has been particularly well documented. In total, 40–50% of arterial injuries have concomitant venous injuries, especially in the popliteal fossa.

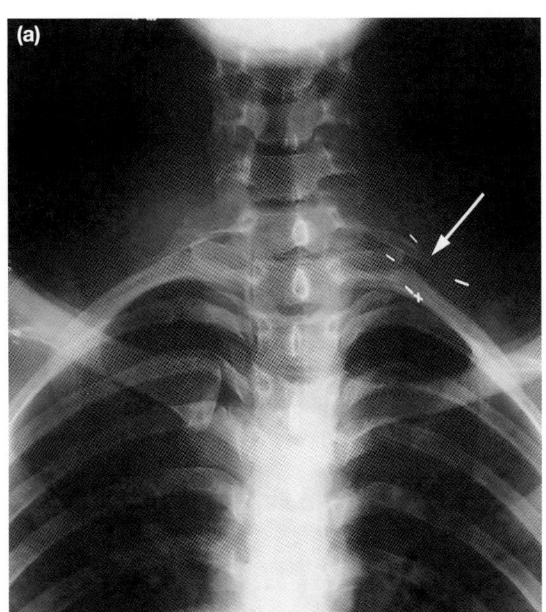

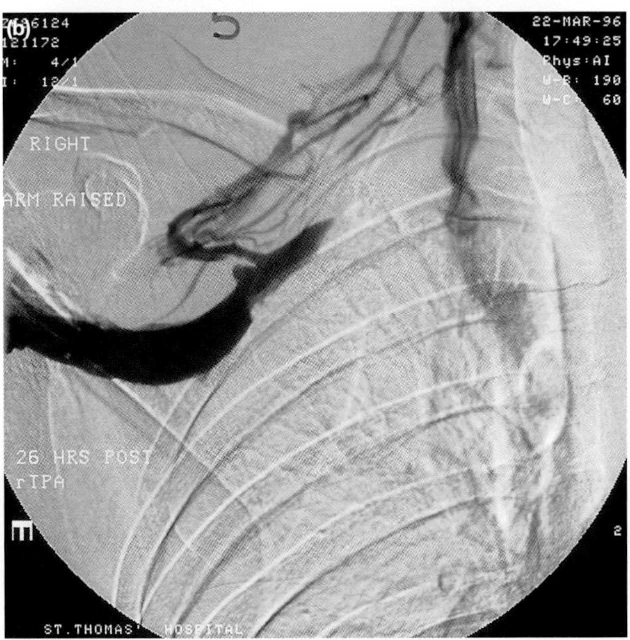

Figure 62.37 Thoracic outlet syndrome: **(a)** cervical ribs on plain radiograph; **(b)** elevation of the arm causes occlusion of the axillary vein with collaterals. The patient has had previous surgery to decompress the left side (arrow in **(a)**).

The mechanism may be laceration, contusion or avulsion (*Figure 62.38*). Iatrogenic injuries result from damage at the time of surgery and from punctures caused by catheter insertion. Thrombosis, haemorrhage and embolisation are all common complications and arteriovenous fistulae may develop when there is a local concomitant arterial injury.

Associated injuries to soft tissue, arteries and bones often overshadow the venous injury. Massive haemorrhage from the pelvic bones or the inferior vena cava can rapidly lead to hypovolaemic shock and death if left untreated. Haematomas are common and engorgement, cyanosis and swelling are also indicative of a major venous injury.

Management

As with all traumatic injuries, the management priorities are the assessment and management of issues affecting the airway, then breathing and then circulation. Venous injuries have the potential to threaten life through massive bleeding and patients require vascular access, circulatory support and blood products. Trauma patients with life-threatening haemorrhage are at risk of hypothermia, acidosis, functional and consumptive coagulopathy and paradoxical thrombosis, and these issues need to be prevented where possible and managed when present.

Venous pressures are low and so, where there is access to the site of injury, pressure will control bleeding and in most cases offer definitive management. Intervention is required where pressure cannot be applied, or where the loss of venous function itself threatens life or limb. Intervention can include reduction and stabilisation of a fracture (e.g. pelvis), endovenous embolisation or stent grafting.

A small proportion of venous injuries will require formal exploration and ligation or repair. Different types of repair are shown in *Figure 62.39*; the type of repair carried out depends on the extent of the venous injury, including how much venous wall has been lost or damaged. Lateral sutures and vein patches are ideal methods of repair and end-to-end anastomosis is satisfactory, provided that it is not carried out under tension. A jump graft may be required.

Vein replacement should be by autogenous tissue whenever possible, using vein harvested from another site, e.g. the internal jugular vein or the GSV from an undamaged limb. Artificial grafts, such as polytetrafluoroethylene (PTFE) grafts, are at risk of infection and have given poor results in recent conflicts. The use of anticoagulants and an arteriovenous fistula to reduce the risk of thrombosis in the vein graft are controversial and depend on the associated injuries that are present. In

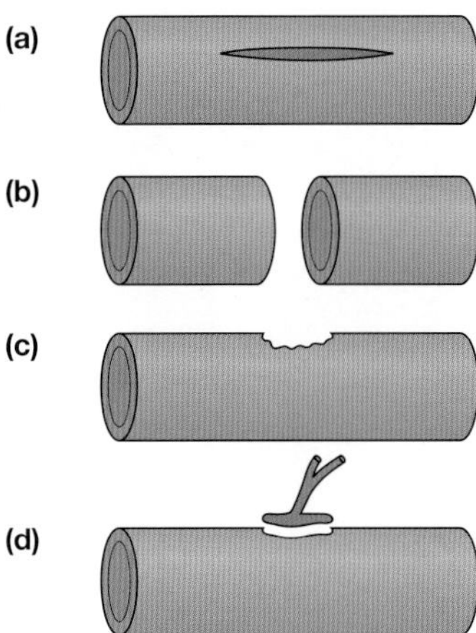

Figure 62.38 Types of venous damage: **(a)** incision; **(b)** transection; **(c)** irregular laceration; **(d)** avulsion of a tributary.

contaminated wounds, tetanus toxoid and antibiotics should be given. A fasciotomy should always be considered if there is a concomitant arterial and venous injury.

Prognosis

It is now recognised that repair of a major vein can be carried out with a 70–80% success rate, reducing the morbidity of a combined arterial and venous injury considerably (especially limb loss). Complex repairs should not, however, be carried out if a patient's life is at risk, when ligation may have to suffice in the short term.

VENOUS TUMOURS

Venous malformation cavernous angioma/haemangioma

These malformations are common, representing one end of a spectrum of arteriovenous malformations. They often affect the skin but also extend into the deep tissues, including bones and joints. They usually present with variable swelling and dilated veins beneath the skin. Occasionally, there is no visible mass and the complaint is one of pain. Haemorrhage and thrombophlebitis may exacerbate the pain. A soft compressible mass, which is venous in colour especially if it is under the skin, is usually present (***Figure 62.40a***). A dark-blue tinge is often apparent, even if the malformation is deeply situated. Nodules within the mass usually represent previous episodes of thrombosis. The size and extent of the haemangioma are best visualised by nuclear MR with a short tau inversion recovery (STIR) sequence (***Figure 62.40b***) or CT scanning with contrast enhancement. Venography rarely shows an abnormality, but direct puncture with contrast injection shows the connections of the malformation.

Treatment is a highly specialised area. Treatment options nowadays rarely initially involve surgical excision as once this is done future embolisation and sclerotherapy are very difficult. No treatment is entirely curative because it is difficult to remove all of the angiomatous tissue or sclerose the angioma completely. Sclerosis can be dangerous when the veins connect to the deep system, particularly near the central nervous system.

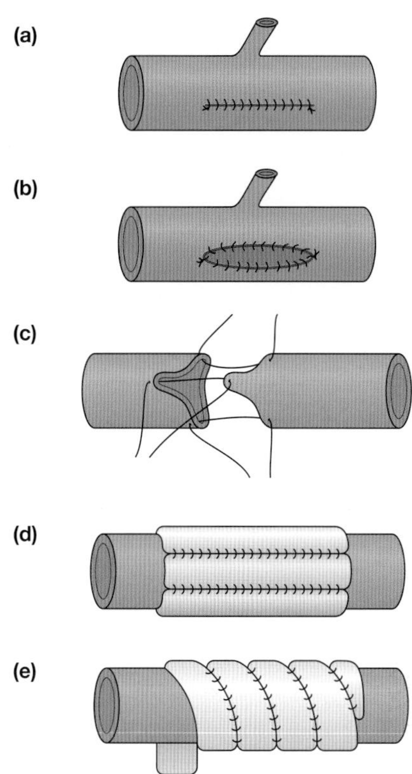

Figure 62.39 Types of venous repair: **(a)** lateral suture (risk of stenosis); **(b)** patch graft; **(c)** Carrel triangulation technique of venous anastomosis; **(d)** panel graft; **(e)** spiral graft.

Leiomyoma and leiomyosarcoma of the vein wall

These are extremely rare tumours that are usually slow growing. They present with pain and a mass with signs of venous obstruction, e.g. oedema and distended veins. Duplex scanning, CT (***Figure 62.41***) and magnetic resonance imaging (MRI) show a filling defect within the vein wall. Treatment is by resection with replacement by autogenous vein taken from another site. Rarely, a PTFE graft is required. When the tumour affects the vena cava it must be resected and replaced with a prosthetic graft.

Cystic degeneration

As in the peripheral arterial system, cystic degeneration of the vein wall is an uncommon cause of venous occlusion. It may be detected by ultrasound. The cyst may be deroofed or the venous segment excised.

Alexis Carrel, 1873–1944, a French surgeon who emigrated to work at the University of Chicago, Chicago, IL, USA. He was awarded the Nobel Prize in Physiology or Medicine in 1912 for pioneering vascular suturing techniques.

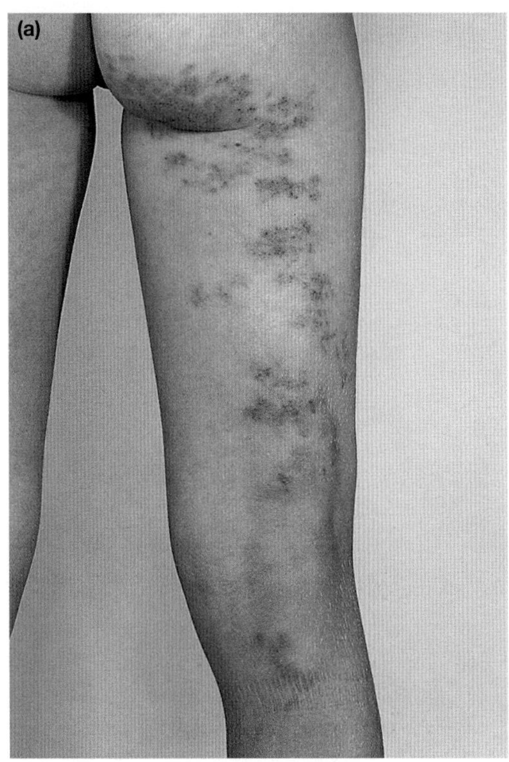

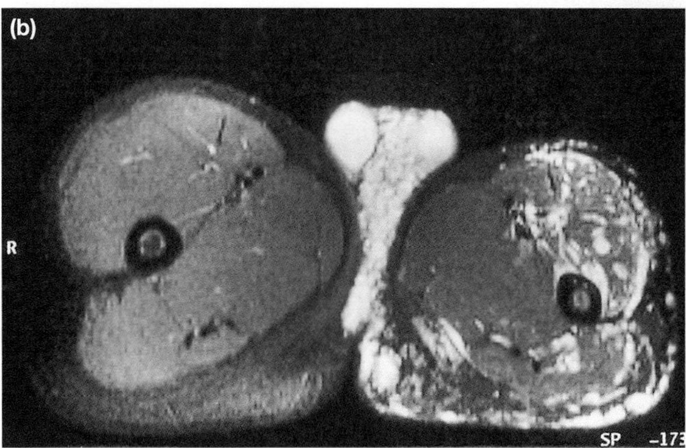

Figure 62.40 **(a)** Venous angioma of the leg; **(b)** magnetic resonance imaging showing extensive angioma (white) throughout the superficial tissues and anterior and posterior compartments of the left leg in a different patient.

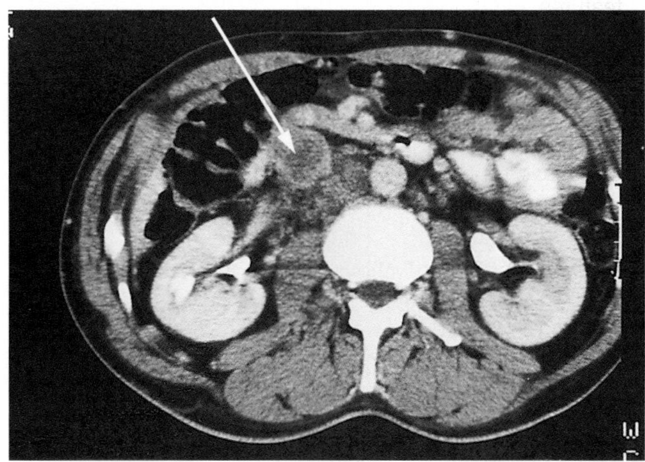

Figure 62.41 Inferior vena cava containing a filling defect from a leiomyosarcoma (arrow).

FURTHER READING

Barwell JR, Davies CE, Deacon J *et al.* Comparison of surgery and compression with compression alone in chronic venous ulceration (ESCHAR study): randomised controlled trial. *Lancet* 2004; **363**: 1857–60.

Brittenden J, Cotton SC, Elders A *et al.* Clinical effectiveness and cost-effectiveness of foam sclerotherapy, endovenous laser ablation and surgery for varicose veins: results from the Comparison of LAser, Surgery and foam Sclerotherapy (CLASS) randomised controlled trial. *Health Technol Assess* 2015; **19**(27): 1–342.

Carradice D, Mekako AI, Mazari FA *et al.* Randomized clinical trial of endovenous laser ablation compared with conventional surgery for great saphenous varicose veins. *Br J Surg* 2011; **98**(4): 501–10.

Carradice D, Mekako AI, Mazari FA *et al.* Clinical and technical outcomes from a randomized clinical trial of endovenous laser ablation compared with conventional surgery for great saphenous varicose veins. *Br J Surg* 2011; **98**(8): 1117–23.

Carradice D, Wallace T, Gohil R, Chetter I. A comparison of the effectiveness of treating those with and without the complications of superficial venous insufficiency. *Ann Surg* 2014; **260**(2): 396–401.

Coleridge-Smith P, Labropoulos N, Partsch K *et al.* Duplex ultrasound investigation of the veins in chronic venous disease of the lower limbs: UIP consensus statement. *Eur J Vasc Endovasc Surg* 2006; **31**: 83–92.

Comerota AJ, Kearon C, Gu CS, *et al.* Endovascular thrombus removal for acute iliofemoral deep vein thrombosis. *Circulation* 2019; **139**(9): 1162-73.

Gohel MS, Epstein DM, Davies AH. Cost-effectiveness of traditional and endovenous treatments for varicose veins. *Br J Surg* 2010; **97**(12): 1815–23.

Gohel MS, Heatley F, Liu X *et al.* A randomized trial of early endovenous ablation in venous ulceration. *N Engl J Med* 2018; **378**: 2105–114.

Lurie F, Passman M, Meisner M, *et al.* The 2020 update of the CEAP classification system and reporting standards. *J Vasc Surg Venous Lymphat Disord* 2020; **8**(3): 342-52. Erratum in: *J Vasc Surg Venous Lymphat Disord* 2021; **9**(1): 288.

Michaels JA, Campbell WB, Brazier JE *et al.* Randomised clinical trial, observational study and assessment of cost-effectiveness of the treatment of varicose veins (REACTIV trial). *Health Technol Assess* 2006; **10**(13): 1–196.

National Institute for Health and Care Excellence. *Venous thromboembolism in over 16s: reducing the risk of hospital-acquired deep vein thrombosis or pulmonary embolism.* NICE Guideline 89. London: NICE, 2018. Available from https://www.nice.org.uk/guidance/ng89.

National Institute for Health and Care Excellence. *Varicose veins: diagnosis and management.* NICE Guideline 168. London: NICE, 2013. Available from https://www.nice.org.uk/guidance/cg168.

Shalhoub J, Lawton R, Hudson J *et al.* Graduated compression stockings as an adjuvant to pharmaco-thromboprophylaxis in elective surgical patients (GAPS study): randomised controlled trial. *BMJ* 2020; **369**: m1309.

'VEIN' supplement. *Phlebology* 2015; **30**(2 suppl): 3–52.

Watson L, Broderick C, Armon MP. Thrombolysis for acute deep vein thrombosis. *Cochrane Database Syst Rev* 2016; Issue 11, Art. No. CD002783.

CHAPTER 63 History and examination of the abdomen

Learning objectives

To learn:
- The art and science of history-taking in a patient with abdominal complaints

To be able to:
- Recognise the organ or system responsible for the clinical features

To understand:
- The pathophysiological basis of common abdominal symptoms and signs as the pathway to clinical diagnosis

To be aware of:
- Leading questions and relevant physical signs based on the organ or system affected

INTRODUCTION

Abdominal symptoms are a frequent cause for surgical consultation. The underlying cause may be acute, presenting with the euphemistically termed 'acute abdomen'; subacute, indicating an evolving disorder; or longstanding, suggesting a functional or degenerative condition. Occasionally symptoms are due to disorders outside the abdomen, in which case the term 'referred' is used; for example, epigastric pain experienced as a result of a myocardial infarction.

At first presentation, a detailed clinical history and careful clinical examination are essential to establish a differential diagnosis, which, in turn, leads to appropriate triage into urgent and non-urgent investigation and subsequent treatment.

The advent of telemedicine and online remote consultation does not alter the basic art and science of consultation; however, the inability to perform a 'physical' examination may hamper arrival at a proper diagnosis. In such a scenario, a patient should be asked to come for a face-to-face consultation, physical examination and necessary investigations. It is vital to not miss a potentially seriously illness that needs urgent attention.

GATHERING INFORMATION

The experienced clinician will recognise the acuity and severity of the patient's condition even before a history has been taken. Initial observation provides clues to the direction that the history should take: general appearance, gait, position in bed, facial expression and tone of speech all provide useful hints. In an acute presentation, it is important to realise that the patient will feel anxious and vulnerable and may well be in severe pain; therefore, clinicians should introduce themselves, try to comfort the patient and gain the patient's confidence. Clinicians should put the patient at ease and seek permission to begin the consultation in ensured privacy. If a patient is still uncomfortable or reticent, the presence of a close family member as a chaperone can help. A tense patient without a relaxed abdominal wall will substantively affect the accuracy of the clinical examination. This is particularly important in a busy emergency department where the patient is only one among many.

Summary box 63.1

Importance of history and examination
- There is no substitute for a detailed history and thorough clinical examination
- The temptation to proceed to a diagnostic investigation such as abdominal ultrasound or computed tomography scan without clinical examination should be resisted

Obtaining a history

Presenting complaint

To establish the presenting complaint one should start with an open question inviting the patient to explain the reason for seeking medical advice. The patient must be allowed to explain the presenting complaint without interruption, after which carefully directed questions are used to further refine the history (Osler). Clues from these will allow identification of a

Sir William Osler, 1849–1919, Canadian Physician, initiated bedside clinical training for medical students at Johns Hopkins School of Medicine, Baltimore, MD, USA. 'Listen to the patient; he is giving you the diagnosis'.

likely organ or system responsible for the patient's symptoms, which then guides subsequent clinical examination and investigation to arrive at a probable diagnosis. History taking can be forwards and backwards, but its record should be structured.

In the acute situation, pain is the most common presenting feature. The classic features of site, nature, onset, duration, radiation and aggravating or relieving features of the pain should be established. In non-acute presentations, anorexia, weight loss, jaundice, altered bowel habit, blood loss and fatigue are all features that should be questioned.

Past medical history

The past history is important because it may have a bearing on the diagnosis and management. A history of previous similar episodes or past abdominal surgery often guides the diagnosis; for example, adhesive small bowel obstruction in a patient with a history of laparotomy or recurrent left iliac fossa pain in a patient with a past history of diverticulitis. Some symptoms and signs may be due to cardiac, respiratory, haematological conditions, such as abdominal pain in sickle cell crisis or acute epigastric pain in diabetic ketoacidosis.

Recurrent right iliac fossa pain may suggest a past history of appendicitis, Crohn's disease or in some regions amoebic typhlitis or ileocaecal tuberculosis. A positive history of tuberculosis can help in differential diagnoses in many patients. Efforts should be made to obtain previous medical records and investigations.

Drug history and allergies

Some drugs will have an effect on the symptoms and signs or may have to be discontinued before surgery. For example, a patient with bleeding who is taking a β-blocker will not have tachycardia proportionate to the blood loss; a patient taking long-term corticosteroids will need intravenous steroid supplementation to prevent an adrenal crisis in the perioperative period; a patient taking anticoagulant drugs may require reversal of the effects before surgical intervention. Patients with diabetes will require strict glycaemic control with sliding scale insulin in the perioperative period. Detailed enquiry about adverse reactions to anaesthetics or medications can prevent such problems later on.

Social history

The use of alcohol and illicit drugs, smoking and occupation are important. A history of family background and domestic support will guide the planning of discharge after surgery.

Family history

It is important to establish a family history of similar or related conditions, particularly cancer, inflammatory bowel disease, endocrine disease (e.g. hyperparathyroidism causing hypercalcaemia or renal calculi) and genetic disorders, including adverse reactions to anaesthetics or medications.

Review of the systems

A systems review should highlight any comorbid disease, such as cardiac, vascular, respiratory or endocrine problems; these have grave implications for the safety of any surgical intervention.

Summary box 63.2

Principles of history taking

- Identify the reason for consultation – the presenting complaint
- Determine the onset, duration and evolution of the symptoms
- Deduce the most likely organ or system affected
- Refine the history with relevant direct questions
- Establish relevant past, social, family, drug and allergy history
- Complete with a thorough review of other systems
- Devise a list of differential diagnoses

CLINICAL PRESENTATION OF ABDOMINAL PROBLEMS

Pain, weight loss, anorexia or vomiting, jaundice, abdominal bloating/distension, presence of a lump, alteration of bowel habit and blood loss or anaemia are the common clinical presentations of abdominal pathology. It is important to be vigilant about insidious presentations of malignancies. Classic examples are right colon cancer presenting with symptoms of anaemia, metastatic liver cancer with weight loss, gastric cancer with loss of appetite, ovarian cancer with abdominal distension and malignant obstruction of the extrahepatic biliary tree presenting with jaundice.

Abdominal pain

Pain is the most common of all abdominal symptoms and may be due to inflammatory, infective, obstructive, neurogenic, neoplastic or ischaemic pathology. Sometimes no organic cause can be found, a situation often labelled as 'functional or non-specific abdominal pain'. Improved understanding of pain pathways and the relationship with the gastrointestinal microbiome is likely to provide a more precise diagnosis, particularly in common 'functional' disorders such as non-ulcer dyspepsia and irritable bowel syndrome (IBS) (see ***Chapter 73***).

It is essential to establish the site, nature and radiation of the pain, the rapidity of onset and associated or relieving features such as food intake and or vomiting. Thus biliary colic will classically result in colicky pain in the right upper quadrant of the abdomen that radiates to the angle of the scapula and is associated with food intake (which results in cholecystokinin release and gallbladder contraction). The pain of acute appendicitis starts around the umbilicus and then shifts and localises to the right iliac fossa. Acute pancreatitis often has an abrupt onset of severe epigastric pain radiating to the back, which may be similar to pain emanating from peptic ulcer perforation or a leaking aortic aneurysm. Intestinal colic is most frequently associated with periumbilical pain and abdominal distension: the more distal in the intestine the pathology, the greater the degree of distension. Vomiting is an early feature of proximal small bowel obstruction, whereas absolute constipation is an early feature of colonic obstruction. Renal or ureteric colic is intense, located in the flanks and radiating towards the lower midline and scrotum. It is usually associated with either macroscopic or microscopic haematuria.

With regard to altered bowel habit, the onset, nature, duration, type of alteration (constipation or diarrhoea) and its relationship to abdominal pain will help to differentiate organic pathology causing obstruction or inflammation (colon cancer or inflammatory bowel disease [IBD]) from functional conditions such as IBS. When patients complain of diarrhoea, they may imply different meanings – some use the term for loose stools, others may mean frequent but normal stools. A longstanding increase in frequency of stools, with left-sided abdominal pain before defecation that eases after defecation, is suggestive of IBS. However, if such symptoms are of recent onset or are associated with blood or mucus in the stools, colonic carcinoma or IBD is more likely. A history of progressive change in bowel habit with an acute presentation with abdominal pain, distension and absolute constipation suggests acute-on-chronic intestinal obstruction, often from a stenotic left colon cancer. Marked distension with tenderness over the caecal area suggests a closed-loop obstruction with impending caecal rupture. Ileocaecal tuberculosis may present as a mass in the right iliac fossa with a ball of wind and gurgle suggestive of ileal stricture.

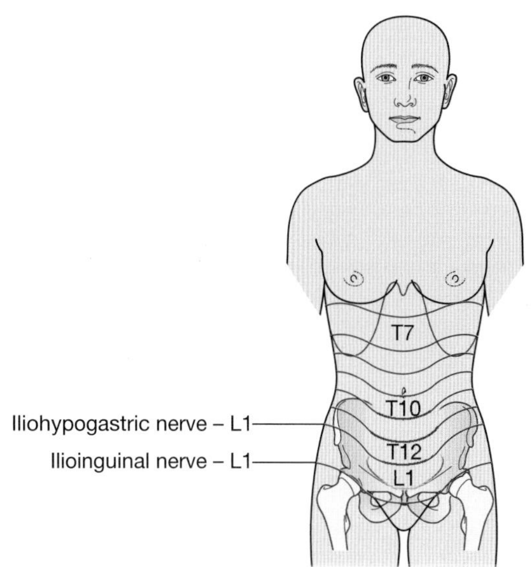

Figure 63.1 Distribution of the anterior abdominal wall dermatome and nerves.

Summary box 63.3

Classic presentations of abdominal pathology

- Obstructive and inflammatory pathology must be excluded in patients with abdominal pain and altered bowel habit as these require urgent care
- Closed-loop obstruction with tenderness in the right iliac fossa is indicative of imminent caecal rupture
- Caecal and ascending colon cancers classically present with anaemia
- Patients who have had previous abdominal surgery may have adhesions
- Check carefully for small incarcerated hernias, particularly femoral in obese patients as these may be hidden by 'abdominal panniculus'

PATHOPHYSIOLOGICAL BASIS OF COMMON ABDOMINAL SYMPTOMS AND SIGNS

The abdominal wall and parietal peritoneum are innervated by the somatic nervous system, whereas the abdominal organs and visceral peritoneum are innervated by the autonomic nervous system. Therefore pain may change in its character and distribution as the underlying pathology evolves. Visceral pain from the foregut is generally felt in the epigastrium, in the periumbilical area from the midgut and in the suprapubic area from the hindgut.

The skin and the muscles of the abdominal wall are supplied by the lateral and anterior cutaneous branches of the lower six intercostal nerves, the iliohypogastric nerve and the ilioinguinal nerve (***Figure 63.1***). The dermatome levels of the xiphoid process, umbilicus and pubis are T7, T10 and T12, respectively. The parietal peritoneum is supplied segmentally by the same nerves that innervate the overlying muscles. The central part of the diaphragmatic peritoneum is supplied by the phrenic nerve (C4); therefore, pain arising in this region is referred to the tip of the shoulder as it has the same segmental supply. The peripheral rim of the diaphragmatic peritoneum is supplied by the intercostal nerves. The obturator nerve is the principal nerve supply of the pelvic parietal peritoneum.

Pain from the viscera is principally due to ischaemia, muscle spasm or stretching of the visceral peritoneum. Unlike somatic pain, autonomic pain is deep and poorly localised. This pain is transmitted via sympathetic fibres and so is referred to the appropriate somatic distribution of that nerve root from T1 to L2. However, when an inflamed organ touches the parietal peritoneum, the pain becomes sharp and localises to the appropriate segmental dermatome of the abdominal wall. Referred pain due to irritation of the undersurface of the diaphragm by blood from a ruptured spleen can be felt at the left shoulder. Pain arising from the parietal peritoneum may radiate to the back or the front along the appropriate dermatome. This referral pattern is classically seen in acute cholecystitis when an inflamed gallbladder touches the parietal peritoneum. Pain then radiates round to the back along the involved dermatome. The overlying muscle and skin are supplied by the same nerve root, so, when the patient takes a deep breath, the tenderness in the right subcostal region is markedly increased, causing the patient to stop breathing; this is Murphy's sign. In children with abdominal pain who hold their right hip in a flexed position to obtain relief from the pain, one should suspect retrocaecal appendicitis causing irritation of the psoas muscle.

John Benjamin Murphy, 1857–1916, Professor of Surgery, Northwestern University, Chicago, IL, USA, described his sign in 1903. He was the son of immigrants fleeing the potato famine in Ireland. He was known as the 'stormy petrel' of American surgery.

Summary box 63.4

Nerves responsible for abdominal pain

- Abdominal wall and parietal peritoneum are supplied by the somatic nerves
- Abdominal organs and the visceral peritoneum are supplied by the autonomic nervous system
- Skin, muscles and parietal peritoneum are supplied by the iliohypogastric and ilioinguinal nerves and the lower six intercostal nerves
- Afferent pain fibres from the abdominal organs and visceral peritoneum travel with sympathetic nerves

Summary box 63.5

Specific characteristics of abdominal pain

- Visceral pain arises from ischaemia, muscle spasm or stretching of the visceral peritoneum
- Autonomic pain, deep and poorly localised, is referred to the equivalent somatic distribution of that nerve root from T1 to L2
- When an inflamed organ touches the parietal peritoneum, pain is then localised to the segmental dermatome of the abdominal wall
- The pain in the parietal peritoneum may radiate to back or front along the dermatome

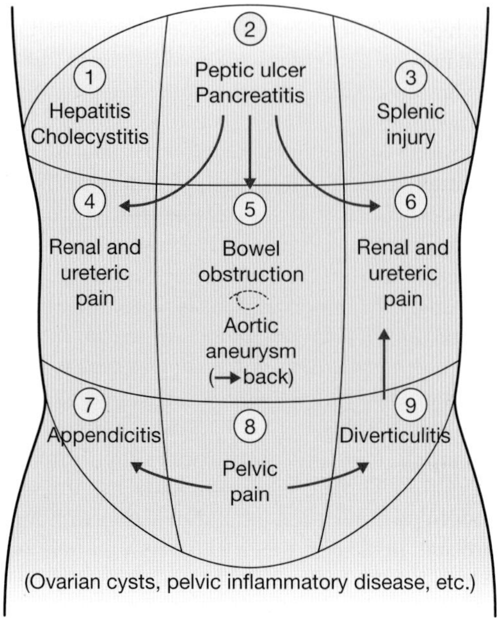

Obstruction

Central colicky abdominal pain is a classic presentation of small bowel obstruction. The central distribution is because of the segmental nerve supply of the midgut. When the peristaltic waves hit an obstruction, the contractions increase to overcome the resistance, producing the colic. The pain reaches a crescendo and then disappears in minutes when the peristaltic wave passes. This is different from that of biliary colic. When the gallbladder contracts against a stone, pain is relatively insidious in onset and reaches its peak in about half an hour and then eases off. A basal pain persists between the bouts of colic. Pain of ureteric colic is intense, lasting 1–2 minutes along the line of the ureter.

Summary box 63.6

Colicky abdominal pain

- Pain of 'small bowel colic' comes in waves and disappears completely in minutes when the peristaltic wave ceases
- Pain of biliary colic is insidious in onset, reaches the peak in half an hour or so and does not ease off completely between spasms
- Pain of ureteric colic is intense, lasting 1–2 minutes

Rupture and perforation of organs

The urinary bladder, gallbladder and gastrointestinal tract are hollow organs that contain fluid. The gastrointestinal system also contains faeces, air and a high concentration of organisms. Trauma, ischaemia or tissue ulceration may cause perforation, with resulting leak of luminal contents with peritonitis and resulting in severe abdominal pain. This may be localised to the area immediately adjacent to the perforation (for example, in a localised perforation of an appendix) or more generalised. The initial site of onset of the pain may give a clue as to the organ involved and so help with the differential diagnosis. For example, the diagnosis of a perforated peptic ulcer is supported by a past history of ulcer-type pain followed by a sudden onset of upper abdominal pain. The urgency of the situation must not be missed as such a patient can deteriorate rapidly with septicaemia.

The abdomen is divided into nine areas for ease of description (*Figure 63.2*). These regions are demarcated by the midclavicular lines in the vertical axis and by the transpyloric and transtubercular lines in the horizontal axis. *Figure 63.2* also indicates some of the organs and pathological processes that commonly cause pain experienced in these regions.

Figure 63.2 Nine sites of abdominal pain: 1, right subcostal; 2, epigastrium; 3, left subcostal; 4, right flank; 5, periumbilical; 6, left flank; 7, right iliac fossa; 8, suprapubic/hypogastrium; 9, left iliac fossa. (From Bailey and Love, 25th edn, courtesy of Mr Simon Paterson-Brown, Consultant Surgeon, Royal Infirmary of Edinburgh.)

EXAMINATION OF THE ABDOMEN

Abdominal examination must be preceded by a detailed general examination of the patient as a whole. Physical examination should be systematic using the following sequence: inspection, palpation, percussion and auscultation.

General examination

The patient must be lying flat with hips and knees extended but without causing distress (this may require provision of a pillow) and the abdomen should be adequately exposed.

While inspection of the abdomen is done in this position, for palpation hips and knees are flexed to ensure relaxation of abdominal muscles.

The examination should be performed sequentially, beginning with general inspection looking for evidence of weight loss, dehydration, pedal oedema, anaemia, jaundice or abnormal pigmentation. Examination of the hands may provide evidence of anaemia or chronic liver disease whereas examination of the head and neck may identify features indicative of liver disease or cervical lymphadenopathy (particularly left supraclavicular) suggestive of intra-abdominal malignancy. The patient's vital signs (heart rate, blood pressure, respiratory rate and body temperature) should be noted. In the elective setting the patient's weight and body mass index are also recorded.

Inspection

Scars, abdominal distension, visible peristalsis or abdominal masses, dilated veins, pulsation or abdominal wall swelling suggestive of hernia should all be carefully sought. The size and location of scars from previous surgery may provide some insight into the nature of the intervention that was performed (see ***Chapter 7***).

In an abdominal emergency look for Grey Turner's sign – skin discoloration of the flanks due to retroperitoneal haemorrhage in severe acute pancreatitis and leaking abdominal aortic aneurysm. Cullen's sign – discoloration around the umbilicus – may indicate severe acute pancreatitis, ruptured ectopic pregnancy or trauma to the liver. In these situations, blood tracks to the umbilicus along the ligamentum teres (***Figure 63.3***). These signs are better appreciated in a fair-skinned patient.

In a patient with acute abdominal pain, it is important to observe whether the abdominal wall moves with respiration. A thin patient with diffuse peritonitis may be unable to lie flat and the abdominal wall will have a 'scaphoid' appearance owing to protective contraction of the rectus abdominis muscles. It is often appropriate to ask the patient to cough gently – this will evoke sudden discomfort in the area of underlying peritoneal irritation (equivalent to eliciting rebound tenderness, but not as distressing for the patient). A visible 'cough impulse' will also help to identify an abdominal wall hernia, if present. A rounded, symmetrical contour of the abdomen with bulging flanks is seen in the presence of ascites. Visible abdominal masses, mobility on respiration and peristalsis are all best observed if the clinician kneels by the patient's bed so that the observer's eye is at the level of the patient's anterior abdominal wall. The same position is useful during palpation for abdominal masses (***Figure 63.4***).

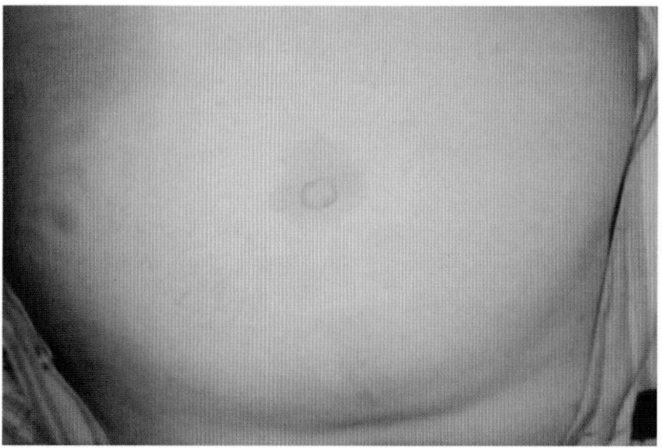

Figure 63.3 Cullen's and Grey Turner's sign of skin discoloration of the flanks and around the umbilicus (courtesy of Mr Pradip Datta, Honorary Consultant Surgeon, Wick, Scotland).

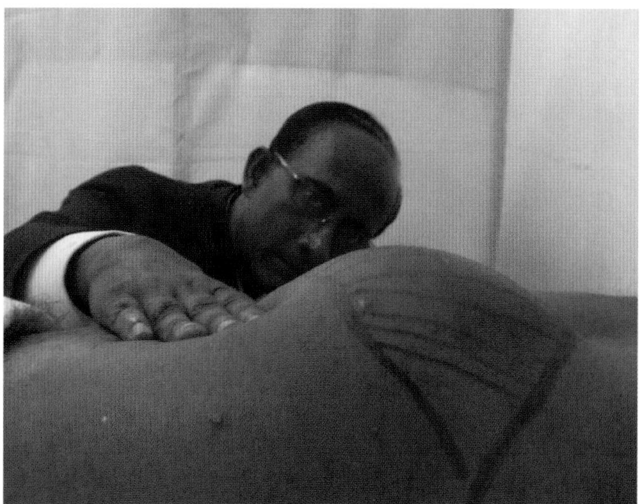

Figure 63.4 Eye at the level of patient's abdominal wall.

In a thin patient, visible bowel loops give clues about the pathology: an overdistended, bean-shaped loop is seen in caecal volvulus, which characteristically points towards the left upper quadrant, and in sigmoid volvulus, which points towards the right upper quadrant.

Palpation

Palpation should be performed in a systematic manner, checking all nine regions of the abdomen (***Figure 63.2***). Palpation should start in the region furthest away from the site of pain and the patient instructed to let the examiner know if tenderness is elicited. The examination should be gentle and the hands warm. The patient's facial expression will immediately reveal discomfort. Superficial palpation is followed by deep palpation if tenderness will allow. To avoid 'poking' during palpation, the forearm is kept horizontal, the whole of the palm is kept lightly on the abdomen and hand movement is made only at the metacarpophalangeal joints; never at the interphalangeal

George Grey Turner, 1877–1951, Professor of Surgery, at the University of Durham (1927–1934) and at the Royal Postgraduate Medical School, Hammersmith Hospital, London, UK (1935–1946).

Thomas Stephen Cullen, 1868–1953, Professor of Gynecology, the Johns Hopkins University, Baltimore, MD, USA, described the sign in ruptured ectopic pregnancy in 1916.

joints of the fingers. Palpation during respiration is performed to identify the lower margins of the liver and spleen as they move with respiration. Palpation of the abdomen in a patient with ascites will often demonstrate a doughy feel in the tubercular abdomen.

Signs of parietal peritoneal irritation (tenderness, guarding, rebound tenderness, rigidity)

In the presence of abdominal pain, the degree of abdominal wall rigidity and involuntary guarding should be assessed. Guarding represents contraction of the abdominal wall muscles over the area of pain. This might occur 'voluntarily' when the patient wishes to avoid the pain from examination or 'involuntarily' when the muscles go into spasm as the inflamed viscus touches the parietal peritoneum. This produces a reflex spasm of the overlying abdominal wall muscles. The presence of rebound tenderness indicates underlying peritoneal inflammation and is examined best using gentle percussion, although pain on coughing is also found when there is rebound tenderness. When the underlying peritoneal inflammation becomes generalised, the abdomen is 'board-like rigid' to palpation, and selective tenderness can no longer be elicited. This sign represents widespread involuntary guarding.

Abdominal masses

A mass arising from the anterior abdominal wall will usually be mobile when the patient is relaxed. On contracting the abdominal wall muscles (ask the patient to lift his or her legs with the knees extended or perform Valsalva's manoeuvre for laterally placed swellings), lumps superficial to the abdominal wall muscles will become more obvious, and those attached to the deep fascia will become less mobile. Those arising within the muscle layer will become fixed and remain unchanged in size. Lumps arising deep to the abdominal wall (i.e. within the peritoneal cavity or behind the peritoneum) will become impalpable or less prominent on tensing the anterior abdominal wall muscles.

An intraperitoneal mass in contact with the diaphragm will move on respiration whereas retroperitoneal masses are usually fixed and do not move with respiration; an enlarged kidney is 'ballotable' and bimanually palpable. Normal aortic pulsations can be both seen and felt in a thin abdomen, but expansile pulsation is characteristic of an abdominal aortic aneurysm. This should be differentiated from transmitted pulsation of a mass sitting on the aorta (e.g. pseudocyst of the pancreas). When 'palpating during inspiration', the examining hand is placed distal to the normal site of the organ and is held there until the edge of the organ descends and touches the examiner's fingers. Liver, spleen, gallbladder and kidneys are best palpated during inspiration. An abdominal mass in a female, the lower limit of which cannot be distinguished, is likely to arise from the pelvis. If the mass can be moved in a transverse direction, it is likely to be a uterine or ovarian mass. The movement of a mesenteric cyst is perpendicular to the direction of attachment of the root of the mesentery.

Spleen

In a healthy patient the spleen is not normally palpable. An enlarged spleen descends downwards, forwards and medially. Palpation for an enlarged spleen is best performed in a supine patient. The examining hand should start in the right lower abdomen, with the tips of the fingers pointing upwards and pressed inwards. The patient is then asked to take a deep breath; if the spleen is enlarged the lower edge with the characteristic notch will touch the fingers. If it is not palpable, then the hand is gradually moved upwards in the direction of the position of the edge of the normal-sized spleen with each breath. If the spleen is still not palpable, the patient is moved to the right lateral position and the examination repeated.

Liver

In a supine patient, the hand is placed in line with the potential enlarged liver edge lateral to the rectus muscle. The patient is then asked to take a deep breath. If the liver is enlarged sufficiently below the costal margin, then surface irregularities can also be felt.

Percussion

Percussion helps to distinguish distension due to bowel gas from solid masses and free fluid in the abdomen. Percussion is most sensitive when the examiner moves from resonant parts of the abdomen to dull areas. In patients with free fluid in the peritoneal cavity, percussion from the centre to the periphery reveals dullness of flanks. Shifting dullness is elicited if the patient is re-examined lying on his or her side. The margin of dullness is then found to shift when the patient has moved. Free fluid can also give rise to 'fluid thrill'; this is feeling the vibrations from a tap in one flank on the other flank while pressure is kept on the midline to prevent vibrations through the abdominal wall.

Percussion is also a very sensitive and refined method of testing for rebound tenderness. If the patient winces with pain on abdominal percussion it denotes underlying peritonitis.

Auscultation

High-pitched bowel sounds are heard during the early stages of mechanical intestinal obstruction. Aortic and iliac bruits are heard when blood flows through a stenosis. A succussion splash is a sound like 'shaking a half-filled bottle with water' and is found most often in patients with gastric stasis due to gastric outlet obstruction. In generalised peritonitis and paralytic ileus, bowel sounds will not be heard or be very few and far between.

Inspection of hernia sites, examination of genitalia, inspection of anal region and digital rectal examination

Abdominal examination is not complete until all external hernia sites and the anal area have been carefully inspected,

Antonio Maria Valsalva, 1666–1723, Professor of Anatomy, Bologna, Italy, of whom Morgagni wrote 'there is nobody of those times who goes ahead of him, very few who are his equals'.

the genitalia, renal angles and the thoracic and lumbar spine are examined and a digital rectal examination performed. A vaginal examination may also be needed in females. Details of these clinical examinations are covered in the respective chapters.

VALUE OF OBSERVATION AND REVIEW

In the case of acute abdominal pain, there will be a subset of patients in whom, after full clinical assessment, the surgeon remains uncertain about the need for an urgent operation. This is probably the most difficult group to deal with compared with those in whom an urgent operation is either clearly required or clearly not required, and undoubtedly the one in which the majority of errors occur. These include rare causes of abdominal pain and vomiting such as metabolic diseases (diabetic ketoacidosis, diabetic gastroparesis, porphyria, hyperparathyroidism etc.), referred pain from the spine, heart and lungs and functional pain. Further urgent investigations are obviously needed in this group and these are discussed in some detail elsewhere in this book. However, while these are taking place, regular review of the patient is essential, preferably by the same clinician who initially examined the patient so as not to miss any subtle changes or worsening of the situation. Such a period of observation is an integral part of the early management of patients with acute abdominal pain.

FURTHER READING

Das S, Das S. *A manual on clinical surgery*, 14th edn. Kolkata: Das Publications, 2019.

Lumley JS, D'Cruz AK, Hoballah JJ, Scott-Connor CE. *Hamilton Bailey's demonstrations of physical signs in clinical surgery*, 19th edn. London: CRC Press, 2016.

PART 11 | Abdominal

CHAPTER 64 The abdominal wall, hernia and umbilicus

Learning objectives

To know and understand:

- Basic anatomy of the abdominal wall and its weaknesses
- Causes of abdominal hernia
- Types of hernia and classifications
- Clinical history and examination findings in hernia
- Complications of abdominal hernia
- Non-surgical and surgical management of hernia, including mesh
- Complications of hernia surgery
- Other abdominal wall conditions

THE ABDOMINAL WALL

Basic anatomy and function related to pathology

The abdominal wall is a complex structure composed primarily of muscle, bone and fascia. Its major function is to protect the enclosed organs but it must also enable mobility and be able to flex, extend, rotate and vary its capacity. Flexibility requires elasticity and stretch, which compromise abdominal wall strength.

The roof of the abdomen is formed by the diaphragm separating the thoracic cavity above, with negative pressure, from the abdomen below, with positive pressure. Weakness of the diaphragm can lead to much of the bowel being drawn into the chest down this pressure gradient. The bony pelvis forms the floor of the cavity but a muscular central portion, the perineum, may also weaken and allow rectum, bladder and gynaecological organs to bulge downwards, a condition called prolapse.

The overall design of the abdominal muscles is best seen on transverse section through the mid-abdomen (***Figure 64.1***). Posteriorly the muscles are strong, further supported by the vertebral column, ribs and pelvis. Two regions called the posterior triangles represent areas of weakness, which can lead to rare lumbar hernias. Laterally there are three thin muscle layers, the fibres of which criss-cross for strength and flexibility.

Anteriorly the two powerful rectus abdominis muscles extend vertically from ribs to pelvis. Herniation through these strong muscles does not occur naturally but their central join, the linea alba, is an area of weakness that may result in epigastric or umbilical herniation. Divarication of the recti is the condition where the linea alba stretches laterally as the two rectus muscles separate. It occurs predominantly in the upper abdomen in middle-aged, overweight men (***Figure 64.2***) and also as a result of pregnancy in women, where it is primarily below the umbilicus. Divarication is not a hernia and does not require treatment, although some surgeons do offer repair for purely cosmetic reasons.

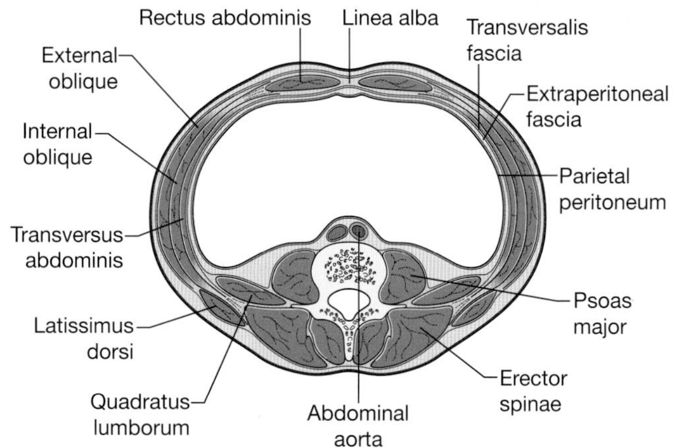

Figure 64.1 A cross-section of the mid-abdomen showing the muscular anatomy.

ABDOMINAL HERNIA

A hernia is an abnormal protrusion of an organ or tissue through an opening in the layer that normally confines it. There are many varieties of hernia arising through areas of weakness in the abdominal wall. Because they 'push' from the inside to the outside, an abdominal hernia takes with it all the coverings of the abdominal wall, although they may be thinned and attenuated. However, not all abdominal hernias have a peritoneal sac: many epigastric hernias, for example, arise in the interstitial layers and only draw peritoneum into the protrusion as a secondary phenomenon when they become larger.

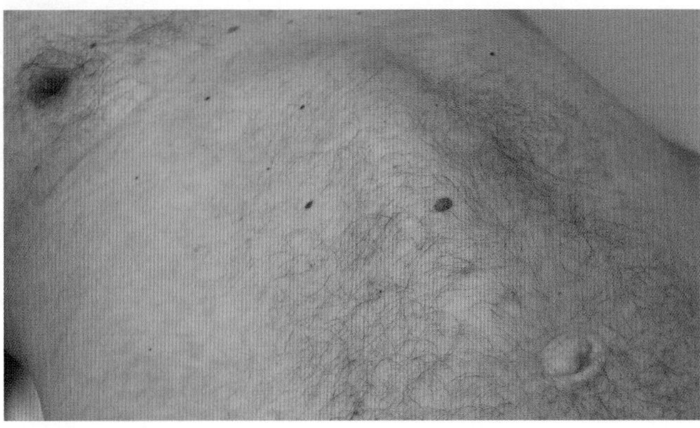

Figure 64.2 Divarication of the recti. Note a coexisting small umbilical hernia.

Anatomical causes of abdominal wall herniation

These may be classified as areas of natural weakness due to absence of muscle, natural defects that allow structures to enter or leave the abdomen, developmental abnormalities and disruptions of the abdominal wall as a result of injury. The only natural weaknesses caused by inadequate muscular strength are the lumbar triangles (see ***Lumbar hernia***) and the posterior wall of the inguinal canal (***Figure 64.3***).

Many structures enter and leave the abdominal cavity, creating weakness that can lead to hernia formation. The most common example is the inguinal canal, along which, in males, the testis and its associated vessels descend from the abdomen to scrotum at the time of birth. In females the round ligament traverses the inguinal canal. The resultant weakness may lead to an indirect inguinal hernia. The risk of inguinal hernia is related to the anatomical shape of the pelvis and is greater in patients with a wider and shorter pelvis. Other examples of inherent areas of weakness include the oesophageal hiatus, the femoral canal and the umbilical cicatrix.

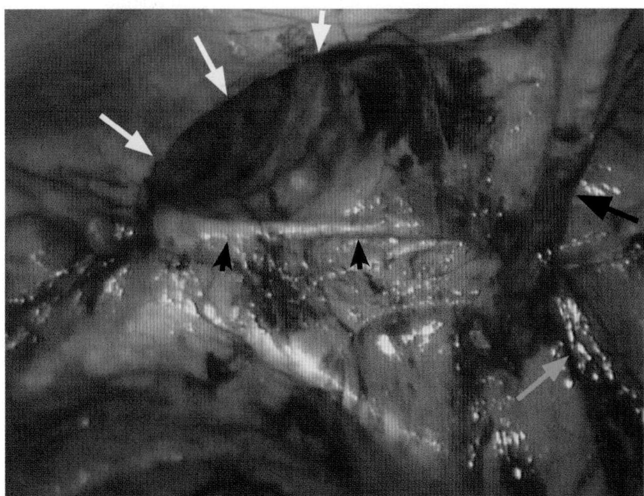

Figure 64.3 A right direct inguinal hernia defect (yellow arrows) is above the inguinal ligament (arrowheads). The round ligament (green arrow) enters the deep inguinal ring just lateral to the inferior epigastric vessels (black arrow).

Failure of normal development may lead to congenital hernias. The most common is an indirect inguinal hernia arising through failure of the processus vaginalis to close. As the testis (or round ligament) descends, it pulls a tube of peritoneum along with it. This tube should naturally fibrose and become obliterated, but, if it fails to do so, a hernia may develop. Recent studies have shown that calcitonin gene-related peptide and hepatocyte growth factor influence the closure of the processus, raising the possibility of a hormonal cause of hernia development.

Other examples of congenital herniation include Morgagni and Bochdalek hernias of the diaphragm and some umbilical hernias. In neonates these are often seen in association with other congenital abnormalities.

Weak areas of the abdominal wall may also arise from direct injury. A surgical scar, even with perfect wound healing, has only 70% of the initial muscle strength, resulting in incisional herniation in at least 10% of laparotomy incisions. Smaller laparoscopic port-site incisions have a hernia rate of 1%. Increasing use of the laparoscopic surgical approach should lead to a fall in the incidence of incisional hernia.

Muscle damage by blunt trauma or tearing of the abdominal muscles is rare but is seen after exceptional force, such as high-speed motor vehicle accidents (***Figure 64.4***).

Summary box 64.1

Causes of hernia

- Anatomical weakness
- Developmental failures
- Genetic weakness of collagen
- Sharp and blunt trauma
- Weakness due to ageing and pregnancy
- Primary neurological and muscle diseases

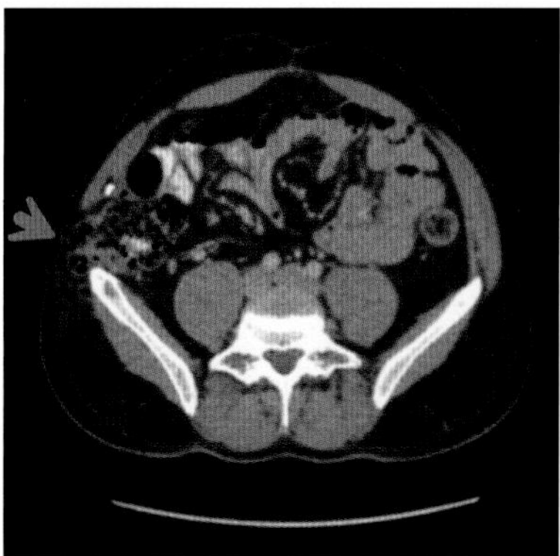

Figure 64.4 Traumatic hernia in the right iliac fossa (arrow) following a motor vehicle accident in which the lateral muscles, along with a tiny sliver of bone, were torn off the iliac crest.

Giovanni Battista Morgagni, 1682–1771, Professor of Anatomy, Padua, Italy.
Vincent Alexander Bochdalek, 1801–1883, Professor of Anatomy, Prague, Czech Republic.

Pathophysiology of hernia formation

A normal abdominal wall has sufficient strength to resist high abdominal pressure and prevent herniation of content. Many patients will first notice a hernia after excessive straining, the strain bringing the hernia to the attention of the patient, rather than being the cause.

There is good evidence that hernia is a 'collagen disease' and is due to an inherited imbalance in the types of collagen. This is supported by histological evidence and relationships between hernia and other diseases related to collagen, such as aortic aneurysm. In extreme collagen disorders, such as Ehlers–Danlos syndrome, successful long-term repair of a hernia can be very difficult. Hernia is more common in smokers as smoking is linked to impaired collagen maturation.

Hernias are more common in elderly people owing to degenerative weakness of muscles and fibrous tissue. Incisional hernias are more common after wound complications and in patients with a high body mass index; however, a major risk factor is the surgeon and the way the abdominal wall was closed.

Common principles in abdominal hernia

An abdominal wall hernia has two essential components: a defect in the wall and the content, i.e. tissue that has been forced outwards through the defect. The weakness may be through fascia and muscle, or through fascia alone, such as an epigastric hernia. It may have a bony component, such as a femoral hernia. The weakness in the wall is usually the narrowest part of the hernia, which expands into the subcutaneous fat outside the muscle. The defect varies in size and may be very small or indeed very large. The nature of the defect is important to understanding the risk of hernia complications. A small defect with rigid walls traps the content and prevents it from freely moving in and out of the defect, increasing the risk of complications.

The content of the hernia may be tissue from the extraperitoneal space alone, such as fat within an epigastric hernia or urinary bladder in a direct inguinal hernia. However, if a hernia enlarges then peritoneum may also be pulled into the hernia secondarily along with intraperitoneal structures such as bowel or omentum; a good example is a '**sliding type**' of inguinal hernia. More commonly, when peritoneum is lying immediately deep to the abdominal wall weakness, pressure forces the peritoneum through the defect and into the subcutaneous tissues. This '**sac**' of peritoneum allows bowel and omentum to pass through the defect. In most cases, the intraperitoneal organs can move freely in and out of the hernia, a '**reducible**' hernia; however, if adhesions form or the defect is small, bowel can become trapped and unable to return to the main peritoneal cavity, an '**irreducible**' hernia, with higher risk of further complications. The narrowest part of the sac, at the abdominal wall defect, is called the '**neck**' of the sac.

When tissue is trapped inside a hernia it is in a confined space. The narrow neck acts as a constriction ring impeding venous return and increasing pressure within the hernia. Resulting tension leads to pain and tenderness. If the hernia contains bowel then it may become '**obstructed**', partially or totally. If the pressure rises sufficiently, arterial blood is not able to enter the hernia and the contents become ischaemic and may infarct. The hernia is then said to have '**strangulated**'. The wall of the bowel perforates, releasing infected, toxic bowel content into the tissues and ultimately back into the peritoneal cavity. The risk of strangulation is highest in hernias that have a small neck of rigid tissue, leading first to irreducibility and on to strangulation. The term '**incarcerated**', literally 'in prison', means that a hernia is not only irreducible but also potentially developing strangulation.

Summary box 64.2

Types of hernia by complexity

- Occult – not detectable clinically
- Reducible – a swelling that appears and disappears
- Irreducible – a swelling that cannot be replaced in the abdomen, at risk of complications
- Incarcerated – irreducible, trapped, risk of strangulation
- Strangulated – acutely painful swelling with tissue ischaemia: requires emergency surgery
- Infarcted – when contents of the hernia have become gangrenous: high mortality

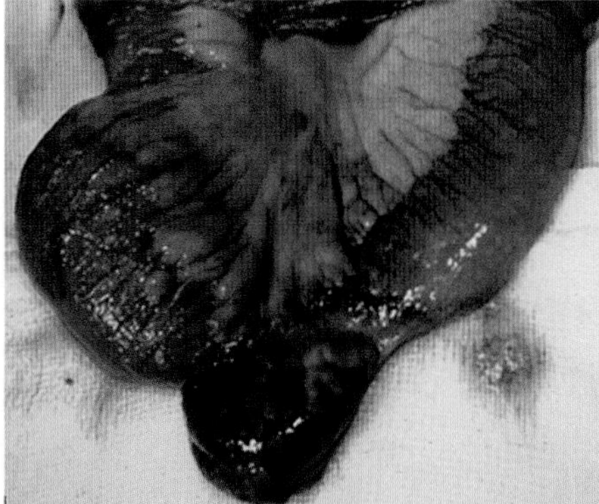

Figure 64.5 A gangrenous Richter's hernia from a case of strangulated femoral hernia.

In a special circumstance (Richter's hernia) only part of the bowel wall enters the hernia (***Figure 64.5***). It may be small and difficult or even impossible to detect clinically. Bowel obstruction may or may not be present but the bowel wall may still become necrotic and perforate with life-threatening consequences. Femoral hernia may present in this way, often with diagnostic delay and high risk to the patient.

Edvard Ehlers, 1863–1937, dermatologist, Frederiks Hospital, Copenhagen, Denmark.
Henri-Alexandre Danlos, 1844–1912, dermatologist, Hôpital Saint Louis, Paris, France.
August Gottlieb Richter, 1742–1812, surgeon, Göttingen, Germany.

An interstitial hernia occurs when the hernia arises entirely between the musculofascial layers of the abdominal wall muscle and does not contain a peritoneal sac. This is commonly seen with small Spigelian hernias (see ***Spigelian hernia***).

An internal hernia describes bowel entrapment within the peritoneal cavity. This can occur in naturally existing spaces such as the foramen of Winslow or the paraduodenal and paracaecal fossae, around adhesive bands or through iatrogenic defects in the mesentery.

Clinical history and diagnosis in hernia cases

Patients are usually aware of a lump on the abdominal wall under the skin. Self-diagnosis is common. The hernia is usually painless but patients may complain of an aching or heavy feeling. Sharp, intermittent pains suggest pinching of tissue at the hernia neck. Severe pain should alert the surgeon to a high risk of strangulation. One should determine whether the hernia reduces spontaneously or needs to be helped. The patient should be asked about symptoms that might suggest bowel obstruction.

Once the clinician is satisfied that a swelling is indeed a hernia, it is important to know if this is a primary hernia, a recurrent hernia or an incisional hernia after previous surgery. Recurrent and incisional hernias are more difficult to treat and may require a different surgical approach.

General questions about the cardiac and respiratory systems are necessary to assess a patient's anaesthetic risk. Intake of anticoagulants such as warfarin and apixaban or antiplatelet medication such as aspirin or clopidogrel is important because this impacts on future surgery. Many hernia operations can be performed as a day case or single overnight stay, so that suitability for such treatment needs to be assessed, including home support, distance from the hospital, mobility levels, etc. (see ***Chapter 22***).

Examination for hernia

The patient should be examined lying down initially and then standing, as this will usually increase hernia size. Some hernias will only be apparent with the patient standing. The patient may be asked to cough or to perform the Valsalva manoeuvre to make the hernia appear. Divarication is best seen by asking a supine patient to simply lift his/her head off the pillow. Finally, it should be remembered that if a patient describes an intermittent swelling but the surgeon finds no hernia on examination, there still may be a hernia present.

The overlying skin is usually of normal colour. If there is overlying cellulitis then the hernia content is strangulating and the case should be treated as an emergency.

In most cases an expansile cough impulse is felt if gentle pressure is applied to the lump and the patient is asked to cough; however, there may be no cough impulse when the neck is tight and the hernia irreducible. This is typical of a femoral hernia, where lack of an impulse leads the clinician to misdiagnose a lymph node. A cough impulse can also be appreciated in a saphena varix (see ***Chapter 62***).

If a groin hernia is found on one side, the other side must also be examined as occult contralateral hernias are present in up to 20% of patients.

If a hernia does not reduce spontaneously, the surgeon should ask the patient to attempt reduction because he/she may be well practised in this task, and the surgeon might cause unnecessary discomfort. If neither the patient nor the surgeon can reduce the hernia, the treatment is more urgent.

Summary box 64.3

Checks
- Reducibility
- Cough impulse
- Tenderness
- Overlying skin colour changes
- Multiple defects/contralateral side
- Signs of previous repair
- Scrotal content for groin hernia
- Associated pathology

Summary box 64.4

Examination
- A swelling with a cough impulse is not necessarily a hernia
- A swelling with no cough impulse may still be a hernia but consider other diagnoses

Investigations for hernia

For most hernias, the diagnosis is made on clinical examination. However, the patient may have symptoms suggesting a hernia but no hernia is found, or the patient may have a swelling suggestive of hernia but with clinical uncertainty. It is important to be certain that any symptoms described are due to a hernia and not to coexisting pathology, particularly when the major symptom is pain. Soft, reducible hernias are rarely painful. There may also be a requirement for more detailed information than can be found by examination alone. An ultrasound scan may be helpful in cases of irreducible hernia when the differential diagnosis includes a mass or fluid collection, enlarged lymph node or saphena varix or when the nature of the hernia content is in doubt. It is non-invasive, dynamic and low cost but highly operator dependent. Ultrasonography may be useful in the early postoperative period to distinguish a haematoma or seroma from an early recurrence.

Computed tomography (CT) is helpful in complex ventral and incisional hernias, determining the number and size of muscle defects, identifying the content, giving some indication

Adriaan van den Spiegel, 1578–1625, Flemish anatomist who practised in Padua, Italy.
Jacob Benignus Winslow, 1669–1764, Danish-born anatomist, Jardin du Roi, Paris, France
Antonio Maria Valsalva, 1666–1723, Professor of Anatomy, Bologna, Italy.

of presence of adhesions and excluding other intra-abdominal pathology such as ascites, occult malignancy and portal hypertension. By showing the surrounding muscle layers CT helps planning abdominal wall reconstruction.

Magnetic resonance imaging (MRI) can help in the diagnosis of sportsman's (Gilmore's) groin, where pain is the presenting feature and the surgeon needs to distinguish an occult hernia from an orthopaedic injury.

Laparoscopy itself may be used. In incisional hernia, initial laparoscopy may determine whether a laparoscopic approach is feasible or not. In inguinal hernia repair by the transabdominal route, initial laparoscopy can determine the presence of an occult contralateral hernia. However, laparoscopy will not identify intraparietal hernias such as lipomas of the spermatic cord and some epigastric and Spigelian hernias.

Summary box 64.5

Investigations

- Plain radiograph – of little value
- Ultrasound scan – low cost, operator dependent
- CT scan – ventral and incisional hernia
- MRI – good in sportsman's groin with pain
- Laparoscopy – useful to identify occult defects but not interstitial hernias

Management principles

An abdominal wall hernia does not necessarily require repair. A patient may request surgery for relief of symptoms or for cosmesis. The surgeon should recommend repair when complications are likely, the most worrying being bowel obstruction and strangulation. These are most likely in narrow-necked hernias; for this reason all femoral hernias should be repaired, as should symptomatic or irreducible hernias unless coexisting medical factors place the patient at very high risk. Increasing difficulty in reduction and increasing size are also indications for surgery. Surgery should be offered to younger adult patients as symptoms and complications are likely over time.

Summary box 64.6

Management

- Not all hernias require surgical repair
- Small hernias can be more dangerous than large
- Pain, tenderness, skin changes and difficulty reducing imply high risk of strangulation
- Femoral hernia should always be repaired

In elderly patients a policy of 'watchful waiting' in asymptomatic inguinal hernia appears generally safe, with an annual crossover to surgery because of symptoms developing of around 10%. A truss can be used to control a hernia but nowadays few surgeons recommend this approach. Small umbilical and epigastric hernias may also be managed conservatively as they cause few symptoms and usually contain fat or omentum with a very low risk of complications.

Large incisional hernias, particularly recurrent, present a major problem. Surgical repair is a complex procedure with significant risk of complications and later recurrence. When the neck is wide, the risk of strangulation is low. In obese and elderly patients, these risks may outweigh the benefits of surgery and it is common for surgeons to adopt a conservative approach.

A patient who presents with acute pain in a hernia, particularly if it is irreducible, should be offered urgent surgery. It may be reducible by taxis (gentle forceful reduction, perhaps requiring analgesia and/or sedation) and sometimes, after admission to hospital and adequate analgesia, the hernia will reduce as a result of muscle relaxation. In either case, the likelihood of similar episodes is very high and surgery should be recommended at the next available opportunity.

Surgical approaches to hernia

In general, modern surgical repairs follow these principles:

- Reduction of the hernia contents into the abdominal cavity with excision of any non-viable tissue and bowel repair if necessary.
- Excision and closure of the peritoneal sac if present (though small sacs may be reduced intact).
- Closure of the hernia defect if possible.
- Reinforcement of the abdominal wall with mesh (though non-mesh repairs are an option).
- If necessary, excise redundant skin to improve cosmetic outcome.

Reduction of hernia content is essential for a successful repair. Excision and closure of the peritoneal sac is ideal but not essential. During intraperitoneal onlay mesh laparoscopic repair of incisional hernia, for example, surgeons will often leave the sac *in situ* after reducing the hernia contents, and simply fix a mesh over the defect. Leaving the peritoneal sac *in situ* risks the accumulation of serous fluid formation within the sac (seroma). This can arise after all forms of hernia repair. In open repair of lateral (indirect) inguinal hernia, most surgeons excise the peritoneal sac but small sacs can be simply pushed back through the deep inguinal ring, which is said to reduce postoperative pain. Similarly, in laparoscopic repair of inguinal hernias, surgeons simply pull the sac back into the abdominal cavity from within and do not excise it.

Closure of the hernial defect is ideal but may not be possible when the defect is large, the surrounding tissues are rigid (such as the femoral canal) or structures traversing the defect must be retained (such as the spermatic cord traversing the deep inguinal ring). Plastic surgical techniques have been developed to 'borrow' tissue from elsewhere in order to cover large muscle defects, but usually at the cost of leaving a weak area elsewhere. The repair of large and complex hernias using a variety of such specialised techniques has led to some surgeons declaring a specialist hernia interest.

Jerry Gilmore, 1942–2019, surgeon, London, UK, gave his name to a syndrome of chronic groin pain in professional footballers.

Closure of the hernia defect alone is associated with a high recurrence rate. Additional reinforcement of the repair with a non-absorbable mesh reduces but does not prevent recurrence. With improved techniques and new meshes it is hoped that recurrence after surgery will fall further. Mesh repair has become so important in hernia surgery that some understanding of mesh technology is essential for the modern surgeon.

Mesh in hernia repair

The term 'mesh' refers to prosthetic material, either a net or a flat sheet, that is used to strengthen a hernia repair. Mesh can be used to:

- bridge a defect: the mesh is simply fixed over the defect as a tension-free patch;
- plug a defect: a plug of mesh is pushed into the defect;
- augment a repair: the defect is closed with sutures and the mesh added for reinforcement.

Simple bridging of a hernia defect relies on a generous overlap of the mesh onto strong tissues around the defect in order to reduce the risk of recurrence. Mesh plug repairs have been used in small defects, especially where tissue overlap is hard to achieve, but have been largely abandoned because collagen deposition often produces a fibrous mass, a 'meshoma', that may cause chronic pain. Other complications include mesh migration, erosion into adjacent organs and fistula formation. Primary closure of the hernia defect with the addition of mesh for reinforcement placed in a tension-free manner is currently regarded as optimal. Suturing a mesh edge to edge into the defect (inlay), with no overlap, is not recommended.

Mesh types

Gross structure

Net meshes are woven or knitted. Sheet meshes are not porous but may be perforated with multiple holes. Net meshes allow native tissue ingrowth between the strands so that the mesh becomes integrated into host tissues within a few months. Initial fixation of such mesh is by glue, sutures or tacks/staples, which may or may not be absorbable; in some cases, such as extraperitoneal repair of inguinal hernias, no mesh fixation may be required at all. 'Sheet' meshes do not allow host tissue ingrowth but eventually become encapsulated by host fibrous tissue. They always require strong, non-absorbable fixation to prevent mesh migration.

Synthetic mesh

Most meshes used today are synthetic polymers of polypropylene, polyester or polytetrafluoroethylene (PTFE), but there may be other chemical additives and meshes may have a composite structure such as those with anti-adhesive barriers. Meshes for hernia repair are generally non-absorbable and designed to provoke tissue ingrowth that leads to the formation of a tissue barrier. Polypropylene is an inert, hydrophobic, monofilament material so does not generate an immune response and tends to resist bacterial ingrowth. Polyester mesh is similar but hydrophilic, and is said to encourage microvascular ingrowth. PTFE meshes are flat sheets, quite inert and resistant to both tissue ingrowth and adhesion formation (***Figure 64.6***).

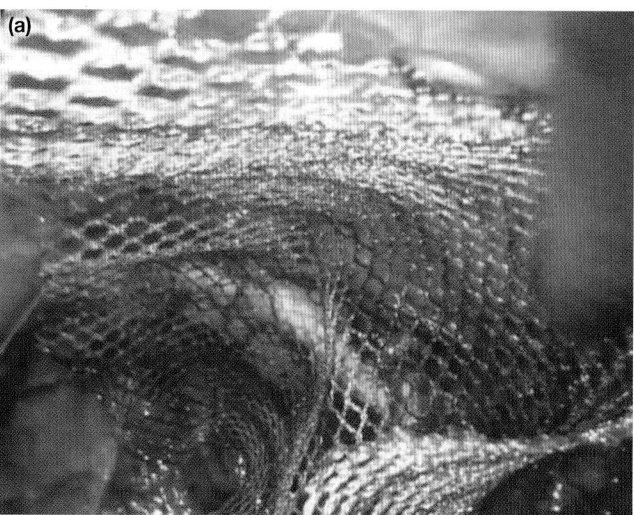

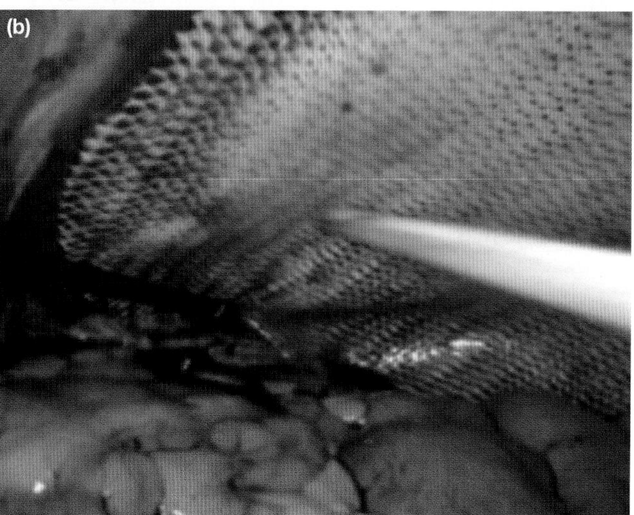

Figure 64.6 (a) Polypropylene mesh in totally extraperitoneal inguinal hernia repair. The blue lines are added purely to help the surgeon orientate the mesh. (b) Polyester mesh in an epigastric hernia repair.

Weight and porosity

Synthetic meshes are very strong; early meshes were much stronger than a human abdominal wall, so they are considered to be 'over-engineered'. All meshes provoke a fibrous reaction. More dense or heavyweight meshes provoke a greater reaction, leading to collagen contraction and mesh stiffening, which is associated with impaired elasticity/mobility of the abdominal wall, foreign body sensation and pain.

The term 'mesh shrinkage' is often used to describe this progressive decrease in mesh size over time, but the mesh itself does not shrink; instead, it is simply the natural progressive contraction of the fibrous tissue that has grown into the mesh. Thus 'mesh contracture' is a more accurate term. This process can lead to hernia recurrence if the mesh no longer covers the defect. Meshes can contract in area by more than 50%. Meshes with thinner strands and larger spaces (pores) between them are preferred because they have better tissue integration, less contracture, less foreign body reaction, more flexibility and improved comfort.

Current opinion avoids the use of stiff, heavyweight mesh and favours a pore size of at least 1 mm in all directions in order to promote collagen ingrowth that is not only strong but also elastic.

Biological mesh

So-called 'biological meshes' are sheets of sterilised, decellularised, connective tissue derived from a variety of sources, including human or animal dermis, bovine pericardium or porcine intestinal submucosa. They provide a 'scaffold' to encourage neovascular ingrowth, fibroblast infiltration and new collagen deposition. In theory host enzymes eventually break down the biological implant and replace it with normal host fibrous tissue. The rates of enzymatic degradation and collagen deposition vary between products and also depend on the local environment of the mesh. In the presence of infection, for example, some biological meshes break down more rapidly and weaken before remodelling can occur, leading to early hernia recurrence. Others are more resistant to breakdown, particularly those with chemical cross-linking between the fibrous strands. The choice of biological mesh depends on the clinical situation for which it is to be used. They are expensive, and their precise role in abdominal wall hernia repair has yet to be fully established.

Absorbable meshes

Synthetic absorbable meshes such as those made from polyglycolic acid, collagen or polyhydroxybutyrate may be used in temporary abdominal wall closure and for short-term buttressing suture lines but are not recommended in hernia repair as they are absorbed too quickly and induce only minimal collagen deposition. In recent years a number of synthetic, slowly absorbable meshes have been developed. These are designed to be gradually degraded by the body and replaced with strong native collagenous fibrosis in order to create a lasting repair. The long-term outcomes of repairs using these meshes are as yet unknown.

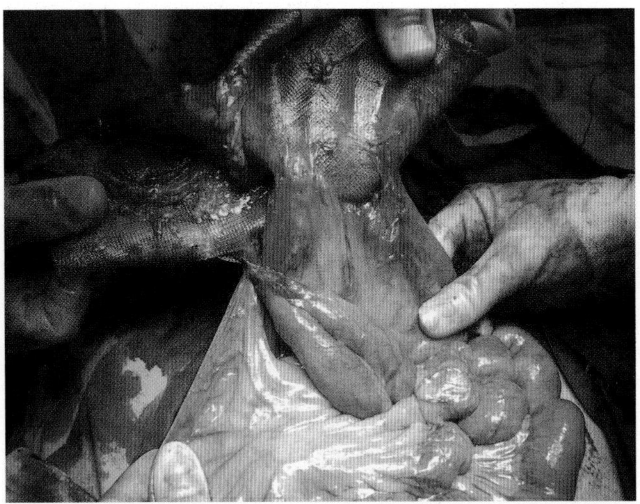

Figure 64.7 Adhesions to intraperitoneal mesh causing bowel obstruction.

Tissue-separating meshes

Most standard meshes induce fibrosis and, if placed within the peritoneal cavity, promote unwanted adhesions. A number of meshes have been designed for intraperitoneal use. Most of these have two very different surfaces, one being sticky and one slippery. Good adherence and host-tissue ingrowth is required on the parietal (fascia/muscle/peritoneum) side of the mesh, but the opposite (bowel) side needs to prevent adhesions to the abdominal contents. Usually, one side of the mesh is coated by material that prevents adhesions, such as polycellulose, collagen or PTFE. However, none of these materials is 100% effective at preventing adhesions and consequently intraperitoneal placement of mesh is associated with bowel obstruction, mesh erosion and fistulation (***Figure 64.7***). Surgeons now try to avoid intraperitoneal mesh placement whenever possible.

Summary box 64.7

Mesh characteristics

- Net (woven or knitted) or sheet
- Synthetic or biological – mainly synthetic
- Large pore, small pore – large pore causes less fibrosis and pain
- If for intraperitoneal use – non-adhesive surface on one side
- Non-absorbable or absorbable – mainly non-absorbable

Positioning the mesh

The strength of a mesh repair depends on host-tissue ingrowth. Meshes should be laid in a tension-free manner on a firm, well-vascularised tissue bed with generous overlap of the hernia zone. The mesh can be placed:

- on top of the muscle/fascia in the subcutaneous space (onlay);
- within the defect (inlay);
- immediately deep to the muscle layers in the abdominal wall (sublay);
- extraperitoneally;
- intraperitoneally.

Each of these planes may be used with both open and laparoscopic techniques (***Figure 64.8***). Onlay meshes may become

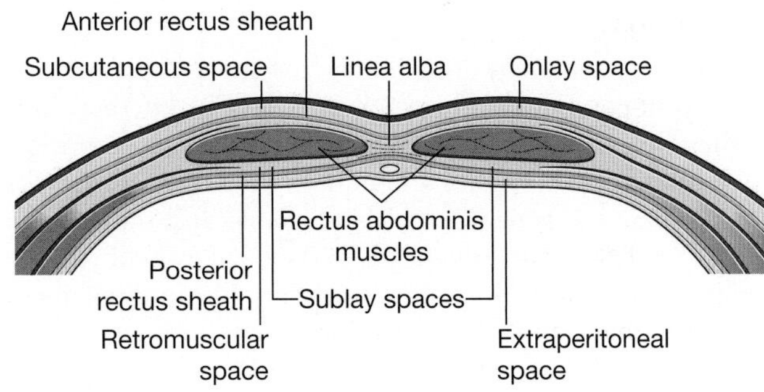

Figure 64.8 Diagrammatic representation of the various layers into which meshes are placed in ventral hernia repair.

exposed in the event of wound breakdown, and the elevation of skin flaps to allow wide overlap can lead to skin ischaemia and/or seroma formation. Inlay meshes are not recommended as they are effectively no more than a suture repair at each mesh–tissue interface. Meshes placed deep to the abdominal wall muscle layers have a mechanical advantage over onlay positioning as the abdominal pressure helps to keep the mesh in place; both sublay and extraperitoneal mesh placement techniques are generally preferred. Intraperitoneal mesh is associated with complications described earlier and many surgeons now try to avoid this.

Limitations to the use of mesh

The presence of infection limits the use of mesh. If a mesh becomes infected then it usually needs to be removed, although some infected situations can be salvaged using a combination of debridement, appropriate antibiotics and modern vacuum-assisted dressings.

Meshes are expensive, especially biological, biodegradable or those for intraperitoneal use. Price or novelty is not always an indicator of quality or safety and a simple, non-absorbable, large-pore synthetic mesh is nowadays seen as the safest implant.

SPECIFIC HERNIA TYPES

Hernia sites are shown in ***Figure 64.9***.

Inguinal hernia

Inguinal hernia, often referred to as a 'rupture' by patients, is the most common hernia in men and is around 10 times more common in men than in women. There are two basic types that are fundamentally different in anatomy, causation and complications. However, they are anatomically very close to each other, the surgical repair techniques are very similar and ultimate reinforcement of the weakened anatomy is identical, so they are often referred to together as inguinal hernia.

Summary box 64.8

Inguinal hernia

- Types – indirect (lateral, or oblique) or direct (medial)
- Origin – congenital or acquired
- Anatomy – inguinal canal
- Diagnosis – usually clinical but radiological in special circumstances
- Surgery – open or minimally invasive (laparoscopic/robot assisted)

Congenital inguinal hernias are of the indirect type, whereas the acquired hernias may be either indirect or direct.

Anatomy of the inguinal canal

As the testis descends from the abdominal cavity to the scrotum it passes through a defect in the transversalis fascia called the deep inguinal ring, just deep to the abdominal muscles. This ring lies midway between the anterior superior iliac spine and the pubic tubercle, approximately 2–3 cm above and marginally lateral to the femoral artery pulse in the groin. The inferior epigastric vessels lie just medial to the deep inguinal ring, passing from the iliac vessels to rectus abdominis. Muscle fibres from the innermost two layers of the lateral abdominal wall, the transversus muscle and the internal oblique muscle, arch over the deep inguinal ring from lateral to medial before descending to become attached to the pubic tubercle. These two muscles fuse and become tendinous, forming the conjoint tendon. Below this arch there is no muscle but only transversalis fascia and external oblique aponeurosis, resulting in an area of weakness (***Figure 64.10***).

The testis proceeds medially and downwards along the inguinal canal. Anterior to the canal is the aponeurosis of the external oblique muscle, the fibres of which run downwards and medially. The testis finally emerges through an inverted V-shaped defect in the aponeurosis, the superficial inguinal ring, and descends into the scrotum.

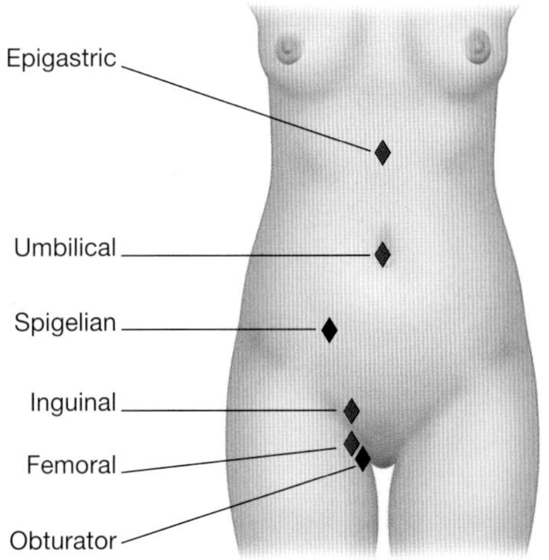

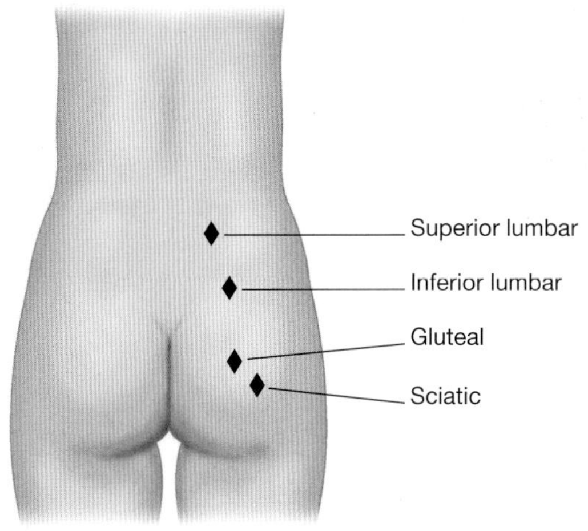

Figure 64.9 Diagram to show the sites of abdominal wall hernias: common in red and rare in black. Incisional and parastomal hernias can be found at various sites.

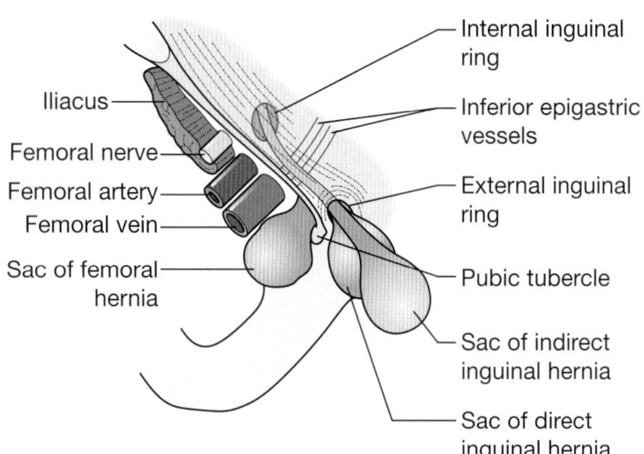

Figure 64.10 The close relationships of direct inguinal, indirect inguinal and femoral hernias.

The inguinal canal is roofed by the conjoint tendon; its posterior wall is transversalis fascia, the anterior wall is the external oblique aponeurosis and the floor is the free inferior edge of the external oblique aponeurosis, rolled inwards thickened to become the inguinal (Poupart's) ligament. The inguinal canal in males contains the testicular artery, veins, lymphatics and the vas deferens all covered in cremasteric muscle. In females, the round ligament descends through the canal to end in the labia majora. Three important nerves, the ilioinguinal, the iliohypogastric and the genital branch of the genitofemoral nerve, also pass through the canal.

As the testis descends, a tube of peritoneum is pulled with the testis and wraps around it ultimately to form the tunica vaginalis. This peritoneal tube should obliterate, possibly under hormonal control, but it commonly fails to do so completely. As a result, bowel within the peritoneal cavity can pass inside the tube towards the scrotum. Inguinal hernias in neonates and children are always of this congenital type. However, in other patients, the muscles around the deep inguinal ring can prevent a hernia from developing until later in life, when, under the constant positive abdominal pressure, the deep inguinal ring and muscles are stretched and a hernia becomes apparent. As the hernia increases in size, the contents are directed down into the scrotum. These hernias can become massive and may be referred to as a scrotal hernia. An indirect hernia is lateral because its origin is lateral to the inferior epigastric vessels. It is also oblique as the hernia passes obliquely from lateral to medial through the abdominal muscle layers. An indirect hernia can pass all the way down to the scrotum, following the line of the processus vaginalis, while this is not possible with a direct hernia.

The second type of inguinal hernia, referred to as direct or medial, is always acquired. It is a result of stretching and weakening of the abdominal wall just medial to the inferior epigastric vessels, an area known as Hesselbach's triangle, the three sides of which are the inferior epigastric vessels laterally, the lateral edge of rectus abdominis muscle medially and the inguinal ligament below (the iliopubic tract) (*Figure 64.11*). This area is weak because the abdominal wall at this point consists of only transversalis fascia covered by the external oblique aponeurosis.

A direct medial hernia is more likely in elderly patients. It is broadly based and therefore unlikely to strangulate. The bladder can be pulled into a direct hernia (*Figure 64.12*).

Inguinal hernias are sometimes referred to as 'sliding' in type. These are acquired indirect hernias arising at the deep inguinal ring lateral to the inferior epigastric vessels. Retroperitoneal fatty tissue is pushed downwards along the inguinal canal. As more tissue enters the hernia, peritoneum is pulled with it, thus creating a sac. However, the sac has formed secondarily, distinguishing it from a classic indirect hernia. On the left side, sigmoid colon may descend into a sliding hernia and

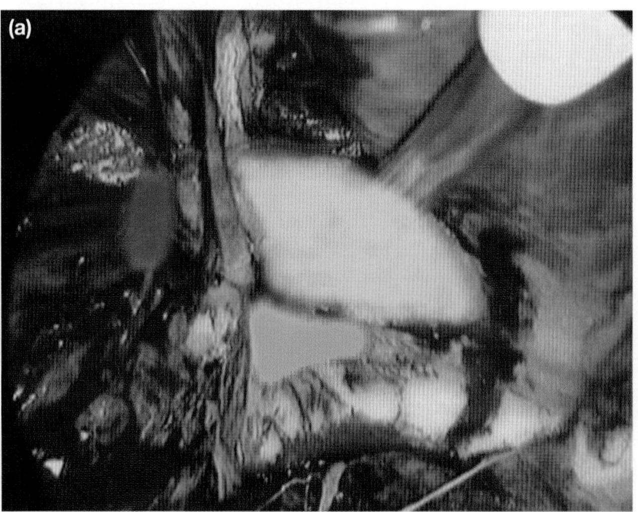

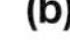

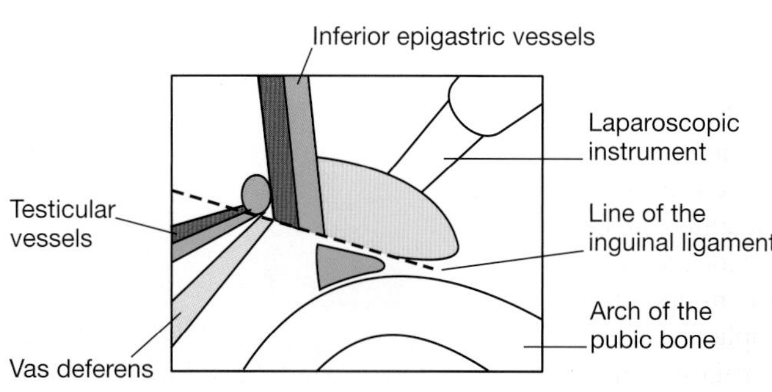

Figure 64.11 (a) Laparoscopic view of the left inguinal region with hernia defects highlighted: yellow, Hesselbach's triangle (medial or direct inguinal); blue, lateral or indirect inguinal; green, femoral. (b) Diagrammatic representation of (a).

Francois Poupart, 1661–1709, physician and anatomist, Hôtel Dieu, Reims, France, described the inguinal ligament in 1705 although it had been described in 1561 by **Gabrielle Fallopius**, 1523–1563, Professor of Anatomy, Padua, Italy.
Franz Kaspar Hesselbach, 1759–1816, surgeon and anatomist, Würzburg, Germany.

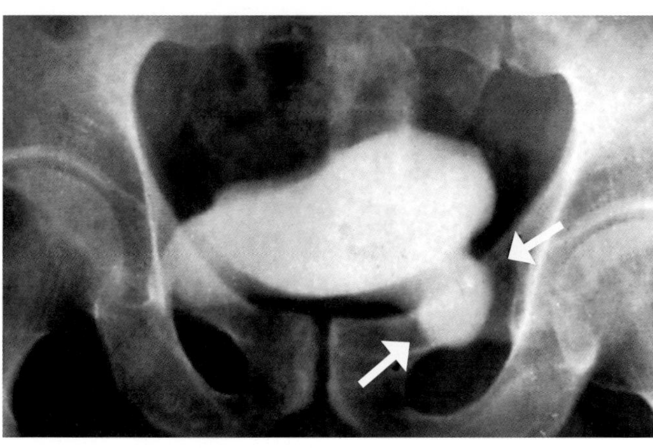

Figure 64.12 A cystogram showing that part of the urinary bladder has descended into a left direct inguinal hernia (arrows).

the caecum may do so on the left. Surgeons need extra caution during repair because the bowel may form part of the sac itself and can be damaged during the dissection.

Occasionally, both lateral and medial hernias are present in the same patient (pantaloon hernia).

Classification

Many ways to classify inguinal (and femoral) hernias have been described. The European Hernia Society has recently suggested a simplified system of:

- primary or recurrent (P or R);
- lateral, medial or femoral (L, M or F);
- defect size in fingerbreadths (assumed to be 1.5 cm), with three sizes of one fingerbreadth or less, between one and three fingerbreadths and three or more fingerbreadths.

A primary indirect inguinal hernia with a 3-cm defect size would be PL2.

Diagnosis of an inguinal hernia

In most cases, the diagnosis of an inguinal hernia is simple. Often the hernia will reduce on lying and reappear on standing. With the patient lying down, the patient is asked to reduce the hernia if it has not spontaneously reduced. If the patient cannot then the surgeon gently attempts to reduce the hernia. Once reduced, the surgeon identifies the bony landmarks of the anterosuperior iliac spine and pubic tubercle, from which the location of the deep inguinal ring can be found just above the midpoint of the inguinal ligament. Gentle pressure is applied at this point and the patient asked to cough. If the hernia is controlled with pressure on the deep inguinal ring then it is likely to be indirect/lateral; if the hernia appears medial to this point despite local pressure, then it is direct/medial. Other examination techniques have been suggested but even experienced surgeons find it difficult to distinguish lateral and medial hernias with certainty (*Figure 64.13*).

Diagnostic difficulties

Confirmation of the diagnosis may not be possible when the patient describes an intermittent swelling but nothing is found on examination. Surgeons will often accept the diagnosis on history alone but re-examination at a later date or investigation by ultrasound scan may be requested.

If an inguinal hernia becomes irreducible and tense there may be no cough impulse. Differential diagnosis would include a groin lymph node mass, psoas abscess, subcutaneous soft tissue mass (e.g. lipoma) or an abdominal mass. Such cases may require investigation by either ultrasonography or CT.

Large scrotal hernias may be misdiagnosed as a hydrocele or other testicular swelling. The surgeon should be able to identify the upper limit of a swelling that arises from within the scrotum, but a large scrotal hernia has no upper limit because it extends back along the inguinal canal to the peritoneal cavity. In cases of doubt, ultrasonography or CT should establish the diagnosis.

As inguinal hernia is so common, less experienced clinicians might suggest this diagnosis when referring cases of femoral hernia or Spigelian hernia. A saphena varix may present as a groin swelling that increases in size on standing and with a definite cough impulse and be misdiagnosed as a hernia, particularly in pregnant women.

It is essential in men to examine the scrotal contents to exclude other pathologies and to check that the patient has both testes. It is also important to examine the opposite side because contralateral hernia is common. A patient with a single hernia has a 50% lifetime risk of developing a hernia on the other side. Some surgeons have suggested that patients should be offered bilateral repair, especially if laparoscopic surgery is planned, but this is not widespread practice at present.

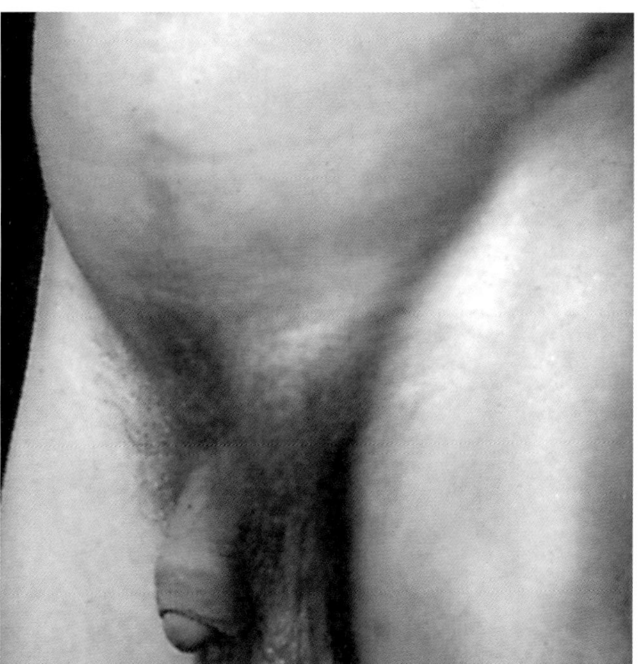

Figure 64.13 Oblique left inguinal hernia that became apparent when the patient coughed and persisted until it was reduced when he lay down.

Investigations for inguinal hernia

Most cases require no diagnostic tests but ultrasonography, CT and MRI are occasionally used and show excellent anatomical detail but may miss groin hernias because they tend to reduce spontaneously in supine patients.

Management of inguinal hernia

It is safe to recommend no active treatment in cases of early asymptomatic direct hernia, particularly in elderly patients who do not wish for surgical intervention. These patients should be warned to seek early advice if the hernia increases in size or becomes symptomatic. Surgical trusses are not recommended. Elective surgery for inguinal hernia can be undertaken under local, regional or general anaesthesia with minimal risk, even in high-risk patients.

Herniotomy

In children who have lateral hernias with a persistent processus vaginalis, it is sufficient just to excise and close the sac. This is called a herniotomy (see ***Chapter 18***). In adult surgery, herniotomy alone has a high recurrence rate and some form of muscle-strengthening repair (herniorrhaphy) is recommended.

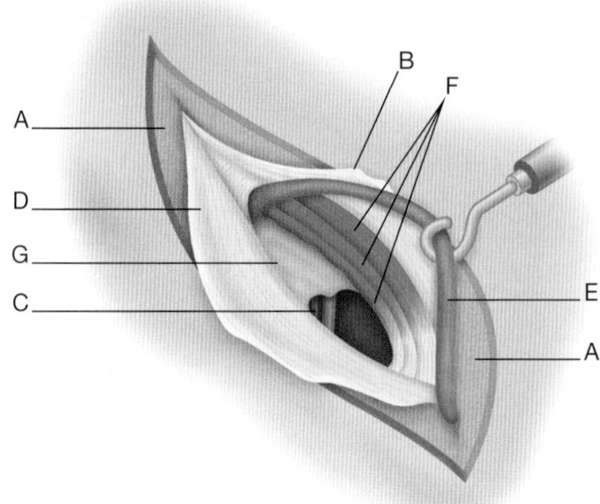

Figure 64.14 Inguinal canal anatomy as shown in Bassini's original diagram (1890). A, subcutaneous fat; B, external oblique aponeurosis (opened); C, inferior epigastric vessels; D, Poupart's (inguinal) ligament; E, spermatic cord retracted; F, the conjoint tendon (triple layer of lesser oblique, transversus abdominis and Cooper's (cremasteric) fascia); G, transversalis fascia.

Open suture repair

In 1890, Edoardo Bassini described a suture repair for inguinal hernia that remained the basis of open repair for over 100 years (***Figure 64.14***). The surgeon enters the inguinal canal by opening its anterior wall, the external oblique aponeurosis. The spermatic cord is dissected free and the presence of a lateral or a medial hernia is confirmed. The sac of a lateral hernia is separated from the cord, opened and any contents reduced. The sac is then sutured closed at its neck and excess sac removed. If there is a medial hernia then the sac is inverted and the transversalis fascia is suture plicated. Sutures are now placed between the conjoint tendon above and the inguinal ligament below, extending from the pubic tubercle to the deep inguinal ring. The posterior wall of the inguinal canal is thus strengthened.

Over 150 modifications to Bassini's operation have been described with little or no benefit except for the Shouldice modification. In this operation, the transversalis fascia is opened by a central incision from the deep inguinal ring to the pubic tubercle and then closed to create a two-layered posterior wall (double breasting). The external oblique is closed in a similar fashion. Expert centres have reported lifetime failure rates of less than 2% after Shouldice repair but it is a technically demanding operation that, in most hands, gives results similar to those of a Bassini repair.

Today, when a Bassini-type operation is done, most surgeons use a continuous, non-absorbable nylon or polypropylene suture that is darned between the conjoint tendon and inguinal ligament (Maloney). This operation gives excellent results and is the most common operation performed in countries where mesh is too expensive.

Desarda has described an operation where a 1- to 2-cm strip of external oblique aponeurosis lying over the inguinal canal is isolated from the main muscle, but left attached both medially and laterally. It is then sutured to the conjoint tendon and inguinal ligament, reinforcing the posterior wall of the inguinal canal. As the abdominal muscles contract, this strip of aponeurosis tightens to add further physiological support to the posterior wall. This operation is currently seen as equivalent to Shouldice repair.

Open flat mesh repair

Synthetic mesh has been used since the 1950s to reinforce hernia repair, and in the 1980s Lichtenstein described a tension-free, simple, flat, polypropylene mesh repair for inguinal hernia (***Figure 64.15***). The initial part of the operation is identical to Bassini's. Once the hernia sac has been removed and any medial defect closed, a piece of mesh measuring 8 × 15 cm is placed over the posterior wall, behind the spermatic cord, and is slit to wrap around the spermatic cord at the deep inguinal ring. Loose sutures hold the mesh to the inguinal ligament and conjoint tendon. Two major advantages are claimed: lower hernia recurrence rates and accelerated postoperative recovery. Randomised trials show that hernia recurrence within the first 2 years is lower but acute pain scores are similar. Recent research comparing Lichtenstein's repair with laparoscopic surgery has identified chronic pain as the most common complication of open flat mesh repair with rates reported as

Edoardo Bassini, 1844–1924, Professor of Surgery, Padua, Italy.
Edward Earle Shouldice, 1890–1965, surgeon, Thornhill, Ont, Canada, established the Shouldice Hernia Hospital in 1945.
Sir Astley Paston Cooper, 1768–1841, surgeon, Guy's Hospital, London, UK.
George Edward Maloney, 1912–1997, born Dunedin, New Zealand, surgeon, the Radcliffe Infirmary, Oxford, UK.
Mohan P Desarda, contemporary, Poona, India.
Irving Lichtenstein, 1920–2000, surgeon, Beverley Hills, CA, USA.

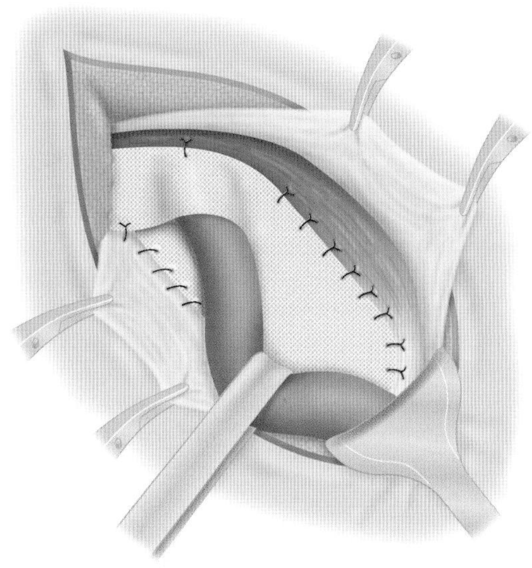

Figure 64.15 Lichtenstein's repair.

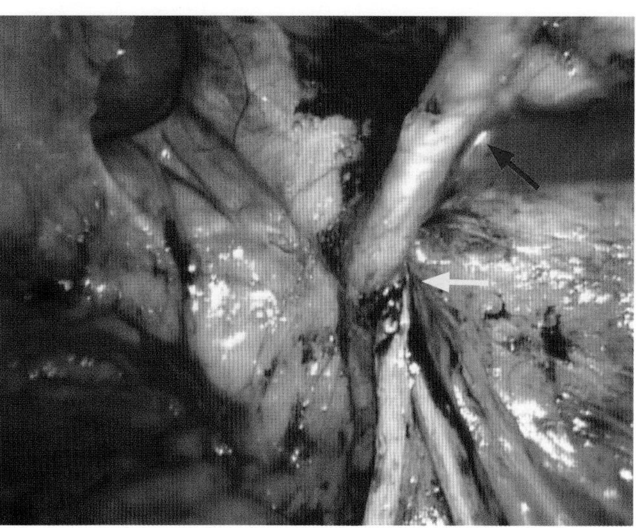

Figure 64.16 Right medial/direct inguinal hernia: laparoscopic view. Note the inferior epigastric vessels (red arrow) and contents of the spermatic cord passing through the deep ring (yellow arrow).

high as 20%. Nevertheless, today, Lichtenstein's repair is the most common operation for inguinal hernia in resource-rich countries.

Open plug/device/complex mesh repair

Shaped mesh plugs have been developed in an attempt to improve on simple flat mesh repair. They are simple to insert and require little if any fixation. However, they can become solid (meshoma) and migrate/erode into adjacent structures such as the urinary bladder. Other meshes have been designed to be placed beneath the transversalis fascia. There is little evidence that any of these techniques are superior to Lichtenstein's operation and use is not recommended in the 2018 European Hernia Society groin hernia guidelines.

Open preperitoneal repair

The preperitoneal approach was first described by Annandale in 1880, but was largely discarded until the 1950s when Stoppa described it with mesh reconstruction through a midline incision. It is useful when multiple attempts at open standard surgery have failed and the hernia(s) keeps recurring. It has been largely superseded by the totally extraperitoneal laparoscopic approach, which is modelled on Stoppa's operation.

Laparoscopic inguinal hernia repair

Two techniques are described and have been extensively studied: the totally extraperitoneal (TEP) and the transabdominal preperitoneal (TAPP) approach. In both, the aim of surgery is to reduce the hernia and hernia sac from within the abdomen and place a 10 × 15 cm mesh (or larger) in the preperitoneal plane, just deep to the abdominal wall extending medially into the retropubic space and at least 5 cm lateral to the deep inguinal ring (***Figure 64.16***). The mesh covers Hesselbach's triangle, the deep inguinal ring and the femoral canal. In TEP, the surgeon develops the extraperitoneal plane just deep to the abdominal muscles, taking care not to enter the peritoneal cavity. In TAPP, the surgeon enters the peritoneal cavity first and incises the peritoneum above the hernia defect to open up the extraperitoneal space as in TEP.

Compared with an open approach, the laparoscopic approach is associated with reduced pain both immediately after surgery and up to 5 years later, more rapid return to full activity and a reduced incidence of wound complications such as infection, bleeding and seroma. Laparoscopic surgery is of particular benefit in bilateral hernias and in patients with hernia recurrence after open surgery. The proportion of cases performed laparoscopically is slowly rising, but there is a long learning curve.

The increasing use of robot-assisted laparoscopic inguinal hernia surgery is evident. To date, little additional patient benefit has been noted, although the enhanced surgical view of the robot and the ergonomic comfort for the surgeon are compelling reasons to utilise this platform. The cost of using a robot for simple inguinal repair remains hard to justify.

Tailored approach

A number of surgical approaches and operations are available, as noted in ***Summary box 64.9***. No one operation suits all hernias. Taking into account the surgeon's skills, equipment available, patient type and hernia characteristics will aid a preoperative discussion as to which repair is best, or indeed whether no operation at all is the best management plan.

Thomas Annandale, 1838–1907, Regius Professor of Surgery, Edinburgh, UK.
Rene Stoppa, 1921–2006, surgeon, Amiens, France.

Summary box 64.9

Operations for inguinal hernia

- Herniotomy
- Open suture repair
  - Bassini
  - Shouldice
  - Desarda
  - Maloney darn
- Open flat mesh repair
  - Lichtenstein
- (Open complex mesh repair – not recommended
  - Mesh plugs
  - Hernia systems)
- Open preperitoneal repair
  - Transinguinal, Stoppa repair
- Laparoscopic/robot-assisted repair
  - TEP
  - TAPP

Emergency inguinal hernia surgery

Approximately 5% of inguinal hernias present as an irreducible, painful lump that may progress to strangulation and possible bowel infarction. Time is critical in the presence of ischaemic bowel. The principles of surgery are the same as in an elective setting. Open or laparoscopic surgery is possible depending on the local facilities, the surgeon's skills and the patient's characteristics. Approximately 20% of patients who present as an emergency require bowel resection. This may require conversion to a midline laparotomy, which adds significantly to postoperative morbidity and mortality. Surgical site infection may complicate emergency cases but, unless there is significant infection/contamination, use of synthetic mesh is acceptable as long as the operation is covered by appropriate antibiotics.

Complications of inguinal hernia surgery

Despite inguinal hernia repair being a common procedure, postoperative complications are common. Immediate complications include bleeding or haematoma (usually from subcutaneous vessels but occasionally from accidental damage to the inferior epigastric or iliac vessels). Urinary retention may require catheterisation. Infusion of local anaesthetic may lead to femoral nerve blockade that will resolve over some hours.

Within the first week, pain, bruising and swelling are common while seroma formation and wound infection are less frequent. Seroma is due to an inflammatory response to dissection, sutures or mesh and is more common if the peritoneal sac is left *in situ*. In most cases the fluid resolves spontaneously but may require aspiration. After laparoscopic surgery, a seroma may be misdiagnosed as an early recurrence. Despite the potential of bacterial contamination of a groin incision and use of mesh, routine use of antibiotics is not recommended in recent guidelines.

In the longer term, hernia recurrence and chronic pain are the main concerns. No operation can be guaranteed to be recurrence free and good centres aim for a 5-year recurrence rate of less than 5%. Mesh repairs have lower recurrence rates than suture repairs, but there is no difference between the various mesh repairs and no difference between open and laparoscopic surgery. There is very strong evidence that specialist hernia surgeons have lower recurrence rates and chronic pain rates whatever technique they use.

Chronic pain, defined as pain persisting for more than 3 months after surgery, is common after all forms of surgery and possibly affects as many as 20% of patients after groin hernia repair. It is less common and less severe after laparoscopic surgery. Different types of pain have been described but the most severe is neuralgic pain due to nerve irritation. This may be the result of nerve injury at the time of operation or chronic irritation of nerves by suture material or mesh. Chronic pain has become one of the main areas of focus when comparing inguinal hernia outcomes. Patients at higher risk of chronic pain include females, the young, those with a painful hernia, those with a chronic pain syndrome, those with an exaggerated response to a heat stimulus and those with certain psychological tendencies. In addition, the handling of the nerves at open surgery is thought to be important. The variation of anatomy of the three nerves should be considered during the dissection, keeping nerves contained within their connective tissue surroundings when possible. In laparoscopic surgery, placing sutures or staples/tacks into the retroperitoneal area should be avoided for fear of causing nerve injury. If a nerve requires to be sacrificed, this should be done as proximally as practicable and the nerve end buried within the muscle belly.

Rarely, damage to the testicular artery can lead to testicular infarction, perhaps the most serious complication of inguinal hernia surgery in a young man. There is no evidence that hernia surgery has an effect on male fertility despite extensive study in this area.

Summary box 64.10

Complications

- Early: pain, bleeding/haematoma, urinary retention
- Medium: seroma, wound infection
- Late: chronic pain, testicular atrophy

Sportsman's groin

This specific entity is well described and presents with severe pain in the groin area, often extending into the upper thigh and the scrotum in men. It is seen in both men and women who play contact sports such as football and rugby. The pain can be debilitating and prevent the patient from exercising. On examination there may be some tenderness in the region of the inguinal canal, over the pubic tubercle and over the insertion of the thigh adductor muscles. Tightening the hip flexor or thigh adductor muscles against resistance may reproduce the pain. Usually no hernia is present.

In most cases, the pain is due to adductor strain or pubic symphysis diastasis. However, some believe that it can be due to muscle tearing (Gilmore's groin) or stretching of the posterior wall of the inguinal canal. Other causes of pain should be excluded, such as hip, pelvic or lumbar spinal disease and bladder/prostate problems. MRI is most likely to detect a musculoligamentous problem but ultrasonography or laparoscopy may be used to exclude an underlying hernia.

Hernia surgery should be a last resort and the patient should be warned of a significant risk of failure to relieve the pain. The same is true for patients with groin pain and no obvious hernia, even if a small hernia is noted on groin ultrasound.

Femoral hernia

Basic anatomy

The external iliac artery and vein pass below the inguinal ligament to become the common femoral vessels in the leg. The vein lies medially and the artery is lateral to the vein, with the femoral nerve lateral to the artery. They are enclosed in a fibrous sheath. Just medial to the vein is a small space containing fat and some lymphatic tissue (node of Cloquet). It is this space, the femoral canal, that is exploited by a femoral hernia. The boundaries of the femoral canal are the femoral vein laterally, the inguinal ligament anteriorly, the pelvic bone covered by the iliopectineal ligament (Astley Cooper's) posteriorly and the lacunar ligament (Gimbernat's) medially. This is a strong curved ligament with a sharp unyielding edge that impedes reduction of a femoral hernia (***Figure 64.17***).

The female pelvis has a different shape from the male, increasing the size of the femoral canal and the risk of hernia. In old age, the femoral defect enlarges further and femoral hernia is commonly seen in thin, elderly women.

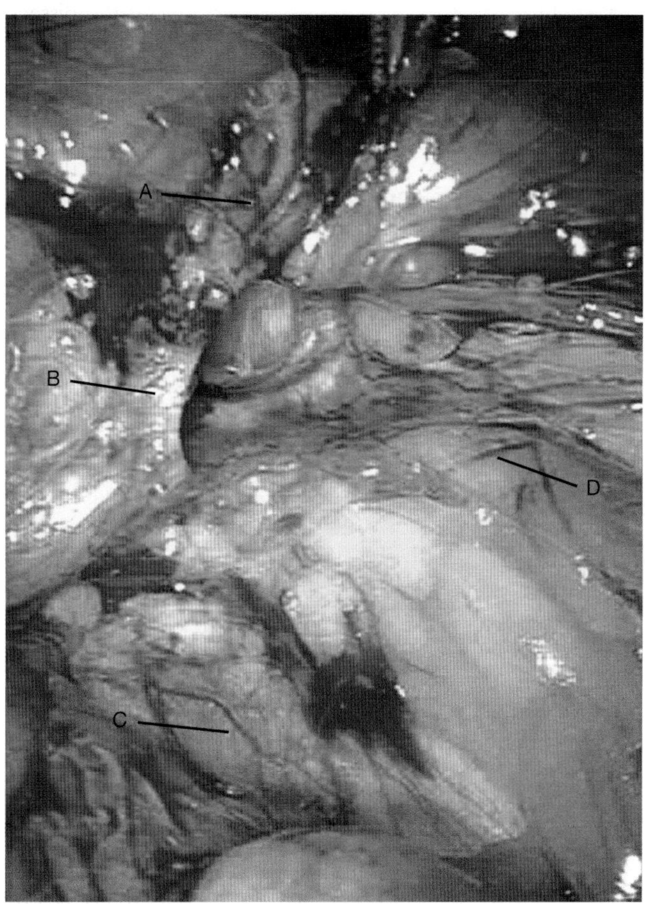

Figure 64.17 Right femoral hernia: laparoscopic view. The slightly oblique inguinal ligament can be seen superolaterally above the defect. The external iliac vein is not seen. A, inguinal ligament; B, lacunar ligament; C, arch of pubic bone; D, fatty tissue overlying iliac vessels.

Summary box 64.11

Femoral hernia

- Less common than inguinal hernia
- More common in women than in men
- Easily missed on examination
- 50% present as an emergency with very high risk of strangulation

Diagnosis of femoral hernia

Diagnostic error is common and often leads to delay in diagnosis and treatment. The hernia appears below and lateral to the pubic tubercle and lies in the upper leg rather than in the lower abdomen. Inadequate exposure of this area during routine examination leads to failure to detect the hernia. The hernia often rapidly becomes irreducible and loses any cough impulse owing to the tightness of the neck. It may only be 1–2 cm in size and can easily be mistaken for a lymph node. As it increases in size, it is reflected superiorly and becomes difficult to distinguish from a medial direct hernia, which arises only a few centimetres above the femoral canal.

Summary box 64.12

Differential diagnosis

- Inguinal hernia
- Lymph node
- Saphena varix
- Femoral artery aneurysm
- Psoas abscess
- Rupture of adductor longus with haematoma

Investigations

In routine cases, no specific investigations are required. However, if there is uncertainty then ultrasonography or CT should be requested. In the emergency patient, bowel obstruction is often present and a plain radiograph is likely to show this. All patients with unexplained small bowel obstruction should undergo careful examination for a femoral hernia.

Jules Germain Cloquet, 1790–1883, Professor of Anatomy and Surgery, Paris, France.
Manoel Louise Antonio don Gimbernat, 1734–1816, Professor of Anatomy, Barcelona, Spain.

It is now common to perform CT scanning in cases of bowel obstruction primarily to exclude malignancy, but it can identify an obstructing femoral hernia missed by clinicians.

Surgery for femoral hernia

There is no alternative to surgery for femoral hernia and it is wise to treat such cases with some urgency. There are three open approaches and appropriate cases can be managed laparoscopically.

Low approach (Lockwood)

This is the simplest operation for a femoral hernia but suitable only when there is no risk of bowel resection. It can easily be performed under local anaesthesia. A transverse incision is made over the hernia. The sac of the hernia is opened and its contents reduced. The sac is also reduced and non-absorbable sutures are placed between the inguinal ligament above and the pectineal ligament overlying the pubic bone below. A small incision can be made in the medial lacunar ligament to aid reduction but there may be an abnormal branch of the obturator artery just deep to it, which can bleed. The femoral vein, lateral to the hernia, needs to be protected. Some surgeons place a mesh plug into the hernia defect for further reinforcement.

The inguinal approach (Lotheissen)

The initial incision is identical to that of Bassini's or Lichtenstein's operation into the inguinal canal. The spermatic cord (or round ligament) is mobilised and the transversalis fascia opened from the deep inguinal ring to the pubic tubercle, avoiding injury to the inferior epigastric vessels. This gains entry into the extraperitoneal space. A femoral hernia lies immediately below this incision and can be reduced by a combination of pulling from above and pushing from below. If necessary, the peritoneum can be opened to deal with the contents. Once reduced, the neck of the hernia is closed with sutures or a mesh plug, protecting the external iliac vein throughout; alternatively, a sheet of flat mesh may be laid over the defect in the extraperitoneal plane. The layers are closed as for inguinal hernia and the surgeon may place a mesh into the inguinal canal to protect against development of an inguinal hernia.

High approach (McEvedy)

This more complex operation is ideal in the emergency situation where the risk of bowel strangulation is high. It requires regional or general anaesthesia. Although McEvedy described a paramedian incision, most surgeons nowadays use the Nyhus modification, which is a transverse incision just above the inguinal canal, centred on the lateral border of the rectus muscle. The anterior rectus sheath is incised and the rectus muscle retracted. The surgeon proceeds deep to the muscle in the preperitoneal space. The femoral hernia is reduced and the sac opened to allow careful inspection of the hernia contents. In dubious cases, the bowel is replaced into the peritoneal cavity for 5 minutes and then re-examined. The femoral defect is then closed with sutures or mesh.

This approach allows a generous incision to be made in the peritoneum, which aids inspection of the bowel and facilitates bowel resection. Bowel resection is not possible via the low (Lockwood) approach because the completed anastomosis will not be able to be returned to the abdominal cavity through the narrow femoral canal. The preperitoneal approach may be extended to gain access to repair bilateral femoral hernias through a single incision (Henry).

Laparoscopic approach

Both the TEP and TAPP approaches can be used for a femoral hernia and a standard mesh inserted in the extraperitoneal plane. This is ideal for reducible femoral hernias presenting electively, but there are increasing reports of the laparoscopic approach in the emergency setting, mainly with the TAPP approach.

In women, the laparoscopic approach is recommended because of the increased early recurrence observed in women, thought to relate more to misdiagnosis of the hernia (inguinal versus femoral) than true recurrence. The laparoscopic approach allows good visualisation of all the hernia orifices, removing any diagnostic uncertainty.

VENTRAL HERNIA

This term refers to hernias of the anterior abdominal wall. Inguinal and femoral hernias are not included, however lumbar hernia is included despite being dorsolateral. The European Hernia Society classification (2009) distinguished primary ventral from incisional hernia but did not include parastomal hernia, which is included in this section.

Summary box 64.13

Primary ventral hernias
- Umbilical
- Epigastric
- Spigelian
- Lumbar
- Traumatic

'Secondary' ventral hernias
- Incisional
- Parastomal

Umbilical hernia

The umbilical defect is present at birth but closes as the stump of the umbilical cord heals, usually within a week of birth. This process may be delayed, leading to the development of herniation in the neonatal period. The umbilical ring may also stretch and reopen in adult life.

Charles Barrett Lockwood, 1856–1914, surgeon, St Bartholomew's Hospital, London, UK.
George Lotheissen, 1868–1941, surgeon, the Kaiser Franz Joseph Hospital, Vienna, Austria.
Peter George McEvedy, 1890–1951, surgeon, Ancoats Hospital, Manchester, UK.
Lloyd Milton Nyhus, 1923–2008, Chief of Surgery, University of Illinois, Chicago, IL, USA.
Arnold K Henry, 1886–1962, Professor of Surgery, Cairo, later Anatomy Professor, Royal College of Surgeons in Ireland, Dublin, Ireland.

Umbilical hernia in children

This common condition occurs in up to 10% of infants, with a higher incidence in premature babies. The hernia appears within a few weeks of birth and is often symptomless, but increases in size on crying and assumes a classic conical shape. Sexes are equally affected but the incidence in black infants is up to eight times higher than in white. Obstruction and/or strangulation is extremely uncommon below the age of 3 years.

Treatment

Conservative treatment is indicated under the age of 2 years when the hernia is symptomless. Parental reassurance is all that is necessary as 95% will resolve spontaneously. If the hernia persists beyond the age of 2 years surgical repair is indicated.

Surgery

A small, curved incision is made immediately below the umbilicus. The neck of the sac is defined, opened and any contents are returned to the peritoneal cavity. The sac is closed and redundant sac excised. The defect in the linea alba is closed with interrupted sutures of slowly absorbable material.

Summary box 64.14

Umbilical hernia in children

- Common in infants and most resolve spontaneously
- Rarely strangulate

Umbilical hernia in adults

Conditions that cause stretching and thinning of the midline raphe (linea alba), such as pregnancy, obesity and liver disease with cirrhosis and ascites, predispose to reopening of the umbilical defect. In adults, the defect can be not only through the umbilicus but also in the median raphe (linea alba) immediately adjacent to (most often above) the true umbilicus. The latter are commonly called 'paraumbilical' hernias; however, under current guidelines, any hernia in the immediate vicinity of the umbilicus can now be called 'umbilical'. Small umbilical hernias often contain extraperitoneal fat or omentum. Larger hernias can contain small or large bowel. Because the hernia neck is relatively narrow in relation to the size of the sac, they are prone to become irreducible, obstructed and strangulated.

Clinical features

Umbilical hernias are commonly seen in overweight men with a thinned and attenuated midline raphe or in postpartum women with a weakened abdominal wall. The bulge is typically slightly to one side of the umbilical depression, creating a crescent-shaped appearance to the umbilicus (***Figure 64.18***). Women are affected more than men. Most patients complain of pain due to tissue tension or symptoms of intermittent bowel obstruction. In large hernias, the overlying skin may become very thin; while overlying skin irritation and ulceration may be seen, spontaneous rupture is extremely rare.

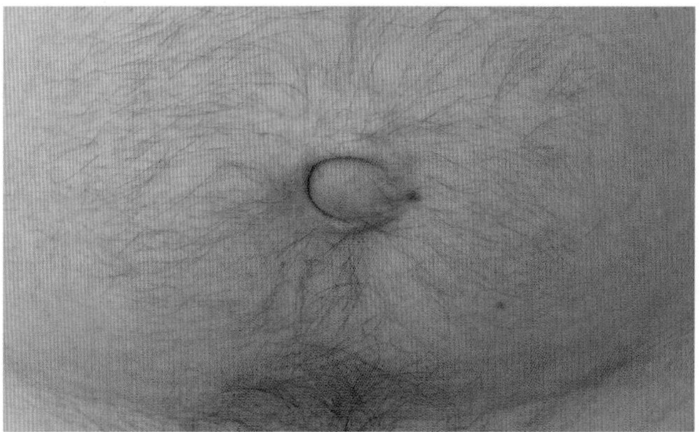

Figure 64.18 A small adult umbilical hernia.

Treatment

As a result of the high risk of strangulation, surgery should be advised in cases where the hernia contains bowel. Small hernias may be left alone if they are asymptomatic, but they may enlarge and require surgery at a later date. Surgery may be performed open or laparoscopically.

Open umbilical hernia repair

Very small defects less than 1 cm in size may be closed with a simple suture repair as long as the fascia is not closed under tension. An alternative technique utilises a darn suture where a non-absorbable, monofilament suture is criss-crossed across the defect and anchored firmly to the fascia all around. For defects up to 2 cm in diameter a transverse incision is made and the hernia sac dissected, opened and its contents reduced. The peritoneum is closed. The defect in the linea alba is extended in a transverse direction and the fascial edges are closed in an overlapping style with the superior flap on top ('waistcoat over trousers') (Mayo). Non-absorbable sutures are used and the skin is closed in a routine manner, but redundant skin may need to be excised to achieve a better cosmetic result. The Mayo repair remains popular for defects up to 2 cm, but the larger the defect the more tissue tension. Current evidence advises the use of mesh even in small defects, and certainly for all defects larger than 2 cm, owing to the high likelihood of recurrence (***Figure 64.19***).

Special circumstances

Women often develop umbilical hernias during pregnancy and may present in the early postpartum period. There is often a degree of rectus divarication. They should be advised to exercise specifically for this condition, lose weight and increase their abdominal muscle tone before operation should be considered as these may resolve completely within a few months. It is strongly recommended to avoid surgery for umbilical hernia repair before or during pregnancy.

William James Mayo, 1861–1939, surgeon, the Mayo Clinic, Rochester, MN, USA, described this operation in 1901. He and his brother **Charles Horace Mayo** (1865–1939) joined their father's (William Worrall Mayo) private practice in Rochester. This practice became the Mayo Clinic.

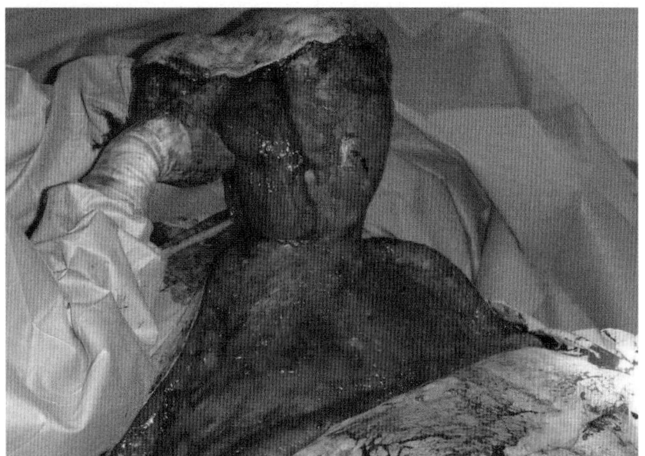

Figure 64.19 A massive umbilical hernia, intraoperative view.

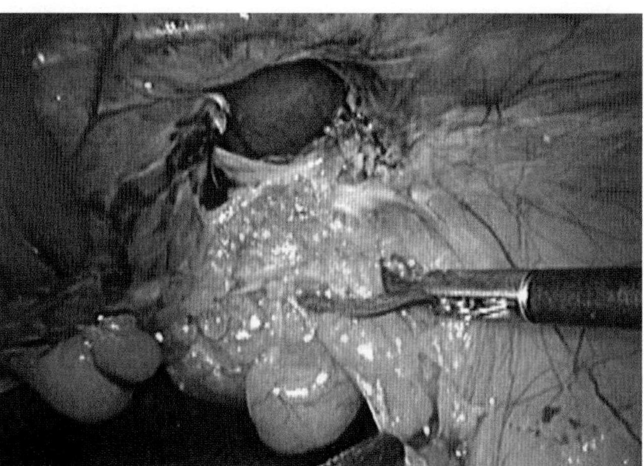

Figure 64.20 Umbilical defect: laparoscopic view, before the bulky falciform ligament has been taken down to create a smoother surface for mesh placement.

Patients with liver cirrhosis have extremely high mortality and morbidity after primary ventral hernia repair, especially with Child's B and C disease. Patient selection is very important, with appropriate hepatology support if surgery is contemplated. Fascial repair is best done with fine continuous sutures to minimise the risk of post-operative ascites leakage.

Laparoscopic umbilical hernia repair

A camera port and two working ports are placed laterally on the abdominal wall, well away from the defect. The contents of the hernia are reduced by traction and external pressure. The falciform ligament above and the median umbilical fold below may need to be taken down to create a smooth, firm surface for mesh placement (***Figure 64.20***). A disc of non-adherent mesh, designed for intraperitoneal use, is introduced and positioned on the undersurface of the abdominal wall, centred on the defect. It is then fixed to the peritoneum and posterior rectus sheaths using staples, tacks or sutures. This is a simple and secure repair, which achieves generous overlap without surgical damage to umbilicus and surrounding fascia. However, it requires specialised equipment and expensive tissue-separating mesh and brings with it all the potential problems of intraperitoneal mesh, including bowel adhesion, erosion and fistulation. Intraperitoneal meshes can cause severe pain lasting for 24–48 hours after surgery, which can mimic peritonitis. The tacks or sutures used to fix the mesh can be a source of chronic or long-lasting pain. However, this approach is associated with fewer wound complications than open repair and allows large pieces of mesh to be used, so should be considered for obese patients, those with concomitant rectus divarication and those with multiple ventral hernia defects.

Emergency repair of umbilical hernia

Incarceration, bowel obstruction and strangulation are frequent because of the narrow neck and the fibrous edge of the defect in the midline raphe. Delay to surgery can lead to gangrene of the omentum or bowel. Large hernias are often multiloculated and there may be strangulated bowel in one component when other areas are clinically soft and a non-tender hernia. Multiloculated hernias are however more common as incisional then primary ventral. Most emergency repairs are performed by open surgery. In the presence of established strangulation mesh should be avoided as the risk of infection is too high; the focus of the operation should be to deal with the strangulated tissue, so a suture repair is advised with a more definite repair to be performed at a later date if necessary.

Epigastric hernia

These hernias arise through the midline raphe (linea alba) anywhere between the xiphoid process and the umbilicus. They begin with a transverse split in the midline raphe so the defect is elliptical and usually less than 1 cm in diameter. The hernia commonly contains only extraperitoneal fat, which gradually enlarges, spreading in the subcutaneous plane to resemble the shape of a mushroom (***Figure 64.21***). When very large they may contain a peritoneal sac but rarely any bowel. More than one hernia may be present. Indeed, the most common cause of 'recurrence' is failure to identify a second defect at the time of original repair.

Clinical features

The patients are often fit, healthy men, but they are also seen in older, overweight men and women especially after multiple pregnancies. The hernia can be very painful even when the swelling is small owing to the fatty contents becoming nipped sufficiently to produce partial strangulation. It may be locally tender. It is unlikely to be reducible because of the narrow neck and may resemble a lipoma. A cough impulse may or may not be felt.

Charles Gardner Child, 1908–1991, Chair of the Departments of Surgery at Cornell University, Ithaca, NY (1947–1953), Tufts University, Boston, MA (1953–1974), and the University of Michigan, Ann Arbor, MI (1978–1983), USA.

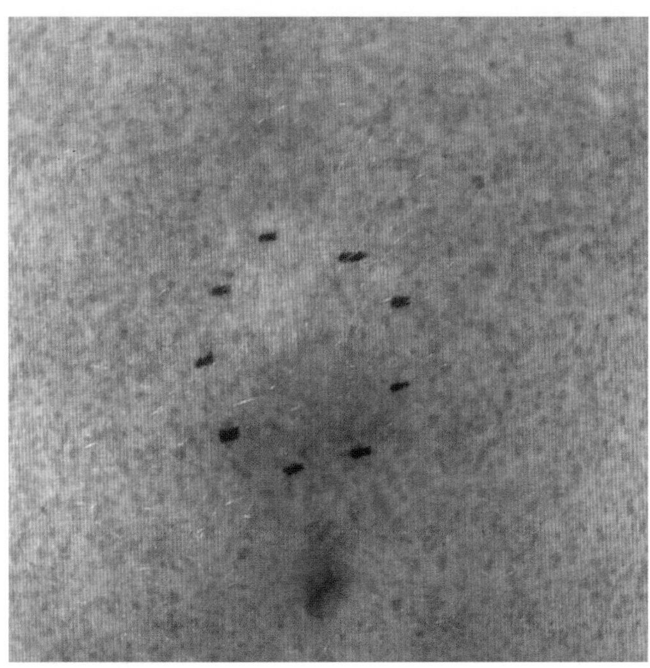

Figure 64.21 Epigastric hernia.

Treatment

Very small epigastric hernias have been known to disappear spontaneously, probably because of infarction of the fat. Small- to moderate-sized hernias without a peritoneal sac are not inherently dangerous and surgery should be offered only if the hernia is sufficiently symptomatic. Hernias containing bowel should always be repaired.

Surgery

This may be open or laparoscopic. At open surgery, a vertical or transverse incision is made over the swelling and down to the linea alba. Protruding extraperitoneal fat can simply be pushed back through the defect or excised. Often a small vessel is present in the hernia content that can cause troublesome bleeding. Small defects in the linea alba may be closed with non-absorbable sutures in adults and absorbable sutures in children; however, in larger hernias and when a peritoneal sac is present, the surgical approach is similar to that described for an umbilical mesh repair.

Laparoscopic repair is also very similar to that for umbilical hernia except that the defect is hidden behind the falciform ligament, which must first be taken down from the undersurface of the abdominal wall to allow the margins of the defect to be exposed. It is very important to fully reduce the fatty contents, as simply placing a mesh under the linea alba may leave the patient with a palpable lump if the hernia contents are extraperitoneal fat.

Spigelian hernia

These hernias are uncommon although probably underdiagnosed. They affect men and women equally and are most common in elderly people. They have also been described in infants, reflecting incomplete differentiation of the mesenchymal layers within the abdominal wall. They arise through a defect in the aponeurosis of transversus abdominis (Spigelian fascia) and may advance through the internal oblique to spread out deep to the external oblique aponeurosis. Most Spigelian hernias appear below the level of the umbilicus near the edge of the rectus sheath, but they can be found anywhere along the Spigelian line (***Figure 64.22***). There is a common misconception that they protrude below the arcuate line as a result of deficiency of the posterior rectus sheath at that level, but in fact the defect is almost always above the arcuate line. In young patients they usually contain extraperitoneal fat only, but in older patients there is often a peritoneal sac and they can become very large.

Clinical features

Young patients usually present with intermittent pain, due to pinching of the fat, similar to an epigastric hernia. A lump may or may not be palpable because the fatty hernia is small and the overlying external oblique is intact. Older patients generally present with a reducible swelling at the edge of the rectus sheath and may have symptoms of intermittent obstruction. The diagnosis should be suspected because of the location of the symptoms and is confirmed by CT. Ultrasonography has the advantage that it can be performed in the upright patient because no defect may be visible with the patient lying down.

Treatment

Surgery is recommended because the narrow and fibrous neck predisposes to strangulation. Surgery can be open or laparoscopic. At open surgery a skin crease is made over the hernia, but no abnormality will be seen until the external oblique is opened. The sac and contents are dealt with and the small defect in the Spigelian fascia is repaired by suture or mesh laid deep to the external oblique aponeurosis. The plane of the mesh can be extended medially into the posterior rectus sheath if required. The external oblique aponeurosis is closed over the mesh.

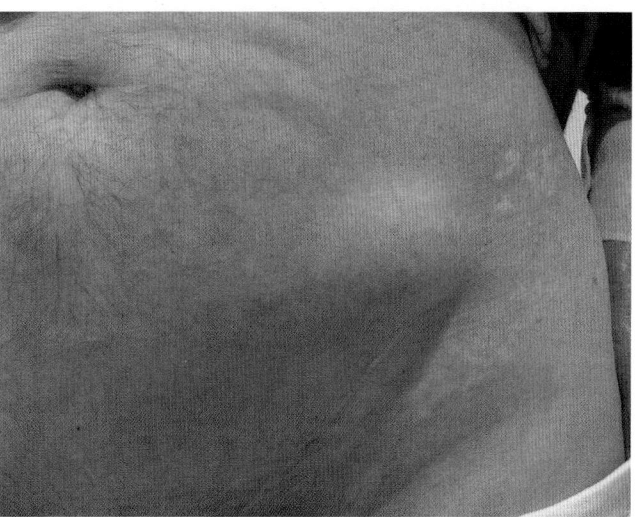

Figure 64.22 Spigelian hernia in the left iliac fossa. Note the scar from a previous left inguinal hernia repair.

Laparoscopy is useful if no sac is palpable, but, in young patients with a hernia containing only extraperitoneal fat, no hernia will be seen from within the peritoneum. In such cases, the peritoneum can be incised and the extraperitoneal plane explored for the small defect, which can then be closed by either suture or mesh. When an intraperitoneal sac is present, laparoscopic repair can be performed using either the intraperitoneal onlay of mesh (IPOM) or, more commonly now because of the risks of intraperitoneal mesh, the TAPP technique.

Summary box 64.15

Spigelian hernia

- Rare
- Often misdiagnosed
- High risk of complications

Lumbar hernia

Most primary lumbar hernias occur through the inferior lumbar triangle of Petit, bounded below by the crest of the ilium, laterally by the external oblique muscle and medially by latissimus dorsi (*Figure 64.23*). Less commonly, the sac comes through the superior lumbar triangle, which is bounded by the twelfth rib above, medially by sacrospinalis and laterally by the posterior border of the internal oblique muscle (*Figure 64.24*). Primary lumbar hernias are rare, but may be mimicked by incisional hernias arising through flank incision operations.

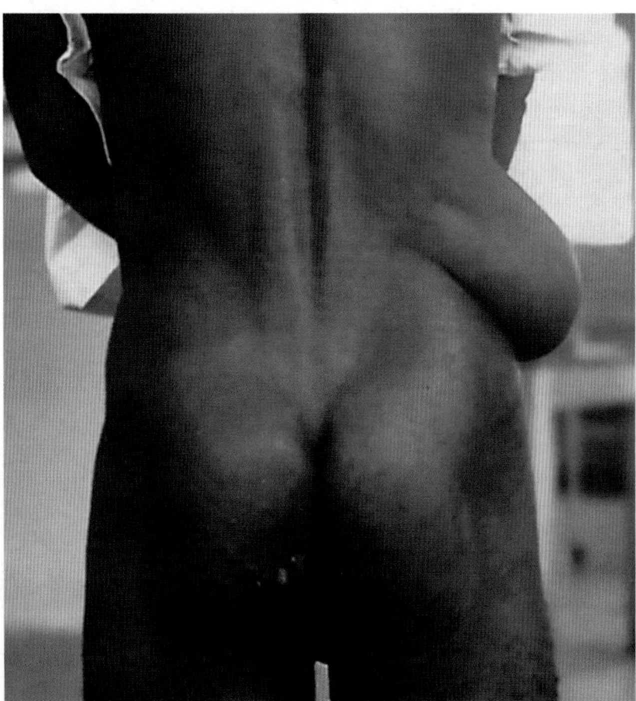

Figure 64.23 Inferior lumbar hernia, which contained caecum, appendix and small bowel. Note the filarial skin rash on the buttocks (courtesy of VJ Hartfield, formerly of south-east Nigeria).

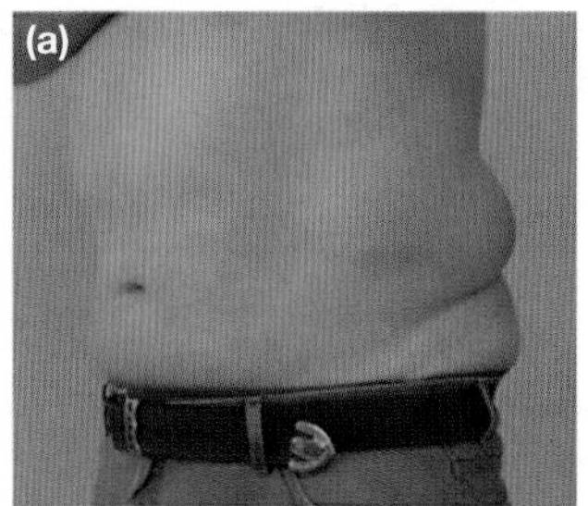

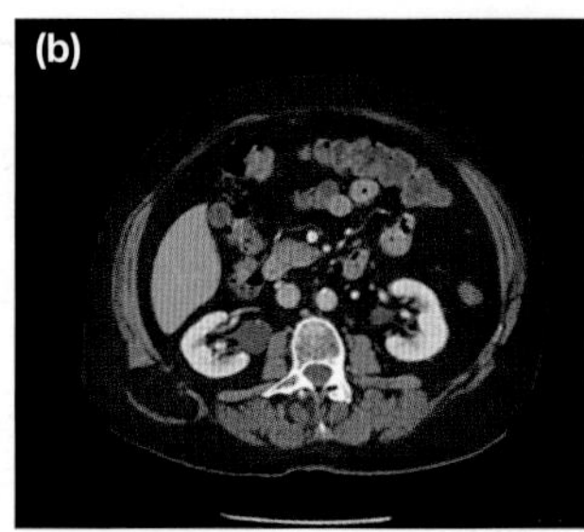

Figure 64.24 (a) Left superior lumbar hernia, containing only extraperitoneal fat. (b) Computed tomography scan of a similar but right-sided superior lumbar hernia. Emerging just below the twelfth rib, it is level with the right kidney and the right lobe of the liver.

Differential diagnosis

A lumbar hernia must be distinguished from:

- a lipoma;
- an incisional hernia, such as from a renal operation;
- a cold (tuberculous) abscess pointing to this position;
- a pseudohernia due to local muscular paralysis. Lumbar pseudohernia can result from any interference with the nerve supply of the affected muscles, the most common cause being injury to the subcostal nerve during a kidney operation.

Treatment

The natural history is for these hernias to increase in size and surgery is recommended. Lumbar hernias can be approached by open or laparoscopic surgery. The defects can be difficult to close with sutures alone and mesh is recommended.

The TAPP laparoscopic approach is gaining popularity for small hernias. With the patient in a semilateral position ports are inserted well away from the defect. The peritoneum is incised above the hernia and dissected back to expose the muscle defect. The content, often extraperitoneal fat, is reduced and a mesh fixed with ample overlap. The peritoneum can then be resutured or tacked back to cover the mesh.

Lumbar incisional hernias can be approached in the same way; however, large ones can be very difficult, especially if there is a component of neuropathic muscle atrophy causing a diffuse bulge (pseudohernia).

Traumatic hernia

These hernias arise through non-anatomical defects caused by injury. They can be classified into three types:

1. Hernias through abdominal stab wound sites. These are effectively incisional hernias.
2. Hernias protruding through splits or tears in the abdominal muscles after blunt trauma (*Figure 64.4*).
3. Abdominal bulging secondary to muscle atrophy that

Jean Louis Petit, 1674–1750, Director of the Academie de Chirurgie, Paris, France.

occurs as a result of nerve injury or other traumatic denervation. Akin to the lumbar pseudohernia seen after open nephrectomy, these can also arise after rib fractures with damage to the intercostal nerves.

Clinical features

Traumatic hernias present as any other hernia. The key to the aetiology is in the history and the non-anatomical location of the hernia.

Treatment

Surgery may be justified if the hernia is sufficiently symptomatic or if investigations suggest a narrow neck and hence a risk of obstruction or strangulation. CT scanning is useful to define the tissue layers that have been damaged in order to plan repair. Stab wound traumatic hernias are straightforward to repair. Diffuse abdominal bulges are more difficult to correct and require some form of plication of the stretched musculofascial layer with mesh reinforcement to prevent further bulging in the future. Some bulging may persist, however.

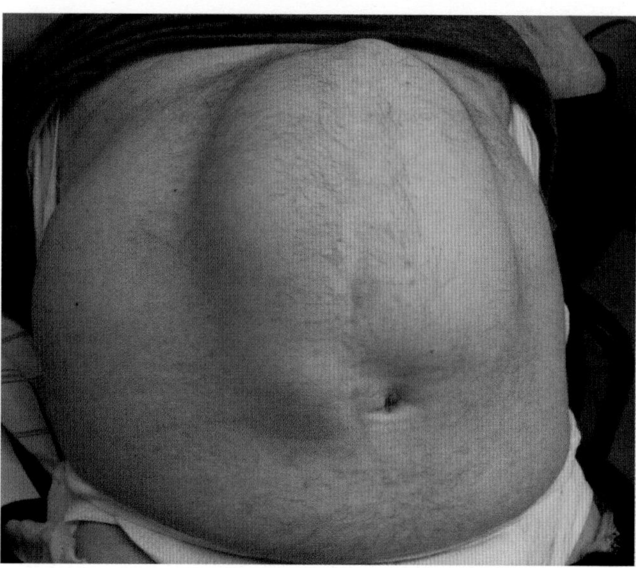

Figure 64.25 A large incisional hernia involving the full length of the incision.

Incisional hernia

These arise through a defect in the musculofascial layers of the abdominal wall at the site of a postoperative scar. Thus, they may appear anywhere where a laparotomy has been made.

Incidence and aetiology

Incisional hernias have been reported in 10–50% of laparotomy incisions and 1–5% of laparoscopic port-site incisions. Factors predisposing to their development include patient factors (genetic collagen disorders, obesity, general poor healing due to malnutrition, immunosuppression or steroid therapy, chronic cough, cancer), wound factors (poor quality tissues, wound tension, wound infection) and surgical factors (inappropriate suture material, poor closure technique).

An incisional hernia usually starts as disruption of the musculofascial layers of a wound in the early postoperative period. This may progress rapidly to full thickness wound dehiscence, usually heralded by a serosanguineous discharge around the sixth postoperative day, but more commonly the event passes unnoticed if the overlying skin wound has healed securely. A visible swelling may take weeks, months or years to appear. Many incisional hernias may be preventable by ensuring healthy wound edges, minimal wound tension and good surgical technique as described by the European Hernia Society abdominal wall closure guidelines. The small-stitch, small-bite technique is recommended, and the role of prophylactic mesh in high-risk patients is also a current area of research.

Clinical features

Incisional hernias commonly appear as a localised swelling involving part of a surgical scar but may present as a diffuse bulging of the whole length of the incision (***Figure 64.25***). Alternatively there may be several discrete hernias along the length of the incision, but even with apparently singular hernias unsuspected defects are frequently found at operation (***Figure 64.26***). Incisional hernias tend to increase steadily in size with time, and the overlying skin may become thin and atrophic. Local trauma and microvascular damage to skin may lead to ulceration. Episodes of intestinal obstruction are common because there are usually coexisting internal

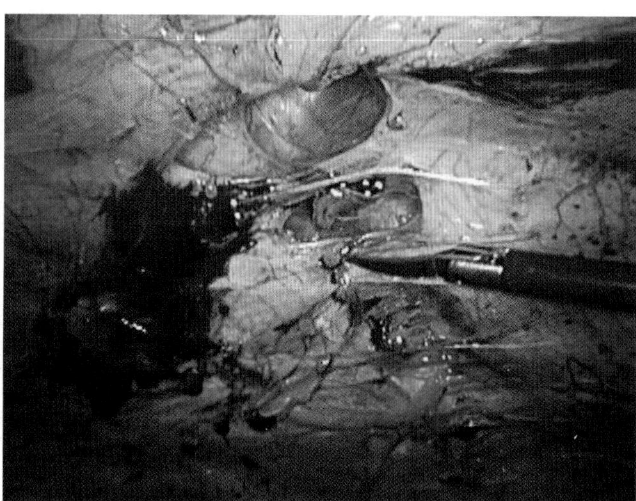

Figure 64.26 Multiple defects along the line of the scar, seen at laparoscopy.

Summary box 64.16

Incisional hernia

- Incidence 10–50% after surgery
- Aetiology includes patient, wound and surgeon factors
- Wide variation in size
- Multiple defects within the same scar are very common
- Obstruction is common but strangulation is rare
- Open and laparoscopic repairs possible

adhesions, but strangulation is less frequent because most incisional hernias are shallow and wide-necked. As with any hernia type, strangulation is most likely when the fibrous defect is small and the sac is large.

Treatment

Asymptomatic incisional hernias may not require treatment. The wearing of an abdominal binder or belt often provides symptomatic relief and may prevent the hernia from increasing in size. Many patients with an incisional hernia have other comorbidities and discussion around the balance of benefits and risks of surgery is important. The decision to operate and choice of technique should always be agreed between the patient and the surgeon and patients' preferences need to be respected. Repair of large and/or complex incisional hernias can be extremely challenging; in such cases advice from, or referral to, a colleague with a special interest in abdominal wall reconstruction should be considered.

Each patient undergoing an elective incisional hernia repair should be optimised for surgery. In many centres, patients undergo formal multidisciplinary team assessment and this is likely to become the standard of care in the coming years. So-called 'prehabilitation' includes weight loss if the patient is obese, smoking cessation, fitness improvement and core strength exercising. Loss of 7% of total bodyweight achieves a significant improvement in metabolic state, and 5 kg of body weight is said to create about one extra litre of space inside the adult male abdomen (0.5 litres in women).

Prevention of incisional hernia

The risk of incisional hernia may be reduced by improving the patient's general condition preoperatively where possible, e.g. smoking cessation, weight loss for obesity or improving nutritional status in undernourished individuals. Closing the fascial layers with good technique and materials is important. For years it has been advised that sutures should be 1 cm back from the wound edge and 1 cm apart, but recent work has shown that lower incisional hernia rates and reduced infection rates are gained when smaller and closer bites are used: 5 mm apart and 5–8 mm back from the wound edge, with care taken to incorporate fascia only in the suture bites (no muscle) and to minimise excessive suture tension. A 2/0 slowly resorbable suture is also recommended rather than traditional heavier and/or non-absorbable materials (see ***Chapter 7***).

There is no evidence that interrupted sutures are better or worse than continuous. However, if continuous suturing is used, the tissue bites must not be too near the fascial edge or pulled too tight because they may cut out. The optimal ratio of suture length to wound length is 4:1. If a ratio of less than this is achieved, the suture bites are likely to be too far apart and/or too tight (and vice versa).

Drains should be brought out through separate incisions and not through the wound itself because this prevents fascial apposition and increases the risk of hernia formation.

Studies in obese patients undergoing bariatric surgery have suggested that placement of a prophylactic mesh in patients at high risk of incisional hernia formation will substantially reduce that risk. Use of prophylactic mesh may reduce the risk of parastomal herniation, which occurs in up to 50% of patients.

Principles of surgical repair

For repair of most incisional hernias, both open and laparoscopic options are available. A number of principles apply, irrespective of the technique used. First, the repair should cover the whole length of the previous incision. Second, approximation of the musculofascial layers should be done with minimal tension; third, prosthetic mesh should be used to reduce the risk of recurrence. Mesh may be contraindicated in a contaminated field, e.g. in the event of perforation of strangulated bowel, but mesh may still be used in a clean-contaminated field, such as after an elective bowel resection, if strict hygiene measures are observed and appropriate prophylactic antibiotics are given.

Open repair

The previous incision is opened along its full length to reveal any clinically unsuspected defects. The hernial sac, its neck and the margins of the defect are fully exposed. The sac can be opened, contents reduced, local adhesions divided and any redundant sac excised to allow safe fascial closure.

Simple suture techniques without the use of prosthetic mesh for reinforcement, even with the overlapping repair of Mayo or the layered closure of da Silva, are not recommended because of the unacceptable risk of recurrence. However, they may be the only option in the presence of gross contamination, where mesh is contraindicated. Mesh should ideally be used in a tension-free manner to augment primary fascial closure and not used to 'bridge' a gap between fascial edges as the unsupported mesh centrally will inevitably bulge outwards postoperatively, giving the appearance of recurrence. However, if the mesh-to-defect area ratio is sufficiently large, i.e. there is sufficient circumferential overlap of mesh in relation to the size of the defect, then a bridging repair is generally secure. Mesh can be placed in one of several planes, as for primary ventral hernia repair. The simplest approach is an onlay mesh but this carries the risk of mesh exposure and contamination in the event of wound infection or wound breakdown. Furthermore, placement of a large onlay mesh requires elevation of large skin flaps, which increases the risk of wound seroma and overlying skin ischaemia. Intraperitoneal mesh placement is difficult at open surgery and mesh in direct contact with the intra-abdominal organs is prone to complications such as adhesive bowel obstruction, erosion into adjacent organs and bowel fistulation. The retromuscular plane is preferred by many surgeons.

Laparoscopic repair

Great advances have been made in applying laparoscopic techniques to incisional hernia repair. Laparoscopy and division of adhesions is initially performed, hernia contents are reduced and the fibrous margins of the hernia defect(s) are exposed. Often the falciform ligament and median umbilical fold need

---

Alcino Lazaro da Silva, contemporary, surgeon, Vitoria, Brazil.

to be taken down. Some surgeons prefer to close the fascial defect(s) with sutures before reinforcing with mesh, while others simply 'bridge' the defect with no attempt at closure. Larger defects are more difficult to close, but bridging large defects is associated with bulging of the mesh postoperatively, often referred to as 'pseudo-recurrence' (***Figure 64.27***). Only small hernias can be safely fixed without closing the defect, as the large mesh to defect area ratio will help to minimise mesh bulging and recurrence.

The mesh is placed directly onto the peritoneum deep to the abdominal wall muscles, fixed in place with tissue glue, sutures or staple/tacks and is known as an IPOM repair. Special meshes with anti-adhesion coatings must be used, so-called 'tissue separating' meshes, and these are generally expensive.

In the presence of dense peritoneal adhesions, the laparoscopic surgeon needs to take great care because injury to the bowel is possible and may not be recognised. If occult bowel injury does occur it can lead to postoperative peritonitis.

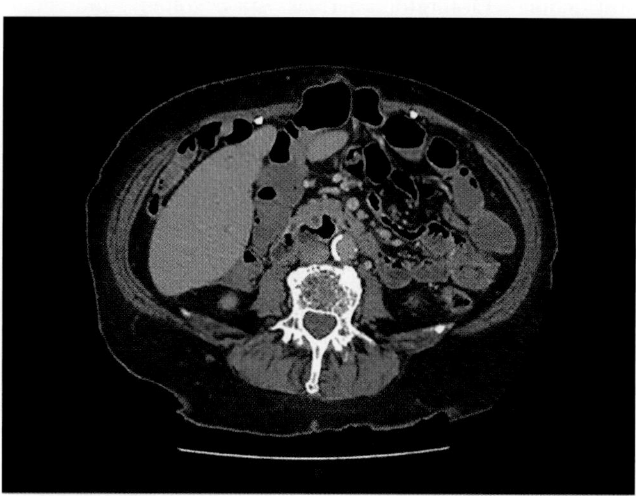

Figure 64.27 Abdominal computed tomography scan showing mesh bulge (pseudo-recurrence) 2 years after a laparoscopic repair of incisional hernia. The two white dots are metal tacks still in place, fixing the mesh to the underside of the abdominal wall.

Parastomal hernia

When surgeons create a stoma, such as a colostomy or ileostomy, they are effectively creating a hernia by bringing bowel out through the abdominal wall. The muscle defect created tends to increase in size over time and can ultimately lead to massive herniation around the stoma. The rate of parastomal hernia is over 50%. For patients, it is very difficult to manage a stoma that is lying adjacent to or atop a large hernia. The stoma may intermittently obstruct and appliance bags fit poorly leading to leakage.

The ideal surgical solution for the patient is to rejoin the bowel and remove the stoma altogether, but this is not always possible. The stoma may be re-sited but parastomal hernia will occur at the same rate at the new location, so it is no longer recommended. Numerous techniques have been described to repair parastomal hernia but failure rates remain high. Mesh repairs are associated with a lower recurrence rate but also with occasional bowel erosion and infection. Meshes are best placed in the retromuscular space but intraperitoneal mesh placement is also popular (Sugarbaker). Laparoscopic repair is also possible, using a modified Sugarbaker technique or by using a large mesh with a central hole ('keyhole' technique).

Recent reports have described the use of prophylactic mesh insertion at the time of formation of the stoma. A large-pore polypropylene mesh is inserted in the retromuscular space so that the bowel passes through a hole in the centre of the mesh. Using this technique, parastomal hernia rates may be reduced significantly.

Rare external hernias

Perineal hernia

Primary perineal hernias are very rare. The majority of perineal hernias encountered are some form of incisional hernia arising after previous pelvic floor surgery or trauma. This type of hernia includes:

- postoperative hernia through a perineal scar, typically after excision of the rectum;
- median sliding perineal hernia, which is a complete prolapse of the rectum;
- anterolateral perineal hernia, which occurs in women and presents as a swelling of the labium majus;
- posterolateral perineal hernia, which passes through the levator ani to enter the ischiorectal fossa.

A combined abdominoperineal operation is generally employed. The hernia is exposed by an incision directly over it. The sac is opened and its contents are reduced. The sac is cleared from surrounding structures and the wound closed. With the patient in semi-Trendelenburg position, either laparoscopically or at open surgery, the abdomen is opened and the mouth of the sac exposed. The sac is inverted, ligated and excised, and the pelvic floor repaired by muscle apposition and, if indicated, buttressing of the repair with prosthetic mesh or tissue flap with the involvement of plastic surgeons.

Obturator hernia

Obturator hernia, which passes through the obturator canal, occurs six times more frequently in women than in men. Most patients are older than 60 years. Any swelling is liable to be overlooked because it is covered by pectineus. It seldom causes a palpable lump but, if the limb is flexed, abducted and rotated outwards, the hernia sometimes becomes apparent. The leg is usually kept in a semiflexed position and movement increases the pain. In more than 50% of cases of strangulated obturator hernia, pain is referred along the obturator nerve by its geniculate branch to the knee. On vaginal or rectal examination the hernia can sometimes be felt as a tender swelling in the region of the obturator foramen.

These hernias are most frequently diagnosed on a CT scan, usually requested to investigate pelvic pain or bowel

Paul H Sugarbaker, contemporary, surgeon, Washington Cancer Institute, Washington, DC, USA.

obstruction. Obturator hernias have often undergone strangulation, frequently of the Richter type, by the time of presentation. Occasionally, asymptomatic obturator hernia defects are noted at laparoscopy on the lateral pelvic wall, under the pubic arch.

Surgery is indicated. The diagnosis is rarely made preoperatively and so it is often approached through a laparotomy incision. The full Trendelenburg position is adopted. The constricting agent is the obturator fascia, which can be stretched by inserting the operator's index finger, or suitable forceps, through the gap in the fascia. The content is reduced. If incision of the fascia is required, it is made parallel to the obturator vessels and nerve. The contents of the sac are dealt with in a standard manner. The defect cannot simply be closed because one margin is bone and the obturator nerve and vessels run through it. It is best repaired using a flat mesh laid over the defect in the extraperitoneal plane. In the absence of mesh or in an infected field, the broad ligament can be sutured over the defect or used as a plug.

Laparoscopic TAPP repair may also be performed again using a mesh. As with other extraperitoneal mesh repairs, mesh fixation is often not required. Alternatively, to avoid nerve injury, tissue glue can be used to fix a mesh over the defect. Note that it can be very difficult to reduce an incarcerated hernia laparoscopically and it is easy to damage the bowel with traction.

Gluteal and sciatic hernias

Both of these hernias are very rare. A gluteal hernia passes through the greater sciatic foramen, either above or below piriformis. A sciatic hernia passes through the lesser sciatic foramen. Differential diagnosis must be made between these conditions and:

- a lipoma or other soft-tissue tumour beneath gluteus maximus;
- a tuberculous abscess;
- a gluteal aneurysm.

All doubtful swellings in this situation can be characterised with CT scanning but, if in doubt, they should be explored by operation. After reduction of the hernia contents, complete closure of the defect may not be possible because of the unyielding bony and ligamentous margins of the hernia orifices. Bridging mesh may be useful but should not be placed directly on top of major nerves or vessels in the vicinity for fear of causing local irritation and neuralgic pain.

UMBILICAL CONDITIONS IN THE ADULT

Chronic infection in the umbilical area is common, particularly in patients with poor hygiene due to a plug of keratin causing chronic irritation. It is often encountered during elective surgery and may complicate the insertion of a laparoscope port at the umbilicus. Occasionally, a rapid-onset, superficial cellulitis occurs even after minor surgery in this region. It is normally due to a streptococcal infection and is treated with appropriate antibiotics. Pre-existing infection should be treated before surgery where possible.

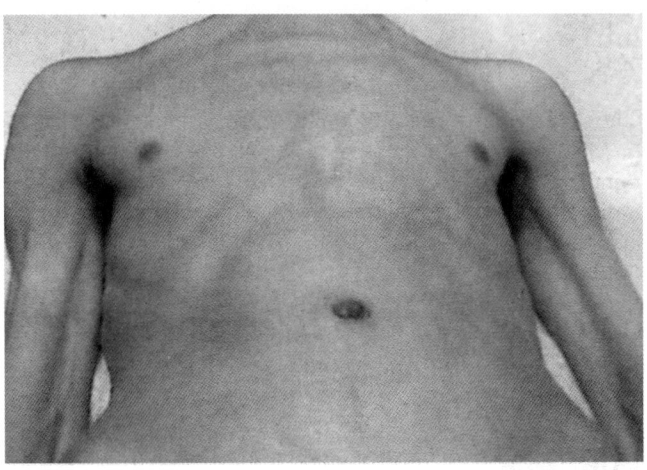

Figure 64.28 Secondary nodule at the umbilicus: Sister Joseph's nodule.

A chronic sinus may arise following umbilical hernia repair owing to infection of a mesh or non-absorbable suture material used. Antibiotics may help but usually the mesh or suture will need to be removed with a risk of recurrence of the hernia.

In utero the umbilicus is connected to the gut by the vitellointestinal duct. In most patients the duct becomes totally obliterated. The bowel end of the duct may persist as Meckel's diverticulum. More rarely, the umbilical end persists, leading to chronic faeculent discharge. Rarely endometriosis can present with cyclical bleeding from the umbilicus.

The urachus is a connection between the urinary bladder and umbilicus. It usually involutes but may present in later life as a result of increased pressure in the bladder usually due to prostatic hypertrophy. The cause of obstruction should be dealt with initially, but if the problem persists then surgical excision of the patent urachus might be considered.

If tumour presents at the umbilicus it is most probably due to spread from the internal organs along internal ligaments, e.g. from the liver along the falciform ligament. A malignant mass at the umbilicus is called a Sister Joseph's nodule. It usually indicates very advanced malignant disease and surgery probably has little to offer (***Figure 64.28***). Malignancy at the umbilicus is rare; however, primary squamous carcinoma may occur and malignancy may develop in a urachal remnant. Local excision is required.

Friedrich Trendelenburg, 1844–1924, Professor of Surgery, successively at Rostock (1875–1882), Bonn (1882–1895) and Leipzig (1895–1911), Germany. The Trendelenburg position was first described in 1885.

Johann Frederick Meckel (the younger), 1781–1833, Professor of Anatomy and Surgery, Halle, Germany, described his diverticulum in 1809 although **Alexis Littre**, 1658–1726, surgeon and lecturer in anatomy, Paris, France, described Meckel's diverticulum in a hernial sac in 1700, 81 years before Meckel was born.

Sister Mary Joseph (nee Julia Dempsey), Nursing Superintendent, St Mary's Hospital, Rochester, MN, USA, observed that patients with terminal cancer sometimes developed a red papular lesion in the umbilicus. She and William Mayo published this observation in 1928; however, it was Hamilton Bailey who coined the term '**Sister Mary Joseph's nodule**' in 1949.

GENERAL INFECTION OF THE ABDOMINAL WALL

The skin of the abdominal wall, similar to all skin, is prone to develop superficial infection that may be spontaneous, due to minor trauma or infection of skin lesions such as an epidermoid cyst. Although antibiotics will suffice in most patients, if an abscess develops then surgical drainage may be required.

The close proximity of bowel and bowel organisms opens the abdominal wall to attack from a wide range of highly virulent bacteria. Most commonly, these are released during abdominal surgery such as appendicectomy and hence the need for appropriate antibiotic prophylactic cover.

Synergistic gangrene

This rare condition is due to the synergistic action of non-haemolytic streptococci and staphylococci causing rapid tissue necrosis and overwhelming systemic infection (***Figure 64.29***). It requires immediate administration of high-dose, broad-spectrum antibiotics in combination with early debridement of any non-viable tissue. Hyperbaric oxygen therapy has been advocated.

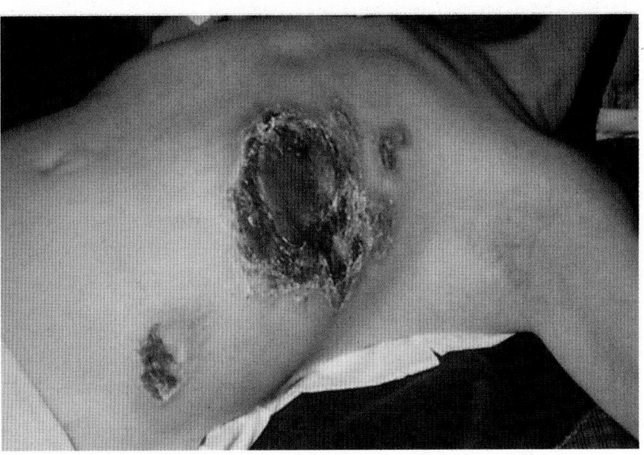

Figure 64.29 Bacterial synergistic gangrene of the chest and abdominal wall. The area has become gangrenous and looks like suede leather.

Other forms of severe abdominal wall infections occur, generally known as necrotising fasciitis (also known as Fournier's gangrene). All of these conditions have a high associated morbidity and mortality. They occur more frequently in diabetic, debilitated or immunocompromised patients but can occasionally occur in healthy patients. The necrosis spreads rapidly through the subcutaneous layers of the abdominal wall and may extend into the chest, axilla, thigh and perineum. Necrotising fasciitis is characterised by systemic features of septic shock, a high temperature, a foul smell and occasionally crepitus in the skin, indicating gas-producing bacteria. Prompt diagnosis and aggressive surgical debridement within hours of onset are the keys to success, with repeated debridements under anaesthesia over several days until all of the necrotic and infected tissues have been cleared. If the patient survives, extensive skin grafting is usually required.

Patients with lymphatic oedema of the abdominal wall may present with redness and tenderness, suspicious for necrotising fasciitis. This important diagnosis needs to be excluded, but cellulitis secondary to lymphatic stasis is more likely to be the cause.

Cutaneous fistula

Because of the thickness of the abdominal wall, it is rare for abdominal inflammatory conditions to discharge spontaneously through the wall to the skin. Chronic intraperitoneal abscesses arising after occult bowel perforation, appendicitis, diverticulitis and cholecystitis are the most likely sources. CT will locate the internal abscess and suggest the likely origin. Treatment is usually by CT- or ultrasonography-guided drainage but the surgeon may be called on to remove the source organ (source control). Malignancy in its later stages can occasionally erode through the abdominal wall. Crohn's disease also has a tendency to fistulate into adjacent organs and may develop an enterocutaneous fistula.

Abdominal compartment syndrome

Surgeons are increasingly aware of the harmful effect of high intra-abdominal pressures that can occur in severe intra-abdominal sepsis, such as pancreatitis and also following aortic aneurysm rupture. High pressure leads to reduced blood flow and tissue ischaemia, which contributes to multiorgan failure. Although the abdominal wall has elasticity, if intra-abdominal volume increases as a result of fluid, gas, pus, tissue oedema, etc., the maximal capacity may be reached and pressure rises to a critical level. Intra-abdominal pressure >20 mmHg, as measured via a catheter in the urinary bladder, is diagnostic and requires intervention to avoid organ failure.

Occasionally, such as after surgery for severe intraperitoneal sepsis, there is so much retroperitoneal swelling and/or oedema of the bowel that the surgeon cannot close the abdomen. In such cases it is often wise to leave the incision open, cover the abdominal contents with mesh or a saline-soaked dressing and plan to return at a future date to close the defect. This is called a laparostomy. Vacuum-assisted dressings assist in managing the large amounts of wound exudate. The patient may require repeated trips to the operating theatre, gaining a little more fascial apposition each time, before the wound can be finally closed.

Neoplasms of the abdominal wall

As the abdominal wall is composed of muscle, fascia and bone, benign and malignant tumours can arise from each, although these are rare.

Jean Alfred Fournier, 1832–1915, French syphilologist and founder of the Venereal and Dermatological Clinic, Hôpital St Louis, Paris, France.
Burrill Bernard Crohn, 1884–1983, gastroenterologist, Mount Sinai Hospital, New York, NY, USA, along with Leon Ginzburg and Gordon Oppenheimer described regional ileitis in 1932.

Desmoid tumour

This is usually considered by pathologists to be a hamartoma and is more common in women. Some, however, believe it to be a fibroma and possibly the result of repeated trauma. Desmoids also occur in familial adenomatous polyposis. Histologically, they contain plasmodial cell masses resembling giant cells. They undergo central myxomatous change. Surgical excision with a wide margin is required to prevent local recurrence, which is a frequent problem.

ACKNOWLEDGEMENT

The authors are grateful to Andrew C de Beaux MBChB MD FRCS FEBS AWS, Consultant General and Upper GI Surgeon, Royal Infirmary of Edinburgh, Edinburgh, UK, for his input to this chapter.

FURTHER READING

Henriksen NA, Montgomery A, Kaufmann R *et al.* Guidelines for treatment of umbilical and epigastric hernias from the European Hernia Society and Americas Hernia Society. *Br J Surg* 2020; **107**: 171–90.

Miserez M, Alexandre JH, Campanelli G *et al.* The European Hernia Society groin hernia classification. *Hernia* 2007; **11**: 113–16.

Muysoms FE, Miserez M, Berrevoet F *et al.* Classification of primary and incisional abdominal wall hernias. *Hernia* 2009; **13**: 407–14.

Muysoms FE, Antoniou SA, Bury K *et al.* European Hernia Society guidelines on the closure of abdominal wall incisions. *Hernia* 2015; **19**: 1–24.

The HerniaSurge Group. International guidelines for groin hernia management. *Hernia* 2018; **22**: 1–165.

CHAPTER 65 The peritoneum, mesentery, greater omentum and retroperitoneal space

Learning objectives

To understand:

- The development and anatomy of the mesentery and peritoneum
- Surgical conditions of the peritoneum, mesentery, greater omentum and retroperitoneal space

DEVELOPMENT OF THE MESENTERY AND PERITONEUM

Early in development, the human abdomen comprises a wall and enclosed space (coelom). A partition (mesentery) subdivides the cavity into left- and right-sided spaces (***Figure 65.1***). The mesentery comprises a cell body (mesodermal mesentery) lined on either side by a sheet of mesothelial cells (***Figure 65.2***). At first the cell body is continuous with the posterior abdominal wall, and the mesothelial covering of the mesentery is continuous with that lining the inner surface of the posterior abdominal wall. Soon after this arrangement has developed, the cell body of the mesentery separates from the posterior abdominal wall but remains in contact with it (*65.1*). The surface mesothelium of the mesentery remains in continuity with that of the posterior abdominal wall (***Figure 65.2***).

The mesentery remains continuous throughout development, following birth and into adult life (*65.2*). Early during development, the mid-region of the mesentery forms a fold that subdivides the mesentery into upper (pre-fold), mid- (fold) and lower (post-fold) regions (***Figure 65.1***). The upper region develops as a sack overlapping the mid-region. As it develops, the spleen, stomach and liver emerge.

The mid-region fold has left and right sides (on either side of the midline). The mid-region nearest the posterior abdominal wall is termed the central zone (***Figure 65.1***). The remainder of the fold is termed the peripheral zone. Soon after the mid-region fold first emerges, the sides of the periphery (but not of the central zone) switch position relative to the superior mesenteric artery (SMA). After the switch, the original right side of the mid-region commences on the right side centrally but continues peripherally on the left of the SMA. The original left side commences peripherally on the right side of the vessel then returns centrally on the left of the SMA (***Figure 65.1***). Failure of switch formation occurs in malrotation (see ***Rotational disorders***).

During development of the upper region of the mesentery, the region of the mesodermal mesentery that is nearest the posterior abdominal wall adheres to the wall (*65.1*). This process progresses from the midline laterally to the left. Adhesion of both displaces the mesothelial junction between the mesentery and the adjacent posterior abdominal wall (***Figure 65.2***). At completion of development the posterior wall of the upper region (the dorsal mesogastrium) is fully adherent to the abdominal wall of the left upper quadrant (LUQ). The spleen is located at the lateral part of the upper region sac, in the LUQ. The original mesothelial junction remains as the peritoneal reflection linking the surface lining the mesenteric domain (in this case the spleen) with the surface lining of the adjacent non-mesenteric domain (in this case the LUQ).

During development of the mid-region fold, the region of the mesodermal mesentery that is nearest the posterior abdominal wall (i.e. the central zone) progressively adheres to the posterior abdominal wall. With continued adhesion, the periphery of the mid-region fold also adheres (*65.2 and 65.3*). Adhesion occurs inferolaterally to the right, and from the central to peripheral zones. The mesothelial junction between the mid-region mesentery and abdominal wall is displaced in tandem, inferolaterally to the right. At completion of development the mid-region fold is adherent to the posterior abdominal wall at the right mesocolon. The original mesothelial junction is at the periphery of the fold and persists as a peritoneal reflection bridging the surface lining of the mesenteric and non-mesenteric domains (***Figure 65.2***) (*65.3*). Incomplete adhesion of the mid-region fold is associated with increased mobility of the ileocaecal region and volvulus (see ***Volvulus of the intestine and adjoining mesentery***).

During development of the lower region of the mesentery, the part nearest the posterior abdominal wall progressively adheres to the wall (*65.1*). This proceeds from the midline laterally to the left. The overlying mesothelial junction is displaced in tandem (***Figure 65.2***). At completion of development, the lower region has fully adhered at the left mesocolon, medial mesosigmoidal and mesorectal levels. The lateral part of the mesosigmoid remains mobile. The mesothelial junction remains as a peritoneal reflection bridging the surface lining of the mesenteric and adjacent non-mesenteric domain

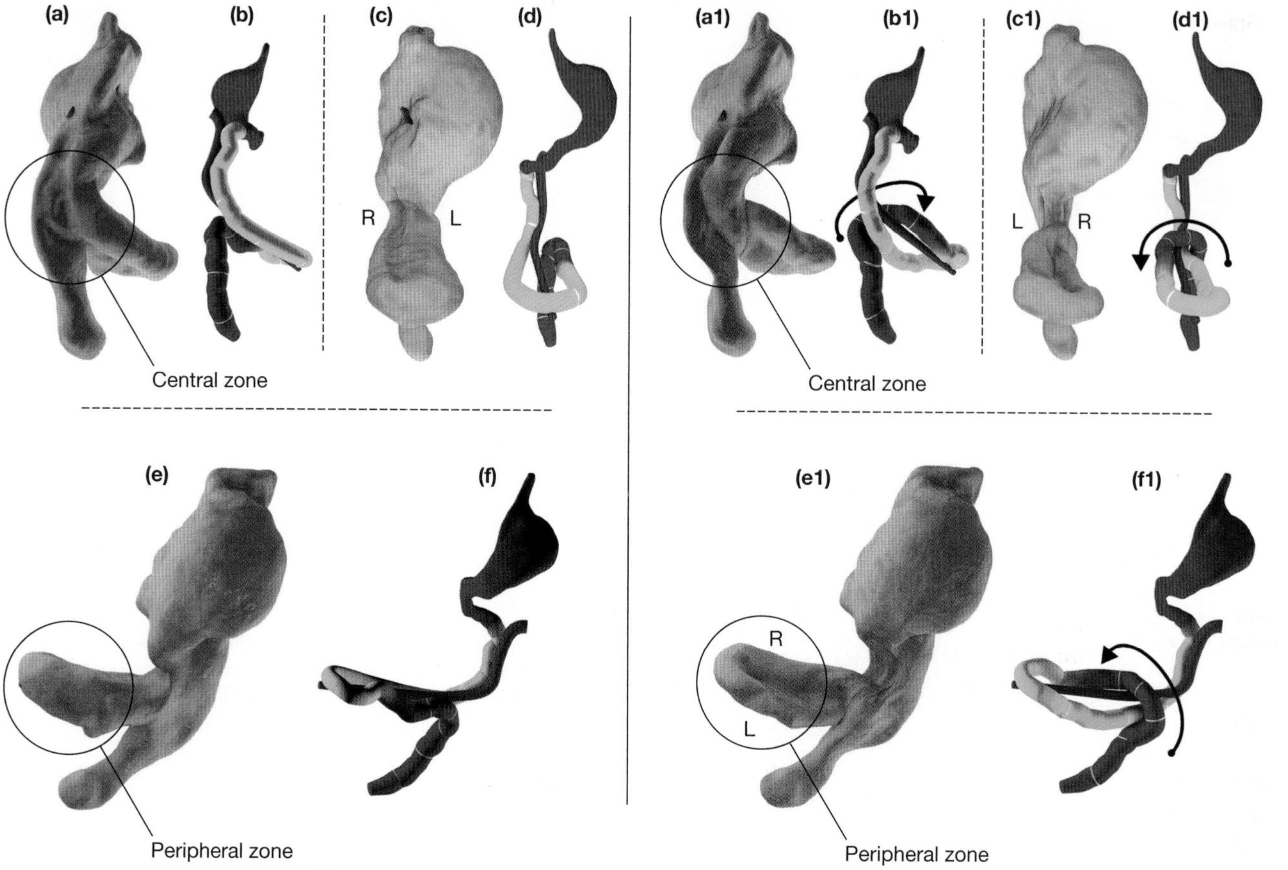

Figure 65.1 Switching of the mid-region of the mesentery during development. (a–f) Digital reconstructions of the developing mesentery prior to switching of the sides of the mid-region fold. (a, c, e) Three-dimensional reconstructions of the mesentery before switching. The intestine develops within the mesentery. (b, d, f) Three-dimensional reconstructions of the intestine. The mesentery has been removed to expose the developing intestine. (a1, c1, e1) Digital reconstructions of the developing mesentery after switching of the sides of the mid-region fold. The mesentery is coloured yellow. (b1, d1, f1) Three-dimensional reconstructions of the intestine after the mid-region switch. The mesentery has been removed to expose the developing intestine. Yellow, the mesentery; red, upper region of intestine; green, developing mid-region; blue, lower region of the intestine. The superior mesenteric artery (blind-ending red tube) has been included for reference.

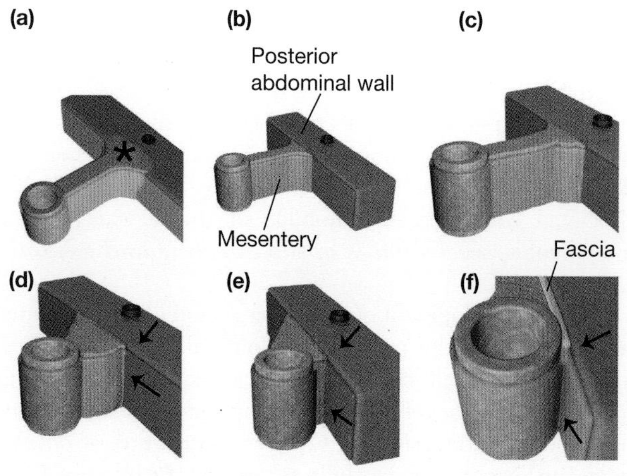

Figure 65.2 (a-f) Adhesion and displacement. Development of the junction between the mesentery (*) and the posterior abdominal wall. The peritoneal reflection (thick arrows) is displaced towards the periphery during adhesion of the mesentery to the abdominal wall.

(*65.3*). Incomplete adhesion (and hence anchorage) of the lower region is associated with sigmoid volvulus (see ***Volvulus of the intestine and adjoining mesentery***).

ANATOMY OF THE MESENTERY AND PERITONEUM

All abdominal digestive organs develop *in* or *on* the mesentery and then remain directly connected to it (***Figure 65.3***). In the adult setting, these collectively comprise a discrete anatomical unit, the mesenteric domain (***Figure 65.4***). All genitourinary organs develop on and remain on the musculoskeletal mainframe of the abdomen. In the adult, these are collectively termed the non-mesenteric domain. Thus, the adult abdomen comprises two discrete anatomical compartments: the mesenteric and non-mesenteric domains (***Figure 65.5***) (*65.2*).

When development is complete, the mesentery and conjoined digestive organs (intestine, pancreas, spleen and liver) have taken shape and adherence to the posterior abdominal wall is nearly complete. The dorsal mesogastrium, mesoduodenum, right and left mesocolon and mesorectum are

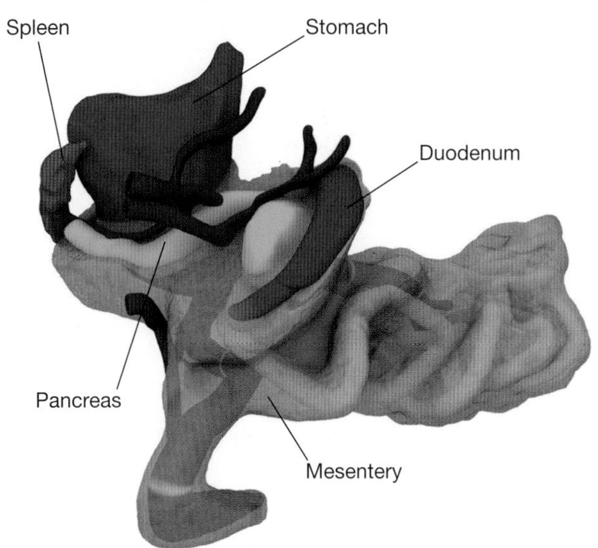

Figure 65.3 The right lateral aspect of the mesentery during development. The mesentery has been sectioned to expose the developing stomach (red), pancreas (light blue) and major blood vessels.

anchored to the subjacent abdominal wall (or pelvic sidewall) (*Figure 65.4*). The small intestinal region of mesentery, transverse mesocolon and lateral mesosigmoidal mesentery are not adherent and thus are mobile.

Adhesion of the mesentery to the abdominal wall anchors the mesenteric to the non-mesenteric domain, maintained by peritoneal reflection at the periphery of the mesenteric domain (*65.1 and 65.3*). At the periphery, the peritoneal reflection bridges the surface lining of the mesenteric and non-mesenteric domains (*Figure 65.6*). The peritoneum thus comprises visceral peritoneum (corresponding to the surface lining of the mesenteric domain), parietal peritoneum (corresponding to the surface lining of the non-mesenteric domain) and the reflection joining both. Peritonitis refers to inflammation of any region (see ***Peritonitis***).

The surface contours generated by the organisation of the domains and the peritoneum explains the sacs, recesses, fossae and pouches in which abnormal fluid collections arise in the abdomen (*65.3*). On completion of development, the free (non-adherent) surface of each organ of the mesenteric domain is peritonealised. The opposing adherent surface is not peritonealised.

In the male, the peritoneal cavity is normally closed. In the female, the peritoneal cavity is open to the environment at the fimbrial entrance to the fallopian tubes. In both sexes (but more frequently in the male) a peritoneal tube (processus vaginalis) can persist at the deep inguinal ring and predispose to inguinal hernia formation.

The interface between adherent regions of the mesenteric and non-mesenteric domains is termed the retroperitoneal space (*65.4*). The retroperitoneal space normally contains connective tissue fascia. The space (and fascia) continues into the thorax superiorly and into the pelvis inferiorly. The retroperitoneum is deep to the retroperitoneal space. It includes the kidneys, ureters, gonadal vessels, lumbosacral plexus and the musculoskeletal frame of the posterior abdominal wall.

The arterial inflow to the mesenteric domain is limited to the coeliac trunk and superior and inferior mesenteric arteries. The venous drainage of the mesenteric domain occurs via the hepatic veins at the junction of these and the inferior vena cava. In between the arterial inflow and venous drainage, the vasculature of the abdominal digestive organs is entirely intramesenteric and aligned with the mesenteric regional anatomy (*65.5*). The limited routes of arterial inflow and venous drainage have significant implications when these are affected by pathology (discussed in ***Vascular abnormalities of the mesentery***).

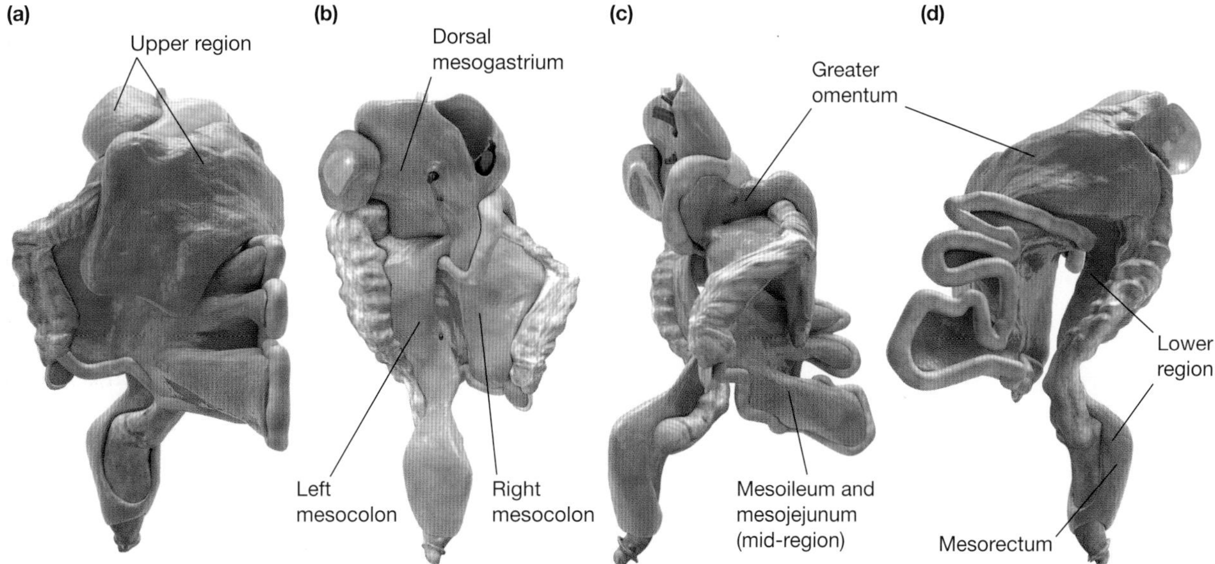

Figure 65.4 The mesentery. (a–d) The adult mesentery (and mesenteric domain) as seen from anterior (a), posterior (b), right posterolateral (c) and left anterolateral (d) perspectives.

(a)

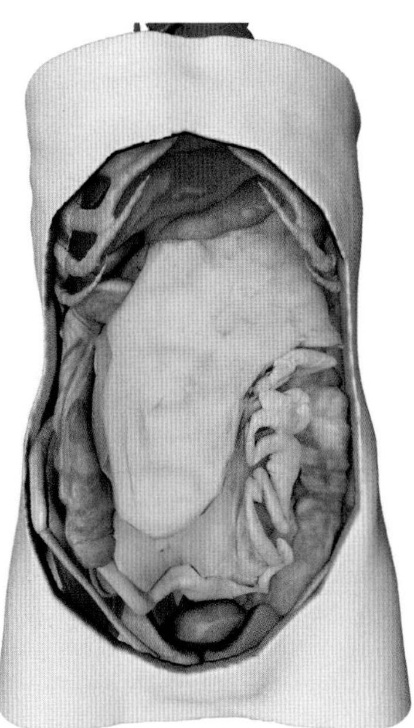

(b)

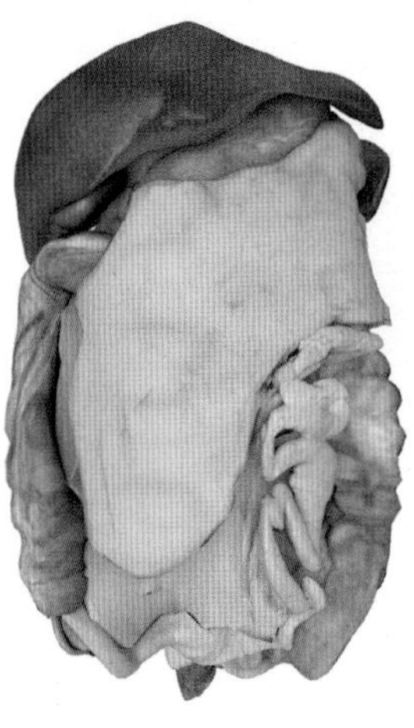

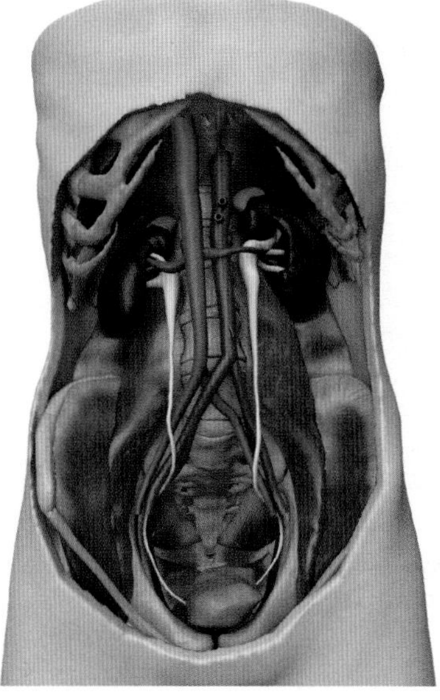

Figure 65.5 The mesenteric and non-mesenteric domains of the abdomen. (a) Intact abdomen. (b) Mesenteric domain (top) and non-mesenteric domain (bottom).

A knowledge of the anatomical relationships between the mesenteric and non-mesenteric domains provides the student of abdominal surgery with a roadmap by which to perform safe and optimal abdominal surgery. The above description is termed the mesenteric model of abdominal anatomy. It is a model that matches observations during development with clinical observations *in vivo* and with radiological depictions of the abdomen. It provides the anatomical context on which surgical diseases of the abdomen and pelvis arise. Given this, it is rapidly substituting the peritoneal model in reference anatomical texts.

THE PERITONEUM

The peritoneal cavity is the largest cavity in the body, the surface area of its lining membrane (2 m^2 in an adult) being nearly equal to that of the skin (*65.3*). The peritoneal membrane is composed of flattened polyhedral cells (mesothelium), one layer thick, resting on a thin layer of fibroelastic tissue. Beneath the peritoneum, supported by a small amount of areolar tissue, lies a network of lymphatic vessels and a rich plexus of capillary blood vessels from which all absorption and exudation must occur. In health, only a few millilitres of peritoneal fluid are found in the peritoneal cavity. The fluid is pale yellow, somewhat viscid and contains lymphocytes and other leukocytes; it lubricates the viscera, allowing easy movement and peristalsis. The parietal portion is richly innervated and, when irritated, causes severe pain that is accurately localised to the affected area. The visceral peritoneum, in contrast, is poorly innervated and irritation causes pain that is usually poorly localised to the midline.

Summary box 65.1

Functions of the peritoneum

In health

- Visceral lubrication
- Fluid and particulate absorption

In disease

- Pain perception (mainly parietal)
- Inflammatory and immune responses
- Fibrinolytic activity

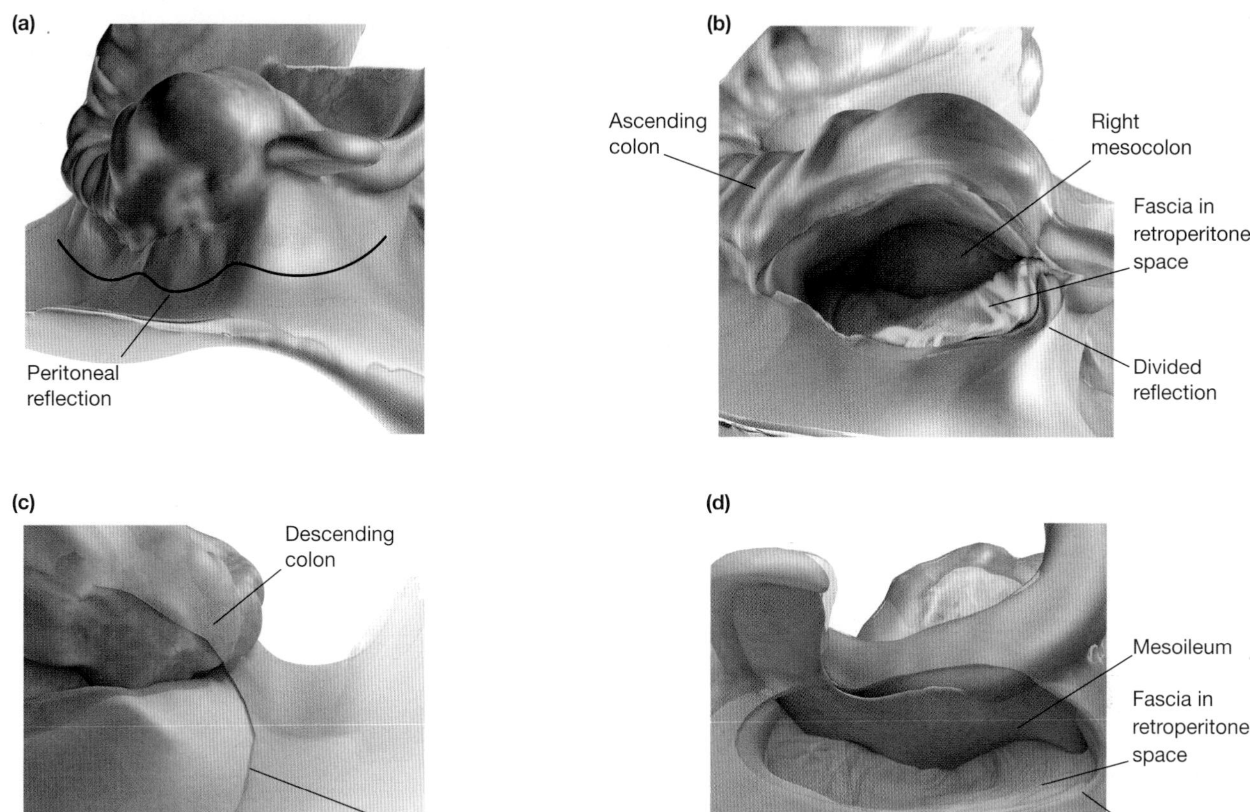

Figure 65.6 The reflection at the periphery of the mesenteric domain, i.e. the junction between the mesenteric and non-mesenteric domains. (Reproduced with permission from Coffey JC, Lavery I, Sehgal R (eds). *Mesenteric principles of gastrointestinal surgery: basic and applied principles*. Boca Raton: CRC Press, 2017.)

The peritoneum has the capacity to absorb large volumes of fluid; however, the peritoneum can also produce large volumes of fluid (ascites) and an inflammatory exudate when injured (seen in peritonitis). During expiration, intra-abdominal pressure is reduced and peritoneal fluid, aided by capillary attraction, travels in an upward direction towards the diaphragm. Particulate matter and bacteria are absorbed within a few minutes into the lymphatic network through a number of 'pores' in the diaphragmatic peritoneum. The circulation of peritoneal fluids may be responsible for the occurrence of abscesses anatomically remote from primary disease. The two sites most prone to collection are the pelvis and subdiaphragmatic areas, reflecting the effects of gravity while standing and lying, respectively.

PERITONITIS

Peritonitis is inflammation of the peritoneum and can be categorised as localised or diffuse, acute or chronic or according to the primary underlying pathology. In the clinical setting, the most useful categorisation of peritonitis is based on whether it is localised or diffuse.

Summary box 65.2

Causes of peritoneal inflammation

- Bacterial, gastrointestinal and non-gastrointestinal
- Chemical, e.g. bile, barium
- Allergic, e.g. starch peritonitis
- Traumatic, e.g. operative handling
- Ischaemia, e.g. strangulated bowel, vascular occlusion
- Miscellaneous, e.g. familial Mediterranean fever

Summary box 65.3

Paths to peritoneal infection

- Gastrointestinal perforation, e.g. perforated ulcer, appendix, diverticulum
- Transmural translocation (no perforation), e.g. pancreatitis, ischaemic bowel, primary bacterial peritonitis
- Exogenous contamination, e.g. drains, open surgery, trauma, peritoneal dialysis
- Female genital tract infection, e.g. pelvic inflammatory disease
- Haematogenous spread (rare), e.g. septicaemia

Localised peritonitis

This is where a localised area of the peritoneum has become inflamed. If the parietal peritoneum is involved, the patient complains of pain (somatic pain) in the area affected. Vital signs may be normal, but tachycardia and pyrexia are common. The characteristic signs are involuntary guarding (reflex abdominal wall contraction to reduce further peritoneal irritation) and rebound tenderness (worsening of pain on lifting the examining hand off the abdominal wall). Collectively these signs and symptoms are termed *peritonism* and the patient is described as *peritonitic* (see ***Chapter 63***).

If inflammation arises under the diaphragm, shoulder tip ('phrenic') pain may be felt. This is referred pain to the C5 dermatome. In cases of pelvic peritonitis, e.g. from an inflamed appendix or salpingitis, abdominal signs may be limited; deep-seated tenderness may be detected by digital rectal or vaginal examination. Signs may be limited in obese patients or in patients on immunosuppressive medications.

The aim is to diagnose the underlying cause and guide treatment. Diagnosis of the underlying condition is made through a combination of history and physical examination, supplemented by laboratory and radiological investigations. Laboratory biomarkers will support a diagnosis of acute inflammation, but are rarely diagnostically specific. The investigation of choice is computed tomography (CT) scanning. Modalities such as ultrasound can be used but lack specificity except in the case of tubo-ovarian pathology (see ***Chapter 87***). Laparoscopy may be required if the above investigations are inconclusive.

The aims of treatment are to remove the underlying cause and to lavage or dilute residual contamination. At surgery the inflamed peritoneum appears reddened, thickened and has a velvety texture. Plaques of yellow/white fibrin may be apparent, causing loops of intestine (and mesentery) to adhere to themselves and to the parietes. There is a reactionary, serous exudate (rich in leukocytes and plasma proteins) that gradually becomes turbid in appearance. The fluid may transform to frank pus if not evacuated.

Diffuse (generalised) peritonitis

This normally signifies the occurrence of a life-threatening pathology. It means that regions (not just focal areas) of the parietes (parietal peritoneum) are inflamed. It normally arises as a result of pressure-related perforation of a viscus (e.g. in the setting of an obstructed colon), when large volumes of blood abruptly enter the peritoneal cavity (ruptured aortic aneurysm) or when substantial volumes pour incessantly (albeit not under pressure) into the peritoneal cavity (e.g. perforated duodenal ulcer or anastomotic leak).

The patient may describe acute or gradual onset abdominal pain of considerable intensity. The pain may be localised at first and then become diffuse. The patient is gravely ill looking (Hippocratic facies) and usually lies as still as possible to minimise fluid movement within the peritoneal cavity. The entirety of the abdominal musculature undergoes a reflex contraction and feels board-like on palpation ('board-like' rigidity). In a thin patient, contraction of the rectus abdominis muscles may be reflected in a scaphoid appearance of the abdomen (see ***Chapter 63***). A generalised ileus occurs and the abdomen may become distended.

Vital signs are usually deranged. In advanced cases the patient is hypotensive, tachycardic and pyrexial. At first the patient may seem confused, drowsy and disoriented. If the underlying pathology is not corrected the patient will lose consciousness. Signs may be limited in obese patients or in patients on immunosuppressive medications.

Investigation and treatment must be undertaken expediently as the time available to salvage may be limited. Investigations aim to identify the underlying cause and to guide treatment. An erect chest radiograph can be useful in identifying subdiaphragmatic gas (***Figure 65.7***). If a patient is particularly unwell and a CT is not available, then a lateral decubitus radiograph serves the same purpose as an erect radiograph (provided the patient has been appropriately positioned for long enough for the gas to rise within the peritoneal cavity).

Summary box 65.4

Clinical features of peritonitis

- Abdominal pain, worse on movement, coughing and deep respiration
- Constitutional upset: anorexia, malaise, fever, lassitude
- Gastrointestinal upset: nausea +/– vomiting
- Pyrexia (may be absent)
- Raised pulse rate
- Tenderness +/– guarding/rigidity/rebound of abdominal wall
- Pain/tenderness on rectal/vaginal examination (pelvic peritonitis)
- Absent or reduced bowel sounds
- 'Septic shock' (systemic inflammatory response syndrome [SIRS] and multiorgan dysfunction syndrome [MODS]) in later stages

Summary box 65.5

Management of peritonitis

General care of patient

- Correction of fluid and electrolyte imbalance
- Insertion of nasogastric drainage tube and urinary catheter
- Broad-spectrum antibiotic therapy
- Analgesia
- Vital system support

Surgical treatment of cause when appropriate

- 'Source control' by removal or exclusion of the cause
- Peritoneal lavage +/– drainage

Hippocrates of Kos, Greek physician and surgeon, and by common consent 'the father of medicine', was born on the island of Kos, off Turkey, about 460 BCE and probably died in 375 BCE.

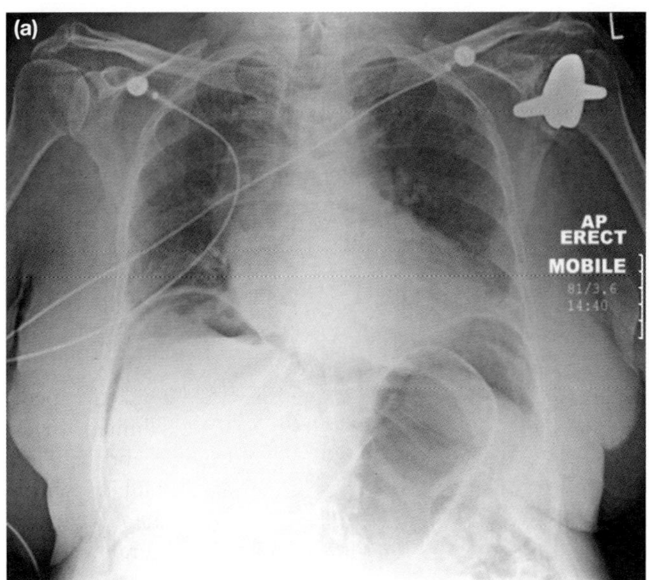

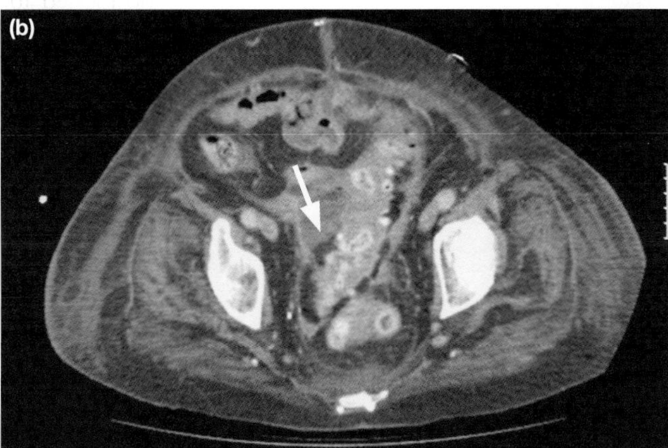

Figure 65.7 Intraperitoneal perforation. **(a)** Erect chest radiograph demonstrating air under the diaphragm on the right side. **(b)** Axial computed tomography image showing a segment of sigmoid diverticulosis with localised perforation (arrow).

Acute bacterial peritonitis

Acute bacterial peritonitis most commonly arises from perforation of a viscus of the alimentary tract. Other routes of infection can include the female genital tract and exogenous contamination. Less common forms involve a primary 'spontaneous' peritonitis due to streptococcal, pneumococcal or *Haemophilus* infection.

Non-gastrointestinal causes of acute bacterial peritonitis

Pelvic infection via the Fallopian tubes is responsible for a high proportion of 'non-gastrointestinal' infections. The most common offending organisms are *Chlamydia* spp. and gonococci. These organisms lead to a thinning of cervical mucus and allow bacteria from the vagina to pass into the uterus and oviducts, causing infection and inflammation. A variant of transperitoneal spread of such organisms is perihepatitis, which can cause scar tissue to form on Glisson's capsule, a thin layer of connective tissue surrounding the liver (Fitz-Hugh–Curtis syndrome). Fungal peritonitis is rare but may complicate severely ill patients.

Biliary peritonitis

Biliary peritonitis is mostly seen after cholecystectomy and arises from slippage of a clip off the cystic duct, drainage of bile from an accessory cystic duct or perforation of the common bile or hepatic duct (see ***Chapter 71***). It can also arise after hepatectomy or duodenal surgery, although this is unusual if a drain has been placed at the time of surgery.

Investigation follows the principles and steps described in ***Peritonitis***. The natural course of biliary peritonism varies depending on the volume of contamination. In severe contamination the patient will be extremely unwell and urgent intervention is required.

Localised collections can be treated by percutaneous insertion of a drain followed by endoscopic retrograde pancreatography (ERCP) to identify the source of bile leak. ERCP enables placement of a stent across the source of the leak. Diffuse or high-volume contamination, or the presence of multiple separate locules, normally mandates surgical exploration with the aim being lavage and drainage.

Spontaneous bacterial peritonitis

Spontaneous bacterial peritonitis (SBP; sometimes called primary bacterial peritonitis) is an acute bacterial infection of ascitic fluid. There is often a history of cirrhosis and ascites. The clinical picture is highly variable as the patient may be asymptomatic. The course can be prolonged.

The diagnosis is made by paracentesis and should be considered in cirrhotic patients and those with ascites even when there is a low index of suspicion. The diagnosis is confirmed by finding an increased neutrophil count of $250/\text{mm}^3$ in aspirated ascitic fluid. Culture of ascites is negative in as many as 60% of patients with clinical manifestations of SBP. When culture is positive the most common pathogens include Gram-negative bacteria, usually *Escherichia coli*, and Gram-positive cocci (mainly streptococci and enterococci).

Empirical treatment of SBP must be initiated immediately after diagnosis and before the results of culture have been received. Although the choice of antibiotic may vary, a third-generation cephalosporin, e.g. cefotaxime, is a reasonable first-line treatment that avoids the renal toxicity of aminoglycosides. Alternatives are amoxicillin/clavulanic acid and quinolones such as ciprofloxacin.

Francis Glisson, 1597–1677, Regius Professor of Medicine, Cambridge, UK.
Fitz-Hugh–Curtis syndrome: named after the two physicians, **Thomas Fitz-Hugh, Jr** 1894–1963, physician, University of Pennsylvania, Philadelphia, PA, USA, and **Arthur Hale Curtis** 1881–1955, gynecologist, Chicago, IL, USA, who first reported this condition in 1934 and 1930, respectively.

Primary pneumococcal peritonitis

The incidence of pneumococcal peritonitis has declined greatly and the condition is now rare. It may complicate nephrotic syndrome or cirrhosis in children; however, otherwise healthy children may also be affected. In girls, the route of infection may be via the vagina and Fallopian tubes, while a blood-borne route secondary to respiratory tract or middle-ear disease is also possible.

The clinical onset is usually sudden, with pain usually localised to the lower half of the abdomen. The temperature is raised to 39°C or more and there is usually frequent vomiting. After 24–48 hours, profuse diarrhoea is characteristic. There is usually increased frequency of micturition. The last two symptoms are caused by severe pelvic peritonitis. On examination, peritonism is usually diffuse but less prominent than in cases of a perforated viscus, leading to peritonitis.

An underlying pathology must always be excluded before primary peritonitis can be diagnosed with certainty. Causative organisms include *Haemophilus* spp., group A streptococci and a few Gram-negative bacteria. Idiopathic streptococcal and staphylococcal peritonitis can also occur in adults.

After starting antibiotic therapy and correcting dehydration and electrolyte imbalance, early surgery is required unless spontaneous infection of pre-existing ascites is strongly suspected, in which case a diagnostic peritoneal tap is useful. Laparotomy or laparoscopy may be used. Assuming that no other cause for the peritonitis is discovered, some of the exudate is aspirated and sent to the laboratory for microscopy, culture and sensitivity tests. Thorough peritoneal lavage is carried out and the incision closed. Antibiotics and fluid replacement therapy are continued and recovery is usual.

Tuberculous peritonitis

Intra-abdominal tuberculosis (TB) is common in resource-poor countries; however, the incidence is rising in resource-rich countries as a consequence of migration and immunosuppression. *Mycobacterium avium intracellulare* is becoming increasingly prevalent with the widespread increase in human immunodeficiency virus (HIV) co-infection. The abdomen is involved in approximately 11% of patients with extrapulmonary TB and includes intraperitoneal, gastrointestinal tract and solid organ disease forms. TB peritonitis requires specific mention because it is often diagnosed late, resulting in undue patient morbidity and mortality.

TB can spread to the peritoneum through the gastrointestinal tract (typically the ileocaecal region) via mesenteric lymph nodes or directly from the blood, usually from the 'miliary' (***Figure 65.8a***) but occasionally from the 'cavitating' form of pulmonary TB, lymph and the Fallopian tubes; 50–80% of patients with abdominal TB can be expected to have peritoneal involvement.

The most common form of TB peritonitis is the wet, ascitic-type disease (90%), which is characterised by generalised or loculated ascites. Multiple tubercle deposits are present on both layers of the peritoneum. In the less common form fibrotic fixed loops of bowel and omentum are matted together and may present with subacute intestinal obstruction. Ascites is not present in the dry, plastic type. Presentation is often insidious with abdominal pain, weight loss and abdominal distension. Distinction from diffuse peritoneal metastases is difficult and may require biopsy.

Diagnosis is via abdominal ultrasonography or CT to detect ascites and lymphadenopathy with/without diffuse thickening of the peritoneum, mesentery and/or omentum (***Figure 65.8b,c***). Ascitic fluid is typically a straw-coloured exudate (protein >25–30 g/L) with white cells >500/mL and lymphocytes >40%. Unfortunately, diagnostic smears for acid-fast bacilli are often not diagnostic and culture may take up to 4–8 weeks. Laparoscopy and peritoneal biopsy may thus be helpful to couple typical appearances with histology. The value of new laboratory investigations such as the Xpert® MTB/RIF assay and the interferon-gamma release assay in diagnosing extrapulmonary TB remains to be determined; however, measurement of adenosine deaminase activity in ascitic fluid has a high sensitivity and specificity in diagnosing peritoneal TB.

TB management is principally supportive (nutrition and hydration) and medical (systemic anti-TB therapy, noting that multidrug resistance may be higher for abdominal than for pulmonary TB), although surgery may be required for specific complications such as intestinal obstruction.

Summary box 65.6

Tuberculous peritonitis

- Acute (may be clinically indistinguishable from acute bacterial peritonitis) and chronic forms
- Abdominal pain, sweats, malaise and weight loss are frequent
- Ascites common, may be loculated
- Caseating peritoneal nodules are common – distinguish from metastatic carcinoma and fat necrosis of pancreatitis
- Intestinal obstruction may respond to anti-TB treatment without surgery

Familial Mediterranean fever

Familial Mediterranean fever (FMF; synonym familial paroxysmal polyserositis) is an autosomal recessive inherited autoinflammatory syndrome characterised by episodic diffuse abdominal pain and tenderness, mild pyrexia and joint pain. Symptoms are usually mild and resolve within 24–72 hours. Rarely pericardial or meningeal inflammation may occur. Amyloidosis is a long-term complication.

FMF is associated with mutations in the *MEFV* (Mediterranean fever) gene most frequently found in Arab, Armenian and Jewish populations. *MEFV* encodes the protein pyrin, which is expressed in neutrophils and is thought to regulate interleukin-1B (a proinflammatory cytokine) release.

Symptoms often present in childhood and may be misdiagnosed as appendicitis. Treatment of an acute episode is symptomatic. Colchicine can be used to reduce the frequency and severity of attacks and to prevent development of amyloidosis.

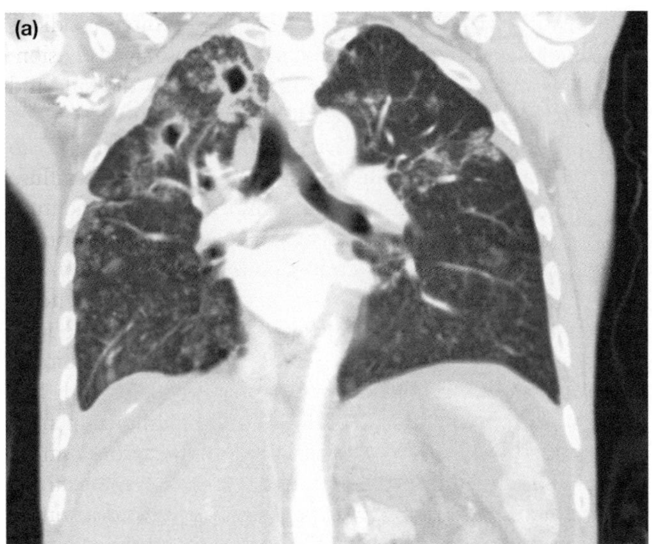

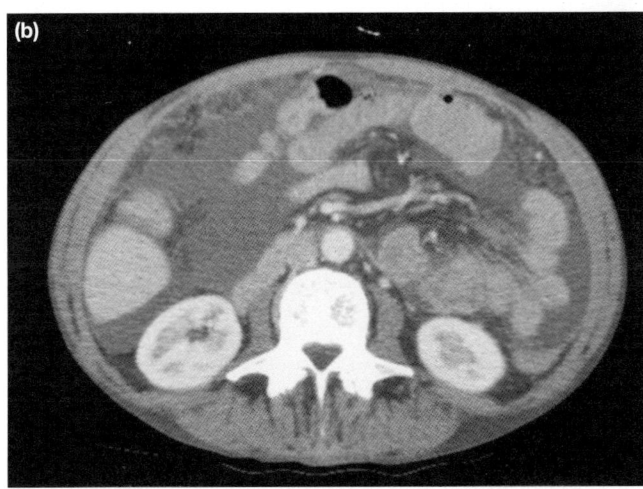

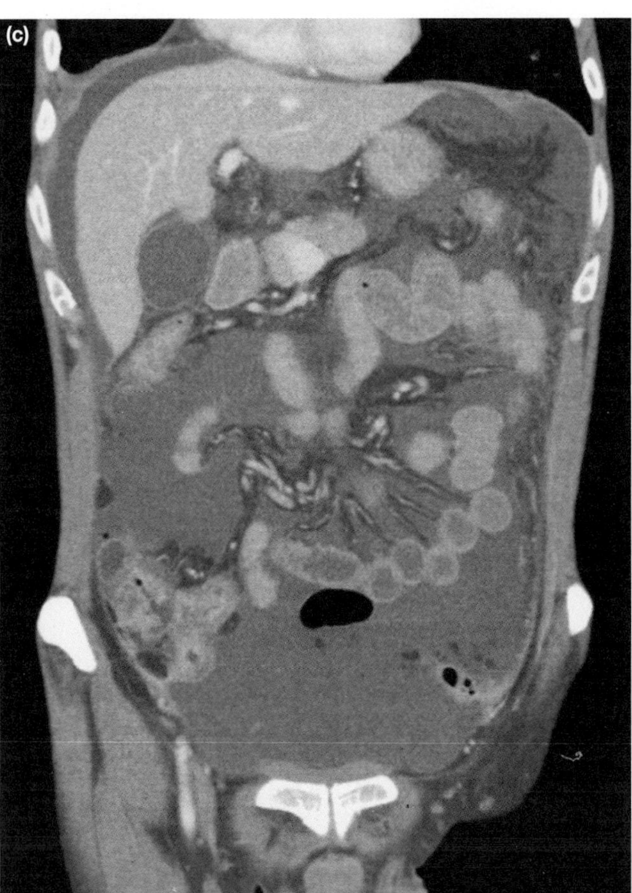

Figure 65.8 (a) Plain chest radiograph from a 55-year-old man showing miliary tuberculosis (TB); (b, c) representative computed tomography images from the same patient showing gross ascites, nodular stranding in the omentum and mesentery, as well as nodular enhancement of the peritoneum – TB peritonitis (courtesy of Dr S Burke, Homerton University Foundation Trust, London, UK).

TUMOURS OF THE PERITONEUM

Primary peritoneal malignancy

Primary tumours of the peritoneum are rare. They arise in the mesothelium of the peritoneum. Mesothelioma of the peritoneum is less frequent than in the pleural cavity but is equally lethal. Asbestos is a recognised cause. It has a predilection for the pelvic peritoneum. Cytoreductive surgery with heated intraperitoneal chemotherapy (HIPEC) or systemic cisplatin-based chemotherapy are the mainstays of treatment.

Secondary peritoneal malignancy

Peritoneal carcinomatosis

Peritoneal carcinomatosis is common and refers to malignant nodules on the surface of the peritoneum. It normally arises in conjunction with ovarian malignancy or malignancy in an organ of the mesenteric domain. It can be localised or diffuse. Any peritoneal surface can be involved. Sometimes the omentum is diffusely involved, forming a mass termed an omental cake.

The symptoms and signs are mainly related to the primary pathology. If the tumour burden is considerable, a mass may be palpable and the accompanying ascites substantial. Radiological cross-sectional imaging with CT or magnetic resonance imaging (MRI) is usually diagnostic; however, histological or cytological confirmation is essential to distinguish it from peritoneal TB. The visceral origin of peritoneal carcinomatosis is important as this can guide chemotherapy and cytoreductive or extirpative surgery.

The visceral origin of peritoneal carcinomatosis is important because if curative resection of the primary tumour is deemed feasible and the peritoneal disease considered resectable, resection with peritonectomy and HIPEC should be considered. HIPEC is a highly concentrated, heated (41–42°C) chemotherapy delivered directly into the abdomen for 90 minutes after cytoreductive surgery. HIPEC is particularly valuable in treatment of pseudomyxoma peritonei and has become the standard of care in carefully selected patients assessed in specialist centres (Sugerbaker) (see ***Chapter 76***).

Paul H Sugerbaker, b. 1941, Director of Surgical Oncology, Washington Cancer Institute, Washington, DC, USA.

In the majority of patients with peritoneal carcinomatosis treatment is palliative. Subacute intestinal obstruction may require intestinal bypass or a defunctioning stoma (see *Chapter 78*). Malignant ascites may be drained externally or via a peritoneovenous shunt (LeVeen).

PERITONEAL INCLUSION CYSTS

Introduction

These are benign cysts lined by peritoneal mesothelium. They can arise at any location of the peritoneum, in continuity with the surface of either parietal or visceral peritoneum. They can gradually expand and rarely rupture. Most are asymptomatic and are identified incidentally on cross-sectional imaging for other indications. There is a loose association with ovarian malignancy and thus MRI evaluation of the ovaries is advisable in the premenopausal context. If symptomatic an inclusion cyst may be drained under imaging control, deroofed or excised. Recurrent rates are high.

Abdominal fluid collections

Abdominal collections are subdivided into intraperitoneal and retroperitoneal collections. Retroperitoneal collections are further subdivided into those limited to the retroperitoneal space (e.g. in pancreatitis) and collections arising in relation to retroperitoneal organs such the kidney. The latter are collections of the retroperitoneum. Collections of the retroperitoneal space and retroperitoneum are considered in the final section of the chapter.

Intraperitoneal collections

Ascites

Peritoneal fluid is constantly secreted and absorbed. Accumulation of peritoneal fluid, termed ascites, occurs when there is excess production or reduced absorption. Production of large volumes of a protein-rich fluid occurs in peritonitis and carcinomatosis peritonei. Reduced absorption occurs when capillary pressure is increased as a result of generalised water retention, cardiac failure, constrictive pericarditis or vena cava obstruction. Capillary pressure is also raised selectively in the portal venous system in the Budd–Chiari syndrome, hepatic cirrhosis or extrahepatic portal venous obstruction. Plasma colloid osmotic pressure may be lowered in patients with reduced nutritional intake, diminished intestinal absorption, abnormal protein losses or defective protein synthesis, such as occurs in cirrhosis. Peritoneal lymphatic drainage may be impaired, resulting in the accumulation of protein-rich fluid.

Hepatic cirrhosis is the most common cause of ascites due to portal venous hypertension secondary to fibrosis of the intrahepatic venous bed. In the Budd–Chiari syndrome (see *Chapter 69*), thrombosis of hepatic veins leads to obstruction of venous outflow from the liver and hence from the mesenteric domain in general. Alternative routes of venous drainage may open up. One such route involves the vestigial umbilical vein at the base of the falciform ligament. Venous drainage via this route may reach the systemic venous drainage at the umbilicus. This is termed a portosystemic shunt and has a characteristic clinical appearance (involving veins) at the umbilicus (caput medusae).

Congestive heart failure increases pressure in the vena cava and resistance to the venous outflow from the liver. In this setting, ascitic fluid is light yellow and has a low specific gravity and low protein concentration (<25 g/L). In constrictive pericarditis there is a diminished capacity of the right heart. This leads to simultaneous peritoneal and pleural effusions due to engorgement of the venae cavae (Pick's disease).

Ascites occurring in peritoneal metastases is due to excessive exudation of fluid and lymphatic blockage. The fluid is dark yellow and frequently blood stained. The specific gravity and protein content (>25 g/L) are high. Rarely, ascites and pleural effusion are associated with solid fibromas of the ovary (Meigs' syndrome). These effusions disappear when the tumour is excised.

Summary box 65.7

Causes of ascites

Transudates (protein <25 g/L)

- Low plasma protein concentrations
  - Malnutrition
  - Nephrotic syndrome
  - Protein-losing enteropathy
- High central venous pressure
  - Congestive cardiac failure
- Portal hypertension
  - Portal vein thrombosis
  - Cirrhosis

Exudates (protein >25 g/L)

- Peritoneal malignancy
- Tuberculous peritonitis
- Budd–Chiari syndrome (hepatic vein occlusion or thrombosis)
- Pancreatic ascites
- Chylous ascites
- Meigs' syndrome

Ascites normally becomes clinically recognisable when greater than 1.5 litres of fluid is apparent (although greater volumes may be required in obese patients). The abdomen is distended evenly with fullness of the flanks, which are dull to percussion. Usually, shifting dullness is present but, when there is a very large accumulation of fluid, this sign is absent. In such cases, flicking the abdominal wall produces a characteristic

---

Harry H LeVeen, 1915–1997, Professor of Surgery, University of South Carolina, Columbia, SC, USA.
George Budd, 1808–1882, Professor of Medicine, King's College Hospital, London, UK.
Hans Chiari, 1851–1916, Professor of Pathological Anatomy, Strasbourg, Germany (Strasbourg was returned to France in 1918 at the end of the First World War).
Caput Medusa (head of Medusa), in Greek mythology depicted as having venomous snakes instead of hair.
Friedel Pick, 1867–1926, physician, Prague, the former Czechoslovakia, described this disease in 1896.
Joe Vincent Meigs, 1892–1963, Professor of Gynecology, Harvard University Medical School, Boston, MA, USA.

fluid thrill on the other side of the abdomen. This is not a reliable clinical sign. In women, ascites must be differentiated from an enormous ovarian cyst.

Investigations

The aims are identification of ascites and determination of the underlying cause. Liver function tests (LFTs), cardiac function, ultrasonography and/or CT scanning (***Figure 65.9***) may help diagnose aetiology, e.g. carcinomatosis or liver disease.

Ascitic aspiration or tap under imaging guidance helps minimise the risk of visceral injury. It can be both diagnostic and therapeutic. After the bladder has been emptied, puncture of the peritoneum is carried out under local anaesthetic using a moderately sized trocar and cannula. A peritoneal drain may be inserted at the time.

In cases where the effusion is caused by cardiac failure, fluid must be evacuated slowly. Fluid is sent for microscopy/cytology, culture, including mycobacteria (see ***Tuberculus peritonitis*** above), and analysis of protein content and amylase. Unless other measures are taken the fluid soon accumulates and repeated tappings remove valuable protein.

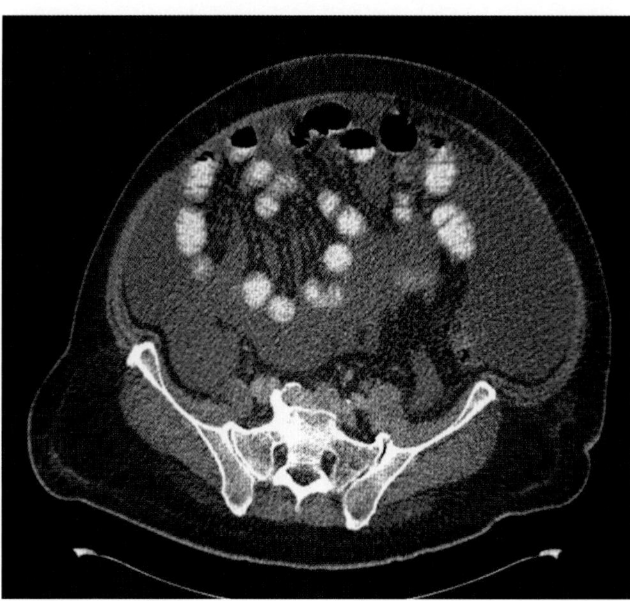

Figure 65.9 Computed tomography axial scan of the abdomen showing gross ascites.

Management

Management aims to address any reversible primary pathology (following which the ascites resolves) or symptom-based management of the ascites itself. If portal venous pressure is raised, it may be possible to lower it by treatment of the primary condition or by transjugular intrahepatic portosystemic shunt or transjugular intrahepatic portosystemic stent shunting (commonly abbreviated as TIPS or TIPSS).

Dietary sodium restriction to 200 mg/day may be helpful, but diuretics are usually required (combination of spironolactone and furosemide). For patients failing to respond to such measures, therapeutic needle paracentesis can be performed. Serial large volume paracentesis (4–6 L/day and up to 8 litres in one session) can be performed safely with colloid replacement and can be performed in patients with cirrhosis and deranged clotting. Guidelines recommend albumin replacement after paracentesis to reduce complications. It may also be possible to leave an indwelling external drain for smaller volume home paracentesis.

Chylous ascites

In some patients, the ascitic fluid appears milky because of an excess of chylomicrons (triglycerides). Most of these cases are associated with malignancy (usually lymphoma). Other causes include cirrhosis, TB, filariasis, nephrotic syndrome, abdominal trauma (including surgery), constrictive pericarditis, sarcoidosis and congenital lymphatic abnormality. The prognosis is poor unless the underlying condition can be cured. In addition to other measures used to treat ascites, patients should be placed on a fat-free diet with medium-chain triglyceride supplements.

INTRAPERITONEAL ABSCESS FORMATION

An intraperitoneal abscess is a collection of pus in the peritoneal cavity (***Figure 65.10***). It normally arises secondary to another pathology. Inflammation of any viscus, if unresolved, will lead to hypersecretion of peritoneal fluid. The nature of the fluid progresses to frank pus unless adsorbed or drained. Hence, abscess formation commonly accompanies inflammation of an abdominal viscus and is usually labelled either according to location (subphrenic, intrapelvic) or with reference to nearby organs (periappendiceal, paracolic, subhepatic).

Intraperitoneal abscess formation is associated with a spectrum of symptoms and signs. At one end, patients may be asymptomatic or may feel somewhat unwell, anorectic, fatigued, with failure to maintain or gain weight. At the opposite end, patients may have significant abdominal symptoms and signs (nausea, vomiting, abdominal pain, diarrhoea) and be extremely unwell. A swinging pyrexia is strongly suggestive of intraperitoneal abscess formation.

Summary box 65.8

Clinical features of an abdominal/pelvic abscess

Symptoms
- Malaise, lethargy – failure to recover from surgery as expected
- Anorexia and weight loss
- Sweats +/– rigors
- Abdominal/pelvic pain
- Symptoms from local irritation, e.g. shoulder tip/hiccoughs (subphrenic), diarrhoea and mucus (pelvic), nausea and vomiting (any upper abdominal)

Signs
- Increased temperature and pulse +/– swinging pyrexia
- Localised abdominal tenderness +/– mass (including on pelvic examination)

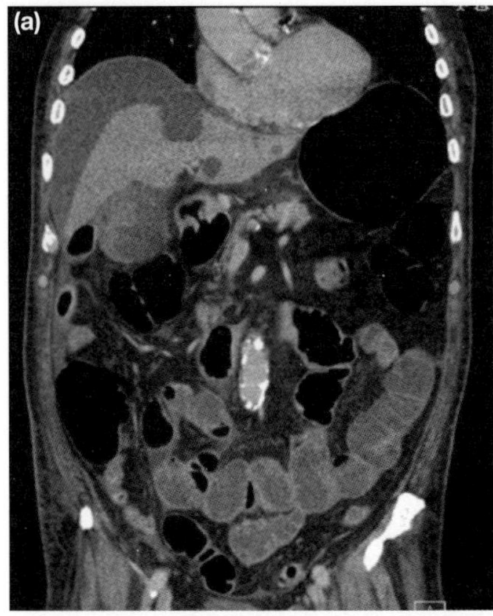
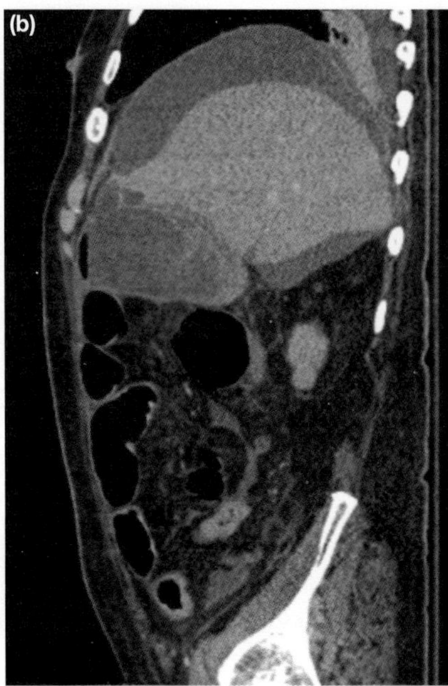
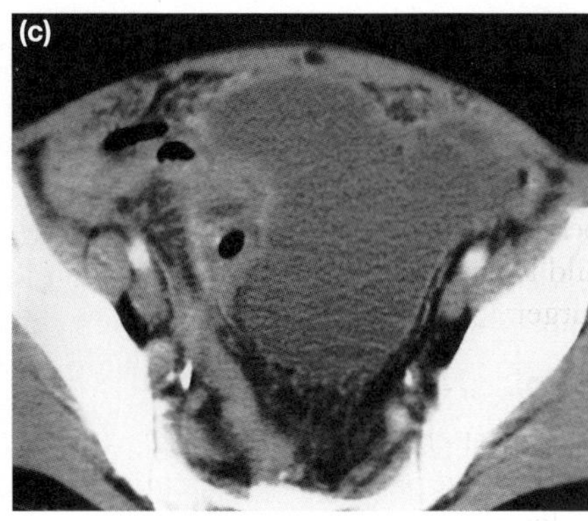

Figure 65.10 Intraperitoneal abscesses. (a) and (b) Subphrenic and subhepatic abscesses seen on computed tomography (CT) scanning. (c) Pelvic abscess seen on CT scanning.

Investigation

The modern diagnosis of an abscess is radiological using CT (*Figure 65.10*). CT imaging can also guide treatment by drain placement or aspiration. Ultrasound is a useful (though non-specific) modality for use in select populations (e.g. paediatric or pregnant patients). Serial imaging is used to monitor treatment efficacy or disease progression. Radiolabelled white cell scanning may occasionally prove helpful if an abscess is suspected but has not been identified by the above means.

Treatment

Abscesses less than 5 cm in diameter normally resolve with intravenous antibiotic treatment. As antibiotics take effect, the magnitude of the swinging pyrexia can decrease with each successive spike in temperature. Serial monitoring of C-reactive protein levels is useful to non-invasively monitor response to treatment.

Abscesses greater than 5 cm require either percutaneous aspiration/drainage or surgical intervention. If percutaneous radiological approaches fail, then operative washout is indicated. This can be conducted laparoscopically (laparoscopic lavage) or via an open approach. The technical challenges involved are such that this should only be undertaken by an experienced surgeon. The bowel may be matted and difficult to separate in order to access the abscess. All regions of the peritoneal cavity should be accessed, with a view to drainage of any residual collections. The entirety of the small intestine and adjoining mesentery should be exposed to ensure that there are no residual interloop abscesses. If a phlegmon is apparent, then only in the setting of life-threatening circumstances should the components of this be separated.

Special considerations: Prevention of abscess formation after appendicitis

During appendectomy, it is important to aspirate the pelvic, paracolic and subhepatic spaces prior to closure of the abdominal wall. This simple measure can reduce the incidence of postoperative abscess, which is common after appendectomy, occurring in up to 30% of patients following appendectomy for a perforated appendix. It can lead to frustration for patients if not forewarned of the possibility.

Special considerations: Abscess formation following intestinal surgery and anastomosis

The development of an abscess following intestinal resection and anastomosis signifies infection of a haematoma or an anastomotic leak. Locules of gas or free contrast (Gastrografin) on CT support anastomotic leak. Pelvic abscess formation is not uncommon following excision of the rectum and formation of a pelvic anastomosis.

Special considerations: Subphrenic abscess

This refers to the presence of pus immediately beneath the diaphragm. Patients may complain of shoulder tip pain. The diaphragm also develops at the same level as the C5 dermatome. If the parietal peritoneum under the diaphragm is irritated, pain is referred to the shoulder tip. This also explains why patients frequently complain of shoulder tip pain following laparoscopic or robotic surgery. In the era preceding that of cross-sectional imaging via CT, the adage 'pus somewhere, pus nowhere, pus under the diaphragm' was useful.

Special considerations: Pelvic abscess

The pelvis is the most common site of abscess formation because the vermiform appendix is often pelvic in position and the Fallopian tubes are also frequent sites of infection. A pelvic abscess can also occur as a sequel to diffuse peritonitis and is common after anastomotic leakage following colorectal surgery.

Clinical features

The most characteristic symptoms are pelvic pain, diarrhoea and passage of mucus in the stools. The patient may complain of lower back pain or a pressure sensation in the pelvis. This symptom can be quite severe in intensity. The abscess may discharge into the anal canal as the pelvic collection points through an anastomotic leak (the point of least resistance). Rectal or vaginal examination can be extremely uncomfortable for the patient.

Investigation and management

If any uncertainty exists, the presence of pus should be confirmed by ultrasonography or CT scanning. Pelvic abscesses can be drained transanally or transgluteally. The past vogue for transintestinal drainage is no longer practised because of the high incidence of complications such as fistulae. Laparotomy may sometimes be indicated.

PERITONEAL (MESOTHELIAL) SAC AND HERNIA FORMATION

The processus vaginalis refers to a peritoneal tube that advances into the inguinal ligament in tandem with migration of the testes. The lumen of the processus vaginalis is in continuity with the peritoneal cavity. Given this, it provides a conduit for herniation of abdominal contents. Even a residual indentation at the ostium of the processus vaginalis represents a mechanical defect at which repeated episodes of raised intraperitoneal pressure can lead to gradual extension of the parietal peritoneum into the inguinal canal.

The mesothelial sac is a near constant feature of incisional and parastomal hernias. In these instances, the peritoneum gradually advances over subcutaneous fat, or the serosal surface of the intestine, bringing that region of anatomy directly in continuity with the peritoneal cavity. Not surprisingly, incisional or parastomal hernias gradually increase in size with time. In addition, they are frequently complicated by parastomal herniation of intestinal contents and intestinal compromise.

THE MESENTERY

GENERAL CONSIDERATIONS

The arterial supply and venous and lymphatic drainage of each digestive organ are located in the mesentery. Thus diseases of individual organs can have significant effects on the adjoining mesentery and its components. The pancreas and the effects of pancreatitis are a good example. The pancreas is positioned on the mesentery (*65.5*). It arches over the SMA and superior mesenteric vein (both of which are intramesenteric). The neck of the pancreas is anterior to the region of the mesentery that contains the portal vein. The body and tail of the pancreas are in the dorsal mesogastrium (i.e. the posterior wall of the upper region sack) and the tip of the tail of the pancreas is located at the hilum of the spleen (see ***Development of the mesentery and peritoneum***). Given these anatomical relations, acute inflammation of the pancreas can affect any of these structures. Complications of acute pancreatitis thus include thrombosis in the portal and splenic vein, gastric outlet obstruction and arterial haemorrhage (see ***Chapter 72***).

The mesentery is remarkably well preserved in most diseases. Although rarely encountered in clinical practice, mesenteric necrosis is mostly seen in advanced necrotising pancreatitis. Primary defects (i.e. non-surgical causes) of the mesentery are rare. These are always accompanied by failure of normal development of the adjoining organ. For example, intestinal atresia arises when a section of the adjoining mesentery fails to develop.

The mesentery comprises adipose, connective tissue, neurological, lymphatic and vascular components. Abnormalities can arise in any of these and lead to either solid (tumour deposits, lymphatic metastases) or cystic lesions. The supportive capacity of the mesentery is reflected in the finding of splenunculi, heterotopic pancreas, ossification, teratomas and even ectopic pregnancies in different regions of the mesentery.

MESENTERIC HAEMATOMA

A mesenteric haematoma can follow abdominal compression in trauma (e.g. seat-belt syndrome) or during abdominal surgery, when the mesentery must be manipulated. The mesenteric stroma is mainly adipose and thus easily damaged. It bleeds readily if disrupted. A haematoma may form and quickly enlarge to compress mesenteric veins. Mesenteric haematoma can sometimes occur during surgery for Crohn's disease.

MESENTERIC ADENITIS

This is inflammation of the lymph nodes of the mesentery (***Figure 65.11***). It mostly occurs in the ileocaecal region because of the volume of lymphatic tissue. It is often the site of viral or infective lymphadenopathy (*Yersinia* spp., *Campylobacter* spp., *Mycobacterium tuberculosis*) and may follow an upper respiratory tract infection with either a viral or bacterial pathogen. Mesenteric adenitis caused by severe acute respiratory syndrome coronavirus 2 (SARS-CoV-2) is not uncommon. Swelling of ileocaecal lymph nodes results in capsular stretch and somatic pain in the right iliac fossa. The patient is frequently pyretic (often the temperature is markedly elevated) and may have enlarged cervical lymph nodes.

During childhood, acute, non-specific mesenteric adenitis is a common condition. The typical history is one of short attacks of central abdominal pain lasting from 10 to 30 minutes, commonly associated with vomiting. The patient seldom looks ill. In more than half of the cases the temperature is elevated. Abdominal tenderness is poorly localised and, when present, shifting tenderness is a valuable sign for differentiating the condition from appendicitis. The neck, axillae and groins should be palpated for enlarged lymph nodes.

Investigation

There is often a leukocytosis of 10 000–12 000/μL (10–12 × 10^9/L) or more on the first day of the attack, but this falls on the second day. Ultrasonography may be helpful in differentiating this from appendicitis. Sometimes a CT or exploratory laparoscopy is required.

Treatment

This is normally supportive. Viral mesenteric adenitis normally resolves spontaneously but can recur. The symptoms in bacterial mesenteric adenitis include cramping pain, vomiting and diarrhoea. They can be severe and require hospitalisation.

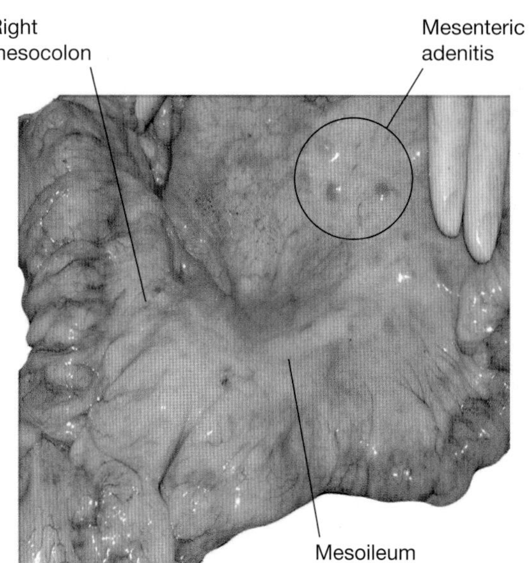

Figure 65.11 Mesenteric adenitis. (Reproduced with permission from Coffey JC, Lavery I, Sehgal R (eds). *Mesenteric principles of gastrointestinal surgery: basic and applied principles*. Boca Raton: CRC Press, 2017: 69–84.)

MESENTERIC ADENITIS AND THE MESENTERY IN CROHN'S DISEASE

Ileocaecal mesenteric adenitis occurs in ileocolic Crohn's disease and the mesentery is thickened, shortened and oedematous with a tendency to bleed readily when handled. The vascular pedicles within the mesentery may not be apparent, thus great care is needed when dividing the mesentery as normal techniques may not be suitable.

In Crohn's disease, the mesentery can extend over adjoining intestine as 'fat wrapping' or 'creeping fat' (***Figure 65.12***). These appear to be specific to Crohn's disease. The mesentery changes from normal to abnormal at the mesenteric transition zone. Conventional surgery for Crohn's disease involves amputation of the intestine at its intersection with adjoining mesentery. The mesentery is thus retained. Increasingly, surgeons are removing the mesentery adjoining the diseased intestine (see ***Chapter 75***).

TUBERCULOSIS OF THE MESENTERIC LYMPH NODES

Tuberculous mesenteric lymphadenitis is considerably less common than acute non-specific lymphadenitis. Tubercle bacilli, usually, but not necessarily, bovine, are ingested and enter the mesenteric lymph nodes by way of Peyer's patches. Sometimes only one lymph node is infected; usually there are several, and occasionally massive involvement occurs. The presentation may be with abdominal pain (a rare differential for appendicitis) or with general constitutional symptoms (pyrexia, weight loss, etc.). Calcified lymph nodes may be demonstrated on a plain radiograph of the abdomen, where they must be distinguished from other calcified lesions, e.g. renal or ureteric stones.

VASCULAR ABNORMALITIES OF THE MESENTERY

Acute mesenteric ischaemia

The arterial inflow to the mesenteric domain is limited to three major vessels: the coeliac trunk and the superior and inferior mesenteric arteries (*65.5*). Additional arterial inflow in the pelvis comes via the middle rectal arteries. The limited number of arterial inputs to the mesenteric domain mean that narrowing or occlusion at the origin of any one vessel can have significant clinical effects. Acute mesenteric ischaemia mostly follows embolisation to the origin of either the coeliac or superior mesenteric arterial trunk. Unless quickly reversed, it can lead to ischaemia and necrosis of most of the intestine. At first, the severity of abdominal pain does not match clinical findings on examination. If ischaemia and necrosis occur, the patient develops peritonism as a result of irritation of the parietal peritoneum by the necrotic intestine.

The inferior mesenteric artery (IMA) is usually divided at open repair of an abdominal aortic aneurysm; however, anastomoses between peripheral branches of the SMA and IMA, referred to as the marginal artery of Drummond, usually prevent critical ischaemia of the sigmoid and descending colon. If ischaemia is limited to the mucosa, the patient may experience cramping suprapubic pain and diarrhoea that normally settles. If ischaemia is transmural the colon may become necrotic and require resection.

Johann Conrad Peyer, 1653–1712, Professor of Logic, Rhetoric and Medicine, Schaffhausen, Switzerland, described the lymph follicles in the intestine in 1677.
Sir David Drummond, 1852–1932, born Dublin, Ireland, pathologist and physician at the Royal Victoria Infirmary, Newcastle (1878–1920), President of the British Medical Association (1921–1922) and vice chancellor of the University of Durham (1920–1922).

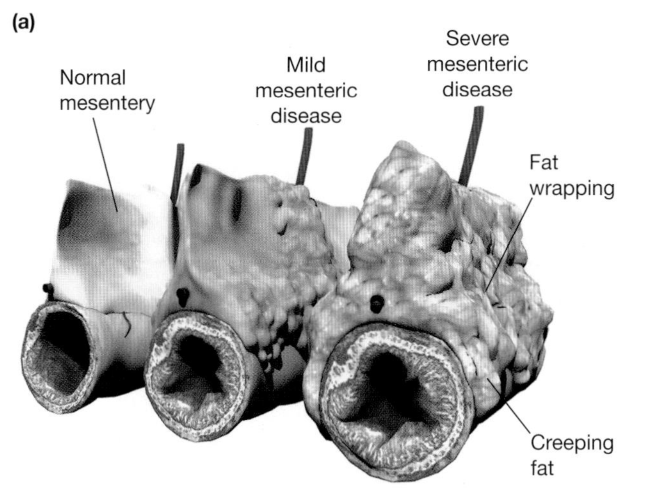

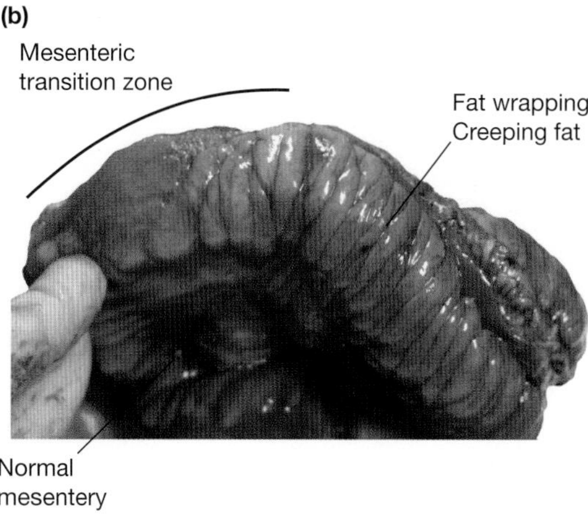

Figure 65.12 The mesentery in Crohn's disease. (a) Levels of mesenteric disease manifestations. (b) The mesenteric transition zone and creeping fat. (Reproduced with permission from Coffey JC, Lavery I, Sehgal R (eds). *Mesenteric principles of gastrointestinal surgery: basic and applied principles*. Boca Raton: CRC Press, 2017: 85–108.)

Chronic mesenteric ischaemia

Chronic mesenteric ischaemia is due to atherosclerotic narrowing at the origin of any of the three arterial trunks. Patients describe postprandial abdominal pain that can be severe, resulting in a fear of eating with progressive weight loss. The diagnosis requires CT angiography. Radiological stent placement may be successful, but surgical endarterectomy of bypass repair may be required.

Venous ischaemia

The venous drainage of the mesenteric domain is limited to the junction between the hepatic veins and the inferior vena cava. Narrowing or blockage of the lumen at this junction occurs in Budd–Chiari syndrome. It has major clinical implications. Most venous drainage of the mesenteric domain returns to the liver via the portal vein. Portal venous thrombosis impedes venous drainage of all abdominal digestive organs unless an alternative drainage route opens (i.e. a portosystemic shunt) or is created (see *Chapter 69*) (*65.5*).

ROTATIONAL DISORDERS

Malrotation

Malrotation refers to a failure of formation of the mid-region switch (described in ***Development of the mesentery and peritoneum***) (***Figure 65.13***) and is the most common abdominal surgical emergency in the neonatal period. Early during development, the right and left side of the mid-region fold of the mesentery are aligned from the central to peripheral zones. Later, the sides switch position at the periphery but not at the central zone. Adjoining intestine similarly changes position to take up the normal conformation. In malrotation, the switch does not occur, and the sides of the mid-region fold remain aligned. This explains why the duodenum, jejunum and ileum are aligned in the right flank of the abdomen. Malrotation in itself is not pathogenic. However, the small intestine and adjoining mesentery are abnormally mobile and can undergo torsion around the superior mesentery artery, which can be life-threatening.

History

The neonate with a volvulus due to malrotation is patently distressed, vomiting and has a distended abdomen.

Investigation

Urgent CT is mandated and clarifies the position of the duodenojejunal junction. Normally the duodenojejunal flexure is positioned at or to the left of the midline. In volvulus due to malrotation, the duodenojejunal junction is on the right of the midline (i.e. the mid-region switch has not occurred).

Treatment

The mainstay of treatment is Ladd's procedure, in which the volvulus is first reversed and then the intestine is secured to the posterior abdominal wall. Although this does not correct the underlying mesenteric abnormality, it does reduce the mobility of the intestine and mesentery and reduces the likelihood of further volvulus. It is possible however to address the underlying mesenteric abnormality by recapitulating the mid-region switch. This returns the intestine and mesentery to a normal conformation. They can then be fixed to the posterior abdominal wall.

Volvulus of the intestine and adjoining mesentery

Volvulus can only be understood if considered in mesenteric terms. Where a section of intestine is curved, the adjoining mesentery is buckle-shaped or folded. If the intestine progresses from a curve to a coil, the adjoining mesentery acquires a

William Edwards Ladd, 1880–1967, Surgeon in Chief, Boston Children's Hospital, Boston, MA, USA.

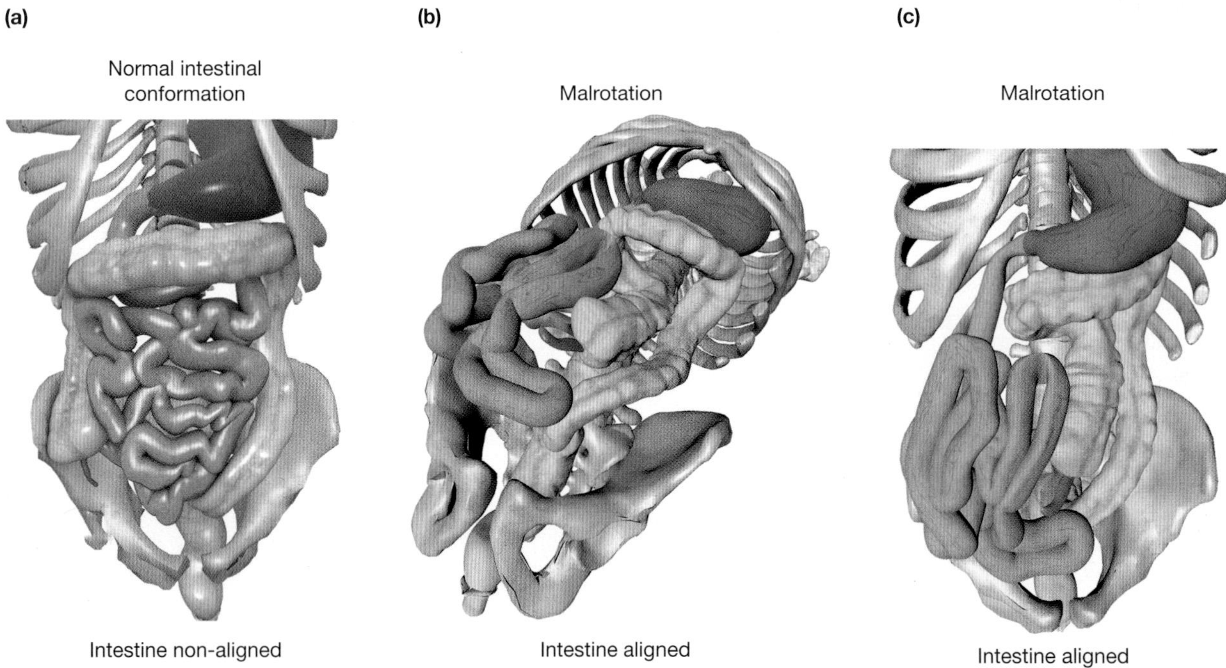

Figure 65.13 Malrotation. (Reproduced with permission from Coffey JC, Lavery I, Sehgal R (eds). *Mesenteric principles of gastrointestinal surgery: basic and applied principles*. Boca Raton: CRC Press, 2017: 85–108.)

spiral shape. The resultant coil/spiral complex of the intestine and mesentery is termed a volvulus. Its formation is normally prevented by adhesion of the mesentery to the posterior abdominal wall during development. Wherever mesenteric adhesion is inadequate, there is a risk of volvulus formation. Sigmoid volvulus is the commonest type, followed by ileocaecal. However, the anatomy of the mesentery is such that volvulus can theoretically arise at any level from the oesophagogastric to anorectal junction.

History

In ileocaecal volvulus the patient often describes a longstanding history of intermittent, colicky abdominal pain associated with distension and vomiting. In between episodes (when the volvulus has detorted) the patient is entirely asymptomatic and repeated CT and endoscopic examinations are normal. The clinical picture is similar to that of irritable bowel syndrome.

Sigmoid volvulus occurs mainly in the elderly as the intestine and mesentery continue to lengthen throughout life.

Investigation

A plain film of the abdomen is frequently diagnostic. CT is recommended when planning operative intervention.

Treatment

Sigmoid volvulus can be quickly reversed with endoscopic decompression, but recurrence is common. Most patients will ultimately require surgery to resect the intestine and adjoining mesentery. These patients often have multiple comorbidities and present challenging anaesthetic and ethical dilemmas (see ***Chapter 77***).

Mesenteric stretch during colonoscopy

Development of pain doing colonoscopy is frequently attributed to distension of the colon and stretch of the colon wall. In reality, substantial volumes of gas would be required to insufflate the colon to the degree at which the colon stretches. Pain during colonoscopy is common and arises mainly because of stretch of the adjoining mesentery. Looping of the intestine is a frequent event during colonoscopy. The loop corresponds to a coil, which means that the mesentery adjoining the loop must form a spiral. It thus resembles the anatomical arrangement seen in volvulus. Attempts to advance the endoscope beyond a coil will place both the intestine and mesentery under stretch. Stretch of the mesentery leads to severe central colicky abdominal pain, often accompanied by bradycardia. An understanding of the anatomical basis of loop formation enables the endoscopist to take appropriate preventative or corrective measures.

Mesenteric sclerosis and panniculitis

Mesenteric sclerosis

This is also termed sclerosing encapsulating peritonitis or abdominal cocoon syndrome (***Figure 65.14***). It occurs mostly in patients on long-term peritoneal dialysis. It is a disease of the mesothelial component of visceral peritoneum (i.e. peritoneum overlying organs of the mesenteric domain). The mesothelium undergoes hypertrophy and the peritoneum becomes thickened. Underlying organs become encapsulated by a peritoneal 'cocoon'. Mesenteric sclerosis may follow intraperitoneal sepsis, when fibrin plaques accumulate along the intestine and mesentery leading to a reactionary mesothelial hypertrophy.

History and investigation

The clinical picture is highly variable, as is the natural history of the condition among individuals. Mesenteric sclerosis can lead to obstruction of the intestine. The diagnosis is normally made based on CT and intraoperative appearances and post-operative surgical histology.

Treatment

Treatment is supportive and surgery is reserved for emergency cases only as surgical intervention may lead to further peritoneal sclerosis.

Mesenteric panniculitis

This is inflammation of the mesodermal mesentery (i.e. the mesenteric stroma). It is always present in Crohn's disease (see ***Mesenteric adenitis and the mesentery in Crohn's disease***). Often it is an incidental finding on cross-sectional imaging of the abdomen by CT ('misty mesentery'; ***Figure 65.14***). Although there are concerns over malignant potential, this is not supported by the general literature. It can arise secondary to inflammation in any digestive organ. It is associated with connective tissue disorders (including Weber–Christian disease). As with mesenteric sclerosis, treatment is normally medical and surgery is rarely required. Serial CT scanning is indicated to ensure resolution.

Sclerosing mesenteritis

Sclerotic (mesothelial) and inflammatory (mesodermal) abnormalities of the mesentery may coexist. Although this can arise *de novo*, it is normally a secondary manifestation of another pathology (i.e. immunoglobulin G4 [IgG4] disease, which is a systemic fibroinflammatory disease).

Adhesions

Pathology

Adhesions are best classified with reference to their appearance. They are subdivided into peritoneal, areolar and dense adhesions.

Peritoneal (sclerotic) adhesions

These are mesothelial adhesions between two mesothelial surfaces (***Figure 65.15a***). They reflect mesothelial proliferation, resemble peritoneum and are generally soft and non-vascular. They are similar in appearance (though not in consistency) to the peritoneal cocoon that occurs in mesenteric sclerosis. These can be band-like. They may occur following laparoscopic surgery, where they form a band linking a viscus to the inner surface of a port site. Band adhesions can lead to focal abdominal pain, internal herniation (through the window created with surrounding related structures) or intestinal torsion around the band.

Areolar adhesions

These flimsy connective tissue adhesions are identical to the connective tissue that fills the retroperitoneal space between the mesentery and posterior abdominal wall (***Figure 65.15b***). Given this appearance they have been called 'angel hairs'. They are generated in a process similar to that involved when the mesentery adheres to the posterior abdominal wall.

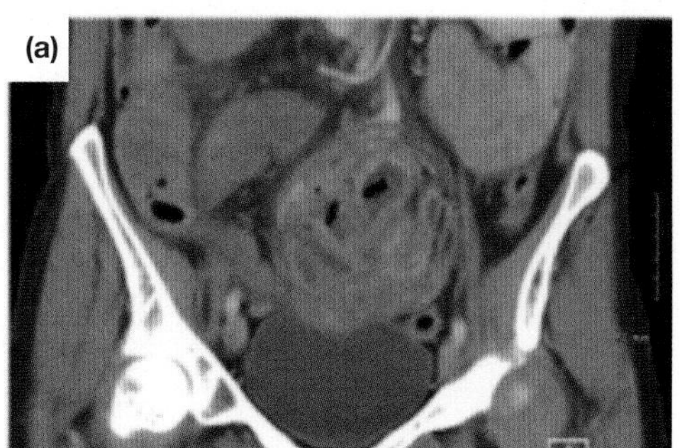

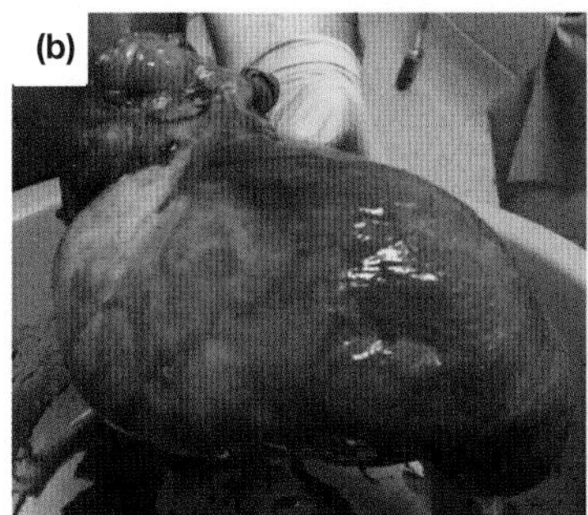

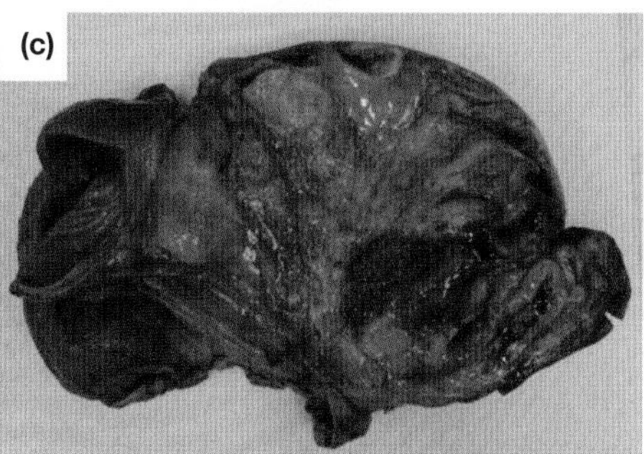

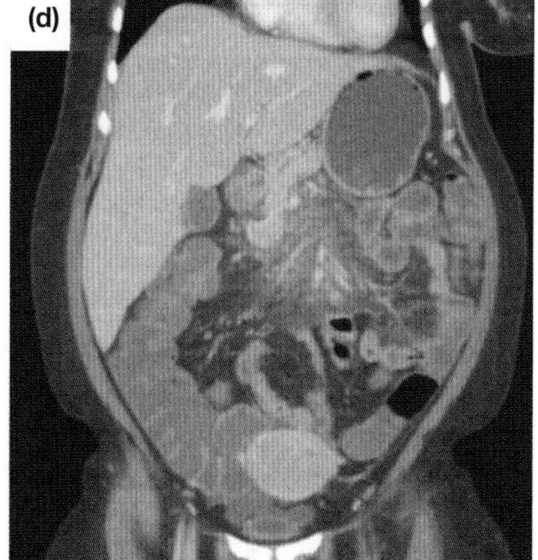

Figure 65.14 Mesenteric sclerosis. **(a)** Coronal section of abdomen on computed axial tomography demonstrating a sclerotic mass. **(b)** Postexcision mass in **(a)**. The intestine is contained in a sclerotic capsule. **(c)** Appearance of the mass in **(b)** after division into halves. The intestine is draped across the surface of a mesenteric tissue mass. **(d)** Mesenteric panniculitis (misty mesentery).

Frederick Parkes Weber, 1863–1962, physician, Mount Vernon Hospital, London, UK.
Henry Asbury Christian, 1876–1951, pathologist, Boston, MA, USA.

(a)
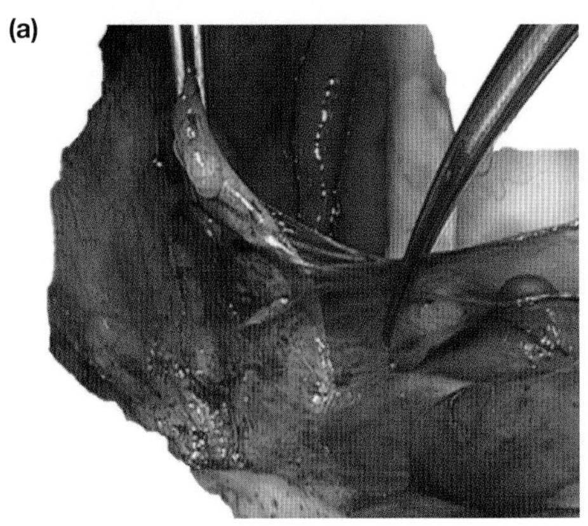

(b)
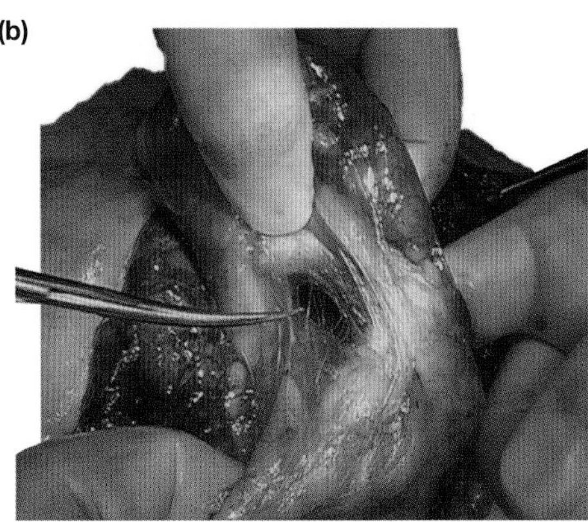

Figure 65.15 Adhesions. (a) Peritoneal (sclerotic) adhesions. (b) Areolar adhesions. (Reproduced with permission from Coffey JC, Lavery I, Sehgal R (eds). *Mesenteric principles of gastrointestinal surgery: basic and applied principles*. Boca Raton: CRC Press, 2017: 333–42.)

The capacity to adhere is shared by all organs of the mesenteric domain. This explains the anatomical relations between the liver, colon, spleen and mesentery on one side and the abdominal wall on the other. The capacity is retained to varying degrees among individuals and explains adhesion formation in the adult setting. Adhesion occurs following abdominal surgery when the intestine and mesentery adhere to the inside surface of the anterior abdominal wall. The resultant anatomical arrangement is similar to that observed during development, except the anterior abdominal wall is involved.

Postoperative adhesion formation occurs to varying degrees. At one end of the spectrum, it may be entirely absent. At the other end, mesenteric, intestinal and other components of the mesenteric domain may adhere over broad areas to the anterior abdominal wall. This normally commences in the midline and extends laterally towards the flanks, displacing the overlying peritoneum. The conformation of the peritoneal cavity changes markedly. In the most extremes cases, the peritoneal cavity may be obliterated or limited to small pockets at the flanks. This generates considerable technical challenges during reoperative surgery.

Dense adhesions

These differ markedly in appearance from peritoneal or areolar adhesions. They can bridge the abdominal wall and intestine, or intestine and mesentery, and lead to fusion of the bridged structures. Surgical division can be challenging. Sometimes it is not possible to separate conjoined organs without disrupting the integrity of one of them. Such dense adhesions arise mostly following severe intraperitoneal contamination (e.g. after perforation) at sites of gross fibrin deposition and are highly variable in terms of vascularity.

Complications of adhesions

The most common adhesion-related problem is small bowel obstruction (SBO). Adhesions are the most frequent cause of SBO in resource-rich countries and are responsible for 60–70% of SBOs (see ***Chapter 74***). Adhesions are also implicated as a major cause of secondary infertility (see ***Chapter 87***). The relationship of adhesions to chronic abdominal and pelvic pain is contentious. Unguided division of adhesions has not been shown to reduce chronic abdominal pain although conscious pain mapping (laparoscopy under local anaesthesia) to direct lysis may improve success rates.

A substantial industry has developed around the prevention of adhesions. To date, no agent or mechanism has been identified that reliably reduces adhesion formation.

Mesenteric cysts

Cysts may occur in any region of the mesentery (***Figure 65.16***). They are most often observed in mesentery adjoining the small intestine (60%) or the colon (40%) and can be classified as follows:

- chylolymphatic;
- enterogenous;
- traumatic;
- hydatid.

Chylolymphatic cysts

Although mesenteric cysts are rare, this is the most common variety, probably arising in congenitally misplaced lymphatic tissue that has no efferent communication with the lymphatic system (most frequently in the mesentery of the ileum). The thin wall of the cyst, which is composed of connective tissue

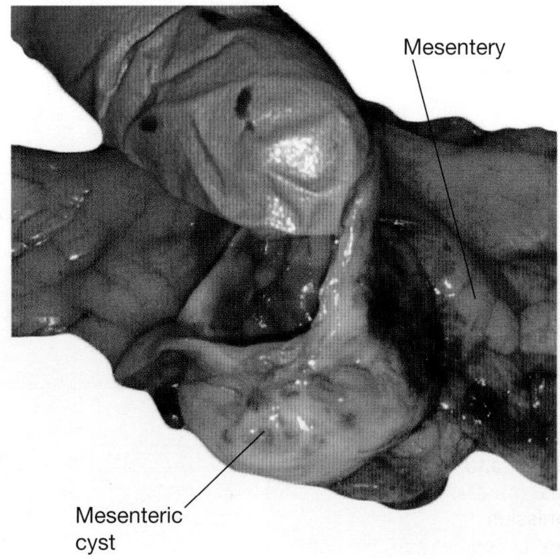

Figure 65.16 Mesenteric cyst. (Reproduced with permission from Coffey JC, Lavery I, Sehgal R (eds). *Mesenteric principles of gastrointestinal surgery: basic and applied principles.* Boca Raton: CRC Press, 2017: 85–108.)

lined by flat endothelium, is filled with clear lymph or, less frequently, with chyle, varying in consistency from watered milk to cream. Occasionally, the cyst attains a large size. More often unilocular than multilocular, a chylolymphatic cyst is almost invariably solitary, although there is an extremely rare variety in which myriads of cysts are found in various regions of the mesentery. A chylolymphatic cyst has a blood supply that is independent from that of the adjacent intestine and, thus, enucleation is possible without the need for resection of the gut.

Enterogenous cysts

These are believed to be derived either from a diverticulum of the mesenteric border of the intestine that has become sequestrated from the intestinal canal during embryonic life or from a duplication of the intestine (see ***Chapter 18***). An enterogenous cyst has a thicker wall than a chylolymphatic cyst and is lined by mucous membrane, which is sometimes ciliated. The content is mucinous and either colourless or yellowish brown as a result of past haemorrhage. The muscle in the wall of an enteric duplication cyst and the bowel with which it is in contact have a common blood supply; consequently, removal of the cyst always entails resection of the related portion of intestine.

Summary box 65.9

Mesenteric cysts: clinical features

- Cysts occur most commonly in adults with a mean age of 45 years
- Twice as common in women as in men
- Rare: incidence around 1 per 140 000
- Approximately a third of cases occur in children younger than 15 years
- The mean age of children affected is 5 years
- The most common presentation is of a painless fluctuant abdominal swelling near the umbilicus
- Other presentations are with recurrent attacks of abdominal pain with or without vomiting (pain resulting from recurring temporary impaction of a food bolus in a segment of bowel narrowed by the cyst or possibly from torsion of the mesentery) and acute abdominal catastrophe due to:
  - torsion of that portion of the mesentery containing the cyst
  - rupture of the cyst, often as a result of a comparatively trivial accident
  - haemorrhage into the cyst
  - infection

Tumours of the mesentery

Primary tumours of the mesentery include carcinoid, lymphoma, sarcoma and desmoid tumours. The mesentery is affected in local lymphatic spread of carcinoma arising from abdominal viscera (***Figure 65.17***). If indicated, a benign tumour of the mesentery may be excised with resection of the adjacent intestine. A malignant tumour of the mesentery requires biopsy confirmation and specific, usually non-surgical, treatment, e.g. chemotherapy for lymphoma.

Diffuse fibromatosis

Fibromatosis is rare, characterised by an abnormal proliferation of myofibroblasts. Although non-metastasising, and said to be benign, it can nevertheless prove widely invasive, compressing and infiltrating surrounding tissues such as the bowel and mesentery with complications thereof. There is an association with familial adenomatous polyposis (FAP).

Summary box 65.10

Mesenteric tumours

Benign
- Lipoma
- Fibroma
- Fibromyxoma
- Desmoid

Malignant
- Lymphoma
- Secondary carcinoma
- Neuroendocrine tumours
- Lymphatic metastases
- Tumour deposits (lymphovascular and perineural)
- Peritoneal carcinomatosis

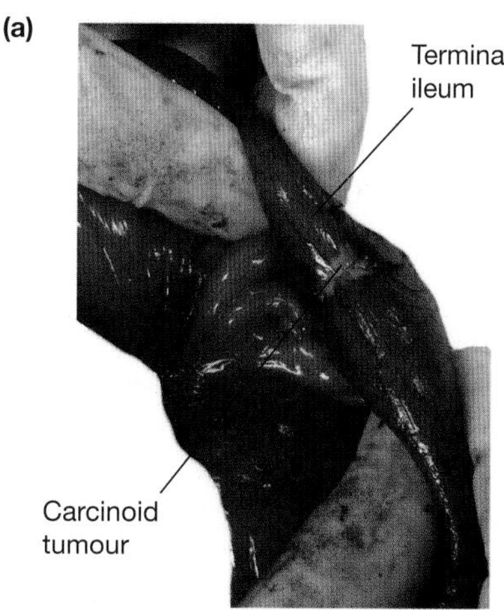

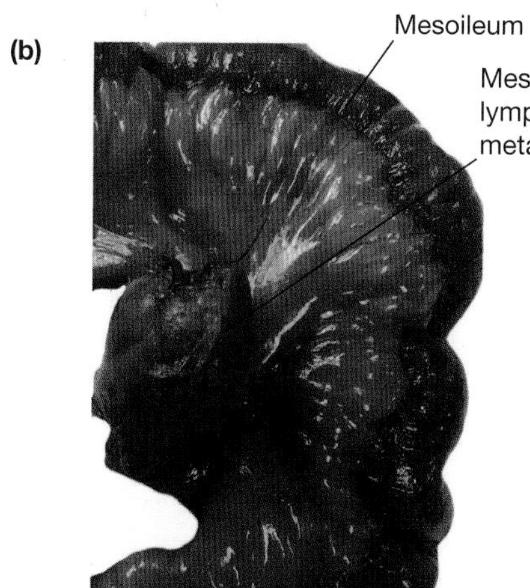

Figure 65.17 Terminal ileal carcinoid **(a)** and lymphatic metastasis **(b)**. (Reproduced with permission from Coffey JC, Lavery I, Sehgal R (eds). *Mesenteric principles of gastrointestinal surgery: basic and applied principles*. Boca Raton: CRC Press, 2017: 85–108.)

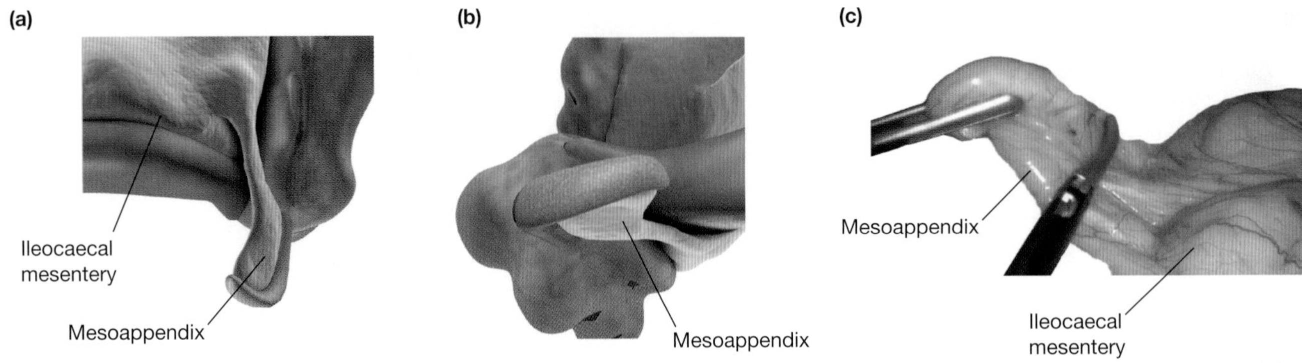

Figure 65.18 The mesoappendix. (Reproduced with permission from Coffey JC, Lavery I, Sehgal R (eds). *Mesenteric principles of gastrointestinal surgery: basic and applied principles*. Boca Raton: CRC Press, 2017: 11–40.)

THE GREATER OMENTUM

The **greater omentum** corresponds to the anterior wall of the upper region of the mesentery. Rutherford Morison called the greater omentum 'the abdominal policeman'. The greater omentum attempts, often successfully, to limit intraperitoneal infective and other noxious processes. For instance, an acutely inflamed appendix is often found wrapped in omentum, and this saves many patients from developing diffuse peritonitis. The omentum often plugs the neck of a hernial sac and prevents a coil of intestine from entering and becoming strangulated. The omentum can also be a cause of obstruction (acting as a large adhesion). The omentum is usually involved in tuberculous peritonitis and carcinomatosis of the peritoneum.

The **mesoappendix** arises from the posterior aspect of the ileocaecal region of the mesentery (*Figure 65.18*). As a result, it often occupies a retrocaecal position, as does the adjoining appendix. The position of the mesoappendix is thus a determinant of the symptoms and signs associated with acute appendicitis (see *Chapter 76*).

A **Meckel's diverticulum** (see *Chapter 74*) resembles the appendix in that it comprises an intestinal diverticulum at the periphery of a flange of mesentery. The latter arises from a nearby small intestinal region of mesentery.

The bloodless fold of Treves, a flange of mesentery at the antimesenteric side of the ileum just proximal to the ileocaecal valve, is a mesenteric remnant that arises after differentiation of the intestine at that level.

THE RETROPERITONEAL SPACE AND RETROPERITONEUM

The non-mesenteric domain is posterior to the mesenteric domain. The space between both is termed the retroperitoneal space (*Figure 65.19*) (*65.4*). It is a conceptual space as it contains areolar connective tissue. Regions of the connective tissue were separately named Toldt's, Waldeyer's, Denonvilliers', Gerota's and Fredet's fascia, as if they are separate entities. These are merely different zones of the same connective tissue layer that is interposed between the mesenteric domain in front and the non-mesenteric domain behind.

The space continues into the thorax and thereafter into the neck. This explains why, on occasion, a patient with an intestinal perforation during colonoscopy develops surgical emphysema and crepitus at the neck level. In these cases, perforation occurs into the retroperitoneal space (*Figure 65.20*). Gas tracks along the space into the thorax and thereafter into the neck, where it accesses subcutaneous tissue to generate surgical emphysema and crepitus. The volume of gas insufflated can be considerable given that the peritoneal cavity will not have been entered and the endoscopist may not recognise the perforation. The space may be obliterated following radiation treatment, in Crohn's disease or in longstanding diverticular inflammation. This presents considerable challenges for the surgeon who needs access to the plane whenever conducting visceral surgery.

James Rutherford Morison, 1853–1939, Professor of Surgery, University of Durham, Durham, UK.
Sir Fredrick Treves, 1853–1923, surgeon, the London Hospital, London, UK, renowned for operating on King Edward VII for appendicitis, resulting in the postponement of the coronation and his care for Joseph Merrick, the 'elephant man'.
Carl Toldt, 1840–1920, Professor of Anatomy in Prague, the former Czechoslovakia, and later Vienna, Austria.
Wilhelm von Waldeyer-Hartz, 1836–1921, Professor of Anatomy, Berlin, Germany.
Charles-Pierre Denonvilliers, 1808–1872, Professor of Surgery and Anatomy, Paris, France.
Dimitrie Gerota, 1867–1939, Professor of Surgical Anatomy, Bucharest, Romania.
Pierre Fredet, 1870–1946, surgeon, Paris, France.

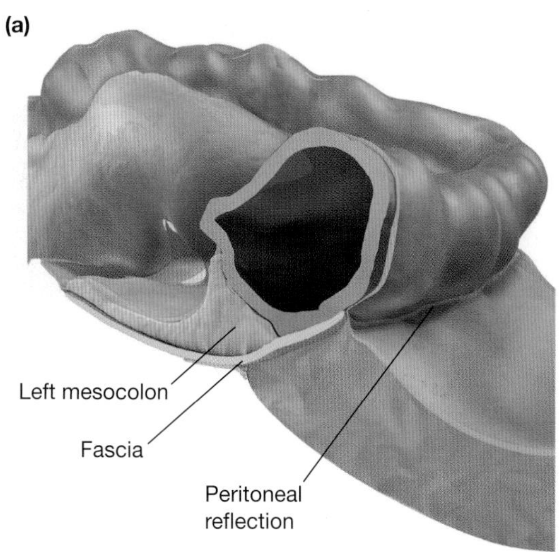

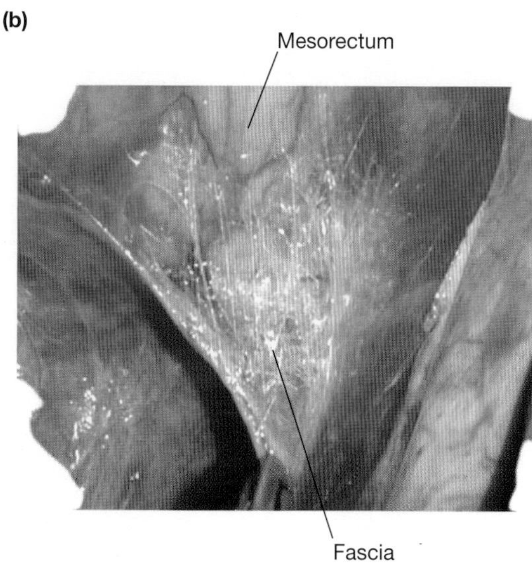

Figure 65.19 The retroperitoneal space. (a) Digital image of the fascia (green) located in the retroperitoneal space. (b) Intraoperative appearance of fascia in the retroperitoneal space. (Reproduced with permission from Coffey JC, Lavery I, Sehgal R (eds). *Mesenteric principles of gastrointestinal surgery: basic and applied principles*. Boca Raton: CRC Press, 2017: 11–40 and 57–68.)

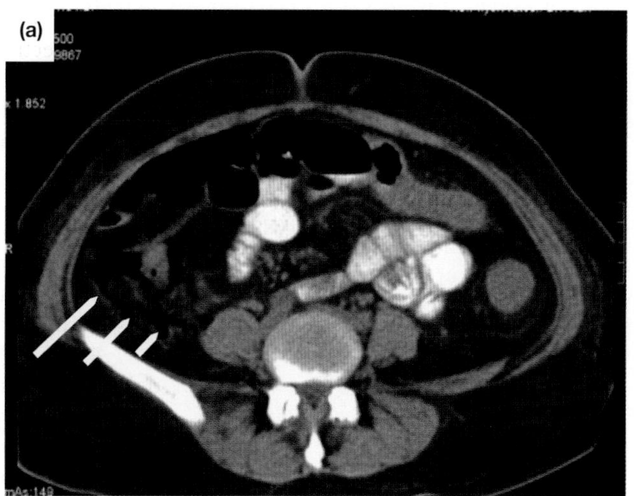

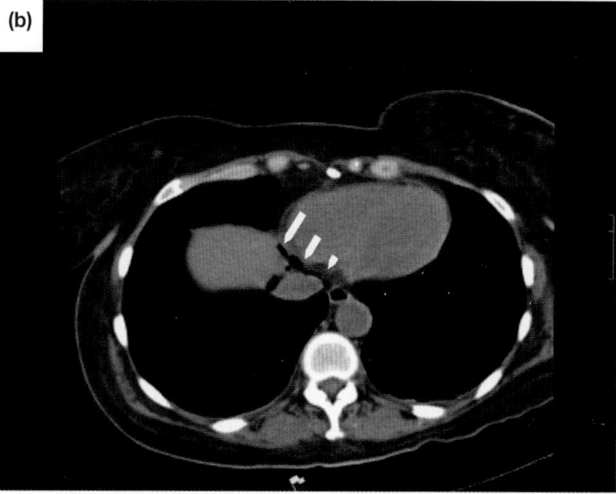

Figure 65.20 Perforation into the retroperitoneal space. Axial computed tomography section of the abdomen demonstrating gas (arrows) in the retroperitoneal space (a) and mediastinum (b).

RETROPERITONEAL SPACE COLLECTIONS

These are fluid collections in the retroperitoneal space and these differ from intraperitoneal collections because of their location (*Figure 65.21*). They are a common finding in moderate to severe acute pancreatitis. Fluid accumulates as a result of pancreatic inflammation, dissecting the left mesocolon off the underlying fascia and posterior abdominal wall. With continued expansion retroperitoneal space collections track subperitoneally around the flanks. A rapidly expanding retroperitoneal collection, such as occurs with a ruptured aortic aneurysm, may rupture intraperitoneally.

THE RETROPERITONEUM

The retroperitoneum is the region of the non-mesenteric domain deep to the retroperitoneal space. It contains the kidneys, adrenal glands, major vessels, ureters and gonadal vessels and is surrounded by adipose tissue.

Swellings in the retroperitoneum include abscess, haematoma, cysts and malignancy from retroperitoneal organs (kidney, ureter, adrenal). The term retroperitoneal tumour refers to primary tumours arising in connective tissues in this region.

Retroperitoneal fibrosis

This is a relatively rare diagnosis characterised by development of a flat grey/white plaque of tissue that usually develops in

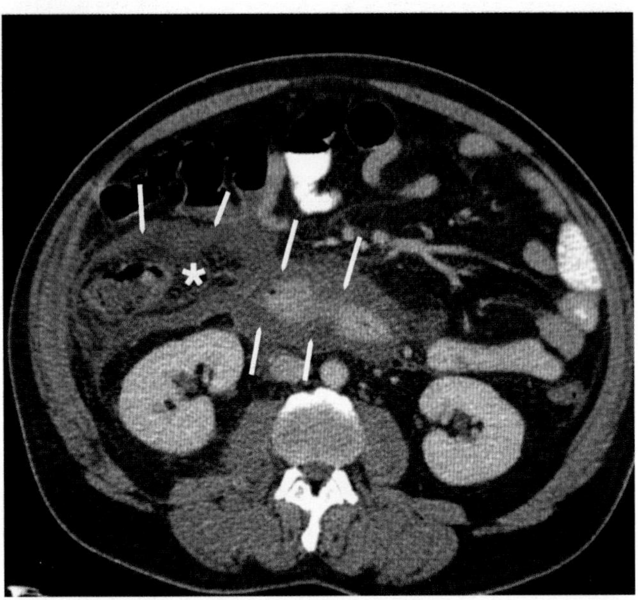

Figure 65.21 Computed tomography scan demonstrating retroperitoneal space collection in acute pancreatitis. The collection (arrows) has dissected the right mesocolon (asterisk) and duodenum, off the underlying retroperitoneum. Fluid is apparent in the retroperitoneal space.

the low lumbar region and later spreads laterally and upwards to encase the common iliac vessels, ureters and aorta. Histological appearances vary from active inflammation with a high cellular content interspersed with bundles of collagen through to one of relative acellularity and mature fibrosis/calcification. Its aetiology is obscure in most cases (idiopathic; synonym Ormond's disease), being allied to other fibromatoses (others being Dupuytren's contracture and Peyronie's disease).

Summary box 65.11

Causes of retroperitoneal fibrosis

Benign

- Idiopathic (Ormond's disease)
- Chronic inflammation
- Extravasation of urine
- Retroperitoneal irritation by leakage of blood or intestinal content
- Aortic aneurysm (inflammatory type)
- Trauma
- Drugs (chemotherapeutic agents and previously methysergide)

Malignant

- Lymphoma
- Carcinoid tumours
- Secondary deposits (especially from carcinoma of stomach, colon, breast and prostate)

Retroperitoneal (psoas) abscess

The psoas abscess is an abscess of the retroperitoneum (***Figure 6.22***). At the start of the twentieth century, psoas abscess was mainly caused by TB of the spine (Pott's disease). With the decline of *M. tuberculosis* as a major pathogen in resource-rich countries, a psoas abscess was mostly found secondary to direct spread of infection from the inflamed digestive or urinary tract with or without perforation. In more recent years it is most commonly seen in advanced Crohn's disease. Rarely, it arises due to haematogenous spread from an occult source in immunocompromised patients and in association with intravenous drug misuse.

History

Clinical presentation is with back pain, lassitude and fever. A swelling may point to the groin as it tracks distally along the iliopsoas muscle, under the inguinal ligament. Pain may be elicited by passive extension of the hip or a fixed flexion of the hip evident on inspection.

Investigation and treatment

Radiological investigation is by CT scanning and treatment is usually by percutaneous CT-guided drainage and appropriate antibiotic therapy. Surgical intervention is required if these are unsuccessful.

Retroperitoneal lipoma

The patient may seek advice on account of a swelling or because of indefinite abdominal pain. The swelling sometimes reaches an immense size. Diagnosis is usually by CT scan. A retroperitoneal lipoma sometimes undergoes myxomatous degeneration, a complication that does not occur in a lipoma

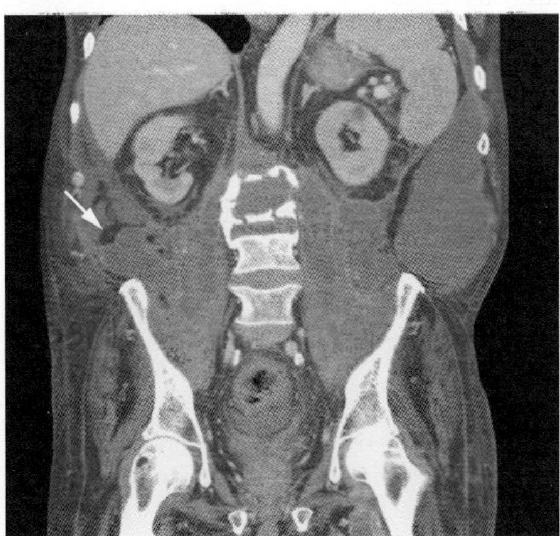

Figure 65.22 Representative sagittal computed tomography reconstruction of a right-sided psoas abscess (arrow) (courtesy of Dr K Patel, Homerton University Foundation Trust, London, UK).

John Kelso Ormond, 1886–1978, urologist, Ann Arbor, MI, USA.
Baron Guillaume Dupuytren, 1777–1835, Surgeon in Chief, Hôtel Dieu, Paris, France.
François Gigot de la Peyronie, 1678–1747, surgeon to King Louis XIV of France.
Percival Pott, 1714–1788, surgeon, St Bartholomew's Hospital, London, UK.

in any other part of the body. A lesion that rapidly increases in size is often malignant (liposarcoma).

Retroperitoneal sarcoma

Retroperitoneal sarcomas are rare tumours accounting for only 1–2% of all solid malignancies (10–20% of all sarcomas are retroperitoneal). The peak incidence is in the fifth decade of life, although they can occur at almost any age. The most frequently encountered cell types are:

- liposarcoma;
- leiomyosarcoma;
- malignant fibrous histiocytoma.

History and examination

Patients with sarcomas present late because these tumours arise in the large potential spaces of the retroperitoneum and can grow to a considerable size without producing symptoms. Moreover, when symptoms do occur, they are non-specific, such as abdominal pain and fullness, and are easily dismissed as being caused by other less serious processes. Retroperitoneal sarcomas are therefore often very large at the time of presentation.

Investigation

Detailed multiplanar imaging (CT and MRI) with reconstructions is required not only for tumour detection, staging and surgical planning but also for guiding percutaneous or surgical biopsy of these tumours.

Treatment

The definitive treatment of primary retroperitoneal sarcomas is surgical resection. Chemotherapy and radiotherapy without surgical debulking have rarely been beneficial, when used alone or in combination. A multidisciplinary treatment approach with imaging review will be required when assessing operability (based on adjacency or involvement of vital structures) and approach. Up to 75% of retroperitoneal sarcoma resections involve resection of at least one adjoining intra-abdominal visceral organ (commonly large or small bowel or kidney). The most common types of vascular involvement precluding resection are involvement of the proximal superior mesenteric vessels or involvement of bilateral renal vessels.

Prognosis

Survival rates are in general poor, even after complete resection, being of the order of 35–50% (excluding low-grade liposarcomas, which may frequently be cured by resection).

ACKNOWLEDGEMENTS

The author would like to acknowledge the artistic support of Dara Walsh, who generated all digital images and videos. He would also like to acknowledge Mr Kevin Byrnes for his work on the development of the mesentery and abdominal digestive system.

FURTHER READING

Byrnes KG, McDermott K, Coffey JC (eds). Mesenteric organogenesis. *Semin Cell Dev Biol* 2019; **92**: 1–138.

Coffey JC, Dockery P. Peritoneum, mesentery and peritoneal cavity. In: Standring S (ed.). *Gray's anatomy: the anatomical basis of clinical practice*, 42nd edn. Elsevier Limited, 2021: 1150–60.

Coffey JC, Lavery I, Sehgal R (eds). *Mesenteric principles of gastrointestinal surgery: basic and applied principles*. Boca Raton: CRC Press, 2017.

de Bakker BS, de Jong KH, Hagoort J *et al.* An interactive three-dimensional digital atlas and quantitative database of human development. *Science* 2016; **354**(6315): aag0053.

Ha CWY, Martin A, Sepich-Poore GD *et al.* Translocation of viable gut microbiota to mesenteric adipose drives formation of creeping fat in humans. *Cell* 2020; **183**(3): 666–83.

Sadler TW. *Langman's medical embryology*, 14th edn. Lippincott Williams & Wilkins, 2019.

World Gastroenterology Organisation. *WGO practice guideline – digestive tract tuberculosis*, 2021. Available from https://www.worldgastroenterology.org/guidelines/digestive-tract-tuberculosis.

CHAPTER 66 The oesophagus

Learning objectives

To understand:

- The anatomy and physiology of the oesophagus and their relationship to disease
- The clinical features, investigations and treatment of benign and malignant disease with particular reference to common adult disorders

APPLIED SURGICAL ANATOMY AND PHYSIOLOGY

The oesophagus is a muscular tube connecting the pharynx to the stomach. It starts at the level of the cricoid cartilage (C6 vertebra) and ends at the oesophagogastric junction (OGJ) (opposite T11 thoracic vertebra). In the neck, it descends behind the trachea and anteriorly to the vertebral column following its curvature into the thorax. At the lower part of the thoracic cavity, it transverses the diaphragmatic hiatus, clasped by the crura of the diaphragm and into the stomach. There are slight curvatures of the oesophagus; in the neck, it leans slightly more towards the left side, while in the mid-chest it curves slightly towards the right and in the lower part of the thorax edges to the left again. Thus, in the neck exposure of the cervical oesophagus is generally easier from the left side. The recurrent laryngeal nerves lie in the tracheo-oesophageal grooves. On the right side, the recurrent laryngeal nerve at the lower neck is often at a small distance from the tracheo-oesophageal groove, while on the left side the nerve is apposed closely to the oesophagus and trachea. This is an important anatomical detail when exposing the oesophagus and when cervical lymphadenectomy is performed. In perforation from Boerhaave's syndrome, the perforation tends to affect the lower oesophagus on the left side, as this part of the oesophagus is less well supported anatomically.

There are multiple relative constrictions along the oesophagus. First is the upper oesophageal sphincter (UOS); second is where the arch of the aorta/left main bronchus crosses the oesophagus; and third is the lower oesophageal sphincter (LOS). Foreign bodies such as food boluses tend to lodge at these sites.

The UOS is a structural sphincter formed by a band of striated muscles of the inferior pharyngeal constrictor and cricopharyngeus. The LOS is much less well defined. It is a complex interplay of the intrinsic muscle tone of the oesophageal wall, as well as the diaphragmatic crura. It is also variably exposed to the negative intrathoracic and positive intra-abdominal pressure. Thus, on oesophageal manometry, it is identified as a high-pressure zone; the diaphragmatic contribution is more obvious in the presence of a hiatus hernia, where two components of the high-pressure zone can be identified. Disorders of the coordination in UOS and pharyngeal function can result in dysphagia or aspiration symptoms. A common example is in elderly patients following a cerebrovascular accident or in those with neurological diseases. Dysfunction of the UOS is also related to the pathogenesis of the pharyngeal pouch/upper oesophageal diverticulum (Zenker's). Weakness of the LOS or inappropriate relaxation can result in oesophagogastric reflux disease (GORD), or tightness (incomplete relaxation) can lead to dysphagia, such as in achalasia.

For clinical purposes, the oesophagus is divided into the cervical, the thoracic and the abdominal oesophagus (***Figure 66.1***). These divisions are relevant for cancer staging purposes. The 'cardia' is the portion of the stomach that lies immediately below the OGJ, but there is no clear definition of its extent. Tumours around this region are often referred to as cancer of the cardia; however, it may be better to refer to 'cancer at the oesophagogastric junction'.

Anatomically the OGJ is defined as the point where the tubular oesophagus becomes the saccular stomach; histologically it is the junction between the squamous mucosa and the columnar mucosa, but these levels will be different in Barrett's oesophagus. The physiological LOS does not correspond to the anatomical OGJ; the LOS is a high-pressure zone defined physiologically but not anatomically. In practice, the most relevant definitions relate to findings on endoscopy. Endoscopically the OGJ is defined as the top of the gastric folds (the oesophagus is tubular and does not have folds while the stomach has rugae). In Japan, it is also commonly recognised as

Hermann Boerhaave, 1668–1738, Professor of Medicine and Botany, the University of Leiden, The Netherlands.
Friedrich Albert Zenker, 1825–1898, Professor of Pathology, Dresden, Germany.
Norman Rupert Barrett, 1903–1979, surgeon, St Thomas' Hospital, London, UK.

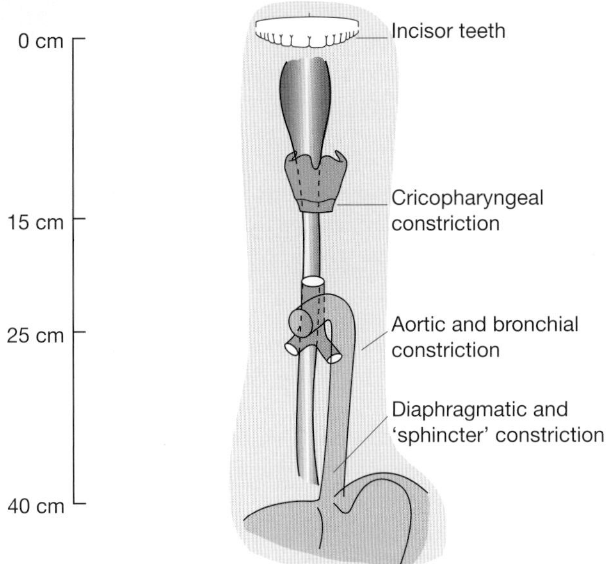

Figure 66.1 Anatomy of the oesophagus, divisions of the oesophagus and measurements endoscopically from the incisors. The three relatively 'narrow' parts of the oesophagus are at the level of the cricopharyngeus muscle (upper oesophageal sphincter), where the left main bronchus and aorta cross the oesophagus and the oesophagogastric junction (lower oesophageal sphincter).

the distal end of the oesophagus where palisading vessels are found (*Figure 66.2*). Which definition used is not so important; rather, it requires experience from the endoscopist to define this point accurately. In a real-life situation, the junction is somewhat dynamic with the patient's breathing excursions; an excessive amount of air insufflation may 'flatten' the gastric folds, making it difficult to define their 'top'. The presence of a hiatus hernia adds to the difficulty. The location of the junction is important in defining hiatus hernia, assessing the presence of Barrett's oesophagus, defining cancers around the OGJ and tumour staging.

Histologically the oesophageal wall has layers: mucosa, submucosa, muscularis propria and adventitia. The mucosa consists of a non-keratinised stratified squamous epithelium, the lamina propria and the muscularis mucosae. The oesophageal wall lacks a serosa; it is the muscularis mucosae and submucosa that give it strength for suture holding. The muscularis propria has an inner circular muscle and external longitudinal muscle layer (*Figure 66.3*). The muscle of the upper third of the oesophagus is made up of striated muscle, the middle third with a mixture of striated and smooth muscle and the lower third with smooth muscle. Connective tissue disease, such as scleroderma, mainly affects smooth muscle, hence the lower oesophagus.

The blood supply of the upper oesophagus is derived from the superior and inferior thyroid arteries. The middle oesophagus receives its supply from direct branches of the aorta and bronchial and intercostal vessels. The distal oesophagus has the arterial supply from the left gastric, left inferior phrenic and splenic vessels. The blood supply is usually excellent, and a long length of the oesophagus can be mobilised without compromising perfusion. An anastomotic leak from oesophageal anastomosis after oesophagectomy is rarely attributed to poor blood supply of the oesophagus; rather, it is the conduit that lacks perfusion. Venous return to the systemic circulation forms a network of vessels within the oesophageal wall. They drain to the inferior thyroid, azygos, hemiazygos and gastric veins. The communications of oesophageal veins and left gastric veins form part of the portal–systemic anastomosis. Cirrhosis leads to their dilatation (varices).

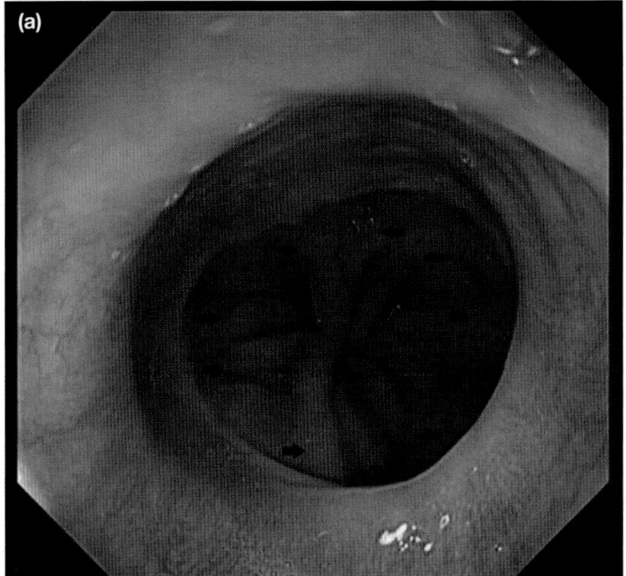

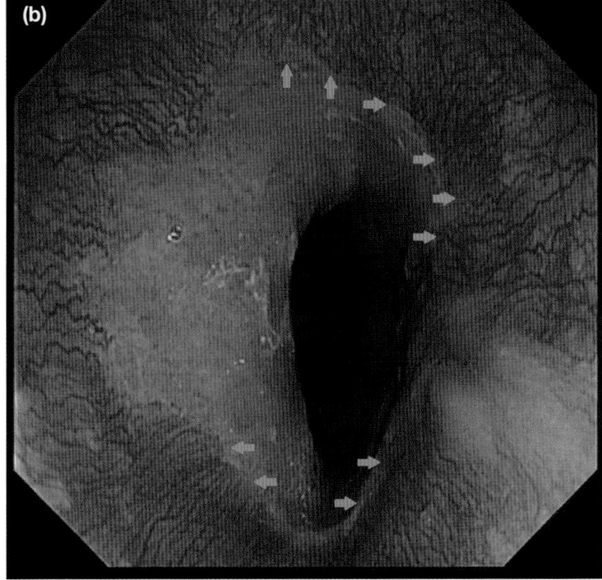

Figure 66.2 (a) Endoscopic image showing the 'top of the gastric folds' (black arrows), indicating that this is the oesophagogastric junction. (b) The distal end of the 'palisading vessels' also indicates the oesophagogastric junction (blue arrows pointing at the end of the palisading vessels).

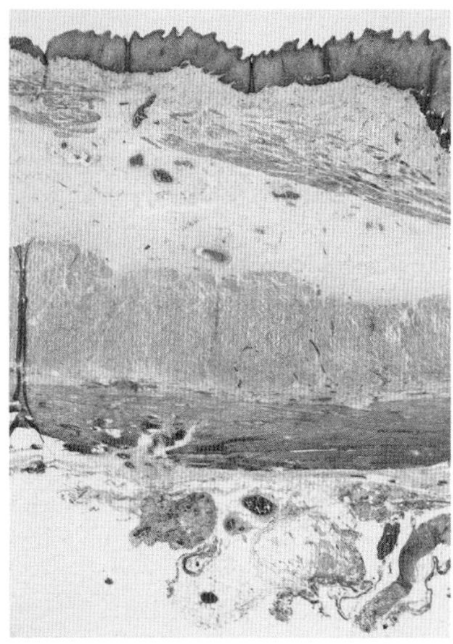

Figure 66.3 Histological layers of the oesophagus (courtesy of Dr Anthony Lo, Department of Pathology, Queen Mary Hospital, Hong Kong SAR, China).

The lymphatic drainage of the oesophagus is important, especially for cancer spread. There is a rich plexus of lymphatics in the submucosa, and direct drainage to the thoracic duct is also demonstrated. Submucosal spread of cancer along the oesophagus proximally and distally is common, and a longer resection margin reduces the chance of local recurrence. In the neck, the cervical oesophagus drains to the deep cervical and paratracheal nodes. In the thoracic oesophagus, lymphatic spread from a tumour can travel widely; potentially, it can spread to the neck, mediastinum and the nodes around the coeliac axis. Although upper third tumours tend to spread upwards and lower oesophageal cancer distally, this can be unpredictable and skip lesions can occur. Of particular importance is lymph node spread along the bilateral recurrent laryngeal nerves. This should be treated as a continuum of lymph node chains along both nerves, and thus they traverse from the chest into the neck. This widespread lymph node spread is the rationale behind the concept of three-field lymphadenectomy, whereby lymph nodes in the cervical region, mediastinum and around the coeliac axis are treated as regional nodes and dissection is recommended in curative surgery. The data mostly come from studies on squamous cell cancers in Japan. The lack of sufficient data for adenocarcinomas (mostly in the lower oesophagus) makes the benefit of such extended lymphadenectomy less certain.

The thoracic duct is the largest lymphatic vessel in the body. It is formed from the abdominal confluence of the left and right lumbar lymph trunks, as well as the left and right intestinal lymph trunks between T12 and L2. The confluence of lymph trunks is saccular and is referred to as cisterna chyli. Through the diaphragmatic hiatus, the thoracic duct is formed as it ascends along the aorta, next to the azygos vein and oesophagus. It then crosses to the left side at T4–T6, going upwards behind the aortic arch and left subclavian artery. In the left neck, it drains into the junction between the left jugular vein and left subclavian vein. Around 75% of the lymph from the entire body (aside from the right upper limb, right breast, right lung and right side of the head and neck) passes through the thoracic duct. The cells of the immune system circulate through the lymphatic system. Also, large molecular products of digestion, such as fats, first need to be absorbed into the lymphatic system, and then reach the systemic circulation through the venous system.

During oesophagectomy, the thoracic duct and its tributaries may be damaged, postoperatively presenting as chylothorax. The thoracic duct may also be injured during cervical lymphadenectomy, leading to a chylous leak from the neck wound after surgery. Prolonged chylous drainage cannot be tolerated because there is loss not only of fluid and electrolytes but also important proteins as well as lymphocytes, which cannot be replaced. The path of drainage of lymph explains the finding of Virchow's node (Troisier's sign), when a metastatic node is found in the left supraclavicular fossa, both from intra-abdominal malignancies as well as from oesophageal cancer.

INVESTIGATIONS OF OESOPHAGEAL DISEASES

Radiography

As a posterior mediastinal structure, the oesophagus is normally obscured on plain radiographs by other structures such as the spine, major vessels, airway and heart. However, this simple imaging test often gives clues of major pathologies, such as a dilated oesophagus with a fluid level in advanced achalasia (***Figure 66.4***) or pneumomediastinum and pleural effusion in oesophageal perforation (***Figure 66.5***). Radio-opaque foreign bodies can also be seen. A barium contrast swallow can demonstrate narrowing, anatomical distortion or abnormal oesophageal motility. It is however inaccurate in the diagnosis of GORD and should not be used for this purpose. Computed tomography (CT) scanning is important in the staging of a malignant neoplasm, delineating the anatomical relationship with other mediastinal structures, or detecting surgical site infection and extraluminal gas densities (***Figure 66.6***). When used in conjunction with oral contrast, CT is sensitive in identifying perforation and leakage.

Endoscopy

Endoscopy is an essential tool with both diagnostic and therapeutic roles. A standard diagnostic upper endoscopy includes the examination of the pharynx, hypopharynx, laryngeal inlet, oesophagus, stomach and part of the duodenum. The risk of the procedure, depending on complexity, is generally low. Extra care should be taken when performing endoscopy for patients with achalasia or obstruction as the oesophagus can be fluid-filled and regurgitation may lead to aspiration. For patients

Rudolf Virchow, 1821–1902, pathologist, Charité Hospital, Berlin, Germany.
Charles Émile Troisier, 1844–1919, pathologist, University of Paris, Paris, France.

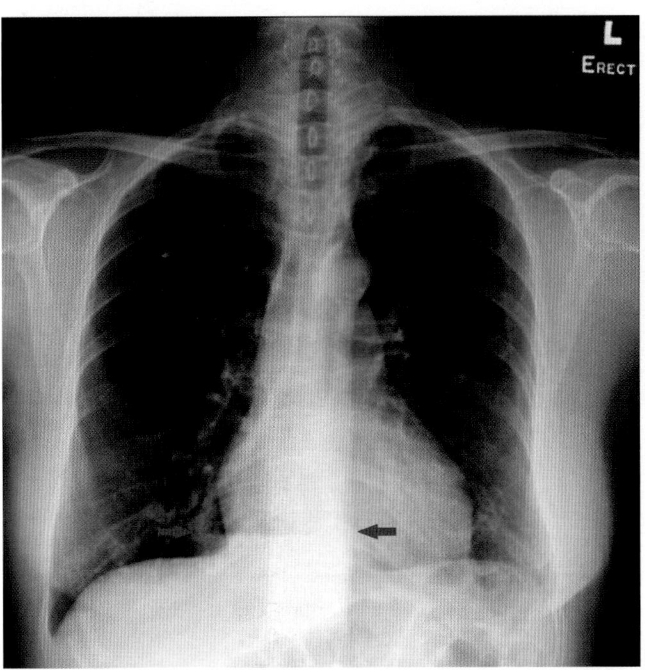

Figure 66.4 A fluid level (arrows) is apparent in a dilated oesophagus in a patient with achalasia.

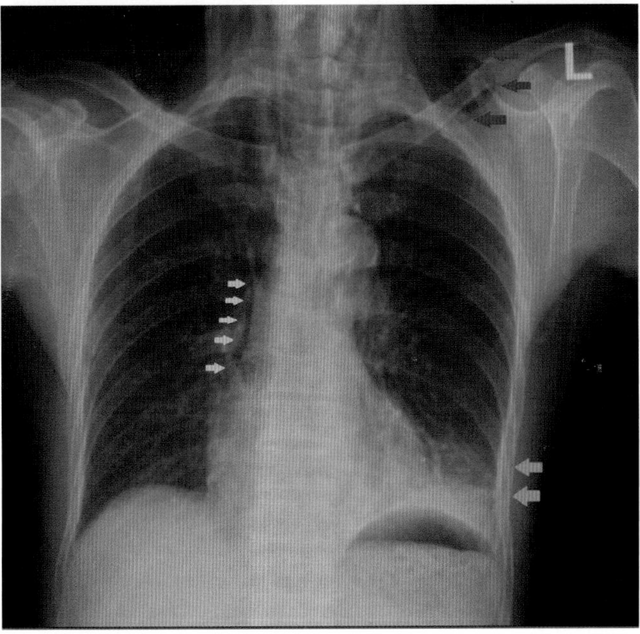

Figure 66.5 Chest radiography showing pleural effusion (blue arrows), subcutaneous emphysema (red arrows) and pneumomediastinum (yellow arrows).

with suspected oesophageal perforation or when the procedure is expected to be prolonged, carbon dioxide should be used for insufflation since it is absorbed more quickly than air. Rigid oesophagoscopy is rarely used nowadays except for unusual circumstances, such as retrieving large or sharp foreign objects. Flexible endoscopy with the use of an overtube is an alternative.

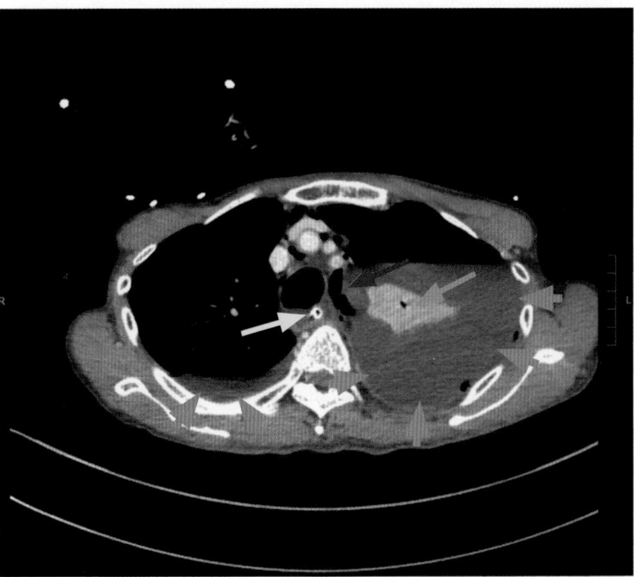

Figure 66.6 Computed tomography scan showing perforation of the oesophagus secondary to Boerhaave's syndrome. There is pneumomediastinum (red arrow), bilateral pleural effusion (blue arrows) and atelectasis of the left lung (orange arrow). A nasogastric tube is in the oesophagus (yellow arrow).

In patients with significant trismus or obstruction, an ultra-thin endoscope could be used, via either the oral or nasal route, to facilitate the diagnostic or therapeutic procedure. Increasingly ultra-thin endoscopy can be used in an outpatient clinic setting.

Image-enhanced endoscopy improves the diagnostic yield and sensitivity of assessment. It should be performed with a high-definition upper gastrointestinal endoscope, equipped with digital image enhancement such as narrow-band imaging (NBI) and magnification. It can be further supplemented by chromoendoscopy, using Lugol's iodine (0.5–1%) to look for any suspicious unstained areas and pink colour sign in squamous neoplasia. Similarly, acetic acid (1–3%) is used to look for any loss of aceto-whitening of the mucosal surface of Barrett's mucosa and neoplasia (***Figure 66.7***). Endocytoscopy is a novel ultra-high-magnification endoscopic technique enabling high-quality *in vivo* assessment of lesions with continuous zoom magnification up to 500 times. However, standardised staining methods and endocytoscopic classification are still lacking. With the aid of machine learning and deep learning by artificial intelligence, it is foreseeable that this technique of pattern recognition will greatly improve the sensitivity and specificity of early neoplasia detection and diagnosis.

Endosonography

Endoscopic ultrasonography (EUS) relies on a high-frequency (5–30 MHz) transducer to provide highly detailed images of the layers of the oesophageal wall and mediastinal structures close to the oesophagus. There are two types of EUS: radial echoendoscope, which has a rotating transducer that creates

Jean Guillaume Auguste Lugol, 1786–1851, physician, Hôpital Saint Louis, Paris, France, suggested that his iodine solution could be used to treat tuberculosis.

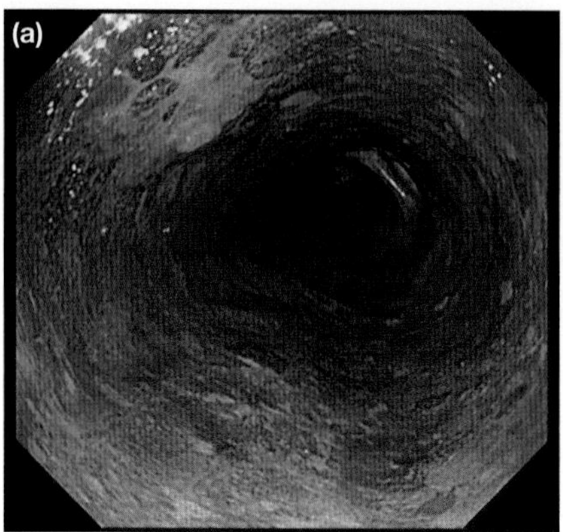

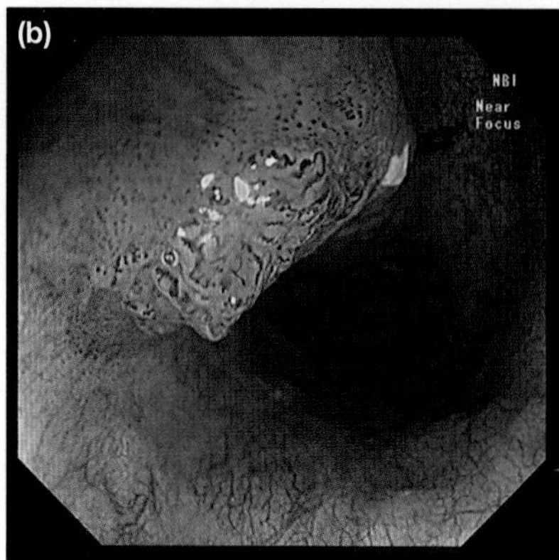

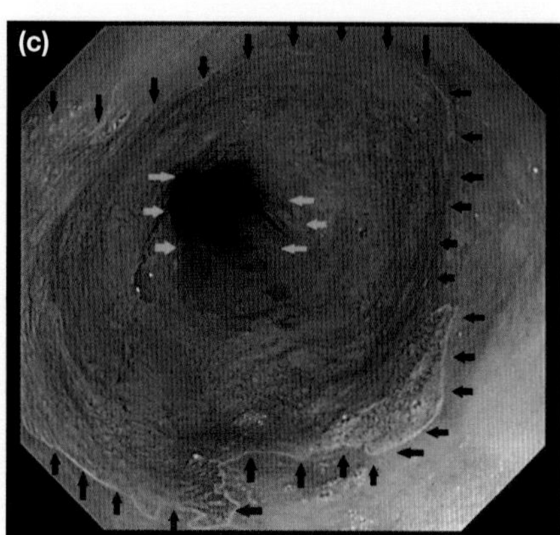

Figure 66.7 Endoscopic pictures of the oesophagus. (a) High-grade dysplasia of the oesophagus stained by Lugol's iodine solution. The unstained area is the abnormal area. (b) Early squamous cell cancer examined using narrow-band imaging. Abnormal intrapapillary capillary loops are seen. (c) Barrett's oesophagus stained by acetic acid (black arrows). Top of gastric fold (green arrows).

a circular image with the endoscope in the centre, and linear echoendoscope, which produces a sectoral image in the line of the endoscope. Mini-ultrasound probes that are around 2.0–2.9 mm in diameter can be inserted through the biopsy channel of an ordinary endoscope to give a simple radial diagnostic assessment within a narrowed lumen. This is useful for obstructive tumour.

The different layers of the oesophageal wall are characterised by its alternating echogenicity (*Figure 66.8*). Different structures can be identified adjacent to the oesophagus and used as landmarks, such as the aorta, the azygos vein and the spine. EUS can also provide a Doppler signal to differentiate index lesions from genuine vascular structures or abnormality before attempting biopsy. Biopsy of submucosal oesophageal lesions or mediastinal masses such as lymph nodes can be performed with linear echoendoscopes for histological diagnosis and staging.

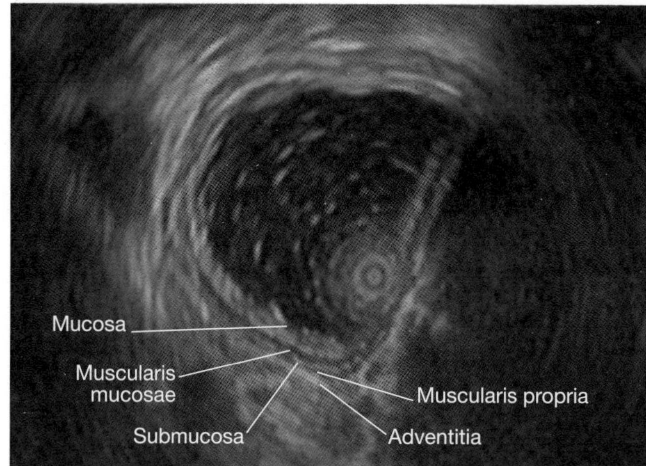

Figure 66.8 Endosonographic picture of an oesophagus. Five layers of the oesophageal wall can be seen.

Oesophageal manometry

Manometry is used to diagnose oesophageal motility disorders and to assess the oesophageal body and LOS function before surgery, such as antireflux operations. Conventional manometry was developed in the 1950s with water-perfused catheters. Recordings were made by passing a multilumen catheter (usually with only eight channels) down the oesophagus and into the stomach. The catheter is withdrawn progressively up the oesophagus and recordings are taken at intervals of 0.5–1.0 cm to measure the length and pressure of the LOS and assess motility in the body of the oesophagus during swallowing water boluses. With the introduction of the colour contour plot by Ray Clouse in 1995, conventional manometry is gradually being replaced by high-resolution manometry (HRM) with solid-state pressure catheters. A typical HRM catheter has 36 circumferential sensors along its length, each spaced 1 cm apart. HRM defines important anatomical landmarks and abnormality of the UOS, LOS and hiatus hernia. It also measures the contractility of the oesophageal body (*Figure 66.9*). Various parameters are measured in response to a standardised protocol of drinking a small volume of water. Other optional evaluations include solid test swallows and/or pharmacological provocation tests. Oesophageal peristalsis that is triggered by the swallow centre in the brain is called primary peristalsis. A hierarchical analysis is established under the Chicago classification to diagnose various oesophageal motility disorders.

Endoluminal functional lumen imaging planimetry

Endoluminal functional lumen imaging planimetry (FLIP) is a volume-controlled distension balloon device. It utilises impedance planimetry to measure the cross-sectional areas along the length of the balloon, and one pressure sensor measures the intra-balloon pressure. When placed inside the oesophagus

Christian Johann Doppler, 1803–1853, Professor of Experimental Physics, Vienna, Austria, enunciated the Doppler principle in 1842.
Ray E Clouse, 1951–2007, gastroenterologist, Washington University, St Louis, MO, USA.

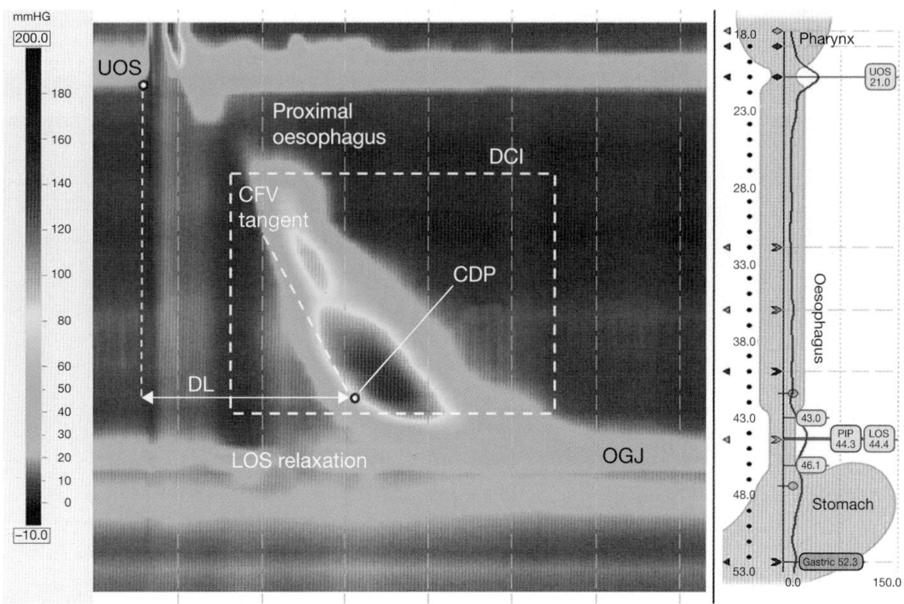

Figure 66.9 High-resolution manometry picture of a typical swallow. The break at the upper oesophageal sphincter (UOS) signifies the beginning of a swallow. The oesophageal body contractility is represented by the distal contractile integral (DCI), calculated by multiplying the pressure (mmHg) and time (seconds) along the whole length (cm) of the oesophageal body. There is a reflex relaxation of the lower oesophageal sphincter (LOS) upon each swallow. The time between the start of a swallow to the contractile deceleration point (CDP) is the distal latency (DL). CFV, contractile front velocity; OGJ, oesophagogastric junction; PIP, pressure inversion point.

spanning across the LOS, it gives a real-time assessment of LOS distensibility (cross-sectional area divided by intra-bag pressure) and oesophageal contractility in response to balloon distension. The device is mostly still investigational but is expected to gain wider clinical use. It can be used to guide the intraoperative end point for completeness of myotomy for achalasia (change in diameter and distensibility of the LOS) or in screening oesophageal function to assess the need for formal HRM (*Figure 66.10*).

Ambulatory reflux and combined pH-impedance monitoring

Ambulatory reflux monitoring is considered one of the most important confirmatory tests for GORD. There are two types of monitoring devices: catheter based and wireless capsule (*Figure 66.11*). Both measure the pH value at 5–6 cm above the upper border of the LOS, as defined by manometry. For the catheter-based device, data are captured conventionally for 24 hours. The wireless capsule device is anchored onto the mucosa of the oesophagus by a pin and can transmit pH data for up to 96 hours. Various parameters are measured, such as the number of reflux episodes (when pH drops below 4) and oesophageal acid exposure time (the percentage of time exposed to pH < 4) (*Figure 66.12*). An oesophageal exposure time of more than 4% can be considered abnormal, and one more than 6% is considered diagnostic. A composite score (Johnson–DeMeester) consists of six parameters that can be calculated. The patient needs to record their symptoms throughout the study period, so that symptom correlation with pH data can be calculated.

The catheter-based pH monitoring device also incorporates measurement of impedance. Impedance is inversely proportional to the electrical conductivity of the luminal contents and the cross-sectional area. Liquid refluxate has high conductivity and therefore low impedance. On the other hand, air has low conductivity and high impedance. With the change in the temporal–spatial patterns in different impedance sensors spreading across different levels of the monitoring catheter, any bolus transit can be assessed in its direction (antegrade or retrograde) as well as by its nature (air or liquid). Thus, acid reflux, aerophagia, belching and liquid passage can be distinguished (*Figure 66.13*).

GASTRO-OESOPHAGEAL REFLUX DISEASE

Aetiology

GORD is defined by the 'Montreal definition' as a condition that develops when the reflux of stomach contents causes troublesome symptoms and/or complications. The aetiology of GORD can be explained by the interaction between the reflux barrier and the pressure difference between the thoracic and abdominal cavity. The reflux barrier consists of the crural diaphragm and the LOS. Physiological relaxation of the LOS in response to stretching of the gastric fundus, particularly after a meal to allow venting of swallowed air, is termed transient

Lawrence F Johnson, contemporary, gastroenterologist, Birmingham, AL, USA.
Tom R DeMeester, contemporary, surgeon, Los Angeles, CA, USA.

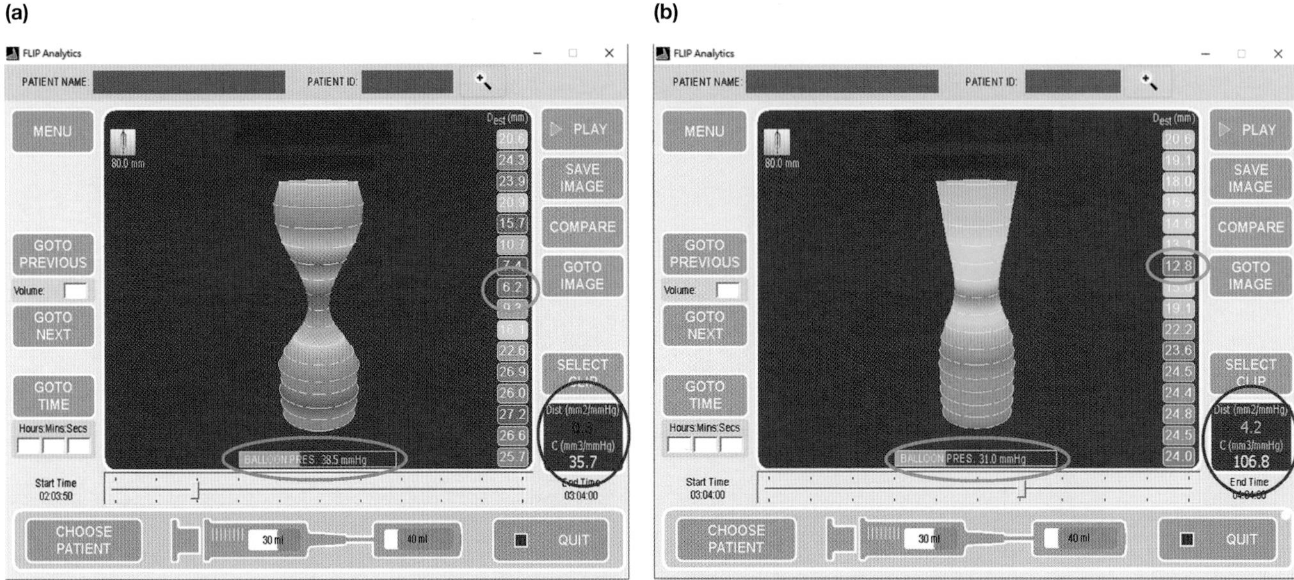

Figure 66.10 Endoluminal functional lumen imaging planimetry reading before **(a)** and after **(b)** peroral endoscopic myotomy (POEM) in a patient with achalasia. The column of numbers on the right-hand side of each panel shows the diameter of each 0.5-cm segment along the catheter (the narrowest segment is indicated by the green circle). This is used to calculate the cross-sectional area. The distensibility index (DI) (red circle) is calculated by dividing the cross-sectional area (mm^3) by the intra-balloon pressure (mmHg) (blue circle). The DI improves from 0.8 mm^3/mmHg to 4.2 mm^3/mmHg after POEM, indicating that the lower oesophageal sphincter has become more 'compliant'.

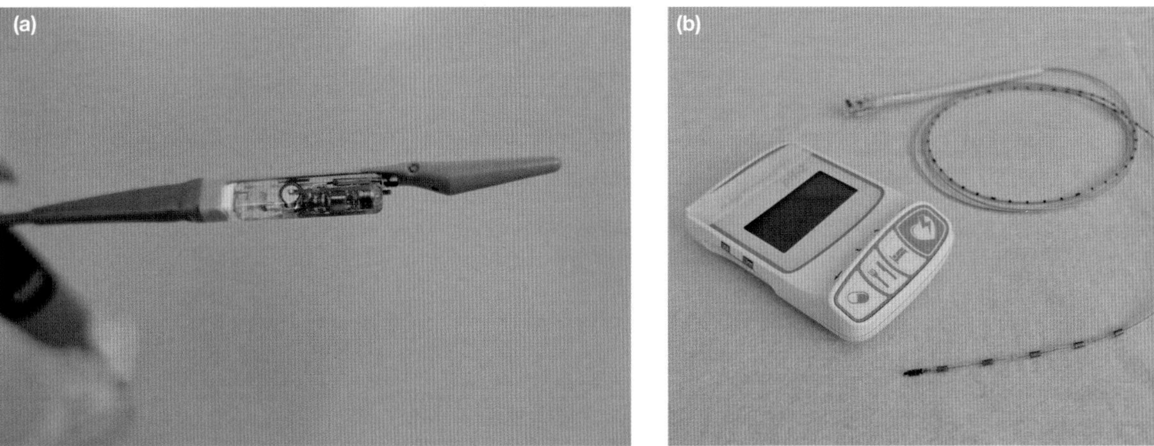

Figure 66.11 **(a)** Wireless capsule used to measure pH data in pH monitoring, with the capsule in the delivery catheter before deployment. **(b)** Catheter used to measure pH as well as impedance. The catheter is placed through the nostril. The most distal sensor is placed 5 cm above the upper border of the lower oesophageal sphincter measured on high-resolution manometry.

LOS relaxations (TLOSRs). An increased number of TLOSRs and a more compliant LOS would increase reflux. Delay in acid refluxate clearance from the oesophagus, as a result of defective oesophageal motility, also contributes to oesophageal exposure.

Hiatus hernia is associated with GORD; it is formed when the weakened phreno-oesophageal ligament and widened crural opening allow the proximal stomach to herniate through the diaphragmatic hiatus. Ageing, connective tissue disease and elevated intra-abdominal pressure (e.g. central obesity, pregnancy, tight garments, chronic straining) will further aggravate the hernia. An acid pocket is an area of unbuffered gastric acid that accumulates in the proximal stomach after meals and serves as a reservoir for acid reflux. Together with a hiatus hernia, it can exacerbate the severity and symptoms of GORD.

The overall global incidence of GORD is increasing and has a predominant regional distribution in the Americas and Europe; up to 33% of the population is affected, compared with <10% in Asia. The increase in GORD incidence is attributed to the global increase in obesity and declining rates of *Helicobacter pylori* infection. This increasing prevalence of GORD coincides with the increased mortality rates from oesophageal adenocarcinoma. Central obesity, independent of body mass index, is a risk factor for developing Barrett's oesophagus and adenocarcinoma, while *H. pylori* may have a preventive role.

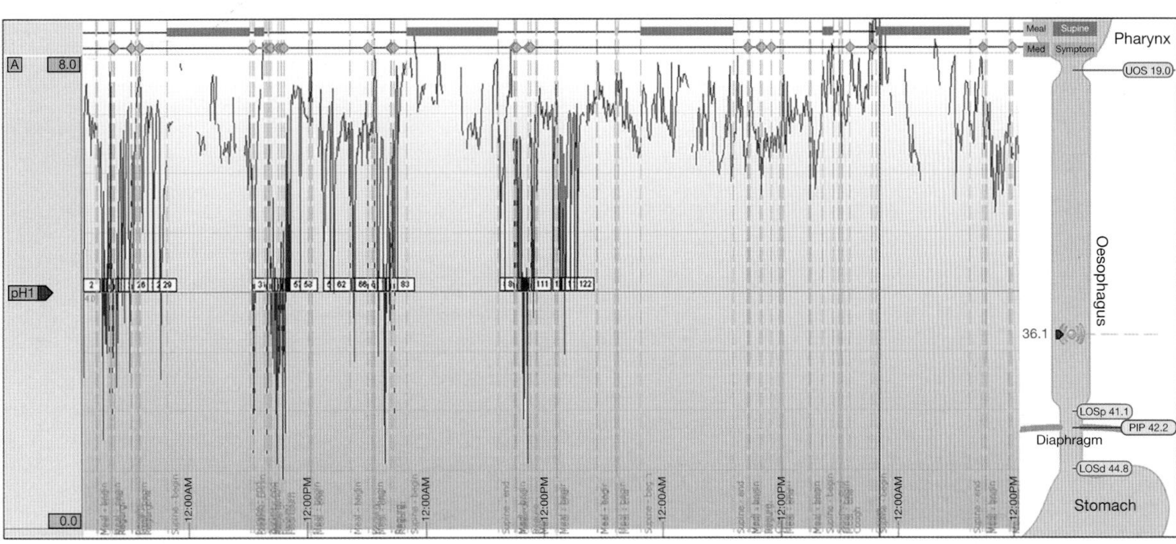

Interpretation / Findings

	DeMeester Score	Acid exposure time	No. of total reflux/post-prandial/supine	SI, SSI, SAP
Day1 off PPI	40.2	2 h 42 min	57/46/1	77.8, 12.3, 100.0
Day2 off PPI	16.9	1 h 17 min	54/48/0	85.7, 11.1, 100.0
Day3 on PPI	4.3	15 min	10/9/0	0
Day4 on PPI	0.3	0	0	0

Overall

- DeMeester Score = 15.9

Figure 66.12 A wireless pH monitoring trace over 4 days. A reflux episode is defined when the pH drops to less than pH 4 (below the horizontal blue line). This patient had stopped taking a proton pump inhibitor (PPI) 2 weeks before the study. He was then given a daily dose of PPI starting on day 3 of the examination. The DeMeester scores were abnormal (>14.7) on days 1 and 2 but returned to the normal range after acid suppression by the PPI. The symptom association probability (SAP) was 100% on days 1 and 2, meaning that every time there was acid reflux the patient experienced symptoms. SI, symptom index; SSI, symptom sensitivity index. LOSd, lower oesophageal sphincter, distal; LOSp, lower oesophageal sphincter, proximal; PIP, pressure inversion point; UOS, upper oesophageal sphincter.

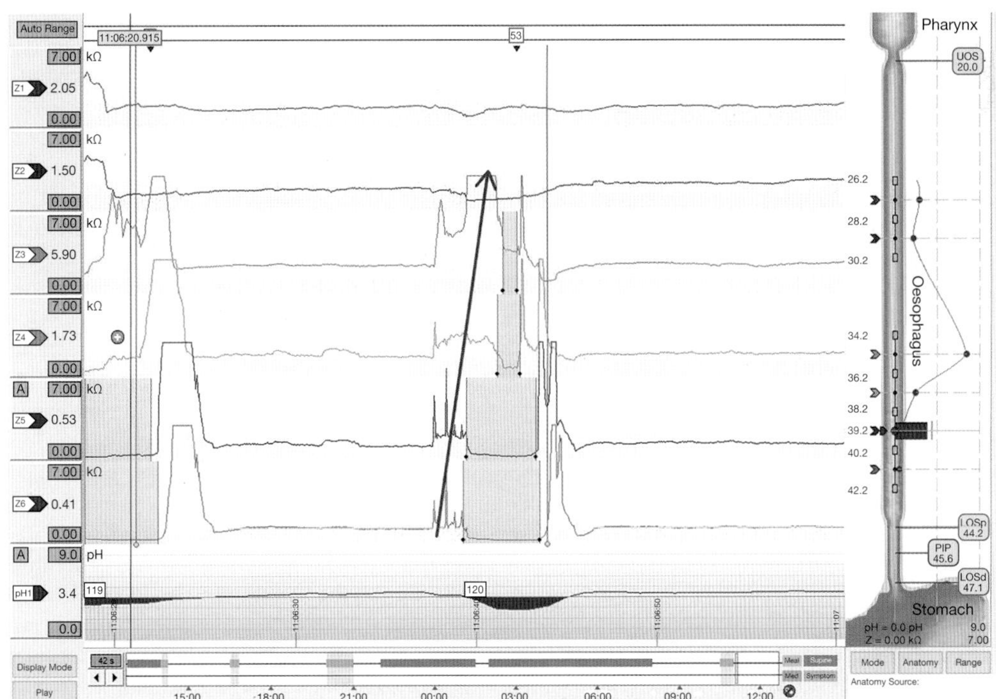

Figure 66.13 pH impedance data tracing. A drop in impedance signifies liquid within the oesophageal lumen while a belch (with air) results in a rise in impedance. In this figure, the x-axis represents time. There is a sequential drop of impedance from the distal sensor (Z6) to the more proximal sensor (Z3) (indicated by the red arrow and the shaded boxes), signifying a liquid reflux episode. At the same time, the pH sensor detected pH < 4 (lowest row), indicating that the reflux episode is an acid reflux. LOSd, lower oesophageal sphincter, distal; LOSp, lower oesophageal sphincter, proximal; PIP, pressure inversion point; UOS, upper oesophageal sphincter.

The postulated mechanism is that decreased acid production as a result of *H. pylori*-related corpus gastritis or gastric atrophy would lead to decreased oesophageal acid exposure.

Clinical features

Symptoms of GORD can be classified into oesophageal or extraoesophageal. Typical oesophageal complaints include heartburn, which is defined as a burning sensation behind the sternum, and regurgitation, which is the perception of the flow of refluxed gastric content into the mouth or hypopharynx. Patients may also complain of epigastric pain, which can be a manifestation of erosive oesophagitis. Symptoms cannot accurately predict the severity of the mucosal injury. Dysphagia can be related to large hiatus hernia, stricture or even oesophageal carcinoma. Bleeding from erosive oesophagitis, Cameron ulcers (gastric ulcers at the level of the diaphragmatic constriction within large hiatus hernias) or tumours can present as coffee-ground vomiting or frank haematemesis. Extraoesophageal symptoms may include chronic cough, laryngitis, asthma and dental erosions (especially on the lingual and palatal tooth surfaces). The causative relationship of extraoesophageal manifestations can sometimes be vague. These problems are usually multifactorial but can be aggravated by GORD. Other conditions with proposed association with GORD include sinusitis, pulmonary fibrosis, pharyngitis and recurrent otitis media.

Symptoms are often provoked by food, particularly after a full meal with increased intragastric pressure or food that delays gastric emptying (e.g. oily, spicy food). The refluxate can cause an unpleasant taste, often described as 'acidic' or 'bitter'. Intensive exercise may sometimes induce GORD in healthy subjects owing to an increase in intra-abdominal pressure. Some patients may complain of nocturnal symptoms especially when lying supine, probably related to the gravitational effect. This may significantly affect patients' sleep. Mild symptoms occurring two or more days a week or moderate/severe symptoms affecting more than one day a week are considered troublesome.

Diagnosis

In most cases, the diagnosis is assumed rather than proven, and treatment is empirical. Proton pump inhibitors (PPIs) are very effective drugs in managing erosive oesophagitis and acid-related symptoms. They are often used empirically as a diagnostic trial. However, there is a significant placebo effect. A positive treatment response with 2 weeks of a PPI can be observed in 69% of GORD patients and 51% of those without GORD (as defined by pH monitoring and endoscopic oesophagitis). This may create a problem of overdiagnosis of GORD and overuse of PPIs.

Endoscopic examination provides anatomical assessment, screening for complications of GORD and potential alternative diagnoses such as eosinophilic oesophagitis (EOO), oesophageal motility disorder or oesophageal cancer (***Figure 66.14***). In practice, many patients will have received PPIs before referral to endoscopy and such information must be available before the procedure because PPIs can heal oesophagitis quickly (***Figure 66.15***). It is worth remembering that the correlation between symptoms and endoscopic appearances is poor.

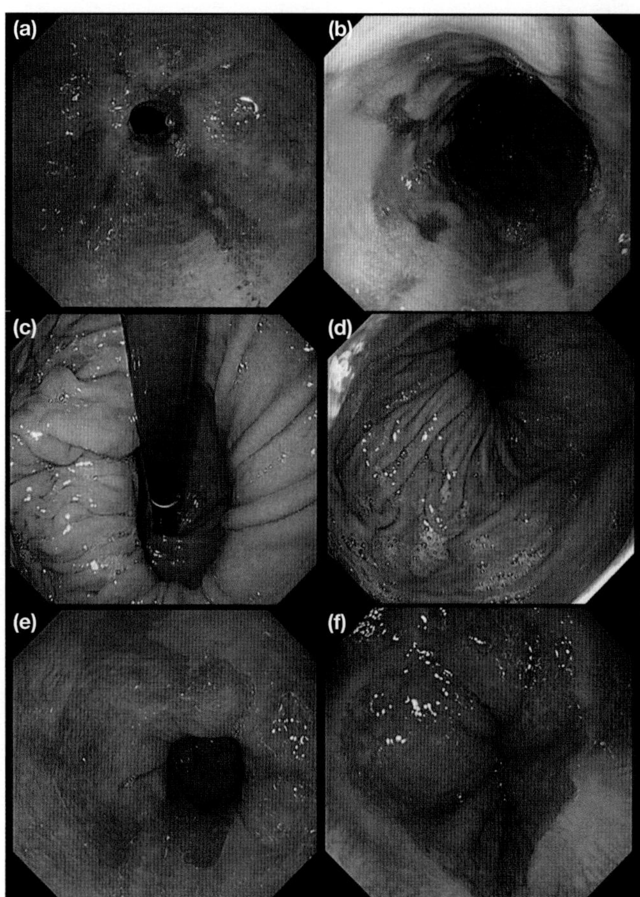

Figure 66.14 Endoscopic appearance of an oesophageal stricture with esophagitis **(a)**; Los Angeles classification grade C oesophagitis **(b)**; retrograde view of a hiatus hernia **(c)**; end view of a hiatus hernia **(d)**; Barrett's oesophagus **(e)**; normal oesophagogastric junction **(f)**.

In patients with atypical or persistent symptoms despite PPI therapy, oesophageal manometry and ambulatory pH recording (with or without impedance measurement) are justified to establish the diagnosis and guide management. In patients considered for surgery, it is also prudent to have objective proof of significant reflux before embarking on a potentially irreversible invasive procedure.

HRM is useful in (i) detecting major oesophageal motility disorder, e.g. achalasia, which can sometimes mimic GORD; (ii) defining the location of the LOS for accurate pH monitoring placement; (iii) assessing the function and morphology of the LOS, including the size of a hiatus hernia; and (iv) assessing oesophageal body motility to tailor intervention, especially the various antireflux procedures.

PPIs are usually stopped for 2 weeks before oesophageal pH recording. For patients with a strong pretest probability of

Alan J Cameron, contemporary, gastroenterologist, Mayo Clinic, Rochester, MN, USA.

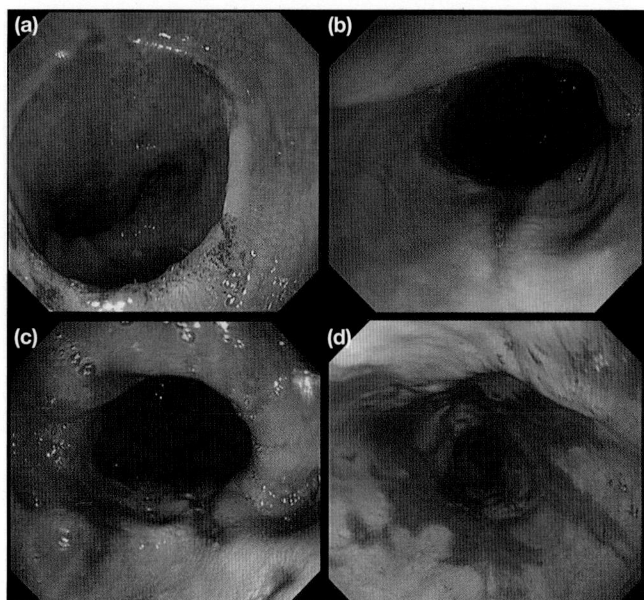

Figure 66.15 Grading of oesophagitis according to the Los Angeles classification. Grade A, one (or more) mucosal breaks no longer than 5 mm that do not extend between the tops of the two mucosal folds (a). Grade B, one (or more) mucosal breaks longer than 5 mm that do not extend between the tops of two mucosal folds (b). Grade C, mucosal breaks that are continuous between the tops of two or more mucosal folds but that involve less than 75% of the circumference (c). Grade D, mucosal break that involves at least 75% of the oesophageal circumference (d).

GORD but refractory to PPI treatment, an 'on-PPI' assessment can be performed to test for breakthrough acid exposure despite PPI therapy. Wireless pH monitoring increases the duration of recording to 96 hours and could potentially increase the test sensitivity and diagnostic yield.

A barium contrast study gives an objective and dynamic assessment of the oesophagogastric anatomy. This may be important in the context of surgery for rolling or mixed hiatus hernias. It is also useful in assessing surgical complications after antireflux surgery, such as a disrupted wrap, slipped fundoplication or wrap herniation. However, it is not mandatory for ordinary and uncomplicated GORD patients.

Management of uncomplicated GORD

Lifestyle modification

Patients are recommended to have a healthy diet, avoid overeating and avoid dietary items (e.g. carbonated drinks, alcohol, tea or coffee) or activities that in the patient's experience would provoke the symptoms. Patients with nocturnal symptoms should have early dinner and avoid recumbence after meals. Elevation of the head of the bed may also help. Smoking cessation reduces severe reflux symptoms in normal-weight individuals on medical treatment. Weight management is recommended for overweight patients.

Medical management

Most patients with GORD self-medicate with over-the-counter medicines such as simple antacids, antacid–alginate preparations and H_2-receptor antagonists. Consultation is more likely when symptoms are severe, prolonged and unresponsive to simple measures and treatments. Pharmacological treatments mainly target acid reduction or neutralisation. With the development of PPIs in the 1980s, they have quickly become the first-line treatment for symptomatic GORD. Given an adequate dose for 8 weeks, most patients have a rapid improvement in symptoms (within a few days), and more than 90% can expect full mucosal healing of oesophagitis (if present) at the end of this time. A policy of 'step-down' medical treatment is advocated after the initial 8 weeks of treatment to a dose that keeps the patient free of symptoms, and this might even mean the cessation of PPI.

Most patients do not make sustained major lifestyle changes and because PPIs are so effective many remain on long-term treatment. Those patients who have an inadequate treatment response may benefit from changing to another PPI, an increased dosage of the same PPI, a twice-a-day regimen or the addition of an H_2-receptor antagonist. PPI is also important in patients with reflux-induced strictures, resulting in significant prolongation of the intervals between endoscopic dilatations. There have been numerous reports on the association between chronic PPI use and a myriad of side effects. Most could not demonstrate a causal relationship except some enteric infections and fundic gland polyps. However, patients are still advised to use the lowest effective dose for symptom control.

Prokinetic agents, e.g. metoclopramide and domperidone, are not particularly useful and have potential safety issues. Other TLOSR inhibitors were also disappointing. Antacid–alginate preparations target the acid pockets and form a polysaccharide barrier at the proximal stomach. A more recent development are the potassium-competitive acid blockers (P-CABs). Compared with PPIs, P-CABs have a more rapid, competitive, reversible inhibition of proton pumps. However, they are available in only limited regions. With pH monitoring, it is possible to identify patients with different phenotypes, especially distinguishing those having pathological versus physiological reflux, and positive versus negative symptom correlations. For patients with discordant reflux activity and symptom association, as in oesophageal hypersensitivity or functional disorder, antireflux therapy is likely to fail. Other treatment options include perception modulators, e.g. tricyclic antidepressants and selective serotonin reuptake inhibitors (SSRIs), or alternative therapies, e.g. hypnosis and behavioural therapy.

Summary box 66.1

Gastro-oesophageal reflux disease

- GORD is common but symptomatology may be confused with other disorders, such as achalasia; both may present with regurgitation
- Sliding hiatus hernia predisposes to GORD
- Heartburn and regurgitation are typical GORD symptoms
- Beware of extraoesophageal manifestations of GORD
- A PPI is the most effective medical treatment, but regurgitation is not well controlled by PPIs

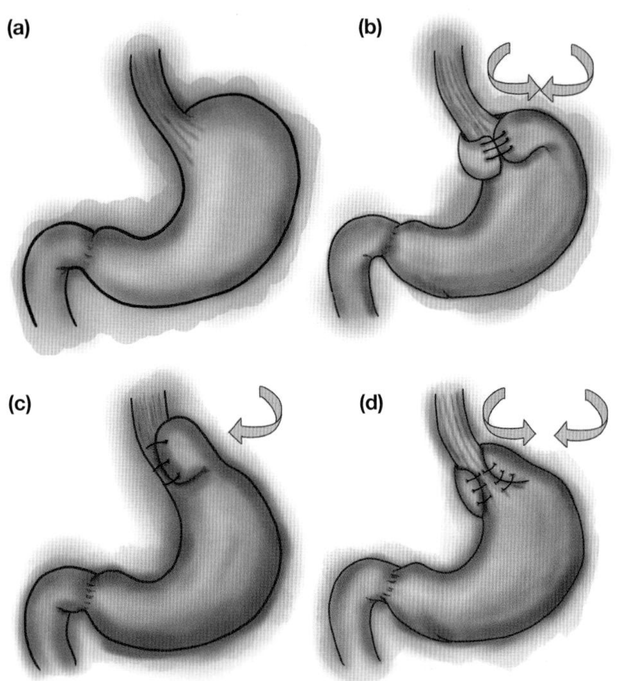

Figure 66.16 Examples of various types of fundoplication. (a) Normal anatomy. (b) Nissen 360° fundoplication. (c) Dor anterior fundoplication. (d) Toupet posterior fundoplication.

Surgical management

While most patients' symptoms are satisfactorily controlled with PPIs and other medications, surgery remains an important option. The indications for surgery include (i) incomplete symptom control with medical management, (ii) intolerance of, or unwillingness to comply with, long-term medical therapy, (iii) regurgitation despite medication (less well amenable to PPI), (iv) presence of a large hiatus hernia, (v) complications arising from GORD, and (vi) extraoesophageal symptoms. The predictors of good surgical outcome include typical GORD symptoms, PPI responders, presence of hiatus hernia and presence of GORD complications, e.g. reflux oesophagitis (grade B or above) and non-dysplastic Barrett's oesophagus. Factors leading to poor surgical outcomes are normal preoperative pH monitoring when performed off PPI, functional heartburn, EOO, connective tissue diseases and extreme obesity.

Careful preoperative counselling is essential. Risks of antireflux surgery include a small mortality rate (0.1–0.5%), failed operation (5–10%) and side effects such as dysphagia, gas bloat or abdominal discomfort (10%). When performed well in appropriately selected patients, 80–90% of patients should be satisfied with the result of the operation.

Which operation?

Antireflux operations have three essential components: (i) restoration of an intra-abdominal segment of the oesophagus, (ii) crural repair, and (iii) some form of reinforcement of the LOS by the upper stomach (fundoplication) or by a prosthesis placed around the intra-abdominal oesophagus.

The major types of antireflux operations were all developed in the 1950s. For many years, the relative merits of thoracic and abdominal approaches were hotly debated. With the introduction of laparoscopy, laparoscopic fundoplication with hiatal reconstruction is the standard approach. The mechanism of fundoplication is to create a 'floppy' valve around the OGJ and to restore the angle of His. It has the effect of increasing LOS basal pressure, lessening TLOSR and reducing the capacity of the gastric fundus, thereby enhancing gastric emptying. The different types of fundoplication have been compared extensively in clinical trials but the superiority of one over the others could not be shown.

Complete fundoplication (Nissen) is associated with a higher incidence of short-term dysphagia but is most durable in reflux control. Partial fundoplication, whether performed posteriorly (Toupet) or anteriorly (Dor, Watson), has fewer short-term side effects, although this is at the expense of a slightly higher long-term failure rate (***Figure 66.16***).

The most common side effect of fundoplication is short-term dysphagia, related presumably to tissue oedema and inflammation. It usually resolves within 3 months of surgery. Some patients may experience 'gas-bloat syndrome', especially after a complete fundoplication. Typically, the patient would complain of gaseous distension of the abdomen and failure to belch or vomit, together with an increase in flatulence.

In the last decade, a magnetic prosthesis has become available to reinforce the LOS after hiatal reconstruction (***Figure 66.17***). This has a similar efficacy to fundoplication in the mid- to long term and has fewer gas-bloat side effects. The magnetic ring prosthesis consists of titanium-coated magnetic beads, connected by titanium wire. The physics of the magnets allows a lower attraction force when the beads are separated. This property of 'relaxation' is a more physiological sphincter to allow food passage and is less likely to create oesophageal outflow obstruction. This device is contraindicated in patients with major motility disorders, ineffective oesophageal motility or connective tissue disease.

Summary box 66.2

Laparoscopic fundoplication

- HRM and pH monitoring are recommended investigations before consideration of surgical treatment
- pH monitoring confirms GORD and HRM assesses oesophageal body function and LOS characteristics
- Surgery should be tailored to oesophageal motility

Wilhelm His, 1831–1904, Professor of Anatomy, Leipzig, Germany.
Rudolph Nissen, 1896–1981, Professor of Surgery, Istanbul, Turkey, and later Basel, Switzerland.
André M Toupet, 1915–2015, surgeon, St Cloud Hospital, Senior Consultant, University of Paris, France, proposed his technique in 1963.
Jacques Dor, 1904–1997, thoracic surgeon, Marseilles, France.
Anthony Watson, contemporary, surgeon, Royal Free Hospital, London, UK.

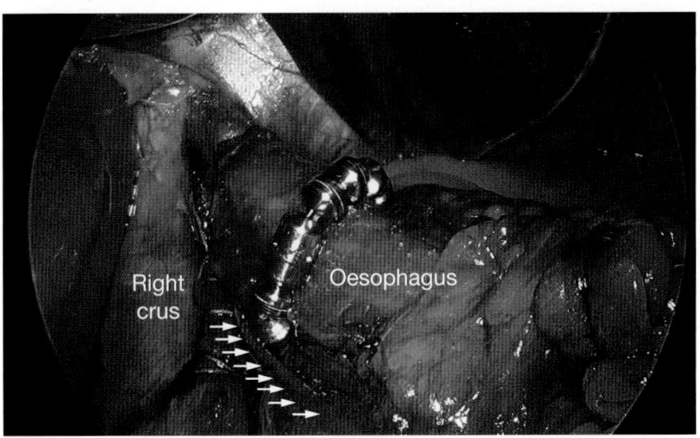

Figure 66.17 Magnetic sphincter augmentation. Intraoperative photograph following hiatus hernia repair. The magnetic sphincter is implanted around the lower oesophagus, in between the posterior vagus nerve (white arrows) and the oesophageal wall.

Complications of antireflux surgery and revisional surgery

Structurally, a wrap can be too tight or too loose. It can also be partially or completely disrupted, herniated or slipped. Structural laxity can give rise to recurrent or persistent GORD. Too long or too tight a fundoplication can give rise to dysphagia and gas-bloat syndrome. Endoscopy, contrast radiography and functional testing can assess the anatomy responsible and guide further management.

Management strategies include a PPI for recurrent acid reflux, endoscopic dilatation of stenosis and surgical revision as a last resort. A tight complete fundoplication can be remedied by conversion to a partial fundoplication. For patients with anatomical failure and refractory symptoms, revisional surgery carries a lower chance of success; in some patients, local revision is technically impossible, as often there will be adhesion formation and altered anatomy. Transient dysphagia is common after both fundoplication and magnetic sphincter augmentation. For the latter, there may be more prolonged dysphagia requiring dilatation or, rarely, migration and erosion (0.15%). Removal of the device is required in 2.7% of patients; the majority can be accomplished endoscopically or laparoscopically.

Endoscopic treatment

Several endoscopic treatments have been tested that attempt to augment a failing LOS. Transoral incisionless fundoplication mimics classic fundoplication by recreating the dynamics of the angle of His using an endoscopic stapling device. Meta-analysis demonstrates improvement in clinical response compared with PPIs; however, oesophageal acid exposure time and reflux episodes are not significantly improved and PPI usage increases with time. Radiofrequency ablation (RFA) is another strategy to remodel the LOS by reducing compliance. Again, it partially improves quality of life but does not normalise pH exposure time and almost 50% of patients still require PPI at follow-up. Antireflux mucosectomy makes use of the endoscopic mucosal resection (EMR) technique to remove subcardiac mucosa while preserving a 1-cm gap at the lesser and greater curves. The contraction and scarring presumably improve the reflux barrier. Small case series have shown improvement in both quality of life and acid reflux. A significant proportion of patients require balloon dilatation for stenosis. These procedures have been applied to patients with only small hiatus hernias or none at all, so only a small proportion of patients are suitable. Recently argon plasma coagulation has been used to accomplish the same subcardiac mucosal injury instead of EMR. Technically this is much less demanding than EMR.

Complex gastro-oesophageal reflux disease

Peptic strictures and dilatation

Reflux-induced strictures are relatively rare in the era of PPIs as most patients will be treated empirically before long-term complications occur. These strictures generally respond well to dilatation and long-term treatment with a PPI. Antireflux surgery is an alternative to long-term PPI treatment, just as in uncomplicated GORD. Most patients do not require anything other than a standard operation.

Hiatus hernia and paraoesophageal ('rolling') hernia

Hiatus hernia is a condition in which the abdominal contents migrate through the hiatal opening of the diaphragm into the mediastinum. There are four types of hiatus hernia (***Figure 66.18***): (i) the sliding hernia (type I), accounting for most hiatus hernias (85–95%), where the OGJ is herniated upwards; (ii) the true paraoesophageal/rolling hernia (type II), where there is asymmetrical herniation of the stomach next to the oesophagus and the OGJ remains in its normal intra-abdominal position (this is relatively uncommon); (iii) the more common mixed sliding and paraoesophageal hernia (type III); and (iv) when abdominal viscera other than the stomach migrate into the hernia sac, it is classified as type IV. Hiatus hernia is closely related to advanced age and obesity.

A sliding hiatus hernia predisposes to GORD and is usually diagnosed in the presence of reflux symptoms. For asymptomatic patients, it can be an incidental finding on plain chest radiographs or CT as an intrathoracic gas bubble or fluid level (***Figure 66.19***). A paraoesophageal hernia, especially when large, presents more with obstructive symptoms. The term 'giant paraoesophageal hernia' is present when more than half of the stomach has herniated into the thoracic cavity (***Figure 66.20***). This may present as a surgical emergency if gastric volvulus occurs. It is more common for the stomach to rotate along its longitudinal axis, termed organoaxial volvulus. When the stomach rotates around the transverse axis, it is called mesentericoaxial volvulus.

Gastric volvulus can produce symptoms such as dysphagia and chest pain. In severe cases, it can cause obstruction, strangulation, ischaemia, perforation and compression on the lungs, leading to impaired lung function. Emergency presentation and operation with any of these complications carries a high morbidity rate on account of a combination of late diagnosis, advanced patient age, comorbidities and the complexity of surgery involved. Therefore, all symptomatic paraoesophageal

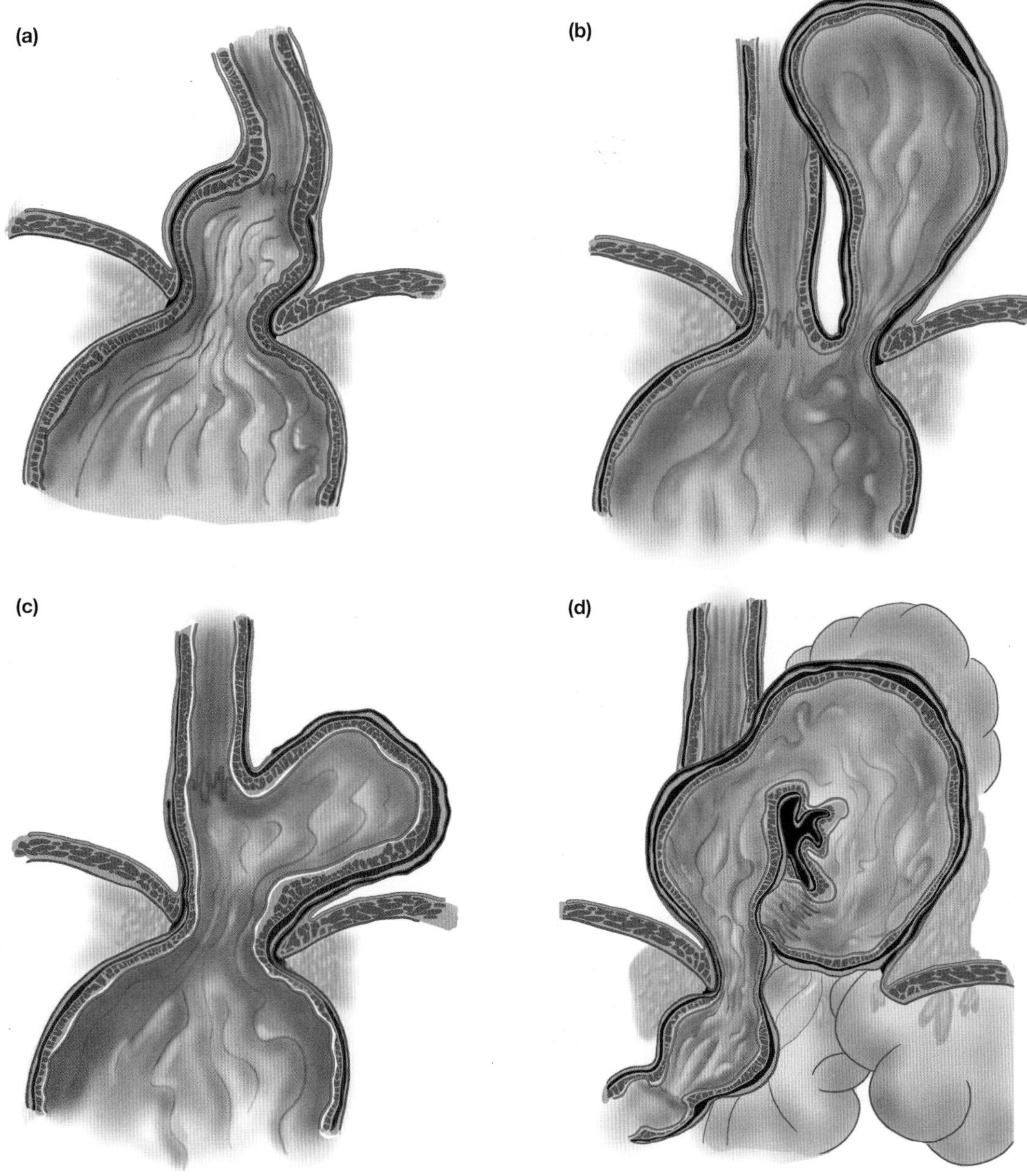

Figure 66.18 Types of hiatus hernias. (a) Type I, sliding hiatus hernia. (b) Type II, true rolling/paraoesophageal hiatus hernia. (c) Type III, mixed paraoesophageal hernia. (d) Type IV, giant hiatus hernia with herniation of another abdominal organ, e.g. colon.

hiatus hernias should be repaired. The decision to repair an asymptomatic paraoesophageal hernia needs to balance risk with the patient's age and comorbidities, as the annual risk of developing acute symptoms requiring emergency surgery is probably less than 2%.

Patients who present acutely should first be resuscitated, followed by nasogastric tube decompression. Immediate surgery is needed if there is suspicion of ischaemia, perforation or unresolved obstruction. The surgical principle is similar to that of sliding hiatus hernia repair but more technically demanding. The steps include reduction of any herniated organ, extensive mediastinal dissection to restore the intra-abdominal length of the oesophagus, excision of the hernia sac to prevent a recurrence, repair of the crura in a tension-free manner and some form of fixation of the stomach in the abdomen.

Summary box 66.3

Hiatus hernia

- Type I sliding hernia predisposes to GORD
- Types II/III/IV paraoesophageal hernia present mainly with obstructive symptoms
- Volvulus and strangulation require emergency surgical treatment

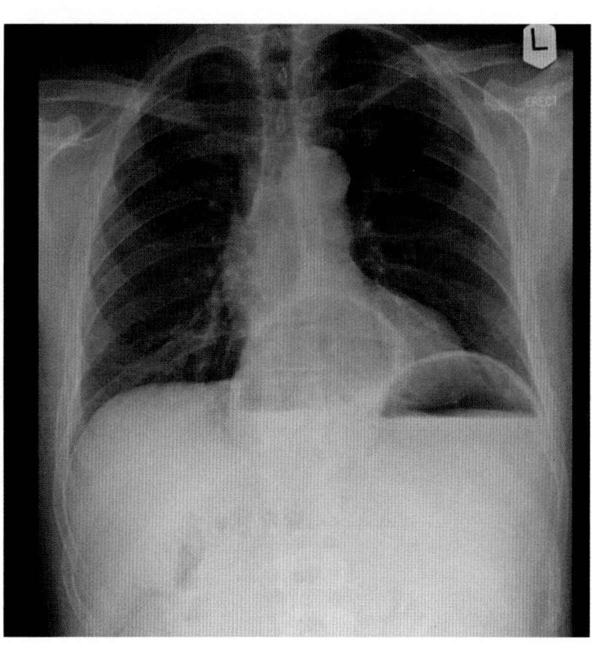

Figure 66.19 Chest radiograph showing a gastric bubble in the lower mediastinum behind the heart corresponding to a hiatus hernia.

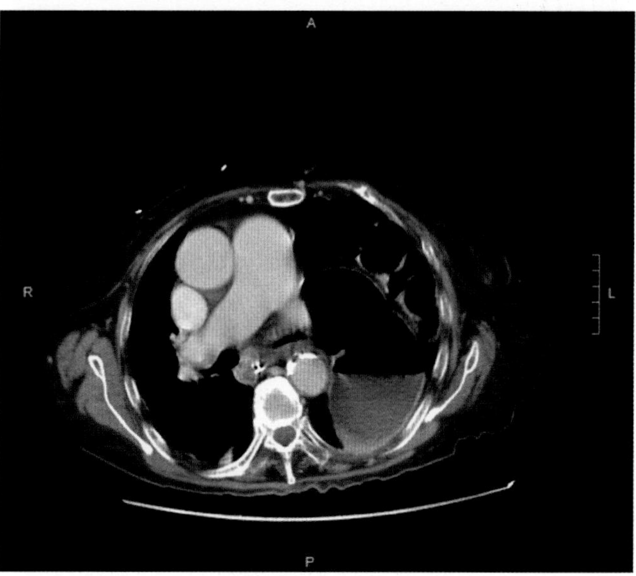

Figure 66.20 Computed tomography scan showing a large type IV paraoesophageal hernia with stomach and intestine in the mediastinum and left thoracic cavity. Mediastinal shift towards the right side is evident.

BARRETT'S OESOPHAGUS

Diagnosis and definitions

Barrett's oesophagus is a known complication of GORD. First described in 1950 as peptic ulceration in a tubular organ lined by columnar epithelium, it was interpreted as an intrathoracic tubular stomach with a congenitally short oesophagus. Later it was correctly identified as 'oesophagus lined with a gastric mucous membrane'. Currently, the commonly agreed definition of Barrett's oesophagus is the proximal migration of columnar epithelium (salmon-coloured mucosa) in the lower oesophagus extending more than 1 cm above the OGJ. The additional criterion of the biopsy-proven presence of mucus-secreting goblet cells or intestinal metaplasia is controversial.

Endoscopically, the OGJ is defined as the proximal end of the longitudinal gastric folds under minimal air insufflation. It should not be confused with the diaphragmatic hiatal pinch or the squamocolumnar junction. The Prague C&M Classification for Barrett's length is based on validated, explicit, consensus-driven criteria, including assessment of the circumferential (C) and maximal (M) extent of the endoscopically visualised Barrett's segment (***Figure 66.21***). The length of Barrett's oesophagus is a risk factor for developing neoplasia.

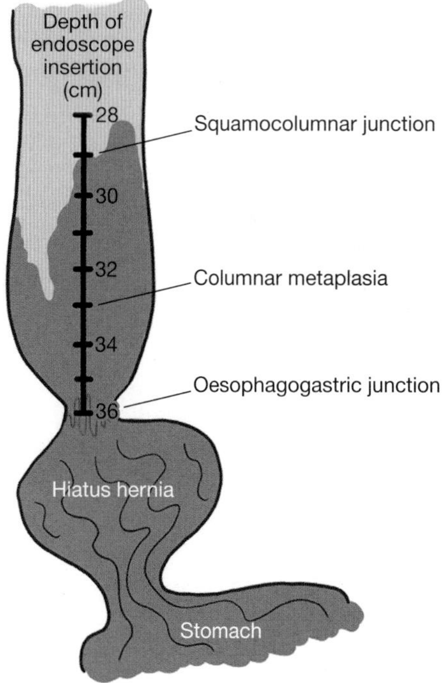

Figure 66.21 Prague C&M criteria to report endoscopic Barrett's oesophagus. The location of the oesophagogastric junction is defined by the top of the gastric folds (36 cm). Prague criteria of Barrett's oesophagus are expressed in C (circumferential), in this case 33–36 cm (3 cm), and M (maximum extent), in this case 28–36 cm (8 cm). This patient therefore has Prague C3 M8 Barrett's oesophagus.

Screening and surveillance

The risk factors for Barrett's oesophagus and related neoplasm include chronic (>5 years) GORD symptoms, advanced age (>50 years), smoking, central obesity and male gender. For non-dysplastic Barrett's, the risk of progression to cancer is around 0.2–0.5% per year. This increases to around 0.7% per year for low-grade dysplasia. For high-grade dysplasia, the risk of cancer progression can be as high as 7%. Therefore, screening and surveillance protocols should be tailored to individuals according to the potential benefit of cancer prevention and the risk and cost-effectiveness of such intervention (***Figure 66.22***). Screening or surveillance aims to identify premalignant lesions and to treat them early.

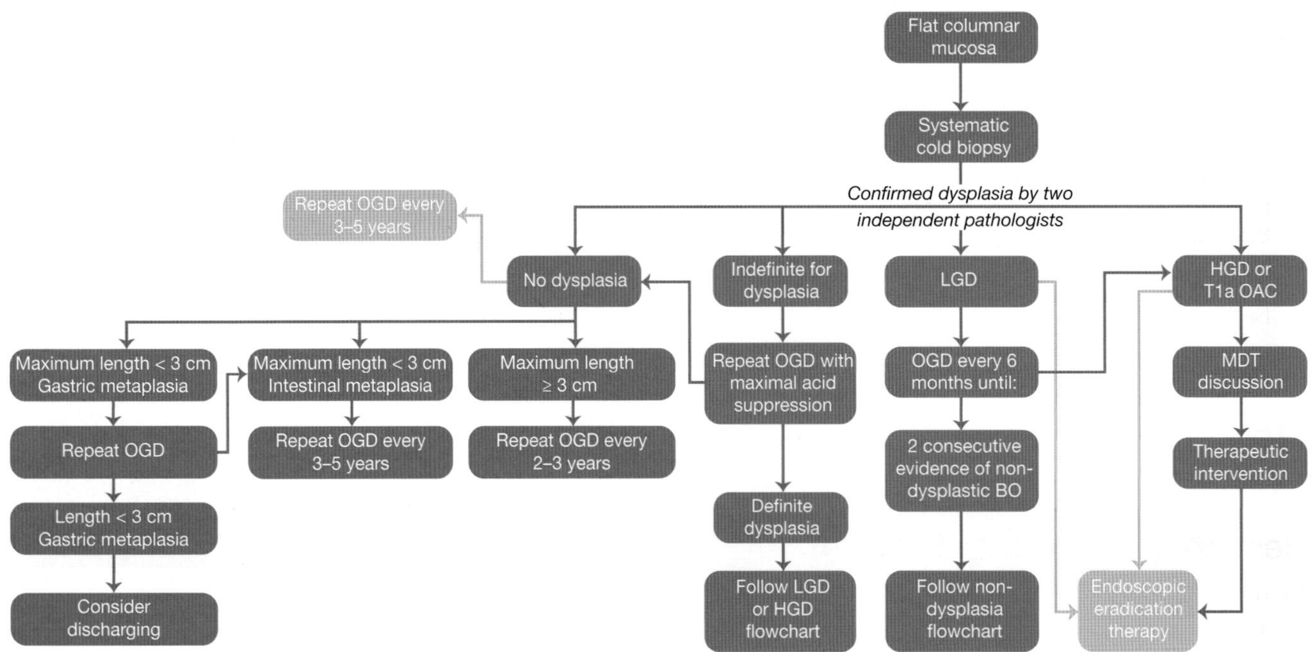

Figure 66.22 Algorithm for managing Barrett's oesophagus, including dysplasia. Summary of guidelines from the American College of Gastroenterology (orange) and the British Society of Gastroenterology (blue). BO, Barrett's oesophagus; HGD, high-grade dysplasia; LGD, low-grade dysplasia; MDT, multidisciplinary team; OAC, oesophageal adenocarcinoma; OGD, oesophagogastroduodenoscopy.

The vast majority of patients with Barrett's oesophagus in the community are asymptomatic; a general population screening programme is considered not to be cost-effective. High-definition white light endoscopy including NBI is used to assess the mucosal and vascular patterns of the Barrett's segment. Additional chromoendoscopy using different agents, e.g. methylene blue, acetic acid or indigo carmine, could aid diagnosis. The histological specimen obtained should be examined by an experienced gastrointestinal pathologist. The sensitivity of the assessment can be improved by increasing the number of biopsies and, when in doubt, endoscopy and biopsy should be repeated. The Seattle biopsy protocol, which includes four-quadrant random biopsies every 2 cm in addition to targeted biopsies on macroscopically visible lesions, is recommended at the time of diagnosis and subsequent surveillance.

Treatment

When Barrett's oesophagus is discovered, the treatment is that of the underlying GORD. Pharmacological therapy generally is the same as treatment of symptomatic GORD patients. Antireflux surgery is indicated if it is associated with GORD symptoms. A randomised trial suggested that aspirin, as a chemoprevention agent, in combination with a high-dose PPI, may improve outcomes in patients with Barrett's oesophagus measured by progression to cancer and mortality.

In patients with dysplastic Barrett's oesophagus without suspicion of invasive cancer, the epithelium can be ablated or resected. Indication for such procedures in non-dysplastic Barrett's oesophagus is controversial. Ablative therapy aims to completely eradicate all intestinal metaplasia. When the mucosa regenerates after ablation in a non-acidic environment (when a high-dose PPI is prescribed), a 'neosquamous' lining is formed. Ablative approaches that are supported by evidence include photodynamic therapy, RFA and cryotherapy. Among these methods, RFA is most popular because there is evidence of its effectiveness, cost and side-effect profile. EMR by the cap method or multiband technique can be done to remove the whole segment of the mucosa. When this is applied to circumferential Barrett's oesophagus, the stricture rate is high when healing occurs. The procedure can be performed in stages, allowing mucosal healing to occur first in one half of the oesophagus before a second stage to remove the other half, thus lessening the chance of stenosis. In contrast, the incidence of stricture formation is low following RFA, because the depth of ablation extends to the muscularis mucosae only.

Endoscopic ablation should only be applied to flat lesions without nodularity, ulceration or irregular contour. Such features are suggestive of invasive neoplasm that should be investigated and treated by EMR or endoscopic submucosal dissection (ESD). ESD, though more technically demanding, provides en bloc resection of the index lesion with better margins for histological diagnosis. EMR is easier and large areas can be resected in a piecemeal manner. If histological examination of the resected tissue demonstrates the absence of invasive cancer, or T1a tumour, only the 'biopsies' can be regarded as curative. When T1b lesions are found on histology, or when the resection margins (lateral or deep) are involved, additional therapy including oesophagectomy should be considered. Regardless of treatment performed, the patient should enter a surveillance programme to detect recurrent or persistent Barrett's oesophagus or neoplasia.

Summary box 66.4

Barrett's oesophagus

- Endoscopic examination and biopsies are crucial in the diagnosis of Barrett's oesophagus
- Dysplasia should be confirmed by at least two experienced pathologists
- Surveillance or ablation are options for low-grade dysplasia
- In patients with high-grade dysplastic Barrett's oesophagus, ablative, endoscopic resection and oesophagectomy should be considered

MOTILITY DISORDERS AND DIVERTICULA

Oesophageal motility disorders

Oesophageal motility disorders are a spectrum of diseases that involve the diminished, overaction or desynchronised neuromuscular function of the oesophageal body or sphincters. The most common presenting symptom is dysphagia. Chest pain, with or without swallowing difficulty, is another frequent complaint. Patients often undergo extensive investigations before the oesophagus is considered the responsible organ. It is important to have a proper diagnostic work-up before treatment is considered.

Manometric classification

Oesophageal motility disorders are classified on HRM under the Chicago classification. A hierarchy diagnostic algorithm is utilised (***Figure 66.23***). Broadly speaking, these disorders can be classified as disorders of OGJ outflow and disorders of peristalsis. Disorders of OGJ outflow are characterised by an elevated integrated relaxation pressure (IRP), which is the relaxation pressure across the OGJ in response to a swallow. Diagnoses include the three types of achalasia and OGJ outflow obstruction (OGJOO). Disorders of peristalsis include absent contractility, distal oesophageal spasm, hypercontractile oesophagus and ineffective oesophageal motility. All motility disorders have to be associated with symptoms or other supporting tests to make them clinically relevant. Various metrics have been developed in HRM; the details are beyond the scope of this chapter and the reader is encouraged to consult the relevant publications.

Achalasia

Pathology and aetiology

The term achalasia originated from the Greek word 'khalasis', meaning 'failure to relax'. It is uncommon, with a prevalence of 1.8–12.6 per 100 000 persons per year. The aetiology remains uncertain but is postulated to be due to loss of the inhibitory ganglion cells in the myenteric (Auerbach's) plexus, possibly related to a virus-induced autoimmune effect. Histology of muscle specimens generally shows a reduction in the number of ganglion cells with a variable degree of chronic inflammation. During a normal swallow, the food bolus will trigger primary peristalsis in the oesophagus by sequential activation of excitatory lower motor neurones. At the same time, relaxation of the LOS allows oesophageal emptying. The mismatch in excitatory and inhibitory activity results in the failure of LOS relaxation and absent peristalsis. With time, the oesophagus dilates and contractions disappear, so that the oesophagus empties mainly by the hydrostatic pressure of its contents. This is nearly always incomplete, leaving residual food and fluid. The air–fluid level in the stomach evidenced on radiography taken in the erect position in normal individuals is frequently absent, as no bolus with its accompanying air passes through the LOS. The oesophagus becomes progressively more tortuous and dilated (megaoesophagus); persistent retention oesophagitis due to fermentation of food residues may predispose to the increased incidence of carcinoma of the oesophagus. In South America, chronic infection with the parasite *Trypanosoma cruzi* causes Chagas' disease and the destruction of the myenteric plexus has marked clinical similarities to achalasia. A rare genetic syndrome (Allgrove syndrome) is associated with familial adrenal insufficiency, alacrimia and achalasia.

Clinical features

The disease is most commonly diagnosed between 30 and 60 years of age. It typically presents with dysphagia (to both solid and liquid), regurgitation and heartburn (often mistaken for GORD), although chest pain/odynophagia is also common in the early stages. Patients often present late and, having had relatively mild symptoms, remain untreated for many years. Patients may or may not have experienced weight loss. Frequently, patients will adjust their diet according to symptoms and can maintain their body weight after an initial drop. An 'Eckardt score' was developed to assess the severity of symptoms and monitor treatment outcome (***Table 66.1***). Aspiration-related respiratory symptoms and pneumonia can also occur when there is significant stasis of food residue in the dilated oesophagus. The retained food substance can cause fermentation and therefore halitosis. Patients may report regurgitating food that they have ingested before.

Diagnosis

A high index of suspicion is needed in the diagnosis of achalasia as symptoms can be mild and chronic and can be easily misdiagnosed as GORD. Endoscopy typically shows frothy saliva pooling in the oesophagus and the presence of food residue. The oesophagus may be dilated and can be tortuous. The OGJ appears tight and spastic but can usually allow an endoscope to

Leopold Auerbach, 1828–1897, neuropathologist, Breslau, Germany (now Wrocław, Poland).
Carlos Chagas, 1879–1934, microbiologist, Rio de Janeiro, Brazil.
Jeremy Allgrove, contemporary, paediatric endocrinologist, London, UK.
Volker F Eckardt, b. 1942, gastroenterologist, Wiesbaden, Germany.

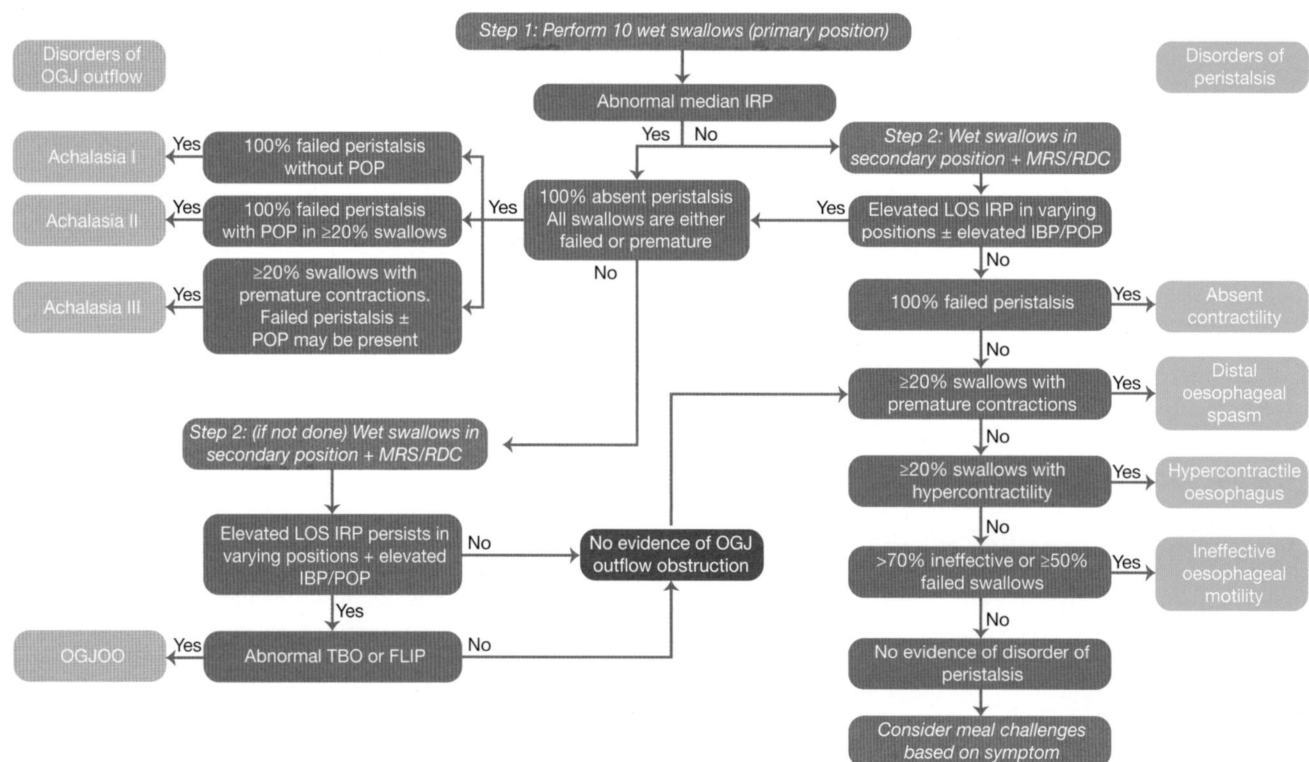

Figure 66.23 Hierarchy diagnostic algorithm of oesophageal motility disorders according to the Chicago classification 4.0. The broad categories of 'disorders of oesophagogastric junction (OGJ) outflow' and 'disorders of oesophageal peristalsis' are differentiated by the integrated relaxation pressure (IRP). FLIP, functional lumen imaging planimetry; IBP, intrabolus pressurisation; LOS, lower oesophageal sphincter; MRS, multiple rapid swallow; OGJOO, oesophagogastric outflow obstruction; POP, pan-oesophageal pressurisation; RDC, rapid drink challenge; TBO, timed barium oesophagram.

Table 66.1 Clinical scoring system for achalasia (Eckardt score).

Score	Symptom			
	Weight loss (kg)	Dysphagia	Retrosternal pain	Regurgitation
0	None	None	None	None
1	<5	Occasionally	Occasionally	Occasionally
2	5–10	Daily	Daily	Daily
3	>10	Each meal	Each meal	Each meal

pass with gentle pressure. A normal endoscopy however does not exclude achalasia, as 30–40% of endoscopies are reported as normal before a final diagnosis of achalasia is made. It is an important investigation to exclude 'pseudo-achalasia', often referring to cancer of the gastric cardia mimicking achalasia (*Figure 66.24*).

Barium contrast study typically shows a hold-up of contrast in the distal oesophagus, abnormal contractions in the oesophageal body and a tapering stricture in the distal oesophagus, described as a 'bird's beak' or 'rat's tail' (*Figure 66.25*). Progressive dilatation leads to a 'sigmoidal'-shaped oesophagus. A timed barium oesophagogram is used to quantify the height of the retained contrast at a specific time after ingestion to determine the severity of the disease. All these investigations are suggestive of achalasia but definitive diagnosis relies on HRM.

Treatment

The treatment goal of achalasia is for symptom palliation since there is no therapy to reverse the neuronal degeneration. Therapies target the LOS, aiming to reduce its contractility by pharmacological means or by destroying the muscle fibres using endoscopic or surgical methods.

Medical therapy

Pharmacological therapy has a limited role. Calcium channel blockers, nitrates or 5′-phosphodiesterase inhibitors are used to reduce the LOS pressure. Most have limited efficacy in symptom improvement. There are also significant side effects, such as headache, oedema and hypotension, after repeated doses. Medical therapy should be reserved for selected patients who are poor candidates for endoscopic or surgical treatments.

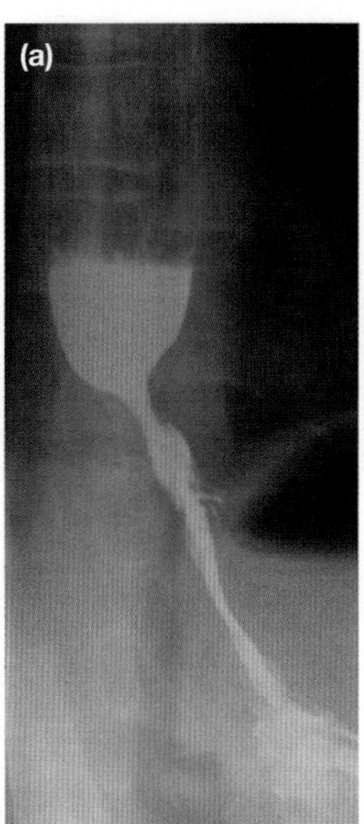

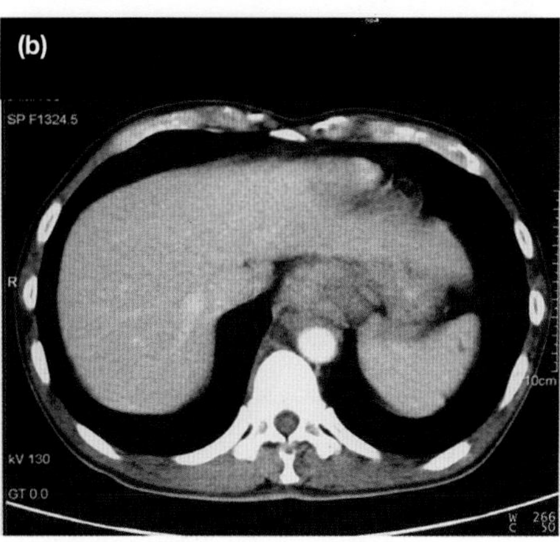

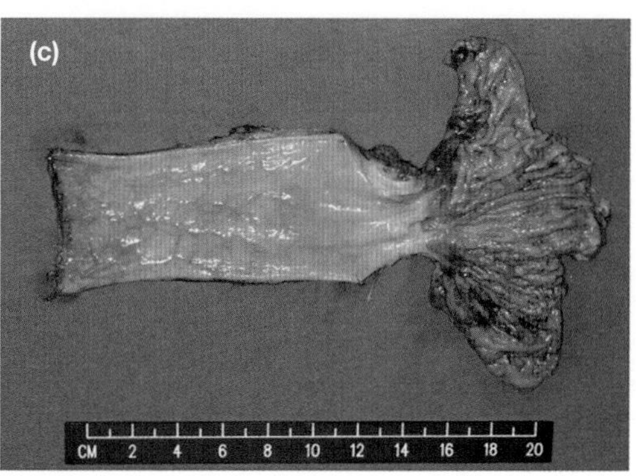

Figure 66.24 Pseudo-achalasia in a patient with cancer of the oesophagogastric junction. The patient was referred as having possible achalasia based on a barium contrast study (a). Endoscopy could not get past the obstruction, prompting a computed tomography scan (b), making a diagnosis of cancer. The resected surgical specimen (c).

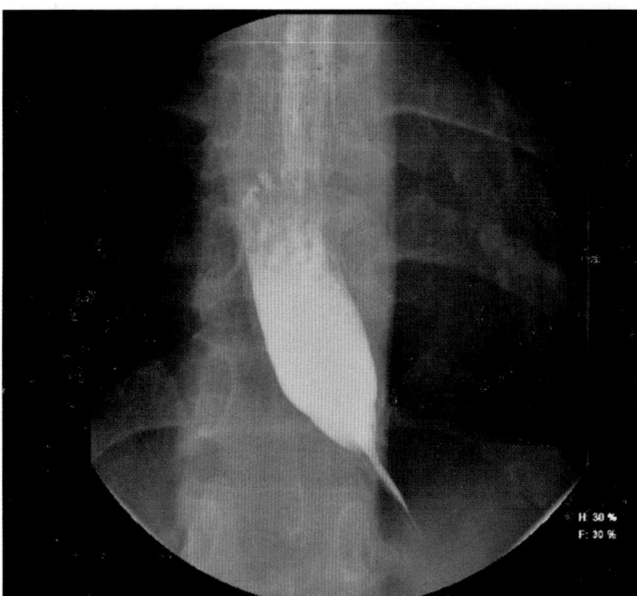

Figure 66.25 Barium contrast study showing the typical 'rat's tail' appearance of achalasia.

Botulinum toxin

Botulinum toxin is a potent presynaptic inhibitor of acetylcholine release from nerve endings. When injected endoscopically into the LOS, it interferes with the LOS cholinergic excitatory neural activity and paralyses the sphincter muscle. The reported symptom relief decreased from 70% in 3 months to around 40% in a year. The injection usually has to be repeated after a few months. Because the effect is temporary, it is sometimes used when the diagnosis of achalasia is in doubt. Repeated injection may result in scarring, making subsequent treatments more difficult. It should not be offered as first-line treatment in patients who are suitable for myotomy or pneumatic dilatation and its indication is usually restricted to elderly patients with comorbidities.

Pneumatic dilatation

This involves stretching the LOS with a non-compliant balloon to disrupt the sphincter muscle and render it less competent. Plastic (polyethene) balloons with a precisely controlled external diameter are used. If the pressure in the balloon is too high, the balloon is designed to split along its length rather than expanding further. Balloons of 30–40 mm in diameter are available and are inserted over a guidewire. There is no standardised dilatation protocol. Generally, it is preferred to have serial dilatations in a graded manner, from 30 mm to 35 mm and 40 mm.

Serial pneumatic dilatation has similar efficacy to surgical myotomy in selected patients. Features that predict optimal response are: patients older than 45 years, female, those with an undilated oesophagus, those who have responded to first dilatation and those with type II achalasia. Perforation is uncommon; the reported incidence averaged about 1.9% (0–16%). With a 30-mm balloon, the chance of perforation should be less than 0.5%. The risk of perforation increases with bigger balloons, which should be used cautiously for progressive dilatation over weeks. It is important to have an experienced endoscopist performing the procedure and surgical back-up in case of perforation.

Heller's myotomy

This involves cutting the muscle of the lower oesophagus and gastric cardia (***Figure 66.26***).Typically, anterior myotomy is

Ernst Heller, 1877–1964, surgeon, St George's Krankenhaus, Leipzig, Germany.

performed for at least 6 cm proximally at the oesophageal side and 2–3 cm distally into the gastric cardia. Transabdominal or transthoracic approaches have been advocated. Currently, the standard procedure is a laparoscopic approach. The major complication is GORD, which can occur in up to 40% of patients. The addition of a partial fundoplication (anterior Dor or posterior Toupet) has been shown to be effective in reducing the incidence of GORD. A complete 360° fundoplication (Nissen) is considered contraindicated because the increase in outflow resistance against an aperistaltic oesophageal body will probably result in postoperative dysphagia. Laparoscopic myotomy is superior to single pneumatic dilatation in efficacy and durability. The surgical outcome is better in types I and II achalasia than in type III. For the latter, a longer extended proximal myotomy is often needed for adequate treatment.

Peroral endoscopic myotomy

Peroral endoscopic myotomy (POEM) involves opening the mucosa at a short distance proximal to the intended myotomy site. Entrance is gained into the submucosal plane, which is extended distally to about 2–3 cm into the gastric cardia. The circular +/– longitudinal muscles are then cut using ESD instruments. Typically, the myotomy extends a minimum of 6 cm in the oesophagus proximally and 2 cm into the gastric cardia distally (***Figure 66.27***). The mucosal opening is then closed with endoclips. In type III achalasia, there is a spastic component at the distal oesophagus that responds less well to pneumatic dilatation and Heller's myotomy. POEM has the advantage in that it can extend the length of the myotomy proximally, tailored to preoperative HRM and barium swallow parameters. POEM can also be utilised to treat other types of 'spastic' oesophageal motility disorders such as distal oesophageal spasm and hypercontractile oesophagus. Randomised controlled trials have demonstrated similar efficacy of POEM to pneumatic dilatation and Heller's myotomy in relieving dysphagia. Without any antireflux procedure, the incidence of GORD is expectedly higher in POEM compared with Heller's myotomy with partial fundoplication. The incidence of oesophagitis at 3 months after POEM can be as high as 57%, which may subject patients to lifelong acid suppression therapy or subsequent antireflux operation.

Oesophagectomy

Oesophagectomy is reserved only for the treatment of patients with 'end-stage' achalasia with a sigmoidal or megaoesophagus that is not responding to other methods (***Figure 66.28***). Depending on the chronicity of the disease, the symptoms of achalasia may be tolerated. However, a grossly dilated oesophagus predisposes to regurgitation and aspiration pneumonia. Balancing the risk of an oesophagectomy with the patient's quality of life and risk of aspiration complication, surgery can be a reasonable option for surgically fit patients.

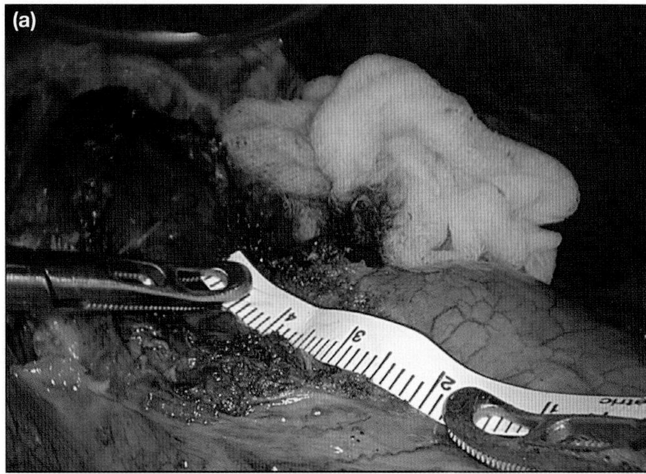

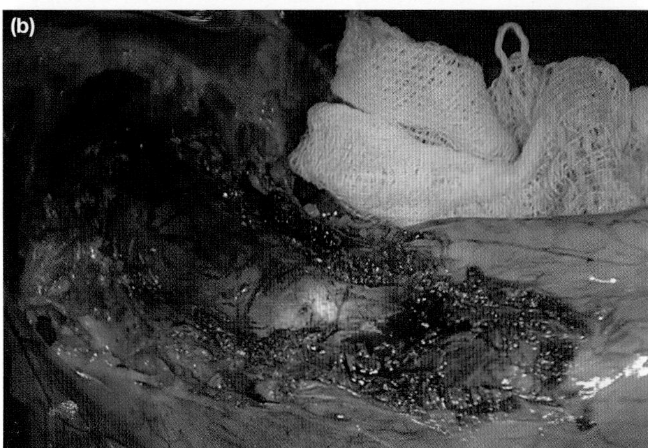

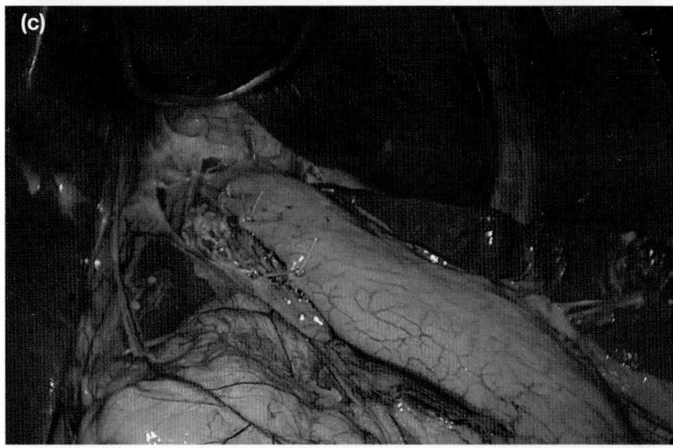

Figure 66.26 Laparoscopic myotomy and Dor hemi-fundoplication. **(a)** The lower oesophageal myotomy extending onto the stomach for at least 2 cm. **(b)** Completion of the myotomy; the light of the endoscope can be seen shining through the thin mucosa. **(c)** Completion of the Dor anterior fundoplication.

Follow-up

Treatment success is usually defined by symptom relief. The Eckardt score is quantified and compared with the preoperative score. Patients should be counselled on a post-treatment diet as the oesophageal body motility remains defective. Ideally, HRM, barium contrast study, endoscopy and 24-hour pH monitoring should be performed postoperatively to objectively assess LOS function, bolus retention, response to treatment, presence of oesophagitis and acid reflux. This depends on the availability of resources and patients' preference.

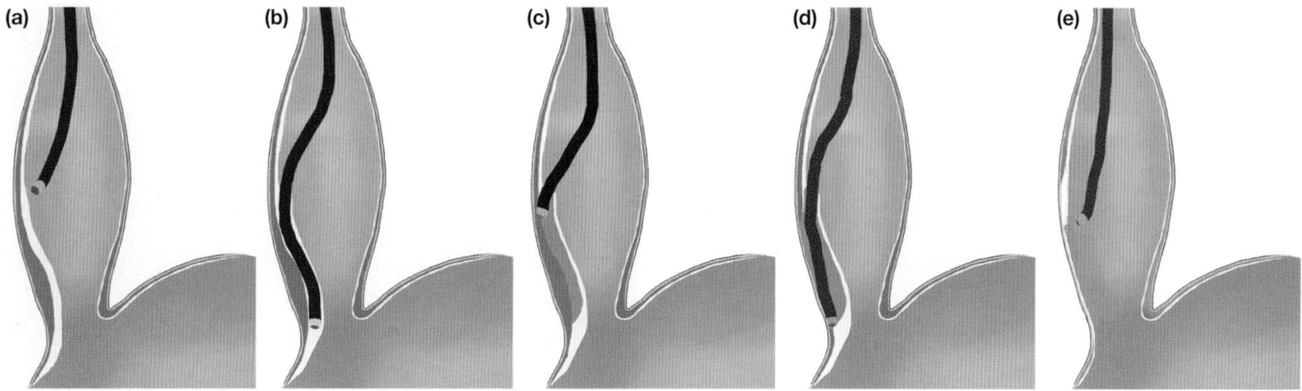

Figure 66.27 The procedure of peroral endoscopic myotomy (POEM). (a) Creation of a mucosal opening. (b) A tunnel is created between the mucosa and the muscle layer down to the stomach. (c) Myotomy starts a short distance below the mucosal opening. (d) Myotomy is carried out into the proximal stomach. (e) The mucosal opening is closed by endoclips.

Summary box 66.5

Achalasia

- Achalasia is the most common oesophageal motility disorder
- A normal endoscopy does not exclude the diagnosis of achalasia
- Beware of pseudo-achalasia
- HRM is the gold standard for the diagnosis of oesophageal motility disorder
- Laparoscopic myotomy, pneumatic balloon dilatation and POEM are effective treatments of achalasia
- Type III achalasia may be better treated with long myotomy by POEM

Other oesophageal motility disorders

Hypercontractile motility disorders

Distal oesophageal spasm is a condition in which there are incoordinate, premature and rapidly propagated contractions of the oesophagus, causing dysphagia and/or chest pain. The condition may be dramatic, with marked hypertrophy of the circular muscle and a corkscrew oesophagus on the barium oesophagogram (***Figure 66.29***). These abnormal contractions are more common in the distal two-thirds of the oesophageal body. Hypercontractile (jackhammer) oesophagus is characterised by high-amplitude contractions and should be differentiated from contractility disorder secondary to outflow obstruction. Patients may present with dysphagia or pain.

There is no well-proven treatment strategy for hypercontractile motility disorders. Patients should avoid any identifiable triggering factors (e.g. dietary or GORD related). Similar to achalasia, medical therapy such as calcium channel blockers, nitrates, 5′-phosphodiesterase inhibitors and pain modulators have been used with limited efficacy. Botulinum toxin injection in the oesophageal body may be useful. Long-segment surgical myotomy has been attempted with good results. POEM with extended myotomy is also advocated as a minimally invasive approach to treat these disorders.

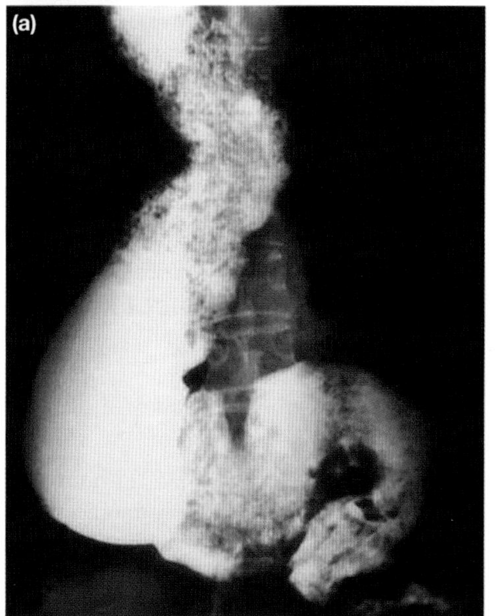

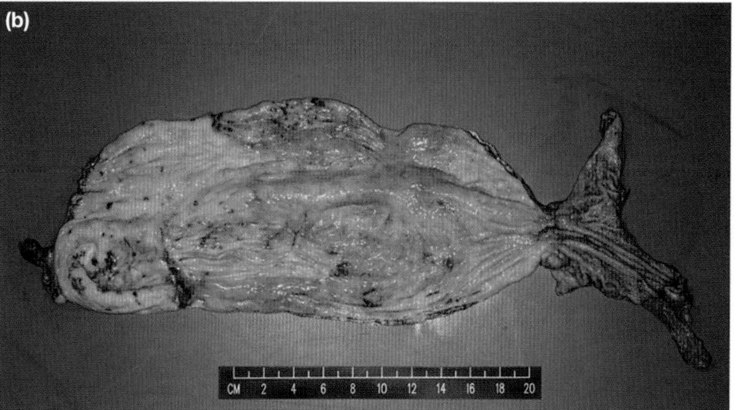

Figure 66.28 End-stage achalasia. A grossly dilated sigmoidal-shaped oesophagus (a). Transected oesophagus (b).

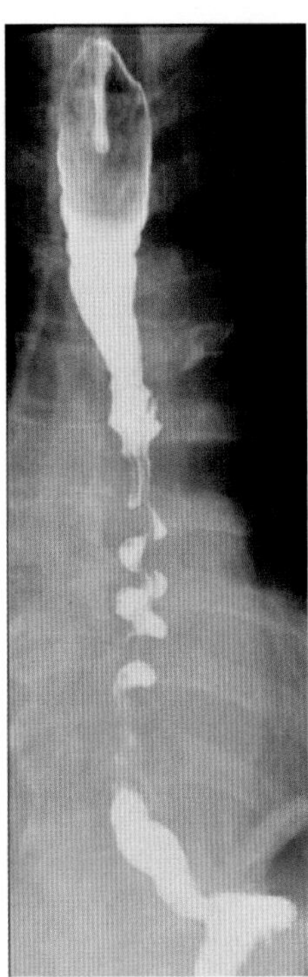

Figure 66.29 Barium contrast study showing a corkscrew oesophagus in a patient with diffuse oesophageal spasm.

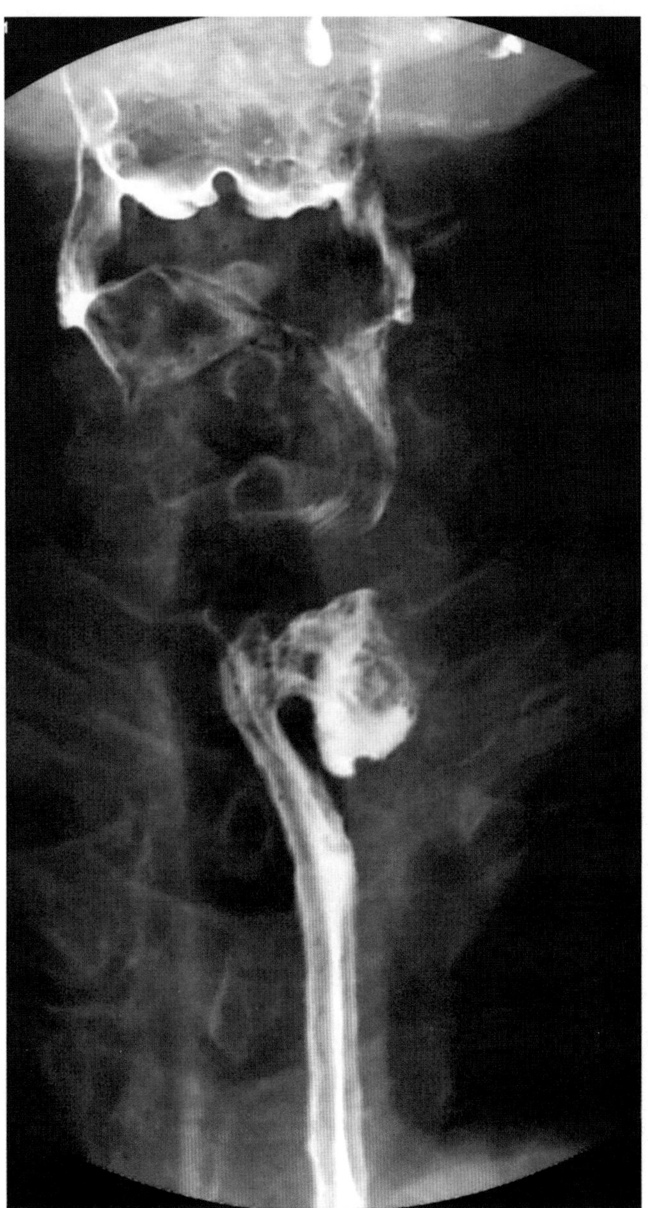

Figure 66.30 Barium contrast study showing a Zenker's diverticulum.

Functional oesophageal disorders

According to the Rome IV classification, functional oesophageal disorders include a variety of oesophageal symptoms (heartburn, chest pain, dysphagia, globus) that are not explained by mechanical obstruction (stricture, tumour, EOO), major motor disorders (achalasia, OGJOO, absent contractility, distal oesophageal spasm, jackhammer oesophagus) or GORD. The mechanisms responsible are unclear but are likely to be more related to visceral hypersensitivity and hypervigilance. The diagnosis is generally by exclusion. Physiological and psychological factors should be considered.

Among all the oesophageal disorders defined under the Rome diagnostic criteria, functional heartburn and reflux hypersensitivity contribute to most diagnostic confusion with genuine GORD. Therefore, patients have to be carefully assessed before antireflux surgery is offered. Pharmacological agents such as PPIs, tricyclic antidepressants, SSRIs and other pain modulators can be part of the treatment strategy. Surgery has a very limited role in the treatment and usually results in a poor outcome.

Pharyngeal and oesophageal diverticula

Oesophageal diverticula can be classified as true diverticula, which involve a full-thickness oesophageal wall, and false diverticula, which involve mucosal outpouching only. Diverticula are usually described by their location as pharyngeal, midoesophageal and epiphrenic. Diverticula alone seldom produce troublesome symptoms unless large or secondary to an underlying oesophageal motility disorder. The most common symptoms are dysphagia, regurgitation, halitosis and recurrent aspiration.

Pharyngeal pouch (Zenker's diverticulum)

Zenker's diverticulum is a false pulsion diverticulum as it protrudes posteriorly above the cricopharyngeal sphincter through the natural weak point (the dehiscence of Killian) between the oblique and horizontal fibres of the inferior pharyngeal constrictor. The pathophysiology is believed to involve loss of coordination between pharyngeal contraction and opening of the upper sphincter (*Figure 66.30*).

Gustav Killian, 1860–1921, Professor of Laryngology, Freiburg and later Berlin, Germany.

When the diverticulum is small, symptoms largely reflect desynchronisation of swallowing with predominantly pharyngeal dysphagia. As the pouch enlarges, it tends to fill with food on eating, and the fundus descends into the mediastinum. Regurgitation of trapped food can occur and lead to aspiration. Another symptom is halitosis. Conventional surgical treatment involves an open left cervical incision (most diverticula point towards the left side) with diverticulectomy and cricopharyngeus myotomy. Another option is diverticular suspension, whereby the diverticulum is dissected and inverted with its apex pointing cranially. This will stop food from entering the pouch. The absence of a suture line lessens the chance of a postoperative leak. A cricopharyngeus myotomy is also an integral part of the surgery. Newer techniques include transoral introduction of a linear stapler to divide the septum in between the diverticulum and the true oesophageal lumen. This creates a common channel, and the myotomy is in effect performed by the stapler transection (***Figure 66.31***).

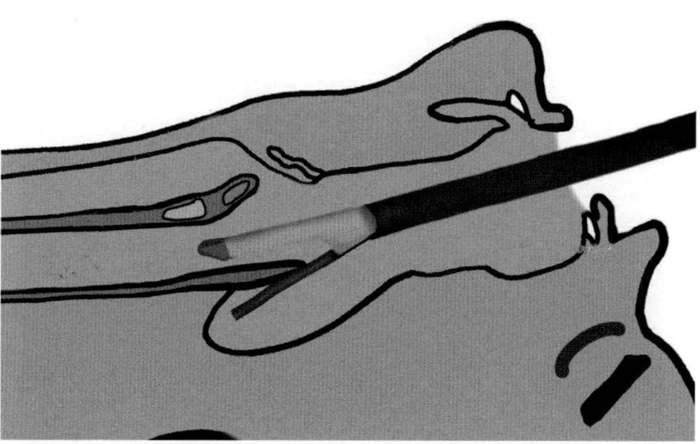

Figure 66.31 A linear stapler is introduced orally and the 'ridge' including the muscle is divided.

Midoesophageal diverticula (Rokitansky diverticulum)

Midoesophageal diverticula are usually small traction diverticula of no particular consequence. In granulomatous diseases with chronic inflammation, fibrosis or lymphadenopathy in the mediastinum can exert traction force onto the oesophageal wall and cause full-thickness outpouching. Rarely it may cause fistulation into the airway in uncontrolled pulmonary tuberculosis. Asymptomatic midoesophageal diverticulum does not warrant any treatment. HRM may be indicated in symptomatic patients to exclude pulsion diverticulum due to oesophageal motility disorder, e.g. hypercontractile oesophagus.

Epiphrenic diverticula

Epiphrenic diverticula are pulsion diverticula typically situated at the distal 10 cm of the oesophagus. They are commonly associated with oesophageal motility disorders, e.g. achalasia, or other causes of oesophageal outflow obstruction. Barium oesophagogram is a useful investigation depicting the size and anatomical relationship of the diverticulum and, at the same time, screening for oesophageal motility disorder (***Figure 66.32***). Large diverticula should be excised combined with a myotomy from the neck of the diverticulum to the cardia to relieve the functional obstruction. Concurrent fundoplication or repair of hiatus hernia may be necessary, depending on the size of the diverticulum or associated conditions. A laparoscopic approach is the preferred option to reduce morbidity.

OESOPHAGEAL PERFORATION

Oesophageal perforation is associated with high morbidity and mortality rates. It is an emergency and prompt treatment should be instituted because delayed diagnosis and treatment are associated with a marked increase in mortality rate.

Aetiology

Iatrogenic perforation secondary to endoscopic procedures such as dilatation of strictures or achalasia is the most common cause. Other endoscopic procedures such as EMR/ESD/POEM may result in leakage if there is transmural disruption and mucosal defects are not closed properly. Spontaneous emetogenic perforation (Boerhaave's syndrome) results from a sudden increase in oesophageal pressure against a closed glottis from vomiting. Perforation from direct penetrating trauma is rare as the oesophagus is a deep-seated organ. Blunt external trauma rarely causes oesophageal perforation. Foreign body ingestion, especially with sharp objects, may perforate the oesophagus. Corrosive ingestion can also lead to transmural necrosis and disruption of the oesophageal wall. Patients with EOO may present with spontaneous perforation. Oesophageal cancer can perforate, and the prognosis is usually poor since it reflects the underlying advanced disease.

Presentation and diagnosis

Sometimes the history is obvious, such as after instrumentation or foreign body ingestion. At other times there may not have been any precipitating cause. Patients with Boerhaave's syndrome may have the classic triad of vomiting, chest pain and subcutaneous emphysema. There may or may not be associated haematemesis. Typically, the site of perforation is the lower oesophagus towards the left pleural cavity. Gastric juice as well as ingested food is forcefully ejected into the left chest. A left pleural effusion rapidly accumulates. Physical examination reveals subcutaneous emphysema on the chest wall, sometimes extending to the cervical region as well. In the presence of sepsis, the patient will run a fever, has tachycardia and appears tachypnoeic. Hamman's sign refers to a crunching sound on auscultation of the heart owing to surgical emphysema. Differential diagnoses usually include pneumonia, myocardial ischaemia or other intra-abdominal pathologies such as a perforated viscus when the pain is referred to the epigastrium.

Baron Carl von Rokitansky, 1804–1878, pathologist, philosopher and politician, Vienna, Austria, classified oesophageal diverticula as either traction or pulsion in 1840.

Louis Hamman, 1877–1946, physician, Johns Hopkins Hospital, Baltimore, MD, USA.

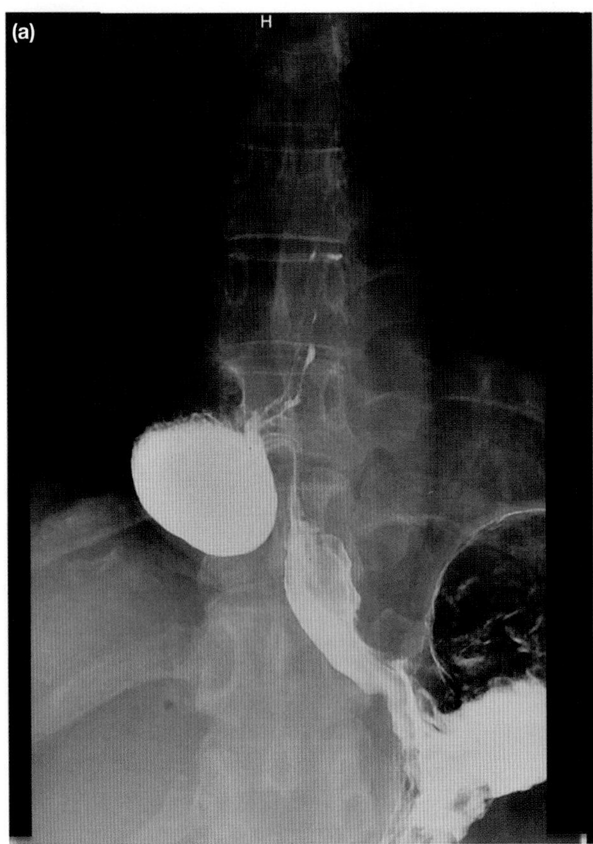

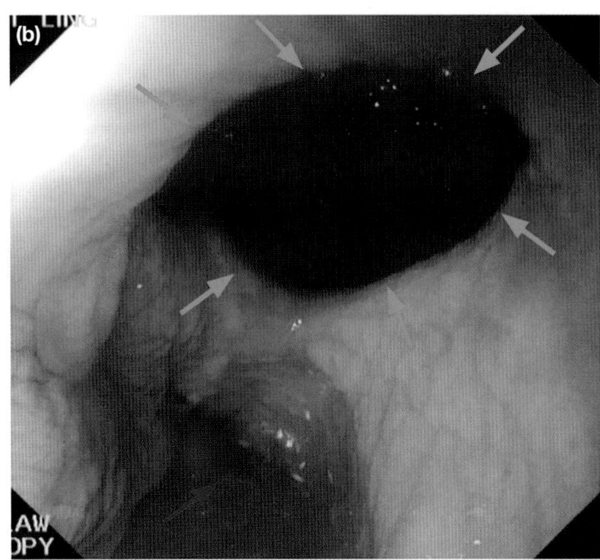

Figure 66.32 Epiphrenic diverticulum on a barium contrast study (a). Endoscopic picture (b) showing the diverticulum (green arrows) and true lumen (red arrow).

Patients with cervical oesophageal or pharyngeal perforation are usually much less septic than those with intrathoracic perforations and mediastinitis. A typical example would be foreign body perforation, such as by a sharp fishbone, having lodged at the postcricoid area and perforated the oesophagus. There may be a history of foreign body ingestion and neck pain and physical examination may reveal tenderness and subcutaneous emphysema.

Subcutaneous and mediastinal air, pneumothorax, hydropneumothorax and a widened mediastinum may be seen on the chest radiograph (***Figure 66.5***). Contrast swallow study using Gastrografin or a non-ionic contrast usually reveals the site of perforation. However, sick patients may not be able to tolerate oral contrast. A CT scan (preferably with intravenous as well as oral contrast) will be able to demonstrate the site (and aetiology) of perforation and the extent of mediastinitis, effusion and collections (***Figure 66.6***).

Management

In stable patients with a clear history and contained perforation, sometimes conservative expectant treatment can be successful. This usually applies to cervical/pharyngeal perforation when patients are much less septic. Antibiotics should be given; patients are kept nil by mouth and should wait for the perforation to heal by itself. In intrathoracic perforations, patients are usually sicker. They should be resuscitated with intravenous fluid and given antibiotics and oxygen supplement. Electrolyte disturbances are corrected if present. Septic shock is treated appropriately. The objectives of treatment are (i) seal the perforation if possible, (ii) adequate drainage, and (iii) supportive measures, including nutrition (alimentary preferred over parenteral), cardiorespiratory support and sepsis control.

In patients with significant pleural fluid and pneumothorax that result in respiratory compromise, a wide-bore chest tube is inserted to the appropriate side for drainage while waiting for more definitive investigations such as a CT scan. Endoscopy can be both diagnostic and therapeutic. The location and size of the perforation site should be ascertained. Foreign bodies are retrieved. Endoscopic sealing of the perforation site with clips and self-expanding metallic stents may be possible (***Figure 66.33***). The stent is usually removed around 4–6 weeks later. Healing is expected to have occurred. A nasogastric tube can be placed at the same time for nutritional support.

Surgical intervention is indicated in the presence of significant sepsis when drainage is not affected by other means (such as interventional radiology), and no effective closure of the perforation can be done otherwise. These conditions are usually present when the perforation is large, when the perforation is in the intrathoracic oesophagus, when the pleura is breached, when there is a large septic load and when the presentation is delayed.

When the diagnosis is delayed, closure of the perforation is unlikely to succeed; conversion of the perforation into a controlled fistula is another option. A simple way would be to place a T-tube through the defect and repair around it, in addition to adjacent drains. With modern supportive treatment, oesophageal diversion (cervical oesophagostomy; often an end

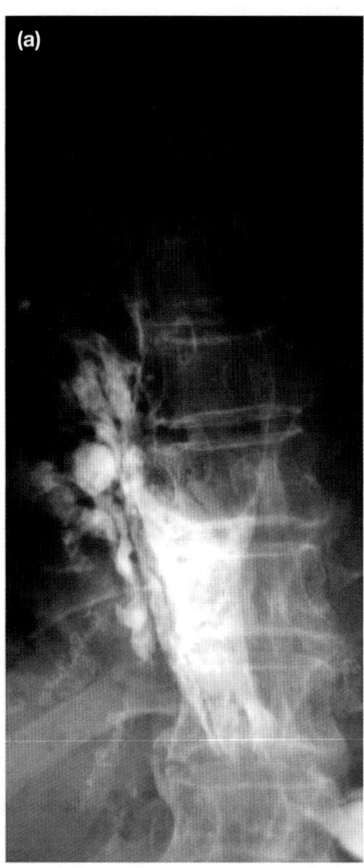

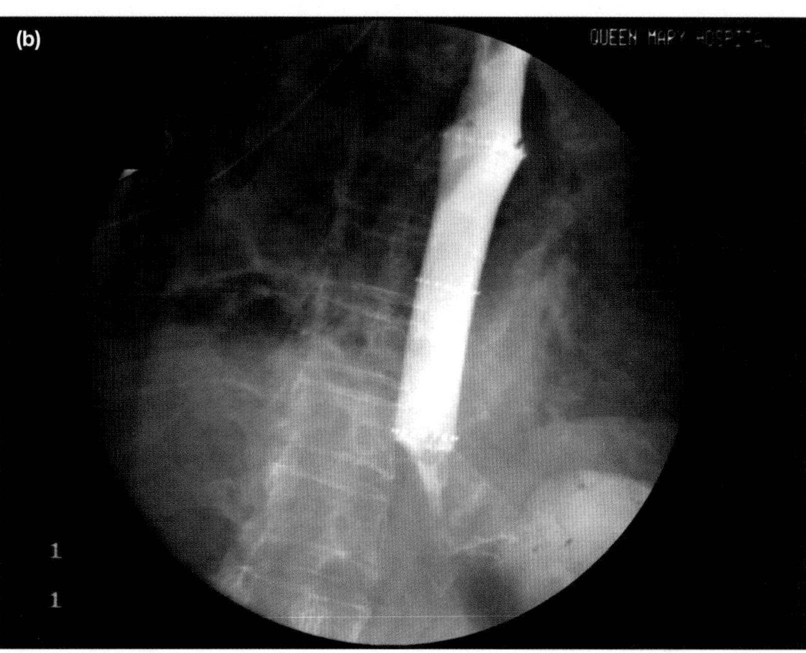

Figure 66.33 Stent for oesophageal perforation. (a) Leakage of oral contrast outside the oesophagus; (b) contrast flowing through the stent, no leakage is seen.

stoma is required for effective diversion and OGJ ligation) with later staged reconstruction is rarely needed. Oesophagectomy is even more uncommonly indicated, perhaps except for extensive caustic burn with perforation when the oesophagus is necrotic.

Summary box 66.6

Oesophageal perforation

- A potentially lethal condition due to sepsis
- Surgical emphysema, chest pain and vomiting constitute the classic triad of Boerhaave's syndrome
- Treatment aims at adequate drainage, closure of the perforation site if possible and supportive measures
- Delayed diagnosis and management lead to high morbidity and mortality rates

MALLORY-WEISS SYNDROME AND INTRAMURAL OESOPHAGEAL HAEMATOMA/DISSECTION

Forceful vomiting may lead to a tear at the OGJ, mostly immediately below the squamocolumnar junction. Patients present with haematemesis. Bleeding is rarely severe, and the diagnosis is readily made with endoscopy. Endoscopically the bleeding can be stopped by adrenaline (epinephrine) injection or endoscopic clips to stop bleeding and close the mucosal defect.

Intramural oesophageal dissection is characterised by the separation of the mucosa and/or submucosa from deeper muscular layers. This most commonly occurs in elderly patients taking anticoagulants or patients with coagulation disorders. It is often precipitated by vomiting. A break in the oesophageal mucosa is followed by an increase in intraoesophageal pressure that causes separation of mucosa and/or submucosa from the muscle layers. The mucosal break can also be caused by trauma such as foreign body impaction or air insufflation during endoscopy.

Patients present with acute onset of chest discomfort or odynophagia. If the haematoma ruptures into the oesophageal lumen haematemesis ensues. When the dissection or haematoma is confined to the oesophageal wall, treatment is conservative. Anticoagulation is corrected and the haematoma usually resolves in 7–14 days.

CAUSTIC INJURY

Caustic injury to the oesophagus can be mild, but also is potentially lethal. Most caustic ingestions occur in children, in whom it is usually accidental, or in adults with suicidal intent. The severity of the injury depends on the type, pH, quantity

George Kenneth Mallory, 1900–1986, pathologist, Boston University, Boston, MA, USA.
Soma Weiss, 1898–1942, Physician in Chief, Peter Bent Brigham Hospital, Boston, MA, USA.

and duration of exposure. The substance ingested can be a strong acid, causing coagulative necrosis with eschar formation, which may limit penetration to deeper layers, or strong alkali, leading to liquefactive necrosis. The latter potentially penetrates deeper into the oesophageal wall, producing a more severe injury pattern.

Diagnosis is usually not difficult. When the injurious agent is identified, it should be tested for its pH, and suicidal attempt considered. Patients may have pain in the neck, throat, chest or even the abdomen. Drooling of saliva, dysphagia and odynophagia can be present. Hoarseness of voice is an important sign to look for as it may signify laryngeal injury and potential airway obstruction. If the airway is judged to be compromised, careful assessment and emergency intubation using fibreoptic guidance, or even a surgical airway, are indicated. There is no role for gastric lavage or attempts to neutralise the acid or alkali. Initial treatment after securing an adequate airway is supportive, with intravenous fluid, oxygen supplementation and cardiorespiratory monitoring.

Once the patient is stabilised, an endoscopy and CT scan with intravenous contrast should be considered. Careful endoscopy allows assessment of the extent of the injury (***Figure 66.34***). The Zargar grading can be used (***Table 66.2***). In general, the longer and more circumferential the injury, the more likely that stricture will form. The stomach is assessed as well for injury, and a nasogastric/duodenal tube can be placed with endoscopic guidance. This can be used for alimentary nutritional support; if a stricture forms, there is still a potential route of access through to the stomach. A CT scan can assess oesophageal oedema and also surrounding soft-tissue infiltration.

Most caustic injuries can be managed conservatively with supportive measures. Deterioration requires surgical treatment, with emergency oesophagectomy. The oesophagus can be mobilised transhiatally or via a thoracoscopic approach. Immediate reconstruction is not recommended. A cervical oesophagostomy and a gastrostomy can be done and future reconstruction planned. A feeding jejunostomy is an alternative for nutritional support if the stomach also requires resection.

Delayed complications include stricture and malignancy. A stricture can form early and may be resistant to dilatation (***Figure 66.35***). There is not enough evidence to support routine use of systemic steroids, intralesional injection of steroid or topical mitomycin C to reduce stricture formation. Endoscopic dilatation should be gradual, as the perforation rate is higher than in other forms of strictures. Long strictures are often resistant to dilatation. Oesophagectomy or bypass surgery may be required. Oesophagectomy has the advantage of removing the oesophagus with its long-term risk of malignancy. However, surgery is difficult because of scarring and adhesions to the mediastinum, thus a bypass operation may be preferable. The gastric conduit is placed in the retrosternal route to reach the neck. When it is also damaged and cannot be used, a colonic interposition is the alternative. The native oesophagus can be left *in situ* as the risk of dilatation and resultant mucocele is low.

Table 66.2 Zargar endoscopic classification of caustic injury to the oesophagus.

Zargar classification grade	Description
0	Normal appearance
1	Oedema and hyperaemia
2a	Superficial ulceration and friability
2b	Deep ulceration or circumferential ulceration
3a	Multiple deep ulceration ad scattered necrosis
3b	Extensive necrosis
4	Perforation

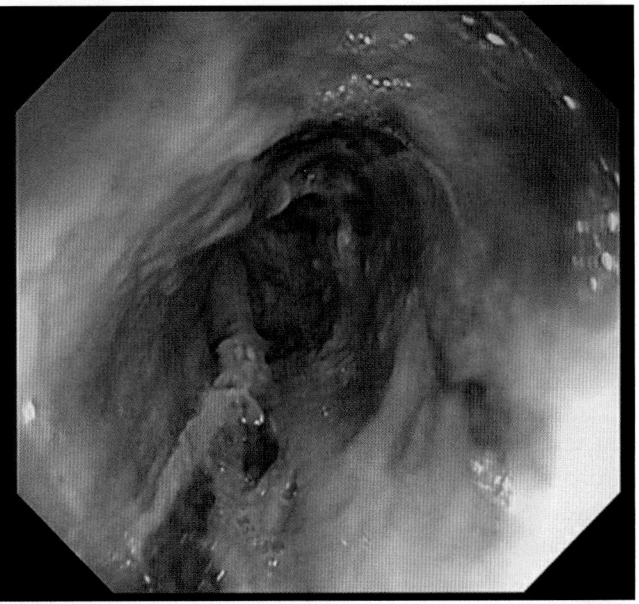

Figure 66.34 Endoscopy picture showing caustic burn to the oesophagus.

EOSINOPHILIC OESOPHAGITIS

EOO is defined as a chronic, immune/antigen-mediated oesophageal disease, characterised clinically by symptoms related to oesophageal dysfunction and histologically by eosinophil-predominant inflammation. However, there is overlap with GORD-related eosinophilia and other pathologies that may also be associated with similar oesophageal eosinophilia, such as achalasia, hypereosinophilic syndrome, Crohn's disease, coeliac disease, vasculitis, pemphigus, graft-versus-host disease and other connective tissue disorders. The incidence of EOO is increasing, ranging from 0.7/100 000 to 10.7/100 000 depending on the population studied. It is predominantly a disease among the white population in Western countries (white versus non-white ratio, 3:1).

Showkat Ali Zargar, contemporary, gastroenterologist, Sher-i-Kashmir Institute of Medical Sciences, Srinagar, India.
Burrill Bernard Crohn, 1884–1983, gastroenterologist, Mount Sinai Hospital, New York, NY, USA, described regional ileitis in 1932.

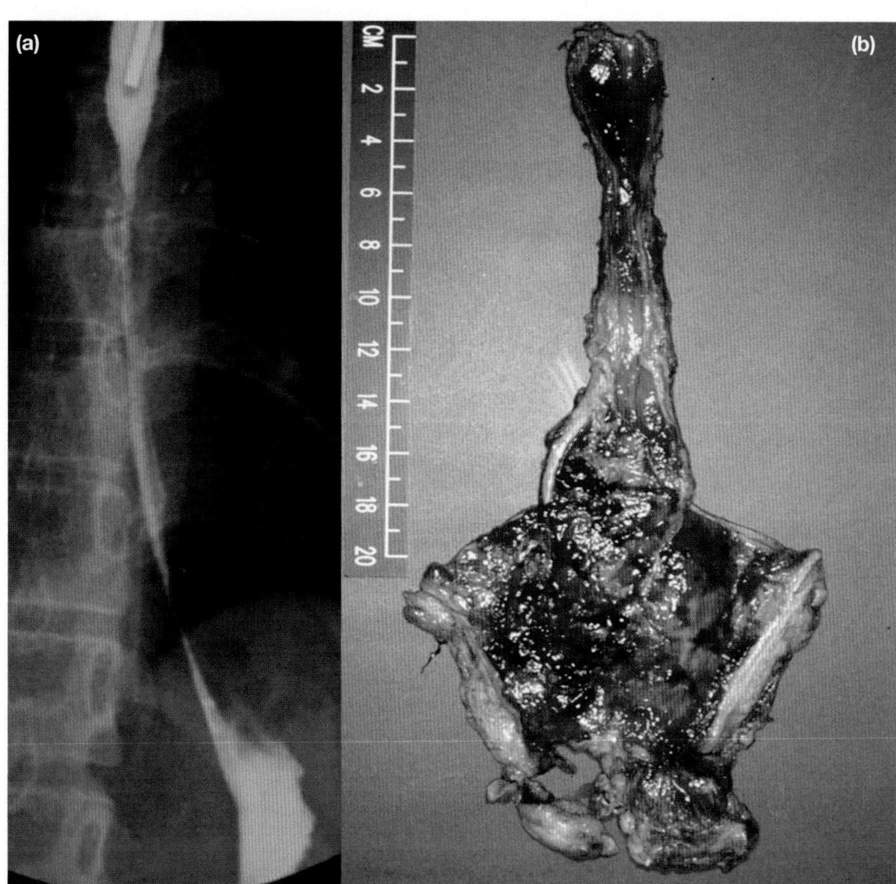

Figure 66.35 Contrast study showing a long undilatable stricture of the oesophagus secondary to caustic burn (a). The patient underwent an oesophagogastrectomy and colonic interposition. Note that the oesophagus and the stomach were scarred (b).

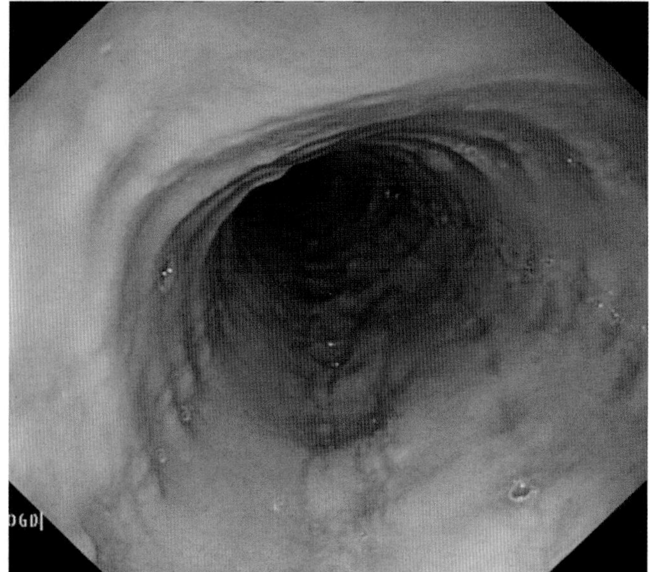

Figure 66.36 Endoscopic appearance of eosinophilic oesophagitis. The linear furrows and circular rings are evident.

EOO is believed to commence with food antigen initiation of cytokine-mediated signals that lead to eosinophilia, inflammation and subsequent remodelling by fibrosis. It is a progressive disease; thus, in infants or toddlers, it may present with irritability, food aversion and failure to thrive. In young children vomiting and regurgitation predominate. In older children or early adolescents, it may present with heartburn and dyspeptic symptoms, while in adults dysphagia and food impaction become the most common symptoms. The peak age of presentation is around 20–30 years. There is a clear association with other atopic disorders such as asthma, atopic rhinitis or dermatitis and food allergies.

Typical findings on endoscopy include the presence of rings, furrows, exudates, oedema, stricture, narrowing and 'crepe paper mucosa' (***Figure 66.36***). Biopsies of the oesophagus show 15 or more eosinophils per high-power field (hpf). The eosinophilic infiltration is isolated to the oesophagus. Biopsies should be taken at a minimum of two separate levels of the oesophagus together with suspicious areas. Usually gastric and duodenal biopsies are also taken to exclude eosinophilia at these sites. Barium contrast study may demonstrate narrowing and assess the diameter of the oesophagus better than endoscopy.

Treatment goals include reduction of oesophageal eosinophilia (to <15/hpf and preferably to <5/hpf), control of symptoms and normalisation of endoscopic findings, although these goals can only be completely achieved in a minority of patients. In children, the disease process is predominantly inflammatory, and associated symptoms such as nausea, vomiting and abdominal pain are relieved with appropriate medical treatments. In adults, reduction in inflammation per se may not relieve the fibrotic component (stricture and small-calibre oesophagus) and dilatation may be required.

Topical corticosteroids are the mainstay medical treatment for EOO; swallowing topically acting corticosteroids such as

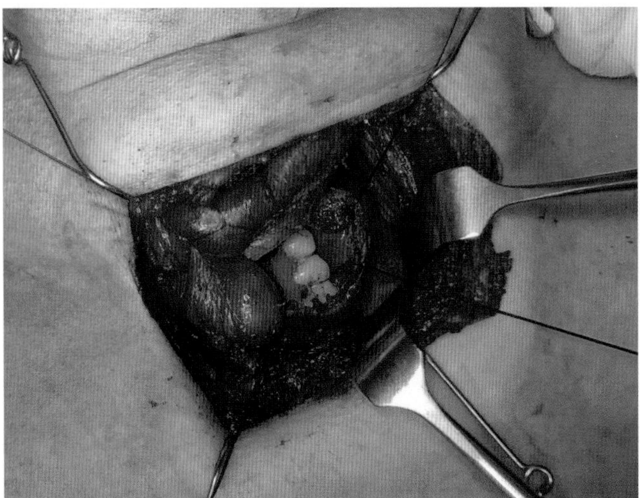

Figure 66.37 Open surgery was required to extract a broken denture stuck in the cervical oesophagus. The oesophagus was repaired in two layers.

budesonide or fluticasone is highly effective in resolving symptoms. Systemic steroids should be avoided. PPIs are effective in 40–50% of adults through blockage of cytokine release rather than acid suppression. Diet therapy is useful, eliminating gluten, milk, soy, egg, nuts and seafood as the most likely antigens.

Endoscopy is used for diagnostic purposes, to monitor treatment progress and therapeutically to deal with strictures. Careful gradual dilatations should be performed, although perforation rates appear similar to other types of strictures.

FOREIGN BODIES IN OESOPHAGUS

Swallowed foreign bodies are common and tend to impact at the three narrow portions of the oesophagus; namely, the cricopharyngeus/pyriform fossa, the midoesophagus where the aorta/left main bronchus crosses the oesophagus and at the OGJ. It is a common problem in children; in adults, it is more prevalent among the elderly with swallowing difficulties, those with dementia, those with unhealthy alcohol use and those with mental health disorders (*Figure 66.37*). Bones from fish, pork and chicken are common offenders. In complete obstruction, patients may not even be able to swallow fluids or their saliva.

A clear history may be volunteered, but in children, the elderly and those with mental health disorders the history may not be clear. Complaints should always be treated seriously even though they may sound implausible. A plain radiograph may reveal radio-opaque bodies and should be taken in two views. If in doubt, a CT scan is the best method to identify a foreign body.

Flexible endoscopy is the mainstay of treatment to extract using forceps, nets, baskets or a balloon inflated distal to the object. Airway protection may be needed. Sharp objects should be retrieved with the sharp end pointing distally to lessen the chance of perforation. An overtube can be used as needed. Batteries should always be removed as they may cause injury by direct electrical burn or by liquefactive necrosis from leaked battery content. A food bolus can usually be broken down and either retrieved or pushed into the stomach. Occasionally open surgery is required for foreign body retrieval.

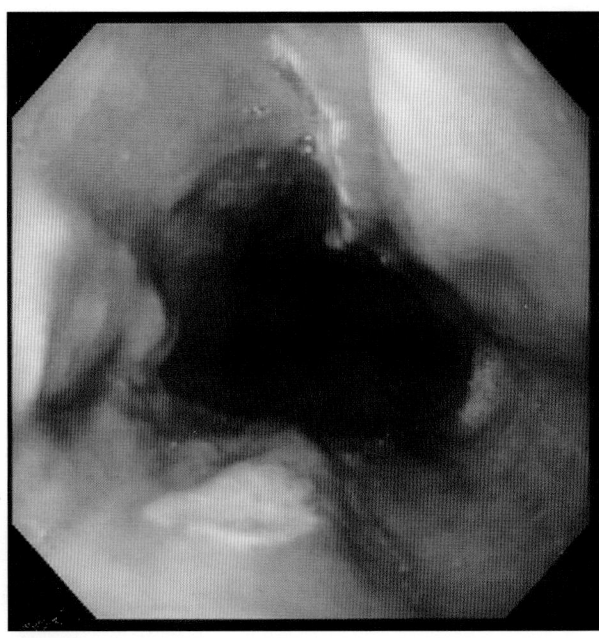

Figure 66.38 Pill-induced ulceration of the oesophagus. Note the 'kissing' ulcers on opposite sides.

Summary box 66.7

Foreign bodies

- Swallowed foreign bodies tend to lodge at the three relative constrictions of the oesophagus: the cricopharyngeus, where the left main bronchus crosses the oesophagus and at the OGJ
- Beware of underlying pathology, such as reflux stricture, eosinophilic oesophagitis and Schatzki's ring (see *Miscellaneous conditions*)
- Flexible endoscopy can remove most foreign bodies successfully

OESOPHAGEAL ULCERATION/ INFECTIONS

GORD is the most common cause of oesophageal ulceration but there are a variety of other reasons, including iatrogenic related to endoscopic procedures, the presence of a nasogastric tube and medications such as tetracyclines, potassium chloride tablets, non-steroidal anti-inflammatory drugs and bisphosphonates. Typically, when a medication is lodged in the oesophagus there may be 'kissing' ulcers with ulceration on opposite sides of the oesophagus. Patients may present with odynophagia (*Figure 66.38*).

Infection of the oesophagus typically occurs in immunocompromised, elderly, debilitated or steroid-dependent patients. Candidiasis is the most common fungal infection, characteristically seen as adherent white pseudo-membranes

Richard Schatzki, 1901–1992, radiologist, Mount Auburn Hospital, Boston, MA, USA.

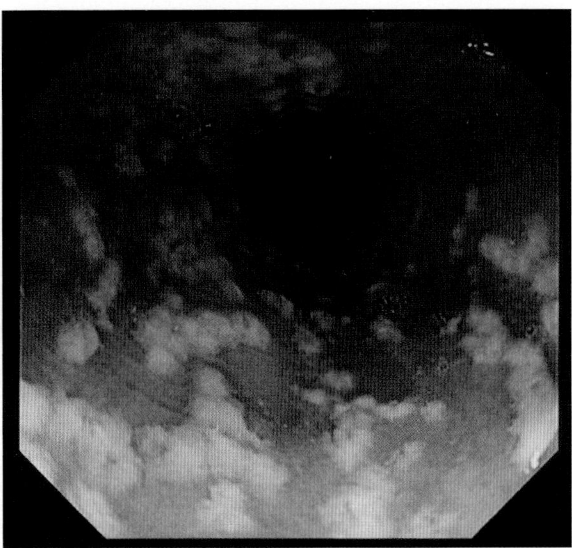

Figure 66.39 Oesophageal candidiasis.

(*Figure 66.39*). Viral infections include herpes simplex virus (HSV) or cytomegalovirus (CMV). HSV gives rise to punched-out ulcers with edges that appear vesicular, while CMV ulcers are more shallow. CMV inclusions can be found histologically. Special immunohistochemical stains are required to make the diagnosis. Tuberculous infection can also occur, such as bovine tuberculosis when infected unpasteurised milk is consumed. Treatment would depend on individual aetiology and underlying predisposing conditions.

OESOPHAGEAL INVOLVEMENT IN SYSTEMIC DISEASE

The oesophagus can be affected by a variety of systemic diseases; examples include systemic sclerosis/scleroderma, polymyositis, dermatomyositis, systemic lupus erythematosus and polyarteritis nodosa. Scleroderma most frequently affects women aged 40–65 years (female to male ratio, 8:2). The oesophagus is the most commonly affected part of the gastrointestinal tract, characterised by the excessive deposit of collagen, resulting in fibrosis. Symptoms are related to GORD (heartburn and regurgitation) as well as dysmotility (dysphagia and chest discomfort). On HRM the classical findings are poor oesophageal motility or even distal oesophageal aperistalsis (smooth muscle portion), with a hypotensive LOS. GORD can be severe because of the combination of dysmotility and hypotensive LOS, and complications such as peptic strictures and Barrett's oesophagus can be found in about one-third of patients. Management is directed at the control of GORD. PPIs remains the mainstay of treatment but standard doses may not be enough. Other medicines such as prokinetics and alginic acid may be added, though efficacy is limited. The results of surgical fundoplication are suboptimal because of poor oesophageal motility. Strictures are treated by standard endoscopic therapy.

Oesophageal varices

Oesophageal varices usually present with sudden, large-volume haematemesis secondary to portal hypertension, which is most commonly due to hepatic cirrhosis. Details of presentation and management can be found in *Chapter 69*.

NEOPLASMS OF THE OESOPHAGUS

Benign pathologies

Benign epithelial lesions include papillomas, fibrovascular polyps, glycogen acanthosis, parakeratosis, lipomas, lymphangiomas and haemangiomas. They are benign, though parakeratosis is associated with malignancy of the oesophagus and head and neck region.

Inlet patches (also referred to as heterotopic gastric mucosa) are common and are most often found within a short distance of the postcricoid region (*Figure 66.40*). They consist of

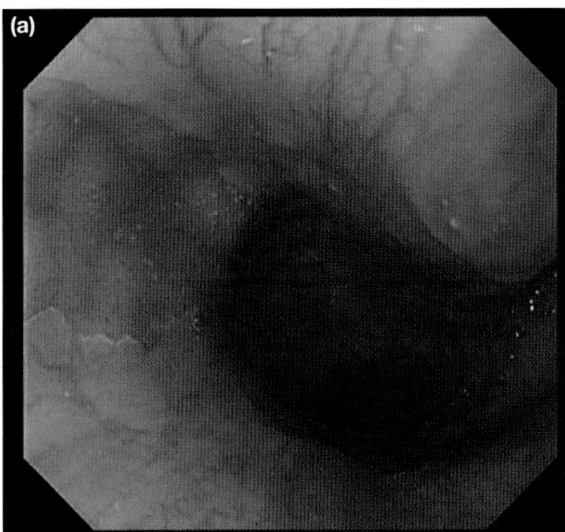

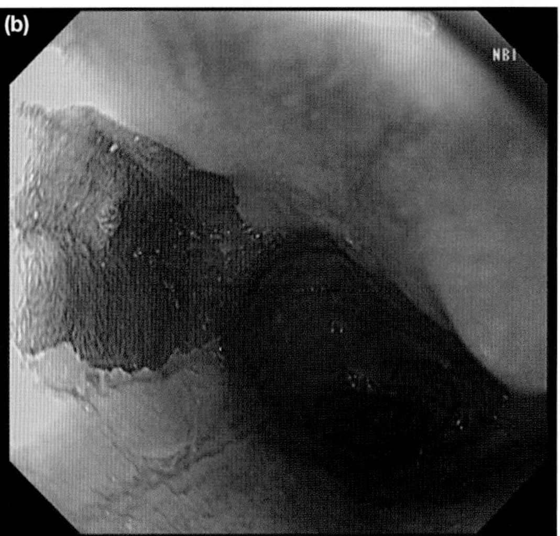

Figure 66.40 Inlet patch or heterotopic gastric mucosa in the upper oesophagus. (a) Inlet patch on white light endoscopy at 9–10 o'clock. (b) Using narrow-band imaging.

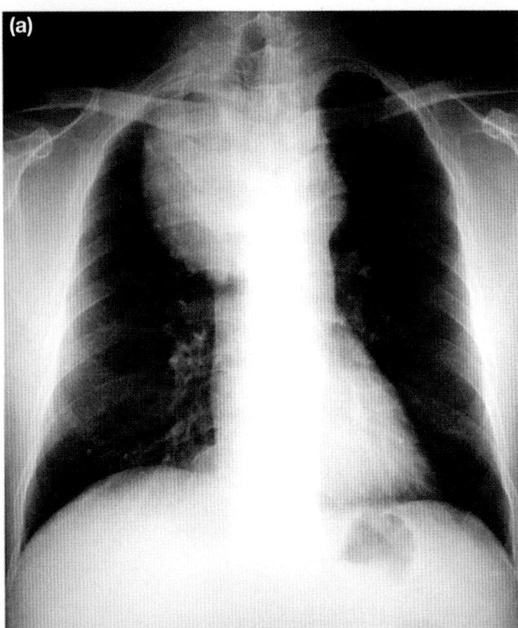

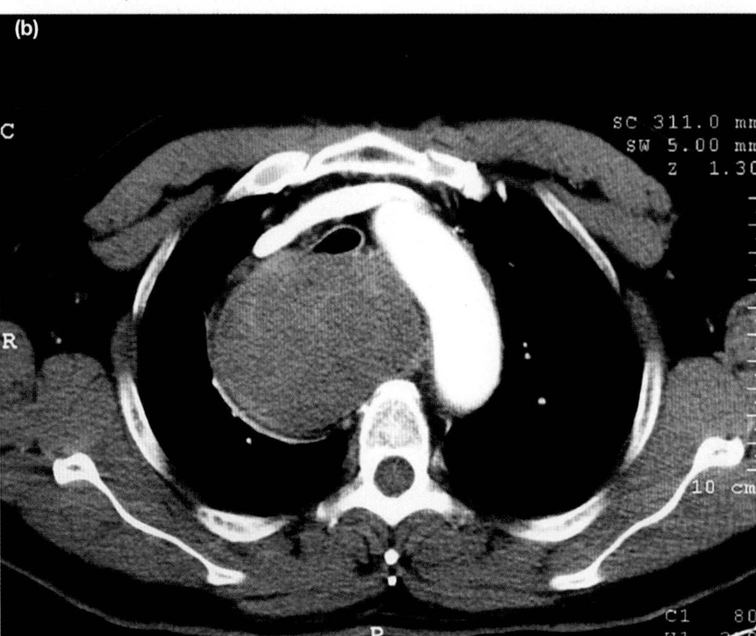

Figure 66.41 Large tumour of the upper oesophagus showing as an opacity on chest radiograph (a). Computed tomography scan shows a homogeneous tumour causing tracheal compression (b). The resected tumour was a Schwannoma.

embryonic gastric mucosa, though there are conflicting views as to whether they are truly embryonic or acquired in origin. The discovery of inlet patches is usually incidental on endoscopy. Biopsies will show corpus- or fundus-type gastric mucosa, sometimes even with parietal cells. Most are incidental and can be observed. An association with globus sensation, chronic cough and laryngopharyngeal reflux has been suggested. The patches can be ablated with RFA, argon plasma coagulation or multipolar electrocoagulation. Resolution of symptoms, however, is unpredictable.

Oesophageal duplication cysts are congenital anomalies that arise during early embryonic development. They are located within the oesophageal wall, covered by two muscle layers, and contain squamous epithelium or a lining compatible with that found in the embryonic oesophagus. Sometimes heterotopic gastric or pancreatic mucosa can be found. Most duplication cysts do not communicate with the oesophageal lumen, run parallel with the oesophagus and are asymptomatic unless large. Symptomatic duplication cysts can be resected.

Granular cell tumours are rare. On endoscopy they are typically sessile, yellowish-white and submucosal. They feel firm when prodded with a biopsy forceps. On EUS, they are hyperechoic and arise from the submucosal layer. They most likely arise from Schwann cells, suggesting a neural origin. Rarely they undergo malignant transformation. Schwannomas are often found incidentally; if large, surgical removal is indicated (***Figure 66.41***).

Leiomyomas are the most common solid benign tumours of the oesophagus (***Figure 66.42***). They are mostly found incidentally as a submucosal mass on endoscopy but may produce compressive symptoms when large. EUS shows a hypoechoic mass arising from the muscularis propria or the submucosal layer. They rarely become malignant; however, resection is indicated if enlarging on serial assessment. Small leiomyomas can be enucleated with a thoracoscopic approach, keeping the mucosa intact. Preoperative biopsy or EUS-guided fine-needle aspiration (FNA) is relatively contraindicated as the consequent scarring will increase the chance of breaching the mucosa during enucleation.

Endoscopic resection is possible using submucosal tunnelling endoscopic resection (STER); this creates a mucosal opening a short distance from the leiomyoma (3–5 cm proximally), allowing a submucosal tunnel to reach the lesion. The lesion is resected using ESD techniques and the specimen retrieved via the mouth. The mucosal opening is closed with clips (***Figure 66.43***). Because of the availability of STER, the threshold of removing smaller leiomyomas is reduced because of its minimal invasiveness. Larger lesions (perhaps larger than 5 cm) are technically challenging and are better removed thoracoscopically.

Leiomyosarcoma is rare and resection offers a chance of cure. Oesophageal gastrointestinal stromal tumours (GISTs) are uncommon and are usually found at the OGJ/proximal stomach. They should be managed along the same principles as GIST in the rest of the gastrointestinal tract.

Theodor Schwann, 1801–1882, physiologist, Berlin, Germany, later Leuven and Liège, Belgium.

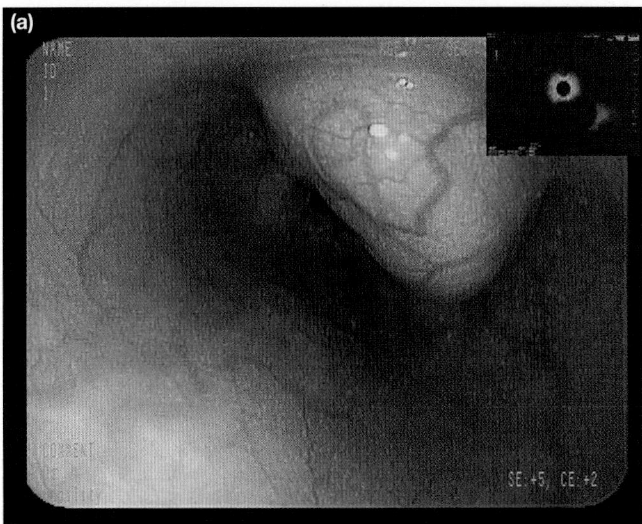

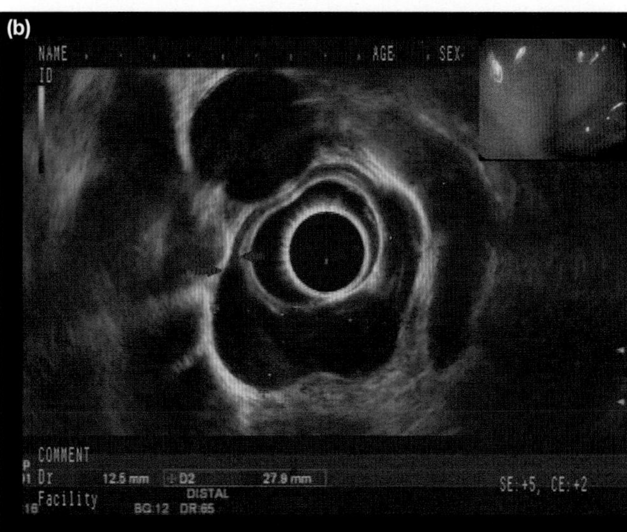

Figure 66.42 Leiomyoma of the oesophagus. **(a)** Endoscopic view of a submucosal lesion with intact mucosa. **(b)** Endoscopic ultrasound finding of a hypoechoic lesion arising from the muscularis propria layer (red arrows).

CARCINOMA OF THE OESOPHAGUS

Epidemiology

Oesophageal cancer is the eighth most common cancer worldwide and the sixth most common cause of cancer death. It most commonly presents in the sixth and seventh decades of life. Squamous cell carcinoma and adenocarcinoma are the most common cell types while other malignancies such as melanoma and small cell carcinomas are rare. Secondary malignancies are likewise rare; however, bronchogenic carcinoma or metastatic lymph nodes can invade the oesophagus.

Squamous cell cancer is the predominant histological cell type but there are significant geographical and ethnic variations, with the incidence of oesophageal cancer 50–100-fold higher in areas of high incidence than in the rest of the world. Squamous cell carcinoma incidence remains steady; however, among white populations, especially in developed Western countries, there has been an epidemiological shift since the 1990s from squamous cell carcinoma to adenocarcinoma such that the incidence of adenocarcinoma has surpassed that of squamous cell cancer.

Aetiology

The aetiological factors for the development of oesophageal cancer vary between the two main cell types (***Table 66.3***). Genetic predisposition may be important in the pathogenesis of oesophageal squamous cell cancer. While smoking and alcohol intake are independent contributing factors, genetic polymorphism is important in individuals with chronic alcohol consumption. Approximately 36% of East Asians show a physiological response to drinking that includes facial flushing, nausea and tachycardia. This facial flushing response is predominantly related to an inherited deficiency in the enzyme aldehyde dehydrogenase 2 (ALDH2). Alcohol is metabolised to acetaldehyde by alcohol dehydrogenase and the acetaldehyde is in turn metabolised by ALDH2 to acetate. Individuals with variants of the *ALDH2* gene may have a suboptimal level of the enzyme, leading to the accumulation of the carcinogen acetaldehyde.

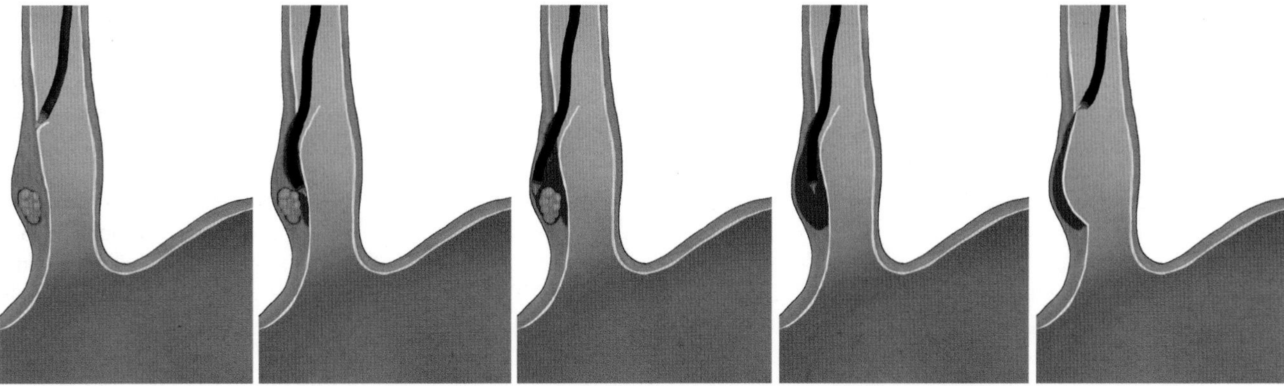

(a) Mucosal incision **(b)** Submucosal tunnelling **(c)** Tumour resection **(d)** Finish resection and haemostasis **(e)** Mucosa closure

Figure 66.43 Submucosal tunnelling endoscopic resection (STER) technique to excise a leiomyoma.

TABLE 66.3 Aetiological factors for oesophageal cancer.

Factor	Squamous cell cancer	Adenocarcinoma
Smoking	+++	+
Alcohol	+++	–
Hot beverages	+	–
N-nitroso-containing food (e.g. pickled vegetables)	+	–
Chewing betel nut	+	–
Drinking yerba mate	+	–
Dietary deficiency of fresh green vegetables, fruits and vitamins	+	–
Low socioeconomic class	+	–
Fungal toxin or virus	+	–
History of radiation to mediastinum	+	+
Lye corrosive stricture	+	–
History of upper aerodigestive malignancy	+++	–
Plummer–Vinson syndrome	+	–
Achalasia	+	–
Obesity	–	++
Gastro-oesophageal reflux	–	+++
Barrett's oesophagus	–	++++

For squamous cell cancer, dietary and environmental factors are important. Nitrosamines and their precursors (nitrate, nitrite and secondary amines), commonly found in preserved food, such as pickled vegetables, have been identified as predisposing factors. Nutritional depletion of certain micronutrients, particularly vitamins A, C and E, niacin, riboflavin, molybdenum, manganese, zinc, magnesium and selenium, as well as dietary deficiencies of fresh fruit and vegetables, together with an inadequate protein intake, predisposes the oesophageal epithelium to neoplastic transformation. Other dietary risk factors include consumption of hot beverages, chewing betel nuts and drinking yerba mate in South American countries.

Patients with other aerodigestive malignancies are at particularly high risk, presumably because of exposure to similar environmental carcinogens. Using oesophageal cancer as the index tumour, multiple primary cancers are found in about 10% of patients, of which 70% are in the aerodigestive tract. The overall incidence of synchronous or metachronous oesophageal cancer in patients with primary head and neck cancer is estimated to be 3%.

The rise in incidence of adenocarcinoma coincides with the increase in obesity, GORD and Barrett's oesophagus in Western populations. GORD affects up to 44% of the general population in the USA and approximately 5–8% will develop Barrett's oesophagus, with an estimated annual rate of neoplastic transformation of 0.2–0.5% per year.

Pathology, clinical features and diagnosis

Oesophageal cancer has a poor prognosis, which is in part related to late presentation; patients with early disease have no symptoms and the cancer tends to metastasise early. Both squamous cell and adenocarcinoma develop from dysplastic mucosa. Most adenocarcinomas are mucin producing with intestinal-type features. Squamous cell cancers tend to be found in the middle and upper part of the oesophagus, while adenocarcinoma predominantly affects the lower oesophagus and OGJ. Both cell types may directly infiltrate adjacent organs and, depending on tumour location, can involve the trachea and bronchi (leading to haemoptysis, airway obstruction and even oesophagus–airway fistula), aorta (though aorto-oesophageal fistula is rare), diaphragmatic crura or pericardium.

The oesophageal wall has a rich network of submucosal lymphatics, and therefore longitudinal submucosal spread of cancer is common. Lymph node metastasis can involve the cervical area, the mediastinum as well as the perigastric/coeliac axis. Distant haematogenous spread can occur to non-regional lymph nodes, lungs, liver, brain and bones. Peritoneal metastasis is an important mode of spread of adenocarcinoma of the OGJ but is rare for squamous cell cancer.

Progressive dysphagia is the most common symptom, related to increasing luminal obstruction by cancer. Early symptoms may include a mild hold-up sensation that, if ignored, will progress from dysphagia to a solid, soft and eventually to a liquid diet. There may often be anorexia, weight loss, odynophagia and regurgitation symptoms. Hoarseness may indicate involvement of either recurrent laryngeal nerve. Aspiration and choking symptoms may be related not only to tumour obstruction but also to the presence of an oesophagus–airway fistula. Choking and cough on drinking water are typical of fistulation and associated haemoptysis is common. Blood loss is less common for squamous cell cancer than adenocarcinoma. Chronic blood loss can lead to iron deficiency anaemia. Acute gastrointestinal bleeding can occur, though it is rarely severe, except for aorto-oesophageal fistula, which usually presents with a smaller sentinel bleed followed by massive bleeding that is invariably fatal.

Early cancers are usually asymptomatic and are only picked up on endoscopy performed for other reasons, except in countries where a screening programme exists. For squamous cell dysplasia and cancer, chromoendoscopy using Lugol's iodine is a useful adjunct (***Figure 66.44***); the normal squamous mucosa will be stained brown, while dysplastic and early cancer remains unstained. NBI light consists of only two wavelengths: 415-nm blue light and 540-nm green light. The differential absorption and reflection of these spectra facilitates detection of mucosal abnormalities (see ***Chapter 9***). A classification of an intraepithelial papillary capillary loop (IPCL) system has been introduced to grade the severity of these early neoplastic changes (***Figure 66.45***).

For patients with advanced cancer, diagnosis is usually not difficult. A barium contrast study may demonstrate the tumour as an ulcerated or stenotic lesion with proximal

Yerba mate is a herbal tea made from the leaves and twigs of the *Ilex paraguariensis* plant.

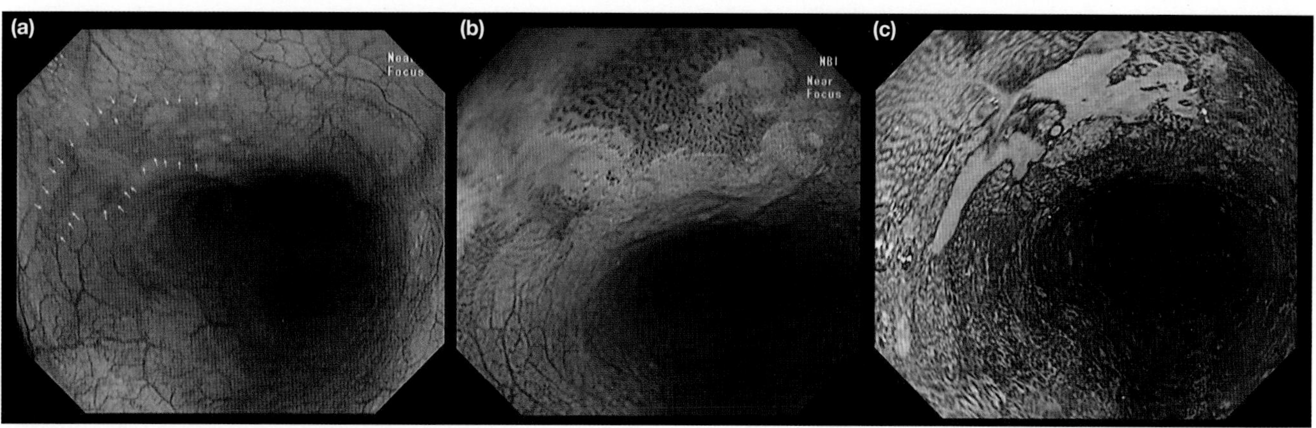

Figure 66.44 Early squamous cell cancer of the oesophagus. **(a)** A suspicious lesion under white light (marked by white arrows); **(b)** the area shown up on narrow-band imaging with magnification (abnormal intraepithelial papillary capillary loops can be seen); **(c)** the lesion is not stained by Lugol's iodine.

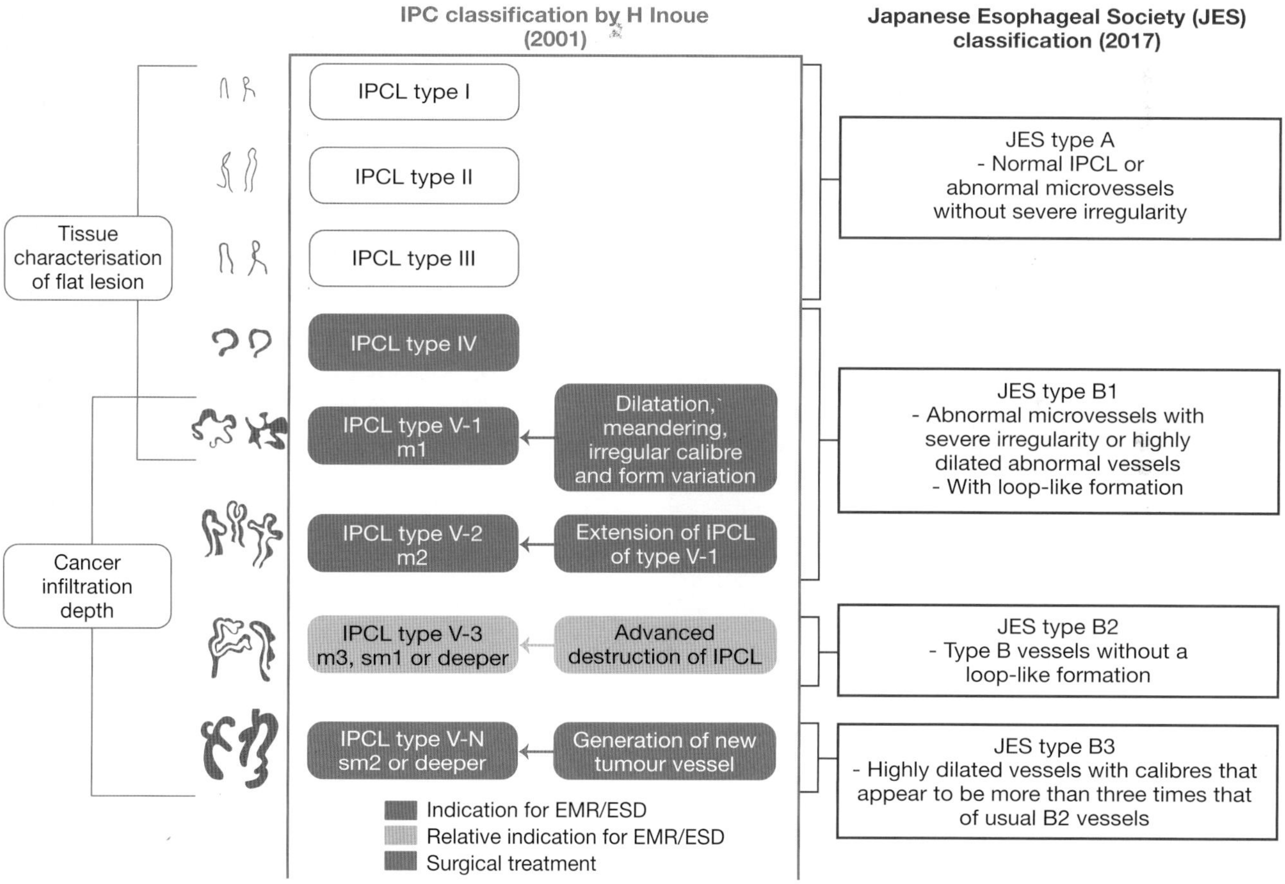

IPC classification by H Inoue (2001)

Japanese Esophageal Society (JES) classification (2017)

Tissue characterisation of flat lesion

Cancer infiltration depth

IPCL type I

IPCL type II

IPCL type III

IPCL type IV

IPCL type V-1 m1 ← Dilatation, meandering, irregular calibre and form variation

IPCL type V-2 m2 ← Extension of IPCL of type V-1

IPCL type V-3 m3, sm1 or deeper ← Advanced destruction of IPCL

IPCL type V-N sm2 or deeper ← Generation of new tumour vessel

Indication for EMR/ESD
Relative indication for EMR/ESD
Surgical treatment

JES type A
- Normal IPCL or abnormal microvessels without severe irregularity

JES type B1
- Abnormal microvessels with severe irregularity or highly dilated abnormal vessels
- With loop-like formation

JES type B2
- Type B vessels without a loop-like formation

JES type B3
- Highly dilated vessels with calibres that appear to be more than three times that of usual B2 vessels

Figure 66.45 Intraepithelial papillary capillary loop (IPCL) classification system. Pictorial diagram showing the appearance of the various types of IPCL correlating with the depth of invasion. EMR, endoscopic mucosal resection; ESD, endoscopic submucosal dissection.

dilatation (***Figure 66.46***). Endoscopy will visualise the tumour (***Figure 66.47***), allowing biopsies or brush cytology to confirm the histology. Attempts can be made to traverse the tumour stenosis. If significant dysphagia and weight loss are present, a nasogastric tube can be placed for nutritional build-up. The stomach is assessed for other pathologies in case it will be used to replace the oesophagus when oesophagectomy is performed.

Care should also be taken to assess the rest of the oesophagus, pharynx and larynx to ensure no synchronous tumours are present. The movement of the vocal cords should be assessed. For cancers of the mid- or upper oesophagus in proximity to the airway, a bronchoscopic examination is required to ensure no airway involvement, in which case oesophagectomy will be contraindicated (***Figure 66.48***).

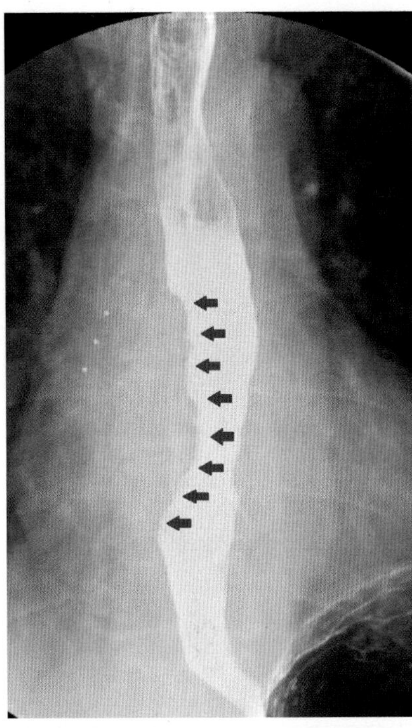

Figure 66.46 Barium contrast study showing midoesophageal cancer. Mucosal irregularity with mild luminal narrowing at the lower third of the oesophagus (arrows).

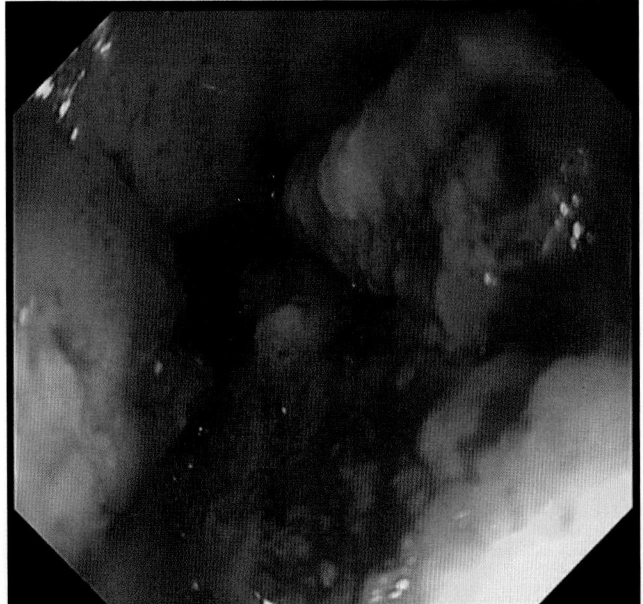

Figure 66.47 Endoscopic picture of an ulcerating cancer of the oesophagus.

Disease staging

Careful disease staging is essential to guide therapy. Current staging classification according to the American Joint Committee on Cancer (AJCC)/Union for International Cancer Control (UICC) (8th edition) is shown in ***Table 66.4***. The T stage advances as the tumour invades from mucosa deep to muscle, adventitia and beyond the oesophagus. Regional nodes

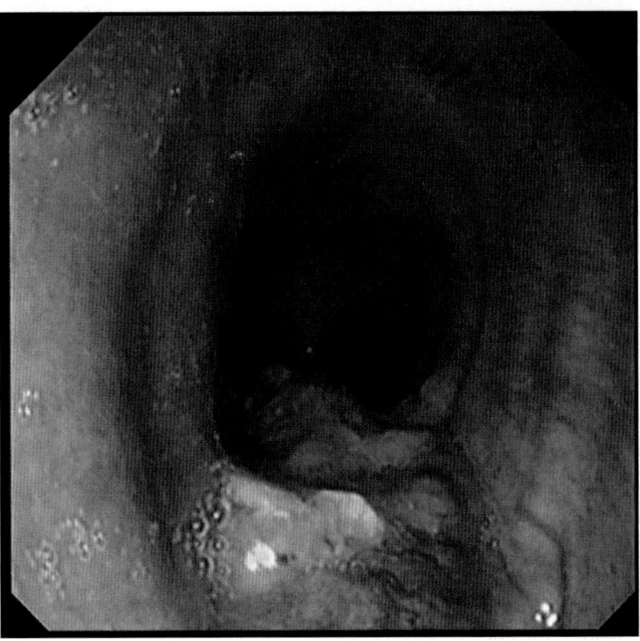

Figure 66.48 Bronchoscopic picture of airway infiltration by oesophageal cancer.

TABLE 66.4 TNM classification of oesophageal cancer.

T: Primary tumour	
Tx	Tumour cannot be assessed
T0	No evidence of primary tumour
Tis	High-grade dysplasia, defined as malignant cells confined to the epithelium by the basement membrane
T1	Tumour invades the lamina propria, muscularis mucosae or submucosa
	T1a: Tumour invades the lamina propria or muscularis mucosae
	T1b: Tumour invades submucosa
T2	Tumour invades the muscularis propria
T3	Tumour invades adventitia
T4	Tumour invades the adjacent structures
	T4a: Tumour invades the pleura, pericardium, azygos vein, diaphragm or peritoneum
	T4b: Tumour invades other adjacent structures, such as the aorta, vertebral body or airway
N: Regional lymph nodes[a]	
Nx	Regional nodal status cannot be assessed
N0	No regional lymph node metastasis
N1	Metastasis in one or two regional lymph nodes
N2	Metastasis in three to six regional lymph nodes
N3	Metastasis in seven or more regional lymph nodes
M: Distant metastases	
M0	No distant metastasis
M1	Distant metastasis

[a]Regional nodes extend from the paratracheal/oesophageal nodes in the neck to the coeliac nodes.

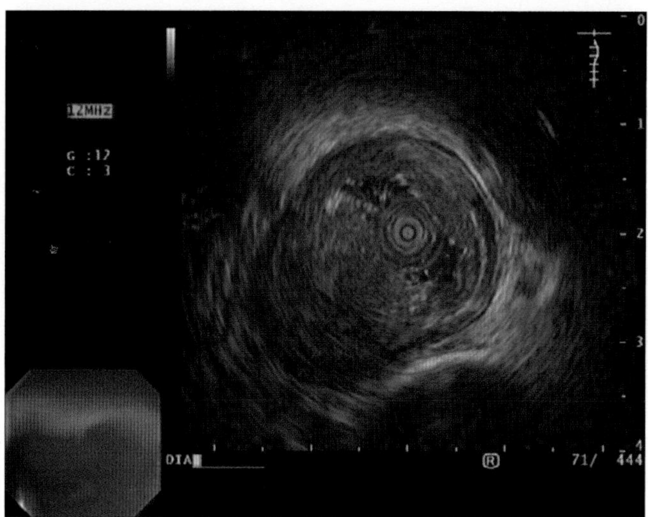

Figure 66.49 Endoscopic ultrasonography (EUS) picture of an oesophageal tumour. The layers of the oesophageal wall on EUS are obliterated. The tumour appears eccentric with extraoesophageal invasion (6 o'clock to 9 o'clock).

encompass the paratracheal nodes from the neck, through the mediastinum to the upper abdomen, including the coeliac nodes. The segregation of N1 to N3 is by the number of involved lymph nodes. Location is defined by the position of the epicentre of the tumour in the oesophagus (***Figure 66.1***). Stage groupings differ among squamous and adenocarcinomas. Separate groupings are assigned for clinical (cTNM), pathological (pTNM) and post-neoadjuvant (ypTNM) systems. Because of the complexity, these are not reproduced in this chapter but readers can refer to the staging manual.

Controversy exists as to whether adenocarcinoma of the OGJ should be staged as oesophageal or gastric cancer. According to the latest staging definitions, a tumour involving the OGJ with its epicentre no more than 2 cm into the gastric cardia is staged as adenocarcinoma of the oesophagus, while those with a centre located at more than 2 cm distal to the anatomical OGJ are staged as gastric cancer.

Endoscopic and percutaneous ultrasonography

The cT stage and paraoesophageal nodes are best staged using EUS. EUS is the only imaging modality able to distinguish the various layers of the oesophageal wall, usually seen as five alternating hyper- and hypoechoic layers using 12-MHz ultrasound (***Figure 66.49***). Infiltration to adjacent structures (cT4) is most accurately assessed. The accuracy of EUS for tumour and nodal staging averages 85% and 75%, respectively. The drawback is that many advanced cancers do not permit passage of a conventional echoendoscope, though most non-traversable tumours are likely to be at least cT3. Miniaturised ultrasonography catheter probes can be used to pass through the working channel of a conventional endoscope. EUS-guided FNA can be used to obtain cytological proof of involved lymph nodes. Bronchoscopic examination can assess airway involvement by the tumour. Percutaneous ultrasonography of cervical nodes is useful, as FNA can be obtained in the same setting.

Computed tomography scan

In diagnosing possible T4 cancer by CT scan, obliteration of the fat plane between the oesophagus and the aorta, trachea and bronchi, and pericardium is suggestive of invasion, but the paucity of fat in cachectic patients makes this criterion unreliable. Diagnosis of paraoesophageal nodes is less accurate than with EUS, but distant nodes are better assessed by CT scan.

Fluorodeoxyglucose-positron emission tomography scans

Squamous cell cancers are usually fluorodeoxyglucose (FDG) avid (***Figure 66.50***). Detection of the primary tumour is useful. Adenocarcinomas of the OGJ sometimes show limited or absent FDG accumulation regardless of tumour volume (FDG non-avidity). Positron emission tomography (PET) does not define the oesophageal wall and thus has no value in cT staging. Its spatial resolution is also insufficient to separate the primary tumour with juxtatumoral nodes because of interference from the primary cancer. It is mostly used for detecting regional and non-regional nodes, as well as distant metastases. The uptake by the tumour may have some prognostic value, and change in uptake after neoadjuvant treatment is similarly useful in predicting histological response and outcome.

Laparoscopy

Laparoscopic staging is useful in adenocarcinomas, especially those of the OGJ, but not for squamous cell cancer. Laparoscopy should be reserved for patients in whom confirmation of metastatic disease that is not otherwise obtainable is essential in deciding on treatment.

Treatment

Stage-directed therapy

Treatment principles depend on the disease stage and physiological reserve of patients. Patients should be discussed in a multidisciplinary team to decide on the best course of management. When distant metastatic disease is identified palliation is the aim.

Endoscopic treatment

The chance of nodal metastasis depends on the depth of infiltration of the primary tumour. Cancers that are confined to the mucosa (T1a) rarely metastasise, but squamous tumours that have infiltrated the submucosa (T1b) have a substantial risk of nodal spread. In adenocarcinoma, the corresponding risk is less. Such early cancers may be amenable to curative endoscopic treatment (***Figure 66.51***). EMR involves the injection of saline (or other solutions such as glycerol or hyaluronic acid) into the submucosal plane to raise the mucosal lesion; it is then sucked into a cap fitted onto the tip of the endoscope, looped by a snare wire and cut by electrocautery. The limitation of this method is the size of the cap, so it is generally recommended for smaller lesions. For larger lesions, if resected by EMR, piecemeal resection is required; therefore, it is associated with higher incomplete resection and recurrence rates. ESD is more complex. It involves first marking the margins

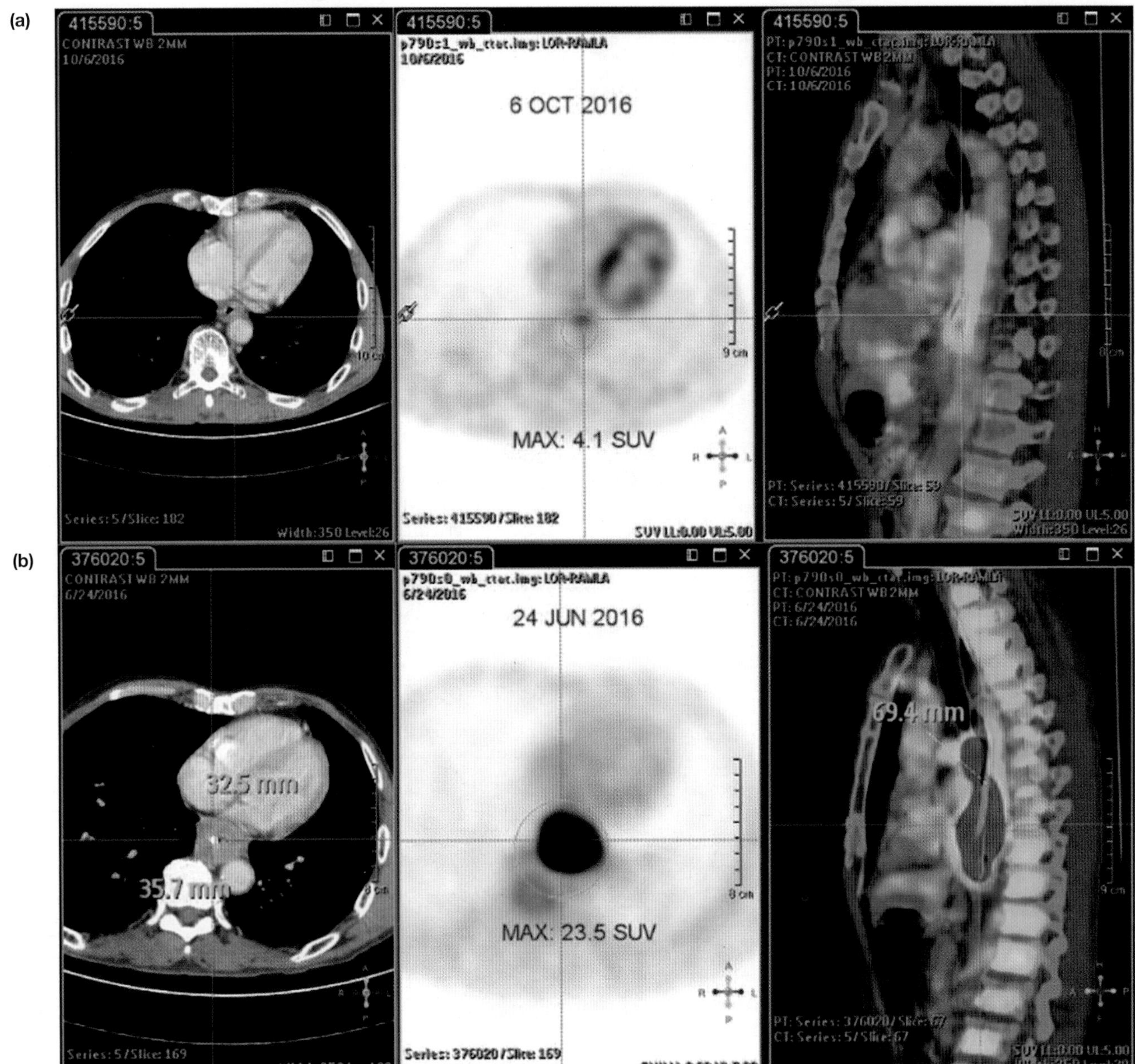

Figure 66.50 Positron emission tomography/computed tomography (CT) scan for staging of oesophageal cancer and assessment of response to neoadjuvant therapy. The patient underwent neoadjuvant chemoradiotherapy. The tumour had high fluorodeoxyglucose uptake (SUV_{max} 23.5) before treatment **(b)**. After chemoradiotherapy the SUV_{max} dropped to 4.1 with a corresponding reduction in size of the cancer seen on CT scan **(a)**.

of the lesion, then submucosal injection, cutting the mucosal edges along the line of marking, submucosal dissection of the tumour from its bed (superficial to the muscle layer) and lastly haemostasis. There are various 'knives' that can be inserted via the biopsy channel of the endoscope to carry out these procedures. Technically ESD is more demanding than EMR but is not limited by the size of the lesion for en bloc resection. There is an increased risk of postresection stricture formation if too much of the circumference of the mucosa (such as over two-thirds) is removed. This chance is somewhat reduced by steroid treatment (often endoscopic injection at the time of EMR/ESD, combined with oral medication for some time).

For early Barrett's cancer, EMR and ESD are options, and additional circumferential resection or ablation of the whole length of Barrett's mucosa can be done. For ablative therapy, RFA is most commonly used. RFA energy is delivered by the bipolar electrode and the energy causes frictional heating of cellular water molecules. After ablation, in the presence of a non-acid milieu (suppressed by a high-dose PPI), the epithelium would regenerate to be squamous cell mucosa. The advantage of RFA is that it is technically easy to operate but the drawback is that no surgical specimen for detailed histopathological examination is available. Other examples of ablative technique include cryotherapy or photodynamic therapy.

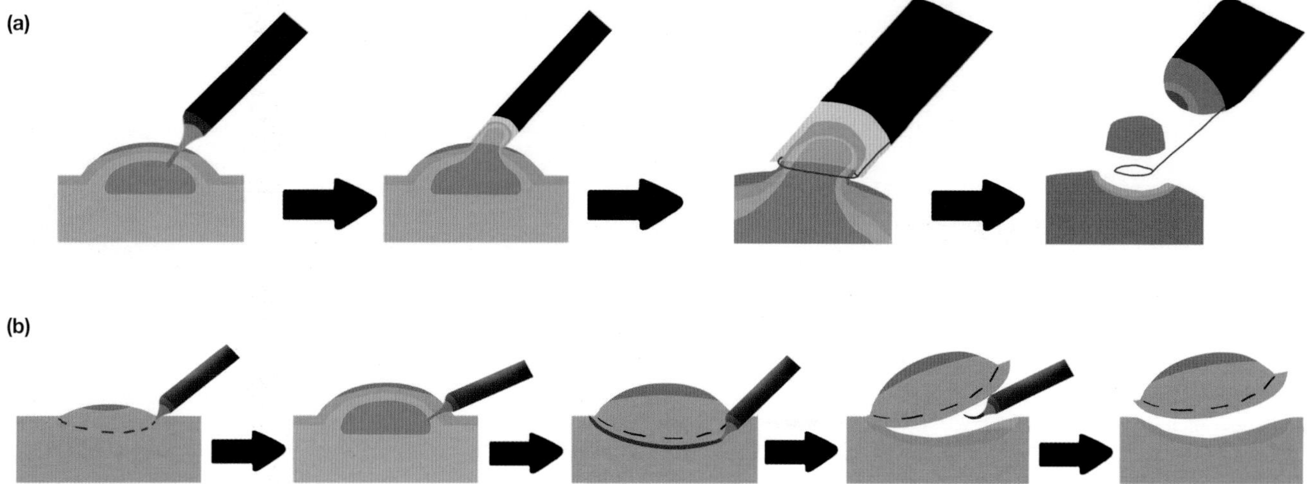

Figure 66.51 Schematic diagrams showing technique of (a) endoscopic mucosal resection – cap with submucosal injection and snare excision; (b) endoscopic submucosal dissection.

Because the pretreatment distinction of T1a and T1b disease may not be accurate, it may be prudent to perform endoscopic resection first in case of uncertain diagnosis. Should the resected specimen be found to be T1a with clear margins and without lymphovascular permeation in the pathological examination, the endoscopic treatment is deemed curative. If the tumour is found to be deeper than expected or if resection margins are not clear, further therapy can be planned.

Surgery

The primary indication for surgical resection is for potential cure, which can be achieved in patients whose tumours are confined to its wall and only limited local/regional disease is found. One should aim to maximise the chance of an R0 resection (macroscopic and microscopic clearance of proximal, distal and lateral margins), a parameter that has consistently been shown to result in the best long-term survival. Surgical resection alone is generally indicated for more advanced cancers when endoscopic treatment is unlikely to be curative (T1b, T2, N0). For patients with more advanced disease (≥T3, N+), multimodality treatment is usually preferred.

Patient selection and preparation

Oesophagectomy is a major procedure; patients should be assessed carefully for operative risk and their physiological status optimised. Cardiorespiratory assessments are essential. Patients must stop smoking and alcohol intake. Chest physiotherapy is instituted, and incentive spirometry is a good preoperative exercise. Patients with high-grade oesophageal tumour stenosis may have lost a substantial amount of weight. A fine-bore nasogastric tube can be placed for nutritional support while work-up is performed. Feeding jejunostomy is an alternative. Enhanced recovery after surgery (ERAS) programmes entail preoperative 'pre-habilitation' as well (***Table 66.5***). All measures are aimed to optimise patients for surgery. Immediate preoperative preparations include prophylactic antibiotics and deep vein thrombosis prophylaxis. Bowel preparation is not necessary unless a colonic interposition is intended.

Surgical techniques

Choice of surgical approach

The choice of the appropriate technique depends mainly on: (i) the location of the tumour, (ii) the intended extent of lymphadenectomy, and (iii) the reconstructive technique. The surgeon should be well versed in the methods adopted to different clinical situations. For ease of description, the following sections discuss the surgical approach by tumour location.

Cervical oesophageal cancer

Surgery involves removing the pharynx, larynx and oesophagus (pharyngo-laryngo-oesophagectomy); a gastric pull-up is used to anastomose with the neo-pharynx. In cases where involvement of the cervical oesophagus is limited, pharyngo-laryngo-cervical oesophagectomy can be carried out without the need for total oesophageal resection. The resultant gap can be bridged using either a free jejunal graft, or various musculocutaneous flaps. Definitive chemoradiotherapy has become the preferred alternative treatment to preserve the larynx. Surgery is therefore mostly reserved for salvage, when there is an incomplete response or for recurrent disease.

Intrathoracic oesophageal cancer

The surgical procedures usually performed are:

- Left thoracoabdominal incision. Via a large incision traversing the chest and upper abdomen, the whole left upper quadrant of the abdomen and left thoracic cavity are accessed at the same time for oesophagectomy, gastroplasty and anastomosis (***Figure 66.52a***).
- Lewis–Tanner (or Ivor Lewis) procedure. This is a two-phase oesophagectomy consisting of laparotomy for gastric mobilisation and tubularisation, followed by a right

Ivor Lewis, 1895–1982, surgeon, North Middlesex Hospital, London, later Rhyl, UK.
Norman Cecil Tanner, 1906–1982, surgeon, Charing Cross Hospital, London, UK.

TABLE 66.5 An enhanced recovery after surgery (ERAS) programme for oesophagectomy.

Preoperative	
Preoperative counselling	
Nutritional assessment	Nasogastric tube feeding for those with significant stenosis of the oesophagus, and oral supplement in those at risk of malnutrition
Preoperative exercise	General and incentive spirometry + pre-habilitation programme
Stop smoking and alcohol intake	
Chest physiotherapy	
Carbohydrate loading on day of surgery	No solid food 6 hours before and fluid 2 hours before surgery. Carbohydrate loading night before and finishes 2 hours before surgery
No need for bowel preparation unless colonic interposition is planned	
Intraoperative	
Prophylactic antibiotics	
DVT prophylaxis	Mechanical +/– pharmacological
Judicious use of intraoperative fluids	
Avoid hypothermia	
Minimally invasive surgery if possible	
Epidural analgesia	
Postoperative	
Nutrition	POD1 carbohydrate drink, gradual advancement to soft diet by POD5 (if no vocal cord palsy and assessment by speech therapist shows no risk of aspiration) PPN/TPN/feeding via jejunostomy in those at nutritional risk and oral intake insufficient
Nasogastric tube	Removal on POD1 (if no vocal cord palsy and assessment by speech therapist shows no risk of aspiration)
Analgesia	Epidural analgesia/patient-controlled analgesia/multimodal analgesia
Chest drain	Single closed small-calibre drain (19Fr Blake drain), removal POD3–4 when output <200–300 mL/day
Early mobilisation	From POD1, supervised by physiotherapist
Urinary catheter	Early removal as soon as close monitoring of urine output is not essential
Intravenous fluid	Balanced intravenous fluid to avoid over- and underhydration
DVT prophylaxis	

DVT, deep vein thrombosis; POD, postoperative day; PPN, peripheral parenteral nutrition; TPN, total parenteral nutrition.

thoracotomy for oesophageal resection. The gastroplasty is delivered into the right thoracic cavity for an oesophago-gastrostomy near the apex of the chest (***Figure 66.52b***).

- McKeown or three-stage oesophagectomy. This consists of the mobilisation of the thoracic oesophagus and lymphadenectomy via a thoracotomy (usually right side), followed by abdominal and neck incisions for preparation of the oesophageal substitute (usually the stomach) and its delivery to the neck for a cervical anastomosis.
- Left thoracic resection (Sweet oesophagectomy). Via a single posterolateral incision on the left chest wall (usually fifth to sixth intercostal space), the oesophagus is mobilised. The diaphragm is opened and the gastroplasty prepared from this opening. The stomach is delivered to the left thoracic cavity for anastomosis.
- Transhiatal oesophagectomy. Through a cervical and abdominal approach, the oesophagus is mobilised via both directions, being stripped out bluntly from its mediastinal bed. The gastric conduit is delivered to the neck for cervical anastomosis (***Figure 66.53***).
- Minimally invasive surgical approaches. Traditional open procedures (described above) are increasingly replaced by minimally invasive methods, by a combination of video-assisted thoracoscopy (VATS) and laparoscopy or robotic techniques (***Figure 66.54***). Both thoracic and abdominal phases can be performed via minimally invasive techniques, or one phase can be minimally invasive and the other by open surgery (hybrid procedures). The anastomosis can be constructed in the chest or the neck.

Kenneth Charles McKeown, 1912–1995, surgeon, Darlington Memorial Hospital, Durham, UK.
Richard H Sweet, 1901–1962, surgeon, Massachusetts General Hospital, Boston, MA, USA.

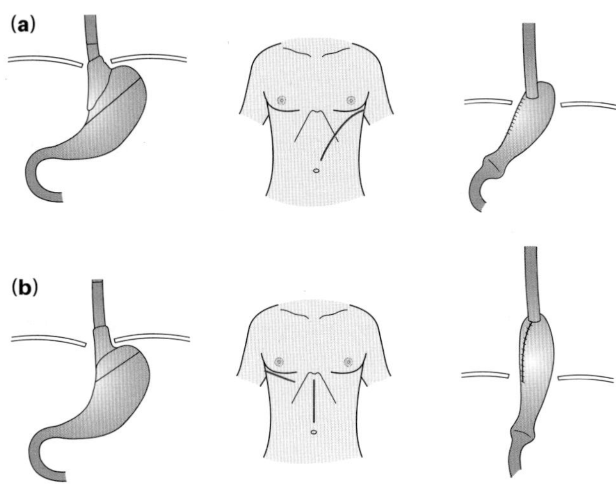

Figure 66.52 The common open approaches for surgery of the oesophagus: **(a)** left thoracoabdominal; **(b)** two-stage Lewis–Tanner (Ivor Lewis) approach. In the McKeown approach a third incision in the neck is made to allow anastomosis to the cervical oesophagus.

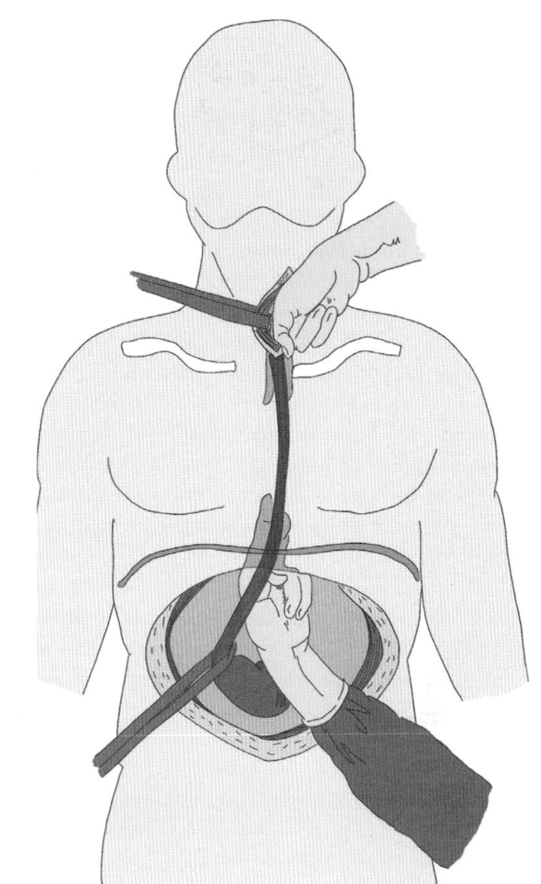

Figure 66.53 Transhiatal oesophagectomy whereby the oesophagus is mobilised blindly using fingers from the neck and hand inserted from the abdomen.

Oesophagogastric junction cancer

The options detailed above for intrathoracic cancers also apply to cancers of the OGJ. Suitability depends in part on the extent of oesophageal and gastric involvement by cancer and the intended extent of resection and lymphadenectomy. In addition, an extended total radical gastrectomy can be performed. The whole stomach and the lower oesophagus (accessed via the oesophageal hiatus from the abdomen) are resected and intestinal continuity is restored with a jejunal Roux loop (Roux-en-y reconstruction). In selected patients with early disease, a proximal gastrectomy can be performed as nodal spread to the distal stomach is rare.

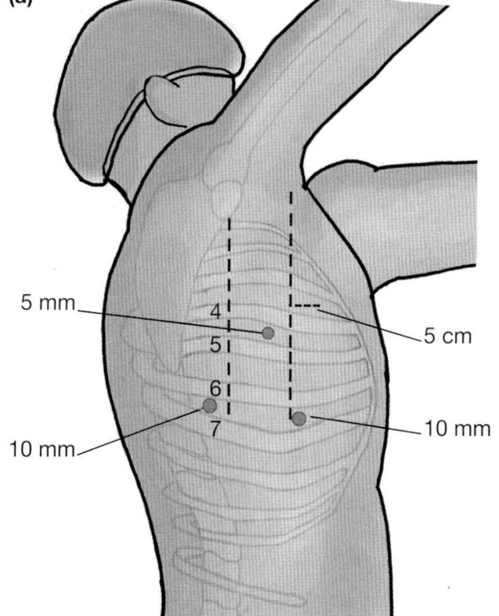

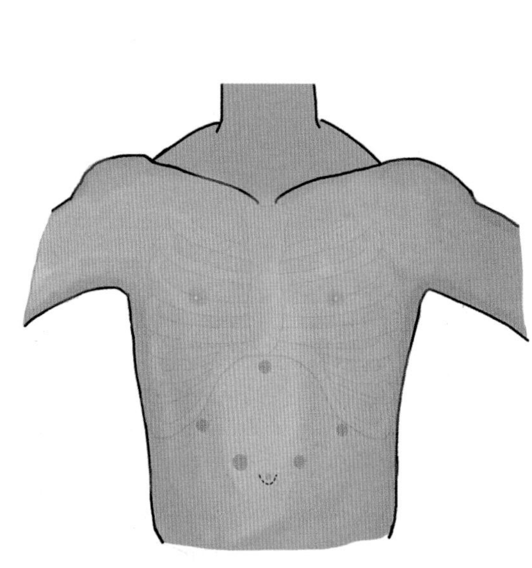

Figure 66.54 Port sites for video-assisted thoracoscopic oesophagectomy in the left lateral position **(a)** and laparoscopic gastric mobilisation **(b)**. Port sites can vary depending on the surgeon's preference.

César Roux, 1857–1934, Professor of Surgery and Gynaecology, Lausanne, Switzerland, described this method of forming a jejunal conduit in 1908.

Extent of lymphadenectomy

Lymphadenectomy ensures adequate nodal sampling for staging, improves local disease control and increasingly there is evidence to show the prognostic impact of extended lymphadenectomy. The most appropriate extent of lymphadenectomy remains somewhat controversial. Transhiatal oesophagectomy does not allow adequate mediastinal nodal dissection (for the mid- and upper thoracic part oesophageal mobilisation is mostly a 'blind' procedure) and thus is often chosen by surgeons who perform only a limited lower mediastinal dissection for OGJ adenocarcinoma. Squamous cell cancers are mostly more proximally located and the transhiatal approach may be dangerous except in early cancers.

The extent of lymphadenectomy can be defined as 'fields'. Two-field dissection refers to lymphadenectomy of the mediastinum and upper abdomen around the coeliac trifurcation. The mediastinal 'field' is further classified as (i) standard: lymphadenectomy below the tracheal bifurcation, (ii) extended: standard lymphadenectomy plus right paratracheal nodal dissection including those around the right recurrent laryngeal nerve, and (iii) total: extended lymphadenectomy plus nodal dissection along the left recurrent laryngeal nerve chain (***Figure 66.55***). The third field refers to bilateral cervical lymphadenectomy, including those in the paratracheal as well as supraclavicular fossae.

The most appropriate extent of lymphadenectomy remains a contentious issue. For patients with squamous cell cancers, most surgeons would perform at least a total two-field lymphadenectomy since lymph node mapping data in Japan showed significant nodal metastases, especially around the bilateral recurrent laryngeal nerves. In selected patients and in particular those with upper thoracic cancers, additional third-field nodal dissection is performed (three-field lymphadenectomy). For oesophageal adenocarcinoma, most surgeons perform an infracarinal two-field lymphadenectomy. For OGJ tumours (in particular those with limited oesophageal extent and centre on the OGJ), surgeons are divided among those who prefer oesophagectomy and those who perform extended total gastrectomy with limited lower oesophageal resection and lymphadenectomy. The issue is unsettled. The extent of resection (and lymphadenectomy) has to be balanced against associated morbidities and physiological reserve of the individual patient.

Reconstruction

Restoration of intestinal continuity after oesophageal extirpation is mostly done using a gastric conduit. The right gastroepiploic vessels are its main blood supply. A pyloric drainage procedure is optional, with some surgeons advocating its use to facilitate gastric emptying, after the inevitable vagotomy. In the case of a previous gastrectomy, or if concomitant pathology (such as gastric cancer) requires its removal, the colon (right ileocolon, left or transverse colon) can be used. The surgery is more extensive and three anastomoses are required. The conduit can be placed in the right thoracic cavity (as in after a Lewis–Tanner oesophagectomy) or the neck for cervical

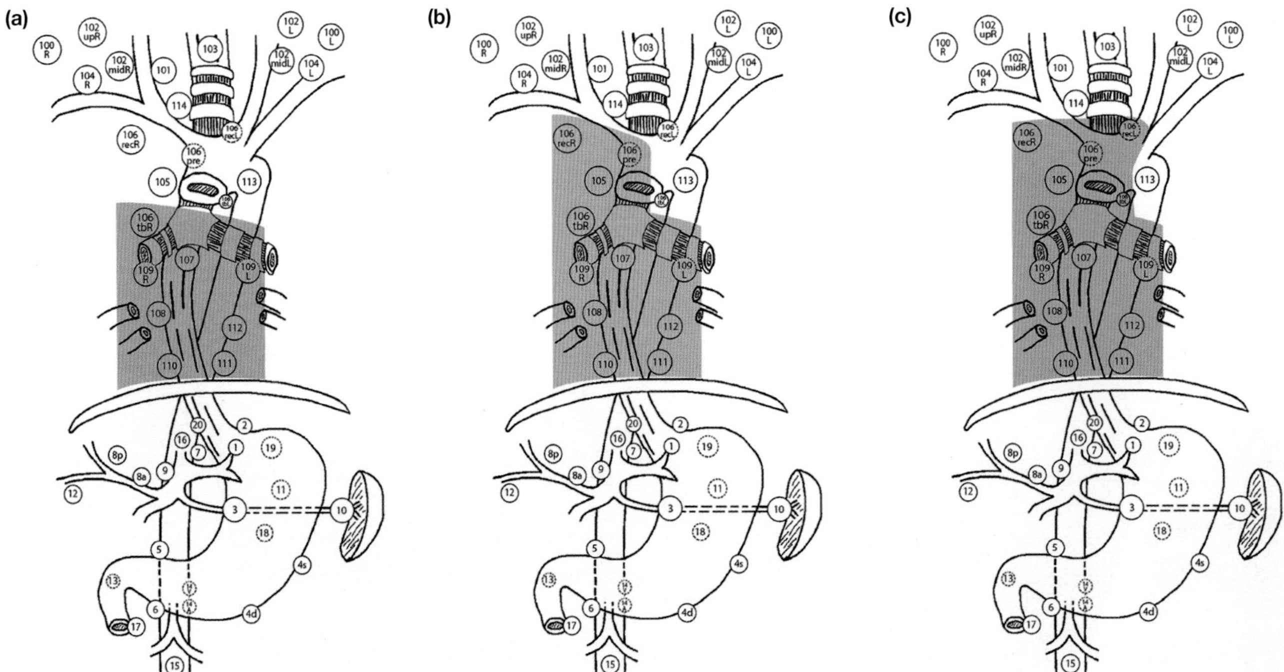

Figure 66.55 The lymph node station nomenclature according to the Japanese classification. Extent of mediastinal lymphadenectomy. (a) Standard mediastinal lymphadenectomy includes stations below the tracheal bifurcation. (b) Extended mediastinal lymphadenectomy includes standard lymphadenectomy + right paratracheal nodal dissection including those around the right recurrent laryngeal nerve. (c) Total mediastinal lymphadenectomy includes extended lymphadenectomy + left paratracheal area and nodes along the left recurrent laryngeal nerve. Two-field lymphadenectomy includes mediastinal dissection plus nodal dissection around the coeliac axis and three-field dissection includes cervical lymphadenectomy.

oesophagogastrostomy. In the case of a neck anastomosis, three choices of routes of reconstruction exist: posterior mediastinal, retrosternal or subcutaneous.

Perioperative care

For most patients, a standardised clinical pathway is helpful, along the lines of the ERAS protocol (***Table 66.5***). ERAS is a global perioperative quality improvement initiative based on attenuation of the stress response to surgical injury. The gastrointestinal system is central to many of the core ERAS elements, including carbohydrate loading, no prolonged fasting, avoidance of mechanical bowel preparation, avoidance of nasogastric intubation, maintaining fluid balance and early feeding. Employing these ERAS care practices leads to improved clinical outcome.

Management of complications

Complications are common as patients are often elderly with pre-existing morbidities and surgery is extensive. Atelectasis and pneumonia are managed by chest physiotherapy, adequate pain relief, avoidance of fluid overload, appropriate antibiotics and, if needed, sputum suction by bronchoscopy. Atrial fibrillation occurs in around 15–20% of patients; it is benign in most and is treated by antiarrhythmic medication. In some patients, it is a reflection of underlying serious complication, such as bronchopneumonia, or more importantly surgical morbidities, such as anastomotic leak or ischaemia of the conduit. Its occurrence should prompt appropriate investigations, such as endoscopy. Recurrent laryngeal nerve injury is not uncommon when superior mediastinal lymphadenectomy or neck nodal dissection is carried out. Postoperatively the patient will experience hoarseness of the voice, coughing becomes less effective and aspiration may be a problem when the diet is introduced. Active chest therapy and delay of oral intake may be necessary. Injection thyroplasty can temporarily improve glottic closure and coughing effort and lower the chance of aspiration. More definitive therapy may be needed if vocal cord function does not return.

Gross ischaemia of the conduit usually presents within the first 2–3 days after the operation and dictates taking down of the conduit, adequate drainage and staged reconstruction later once sepsis is under control (***Figure 66.56***). In selected cases immediate reanastomosis is an option if the patient is haemodynamically stable and an adequate length of healthy stomach remains.

Clinically apparent thoracic anastomotic leaks usually occur within the first week. Signs of sepsis and excessive output from the chest drain, which may be turbid in colour, may lead to the diagnosis. The location and magnitude of the leak can be visualised by a water-soluble contrast study. A carefully performed flexible endoscopic examination is also helpful and will not worsen the leak. For small, contained leaks, CT-guided drainage or use of a luminal vacuum Endo-Sponge™ may suffice. In septic patients with a sizeable leak, exploration is warranted to establish drainage. Direct repair is seldom possible.

For cervical anastomosis, leakage is suspected when there is inflammation and pain of the neck wound. Turbid infected discharge is found when the skin stitches are removed. Leaks that are truly confined to the neck are simply treated by laying the wound open with daily washing and frequent changes of dressing. Leaks that communicate with the mediastinum may require formal exploration and placement of mediastinal drains.

In all leaks, treatment with broad-spectrum antibiotics is required, guided by microbial culture and sensitivity. Nutritional support is essential. With an intrathoracic stomach, careful endoscopic placement of a fine-bore feeding tube into the duodenum for enteral feeding is useful. Injection of fibrin glue, placement of intraluminal stents, use of a luminal vacuum

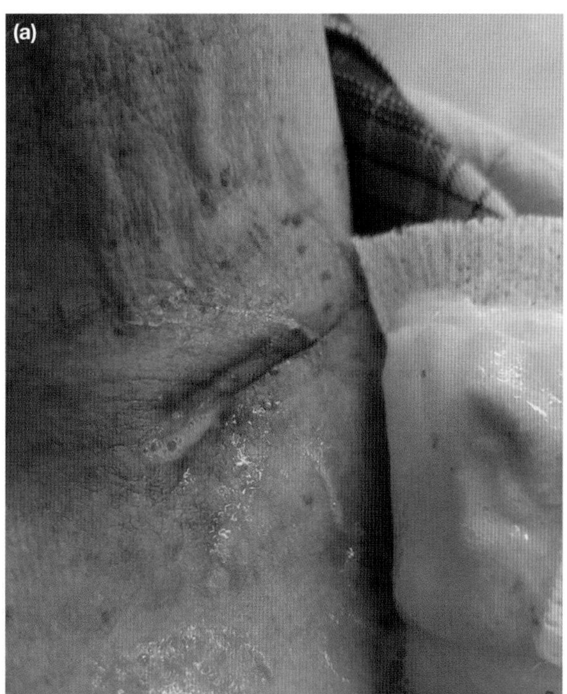

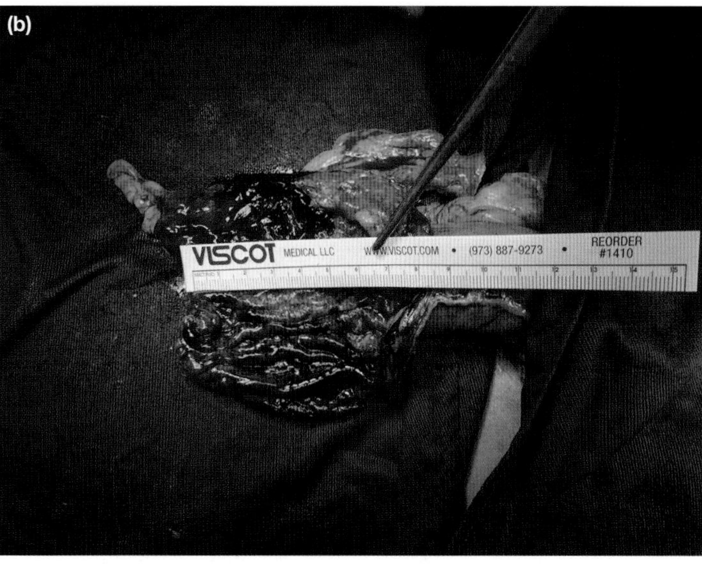

Figure 66.56 **(a)** Cervical wound with erythema, swelling and discharge of purulent material, typical of a cervical anastomotic leak. **(b)** An ischaemic gastric conduit; 5 cm of the stomach appeared unhealthy and required resection.

Endo-Sponge™ or endoscopic clip closure of the defect are increasingly used to treat leaks; sealing of the leak allows early control of sepsis and resumption of oral alimentation. The stent can be removed afterwards, depending on the severity of the leak in the first place. Usually, 4–6 weeks will suffice for adequate healing.

A chylous leak is suspected when there is excessive chest drainage. A milk challenge, looking at the colour of the effluent before and after taking milk by mouth or via the nasogastric tube, will usually be obvious. This can be aided by biochemical testing of the drain fluid, measuring triglyceride level or chylomicrons. In a low-output fistula of less than 0.5–1 litre per day, conservative management with total parenteral nutrition or a mid-chain triglyceride diet may suffice. In case of persistence or if the output is more than 1 litre per day, prolonged conservative treatment is not recommended and early re-exploration is warranted. A lymphangiogram preoperatively will help locate the site of leakage, and intraoperative milk feed will also serve the same purpose. The site of the leak can then be clipped or sutured. Increasingly, however, the interventional radiological method of percutaneous embolisation has gained success and has reduced the need for surgical re-exploration.

Multimodality treatment strategies

Results from surgical resection alone have improved. Mortality from surgery is less than 5% in dedicated centres. The long-term prognosis remains suboptimal. Since the 1990s, multimodality treatment has gained impetus and is now routine for advanced disease. Neoadjuvant therapy is more popular than postoperative therapy, in the form of either neoadjuvant chemotherapy or chemoradiotherapy. In OGJ cancers, perioperative (pre- and postoperative chemotherapy) has advocates. The optimal regimen remains controversial. Recent advances in immunotherapy add to the armamentarium. Overall, after treatment in a multimodality programme, a 5-year survival rate of 40–50% is expected. The disease stage and the ability to perform an R0 resection are the most powerful predictors of outcome.

Palliation

In the presence of distant metastases, palliation is the aim. Dysphagia is the main symptom to relieve. Placement of a self-expanding metallic stent is simple and effective and allows immediate relief of dysphagia (***Figure 66.57***). The risks are stent migration, tumour ingrowth, airway compression and tracheal erosion if placed in the mid- and upper oesophagus. Other endoscopic methods, such as dilatation, laser treatment and photodynamic therapy, can be used.

Chemotherapy/radiotherapy/brachytherapy can help restore luminal patency; in case of bleeding from OGJ tumours, radiotherapy can be haemostatic. Immunotherapy has promise in selected patients.

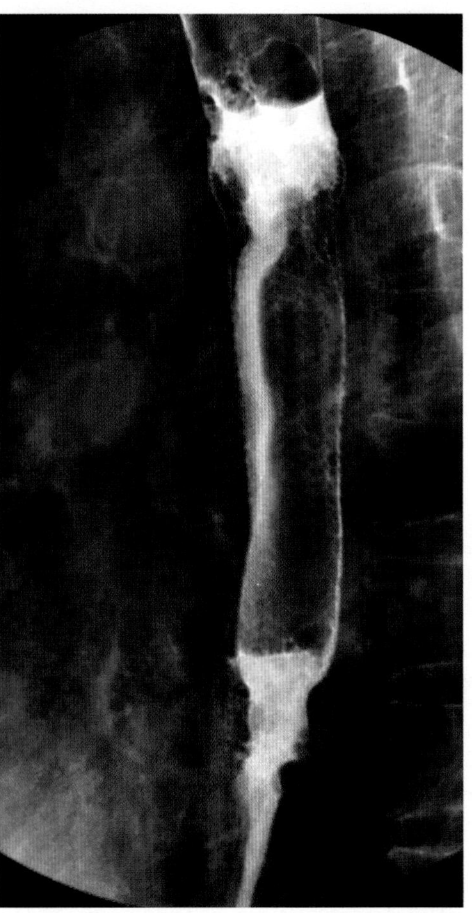

Figure 66.57 Self-expanding metallic stent in palliation of oesophageal cancer.

Summary box 66.8

Oesophageal cancer

- Squamous cell cancer still predominates in the East, while Barrett's adenocarcinoma is more common in the West
- Late presentation and early spread are reasons for poor prognosis
- Early diagnosis has the best chance of cure
- Lymphatic spread can be widespread, from the neck to the mediastinum and coeliac axis
- Adenocarcinomas around the OGJ are sometimes regarded as proximal gastric cancer and treatment is particularly controversial

MISCELLANEOUS CONDITIONS

Plummer–Vinson (in the USA) or Paterson–Brown-Kelly syndrome (UK) refers to the findings of a cervical oesophageal web, iron deficiency anaemia and dysphagia. It is also known as

Henry Stanley Plummer, 1874–1937, physician, Mayo Clinic, Rochester, MN, USA.
Porter Paisley Vinson, 1890–1959, surgeon, Mayo Clinic, Rochester, MN, USA.
Donald Ross Paterson, 1863–1939, ENT surgeon, Cardiff Royal Infirmary, Cardiff, UK.
Adam Brown-Kelly, 1865–1941, ENT surgeon, Victoria Infirmary, Glasgow, UK.

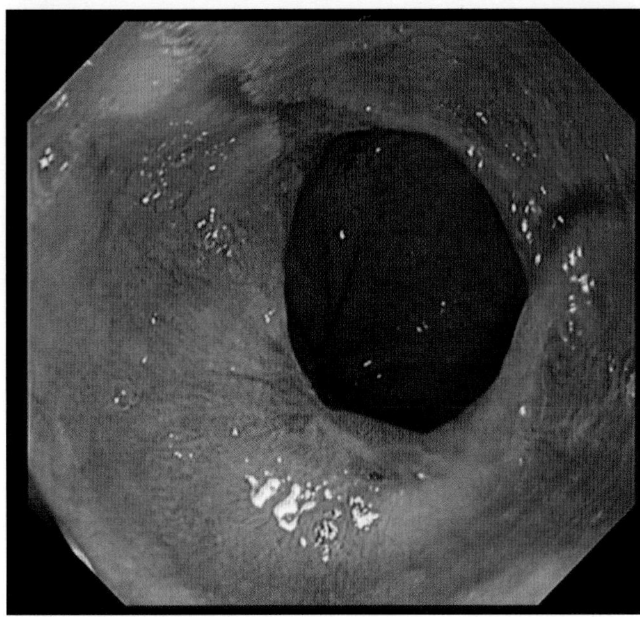

Figure 66.58 Schatzki's ring found on endoscopy. Note there is also oesophagitis.

sideropenic dysphagia. The pathophysiology remains elusive, and the association of iron deficiency is also controversial. Possible mechanisms include iron and nutritional deficiencies, genetic predisposition and autoimmunity. It is a rare disease, mainly affecting middle-aged women. There is a predisposition to postcricoid, cervical oesophageal cancer. A web is distinguished from a Schatzki's ring in that both the proximal and distal surfaces of the web are lined by squamous mucosa; in a Schatzki's ring, the proximal side is lined with squamous mucosa and the distal side by columnar mucosa, coinciding with its location at the squamocolumnar junction. Treatment is with iron therapy, diet modification and, if necessary, endoscopic dilatation of the cervical web.

A Schatzki's ring (also known as oesophageal B ring; an A ring is located a few centimetres proximal to the B ring, if found) is a mucosal band found at the squamocolumnar junction and is not an uncommon cause of food impaction in adults (***Figure 66.58***). Radiological studies using barium contrast by Schatzki demonstrated that, in individuals with a ring size of less than 13 mm, the symptom of dysphagia may occur. The exact aetiology of Schatzki's ring is uncertain but is believed to be related to GORD; hiatus hernia is more common. Treatment is by endoscopic dilatation if symptomatic with dysphagia.

FURTHER READING

Bennett RD, Starghan DM, Velanocivh V. Gastroesophageal reflux disease, hiatal hernia, and Barrett esophagus. In: Zinner MJ, Ashley SW, Hines OJ (eds). *Maingot's abdominal operations*, 13th edn. New York: McGraw-Hill, 2019: 393–422.

Hölscher AH, Law S. Esophagogastric junction adenocarcinomas: individualization of resection with special considerations for Siewert type II, and Nishi types EG, E=G and GE cancers. *Gastric Cancer* 2020; **23**(1): 3–9.

Katzka DA. Eosinophilic esophagitis. *Ann Intern Med* 2020; **172**(9): ITC65–ITC80.

Law S. Esophagogastrectomy for carcinoma of the esophagus. In: Fischer JE (ed.). *Mastery of surgery*, 7th edn. Philadelphia: Wolters Kluwer, 2019: 983–99.

Low DE, Allum W, De Manzoni G *et al.* Guidelines for perioperative care in esophagectomy: Enhanced Recovery After Surgery (ERAS®) Society Recommendations. *World J Surg* 2019; **43**(2): 299–330.

Tong DKH, Law S. Cancer of the oesophagus. In: Zinner MJ, Ashley SW, Hines OJ (eds). *Maingot's abdominal operations*, 13th edn. New York: McGraw-Hill, 2019: 443–74.

Yadlapati R, Kahrilas PJ, Fox MR *et al.* Esophageal motility disorders on high-resolution manometry: Chicago classification version 4.0©. *Neurogastroenterol Motil* 2021; **33**(1): e14058.

Zaninotto G, Bennett C, Boeckxstaens G *et al.* The 2018 ISDE achalasia guidelines. *Dis Esophagus* 2018; **31**(9).

Zundel N, Melvin WS, Patti MG, Camacho D (eds). *Benign esophageal disease. Modern surgical approaches and techniques*. Cham: Springer, 2021.

CHAPTER 67 The stomach and duodenum

Learning objectives

To understand:
- The gross and microscopic anatomy and pathophysiology of the stomach and duodenum
- The critical importance of gastritis and *Helicobacter pylori* in upper gastrointestinal disease
- The causes of duodenal obstruction and the presentation of duodenal tumours

To be able to:
- Decide on the most appropriate investigation of patients with complaints relating to the stomach and duodenum
- Treat peptic ulcer disease and its complications
- Recognise the presentation of gastric cancer and understand the principles involved in treatment

INTRODUCTION

The stomach acts as a reservoir for ingested food, where it is mechanically broken down and the process of digestion begins before the ingested content passes into the duodenum.

ANATOMY OF THE STOMACH AND DUODENUM

Blood supply

Arteries

The stomach has an arterial supply on both the lesser and greater curves (*Figure 67.1*). On the lesser curve, the left gastric artery, a branch of the coeliac axis, forms an anastomotic arcade with the right gastric artery, which arises from the common hepatic artery. Branches of the left gastric artery pass up towards the cardia. The gastroduodenal artery, also a branch of the hepatic artery, passes behind the first part of the duodenum, which is highly relevant with respect to a bleeding duodenal ulcer. Here it divides into the superior pancreaticoduodenal artery and the right gastroepiploic artery. The superior pancreaticoduodenal artery supplies the duodenum and pancreatic head and forms an anastomosis with the inferior pancreaticoduodenal artery, a branch of the superior mesenteric artery. The right gastroepiploic artery runs along the greater curvature of the stomach, eventually forming an anastomosis with the left gastroepiploic artery, a branch of the splenic artery. This vascular arcade, important during construction of a gastric conduit in oesophageal resection (see *Chapter 66*), is often variably incomplete. The fundus of the stomach is supplied by the vasa brevia (or short gastric arteries), which arise from near the termination of the splenic artery.

Veins

In general, the veins accompany the arteries; those along the lesser curve drain into the portal vein and those on the greater curve drain into the splenic vein. On the lesser curve, the coronary vein is particularly important. It runs along the lesser curve towards the oesophagus and then passes left to right to join the portal vein. This vein becomes markedly dilated in portal hypertension.

Lymphatics

The lymphatics of the stomach are of considerable importance in surgery for gastric cancer and are described in detail in that section.

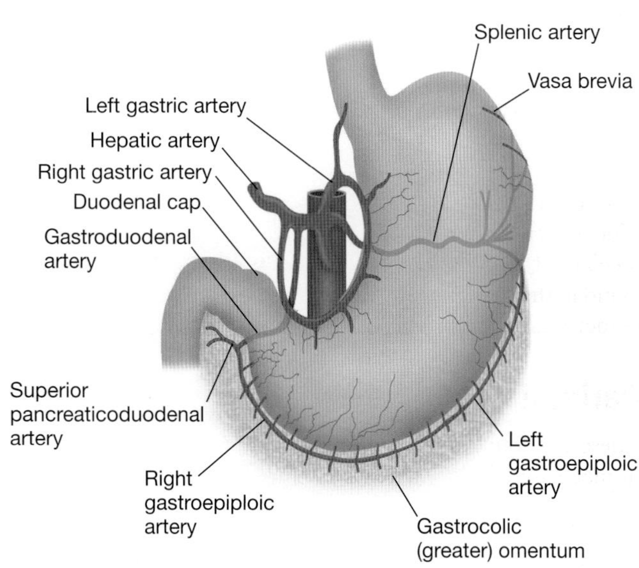

Figure 67.1 The arterial blood supply of the stomach.

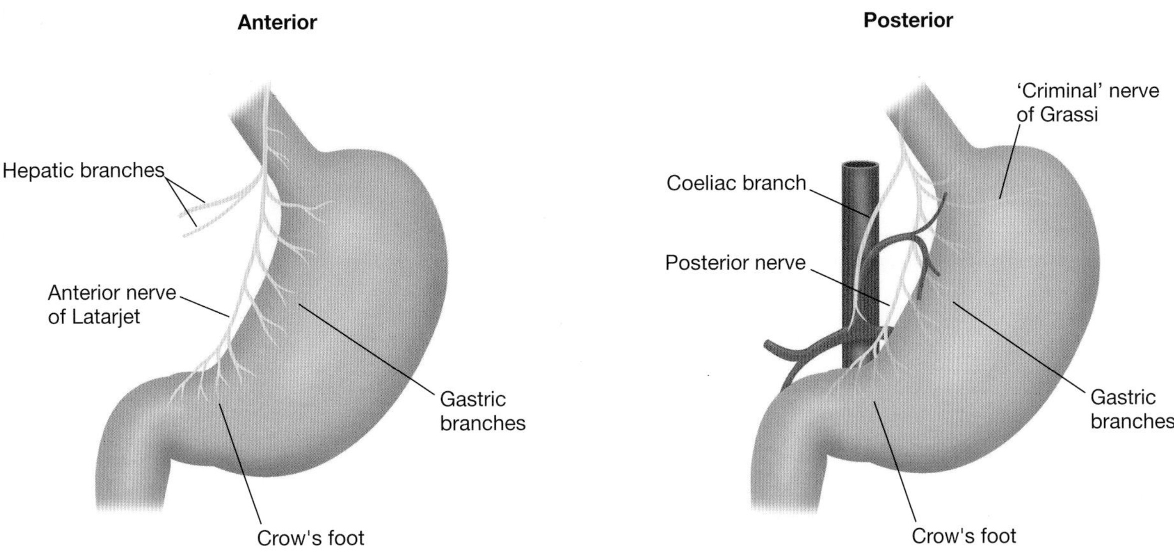

Figure 67.2 The anatomy of the anterior and posterior vagus nerves in relation to the stomach.

Nerves

The stomach and duodenum possess both intrinsic and extrinsic nerve supplies. The intrinsic nerves exist principally in two plexuses, the myenteric plexus of Auerbach and the submucosal plexus of Meissner. Compared with the rest of the gut, the submucosal plexus of the stomach contains relatively few ganglionic cells, as does the myenteric plexus in the fundus. However, in the antrum the ganglia of the myenteric plexus are well developed. The extrinsic supply is derived mainly from the vagus nerves (cranial nerve X), fibres of which originate in the brainstem. The vagal plexus around the oesophagus condenses into bundles that pass through the oesophageal hiatus (***Figure 67.2***), the posterior bundle being usually identifiable as a large nerve trunk. Vagal fibres are both afferent (sensory) and efferent. The efferent fibres are involved in the receptive relaxation of the stomach and the stimulation of gastric motility, as well as having the well-known secretory function. The sympathetic supply is derived mainly from the coeliac ganglia.

MICROSCOPIC ANATOMY OF THE STOMACH AND DUODENUM

The gastric surface epithelial cells are mucus producing. Mucus-secreting glands are found also in the duodenum. The specialised cells of the stomach (parietal and chief cells) are found in the gastric crypts (***Figure 67.3***). The stomach also has numerous endocrine cells.

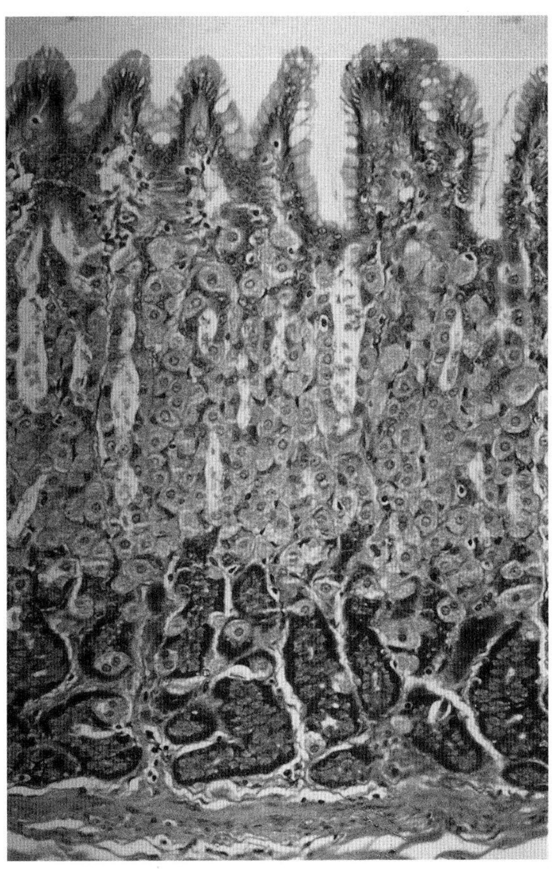

Figure 67.3 The histological appearance of a gastric gland. The mucus-secreting cells are seen at the mucosal surface, the eosinophilic parietal cells superficially in the glands and the basophilic chief cells in the deepest layer.

Parietal cells

These are found in the body (acid-secreting portion) of the stomach and line the gastric crypts, being more abundant

Leopold Auerbach, 1828–1897, Professor of Neuropathology, Breslau, Germany (now Wrocław, Poland).
George Meissner, 1829–1905, Professor of Pathology, Gottingen, Germany.
André Latarjet, 1877–1947, anatomist, Lyon, France.
Guiseppe Grassi, 1913–1980, surgeon, San Giovanni Hospital, Rome, Italy.

distally. They are responsible for the production of the hydrogen ions that form hydrochloric acid. The hydrogen ions are actively secreted by a hydrogen–potassium-ATPase proton pump, which exchanges intraluminal potassium for hydrogen ions. The potassium ions enter the lumen of the crypts passively, but the hydrogen ions are pumped against an immense concentration gradient (1 000 000:1). Proton pump inhibitors (PPIs) act by blocking the H^+/K^+ ATPase and thereby significantly reduce gastric acid secretion (see ***Gastric acid secretion***).

Chief cells

These lie proximally in the gastric crypts and produce pepsinogen. Two forms of pepsinogen are described: pepsinogen I and pepsinogen II. The ratio between pepsinogens I and II in the serum decreases with gastric atrophy. Pepsinogen is activated in the stomach to produce the digestive protease pepsin.

Endocrine cells

The stomach has numerous endocrine cells that are critical to its function. In the gastric antrum, the mucosa contains G cells, which produce gastrin. Throughout the body of the stomach, enterochromaffin-like (ECL) cells are abundant and produce histamine, a key factor in driving gastric acid secretion. In addition, there are large numbers of somatostatin-producing D cells throughout the stomach. Somatostatin has a negative regulatory role. The peptides and neuropeptides produced in the stomach are discussed in ***Gastric acid secretion***.

Duodenum

The duodenum is lined by a mucus-secreting columnar epithelium. In addition, Brunner's glands lie beneath the mucosa and are similar to the pyloric glands in the pyloric part of the stomach. Endocrine cells in the duodenum produce cholecystokinin and secretin.

PHYSIOLOGY OF THE STOMACH AND DUODENUM

The stomach mechanically breaks down ingested food and, together with the actions of acid and pepsin, forms chyme that passes into the duodenum. In contrast with the acidic environment of the stomach, the environment of the duodenum is alkaline, owing to secretion of bicarbonate ions from both the pancreas and the duodenum. This neutralises the acid chyme and adjusts the luminal osmolarity to approximately that of plasma. Endocrine cells in the duodenum produce cholecystokinin, which stimulates the pancreas to produce trypsin and the gallbladder to contract. Secretin is also produced by the endocrine cells of the duodenum. This hormone inhibits gastric acid secretion and promotes production of bicarbonate by the pancreas.

Summary box 67.1

Anatomy and physiology of the stomach

- The stomach acts as a reservoir for food and commences the process of digestion
- Gastric acid is produced by a proton pump in the parietal cells, which in turn is controlled by histamine acting on H_2-receptors
- The histamine is produced by the endocrine gastric ECL cells in response to a number of factors, particularly gastrin and vagus nerve stimulation
- PPIs abolish gastric acid production, whereas H_2-receptor antagonists only markedly reduce it
- The gastric mucous layer is essential to the integrity of the gastric mucosa

Gastric acid secretion

Secretion of gastric acid and pepsin tends to run in parallel, although the understanding of the mechanisms of gastric acid secretion is considerably greater than that of pepsin. Numerous factors are involved to some degree in the production of the gastric acid. These include neurotransmitters, neuropeptides and peptide hormones. This complexity need not detract from the fact that there are basic principles that are relatively easily understood (***Figure 67.4***). Hydrogen ions are produced in the parietal cell by the proton pump. Although numerous factors can act on the parietal cell, the most important of these is histamine, which acts via the H_2-receptor. Histamine is produced, in turn, by the ECL cells of the stomach and acts in a paracrine (local) fashion on the parietal cells. These relationships explain why PPIs can abolish gastric acid secretion, as they act on the final common pathway – hydrogen ion secretion. H_2-receptor antagonists have profound effects on gastric acid secretion, but this is not insurmountable. The ECL cell produces histamine

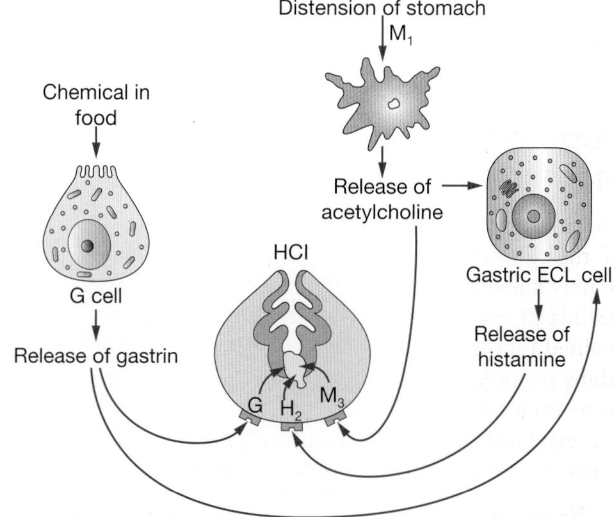

Figure 67.4 The parietal cell in relation to the mechanism of gastric acid secretion. ECL, enterochromaffin-like; G, gastrin receptor; H, histamine receptor; HCl, hydrochloric acid; M, muscarinic receptor.

Johann Conrad Brunner, 1653–1729, Professor of Anatomy, Heidelberg, Germany, and later Strasburg, France.

in response to a number of stimuli, which include the vagus nerve and gastrin. Gastrin is released by the G cells in response to the presence of food in the stomach. The production of gastrin is inhibited by acid, creating a negative feedback loop. Various other peptides, including secretin, inhibit gastric acid secretion.

Classically, three phases of gastric secretion are described. The **cephalic phase** is mediated by vagal activity, secondary to sensory arousal as first demonstrated by Pavlov. The **gastric phase** is a response to food within the stomach, which is mediated principally, but not exclusively, by gastrin. In the **intestinal phase**, the presence of chyme in the duodenum and small bowel inhibits gastric emptying, and acidification of the duodenum leads to the production of secretin, which inhibits gastric acid secretion, along with numerous other peptides originating from the gut. The stomach also possesses somatostatin-containing D cells. Somatostatin is released in response to a number of factors, including acidification. This peptide acts probably on the G cell, the ECL cell and the parietal cell itself to inhibit the production of acid.

Gastric mucus and the gastric mucosal barrier

The gastric mucous layer is essential to the integrity of the gastric mucosa. It is a viscid layer of mucopolysaccharides produced by the mucus-producing cells of the stomach and the pyloric glands. Gastric mucus is an important physiological barrier that protects the gastric mucosa from mechanical damage and also the effects of acid and pepsin. It has considerable buffering capacity, enhanced by the presence of bicarbonate ions within the mucus. Many factors can lead to the breakdown of this gastric mucous barrier. These include bile, non-steroidal anti-inflammatory drugs (NSAIDs), alcohol, trauma and shock. Tonometry studies have shown that, of the entire gastrointestinal tract, the stomach is the most sensitive to ischaemia following a hypovolaemic insult and also the slowest to recover. This may explain the high incidence of stress ulceration in the stomach.

Peptides and neuropeptides in the stomach and duodenum

As with most of the gastrointestinal tract, the endocrine cells of the stomach produce peptide hormones and neurotransmitters. Previously, nerves and endocrine cells were considered distinct in terms of their products. However, it is increasingly realised that there is enormous overlap within these systems. Many peptides recognised as hormones may also be produced by neurones, hence the term neuropeptides. The term 'messenger' can be used to describe all such products. There are three conventional modes of action that overlap.

1 **Endocrine**. The messenger is secreted into the circulation, where it affects tissues that may be remote from the site of origin.
2 **Paracrine**. Messengers are produced locally and have local effects on tissues. Neurones and endocrine cells both act in this way.
3 **Neurocrine** (classical neurotransmitter). Messengers are produced by the neurone via the synaptic knob and pass across the synaptic cleft to the target.

Many peptide hormones act on the intrinsic nerve plexus of the gut (see ***Gastroduodenal motor activity***) and influence motility. Similarly, neuropeptides may influence the structure and function of the mucosa. Some of these peptides, neuropeptides and neurotransmitters are listed in ***Table 67.1***. The stomach is vital to regulation of appetite and weight control through a combination of mechanical and hormonal mechanisms (see ***Chapter 68***).

Gastroduodenal motor activity

The motility of the gastrointestinal tract is modulated by its intrinsic nervous system. Critical in this process is the migrating motor complex (MMC). In the fasting state, and after food has cleared, there is a period of quiescence in the small bowel lasting in the region of 40 minutes (phase I). There follows a series of waves of electrical and motor activity, also lasting about 40 minutes, propagated from the fundus of the stomach in a caudal direction at a rate of about three per minute (phase II). These pass as far the pylorus, but not beyond. Duodenal slow waves are generated in the duodenum at a rate of about 10 per minute, which potentiate into the small bowel. The amplitude of these contractions increases to a maximum in phase III, which lasts for about 10 minutes. This 90-minute cycle of activity is then repeated. From the duodenum, the MMC moves distally at 5–10 cm/min, reaching the terminal ileum after 1.5 hours.

Following a meal, the stomach exhibits receptive relaxation, which allows the proximal stomach to act as a reservoir. Most of the peristaltic activity is found in the distal stomach (the antral mill) and the proximal stomach demonstrates only tonic activity. The pylorus, which is most commonly open, contracts with the peristaltic wave and allows only a few millilitres of chyme to pass into the duodenum at a time. The antral contraction against the closed pylorus is important in the milling activity of the stomach. Although the duodenum is capable of generating 10 waves per minute, after a meal it only contacts after an antral wave reaches the pylorus. Coordination of the motility of the antrum, pylorus and duodenum means that only small quantities of food reach the small bowel at a time. This control of gastric emptying can be abolished after gastric surgery, leading to significant symptoms (discussed in ***Sequelae of peptic ulcer surgery***).

INVESTIGATION OF THE STOMACH AND DUODENUM

Flexible endoscopy

Flexible endoscopy is more sensitive than conventional radiology in the assessment of the majority of gastroduodenal

Ivan Petrovitch Pavlov, 1849–1936, Professor of Physiology, St Petersburg, Russia.

TABLE 67.1 Function and source of peptides and neuropeptides in the stomach.

Function	Source
Stimulate secretion	
Gastrin	G cells
Histamine	ECL cells
Acetylcholine	Neurones
Gastrin-releasing peptide	Neurones and mucosa
CCK	Duodenal endocrine cells
Inhibit secretion	
Somatostatin	D cells and neurones
Secretin	Duodenal endocrine cells
Enteroglucagon	Small intestinal endocrine cells
Prostaglandins	Mucosa
Neurotensin	Neurones
GIP	Duodenal and jejunal endocrine cells
PYY	Small intestinal endocrine cells
Stimulate motility	
Acetylcholine	Neurones
5-HT	Neurones
Histamine	ECL cell
Substance P	Neurones
Substance K	Neurones
Motilin	Neurones
Gastrin	G cells
Angiotensin	
Inhibit motility	
Somatostatin	D cells and neurones
VIP	Neurones
Nitric oxide	Neurones and smooth muscle
Noradrenaline (norepinephrine)	Neurones
Encephalin	Neurones
Dopamine	Neurones

CCK, cholecystokinin; ECL, enterochromaffin-like cells; G, gastrin receptor; GIP, gastric inhibitory polypeptide; 5-HT, 5-hydroxytryptamine; PYY, peptide YY; VIP, vasoactive intestinal peptide.

conditions, particularly peptic ulceration, gastritis and duodenitis. In upper gastrointestinal bleeding, endoscopy is far superior to any other investigation and offers the possibility of endoscopic therapy. In most circumstances it is the only investigation required.

It is generally a safe investigation, but it is important that all personnel undertaking these procedures are adequately trained. Careless and rough handling of the endoscope during intubation of a patient may result in perforations of the pharynx and oesophagus. Any other part of the upper gastrointestinal tract may also be perforated. An inadequately performed endoscopy is also dangerous as a serious condition may be overlooked. This is particularly the case in respect of early and curable gastric cancer, the appearances of which may often be extremely subtle and may be missed by inexperienced endoscopists. Spraying the mucosa with dye endoscopically may allow better discrimination between normal and abnormal mucosa, so allowing a small cancer to be more easily seen. In the future, advances in technology may allow 'optical biopsy' to determine the nature of mucosal abnormalities in real time (see *Chapter 9*).

Summary box 67.2

Investigation of gastroduodenal symptoms

- Flexible endoscopy is the most commonly used and sensitive technique
- Great care is needed to avoid complications and missing important pathology
- Axial imaging, particularly multislice computed tomography (CT), is useful in staging gastric cancer
- Endoscopic ultrasonography is the most sensitive technique for evaluation of the 'T' stage of gastric cancer and assessment of duodenal tumours
- Laparoscopy is very sensitive in detecting peritoneal metastases, and laparoscopic ultrasound provides an accurate evaluation of lymph node and liver metastases

Upper gastrointestinal endoscopy can be performed without sedation, but when sedation is required incremental doses of a benzodiazepine are usually administered. Sedation is of particular concern in the case of gastrointestinal bleeding as it may have a more profound effect on the patient's cardiovascular stability. It has now become the standard to use pulse oximetry to monitor patients during upper gastrointestinal endoscopy, and nasal oxygen is often also administered. Hyoscine butylbromide (Buscopan) is useful to abolish duodenal motility for examinations of the second and third parts of the duodenum. Examinations of this type are best carried out using a side-viewing endoscope such as is used for endoscopic retrograde cholangiopancreatography.

Some patients are relatively resistant to sedation with benzodiazepines, particularly those who are accustomed to drinking alcohol. Increasing the dose of benzodiazepines in these patients may not result in any useful sedation, but merely make the patient more restless and confused. Such patients are better endoscoped fully awake using a local anaesthetic throat spray and a narrow-gauge endoscope. Whatever the circumstances, it is important that resuscitation facilities are available including agents that reverse the effects of benzodiazepines, such as flumazenil.

The technology associated with upper gastrointestinal endoscopy is continuing to advance. Instruments that allow both endoscopy and endoluminal ultrasonography to be performed simultaneously (see ***Ultrasonography***) are used routinely. Bleeding from the stomach and duodenum can be treated using a number of haemostatic measures, including injection with adrenaline (epinephrine), diathermy, heater probes, lasers and clip application.

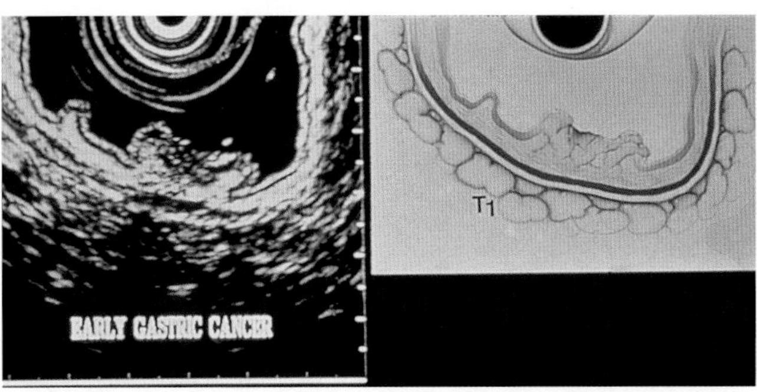

Figure 67.5 Endoscopic ultrasonography of the stomach. Five layers can be identified in the normal stomach. A gastric cancer is shown invading the muscle of the gastric wall (courtesy of KeyMed (Medical and Industrial Equipment Ltd)).

Contrast radiology

Upper gastrointestinal radiology is not used as much as in previous years, as endoscopy is a more sensitive investigation. Computed tomography (CT) imaging with oral contrast has replaced contrast radiology in many of the areas where anatomical information is sought, e.g. large hiatus hernias of the rolling type and chronic gastric volvulus. In these conditions it may be difficult for the endoscopist to determine exactly the anatomy or, indeed, negotiate the deformity to see the distal stomach (see ***Chapter 66***).

Ultrasonography

Standard ultrasonography can be used to investigate the stomach but used conventionally it is less sensitive than other modalities. In contrast, endoluminal ultrasonography and laparoscopic ultrasonography are probably the most sensitive techniques available in preoperative local staging of gastric cancer. In endoluminal ultrasonography, the transducer is usually attached to the distal tip of the instrument. Five layers (***Figure 67.5***) of the gastric wall may be identified on endoluminal ultrasonography and the depth of invasion of a tumour can be assessed (90% accuracy for the 'T' component of the staging). Enlarged lymph nodes can also be identified and the accuracy of the technique is about 80% in this situation. Laparoscopic ultrasonography is also a very sensitive imaging modality, to a large measure because of the laparoscopy itself (see ***Laparoscopy***).

Ultrasonography can be used to assess gastric emptying. Swallowed contrast that is designed to be easily seen using an ultrasound transducer is used. Emptying of the contrast is followed directly. The accuracy of the technique is similar to that of radioisotope gastric emptying studies (see ***Gastric emptying studies***).

Computed tomography scanning and magnetic resonance imaging

CT is increasingly used in the investigation of the stomach, especially in the context of gastric malignancies. Although it is much less accurate in 'T' staging than endoluminal ultrasonography (***Figure 67.6***), lymph node enlargement can be easily detected and is reasonably accurate in detecting nodal involvement with tumour. However it is important to understand that microscopic tumour deposits in lymph nodes cannot be detected and lymph nodes may undergo reactive enlargement but not contain tumour.

Hepatic metastases from gastric cancer may be difficult to identify as they are often of the same density as liver and may not handle the intravenous contrast differently. At present, magnetic resonance imaging (MRI) scanning does not offer any specific advantage in assessing the stomach, although it has a higher sensitivity for the detection of gastric cancer liver metastases than conventional CT imaging.

Computed tomography/positron emission tomography

Positron emission tomography (PET) is increasingly being used in the preoperative staging of gastro-oesophageal cancer as it will detect otherwise occult tumour spread in up to 10% of patients who might otherwise have undergone a major surgical resection (***Figure 67.7***). PET/CT may also be used to determine the response to neoadjuvant chemotherapy in oesophagogastric malignancies, although this is the subject of ongoing studies (see ***Chapter 8***).

Laparoscopy

Laparoscopy is routine in the assessment of patients with gastric cancer. Its particular value is in the detection of peritoneal disease, which is difficult by any other technique, unless the patient has ascites or bulky intraperitoneal deposits. The main limitation is evaluation of posterior extension but CT and endoluminal ultrasonography can provide this information. Samples are usually taken for peritoneal cytology unless laparotomy follows immediately.

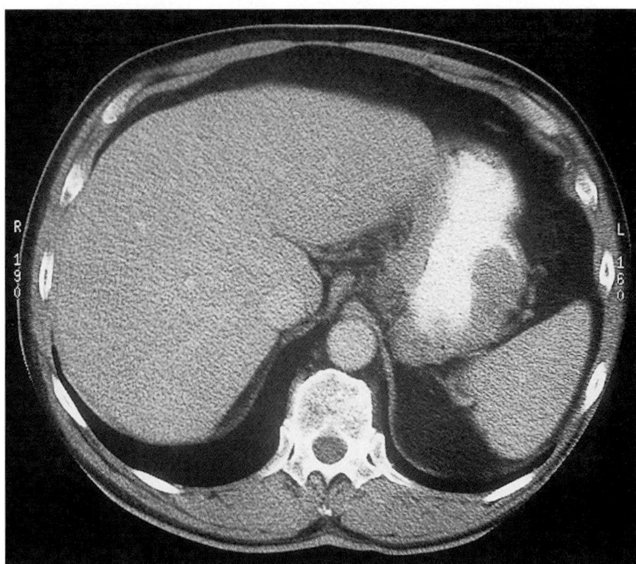

Figure 67.6 A computed tomography scan of the abdomen showing a gastric cancer arising in the body of the stomach.

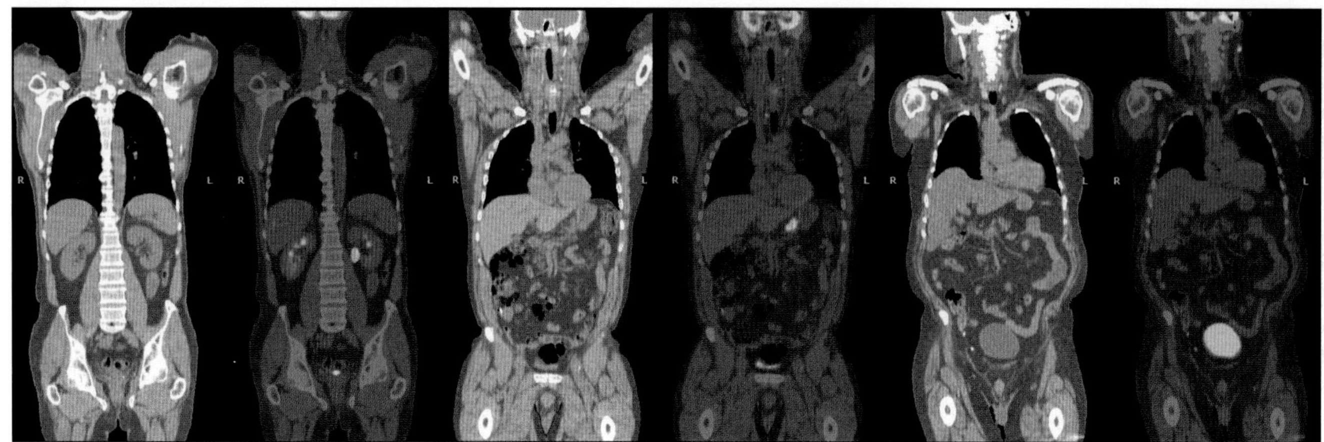

Figure 67.7 Computed tomography/positron emission tomography of a patient with gastric cancer. The middle pair of images shows the primary tumour. The two images on the left show unsuspected liver metastases, whereas the two on the right show a left cervical node positive for metastases.

Gastric emptying studies

These are useful in the study of gastric dysmotility problems, particularly those that follow gastric surgery. The principle is that a radioisotope-labelled liquid and solid meal is ingested by the patient and emptying of the stomach is followed on a gamma camera. This allows the proportion of activity in the remaining stomach to be assessed. It is possible to follow liquid and solid gastric emptying independently (***Figure 67.8***).

Angiography

Angiography is used most commonly in the investigation of upper gastrointestinal bleeding not identified using endoscopy. Therapeutic embolisation may also be of value in the treatment of bleeding; in some centres, embolisation has replaced surgery in the majority of cases.

HELICOBACTER PYLORI

H. pylori is involved in the aetiology of a number of common gastroduodenal diseases, such as chronic gastritis, peptic ulceration and gastric cancer. Although Bizzozero identified the presence of spirochaetal organisms in gastric mucosa, it was not until the early 1980s that Warren and Marshall confirmed Koch's postulates with respect to *H. pylori* and gastritis. Both received the Nobel Prize in Medicine or Physiology in 2005.

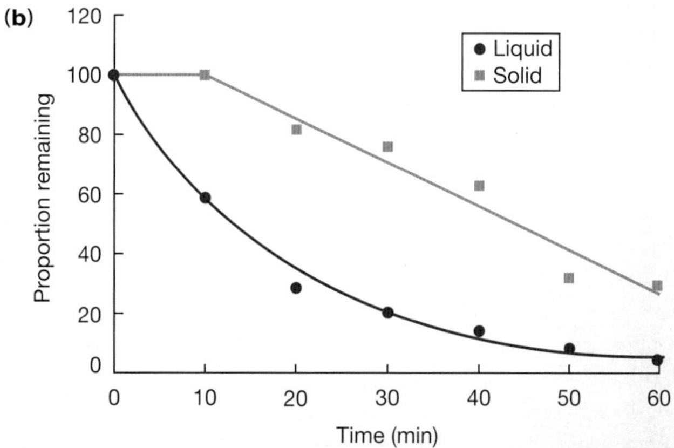

Figure 67.8 Dual-phase solid and liquid gastric emptying. The use of two isotopic labels allows the liquid and solid phases of the emptying to be followed separately. (a) Image acquisition. (b) Gastric emptying curves in a normal individual showing a typical lag period in the solid phase before linear emptying (courtesy of Dr V Lewington, Southampton, UK).

Giulio Bizzozero, 1846–1901, pathologist, University of Turin, Italy.
John Robin Warren, b. 1937, pathologist, Royal Perth Hospital, WA, Australia.
Barry Marshall, b. 1951, physician, University of Western Australia, WA, Australia.
Robert Koch, 1843–1910, Professor of Hygiene and Bacteriology, Berlin, Germany, stated his 'postulates' in 1882 that define the conditions that must be met before an organism can be shown to be causative of a particular condition.

One of the characteristics of *H. pylori* is its ability to hydrolyse urea, resulting in the production of ammonia, a strong alkali. The effect of ammonia on the antral G cells is to cause release of gastrin via a negative feedback that is responsible for the modest, but inappropriate, hypergastrinaemia in patients with peptic ulcer disease, which, in turn, may result in gastric acid hypersecretion. The organism's obligate urease activity is utilised by various tests used to detect the presence of the organism, including the ^{13}C and ^{14}C breath tests and the CLO test (a commercially available urease test kit), which is performed on gastric biopsies. The organism can also be detected histologically (***Figure 67.9***), using the Giemsa or the Ethin–Starry silver stains, and cultured using appropriate media. Previous or current infection with the organism may also be detected serologically. Breath tests or faecal antigen tests are recommended for the pretreatment diagnosis of *H. pylori* infection in the community. Less accurate, hospital-based serology tests have a place within a non-invasive test-and-treat strategy.

Infection with *H. pylori* leads to disruption of the gastric mucous barrier by the enzymes produced by the organism, and the inflammation induced in the gastric epithelium is the basis of many of the associated disease processes. The association of the organism with chronic (type B) gastritis is not in doubt. Some strains of *H. pylori* produce cytotoxins, notably the Cag A and Vac A products. Production of cytotoxins seems to be associated with the ability to cause gastritis, peptic ulceration and gastric cancer. The effect of the organism on the gastric epithelium is to incite a classical inflammatory response that involves the migration and degranulation of acute inflammatory cells, such as neutrophils, and also the accumulation of chronic inflammatory cells, such as macrophages and lymphocytes.

It is evident how *H. pylori* infection results in chronic gastritis and also how this may progress to gastric ulceration, but for a while it remained unclear how the organism could be involved in duodenal ulceration, as the normal duodenum is not colonised. As mentioned above, the production of ammonia does increase the level of circulating gastrin and it has been shown subsequently that eradication of the organism in patients with duodenal ulcer disease will reduce the acid levels to normal.

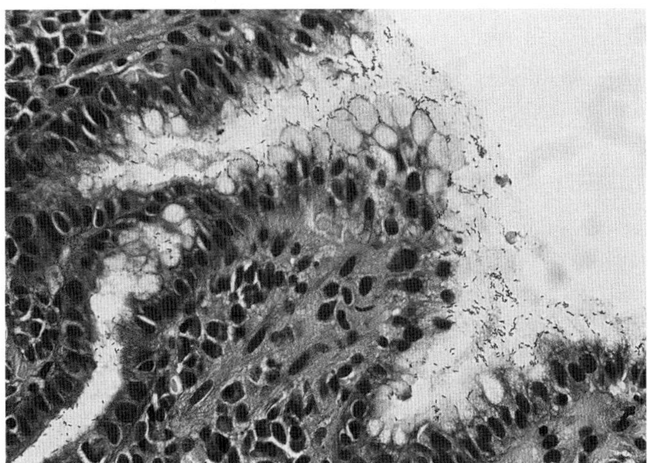

Figure 67.9 Antral mucosa showing colonisation with *Helicobacter pylori* (modified Giemsa stain).

However, the overlap in gastric acid secretion between normal subjects and those with duodenal ulcers is considerable and the modestly increased acid levels in patients with *Helicobacter*-associated antral gastritis are insufficient to explain the aetiology of duodenal ulceration.

The explanation can probably be found in the phenomenon of duodenal gastric metaplasia. Gastric metaplasia is the normal response of the duodenal mucosa to excess acidity. It can be thought of in the same way as any other metaplasia in the gastrointestinal tract: an attempt by the mucosa to resist an injurious stimulus. Although normal duodenal mucosa cannot be infected with *H. pylori*, gastric metaplasia in the duodenum is commonly infected and this infection results in the same inflammatory process that is observed in the gastric mucosa. The result is duodenitis, which is almost certainly the precursor of duodenal ulceration.

Infection with *H. pylori* may be the most common human infection. The incidence of infection within a population increases with age, and in many populations infection rates of 80–90% are not unusual. Up to 50% of the world's population may be infected with *Helicobacter*. It appears that most infection is acquired in childhood and the possibility of infection is inversely related to socioeconomic group. The means of spread has not been identified, but the organism can occur in the faeces and faecal–oral spread seems most likely. The organism is not normally found in saliva or dental plaque. There is evidence in different environments and in different population groups that the manifestations of the infection may be different. Predominantly antral gastritis, which is commonly seen in the West, results initially in increased levels of acid production and peptic ulcer disease, whereas gastritis affecting the body, common in the developing world, may lead to hypochlorhydria and gastric neoplasia.

It has been known since 1984 that *Helicobacter* infection is amenable to treatment with antibiotics. The profound hypochlorhydria produced by PPIs combined with antibiotics is also effective in eradicating the organism. Commonly used eradication regimes include a PPI and two antibiotics, such as metronidazole and amoxicillin. Very high eradication rates, in the region of 90%, can be achieved with combinations that include the antibiotic clarithromycin, although it may be that in the future antibiotic resistance will become a problem. Reinfection following successful eradication appears rare (<0.5%) but incomplete eradication is a more important clinical problem.

At present, eradication therapy is recommended for patients with duodenal ulcer disease, but not for patients with non-ulcer dyspepsia or in asymptomatic patients who are infected. However, recent data show that a proportion of patients with non-ulcer dyspepsia do respond to treatment. *H. pylori* is now classified by the World Health Organization as a class 1 carcinogen, and it may be that the further epidemiological studies on the risk of gastric cancer change current advice on treatment.

GASTRITIS

The great variety of names and classification systems used in gastritis is confusing. Thankfully, the understanding of gastritis has increased markedly following elucidation of the role of

H. pylori in chronic gastritis and there is broad agreement that gastritis should be classified according to the underlying aetiology. Gastritis describes any histologically confirmed inflammation of the gastric mucosa. In most modern classification systems, the amount of inflammatory infiltrate and the degree of gastric atrophy will be included.

Summary box 67.3

Helicobacter and gastritis

- *Helicobacter pylori* is critical in the development of gastritis, peptic ulceration and gastric cancer
- Infection appears to be acquired mainly in childhood and the infection rate is inversely associated with socioeconomic status
- Eradication, recommended specifically in patients with peptic ulcer disease, can be achieved in up to 90% of patients with a combination of a PPI and antibiotics, and reinfection is uncommon (<0.5%)
- Erosive gastritis is usually related to the use of NSAIDs
- Autoimmune gastritis is associated with development of pernicious anaemia and gastric cancer

Autoimmune gastritis

This is an autoimmune condition in which there are circulating antibodies to parietal cells that results in atrophy of the parietal cell mass, hence hypochlorhydria and ultimately achlorhydria. As intrinsic factor is also produced by parietal cells there is malabsorption of vitamin B_{12}, which, if untreated, may result in pernicious anaemia. The antrum is not affected; thus, hypochlorhydria leads to production of high levels of gastrin from antral G cells, resulting in chronic hypergastrinaemia with consequent hypertrophy of ECL cells in the body of the stomach not affected by autoimmune damage. Over time, microadenomas develop in the ECL cells, sometimes becoming identifiable tumour nodules that rarely can become malignant; endoscopic screening of such patients may be appropriate.

Helicobacter pylori gastritis

H. pylori gastritis, previously described as type B gastritis, affects the antrum and predisposes to peptic ulcer disease. *Helicobacter*-associated pangastritis is common, but gastritis affecting the corpus alone is not. Chronic pangastritis with atrophy is associated with intestinal metaplasia and has significant malignant potential when associated with dysplasia. Endoscopic screening may be appropriate.

Reflux gastritis

This is caused by enterogastric reflux. Its histological features are distinct from other types of gastritis. Although commonly seen after gastric surgery, it is occasionally found in patients with no previous surgical intervention or those who have had a cholecystectomy. Bile chelating or prokinetic agents may be useful in treatment and as a temporising measure to avoid revisional surgery that should be reserved for severe cases.

Erosive gastritis

This is caused by agents that disturb the gastric mucosal barrier; NSAIDs and alcohol are common causes. The NSAID-induced gastric lesion is associated with inhibition of cyclo-oxygenase type 1 (COX-1) receptor enzyme, reducing production of cytoprotective prostaglandins. Many of the anti-inflammatory activities of NSAIDs are mediated by COX-2 and use of specific COX-2 inhibitors reduces the incidence of gastritis.

Stress gastritis

This is a common sequel of serious illness or injury and is characterised by a reduction in the blood supply to the gastric mucosa. Although common, this is not usually recognised unless stress ulceration and bleeding supervene, in which case treatment can be difficult. Prevention is much easier than treating it, hence routine use of H_2 antagonists with or without barrier agents, such as sucralfate, in patients who are on intensive care. These measures have been shown to reduce the incidence of bleeding from stress ulceration.

Ménétrier's disease

This is an unusual condition characterised by gross hypertrophy of the gastric mucosal folds, mucus production and hypochlorhydria. The condition is premalignant and may present with hypoproteinaemia and anaemia. There is no treatment other than a gastrectomy. The disease seems to be caused by overexpression of transforming growth factor alpha (TGF-α). Like epidermal growth factor (EGF), this peptide also binds to the EGF receptor. The histological features of Ménétrier's disease may be reproduced in transgenic mice overexpressing TGF-α.

Lymphocytic gastritis

This type of gastritis is rare. It is characterised by the infiltration of the gastric mucosa by T cells and is probably associated with *H. pylori* infection. The pattern of inflammation resembles that seen in coeliac disease or lymphocytic colitis.

Other forms of gastritis

Eosinophilic gastritis appears to have an allergic basis and is treated with steroids and cromoglycate. Granulomatous gastritis is seen rarely in Crohn's disease and also may be associated with tuberculosis. Acquired immunodeficiency syndrome (AIDS) gastritis is secondary to infection with cryptosporidiosis. Phlegmonous gastritis is a rare bacterial infection of the stomach found in patients with severe intercurrent illness. It is usually an agonal event.

Pierre Eugène Ménétrier, 1859–1935, pathologist, Paris, France.
Burrill Bernard Crohn, 1884–1983, gastroenterologist, Mount Sinai Hospital, New York, NY, USA, described regional ileitis in 1932 along with Leon Ginzburg and Gordon Oppenheimer.

PEPTIC ULCER

Although the name 'peptic' ulcer suggests an association with pepsin, this is essentially unimportant as, in the absence of acid, peptic ulcers do not occur. Nearly all peptic ulcers can be healed by using PPIs, which can render a patient virtually achlorhydric.

Common sites for peptic ulcers are the first part of the duodenum and the lesser curve of the stomach, but they also occur on the stoma following gastric surgery, in the oesophagus and even in a Meckel's diverticulum, which contains ectopic gastric epithelium. In general, the ulcer occurs at a junction between different types of epithelia, in the epithelium least resistant to acid damage.

In the past, much distinction has been made between acute and chronic peptic ulcers, but this difference can sometimes be difficult to determine clinically. It is probably best to consider that there is a spectrum of disease from the superficial gastric and duodenal ulceration, frequently seen at endoscopy, to deep chronic penetrating ulcers. This does not minimise the importance of acute stress ulceration. These ulcers can both perforate and bleed.

For many years, the cause of peptic ulceration remained an enigma. When comparing groups of patients with duodenal and prepyloric peptic ulcers with normal subjects, gastric acid levels are higher, but the overlap is considerable. Patients with gastric ulceration have relatively normal levels of gastric acid secretion. It is clear that acid is important as peptic ulceration occurs in the presence of very high acid levels, such as those found in patients with a gastrinoma (Zollinger–Ellison syndrome), and ulcers heal in the absence of acid. In patients with a gastrinoma it may be the only aetiological factor, but this is not the case in the majority of patients.

Summary box 67.4

Peptic ulceration

- Most peptic ulcers are caused by *H. pylori* or NSAIDs and changes in epidemiology mirror changes in these principal aetiological factors
- Duodenal ulcers are more common than gastric ulcers, but the symptoms are indistinguishable
- Gastric ulcers may be malignant and an ulcerated gastric cancer may mimic a benign ulcer
- Gastric antisecretory agents and *H. pylori* eradication therapy are the mainstays of treatment, and elective surgery is very rarely performed
- The long-term complications of peptic ulcer surgery may be difficult to treat
- The common complications of peptic ulcers are perforation, bleeding and stenosis
- The treatment of the perforated peptic ulcer is primarily surgical, although some patients may be managed conservatively

It is now widely accepted that infection with *H. pylori* and consumption of NSAIDs are the most important factors in the development of peptic ulceration. Cigarette smoking predisposes to peptic ulceration and increases the relapse rate after treatment.

Duodenal ulceration

Incidence

There have been marked changes in the demography of patients presenting with duodenal ulceration in the West. In part, this may relate to the widespread use of gastric antisecretory agents and *H. pylori* eradication therapy in patients with dyspepsia. Second, the peak incidence is now in a much older age group and, although still more common in men, gender difference is less marked. These changes mirror the changes, at least in part, in the epidemiology of *H. pylori* infection. In eastern Europe, the disease remains common, and the incidence is rising in resource-poor nations.

Pathology

Most ulcers occur in the first part of the duodenum (***Figures 67.10 and 67.11***). A chronic ulcer penetrates the mucosa into the muscle coat, leading to fibrosis. The resulting scarring may cause a deformity such as pyloric stenosis. When an ulcer heals, a residual scar can be observed in the mucosa. Sometimes there may be more than one duodenal ulcer. The situation in which there is both a posterior and an anterior duodenal ulcer is referred to as 'kissing ulcers'. Anterior ulcers tend to perforate

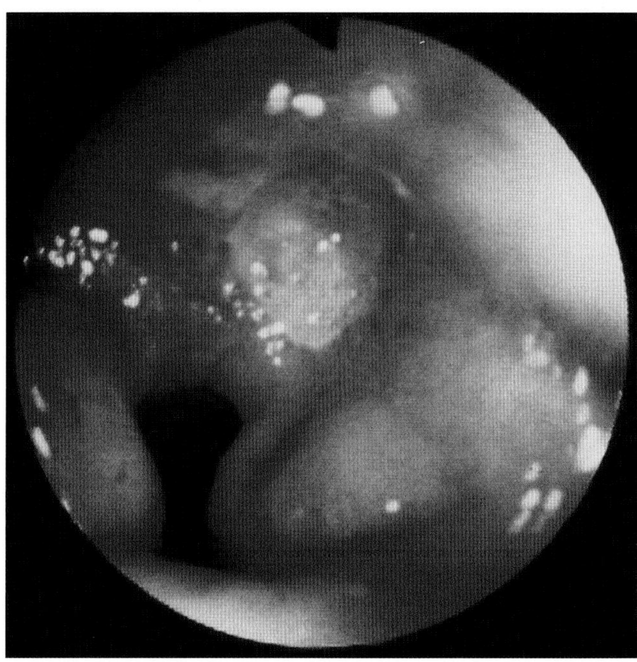

Figure 67.10 Duodenal ulcer at gastroduodenoscopy (courtesy of Dr GNJ Tytgat, Amsterdam, The Netherlands).

Johann Friedrich Meckel (the younger), 1781–1833, Professor of Anatomy and Surgery, Halle, Germany, described the diverticulum in 1809.
Robin Milton Zollinger, 1903–1992, Professor of Surgery, Iowa State University, Columbus, OH, USA.
Edwin Homer Ellison, 1918–1970, Professor of Surgery, Marquette University, Milwaukee, WI, USA.

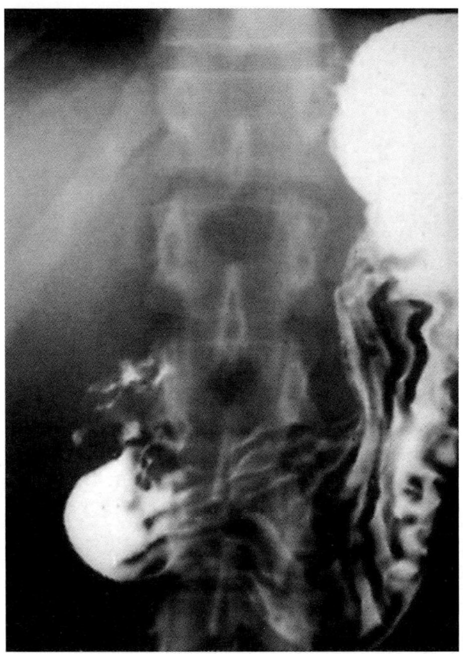

Figure 67.11 Duodenal ulcer shown by barium meal.

while posterior duodenal ulcers tend to bleed, sometimes by eroding into the gastroduodenal artery. Occasionally, the ulceration may be so extensive that the entire duodenal cap is ulcerated and devoid of mucosa. With respect to the giant duodenal ulcer, malignancy in this region is so uncommon that under normal circumstances surgeons can be confident that they are dealing with benign disease, even though from external palpation it may not appear so. In the stomach the situation is different.

Histopathology

Microscopically, the base of the ulcer is covered with granulation tissue and there may be evidence of endarteritis obliterans. The pathological appearances of the healing ulcer must be carefully interpreted as some of the epithelial down growth can be misinterpreted as invasion.

Gastric ulcers

Incidence

As with duodenal ulceration, *H. pylori* and NSAIDs are the important aetiological factors. Gastric ulceration is also associated with smoking. Gastric ulceration is much less common than duodenal ulceration. The gender incidence is equal and patients with gastric ulcers tend to be older. Gastric ulceration is more prevalent in low socioeconomic groups and is considerably more common in resource-poor than in resource-rich countries.

Pathology

Gastric ulcers have similar features to duodenal ulcers but tend to be larger. Fibrosis may result in an 'hourglass' deformity of the stomach. Chronic ulcers may erode posteriorly into the pancreas, major vessels such as the splenic artery or rarely into other organs such as the transverse colon. Chronic gastric ulcers are more common on the lesser curve (especially at the incisura angularis; ***Figures 67.12 and 67.13***) than on the greater curve and, even when high on the lesser curve, they tend to be at the boundary between the acid-secreting and the non-acid-secreting epithelia. With atrophy of parietal cell mass, non-acid-secreting epithelium migrates up the lesser curvature.

Malignancy in gastric ulcers

In contrast to chronic duodenal ulcers, gastric ulcers are associated with malignancy. There are two clinical scenarios that should be distinguished: one in which a benign chronic gastric ulcer undergoes malignant transformation (rare) and the more common scenario in which a gastric ulcer is assessed as benign either endoscopically or on contrast radiology but biopsies reveal malignancy. In this situation, the patient has

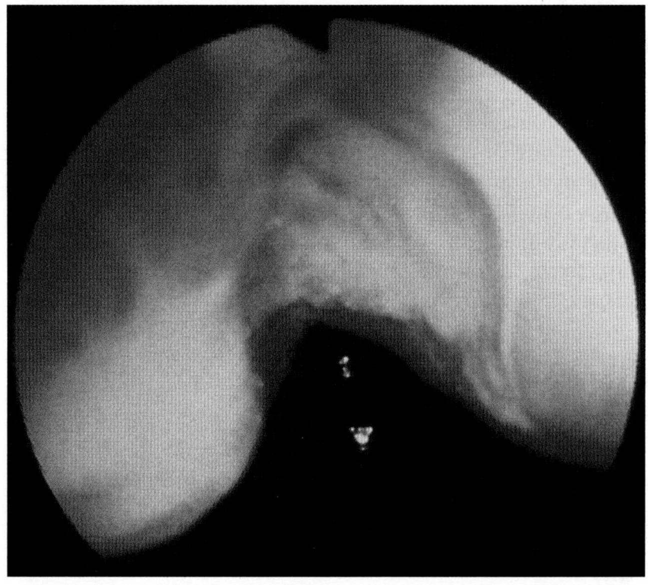

Figure 67.12 Benign incisural gastric ulcer shown at gastroscopy (courtesy of Dr GNJ Tytgat, Amsterdam, The Netherlands).

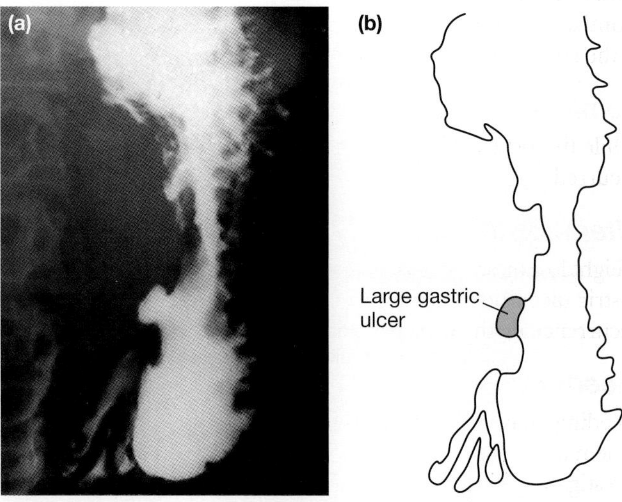

Figure 67.13 Benign gastric ulcer shown on barium meal. (a) Radiograph; (b) diagrammatic outline.

in fact presented with an ulcerated cancer and not a chronic peptic ulcer. Therefore, all gastric ulcers should be regarded as being malignant, no matter how classical the features of a benign gastric ulcer. Multiple biopsies should always be taken, perhaps as many as 10 well-targeted biopsies, before an ulcer can be tentatively accepted as being benign. Even then it is important that further biopsies are taken while the ulcer is healing and when healed. Modern antisecretory agents can frequently heal the ulceration associated with gastric cancer but, clearly, are ineffective in treating the malignancy itself.

At operation, even experienced surgeons may have difficulty distinguishing between the gastric cancer and a benign ulcer. Operative strategies differ so radically that it is essential that a confident diagnosis be made before operation. At operation for a perforated gastric ulcer, even if it is considered that the ulcer is benign, the ulcer should be excised and submitted for histological examination.

Other peptic ulcers

A prepyloric gastric ulcer was in the past difficult to treat, a problem overcome with the introduction of PPIs. Pyloric channel ulcers are similar to duodenal ulcers. Both prepyloric and pyloric ulcers may be malignant and biopsy is essential. Stomal ulcers occur after a gastroenterostomy (now most commonly found after bariatric surgery; see ***Chapter 68***) or a gastrectomy of the Billroth II type. The ulcer is usually found on the jejunal side of the stoma.

Clinical features of peptic ulcers

The clinical features of gastric and duodenal ulceration cannot be differentiated on the basis of symptoms. The demographic characteristics of groups of patients with gastric and duodenal ulceration do differ but this does not allow discrimination.

Pain

Epigastric pain, often described as gnawing and sometimes radiating to the back, is characteristic. Eating may sometimes relieve the discomfort. The pain is normally intermittent rather than intractable. Symptoms may disappear for weeks or months only to return again. This periodicity may be related to the spontaneous healing of the ulcer.

Vomiting

While this occurs, it is not a notable feature unless stenosis has occurred.

Alteration in weight

Weight loss or, sometimes, weight gain may occur. Patients with gastric ulceration are often underweight but this may precede occurrence of the ulcer.

Bleeding

Bleeding may be chronic and presentation with microcytic anaemia is not uncommon. All such patients should be investigated with endoscopy. Acute presentation with haematemesis and melaena is discussed in ***Haematemesis and melaena***.

Clinical examination

Examination of the patient may reveal epigastric tenderness but, except in gastric outlet obstruction, there is unlikely to be much else to find (see ***Chapter 63***).

Investigation of the patient with suspected peptic ulcer

Gastroduodenoscopy

In the stomach, any abnormal lesion should be biopsied, and in the case of a suspected benign gastric ulcer numerous biopsies must be taken in order to exclude, as far as possible, the presence of a malignancy. Commonly, biopsies of the antrum will be taken to see whether there is histological evidence of gastritis and a *Campylobacter*-like organism (CLO) test performed to determine the presence of *H. pylori*. A 'U' manoeuvre should be carried out to inspect the incisura, lesser curve and gastro-oesophageal junction (GOJ), given the increasing incidence of cancer at the GOJ (see ***Chapter 66***). Similarly, if a stoma is present, for instance after gastroenterostomy or Billroth II gastrectomy, it is important to enter both afferent and efferent loops. Almost all stomal ulcers will be close to the junction between the jejunal and gastric mucosa. Attention should be given to the pylorus to note whether there is any prepyloric or pyloric channel ulceration, and also whether it is deformed, which is often the case with chronic duodenal ulceration. In the duodenum, care must be taken to view all of the first part and the endoscope advanced into the second part.

Treatment of peptic ulceration

The vast majority of uncomplicated peptic ulcers are treated medically. Surgical treatment of uncomplicated peptic ulceration has decreased markedly and is now seldom performed. Surgical treatment was aimed principally at reducing gastric acid secretion and, in the case of gastric ulceration, removing the diseased mucosa. When originally devised, medical treatment also aimed to reduce gastric acid secretion, initially using the highly successful H_2-receptor antagonist and, subsequently, PPIs. This has now largely given way to *H. pylori* eradication therapy.

Medical treatment

It is reasonable to suggest modifications to the patient's lifestyle, particularly the cessation of cigarette smoking; however, pharmacological measures form the mainstay of treatment.

H_2-receptor antagonists and proton pump inhibitors

H_2-antagonists revolutionised the management of peptic ulceration. Most duodenal ulcers and gastric ulcers can be healed by a few weeks of treatment. There remained, however,

Christian Albert Theodor Billroth, 1829–1894, Professor of Surgery, Vienna, Austria.

a group of patients who were relatively refractory to conventional doses of H_2-receptor antagonists. This is largely now irrelevant as PPIs can effectively render a patient achlorhydric and all benign ulcers will heal using these drugs, the majority within 2 weeks. Symptom relief is rapid, most patients being asymptomatic within a few days. Like H_2-antagonists, PPIs are safe and relatively devoid of serious side effects. The problem with all gastric antisecretory agents is that, following cessation of therapy, relapse is almost universal.

Eradication therapy

Eradication therapy is now routinely given to patients with peptic ulceration. If *H. pylori* is the principal aetiological factor (essentially in patient not taking NSAIDs) then complete eradication of the organism will cure the disease. Reinfection as an adult is uncommon. Eradication therapy is therefore the mainstay of treatment for peptic ulceration. It is extremely economical by comparison with prolonged courses of antisecretory agents or surgery. It is also considerably safer than surgical treatment.

There are some patients with peptic ulcers in whom eradication therapy may not be appropriate, and this includes patients with NSAID-associated ulcers. Such patients should avoid these drugs if possible; if not, they should be co-prescribed with a potent antisecretory agent. Similarly, patients with stomal ulceration are not effectively treated with eradication therapy and require prolonged prescription of antisecretory agents. Patients with Zollinger–Ellison syndrome should be treated in the long term with PPIs unless the tumour can be adequately managed by surgery.

Ulcers that fail to heal

The introduction of antisecretory agents and effective treatments for *H. pylori* have revolutionised the management of peptic ulcers. Despite these advances, peptic ulceration fails to heal in a small minority of patients. Endoscopic re-evaluation should be regarded as mandatory to confirm healing of all gastric ulcers. Furthermore, endoscopy permits the differentiation between a refractory ulcer and persistent symptoms despite ulcer healing. The most common cause of failed healing is persistent *H. pylori* infection. Biopsies should be repeated at the time of endoscopy as false-negative results with breath tests may be expected soon after eradication therapy and serum antibody titres may not fall for 6 months after successful eradication. Failure of eradication is usually due to poor compliance or bacterial resistance and bacteriological culture will guide further attempts at *H. pylori* eradication. The ingestion of NSAIDs should once again be addressed. A diagnosis of Zollinger–Ellison syndrome (described in detail in ***Zollinger–Ellison syndrome***) should be suspected in *H. pylori*-negative, non-NSAID-related peptic ulceration and serum gastrin levels should be measured. Very rarely a recently described autoimmune immunoglobulin G4-related (IgG4) phenomenon is the cause of resistant and recurrent gastric ulceration.

Operations for duodenal ulceration

Procedures for the treatment of duodenal ulcers have the common aim of excluding acid from the duodenum. This is achieved by diversion of acid away from the duodenum, reducing the secretory potential of the stomach or both. All procedures achieve this aim to some extent, but with varying degrees of morbidity and postoperative side effects. There is now no role for acid-reducing operations in the routine management of peptic ulcer disease, but occasionally operations that involve gastrectomy have to be performed in the emergency situation.

Gastrectomy-based procedures

Gastrectomy in the form of either Billroth I (***Figure 67.14***) or Billroth II/Pólya (***Figure 67.15***) has been performed for

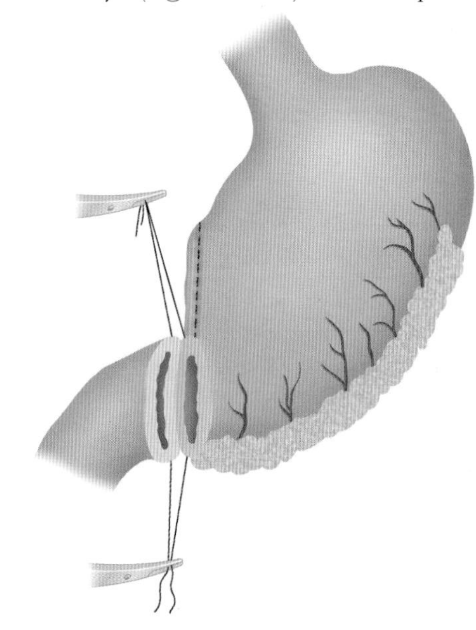

Figure 67.14 Billroth I gastrectomy. The lower half of the stomach is removed and the cut stomach anastomosed to the first part of the duodenum.

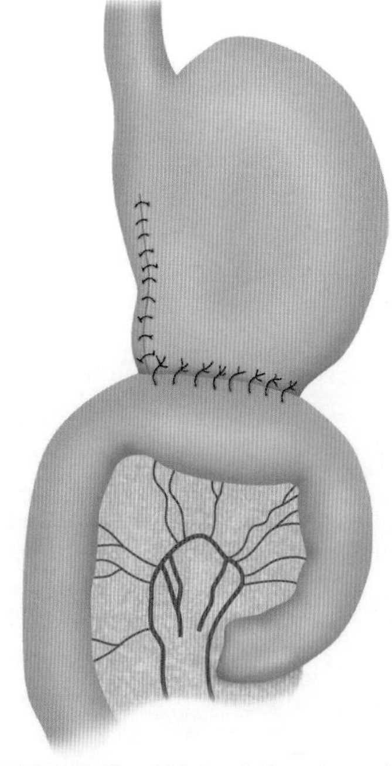

Figure 67.15 Billroth II. Two-thirds of the stomach is removed, the duodenal stump is closed and the stomach anastomosed to the jejunum.

duodenal ulcer since the end of the nineteenth century. Both operations remove the gastric antrum, hence reducing acid. The Pólya gastrectomy diverts the gastric secretions away from the duodenum. There is no elective role for these procedures in the treatment of duodenal ulcer, but the safer Pólya procedure is occasionally needed in the management of complex ulcer disease presenting as an emergency.

Gastrojejunostomy

Gastrojejunostomy (***Figure 67.16***) was developed as an operation for duodenal ulcer, in which role it was very unsuccessful. Although reflux of alkali into the stomach allowed healing in some cases, the exposure of jejunal mucosa to acid resulted in stomal ulceration. Gastroenterostomy, however, remains a commonly performed operation, usually to bypass malignant obstruction due to tumours in the distal stomach, duodenum or pancreas. This is performed through opening the lesser sac and performing an anastomosis between the most dependent part of the antrum and the first jejunal loop. An isoperistaltic anastomosis is most commonly performed.

Vagotomy-based procedures

The principle of the operation is that section of the vagus nerves, which are critically involved in the secretion of gastric acid, reduces the maximal acid output by approximately 50%. Truncal vagotomy (cutting the vagal verves at the lower oesophagus) was first introduced in the mid-twentieth century and, for many years, combined with a gastric drainage procedure, was the mainstay of treatment of duodenal ulceration (***Figure 67.17***). Because the vagal nerves are motor to the stomach, denervation of the antropyloroduodenal segment results in gastric stasis in a substantial proportion of patients on whom truncal vagotomy alone is performed. The most popular drainage procedure was the Heineke–Mikulicz pyloroplasty (***Figure 67.18***). It is simple to perform and involves longitudinal division of the pyloric ring. The incision is closed transversely. Gastrojejunostomy (***Figure 67.16***) is an alternative drainage procedure to pyloroplasty. In highly selective vagotomy, only the parietal cell mass of the stomach is denervated (***Figure 67.19***).

Operations for gastric ulcer

In contrast to surgery for duodenal ulcer, where the principal objective is to reduce duodenal exposure to gastric acid, in gastric ulcer surgery the ulcer is usually excised so that malignancy can then be confidently excluded. The standard operation is the Billroth I (***Figure 67.14***) but as with duodenal ulceration such surgery is now performed only for complications of gastric ulcer.

Sequelae of peptic ulcer surgery

There are a number of sequelae of peptic ulcer surgery, which include recurrent ulceration, small stomach syndrome, bilious vomiting, early and late dumping, diarrhoea and malignant transformation. These sequelae principally follow from the more destructive operations that are now seldom performed. However, a substantial number of patients have side effects from operations undertaken in the past. Approximately 30% of patients can expect to suffer a degree of dysfunction following peptic ulcer surgery (***Table 67.2***); in about 5% of such patients, the symptoms will be intractable.

TABLE 67.2 Operative mortality, side effects and incidence of recurrence following duodenal ulcer operations.

Operation	Operative mortality (%)	Significant side effects (%)	Recurrent ulceration (%)
Gastrectomy	1–2	20–40	1–4
Gastroenterostomy alone	<1	10–20	50
Truncal vagotomy and drainage	<1	10–20	2–7
Selective vagotomy and drainage	<1	10–20	5–10
Highly selective vagotomy	<0.2	<5	2–10
Truncal vagotomy and antrectomy	1	10–20	1

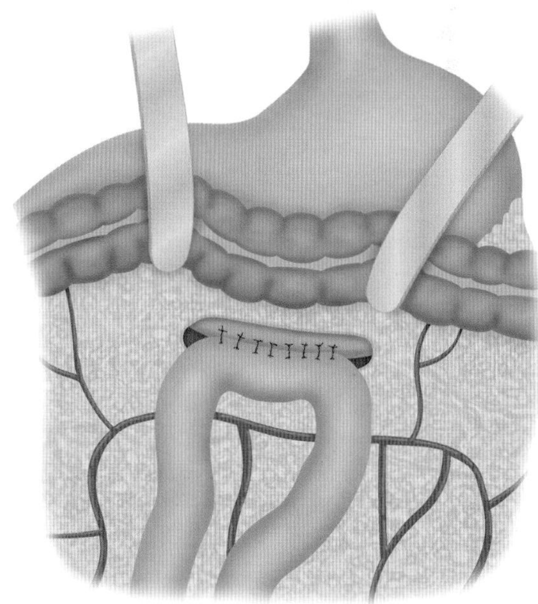

Figure 67.16 Gastroenterostomy. The jejunum is anastomosed to the posterior, dependent, wall of the stomach.

Eugen (Jeno) Alexander Pólya, 1876–1944, surgeon, St Stephen's Hospital, Budapest, Hungary.
Walther Hermann Heineke, 1834–1901, surgeon, Erlangen, Germany.
Johann von Mikulicz-Radecki, 1850–1905, Professor of Surgery, Breslau, Germany (now Wrocław, Poland).

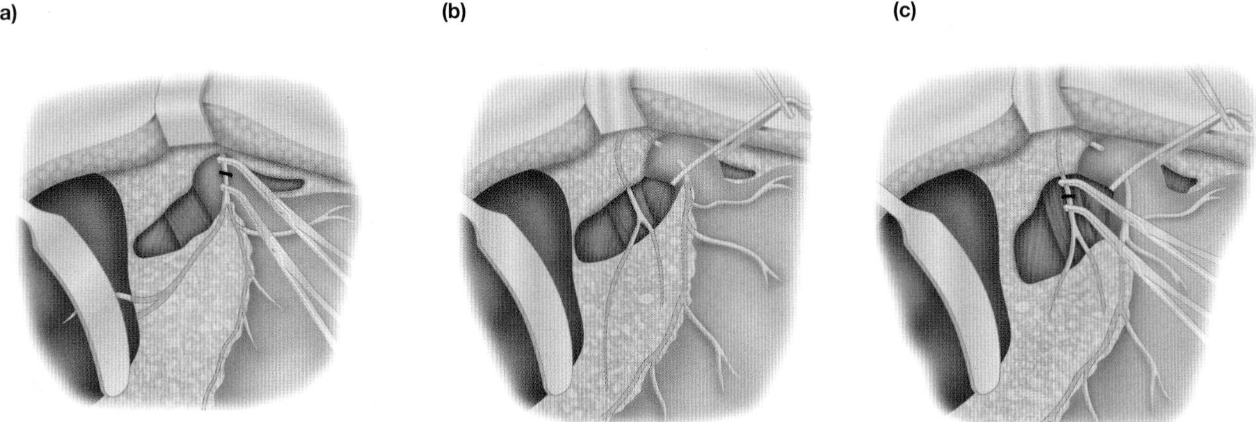

Figure 67.17 Truncal vagotomy: (a) division of the anterior vagus; (b) mobilisation of the oesophagus; (c) division of the posterior vagus.

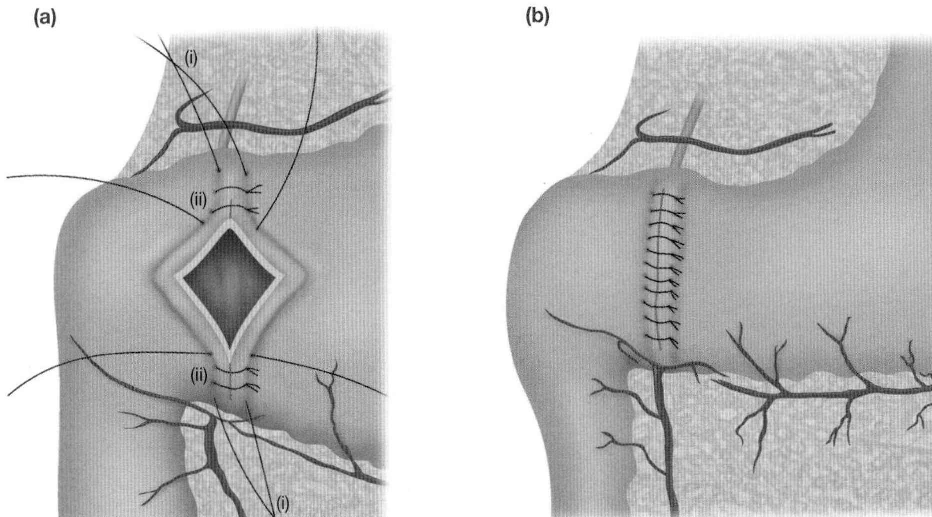

Figure 67.18 Heineke–Mikulicz pyloroplasty in which (a) a full-thickness longitudinal incision traversing the pylorus is retracted by stay sutures (i) and closed transversely with full-thickness sutures (ii). (b) Completed transverse closure.

Recurrent ulceration and gastrocolic fistula

As with other peptic ulcers, recurrent ulcers may present with complications, particularly bleeding and perforation. In this respect, the complication of gastrojejunal–colic fistula requires particular mention. In this rare condition, an anastomotic ulcer in the gastrojejunostomy penetrates into the transverse colon. Patients suffer from diarrhoea that is severe and follows every meal. They have foul breath and may vomit formed faeces. Severe weight loss and dehydration are rapid in onset; for this reason the condition may be mistaken for malignancy. The major factor producing the nutritional disturbance is the severe contamination of the jejunum with colonic bacteria. A number of imaging techniques can be used to detect the fistula, most commonly CT with oral contrast or indeed a barium enema. Endoscopy may not convincingly demonstrate the fistula and, in about one-half of such cases, the barium meal will not reveal the problem. The treatment of gastrocolic fistula consists of first correcting the dehydration and malnutrition and then performing revisional surgery.

Small stomach syndrome

Early satiety follows most ulcer operations to some degree, including highly selective vagotomy. In this latter circumstance, although there is no anatomical disturbance of the stomach there is loss of receptive relaxation. Fortunately, this problem does tend to get better with time and revisional surgery is not necessary.

Bile vomiting

Bile vomiting can occur after any form of vagotomy with drainage or gastrectomy. Commonly, the patient presents with vomiting a mixture of food and bile or sometimes some bile alone after a meal. Often eating will precipitate abdominal pain and reflux symptoms are common. Bile-chelating agents can be tried but are usually ineffective. In intractable cases, revisional surgery may be indicated. The nature of that revisional surgery depends very much on the original operation. Following gastrectomy, Roux-en-Y diversion is probably the best treatment. In patients with a gastroenterostomy, this can

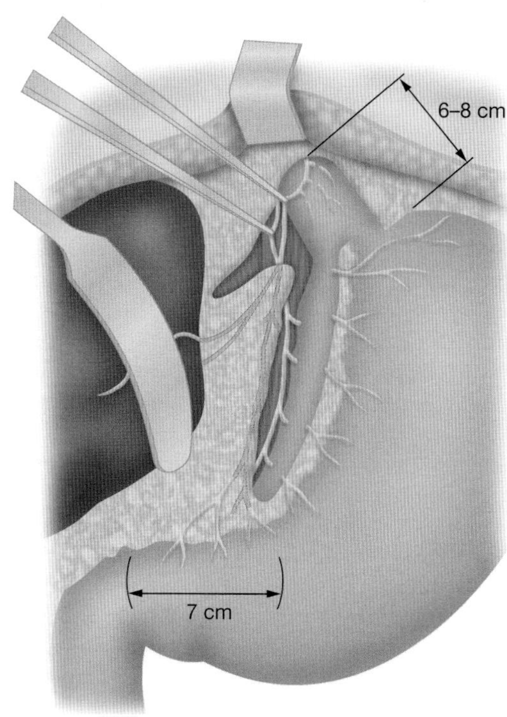

Figure 67.19 Highly selective vagotomy. The anterior and posterior vagus nerves are preserved but all branches to the fundus and body of the stomach are divided.

be taken down and, in most circumstances, a small pyloroplasty can be performed. In patients with a pyloroplasty, reconstruction of the pylorus has been attempted but, in general terms, the results of this operation have been rather poor. Antrectomy and Roux-en-Y reconstruction may be the better option.

Early and late dumping

Although considered together because the symptoms are similar, early and late dumping have different aetiologies A common feature, however, is early rapid gastric emptying. Many patients have both early and late dumping.

Early dumping

Early dumping consists of abdominal and vasomotor symptoms that are found in about 10% of patients following gastrectomy or vagotomy and drainage. It also affects a small percentage of patients following highly selective vagotomy owing to the loss of receptive relaxation of the stomach. The small bowel is filled with foodstuffs from the stomach, which have a high osmotic load that leads to the sequestration of fluid from the circulation into the gastrointestinal tract. This can be observed by the rise in the packed cell volume while the symptoms are present. All of the symptoms shown in ***Table 67.3*** can be related to this effect on the gut and the circulation.

The principal treatment is dietary manipulation. Small, regular meals based on fat and protein are best. Avoiding fluids with a high carbohydrate content also helps. Fortunately, the

TABLE 67.3 Features of early and late dumping.

	Early	Late
Incidence	5–10%	5%
Relation to meals	Almost immediate	Second hour after meal
Durations of attack	30–40 minutes	30–40 minutes
Relief	Lying down	Food
Aggravated by	More food	Exercise
Precipitating factor	Food, especially carbohydrate rich and wet	As early dumping
Major symptoms	Epigastric fullness, sweating, light-headedness, tachycardia, colic, sometimes diarrhoea	Tremor, faintness, prostration

syndrome tends to improve with time; however, a group of patients have intractable dumping. The somatostatin analogue octreotide given before meals is useful in some individuals and the long-acting preparation may also be useful; however, it does not help diarrhoea, which many patients with dumping also suffer.

Revisional surgery may be occasionally required. In patients with a gastroenterostomy, the drainage may be taken down or, in the case of a pyloroplasty, repaired. Alternatively, antrectomy with Roux-en-Y reconstruction is often effective, although the procedure is of greater magnitude; following gastrectomy, it is the revisional procedure of choice (***Figure 67.20***).

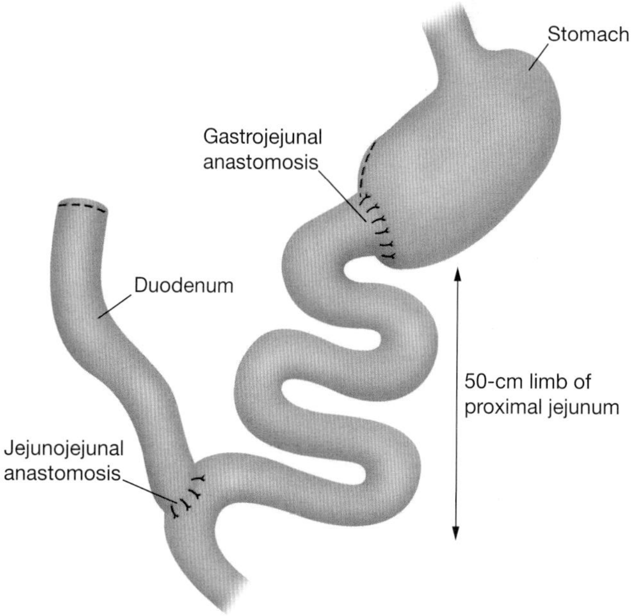

Figure 67.20 Roux-en-Y reconstruction following Billroth I gastrectomy. Note the length of the proximal jejunal limb required to minimise bilious reflux.

César Roux, 1857–1934, Professor of Surgery and Gynecology, Lausanne, Switzerland.

Late dumping

This is due to reactive hypoglycaemia. The carbohydrate load in the small bowel causes a rise in the plasma glucose, which, in turn, causes insulin levels to rise, causing a secondary hypoglycaemia. This can be easily demonstrated by serial measurements of blood glucose in a patient following a test meal. The treatment is essentially the same as for early dumping. Octreotide is very effective in dealing with this problem.

Postvagotomy diarrhoea

This can be the most devastating symptom to afflict patients having peptic ulcer surgery. Most patients will have some looseness of bowel action (with the exception of highly selective vagotomy), but it may be intractable in approximately 5%. The cause is uncertain but is related to rapid gastric emptying, denervation of the upper gastrointestinal tract and an exaggerated gastrointestinal peptide response. Many patients with severe diarrhoea do not have other symptoms of dumping and likewise some patients with dumping do not experience significant diarrhoea. In general, patients should be managed as for early dumping and antidiarrhoeal preparations may be of value. Octreotide is not effective and the results of revisional surgery are unpredictable.

Malignant transformation

Partial gastrectomy or vagotomy and drainage are independent risk factors for development of gastric cancer as bile reflux gastritis, intestinal metaplasia and gastric cancer are linked. The lag phase between operation and the development of malignancy is at least 10 years. Highly selective vagotomy does not seem to be associated with an increased long-term incidence of gastric cancer.

Nutritional consequences

Nutritional disorders are more common after gastrectomy than after vagotomy and drainage. Weight loss is common after gastrectomy and patients may never return to their original weight. Taking more frequent small meals is often useful.

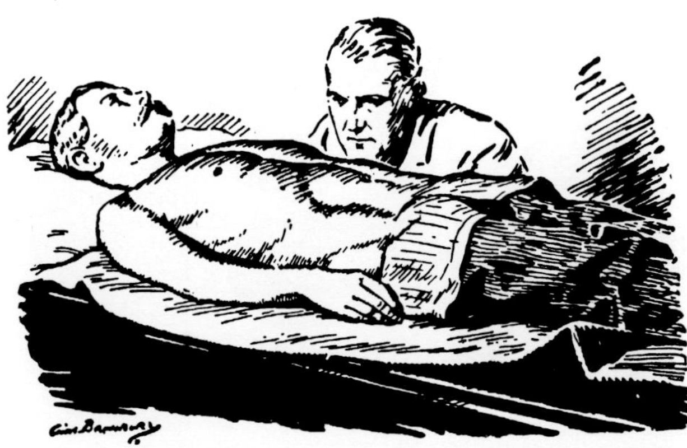

Figure 67.21 A sketch of Mr Hamilton Bailey watching for abdominal movement on respiration. In the case of a classically presenting perforated ulcer, the abdominal movement is restricted or absent.

Iron deficiency anaemia occurs after both gastrectomy and vagotomy and drainage. Reduced iron absorption is probably the most important factor. Vitamin B_{12} deficiency occurs after total gastrectomy; however, it may be years before megaloblastic anaemia is clinically apparent. Vitamin B_{12} supplementation after total gastrectomy is essential. Rarely, vitamin B_{12} deficiency may occur after lesser forms of gastrectomy. In such patients the cause is probably a combination of reduced intrinsic factor production and bacterial colonisation, which results in vitamin B_{12} being metabolised in the gut, preventing absorption.

Bone disease is seen principally after gastrectomy and mainly in women. The condition is essentially indistinguishable from the osteoporosis commonly seen in postmenopausal women. It is only the frequency and magnitude of the disorder that distinguish it. Treatment is with dietary supplementation, calcium and vitamin D, and exercise.

Gallstones

Following truncal vagotomy, the biliary tree is denervated, leading to cholestasis and gallstone formation. Symptomatic patients require cholecystectomy; however, this may induce or worsen other postpeptic ulcer surgery syndromes such as bilious vomiting and postvagotomy diarrhoea.

Complications of peptic ulceration

The common complications of peptic ulcer are perforation, bleeding and stenosis. Bleeding and stenosis are considered below in the relevant sections.

Perforated peptic ulcer

Epidemiology

Despite the widespread use of gastric antisecretory agents and eradication therapy, the incidence of perforated peptic ulcer has changed little. However, there has been a steady increase in the age of the patients with this complication and an increase in the numbers of females, such that perforations now occur most commonly in elderly female patients. NSAIDs appear to be responsible for most of these perforations.

Clinical features

The classical presentation of perforated duodenal ulcer is instantly recognisable (***Figure 67.21***). The patient, who may have a history of peptic ulceration, develops sudden-onset severe generalised abdominal pain due to the irritant effect of gastric acid on the peritoneum. Although the contents of an acid-producing stomach are relatively low in bacterial load, bacterial peritonitis supervenes over a few hours, usually accompanied by a deterioration in the patient's condition. Initially, the patient may be shocked with a tachycardia, but a pyrexia is not usually observed until some hours after the event. The abdomen exhibits a board-like rigidity, and the patient is disinclined to move because of the pain. The abdomen does not move with respiration. Patients with this form of presentation need an operation, without which the patient will deteriorate with a septic peritonitis.

Henry Hamilton Bailey, 1894–1961, surgeon, The Royal Northern Hospital, London, UK.

This classical presentation of the perforated peptic ulcer is observed less commonly than in the past. Very frequently the elderly patient will have a less dramatic presentation, perhaps because of the use of potent anti-inflammatory drugs (steroids). The board-like rigidity seen in the abdomen of younger patients may also not be observed and a higher index of suspicion is necessary to make the correct diagnosis. In other patients, the leak from the ulcer may be contained such that they present with pain in the epigastrium and right iliac fossa as the fluid may track down the right paracolic gutter. Sometimes perforations will seal owing to the inflammatory response and adhesion within the abdominal cavity, and so the perforation may be self-limiting. All of these factors may combine to make the diagnosis of perforated peptic ulcer difficult.

Investigations

An erect chest radiograph will reveal free gas under the diaphragm in more than 50% of cases with perforated peptic ulcer (***Figure 67.22***), but CT imaging is now most commonly used and is more accurate. All patients should have serum amylase performed, as distinguishing between peptic ulcer, perforation and pancreatitis can be difficult. Measuring the serum amylase, however, may not remove the diagnostic difficulty. It can be elevated following perforation of a peptic ulcer, although, fortunately, the levels are not usually as high as the levels commonly seen in acute pancreatitis. A CT scan will normally be diagnostic in both conditions.

Treatment

The initial priorities are resuscitation and analgesia. Analgesia should not be withheld for fear of removing the signs of an intra-abdominal catastrophe. In fact, adequate analgesia makes the clinical signs more obvious. It is important, however, to titrate the analgesic dose. Following resuscitation, the treatment is principally surgical. Laparotomy is performed, usually through an upper midline incision if the diagnosis of perforated peptic ulcer can be made with confidence. Alternatively, laparoscopy may be used. The most important component of the operation is a thorough peritoneal toilet to remove all of the fluid and food debris. If the perforation is in the duodenum, it can usually be closed by several well-placed sutures, closing the ulcer in a transverse direction as with a pyloroplasty. It is important that sufficient tissue is taken in the suture to allow the edges to be approximated, and the sutures should not be tied so tight that they tear out. It is common to place an omental patch over the perforation in the hope of enhancing the chances of the leak sealing. If the perforation is difficult to close primarily it is frequently possible to seal the leak with an omental patch alone, and many surgeons now employ this strategy for all perforations.

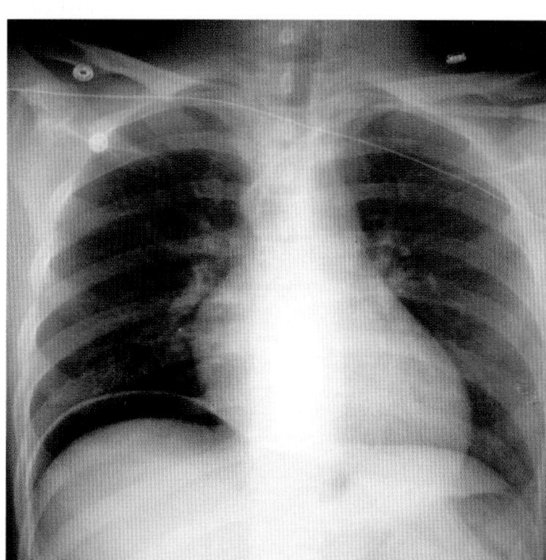

Figure 67.22 Erect chest radiograph showing air under the right diaphragm in a patient with a perforated duodenal ulcer.

When securing the omental patch, it is important not to tie the sutures too tight so as to obliterate the omental blood supply. Gastric ulcers should, if possible, be excised and closed, so that malignancy can be excluded. Occasionally a patient is seen who has a massive duodenal or gastric perforation such that simple closure is impossible; in these patients a distal gastrectomy with Roux-en-Y reconstruction is the procedure of choice (***Figure 67.20***).

Perforated peptic ulcers can often be managed by minimally invasive techniques if the expertise is available. The principles of operation are the same: thorough peritoneal toilet and closure of the perforation by intracorporeal suturing.

Following operation, it is important that the stomach is kept empty postoperatively by nasogastric suction, and that gastric antisecretory agents are commenced to promote healing in the residual ulcer. *H. pylori* eradication is mandatory.

A minority of patients who have small leaks from a perforated peptic ulcer and relatively mild peritoneal contamination may be managed with intravenous fluids, nasogastric suction and antibiotics. Any deterioration should prompt immediate surgical intervention.

Patients who have had one perforation may have another. Therefore, they should be managed aggressively to ensure that this does not happen. Lifelong treatment with PPIs is a reasonable option, especially in those who have to continue with NSAID treatment.

HAEMATEMESIS AND MELAENA

Upper gastrointestinal haemorrhage remains a major medical problem with an incidence of over 100/100 000 per year in Western practice. The incidence increases with age. Haemorrhage is strongly associated with NSAID use. Despite improvements in diagnosis and the proliferation in treatment modalities over the last few decades, an in-hospital mortality of 5–10% can be expected. This rises to 33% when bleeding is first observed in patients who are hospitalised for other reasons. In patients in whom the cause of bleeding can be found, the most common causes are peptic ulcer, erosions, Mallory–Weiss tear and bleeding oesophageal varices (***Table 67.4***).

Whatever the cause, the principles of management are identical. First, the patient should be adequately resuscitated

George Kenneth Mallory, 1900–1986, Professor of Pathology, Boston, MA, USA.
Soma Weiss, 1899–1942, Professor of Medicine, Boston, MA, USA.

TABLE 67.4 Causes of upper gastrointestinal bleeding

Condition	Percentage
Ulcers	60
Oesophageal	6
Gastric	21
Duodenal	33
Erosions	26
Oesophageal	13
Gastric	9
Duodenal	4
Mallory–Weiss tear	4
Oesophageal varices	4
Tumour	0.5
Vascular lesions	0.5
Others	5

and, following this, should be investigated urgently to determine the cause of the bleeding. Intravenous access should be established and, for those with severe bleeding, central venous pressure monitoring should be established and bladder catheterisation performed. Blood should be cross-matched and the patient transfused as clinically indicated, usually when >30% of blood volume has been lost (see ***Chapter 2***). There is no evidence for the use of intravenous PPI prior to endoscopy. As a general rule, most gastrointestinal bleeding will stop, albeit temporarily, but there are sometimes instances when this is not the case. In these circumstances, resuscitation, diagnosis and treatment should be carried out simultaneously. There are occasions when life-saving manoeuvres have to be undertaken without the benefit of an absolute diagnosis. In some patients, bleeding is secondary to a coagulopathy. The most important current causes are liver disease and anticoagulation therapy. In these circumstances the coagulopathy should be corrected, if possible, with fresh-frozen plasma or concentrated clotting factors with haematology advice.

Upper gastrointestinal endoscopy should be carried out by an experienced operator as soon as practicable after the patient has been stabilised. In patients in whom the bleeding is relatively mild, endoscopy may be carried out on the morning after admission; this is usually guided by local policy. In all cases of severe bleeding, it should be carried out immediately. A number of scoring systems have been advocated for the assessment of rebleeding and death after upper gastrointestinal haemorrhage. The Rockall score (***Table 67.5***) can be used in a pre-endoscopy format to stratify patients to safe early discharge and, post endoscopy, it can relatively accurately predict rebleeding and death.

Bleeding peptic ulcers

The epidemiology of bleeding peptic ulcers mirrors that of perforated ulcers. In recent years, the population affected has become older and bleeding is commonly associated with the ingestion of NSAIDs. Diagnosis can normally be made endoscopically, although occasionally the nature of the blood loss precludes accurately identifying the lesion. However, the more experienced the endoscopist, the less likely this is to be a problem.

Medical and minimally interventional treatments

Medical treatment has limited efficacy. All patients are commonly started on either an H_2 antagonist or a proton pump inhibitor, and recent evidence confirms the benefit of PPI administration to prevent rebleeding after endoscopy. Meta-analysis of studies suggests that tranexamic acid, an inhibitor of fibrinolysis, may reduce overall mortality.

Therapeutic endoscopy can achieve haemostasis in approximately 70% of cases, with the best evidence supporting a combination of adrenaline injection with heater probe and/or clips. Therapeutic endoscopy will probably never be effective

TABLE 67.5 The Rockall scoring system of bleeding severity.

	Score			
	0	1	2	3
Age	<60	60–79	>80	
Shock	Pulse <100 bpm Systolic BP >100 mmHg	Pulse >100 bpm Systolic BP <100 mmHg	Pulse >100 bpm Systolic BP <100 mmHg	
Comorbidities	None		Circulatory failure/coronary artery disease	Renal failure Liver failure Disseminated malignancy
Endoscopic signs of bleeding	None/dark spot		Blood/adherent clot/visible or spurting vessel	
Diagnosis	Mallory–Weiss syndrome/no pathology	All other diagnoses	Malignancy of the upper gastrointestinal tract	

BP, blood pressure; bpm, beats per minute.

Timothy Alexander Rockall, contemporary, Royal Surrey County Hospital, Guilford, Surrey, UK.

in patients who are bleeding from large vessels and with which the majority of the mortality is associated.

In patients where the source of bleeding cannot be identified or in those who rebleed after endoscopy, angiography with transcatheter embolisation may offer a valuable alternative to surgery in expert centres. The risk of significant ischaemia following embolisation is low because of the rich collateral blood supply of the stomach and duodenum. The surgeon should be mindful that rescue surgery after failed embolisation is associated with poor outcome and it may be advantageous to proceed directly to surgery.

Surgical treatment

Patients who continue to bleed require surgery except in expert centres with experience of angiographic embolisation where attempts may be made to arrest bleeding and avoid surgery. The surgical team should be immediately available, and an operation should not be delayed if bleeding persists. Patients with a visible vessel in the ulcer base, a spurting vessel or an ulcer with a clot in the base are likely to require surgical treatment. Frail and elderly patients are more likely to die as a result of bleeding than younger patients; thus, paradoxically, they should have early surgery. In general, a patient who has required more than six units of blood needs surgical treatment.

The aim of the operation is to stop the bleeding. Preoperative endoscopy can usually identify the site of bleeding, which is most often from a peptic ulcer in the duodenum. At operation it is important that the duodenum is fully mobilised before it is opened as it makes the ulcer much more accessible and also allows the surgeon's hand to be placed behind the gastroduodenal artery, which is commonly the source of major bleeding. Following mobilisation, the duodenum, and usually the pylorus, is opened longitudinally as in a pyloroplasty. This allows good access to the ulcer, which is usually found posteriorly or superiorly. Accurate haemostasis is important and can be achieved initially by direct pressure. It is the vessel within the ulcer that is bleeding and this should be controlled using well-placed sutures on a small round-bodied needle that underrun the vessel. The pyloroplasty is then closed with interrupted sutures in a transverse direction in the usual fashion. In the case of a large ulcer, the first part of the duodenum may be destroyed, making primary closure impossible. In this circumstance one should proceed to distal gastrectomy with Roux-en-Y reconstruction. The duodenal stump may then be closed with T-tube drainage or around a drain to create a controlled fistula.

The management of bleeding gastric ulcers is essentially the same. The stomach is opened at an appropriate site anteriorly and the vessel in the ulcer under-run. Consideration is then given to local excision of the ulcer. If the ulcer is not excised, the ulcer margins must be biopsied to exclude malignancy. Gastrectomy for bleeding is associated with a high perioperative mortality, even if the incidence of recurrent bleeding is less.

Bearing in mind that most patients nowadays are elderly and unfit, the minimum surgery that stops the bleeding is probably optimal (damage control surgery). Acid can be inhibited by pharmacological means and appropriate eradication therapy will prevent ulcer recurrence. Definite acid-lowering surgery is not now required. Patients on long-term NSAIDs can be managed as outlined in ***Treatment of peptic ulceration***.

Stress ulceration

This commonly occurs in patients with major injury or illness who have undergone major surgery or who have major comorbidity. Many such patients are found in intensive care units. The incidence has reduced in recent years owing to the widespread use of prophylactic acid inhibition and nasogastric or oral administration of sucralfate. Endoscopic means of treating stress ulceration may be ineffective and operation may be required. The principles of management are the same as for a chronic ulcer.

Gastric erosions

Erosive gastritis has a variety of causes, especially NSAIDs. Fortunately, most such bleeding settles spontaneously, but it can be a major problem to treat. In general terms, although there is a diffuse erosive gastritis, there is one (or more) specific lesion that has a significant-sized vessel within it. This should be dealt with appropriately, preferably endoscopically, but sometimes surgery is necessary.

Mallory-Weiss tear

This is a longitudinal tear at the GOJ, which is induced by repetitive and strenuous vomiting. Doubtless, many such lesions occur and do not cause bleeding. When it is a cause of haematemesis, the lesion may often be missed as it can be difficult to see because it is just below the GOJ, a position that can be difficult for the inexperienced endoscopist. Occasionally these lesions continue to bleed and require surgical treatment (see also ***Chapter 66***).

Dieulafoy lesion

This is essentially a gastric arterial venous malformation that has a characteristic histological appearance. Bleeding due to this malformation is one of the most difficult causes of upper gastrointestinal bleeding to treat. The lesion itself is covered by normal mucosa and, when not bleeding, it may be invisible. If it can be seen while bleeding, all that may be visible is profuse bleeding coming from an area of apparently normal mucosa. If this occurs, the cause is instantly recognisable. If the lesion can be identified endoscopically (***Figure 67.23***) bleeding can be stopped by injection of sclerosant or application of endoscopic clips. If it is identified at operation, only local excision is necessary.

Tumours

All gastric neoplasms may present with chronic or acute upper gastrointestinal bleeding. Bleeding is not normally torrential

Georges Dieulafoy, 1851–1919, physician and surgeon, Hôtel-Dieu de Paris, Paris, France, later President of the French Academy of Medicine (1910).

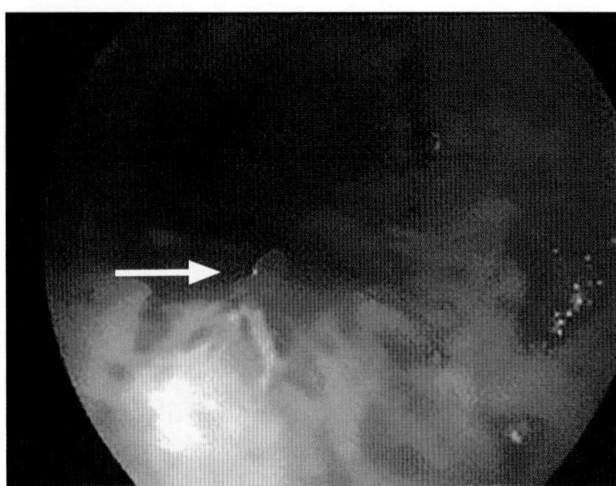

Figure 67.23 Endoscopic view of actively bleeding Dieulafoy lesion in the gastric fundus.

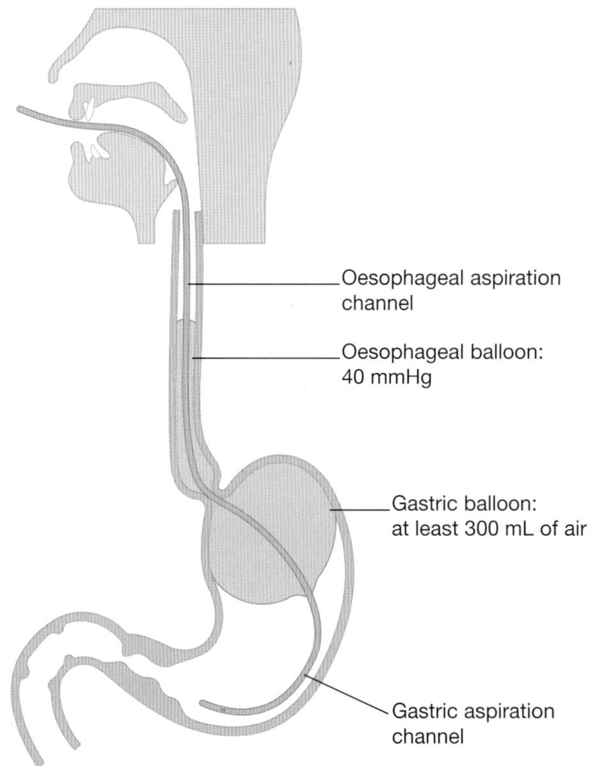

Figure 67.24 Balloon tamponade of gastric and oesophageal varices with a Sengstaken–Blakemore tube. The balloons should be deflated every 12 hours to prevent pressure necrosis.

but can be unremitting. Treatment is that of the underlying tumour as discussed in ***Gastric cancer***.

Portal hypertension and portal gastropathy

The management of bleeding gastric varices is very challenging. Fortunately, most bleeding from varices is oesophageal and is much more amenable to sclerotherapy, banding and balloon tamponade. Gastric varices may also be injected, although this is technically more difficult. Banding can also be used, again with difficulty. The gastric balloon of the Sengstaken–Blakemore tube can be used to arrest the haemorrhage from the fundus of the stomach or GOJ (***Figure 67.24***). Intravenous infusion of octreotide (somatostatin analogue) or terlipressin (Glypressin), a vasopressin analogue, reduces portal pressure in patients with varices and is of value in arresting haemorrhage.

Acute surgery on bleeding varices should be avoided, if possible, because of high operative mortality; it has been superseded in most centres by transjugular intrahepatic portosystemic shunt (TIPSS) insertion (see ***Chapter 69***).

Portal gastropathy

Portal gastropathy refers to changes in the gastric mucosa as a result of portal hypertension. The mucosa is friable and may exude blood, even in the absence of well-developed visible varices. The treatment is as for portal hypertension.

Aortic enteric fistula

This diagnosis should be considered in any patient with haematemesis and melaena that cannot be otherwise explained. Contrary to expectation, the bleeding from such patients is not always massive. Very often there is nothing much to distinguish between the bleeding from the aortic enteric fistula and any other recurrent upper gastrointestinal bleeding. The vast majority of patients will have had an aortic graft; however, it is occasionally seen in patients with an untreated aortic aneurysm. A CT scan with intravenous contrast will confirm the diagnosis. Treatment requires aortic aneurysm or aortic graft excision/replacement and carries a high mortality (see ***Chapter 61***).

GASTRIC OUTLET OBSTRUCTION

The two common causes of gastric outlet obstruction are gastric cancer (see ***Gastric cancer***) and pyloric stenosis secondary to peptic ulceration. With the decreasing incidence of peptic ulceration gastric outlet obstruction should be considered malignant until proven otherwise. In this circumstance the metabolic consequences may be somewhat different from those of benign pyloric stenosis because of the relative hypochlorhydria found in patients with gastric cancer.

Clinical features

In benign gastric outlet obstruction, there is usually a long history of peptic ulcer disease. The vomitus is characteristically of undigested food and is totally lacking in bile. Weight loss is a feature, and the patient appears unwell and dehydrated. On examination the distended stomach may be visible and a succussion splash may be audible.

Robert William Sengstaken Sr, 1923–1978, surgeon, Garden City, New York, NY, USA.
Arthur Blakemore, 1897–1970, surgeon, The Columbia College of Physicians and Surgeons, New York, NY, USA.

Summary box 67.5

Gastric outlet obstruction

- Gastric outlet obstruction is most commonly associated with longstanding peptic ulcer disease and gastric cancer
- The metabolic abnormality of hypochloraemic alkalosis is usually only seen with peptic ulcer disease and should be treated with isotonic saline with potassium
- Endoscopic biopsy is essential to exclude malignancy
- Aggressive medical therapy for peptic ulcer disease often leads to resolution
- Endoscopic dilatation of the gastric outlet may be effective in benign stenosis
- Operation is frequently required, with a drainage procedure being performed for benign disease or appropriate resection of malignancy

Metabolic effects

Vomiting hydrochloric acid results in hypochloraemic alkalosis. Initially the sodium and potassium may be relatively normal; however, as dehydration progresses, more profound metabolic abnormalities arise, partly related to renal dysfunction. Initially, the urine has a low chloride and high bicarbonate content, reflecting the primary metabolic abnormality. With time the patient becomes progressively hyponatraemic and more profoundly dehydrated. Because of the dehydration, sodium is retained and potassium and hydrogen ions are excreted. This results in the urine becoming paradoxically acidic and hypokalaemia ensues. Alkalosis leads to a lowering in the circulating ionised calcium, and tetany can occur.

Management

Treating the patient involves correcting the metabolic abnormalities and dealing with the mechanical obstruction. The patient should be rehydrated with intravenous isotonic saline with potassium supplementation. Replacing the sodium chloride and water allows the kidney to correct the acid–base abnormality. The metabolic abnormalities may be less if the obstruction is due to malignancy, as the acid–base disturbance is less pronounced.

The stomach should be emptied using a wide-bore tube. A large nasogastric tube may not be sufficiently large to deal with the contents of the stomach, and it may be necessary to pass an orogastric tube and lavage the stomach until it is completely emptied. This allows investigation with endoscopy and contrast radiology. Biopsy of the area around the pylorus is essential to exclude malignancy.

Early cases may settle with conservative treatment, as oedema around the ulcer diminishes as the ulcer is healed. Traditionally, severe cases are treated surgically, usually with a gastroenterostomy rather than a pyloroplasty. Endoscopic treatment with balloon dilatation may be most useful in early cases and may have to be repeated several times. A duodenal stent insertion may be considered in patients with unresectable malignancy.

GASTRIC POLYPS

A number of conditions manifest as gastric polyps. Their main importance is that they may actually represent early gastric cancer. Biopsy is essential.

The most common type of gastric polyp is metaplastic. These are associated with *H. pylori* infection and regress following eradication therapy. Inflammatory polyps are also common. Fundic gland polyps deserve particular attention. They are associated with use of PPIs and are also found in patients with familial adenomatous polyposis (FAP). Neither metaplastic nor fundic gland polyps have proven malignant potential; however, true adenomas do and should be removed.

GASTRIC CANCER

Carcinoma of the stomach is a major cause of mortality worldwide. Its prognosis tends to be poor, with cure rates little better than 5–10%, although better results are obtained in Japan, where the disease is common. Gastric cancer is actually an eminently curable disease and early diagnosis is key to success. Unfortunately, late presentation is common and the cause of poor overall survival figures. The only curative treatment is resectional surgery.

Summary box 67.6

Gastric cancer

- Gastric cancer is one of the most common causes of cancer death
- The outlook is generally poor, owing to the advanced stage at presentation
- Better results are obtained in Japan, which has a high population incidence, screening programmes and high-quality surgical treatment
- The aetiology of gastric cancer is multifactorial
- *H. pylori* is important in distal but not proximal gastric cancer
- Early gastric cancer is associated with high cure rates
- Gastric cancer can be classified into intestinal and diffuse types, the latter having a worse prognosis
- Spread may be by lymphatics, blood, transcoelomic or direct
- Distant metastases are uncommon in the absence of lymph node involvement
- Radical surgery and removal of second tier of nodes (around the principal arterial trunks) may be advantageous
- Chemotherapy improves survival in patients having surgery and in advanced disease

Incidence

There are marked variations in the incidence of gastric cancer worldwide. In the UK, it is approximately 15 per 100 000 per year; in the USA, 10 per 100 000 per year; and in Eastern Europe, 40 per 100 000 per year. In Japan, the disease is much more common, with an incidence of approximately 70 per 100 000 per year. There are areas in China where the incidence even higher. These underlying epidemiological data make it clear that this is an environmental disease. In general, men are more affected by the disease than women and, as with most solid organ malignancies, the incidence increases with age.

At present, marked changes are being observed in the West in terms of the incidence and site of gastric cancer and the population affected, changes that to date have not been observed in Japan. First, the incidence of gastric cancer is continuing to fall at about 1% per year. This reduction exclusively affects carcinoma arising in the body and distal stomach. In contrast, there appears to be an increase in the incidence of carcinoma in the proximal stomach, particularly the GOJ. Carcinoma of the distal stomach and body of the stomach is most common in low socioeconomic groups, whereas the increase in proximal gastric cancer seems to affect principally higher socioeconomic groups. Proximal gastric cancer does not seem to be associated with *H. pylori* infection, in contrast with carcinoma of the body and distal stomach.

Aetiology

Gastric cancer is a multifactorial disease. Epidemiological studies point to a role for *H. pylori*; however, there is insufficient evidence to support eradication programmes in asymptomatic patients. *H. pylori* seems to be principally associated with carcinoma of the body, stomach and distal stomach rather than the proximal stomach.

Patients with pernicious anaemia and gastric atrophy are at increased risk, as are those with gastric adenomatous polyps. Patients who have had peptic ulcer surgery, particularly those who have had drainage procedures such as Billroth II or Pólya gastrectomy, gastroenterostomy or pyloroplasty, are at approximately four times the average risk; this is thought to be related to bile reflux and intestinal metaplasia. Carcinoma is associated with cigarette smoking and dust ingestion from a variety of industrial processes. Diet appears to be important, as illustrated by the example of the decline in the incidence of gastric cancer among Japanese families living in the USA. The high incidence of gastric cancer in some pockets in China is probably environmental and probably diet related. Excessive salt intake, deficiency of antioxidants and exposure to *N*-nitroso compounds are also related. The aetiology of proximal gastric cancer remains an enigma. It is not associated with *H. pylori* but is associated with obesity and higher socioeconomic status. Genetic factors are also important but not fully elucidated (see ***The molecular pathology of gastric cancer***).

Clinical features

The features of advanced gastric cancer are usually obvious. Unfortunately, early gastric cancer has no specific features to distinguish it from benign dyspepsia and a high index of suspicion is necessary.

In advanced cancer, early satiety, bloating, distension and vomiting may occur. The tumour frequently bleeds, resulting in iron deficiency anaemia. Obstruction leads to dysphagia, epigastric fullness or vomiting. Weight loss can be profound. With pyloric involvement the presentation may be of gastric outlet obstruction, although the alkalosis is usually less pronounced than when duodenal ulceration leads to obstruction. Non-metastatic effects of malignancy are seen, particularly thrombophlebitis (Trousseau's sign) and deep venous thrombosis. These features result from the effects of the tumour on thrombotic and haemostatic mechanisms.

Site

The proximal stomach is now the most common site for gastric cancer in the West. Because the lower oesophagus is also a very common site of adenocarcinoma approximately 60% of all malignancies in the upper gastrointestinal tract occur in proximity to the GOJ (see ***Chapter 66***). Adenocarcinoma at this site has doubled in incidence in the UK over the last 30 years. This high prevalence of proximal gastric cancer is not seen in Japan, where distal cancer still predominates, as it does in most of the rest of the world.

Pathology

The most useful clinicopathological classification of gastric cancer is the Laurén classification. In this system there are principally two forms of gastric cancer: intestinal gastric cancer and diffuse gastric cancer (often with signet ring cells). In intestinal gastric cancer, the tumour resembles a carcinoma elsewhere in the tubular gastrointestinal tract and forms polypoid tumours or ulcers; it probably arises in areas of intestinal metaplasia. In contrast, diffuse gastric cancer infiltrates deeply into the stomach without forming obvious mass lesions but spreads widely in the gastric wall. Not surprisingly, this has a much worse prognosis. A small proportion of gastric cancers are of mixed morphology.

Gastric cancer can be divided into early gastric cancer and advanced gastric cancer. Early gastric cancer is defined as cancer limited to the mucosa and submucosa with or without lymph node involvement (T1, any N); it can be protruding, superficial or excavated as described in the Japanese classification (***Figures 67.25 and 67.26***). This type of cancer is eminently curable with 5-year survival rates in the region of 90%. In Japan, approximately one-third of gastric cancers diagnosed are in this stage. However, early gastric cancer diagnosis in the UK is relatively uncommon as dyspeptic patients are not always referred for endoscopy at an appropriate stage.

Advanced gastric cancer involves the muscularis. Its macroscopic appearances have been classified by Borrmann into four types (***Figures 67.27 and 67.28***). Types III and IV are commonly incurable.

The molecular pathology of gastric cancer

Understanding of the molecular pathology of gastric cancer has been revolutionised by the application of next-generation

---

Armand Trousseau, 1801–1867, physician, Hôtel-Dieu de Paris, Paris, France. The sign led him to suspect that he personally had gastric cancer, however it proved to be pancreatic cancer on post-mortem.
Pekka August Laurén, 1922–2016, pathologist, University of Turku, Finland.
Robert Borrmann, 1870–1943, pathologist, Bremen, Germany.

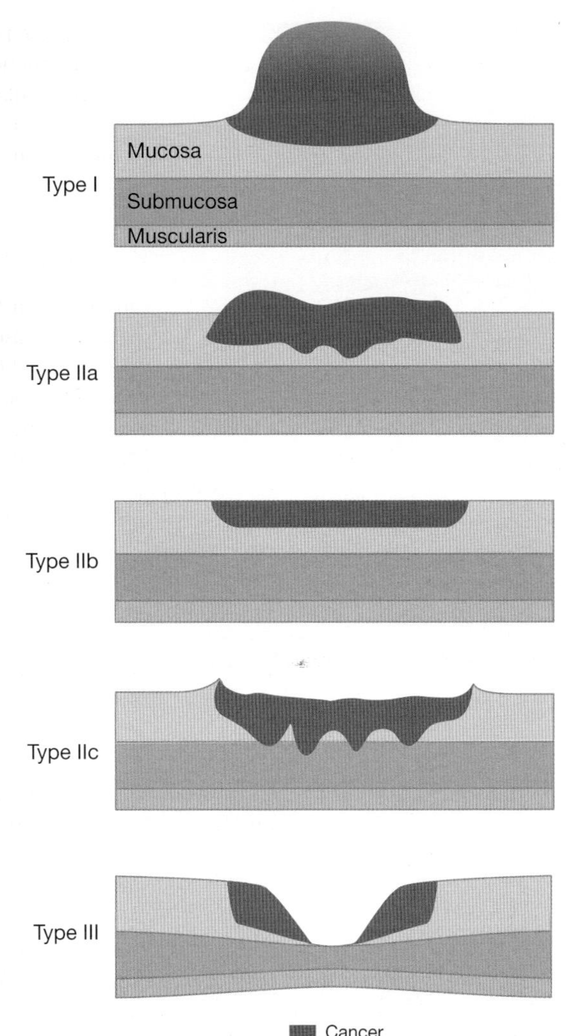

Figure 67.25 Japanese classification of early gastric cancer: type I, protruding; type II, superficial, a, elevated, b, flat, c, depressed; type III, ulcerated.

sequencing platforms to the disease. The Cancer Genome Atlas (TCGA) group described four molecular subtypes of gastric cancer: Epstein–Barr virus positive, microsatellite unstable, genomically stable and chromosomal instability. Recognition of these subgroups and their underlying common gene mutations and driver events is leading to the development of targeted therapies, including immunotherapies. Similar genetic classifications are now available for other tumours of the gastrointestinal tract, meaning that novel treatments can be applied across tumour types.

A range of mutations in genes related to genome integrity (e.g. *BRCA2, TP53, ARID1A*), chromatin remodelling (e.g. *SMARCA1, CHD3, CHD4*) and cell–cell adhesion and motility (e.g. *RHOA, CDH1*) have been described in gastric cancer. In addition, cell signalling pathways commonly mutated in other solid organ tumours are also often found perturbed in gastric cancer. For example, the Wnt pathway may be amenable to specific small-molecule inhibitors. Unsurprisingly gastric cancer exhibits a range of mutations in receptor tyrosine kinases and PI3K/MAPK signalling (see ***Chapter 11***).

The rapid development of sequencing technologies, including single-cell platforms and the development of real-time sequencing, offers the promise of precision therapy for gastric cancer in the future, but currently treatment is still based on surgery with or without conventional chemo/radiotherapy.

Staging

The International Union Against Cancer (UICC) staging system is shown in ***Table 67.6***. Important changes have been made in the seventh and eighth editions of the TNM staging system that are worthy of discussion. In an attempt to reflect the current evidence base and to improve outcome prediction for individual patients, all gastric tumours whose epicentre is within 5 cm of the GOJ and extend into the oesophagus are now classified according to the oesophageal system. Tumours whose epicentre is within 5 cm of the GOJ but do not extend into the oesophagus, and all other gastric cancers, are staged using the revised gastric staging system. In addition, any tumour that perforates the serosa is now classified as T4 disease.

Spread of carcinoma of the stomach

Gastric cancer is an excellent example of the various distant metastases that are uncommon in the absence of lymph node metastases. The intestinal and diffuse types of gastric cancer spread differently. The diffuse type spreads via the submucosal and subserosal lymphatic plexus and penetrates the gastric wall at an early stage.

Direct spread

The tumour penetrates the muscularis, serosa and ultimately adjacent organs such as the pancreas, colon and liver.

Lymphatic spread

This is by both permeation and emboli to the affected tiers (see ***Lymphatic drainage of the stomach***) of nodes. This may be extensive, the tumour even appearing in the supraclavicular nodes (Troisier's sign). Unlike malignancies such as breast cancer, nodal involvement does not imply systemic dissemination.

Blood-borne metastases

This occurs first to the liver and subsequently to other organs, including lung and bone. This is uncommon in the absence of nodal disease.

Transperitoneal spread

This is a common mode of spread once the tumour has reached the serosa of the stomach and indicates incurability. Tumours can manifest anywhere in the peritoneal cavity and

Michael Anthony Epstein, b. 1921, Professor of Pathology, University of Bristol, Bristol, UK.
Yvonne Barr, 1931–2016, virologist who emigrated to Australia. Epstein and Barr discovered this virus in 1964.
Charles Emile Troisier, 1844–1919, Professor of Pathology, Paris, France.

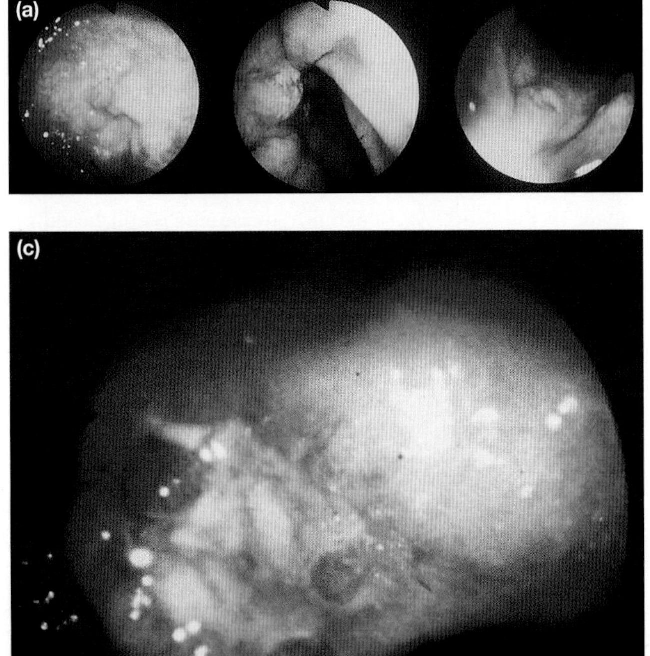

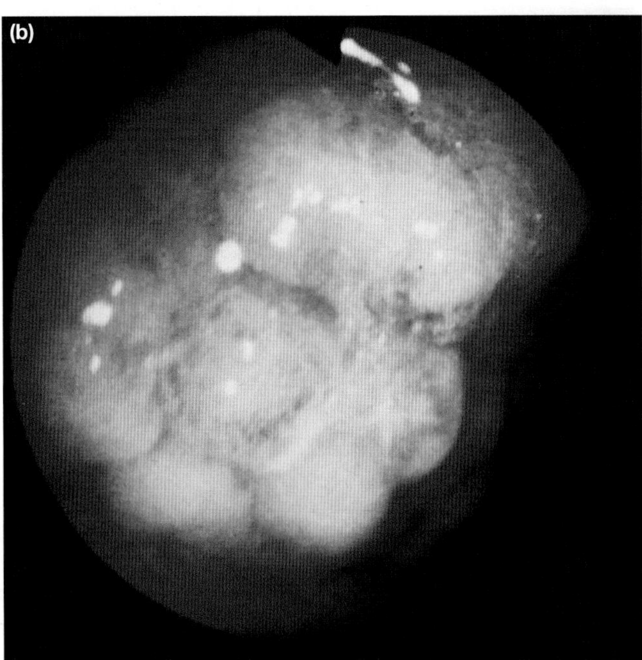

Figure 67.26 Early gastric cancer: (a) type I; (b) type IIa; (c) type III (courtesy of Dr GNJ Tytgat, Amsterdam, The Netherlands).

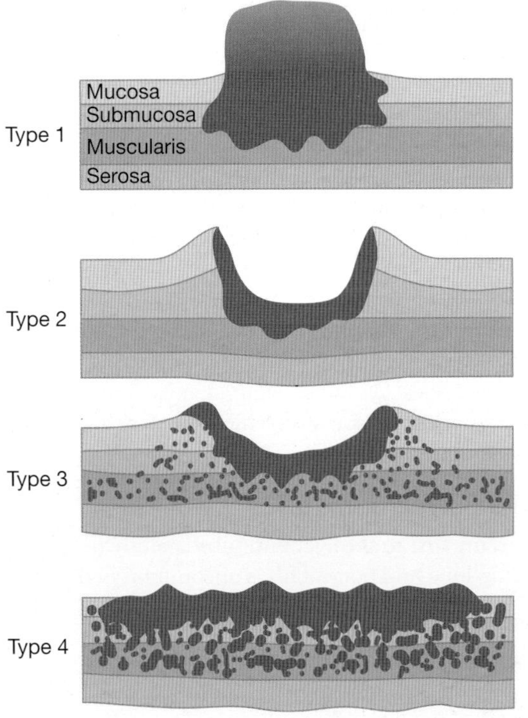

Figure 67.27 Borrmann classification of advanced gastric cancer: type 1, polypoid; type 2, ulcerating; type 3, infiltrating/ulcerating; type 4, infiltrating/linitis plastica.

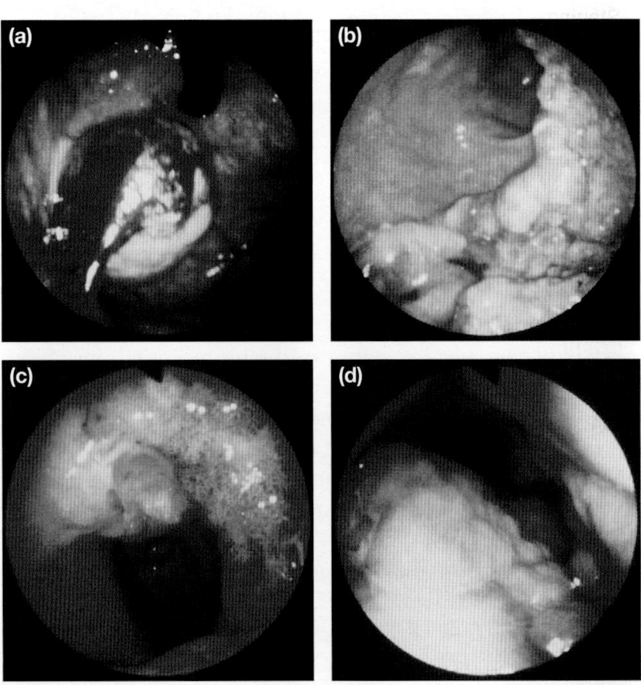

Figure 67.28 Advanced gastric cancer: (a) type I; (b) type II; (c) type III; (d) type IV (linitis plastica) (courtesy of Dr GNJ Tytgat, Amsterdam, The Netherlands).

TABLE 67.6 International Union Against Cancer (UICC) staging of gastric cancer (8th edition).

Tx	Primary tumour cannot be assessed		
T0	No evidence of primary tumour		
Tis	Carcinoma *in situ*: intraepithelial tumour without invasion of the lamina propria, high-grade dysplasia		
T1	Tumour involves lamina propria, muscularis mucosae or submucosa		
	T1a Tumour invades lamina propria or muscularis mucosae		
	T1b Tumour invades submucosa		
T2	Tumour invades muscularis propria		
T3	Tumour involves subserosa		
T4	Tumour perforates serosa (visceral peritoneum) or invades adjacent structures		
	T4a Tumour perforates serosa		
	T4b Tumour invades adjacent structures		
Nx	Regional lymph nodes cannot be assessed		
N0	No regional lymph node metastasis		
N1	Metastasis in 1 or 2 regional lymph nodes		
N2	Metastasis in 3–6 regional lymph nodes		
N3	Metastasis in 7 or more regional lymph nodes		
	N3a Metastasis in 7–15 regional lymph nodes		
	N3b Metastasis in 16 or more regional lymph nodes		
M0	No distant metastasis		
M1	Distant metastasis Involvement of non-regional intra-abdominal lymph nodes such as retropancreatic, mesenteric and para-aortic groups is considered to be distant metastasis (M1) Involvement of the liver or the presence of peritoneal seedlings is also staged as M1		
Staging			
IA	T1	N0	M0
IB	T1	N1	M0
	T2	N0	M0
IIA	T1	N2	M0
	T2	N1	M0
	T3	N0	M0
IIB	T1	N3	M0
	T2	N2	M0
	T3	N1	M0
	T4a	N0	M0
IIIA	T2	N3	M0
	T3	N2	M0
	T4a	N1	M0
IIIB	T3	N3	M0
	T4a	N2	M0
	T4b	N0–1	M0
IIIC	T4a	N3	M0
	T4b	N2–3	M0
IV	Any T	Any N	M1

commonly give rise to ascites. Advanced peritoneal disease may be palpated either abdominally or rectally as a tumour 'shelf'. The ovaries may sometimes be the sole site of transcoelomic spread (Krukenberg's tumours). Tumour may spread via the abdominal cavity to the umbilicus (Sister Joseph's nodule). Transperitoneal spread of gastric cancer can be detected most effectively by laparoscopy and cytology.

Lymphatic drainage of the stomach

Understanding the lymphatic drainage of the stomach is the key to understanding radical surgery for gastric cancer. The lymphatics of the antrum drain into the right gastric lymph node superiorly and right gastroepiploic and subpyloric lymph nodes inferiorly. The lymphatics of the pylorus drain to the right gastric suprapyloric nodes superiorly and the subpyloric lymph nodes situated around the gastroduodenal artery inferiorly. The efferent lymphatics from suprapyloric lymph nodes converge on the para-aortic nodes around the coeliac axis, whereas the efferent lymphatics from the subpyloric lymph nodes pass to the main superior mesenteric lymph nodes situated around the origin of the superior mesenteric artery. The lymphatic vessels related to the cardia communicate freely with those of the oesophagus.

The prognosis of operable cases of carcinoma of the stomach depends on whether or not there is histological evidence of regional lymph node involvement. Retrograde (downwards) spread may occur if the upper lymphatics are blocked. In Japan, lymph node dissection is highly advanced and the Japanese Research Society for Gastric Cancer has assigned a number to each lymph node station to aid pathological staging (***Figure 67.29***).

Operability

Patients with incurable disease should not subjected to futile radical surgery, hence the value of preoperative CT/PET and laparoscopic staging. Haematogenous metastases, involvement of the distant peritoneum, M1 nodal disease and fixation to structures that are not resectable are unequivocal features of incurable disease. Involvement of another organ per se does not imply incurability, provided it can be excised.

Neoadjuvant chemotherapy

Most operable patients should have neoadjuvant chemotherapy as there is level 1 evidence of improved survival. Since the early 2000s a platinum-based triplet regime containing epirubicin (e.g. epirubicin, cisplatin and 5-fluorouracil [5-FU]; ECF) has been the standard of care. Recently epirubicin has been replaced by docetaxel after publication of the FLOT4 trial; this was a direct comparison of ECF with FLOT (fluorouracil, leucovorin, oxaliplatin, docetaxel) chemotherapy that showed a significant survival advantage for FLOT (50 months versus 35 months). Unfortunately, only a minority of patients receive a clinically meaningful survival advantage and mechanisms to predict response are urgently required to prevent the ineffective and harmful treatment of the majority. Evidence for the use of perioperative (before and after surgery) chemotherapy is less robust, as in all major trials (MRC-MAGIC and FLOT4) fewer than 50% of patients received the postoperative component.

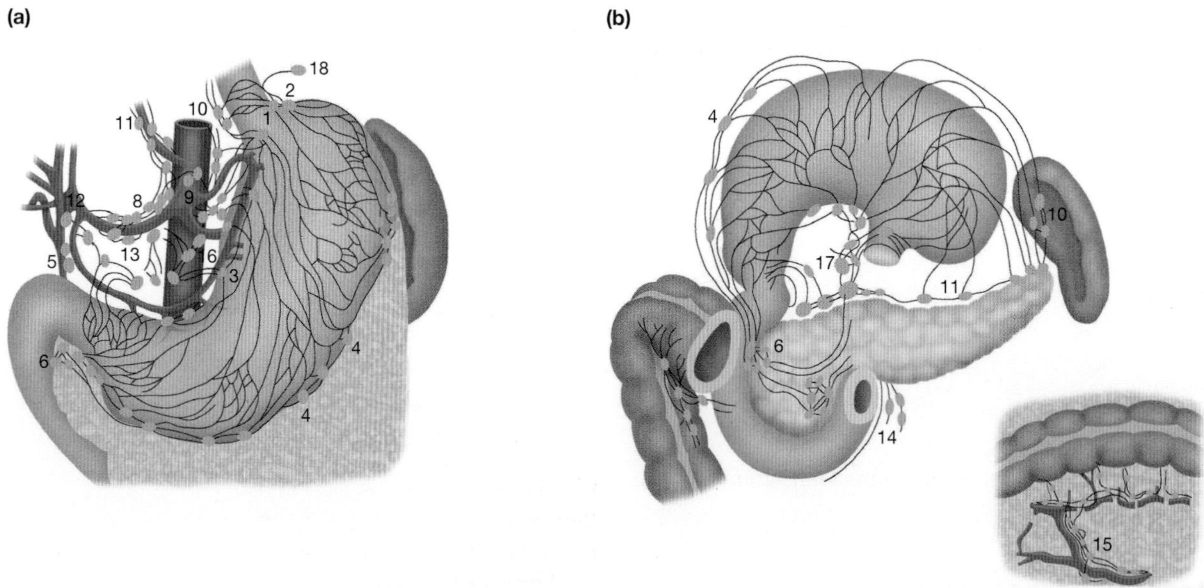

Figure 67.29 Lymphatic drainage of the stomach and nodal stations by the Japanese classification: (a) the anterior view of the stomach; (b) the posterior view.

Friedrich Ernest Krukenberg, 1870–1946, ophthalmologist, Halle, Germany, wrote a classic paper on malignant tumours of the ovary in 1896.
Sister Mary Joseph (Julia Dempsey), 1856–1939, Nursing Superintendent, St Mary's Hospital, Rochester, MN, USA, noted the presence of umbilical nodules in many patients with advanced gastric cancer. She drew this to the attention of Dr William Mayo, founder of the Mayo Clinic.

Total gastrectomy

This is best performed through a long upper midline incision. The stomach is removed en bloc, including the tissues of the entire greater omentum and lesser omentum (*Figure 67.30*). In commencing the operation, the transverse colon is completely separated from the greater omentum. The dissection may then be commenced proximally or, more usually, distally. The subpyloric nodes are dissected, and the first part of the duodenum is divided, usually with a surgical stapler. The hepatic nodes are dissected to clear the hepatic artery; this dissection also includes the suprapyloric nodes. The right gastric artery is divided at its origin from the hepatic artery. The lymph node dissection is continued to the origin of the left gastric artery, which is divided at its origin. Dissection is continued along the splenic artery, removing all nodes on the superior aspect of the pancreas and accessible nodes in the splenic hilum.

Separation of the stomach from the spleen, if it is not going to be removed, allows access to the nodal tissues around the upper stomach and GOJ. The oesophagus can then be divided at an appropriate point using a combination of stay sutures and a soft non-crushing clamp, usually of the right-angled variety. It is important that the resection margins are well clear of the tumour (>5 cm). Frozen section should be performed if involvement of either proximal or distal resection margin is in doubt.

Gastrointestinal continuity is reconstituted by means of a Roux loop. The alimentary limb of the Roux loop should be at least 50 cm long to avoid bile reflux oesophagitis. The simplest means of effecting the oesophagojejunostomy is to place a purse-string suture in the cut end of the oesophagus and, using a circular stapler introduced through the blind end of the Roux loop, staple the end of the oesophagus onto the side of the Roux loop. The blind open end of the Roux loop may then be closed either with sutures or with a linear stapler. Recent evidence supports long-term intestinal and nutritional benefits of construction of a jejunal pouch. The anastomosis can also be fashioned end to end. The Roux loop may be placed in either an antecolic or retrocolic position. The end-to-side jejunojejunostomy is undertaken at a convenient point (*Figure 67.31*).

The differentiation between a D1 and a D2 operation depends upon the tiers of nodes removed. Different tiers need to be removed depending on the positions of primary tumour (*Table 67.7*). In general, a D1 resection involves the removal of the perigastric nodes and a D2 resection involves the clearance of the major arterial trunks. In practice the majority of specialist centres will perform a radical total gastrectomy, conserving the spleen and pancreas, with D2 lymphadenectomy sparing station 10 lymph nodes.

Subtotal gastrectomy

For tumours in the distal stomach, it is unnecessary to remove the whole stomach. However, the operation is very similar to that of a total gastrectomy except that the proximal stomach is preserved, the blood supply being derived from the short gastric arteries. Following the resection, the simplest form of reconstruction is to close the stomach from the lesser curve, near the GOJ, with either sutures or staples and then perform an anastomosis of the greater curve to the jejunum. Although this can be performed as in a Billroth II/Pólya-type gastrectomy, this reconstruction may result in quite marked enterogastric reflux and bile reflux oesophagitis; the preferred reconstruction is to use a Roux loop.

Palliative surgery

In patients with significant symptoms of either obstruction or bleeding, palliative resection is appropriate. A palliative gastrectomy need not be radical as it is sufficient to remove the tumour and reconstruct the gastrointestinal tract. Sometimes it is impossible to resect an obstructing tumour in the distal stomach and other palliative procedures need to be considered. A high gastroenterostomy is a poor operation that very frequently does not allow the stomach to empty adequately and may produce the additional problem of bile reflux. A Roux loop with a wide anastomosis between the stomach and jejunum may be a better option, although even this may not allow the stomach to empty well. For inoperable tumours situated in the cardia, palliative intubation or stenting can be used (see *Chapter 66*).

Postoperative complications of gastrectomy

Radical gastrectomy is complex major surgery and predictably there is a large number of potential complications of the operation. Leakage of the oesophagojejunostomy can often be managed conservatively as the Roux-en-Y reconstruction means that it is mainly saliva and ingested food that leaks. Some patients may establish a fistula from the wound or drain site and others may need radiologically or surgically placed drains. It is unusual to detect a major anastomotic leak in the absence of clinical signs and the use of postoperative water-soluble contrast swallows is no longer routine in most centres.

Leakage from the duodenal stump is usually due to a degree of distal obstruction and care must be taken to avoid kinking when performing the Roux-en-Y anastomosis. Paraduodenal collections can be drained radiologically, which may convert the collection into an external fistula. Biliary peritonitis requires a laparotomy and peritoneal toilet. In this circumstance it is best to leave a Foley catheter in the duodenum to establish a controlled duodenal fistula. If it is established that there is no distal obstruction, or if any such obstruction is managed, then the fistula will close with time.

The presence of septic collections along with a radical vascular dissection may lead to catastrophic secondary haemorrhage from the exposed or divided blood vessels. This situation may be very difficult to manage, whether or not reoperation or interventional radiology is employed.

Frederick Eugene Basil Foley, 1891–1966, urologist, St Paul Ramsey Medical Center, St Paul, MN, USA.

(a)

(b)

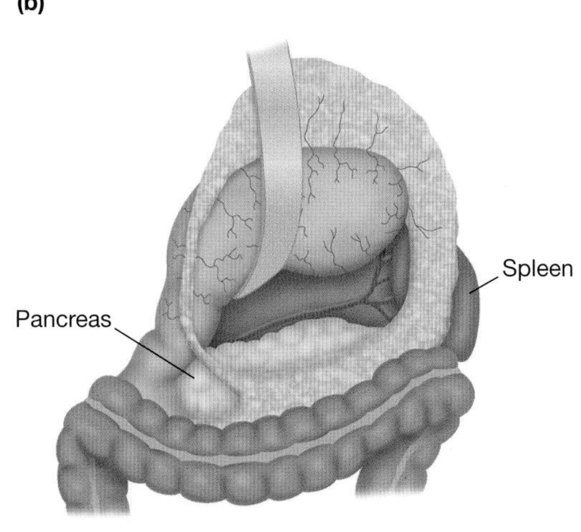

(c)

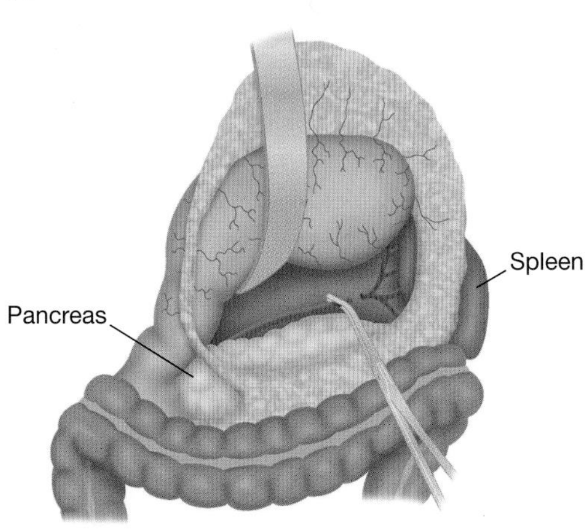

(d)

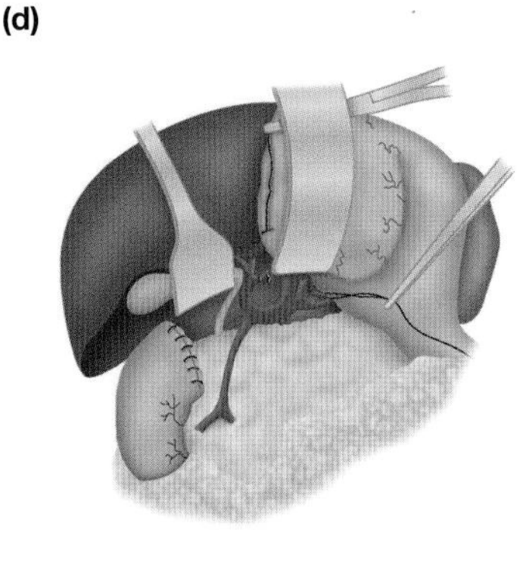

(e)

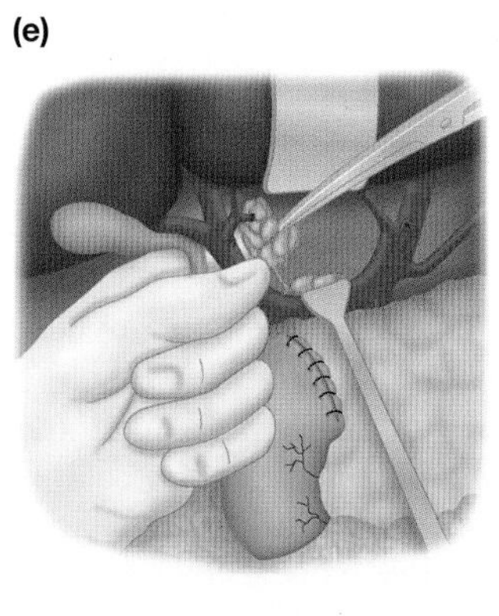

(f)

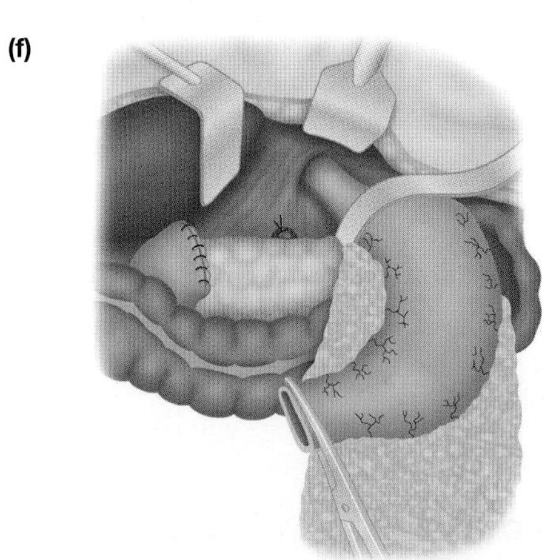

Figure 67.30 Radical total gastrectomy: (a) dissection of omentum off the transverse colon; (b) exposure of the lesser sac; (c) splenectomy; (d) division and oversewing of the duodenum; (e) dissection of the left gastric artery nodes (group 17); (f) mobilisation of the oesophagus.

Long-term complications of surgery

There is very little functional difference between patients who have a total gastrectomy and those who have a subtotal gastrectomy. Patients need to be given detailed nutritional advice, the substance of which is to eat small meals and often, while the jejunum or small gastric remnant adapts. Nutritional deficiencies may occur and loss of the parietal mass leads to vitamin B_{12} deficiency that requires replacement routinely.

TABLE 67.7 The lymph node stations (see *Figure 67.30*) that need to be removed in a D1 (N1 nodes removed) or a D2 (N2 nodes removed) resection.

		Site of cancer			
Lymph node number		**Antrum**	**Middle**	**Cardia**	**Cardia and oesophagus**
1	Right cardia	N2	N1	N1	N1
2	Left cardia		N1	N1	N1
3	Lesser curve	N1	N1	N1	N1
4sa	Short gastric	N1	N1	N1	N1
4sb	Left gastroepiploic	N1	N1	N1	N1
4d	Right gastroepiploic	N1	N1	N2	N2
5	Suprapyloric	N1	N1	N2	N2
6	Infrapyloric	N1	N1	N2	N2
7	Left gastric artery	N2	N2	N2	N2
8a	Anterior hepatic artery	N2	N2	N2	N2
9	Coeliac artery	N2	N2	N2	N2
10	Splenic hilum		N2	N2	N2
11	Splenic artery		N2	N2	N2
19	Infradiaphragmatic				N2
20	Oesophageal hiatus			N2	N1
110	Lower oesophagus				N2
111	Supradiaphragmatic				N2

The nodes in stations 12–18 are not routinely removed in a D1 or D2 gastrectomy.

Outlook after surgical treatment

The outlook after surgical treatment varies considerably between the West and Japan. In Japan, approximately 75% of patients will have a curative resection and, of these, the overall 5-year survival rate is 50–70%. In contrast, in the West most series show that only 25–50% of patients undergoing surgery will have a curative operation and the 5-year survival rate in such patients is only about 25–30%, although in some series it approaches Japanese levels. A combination of differences in staging and a higher standard of surgery in Japan probably accounts for the differences. Staging is clearly crucial when survival figures are being compared and, therefore, stage for stage the outcome seems better in patients who are adequately staged pathologically. This phenomenon is termed 'stage migration'.

Other treatment modalities

Because of the failure of radical surgery to cure advanced gastric cancer, there has been an interest in the use of radiotherapy and chemotherapy.

Palliative radiotherapy

The routine use of radiotherapy is controversial as the results of clinical trials are inconclusive. There are a number of radiosensitive tissues in the region of the gastric bed, which limits the dose that can be given. Radiotherapy has a role in the palliative treatment of painful bony metastases.

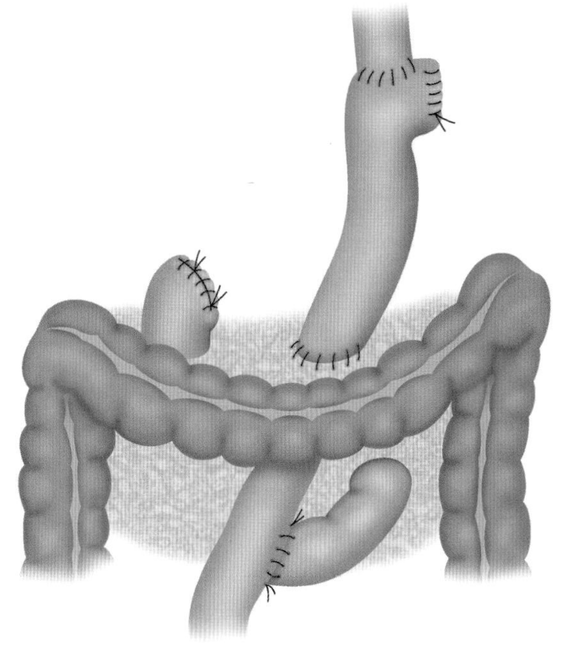

Figure 67.31 Oesophagojejunostomy Roux-en-Y.

Palliative chemotherapy

There are a number of regimes, but the best results are currently obtained using either platinum-containing triplet combinations or FLOT. Second-line treatment using combinations that include docetaxel are increasingly being used. Chemotherapy for advanced disease is palliative. Newer biological agents such as trastuzumab (Herceptin) offer potential advantages to survival in the minority of patients (<20%) with *HER2*-positive gastric cancer. However, the absolute survival advantages are small (~4 months) and the cost of treatment is high. Nevertheless trastuzumab has been approved for use in metastatic *HER2*-positive gastric cancer in the UK and European Union.

Pattern of relapse following surgical treatment

The most common site of relapse following radical gastrectomy is the gastric bed, representing inadequate extirpation of the primary tumour. Widespread nodal intraperitoneal metastases, distant nodal metastases and liver metastases are all common. Dissemination to the lung and bones usually only occurs after liver metastases are already established.

GASTROINTESTINAL STROMAL TUMOURS

Gastrointestinal stromal tumours (GISTs) may arise in any part of the gastrointestinal tract but 50% will be found in the stomach. Previously named leiomyoma and leiomyosarcoma, the term GIST is now used, recognising the distinct phenotype. They are tumours of mesenchymal origin and are observed equally commonly in males and females. The tumours are universally associated with a mutation in the tyrosine kinase *c-kit* oncogene. These tumours are sensitive to the tyrosine kinase antagonist imatinib, and an 80% objective response rate can be observed. Tumours with mutations in exon 11 of *c-kit* are particularly sensitive to this drug. The biological behaviour of these tumours is unpredictable but size and mitotic index are the best predictors of metastasis. Peritoneal and liver metastases are most common but spread to lymph nodes is extremely rare.

The incidence of the condition is uncertain as small stromal tumours of the stomach are probably quite common and remain unnoticed. Clinically obvious tumours are considerably less common than gastric cancer. GISTs constitute 1–3% of all gastrointestinal neoplasia.

Many GISTs are noticed incidentally at endoscopy or diagnosed if the overlying mucosa ulcerates with bleeding and anaemia (***Figure 67.32***). Because the mucosa overlying the tumour is normal, endoscopic biopsy can be uninformative unless the tumour has ulcerated. Targeted biopsy by endoscopic ultrasonography is more helpful. Larger tumours present with non-specific gastric symptoms, and, in many instances, they may be thought to be gastric cancer initially (***Figure 67.33***).

As the biological behaviour is difficult to predict, the best guide is to consider the size of the tumour. Tumours over 5 cm in diameter should be considered to have metastatic potential. If easily resectable surgery is the primary mode of treatment. Smaller tumours can be treated by wedge excision although the appropriate management of asymptomatic diminutive tumours found incidentally at endoscopy is unclear. Larger tumours may require a gastrectomy or duodenectomy, but lymphadenectomy is not required. Larger tumours that require multivisceral resection may be better treated with 3–6 months of imatinib prior to operation as this will usually radically reduce the size and vascularity of the tumours. Adjuvant imatinib for resected tumours of high malignant potential should probably be continued indefinitely.

The prognosis of advanced metastatic GISTs has been dramatically improved with imatinib chemotherapy but resection of metastases has an important role.

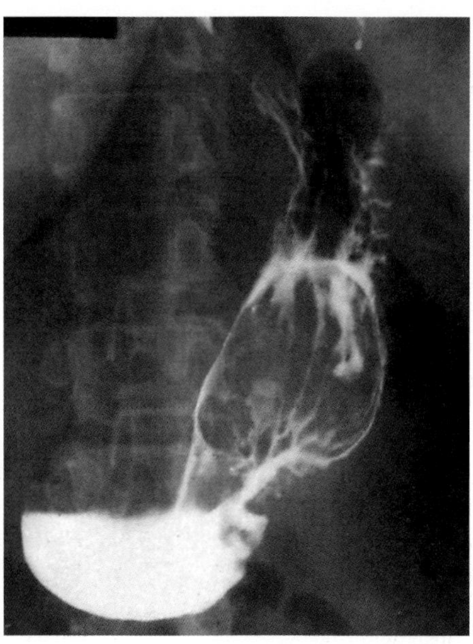

Figure 67.32 Gastrointestinal stomal tumour (GIST) on the greater curve of the stomach with ulceration.

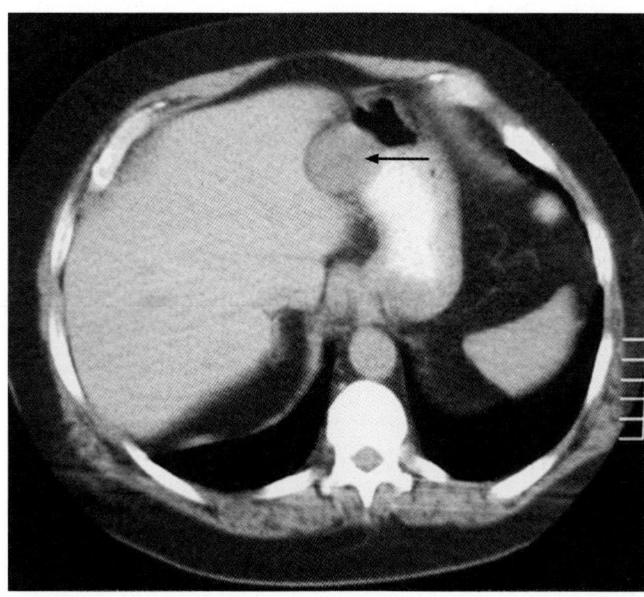

Figure 67.33 Computed tomography scan of the upper abdomen showing a 3.5-cm gastrointestinal stromal tumour arising from the gastric wall.

GASTRIC LYMPHOMA

Unlike gastric carcinoma, the incidence of lymphoma seems to be increasing. It is most common in the sixth decade and presentation is similar to that of gastric cancer. Acute presentation with haematemesis, perforation or obstruction is uncommon. Primary gastric lymphoma accounts for approximately 5% of all gastric neoplasms. It is important to distinguish primary gastric lymphoma from the more common involvement of the stomach in a diffuse lymphoma.

Primary gastric lymphomas are B-cell derived, the tumour arising from mucosa-associated lymphoid tissue (MALT). Primary gastric lymphoma remains in the stomach for a prolonged period before involving lymph nodes. At an early stage, the disease takes the form of a diffuse mucosal thickening, which may ulcerate. Diagnosis is made as a result of the endoscopic biopsy and seldom on the basis of the endoscopic features alone, which are not specific.

Following diagnosis, adequate staging is necessary, primarily to establish whether the lesion is a primary gastric lymphoma or part of a more generalised process. CT scans of the chest and abdomen and bone marrow aspirate are required.

Although the treatment of primary gastric lymphoma is somewhat controversial, it seems most appropriate to use surgery alone for localised disease. Chemotherapy is appropriate for patients with systemic disease. Lymphocytes are not found to any degree in normal gastric mucosa but are found in association with *Helicobacter* infection. Early gastric lymphomas may regress and disappear when the *Helicobacter* infection is treated. Patients with gastric involvement of a diffuse lymphoma are treated with chemotherapy, sometimes with dramatic and rapid responses. The two common surgical complications are bleeding and perforation. Both may follow the chemotherapy when there is rapid regression and necrosis of the tumour and normally require gastrectomy.

DUODENAL TUMOURS

Benign duodenal tumours

Duodenal villous adenomas occur principally in the periampullary region. Although generally uncommon, they are often found in patients with FAP. The appearances are similar to those adenomas arising in the colon and, as they have malignant potential, they should be locally excised with histologically clear margins.

Duodenal adenocarcinoma

Most duodenal tumours originate in the periampullary region and commonly arise in pre-existing villous adenomas. Patients present with anaemia due to ulceration of the tumour or obstruction. Direct involvement in the ampulla leads to obstructive jaundice. Histologically, the lesion is an adenocarcinoma. Metastases are commonly to regional lymph nodes and the liver. At presentation, about 70% of patients have resectable disease with an expected 5-year survival rate of approximately 20%. Poor prognostic features include regional lymph node metastases, transmural involvement and perineural invasion. Curative surgical treatment will normally involve a pancreaticoduodenectomy (Whipple's procedure). Patients with FAP, which is due to a mutation in the *APC* gene on chromosome 5, are predisposed to periampullary cancer, which is one of the most common causes of death in patients who have had their colon removed. Other duodenal malignancies include GISTs (see ***Gastrointestinal stromal tumours***) and neuroendocrine tumours.

Summary box 67.7

Duodenal tumours

- Duodenal villous adenomas are commonly found around the ampulla of Vater and are premalignant
- The duodenum is the most common site for adenocarcinoma of the small intestine
- Regular endoscopic screening is advisable in patients with FAP
- Pancreatic cancer is the most common cause of duodenal obstruction

Neuroendocrine tumours

A number of neuroendocrine neoplasms occur in the duodenum. It is a common site for primary gastrinoma (Zollinger–Ellison syndrome). Non-functioning neuroendocrine tumours (usually called carcinoid tumours) also occur but uncommonly in comparison with the ileum.

Zollinger-Ellison syndrome

This syndrome is mentioned here because the gastrin-producing endocrine tumour is often found in the duodenal loop, although it also occurs in the pancreas, especially the head. It is a cause of persistent peptic ulceration. Before the development of potent gastric antisecretory agents, the condition was recognised by sometimes fulminant peptic ulceration that did not respond to gastric surgery short of total gastrectomy. The advent of PPIs such as omeprazole has rendered this extreme endocrine condition fully controllable, but also less easily recognised.

Gastrinomas may be either sporadic or associated with the autosomal dominantly inherited multiple endocrine neoplasia (MEN) type I (in which a parathyroid adenoma is almost invariable). The tumours are most commonly found in the 'gastrinoma triangle', which is defined by the junction of the cystic duct and common bile duct superiorly, the junction of the second and third parts of the duodenum inferiorly and the junction of the neck and body of the pancreas medially (essentially the superior mesenteric artery). Many are found in the duodenal loop, presumably arising in the G cells found in Brunner's glands. It is extremely important that the duodenal wall is carefully inspected endoscopically and at operation.

Abraham Vater, 1684–1751, Professor of Anatomy and Biology, Wittenberg, Germany.
Allen Oldfather Whipple, 1881–1963, surgeon, Columbia-Presbyterian Medical Center, New York, NY, USA.

Very often all that can be detected is a small nodule that projects into the medial wall of the duodenum.

Even malignant sporadic gastrinomas may have a very indolent course. The palliative resection of liver metastases may be beneficial and, as for other gut endocrine tumours, liver transplantation is practised in some centres with reasonable long-term results. However, a minority of tumours found to the left of the superior mesenteric artery (outside the 'triangle') seem to have a worse prognosis, with more having liver metastases at presentation. In MEN type I, the tumours may be multiple and the condition is incurable. Even in this situation, surgical treatment should be employed to remove any obvious tumours and associated lymphatic metastases, as good palliation may be achieved (see *Chapter 57*).

DUODENAL OBSTRUCTION

Duodenal obstruction in adults is usually due to malignancy, and cancer of the pancreas is the most common cause. Treatment is usually by gastroenterostomy, but duodenal stenting is increasingly being used. In patients having a surgical biliary bypass for pancreatic cancer, gastric drainage may be necessary.

A variety of other malignancies can cause duodenal obstruction, including metastases from colorectal and gastric cancer. Primary duodenal cancer is much less common as a cause of obstruction than these other malignancies.

Annular pancreas may rarely cause duodenal obstruction. Obstruction usually follows an attack of pancreatitis, and, on occasions, the obstruction may be mistaken for malignancy.

Arteriomesenteric compression is an ill-defined condition in which it is proposed that the fourth part of the duodenum is compressed between the superior mesenteric artery and the vertebral column; when it is convincingly demonstrated and causing weight loss, duodenojejunostomy may be performed.

OTHER GASTRIC CONDITIONS

Acute gastric dilatation

This condition usually occurs in association with pyloroduodenal disorders or following abdominal surgery. The stomach dilates enormously. The patient may be dehydrated and have electrolyte disturbances. Failure to treat can result in a sudden vomit with aspiration into the lungs. Treatment is nasogastric suction with a large-bore tube, fluid replacement and treatment of the underlying condition.

Trichobezoar and phytobezoar

Trichobezoar (hair balls) (*Figure 67.34*) are unusual and are virtually exclusively found in young psychiatric patients. It is caused by the ingestion of hair, which remains undigested in the stomach. The hair ball can lead to ulceration and gastrointestinal bleeding, perforation or obstruction. The diagnosis is made easily at endoscopy. Treatment consists of removal of the bezoar, which may require open surgical treatment. Phytobezoars are made of vegetable matter and are found principally in patients who have gastric stasis, usually following gastric surgery.

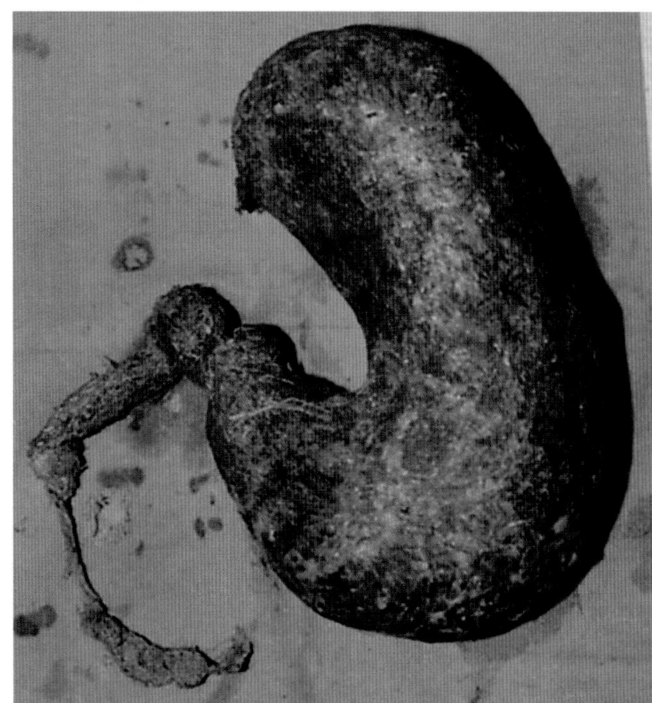

Figure 67.34 Trichobezoar of the stomach in a girl aged 15 years.

Foreign bodies in the stomach

A variety of ingested foreign bodies reach the stomach, and very often these can be seen on a plain radiograph. If possible, they should be removed endoscopically but, if not, most can be left to pass normally. Even objects such as needles, with which there is understandable anxiety, will seldom cause harm. In general, an object that leaves the stomach will pass spontaneously. In contrast, attempted removal at laparotomy can be very difficult as the object may be much more difficult to find than might be expected. Most adults who swallow foreign bodies have psychiatric problems and may appear to relish the attention associated with serial laparotomies. The treatment should therefore be expectant, and intervention reserved for patients with symptoms in whom the foreign body is failing to progress.

Volvulus of the stomach

Rotation of the stomach usually occurs around the axis and between its two fixed points, i.e. the cardia and the pylorus. In theory, rotation can occur in the horizontal (organoaxial) or vertical (mesenteroaxial) direction, but the former is more common. Volvulus is usually associated with a large diaphragmatic defect around the oesophagus (paraoesophageal herniation) (*Figure 67.35*). Commonly the transverse colon moves upwards to lie under the left diaphragm, taking the stomach with it. The stomach and colon may both enter the chest through the eventration of the diaphragm. The condition is commonly chronic, the patient presenting with difficulty in eating. An acute presentation with ischaemia may occur. Endoscopically, it can be extremely difficult to identify the anatomy, and this is one situation in which the contrast radiograph is superior.

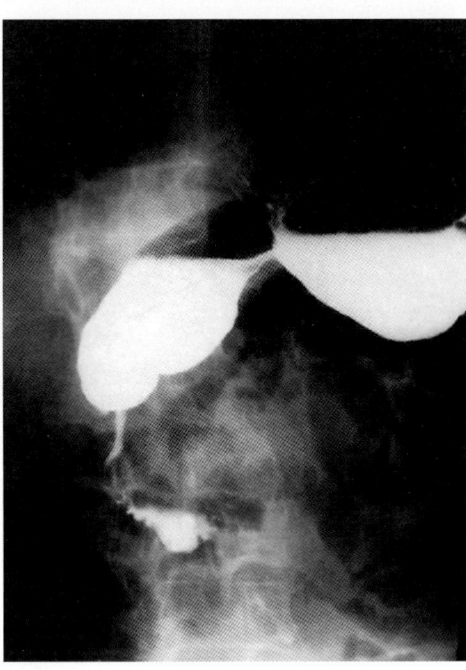

Figure 67.35 Barium meal showing organoaxial volvulus of the stomach associated with eventration of the diaphragm.

Treatment

If symptomatic, surgical treatment is required increasingly by a laparoscopic approach. If there is a hernia, the sac and its contents (usually the stomach) should be reduced. The defect in the diaphragm should be closed, if necessary, with a mesh. It is advisable to separate the stomach from the transverse colon and to perform an anterior gastropexy to fix the stomach to the anterior abdominal wall.

FURTHER READING

Al-Batran S-E, Homann N, Schmalenberg H *et al.* Perioperative chemotherapy with docetaxel, oxaliplatin, and fluorouracil/leucovorin (FLOT) versus epirubicin, cisplatin, and fluorouracil or capecitabine (ECF/ECX) for resectable gastric or gastroesophageal junction (GEJ) adenocarcinoma (FLOT4-AIO): a multicenter, randomized phase 3 trial. *J Clin Oncol* 2017; **35**(15 suppl): 4004.

Cristescu R, Lee J, Nebozhyn M *et al.* Molecular analysis of gastric cancer identifies subtypes associated with distinct clinical outcomes. *Nat Med* 2015; **21**(5): 449–56.

Lee SS, Chung HY, Kwon OK, Yu W. Long-term quality of life after distal subtotal and total gastrectomy: symptom- and behaviour-oriented consequences. *Ann Surg* 2016; **263**(4): 738–44.

Smyth EC, Nilsson M, Grabsch HI *et al.* Gastric cancer. *Lancet* 2020; **396**(10251): 635–48.

Wilson MS, Blencowe NS, Boyle C *et al.*; AUGIS. A modified Delphi process to establish future research priorities in malignant oesophagogastric surgery. *Surgeon* 2020; **18**(6): 321–6.

CHAPTER 68 Bariatric and metabolic surgery

Learning objectives

To know and understand:

- How to treat obesity as a disease
- Rationale for surgery and the concept of metabolic surgery
- Eligibility and NICE guidelines
- Multidisciplinary assessment and multimodal treatment
- The common operations and how they work
- How to assess and treat perioperative complications
- Follow-up, nutritional supplements and biochemical monitoring

INTRODUCTION

Obesity is becoming the plague of the twenty-first century. With overweight becoming the norm in most Western countries and developing countries, two-thirds of adults suffer from overweight or obesity (***Table 68.1***). Every clinician and definitely every surgeon faces the condition and its associated diseases, such as type 2 diabetes, as part of their practice. According to the World Health Organization (WHO), overweight and obesity are defined as abnormal or excessive fat accumulation that may impair health. For adults, WHO defines overweight as a body mass index (BMI) of 25 kg/m^2 or more and obesity as a BMI of 30 kg/m^2 or more. Severe obesity increases the risk of cancer, is associated with multiple other diseases, affects quality of life and reduces life expectancy by 5–20 years. Severe and complex obesity is a phrase commonly used for patients with BMI ≥35 kg/m^2 and obesity-related disease, or BMI ≥40 kg/m^2 by itself (***Table 68.2***).

Overweight and obesity can be considered normal physiological responses to the current food environment. Few people with obesity have a single identifiable genetic or hormonal basis. *MC4R* deficiency represents the most common genetic form of severe obesity, with heterozygous mutations in *MC4R* detected in up to 5% of patients with severe, early-onset obesity. Surgeons encounter the challenge of obesity on a daily basis as it affects the treatment of nearly every abdominal pathology in terms of approach and outcomes.

Obesity is a heterogeneous disease and the response of individuals seeking treatment to different therapeutic modalities is variable. Currently there are no available robust tools to predict this response. Therefore a trial of options is required. The principles of therapeutic interventions for all other diseases are applicable, including escalation of treatment, cessation of modalities that are not effective and addition of therapy when the response is insufficient or transient. Lifestyle modifications, supervised interventions, pharmacotherapy, bariatric surgery and bariatric surgery combined with pharmacotherapy are available interventions. It is important to stress that the response is a biological phenomenon and not a volitional one.

TABLE 68.1 Definitions of overweight and obesity.[a,b]

Adult weight status	BMI (kg/m^2)
Normal	18.5–24.9
Overweight	25.0–29.9
Class 1 obesity	30.0–34.9
Class 2 obesity	35.0–39.9
Class 3 obesity	≥40.0

Body mass index (BMI) = weight (kg)/height (m)^2
[a]Obesity for children is defined as BMI at or above the 95th centile.
[b]'Super-obesity' is a term commonly used to describe BMI ≥49.9 kg/m^2.

TABLE 68.2 Conditions that are associated with severe and complex obesity.

Condition
Type 2 diabetes
Hypertension
Dyslipidaemia
Obstructive sleep apnoea
Arthritis and functional impairment
Gastro-oesophageal reflux disease
Non-alcoholic fatty liver disease/non-alcoholic steatohepatosis
Polycystic ovary syndrome
Clinical depression
Various cancers, in particular endometrial cancer

Bariatric surgery comes from the Greek 'baros' (meaning weight/pressure) and 'iatric' (the medicine or surgery thereof).

Bariatric surgery is the branch of surgery involving manipulation of the stomach and/or small bowel to achieve weight loss and control of obesity-related disease.

RATIONALE

Bariatric surgery leads to weight loss of 25–35% of body weight (usually at least 15 kg) after 1 year, and sustained weight loss maintenance at 15–25% after 20 years. Additional benefits are that most or all of the obesity-related diseases improve as weight is lost and even independently of weight loss. Quality of life improves. A number of randomised controlled trials (RCTs) have reported on the outcomes of bariatric surgery versus intensive lifestyle interventions, and all favour surgery. The longest follow-up in an RCT is 5 years. However, the non-randomised Swedish Obese Subjects (SOS) study has now shown sustained weight loss and improvement in obesity-related disease up to 20 years after surgery. In this study 2010 patients who chose to have surgery were compared with 2037 controls who did not.

When the SOS study was conceived in 1987 all surgery was done by laparotomy and it was considered unethical to attempt to randomise patients between best medical therapy and bariatric surgery. All had best medical care throughout and follow-up was better than 99%. The SOS study was among the first to demonstrate that bariatric surgery also leads to survival benefit. The primary end point was overall mortality and a significant difference was found at a mean follow-up of 10 years. Many other studies have now found similarly, including one of nearly 8000 operated patients from Utah.

The Utah study was the first large study to show improved survival after gastric bypass surgery compared with matched population controls. The SOS study also reported a lower incidence of both microvascular and macrovascular complications at 15 years of follow-up in the surgical group. The Swedish registry (SOREG) data indicate lower mortality within only 3–4 years after surgery in patients with type 2 diabetes. Both the SOS and Utah studies have shown that bariatric surgery also effectively reduces cancer risk in large patient cohorts.

Rationale for surgery

Owing to the tendency for basal metabolic rate to decrease with dietary calorie restriction most people will regain all their weight, returning to the previous homeostatic set point. Bariatric surgery appears to alter this mechanism and 'reset' this point, with 15–25% weight loss maintenance for up to 20 years. Despite the fact that bariatric surgery leads to long-term survival benefit and improves obesity-related disease and quality of life, it is available to only a fraction of the individuals who could potentially benefit. This is largely because of inequalities in healthcare prioritisation, misconceptions and obesity stigma. Person-first language should always be used ('patient with obesity' or 'patient with diabetes') to avoid categorising patients as the disease, to reduce stigma.

Summary box 68.1

Rationale for surgery

- Because of the tendency for basal metabolic rate to decrease with dieting, most people will regain all their weight, returning to the previous homeostatic set point
- Bariatric surgery appears to alter this mechanism and 'reset' this point, with 15–25% weight loss maintenance for up to 20 years
- Bariatric surgery leads to long-term survival benefit and improves obesity-related disease and quality of life

METABOLIC SURGERY

The phrases 'metabolic' or 'diabetes' surgery are increasingly being used in conjunction with, or instead of, 'bariatric surgery' owing to the highly effective way that surgery improves the metabolic syndrome, with weight loss being a welcome additional effect. Type 2 diabetes is part of the 'metabolic syndrome', which includes high blood pressure, dyslipidaemia and polycystic ovary syndrome.

Control of type 2 diabetes improves with weight loss owing to an improvement in insulin resistance. Remarkably, diabetes control appears to improve after several types of bariatric surgery *before* meaningful weight loss occurs. Some of the effects on glucose metabolism can be attributed to caloric restriction, but changes in gut hormones levels, particularly glucagon-like-peptide 1 (GLP-1), have provoked much interest. GLP-1 is an incretin, a gut hormone that stimulates the beta cells in the pancreas to restore the normal first-phase insulin response after eating. Bile acids are also involved in this.

Although type 2 diabetes is a chronic disease and bariatric surgeons in the early 2000s initially claimed to 'cure' it, the emphasis has now changed to improving glycaemic control by lowering glycated haemoglobin (HbA1c) and improving insulin resistance, with the ultimate goal of reducing cardiovascular risk and improving survival. The term diabetes 'remission' is now commonly used by bariatric surgeons and endocrinologists, and is defined as patients being off all medication with normal glucose homeostasis. In the SOS study, patients with diabetes went into remission after surgery, and in patients without diabetes there was a decreased incidence of patients developing diabetes.

Summary box 68.2

Metabolic surgery

- The term **metabolic surgery** refers to the marked effects of surgery on diabetes and the metabolic syndrome, which may have a more important impact than weight loss itself
- Improvement in type 2 diabetes may be additional to weight loss
- Surgery is very cost-effective

COST-EFFECTIVENESS

A 2009 Health Technology Assessment report in the UK showed bariatric surgery to be cost-effective compared with non-surgical options. The incremental cost-effectiveness ratio (ICER) compared with no surgery was between £2000 and

£4000 per quality-adjusted life year (QALY) gained for patients with BMI ≥40 kg/m^2 over 20 years. For patients with BMI between 30 and <40 kg/m^2 the ICER was £1367 per QALY gained. Regarding maximum willingness to pay, compared with non-surgical interventions, if a decision-maker is willing to pay £20 000 for an additional QALY, then the probability of surgery being cost-effective over a 20-year time horizon was reported as 100%. The ICERs are similar to the cost-effectiveness of stopping smoking and routine statin therapy for the primary prevention of cardiovascular disease. In practice it means that the cost of the operation is recouped within 1–2 years after surgery from reduced medication costs. All the cost-effectiveness studies assess direct or indirect healthcare costs but not the additional benefits of surgery. Thus, return to paid work, coming off state benefits, improved functional capacity and quality of life are 'add-ons' that incur no cost. A systematic review including studies up to 2018 confirmed that bariatric surgery is cost saving over a lifetime. Medication costs for obesity-related comorbidities are substantially reduced after bariatric surgery in the shorter term.

ELIGIBILITY

Eligibility criteria were first proposed by the US National Institutes of Health in 1991, when the obesity epidemic was first recognised. All bariatric surgery was done by open laparotomy, and the safety profile was very different. The National Institute for Health and Care Excellence (NICE) in the UK recommends consideration of bariatric surgery for people with severe obesity in whom all non-surgical measures have been tried with no adequate weight loss achieved or maintained. Commitment to long-term follow-up and behaviour change are also advised. After a review of recent RCTs, NICE updated its guidance and lowered the BMI threshold to 30 kg/m^2 for recent-onset type 2 diabetes (***Table 68.3***). The criteria according to the International Federation for the Surgery of Obesity and Metabolic Disorders (IFSO) Asia Pacific chapter for Asian patients include lower BMI thresholds because of the susceptibility of Asian populations to type 2 diabetes at a lower BMI.

TABLE 68.3 Summary of updates to National Institute for Health and Care Excellence (NICE) guidance on bariatric surgery, 2014 (CG189).

Bariatric surgery is a treatment option for anyone with BMI ≥40 kg/m^2
Offer an expedited assessment for people with BMI ≥35 kg/m^2 with onset of type 2 diabetes in past 10 years
Consider an assessment for people with BMI of 30–34.9 kg/m^2 with onset of type 2 diabetes within 10 years
Consider an assessment for people of Asian origin with onset of type 2 diabetes at a lower BMI than other populations
Bariatric surgery is the option of choice for adults with BMI >50 kg/m^2 when other interventions have not been effective
People fitting the above criteria are also required to be receiving or to receive assessment in a specialist weight management service before referral to a surgical team

BMI, body mass index.

TABLE 68.4 National Institute for Health and Care Excellence (NICE)-accredited guidance on the make-up of the medical and surgical bariatric multidisciplinary team.

Bariatric physician in primary (can be the general practitioner) or secondary care (usually a diabetologist)
Dietician
Specialist nurse
Appropriately trained mental health professional
Bariatric surgeon
Anaesthetist
Radiologist
± Exercise therapists
Other secondary care specialties, e.g. respiratory/sleep medicine, cardiology

NICE estimated that about 80% of people fulfilling the eligibility criteria would have no medical or psychological reason why they would not be fit for surgery. An estimate is that perhaps 10% of these might want it, if bariatric/metabolic surgery were to be promoted or recommended by physicians to patients.

PRINCIPLES OF SETTING UP A BARIATRIC/METABOLIC SURGERY SERVICE

As for gastrointestinal cancer surgery where a number of different specialists routinely work together, it is now agreed that 'bariatric physicians/internists', dieticians, mental health professionals and nurse practitioners should be part of the team assessing and managing long-term care after bariatric surgery (***Table 68.4***). The perioperative risk of surgery is low; however, outcomes can be improved further with appropriate multidisciplinary team (MDT) work-up. Using risk scores such as the Edmonton Obesity Staging System (EOSS) and the Obesity Surgery–Mortality Risk Score (OS-MRS) can help the team discuss with patients the likely prognosis without surgery, and the risk of complications. The OS-MRS scores one point for each of: age 45 or more; BMI 50 kg/m^2 or more; male gender (owing to central obesity); hypertension (owing to central obesity); and increased deep vein thrombosis (DVT)/pulmonary embolism (PE) risk. The more points that are present, the greater the risk. Swedish registry data indicate that obstructive sleep apnoea (OSA) is a risk factor for anastomotic leak. Therefore OSA should be actively investigated as treatment with continuous positive airway pressure might reduce risk. Poorly controlled diabetes must also be considered a risk factor, as it is for all other operations.

Better surgical results are likely in high-volume surgical units. IFSO and the American Society for Metabolic and Bariatric Surgery (ASMBS) recommended 100–125 cases per year, and there should be at least two surgeons each performing 50 or more cases. Surgeons early in the learning curve (about 100 for gastric bypass) need to be mentored before independent practice. Irrespective of the technical expertise of each surgeon, higher volumes usually mean that there are sufficient

MDT members available to provide support and follow-up. Each unit should have expertise in a variety of surgical procedures, including revisions.

It is routine to put patients on a 'liver shrinkage diet' for at least 2 weeks before surgery, especially when there is central obesity, as this is associated with a large liver that can make surgery impossible. Male patients, especially those with central obesity, a very dense/hard abdomen, OSA/diabetes and BMI >50 kg/m^2, may need more, supervised, mandatory weight loss to make surgery safe.

Although not stipulated in any national guidance, every successful bariatric unit depends on active patient support groups and preoperative education sessions, which are best run by bariatric nurses and dieticians. These are invaluable in preparing patients for surgery, and it is difficult to conceive how a programme can run without them. Also, the ward and outpatient environment must be suitably equipped for patients with severe obesity.

Summary box 68.3

Multidisciplinary assessment

- Every patient should be assessed and managed by a coherent and well-functioning team of healthcare professionals with varied backgrounds and expertise
- Improved outcomes are usually achieved in high-volume specialised units
- Data collection and submission to national registries are recommended to provide quality assurance and long-term outcomes

Laparoscopic surgery and enhanced recovery

Bariatric surgery has been transformed by its amenability to laparoscopic techniques, including intracorporeal suturing and modern laparoscopic stapling devices. Probably equally important is the adoption of enhanced recovery after surgery (ERAS) protocols, with preoperative education, avoidance of catheters, central venous and arterial lines and early mobilisation. Free access to fluids is routine immediately after surgery and, because of the relative lack of pain, patients can mobilise straightaway. It is usual for gastric bypass and sleeve gastrectomy patients to go home on postoperative day 2 or 3. Gastric banding patients can be treated as day cases or can go home within 24 hours. The main cause of death after surgery is DVT/PE rather than anastomotic leakage or bleeding; appropriate prophylaxis is usually used for at least a week.

Randomised controlled trial evidence for the different types of surgery

Some evidence suggests that weight loss is more with a Roux-en-Y gastric bypass than sleeve gastrectomy. However, bariatric surgery needs more RCTs comparing different procedures with long-term follow-up. One of the challenges is keeping the research question relevant given the rapidity with which surgeons adopt different techniques. Long-term, large-scale, pragmatic RCTs with good follow-up are needed to inform practice. The By-Band-Sleeve study is an ongoing pragmatic, multicentre, three-arm RCT in the UK assessing weight loss and quality of life at 3 years between gastric bypass, gastric banding and sleeve gastrectomy in 1341 patients; it is expected to report in 2023.

Summary box 68.4

Evidence for the different operations

- Usually the operation choice is guided by patient, surgeon and unit preference
- Well-conducted RCTs comparing the different operations, with comprehensive follow-up, are needed
- Bariatric surgeons and bariatric surgical units should be recording their outcomes, ideally in a registry

The common operations

According to the IFSO Global Registry, in 2018 sleeve gastrectomy constituted 46%, gastric bypass 38%, one-anastomosis gastric bypass procedures 7.6% and gastric banding 5% of procedures. Other procedures include the biliopancreatic diversion (BPD) procedure and its duodenal switch variant (BPD/DS). The variety of procedures usually reflects surgeons' expertise and surgeons' and patients' preferences, as there are no RCTs beyond 5 years comparing different operations. Sleeve gastrectomy is now the most common operation and has gained rapid popularity at the expense of gastric banding and to a lesser extent gastric bypass. Some clinical outcomes are shown (***Table 68.5***). The mechanism of action of most weight-loss procedures remains incompletely understood.

TABLE 68.5 Malabsorption, per cent excess weight loss (% EWL)[a] and diabetes remission after bariatric surgery.

	Protein/ calorie malabsorption	3-year % EWL	3-year % diabetes remission
Sleeve gastrectomy	No	50–60%	50%
Gastric bypass	No	50–60%	50%
OAGB	Yes	60–80%	80%
Gastric band	No	40–50%	20%
BPD/DS, SADI-S	Yes	70–80%	80%

BPD, biliopancreatic diversion; DS, duodenal switch; OAGB, one-anastomosis gastric bypass; SADI-S, single-anastomosis duodenoileal bypass with sleeve gastrectomy.

[a] %EWL refers to the excess weight lost above a notional upper normal body mass index of 25 kg/m^2. Per cent weight loss is another way of measuring weight change, preferred by physicians.

César Roux, 1857–1934, surgeon, Lausanne, Switzerland.

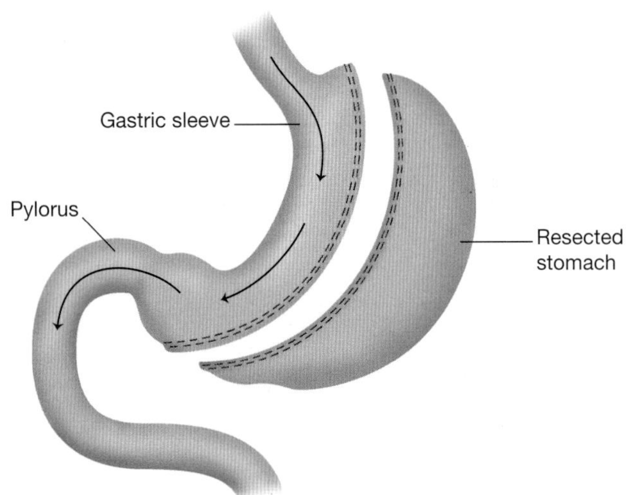

Figure 68.1 Sleeve gastrectomy. (Adapted from Griffin SM, Raimes SA, Shenfine J. *Oesophagogastric surgery*, 5th edn. London: Saunders Elsevier, 2013.)

Reduced appetite and early satiety are common features that are potentially explained by changes in levels of gut hormones such as peptide YY (PYY) and GLP-1 and how these interact with the brain.

Sleeve gastrectomy

Sleeve gastrectomy (***Figure 68.1***) is less challenging to perform than gastric bypass. It evolved from the magenstrasse and mill operation, in which the divided fundus (the 'mill') was left in continuity with the lesser curve-based tube (the 'main street'). Initially, it was done as the first step of a duodenal switch operation; however, it was found to be effective on its own without the switch (see ***Biliopancreatic diversion/duodenal switch***).

The lesser curve-based gastric tube is constructed over a size 32–36Fr bougie, although some surgeons advocate use of larger sizes to reduce the risk of staple line leakage. Linear stapling devices are used. There is variation in the techniques employed between how wide the staplers should be and whether reinforcement strips should be used. The Achilles heel of the sleeve is the risk of a staple line leak at the angle of His, which can take months to heal owing to the high-pressure system in the stomach with an intact pylorus. Another concern in the long term is symptomatic reflux and *de novo* Barrett's oesophagus (see ***Chapter 66***). A proportion of patients will need revisional surgery in future for weight regain.

The mechanism of action is still being investigated. The initial belief that sleeve gastrectomy acts as a restrictive procedure has been challenged by studies which that show gastric emptying is accelerated rather than delayed after sleeve gastrectomy. A change in satiety gut hormones and bile salt metabolism, similar to those described after gastric bypass, may explain some of the phenomena observed.

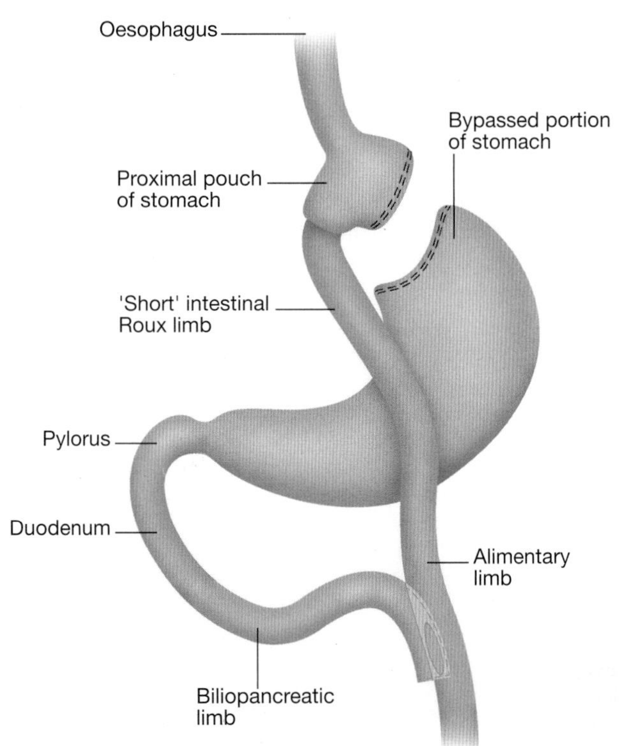

Figure 68.2 Gastric bypass showing a short vertical lesser curve-based gastric pouch with a Roux-en-Y jejunojejunostomy reconstruction. (Adapted from Griffin SM, Raimes SA, Shenfine J. *Oesophagogastric surgery*, 5th edn. London: Saunders Elsevier, 2013.)

Roux-en-Y gastric bypass

Despite the variety in laparoscopic techniques described and the lack of standardisation, most agree that Roux-en-Y gastric bypass (***Figure 68.2***) should include a short vertical lesser curvature-based gastric pouch. The techniques available for construction of the pouch-jejunostomy are linear stapler with suture closure of the defect, circular stapler and entirely hand sewn. It is routine to perform a leak test. The Roux limb can be retro- or antecolic. There is no standard length of the biliary and Roux limbs; however, the biliary limb is usually kept short to reduce vitamin and mineral deficiencies and the Roux limb length is varied between 100 and 150 cm. There are no consistent data regarding the effect of different limb lengths on weight loss. Bowel continuity is restored by a 'Y' jejunojejunostomy, which is either stapled with suture closure of the defect or stapled in its entirety.

It is now recognised that the mechanism of action is complex. Patients lose weight, at least in part, because they eat less owing to a change in appetite, which is facilitated by a change in satiety gut hormones. Other mechanisms such as changes in energy expenditure and change in food preferences may also play a role.

Wilhelm His, 1831–1904, Professor of Anatomy, Leipzig, Germany.
Norman Rupert Barrett, 1903–1979, surgeon, St Thomas' Hospital, London, UK.

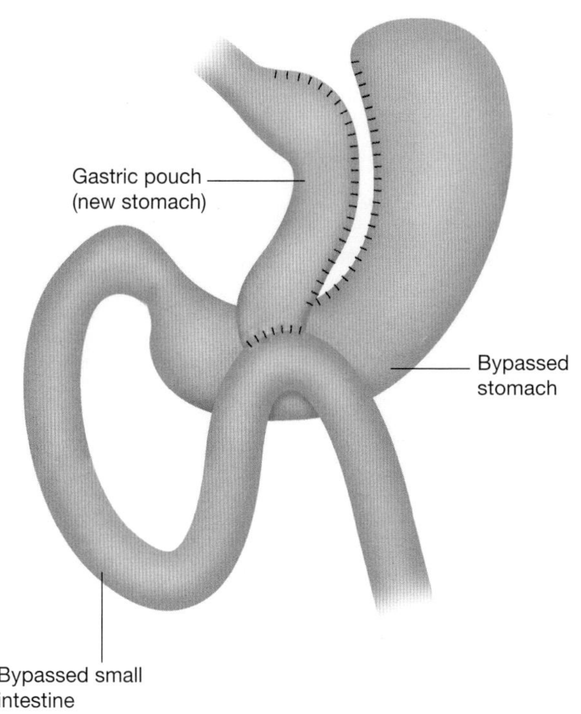

Figure 68.3 Gastric bypass showing a longer vertical lesser curve-based gastric pouch with gastrojejunostomy reconstruction (one-anastomosis gastric bypass).

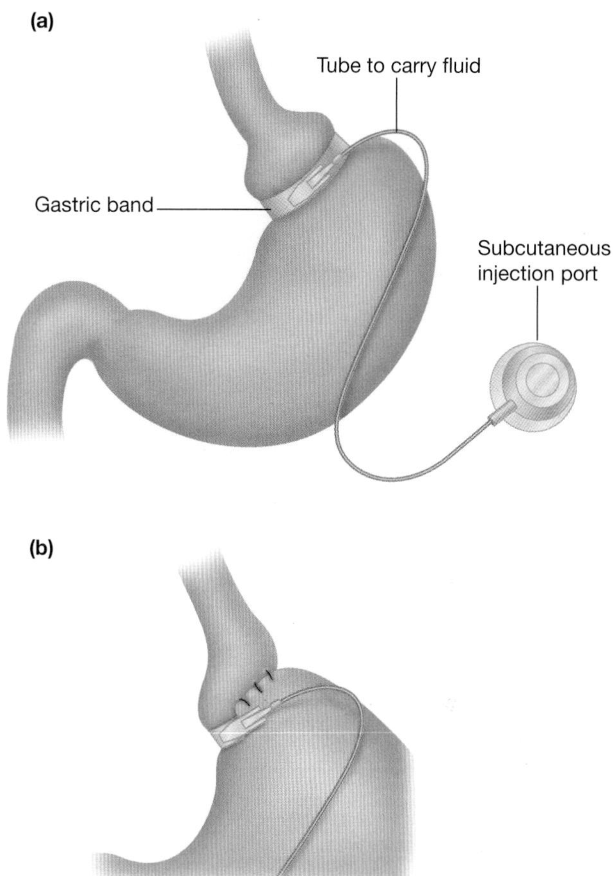

Figure 68.4 Adjustable gastric band. Gastric band surgery showing (a) a small 'virtual' pouch of stomach below the gastro-oesophageal junction and (b) gastrogastric tunnelling sutures. (Adapted from Griffin SM, Raimes SA, Shenfine J. *Oesophagogastric surgery*, 5th edn. London: Saunders Elsevier, 2013.)

One-anastomosis gastric bypass

One-anastomosis gastric bypass (OAGB) (***Figure 68.3***), previously known as a mini-gastric bypass, was first described by Rutledge. The objective was to develop a technique that is technically less demanding with only one anastomosis (antecolic loop gastrojejunostomy without a Roux-en-Y configuration) and a longer gastric pouch than for standard gastric bypass. Similar weight loss outcomes have been reported but there is concern regarding symptomatic biliary reflux causing gastritis or oesophagitis, marginal ulcers and the management of anastomotic leaks owing to a potentially high volume of biliary and pancreatic secretions. With the Roux-en-Y historically being the standard in surgery of the stomach for ulcer disease and cancer, there is further concern owing to possibly increased risk of Barrett's oesophagus and gastric or oesophageal cancer associated with biliary reflux. These outcomes will need long-term investigation.

Gastric banding

Although use of adjustable gastric banding (***Figure 68.4***) is declining, it did boost the popularity of bariatric surgery because of perioperative safety, lack of nutritional complications and relative ease and availability. The pars flaccida technique (through the window of the lesser omentum) is now standard practice with a band placed just below the oesophagogastric junction, making a small 'virtual' gastric pouch. The band is sutured into place anteriorly with gastrogastric tunnelling sutures to reduce slippage. The access port is routinely sutured to the rectus sheath in the upper abdomen for ease of access by a non-coring, Huber needle for band adjustments.

The operation appears to work by reducing hunger, probably vagally mediated. The initial surgical placement is only the beginning of the treatment. Specialist nurses, physicians and surgeons do 'band consultations' to assess eating habits and then perform an adjustment with injection or aspiration of saline if indicated. The objective is to reach the so-called 'sweet spot' of optimal appetite control. Follow-up should be monthly to begin with as needed during the first year, with full MDT support to help patients get the best use out of their bands. Lack of appropriate follow-up is why results in the literature vary so much, with a consequent high band removal rate.

Biliopancreatic diversion/duodenal switch

BPD, described by Scopinaro, produces greater weight loss than other procedures but is associated with a higher

Robert Rutledge, contemporary, surgeon, Las Vegas, NV, USA.
Nicola Scopinaro, 1945–2020, Professor of Surgery, Genoa, Italy.

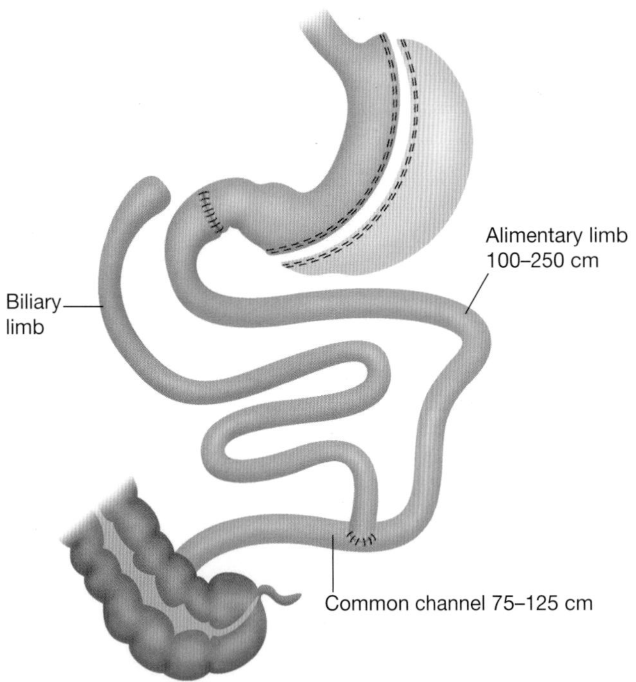

Figure 68.5 Biliopancreatic diversion with duodenal switch variant (BPD/DS).

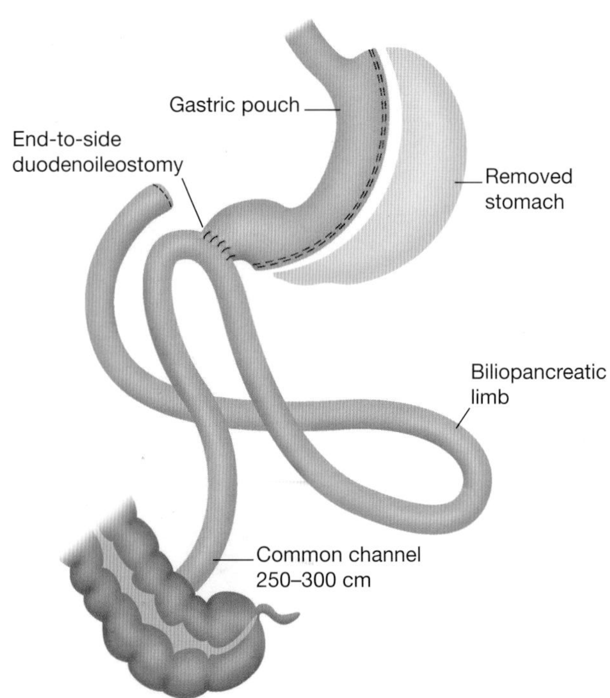

Figure 68.6 Single-anastomosis duodenoileal bypass with sleeve gastrectomy (SADI-S).

nutritional complication rate. The mechanism of action appears to be mainly malabsorption of calories. BPD/DS is the version mainly performed (***Figure 68.5***). A sleeve gastrectomy is followed by division of the duodenum just distally to the pylorus. The ileum is divided with a linear stapler, followed by a duodenoileostomy and ileoileostomy with the objective of creating a common channel of 75–125 cm and an alimentary channel of 100–250 cm. The long remaining biliary limb is not measured.

BPD/DS is increasingly seen as a definitive procedure, particularly after significant weight regain following sleeve gastrectomy. A high-protein diet and regular vitamin and mineral supplements with lifelong monitoring and patient commitment, to avoid malnutrition, is essential postoperatively. Only a few centres offer these procedures.

Single-anastomosis duodenoileal bypass with sleeve gastrectomy

Single-anastomosis duodenoileal bypass with sleeve gastrectomy (SADI-S) is a novel procedure based on the BPD/DS. A sleeve gastrectomy is followed by an end-to-side duodenoileal anastomosis (***Figure 68.6***). The length of the common channel–alimentary limb is 250–300 cm. Potential advantages include the preservation of the pylorus, elimination of one anastomosis compared with the duodenal switch and reducing operating time and risk of perioperative complications.

Complications

The common complications are shown in ***Table 68.6***. In sleeve gastrectomy, a staple line leak at the angle of His usually presents any time *after* discharge up to 30 days, and patients can also deteriorate rapidly with sepsis. Urgent computed tomography (CT) scanning and relaparoscopy is indicated, with source control by drainage the major goal. Patients are typically in hospital for months and need multiple reinterventions, including any of: endoscopic interventions (stenting, endoscopic vacuum therapy), making a controlled fistula, conversion to gastric bypass and fistula enterostomy. Long-term nutritional support is needed as patients are severely catabolic after complications from both bypass and sleeve surgery.

Anastomotic leakage, bleeding and closed loop obstruction after Roux-en-Y or one-anastomosis gastric bypass can be life-threatening. If a bypass patient is not well after 24 hours urgent consideration should be given to oral contrast X-ray swallow or CT scanning and/or relaparoscopy. Other than a feeling of 'impending doom' patients may have few overt features of sepsis and abdominal examination can be very misleading. Deterioration after an anastomotic leak can be very rapid and there is no time for delay.

Very few patients with gastric bands develop early intra-abdominal complications. Unfortunately a large number of patients have their bands removed later on if there is inadequate follow-up, a late complication or the patient is unable to tolerate the device.

The incidence of late complications is difficult to estimate as so many patients are lost to follow-up. Internal hernias develop as weight is lost and hernia spaces open up after gastric bypass. CT scanning has a high rate of false negatives for internal hernia, so anyone presenting with severe, cramping abdominal pain 2–3 years after surgery needs to be

TABLE 68.6 Estimated early surgical complication rates, operative mortality after sleeve gastrectomy, Roux-en-Y or one-anastomosis gastric bypass, and gastric banding, and late complications.

	Early	Mortality	Late
Sleeve gastrectomy	Leak at angle of His (1–2%)	0.1%	Gastro-oesophageal reflux
	Intra-abdominal bleed (2–3%)		Barrett's oesophagus
	DVT/PE (<1%)		Weight regain
Gastric bypass	Anastomotic leak (<1%)	0.1%	Internal hernia
	Intra-abdominal bleed (2–3%)		Chronic abdominal pain
	Unspecified obstruction (1–2%)		Malnutrition if long limb bypass
	DVT/PE (<1%)		Anastomotic ulcer/stricture
			Weight regain
Gastric band	Access port infection (1%)	0.05–0.1%	Band infection
	DVT/PE (<0.1%)		Tubing leak
			Slippage
			Erosion into stomach
			Band intolerance
			Failure to lose weight/weight regain

high priority for investigation by laparoscopy. Closure of the internal hernia spaces is now standard of care in Roux-en-Y gastric bypass.

Summary box 68.5

Acute complications

- Anastomotic leak and staple line dehiscence can be rapidly fatal and require emergency laparoscopy
- Internal hernias developing after surgery are very difficult to diagnose other than by prompt laparoscopy; they require a high index of suspicion

Outcomes reported

There is wide variation in how surgeons report the results of surgery, which means that it is often difficult to compare studies. There is a need to standardise clinician-reported outcomes and patient-reported outcome measures (PROMs) into an agreed core outcome set that includes risk stratification. Obvious PROMs include quality of life.

Follow-up and a shared care model of chronic disease

Shared care arrangements with surgeons/physicians and primary care need to be in place so that diabetes and hypertension medications and dosage can be appropriately reduced as weight is lost. Every patient with diabetes needs at least an annual review.

Although sleeve gastrectomy, short-limb forms of gastric bypass and gastric banding do not cause protein-calorie malabsorption, bariatric surgery can cause severe vitamin and mineral deficiencies, amplifying pre-existing deficiencies caused by obesity. All patients should have lifelong routine metabolic and nutritional monitoring (***Table 68.7***). Patients need regular multivitamins/trace element supplements (***Table 68.8***). The minimum frequency of assessment is 3–6 monthly in the first postoperative year, 6–12 monthly in the second year and at least annually thereafter. Folic acid supplementation should be considered in all sexually active women of childbearing age because of the risk of neural tube defects. This is especially important as fertility often improves after surgery. The MDT also needs to support the small number of patients who develop severe mental health issues after surgery as there is a slightly increased risk of suicide after gastric bypass.

TABLE 68.7 Summary of British Obesity and Metabolic Surgery Society (BOMSS) biochemical guidance after bariatric surgery.

Blood tests all patients should have at baseline
Full blood count, including haemoglobin, ferritin, folate and vitamin B12 levels, urea and electrolytes, liver function tests, vitamin D, Ca^{2+}, parathormone, HbA1c, lipid profile
Postoperatively
After gastric banding: Annual full blood count, urea and electrolytes, HbA1c, fasting glucose, lipids as appropriate *After sleeve gastrectomy, forms of gastric bypass, BPD/DS, SADI-S:* As for banding + liver function tests, ferritin, folate, vitamin D, Ca^{2+}, parathormone at 3, 6, 12 months then annually; vitamin B12 at 6, 12 months then annually; zinc, copper annually; vitamins A, E, K, selenium if concern (e.g. steatorrhoea, night blindness, unexplained fatigue, anaemia, metabolic bone disease, chronic diarrhoea, heart failure)

BPD, biliopancreatic diversion; DS, duodenal switch; HbA1c, glycated haemoglobin; SADI-S, single-anastomosis duodenoileal bypass with sleeve gastrectomy.

TABLE 68.8 Summary of British Obesity and Metabolic Surgery Society (BOMSS) nutritional and micronutrient guidance after bariatric surgery.

After gastric banding
Multivitamin and mineral supplement, thiamine if vomiting, vitamin D, iron
After sleeve gastrectomy, forms of gastric bypass, BPD/DS, SADI-S
As for banding + selenium, copper, zinc, folic acid, vitamins B12, A, E, K BPD/DS, SADI-S may require higher doses

BPD, biliopancreatic diversion; DS, duodenal switch; SADI-S, single-anastomosis duodenoileal bypass with sleeve gastrectomy.

Summary box 68.6

Shared care model of chronic disease

- Close collaboration between surgeons, physicians and primary care doctors is needed to enable seamless follow-up before and after surgery with a focus on the long-term care of patients
- Patients should be committed to lifelong vitamin and micronutrient monitoring and replacement

FUTURE CHALLENGES

Patients with obesity suffer from widespread prejudice. Understanding that the obesity epidemic currently experienced in different parts of the world is driven by a change in the environment towards becoming 'obesogenic' and not a lack of willpower would be the first step in removing the barriers to more surgery.

All surgeons should contribute their results to national registries so that safety can be monitored and operation trends established. Ideally registries should also link to other national healthcare records, e.g. diabetes databases, so that long-term outcomes data can be collected outside of funded RCTs.

FURTHER READING

Adams TD, Gress RE, Smith SC *et. al.* Long-term mortality after gastric bypass surgery. *N Engl J Med* 2007; **357**: 753–61.

Mingrone G, Panunzi S, De Gaetano A *et al.* Bariatric–metabolic surgery versus conventional medical treatment in obese patients with type 2 diabetes: 5 year follow-up of an open-label, single-centre, randomised controlled trial. *Lancet* 2015; **386**: 964–73.

National Institute for Health and Care Excellence. *Obesity: identification, assessment and management.* NICE Clinical Guideline 189. London: NICE, 2014. Available from https://www.nice.org.uk/guidance/cg189.

O'Kane M, Parretti HM, Pinkney J *et al.* British Obesity and Metabolic Surgery Society Guidelines on perioperative and postoperative biochemical monitoring and micronutrient replacement for patients undergoing bariatric surgery: 2020 update. *Obes Rev* 2020; **21**: e13087.

Sjöström L. Review of the key results from the Swedish Obese Subjects (SOS) trial – a prospective controlled intervention study of bariatric surgery. *J Int Med* 2013; **273**: 219–34.

Welbourn R, Dixon J, Barth JH *et al.* NICE-accredited commissioning guidance for weight assessment and management clinics: a model for a specialist multidisciplinary team approach for people with severe obesity. *Obes Surg* 2016; **26**: 649–59.

Welbourn R, le Roux CW, Owen-Smith A *et al.* Why the NHS should be doing more bariatric surgery; how much should we do? *BMJ* 2016; **353**: i1472.

Welbourn R, Pournaras DJ, Dixon J *et al.* Bariatric surgery worldwide: baseline demographic description and one-year outcomes from the second IFSO Global Registry Report 2013–2015. *Obes Surg* 2018; **28**: 313–22.

CHAPTER 69 The liver

Learning objectives

To understand:

- The anatomy of the liver
- The signs of acute and chronic liver disease
- The investigation of liver disease
- The management of liver trauma
- The management of liver infections
- The management of benign and cystic liver lesions
- The management of intrahepatic cholangiocarcinoma
- The management of hepatocellular carcinoma
- The management of colorectal liver metastases

INTRODUCTION

The liver is a highly complex organ found only in vertebrates that is responsible for over 500 individual functions. It is located in the right upper quadrant, protected by the ribs, and weighs on average 1.5 kg (970–1860 g). It is wedge shaped in both the coronal and axial planes and is divided by the middle hepatic vein into two lobes, with the larger right lobe generally representing 60% by volume. The parenchyma is covered by a thin capsule (Glisson's capsule) and visceral peritoneum apart from the posterior surface, the 'bare area'. Surgery for hepatic disease evolved slowly because of the complexity of hepatic function and anatomy. Remarkable progress has been made since the first formal resection in 1952 with the advent of cross-sectional imaging, liver transection technology and low central venous pressure anaesthesia. Progress continues with the incorporation of laparoscopic and robotic surgery and training techniques, including virtual reality.

ANATOMY OF THE LIVER

Embryology

Liver development begins at 3–4 weeks' gestation when a hepatic foregut diverticulum buds into the ventral wall of the primitive midgut. This diverticulum is the anlage for the liver, extrahepatic biliary ducts, gallbladder and ventral pancreas, which develop over the next week. The basement membrane surrounding the liver bud is then lost and cords of bipotential hepatoblasts invade the septum transversum and differentiate into hepatocytes and cholangiocytes.

Ligaments and peritoneal reflections

The liver is covered by visceral peritoneum (serosa), with a layer of connective tissue, the Glisson capsule, underneath. At the porta hepatis, the capsule envelops and travels along the portal tracts (triads) into the liver, carrying branches of the hepatic artery, portal vein and bile ducts. The liver is fixed in the right upper quadrant by the hepatic veins and ligaments formed from the peritoneal reflections. Division of the left triangular ligament on the superior surface of the left lobe mobilises the liver from the diaphragm, exposing the left lateral wall of the inferior vena cava (IVC). The right triangular ligament similarly fixes the right lobe to the undersurface of the right hemidiaphragm, and division mobilises the liver sufficiently to allow it to be rotated to the left. Another major supporting structure is the falciform ligament (the remnant of the umbilical vein), which runs cephalad from the umbilicus, enters the liver at the interlobar fissure and passes anteriorly on the surface of the liver, attaching it to the anterior abdominal wall. Dividing the cephalad leaves of the falciform ligament exposes the suprahepatic IVC within a thin fibrous sheath. The final peritoneal reflection is the lesser omentum between the stomach and the liver, which contains the hilar structures in its right free edge.

The blood supply to the liver

The liver is composed of eight segments (***Figure 69.1***), each supplied by terminal branches of the portal vein (80% of the blood flow) and hepatic artery (20%) and drained by bile ducts and hepatic veins. The shape of the segments varies among individuals, but the configuration remains relatively constant.

Francis Glisson, 1597–1697, Regius Professor of Physic, Cambridge, UK, described the capsule of the liver and its blood supply in his book *Anatomia hepatis* (1654).

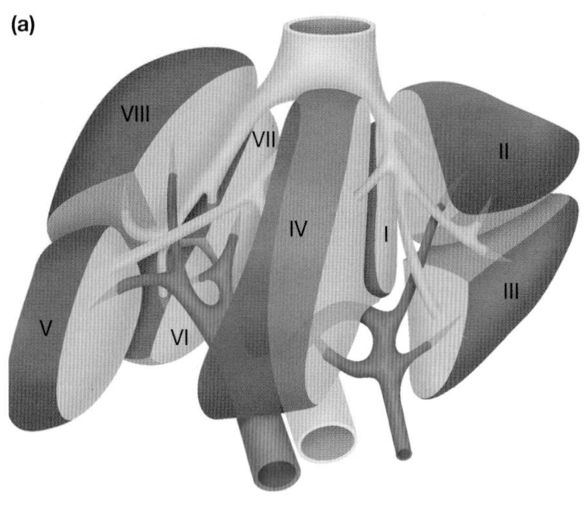

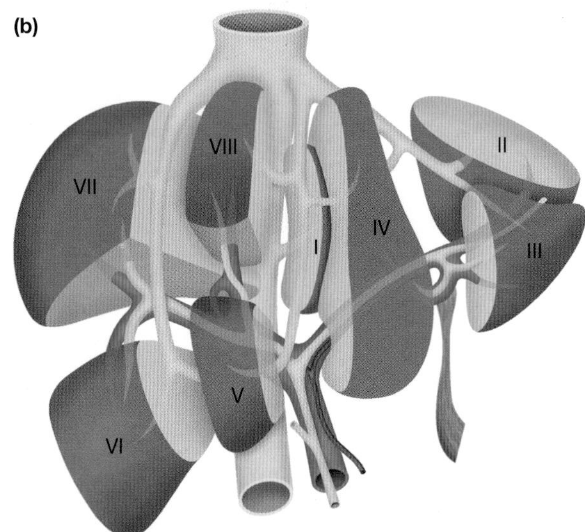

Figure 69.1 The functional division of the liver and of the liver segments according to Couinaud's nomenclature. (a) As seen in the patient. (b) In the *ex vivo* position.

The arterial blood supply is variable in origin and course but in most individuals is derived from the coeliac trunk, which usually divides into left gastric, common hepatic and splenic arteries.

After supplying the gastroduodenal artery, the hepatic artery branches at a variable level to produce the right and left hepatic arteries, the larger right branch supplying the right lobe. The right lobe may be partly or completely supplied by a right hepatic artery arising directly from the superior mesenteric artery running to the liver on the posterior wall of the bile duct after passing behind the uncinate process and head of the pancreas. Similarly, the left lobe artery may be augmented or replaced by a branch of the left gastric artery running in the lesser omentum from the lesser curve of the stomach.

The hilum of the liver

The porta hepatis is a pronounced transverse fissure on the visceral surface of the liver running between the cephalad end of the fissure for the ligamentum teres and the gallbladder fossa. The neurovascular structures and lymphatics running in the right free edge of the lesser omentum (the hepatoduodenal ligament) enter at this point and the right and left hepatic ducts emerge. There are numerous variations of the hilar structures which are important in the planning and performance of operations on the liver (***Figure 69.2***).

In the most common arrangement, the bile duct runs in the free edge of the hepatoduodenal ligament with the hepatic artery medially and the portal vein posteriorly, each dividing into two branches at the hilum. The right and left hepatic ducts arise from the hepatic parenchyma and form the common hepatic duct. The cystic duct draining the gallbladder enters the ligament at a variable level, joining the common hepatic duct to form the common bile duct (CBD). The right hepatic artery crosses the bile duct anteriorly or posteriorly before giving rise to the cystic artery, and multiple branches predominantly from the right hepatic artery supply the bile duct. The portal vein is formed by the confluence of the splenic and superior mesenteric veins behind the neck of the pancreas, with the left branch having a longer (approximately 2 cm) extrahepatic course. The portal vein often has two large branches to the right lobe, which are usually outside the liver for a short length, before giving a left portal vein branch that runs behind the left hepatic duct.

The venous drainage

The IVC occupies a groove on the posterior surface of the liver that drains into it via three large veins immediately below the diaphragm. The suprahepatic IVC immediately traverses the diaphragm to enter the right atrium, but below the liver there is a short clear segment above the insertion of the renal veins. A variable number of short inferior hepatic veins pass directly from the liver to the anterior wall of the IVC. The right hepatic vein can be exposed fully outside the liver parenchyma, but the middle and left veins usually terminate in a short common trunk before entering the IVC. The right adrenal gland is adjacent to the retrohepatic IVC and drains into it, usually by a single vein.

Segmental anatomy

The liver is divided into functional right and left 'units' along the line between the gallbladder fossa and the middle hepatic vein (Cantlie's line). Understanding the internal anatomy of the liver facilitated safe liver surgery and Couinaud, a French anatomist, described the liver *as being divided into eight segments* (***Figure 69.1***). Each segment can be considered a functional

A **hilum** is a depression or fissure where nerves, vessels or ducts enter a bodily organ.

Sir James Cantlie, 1851–1926, Scottish-born physician who cofounded the Hong Kong College of Medicine for Chinese (now Hong Kong University School of Medicine).

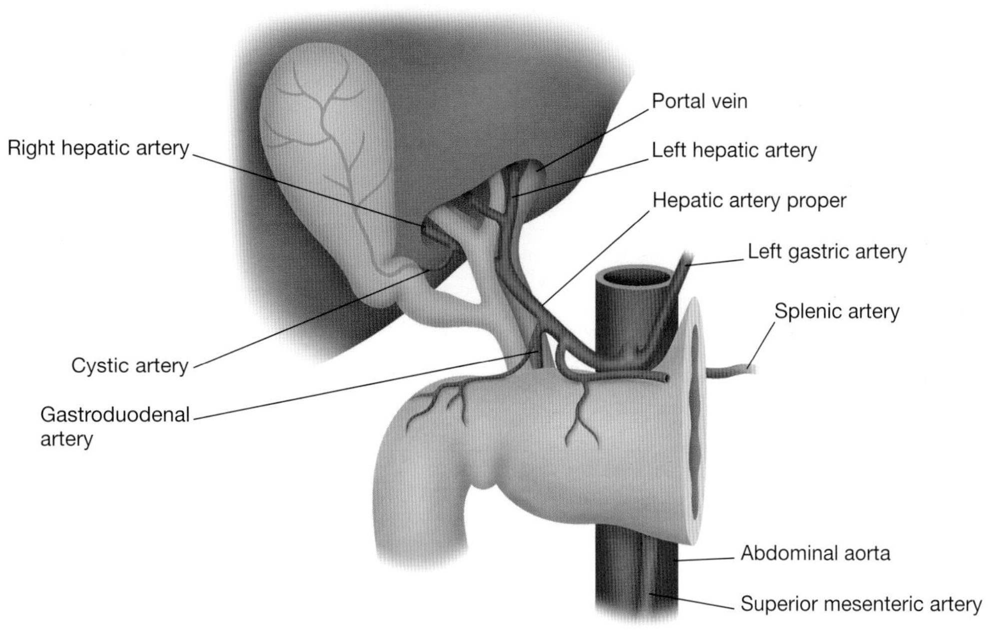

Figure 69.2 Anatomy of the liver hilum.

unit supplied by a branch of the hepatic artery, portal vein and bile duct, and drained by a hepatic vein tributary; this concept facilitates 'anatomical' liver resection. Liver segments V–VIII to the right of Cantlie's line are supplied by the right hepatic artery and the right branch of the portal vein and biliary drainage is via the right hepatic duct. To the left of Cantlie's line segments, I–IV are supplied by the left hepatic artery and left portal vein and drain via the left hepatic duct. Resections of individual segments, the whole of the left or the right hemiliver or combinations are possible.

Microscopic anatomy and structure

The liver comprises approximately 100 000 hexagonal functional units known as lobules with a central vein surrounded by six hepatic portal veins and six hepatic arteries. These vessels are connected by capillary-like tubes called sinusoids, which extend to meet the central vein. Lobules are separated by hepatic sinusoids, which are large-diameter capillaries lined by endothelial cells between rows of plates or cords of hepatocytes. Each sinusoid contains Kupffer cells, a type of macrophage that captures and breaks down effete red blood cells, and hepatocytes, which are cuboidal epithelial cells making up the majority of cells in the liver. Hepatocytes perform most liver functions, including metabolism, storage, digestion and bile production. Tiny bile canaliculi run parallel to the sinusoids on the contralateral side to the hepatocytes and drain bile in the opposite direction to the blood flow via the bile duct tributaries within the portal tracts.

Summary box 69.1

Liver anatomy

- There are two anatomical lobes with a separate blood supply, bile duct and venous drainage
- There is a dual blood supply; 80% portal vein and 20% hepatic artery
- The liver regenerates to 90–100% of its previous volume following resection
- Resection is based on anatomical lines to preserve maximal functioning liver and blood supply

ACUTE AND CHRONIC LIVER DISEASE

Liver blood tests

The liver performs a myriad of biochemical, metabolic and immunological functions. Anhepatic humans survive for 24–48 hours. It is the only organ in the body that regenerates. Awareness of currently available liver blood tests and their significance is essential (***Table 69.1***).

Karl Wilhelm von Kupffer, 1829–1902, Professor of Anatomy at Kiel (1869), Königsberg (1875) and Munich (1880), Germany, described these 'stellate cells' in 1880.

Summary box 69.2

Main functions of the liver

- Maintaining core body temperature
- pH balance and correction of lactic acidosis
- Synthesis of clotting factors
- Glucose metabolism, glycolysis and gluconeogenesis
- Urea formation from protein catabolism
- Bilirubin formation from haemoglobin after breakdown of effete red cells in the spleen
- Drug and hormone metabolism and excretion
- Removal of gut endotoxins and foreign antigens
- Vitamin and mineral storage, including A, D, E, K and B12
- Immunological function as part of the mononuclear phagocyte system
- Albumin production for transport of fatty acids, steroids and waste products
- Angiotensin synthesis
- Body temperature through heat production
- Cytochrome P450 detoxifies contaminants and pollutants, insecticides, food additives and alcohol

Clinical signs

Depending on the severity of liver dysfunction, the aetiology and acute or chronic development, symptoms vary and combinations occur. The most common include jaundice, drowsiness, abdominal pain/swelling, nausea, tremors, vomiting, malaise, confusion and disorientation, bruising, peripheral oedema and foetor hepaticus (strong musty smell to the breath).

Acute liver failure

Causes of acute liver failure

Acute liver failure is the development of sudden, severe hepatic dysfunction from an acute insult associated with the onset of hepatic encephalopathy and coagulation abnormalities. The most widely accepted definition, from the American Association for the Study of Liver Diseases, is:

> ***evidence of coagulation abnormality, usually an international normalized ratio above 1.5, and any degree of mental alteration (encephalopathy) in a patient without pre-existing liver disease and with an illness of less than 26 weeks' duration.***

Treatment of acute liver failure

Acute liver failure is rare in the developed world, with an annual incidence of <10 cases per million and a current mortality of 30–40%. In the early stages, there may be no objective signs, but with severe dysfunction clinical jaundice may be associated with neurological signs of liver failure (hepatic encephalopathy), consisting of a liver flap, drowsiness, confusion and eventually coma.

Liver transplantation is appropriate for some patients, although the short-term results are poor compared with transplantation for chronic liver disease and suitable donor livers are frequently not available in a suitable time frame owing to the precipitate deterioration.

TABLE 69.1 Routinely available blood tests for the assessment of liver function.

Test	Normal range	Significance
Bilirubin	5–17 μmol/L (0.3–1.2 mg/dL)	Bilirubin is synthesised in the liver and excreted in bile. Increased levels may be associated with increased haemoglobin breakdown, hepatocellular dysfunction resulting in impaired bilirubin transport and excretion or mechanical biliary obstruction. In patients with known parenchymal liver disease, progressive elevation of bilirubin in the absence of a secondary complication suggests deterioration in liver function
Alkaline phosphatase (ALP)	30–140 IU/L	The serum ALP is particularly elevated with cholestatic liver disease or biliary obstruction. It is important to note that routine laboratory analysis of ALP is not isoform specific and so ALP from a skeletal source may also lead to elevation, particularly Paget's disease and prostate cancer
Aspartate transaminase (AST)	5–40 IU/L	Although significant liver injury does occur in the presence of normal liver blood tests, levels of the transaminase (AST, ALT and GGT) usually reflect acute hepatocellular damage and GGT is a useful marker of alcohol intake
Alanine transaminase (ALT)	5–40 IU/L	
Gamma-glutamyl transpeptidase (GGT)	10–48 IU/L	
Albumin	35–50 g/L (3.5–5 g/dL)	The synthetic functions of the liver are indicated by the ability to synthesise proteins (albumin level) and clotting factors (PT) and the standard method of monitoring liver function in patients with chronic liver disease is serial measurement of bilirubin, albumin and PT
Total protein	60–85 g/L (6–8.5 g/dL)	
Prothrombin time (PT)	12–16 s	

Chronic liver disease

Liver disease is the third leading cause of premature death in the UK, and since 1970 deaths have increased by 400%. Liver disease is potentially preventable in 90% of cases, and 75% of patients present with late-stage disease. Lethargy and weakness are common features, irrespective of the aetiology, and often precede clinical jaundice. In advanced cirrhosis, glucuronyl conjugation of bilirubin and biliary excretion of conjugated

Sir James Paget, 1814–1899, Surgeon, St Bartholomew's Hospital, London, UK.

Summary box 69.3

Causes of acute liver failure

- Viral hepatitis (hepatitis A, B, C, D, E)
- Drug reactions (halothane, isoniazid–rifampicin, antidepressants, non-steroidal anti-inflammatory drugs [NSAIDs], valproic acid)
- Paracetamol overdose
- Prescription medicines, including antibiotics, NSAIDs, anticonvulsants and statins
- Herbal supplements
- Mushroom poisoning
- Toxins, including carbon tetrachloride in refrigerants, solvents for industrial use and varnishes
- Shock and multiorgan failure
- Autoimmune disease
- Acute Budd–Chiari syndrome
- Rare metabolic disorders, including Wilson's disease
- Cancer
- Fatty liver of pregnancy
- Heat stroke
- Reye's syndrome in children following a viral infection including
- Chickenpox
- Severe acute respiratory syndrome coronavirus (SARS-CoV-2) can cause liver failure in up to 20% of patients with a severe episode

Summary box 69.4

Supportive therapy for acute liver failure

- Fluid balance and electrolytes
- Acid–base balance and blood glucose monitoring
- Nutrition
- Renal function (haemofiltration)
- Respiratory support (ventilation)
- Monitoring and treatment of cerebral oedema
- Treat bacterial and fungal infection
- Extracorporeal liver support devices (principally as a bridge to transplantation)

bilirubin are impaired and jaundice develops. Progressive deterioration in liver function is associated with a hyperdynamic circulation with a high cardiac output, large pulse volume, low blood pressure and flushed warm extremities. Fever is common and may be related to underlying inflammation and cytokine release or bacterial infection due to innate immune dysfunction in acute and chronic liver disease. Skin changes include spider naevi (cutaneous vascular abnormalities that blanch on pressure), palmar erythema and white nails (leukonychia) and endocrine abnormalities produce hypogonadism and gynaecomastia. Hepatic encephalopathy is responsible for the mental derangement with memory impairment, confusion, personality changes, altered sleep patterns and slow, slurred speech. The most useful clinical sign is a flapping tremor when

Summary box 69.5

King's College selection criteria for liver transplantation in acute liver failure: paracetamol (acetaminophen) and non-paracetamol induced

Paracetamol toxicity	Non-paracetamol toxicity
Criteria met if arterial pH <7.30 OR/AND All three of the following present: • INR >6.5 (PT >100 s) • Serum creatinine 3.4 mg/dL (301 μmol/L) • Grade III or IV encephalopathy[a] Additionally,[b] • Hyperlactaemia or hyperphosphataemia are strong predictors of poor prognosis for survival without transplantation	Criteria met if INR >6.5 (PT >100 s) OR/AND Three out of five of the following present: • Age less than 10 or greater than 40 • Aetiology non-A, non-B hepatitis, idiosyncratic drug reactions • Duration of jaundice before development of encephalopathy >7 days • PT greater than 50 s (approximate INR >3.5) • Serum bilirubin >18 mg/dL (300 μmol/L)

INR, international normalised ratio; PT, prothrombin time.

[a]Hepatic encephalopathy grades can be described as:

- Grade 1: inverted sleep pattern, agitation, forgetfulness, irritability, apraxia
- Grade 2: lethargy, time and/or place disorientation, personality change, ataxia
- Grade 3: somnolence to semistupor but responds to verbal stimuli, place disorientation, asterixis, hyperactive reflexes
- Grade 4: coma

[b]The addition of lactate or phosphate thresholds to the criteria may improve sensitivity and negative predictive value.

the patient extends their arms while hyperextending the wrist joints. Ascites is a common late feature causing abdominal distension, detected clinically by the demonstration of a fluid thrill or shifting dullness. Protein catabolism produces sarcopenia and wasting, and bruising suggests a coagulopathy.

Summary box 69.6

Features of chronic liver disease

- Lethargy
- Fever
- Jaundice
- Protein catabolism (wasting)
- Coagulopathy (bruising)
- Cardiac (hyperdynamic circulation)
- Neurological (hepatic encephalopathy)
- Portal hypertension
  - Ascites
  - Oesophageal varices
  - Splenomegaly and hypersplenism
- Cutaneous
  - Spider naevi
  - Palmar erythema

SA Kinnier Wilson, 1878–1937, Professor of Neurology, King's College, London, UK.
Ralph Douglas Reye, 1912–1977, pathologist, Royal Alexandra Hospital for Children, Sydney, Australia.

Assessment of chronic liver disease

A number of parameters are required to accurately assess the degree of liver dysfunction, enable predictions about a patient's ability to tolerate surgical or radiological procedures and assess the prognosis following transplantation. Two prognostic models commonly used are the Child–Turcotte–Pugh (CTP) classification (***Table 69.2***) and the Model for End-Stage Liver Disease (MELD) score. The original Child classification was developed to predict mortality following shunt surgery in patients with cirrhosis, with the CTP classification modified to predict mortality after any surgery. The MELD score was devised to predict the short-term prognosis following transjugular intrahepatic portosystemic stent shunt (TIPSS) but has been adopted to prioritise patients on liver transplant waiting lists. In the MELD model survival probability is calculated based on the patient's international normalised ratio (INR), serum bilirubin and creatinine.

TABLE 69.2 Child–Turcotte–Pugh (CTP) classification of hepatocellular function in cirrhosis.

Points	1 point each	2 points each	3 points each
Bilirubin (μmol/L)	<34	34–50	>50
Albumin (g/L)	>35	25–35	<25
Ascites	None	Easily controlled	Poorly controlled
Encephalopathy	None	Grade I or II	Grade III or IV
INR	<1.7	1.7–2.2	>2.2

CTP-A, 5 or 6 points; CTP-B, 7–9 points; CTP-C, 10–15 points.
INR, international normalised ratio.

Operating in the presence of chronic liver disease

Surgical and anaesthetic complications are increased in chronic liver disease, with the risk dependent on the magnitude of the procedure, degree of liver impairment and type of anaesthesia. Overall surgical mortality rates are increased by 10% in CTP-A disease, 30% in CTP-B and 75–80% in CTP-C (***Table 69.2***). MELD scores correlate with operative mortality: 1% increase for each MELD point up to 20 and a further 2% for each point above 20, with rates considerably higher following emergency presentation.

INVESTIGATING LIVER DISEASE

Imaging modalities

Major advances in surgical approaches to the liver required improvements in preoperative imaging. The choice of imaging modality is determined by the likely pathology and locally available equipment and expertise (***Table 69.3***).

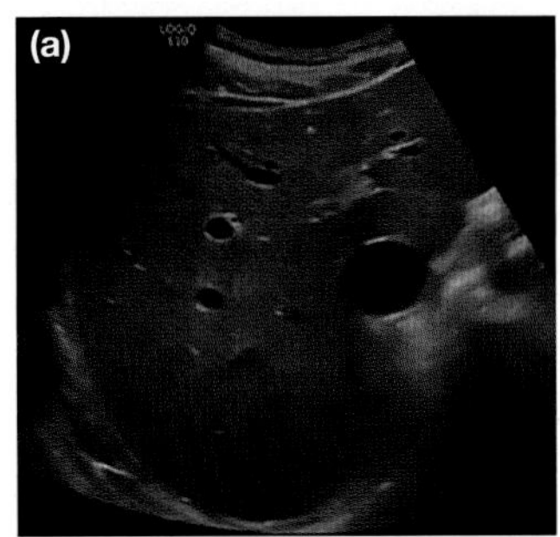

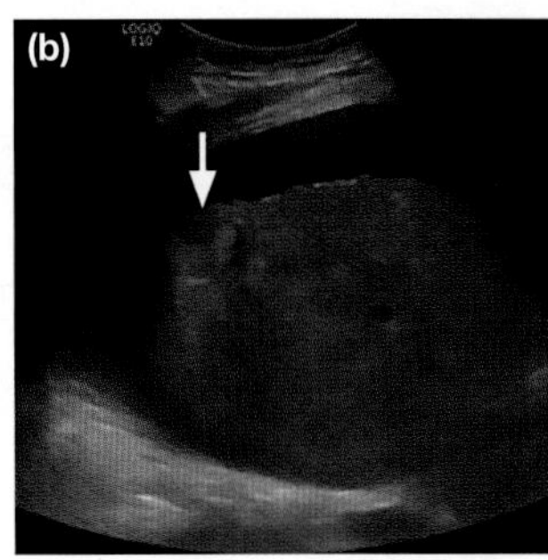

Figure 69.3 Ultrasound scans of the liver. **(a)** Normal liver and **(b)** surveillance for a patient with cirrhosis demonstrating hepatocellular carcinoma (arrow).

Ultrasonography

Ultrasonography (US) is traditionally the first imaging modality for the investigation of jaundice and right upper quadrant pain (***Figure 69.3***). Good quality US can characterise benign cystic lesions but is operator dependent; accurate characterisation of malignant pathologies is not possible. Body habitus and anatomical variations frequently prevent detailed examination, with steatosis reducing liver penetration; US should not be used when malignancy is suspected.

US can reliably identify biliary dilatation but not the aetiology, and overlying air-containing viscera often prevent complete examination. Contrast-enhanced ultrasonography (CEUS), introduced in the early 1990s, uses transient intravascular bubbles to differentiate normal liver parenchyma from solid tumours. CEUS increases US sensitivity and specificity by assessing real-time lesion vascularity with an accuracy for focal liver lesions of 90%.

Computed tomography

Modern spiral computed tomography (CT) technology has increased the accuracy of diagnosis and staging of liver lesions, and contrast-enhanced CT is currently the most widely used and best validated modality. Fine detail of liver lesions with resolutions of 6–8 mm is possible, liver algorithms allow characterisation and density data identify cystic lesions (***Figure 69.4a***). The early arterial phase following intravenous contrast detects small hepatocellular carcinomas (HCCs) owing to their predominantly arterial blood supply. The venous phase demonstrates branches of the intrahepatic portal vein and the hepatic veins. Inflammatory liver lesions often exhibit rim enhancement with intravenous contrast, whereas haemangiomas characteristically show late venous enhancement. CT is extremely accurate when assessing the stage and resectability of liver tumours apart from peritoneal metastases.

Magnetic resonance imaging

Magnetic resonance (MR) of the liver is superior to CT in characterising focal lesions (***Figure 69.4b***). The resolution for small metastases is superior and is further improved by liver-specific

Charles Gardner Child, 1908–1991, surgeon, Michigan, USA. **Child** and **Jeremiah G Turcotte** first proposed the scoring system in 1964. In 1972, **RN Pugh** and colleagues from King's College Hospital, London, UK, modified the scoring system by replacing nutritional status with prothrombin time or international normalised ratio.

TABLE 69.3 Modalities employed for imaging of the liver.

Imaging modality	Principal indication
Ultrasonography	• Standard first-line investigation • CEUS 90% accurate for focal lesions
Spiral CT	• Investigation of malignancy • Cancer surveillance • Anatomical planning for liver surgery
MRI	• Alternative to spiral CT • Characterisation of liver lesions • Liver-specific contrast agents are taken up by hepatocytes, which are absent in malignant lesions, which consequently contrast with the enhanced background liver
MRCP	• First-line, non-invasive cholangiography • Investigation and surveillance of parenchymal liver disease (sclerosing cholangitis, autoimmune cholangitis) for the development of malignancy
ERCP	• Therapeutic procedure only • Imaging the biliary tract when endoscopic intervention is required (stones, strictures, iatrogenic and traumatic injury)
PTC	• Biliary tract imaging when ERCP not possible or failed
EUS	• Generally for examination of the extrahepatic biliary tree and pancreas • Caudate lobe, hilar nodes and liver parenchyma can be assessed
Octreotide scanning	• Form of scintigraphy used to identify and localise NETs and carcinoid tumours • Particularly useful to exclude metastatic disease
HIDA scanning	• Determination of the patency of the intra- and extrahepatic biliary system and investigation of biliary atresia and jaundice following liver transplantation
Angiography	• To detect vascular involvement by tumour • Treatment of vascular pathology (pseudotumours, haemobilia, iatrogenic injuries, trauma)
PET scanning	• To quantify tumour spread • Differentiate benign and malignant pathologies
Laparoscopy ± laparoscopic ultrasonography	• To detect peritoneal and serosal disease, assess the extent of tumours and spread • Ultrasonography to determine the relationship of tumours to vascular structures and biopsy of liver tumours and superficial lesions

CEUS, contrast-enhanced ultrasonography; CT, computed tomography; ERCP, endoscopic retrograde cholangiopancreatography; EUS, endoscopic ultrasonography; HIDA, hepatobiliary iminodiacetic acid; MRCP, magnetic resonance cholangiopancreatography; MRI, magnetic resonance imaging; NET, neuroendocrine tumour; PET, positron emission tomography; PTC, percutaneous transhepatic cholangiography.

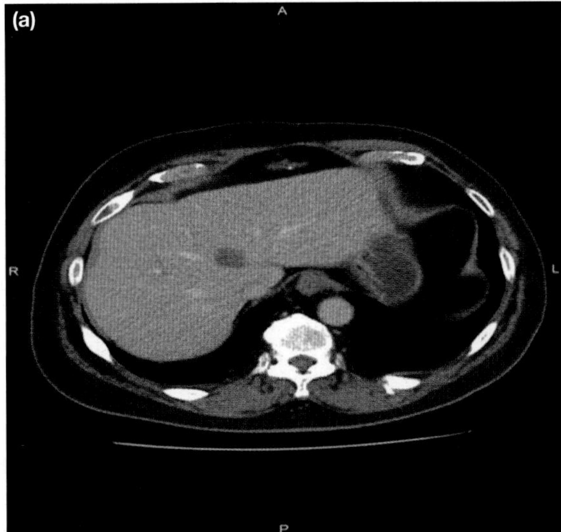

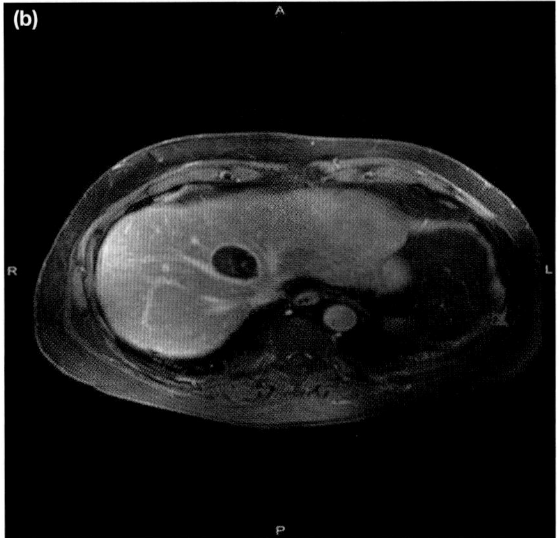

Figure 69.4 Computed tomography (CT) and magnetic resonance imaging (MRI) scans of the same patient following a road traffic accident and fall from a motorcycle. CT scan **(a)** was interpreted as a traumatic haematoma, but the MRI scan **(b)** demonstrated an incidental hepatocellular carcinoma.

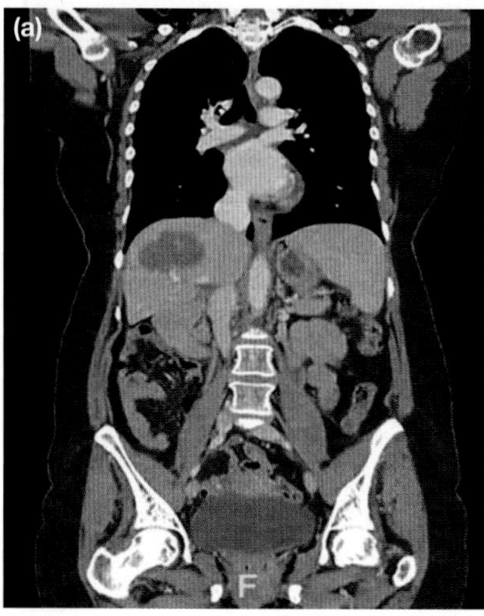
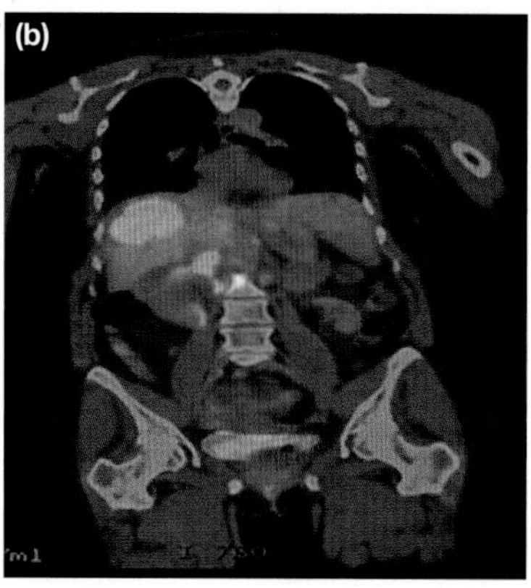

Figure 69.5 Computed tomography scan (a) and positron emission tomography scan (b) of a patient with a large colorectal metastasis and hilar lymphadenopathy.

contrast agents, particularly in differentiating between small HCCs and regenerative nodules. Magnetic resonance cholangiopancreatography (MRCP) provides excellent, non-invasive imaging of the intra- and extrahepatic biliary tract with an accuracy comparable to direct cholangiography.

Positron emission tomography

Positron emission tomography (PET) scanning is a functional test that demonstrates the metabolic activity of a tissue. A variety of tracers are available depending on the process being investigated. For the investigation of malignancy ^{18}F-2-fluoro-2-deoxy-d-glucose is commonly used, and detection depends on the avid uptake of glucose by malignant cells compared with benign or inflammatory tissue. Deoxyglucose is labelled with the positron emitter fluorine-18 (^{18}F-FDG) which is administered prior to PET imaging. A three-dimensional image of the whole body is obtained, highlighting areas of increased glucose metabolism (***Figure 69.5***). A positive PET scan result does not always indicate malignant disease (inflammation being the most common cause of a false-positive result), and conversely false-negative results occur. A critical mass is required for adequate uptake to be detectable, and resolution is similar to CT and MRI. PET scanning is particularly useful for the detection of metastatic disease and confirmation of lymph node involvement, serving as 'its own control' if some lesions prove to be FDG avid and some are cold.

Angiography

Angiography is almost exclusively employed when therapeutic intervention is considered; occlusion of arteriovenous malformations, embolisation of bleeding sites in the liver and the treatment of liver tumours by transarterial chemoembolisation (TACE).

Octreotide scan

Octreotide scanning is a form of scintigraphy in which radioisotopes attached to drug carriers are taken up by specific tissues or processes (***Figure 69.6***). Octreotide is an octapeptide that pharmacologically mimics somatostatin. When radiolabelled with indium-111 and administered intravenously it is taken up by tumour cells containing somatostatin receptors; emitted gamma radiation is detected by a scintillation camera and a whole-body image constructed. It is particularly useful for the identification of carcinoid and neuroendocrine tumours (NETs) and metastatic disease, with a 75–100% sensitivity for detecting pancreatic NETs.

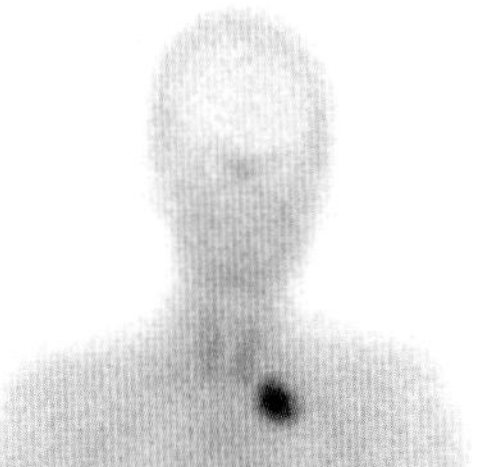
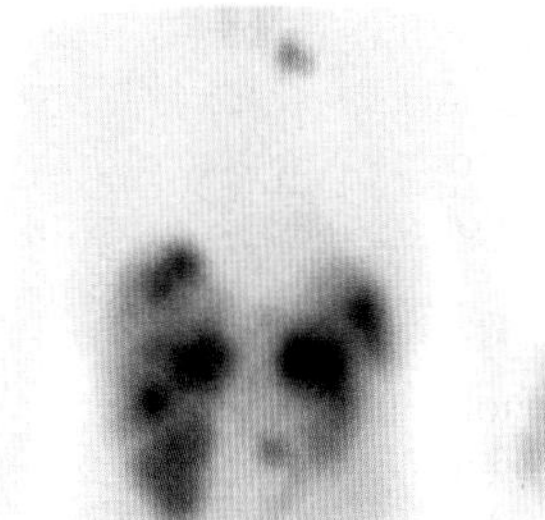

Figure 69.6 Octreotide scan demonstrating liver metastases from a neuroendocrine tumour with additional metastatic disease in mediastinal lymph nodes.

Hepatobiliary iminodiacetic acid

Hepatobiliary iminodiacetic acid (HIDA) labelled with technetium-99m (^{99m}Tc-HIDA) is concentrated by hepatocytes and excreted with bile, visualising intrahepatic uptake, the extrahepatic biliary system and the gallbladder. Under normal circumstances HIDA enters the duodenum within 30 minutes and scintigraphy produces an image together with an activity–time curve. HIDA scanning is useful because biliary excretion occurs despite hyperbilirubinaemia (<85 µmol/L). It is most commonly used to investigate biliary atresia, to investigate jaundice in liver transplant patients and to demonstrate patency of the biliary tract.

Endoscopic retrograde cholangiopancreatography

Endoscopic retrograde cholangiopancreatography (ERCP) is performed in patients with obstructive jaundice when a therapeutic endoscopic procedure is indicated (see ***Chapter 9***). It provides definitive views of Klatskin tumours (hilar

Gerald Klatskin, 1910–1986, pathologist, Yale School of Medicine, New Haven, CT, USA.

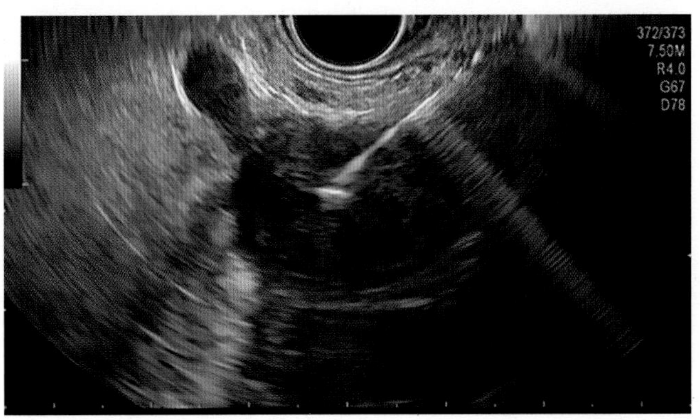

Figure 69.7 Endoscopic ultrasonography demonstrating liver parenchyma and a caudate lobe metastasis being biopsied.

cholangiocarcinoma) and facilitates staging by defining the extent of involvement of intrahepatic ducts. ERCP also provides clear images of the intrahepatic ducts in primary sclerosing cholangitis (PSC) and facilitates stenting and drainage of obstructed, infected segments.

Endoscopic (peroral) cholangiography

Cholangioscopy enables direct visualisation of the bile ducts, either operatively or endoscopically. The original 'mother and baby' ERCP cholangioscopy has been superseded by SpyGlass™ (Boston Scientific) cholangioscopy, which enables a single operator to examine the biliary mucosa. The inclusion of a working channel facilitates visualised biopsies and targeted therapy. Targeted biopsies improve diagnostic yields, with an overall accuracy of 85–95% in patients with indeterminate biliary strictures compared with 55–90% for brush cytology.

Endoscopic ultrasonography

Endoscopic ultrasonography (EUS) is predominantly used to evaluate the extrahepatic biliary tree and pancreas, but linear and radial instruments enable visualisation of hilar lymph nodes and the caudate lobe and assessment of the liver parenchyma (***Figure 69.7***).

Percutaneous transhepatic cholangiography

Percutaneous transhepatic cholangiography (PTC) is indicated where endoscopic cholangiography has failed or is impossible because of anatomical constraints from previous surgery or malignant involvement of the duodenum. Tumour extent in patients with hilar tumours can be assessed and combined percutaneous/endoscopic or antegrade metal stent placement is facilitated.

Laparoscopy and laparoscopic ultrasonography

Laparoscopy is useful to stage primary hepatopancreatobiliary cancers. Unrecognised peritoneal metastases, superficial liver tumours and peritoneal disease can be identified and biopsied, avoiding an inappropriate laparotomy. Routine biopsy of resectable lesions is contraindicated to avoid tumour seeding.

Summary box 69.7

Management of liver trauma

- Remember associated injuries
- At-risk groups
  - Stabbing or gunshot to lower chest or upper abdomen
  - Crush injury with multiple rib fractures
  - High-speed road traffic accident
- Resuscitate
  - Airway
  - Breathing
  - Circulation
- Assessment of the injury
  - CT chest and abdomen with contrast
  - Laparotomy if haemodynamically unstable
- Treatment
  - Correct coagulopathy
  - Suture lacerations
  - Resect if major vascular injury
  - Packing if diffuse parenchymal injury

LIVER TRAUMA

Liver injury due to blunt or penetrating abdominal trauma is second in frequency only to that of the spleen. Blunt injury produces contusion, laceration and avulsion, often associated with splenic, mesenteric or renal injuries. Penetrating injuries, including stab and gunshot wounds, are often associated with chest or pericardial involvement. Blunt injuries are more common and have a higher mortality (***Table 69.4***).

TABLE 69.4 Mortality from liver trauma.

Type of injury	Mortality
Blunt abdominal trauma	Overall mortality 10–30%
Severe and high-velocity injuries	Up to 60%
Injury to main hepatic veins or retrohepatic inferior vena cava	50–100%
Penetrating injuries	12–20%
Penetrating injuries with associated duodenal, pancreatic or chest involvement; multiple stab wounds	20–40%

Diagnosis and grading of liver injury

The liver is an extremely well-vascularised organ and blood loss is the major early complication following injury. A high index of suspicion is essential with any chest or upper abdominal stab wound, especially where significant blood loss is obvious. Severe crushing injuries to the lower chest or upper abdomen frequently result in rib fractures, haemothorax and splenic and/or liver injury. Focused assessment sonography in trauma (FAST) performed by an experienced operator will identify free intraperitoneal fluid. In haemodynamically unstable patients with penetrating wounds a laparotomy and/or thoracotomy is indicated once active resuscitation has commenced. Penetrating injuries are frequently associated with massive, continued blood loss and coagulopathies; transfer to the operating theatre should occur while blood products are obtained and resuscitation continues. In haemodynamically stable patients, urgent contrast-enhanced CT scan of the chest and abdomen is performed to look for parenchymal injury and concomitant damage to other thoracic or abdominal organs.

The American Association for the Surgery of Trauma liver injury scale was revised in 2018 to incorporate vascular injury such as pseudoaneurysm and arteriovenous fistula. The guidelines recommend dual arterial/portal venous phase imaging (*Table 69.5*).

TABLE 69.5 Grading of liver injuries according to American Association for the Surgery of Trauma.

Grade 1	• Haematoma: subcapsular, <10% surface area • Laceration: capsular tear, <1 cm parenchymal depth
Grade 2	• Haematoma: subcapsular, 10–50% surface area • Haematoma: intraparenchymal, <10 cm diameter • Laceration: capsular tear 1–3 cm parenchymal depth, <10 cm length
Grade 3	• Haematoma: subcapsular, >50% surface area of ruptured subcapsular or parenchymal haematoma • Haematoma: intraparenchymal, >10 cm • Laceration: capsular tear, >3 cm parenchymal depth • Vascular injury with active bleeding contained within liver parenchyma
Grade 4	• Laceration: parenchymal disruption involving 25–75% hepatic lobe or involves 1–3 Couinaud segments • Vascular injury with active bleeding breaching the liver parenchyma into the peritoneum
Grade 5	• Laceration: parenchymal disruption involving >75% of hepatic lobe • Vascular: juxtahepatic venous injuries (retrohepatic vena cava/central major hepatic veins)

Additional points:
- Advance one grade for multiple injuries up to grade III.
- 'Vascular injury' (i.e. pseudoaneurysm or arteriovenous fistula): appears as a focal collection of vascular contrast that decreases in attenuation on delayed images.
- 'Active bleeding': focal or diffuse collection of vascular contrast that increases in size or attenuation on a delayed phase.

Initial management of liver injuries

Penetrating injuries

Modern approaches to liver trauma are based on conservative management where possible. The initial management is maintenance of airway patency, breathing and circulation (ABC), following the principles of advanced trauma life support (ATLS). Peripheral venous access requires two large-bore cannulae and blood is sent for cross-match of 10 units of blood, full blood count, urea and electrolytes, liver function tests, clotting screen, glucose and amylase. Initial volume replacement should be with blood; arterial blood gases should be obtained; and the patient intubated and ventilated if gas exchange is inadequate. Intercostal chest drains are indicated if an associated pneumothorax or haemothorax is suspected. Once resuscitation has commenced, the patient should be transferred to the operating theatre, with further resuscitation performed on the operating table. The necessity for fresh-frozen plasma (FFP) and cryoprecipitate should be discussed with the blood transfusion service immediately the patient arrives in the hospital (often by activation of a major transfusion protocol), as these patients rapidly develop irreversible coagulopathies due to a lack of fibrinogen and clotting factors. Standard coagulation profiles are inadequate to evaluate this acute loss of clotting factors, and products should be given empirically aided by the results of thromboelastography if available (see *Chapter 2*).

Blunt trauma

Enhanced resuscitation, anaesthesia and intensive care have contributed to reduced mortality rates. Optimum results are obtained with specialist teams that include experienced liver surgeons, anaesthetists, endoscopists and interventional radiologists (*Figure 69.8*).

Initial resuscitation and management are as outlined for penetrating injuries. Unstable patients require immediate laparotomy, but the majority of haemodynamically stable patients should be managed non-surgically (management depends on haemodynamic stability not the grade of injury).

Haemodynamic instability and signs of generalised peritonitis mandate surgical intervention. Interventional radiology with embolisation for hepatic arterial bleeding is safe and

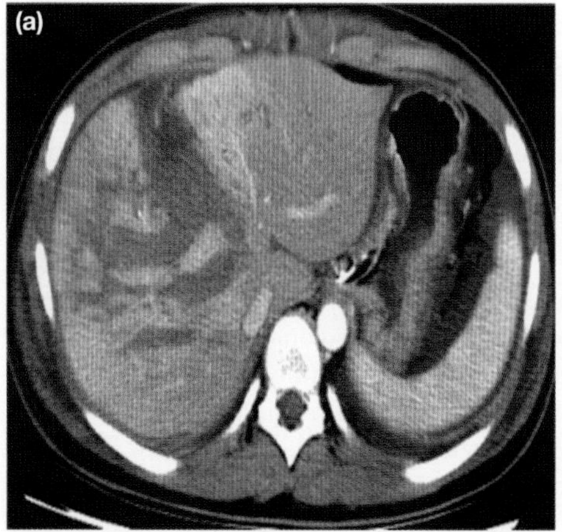

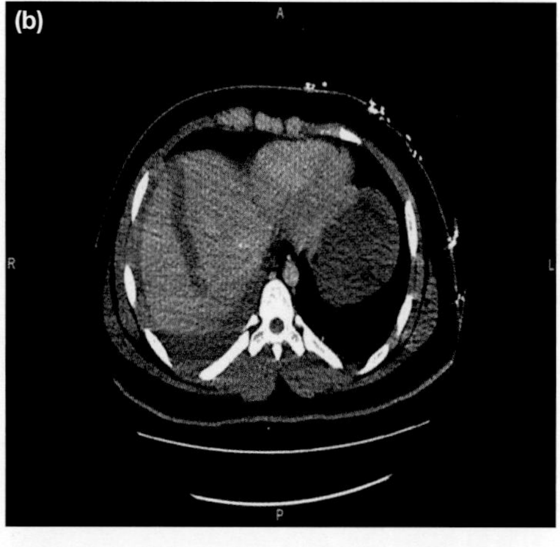

Figure 69.8 Computed tomography scans demonstrating the significant differences between blunt **(a)** and penetrating **(b)** trauma (assault with a kitchen knife).

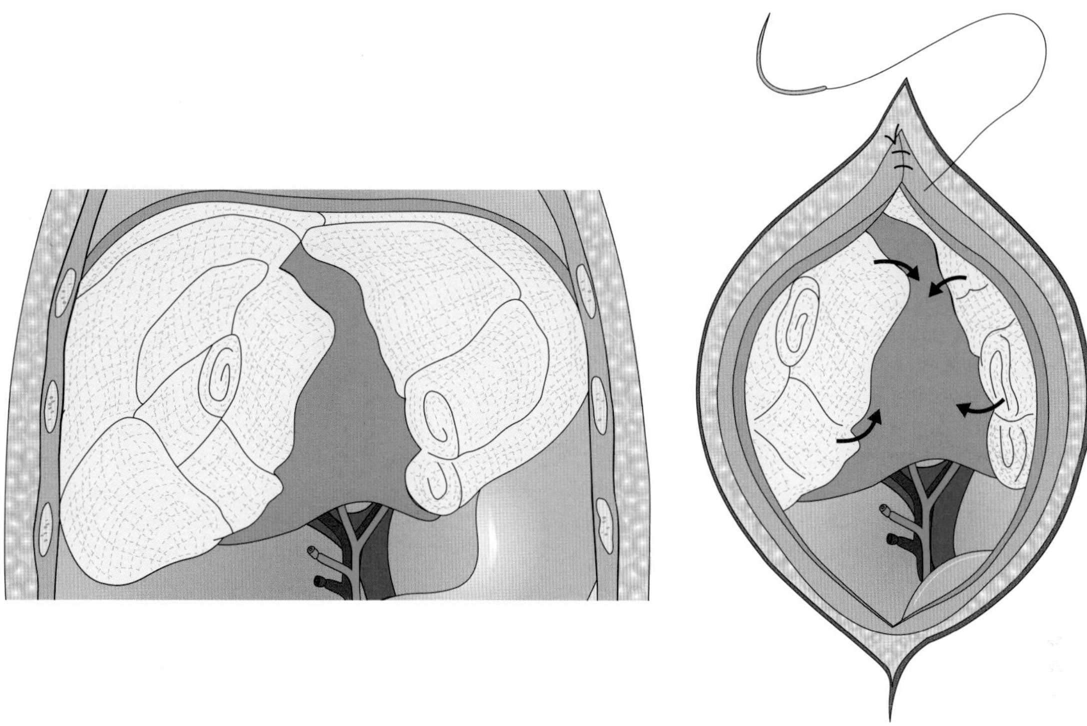

Figure 69.9 Packing the liver to achieve haemostasis. The abdomen can then be closed and the patient transferred to critical care for stabilisation prior to relook laparotomy 24–48 hours later. (Adapted from Poston GJ, D'Angelica M, Adam R (eds). *Surgical management of hepatobiliary and pancreatic disorders*. Boca Raton: CRC Press, 2010.)

effective in stable patients. If conservative management is successful patients are discharged after 8–10 days, advised to avoid abdominal trauma and rescanned after 6–8 weeks. If fever, bleeding or pain occurs prompt readmission is required.

Surgical approaches to liver trauma

When a laparotomy is indicated, especially when CT scanning is not possible, a 'rooftop' incision (see ***Figure 69.19***) with midline extension to the xiphisternum and retraction of the costal margins gives excellent access to the liver and spleen. If a midline incision is made initially a transverse right lateral extension will improve access. Required operative techniques include resectional debridement, hepatotomy with direct suture ligation and perihepatic packing. Anatomical resection, hepatic artery ligation and bypass techniques are possible following transfer of patients to tertiary hepatobiliary centres. Major complications include recurrent haemorrhage, sepsis and bile leak.

Packing or manual pressure intended to compress the parenchyma without causing caval compression is the initial aim (***Figure 69.9***); if additional intra-abdominal bleeding is found the source needs to be identified.

Care should be taken to avoid overzealous packing, which may produce pressure necrosis of the liver parenchyma or abdominal compartment syndrome. Packing is effective for the majority of liver injuries if the liver is packed against the natural contour of the diaphragm. If control is not achieved a Pringle manoeuvre should be performed (***Figure 69.10***). Large abdominal packs should be used to ease their removal, and the abdomen closed to facilitate compression.

Continued bleeding implies damage to the hepatic veins and/or the IVC but exploration of a liver laceration should only be attempted if control is not possible. If insufficient facilities or assistance are available and packing controls the situation, the abdomen should be closed and the patient transferred to a tertiary centre.

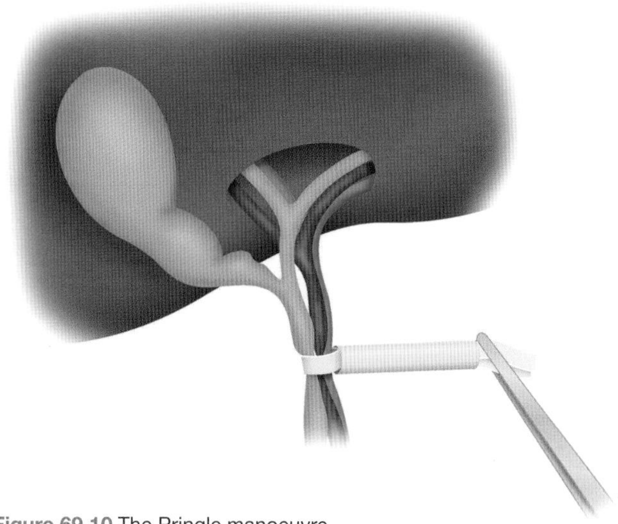

Figure 69.10 The Pringle manoeuvre.

James Hogarth Pringle, 1863–1941, surgeon, The Royal Infirmary, Glasgow, UK.

Crush injuries to the liver may produce large parenchymal haematomas and diffuse capsular lacerations (***Figure 69.8a***). Suturing is ineffective, and perihepatic packing is frequently the only option. Necrotic tissue should be removed but poorly perfused but viable liver left *in situ*. If packing is necessary, this should be removed after 48–72 hours; usually, no further intervention is required. Antibiotic cover is advisable and full reversal of any coagulopathy essential. If a major vascular injury (hepatic vein or vena cava, grade V or VI) is suspected then packing and referral to a specialist centre should be considered as venovenous bypass is often required. Following transfer, a further laparotomy is performed, the liver fully mobilised and, after a Pringle manoeuvre and IVC occlusion above the renal veins and at the level of the diaphragm using atraumatic vascular clamps (with/without venovenous bypass), caval or hepatic vein damage is repaired. Warm ischaemia of the liver is tolerated for up to 45 minutes.

Complications of liver trauma

A subcapsular or intrahepatic haematoma requires no specific intervention and should be allowed to resolve spontaneously. Abscesses may form as a result of secondary infection of an area of parenchymal ischaemia and treatment is systemic antibiotics and US-guided aspiration once liquefaction has occurred. Bile collections require US-guided aspiration with/without drain insertion and biliary fistulae are investigated by endoscopic or percutaneous cholangiography with/without stent insertion for biliary decompression. If a fistula persists liver resection may be required.

Late vascular complications include hepatic artery aneurysms and arteriovenous fistulae (hepatic artery to hepatic vein, producing heart failure; arterioportal, causing portal hypertension) and arteriobiliary fistulae indicated by haemobilia are treated by embolisation. Hepatic insufficiency may occur following extensive liver trauma but usually recovers following supportive treatment if the blood supply and biliary drainage to an adequate liver remnant are preserved (***Figure 69.11***).

Summary box 69.8

Complications of liver trauma

- Intrahepatic haematoma
- Liver abscess
- Bile collection
- Biliary fistula
- Haemobilia
- Ascites
- Biliary strictures
- Intra-abdominal collections
- Hepatic artery aneurysm
- Arteriovenous fistulae
- Arteriobiliary fistulae
- Liver failure

Long-term problems following liver trauma and their management

Late complications are rare, but biliary strictures occur many years after liver trauma and treatment depends on the extent and site of stricturing. A segmental or lobar stricture with atrophy of the corresponding area of liver parenchyma and compensatory contralateral hypertrophy is treated expectantly. A dominant extrahepatic bile duct stricture associated with obstructive jaundice should be treated endoscopically but may require surgical correction with a Roux-en-Y hepatodochojejunostomy.

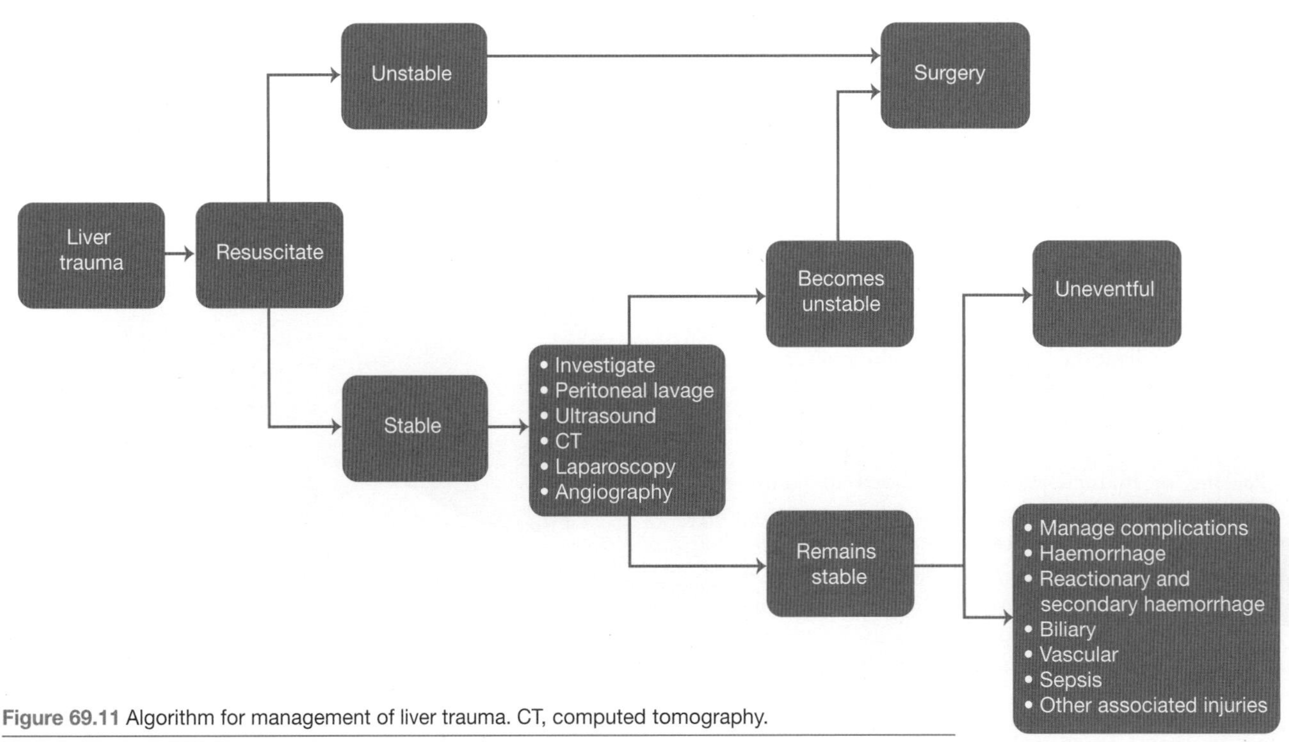

Figure 69.11 Algorithm for management of liver trauma. CT, computed tomography.

César Roux, 1857–1934, Professor of Surgery and Gynaecology, Lausanne, Switzerland. Described the Roux-en-Y loop in 1908.

PORTAL HYPERTENSION

Portal hypertension is most commonly due to liver cirrhosis, although it also occurs with extrahepatic portal vein occlusion, intrahepatic veno-occlusive disease and occlusion of the main hepatic veins (Budd–Chiari syndrome). The condition is common in clinical practice and portal hypertension represents a significant clinical challenge, with patients who have often been ill for long periods repeatedly presenting as emergencies. Many symptoms are intractable, surgery is technically difficult and procedures and timing must be chosen with extreme care. Portal hypertension *per se* produces no symptoms and is generally diagnosed following presentation with decompensated chronic liver disease causing encephalopathy, ascites or variceal bleeding (***Figure 69.12***).

Surgical involvement occurs in four situations:

1. ascites;
2. oesophageal varices;
3. portosystemic shunting for problems not managed by other methods;
4. left-sided portal hypertension and hypersplenism.

Management of variceal bleeding

Resuscitation

Varices are ubiquitous in patients with portal hypertension irrespective of the aetiology and usually present with an acute, large-volume haematemesis associated with a high morbidity and significant mortality. The lower oesophagus is the most common site and the diagnosis should be suspected in a patient known to have cirrhosis, but confirmation of the source is required following initial resuscitation. Variceal haemorrhage is a medical emergency and failure to control variceal bleeding with current medical management occurs in 10–20% of cases.

Patients with massive haemorrhage should be admitted to an intensive therapy unit, venous access obtained through two

Summary box 69.9

Causes of portal hypertension

- Pre-sinusoidal
  - Extrahepatic: portal vein thrombosis, splenic vein thrombosis (pancreatitis, pancreatic tumour), myelofibrosis, arterioportal shunt, tropical splenomegaly
  - Intrahepatic: schistosomiasis, congenital hepatic fibrosis and portal infiltration (sarcoidosis), drugs and toxins, veno-occlusive disease
- Sinusoidal
  - Cirrhosis
- Post-sinusoidal
  - Hepatic vein occlusion (Budd–Chiari syndrome), veno-occlusive disease, congestive cardiac failure

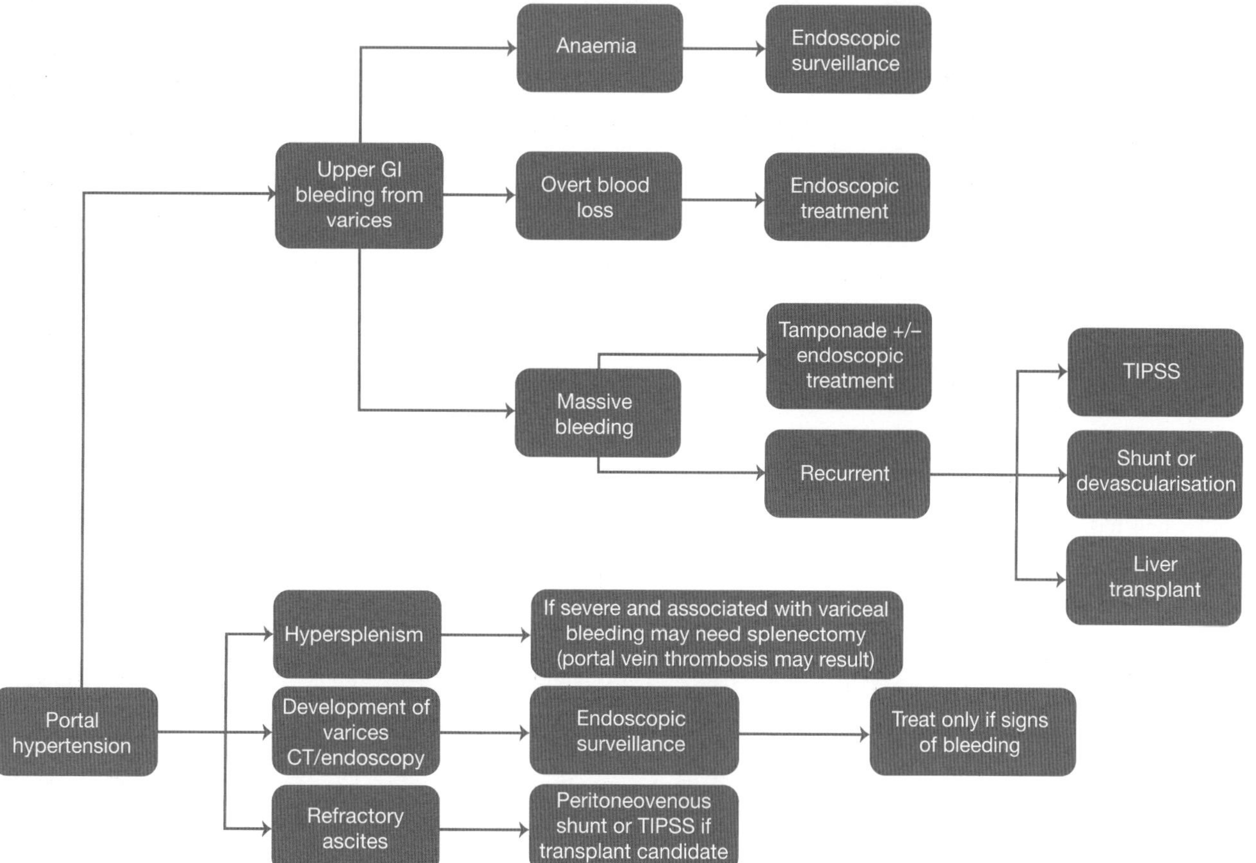

Figure 69.12 Management of complications of portal hypertension. CT, computed tomography; GI, gastrointestinal; TIPSS, transjugular intrahepatic portosystemic stent shunt.

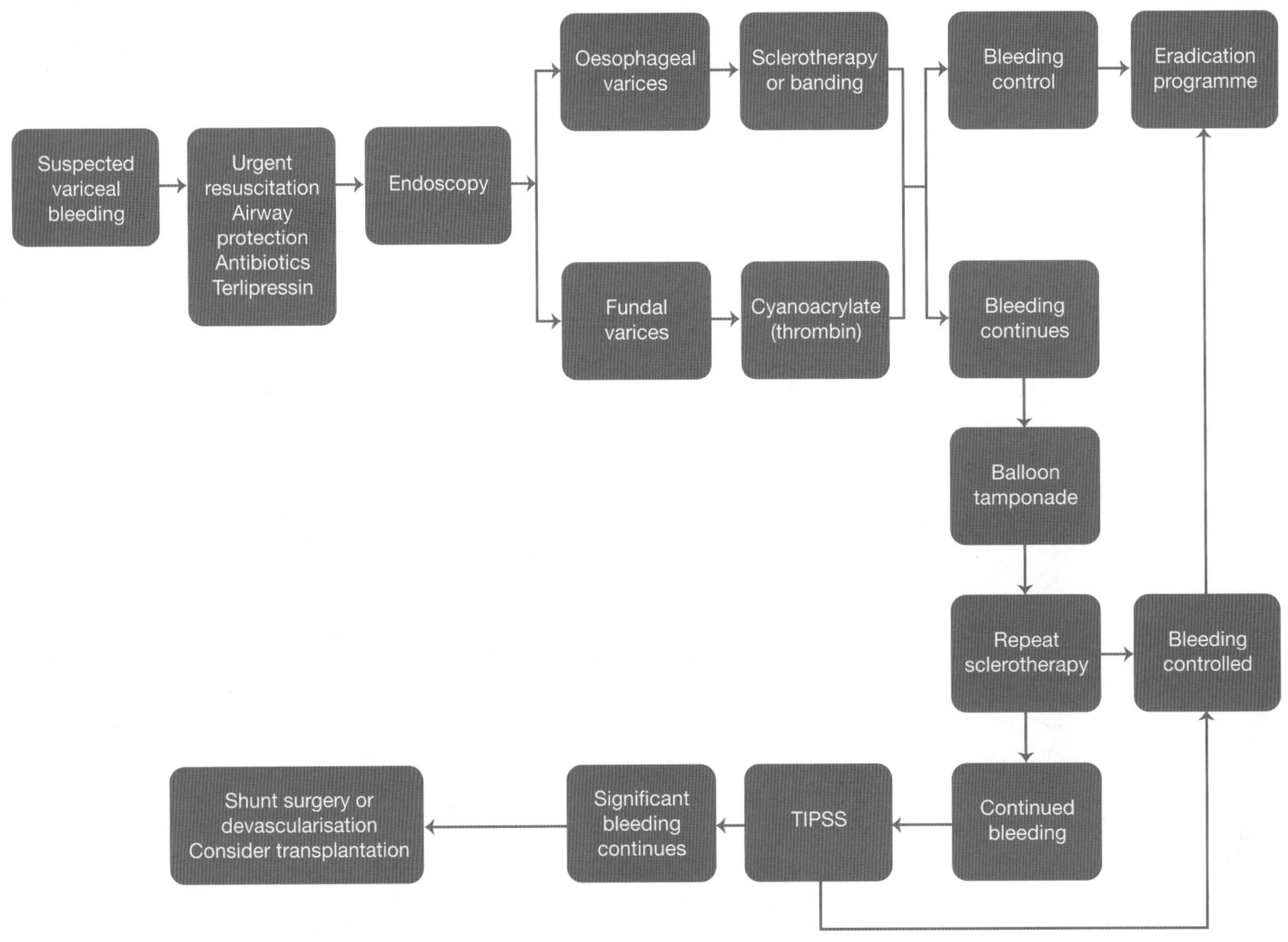

Figure 69.13 The management of variceal bleeding. TIPSS, transjugular intrahepatic portosystemic stent shunt.

large-bore peripheral cannulae and resuscitation commenced, ideally with blood. Liver function tests will reveal underlying liver disease and a coagulation profile will identify any coagulopathy. Hypervolaemia may increase portal pressure and exacerbate bleeding. Ten milligrams of vitamin K are administered intravenously but a coagulopathy requires FFP and activation of a major transfusion protocol. Thrombocytopenia secondary to hypersplenism is treated if the platelet count is $<50 \times 10^9$/L. Treatment protocols include the use of splanchnic vasoconstrictors, such as terlipressin, octreotide and somatostatin, and prophylactic antibiotics. When bleeding continues treatment options are sclerotherapy, banding, balloon tamponade and TIPSS. The use of oesophageal balloons should be avoided, which is usually possible when experienced endoscopists are available. As soon as the patient is haemodynamically stable the diagnosis should be confirmed endoscopically as 30% will have a non-variceal source of bleeding. Variceal bleeding is often associated with hepatic encephalopathy and endotracheal intubation may be required prior to endoscopy to protect the airway and prevent aspiration (***Figure 69.13***).

Balloon tamponade and self-expanding stents

Balloon tamponade is effective for massive or refractory variceal bleeding but is only recommended as a 'bridge' to definitive treatment. If the rate of blood loss prohibits endoscopic evaluation, a Sengstaken–Blakemore tube (originally described in 1950) or a Minnesota tube (addition of an oesophageal aspiration port) can be inserted to provide temporary haemostasis (***Figure 69.14***).

Once inserted, the gastric balloon is inflated with 300 mL of air and retracted to the gastric fundus and the oesophagogastric varices tamponaded by inflation of the oesophageal balloon to 60 mmHg. The two remaining channels allow gastric and oesophageal aspiration, and the position of the tube is confirmed radiologically. A strict protocol for the management of balloon tamponade is important to avoid complications particularly oesophageal pressure necrosis.

Recently, self-expanding covered metal oesophageal stents have also been employed for the emergency treatment of oesophageal varices and results are equivalent to balloon tamponade unless the bleeding site is intragastric.

Robert William Sengstaken Sr, 1923–1978, neurosurgeon, Garden City, New York, NY, USA.
Arthur Blakemore, 1897–1970, surgeon, the Columbia College of Physicians and Surgeons, New York, NY, USA

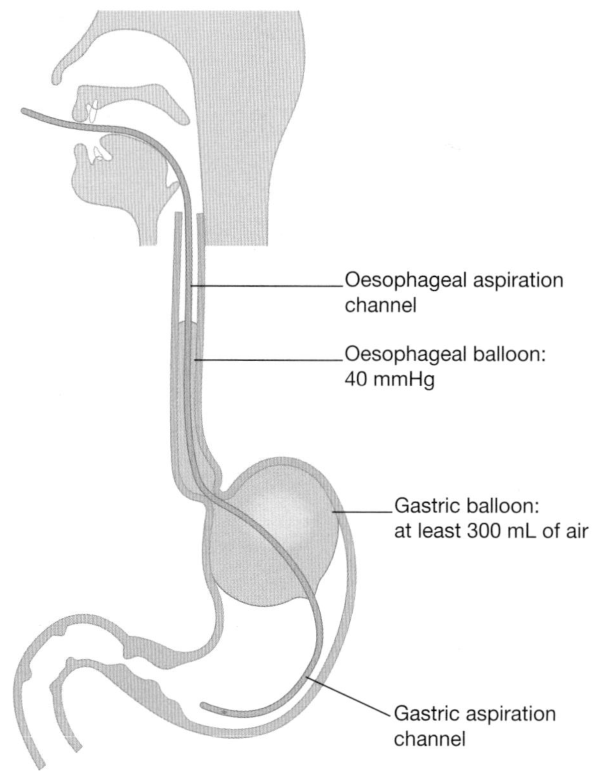

Figure 69.14 Oesophageal and gastric balloon tamponade with a Sengstaken–Blakemore or Minnesota tube. The tube must be carefully managed.

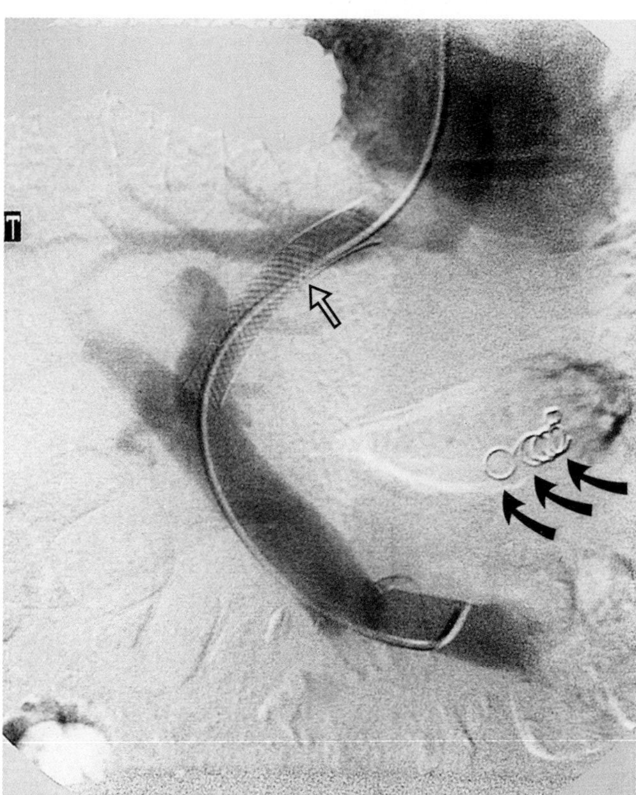

Figure 69.15 An angiogram following insertion of a transjugular intrahepatic portosystemic stent shunt (TIPSS) (open arrow). Contrast in the portal vein flows through the metallic stent and outlines the right hepatic vein. Pressure measurements are taken from within the portal vein before and after insertion. Solid arrows indicate coils placed at the site of previous embolisation.

Endoscopic treatment

The two most commonly used endoscopic techniques are endoscopic band ligation to the base of the varix and injection of a sclerosant into or around the varix. Following resuscitation, endoscopy is performed in a head-down position with good suction available. A double-channel endoscope with a bridge is essential to facilitate suction during injection and provide manoeuvrability of the needle, and power washers dramatically improve visualisation. Some time should be spent assessing the bleeding, confirming it is variceal and obtaining a stable position. When the bleeding varix or varices are identified only the source should be treated. Sclerotherapy or banding both achieve effective control with banding reducing rebleeding; a single treatment is usually sufficient.

Transjugular intrahepatic portosystemic stent shunts

The emergency management of variceal haemorrhage is extremely difficult when pharmacological and endoscopic therapies have failed. Treatment of these patients now relies on TIPSS, a radiological procedure first described in 1969 but not widely available until the development of endovascular stents in 1985. TIPSS has replaced surgical portocaval shunt and is now accepted as the preferred method for treating refractory portal hypertension. A TIPSS is inserted under local anaesthetic, analgesia and sedation using fluoroscopic guidance and ultrasonography. Via the internal jugular vein, superior vena cava and hepatic vein, a guidewire is inserted through the hepatic parenchyma into a branch of the portal vein. The tract is dilated; a metallic stent is then inserted and expanded, forming a portovenous channel (***Figure 69.15***). A satisfactory drop in portal venous pressure is usually associated with good control of the variceal haemorrhage. The main early complication is perforation of the liver capsule, with potentially fatal intraperitoneal haemorrhage. TIPSS occlusion may produce further variceal haemorrhage and occurs more commonly in patients with well-compensated liver disease and good synthetic function. The incidence of post-TIPSS encephalopathy is comparable to that following surgical shunts (40%) and due to portal blood avoiding hepatic detoxification, if severe, flow is reduced by inserting a smaller stent. The main contraindication to TIPSS is portal vein occlusion, and long-term stenosis occurs in 50% of patients at 1 year.

Surgical shunts

The increasing availability of liver transplantation and TIPSS has greatly reduced the indications for surgical portosystemic shunts, which, because of their high morbidity and mortality, are now rarely considered for variceal haemorrhage. The current indication is the failure of medical management in non-cirrhotic patients with extrahepatic portal vein occlusion. Surgical shunts effectively prevent rebleeding from oesophageal

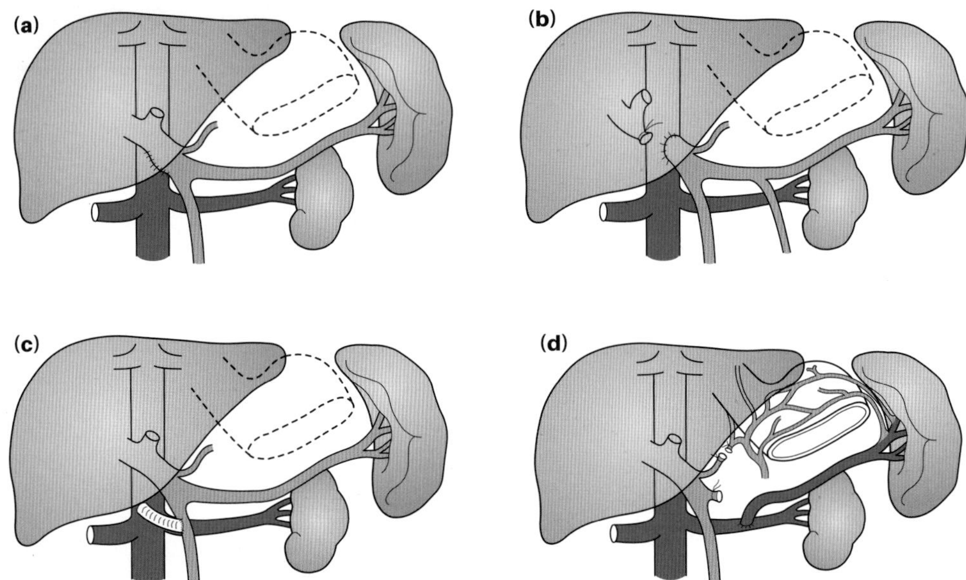

Figure 69.16 Surgical shunts for portal hypertension involve shunting portal blood into the systemic veins. This commonly involves a side-to-side portocaval anastomosis (a) or end-to-side portocaval (b), mesocaval 'H graft' (c) or splenorenal (d) anastomoses.

or gastric varices by reducing portal pressure and are divided into selective, splenorenal and non-selective portocaval. Selective shunts attempt to preserve hepatoportal blood flow while decompressing the left side of the portal circulation, which is responsible for oesophageal and gastric varices (*Figure 69.16*). Selective shunts have a lower incidence of encephalopathy but there is no evidence that prophylactic shunting is beneficial.

Recurrent or refractory variceal bleeding

Sugiura procedure

The Sugiura procedure for oesophageal varices combines splenectomy with oesophagogastric devascularisation, permanently interrupting the intraoesophageal portacaval shunt while preserving perioesophageal varices. The surgery is performed on the stomach wall and all venous tributaries are divided as for highly selective vagotomy except on both the lesser and greater curves. The upper half of the stomach and 8–10 cm of oesophagus are cleared (less than originally described but avoiding entering the chest). After devascularisation with careful preservation of the collateral channels and the vagus, a large oesophageal stapler is introduced into the lower oesophagus, which is transected just above the cardia.

Liver transplantation

Liver transplantation is the only therapy that treats portal hypertension and the underlying liver disease and may ultimately be required in patents with variceal bleeding. Previous surgical shunts increase the complexity and morbidity of orthotopic liver transplantation and TIPSS should be the preferred management (see *Chapter 89*).

Summary box 69.10

Management of bleeding oesophageal varices

- Blood transfusion
- Correct coagulopathy
- Oesophageal balloon tamponade (Sengstaken–Blakemore or Minnesota tube)
- Drug therapy (terlipressin)
- Endoscopic sclerotherapy or banding
- Assess portal vein patency (Doppler ultrasonography or CT)
- TIPSS
- Surgery
- Portosystemic shunts
- Splenectomy and gastric devascularisation
- Sugiura procedure

Ascites

Accumulation of ascites is a common feature of advanced liver disease irrespective of the aetiology. Development is usually insidious and fluid accumulation is associated with abdominal discomfort and a dragging sensation. CT will confirm the aetiology of the ascites and demonstrate the irregular, shrunken cirrhotic liver, associated portal hypertension and splenomegaly. Intravenous contrast will demonstrate abdominal varices and assess patency of the portal vein. Portal vein occlusion is a common finding and in non-cirrhotic patients malignancy is usually responsible. The protein content and amylase levels will exclude pancreatic ascites and determine the serum–ascites albumin gradient (SAAG), with a high gradient (>1.1 g/dL) indicating portal hypertension. Cytology may confirm the presence of malignant cells, and microscopy and culture will

Mitsuo Sugiura, 1925–1988, surgeon, University of Juntendo, Tokyo, Japan.

exclude primary bacterial and tuberculous peritonitis (see *Chapter 65*).

Summary box 69.11

Determining the cause of ascites

- Imaging, ultrasonography or CT
  - Irregular cirrhotic liver
  - Portal vein patency
  - Splenomegaly of cirrhosis
- Aspiration
  - Culture and microscopy
  - Protein content
  - Cytology
  - Amylase level

Management of ascites in chronic liver disease

The initial treatment is to restrict salt intake and commence diuretics (spironolactone or frusemide), together with advice on avoiding precipitating factors, including alcohol intake, infection and causes of hypoproteinaemia. Patients on diuretics require regular biochemical monitoring.

Summary box 69.12

Treatment of ascites in chronic liver disease

- Salt restriction
- Diuretics
- Abdominal paracentesis
- Peritoneovenous shunts
- TIPSS
- Liver transplantation

CHRONIC LIVER DISEASE

Several rare chronic liver conditions are important because they require a specific investigation plan and treatment and may imitate more common clinical conditions (*Table 69.6*).

TABLE 69.6 Important chronic liver conditions.

Condition	Common presentations
Primary sclerosing cholangitis	Abnormal LFTs, pruritus or jaundice
Primary biliary cirrhosis	Malaise, lethargy, pruritus, abnormal LFTs
Budd–Chiari syndrome	Ascites, pain, abdominal distension
Caroli's disease	Abdominal pain, sepsis, biliary obstruction
Simple liver cysts	Coincidental finding, pain, palpable mass
Polycystic liver disease	Hepatomegaly, pain

LFT, liver function test.

Primary sclerosing cholangitis

PSC is a chronic cholestatic liver disease of unknown aetiology, although a genetic predisposition is likely owing to its association with ulcerative colitis. It produces diffuse, progressive inflammation and fibrosis with structuring of the intra- and extrahepatic biliary tree and mainly affects young men in their thirties. The exact worldwide prevalence is unclear, but it appears to affect 1.5/100 000 men and 0.5/100 000 women.

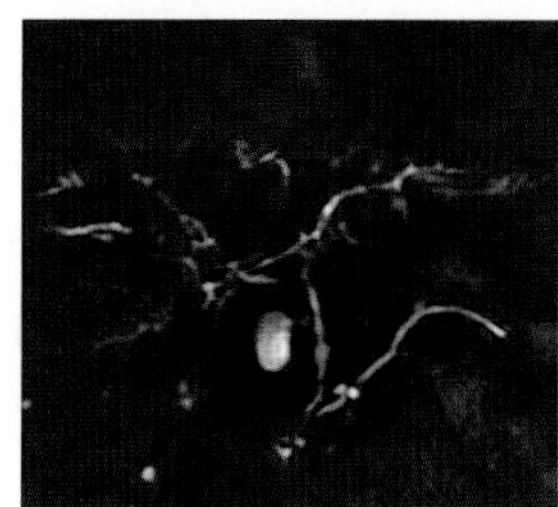

Figure 69.17 Typical appearance of primary sclerosing cholangitis with a 'beaded' appearance of the intrahepatic ducts and diffuse widespread strictures. The intrahepatic ducts usually do not dilate owing to the pathological process involving the whole of the biliary tract.

In patients with PSC and ulcerative colitis, the condition usually progresses even following colectomy. The diagnosis is principally based on the finding of irregular, narrowed bile ducts at cholangiography involving both the intra- and extrahepatic biliary tree (*Figure 69.17*), but if the radiological appearances are equivocal a liver biopsy is required. There is no specific treatment and patients usually progress inexorably with progressive cholestasis and fatal liver failure. Isolated areas of intrahepatic sclerosing cholangitis can occasionally be resected but diffuse disease usually requires liver transplantation. There is a strong predisposition to cholangiocarcinoma and gallbladder cancer, which should be considered when a new or dominant stricture is demonstrated on cholangiography or when gallbladder 'polyps' are identified.

The difficulty in the clinical setting is distinguishing sclerosing cholangitis from a malignant process, particularly multifocal cholangiocarcinoma. Imaging cannot reliably differentiate between inflammatory and malignant strictures and rarely demonstrates a mass lesion even in patients with advanced cholangiocarcinoma. Diagnosis often requires biliary brush cytology or direct endoscopic inspection (SpyGlass™). Serum cancer antigen (CA) 19-9 levels may be increased but the sensitivity of CA 19-9 in detecting cholangiocarcinoma in PSC is only 60%. Temporary relief of obstructive jaundice owing to a dominant bile duct stricture can be achieved by biliary stenting, although there is considerable risk of cholangitis. Patients with good liver function, no dominant strictures and negative biliary cytology are monitored for disease progression. Liver transplantation produces excellent results if performed before the development of malignancy.

Primary biliary cirrhosis

As with PSC, patients with primary biliary cirrhosis often present insidiously with malaise, lethargy and pruritus or abnormal liver function tests prior to becoming clinically jaundice. The condition is largely confined to females and the diagnosis is suggested by circulating anti-smooth muscle antibodies with/without liver biopsy. As the condition progresses liver function deteriorates, and portal hypertension, ascites and variceal bleeding may occur. The definitive treatment is liver transplantation when a normal lifestyle is not possible.

Non-alcoholic steatohepatitis, non-alcoholic fatty liver disease and chemotherapy-associated hepatitis

Non-alcoholic steatohepatitis (NASH) is the inflammatory subtype of non-alcoholic fatty liver disease (NAFLD) and is associated with disease progression, the development of cirrhosis and frequently the need for liver transplantation. NAFLD is now recognised as the most prevalent chronic liver disease worldwide and this is expected to increase 60% by 2030. Presently the prevalence of NAFLD is 25% and NASH 1.5–6%, with an estimated 20% of patients with NASH developing cirrhosis.

Some drugs may induce hepatotoxic lesions, such as steatosis or steatohepatitis found in NAFLD. Among these drugs there are some antitumoral molecules, such as methotrexate, 5-fluorouracil, irinotecan, tamoxifen and l-asparaginase. The hepatotoxic phenotype developed from treatment with such drugs is known as chemotherapy-associated, chemotherapy-induced acute steatohepatitis or chemotherapy-associated hepatitis (CASH). The parenchymal consequences of CASH are important surgically and must be considered when predicting future liver remnant (FLR) function.

Budd-Chiari syndrome

The Budd–Chiari syndrome affects 1/1 000 000 adults and is a collective term for conditions that impede hepatic venous outflow at any level from the small hepatic veins to the junction of the IVC with the right atrium. Cardiac and pericardial diseases and sinusoidal obstruction syndrome are excluded from this definition. It principally affects young women, who present the classic triad of abdominal pain, ascites and hepatomegaly. A hypercoagulable condition such as antithrombin 3, protein C or protein S deficiency is identified in 75% of patients, extrinsic compression in 25% and rarely congenital or acquired IVC webs.

The liver becomes acutely congested, with impaired liver function and portal hypertension; ascites and oesophageal varices develop. Fulminant hepatic failure may result from acute thrombosis but in the majority of cases abdominal discomfort and ascites are the main presenting features. If chronic, the liver progresses to established cirrhosis. Colour and pulsed Doppler ultrasonography and CT scanning together with detailed haematological studies will usually identify the cause. The diagnosis should be suspected in patients with ascites where a CT scan demonstrates a large, congested liver or cirrhosis with gross enlargement of the caudate lobe resulting from preservation and hypertrophy of the segment due to direct venous drainage to the IVC. Further IVC compression or occlusion and portal vein thrombosis are common consequences of caudate lobe hypertrophy.

Treatment of Budd–Chiari syndrome depends on the stage of disease at presentation and the specific findings in each patient. Fulminant liver failure, established cirrhosis and complications of portal hypertension may require liver transplantation. If the liver parenchyma is relatively normal TIPSS or a side-to-side portocaval shunt should be considered and IVC compression relieved by the insertion of a retrohepatic expandable metallic stent. With effective Budd–Chiari syndrome treatment prognosis depends on whether it is possible to treat the underlying pathology. Patients usually require lifelong anticoagulation.

Caroli's disease

Caroli's disease is a rare congenital dilatation of the intrahepatic biliary tree with an incidence of <1/100 000. It is often complicated by intrahepatic stone formation and presentation is usually with abdominal pain or sepsis. Imaging is diagnostic with ultrasonography or CT demonstrating intrahepatic biliary lakes containing stones which predispose to potentially life-threatening biliary sepsis. Acute infective episodes are treated with antibiotics and obstructed and infected bile ducts may be drained radiologically, endoscopically or surgically. Ductal dilatation is usually diffuse but if segmental may be treated by resection of the affected part. Cholangiocarcinoma is more common than for other forms of biliary ectasia and treatment by liver transplantation is described.

INFECTIVE CONDITIONS OF THE LIVER

Ascending cholangitis

Ascending cholangitis is a potentially life-threatening emergency associated with infection of the biliary tree and usually associated with obstruction. It presents with clinical jaundice, rigors and a tender right upper quadrant (Charcot's triad). The most common bacteria linked to ascending cholangitis are gram-negative bacilli: *Escherichia coli* (25–50%), *Klebsiella* (15–20%) and *Enterobacter* (5–10%). The diagnosis is confirmed by the finding of dilated bile ducts on ultrasonography, an obstructive picture of liver function tests and organisms identified from blood cultures. Delay in appropriate treatment may result in multiorgan failure secondary to sepsis and broad-spectrum antibiotics, rehydration, and endoscopic or percutaneous transhepatic drainage are urgently required. Biliary stone disease is a common predisposing factor although strictures, pancreatitis, pancreatic tumours and parasites may also be responsible. If an obstructive cause is identified it must be urgently treated by ERCP, sphincterotomy (± stent) or percutaneous drainage.

George Budd, 1808–1882, Professor of Medicine, King's College Hospital, London, UK.
Hans Chiari, 1851–1916, Austrian pathologist, later Professor at the University of Strasbourg, France.
Christian Johann Doppler, 1803–1853, Professor of Experimental Physics, Vienna, Austria, enunciated the 'Doppler principle' in 1842.
Jacques Caroli, 1902–1979, Professor of Medicine, Hôpital St Antoine, Paris, France, described the disease in 1958.
Jean-Martin Charcot, 1825–1893, French neurologist and Professor of Pathology, Hôpital Pitié-Salpêtrière, Paris, France.

Liver abscess

Microbial contamination of the liver leading to a liver abscess continues to occur at a fairly constant rate of approximately 1/5000 hospital admissions. The incidence of causative organisms varies and reflects changes in aetiology and geographical distribution. Bacterial, parasitic and fungal organisms can cause liver abscess but, worldwide, bacteria remain the most common; although infection is usually polymicrobial *Klebsiella*, *Escherichia coli* and the *Streptococcus milleri* group are the usual organisms identified.

There is an increased incidence in the elderly, those with diabetes and the immunosuppressed and presentation is usually with anorexia, fever, malaise and right upper quadrant discomfort. The overall mortality has declined because of improved imaging and effective antimicrobial therapy and the outcome is increasingly dependent on the underlying cause and the presence of comorbidities.

Biliary tract pathology is the most common source (35%), followed by portal spread from the gastrointestinal tract, including diverticulitis and appendicitis (20%). Other unusual aetiologies include contiguous spread from subphrenic or intra-abdominal collections, bacteraemia secondary to trauma or infected cysts and necrotic tumours following chemotherapy. The cause is not identified in 10% of cases and a number of liver abscesses become recurrent (12–38% depending on whether the responsible organism is identified and whether the patient has diabetes). The diagnosis is suggested by the finding of a multiloculated cystic mass on ultrasonography or CT scan (***Figure 69.18***) and is confirmed by aspiration.

Treatment of liver abscesses initially requires identification of the source, if possible, aspiration of the lesion for microbiology and culture (repeated aspirations may be required) and treatment with appropriate antibiotics. Simple cysts containing debris, hydatid cysts, necrotic tumours and non-infected haematomas (after unrecognised or occasional trivial trauma) can all be mistaken for abscesses. Antibiotic treatment using a combination of two or more antibiotics is recommended. Metronidazole and clindamycin provide wide anaerobic coverage and excellent penetration into the abscess cavity. Third-generation cephalosporins and aminoglycosides are very effective against most Gram-negative organisms.

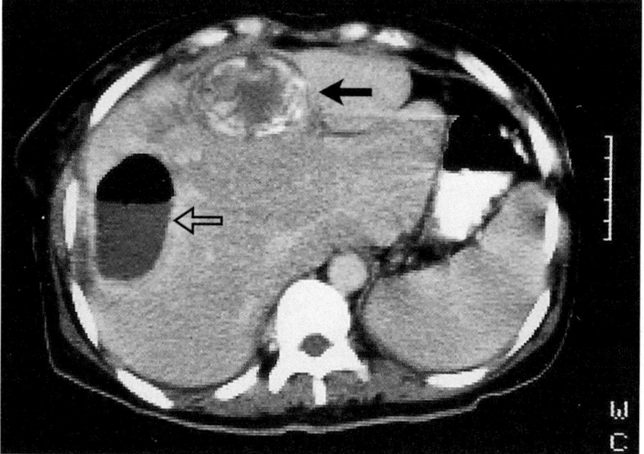

Figure 69.18 Liver abscess. Computed tomography scan showing an air–fluid level and rim enhancement (open arrow). The second lesion seen is a haemangioma (closed arrow).

Recurrent or refractory abscesses

Recurrent abscesses usually occur when the initial lesion was large, abscesses were multiple or there is continued communication with the biliary tract. It can be difficult to confirm whether a liver abscess is recurrent or new, but it is important as treatment differs. Recurrent lesions which were aspirated and treated with antibiotics can be re-aspirated, but a drain is often required. Refractory lesions should have microbiology repeated and a drain inserted, and recurrences are rare if left until resolution is complete. If unsuccessful occasionally surgery is required, and laparoscopy which allows a full examination of the peritoneal cavity (especially valuable when the source has not been identified) has replaced laparotomy.

Parasitic diseases of the liver

The liver is frequently affected by parasitic infections, which, owing to the worldwide prevalence of these organisms, are responsible for considerable morbidity and mortality (see ***Chapter 6***).

Hydatid disease

Human echinococcosis (hydatidosis, hydatid disease) is a parasitic disease caused by the larval stages of cestodes (tapeworms) of the genus *Echinococcus*. Medical treatment and diagnosis are discussed in ***Chapter 6***. Surgical intervention is occasionally required when medical management fails, and options range from liver resection or local excision of the cysts to deroofing with evacuation of the contents. Contamination of the peritoneal cavity at the time of surgery with active hydatid daughters should be avoided by continuing drug therapy with albendazole and adding preoperative praziquantel. This should be combined with packing of the peritoneal cavity with 20% hypertonic saline-soaked packs and instilling 20% hypertonic saline into the cyst before it is opened. A biliary communication should be actively sought and sutured. Infection and

Summary box 69.13

Infections of the liver

- Pyogenic liver abscesses 1/5000 admissions
- Worldwide billions of people have parasitic infections
- Parasitic infections cause live abscess and biliary tract damage
- Biliary tract involvement predisposes to cholangiocarcinoma
- Parasitic infections mimic pyogenic abscesses
- Obstructive jaundice from calcified flukes or involvement of the biliary tract

Theodor Albrecht Edwin Klebs, 1834–1913, Professor of Bacteriology successively at Prague, Czechoslovakia, Zurich, Switzerland, and the Rush Medical College, Chicago, IL, USA.

bile leaks can be reduced by packing the space with pedicled greater omentum (an omentoplasty). Calcified cysts may be dead; however, if doubt exists as to whether a suspected cyst is active, it can be followed on ultrasonography as active cysts gradually enlarge and become more superficial.

LIVER TUMOURS

Liver resection continues to evolve, and the safety has been established with a mortality of 1–2% and a 5-year survival following resection of colorectal metastases of 50%. Early surgical approaches involved a formal left or right hepatectomy and the presence of bilobar disease or more than three or four metastases were considered inoperable. Advances in surgery and anaesthesia, including combinations of staged procedures, portal vein embolisation (PVE), ablation and local resections, increased the number of potentially curative procedures. Concurrent progress in oncology has increased the ability of chemotherapy to 'downstage' disease sufficiently to operable lesions that would have been formerly considered inoperable.

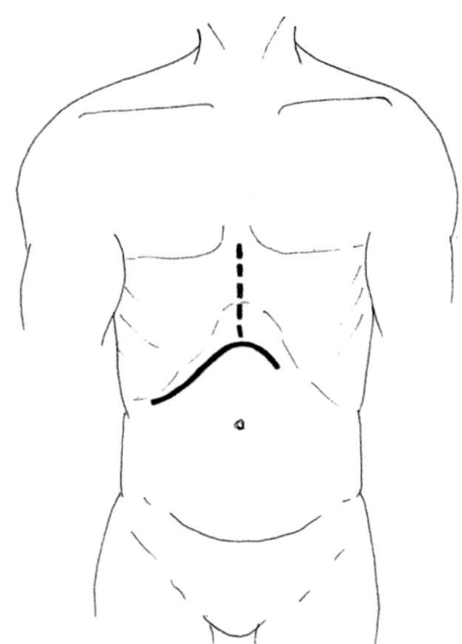

Figure 69.19 Access for liver surgery. Rooftop incision with optional vertical extension.

Surgical approaches to resection of liver tumours

Parenchyma-preserving resections that achieve adequate oncological clearance have emerged from an understanding of oncological principles and the impact of chemotherapy on hepatic function. Such resections preserve functioning liver volume, improving postoperative recovery, reducing morbidity and facilitating re-do surgery for recurrent metastases. Limited extrahepatic disease is also no longer an absolute contraindication and pulmonary and adrenal metastases and contiguous portal vein lymph nodes are increasingly resected.

Mobilisation of the liver

Incision

A roof top incision is performed 2–3 cm below the costal margin (***Figure 69.19***) with a vertical extension (Mercedes-Benz) if required. Fixed retraction under the ribs provides adequate access and thoracoabdominal incisions are no longer required. If doubt exists about operability a small right subcostal incision is used initially, and a thorough examination performed, including the caudate lobe. Intraoperative ultrasonography (IUS) is the standard of care for hepatobiliary surgery and is used with bimanual palpation to assess the extent of the tumour(s). IUS detects only an additional 10% compared with palpation alone.

The hepatic pedicle

Hilar dissection

Having determined that tumour does not directly involve the hilar structures a standard cholecystectomy is performed. The CBD is identified in the free edge of the lesser omentum, facilitated by following the cystic duct to its junction, dissected free and slung. The tissue in the right free border of the hepatoduodenal ligament is dissected and removed by ligation and division to avoid lymphatic leaks and the portal vein identified and slung. Developing the plane anterior to the vein allows the bile duct and artery to be mobilised forwards and the bifurcation of the vein to be identified (the branch to the side to be retained must be clearly identified). At this point anterior tissue (the hilar plate) should be freed from the base of the liver, lowering the structures that bifurcate. The artery and duct are separated at the bifurcation and slung just below it. The vascular anatomy is then confirmed, and the possibility of a replaced right hepatic artery arising from the superior mesenteric artery and lying posterior to the bile duct (25% of people) and an accessory left hepatic artery from the left gastric artery in the lesser omentum (25% of people) considered. Hilar arterial and biliary anatomy in the hepatoduodenal ligament and at the hilum is so variable that careful dissection is required even if the pattern appears to be one of the recognised variants. A standard approach is important in the event of unexpected intraoperative findings. The approach to the hilum allows different conditions and pathologies to be approached with confidence, including formal resections (metastases and primary liver tumours), hilar cholangiocarcinoma, bile duct injuries and penetrating trauma.

Methods of parenchymal transection

An array of techniques and technologies have been developed to aid parenchymal dissection by facilitating identification of vascular and biliary structures to enable accurate diathermy, ligation or clipping. They also allow safe resection with adequate clearance of centrally placed tumours near the confluence of the hepatic veins and the IVC or the inflow sheaths. Safe transection with minimal blood loss and an adequate tumour clearance can be achieved using a crushing clamp, cavitating

The Mercedes-Benz sign takes its name from the insignia displayed on the bonnet of a Mercedes-Benz car.

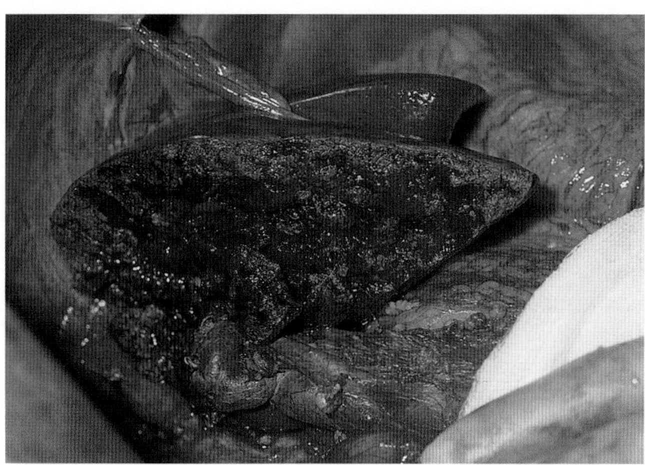

Figure 69.20 Hepatectomy post resection. Cut surface of the residual liver following a right hepatectomy in which segments V–VIII have been removed. On the lower edge, the portal vein and bile duct can be seen.

ultrasonic suction and aspiration (CUSA), harmonic scalpel or radiofrequency ablation (RFA) and is a matter of personal preference with no evidence that any method is superior (***Figure 69.20***). Hepatic veins and the Glissonian sheath are now routinely stapled with an endoscopic vascular stapler.

The parenchyma is divided after diathermy of the liver capsule along the plane of demarcation 5 mm into the devascularised liver. As the parenchyma is divided, vessels and bile ducts are diathermised, clipped or ligated depending on their size. The hepatic veins can be divided outside the liver at the time of mobilisation or parenchymal dissection continued until they are encountered, when they are ligated or stapled then divided.

Resection options

Segmental resections

Hepatic resection traditionally involved the formal removal of the right (segments V–VIII) or left (segments II–IV with/without I) hemiliver to ensure the largest possible clearance. Although anatomical resection remains the treatment of choice for patients with HCC, a parenchyma-sparing non-anatomical approach involving multiple segmentectomies and/or metastectomies is now the standard of care for colorectal liver metastasis (***Figure 69.21***).

Staged procedures

Extensive resection of the liver in two stages was first described in 1965. The aim is to 'clear' one lobe of the liver of all known disease followed 4–6 weeks later by a formal major resection to clear all residual disease. Staged resections are usually only possible if the left side can be cleared first by local resections, something that is usually not possible on the right because of the need to remove as little normal parenchyma as possible to avoid stimulating too much regeneration. The stimulus for regeneration following resection of too much liver may accelerate growth of the tumour, which despite chemotherapy may become inoperable.

ALPPS procedure for extended liver resections

'ALPPS' stands for Associating Liver Partition and Portal vein Ligation for Staged hepatectomy and was first described in 2011. It is the most recent modification of techniques developed to facilitate two-stage hepatectomies for resection of widespread or extensive liver tumours and employs the remarkable capacity of the liver to regenerate. ALPPS involves two stages. Initially the right portal vein is ligated and, depending on the distribution of the tumour within the liver, transection is performed as for a formal hemihepatectomy or left lateral segmentectomy (*in situ* splitting). In contrast to a classical hepatectomy, the liver containing the tumour(s) is left *in situ* and remains vascularised by the right hepatic artery and the biliary and systemic venous drainage, represented by the right bile duct and hepatic veins, preserved. The second stage of the procedure is performed 1–2 weeks after the first stage following CT demonstration of adequate hypertrophy; the involved liver is resected after division of the right hepatic artery, bile duct and hepatic vein. Initially ALPPS was associated with significant morbidity and mortality but modifications of the technique, particularly a reduction in the amount of liver transected, improved results.

Portal vein embolisation

Preoperative PVE induces hypertrophy of one side of the liver prior to a planned resection of the other side. The procedure

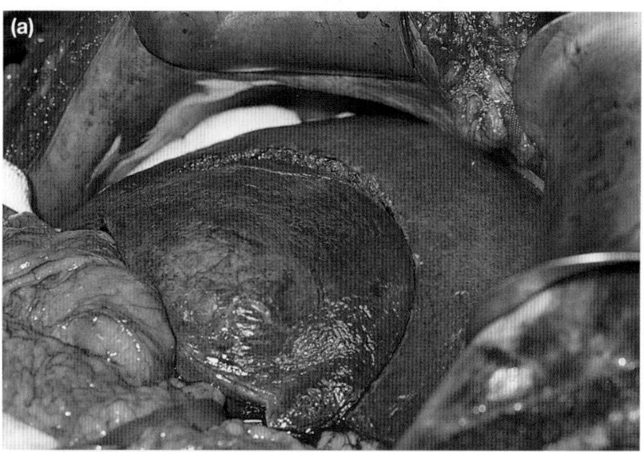

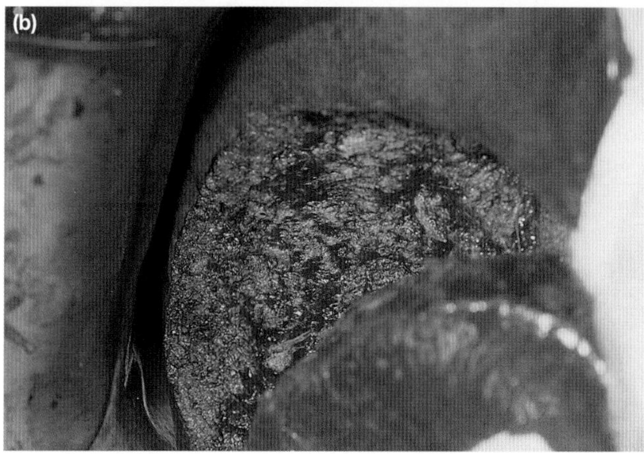

Figure 69.21 (a, b) Segmental resection. Removal of a primary liver tumour by resection of liver segment VI in a patient with well-compensated liver cirrhosis.

is frequently used for HCC and colorectal liver metastases and was first described by Makuuchi in 1984 before an extended hepatectomy for bile duct carcinoma. Several techniques for PVE have been reported, including intraoperative ligation, transileocolic PVE and the percutaneous transhepatic ipsilateral or contralateral PVE techniques. The underlying principle is to block the portal venous blood flow to the liver segments that require resection. This induces atrophy of the ipsilateral liver segments and compensatory hypertrophy of the contralateral liver segments, resulting in an increase in the size of the proposed FLR. In addition to the different techniques, different embolisation materials are used, including polyvinyl alcohol particles, coils, gelatin sponge, *n*-butyl cyanoacrylate and lipiodol, or fibrin glue. Indications for PVE depend on the ratio of the proposed FLR to total estimated liver volume (TELV) and the condition of the liver. There is no clear consensus about the volume required for adequate postresection liver function but an FLR/TELV ratio of at least 25% is recommended with a normal liver and 40% in the presence of cirrhosis. Patients who have received extensive chemotherapy with an FLR/TELV ratio less than 30% should also receive PVE prior to resection.

Laparoscopic liver resections

The development of laparoscopic liver resection (LLR) following its first performance in the USA in 1991 for a benign tumour on the edge of the liver has been one of the most impressive in the field of hepatobiliary surgery. Technical innovation has made LLR a safe and effective procedure with significantly improved postoperative recovery. The potential advantages of LLR mean that it is gradually replacing conventional open liver resection. Indications have expanded from local resections to include major liver resection, isolated resection of the caudate lobe, living donor liver resection and ALPPS. For some procedures such as laparoscopic local resection and left lateral segmentectomy LLR is the approach of choice and formal hepatectomies are now routinely performed laparoscopically in high-volume centres.

Robotic surgery

With the safe and effective development of laparoscopic liver surgery, robotic surgery, which obviates some of the technical issues, was welcomed and the first robotic liver resection was performed in 2007 for a 2.4-cm HCC. Indications for robotic surgery will expand but are presently limited by cost, time constraints, the lengthy learning curve, the lack of haptic feedback and the availability of dedicated instruments for parenchymal transection (see ***Chapter 10***).

Blood loss and transfusion

The reduction of blood loss during liver surgery has developed such that resection is often possible without blood transfusion. Better understanding of the segmental anatomy of the liver and patient selection, low central venous pressure anaesthesia and the routine availability of thromboelastography has facilitated better control of the coagulation cascade and significantly reduced bleeding in patients with liver disease and underlying coagulopathies.

The Pringle manoeuvre can reduce blood loss during parenchymal transection and improves the effectiveness of other techniques used to treat oozing from the resected surface of the remnant liver. These include the topical application of fibrin glue or fibrin-impregnated collagen fleece and non-contact electrosurgical technique such as argon plasma coagulation.

Ablation for liver tumours

Ablative therapies destroy tumour by the direct application of energy or toxic substances to discrete lesions. The basic technique for RFA was described in 1891 by d'Arsonval, who first demonstrated that heat was produced when radiofrequency waves passed through tissue. Ablation techniques now include RFA, microwave ablation, cryoablation, laser ablation, irreversible electroporation (IRE) and alcohol injection, all of which can be performed percutaneously, laparoscopically or at open surgery. There is wide variation in overall survival and local recurrence rates following ablation and surgery remains the gold standard treatment for resectable disease. Despite these concerns, ablation still has a role as an adjunct to resection and for combined approaches. Patients with small-volume resectable lesions who are not sufficiently fit to undergo liver resection should be considered for ablation, as should those with liver metastases where predicted FLR precludes resection.

RFA and microwave ablation, which rely on the generation of heat, are the most widely used techniques. Increasing lesion size exponentially increases impedance, limiting the size of the effective ablation zone and increasing the risk of local recurrence. Microwave ablation has been designed to overcome these issues with higher intratumoral temperatures, larger tumour ablation volumes and faster ablation times. Newer microwave technologies include the use of cooled applicators and multiple antennae, such that tumours adjacent to large vascular structures can be effectively treated. Local recurrence after RFA and microwave ablation is 5–15%.

Benign tumours

A number of pathologies produce focal liver lesions, and the three most common benign hepatic tumours are haemangiomas, focal nodular hyperplasia (FNH) and hepatic adenomas. These lesions are common and often discovered incidentally on cross-sectional imaging. The main clinical challenge is confirming the benign nature non-invasively where possible.

Hepatic adenoma

Adenomas are benign liver tumours seen almost exclusively in women aged between 25 and 50 years. These well-defined and vascular lesions are classically associated with use of the oral

---

Masatoshi Makuuchi, b. 1946, surgeon, Koto Hospital, Tokyo, Japan. In 1990 described preoperative portal embolisation to increase the safety of major hepatectomy for hilar bile duct carcinoma.
Jacques-Arsène d'Arsonval, 1851–1940, physician and physicist, Collège de France, Paris, France.

contraceptive pill and are generally solitary. The majority are found incidentally on imaging, although up to one-third may present with pain because of rupture or bleeding. Adenomas are recognised as having malignant potential, with up to 10% developing into HCC. The risk of rupture and malignancy means that surgical excision is generally recommended if >5 cm in size, although some lesions may regress after discontinuation of the oral contraceptive pill.

Focal nodular hyperplasia

FNH is an unusual but not uncommon benign condition of unknown aetiology, in which there is a focal overgrowth of functioning liver tissue supported by fibrous stroma. Patients are usually middle-aged women, and there is no association with underlying liver disease. Ultrasonography shows a solid tumour mass. Contrast CT or MRI may show central scarring and a hypervascular lesion. FNH contains both hepatocytes and Kupffer cells. MRI using liver-specific contrast agents may be useful in determining the hepatocellular origin of FNH and allowing differentiation of FNH from metastatic cancer. FNH does not have any malignant potential and, once the diagnosis is confirmed, does not require any treatment or follow-up.

Haemangiomas

These are the most common benign liver lesions, and the reported incidence has increased with the widespread availability of diagnostic ultrasonography. They consist of an abnormal plexus of vessels, and their nature is usually apparent on ultrasonography. If diagnostic uncertainty exists, CT scanning with delayed contrast enhancement shows the characteristic appearance of slow contrast enhancement owing to small vessel uptake in the haemangioma. Often, haemangiomas are multiple. Lesions found incidentally require radiological confirmation of their nature and no further treatment. Diagnosis is usually incidental, and surgical resection is only recommended if patients are significantly symptomatic or significant diagnostic uncertainty remains after multimodal imaging.

Biopsy of liver lesions

Liver biopsy is generally considered a safe procedure but is not without risk of mechanical complications, which although minor (pain and subcapsular or intrahepatic haematoma) occur in 6–25% of patients. Significant complications, including bile leak, sepsis, pancreatitis, local infections or pneumothorax, occur in 0.25% and haemobilia in 0.05% of cases. Mortality specifically related to liver biopsy is mainly caused by haemorrhage and varies from 0.1% to 0.3%.

Lesions found within the liver that are likely to be malignant will need resection; if surgery is possible then FNA or true cut biopsy should not be performed. Biopsy of malignant liver lesions results in poorer long-term survival following resection and confers no diagnostic advantage over non-invasive imaging and tumour markers. Needle tract seeding also occurs (1000–100 000 cells/tract) or peritoneal spread, particularly with HCC.

Summary box 69.14

Benign liver lesions

- May present with symptoms or be found incidentally on imaging for another condition
- Significant symptoms (pain or pressure effects) justify surgery
- If imaging is equivocal biopsy may be necessary to exclude a primary or metastatic lesion
- If observation for 3–6 months demonstrates a stable lesion malignancy is unlikely

Cystic lesions

Simple liver cysts

Simple cysts of the liver are usually asymptomatic and were thought to be uncommon before the routine use of ultrasonography. The exact prevalence and incidence are not known but they are estimated to occur in 5% of the population with 10–15% presenting because of symptoms. Fortunately, their appearance on ultrasonography and MRI scanning generally allows them to be dismissed; confusion usually only occurs when CT scanning was the initial investigation. Cysts are more common in females (1.5:1) and are larger in patients over 50 years of age. The situation is different for very large symptomatic or complex cysts, which are 10 times more common in women, and huge cysts requiring treatment in men are rare. Most cysts only cause problems and require treatment when they increase in size or become complex or infected. Prior to treatment it is important to exclude other causes, particularly parasitic infections.

Polycystic liver disease

Multiple liver cysts are frequently associated with adult polycystic kidney disease (PKD) but may occur alone. PLD is a term for a heterogeneous group of patients; it is an inherited disorder estimated to affect around 1 in 100 000 people and 10% have cerebral aneurysms. It is characterised by the progressive growth of cysts of various sizes that are widely and randomly distributed throughout the liver. In many patients the cysts are asymptomatic but when extensive they produce mechanical symptoms from stretching of the liver capsule, pressure effects on the stomach when the left side is involved and gross abdominal distension related to the large increase in the size of the liver. Cysts can become infected, but this normally follows ill-advised aspiration of what is felt to be a symptomatic cyst. Biliary obstruction occurs as a result of distortion or compression and must be treated endoscopically as there is no surgical option. Surgical treatment is usually employed for bulk reduction or a mechanical problem and, when planning surgery, it is important to remember that biliary radicals and vessels run between cysts and are difficult to differentiate from the wall.

Hepatic cystadenomas and cystadenocarcinomas

The prevalence of hepatic cystadenomas is low, with fewer than 200 cases reported. Of the two types, cystadenomas with mesenchymal (ovarian-like) stroma occur only in females and cystadenomas without mesenchymal stroma predominate in men.

Cystadenomas are often multilocular, septated, non-calcified and surrounded by compressed liver tissue. Upper abdominal pain and an abdominal mass can occur, but patients are usually asymptomatic. Cystadenomas are slow growing but have malignant potential and must be distinguished from simple hepatic cysts, polycystic liver disease, hydatid cysts and complex non-neoplastic cystic lesions. Serum and cyst fluid CA 19-9 levels may be elevated in cases of cystadenoma with mesenchymal stroma, but serum carcinoembryonic antigen (CEA) is unhelpful although it may be raised in cyst fluid. Cyst fluid cytology is unreliable.

Ultrasonography may demonstrate an anechoic mass with internal septations. CT scanning generally demonstrates the multilocular nature with internal septations. In the contrast phase, the wall of the cyst enhances and nodules may be seen. MRI also demonstrates septations and a hyperintense signal on T2-weighted images. The risk of recurrence and the potential for malignant transformation mandates complete anatomical resection. If the lesions are technically irresectable or cannot be separated from major venous or arterial structures liver transplantation may be required. Biliary cystadenocarcinomas account for 0.4% of malignant epithelial hepatic lesions.

Malignant liver tumours

Neuroendocrine/carcinoid tumours

Carcinoids are the most common NETs affecting men and women equally. The overall incidence is steadily increasing, estimated at 1.5–1.9 clinical cases per 100 000 population, although in autopsy series this reaches 650/100 000 population. Primary carcinoid tumours in the liver are rare and hepatic lesions are almost invariably metastases from small bowel or colon. Approximately 20% of small intestine carcinoids develop metastases and 30% of these patients develop carcinoid syndrome.

If the primary has been resected, liver metastases can be observed unless carcinoid syndrome develops. Hepatic carcinoid disease that is resectable should be treated but this must be preceded by a thin-slice CT scan and laparoscopy with intraoperative ultrasonography if doubt remains to exclude small-volume disease. Carcinoid syndrome is a difficult clinical problem, especially when pharmacological approaches are ineffective; in these patients, debulking should be considered. Some patients will develop a small number of lesions of similar sizes that can often be resected with curative intent. A significant proportion will develop recurrence(s), but this may take 18–36 months and further surgery is often possible. When lesions are numerous and of different generations (sizes) there are no surgical options and ablative, transarterial embolisation or targeted treatment with somatostatin analogues should be considered.

Hepatocellular carcinoma

HCC is a malignant tumour arising from hepatocytes and is the most common primary liver cancer. There is a steadily rising global burden. In 2016 there were 1 million incident cases of liver cancer globally and 829 000 deaths. It ranks as the fifth most common cause of cancer in men and the seventh in women, representing a third of all cancer-related deaths. HCC is the leading cause of death in patients with cirrhosis, affecting three times more men than women.

There is wide variation in geographical incidence. More than 80% of cases occur in Asia and sub-Saharan Africa, with an incidence of 99/100 000 compared with 5/100 000 in Europe. Geographical variation reflects the incidence of aetiological factors. Chronic hepatitis B virus (HBV) infection accounts for >50% of cases worldwide and HBV vaccination programmes reduce the incidence in high-risk areas. Hepatitis C virus (HCV) increases the risk of HCC 17-fold by promoting end-stage liver disease. Aflatoxin contamination of rice in some parts of the world is probably responsible for seasonal variations. Lifetime alcohol exposure remains an intractable risk factor and correlates with the incidence of HCC. Obesity and diabetes mellitus are additional independent risk factors.

Cancer-related causes are fatal in 60% of patients and 40% die of underlying parenchymal disease. HCC is typically diagnosed at a late stage and prognosis even in developed countries is limited with median survivals following diagnosis of 6–20 months and overall survival of less than 50% at 2 years and 10% at 5 years, with worse results in developing countries.

Staging of hepatocellular carcinoma

Clinical staging systems for HCC are designed to guide management. The Barcelona Clinic Liver Group (BCLC) staging system, initially designed to define both prognosis and optimal treatment for patients with HCC, is the most commonly used (***Figure 69.22***). As patients with HCC usually have underlying liver disease that has a marked impact on prognosis, the BCLC system was designed to reflect underlying liver function and performance status together with tumour characteristics. Underlying liver function is assessed using the CTP system.

Treatment of hepatocellular carcinoma

Surgical resection for hepatocellular carcinoma

Only 20–40% of patients with HCC are candidates for surgery, but with surveillance programmes in at-risk patients, improved imaging and advances in perioperative management resection is increasingly possible. Selecting suitable patients remains controversial and although tumour size, vascular invasion and multifocal disease are poor prognostic indicators they are not absolute contraindications. Multinodular lesions may represent multiple discrete lesions occurring independently against a background of procarcinogenic parenchymal damage or aggressive tumour biology with intrahepatic metastases. Oncological contraindications include extrahepatic metastasis, multiple/bilobar tumours, main bile duct involvement and tumour thrombus in the main portal vein/vena cava.

Preoperative evaluation of patients with hepatocellular carcinoma

Achieving good outcomes for patients undergoing surgical resection requires accurate assessment of tumour stage, comorbidities and liver function. This is particularly important

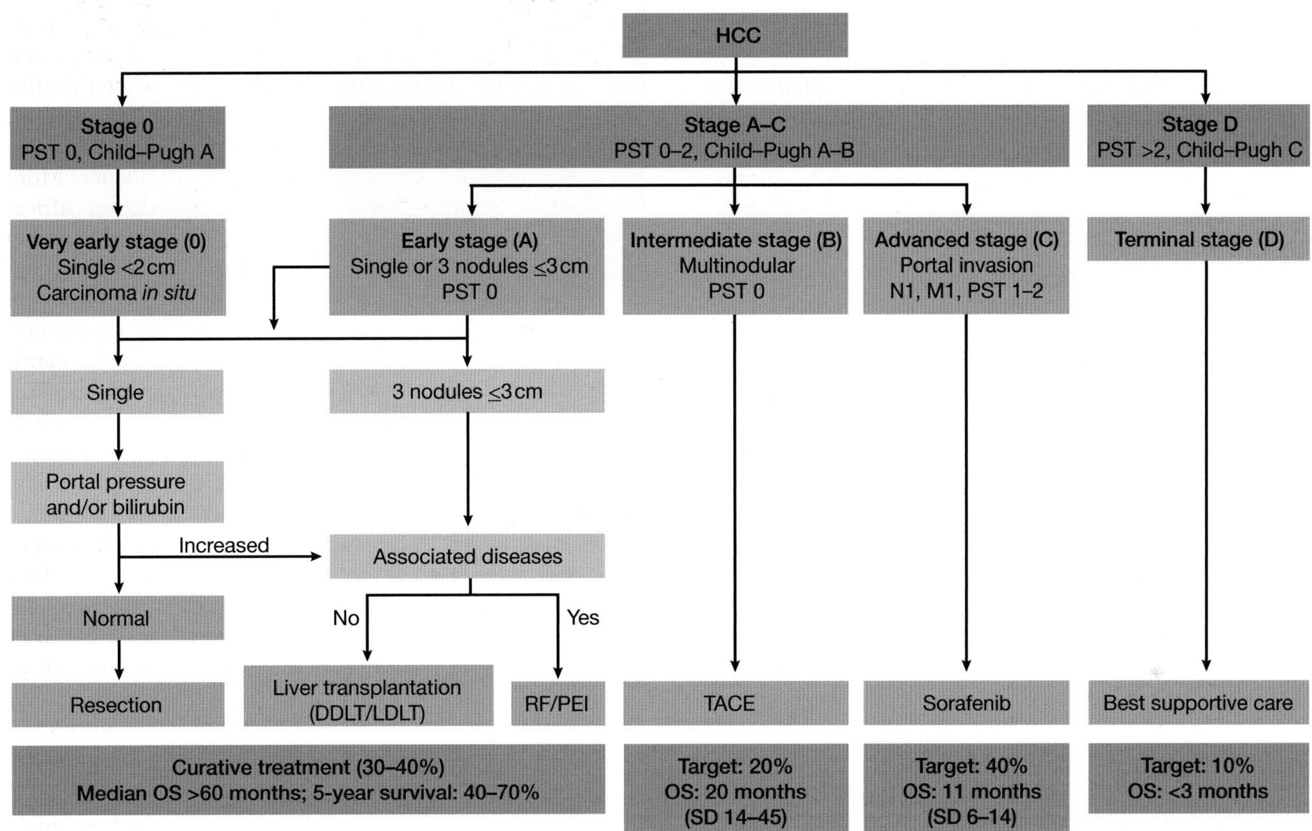

Figure 69.22 The Barcelona Clinic Liver Group staging system for the management of hepatocellular carcinoma (HCC). Patients with asymptomatic early tumours (stage 0–A) are candidates for curative therapies (resection, transplantation or local ablation). Asymptomatic patients with multinodular HCC (stage B) are suitable for chemoembolisation (TACE), whereas patients with advanced symptomatic tumours and/or an invasive tumoral pattern (stage C) are candidates for sorafenib. End-stage disease (stage D) includes patients with grim prognosis who should be treated by best supportive care. DDLT, deceased donor liver transplantation; LDLT, living donor liver transplantation; OS, overall survival; PEI, percutaneous ethanol injection; PST, ECOG performance status; RF, radiofrequency ablation; SD, standard deviation; TACE, transcatheter arterial chemoembolisation. (Reproduced with permission from Villanueva A. Medical therapies for hepatocellular carcinoma: a critical view of the evidence. *Nat Rev Gastroenterol Hepatol* 2013; **10**: 34–42.)

when planning larger resections, where the function of the FLR becomes critical. Postoperative morbidity and mortality increase with higher CTP scores, and major liver resection is usually only possible in patients with CTP-A disease. Minor liver resection may be considered in those with CTP-B disease but remains a high-risk procedure, and CTP-C patients are not candidates for liver resection. If inadequate FLR is the only contraindication preoperative radiological PVE should be performed.

Preoperative imaging for hepatocellular carcinoma

Imaging is a critical part of the preoperative assessment of HCC and accurate tumour staging and anatomical assessment is essential to determine technical and oncological resectability and exclude metastatic disease. Triple-phase CT chest/abdomen/pelvis and MRI of the liver is the standard of care, although MRI and CT have limited sensitivity and specificity for lesions <1 cm (improved with liver-specific contrast agents). FDG-PET does not appear to confer any benefit over standard imaging.

Surgical principles for hepatocellular carcinoma

Surgical resection is a compromise requiring resection of the tumour while preserving sufficient functional parenchyma. HCC spreads within the liver by direct invasion of portal and hepatic venous systems. Anatomical resections that include removal of the entire venous drainage of a tumour, including occult micrometastases, is the optimal approach. There are clear long-term survival benefits for anatomical versus non-anatomical resections, with anatomical resection now considered the standard of care when underlying liver function allows. Improvements in patient selection and surgical technique have reduced the 30-day mortality to <5%.

Disease recurrence after resection

Intrahepatic recurrence occurs in 80% of cases within 5 years and neoadjuvant or adjuvant options do not reduce the risk. Intrahepatic recurrence is thought to result from missed micrometastases or the development of new lesions and the most effective approach to reducing intrahepatic recurrence is liver transplantation.

Liver transplantation

Liver transplantation that definitively treats the tumour and underlying cirrhosis represents an attractive option, but organ shortages mandate careful selection of patients and early experience with transplantation was disappointing. Transplantation for HCC, first described by Mazzaferro in 1996 for patients with tumours ≤5 cm or up to three nodules ≤3 cm, achieved 4-year overall survivals of 75% and recurrence-free survivals of 83%. These inclusion criteria were adopted as the Milan criteria, with angioinvasion and extrahepatic involvement as additional exclusion criteria, and are now universally accepted. Liver transplantation criteria, however, continue to evolve and 'expanded' criteria remain debated. Locoregional therapies such as ablation may downstage HCC from beyond to within the Milan criteria and following a period of observation these patients may be considered as candidates for transplantation.

Intrahepatic cholangiocarcinoma

Cholangiocarcinomas develop in the bile duct and demonstrate considerable variation in origin, behaviour and pathophysiology. Twenty per cent of cholangiocarcinomas are intrahepatic (ICC), representing 5–30% of primary liver tumours, which is second only to HCC. They are rare in the West with an incidence of 0.5–2/100 000, although the incidence is increasing and is significantly higher in South East Asia, where *Clonorchis sinensis* infection is endemic, and in Thailand the rate is 60/100 000. There are three morphological subtypes – infiltrating periductal (***Figure 69.23a***), mass-forming (***Figure 69.23b***) and intraductal – and ICC is now considered to have multiple cellular origins. Ultrasonography will confirm intrahepatic biliary obstruction and MRCP is preferred for diagnosis. ERCP will delineate tumour extent and with brush cytology or SpyGlass™ can achieve pathological confirmation of malignancy.

ICC was originally staged with HCC but is now classified separately. Prognostic pathological features include vascular invasion, tumour multiplicity, local extension, periductal infiltration and lymph node metastasis. CT scanning is the best staging modality to identify distant metastases and confirm that the lesion is primary and not metastatic. Angiography is sometimes required preoperatively to assess vascular involvement. The sensitivity and specificity of PET-CT for diagnosis of cholangiocarcinoma varies by location, being higher for intrahepatic (>90%) than for extrahepatic (60%) tumours, although detection rates for distant metastases approach 100%.

ICC is an aggressive tumour and, even when confined to the liver, only 30% of patients are suitable for resection at the time of presentation. If surgical resection is considered, biopsy should be avoided; in borderline cases diagnostic laparoscopy and intraoperative ultrasonography will exclude additional hepatic or peritoneal disease. Lymph node status (porta hepatis, common hepatic artery and the gastroduodenal ligament) remains an important prognostic factor and should be sampled. One-year survival rates have improved to 25%, although

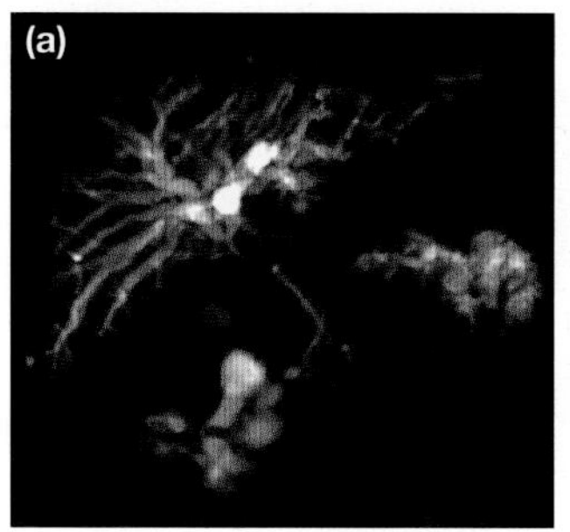

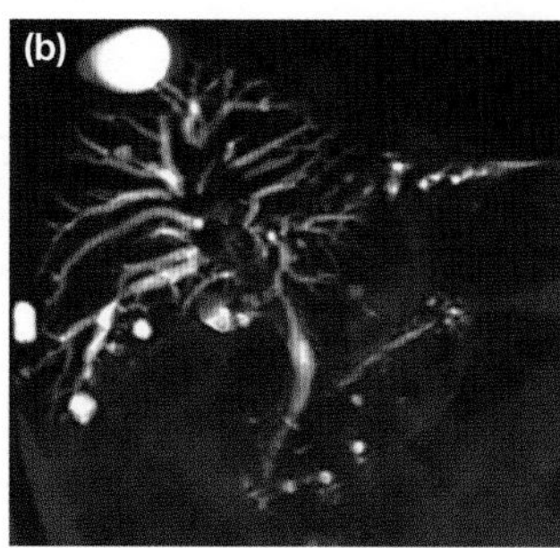

Figure 69.23 Hilar cholangiocarcinoma (Klatskin tumour) demonstrating tight stricture and intrahepatic dilatation of intrahepatic ducts due to infiltrating tumour (a) and an apparent space-occupying lesion due to the mass-forming variety (b).

5-year survival of 3% remains unchanged. Unfortunately, conventional chemotherapy offers limited survival benefit for unresectable or metastatic disease.

Colorectal liver metastases

Worldwide colorectal cancer (CRC) is the third most common solid organ malignancy and the fourth most common cause of cancer-related deaths. Up to 70% of patients with CRC develop synchronous (15–25%) or metachronous (20–45%) liver metastases. Thirty years ago, metastatic CRC was associated with a 5-year survival of less than 3%; however, liver resection in selected patients with liver-only metastatic disease demonstrated 5-year survivals of 50%, so the potential benefits were recognised. Despite recent advances in chemotherapeutic agents, resection remains the only potentially curative option, but only 20% of patients will be candidates at presentation. A further 20–30% will become operable following chemotherapy, the 5-year overall survival rate following resection is 50% and tumour recurs in 65% with the recurrent disease limited to the liver in 40%.

Defining resectability for colorectal liver metastases

Previously, patients with synchronous metastases, a rectal primary, multiple diffuse metastases, metastases larger than 5 cm, disease-free intervals of less than 1 year from the diagnosis of primary disease or a high serum CEA were considered irresectable and suitable only for palliative treatment. Modern surgical techniques and chemotherapy regimes now mean that resection with curative intent is defined as the ability to successfully remove all residual disease from the liver with clear surgical margins, leaving adequate disease-free viable liver. Technical contraindications to resection are related to the anatomical location of metastases, principally the involvement of major vascular or biliary structures.

An R0 resection with a negative surgical margin of 1 cm is considered the gold standard, but with effective modern chemotherapy patients with an R1 resection (≥1-mm margin

Vincenzo Mazzaferro, b. 1957, surgeon, Istituto Nazionale dei Tumori, Milan, Italy.

microscopically negative), which occurs in 10–30% of patients, have similar survivals to those with R0 resections. An FLR of 25% of preoperative volume is considered sufficient to prevent postoperative hepatic failure (see ***Portal vein embolisation***). Historically, extrahepatic metastatic disease was considered a contraindication to liver surgery, but long-term survival is now possible in selected patients. Survival after lung resection for colorectal metastases is similar to that seen after liver resection (40–50%) with low morbidity and mortality.

Staging and selection of patients for liver surgery

A specialist multidisciplinary team should coordinate the staging of patients with colorectal liver metastases and the treatment plan. Routine staging involves triple-phase CT chest/abdomen/pelvis, contrast MRI scan of the liver, whole-body PET-CT to identify metastatic disease with/without laparoscopy and intraoperative ultrasonography.

Chemotherapy for colorectal liver metastases

Despite new chemotherapeutic agents and locoregional therapies (embolisation, percutaneous ablation, hepatic artery-directed infusion chemotherapy, internal radiation) the role of adjuvant and neoadjuvant chemotherapy remains unclear. The traditional approach was to resect an operable colonic primary followed by routine postoperative chemotherapy or holding chemotherapy 'in reserve' in case of metastases. Neoadjuvant chemotherapy is now recommended by some groups for the majority of patients even if the liver disease is resectable. The aim is to reduce lesion size and improve resectability while treating occult disease and revealing the tumour biology where progression despite chemotherapy signifies a poor prognosis.

A major development with advanced disease was the recognition that a subgroup of patients may become resectable after systemic chemotherapy. Although resectability rates after chemotherapy for initially irresectable disease vary, when successful 5-year survivals of 35–50% are similar to disease resectable at presentation. Chemotherapy with 5-fluorouracil and folinic acid produces a response rate of approximately 30% but combination with oxaliplatin increases this to 50–60%. Combination chemotherapy with monoclonal antibodies that recognise vascular endothelial growth factor receptor (VEGFR) or epidermal growth factor receptor (EGFR) provide additional benefit (see also ***Chapters 12 and 77***).

Synchronous colon and liver resection

Synchronous resectable liver metastases are frequently identified at the time of diagnosis. Treatment options include sequential, delayed and simultaneous resection strategies. Resection of the colonic primary followed by chemotherapy, restaging and resection of the liver disease, if appropriate, is the standard approach. It is occasionally possible with low-volume, accessible liver disease to perform synchronous liver and colonic resections, but this is contraindicated when both procedures represent a major undertaking per se.

Liver-first approach

The traditional surgical strategy for resectable synchronous colorectal liver metastases (CRLMs) is colonic resection followed by chemotherapy and a delayed liver resection. This may allow progression of the liver disease and render the CRLM unresectable, which is a particular concern in patients who develop postoperative complications following their colon resection that delay or prevent chemotherapy. The liver-first approach or reverse strategy is a downstaging regimen consisting of systemic chemotherapy, chemoradiotherapy and/or biological agents, followed by resection of the CRLM prior to removal of the colonic primary. The approach is valuable in the subset of patients in whom failure to respond to systemic treatment potentially renders CRLMs non-resectable.

Follow-up

Optimal follow-up remains controversial, and protocols vary. Close observation will identify patients who may benefit from further surgery and at least a yearly scan should be performed for the first 5 years. Tumour markers are measured if initially elevated and patients seen if symptoms develop. Recurrence within 12 months has a poor prognosis.

Re-do surgery

Close follow-up identifies recurrent isolated liver metastases and if CT and PET exclude additional disease repeat resection is appropriate when possible. The operative approach must take into account the consequences of previous surgery and hypertrophy following a major resection. Left lobe resections may produce a more inferiorly based and medially shifted portal triad, making the origin of the right hepatic pedicle deeper and more medial than expected, and a right hepatectomy will often rotate the hilum more anteriorly.

Non-colorectal, non-neuroendocrine metastases

Although metastases from non-CRCs do not spread via the portal circulation and are rarely confined to the liver, with the low mortality associated with liver resection palliative or potentially curative surgery for metastases from renal, breast, gastric and lung metastases together with deposits from melanoma, sarcoma and a range of rarer tumours is reported.

Management of metastatic gastrointestinal stromal cell tumours

Gastrointestinal stromal tumours (GISTs) are non-epithelial tumours originating in interstitial Cajal cells of the autonomic nervous system, which metastasise in 20–25% of patients. Management has changed with the effective chemotherapy

Santiago Ramón y Cajal, 1852–1934, neurophysiologist and director Instituto Nacional de Hygiene, Madrid, Spain.

imatinib mesylate, which often produces dramatic responses. The primary bowel tumour should be removed if possible and the liver assessed to identify potentially resectable disease. If metastases respond to postoperative imatinib, surveillance is recommended; however, when metastases escape imatinib control debulking has no role and surgical resection is performed only if extirpation of all disease is possible.

FURTHER READING

Banale JM, Cardinale V, Carpino G *et al.* Expert consensus document: Cholangiocarcinoma: current knowledge and future perspectives consensus statement from the European Network for the Study of Cholangiocarcinoma (ENS-CCA). *Nat Rev Gastroenterol Hepatol* 2016; **13**: 261–80.

Benson AB, D'Angelica MI, Abbott DE *et al.* Guidelines insights: hepatobiliary cancers, version 2.2019. *J Natl Compr Canc Netw* 2019; **17**: 302–10.

Coccolini F, Coimbra R, Ordonez C *et al.* Liver trauma: WSES 2020 guidelines. *World J Emerg Surg* 2020; **15**: 24.

Couinaud C. *Le foie: études anatomiques et chirurgicales* [*The liver: anatomical and surgical studies*]. Paris: Masson, 1957.

Dennison A, Maddern G. *Operative solutions in hepatobiliary and pancreatic surgery*. Oxford: Oxford University Press, 2010.

Dhir M, Melin AA, Douaiher J *et al.* A review and update of treatment options and controversies in the management of hepatocellular carcinoma. *Ann Surg* 2016; **263**: 1112–25.

Healey JE, Schroy PC. Anatomy of the biliary ducts within the human liver. An analysis of the prevailing patterns of branching and their major variants. *Arch Surg* 1953; **66**: 599–616.

Mak LY, Cruz-Ramon V, Chinchilla-Lopez P *et al.* Global epidemiology, prevention, and management of hepatocellular carcinoma. *Am Soc Clin Oncol Educ Book* 2018; **38**: 262–79.

Mavilia MG, Pakala T, Molina M, Wu GY. Differentiating cystic liver lesions: a review of imaging modalities, diagnosis and management. *J Clin Trans Hepatol* 2018; **6**: 208–16.

Serraino C, Elia C, Bracco C *et al.* Characteristics and management of pyogenic liver abscess. *Medicine (Baltimore)* 2018; **97**(19): e0628.

Van Cutsem E, Cervantes A, Adam R *et al.* ESMO consensus guidelines for the management of patients with metastatic colorectal cancer. *Ann Oncol* 2016; **2**: 1386–422.

CHAPTER 70 The spleen

Learning objectives

To understand:
- The function of the spleen
- The common pathologies involving the spleen
- The principles and potential complications of splenectomy
- The potential advantages of laparoscopic splenectomy
- The benefits of splenic conservation
- The importance of prophylaxis against infection following splenectomy

EMBRYOLOGY, ANATOMY AND PHYSIOLOGY

Embryology

Fetal splenic tissue develops from condensations of mesoderm in the dorsal mesogastrium. This peritoneal fold attaches the dorsal body wall to the fusiform swelling in the foregut that develops into the stomach. This condensation divides the mesogastrium into two parts, one between the fetal splenic tissue and the stomach to form the gastrosplenic ligament and the other between it and the left kidney to form the lienorenal ligament.

Anatomy

The weight of the normal adult spleen is 75–250 g and it measures up to 10 × 7 × 3 cm. It lies in the left hypochondrium between the gastric fundus and the left hemidiaphragm, with its long axis lying along the 10th rib. The spleen is connected to the stomach and kidney by a double fold of peritoneum that originates from the stomach as a part of the greater omentum. The gastrosplenic (gastrolienal) ligament is anterior to the splenic hilum and connects the spleen to the greater curvature of the stomach. The splenorenal (lienorenal) ligament lies posterior to the splenic hilum and connects the hilum of the spleen to the left kidney. The splenic vessels and the tail of the pancreas lie within this ligament (***Figure 70.1***). The hilum of the spleen sits in the angle between the stomach and the kidney and is in contact with the tail of the pancreas. The concave visceral surface lies in contact with these structures, and the lower pole extends no further than the midaxillary line. There is a notch on the inferolateral border, and this may be palpated only when the spleen is enlarged. The tortuous splenic artery arises from the coeliac axis and runs along the upper border of the body and tail of the pancreas, to which it gives small branches. The short gastric and left gastroepiploic branches pass between the layers of the gastrosplenic ligament. These arteries are divided whenever the greater curvature of the stomach has to be excised. The main splenic artery generally divides into superior and inferior branches, which, in turn, subdivide into several segmental branches. The splenic vein is formed from several tributaries that drain the hilum and runs behind the pancreas, receiving several small tributaries from the pancreas before joining the superior mesenteric vein at the neck of the pancreas to form the portal vein (***Figure 70.2***).

The splenic pulp is invested by an external serous and internal fibroelastic coat, which is reflected inwards at the hilum onto the vessels to form vascular sheaths. The lymphatic drainage comprises efferent vessels in the white pulp that run with the arterioles and emerge from nodes at the hilum. These nodes and lymphatics drain via retropancreatic nodes to the coeliac nodes.

Physiology

The splenic parenchyma consists of white and red pulp that is surrounded by serosa and a collagenous capsule with smooth muscle fibres. These penetrate the parenchyma as trabeculae of dense connective tissue fibres rich in collagen and elastic tissue. These, with the reticular framework, support the cells of the spleen and surround the vessels in the splenic pulp. The white pulp comprises a central trabecular artery surrounded by nodules with germinal centres and periarterial lymphatic sheaths that provide a framework filled with lymphocytes and macrophages. Arteries from the central artery and the peripheral 'penicillar' arteries pass into the marginal zone that lies at the edge of the white pulp. Plasma-rich blood that has passed through the central lymphatic nodules is filtered as it passes through the sinuses within the marginal zone, and particles are phagocytosed.

Immunoglobulins produced in the lymphatic nodules enter the circulation through the sinuses in the marginal zone,

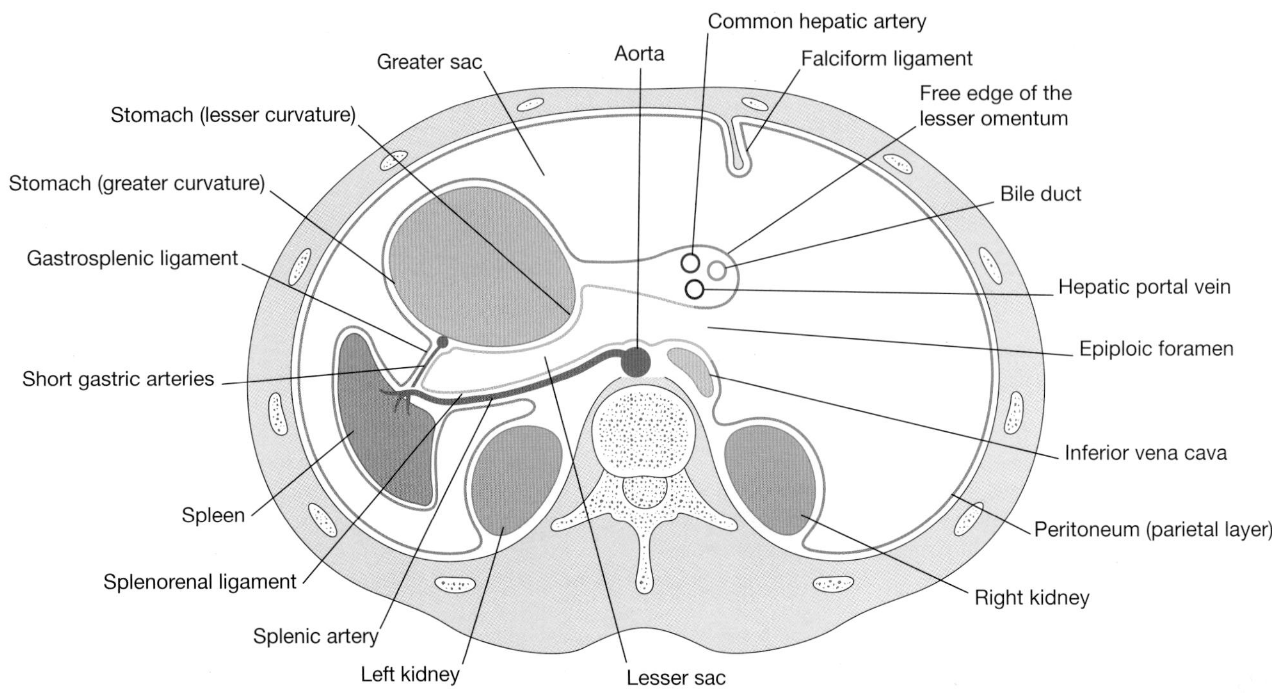

Figure 70.1 Transverse section (craniocaudal view) showing the important ligaments of the spleen containing the blood vessels (courtesy of Dr Tusharindra Lal, Chennai, India).

beyond which lies the red pulp, which consists of cords and sinuses. Cell-concentrated blood passes in the trabecular artery through the centre of the white pulp to the red pulp cords. Red cells must elongate and become thinner to pass from the cords to the sinuses, a process that removes abnormally shaped cells from the circulation (***Figure 70.3***). As 90% of the blood passing through the spleen moves through an open circulation in which blood flows from arteries to cords, and thence sinuses, splenic pulp pressure reflects the pressure throughout the portal system. The remaining 10% of the blood flow through the spleen bypasses the cords and sinuses by direct arteriovenous communications. The overall flow rate of blood is about 300 mL/min.

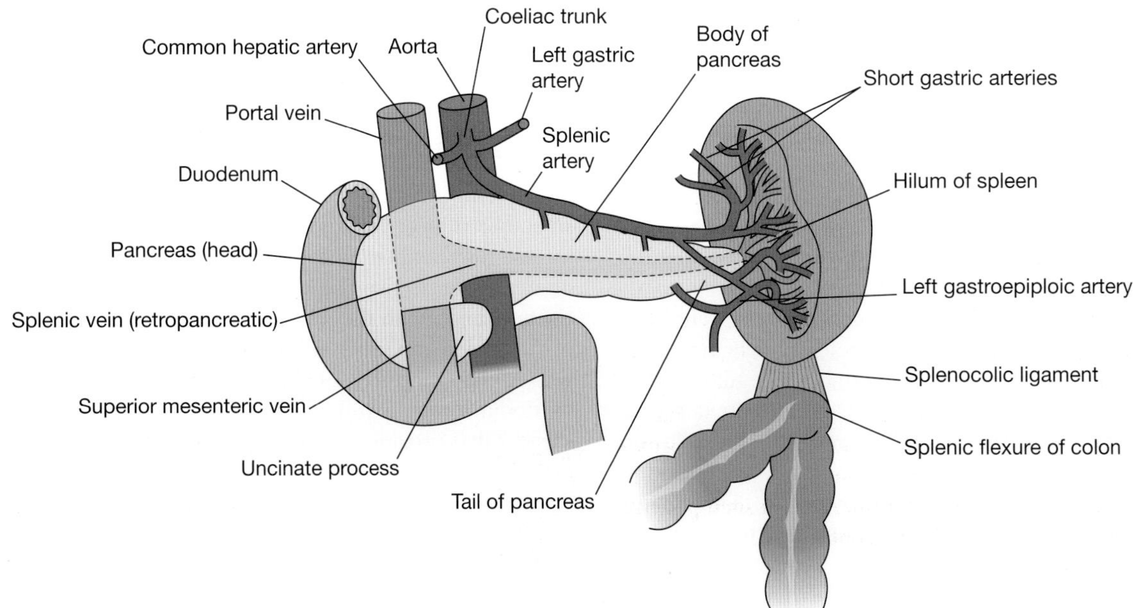

Figure 70.2 Schematic representation showing relations at the hilum of the spleen with the blood supply and venous drainage. Note the avascular splenocolic ligament that needs to be divided carefully to free the inferior pole of the spleen from the splenic flexure (courtesy of Dr Tusharindra Lal, Chennai, India).

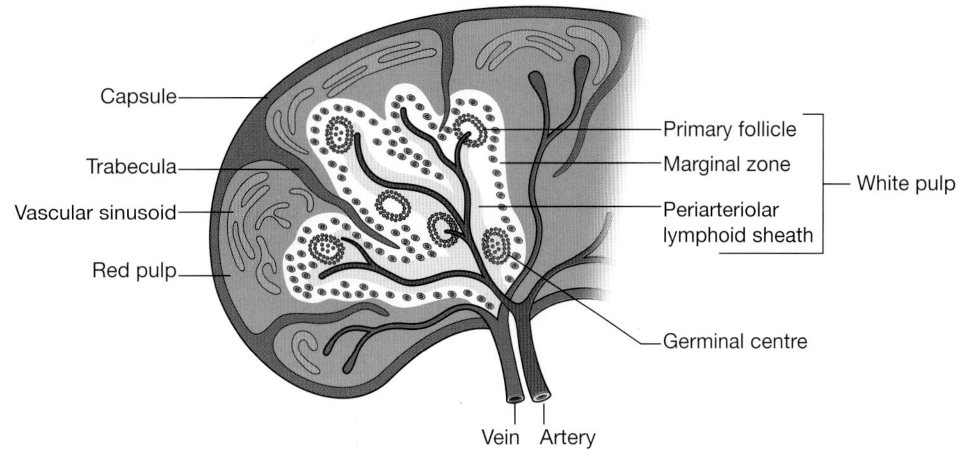

Figure 70.3 Functional anatomy of the spleen. Blood from a central trabecular artery passes through the white pulp into the surrounding red pulp and hence to the vascular cords and sinuses that drain into the trabecular vein.

FUNCTIONS OF THE SPLEEN

Although the spleen was previously thought to be dispensable, it is now recognised that an incidental splenectomy during the course of another operative procedure increases the risk of complications and death. The surgeon should therefore normally endeavour to preserve the spleen to maintain the following functions.

- **Immune function**. The spleen contains 70.5% and 10–15% of the body's total T and B lymphocyte population, respectively. It processes foreign antigens and is the major site of specific immunoglobulin (Ig) M production. The non-specific opsonins, properdin and tuftsin, are synthesised. These antibodies are of B- and T-cell origin and bind to the specific receptors on the surface of macrophages and leukocytes, stimulating their phagocytic, bactericidal and tumoricidal activity. Loss of this function necessitates vaccination against capsulated microorganisms such as pneumococci in splenectomised patients.
- **Filter function**. Macrophages in the reticulum capture cellular and non-cellular material from the blood and plasma. This will include the removal of effete platelets and red blood cells. This process takes place in the sinuses and the splenic cords by the action of the endothelial macrophages. Iron is removed from the degraded haemoglobin during red cell breakdown and is returned to plasma. Removed non-cellular material may include bacteria and, in particular, pneumococci. This occurs in the red pulp of the spleen and needs red cells with the capability to change shape and traverse through the sinusoids. As the deformability is reduced in spherocytosis, the cells get removed in the spleen. Splenectomy is recommended in such patients to maintain the haemoglobin concentration.
- **Pitting**. Distorted red cells in sickle cell disease result in slowing of circulation with multiple splenic infarcts, leading to loss of splenic function – autosplenectomy. This leads to the appearance of circulating red cells with Howell–Jolly and Heinz bodies, which represent nuclear remnants and precipitated haemoglobin or globin subunits, respectively, and appear as target cells on a smear. These particulate inclusions within the red cells are removed, and the repaired red cells are returned to the circulation in the process of pitting.
- **Reservoir function**. This function in humans is less marked than in other species, but the spleen does contain approximately 8% of the red cell mass. An enlarged spleen may contain a much larger proportion of the blood volume. Massive splenic enlargement will be associated with a larger proportion of blood volume in the spleen, leading to pancytopenia, which can be corrected by splenectomy.
- **Cytopoiesis**. From the fourth month of intrauterine life, some degree of haemopoiesis occurs in the fetal spleen. Stimulation of the white pulp may occur following antigenic challenge, resulting in the proliferation of T and B cells and macrophages. This may also occur in myeloproliferative disorders, thalassaemias and chronic haemolytic anaemias.

Summary box 70.1

Functions of the spleen

- Immune
- Filter function
- Pitting
- Reservoir
- Cytopoiesis

William Henry Howell, 1860–1945, Professor of Physiology, Johns Hopkins University, Baltimore, MD, USA.
Justin Marie Jules Jolly, 1870–1953, Professor of Histopathology, Collège de France, Paris, France.
Robert Heinz, 1865–1962, Professor of Pharmacology and Toxicology, Erlangen, Germany.

INVESTIGATION OF THE SPLEEN

Conditions that result in splenomegaly can be diagnosed on the basis of the history and examination and laboratory examination. In haemolytic anaemia, a full blood count, reticulocyte count and tests for haemolysis will determine the cause of the anaemia. Splenomegaly associated with portal hypertension caused by cirrhosis is diagnosed on history, physical signs of liver dysfunction including ascites, abnormal tests of liver function, often anaemia, leukopenia and thrombocytopenia, as well as endoscopic evidence of oesophageal varices. Non-cirrhotic portal fibrosis, a condition common in tropical countries, is associated with massive splenomegaly and pancytopenia without stigmata of liver dysfunction. Sinistral or segmental portal hypertension may result from isolated occlusion of the splenic vein by thrombosis, pancreatic inflammation or tumour infiltration. As many conditions that cause splenomegaly are associated with lymphadenopathy, investigation should be directed at those disease processes known to be associated with both physical signs. Lymph node biopsy may be required.

Radiological imaging

Plain radiology is rarely used in investigation, but the incidental finding of calcification of the splenic artery or spleen may raise the possible diagnosis of a splenic artery aneurysm, an old infarct, a benign cyst or hydatid disease. Multiple areas of calcification may suggest splenic tuberculosis. Ultrasonography can determine the size and consistency of the spleen and whether a cyst is present. However, computed tomography (CT) with contrast enhancement is more commonly undertaken to better characterise the nature of the suspected splenic pathology and to exclude other intra-abdominal pathology. Magnetic resonance imaging (MRI) may be similarly useful, especially as T2-weighted images allow cystic lesions to be distinguished.

CONGENITAL ABNORMALITIES OF THE SPLEEN

Splenic agenesis is rare but is present in 5% of children with congenital heart disease. Polysplenia is a rare condition resulting from failure of splenic fusion.

Splenunculi are single or multiple accessory spleens that are found in approximately 10–30% of the population. They are located near the hilum of the spleen in 50% of cases and are related to the splenic vessels, or behind the tail of the pancreas in 30%. The remainder are located in the mesocolon, greater omentum or the splenic ligaments. Their significance lies in the fact that failure to identify and remove these at the time of splenectomy may give rise to persistent disease.

Hamartomas are rarely found in life and vary in size from 1 cm in diameter to masses large enough to produce an abdominal swelling. One form is mainly lymphoid and resembles the white pulp, whereas the other resembles the red pulp.

Non-parasitic **splenic cysts** are rare. Splenic cysts are classified as primary cysts (true) or pseudocysts (secondary) on the basis of the presence or absence of lining epithelium. True cysts form from embryonal rests and include dermoid and mesenchymal inclusion cysts (***Figure 70.4***). Rarely, the entire spleen may be replaced by a cystic mass (***Figure 70.5***). True cysts of the spleen are very rare and are frequently classified as cystic haemangiomas, cystic lymphangiomas and epidermoid and dermoid cysts. Splenectomy or partial splenectomy is usually considered for cysts larger than 5 cm in diameter. These should be differentiated from false or secondary cysts that may result from trauma and contain serous or haemorrhagic fluid. The walls of such degenerative cysts may be calcified and therefore resemble the radiological appearances of a hydatid cyst (***Figure 70.6***). The spleen is also a common site for pseudocyst development following a severe attack of pancreatitis (***Figure 70.7***). Pseudocysts can easily be diagnosed on scanning; intervention is normally required for symptomatic lesions that persist following a period of observation.

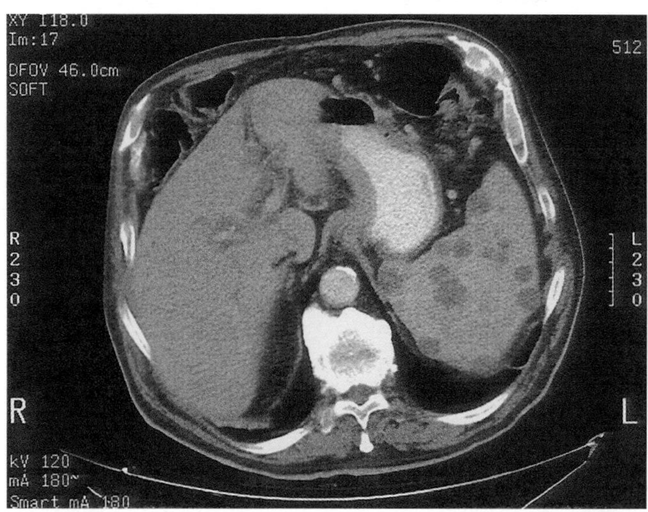

Figure 70.4 Computed tomography scan showing multiple low-density areas in the spleen consistent with multiple benign splenic cysts.

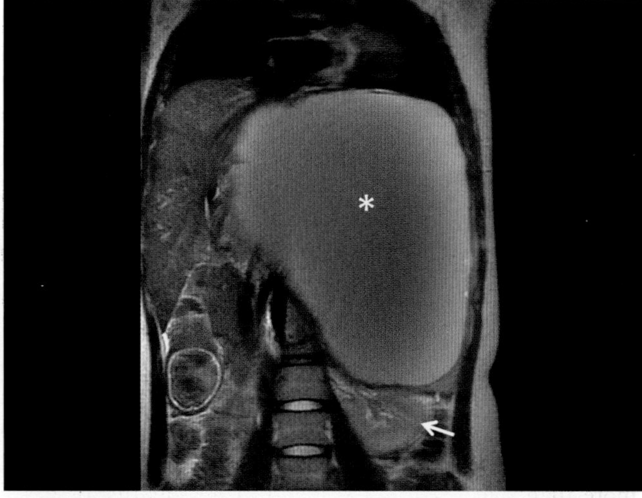

Figure 70.5 T2-weighted coronal magnetic resonance image showing a large, homogeneously hyperintense lesion (asterisk) in the region of the spleen displacing the left kidney inferiorly (arrow). Note that the normal splenic parenchyma is completely replaced by the cyst (courtesy of Dr Amit Kumar Sahu, New Delhi, India).

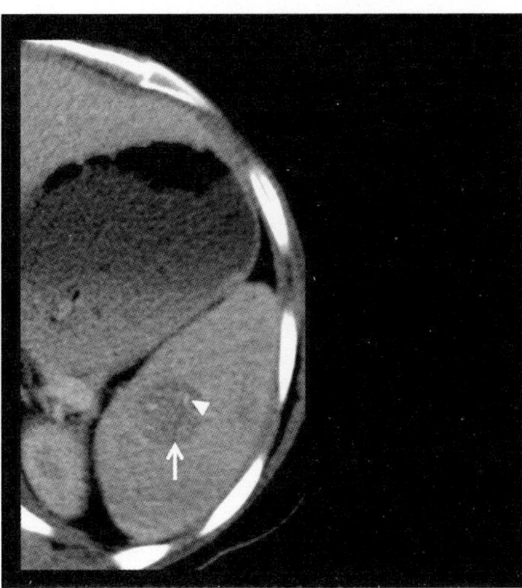

Figure 70.6 Axial contrast-enhanced computed tomography scan shows a well-defined hypodense lesion (arrow) in the spleen with mild internal calcification suggestive of splenic hydatid (arrowhead) (courtesy of Dr Amit Kumar Sahu, New Delhi, India).

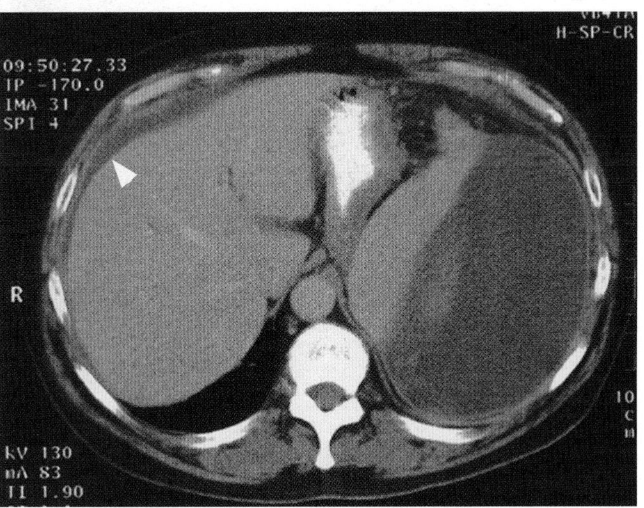

Figure 70.7 Computed tomography scan showing a large pseudocyst involving the spleen. There is displacement of the stomach medially and a trace of ascitic fluid (arrowhead) is present above the liver.

SPLENIC ARTERY ANEURYSM, INFARCT AND RUPTURE

Splenic artery aneurysm

Aneurysms involving the splenic artery are estimated to be identified at 0.04–1% of postmortem examinations. They are twice as common in women and are usually situated in the main arterial trunk. Although these are generally single, more than one aneurysm is found in one-quarter of cases. These may be a consequence of intra-abdominal sepsis and pancreatic necrosis, in particular. They are more likely to be associated with arteriosclerosis in elderly patients.

The aneurysm is symptomless unless it ruptures and is more likely to be detected on a plain abdominal radiograph

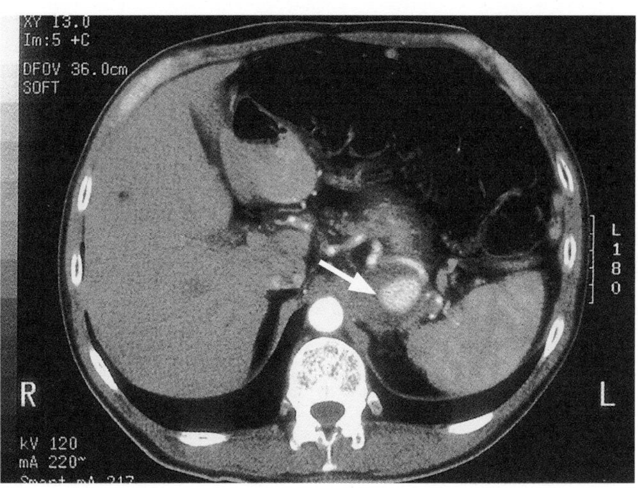

Figure 70.8 Computed tomography scan showing a pool of contrast in a pseudoaneurysm (arrow) situated in the tail of the pancreas adjacent to the spleen.

or scan. It is unlikely to be palpable, although a bruit may be present. Rupture is unsuspected in the majority of cases and, as it will generally rupture into the peritoneal cavity, the symptoms mimic those of splenic rupture. Almost half the cases of rupture occur in patients younger than 45 years of age and one-quarter are in pregnant women, usually in the third trimester of pregnancy or at labour. Aneurysmal rupture carries a high mortality rate and this increases disproportionately in pregnant women, with almost inevitable fetal death.

The treatment of choice previously consisted of splenectomy and removal of the diseased artery. Embolisation or endovascular stenting following selective splenic artery angiography can be considered and is now more commonly undertaken. In younger patients with an asymptomatic splenic artery aneurysm, surgery or interventional radiology is indicated, depending on local expertise, after CT scan, MRI or selective coeliac angiography has confirmed the diagnosis (***Figure 70.8***). In elderly patients with a calcified aneurysm, there is less risk of rupture and observation may be preferred.

Splenic infarction

This condition commonly occurs in patients with a massively enlarged spleen from myeloproliferative syndrome, portal hypertension or vascular occlusion produced by previous surgical intervention (such as spleen-preserving distal pancreatectomy), pancreatic disease, splenic vein thrombosis or sickle cell disease. The infarct may be asymptomatic or give rise to left upper quadrant and left shoulder tip pain. Contrast-enhanced CT will show the characteristic perfusion defect in the enlarged spleen (***Figure 70.9***). Treatment is conservative and splenectomy should be considered only when a septic infarct causes an abscess.

Splenic rupture due to trauma

The spleen is the most commonly injured intra-abdominal organ followed by the liver. Splenic rupture should be considered in any case of blunt abdominal trauma, particularly when

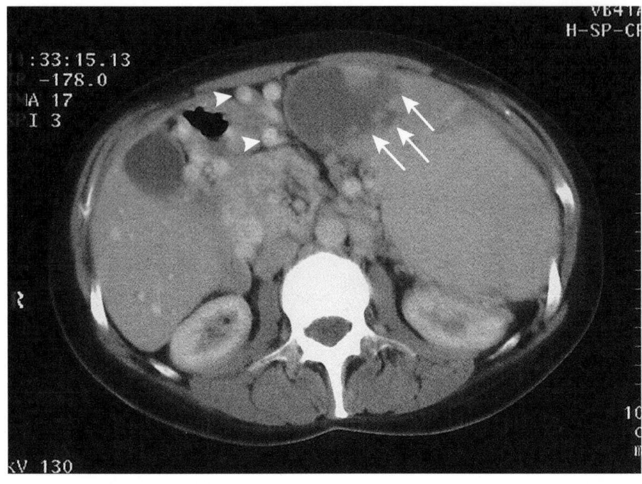

Figure 70.9 Computed tomography scan showing a splenic infarct (arrows) in a patient with splenomegaly and hypersplenism secondary to portal hypertension and portal vein thrombosis. Varices are evident at the hilus and at the greater curvature of the stomach (arrowheads).

the injury occurs to the left upper quadrant of the abdomen. Iatrogenic injury to the spleen remains a frequent complication of any surgical procedure, particularly those in the left upper quadrant when adhesions are present.

Based upon the extent of injury, spleen rupture is classified into five grades on the basis of CT, which is considered to be the most important investigation for assessment of abdominal trauma in a haemodynamically stable patient (***Table 70.1***). Vigorous resuscitation remains the key to management of blunt trauma. Splenectomy should be performed for severe grades of injury where control of bleeding takes precedence over measures to salvage the spleen. Splenic angiography with embolisation of actively bleeding vessels may obviate the need for splenectomy but should not delay laparotomy in a haemodynamically unstable patient.

TABLE 70.1 Criteria for grading of splenic injury based on computed tomography.

Grade 1	Subcapsular haematoma <10% of surface area Parenchymal laceration <1 cm depth Capsular tear
Grade 2	Subcapsular haematoma 10–50% of surface area; intraparenchymal haematoma <5 cm Parenchymal laceration 1–3 cm
Grade 3	Subcapsular haematoma >50% surface area; ruptured subcapsular or intraparenchymal haematoma ≥5 cm Parenchymal laceration >3 cm depth
Grade 4	Any injury in the presence of a splenic vascular injury or active bleeding confined within the splenic capsule Parenchymal laceration involving segmental or hilar vessels producing >25% devascularisation
Grade 5	Any injury in the presence of splenic vascular injury[a] with active bleeding extending beyond the spleen into the peritoneum – shattered spleen

[a]Vascular injury is defined as a pseudoaneurysm or arteriovenous fistula and appears as a focal collection of vascular contrast that decreases in attenuation with delayed imaging. Active bleeding from a vascular injury presents as vascular contrast, focal or diffuse, that increases in size or attenuation in the delayed phase.

Rupture of a malarial spleen

In tropical countries, rupture of a spleen enlarged as a result of malaria is not uncommon (see ***Tropical splenomegaly***). Delayed presentation following a 'trivial' injury is not infrequent. In such patients, radiological embolisation may be performed if available, and splenectomy should be considered before a perisplenic haematoma ruptures, a complication that is associated with a worse prognosis.

Surgery in such patients is challenging and early ligation of the splenic vessels along the superior border of the pancreatic body should be considered before disturbing the haematoma.

SPLENOMEGALY AND HYPERSPLENISM

Splenomegaly is a common feature of many disease processes, although the spleen has to enlarge threefold before it is palpable (***Table 70.2***). It should be borne in mind that many conditions affecting the spleen, such as idiopathic thrombocytopenic purpura (ITP), may be associated with enlargement but the spleen is seldom palpable. Few conditions that cause splenomegaly will require splenectomy as part of treatment.

Hypersplenism is an indefinite clinical syndrome that is characterised by splenic enlargement, any combination of anaemia, leukopenia or thrombocytopenia, compensatory bone marrow hyperplasia and improvement after splenectomy. Careful clinical judgement is required to balance the long- and short-term risks of splenectomy against continued conservative management.

Splenic abscess

Splenic abscess may arise from an infected splenic embolus or in association with typhoid and paratyphoid fever, osteomyelitis, otitis media and puerperal sepsis. In general surgical practice, it may be associated with pancreatic necrosis or other intra-abdominal infection (***Figure 70.10***). An abscess may rupture and form a left subphrenic abscess or result in diffuse peritonitis. Treatment involves that of the underlying cause; percutaneous drainage of the splenic abscess under radiological guidance is normally required, with splenectomy being reserved when interventional radiology is not available.

Tuberculosis

The diagnosis of tuberculosis should be considered in young adults with splenomegaly presenting with asthenia, loss of weight and fever. Tuberculosis of the spleen may produce portal hypertension or, rarely, cold abscess. CT shows small low-attenuation areas with central enhancement in the acute stage and MRI shows hypointense lesions (***Figure 70.11***). Multidrug chemotherapy with four drugs in the intensive phase of 2 months followed by two drugs in the maintenance

TABLE 70.2 Causes of splenic enlargement.

Infective	Bacterial	Typhoid and paratyphoid
		Typhus
		Tuberculosis
		Psittacosis
		Septicaemia
		Splenic abscess
	Spirochaetal	Weil's disease
		Syphilis
	Viral	Infectious mononucleosis
		HIV-related thrombocytopenia
	Protozoal and parasitic	Malaria
		Schistosomiasis
		Trypanosomiasis
		Kala-azar
		Hydatid cyst
		Tropical splenomegaly
Blood disease	Acute leukaemia	Idiopathic thrombocytopenic purpura
	Chronic leukaemia	Hereditary spherocytosis
	Pernicious anaemia	Autoimmune haemolytic anaemia
	Polycythaemia vera	Thalassaemia
	Erythroblastosis fetalis	Sickle cell disease
Metabolic	Rickets	
	Amyloid	
	Porphyria	
	Gaucher's disease	
Circulatory	Infarct	
	Portal hypertension	
	Segmental portal hypertension	(Pancreatic carcinoma, splenic vein thrombosis)
Collagen disease	Still's disease	
	Felty's syndrome	
Non-parasitic cysts	Congenital	
	Acquired	
Neoplastic	Angioma	
	Primary fibrosarcoma	
	Hodgkin's lymphoma	
	Other lymphomas	
	Myelofibrosis	

HIV, human immunodeficiency virus.

Adolph Weil, 1848–1916, physician, Dorpat (now Tartu), Estonia, described leptospirosis icterohaemorrhagica in 1886.
Philippe Charles Ernest Gaucher, 1854–1918, dermatologist, Paris, France.
Sir George Frederic Still, 1868–1941, Professor of Diseases of Children, King's College Hospital, London, UK, described chronic articular rheumatism in children in 1896.
Augustus Roy Felty, 1895–1964, physician, Hartford, CT, USA, described the combination of arthritis, splenomegaly and leukopenia in 1924 while still a medical student at Johns Hopkins School of Medicine, Baltimore, MD, USA.
Thomas Hodgkin, 1798–1870, lecturer in morbid anatomy and curator of the museum, Guy's Hospital, London, UK, described lymphadenoma in 1836.

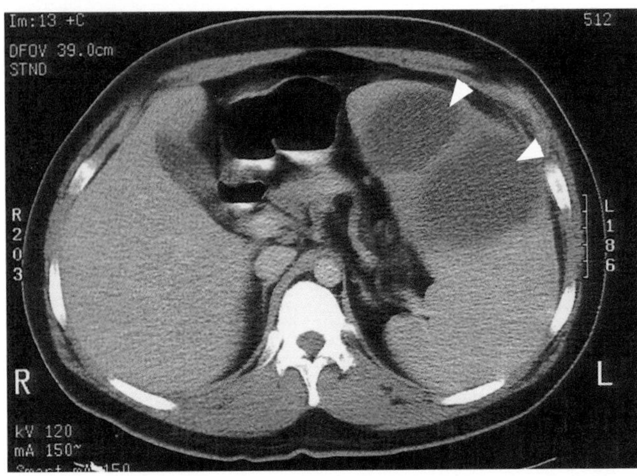

Figure 70.10 Computed tomography scan showing a multiloculated abscess (arrowheads) in the enlarged spleen. This was managed successfully by percutaneous drainage under ultrasound guidance.

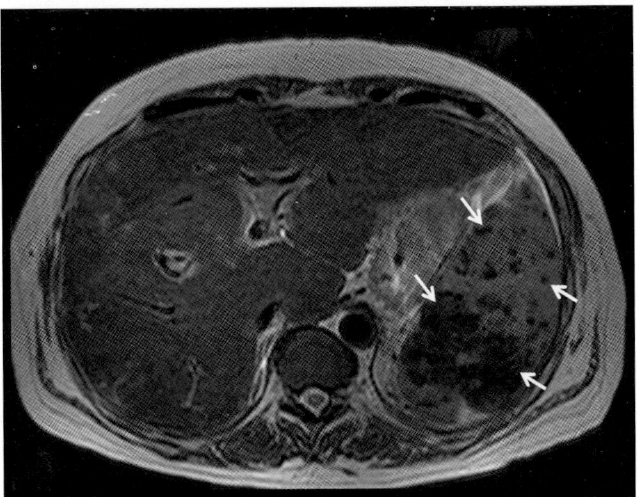

Figure 70.11 T2-weighted axial magnetic resonance image showing multiple hypointense lesions (arrows) of varying sizes in the spleen, suggestive of tuberculosis (courtesy of Dr Ruchi Rastogi, New Delhi, India).

phase for a total duration of 12–18 months is preferred for treatment of extrapulmonary tuberculosis. Splenectomy is not normally required and is made difficult by inflammatory adhesions. Typical epithelioid cell granulomas are seen in the histopathology of the spleen only if splenectomy had to be performed (***Figure 70.12***).

Tropical splenomegaly

Massive splenic enlargement frequently occurs in the tropics from malaria, kala-azar and schistosomiasis. Occasionally, splenomegaly cannot be fully attributed to these diseases and may result from occult infection or be related to malnutrition. Massive splenomegaly may require removal because of anaemia, hypersplenism, local symptoms or the threat of rupture. Lifelong antimalarial therapy is indicated in endemic areas.

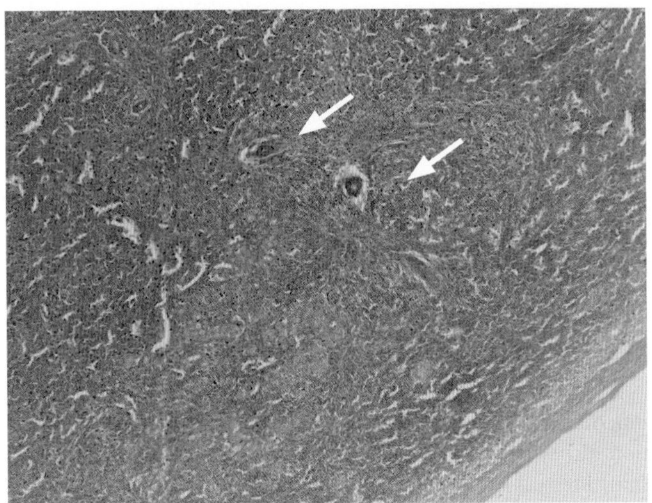

Figure 70.12 Splenic parenchyma showing epithelioid cell granulomas (arrows) in a human immunodeficiency virus-positive patient with disseminated cryptococcosis who presented with spontaneous splenic rupture necessitating splenectomy; haematoxylin and eosin; ×200 (courtesy of Dr Nita Khurana, New Delhi, India).

Schistosomiasis

This condition is prevalent in Africa, Asia and South America. It is caused by infection with *Schistosoma mansoni* in 75% of cases and by *Schistosoma haematobium* in the remainder. Splenic enlargement may result from portal hypertension associated with hepatic fibrosis, but can also result from hyperplasia induced by the phagocytosis of disintegrated worms, ova and toxin. Splenomegaly can occur at any age. The diagnosis is based on examination of the urine and faeces for ova, abnormal liver function tests and the presence of hypochromic anaemia.

Successful medical treatment does not result in the regression of splenomegaly. Removal of a painful spleen may be indicated or as part of a devascularisation procedure in patients with associated portal hypertension.

Leukaemia

Leukaemia should be considered in the differential diagnosis of splenomegaly. The diagnosis is made by examining a blood or bone marrow film. Splenectomy is reserved for hypersplenism that occurs during the chronic phase of chronic granulocytic leukaemia.

Idiopathic thrombocytopenic purpura

ITP, also known as immune and autoimmune thrombocytopenic purpura, results from antibodies to specific platelet membrane glycoproteins (antiplatelet IgG autoantibodies) that result in isolated thrombocytopenia in the presence of normal bone marrow and the absence of other causes of thrombocytopenia. Two distinct clinical types are evident: an

Sir Patrick Manson, 1844–1922, practised in Formosa (now Taiwan) and Hong Kong before becoming physician to the Dreadnought Hospital, Greenwich, London, UK. He is regarded as 'the father of tropical medicine'.

acute condition in children and a chronic condition in adults. Acute ITP often follows an acute infection and usually resolves spontaneously. Chronic ITP persists longer than 6 months without a specific cause being identified.

Clinical features

The adult form normally affects females between the ages of 15 and 50 years, although it can be associated with other conditions, including systemic lupus erythematosus, chronic lymphatic leukaemia and Hodgkin's disease. The childhood form is distributed equally between males and females and commonly presents before the age of 5 years.

Purpuric patches (ecchymoses) occur on the skin and mucous membranes. Following trauma or pressure, examination often reveals numbers of petechial haemorrhages in the skin. There is a tendency to spontaneous bleeding from mucous membranes (e.g. epistaxis); menorrhagia in women and prolonged bleeding of minor wounds are common. Haemorrhage from the urinary and gastrointestinal tracts and haemarthrosis are rare. Although intracranial haemorrhage is also uncommon, it is the most frequent cause of death. The diagnosis is indicated by the presence of cutaneous ecchymoses and a positive tourniquet test. The spleen is palpable in fewer than 10% of patients. The presence of gross splenic enlargement should raise suspicion of an alternative diagnosis.

Investigations

Coagulation studies are normal and a bleeding time is not helpful in diagnosis. Platelet count in the peripheral blood film is reduced (usually $<60 \times 10^9/L$). Bone marrow aspiration reveals a plentiful supply of platelet-producing megakaryocytes.

Treatment

The course of the disease differs in children and adults. The disease usually regresses spontaneously in paediatric cases. Short courses of corticosteroids in both adults and children are usually followed by recovery. Steroid therapy should not be prolonged.

Splenectomy is usually recommended for refractory or relapsing ITP. Up to two-thirds of patients will be cured by surgical intervention and 15% will be improved, but no benefit will be derived in the remainder. The response to steroids predicts a good response to splenectomy if the disease relapses.

Laparoscopic splenectomy is rapidly becoming the mainstay of treatment since the size of the spleen is usually normal or slightly enlarged and the spleen is not friable. It is important to identify and remove splenunculi as they have the potential to enlarge with time and lead to recurrence of symptoms.

In the acute setting, fresh blood transfusion or transfusion with platelet concentrates before operation may be necessary, although these are generally withheld until the splenic vessels have been controlled.

Haemolytic anaemias

There are four causes of haemolytic anaemia that are generally amenable to splenectomy.

Hereditary spherocytosis

Hereditary spherocytosis is an autosomal dominant hereditary disorder characterised by the presence of spherocytic red cells, caused by various molecular defects in the genes that code for alpha- and beta-spectrin, ankyrin, band 3 protein, protein 4.2 and other erythrocyte membrane proteins. These proteins are necessary to maintain the normal biconcave shape of the erythrocyte.

Spherocytosis arises essentially from an increase in permeability of the red cell membranes to sodium. As this ion leaks into the cell, the osmotic pressure rises, resulting in swelling and increased fragility of the spherocyte. As the sodium pump has to work harder to rid the cells of sodium, there is greater loss of membrane phospholipid, resulting in an increased fragility of the membrane, and the energy and oxygen requirements increase. A large number of red cells are destroyed in the spleen, where there is a relative deficiency of both glucose and oxygen.

The clinical presentation is generally in childhood but may be delayed until later life. Mild intermittent jaundice is associated with mild anaemia, splenomegaly and gallstones. Circulating bilirubin is not conjugated with glucuronic acid and is not therefore excreted in the urine as it is bound to albumin. Excretion of the resulting bilirubin complex by the liver favours formation of pigment gallstones. Once the disease manifests itself, spontaneous remissions are uncommon; the patient is often pale and jaundiced at presentation and, in established cases, lassitude and undue fatigue are present.

In some families, the disease is characterised by a severe crisis of red blood cell destruction, during which the erythrocyte count may fall from $4.5 \times 10^6/mL$ to $1.5 \times 10^6/mL$ within 1 week. Such crises are characterised by the onset of pyrexia, abdominal pain, nausea, vomiting and extreme pallor, followed by increasing jaundice. These episodes may be precipitated by acute infection. Any child with gallstone disease should be investigated for hereditary spherocytosis and a family history sought.

Examination reveals splenomegaly and the liver may also be palpable. Chronic leg ulcers may arise in adults.

Haematological investigations include the fragility test. Erythrocytes begin to haemolyse in 0.47% saline solution but, in this condition, haemolysis may occur in 0.6% or even stronger solutions. Immature red blood cells (reticulocytes), which differ from adult cells by possessing a reticulum, are discharged into the circulation by the bone marrow to compensate for the loss of erythrocytes by haemolysis.

Faecal urobilinogen is increased as this route excretes most of the urobilinogen.

Radioactive chromium (^{51}Cr) labelling of the patient's own red cells will demonstrate the severity of red cell destruction. Daily scanning over the spleen will show the degree of red cell sequestration by the spleen. The presence of high levels of splenic radioactivity generally predicts a good response to splenectomy.

All patients with hereditary spherocytosis should be treated by splenectomy but, in juvenile cases, this is generally delayed until 6 years of age to minimise the risk of postsplenectomy infection, but before gallstones have had time to form. Ultrasonography should be performed preoperatively to determine the presence of gallstones.

Acquired autoimmune haemolytic anaemia

This condition is divided into immune- and non-immune-mediated forms. It may arise following exposure to agents such as chemicals, infection or drugs, e.g. alpha-methyldopa, or be associated with another disease (e.g. systemic lupus erythematosus). In most instances, the cause is unknown, and red cell survival is reduced because of an immune reaction triggered by immunoglobulin or complement on the red cell surface. The condition is more common in women after the age of 50 years. The spleen is enlarged in about half the patients and pigment gallstones are present in about 20%.

Anaemia is invariably present and may be associated with spherocytosis because of red cell membrane damage. In the immune type, antibody, which coats the red cells, can be detected by agglutination when anti-human globulin is added to a suspension of the patient's erythrocytes (Coombs' test positive). The disease runs an acute self-limiting course and no treatment is necessary. Splenectomy should, however, be considered if corticosteroids are ineffective, when the patient is developing complications from long-term steroid treatment or if corticosteroids are contraindicated; 80% of patients respond to splenectomy.

Thalassaemia (synonyms: Cooley's anaemia, Mediterranean anaemia)

This condition results from a defect in haemoglobin peptide chain synthesis and is transmitted most commonly as a recessive trait. The disease is really a group of related diseases, alpha, beta and gamma, depending upon which haemoglobin peptide chain rate of synthesis is reduced. Most patients have beta-thalassaemia, in which a reduction in the rate of beta-chain synthesis results in a decrease in haemoglobin A. Intracellular precipitates (Heinz bodies) contribute to premature red cell destruction.

Graduations of the disease range from heterozygous thalassaemia minor to homozygous thalassaemia major, which is associated with chronic anaemia, jaundice and splenomegaly. Patients with homozygous thalassaemia major frequently develop clinical signs in the first year of life, and these include retarded growth, enlarged head with slanting eyes and depressed nose, leg ulcers, jaundice and abdominal distension secondary to splenomegaly.

Red cells are small, thin and misshapen and have a characteristic resistance to osmotic lysis. In the more severe forms, nucleated red cells and other immature blood cells are seen. The diagnosis is confirmed by haemoglobin electrophoresis.

Blood transfusion may be required to correct profound anaemia, but the patient may become transfusion dependent because of hypersplenism. Splenectomy is therefore of benefit in patients who require frequent blood transfusion or if haemolytic antibodies have developed.

Sickle cell disease

Sickle cell disease is a hereditary, autosomal recessive haemolytic anaemia occurring mainly among those of African origin, in whom the normal haemoglobin A is replaced by haemoglobin S (HbS). The HbS molecule crystallises when blood oxygen tension is reduced, thus distorting and elongating the red cell. The resulting increased blood viscosity may obstruct the flow of blood in the spleen. Splenic microinfarcts are therefore common.

The sickle cell trait can be detected in 9% of those of African origin, but most are asymptomatic; sickle cell disease occurs in about 1% of Africans. Depending upon the vessels affected by vascular occlusion, patients may complain of bone or joint pain, priapism, neurological abnormalities, skin ulcers or abdominal pain due to visceral blood stasis. The diagnosis is made by finding characteristic sickle-shaped cells on blood film, although this investigation has largely been replaced by haemoglobin electrophoresis.

Hypoxia that provokes a sickling crisis should be avoided and is particularly relevant in patients undergoing general anaesthesia. Adequate hydration and partial exchange transfusion may help in a crisis. Splenectomy is of benefit in a few patients in whom excessive splenic sequestration of red cells aggravates the anaemia. Chronic hypersplenism usually occurs in late childhood or adolescence, although *Streptococcus pneumoniae* infection may precipitate an acute form in the first 5 years of life.

Porphyria

Porphyria is a hereditary error of haemoglobin catabolism in which porphyrinuria occurs. The urine may be orange and develops a port-wine colour after a few hours of exposure to the air. Splenectomy has little role to play in the management.

Gaucher's disease

This lipid storage disease is characterised by storage of glucocerebroside in the reticuloendothelial system and in the spleen. Enormous splenic enlargement may be associated with yellowish brown discoloration of the skin on the hands and face, anaemia and conjunctival thickening (pinguecula). Slavonic and Jewish races are more prone to the disease, and the detection of Gaucher cells in the bone marrow confirms the diagnosis. Splenectomy is indicated only for severe symptoms related to the splenomegaly.

Hypersplenism due to portal hypertension

Splenomegaly is an invariable feature of portal hypertension (***Figure 70.13***) and results in the thrombocytopenia and granulocytopenia observed in these patients. These may be improved if the portal hypertension is relieved by shunt surgery or liver transplantation. Splenectomy would normally be required only in those patients whose segmental portal hypertension has

Robin Royston Amos Coombs, 1921–2006, Quick Professor of Biology, University of Cambridge, Cambridge, UK, described this test in 1945.
Thomas Benton Cooley, 1871–1945, Professor of Pediatrics, Wayne University, Detroit, MI, USA, described this type of anaemia in 1927.

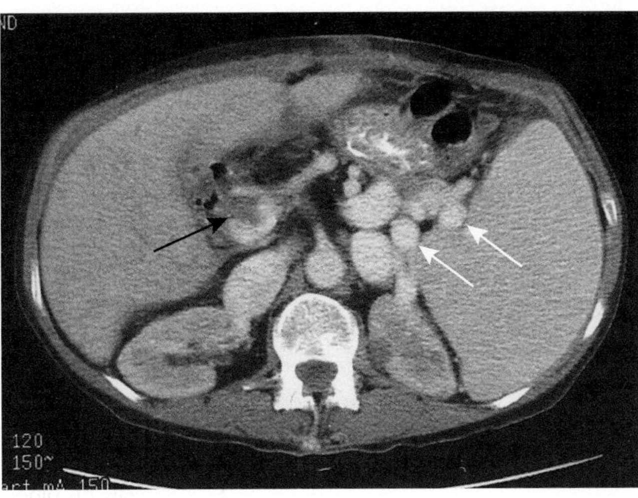

Figure 70.13 Computed tomography scan showing an enlarged spleen in a patient with portal hypertension secondary to portal vein thrombosis. Clot is evident within the lumen of the portal vein (black arrow) and large vessels of portosystemic shunts (white arrows) are present at the splenic hilus.

resulted in symptomatic oesophagogastric varices either as a standalone procedure in cases with massive splenomegaly due to extrahepatic portal vein obstruction or in combination with proximal lienorenal shunt (see ***Chapter 69***).

Felty's syndrome

Patients with rheumatoid arthritis may develop leukopenia. This is referred to as Felty's syndrome if it is extreme and associated with splenomegaly. Splenectomy produces only a transient improvement in the blood picture, but rheumatoid arthritis may respond to steroid therapy to which it had previously become resistant.

NEOPLASMS

Haemangioma is the most common benign tumour of the spleen. It may rarely develop into a haemangiosarcoma. The spleen is rarely the site of metastatic disease. Lymphoma is the most common cause of neoplastic enlargement and splenectomy may play a part in its management.

Splenectomy may be required to achieve a diagnosis in the absence of palpable lymph nodes or to relieve the symptoms of gross splenomegaly. However, the need for staging laparotomy or laparoscopy has largely receded with the advent of CT and guided biopsy. Its use has been restricted to those patients in whom a definite histological diagnosis of intra-abdominal disease will affect management. In the absence of obvious liver or intra-abdominal nodal disease, splenectomy is an integral part of the staging procedure to exclude splenic involvement, which would alter the method of treatment.

Myelofibrosis results from an abnormal proliferation of mesenchymal elements in the bone marrow, spleen, liver and lymph nodes. Most patients present over the age of 50 years, and the spleen may produce pain owing to its gross enlargement (***Figure 70.14***) or to splenic infarcts. Splenectomy reduces the need for transfusion and may relieve the discomfort resulting from the splenomegaly.

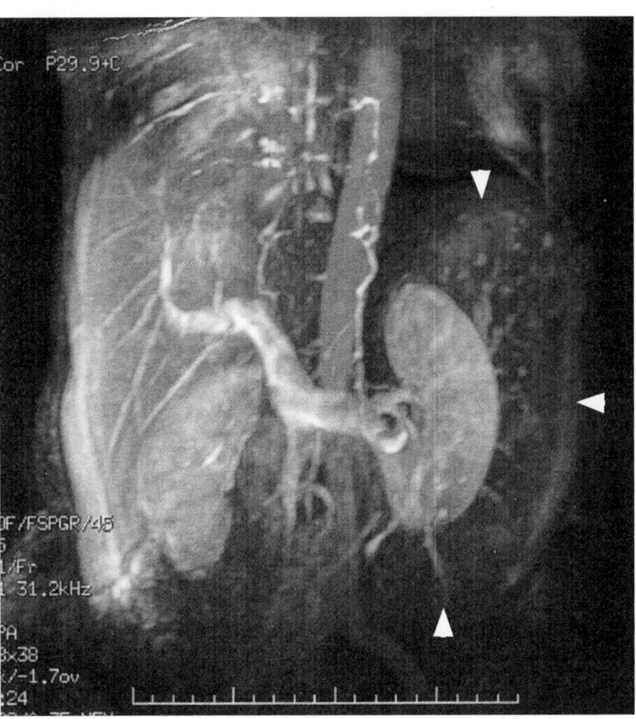

Figure 70.14 Magnetic resonance imaging scan showing massive hepatosplenomegaly secondary to myelofibrosis. Note the prominent portal system and the left kidney, which is superimposed over the grossly enlarged spleen (arrowheads).

SPLENECTOMY

The common indications for splenectomy are:

- trauma resulting from an accident or iatrogenic during a surgical procedure; for example, during mobilisation of the oesophagus, stomach, distal pancreas or splenic flexure of the colon;
- removal en bloc with the stomach as part of a radical gastrectomy or with the pancreas as part of a distal or total pancreatectomy;
- to treat anaemia or thrombocytopenia in spherocytosis, ITP or hypersplenism;
- in association with shunt or variceal surgery for portal hypertension.

Summary box 70.2

Indications for splenectomy

Trauma
- Accidental
- Iatrogenic

Oncological
- Part of *en bloc* resection
- Diagnostic
- Therapeutic

Haematological
- Spherocytosis
- Purpura (ITP)
- Hypersplenism

Portal hypertension
- Variceal surgery

Preoperative preparation

In the presence of a bleeding tendency, transfusion of blood, fresh-frozen plasma, cryoprecipitate or platelets may be required. Coagulation profiles should be as near normal as possible at operation, and platelets should be available for patients with thrombocytopenia during operation and in the early postoperative period.

Antibiotic prophylaxis appropriate to the operative procedure should be given, and consideration should be given to the risk of postsplenectomy sepsis (see ***Postoperative complications***).

Technique of open splenectomy

Most surgeons use a midline or transverse left subcostal incision for open splenectomy with the patient in the supine position. Rarely, a thoracoabdominal incision may be necessary for a massive spleen that is adherent to the diaphragm. Passage of a nasogastric tube following induction of the anaesthetic enables the stomach to be emptied.

In elective splenectomy, the gastrosplenic ligament is opened and the short gastric vessels are divided. The splenic vessels at the superior border of the pancreas are suture ligated. Division of the posterior leaf of the lienorenal ligament with long curved scissors on the posterior surface of the spleen helps to rotate and deliver the spleen medially into the laparotomy wound along with the tail and body of the pancreas. The posterior surface of the spleen is exposed and the spleen rotated medially along with the tail and body of the pancreas (***Figure 70.15***). The pancreas is separated from the hilar vessels, which are normally doubly ligated separately and divided. Accessory splenic tissue in the splenic hilum or omentum should be excluded by a careful search at operation. There is no need to drain the wound.

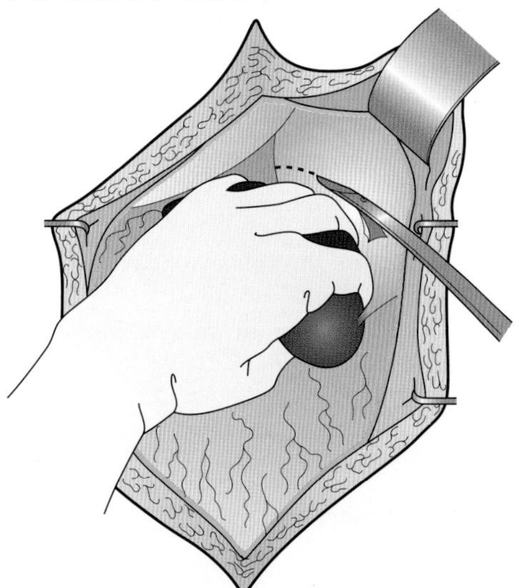

Figure 70.15 Diagrammatic view of the approach to mobilise the spleen at open surgery with division of the peritoneal fold of the lienorenal ligament posteriorly using Metzenbaum scissors, enabling delivery of the spleen into the laparotomy wound.

The segmental vasculature of the spleen does make it possible to undertake limited resection of the parenchyma. Haemostasis can be achieved by ligation of, or application of metal clips to, intrasplenic vessels and by careful application of topical haemostatic agents. Conservative splenic surgery is therefore possible in some cases of splenic trauma and other pathology such as splenic cysts.

Technique of laparoscopic splenectomy

The patient is placed on the right side with the space between the left ilium and costal margin exposed. Placement of access ports is often determined by the size of the patient and the spleen. Insufflation of the abdomen can be performed once access is obtained through an incision 1 cm from the costal margin at the left midclavicular line. A further trocar is inserted close to the costal margin below the xiphoid. A 12-mm trocar is inserted at a similar distance from the costal margin at the posterior axillary line. The splenocolic ligament is divided to give access to the lower splenic pole. The spleen is separated from the kidney and diaphragm before the gap between the splenic hilum and the tail of the pancreas is enlarged. The spleen is elevated to expose the splenic hilum, which is secured and divided with an endoscopic vascular stapler (***Figure 70.16***). Two or three applications of the instrument may be required to secure the hilum and the short gastric vessels. Any remaining attachments to the diaphragm are divided before a self-retaining opening bag is introduced through the incision of the open laparoscopy, after removal of the 12-mm port.

Postoperative complications

Immediate complications specific to splenectomy include haemorrhage resulting from a slipped ligature. Left basal

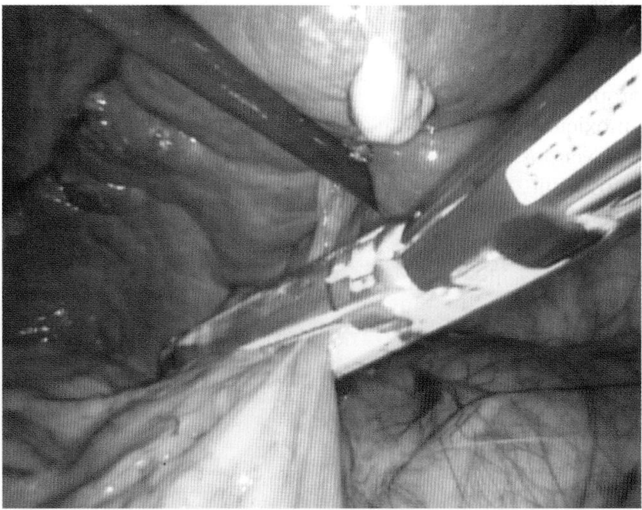

Figure 70.16 Photograph showing a stapling device across the splenic hilus for division of the splenic vessels during laparoscopic splenectomy.

Myron Firth Metzenbaum, 1876-1944, surgeon, Cleveland, OH, USA.

atelectasis is common and a pleural effusion may be present. Adjacent structures at risk during the procedure include the stomach and pancreas. A fistula may result from damage to the greater curvature of the stomach during ligation of the short gastric vessels. Damage to the tail of the pancreas during ligation of the splenic vessels at the hilum may result in pancreatitis, a localised abscess or a pancreatic fistula. Haematemesis from gastric mucosal damage and gastric dilatation are uncommon.

Postoperative thrombocytosis may arise and, if the blood platelet count exceeds 1×10^6/mL, prophylactic aspirin is recommended. Long-term surveillance programmes have emphasised an increased risk of deep vein thrombosis and pulmonary embolism. The relative risk and benefit of thromboprophylaxis in this setting has not been assessed adequately.

Postsplenectomy septicaemia may result from *S. pneumoniae, Neisseria meningitides, Haemophilus influenzae* or *Escherichia coli*. Long-term surveillance programmes have suggested that the risk of pneumonia, meningitis and major sepsis following splenectomy is increased threefold. However, the risk is greater in the young patient, in splenectomised patients treated with chemoradiotherapy and in patients who have undergone splenectomy for thalassaemia, sickle cell disease and autoimmune anaemia or thrombocytopenia.

Opportunist postsplenectomy infection (OPSI) is a major concern. Published guidelines emphasise that most infections after splenectomy could be avoided through measures that include offering patients appropriate and timely immunisation, antibiotic prophylaxis, education and prompt treatment of infection. The benefit of prophylactic antibiotics in this setting remains controversial. It is thought that children who have undergone splenectomy before the age of 5 years should be treated with a daily dose of penicillin until the age of 10 years. Prophylaxis in older children should be continued at least until the age of 16 years, but its use is less well defined in adults. Furthermore, compliance is problematic in the long term but, as the risk of overwhelming sepsis is greatest within the first 2–3 years after splenectomy, it seems reasonable to give prophylaxis during this time. However, all patients with compromised immune function should receive prophylaxis. Satisfactory oral prophylaxis can be obtained with penicillin, erythromycin, amoxicillin or co-amoxiclav. Suspected infection can be treated intravenously with these same antibiotics and cefotaxime or ceftriaxone, or chloramphenicol in patients allergic to penicillin and cephalosporins.

If elective splenectomy is planned, consideration should be given to vaccinating against pneumococcus, meningococcus C (both repeated every 5 years) and *H. influenzae* type b (Hib) (repeated every 10 years). The last two vaccines are commonly delivered as a combined preparation. Yearly influenza vaccination has been recommended, as there is some evidence that it may reduce the risk of secondary bacterial infection. Such vaccinations should be administered at least 2 weeks before elective surgery or as soon as possible after recovery from surgery but before discharge from hospital. Pneumococcal vaccination is recommended in those patients aged over 2 years. Hib vaccination is recommended irrespective of age. Asplenic patients should carry a medical alert and an up-to-date vaccination card. They require specific advice regarding travel and animal handling. OPSI due to *Capnocytophaga canimorsus* may result from dog, cat or other animal bites.

Vaccination can be given in the postoperative period following splenectomy for trauma, and the resulting antibody levels will be protective in the majority of cases. Antibody levels are, however, less than 50% of those achieved if vaccination is given in the presence of an intact spleen. Protection following vaccination is not always guaranteed.

Summary box 70.3

Splenectomy

- Remember preoperative immunisation
- Prophylactic antibiotics in children and immune compromised adults
- Opportunistic postsplenectomy infection is a real clinical danger
- Splenic conservation should be considered

FURTHER READING

Boyle S, White RH, Brunson A, Wun T. Splenectomy and the incidence of venous thromboembolism and sepsis in patients with immune thrombocytopenia. *Blood* 2013; **121**: 4782–90.

Di Sabatino A, Carsetti R, Corazza GR. Post splenectomy and hyposplenic states. *Lancet* 2011; **378**: 86–97.

Easow MM, Sharma A, Aravindakshan R. Splenectomy for people with thalassaemia major or intermedia. *Cochrane Database Syst Rev* 2014; Issue 6, Art. No. CDO10517.

Edgren G, Almqvist R, Hartman M, Utter GH. Splenectomy and the risk of sepsis: a population-based cohort study. *Ann Surg* 2014; **260**: 1081–7.

Glasgow RE, Mulvihill SJ. Laparoscopic splenectomy. *World J Surg* 1999; **23**: 384–8.

Kozar RA, Crandall M, Shanmuganathan K *et al.* Organ injury scaling 2018 update: spleen, liver, and kidney. *J Trauma Acute Care Surg* 2018; **85**(6): 1119–22.

Mourtzoukou EG, Mikhael J, Northridge K *et al.* Short-term and long-term failure of laparoscopic splenectomy in adult immune thrombocytopenic purpura patients: a systematic review. *Am J Hematol* 2009; **84**(11): 743–8.

Pappas G, Peppas G, Falagas ME. Vaccination of asplenic or hyposplenic adults. *Br J Surg* 2008; **95**(3): 273–80.

Sarin SK, Kumar A, Chawla YK *et al.* Noncirrhotic portal fibrosis/idiopathic portal hypertension: APASL recommendations for diagnosis and treatment. *Hepatol Int* 2007; **1**(3): 398–413.

Weatherall DJ. The hereditary anaemias. *Br Med J* 1997; **314**: 492–6.

Albert Ludwig Siegmund Neisser, 1855–1916, Director of the Dermatological Institute, Breslau, Germany (now Wroclaw, Poland).
Theodor Escherich, 1857–1911, Professor of Paediatrics, Vienna, Austria.

CHAPTER 71 The gallbladder and bile ducts

Learning objectives

- To understand the surgical anatomy and physiology of the gallbladder and bile ducts
- To be familiar with the pathophysiology and management of gallstones
- To be aware of unusual disorders of the biliary tree
- To be aware of malignant disease of the gallbladder and bile ducts

SURGICAL ANATOMY AND PHYSIOLOGY

The gallbladder is a pear-shaped structure, 7.5–12 cm long, with a normal capacity of about 25–30 mL. Its anatomical divisions are fundus, body and neck, which terminates in a narrow infundibulum. The gallbladder lies on the underside of the liver in the main liver scissura at the junction of the right and left lobes. Its relationship to the liver varies from being embedded within the liver substance to being suspended by a mesentery. The muscle fibres in the wall of the gallbladder are arranged in a criss-cross manner, being particularly well developed in its neck. The mucous membrane contains indentations (crypts of Luschka) that sink into the muscle coat.

The cystic duct is about 3 cm in length, but this is variable. Its lumen is 1–3 mm in diameter; its mucosa is arranged in spiral folds (valves of Heister); and the wall is surrounded by the sphincter of Lütkens. The cystic duct joins the supraduodenal segment of the common hepatic duct in 80% of cases; however, the junction may be much lower in the retroduodenal or even retropancreatic part of the bile duct. Occasionally, the cystic duct may join the right hepatic duct or even a right hepatic sectorial duct (see ***Low insertion of the cystic duct***).

The common hepatic duct is usually less than 2.5 cm long and is formed by the union of the right and left hepatic ducts. The common bile duct (CBD) is about 7.5 cm long and is formed by the junction of the cystic and common hepatic ducts. It is divided into four parts:

1 supraduodenal portion, about 2.5 cm long, runs in the free edge of the lesser omentum;
2 retroduodenal portion;
3 infraduodenal portion, lies in a groove, at times in a tunnel, on the posterior surface of the pancreas;
4 intraduodenal portion, passes obliquely through the wall of the second part of the duodenum, where it is surrounded by the sphincter of Oddi and terminates by opening on the summit of the ampulla of Vater.

The cystic artery, a branch of the right hepatic artery, usually arises behind the common hepatic duct (***Figure 71.1***). Occasionally, an accessory cystic artery arises from the gastroduodenal artery. In 15% of cases the right hepatic artery and/or cystic artery cross in front of the common hepatic duct and cystic duct.

Calot's triangle, or the hepatobiliary triangle, was initially described by Calot as the space bordered by the cystic duct inferiorly, the common hepatic duct medially and the superior border of the cystic artery.

This has been modified in contemporary literature as the area bound superiorly by the inferior surface of the liver, laterally by the cystic duct and the medial border of the gallbladder and medially by the common hepatic duct ('hepatocystic triangle'). It is an important surgical landmark as the cystic artery usually can be found within its boundaries (***Figure 71.2a***). The cystic lymph node often lies superficial to the cystic artery and acts as a landmark to locate this artery in difficult cases.

The cystic plate is a flat ovoid fibrous sheet continuous with the liver capsule of segments IV (medially) and V

Hubert Luschka, 1820–1875, Professor of Anatomy, Tübingen, Germany.
Lorenz Heister, 1683–1758, Professor of Surgery and Botany, Helmstädt, Germany.
Ulrich Lütkens, b. 1894, surgeon, University Clinic, Berlin, Germany, published a monograph on the structure and function of the extrahepatic biliary tract in 1926.
Ruggero Oddi, 1845–1906, physiologist, Perugia, Italy.
Abraham Vater, 1684–1751, Professor of Anatomy and Botany, Wittenberg, Germany.
Jean François Calot, 1861–1944, surgeon, Paris, France.

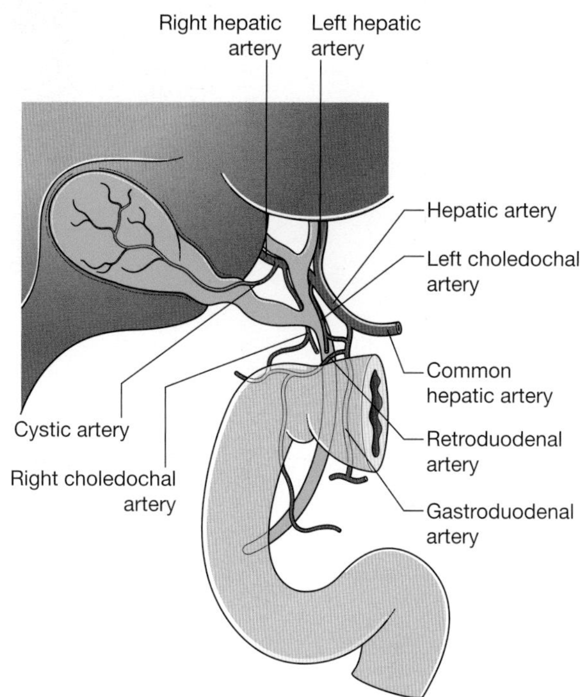

Figure 71.1 Anatomy of the gallbladder and bile ducts. Note the arrangement of the arterial tree.

(laterally). It is located in the gallbladder bed and needs to be exposed to achieve the critical view of safety (CVS) during cholecystectomy. Rouvière's sulcus on the undersurface of the right lobe of the liver running to the right of the hepatic hilum marks the position of the right posterior sectoral pedicle. The advantage of identifying Rouvière's sulcus and the line joining the roof of the sulcus to the base of segment IV (R4U line) (Rouvière's sulcus→segment IV→umbilical fissure) is that the cystic duct and the cystic artery lie ventral (anterosuperior) to the line and the CBD lies below the line. CBD injury can be minimised by maintaining the dissection ventral to the line during cholecystectomy. In the case of difficulty, all dissection during laparoscopic cholecystectomy should be performed ventral to the R4U line (***Figure 71.3***).

Blood supply to the bile ducts

The supraduodenal CBD is supplied by the left and right choledochal arteries, arising from the posterior superior pancreaticoduodenal artery below and the right (RHA) and left (LHA) hepatic arteries and cystic arteries above (***Figure 71.1***). The choledochal arteries give small branches that form the epicholedochal plexus. The communicating arcade connects the RHA and LHA and lies cranial to the confluence of the right and left hepatic ducts.

The venous drainage of the extrahepatic bile ducts consists of the epicholedochal venous plexus that drains into two marginal veins that drain into the right gastric vein, posterior superior pancreaticoduodenal vein and superior mesenteric vein and connect to the hilar plexus.

Anatomical variations

The right hepatic artery can be tortuous (caterpillar turn/ Moynihan's hump) and may lie very close to the gallbladder and the cystic duct before giving off a short cystic artery (***Figure 71.2b,c***).

Biliary and ductal anomalies include double cystic duct, separate insertion into the duodenum and anomalous low insertion of a right sectional duct (usually the posterior one, which puts this sectional duct at higher risk of injury).

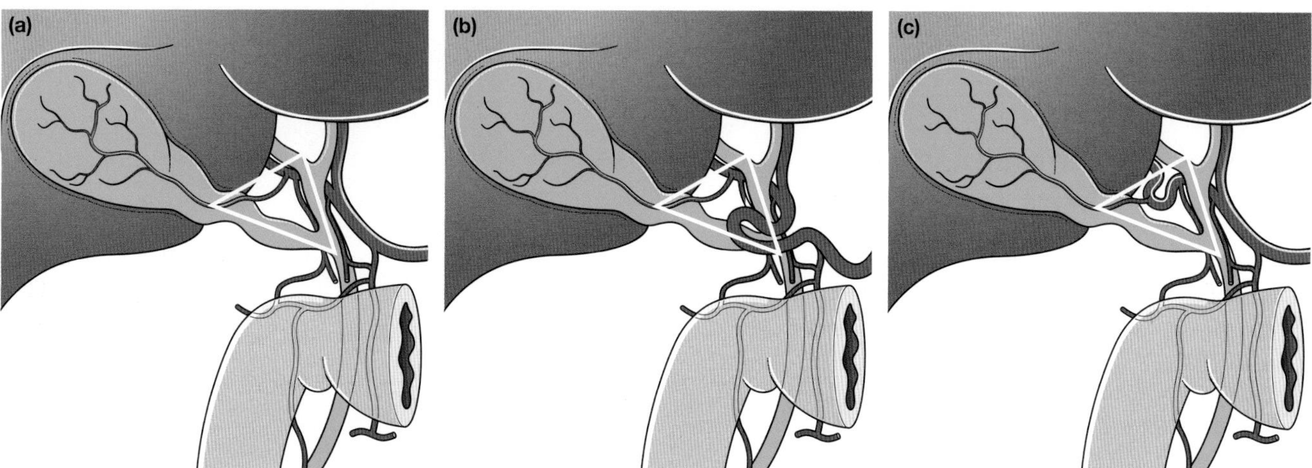

Figure 71.2 **(a)** The usual anatomy of the 'hepatocystic triangle'; **(b)** tortuous common hepatic artery; **(c)** tortuous right hepatic artery with a short cystic artery. **(b)** and **(c)** are examples of the 'caterpillar turn' or 'Moynihan's hump', which can lead to inadvertent arterial injury or bleeding during cholecystectomy.

M. Henri Rouvière, 1876–1952, Professor of Anatomy, LeBleymard, France.
Berkeley George Andrew Moynihan (Lord Moynihan), 1865–1936, Professor of Clinical Surgery, Leeds, UK.

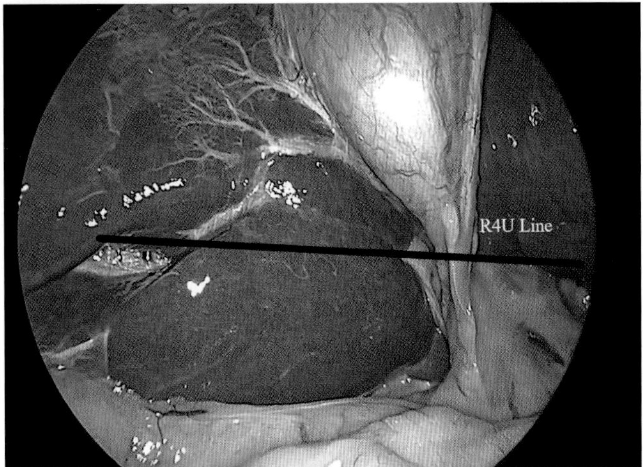

Figure 71.3 Rouvière's sulcus. R4U line, Rouvière's sulcus→segment IV→umbilical fissure.

Lymphatics

The subserosal and submucosal lymphatic vessels of the gallbladder drain into the cystic lymph node of Lund (the sentinel lymph node), which lies in the fork created by the junction of the cystic and common hepatic ducts. Efferent vessels from this lymph node go to the hilum of the liver and to the coeliac lymph nodes. The subserosal lymphatics also connect with the subcapsular lymph channels of the liver; this accounts for the frequent spread of carcinoma of the gallbladder to the liver.

Surgical physiology

Bile is produced by the liver and stored in the gallbladder before being released into the duodenum. The liver excretes bile at approximately 40 mL/h. As it leaves the liver its composition is 97% water; the remaining 3% consists of bile salts (cholic and chenodeoxycholic acids, deoxycholic and lithocholic acids), phospholipids, cholesterol and bilirubin. About 95% of bile salts are reabsorbed in the terminal ileum and returned to the liver (enterohepatic circulation).

Functions of the gallbladder

The gallbladder is a reservoir for bile. During fasting, the resistance to flow through the sphincter of Oddi is high, and bile excreted by the liver is diverted to the gallbladder. After feeding, the resistance to flow through the sphincter is reduced, the gallbladder contracts and bile enters the duodenum. The motor responses of the biliary tract are in part affected by the hormone cholecystokinin. An additional function of the gallbladder is the concentration of bile by 5–10 times by active absorption of water, sodium chloride and bicarbonate via the mucous membrane. The gallbladder mucosa also secretes approximately 20 mL of mucus per day. If the cystic duct is completely obstructed in an otherwise healthy gallbladder, a mucocele may develop as a result of ongoing mucus secretion.

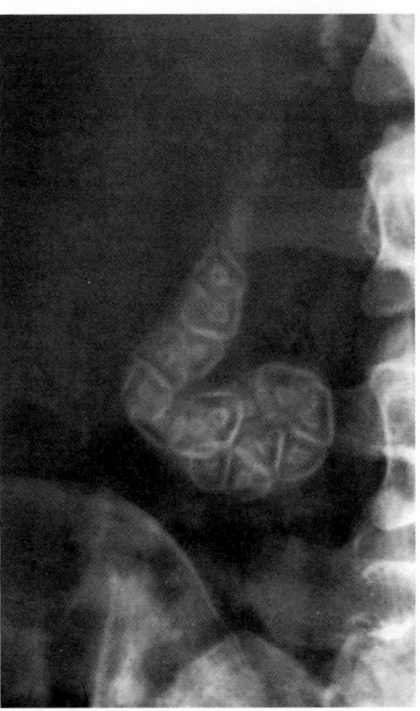

Figure 71.4 Plain radiograph showing radio-opaque stones with the centre containing radiolucent gas in a triradiate or biradiate fissure ('Mercedes-Benz' or 'seagull' sign).

IMAGING

Plain radiographs

A plain radiograph of the gallbladder will show radio-opaque stones in 10% (***Figure 71.4***). It may also show calcification of the gallbladder – the rare 'porcelain' gallbladder (***Figure 71.5***).

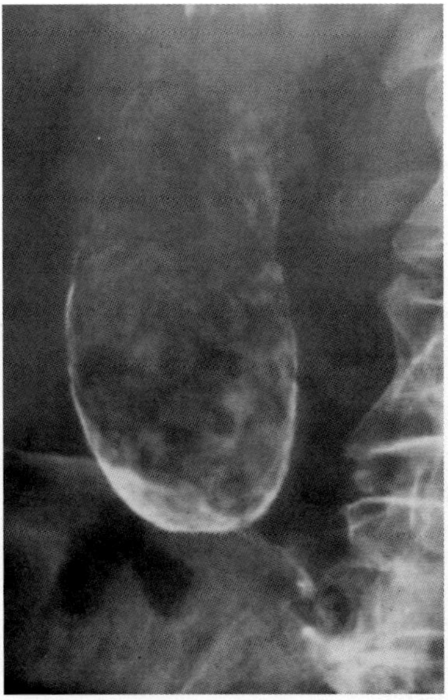

Figure 71.5 Porcelain gallbladder.

Fred Bates Lund, 1865–1950, surgeon, Boston, MA, USA. The node was also named after the Italian anatomist and physician **Paolo Mascagni**, 1752–1815, who first identified the node around 1787.

The **Mercedes-Benz** sign takes its name from the insignia on the bonnet of a Mercedes-Benz car

Gas may be seen in the wall of the gallbladder (emphysematous cholecystitis) (***Figure 71.6***). Gas in the biliary tree may also be seen after endoscopic sphincterotomy or following a surgical anastomosis.

Cholecystography

Oral and intravenous cholecystography have been replaced by more accurate imaging modalities.

Ultrasonography

Transabdominal ultrasonography (USG) (***Figure 71.7***) is the initial imaging modality of choice as it is accurate, readily available, inexpensive and quick to perform. However, it is operator dependent and may be compromised by excessive body fat and intraluminal bowel gas. The size of the gallbladder and presence of stones or polyps can be determined. Acute calculous cholecystitis is diagnosed radiologically (sensitivity 90–95%) by thickening of the gallbladder wall (>3 mm), presence of pericholecystic fluid or direct tenderness when the probe is pushed against the gallbladder (ultrasonographic Murphy's sign). Additionally, the presence of inflammation around the gallbladder, the size of the CBD and, occasionally, the presence of stones within the extrahepatic biliary tree can be determined.

In a patient with obstructive jaundice, USG can identify intra- and extrahepatic biliary dilatation, the level of the obstruction and the cause of the obstruction – stones, common hepatic duct or CBD, lesions within the wall of the CBD suggestive of cholangiocarcinoma, gallbladder cancer or mass lesions in the pancreatic head.

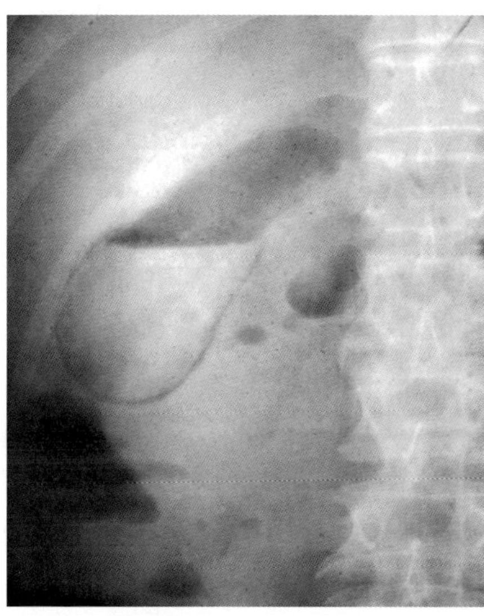

Figure 71.6 Gas in gallbladder and gallbladder wall (*Clostridium perfringens* infection). Emergency cholecystectomy is indicated.

Endoscopic ultrasonography

Endoscopic ultrasonography (EUS) utilises an endoscope with an ultrasound transducer at its tip, which allows the endoscopist to visualise the liver and biliary tree from within the stomach and duodenum (***Figure 71.8***). It is accurate in detecting choledocholithiasis and in the diagnosis and staging of pancreatic and periampullary cancers. Biopsies can be taken from suspicious areas for cytological and histological analysis.

Cholescintigraphy

Technetium-99m (^{99m}Tc)-labelled derivatives of iminodiacetic acid (hepatobiliary iminodiacetic acid [HIDA]; the utility of a hepatobiliary IDA or HIDA scan is that the radiotracer follows

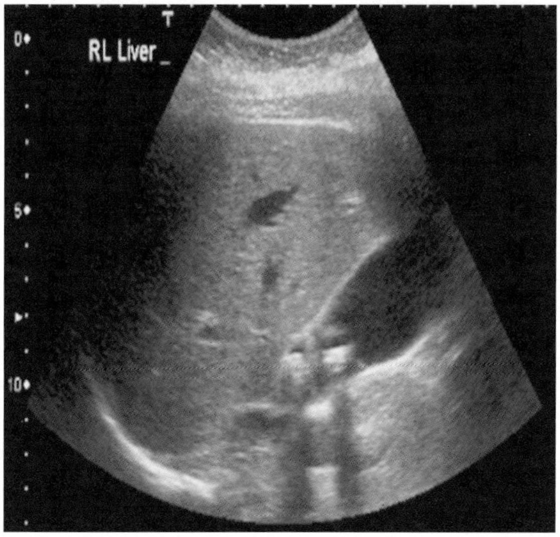

Figure 71.7 Ultrasound examination. Gallstones in neck of gallbladder with acoustic shadowing.

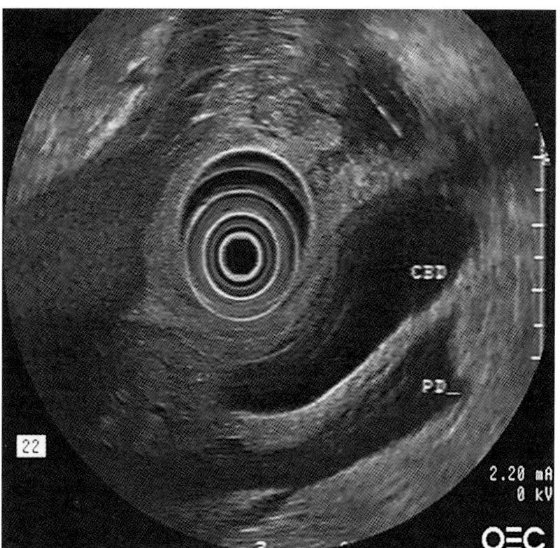

Figure 71.8 Endoscopic ultrasonography. CBD, common bile duct; PD, pancreatic duct.

John Benjamin Murphy, 1857–1916, surgeon, Mercy Hospital, Chicago, IL, USA.

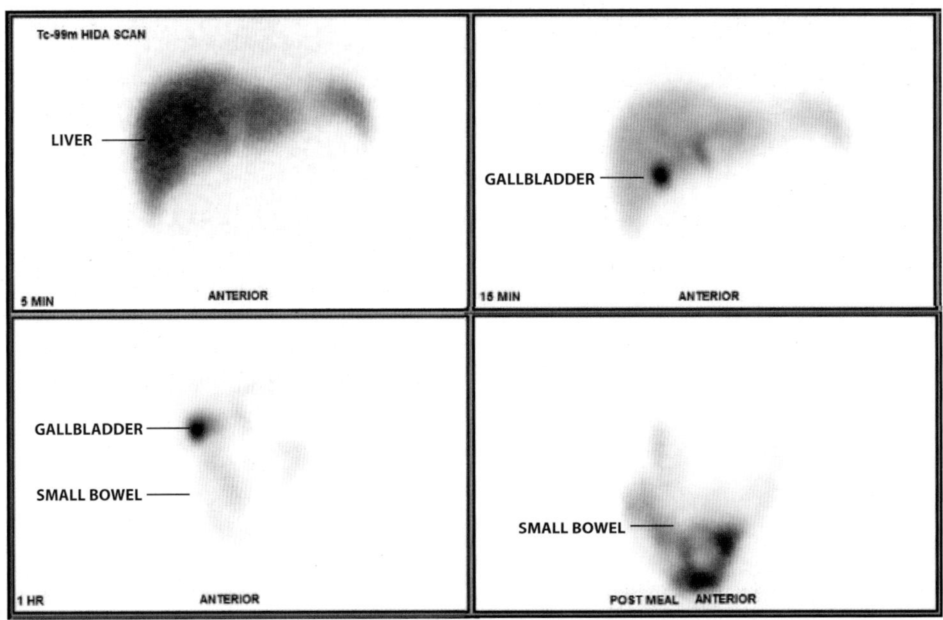

Figure 71.9 Dimethyl iminodiacetic acid (HIDA) scan before and after a meal to evaluate gallbladder function (courtesy of the Department of Nuclear Medicine, KEM Hospital, Mumbai, India).

the bilirubin metabolic pathway) are excreted into the bile. This allows visualisation of the biliary tree and gallbladder. In 90% of normal individuals the gallbladder is visualised within 30 minutes following injection, with 100% being seen within 1 hour (*Figure 71.9*). The bowel is seen usually within an hour in the majority of patients.

Non-visualisation of the gallbladder is suggestive of acute cholecystitis. If the patient has a contracted gallbladder, as often occurs in chronic cholecystitis, visualisation may be reduced or delayed. An abnormally low gallbladder ejection fraction may be suggestive of gallbladder dyskinesia; however, interpretation of cholescintigraphy in this context is controversial. Biliary scintigraphy may also be helpful in diagnosing bile leaks, biliary obstruction and in testing the patency of a bilioenteric anastomosis.

Computed tomography

Unlike USG, computed tomography (CT) is less affected by body habitus and is not operator dependent. It allows visualisation of the liver, bile ducts, gallbladder and pancreas. CT findings in acute cholecystitis include gallbladder distension, gallbladder wall thickening, subserosal oedema, pericholecystic fat stranding and pericholecystic fluid collection. It is particularly useful in detecting hepatic and pancreatic lesions and is the modality of choice in the staging of cancers of the liver, gallbladder, bile ducts and pancreas. It can identify the extent of the primary tumour, define the relationship of the tumour to other organs and blood vessels (*Figure 71.10*) and detect the presence of enlarged lymph nodes or metastatic disease. However, as only 75% of gallstones are identified by CT, it is not used as a screening modality for uncomplicated gallstones.

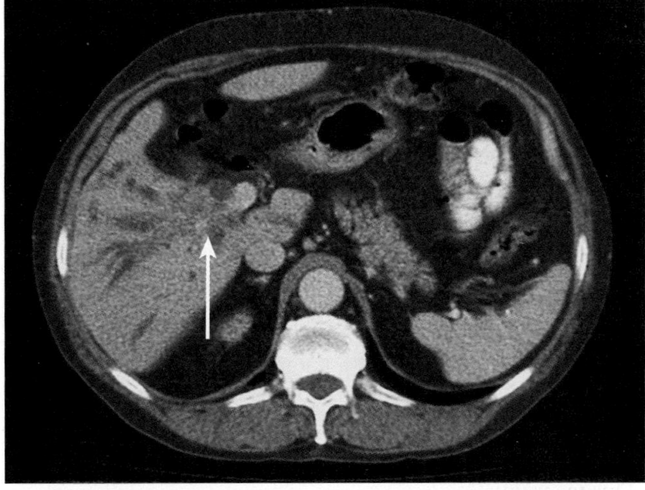

Figure 71.10 Computed tomography showing hilar mass (arrow).

Magnetic resonance cholangiopancreatography

Magnetic resonance cholangiopancreatography (MRCP) is a non-invasive modality that provides excellent images of the gallbladder and biliary system (*Figures 71.11 and 71.12*). These images are comparable to those obtained at endoscopic retrograde cholangiopancreatography (ERCP) or percutaneous transhepatic cholangiography (PTC) (see ***Percutaneous transhepatic cholangiography*** and ***Endoscopic retrograde cholangiopancreatography***) without the potential complications of the latter; they can demonstrate ductal abnormalities, including obstruction/stricture, stones and tumours.

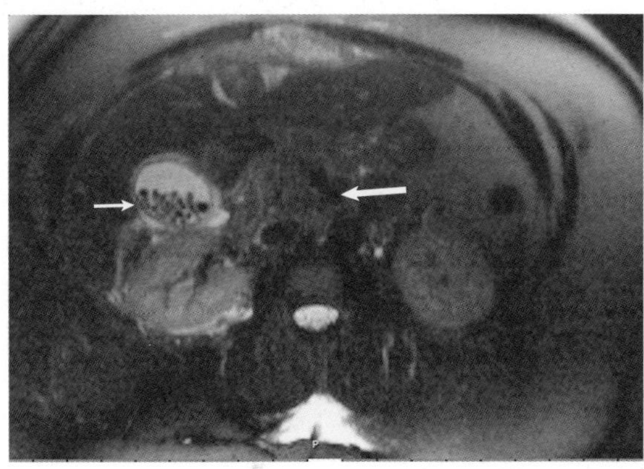

Figure 71.11 Magnetic resonance cholangiopancreatography: cross-sectional image demonstrating hilar mass (thick arrow) and gallstones (thin arrow).

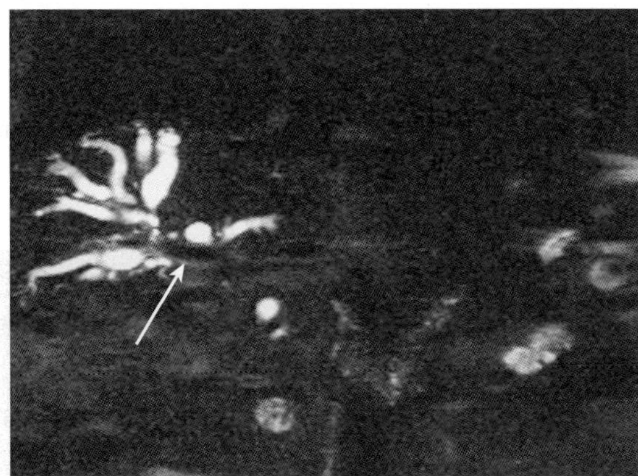

Figure 71.12 Magnetic resonance cholangiopancreatography: projectional images demonstrating stones and hilar obstruction (arrow).

Endoscopic retrograde cholangiopancreatography

This technique is now used only as a therapeutic modality in patients with obstructive jaundice; USG and MRCP have taken over the diagnostic aspect. Using a side-viewing endoscope the ampulla of Vater is identified and cannulated. Injection of water-soluble contrast into the bile duct provides excellent images of the ductal anatomy (*Figure 71.13*) and can identify causes of obstruction such as calculi (*Figure 71.14*) and malignant strictures (*Figure 71.15*). Bile aspirates can be obtained and sent for cytological and microbiological examination and brushings can be taken from strictures for cytology. Therapeutic interventions such as stone removal or stent placement to relieve obstruction can be performed simultaneously.

Cholangioscopy is a relatively new technique in which a thin scope is inserted through the channel of an ERCP scope to visually inspect the bile duct. The main indications include indeterminate or unexplained biliary strictures, nodules or masses and crushing difficult-to-remove bile duct stones with lithotripsy.

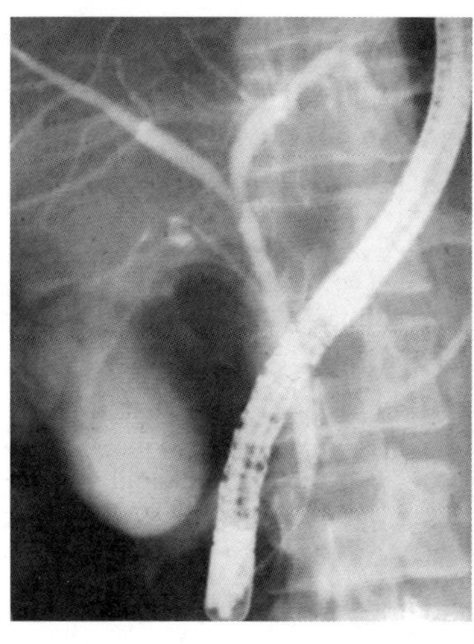

Figure 71.13 Endoscopic retrograde cholangiopancreatography: normal cholangiogram.

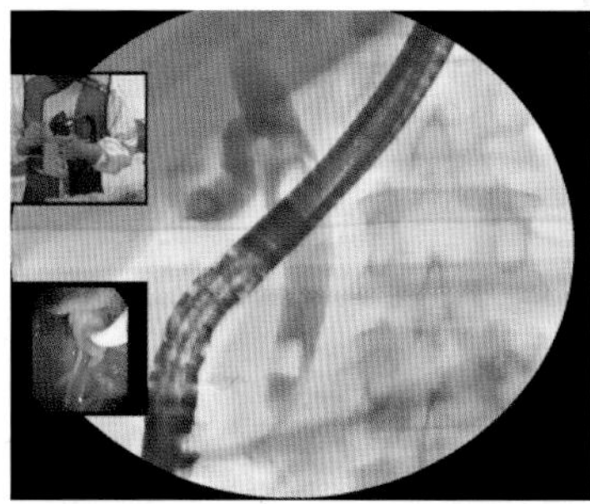

Figure 71.14 Endoscopic retrograde cholangiopancreatography: common duct obstruction due to stone (courtesy Dr Amit Maydeo, Mumbai, India).

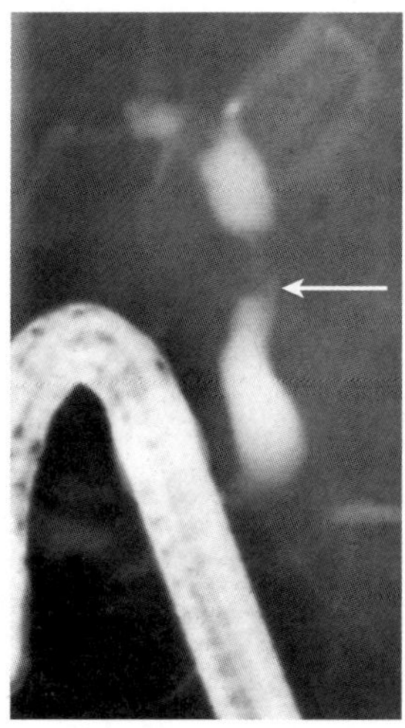

Figure 71.15 Endoscopic retrograde cholangiopancreatography: partial occlusion of bile duct by malignant stricture (arrow).

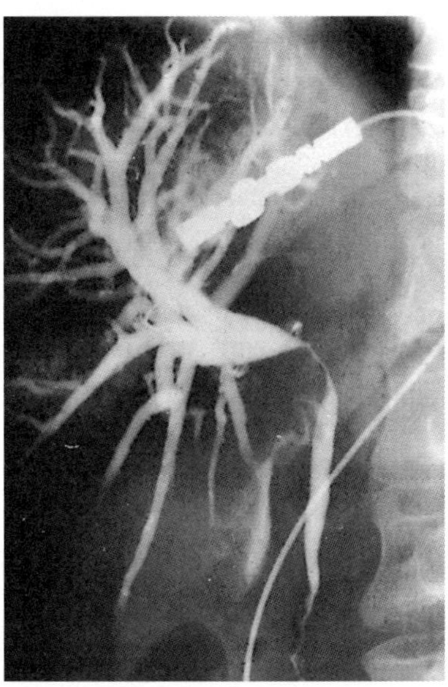

Figure 71.16 Transhepatic cholangiogram showing stricture of common hepatic duct (courtesy of Ms Phyllis George, FRCS, London, UK).

Percutaneous transhepatic cholangiography

This is an invasive technique in which the bile ducts are cannulated percutaneously. The main indication is to drain intrahepatic ducts when strictures cannot be accessed at ERCP. The procedure is undertaken after confirming normal coagulation parameters; antibiotics should be given prior to the procedure. Under fluoroscopic or sonographic control, a slender (Chiba or Okuda) needle is introduced percutaneously into the liver substance. Successful entry into the bile duct is confirmed by contrast injection or aspiration of bile. Water-soluble contrast medium is injected to visualise the biliary system and images are taken to demonstrate strictures or obstruction (*Figure 71.16*). Bile can be sent for cytology. This technique enables placement of a catheter into the bile ducts to provide external or internal biliary drainage and insertion of indwelling stents. The drainage catheter can be left *in situ* for a number of days and the track dilated sufficiently for the introduction of a fine flexible choledochoscope to diagnose strictures, take biopsies and remove stones.

Summary box 71.1

Radiological investigation of the biliary tree

- Plain radiograph: calcification, air within the biliary system
- USG: stones and biliary dilatation
- MRCP: anatomy and stones
- CT scan: anatomy, and liver, biliary and pancreatic cancer
- Radioisotope scanning (HIDA scan): function
- ERCP: anatomy, stones and biliary strictures, with or without cholangioscopy
- PTC: anatomy and biliary strictures
- EUS: anatomy, stones

Intraoperative imaging techniques

Peroperative cholangiography

During open or laparoscopic cholecystectomy, a catheter can be placed in the cystic duct and contrast injected directly into the biliary tree. The technique defines the anatomy and is used mainly to exclude the presence of stones within the bile ducts (*Figures 71.17–71.19*). A radiographic plate or image intensifier can be used to obtain and review the images intraoperatively. The operating table should be tilted head-down by approximately 20° to facilitate filling of the intrahepatic ducts.

Care should be taken when injecting contrast not to introduce air bubbles into the system as these may mimic the appearance of stones.

Operative biliary endoscopy (choledochoscopy)

At operation, a flexible fibreoptic endoscope can be passed either via the cystic duct or directly via a choledochotomy (open or laparoscopic) into the CBD, enabling stone identification and removal under direct vision. After exploration of

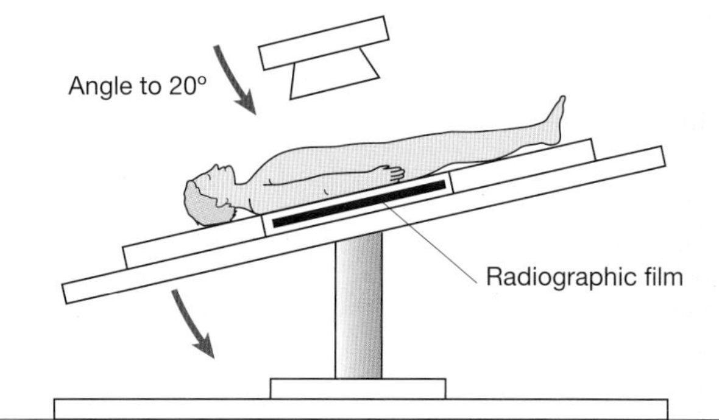

Figure 71.17 Peroperative cholangiography using a radiolucent tabletop.

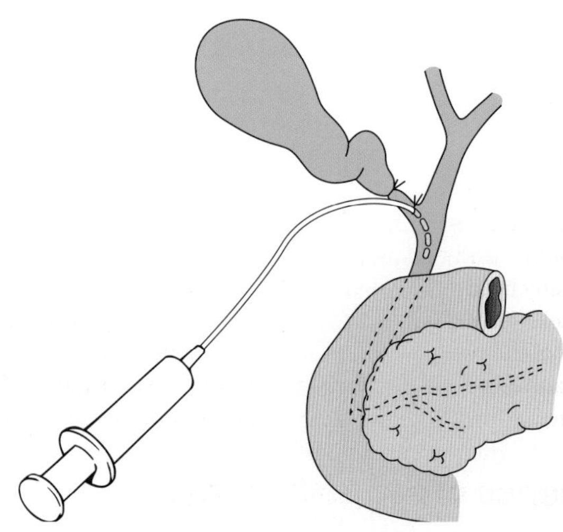

Figure 71.18 Peroperative cholangiography. Technique of introducing contrast.

Kunio Okuda, 1921–2003, Professor of Medicine, Chiba University, Chiba, Japan.

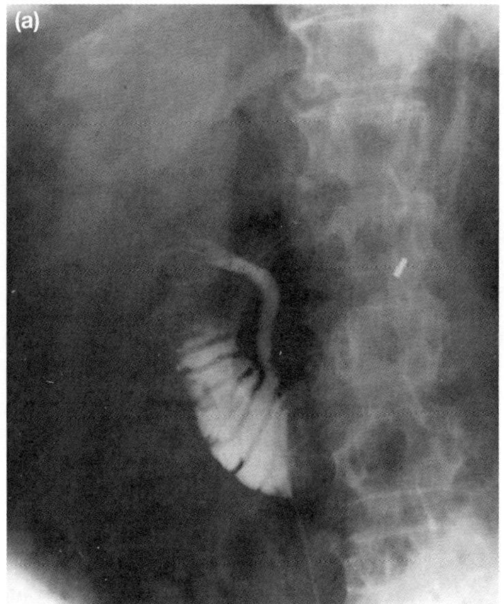

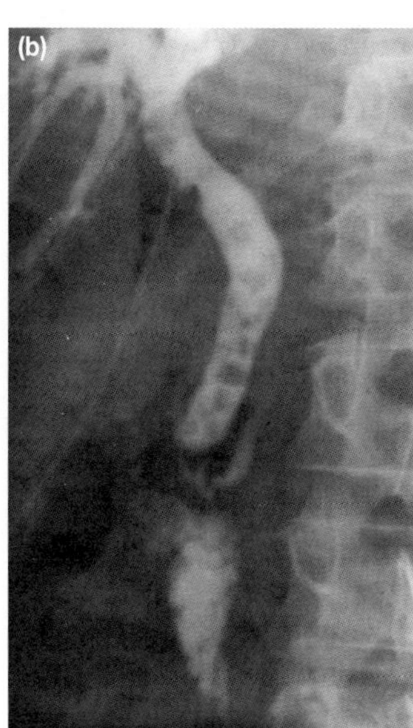

Figure 71.19 Peroperative cholangiography. (a) Gentle infusion of contrast, passing without hindrance into the duodenum. A normal duct. (b) Dilated duct containing multiple stones; there is a delay in contrast passing into the duodenum.

the bile duct, a tube can be left in the cystic duct remnant or in the CBD (T tube) and drainage of the biliary tree established. After 7–10 days, a track will be established. This track can be used subsequently for the passage of a choledochoscope or radiologically guided stone retrieval catheter (Burhenne technique) to remove residual stones.

Laparoscopic ultrasonography

At laparoscopy, a laparoscopic ultrasound probe can be used to closely image the extrahepatic biliary system. This technique is useful in biliary and pancreatic tumour staging as it can determine the relationship of the tumour to major vessels such as the hepatic artery, superior mesenteric artery, portal vein and superior mesenteric vein.

CONGENITAL ABNORMALITIES OF THE GALLBLADDER AND BILE DUCTS

Embryology

The hepatic diverticulum arises from the ventral wall of the foregut and elongates into a stalk to form the choledochus. A lateral bud is given off, which is destined to become the gallbladder and cystic duct. The embryonic hepatic duct sends out many branches that join up with the canaliculi between the liver cells. As is usual with embryonic tubular structures, hyperplasia obliterates the lumina of this ductal system; normally recanalisation occurs subsequently and bile begins to flow. During early fetal life the gallbladder is entirely intrahepatic.

Absence of the gallbladder

Rarely, the gallbladder is absent; failure to visualise it should not be mistaken for pathology.

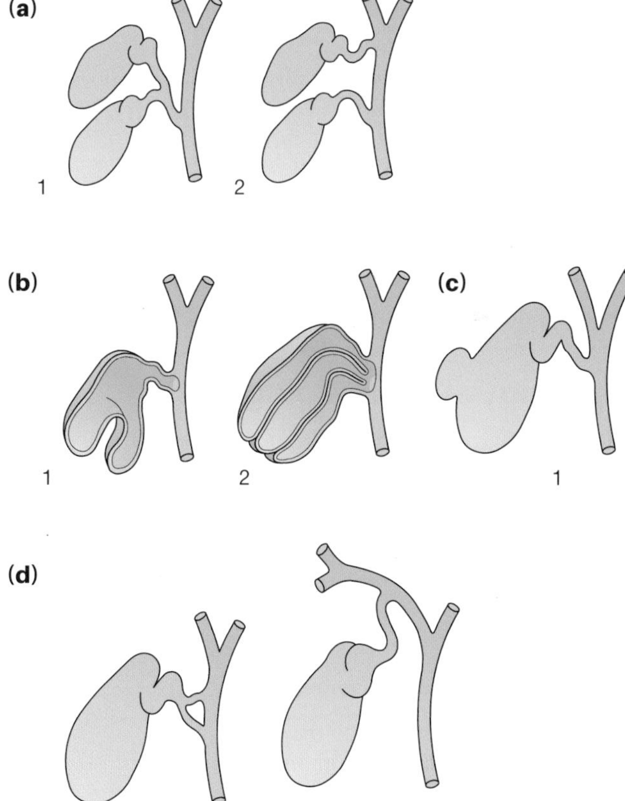

Figure 71.20 The main variations in gallbladder and cystic duct anatomy. (a) Double gallbladder. (b) Septum of the gallbladder: (1) is the most common ('Phrygian cap'). (c) Diverticulum of the gallbladder. (d) Variations in cystic duct insertion.

H Joachim Burhenne, 1925–1996, radiologist, Vancouver, Canada, described this technique in 1973.

The Phrygian cap

The Phrygian cap (*Figure 71.20*) is present in 5% of gallbladders and may be mistaken for a pathological deformity.

Floating gallbladder

The gallbladder may hang on a mesentery, which makes it liable to undergo torsion.

Absence of the cystic duct

This 'anomaly' is usually pathological, indicating the recent passage of a stone or, in the presence of jaundice, a stone at the lower end of the cystic duct ulcerating into the CBD (Mirizzi syndrome). The main danger at surgery is damage to the bile duct; care is essential before division of any duct.

Low insertion of the cystic duct

The operating surgeon must identify variations in the anatomy (*Figure 71.21*) to avoid inadvertent damage to the common hepatic duct or CBD. Complete dissection of the cystic duct (*Figure 71.22*) should be avoided because there is a potential to devascularise the CBD, which could result in stricture formation.

Accessory cholecystohepatic duct

Ducts passing directly into the gallbladder from the liver are not uncommon. Larger ducts should be closed, but before doing so the precise anatomy should be carefully ascertained to ensure that the right hepatic duct is not being ligated (*Figure 71.21*).

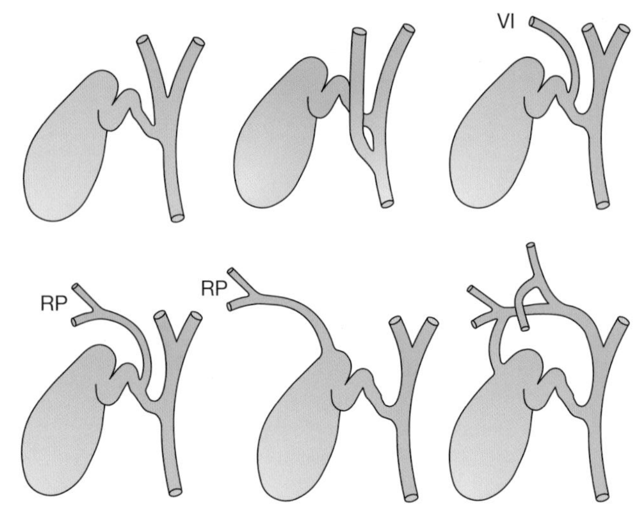

Figure 71.21 Patterns of cystic duct anatomy. Note segment VI drainage into the cystic duct and drainage of the right posterior sectorial duct (RP) into the neck of the gallbladder or an accessory duct (duct of Luschka).

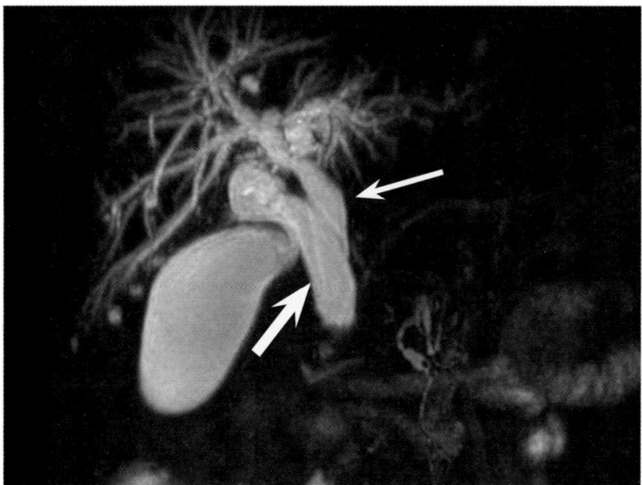

Figure 71.22 Magnetic resonance cholangiopancreatography demonstrating low insertion of the cystic duct (thick arrow) into the common bile duct (thin arrow).

EXTRAHEPATIC BILIARY ATRESIA

Aetiology and physiology

Biliary atresia is present in approximately 1 in 12 000 live births and affects males and females equally. The aetiology is unclear; the extrahepatic bile ducts are progressively destroyed by an inflammatory process that starts around the time of birth. Intrahepatic changes also occur and eventually result in biliary cirrhosis and portal hypertension. Untreated, death from the consequences of liver failure occurs before the age of 3 years.

The Japanese and Anglo-Saxon classification describes three main types (Kasai) (*Figure 71.23*):

- type I: atresia restricted to the CBD;
- type II: atresia of the common hepatic duct:
  - type IIa: a patent gallbladder and a patent CBD are present;
  - type IIb: the gallbladder, cystic duct and CBD are also obliterated;
- type III: atresia of the right and left hepatic ducts and the entire extrahepatic biliary tree.

Clinical features

About one-third of patients are jaundiced at birth; in all affected babies, jaundice is present by the end of the first week and deepens progressively. The meconium may be a little bile-stained, but later the stools are pale and the urine is dark. Pruritus is severe. Clubbing and skin xanthomas, probably related to raised serum cholesterol, may be present. Prolonged steatorrhea gives rise to osteomalacia (biliary rickets). Liver function tests show an obstructive pattern with elevated bilirubin and alkaline phosphatase (ALP). Associated anomalies occur in about 20% of cases and include cardiac lesions,

Hats worn by the **people of Phrygia**, an ancient country in Asia Minor; they resemble the liberté cap of the French Revolution.
Pablo Luis Mirizzi, 1893–1964, surgeon, Córdoba, Argentina.
Morio Kasai, 1922–2008, Professor of Surgery, Tokyo University, Tokyo, Japan.

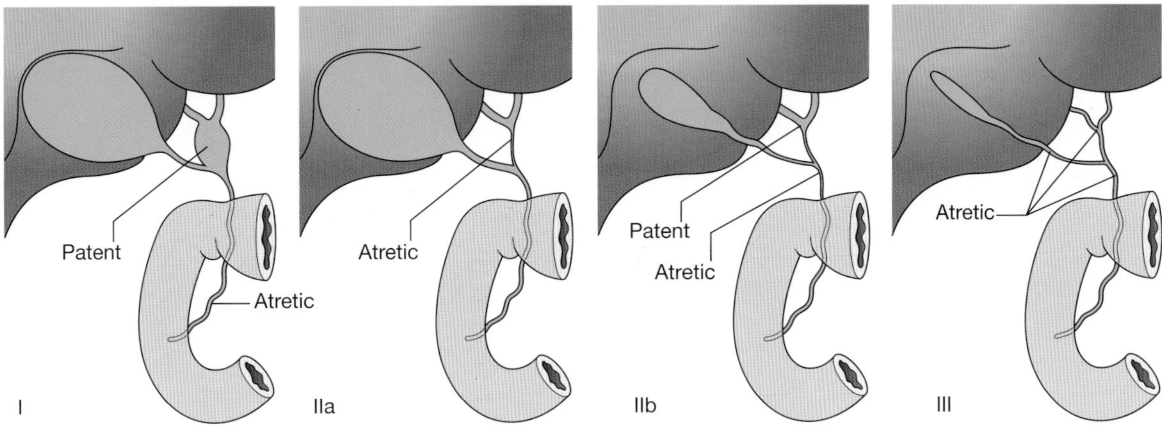

Figure 71.23 Classification of biliary atresia. Gallbladder filling provides a clue to the type of atresia.

polysplenia, situs inversus, absent vena cava and preduodenal portal vein. Biliary atresia may be suspected prenatally, when a cystic structure is observed in the porta hepatis on fetal USG.

Imaging studies and biopsy

Fasting USG is the gold standard when biliary atresia is suspected. A shrunken gallbladder, a hyperechogenic liver hilum ('triangular cord sign') or a cyst at the liver hilum without bile duct dilatation with associated anomalies support the diagnosis. Hepatobiliary scintigraphy may reveal the diagnosis but MRCP is highly sensitive and specific in the diagnosis. Inflammatory cells, a fibrotic liver parenchyma exhibiting signs of cholestasis and biliary neoductal structures establishes the definite diagnosis on liver biopsy. Cholangiography is required to define the surgical anatomy.

Differential diagnosis

This includes all causes of cholestatic jaundice in a neonate; namely, α_1-antitrypsin deficiency, cholestasis associated with intravenous feeding, choledochal cyst and inspissated bile syndrome. The most common differential diagnoses are Alagille syndrome (biliary atresia, congenital heart disease, skeletal and other abnormalities), progressive familial intrahepatic cholestasis and cystic fibrosis. Neonatal hepatitis is the most difficult to differentiate. Liver biopsy and radionuclide excretion scans are helpful.

Treatment

For breast-fed infants, introducing supplemental formula feeds using a medium-chain triglyceride-based feed and fat-soluble vitamin supplementation (titrated according to growth) is a priority.

Patent segments of proximal bile duct are found in 10% of type I lesions. A direct Roux-en-Y hepaticojejunostomy will achieve bile flow in 75%, but progressive fibrosis results in disappointing long-term results. A simple biliary–enteric anastomosis is not possible in the majority of cases in which the proximal hepatic ducts are either very small (type II) or atretic (type III). These are treated by the Kasai procedure, in which radical excision of all bile duct tissue up to the liver capsule is performed. A Roux-en-Y loop of jejunum is anastomosed to the exposed area of liver capsule above the bifurcation of the portal vein, creating a portoenterostomy. The chances of achieving effective bile drainage after portoenterostomy are maximal when the operation is performed before the age of 8 weeks, and approximately 90% of children whose bilirubin falls to normal can be expected to survive for 10 years or more. Early referral for surgery is critical.

Postoperative complications include bacterial cholangitis, which occurs in 40% of patients. Repeated attacks lead to hepatic fibrosis, and 50% of long-term survivors develop portal hypertension, with one-third having variceal bleeding.

Liver transplantation should be considered in children in whom a portoenterostomy is unsuccessful. Results are improving, with 70–80% alive 2–5 years following transplant.

CONGENITAL DILATATION OF INTRAHEPATIC DUCTS (CAROLI'S DISEASE)

This rare congenital condition is characterised by multiple irregular saccular dilatations of the intrahepatic ducts, separated by segments of normal or stenotic ducts, with a normal extrahepatic biliary system. In Caroli's syndrome, the biliary dilatation is associated with congenital hepatic fibrosis. The presentation is varied, with most patients presenting with abdominal pain, cholangitis or end-stage liver disease. The majority of patients present before the age of 30 years. The sex distribution is equal. Malignancy is a complication of longstanding disease.

Daniel Alagille, 1925–2005, paediatric hepatologist, Hôpital Bicêtre, Paris, France.
César Roux, 1857–1934, Professor of Surgery and Gynaecology, Lausanne, Switzerland, described the Roux-en-Y loop in 1908.
Jacques Caroli, 1902–1979, gastroenterologist, Hôpital St Antoine, Paris, France, described cavernous ectasia in the biliary tree in 1958.

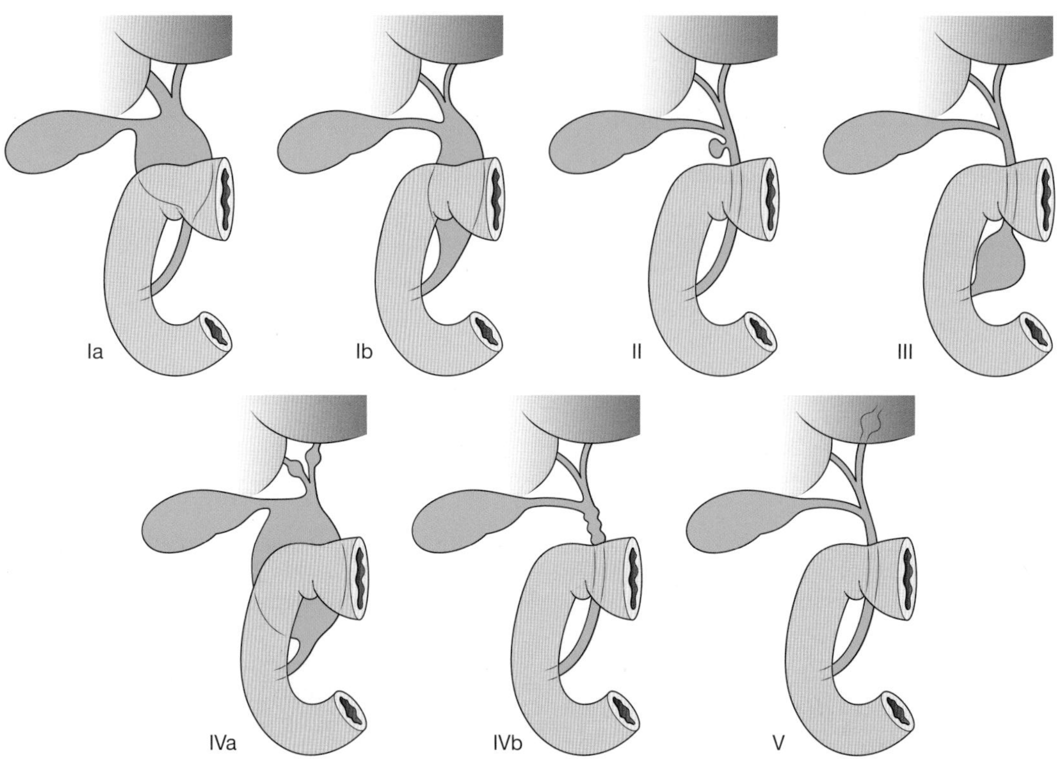

Figure 71.24 Classification of choledochal cysts. Type Ia and Ib (80–90%): diffuse cystic dilatation; note the extension into the intrapancreatic portion in type Ib. Type II (3%): diverticulum of the common bile duct. Type III (5%): diverticulum within the intrapancreatic portion. Type IV (10%): extension into the liver; type IVa: fusiform dilatation of the entire extrahepatic bile duct with extension into the intrahepatic ducts; type IVb: multiple cystic dilatations involving only the extrahepatic bile duct. Type V: cystic dilatation only of the intrahepatic ducts.

Management is multidisciplinary: cholangitis or jaundice are treated with appropriate antibiotic therapy and endoscopic or interventional stenting. Hepatic resection may be considered in patients with limited disease. Patients with diffuse disease and concomitant hepatic fibrosis are candidates for liver transplantation. Recurrence is common, particularly after resection, and long-term surveillance is required.

CHOLEDOCHAL CYST

Choledochal cysts are congenital dilatations of the intra- and/or extrahepatic biliary system. The pathogenesis is unclear. Anomalous insertions of the biliary–pancreatic junction are frequently observed, but whether or not these play a role in the pathogenesis of the condition is unclear. Todani and colleagues proposed a classification of cystic disease of biliary tract (*Figure 71.24*).

Patients may present at any age with jaundice, fever, abdominal pain and a right upper quadrant mass on examination; 60% of cases are diagnosed before the age of 10 years. Pancreatitis is not an infrequent presentation in adults. Patients with choledochal cysts have an increased risk of developing cholangiocarcinoma, with the risk varying directly with the age at diagnosis.

USG confirms the presence of an abnormal cyst and magnetic resonance imaging (MRI)/MRCP will reveal the anatomy, in particular the relationship between the lower end of the bile duct and the pancreatic duct. CT is also useful for delineating the extent of intra- or extrahepatic dilatation.

Radical excision of the cyst is the treatment of choice, with reconstruction of the biliary tract using a Roux-en-Y loop of jejunum. Complete resection is important because of an association with the later development of cholangiocarcinoma. Resection and Roux-en-Y reconstruction is also associated with a reduced incidence of stricture formation and recurrent cholangitis. Type III needs endoscopic management with sphincterotomy. It should be accompanied by biopsy of the cyst epithelium to exclude dysplasia in symptomatic cases and in young patients without symptoms.

TRAUMA

Injury to the gallbladder and extrahepatic biliary tree is rare and may occur as a result of blunt or penetrating abdominal trauma. Iatrogenic injury is perhaps more frequent than external trauma. Physical signs are those of an acute abdomen. Management depends on the location and extent of biliary and associated injury. In a stable patient, a transected bile duct

Takuji Todani, b. 1931, Department of Surgery, Okayama University Medical School, Okayama, Japan, modified Alonso-Lej's classification of choledochal cysts in 1977.

is best repaired by Roux-en-Y choledochojejunostomy. Injuries to the gallbladder can be dealt with by cholecystectomy.

TORSION OF THE GALLBLADDER

This is a very rare complication, requires a long mesentery and therefore occurs most often in an older patient with a mucocele of the gallbladder. Presentation is with extreme right upper quadrant abdominal pain. Urgent exploration is indicated, with cholecystectomy as the only treatment.

GALLSTONES (CHOLELITHIASIS)

Gallstones are the most common biliary pathology. It is estimated that gallstones affect 10–15% of the population in western societies. In the UK, the prevalence of gallstones at the time of death is estimated to be 17%. Gallstones are asymptomatic in the majority of cases (>80%). Approximately 1–2% per year will develop symptoms requiring surgery, making cholecystectomy one of the most common operations performed.

Causal factors

Gallstones can be divided into three main types: cholesterol, pigment (brown/black) and mixed stones. In the USA and Europe, 80% of gallstones are cholesterol or mixed stones, whereas in parts of Asia 80% are pigment stones. Cholesterol or mixed stones contain 50–99% pure cholesterol plus an admixture of calcium salts, bile acids, bile pigments and phospholipids.

Cholesterol is insoluble in water and is secreted from the canalicular membrane in phospholipid vesicles. Whether cholesterol remains in solution depends on the type and relative concentrations of phospholipids and bile acids in the bile. When bile is supersaturated with cholesterol and/or bile acid concentrations are low, unstable unilamellar phospholipid vesicles form, from which cholesterol crystals may nucleate. Obesity, a high-calorie diet and certain medications (e.g. oral contraceptives) can increase the secretion of cholesterol, while ileal disease or resection can deplete the bile acid pool and result in lithogenic bile (***Figure 71.25***). Nucleation of cholesterol monohydrate crystals from multilamellar vesicles is a crucial step in gallstone formation. Abnormal emptying of the gallbladder may aid the aggregation of nucleated cholesterol crystals; thus, removing gallstones without removing the gallbladder will inevitably lead to gallstone recurrence.

Pigment stones contain <30% cholesterol. Overall, 20–30% of pigment stones are black; the incidence rises with age. For reasons that are unclear, patients with cirrhosis have a higher incidence of pigment stones. Black pigment stones are composed largely of an insoluble bilirubin pigment polymer mixed with calcium phosphate and calcium bicarbonate. These stones are associated with haemolysis, as in hereditary spherocytosis and sickle cell disease.

Brown pigment stones contain calcium bilirubinate, calcium palmitate and calcium stearate, as well as cholesterol. Brown stones are more common in the bile ducts and are related to bile stasis and infection secondary to deconjugation of bilirubin glucuronide by bacterial β-glucuronidase. Insoluble unconjugated bilirubinate precipitates. Brown pigment stones are also associated with the presence of foreign bodies within the bile ducts, such as endoprostheses (stents) or parasites such as *Clonorchis sinensis* and *Ascaris lumbricoides*.

Clinical presentation

Gallstones are being increasingly detected incidentally during imaging for other symptoms. Prophylactic cholecystectomy is not usually indicated since the risk of developing serious complications is low. Longitudinal follow-up study of individuals with silent gallstones has shown that over 20 years only 18% developed biliary pain; the mean yearly probability was 2% during the first 5 years, 1% during the second 5 years and 0.5% during the third 5 years.

If symptoms occur, patients typically complain of right upper quadrant or epigastric pain, which may radiate to the back. This may be described as colicky but the typical biliary 'colic' more often is dull, continuous and severe, lasting for several minutes or even hours, with associated nausea and vomiting (***Chapter 63***). Frequently, pain starts during the night and wakes the patient; minor episodes may occur intermittently during the day. In the majority of cases the process is limited by the stone slipping back into the body of the gallbladder. The development of acute cholecystitis is marked by fever. Associated symptoms that have a questionable relation to gallstones include dyspepsia, flatulence, food intolerance, particularly to fats, and some alteration in bowel frequency. As pain resolves (spontaneously or with medications) the patient improves and is able to eat and drink again, often only to suffer further episodes. A patient may have several such episodes over a few weeks and then no symptoms for some months. This may culminate in a contracted non-functioning gallbladder with the

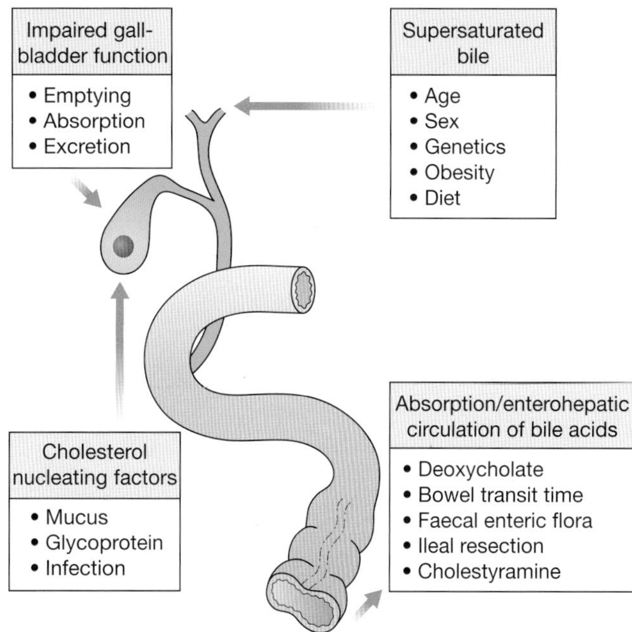

Figure 71.25 Factors associated with gallstone formation.

development of chronic cholecystitis. The differential diagnosis is given in *Summary box 71.3*.

In acute cholecystitis the right upper quadrant tenderness is exacerbated during inspiration by palpation in the right subcostal region (Murphy's sign). A mass may become palpable as the omentum walls off an inflamed gallbladder. If resolution does not occur, empyema of the gallbladder may result. The wall may become necrotic and perforate, with the development of localised peritonitis (*Table 71.1*). Occasionally, complete obstruction of the cystic duct leads to reabsorption of bile salts by the gallbladder epithelium and secretion of uninfected mucus, resulting in a mucocele of the gallbladder.

Jaundice may ensue if the gallstone migrates from the gallbladder and obstructs or compresses the CBD (Mirizzi). Rarely, a large solitary gallstone may erode the gallbladder wall, causing a cholecystoduodenal fistula and subsequent bowel obstruction, known as gallstone ileus.

A palpable, non-tender gallbladder in the presence of jaundice may portend a more sinister diagnosis as a palpable gallbladder in the presence of jaundice is unlikely to be due to gallstones (Courvoisier) and usually results from a distal common duct obstruction secondary to periampullary malignancy.

Summary box 71.2

Effects and complications of gallstones

- Biliary colic
- Acute cholecystitis
- Chronic cholecystitis
- Empyema of the gallbladder
- Mucocele of the gallbladder
- Perforation of the gallbladder
- Biliary obstruction (jaundice)
- Acute cholangitis
- Acute pancreatitis
- Intestinal obstruction (gallstone ileus)

Summary box 71.3

Differential diagnosis of acute cholecystitis

Common	Uncommon
• Appendicitis	• Acute pyelonephritis
• Perforated peptic ulcer	• Myocardial infarction
• Acute pancreatitis	• Pneumonia – right lower lobe

Diagnosis

A clinical diagnosis of acute cholecystitis must be confirmed with radiological and laboratory investigations. USG is the first choice for imaging; however, the sensitivity and specificity of diagnosing acute cholecystitis is increased when combined with positive clinical and/or laboratory findings (*Table 71.1*).

TABLE 71.1 Tokyo Consensus Guidelines diagnostic criteria for acute cholecystitis.

A. Local signs of inflammation, etc. 1) Murphy's sign 2) Right upper quadrant pain/tenderness/mass
B. Systemic signs of inflammation, etc. 1) Fever 2) Elevated CRP 3) Elevated WBC count
C. Imaging findings
Imaging findings characteristic of acute cholecystitis:
Suspected diagnosis: 1 item in A + 1 item in B
Definite diagnosis: 1 item in A + 1 item in B + C

CRP, C-reactive protein; WBC, white blood cell.

Reproduced with permission from Yokoe M *et al*. Tokyo Guidelines 2018: diagnostic criteria and severity grading of acute cholecystitis (with videos). *J Hepatobiliary Pancreat Sci* 2018; **25**(1) 41–54.

Treatment

Asymptomatic gallstones do not need intervention, however prophylactic cholecystectomy may be performed for asymptomatic cholelithiasis in the following situations:

- large (>3 cm) gallstones;
- choledocholithiasis;
- chronic haemolytic conditions (sickle cell disease, hereditary spherocytosis);
- gallbladder polyps >1 cm in diameter;
- suspicion/risk of malignancy (anomalous pancreatic ductal drainage);
- calcification of the wall (porcelain gallbladder);
- some ethnic groups or subjects living in areas with a high prevalence of gallbladder cancer associated with gallstones (some parts of northern India, Native Americans, Mexican Americans, Colombia, Chile, Bolivia);
- transplant patients (during transplantation);
- bariatric surgery.

For patients with symptomatic gallstones, cholecystectomy is the treatment of choice if there are no medical contraindications. The initial non-operative treatment is based on four steps:

1. Nil by mouth and intravenous fluid administration until the pain resolves.
2. Analgesics.
3. Antibiotics. As the cystic duct is blocked in most instances, the concentration of antibiotic in the serum is more important than the concentration in the bile. A broad-spectrum antibiotic effective against Gram-negative aerobes is most appropriate (e.g. cefazolin, cefuroxime or ciprofloxacin).
4. Subsequent management. When the temperature, pulse and other physical signs show that the inflammation is subsiding, oral fluids are reinstated, followed by a regular diet.

Ludwig Georg Courvoisier, 1843–1918, surgeon, Basel, Switzerland, made his observation in 1890. No mention was made of either gallbladder tenderness or malignancy.

USG is performed to confirm the diagnosis (***Table 71.1***). If jaundice with deranged ALP and enzyme levels is present, MRCP should be performed to exclude choledocholithiasis. If there is any concern regarding the diagnosis or the presence of complications such as perforation, CT should also be performed.

The timing of surgery in acute cholecystitis remains controversial. Early cholecystectomy, undertaken by an experienced surgeon with excellent operating facilities within 5–7 days of the onset of the attack, is safe and shortens total hospital stay. Nevertheless, the conversion rate in laparoscopic cholecystectomy is higher in acute than in elective surgery. If early operation is not indicated, one should wait approximately 6 weeks for the inflammation to subside before operating. The Tokyo Guidelines (2013/2018) allow the assessment of severity and grading of acute cholecystitis (***Table 71.2***) and provide a consensus-derived treatment algorithm based on grading, patient comorbidity and the facilities and expertise available (***Figure 71.26***).

TABLE 71.2 Tokyo Consensus Guidelines for severity grading of acute cholecystitis.

Grade III (severe) acute cholecystitis	
Associated with dysfunction of any one of the following organs/systems:	
1 Cardiovascular dysfunction	Hypotension requiring treatment with dopamine ≥5 μg/kg/min, or any dose of epinephrine
2 Neurological dysfunction	Decreased level of consciousness
3 Respiratory dysfunction	PaO_2/F_iO_2 ratio <300
4 Renal dysfunction	Oliguria; creatinine >2.0 mg/dL
5 Hepatic dysfunction	Prothrombin time (PT-INR) >1.5
6 Haematological dysfunction	Platelet count <100 000/mm^3
Grade II (moderate) acute cholecystitis	
Associated with any one of the following conditions:	
1 Elevated white cell count (>18 000/mm^3)	
2 Palpable tender mass in the right upper abdominal quadrant	
3 Duration of complaint >72 hours	
4 Marked local inflammation (gangrenous cholecystitis, pericholecystic abscess, hepatic abscess, biliary peritonitis, emphysematous cholecystitis)	
Grade I (mild) acute cholecystitis	
Does not meet the criteria of grade II or grade III acute cholecystitis. Grade I can also be defined as acute cholecystitis in a healthy person with no organ dysfunction and mild inflammatory changes in the gallbladder, making cholecystectomy a safe and low-risk operative procedure	

PaO_2/F_iO_2 ratio is the ratio of arterial oxygen partial pressure (PaO_2 in mmHg) to fractional inspired oxygen (F_iO_2) expressed as a fraction (not a percentage) at sea level, the normal PaO_2/F_iO_2 ratio is ~400–500 mmHg (~55–65 kPa); PT-INR, prothrombin time–international normalised ratio.

Reproduced with permission from Yokoe M *et al.* Tokyo Guidelines 2018: diagnostic criteria and severity grading of acute cholecystitis (with videos). *J Hepatobiliary Pancreat Sci* 2018; **25**(1) 41–54.

Acalculous cholecystitis

Acute and chronic inflammation of the gallbladder can occur in the absence of stones and give rise to a clinical picture similar to that of calculous cholecystitis. Some patients have non-specific inflammation of the gallbladder, whereas others have one of the cholecystoses. Acute acalculous cholecystitis is particularly seen in critically ill patients and those recovering from major surgery, trauma and burns. The diagnosis is often missed and the mortality rate is high. The treatment is cholecystectomy for patients who are able to tolerate surgery. In selected patients, non-surgical treatment (such as antibiotics or percutaneous cholecystostomy) may be an effective alternative to surgery.

CHOLECYSTOSES (CHOLESTEROLOSIS, POLYPOSIS, ADENOMYOMATOSIS AND CHOLECYSTITIS GLANDULARIS PROLIFERANS)

This is a relatively uncommon group of conditions affecting the gallbladder, in which there are chronic inflammatory changes with hyperplasia of all tissue elements.

Cholesterolosis ('strawberry gallbladder')

Cholesterolosis (cholesterosis) is characterised by the accumulation of lipids (triglycerides, cholesterol precursors and cholesterol esters) in the mucosa of the gallbladder wall. These nodules are less than 1 mm in diameter in about two-thirds of cases, which gives the mucosa a coarse and granular appearance. The nodules in the remaining one-third of cases are larger and polypoid in appearance (polypoid form). The lipid accumulation creates yellow deposits on a background of hyperaemic mucosa ('strawberry gallbladder'). It may be associated with cholesterol stones (***Figure 71.27***).

Cholesterol polyposis of the gallbladder

USG may show a non-mobile defect in the gallbladder lumen with no acoustic shadow. The differential is an adenomatous polyp, and interval follow-up is indicated to ensure stability. Surgery is advised only if there is a diagnostic dilemma.

Cholecystitis glandularis proliferans (adenomyomatosis)

Adenomyomatosis is an abnormality of the gallbladder characterised by overgrowth of the mucosa and thickening of the muscle wall, leading to cyst-like structures in the gallbladder wall or polypoid projections from the mucosa of the gallbladder and intramural diverticulae (*diffuse* adenomyomatosis). While generally not considered to be a premalignant condition, there is a clear association of adenomyomatosis with cholelithiasis.

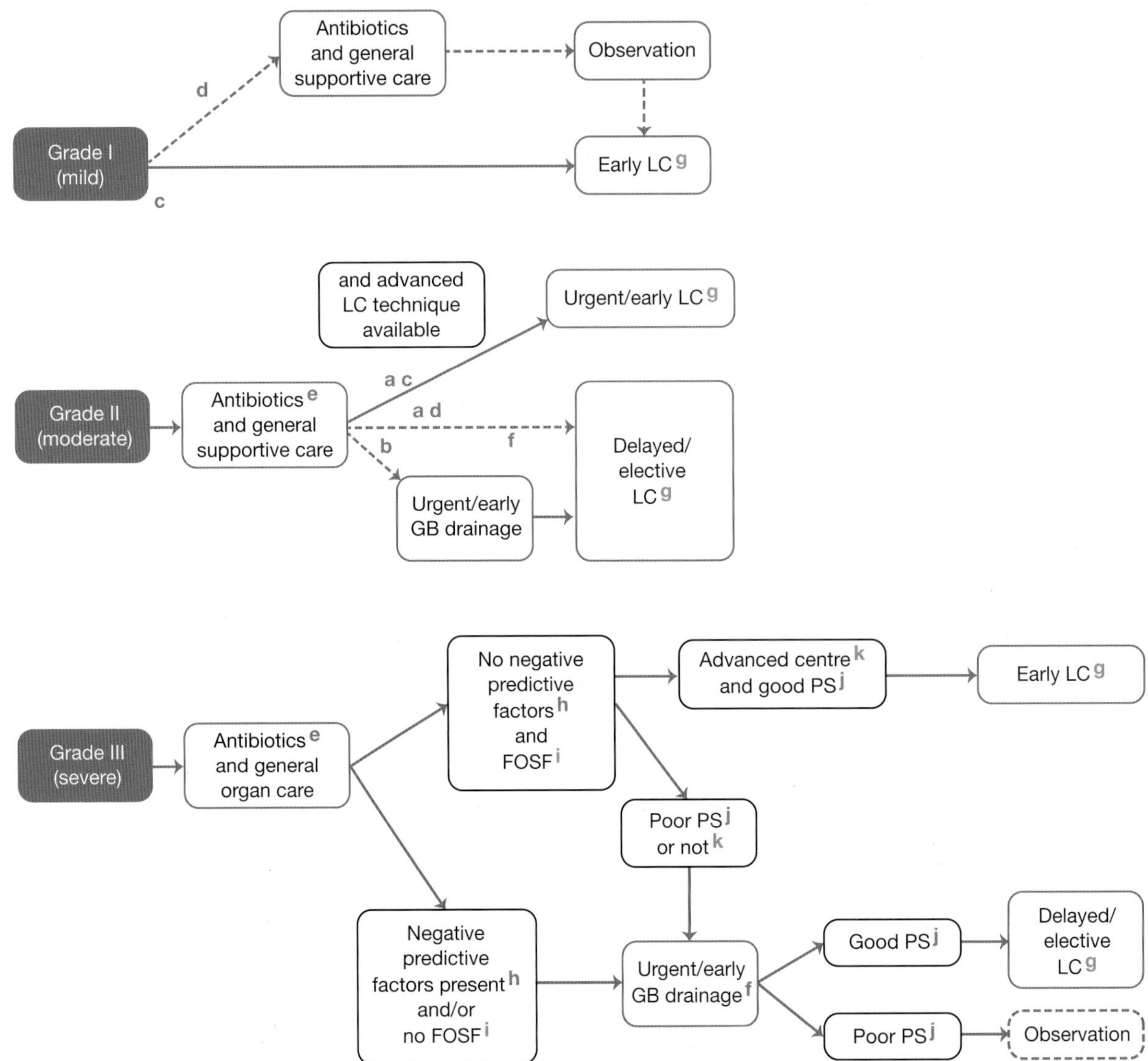

Figure 71.26 Tokyo Guidelines for the management of acute cholecystitis. [a]Antibiotics and general supportive care successful. [b]Antibiotics and general supportive care fail to control inflammation. [c]CCI 5 or less and/or ASA-PS class II or less (low risk). [d]CCI 6 or greater and/or ASA-PS class III or greater (not low risk). [e]Blood culture should be taken before initiation of administration of antibiotics. [f]A bile culture should be performed during GB drainage. [g]In cases of serious operative difficulty, bail-out procedures including conversion should be considered. [h]Negative predictive factors: jaundice (TBil ≥2 mg/dL), neurological dysfunction, respiratory dysfunction. [i]FOSF: favourable organ system failure = rapidly reversible after admission and before early LC. [j]CCI 4 or greater, ASA-PS 3 or greater are high risk. [k]Advanced centre = intensive care and advanced laparoscopic techniques are available. ASA-PS, American Society of Anesthesiologists physical status; CCI, Charlson comorbidity index; GB, gallbladder; LC, laparoscopic cholecystectomy; PS, performance status; TBil, total bilirubin. (Reproduced with permission from Okamoto K *et al*. Tokyo Guidelines 2018: flowchart for the management of acute cholecystitis. *J Hepatobiliary Pancreat Sci* 2018; **25**(1): 55–72.)

These can be complicated by intramural, and later extramural, abscess and potentially fistula formation. If symptomatic, the patient is treated by cholecystectomy (***Figure 71.28***).

Diverticulosis of the gallbladder

Diverticulosis of the gallbladder is usually manifest as black pigment stones impacted in the outpouchings of the lacunae of Luschka. This may be demonstrated by cholecystography, especially when the gallbladder contracts after a fatty meal. There are small dots of contrast medium within and outside the gallbladder wall (***Figure 71.29***). The treatment is cholecystectomy.

Typhoid infection of the gallbladder

Salmonella Typhi or *Salmonella* Typhimurium can infect the gallbladder. Acute or, more frequently, chronic cholecystitis

Mary E Charlson, contemporary, Clinical Epidemiologist, Weill Cornell Medical Center, New York, NY, USA.
Daniel Elmer Salmon, 1850–1914, veterinary pathologist, Chief of the Bureau of Animal Industry, Washington, DC, USA.

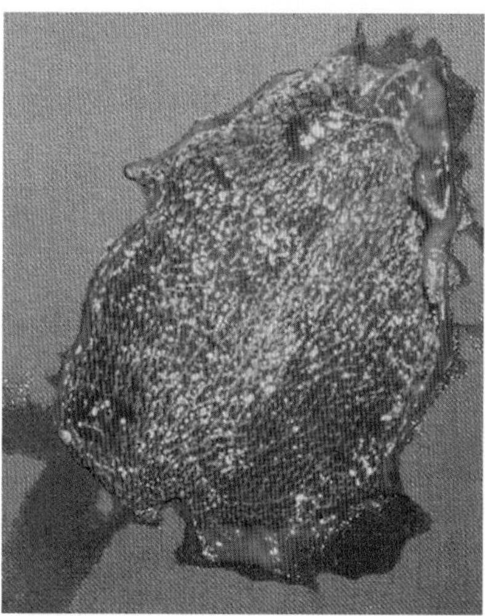

Figure 71.27 The interior of a strawberry gallbladder (cholesterosis) (courtesy of Dr Sanjay P Thakur, Patna, India).

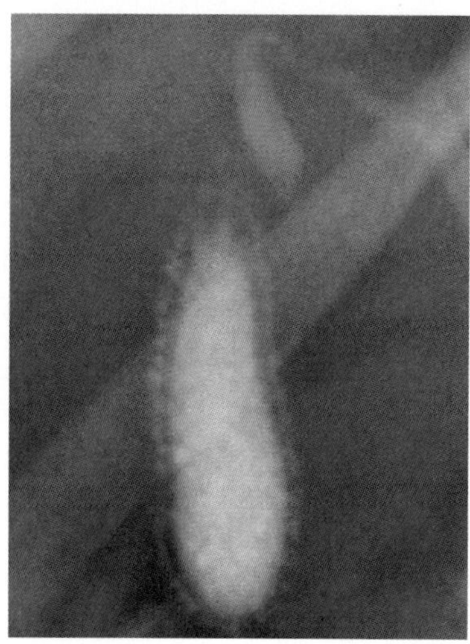

Figure 71.29 Cholecystogram showing diverticulosis with dots of contrast medium in the gallbladder wall.

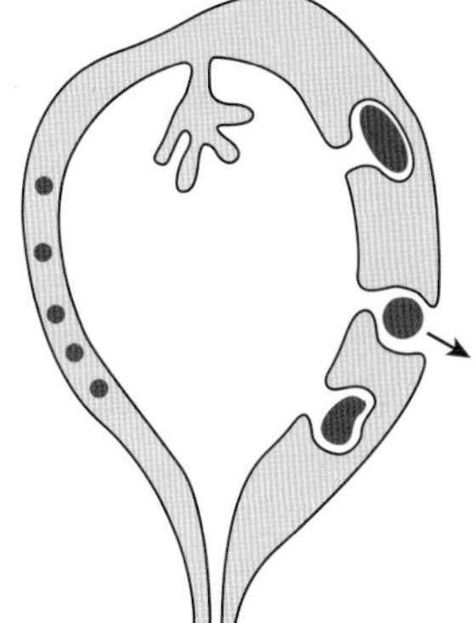

Figure 71.28 Types of cholecystitis glandularis proliferans (polyps, intramural or diverticular stones and fistula).

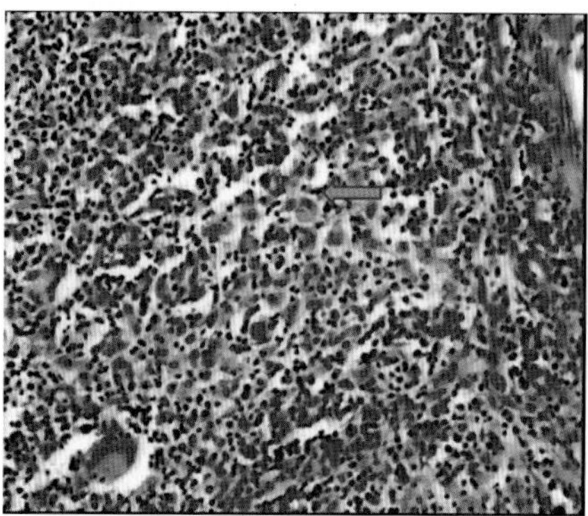

Figure 71.30 Xanthogranulomatous cholecystitis. Infiltrates in the wall of the gallbladder show foamy macrophages (arrow), giant cells and lymphoplasma cells in the background (courtesy of Dr Amita Joshi, Mumbai, India).

occurs, with the patient becoming a typhoid carrier excreting the bacteria in the bile. Gallstones may be present (surgeons should not give patients their stones after their operation if there is any suspicion of typhoid). It is debatable whether the stones are secondary to the *Salmonella* cholecystitis or whether pre-existing stones predispose the gallbladder to chronic infection. Treatment with ampicillin and cholecystectomy are indicated. In the case of penicillin allergy, a quinolone antibiotic can be used.

Gallbladder polyps

Polyps of the gallbladder are incidental findings during radiological imaging of the abdomen. The polyps are more often benign (cholesterol polyps, adenomyomas, inflammatory, adenomas or miscellaneous) but may be malignant (adenocarcinoma [80%] or squamous cell carcinoma, or cystadenomas).

A majority of polyps remain stable. Cholecystectomy should be considered in symptomatic patients or as prophylaxis to prevent malignant transformation in those who also have gallstones, primary sclerosing cholangitis (PSC), biliary colic or pancreatitis. Polyps in patients older than 50 years, sessile polyps with wall thickening greater than 4 mm and polyps larger than 10 mm merit cholecystectomy. Smaller polyps should be kept under observation and need surgery if the size is increasing.

Xanthogranulomatous cholecystitis

Xanthogranulomatous cholecystitis (***Figure 71.30***) is an uncommon inflammation of the gallbladder, more frequently seen in India and Japan. It is more common in females. It is caused by extravasation of bile into the gallbladder wall from rupture of the Rokitansky–Aschoff sinuses or by mucosal ulceration as a result of a focal or diffuse destructive inflammatory process, with accumulation of lipid-laden macrophages (xanthoma cells), fibrous tissue and acute and chronic inflammatory cells. USG shows gallbladder wall

Carl Freiherr von Rokitansky, 1804–1878, pathologist, Vienna, Austria.
Karl Albert Ludwig Aschoff, 1866–1942, pathologist, Freiburg, Germany.

thickening (diffuse or focal, with intact mucosal lining), intramural hypoechoic nodules or bands and often the presence of gallstones. CT shows 5- to 20-mm intramural hypoattenuating nodules and poor/heterogeneous contrast enhancement. As with acute cholecystitis, early enhancement of the adjacent liver parenchyma may occur. Extension into the liver along with enlarged hepatoduodenal lymph nodes closely mimics gallbladder carcinoma. Diagnosis is difficult and depends on pathological examination. Intraoperatively, frozen-section examination should be carried out to differentiate xanthogranulomatous cholecystitis from carcinoma of the gallbladder (coexistence of gallbladder cancer 2.3–13.3%). Because of diagnostic difficulties if there is preoperative suspicion of xanthogranulomatous cholecystitis open cholecystectomy should be considered.

Gallstones in pregnancy

Acute cholecystitis is the second most common non-obstetric indication for surgery in pregnant women. Hormonal (oestrogen) changes during pregnancy increase cholesterol secretion and progesterone reduces bile acid secretion, reducing the ability of bile to solubilise cholesterol; bile becomes supersaturated with cholesterol. Progesterone also slows gallbladder emptying, which further promotes the formation of stones owing to bile stasis. Prepregnancy obesity, multiparity, increasing age and genetic predisposition are risk factors.

Acute right upper quadrant/epigastric pain in pregnancy may be due to severe pre-eclampsia and the HELLP syndrome (haemolysis, elevated liver enzymes, low platelet count), acute fatty liver, abruptio placentae, uterine rupture or intra-amniotic infection. USG and non-contrast MRI are acceptable diagnostic modalities.

For women in their first trimester, the mainstay of treatment for mild cases is conservative. Non-steroidal anti-inflammatory drugs are effective analgesics but are generally avoided in pregnancy, especially after 32 weeks of gestation, because of potential adverse fetal effects, e.g. premature closure of the ductus arteriosus.

In the second trimester, with moderate or severe disease, good surgical candidates (American Society of Anesthesiologists [ASA] I or II) should undergo cholecystectomy during their initial hospitalisation as there is a high risk of recurrence or serious complications. In the third trimester, non-operative medical management with antibiotics and fluid therapy should be initiated. The patient should be re-evaluated after delivery. Generally, a waiting period of 6 weeks following delivery is preferred to allow the mother to recover from the delivery, bond with the infant and regain her strength.

Gallstone ileus

Gallstone ileus is an infrequent complication (0.4%) of cholelithiasis, occurring as a result of impaction of one or more gallstones within the gastrointestinal tract. It is seen more frequently in the elderly and in women. Frequently an episode of acute cholecystitis leads to erosion of inflamed tissues, resulting in a cholecystointestinal fistula.

A majority of small gallstones pass through the intestines spontaneously. However, gallstones of size 2–5 cm get impacted, usually in the terminal ileum or at the ileocecal valve owing to the relatively narrow lumen and less active peristalsis here. Less common locations include the stomach and the duodenum (Bouveret's syndrome). Impacted stones may lead to necrosis and perforation followed by peritonitis.

Clinical manifestations include acute, intermittent or chronic episodes of partial or complete gastrointestinal obstruction. Physical examination may be non-specific or may show signs of obstruction: dehydration, abdominal distension and tenderness, with high-pitched bowel sounds, and obstructive jaundice. A plain abdominal radiograph shows:

- partial or complete intestinal obstruction;[a]
- pneumobilia or contrast material in the biliary tree;[a]
- an aberrant rim-calcified or total-calcified gallstone;[a]
- a change in the position of such a gallstone on serial films ('tumbling sign').

CT is considered superior to plain radiographs or USG, with a sensitivity of up to 93%. It additionally shows an abnormal gallbladder with air, an air–fluid level or fluid accumulation with an irregular wall.

In addition to the management of intestinal obstruction, enterolithotomy has been the most common surgical procedure performed. A longitudinal incision is made on the antimesenteric border proximal to the site of gallstone impaction, and the gallstone is brought proximally to a non-oedematous segment of the bowel by gentle manipulation and extracted. A cholecystoenteric fistula should not be resected unless the patient is stable and there are residual gallstones that may cause infection or recurrent ileus (see ***Chapter 78***).

CHOLECYSTECTOMY

Preparation for operation

After appropriate history taking and assessment of the patient's fitness for the procedure, routine laboratory investigations including a coagulation screen and liver function tests should be checked. The patient must sign a consent form to indicate that he or she is fully aware of the procedure being undertaken, the alternative options and the risks involved including complications that may occur. Prophylactic antibiotics should be administered at the time of induction of anaesthesia. A second-generation cephalosporin is appropriate. Subcutaneous heparin and antiembolic stockings should be prescribed (***Summary box 71.4***).

The various factors identified as predictors of difficult cholecystectomy are listed in ***Table 71.3***, and the risk factors for the presence of CBD stones are listed in ***Table 71.4***.

Leon Bouveret, 1850–1929, physician, Lyon, France.

[a]These three constitute Rigler's triad.

Leo George Rigler, 1896–1979, Professor of Radiology, University of California, Los Angeles, CA, USA.

Summary box 71.4

Preparation for cholecystectomy

- Appropriate history taking (jaundice) and assessment
- Full blood count
- Renal and liver function tests
- Prothrombin time
- Chest radiograph and electrocardiogram (if medically indicated)
- Antibiotic prophylaxis, second-generation cephalosporin at the time of induction
- Deep vein thrombosis prophylaxis
- Informed consent: patient is aware of the procedure being undertaken, the alternative options and the risks involved

TABLE 71.3 Risk factors of difficult cholecystectomy.

History
Male gender, >65 years, interval between onset and presentation (>72–96 hours) in acute cholecystitis, previous multiple attacks, previous upper abdominal surgery, prior attempt at cholecystectomy (cholecystostomy)
Physical examination
Morbid obesity, high ASA score
Laboratory tests
Abnormal liver function tests
Imaging (USG/CT/MRI–MRCP)
Thick-walled gallbladder (>4–5 mm) Contracted gallbladder Distended gallbladder with impacted stone in the neck Gangrenous gallbladder/gallbladder perforation Mirizzi's syndrome/cholecystoenteric fistula Cirrhosis/extrahepatic portal vein obstruction (portal cavernoma) with portal hypertension
Intraoperative
Shrunken gallbladder, liver edge retracted with fissure/depression/ puckering near the fundus, fatty/firm cirrhotic liver (difficulty in retraction)

ASA, American Society of Anesthesiologists; CT, computed tomography; MRCP, magnetic resonance cholangiopancreatography; MRI, magnetic resonance imaging; USG, ultrasonography.

TABLE 71.4 Risk factors for common bile duct (CBD) stones.

Risk of CBD stones	History of cholangitis or pancreatitis	Liver function tests	Abdominal USG: CBD diameter	Further evaluation required
Low, 2–3%	Absent	Normal	≤6 mm	None
Medium, 20–40%	Present	2× normal	8–10 mm	MRCP +/– ERCP stone extraction
High, 50–80%	Present, with jaundice	2× normal	≥10 mm	MRCP +/– ERCP stone extraction

ERCP, endoscopic retrograde cholangiopancreatography; MRCP, magnetic resonance cholangiopancreatography; USG, ultrasonography.

Laparoscopic cholecystectomy

Laparoscopic cholecystectomy is the procedure of choice for the majority of patients. The indications and preparation for cholecystectomy are the same whether it is performed by laparoscopy or by open technique.

The patient is placed supine on the operating table. Following induction and maintenance of general anaesthesia, the abdomen is prepared in a standard fashion. Pneumoperitoneum is established. The authors' preference is to use an open subumbilical cut down with direct visualisation of the peritoneum to place the initial port. This port will function as the camera port. An angled telescope (30°) is preferred. Many surgeons prefer a 'closed' technique using a Verres needle to establish pneumoperitoneum (see ***Chapter 7***). Recently, single-port laparoscopic cholecystectomy has been described. Proponents report decreased postoperative pain and improved cosmesis. However, systematic reviews have reported a higher failure rate, longer operative time and increased blood loss without any substantive benefits with the technique.

Additional operating ports are inserted in the subxiphoid area and in the right subcostal area. The patient is placed in a reverse Trendelburg position slightly rotated to the left. This exposes the fundus of the gallbladder, which is retracted towards the diaphragm. The neck of the gallbladder is then retracted towards the right iliac fossa, exposing Calot's triangle. The key, as in open surgery, is the identification and safe dissection of Calot's triangle (***Table 71.5***). This area is laid wide open by dividing the peritoneum on the posterior and anterior aspects. The cystic duct is carefully defined, as is the cystic artery. The gallbladder is separated from the liver bed for about 2 cm to allow confirmation of the anatomy. Unless there are specific indications, routine cholangiogram is not performed. However, if doubt exists regarding the anatomy, cholangiogram is warranted. Real-time intraoperative imaging using indocyanine green (ICG) fluorescence cholangiography (with special scopes and imaging system) improves visualisation of the biliary tree during laparoscopic cholecystectomy and enables better visualisation and identification of the biliary tree. It can be considered a means of increasing the safety of laparoscopic cholecystectomy. This is likely to reduce risk of biliary duct injury. Once the anatomy is clearly defined and the triangle of Calot has been laid wide open, the cystic duct and artery are clipped and divided. The gallbladder is then removed from its bed by sharp or cautery dissection and, once free, removed via the umbilicus in a retrieval bag.

Open cholecystectomy

For patients in whom a laparoscopic approach is not indicated or in whom conversion from a laparoscopic approach is required, open cholecystectomy is performed.

Janos Verres, 1903–1979, chest physician and chief of the Department of Internal Medicine, The Regional Hospital, Kapuvar, Hungary.

TABLE 71.5 Important operative steps during cholecystectomy.

Operative steps	Purpose
Retraction (*Figure 71.31a*) Proper retraction in the correct direction: the fundus is retracted towards the patient's right shoulder and the infundibulum is retracted inferolaterally towards the patient's right side	• Opens the hepatocystic triangle • Increases the angle between the cystic duct and the CBD • Limits the dissection above Rouvière's sulcus • Mental and spatial orientation of the anatomy, variation and landmarks
Look out for red flag signs • Failure of timely progression of the dissection • Anatomical disorientation • Difficulty in visualisation of the operative field	**Time out** The surgeon should recognise these clues, stop dissection and decide on the strategy for safe operation before proceeding **Do not hesitate to seek a second opinion**
Achieve CVS (*Figure 71.31b*) Clearance of the hepatocystic triangle of all fibrofatty and soft areolar tissue to see **only 2 structures enter the gallbladder** (cystic artery and duct) **Exposure of the cystic plate** (*Figure 71.31c*) This is done by separating the gallbladder from its liver bed to expose at least the medial third of the cystic plate	Difficulty achieving CVS is a **warning** • Further dissection may be hazardous, with an increased risk of biliary and/or vascular injury • **Stop and reconfirm** (with the team/second surgeon) that CVS has been achieved May be documented by photographs and/or video recordings
Separate the gallbladder from the fossa This is done by leaving the cystic plate attached to liver	To avoid bleeding from the liver sinuses and bile leak

CBD, common bile duct; CVS, critical view of safety.

An upper midline, short subcostal (Kocher) or right upper transverse incision is made, centred over the lateral border of the rectus muscle. The gallbladder is appropriately exposed and packs are placed on the hepatic flexure of the colon, the duodenum and the lesser omentum to ensure a clear view of the anatomy of the porta hepatis. These packs may be retracted by the assistant's hand ('It is the left hand of the assistant that does all the work' – Moynihan).

An artery or Duval forceps is placed on the infundibulum of the gallbladder and the peritoneum overlying Calot's triangle is placed on a stretch. The peritoneum is then divided close to the wall of the gallbladder and the fat in the triangle of Calot carefully dissected away to expose the cystic artery and the cystic duct. The cystic duct is cleaned down to the CBD, whose position is clearly ascertained. The cystic artery is tied and divided. The whole of the triangle of Calot is displayed to ensure that the anatomy of the ducts is clear and the cystic duct is then divided between ligatures (*Figure 71.32*). The gallbladder is then dissected away from its bed.

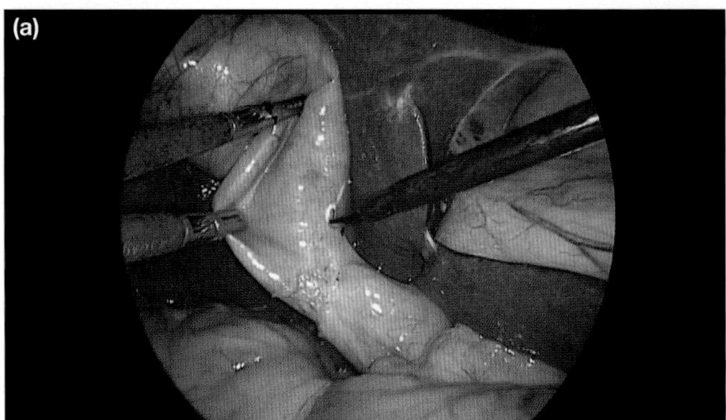

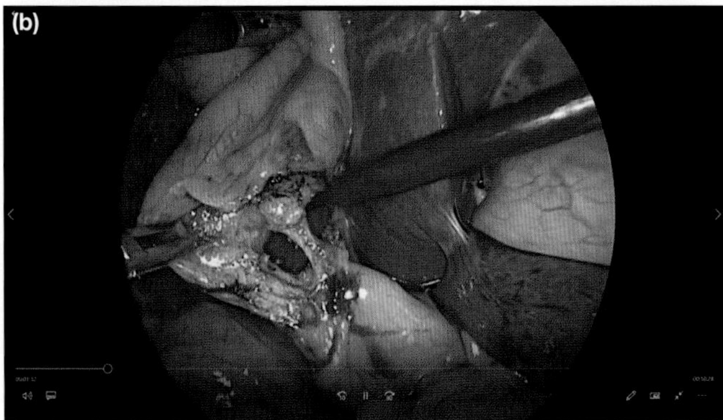

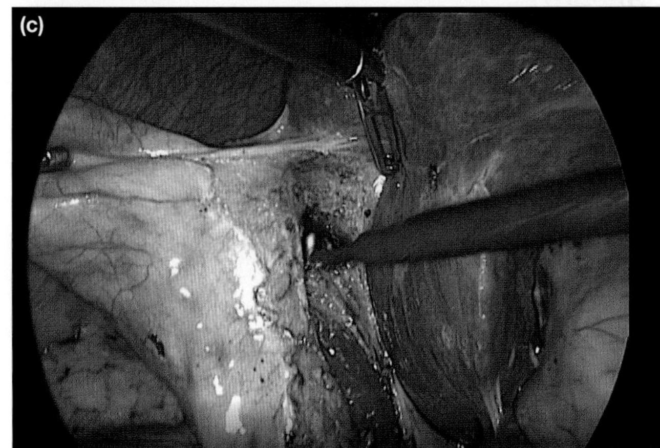

Figure 71.31 (a–c) Operative images of laparoscopic cholecystectomy. See *Table 71.5* for the important steps during operation (courtesy of Dr Sameer Rege, Mumbai, India).

Tenets for safe cholecystectomy (*Table 71.5*)

Safe zone of dissection

The safe zone of dissection lies cephalad to a line extending from the roof of Rouvière's sulcus to the umbilical fissure across the base of segment IV (R4U line). The operating surgeon tends to zoom the laparoscope closer to the surgical field to get a better view during difficulty, but this results in

Emil Theodor Kocher, 1841–1917, Professor of Surgery, Bern, Switzerland, first surgeon to win the Nobel Prize in Physiology or Medicine (1909) for his work on the physiology and surgery of the thyroid gland.
Pierre Alfred Duval, 1874–1941, Professor of Surgery, Paris, France

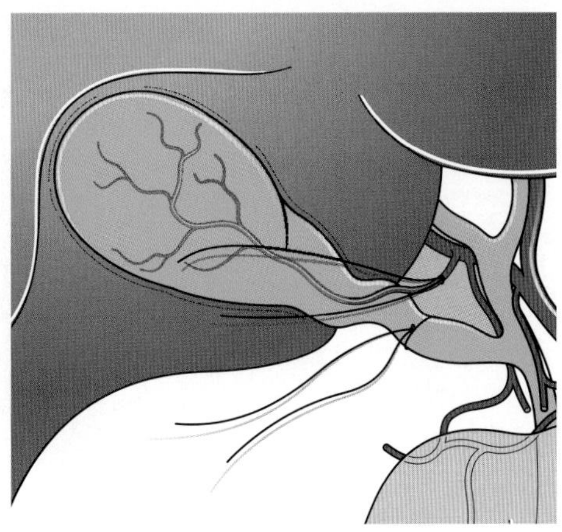

Figure 71.32 Ligatures are passed and tied around the cystic artery and cystic duct. The grey shaded area represents Calot's triangle.

non-visualisation of the normal clues/landmarks necessary for correct orientation. Dissection on the posterior aspect of the hepatocystic triangle can be safely started immediately ventral and cephalad to the sulcus. The **B-SAFE method** uses five anatomical landmarks (B, bile duct; S, sulcus of Rouvière; A, hepatic artery; F, umbilical fissure; E, enteric/duodenum) to correctly place a cognitive map during dissection.

Concept of 'time out'

During difficult gallbladder surgery, the surgeon may become disoriented and enter the zone of danger. To avoid this, the concept of time out has been introduced as it serves as a procedural cognitive aid to recall and apply essential safety measures.

Judicious use of energy sources

With a monopolar energy device (mostly hook cautery), it is important to:

- keep a low setting (approximately 30 W) to avoid arcing of the current to the bile duct;
- divide small amounts of the tissue at a time after a gentle pull to avoid injury to the deeper structures by the heel of the cautery hook;
- use intermittent short bursts of current at intervals to avoid thermal lateral spread;
- avoid blind use of cautery in brisk bleeding.

Lateral thermal spread occurs less with an ultrasonic energy source, but it may be cumbersome to use the long and straight jaws to dissect in the hepatocystic triangle.

Concept of the critical view of safety

The aim of the CVS is the conclusive identification of the cystic duct and cystic artery to avoid misidentification injury.

'Stopping rules'

With the help of red flag signs (severe adhesions, severe acute inflammation, large impacted stone in the neck of the gallbladder, Mirizzi syndrome, chronic inflammation with fibrosis or scarring), the operating surgeon should be able to identify or pre-empt difficult situations that increase the risk of biliary/vascular injury and to stop in time.

Call for help/second opinion

The operating surgeon should not hesitate to seek a second opinion whenever needed, and this should be considered a sign of good clinical practice rather than of surgical ineptitude.

Bailout techniques/strategies

The primary aim is the safety of the patient from biliary/vascular injury. It is important to perform an alternative procedure (bailout technique) that allows the surgeon to complete the operation in a safe manner. There are five bailout strategies:

1. abort the procedure altogether;
2. convert to an open procedure;
3. carry out a tube cholecystostomy using a 14 Fr Foley catheter (a simple procedure to provide symptomatic relief until a definitive procedure can be performed);
4. carry out a subtotal cholecystectomy (open/laparoscopic): leaving behind a part of the gallbladder is safer than a difficult dissection in the hepatocystic triangle with a potential for bile duct injury in an attempt to remove the entire gallbladder;
5. fundus-first approach.

The choice of bailout procedure depends on the clinical situation and the experience/expertise of the surgeon. Conversion to open cholecystectomy should be 'by choice' at an early stage in a difficult cholecystectomy, e.g. the anatomy is not clear, the pathology is too difficult or no progress is being made, rather than the surgeon having to convert because of a complication, e.g. bleeding or bile duct injury.

Complications of cholecystectomy

Recovery after laparoscopic cholecystectomy is associated with less pain and faster return to normal activity than open cholecystectomy. The majority of elective patients can have this performed as a day case; however, any patient looking unwell in the postoperative period, with untoward symptoms such as fever, chills or abdominal pain, should be kept under observation.

Complications can occur in 10–15% of cases. Serious complications fall into two major areas: access complications and bile duct injuries. The latter are rare, occurring in approximately 0.5% following laparoscopic cholecystectomy. In the main, biliary injury results from poor dissection and a failure to define the surgical anatomy adequately. Controversy exists as to whether operative cholangiography reduces the incidence of bile duct injury. The majority of surgeons use cholangiography only in selected cases. The operative mortality for cholecystectomy is less than 1%. Factors increasing the risk for postoperative mortality include advanced age, comorbid conditions and an acute presentation.

Patients who develop jaundice in the postoperative period need urgent investigation. This is especially true if the jaundice

Frederic Eugene Basil Foley, 1891–1965, urologist, The Miller and Anker Hospitals, St. Paul, MN, USA.

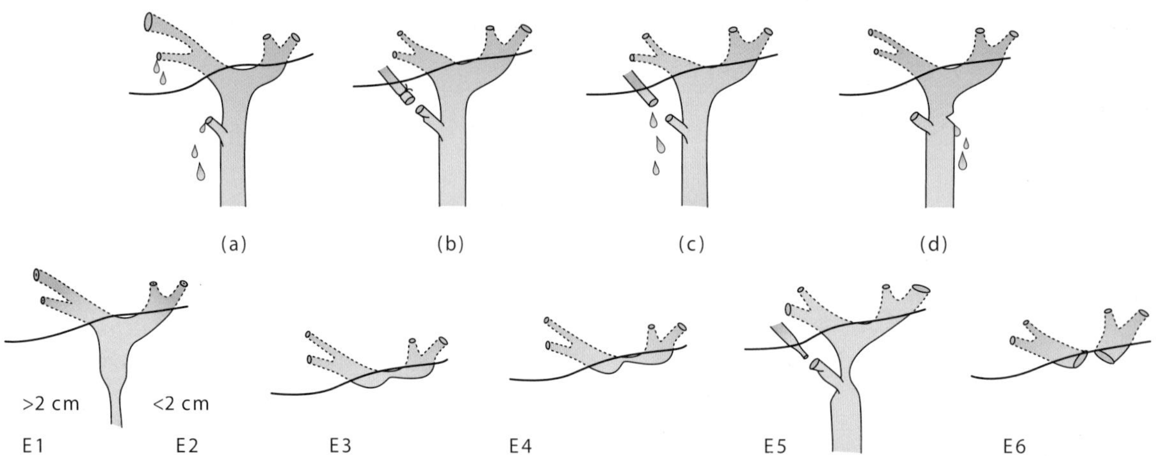

Figure 71.33 Schematic representation of the Strasberg classification of bile duct injuries. **(a)** A bile leak from the cystic duct stump or minor biliary radical in the gallbladder fossa. **(b)** An occluded right posterior sectoral duct. **(c)** A bile leak from the divided right posterior sectoral duct. **(d)** A bile leak from the main bile duct without any major tissue loss. **E1**, transected main bile duct with a stricture more than 2 cm from the hilus. **E2**, transected main bile duct with a stricture less than 2 cm from the hilus. **E3**, stricture of the hilus with the right and left ducts in communication. **E4**, stricture of the hilus with separation of the right and left hepatic ducts. **E5**, stricture involving the right aberrant sectoral duct and the main bile duct. **E6**, complete excision of the extrahepatic ducts involving the confluence (this injury is not described in Strasberg's classification). (After Connor S, Garden OJ. Bile duct injury in the era of laparoscopic cholecystectomy. *Br J Surg* 2006; **93**(2): 158–68.)

is attributed to infection and cholangitis. The first step following resuscitation and administration of appropriate antibiotics is to undertake urgent USG. This will demonstrate whether there is intra- or extrahepatic ductal dilatation. The anatomy may need to be defined by MRCP or ERCP. The latter is undertaken when therapeutic manoeuvres are planned, such as the removal of an obstructing stone or the insertion of a stent across a biliary leak. If a fluid collection is present in the subhepatic space, drainage catheters may be required. These can be inserted under radiological control or, if this expertise is not available, at open operation. Small biliary leaks will usually resolve spontaneously, especially if there is no distal obstruction. If the CBD is damaged, the patient should be referred to an appropriate expert for reconstruction.

Bile duct injuries

About 15% of injuries to the bile ducts are recognised at the time of operation; in the remainder, the injury declares itself postoperatively either by profuse and persistent leakage of bile (if drainage has been provided; bile peritonitis if no drainage provided) or by deepening obstructive jaundice. When the obstruction is incomplete, jaundice is delayed until subsequent fibrosis renders the lumen of the duct inadequate.

Any postoperative elevation in the serum bilirubin or suggestion of duct damage requires investigation to determine the nature of the injury. Abdominal USG may show collections, dilatation of the CBD and any associated vascular lesions. Abdominal CT defines the presence of focal fluid collections, ascites, biliary obstruction with an upstream dilatation in the acute phase or long-term sequelae of longstanding bile stricture, such as hepatic atrophy or signs of secondary biliary cirrhosis. CT may identify an associated vascular injury, such as to the right hepatic artery.

MRCP is the 'gold standard' for complete morphological evaluation of the biliary tree as it offers detailed information about the integrity of the biliary tract. It is helpful in determining the level and degree of injury. MRCP with magnetic resonance angiography is more informative as it may identify associated vascular injuries.

A HIDA scan can confirm the presence of a bile leak or biliary obstruction. If available, ERCP should be considered because this is diagnostic of a bile leak, demonstrates ductal continuity, detects the site and type of injury, identifies residual/retained CBD stones and is potentially therapeutic. The most common bile leak following cholecystectomy is from the cystic duct. This can be treated by placing a biliary endoprosthesis (stent) in the CBD across the origin of the cystic duct.

Surgical repair and the subsequent outcome are related to the level and degree of injury, in conjunction with the presence or absence of concomitant vascular injury. A number of classification systems have been proposed, with the Strasberg classification being commonly used (***Figure 71.33***).

In a debilitated patient, temporary external biliary drainage may be achieved by passing a catheter percutaneously into an intrahepatic duct. Also, stents may be passed through strictures at the time of ERCP and left to drain into the duodenum. When the general condition of the patient improves, definitive surgery can be undertaken. The principles of surgical repair are the maintenance of the duct length and the restoration of biliary drainage. For a stricture of recent onset through which a guidewire can be passed, balloon dilatation with insertion of a stent is an acceptable option, provided the services of an experienced endoscopist are available. For benign stricture or duct transection, the preferred treatment is a Roux-en-Y hepaticojejunostomy performed by an experienced hepatobiliary surgeon. Biliary reconstruction in the presence of peritonitis, combined vascular and bile duct injuries and injury at or above the level of the biliary bifurcation are significant predictors of poor surgical outcome. The long-term impact of bile duct injury is a significant decrease in the patient's quality of life and work-related limitations.

Late symptoms after cholecystectomy

In up to 15% of patients, cholecystectomy fails to relieve the symptoms for which the operation was performed. Such patients may be considered to have a 'postcholecystectomy' syndrome. In most such cases, this is merely a continuation of earlier symptoms. A detailed history with full investigation should be undertaken to confirm the diagnosis and exclude the presence of a stone in the bile duct, a stone in the cystic duct stump or operative damage to the biliary tree. This is best performed by MRCP or ERCP, the latter having the advantage that a stone in the CBD can be removed.

Postcholecystectomy choledocholithiasis

Any obstruction to the flow of bile can give rise to stasis, with the formation of stones within the duct. Duct stones may be detected many years after cholecystectomy and may also be related to the development of new pathology, such as infection of the biliary tree or infestation by *Ascaris lumbricoides* or *Clonorchis sinensis*. The consequence of duct stones is either obstruction to bile flow or infection. Stones in the bile ducts are more often (80%) associated with infected bile than with stones in the gallbladder.

Symptoms

The individual may be asymptomatic; symptomatic patients with cholangitis have bouts of pain, jaundice and fever ('Charcot's triad').

Signs

Febrile, icteric tenderness may be elicited in the epigastrium and right hypochondrium.

Management

It is essential to confirm that the jaundice is due to duct obstruction. Liver function tests and USG are the initial tests, and MRCP will identify the nature of the obstruction.

Pus may be present within the biliary tree and liver abscesses may develop. Measures required include rehydration, attention to clotting, exclusion of diabetes and the administration of appropriate broad-spectrum antibiotics. Once resuscitation has taken place, relief of the obstruction is essential. Endoscopic papillotomy/sphincterotomy is the preferred technique, followed by removal of the stones using a Dormia basket or placement of a stent or a nasobiliary drain for flushing if stone removal is not possible (***Figures 71.34 and 71.35***). If this fails, PTC drainage can be done, with subsequent percutaneous choledochoscopy. Surgery, in the form of choledochotomy, is now rarely used for this situation as most patients can be managed by minimally invasive techniques.

Choledochotomy

When faced with a patient with cholangitis due to stones in the CBD, and minimally invasive techniques for stone extraction are not possible, the surgeon must undertake laparotomy, drain the CBD and remove the stones through a longitudinal incision in the duct. When the duct is clear of stones, on-table

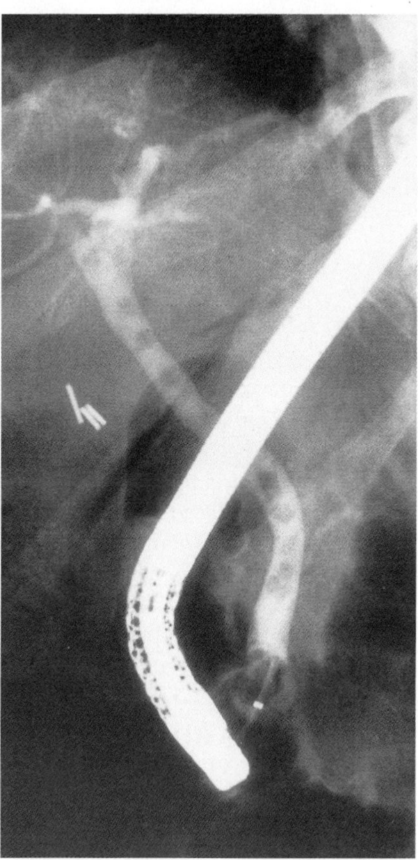

Figure 71.34 This patient presented with jaundice 4 days after laparoscopic cholecystectomy. The duct contained multiple stones.

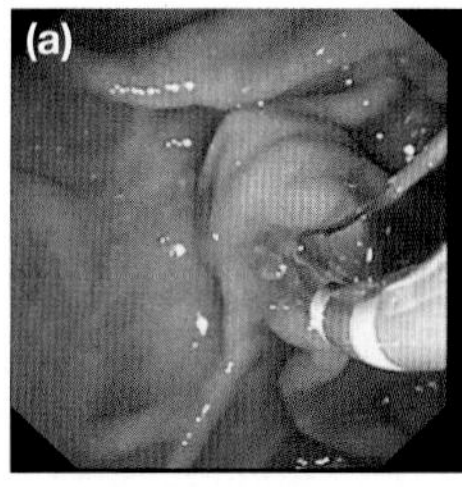

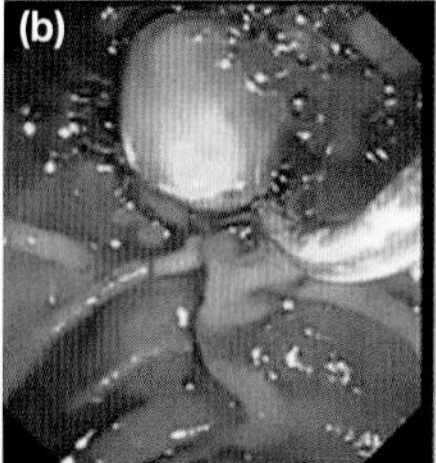

Figure 71.35 (a) Endoscopic sphincterotomy; **(b)** extraction of a stone from the bile duct through an ampulla (courtesy of Dr Amit Maydeo, Mumbai, India).

Jean Martin Charcot, 1825–1893, physician, La Salpêtrière, Paris, France.
Enrico Dormia, 1928–2009, Professor of Urology, University of Milan and Chief of the Department of Urology, S Carlo Hospital, Milan, Italy.

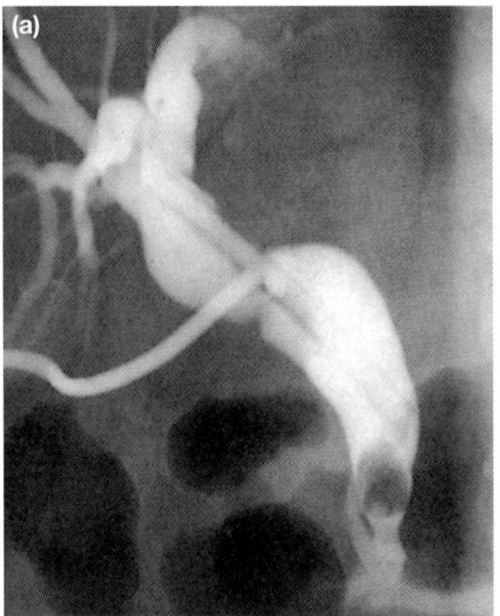

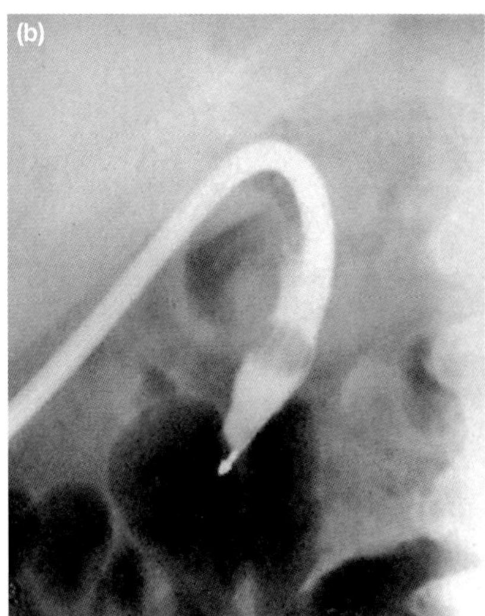

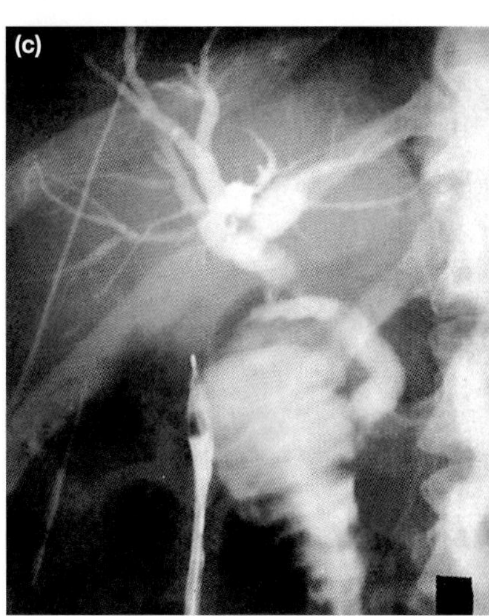

Figure 71.36 Extraction of a stone from the common bile duct by the Burhenne technique. (a) A T-tube *in situ* with a stone in the bile duct. (b) A steerable catheter is manipulated into the duct and a basket placed around the stone. (c) The stone is extracted from the duct along the T-tube track.

choledochoscopy should be performed to confirm clearance. A T-tube is inserted and the duct closed around it; the long limb is brought out on the right side and bile is allowed to drain externally. When the bile becomes clear and the patient has recovered, a cholangiogram is performed. If residual stones are found, the tube is left in place for 6 weeks so that the track is 'mature'. The radiologist can then use the track for percutaneous removal of the stones (Burhenne) (***Figure 71.36***). Once the radiologist has removed the tube, the track will close and the patient will recover. Such residual small stones are now usually managed with endoscopic methods.

Stricture of the bile duct

The causes of benign biliary stricture are given in ***Summary box 71.5***. Bile duct strictures may be investigated radiologically as described in ***Summary box 71.6***.

Summary box 71.5

Causes of benign biliary stricture

Congenital
- Biliary atresia

Bile duct injury at surgery
- Cholecystectomy
- Choledochotomy
- Gastrectomy
- Hepatic resection
- Transplantation

Inflammatory
- Stones
- Cholangitis
- Parasitic
- Pancreatitis
- Sclerosing cholangitis
- Radiotherapy

Trauma

Idiopathic

Summary box 71.6

Radiological investigation of biliary strictures
- USG
- MRCP
- ERCP (with brush cytology in cases of a dominant stricture)
- PTC
- CT

PRIMARY SCLEROSING CHOLANGITIS

PSC is a rare idiopathic and progressive biliary tract disease characterised by inflammation and destruction of the intrahepatic and extrahepatic bile ducts that can lead to liver fibrosis and cirrhosis. Association with hypergammaglobulinaemia and markers such as anti-smooth muscle antibodies and anti-nuclear factor suggest an immunological basis; *cystic fibrosis* transmembrane conductance regulator (*CFTR*) gene mutations have been associated with the development of PSC. The majority of patients are between 30 and 60 years of age. There appears to be a male predominance and a strong association with inflammatory bowel disease (IBD), especially ulcerative colitis (IBD in PSC, 80%; PSC in IBD, 5%).

Patients may be asymptomatic, but common symptoms include pruritus, fever, fatigue, right upper quadrant discomfort, jaundice and weight loss. Liver function tests reveal a cholestatic pattern, elevated serum ALP and gamma-glutamyl transpeptidase (GGTP) and smaller rises in the aminotransferases; bilirubin values can be variable. MRCP (or ERCP) may demonstrate stricturing and beading of the bile ducts (***Figure 71.37***). Liver biopsy is helpful to confirm the diagnosis (concentric periductal 'onion skinning') and may help guide therapy by excluding cirrhosis. Important differential diagnoses are secondary sclerosing cholangitis, immunoglobulin G4 (IgG4) cholangitis, autoimmune hepatitis, human immunodeficiency

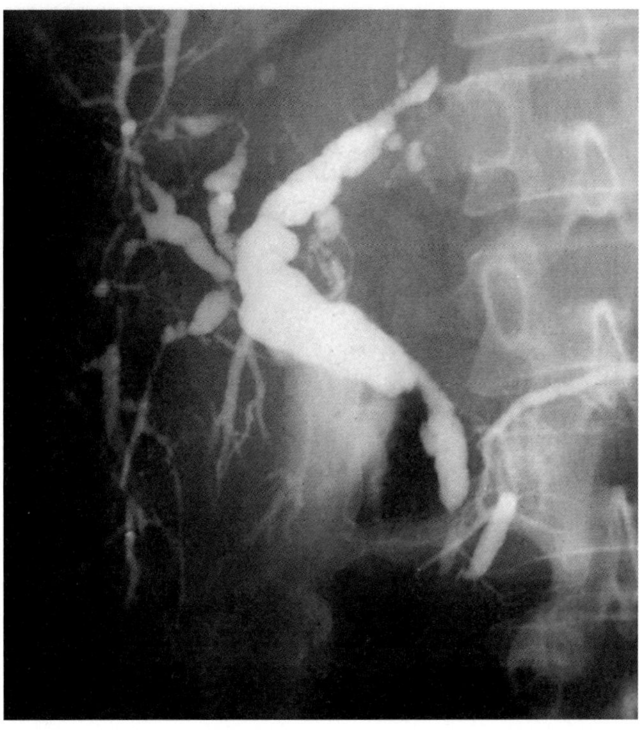

Figure 71.37 Sclerosing cholangitis in a patient with ulcerative colitis, visualised by endoscopic retrograde cholangiopancreatography.

virus (HIV) cholangiopathy and cholangiocarcinoma. The last may arise in patients with PSC and is difficult to diagnose; a high index of suspicion is required, especially in the setting of unexplained clinical deterioration.

Patients with PSC are at increased risk for cholangiocarcinoma and gallbladder cancer, as well as colon cancer in those with concurrent IBD. Medical management with antibiotics, vitamin K, cholestyramine, steroids and immunosuppressant drugs may not relieve symptoms. Endoscopic stenting of dominant strictures and, in selected patients with predominantly extrahepatic disease, operative resection may be worthwhile. For patients with cirrhosis, liver transplantation is the best option; 5-year survival following transplantation in high-volume centres is in excess of 80%. Screening for malignancies involving the gallbladder (polyp) and bile ducts and colonoscopy for IBD or malignancy are therefore critical, and bone densitometry for bone density is mandatory.

Immunoglobulin G4-related cholangitis

This recently recognised entity presents with diffuse or segmental narrowing of the intra- or extrahepatic bile ducts. Its features may make differentiation from PSC, cholangiocarcinoma and pancreatic cancer difficult. However, patients often have elevated serum IgG4 levels and concomitant autoimmune pancreatitis, IgG4-related sialadenitis or retroperitoneal fibrosis. Biliary biopsies show lymphoplasmacytic sclerosing cholangitis. Treatment is with systemic steroids. Failure to respond to steroid therapy should make one reconsider the diagnosis and exclude an underlying malignancy.

PARASITIC INFESTATION OF BILIARY TRACT

Biliary ascariasis

The roundworm *Ascaris lumbricoides* commonly infests the intestines of inhabitants in Asia, Africa and Central America. It may enter the biliary tree through the ampulla of Vater and cause biliary pain. Complications include obstruction, strictures, suppurative cholangitis, liver abscesses and empyema of the gallbladder. In uncomplicated cases, antispasmodics can be given to relax the sphincter of Oddi and the worms may return to the intestine to be dealt with by anthelminthic drugs. Worms can be extracted by ERCP. Operation may be necessary to remove the worms or deal with complications.

Clonorchiasis (Asiatic cholangiohepatis)

This disease is endemic in the Far East. The fluke inhabits the bile ducts, including the intrahepatic ducts. Fibrous thickening of the duct walls occurs. Many cases are asymptomatic. Complications include biliary pain, stones, cholangitis, cirrhosis and bile duct carcinoma. Because a process of recurrent stone formation is established, choledochojejunostomy with a Roux loop fixed to the adjacent abdominal wall is performed in some centres to allow easy subsequent access to the duct system.

Hydatid disease

A large hydatid cyst may obstruct the hepatic ducts. Sometimes, a cyst will rupture into the biliary tree and its contents cause obstructive jaundice or cholangitis, requiring appropriate surgery (see ***Chapter 6***).

TUMOURS OF THE BILE DUCT

Benign tumours of the bile duct

Benign neoplasms such as papilloma, adenoma, papillomatosis, leiomyoma and neural and endocrine tumours causing biliary obstruction are uncommon and may be an incidental finding. For symptomatic patients, the duration of symptoms may vary from a few days to months.

Intraductal papillary neoplasm of the bile duct

Intraductal papillary neoplasm of the bile duct (IPNB) is a rare variant of bile duct tumours characterised by papillary growth within the bile duct lumen with ductal dilatation. It is regarded as the biliary counterpart of an intraductal papillary mucinous neoplasm of the pancreas. IPNBs display a spectrum from premalignant lesions to invasive cholangiocarcinoma. The most common radiological findings are bile duct dilatation and intraductal masses. USG, CT and MRI are usually performed to assess tumour location and extension. Cholangioscopy can confirm the histology and assess the extent of the tumour, including superficial spread along the biliary epithelium. Patients without distant metastasis are considered for surgical resection in a manner similar to that for other types of intrahepatic cholangiocarcinomas and extrahepatic bile duct carcinomas, i.e. major hepatectomy with or without extrahepatic bile duct resection.

Malignant tumours of the bile duct

Summary box 71.7

Bile duct cancer (cholangiocarcinoma)

- Malignancy arising from the biliary epithelium; histologically of three types: mass forming, intraductal growing and periductal infiltrating
- Rare, but incidence increasing
- Most patients present with abnormal liver function tests or frank jaundice
- Diagnosis by USG, CT or MRI
- Majority of patients receive palliative care only
- Complete surgical excision possible in <10%
- Prognosis poor: 90% die within 1 year from liver failure or biliary sepsis
- Adjuvant chemoradiation therapy has a limited role

Cholangiocarcinoma

Incidence

Cholangiocarcinoma is an uncommon malignancy. The overall annual incidence is 1–1.5 per 100 000 with the peak incidence in the eighth decade. The male-to-female ratio is approximately 1.5:1. Anatomically, tumours involving the biliary confluence (hilar cholangiocarcinoma or Klatskin tumours) account for 60% of cases, with the remainder involving the distal bile duct (20–30%) or intrahepatic ducts (10–20%).

Risk factors

A minority of patients have a known risk factor; the major risk factor in western practice is PSC. It is estimated that a longstanding history of PSC increases the risk of developing biliary tract cancer 20-fold compared with the normal population; those with concomitant IBD are at significantly higher risk. Cholangiocarcinoma appears to occur at an earlier age in patients with PSC (30–50 years of age) than in the general population. In addition, disease is usually multifocal and detected at an advanced stage with a resultant poor prognosis compared with the general population.

Congenital cystic disease, hepatolithiasis, oriental cholangiohepatitis, hepatitis C virus infection and infestation with liver flukes have also been associated with an increased risk of cholangiocarcinoma. While the pathophysiology is unclear, it is thought that these parasites cause chronic inflammation that leads to DNA mutations through production of carcinogens and free radicals; the latter can stimulate cellular proliferation in the intrahepatic bile ducts and ultimately lead to invasive cancer (***Summary box 71.8***).

Clinical features

Early symptoms are often non-specific, with abdominal pain, early satiety, anorexia and weight loss commonly seen. Symptoms associated with biliary obstruction (pruritus and jaundice) may be present in a minority of patients. In these patients, examination often demonstrates clinical signs of jaundice, cachexia is often noticeable and the gallbladder is palpable if the obstruction is in the distal CBD (Courvoisier's sign).

Summary box 71.8

Risk factors for cholangiocarcinoma

Chronic inflammatory conditions
- PSC
- Oriental cholangiohepatitis
- Hepatitis C infection

Parasitic infections
- *Opisthorchis viverrini*
- *C. sinensis*

Congenital
- Choledochal cysts
- Caroli's disease

Chemical agents
- Thorium dioxide (Thorotrast)
- Vinyl chloride
- Dioxin
- Asbestos

Post surgical
- Biliary–enteric anastomosis

Non-alcoholic fatty liver disease

Investigations

Biochemical investigations (elevated bilirubin, ALP and GGTP) will confirm obstructive jaundice. The tumour marker carbohydrate 19-9 (CA19-9) may also be elevated. Imaging studies such as USG, CT and MRI/MRCP are essential for diagnosis, staging and assessing the anatomical relationship between the tumour and the major perihilar vascular structures (***Figure 71.38***). These studies allow the level of biliary obstruction to be defined and determine the locoregional extent of disease and the presence of metastases. Direct cholangiography using ERCP or PTC is also used following non-invasive studies. Both can define the level of obstruction and allow biopsy (non-diagnostic in 40–80% of patients) and placement of endobiliary stents for biliary drainage. The choice between the modalities depends on local availability and the anatomical site of the tumour, with PTC preferred for more proximal lesions and ERCP favoured for distal tumours. Despite a higher incidence of postoperative infection with stenting, patients undergoing anticipated major liver resection need preoperative biliary drainage as hyperbilirubinaemia (bilirubin level >6 mg/dL) may impair hepatic regeneration and hypertrophy. Cholangioscopy is an adjunct to ERCP, with diagnostic accuracy increased from 78% to 93% and sensitivity from 58% to 100%.

Positron emission tomography (PET) is useful in detecting lymph node and distant metastases but has limited value in the assessment of local resectability.

Gerald Klatskin, 1910–1986, hepatologist, VA Hospital, Newington, CT, USA.

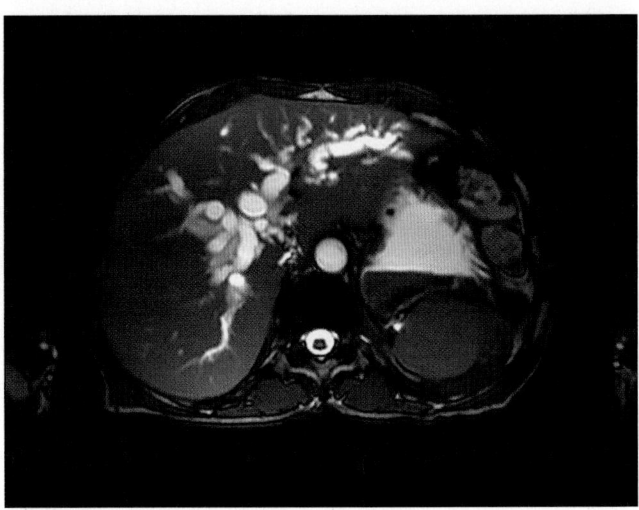

Figure 71.38 Magnetic resonance imaging scan showing a hilar cholangiocarcinoma with dilatation of the intrahepatic biliary tree.

The anatomical extent of the disease is classified according to either the Bismuth–Corlette (***Figure 71.39***) or the Memorial Sloan Kettering Cancer Center (MSKCC) classification.

The MSKCC classification T-stage criteria for hilar cholangiocarcinoma are as follows:

- T1 tumour involving the biliary confluence without extension to second-order biliary radicles.
- T2 tumour involving the biliary confluence with unilateral extension to second-order biliary radicles and ipsilateral portal vein involvement or ipsilateral hepatic atrophy.
- T3 tumour involving the biliary confluence with bilateral extension to second-order biliary radicles; or unilateral extension to second-order biliary radicles with contralateral portal vein involvement; or unilateral extension to second-order biliary radicles with contralateral hepatic lobar atrophy; or main or bilateral portal venous involvement.

Treatment

A multidisciplinary approach is required. The choice of treatment depends on the site and extent of the disease. Unfortunately, the majority of patients present with advanced disease. However, 10–15% are suitable for surgical resection, which offers the only hope for long-term survival. The aim of surgical resection is to achieve complete resection with negative pathological margins (R0 resection) and safely restore biliary–enteric continuity.

Whether or not the disease is resectable depends on patient factors (comorbidities, presence or absence of chronic liver disease) and tumour factors (extent of disease within the biliary tree, vascular involvement, remnant liver volume, increase in the remnant after portal vein embolisation, presence or absence of metastatic disease). Depending on the site of disease, surgery involves either a standard or extended hepatic resection with caudate lobe excision with en bloc lymphadenectomy and reconstruction of the biliary tree. Distal common duct tumours may require pancreaticoduodenectomy (Whipple procedure). Local resection should be avoided.

In selected patients, liver transplantation has been recommended for those with locally unresectable disease without evidence of distant metastases. Transplantation is often preceded by neoadjuvant chemoradiation therapy and staging laparoscopy. While emerging data are encouraging, this aggressive approach remains controversial and is reserved for selected patients in specialised centres (Mayo protocol).

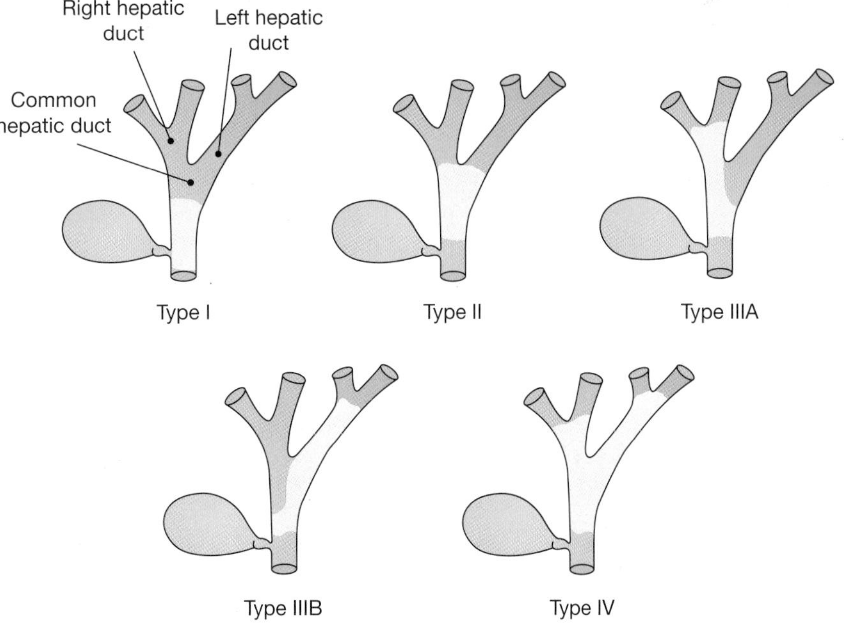

Figure 71.39 Bismuth–Corlette classification of cholangiocarcinoma.

Henri Bismuth, b. 1934, surgeon, Hôpital Paul Bruce, Villejif, France, and **Marvin Corlette** described the classification of cholangiocarcinoma in 1975.
Allen Oldfather Whipple, 1881–1963, surgeon, Columbia-Presbyterian Medical Center, New York, NY, USA.
Mayo Clinic, Rochester, MN, USA, established in the 1880s by Dr William Worral Mayo and his sons William and Charles, both surgeons.

Following resection, disease-specific survival is related to the T-stage, margin status, metastatic lymph node spread, perineural and perivascular invasion, non-papillary tumour subtypes and poor tumour differentiation. Of these, the only variable in which the surgeon plays a major role is margin-negative resection, and emphasis needs to be placed on achieving R0 resection. Approximately 35% of patients will survive 5 years after surgery. Adjuvant chemotherapy and radiotherapy have a limited role and have not been demonstrated to add survival benefit following surgical resection. However, patients at high risk for recurrence (positive surgical margins or node positive) may benefit from adjuvant therapy and should be referred for medical or radiation oncology opinion. The majority of patients who present with unresectable disease are candidates for palliative chemotherapy – gemcitabine with cisplatin. The aim is to maintain or improve quality of life by relieving symptoms and preventing cholestatic liver failure. Biliary obstruction can be relieved by endoscopic (ERCP) or percutaneous (PTC) methods. Surgical bypass rarely has a role apart from in patients with a distal bile duct lesion found to have unresectable disease at operation.

Cancer of the gallbladder

Incidence

Gallbladder cancer is extremely variable by geographical region and racial–ethnic groups; the highest incidence is among Chileans, Native Americans and residents in parts of northern India, where it accounts for as much as 9% of all biliary tract disease. Women appear to have a higher incidence across all geographical areas. In western practice, gallbladder cancer accounts for less than 1% of new cancer diagnoses. The disease usually presents in the seventh or eighth decade. The aetiology is unclear but there is a suggested association with pre-existing gallstone disease, implying that chronic inflammation may play a role. Calcification of the gallbladder wall, presumably due to chronic inflammation (porcelain gallbladder), is also associated with a small increased risk of cancer (***Figure 71.5***). Chronic infection may promote the development of cancer and the risk in typhoid carriers is significantly increased over that of the general population. Patients with PSC, especially with concomitant IBD, and those with an abnormal pancreatic–biliary junction are at greater risk of gallbladder cancer.

In patients with gallbladder polyps (***Figure 71.40***) the risk of malignant transformation increases with increasing size of the polyp.

Summary box 71.9

Gallbladder cancer

- Rare
- Similar presentation to benign biliary disease (gallstones)
- Diagnosis by USG, CT, MRI/MRCP
- Most patients present with advanced disease
- Surgical resection in less than 10% – remainder receive palliative treatment
- Prognosis is poor

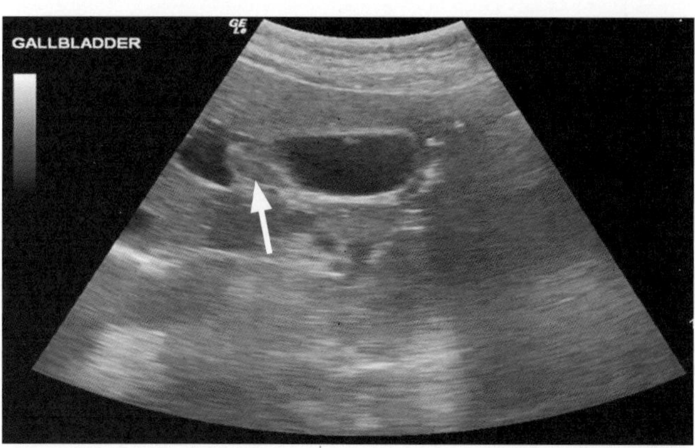

Figure 71.40 Ultrasonography demonstrating a gallbladder polyp. Note the absence of an acoustic shadow (arrow).

Pathology

The majority (90%) of tumours are adenocarcinomas. Squamous carcinomas may arise from areas of mucosal squamous metaplasia.

At operation, localised carcinomas are difficult to differentiate from chronic cholecystitis; the tumour most commonly is nodular and infiltrative, with thickening of the gallbladder wall, often extending to the whole gallbladder. The tumour spreads by direct extension into the liver, seeding of the peritoneal cavity and involvement of the perihilar lymphatics and neural plexuses. At the time of presentation, the majority of tumours are advanced.

Clinical features

Patients may be asymptomatic; symptoms, if present, are usually indistinguishable from those of benign gallbladder disease such as biliary colic or cholecystitis, particularly in older patients. Jaundice and anorexia are late features, heralding a low resectability rate and even fewer negative margins. A palpable mass is a late sign.

Investigation

Laboratory findings are generally non-specific but may be consistent with biliary obstruction. Non-specific findings include anaemia, leukocytosis and a mild elevation in transaminases. Serum CA19-9 and carcinoembryonic antigen may be elevated in approximately 80% of patients.

The preoperative diagnosis is often made on USG and confirmed by CT thorax, abdomen and pelvis or MRI/MRCP. Preoperative staging should aim to determine the local extent of disease and exclude the presence of distant metastases. Percutaneous biopsy under radiological guidance may be considered to obtain tissue for pathological examination, but only in unresectable disease prior to palliative treatment. Laparoscopic examination is useful in staging the disease. Laparoscopy can detect peritoneal or liver metastases, which would preclude further surgical resection (***Figure 71.41***). PET scanning has a role in detecting metastatic disease.

Treatment and prognosis

The majority of patients have advanced disease at presentation and are not candidates for surgical therapy. Staging

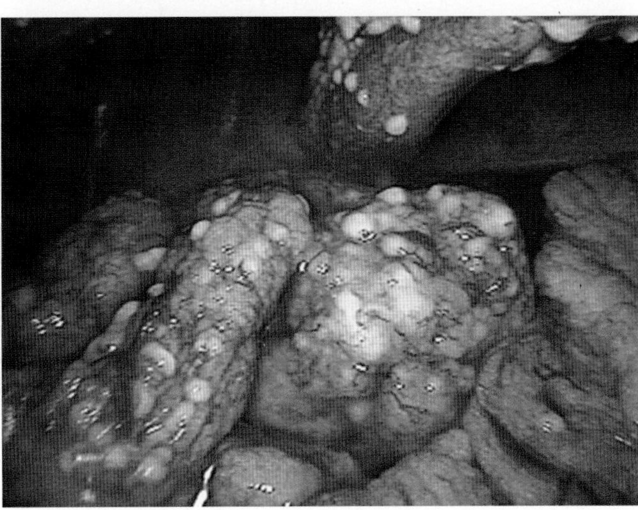

Figure 71.41 Laparoscopic staging in a patient with gallbladder cancer demonstrating gross peritoneal metastases.

laparoscopy is mandatory prior to formal laparotomy to detect occult metastases not picked up on imaging. Radical en bloc resection includes the gallbladder, wedge hepatectomy (2 cm of liver in the gallbladder bed or segments IVb and V if there is concomitant liver infiltration) or extended hepatectomy and bile duct resection if the bile duct is involved or the cystic duct margin is positive on intraoperative frozen section. Regional lymphadenectomy (paracholedochal portal, along the right hepatic artery and retroduodenal nodes) should be considered. The aim is to remove the tumour entirely and achieve negative histopathological margins.

Some patients have the disease diagnosed following histopathological examination of the gallbladder after it has been removed for presumed benign disease (incidental gallbladder cancer). In these cases, the need for further surgery is determined by the stage of disease. For early-stage disease confined to the mucosa of the gallbladder with a negative cystic duct margin and no evidence of recurrence on imaging, no further treatment is indicated. However, for transmural disease, a radical en bloc resection of the gallbladder fossa and surrounding wedge of liver along with the regional lymph nodes should be performed. If the initial procedure was performed laparoscopically, the surgeon should examine the laparoscopic port sites. Routine resection of port sites is no longer recommended. However, it is recognised that the finding of disease at the port sites is a sign of generalised peritoneal disease and carries a very poor prognosis. Adjuvant oral chemotherapy (capecitabine alone is preferred or in combination with gemcitabine/oxaliplatin) may derive survival benefit.

Gallbladder cancer is a lethal disease with a grim prognosis; the median survival is less than 6 months and 5-year survival figures of 50% for localised gallbladder cancer (with chemotherapy) and 2-5% in patients with distant metastasis have been reported.

For the majority of patients with advanced disease a non-operative approach to palliation is best. Obstructive jaundice can be relieved by endoscopic and/or percutaneous methods after discussion in the multidisciplinary team.

Summary box 71.10

Aims of staging gallbladder cancer

- Assessment of local disease
- Detection of metastatic disease:
  - Liver
  - Peritoneum
  - Lymphatics
  - Extra-abdominal disease

FURTHER READING

Carter DC, Russell RCG, Pitt HA, Bismuth H (eds). *Rob and Smith's operative surgery: hepatobiliary and pancreatic surgery.* London: Chapman & Hall, 1996.

Dooley JS, Lok A, Burroughs A, Heathcoate J (eds). *Sherlock's diseases of the liver and biliary system*, 12th edn. Oxford: Wiley-Blackwell, 2011.

Garden OJ, Parks RW. *Hepatobiliary and pancreatic surgery: a companion to specialist practice*, 5th edn. New York: Saunders Elsevier, 2013.

Jarnagin W. *Blumgart's surgery of the liver, pancreas and biliary tract*, 5th edn. New York: Elsevier, 2012.

Rocha FG, Matsuo K, Blumgart LH, Jarnagin WR. Hilar cholangiocarcinoma: the Memorial Sloan-Kettering Cancer Center experience. *J Hepatobiliary Pancreat Sci* 2010; **17**(4): 490–6.

Society of American Gastrointestinal and Endoscopic Surgeons. *The SAGES safe cholecystectomy program*, 2015. Available from: https://www.sages.org/safe-cholecystectomy-program (accessed October 2020).

Takada T (ed.). Tokyo Guidelines 2018: updated Tokyo Guidelines for the management of acute cholangitis/acute cholecystitis. *J Hepatobiliary Pancreat Sci* 2018; **25**(1): 1–114.

CHAPTER

72 The pancreas

Learning objectives

To understand:

- The anatomy and physiology of the pancreas
- Investigations of the pancreas
- Congenital abnormalities of the pancreas
- Assessment and management of pancreatitis
- Diagnosis and treatment of pancreatic cancer

ANATOMY AND PHYSIOLOGY

Anatomy

The name 'pancreas' is derived from the Greek 'pan' (all) and 'kreas' (flesh). For a long time, its glandular function was not understood and it was thought to act as a cushion for the stomach. The pancreas is situated in the retroperitoneum. It is divided into a head, which occupies 30% of the gland by mass, and a body and tail, which together constitute 70%. The head lies within the curve of the duodenum, overlying the body of the second lumbar vertebra and the vena cava. The aorta and the superior mesenteric vessels lie behind the neck of the gland. Coming off the side of the pancreatic head and passing to the left and behind the superior mesenteric vein is the uncinate process of the pancreas. Behind the neck of the pancreas, near its upper border, the superior mesenteric vein joins the splenic vein to form the portal vein (***Figures 72.1 and 72.2***). The tip of the pancreatic tail extends up to the splenic hilum.

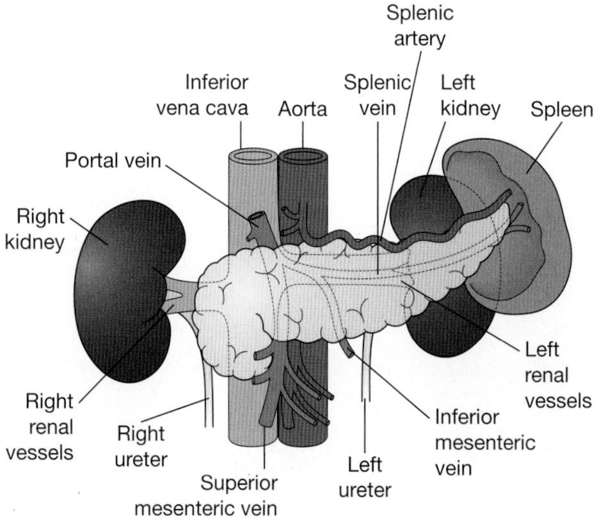

Figure 72.1 The posterior relations of the pancreas.

The pancreas weighs approximately 80 g. Of this, 80–90% is composed of exocrine acinar tissue, which is organised into lobules. The main pancreatic duct branches into interlobular and intralobular ducts, ductules and, finally, acini. The main duct is lined by columnar epithelium, which becomes cuboidal in the ductules. Acinar cells are clumped around a central lumen, which communicates with the duct system. Clusters of endocrine cells, known as islets of Langerhans, are distributed throughout the pancreas. Islets consist of different cell types: 75% are B cells (producing insulin); 20% are A cells (producing glucagon); and the remainder are D cells (producing somatostatin) and a small number of pancreatic polypeptide cells. Within an islet, the B cells form an inner core surrounded by the other cells. Capillaries draining the islet cells drain into the portal vein.

There are nine key processes that occur during pancreatic embryogenesis (***Table 72.1***). Malrotation of the ventral bud in the fifth week results in an annular pancreas, while the mode of

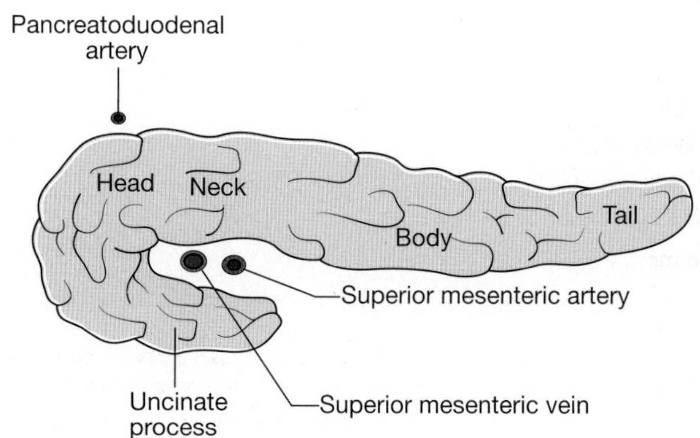

Figure 72.2 Transverse section of the pancreas. Note the position of the uncinate process behind the vessels.

Paul Langerhans, 1847–1888, Professor of Pathological Anatomy, Freiberg, Germany, described the islets in 1869, in his doctoral thesis.

ductule fusion in the seventh week produces the various possible ductular patterns. Between the 12th and 40th weeks of fetal life, the pancreas differentiates into exocrine and endocrine elements. The primitive ducts and their ductules are responsible for the lobular arrangement of the pancreas. Congenital anomalies of the pancreas are varied and arise during the early phase of development. The anatomy of the pancreatic duct is variable as a result of the primordial bud development. The dorsal duct is expressed in a variable manner in the adult, as outlined in *Figure 72.3*. Approximately 10% of patients will have a significant flow from the main duct through the accessory papilla. The anatomy of the main duodenal papilla, also known as the ampulla of Vater, is also variable (*Figure 72.4*).

The outlet of each duct is protected by a complex sphincter mechanism (sphincter of Oddi) (*Figure 72.5*).

TABLE 72.1 Steps in the development of the pancreas.

1	Day 26	Dorsal pancreatic duct arises from the dorsal side of the duodenum
2	Day 32	Ventral bud arises from the base of the hepatic diverticulum
3	Day 37	Contact occurs between the two buds. Fusion by the end of week 6
4	Week 6	Ventral bud produces the head and uncinate process
5	Week 6	Ducts fuse
6	Week 6	Ventral duct and distal portion of the dorsal duct form the main duct (duct of Wirsung)
7	Week 6	Proximal dorsal duct forms the duct of Santorini
8	Month 3	Acini appear
9	Months 3–4	Islets of Langerhans appear and become biologically active

Summary box 72.1

Anomalies of the pancreas

- Aplasia
- Hypoplasia
- Hyperplasia
- Hypertrophy
- Dysplasia
- Variations and anomalies of the ducts[a]
  - Pancreas divisum
  - Rotational anomalies
- Annular pancreas[a]
- Pancreatic gallbladder
- Polycystic disease[a]
- Congenital pancreatic cysts
  - Cystic fibrosis[a]
  - von Hippel–Lindau syndrome
- Ectopic pancreatic tissue, accessory pancreas[a]
- Vascular anomalies
- Choledochal cysts[a]
- Horseshoe pancreas

[a]The more frequent anomalies encountered in surgical practice.

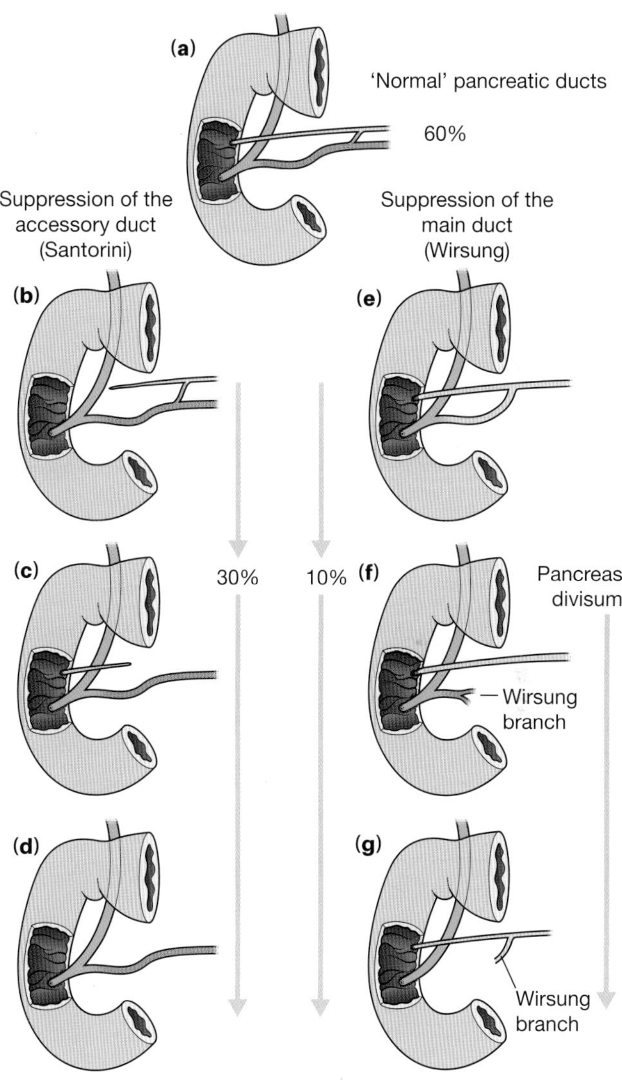

Figure 72.3 Variations in the pancreatic ducts. (a) Normal. (b–d) Progressive suppression of the accessory duct (30%). (e–g) Progressive suppression of the main duct (10%). (f, g) Pancreas divisum.

Abraham Vater, 1704–1751, Professor of Anatomy and Botany, and later of Pathology and Therapeutics, Wittenberg, Germany.
Johann Georg Wirsung, 1589–1643, Professor of Anatomy, Padua, Italy.
Giovanni Domenico Santorini, 1701–1737, Professor of Anatomy and Medicine, Venice, Italy. His drawings of the accessory pancreatic duct were published after his death.
Eugen von Hippel, 1866–1939, Professor of Ophthalmology, Göttingen, Germany.
Arvid Lindau, 1892–1958, pathologist, Lund, Sweden, established the link between the retinal angiomatosis described by von Hippel and the cerebellar and visceral components of the syndrome.
Ruggero Oddi, 1866–1913, anatomist and physiologist, Perugia, Italy.

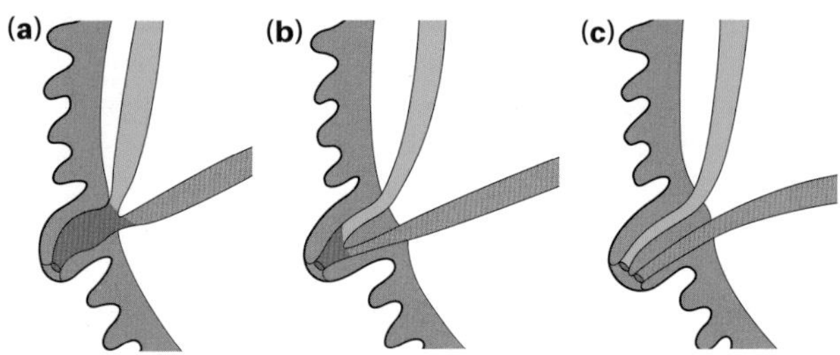

Figure 72.4 Variations in the relation of the common bile duct and main pancreatic duct at the main duodenal papilla. In (a) there is a common channel with no sphincter mechanism protecting flow between the ducts. In (b) there is a partial common channel, while in (c) there is separation of the two channels. Gallstone pancreatitis is more likely with (a) and (b).

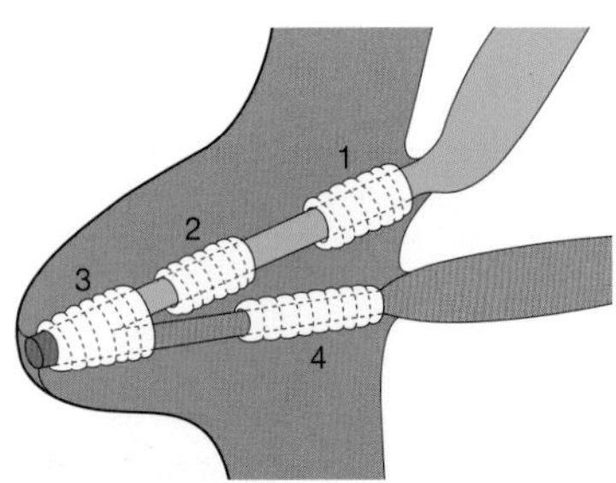

Figure 72.5 The complexity of the sphincter of Oddi. (1) Superior choledochal sphincter; (2) inferior choledochal sphincter; (3) ampullary sphincter; (4) pancreatic sphincter.

Physiology

In response to a meal, the pancreas secretes digestive enzymes in an alkaline (pH 8.4) bicarbonate-rich fluid. Spontaneous secretion is minimal; the hormone secretin, which is released from the duodenal mucosa, evokes a bicarbonate-rich fluid. Cholecystokinin (CCK) (synonym: pancreozymin) is released from the duodenal mucosa in response to food. CCK is responsible for enzyme release. Vagal stimulation increases the volume of secretion. Protein is synthesised at a greater rate (per gram of tissue) in the pancreas than in any other tissue, with the possible exception of the lactating mammary gland. About 90% of this protein is exported from the acinar cells as a variety of digestive enzymes. Approximately 6–20 g of digestive enzymes enters the duodenum each day. Nascent proteins are synthesised as preproteins and undergo modification in a sequence of steps. The proteins move from the rough endothelial endoplasmic reticulum to the Golgi complex, where lysosomes and mature zymogen storage granules containing proteases are stored, and then to the ductal surface of the cell, from which they are extruded by exocytosis. During this phase, the proteolytic enzymes are in an inactive form, which is important in preventing pancreatitis.

TABLE 72.2 Investigation of the pancreas.
Serum enzyme levels
Pancreatic function tests
Morphology
Ultrasonography
Computed tomography
Magnetic resonance imaging
Endoscopic retrograde cholangiopancreatography
Endoscopic ultrasonography
Plain radiography
Chest
Upper abdomen

INVESTIGATIONS

Estimation of pancreatic enzymes in body fluids

Investigations of the pancreas are listed in *Table 72.2*.

When the pancreas is damaged, enzymes such as amylase, lipase, trypsin, elastase and chymotrypsin are released into the serum. Measurement of serum amylase is the most widely used test of pancreatic damage (serum lipase is more sensitive and specific but is not widely available). The serum amylase rises within a few hours of pancreatic damage and declines over the next 4–8 days. A markedly elevated serum level is highly suspicious but not diagnostic of acute pancreatitis. Urinary amylase and amylase–creatinine clearance ratios add little to diagnostic accuracy. If confirmation of the diagnosis is required, computed tomography (CT) of the pancreas is of greater value.

Summary box 72.2

Causes of raised serum amylase level other than acute pancreatitis

- Upper gastrointestinal tract perforation
- Mesenteric infarction
- Torsion of an intra-abdominal viscus
- Retroperitoneal haematoma
- Ectopic pregnancy
- Macroamylasaemia
- Renal failure
- Salivary gland inflammation

Pancreatic function tests

Pancreatic exocrine function can be assessed by directly measuring pancreatic secretion in response to a standardised stimulus. The stimulus to secretion can be physiological, e.g. ingestion of a test meal, as in the Lundh test, or pharmacological, e.g. intravenous injection of a hormone such as secretin

Camillo Golgi, 1844–1926, Professor of Anatomy and Histology at Pavia, and later at Siena, Italy, developed silver staining of neural tissue and received the Nobel Prize in 1906 (with Ramón y Cajal).
Göran Lundh, 1926–1999, surgeon, Södersjukhuset, Stockholm, Sweden.

or CCK. Duodenal intubation has to be performed with a triple-lumen tube so that the gastric and duodenal juices can be aspirated, and a non-absorbable marker such as polyethylene glycol is used to assess the completeness of the aspiration. The nitroblue tetrazolium–para-aminobenzoic acid (NBT–PABA) test provides an indirect measure of pancreatic function. The substance is administered orally and degraded in the gut by a pancreatic enzyme, and the breakdown product (PABA) is absorbed by the intestine and excreted in the urine; its urinary level is measured. The pancreolauryl test works on a similar principle. These tests are cheap and easy to perform but are non-specific, especially following gastrectomy and in conditions that may alter gastrointestinal transit and intestinal absorptive capacity. They are rarely used now in the clinical setting. Measurement of the enzyme elastase in stool is simple, specific and now used widely. A low level of faecal elastase indicates exocrine insufficiency.

Imaging investigations

Ultrasonography

Ultrasonography is the initial investigation of choice in patients with jaundice to determine whether or not the bile duct is dilated, the coexistence of gallstones or gross disease within the liver such as metastases. It may also define the presence or absence of a mass in the pancreas (***Figure 72.6***). However, obesity and overlying bowel gas often make interpretation of the pancreas itself unsatisfactory.

Computed tomography

Most significant pathologies within the pancreas can be diagnosed on high-quality CT scans, with three-dimensional reconstruction if necessary. A specific pancreatic protocol should be followed. An initial unenhanced CT scan is essential to determine the presence of calcification within the pancreas and gallbladder (***Figure 72.7***). Then, following rapid injection of intravenous contrast, scanning is performed in the arterial and venous phases. The stomach and duodenum should be outlined with water and distended to define the duodenal loop.

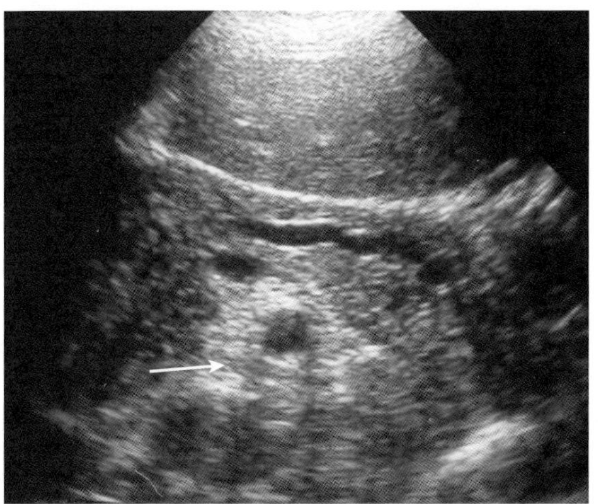

Figure 72.6 Ultrasound scan showing a mass in the head of the pancreas (marked by an arrow) and a dilated pancreatic duct in the body of the gland (courtesy of Dr Alison McLean).

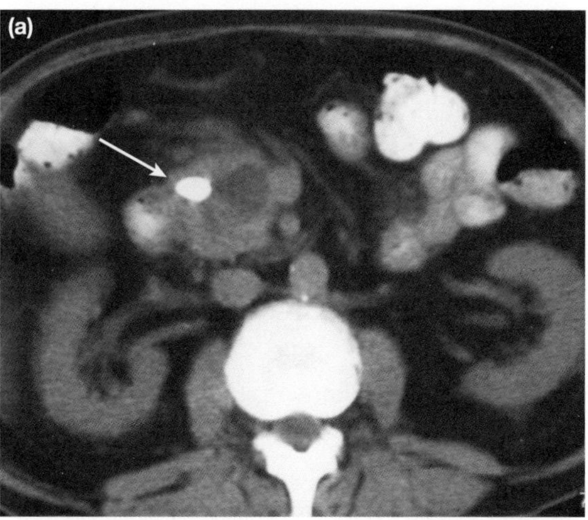

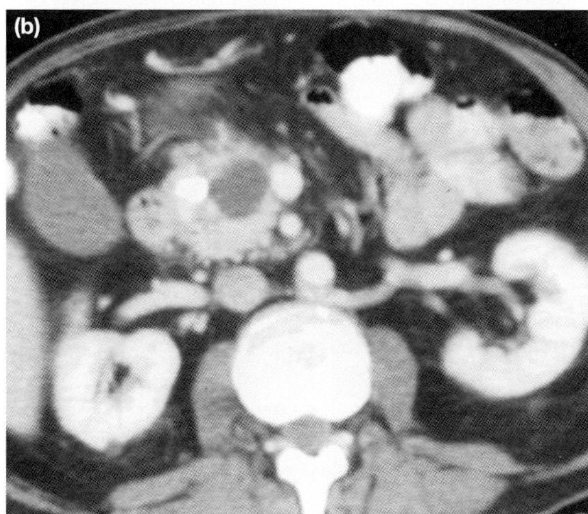

Figure 72.7 (a) Unenhanced computed tomography scan of a man with chronic pancreatitis, showing a focus of calcification (marked by an arrow) in the head of the pancreas and a cyst adjacent to that. Oral contrast has been administered. (b) The same area after injection of intravenous contrast.

Pancreatic carcinomas of 1–2 cm in size can usually be demonstrated (***Figure 72.8***). Endocrine tumours are also well imaged on CT (***Figure 72.9***). In patients with pancreatitis, necrotic areas within the gland can be identified by the absence of contrast enhancement on CT. Inflammatory collections and pseudocysts can be seen (***Figure 72.10***). CT-guided drainage is helpful in the treatment of pancreatic collections, cysts and pseudocysts, and facilitates percutaneous fine-needle or Trucut biopsy.

Magnetic resonance imaging

With magnetic resonance imaging (MRI) the pancreas can be clearly identified, and the anatomy of the bile duct and the pancreatic duct, together with fluid collections, can be defined. Magnetic resonance cholangiography and pancreatography (MRCP) has largely replaced diagnostic endoscopic cholangiography and pancreatography (ERCP) as it is non-invasive and less expensive (***Figure 72.11***). Using the technique in conjunction with intravenous injection of secretin, emptying of the pancreatic duct can be demonstrated to show the absence or presence of obstruction.

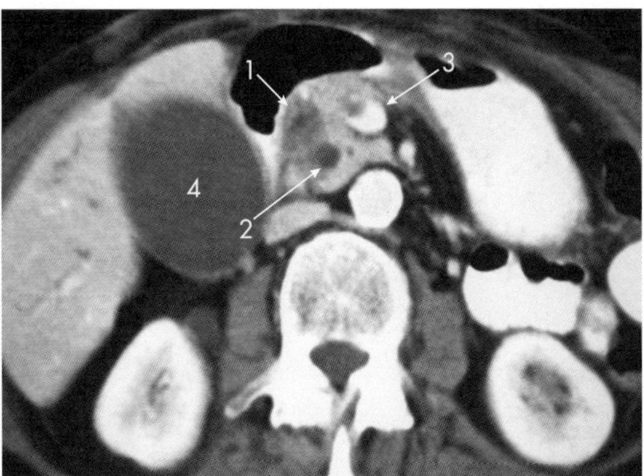

Figure 72.8 Contrast-enhanced computed tomography scan of a patient with a carcinoma of the pancreatic head. The main bulk of the tumour lies inferior to the section shown here. The dilated bile duct (1) and main pancreatic duct (2) can be seen, with tumour infiltration around them. There is a thrombus in the superior mesenteric vein (3). The gallbladder is distended (4).

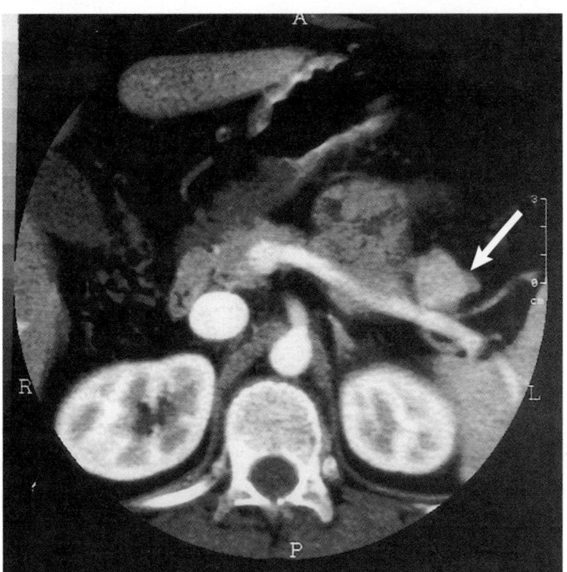

Figure 72.9 Computed tomography scan showing a hypervascular insulinoma (arrow) adjacent to the splenic vein. Local excision of the tumour resulted in normoglycaemia.

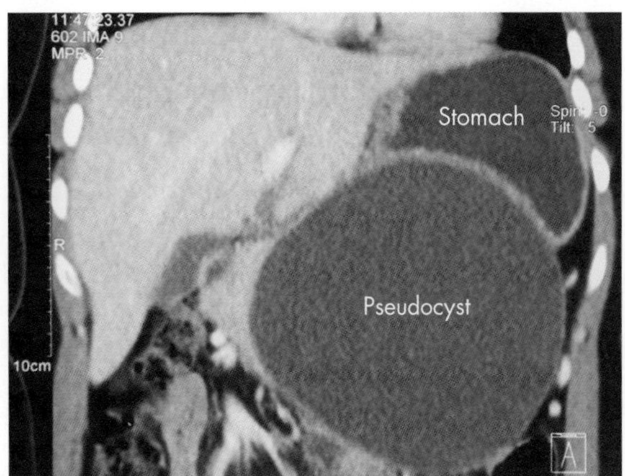

Figure 72.10 Computed tomography scan of a large pseudocyst in relation to the body and tail of the pancreas.

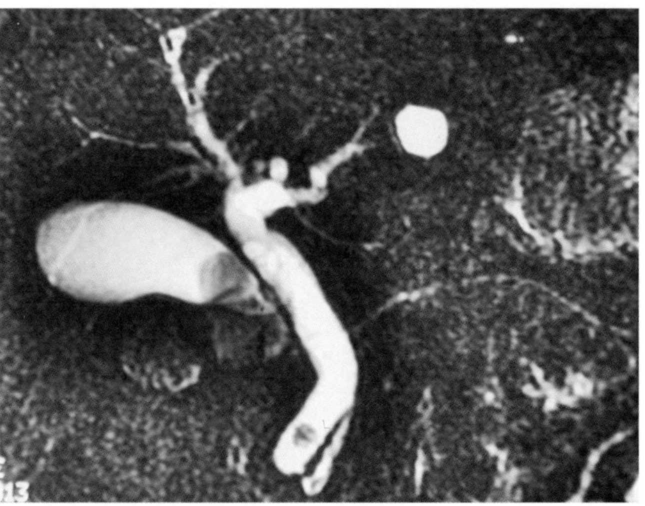

Figure 72.11 Magnetic resonance cholangiopancreatography in a patient with obstructive jaundice. A dilated common bile duct was seen on ultrasonography, but no pancreatic mass lesion was visible on computed tomography. The bile duct and the main pancreatic duct are seen very well, with a stone visible in the lower part of the bile duct and another in the neck of the gallbladder.

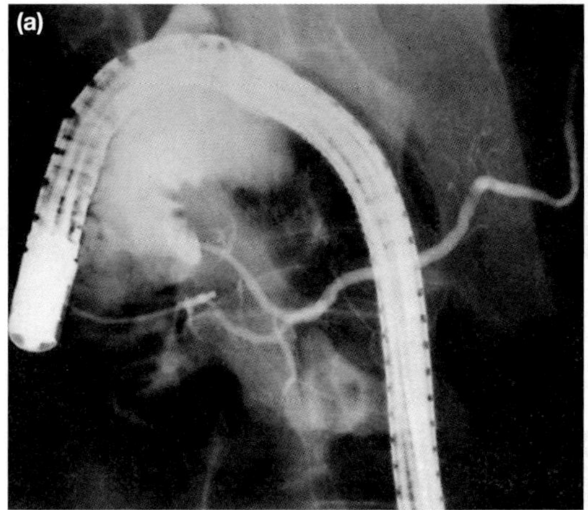

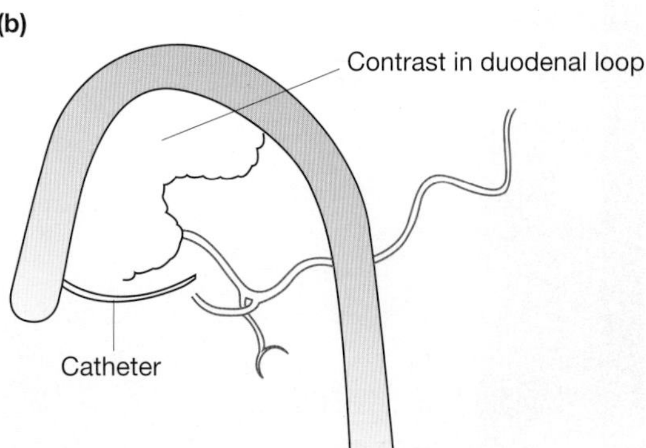

Figure 72.12 Endoscopic retrograde cholangiopancreatography. (a) Normal pancreatic duct with filling of the duct of Santorini from the duct of Wirsung. (b) Diagrammatic outline of (a).

Endoscopic retrograde cholangiopancreatography

ERCP is performed using a side-viewing fibreoptic duodenoscope. The ampulla of Vater is intubated, and contrast is injected into the biliary and pancreatic ducts to display the anatomy radiologically (*Figure 72.12*). In pancreatic carcinoma, the main pancreatic duct may be narrowed or completely obstructed at the site of the tumour (*Figure 72.13*), or the distal bile duct may be narrowed. Concurrent narrowing of both ducts results in the so-called double duct sign (*Figure 72.14*). Changes seen in chronic pancreatitis include the presence of pancreatic duct strictures, dilatation of the main pancreatic duct with stones, abnormalities of pancreatic duct side branches, communication of the pancreatic duct with cysts and bile duct strictures (*Figures 72.15–72.17*). A plain radiograph before contrast studies is essential to delineate calcification (*Figure 72.18*). In addition to imaging, bile or pancreatic fluid and brushings from duct strictures can yield cells that confirm the suspected diagnosis of carcinoma (*Figure 72.19*). Brush cytology taken from malignant strictures at the time of ERCP yields a positive diagnosis in 40–50% of patients. ERCP also allows the placement of biliary and pancreatic stents.

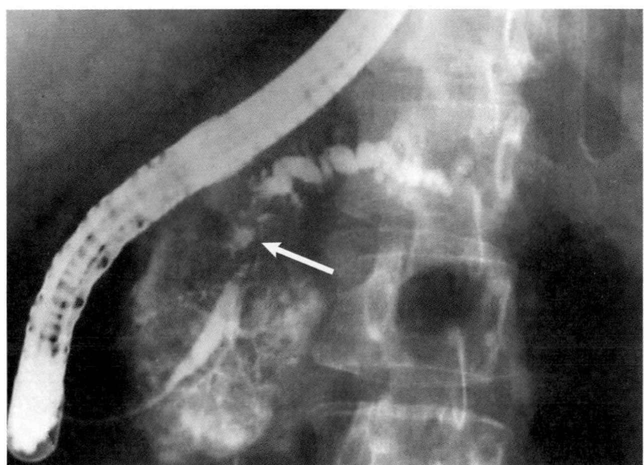

Figure 72.13 Endoscopic retrograde cholangiopancreatography: pancreatic carcinoma. Irregular stricture of the main pancreatic duct (arrow) with dilatation distal to the obstruction.

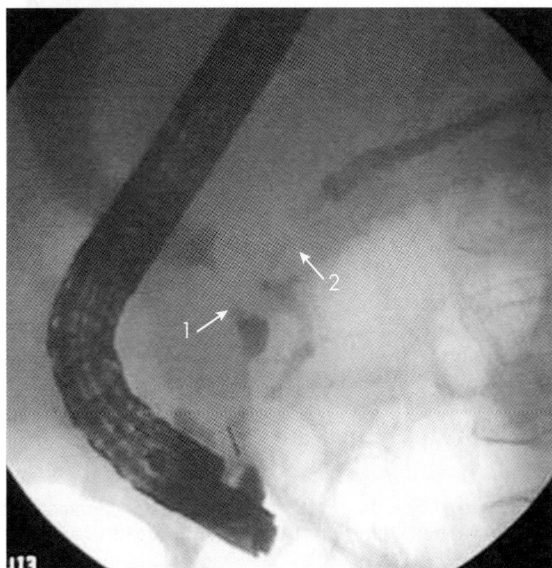

Figure 72.14 Endoscopic retrograde cholangiopancreatography depicting a malignant stricture in the lower part of the common bile duct (1) and in the main pancreatic duct (2), an appearance referred to as the double duct sign (courtesy of Dr George Webster).

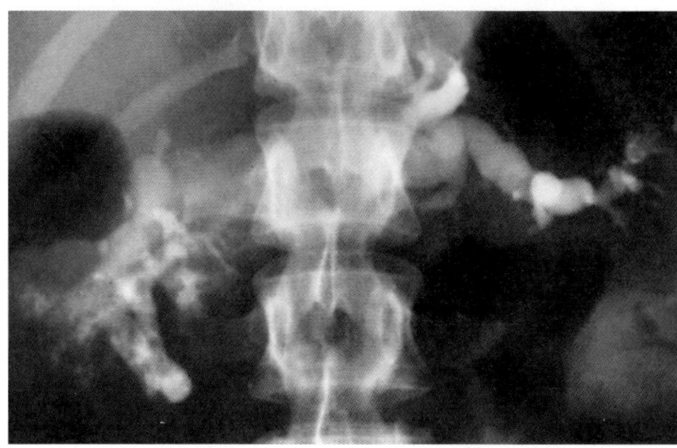

Figure 72.15 Endoscopic retrograde cholangiopancreatography: chronic pancreatitis. Most of the opacities lie within the duct system and are stones. Gross dilatation of ducts in the body and tail are due to obstruction by stones in the head of the pancreas.

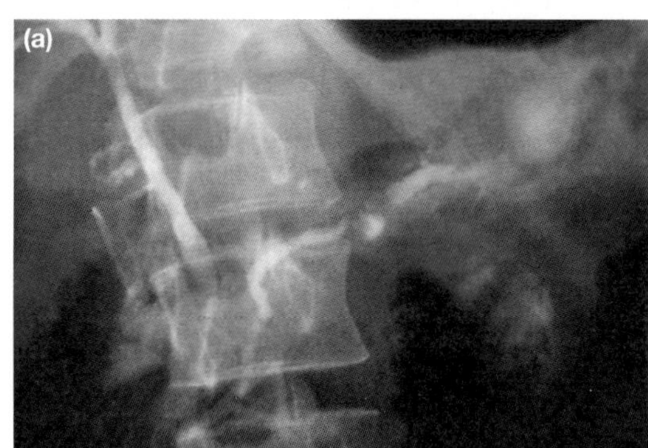

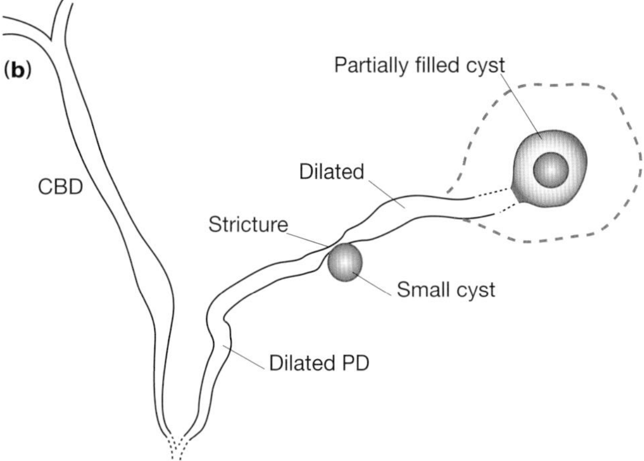

Figure 72.16 (a) Endoscopic retrograde cholangiopancreatography: relapsing acute pancreatitis. Normal biliary tree. Pancreatogram shows stricture of the main duct in the body with distal dilatation and cyst formation. (b) Diagrammatic outline of (a). CBD, common bile duct; PD, pancreatic duct.

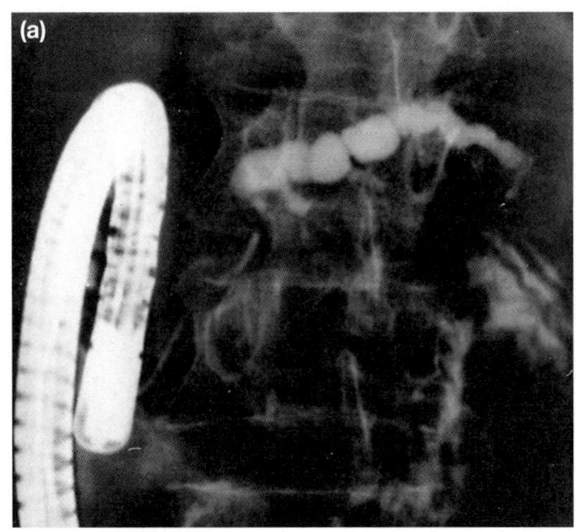

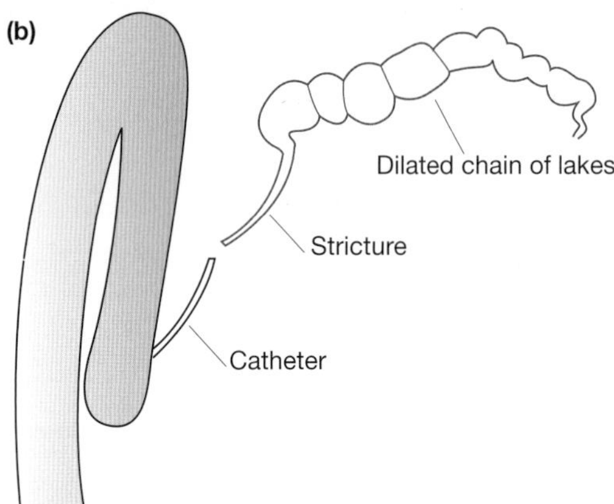

Figure 72.17 **(a)** Endoscopic retrograde cholangiopancreatography: chronic pancreatitis. Long stricture of the pancreatic duct in the head; distal pancreatic duct shows sacculation with intervening short strictures, 'chain of lakes'. **(b)** Diagrammatic outline of **(a)**.

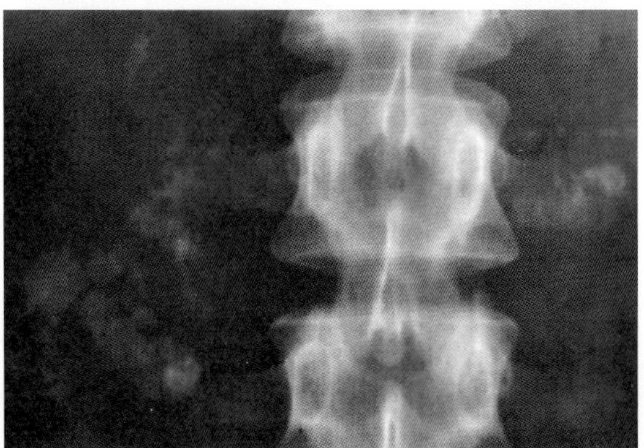

Figure 72.18 Plain abdominal radiograph: chronic pancreatitis. Multiple opacities can be seen in the region of the head and tail of the pancreas.

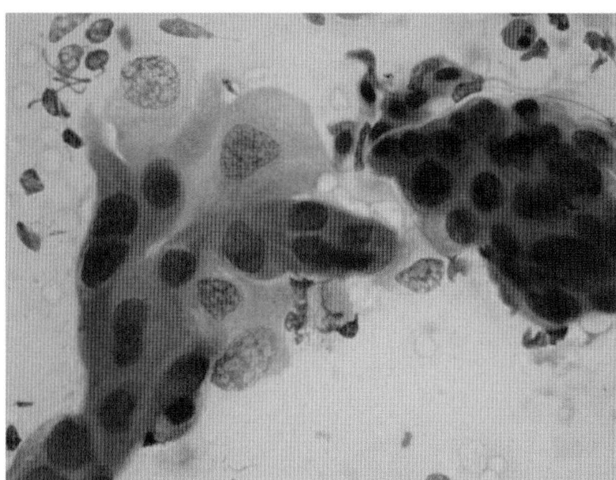

Figure 72.19 Adenocarcinoma cells identified in pancreatic juice collected at the time of endoscopic retrograde cholangiopancreatography (courtesy of Professor Roger Feakins).

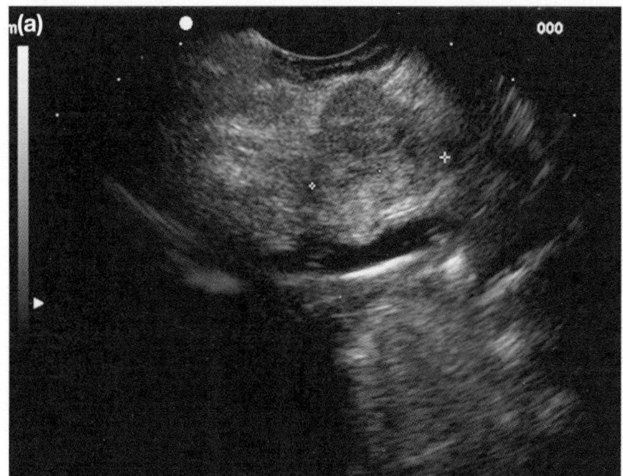

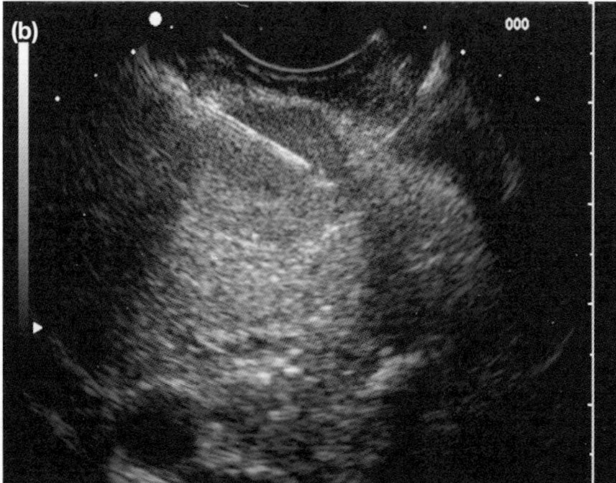

Figure 72.20 **(a)** Carcinoma of the pancreatic head as seen with endoscopic ultrasonography (EUS). **(b)** Aspiration biopsy carried out under EUS guidance: needle seen entering the tumour (courtesy of Dr Peter Fairclough).

Endoscopic ultrasonography

Endoscopic ultrasonography (EUS) is performed using a special endoscope that has a high-frequency ultrasonic transducer at its tip. When the endoscope is in the lumen of the stomach or duodenum, the pancreas and its surrounding vasculature and lymph nodes can be assessed (***Figure 72.20***). This is particularly useful in identifying small tumours that may not show up well on CT or MRI, and in demonstrating the relationship of a pancreatic tumour to major vessels nearby. EUS can clarify the relationship of a neuroendocrine tumour to the main pancreatic duct (important if enucleation is being considered).

It helps to distinguish cystic tumours from pseudocysts. Transduodenal or transgastric fine-needle aspiration (FNA) or Trucut biopsy performed under endoscopic ultrasound guidance avoids spillage of tumour cells into the peritoneal cavity.

CONGENITAL ABNORMALITIES

Cystic fibrosis

This is inherited as an autosomal recessive condition. It occurs most frequently among white people, in whom it is the most common inherited disorder (incidence of 1:2000 live births in the UK). Cystic fibrosis (CF) develops when there is a mutation in the CFTR (cystic fibrosis transmembrane conductance regulator) gene on chromosome 7. This gene creates a cell membrane protein that helps to control the movement of chloride across the cell membrane.

CF is a multisystem disorder of exocrine glands that affects the lungs, intestines, pancreas and liver and is characterised by elevated sodium and chloride ion concentrations in sweat. The mother may notice that the child is salty when kissed.

Most of the organ damage is due to blockage of narrow passages by thickened secretions. Chronic pulmonary disease arises from plugging of bronchi and bronchioles. CF is the most common cause of chronic lung disease among children in resource-rich countries. Cor pulmonale may develop later. At birth, the meconium may set in a sticky mass and produce intestinal obstruction (meconium ileus) (see ***Chapter 18***). Secretions precipitate in the lumen of the pancreatic duct causing blockage, which results in duct ectasia and fatty replacement of exocrine acinar tissue. Pancreatic exocrine insufficiency leads to fat malabsorption. Steatorrhoea is usually present from birth, resulting in stools that are bulky, oily and offensive. The islets of Langerhans usually appear normal, but diabetes mellitus can occur in older patients. The liver may become cirrhotic as a result of bile duct plugging, and signs of portal hypertension may appear. Infertility is common owing to the absence of the vas deferens in men and thick cervical mucus in women.

Outside the newborn period, the earliest clinical signs of CF are poor growth, poor appetite, rancid greasy stools, abdominal distension, chronic respiratory disease and finger clubbing. The appearance of secondary sexual characteristics may be delayed. The diagnosis can be made by prenatal genetic testing, by the newborn blood spot (heel prick) test done on newborns in the UK and by the sweat test. Levels of sodium and chloride ions in the sweat above 90 mmol/L confirm the diagnosis.

Treatment is aimed at control of the secondary consequences of the disease. Pulmonary function is preserved with aggressive physiotherapy and antibiotics. Malabsorption is treated by administration of oral pancreatic enzyme preparations. The diet should be low in fat but contain added salt to replace the high losses in the sweat. With early diagnosis and optimal treatment, patients in resource-rich countries can now expect to survive to their mid-thirties. Those with end-stage lung disease may be considered for lung transplantation. Heterozygous carriers of the various gene mutations are asymptomatic but can be identified by DNA analysis. There is a suggestion that such patients may develop pancreatitis later in life.

Pancreas divisum

Pancreas divisum occurs when the embryological ventral and dorsal parts of the pancreas fail to fuse (***Figure 72.3***). The dorsal pancreatic duct becomes the main pancreatic duct and drains most of the pancreas through the minor or accessory papilla. The incidence of pancreas divisum ranges from 5% in autopsy series to 10% in some ERCP and MRCP series. Pancreas divisum found incidentally in an asymptomatic person does not warrant intervention; however, the incidence of pancreas divisum ranges from 25% to 50% in patients with recurrent acute pancreatitis, chronic pancreatitis and pancreatic pain. The minor papilla is substantially smaller than the major papilla, thus large volumes of secretions flowing through a narrow papilla leads to incomplete drainage, which may in turn cause obstructive pain or pancreatitis. Certainly, pancreas divisum should be excluded in patients with idiopathic recurrent pancreatitis. The diagnosis can be arrived at by MRCP, EUS or ERCP, augmented by injection of secretin if necessary. There may be changes indicative of obstruction or chronic inflammation in the dorsal duct system. Endoscopic sphincterotomy and stenting of the minor papilla may relieve the symptoms. Surgical intervention can take the form of sphincteroplasty, pancreatojejunostomy or even resection of the pancreatic head.

Annular pancreas

This is the result of failure of complete rotation of the ventral pancreatic bud during development, so that a ring of pancreatic tissue surrounds the second or third part of the duodenum. It is most often seen in association with congenital duodenal stenosis or atresia and is therefore more prevalent in children with Down syndrome. Duodenal obstruction typically causes vomiting in the neonate (see ***Chapter 18***). The usual treatment is bypass (duodenoduodenostomy). The diagnosis may be made in later life as a cause of pancreatitis, in which case resection of the head of the pancreas should be considered.

Ectopic pancreas

Islands of ectopic pancreatic tissue can be found in the submucosa in parts of the stomach, duodenum or small intestine (including Meckel's diverticulum), the gallbladder, adjoining the pancreas, in the hilum of the spleen and within the liver. Ectopic pancreas may also be found in the wall of an alimentary tract duplication cyst.

John Langdon Haydon Down (sometimes given as Haydon-Down), 1828–1896, physician, The London Hospital, London, and Superintendent, Earlswood Asylum for Idiots, Redhill, UK, described this syndrome in 1866.

Johann Friedrich Meckel (the younger), 1781–1833, Professor of Anatomy and Surgery, Halle, Germany, described the embryological origin of the eponymous diverticulum in 1809.

Congenital cystic disease of the pancreas

This sometimes accompanies congenital disease of the kidneys and liver and occurs as part of the von Hippel–Lindau syndrome.

INJURIES TO THE PANCREAS

External injury

Presentation and management

The pancreas is not frequently damaged in blunt abdominal trauma but when it occurs it is often associated with injuries to other viscera, especially the liver, the spleen and the duodenum. Occasionally, a forceful blow to the epigastrium (such as from the steering wheel in a car accident) may crush the body of the pancreas against the vertebral column. Penetrating trauma to the upper abdomen or the back carries a higher chance of pancreatic injury. Pancreatic injuries may range from a contusion or laceration of the parenchyma without duct disruption to major parenchymal destruction with duct disruption (sometimes complete transection) and, rarely, massive destruction of the pancreatic head. The most important factor that determines treatment is whether the pancreatic duct has been disrupted.

Blunt pancreatic trauma usually presents with epigastric pain, which may be minor at first, with the progressive development of more severe pain due to the sequelae of leakage of pancreatic fluid into the surrounding tissues. The clinical presentation can be quite deceptive; careful serial assessments and a high index of suspicion are required. A rise in serum amylase occurs in most cases. A CT scan of the pancreas will delineate the damage that has occurred to the pancreas (***Figure 72.21***). If there is doubt about duct disruption, an urgent ERCP should be sought. MRCP may also provide the answer, but the images can be difficult to interpret. Support with intravenous fluids and a 'nil by mouth' regimen should be instituted while these investigations are performed. There is no need to rush to a laparotomy if the patient is haemodynamically stable, without peritonitis. It is preferable to manage conservatively at first, investigate and, once the extent of the damage has been ascertained, undertake appropriate action. Operation is indicated if there is disruption of the main pancreatic duct; in almost all other cases, the patient will recover with conservative management.

In penetrating injuries, especially if other organs are injured and the patient's condition is unstable, there is a greater need to perform an urgent surgical exploration. Assessment of pancreatic damage and duct disruption at the time of surgery can be difficult because the bruising associated with the retroperitoneal damage prevents clear visualisation of the pancreas. A patient and thorough examination of the gland should be carried out. Haemostasis and closed drainage are adequate for minor parenchymal injuries. If the gland is transected in the body or tail, a distal pancreatectomy should be performed, with or without splenectomy. If damage is purely confined to the head of the pancreas, haemostasis and external drainage are normally effective. In the emergency setting, in an unstable patient with concomitant injuries, a surgeon unaccustomed to pancreatic surgery should refrain from trying to ascertain whether the duct in the pancreatic head is intact or embarking on a major resection. However, if there is severe injury to the pancreatic head and duodenum, then a pancreatoduodenectomy may be necessary.

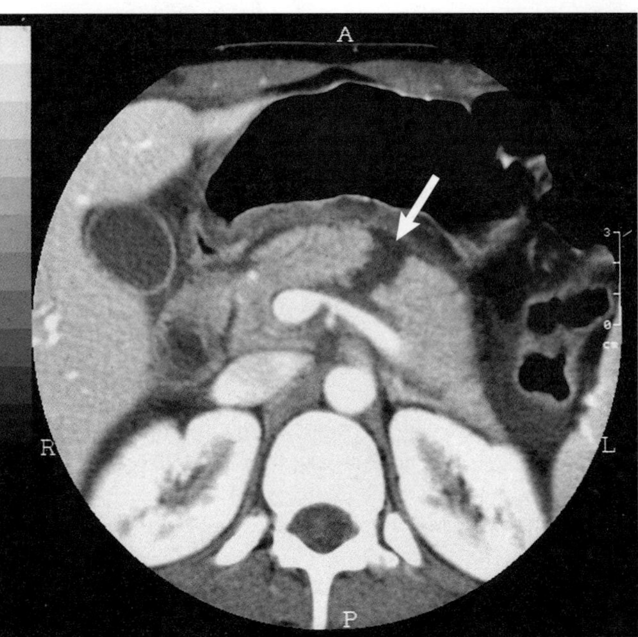

Figure 72.21 Computed tomography scan showing a pancreatic transection due to a bicycle handlebar injury. A distal pancreatectomy was performed.

Summary box 72.3

External injury to the pancreas

- Other organs are likely to be injured
- It is important to ascertain if the pancreatic duct has been disrupted
- CT and ERCP are the most useful tests
- Surgery is indicated if the main pancreatic duct is disrupted

Prognosis

The most common cause of death in the immediate period is bleeding, usually from associated injuries. Once the acute phase has passed, the morbidity related to the pancreatic injury itself is treatable, with a complete return to normal activity being the usual outcome.

Persistent drain output occurs in up to a third of patients (see ***Pancreatic fistula***). Sometimes, in the aftermath of trauma that has been treated conservatively, duct stricturing develops, leading to recurrent episodes of pancreatitis. The appropriate treatment in such cases is resection of the tail of the pancreas distal to the site of duct disruption.

A pancreatic pseudocyst may develop. If the main duct is intact, the cyst can be aspirated percutaneously in the first instance; it may not be necessary to undertake a cyst gastrostomy. If the cyst develops in the presence of complete disruption of the pancreas, there is no alternative but to undertake a distal resection or, occasionally, a pancreatojejunostomy with a Roux-en-Y loop. In a patient who presents with a peripancreatic cyst and a history of previous blunt abdominal trauma, do not assume that it is a post-traumatic pseudocyst. The possibility of a cystic neoplasm should be considered and excluded.

Iatrogenic injury

This can occur in several ways:

- Injury to the tail of the pancreas during splenectomy, resulting in a pancreatic fistula.
- Injury to the pancreatic head and the accessory pancreatic duct (Santorini), which is the main duct in 7% of patients, during Billroth II gastrectomy. A pancreatogram performed by cannulating the duct at the time of discovery of such an injury will demonstrate whether it is safe to ligate and divide the duct. If no alternative drainage duct can be demonstrated, then the duct should be reanastomosed to the duodenum or alternatively resection of the pancreatic head should be considered.
- Enucleation of islet cell tumours of the pancreas can result in fistulae.
- Duodenal or ampullary bleeding following sphincterotomy. This injury may require duodenotomy to control the bleeding.

Pancreatic fistula

Pancreatic fistula usually follows operative trauma to the gland or occurs as a complication of acute or chronic pancreatitis. It is important to define the site of the fistula and the epithelial structure with which it communicates (e.g. externally to skin or internally to bowel). If there is uncertainty about whether the fluid issuing from a drain site or a wound is pancreatic juice, measurement of the amylase content will be diagnostic.

Management includes correction of metabolic and electrolyte disturbances and adequate drainage of the fistula into a stoma bag with protection of the skin. Investigation of the cause of the fistula is required as the underlying cause must be treated before the fistula will close. Frequently, the cause is related to obstruction within the pancreatic duct, which can be overcome by endoscopic insertion of a stent or catheter into the pancreatic duct. While waiting for closure of the fistula, the patient should be given parenteral or nasojejunal nutritional support (as opposed to nasogastric or oral feeding; the rationale is that parenteral or nasojejunal feeding reduces the volume of pancreatic secretion). The use of octreotide will also suppress pancreatic secretion.

Summary box 72.4

Management of pancreatic fistulae

Tests

- Measure amylase level in fluid
- Determine the anatomy of the fistula
- Check if the main pancreatic duct is blocked or disrupted

Measures

- Correct fluid and electrolyte imbalances
- Protect the skin
- Drain adequately
- Parenteral or nasojejunal feeding
- Octreotide to suppress secretion
- Relieve pancreatic duct obstruction if possible (ERCP and stent)
- Treat underlying cause

PANCREATITIS

Pancreatitis is inflammation of the pancreatic parenchyma. For clinical purposes, it is useful to divide pancreatitis into acute, which presents as an emergency, and chronic, which is a prolonged and frequently lifelong disorder resulting from the development of fibrosis within the pancreas. It is possible that acute and chronic pancreatitis are different phases of the same process.

Acute pancreatitis is defined as an acute condition presenting with abdominal pain, a threefold or greater rise in the serum levels of the pancreatic enzymes amylase or lipase and/or characteristic findings of pancreatic inflammation on contrast-enhanced CT. Acute pancreatitis may recur.

The underlying mechanism of injury in pancreatitis is thought to be premature activation of pancreatic enzymes within the pancreas, leading to a process of autodigestion. Anything that injures the acinar cells and impairs the secretion of zymogen granules or damages the duct epithelium, and thus delays enzymatic secretion, can trigger acute pancreatitis. Once cellular injury has been initiated, the inflammatory process can lead to pancreatic oedema, haemorrhage and, eventually, necrosis. As inflammatory mediators are released into the circulation, systemic complications can arise, such as haemodynamic instability, bacteraemia (due to translocation of gut flora), acute respiratory distress syndrome and pleural effusions, gastrointestinal haemorrhage, renal failure and disseminated intravascular coagulation (DIC).

Acute pancreatitis may be categorised as mild (interstitial oedematous pancreatitis) or severe (necrotising pancreatitis). The former is characterised by interstitial oedema of the gland and minimal organ dysfunction. The majority of patients will have a mild attack of pancreatitis, the mortality from which is around 1%. Severe acute pancreatitis is seen in 5–10% of patients and is characterised by pancreatic necrosis, a severe

César Roux, 1857–1934, Professor of Surgery and Gynaecology, Lausanne, Switzerland.
Christian Albert Theodor Billroth, 1829–1894, Professor of Surgery, Vienna, Austria.

systemic inflammatory response and often multiorgan failure. In those who have a severe attack of pancreatitis, the mortality varies from 20% to 50%.

Acute pancreatitis has an early phase that usually lasts a week. It is characterised by a systemic inflammatory response syndrome (SIRS), which – if severe – can lead to transient or persistent organ failure (deemed persistent if it lasts for over 48 hours). About one-third of deaths occur in the early phase of the attack, from multiple organ failure. The late phase is seen typically in those who suffer a severe attack and can run from weeks to months. It is characterised by persistent systemic signs of inflammation and/or local complications, particularly fluid collections and peripancreatic sepsis. Deaths occurring after the first week of onset are often due to septic complications.

Chronic pancreatitis is defined as a continuing inflammatory disease of the pancreas characterised by irreversible morphological change typically causing pain and/or permanent loss of function. Many patients with chronic pancreatitis have painful exacerbations, but the condition may be completely painless.

Acute pancreatitis

Incidence

Acute pancreatitis accounts for 3% of all cases of abdominal pain among patients admitted to hospital in the UK. The hospital admission rate for acute pancreatitis is 9.8 per year per 100 000 population in the UK, although worldwide the annual incidence may range from 5 to 50 per 100 000. The disease may occur at any age, with a peak in young men and older women.

Summary box 72.5

Possible causes of acute pancreatitis

- Gallstones
- Alcoholism
- Post ERCP
- Abdominal trauma
- Following biliary, upper gastrointestinal or cardiothoracic surgery
- Ampullary tumour
- Drugs (corticosteroids, azathioprine, asparaginase, valproic acid, thiazides, oestrogens)
- Hyperparathyroidism
- Hypercalcaemia
- Hypertriglyceridaemia
- Pancreas divisum
- Sphincter of Oddi dysfunction
- Autoimmune pancreatitis
- Hereditary pancreatitis
- Viral infections (mumps, coxsackie B)
- Malnutrition
- Scorpion bite
- Idiopathic

Aetiology

The two major causes of acute pancreatitis are biliary calculi, which occur in 50–70% of patients, and alcohol abuse, which accounts for 25% of cases. Gallstone pancreatitis is thought to be triggered by the passage of gallstones down the common bile duct. If the biliary and pancreatic ducts join to share a common channel before ending at the ampulla, then obstruction of this passage may lead to reflux of bile or activated pancreatic enzymes into the pancreatic duct. Patients who have small gallstones and a wide cystic duct may be at a higher risk of passing stones. The proposed mechanisms for alcoholic pancreatitis include the effects of diet, malnutrition, direct toxicity of alcohol, concomitant tobacco smoking, hypersecretion, duct obstruction or reflux, and hyperlipidaemia. The remaining cases may be due to rare causes or may be idiopathic.

Among patients who undergo ERCP, 1–3% develop pancreatitis, probably as a consequence of duct disruption and enzyme extravasation. Patients with sphincter of Oddi dysfunction or a history of recurrent pancreatitis, and those who undergo sphincterotomy or balloon dilatation of the sphincter, carry a higher risk of developing post-ERCP pancreatitis. Patients who have undergone upper abdominal or cardiothoracic surgery may develop acute pancreatitis in the postoperative phase, as may those who have suffered blunt abdominal trauma.

Hereditary pancreatitis is a rare familial condition associated with mutations of the cationic trypsinogen gene. Patients have a tendency to suffer acute pancreatitis while in their teens, progress to chronic pancreatitis in the next two decades and have a high risk (possibly up to 40%) of developing pancreatic cancer by the age of 70 years. Hypertriglyceridaemia should be excluded.

Occasionally, tumours at the ampulla of Vater may cause acute pancreatitis. It is important to check the serum calcium level, a fasting lipid profile, autoimmune markers and viral titres in patients with so-called idiopathic acute pancreatitis. It is equally important to take a detailed drug history and remember the association of corticosteroids, azathioprine, asparaginase and valproic acid with acute pancreatitis. Statins (taken over a long time) and gliptins have been linked with pancreatitis, but the evidence is slim. It is essential to exclude tiny gallstones. A careful search for the aetiology must be made in all cases, and no more than 20% of cases should fall into the idiopathic category.

Summary box 72.6

Aetiology of acute pancreatitis

- It is essential to establish the aetiology
- Investigate thoroughly before labelling it as 'idiopathic'
- If due to gallstones, cholecystectomy is desirable during the same admission

Clinical presentation

Pain is the cardinal symptom. It characteristically develops quickly, reaching maximum intensity within minutes rather than hours and persists for hours or even days. The pain is frequently severe, constant and refractory to the usual doses of analgesics. Pain is usually experienced first in the epigastrium but may be localised to either upper quadrant or felt diffusely throughout the abdomen. There is radiation to the back in about 50% of patients, and some patients may gain relief by sitting or leaning forwards. The suddenness of onset may simulate a perforated peptic ulcer, while biliary colic or acute cholecystitis can be mimicked if the pain is maximal in the right upper quadrant. Radiation to the chest can simulate myocardial infarction, pneumonia or pleuritic pain. In fact, acute pancreatitis can mimic most causes of the acute abdomen and should seldom be discounted in differential diagnosis.

Nausea, repeated vomiting and retching are usually marked. The retching may persist despite the stomach being kept empty by nasogastric aspiration. Hiccoughs can be troublesome and may be due to gastric distension or irritation of the diaphragm.

On examination, the appearance may be that of a patient who is well or, at the other extreme, one who is gravely ill with profound shock, toxicity and confusion. Tachypnoea is common, tachycardia is usual and hypotension may be present. The body temperature is often normal or even subnormal, but frequently rises as inflammation develops. It is useful to reiterate here that SIRS is defined by the presence of two or more of the following criteria: heart rate >90/min, core temperature <36°C or >38°C, respirations >20/min or PCO_2 <32 mmHg, and white blood cell count <4000 or >12 000/mm^3 (see also ***Chapter 2***). Mild icterus can be caused by biliary obstruction in gallstone pancreatitis, and an acute swinging pyrexia suggests cholangitis. Bleeding into the fascial planes can produce bluish discoloration of the flanks (Grey Turner's sign) or umbilicus (Cullen's sign). Subcutaneous fat necrosis may produce small, red, tender nodules on the skin of the legs.

Abdominal examination may reveal distension due to ileus or, more rarely, ascites with shifting dullness. A mass can develop in the epigastrium owing to inflammation. There is usually muscle guarding in the upper abdomen, although marked rigidity is unusual. A pleural effusion is present in 10–20% of patients. Pulmonary oedema and pneumonitis are also described and may give rise to the differential diagnosis of pneumonia or myocardial infarction. The patient may be confused and exhibit the signs of metabolic derangement together with hypoxaemia.

Investigations

Typically, the diagnosis is made on the basis of the clinical presentation and an elevated serum amylase level. A serum amylase level three times above normal is indicative of the disease. A normal serum amylase level does not exclude acute pancreatitis, particularly if there is delay in presentation. The serum lipase level provides a more sensitive and specific test than amylase. If there is doubt, and other causes of acute abdomen have to be excluded, contrast-enhanced CT is the best single imaging investigation.

Summary box 72.7

Investigations in acute pancreatitis should be aimed at answering three questions:

- Is a diagnosis of acute pancreatitis correct?
- How severe is the attack?
- What is the aetiology?

Assessment of severity

It is important to identify those patients who will develop severe pancreatitis as they require aggressive early management and possibly transfer to a specialist unit. A severe attack may be heralded by an initial clinical impression of a very ill patient and a worsening physiological state at 24–48 hours. Various prognostic scoring systems have been used, all aimed at predicting persistent organ failure, particularly respiratory, cardiac and renal. Severity stratification assessments should be performed in patients at 24 hours, 48 hours and 7 days after admission. The Ranson and Glasgow scoring systems are specific for acute pancreatitis, and a score of 3 or more at 48 hours indicates a severe attack (***Table 72.3***). Several other systems that are used in intensive care units can also be applied. These include the APACHE, SAPS, SOFA, MODS and modified Marshall scoring systems (the latter has the advantage of simplicity). Regardless of the system used, persisting organ failure indicates a severe attack. A serum C-reactive protein level >150 mg/L at 48 hours after the onset of symptoms is also an indicator of severity. Patients with a body mass index over 30 are at higher risk of developing complications. A revision in 2013 of the Atlanta classification of acute pancreatitis (1992) recommends that patients with acute pancreatitis be stratified into three groups:

- Mild acute pancreatitis:
  - no organ failure;
  - no local or systemic complications.
- Moderately severe acute pancreatitis:
  - organ failure that resolves within 48 hours (transient organ failure); and/or
  - local or systemic complications without persistent organ failure.
- Severe acute pancreatitis:
  - persistent organ failure (>48 hours);
  - single organ failure;
  - multiple organ failure.

George Grey Turner, 1877–1951, Professor of Surgery, Durham University, Durham (1927–1934), and at the Postgraduate Medical School, Hammersmith, London, UK (1934–1945).

Thomas Stephen Cullen, 1870–1953, Professor of Gynecology, Johns Hopkins University, Baltimore, MD, USA. Described bluish discoloration of the periumbilical skin as a sign of ruptured ectopic pregnancy.

John HC Ranson, 1938–1995, Professor of Surgery, New York University School of Medicine, New York, NY, USA.

John C Marshall, contemporary, trauma surgeon and intensivist, St Michael's Hospital, Toronto, Canada.

TABLE 72.3 The Ranson and Glasgow scoring systems to predict the severity of acute pancreatitis: in both systems, disease is classified as severe when three or more factors are present.

Ranson score	Glasgow score
On admission	Within 48 hours
Age >55 years	Age >55 years
White blood cell count >16 × 10^9/L	White blood cell count >15 × 10^9/L
Blood glucose >11 mmol/L (>200 mg/dL)	Blood glucose >10 mmol/L (no history of diabetes)
LDH >350 units/L	LDH >600 units/L or AST >200 units/L
AST >250 units/L	Serum urea >16 mmol/L (no response to intravenous fluids)
Within 48 hours	Arterial oxygen saturation (PaO_2) <8 kPa (60 mmHg)
Haematocrit fall of 10% or greater	Serum calcium <2.0 mmol/L
Blood urea nitrogen rise >5 mg/dL (1.8 mmol/L) despite fluids	Serum albumin <32 g/L
Arterial oxygen saturation (PaO_2) <8 kPa (60 mmHg)	
Serum calcium <8 mg/dL (2.0 mmol/L)	
Base deficit >4 mmol/L	
Fluid sequestration >6 litres	

AST, aspartate aminotransferase; LDH, lactate dehydrogenase; PaO_2, arterial oxygen tension.

Imaging

Plain erect chest and abdominal radiographs are not diagnostic of acute pancreatitis but are useful in the differential diagnosis. Non-specific findings in pancreatitis include a generalised or local ileus (sentinel loop), a colon cut-off sign and a renal halo sign. Occasionally, calcified gallstones or pancreatic calcification may be seen. A chest radiograph may show a pleural effusion and, in severe cases, a diffuse alveolar interstitial shadowing may suggest acute respiratory distress syndrome.

Ultrasonography does not establish a diagnosis of acute pancreatitis. The swollen pancreas may be seen, but ultrasonography should be performed within 24 hours in all patients to detect gallstones as a potential cause, rule out acute cholecystitis as a differential diagnosis and determine whether the common bile duct is dilated.

CT is not necessary for all patients, particularly those deemed to have a mild attack on prognostic criteria. But a contrast-enhanced CT is indicated in the following situations:

- If there is diagnostic uncertainty.
- In patients with severe acute pancreatitis to distinguish interstitial from necrotising pancreatitis (*Figure 72.22*). In the first 72 hours, CT may underestimate the extent of necrosis. The severity of pancreatitis detected on CT may be staged according to the Balthazar criteria.
- In patients with organ failure, signs of sepsis or progressive clinical deterioration.
- When a localised complication is suspected, such as fluid collection, pseudocyst or a pseudoaneurysm.

Cross-sectional MRI can yield similar information to that obtained by CT. EUS and MRCP can help in detecting stones in the common bile duct and directly assessing the pancreatic parenchyma but are not widely available. ERCP allows the identification and removal of stones in the common bile duct in gallstone pancreatitis. In patients with severe acute gallstone pancreatitis and signs of ongoing biliary obstruction and cholangitis, an urgent ERCP should be sought.

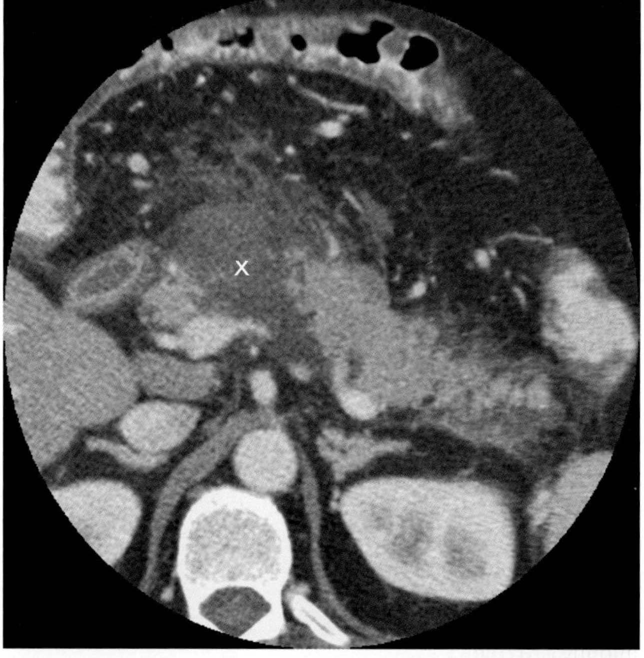

Figure 72.22 Contrast-enhanced computed tomography scan showing acute necrotising pancreatitis. Note the area of reduced enhancement in the pancreas (marked X), the peripancreatic oedema and stranding of the fatty tissues (courtesy of Dr Niall Power).

The presentation is so variable that sometimes even an experienced clinician can be mistaken. While this is not desirable, occasionally the diagnosis is only made at laparotomy. The appearances at laparotomy are characteristic (*Figure 72.23*).

Emil J Balthazar, contemporary, Professor Emeritus, Department of Radiology, New York University, New York, NY, USA.

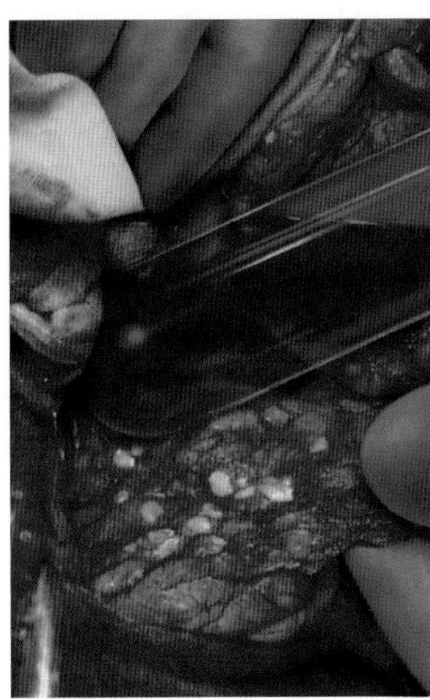

Figure 72.23 Widespread fat necrosis of the omentum. A test tube has been filled with blood-stained peritoneal fluid. This specimen was rich in amylase. Fat necroses are dull, opaque, yellow-white areas suggestive of drops of wax. They are most abundant in the vicinity of the pancreas but are widespread in the greater omentum and the mesentery. Fat necroses consist of small islands of saponification caused by the liberation of lipase, which splits into glycerol and fatty acids. Free fatty acids combine with calcium to form soaps (fatty necrosis) (courtesy of Dr GD Adhia, Mumbai, India).

TABLE 72.4 Early management of severe acute pancreatitis.
Admission to HDU/ICU
Analgesia
Aggressive fluid rehydration
Supplemental oxygen
Invasive monitoring of vital signs, central venous pressure, urine output, blood gases
Frequent monitoring of haematological and biochemical parameters (including liver and renal function, clotting, serum calcium, blood glucose)
Nasogastric drainage (only initially)
Antibiotics if cholangitis suspected; prophylactic antibiotics can be considered
CT scan essential if organ failure, clinical deterioration or signs of sepsis develop
ERCP within 72 hours for severe gallstone pancreatitis or signs of cholangitis
Supportive therapy for organ failure if it develops (inotropes, ventilatory support, haemofiltration, etc.)
If nutritional support is required, consider enteral (nasogastric) feeding

CT, computed tomography; ERCP, endoscopic retrograde cholangiopancreatography; HDU, high-dependency unit; ICU, intensive care unit.

Management

If after initial assessment a patient is considered to have a mild attack of pancreatitis, a conservative approach is indicated with intravenous fluid administration and frequent, but non-invasive, observation. A brief period of fasting may be sensible in a patient who is nauseated and in pain, but there is little physiological justification for keeping patients on a prolonged 'nil by mouth' regimen. Antibiotics are not indicated. Apart from analgesics and antiemetics, no drugs or interventions are warranted, and CT scanning is unnecessary unless there is evidence of deterioration. However, if a stable patient meets the prognostic criteria for a severe attack of pancreatitis, then a more aggressive approach is required, with admission to a high-dependency or intensive care unit and invasive monitoring (***Table 72.4***).

Adequate analgesia should be administered. Aggressive fluid resuscitation is important, guided by frequent measurement of vital signs, urine output and central venous pressure. Supplemental oxygen should be administered and serial arterial blood gas analysis performed. The haematocrit, clotting profile, blood glucose and serum levels of calcium and magnesium should be closely monitored.

A nasogastric tube is not essential but may be of value in patients with vomiting. Specific treatments such as aprotinin, somatostatin analogues, platelet-activating factor inhibitors and selective gut decontamination have failed to improve outcome in numerous clinical trials. There are no data to support a practice of 'resting' the pancreas and feeding only by the parenteral or nasojejunal routes. If nutritional support is felt to be necessary, enteral nutrition (e.g. feeding via a nasogastric tube) should be used.

There is some evidence to support the use of prophylactic antibiotics in patients with severe acute pancreatitis but there is no consensus. The rationale is to prevent local and other septic complications. The regimens used include intravenous cefuroxime, or imipenem, or ciprofloxacin plus metronidazole. The duration of antibiotic prophylaxis should not exceed 14 days. Additional antibiotic use should be guided by microbiological cultures. If, however, there is evidence of cholangitis or concomitant respiratory or urinary infection then antibiotics should be given promptly.

If gallstones are the cause of an attack of predicted or proven severe pancreatitis, or if the patient has jaundice, cholangitis or a dilated common bile duct, ERCP should be carried out within 72 hours of the onset of symptoms as sphincterotomy and clearance of the bile duct can reduce the incidence of infective complications. In patients with cholangitis, sphincterotomy should be carried out or a biliary stent placed to drain the duct; however, ERCP is an invasive procedure and carries a small risk of worsening the pancreatitis.

Systemic complications

Pancreatitis may involve all organ systems (***Table 72.5***) and should be managed by a multidisciplinary team including intensive care specialists. When there is organ failure, appropriate supportive therapies may include inotropic support for haemodynamic instability, haemofiltration in the event of renal failure, ventilatory support for respiratory failure and correction of coagulopathies (including DIC). Surgery has no role during the initial period of resuscitation and stabilisation and is reserved for the patient who deteriorates following successful stabilisation.

Local complications and their management

Once the patient survives the acute phase and major organ failure is controlled, local complications become pre-eminent as they carry a significant mortality. A CT scan should be performed if pain persists, signs of sepsis develop, organ dysfunction worsens or there is a further spike in the serum amylase level. The management is conservative with surgery only when conservative management has failed. Definitions are important. Terms such as 'phlegmon', which may refer to an abscess or to an inflammatory mass in the pancreas, are best avoided.

TABLE 72.5 Complications of acute pancreatitis.

Systemic	Local
(More common in the first week)	*(Usually develop after the first week)*
Cardiovascular	Peripancreatic fluid collection
Shock	Sterile pancreatic necrosis
Arrhythmias	Infected pancreatic necrosis
Pulmonary	Pancreatic abscess
ARDS	Pseudocyst
Renal failure	Pancreatic ascites
Haematological	Pleural effusion
DIC	Portal/splenic vein thrombosis
Metabolic	Pseudoaneurysm
Hypocalcaemia	
Hyperglycaemia	
Hyperlipidaemia	
Gastrointestinal	
Ileus	
Neurological	
Visual disturbances	
Confusion, irritability	
Encephalopathy	
Miscellaneous	
Subcutaneous fat necrosis	
Arthralgia	

ARDS, acute respiratory distress syndrome; DIC, disseminated intravascular coagulation.

Acute peripancreatic fluid collection

Acute peripancreatic fluid collection (APFC) occurs early in the course of mild pancreatitis without necrosis and is located adjacent to the pancreas. It has no encapsulating wall and is confined within normal fascial planes. The fluid is sterile and most such collections resolve. No intervention is necessary unless a large collection causes symptoms or pressure effects, in which case it can be percutaneously aspirated under ultrasound or CT guidance. Transgastric drainage under endoscopic ultrasound guidance is another option.

Sterile and infected pancreatic necrosis

The term 'pancreatic necrosis' refers to a diffuse or focal area of non-viable parenchyma. This can be identified by an absence of parenchymal enhancement on CT with intravenous contrast. Pancreatic necrosis is typically associated with lysis of peripancreatic fat. This may lead to an *acute necrotic collection* (ANC). This is typically an intra- or extrapancreatic collection containing fluid and necrotic material, with no definable wall. Gradually, over a period of over 4 weeks, this may develop a well-defined inflammatory capsule and evolve into *walled-off necrosis* (WON).

Collections associated with necrotising pancreatitis are sterile to begin with but often become subsequently infected, probably because of translocation of gut bacteria. Infected necrosis is associated with a mortality rate of up to 50%. Sterile necrotic material should not be drained or interfered with. However, if the patient shows signs of sepsis, then one should determine whether the collection is infected (***Figure 72.24***). Aspiration fluid with a fine needle, percutaneously under CT or ultrasound guidance, can provide the answer. If the aspirate is purulent, drainage of the infected fluid should be carried out. Internal drainage into the stomach under endoscopic ultrasound guidance should be considered first. A plastic or covered metal stent can be used to create a communication between the collection and the gastric lumen. The stent may be left in for weeks if necessary and may need to be changed if blocked. If endoscopic internal drainage is not possible, then percutaneous drainage should be considered. The tube drain inserted should have the *widest* bore possible. The aspirate should be sent for microbiological assessment and appropriate antibiotic therapy should be commenced as per the sensitivity report. The fluid can be quite viscous with particulate matter, and the drain may need regular flushing with full aseptic

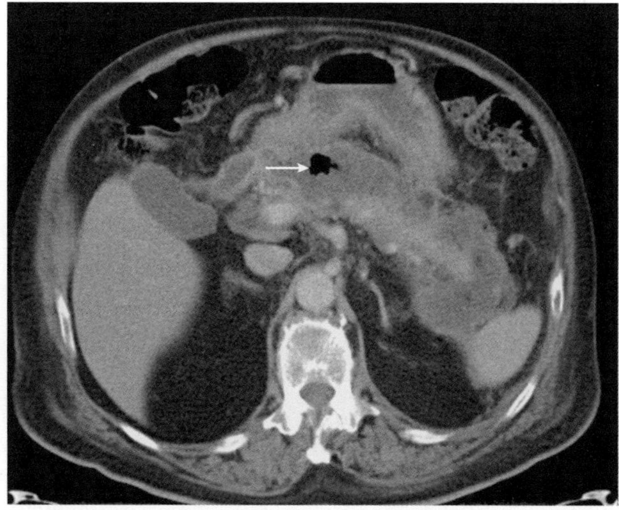

Figure 72.24 Infected pancreatic necrosis. Note the areas of reduced enhancement in the pancreas and the peripancreatic fluid collection with pockets of gas within it (arrow). This resolved after percutaneous drainage and antibiotic therapy.

precautions. Often, repeated imaging and repeated insertion of progressively wider drains is necessary.

Pancreatic necrosectomy should be considered if sepsis worsens despite conservative measures. This is a challenging operation that carries a high morbidity and mortality; it is best carried out in a specialist unit and is necessary only in a very small proportion of patients. The surgical approach may be through a midline laparotomy, especially if the area involved is around the pancreatic head. The duodenocolic and gastrocolic ligaments should be divided and the lesser sac opened. Thorough debridement of the dead tissue around the pancreas should be carried out. If the body and tail of the gland are primarily involved (*Figure 72.25*), a retroperitoneal approach through a left flank incision may be more appropriate. The tissues are inevitably friable, and one should be careful not to precipitate excessive bleeding or inadvertently breach the bowel wall. Blunt dissection is preferable to sharp dissection. A feeding jejunostomy may be a useful adjunct to the procedure. If gallstones are the precipitating factor of the pancreatitis, a cholecystectomy should be included. Some prefer a minimally invasive approach to a formal laparotomy. A rigid laparoscope is inserted into the peripancreatic area through a retroperitoneal approach, and vigorous irrigation and suction is combined with a gradual nibbling away of the necrotic debris.

Once a necrosectomy has been completed, further necrotic tissue may form. There are several possible ways of dealing with this (listed below), none of which has been proved to be more effective than the others. The last two approaches make greater logistic demands as one is committed to a re-exploration every 48–72 hours.

- **Closed continuous lavage.** Tube drains are left in and the raw area flushed (Beger) (*Figure 72.26*).
- **Closed drainage.** The incision is closed, but the cavity is packed with gauze-filled Penrose drains and closed suction drains. The Penrose drains are brought out through the flank and slowly pulled out and removed after 7 days.
- **Open packing.** The incision is left open, and the cavity is packed with the intention of returning to the operating room at regular intervals and repacking until there is a clean granulating cavity.
- **Closure and relaparotomy.** The incision is closed with drains with the intention of performing a series of planned relaparotomies every 48–72 hours until the raw area granulates (Bradley).

There is a subgroup of patients who respond initially to percutaneous treatment but then develop recurrent sepsis that requires repeated insertion of drains and fail to thrive. Necrosectomy should be considered in these patients, but it can be a difficult judgement call.

Patients with peripancreatic sepsis are ill for long periods of time and may require management in an intensive care unit. Nutritional support is essential. The parenteral and nasojejunal approaches are more popular (on the assumption that they rest the pancreas), although there is little evidence to show that nasogastric feeding, if tolerated, is harmful in any way.

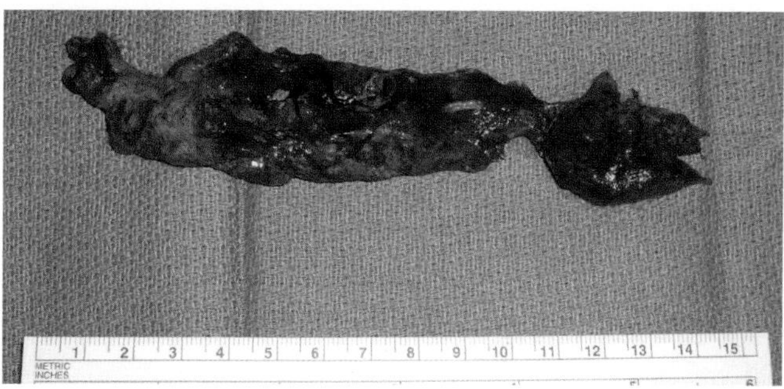

Figure 72.25 Necrotic body and tail of the pancreas removed as an intact specimen rather than piecemeal. The patient had suffered severe necrotising gallstone pancreatitis complicated by persistent pancreatic sepsis. Necrosectomy was carried out through a left flank retroperitoneal approach.

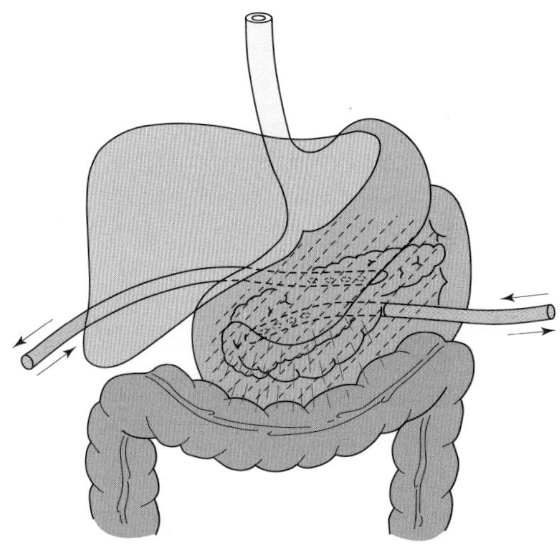

Figure 72.26 Continuous postoperative closed lavage of the lesser sac as advised by Beger. Lavage is carried out through several double-lumen and single-lumen catheters. Each time, 1 litre of saline is infused through and then drained over a period of hours, and the process is repeated.

Pancreatic abscess

This is a circumscribed intra-abdominal collection of pus, usually in proximity to the pancreas. It may be an ANC or a WON that has become infected. The principles of diagnosis and management are as outlined above for infected pancreatic necrosis. Endoscopic internal drainage or, failing that, percutaneous drainage with the widest possible drains is the treatment, along with appropriate antibiotics and supportive care. Repeated scans may be required depending on the progress of the patient, and drains may need to be flushed, repositioned or reinserted. Very occasionally, open drainage of the abscess may be necessary.

Hans Günter Beger, b. 1936, Emeritus Professor of Surgery, Ulm, Germany.
Charles Bingham Penrose, 1862–1925, Professor of Gynecology, University of Pennsylvania, Philadelphia, PA, USA.
Edward Bradley III, contemporary, Emeritus Professor of Surgery, Florida State University College of Medicine, FL, USA.

Pancreatic ascites

This is a chronic, generalised, peritoneal, enzyme-rich effusion usually associated with pancreatic duct disruption. Paracentesis will reveal turbid fluid with a high amylase level. Adequate drainage with wide-bore drains placed under imaging guidance is essential. Measures that can be taken to suppress pancreatic secretion include parenteral or nasojejunal feeding and administration of octreotide. An ERCP may demonstrate duct disruption and allow placement of a pancreatic stent.

Pancreatic effusion

This is an encapsulated collection of fluid in the pleural cavity, arising as a consequence of acute pancreatitis. Concomitant pancreatic ascites may be present or there may be a communication with an intra-abdominal collection. Percutaneous drainage under imaging guidance is necessary.

Haemorrhage

Bleeding may occur into the gut, the retroperitoneum or peritoneal cavity. Possible causes include bleeding into a pseudocyst cavity, diffuse bleeding from a large raw surface or a pseudoaneurysm. The last is a false aneurysm of a major peripancreatic vessel confined as a clot by the surrounding tissues and often associated with infection. Recurrent bleeding is common, often culminating in fatal haemorrhage. CT, angiography or magnetic resonance angiography helps to make the diagnosis. Treatment involves embolisation or surgery.

Portal or splenic vein thrombosis

This may develop silently and is identified on a CT scan. A marked rise in the platelet count should raise suspicions. In the context of acute pancreatitis, treatment is usually conservative. The patient should be screened for procoagulant tendencies. If varices or other manifestations of portal hypertension develop, they will require treatment, such as endoscopic injection or banding, β-blockade, etc. Thrombocytosis may mandate the use of aspirin or other antiplatelet drugs for a period. Systemic anticoagulation, if instituted early in the process, may achieve recanalisation of the vein but it is not routinely used as it carries considerable risks in a patient with ongoing pancreatitis.

Pseudocyst

A pseudocyst is a collection of amylase-rich fluid enclosed in a well-defined wall of fibrous or granulation tissue. Pseudocysts typically arise following an attack of mild acute pancreatitis, lie outside the pancreas and represent an APFC that has not resolved and matured. Formation of a pseudocyst requires 4 weeks or more from the onset of acute pancreatitis. The term 'pseudocyst' is often used more loosely to include sterile WON that has failed to resolve or a collection that has developed in the context of chronic pancreatitis or after pancreatic trauma. (***Figure 72.27***; see also ***Figure 72.10***). More than half have a communication with the main pancreatic duct. Pseudocysts are often single but are occasionally multiple.

It is important to differentiate a pseudocyst from an APFC; the clinical scenario and radiological appearances should allow that distinction to be made. Occasionally, a cystic neoplasm may be confused with a chronic pseudocyst. EUS and aspiration of the cyst fluid are very useful in such a situation. The fluid should be sent for measurement of carcinoembryonic antigen (CEA) levels, amylase levels and cytology. Fluid from a pseudocyst typically has a low CEA level, and levels above 400 ng/mL are suggestive of a mucinous neoplasm. Pseudocyst fluid usually has a high amylase level, but that is not diagnostic as a tumour that communicates with the duct system may yield similar findings. Cytology typically reveals inflammatory cells in pseudocyst fluid. If there is no access to EUS, then percutaneous FNA is acceptable (just aspiration, *not* percutaneous insertion of a drain). ERCP and MRCP may demonstrate communication of the cyst with the pancreatic duct system, demonstrate ductal anomalies or diagnose chronic pancreatitis, and thus help in planning treatment.

Pseudocysts usually resolve spontaneously, but complications can develop (***Table 72.6***). Pseudocysts that are thick walled or large (>6 cm in diameter), have lasted for a long time (over 12 weeks) or have arisen in the context of chronic pancreatitis are less likely to resolve spontaneously. Therapeutic intervention is advised only if the pseudocyst causes symptoms, complications develop or distinction has to be made between a pseudocyst and a tumour.

There are three possible approaches to draining a pseudocyst: percutaneous, endoscopic and surgical. Percutaneous drainage to the exterior under radiological guidance should be avoided. It carries a very high likelihood of recurrence. Moreover, it is not advisable unless one is absolutely certain that the cyst is not neoplastic and that it has no communication with the pancreatic duct (or else a pancreaticocutaneous fistula will develop). A percutaneous transgastric cystgastrostomy can be performed under imaging guidance, and a double-pigtail drain placed with one end in the cyst cavity and the other end in the gastric lumen. In experienced hands, recurrence rates are no more than 15%. Endoscopic drainage usually involves

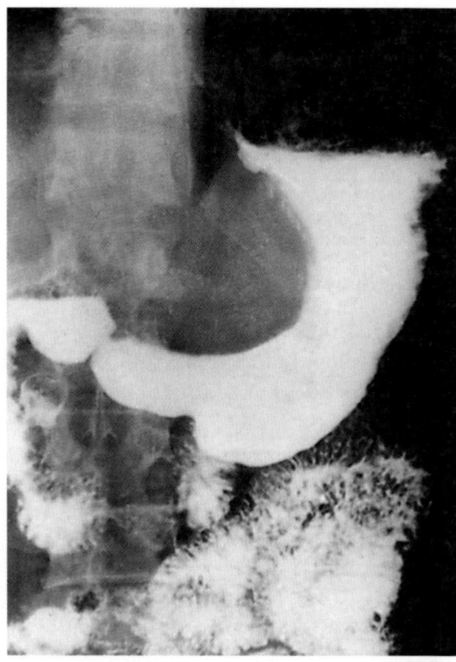

Figure 72.27 Barium meal. Pseudocyst displacing the stomach (courtesy of Professor VK Kapoor, Lucknow, India).

TABLE 72.6 Possible complications of a pancreatic pseudocyst.

Process	Outcomes
Infection	Abscess
	Systemic sepsis
Rupture	
Into the gut	Gastrointestinal bleeding
	Internal fistula
Into the peritoneum	Peritonitis
Enlargement	
Pressure effects	Obstructive jaundice from biliary compression
	Bowel obstruction
Pain	
Erosion into a vessel	Haemorrhage into the cyst
	Haemoperitoneum

puncture of the cyst through the stomach or duodenal wall under endoscopic ultrasound guidance, and placement of a tube drain with one end in the cyst cavity and the other end in the gastric lumen. The success rates depend on operator expertise. Occasionally, ERCP and placement of a pancreatic stent across the ampulla may help to drain a pseudocyst that is in communication with the duct. Surgical drainage involves internally draining the cyst into the gastric or jejunal lumen (*Figure 72.28*). Recurrence rates should be no more than 5%, and this still remains the standard against which the evolving radiological and endoscopic approaches are measured. The approach is conventionally through an open incision but laparoscopic cystgastrostomy is also feasible. Pseudocysts that have developed complications are best managed surgically.

There is a small group of patients who, having suffered an attack of necrotising pancreatitis with duct disruption, go on to suffer repeated complications in the form of recurrent fluid collections, pseudocysts, pleural effusions or pancreatic ascites. Very often disruption of the main pancreatic duct in the neck, body or tail is compounded by a stricture or a stone in the head that cannot be treated endoscopically. In such patients, some form of surgical resection and/or a drainage procedure – even though it may be technically challenging – may be the only way to achieve lasting resolution.

Summary box 72.8

Distinguishing a pseudocyst from a cystic neoplasm

- History
- Appearance on CT and ultrasonography
- FNA of fluid, preferably under endoscopic ultrasound guidance:
  - CEA (high level in mucinous tumours)
  - Amylase (level usually high in pseudocysts but occasionally in tumours)
  - Cytology

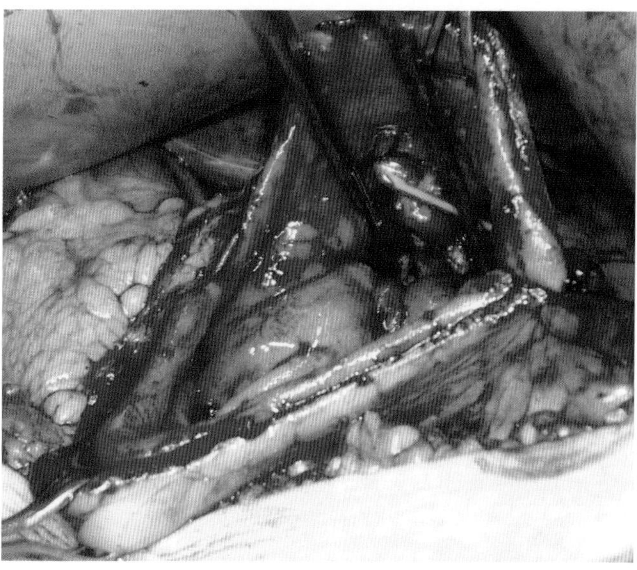

Figure 72.28 Cystgastrostomy for the pancreatic pseudocyst shown in *Figure 72.10*. The anterior wall of the stomach has been opened and the edges drawn back, held by Babcock's forceps. An opening has been made through the posterior wall of the stomach into the pseudocyst and the tips of the dissecting forceps are in the cavity of the pseudocyst, which is lined by slough and granulation tissue. The tip of a nasogastric tube is visible. A running stitch will next be placed along the edges of this opening, suturing the full thickness of the posterior gastric wall to the capsule of the pseudocyst.

Outcomes and follow-up of acute pancreatitis

The overall mortality from acute pancreatitis has remained at 10–15% over the past 20 years. There is a clear responsibility before the patient is discharged to determine the aetiology of the attack of pancreatitis and the causes listed in *Summary box 72.5* must be looked for and excluded. Failure to remove a predisposing factor could lead to a second attack of pancreatitis, which could be fatal. A proportion of patients in the idiopathic group who suffer repeated attacks may prove to have biliary microlithiasis, which can be identified only by bile sampling at ERCP or by EUS. In a patient who has gallstone pancreatitis, the gallbladder and gallstones should be removed as soon as the patient is fit to undergo surgery and, preferably, before discharge from hospital.

Chronic pancreatitis

Chronic pancreatitis is a progressive inflammatory disease in which there is irreversible destruction of pancreatic tissue. Its clinical course is characterised by severe pain and, in the later stages, exocrine and endocrine pancreatic insufficiency. In the early stages of its evolution, it is frequently complicated by attacks of acute pancreatitis, which are responsible for the recurrent pain that may be the only clinical symptom. The incidence of chronic pancreatitis in several European, North American and Japanese studies ranges from 2 to 10 new cases per 100 000 population per year, with a prevalence of around 13 cases per 100 000, although there are suspicions that the prevalence is actually higher. In certain parts of the world, such

William Wayne Babcock, 1872–1963, surgeon, Philadelphia, PA, USA.

as southern India, the prevalence is much higher (100–200 per 100 000). The disease occurs more frequently in men (male-to-female ratio of 4:1) and the mean age of onset is about 40 years.

Aetiology and pathology

High alcohol consumption is the most frequent cause of chronic pancreatitis, accounting for 60–70% of cases, but only 5–10% of people with alcoholism develop chronic pancreatitis. The exact mechanism of how alcohol causes chronic inflammation in these patients is unclear; genetic and metabolic factors may be at play.

Other causes include pancreatic duct obstruction resulting from stricture formation after trauma, after acute pancreatitis or even occlusion of the duct by pancreatic cancer. Congenital abnormalities, such as pancreas divisum and annular pancreas, if associated with papillary stenosis, are rare causes of chronic pancreatitis.

Hereditary pancreatitis, CF, infantile malnutrition and a large unexplained idiopathic group make up the remainder. Normally, if trypsinogen becomes prematurely activated within the pancreas, it is inhibited by *SPINK1* and is destroyed. Hereditary pancreatitis is an autosomal dominant disorder with an 80% penetrance; it is associated with a gain-of-function mutation in the cationic trypsinogen gene (*PRSS1*) on chromosome 7, which leads to production of a degradation-resistant form of trypsin. A loss-of-function mutation in *SPINK1* also predisposes to idiopathic pancreatitis. Some patients with idiopathic chronic pancreatitis have mutations in the *CFTR* gene. Idiopathic chronic pancreatitis accounts for approximately 30% of cases and has been subdivided into early-onset and late-onset forms.

The importance of hereditary pancreatitis and pancreatitis occurring at a young age is that there is a markedly increased risk of developing pancreatic cancer, particularly if the patient smokes tobacco. Hyperlipidaemia and hypercalcaemia can lead to chronic pancreatitis.

Tropical pancreatitis is a form of idiopathic pancreatitis that begins at a young age and is associated with a high incidence of diabetes mellitus and stone formation. This has been described in resource-poor countries in Asia, Africa and central America. Malnutrition, ingestion of cyanogenic glycosides in cassava and exposure to hydrocarbons released by kerosene or paraffin lamps have been proposed as possible mechanisms for tropical pancreatitis.

Autoimmune pancreatitis has been described relatively recently. Features include diffuse enlargement of the pancreas and diffuse and irregular narrowing of the main pancreatic duct. It may occur in association with other autoimmune diseases, as a multisystem disorder, or may affect the pancreas alone. There may be changes in the biliary tree (autoimmune cholangiopathy) as well. The changes may be confused with neoplasia. Autoantibodies may be present and levels of the immunoglobulin subtype IgG4 are elevated.

At the onset of the disease when symptoms have developed, the pancreas may appear normal. Later, the pancreas enlarges and becomes hard as a result of fibrosis. The ducts become distorted and dilated with areas of both stricture formation and ectasia. Calcified stones weighing from a few milligrams to 200 mg may form within the ducts. The ducts may become occluded with a gelatinous proteinaceous fluid and debris and inflammatory cysts may form. Histologically, the lesions affect the lobules, producing ductular metaplasia and atrophy of acini, hyperplasia of duct epithelium and interlobular fibrosis.

Clinical features

Pain is the outstanding symptom in the majority of patients. The site of pain depends to some extent on the main focus of the disease. If the disease is mainly in the head of the pancreas then epigastric and right subcostal pain is common, whereas if it is limited to the left side of the pancreas left subcostal and back pain are the presenting symptoms. In some patients, the pain is more diffuse. Radiation to the shoulder can occur. Nausea is common during attacks and vomiting may occur. The pain is often dull and gnawing. Severe flare-ups of pain may be superimposed on background discomfort.

All the complications of acute pancreatitis can occur with chronic pancreatitis. Weight loss is common because the patient does not feel like eating. The pain prevents sleep and time off work is frequent. The number of hospital admissions for acute exacerbations is a pointer towards the severity of the disease. Analgesic use and abuse are frequent. This, too, gives an indication of the severity of the disability. The patient's lifestyle is gradually destroyed by pain, analgesic dependence, weight loss and inability to work. Loss of exocrine function leads to steatorrhoea in more than 30% of patients with chronic pancreatitis. Loss of endocrine function and the development of diabetes are not uncommon, and the incidence increases as the disease progresses. Complications frequently bring the patient to the attention of the surgeon. Infection is not infrequent, possibly related to the diabetes mellitus.

Investigations

Only in the early stages of the disease will there be a rise in serum amylase. Tests of pancreatic function merely confirm the presence of pancreatic insufficiency or that more than 70% of the gland has been destroyed.

Pancreatic calcifications may be seen on abdominal radiographs (***Figure 72.18***). CT or MRI scan will show the outline of the gland, the main area of damage and the possibilities for surgical correction (***Figure 72.29***; see also ***Figure 72.7***). Calcification is seen very well on CT but not on MRI. An MRCP will identify the presence of biliary obstruction and the state of the pancreatic duct (***Figure 72.30***). The use of intravenous secretin during the study may demonstrate a pancreatic duct stricture not apparent on standard MRCP, but a normal-looking pancreas on CT or MRI does not rule out chronic pancreatitis. ERCP is the most accurate way of elucidating the anatomy of the duct and, in conjunction with the whole organ morphology, can help to determine the type of operation required, if operative intervention is indicated. Histologically proven chronic pancreatitis can, however, occur in the setting of normal findings on pancreatography. Sonographic findings characteristic of chronic pancreatitis include the presence of stones, visible side branches, cysts, lobularity, an irregular main pancreatic duct, hyperechoic foci and strands, dilatation of the main pancreatic duct and hyperechoic margins of the main pancreatic duct. The presence of four or more of these features is highly suggestive of chronic pancreatitis.

Treatment

Most patients can be managed with medical measures. There is no single therapeutic agent that has been shown to relieve symptoms (*Summary box 72.9*).

Endoscopic, radiological or surgical interventions are indicated mainly to relieve obstruction of the pancreatic duct, bile duct or the duodenum, or in dealing with complications (e.g. pseudocyst, abscess, fistula, ascites or variceal haemorrhage). Decompressing an obstructed pancreatic duct can provide pain relief in some patients (the assumption is that ductal hypertension causes the pain).

Endoscopic pancreatic sphincterotomy might be beneficial in patients with papillary stenosis and a high sphincter pressure and pancreatic ductal pressure. Patients with a dominant pancreatic duct stricture and upstream dilatation may benefit by placement of a stent across the stricture. The stent should be left in for no more than 4–6 weeks as it will block. The complication rate is high and less than two-thirds of patients experience pain relief, but those who do get relief may benefit from a surgical bypass. Pancreatic duct stones may be extracted at ERCP; this may sometimes be combined with extracorporeal shock wave lithotripsy. Pseudocysts may be drained internally under endoscopic ultrasound guidance. Percutaneous or transgastric drainage of pseudocysts under ultrasound or CT guidance may be performed.

The role of surgery is to overcome obstruction and remove mass lesions. Some patients have a mass in the head of the pancreas, for which either a pancreatoduodenectomy or a Beger procedure (duodenum-preserving resection of the pancreatic head) is appropriate. If the duct is markedly dilated, then a longitudinal pancreatojejunostomy or Frey procedure can be of value (*Figure 72.31*). The natural evolution of the disease may not be altered significantly, but around half the patients get long-term pain relief. The rare patient with disease limited to the tail will be cured by a distal pancreatectomy. Patients with intractable pain and diffuse disease may plead for a total pancreatectomy in the expectation that removing the

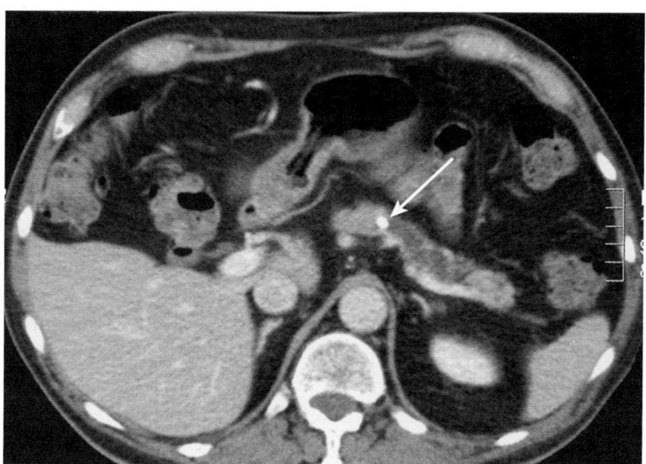

Figure 72.29 Computed tomography scan in a patient with chronic pancreatitis. A stone (arrow) is obstructing the main pancreatic duct in the body of the gland. The duct is markedly dilated upstream of the obstruction.

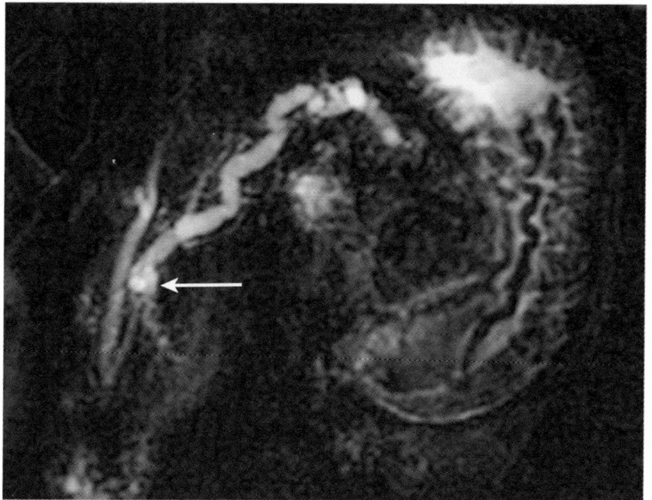

Figure 72.30 Magnetic resonance cholangiopancreatography in a patient with chronic pancreatitis, showing a stricture of the pancreatic duct in the body of the gland (arrow), with dilatation upstream.

Summary box 72.9

Medical treatment of chronic pancreatitis

Treat the addiction
- Help the patient to stop alcohol consumption and tobacco smoking
- Involve a dependency counsellor or a psychologist

Alleviate abdominal pain
- Eliminate obstructive factors (duodenum, bile duct, pancreatic duct)
- Escalate analgesia in a stepwise fashion
- Refer to a pain management specialist
- For intractable pain, consider CT/EUS-guided coeliac axis block

Nutritional and pharmacological measures
- Diet: low in fat and high in protein and carbohydrates
- Pancreatic enzyme supplementation with meals
- Correct malabsorption of the fat-soluble vitamins and vitamin B12
- Micronutrient therapy with methionine, vitamins C and E, selenium (may reduce pain and slow disease progression)
- Steroids (only in autoimmune pancreatitis, for relief of symptoms)
- Medium-chain triglycerides in patients with severe fat malabsorption (they are directly absorbed by the small intestine without the need for digestion)
- Reducing gastric secretions may help

Treat diabetes mellitus

Charles Frederick Frey, b. 1929, Professor of Surgery, University of California, Davis, CA, USA.

offending organ will relieve their pain. However, one should keep in mind that pancreatic function and quality of life are significantly impaired after this procedure, and the operative mortality rate is not trivial. Moreover, there is no guarantee of pain relief (approximately a third of patients get resolution, a third show some benefit and a third see no benefit at all). Total pancreatectomy and islet autotransplantation have been reported in selected patients, but it is difficult to demonstrate any overall benefit.

Prognosis

Chronic pancreatitis is a difficult condition to manage. Patients often suffer a gradual decline in their professional, social and personal lives. The pain may abate after a surgical or percutaneous intervention but tends to return over a period of time. In a proportion of patients, the inflammation may gradually burn out over a period of years, with disappearance of the pain, leaving only the exocrine and endocrine insufficiencies. Development of pancreatic cancer is a risk in those who have had the disease for more than 20 years. New symptoms or a change in the pattern of symptoms should be investigated and malignancy excluded.

Sphincter of Oddi dysfunction

Sphincter of Oddi dyskinesia or dysfunction (SOD) is a clinical syndrome in which pain, biochemical abnormalities and dilatation of the bile duct and/or pancreatic duct are attributed to abnormal function of the sphincter of Oddi. The true incidence of SOD is unknown. Females are more commonly affected than males. SOD may result from stenosis of the sphincter or from dysmotility. Scarring or stenosis of the sphincter can result from passage of stones, pancreatitis or prior endoscopic sphincterotomies.

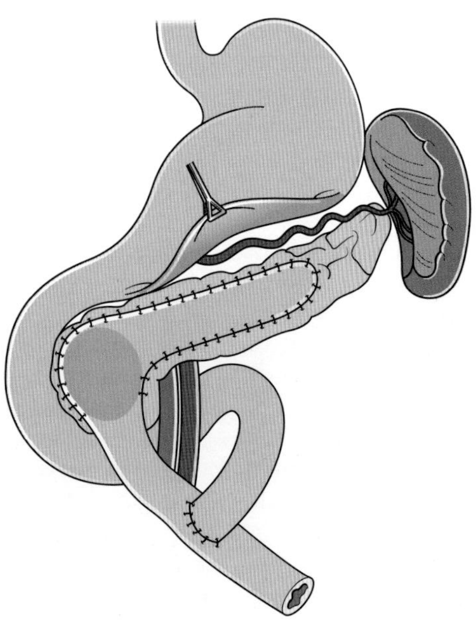

Figure 72.31 Pancreatojejunostomy. The pancreatic duct is opened longitudinally and a loop of jejunum is sutured to the duct. In the Frey procedure, the superficial part of the head of the pancreas is removed to achieve drainage.

There are two clinical types of SOD. Biliary-type SOD is characterised by biliary pain, which may be accompanied by abnormally raised liver enzymes and/or dilatation of the bile duct and/or evidence of delayed emptying on biliary scintigraphy. It may be a cause of persistent postcholecystectomy symptoms. A predominance of pancreatic problems, especially recurrent episodes of acute pancreatitis, is known as pancreatic-type SOD. Each type of SOD is further divided into types I, II and III (*Table 72.7*). This classification helps to predict the underlying pathology and the likelihood of successful treatment. Type I disease is thought to result from a fixed stenosis and responds best to therapy. An episodic dysmotility is the presumed underlying abnormality in the other types and often does not respond as well to treatment.

Biliary-type SOD should be considered and excluded in patients with the postcholecystectomy syndrome. Pancreatic-type SOD should be excluded in patients with recurrent acute pancreatitis of unexplained aetiology. The role of SOD in chronic pancreatitis is unclear. A careful history is essential. CT and MRCP can demonstrate dilatation of the biliary and pancreatic ducts. MRCP with intravenous secretin injection can particularly demonstrate pancreatic duct dilatation due to raised sphincter pressures. EUS may achieve the same end. Quantitative cholescintigraphy (hepatobiliary iminodiacetic acid [HIDA] scan) may demonstrate delayed biliary transit. ERCP with manometry is indicated to confirm the diagnosis if the pain is disabling, non-invasive investigations have not shown structural abnormalities and conservative therapy has

TABLE 72.7 Milwaukee classification of sphincter of Oddi (SOD) dysfunction.

1. Biliary-type SOD
Type I: Typical biliary-type pain Liver enzymes (AST, ALT or ALP) >2 times normal limit documented on at least two occasions during episodes of pain Dilated CBD >12 mm in diameter Prolonged biliary drainage time (>45 min)[a]
Type II: Biliary-type pain, and One or two of the above criteria
Type III: Biliary-type pain only
2. Pancreatic-type SOD
Type I: Pancreatic-type pain Amylase and/or lipase >2 times upper normal limit on at least two occasions during episodes of pain Dilated pancreatic duct (head >6 mm, body >5 mm) Prolonged pancreatic drainage time (>9 min)[a]
Type II: Pancreatic-type pain, and one or two of the above criteria
Type III: Pancreatic-type pain only

AST, aspartate aminotransferase; ALT, alanine aminotransferase; ALP, alkaline phosphatase; CBD, common bile duct.

[a]Difficult to measure and often eschewed in clinical practice.

not helped. A basal sphincter pressure higher than 40 mmHg is the manometric criterion used to diagnose SOD.

Endoscopic sphincterotomy is the treatment of choice for type I SOD. The question of whether dual sphincterotomies (biliary and pancreatic) should be carried out remains unanswered. There is however a particularly high risk of post-ERCP pancreatitis (30% or more), though placement of a pancreatic stent at the time of the procedure appears to reduce this risk. For patients with type II SOD, manometry should be done before considering sphincterotomy, and the results of sphincterotomy are less consistent. Patients with type III SOD are even more difficult, with response rates to sphincterotomy ranging from 8% to 65%. Medical therapy should be tried before proceeding to manometry. Proton pump inhibitors, spasmolytic drugs, calcium blockers (nifedipine) and psychotropic agents have all been tried with varying degrees of success. Injection of botulinum toxin (which can cause a chemical sphincterotomy for up to 3 months) or placement of a pancreatic stent (these are usually removed after 6 weeks) do not provide lasting relief but can be used to identify patients who may benefit from a sphincterotomy.

In a small subgroup of patients who have experienced significant but short-lived relief with sphincterotomy or stenting, surgical transduodenal sphincteroplasty may be considered but the long-term results are often poor. In exceptional circumstances, where the pancreatic head is badly scarred after repeated stenting and numerous attacks of pancreatitis and sphincteroplasty has failed or is unlikely to succeed, one should consider surgical resection of the pancreatic head.

TABLE 72.8 Risk factors for the development of pancreatic cancer.

Demographic factors
Age (peak incidence 65–75 years)
Male gender
Black ethnicity
Environment/lifestyle
Cigarette smoking
Genetic factors and medical conditions
Family history
Two first-degree relatives with pancreatic cancer: relative risk increases 18- to 57-fold
Germline *BRCA2* mutations in some rare high-risk families
Hereditary pancreatitis (50- to 70-fold increased risk)
Chronic pancreatitis (5- to 15-fold increased risk)
Lynch syndrome (HNPCC)
Ataxia telangiectasia
Peutz–Jeghers syndrome
Familial breast–ovarian cancer syndrome
Familial atypical multiple mole melanoma
Familial adenomatous polyposis – risk of ampullary/duodenal carcinoma
Diabetes mellitus
Obesity

HNPCC, hereditary non-polyposis colorectal cancer.

CARCINOMA OF THE PANCREAS

Pancreatic cancer is the seventh leading cause of cancer deaths in men and women worldwide. In the USA it follows lung cancer and colorectal cancer as the third most common cause of cancer death. In the UK, it is the tenth most common cancer and its incidence has increased slightly over the last 10 years. Nearly 85% of patients present with unresectable or metastatic disease. Even among those who undergo surgery, 5-year survival is around 20%. There is no simple screening test. Patients with an increased inherited risk of pancreatic cancer (***Table 72.8***) should be referred to specialist units for screening and counselling.

Pathology

More than 85% of pancreatic cancers are ductal adenocarcinomas. The remaining tumours constitute a variety of pathologies with individual characteristics. Endocrine tumours of the pancreas are rare. These are covered in ***Chapter 57***.

Ductal adenocarcinomas arise most commonly in the head of the gland. They are solid, scirrhous tumours, characterised by neoplastic tubular glands within a markedly desmoplastic fibrous stroma. Fibrosis is also a characteristic of chronic pancreatitis, and histological differentiation between tumour and pancreatitis can cause diagnostic difficulties. Ductal adenocarcinomas infiltrate locally, typically along nerve sheaths, along lymphatics and into blood vessels. Liver and peritoneal metastases are common. Proliferative lesions in the pancreatic ducts can precede invasive ductal adenocarcinoma. These are termed pancreatic intraepithelial neoplasia or PanIN, and can demonstrate a range of structural complexity and cellular atypia.

Cystic tumours of the pancreas may be serous or mucinous. Serous cystadenomas are typically found in older women and are large aggregations of multiple small cysts, almost like bubble wrap. They are benign. Mucinous tumours, on the other hand, have the potential for malignant transformation. They include mucinous cystic neoplasms (MCNs) and intraductal papillary mucinous neoplasms (IPMNs). MCNs are seen in perimenopausal women, show up as multilocular thick-walled cysts in the pancreatic body or tail and, histologically, contain an ovarian-type stroma. IPMNs are more common in the pancreatic head and in older men, but an IPMN arising from a branch duct can be difficult to distinguish from an MCN. IPMNs arising within the main duct are often multifocal and have a greater tendency to prove malignant. Thick mucus seen extruding from the ampulla at ERCP is diagnostic of a main duct IPMN. Mucinous tumours can be confused with pseudo-

Henry T Lynch, 1928–2019, Professor of Preventative Medicine, Creighton University, Omaha, NE, USA.
John Law Augustine Peutz, 1886–1970, Chief Specialist for Internal Medicine, St John's Hospital, The Hague, The Netherlands.
Harold Joseph Jeghers, 1904–1990, Professor of Internal Medicine, The New Jersey College of Medicine and Dentistry, Jersey City, NJ, USA.

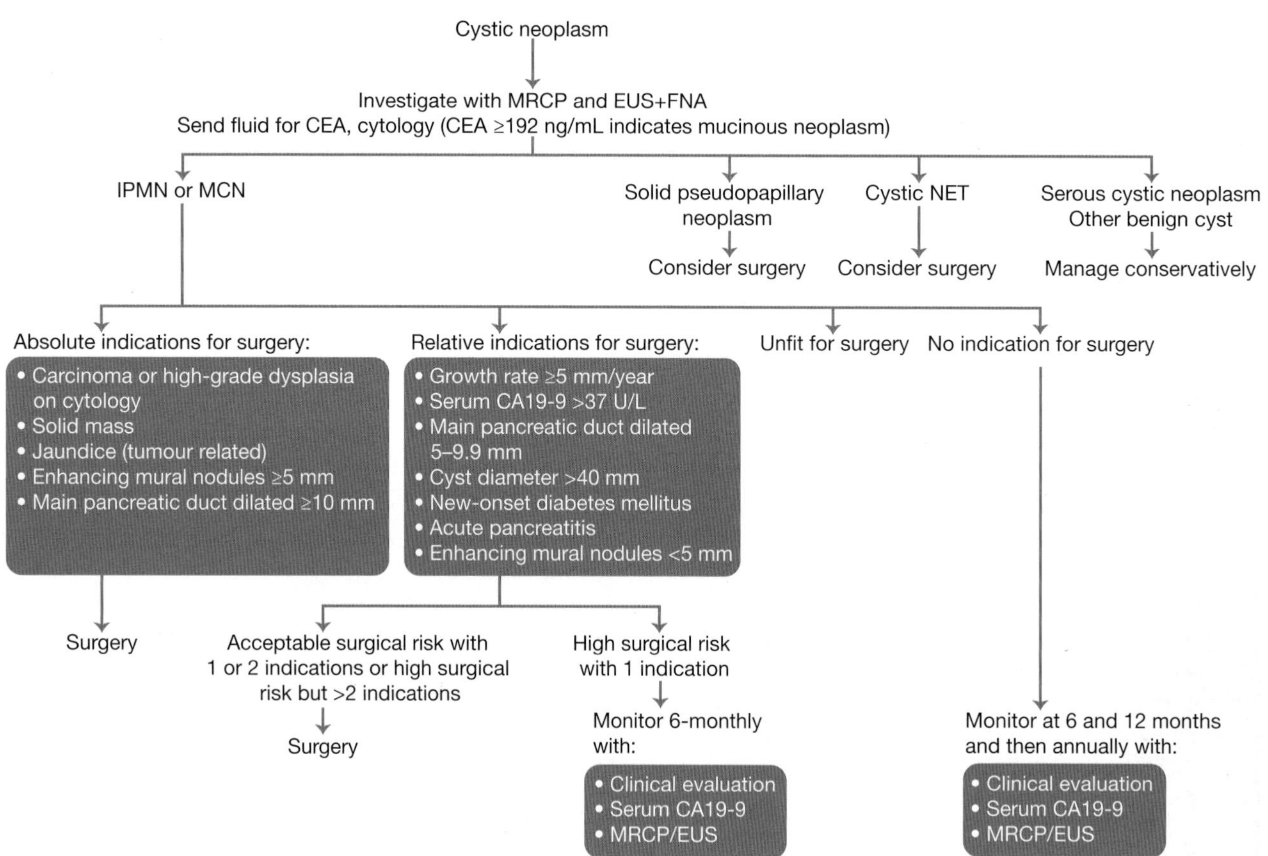

Figure 72.32 Management algorithm for cystic neoplasms of the pancreas. CA19-9, carbohydrate antigen 19-9; CEA, carcinoembryonic antigen; EUS, endoscopic ultrasonography; FNA, fine-needle aspiration; IPMN, intraductal papillary mucinous neoplasm; MCN, mucinous cystic neoplasm; MRCP, magnetic resonance cholangiography and pancreatography; NET, neuroendocrine tumour. (Adapted from The European Study Group on Cystic Tumours of the Pancreas. European evidence-based guidelines on pancreatic cystic neoplasms. *Gut* 2018; **67**: 789–804.)

cysts (***Summary box 72.8 and Figure 72.32***). Occasionally, lymphoepithelial cysts, lymphangiomas, dermoid cysts and intestinal duplication cysts can show up in the pancreas. Solid pseudopapillary neoplasms are rare, slowly progressive but malignant lesions seen in women of childbearing age, and manifest as large, part-solid, part-cystic tumours.

Tumours arising from the ampulla or from the distal common bile duct can present as a mass in the head of the pancreas and constitute around a third of all tumours in that area. Adenomas of the ampulla of Vater are diagnosed at endoscopy as polypoid submucosal masses covered by a smooth epithelium. They can harbour foci of invasive carcinoma; the larger the adenoma, the greater the risk. Biopsies taken at endoscopy may not always include the malignant focus. Endoscopic surveillance, endoscopic resection or even surgical transduodenal ampullary excision should be considered (***Figure 72.33***). Patients with familial adenomatous polyposis (FAP) can present with multiple duodenal polyps. Malignant transformation in a duodenal polyp is a significant cause of mortality in these patients, mandating endoscopic follow-up and pancreatoduodenectomy in selected patients with high-grade dysplasia within the polyp.

Ampullary adenocarcinomas often present early with biliary obstruction. Their natural history is distinctly more favourable than that of pancreatic ductal adenocarcinoma. Ampullary carcinomas are relatively small when diagnosed, which may account for their better prognosis. Occasionally, other malignant neoplasms can arise at the ampulla, such as carcinoid tumours and high-grade neuroendocrine carcinomas.

Clinical features

Jaundice secondary to obstruction of the distal bile duct is the most common symptom that draws attention to ampullary and pancreatic head tumours. It is characteristically painless jaundice but may be associated with nausea and epigastric discomfort. Pruritus, dark urine and pale stools with steatorrhoea are common accompaniments of jaundice. In the absence of jaundice, symptoms are often non-specific, namely vague discomfort, anorexia and weight loss, and are frequently dismissed by both patient and doctor. Upper abdominal symptoms in a patient recently diagnosed with diabetes, especially in one above 50 years of age with no family history or obesity, should raise suspicion. Occasionally, a patient will present with an unexplained attack of pancreatitis; all such patients should have follow-up imaging of the pancreas. Tumours of the body and tail of the gland often grow silently and present at an advanced unresectable stage.

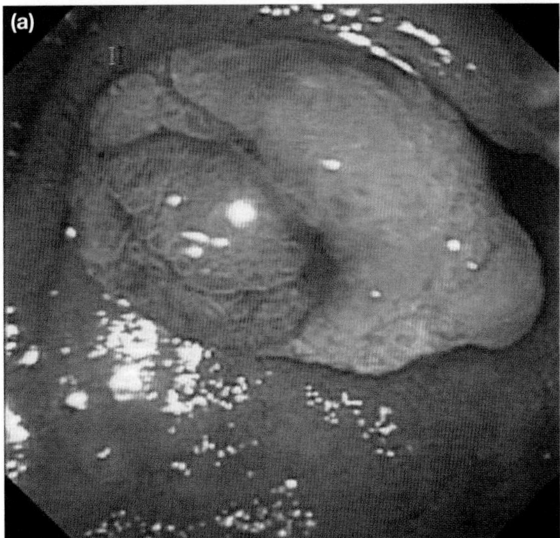

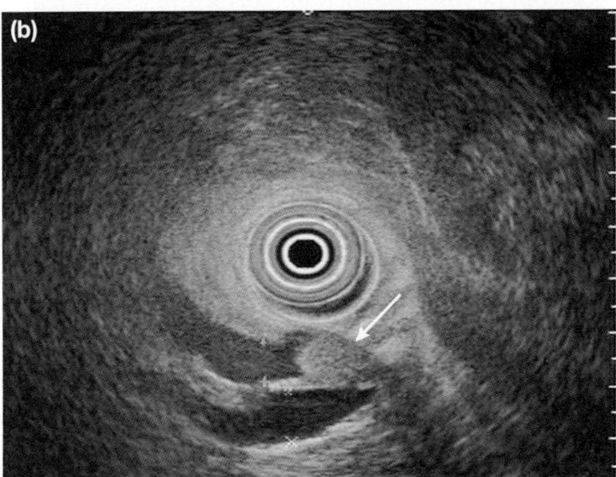

Figure 72.33 (a) Carcinoma of the ampulla as seen at endoscopy. (b) Appearance of the same tumour (arrow) on endoscopic ultrasonography (courtesy of Dr Peter Fairclough).

Back pain is a worrying symptom, raising the possibility of retroperitoneal infiltration.

On examination, there may be evidence of jaundice, weight loss, a palpable liver and a palpable gallbladder. Courvoisier first drew attention to the association of an enlarged gallbladder and a pancreatic tumour in 1890, when he noted that, when the common duct is obstructed by a stone, distension of the gallbladder (which is likely to be chronically inflamed) is rare; when the duct is obstructed in some other way, such as a neoplasm, distension of the normal gallbladder is common. Other signs of intra-abdominal malignancy should be looked for with care, such as a palpable mass, ascites, supraclavicular nodes and tumour deposits in the pelvis; when present, they indicate a grim prognosis.

Investigations

In a jaundiced patient, the usual blood tests and ultrasound scan should be performed. Ultrasonography will determine if the bile duct is dilated. If it is, and there is a genuine suspicion of a tumour in the head of the pancreas, the preferred test is a contrast-enhanced CT scan (***Figure 72.8***). In the majority of instances, this should establish if there is a tumour in the pancreas and if it is resectable. The presence of hepatic or peritoneal metastases, lymph node metastases distant from the pancreatic head or encasement of the superior mesenteric, hepatic or coeliac artery by tumour are clear contraindications to surgical resection. Tumour size, continuous invasion of the duodenum, stomach or colon and lymph node metastases within the operative field are not contraindications. If the tumour abuts or minimally invades the portal or superior mesenteric vein, this is not a contraindication to surgery (as part of the vein can be resected if necessary); however, complete encasement and occlusion of the vein and any degree of arterial involvement remain contraindications to surgical resection. MRI and magnetic resonance angiography can provide information comparable to CT.

ERCP and biliary stenting should be carried out if there is any suggestion of cholangitis, if there is diagnostic doubt or if there is likely to be a delay between diagnosis and surgery in a deeply jaundiced patient with distressing pruritus. It relieves the jaundice and can also provide a brush cytology or biopsy specimen to confirm the diagnosis (***Figures 72.13, 72.14 and 72.19***). Otherwise, preoperative ERCP and biliary stenting is not routine in patients with resectable disease as it is associated with a higher incidence of infective complications after surgery.

The prothrombin time should be checked, and clotting abnormalities should be corrected with vitamin K or fresh-frozen plasma prior to ERCP. If a stent is placed in a patient who may undergo resection, it should be a plastic stent or a covered metal stent, as these can be easily removed during surgery.

EUS is useful if CT fails to demonstrate a tumour, if tissue diagnosis is required prior to surgery (e.g. a mass has developed on a background of chronic pancreatitis and a distinction needs to be made between inflammation and neoplasia), if vascular invasion needs to be confirmed or if separating cystic tumours from pseudocysts (***Figure 72.33***; see also ***Figure 72.20***). Transduodenal or transgastric FNA or Trucut biopsy performed under endoscopic ultrasound guidance avoids spillage of tumour cells into the peritoneal cavity. Percutaneous transperitoneal biopsy of potentially resectable pancreatic tumours should be avoided as far as possible. Histological confirmation of malignancy is desirable but not essential, particularly if the imaging clearly demonstrates a resectable tumour. The lack of a tissue diagnosis should not delay appropriate surgical therapy. In patients judged to have unresectable disease, tissue diagnosis should be obtained prior to starting palliative therapy. A CT scan of the chest and a fluorodeoxyglucose–positron emission tomography (FDG-PET) scan are routinely used to complete the staging.

Diagnostic laparoscopy prior to an attempt at resection can spare a proportion of patients an unnecessary laparotomy by identifying small peritoneal and liver metastases. It can be combined with laparoscopic ultrasonography. The tumour marker carbohydrate antigen 19-9 (CA19-9) is not highly specific or sensitive, but a baseline level should be

Ludwig Courvoisier, 1843–1918, surgeon, Basel, Switzerland, was one of the first surgeons to remove stones from the common bile duct.

established; if it is initially raised, it can be useful later in identifying recurrence.

Management

At presentation, more than 85% of patients with ductal adenocarcinoma are unsuitable for resection because of advanced disease. If imaging shows that the tumour is potentially resectable, the patient should be considered for surgical resection, as that offers the only (albeit small) chance of a cure. Every patient with pancreatic cancer should ideally be discussed in a multidisciplinary forum. Comorbidities should be taken carefully into account. Biological rather than chronological age should be the consideration. In patients with locally advanced or metastatic disease the primary objective should be to relieve symptoms, improve quality of life and extend survival, rather than achieve a cure. Patients will broadly fall into four categories.

1 Resectable: these patients should be offered surgery, to be followed by adjuvant chemotherapy. Some centres have begun to suggest that neoadjuvant chemotherapy be used prior to resection, but the evidence is not strong.
2 Borderline resectable (usually because of significant venous occlusion or arterial abutment): these patients may be offered neoadjuvant chemotherapy with/without chemoradiotherapy, to be followed by surgical resection if the disease has been downstaged. Adjuvant therapy should follow.
3 Locally advanced and unresectable: offer systemic chemotherapy. Surgery may subsequently be possible in a small cohort who get downstaged.
4 Metastatic: offer systemic chemotherapy

If a cystic tumour is encountered, no matter how large, surgical resection should be considered as it carries a reasonable chance of cure. Tumours of the ampulla have a good prognosis and should, if at all possible, be resected. Some of the rare tumours and the neuroendocrine lesions should also be resected if at all possible.

Surgical resection

The standard resection for a tumour of the pancreatic head or the ampulla is a pylorus-preserving pancreatoduodenectomy (PPPD). This involves removal of the duodenum and the pancreatic head, including the distal part of the bile duct. The original pancreatoduodenectomy as proposed by Whipple included resection of the gastric antrum. Preserving the antrum and the pylorus is thought to result in a more physiological outcome with no difference in survival or recurrence rates. The Whipple procedure is now reserved for situations in which the entire duodenum has to be removed (e.g. in FAP) or in which the tumour encroaches on the first part of the duodenum or the distal stomach and a PPPD would not achieve a clear resection margin. Total pancreatectomy is warranted only in situations where one is dealing with a multifocal tumour (e.g. a main duct IPMN) or the body and tail of the gland are too inflamed or too friable to achieve a safe anastomosis with the bowel. The PPPD procedure includes a local lymphadenectomy. Extended lymphadenectomy has not been shown to be beneficial in improving survival and is associated with increased morbidity. If the tumour is adherent to the portal or superior mesenteric vein but can still be removed by including a patch or a short segment of vein in the resection, with an appropriate reconstruction of the vessel, then that should be done. This is not associated with an increase in the morbidity or mortality of the procedure and the outcomes are similar. Arterial resections are not recommended unless carried out within the context of a trial. If performed outside a trial, they should be preceded by multidisciplinary discussion and careful counselling of the patient, and be carried out in a specialist unit.

For tumours of the body and tail, distal pancreatectomy with splenectomy is the standard. Infiltration of the splenic artery or vein by the tumour is not a contraindication to resection. When resecting the pancreatic tail for a benign lesion, one may attempt to preserve the spleen if possible. When removing the spleen, prior vaccinations against pneumococci, meningococci and *Haemophilus influenzae* B should be administered, and subsequent antibiotic prophylaxis given (see ***Chapter 70***).

While the majority of pancreatic resections continue to be performed via an open approach, minimally invasive approaches – laparoscopic and robotic – are feasible and may yield comparable results. Minimally invasive pancreatic resections are technically challenging, pose additional demands on operating room time and equipment and involve a significant learning curve for the surgeon and the entire team. They should be restricted to specialist centres and surgeons who have experience in doing them. Distal pancreatectomy, especially for smaller tumours, lends itself more easily to the laparoscopic or robotic approach than a pancreatic head resection. Robotic surgery may carry greater ergonomic benefit for the surgeon (see ***Chapter 10***).

Pancreatoduodenectomy

The patient's coagulation screen should be checked preoperatively and adequate hydration ensured. The patient should be aware of the diagnosis, the gravity of the operation and the risks involved. The operation has three distinct phases:

- exploration and assessment;
- resection;
- reconstruction.

A cholecystectomy is performed. The bile duct and hepatic artery are exposed, removing the lymphatic tissue in this area. Exposure of the hepatic artery enables division of the gastroduodenal artery and visualisation of the portal vein. The distal part of the gastric antrum is mobilised. The duodenum and right colon are mobilised from the retroperitoneal tissues. The superior mesenteric vein is exposed inferior to the pancreatic

---

Allen Oldfather Whipple, 1881–1963, Director of Surgical Services, The Presbyterian Hospital, and Professor of Surgery, Columbia University, New York, NY, USA, began to perform two-stage pancreatoduodenectomies in 1934 and shortened the procedure into a one-stage process in 1940. **Alessandro Codivilla** (1861–1912) and **Walter Kausch** (1867–1928) had performed the operation before him, but Whipple was the surgeon who established pancreatoduodenectomy as an operation.

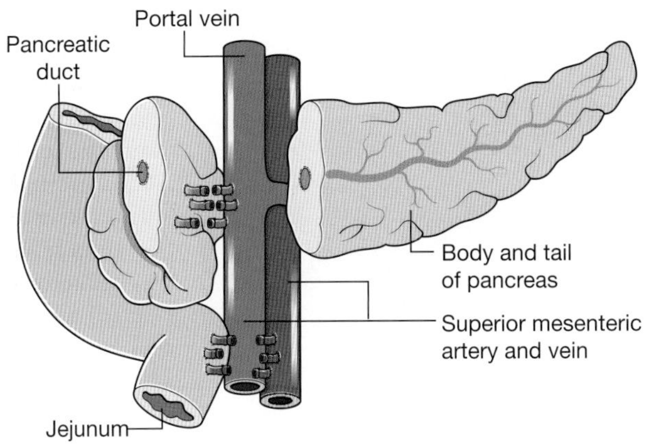

Figure 72.34 Resection of the head of the pancreas in a pylorus-preserving pancreatoduodenectomy.

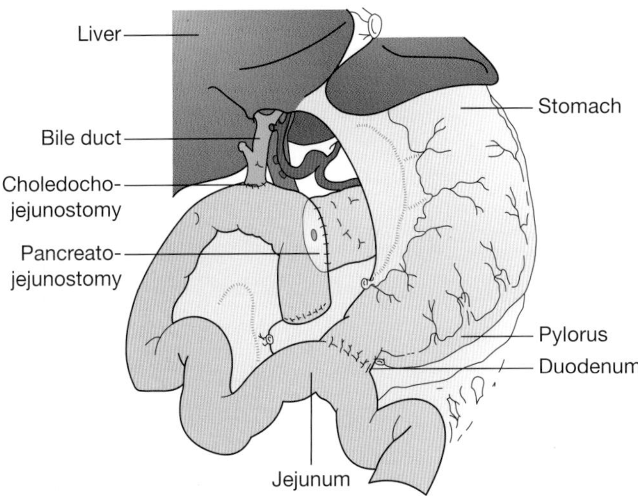

Figure 72.35 Reconstruction after a pylorus-preserving pancreatoduodenectomy.

neck. Careful dissection into the plane between the vein and the pancreatic substance (***Figure 72.2***) will reveal whether the tumour is adherent to the vein. At this juncture, a decision has to be made whether to proceed to the next phase of resection or not. If resection is to be performed, the fourth part of the duodenum is dissected and freed from the ligament of Treitz so that the upper jejunum can be brought into the supracolic compartment. The jejunum is divided 20–30 cm downstream from the duodenojejunal flexure, and the mesentery of the proximal jejunum is detached. The first part of the duodenum is divided. The neck of the pancreas is divided, and then the uncinate process is separated from the superior mesenteric vein and artery working up towards the upper bile duct, which is divided, releasing the specimen (***Figure 72.34***). Retroperitoneal lymph nodes within the operative field are completely removed with the specimen. Reconstruction is carried out as in ***Figure 72.35***. The pancreatic stump, the divided bile duct and the duodenal stump are anastomosed onto the jejunum, in that order. Some surgeons prefer to anastomose the pancreas to the posterior wall of the stomach instead; others prefer to create a separate Roux loop of the jejunum and anastomose the pancreas to that. The operation should take between 3 and 6 hours. Blood loss should be low and transfusion is often not necessary. Patients are usually nursed in a high-dependency area for the first 24–48 hours after surgery. Prolonged nasogastric drainage is unnecessary and early feeding can be commenced. Enhanced recovery after surgery (ERAS) protocols should be applied to pancreatic resections as with other types of gastrointestinal surgery.

Resection for pancreatic cancer should be carried out in specialist units. There is a clear correlation between higher caseload volume and lower hospital mortality and morbidity. PPPD should carry a mortality of no more than 3–5%. The morbidity remains high, with some 30–40% of patients developing a complication in the postoperative period. These complications are usually infective, but a leak from the anastomosis between the pancreas and the bowel is known to occur in at least 10% of patients, and this may give rise to the major complication of a postoperative pancreatic fistula (POPF). Octreotide may be administered in the perioperative period to suppress secretion and reduce the likelihood of a leak, but the evidence for its efficacy is still debatable. Following surgical resection, the pathological tumour–node–metastasis stage should be documented.

Adjuvant therapy

At the beginning of this century, the reported 5-year survival following resection of a pancreatic adenocarcinoma ranged from 7% to 25% (around 10% for most centres). The median survival was 11–20 months. Considering that, at best, 15% of patients had resectable disease to begin with, this meant only two or three out of 100 patients with this disease could expect to survive to 5 years. Moreover, recurrences could and did show up even beyond the 5-year cut-off. The high recurrence rate following resection inevitably led to the consideration of adjuvant treatments to improve outcome. Starting with the large multicentre European study (ESPAC-1) in 2004, which showed an improvement in median survival after adjuvant chemotherapy with 5-fluorouracil (5-FU) but no advantage with adjuvant radiotherapy, there have been several further studies that have looked at gemcitabine alone, gemcitabine with capecitabine and most recently modified fluorouracil plus leucovorin, oxaliplatin and irinotecan (mFOLFIRINOX). The latter has been associated with disease-free survival of over 21 months and median overall survival of over 54 months. Most patients with resected ductal adenocarcinoma are now offered 6 months of adjuvant chemotherapy with mFOLFIRINOX. Those with a poor functional status or a contraindication to mFOLFIRINOX are offered gemcitabine with/without capecitabine. Some centres continue to offer chemoradiotherapy, particularly in patients with involved (R1) resection margins, and further trials of adjuvant chemoradiation are in progress.

Wenzel Treitz, 1819–1872, Professor of Anatomy and Pathology, at Kraków, Poland, and later at Prague, Czech Republic.

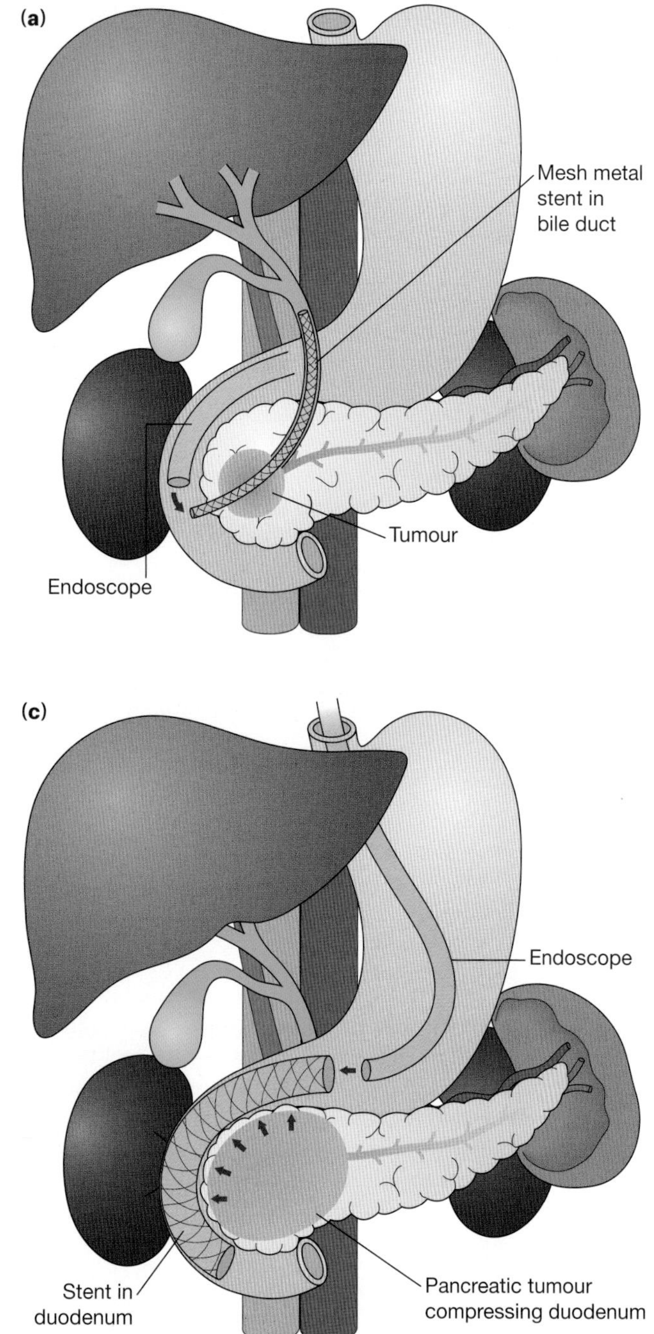

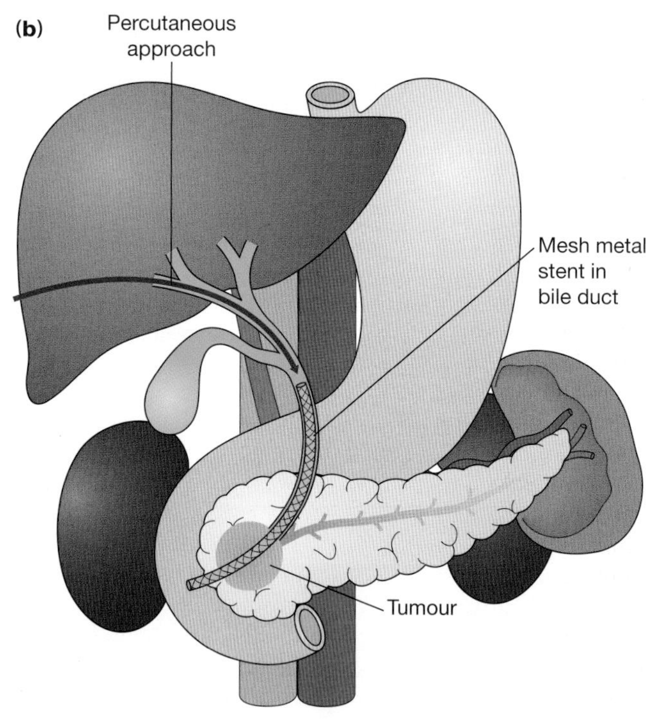

Figure 72.36 Approaches to biliary and duodenal stenting. (a) Endoscopic retrograde cholangiography and placement of a biliary stent; (b) percutaneous transhepatic cholangiography followed by cannulation of the biliary system and percutaneous placement of a biliary stent (mesh metal in this instance); (c) endoscopic placement of a duodenal stent (mesh metal).

It should be emphasised, however, that these depressing statistics apply to ductal adenocarcinomas. Patients with resected ampullary tumours have a 5-year survival of 40%, and cystic tumours and neuroendocrine tumours can often be cured by surgical resection.

Palliation

The median survival of patients with unresectable, locally advanced, non-metastatic pancreatic cancer is 6–10 months and, in patients with metastatic disease, it is 2–6 months.

If unresectable disease is found in the course of a laparotomy that was commenced with the intent to resect, a choledochoenterostomy and a gastroenterostomy should be carried out to relieve (or pre-empt) jaundice and duodenal obstruction. The bile duct may be anastomosed to the duodenum or to a loop of jejunum. It is preferable to use the bile duct rather than the gallbladder. Cholecystojejunostomy is easier to perform, but the bile must then drain through the cystic duct, which is narrow and, if inserted low into the bile duct, is vulnerable to occlusion by tumour growth. A coeliac plexus block can also be administered. A transduodenal Trucut biopsy of the tumour should be obtained.

In patients found to have unresectable disease on imaging, jaundice is relieved by stenting at ERCP (***Figure 72.36a***).

Stents may be made of plastic or self-expanding metal mesh. Plastic stents are cheaper but tend to occlude faster and, if the patient is likely to have a longer life expectancy, a metal stent can be used. If the patient is not a suitable candidate for endoscopic biliary stenting, a percutaneous transhepatic stent can be placed (***Figure 72.36b***). Obstruction of the duodenum occurs in approximately 15% of cases. If this occurs early in the course of the disease, surgical bypass by gastrojejunostomy is appropriate but, if it is late in the course of the disease, then the use of expanding metal stents inserted endoscopically is preferable, as many of these patients have prolonged delayed gastric emptying following surgery (***Figure 72.36c***). If both biliary and duodenal metal stents are to be placed endoscopically, the biliary one should be placed first.

If no operative procedure is undertaken, an EUS-guided or percutaneous biopsy of the tumour should be performed before consideration of chemotherapy or chemoradiation. Lymphomas of the pancreas are rare and constitute less than 3% of all pancreatic cancers. These respond to chemoradiotherapy and surgical resection is not indicated. For patients with ductal adenocarcinoma who have locally advanced or metastatic disease, mFOLFIRINOX or alternatively gemcitabine plus albumin-bound paclitaxel particles (nab-paclitaxel) should be considered if the functional status is good. However, the 2–5 months' increase in median survival with these regimens has to be offset against the higher toxicity and cost. No long-term cures have been described with chemotherapy or radiotherapy.

There is no role for surgical resection if metastases are present at the time of the initial presentation. In a very small proportion of patients who have been deemed unresectable owing to major vascular involvement and do not have metastatic disease, attempts have been made to downstage the tumour with one of the newer combination chemotherapy regimens, sometimes with chemoradiation added in, to try to render them resectable. Such neoadjuvant therapies are only very occasionally successful and should ideally be considered within a clinical trial.

Steatorrhoea is treated with enzyme supplementation. Diabetes mellitus, if it develops, is treated with oral hypoglycaemics or insulin as appropriate, and pain with either analgesics or an appropriate nerve block.

Summary box 72.10

Palliation of pancreatic cancer

Relieve jaundice and treat biliary sepsis
- Surgical biliary bypass
- Stent placed at ERCP or percutaneous transhepatic cholangiography

Improve gastric emptying
- Surgical gastroenterostomy
- Duodenal stent

Pain relief
- Stepwise escalation of analgesia
- Coeliac plexus block
- Transthoracic splanchnicectomy

Symptom relief and quality of life
- Encourage normal activities
- Enzyme replacement for steatorrhoea
- Treat diabetes

Consider chemotherapy

FURTHER READING

Braganza JM, Lee SH, McCloy RF, McMahon MJ. Chronic pancreatitis. *Lancet* 2011; **377**: 1184–97.

Conroy T, Hammel P, Hebbar M *et al.* FOLFIRINOX or gemcitabine as adjuvant therapy for pancreatic cancer. *N Engl J Med* 2018; **379**: 2395–406.

Jarnagin W. *Blumgart's surgery of the liver, biliary tract and pancreas*, 6th edn. Philadelphia, PA: Elsevier, 2016.

Leppäniemi A, Tolonen M, Tarasconi A *et al.* WSES guidelines for the management of severe acute pancreatitis. *World J Emerg Surg* 2019; **14**: 27.

Mizrahi JD, Surana R, Valle JW, Shroff RT. Pancreatic cancer. *Lancet* 2020; **395**: 2008–20.

National Institute for Health and Care Excellence. *Pancreatitis.* NICE Clinical Guideline 104. London: NICE, 2020. Available from https://www.nice.org.uk/guidance/ng104.

The European Study Group on Cystic Tumours of the Pancreas. European evidence-based guidelines on pancreatic cystic neoplasms. *Gut* 2018; **67**: 789–804.

CHAPTER 73 Functional disorders of the intestine

Learning objectives

To recognise and understand:

- The spectrum of intestinal disorders resulting from abnormal neuromuscular functions
- The management of relatively common acute motility disturbances
- The management of common chronic disorders that present to surgeons such as chronic constipation and irritable bowel syndrome
- The existence of several rare neuromuscular diseases that may affect the intestine
- The limited role of surgery in the treatment of most of these disorders

APPLIED ANATOMY AND PHYSIOLOGY

The intestine must subserve basic functions of moving contents from proximal to distal in a rhythmical fashion to allow mixing, digestion and absorption of contents. The motility of the intestine has been studied for more than a century and all readers should know of the seminal experiments of Bayliss and Starling in their 1899 paper 'The movements and innervation of the small intestine', which led to adoption of the term 'peristalsis'. In the small intestine, fasting motility can be described by the three phases of the migrating motor complex (MMC), with fed activity resembling phase II. Colonic motility is much more complicated and still poorly understood with some features akin to the MMC but also specific phenomena such as retrograde movements (presumed to allow greater resident time and therefore fluid and electrolyte absorption). The main characteristics of intestinal motility are shown in ***Table 73.1***.

The intestine, like the heart, is autonomous in generating its own rhythmical electrical, and therefore local motor, activity by intrinsic pacemaker activity generated by small fibroblast-like cells called the interstitial cells of Cajal. These cells, which are mainly resident within the muscularis propria, have several key functions, including setting the membrane potential of smooth muscle cells so that they are primed to contract and connecting smooth muscle cells electrically so that synchronous

TABLE 73.1 Contractile activity of the intestine.

Region	Broad category	
Small intestine	Phase I	Quiescence (40–60% of total time)
	Phase II	High-frequency contractions allowing mixing and absorption (20–30% of total time)
	Phase III	High-amplitude propagated activity (5–10 minutes)
Large intestine	Phasic contractions	Low-amplitude propagated pressure waves
		High-amplitude propagated pressure waves[a]
		Retrograde pressure waves
		Simultaneous pressure waves
		Periodic colonic and rectal motor activity (localised bursts)
	Tonic contractions	Sustained activity responsible for tone

[a]Most akin to phase III of the migrating motor complex and responsible for mass movements of faecal content.

Sir William Bayliss, 1860–1924, physiologist, and **Ernest Henry Starling**, 1866–1927, University College London, London, UK. Starling's contributions to medicine also included Starling's principle (capillary pressures) and filling of the heart (Frank–Starling law).

Santiago Ramon y Cajal, 1852–1934, Spanish neuroscientist, pathologist and Nobel prize winner (1906) for studies of cellular anatomy of the nervous system.

contraction occurs. Also akin to the heart, this activity is affected by a hierarchy of external control systems but mainly by the enteric nervous system (ENS) via the myenteric plexus. The myenteric plexus is one of the two intramural plexuses of the ENS (the other being the submucosal plexus). The former has the major role in motor functions while the latter has roles in sensing, mucosal blood flow regulation and secretion. Both are composed of small groups of enteric neurones that congregate with glial cells to form ganglia, these being connected in a lattice-type network of axons (*Figure 73.1*). The ENS has a neurochemical complexity and number of neurones (five times the number in the spinal cord) that has led to it being called the 'little brain' (*Summary box 73.1*). Thus, although higher control mechanisms including the autonomic nervous system (ANS) and brain allow the intestinal motility to respond to wider environmental cues, e.g. waking, exercise, the smell and taste of food and stress, the intestine can initiate and sustain peristalsis without any external inputs.

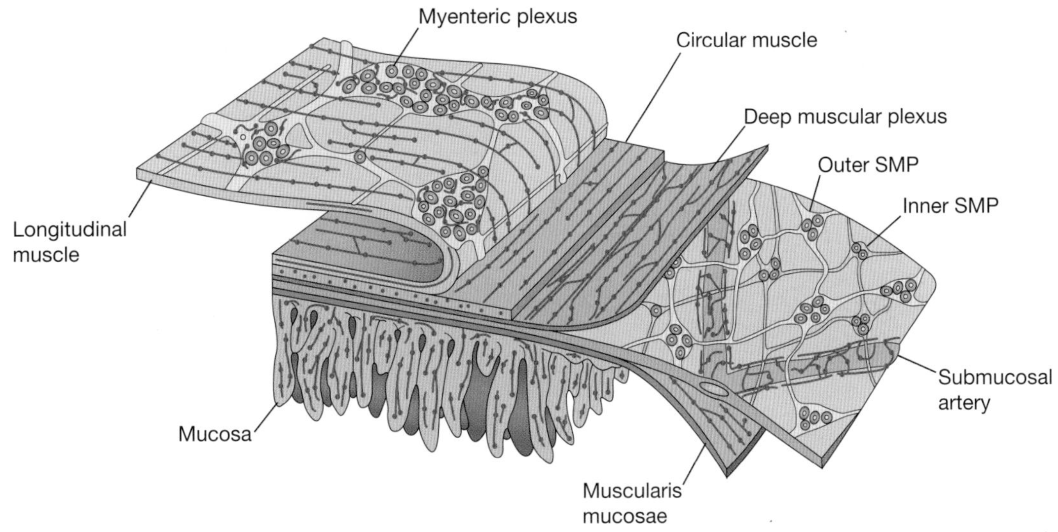

Figure 73.1 Schematic diagram of the enteric nervous system. SMP, submucosal plexus. (Reproduced by permission from Springer Nature. Furness JB. The enteric nervous system and neurogastroenterology. *Nat Rev Gastroenterol Hepatol* 2012; **9**: 286–94. © 2012.)

Summary box 73.1

Regulation of intestinal contractile activity

Myogenic control mechanisms
- Interstitial cells of Cajal generating slow wave activity

Neurogenic control mechanisms
- ENS (a variety of cells in myenteric and submucosal ganglia)
- ANS (sympathetic and parasympathetic mainly via ENS ganglia)
- Central nervous system (CNS) (brain–gut interactions)

Chemical control mechanisms
- Local paracrine (especially from mucosal enteroendocrine cells)
- Endocrine

The rectum constitutes a final and specialised end to the intestine. Its role is mainly for temporary storage of faeces prior to defecation. This role permits both further water absorption and the ability of higher mammals to socially defecate (an ability shared with small rodents as well as many larger species). To this end, the wall of the rectum is specialised in terms of compliance and of having nerve endings that provide conscious perception of filling. In concert with the upper anal canal, the rectum is also capable of distinguishing solid, liquid and gas by the 'sampling' reflex. Together the act of defecation requires complex neuromuscular functions and it is no surprise that it goes wrong with sufficient regularity to cause much human misery in the form of constipation and incontinence (see *Chapter 80*).

TESTS OF INTESTINAL FUNCTION

Subsequent chapters address diagnostic tests specific to the rectum (see *Chapter 79*) and anus (see *Chapter 80*). Here the focus is on tests that may be relevant to studying the motility of the small intestine and colon. A general proviso in reading this section is that our current ability to understand the physiology of the intestine in humans is limited by both access and understanding. In general, we measure what can be measured and all tests have inherent limitations to interpretation. *Summary box 73.2* provides an overview of all tests, denoting those that have general clinical application versus those that are the preserve of highly specialised units or research studies.

Summary box 73.2 makes clear that few tests are in general use. Small bowel contrast studies, e.g. barium follow-through, although available, have poor sensitivity for detecting much other than visceral distension (superseded by axial imaging with computed tomography [CT] or MRI) or grossly retarded transit. Breath hydrogen testing assesses the presence

Summary box 73.2

Tests of small intestinal function

Transit
- Small bowel barium contrast study[a]
- Breath hydrogen small bowel transit tests (lactulose or lactose ^{13}C-ureide)[a]
- Wireless motility capsule small bowel transit study[b]

Contractile activity
- Antroduodenal manometry (ideally prolonged [24 hours] ambulatory study)
- Dynamic magnetic resonance imaging (MRI) studies

Tests of colonic function

Transit
- Radio-opaque marker studies[a]
- Isotope scintigraphy
- Wireless motility capsule whole-gut transit study[b]

Contractile activity
- Colonic manometry
- Dynamic MRI studies

[a]Denotes general availability.
[b]Adopted by some highly funded health systems.

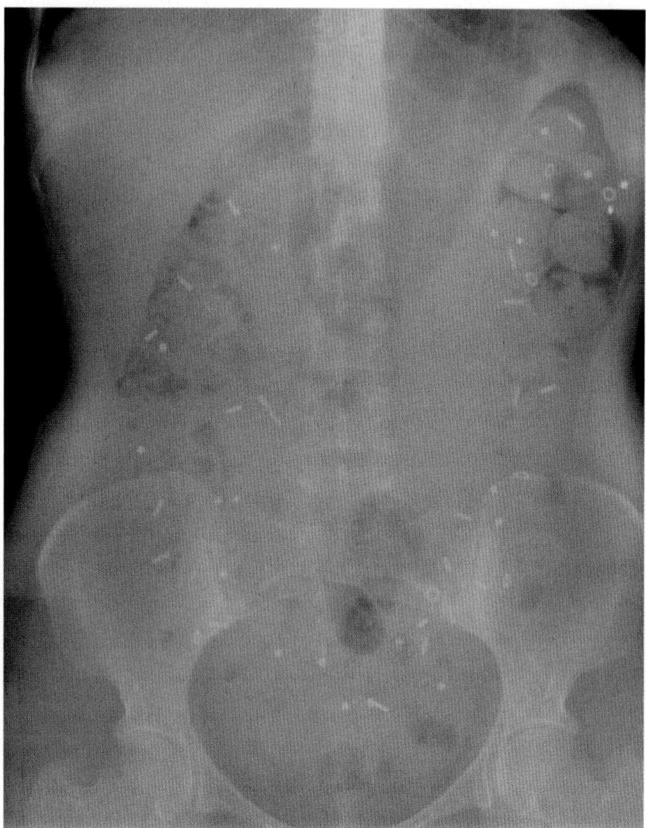

Figure 73.2 Radio-opaque marker transit study in a woman. All 50 markers are retained, indicating slow-transit constipation.

of carbohydrate malabsorption and is an indirect measure of transit because stagnated content allows some degree of bacterial overgrowth and fermentation products (hydrogen, methane and carbon dioxide). Although frequently used in patients with unexplained chronic abdominal symptoms such as irritable bowel syndrome (IBS), its utility in reliably measuring transit or detecting bacterial overgrowth is limited by issues of reproducibility.

The wireless motility capsule measures pH, temperature and pressure as it traverses the whole gastrointestinal tract; changes in these variables can be used to determine timings as it migrates from stomach to small bowel and large bowel. While it offers a number of advantages over and above current techniques, especially with respect to patient tolerability, safety and standardisation, it is not widely available owing to cost.

Prolonged measurement of small bowel contractile activity can be performed using multichannel pressure recordings called manometry that show phases of the MMC. Some findings may be indicative of underlying small bowel neuromuscular diseases such as myopathies and neuropathies (see ***Chronic impairment of intestinal motility with dilatation of the small intestine: intestinal pseudo-obstruction***) but these findings have issues of specificity and the technology itself is only available in a small number of centres worldwide. Dynamic MRI (long sequences of image acquisition with computer analysis) is currently a research tool but may well represent the future.

The radio-opaque marker study is the mainstay of evaluation of colonic transit. Though variations in technique exist in terms of the number of markers, interval to radiograph and definition of slow transit, the basic premise is that a number of markers (small pieces of plastic tubing, prepackaged in gelatin capsules) are ingested and an abdominal radiograph (which includes the pelvis) taken at an interval. The patient abstains from laxatives for the duration of the study. In patients with significant numbers of retained markers (based on control data), slow-transit constipation is diagnosed (***Figure 73.2***). Other studies of colonic transit, e.g. isotope scintigraphy and direct measurements of colonic contractile activity, are restricted to a very small number of specialist centres worldwide.

SCOPE OF DISEASE

A functional diagnosis is usually made when *routine* investigations fail to find an easy explanation (e.g. a structural or biochemical cause) for a combination of typical symptoms. For instance, in a patient with lower abdominal pain, constipation and bloating if routine investigation finds a morphological abnormality, e.g. sigmoid diverticulosis, then the patient will be given a diagnosis of diverticular disease. However, if all usual tests, including colonoscopy, yield no findings then the same patient might be described as having IBS – a functional intestinal disorder. Like much of medicine, there are however grey areas. Further, understanding is not aided by historic nomenclature where terms such as pseudo-obstruction describe different entities in the small and large intestine (***Table 73.2***). This chapter considers the main disorders using this classification with a focus on those most pertinent to the surgical reader.

TABLE 73.2 Scope of functional intestinal diseases.

History of onset	Visceral diameter	Region predominantly affected	Nomenclature
Acute	Dilated	Small intestine	Ileus (including postoperative ileus)
		Large intestine	Acute colonic pseudo-obstruction
Chronic	Dilated	Small intestine	Intestinal pseudo-obstruction
		Large intestine	Megacolon
Chronic	Normal	Intestine	Constipation and irritable bowel syndrome

ACUTE ADYNAMIC NEUROMUSCULAR STATES OF THE SMALL INTESTINE WITH DILATATION: ILEUS

Definition

Ileus can be defined as:

> ***a disruption of the normal propulsive ability of the intestine due to a malfunction of contractile activity in the absence of mechanical obstruction.***

This definition excepts certain older terms such as 'meconium ileus' and 'gallstone ileus' (see ***Chapters 17 and 78***) that persist in usage, although they are technically misnomers (i.e. there is mechanical obstruction). The term 'paralytic ileus', although descriptive for the student, is outdated and not entirely correct since studies show that motor activity is not abolished but rather dysregulated.

Causes and risk factors

The risk factors for ileus are listed in ***Summary box 73.3***. Postoperative ileus (POI) occurs in 10–20% of patients undergoing elective major abdominal surgery and is usually defined by a failure to tolerate oral intake or pass stool 72 hours after surgery.

Summary box 73.3

Risk factors for ileus

- Recent surgery: POI
- Local inflammation (peritonitis, severe acute pancreatitis)
- Systemic inflammation by any cause, e.g. sepsis, trauma
- Electrolyte disturbance (especially hypokalaemia and hypercalcaemia)
- Acute endocrine disturbance (hypothyroidism, diabetic ketoacidosis)
- Medications, e.g. opioids
- Acute CNS disease (especially high spinal transections)
- Intestinal ischaemia (mesenteric vascular disease)

Pathophysiology

Classic teaching points to a reflex inhibition of intestinal motility caused by deranged ANS inputs. This teaching, which fits nicely with basic 'fight and flight' concepts of increased sympathetic signalling and parasympathetic withdrawal during trauma (including surgery), has been superseded by the concept of a two-phase response. First, an immediate stress response, mediated by spinal reflexes and activation of the hypothalamic–pituitary–adrenal axis (HPA) axis, leads to a decrease or abolition of motility. This is then followed very rapidly by evolution of a more prolonged inflammatory response in the bowel wall itself, mediated first by mast cell activation and thence recruitment and activation of macrophages and neutrophils (***Figure 73.3***). These lead to inhibition of enteric neuronal and smooth muscle function as well as further effects on spinal reflexes.

Clinical features

Symptoms include abdominal distension and vomiting akin to mechanical small bowel obstruction (see ***Chapter 78***); however, colicky pain is less of a feature. On examination, other than evidence of the cause, e.g. recent surgery, the abdomen will be distended, tympanic and have reduced or absent bowel sounds.

Diagnosis

CT scanning is frequently required to exclude both mechanical obstruction and any local driver of ileus in the peritoneum such as inflammation or infection (***Figure 73.4***). In instances of POI this is required to exclude local complications of surgery. Blood tests should be used to detect any drivers of ileus such as metabolic abnormalities (especially hypokalaemia).

Management

Ileus may be managed by nasogastric drainage and restriction of oral intake until there is evidence of improvement. Supportive care such as attention to fluid and electrolyte balance and nutrition is also important, especially if ileus persists. Underlying drivers of ileus, e.g. abscess or peritonitis, should be managed on their merits. Regrettably, despite improved knowledge of the pathophysiology, specific drugs aimed at blocking inflammation or stimulating local neuromuscular function, e.g. prokinetics, have not proved sufficiently effective yet to be adopted for routine use.

In patients with POI, if prolonged, CT scanning is the most effective investigation; it will demonstrate any intra-abdominal sepsis or mechanical obstruction and therefore guide any

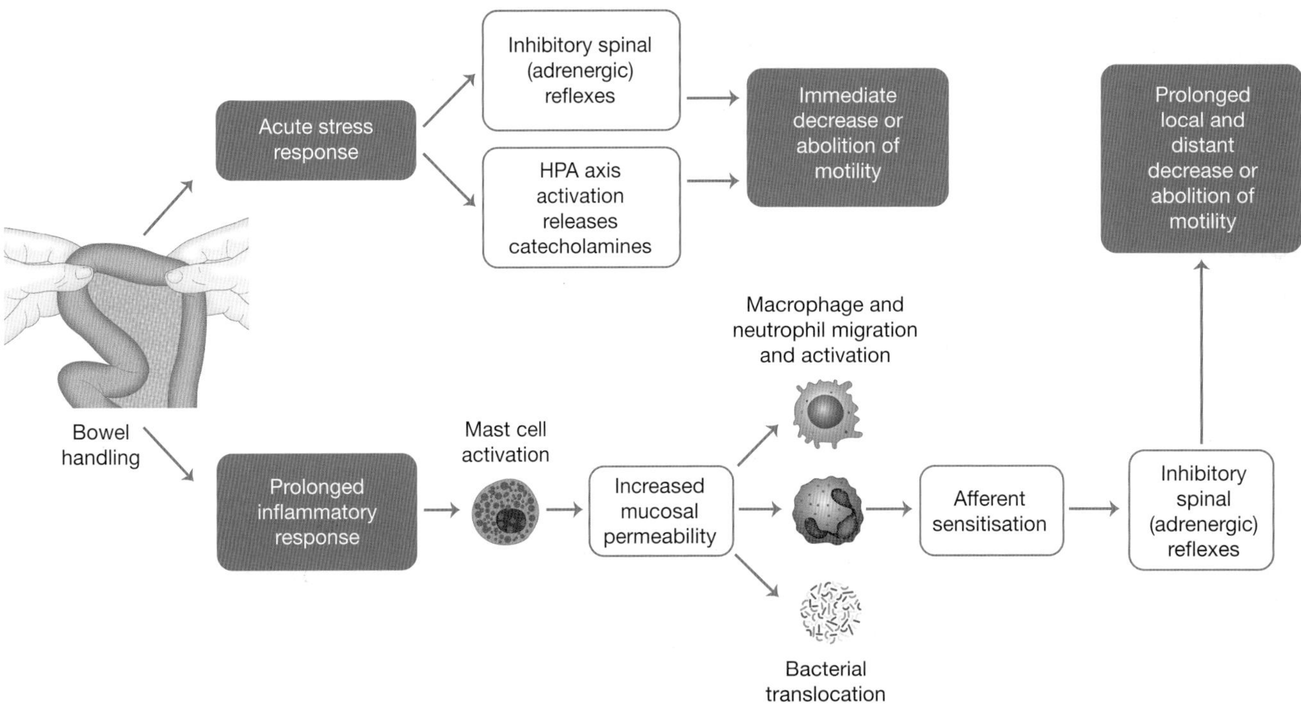

Figure 73.3 Pathophysiology of postoperative ileus. HPA, hypothalamic–pituitary–adrenal axis.

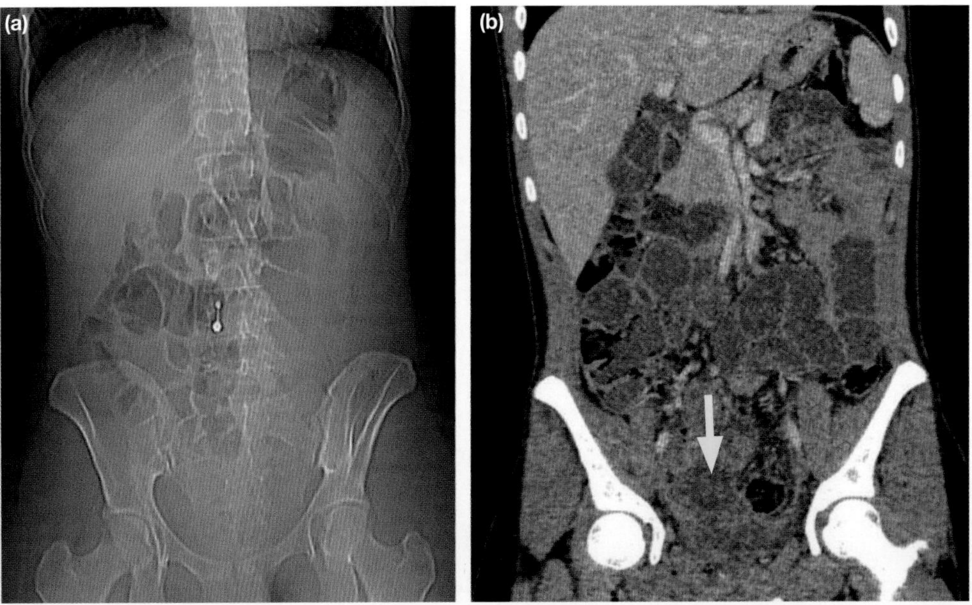

Figure 73.4 Computed tomography abdomen scout film (a) and representative coronal image (b) of a 22-year-old woman showing widespread dilatation of the small intestine (ileus) secondary to a driving inflammatory focus (pelvic collection, arrow) (courtesy of Dr Arman Parsai, Barts Health NHS Trust, London, UK).

requirement for laparotomy. Otherwise the decision to take a patient back to theatre in these circumstances is always difficult. The need for a laparotomy becomes increasingly likely the longer the bowel inactivity persists, particularly if it lasts for more than 7 days or if bowel activity recommences following surgery and then stops again.

Prevention

Minimally invasive surgical approaches have reduced risks of POI for many operations. The enhanced recovery programme (see *Chapter 74*) seeks to further reduce risk of POI by avoidance of opioid-containing drugs and suppression of the inflammatory response.

ACUTE ADYNAMIC NEUROMUSCULAR STATES OF THE LARGE INTESTINE WITH DILATATION: ACUTE COLONIC PSEUDO-OBSTRUCTION

Definition

The term acute colonic pseudo-obstruction (ACPO) is defined as:

> ***Acute massive dilatation of the colon with obstructive symptoms but in the absence of mechanical obstruction.***

ACPO was first described by Sir William Ogilvie, who in 1948 recognised this syndrome in two patients with sudden onset of abdominal pain, constipation and large bowel dilatation (hence the eponym Ogilvie's syndrome). It is one of the three common diagnoses in patients evaluated for a clinical presentation of large bowel obstruction (see ***Chapter 78***), the other two being colorectal cancer and volvulus (remember the three Ts: tumour, torsion and 'tired out'). Toxic megacolon (see ***Chapter 75***), although conveniently being a fourth 'T', should be considered as a different condition entirely although the end point is also one of acute dilatation.

Risk factors

In Ogilvie's original report, the clinical picture was associated with a retroperitoneal neoplasm infiltrating and destroying prevertebral ganglia. This is actually a very rare cause. The main risks are shown in ***Summary box 73.4***.

Summary box 73.4

Risk factors for acute colonic pseudo-obstruction

- Frailty and senility
  - Neurological
  - Neurodegenerative diseases
  - Stroke
  - Spinal cord injury
  - Retroperitoneum tumour infiltration
- Trauma/surgical
  - Major orthopaedic injuries or surgery, e.g. vertebral, pelvic and femoral
  - Major gynaecological surgery
  - Obstetrics, including caesarean section
- Systemic inflammation by any cause, e.g. sepsis, trauma, especially with multiorgan failure
- Localised infective conditions, e.g. respiratory, urinary
- Myocardial infarction
- Metabolic and electrolyte disturbances
- Medications, e.g. opioids and any with anticholinergic actions (e.g. psychiatric and Parkinson's), calcium channel antagonists

The majority of patients fall into two categories: those that have a high background risk and a small acute event (e.g. the elderly patient with Parkinson's disease and a urinary tract infection [UTI]) – the colon has little 'reserve' and a small insult tips the balance into one of progressive abolition of motility and tone with consequent gaseous dilatation; and those with little background risk and a large acute event, e.g. major surgery/trauma.

Pathophysiology

This is poorly understood. It can however be appreciated that, like ileus, risk factors reflect both 'imbalanced' extrinsic autonomic innervation and an 'inflammatory' state. Evidence to support the former is provided by the response to anticholinesterase pharmacological therapy.

Clinical features

Symptoms include abdominal distension, absolute constipation and, as a later feature, vomiting akin to mechanical large bowel obstruction (see ***Chapter 78***); however, colicky pain is less of a feature. The history is very important to establish risk factors, some of which may be modifiable. On abdominal examination, the abdomen is usually grossly distended and tympanic. In uncomplicated cases, the abdomen should not be tender. Tenderness and especially any evidence of peritonism indicate that massive colonic dilatation may have led to ischaemia with/without perforation – a surgical emergency. Such complications occur in 3–15% of patients with advanced age and increased caecal diameter, with a delay in decompression increasing risk.

Diagnosis relies upon accurate clinical observation and plain abdominal radiography showing degrees of colonic dilatation, mainly involving the proximal colon. CT is however the definitive investigation (***Figure 73.5***) to differentiate mechanical from pseudo-obstruction, to provide a caecal diameter and to show any evidence of complications (e.g. perforation). A CT scan will also differentiate pseudomembranous colitis with toxic dilatation, which is a further differential diagnosis in hospitalised or institutionalised patients due to *Clostridium difficile* infection.

Management

The management of ACPO depends on whether complications are evident or considered imminent. In patients with clinical and radiological features of caecal ischaemia or perforation, emergency surgery will be required and usually necessitates a subtotal colectomy and end ileostomy (with high levels of morbidity and mortality). The majority of patients can however follow a more stepwise approach, starting with conservative measures (***Table 73.3***). Clearly the underlying cause where relevant, e.g. UTI, respiratory tract infection or myocardial infarction, should also be managed in parallel. It is reasonable to wait before progressing from one stage to the

Sir William Heneage Ogilvie, 1887–1973, surgeon, Royal Army Medical Corps (First World War), Oxford, and Guy's Hospital, London, UK.
James Parkinson, 1755–1824, general practitioner of Shoreditch, London, UK, published 'An essay on the shaking palsy' in 1817.

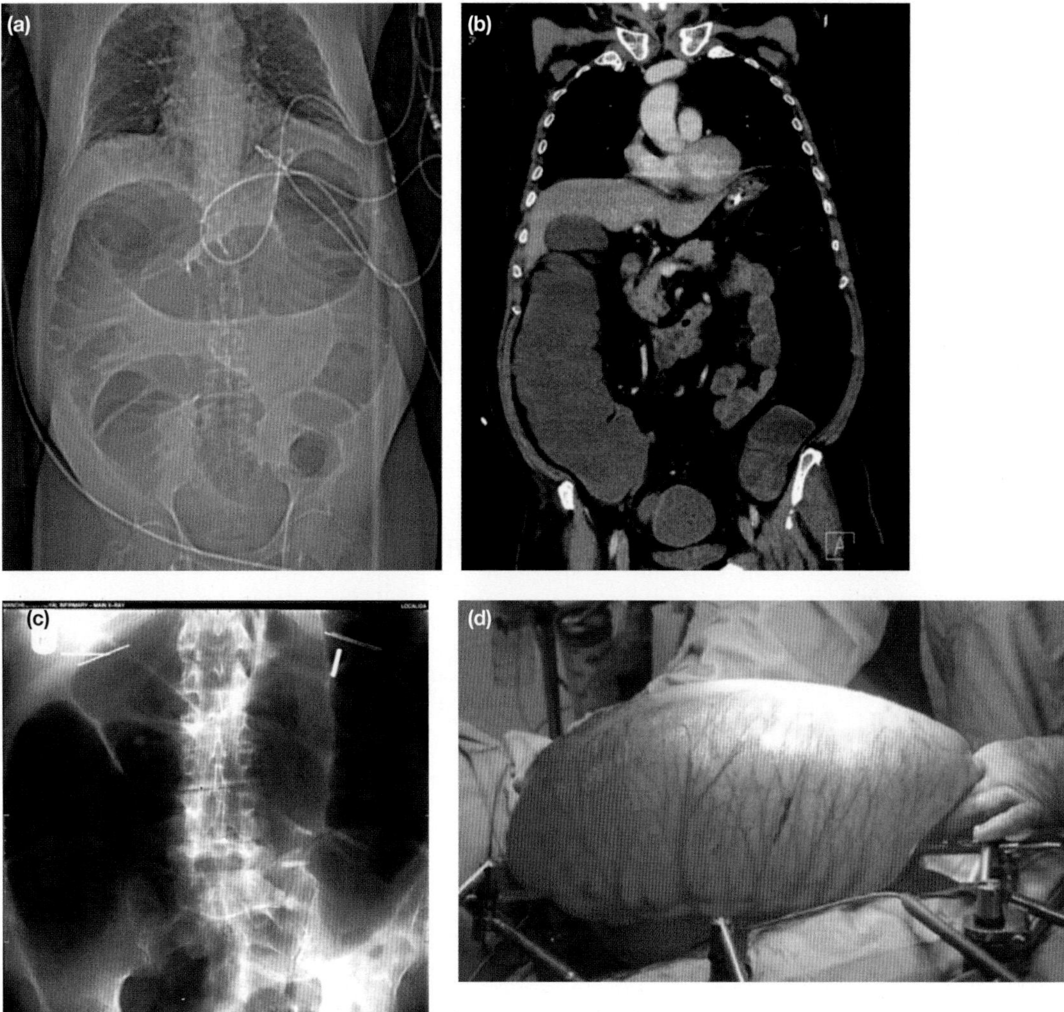

Figure 73.5 Scout film (a) and representative coronal computed tomography image (b) of a patient with acute colonic pseudo-obstruction. The entire colon and rectum is variably distended with fluid and gas. (c) Plain abdominal radiograph (courtesy of James Hill) and (d) intraoperative photograph of the colon during surgery for acute colonic pseudo-obstruction (courtesy of James Hill).

TABLE 73.3 Management of acute colonic pseudo-obstruction.

Reversal of risk factors	Correct fluid and electrolyte imbalances
	Stop or reduce offending drugs, e.g. opioids, anticholinergics, calcium channel blockers (where possible)
	Empty the rectum by enemas and/or flatus tube
Endoscopic decompression	Colonoscopy +/– flatus tube
Pharmacological decompression	Intravenous neostigmine unless contraindicated (risk of arrhythmia and bronchospasm[a])
Surgery	Subtotal colectomy (usually with ileostomy)
	Venting stoma, e.g. caecostomy, in very unfit patients

[a]Requires high-dependency unit-level monitoring and support on hand for cardiorespiratory complications.

next but caecal diameters of 12 cm or above warrant rapid decompression to reduce perforation risk.

The decision of whether to use intravenous neostigmine is difficult and is usually reserved for patients in whom supportive measures and colonic decompression have failed. Treatment is associated with profound autonomic effects (salivation, bradycardia, bronchospasm and hypotension) as well as abdominal cramps, followed often by a massive evacuation of flatus and faeces. Cardiac monitoring and a health professional competent in the emergency administration of resuscitative drugs (especially atropine) are essential. Contraindications to the use of neostigmine include renal insufficiency, recent myocardial infarct, arrhythmias and asthma.

Surgery is associated with high morbidity and mortality and should be reserved for those with impending perforation when other treatments have failed or perforation has occurred.

Prognosis

ACPO is a life-threatening condition in which prompt diagnosis and appropriate management can limit the occurrence of complications (e.g. ischaemia or perforation). Such complications occur in about 5–10% of patients and require emergency surgery with mortality rates between 30% and 60%. Recurrence is an issue in some patients with unmodifiable risk factors, e.g. senility and neurological disease. Such patients should have chronic modification of polypharmacy to avoid offending drugs and keep the rectum empty by regular enemas. Prokinetic medications, such as those used for chronic constipation, may have a role in such patients, although none are licensed for this indication.

CHRONIC IMPAIRMENT OF INTESTINAL MOTILITY WITH DILATATION OF THE SMALL INTESTINE: INTESTINAL PSEUDO-OBSTRUCTION

Definition

Intestinal pseudo-obstruction (IPO) is defined as:

> ***A clinical syndrome caused by severe impairment of intestinal motility leading to small intestinal dilatation in the absence of a mechanical cause.***

The term 'chronic' is sometimes added for clarity.

Causes

IPO is a rare disease. Approximately half of cases arise shortly after birth or in infancy, caused by a number of very rare enteric neuropathies and myopathies, including genetic and familial, inflammatory and degenerative forms. Other cases arise later in life when a secondary aetiology is more common. In some patients, a cause is not found and these are termed idiopathic. The full list of causes is given in ***Summary box 73.5***.

Summary box 73.5

Causes of intestinal pseudo-obstruction

Primary

- Several very rare enteric myopathies and neuropathies
- Unknown (termed 'idiopathic')

Secondary

- Connective tissue disease, especially scleroderma
- Radiation injury
- Amyloidosis
- Autonomic neuropathies including diabetes and paraneoplasia
- Infections: Chagas' disease (South American trypanosomiasis)

Diagnosis

IPO presents clinically with the symptoms and signs of small bowel obstruction with pain, distension and vomiting. After clinical evaluation and plain radiology, a degree of suspicion is helpful to avoid unnecessary and potentially harmful surgery. Such suspicion is merited when there is no obvious cause for mechanical obstruction, i.e. no known bowel disease, previous surgery or hernia, and on the length of history. Here, knowing the list of secondary causes becomes helpful. For instance, in someone who is a smoker with finger clubbing, a small cell carcinoma of the lung may be the cause of paraneoplastic pseudo-obstruction; alternatively, the patient may have clinical signs of scleroderma. Axial imaging is essential to exclude mechanical obstruction. Adjunctive blood and imaging tests may help define a cause and these can include MRI of the brain and skeletal muscle biopsy for rare diagnoses such as mitochondrial myopathies.

Primary neuropathies and myopathies can be diagnosed histologically, but this requires full-thickness tissue and a variety of special stains (available only in specialist centres). Since laparotomy and bowel resections are best avoided, a laparoscopic or minilaparotomy full-thickness biopsy may be warranted for diagnosis (***Figures 73.6 and 73.7***).

Management

The main lines of management are shown in ***Summary box 73.6***, noting that for most patients there is no cure. Surgery, with the exception of placing feeding tubes or formation of a venting stoma, is impotent for a condition that is a diffuse neuromuscular disease. Further, surgery worsens the prognosis by adding the risk of adhesions into the diagnosis and, if resections or complications occur, speeding the patient towards intestinal failure. Small bowel (or multivisceral) transplantation is an option in selected patients.

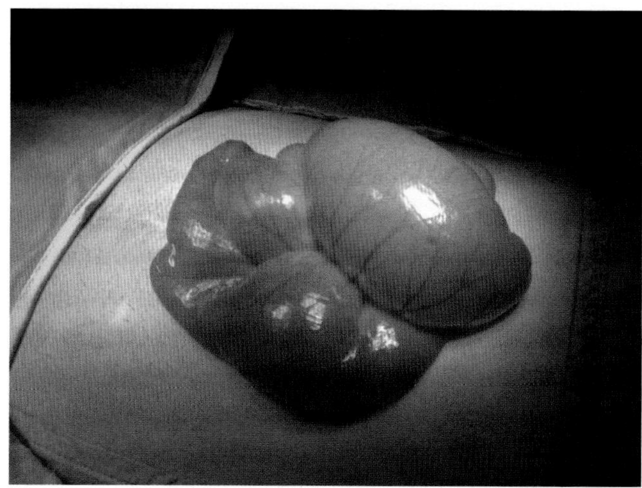

Figure 73.6 Intestinal pseudo-obstruction in a young male patient. A full-thickness biopsy was undertaken from the proximal jejunum at minilaparotomy.

Carlos Justiniano Ribeiro Chagas, 1879–1934, Director of the Oswaldo Cruz Institute and Professor of Tropical Medicine, University of Rio de Janeiro, Brazil.

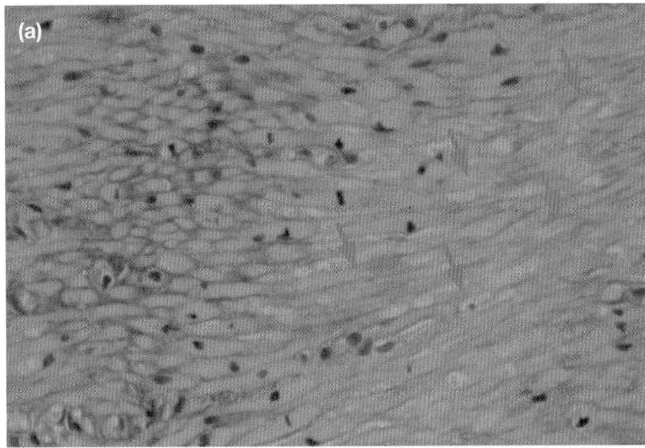

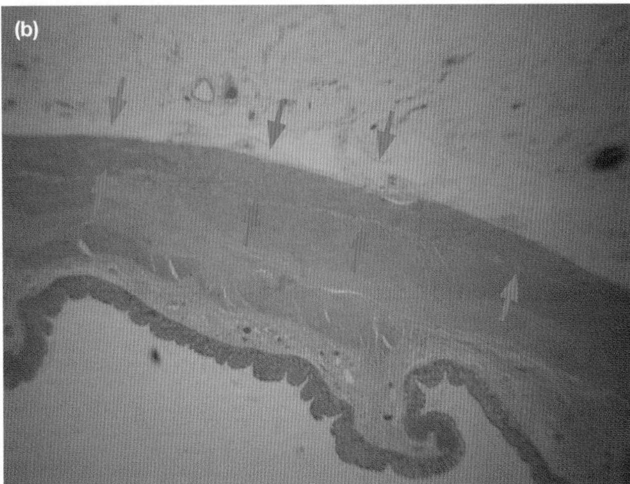

Figure 73.7 Two examples of myopathy: (a) hollow visceral myopathy (note the vacuolation of the smooth muscle, arrows); (b) extra muscle layer in the muscularis propria (arrows).

Summary box 73.6

Management of intestinal pseudo-obstruction

- Nutrition (enteral/parenteral)
- Analgesia (but try to avoid opioids)
- Prokinetics (generally disappointing)
- Antibiotics (overgrowth)
- Immunotherapy – specific inflammatory cases (limited data)
- Psychological support, including specific patient support groups
- Palliative care
- Surgery (very selected cases)

Prognosis

Prognosis is poor – sometimes considered the 'motor neurone disease' of the gut. Infantile forms have a mortality of approximately 50%. This is generally lower in adult forms depending on cause and avoiding repeated surgery and overuse of opioid drugs. Together these cause a vicious spiral of declining motility and progression to type II/III intestinal failure with the need for lifelong parenteral nutrition.

CHRONIC IMPAIRMENT OF INTESTINAL MOTILITY WITH DILATATION OF THE LARGE INTESTINE: MEGACOLON AND MEGARECTUM

Definition

Chronic dilatation in the absence of a mechanically obstructing cause can be focused in the colon (megacolon) or rectum (megarectum), although in practice these commonly overlap (***Figure 73.8***). Megacolon may also accompany some forms of IPO in patients found to have chronic small and large intestinal dilatation. Toxic megacolon refers to an acute condition in which acute inflammation leads to a loss of compliance and rapid dilatation (it has nothing in common other than the name).

Causes of megacolon and megarectum

Primary and secondary causes (***Table 73.4***) vary between megarectum and megacolon. The most common disease to use the term megacolon is Hirschsprung's disease (occurring in 1 in 5000 live births) (see ***Chapter 17***). Actually, in this instance, it can be argued that the so-called 'congenital megacolon' does in fact reflect a degree of distal obstruction from the distal contracted aganglionic segment. This leads to the absence of passage of meconium at birth and is generally incompatible with life without urgent surgery. Adult Hirschsprung's disease is a very rare disease and leads to a megarectum because the affected segment is 'ultrashort', affecting only the transition zone of the anus. Histologically, this is very difficult to diagnose with certainty and some challenge its existence at all.

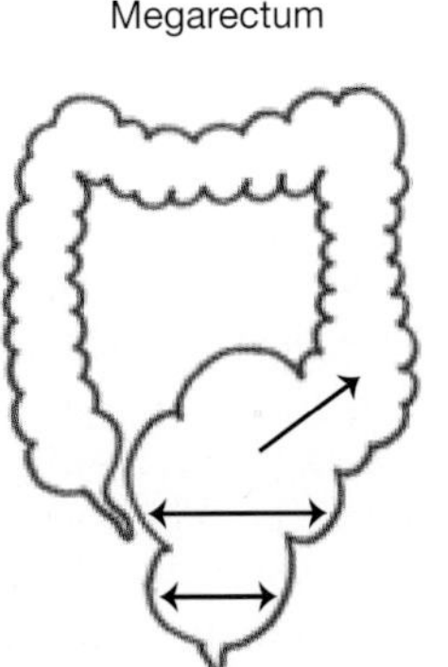

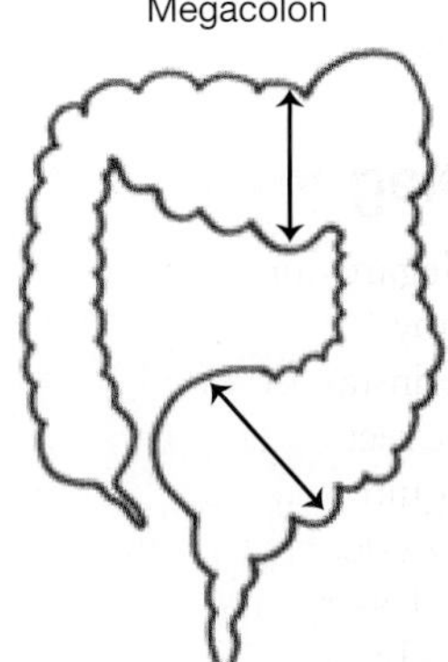

Figure 73.8 Schematic drawing of the distribution of bowel dilatation in megacolon and megarectum.

Harald Hirschsprung, 1830–1916, physician, The Queen Louise Hospital for Children, Copenhagen, Denmark, described congenital megacolon in 1887.

TABLE 73.4 Causes of megacolon and megarectum.

Megacolon	*Primary*	Congenital	Classic (rectosigmoid) Hirschsprung's disease
			Rare early-onset (some genetic) myopathies and neuropathies
		Acquired	Rare late-onset (some genetic mitochondrial) myopathies and neuropathies
			Unknown (termed 'idiopathic')
	Secondary	Genetic	Muscular dystrophy and other rare genetic muscle diseases
			MEN type 2B with ganglioneuromatosis
			Rare genetic autonomic neuropathies
		Acquired	CNS diseases, including senility, Parkinson's, dementias, amyloid and spinal cord injury
			Connective tissue disease, especially scleroderma
			Infections: Chagas' disease (South American trypanosomiasis)
			Autonomic neuropathies secondary to diabetes and paraneoplasia
Megarectum	*Primary*	Congenital	Ultrashort-segment Hirschsprung's disease (congenital megarectum)
			Inadequately resected Hirschsprung's disease (post reconstruction)
			Anorectal malformations (post reconstruction)
	Secondary	Congenital	Severe psychobehavioural + cognitive impairment (+ genetic)
		Acquired	Later-onset behavioural (autistic spectrum) disorders
			Sexual abuse; neglect; parental negativism

CNS, central nervous system; MEN, multiple endocrine neoplasia.

More common causes of megacolon include extreme senility and CNS neurodegenerative disease, resembling an attenuated form of ACPO. Others are denoted 'idiopathic' to reflect that no cause is established; this group, who are predominantly female, phenotypically resemble a severe form of slow-transit constipation (see ***Constipation***). All are rare.

Patients with megarectum are usually divided into two groups by clinicians. The first are those who have had previous surgery for Hirschsprung's disease or anorectal malformations in whom ongoing problems are common – due perhaps to surgical reconstruction or an as yet undetermined neuromuscular disease. The second, predominantly male, group are sometimes described as 'idiopathic'; however, nearly all, if assessed carefully, will have some form of psychobehavioural disorder. The pathogenesis is considered to be stool withholding in infancy or childhood, leading to chronic distension and loss of compliance.

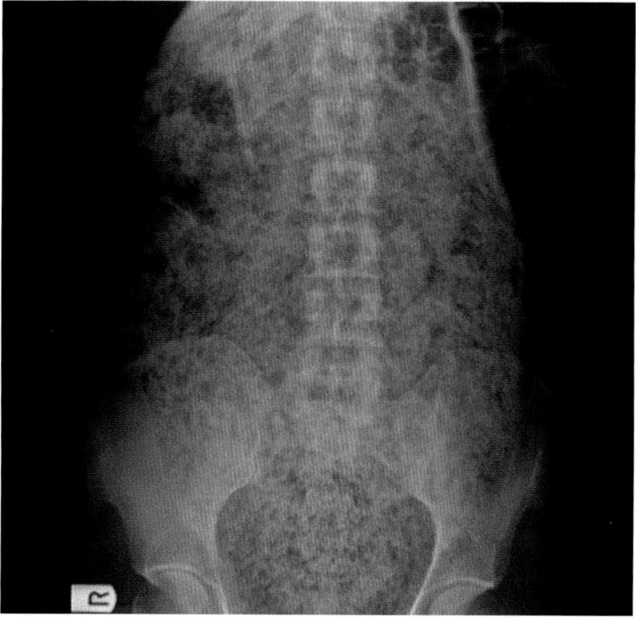

Figure 73.9 Plain abdominal radiograph of a teenage male with megarectum.

Diagnosis and management

Megarectum may present with a mass the size of a full-term baby (***Figure 73.9***) but diagnosis is mainly radiological. The mainstay of management of both (in brief) requires getting the rectum empty. In some patients with megarectum this may require manual disimpaction under anaesthesia. Thereafter, high doses of regular osmotic and simulant laxatives orally as well as regular enemas (or high-volume transanal irrigation (TAI); see ***Constipation***) are required to keep it empty. Prokinetics may also have a role. Compliance with medication is often an issue in young patients with psychobehavioural problems. Surgery has an important role in patients who fail medical management. Colectomy or subtotal colectomy is generally required for megacolon. A variety of options exist for megarectum. A first step may be an anterograde colonic enema (ACE) procedure (see ***Constipation***). If this fails, definitive surgery includes pull-through procedures, low anterior resection, restorative proctocolectomy and rectum-reducing procedures, e.g. vertical reduction rectoplasty. All should be undertaken with covering loop ileostomy and many advocate performing an ileostomy for 6 months to 1 year prior to surgery. This allows the rectum to shrink and reduce in vascularity, making eventual surgery safer; some patients may also simply choose to live with the ileostomy rather than risk pelvic surgery. The hazard of operating on a rectum that occupies the whole pelvis with serosal veins that sometimes resemble the iliac veins cannot be underestimated and surgery should be performed in specialist centres.

CHRONIC IMPAIRMENT OF INTESTINAL MOTILITY WITHOUT DILATATION

Constipation and IBS are very common conditions and collectively represent about a third of patients presenting to the average colorectal clinic in the Western world. They are presented here as separate entities to reflect the general approach of most physicians; however, the reader should be aware that there is very considerable overlap, especially between constipation and the constipation-predominant form of IBS (C-IBS). Patients can fulfil the criteria for both diagnoses concurrently or move between diagnoses over time.

Constipation

Definitions

'Constipation' is not a disease but rather a term often used by patients to describe dissatisfaction with their bowel function or their ability to defecate. As such it means different things to different patients (and different doctors) and can describe symptoms that directly relate to defecation, e.g. straining, or those considered consequent in the abdomen, e.g. pain and bloating. More formal definitions such as that of the American College of Gastroenterologists – 'unsatisfactory defecation, characterized by infrequent stools, difficult stool passage or both for at least 3 months' – cover most symptoms and introduce a time criterion to exclude patients with transient symptoms (sometimes called 'simple constipation'). Stricter definitions of 'chronic constipation' include a measure of resistance to treatment – 'unsatisfactory defecation characterized by infrequent stools, difficult stool passage or both for at least 6 months where this has proven unresponsive to lifestyle alterations and basic laxative therapy'.

Epidemiology

Self-reported constipation is very common, with a worldwide prevalence of about 10% (making it one of the commonest ailments in humans). Fortunately, patients with chronic constipation (based on 6 months of symptoms and failure of at least two laxatives) are much less common (approximately 0.5%). Most studies report a higher prevalence of self-reported constipation in women than in men with a ratio of 2:1. The ratio is much higher for chronic constipation at approximately 9:1 female to male.

Risk factors

The vast majority of patients with chronic constipation lack a single unifying cause for their problems. The main associated medical conditions and diseases within the gastrointestinal tract itself are listed in ***Table 73.5***.

Diagnosis

Clinical history

A thorough history will determine whether constipation represents a new complaint, i.e. one indicative of a change

TABLE 73.5 Risk factors for constipation.

Gastrointestinal causes	
Mechanical obstruction	Benign and malignant strictures
Functional obstruction	Pelvic organ prolapse syndromes (dynamic obstruction at the level of the anorectum)
	Megarectum
	Anal pain, e.g. chronic fissure
Medical causes	
Metabolic disorders	Hypercalcaemia, uraemia, hypokalaemia, hypomagnesaemia
Endocrine disorders	Hypothyroidism, diabetes, pregnancy
Neurological disorders	Degenerative CNS diseases, e.g. multiple sclerosis, Parkinson's, cerebrovascular disease, spinal or pelvic nerve lesions, autonomic neuropathies, cognitive impairment
Drugs	Opioids
	Anticholinergics
	Calcium channel blockers
Psychological	Severe endogenous depression
	Eating disorders
	Cognitive behavioural disorders
Other	Connective tissue diseases
	Joint hypermobility
	Causes of immobility, e.g. degenerative joint disease

CNS, central nervous system.

in bowel habit. The patient should be asked specifically about the frequency and consistency of bowel movements and the progress of such changes over time (as well as other alarm symptoms such as rectal bleeding and weight loss). With additional information regarding family history, previous colon cancer screening and other gastrointestinal investigations, an informed decision can be made whether intraluminal investigation of the colon is required. Other organic causes of constipation may be deduced by appropriate history taking and biochemical investigation. With the exclusion of treatable secondary causes, if the history is short and multiple previous therapies have not already been tried, the patient may be first considered to have 'simple' constipation that can be managed with reassurance and lifestyle advice (fibre, fluids and exercise) with/without simple laxative therapy.

In patients with chronic symptoms, after exclusion of a secondary cause, the focus should shift to the investigation and management of chronic constipation. Many patients may attribute the start of symptoms to a major life event. Common among these are hysterectomy and childbirth, other abdominal surgeries or trauma. Constipation can also be associated with previous abuse and it may sometimes be necessary to tactfully seek a history of physical or sexual abuse. Other patients will have no such triggers, having had symptoms from childhood and on occasion from infancy. Such patients are overwhelmingly female (>95%) and on investigation are often found to have generalised slow-transit constipation as opposed to other pathophysiological findings (this group, who represent 5–10% of patients with chronic constipation, are variably referred to in the literature are 'idiopathic slow-transit constipation' or 'colonic inertia'). It is helpful to systematically document the main symptoms that in the patient's mind constitute a problem since this has some bearing on treatment decisions and subsequent monitoring of effectiveness. Several questions form detailed scoring systems to systematically facilitate this in a research context. However, in routine practice it is sufficient to list in the patient's record the presence or absence of several common symptoms (***Summary box 73.7***). The presence of prolapse symptoms reflects the overlap between diagnoses in patients with pelvic floor disorders (see ***Chapter 80***). The remaining history should document prescribed and self-administered laxatives (and therapeutic benefit thereof) and also gain an impression of the quality of diet in respect of fibre and fluid intake.

Summary box 73.7

Symptoms to directly question in patients with constipation

Abdominal symptoms
- Abdominal pain
- Bloating

Defecatory symptoms
- Frequency of spontaneous or assisted bowel opening
- Painful defecation
- Stool consistency (can use Bristol stool scale)
- Digitation (vaginal or anal)
- Straining
- Incomplete/unsuccessful evacuation
- Leakage/incontinence
- Prolapse

Other pelvic symptoms
- Vaginal bulging or prolapse
- Urinary incontinence

Clinical examination

Poor nutritional status should prompt a search for a secondary cause, including occult carcinoma, more widespread intestinal motility disorders such as IPO (see ***Chronic impairment of intestinal motility with dilatation of the small intestine: intestinal pseudo-obstruction***) and eating disorders. An abdominal examination should be conducted to look for scars, any significant abdominal distension, tenderness or masses. Bloating is a common and expected finding with chronic constipation, but significant distension, tenderness or masses should prompt a full investigation.

All patients presenting with constipation should undergo a rectal examination. The perineum and anus should be examined for evidence of faecal incontinence that may indicate impaction and overflow. Some degree of faecal incontinence and chronic constipation coexists in 40% of patients; marked soiling of the underwear is especially associated with the rarer diagnosis of megarectum. Scarring, e.g. from episiotomy, sentinel pile formation secondary to an underlying anal fissure, external haemorrhoids or prolapse, may also be present. The degree of perineal descent on straining, indicative of pelvic floor weakness, should also be determined visually (>3 cm is usually considered abnormal). A digital rectal examination will diagnose impaction, gain a rough measure of anal tone at rest and on squeeze and ascertain obvious sphincter defects. An effort should be made to look for any anterior defect in the rectovaginal septum leading to a rectocele. Anoscopy and proctoscopy should be performed if there is any history of rectal bleeding and may indicate fissure or internal piles. A urogynaecological examination is desirable in all patients with suspected pelvic multi-organ prolapse.

Investigations

While findings from history or physical examination may indicate a secondary cause of constipation, making further investigation mandatory, it is also typical practice in patients with chronic constipation to exclude certain secondary causes by investigation even though the diagnostic utility of such investigations is acknowledged to be low (the commonest undiagnosed systemic disease is hypothyroidism). Thus, serum electrolyte, creatinine, calcium, glucose, haemoglobin levels and thyroid function tests are usually performed. The approach taken to structural investigation of the colon when patients have no suspected intraluminal pathology varies on the basis of available resource and may include colonoscopy.

In patients with chronic constipation in whom basic laxatives have failed, further specialist investigative tests may be warranted. Colonic transit can be investigated by a radio-opaque marker study (***Figure 73.2***). In addition, rectal sensory testing and evacuation proctography will determine if the patient has a functional or dynamic structural cause of evacuation disorder. Problems such as dyssynergic defecation (functional) and intussusception/rectocele (structural) may occur in isolation or coexist with transit disturbances (*Figure 73.10*).

Management

The treatment of chronic constipation follows a stepwise progression from lifestyle changes through potentially to major surgery in a small minority of patients. *Table 73.6* lists the main available approaches, noting where some apply only to certain diagnoses derived from the results of specialist tests of colonic and anorectal function. *Figure 73.11* provides a basic algorithm to accompany *Table 73.6*.

Patients with chronic constipation have generally had symptoms for many years and will have tried a number of remedies and prescribed laxatives. They will also usually have tried to address lifestyle modifications. Before resorting to specialist tests, it is possible to try and rationalise laxative therapy and provide a programme of nurse-led behavioural interventions. In regard to laxatives, current advice is to stop current laxatives (unless these are working well) and then titrate an oral osmotic laxative, e.g. polyethylene glycol (PEG), until the stool form is soft or liquid. If this is insufficient then a stimulant laxative such as bisacodyl may be added. If symptoms of obstructed defecation predominate then rectal laxatives in the form of suppositories or enemas may be tried with or without continuation of oral laxatives. The failure of such drugs should then prompt a trial of one of the newer prokinetic or secretagogue

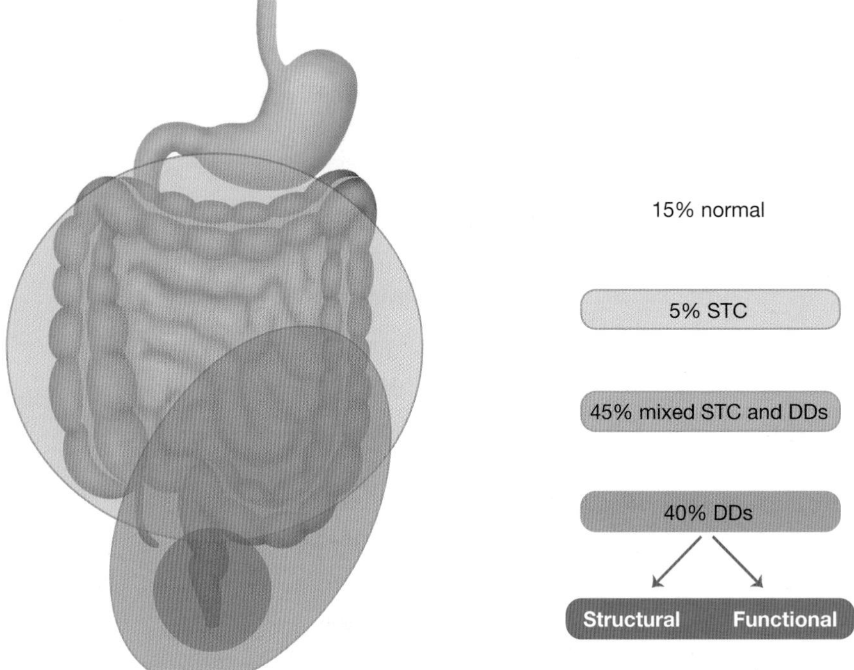

Figure 73.10 Schematic overview of pathophysiology of chronic constipation. DD, defecation disorder; STC, slow-transit constipation.

TABLE 73.6 Treatment options in patients with chronic constipation.

Lifestyle	Increase fluid intake
	Dietary modification, e.g. increased fibre
	Increase exercise
	Reduce body mass (pelvic floor prolapse syndromes)
Drugs	Oral laxatives (favoured for slow transit)
	Rectal laxatives (favoured for rectal evacuation disorders)
	Prokinetics, e.g. prucalopride
	Secretagogues, e.g. linaclotide
Behavioural therapies	Habit training
	Habit training with direct visual biofeedback (favoured for dyssynergic defecation)
	Pelvic floor muscle training (favoured for pelvic floor prolapse syndromes)
Transanal irrigation	High- or low-volume systems available
Surgery	See *Summary box 73.8*

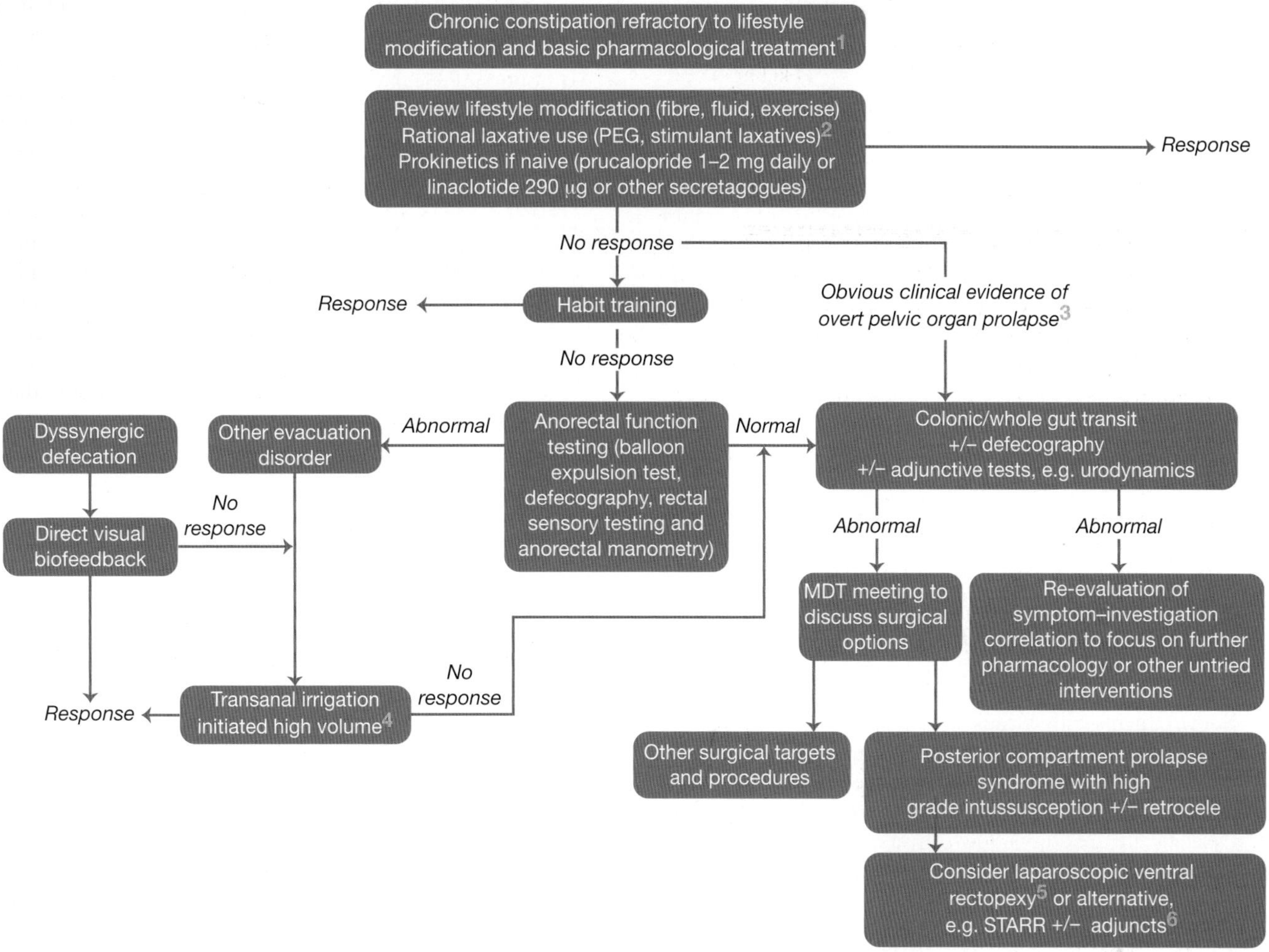

Chronic constipation refractory to lifestyle modification and basic pharmacological treatment[1]

Review lifestyle modification (fibre, fluid, exercise)
Rational laxative use (PEG, stimulant laxatives)[2]
Prokinetics if naive (prucalopride 1–2 mg daily or linaclotide 290 μg or other secretagogues)

Response

No response

Habit training

Response

No response

Obvious clinical evidence of overt pelvic organ prolapse[3]

Anorectal function testing (balloon expulsion test, defecography, rectal sensory testing and anorectal manometry)

Abnormal

Normal

Dyssynergic defecation

Other evacuation disorder

Direct visual biofeedback

No response

Transanal irrigation initiated high volume[4]

Response

No response

Colonic/whole gut transit +/– defecography +/– adjunctive tests, e.g. urodynamics

Abnormal

Abnormal

MDT meeting to discuss surgical options

Re-evaluation of symptom–investigation correlation to focus on further pharmacology or other untried interventions

Other surgical targets and procedures

Posterior compartment prolapse syndrome with high grade intussusception +/– retrocele

Consider laparoscopic ventral rectopexy[5] or alternative, e.g. STARR +/– adjuncts[6]

Figure 73.11 Algorithm of chronic constipation management. MDT, multidisciplinary team; PEG, polyethylene glycol. 1, alarm features excluded and secondary causes treated appropriately; 2, in constipation-predominant irritable bowel syndrome, consider antispasmodics or neuromodulators in case constipation improves but abdominal pain persists and is dominant symptom; 3, examples of overt prolapse include anterior (stage 3 cystocele), middle (stage 3 rectocele, uterovaginal prolapse) and posterior compartments (grade IV/V intussusception); 4, unless patient preference for low volume or specific contraindications to high volume; 5, may reduce specific symptoms but not have overall effect on quality of life; 6, common adjuncts include sacrocolpopexy, hysterectomy, transvaginal tape and cystocele repair.

drugs. These drugs are successful in a proportion of patients but do have some unwanted side effects (that the patient should be warned about). All drugs should be tried daily for a minimum of 4 weeks before concluding that they are ineffective and the reactionary use of laxatives, i.e. in response to being constipated, rather than their preventative use, should be strongly discouraged.

The most common form of behavioural intervention is often described by the term 'habit training'. This involves optimising dietary patterns to maximise gastrocolic response and the morning clustering of colonic high-amplitude propagated contractions that propel contents towards the rectum for subsequent evacuation. Dietary advice to optimise intake of liquid and fibre is given as well as advice about frequency and length of toilet visits and posture (***Figure 73.12***). Patients are also instructed on basic gut anatomy and function and gain an appreciation of how psychological and social stresses may influence gut functioning. Simple pelvic floor and balloon expulsion exercises are often included. Such appointments also

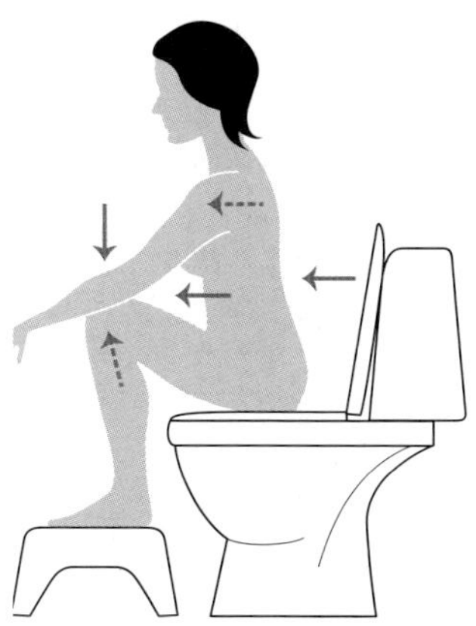

Figure 73.12 Correct posture for defecation.

offer an opportunity to further rationalise and monitor laxative therapy.

If this fails, there may be recourse to the specialist tests to assess colonic transit and also anorectal function (see *Chapter 80*). Armed with the results of these tests, the patient may have a more targeted approach relative to their observed pathophysiology. One example of this approach is for patients with a condition termed 'dyssynergic defecation', where there is a failure to relax, or even paradoxical contraction of the pelvic floor muscles (especially puborectalis) during defecatory efforts. In such patients, instrument-based biofeedback learning techniques provide direct visual computer-based biofeedback of pelvic floor activity. The aim is to retrain the patient to appropriately contract abdominal and relax pelvic floor muscles during defecation with the patient receiving feedback of anal and pelvic floor muscle activity as recorded by surface electromyographic anal pressure sensors or digital examination by the therapist.

Transanal irrigation (TAI) may be used for any patient with an evacuation disorder when habit training and/or biofeedback have failed. A number of devices are available that administer a low (approximately 50–100 mL) or high volume (approximately 500 mL) of irrigant fluid into the rectum. The patient sits on the toilet to evacuate the fluid and faecal material.

Some patients with chronic refractory symptoms may seek a surgical solution to their problem. Surgical procedures can be broadly divided into those addressing dynamic structural problems of the pelvic floor (prolapse procedures), those that seek specifically to address slow-transit constipation and those that may have a role for both (*Summary box 73.8*).

Summary box 73.8

Surgical options in patients with chronic constipation

Prolapse procedures for dynamic structural causes of obstructed defecation

- Hitching procedures, e.g. rectopexy
- Rectal wall excisional procedures, e.g. stapled transanal rectal resection (STARR)
- Rectovaginal reinforcement procedures, e.g. posterior vaginal repair, intra-anal Delorme's procedure

Procedures for slow-transit constipation

- Colectomy and ileorectal anastomosis
- Other variants of subtotal colectomy

Procedures for refractory chronic constipation in general

- Stoma: ileostomy or colostomy
- ACE procedures
- Neuromodulation

All surgery should be undertaken in the knowledge that none of the above-listed operations is perfect. All represent a trade-off between benefits and short-term harms and poor long-term functional outcomes. On this basis, the following are essential requirements before surgery is undertaken:

- pathophysiological findings from specialist tests concur with the symptomatology and findings on clinical examination;
- conservative (non-surgical) treatment options have been tried;
- the patient's case has been reviewed at a multidisciplinary team (MDT) meeting and surgery recommended;
- the patient has been consented in the very clear knowledge of the range of possible outcomes;
- surgery is undertaken in a centre with expertise in managing functional conditions.

The range of procedures for rectal prolapse are covered in detail in *Chapter 79*. Those primarily targeting the intestine are covered briefly here.

Colectomy

Colectomy is a radical and clearly irreversible final solution for patients with refractory slow-transit constipation. Its use should be very highly selective, not least because it is not actually a solution for many patients even when the surgery itself passes without complication. Removal of the whole colon with ileorectal anastomosis (as performed for inflammatory bowel disease) is best studied; subtotal resections with ileosigmoid or caecorectal anastomosis are alternatives. Outcomes vary greatly and are often compromised by early problems of ileus and a higher than expected rate of adhesional small bowel obstruction. Later problems include ongoing constipation and obstructive symptoms, diarrhoea and urgency, abdominal pain and bloating. Embarking on this procedure requires very careful MDT review, documentation of generalised slow-transit constipation and exclusion of a long list of relative contraindications.

Stoma

A stoma may be used as a definitive procedure, as a guide to further treatment or as salvage from a failed or complicated prior surgical intervention. There are few published data to support evidence-based use; however, an ileostomy may be employed as a guide to colectomy with subsequent resection avoided if ileostomy output is unsatisfactorily high or symptoms such as pain and bloating are untouched by diversion. As a definitive procedure, there is little evidence in adults to guide the choice of ileostomy or colostomy; however, it is generally considered that slow-transit constipation is unsatisfactorily treated by colostomy.

Anterograde colonic enema procedures

The formation of a conduit to introduce irrigant into the colon is best established in children and in patients with neurological disease. A variety of methods have been proposed to access the caecum either directly, e.g. with a Chait tube caecostomy, or indirectly via the appendix (appendicostomy). The latter is almost certainly preferable although only possible when the

Edmond Delorme, 1847–1929, French military surgeon and Professor of Surgery, Val-de-Grace Military Hospital, Paris, France.
Peter Graham Chait, contemporary, radiologist, Toronto, Canada.

native appendix is still present and the patient is not obese. The appendix can be reversed (Malone anterograde continent enema technique) or used in its native orientation (much simpler). Outcomes in adults with chronic constipation are variable but generally this is a good option in patients considering colectomy or stoma as the only alternative.

Neuromodulation

The attraction of being able to treat chronic constipation with a minimally invasive and safe approach such as sacral neuromodulation is supported by research data showing that stimulation improves motility and also some observational data. It is now clear from randomised trials that it has no role for slow-transit constipation but it may yet have a place in modifying anorectal function in some patients with severe functional syndromes leading to obstructed defecation (as it does for the bladder).

Irritable bowel syndrome

Surgery has no role in treating IBS. Nevertheless, patients with chronic abdominal pain and a change in their bowels are very common in surgical clinics and all surgeons should at least have a passing familiarity with a disorder that is a source of misery to millions of people worldwide.

Definitions

IBS is a functional bowel disorder characterised by abdominal pain or discomfort, stool irregularities and bloating. The term replaced nineteenth century descriptions such as 'irritable' or 'spastic' colon in 1979 to reflect the fact that the colon is not the only site of the problem. Diagnostic criteria have evolved to the now used Rome IV Foundation definition:

> ***Recurrent abdominal pain on average at least 1 day/week in the last 3 months, associated with two or more of three criteria: (1). related to defecation; (2). associated with a change in the frequency of stool and (3). associated with a change in the form (appearance) of stool. These criteria should be fulfilled for the last 3 months with symptom onset at least 6 months prior to diagnosis.***

The change in frequency and form of the stool dictates subdivisions of IBS into constipation-predominant (IBS-C), diarrhoea-predominant (IBS-D) and mixed (IBS-M) subclasses (***Figure 73.13***).

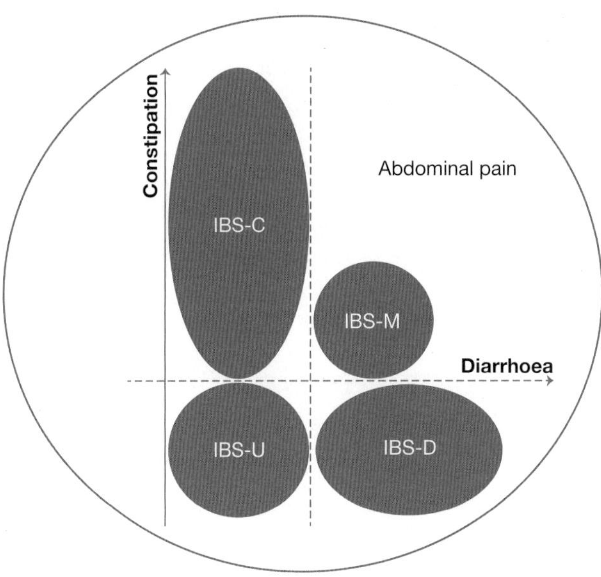

Figure 73.13 Irritable bowel syndrome (IBS) subtypes according to the Rome criteria. All patients have abdominal pain but subtypes vary according to bowel form at presentation such as to meet criteria for IBS with constipation (IBS-C), IBS with diarrhoea (IBS-D), mixed-type IBS (IBS-M) and unsubtyped (IBS-U).

Aetiology and risk factors

Regardless of exact definition, the cardinal symptoms of chronic abdominal pain and 'deranged digestion' favour a 'biopsychosocial model' (***Figure 73.14***) that encompasses the role of stressful life events and brain–gut interactions in symptom generation. Several common life events are particularly well documented; these include postinfective IBS, where a seemingly discrete attack of gastroenteritis (viral, bacterial or otherwise) is followed by chronic ongoing symptoms; physical and/or sexual abuse (and neglect); surgery; and trauma. One implication of the model is that IBS has much overlap with other medical conditions that have similar or nearly identical biopsychosocial determinants (***Summary box 73.9***).

Summary box 73.9

IBS-associated comorbidities

General

- Fibromyalgia syndrome
- Chronic fatigue syndrome
- Chronic pelvic pain, chronic prostatitis and bladder pain syndromes
- Chronic back pain
- Migraines
- Depression
- Anxiety
- Somatisation
- Sleep disturbance

Gastrointestinal disorders[a]

- Eating disorders
- Dyssynergic defecation
- Levator ani syndrome and proctalgia fugax
- Food intolerances

[a]The overlap of IBS with other Rome-defined functional gastrointestinal disorders should also be noted, including functional dyspepsia and functional constipation.

Patrick Malone, contemporary, surgeon, Southampton, UK.

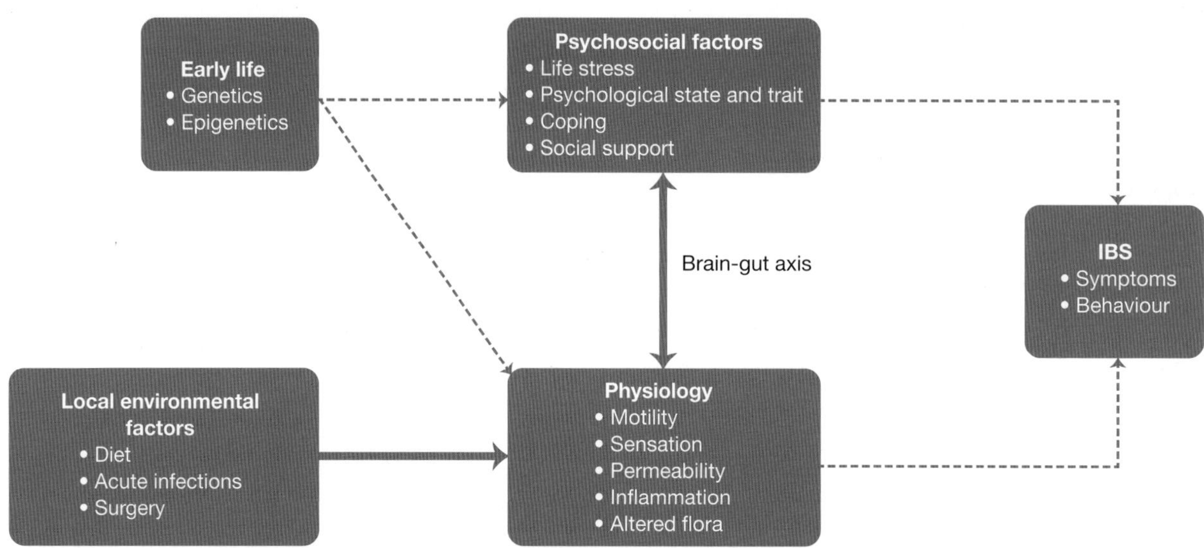

Figure 73.14 Biopsychosocial model of irritable bowel syndrome (IBS). The scheme is a conceptualisation of the pathogenesis and clinical expression of IBS showing interrelationships between various risk factors and changes in physiology.

Diagnosis

Clinical history

Besides symptoms required by the diagnostic criteria, other symptoms may be present. Common associated symptoms include bloating (very common), straining at defecation, excessive flatulence and postprandial indigestion. A history of precipitating events (as per the model) and of comorbidities (*Summary box 73.7*) should also be sought to support the diagnosis. The patient may also have a history of multiple operations, which on reflection may have been directed to chronic abdominal pain, e.g. appendicectomy, cholecystectomy or hysterectomy.

Clinical examination

Physical examination helps to reassure patients and also to exclude another organic cause for symptoms. However, abdominal examination rarely discloses a specific diagnosis (abdominal tenderness is often present but non-specific); the absence of objective findings supports a diagnosis of IBS. A digital rectal examination may identify patients with dyssynergic defecation and other causes of constipation.

Investigations

There are no valid laboratory biomarkers of IBS. Routine blood panels, including inflammatory markers, are generally

TABLE 73.7 Treatments for irritable bowel syndrome.

Nutrition	Increased (constipation) or reduced (bloating) fibre
	Gluten-free diet (especially if equivocal diagnosis of coeliac disease)
	FODMAP diet
	Probiotics
	Consider dietary supplements, prebiotics
Drugs	Antispasmodics: peppermint oil, hyoscine butylbromide (Buscopan)
	Laxatives, e.g. stool softeners, osmotic and stimulant (avoid lactulose because of bloating and pain)
	Antidiarrhoeals: loperamide (μ-opioid receptor agonist); 5-HT_3 receptor antagonists, such as alosetron, ondansetron
	Motility accelerants, e.g. linaclotide (guanylyl cyclase C agonist), prucalopride (5-HT_4 receptor agonist)
	Low-dose antidepressants: tricyclics and selective serotonin reuptake inhibitors
	Manipulation of the microbiota by non-absorbable antibiotics, e.g. rifaximin
	Neuromodulators, e.g. gabapentin and pregabalin
Psychotherapy	Cognitive–behavioural therapy
	Gut-directed hypnosis
	Guided self-help interventions

5-HT, 5-hydroxytryptamine; FODMAP, fermentable oligosaccharides, disaccharides, monosaccharides and polyols.

performed to reassure that there are no indicators of organic disease, e.g. cancer, inflammatory bowel disease or diverticular disease. Specific tests include serological tests for coeliac disease, faecal calprotectin and stool microbiology in cases of diarrhoea predominance. Invasive procedures are generally not warranted unless alarm features are present that mandate endoscopy. That noted, it is quite common practice to perform colonoscopy, not least to reassure the patient that their chronic symptoms do not have an organic basis. In patients with IBS-D, colonoscopy with random biopsies is warranted to exclude microscopic colitis. Other tests that may be relevant include (75Se-homocholic acid taurine [^{75}SeHCAT] test or serum serum 7-α-hydroxy-4-cholesten-3-one (C4) levels) for bile salt malabsorption, breath testing for carbohydrate malabsorption, gastrointestinal physiology for constipation and upper gastrointestinal endoscopy for associated dyspeptic symptoms.

Management

Only a fraction of patients with IBS-like symptoms seek medical care and most will initially consult primary care physicians for their symptoms. The factors that drive this consultation are symptom severity, especially pain, and concerns that symptoms might indicate an underlying severe disease, e.g. cancer. Therefore, in many cases, the doctor's role is to exclude diseases that can mimic IBS symptoms by relevant investigations such as endoscopy.

When a positive diagnosis of IBS has been made, management requires an integrated approach, including education, reassurance, dietary alterations, pharmacotherapy and behavioural or psychological interventions/support. The initial treatment strategy should be based on predominant symptoms and includes antispasmodics for abdominal pain, antidiarrhoeals for IBS-D and laxatives for IBS-C, whereas nutritional interventions and psychotherapy can be used in all subtypes. ***Table 73.7*** provides a list of potential management strategies for IBS. This list is not all encompassing, nor does it provide weighting to one treatment over another in terms of effectiveness in clinical trials. Some treatments are popular, e.g. low-dose antidepressants but such use is off-label; others may be tried over the counter by patients, e.g. prebiotics, although there is no trial evidence.

A key point in the management of IBS rests with notable exclusions from ***Table 73.7***. Thus the table makes no reference to standard analgesics and surgery. Opioid analgesia should be avoided in IBS because the further disturbance to motility worsens the prognosis and in extreme use can lead to narcotic bowel syndrome (an opioid-induced state of hyperalgesia whose main driver is the activation of glial cells). Surgery has a well-documented association with symptom onset of IBS (cholecystectomy, appendicectomy, hysterectomy and back surgery); further surgery leads not only to greater potential visceral sensitisation (via injury) but also serves to confuse subsequent diagnosis, e.g. adhesional versus functional cause for symptoms. There is also a body of evidence to suggest that surgery perpetuates a search for an 'organic' diagnosis that hinders patient acceptance and adaption to their chronic problem. For the surgeon, the key is to exclude any surgical cause of pain and then prevent further harm by avoiding surgery.

SUMMARY

Functional intestinal disorders range from the very common – constipation and IBS – through to the very rare, e.g. various genetic and familial neuropathies and myopathies causing IPO. The surgeon will almost certainly encounter acute problems such as POI and ACPO. This chapter provides an overview that can be supplemented by the recommended further reading.

FURTHER READING

Bharucha A, Knowles CH. Chronic constipation. In: Sagar PM, Hill AG, Knowles CH *et al.* (eds). *Keighley & Williams' surgery of the anus, rectum and colon*, 4th edn. Boca Raton, FL: Taylor & Francis, 2019: 305–46.

Enck P, Aziz Q, Barbara G *et al.* Irritable bowel syndrome. *Nat Rev Dis Primers* 2016; **2**: 16014.

van Bree SHW, Nemethova A, Cailotto C *et al.* New therapeutic strategies for postoperative ileus. *Nat Rev Gastroenterol Hepatol* 2012; **9**: 675–83.

CHAPTER 74 The small intestine

Learning objectives

To appreciate:
- The basic anatomy and physiology of the small intestine
- The range of conditions that may affect the small intestine

To understand:
- The aetiology and pathology of common small intestinal conditions
- The principles of investigation of small intestinal symptoms
- The importance of non-surgical management of small intestinal problems
- The principles of small intestinal surgery
- That complex intestinal problems are best managed by a multidisciplinary team

ANATOMY OF THE SMALL INTESTINE

Although the duodenum is anatomically indistinguishable from the rest of the small intestine, in surgical terms it may be regarded as a distinct structure and is discussed in ***Chapter 67***. The small intestine lies between the duodenojejunal (DJ) flexure and the ileocaecal valve (***Figure 74.1***). It is difficult to establish the length of the small intestine. It varies widely between subjects (it is said to be longer in men) and estimates gathered at surgery, at postmortem and during radiological investigations have been noted to vary widely, even in the same individual. Most studies however describe a range between 300 and 850 cm.

The proximal 40% of the small intestine is referred to as the jejunum and the remainder is the ileum. There is no clear demarcation between jejunum and ileum, as the character of the small intestine changes gradually from proximal to distal. The jejunum tends to have a wider diameter and a thicker wall, with more prominent mucosal folds (valvulae conniventes), while the ileum has a thicker, more fatty mesentery with more complex arterial arcades. The ileum also contains larger aggregates of lymph nodes (Peyer's patches), which can occasionally become the lead points in childhood intussusception.

The small intestine has a rich blood supply, derived from the superior mesenteric artery (SMA), while venous drainage is via the portal venous system. The superior mesenteric vein joins the splenic vein to form the portal vein, which drains into the liver, carrying absorbed nutrients from the bowel for processing. The lymphatic drainage of the small intestine follows the arterial supply.

The small intestine has a rich autonomic innervation arising from the splanchnic nerves, which contribute a dense network of sympathetic fibres around the SMA and its branches. Referred pain from the small intestine is usually felt in the periumbilical region (T10). The blood and nerve supplies to the small intestine run in its mesentery, which is attached to the posterior abdominal wall and runs obliquely downwards to the right between the DJ flexure to the left of the second lumbar vertebra and the right sacroiliac joint (***Summary box 74.1***; see ***Chapter 65***).

Summary box 74.1

Important features of small bowel anatomy
- Comprises jejunum and ileum
- Has valvulae conniventes
- Blood supply from SMA

PHYSIOLOGY OF THE SMALL INTESTINE

The principal function of the small intestine is the digestion of food and absorption of nutrients, water and electrolytes. Carbohydrates and proteins are broken down in the intestinal lumen by pancreatic enzymes, but the final hydrolysis takes place at the brush border of the jejunum, after which these nutrients are absorbed. Fats are digested chiefly by the actions of pancreatic lipase and bile salts. The products of fat digestion, fatty acids and monoglycerides, separate from bile salts in the jejunum and are absorbed for further processing. The jejunum is the principal site for digestion and absorption of fluid, electrolytes, iron, folate, fat, protein and carbohydrate,

Valvulae conniventes describes a fold of mucous membrane that passes across two-thirds of the bowel circumference.

Johann Conrad Peyer, 1653–1712, Professor of Logic, Rhetoric and Medicine, Schaffhausen, Switzerland, described the lymph follicles in the intestine in 1677.

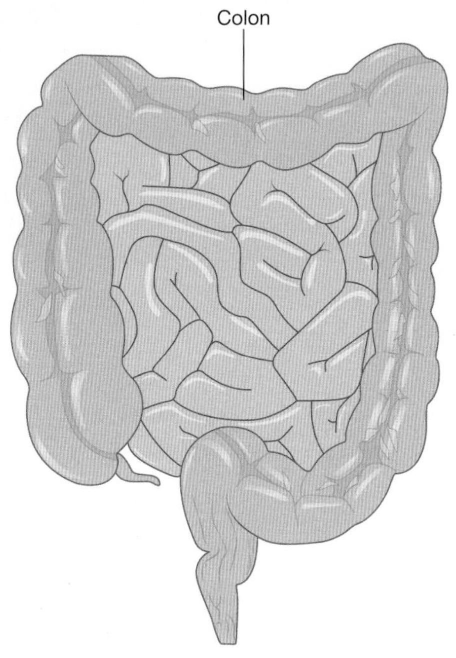

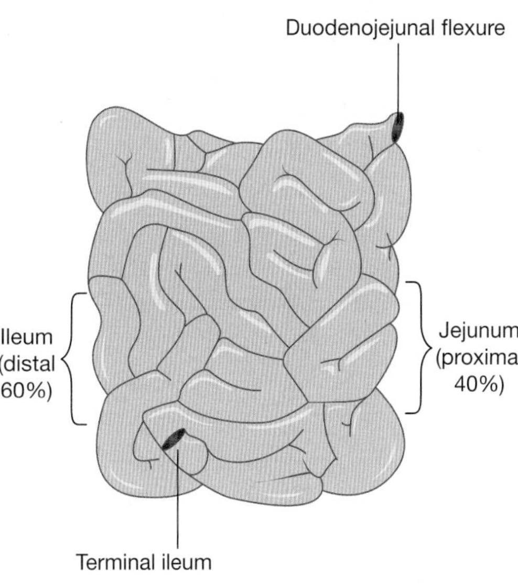

Figure 74.1 Portions of the small bowel and their relationship to the colon.

but the absorption of bile salts and vitamin B12 only occurs in the terminal ileum, where there are specific transporters. If the jejunum is resected, the ileum can assume all the required absorptive functions, but resection of the terminal ileum will result in a diminished bile salt pool, vitamin B12 deficiency and may lead to deficiency of the fat-soluble vitamins A, D, E and K. The ileum also plays an important role in water absorption, possibly because the tightness of the intercellular junctions supports a concentration gradient across its lumen. Significant ileal resection therefore commonly results in very troublesome diarrhoea.

The small intestine plays an important role in the metabolism of plasma lipoproteins, as it is the main site of synthesis of high-density, low-density and very low-density lipoproteins (HDL, LDL, VLDL). These particles transport most of the absorbed dietary fat to the systemic circulation via the lymph. The small bowel also synthesises intestinal hormones such as glucagon-like peptides GLP-1 and 2, peptide YY and motilin, which interact with the enteric nervous system to modulate intestinal function, growth and differentiation.

INFLAMMATORY BOWEL DISEASE

The term 'inflammatory bowel disease' is reserved for conditions characterised by the presence of idiopathic intestinal inflammation; conditions such as infective or ischaemic enteritis are, by definition, excluded. Crohn's disease (CD) is the only known 'inflammatory bowel disease' that affects the small intestine and is covered in detail in ***Chapter 75***.

INFECTIVE ENTERITIS

Campylobacter

Infection with *Campylobacter jejuni* (a Gram-negative rod with a distinctive spiral shape) is the most common form of bacterial gastroenteritis in the UK, typically acquired from eating infected poultry. It causes diarrhoea and abdominal pain and may mimic an acute abdomen. Severe cases may resemble ulcerative colitis, with rectal bleeding and colorectal ulceration, causing diagnostic difficulty. The organism is fastidious in culture and may take several days to isolate in the laboratory. Toxic dilatation and even disintegrative colitis have rarely been reported to occur. Treatment is generally supportive as the condition usually resolves without antibiotics. It is a notifiable disease.

Yersinia

Yersinia enterocolitica is a Gram-negative rod that can infect the terminal ileum, appendix, ascending colon and mesenteric lymph nodes, and can cause a granulomatous inflammatory process that may mimic CD. *Yersinia* typically causes a fever and gastroenteritis, but may persist and cause a terminal ileitis, which, on occasion, may perforate. The diagnosis may be made on stool culture, but is more often confirmed serologically. If discovered at laparotomy, the terminal ileum and mesenteric nodes will look thickened and inflamed and a lymph node biopsy can be taken for diagnostic purposes. The disease is normally self-limiting, but responds to treatment with co-trimoxazole or chloramphenicol antibiotics.

Burrill Bernard Crohn, 1884–1983, gastroenterologist, Mount Sinai Hospital, New York, NY, USA, along with Leon Ginzburg and Gordon Oppenheimer, described regional ileitis in 1932.

Salmonella, typhoid and paratyphoid

Salmonella are a family of Gram-negative rods that can cause a range of enteric infections. *Salmonella* gastroenteritis is typically caused by *Salmonella enteritidis* from poultry and is most often a self-limiting illness comprising headache, fever and watery diarrhoea. When severe, antibiotics and hospitalisation and intravenous fluids may be needed. The diagnosis is based on stool culture. *Shigella* and enteropathogenic strains of *Escherichia coli* may cause similar diarrhoeal illnesses.

Typhoid fever is caused by *Salmonella enterica* and presents with fever and abdominal pain after an incubation period of 10–20 days. Over the next week, the patient can develop distension, diarrhoea, splenomegaly and characteristic 'rose spots' on the abdomen caused by a vasculitis. Typhoid is a systemic infection and diagnosis of typhoid is confirmed by culture of blood or stool. Treatment is by antibiotics, usually chloramphenicol. A number of surgical complications can result, including paralytic ileus, intestinal haemorrhage, free ileal perforation and cholecystitis.

Invasion of the systemic circulation, which is a characteristic feature of salmonellosis, may cause severe Gram-negative sepsis, resulting in septic shock. Some patients develop metastatic sepsis, including septic arthritis and osteomyelitis, meningitis, encephalitis, disseminated intravascular coagulation and pancreatitis.

Perforation of a typhoid ulcer characteristically occurs during the third week of the illness, although it is sometimes the first clinical sign of the disease. The ulcer is parallel to the long axis of the gut and is usually situated in the distal ileum. Perforation requires surgery to wash out and close the ulcer and intestinal resection is usually avoided. In unstable patients, notably with evidence of septic shock, the bowel should be exteriorised and the perforation closed after recovery. Paratyphoid infection (with *Salmonella* Paratyphi A) resembles typhoid fever and is treated in a similar manner (see ***Chapter 6***).

Tuberculosis of the intestine

Tuberculosis, like CD, can affect any part of the gastrointestinal tract. The sites affected most often are the ileum, proximal colon and peritoneum. There are two principal disease presentations.

Ulcerative tuberculosis

Ulcerative tuberculosis develops secondary to pulmonary tuberculosis and arises as a result of swallowing tubercle bacilli. Multiple ulcers, lying transversely, develop in the terminal ileum and the overlying serosa is thickened, reddened and covered in tubercles. Patients typically present with diarrhoea and weight loss, although subacute obstruction and even local perforation and fistula formation can occur. A barium follow-through or computed tomography (CT) examination fails to show filling of the distal ileum, caecum and the ascending colon as a result of narrowing of the ulcerated segment (***Figure 74.2***).

A course of antituberculous chemotherapy usually leads to cure, provided the pulmonary tuberculosis is adequately treated. Surgery is usually undertaken only in the rare event of a perforation or complete intestinal obstruction.

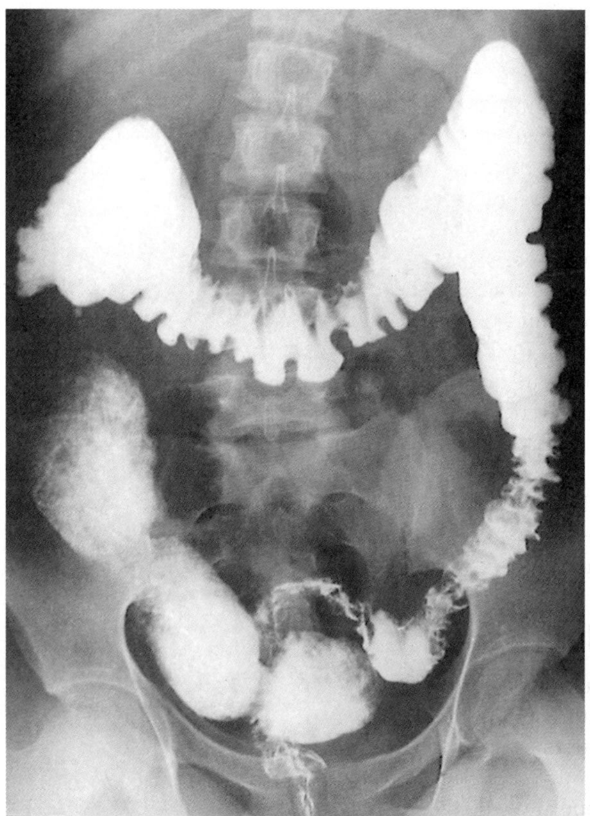

Figure 74.2 Ileocaecal tuberculosis showing dilatation of the distal ileum and stricturing of the terminal ileum and caecum (courtesy of Dr. VK Kapoor, Delhi, India).

Hyperplastic tuberculosis

This is caused by the ingestion of *Mycobacterium tuberculosis* by patients with a high resistance to the organism. The infection usually occurs in the ileocaecal region, although solitary and multiple lesions in the distal ileum are also sometimes seen. The infection establishes itself in lymphoid follicles, and the resulting chronic inflammation causes thickening of the intestinal wall and narrowing of the lumen. There is early involvement of the regional lymph nodes, which may caseate. Unlike in CD, abscess and fistula formation are uncommon.

Patients usually present with attacks of abdominal pain and intermittent diarrhoea. There is incomplete ileal obstruction, leading to stasis and bacterial overgrowth. This in turn causes steatorrhoea, anaemia and loss of weight. Patients may present with a mass in the right iliac fossa and vague ill health. The differential diagnosis is that of an appendix mass, lymphoma, carcinoma of the caecum, CD, tuberculosis or actinomycosis. A barium follow-through or small bowel enema will show a long narrow filling defect in the terminal ileum (which may result in a differential diagnosis of CD). CT will also demonstrate the narrowed segment with proximal distension and the associated lymphadenopathy. When the diagnosis is clear and the patient has not yet developed obstructive symptoms, treatment with antituberculous medication is advised and may be curative. Where obstruction is present, or the possibility of CD or lymphoma requires clarification, ileocaecal resection is often required (see ***Chapters 6 and 65***).

Actinomycosis

Abdominal actinomycosis is rare. It is caused by infection with *Actinomyces israelii* and usually develops several weeks after an apparently straightforward perforated appendicitis. An abscess develops and spreads to the retroperitoneal tissues and the adjacent abdominal wall, eventually becoming the seat of multiple indurated discharging sinuses. At first, the discharge from the sinuses is thin, watery and inoffensive, but it may later become thicker and malodorous. Secondary fistulation may occur and the tissues may become extensively indurated and woody. In contrast to tuberculosis, however, mesenteric lymph nodes are not involved and the lumen of the intestine is not narrowed. Haematogenous spread via the portal vein may lead to multiple liver abscesses.

Pus should be sent for bacteriological examination, which will reveal the characteristic sulphur granules. Penicillin or co-trimoxazole treatment is required and should be prolonged and in high dosage.

Human immunodeficiency virus

Human immunodeficiency virus (HIV) infection is associated with a number of proctological problems (see ***Chapter 80***). Intestinal complications are common after the development of acquired immunodeficiency syndrome (AIDS), when opportunistic organisms can cause gastroenteritis (***Summary box 74.2***). HIV may also cause a specific enteropathy. Treatment is directed towards the relevant organism and surgery should be avoided if possible.

Summary box 74.2

Opportunistic intestinal infections in patients with AIDS

- Bacterial
  - *Salmonella*
  - *Shigella*
  - *Yersinia*
  - *Campylobacter*
  - *Mycobacterium avium–intracellulare* (MAI)
- Viral
  - *Cytomegalovirus*
- Protozoal
  - *Cryptosporidium*
  - *Giardia*
- Fungal
  - *Candida albicans*

TUMOURS OF THE SMALL INTESTINE

Small bowel tumours are rare and in total account for less than 10% of gastrointestinal neoplasia.

Benign

The majority of small bowel neoplasms are benign, comprising adenomas, lipomas, haemangiomas and neurogenic tumours. They are frequently asymptomatic and identified incidentally, but can present with intussusception, small bowel obstruction and bleeding that may cause anaemia or may even be overt. Where these lesions do cause anaemia, the cause can be difficult to diagnose, as CT or small bowel contrast studies do not show them easily. Capsule endoscopy or small bowel endoscopy have been used successfully where the facilities exist. Symptomatic lesions can be treated by small bowel resection.

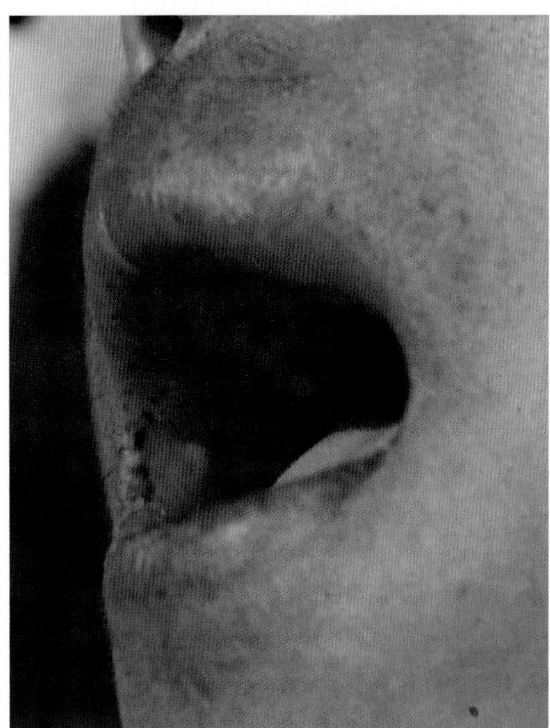

Figure 74.3 Melanin spots on the lips of a patient with Peutz–Jeghers syndrome (courtesy of Major PCM Manta, Indian Medical Service).

Peutz-Jeghers syndrome

This is an autosomal dominant condition characterised by melanosis of the mouth and lips, with multiple hamartomatous (benign tumour-like malformations resulting from faulty development in an organ) polyps in the small bowel and colon (***Figure 74.3***). Melanin spots can also occur on the digits and perianal skin. Mutation of the *STK11* gene on chromosome 19 has been found in a proportion of patients. Long-term follow-up of the original family described by Peutz has shown reduced survival as a consequence of complications of bowel obstruction and the development of a range of cancers. Regular colonic surveillance should be performed and female patients should attend breast and cervical screening. Despite the increased risk of malignancy in general, malignant change in the polyps themselves is uncommon. Resection may be indicated, however, for heavy and persistent or recurrent bleeding or intussusception. Polyps may be removed by enterotomy or, at laparotomy, snared via a colonoscope introduced via an enterotomy. Heavily involved segments of small intestine may occasionally be resected.

James Israel, 1848–1926, first found sulphur granules in pus from a discharging sinus in a man's neck. Later, he became a famous Berlin urologist.
John Law Augustine Peutz, 1886–1968, Chief Specialist for Internal Medicine, St. John's Hospital, The Hague, The Netherlands.
Harold Joseph Jeghers, 1904–1990, Professor of Internal Medicine, The New Jersey College of Medicine and Dentistry, Jersey City, NJ, USA.

Malignant

Small bowel malignancy is rare, classically presents late and is most often diagnosed after surgery for small bowel obstruction. Four types will be considered, which account for over 99% of small bowel malignancies: adenocarcinoma, neuroendocrine tumours (NETs), lymphomas and gastrointestinal stromal tumours (GISTs).

Adenocarcinoma

Small bowel adenocarcinoma is more often found in the jejunum than in the ileum and, although the aetiology is unknown, it is more common in patients with CD, coeliac disease, familial adenomatous polyposis, hereditary non-polyposis colon cancer and Peutz–Jeghers syndrome. The tumours present with anaemia, overt gastrointestinal bleeding, intussusception or obstruction. Prognosis is poor, particularly in patients with CD, in whom these tumours often present late because the symptoms are commonly mistaken for those of CD and treated conservatively. When diagnosed, surgical treatment is a resection of 5 cm of non-involved bowel either side of the lesion and the affected mesentery (***Figure 74.4***). A right hemicolectomy is likely to be required for tumours of the distal ileum.

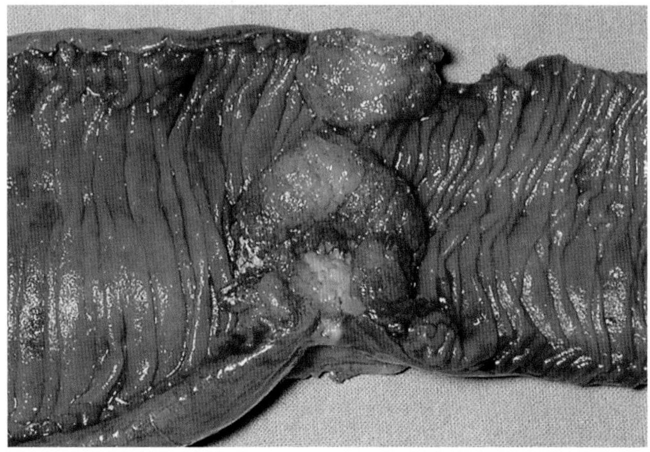

Figure 74.4 Small bowel adenocarcinoma.

Neuroendocrine tumours

NETs (previously known as carcinoid tumours) occur throughout the gastrointestinal tract, most commonly in the appendix, ileum and rectum in decreasing order of frequency. They arise from Kulchitsky cells at the base of intestinal crypts (of Lieberkuhn). The primary is usually small, although significant lymph node metastases can occur. In up to one-third of cases of small bowel NETs, the tumours are multiple. They may produce dense fibrosis in the surrounding tissues, resulting in distortion and scarring of the bowel and associated mesentery, giving them a characteristic radiological appearance. NETs can produce a number of vasoactive peptides, most commonly 5-hydroxytryptamine (serotonin), but also histamine, prostaglandins and kallikrein. When they metastasise to the liver, the 'carcinoid syndrome' can become evident because the vasoactive substances escape the filtering actions of the liver. The clinical syndrome itself consists of reddish-blue cyanosis, flushing attacks, diarrhoea, borborygmi, asthmatic attacks and, eventually, pulmonary and tricuspid stenosis (***Summary box 74.3***). Classically, the flushing attacks are induced by alcohol.

Surgical resection is usually sufficient for patients with primary disease, but the incidence of recurrence is significant. The extent of disease can be assessed preoperatively using octreotide scanning (somatostatin receptor scintigraphy), which may detect otherwise clinically unapparent primary and secondary tumours. Plasma markers of tumour bulk, such as chromogranin A concentrations, may be useful markers of disease recurrence, as well as of prognostic value.

Hepatic resection can be carried out in patients with metastatic disease. The treatment has been transformed by the use of octreotide (a somatostatin analogue), which reduces both flushing and diarrhoea, and octreotide cover is usually used in patients with a carcinoid syndrome who have surgery to prevent a carcinoid crisis resulting from liberation of vasoactive substances following handling of the tumour. NETs generally grow more slowly than most metastatic malignancies and patients may live with metastatic disease for many years. The tumour is not usually sensitive to chemo- or radiotherapy (see ***Chapter 69***).

Summary box 74.3

Carcinoid syndrome

- Diarrhoea
- Bronchospasm
- Facial/upper chest flushing
- Palpitations
- Tricuspid regurgitation

Lymphoma

Small bowel lymphoma may be primary or, more commonly, secondary to systemic lymphoma. The incidence of small bowel lymphoma is increased in patients with CD and immunodeficiency syndromes. The classification of lymphoma is beyond the scope of this chapter but a number of points are worth noting briefly. It is rare for Hodgkin's lymphoma to affect the small bowel and most Western-type lymphomas are non-Hodgkin's B-cell lymphomas. They usually present with anaemia, bleeding, perforation, anorexia and weight loss.

Small bowel T-cell lymphoma can develop in patients with coeliac disease. It usually presents with worsening of the patient's diarrhoea, pyrexia of unknown origin and local obstructive symptoms. Mediterranean lymphoma is found mostly in North Africa and the Middle East and is often widespread at diagnosis. Burkitt's lymphoma can aggressively affect the ileocaecal region, particularly in children. The mainstay of treatment for these conditions is chemotherapy; however, surgery may be required for obstruction, perforation or bleeding.

Nikolai Kulchitsky, 1856–1925, Professor of Histology, Kharkov, Ukraine, who left Russia after the Revolution of 1917 and later worked at University College, London, UK. He described these cells in 1897.

Johann Nathaniel Lieberkühn, 1711–1756, physician and anatomist, Berlin, Germany, described these glands in 1745.

Thomas Hodgkin, 1798–1866, lecturer in morbid anatomy and curator of the museum, Guy's Hospital, London, UK, described lymphadenoma in 1832.

Denis Parsons Burkitt, 1911–1993, Irish-born surgeon who worked in Kampala, Uganda.

Gastrointestinal stromal tumours

GISTs are mesenchymal tumours and the distinction between benign and malignant types is difficult even on histological examination. Increased size and high levels of *c-kit* (CD117) staining are associated with malignant potential. GISTs are found most commonly in the stomach but can be found in other parts of the gut. They occur most commonly in the 50- to 70-year age group. Although the cause is unknown, patients with neurofibromatosis have an increased risk of developing these types of tumour. Patients may be asymptomatic and the tumour may present as an incidental mass on a CT scan. Symptoms include lethargy, pain, nausea, haematemesis or melaena. Surgery is the most effective way of treating GISTs as the tumour is radioresistant and is not sensitive to conventional chemotherapy. Imatinib is a tyrosine kinase inhibitor that has been shown to be effective in advanced cases and may also have a role in adjuvant treatment. It may be used preoperatively to reduce tumour size; however, the involuting tumour may perforate, precipitating a surgical crisis (see ***Chapters 11 and 67***).

CONNECTIVE TISSUE DISORDERS

Intestinal diverticula

Diverticula (hollow outpouchings) are a common structural abnormality that can occur from the oesophagus to the rectosigmoid junction. Small bowel diverticula may be congenital or acquired. In congenital diverticula all three coats of the bowel are present in the wall of the diverticulum (e.g. Meckel's diverticulum).

Acquired diverticula

These often develop in the jejunum and arise from the mesenteric side of the bowel as a result of mucosal herniation at the point of entry of the blood vessels, where there is a potential defect in the muscularis layer. Jejunal diverticula can vary in size and are frequently multiple. They are commonly asymptomatic and present as an incidental finding at surgery or on radiological imaging. However, they can result in malabsorption, due to bacterial overgrowth, or present as an acute abdominal emergency if they become inflamed or perforate. Bleeding from a jejunal diverticulum is a rare complication (compared with sigmoid diverticular disease). Elective resection of an affected small bowel segment causing malabsorption can be effective, provided there is only a limited amount of jejunum involved. If perforated jejunal diverticulitis is found at emergency laparotomy, a small bowel resection should be performed and a decision made between primary anastomosis and stoma formation. This will depend on the degree of contamination, physiological stability and local resources for managing a patient with a high-output jejunostomy.

Complications resulting from extensive jejunal diverticulosis can be extremely difficult to treat. In severe cases, much of the proximal small intestine may be involved, effectively precluding resection. Prolonged antibiotic therapy for bacterial overgrowth may be preferable, and antibiotics (metronidazole, ciprofloxacin, rifaximin) may be rotated in an attempt to avoid antibiotic resistance. Limited resection, leaving remaining segments of affected jejunum, may be feasible, but may also fail to deal adequately with bacterial overgrowth, recurrent attacks of inflammation or bleeding.

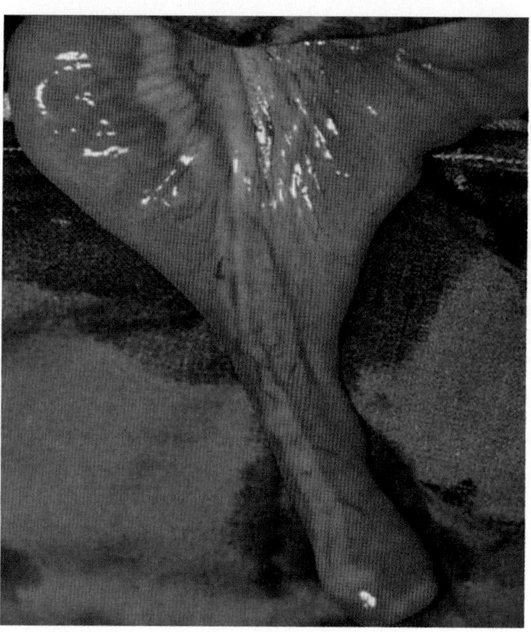

Figure 74.5 Meckel's diverticulum.

Meckel's diverticulum

A Meckel's diverticulum is a persistent remnant of the vitello-intestinal duct and is present in about 2% of the population. It is found on the antimesenteric side of the ileum approximately 60 cm from the ileocaecal valve and is classically 5 cm long (2% prevalence; 2 feet [60 cm] from ileocaecal valve; 2 inches [5 cm] long). A Meckel's diverticulum is a congenital diverticulum (***Figure 74.5***). It contains all three coats of the bowel wall and has its own blood supply. It may be vulnerable to obstruction and inflammation in the same way as the appendix; indeed, when a normal appendix is found at surgery for suspected appendicitis, a Meckel's diverticulum should be looked for by examining the small bowel, particularly if free fluid or pus is found (see ***Chapter 76***). In approximately 20% of cases, the mucosa of a Meckel's diverticulum contains heterotopic epithelium of gastric, colonic or pancreatic type. The presence of heterotopic mucosa may predispose to the development of complications (***Summary box 74.4***).

The vast majority of Meckel's diverticula are asymptomatic and a Meckel's diverticulum is notoriously difficult to visualise with contrast radiology. Meckel's diverticulum may however present clinically in the following ways.

Haemorrhage. If gastric mucosa is present, peptic ulceration can occur and present as painless dark rectal bleeding or melaena. If the stomach, duodenum and colon are excluded as a source of bleeding by endoscopy, radioisotope scanning with technetium-99m may demonstrate a Meckel's diverticulum.

Johann Friedrich Meckel (the younger), 1781–1833, Professor of Anatomy and Surgery, Halle, Germany, described the diverticulum in 1809.

Diverticulitis. Meckel's diverticulitis presents like appendicitis, although if perforation occurs the presentation may resemble a perforated duodenal ulcer.

Intussusception. A Meckel's diverticulum can be the lead point for ileoileal or ileocolic intussusception.

Chronic ulceration. Pain is felt around the umbilicus, as the site of the diverticulum is midgut in origin.

Intestinal obstruction. A band between the apex of the diverticulum and the umbilicus (also part of the vitello-intestinal duct) may cause obstruction directly, or by predisposing to the development of a volvulus around it.

Perforation. (*Figure 74.6*).

When found in the course of abdominal surgery, a Meckel's diverticulum can safely be left alone, provided it has a wide mouth and is not thickened. When there is doubt, it can be resected. The finding of a Meckel's diverticulum in an inguinal or femoral hernia has been described as 'Littre's hernia'.

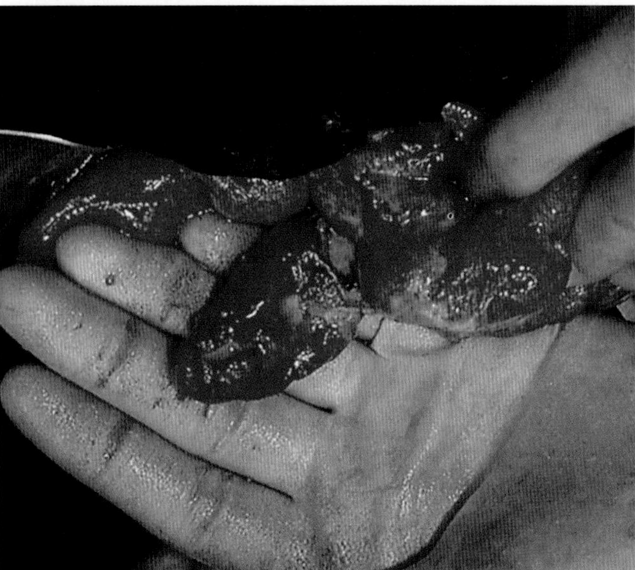

Figure 74.6 Gangrenous Meckel's diverticulitis.

Summary box 74.4

Features of Meckel's diverticulum

- Remnant of vitellointestinal duct
- Occurs in 2% of patients, 5 cm (2 inches) long, 60 cm (2 feet) from the ileocaecal valve, 20% heterotopic epithelium
- Should be looked for when a normal appendix is found at surgery for suspected appendicitis
- If a Meckel's diverticulum is found incidentally at surgery, it can be left provided it has a wide mouth and is not thickened
- Can be a source of gastrointestinal bleeding if it contains ectopic gastric mucosa

Meckel's diverticulectomy

A broad-based Meckel's diverticulum should not be amputated at its base and invaginated (as for an appendix), as there is the risk of stricture and of leaving heterotopic epithelium behind. It is safer simply to excise the diverticulum, either by resecting the diverticulum and suturing the defect at its base or by performing a limited small bowel resection with anastomosis. This can also be achieved with a linear stapler–cutter. If the base of the diverticulum is indurated, it is on balance safer to perform a limited small bowel resection of the entire involved segment, followed by an anastomosis.

VASCULAR ANOMALIES OF THE INTESTINE

Mesenteric ischaemia

Mesenteric vascular disease may be classified as acute intestinal ischaemia – with or without occlusion – venous, chronic arterial, central or peripheral. The superior mesenteric vessels are the visceral vessels most likely to be affected by embolisation or thrombosis. Occlusion at the origin of the SMA is almost invariably the result of thrombosis, whereas emboli tend to lodge at the origin of the middle colic artery. Inferior mesenteric artery involvement is usually clinically silent because of a rich collateral circulation.

SMA emboli may be carried from the left atrium in atrial fibrillation, the left ventricle after mural myocardial infarction, vegetations on mitral and aortic valves associated with endocarditis or an atheromatous plaque from an aortic aneurysm. Primary thrombosis is associated with atherosclerosis and vasculitides, including conditions such as thromboangitis obliterans and polyarteritis nodosa. Primary thrombosis of the superior mesenteric veins may occur in association with factor V Leiden disorder, portal hypertension, portal pyaemia, sickle cell disease and in women taking the oral contraceptive pill. A specific form of 'non-occlusive mesenteric ischaemia' (in which the vessels are normal but flow is critically reduced) may complicate critical illness, possibly because of alterations in splanchnic blood flow.

Irrespective of whether the occlusion is arterial or venous, haemorrhagic infarction occurs. The mucosa is especially sensitive to ischaemic injury because of its high metabolic activity. The intestine and its mesentery become swollen and oedematous, especially with venous occlusion. Bloodstained fluid exudes into the peritoneal cavity and bowel lumen. The changes develop rapidly and irreversible injury, ranging in severity from mucosal necrosis and sloughing to full-thickness infarction, usually occurs within 6 hours at most. If the main trunk of the SMA is involved, the infarction usually covers an area from just distal to the DJ flexure to the splenic flexure. Usually, a branch of the main trunk is implicated and the area of infarction is smaller.

Clinical features

The most important clue to an early diagnosis of acute mesenteric ischaemia is sudden onset of severe abdominal pain in a

Alexis Littre, 1658–1746, surgeon and Lecturer in Anatomy, Paris, France, described Meckel's diverticulum in a hernial sac in 1700, 81 years before Meckel was born.

patient with atrial fibrillation or atherosclerosis. The pain is typically in the central abdomen and is out of all proportion to the physical findings. Persistent vomiting and defecation occur early, with the subsequent passage of altered blood. Abdominal tenderness may be mild initially, with rigidity being a late feature. Shock, with features of both hypovolaemia and sepsis, rapidly ensues.

Investigation

Investigation will usually reveal a profound neutrophil leukocytosis, a severe metabolic acidosis and raised blood lactate. A contrast-enhanced CT scan will show bowel wall enhancement absent or reduced and there may be free fluid in the abdomen. Gas may be present within the intestinal wall and occasionally in the mesenteric and portal vein, a late and ominous sign.

Treatment

Mesenteric venous thrombosis may be treated by anticoagulation with close monitoring. An immediate laparotomy with embolectomy or revascularisation of the SMA by vascular bypass may be considered in early cases of arterial ischaemia, followed by postoperative anticoagulation. However, the condition is usually diagnosed late in the disease process and the mortality rate is extremely high. In the young, all affected bowel should be resected, whereas in the elderly or infirm the situation may be deemed incurable. Where the demarcation between viable and non-viable bowel is uncertain a planned relook laparotomy may be useful.

After extensive enterectomy, it is usual for patients to require intravenous nutrition. The young, however, may sometimes develop sufficient intestinal digestive and absorptive function to lead relatively normal lives. In selected cases, consideration may be given to small bowel transplantation (see ***Chapter 91***).

Chronic small intestinal ischaemia

Chronic small intestinal ischaemia almost invariably results from atherosclerosis and affects the proximal superior mesenteric and coeliac vessels. Patients classically present with symptoms of severe central abdominal pain that comes on within 30–60 minutes of eating (mesenteric angina). Weight loss and diarrhoea due to malabsorption may also occur. The condition may be difficult to diagnose and is often overlooked. The presence of significant vascular disease on CT is common in elderly patients and in those with severe vascular disease and should not necessarily be assumed to indicate that abdominal symptoms are attributable to chronic ischaemia. Treatment is usually by selective visceral angiography, with stenting/angioplasty and, where this is not possible, bypass surgery. Smoking cessation is imperative and patients are usually anticoagulated.

STOMAS

A stoma is an artificial opening made in the bowel to divert faeces and flatus outside the abdomen, where they can be collected in an external appliance. Depending on the purpose for which the diversion has been necessary, a stoma may be temporary or permanent (***Summary box 74.5***).

Summary box 74.5

Stomas

- May be colostomy or ileostomy
- May be temporary or permanent
- Temporary or defunctioning stomas are usually fashioned as loop stomas
- An ileostomy is spouted; a colostomy is flush
- Ileostomy effluent is usually liquid, whereas colostomy effluent is usually solid
- Ileostomy patients are more likely to develop fluid and electrolyte problems
- An ileostomy is usually sited in the right iliac fossa
- End-colostomy is usually sited in the left iliac fossa
- Whenever possible, patients should be counselled and sited by a stoma care nurse before operation

Loop ileostomy

A loop ileostomy is often used for defunctioning a low rectal anastomosis or an ileal pouch. A knuckle of ileum is exteriorised through a skin trephine in the right iliac fossa. An incision is made in the distal part of the knuckle, and this is then pulled over the top of the more proximal part to create a spout on the proximal side of the loop with a flush distal side still in continuity. This allows near perfect defunctioning, but also the possibility of restoration of continuity, by taking down the spout and reanastomosing the partially divided ileum.

The advantage of a loop ileostomy over a loop colostomy is the ease with which the bowel can be brought to the surface. Care is needed when the ileostomy is closed such that suture line obstruction does not occur. Closure of a loop ileostomy can be a technically challenging procedure, particularly if there are dense adhesions resulting from previous surgery.

End-ileostomy

An end-ileostomy is formed after a colectomy without anastomosis, when it may later be reversed, or after panproctocolectomy, when it is permanent. The ileum is normally brought through the rectus abdominis muscle. Careful attention should be paid to the terminal ileal mesentery to ensure that it is not too bulky. The use of a spout was originally described by Brooke; this should project some 2–4 cm from the skin surface (***Figure 74.7***). A disposable appliance is placed over the ileostomy so that it is a snug fit at skin level.

There may be an 'ileostomy flux' while the ileum adapts to the loss of the colon. While ileostomy output can amount to 4–5 litres per day, losses of 1–2 litres are more common. A consistent ileostomy output in excess of 1.5 litres is usually associated with dehydration and sodium depletion in the absence of intravenous therapy. Up to 20% of patients may require readmission for the treatment of dehydration after creation of

Bryan Nicholas Brooke, 1915–1998, Professor of Surgery, St George's Hospital, London, UK.

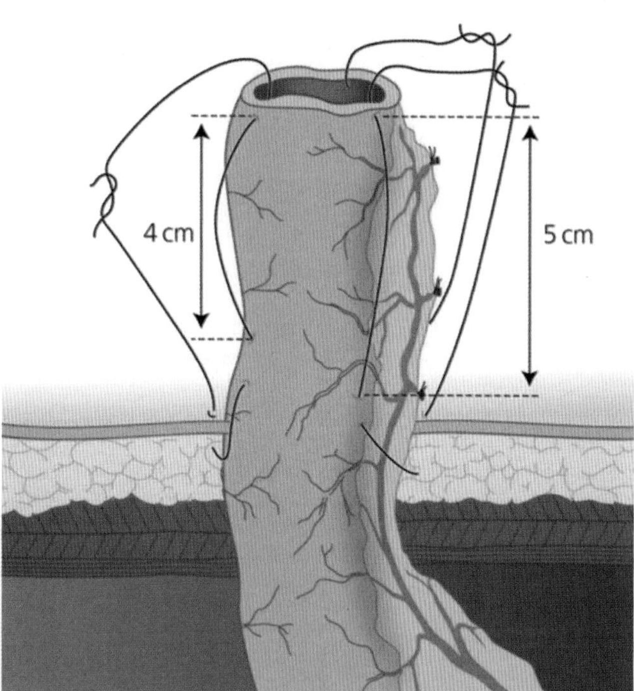

Figure 74.7 Construction of an end-ileostomy. The diagram is orientated such that the upper aspect of the stoma is to the right, thus when the sutures are tied the everted stoma is angled slightly inferiorly. (Reproduced with permission from O'Connell PR, Madoff RD, Solomon MJ (eds). *Operative surgery of the colon rectum and anus*, 6th edn. Boca Raton, FL: CRC Press, 2015.)

an ileostomy but the stools thicken in a few weeks and are usually semisolid in a few months. The help, skill and advice of the stoma care nurse specialist are essential. Modern appliances have transformed stoma care and skin problems are unusual (***Figure 74.8***). Complications of an ileostomy include prolapse, retraction, stenosis, bleeding, fistula and parastomal hernia.

Stoma bags and appliances

Stoma output is collected in a disposable adhesive bag. Ileostomy appliances tend to be drainable bags that are left in place for 48 hours, while colostomy appliances are simply changed two or three times each day. A wide range of such bags is currently available. Many now incorporate an adhesive backing, which can be left in place for several days. In most hospitals, a stoma care service is available to offer advice to patients, to acquaint them with the latest appliances and to provide the appropriate psychological and practical help.

Complications of stomas

Stoma complications are underestimated and common (***Summary box 74.6***). On occasion, these complications require surgical revision. Sometimes, this can be achieved with an incision immediately around the stoma, but on occasion reopening the abdomen and freeing up the stoma may be necessary. Repair of parastomal hernias is particularly technically challenging and the recurrence rate is high. Simple suture of the parastomal hernia is associated with an almost 100% risk of recurrence and transfer to the opposite side of the abdomen, or insertion of a piece of prosthetic material within the abdominal wall around the stoma may be necessary (see ***Chapter 64***).

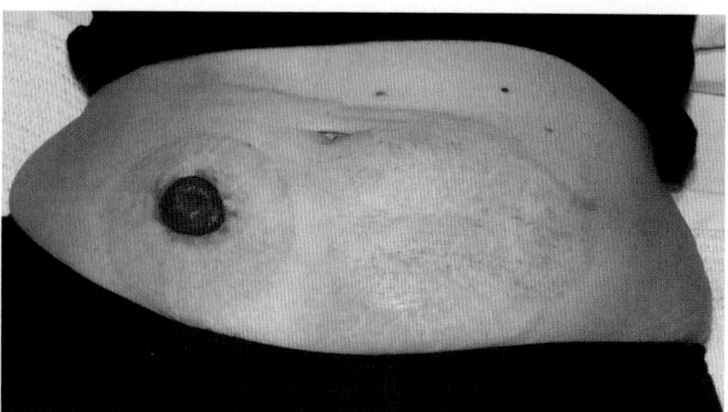

Figure 74.8 Spouted ileostomy in the right iliac fossa.

Summary box 74.6

Stoma complications

- Skin irritation
- Prolapse
- Retraction
- Ischaemia
- Stenosis
- Parastomal hernia
- Bleeding
- Fistulation

CONDITIONS CAUSING MALABSORPTION

Coeliac disease

Coeliac disease is the most common cause of malabsorption in the UK with a reported prevalence of 1:1800, although this may be an underestimate. It is characterised by a hypertrophic small bowel mucosa with atrophic villi and deep crypts. Loss of surface area and brush border enzymes results in malabsorption.

Coeliac disease is caused by an abnormal immune response to gluten, a cereal protein, although the exact mechanism remains unclear. There is a genetic component, as the disease is more common in first-degree relatives and has an association with HLA-B8. In children, coeliac disease presents with steatorrhoea and growth retardation. In adults, it may result in diarrhoea and weight loss but many patients simply present with iron deficiency anaemia. Some patients develop a characteristic skin rash (dermatitis herpetiformis).

The diagnosis is usually made after an endoscopic duodenal biopsy allows pathological examination of the mucosa. A blood test for immunoglobulin A anti-tissue transglutaminase (IgA tTGA) is relatively sensitive and specific for diagnosing coeliac disease, making it the preferred test for detection. Measurement of IgA antiendomysial antibodies (anti-EMA) should be used as a confirmatory test. A duodenal biopsy is usually indicated to confirm the diagnosis. The biopsy usually shows

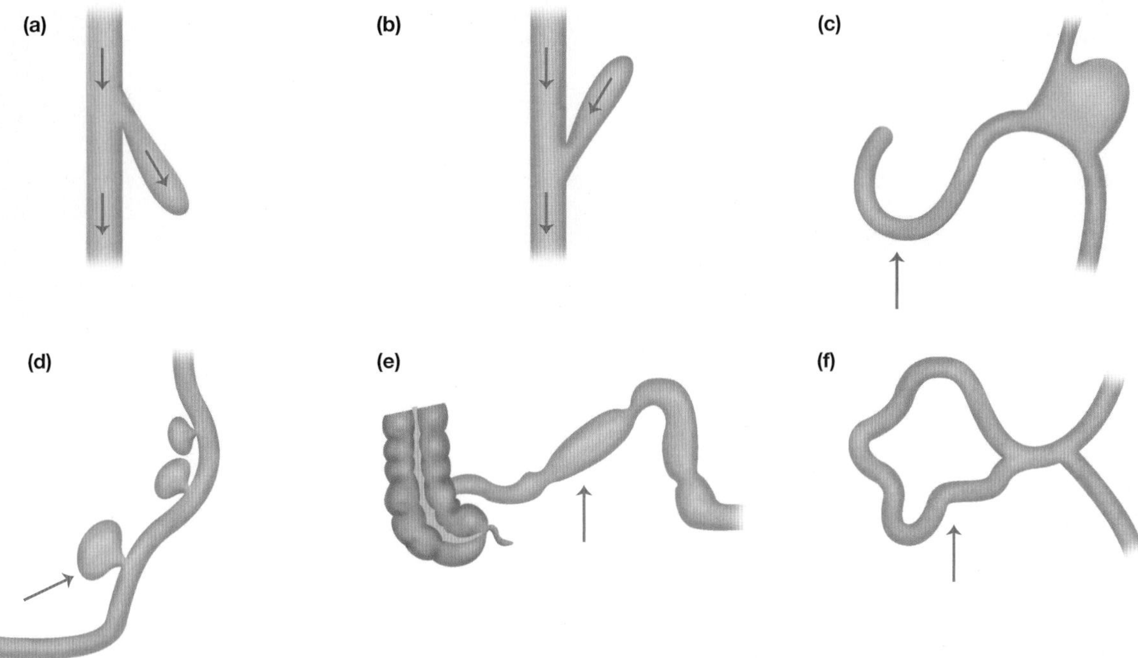

Figure 74.9 Common types of blind loop: (a) self-filling: deficiency occurs; (b) self-emptying: no deficiency occurs; (c) long afferent loop stasis in Pólya gastrectomy; (d) jejunal diverticula; (e) intestinal stricture causing stasis; (f) 'stenosis–anastomosis loop' syndrome.

flattening of the mucosa, marked inflammatory changes and characteristic findings of intraepithelial lymphocytes. All tests should be performed while the patient is on a gluten-containing diet as false-negative tests may occur if on a gluten-free diet.

Patients with coeliac disease may develop an acute inflammatory condition of the small intestine (ulcerative jejunoileitis) and have an increased risk of small bowel lymphoma and adenocarcinoma.

The main treatment for coeliac disease is the withdrawal of gluten from the diet by avoiding wheat, rye and barley. Surgery does not usually play a role in the management of coeliac disease and is primarily reserved for resection of malignancy.

Bacterial overgrowth

The small intestine can become colonised with bacteria normally confined to the colon if there is stasis resulting in delayed bacterial clearance (blind loop syndrome; *Figure 74.9*). Similar complications may result from chronic small bowel obstruction, jejunal diverticulosis and ileocolic fistulation. Overgrowth in the upper small intestine results in fat malabsorption due to the deconjugation of bile salts, while vitamin B12 deficiency results from overgrowth more distally. There is usually relatively little effect on carbohydrate or protein metabolism. If steatorrhoea occurs, other serious malabsorption features may follow, including glossitis, osteomalacia, paraesthesia and peripheral neuropathy.

Improvement normally follows after intermittent therapy with oral antibiotics; metronidazole, ciprofloxacin, tetracycline and rifaximin are commonly used. Definitive treatment is surgical if the anatomical abnormality can be corrected, but this is not always possible.

ENTEROCUTANEOUS FISTULA

An abnormal connection between the small intestine and the skin can occur as a result of CD, radiotherapy or abdominal trauma, but the condition most commonly follows a surgical complication – either a leak from an anastomosis or an inadvertent enterotomy. At least 50% of small bowel enterocutaneous fistulae develop after surgery in which no small bowel has been resected as a result of injury to the intestine during division of adhesions. The frequency of this complication has been shown to increase with the number of previous laparotomies. Management of patients with an enterocutaneous fistula can be very challenging, especially when the fistula output is high (defined as >500 mL of effluent/day). The majority of low-output fistulae can be expected to heal spontaneously, provided there is no distal obstruction or disease at the fistula site. Reasons for failure of spontaneous healing also include epithelial continuity between the gut and the skin and an associated complex abscess.

The management of fistulae is based on well-established principles ('SNAP'; see *Summary box 74.7*). An early return to theatre to try to treat the problem definitively (i.e. by

Eugen (Jeno) Alexander Pólya, 1876–1944, surgeon, St Stephen's Hospital, Budapest, Hungary.

attempting to restore bowel continuity) in a septic, malnourished patient is doomed to failure.

Summary box 74.7

Principles of management of enterocutaneous fistulae (SNAP)

- S, elimination of Sepsis and skin protection
- N, Nutrition – a period of parenteral nutrition may well be required
- A, Anatomical assessment
- P, definitive Planned surgery

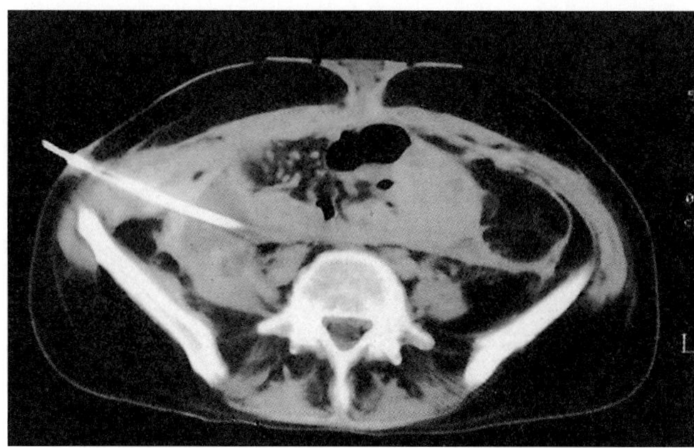

Figure 74.10 Computed tomography (CT) scan in a patient with a complex enterocutaneous fistula and an intra-abdominal abscess being drained with a CT-guided catheter.

Infected collections are best identified at CT (***Figure 74.10***) and can be drained percutaneously. Skin protection is important as small bowel effluent is caustic. Nutritional support must include fluid and electrolytes, which can be lost in high quantities from a proximal fistula, as well as carbohydrates, protein, fat and vitamins. Judgements have to be made between enteral and parenteral feeding: enteral feeding has advantages, but if the fistula is proximal or high output total parenteral nutrition will be required. Defining fistula anatomy is best done after careful discussion with the radiologist; a sequence of contrast studies (follow-through, fistulogram and enema) may well be required to define bowel length and plan a surgical strategy. Surgery can be extremely technically demanding and an anastomosis should be avoided in the presence of continuing intra-abdominal sepsis or when the patient is hypoalbuminaemic (<32 g/dL).

SHORT BOWEL SYNDROME/ INTESTINAL FAILURE

Intractable diarrhoea with impaired absorption of nutrients following resection or bypass of the small intestine, ultimately leading to progressive malnutrition, is referred to as short bowel syndrome. When a patient is unable to maintain satisfactory fluid, electrolyte or nutritional homeostasis without intravenous administration of fluid, electrolytes or nutrients they are said to have intestinal failure. The mainstay of treatment for intestinal failure is parenteral nutrition.

The most common causes of short bowel syndrome are resection resulting from the management of CD and its complications (which accounts for almost half of cases), mesenteric vascular thrombosis, radiation enteritis and tumours. Although features of short bowel syndrome usually appear when there is less than 200 cm of small bowel, the length and nature of the remaining intestine are also important. In general, diseases that result in short bowel syndrome tend to preferentially affect the distal small intestine, and there is some evidence that the ileum, with its tighter intercellular junctions and consequently better fluid absorptive capacity, can assume the functions of a missing jejunum, but not *vice versa*. While the ileocaecal valve used to be considered important with regard to preservation of absorptive function, it is more likely that this is a reflection of the associated preservation of the distal ileum and right colon than the valve itself.

Patients with an intact colon are relatively protected from the effects of massive small bowel resection because of the ability of the colon to absorb not only fluid and electrolytes but also a modest amount of nutrient energy. Patients with as little as 100–200 cm of jejunum anastomosed to an intact colon may therefore be able to maintain satisfactory macronutrient, fluid and electrolyte status, although they will, of course, be at risk of fat-soluble and B12 vitamin deficiencies and will also generally need oral nutritional supplements of trace elements, vitamins and minerals. Some (but not all) patients with 50–100 cm of small intestine and an intact colon will have intestinal failure, as will almost all patients with 50 cm or less of jejunum anastomosed to an intact colon. In contrast, most patients with less than 200 cm and virtually all with less than 100 cm of small intestine ending in a stoma will have intestinal failure and will require long-term parenteral nutrition.

Medical management of patients with short bowel syndrome relies on the use of antidiarrhoeal agents (loperamide and codeine phosphate), drugs to reduce diarrhoea related to bile-salt malabsorption (cholestyramine), drugs to reduce the increased gastric acid secretion resulting from the loss of the small bowel 'brake' on gastric acid production (proton pump inhibitors) and enteral and parenteral vitamin and trace element supplements. Although there has also been interest in the use of drugs to promote intestinal adaptation, such as growth hormone, glutamine and, most recently, glucagon-like peptide 2 agonists, the mainstay of treatment for short bowel syndrome remains home parenteral nutrition (HPN). The development of this treatment in the late 1960s enabled the majority of patients with short bowel syndrome to enjoy a reasonably good quality of life, with long-term survival related principally to the underlying disease. HPN is, however, expensive and demanding and patients are at risk from catheter-related complications (notably catheter-related sepsis and occlusion), as well as metabolic complications (fibrotic liver disease, gallstones, metabolic bone disease and kidney stones).

Surgical procedures designed to improve the surface area or reduce the speed of transit of the remaining small intestine (and thus improve absorptive capacity) have shown some promise in children, but their place in managing adults with established short bowel syndrome currently remains unclear. In some patients, the loss of venous access resulting from the complications of long-term intravenous feeding or the development of progressive liver dysfunction may represent indications for small bowel transplantation. The results of small bowel transplantation have progressively improved and 5-year patient survival now exceeds 80% in some centres (see ***Chapter 91***).

FURTHER READING

Bland KI, Sarr MG, Büchler MW *et al.* (eds.) *Surgery of the small bowel.* Handbooks in General Surgery. London: Springer-Verlag, 2011.

Keighley MRB, Williams NS. *Keighley & Williams' surgery of the anus rectum and colon,* 4th edn. Boca Raton, FL: CRC Press, 2018.

Slade DAJ, Carlson GL. Takedown of enterocutaneous fistula and complex abdominal wall reconstruction. *Surg Clin North Am* 2013; **93**: 1163–83.

Soop M, Carlson GL. Intestinal failure: In: Herold A, Lehur P-A, Matzel KE, O'Connell PR (eds). *European manual of medicine: coloproctology*, 2nd edn. Berlin: Springer, 2017.

CHAPTER 75 Inflammatory bowel disease

Learning objectives

To understand:

- The aetiology and pathology underlying inflammatory bowel disease
- The distinguishing features of ulcerative colitis and Crohn's disease
- The principles of medical management
- The role of surgery in acute and elective settings
- The management of postoperative complications and long-term outcomes

INTRODUCTION

The term inflammatory bowel disease (IBD) is reserved for conditions characterised by the presence of idiopathic intestinal inflammation. Conditions such as infective or ischaemic enteritis are covered in ***Chapters 6, 74 and 77***.

Crohn's disease (CD) may affect any portion of the gastrointestinal tract from mouth to anus, most typically the distal ileum, the anal canal and the large bowel, whereas ulcerative colitis (UC) is confined to the large intestine. UC is characterised primarily by mucosal inflammation, whereas CD most typically involves transmural inflammation. On occasion there may be difficulty distinguishing UC from CD in the colon. This occurs in approximately 10% of patients with colitis; in such instances the term indeterminate colitis (IC) may be used.

The incidence and prevalence of IBD is highest in Europe and North America, where it affects around 3 in 1000 people. The overall incidence is steadily rising worldwide, linked to improved public hygiene, dietary changes and industrialisation. Both UC and CD occur in individuals who may have a genetic predisposition and who are exposed to environmental factors that trigger abnormal immune responses that lead to intestinal inflammation. Microscopic colitis includes two main subtypes: lymphocytic colitis and collagenous colitis (CC). The aetiology is uncertain but may reflect inappropriate immune responses to alterations in the gut microenvironment consequent to oral drug ingestion, particularly non-steroidal anti-inflammatory drugs.

UC is characterised by mucosal inflammation of the large bowel, always involving the rectum (proctitis) and extending to involve varying degrees of more proximal colon (colitis). When the entire colon and rectum are involved (pancolitis), some patients may also have a degree of 'backwash ileitis', in which there is secondary inflammation in the terminal ileum.

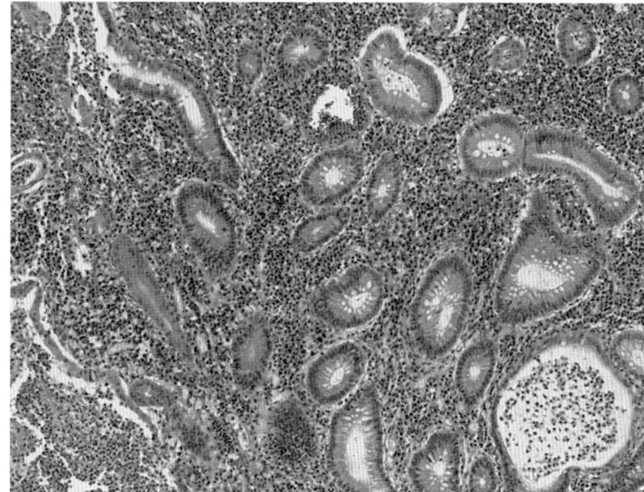

Figure 75.1 Mucosal biopsy in ulcerative colitis illustrating inflammatory infiltrate and crypt abscess formation.

UC is a chronic condition that tends to be relapsing and remitting. Early relapse and persistent disease within the first 2 years of diagnosis are both predictors of a severe disease course. The extent of disease may also change after initial diagnosis; half of patients with UC affecting the rectum or rectosigmoid progress to develop more proximal disease.

Histological hallmarks of UC typically include atrophy and distortion of the crypts, irregularity of the mucosal villi, marked infiltration of plasma cells within the deep lamina propria (basal plasmacytosis) and mucus depletion, but none of these is pathognomonic; the diagnosis ultimately depends on clinical correlation, disease course and elimination of other potential causes, especially infection (***Figure 75.1***). Pseudopolyposis occurs in almost one-quarter of cases. Stricturing in

Burrill Bernard Crohn, 1884–1983, gastroenterologist, Mount Sinai Hospital, New York, NY, USA.

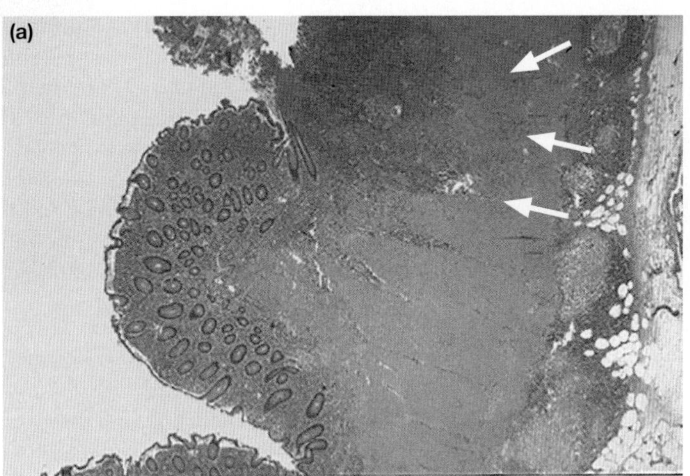

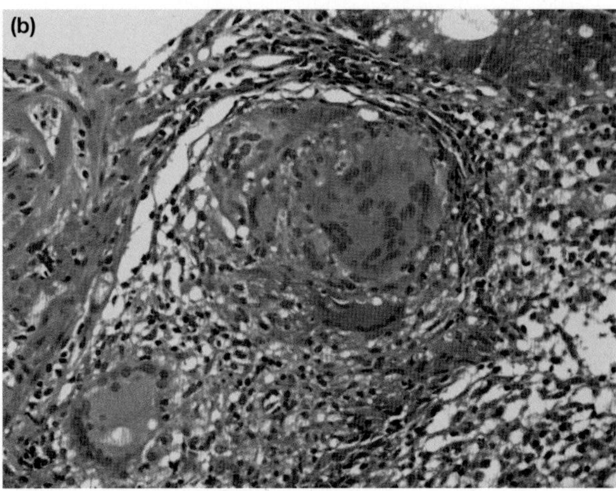

Figure 75.2 Photomicrographs of Crohn's disease illustrating mucosal ulceration and transmural inflammation (arrows) (a); high-power view of non-caseating granulomas (b) (courtesy of Professor Kieran Sheahan, St Vincent's University Hospital, Dublin, Ireland).

UC is very unusual (unlike in CD) and should prompt urgent assessment because of the possibility of coexisting carcinoma. A small proportion of patients develop irregular mucosal swellings (dysplasia-associated lesions or mass [DALMs]), which are highly predictive of coexisting carcinoma.

CD (see ***Crohn's disease (regional enteritis)***) is characterised by discontinuous transmural inflammation of the bowel caused by transmural inflammation of any part of the gastrointestinal tract from mouth to anus, but most commonly the ileocaecal region, colon and anus. There is often a degree of rectal sparing when the colon is involved. The transmural inflammation may be patchy (rather than diffuse) and crypt distortion is commonly seen. Histology typically demonstrates discontinuous segments of disease or 'skip lesions', involvement of the terminal ileum and the presence of granulomas with a tendency for more marked inflammation in the proximal colon (***Figure 75.2***). Clinical correlation of histopathology with endoscopic and radiological findings is key to clinching the diagnosis of CD. Stricturing in the colon, while usually benign in CD, may mask an underlying neoplasm.

When endoscopic and histological appearances do not categorically confirm either UC or CD, and the term IC is used, the clinical phenotype may help define the diagnosis, especially if there are features of small bowel or perianal disease suggestive of CD. Patients with IC may later come to a definitive diagnosis of UC or CD, depending on the disease course.

CLINICAL MANIFESTATIONS

The clinical manifestations of IBD primarily depend on the diagnosis (either CD or UC), the location (small or large intestine, or both) and the extent of the disease. In the large bowel, the clinical presentation depends in large part on the extent of disease. If inflammation is confined to the rectum (proctitis), there is usually no systemic upset and extra-alimentary manifestations are rare. The main symptoms are rectal bleeding, tenesmus and mucous discharge. The disease often remains confined to the rectum, usually with a benign course. Colitis is almost always associated with bloody diarrhoea and urgency. Severe and/or extensive colitis may result in anaemia, hypoproteinaemia and electrolyte disturbances. Pain is unusual. Children with poorly controlled colitis may have impaired growth. The more extensive the disease, the more likely extraintestinal manifestations are to occur. Extensive colitis is also associated with systemic illness, characterised by malaise, loss of appetite and fever.

CLASSIFICATION OF SEVERITY

The assessment of the severity of colitis is determined by the frequency of bowel action and the presence of systemic signs of illness, as originally proposed by Truelove and Witts:

- **Mild disease** is characterised by fewer than four stools daily, with or without bleeding. There are no systemic signs of toxicity.
- **Moderate disease** corresponds to more than four stools daily, but with few signs of systemic illness. There may be mild anaemia. Abdominal pain may occur. Inflammatory markers, including erythrocyte sedimentation rate and C-reactive protein, are often raised.
- **Severe disease** corresponds to more than six bloody stools a day and evidence of systemic illness, with fever, tachycardia, anaemia and raised inflammatory markers. Hypoalbuminaemia is common and an ominous finding.
- **Fulminant disease** is associated with more than 10 bowel movements daily, fever, tachycardia, continuous bleeding, anaemia, hypoalbuminaemia, abdominal tenderness and distension, the need for blood transfusion and, in the most severe cases, progressive colonic dilation (toxic megacolon). This is a very significant finding, suggestive of disintegrative colitis, and an indication for emergency surgery if colonic perforation is to be avoided.

Sidney Charles Truelove, 1913–2002, gastroenterologist, Oxford, UK.
Leslie John Witts, 1898–1982, Nuffield Professor of Medicine, Oxford, UK.

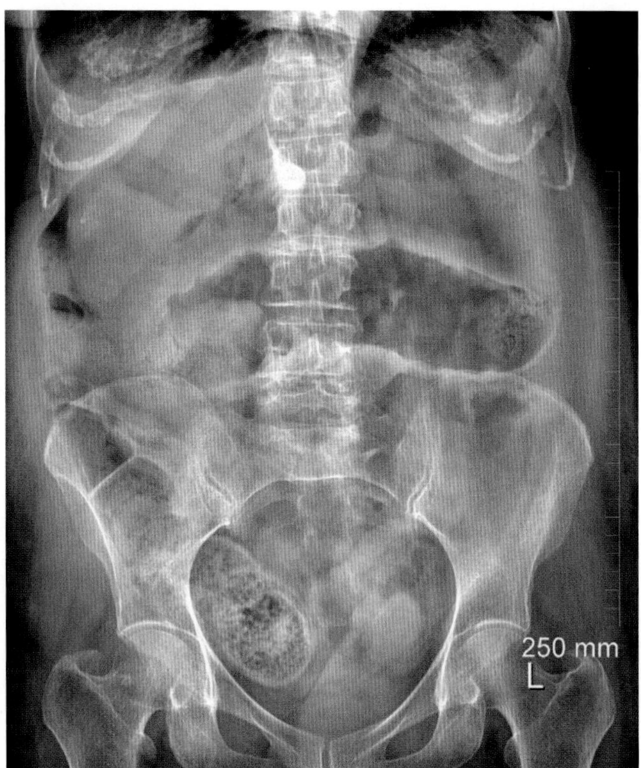

Figure 75.3 Supine abdominal radiograph of a patient with acute colitis showing toxic dilatation of the transverse colon with classical mucosal 'thumbprinting' of the colonic mucosa (courtesy of Mr Sean Martin FRCSI, St Vincent's University Hospital, Dublin, Ireland).

EXTRAINTESTINAL MANIFESTATIONS

Arthritis occurs in around 15% of patients and is typically an asymmetrical large joint polyarthropathy, affecting knees, ankles, elbows and wrists. Sacroiliitis and ankylosing spondylitis are 20 times more common in patients with UC than in the general population and are associated with the HLA-B27 genotype. Sclerosing cholangitis is associated with UC and can progress to cirrhosis and hepatocellular failure. Cholangiocarcinoma is a rare association, but its frequency is not influenced by colectomy (see ***Chapter 71***). The skin lesions erythema nodosum and pyoderma gangrenosum are associated with UC and both normally resolve with good colitis control. The eyes can be affected by uveitis and episcleritis.

ACUTE COLITIS

Approximately 5% of patients present with acute severe (fulminant) colitis. Intensive medical treatment leads to remission in 70% but the remainder require urgent surgery. Toxic dilatation should be suspected in patients who develop severe abdominal pain and confirmed by the presence on a plain abdominal radiograph of a colon with a diameter of more than 6 cm (***Figure 75.3***). A reduction in stool frequency is not always a sign of improvement in patients with acute severe colitis, and a falling stool frequency, abdominal distension and abdominal pain (resulting from progression of the inflammatory process through the colonic wall) are strongly suggestive of fulminant colitis and impending perforation. Plain abdominal radiographs or abdominal computed tomography (CT) may help monitor disease progression in patients with acute severe colitis, and a progressive increase in colon diameter despite medical therapy is an indication for urgent surgery. Colonic perforation is a grave complication with a mortality rate of 40%. Steroids may mask the physical signs. Severe haemorrhage is uncommon (1–2%) but may occasionally require urgent surgical intervention.

CANCER RISK IN COLITIS

The risk of cancer in ulcerative colitis increases with duration of disease. At 10 years from diagnosis, it is approximately 1%, increasing to 10–15% at 20 years and 20% at 30 years. Patients with pancolitis (defined as the presence of inflammation proximal to the splenic flexure) of more than 10 years' duration should be entered into endoscopic screening programmes in order to detect clinically silent dysplasia, which is predictive of increased cancer risk. The value of screening programmes remains somewhat controversial, as most patients with UC who develop cancer (approximately 3.5% of all patients) present between attendances for screening colonoscopy. Malignant change, often atypical and high grade, may be multifocal or submucosal (***Figure 75.4***). Colonoscopic surveillance with dye spray (chromoendoscopy) or multiple biopsies every 10 cm should look for subtle mucosal abnormalities, which can occur in flat mucosa or a DALM. Patients with UC and sclerosing cholangitis are also at a significantly greater risk of development of large bowel cancer.

INVESTIGATIONS

Endoscopy and biopsy

Rigid/flexible sigmoidoscopy can detect proctitis in the clinic; the mucosa is hyperaemic, bleeds on touch and there may be a

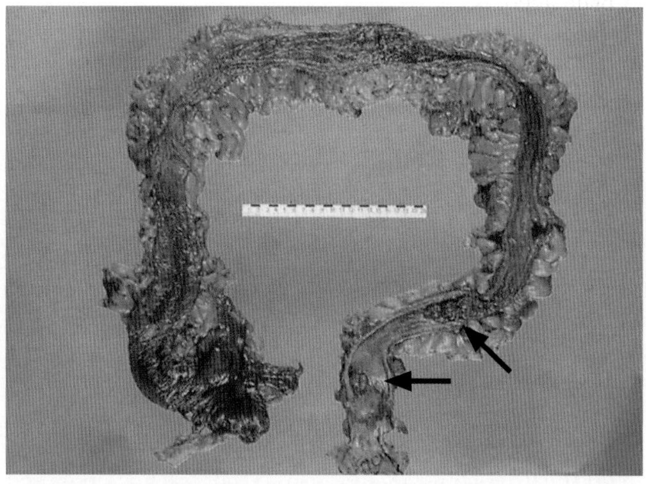

Figure 75.4 Resection specimen from a patient with longstanding ulcerative colitis showing a narrow tubular colon with areas of cancerous change in the rectum and sigmoid (arrows) (courtesy of the late Professor Brian Warren, John Radcliffe Hospital, Oxford, UK).

TABLE 75.1 Distinguishing ulcerative colitis (UC) and Crohn's disease (CD).

	UC	CD
Macroscopic		
Distribution	Colon/rectum	Anywhere in the gastrointestinal tract
Rectum	Always involved	Often spared
Perianal disease	Rare	Common
Fistula formation	Rare	Common
Stricture	Rare	Common
Microscopic		
Layers involved	Mucosa/submucosa	Full thickness
Granulomas	No	Common
Fissuring	No	Common
Crypt abscesses	Common	Rare

purulent exudate. Where there has been remission and relapse, there may be regenerative mucosal nodules or pseudopolyps. Later, tiny ulcers may be seen that appear to coalesce. Colonoscopy with biopsy has a key role in diagnosis and management:

- to establish the extent of inflammation, although colonoscopy is contraindicated in severe acute colitis because of the risk of colonic perforation;
- to distinguish between UC and Crohn's colitis (***Table 75.1***);
- to monitor the response to treatment;
- to assess longstanding cases for malignant change.

Endoscopic findings can be combined with clinical features and the physician's assessment to produce a disease activity score. The most widely used is the Mayo score, which provides a useful tool for measuring disease progression or response to treatment (***Table 75.2***).

Radiology

A plain abdominal film may indicate the severity of disease in the acute setting and is particularly valuable in demonstrating the development of toxic megacolon. Barium enema has been replaced by CT, although a contrast study will show a featureless colon. CT findings in pancolitis may show significant thickening of the colonic wall, as well as inflammatory stranding in the colonic mesentery (***Figure 75.5***).

Bacteriology

A stool specimen should be sent for microbiological analysis when UC is suspected in order to exclude infective colitides, notably *Campylobacter*, which may be very difficult to distinguish from acute severe UC. *Clostridium difficile* colitis may need to be considered in populations at risk of this disease (see ***Chapter 77***). Cytomegalovirus infection is a major pathogen in immunocompromised patients and can be difficult to distinguish from UC. Superimposed infection may precipitate fulminant colitis.

TREATMENT

Effective treatment of UC requires a multidisciplinary approach to management. Members of the IBD multidisciplinary team typically include specialists in IBD gastroenterology, colorectal surgery, IBD nursing, stoma therapy, gastrointestinal and interventional radiology, pathology, dieticians and nutritional support services, clinical psychologist and other specialties according to the individual patient's need.

Summary box 75.1

Principles of management of ulcerative colitis

- Most patients are maintained on optimised medical therapy
- Acute severe colitis (ASC) requires multidisciplinary management
- Toxic dilatation or impending complication should be suspected if the patient develops abdominal tenderness or distension, or deteriorates clinically
- Patients with colitis are at increased risk of developing cancer; those with pancolitis of long duration are most at risk

TABLE 75.2 Scoring system for assessment of ulcerative colitis activity.

Finding							
Stool frequency	Sub-score	Rectal bleeding	Sub-score	Disease activity on flexible sigmoidoscopy	Sub-score	Global assessment	Sub-score
Normal	0	None	0	Normal	0	Normal	0
1 or 2 more than normal	1	Streaks of blood <50% of the time	1	Mild	1	Mild	1
3 or 4 more than normal	2	Obvious blood >50% of the time	2	Moderate	2	Moderate	2
5+ more than normal	3	Blood alone passed	3	Severe	3	Severe	3

Adapted from Schroeder KW, Tremaine WJ, Ilstrup DM. Coated oral 5-aminosalicylic acid therapy for mildly to moderately active ulcerative colitis. *N Engl J Med* 1987; **317**(26): 1625–9.

Mayo score named after the Mayo Clinic, Rochester MN, USA.

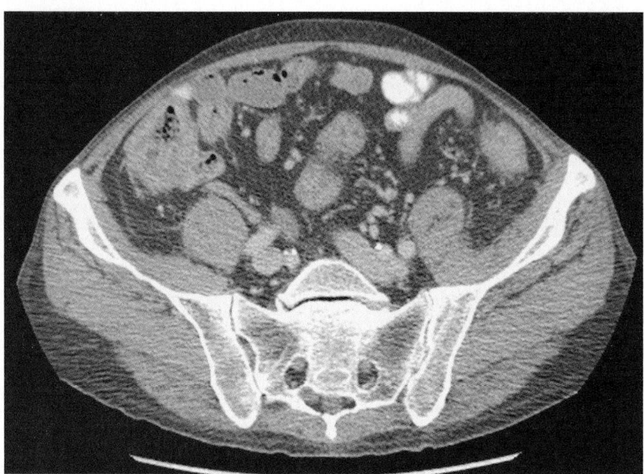

Figure 75.5 Computed tomography scan demonstrating colitis with a thickened colonic wall and inflammatory stranding in the mesentery (courtesy of Dr D Kasir, Hope Hospital, Salford, UK).

Medical treatment

Improved understanding of the complex cell signalling pathways that underlie aberrant immune responses in both UC and CD has radically changed treatment algorithms. The focus is now on both clinical and endoscopic remission end points with the aim of controlling symptoms and preventing disease progression. The particular choice of anti-inflammatory agent or immunosuppressive drug, the sequence and combination of use must take into account individual disease phenotypes, coexisting conditions, patient preferences, response to treatment, side effects and treatment availability. There has been a paradigm shift in treatment algorithms from escalation therapy in response to treatment failure to a top-down approach predicated on achieving clinical and endoscopic remission with subsequent de-escalation of treatment to maintain remission.

Conventional first-line treatment has been 5-aminosalicylic acid (5-ASA) derivatives given topically (per rectum) or systemically. These act as inhibitors of the cyclo-oxygenase enzyme system and are formulated to protect the aspirin-related drug from degradation before reaching the colon. Used as a single agent, 5-ASA is useful in treating ulcerative proctitis and as maintenance therapy following induction of remission.

Corticosteroids have been the mainstay of treatment used either topically or systemically. They have a widespread anti-inflammatory action and are frequently used in combination with 5-ASA derivatives to deliver prompt relief of symptoms.

The immunosuppressive drugs azathioprine and ciclosporin can be used to maintain remission and as steroid-sparing agents should maintenance therapy be required. Azathioprine is a purine analogue that is metabolised to 6-mercaptopurine (6-MP) and works by inhibiting cell-mediated immune responses. 6-MP may be given directly for the same effects. Approximately 10% of people have deficient thiopurine methyltransferase (TPMT) and 1 in 300 people have no enzyme activity, causing inefficient metabolism of 6-MP. The resulting high pharmacological concentrations may cause adverse effects such as myelosuppression. Testing of TPMT activity should be undertaken before commencing treatment.

Ciclosporin acts by inhibiting cell-mediated immunity. Short-course intravenous ciclosporin treatment is associated with remission in 80% of patients; however, many patients relapse after completion of treatment.

The monoclonal antibodies infliximab and adalimumab both act as antagonists to tumour necrosis factor alpha (TNFα), which has a central role in inflammatory cascades. Infliximab, a murine chimeric monoclonal antibody, was the first available monoclonal antibody for the treatment of CD. It is administered as an intravenous infusion most frequently to induce remission in moderate to severe disease and may be used as maintenance treatment once remission has been achieved. Adalimumab, an entirely human monoclonal antibody, is an alternative to infliximab that also targets TNFα. It can be self-administered by patients, which is advantageous in long-term maintenance. Trough levels and antibodies to anti-TNFα monoclonal antibodies should be monitored to ensure optimal dosing and efficacy of treatment.

Recently, ustekinumab, a monoclonal antibody against interleukin-12/23; vedolizumab and etrolizumab, anti-integrin monoclonal antibodies; tofacitinib, a JAK (Janus kinase) inhibitor; and ozanimod, an S1P (sphingosine-1-phosphate) receptor modulator have received regulatory approval for treatment of IBD. The complexity and best sequencing of treatment options requires multidisciplinary specialist input and is beyond the remit of this chapter (see ***Further reading***).

Nutritional support

It is essential that nutritional status is evaluated in all patients with IBD. Nutritional support is frequently required. Patients with moderate nutritional impairment will require nutritional supplementation and severely malnourished patients may require enteral tube or even intravenous feeding. Anaemia, hypoproteinaemia and electrolyte, vitamin and metabolic bone problems must all be addressed. Nutritional optimisation has been shown to improve surgical outcomes but it is important to recognise that a significant improvement in nutritional status is very unlikely in the setting of active infection; in patients with abscesses, effective drainage remains the overwhelming priority.

Acute severe colitis

Patients with a mild attack usually respond to a course of oral prednisolone. A moderate attack often responds to oral prednisolone, twice-daily steroid enemas and 5-ASA. Failure to achieve remission as an outpatient is an indication for admission. Acute severe colitis occurs in up to 10% of patients, who require hospital admission. Regular assessment of vital signs, weight and the abdomen are required. A stool chart should be kept, regular clinical review is required and supine abdominal radiographs should be done when there is clinical concern for toxic megacolon. The presence of mucosal islands or intramural gas on plain radiographs, increasing colonic diameter or a sudden increase in pulse and temperature may indicate impending colonic perforation. Limited endoscopic assessment and reassessment is useful in monitoring response to treatment. Fluid and electrolyte balance must be maintained, anaemia corrected and adequate nutrition provided, often parenterally.

Initial treatment is with intravenous steroids. Regular and joint review by a gastroenterologist and a colorectal surgeon is essential to identify patients who are failing to make anticipated progress and to ensure that surgery is neither inappropriately delayed nor inappropriately undertaken. Patients should be supported by IBD specialist nurses and early introduction to a stoma therapist is considered best practice.

Instigation of immunosuppressive therapy with either intravenous ciclosporin A or an anti-TNFα agent may be appropriate; however, surgery should be considered if rescue therapy does not result in rapid clinical improvement for the patient. Clinical deterioration requires urgent colectomy.

Indications for surgery

Surgery has a significant role in managing complications of IBD and in improving quality of life for patients with IBD. Current best practice ensures that surgeons and stoma therapists are an integral part of the multidisciplinary team throughout a patient's journey and that surgery is not presented as a last resort. Patients are then more likely to accept timely surgical intervention when indicated and be better prepared for life with a temporary or permanent stoma.

The overall lifetime risk of colectomy for a patient with UC is about 20%. Common indications for surgery in the emergency setting include refractory acute severe colitis or its complications, including perforation, toxic megacolon or, rarely, colonic haemorrhage not controlled by endoscopic or interventional radiological means.

The indications for surgery in UC are:

- severe or fulminating disease failing to respond to medical therapy;
- chronic disease with anaemia, frequent stools, urgency and tenesmus;
- steroid-dependent disease where remission cannot be maintained without substantial doses of steroids with harmful side effects;
- intolerance or side effects of medical therapy required to control the disease, e.g. steroid psychosis, azathioprine-induced pancreatitis;
- growth retardation in children or adolescents;
- neoplastic change: patients who have severe dysplasia or carcinoma;
- associated sclerosing cholangitis;
- extraintestinal manifestations;
- rarely, severe haemorrhage or stenosis causing obstruction.

Operative treatment

Emergency

In the emergency situation (or for a patient who is malnourished or on high-dose steroids), the safest procedure is subtotal colectomy and end-ileostomy. The rectosigmoid remnant may be left long and can either be brought out as a formal mucous fistula or closed just beneath the skin as a subcutaneous mucous fistula (***Figure 75.6***); alternatively, it can be closed off with staples across the upper rectum at the pelvic brim and rectal decompression achieved via a transanal catheter. This operation has the advantage that the patient avoids the risks of pelvic dissection while unwell and that colonic histology can be assessed to distinguish between UC and CD. Restorative surgery can be contemplated at a later date when the patient is no longer on steroids and has fully recovered. The mesentery should be divided where convenient and there is no evidence for or against preservation of the omentum in the laparoscopic era, when resection or preservation is a matter of surgical convenience. Most surgeons would recommend close dissection for UC and a greater degree of mesocolic resection for CD given the potential role for the mesentery

(a)

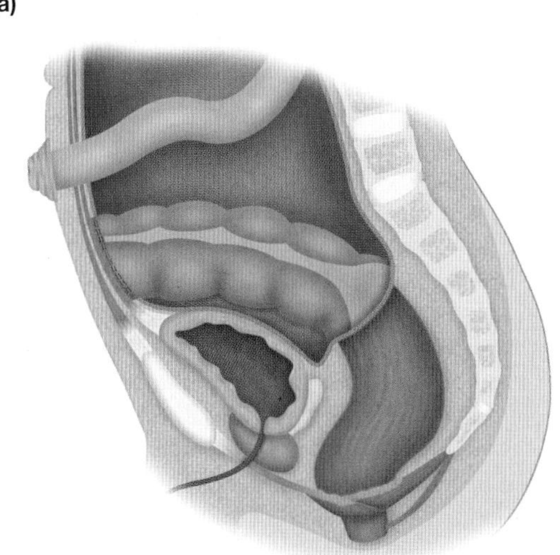

(b)

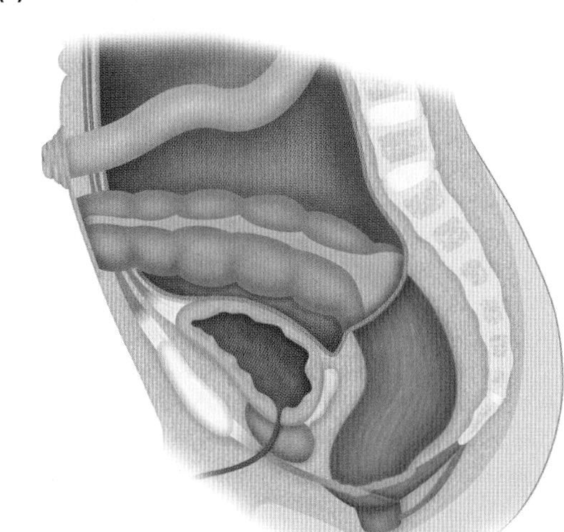

Figure 75.6 Subfascial closure of the rectal remnant following subtotal colectomy and end-ileostomy for acute ulcerative colitis **(a)**. The rectal remnant can alternatively be brought to the skin as a mucus fistula **(b)**.

postulated in CD. Dissection of the left colon is continued to divide the sigmoid at a level that will comfortably reach the skin as a mucous fistula unless this part of the bowel is severely diseased, in which case resection at the sacral promontory is the preferred approach.

Urgent subtotal colectomy for acute severe colitis can be performed laparoscopically, provided the surgeon and theatre team have adequate experience, with care to avoid perforation when handling friable bowel with laparoscopic instruments. Emergency colectomy for septic complications of acute severe colitis should be carried out in a timely fashion and should not be delayed pending availability of laparoscopic colorectal expertise.

Proctectomy is rarely needed in the urgent or emergency situation and should be avoided as pelvic dissection of the diseased rectum is difficult, carries risks to bladder and sexual function, prolongs the surgery in a critically ill patient, increases the risk of mortality and reduces the potential for later restorative surgery.

Fulminant colitis or toxic megacolon can also occur in CD, but less frequently than in UC. Without a pre-established diagnosis, distinction is usually not possible unless there is clear radiological evidence of small bowel CD or clinically apparent perianal CD. In the urgent setting subtotal colectomy for pancolitis should be performed as for UC, preferably with omental resection and a more radical approach to the mesentery. In situations where a diagnosis of colonic CD is established a more tailored segmental resection may be considered in highly selected patients. Primary anastomosis should be avoided in the acute setting and in immunosuppressed patients.

Elective

In the elective setting the following operations are available – all of these can be successfully performed laparoscopically in experienced hands:

- subtotal colectomy and ileostomy (as in an urgent colectomy);
- proctocolectomy and permanent end-ileostomy;
- restorative proctocolectomy with ileal pouch–anal anastomosis (IPAA);
- subtotal colectomy and ileorectal anastomosis;
- segmental colectomy (Crohn's colitis only).

Segmental resections are not recommended for UC as, even when the right colon is not obviously involved, there is a high recurrence rate in the remaining colon. Segmental colonic resection may be considered in selected patients with isolated CD. Subtotal colectomy with ileostomy is performed electively in frail patients, patients who cannot be weaned from steroids and when there is doubt as to the underlying diagnosis. In such situations, restorative surgery or completion proctectomy can be considered at a future date.

Complications of CD including fibrotic strictures not amenable to endoscopic dilatation and enteric fistulae are common indications for elective surgery in patients with CD. Patients who have previously undergone emergency resection and stoma formation will also require follow-up for counselling about restoration of bowel continuity.

Preoperative optimisation and timing of surgery

For many patients who require surgical intervention for colitis, the timing of surgery will be a critical part of shared decision making between clinicians and patient. In the elective setting, patients will want to plan surgery around social, educational, family and work commitments to minimise the impact of surgery and postoperative recovery on their lives. As proctectomy carries small but recognised risks to sexual function and fertility, patients may choose to defer surgery until after completing their families or consider sperm, oocyte or embryo storage to allow assisted fertility at a later date.

Steroid therapy in both UC and Crohn's colitis increases the risk of postoperative complications, although it is difficult to quantify this effect. Patients treated with steroids have an increased risk of infectious complications and poor healing. It is likely that there is a dose-related aspect to this phenomenon. In view of this, steroid use should be reduced as much as possible prior to surgery, preferably below 10 mg prednisolone per day, particularly if an anastomosis is planned. Both anti-TNFα and anti-integrin biological therapies also increase the risk of postoperative complications and should be discontinued wherever possible between 14 and 30 days prior to surgery.

Venous thromboembolism prophylaxis

Patients with IBD have a threefold increased risk of venous thromboembolism compared with the general population and this risk increases in patients who require surgery. The rate of thromboembolic events after surgery for IBD is around 3%, with the strongest predictors of thromboembolic complications being stoma formation, preoperative steroid therapy, ileoanal pouch formation and increased length of stay. The risk of venous thromboembolism is higher in patients with UC than in those with CD. Because of the increased risk of venous thromboembolism, extended chemoprophylaxis has been recommended with low-molecular-weight heparin used for up to 28 days after any abdominal procedure for IBD.

Panproctocolectomy and ileostomy

This operation removes the entire colon and rectum and, by doing so, removes any risk of colorectal neoplasia or colitic symptoms; it results in a permanent ileostomy. It has a lower complication rate than an ileal pouch procedure, although the perineal wound can be problematic (10% fail to heal) and stoma problems are common. It is indicated for patients who are not candidates for restorative surgery owing to impaired anal sphincter function, comorbidities or patient preference. The colectomy is performed as above. In UC, provided there is no concern regarding rectal cancer, a close rectal dissection may be performed to minimise damage to the pelvic nerves, avoiding erectile and bladder dysfunction. Recent evidence suggests that the mesorectum should be excised when proctectomy is performed in CD as the mesentery itself may be involved in the inflammatory process and delay perineal healing.

In UC without dysplasia or cancer present, an intersphincteric dissection of the anal canal should be performed. This results in a smaller perineal wound and fewer healing problems. In CD, wider excision of the anal canal and diseased perineum may be required if perianal disease is present. A permanent end-ileostomy is formed. The position of the ileostomy should be carefully sited preoperatively with the expert guidance of a stoma nurse specialist.

Restorative proctocolectomy with ileal pouch-anal anastomosis

Although restoration of bowel continuity by ileoanal anastomosis was first performed by Nissen in 1933 and later by Ravitch and Sabiston, the functional outcomes were poor and the operation was rarely performed. The combination of improved surgical techniques, better understanding of the physiology of faecal continence and the relative success of the continent ileostomy operation (Kock pouch) led Parks and Nicholls in the 1970s to reintroduce the concept of IPAA first promulgated by Bacon in the 1950s. Parks and Nicholls devised an 'S' pouch and later a 'W' pouch configuration; however, these have been generally superseded by the 'J' pouch described by Utsunomiya, which is technically easier to construct and avoids a potentially obstructing efferent limb from the pouch reservoir (***Figure 75.7***).

Early pouch surgery included dissection of the rectal muscularis propria (mucosal proctectomy) but it is now clear that continence is better if the mucosa immediately above the dentate line (anal transitional zone) is preserved. A distal mucosectomy to the upper anal canal with anastomosis at the dentate line is now reserved for patients with rectal mucosal dysplasia and selectively for patients in whom the operation is performed for familial adenomatous polyposis (FAP) (see ***Chapter 77***). Usually the anastomosis is double-stapled to the top of the anal canal, preserving the upper anal mucosa (***Figure 75.8***), although a hand-sewn pull-through anastomosis is also possible. Care must be taken to ensure that the anastomosis is to the anal canal and not the distal rectum as residual inflamed mucosa behind may cause persistent symptoms, so-called cuffitis.

IPAA is usually performed as a two-stage procedure with a covering loop ileostomy that may be closed at an interval once pouch healing has been confirmed, usually by means of a Gastrografin (water soluble) contrast enema radiograph. In patients who have previously undergone an urgent colectomy or those with IC in whom a colectomy had provided a definitive diagnosis of UC, the operation is considered to have been a three-stage procedure. In highly selected individuals whose operation is elective and immunosuppressive medication has been discontinued a one-stage operation without ileostomy may be considered. The modified two-stage approach of initial subtotal colectomy and end-ileostomy followed by proctectomy with pouch formation and without diversion is the standard of practice in many specialist centres.

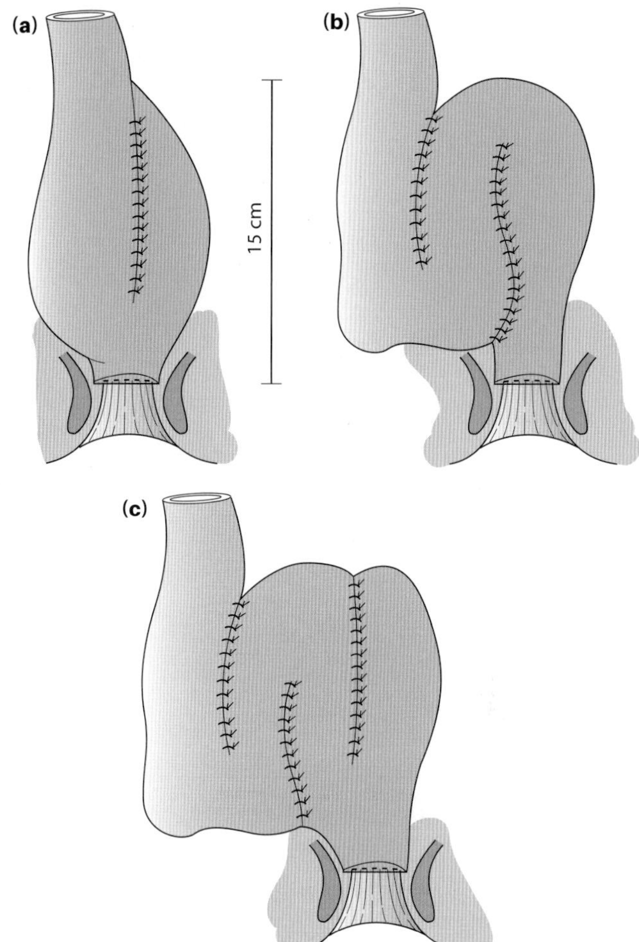

Figure 75.7 Ileoanal anastomosis with a pouch. A substitute rectum is made from joined folds of ileum to form an expanded pouch of small intestine. The pouch is then joined directly to the anus at the level of the dentate line, all other rectal mucosa having been removed. Three ways of forming a pouch are illustrated: **(a)** a simple reversed 'J'; **(b)** an 'S' pouch; **(c)** a 'W' pouch.

Postoperative complications include pelvic infection (usually resulting from a leak at the ileoanal anastomosis or, in a 'J' pouch, from the top of the 'J'), postoperative small bowel obstruction (which may occur in as many as 10–15% of patients) and pouch–vaginal fistula.

The frequency of evacuation is determined by pouch volume, completeness of emptying, reservoir inflammation and intrinsic small bowel motility, but is typically between three and eight evacuations in each 24-hour period, of which at least one evacuation is nocturnal. Stool frequency, urgency and minor faecal incontinence are common, but usually reduce with time

Rudolph Nissen, 1896–1981, surgeon, Istanbul, Turkey, later Jewish Hospital, New York, NY, USA, and University of Basel, Switzerland.
Mark Mitchell Ravitch, 1911–1989, surgeon, Montefiore Hospital, Pittsburgh, PA, USA.
David Sabiston, 1925–2009, surgeon, Duke University, Durham, NC, USA.
Nils G Kock, 1924–2011, Professor of Surgery, University of Gothenburg, Sweden.
Sir Alan Guyatt Parks, 1920–1982, surgeon, St Mark's Hospital, London, UK.
Ralph John Nicholls, b. 1943, surgeon, St Mark's Hospital, London, UK.
Harry Ellicott Bacon, 1900–1981, surgeon, Temple University, Philadelphia, PA, USA.
Joyi Utsunomiya, surgeon, Hyogo College of Medicine, Hyogo, Japan.

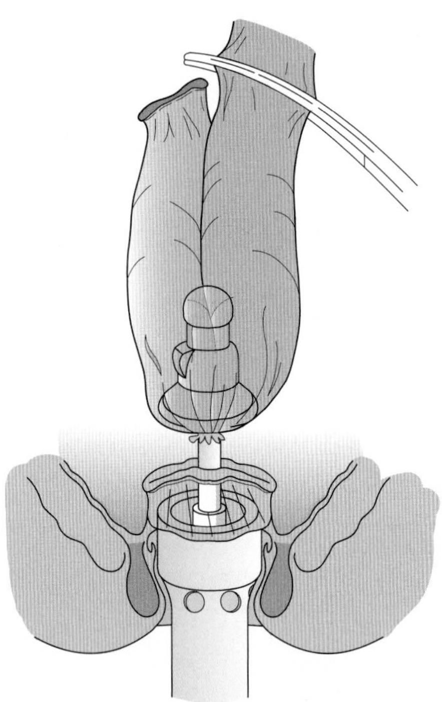

Figure 75.8 Stapled 'J' pouch with the stapler creating an ileal pouch–anal anastomosis

as ileal pouch capacity increases. The majority of patients with IPAA have a very good quality of life. The main reasons for pouch failure are pelvic infection, poor functional outcome and pouchitis (see below). Follow-up of patients with IPAA shows that, although the functional outcome may deteriorate with ageing, between 85% and 90% of patients retain their IPAA in the long term.

Women of reproductive age should be advised of potentially reduced fertility, as well as vaginal dryness, owing to denervation of the secretory glands of the vaginal mucosa. Laparoscopic or robotic techniques may reduce this effect; however, women who have not completed their family may elect for a colectomy with ileostomy and IPAA at a later date.

Pouchitis is inflammation of the ileal pouch mucosa that occurs to varying degrees in up to 50% of patients who undergo IPAA for UC. Interestingly, pouchitis is exceedingly rare after IPAA for FAP, suggesting that there is an inherent enteric mucosal proinflammatory response to an altered gut-associated microbiome following IPAA for UC. Pouchitis usually responds to a short course of antibiotic therapy, notably with metronidazole or ciprofloxacin, and can be followed by maintenance with probiotics. In a small percentage of patients (3–5%), pouchitis is recurrent or persistent such that pouch excision may be necessary. In such cases, previously undiagnosed CD and pouch ischaemia should be considered as alternative diagnoses.

Kock ileal pouch reservoir

The Kock pouch was originally designed as a continent urostomy but later adapted as a continent ileostomy for patients following proctocolectomy for IBD. The technique confirmed the safety of a small bowel reservoir, but difficulties with prolapse of the nipple valve mechanism required for continence and the success of IPAA as a mechanism to retain continence and anatomical continuity has meant that the operation is now rarely performed.

Colectomy and ileorectal anastomosis

This procedure is occasionally performed in UC if there is minimal rectal inflammation. A very considerable percentage (at least 50%) of patients with a quiescent rectum after total colectomy will develop significant mucosal inflammation in the rectum once the faecal stream has been re-established. Although rectal inflammation can be controlled with medical treatment, functional results may be disappointing. If the rectum is preserved, then annual rectal inspection is advocated. This procedure has the advantage of avoiding a stoma and the risk to sexual function associated with rectal dissection, and so may provide a useful transition in highly selected patients.

INDETERMINATE COLITIS

Approximately one in 10 patients with colitis presents with histological features that make their disease difficult to characterise. While the clinical history may suggest the diagnosis in some cases (for example, a history of recurrent perianal sepsis and fistulation would make a diagnosis of CD more likely), in others it may remain unclear whether a patient has UC or CD. In such cases, it may still be appropriate to offer IPAA after detailed informed consent, but the risks of pouch failure appear to be significantly higher (up to 25–30%) and patients should be advised accordingly.

CROHN'S DISEASE (REGIONAL ENTERITIS)

Chronic inflammatory disease of the ileum, possibly first recognised by Morgagni in 1761 and described separately by Leśniowski and Dalziel in the early twentieth century, is known as Crohn's disease after a key publication by Crohn, Ginzburg and Oppenheimer in 1932. It is characterised by a chronic full-thickness inflammatory process that can affect any part of the gastrointestinal tract from the lips to the anal margin. It is most common in North America and northern Europe, with an annual incidence of 8 per 100 000. CD is slightly more common in women and is most frequently diagnosed between the ages of 25 and 40 years. There is a second peak of incidence around the age of 70 years. The prevalence is highest among white people, notably in North America and north-western Europe. CD is less common in central Europe

Giovanni Battista Morgagni, 1682–1771, Professor of Anatomy, Padua, Italy.
Antoni Leśniowski, 1867–1940, Professor of Surgery, Warsaw University, Warsaw, Poland.
Thomas Kennedy Dalziel, 1861–1924, surgeon, Western Infirmary, Glasgow, UK.
Leon Ginzburg, 1989–1988, surgeon, Mount Sinai Hospital, New York, NY, USA.
Gordon D Oppenheimer, 1900–1974, surgeon, Mount Sinai Hospital, New York, NY, USA.

and less prevalent still in South America and Africa. The incidence is rising in Asia, which is attributed to increased urbanisation. There are differences in clinical manifestations in Asian populations, with a higher male predominance, more perianal involvement, fewer extraintestinal manifestations and worse clinical outcomes. The prevalence of CD seems to be three to five times higher in the Ashkenazi Jewish population, although it is lower in the Jewish population in Israel, suggesting the importance of environmental factors.

Aetiology

The aetiology of CD remains incompletely understood but is thought to involve a complex interplay of genetic and environmental factors. Although CD shares some features with chronic infections, particularly tuberculosis, no causative organism has ever been demonstrated. There is an intriguing similarity to Johne's disease of cattle, a chronic inflammatory enteropathy resulting from infection with *Mycobacterium paratuberculosis*, suggesting that CD may have a related aetiology. Some studies have identified mycobacterial DNA more frequently in tissue from patients with CD than in tissue from controls, but trials have not demonstrated any therapeutic benefit of treating CD with antituberculous drugs.

A wide variety of foods and a highly refined diet have been implicated in CD; however, no conclusive link has been proven. There is considerable recent interest in food additives, particularly preservatives that may support a proinflammatory dysbiosis in the gut microbiome. An association with high levels of sanitation in childhood has also been implicated. Smoking increases the relative risk of CD threefold and is an exacerbating factor after diagnosis, contrary to the protective effect seen in UC. Smoking cessation has a beneficial effect on disease activity comparable to that of medical therapies and is therefore an essential component in the effective management of CD.

Genetic factors are important in CD. Approximately 10% of patients have a first-degree relative with the disease, and concordance approaches 50% in monozygotic twins. Inheritance is thought to involve multiple genes with low penetrance. Variants of NOD2/CARD15, a gene involved in intracellular recognition of bacteria, have been shown to have a strong association with CD. Recent genome-wide association studies have identified activation of over 200 genes in IBD, some of which are associated with CD and others with UC. Most patients have no identifiable germline mutational signature, and epigenetic mutations are more likely to be involved.

Both UC and CD are associated with alterations in the gut microbiome, with generally decreased microbial diversity. New techniques including next-generation 16S ribosomal RNA sequencing allow detailed analysis of individual microbial communities within the gut with sequential studies informing changes that might be associated with disease activity. Despite over a decade of intense study, no definitive signature of either CD or UC has been established, other than reduced microbial diversity, particularly in CD.

Pathogenesis

In both CD and UC increased gut mucosal permeability appears to develop at a relatively early stage and may lead to increased passage of luminal antigens that induce a cell-mediated inflammatory response. Proinflammatory cytokines, such as interleukin-2 and tumour necrosis factor, are then released. It has been suggested that CD is associated with a defect in suppressor T cells. It is unclear whether the proposed increase in intestinal permeability is a cause or consequence of the disease process. Animal studies have suggested that the increase in gut permeability develops because of changes in bacterial recognition proteins and an increase in inflammatory gene activation before macroscopic evidence of inflammation develops. Studies of healthy and apparently unaffected first-degree relatives of patients with CD suggest that gut permeability is increased, which in turn suggests that a genetically determined increase in gut permeability, perhaps combined with an abnormal immune-mediated response to colonisation of the gut with enteric microflora, may initiate the disease.

Pathology

The terminal ileum is the most commonly affected segment of bowel in patients with CD, often occurring in combination with other areas of disease. More proximal small bowel is less frequently involved. Colitis alone occurs in up to one-third of cases, the stomach and duodenum are affected in around 5% of cases, but perianal lesions are common, affecting up to 50% of patients. Perianal disease occurs in 25% of patients with small bowel disease and in 75% of patients with Crohn's colitis.

Macroscopically CD is characterised by fibrotic thickening of the intestinal wall with narrowing (stricturing) of the lumen and fat wrapping (encroachment of mesenteric fat around the bowel) (***Figure 75.9***). There is usually dilated bowel just proximal to the stricture and deep mucosal ulcerations with linear or serpiginous (snake-like) patterns in the strictured area itself. Oedema between ulcers gives rise to a characteristic cobblestone appearance of the mucosa (***Figure 75.10***). The transmural inflammation (a pathognomonic feature of CD) may lead to segments of bowel becoming adherent to each other and to surrounding structures, forming inflammatory masses with mesenteric abscesses and fistulation into adjacent organs (***Figure 75.11***). The serosa is usually opaque, with thickening of the mesentery and enlarged mesenteric lymph nodes. CD is characteristically discontinuous, with inflamed areas separated by apparently normal intestine, so-called skip lesions.

Microscopically focal areas of chronic inflammation involving all layers of the intestinal wall with lymphoid aggregates are characteristic of CD. Non-caseating giant cell granulomas found in 60% of patients are pathognomonic of CD (***Figure 75.2***). They are most commonly seen in anorectal disease. Multifocal arterial occlusions are found in thickened muscularis propria. There may be nerve cell hyperplasia and deep, fissuring ulceration within affected areas. Characteristically, and unlike in UC, there may be completely normal areas immediately next to areas of severe inflammation.

Heinrich Albert Johne, 1839–1910, pathologist, Dresden, Germany.

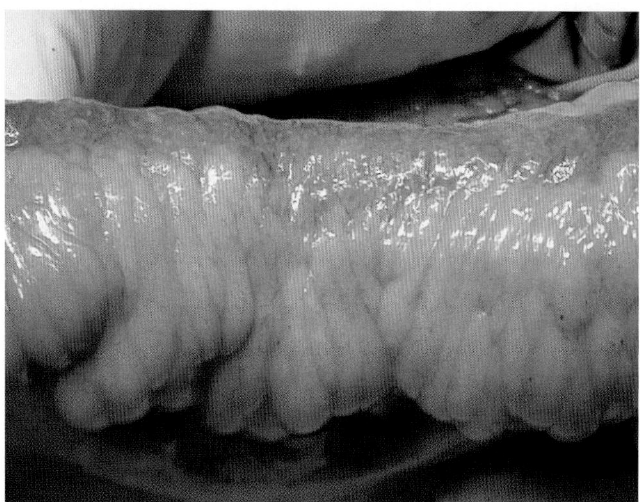

Figure 75.9 Crohn's disease of the ileocaecal region showing typical thickening of the wall of the terminal ileum with encroachment of mesenteric fat.

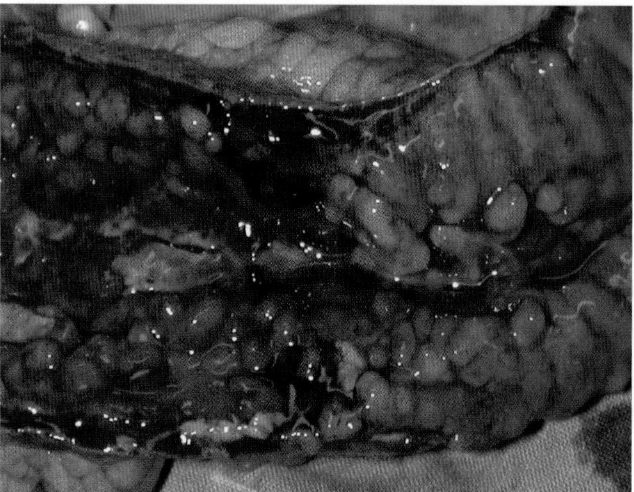

Figure 75.10 Crohn's disease of the terminal ileum illustrating longitudinal ulceration and cobblestone mucosa.

Clinical features

The clinical presentation depends on the pattern of disease. Occasionally, CD presents acutely with ileal inflammation and symptoms and signs resembling those of acute appendicitis or, much less commonly, free perforation of the small intestine resulting in a local or diffuse peritonitis. CD may present with acute severe colitis but this is considerably less common than in UC.

Small bowel CD often presents with bouts of abdominal pain and mild diarrhoea. A tender mass may be palpable in the right iliac fossa. Intermittent fever, anaemia and weight loss are common. After months of repeated attacks characterised by acute inflammation, the affected area of intestine stenoses with fibrosis, causing chronic obstructive symptoms. Children developing the illness before puberty may have retarded growth and sexual development. As CD progresses, transmural fissuring, intra-abdominal abscesses and fistulae may develop.

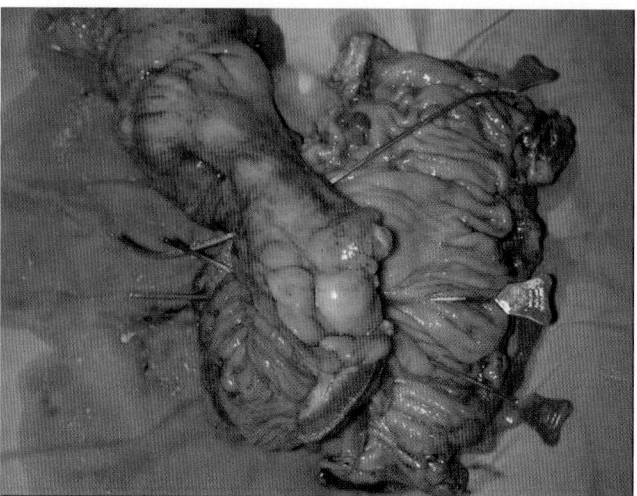

Figure 75.11 Resected specimen of terminal ileum and sigmoid colon illustrating Crohn's disease of the terminal ileum with multiple enterocolic fistulae.

Fistulation may occur into adjacent loops of bowel (entero-enteric or interloop fistulae). Occasionally, a mobile loop of sigmoid loop may become adherent to the affected terminal ileum, resulting in ileosigmoid fistulation (*Figure 75.11*). The fistula tracks in such cases are usually small and the profuse diarrhoea that results from ileosigmoid fistulation is due primarily to bacterial overgrowth (attributable to colonisation of the small bowel with colonic flora) rather than passage of small bowel content into the colon. Fistulation may also occur into the bladder (enterovesical), the female genital tract or, less commonly, the duodenum. Fistulation to the abdominal wall (enterocutaneous fistula) may also develop spontaneously or following appendicectomy in unrecognised CD, but more commonly presents as a complication of abdominal surgery.

Colonic Crohn's disease

Colonic involvement is found in 30% of patients with CD, frequently in association with perianal disease, and may coexist with small bowel pathology. Colonic CD presents with symptoms of colitis and proctitis as described for UC, although toxic megacolon is much less common. Colonic strictures may form just as are seen in small bowel CD. Endoscopic dilatation may be performed in expert hands as an alternative to surgical resection. Distinguishing between CD and UC is often difficult and requires clinical and pathological patterns to be combined. The presence of skip lesions, rectal sparing, non-caseating granulomas or perianal disease will point to CD (*Figure 75.12*).

Many patients with CD present with perianal problems. In the presence of active disease, the perianal skin can have a bluish tinge. Large, oedematous and inflamed skin tags are common. Fissures and superficial ulcers with undermined edges are relatively painless and can heal with bridging of epithelium. Deep cavitating ulcers are usually found in the upper anal canal; they can be painful and cause perianal abscesses and fistulae. Fistulation through the posterior wall of the vagina may lead to rectovaginal fistula and continuous leakage of gas and/or faeces per vagina (see *Chapter 80*).

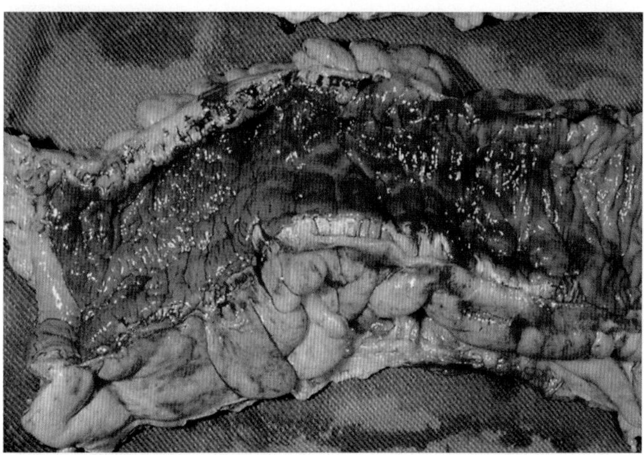

Figure 75.12 Colonic Crohn's disease. Note the normal mucosa on either side of the inflammatory stricture (courtesy of Professor Brian Warren, John Radcliffe Hospital, Oxford, UK).

The rectal mucosa is often spared in CD and will feel normal on rectal examination. If involved, it may feel thickened, nodular and irregular. Severe CD proctitis may occasionally be mistaken for cancer. Perianal disease is frequently associated with dense, fibrous stricturing (stenosis) at the anorectal junction. Incontinence may develop because of destruction of the anal sphincter musculature owing to inflammation, abscess formation, fibrosis and repeated surgical drainage. In severe cases, the perineum may become densely fibrotic, rigid and covered with multiple discharging openings (watering-can perineum).

Each patient with CD should have their disease phenotype (manifestations) classified according to the Montreal classification (*Table 75.3*). This is important as it allows an overview of disease progression in the individual patient over time, and enables group comparisons and evaluations. The Montreal classification specifies age at diagnosis, behaviour and disease location.

TABLE 75.3 The Montreal classification of Crohn's disease.

A: age at diagnosis	A1	≤16 years old
	A2	17–40 years old
	A3	>40 years old
B (behaviour): progression	B1	Inflammatory
	B2	Stenosing
	B3	Penetrating
	p	Perianal (can exist with any of the above)
L: location	L1	Ileal
	L2	Colonic
	L3	Ileocolonic
	L4	Upper digestive tract; can be added to any of the three above

After Silverberg MS, Daly MJ, Moskovitz DN *et al*. Diagnostic misclassification reduces the ability to detect linkage in inflammatory bowel disease genetic studies. *Gut* 2001; **49**: 773–6.

Extraintestinal manifestations

The extraintestinal manifestations of CD are similar to those that occur in UC. Primary sclerosing cholangitis is relatively rare in CD, compared with UC. Gallstones are common, as an inflamed or absent (because of resection) terminal ileum leads to reduced absorption of bile salts. Amyloidosis is common but is rarely symptomatic. Metastatic CD can occur in the vagina and/or skin with nodular ulcers, which demonstrate non-caseating granulomas when biopsied. Such cutaneous CD can be virtually indistinguishable macroscopically from hidradenitis suppurativa.

Investigations

Laboratory

A full blood count should be performed as anaemia is common, resulting from iron deficiency owing to blood loss, malabsorption or chronic disease. Vitamin B12 and folate deficiency may occur as a consequence of terminal ileal disease or resection. Active inflammatory disease is usually associated with low serum albumin, magnesium, zinc and selenium. Acute-phase protein measurements (C-reactive protein) and erythrocyte sedimentation rate may correlate with disease activity.

An elevated faecal concentration of calprotectin, a protein marker of mucosal inflammation, may support a diagnosis of CD in patients with new onset of persistent gastrointestinal symptoms. It can also be used to monitor disease activity in the long-term management of established CD.

Endoscopy

Colonoscopic examination may be normal or show patchy inflammation. Characteristically, there are areas of normal mucosa in between areas of inflammation that are irregular and ulcerated, with a mucopurulent exudate. The earliest findings are often aphthous ulcers surrounded by a rim of erythematous mucosa. These become larger and deeper with increasing severity of disease. There may be stricturing, and it is important to exclude malignancy at these sites by multiple and often repeated mucosal biopsies. An irregular Crohn's stricture with polypoid mucosa may be almost macroscopically indistinguishable from malignancy. The terminal ileum may be ulcerated and strictured. In patients who have had previous ileocaecal resection and anastomosis, recurrent disease usually presents first with aphthous ulceration just proximal to the anastomosis. Interval colonoscopy is therefore important in the follow-up after surgery for CD.

Upper gastrointestinal symptoms may require upper gastrointestinal endoscopy, which may reveal deep longitudinal ulcers and cobblestoning of the mucosa in the duodenum, stomach or, rarely, in the oesophagus or mouth. Enteroscopy may reveal jejunal ulceration and stricturing. Capsule endoscopy, which allows visualisation of the entire small intestinal mucosa by telemetry, has a useful role in those patients with evidence of chronic gastrointestinal symptoms or blood loss and where no evidence of ulceration can be found with more

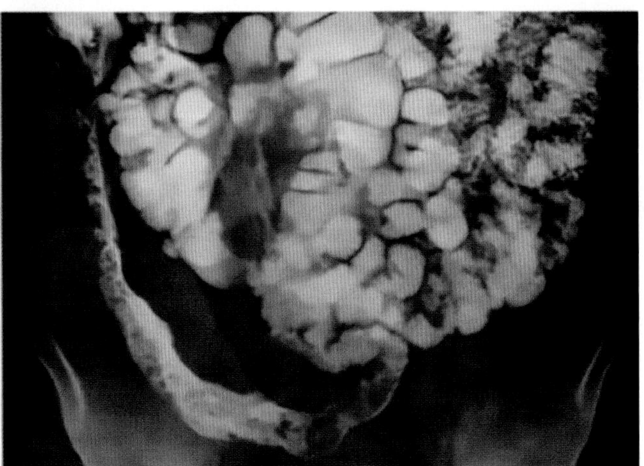

Figure 75.13 Radiograph showing a small bowel enema illustrating a long, strictured segment of terminal ileum due to Crohn's disease (string sign of Kantor).

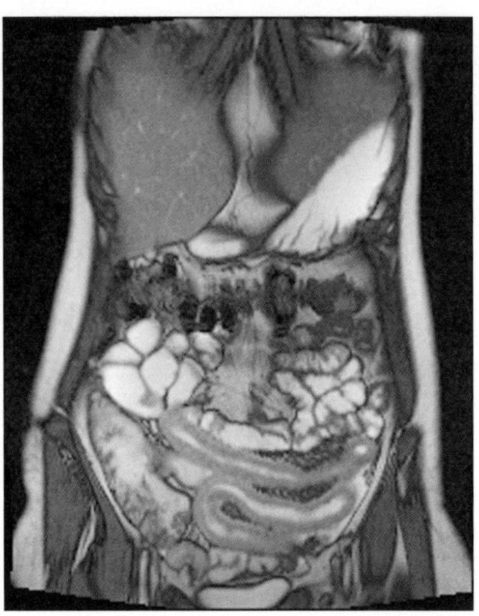

Figure 75.14 Magnetic resonance enteroclysis demonstrating small bowel inflammation (courtesy of Dr D Kasir, Hope Hospital, Salford, UK).

conventional endoscopic assessment. Investigation of the small intestine by capsule endoscopy should not be undertaken when there is a suspicion of stricture because of the possibility of the capsule becoming impacted in the narrow segment. A biodegradable test capsule can be used if this is a source of concern.

Imaging

High-resolution ultrasound in expert hands can demonstrate inflamed and thickened bowel loops as well as fluid collections and abscesses – the string sign of Kantor (*Figure 75.13*).

CT scans with oral contrast are widely used in the investigation of abdominal symptoms and can demonstrate fistulae, intra-abdominal abscesses and bowel thickening or dilatation. Magnetic resonance imaging (MRI) is useful in assessing complex perianal disease and has been shown to be an excellent method for investigating the small bowel. Magnetic resonance enterography (oral contrast) or enteroclysis (contrast administered via nasoduodenal tube) is particularly effective at demonstrating small bowel stricturing, including the string sign of Kantor, and avoids the need for repeated exposure to large doses of ionising radiation in young patients (*Figure 75.14*). A labelled white cell scan is occasionally of value to determine whether or not a segment of bowel is actively inflamed and to guide decisions on medical treatment.

In patients with an enterocutaneous fistula, fistulography may help to demonstrate the anatomy and complexity of the fistula and allow adequate planning for future surgery.

Medical treatment

Steroids

Corticosteroids are widely used to treat acute flares of CD. They induce remission in 70–80% of cases of moderate to severe disease. They should be used in short courses and tapered once a response has been achieved. They reduce inflammation and are therefore ineffective in established fibrostenotic disease. Steroid enemas may be used in the rectum, where the benefits include reduced systemic bioavailability, although long-term use may still cause adrenal suppression. Oral steroid formulations such as budesonide have been devised, where the steroid moiety is removed in the portal circulation, thus reducing systemic side effects. Steroids should not be used as maintenance therapy and are usually replaced with immunomodulatory agents to minimise the risk of side effects associated with long-term steroid use.

Aminosalicylates

Colonic symptoms can be treated by 5-ASA agents in a similar manner to those in UC. These agents have limited efficacy in small bowel CD.

Antibiotics

Metronidazole and ciprofloxacin may be used, particularly for periods of a few weeks at a time, especially in perianal disease. Long-term use of metronidazole should be avoided as there is a risk of peripheral neuropathy. Ciprofloxacin also has significant side effects when used in the long term, including tendinitis and tendon rupture. Antibiotics may be used to treat an inflammatory mass or an abscess. In general, however, a confirmed abscess should be treated by percutaneous drainage and/or surgery as antibiotics alone will not treat a Crohn's mass effectively.

Immunomodulatory agents

Azathioprine is used for its additive and steroid-sparing effects and currently represents standard maintenance therapy. It is a purine analogue, which is metabolised to 6-MP, and works by inhibiting cell-mediated immune responses (see ***Medical treatment of ulcerative colitis***).

John Leonard Kantor, 1890–1947, gastroenterologist, Presbyterian Hospital, New York, NY, USA, described his string sign in 1934.

Ciclosporin acts by inhibiting cell-mediated immunity. Short-course intravenous ciclosporin treatment is associated with remission in 80%; however, there is relapse after completion of treatment in many cases. Methotrexate is a drug that has a wide effect on DNA synthesis and immune signalling and can also be used in CD, although it is used less frequently in the biological era.

Monoclonal antibody (biologic) therapy

Infliximab, a murine chimeric anti-TNFα monoclonal antibody, and adalimumab, an entirely human anti-TNFα monoclonal antibody, are widely used to induce remission in moderately severe and severe CD. Third-generation monoclonal antibody therapies vedolizumab and etrolizumab prevent leukocyte migration preferentially in the gastrointestinal tract and may therefore have fewer side effects. More recently ustekinumab has entered widespread use as a CD therapy. It targets interleukin-12/23 to dampen the autoimmune system.

Monoclonal antibody therapy is currently widely used for induction and maintenance of remission. Early and aggressive use in patients at high risk for early recrudescent disease after surgery (for example, penetrating phenotype, early mucosal inflammation or aphthous ulceration at follow-up colonoscopy) may reduce (or at least postpone) the need for subsequent surgery. Perforation and abscess formation are usually regarded as contraindications to the use of biological therapy, although biologicals may be safely used after percutaneous drainage. While biologicals may reduce inflammation and may occasionally achieve healing of fistula openings in anal disease, the fistula tracks may remain patent and cessation of therapy is associated with a high risk of reactivation. Care must be taken before starting biological therapy to ensure that there is no active sepsis and that a diagnosis of intestinal tuberculosis has been excluded (see ***Chapter 65***).

Nutritional support

Nutritional support is frequently required in CD. Patients with moderate nutritional impairment will require nutritional supplementation and severely malnourished patients may require enteral tube or even parenteral nutrition. Anaemia, hypoproteinaemia and electrolyte, vitamin and metabolic bone problems must all be addressed. Elemental diet or parenteral nutrition can induce remission in up to 80% of patients, an effect comparable to steroids, but almost all patients relapse rapidly after cessation of therapy. Nutritional optimisation has been shown to improve surgical outcomes, but it is important to recognise that a significant improvement in nutritional status is unlikely in the setting of active infection and, in patients with abscesses, effective drainage remains the overwhelming priority.

Endoscopic dilatation in Crohn's disease

Although penetrating disease will often require surgical resection, stricturing may be amenable to endoscopic treatment. This may be accomplished by enteroscopy or colonoscopy, depending on the site of the stricture. Dilatation of an inflamed or ulcerated stricture is contraindicated because of the risks of perforation, but balloon dilatation of fibrostenotic disease may result in substantial symptomatic improvement and obviate the need for surgery in selected cases. It is most suited for short (<5 cm) fibrostenotic strictures, including those seen at a previous anastomosis.

Indications for surgery

Population-based studies show that approximately 70% of patients with CD will require a bowel resection in the first decade after diagnosis, and 40% will require a further resection in the decade after their index resection. Recent population-based data in the era of monoclonal antibodies suggest that the incidence of surgery may be falling, but surgery nevertheless remains a key component of treatment.

Surgical resection will not cure CD. Surgery therefore focuses on managing the complications of the disease (***Summary box 75.2***). As many of these indications for surgery may be relative, joint management by an aggressive physician and a conservative surgeon is ideal and decisions regarding surgical intervention are best made by a multidisciplinary team in consultation with the patient and recognising their preferences. The fundamental principle is to preserve healthy gut and to maintain adequate function. Intestinal resection should be kept to the minimum required to treat the local consequences of disease to mitigate against the potential for short bowel syndrome (see ***Chapter 91***).

In laparoscopic surgery it may be more difficult to assess the full length of the small intestine, so up-to-date preoperative small bowel imaging is important. While surgery carries perioperative risks, it also carries significant benefits, notably in patients with isolated terminal ileal disease, in whom a prolonged period of good health may be achieved. The relative benefits of surgical resection and long-term medical therapy in CD can be very finely balanced and require careful consideration and discussion with the patient within the setting of a combined gastroenterological and surgical IBD clinic.

Summary box 75.2

Principles of management of CD

- Close liaison between physician and surgeon is crucial
- Both medical and surgical treatment options should be considered; however, surgery should not be delayed when there is a clear indication
- Patients must be optimised prior to surgery; this may include radiological drainage of sepsis, antibiotic treatment and nutritional support
- CD is a chronic relapsing disease with a high likelihood of reoperation; the surgeon must take every reasonable effort to preserve bowel length and sphincter function
- Shared decision making with patients to accommodate their treatment preferences

Occasionally unsuspected ileal inflammation is found during emergency appendicectomy. Determining whether or not to resect the ileum in this situation is a complex clinical decision that should be made by a senior surgeon.

This decision involves an assessment of the likelihood that the ileitis is an expression of CD rather than another aetiology such as *Yersinia* infection; an assessment of the likelihood of remission with medical therapy rather than surgery; risk of enterocutaneous fistulation from appendiceal base leakage; and an assessment of the rest of the small bowel for the presence of additional sites of inflammation. In the current era of monoclonal therapy, it would be controversial to resect uncomplicated terminal ileitis found during an emergency procedure for suspected appendicitis, as this is likely to respond to medical therapy. If reasonably safe, appendicectomy is now encouraged for histological confirmation in limited previously undiagnosed disease, with appendicectomy carried out using a laparoscopic stapler to reduce the risk of enterocutaneous fistula (see ***Chapter 76***).

The course of CD after surgery is unpredictable, but recrudescence (a better term than recurrence) is common. Symptomatic recrudescence does not seem to be related to the presence of disease at the resection line. The cumulative probability of recrudescence requiring surgery for ileal disease is approximately 20%, 40%, 60% and 80% at 5, 10, 15 and 20 years, respectively, after a previous resection.

Surgery for CD is technically demanding as the involved mesentery is thickened and oedematous and healing may be impaired (see ***Chapter 65***). The patient may be malnourished, on immunosuppressants or have active infection/sepsis, or potentially all three. Decision making regarding the timing and nature of surgery to be undertaken is key to a satisfactory outcome of surgical treatment, and frequently requires experience and multidisciplinary discussion with other healthcare professionals and, most importantly, the patient. A key decision must be made whether to anastomose the apparently healthy bowel ends after macroscopically apparent disease has been resected, as anastomotic leaks and fistulation represent a considerable problem after surgery for CD. Intra-abdominal septic complications are more common if one or more of the following risk factors are present:

- current high-dose steroid therapy (>10 mg prednisolone for >4 weeks before surgery);
- current or very recent (<14 days) preoperative monoclonal antibody therapy;
- preoperative significant weight loss (>10% premorbid weight);
- coexisting abdominal sepsis (notably an abscess or fistula);
- low serum albumin <30 g/L.

If any risk factors are present (and particularly if more than one risk factor is present as the risks appear to be additive), one should consider exteriorising the bowel to create a stoma, with distal segment closure left close to the ileostomy site, and plan a delayed anastomosis when the risk factors have been corrected.

Ileocaecal or colonic resections can be undertaken laparoscopically, with the potential advantage of smaller incisions and potentially shorter recovery time. Reoperative surgery is technically demanding and ileosigmoid or ileoduodenal adhesions and fistulae can be difficult to safely dissect laparoscopically. Laparotomy should be considered in this setting. Although CD is usually regarded as a contraindication to ileal pouch surgery, the other options (panproctocolectomy or total colectomy with ileorectal anastomosis) are frequently appropriate and there may be considerable rectal sparing in CD, justifying the latter. Where the diagnosis of CD is firmly established, segmental rather than total colectomy may be appropriate.

The range of operations performed for CD depends on the pattern of disease; the most common are outlined below:

- **Ileocaecal resection** is the usual procedure for terminal ileal disease, with a primary anastomosis between the ileum and the ascending or transverse colon, depending on the extent of the disease. Ileostomy without primary anastomosis is indicated if the patient is unwell, has active infection or is nutritionally depleted.
- **Segmental resection** of short segments of small or large bowel strictures can be performed.
- **Colectomy and ileorectal anastomosis** may be undertaken for colonic CD with rectal sparing and a normal anus.
- **Subtotal colectomy and ileostomy** for Crohn's colitis accounts for 8% of such procedures for acute colonic disease. The indications are similar to those for UC.
- **Temporary loop ileostomy**. This can be used either in patients with acute distal CD, allowing remission and later restoration of continuity, or in patients with severe perianal or rectal disease.
- **Panproctocolectomy**. Many patients with severe anal disease failing to respond to medical treatment will eventually require a permanent colostomy. When this occurs in a setting of severe colonic disease, proctocolectomy and permanent ileostomy may be required.
- **Strictureplasty**. Strictured areas of CD (***Figure 75.15a***) can be treated by strictureplasty, a local widening procedure, to avoid small bowel resection and is thus an important bowel-sparing technique. Strictureplasty is particularly useful for the treatment of fibrostenotic disease when there is little or no active inflammation in the involved segment. Strictureplasty is contraindicated in the presence of a phlegmon, Crohn's associated cancer or haemorrhage due to mucosal ulceration. If there is any concern about malignancy at the site of a stricture, then frozen biopsy carried out intraoperatively may allow a strictureplasty to take place rather than resection, although resection and formal histological assessment remains the better option if there is any doubt. Multiple strictureplasties can be performed and strictureplasty can be combined with resection. The Heineke–Mikulicz technique of an antimesenteric longitudinal incision that is closed transversely is the most common technique. A Finney antimesenteric side-to-side anastomosis is used to treat long segments of stenosis when preservation of bowel length is important (***Figure 75.15b***).

Walter Hermann von Heineke, 1834–1901, Professor of Surgery, Erlangen, Germany.
Jan Mikulicz-Radecki, 1850–1905, surgeon, Kraków and later Königsberg and Wrocław, Poland.
John Miller Turpin Finney, 1863–1942, surgeon, Johns Hopkins Medical School, Baltimore, MD, USA.

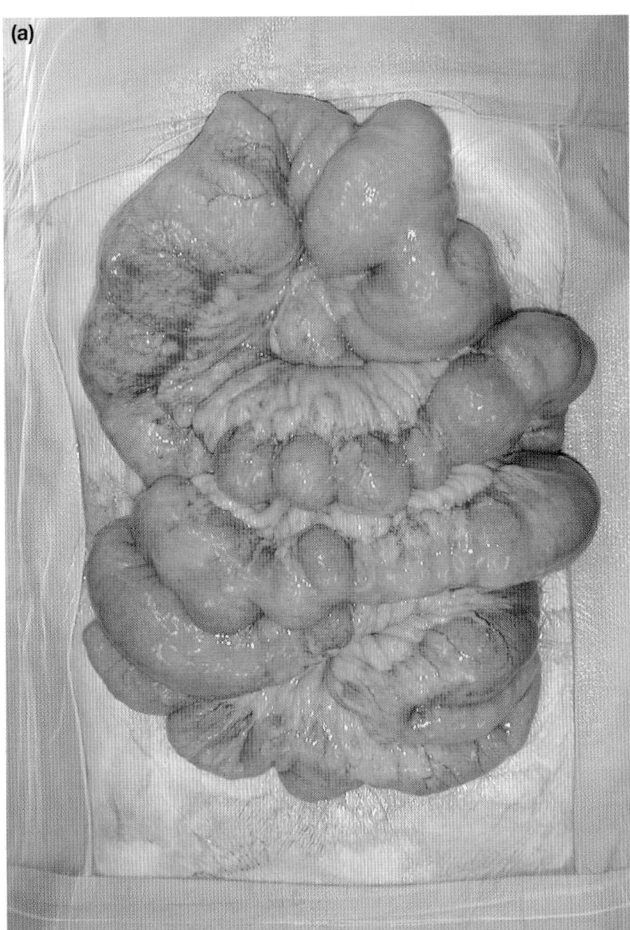

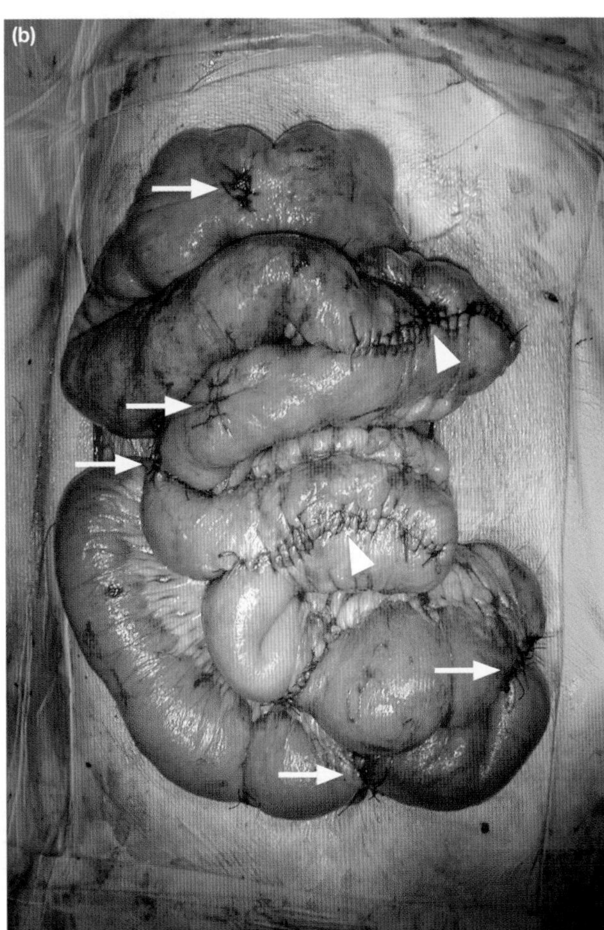

Figure 75.15 (a) Crohn's disease affecting the jejunum and ileum (jejunoileitis) with multiple strictures and bowel dilatation between skip lesions. (b) Same patient following multiple strictureplasties: Heineke–Mikulicz (arrows) and Finney (arrowheads).

Recent clinical research has pointed towards the importance of the mesentery in disease recurrence following resection (see *Chapter 65*). Complete excision of macroscopically diseased mesentery may reduce the incidence of recurrence, as may anastomotic techniques that ensure that an anastomosis is fashioned on the antimesenteric aspect of the bowel (Kono-S procedure).

Irrespective of the site of resection or anastomotic technique used, it is important to follow patients closely in the postoperative months to ensure that recrudescence of CD is identified at a very early stage and medical treatment reinstituted. A strong case can be made for restarting prophylactic biological treatment subject to endoscopic review at 6 months following resection.

Perianal Crohn's disease

Perianal CD is distressing and often debilitating for patients. The most common presentation is with a perianal abscess: perianal swelling, redness and pain, followed by discharge of pus or faecal drainage to perianal skin or vagina, representing a fistulous connection. Management requires a combination of medical and surgical treatments. The role of surgery is to control infection in the first instance, and later to minimise recurrent infection, reduce drainage and to offer potential for fistula cure. If a fistula is seen at the time of abscess drainage, a seton may be placed. Otherwise, further examination under anaesthesia will be required for placement of draining seton(s) by an experienced colorectal surgeon.

MRI may aid identification of occult fistulae or sources of ongoing sepsis. Long-term drainage with setons prevents further tissue loss from undrained infection but also allows safe initiation of biological therapy. Infliximab or adalimumab therapy may be combined with seton insertion in the early phase of management of perianal fistulae. Once fistula discharge has reduced, typically after two or three doses, the seton can be removed. Laying open of fistulae (fistulotomy), commonly performed for fistulae resulting from the more common cryptoglandular perianal abscess, should generally be avoided in CD as the wound edges heal poorly.

Potentially curative surgical options include advancement flaps, fibrin glue, fistula plugs, ligation of the intersphincteric

Toru Kono, 1955–2021, Sapporo Higashi Tokushukai Hospital, Higahi-ku, Sapporo, Hokkaido, Japan.

fistula track (LIFT) and adipose-derived stem cell injection coupled with sutured closure of the internal fistula opening. The over-the-scope clip (OTSC®) and video-assisted anal fistula treatment (VAAFT) have only been used in small numbers of patients (see ***Chapter 80***).

Injection of adipose-derived mesenchymal stem cells into tissue surrounding complex anal fistula tracts is well tolerated and when used in combination with established treatments may increase fistula healing rates. The mechanisms of action are uncertain but are thought to relate to regenerative and anti-inflammatory cytokines produced by stem cells. The treatment is expensive and further trials are needed.

A diverting stoma may offer significant quality of life benefit in selected patients and should be offered to symptomatic patients in the presence of intractable symptomatic perianal disease or proctitis, or failure to control perianal sepsis. Proctectomy is a good option for some patients and a permanent stoma should not be viewed as a treatment failure as it may again offer significant improvement in quality of life in selected patients. Rectovaginal fistulae hardly ever close with medical management alone, and surgery to repair rectovaginal fistulae has relatively low success rates. Failure of surgical repair may result in further deterioration in symptoms if there is additional loss of functional anorectal, vaginal or perineal tissue, and ultimately stoma rates are high in this group of patients.

Ileal pouch–vaginal fistula

Ileal pouch–vaginal fistula is most commonly due to an anastomotic complication; however, a delayed presentation may reflect an underlying diagnosis of CD rather than UC. Management depends on cause: biological therapy for CD, diverting ileostomy if there is complex sepsis, and definitive repair with interposition of native tissue if the sepsis resolves and CD has been excluded.

Duodenal Crohn's disease

The duodenum is an uncommon site for CD and involvement is more commonly the result of inflammation in another part of the bowel as a bystander effect (secondary). This can often be managed by resection of the source of the fistula with direct duodenal repair if the defect is small or closure using an omental patch or duodenojejunostomy if the defect is sizeable. Duodenal strictures may be amenable to endoscopic balloon dilatation; however, strictureplasty, bypass gastrojejunostomy or gastroduodenostomy may be required.

SPECIALISATION IN INFLAMMATORY BOWEL DISEASE SURGERY

Many general surgeons have relatively little experience in managing patients with IBD. High-volume centres have lower morbidity and mortality rates after colectomy for emergency surgery for IBD and after primary ileocaecal resection for CD. Specialist units also have a lower failure rate following IPAA and are more likely to offer subsequent restorative surgery, rather than permanent stoma, for patients who have required emergency colectomy.

Less common aspects of IBD surgery, including the need for revision or excision pouch surgery, rectovaginal fistula management, Kock pouch formation or care of adolescent patients, require specialist expertise to achieve good outcomes.

FURTHER READING

Baumgart DC, LeBerre C. Newer biologic and small-molecule therapies for inflammatory bowel disease. *N Engl J Med* 2021; **385**: 1302–15.

Brown SR, Fearnhead NS, Faiz OD *et al.* The Association of Coloproctology of Great Britain and Ireland consensus guidelines in surgery for inflammatory bowel disease. *Colorectal Dis* 2018; **20**(Suppl 8): 3–117.

Colombel JF, Sandborn WJ, Rutgeerts P *et al.* Adalimumab for maintenance of clinical response and remission in patients with Crohn's disease: the CHARM trial. *Gastroenterology* 2007; **132**(1): 52–65.

Cottrill M. BSG updates guidance on ulcerative colitis and Crohn's disease. Available from https://www.guidelinesinpractice.co.uk/gastrointestinal/bsg-updates-guidance-on-ulcerative-colitis-and-crohns-disease/300702.article (accessed 7 October 2021).

Dinesen LC, Walsh AJ, Protic MN *et al.* The pattern and outcome of acute severe colitis. *J Crohns Colitis* 2010; **4**(4): 431–7.

Panés J, Garcia-Olmo D, van Assche G *et al.* Long-term efficacy and safety of stem cell therapy (Cx601) for complex perianal fistulas in patients with Crohn's disease. *Gastroenterology* 2018; **154**: 1334–1342.e4.

Ran Z, Wu K, Matsuoka K *et al.* Asian Organization for Crohn's and Colitis and Asia Pacific Association of Gastroenterology practice recommendations for medical management and monitoring of inflammatory bowel disease in Asia. *J Gastroenterol Hepatol* 2021; **36**: 637–45.

Sands BE, Anderson FH, Bernstein CN *et al.* Infliximab maintenance therapy for fistulizing Crohn's disease. *N Engl J Med* 2004; **350**(9): 876–85.

Wasmann K, de Groof EJ, Stellingwerf ME *et al.* Treatment of perianal fistulas in Crohn's disease, seton versus anti-TNF versus surgical closure following anti-TNF (PISA): a randomised controlled trial. *J Crohns Colitis* 2020; **14**: 1049–56.

CHAPTER

76 The vermiform appendix

Learning objectives

To understand:

- The aetiology and surgical anatomy of acute appendicitis
- The clinical signs and differential diagnoses of appendicitis
- The investigation of suspected appendicitis
- Evolving concepts in the management of acute appendicitis
- Basic surgical techniques, both open and laparoscopic
- The management of postoperative problems
- Tumours of the appendix and pseudomyxoma peritonei

INTRODUCTION

The importance of the vermiform appendix in surgery arises primarily from its propensity for inflammation, which results in the clinical syndrome known as acute appendicitis. Acute appendicitis is the most common cause of an 'acute abdomen' in young adults and, as such, the associated symptoms and signs have become a paradigm for clinical teaching. Appendicitis is sufficiently common that appendicectomy (termed appendectomy in North America) is the most frequently performed urgent abdominal operation and is often the first major procedure performed by a surgeon in training. Advances in modern radiographic imaging have improved diagnostic accuracy; however, the diagnosis of appendicitis remains essentially clinical, requiring a mixture of observation, clinical acumen and surgical science and as such it remains an enigmatic challenge and a reminder of the art of surgical diagnosis. Although much more uncommon, the appendix also has a propensity to the formation of tumours, which, despite humble and innocuous beginnings, may disseminate widely with dramatic clinical consequences.

Aside from its tendency to cause surgical pathology, the appendix, long thought to be a vestigial organ, may also have important roles in both immune function and maintaining the gut microbiota. The putative role of the appendix in the pathogenesis of ulcerative colitis (appendicectomy seems to be protective), for example, may be explained by its interaction with the intestinal flora and gut immune function.

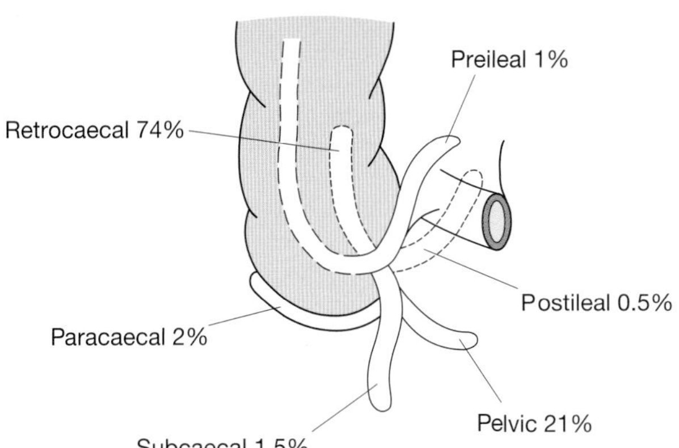

Figure 76.1 The various positions of the appendix (after Sir C Wakeley, London).

ANATOMY

The vermiform appendix is present only in humans, certain anthropoid apes and the wombat. It is a blind muscular tube with mucosal, submucosal, muscular and serosal layers. Morphologically, it is the undeveloped distal end of the large caecum found in many lower animals. At birth, the appendix is short and broad at its junction with the caecum, but differential growth of the caecum produces the typical tubular structure by about the age of 2 years (Condon). During childhood, continued growth of the caecum commonly rotates the appendix into a retrocaecal but intraperitoneal position (***Figure 76.1***). In approximately one-quarter of cases, rotation of the appendix does not occur, resulting in a pelvic, subcaecal or paracaecal position. Occasionally, the tip of the appendix becomes extraperitoneal, lying behind the caecum or ascending colon. Rarely, the caecum does not migrate during development to its normal position in the right lower quadrant of the abdomen. In these circumstances, the appendix can be found near the gallbladder or, in the case of intestinal malrotation, in the left iliac fossa, causing diagnostic difficulty if appendicitis develops (***Figure 76.2***).

A wombat is a nocturnal, burrowing Australian marsupial.
Robert E Condon, 1929–2015, Emeritus Professor of Surgery, Medical College of Wisconsin, WI, USA.

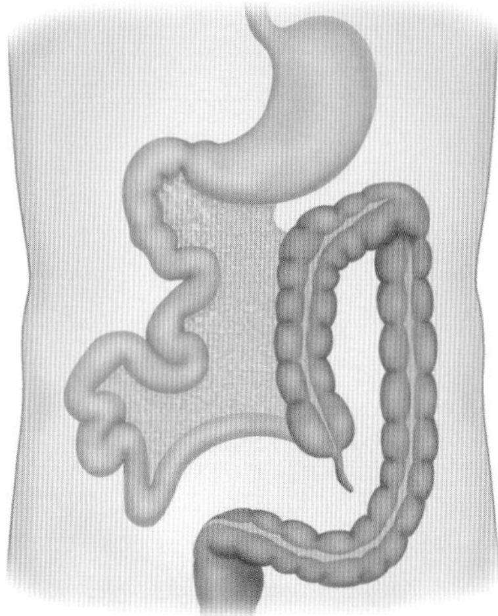

Figure 76.2 Left-sided caecum and appendix due to intestinal malrotation.

Gross anatomy

The position of the base of the appendix is constant, being found at the confluence of the three taeniae coli of the caecum, which fuse to form the outer longitudinal muscle coat of the appendix. At operation, use can be made of this to find an elusive appendix, as gentle traction on the taeniae coli, particularly the anterior taenia, will lead the operator to the base of the appendix. The mesentery of the appendix or mesoappendix arises from the lower surface of the mesentery of the terminal ileum and is itself subject to great variation. Sometimes, as much as the distal one-third of the appendix is bereft of mesoappendix. Especially in childhood, the mesoappendix is so transparent that the contained blood vessels can be seen (***Figure 76.3***). In many adults, it becomes laden with fat, which obscures these vessels. The appendicular artery, a branch of the lower division of the ileocolic artery, passes behind the terminal ileum to enter the mesoappendix a short distance from the base of the appendix. It then comes to lie in the free border of the mesoappendix. An accessory appendicular artery may be present but, in most people, the appendicular artery is an 'end-artery', thrombosis of which results in necrosis of the appendix (synonym: gangrenous appendicitis). Four, six or more lymphatic channels traverse the mesoappendix to empty into the ileocaecal lymph nodes.

Microscopic anatomy

The appendix varies considerably in length and circumference. The average length is between 7.5 and 10 cm. The lumen is irregular, being encroached on by multiple longitudinal folds of mucous membrane lined by columnar cell intestinal mucosa of colonic type (***Figure 76.4***). Crypts are present but are not numerous. In the base of the crypts lie argentaffin cells (Kulchitsky cells), which may give rise to neuroendocrine tumours (NETs) (see ***Neuroendocrine tumours of the appendix***). The submucosa contains numerous lymphatic aggregations or follicles. While no discernible change in immune function results from appendicectomy, the prominence of lymphatic tissue in the appendix of young adults seems to be important in the aetiology of appendicitis (see ***Acute appendicitis***).

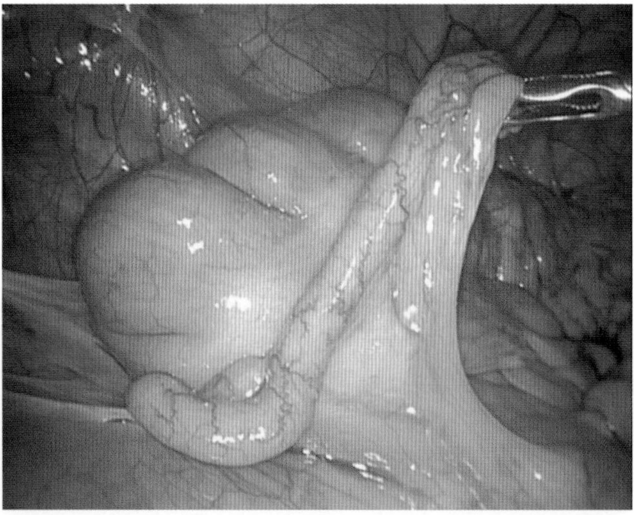

Figure 76.3 Laparoscopic view of a normal appendix with mesoappendix displaying the appendicular artery.

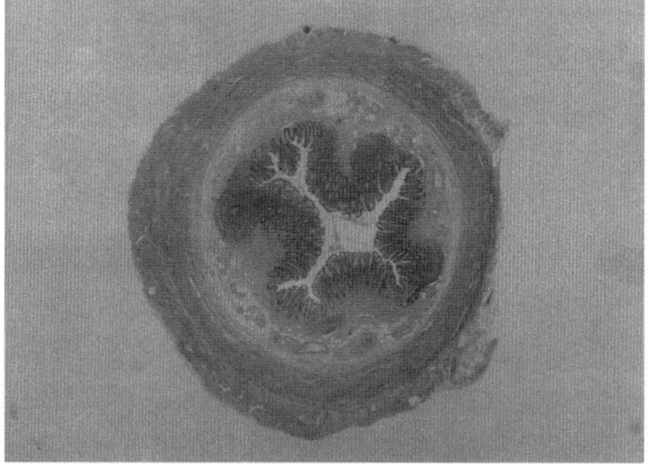

Figure 76.4 Normal vermiform appendix. The narrow lumen is bounded by mucosa, which may be arranged in folds. There is usually abundant lymphoid tissue in the mucosa, especially in younger individuals. This may encroach on and further narrow the lumen. The mucosa is bounded by a relatively thin muscularis mucosa (courtesy of Dr P Kelly, FRCPath, Dublin, Ireland).

Nikolai Kulchitsky, 1856–1925, Professor of Histology, Kharkov, Ukraine, who left Russia after the Revolution of 1917 and later worked at University College, London, UK. He described these cells in 1897.

ACUTE APPENDICITIS

While there are isolated reports of perityphlitis (fatal inflammation of the caecal region) from the late 1500s, recognition of acute appendicitis as a clinical entity is attributed to Reginald Fitz, who presented a paper to the first meeting of the Association of American Physicians in 1886 entitled 'Perforating inflammation of the vermiform appendix'. Soon afterwards, Charles McBurney described the clinical manifestations of acute appendicitis, including the point of maximum tenderness in the right iliac fossa that now bears his name.

The incidence of appendicitis seemed to rise greatly in the first half of the twentieth century, particularly in Europe, America and Australasia, with up to 16% of the population undergoing appendicectomy. In the past 30 years, the incidence has fallen dramatically in these countries, such that the individual lifetime risk of appendicectomy is 8.6% and 6.7% among males and females, respectively.

Acute appendicitis is relatively rare in infants and becomes increasingly common in childhood and early adult life, reaching a peak incidence in the teens and early twenties. After middle age, the risk of developing appendicitis is quite small. The incidence of appendicitis is equal among males and females before puberty. In teenagers and young adults, the male-to-female ratio increases to 3:2 at age 25; thereafter, the greater incidence in males declines.

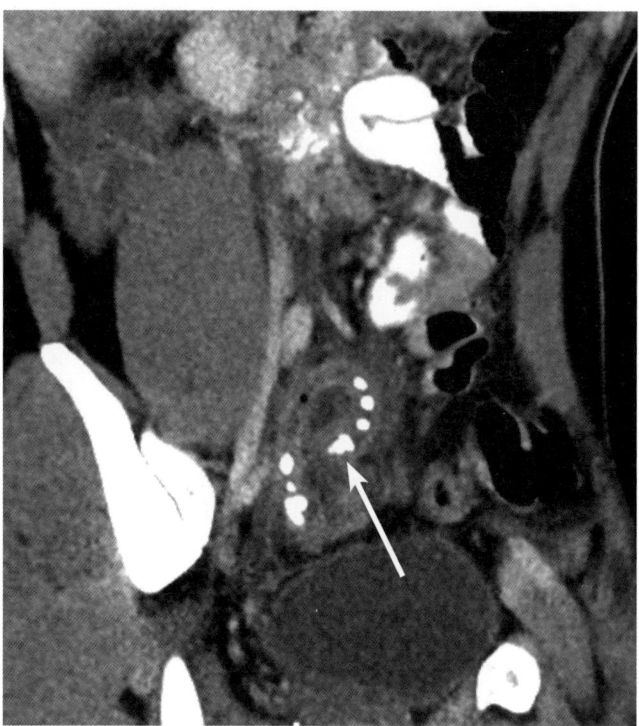

Figure 76.5 Coronal reformat of a computed tomography scan of the abdomen obtained with oral and intravenous contrast, demonstrating an inflamed, enhancing and enlarged appendix that is curled in the midline extending towards the pelvis (arrow). It contains multiple radiopaque appendicoliths. There is extensive periappendiceal fat stranding (courtesy of Professor P MacMahon, FRCR, Dublin, Ireland).

Aetiology

There is no unifying hypothesis regarding the aetiology of acute appendicitis. Decreased dietary fibre and increased consumption of refined carbohydrates may be important. As with colonic diverticulitis, the incidence of appendicitis is lowest in societies with a high dietary fibre intake. In resource-poor countries that are adopting a more refined Western-type diet, the incidence continues to rise. This is in contrast to the dramatic decrease in the incidence of appendicitis in Western countries observed in the past 30 years. No reason has been established for these paradoxical changes; however, improved hygiene and a change in the pattern of childhood gastrointestinal infection related to the increased use of antibiotics may be responsible.

While appendicitis is clearly associated with bacterial proliferation within the appendix, no single organism is responsible. A mixed growth of aerobic and anaerobic organisms is usual. The initiating event causing bacterial proliferation is controversial. Obstruction of the appendix lumen has been widely held to be important, and some form of luminal obstruction, either by a faecolith (***Figure 76.5***) or by a stricture, is found in the majority of cases.

A faecolith (sometimes referred to as an appendicolith) is composed of inspissated faecal material, calcium phosphates, bacteria and epithelial debris. Rarely, a foreign body is incorporated into the mass. The incidental finding of a faecolith is a relative indication for prophylactic appendicectomy or an interval appendicectomy in a patient treated conservatively. A fibrotic stricture of the appendix usually indicates previous appendicitis that resolved without surgical intervention. Obstruction of the appendiceal orifice by tumour, particularly carcinoma of the caecum, is an occasional cause of acute appendicitis in middle-aged and elderly patients. Intestinal parasites, particularly *Enterobius vermicularis* (pinworm), can proliferate in the appendix and occlude the lumen.

Pathology

Obstruction of the appendiceal lumen seems to be essential for appendiceal perforation. However, in many cases of early appendicitis, the appendix lumen is patent despite the presence of mucosal inflammation and lymphoid hyperplasia. Occasional clustering of cases among children and young adults suggests an infective agent, possibly viral, which initiates an inflammatory response. Seasonal variation in the incidence is also observed, with more cases occurring between May and August in northern Europe than at other times of the year.

Lymphoid hyperplasia narrows the lumen of the appendix. Once obstruction occurs, continued mucus secretion and inflammatory exudation increase intraluminal pressure, obstructing lymphatic drainage. Oedema and mucosal

Reginald Heber Fitz, 1843–1913, Professor of Medicine, Harvard University, Boston, MA, USA.

Charles McBurney, 1854–1913, Professor of Surgery, Columbia College of Physicians and Surgeons, New York, NY, USA. In 1889 McBurney published a paper on appendicitis in which he stated, 'I believe that in every case the seat of greatest pain "determined by the pressure of one finger" has been very exactly between an inch and a half and two inches from the anterior spinous process of the ilium on a straight line drawn from that process to the umbilicus.'

ulceration develop with bacterial translocation to the submucosa. Resolution may occur at this point either spontaneously or in response to antibiotic therapy. If the condition progresses, further distension of the appendix may cause venous obstruction and ischaemia of the appendix wall. With ischaemia, bacterial invasion occurs through the muscularis propria and submucosa, producing acute appendicitis (***Figure 76.6***). Finally, ischaemic necrosis of the appendix wall produces gangrenous appendicitis, with free bacterial contamination of the peritoneal cavity. Alternatively, the greater omentum and loops of small bowel become adherent to the inflamed appendix, walling off the spread of peritoneal contamination and resulting in a phlegmonous mass or paracaecal abscess. Rarely, appendiceal inflammation resolves, leaving a distended mucus-filled organ termed a mucocele of the appendix.

Peritonitis occurs as a result of free migration of bacteria through an ischaemic appendicular wall, frank perforation of a gangrenous appendix or delayed perforation of an appendix abscess. Factors that promote this process include extremes of age, immunosuppression, diabetes mellitus, faecolith obstruction of the appendix lumen, a free-lying pelvic appendix and previous abdominal surgery that limits the ability of the greater omentum to wall off the spread of peritoneal contamination. In these situations, a rapidly deteriorating clinical course is accompanied by signs of diffuse peritonitis and systemic sepsis syndrome.

Clinical diagnosis

History

Appendicitis is relatively rare in infants under 36 months of age and, for obvious reasons, the patient is unable to give a history. Because of this, diagnosis is often delayed, and thus the incidence of perforation and postoperative morbidity is considerably higher than in older children.

In older age groups the classical features of acute appendicitis begin with poorly localised colicky abdominal pain. This is due to midgut visceral discomfort in response to appendiceal inflammation and obstruction. The pain is frequently first noticed in the periumbilical region and is similar to, but less intense than, the colic of small bowel obstruction. Central abdominal pain is associated with anorexia, nausea and usually one or two episodes of vomiting that follow the onset of pain (Murphy). Anorexia is a useful and constant clinical feature, particularly in children, who invariably also have vomiting. The patient often gives a history of similar discomfort that settled spontaneously. A family history is also useful as up to one-third of children with appendicitis have a first-degree relative with a similar history. In women of childbearing age pelvic disease can mimic acute appendicitis and a careful gynaecological history should be taken, concentrating on menstrual cycle, vaginal discharge and possible pregnancy.

Summary box 76.1

Risk factors for perforation of the appendix

- Extremes of age
- Immunosuppression
- Diabetes mellitus
- Faecolith obstruction
- Pelvic appendix
- Previous abdominal surgery

Summary box 76.2

Symptoms of appendicitis

- Periumbilical colic
- Pain shifting to the right iliac fossa
- Anorexia
- Nausea

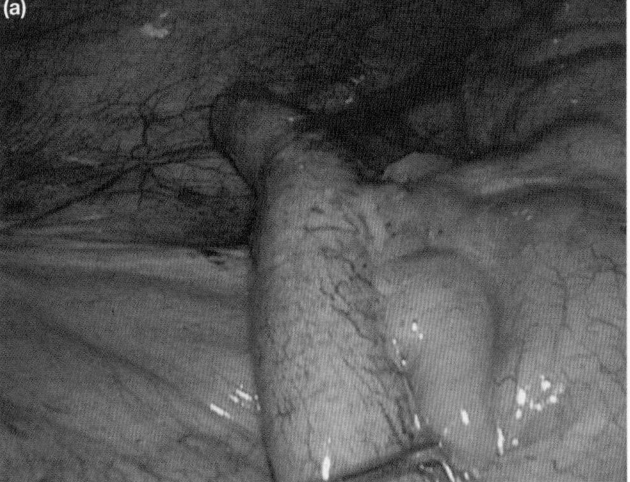

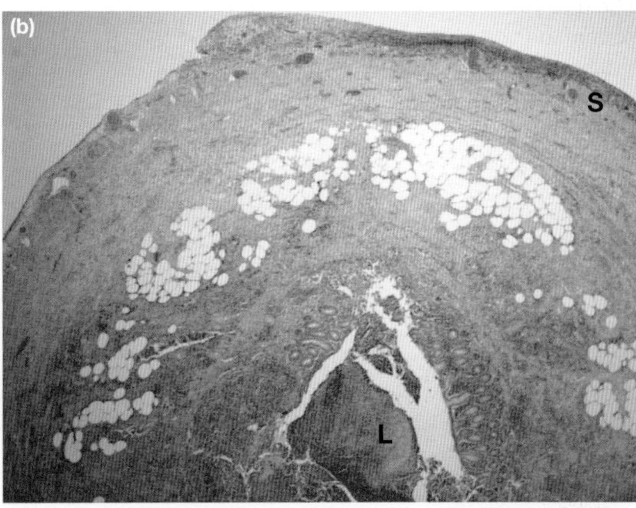

Figure 76.6 Acutely inflamed appendix with purulent exudate extending to the mesoappendix in a 28-year-old man as seen at laparoscopy **(a)** and a photomicrograph (original magnification ×20) **(b)** from the same patient showing the appendix with pus-filled lumen (L) and inflammation extending to inflamed serosa (S) (courtesy of Professor C O'Keane, FFPath, FRCPI, Dublin, Ireland).

John Benjamin Murphy, 1857–1916, Professor of Surgery, Northwestern University, Chicago, IL, USA.

With progressive inflammation of the appendix, the parietal peritoneum in the right iliac fossa becomes irritated, producing more intense, constant and localised somatic pain that begins to predominate. Patients often report this as an abdominal pain that has shifted and changed in character. Typically, coughing or sudden movement exacerbates the right iliac fossa pain.

The classic visceral–somatic sequence of pain is present in only about half of those patients subsequently proven to have acute appendicitis. A typical presentation includes pain that is predominantly somatic or visceral and poorly localised. Atypical pain is more common in the elderly, in whom localisation to the right iliac fossa is unusual. An inflamed appendix in the pelvis may not produce somatic pain involving the anterior abdominal wall, but instead cause suprapubic discomfort and tenesmus. In this circumstance, tenderness may be elicited only on rectal examination and is the basis for the recommendation that a rectal examination should be performed on every patient who presents with acute lower abdominal pain.

During the first 6 hours, there is rarely any alteration in temperature or pulse rate. After that time, slight pyrexia (37.2–37.7°C) with a corresponding increase in the pulse rate to 80–90 beats per minute is usual. However, in 20% of patients there is no pyrexia or tachycardia in the early stages. In children, a temperature greater than 38.5°C suggests other causes (e.g. mesenteric adenitis; see ***Differential diagnosis, Children***).

Typically, two clinical syndromes of acute appendicitis can be discerned: acute catarrhal (non-obstructive) appendicitis and acute obstructive appendicitis, the latter characterised by a more acute course. The onset of symptoms is abrupt and there may be generalised abdominal pain from the start. The temperature may be normal and vomiting is common, so the clinical picture may mimic acute intestinal obstruction.

Signs

The diagnosis of appendicitis rests more on thorough clinical examination of the abdomen than on any aspect of the history or laboratory investigation. The cardinal features are those of an unwell patient with low-grade pyrexia, localised abdominal tenderness, muscle guarding and rebound tenderness. Inspection of the abdomen may show limitation of respiratory movement in the lower abdomen. The patient is then asked to point to where the pain began and where it moved (pointing sign). Gentle superficial palpation of the abdomen, beginning in the left iliac fossa and moving anticlockwise to the right iliac fossa, will detect muscle guarding over the point of maximum tenderness, classically McBurney's point. Asking the patient to cough or gentle percussion over the site of maximum tenderness will elicit rebound tenderness (see ***Chapter 63***).

Deep palpation of the left iliac fossa may cause pain in the right iliac fossa, Rovsing's sign, which is helpful in supporting a clinical diagnosis of appendicitis. Occasionally, an inflamed appendix lies on the psoas muscle, and the patient, often a young adult, will lie with the right hip flexed for pain relief (the psoas sign). Spasm of the obturator internus is sometimes demonstrable when the hip is flexed and internally rotated. If an inflamed appendix is in contact with the obturator internus, this manoeuvre will cause pain in the hypogastrium (the obturator test; Zachary Cope). Cutaneous hyperaesthesia may be demonstrable in the right iliac fossa, but is rarely of diagnostic value.

Summary box 76.3

Clinical signs in appendicitis

- Pyrexia
- Localised tenderness in the right iliac fossa
- Muscle guarding
- Rebound tenderness

Summary box 76.4

Signs to elicit in appendicitis

- Pointing sign
- Rovsing's sign
- Psoas sign
- Obturator sign

Special features, according to position of the appendix

Retrocaecal

Rigidity is often absent, and even application of deep pressure may fail to elicit tenderness (silent appendix), the reason being that the caecum, distended with gas, prevents the pressure exerted by the hand from reaching the inflamed structure. However, deep tenderness is often present in the loin, and rigidity of the quadratus lumborum may be in evidence. Psoas spasm, due to the inflamed appendix being in contact with that muscle, may be sufficient to cause flexion of the hip joint. Hyperextension of the hip joint may induce abdominal pain when the degree of psoas spasm is insufficient to cause flexion of the hip.

Pelvic

Occasionally, early diarrhoea results from an inflamed appendix being in contact with the rectum. When the appendix lies entirely within the pelvis, there is usually complete absence of abdominal rigidity, and often tenderness over McBurney's point is also lacking. In some instances, deep tenderness can be made out just above and to the right of the symphysis pubis. In either event, a rectal examination reveals tenderness in the rectovesical pouch or the pouch of Douglas, especially on the right side. Spasm of the psoas and obturator internus muscles may be present when the appendix is in this position. An inflamed appendix in contact with the bladder may cause frequency of micturition. This is more common in children.

Neils Thorkild Rovsing, 1862–1937, Professor of Surgery, Copenhagen, Denmark.
Sir Vincent Zachary Cope, 1881–1975, surgeon, St Mary's Hospital, London, UK
James Douglas, 1715–1742, anatomist and midwife who practised in London, UK, described this pouch in 1730.

TABLE 76.1 Differential diagnosis of acute appendicitis.

Children	Adult	Adult female	Elderly
Gastroenteritis	Regional enteritis	Mittelschmerz	Diverticulitis
Mesenteric adenitis	Ureteric colic	Pelvic inflammatory disease	Intestinal obstruction
Meckel's diverticulitis	Perforated peptic ulcer	Pyelonephritis	Colonic carcinoma
Intussusception	Torsion of testis	Ectopic pregnancy	Torsion appendix epiploicae
Henoch–Schönlein purpura	Pancreatitis	Torsion/rupture of ovarian cyst	Mesenteric infarction
Lobar pneumonia	Rectus sheath haematoma	Endometriosis	Leaking aortic aneurysm

Postileal

In this case, the inflamed appendix lies behind the terminal ileum. It presents the greatest difficulty in diagnosis because the pain may not shift, diarrhoea is a feature and marked retching may occur. Tenderness, if any, is ill defined, although it may be present immediately to the right of the umbilicus.

Differential diagnosis

Although acute appendicitis is the most common abdominal surgical emergency, the diagnosis can be extremely difficult at times. There are a number of common conditions that it is wise to consider carefully and, if possible, exclude. The differential diagnosis differs in patients of different ages; in women, additional differential diagnoses are diseases of the female genital tract (***Table 76.1***).

Children

The diseases most commonly mistaken for acute appendicitis are **acute gastroenteritis** and **mesenteric lymphadenitis**. In mesenteric lymphadenitis, the pain is colicky in nature and cervical lymph nodes may be enlarged. It may be impossible to clinically distinguish **Meckel's diverticulitis** from acute appendicitis. The pain is similar; however, signs may be central or left sided. Occasionally, there is a history of antecedent abdominal pain or intermittent lower gastrointestinal bleeding.

It is important to distinguish between acute appendicitis and **intussusception**. Appendicitis is uncommon before the age of 2 years, whereas the median age for intussusception is 18 months. A mass may be palpable in the right lower quadrant, and the preferred treatment of intussusception is reduction by careful barium enema.

Henoch–Schönlein purpura is often preceded by a sore throat or respiratory infection. Abdominal pain can be severe and can be confused with intussusception or appendicitis. There is nearly always an ecchymotic rash, typically affecting the extensor surfaces of the limbs and on the buttocks. The face is usually spared. The platelet count and bleeding time are within normal limits. Microscopic haematuria is common.

Lobar pneumonia and pleurisy, especially at the right base, may give rise to right-sided abdominal pain and mimic appendicitis. Abdominal tenderness is minimal, pyrexia is marked and chest examination may reveal a pleural friction rub or altered breath sounds on auscultation. A chest radiograph is diagnostic.

Adults

Terminal ileitis in its acute form may be clinically indistinguishable from acute appendicitis unless a doughy mass of inflamed ileum can be felt. An antecedent history of abdominal cramping, weight loss and diarrhoea suggests regional ileitis rather than appendicitis. The ileitis may be non-specific, due to Crohn's disease (***Figure 76.7***) or *Yersinia* infection. *Yersinia enterocolitica* causes inflammation of the terminal ileum, appendix and caecum with mesenteric adenopathy. If suspected, serum antibody titres are diagnostic, and treatment with intravenous tetracycline is appropriate. If *Yersinia* infection is suspected at operation, a mesenteric lymph node should be excised and divided, with half submitted for microbiological culture (including tuberculosis) and half for histological examination.

Ureteric colic does not commonly cause diagnostic difficulty, as the character and radiation of pain differs from that of appendicitis. Urinalysis should always be performed, and the presence of red cells should prompt a supine abdominal radiograph. A renal ultrasound or urogram will provide the diagnosis.

Right-sided acute **pyelonephritis** is accompanied and often preceded by increased frequency of micturition. It may cause difficulty in diagnosis, especially in women. The leading features are tenderness confined to the loin, fever (temperature 39°C) and possibly rigors and pyuria.

In **perforated peptic ulcer**, the duodenal contents pass along the paracolic gutter to the right iliac fossa. As a rule there is a history of dyspepsia and a very sudden onset of pain that starts in the epigastrium and passes down the right paracolic gutter. In appendicitis, the pain starts classically in the umbilical region. Rigidity and tenderness in the right iliac fossa are present in both conditions but, in perforated duodenal ulcer, the rigidity is usually greater in the right hypochondrium.

Johann Friedrich Meckel (the younger), 1781–1883, Professor of Anatomy and Surgery, Halle, Germany, described the diverticulum in 1809.
Eduard Heinrich Henoch, 1820–1910, Professor of Diseases of Children, Berlin, Germany, described this form of purpura in 1868.
Johann Lucas Schönlein, 1793–1864, Professor of Medicine, Berlin, Germany, described this form of purpura in 1837.
Burrill Bernard Crohn, 1884–1983, gastroenterologist, Mount Sinai Hospital, New York, NY, USA.
Alexandre Emile Yersin, 1863–1943, bacteriologist, Paris, France.

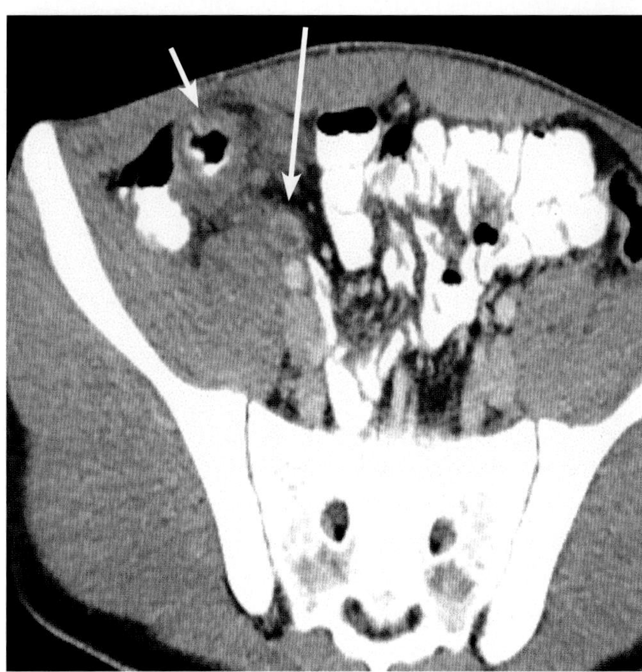

Figure 76.7 First presentation in a 19-year-old man with terminal ileitis, later confirmed to be Crohn's disease. Short arrow demonstrates abnormally thickened and inflamed terminal ileum. Long arrow indicates wall enhancement and enlargement of the appendix, indicating secondary acute appendicitis (courtesy of Professor P MacMahon, FRCR, Dublin, Ireland).

An erect chest radiograph will show gas under the diaphragm in 70% of patients. An abdominal computed tomography (CT) examination is valuable when there is diagnostic difficulty. **Testicular torsion** in a teenage or young adult male is easily missed. Pain can be referred to the right iliac fossa, and shyness on the part of the patient may lead the unwary to suspect appendicitis unless the scrotum is examined in all cases.

Acute pancreatitis should be considered in the differential diagnosis of all adults suspected of having acute appendicitis and, when appropriate, should be excluded by serum or urinary amylase measurement.

Rectus sheath haematoma is a relatively rare but easily missed differential diagnosis. It usually presents with acute pain and localised tenderness in the right iliac fossa, often after an episode of strenuous physical exercise. Localised pain without gastrointestinal upset is the rule. Occasionally, in an elderly patient, particularly one taking anticoagulant therapy, a rectus sheath haematoma may present as a mass and tenderness in the right iliac fossa after minor trauma.

Pelvic inflammatory disease comprises a spectrum of diseases that include salpingitis, endometritis and tubo-ovarian sepsis. The incidence of these conditions is increasing, and the diagnosis should be considered in every young adult female. Typically, the pain is lower than in appendicitis and is bilateral. A history of vaginal discharge, dysmenorrhoea and burning pain on micturition is a helpful differential diagnostic point. The physical findings include adnexal and cervical tenderness on vaginal examination. When suspected, a high vaginal swab should be taken for *Chlamydia trachomatis* and *Neisseria gonorrhoeae* culture, and the opinion of a gynaecologist should be obtained (see ***Chapter 87***).

Midcycle rupture of a follicular cyst with bleeding produces lower abdominal and pelvic pain, typically midcycle, which is characteristic of **mittelschmerz**. Systemic upset is rare, a pregnancy test is negative and symptoms usually subside within hours. Occasionally, diagnostic laparoscopy is required. Retrograde menstruation may cause similar symptoms.

Torsion or haemorrhage of an ovarian cyst can prove a difficult differential diagnosis. When suspected, pelvic ultrasound and a gynaecological opinion should be sought.

It is unlikely that a ruptured **ectopic pregnancy**, with its well-defined signs of haemoperitoneum, will be mistaken for acute appendicitis, but the same cannot be said for a right-sided tubal abortion or, still more, for a right-sided unruptured tubal pregnancy. In the latter, the signs are very similar to those of acute appendicitis except that the pain commences on the right side and stays there. The pain is severe and continues unabated until operation. Usually, there is a history of a missed menstrual period, and a urinary pregnancy test may be positive. Severe pain is felt when the cervix is moved on vaginal examination. Signs of intraperitoneal bleeding usually become apparent and the patient should be questioned specifically regarding referred pain in the shoulder. Pelvic ultrasonography should be carried out in all cases in which an ectopic pregnancy is a possible diagnosis.

In some patients with a long sigmoid loop, the colon lies to the right of the midline and it may be impossible to differentiate between **diverticulitis** and appendicitis. Abdominal CT scanning is particularly useful in this setting and should be considered in the management of all patients over the age of 60 years. Right-sided diverticulitis is more common in Asia and may be clinically indistinguishable from appendicitis. Abdominal CT scanning is particularly useful in making the distinction. As with left-sided diverticulitis, treatment should be conservative with intravenous antibiotics with recourse to laparoscopy or laparotomy in the face of clinical deterioration.

The diagnosis of **intestinal obstruction** is usually clear; the subtlety lies in recognising acute appendicitis as the occasional cause in the elderly. An abdominal CT scan will clarify the diagnosis.

When obstructed or locally perforated, **carcinoma of the caecum** may mimic or cause obstructive appendicitis in adults. A history of antecedent discomfort, altered bowel habit or unexplained anaemia should raise suspicion. A mass may be palpable and an abdominal CT scan diagnostic.

Rare differential diagnoses

Preherpetic pain of the right 10th and 11th dorsal nerves is localised over the same area as that of appendicitis. It does not shift and is associated with marked hyperaesthesia. There is no intestinal upset or rigidity. The herpetic eruption may be delayed for 3–8 hours.

Spinal conditions are sometimes associated with acute abdominal pain, especially in children and the elderly. These may include tuberculosis of the spine, metastatic carcinoma, osteoporotic vertebral collapse and multiple myeloma. The pain is due to compression of nerve roots and may be aggravated by movement. There is rigidity of the lumbar spine and intestinal symptoms are absent.

The abdominal crises of porphyria and diabetes mellitus need to be remembered. A urinalysis should be undertaken in every abdominal emergency. In cyclical vomiting of infants or young children, there is a history of previous similar attacks and abdominal rigidity is absent. Acetone is found in the urine but is not diagnostic as it may accompany starvation.

Typhlitis or leukaemic ileocaecal syndrome is a rare but potentially fatal enterocolitis occurring in immunosuppressed patients. Gram-negative or clostridial (especially *Clostridium septicum*) septicaemia can be rapidly progressive. Treatment is with appropriate antibiotics and haematopoietic factors. Surgical intervention is rarely indicated.

Investigation

The diagnosis of acute appendicitis is essentially clinical; however, a decision to operate based on clinical suspicion alone can lead to the removal of a normal appendix in 15–30% of cases. The premise that it is better to remove a normal appendix than to delay diagnosis does not stand up to close scrutiny, particularly in the elderly. A number of clinical and laboratory-based scoring systems have been devised to assist diagnosis. The most widely used is the Alvarado score (***Table 76.2***). A score of 7 or more is strongly predictive of acute appendicitis.

In patients with an equivocal score (5 or 6), abdominal ultrasonography or contrast-enhanced CT examination further reduces the rate of negative appendicectomy. Abdominal ultrasonography is more useful in children and thin adults, particularly if gynaecological pathology is suspected, with a diagnostic accuracy in excess of 90% (***Figure 76.8***). Modern CT is both sensitive and specific (approximately 95%) in the diagnosis of acute appendicitis (***Figure 76.9***) and worldwide there has been a steady increase in its use for this purpose. CT has been shown to reduce the rate of negative appendicectomy without an associated increased perforation rate (due to delay in diagnosis) and may be cost-effective as a result of shorter hospital stay. While the diagnostic accuracy of modern CT scanning for appendicitis is well established, radiation exposure and the theoretical carcinogenic effect are a concern. Low-dose protocols, which reduce the radiation dose to the patient by up to 80%, can be as reliable as standard dose scanning and may be more appropriately applied when considering a diagnosis of acute appendicitis, particularly in the younger adult.

Contrast-enhanced standard dose CT is especially useful in patients in whom there is diagnostic uncertainty, particularly older patients, where acute diverticulitis, intestinal obstruction and neoplasm are likely differential diagnoses.

Summary box 76.5

Preoperative investigations in appendicitis

- Routine
  - Full blood count
  - Urinalysis
- Selective
  - Pregnancy test
  - Urea and electrolytes
  - C-reactive protein
  - Supine abdominal radiograph
  - Ultrasound of the abdomen/pelvis
  - Contrast-enhanced abdomen and pelvic CT scan (consider low-dose protocol in young adults)

TABLE 76.2 The Alvarado (MANTRELS) score.

	Score
Symptoms	
Migratory RIF pain	1
Anorexia	1
Nausea and vomiting	1
Signs	
Tenderness (RIF)	2
Rebound tenderness	1
Elevated temperature	1
Laboratory	
Leukocytosis	2
Shift to left	1
Total	10

RIF, right iliac fossa.

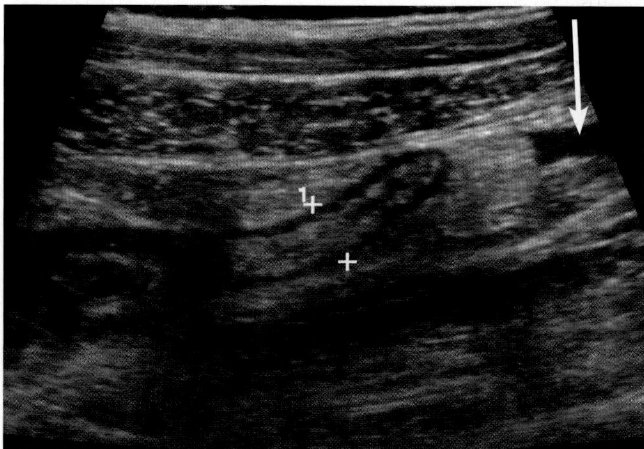

Figure 76.8 Ultrasound image of the right iliac fossa (RIF) demonstrating a mildly enlarged appendix, measuring 8 mm in diameter, consistent with acute appendicitis in a 40-year-old man. Arrow indicates a small pocket of free fluid more inferiorly in the RIF (courtesy of Dr D Byrne, Dublin, Ireland).

Treatment

Non-operative management

There are two scenarios in which patients with acute appendicitis may be considered for non-operative treatment.

Uncomplicated appendicitis

While surgery remains the standard teaching, there is evidence to support a trial of conservative management in patients

Alfredo Alvarado, contemporary, surgeon, Plantation, FL, USA.

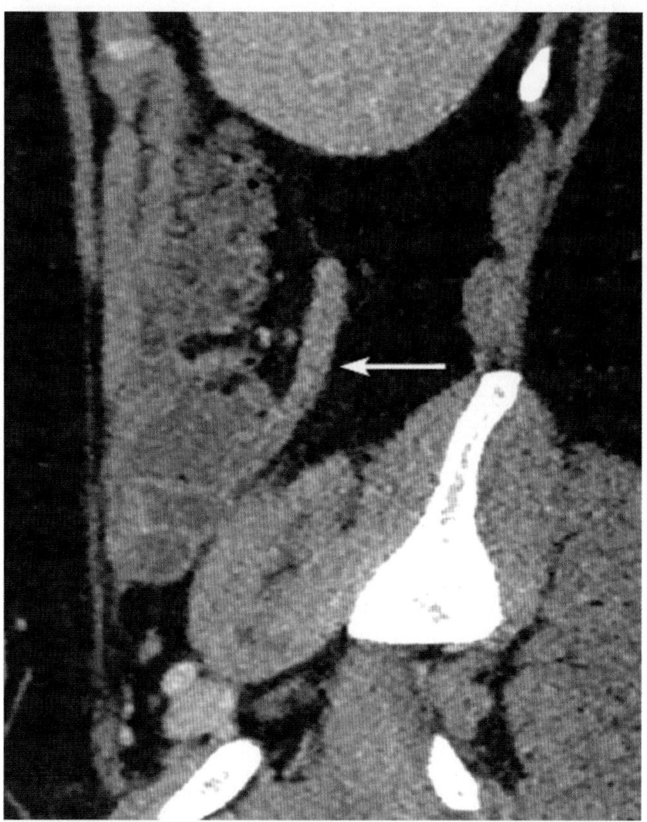

Figure 76.9 Sagittal reformat of a computed tomography scan of the abdomen obtained with oral and intravenous contrast, demonstrating an enlarged (10 mm), enhancing retrocaecal appendix with periappendiceal fat stranding. There is no evidence of necrosis, perforation or collection. No radiopaque appendicolith can be seen. Figure 76.6 refers to the same patient (courtesy of Professor P MacMahon, FRCR, Dublin, Ireland).

with uncomplicated (absence of appendicolith, perforation or abscess) appendicitis. Treatment is bowel rest and intravenous antibiotics, often metronidazole and a third-generation cephalosporin. The available data indicate initial successful outcomes in approximately 85% of patients; however, between one-quarter and one-third of patients initially treated conservatively will require surgery within 1 year for recurrent symptoms. Subsequent surgery, if needed, tends to be uncomplicated and the overall postoperative complication rate is similar when patients treated conservatively and later needing surgery are compared with those undergoing surgery at the outset. Overall hospital length of stay is also similar when comparing patients in each group. Thus, antibiotic treatment of acute uncomplicated appendicitis appears to be safe and it allows a large number of patients to avoid invasive treatment; however, this information must be balanced by the high treatment failure rate and need for interval intervention.

Conservative treatment may be considered in the well patient with limited signs or those with high operative risk (multiple comorbidities); the patients must be aware of the high failure rate. As with conservative treatment of an appendix mass, patients over the age of 40 should be followed up to ensure that there is no underlying malignancy (see ***Neoplasms of the appendix and pseudomyxoma peritonei***).

In children, conservative treatment of uncomplicated appendicitis also appears to be safe in the short term with resolution of acute symptoms in approximately 90% of patients. Re-presentation with complicated appendicitis appears to be very rare; however, recurrent symptoms requiring surgery have been reported in up to 46% of patients. Notably, histological features of acute appendicitis may be present in only one-fifth of patients needing interval surgery.

Appendix mass

If an appendix mass is present and the condition of the patient is satisfactory, the standard treatment is the conservative Ochsner–Sherren regime. This strategy is based on the premise that the inflammatory process is already localised and that inadvertent surgery is difficult and may be dangerous. It may be impossible to find the appendix and, occasionally, a faecal fistula may form. For these reasons, it is wise to observe a non-operative programme but to be prepared to operate should clinical deterioration occur.

Summary box 76.6

Criteria for stopping conservative treatment of an appendix mass

- A rising pulse rate
- Increasing or spreading abdominal pain
- Increasing size of the mass

Careful recording of the patient's condition and the extent of the mass should be made and the abdomen regularly re-examined. It is helpful to mark the limits of the mass on the abdominal wall using a skin pencil. A contrast-enhanced CT examination of the abdomen should be performed and antibiotic therapy instigated. An abscess, if present, should be drained radiologically. Temperature and pulse rate should be recorded 4-hourly and a fluid balance record maintained. Clinical deterioration or evidence of peritonitis is an indication for early laparotomy. Clinical improvement is usually evident within 24–48 hours. Failure of the mass to resolve should raise suspicion of a carcinoma or Crohn's disease. Using this regime, approximately 90% of cases resolve without incident.

The need for interval appendicectomy in this cohort is much debated. The majority of patients will not develop recurrent appendicitis; however, recently published studies have identified higher than expected rates of underlying appendiceal neoplasm in those patients who do go on to interval appendicectomy, particularly those patients over the age of 40. A recent randomised clinical trial was terminated early owing to the unexpected finding of appendiceal tumour during follow-up in 29% (12/41) of patients aged more than 40 years who initially presented with periappendicular abscess. Low-grade appendiceal mucinous neoplasms (LAMNs)

Albert John Ochsner, 1858–1925, Professor of Clinical Surgery, The University of Illinois College of Medicine, Chicago, IL, USA.
James Sherren, 1876–1945, surgeon, The London Hospital, London, UK.

accounted for 42% of the unexpected tumours. This rate of incidental appendix tumour in patients presenting with abscess appears to be much higher than in the general population undergoing appendicectomy, suggesting a different pathogenesis in the former group. Careful consideration should be given to interval appendicectomy in this cohort of patients. At the very least, follow-up CT or magnetic resonance imaging (MRI) should be performed to ensure complete resolution of findings and patients should undergo colonoscopy.

Operative management

General principles

The traditional treatment for acute appendicitis is appendicectomy. While there should be no unnecessary delay, all patients, particularly those most at risk of serious morbidity, benefit by a short period of intensive preoperative preparation. Intravenous fluids, sufficient to establish adequate urine output (catheterisation is needed only in the very ill), and appropriate antibiotics should be given. Risk factors for venous thromboembolism should be considered and appropriate prophylaxis (mechanical and/or pharmacological) initiated. There is evidence that, in the absence of purulent peritonitis, a single perioperative dose of antibiotics reduces the incidence of postoperative wound infection. When peritonitis is suspected, therapeutic intravenous antibiotics to cover Gram-negative bacilli as well as anaerobic cocci should be given. Hyperpyrexia in children should be treated with salicylates in addition to antibiotics and intravenous fluids. With appropriate use of intravenous fluids and parenteral antibiotics, a policy of deferring appendicectomy after midnight to the first case on the following morning does not increase morbidity. However, when acute obstructive appendicitis is recognised, operation should not be deferred longer than it takes to optimise the patient's condition.

Appendicectomy should be performed under general anaesthetic with the patient supine on the operating table and may be undertaken using either an open or laparoscopic approach. When the appropriate equipment and expertise are available and cost allows, the laparoscopic approach is advantageous. The initial laparoscopy allows the diagnosis to be established and may reduce the negative appendicectomy rate. Furthermore, the patient may benefit from the quicker recovery afforded by a minimally invasive approach, the rate of wound infection is lower (when compared with open surgery) and, contrary to initial concerns, the incidence of postoperative pelvic collection does not appear to be increased.

When a laparoscopic technique is used, the bladder must be empty (ensure that the patient has voided before leaving the ward). Prior to preparing the entire abdomen with an appropriate antiseptic solution, the right iliac fossa should be palpated for a mass. If a mass is felt, it may, on occasion, be preferable to adopt a conservative approach. Draping of the abdomen is in accordance with the planned operative technique, taking account of any requirement to extend the incision or convert a laparoscopic technique to an open operation.

Surgical technique: conventional appendicectomy

When the preoperative diagnosis is considered reasonably certain, the incision that is widely used for appendicectomy is the so-called gridiron incision. The gridiron incision (described first by McArthur) is made at right angles to a line joining the anterior superior iliac spine to the umbilicus, its centre being along the line at McBurney's point (***Figure 76.10***). If better access is required, it is possible to convert the gridiron to a Rutherford Morison incision (see below) by cutting the internal oblique and transversus muscles in the line of the incision.

In recent years, a transverse skin crease (Lanz) incision has become more popular, as the exposure is better and extension,

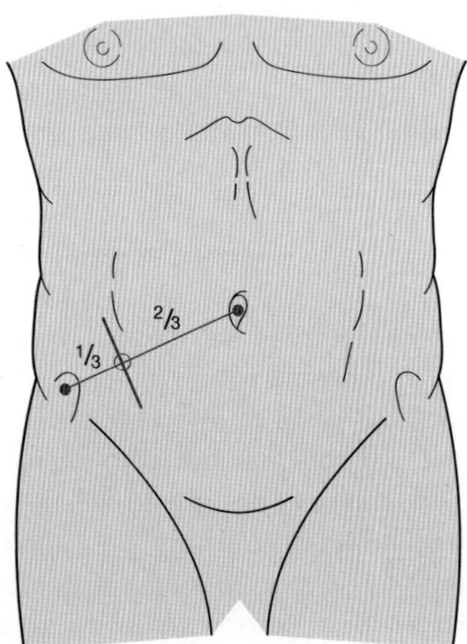

Figure 76.10 Gridiron incision for appendicitis, at right angles to a line joining the anterior superior iliac spine and umbilicus, centred on McBurney's point (courtesy of Professor M Earley, FRCSI, Dublin, Ireland).

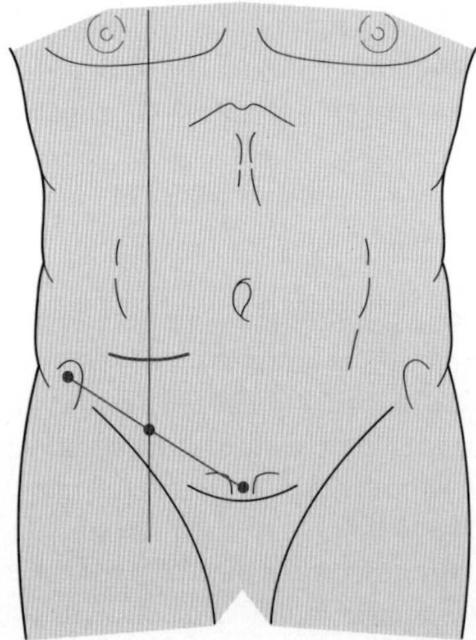

Figure 76.11 Transverse or skin crease (Lanz) incision for appendicitis, 2 cm below the umbilicus, centred on the midclavicular–midinguinal line (courtesy of Professor M Earley, FRSCI, Dublin, Ireland).

Gridiron, a frame of crossbeams to support a ship during repairs.
Lewis Linn McArthur, 1858–1934, surgeon, St. Luke's Hospital, Chicago, IL, USA.
James Rutherford Morison, 1853–1939, Professor of Surgery, Durham University, Durham, UK.
Otto Lanz, 1865–1935, surgeon, Amsterdam, The Netherlands.

when needed, is easier. The incision, appropriate in length to the size and obesity of the patient, is made approximately 2 cm below the umbilicus centred on the midclavicular–midinguinal line (*Figure 76.11*). When necessary, the incision may be extended medially, with retraction or suitable division of the rectus abdominis muscle.

When the diagnosis is in doubt, particularly in the presence of intestinal obstruction, a lower midline abdominal incision is to be preferred over a right lower paramedian incision. The latter, although widely practised in the past, is difficult to extend, more difficult to close and provides poorer access to the pelvis and peritoneal cavity.

Rutherford Morison's incision is useful if the appendix is para- or retrocaecal and fixed. It is essentially an oblique muscle-cutting incision with its lower end over McBurney's point and extending obliquely upwards and laterally as necessary. All layers are divided in the line of the incision.

The caecum is identified by the presence of taeniae coli and, using a finger or a swab, the caecum is withdrawn. A turgid appendix may be felt at the base of the caecum. Inflammatory adhesions must be gently broken with a finger, which is then hooked around the appendix to deliver it into the wound. The appendix is conveniently controlled using a Babcock or Lane's forceps applied in such a way as to encircle the appendix and yet not damage it. The base of the mesoappendix is clamped in artery forceps, divided and ligated (*Figure 76.12a*). When the mesoappendix is broad, the procedure must be repeated with a second or, rarely, a third artery forceps. The appendix, now completely freed, is clamped with an artery forceps near its base and then ligated close to the junction with the caecum using an absorbable 2/0 ligature. The appendix is amputated between the artery forceps and the ligature (*Figure 76.12b*). When the appendix is retrocaecal and adherent, it may be an advantage to divide the base first. The appendiceal vessels are then ligated and gentle traction on the caecum will enable the surgeon to deliver the body of the appendix, which is then removed from base to tip. Occasionally, this manoeuvre requires division of the lateral peritoneal attachments of the caecum.

An absorbable 2/0 or 3/0 purse-string or 'Z' suture may then be inserted into the caecum about 1.25 cm from the base (*Figure 76.12c*). The stitch should pass through the muscle coat, picking up the taeniae coli. The stump of the appendix is invaginated (*Figure 76.12d*) while the purse-string or 'Z' suture is tied, thus burying the appendix stump.

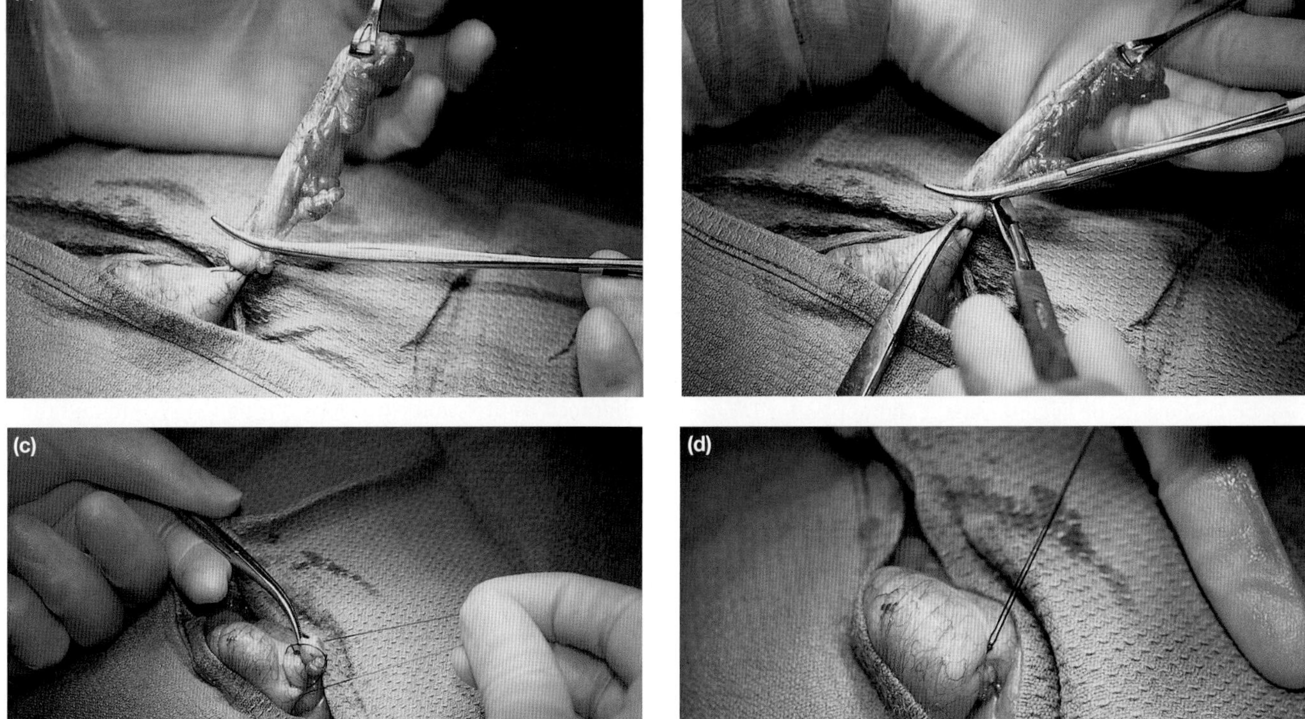

Figure 76.12 Appendicectomy. (a) The mesoappendix divided between artery forceps and ligated. (b) The appendix is ligated at its base and about to be divided. (c) 'Z' suture inserted prior to inversion of the appendiceal stump. (d) The appendiceal stump inverted, the 'Z' suture having been tied.

William Wayne Babcock, 1876–1963, surgeon, Philadelphia, PA, USA.
Sir William Arbuthnot Lane, 1856–1943, surgeon, Guy's Hospital, London, UK

When the caecal wall is oedematous, the purse-string suture is in danger of cutting out. If the oedema is of limited extent, this can be overcome by inserting the purse-string suture into more healthy caecal wall at a greater distance from the base of the appendix. Occasions may arise when, because of the extensive oedema of the caecal wall, it is better not to attempt invagination. Many surgeons believe invagination of the appendiceal stump is unnecessary.

Should the base of the appendix be gangrenous, ligation should not be attempted. Two stitches are placed through the caecal wall close to the base of the gangrenous appendix, which is amputated flush with the caecal wall, after which these stitches are tied. Further closure is effected by means of a second layer of interrupted seromuscular sutures. An alternative but more costly option when the appendix base is compromised is to resect the appendix with a cuff of healthy caecum using a single firing of a linear stapling device.

Surgical technique: laparoscopic appendicectomy

The most valuable aspect of laparoscopy in the management of suspected appendicitis is as a diagnostic tool, particularly in women of childbearing age. The placement of operating ports may vary according to operator preference and previous abdominal scars. Typically, a pneumoperitoneum is established using an open infraumbilical approach. This umbilical port serves as the camera port with two working ports inserted under direct vision, the first suprapubically and the second in the left lower quadrant. A moderate Trendelenburg tilt with elevation of the right side of the operating table improves exposure and assists delivery of loops of small bowel from the pelvis. The appendix is found in the conventional manner by identification of the caecal taeniae and is controlled using a laparoscopic tissue-holding forceps. Occasionally, it is necessary to divide the peritoneal attachments and mobilise the caecum in order to adequately expose the appendix. By elevating the appendix, the mesoappendix is then displayed. A dissecting forceps, hook or scissors diathermy is used to dissect the mesoappendix (***Figure 76.13a***) and expose the appendicular vessels, which may be coagulated or ligated using a clip applicator (***Figure 76.13b***). The appendix, free of its mesentery, can be ligated at its base with an absorbable loop ligature (***Figure 76.13c***) or a linear stapling device, divided (***Figure 76.13d***) and removed in a specimen bag through one of the operating ports. It is not usual to invert the stump of the appendix. Absorbable sutures are used to close the fascia at the umbilicus and at any port sites greater than 5 mm, and the small skin incisions may be closed with subcuticular sutures.

Problems encountered during appendicectomy

The finding of a normal appendix demands careful exclusion of other possible diagnoses, particularly terminal ileitis, Meckel's diverticulitis and tubal or ovarian causes in women. It is usual to remove the appendix to avoid future diagnostic difficulties, even though the appendix is macroscopically normal, particularly if a skin crease or gridiron incision has been made. A case can be made for preserving the macroscopically normal appendix seen at diagnostic laparoscopy, although approximately one-quarter of seemingly normal appendices show microscopic evidence of inflammation.

If the appendix cannot be found, the caecum should be mobilised and the taeniae coli should be traced to their confluence on the caecum before the diagnosis of 'absent appendix' is made.

If an appendix mass is found at operation, particularly at laparoscopy, it may be safer to abandon the procedure rather than risk bowel injury during attempted mobilisation. Any abscess should be drained, intravenous antibiotics administered and the patient carefully monitored during the postoperative period. Very rarely in the face of a frankly necrotic appendix, a caecectomy or partial right hemicolectomy is required.

Occasionally, a patient undergoing surgery for acute appendicitis is found to have concomitant Crohn's disease of the ileocaecal region. Providing that the caecal wall is healthy at the base of the appendix, appendicectomy can be performed without increasing the risk of an enterocutaneous fistula. Rarely, the appendix is involved with the Crohn's disease. In this situation, a conservative approach may be warranted; a trial of intravenous corticosteroids and systemic antibiotics can be used to resolve the acute inflammatory process.

Appendicitis in pregnancy

Appendicitis appears to be less common in pregnant than in non-pregnant females; however, it is the most common extrauterine acute abdominal condition in pregnancy, with an incidence of 0.5–1 per 1000 pregnancies. Appendicitis is slightly more common in the second trimester and, when compared with the non-pregnant population, presentation during pregnancy is more likely to be complicated. The diagnosis is often complicated by a delay in presentation as early non-specific symptoms are often attributed to the pregnancy. Obstetric teaching has been that the caecum and appendix are progressively pushed to the right upper quadrant of the abdomen as pregnancy develops during the second and third trimesters. However, pain in the right lower quadrant of the abdomen remains the cardinal feature of appendicitis in pregnancy.

Every attempt should be made to establish the diagnosis preoperatively as negative appendicectomy is associated with fetal loss in 4% and preterm labour in 10% of patients. Clinical diagnosis can be difficult and may be facilitated by ultrasound scanning, which carries no risk to the fetus and is highly specific; however, sensitivity in some series is low and its reliability varies according to the trimester. MRI scanning carries greater sensitivity but is more expensive and may not be widely available.

Delays in diagnosis or in the initiation of definitive treatment pose the greatest risk to the mother and pregnancy. Fetal loss occurs in 3–5% of cases of acute appendicitis in pregnancy but increases to 20% or more in the presence

Friedrich Trendelenburg, 1844–1924, Professor of Surgery successively at Rostock (1875–1882), Bonn (1882–1895), Leipzig (1895–1911), Germany. The Trendelenburg position was first described in 1885.

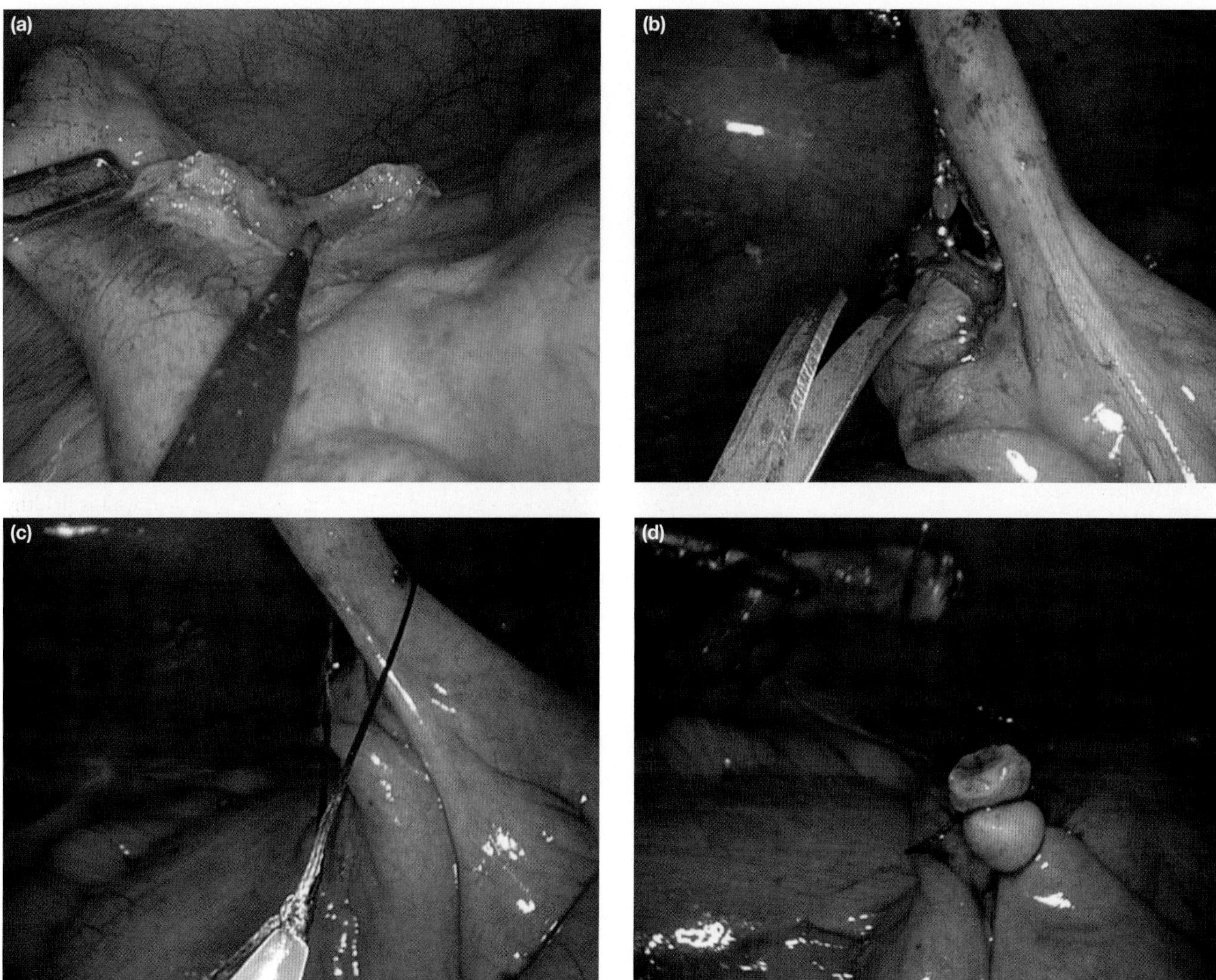

Figure 76.13 Laparoscopic appendicectomy. (a) Hook diathermy dissection of the mesoappendix. (b) The appendicular artery, ligated with clips, is divided. (c) The appendix base is ligated with absorbable ties. (d) Appendicectomy complete.

of perforation. There is insufficient evidence to support a non-operative approach and the pregnant patient with acute appendicitis should proceed to surgery. If the fetus is at a viable gestational age (23 weeks or more), appropriate obstetric and neonatal support should ideally be available. A laparoscopic approach is now considered to be safe in any trimester and, if used, should be initiated via the open Hasson technique. Data from a large series of pregnant women undergoing abdominal surgery (appendicectomy or cholecystectomy) reported a rate of obstetric complications of approximately 5%.

Postoperative complications

Postoperative complications following appendicectomy are relatively uncommon and reflect the degree of peritonitis that was present at the time of operation and intercurrent diseases that may predispose to complications.

Summary box 76.7

Checklist for unwell patients following appendicectomy

- Examine the wound and abdomen for an abscess
- Consider a pelvic abscess and perform a rectal examination
- Examine the lungs – consider pneumonitis or collapse
- Examine the legs – consider venous thrombosis
- Examine the conjunctivae for an icteric tinge and the liver for enlargement, and enquire whether the patient has had rigors (pylephlebitis)
- Examine the urine for organisms (pyelonephritis)
- Suspect subphrenic abscess

Wound infection

Wound infection is the most common postoperative complication, occurring in 5–10% of all patients. This usually presents with pain and erythema of the wound on the fourth or fifth

Harrith Hasson, 1931–2012, Professor of Gynecology, Chicago, IL, USA.

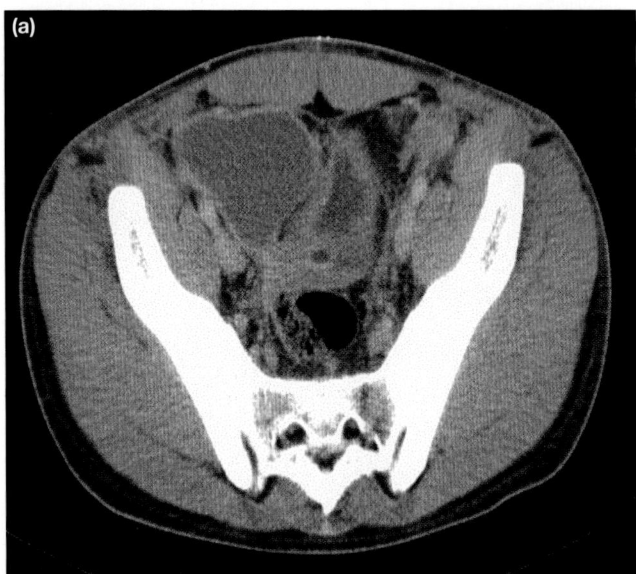

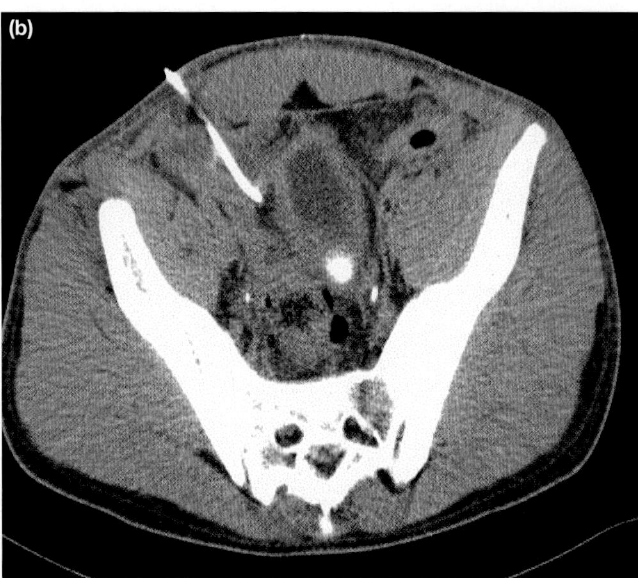

Figure 76.14 (a) Rim-enhancing collection in the right iliac fossa, 1 week after open appendicectomy for perforated appendicitis. (b) Successful radiological drainage with resolution of the abscess (courtesy of Professor P MacMahon, FRCR, Dublin, Ireland).

postoperative day, often soon after hospital discharge. Treatment is by wound drainage and antibiotics when required. The organisms responsible are usually a mixture of Gram-negative bacilli and anaerobic bacteria, predominantly *Bacteroides* species and anaerobic streptococci.

Intra-abdominal abscess

Approximately 8% of patients following appendicectomy will develop a postoperative intra-abdominal abscess. In an era of hospital discharge 24–48 hours following appendicectomy, patients should be advised prior to discharge that a spiking fever, malaise and anorexia developing 5–7 days after operation is suggestive of an intraperitoneal collection and that urgent medical advice should be obtained. Interloop, paracolic, pelvic and subphrenic sites should be considered. Abdominal ultrasonography and CT scanning greatly facilitate diagnosis and allow percutaneous drainage (***Figure 76.14***). Surgical exploration should be considered in patients suspected of having intra-abdominal sepsis but in whom imaging fails to show a collection, particularly those with continuing ileus.

Ileus

A period of adynamic ileus is to be expected after appendicectomy, and this may last a number of days following removal of a gangrenous appendix. Ileus persisting for more than 4 or 5 days, particularly in the presence of a fever, is indicative of continuing intra-abdominal sepsis and should prompt further investigation. Rarely, early during postoperative recovery, a Richter's type of hernia may occur at the site of a laparoscopic port insertion and may be confused with a postoperative ileus. A CT scan is usually definitive.

Respiratory

In the absence of concurrent pulmonary disease, respiratory complications are rare following appendicectomy. Adequate postoperative analgesia and physiotherapy, when appropriate, reduce the incidence.

Venous thrombosis and embolism

These conditions are rare after appendicectomy. Patients should undergo preoperative assessment of risk factors for venous thromboembolism and appropriate prophylactic measures should be taken.

Portal pyaemia (pylephlebitis)

This is a rare but very serious complication of gangrenous appendicitis associated with high fever, rigors and jaundice. It is caused by septicaemia in the portal venous system and leads to the development of intrahepatic abscesses (often multiple). Treatment is with systemic antibiotics and percutaneous drainage of hepatic abscesses as appropriate.

Faecal fistula

Leakage from the appendicular stump occurs rarely, but may follow if the encircling stitch has been put in too deeply or if the caecal wall was involved by oedema or inflammation. Occasionally, a fistula may result following appendicectomy in Crohn's disease.

Adhesive intestinal obstruction

This is the most common late complication of appendicectomy. At operation, a single band adhesion is often found to be responsible. Occasionally, chronic pain in the right iliac fossa is attributed to adhesion formation after appendicectomy. In such cases, laparoscopy is of value in confirming the presence of adhesions and allowing division.

August Gottlieb Richter, 1742–1812, lecturer in surgery, Göttingen, Germany.

RECURRENT ACUTE APPENDICITIS

Rarely, inflammation of the appendix may present as a chronic condition characterised by recurrent episodes of lower abdominal pain. Recurrent appendicitis is thought to arise as a consequence of incomplete self-limiting obstruction of the appendix lumen. The attacks vary in intensity and may occur every few months, and the majority of cases ultimately culminate in severe acute appendicitis. If a careful history is taken from patients with acute appendicitis, many remember having had milder but similar attacks of pain. The appendix in these cases is thickened and shows fibrosis indicative of previous inflammation.

NEOPLASMS OF THE APPENDIX AND PSEUDOMYXOMA PERITONEI

Tumours of the appendix may occur in up to 0.97 per 100 000 of the population. NETs account for approximately 30% of appendix neoplasms while epithelial tumours account for most other cases. Epithelial tumours may show mucinous or non-mucinous features and range in the aggressiveness of their behaviour from low grade to high-grade invasive with signet ring features (***Table 76.3***). A small percentage of appendix neoplasms fall into a third category known as mesenchymal tumours and include lymphoma, neuroma, GIST, Kaposi's sarcoma and granular cell tumour of the appendix.

Most patients with appendix neoplasms are asymptomatic at diagnosis and the appendix tumour is commonly an incidental finding at appendicectomy. Perforation of a mucinous appendix tumour with dissemination of epithelial cells and mucin production leads to a condition known as pseudomyxoma peritonei (PMP) (***Figure 76.15***).

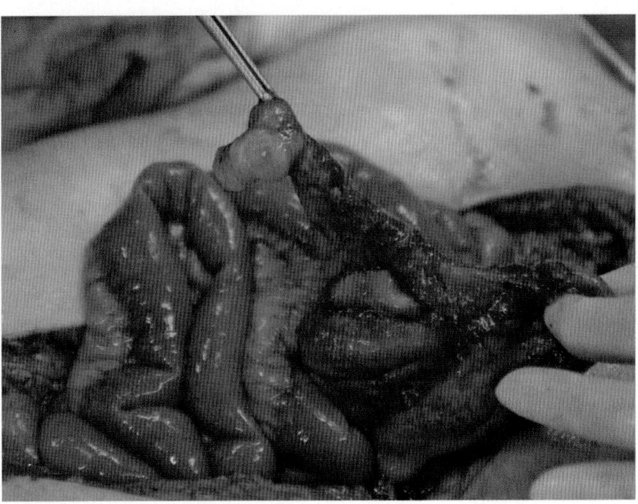

Figure 76.15 A low-grade mucinous tumour of the appendix with mucinous ascites and low-volume pseudomyxoma peritonei.

Neuroendocrine tumours of the appendix

NETs of the appendix are slightly more common in females and have an overall incidence of 0.15–0.6 per 100 000 per year. They arise in subepithelial neuroendocrine cells (***Figure 76.16***) and the majority (70%) are located in the appendix tip. The average age at presentation is 40–50 years and most patients are asymptomatic with early-stage disease typically found at appendicectomy for acute appendicitis. Uncommonly, patients may present with symptoms due to a mass or metastatic disease. Carcinoid syndrome is extremely rare. A diagnosis of NET is based on immunohistochemical staining for synaptophysin and chromogranin A and tumours are classified as grade 1–3 according to their proliferative capacity (determined by the Ki-67 index and mitotic rate).

Treatment

The treatment and prognosis of NETs of the appendix is governed by their grade, the tumour size and the extent of tumour invasion. Fully resected low-grade tumours less than 1 cm in size with minimal serosal or mesoappendix invasion are considered fully treated by appendicectomy alone and no further treatment or follow-up is required. The optimum treatment of patients with tumours 1–2 cm in size that have been fully resected is less clear as metastases may occur, albeit rarely. Current guidelines recommend a single CT or MRI of the abdomen to out rule regional or distant metastatic disease. Further surgery in the form of oncological resection of the right colon should be considered in patients with larger tumours (>2 cm), in the case of incomplete resection at appendicectomy or for higher tumour grade (2 or 3), T4 disease or vascular invasion. In these patients the risk of regional lymph node involvement is increased; however, the potential benefit of further surgery must be weighed against the increased operative risk. No further follow-up is required when the completion hemicolectomy shows no evidence of residual disease. The presence of nodal disease or high-grade tumour mandates subsequent follow-up, typically with CT or

TABLE 76.3 Classification of epithelial neoplasia of the appendix.
Adenoma (tubular, tubulovillous, villous)
Serrated polyp
Non-mucinous adenocarcinoma
Mucinous neoplasm
Low-grade appendiceal mucinous neoplasm
High-grade appendiceal mucinous neoplasm
Mucinous adenocarcinoma
Adenocarcinoma with signet ring cells (<50%)
Signet ring (>50%) carcinoma

Adapted from Carr NJ, Cecil TD, Mohamed F *et al.* A consensus for classification and pathologic reporting of pseudomyxoma peritonei and associated appendiceal neoplasia. The results of the Peritoneal Surface Oncology Group International (PSOGI) modified Delphi process. *Am J Surg Pathol* 2016; **40**: 14–26.

Moritz Kaposi, 1837–1902, dermatologist, Vienna, Austria.

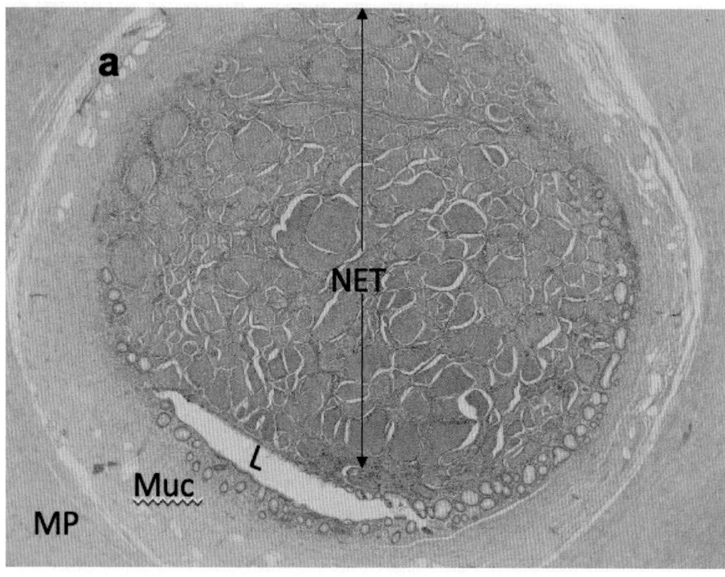

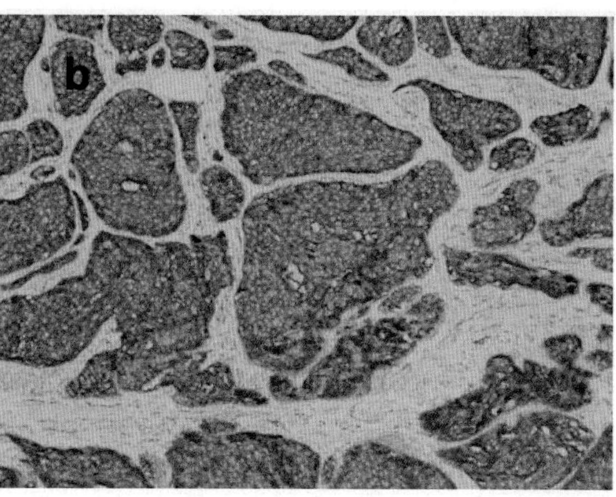

Figure 76.16 **(a)** Cross-sectional view of the appendix with outer, pink, muscularis propria (MP) and inner paler mucosa (Muc). The lumen of the appendix **(L)** has been compressed by an adjacent well-differentiated neuroendocrine tumour (NET). Haematoxylin and eosin stain, ×20. **(b)** Higher power view of synaptophysin immunohistochemical stain showing characteristic positive staining (brown) within tumour cells. Synaptophysin immunohistochemistry, ×100 (courtesy of Dr J Aird, FRCPath, Dublin, Ireland).

MRI at 6 and 12 months and then annually. For patients with early-stage NET the prognosis is excellent with 5-year survival of close to 100%. For those with advanced disease or distant metastases 5-year survival is typically less than 25%.

Goblet cell carcinoma

Goblet cell carcinomas (GCCs) of the appendix are a rare variant, accounting for less than 5% of appendix tumours. They display both neuroendocrine and glandular differentiation and are not considered true NETs. They may be classified as typical GCC or adenocarcinoma ex-GCC (Tang classification), with the latter group carrying a worse prognosis. GCCs display higher grade features than typical NETs and have a greater propensity for nodal and peritoneal dissemination; they should be treated in a similar fashion to appendix adenocarcinoma.

Epithelial tumours of the appendix

Epithelial neoplasms are found in 0.6% of appendicectomy specimens. Numerous classification systems have been proposed, leading to much confusion and difficulty when comparing treatment modalities and outcomes. Following a modified Delphi consultation process, a group of international experts proposed an updated classification system for appendiceal epithelial neoplasms. Tumours may be classified as mucinous or non-mucinous (intestinal type) and according to the degree of cytological atypia and architectural features (infiltrative versus pushing invasion) (***Table 76.3***).

Low-grade neoplasms

Most epithelial tumours of the appendix are classified as LAMNs. These lesions demonstrate minimal cytological atypia and are characterised by pushing rather than infiltrative invasion without evidence of destruction. In the case of appendix perforation, mucin may be found outside the appendix, the significance of which is increased when accompanied by the presence of epithelial cells. Low-grade tumours do not typically metastasise to regional lymph nodes and as such right hemicolectomy is not required. The importance of these lesions lies in their propensity to disseminate throughout the peritoneal cavity, causing the syndrome known as PMP. Patients with low-grade epithelial neoplasms and no evidence of mucin or epithelial cells beyond the appendix are thought to be at low risk of future PMP development. A colonoscopy should be performed to exclude associated colonic epithelial lesions and patients entered into a surveillance protocol for at least 5 years. Surveillance may take the form of clinical review, annual low-dose abdominopelvic CT scan and monitoring of appendix-related tumour markers (carcinoembryonic antigen [CEA], CA-19-9, CA-125). In patients with perforated tumours, particularly when extraluminal mucin contains epithelial cells, the risk of PMP is higher. In some experienced centres these patients may be considered for cytoreductive surgery with hyperthermic intraperitoneal chemotherapy (HIPEC), although a common approach is regular monitoring for the appearance of clinical or radiological features of PMP, which would then warrant surgery.

High-grade and invasive neoplasms

Appendiceal mucinous tumours displaying high-grade dysplasia are classified as high-grade appendiceal mucinous neoplasm (HAMN). Mucinous tumours with infiltrative invasion are classified as mucinous adenocarcinoma and may be well, moderately or poorly differentiated with or without the

Laura H Tang, contemporary, pathologist, Memorial Sloan Kettering Hospital, New York, NY, USA.

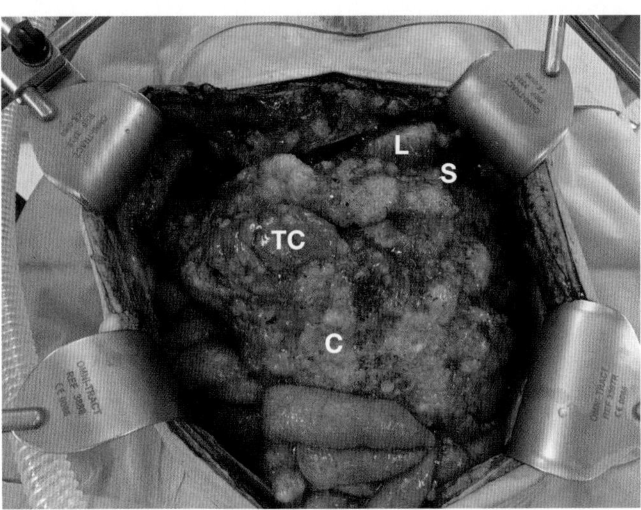

Figure 76.17 Pseudomyxoma peritonei with characteristic omental cake (C) encasing the transverse colon (TC) and extending to the greater curvature of the stomach (S). Tumour is seen to replace the lesser omentum (L).

presence of signet ring cells. Non-mucinous adenocarcinoma is considered to be similar to typical colorectal cancer.

Patients with high-grade tumour or invasive adenocarcinoma are at risk of lymph node involvement. According to current paradigms, they should undergo right hemicolectomy. Because of the risk of peritoneal metastases, cytoreductive surgery (CRS), to include right hemicolectomy with regional (right parietal) peritonectomy, omentectomy and HIPEC, may also be appropriate when the necessary expertise and experience are available. Consideration may also be given to performing bilateral salpingo-oophorectomy because of the risk of tumour seeding to the ovaries, although in patients of childbearing age the decision making is complex.

Pseudomyxoma peritonei

PMP is a rare condition typified by progressive peritoneal tumour deposits, mucinous ascites, omental cake (***Figure 76.17***) and ovarian involvement in females. The vast majority of cases arise as a result of perforation of a mucinous appendiceal tumour. Patients typically present with progressive and massive abdominal distension, anorexia and symptoms of bowel dysfunction. The condition is invariably fatal without intervention. Traditionally, PMP was thought to have an incidence of 1 per 1 000 000 per year, but it is now thought to be at least double that with recent estimates of 3.2 cases per 1 000 000 per year. The overall risk of developing pseudomyxoma following removal of an appendix harbouring epithelial tumour is approximately 9%, with the risk varying according to the tumour subtype and the mode of presentation, while it may be as high as 30–50% in the case of a mucinous adenocarcinoma of the appendix (***Figure 76.18***).

PMP is classified according to the degree of cytological atypia within the peritoneal deposits (***Table 76.4***) and its grading may differ from that of the causative primary appendiceal tumour. Elevated tumour markers (CEA, CA-125, CA-19-9)

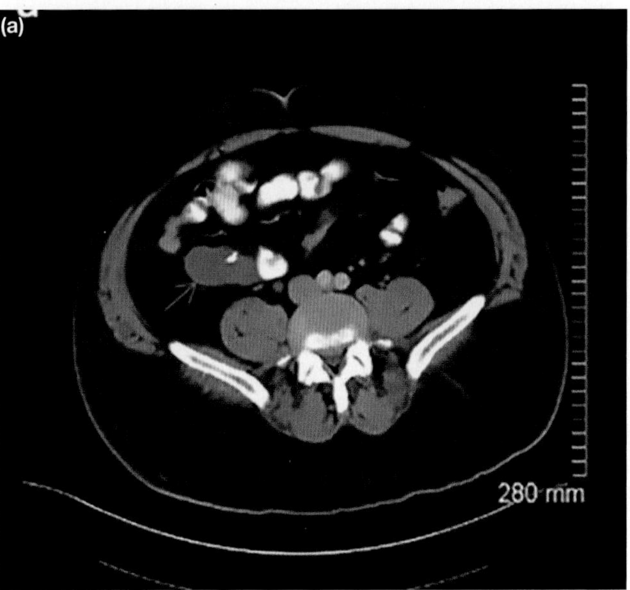

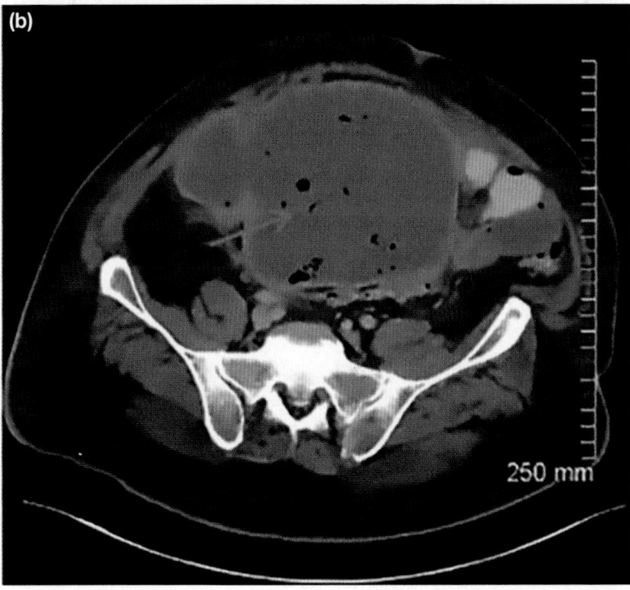

Figure 76.18 **(a)** Contrast-enhanced axial computed tomography (CT) image demonstrates a tubular cystic structure with calcification adjacent to the caecum compatible with an abnormally distended appendix (arrow). **(b)** Six-year follow-up postcontrast axial CT image demonstrated a 19 × 10 × 17 cm complex cystic mass in the right lower quadrant (arrow) highly suspicious for a mucinous tumour of the appendix with extensive peritoneal involvement and pseudomyxoma peritonei (courtesy of Professor Helen Fenlon, Dublin, Ireland).

TABLE 76.4 Classification of pseudomyxoma peritonei.
Acellular mucin
Low-grade mucinous carcinoma peritonei
High-grade mucinous carcinoma peritonei
High-grade mucinous carcinoma peritonei with signet ring cells

Adapted from Carr NJ, Cecil TD, Mohamed F *et al*. A consensus for classification and pathologic reporting of pseudomyxoma peritonei and associated appendiceal neoplasia. The results of the Peritoneal Surface Oncology Group International (PSOGI) modified Delphi process. *Am J Surg Pathol* 2016; **40**: 14–26.

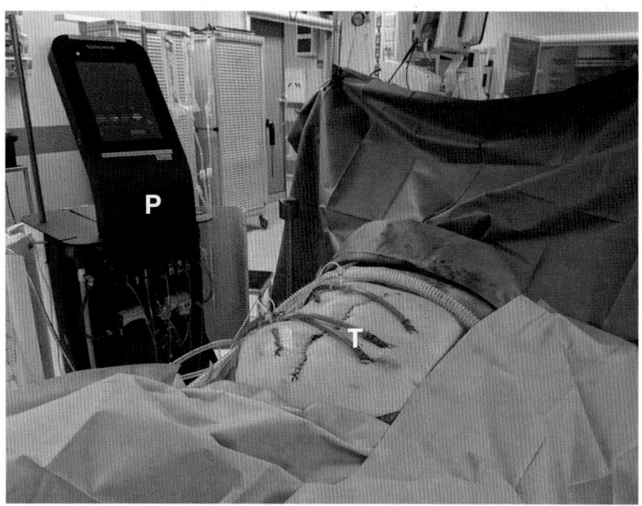

Figure 76.19 Hyperthermic intraperitoneal chemotherapy (HIPEC) delivery following cytoreductive surgery using a closed abdomen technique. The perfusion pump (P) heats and circulates chemotherapy throughout the abdominal cavity via inflow and outflow tubing (T), typically for 60–90 minutes.

predict a more aggressive phenotype and are associated with a worse prognosis.

Investigations

The investigation of a patient with PMP should include a high-resolution CT scan of the abdomen and pelvis with oral and intravenous contrast. A full colonoscopy should be performed to exclude a primary colorectal cancer. Laparoscopy may provide additional staging information by allowing direct visualisation of the small bowel where radiologically occult miliary disease may be found. Ideally laparoscopy should be performed at a centre where subsequent CRS would be undertaken. Laparoscopy also facilitates tissue diagnosis, although this is not always necessary. In experienced centres the clinical and radiological features are often sufficient to establish a diagnosis of PMP.

Treatment

Patients with PMP should be referred to a specialist centre with multidisciplinary expertise in the assessment and management of patients with peritoneal malignancy.

The accepted treatment is CRS combined with HIPEC (Sugarbaker). This approach combines multiple peritonectomy procedures with multivisceral resections as required to achieve a complete surgical clearance of the tumour (complete cytoreduction), which is augmented by HIPEC (typically mitomycin C or oxaliplatin) to eradicate presumed residual microscopic disease (***Figure 76.19***). The combined operation can take in excess of 10 hours and may require total abdominopelvic peritonectomy, greater and lesser omentectomy, bilateral salpingo-oophorectomy, hysterectomy, cholecystectomy, splenectomy, partial gastrectomy, colectomy and anterior resection of the rectum. The largest reported series of CRS/HIPEC for PMP comes from Basingstoke, UK (Moran). In their experience involving more than 1000 patients, a complete cytoreduction was achieved in approximately 75% of patients, with the remainder undergoing maximal tumour debulking. Although a potentially morbid procedure, in experienced centres the operative mortality rate following CRS/HIPEC is less than 2% with major postoperative morbidity in 15% of patients. Appropriate patient selection is critical and patients must have a sufficient performance status and be without major comorbidity in order to withstand the surgery. Preoperative evaluation, including nutritional assessment and optimisation, is paramount.

Following a complete cytoreduction 5- and 10-year survival rates of 87% and 70%, respectively, can be achieved. Poorer outcomes are seen in males, patients with elevated tumour markers and following resection of tumour showing high-grade or invasive features. Follow-up typically comprises at least annual clinical evaluation, monitoring of tumour markers and CT scan. Surveillance should be continued for at least 10 years as late recurrence is documented.

Systemic chemotherapy may be considered as first-line treatment in patients with high-grade or invasive unresectable disease or in the adjuvant setting following CRS/HIPEC, again in patients with high-grade tumour. Chemotherapy is not typically considered in patients with low-grade PMP.

Management of an incidental or unexpected tumour of the appendix

Incidental neoplasm in appendicectomy specimen

In a patient with an incidental finding of an appendix neoplasm and no current evidence of metastatic disease or PMP, subsequent treatment is dependent on the degree of cytological atypia within the primary tumour, the estimated risk of lymph node metastases and the future risk of developing PMP. In general, small low-grade tumours require surveillance only, whereas patients with larger tumour or adverse features may need further surgery.

Unexpected appendix tumour encountered at surgery

An inspection of the abdominal cavity should be performed to establish the presence of metastases or PMP. The appendix should be removed, with care taken to avoid spillage of its contents, to allow a pathological diagnosis, which will determine the need for subsequent intervention. In most cases the tumour can be removed by appendicectomy alone, with or without a cuff of caecum.

Paul H Sugarbaker, contemporary, surgeon, Washington DC, USA.
Brendan J Moran, contemporary, surgeon, Basingstoke, UK.

Incidental finding of pseudomyxoma peritonei encountered at surgery

The surgeon should perform a careful inspection of the abdominal cavity and record the extent and distribution of disease. A peritoneal or omental biopsy can be performed; however, care should be taken to minimise disruption of the anatomical planes. If the appendix is abnormal, an appendicectomy should be performed to allow a histological diagnosis. Ideally the planned procedure should then be aborted with a view to referring the patient to a centre experienced in the management of peritoneal malignancy.

FURTHER READING

Ansari N, Chandrakumaran K, Dayal S *et al.* Cytoreductive surgery and hyperthermic intraperitoneal chemotherapy in 1000 patients with perforated appendiceal epithelial tumours. *Eur J Surg Oncol* 2016; **42**: 1035–41.

Carr NJ, Cecil TD, Mohamed F *et al.* A consensus for classification and pathologic reporting of pseudomyxoma peritonei and associated appendiceal neoplasia. The results of the Peritoneal Surface Oncology Group International (PSOGI) modified Delphi process. *Am J Surg Pathol* 2016; **40**: 14–26.

Govaerts K, Lurvink RJ, DeHingh IHJT *et al.* Appendiceal tumours and pseudomyxoma peritonei: literature review with PSOGI/EU-RACAN clinical practice guidelines for diagnosis and treatment. *Eur J Surg Oncol* 2021; **47**: 11–35.

Harnoss JC, Zelienka I, Probst P *et al.* Antibiotics versus surgical therapy for uncomplicated appendicitis: systematic review and meta-analysis of controlled trials (PROSPERO). *Ann Surg* 2017; **265**: 889–900.

Ingraham AM, Cohen ME, Bilimoria KY *et al.* Effect of delay to operation on outcomes in adults with acute appendicitis. *Arch Surg* 2010; **145**: 886–92.

Jaschinski T, Mosch CG, Eikermann M *et al.* Laparoscopic versus open surgery for suspected appendicitis. *Cochrane Database Syst Rev* 2018; Issue 11, Art. No. CD001546.

Kim K, Kim YH, Kim SY *et al.* Low-dose abdominal CT for evaluating suspected appendicitis. *N Engl J Med* 2012; **366**: 1596–605.

Mällinen J, Rautio T, Grönroos J *et al.* Risk of appendiceal neoplasm in periappendicular abscess in patients treated with interval appendectomy vs follow-up with magnetic resonance imaging. 1-year outcomes of the Peri-Appendicitis Acuta randomized controlled trial. *JAMA Surg* 2019; **154**: 200–7.

Mennie N, Panabokke G, Chang A *et al.* Are post-operative intravenous antibiotics indicated after laparoscopic appendicectomy for simple appendicitis? A prospective double-blinded randomized controlled trial. *Ann Surg* 2020; **276**: 248–52.

Pape UF, Niederle B, Costa F *et al.* ENETS Consensus guidelines for neuroendocrine neoplasms of the appendix (excluding goblet cell carcinomas). *Neuroendocrinology* 2016; **103**: 144–52.

Patkova B, Svenningsson A, Almström M *et al.* Non-operative treatment versus appendectomy for acute nonperforated appendicitis in children: five year follow-up of a randomized controlled pilot trial. *Ann Surg* 2020; **271**: 1030–5.

Rud B, Vejborg TS, Rappeport ED *et al.* Computed tomography for diagnosis of acute appendicitis in adults. *Cochrane Database Syst Rev* 2019; Issue 11, Art. No. CD009977.

van Rossem CC, Bolmers MD, Schreinemacher MH *et al.* Prospective nationwide outcome audit of surgery for suspected acute appendicitis. *Br J Surg* 2016; **103**: 144–51.

Weinstein M, Feuerwerker S, Baxter S. Appendicitis and cholecystitis in pregnancy. *Clin Obstet Gynaecol* 2020; **63**: 405–15.

CHAPTER 77 The large intestine

Learning objectives

To appreciate:
- The basic anatomy and physiology of the large intestine
- The range of conditions that may affect the large intestine

To understand:
- The aetiology and pathology of common large intestinal conditions
- The principles of investigation of large intestinal symptoms
- The importance of non-surgical management of large intestinal problems
- The principles of colonic surgery
- That complex intestinal problems are best managed by a multidisciplinary team
- The management of acute surgical problems of the large intestine

ANATOMY OF THE LARGE INTESTINE

The large intestine begins at the ileocaecal valve and extends to the anus. It is divided into the caecum, ascending colon, hepatic flexure, transverse colon with attached greater omentum, splenic flexure, descending colon, sigmoid colon and rectum. The large intestine is approximately 1.5 m long, but it can be concertinaed over an endoscope so the caecum can be reached with 70–90 cm of a colonoscope.

The external appearance of the colon is distinguished from the small bowel by the presence of taenia coli, three bands of longitudinal muscle that run from the appendix base to the rectosigmoid junction and fat-filled peritoneal tags known as appendices epiploicae found principally on the left side of the colon. The taenia coli act to pull the colon into its sacculated state, producing a series of haustrations that may be visible on abdominal radiograph and allowing distinction from distended small intestine, which has complete transverse markings caused by the valvulae conniventes (see ***Chapter 74***). The important posterior relations of the caecum and ascending colon are the right ureter, right gonadal vessels and duodenum and these must be protected at surgery. The left ureter, left gonadal vessels and tail of the pancreas must be protected when operating on the left colon.

The blood supply of the large intestine from the caecum to the distal transverse colon is derived from branches of the superior mesenteric artery and from the inferior mesenteric artery and its branches more distally. The middle colic artery is a prominent branch of the superior mesenteric artery arising soon after the origin, which divides almost immediately into two or three large arcades to supply the transverse colon. The precise vascular anatomy is variable and needs to be taken into account when performing colectomy, particularly total mesocolic excision for cancer (see ***Chapter 65***). Peripheral branches of the superior and inferior mesenteric vessels usually anastomose, resulting in a continuous vascular supply along the colon, referred to as the marginal artery of Drummond. This vessel is often the key blood supply to the vascular arcades, ensuring adequate perfusion of a colonic anastomosis; however, blood flow in the 'watershed' area of the splenic flexure representing the junction of the embryological mid- and hindgut may be tenuous. Sudden occlusion of the inferior mesenteric artery may leave the area of the splenic flexure poorly perfused, leading to an ischaemic colitis. Venous and lymphatic drainage of the colon follows the arterial supply and venous drainage is into the portal system. High ligation of the artery supplying a segment of colon will therefore also remove the lymphatic vessels and nodes, a key technical point in cancer surgery. The nerve supply to the large intestine is derived from the splanchnic nerves via sympathetic plexuses surrounding the superior (midgut) and inferior (hindgut) mesenteric arteries. Visceral pain from the part of the colon supplied by the superior mesenteric artery is thus felt, like that of the small intestine, in the periumbilical region, while pain from the colon distal to that point is felt suprapubically.

PHYSIOLOGY OF THE LARGE INTESTINE

The principal function of the colon is absorption of water; approximately 1000 mL of ileal content enters the caecum

---

Valvulae conniventes describes a fold of mucous membrane that passes across two-thirds of the bowel circumference.
Sir David Drummond, 1852–1932, born Dublin, Ireland, pathologist and physician at the Royal Victoria Infirmary, Newcastle (1878–1920), President of the British Medical Association (1921–1922) and vice chancellor of Durham University (1920–1922).

every 24 hours, of which only approximately 200 mL is excreted in faeces. Sodium absorption is efficiently accomplished by an active transport system, while chloride and water are absorbed passively. Fermentation of dietary fibre in the colon by the normal colonic microflora leads to the generation of short chain fatty acids, which are an important metabolic substrate for colonic mucosa. Diversion of the faecal stream, denying the mucosa of this nutrition, may lead to inflammatory changes in the colon downstream (diversion colitis). Absorption of nutrients, including glucose, fatty acids, amino acids and vitamins, can also take place in the colon.

Colonic motility is variable. In general, faecal residue reaches the caecum 4 hours after a meal and the rectum after 24 hours. Passage of stool is not orderly because of mixing within the colon (see *Chapter 73*).

TUMOURS OF THE LARGE INTESTINE

Benign

The term 'polyp' is a clinical description of any protrusion of the mucosa. It encompasses a variety of histologically different tumours (*Table 77.1*). Polyps can occur singly, synchronously in small numbers or as part of a polyposis syndrome.

Metaplastic polyps

Metaplastic or hyperplastic polyps are common and are generally considered benign. Recently certain subtypes have been recognised to have malignant potential. Sessile serrated lesions and hyperplastic polyps ≥10 mm in diameter are associated with *KRAS*/*BRAF* mutation that may lead to methylation of tumour-suppressing genes, dysplasia and malignancy along what is termed the 'serrated pathway'. Such polyps should be removed and follow-up colonoscopy arranged (*Figure 77.1*).

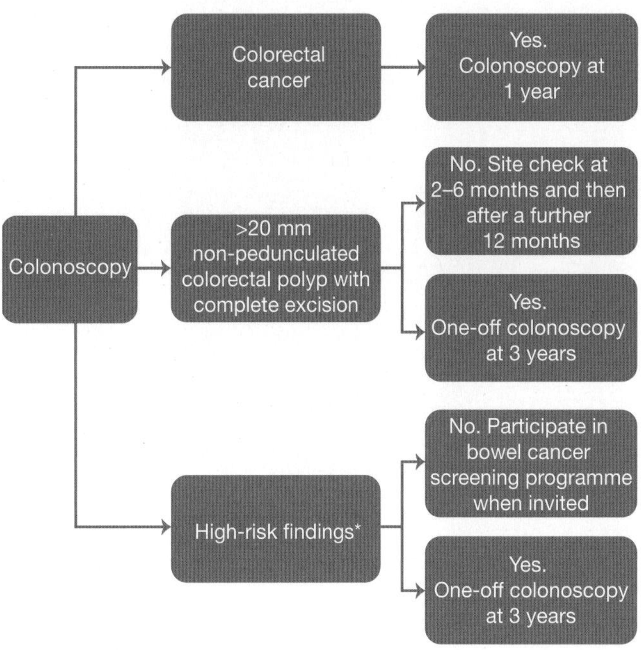

Figure 77.1 Recommendations for polyp follow-up. *Two or more premalignant polyps including at least one advanced polyp (serrated polyp >10 mm or with dysplasia, adenoma more than 10 mm in size or with high-grade dysplasia); or five or more premalignant polyps. (Adapted from Rutter MD, East J, Rees CJ *et al*. British Society of Gastroenterology/Association of Coloproctology of Great Britain and Ireland/Public Health England post-polypectomy and post-colorectal cancer resection surveillance guidelines. *Gut* 2020; **69**: 201–23.)

TABLE 77.1 Classification of intestinal polyps.

Inflammatory	Inflammatory polyps (pseudopolyps in ulcerative colitis) (see *Chapter 75*)
Hamartomatous	Peutz–Jeghers polyp
	Juvenile polyp
Serrated polyps (serrated lesions)	Hyperplastic polyp
	Sessile serrated lesion
	Sessile serrated lesion with dysplasia
	Traditional serrated adenomas
	Mixed polyp
Adenoma	Tubular
	Tubulovillous
	Villous
Malignant polyp	Adenocarcinoma

Adenomatous polyps

Adenomatous polyps are the most common polyps with malignant potential. The risk of malignancy is dependent on histology, morphology and size. Tubular adenomas have the lowest risk, with increasing risk as villous features predominate. Sessile and particularly depressed lesions have more malignant potential than pedunculated lesions (*Figure 77.2*). The risk of malignant change increases with size, almost one-third of large (>3 cm) colonic adenomas will have an area of invasive malignancy. Size is easily assessed endoscopically, which, alongside pit pattern and morphological classification, aids management. If felt appropriate and safe to resect endoscopically, various techniques are available, including hot or cold snare polypectomy for the most common smaller pedunculated lesions. Larger or flatter polyps may require infiltration of a solution to 'raise' the polyp before snare resection. The area of the polyp should be tattooed to facilitate later endoscopic or laparoscopic localisation of the site of the polyp. Failure of submucosal injection to elevate a polyp is suggestive of malignancy. In these circumstances, the site should be tattooed. A biopsy should not be taken if referral for endoscopic mucosal resection or endoscopic submucosal dissection is being considered. Such techniques carry a risk of colonic perforation and should only

John Law Augustine Peutz, 1886–1968, Chief Specialist for Internal Medicine, St John's Hospital, The Hague, The Netherlands.
Harold Joseph Jeghers, 1904–1990, Professor of Internal Medicine, New Jersey College of Medicine and Dentistry, Jersey City, NJ, USA.

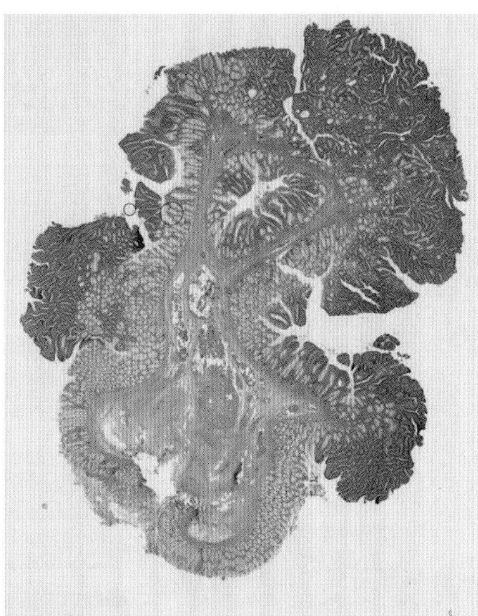

Figure 77.2 Pedunculated polyp of the large intestine showing tubulovillous changes at the apex and normal colonic mucosa at the base (courtesy of Dr Philip Kaye, Nottingham University Hospitals, Nottingham, UK).

be performed by an experienced endoscopist. Rectal adenomas may also be treated by endoscopic or transanal resection (see *Chapter 79*).

Polyp surveillance

After successful endoscopic removal of polyps, there is a risk of further polyp development; however, the risk of subsequent development of colorectal cancer is low. The need for and frequency of follow-up surveillance endoscopy is dependent on polyp morphology, number and size, age and comorbidity of the patient, presence of a family history and accuracy and completeness of the index test. These factors allow polyps to be divided into low, intermediate and high risk. Recent guidelines (*Figure 77.1*) published by the British Society of Gastroenterology have identified patients at high risk needing follow-up colonoscopy as those with either:

- two or more premalignant polyps, including at least one advanced colorectal polyp (defined as a serrated polyp ≥10 mm in size or containing any grade of dysplasia or as an adenoma ≥10 mm in size or containing high-grade dysplasia); or
- five or more premalignant polyps.

Polyposis syndromes

Polyposis syndromes can be divided into familial adenomatous polyposis (FAP), attenuated familial adenomatous polyposis (AFAP), *MUTYH*-associated polyposis (MAP) and *NTHL1*-associated polyposis (NAP).

Familial adenomatous polyposis

FAP is defined clinically by the presence of more than 100 colorectal adenomas but is also characterised by duodenal adenomas and multiple extraintestinal manifestations (*Summary boxes 77.1 and 77.2*). Over 80% of cases come from those with a positive family history. The remainder arise as a result of new mutations in the adenomatous polyposis coli (*APC*) gene on the long arm of chromosome 5. FAP is inherited as an autosomal dominant condition and is consequently equally likely in men and women. The lifetime risk of colorectal cancer is up to 100% in those with an *APC* gene mutation. FAP can also be associated with benign mesodermal tumours such as desmoid tumours and osteomas. Epidermoid cysts can also occur (Gardner's syndrome); desmoid tumours in the abdomen spread locally to involve the intestinal mesentery and, although non-metastasising, they may become unresectable. Up to 50% of people with FAP have congenital hypertrophy of the retinal pigment epithelium (CHRPE), which can be used to screen affected families if genetic testing is unavailable.

Clinical features

Polyps are usually visible on sigmoidoscopy by the age of 15 years and will almost always be visible by the age of 30 years. Regular endoscopic surveillance in a suspected family member should therefore commence at the age of 12–14 years, even if a genetic mutation has not been identified. Patients with mutations located between codons 1286 and 1513 of the *APC* gene generally have a worse prognosis with earlier disease onset than those with mutations outside this region. Germline mutations at codon 1309 are associated with the most severe disease. AFAP, also associated with *APC* gene mutation, is associated with fewer than 100 polyps and may not present until the fourth decade.

If the diagnosis is made during adolescence, surgery is usually deferred to the age of 17 or 18 years unless symptoms develop. Malignant change is unusual before the age of 20 years. Examination of blood relatives, including cousins, nephews and nieces, is essential; a family tree should be constructed, and a register of affected families maintained. Referral to a medical geneticist is essential. If over 100 adenomas are present at colonoscopy, the diagnosis can be made confidently (*Figure 77.3*).

Summary box 77.1

Features of FAP

- Autosomal dominant inherited disease due to mutations of the *APC* gene
- More than 100 colonic adenomas are diagnostic
- Prophylactic surgery is indicated to prevent colorectal cancer
- Polyps and malignant tumours can develop particularly around the duodenal ampulla

Eldon John Gardner, 1909–1989, geneticist, The University of Utah, Salt Lake City, UT, USA, described this syndrome in 1950.

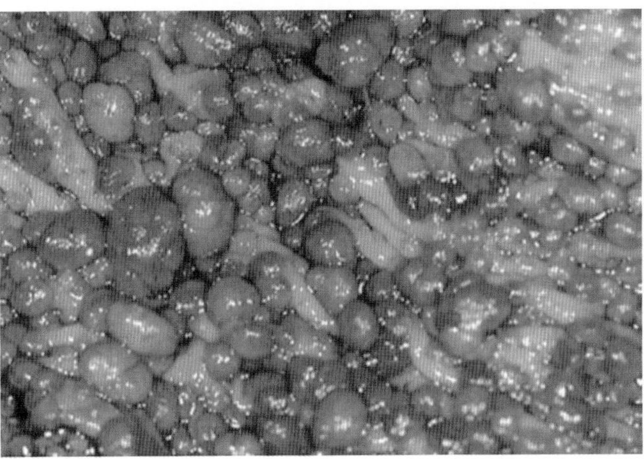

Figure 77.3 Familial adenomatous polyposis showing hundreds of adenomatous polyps.

Summary box 77.2

Extracolonic manifestations of FAP

- Endodermal derivatives
  - Adenomas and carcinomas, particularly around the duodenal ampulla but also stomach, small intestine, thyroid and biliary tree
  - Gastric fundic gland polyps
  - Hepatoblastoma
- Ectodermal derivatives
  - Epidermoid cysts
  - Pilomatrixoma
  - Congenital hypertrophy of the retinal pigment epithelium (CHRPE)
  - Brain tumours
- Mesodermal derivatives
  - Desmoid tumours
  - Osteomas
  - Dental problems

Treatment

The aim of surgery in FAP is to prevent the development of colorectal cancer. The surgical options are:

1 restorative proctocolectomy with an ileal pouch–anal anastomosis;
2 colectomy with ileorectal anastomosis (IRA);
3 total proctocolectomy and end-ileostomy.

As patients are often young, most prefer to avoid a stoma, restorative proctocolectomy with ileal pouch–anal anastomosis has the advantage of removing the whole colon and rectum without the need for a permanent stoma (see *Chapter 75*). However, there is a pouch failure rate of approximately 10%. In addition, and particularly when a stapled anastomosis has been created, endoscopic surveillance is still required as malignant change can occur in the 'rectal cuff' (the small strip of rectal mucosa between the pouch and the dentate line). Some advocate complete mucosectomy of this residual cuff and a transanal anastomosis, although this may result in worse function. In experienced hands, a laparoscopic approach is associated with swifter recovery, improved cosmesis and perhaps increased fecundity in women.

For patients with relative rectal sparing (<20 polyps), total colectomy and IRA is an option to be considered, particularly as it is associated with less risk of sexual dysfunction in males and less infertility in females. However, the rectum requires regular endoscopic surveillance as up to 10% of patients will develop invasive malignancy in the rectum. In AFAP, patients may consider rectal preservation surgery on the understanding that their cancer risk is lower (around 2%) but still present.

Proctocolectomy and ileostomy is the recommended option for patients with poor anal sphincter function, those who have already developed a rectal cancer or those who wish to have a definitive single-stage procedure.

Postoperative surveillance

Because of the ongoing cancer risk, regular lifelong endoscopic surveillance of the rectum/pouch is important with biopsy of the rectal cuff unless mucosal proctectomy has been performed. Endoscopy is also carried out to detect upper gastrointestinal tumours, particularly around the duodenal ampulla (see *Chapter 67*). A side-viewing duodenoscope is required. Despite surveillance, life expectancy is reduced because of extracolonic cancers and complications of desmoid tumours.

MUTYH-associated polyposis

The appearances of MAP can be similar to FAP but it is inherited as an autosomal recessive phenotype and predisposes individuals to multiple colonic polyps. If an *APC* pathogenic variant is not identified in an individual with colonic polyposis, molecular genetic testing of *MUTYH* should be considered. There is an increased risk of colorectal cancer of between three- and sixfold depending on the particular *MUTYH* mutation. Colonoscopy should be performed every 2 years. Colectomy is required when the number and/or characteristics of the polyps do not allow complete endoscopic resection or malignancy is diagnosed. Surveillance for duodenal adenomas is recommended.

NTHL1 tumour syndrome

NTHL1 tumour syndrome is a rare autosomal recessive cause of colorectal polyposis and increased lifetime risk for colorectal cancer. Colorectal polyps can be adenomatous, hyperplastic or sessile serrated. Management is similar to MAP.

Peutz-Jeghers and juvenile polyposis syndrome

Peutz–Jeghers syndrome (PJS) is an autosomal dominant genetic disorder characterised by the development of benign hamartomas in the gastrointestinal tract along with hyperpigmented lesions on the lips and oral mucosa. The main clinical risks are small bowel intussusception in children and increased incidence of gastrointestinal malignancy in adult life (see *Chapter 74*).

Juvenile polyposis (JPS) is an autosomal dominant inherited condition that presents with hamartomatous polyps due to mutations in the *BMPR1A*, *SMAD4* or *ENG* genes. Pigmentation characteristic of PJS is not present.

Lynch syndrome (hereditary non-polyposis colorectal cancer)

Lynch syndrome, previously known as hereditary non-polyposis colorectal cancer (HNPCC), is characterised by an increased risk of colorectal cancer and also cancers of the endometrium, ovary, stomach and small intestine, urinary tract, pancreas, prostate and kidney. It is an autosomal dominant condition caused by a mutation in one of four DNA mismatch repair genes (*MLH1*, *MSH2*, *MSH6* and *PMS2*). These genes, when functioning normally, code for mismatch repair (MMR) proteins, which repair sporadic mutations that occur in other genes. If faulty, mutations accumulate in other key genes, leading to characteristic repeat sequences of DNA, termed microsatellite instability (MSI), and acceleration of the adenoma–carcinoma sequence. Thus individuals with an MMR gene mutation tend to develop colorectal polyps at an early age (before the age of 50 years) that quickly become cancerous. Not everyone with a mutation develops cancer; the lifetime risk is 80%. Most cancers develop in the proximal colon. Females have a 30–50% lifetime risk of developing endometrial cancer.

Diagnosis

Lynch syndrome was historically diagnosed based on a family history of cancer and the clinical parameters set out in the Amsterdam (***Summary box 77.3***) and Bethesda criteria. Recent advances in immunohistochemistry allow for MMR proteins or MSI to be accurately identified in all colorectal tumours with subsequent genetic testing in patients and families of those proven positive.

Summary box 77.3

Amsterdam II criteria

- Three or more family members with a Lynch syndrome-related cancer (colorectal, endometrial, small bowel, ureter, renal pelvis), one of whom is a first-degree relative of the other two
- Two or more successive affected generations
- At least one tumour diagnosed before the age of 50 years
- FAP excluded
- Tumours verified by pathological examination

Because of the accelerated pathway from adenoma to cancer in Lynch syndrome those with a gene mutation should be offered 2-yearly endoscopic surveillance from age 25 years (*MLH1* and *MSH2* carriers) or 35 years (*MSH6* carriers). *PMS2* carriers should be offered 5-yearly screening beginning at age 35 years (see ***Further reading***). For patients with polyps that cannot be managed with endoscopic polypectomy or those who develop a cancer, an extended colectomy (*MLH1* and *MSH2* carriers) should be considered. The benefit of screening other areas of the gastrointestinal tract is unclear but gynaecological screening is recommended in accordance with the 2019 Manchester Consensus (see ***Further reading***).

Malignant: colorectal carcinoma

Epidemiology

In the UK, colorectal cancer is the second most common cause of cancer death. Approximately 42 000 patients are diagnosed with colorectal cancer every year in the UK. Approximately one-third of these tumours are in the rectum and two-thirds in the colon. The burden of disease is greater in men than in women (56% versus 44%). Colorectal cancer occurs less frequently in resource-poor than in resource-rich countries.

Aetiology

Most colorectal cancers are thought to develop from adenomatous polyps through a sequence of genetic mutations influenced by environmental factors. This adenoma–carcinoma sequence is based on strong observational evidence (***Summary box 77.4***). The adenoma–carcinoma sequence is not a simple stepwise progression of mutations but a complicated array of multiple genetic alterations, ultimately resulting in an invasive tumour. Mutations of the *APC* gene occur in two-thirds of colonic adenomas and are thought to develop early in the carcinogenesis pathway. *K-ras* mutations result in activation of cell signalling pathways and are more common in larger lesions, suggesting that that they are later events in mutagenesis. The *p53* gene is frequently mutated in carcinomas but not in adenomas and therefore thought to be a marker of invasion. A recent international consortium has identified four consensus molecular subtypes (CMSs) of colorectal cancer based on bioinformatic analysis of gene expression in more than 4000 patients. MSI, a feature of Lynch syndrome, may occur sporadically, particularly in right-sided tumours (CMS1), while others show *WNT* and *MYC* signalling activation (CMS2), metabolic dysregulation (CMS3) and transforming growth factor beta activation (CMS4). The value of this classification in interpreting tumour aetiology, biology and targeted treatment remains to be determined.

Summary box 77.4

Evidence for adenoma-carcinoma sequence

- The distribution of adenomas is similar to that of cancers (70% left sided)
- Larger adenomas are more likely to be dysplastic than small adenomas
- The majority of early cancers have adjacent adenomatous tissue
- Adenomas are found in one-third of specimens resected for colorectal cancer
- Incidence of colorectal cancer decreases within a screening programme that involves colonoscopy and polypectomy

---

Henry Thompson Lynch, 1928–2019, physician and geneticist, Omaha, NE, USA, first presented his findings of a family with a strong history of colorectal cancer without polyposis in 1964.

Worldwide, the prevalence of colorectal cancer is closely associated with intake of red meat and particularly processed meat products (haem and *N*-nitroso compounds). A protective effect of dietary fibre is also suggested by epidemiological studies. A long-held hypothesis is that increased roughage is associated with reduced colonic transit times that in turn reduce exposure of the mucosa to dietary carcinogens. However, there is increasing evidence associating the colonic microbiota with inflammation, gene methylation and dysplastic changes. Increased risks for colorectal cancer have also been associated with smoking and alcohol. Conversely, high magnesium and calcium intake may be protective. A protective potential for antioxidants such as vitamin E and selenium is as yet unproven.

The epidemiological evidence supporting prostaglandin inhibitors, particularly aspirin, in preventing colorectal cancer is substantial. Given the potential hazards of taking long-term aspirin, the challenge is to identify individuals for whom the protective benefits outweigh the harm. Other factors that increase the risk of developing colorectal cancer include inflammatory bowel disease (IBD) (see ***Chapter 75***). Cholecystectomy may marginally increase the risk of right-sided colon cancer.

Pathology

Macroscopically, the tumour may take one of several forms: annular cancers tend to give rise to obstructive symptoms whereas ulcerating cancers tend to present with bleeding. Most large bowel cancers (***Figure 77.4***) arise from the left colon, notably the rectum (38%), sigmoid (21%) and descending colon (4%). Cancer of the caecum (12%) and ascending colon (5%) is less common but may be gradually increasing in incidence. Cancer of the transverse colon (5.5%), flexures (2–3%) and appendix (0.5%) are relatively uncommon. Microscopically, the neoplasm is a columnar cell adenocarcinoma.

Spread

Colonic cancer can spread locally, via the lymphatics, bloodstream (haematogenous) or across the peritoneal cavity (transcoelomic spread). Direct spread may be longitudinal or radial. Radial spread may be retroperitoneal into the ureter, duodenum and posterior abdominal wall muscles or intraperitoneal into adjacent organs or the anterior abdominal wall.

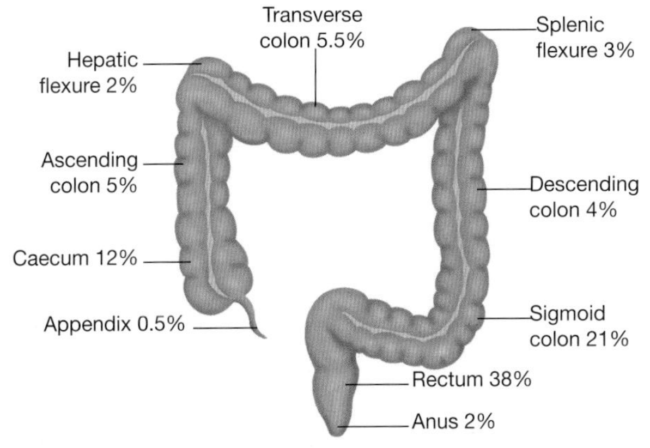

Figure 77.4 Distribution of colorectal cancer by site.

In general, involvement of the lymph nodes by tumour progresses from those closest to the bowel along the course of lymphatics to central nodes. However, this orderly process does not always occur. Haematogenous spread is most commonly to the liver via the portal vein. One-third of patients will have liver metastases at the time of diagnosis and 50% will develop metastases at some point, accounting for the majority of deaths. The lung is the next most common site of metastatic disease whereas spread to the ovaries, brain, kidney and bone is less common. Colorectal cancer can spread from the serosa of the bowel or via subperitoneal lymphatics to other structures within the peritoneal cavity, including peritoneum, ovary and omentum.

Staging colon cancer

Preoperative staging is important to decide whether patients can be managed with curative intent and whether they should have neoadjuvant therapy, undergo palliative interventions including colonic stenting or have symptomatic treatment. Additional interventions include ureteric stenting, en bloc resection for locally advanced disease, intraoperative chemotherapy (hyperthermic intraperitoneal chemotherapy [HIPEC]) for peritoneal disease or synchronous organ resection (e.g. liver, ovaries [Krukenberg tumour]). Information is collated, including patient characteristics (age, frailty, symptoms and comorbidities), endoscopic assessment, histological analysis of biopsies and imaging studies. These factors should be discussed in a dedicated preoperative multidisciplinary meeting. Postoperative pathological staging should also be discussed in the same forum, allowing for decisions about adjuvant therapy.

A variety of staging systems are described for colorectal cancer. Dukes' classification was originally described for rectal tumours but has been adopted for histopathological reporting of colon cancer. Although it is simple and widely recognised (***Summary box 77.5***) the more detailed TNM system is regarded as the international standard (***Summary box 77.6***).

Summary box 77.5

Dukes' staging for colorectal cancer

- A: Invasion of but not breaching the muscularis propria
- B: Breaching the muscularis propria but not involving lymph nodes
- C: Lymph nodes involved

Dukes himself never described a stage D, but this is often used to describe metastatic disease

Friedrich Ernst Krukenberg, 1871–1946, Professor of Gynaecology, Bonn, Germany
Cuthbert Esquire Dukes, 1890–1977, pathologist, St Mark's Hospital, London, UK. The original Dukes' classification in 1932 gave three stages, A–C.

Summary box 77.6

TNM classification for colonic cancer

(note the prefix y refers to neoadjuvant radio- or chemotherapy, p refers to pathological confirmation of stage; Union for International Cancer Control, 8th edn)

- T Tumour stage
  - T1 Tumour invades into submucosa
  - T2 Tumour invades into muscularis propria
  - T3 Tumour invades into non-peritonealised pericolic tissues or subserosa
  - T4a Tumour breaches visceral peritoneum
  - T4b Tumour directly invades another organ/structure
- N Nodal stage
  - N0 No nodes involved
  - N1 1–3 nodes involved (N1a, 1 regional lymph node involved; N1b, 2 or 3 regional lymph nodes involved; N1c, satellite extranodal tumour deposits)
  - N2 4 or more nodes involved (N2a, 4–6 regional lymph nodes involved; N2b, 7 or more regional lymph nodes involved)
- M Metastases
  - M0 No metastases
  - M1 Metastases (M1a, metastasis confined to 1 organ; M1b, metastasis to more than 1 organ; M1c, metastasis to the peritoneum)

Clinical features

Carcinoma of the colon typically occurs in patients over 50 years of age and is most common in the eighth decade of life. Emergency presentation occurs in 20% of cases and is associated with a considerably worse prognosis, even when matched for disease stage. A careful family history should be taken. A first-degree relative who has developed colorectal cancer before the age of 50 years may indicate one of the colorectal cancer familial syndromes. Tumours of the left side of the colon usually present with a change in bowel habit or rectal bleeding, while proximal lesions typically present with iron deficiency anaemia or a mass (*Figure 77.5*). Patients may present with metastatic disease.

Investigation of colon cancer

Screening

Colon cancer is suited to screening as the prognosis is better the earlier stage the disease is diagnosed and polypectomy allows the prevention of cancer development. In the UK screening is offered every 2 years to men and women aged 60–74 years, followed by colonoscopy in those who test positive. Originally a guaiac-based test was used, which detects peroxidase-like activity of faecal haematin. Studies suggested a 15–20% reduction in colorectal cancer-specific mortality in the screened population. More recently the faecal immunochemical test (FIT) has been introduced. This test is more accurate and easier to complete than the old faecal occult blood test. A one-off flexible sigmoidoscopy for people aged 55 was offered as a screening tool in the UK. It was shown to reduce colorectal cancer-specific mortality but is now being replaced with FIT screening.

Endoscopy

For symptomatic patients with rectal bleeding, direct referral from primary care for a flexible sigmoidoscopy is increasingly used. The patient is prepared with an enema and sedation is not usually necessary. The bowel can be assessed as far as the splenic flexure, allowing detection of up to 70% of cancers and almost all that cause fresh rectal bleeding. Finding left-sided colonic polyps or cancer mandates subsequent completion colonoscopy.

Colonoscopy is the investigation of choice if colorectal cancer is suspected (*Figure 77.5*). It has the advantage of not only securing histological diagnosis of a primary cancer but also detecting synchronous polyps or carcinomas, which occur in 3–5% of cases. There is a small risk of perforation (1:1000).

Radiology

Double-contrast barium enema has now been largely replaced by computed tomography (CT) colonography, which is extremely sensitive in picking up polyps to a size of 6 mm (*Figure 77.6*). It has the advantage of being less invasive than colonoscopy but, if a biopsy is required, an endoscopy will still be needed. CT is used as a diagnostic tool in patients with a palpable abdominal mass. CT of the thorax, abdomen and pelvis now represents the standard means of staging colorectal cancer; patients with rectal cancer require magnetic resonance imaging (MRI) for local staging (see *Chapter 79*).

Surgical treatment

Preoperative preparation

With the advent of perioperative enhanced recovery after surgery (ERAS) protocols, mechanical bowel preparation fell out of favour. However, there is evidence that preoperative mechanical bowel preparation in combination with preoperative oral antibiotics not only reduces surgical site infection rates but also rates of anastomotic leak, postoperative ileus, reoperation and even mortality. Further research is required

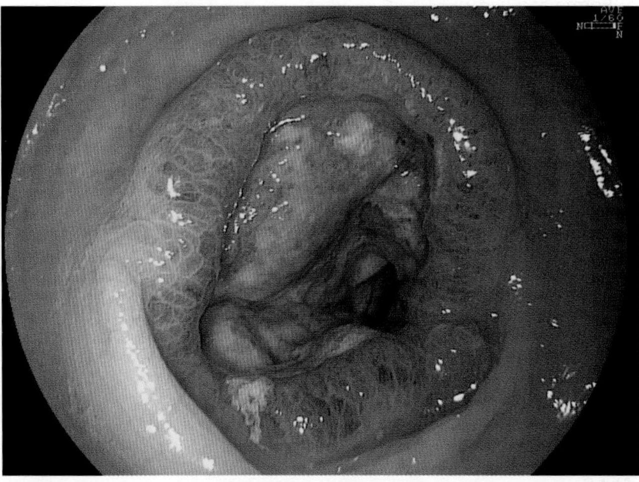

Figure 77.5 Colon cancer seen at colonoscopy (courtesy of Dr Adolfo Parra-Blanco, Nottingham University Hospitals, Nottingham, UK).

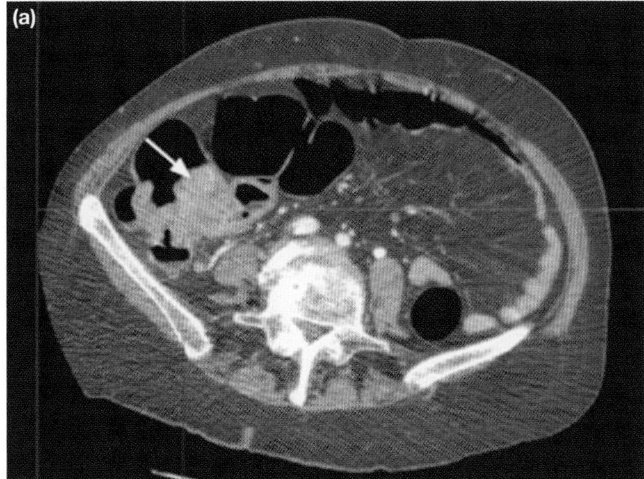

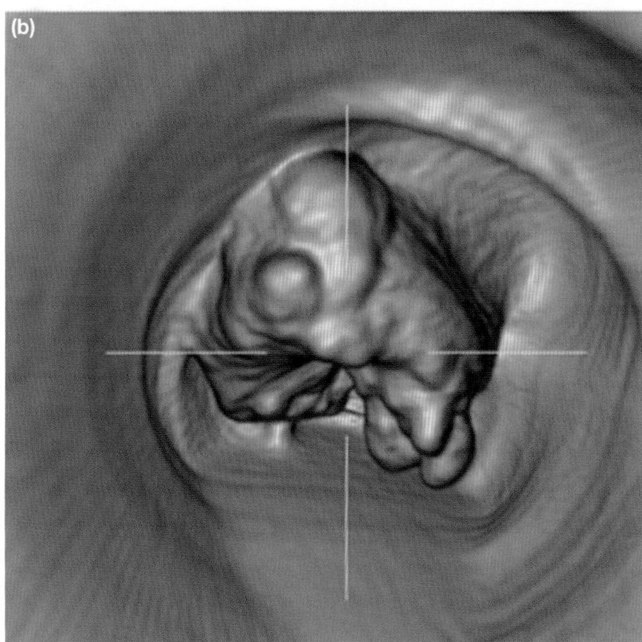

Figure 77.6 Virtual colonoscopy of the right colon. (a) Computed tomography scan of the abdomen showing a caecal tumour (arrow). (b) Formatted 'virtual' image of the same lesion as in (a) (courtesy of Dr A Slater, John Radcliffe Hospital, Oxford, UK).

but mechanical bowel preparation with oral antibiotics appears safe and could reasonably be used in combination with a surgical site infection bundle. This bundle should contain common and variable components such as preoperative bathing, intravenous prophylactic antibiotics given before surgical incision, maintenance of normoglycaemia and normothermia and use of wound protection devices. Antithrombotic stockings should be fitted, and the patient started on prophylactic subcutaneous low-molecular-weight heparin. Manual compression boots may be used perioperatively. In all cases where a stoma is anticipated, careful preoperative counselling and marking of an appropriate site by an enterostomal therapist is essential. ERAS programmes are widely used to reduce the physiological insult of surgery and improve postoperative outcomes (*Summary box 77.7*).

Summary box 77.7

Key elements of an ERAS programme

- Preadmission counselling
- Preoperative carbohydrate loading
- Avoidance of preoperative dehydration
- Avoidance of nasogastric tubes
- Short, transverse incisions (or laparoscopic procedure)
- Short-acting anaesthetic drugs
- Avoidance of perioperative fluid/salt overload
- Avoidance of opiate analgesia
- Maintenance of perioperative temperature
- Prevention of postoperative nausea and vomiting
- Early mobilisation
- Early introduction of oral fluids/diets/supplements
- Early removal of urinary catheters
- Continual audit of outcomes

Operations

The operations described are designed to remove the primary tumour and its draining locoregional lymph nodes. It is unusual to find unsuspected metastases at laparotomy (or laparoscopy) after CT staging, but the presence of peritoneal metastases may predicate a palliative strategy with a segmental resection and less aggressive lymphadenectomy. Similarly, a complete preoperative colonoscopy or CT colonography will have excluded synchronous bowel lesions. The use of stapling and hand-suturing techniques for colonic anastomoses have been compared, and there is probably little difference in leak rate. It is more important that healthy bowel, free of tension or distal obstruction, is used to construct an anastomosis and that patients are adequately nourished and free from active infection if anastomotic leakage is to be avoided.

Right hemicolectomy Carcinoma of the caecum or ascending colon (*Figure 77.7*) is treated by right hemicolectomy (*Figure 77.8*). At open surgery the peritoneum lateral to the ascending colon is incised, and the incision is continued

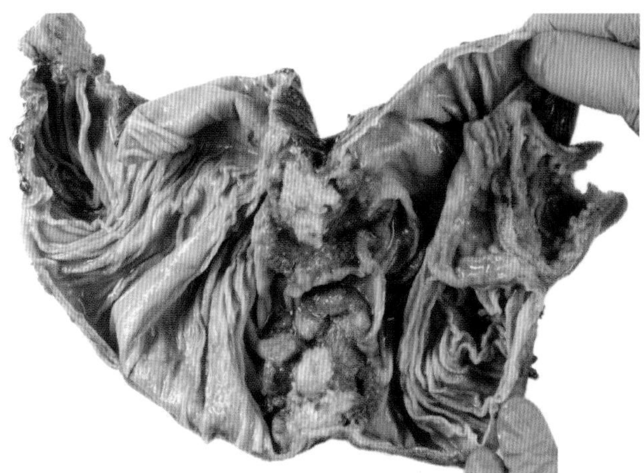

Figure 77.7 Right hemicolectomy specimen showing an ascending colon cancer (courtesy of Dr Philip Kaye, Nottingham University Hospitals, Nottingham, UK).

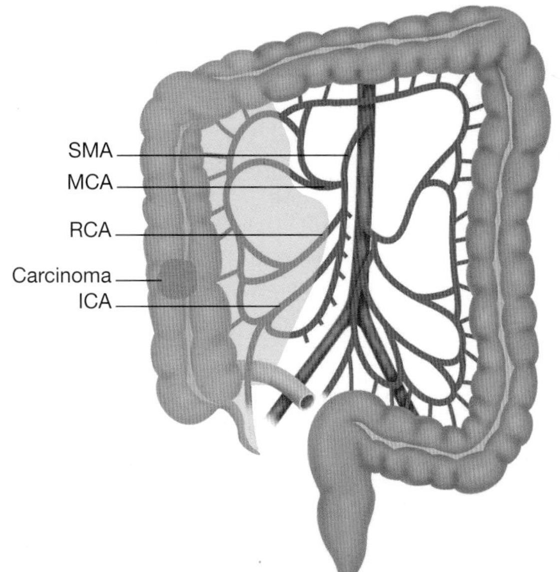

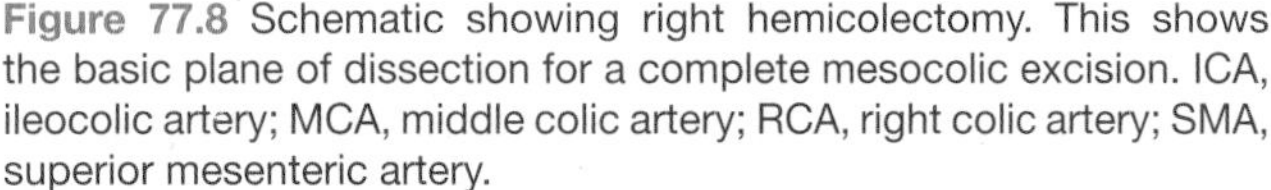
Figure 77.8 Schematic showing right hemicolectomy. This shows the basic plane of dissection for a complete mesocolic excision. ICA, ileocolic artery; MCA, middle colic artery; RCA, right colic artery; SMA, superior mesenteric artery.

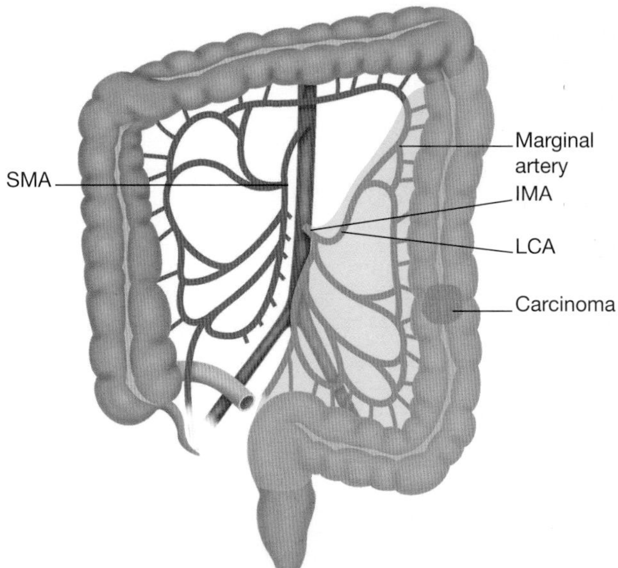

Figure 77.9 Schematic showing left hemicolectomy. This shows the basic plane of dissection for a complete mesocolic excision. IMA, inferior mesenteric artery; LCA, left colic artery; SMA, superior mesenteric artery.

around the hepatic flexure. The right colon and mesentery are elevated, taking care not to injure the ureter, gonadal vessels or the duodenum. The ileocolic artery is ligated close to its origin from the superior mesenteric artery ('high-tie') and divided. Complete mesocolic excision with dissection along embryological planes (see ***Chapter 65***) and removal of the lymphovascular supply of the resected colon with flush ligation of the ileocolic and right colic vessels at their origin from the superior mesenteric artery may improve survival in node-positive disease (Hohenburger). The mesentery of the distal 10 cm of the ileum and the mesocolon as far as the proximal third of the transverse colon is divided. The greater omentum is divided up to the point of intended division of the transverse colon. When it is clear that there is an adequate blood supply at the resection margins, the right colon is resected and an anastomosis is fashioned between the ileum and the transverse colon. If the tumour is at the hepatic flexure the resection must be extended further along the transverse colon and will involve dividing the right branch of the middle colic artery.

Extended right hemicolectomy Carcinomas of the transverse colon and splenic flexure are most commonly treated by an extended right hemicolectomy. The mobilisation is as for a right hemicolectomy but dissection continues to include the tumour, this may include taking down the splenic flexure and excising the whole transverse mesocolon. Some surgeons prefer to perform a left hemicolectomy for a splenic flexure cancer.

Left hemicolectomy This is the operation of choice for descending colon and sigmoid cancers (***Figure 77.9***). The left half of the colon is mobilised completely along the 'white line' that marks the lateral attachment of the mesocolon (see ***Chapter 65***). As the sigmoid mesentery is mobilised, the left ureter and gonadal vessels must be identified and protected. The splenic flexure may be mobilised by extending the lateral dissection from below and completed by entering the lesser sac. The inferior mesenteric artery below its left colic branch, together with the related paracolic lymph nodes, is included in the resection by ligating the inferior mesenteric artery close to its origin ('high-tie'). For full mobility the inferior mesenteric vein is also ligated and divided at the lower border of the pancreas. The bowel and mesentery can then be resected to allow a tension-free anastomosis. A temporary diverting stoma may be fashioned proximally, usually by formation of a loop ileostomy. This is usually undertaken if the anastomosis is below the peritoneal reflection of the rectum, because of the greater risk of anastomotic leakage.

Laparoscopic surgery

Laparoscopic surgery for colon cancer has been shown to have equivalent overall and cancer-related outcomes to open surgery. Lymph node harvests are equivalent to open surgery and initial concerns about reports of port-site recurrence have been dispelled as world experience has grown. In the UK, the National Institute for Health and Care Excellence (NICE) has stated that laparoscopic colorectal surgery should be offered to suitable patients. Operation times are longer but wound infection rates, blood loss and postoperative pain scores are lower than for open surgery. The costs of laparoscopic surgery are, however, generally higher and this may be particularly relevant where funds are limited.

Werner Hohenburger, contemporary, surgeon, Erlangen, Germany.

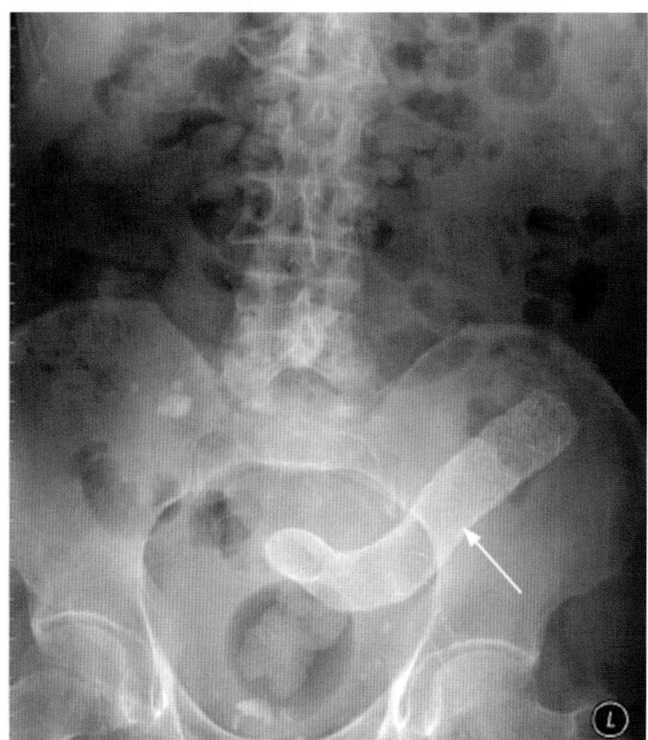

Figure 77.10 Abdominal radiograph demonstrating a colonic stent in position (arrow) (courtesy of Dr D Kasir, Hope Hospital, Salford, UK).

If laparoscopic surgery is planned it is useful to tattoo the lesion at prior colonoscopy as it not possible to locate lesions by palpation. The laparoscopic operation has particular advantages if performed in a medial to lateral manner, i.e. starting the dissection by controlling and dividing the major vascular pedicles and only taking the lateral peritoneal reflection once the mesocolon is completely free. Specimen retrieval and bowel anastomosis can then be performed via a small incision. Dedicated training in laparoscopic colorectal surgery is important as there is a relatively long learning curve.

Emergency surgery

In the UK, 20% of patients with colonic cancer will present as an emergency, the majority with obstruction, but occasionally with haemorrhage or perforation. If the lesion is right sided, it is usually possible to perform a right hemicolectomy and anastomosis in the usual manner. If there has been perforation with substantial contamination or if the patient is unstable, it may be advisable to bring out an ileocolostomy following resection of the lesion rather than forming an anastomosis. For a left-sided lesion the decision lies between a Hartmann's procedure and a resection and anastomosis. An on-table washout may be necessary to remove residual faecal content in the proximally obstructed bowel. Alternatively, removal of the whole proximal bowel may be required if the colon is markedly distended or if there is concern regarding its viability. Where endoscopic and radiological facilities are present an obstructing left-sided lesion can often be treated initially with an expanding metal stent (***Figure 77.10***). This allows decompression of the obstructed bowel and may allow conversion of an emergency operation with a high chance of a stoma to a situation that can be managed semielectively by resection and anastomosis. Although early studies cast doubt on the benefits of colorectal stenting, more recently evidence has emerged that stenting leads to a reduction in stoma rates.

Postoperative care

Patients should be closely monitored after colonic resection as there is a small incidence of postoperative bleeding. Antithrombosis measures should be continued and as currently recommended for 28 days postoperatively. There is no advantage to placing intra-abdominal drains after colonic surgery. Wound infections are relatively common after colonic surgery and may well be more frequent than the 10% usually quoted. Anastomotic leaks occur in 4–8% of ileocolic or colocolic anastomoses. The possibility should be borne in mind in any patient not progressing as expected or with unexplained cardiac abnormalities, fever or worsening abdominal pain. Early investigation with contrast-enhanced CT scan is appropriate. In the presence of sepsis or peritonitis, early return to theatre and taking down the leaking anastomosis with the formation of stomas is usually advised.

Prolonged nasogastric drainage, intravenous fluid therapy and cautious introduction of oral fluid and diet represented traditional postoperative practice. ERAS programmes that include preoperative, intraoperative and postoperative components have been shown to reduce length of hospital stay from 10–14 days to as little as 3–5 days by modulating the surgical stress response and reducing postoperative ileus (***Summary box 77.7***). It is important to appreciate that these programmes require multiple interventions and considerable time, effort and education from the surgical, anaesthetic and ward teams.

Adjuvant therapy

In most patients with colon cancer preoperative chemotherapy is not required; however, a recent research study (FOxTROT) has shown that it is safe and further work on case selection has been recommended. Adjuvant chemotherapy improves survival after surgery in patients with node-positive colon cancer (stage III/Dukes' C). Fluoropyrimidine regimes are often used, with the addition of oxaliplatin in patients who are otherwise fit and have high-risk stage III disease. Patients with stage II disease show less benefit in overall survival with adjuvant chemotherapy, thus it is reserved for those with high-risk stage II disease. Presence of MSI (in the tumour histology) also affects tumour recurrence and is taken into account when making decisions with patients about chemotherapy (see ***Chapter 12***).

Metastatic disease

Hepatic and pulmonary metastases can be resected and series have demonstrated 5-year survival of around 40% in resectable disease. CT, MRI and positron emission tomography (PET) scanning are all used to identify colorectal metastases and assess patients' suitability for further resection (***Figure 77.11***).

Henri Albert Antoine Hartmann, 1860–1952, Professor of Clinical Surgery in the Faculty of Medicine, University of Paris, Paris, France.

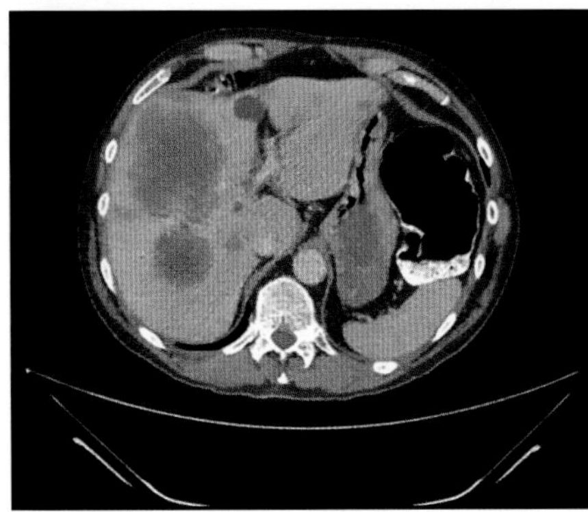

Figure 77.11 Computed tomography scan of the liver showing multiple metastases from carcinoma of the colon (courtesy of Dr Rajpal Dhingsa, Nottingham University Hospitals, Nottingham, UK).

The role of chemotherapy and the timing of colonic and hepatic surgery in synchronous metastases is still a matter of debate and such cases should be carefully discussed by a multidisciplinary team. Many centres offer adjuvant chemotherapy as standard and neoadjuvant therapy also in those with high-risk disease.

Isolated lung metastases may be suitable for resection or stereotactic radiofrequency ablation, but they are more commonly accompanied by metastases elsewhere. In patients with widespread disease, palliative chemotherapy is offered alongside symptomatic treatment and support by a palliative care team.

Prognosis

Overall 5-year survival for colorectal cancer is approximately 58%. While there are numerous factors that may predict prognosis (*Summary box 77.8*) the most important determinant is tumour stage and, in particular, lymph node status. Patients with disease confined to the bowel wall (TNM stage 1, Dukes' stage A) will usually have cure by surgical resection alone and around 95% will have disease-free survival at 5 years. Spread beyond the bowel wall (TNM stage 2, Dukes' B) reduces 5-year disease-free survival to approximately 85% with surgery alone. Patients with lymph node metastases (TNM stage 3, Dukes' C) have a 5-year disease-free survival of around 45–50% with surgery alone.

Adjuvant chemotherapy based on 5-fluorouracil (5-FU) and folinic acid (leucovorin) usually in combination with oxaliplatin (FolFox) is used on an individual basis for those with stage II disease (Dukes' stage B), although the benefit is uncertain. In those with stage III disease adjuvant chemotherapy increases the chance of 5-year disease-free survival by approximately 20% to 67–70%. Those presenting with unresectable metastatic disease at diagnosis have a 5-year survival of approximately 10%.

In metastatic disease chemotherapy based on 5-FU and folinic acid in combination with irinotecan (FolFiri) is often used as first-line treatment. Second-line therapy may include introduction of a monoclonal antibody such as a vascular endothelial growth factor (VEGF) inhibitor (bevacizumab) or an epidermal growth factor receptor (EGFR) inhibitor in *KRAS* wild-type tumours (cetuximab, panitumumab). Recently immunotherapy (pembrolizumab) has been shown to have a role in MSI tumours. Tumours exhibiting the *BRAF* V660E mutation (approximately 10%) have a poor prognosis but may respond to treatment with combined BRAF (encorafenib) and MAP kinase (binimetinib) inhibitors.

Summary box 77.8

Histopathological factors that influence prognosis

- Tumour stage
- Histological grade
- Degree of mucin secretin
- Presence of signet cells
- Venous invasion
- Perineural invasion
- Pushing versus infiltrative margin
- Tumour infiltrating lymphocytes
- Presence of MSI

Colorectal cancer follow-up

Since the advent of safe liver resection for metastases the outcome benefit of follow-up has been clearly demonstrated. Follow-up aims to identify synchronous bowel tumours (present in 3%) that were not identified at the time of original diagnosis. Similarly, 3% of patients will develop a metachronous (at a different time) colonic cancer. Up to a half of all patients with colorectal cancer will develop liver metastases at some point. Regular imaging of the liver (CT scan) and measurement of carcinoembryonic antigen (CEA) is designed to diagnose this early, in order to allow curative metastectomy. Optimum follow-up pathways continue to be developed. NICE guidelines recommend CT scans of the abdomen, pelvis and thorax as well as CEA measurements during the first 3 years after treatment of colon cancer with curative intent but identified no clinically important difference in colorectal cancer-specific survival with a more intensive follow-up schedule compared with a less intensive follow-up.

Palliative care

About 20% of patients present with metastatic disease and about one-fifth of these patients are suitable for potentially curative management. For the rest, quality of residual life is the main outcome but it should be borne in mind that with the combination of interventions including chemotherapy, metastectomy, cytoreductive surgery and intraperitoneal chemotherapy some colonic disease may 'convert to resectable'. For those whose disease remains incurable colonic surgery may still be offered, particularly if symptomatic. This may be non-resectional (defunctioning stoma or internal bypass) or resectional (procedures detailed earlier but with a smaller segmental resection and less aggressive lymphadenectomy). Non-surgical techniques include palliative chemotherapy, stenting for obstruction, intraluminal laser, argon plasma coagulation and radiotherapy for bleeding and pain (especially in rectal cancers).

Malignant: miscellaneous cancers

Gastrointestinal stromal tumours

Gastrointestinal stromal tumours (GISTs) are extremely rare, constituting less than 0.1% of all colorectal tumours. They appear to arise from the interstitial cells of Cajal and are mainly due to a mutation in a specific gene called *c-kit*. This allows a specific marker to be used to diagnose most tumours as well as targeted chemotherapy with imatinib. Thirty per cent are malignant with mitotic rate, Ki-67 (>10%), size (>5 cm), local invasion and cellularity the best indicators of malignant potential. Diagnosis is by CT or MRI and endoscopic biopsy. Surgical resection is the mainstay of treatment with imatinib for those tumours that are unresectable, have metastasised or recurred. Adjuvant imatinib may be used for tumours felt to be at high risk of recurrence.

Carcinoid

'Carcinoids' are well-differentiated neuroendocrine tumours of the colon and are part of a spectrum of disease with poorly differentiated neuroendocrine carcinomas at the most aggressive end of this spectrum.

They constitute around 50% of all neuroendocrine tumours of the gut and about 5% of all colonic tumours. Fewer than 10% of colonic carcinoid tumours present with carcinoid syndrome (skin erythema, diarrhoea, cardiorespiratory symptoms) owing to release of hormones. Surgery remains the only potentially curative treatment and, since the possibility of metastatic disease is directly related to the size of the primary tumour, the extent of resection should be determined accordingly. Tumours greater than 2 cm require en bloc resection of adjacent mesenteric lymph nodes. In the midgut (the area receiving its blood supply from the superior mesenteric artery) even lesions less than 1 cm have been shown to metastasise and radical resection is also indicated. Small (<1 cm) hindgut tumours (the area receiving its blood supply from the inferior mesenteric artery) can be safely locally excised (see ***Chapters 74 and 76***).

Lymphoma

Primary lymphoma of the colon is rare, accounting for less than 1% of all colonic malignancies. The caecum is the most common site of occurrence, usually with non-Hodgkin's type lymphoma (NHL). Patients present with abdominal pain, a mass, change in bowel habit, per rectal bleeding, obstruction or intussusception. These tumours may occasionally perforate. The lack of specific complaints and rarity of intestinal obstruction probably accounts for the often delayed diagnosis. CT and colonoscopy with submucosal biopsy are required for diagnosis. Treatment is combination surgery with systemic chemotherapy, although surgery alone may be considered adequate treatment for low-grade NHL disease that does not infiltrate beyond the submucosa.

Metastatic disease to colon

Metastatic disease to the colon from other primary sites constitutes about 1% of all colorectal cancers. There is often a known primary, usually lung, ovary, breast, kidney, skin, stomach or hepatobiliary system tumours. In most cases multiple lesions are seen and one-third may be asymptomatic. The most common pathway of spread is through peritoneal seeding (typical of ovarian cancer), although haematological and lymphatic dissemination is described in breast and lung cancer and melanoma. Patients may present with obstruction, per rectal bleeding (especially melanoma), anaemia and weight loss. CT and colonoscopic biopsy are required for diagnosis and treatment should be individualised to patient symptoms and prognosis.

COLITIS

There are two types of colitides: IBD (discussed in ***Chapter 75***) and non-IBD. The non-IBD causes can be grouped into infective and non-infective causes, with infective being by far the most common. The majority of non-IBD colitides present acutely with severity ranging from a self-limiting illness to severe disease necessitating emergency colectomy.

A careful history of acute onset and potential predisposing factors, including the use of antibiotics, is often key. Investigations include stool culture, serology and inflammatory markers. Supine abdominal radiographs may demonstrate bowel oedema, colonic distension or, in severe cases, gas in the bowel wall. CT may determine the extent of disease, presence of alternative pathology or resultant complications. In a deteriorating patient awaiting cultures, endoscopic biopsies may also be helpful.

Infective colitides

Infective causes may be classified as bacterial, protozoal, viral and fungal. Common infections include the following.

Escherichia coli

E. coli is a Gram-negative bacillus transmitted via the faeco-oral route from contaminated food or water. Symptoms vary according to strain, with the most common form – enterotoxigenic *E. coli* – causing 'traveller's' diarrhoea (diarrhoea, vomiting and colicky pain). In adults, infection is usually brief and self-limiting. A more severe form – enteroinvasive *E. coli* – causes a more systemic illness and haematochezia. A very severe form – enterohaemorrhagic *E. coli* – results in colonic oedema, ulceration and haemorrhage with the very ill requiring colectomy.

Campylobacter

Infection with *Campylobacter jejuni* (a Gram-negative rod with a distinctive spiral shape) is the most common form of gastroenteritis in resource-rich countries, typically acquired from eating infected poultry. It causes diarrhoea and abdominal pain. Severe cases may resemble ulcerative colitis. The organism

Santiago Ramon y Cajal, 1852–1934, Spanish neuroscientist, pathologist and Nobel prize winner (1906) for studies of cellular anatomy of the nervous system.
Thomas Hodgkin, 1798–1866, pathologist, Guy's Hospital, London, UK, described 'Morbid appearances of the absorbent glands and spleen' in 1832.

may take several days to isolate on stool culture. Treatment is supportive as it usually resolves without antibiotics, but severe colitis and even perforation may occur.

Salmonellosis, typhoid and paratyphoid

Salmonella are a family of Gram-negative rods that can cause a range of enteric infections. Salmonella gastroenteritis is typically caused by *Salmonella enteritidis* from poultry and is most often a self-limiting illness comprising headache, fever and watery diarrhoea. When severe, antibiotics, hospitalisation and intravenous fluids may be needed. The diagnosis is based on stool culture. *Shigella* and enteropathogenic strains of *E. coli* may cause similar diarrhoeal illnesses.

Typhoid fever is caused by *Salmonella enterica* Typhi and paratyphoid fever by *Salmonella enterica* Paratyphi A, B or C. The clinical differences between these infections are subtle. They present with fever and abdominal pain after a 10- to 20-day incubation period. Over the next week, the patient can develop distension, diarrhoea, splenomegaly and characteristic 'rose spots' on the abdomen caused by a vasculitis. A number of surgical complications can result:

- paralytic ileus;
- intestinal haemorrhage;
- perforation;
- cholecystitis.

In addition, invasion of the systemic circulation, which is a characteristic feature of salmonellosis, can cause severe Gram-negative sepsis and septic shock may develop. Occasionally patients develop metastatic sepsis, including septic arthritis, osteomyelitis, meningitis, encephalitis and pancreatitis.

Yersinia

Yersinia, Gram-negative coccobacilli, infection results from ingestion of contaminated food, typically meat, water and dairy products. Invasion typically occurs in the ileocaecal region and may mimic Crohn's disease. Treatment is usually supportive with antibiotics reserved for severe infection or in the immunocompromised.

Shigella (bacillary dysentery)

Dysentery results from the ingestion of contaminated food or water, with only a small dose of infective agent required. The Gram-negative bacilli invade the colonic epithelium, causing cell death, ulceration and necrosis. Exotoxins cause a brief period of watery diarrhoea before the onset of classical severe, bloody diarrhoea.

Clostridium difficile

Clostridium difficile is a toxin-producing Gram-positive bacillus that is of increasing concern in many hospitals. Although normally present in around 2% of the population, it proliferates after antibiotic treatment (especially with cephalosporins). Clinically, *C. difficile* infection presents with diarrhoea, abdominal pain and fever. Infection may progress to pseudomembranous colitis, so called because on endoscopic visualisation of the bowel plaques of inflammatory exudate between oedematous mucosa are seen. Diagnosis is usually made by detection of the toxin in stool samples, rather than by culture. Treatment is by metronidazole or vancomycin alongside supportive care. In refractory cases, faecal transplantation to restore a healthy microbiota may be tried. If toxic dilatation occurs, an emergency subtotal colectomy and ileostomy may be necessary.

Recently more virulent strains have stressed the importance of prevention. Suspicion of the disease should prompt source isolation, protective equipment for health staff, vigorous disinfection and scrupulous hand washing.

Intestinal amoebiasis

Entamoeba histolytica has a worldwide distribution and is transmitted mainly in contaminated drinking water. It can cause colonic ulcers, described as 'bottlenecked' because they have considerably undermined edges. The ulcers typically also have a yellow necrotic floor, from which blood and pus exude. In the majority they are confined to the distal sigmoid colon and the rectum. Clinically amoebiasis can mimic ulcerative colitis, most commonly causing bloody diarrhoea. Severe colonic complications can occur, including haemorrhage, stricture formation or perforation. A pericolitis is not uncommon and results in adhesions that may cause intestinal obstruction. Amoebiasis may cause liver abscesses or an amoebic mass ('amoeboma') of the caecum or sigmoid, which is difficult to distinguish from a carcinoma. Surgery is fraught with danger as the bowel is extremely friable.

Endoscopic biopsies or fresh stools are examined to look for the presence of amoebae (***Figure 77.12***). It is important to emphasise, however, that the presence of the parasite does not indicate that it is pathogenic. It is especially important to exclude amoebic infection in patients suspected of having ulcerative colitis. Treatment is by metronidazole in the acute phase. Diloxanide furoate is effective against chronic infections associated with the passage of cysts in stools.

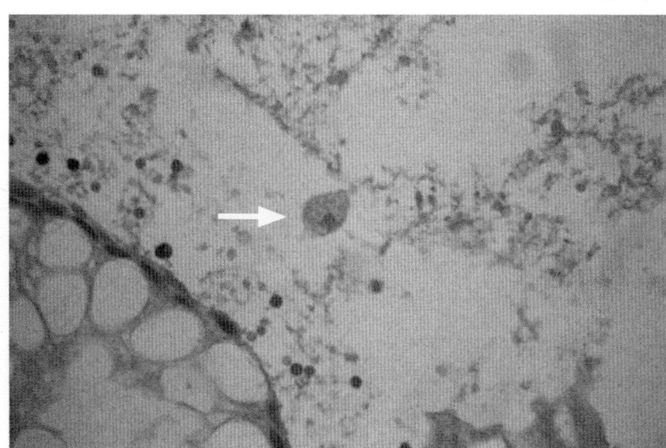

Figure 77.12 An amoeba in a rectal biopsy (arrow).

Burrill Bernard Crohn, 1884–1983, gastroenterologist, Mount Sinai Hospital, New York, NY, USA, described regional ileitis in 1932 along with Leon Ginzburg and Gordon Oppenheimer.

Cytomegalovirus

Cytomegalovirus (CMV) is present asymptomatically in 40–100% of adults. It usually remains latent within the host but can reactivate in immunocompromised patients. Commonly affected are those with acquired immunodeficiency syndrome (AIDS) (where it is the most common indication for colectomy) and patients on immunosuppressive therapy for IBD. Symptoms include profuse bloody diarrhoea and colicky pain. Severe disease may lead to perforation. Treatment is with ganciclovir with surgery necessary for severe disease or complications.

Human immunodeficiency virus

Intestinal complications are common after the development of AIDS when opportunistic organisms can cause gastroenteritis (***Summary box 77.9***). Human immunodeficiency virus 1 (HIV1) may also cause a specific enteropathy. Treatment is directed towards the responsible organism and surgery should be avoided.

Summary box 77.9

Opportunistic intestinal infections in patients with AIDS

- Bacteria
  - *Salmonella*
  - *Shigella*
  - *Yersinia*
  - *Campylobacter*
  - *Mycobacterium avium–intracellulare* (MAI)
- Viral
  - *Cytomegalovirus*
- Protozoa
  - *Cryptosporidium*
  - *Giardia*
- Fungal
  - *Candida albicans*

Non-infective colitides

Diverticular colitis

Diverticular colitis is a clinicopathological entity distinct from acute diverticulitis (see ***Diverticular disease***). The term refers to colonic mucosal inflammation, resembling IBD, in a segment of colon affected by diverticula. Symptoms of diarrhoea, pain and bleeding may occur, and the histology overlaps with that of IBD. It is usually self-limiting, with a short clinical course and low rate of recurrence. It is important to differentiate diverticular colitis from IBD to avoid further unnecessary tests and treatment. Localisation near to diverticula, a previous history of diverticulitis and rectal sparing should raise suspicion.

Diversion colitis

Diversion colitis is an iatrogenic process that occurs when a colon/rectum is defunctioned with a proximal stoma. Although the majority of patients with defunctioned bowel will develop typical changes of diffuse inflammation with friable mucosa and spontaneous bleeding, less than 50% will develop symptoms of lower abdominal pain, blood and mucus per rectum. The aetiology is likely to be multifactorial with alteration of the bacterial flora and a reduction in the bioavailability of short chain fatty acids (the predominant metabolic substrate of colonic mucosa). Diagnosis is by endoscopy and treatment includes reassurance and, if feasible, restoration of the bowel continuity.

Microscopic colitis

See ***Chapter 75***.

Radiation colitis

Radiation colitis refers to the characteristic acute and chronic morphological changes that occur following radiation treatment. Although most commonly occurring in the rectum (proctitis) these changes can affect the colon if any portion falls within the radiation field. Acute inflammatory changes manifest a few days to 6 weeks after treatment, whereas chronic colonic changes leading to fibrosis and stenosis occur up to years later. Obstructive symptoms require appropriate radiological and possibly endoscopic assessment and may lead to resectional surgery. After resection care must be taken to ensure healthy non-irradiated bowel is used for any anastomosis. As the rectum is the most commonly affected part of the large bowel, further details are given in ***Chapter 79***.

Graft-versus-host disease colitis

Graft-versus-host disease colitis (GVHD) is a common complication occurring about 3–6 weeks after haematopoietic stem cell transplantation and is the result of severe immune-mediated toxicity against host cells. The patient develops diarrhoea and vomiting with colicky abdominal pain. Inflammation is evident on endoscopy. Treatment is complex and difficult. Once established the prognosis is poor.

Drug-induced colitis

A wide range of medications may induce colitis (***Summary box 77.10***) and recognition is essential as cessation of the medication often leads to prompt resolution of symptoms. Patients with the *DPYD* (*dihydropyrimidine dehydrogenase*) gene mutation are particularly prone to colitis if treated with 5-FU during treatment for colon cancer. Dose reduction should be employed.

Summary box 77.10

Drugs that may result in colitis

- Non-steroidal anti-inflammatory drugs
- Proton pump inhibitors and H2 antagonists
- Cardiac drugs (digoxin, diuretics, dopamine)
- Immunosuppressants
- Antibiotics (owing to increasing the likelihood of *C. difficile* infection)
- Statins
- Chemotherapy
- Antidepressants (selective serotonin reuptake inhibitors)
- Anti-migraine drugs (ergotamine)
- Cocaine

Ischaemic colitis

Ischaemia of the colon typically results from thrombosis or embolism. Sudden embolic events leading to acutely ischaemic bowel present with severe pain out of proportion to the degree of peritonism, bloody diarrhoea, haemodynamic instability and shock. Resuscitation and laparotomy are required with resection of gangrenous bowel and exteriorisation of viable bowel ends. Mortality is extremely high.

Thrombotic occlusion usually occurs in the context of global atherosclerosis. The presentation of this ischaemic colitis tends to be less dramatic with abdominal pain, a raised white cell count and rectal bleeding. A plain abdominal radiograph may show 'thumb-printing' and endoscopy may demonstrate haemorrhagic oedema. The left colon and, in particular, the splenic flexure are usually the worst affected (the 'watershed' area of blood flow). Symptoms usually settle spontaneously. In some cases, ulceration at the splenic flexure associated with ischaemic colitis may heal with stricturing and present with subsequent large bowel obstruction.

Bowel ischemia is a well-known but uncommon complication following both open and endovascular abdominal aortic aneurysm repair due to sacrifice of the inferior mesenteric artery.

DIVERTICULAR DISEASE

Diverticula (hollow outpouchings) are a common structural abnormality of the gastrointestinal tract. They can be classified as:

- **congenital**: all three coats of the bowel are present in the wall of the diverticulum (e.g. Meckel's diverticulum).
- **acquired**: there is no muscularis layer present in the diverticulum (e.g. sigmoid diverticular disease).

Diverticula are found in the left colon in around 75% of those over 70 years of age in the Western world. The condition is overwhelmingly found in the sigmoid colon but can affect the whole colon. In South East Asia right-sided diverticular disease is more common. Diverticula are most often asymptomatic (diverticulosis) and found incidentally, but they can present clinically with sepsis or haemorrhage.

Aetiology

Epidemiological studies suggest that diverticular disease is a consequence of a refined Western diet, deficient in dietary fibre. The combination of altered collagen structure with ageing, disordered motility and increased intraluminal pressure, most notably in the narrow sigmoid colon, results in herniation of mucosa through the circular muscle at the points where blood vessels penetrate the bowel wall. The rectum has a complete muscular coat and a wider lumen and is thus very rarely affected. Diverticular disease is rare in Africa and Asia, where the diet is high in natural fibre (Burkitt).

Complications of diverticular disease

The majority of patients with diverticulosis are asymptomatic but historical studies suggest that somewhere between 10% and 30% will have symptomatic complications (***Summary box 77.11***).

Summary box 77.11

Complications of diverticular disease

- Diverticulitis
- Abscess
- Peritonitis
- Intestinal obstruction
- Haemorrhage
- Fistula formation

Clinical features

In mild cases, symptoms such as distension, flatulence and a sensation of heaviness in the lower abdomen may be indistinguishable from those of irritable bowel syndrome. These symptoms are thought to result from a combination of increased luminal pressure affecting wall tension and increased visceral hypersensitivity. Surgical treatment is rarely, if ever, appropriate for diverticular disease in the absence of complications.

Diverticulitis typically presents as persistent lower abdominal pain. There may be accompanying diarrhoea or constipation. The lower abdomen is tender, especially over the left iliac fossa, but occasionally also on the right side if the sigmoid loop lies across the midline. The sigmoid colon may be tender and thickened on palpation and rectal examination may reveal a tender mass if an abscess has formed. Distinguishing between diverticulitis and abscess formation is difficult on clinical grounds alone and radiological imaging is essential. Generalised peritonitis as a result of free perforation presents in the typical manner with systemic upset and generalised tenderness and guarding.

Classification of contamination

The degree of infection has a major impact on outcome in acute diverticulitis. Patients with inflammatory masses have a lower mortality than those with perforation (3% versus 33%). Classification systems have been developed for complicated diverticulitis to try to rationalise the literature, the most commonly used being the Hinchey classification (***Table 77.2***).

Haemorrhage from colonic diverticula is typically painless and profuse. Bleeding from the sigmoid will be bright red with

TABLE 77.2 Hinchey classification of complicated diverticulitis.

Grade I	Mesenteric or pericolic abscess
Grade II	Pelvic abscess
Grade III	Purulent peritonitis
Grade IV	Faecal peritonitis

Johann Friedrich Meckel (the younger), 1781–1833, Professor of Anatomy and Surgery, Halle, Germany, described the diverticulum in 1809.
Denis Parsons Burkitt, 1911–1993, Irish surgeon who practised in Uganda, observed that many Western diseases were rare in Africa as a result of diet and lifestyle.
Edward John Hinchey, b. 1934, surgeon, Montreal General Hospital, Montreal, Canada.

clots, whereas right-sided bleeding will be darker. Torrential bleeding is fortunately rare and, in fact, more commonly due to angiodysplasia, but diverticular bleeding may persist or recur, requiring transfusion and resection. The presentation of a fistula resulting from diverticular disease depends on the site. The most common colovesical fistula results in recurrent urinary tract infections and pneumaturia (flatus in the urine) or even faeces in the urine. Colovaginal fistulae are more common after hysterectomy. Colocutaneous fistulation is unusual in the absence of prior intervention (e.g. radiological drainage). Rarely, diverticular disease may perforate into the retroperitoneum, leading to a psoas abscess, and even fistulation to the groin.

Investigation

Radiology

Plain radiographs can demonstrate a pneumoperitoneum. Spiral CT has excellent sensitivity and specificity for identifying bowel wall thickening, abscess formation and extraluminal disease and has revolutionised the assessment of complicated diverticular disease (***Figure 77.13***). On identification of abscesses in stable patients, drainage, under interventional radiology guidance, may be carried out percutaneously, avoiding the need for laparotomy/laparoscopy. Contrast studies and endoscopy are usually avoided for 6 weeks after an acute attack for fear of causing perforation. They are used subsequently, however, to exclude a coexisting carcinoma and assess the extent of diverticular disease. Contrast examination or CT can demonstrate a fistula.

Colonoscopy

Endoscopic assessment may demonstrate the necks of diverticula within the bowel lumen (***Figure 77.14***). A narrowed area of diverticular disease may be impassable because of the severity of disease and there is a significant risk of endoscopic perforation. Colonoscopy in these circumstances requires judgement and experience. Biopsies may be taken if possible and corroboration with CT virtual colonoscopy or occasionally contrast enema is required. Excluding a carcinoma may not always be possible and may represent an indication for resection.

Management

Patients are frequently recommended a high-fibre diet and bulk-forming laxatives, although the evidence for their effectiveness in diverticulosis or after an attack of diverticulitis is limited. Antispasmodics may have a role if recurrent pain is a problem. Acute diverticulitis has been traditionally treated with intravenous antibiotics and bowel rest. More recently, in recognition that diverticulitis may be a more inflammatory process than an infective one, many have advocated selective use of antibiotics. Essentially, antibiotic therapy may not be needed in immunocompetent people with uncomplicated diverticulitis who have no signs of systemic infection, as this may be a self-limiting condition. Uncomplicated disease should be confirmed by CT. For disease complicated by a localised abscess, intravenous antibiotics and image-guided drainage is indicated.

Operative procedures for diverticular disease

The aim of emergency surgery is to control peritoneal infection; indications are generalised peritonitis and failure to respond to optimum medical management. Laparotomy for diverticular disease in the acute setting has considerable risk with mortality in most series of 15%; in the case of faecal peritonitis, mortality approaches 50%.

Traditionally laparotomy and thorough washout of contamination are performed and then a choice has to be made between a Hartmann's procedure (sigmoid resection with formation of a left iliac fossa colostomy and closure of the rectal stump; ***Figure 77.15***) and resection with colonic washout and primary anastomosis (with consideration of a defunctioning

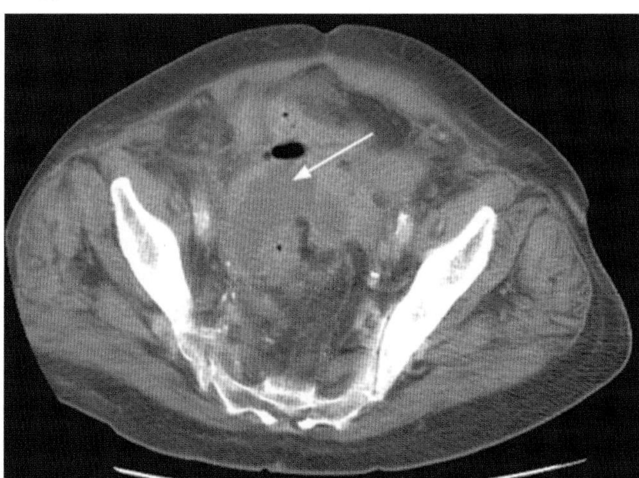

Figure 77.13 Computed tomography scan demonstrating an abscess associated with diverticulitis (arrow) (courtesy of Dr D Kasir, Hope Hospital, Salford, UK).

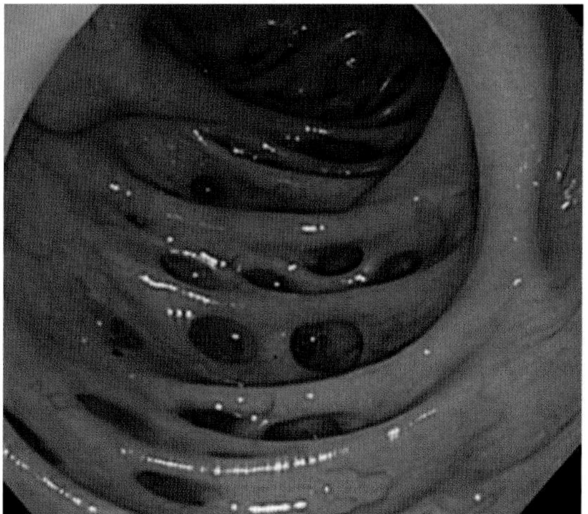

Figure 77.14 Colonoscopic view of right-sided diverticula. (From Niikura R, Nagata N, Akiyama J *et al*. Hypertension and concomitant arteriosclerotic diseases are risk factors for colonic diverticular bleeding: a case–control study. *Int J Colorectal Dis* 2012; **27**: 1137–43.)

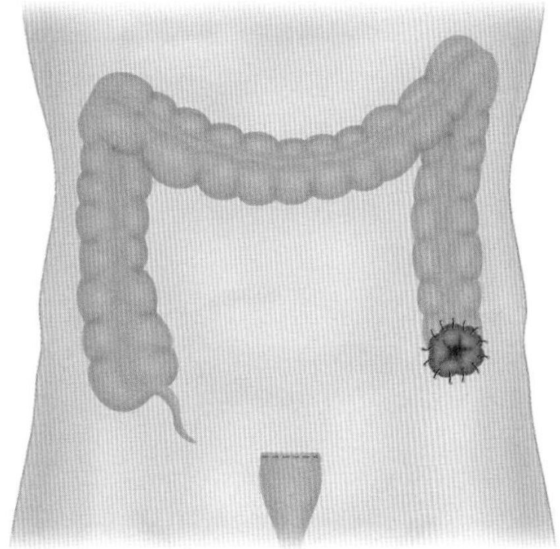

Figure 77.15 Hartmann's procedure with an oversewn rectal stump and an end left-sided colostomy following resection of the diseased segment of sigmoid colon.

loop ileostomy). Primary anastomosis should be used selectively but is appealing in a young fit patient without gross contamination or overwhelming sepsis. There is evidence that simple defunctioning with a proximal stoma is associated with higher mortality than a resection of the affected colon.

There may be a role for emergency laparoscopy in diverticular disease in expert hands. It allows assessment of the disease and in very selected cases a simple but thorough washout and drainage. The patient must have minimal comorbidity, be relatively stable, have no visible perforation and no gross faecal contamination. While this may avoid sigmoid resection in a select few, it remains controversial.

Elective surgery is usually undertaken for management of complications. Diverticular fistulae can only be cured by resecting the affected bowel, although a defunctioning stoma can ameliorate symptoms. In a colovesical fistula, once cancer has been excluded, the sigmoid can often be pinched off the bladder, the sigmoid colon resected and the bladder drained with an indwelling catheter for 7–10 days. If an anastomosis is performed, it is wise to place an omental pedicle between the bowel and bladder to prevent recurrent fistulation. These procedures can be technically challenging and ureteric stents may be advisable to reduce the risk of ureteric injury. Partial cystectomy may be required and assistance from a urological surgeon is often very helpful.

Haemorrhage from diverticular disease should be distinguished from angiodysplasia. It usually responds to conservative management and only occasionally requires resection. Where available, CT angiography is helpful to localise bleeding points and selective embolisation may control active bleeding. Rarely, colonoscopy may be necessary to localise the bleeding site. If the source cannot be located and bleeding continues, subtotal colectomy and ileostomy is the safest option.

Indications for surgery in an elective setting, in the absence of complications of the disease, are controversial. There is undoubtedly a small number of patients with recurrent attacks who should be offered an elective sigmoid colectomy (with anastomosis). This could be performed laparoscopically in experienced hands with a likely swifter recovery as well as improved cosmesis. Cohort studies suggest that of patients under 50 years old admitted with diverticulitis, 25% will have a further episode. The data may be used as an argument for offering elective resection but equally indicate that 75% will not get another severe attack. Many surgeons would discuss the pros and cons of elective surgery after two emergency admissions, although comorbidities must be carefully considered. However, there is an increasing tendency to treat even patients with recurrent attacks of diverticulitis conservatively in the absence of complications.

Summary box 77.12

Principles of surgical management of diverticular disease

- Hartmann's procedure is often the safest option in an emergency setting
- Primary anastomosis (with or without proximal diversion) can be considered in selected patients
- Elective resection may be considered for recurrent attacks or complications
- Laparoscopy has advantages in the elective setting but use in the emergency setting is more controversial

VASCULAR ANOMALIES OF THE INTESTINE

Angiodysplasia

Angiodysplasia is a vascular malformation that commonly causes haemorrhage from the colon in patients over the age of 60. The malformations consist of dilated tortuous submucosal veins.

Clinical features

In the majority of cases, the symptoms are subtle and patients can present with anaemia. About 10–15% have brisk bleeds, which may present as melaena or significant rectal bleeding. Many patients in whom rectal bleeding has been attributed to diverticular disease have probably bled from angiodysplasia. There is an association with aortic stenosis (Heyde's syndrome).

Investigation

Colonoscopy may show the characteristic lesion in the right colon. The lesions are only a few millimetres in size and appear as reddish, raised areas at endoscopy. CT angiography shows the site and extent of the lesion by a 'blush' of contrast, provided bleeding is more rapid than 1 mL/min. If this fails, a ^{99m}Tc-labelled red cell scan may confirm and localise the source of haemorrhage.

Edward Heyde, 1911–2004, American internist, published his findings on the association between aortic valve stenosis and angiodysplasia in a letter to the *New England Journal of Medicine* in 1958.

Treatment

In the context of a massive lower gastrointestinal bleed the first principle is to stabilise the patient. Following this, the bleeding needs to be localised. CT angiography allows not only localisation if bleeding is rapid but also therapeutic embolisation. If angiography fails or is unavailable careful colonoscopy (with copious lavage) may allow cauterisation to be carried out and an argon laser can be helpful. In severe uncontrolled bleeding, surgery becomes necessary. If preoperative localisation has not been successful, on-table colonoscopy is carried out to confirm the site of bleeding. Angiodysplastic lesions are sometimes demonstrated by transillumination through the caecum. If it is still not clear exactly which segment of the colon is involved a subtotal colectomy may be necessary. The management algorithm in ***Summary box 77.13*** is adapted from the diagnosis and management acute lower gastrointestinal bleeding guidelines from the British Society of Gastroenterology.

Summary box 77.13

Management of acute lower gastrointestinal bleeding

Patients with active bleeding and features of hypovolaemic shock

- CT angiogram and embolisation
- Bleeding treated: inpatient colonoscopy
- Bleeding continues: consider therapeutic endoscopy or surgery

Patients without features of hypovolaemic shock

- Significant bleeding: inpatient colonoscopy and consider oesophagogastroduodenoscopy; if normal consider capsule endoscopy, CT angiogram, nuclear medicine scanning
- Minor bleeding: arrange outpatient investigations

All patients: consider withholding anticoagulants and transfuse blood products as required

VOLVULUS

A volvulus is a twist of the intestine and the mesentery that supplies it (***Figure 77.16***). It is most commonly seen in the sigmoid colon, where elongation of the colon and mesentery with a narrow posterior attachment exists in some patients. It can, however, occur in patients with a hypermobile caecum and rarely in the transverse colon. Patients with sigmoid volvulus tend to be elderly and institutionalised; however, in West African countries it is more commonly seen in younger patients. Patients presenting with a caecal volvulus are usually younger and otherwise well. Predisposing factors include adhesions, gastric banding, pelvic masses and pregnancy.

Clinical features

Given the frailty of typical patients with sigmoid volvulus a history is not always forthcoming. Massive distension is key but pain is unusual and if present is a warning sign of ischaemia.

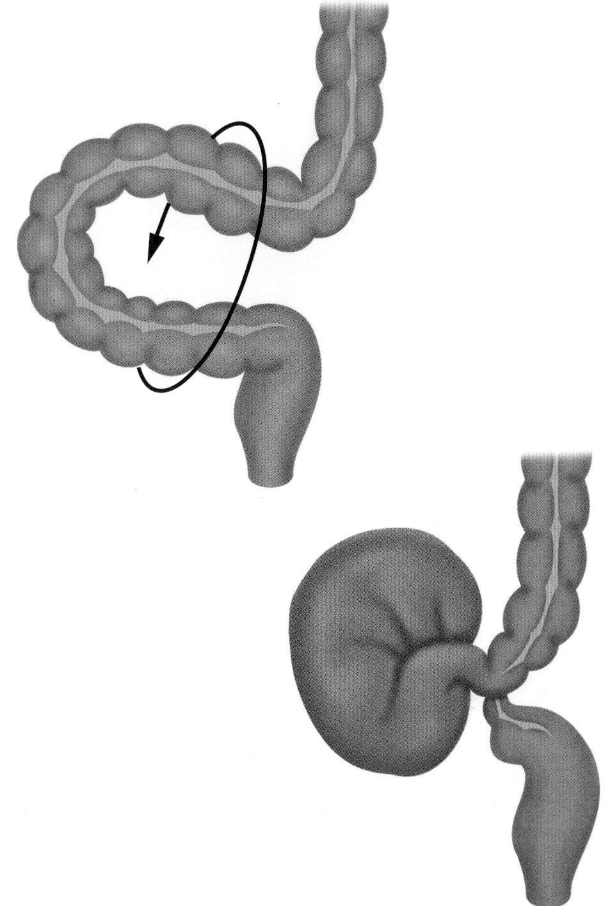

Figure 77.16 A sigmoid volvulus.

Investigation

A supine abdominal radiograph is useful but not always diagnostic (***Figure 77.17***). CT is the mainstay of diagnosis.

Treatment

For sigmoid volvulus the initial management is non-operative decompression using either a rigid sigmoidoscope or a colonoscope. Direct vision allows assessment of mucosal viability and derotation. With successful derotation a well-lubricated flatus tube should be inserted and left for 2–5 days. Bloody bowel contents or discoloured mucosa suggest ischaemia and the need for urgent surgery. Attempted derotation in this situation should be abandoned as it could lead to circulatory collapse and death.

Careful consideration of definitive surgery on a case-by-case basis in this, often elderly and frail, patient group is required. Although they would be subject to significant perioperative risk there is a very high recurrence rate for sigmoid volvulus. Such surgery should involve at least resection of the whole of the sigmoid colon and can be carried out laparoscopically. Given that there is very little need for colonic mobilisation and a large utility incision is required because of the bowel size, some of the benefits of a laparoscopic approach are negated. It is therefore reasonable to carry out surgery through a minilaparotomy

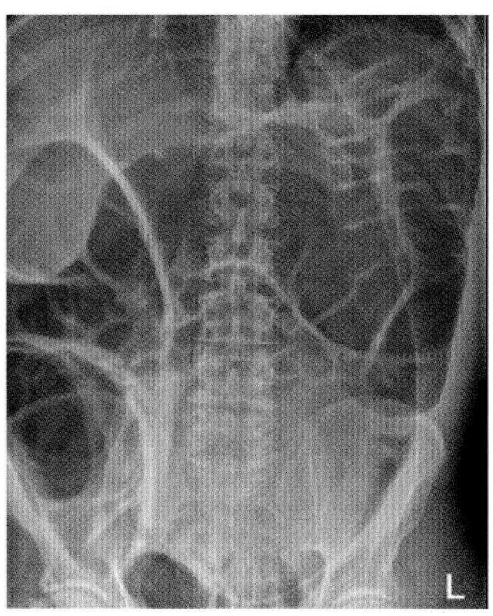

Figure 77.17 Plain abdominal radiograph showing colonic distension associated with a sigmoid volvulus (courtesy of Dr Rajpal Dhingsa, Nottingham University Hospitals, Nottingham, UK).

incision with the same recovery outcomes. An alternative to surgical resection in the very unfit patient is a percutaneous endoscopic colostomy, using a colonoscope to place a drainage tube through the abdominal wall into the sigmoid to fix the bowel in an untwisted position.

In the emergency situation where there is evidence of necrosis it may be wise to ligate the mesenteric vessels before untwisting the volvulus to theoretically avoid the systemic release of ischaemic toxins. It may also be prudent to avoid anastomosis. Instead, a Hartmann's-type approach or a Paul–Mikulicz double-barrelled stoma should be considered. For caecal volvulus endoscopic decompression is often unsuccessful and leads to treatment delay. Instead, urgent right hemicolectomy is indicated.

ENDOMETRIOSIS

This is mainly covered in *Chapter 87*. It tends to be found deep in the pelvis and therefore relates more to the rectum. On the rare occasion it is found in the colon, it may be a cause of fibrosis and obstruction.

COLOSTOMIES

A colostomy is a planned opening made in the colon to divert faeces and flatus through the abdominal wall, where they can be collected in an external appliance. Ileostomies are discussed in *Chapter 74*. Depending on the purpose for which the diversion has been necessary, a stoma may be temporary or permanent. Indications for stomas are shown in *Summary box 77.14*.

In elective surgery stoma counselling and siting should be performed by a trained stoma nurse. The patient should be examined lying, standing and sitting to determine the optimum site, which should be away from scars, skin creases and bony prominences. In obese patients the stoma should be sited higher so that it can be easily seen. Clothing preference and patient disability (hand dexterity and vision) should also be considered. In the emergency setting siting may be difficult with a sick and immobile patient, particularly if the abdomen is distended.

Summary box 77.14

Indications for colostomy formation

- To protect a distal anastomosis or allow healing away from the faecal flow
- Following resection when anastomosis is unsafe or not possible
- To relieve obstruction when resection is not feasible
- To reduce disease activity (e.g. Crohn's disease)
- To allow alternative bowel control (incontinence)

Types of colostomy

Loop colostomy

Loop stomas are most commonly used to temporarily divert the faecal stream; for instance, to protect an anastomosis (usually by a loop ileostomy) following traumatic injury to the rectum, to facilitate the operative treatment of a high anal fistula, for incontinence and to defunction an obstructing low rectal cancer prior to long-course chemoradiotherapy. A mobilised loop of colon is brought out onto the anterior abdominal wall. Once the abdomen has been closed, the colostomy is opened and the edges of the colonic incision are sutured to the adjacent skin margin (*Figure 77.18*). A rod or bridge is sometimes placed under the loop to prevent retraction in the early postoperative period, being removed after a few days. Colostomy function should be expected in 2–7 days after operation.

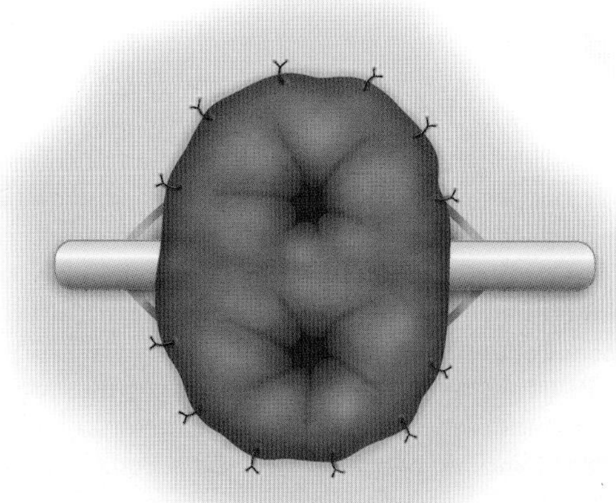

Figure 77.18 Loop colostomy with a bridge.

Frank T Paul, 1851–1941, surgeon, Liverpool, UK.
Johannes von Mikulicz-Radecki, 1850–1905, Professor of Surgery, Breslau, Poland.

If there is resolution of the indication for which the temporary stoma was constructed, the colostomy can usually be closed without recourse to a laparotomy/laparoscopy. Conventionally a water-soluble contrast enema is performed to assess the distal bowel before closure, particularly for pelvic anastomoses. Approximately 25% of temporary diverting stomas are never closed because of complications or changes in medical comorbidity.

End-colostomy

This is formed after an abdominoperineal excision of the rectum or as part of a Hartmann's procedure, bringing the divided colon through a left iliac fossa trephine in rectus abdominis and the skin. The colonic margin is then sutured usually flush or slightly everted on the adjoining skin (***Figure 77.19***).

Double-barrelled colostomy (Paul-Mikulicz)

Occasionally, when resection of a section of colon has occurred but the patient is too ill to undergo a safe reanastomosis it is possible and appropriate to bring up both ends of the bowel to the abdominal wall (see ***Volvulus***). This aids subsequent closure as the ends can simply be mobilised locally and reanastomosed rather than the patient requiring a relaparotomy.

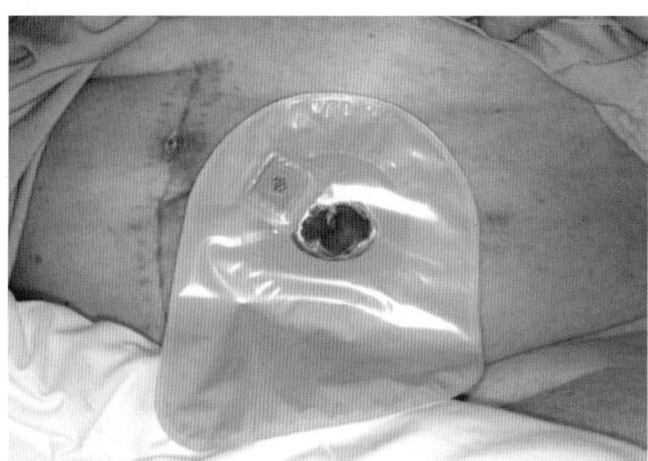

Figure 77.19 A colostomy in the left iliac fossa.

Summary box 77.15

Stomas

- May be colostomy or ileostomy
- May be temporary or permanent
- Temporary or defunctioning stomas are usually fashioned as loop stomas
- An ileostomy is spouted; a colostomy is flush or slightly everted
- Ileostomy effluent is usually liquid whereas colostomy effluent is usually solid
- Ileostomy patients are more likely to develop fluid and electrolyte problems
- An ileostomy is usually sited in the right iliac fossa
- End-colostomy is usually sited in the left iliac fossa
- Whenever possible patients should be counselled and sited by a stoma care nurse before their operation

Stoma bags and appliances

Stoma output is collected in disposable adhesive bags. Colostomy appliances are simply changed as necessary. A wide range of such bags is currently available. In most hospitals, a stoma care service is available to offer advice to patients, to acquaint them with the latest appliances and to provide the appropriate psychological and practical help.

Complications of stomas

Stoma complications are common (***Summary box 77.16***). The vast majority of these complications can be dealt with by a suitably experienced stoma nurse but on occasion revision surgery is needed. Stoma ischaemia is usually evident in the early postoperative period and it is essential to inspect the stoma the day after surgery to assess mucosal viability. If the stoma looks ischaemic a proctoscope is useful to assess viability below the fascia. Urgent surgery is required if the mucosa below the fascia is also ischaemic. Conversely if the mucosa of the bowel immediately proximal to the stoma is viable, the patient can be managed expectantly in the hope that the non-viable mucosa will slough and the worst late result is a stenosis that can be managed with a more local procedure. This may be preferable to an immediate, difficult relaparotomy. Mucocutaneous separation can usually be managed conservatively with intensive stoma care.

Prolapse is more common in loop stomas, particularly transverse colon loop stomas. If recurrent and causing problems with stoma care the most effective solution is reversal. Other options include conversion to an end-stoma and/or resection of redundant bowel. Retraction is mostly a problem in obese patients and may require, what can sometimes be difficult, revision. Minor degrees of stenosis may respond to simple dilatation with more severe or recurrent issues requiring revision surgery.

Repair of parastomal hernias is particularly technically challenging and the recurrence rate is high. Simple sutured repair is associated with an almost 100% risk of recurrence and transfer to the opposite side of the abdomen, or insertion of a piece of prosthetic material within the abdominal wall around the stoma may be necessary. There is some evidence that stoma trephine reinforcement with mesh at the time of initial stoma formation may reduce the incidence of parastomal herniation, which may be as high as 50% over the long term. There are however complications associated with parastomal meshes including recurrence, mesh infection, fistulation and bowel obstruction.

Summary box 77.16

Stoma complications

- Skin irritation
- Prolapse
- Retraction
- Ischaemia
- Stenosis
- Parastomal hernia
- Bleeding
- Fistulation

FURTHER READING

Chakrabarti S, Peterson CY, Sriram D, Mahipal A. Early stage colon cancer: current treatment standards, evolving paradigms, and future directions. *World J Gastrointest Oncol* 2020; **12**(8): 808–32.

Clark S. *Colorectal surgery: a companion to specialist surgical practice*, 6th edn. Edinburgh: Elsevier, 2019.

Crosbie EJ, Ryan NAJ, Arends MJ *et al.* The Manchester International Consensus Group recommendations for the management of gynecological cancers in Lynch syndrome. *Genet Med* 2019; **21**: 2390–400.

Herold A, Lehur P-A, Matzel KE, O'Connell PR (eds). *European manual of medicine: coloproctology*, 2nd edn. New York: Springer, 2017.

Moran B, Cunningham C, Singh T *et al.* Association of Coloproctology of Great Britain and Ireland (ACPGBI). Guidelines for the management of cancer of the colon, rectum and anus. *Colorectal Dis* 2017; **19**(Suppl 1): 18–36.

National Institute for Health and Care Excellence. *Follow-up to detect recurrence after treatment for non-metastatic colorectal cancer.* NICE Clinical Guideline 151. London: NICE, 2020. Available from https://www.nice.org.uk/guidance/ng151.

Oakland K, Chadwick G, East JE *et al.* Diagnosis and management of acute lower gastrointestinal bleeding: guidelines from the British Society of Gastroenterology. *Gut* 2019; **68**: 776–89.

O'Connell PR, Madoff RD, Solomon MJ (eds). *Operative surgery of the colon, rectum and anus*, 6th edn. Bacon Rota, FL: CRC Press, 2015.

Rutter MD, East J, Rees CJ *et al.* British Society of Gastroenterology/Association of Coloproctology of Great Britain and Ireland/Public Health England post-polypectomy and post-colorectal cancer resection surveillance guidelines. *Gut* 2020; **69**: 201–23.

Seppälä TT, Latchford A, Negoi I, *et al.* European guidelines from the EHTG and ESCP for Lynch syndrome: an updated third edition of the Mallorca guidelines based on gene and gender. *Br J Surg* 2020. https://doi.org/10.1002/bjs.11902

CHAPTER 78 Intestinal obstruction

Learning objectives

To understand:

- The pathophysiology of dynamic and adynamic intestinal obstruction
- The cardinal features on history and examination
- The causes of small and large bowel obstruction
- The indications for surgery and other treatment options in bowel obstruction

CLASSIFICATION

Intestinal obstruction may be classified into two types:

- **Dynamic**, in which peristalsis is working against a mechanical obstruction. It may occur in an acute or a chronic form (***Figure 78.1***).
- **Adynamic**, in which there is no mechanical obstruction; peristalsis is absent or inadequate (e.g. paralytic ileus or pseudo-obstruction).

Summary box 78.1

Causes of intestinal obstruction

Dynamic

- Intraluminal
  - Faecal impaction
  - Foreign bodies
  - Bezoars
  - Gallstones
- Intramural
  - Stricture
  - Malignancy
  - Intussusception
  - Volvulus
- Extramural
  - Bands/adhesions
  - Hernia

Adynamic

- Paralytic ileus
- Pseudo-obstruction

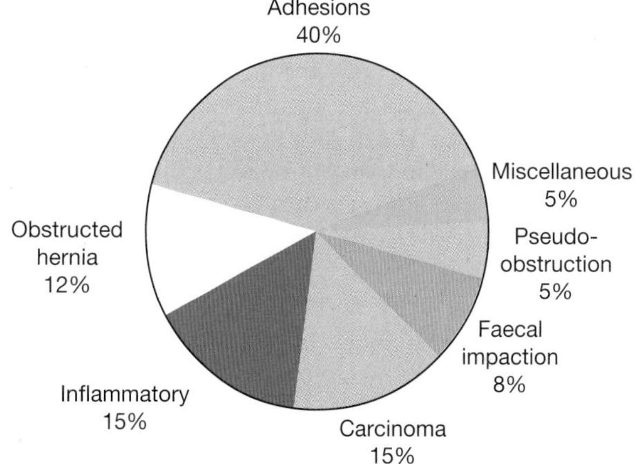

Figure 78.1 Pie chart showing the common causes of intestinal obstruction and relative frequencies.

PATHOPHYSIOLOGY

Irrespective of aetiology or acuteness of onset, in dynamic (mechanical) obstruction the bowel proximal to the obstruction dilates and the bowel below the obstruction exhibits normal peristalsis and absorption until it becomes empty and collapses. Initially, proximal peristalsis is increased in an attempt to overcome the obstruction. If the obstruction is not relieved, the bowel continues to dilate; ultimately there is a reduction in peristaltic strength, resulting in flaccidity and paralysis.

The distension proximal to an obstruction is caused by two factors:

- **Gas**: there is a significant overgrowth of both aerobic and anaerobic organisms, resulting in considerable gas production. Following the reabsorption of oxygen and carbon dioxide, the majority is made up of nitrogen (90%) and hydrogen sulphide.
- **Fluid**: this is made up of the various digestive juices (saliva, 500 mL; bile, 500 mL; pancreatic secretions, 500 mL; gastric secretions, 1 litre; all per 24 hours). This accumulates in the gut lumen as absorption by the obstructed gut is retarded. Dehydration and electrolyte loss are therefore due to:
  - reduced oral intake;
  - defective intestinal absorption;
  - losses as a result of vomiting;
  - sequestration in the bowel lumen;
  - transudation of fluid into the peritoneal cavity.

STRANGULATION

It is important to appreciate that the consequences of intestinal obstruction are not immediately life-threatening unless there is superimposed strangulation. When strangulation occurs, the blood supply is compromised and the bowel becomes ischaemic.

Summary box 78.2

Causes of strangulation

Direct pressure on the bowel wall
- Hernial orifices
- Adhesions/bands

Interrupted mesenteric blood flow
- Volvulus
- Intussusception

Increased intraluminal pressure
- Closed-loop obstruction

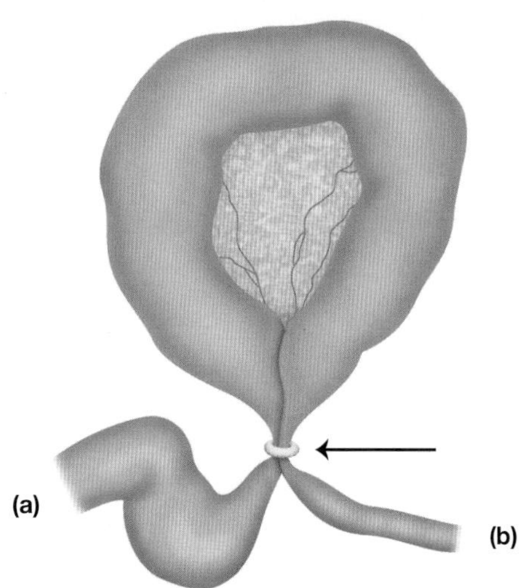

Figure 78.2 Distension. Closed-loop obstruction around a constricting band (arrow) with impending strangulation, mild distension of the proximal limb (a) and collapse of the distal limb (b) of small bowel.

Ischaemia from direct pressure on the bowel wall from a constricting band such as a hernial orifice is easy to understand.

Distension of the obstructed segment of bowel results in high pressure within the bowel wall. This can happen when only part of the bowel wall is obstructed, as seen in a Richter's hernia (see *Chapter 64*). Venous return is compromised before the arterial supply. The resultant increase in capillary pressure leads to impaired local perfusion and, once the arterial supply is impaired, haemorrhagic infarction occurs. As the viability of the bowel is compromised, translocation and systemic exposure to anaerobic organisms and endotoxin occurs.

The morbidity and mortality associated with strangulation are largely dependent on the duration of the ischaemia and its extent. Elderly patients and those with comorbidities are more vulnerable to its effects. Although in strangulated external hernias the segment involved is often short, any length of ischaemic bowel can cause significant systemic effects secondary to sepsis. Bowel distension and fluid sequestration proximal to the obstruction can result in significant dehydration. When bowel involvement is extensive circulatory failure is common.

Closed-loop obstruction

This occurs when the bowel is obstructed at both the proximal and distal points (*Figure 78.2*). The distension is principally confined to the closed loop; distension proximal to the obstructed segment is not typically marked.

A classic form of closed-loop obstruction is seen in the presence of a malignant stricture of the colon with a competent ileocaecal valve (present in up to one-third of individuals). This can occur with lesions as far distally as the rectum. The inability of the distended colon to decompress itself into the small bowel results in an increase in luminal pressure, which is greatest at the caecum, with subsequent impairment of blood flow in the wall. Unrelieved, this results in necrosis and perforation (*Figure 78.3*).

SPECIAL TYPES OF MECHANICAL INTESTINAL OBSTRUCTION

Internal hernia

Internal herniation occurs when a portion of the small intestine becomes entrapped in one of the retroperitoneal fossae or in a congenital mesenteric defect.

The following are potential sites of internal herniation (all are very rare):

- the foramen of Winslow;
- a defect in the mesentery;
- a defect in the transverse mesocolon;
- defects in the broad ligament;
- congenital or acquired diaphragmatic hernia;
- duodenal retroperitoneal fossae;
- caecal/appendiceal retroperitoneal fossae;
- intersigmoid fossa.

Internal herniation in the absence of adhesions is rare and a preoperative diagnosis is unusual. The standard treatment of an obstructed hernia is to release the constricting agent by division. This should not be undertaken in cases of herniation involving the foramen of Winslow, mesenteric defects and paraduodenal/duodenojejunal fossae as major blood vessels run in the edge of the constriction ring. The distended loop in such circumstances must first be decompressed (minimising contamination) and then reduced.

August Gottlieb Richter, 1742–1812, lecturer in surgery, Göttingen, Germany, described this form of hernia in 1777.
Jacob Benignus Winslow, 1669–1760, Professor of Anatomy, Physic and Surgery, Paris, France.

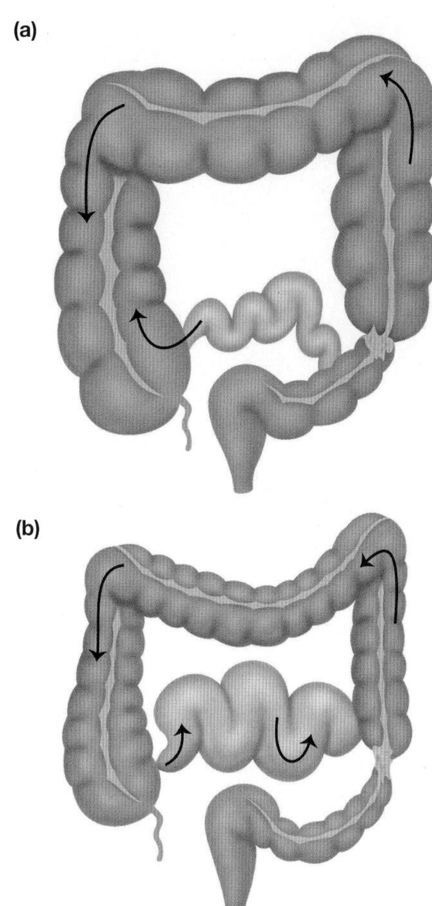

Figure 78.3 Obstructing stricture of the distal descending colon in the presence of (a) a competent ileocaecal valve, resulting in gross caecal distension, and (b) an incompetent ileocaecal valve, allowing decompression into the distal small bowel without gross caecal distension.

Obstruction from enteric strictures

Small bowel strictures usually occur secondary to tuberculosis or Crohn's disease. Malignant strictures associated with lymphoma are uncommon; carcinoma and sarcoma are rare. Presentation is usually subacute or chronic. Standard surgical management consists of resection and anastomosis. Resection is important to establish a histological diagnosis as this can be uncertain clinically. In Crohn's disease, strictureplasty may be considered in the presence of short multiple strictures without active sepsis (see ***Chapter 75***).

Bolus obstruction

Bolus obstruction in the small bowel may be caused by gallstones, food, trichobezoar, phytobezoar, stercoliths and worms.

Gallstones

This type of obstruction tends to occur in the elderly secondary to erosion of a large gallstone directly through the gallbladder into the duodenum. Classically, there is impaction about 60 cm proximal to the ileocaecal valve. The patient may have recurrent attacks as the obstruction may be incomplete or relapsing as a result of a ball-valve effect. The characteristic radiological sign of gallstone ileus is Rigler's triad, comprising: small bowel obstruction, pneumobilia and an atypical mineral shadow on radiographs of the abdomen. The presence of two of these radiological signs has been considered pathognomonic of gallstone ileus and is encountered in 40–50% of the cases (note that pneumobilia is a common finding following endoscopic retrograde cholangiopancreatography with sphincterotomy). At laparotomy, the stone should be milked proximally away from the site of impaction. It may be possible to crush the stone within the bowel lumen; if not, the intestine is opened at this point and the gallstone removed. If the gallstone is faceted, a careful check for other enteric stones should be made. The region of the gallbladder should not be explored (see ***Chapter 71***).

Food

Bolus obstruction may occur after partial or total gastrectomy when unchewed articles can pass directly into the small bowel. Fruit and vegetables are particularly liable to cause obstruction. The management is similar to that for gallstones, with intraluminal crushing usually being successful.

Trichobezoars and phytobezoars

These are firm masses of undigested hair ball and fruit/vegetable fibre, respectively. The former is due to persistent hair chewing or sucking and may be associated with an underlying psychiatric abnormality. Predisposition to phytobezoars results from a high fibre intake, inadequate chewing, previous gastric surgery, hypochlorhydria and loss of the gastric pump mechanism. When possible, the lesion may be kneaded into the caecum; otherwise, open removal is required. A preoperative diagnosis is difficult even with high-resolution computed tomography (CT) scanning.

Stercoliths

These are usually found in the small bowel in association with a jejunal diverticulum or ileal stricture. Presentation and management are identical to that of gallstones.

Worms

Ascaris lumbricoides may cause low small bowel obstruction, particularly in children, the institutionalised and those near the tropics. An attack may follow the initiation of anthelminthic therapy. Debility is frequently out of proportion to that produced by the obstruction. If worms are not seen in the stool or vomitus the diagnosis may be indicated by eosinophilia or the sight of worms within gas-filled small bowel loops on a plain radiograph. At laparotomy it may be possible to knead the tangled mass into the caecum; if not, it should be removed. Occasionally, worms may cause a perforation and peritonitis, especially if the enteric wall is weakened by such conditions as amoebiasis (see ***Chapter 6***).

Burrill Bernard Crohn, 1884–1983, gastroenterologist, Mount Sinai Hospital, New York, NY, USA, described regional ileitis in 1932.
Leo George Rigler, 1896–1979, Professor of Radiology, University of California, Los Angeles, CA, USA.

Obstruction by adhesions and bands

Adhesions

In western countries adhesions and bands are the most common cause of intestinal obstruction. The lifetime risk of requiring an admission to hospital for adhesional small bowel obstruction subsequent to abdominal surgery is approximately 4% and the risk of requiring a laparotomy around 2%. Adhesions start to form within hours of abdominal surgery. In the early postoperative period, the onset of such a mechanical obstruction may be difficult to differentiate from paralytic ileus.

The causes of intraperitoneal adhesions are shown in ***Table 78.1***. Any source of peritoneal irritation results in local fibrin production, which produces adhesions between apposed surfaces. Early fibrinous adhesions may disappear when the cause is removed or they may become vascularised and be replaced by mature fibrous tissue.

There are several factors that may limit adhesion formation.

TABLE 78.1 The common causes of intra-abdominal adhesions.

Acute inflammation	Sites of anastomoses, reperitonealisation of raw areas, trauma, ischaemia
Foreign material	Talc, starch, gauze, silk
Infection	Peritonitis, tuberculosis
Chronic inflammatory conditions	Crohn's disease
Radiation enteritis	

Summary box 78.3

Prevention of adhesions

Factors that may limit adhesion formation include:

- Good surgical technique
- Washing of the peritoneal cavity with saline to remove clots
- Minimising contact with gauze
- Covering anastomoses and raw peritoneal surfaces

Numerous substances have been instilled in the peritoneal cavity to prevent adhesion formation, including hyaluronidase, hydrocortisone, silicone, dextran, polyvinylpropylene (PVP), chondroitin, streptomycin, anticoagulants, antihistamines, non-steroidal anti-inflammatory drugs and streptokinase. Currently, no single agent or combination of agents has been convincingly shown to be effective. It is hoped that with more widespread use of laparoscopic surgery the incidence of intra-abdominal adhesions will reduce.

Adhesions may be classified into various types by virtue of whether they are early (fibrinous) or late (fibrous) or by underlying aetiology. From a practical perspective there are only two types: 'easy' flimsy ones and 'difficult' dense ones (***Figure 78.4***).

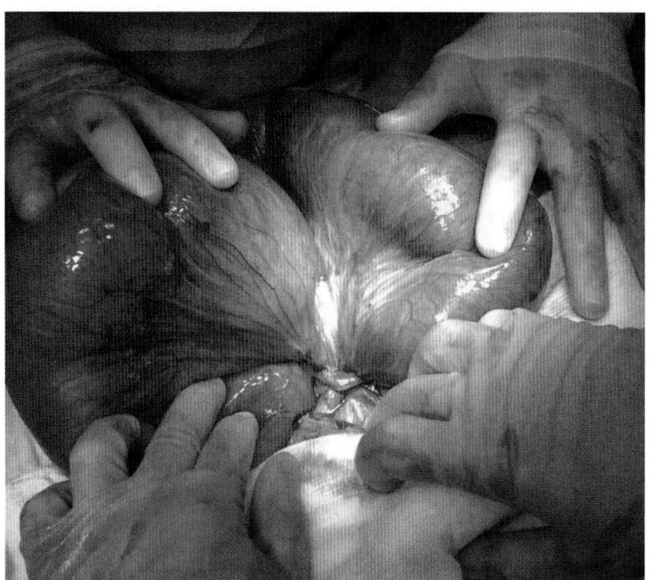

Figure 78.4 Band adhesion causing a closed-loop obstruction.

Postoperative adhesions giving rise to intestinal obstruction usually involve the lower small bowel and less commonly the large bowel.

Bands

Usually only one band is culpable. This may be:

- congenital, e.g. obliterated vitellointestinal duct;
- a string band following previous abdominal surgery or peritoneal inflammation;
- a portion of greater omentum, usually adherent to the parietes.

Acute intussusception

This occurs when one portion of the gut invaginates into an immediately adjacent segment; almost invariably, it is the proximal into the distal.

The condition is encountered most commonly in children, with a peak incidence between 5 and 10 months of age. About 90% of cases are idiopathic but an associated upper respiratory tract infection or gastroenteritis may precede the condition. It is believed that hyperplasia of Peyer's patches in the terminal ileum may be the initiating event. Weaning, loss of passively acquired maternal immunity and common viral pathogens have all been implicated in the pathogenesis of intussusception in infancy (see ***Chapter 17***).

Children with intussusception associated with a pathological lead point such as Meckel's diverticulum, polyp, duplication, Henoch–Schönlein purpura or appendix are usually older than those with idiopathic disease. After the age of 2 years, a

Johann Conrad Peyer, 1653–1782, Professor of Logic, Rhetoric and Medicine, Schaffhausen, Switzerland, described the lymph follicles in the intestine in 1677.
Johann Friedrich Meckel (the younger), 1781–1833, Professor of Anatomy and Surgery, Halle, Germany, described the diverticulum in 1809.
Eduard Heinrich Henoch, 1820–1910, Professor of Diseases of Children, Berlin, Germany, described this form of purpura in 1868.
Johann Lucas Schönlein, 1793–1864, Professor of Medicine, Berlin, Germany, gave his account of this disease in 1837.

(a)

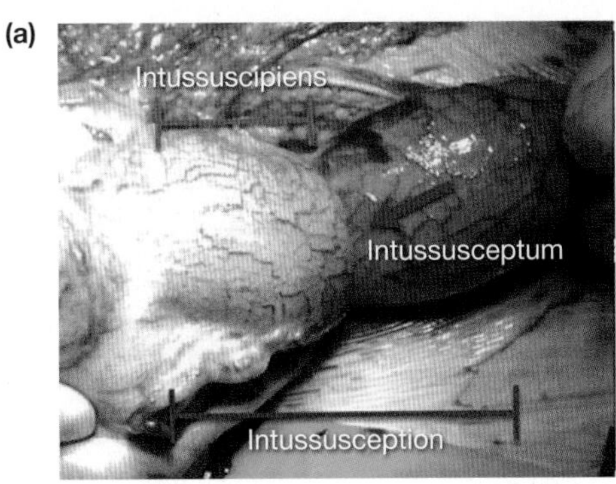

(b)

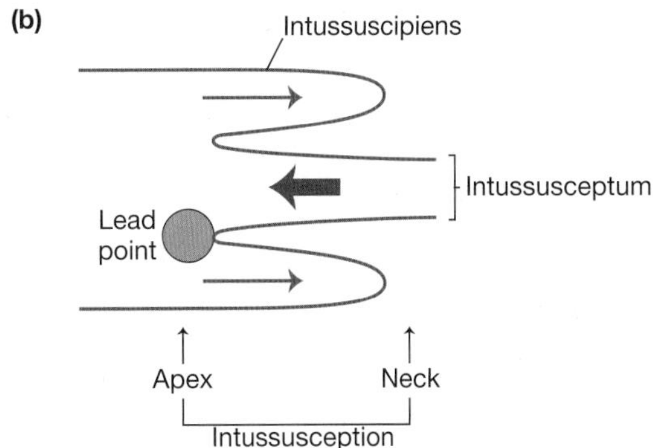

Figure 78.5 Small bowel intussusception showing components: intussusceptum (purple arrow); intussuscipiens; lead point; middle tube (red arrows).

pathological lead point is found in at least one-third of affected children. In adults, cases are almost invariably associated with a lead point, which is usually a polyp (e.g. Peutz–Jeghers syndrome), a submucosal lipoma or other tumour.

The phenomenon of transient intussusception in younger patients is now recognised. Imaging of the small bowel (with CT scanning, capsule endoscopy or enteroscopy) is required to exclude intraluminal disease.

Pathology

An intussusception is composed of three parts (*Figure 78.5*):

- the entering or inner tube (intussusceptum);
- the returning or middle tube;
- the sheath or outer tube (intussuscipiens).

The part that advances is the apex, the mass is the intussusception and the neck is the junction of the entering layer with the mass.

Intussusception may be anatomically defined according to the site and extent of invagination (*Table 78.2*). In most children, the intussusception is ileocolic. In adults, colocolic intussusception is more common. The degree of ischaemia is dependent on the tightness of invagination, which is usually greatest as it passes through the ileocaecal valve.

TABLE 78.2 Types of intussusception in children (after RE Gross) (n = 702).

	Percentage of series
Ileoileal	5
Ileocolic	77
Ileoileocolic	12
Colocolic	2
Multiple	1
Retrograde	0.2
Others	2.8

On CT scanning the target sign may be evident and, if present, is pathognomonic (*Figure 78.6*). It is worth noting that occasionally an asymptomatic intussusception can be observed on CT scanning in adults. This may be transient or intermittent.

Summary box 78.4

Intussusception

- Most common in children
- Adult cases are secondary to intestinal pathology, e.g. polyp, Meckel's diverticulum
- Ileocolic is the most common variety
- Can lead to an ischaemic segment
- Radiological reduction is indicated in most paediatric cases
- Adults who present acutely require surgery

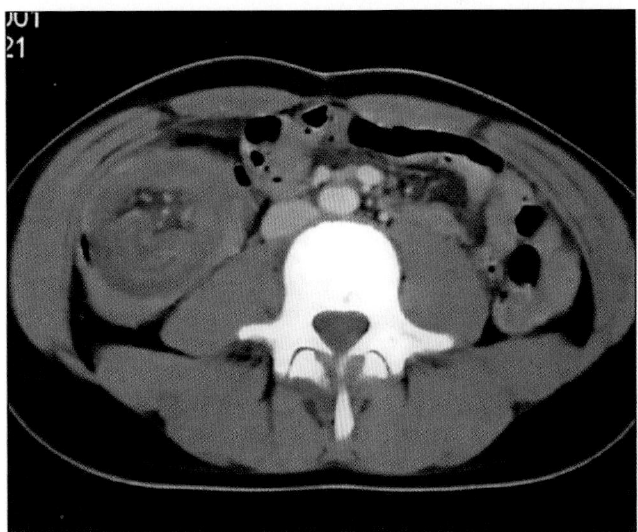

Figure 78.6 Abdominal computed tomography scan illustrating the 'target sign' of the ileocolic intussusception seen in *Figure 78.5*.

John Law Augustine Peutz, 1886–1968, Chief Specialist for Internal Medicine, St John's Hospital, The Hague, The Netherlands.
Harold Joseph Jeghers, 1904–1990, Professor of Internal Medicine, New Jersey College of Medicine and Dentistry, Jersey City, NJ, USA.
Robert Edward Gross, 1905–1988, paediatric surgeon, Harvard Medical School, Boston, MA, USA.

Volvulus

A volvulus is a twisting or axial rotation of a portion of bowel about its mesentery. The rotation causes obstruction to the lumen (>180° torsion) and if tight enough also causes vascular occlusion in the mesentery (>360° torsion). Bacterial fermentation adds to distension and increasing intraluminal pressure impairs capillary perfusion. Mesenteric veins become obstructed as a result of the mechanical twisting; thrombosis results and contributes to ischaemia.

Volvuli may be primary or secondary. The primary form is caused by congenital malrotation of the gut, abnormal mesenteric attachments or congenital bands. Examples include volvulus neonatorum, caecal volvulus and sigmoid volvulus (see *Chapter 65*). A secondary volvulus, which is the more common variety, is due to rotation of a segment of bowel around an acquired adhesion or stoma.

Summary box 78.5

Volvulus

- May involve the small intestine, caecum or sigmoid colon
- Neonatal midgut volvulus secondary to midgut malrotation is life-threatening
- The most common spontaneous type in adults is sigmoid volvulus
- Sigmoid volvulus can be relieved by decompression per anum
- Surgery may be required to prevent or relieve ischaemia

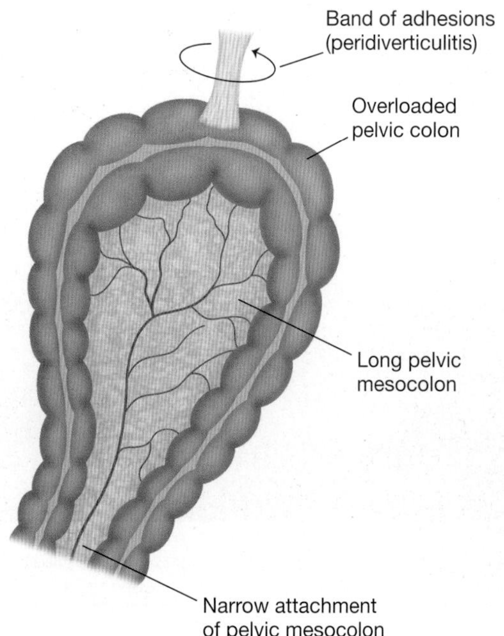

Figure 78.7 Causes predisposing to volvulus of the sigmoid colon. Idiopathic megacolon usually precedes the volvulus in African people.

Volvulus neonatorum

This occurs secondary to intestinal malrotation (see *Chapters 17 and 65*) and is potentially catastrophic.

Sigmoid volvulus

This is uncommon in Europe and the USA but more common in eastern Europe and Africa. Indeed, it is the most common cause of large bowel obstruction in the indigenous black African population. Rotation nearly always occurs in the anticlockwise direction. The predisposing clinical features are summarised in *Figure 78.7*. Other predisposing factors include a high-residue diet and constipation. In western populations, the condition is seen most often in elderly patients with chronic constipation; comorbidities are common and chronic psychotropic drug use is associated with this condition. Younger patients present earlier and the prognosis is inversely related to the duration of symptoms.

Presentation with volvulus can be classified as:

- **fulminant**: sudden onset, severe pain, early vomiting, rapidly deteriorating clinical course;
- **indolent**: insidious onset, slow progressive course, less pain, late vomiting.

Compound volvulus

This is a rare condition that is also known as ileosigmoid knotting. The long pelvic mesocolon allows the ileum to twist around the sigmoid colon, resulting in gangrene of either or both segments of bowel. The patient presents with acute intestinal obstruction, but distension is comparatively mild. Plain radiography reveals distended ileal loops in a distended sigmoid colon. At operation, decompression, resection and anastomosis are required.

CLINICAL FEATURES OF INTESTINAL OBSTRUCTION

Dynamic obstruction

The diagnosis of dynamic intestinal obstruction is based on the classic quartet of pain, distension, vomiting and absolute constipation. Obstruction may be classified clinically into two types:

- small bowel obstruction – high or low;
- large bowel obstruction.

The nature of the presentation will also be influenced by whether the obstruction is:

- complete;
- incomplete.

A complete small bowel obstruction has all the cardinal features. In cases of complete large bowel obstruction there is often a surprising lack of preceding symptoms. Both small and large bowel obstruction can present with more chronic symptoms in which the symptoms and signs are intermittent or the obstruction is incomplete. Incomplete obstruction is also referred to as partial or subacute.

Summary box 78.6

Features of obstruction

- In **high small bowel obstruction**, vomiting occurs early, is profuse and causes rapid dehydration. Distension is minimal with little evidence of dilated small bowel loops on abdominal radiography
- In **low small bowel obstruction**, pain is predominant with central distension. Vomiting occurs later. Multiple dilated small bowel loops are seen on radiography
- In **large bowel obstruction**, distension is early and pronounced. Pain is less severe and vomiting and dehydration are later features. The colon proximal to the obstruction is distended on abdominal radiography. The small bowel will be dilated if the ileocaecal valve is incompetent (*Figure 78.3*)

Summary box 78.7

Cardinal clinical features of acute obstruction

- Abdominal pain
- Distension
- Vomiting
- Absolute constipation

Presentation will be further influenced by whether the obstruction is:

- simple – in which the blood supply is intact;
- strangulating/strangulated – in which there is interference to blood flow.

The common causes of intestinal obstruction in western countries and their relative frequencies are shown in *Figure 78.1*. The underlying mechanisms are shown in *Summary box 78.2*.

The clinical features vary according to:

- the location of the obstruction;
- the duration of the obstruction;
- the underlying pathology;
- the presence or absence of intestinal ischaemia.

Late manifestations of intestinal obstruction that may be encountered include dehydration, oliguria, hypovolaemic shock, pyrexia, septicaemia, respiratory embarrassment and peritonism. In all cases of suspected intestinal obstruction, the hernial orifices must be examined.

Pain

Pain is the first symptom encountered; it occurs suddenly and is usually severe. It is colicky in nature and usually centred on the umbilicus (small bowel) or lower abdomen (large bowel) (see *Chapter 63*). The pain coincides with increased peristaltic activity. With increasing distension, the colicky pain is replaced by a more constant diffuse pain. If there is no ischaemia and the obstruction persists over several days, pain reduces and can disappear.

The development of severe pain is suggestive of strangulation, especially if the pain is continuous. Beware the patient whose pain is not controlled with intravenous opiates. Colicky pain may not be a significant feature in postoperative simple mechanical obstruction and colicky pain does not usually occur in paralytic ileus.

Vomiting

The more distal the obstruction, the longer the interval between the onset of symptoms and the appearance of nausea and vomiting. As obstruction progresses the character of the vomitus alters from digested food to faeculent material, as a result of enteric bacterial overgrowth.

Distension

In the small bowel the degree of distension is dependent on the site of the obstruction and is greater the more distal the lesion. Visible peristalsis may be present in thin patients (*Figure 78.8*). This can sometimes be provoked by 'flicking' the abdominal wall. Distension is a later feature in colonic obstruction and may be minimal or absent in the presence of mesenteric vascular occlusion.

Constipation

This may be classified as absolute (i.e. neither faeces nor flatus is passed) or relative (where only flatus is passed). Absolute constipation is a cardinal feature of complete intestinal obstruction. Some patients may pass flatus or faeces after the onset of obstruction as a result of the evacuation of the distal bowel contents. The administration of enemas should be avoided in cases of suspected obstruction. This merely stimulates evacuation of bowel contents distal to the obstruction and confuses the clinical picture.

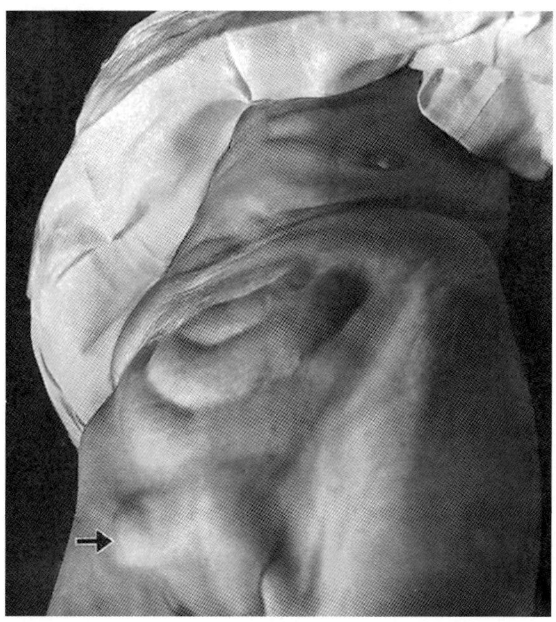

Figure 78.8 Visible peristalsis. Intestinal obstruction due to a strangulated right femoral hernia (arrow).

The rule that absolute constipation is present in intestinal obstruction does not apply in:

- Richter's hernia;
- gallstone ileus;
- mesenteric vascular occlusion;
- functional obstruction associated with pelvic abscess;
- all cases of partial obstruction (in which diarrhoea may occur).

Other manifestations

Dehydration

Dehydration is seen most commonly in small bowel obstruction because of repeated vomiting and fluid sequestration. It results in dry skin and tongue, poor venous filling and sunken eyes with oliguria. The blood urea level and haematocrit rise, giving a secondary polycythaemia.

Hypokalaemia

Hypokalaemia is not a common feature in simple mechanical obstruction. An increase in serum potassium, amylase or lactate dehydrogenase may be associated with the presence of strangulation, as may leukocytosis or leukopenia.

Pyrexia

Pyrexia in the presence of obstruction may indicate:

- the onset of ischaemia;
- intestinal perforation;
- inflammation or abscess associated with the obstructing disease.

Hypothermia indicates septicaemic shock or neglected cases of long duration.

Abdominal tenderness

Localised tenderness indicates impending or established ischaemia. The development of peritonism or peritonitis indicates impending or established infarction and/or perforation. In cases of large bowel obstruction, it is important to elicit these findings in the right iliac fossa as the caecum is most vulnerable to ischaemia.

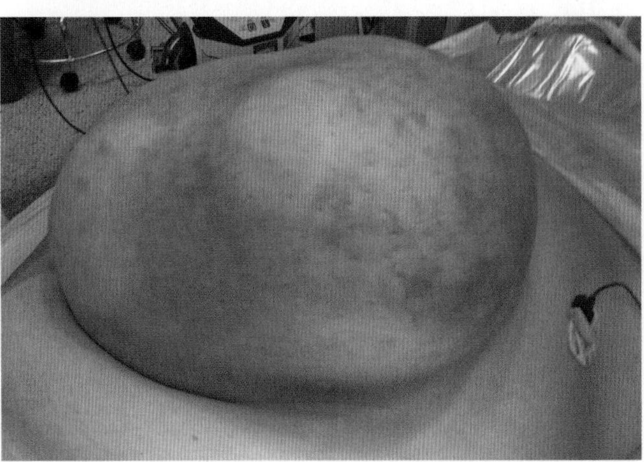

Figure 78.9 Skin discoloration over a strangulated incisional hernia.

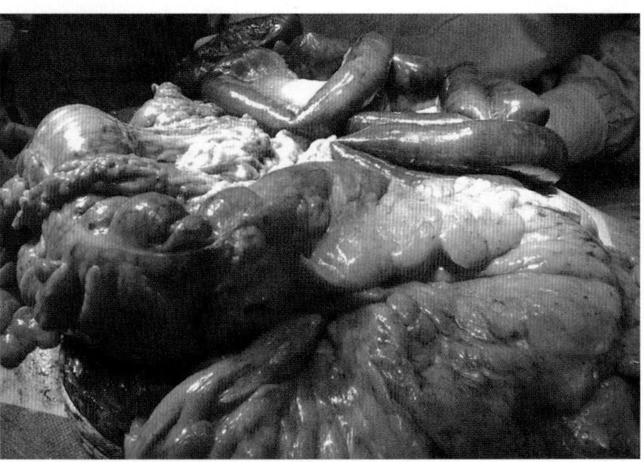

Figure 78.10 Ischaemic small and large bowel in a strangulated incisional hernia.

Bowel sounds

High-pitched bowel sounds are present in the vast majority of patients with intestinal obstruction. Normal bowel sounds are of negative predictive value. Bowel sounds may be scanty or absent if the obstruction is longstanding and the small bowel has become inactive.

Clinical features of strangulation

It is vital to distinguish strangulating from non-strangulating intestinal obstruction because the former is a surgical emergency. The diagnosis is clinical but may be aided by CT scanning as long as this does not delay surgical intervention.

Summary box 78.8

Clinical features of strangulation

- Constant pain, severe pain
- Tenderness with rigidity and peritonism
- Shock

In addition to the features in ***Summary box 78.8***, it should be noted that:

- The presence of shock suggests underlying ischaemia.
- In impending or established strangulation, pain is never completely absent.
- The presence and character of any local tenderness are of great significance and, however mild, tenderness requires frequent reassessment.
- Generalised tenderness and the presence of rigidity indicates the need for early laparotomy.
- When pain persists despite conservative management, even in the absence of the above signs, strangulation should be presumed.
- When strangulation occurs in an external hernia, the lump is tense, tender and irreducible and there is no expansile cough impulse. Skin changes with erythema or purplish discoloration are associated with underlying ischaemia (***Figures 78.9 and 78.10***).

Clinical features of intussusception

The classic presentation of intussusception is with episodes of screaming and drawing up of the legs in a previously well male infant. The attacks last for a few minutes and recur repeatedly. During attacks the child appears pale and between episodes may be listless. Vomiting may or may not occur at the outset but becomes conspicuous and bile-stained with time. Initially, the passage of stool may be normal, whereas, later, blood and mucus are evacuated – the 'redcurrant jelly' stool.

Whenever possible, examination should be undertaken between episodes of colic, without disturbing the child. Classically, the abdomen is not initially distended; a lump that hardens on palpation may be discerned but this is present in only 60% of cases (*Figure 78.11*). There may be an associated feeling of emptiness in the right iliac fossa (the sign of Dance). On rectal examination, blood-stained mucus may be found on the finger. Occasionally, in extensive ileocolic or colocolic intussusception, the apex may be palpable or even protrude from the anus.

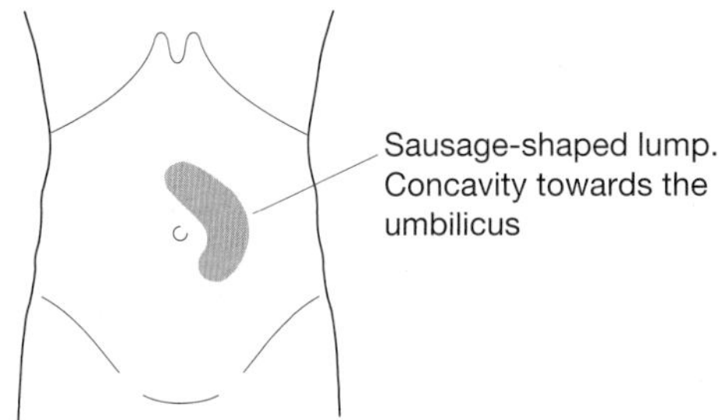

Figure 78.11 The physical signs as recorded by Hamilton Bailey in a typical case of intussusception in an infant.

Unrelieved, progressive dehydration and abdominal distension from small bowel obstruction will occur, followed by peritonitis secondary to gangrene. Rarely, natural cure may occur as a result of sloughing of the intussusception.

Differential diagnosis

Acute gastroenteritis

Although abdominal pain and vomiting are common in acute gastroenteritis, with occasional blood and mucus in the stool, diarrhoea is a leading symptom and faecal matter or bile is always present in the stool.

Henoch-Schönlein purpura

Henoch–Schönlein purpura is associated with a characteristic rash and abdominal pain; intussusception may occur.

Clinical features of volvulus

Volvulus of the small intestine

This may be primary or secondary and usually occurs in the lower ileum. It may occur spontaneously in African people, particularly following the consumption of a large volume of vegetable matter, whereas in western countries it is usually secondary to adhesions passing to the parietes or female pelvic organs.

Caecal volvulus

This may occur as part of volvulus neonatorum or *de novo* and is usually a clockwise twist. It is more common in females in the fourth and fifth decades and usually presents acutely with the classic features of obstruction. Ischaemia is common. At first the obstruction may be partial, with the passage of flatus and faeces. In 25% of cases, examination may reveal a palpable tympanic swelling in the midline or left side of the abdomen. The volvulus typically results in the caecum lying in the left upper quadrant. The diagnosis is not usually made preoperatively.

Sigmoid volvulus

The symptoms are of large bowel obstruction. Presentation varies in severity and acuteness, with younger patients appearing to develop the more acute form. Abdominal distension is an early and progressive sign, which may be associated with hiccough and retching. Constipation is absolute. In the elderly, a more chronic form may be seen. In some patients the grossly distended torted left colon is visible through the abdominal wall.

IMAGING

Erect abdominal films are no longer routinely obtained and the radiological diagnosis is based on a supine abdominal film (*Figure 78.12*). An erect film may subsequently be requested when further doubt exists.

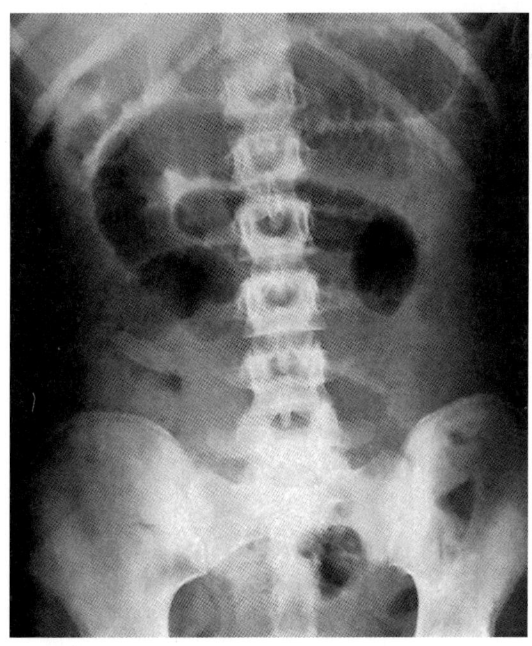

Figure 78.12 Gas-filled small bowel loops illustrating valvulae conniventes; patient supine.

Henry Hamilton Bailey, 1894–1961, surgeon, The Royal Northern Hospital, London, UK.
Jean Baptiste Hippolyte Dance, 1797–1832, physician, Hôpital Cochin, Paris, France.

When distended with gas, the jejunum, ileum, caecum and remaining colon have a characteristic appearance in adults and older children that allows them to be distinguished radiologically.

Summary box 78.9

Radiological features of obstruction (on plain radiograph)

- The obstructed small bowel is characterised by straight segments that are generally central and lie transversely. No/minimal gas is seen in the colon
- The jejunum is characterised by its valvulae conniventes, which completely pass across the width of the bowel and are regularly spaced, giving a 'concertina' or ladder effect
- Ileum – the distal ileum is featureless
- A distended caecum appears as a rounded gas shadow in the right iliac fossa
- Large bowel, except for the caecum, shows haustral folds, which, unlike valvulae conniventes, are spaced irregularly, do not cross the whole diameter of the bowel and do not have indentations placed opposite one another
- Small bowel fluid levels may be seen on an erect abdominal radiograph

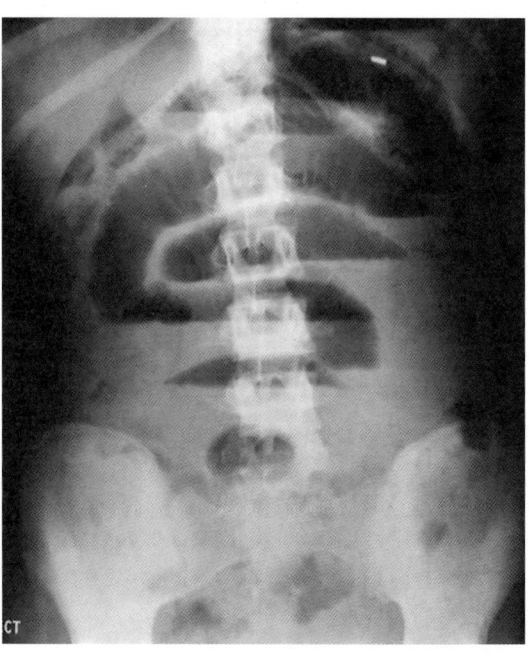

Figure 78.13 Fluid levels with gas above; 'stepladder pattern'. Ileal obstruction caused by adhesions (erect abdominal radiograph).

Fluid levels seen radiologically appear later than gas shadows as it takes time for gas and fluid to separate (***Figure 78.13***). These are most prominent on an erect abdominal radiograph or cross-sectional imaging. In adults, two inconstant fluid levels – one at the duodenal cap and the other in the terminal ileum – may be regarded as normal. In infants (less than 1 year old), a few fluid levels in the small bowel may be physiological. In this age group it is difficult to distinguish large from small bowel in the presence of obstruction because the characteristic features seen in adults are not present or are unreliable.

During the obstructive process, fluid levels become more conspicuous and more numerous when paralysis has occurred. When fluid levels are pronounced, the obstruction is advanced. In the small bowel, the number of fluid levels is directly proportional to the degree of obstruction and to its site, the number increasing the more distal the lesion.

In patients without evidence of strangulation there is a role for other imaging modalities. The appearance of contrast in the colon 4–24 hours after administration of 50–100 mL of water-soluble contrast agent had a sensitivity of 96% and a specificity of 98% in predicting resolution of small bowel obstruction. If contrast does not reach the colon, surgery is required in approximately 90% of patients. Administration of a water-soluble agent was also effective in reducing the need for surgery and shortening the duration of hospital stay.

Low colonic obstruction does not commonly give rise to small bowel fluid levels unless advanced, whereas high colonic obstruction may do so in the presence of an incompetent ileocaecal valve. Colonic obstruction is usually associated with a large amount of gas in the caecum. A limited water-soluble enema can be undertaken to differentiate large bowel obstruction from pseudo-obstruction. A barium follow-through is contraindicated in the presence of acute obstruction and may be life-threatening.

CT scanning is now used very widely to investigate all forms of intestinal obstruction. It is highly accurate and its only limitations are in diagnosing ischaemia. Two features may be helpful when looking for intestinal ischaemia: reduced enhancement of the bowel wall and absence of mesenteric oedema. It is important to remember that, even with the best imaging techniques, the diagnosis of strangulation remains primarily clinical.

Summary box 78.10

CT features of strangulation

- Reduced bowel wall enhancement on CT increases the probability of strangulation
- Absence of mesenteric fluid on CT decreases the probability of strangulation
- The clinical reliability of other CT signs is doubtful for predicting strangulation

Impacted foreign bodies may be seen on abdominal radiographs. It is noteworthy that gas-filled loops and fluid levels in the small and large bowel can also be seen in established paralytic ileus and pseudo-obstruction (see ***Chapter 73***). The former can, however, normally be distinguished on clinical grounds whereas the latter can be confirmed radiologically. Fluid levels may also be seen in non-obstructing conditions such as gastroenteritis, acute pancreatitis and intra-abdominal sepsis.

Imaging in intussusception

A plain abdominal field usually reveals evidence of small or large bowel obstruction with an absent caecal gas shadow in ileocolic cases. A soft-tissue opacity is often visible in children. A barium enema may be used to diagnose the presence of an ileocolic intussusception but does not demonstrate small bowel intussusception. Abdominal ultrasonography has a high diagnostic sensitivity in children, demonstrating the typical doughnut appearance of concentric rings in transverse section. CT scanning is currently considered the most sensitive radiological method to confirm intussusception, with a reported diagnostic accuracy of 58–100%. The characteristic features of CT scan include a 'target'- or 'sausage'-shaped soft-tissue mass with a layering effect (***Figure 78.6***); mesenteric vessels within the bowel lumen are also typical.

Imaging in volvulus

- In caecal volvulus, radiological abnormalities are identifiable in nearly all patients but are often non-specific, with caecal dilatation (98–100%), a single air–fluid level (72–88%), small bowel dilatation (42–55%) and absence of gas in distal colon (82–91%) reported as the most common abnormalities. A barium enema may be used to confirm the diagnosis if there are no concerns about ischaemia, with an absence of barium in the caecum and a bird's beak deformity. CT scanning is now the imaging of choice.
- In sigmoid volvulus, a plain radiograph shows massive colonic distension. The classic appearance is of a dilated loop of bowel; the two limbs are seen running diagonally across the abdomen from right to left (***Figure 78.14***) with two fluid levels seen, one within each loop of bowel (if an erect film is taken).
- In volvulus neonatorum, the abdominal radiograph shows a variable appearance. Initially, it may appear normal or show evidence of duodenal obstruction but, as the intestinal strangulation progresses, the abdomen becomes relatively gasless.

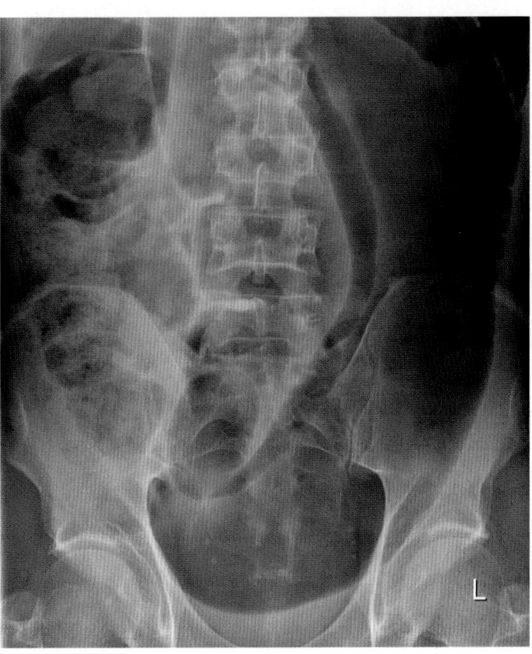

Figure 78.14 Supine abdominal radiograph showing sigmoid volvulus.

TREATMENT OF ACUTE INTESTINAL OBSTRUCTION

There are three main measures used to treat acute intestinal obstruction.

Summary box 78.11

Treatment of acute intestinal obstruction

- Gastrointestinal drainage via a nasogastric tube
- Fluid and electrolyte replacement
- Relief of obstruction
- Surgical treatment is necessary for most cases of intestinal obstruction but should be delayed until resuscitation is complete, provided there is no sign of strangulation or evidence of closed-loop obstruction

The first two steps are always necessary before attempting surgical relief of obstruction and are the mainstay of postoperative management.

Summary box 78.12

Principles of surgical intervention for obstruction

Management of:

- The segment at the site of obstruction
- The distended proximal bowel
- The underlying cause of obstruction

Supportive management

Nasogastric decompression is achieved by the passage of a non-vented (Ryle) or vented (Salem) tube. The tubes are normally placed on free drainage with 4-hourly aspiration but may be placed on continuous or intermittent suction. As well as facilitating decompression proximal to the obstruction, they are essential to reducing the risk of subsequent aspiration during induction of anaesthesia and after extubation.

The basic biochemical abnormality in intestinal obstruction is sodium and water loss, and therefore the appropriate replacement is Hartmann's solution or normal saline. The volume required varies and should be determined by clinical haematological and biochemical criteria.

John Alfred Ryle, 1889–1950, Regius Professor of Physic, University of Cambridge, and later Professor of Social Medicine, University of Oxford, UK, introduced the Ryle's tube in 1921.
Henri Albert Charles Antoine Hartmann, 1860–1952, Professor of Clinical Surgery, University of Paris, Paris, France.

Surgical treatment

The timing of surgical intervention is dependent on the clinical picture. There are several indications for early surgical intervention.

> **Summary box 78.13**
>
> **Indications for early surgical intervention**
> - Obstructed external hernia
> - Clinical features of intestinal strangulation
> - Obstruction in a previously unoperated abdomen

The classic clinical advice that 'the Sun should not both rise and set' on a case of unrelieved acute intestinal obstruction was based on the concern that intestinal ischaemia would develop while the patient was waiting for surgery. If there is complete obstruction, but no evidence of intestinal ischaemia, it is reasonable to defer surgery until the patient has been adequately resuscitated. Where obstruction is likely to be secondary to adhesions, conservative management may be continued for up to 72 hours in the hope of spontaneous resolution.

If the site of obstruction is unknown, adequate exposure is best achieved by a midline laparotomy incision. Assessment is directed to:

- the site of the obstruction;
- the nature of the obstruction;
- the viability of the gut.

In cases of small bowel obstruction, the first manoeuvre is to deliver the distended small bowel into the wound. This permits access to the site of obstruction. The small bowel should be covered with moist swabs and the weight of the fluid-filled bowel supported such that the blood supply to the mesentery is not impaired.

Operative decompression should be performed whenever possible. The simplest and safest method is to insert a large-bore orogastric tube and to milk the small bowel contents in a retrograde manner to the stomach for aspiration. Great care must be taken not to tear the mesentery or injure the small bowel, which will be distended and oedematous. It is important to ensure that the stomach is empty at the end of the procedure to reduce the incidence of postoperative aspiration. Decompression using Savage's decompressor within a seromuscular purse-string suture may be required. Its benefits should be balanced against the potential risk of septic complications from spillage and the risk of leakage from the suture line postoperatively.

The type of surgical procedure required will depend upon the cause of obstruction: division of adhesions (enterolysis), excision, bypass or proximal decompression. If resection is performed, Savage's decompressor can be inserted into this segment to obviate the risk of a suture line.

Following relief of obstruction, the viability of the involved bowel should be carefully assessed (***Table 78.3***). Although frankly infarcted bowel is obvious, viability in many cases may be difficult to discern. If in doubt, the bowel should be wrapped in hot packs for 10 minutes and then reassessed. The state of the mesenteric vessels and pulsation in adjacent arcades should be sought. Viability is also confirmed by colour, sheen and peristalsis. If, at the end of this period, there is still uncertainty about bowel viability, it should be resected unless there is concern that the extent of resection may lead to short bowel syndrome (see ***Chapter 74***). In which case, or in the case of a critically unwell patient, consideration should be given to resecting necrotic bowel and raising both residual ends as stomas. This avoids anastomosis in unfavourable circumstances. When no resection has been undertaken or there are multiple ischaemic areas (mesenteric vascular occlusion), a second-look laparotomy at 24–48 hours may be required.

Intestinal ischaemia/reperfusion injury has been described following reperfusion of ischaemic bowel with remote lung injury resulting from the release of inflammatory mediators. This should be borne in mind when dealing with ischaemic bowel. For example, if there is a volvulus with established infarction, detorsion should be avoided until the affected mesentery has been clamped and thus reperfusion injury prevented.

TABLE 78.3 Differentiation between viable and non-viable intestine.

	Viable	Non-viable
Circulation	Dark colour becomes lighter Visible pulsation in mesenteric arteries	Dark colour remains No detectable pulsation
General appearance	Shiny	Dull and lustreless
Intestinal musculature	Firm	Flabby, thin and friable
	Peristalsis may be observed	No peristalsis

Special attention should always be paid to the sites of constriction at each end of an obstructed segment. If of doubtful viability, they should be infolded using a seromuscular suture (***Figure 78.15***).

The surgical management of massive infarction is dependent on the patient's overall prognostic criteria. In the elderly, infarction of the small bowel from the duodenojejunal flexure to the right colon may be considered incurable, whereas in the young, with the potential for long-term intravenous alimentation and small bowel transplantation, a policy of excision may be justified.

Whenever the small bowel is resected, the exact site of resection, the length of the resected segment and that of the residual bowel should be recorded.

As laparoscopic surgery is now so common, it is important to note that small bowel obstruction and strangulation occur in relation to port-site hernias. The risk of port-site herniation is related to older age, higher body mass, trocar diameter and extension of the port site for tissue extraction.

Paul Thwaites Savage, 1916–2013, surgeon, Whittington Hospital, London, UK.

For laparoscopic cholecystectomy, the hernia rate is reported to be around 2%. Obstruction and strangulation have even been reported through 5-mm port sites. Complications from these hernias may present in the early postoperative period and as a Richter's hernia. They can be easily overlooked and careful examination of port sites in patients with small bowel obstruction is essential.

Treatment of adhesions

Initial management is based on intravenous rehydration and nasogastric decompression; occasionally, this treatment is curative. Although an initial conservative regimen is considered appropriate, regular assessment is mandatory to ensure that strangulation does not occur. Conservative treatment should not usually be prolonged beyond 72 hours.

When laparotomy is required, although multiple adhesions may be found, only one may be causative. If there is absolute certainty that this is the cause of the obstruction, this should be divided and the remaining adhesions can be left *in situ* unless severe angulation is present. Division of these adhesions will only cause further adhesion formation.

When obstruction is caused by multiple adhesions, the adhesions should be freed by sharp dissection from the duodenojejunal junction to the caecum. Following the release of band obstruction, the constriction sites that have suffered direct compression should be carefully assessed and, if they show residual colour changes, invaginated with a seromuscular suture (***Figure 78.15***).

Laparoscopic adhesiolysis may be considered in highly selected cases of small bowel obstruction. This is classed as an advanced laparoscopic procedure and should only be undertaken by surgeons with advanced laparoscopic skills.

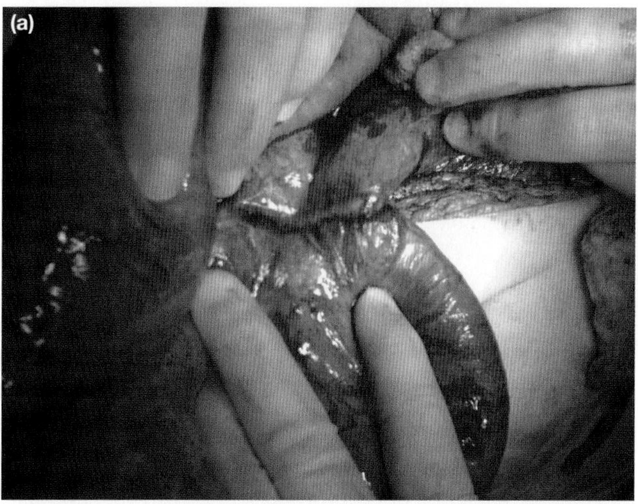

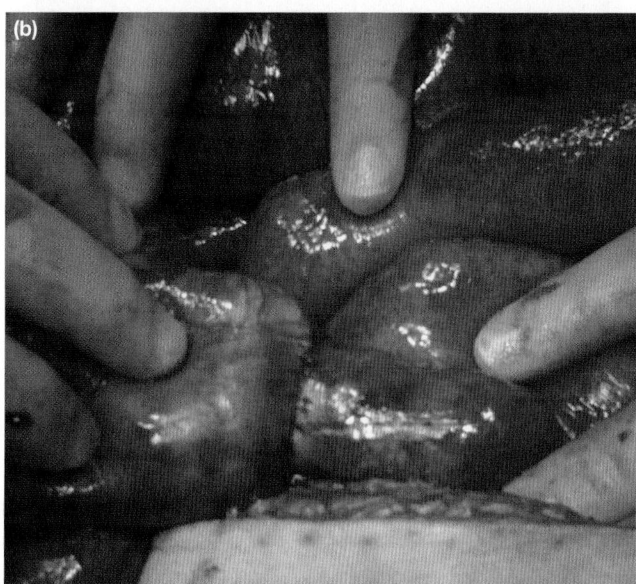

Figure 78.15 (a, b) Wall injury resulting from band compression, oversewn with an absorbable seromuscular suture.

Summary box 78.14

Treatment of adhesive obstruction

- Initially treat conservatively provided there are no signs of strangulation; should rarely continue conservative treatment for longer than 72 hours
- At operation, divide only the causative adhesion(s) and limit dissection
- Repair serosal tears; invaginate (or resect) areas of doubtful viability
- Laparoscopic adhesiolysis should only be performed by surgeons with advanced laparoscopic skills

Treatment of recurrent intestinal obstruction caused by adhesions

Several procedures may be considered in the presence of recurrent obstruction including:

- repeat adhesiolysis (enterolysis) alone;
- Noble's plication operation;
- Childs–Phillips transmesenteric plication;
- intestinal intubation.

The last three operations are now very rarely performed and can probably be consigned to the history books (they have never been required by the author).

Postoperative intestinal obstruction

Differentiation between persistent paralytic ileus and early mechanical obstruction may be difficult in the early postoperative period. Mechanical obstruction is more likely if the patient has regained bowel function postoperatively that subsequently stops. Obstruction is usually incomplete and the majority settle with continued conservative management. Postoperative

Thomas Benjamin Noble, 1895–1965, surgeon, The Community Hospital, Indianapolis, IN, USA.
Wesley A Childs, 1915–2005, surgeon, University of Colorado, Denver, CO, USA.
Richard B Phillips, surgeon, Albuquerque, NM, USA.

intra-abdominal sepsis is a potent cause of postoperative obstruction; CT scanning with oral contrast is of particular value in the assessment of the postoperative abdomen.

Treatment of intussusception

In the infant with ileocolic intussusception, after resuscitation with intravenous fluids, broad-spectrum antibiotics and nasogastric drainage, non-operative reduction can be attempted using an air or barium enema. Successful reduction can only be accepted if there is free reflux of air or barium into the small bowel, together with resolution of symptoms and signs in the patient. Non-operative reduction is contraindicated if there are signs of peritonitis or perforation, there is a known pathological lead point or in the presence of profound shock. In experienced units, more than 70% of intussusceptions can be reduced non-operatively. Strangulated bowel and pathological lead points are unlikely to reduce. Perforation of the colon during pneumatic or hydrostatic reduction is a recognised hazard but is rare. Recurrent intussusception occurs in up to 10% of patients after non-operative reduction.

Surgery is required when radiological reduction has failed or is contraindicated. After resuscitation, a transverse right-sided abdominal incision provides good access. Reduction is achieved by gently compressing the most distal part of the intussusception towards its origin, making sure not to pull. The last part of the reduction is the most difficult (***Figure 78.16***). After reduction, the terminal part of the small bowel and the appendix will be seen to be bruised and oedematous. The viability of the whole bowel should be checked carefully. An irreducible intussusception or one complicated by infarction or a pathological lead point requires resection and primary anastomosis.

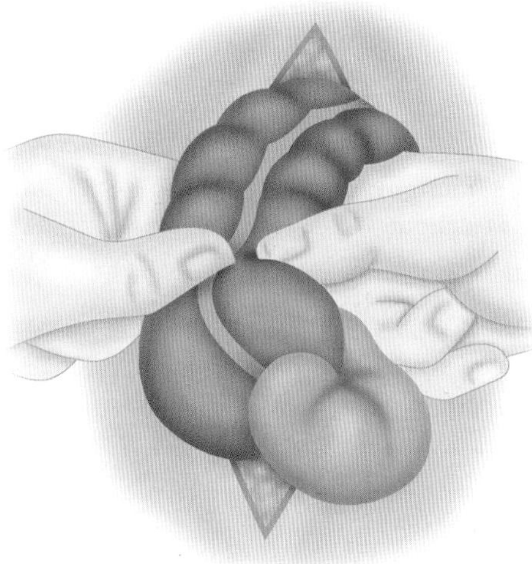

Figure 78.16 Reducing the terminal part of the intussusception (after RE Gross).

Acute intestinal obstruction of the newborn

Neonatal intestinal obstruction has many potential causes. Congenital atresia and stenosis are the most common. Intestinal malrotation with midgut volvulus, meconium ileus, Hirschsprung's disease, imperforate anus, necrotising enterocolitis and an incarcerated inguinal hernia may also be responsible. Many of these conditions are discussed in ***Chapters 17 and 18***.

Intestinal atresia

Duodenal atresia and stenosis are the most common forms of intestinal obstruction in the newborn (see ***Chapter 18***). Jejunal or ileal atresias are next in frequency whereas colonic atresia is rare. The possibility of multiple atresias makes intraoperative assessment of the whole small and large bowel mandatory. As with all congenital anomalies, associated malformations are common and should be excluded.

There are four main types of jejunal/ileal atresia, ranging from an obstructing membrane with continuity of the bowel wall through blind-ended segments of bowel separated by a fibrous cord or V-shaped mesenteric defect (including the so-called apple-peel atresia) (***Figure 78.17***), to multiple atresias ('string of sausages'). The obstructed proximal bowel is at risk of perforation, which may happen prenatally, causing meconium peritonitis in the fetus.

Small bowel atresias present with intestinal obstruction soon after birth. Bilious vomiting is the dominant feature in jejunal atresia whereas abdominal distension is more prominent with ileal atresia. A small amount of pale meconium may be passed despite the atresia.

Plain abdominal radiographs show a variable number of dilated loops of bowel and fluid levels according to the level of obstruction. In a stable infant, a contrast enema may be required to clarify the cause of a distal bowel obstruction.

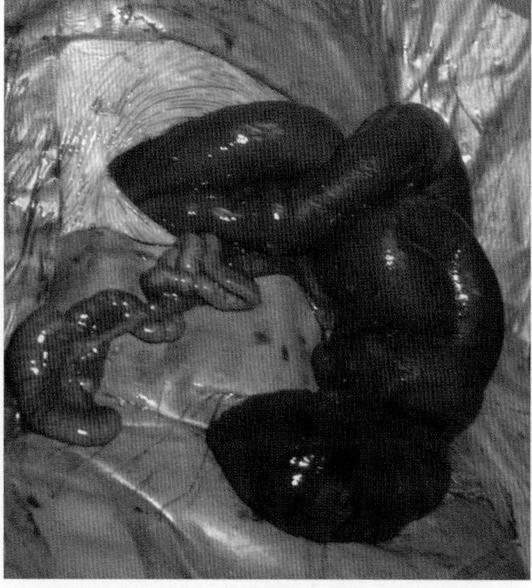

Figure 78.17 Apple-peel jejunal bowel atresia with obstructed proximal jejunum and collapsed distal ileum coiled round a remnant ileocolic artery (courtesy of MD Stringer, Leeds, UK).

Harald Hirschsprung, 1830–1916, physician, The Queen Louise Hospital for Children, Copenhagen, Denmark, described congenital megacolon in 1887.

Surgery

Duodenal atresia is corrected by a duodenoduodenostomy. In most cases of jejunal/ileal atresia, the distal end of the dilated proximal small bowel is resected and a primary end-to-end anastomosis is possible. If the proximal bowel is extremely dilated it may need to be tapered to the distal bowel before anastomosis. Occasionally, a temporary stoma is required before definitive repair.

Meconium ileus

Cystic fibrosis is almost always the underlying cause of this condition. Meconium is normally kept fluid by the action of pancreatic enzymes. In meconium ileus the terminal ileum becomes filled with thick viscid meconium, resulting in progressive intestinal obstruction. A sterile meconium peritonitis may have occurred *in utero*.

Visibly dilated loops of bowel are often palpable in the newborn with meconium ileus. An abdominal radiograph may show a dilated small intestine with mottling. Fluid levels are generally not seen. Unlike ileal atresia there is no abrupt termination of the gas-filled intestine. A contrast enema shows an unused microcolon. As the condition is caused by an autosomal recessive genetic defect, a family history may be present. Further assessment includes gene mutation analysis and, beyond the neonatal period, a sweat test, which shows elevated sodium and chloride levels (>70 mmol/L).

Uncomplicated meconium ileus may respond to treatment with a hyperosmolar Gastrografin enema; this draws fluid into the gut lumen and also has detergent properties, which help to liquefy the meconium. Infants treated in this way need extra intravenous fluids to compensate for fluid shifts. Meconium ileus complicated by intestinal perforation, volvulus or atresia, or unresponsive to enemas, demands surgery. Various surgical procedures are used, including intestinal resection and temporary stoma formation, resection and primary anastomosis, and, in uncomplicated cases, enterotomy and irrigation of the bowel. The Bishop–Koop operation (***Figure 78.18***) with its irrigating stoma is now rarely used.

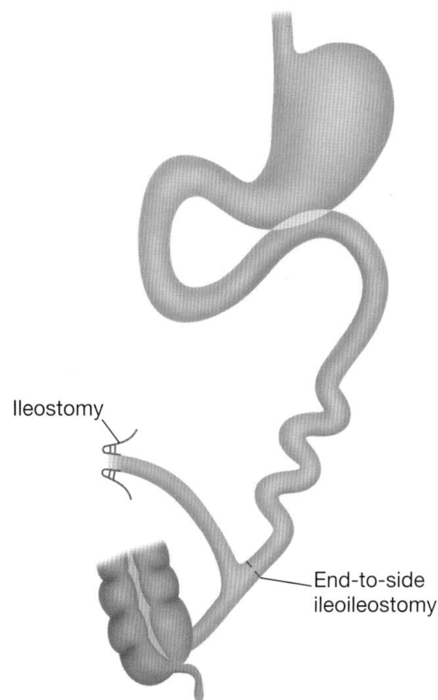

Figure 78.18 Bishop–Koop operation. This shows the completed procedure after a grossly distended ileum has been resected. Because intestinal continuity is preserved, early closure of the ileostomy is not essential.

TREATMENT OF ACUTE LARGE BOWEL OBSTRUCTION

Large bowel obstruction is caused by an underlying carcinoma or less commonly diverticular disease and presents in an acute or chronic form. The condition of pseudo-obstruction should always be considered and excluded by a limited contrast study or CT scan to confirm mechanical obstruction.

After full resuscitation, the abdomen should be opened through a midline incision. Care should be taken to ensure that the loss of tamponade of the abdominal wall does not lead to increased caecal distension and rupture (this starts with splitting along the line of the taenia coli on the antimesenteric border). Distension of the caecum will confirm large bowel involvement. Identification of a collapsed distal segment of the large bowel and its sequential proximal assessment will readily lead to identification of the cause. As surgery for malignant bowel cancer is technically challenging, wherever possible a suitably trained surgeon should perform the procedure. When a removable lesion is found in the caecum, ascending colon, hepatic flexure or proximal transverse colon, an emergency right hemicolectomy should be performed. A primary anastomosis is safe if the patient's general condition is reasonable (see ***Chapter 77***). If the lesion is not resectable a proximal stoma (colostomy or ileostomy if the ileocaecal valve is incompetent) or ileotransverse bypass should be considered. Obstructing lesions at the splenic flexure should be treated by an extended right hemicolectomy with ileo-descending colonic anastomosis.

For obstructing lesions of the left colon or rectosigmoid junction, immediate resection should be considered unless there are clear contraindications. In rare instances or when caecal perforation is imminent, additional time to improve the patient's clinical condition can be bought by performing an emergency caecostomy or loop transverse colostomy (loop ileostomy in the presence of an incompetent ileocaecal valve).

In the absence of senior clinical staff, it is safest to bring the proximal colon to the surface as a colostomy. When possible the distal bowel should be brought out at the same time (Paul–Mikulicz procedure) to facilitate subsequent closure. In the majority of cases, the distal bowel will not reach and is

Harry C Bishop, 1921–2009, Professor of Surgery, University of Philadelphia, Philadelphia, PA, USA.
Charles Everett Koop, 1916–2013, paediatric surgeon and public health administrator, served as the 13th Surgeon General of the USA (1982–1989).
Frank Thomas Paul, 1851–1941, surgeon, The Royal Infirmary, Liverpool, UK.
Johann von Mikulicz-Radecki, 1850–1905, Professor of Surgery, Breslau, Germany (now Wrocław, Poland).

closed and returned to the abdomen (Hartmann's procedure). A second-stage colorectal anastomosis can be planned when the patient is fit.

If an anastomosis is to be considered using the proximal colon, it may be decompressed and cleaned by an on-table colonic lavage.

In a palliative situation or if a patient is unfit for major surgery insertion of a self-expanding metal stent may be preferable as it offers reduced mortality and morbidity and stoma formation (see ***Chapter 77***). Technical and clinical success rates for stenting are of the order of 80–90% (***Figure 78.19***).

For patients with potentially curative disease, stenting as a bridge to surgery (usually performed 1–4 weeks post stenting) has been shown to reduce stoma formation but not to reduce postoperative mortality. Recent guidelines from the European Society of Gastrointestinal Endoscopy recommend stenting as a bridge to surgery to be discussed, within a shared decision-making process, as a treatment option in patients with potentially curable left-sided obstructing colon cancer as an alternative to emergency resection. This is a strong recommendation based on high-quality evidence. Colonic stenting should be performed or directly supervised by an operator who can demonstrate competence in both colonoscopy and fluoroscopic techniques and who performs colonic stenting on a regular basis. A time interval of 2–4 weeks is generally employed prior to definitive surgery. This period allows treatment of comorbidities and completion of staging investigations. A decompressing stoma as a bridge to elective surgery is a valid option if the patient is not a candidate for colonic stenting or when stenting expertise is not available.

Treatment of caecal volvulus

At operation the volvulus is frequently found to be ischaemic and needs resection. If viable, the volvulus should be reduced. Sometimes, this can only be achieved after decompression of the caecum using a needle. Further management consists of either resection or fixation of the caecum to the right iliac fossa (caecopexy) and/or a caecostomy in those considered unfit for resection. Recurrence of volvulus after caecopexy has been reported in up to 40% of cases.

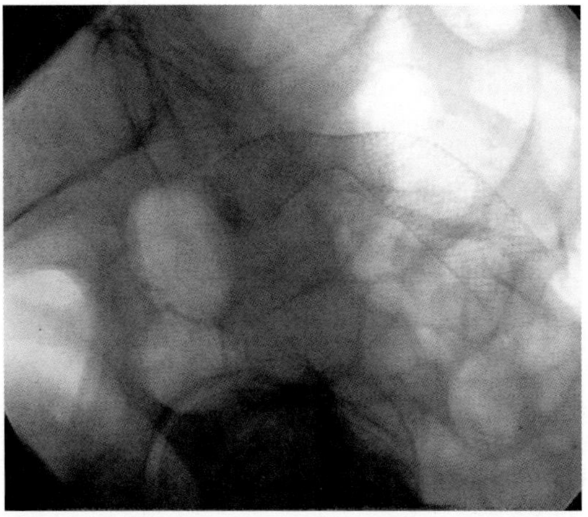

Figure 78.19 Radiograph of a stent inserted for malignant colonic obstruction.

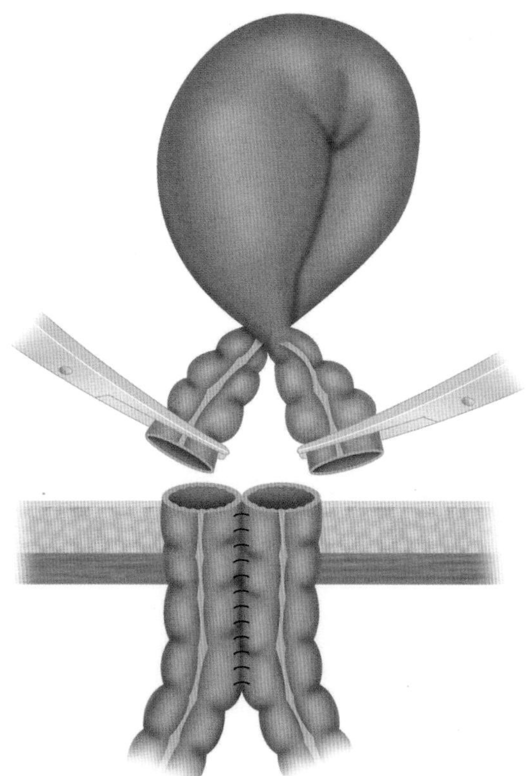

Figure 78.20 The Paul–Mikulicz operation applied to volvulus of the pelvic colon.

Treatment of sigmoid volvulus

Flexible sigmoidoscopy or rigid sigmoidoscopy and insertion of a flatus tube should be carried out to allow deflation of the gut. The tube should be secured in place with tape for 24 hours and a repeat radiograph taken to ensure that decompression has occurred. Success, as long as ischaemic bowel is excluded, will resolve the acute problem.

In fit patients, an elective sigmoid colectomy is required. It may not be reasonable to offer any further treatment following successful endoscopic decompression in elderly or unfit patients; however, if there are recurrent episodes of volvulus, the options are resection or two-point fixation with combined endoscopic/percutaneous tube insertion (gastrostomy tubes are frequently used for this purpose).

When the bowel is viable, fixation of the sigmoid colon to the posterior abdominal wall may be a safer manoeuvre in inexperienced hands. Resection is preferable if it can be achieved safely. A Paul–Mikulicz procedure is useful, particularly if there is suspicion of impending gangrene (***Figure 78.20***); an alternative procedure is a sigmoid colectomy and, when anastomosis is considered unwise, a Hartmann's procedure with subsequent reanastomosis can be carried out.

CHRONIC LARGE BOWEL OBSTRUCTION

The symptoms of chronic intestinal obstruction may arise from two sources: the cause and the subsequent obstruction.

The causes of obstruction may be organic:

- intraluminal (rare) – faecal impaction;
- intrinsic intramural – strictures (Crohn's disease, ischaemia, diverticular), anastomotic stenosis;
- extrinsic intramural (rare) – metastatic deposits (ovarian), endometriosis, stomal stenosis;

or functional:

- Hirschsprung's disease, idiopathic megacolon, pseudo-obstruction.

The symptoms of chronic obstruction differ in their predominance, timing and degree from acute obstruction. In functional cases, the symptoms may have been present for months or years. Constipation appears first. It is initially relative and may become absolute, associated with distension. In the presence of large bowel disease, the point of greatest distension is in the caecum, and this is heralded by the onset of pain. Vomiting is a late feature and therefore dehydration is less severe. Examination is unremarkable, save for confirmation of distension, which can be profound (***Figure 78.21***) and the onset of peritonism in late cases. Rectal examination may confirm the presence of faecal impaction or a tumour.

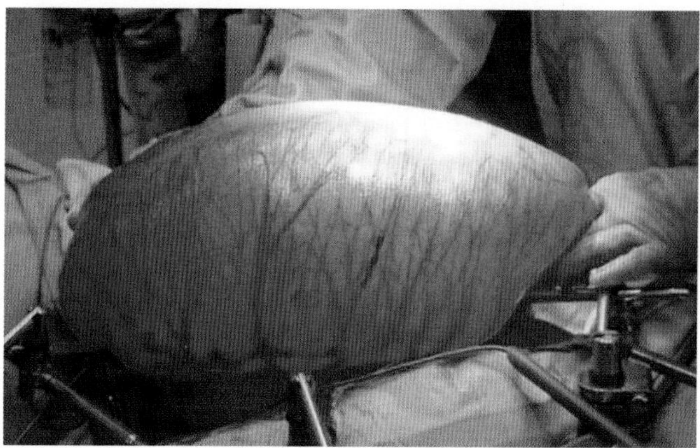

Figure 78.21 Gross functional colonic distension.

Investigation

Plain abdominal radiography confirms the presence of large bowel distension. All such cases should be investigated by a subsequent single-contrast water-soluble enema study, CT scan or endoscopic assessment to rule out functional disease.

Organic disease requires decompression with either a laparotomy or stent. Stomal stenosis can usually be managed at the abdominal wall level. Surgical management after resuscitation depends on the underlying cause and the relevant chapters in this book should be consulted.

Functional disease requires colonoscopic decompression in the first instance and conservative management. Intestinal perforation can occur in patients with functional obstruction (see ***Chapter 73***).

ADYNAMIC OBSTRUCTION

Paralytic ileus

This may be defined as a state in which there is failure of transmission of peristaltic waves secondary to neuromuscular failure (i.e. in the myenteric [Auerbach's] and submucous [Meissner's] plexuses). The resultant stasis leads to accumulation of fluid and gas within the bowel, with associated distension, vomiting, absence of bowel sounds and absolute constipation.

Varieties

The following varieties are recognised:

- **Postoperative**: a degree of ileus usually occurs after any abdominal procedure and is self-limiting, with a variable duration of 24–72 hours. Postoperative ileus may be prolonged in the presence of hypoproteinaemia or metabolic abnormality.
- **Infection**: intra-abdominal sepsis may give rise to localised or generalised ileus.
- **Reflex ileus**: this may occur following fractures of the spine or ribs, retroperitoneal haemorrhage or even the application of a plaster jacket.
- **Metabolic**: uraemia and hypokalaemia are the most common contributory factors.

Clinical features

Paralytic ileus takes on a clinical significance if, 72 hours after laparotomy:

- there has been no return of bowel sounds on auscultation;
- there has been no passage of flatus.

Abdominal distension becomes more marked and tympanitic. Colicky pain is not a feature. Distension increases pain from the abdominal wound. In the absence of gastric aspiration, effortless vomiting may occur. Radiologically, the abdomen shows gas-filled loops of intestine with multiple fluid levels (if an erect film is felt necessary).

Management

Nasogastric tubes are not required routinely after elective intra-abdominal surgery. Paralytic ileus is managed with the use of nasogastric suction and restriction of oral intake until bowel sounds and the passage of flatus return. Electrolyte balance must be maintained. The use of an enhanced recovery programme with early introduction of fluids and solids is, however, becoming increasingly popular (see ***Chapter 73***).

Specific treatment is directed towards the cause, but the following general principles apply:

- If a primary cause is identified this must be treated.
- Gastrointestinal distension must be relieved by decompression.

Leopold Auerbach, 1828–1897, Professor of Neuropathology, Breslau, Germany (now Wrocław, Poland), described the myenteric plexus in 1862.
Georg Meissner, 1829–1905, Professor of Physiology, Göttingen, Germany, described the submucous plexus of the alimentary tract in 1852.

- Close attention to fluid and electrolyte balance is essential.
- There is no convincing evidence for the use of prokinetic drugs to treat postoperative adynamic ileus.
- If paralytic ileus is prolonged CT scanning will demonstrate any intra-abdominal sepsis or mechanical obstruction and therefore guide any requirement for laparotomy.

The decision to take a patient back to theatre in these circumstances is always difficult. The need for a laparotomy becomes increasingly likely the longer the bowel inactivity persists, particularly if it lasts for more than 7 days or if bowel activity recommences following surgery and then ceases.

Pseudo-obstruction

This condition describes an obstruction, usually of the colon, that occurs in the absence of a mechanical cause or acute intra-abdominal disease. It is associated with a variety of syndromes in which there is an underlying neuropathy and/or myopathy and a range of other factors.

Small intestinal pseudo-obstruction

This condition may be primary (i.e. idiopathic or associated with familial visceral myopathy) or secondary. The clinical picture consists of recurrent subacute obstruction. The diagnosis is made by the exclusion of a mechanical cause. Treatment consists of initial correction of any underlying disorder. Metoclopramide and erythromycin may be of use.

Colonic pseudo-obstruction

This may occur in an acute or a chronic form. The former, also known as Ogilvie's syndrome, presents as acute large bowel obstruction. Abdominal radiographs show evidence of colonic obstruction, with marked caecal distension being a common feature. Indeed, caecal perforation is a well-recognised complication. The absence of a mechanical cause requires urgent confirmation by colonoscopy or a single-contrast water-soluble barium enema or CT. The aetiology, investigation and management are covered in detail in ***Chapter 73***.

FURTHER READING

Alavi K, Poylin V, Davids JS *et al.* American Society of Colon and Rectal Surgeons clinical practice guidelines for the management of colonic volvulus and acute colonic pseudo-obstruction. *Dis Colon Rectum* 2021; **64**: 1046–57.

Bickell NA, Federman AD, Aufses AH. Influence of time on risk of bowel resection in complete small bowel obstruction. *J Am Coll Surg* 2005; **201**: 847–54.

Ceresoli M, Coccolini F, Catena F *et al.* Water-soluble contrast agent in adhesive small bowel obstruction: a systematic review and meta-analysis of diagnostic and therapeutic value. *Am J Surg* 2016; **211**(6): 1114–25.

Fevang BT, Fevang J, Lie S *et al.* Long-term prognosis after operation for adhesive small bowel obstruction. *Ann Surg* 2004; **240**: 193–201.

Finan PJ, Campbell S, Verma R *et al.* The management of malignant large bowel obstruction: ACPGBI position statement. *Colorectal Dis* 2007; **9**(Suppl 4): 1–17.

Ha GW, Lee MR, Kim JH. Adhesive small bowel obstruction after laparoscopic and open colorectal surgery: a systematic review and meta-analysis. *Am J Surg* 2016; **212**(3): 527–36.

Miller AS, Boyce K, Box B *et al.* The Association of Coloproctology of Great Britain and Ireland consensus guidelines in emergency colorectal surgery. *Colorectal Dis* 2021; **23**: 476–547.

ten Broek RP, Stommel MW, Strik C *et al.* Benefits and harms of adhesion barriers for abdominal surgery: a systematic review and meta-analysis. *Lancet* 2014; **383**(9911): 48–59.

van Hooft JE, Veld J, Arnold D *et al.* Self-expandable metal stents for obstructing colonic and extracolonic cancer: European Society of Gastrointestinal Endoscopy (ESGE) Guideline – Update 2020. *Endoscopy* 2020; **52**: 389–407.

Vogel JD, Feingold DL, Stewart DB *et al.* Clinical practice guidelines for colonic volvulus and acute colonic pseudo-obstruction. *Dis Colon Rectum* 2016; **59**: 589–600.

Williams SB, Greenspon J, Young HA, Orkin BA. Small bowel obstruction: conservative vs. surgical management. *Dis Colon Rectum* 2005; **48**: 1140–6.

Wolthuis AM, Bislenghi G, Fieuws S *et al.* Incidence of prolonged postoperative ileus after colorectal surgery: a systematic review and meta-analysis. *Colorectal Dis* 2016; **18**: O1–9.

Sir William Heneage Ogilvie, 1887–1978, surgeon, Guy's Hospital, London, UK.

CHAPTER

79 The rectum

Learning objectives

To understand:
- The anatomy of the rectum and its relationship to surgical disease and its treatment
- The pathology, clinical presentation, investigation, differential diagnosis and treatment of diseases that affect the rectum

To appreciate:
- That carcinoma of the rectum is common and can present with symptoms similar to benign disease. Careful evaluation is required
- The principles involved in the management of rectal pathologies

ANATOMY

Surgical anatomy

The rectum begins where the tinea coli of the sigmoid colon join to form a continuous outer longitudinal muscle layer at the level of the sacral promontory. The rectum follows the curve of the sacrum and ends at the anorectal junction. The puborectalis muscle encircles the posterior and lateral aspects of the junction, creating the anorectal angle (normally 120°). The rectum has three lateral curvatures; the upper and lower are convex to the right, and the middle is convex to the left. On the luminal aspect, these three curves are marked by semicircular folds (valves of Houston).

The adult rectum is approximately 12–18 cm in length and is conventionally divided into three equal parts: the upper third, which is mobile and has a peritoneal covering anteriorly and laterally; the middle third, where the peritoneum covers only the anterior and part of the lateral surfaces; and the lowest third, which lies deep in the pelvis below the peritoneal reflection.

The lower third of the rectum is separated by distinct fascial layers from the prostate/vagina anteriorly (Denonvilliers' fascia), and from the coccyx and lower two sacral vertebrae posteriorly (Waldeyer's fascia) (***Table 79.1***). These fascial layers are surgically important as they act as barriers to malignant invasion and form the anatomical envelope for total mesorectal excision (TME) to achieve complete oncological clearance of rectal cancer.

Summary box 79.1

Anatomy of the rectum
- The rectum measures approximately 15 cm in length
- It is divided into lower, middle and upper thirds
- The blood supply consists of superior, middle and inferior rectal vessels
- The lymphatic drainage follows the blood supply. The principal route of drainage is upwards along the superior rectal vessels to the para-aortic nodes, although the lower rectum can drain to lymphatics along the internal iliac pedicle and lateral pelvic side walls

TABLE 79.1 Anatomical relations of the rectum.

	Relation
Anterior	Bladder Seminal vesicles and prostate (males) Denonvilliers' fascia Pouch of Douglas and rectovaginal septum (females) Uterus and cervix (females) Ureters
Lateral	Lateral ligaments and middle rectal artery Obturator internus muscle and side wall of pelvis Pelvic autonomic plexus Levator ani muscle
Posterior	Sacrum and coccyx Waldeyer's fascial condensation Superior rectal artery and lymphatics Hypogastric nerves

John Houston, 1802–1845, physician, City of Dublin Hospital and Lecturer in Surgery, Dublin, Ireland.
Charles-Pierre Denonvilliers, 1808–1872, Professor of Anatomy and later of Surgery, Paris, France.
Heinrich Wilhelm Gottfried Waldeyer-Hartz, 1836–1921, Professor of Pathological Anatomy, Berlin, Germany.
James Douglas, 1675–1742, Scottish anatomist and Physician Extraordinary to Queen Caroline.

Embryology

The embryological hindgut forms the upper rectum, while the lower rectum is derived from the cloaca and is surrounded by extraperitoneal connective tissue. The primitive gut tube is suspended dorsally by a mesentery throughout its length, to form the mesorectum. The muscular layers of the rectum are derived from the mesenchyme that accompanies the endodermal part of the anorectum, with the inner circular layer preceding the outer longitudinal layer in the seventh week of embryonic development.

The levator ani muscles and external anal sphincter muscles form within the surrounding mesenchyme and grow to make contact with each other and with bundles of smooth muscle cells from the outer longitudinal layer of the rectal wall. A layer of undifferentiated mesenchyme separates the rectal muscle layers from the levator ani muscle and the muscle layer of the future anal canal.

Blood supply

The superior rectal artery is the direct continuation of the inferior mesenteric artery and is the main arterial supply of the rectum (***Figure 79.1***). The arteries and their accompanying lymphatics lie within the loose fatty tissue in the mesorectum, surrounded by a sheath of connective tissue (the mesorectal fascia). The middle rectal artery arises on each side from the internal iliac artery and passes to the rectum in the lateral ligaments. It is usually small and often only present on one side, and divides into several branches. The inferior rectal artery arises on each side from the internal pudendal artery as it enters Alcock's canal. It hugs the inferior surface of the levator ani muscle as it crosses the roof of the ischiorectal fossa to enter the anal muscles.

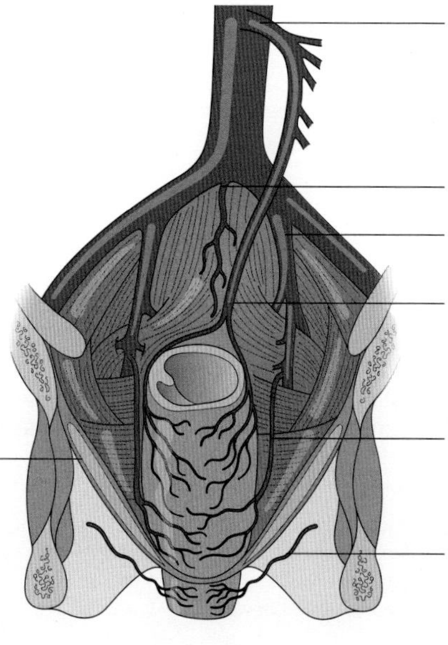

Figure 79.1 Blood supply to the rectum. The main blood supply comes from the superior rectal arteries, supplemented by middle rectal arteries in 20% of cases. The inferior rectal arteries are derived from the pudendal vessels and supply the anal canal and lower rectum.

Venous drainage

The superior haemorrhoidal veins draining the upper half of the anal canal above the dentate line pass upwards to become the rectal veins; these unite to form the superior rectal vein, which later becomes the inferior mesenteric vein. This forms part of the portal venous system and ultimately drains into the splenic vein. Middle rectal veins exist but are small, unimportant channels unless the normal paths are blocked.

Lymphatic drainage

The lymphatics of the rectal mucosa communicate freely with those of the muscle layers. The usual drainage flow is upwards, and only to a limited extent laterally and downwards. For this reason, surgical clearance of malignant disease concentrates mainly on achieving wide resection of proximal lymph nodes. However, if the usual upward routes are blocked, for example by metastatic disease, the flow can reverse and it is possible to find involved lymph nodes on the side walls of the pelvis (along the middle rectal vessels) or even in the inguinal region (along the inferior rectal artery).

CLINICAL FEATURES OF RECTAL DISEASE

Symptoms

Rectal diseases are common and can occur at any age. The symptoms of many of them overlap. In general, inflammatory conditions affect younger age groups, while tumours occur in the middle-aged and elderly.

Summary box 79.2

Main symptoms of rectal disease

- Fresh bleeding per rectum
- Altered bowel habit with loose stool
- Mucus discharge
- Tenesmus
- Prolapse
- Proctalgia (pain)

Bleeding

This is often painless and bright red in colour and should be carefully investigated at any age.

Altered bowel habit

Early morning stool frequency (spurious diarrhoea) is a symptom of rectal carcinoma, while blood-stained, frequent, loose stools characterise the inflammatory diseases.

Benjamin Alcock, 1801–?, first Professor of Anatomy, Queen's College (now University College), Cork, Ireland. Emigrated in 1859 following a resignation dispute over procurement of corpses for dissection.

Discharge

Mucus and pus are associated with rectal inflammation.

Tenesmus

Often described by the patient as 'I feel I want to go but nothing happens', this is normally an ominous symptom of rectal cancer, but can occur with other rectal conditions and is a common symptom of rectal prolapse.

Prolapse

This usually indicates either mucosal or full-thickness rectal wall protrusion from the anus. Internal prolapse or intussusception refers to a telescoping of the rectum into itself without protrusion from the anus.

Pain: 'proctalgia'

This is usually a severe and episodic pain resulting from spasm of the levator ani muscle. It may last for a few seconds to minutes then recur, or it can be constant (see ***Chapter 80***).

Signs

To examine the rectum the patient is most conveniently positioned in the left lateral or semi-prone (Sims) position.

Inspection

Visual examination of the anus precedes rectal examination to exclude the presence of anal disease, e.g. fissure or fistula. Evidence of rectal prolapse or abnormal pelvic floor descent can be elicited by asking the patient to strain.

Digital examination

The index finger used with gentleness and precision remains a valuable test for rectal disease (***Figure 79.2***). The anal sphincters are assessed for anatomical integrity, resting tone and squeeze. In females, a rectocele may be palpable as a herniation of the anterior rectal wall into the vagina. Tumours in the lower and middle thirds of the rectum can usually be felt. On removal, the finger should be examined for mucus, pus or blood. It is useful to note the normal, as well as the abnormal, findings on digital examination, e.g. the prostate in the male. Digital findings can be recorded as intraluminal (e.g. blood, pus), intramural (e.g. tumours, granular areas, strictures) or extramural (e.g. enlarged prostate, uterine fibroids). Intramural lesions can be described as fixed, tethered or mobile.

Proctoscopy

This procedure can be used to inspect the anus, anorectal junction and lower rectum. A lubricated proctoscope is inserted through the anus to provide views of the lower rectum and anal canal (***Figure 79.3***). Biopsy can be performed of any suspicious areas, provided it is above the sensitive anoderm. Proctoscopy is particularly useful for assessing the presence of haemorrhoids.

Sigmoidoscopy

In the past, the sigmoidoscope was a rigid stainless steel instrument of variable diameter and normally 25 cm in length, but this has been replaced by disposable plastic instruments. The rectum must be empty for proper inspection. Direct inspection of the rectal mucosa may alert the clinician to inflammation or tumours. This procedure can be performed in the outpatient setting.

Flexible sigmoidoscope

This is used as a supplement to rigid sigmoidoscopy or when views proximal to the rectum are required (***Figure 79.4***). The lower bowel needs to be cleaned out with preliminary enemas. In addition to the rectum, the whole sigmoid colon up to the splenic flexure is within visual reach. Flexible sigmoidoscopy

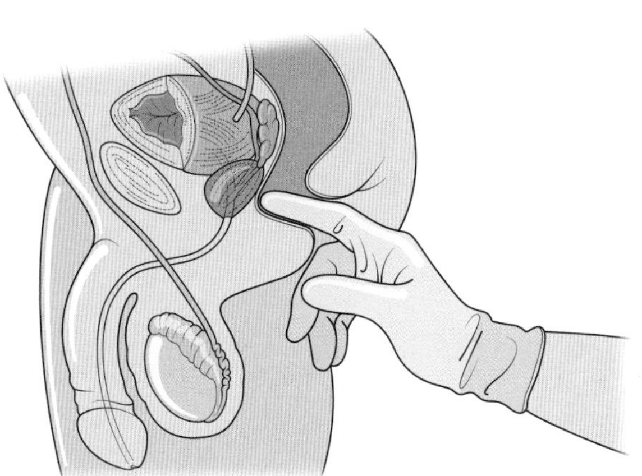

Figure 79.2 Digital rectal examination in the male. Assessment of the anal sphincter complex, lower rectum and prostate.

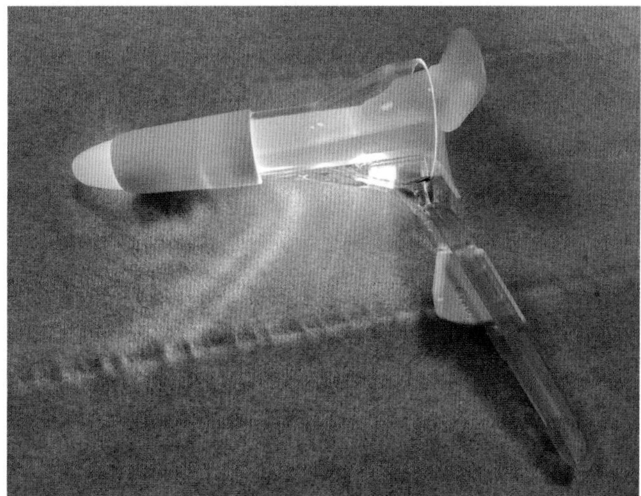

Figure 79.3 Proctoscope for visualisation of the anorectum.

James Marion Sims, 1813–1883, gynaecological surgeon, the State Hospital for Women, New York, NY, USA, introduced this position to give access to the anterior vaginal wall during operations for the closure of vesicovaginal fistula.

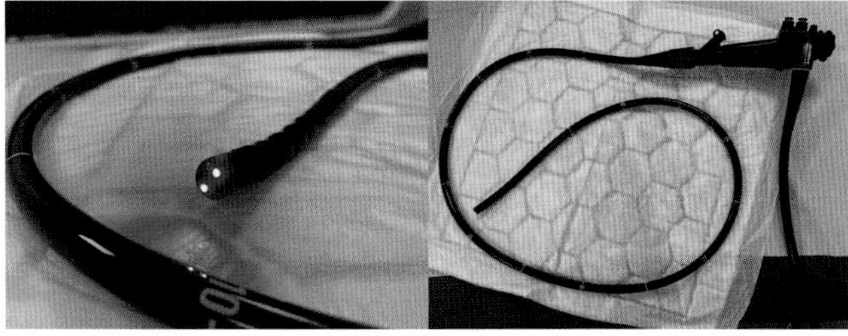

Figure 79.4 Flexible colonoscope.

is indicated to investigate underlying causes of fresh rectal bleeding or other bowel symptoms when full visualisation of the colon by colonoscopy is not required.

Summary box 79.3

Examination of the rectum

- Visual inspection of the perineum
- Digital examination
- Proctoscopy
- Sigmoidoscopy – rigid and/or flexible

INJURIES

The rectum or anal canal may be injured in a number of ways, all of which are uncommon:

- by falling in a sitting posture onto a pointed object;
- penetrating injury (including gunshots) to the buttocks;
- sexual assault or sexual activity involving anal penetration;
- by the fetal head during childbirth, especially forceps assisted.

Diagnosis

The anus should be inspected and the abdomen palpated. If abdominal rigidity or tenderness is present, early laparoscopy or laparotomy is indicated. A water-soluble contrast enema may help in delineating the injury, but a computed tomography (CT) scan is often preferred and will provide additional information on other pelvic injuries, such as accompanying urethral injury.

Treatment

The rectum is examined under general anaesthetic with a finger and a sigmoidoscope. If penetrating injury is confirmed, laparotomy or laparoscopy is required. If an intraperitoneal rupture of the rectum is found, the perforation is closed with sutures and the rectum defunctioned with a stoma. The defunctioned distal segment should be irrigated to remove all residual faecal matter. In the event that the rectal injury cannot be repaired, a Hartmann's procedure may be needed. If the rectal injury is below the peritoneal reflection, wide drainage from below is indicated, with rectal washout and a defunctioning colostomy. Care must be taken to preserve or restore anal sphincter integrity during debridement of the perineal wounds. Antibiotic cover must be provided against both aerobic and anaerobic organisms.

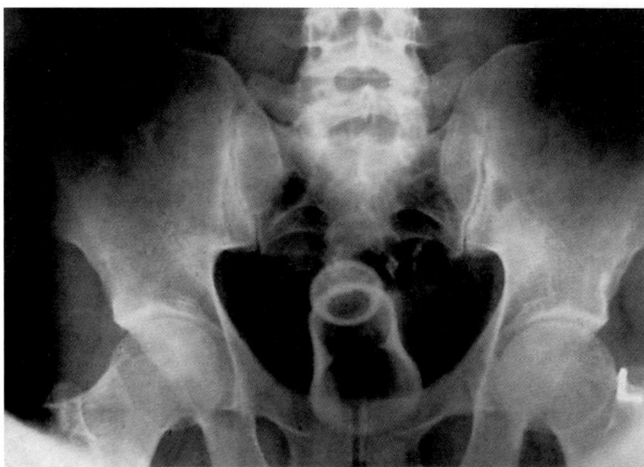

Figure 79.5 Foreign body in the rectum as seen on plain abdominal radiograph.

FOREIGN BODIES IN THE RECTUM

The variety of foreign bodies that have found their way into the rectum is hardly less remarkable than the ingenuity displayed in their removal (***Figure 79.5***). The difficulty lies in the creation of a vacuum effect when trying to extract the object through the anus. If insurmountable difficulty is experienced in grasping any foreign body in the rectum, laparotomy or laparoscopy is usually necessary. The object can be pushed from above into the assistant's fingers in the rectum or removed by means of a rectotomy in a proximal area of the rectum. If there is considerable laceration of the mucosa, a temporary colostomy is advisable.

Summary box 79.4

Injuries to the rectum are serious and invariably require surgery

- A temporary colostomy is often necessary
- There is a serious risk of associated necrotising fasciitis, and broad-spectrum antibiotics are mandatory
- There may be associated bladder or urethral damage

PROLAPSE

Mucosal prolapse

The mucosa and submucosa of the rectum may protrude outside the anus for approximately 1–4 cm. When the prolapsed mucosa is palpated between the finger and the thumb, it is evident that it is composed of no more than a double layer of mucosa. This distinguishes mucosal prolapse

Henri Albert Hartmann, 1860–1952, Chief of Surgery, Hôtel Dieu, Paris, France.

from full-thickness rectal prolapse, in which the entire wall of the rectum protrudes through the anal canal.

In infants

The direct downward course of the rectum, owing to the as-yet undeveloped sacral curve, predisposes infants to this condition.

In children

Mucosal prolapse often commences after an attack of diarrhoea or from loss of weight and consequent loss of fat in the ischiorectal fossa. It may also be associated with cystic fibrosis, neurological disorder, Hirschsprung's disease, rectal polyps and maldevelopment of the pelvis.

Summary box 79.5

Rectal prolapse

- It may be mucosal or full thickness
- If full thickness, the whole wall of the rectum is included
- It may begin as a rectal intussusception (internal rectal prolapse)
- In children, the prolapse is usually mucosal and should be treated conservatively
- In adults, the prolapse is often full thickness and is frequently associated with constipation and incontinence
- Surgery is almost always necessary for full-thickness rectal prolapse
- The operation is performed either via the perineum or via the abdomen

In adults

Mucosal prolapse in adults is often associated with third-degree haemorrhoids, when it is referred to as mucohaemorrhoidal prolapse (***Figure 79.6***). In the female a perineum damaged at childbirth and in the male straining from urethral obstruction predispose to mucosal prolapse. In old age, both mucosal and full-thickness prolapse are associated with weakness of the pelvic floor and anal sphincters. Partial prolapse may follow an operation for fistula-*in-ano* where a large portion of muscle has been divided. Here, the prolapse is usually localised to the damaged quadrant and is seldom progressive.

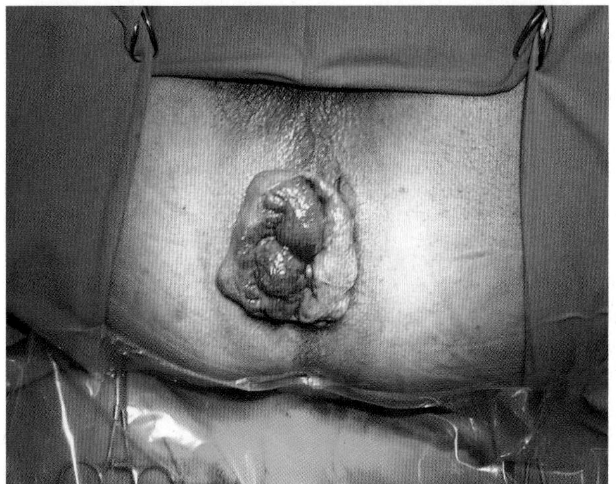

Figure 79.6 Mucohaemorrhoidal prolapse of the anorectum.

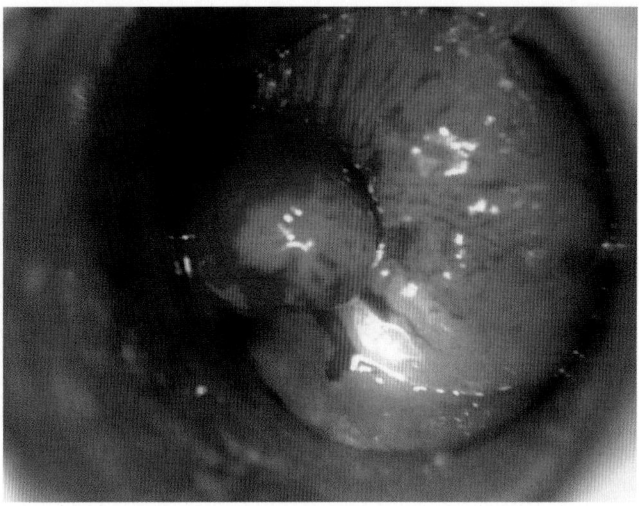

Figure 79.7 Through a proctoscope, a rubber band is applied to an area of mucohaemorrhoidal prolapse.

Treatment

In infants and young children

- **Digital repositioning**. The parents are taught to replace the protrusion, and any underlying causes are addressed.
- **Submucosal injection or banding**. If digital repositioning fails after a 6-week trial, injection of 5% phenol in almond oil or rubber band ligation under general anaesthetic can be tried (***Figure 79.7***).

In adults

- **Local treatments**. Submucosal injections of phenol in almond oil or the application of rubber bands may be successful in cases of mucosal prolapse.
- **Excision of the prolapsed mucosa**. When the prolapse is unilateral, the redundant mucosa can be excised or, if circumferential, an endoluminal stapling technique or internal Delorme's procedure can be used.

Internal rectal prolapse and solitary rectal ulcer syndrome

Internal rectal prolapse, or intussusception, refers to the invagination of the rectal tube during defecation. The prolapse descends towards the anal canal, where it can act as a blockage to defecation; a condition referred to as obstructed defecation. The patient describes the normal desire to defecate but an inability to satisfactorily evacuate the rectum, having to resort to excessive straining and sometimes digitation. Incomplete evacuation leads to a sensation of tenesmus, requiring repeated

Harald Hirschsprung, 1830–1916, Professor of Paediatrics, The Queen Louise Hospital for Children, Copenhagen, Denmark.
Edmond Delorme, 1847–1929, Professor of Surgery, Val-de-Grace Military Hospital, Paris, France.

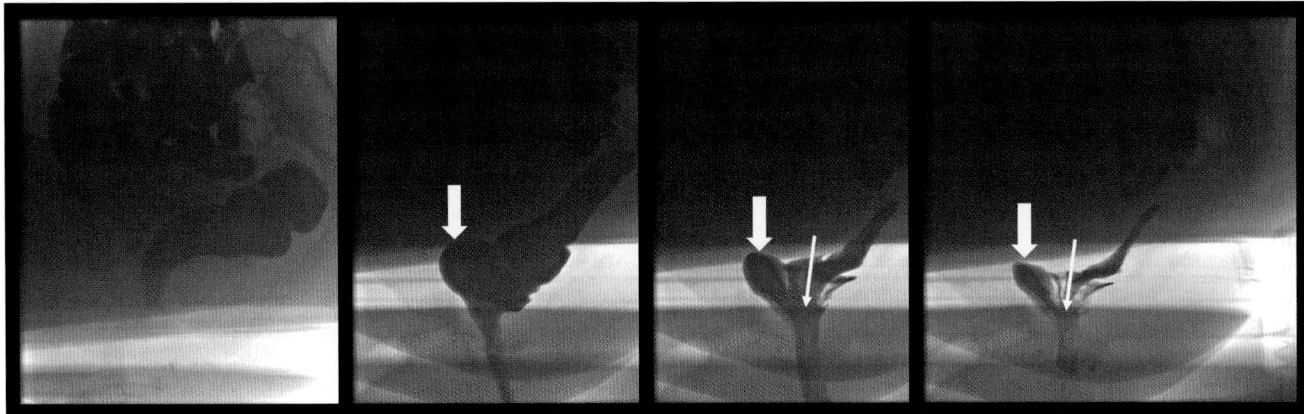

Figure 79.8 Defecating proctogram with selected images from left to right showing normal pelvic floor position at rest with development of a small anterior rectocele on evacuation (thick arrow) and a rectoanal intussusception entering the anal canal (thin arrow) (courtesy of Dr Damian Tolan, St James's Hospital, Leeds, UK).

returns to the toilet. Intussusception is often accompanied by other structural abnormalities of the rectum, including rectocele and enterocele, which can further add to evacuatory difficulty (***Figure 79.8***).

Treatment of internal rectal prolapse is indicated if it can be demonstrated on proctography and correlates with the patient's symptoms of obstructed defecation. Surgical options for treating internal rectal prolapse are the same as those for external rectal prolapse, namely internal Delorme's procedure (perineal approach) or laparoscopic ventral mesh rectopexy (LVMR) (abdominal approach).

Solitary rectal ulcer syndrome (SRUS) may also be another associated manifestation of obstructed defecation syndrome. Classically, SRUS takes the form of an ulcer on the anterior wall of the rectum, situated 6–8 cm from the anal verge. In this form, it can be mistaken for rectal carcinoma or inflammatory bowel disease, particularly Crohn's disease. It may heal, leaving a polypoid appearance. Proctographic studies may indicate accompanying rectal intussusception or anterior rectal wall prolapse. Histology will confirm the diagnosis. The condition is difficult to treat. Symptomatic relief from bleeding and discharge may sometimes be achieved by controlling any associated straining with re-coordination of defecation using biofeedback therapy. Transanal stapled resection of the intussusception (STARR procedure) or resuspension of the rectum by abdominal rectopexy may be beneficial, but the results are not as good as for internal or external rectal prolapse. In rare cases, rectal excision may be required with or without stoma.

Full-thickness prolapse

Complete rectal prolapse (synonym: procidentia) is less common than the mucosal variety. The protrusion consists of all layers of the rectal wall and is usually associated with a weak pelvic floor and/or chronic straining. The prolapse often commences as an intussusception of the rectum, which descends to protrude outside the anus. The process starts with the anterior wall of the rectum, where the supporting tissues are weakest, especially in women. It is more than 4 cm and commonly as much as 10–15 cm in length (***Figure 79.9***). On palpation between the finger and thumb, the prolapse feels much thicker than mucosal prolapse and consists of a double thickness of the entire wall of the rectum. Any prolapse over 5 cm in length will contain anteriorly, between its layers, a pouch of peritoneum. When large, the peritoneal pouch may contain small intestine or bladder. The anal sphincter is characteristically patulous and gapes widely on straining to allow the rectum to prolapse. Complete prolapse is uncommon in children but may occur as a result of malnutrition. In adults, it can occur at any age, but it is more common in the elderly and sometimes in patients with anorexia nervosa. Women are affected six times more often than men, and it is commonly associated with other pelvic organ prolapse. In approximately 50% of adults, faecal incontinence is also a feature. Complications of rectal prolapse include rectal ulceration and bleeding, incontinence and even incarceration with ischaemia and necrosis of the rectum.

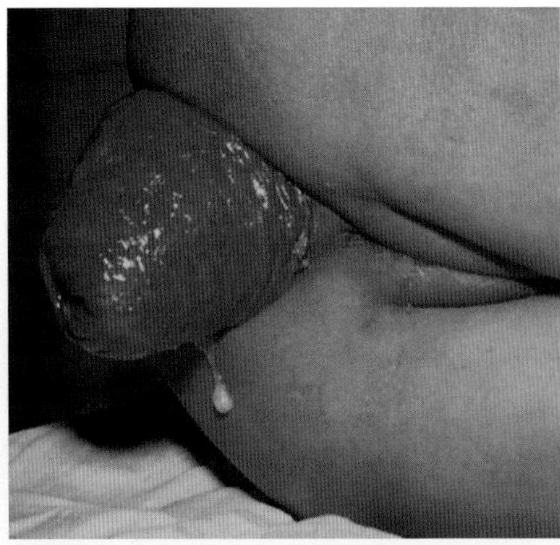

Figure 79.9 Full-thickness rectal prolapse. The whole bowel wall protrudes through the anus.

Burrill Bernard Crohn, 1884–1983, gastroenterologist, Mount Sinai Hospital, New York, NY, USA.

Differential diagnosis

In the case of a child with abdominal pain, the anus should be examined to exclude rectal prolapse as a cause. This should also be distinguished from intussusception protruding from the anus.

Treatment

Surgery is required for full-thickness rectal prolapse, and the operation can be performed via a perineal or abdominal approach. Abdominal operations can be by an open or laparoscopic approach. Abdominal rectopexy, either laparoscopic or open, has a lower rate of recurrence (<10%), but when the patient is elderly and very frail a perineal operation is usually safer and, if necessary, can be performed under regional anaesthetic blockade. As an abdominal procedure risks damage to the pelvic autonomic nerves, resulting in possible sexual dysfunction, a perineal approach may be preferred in young men.

Perineal approach

These procedures have been used most frequently:

- **Thiersch's operation**. In this procedure, a steel wire, or silastic or nylon tape, is placed around the anal canal. It has become largely obsolete owing to problems with chronic perineal sepsis, anal stenosis and obstructed defecation, but may be used to augment perineal repair in cases of severe pelvic floor weakness.
- **Delorme's operation**. In this procedure, the rectal mucosa is stripped circumferentially from the rectum over the length of the prolapse (***Figure 79.10***). The underlying muscle is plicated with a series of sutures, so that the rectal muscle is concertinaed towards the anal canal. The excess rectal mucosa is excised and a mucosal anastomosis performed. The resulting effect is to reduce the prolapse as a plicated ring of muscle above the anal canal. This operation may be preferred in patients with short segment full rectal prolapse, but recurrence rates are high, in the region of 30% over 5 years.

(a)

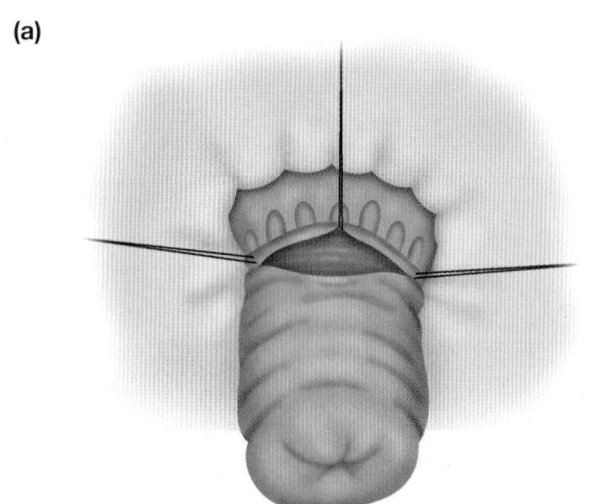

(b)

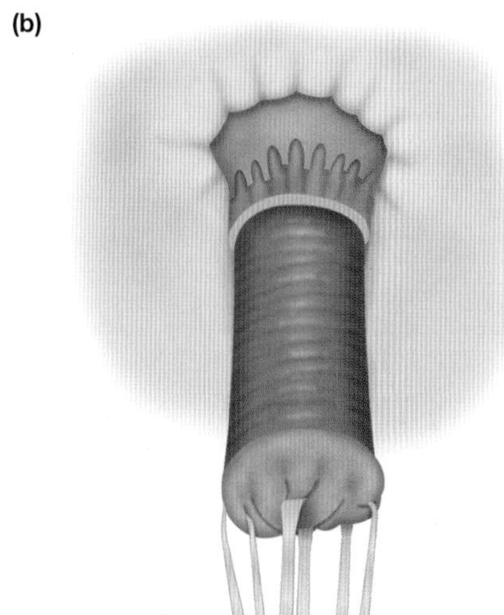

(c)

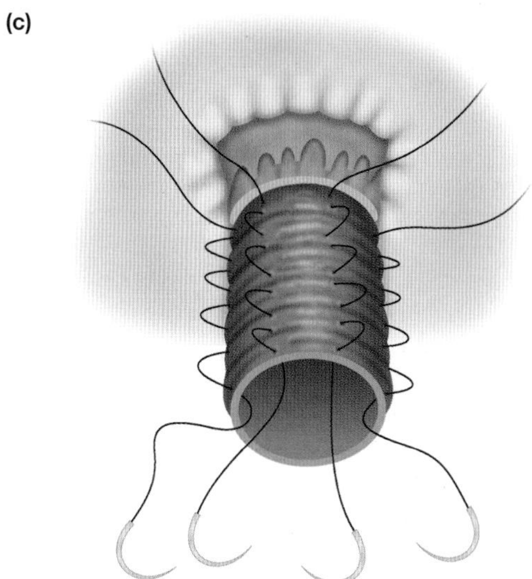

(d)

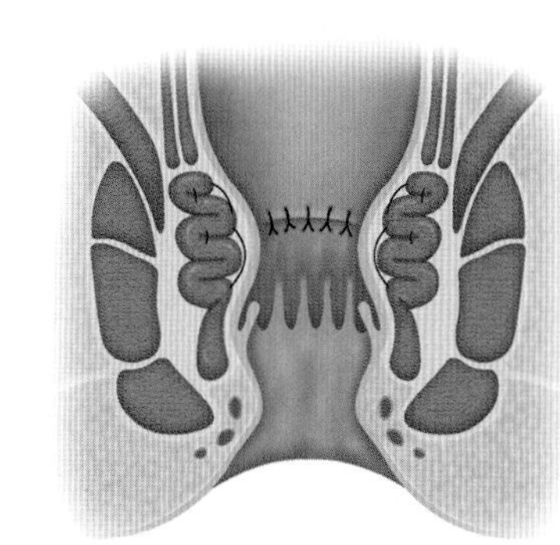

Figure 79.10 Delorme's procedure for rectal prolapse. (a, b) The mucosa is stripped from the muscular gut tube. (c, d) Interrupted sutures are used to plicate the muscular gut tube and reduce the prolapse. The operation is concluded by suturing the mucosa.

Karl Thiersch, 1822–1895, Professor of Surgery, Leipzig, Germany.

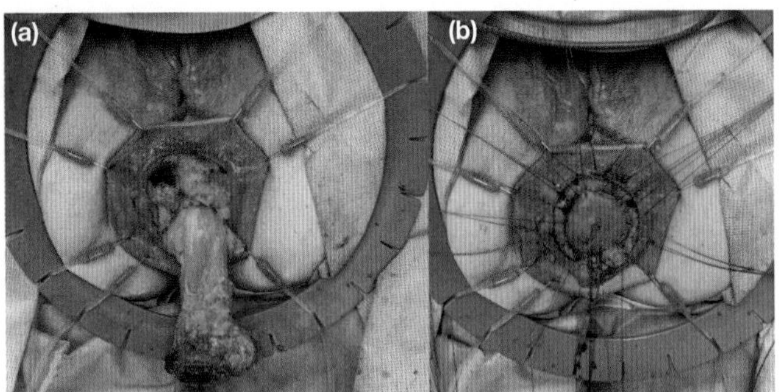

Figure 79.11 Altemeier's procedure showing (a) a full-thickness mobilisation of the prolapse and (b) a hand-sewn coloanal anastomosis following prolapse resection (courtesy of Ms Ann Hanly, FRCSI, Dublin, Ireland).

- **Altemeier's procedure**. In this procedure, the rectum is prolapsed through the anal canal and a full-thickness resection performed, incorporating any associated colonic prolapse (***Figure 79.11***). Restoration of colorectal continuity can be performed by either a hand-sewn or stapled anastomosis. This is the procedure of choice in patients presenting with incarcerated and strangulated prolapse. It is a good alternative perineal procedure to the Delorme's operation, particularly following recurrence. However, it is often complicated by poor bowel control with faecal soiling secondary to loss of the rectal reservoir. Recurrence rates range from 0% to 20%.

The advantages of a perineal approach include minimal postoperative pain, early mobility and low levels of morbidity. However, given the higher recurrence rates when compared with the abdominal operations, it is best reserved for patients at high risk of complications when undergoing a major operation.

Abdominal approach

The principle of all abdominal operations for rectal prolapse is to fix the rectum in its normal anatomical position. Many variations have been described, including inserting a sheet of polypropylene mesh between the rectum and the sacrum, hitching up the rectosigmoid junction with a Teflon sling to the front of the sacrum or simply suturing the mobilised rectum to the sacrum using four to six interrupted non-absorbable sutures – so-called 'sutured rectopexy' (Goldberg). Currently, the technique is most often performed laparoscopically, reducing the operative trauma, limiting the time in hospital and broadening its indication for higher risk patients.

As an abdominal rectopexy may lead to worsening constipation, some surgeons recommend combining this procedure with resection of the sigmoid colon, so-called 'resection rectopexy', but this adds an additional risk because of the anastomosis. An alternative is LVMR, which has become increasingly popular in western practice (D'Hoore). In this procedure, the plane between the rectum and vagina (or prostate) is dissected, and a strip of mesh sutured to the anterior rectum and posterior vaginal vault. The upper end of the mesh is secured to the sacral promontory with sutures or tacks, thus resuspending the rectum and preventing prolapse (***Figure 79.12***).

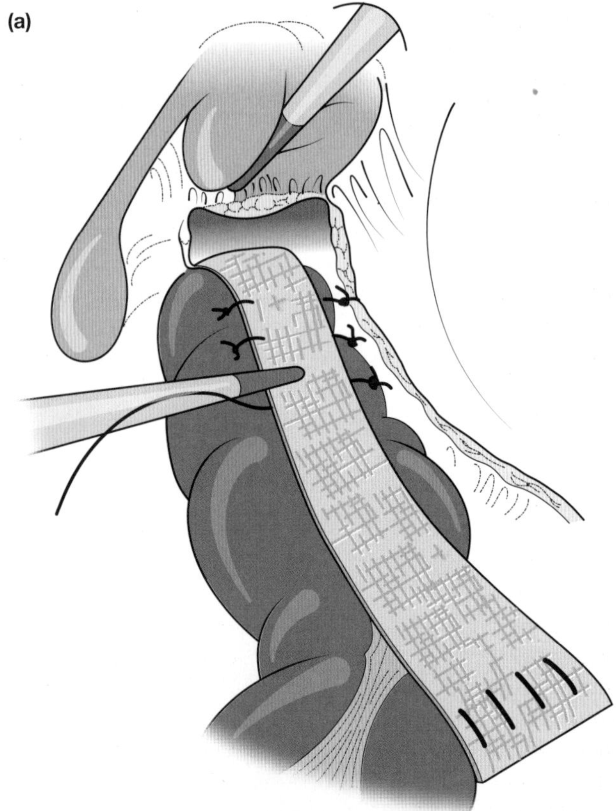

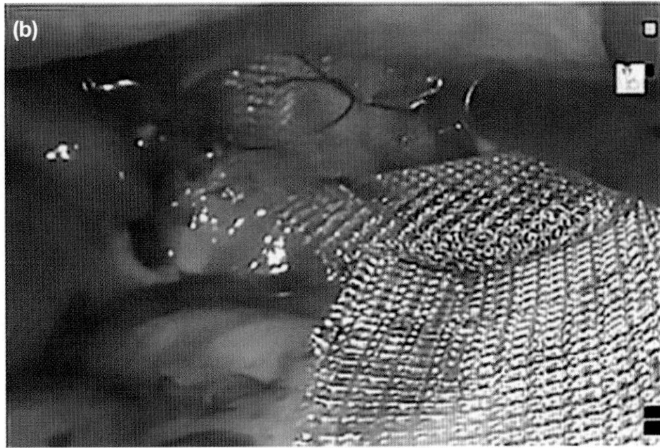

Figure 79.12 (a) Laparoscopic ventral mesh rectopexy: a prosthetic mesh is sutured to the front of the lower rectum and used to resuspend the rectum by securing the proximal end of the mesh to the sacral promontory. (b) Intraoperative image of a robotic ventral mesh rectopexy showing suturing of the mesh to the anterior rectum after dissection of the rectovaginal septum.

William Altemeier, 1910–1983, Professor of Surgery, Cincinnati, OH, USA.
Stanley M Goldberg, b. 1923, Emeritus Professor of Surgery, University of Minnesota, Minneapolis, MN, USA.
André D'Hoore, contemporary, Professor of Surgery, Catholic University Leuven, Leuven, Belgium.

The success of LVMR in treating external rectal prolapse and rectal intussusception has been variously reported between 70% and 80%, with improvement in both constipation and incontinence scores. It is a relatively safe procedure (overall complication rate 10%) with a quick recovery because of the laparoscopic approach. Possible complications include prolapse recurrence, bleeding, pelvic pain and dyspareunia. More recently, there has been concern regarding mesh complications when used more generally for pelvic organ prolapse surgery, culminating in the 2020 publication of the Cumberlege Report in the UK. As a result, the use of mesh for vaginal surgery has been restricted. When used for LVMR, mesh complications (infection and erosion) have been reported in 2–4% of cases and are higher when a polyester mesh is used.

PROCTITIS

The patient is usually middle-aged and complains of defecatory frequency with the passage of loose motions, often with blood mixed in the stools. Inflammation is sometimes limited to the rectum; in other cases, it is associated with a similar condition in the colon (proctocolitis). The inflammation can be acute or chronic. Although the patient has a frequent, intense desire to defecate, the amount of faeces passed at any time is small. Acute proctitis is usually accompanied by malaise and pyrexia. On rectal examination, there may be tenderness and blood on the glove. Proctoscopy is seldom sufficient and sigmoidoscopy is the more valuable method of examination. If the diagnosis is confirmed, colonoscopy with multiple biopsies is mandatory to determine the extent of the inflammatory process. Skilled pathological assessment is required to establish and classify the underlying pathology. Stool cultures should be sent routinely to exclude infective causes. If biopsy and histology are unable to establish an underlying inflammatory aetiology, the condition is frequently termed non-specific proctitis but may herald a subsequent diagnosis of inflammatory bowel disease (ulcerative colitis or Crohn's disease).

Treatment is usually medical and tailored to the underlying pathology. Non-specific colitis may be self-limiting, but treatment with topical 5-aminosalicylic acid (5-ASA) compounds in the form of suppositories or foam enemas is usually effective. In resistant cases, oral steroids may have to be used.

Summary box 79.6

Proctitis

- May be non-specific or related to a specific infective agent
- Non-specific proctitis usually remains confined to the distal bowel but can involve the proximal colon
- Symptoms include defecatory frequency, loose stools, bleeding and tenesmus
- Endoscopic assessment with biopsy is required to establish the diagnosis
- Treatment usually involves medical management

Ulcerative proctocolitis

Proctitis is present in most cases of ulcerative colitis, and the degree of rectal involvement may influence the type of operative procedure (see ***Chapter 75***).

Proctitis due to Crohn's disease

Crohn's disease can occasionally affect the rectum, although classically it is spared. Sigmoidoscopic appearances differ from those in non-specific proctitis. The inflammatory process tends to be patchy rather than confluent, and there may be fissuring, ulceration or even a cobblestone appearance. Rectal Crohn's disease is often associated with severe perineal disease characterised by fistulation, fissuring and haemorrhoids. Coexistent disease is often present in the rest of the colon or small bowel, or both (see ***Chapter 75***).

Radiation proctitis

Radiation therapy is used in the treatment of cervical, prostate and rectal cancers. It can produce acute radiation proctitis with bleeding, pain, diarrhoea and defecatory frequency. Most symptoms settle within a few weeks, but some patients develop chronic proctitis with symptoms appearing months or even decades after the radiation exposure. Bleeding may require treatment with argon laser photocoagulation performed using a flexible sigmoidoscope.

Proctitis due to specific infections

Clostridium difficile

An acute form of proctocolitis caused by infection with *C. difficile* can follow broad-spectrum antibiotics. A membrane can sometimes be seen on sigmoidoscopy ('pseudomembranous' colitis).

Bacillary dysentery

The appearance is that of an acute purulent proctitis with multiple small, shallow ulcers.

Amoebic dysentery

The infection is more likely to be chronic, with exacerbations after a long period of symptom improvement. Proctoscopy and sigmoidoscopy are not painful.

Tuberculous proctitis

This is nearly always associated with active pulmonary tuberculosis or tuberculous ulceration of the anus. Submucous rectal abscesses burst and leave ulcers with an undermined edge. A hypertrophic type of tuberculous proctitis occurs in association with tuberculous peritonitis or tuberculous salpingitis. This type of tuberculous proctitis requires biopsy for confirmation of the diagnosis.

Gonococcal proctitis

Gonococcal proctitis occurs in both sexes as the result of rectal coitus and, in the female, from direct spread from the vulva.

In the acute stage, the mucous membrane is hyperaemic, and thick pus can be expressed as the proctoscope is withdrawn. In the early stages, the diagnosis can be readily established by bacteriological examination but later, when the infection is mixed, it is more difficult to recognise. Systemic treatment is so effective that local treatment is unnecessary.

Lymphogranuloma venereum

The modes of infection are similar to those of gonococcal proctitis but, in the female, chlamydial infection spreading from the cervix uteri via lymphatics to the pararectal lymph nodes is common. The proctological findings are similar to those of gonococcal proctitis. The diagnosis of lymphogranuloma venereum should be suspected when the inguinal lymph nodes are greatly enlarged, although nodal enlargement may be subsiding by the time proctitis commences.

Acquired immunodeficiency syndrome

Acquired immunodeficiency syndrome due to human immunodeficiency virus may present with a particularly florid type of proctitis. In such patients, unusual organisms including *Cytomegalovirus*, herpes simplex virus and parasites such as *Cryptosporidium* are often found.

Rectal bilharziasis

Rectal bilharziasis is caused by *Schistosoma mansoni*, which is endemic in many tropical and subtropical countries and particularly in the Nile Delta. In stage 1, a cutaneous lesion develops at the site of entrance of the cercariae (parasites of freshwater snails). Stage 2 is characterised by pyrexia, urticaria and a high eosinophilia. Both these stages are frequently overlooked. Stage 3 results from deposition of the ova in the rectum (much more rarely in the bladder; see **Chapter 83**) and is manifested by bilharzial dysentery. On examination in the later stages, papillomas are frequently seen. The papillomas, which are sessile or pedunculated, contain the ova of the trematode, the life cycle of which resembles that of *Schistosoma haematobium*. Untreated, the rectum becomes festooned and prolapse of the diseased mucous membrane is usual. Multiple fistulae-*in-ano* are prone to develop. The primary treatment is systemic and should be undertaken by a specialist in tropical medicine.

RECTAL POLYPS

The rectum, along with the sigmoid colon, is the most frequent site of polyps (and cancers) in the gastrointestinal tract. Adenomatous polyps of the colon and rectum have the potential to become malignant. The chance of developing invasive cancer is enhanced if the polyp is more than 1 cm in diameter. Removal of all polyps is recommended to allow complete histological diagnosis and exclude carcinoma. This is best done using endoscopic biopsy or snare polypectomy techniques. If one or more rectal polyps are discovered on sigmoidoscopic examination, a colonoscopy must be performed because further polyps are frequently found in the colon.

The rectum shares the same spectrum of polyps as the colon. Polyps are described in terms of their appearance (pedunculated, sessile, flat) or histological composition (tubular, villous, tubulovillous).

Polyps relevant to the rectum

Hyperplastic polyps

These are small, pinkish, sessile polyps, 2–4 mm in diameter and frequently multiple. They are usually an incidental finding, unless larger in size, when full colonoscopy is warranted to exclude hyperplastic polyposis syndrome.

Tubular adenomas

Tubular adenomas, or mixed tubulovillous adenomas, are the most common type of polyp. They have the potential to turn malignant, particularly if over 1 cm in diameter.

Villous adenomas

These have a characteristic frond-like appearance. They may be very large, occupying much of the circumference of the rectum. These tumours have an increased tendency to become malignant. Rarely, the profuse mucus discharge from these tumours, which is rich in potassium, causes electrolyte and fluid losses.

Serrated adenomas

These polyps are more commonly found in the right colon but may be present in the rectum. They are typically sessile lesions that have a distinct microscopic architecture and can give rise to cancers through an alternative 'serrated' pathway.

Familial adenomatous polyposis

Familial adenomatous polyposis (FAP) is an autosomal dominant inherited condition characterised by the development of multiple rectal and colonic adenomas around puberty. It is due to mutation in the adenomatous polyposis coli (*APC*) gene, allowing genetic testing in the 75% of families in which a mutation can be identified. A colonoscopy and biopsy will confirm the diagnosis. As this condition is premalignant, total colectomy is usually recommended within 10 years of disease onset. This may take the form of panproctocolectomy with permanent ileostomy. Rectal preservation may be an option if the rectal polyp load is not too severe, with colectomy and ileorectal anastomosis, but continuous rectal surveillance for synchronous polyps will be required. The alternative, if restoration of gastrointestinal continuity is desired, is to undertake restorative proctocolectomy with ileal pouch–anal anastomosis (see **Chapter 77**).

Inflammatory pseudopolyps

These are oedematous islands of mucosa. They are usually associated with colitis in the UK, but most inflammatory diseases (including tropical diseases) can cause them. They are more likely to cause radiological difficulty, as the sigmoidoscopic appearance is usually associated with obvious signs of active or quiescent inflammation.

Theodor Maximilian Bilharz, 1825–1862, Professor of Zoology, Cairo, Egypt.

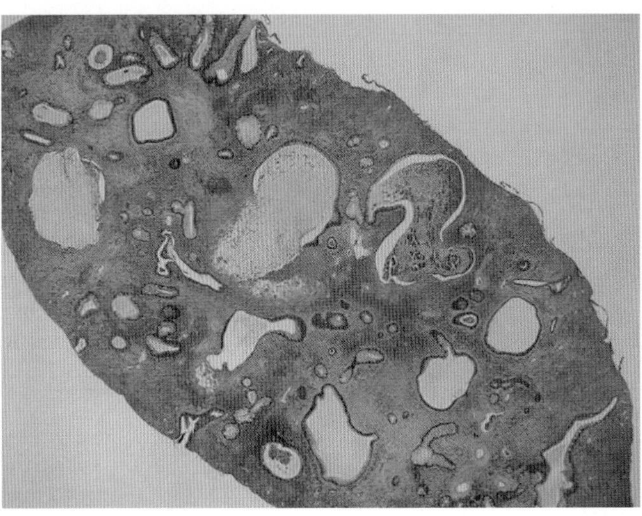

Figure 79.13 Microscopic appearance of a juvenile polyp (courtesy of Professor Kieran Sheahan, St Vincent's University Hospital, Dublin, Ireland).

Juvenile polyp

This is a bright red, glistening pedunculated sphere ('cherry tumour') that is found in infants and children that may persist into adult life. It can cause bleeding or pain if it prolapses during defecation. It often separates spontaneously but can be removed easily with forceps or a snare. A solitary juvenile polyp has virtually no tendency to malignant change but should be treated if symptomatic. Histological features typically consist of large mucus-filled spaces covered by a smooth surface of thin rectal cuboidal epithelium (***Figure 79.13***). The rare autosomal dominant inherited syndrome juvenile polyposis does carry an increased risk of malignancy. It is characterised by multiple polyps and a positive family history.

Treatment of rectal polyps

All rectal polyps should be biopsied or removed for histological analysis. A range of techniques can be used, depending on polyp size and location. The majority are less than 1 cm in size, benign and amenable to endoscopic polypectomy. Polyps greater than 1 cm in size have a 10% chance of malignancy. The difficult polyp can be defined by a range of variables, including the number of polyps, a size greater than 15 mm or a certain shape, whether with a large pedicle or a flat appearance (see ***Chapter 72***). Endomucosal resection (EMR) and endoscopic submucosal dissection (ESD) are techniques to consider when use of biopsy forceps or a snare is not optimal. The resection plane for both EMR and ESD is the superficial submucosal layer. Both techniques utilise an injection into the submucosal layer (***Figure 79.14***). Importantly, if the mucosa does not lift, this may indirectly indicate deeper invasion of the lesion. A 'non-lift' sign may also occur because of fibrosis from previous resection attempts or tattooing (see ***Chapter 9***).

EMR is typically used for lesions up to 20 mm in size, although the piecemeal resection for lesions greater than 20 mm may obviate surgery at the risk of a higher recurrence rate. ESD was created to counter the shortcomings of EMR as en bloc resection allows assessment of both horizontal and

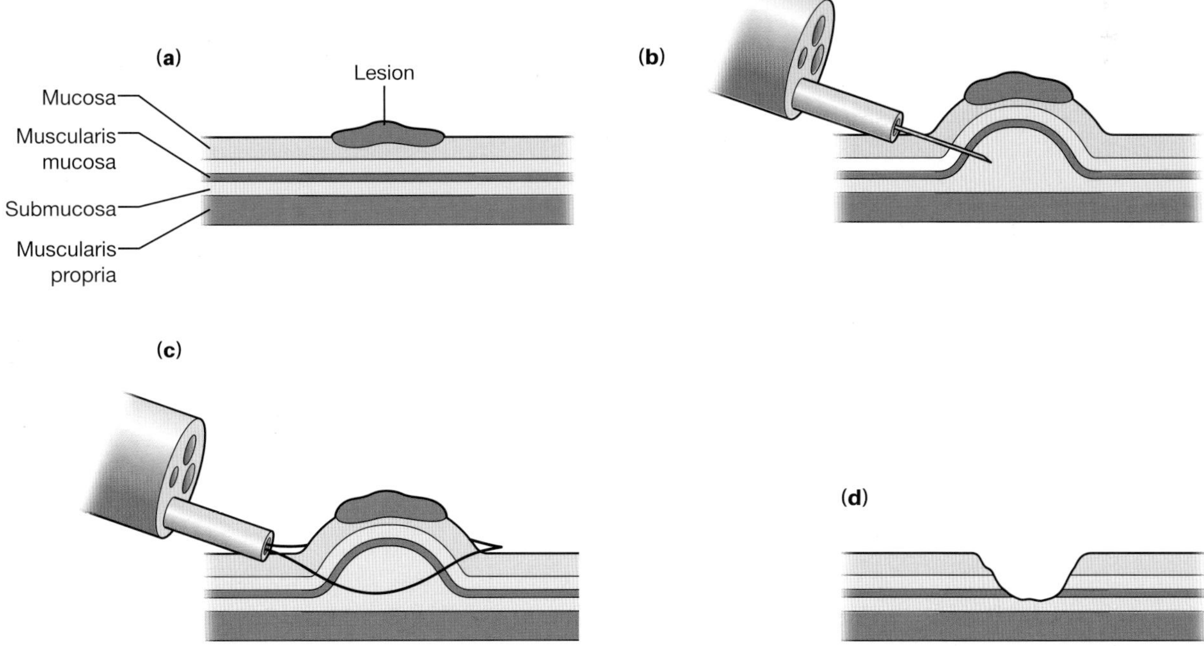

Figure 79.14 Endoscopic mucosal resection. The polyp is identified (a) and infiltration performed (b) to lift it from the underlying muscle layer. A diathermy snare is passed over the raised lesion (c) to achieve complete excision (d).

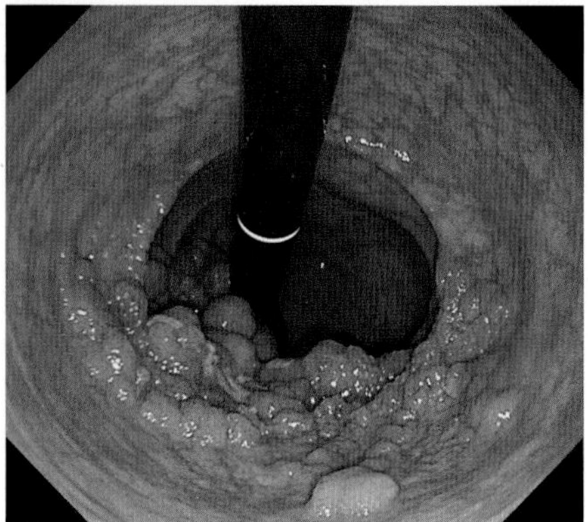

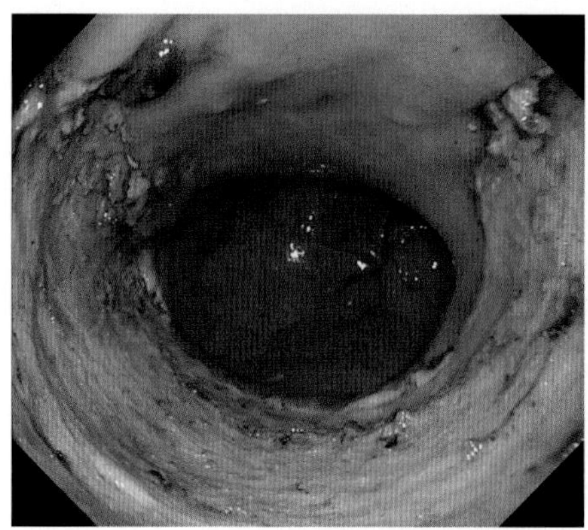

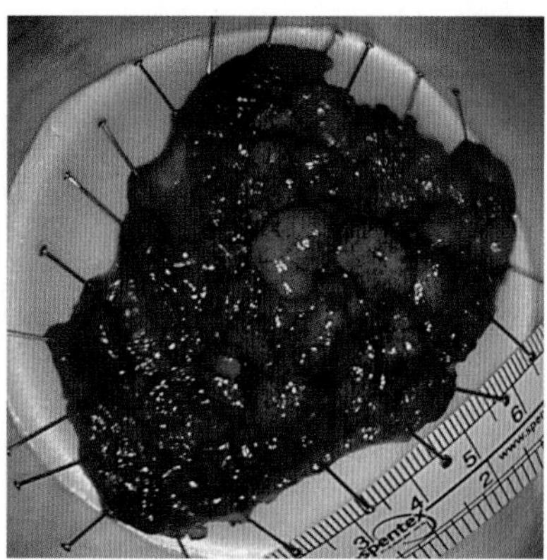

Figure 79.15 Endoscopic submucosal dissection of a rectal polyp (courtesy of Dr Noor Mohammed, St James's Hospital, Leeds, UK).

deep margins, which is not possible with a piecemeal resection (***Figure 79.15***). The submucosal injection is performed at the proximal border of the lesion, after which endoscopic knives are used to create an incision and dissect the submucosal layer free. ESD is informally indicated for lesions larger than 20 mm, when high-grade dysplasia or superficial submucosal invasion is suspected and when other endoscopic techniques have failed. The bleeding risks for EMR and ESD are roughly similar, whether immediate or delayed, with a reported incidence of 1–10%. Larger polyps are more difficult to remove by EMR and may require a transanal procedure, such as transanal endoscopic microsurgery (TEMS).

Summary box 79.7

Polyps in the rectum

- Adenomas are the most frequent histological type
- Villous adenomas may be extensive and undergo malignant change more commonly than tubular adenomas
- All adenomas must be removed to avoid malignant change
- All patients must undergo colonoscopy to determine whether further polyps are present
- Most polyps can be removed by endoscopic techniques, but sometimes major surgery is required

BENIGN RECTAL LESIONS

Endometrioma

Endometrioma is rare and may be misdiagnosed as a carcinoma. The focus of the ectopic endometrial tissue produces either a constricting lesion of the rectosigmoid or a tumour invading the rectum from the rectovaginal septum. The latter variety gives rise to a tender submucous elevation of the rectal wall. Endometrioma usually occurs between 20 and 40 years of age. Dysmenorrhoea and rectal bleeding (particularly coinciding with the menses) are the main symptoms. On sigmoidoscopy, endometriosis involving the rectosigmoid junction usually presents as a stricture, with the mucous membrane intact. Hormonal manipulation is the first-line therapy, but sometimes total abdominal hysterectomy and bilateral salpingo-oophorectomy and even bowel resection are required. The laparoscopic approach for resecting deep rectal endometriosis is becoming popular. Isolated endometrial deposits may be treated by diathermy ablation or local 'discectomy' incorporating the rectal wall.

Haemangioma

Haemangioma of the rectum is an uncommon cause of serious haemorrhage. The symptoms may mimic ulcerative colitis, and the diagnosis is often delayed, or it may be mistaken for a carcinoma. Selective angiography and embolisation may be helpful, but excision of the rectum is sometimes required.

Gastrointestinal stromal tumour

Smooth muscle tumours of the rectum are rare. If the mitotic rate is high, and if there is variation in nuclear number, size and shape, hyperchromasia and frequent bizarre cells, these tumours are likely to metastasise. In these circumstances, they should be classified as malignant gastrointestinal stromal tumours (GISTs) (formerly leiomyosarcomas). The uncertainty in their behaviour means that treatment should, whenever possible, be radical excision.

Neuroendocrine tumours

Neuroendocrine tumours (NETs) of the rectum constitute 19% of all gastrointestinal NETs. They are classified into well-differentiated (grades 1 and 2) and poorly differentiated (grade 3) tumours. Both tumour mitotic index and Ki-67 expression are important factors for histopathological classification. Grade 3 tumours include both small- and large-cell NETs. The majority of rectal NETs are grade 1, also known as carcinoid tumours, with a relatively good prognosis. These tumours are usually small (1–2 cm), solitary and clinically indolent; however, grade 3 NETs, while rare, metastasise at an early stage. Treatment depends on the size of the tumour, depth of tumour invasion and the presence or absence of metastasis. Small lesions (1 cm) can often be treated locally, either endoscopically or transanally. However, larger lesions (>2 cm) require formal oncological resection. Adjuvant therapy is indicated only for metastatic disease.

CARCINOMAS

Globally, colorectal cancer is the second most common malignancy, being the second most common cancer in women and the third most common cancer in men. It is the fourth most common cause of cancer death after lung, gastric and liver cancer. In western countries the incidence is rising, with an overall 14% increase since the 1970s, with the largest increase (20%) seen in males. Risk factors include diet, obesity, smoking and lack of physical exercise. Most colorectal cancers are due to old age, with around 60% of cases affecting patients 70 years or older. The rectum is the most frequently involved site, accounting for approximately one-third of the cancers.

Pathogenesis

Colorectal cancer originates from premalignant precursor lesions in the epithelial lining of the colon or rectum in a stepwise progression that results in increasing dysplasia due to an accumulation of genetic abnormalities. In spontaneous colorectal cancer, as compared with hereditary cancers, this is referred to as the adenoma–carcinoma sequence. Up to 80% of colorectal cancers occur in people with little or no genetic risk. People with inflammatory bowel disease are at an increased risk, which increases with the duration of the disease, and accounts for 2% of cancers each year. Those with a family history in two or more first-degree relatives have a two- to threefold greater risk of disease and this group accounts for about 20% of all cases. A number of genetic syndromes are also associated with higher rates of colorectal cancer. The most common is hereditary non-polyposis colorectal cancer (HNPCC or Lynch syndrome), which accounts for 3% of people with colorectal cancer. Other syndromes include Gardner syndrome and FAP.

The most common abnormality found in colorectal cancer is mutation in the *Wnt* signalling pathway, which increases cell signalling activity. The mutations can be inherited or acquired. The most commonly mutated gene is the *APC* gene, which results in accumulation of the β-catenin protein. β-catenin activates the transcription of various proto-oncogenes that are responsible for normal cell renewal and differentiation, but when overexpressed can cause cancer. Many other mutations, other than in the *Wnt* signalling pathway, are also found in colorectal cancer. They include mutations in the *TP53* gene, which controls normal cell division and death, and in genes responsible for programmed cell death, such as the gene encoding transforming growth factor (TGF)-β and *DCC* (deleted in colorectal cancer) gene. Other genetic abnormalities include overexpression of oncogenes, including genes encoding the proteins KRAS (Kirsten rat sarcoma homologue), RAF (rapidly accelerated fibrosarcoma) and PI3K (phosphoinositide 3-kinase), which lead to increased cell proliferation, and inactivation of tumour suppressor genes, such as *PTEN* (phosphatase and tensin homologue), which normally inactivates the PI3K signalling pathway.

In addition to gene mutations, colorectal cancers frequently exhibit epigenetic alterations – cellular or physiological effects resulting from external or environmental factors that switch genes on or off. Epigenetic alterations can affect hundreds of genes and include changes in the expression of microRNAs, hypermethylation or hypomethylation of CpG islands of protein-encoding genes and alterations in histones and chromosomal architecture, all of which can influence gene expression (see ***Chapter 77***).

Clinical features

Carcinoma of the rectum can occur early in life, but the age of presentation is usually above 55 years, when the incidence rises rapidly. Often, the early symptoms are so insignificant that the patient does not seek advice for 6 months or more, and the diagnosis is often delayed in younger patients as the symptoms are attributed to benign causes. Initial rectal examination and a low threshold for investigating persistent symptoms are essential.

Summary box 79.8

Early symptoms of rectal cancer

- Bleeding per rectum
- Tenesmus
- Early morning diarrhoea

Bleeding

Bleeding is the earliest and most common symptom. Typically, the bleeding is bright red in colour and painless. It can be mixed with the motions or separate in the toilet bowel. It can be indistinguishable from haemorrhoidal bleeding, which is the most common differential diagnosis, particularly in younger patients.

Tenesmus

The patient experiences a sensation of needing to evacuate the rectum but is unable to pass a motion. This is an important early symptom and is almost invariably present in patients with tumours of the lower half of the rectum. The patient may endeavour to empty the rectum several times a day (spurious diarrhoea), often with the passage of flatus and a little bloodstained mucus ('bloody slime').

Alteration in bowel habit

There is frequently a change in bowel habit, with a tendency to more frequent defecation and the passage of looser stool. A patient who has to get up early in order to defecate, or one who passes blood and mucus in addition to faeces ('early morning bloody diarrhoea'), is usually found to have carcinoma of the rectum. Although a change to looser stools is more common,

---

Henry Thompson Lynch, 1928–2019, physician and geneticist, Omaha, NE, USA, first presented his findings of a family with a strong history of colorectal cancer without polyposis in 1964.

Eldon John Gardner, 1909–1989, geneticist, The University of Utah, Salt Lake City, UT, USA, described this syndrome in 1950.

patients with a stenosing carcinoma at the rectosigmoid junction may complain of increasing constipation.

Pain

Pain is a late symptom, but pain of a colicky character may accompany advanced tumours of the rectosigmoid, owing to a degree of obstruction. Advanced cancers invading outside the mesorectum may infiltrate the prostate or bladder anteriorly or the sacral plexus posteriorly, giving rise to severe, intractable pain.

Weight loss

Weight loss is also a late symptom and is almost always associated with metastatic disease.

Investigation

Abdominal examination

Abdominal examination is normal in early cases. Occasionally, in patients with stenosing tumours at the rectosigmoid junction, signs of subacute large bowel obstruction may be present, with abdominal distension. If large volume liver metastases are present, an enlarged liver may be palpable along with other signs, such as cachexia. Occasionally, it may be possible to elicit ascites if there is widespread peritoneal dissemination.

Rectal examination

In many cases where the neoplasm is situated within 7–8 cm of the anal verge it can be felt on digital rectal examination as an elevated, irregular and hard endoluminal mass. When the centre ulcerates, a shallow depression will be felt with raised and everted edges. An attempt should be made to determine whether the neoplasm is mobile, tethered or fixed, and to estimate the distance of the lower margin from the top of the anal sphincter complex: these factors are important in assessing resectability and methods of reconstruction following excisional surgery. In females, a vaginal examination may be useful if involvement of the posterior vaginal wall is suspected. Digital rectal examination also affords the opportunity to evaluate the anal sphincter complex, which is important in cases where resection and low anastomosis is being considered.

Rigid sigmoidoscopy

Rigid sigmoidoscopy can be performed in the outpatient clinic and is useful to identify the neoplasm and possibly obtain biopsies. However, it requires the rectum to be empty of faeces and may require a prior rectal enema, which may not be practical in the outpatient setting. As colonoscopy is almost always required to visualise the whole colorectum, it is often easier and safer to obtain biopsies at this time.

Colonoscopy

A colonoscopy is required in most patients to exclude a synchronous tumour, be it an adenoma or carcinoma. If a proximal adenoma is found, it can be conveniently snared and removed via the colonoscope. If a synchronous carcinoma is present, the operative strategy is likely to change. If a full colonoscopy is not possible, for example when there is a stenosing cancer, a CT colonography or barium enema can be performed.

Differential diagnosis

Many colorectal lesions can give rise to diagnostic difficulty. For example, it may be difficult to distinguish an inflammatory stricture or amoebic granuloma on macroscopic appearance. Similarly, endometriomas, carcinoid tumours and solitary rectal ulcers can be mistaken for adenocarcinoma. Benign adenomas can be distinguished from malignant lesions based on the appearance of their mucosal 'pit patterns', as highlighted with the 'dye spray' colonoscopy technique (see ***Chapter 9***). Biopsy and histological analysis remain the mainstay of diagnosis, accepting that there may be diagnostic limitations caused by sampling errors owing to small biopsy samples being unrepresentative of the larger lesion.

Summary box 79.9

Diagnosis and assessment of rectal cancer

All patients with suspected rectal cancer should undergo:

- Digital rectal examination
- Full colorectal visualisation, preferably by colonoscopy with biopsy or CT colonography or barium enema

All patients with proven rectal cancer require staging by:

- Imaging of the chest, abdomen and pelvis, preferably by CT
- Local pelvic imaging by magnetic resonance imaging (MRI) and/or endoluminal ultrasonography

Types of carcinoma spread

Local spread

Local spread occurs circumferentially rather than in a longitudinal direction. After the muscular coat has been penetrated, the growth spreads into the surrounding mesorectum, but is initially limited by the mesorectal fascia. If penetration occurs anteriorly, the prostate, seminal vesicles or bladder become involved in the male; in the female, the vagina or the uterus is invaded. In either sex, if the penetration is lateral, a ureter may become involved, while posterior penetration may reach the sacrum and the sacral plexus. Downward spread for more than a few centimetres is rare.

Lymphatic spread

Lymphatic spread from a carcinoma of the rectum above the peritoneal reflection occurs almost exclusively in an upward direction. Below that level, the lymphatic spread is still upwards, but when the neoplasm lies within the field of the middle rectal artery, primary lateral spread to the pelvic wall lymphatics occurs in around 20% of cases. Downward spread is exceptional, with drainage along the subcutaneous lymphatics to the groins being confined, for practical purposes, to the lymph nodes draining the perianal rosette and the epithelial lining of the distal 1–2 cm of the anal canal.

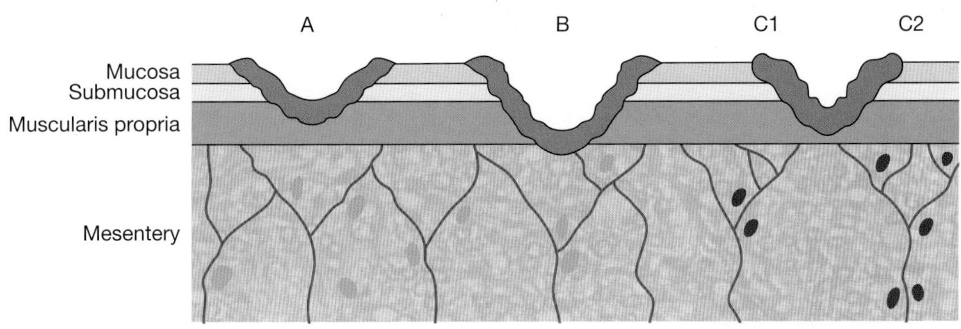

Figure 79.16 Dukes' classification of colorectal cancer. A, the cancer is confined to the bowel wall. B, the cancer penetrates the muscularis propria. C, involvement of the draining lymph nodes. Stage C was later modified: C1, pararectal nodes involved; C2, apical nodes involved.

Metastasis at a higher level than the main trunk of the superior rectal artery occurs late in the disease. A radical operation should ensure that the high-lying lymph nodes are removed by ligating the inferior mesenteric artery at its origin from the aorta. Atypical and widespread lymphatic permeation can occur with highly undifferentiated neoplasms.

Venous spread

The principal sites for blood-borne metastases are liver (34%), lungs (22%) and adrenals (11%). The remaining 33% are divided among the many other locations where secondary carcinomatous deposits tend to lodge, including the brain.

Peritoneal dissemination

This may follow penetration of the peritoneal coat by a high-lying rectal carcinoma.

Stages of progression

Dukes classified carcinoma of the rectum into three stages (*Figure 79.16*).

Dukes' staging

- A: The growth is limited to the rectal wall (15%). The prognosis is excellent (>90% 5-year survival).
- B: The growth extends to the extrarectal tissues, but without metastasis to the regional lymph nodes (35%). The prognosis is reasonable (70% 5-year survival).
- C: There are secondary deposits in the regional lymph nodes (50%). These are subdivided into C1, in which the local pararectal lymph nodes alone are involved, and C2, in which the nodes accompanying the supplying blood vessels to their origin from the aorta are involved. This does not take into account cases that have metastasised beyond the regional lymph nodes or by way of the venous system. The prognosis is poor (40% 5-year survival).

A stage D is often included, which was not described by Dukes. This stage signifies the presence of widespread metastases, usually hepatic. Other staging systems have been developed (e.g. Astler–Coller, TNM) to improve prognostic accuracy, with the tumour–node–metastasis (TNM) classification now recognised internationally as the optimum staging classification (*Table 79.2*).

TABLE 79.2 TNM staging of rectal cancer.

Tx:	Primary tumour cannot be assessed
T0:	No evidence of primary tumour
Tis:	Carcinoma *in situ*, intraepithelial or invasion of lamina propria
T1:	Tumour invading submucosa
T2:	Tumour invading the muscularis propria
T3:	Tumour penetrating the muscularis propria into perirectal fat (mesorectum)
T4a:	Tumour penetrating visceral peritoneum
T4b:	Tumour directly invading or adhering to other organs or structures
Nx:	Regional lymph nodes cannot be assessed
N0:	No lymph node metastasis and no TD
N1:	1–3 lymph node metastases
	N1a: 1 lymph node metastasis
	N1b: 2 or 3 lymph node metastases
	N1c: Submucosal, mesangial or peritoneum-covered paracolorectal TDs in the absence of regional lymph node metastases
N2:	≥ 4 lymph node metastases
	N2a: 4–6 regional lymph node metastases
	N2b: ≥ 7 lymph node metastases
M1:	There are distant metastases
	M1a: Metastases are limited to 1 organ or site (e.g. liver, lung, ovary and extraregional lymph node metastases)
	M1b: Metastases to more than 1 organ or site
	M1c: Peritoneal metastases with or without metastases to other organs

TD, tumour deposits.

Cuthbert Esquire Dukes, 1890–1977, pathologist, St Mark's Hospital, London, UK. The original Dukes' classification in 1932 gave three stages, A–C.
Vernon B Astler, surgeon, University of Michigan Medical School, Ann Arbor, MI, USA.
Frederick A Coller, 1887–1964, pathologist, University of Michigan Medical School, Ann Arbor, MI, USA.

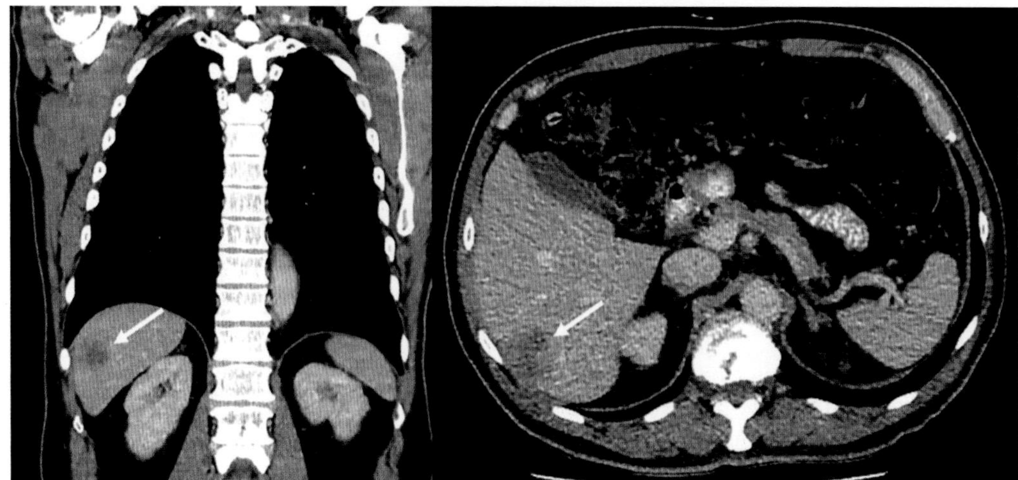

Figure 79.17 Coronal and axial images from surveillance computed tomography showing a solitary 2.5-cm metastasis in segment 6 of the liver (arrow) in a patient with rectal cancer.

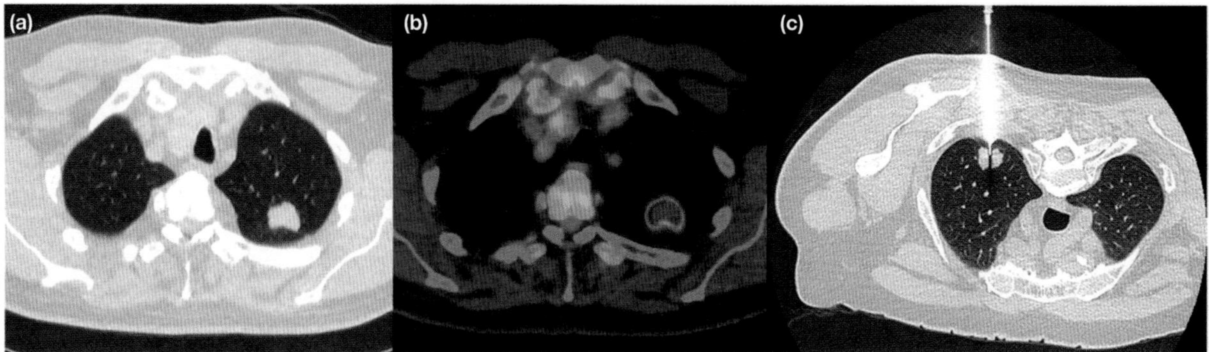

Figure 79.18 (a) Initial screening computed tomography (CT) showing a 1.5-cm diameter solid lesion in the right lung, with **(b)** positron emission tomography–CT indicating increased metabolic uptake and **(c)** later CT-guided biopsy that confirmed adenocarcinoma from a lower gastro-intestinal origin (courtesy of Dr Damian Tolan, St James's Hospital, Leeds, UK).

Radiological staging

All patients with a diagnosis of rectal cancer should undergo staging CT of the thorax, abdomen and pelvis (TAP) to stage both local and metastatic disease (***Figure 79.17***). Positron emission tomography (PET) scanning can be helpful in identifying metastases if imaging is otherwise equivocal or to identify multiple metastatic foci (***Figure 79.18***).

MRI is the best modality to assess soft-tissue extent of the tumour, the degree of infiltration of the mesorectum and mesorectal lymph node involvement and to ascertain whether the mesorectal fascia is potentially involved (***Figure 79.19***). These determinations are of great importance in guiding both surgical and oncological management.

Histological grading

In the great majority of cases, carcinoma of the rectum is an adenocarcinoma, derived from malignant transformation of the columnar rectal epithelium. The more the tumour cells retain normal shape and arrangement (well differentiated), the less aggressive the behaviour. Conversely, the more cells of an undifferentiated type, the more aggressive the behaviour. Other poor prognostic features include vascular and perineural invasion, the presence of an infiltrating (rather than pushing) margin and tumour budding. In a small number of cases, the tumour is a primary mucoid carcinoma. The mucus lies within the cells, displacing the nucleus to the periphery, like the seal of a signet ring. Signet ring carcinomas grow rapidly, metastasise early and have a poor prognosis.

Summary box 79.10

Pathology and staging of rectal cancer

- Tumours are adenocarcinomas and are well, moderately or poorly differentiated
- They spread by local, lymphatic, venous and transperitoneal routes
- Circumferential local spread is the most important and dictates management
- Lymphatic spread follows the blood supply of the rectum in a cephalad direction via the superior rectal vessels to the para-aortic nodes, but in low rectal cancer it can also involve the lateral pelvic lymph nodes
- The TNM classification is the internationally recognised staging system

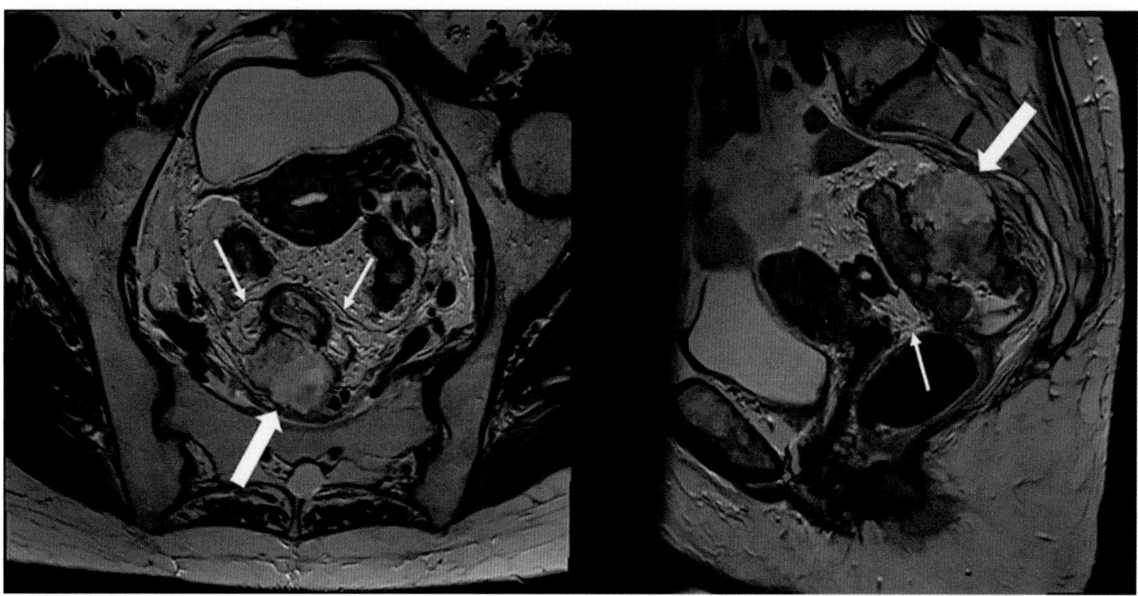

Figure 79.19 Axial and sagittal T2-weighted magnetic resonance images showing a locally advanced high-signal T3 mucinous rectal cancer with involvement of the posterior circumferential resection margin (thick arrows) anterior to the second sacral segment. Note the position of the peritoneal reflection and the peritoneum in relation to the tumour (thin arrows) (courtesy of Dr Damian Tolan, St James's Hospital, Leeds, UK).

Treatment

Surgical excision of the tumour is the conventional treatment, provided this can be achieved with clear oncological margins and acceptable risk of morbidity and mortality. However, the management of rectal cancer has become increasingly complex because of the various surgical techniques available and the range of neoadjuvant and adjuvant options. Before treatment can be planned, it is necessary to assess both the fitness of the patient and the extent of spread of the tumour. The management needs to be discussed within a multidisciplinary team (MDT) setting involving surgeons, radiologists, oncologists, pathologists and specialty nurses. It is particularly important that the recommendation be documented and discussed with the patient. The ultimate treatment decision is made jointly with the patient, taking their wishes and expectations fully into account.

Principles of surgical treatment

Radical excision of the rectum, together with the mesorectum and associated lymph nodes, should be the aim in most cases. In the presence of widespread metastases, other means of palliation should be considered, such as endoluminal stenting or external beam radiotherapy, although there may still be a role for palliative resection. The presence of liver metastases does not necessarily rule out the feasibility of cure: the results of surgery for liver metastases have greatly improved, with long-term survival being achieved in over a third of patients (see ***Chapter 69***).

When a tumour appears to be locally advanced (i.e. invading a neighbouring structure or threatening to breach the circumferential resection margin), the use of neoadjuvant (preoperative) radiotherapy or chemoradiotherapy is usually considered. Long-course chemoradiotherapy is given as five fractions of radiotherapy combined with chemotherapy over a 6-week period. The aim is to downstage the cancer and increase the chances of a complete resection with clear oncological margins. Alternatively, preoperative 'short-course' (5 days) radiotherapy can be used if the resection margins are not threatened but the cancer is still at high risk for local recurrence (e.g. perirectal lymph node involvement).

Approximately 20% of rectal cancers treated by neoadjuvant chemoradiotherapy show a complete clinical response with no evidence of residual cancer on clinical examination, biopsy or radiological imaging. There is an increasing trend for such patients to be offered the option of 'watch and wait' (Habr-Gama) in the hope that they may have been cured of the disease and spared the morbidity of resectional surgery. Some 30% of cases will recur on a 'watch-and-wait' policy, but most can be salvaged by surgical resection (***Figures 79.20 and 79.21***).

There is also growing enthusiasm for 'organ-preserving' surgical techniques in early T1 and even T2 cancers with good prognostic features. This usually involves full-thickness excision of the cancer using TEMS (***Figure 79.22***). Alternative 'organ-preserving' techniques involve the use of brachytherapy and contact radiotherapy, but these are currently reserved for patients unfit for radical resection or as a means of palliation.

When radical excision is possible, the aim should be to restore gastrointestinal continuity and continence by preserving the anal sphincter whenever feasible. A sphincter-saving operation (anterior resection) is usually possible for tumours whose lower margin is ≥2 cm above the anorectal junction. Although in the past removal of the rectum and anus with a

Angelita Habr-Gama, b. 1934, surgeon, Sao Paolo, Brazil.

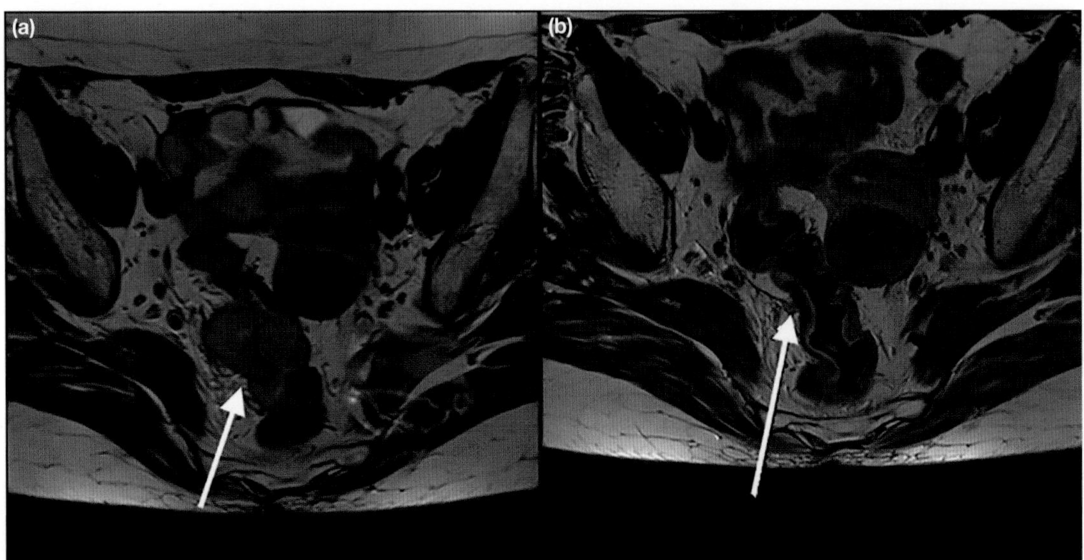

Figure 79.20 T2-weighted magnetic resonance images showing complete response to chemoradiotherapy in a T3 rectosigmoid cancer involving the circumferential resection margin (arrows). Axial images before (a) and after (b) treatment showing normalisation of the rectal wall layer structure and only minimal extramural fibrosis in place of the large tumour (courtesy of Dr Damian Tolan, St James's Hospital, Leeds, UK).

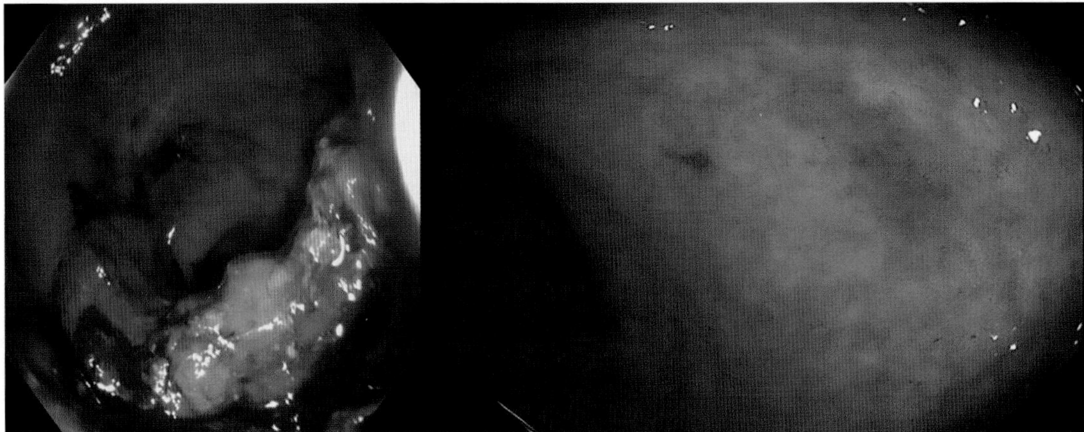

Figure 79.21 Endoscopic view of rectal cancer showing complete response after neoadjuvant chemoradiotherapy. Endoscopic view (a) at the time of diagnosis. Following neoadjuvant treatment (b) with the site of a tattoo only visible (courtesy of Julian Hance, St James's Hospital, Leeds, UK).

permanent colostomy (abdominoperineal excision) was often required for tumours, the introduction of the stapled anastomosis and chemoradiotherapy downstaging has enabled many more patients to be treated by a sphincter-saving procedure.

The principles of anterior resection involve radical excision of the cancer along with its complete mesorectal envelope, combined with high proximal ligation of the inferior mesenteric lymphovascular pedicle. Once the left colon and rectum have been mobilised, the distal rectum is divided at least 1 cm (and preferably more) below the distal cancer margin and the specimen removed. Rectosigmoid cancers and those in the upper third of the rectum are removed by 'high anterior resection', in which the rectum and mesorectum are taken to a margin of at least 3 cm distal to the tumour and a colorectal anastomosis is performed. For tumours in the middle and lower thirds of the rectum, complete removal of the rectum and mesorectum is required, i.e. TME (Heald). Restoration of continuity is usually performed using a stapling technique, which might involve an end-to-end, side-to-end or colopouch construction in low cancers (***Figure 79.23***). The retention of at least a part of the rectum in high anterior resection results in better postoperative function, with less risk of anterior resection syndrome, a condition characterised by defecatory urgency, incontinence and incomplete evacuation, secondary to removal of the normal rectal reservoir. In cancers situated below the peritoneal reflection it is usual practice to defunction the anastomosis with a temporary stoma because of the higher risk of anastomotic leak. Although a defunctioning stoma does not prevent anastomotic leak, it does mitigate against septic complications should a leak occur.

RJ (Bill) Heald, contemporary, surgeon, Basingstoke, UK, and Champalimaud Foundation, Lisbon, Portugal.

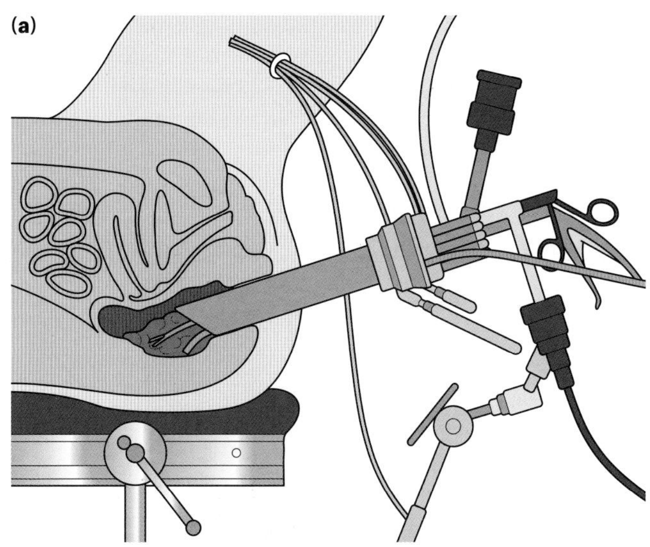

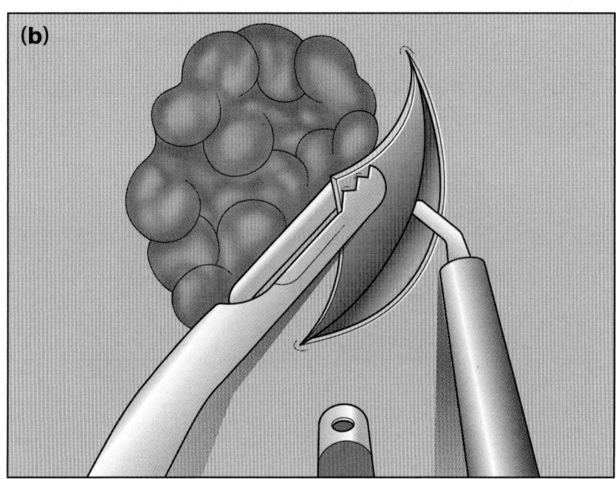

Figure 79.22 Transanal endoscopic microsurgery. (a) An operating sigmoidoscope is inserted through the anal canal to visualise the lesion and enable passage of a laparoscope and instruments. (b) A full-thickness local excision is performed. The defect is closed or, alternatively, may be left open if the peritoneum is not breached.

Summary box 79.11

Surgery for rectal cancer

- Surgery is the mainstay of curative therapy
- The primary resection consists of rectal resection performed by TME
- Early cancers (stages T1 and selected T2) may be suitable for local excision
- Most cases can be treated by anterior resection, with a colorectal or coloanal anastomosis being achieved with a circular stapling device
- Low, extensive tumours require an abdominoperineal excision with a permanent colostomy
- Neoadjuvant chemoradiotherapy can be used to downstage the cancer and reduce local recurrence
- 'Watch and wait' non-operative management is an option for the 20% who have a complete clinical response to neoadjuvant chemoradiotherapy

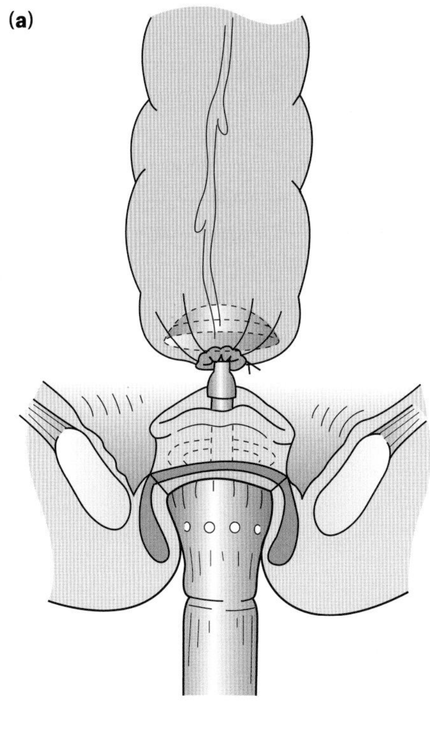

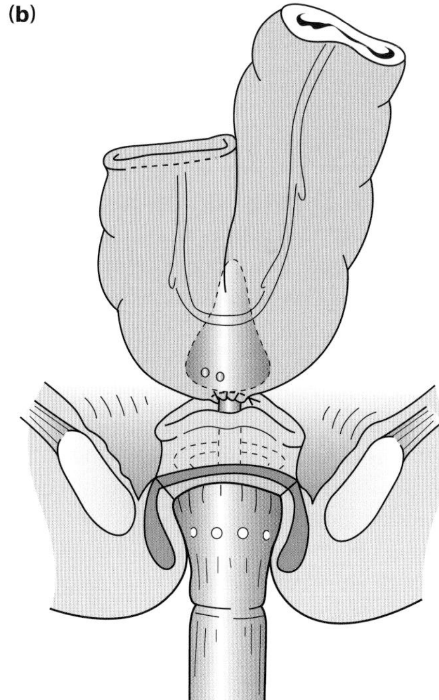

Figure 79.23 Low anterior resection by the double stapling method. The rectum has been excised and the distal anorectal stump has been transected with a transverse stapling device. A circular stapling device is used to construct either (a) a straight low coloanal anastomosis or (b) a colopouch–anal anastomosis.

Preoperative preparation

The bowel is usually prepared by mechanical cleansing using a combination of diet, purgatives and enemas to reduce intraoperative contamination and the risk of surgical site infection. While this approach has been used selectively, recent guidelines recommend preoperative bowel preparation.

Prophylactic systemic antibiotics are usually given perioperatively to reduce the risk of surgical site infection. In Europe, this usually takes the form of broad-spectrum antibiotics given intravenously at induction of anaesthesia. In the USA, antibiotic prophylaxis is more frequently administered as a course of oral antibiotics (neomycin and metronidazole) given preoperatively in addition to intravenous antibiotics at the induction of anaesthesia. There is evidence to suggest that this may reduce the risk of septic complications, including anastomotic leak.

All patients should be seen by a stoma care nurse preoperatively and be sited for a temporary or permanent ileostomy and/or colostomy. They must also be counselled as to the complications of the procedure, and particularly about the risks of pelvic autonomic nerve damage causing bladder and sexual disturbance, especially impotence in males.

Summary box 79.12

Preoperative preparation

- Counselling and siting of stomas
- Correction of anaemia and electrolyte disturbance
- Type and screen for blood transfusion
- Bowel preparation
- Deep vein thrombosis prophylaxis
- Prophylactic antibiotics

Local operations

Early rectal cancers (T1 and good prognosis T2) may be amenable to local transanal excision, preserving much of the rectal reservoir and therefore near normal function. Histological analysis of the specimen is then used to assess the adequacy of excision with respect to the probability of positive lymph nodes being left behind. This may range from 10% in T1 cancers to 20% in T2 cancers and clinical judgement, along with in-depth conversation with the patient, is required to determine whether local excision has achieved a sufficient chance of oncological cure or whether a further radical resection is required.

Local excision is usually performed with one of the commercially available transanal laparoscopic systems or with equipment modified from transanal total mesorectal excision (taTME) procedures (see ***Transanal total mesorectal excision***). A full-thickness excision of the lesion is performed and the defect closed with sutures or else left open. There is a limit to the height of lesion that can be resected, with more proximal lesions in the upper rectum being difficult.

Anterior resection

There has been a move to extend sphincter-saving operations to treat most tumours of the middle and lower thirds of the rectum, thus reducing the abdominoperineal excision rate and the need for permanent colostomy. There is also an increasing trend to use laparoscopic techniques for anterior resection, with patient benefits including less pain, quicker recovery from surgery and improved cosmesis. The evidence suggests that laparoscopic anterior resection is as safe as open surgery in terms of short- and long-term complications and oncological outcomes. More recently, robotic assistance has been employed with the da Vinci robotic surgical system (Intuitive Surgical Inc., Sunnyvale, CA, USA) (***Figure 79.24***). Although this adds significant cost to the procedure, there may be some benefit in terms of a reduced need to convert to open surgery, and

(a)

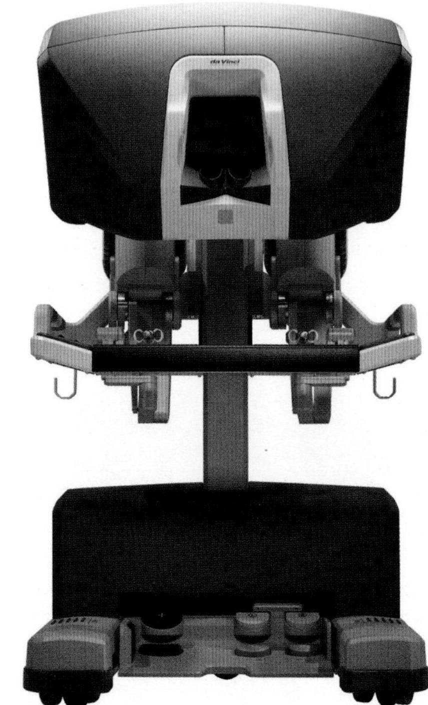

(b)

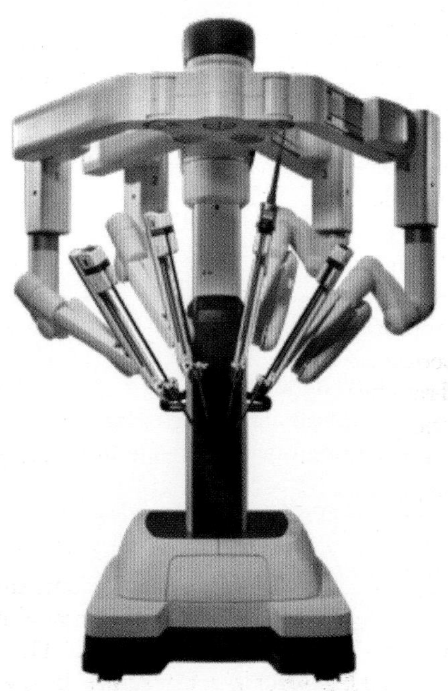

Figure 79.24 da Vinci Xi Robotic Surgical System: **(a)** surgeon console; **(b)** patient cart. (Reproduced with kind permission from Intuitive Surgical Inc. https://www.intuitive.com/en-us/products-and-services/da-vinci/systems/.)

therefore more patients benefiting from a minimally invasive approach. The operation performed is the same whether the procedure is undertaken by open, laparoscopic or robotic surgery, with the difference being in the extent of abdominal access trauma (laparotomy wound versus 'keyhole' incisions).

In open surgery, a midline abdominal incision is made and full laparotomy performed to detect synchronous pathologies, including evidence of intra-abdominal cancer spread. The sigmoid and descending colon are freed by dividing the peritoneal reflection on the left side and then mobilising them to the midline on their mesentery, protecting the left ureter and testicular/ovarian vessels. The splenic flexure is mobilised to gain sufficient left colonic length to allow tension-free colorectal anastomosis. Rectal dissection is performed in the embryological planes (TME) with preservation of the autonomic nerves, which course over the pelvic brim (sympathetic nerves) and exit from the pelvic plexuses (parasympathetic nerves) to supply the pelvic floor and the urogenital organs (***Figure 79.25***). Once rectal dissection has reached the anorectal junction (low anterior resection), or at least 3 cm below the cancer (high anterior resection), the rectum is divided, usually with the aid of a stapling device.

The mesocolon is divided at the site of the proposed division of the colon and the trunk of the inferior mesenteric artery is ligated and divided at its origin from the aorta (high tie). Resection of the specimen is completed by division of the bowel at the point to be used for the proximal anastomosis.

Restoration of bowel continuity is usually achieved by means of a stapled anastomosis. The simplest way of achieving this is by using a 'double stapling' technique, whereby a circular stapling device (***Figure 79.23***) is passed transanally to anastomose the stapled ends of the proximal colon and rectal stump. Alternatively, a 'single stapled' anastomosis may be performed in which purse-string sutures are applied to the proximal colon and rectal stump and anastomosed using a single firing of a circular stapling device inserted transanally. In cases where the anastomosis is very low (coloanal anastomosis) it may be necessary to perform a hand-sewn anastomosis.

Laparoscopic and robotic anterior resection follow the above general principles, but with abdominal access through the use of four or five abdominal ports and carbon dioxide pneumoperitoneum. The dissection usually follows a medial-to-lateral approach, i.e. dissection and high ligation of the vascular pedicle followed by lateral mobilisation of the colon, then rectal resection. A small laparotomy wound is still required to extract the specimen, unless transanal specimen extraction is possible, and restoration of bowel continuity is performed by the usual stapling techniques.

Transanal total mesorectal excision

taTME builds on the principles of laparoscopic surgery, with an airtight anal device used to provide transanal insufflation and access for laparoscopic instruments. The operation proceeds by placing a purse-string suture below the distal level of the tumour and incising the bowel wall to enter the mesorectal plane. Dissection then proceeds using a 'bottom-up' approach to accomplish TME. It is usual for this procedure to be undertaken as a combined operation, with synchronous 'top-down' laparoscopic resection by an abdominal operator who mobilises the left colon, takes down the splenic flexure and does some of the upper rectal dissection.

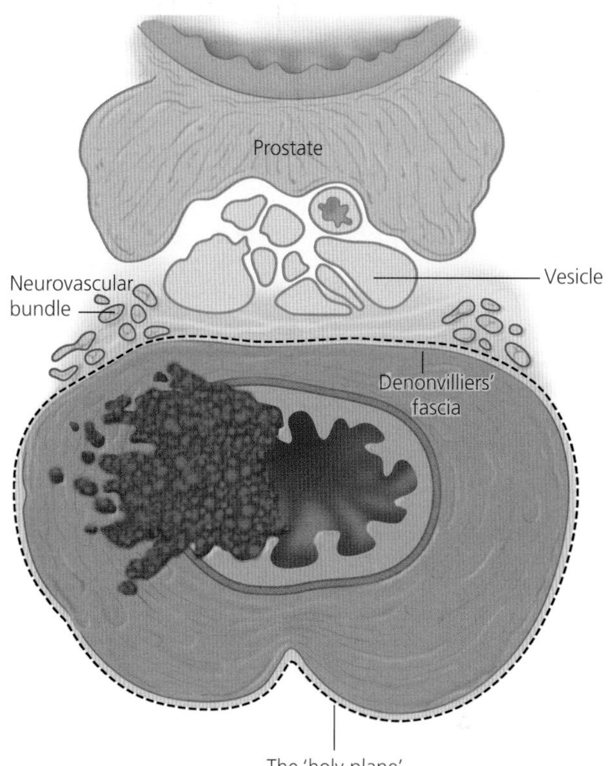

Figure 79.25 Plane of dissection for total mesorectal excision in a male with midrectal cancer. (Reproduced with permission from O'Connell PR, Madoff RD, Solomon MJ (eds). *Operative surgery of the colon, rectum and anus*, 6th edn. Boca Raton, FL: CRC Press, 2015.)

Initial results have demonstrated that taTME is safe, with short-term oncological outcomes, in terms of pathological quality of the resection specimen and circumferential resection margins, comparable to those of traditional laparoscopic and open techniques. However, concerns have been raised regarding the increased incidence of urethral injuries and the development of multifocal local recurrences. These concerns highlight the critical importance of adequate taTME training, proper case selection, and proctorship with maintenance of high procedural volumes in an MDT setting to help ensure optimal outcomes. Meanwhile, several multicentre randomised controlled trials such as COLOR III and TaLaR are well under way to confirm the long-term oncological safety of taTME.

Hartmann's operation

This is an option in elderly and frail patients in whom there is concern about poor anal sphincter function and postoperative incontinence or the viability of an anastomosis. Colorectal excision follows the same principles as outlined above, but the rectal stump is stapled closed and the proximal colon exteriorised as a permanent end-colostomy.

Abdominoperineal excision of the rectum

This operation is still required for some tumours of the lower third of the rectum that are unsuitable for a sphincter-saving

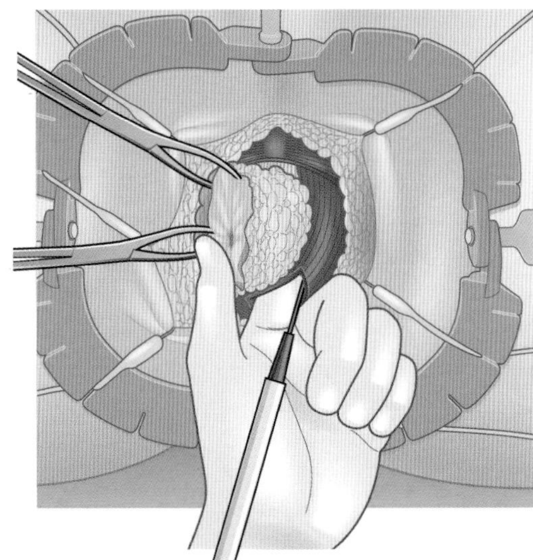

Figure 79.26 Separation and division of the pubococcygeus and puborectalis muscles in the course of the perineal phase of an abdominoperineal excision of the rectum. (Reproduced with permission from O'Connell PR, Madoff RD, Solomon MJ (eds). *Operative surgery of the colon, rectum and anus*, 6th edn. Boca Raton, FL: CRC Press, 2015.)

procedure. Traditionally, the procedure was performed by two surgeons operating simultaneously, one via the abdomen and the other via the perineum, with the patient in the Trendelenburg lithotomy position. More recently, there has been a shift to completing the abdominal procedure first (with the patient in the Lloyd-Davies position, in which the legs are in supports set lower than the lithotomy position), and then placing the patient either in a prone jack-knife or Lloyd-Davies position and completing the operation via the perineum. The aim is to produce a complete resection of the rectum and mesorectum along with cylindrical excision of the extralevator component. This achieves wide excision at the level of the pelvic floor, increasing complete resection rates and reducing local perforation and the risk of local recurrence.

The abdominal procedure is carried out laparoscopically or via a midline laparotomy and is performed in the same way as an anterior resection, except that dissection stops before the pelvic floor is reached (at the level of the seminal vesicles in men or the cervix in women) to avoid 'coning down' onto the tumour at the level of the pelvic floor. Perineal dissection is achieved through a circumanal incision, which is deepened into the ischiorectal fossae and out towards the attachment of the levator muscles to the pelvic side wall (***Figure 79.26***). The dissection is extended posteriorly by incising Waldeyer's fascia, which is a thick condensation of pelvic fascia lying between the rectum and the sacrum. Some surgeons routinely remove the coccyx to improve access and surgical margins. Anteriorly, the plane between the rectum and the prostate in the male or between the rectum and the vagina in the female is developed, with particular care to avoid the membranous urethra in the male. A catheter within it should be palpated so that it can be avoided.

The posterior wall of the vagina can be excised with the rectum if an advanced anterior tumour is present. Resection is completed when the perineal dissection reaches the abdominal dissection, with the specimen retrieved through the perineal wound. An end-colostomy is formed in the left iliac fossa and the wounds closed with drains to the pelvis.

Endoluminal stenting

An increasingly used alternative for patients with an obstructing carcinoma is placement of an endoluminal stent, which can be done endoscopically, often with fluoroscopic guidance. This can be used either as a palliative procedure or to relieve obstruction and permit elective rather than emergency surgery to be undertaken. Only rectosigmoid and upper rectal tumours are suitable for stenting because stent impingement on the anorectum in low cancers causes symptoms of tenesmus (see ***Chapter 77***).

Palliative colostomy

This is indicated only in cases giving rise to intestinal obstruction, or where the rectal cancer is not resectable. It can be performed by either an open or laparoscopic approach. In some cases, a defunctioning colostomy is required in advanced cancers to prevent obstruction during downstaging chemoradiotherapy.

Pelvic exenteration

When carcinoma of the rectum has spread to contiguous organs, a more radical operation known as pelvic exenteration can remove these structures en bloc. Thus, in the male, in whom spread is usually to the bladder or prostate, a cystectomy or prostatectomy may be required in combination with anterior resection to achieve complete oncological clearance. In the female, the uterus acts as an oncological barrier, preventing spread from the rectum to the bladder. Accordingly, a hysterectomy can be undertaken in addition to excision of the rectum.

The aim is to remove pelvic organs involved in the malignant process and may involve a partial (posterior exenteration, including rectum and posterior vagina/uterus) or complete (including rectum and urogenital organs) exenteration (***Figure 79.27***).

Total pelvic exenteration may also be necessary for local disease recurrence. It involves a large excision of the pelvic floor, leaving a sizeable perineal defect that has to be reconstructed using rectus abdominus or gluteal flaps to fill the empty pelvis. Excision of the bladder will require the formation of an ileal conduit in addition to a colostomy. Following such radical surgery, quality of life (QoL) is a crucial postoperative consideration, and therefore detailed preoperative discussion with patients regarding QoL post procedure is required.

Liver resection

Single or multiple well-localised liver metastases can now be resected with relatively low mortality and morbidity. Provided

Friedrich Trendelenburg, 1844–1924, Professor of Surgery, successively at Rostock (1875–1882), Bonn (1882–1895) and Leipzig (1895–1911), Germany. The Trendelenburg position was first described in 1885.

Oswald Vaughan Lloyd-Davies, 1905–1987, surgeon, St Mark's Hospital, London, UK.

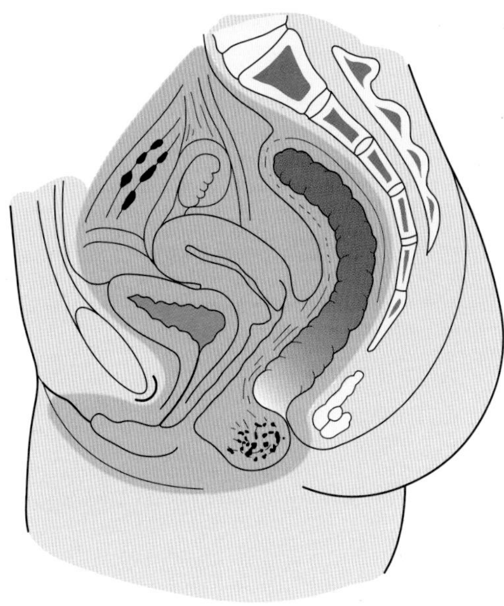

Figure 79.27 Radical pelvic exenteration, indicating the extent of the dissection and the viscera removed (shaded dark pink). (Redrawn with permission from Keighley MRB, Williams NS. *Surgery of the anus, rectum and colon*. London: WB Saunders, 1999.)

the patients are carefully selected, a reasonable long-term survival rate can be achieved (approximately 40%). Such surgery is usually carried out in a specialised liver unit and may be performed synchronously at the time of anterior resection or as a delayed procedure (see ***Chapter 69***).

Radiotherapy

Radiotherapy is now commonly used and may be given preoperatively (neoadjuvant) and less commonly postoperatively (adjuvant). In the neoadjuvant setting, radiotherapy is used to either 'sterilise' the operative field in cancers with suspected lymphovascular involvement, or to downstage locally advanced cancers with threatened circumferential resection margins. In the former instance, radiotherapy is often given as a 'short course' over 5 days with immediate surgery some 7–10 days later. On occasion, short-course radiotherapy can be combined with a delay before surgery (up to 12 weeks) to allow cancer regression.

When radiotherapy is used to downstage a cancer, it is often combined with chemotherapy (chemoradiotherapy) and given over a period of 6 weeks with a 6-week recovery period before surgery. Some 20% of cancers treated with chemoradiotherapy will show a complete pathological response, with a further 25–30% showing a partial response. Unfortunately, it is not yet possible to determine prior to treatment which patients will respond and therefore to tailor treatment accordingly.

Occasionally, radiotherapy is used to palliate unresectable cancers that are causing symptoms due to pain, obstruction or bleeding.

Alternative radiotherapy regimens include the Papillon technique, in which intracavity radiation is directed to the cancer in the form of 'contact radiotherapy' or else delivered by brachytherapy techniques. To date, the application of these techniques has been restricted to selected cases, usually in patients unfit for more radical surgery.

Chemotherapy

Chemotherapy is given either in combination with radiotherapy (chemoradiotherapy) to downstage a cancer prior to surgical resection or else in the postoperative setting to reduce the risk of disseminated disease. 5-Fluorouracil (5-FU)-based regimens remain the first-line therapy and are associated with a 10% improvement in disease-free survival in patients with node-positive rectal cancer. Second-line therapies include oxaliplatin and irinotecan, and biological agents such as cetuximab (see ***Chapter 12***).

Results of surgery for rectal cancer

In specialised centres, the resectability rate for rectal cancer may be as high as 95%, with an operative mortality of less than 5%. Overall, the 5-year survival rate is about 50% and has not changed appreciably over the last decade. Survival rates are influenced by TNM/Dukes' stage, with node-positive patients doing worse than those with node-negative lesions. However, with the introduction of national bowel cancer screening programmes, there is a shift to an earlier stage of disease presentation and consequently improved survival.

Local recurrence

Local recurrence after rectal excision represents a complex problem. The patient may be asymptomatic with recurrence diagnosed as part of a surveillance programme, including regular measurements of blood carcinoembryonic antigen and cross-sectional radiological imaging. The presence of symptoms is often a poor prognostic feature. Persistent pelvic pain, which may radiate down the legs, is indicative of nerve root involvement. Bladder symptoms may occur or there may be fistulating disease onto the perineum. Most local recurrences are situated extrarectally and are therefore not readily diagnosed on endoscopy examination and biopsy. CT and MRI scan are the best means for detecting local recurrence, but PET-CT is increasingly being used to differentiate metabolically active cancer recurrence from metabolically inactive scar tissue. Local recurrence rates vary between 2% and 25% and are higher after abdominoperineal excision than after sphincter-saving resection. High-quality primary surgery with preservation of the mesorectal 'package' and a clear circumferential resection margin are the most important factors in preventing local recurrence.

Overall, 80% of local recurrences develop within 2 years following surgery, are very difficult to treat and should be referred to a centre specialising in exenterative surgery. If the patient is radiotherapy naive then preoperative chemoradiotherapy may be of help. Surgical exenteration offers the only hope of cure.

Jean Papillon, d. 1993, radiation oncologist, Centre Léon Bérard, Lyon, France.

FURTHER READING

Association of Coloproctology of Great Britain and Ireland. Guidelines for the management of cancer of the colon, rectum and anus (2017). *Colorectal Dis* 2017; **19**(S1): 1–97.

Baxter NN, Garcia-Aguilar J. Organ preservation for rectal cancer. *J Clin Oncol* 2007; **25**: 1014–20.

Brown PJ, Hyland R, Quyn AJ *et al.* Current concepts in imaging for local staging of advanced rectal cancer. *Clin Radiol* 2019; **74**(8): 623–36.

Cancer Research UK. *Bowel cancer statistics.* Available from www.cancerresearchuk.org/health-professional/cancer-statistics/statistics-by-cancer-type/bowel-cancer

Tou S, Brown SR, Nelson RL. Surgery for complete (full-thickness) rectal prolapse in adults. *Cochrane Database Syst Rev* 2015; Issue 11, Art. No. CD001758.

Wolthuis AM, Bislenghi G, de Buck van Overstraeten A, D'Hoore A. Transanal total mesorectal excision: towards standardization of technique. *World J Gastroenterol* 2015; **21**(44): 12686–95.

Wright JP, Albert MR. A current review of robotic colorectal surgery. *Ann Laparosc Endosc Surg* 2020; **5**. https://ales.amegroups.com/article/view/5613

CHAPTER

80 The anus and anal canal

Learning objectives

To understand:

- The anatomy and physiology of the anus and anal canal with special reference to clinical presentation, investigation and differential diagnosis
- Anal disease is common and treatment is often conservative
- Aggressive or inappropriate surgery may render the patient disabled

ANATOMY AND PHYSIOLOGY OF THE ANAL CANAL

Surgical anatomy

The anal canal starts at the level where the rectum passes through the pelvic diaphragm, where the rectal ampulla suddenly narrows, and ends at the anal verge. The muscular junction between the rectum and anal canal can be felt with the finger as a thickened ridge called the anorectal ring (***Figure 80.1***).

Anal canal anatomy

The anus is 3–4 cm long in adults, being longer in the adult male than in the female. Posterior is the anococcygeal ligament, which separates it from the tip of the coccyx, while anteriorly it is separated by the perineal body from the membranous urethra and penile bulb or the lower vagina. Laterally are the ischiorectal fossae. The anal canal is lined by mucosa and the sphincter muscles constitute the muscular wall. The anorectal ring is formed by fusion of the puborectalis muscle and the deep external anal sphincter. It can be clearly felt on a digital rectal examination, particularly posteriorly and laterally.

The puborectalis muscle

The puborectalis muscle maintains the angle between the anal canal and rectum (the anorectal angle) and is an important component in the continence mechanism (***Figure 80.2***). The muscle derives its nerve supply from the sacral somatic nerves. The position and length of the anal canal, as well as the angle of the anorectal junction, depend to a major extent on the integrity and strength of the puborectalis muscle sling.

The external anal sphincter

The external sphincter forms the bulk of the anal sphincter complex and, although traditionally it has been subdivided

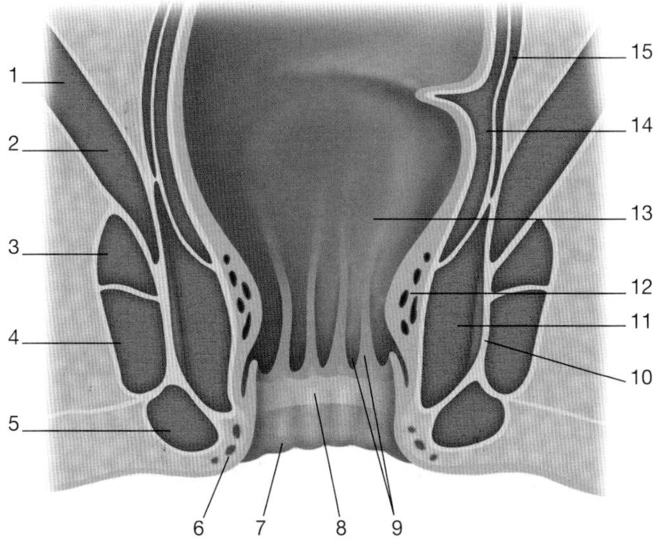

1 Levator ani muscle (iliococcygeal muscle)
2 Levator ani muscle (puborectal muscle)
3–5 External anal sphincter (deep, superficial, subcutaneous)
6 Inferior haemorrhoidal plexus
7 Perianal skin
8 Anoderm
9 Anal columns and crypts
10 Conjoined longitudinal muscle (corrugator ani muscle)
11 Internal anal sphincter
12 Superior haemorrhoidal plexus
13 Anorectal junction
14 Circular rectal muscle layer
15 Longitudinal rectal muscle

Figure 80.1 Anatomy of the anal canal. (Adapted from Anatomy of the colon, rectum, anus, and pelvic floor. In Herold A, Lehur PA, Matzel KE, O'Connell PR (eds). *Coloproctology*. Heidelberg: Springer-Verlag, 2008.)

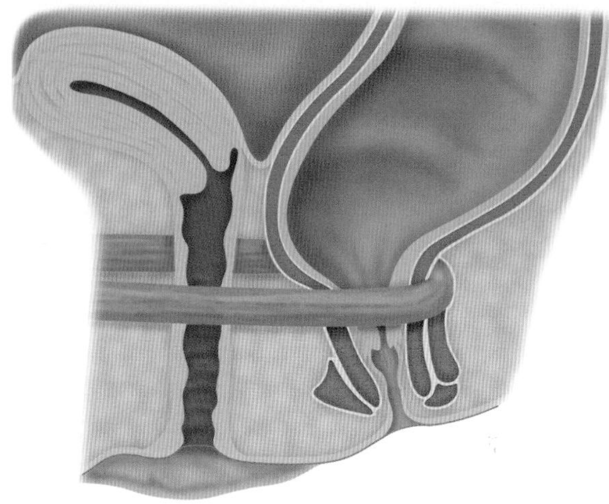

Figure 80.2 The puborectalis muscle. Note how it maintains the rectoanal angle.

into deep, superficial and subcutaneous portions, it is a single muscle (Goligher), which is variably divided by lateral extensions from the longitudinal muscle layer. Some of the fibres are attached to the coccyx posteriorly, whereas anteriorly they fuse with the perineal muscles. Being a somatic voluntary muscle, the external sphincter is red in colour. It is innervated by the pudendal nerve.

The internal sphincter

The internal sphincter is the thickened (2–5 mm) distal continuation of the circular muscle layer of the rectum. This involuntary muscle commences where the rectum passes through the pelvic diaphragm and ends above the anal orifice, its lower border palpable at the intersphincteric groove, below which lie the most medial fibres of the subcutaneous external sphincter, and separated from it by the anal intermuscular septum. When exposed during life, it is pearly-white in colour and its circumferentially placed fibres can be seen clearly. Although innervated by the autonomic nervous system, it receives intrinsic non-adrenergic and non-cholinergic fibres, stimulation of which causes release of the neurotransmitter nitric oxide, which induces internal sphincter relaxation.

The longitudinal muscle

The longitudinal muscle is a direct continuation of the smooth muscle of the outer muscle coat of the rectum, augmented in its upper part by striated muscle fibres originating from the medial components of the pelvic floor. The muscle passes caudally between the external and internal sphincters before splitting into multiple terminal septa that surround the muscle bundles of the subcutaneous portion of the external sphincter, to insert into the skin of the lowermost part of the anal canal and adjacent perianal skin. The most medial of these septa, passing around the inferior border of the internal sphincter, have been termed the 'anal intermuscular septum'. Distally the septum gives off fibres that pass medially across the internal sphincter to reach the submucosal space and laterally across the external sphincter and ischiorectal space to reach the fascia of the pelvic side walls. As well as providing support for the anal canal the septa created provide potential pathways for the spread of infection.

During defecation, contraction of the longitudinal muscle widens the anal lumen, flattens the anal cushions, shortens the anal canal and everts the anal margin; subsequent relaxation allows the anal cushions to distend and thus contribute to an airtight seal.

The intersphincteric plane

Between the external sphincter muscle laterally and the longitudinal muscle medially exists a potential space, the intersphincteric plane. This is important as it contains intersphincteric anal glands (see ***The epithelium and subepithelial structures***) and is also a route for the spread of infection, which occurs along the extensions from the longitudinal muscle layer. This plane can be surgically explored to gain access to sphincter muscles.

The epithelium and subepithelial structures

The pink columnar epithelium lining the rectum extends through the anorectal ring into the upper anal canal. Passing downwards the columnar mucosa becomes a cuboidal 'transitional zone' characterised by 8–12 vertical columns separated by anal sinuses that form folds at their lower ends, the anal valves or crypts (of Morgagni). The row of alternating columns and crypts gives a serrated appearance known as the **dentate line**, which is considered to be the embryological junction between the endodermal and ectodermal parts of the anal canal (the proctodaeum) (***Figure 80.1***). Below the dentate line the anoderm is lined by non-keratinised stratified squamous epithelium that is devoid of glands and hair but richly innervated by somatic sensory nerve endings (Wedel).

Between the epithelial layer and the internal sphincter lies the submucosa, consisting of vascular, muscular and connective tissue supportive elements. From the longitudinal muscle, medial extensions cross the internal anal sphincter and form part of the supporting meshwork of the submucosa, blending with the true submucosal smooth muscle layer supporting the mucosa itself, termed the 'mucosal suspensory ligament'. This separates the superior (portal) and inferior (systemic) haemorrhoidal plexuses. Here the mucosa is more firmly tethered to underlying tissues than above. It is important to appreciate that the meshwork of supporting tissues (muscle fibres and connective tissue) within the subepithelial space is intimately linked to deeper structures within the anal sphincter complex, including the internal sphincter, longitudinal muscle layer and external anal sphincter. With age, the smooth muscle component of this mesh is gradually replaced with fibroelastic connective tissue, which in turn becomes fragmented.

John Cedric Goligher, 1912–1998, Professor of Surgery, University of Leeds, Leeds, UK.
Giovani Battista Morgagni, 1682–1771, Professor of Anatomy, Padua, Italy, regarded as the founder of morbid anatomy.
Thilo Wedel, contemporary, anatomist, University of Kiel, Germany.

Blood supply

The subepithelial space contains venous dilatations supported by the fibroelastic connective tissue and smooth muscle scaffolding. Debate has centred on the nature of the vascular component of haemorrhoids. Thomson demonstrated that the divisions of the superior rectal artery were not constant and that the anal submucosa also receives a blood supply from the middle and inferior rectal arteries. In addition, there is free communication between tributaries of the superior, middle and inferior rectal veins, as well as direct arteriovenous communications with the submucosal venous dilatations. These communications have been shown both histologically and radiologically, and the oxygen tension of the blood contained within the venous dilatations is more arterial than venous. This explains the bright red colour of haemorrhoidal bleeding rather than the darker venous blood that might be expected.

Venous drainage

The anal veins are distributed in a similar fashion to the arterial supply. The upper half of the anal canal is drained by the superior rectal veins, tributaries of the inferior mesenteric vein and thus the portomesenteric venous system, and the middle rectal veins, which drain into the internal iliac veins. The inferior rectal veins drain the lower half of the anal canal and the subcutaneous perianal plexus of veins; they eventually join the internal iliac vein on each side.

Lymphatic drainage

Lymph from the upper half of the anal canal flows upwards to drain into the mesorectal lymph nodes and from there goes to the para-aortic nodes via the inferior mesenteric chain. Lymph from the lower half of the anal canal drains on each side, first into the superficial and then into the deep inguinal group of lymph glands.

Summary box 80.1

Anatomy and physiology of the anal canal

- The internal sphincter is composed of circular, non-striated involuntary muscle supplied by autonomic nerves
- The external sphincter is composed of striated voluntary muscle supplied by the pudendal nerve
- Extensions from the longitudinal muscle layer support the sphincter complex
- The space between sphincters is known as the intersphincteric plane
- The superior part of the external sphincter fuses with the puborectalis muscle, which is essential for maintaining the anorectal angle, necessary for continence
- The lower part of the anal canal is lined by sensitive squamous epithelium
- Blood supply to the anal canal is via superior, middle and inferior rectal vessels
- Lymphatic drainage of the lower half of the anal canal goes to inguinal lymph nodes

EXAMINATION OF THE ANUS

Careful clinical examination will be diagnostic in the vast majority of patients complaining of anal symptoms, but it requires a relaxed patient who is informed of what the examination will entail, a private environment, a chaperone (for the security of both parties) and good light. Most commonly, the patient is examined in the left lateral (Sims) position with the buttocks overlying the edge of the examination couch and with the axis of the torso crossing, rather than parallel with, the edge of the couch. Alternatively, in younger patients, the prone jack-knife or knee–elbow positions may be used (***Figure 80.3***). Some units with access to a gynaecology couch may place the patient supine with legs in stirrups. The examining couch should be of sufficient height to allow easy inspection and access for any necessary manoeuvres. Personal protective equipment should be worn.

Inspection

The buttocks are gently parted to allow inspection of the anus and perineum: the presence of any skin lesions and whether they are confined to the perineum or evident elsewhere on general examination, e.g. psoriasis, lichen planus, or on genital examination, e.g. warts, candidiasis, lichen sclerosus, the vesicles of herpes simplex virus (HSV); evidence of anal leakage; whether the anus is closed or patulous; and the position of the anus and perineum at rest and on bearing down (the latter may reveal prolapse of haemorrhoids or even the rectum). Pain on parting the buttocks, perhaps together with the presence of a sentinel tag, may indicate the presence of an underlying fissure, but may also prompt the need for endoluminal examination under anaesthesia to exclude more suspicious pathology, for example squamous cell carcinoma (SCC) of the anal canal.

Digital examination with the index finger

With an adequately lubricated index finger, the soft tissues around the anus are palpated for induration, tenderness and subcutaneous lesions. The index finger is then introduced gently into the anal canal along its posterior aspect. At the apex of the canal, the sling of puborectalis is felt posteriorly; supralevator induration feels bony hard and is more easily appreciated if unilateral. The posterior surface of the prostate gland with its median sulcus can be palpated anteriorly in male patients; in female patients, the uterine cervix can be palpated. The presence of any distal intrarectal, intra-anal or extraluminal mass is recorded. Sphincter length, resting tone and voluntary squeeze are assessed. On withdrawal, the examining finger

William Hamish Fearon Thomson, contemporary, surgeon, Gloucestershire Royal Hospital, Gloucester, UK.
James Marion Sims, 1813–1883, gynaecological surgeon, State Hospital for Women, New York, NY, USA, introduced this position to give access to the anterior vaginal wall during operations for the closure of vesicovaginal fistulae.

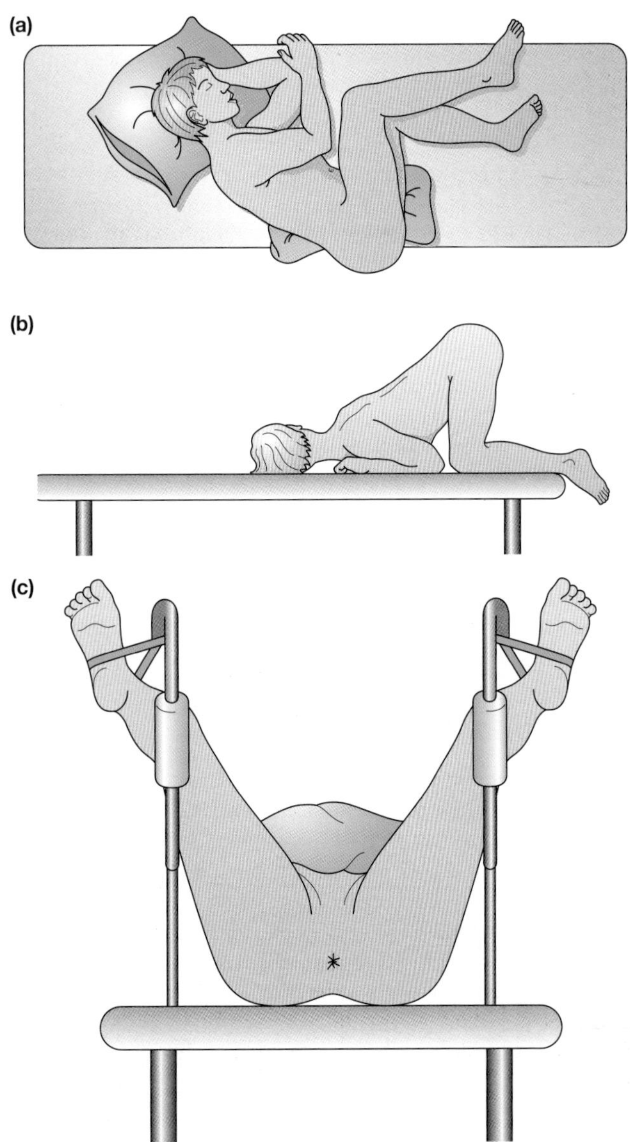

Figure 80.3 (a) The left lateral, (b) knee–elbow and (c) lithotomy positions for examination. (Redrawn with permission from Mann CV. *Surgical treatment of haemorrhoids*. London: Springer, 2002.)

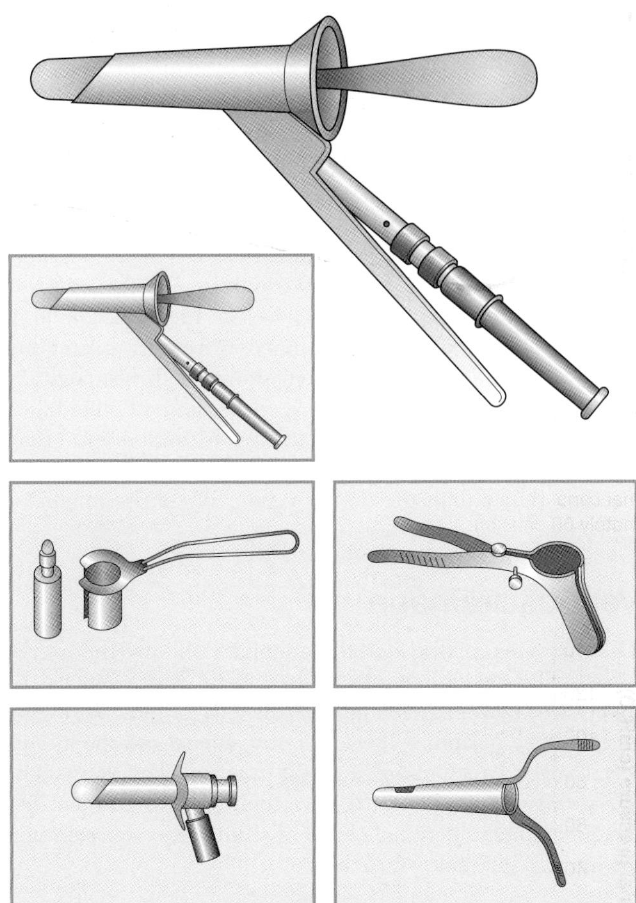

Figure 80.4 Various types of proctoscope. (Redrawn with permission from Mann CV. *Surgical treatment of haemorrhoids*. London: Springer, 2002.)

is inspected for the presence of mucus, blood or pus and to identify stool colour.

Proctoscopy

Proctoscopy, performed with the patient in the same position, allows a detailed inspection of the distal rectum and anal canal (***Figure 80.4***). Minor procedures can also be carried out through this instrument, e.g. treatment of haemorrhoids by injection or banding (see ***Haemorrhoids***) and biopsy. Asking the patient to bear down on slow withdrawal of the proctoscope may reveal a descending intussusception.

Sigmoidoscopy

Although sigmoidoscopy is strictly an examination of the rectum, it should always be performed as rectal pathology is frequently associated with an anal lesion (e.g. anal fistula); not infrequently, rectal pathology is found independent of the anal lesion.

Summary box 80.2

Examination of the anus

- A rectal examination is essential for any patient with anorectal and/or bowel symptoms – 'If you don't put your finger in, you might put your foot in it'
- A proctosigmoidoscopy (rigid or flexible) is essential in any patient with bowel symptoms

PHYSIOLOGICAL ASPECTS OF THE ANAL SPHINCTERS AND PELVIC FLOOR

Anal continence and defecation are highly complex processes that necessitate the structural and functional integrity of the cerebral, autonomic and enteric nervous systems, the gastrointestinal tract (especially the rectum) and the pelvic floor and anal sphincter complex, any of which may be compromised and lead to disturbances of function of varying severity.

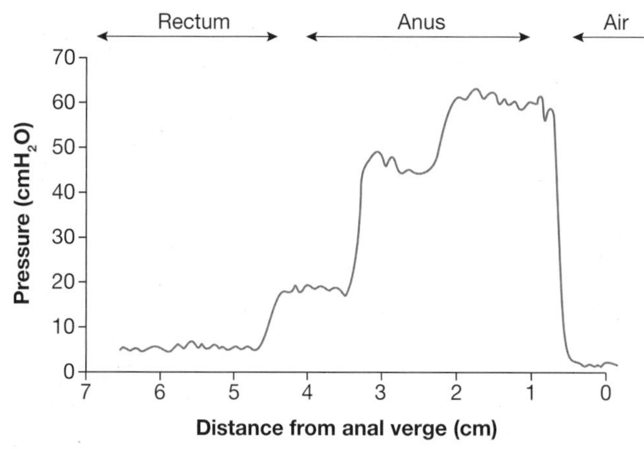

Figure 80.5 A typical normal 'pull-through' manometric study of the anal canal (3.5 cm long; maximal resting anal canal pressure approximately 60 cmH_2O).

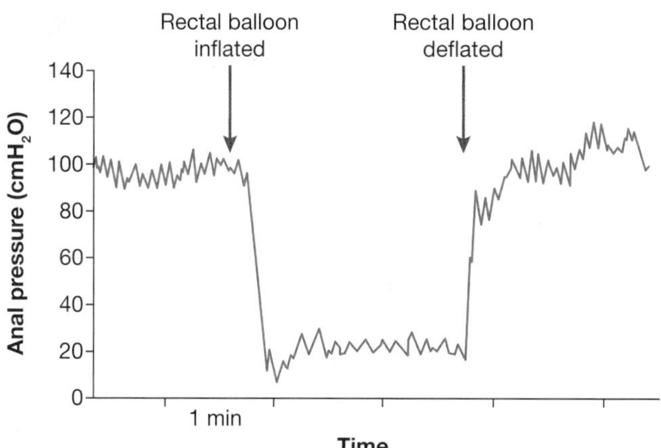

Figure 80.6 Anal manometry tracing demonstrating a normal rectoanal inhibitory reflex when the rectal balloon is inflated with 50 mL of air.

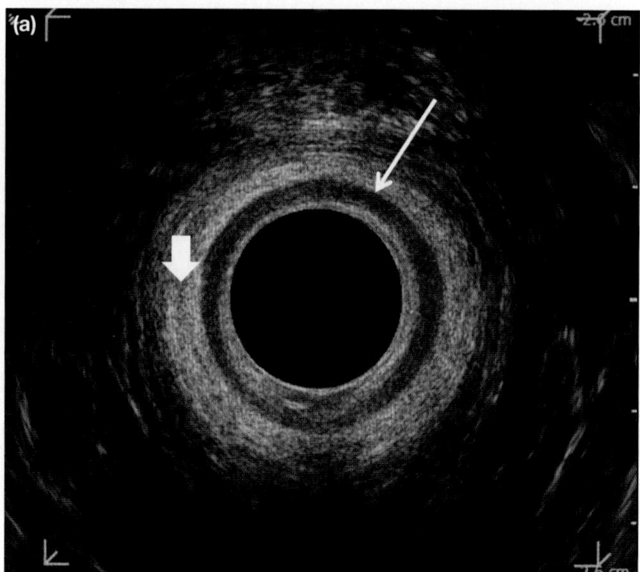

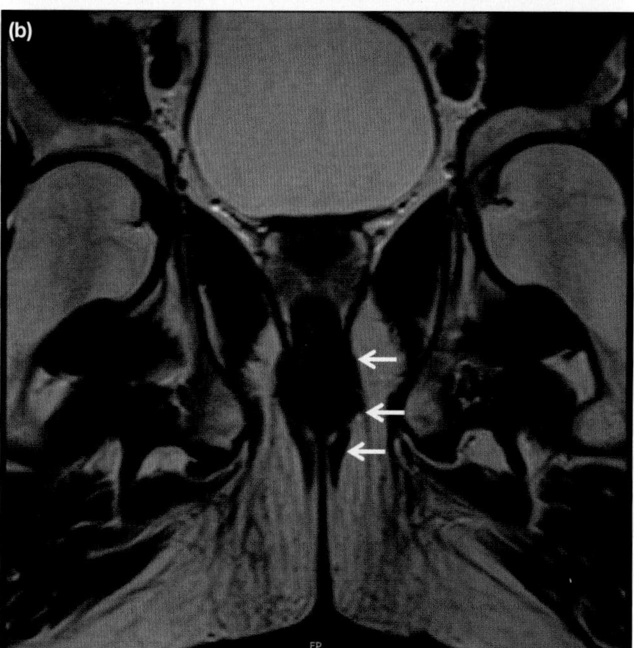

Figure 80.7 **(a)** Axial view of endoanal ultrasonography through the mid-anal canal of a female patient. Normal intact fibres of the internal (thin arrow) and external (thick arrow) anal sphincter complex. **(b)** Coronal T2-weighted magnetic resonance imaging through the anal canal of a male patient showing the three distinct zones of the low-signal external anal sphincter complex (arrows) (courtesy of Dr Alison Corr, Consultant Radiologist, St Mark's Hospital, London, UK).

The sphincter mechanism provides the ultimate barrier to leakage and its integrity can be assessed fairly simply and objectively in the physiology laboratory. Perineal position and degree of descent on straining (markers of pelvic floor and pudendal nerve function) can be quantified, and functional anal canal length, resting tone (reflective predominantly of internal sphincter activity) and squeeze increment (reflective of external sphincter function) can be measured by a variety of simple manometric techniques (*Figure 80.5*). Distension of the rectum produces reflex relaxation of the internal sphincter, which allows rectal contents to come into contact with the anal transition zone mucosa. This allows discrimination of solid, liquid and gas contents. The rate of recovery of sphincter tone after relaxation differs between the proximal and distal anal canal (*Figure 80.6*). This is an important continence mechanism.

The structural integrity of the sphincters can be visualised with endoluminal ultrasonography (*Figure 80.7a*), which usually consists of high-resolution three-dimensional images constructed from standard two-dimensional images. Magnetic resonance imaging (MRI) provides excellent tissue differentiation, although spatial resolution of the anal sphincters using a body coil is reduced (*Figure 80.7b*).

The dynamics of defecation can be assessed radiologically by evacuation proctography, in which radio-opaque pseudostool is inserted into the rectum and the patient asked to rest, squeeze and then bear down to evacuate the rectal contents under real-time imaging (*Figure 80.8 and* 80.1). The procedure may also be performed with oral contrast to outline the small bowel and in females following insertion of a

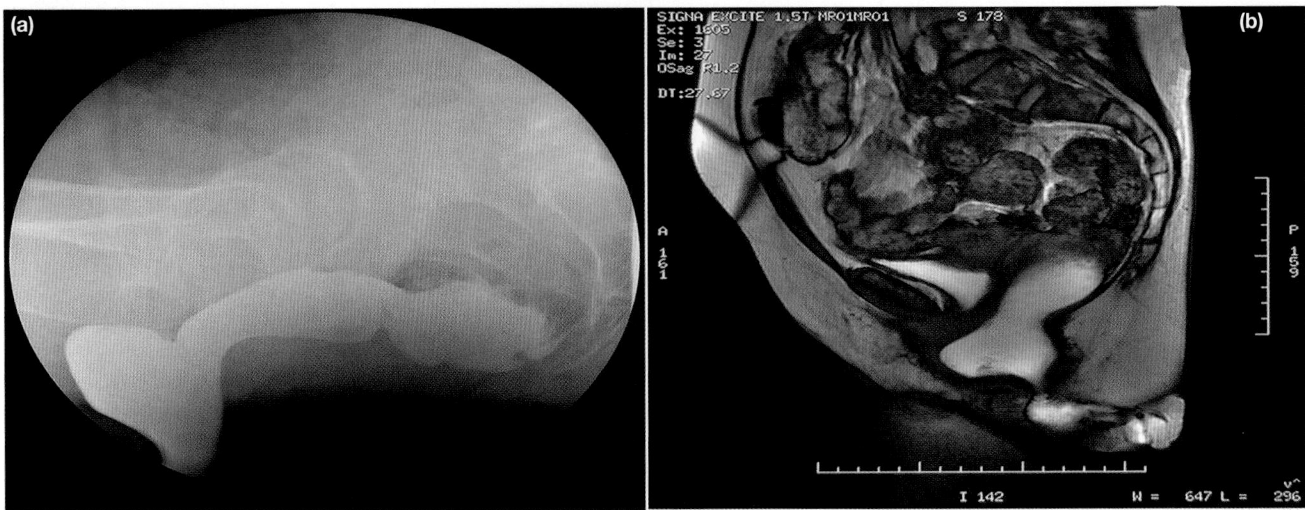

Figure 80.8 Visualisation of the rectum is achieved with barium-impregnated 'synthetic stool' using conventional defecating proctography (a) or magnetic resonance proctography (b). A large rectocele is apparent.

radio-opaque vaginal tampon that will allow anatomical changes during defecation (e.g. rectocele, enterocele) to be identified. Dynamic magnetic resonance (MR) proctography provides more details of other pelvic organs; however, evacuation in the supine position may be less physiological than the sitting position that can be achieved within an open magnet (*Figure 80.8*). Interobserver agreement for MR proctography is better than for barium defecography; however, imaging must be interpreted in the context of the patient's symptoms and used to guide rational rather than empirical treatment strategies.

CONGENITAL ABNORMALITIES

Early in embryonic life there is a common chamber – the cloaca – into which the hind gut and the allantois open. This endoderm-lined chamber is separated from the surface ectoderm of the embryo by the cloacal membrane. The cloaca becomes divided into two parts – dorsal (rectum) and ventral (urogenital sinus) – by the downgrowth of a septum. The dorsal part of the cloacal membrane, known as the anal membrane, is thus composed of an outer layer of ectoderm and an inner layer of endoderm. Resorption of this anal membrane by the eighth week of embryonic life creates the anal canal.

Imperforate anus

Imperforate anus (strictly, it should be anal 'agenesis' or 'atresia') has historically been divided into two main groups – high and low – depending on the level of termination of the rectum in relation to the pelvic floor. Treatment and prognosis are influenced by any associated abnormalities of the sacrum and genitourinary systems (see *Chapter 18*).

Postanal dermoid

The space in front of the lower part of the sacrum and coccyx may be occupied by a soft, cystic swelling – a postanal dermoid cyst. Hidden in the hollow of the sacrum it is unlikely to be discovered unless a sinus communicating with the exterior is present or it develops as a result of inflammation. Such a cyst usually remains asymptomatic until adult life, when it is prone to becoming infected. Exceptionally, because of its size, it gives rise to difficulty in defecation. The cyst is easily palpable on rectal examination.

Differential diagnosis

An anterior sacral meningocele must be excluded, particularly in the presence of bony abnormality of the sacrum. This enlarges when the child cries and is frequently associated with paralysis of the lower limbs and incontinence. When a discharging sinus is present, a postanal dermoid will probably be mistaken for a pilonidal sinus or even an anal fistula. Pressure over the sacrococcygeal region with a finger in the rectum may cause a flow of sebaceous material, and injection of contrast medium followed by radiography reveals a bottle-necked cyst in front of the coccyx.

Treatment

Treatment involves complete excision of the cyst and, if present, the sinus. In the case of large cysts, it is necessary to remove the coccyx to gain access. The coccyx should also be removed en bloc in any child with a presacral dermoid because of the risk of sacrococcygeal teratoma. Care must be taken to exclude the Currarino triad, an autosomal dominant hereditary condition characterised by sacral malformation, anorectal malformation (often stenosis) and a presacral mass consisting of a dermoid cyst/teratoma and/or anterior meningocele.

Guido Carlo Currarino, 1920–2015, radiologist, Southwestern Medical School and Children's Medical Center, Dallas, TX, USA.

Postanal dimple (synonym: fovea coccygea)

A dimple in the skin beneath the tip of the coccyx, sometimes amounting to a short blind pit, is noticed from time to time in the course of a clinical examination and is of no consequence.

Pilonidal sinus

The term pilonidal sinus describes a condition found in the natal cleft overlying the coccyx, consisting of one or more, usually non-infected, midline openings, which communicate with a fibrous track lined by granulation tissue and containing hair lying loosely within the lumen.

Aetiology and pathology

Although acquired theories of development are better accepted than the more historical congenital theories, exact mechanisms of development are speculative. Evidence that supports the theory of the origin of pilonidal sinuses as acquired can be summarised as follows:

- Interdigital pilonidal sinus is an occupational disease of hairdressers.
- The age of the appearance of a pilonidal sinus is older than expected of a congenital lesion.
- Hair follicles are rarely present in the walls of the sinus.
- The pointed hair ends are directed towards the blind end of the sinus.
- The disease mostly affects hirsute men.
- Recurrence is common, even though adequate excision of the track is carried out.

It is thought that the combination of buttock friction and shearing forces in that area allows shed hair or broken hairs that have collected there to drill through the midline skin, or that infection in relation to a hair follicle allows hair to enter the skin by the suction created by movement of the buttocks, so creating a subcutaneous, chronically infected, midline track. From this primary sinus, secondary tracks may spread laterally, which may emerge at the skin as granulation tissue-lined, discharging openings. Usually, but not invariably (when diagnosis may be confused with anal fistula or hidradenitis suppurativa [HA]), the sinus runs cephalad. Carcinoma arising in chronic pilonidal disease is exceedingly rare.

Clinical features

The condition is seen much more frequently in men than in women, usually after puberty and before the fourth decade of life and is characteristically seen in dark-haired individuals rather than those with softer blond hair. Patients complain of intermittent pain, swelling and discharge at the base of the spine but little in the way of constitutional symptoms. There is often a history of repeated abscesses that have burst spontaneously, or that have been incised, usually away from the midline. The primary sinus may have one or many openings, all of which are strictly in the midline between the level of the sacrococcygeal joint and the tip of the coccyx. If no primary pits are seen or if the sinus either drains lateral to the sacrum or appears caudal to the primary pits, other diagnoses should be considered. These might include HA, complex anal fistula, osteomyelitis with draining skin sinuses or infective conditions such as tuberculosis or actinomycosis.

Conservative treatment

The natural history is to regress over time. For those with minimal symptoms, simple cleaning of the tracks and removal of all hair, with regular hair exfoliation of the area and strict hygiene, may be recommended. Local techniques to cauterise the tracks using silver nitrate or laser coagulation may be useful in less complex disease.

Treatment of an acute exacerbation (abscess)

The abscess should be drained through a small longitudinal incision made over the abscess and off the midline, with thorough curettage of granulation tissue and hair. This may result in complete resolution.

Surgical treatment of chronic pilonidal disease

There are a multitude of surgical procedures advocated to eradicate pilonidal disease, which attests to the lack of overall superiority of one surgical technique. Time spent off work, recurrence rates and surgeon preference influence the choice of technique. Options include laying open of all tracks with or without marsupialisation, excision of all tracks with or without primary closure and excision of all tracks with closure by some other means designed to avoid a midline wound (Limberg procedure, Z-plasty, Karydakis procedure (***Figure 80.9***). Bascom's procedure involves an incision lateral to the midline to gain access to the sinus cavity, which is rid of hair and granulation tissue (***Figure 80.10***), and excision and closure of the midline pits. The lateral wound is left open to heal secondarily. Failure to heal or recurrence is treated by a flap or cleft lift procedure, also described by Bascom.

Irrespective of procedure, postoperative wound care is important and centres around elimination of hair (ingrown, local or other) from the wound. Recurrence rates are less but healing times slower after open healing compared with primary closure techniques. For primary closure, recurrence rates are lower and healing time faster after off-midline compared with midline closure techniques.

INCONTINENCE

Aetiology

Continence is dependent upon the structural and functional integrity of both the neurological pathways and the gastrointestinal tract. The risk factors for incontinence are many (***Table 80.1***). Patients complaining of the involuntary loss of rectal contents require a comprehensive assessment of

Alexander A Limberg, 1894–1974, plastic surgeon, Leningrad, former Soviet Union.
George E Karydakis, surgeon, Athens, Greece.
John U Bascom, 1925–2013, surgeon, Eugene, OR, USA.

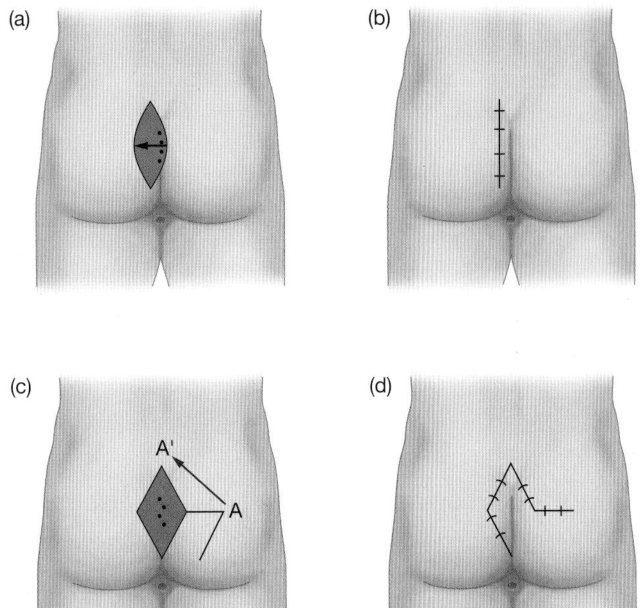

Figure 80.9 Off-midline closure techniques for pilonidal sinus. Karydakis's operation **(a)**: an off-midline incision is made around the sinus complex, which is excised, and a contralateral flap is mobilised to allow tension-free off-midline closure **(b)**. The Limberg flap **(c)**: the sinus complex is excised using a rhomboid incision and a measured flap is rotated (A) to (A') to achieve tension-free closure **(d)**.

the nature and severity of symptoms; past history, especially of gastrointestinal disease, neurological conditions, obstetric events and anorectal surgery; and clinical examination including sigmoidoscopy and/or colonoscopy as indicated. A combination of history and examination will usually be diagnostic, but special investigations are then usually required to clarify the exact cause, including exclusion of an underlying malignancy, and to direct management. Faecal incontinence is a symptom not a diagnosis and an underlying cause should be sought.

Faecal loading or impaction is a major contributor to incontinence in the elderly. A rectum impacted with faeces can result in 'overflow incontinence'. This is easily diagnosed on digital examination and rectally administered treatment to clear the bowel, followed by regular checking to avoid recurrence. When 'empty' on digital examination or when there is no relief from incontinence after evacuation of faeces, the three main mechanisms (sometimes acting in combination) that contribute to incontinence are: loose stool, reduced rectal volume/compliance and anatomical and/or functional injuries to the anal sphincter complex.

Sphincteric causes of incontinence may be classified as structural, in which there is disruption (or atrophy) of part of the sphincter muscles; neuropathic (previously termed idiopathic), in which the nerve supply to the sphincters is damaged, usually by chronic straining or complicated vaginal delivery (prolonged second stage); or a combination of the two. The most common causes of sphincteric disruption are obstetric damage, anal surgery (following haemorrhoidectomy, dilatation or sphincterotomy for anal fissure, and fistulotomy for anal fistula) and trauma (including anal intercourse, forced or otherwise). Incontinence may also arise following major colorectal resection with a colorectal or coloanal anastomosis owing to the reduction or loss of the rectal reservoir and disruption of intramural nerve pathways. Function can be further adversely affected by radiation. This is now known as low anterior resection syndrome (LARS) (Laurberg).

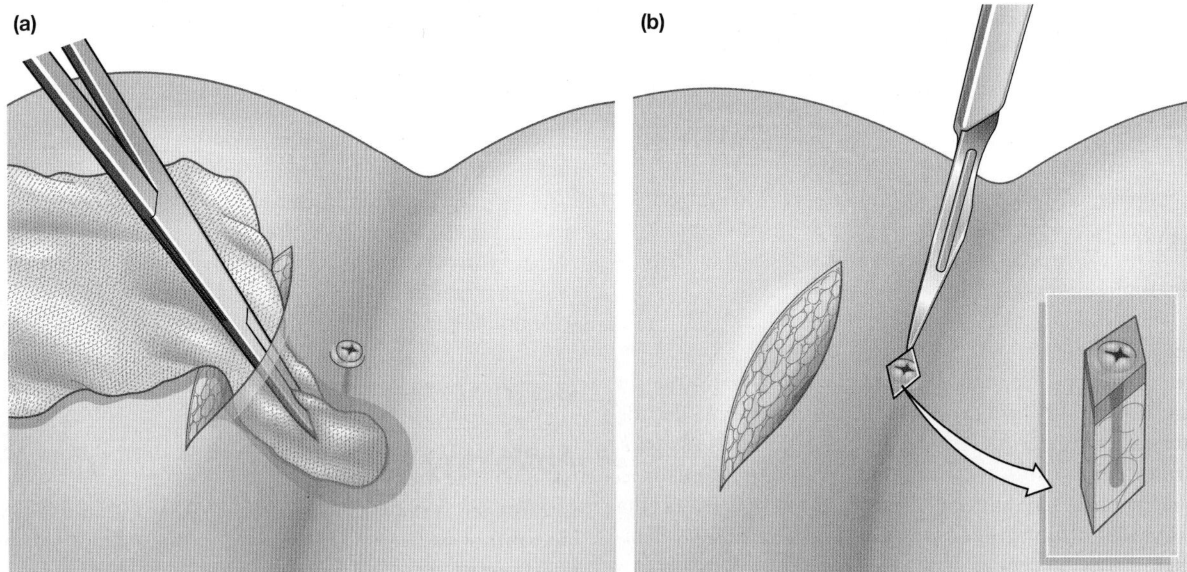

Figure 80.10 (a, b) Bascom's technique for pilonidal sinus **(a)**; lateral incision and curetting cavity **(b)**; excision midline pits. (Reproduced with permission from O'Connell PR, Madoff RD, Solomon MJ (eds). *Operative surgery of the colon, rectum and anus*, 6th edn. Boca Raton, FL: CRC Press, 2015.)

Soren Laurberg, contemporary, Professor of Surgery, Aarhus, Denmark.

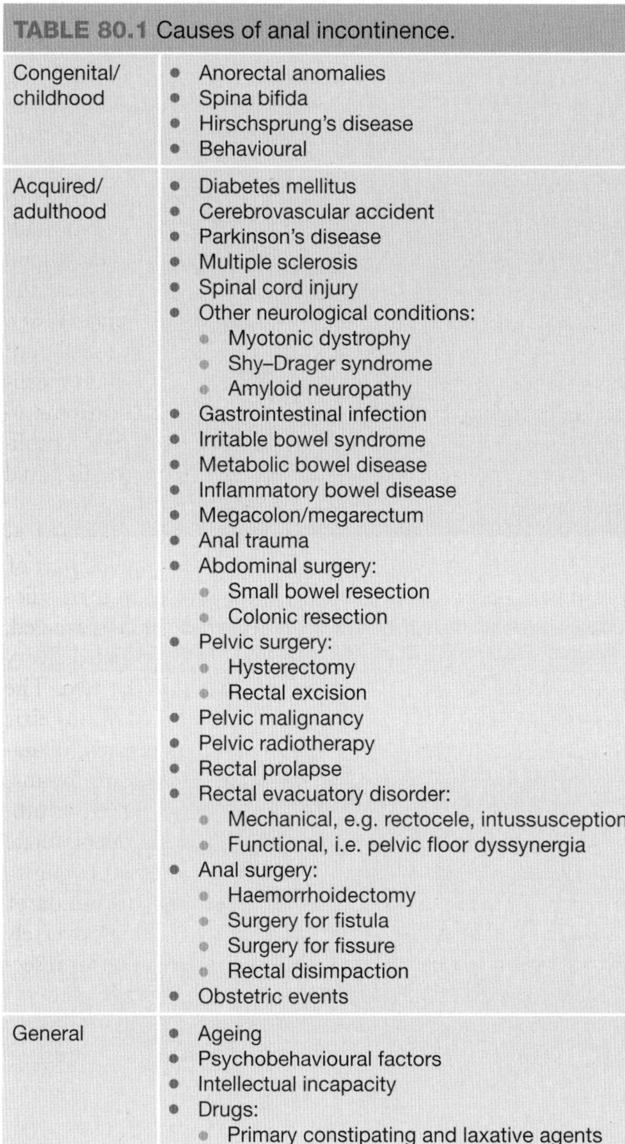

TABLE 80.1 Causes of anal incontinence.

Congenital/ childhood	• Anorectal anomalies • Spina bifida • Hirschsprung's disease • Behavioural

Acquired/ adulthood	• Diabetes mellitus
	• Cerebrovascular accident
	• Parkinson's disease
	• Multiple sclerosis
	• Spinal cord injury
	• Other neurological conditions:
	  ◦ Myotonic dystrophy
	  ◦ Shy–Drager syndrome
	  ◦ Amyloid neuropathy
	• Gastrointestinal infection
	• Irritable bowel syndrome
	• Metabolic bowel disease
	• Inflammatory bowel disease
	• Megacolon/megarectum
	• Anal trauma
	• Abdominal surgery:
	  ◦ Small bowel resection
	  ◦ Colonic resection
	• Pelvic surgery:
	  ◦ Hysterectomy
	  ◦ Rectal excision
	• Pelvic malignancy
	• Pelvic radiotherapy
	• Rectal prolapse
	• Rectal evacuatory disorder:
	  ◦ Mechanical, e.g. rectocele, intussusception
	  ◦ Functional, i.e. pelvic floor dyssynergia
	• Anal surgery:
	  ◦ Haemorrhoidectomy
	  ◦ Surgery for fistula
	  ◦ Surgery for fissure
	  ◦ Rectal disimpaction
	• Obstetric events

General	• Ageing • Psychobehavioural factors • Intellectual incapacity • Drugs: ◦ Primary constipating and laxative agents

Investigations

Anorectal physiology studies provide objective assessment of the anorectal function. Manometry is a simple method for measuring internal (resting) and external (squeeze) anal sphincter tone. Endoanal ultrasonography (EAUS) provides a dynamic assessment of the thickness and structural integrity of the external and internal sphincters (*Figure 80.11*). Dynamic standard or MRI defecography is not routine in patients with incontinence; however, in select cases they can be useful when obstructive or prolapse symptoms are mixed in with incontinence symptoms.

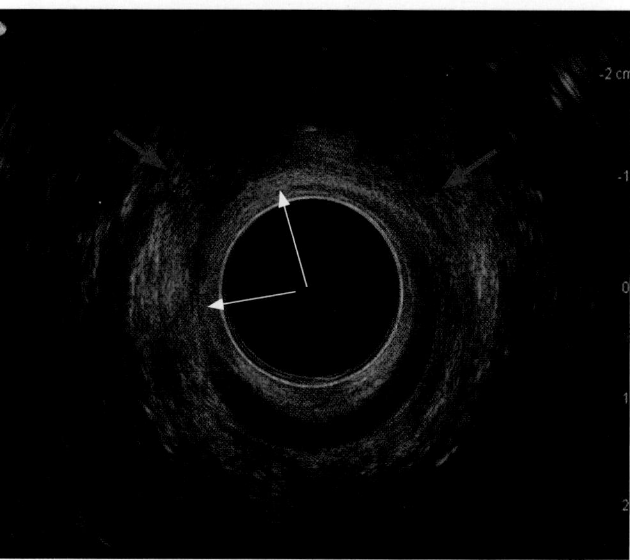

Figure 80.11 Axial view of endoanal ultrasonography through the mid-anal canal of a female patient with faecal incontinence following vaginal delivery. The study demonstrates a defect in the internal (white arrows) and external (red arrows) anal sphincter fibres in keeping with an obstetric anal sphincter injury (courtesy of Dr Alison Corr, Consultant Radiologist, St Mark's Hospital, London, UK)

Management

Most patients with incontinence can be managed conservatively with dietary advice, stool bulking or constipating agents, cleansing enemas, rectal irrigation, nurse-led bowel retraining, including specific biofeedback programmes, or anal plugs, which expand within and thus seal the anal canal. Failure of such measures and the severity of symptoms may result in selection for surgery.

Anal sphincter surgery

In situations where conservative treatment has failed, and where a discrete disruption of the sphincters exists, the ends of the divided muscle are found and reunited by an overlap repair (Parks) (*Figure 80.12*). Short-term results are good, with reports of 75–80% improvement in symptoms at first follow-up. This reduces with time to 50% or less 5–10 years after surgery. Pelvic floor repairs (postanal, preanal or total) are of historical interest only. Sphincter reconstruction (non-stimulated or stimulated) with muscle transposition has been devised to replace the anal sphincter when local repair has failed. 'Gluteoplasty' or 'graciloplasty', especially stimulated muscle transposition, has been performed; however, initial positive results were not maintained in the medium to long term. Artificial sphincters have been implanted to replace or reinforce native sphincters but devices are no longer commercially available.

Harald Hirschsprung, 1830–1916, physician, The Queen Louise Hospital for Children, Copenhagen, Denmark, described congenital megacolon in 1887.
James Parkinson, 1755–1824, general practitioner, Shoreditch, London, UK.
G Milton Shy, 1919–1967, neurologist, National Institute of Neurological Diseases and Blindness, National Institutes of Health, Bethesda, MD, USA.
Glen Drager, 1917–1967, Baylor College of Medicine, Houston, TX, USA.
Sir Alan Guyatt Parks, 1920–1982, surgeon, St Mark's Hospital and The London Hospital, London, UK.

(a)

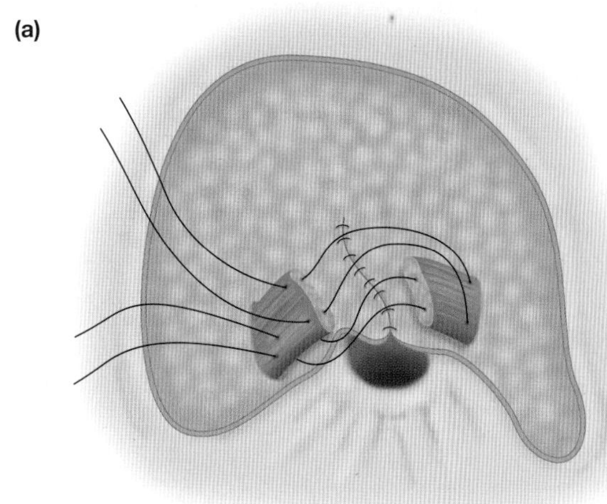

(b)

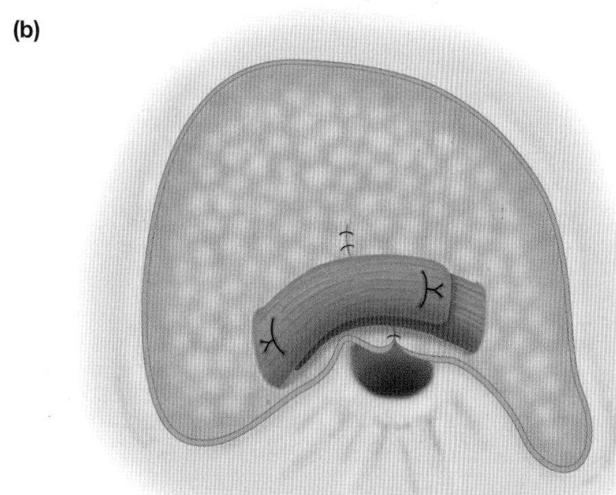

Figure 80.12 Direct sphincter repair in which **(a)** the sphincter defect is excised and **(b)** the remaining muscle is overlapped. (Redrawn with permission from Mann CV, Glass RE. *Surgical treatment of anal incontinence*. New York: Springer, 1991.)

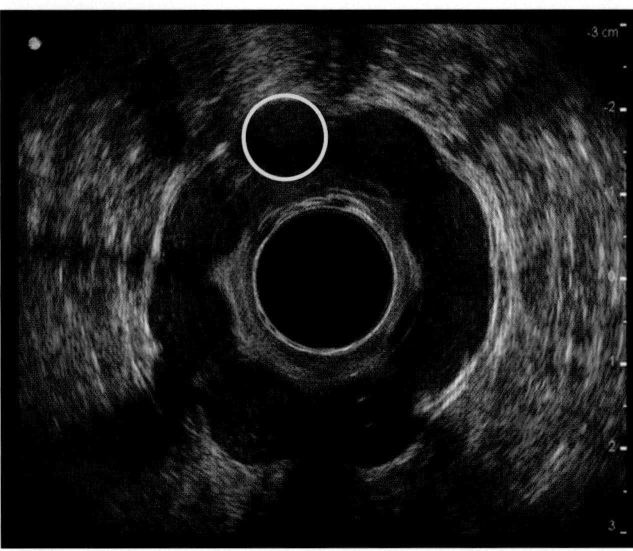

Figure 80.13 Endoanal ultrasonography evaluation of a surgically placed expandable sphincter prosthesis 'SphinKeeper®' (circle) radially within the intersphincteric space. (Courtesy of Dr Alison Corr, Consultant Radiologist, St Mark's Hospital, London, UK).

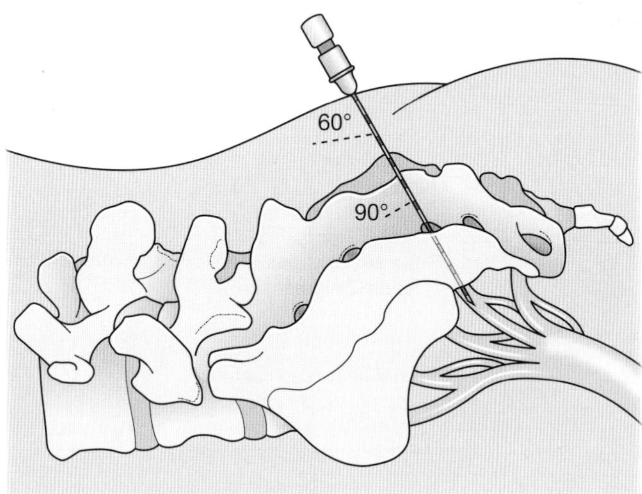

Figure 80.14 Diagram showing placement of the electrode through a sacral foramen.

Injectable biomaterials

Injectable biomaterials to add bulk to the anal canal and thereby augment faecal continence were first introduced by Shafik, who injected polytetrafluoroethylene paste into the anal submucosa. The ideal agent should be biocompatible, easy to deploy and should not migrate. Many materials have been investigated.

Recently the SphinKeeper® (Ratto) has been shown to restore sphincter function through placement of self-expanding prostheses into the intersphincteric space, adding bulk to the sphincter complex (***Figure 80.13***).

Sacral nerve stimulation (SNS) is a novel technique that uses low-voltage electrical stimulation to the S3 or S4 nerve roots to augment continence (***Figure 80.14***). It is thought to work primarily by activation of autonomic sensory pathways in patients with pelvic neuropathy, which principally occurs after childbirth. The technique consists of a *screening* phase of peripheral nerve evaluation, followed by a *therapeutic* phase of permanent neurostimulator implantation (Matzel) (***Figure 80.15***). SNS is sustainable with long-term improvement in symptoms. Postoperative complication rates are low; however, infection or loss of efficacy may require device explantation. **Percutaneous posterior tibial nerve stimulation** (PTNS) is a less expensive neuromodulation technique; however, results from prospective studies suggest only modest improvement in outcome.

Ahmed Shafik, 1933–2007, surgeon, Cairo University, Cairo, Egypt.
Carlo Ratto, contemporary, surgeon, Gemelli University Hospital, Rome, Italy.
Klaus E Matzel, contemporary, surgeon, University of Erlangen, Erlangen, Germany.

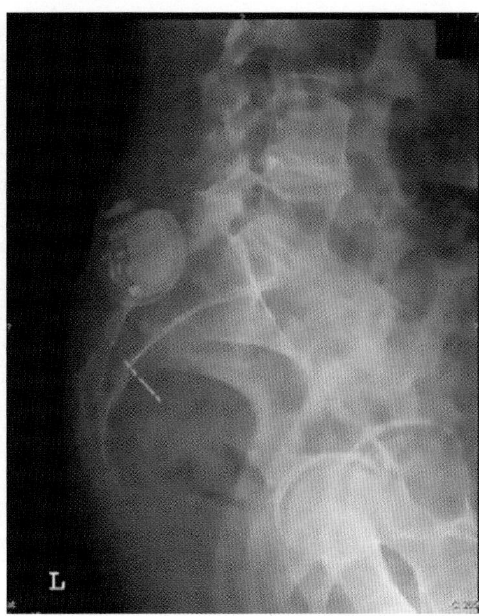

Figure 80.15 Radiograph of sacral nerve stimulation electrode placement in the line of the S3 root. The implanted nerve stimulator is visible in the gluteal area. (Reproduced with permission from O'Connell PR, Madoff RD, Solomon MJ (eds). *Operative surgery of the colon, rectum and anus*, 6th edn. Boca Raton, FL: CRC Press, 2015.)

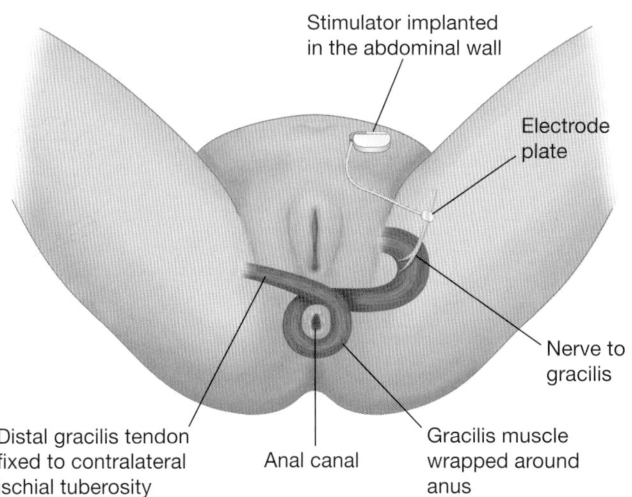

Figure 80.16 The electrically stimulated gracilis neosphincter or dynamic graciloplasty.

Operations to augment the anal sphincters

If the degree of sphincter disruption or weakness is such that restoration of function cannot be achieved by direct means, the sphincter can be augmented by using muscle transposed from nearby (gluteus maximus or gracilis) or by using an artificial sphincter. Transposition of the gracilis muscle around the anal canal is followed by electrical stimulation, with conversion from a fast-twitch to a less fatigable slow-twitch muscle by an implanted pacemaker (Williams) (***Figure 80.16***). Because of its magnitude this technique is performed only in highly selected and motivated patients, most of whom have had more conventional treatment that has failed to cure their incontinence.

Despite all currently available treatments presented and discussed above, each patient requires individualised management. The evidence unfortunately is not robust, and decision making relies on expert opinion. The surgeon is only a small part of the multidisciplinary team of specialists necessary to manage these patients. An end-stoma may be appropriate for patients with severe end-stage incontinence in whom all available treatments have failed. While a stoma is associated with significant psychosocial issues and stoma-related complications, it can allow patients to resume normal activities and improve their quality of life.

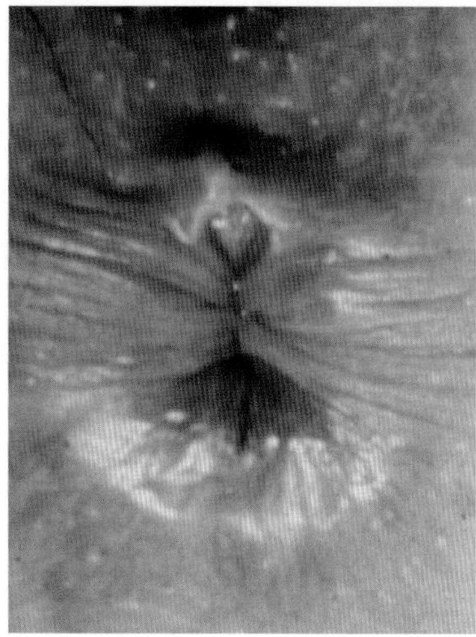

Figure 80.17 The appearance of an anal fissure. If the buttocks are gently parted, the presence of an anal fissure can usually be detected as an ulcer of variable depth with the skin tag and an anal papilla.

ANAL FISSURE

Definition

An anal fissure (synonym: fissure-*in-ano*) is a longitudinal ulcer in the anoderm of the distal anal canal (***Figure 80.17***), which extends from the anal verge proximally towards, but not beyond, the dentate line.

Aetiology

The cause of an anal fissure, and particularly the reason why the posterior midline is so frequently affected, is not completely understood. The location in the posterior midline may relate to the shearing forces acting at that site at defecation, combined with a less elastic anoderm endowed with an increased density of longitudinal muscle extensions in that region of the anal circumference. Anterior anal fissure is more common in women and may arise following vaginal delivery. Affected

Sir Norman S Williams, contemporary, Emeritus Professor of Surgery, The Royal London Hospital, London, UK.

patients frequently present with internal anal sphincter hypertonia, which, in turn, enhances the traumatic effect of the hard stool and perpetuates relative tissue ischaemia with a decrease in blood supply to the anal mucosa. After the initial tear, a vicious cycle of non-healing and repeated trauma leads to the development of chronic deep fissures. Local pain increases sphincter hypertonia, which worsens hard stool and local tissue ischaemia.

Clinical features

Although superficial, acute anal fissures are characterised by severe anal pain during defecation ('passing glass' or 'a knife cutting'), which usually resolves only to recur at the next evacuation. Frequently a trace of fresh blood is noticed on tissue paper after wiping. Chronic fissures are characterised by a hypertrophied anal papilla internally and a sentinel tag externally (both consequent on repeated healing and breakdown), between which lies an indurated anal ulcer that exposes fibres of the internal sphincter. Patients may also complain of itching secondary to irritation from the sentinel tag, discharge from the ulcer or discharge from an associated intersphincteric fistula, which has arisen through infection penetrating via the fissure base. Although most sufferers are young adults, the condition can affect any age, from infants to the elderly. A fissure that is not midline or one with atypical features should raise the suspicion of a specific aetiology. The inability to be able to conduct an adequate examination in the clinic should prompt early examination under anaesthesia, with biopsy and culture to exclude Crohn's disease, tuberculosis, sexually transmitted or human immunodeficiency virus (HIV)-related ulcers (syphilis, *Chlamydia*, chancroid, lymphogranuloma venereum, HSV, cytomegalovirus, Kaposi's sarcoma, B-cell lymphoma) and SCC.

Treatment

After confirmation of the diagnosis and exclusion of secondary causes of anal ulceration, conservative management should result in the healing of almost all acute and the majority of chronic fissures. Emphasis must be placed on normalisation of bowel habits. The addition of fibre to the diet to bulk up the stool, stool softeners and adequate water intake are simple and helpful measures. Warm baths and topical local anaesthetic agents relieve pain. Patients with normal bowel function and excessive straining at defecation might benefit from anorectal biofeedback to correct it. The mainstay of current conservative management is the topical application of pharmacological agents that relax the internal sphincter. If simple measures fail, treatment can be escalated to 'chemical sphincterotomy' using agents that induce smooth muscle (internal sphincter) relaxation. Glyceryl trinitrate (GTN) (0.2% applied two or three times per day to the anal margin) is a nitric oxide donor while diltiazem (2% applied twice daily) is a calcium channel antagonist. Botulinum toxin (10–100 units) injected into the internal sphincter in either divided or a single dose reduces anal canal pressure by blocking the release of acetylcholine at neuromuscular junctions. Temporary incontinence occurs in up to 10% of patients. The cure rate is approximately 50%, although GTN can be associated with headaches, which limits its acceptability to patients. Diltiazem and botulinum toxin have similar efficacy with fewer side effects.

Summary box 80.3

Anal fissure
- Acute or chronic ulcer in the midline of the anal canal
- Ectopic site suggests a more sinister cause

Symptoms:
- Pain on defecation
- Bright-red bleeding
- Mucus discharge
- Constipation

Operative measures

Anal sphincter dilatation has been used to reduce sphincter tone; however, this potentially disrupts the anal sphincters at multiple sites with an associated risk of incontinence such that it is rarely indicated.

Lateral anal sphincterotomy

In this operation, the internal sphincter is divided away from the fissure itself – usually either in the right or the left lateral positions. The procedure can be carried out using an open or a closed method, under local, regional or general anaesthesia, and with the patient in the lithotomy or prone jack-knife position. The distal internal sphincter is palpated with a bivalved speculum at the intersphincteric groove. In the closed method, a small longitudinal incision is made over this, and the submucosal and intersphincteric planes are carefully developed to allow precise division of the internal sphincter with a knife or scissors to the level of the apex of the fissure (***Figure 80.18***); the wound is then closed with absorbable sutures. Alternatively, either plane can be entered using a scalpel (no. 11 blade), with the blade advanced parallel to the sphincter and then rotated such that the sharp edge faces the internal sphincter, which can then be divided along its distal third. Pressure should be applied to the wound for a few minutes to prevent haematoma formation. In the open technique, the anoderm overlying the distal internal sphincter is divided longitudinally to expose the sphincter, which is divided, and the wound is closed with absorbable sutures. Although the fissure needs no specific attention, problematic papillae and external tags can be excised. The optimal amount of sphincter to be divided is a matter of debate, and additional factors have to be considered such as patient age, sex, previous vaginal delivery and operations on the anal canal. Early complications of sphincterotomy include

Burrill Bernard Crohn, 1884–1983, gastroenterologist, Mount Sinai Hospital, New York, NY, USA.
Moritz Kaposi, 1837–1902, Professor of Dermatology, Vienna, Austria, described pigmented sarcoma of the skin in 1872.

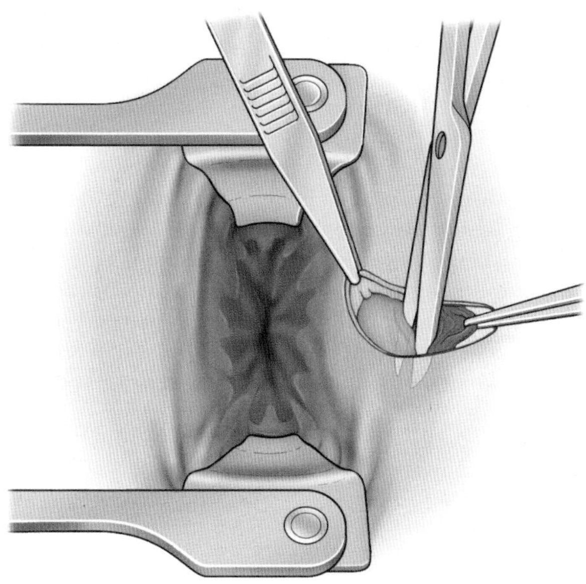

Figure 80.18 Lateral internal sphincterotomy. A dissecting scissors is used to open the intersphincteric space and divide the internal anal sphincter. (Reproduced with permission from O'Connell PR, Madoff RD, Solomon MJ (eds). *Operative surgery of the colon, rectum and anus*, 6th edn. Boca Raton, FL: CRC Press, 2015.)

haemorrhage, haematoma, bruising, perianal abscess and fistula. Healing rates are in the range of 85%, but there is also a significant risk of altered continence (9% flatus incontinence, 6% soiling, <1% solid stool incontinence).

Fissurectomy

Surgical excision of a fissure involves excising of the fibrotic edge, curettage of the base and excision of the sentinel tag and/or anal papilla. Fissurectomy is an alternative to lateral internal sphincterotomy and is used if there are contraindications to lateral internal sphincterotomy. It is frequently combined with an advancement flap anoplasty.

Anal advancement flap

An anal advancement flap to cover the anal fissure should be considered in those with an increased risk of altered continence following lateral internal sphincterotomy, especially in postpartum women and those with normal or low resting anal pressures. After fissurectomy an inverted house-shaped flap of perianal skin is carefully mobilised on its blood supply and advanced without tension to cover the fissure; it is then sutured with interrupted absorbable sutures (***Figure 80.19***). The patient is maintained on stool softeners and bulking agents postoperatively. Minor breakdown of one anastomotic edge does not herald ultimate failure.

Summary box 80.4

Treatment of an anal fissure

- Conservative initially, consisting of stool-bulking agents and softeners, and chemical agents in the form of ointments that are designed to relax the anal sphincter and improve blood flow
- Surgery if above fails, consisting of lateral internal sphincterotomy or anal advancement flap

Hypertrophied anal papilla

Anal papillae occur at the dentate line and are remnants of the ectodermal membrane that separated the hindgut from the proctodaeum. As these papillae are present in 60% of patients examined proctologically, they should be regarded as normal structures. Anal papillae can become elongated in the presence of an anal fissure. Occasionally, an elongated anal papilla may be the cause of pruritus. An elongated anal papilla associated with pain and/or bleeding at defecation is sometimes encountered in infancy. Haemorrhage into a hypertrophied anal papilla can cause sudden rectal pain. A prolapsed papilla may become nipped by contraction of the sphincter mechanism after defecation. Occasionally, a red oedematous papilla is encountered, with local pain and a purulent discharge from the associated crypt. This condition of 'cryptitis' may be cured by laying open the mouth of the infected anal gland and excising the papilla. Troublesome papillae may be simply excised.

Proctalgia fugax

This problem is characterised by attacks of severe pain arising in the rectum, recurring at irregular intervals and apparently unrelated to organic disease. The pain is described as cramp-like, often occurring at night, lasting minutes and disappearing spontaneously. It seems to occur more commonly in patients suffering from anxiety or undue stress. The pain may be intense but gradually subsides. It may be caused by cramp in the pubococcygeus muscle. A salbutamol inhaler can be used to treat acute attacks while amitriptyline may reduce the frequency. A more chronic form of the disease has been termed the 'levator syndrome' and can be associated with

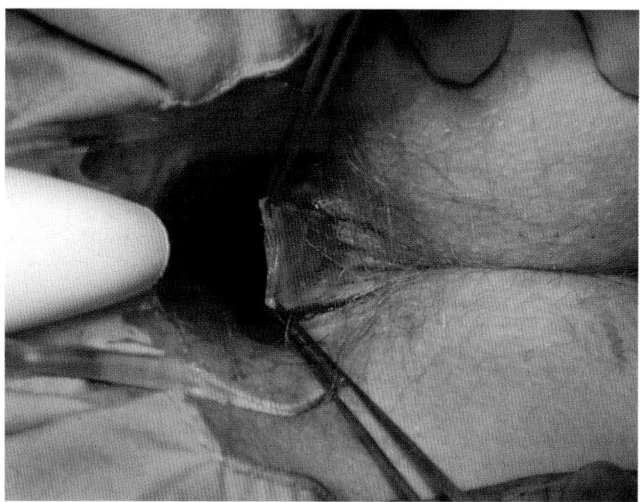

Figure 80.19 Mobilised skin flap prior to suturing intra-anally over the debrided and freshened posterior fissure base.

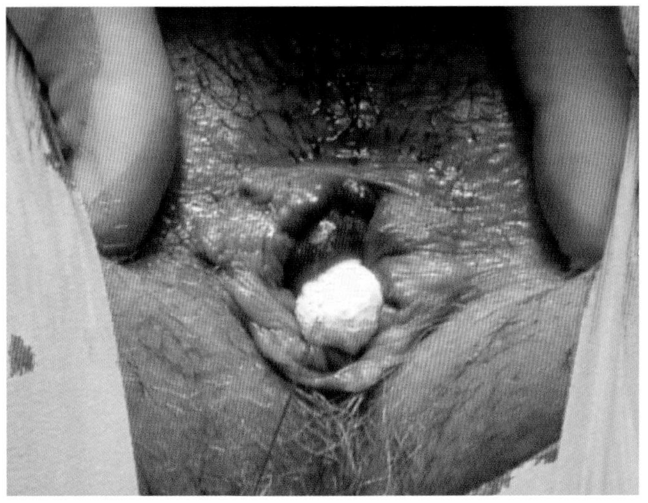

Figure 80.20 'Mixed' haemorrhoids; third-degree internal haemorrhoids become visible when the patient strains. This can be reproduced by withdrawal of a small swab inserted into the anal canal.

severe evacuatory dysfunction (see *Chapter 73*). Biofeedback techniques have been used to help such patients.

HAEMORRHOIDS

Haemorrhoids are symptomatic enlargements of the internal haemorrhoidal venous plexus (Greek: *haima* = blood, *rhoos* = flowing; synonym: piles, Latin: *pila* = a ball). Internal haemorrhoids characteristically lie in the 3, 7 and 11 o'clock positions (with the patient in the lithotomy position). Secondary haemorrhoids may develop between the primary positions. External haemorrhoids relate to venous channels of the inferior haemorrhoidal plexus deep in the skin surrounding the anal verge and are frequently confused with anal skin tags that are not true haemorrhoids.

The internal haemorrhoidal plexus constitutes the submucosal component of the anal cushions that are important in sealing the anal canal. Man's upright posture, the absence of valves in the portal venous system and raised abdominal pressure due to pregnancy or particularly through straining during defecation contribute to venous plexus engorgement and development of varicosities. Shearing forces lead to mucosal trauma (bleeding) and caudal displacement of the anal cushions (prolapse). This in turn leads to impaired venous drainage, progressive venous engorgement, local stasis and transudation of fluid (pruritus). With time, fragmentation of the supporting structures (a normal consequence of ageing but perhaps accelerated in those with haemorrhoids) leads to loss of elasticity of the cushions such that they no longer retract following defecation.

Clinical features

Bleeding is the earliest symptom. The nature of the bleeding is characteristically separate from the motion and is seen either on the paper on wiping or as a fresh splash in the pan. The bleeding is rarely sufficient to cause anaemia and other causes should be excluded. The bleeding is usually painless, although pruritus (skin irritation) is common due to mucus discharge. Pain should alert to the possibility of another diagnosis (e.g. anal fissure). Internal haemorrhoids associated with bleeding alone are called **first-degree** haemorrhoids. Patients may complain of lumps ('piles') that appear at the anal orifice during defecation and that return spontaneously afterwards (**second-degree** haemorrhoids), that have to be replaced manually (**third-degree** haemorrhoids) (*Figure 80.20*) or that lie permanently outside (**fourth-degree** haemorrhoids). By this stage there is often a significant cutaneous component to the haemorrhoidal prolapse, termed '**mixed**' haemorrhoids, which may be best considered as external extensions of internal haemorrhoids that arise through repeated congestion and oedema.

Summary box 80.5

Haemorrhoids: clinical features

- Haemorrhoids ('piles') are symptomatic enlargements of anal cushions
- More common when intra-abdominal pressure is raised, e.g. constipation and pregnancy
- Classically occur in the 3, 7 and 11 o'clock positions with the patient in the lithotomy position
- Symptoms: bright-red, painless bleeding, pruritus, mucus discharge, prolapse

Summary box 80.6

Four degrees of haemorrhoids

- First degree – bleed only, no prolapse
- Second degree – prolapse but reduce spontaneously
- Third degree – prolapse but have to be manually reduced
- Fourth degree – permanently prolapsed

Summary box 80.7

Complications of haemorrhoids

- Strangulation and thrombosis
- Ulceration
- Gangrene
- Portal pyaemia

Treatment of complications

Strangulation and thrombosis are relatively uncommon. The patient presents in severe discomfort with often circumferential haemorrhoidal prolapse with impending mucosal necrosis. Distinction must be made from rectal prolapse and external haemorrhoidal thrombosis. Urgent haemorrhoidectomy (see *Operations*) may expedite symptom resolution, but great care is needed to avoid later anal stenosis. Many surgeons adopt a conservative approach, ensuring adequate pain relief, bed rest, cold saline compresses and laxatives. Resolution usually occurs in 3–4 days. Systemic antibiotics are usually given to reduce the risk of portal pyaemia.

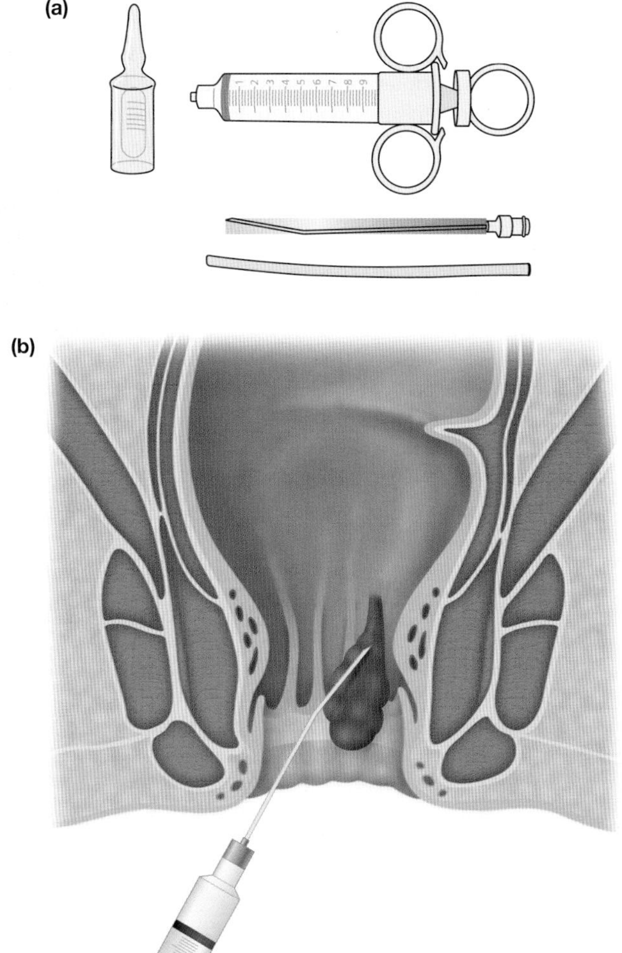

Figure 80.21 (a) Disposable kit for injection of haemorrhoids. (Reproduced with permission from O'Connell PR, Madoff RD, Solomon MJ (eds). *Operative surgery of the colon, rectum and anus*, 6th edn. Boca Raton, FL: CRC Press, 2015.) (b) Correct injection site at the apex of the haemorrhoidal complex.

Severe haemorrhage is usually associated with a bleeding diathesis or anticoagulation. If such causes are excluded, a local compress containing adrenaline (epinephrine) solution will usually suffice with blood transfusion if necessary. After adequate blood product replacement, examination under anaesthesia, ligation and excision of the piles may be required.

Management

Exclusion of other causes of rectal bleeding, especially colorectal malignancy, is the first priority. In the absence of a specific predisposing cause, important measures include improving bowel and defecatory habits, adopting a defecatory position to minimise straining (see ***Chapter 73***) and the addition of stool softeners and bulking agents. Various proprietary creams can be applied at night and before defecation. Suppositories of phlebotonics (plant-based flavonoid extracts) and synthetic compounds (calcium dobesilate) may reduce capillary permeability and increase lymphatic drainage.

In patients with first- or second-degree internal haemorrhoids whose symptoms are not improved by conservative measures, injection sclerotherapy with submucosal injection of 5% phenol in arachis oil or almond oil may be used (***Figure 80.21***). The aim is to cause fibrosis that obliterates the vascular channels and a scar that supports prolapsing anorectal mucosa. It is important to inject about 3–5 mL of sclerosant into the apex of the pedicle and *not* into the haemorrhoid itself using a disposable needle and syringe. The procedure is repeated for each haemorrhoid complex and the patient reassessed after 8 weeks; if necessary, the injections are repeated. Pain upon injection means that the needle is in the wrong place and should be withdrawn. Injections that are too superficial are heralded by the rapid bulging of the mucosa, which turns white; this leads to superficial ulceration but rarely serious septic sequelae. However, injections placed too deeply can have serious consequences, including prostatitis and pelvic sepsis. For this reason, haemorrhoidal injection has largely been superseded by rubber band ligation. The Barron's bander is a commonly available device used to slip tight elastic bands onto the base of the pedicle of each haemorrhoid (***Figure 80.22***). It is essential that the band is applied above the dentate line as below can cause intense pain. The bands cause ischaemic necrosis of the piles, which slough off within 10 days; this may be associated with bleeding, about which the patient must be warned. The resulting fibrosis supports the remaining anal cushions. All three primary haemorrhoids may be treated at one session, and the process may be repeated after several weeks. Other ablative techniques such as cryotherapy and infrared photocoagulation are not commonly used.

Operations

Indications

The indications for haemorrhoidectomy include:

- third- and fourth-degree haemorrhoids;
- second-degree haemorrhoids that have not been cured by non-operative treatments;
- 'mixed' haemorrhoids when the external haemorrhoid is well defined;
- bleeding causing anaemia.

If there is any doubt about the diagnosis of haemorrhoids, examination under anaesthesia and/or endoscopic visualisation are necessary. The indications are more relative than absolute, as surgery aims simply to improve symptoms and is not without risk of complication.

Technique

It is usual for the patient to have been taking stool softeners in the days before surgery and a preoperative enema to empty the rectum. The procedure is usually performed under general or regional anaesthesia with the patient in the lithotomy or prone jack-knife position. Haemorrhoidectomy can be performed using an open or a closed technique. The open technique is

James Barron, 1914–1996, surgeon, Henry Ford Hospital, Detroit, MI, USA.

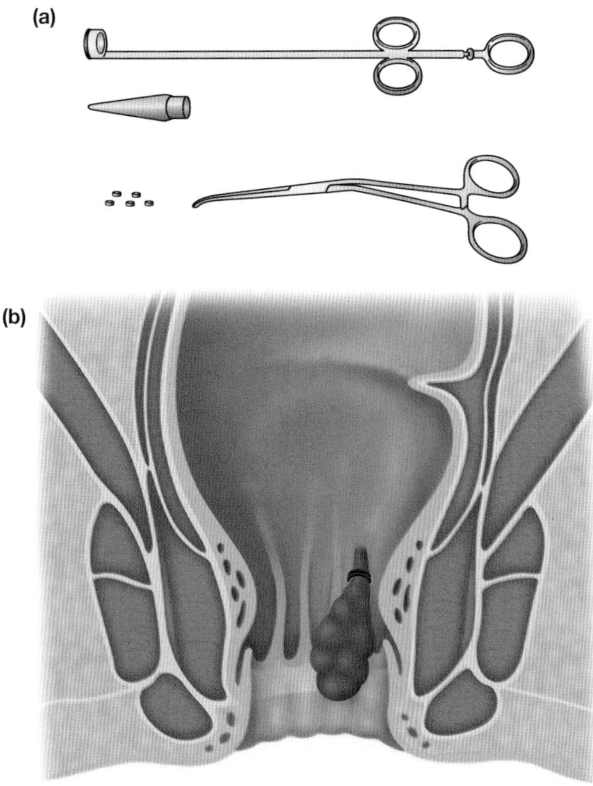

Figure 80.22 (a) Barron's banding apparatus. (Reproduced with permission from O'Connell PR, Madoff RD, Solomon MJ (eds). *Operative surgery of the colon, rectum and anus*, 6th edn. Boca Raton, FL: CRC Press, 2015.) (b) The appearance of a typical 'banded' haemorrhoid.

most commonly used in the UK and is known as the Milligan–Morgan operation – named after the surgeons who described it. The closed technique (Ferguson) is the popular technique in the USA. Both involve ligation and excision of the haemorrhoid, but in the open technique the anal mucosa and skin are left open to heal by secondary intention, and in the closed technique the wound is sutured.

- **Open technique**. The anoderm and subcutaneous tissues between the haemorrhoids may be injected with dilute adrenaline (1:300 000 dilution) to reduce bleeding and aid preservation of the skin bridges left following excision. Artery forceps are applied to the skin-covered external components of the haemorrhoids and traction exerted to reveal the internal components, which are also grasped by artery forceps. With scissors or cutting diathermy, a V-shaped cut is made through the skin (***Figure 80.23a***). Traction by both operator and assistant, combined with careful dissection, will expose the lower border of the internal sphincter. The dissection proceeds up the anal canal, with the sides of the mucosal dissection converging towards the pile apex and with the internal sphincter visible and separate from the dissected pile (***Figure 80.23b***). A transfixion ligature of strong Vicryl is applied to the pedicle at this level (***Figure 80.23c***), the pile is excised well distal to the ligature and, after ensuring haemostasis, the ligature is cut long. Each haemorrhoid is dealt with in this manner, taking care to leave mucocutaneous bridges. If there are significant secondary haemorrhoids under these bridges they can be excised out by submucosal dissection (Parks). Careful haemostasis is important. A soft absorbable anal dressing is inserted.
- **Closed technique**. The haemorrhoid is excised, together with the overlying mucosa, as illustrated in ***Figure 80.24***. The pedicle is transfixed with a 3/0 polyglactin suture and the mucosal defect is closed with a continuous suture, using the same stitch. The remaining haemorrhoids are excised and ligated in a similar fashion, ensuring that there are adequate mucosal and skin bridges between each area of excision to avoid a subsequent stenosis.
- **Stapled technique**. Stapled haemorrhoidopexy, also known as PPH (procedure for prolapse and haemorrhoids) (Longo), utilises a bespoke circular stapling device to excise a cylinder of mucosa and submucosa (together with the vessels within) above the dentate line while simultaneously stapling the mucosal ends together (***Figure 80.25***). Great care

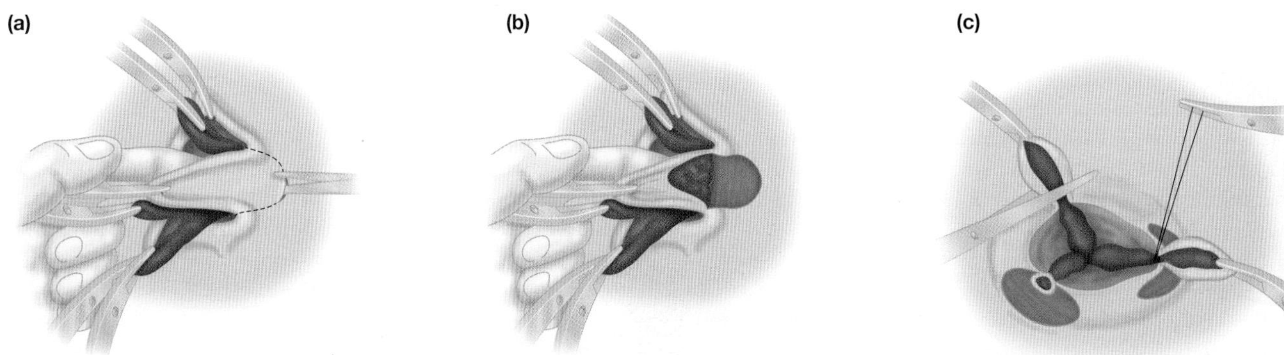

Figure 80.23 Ligation and excision of haemorrhoids. Open technique: (a) artery forceps have been applied; (b) dissection of the left lateral pedicle; (c) transfixion of the pedicle. (Adapted with permission from O'Connell PR, Madoff RD, Solomon MJ (eds). *Operative surgery of the colon, rectum and anus*, 6th edn. Boca Raton, FL: CRC Press, 2015.)

Edward Thomas Campbell Milligan, 1886–1972, surgeon, St Mark's Hospital, London, UK.
Sir Clifford Naughton Morgan, 1901–1986, surgeon, St Mark's and St Bartholomew's Hospitals, London, UK.
James A Ferguson, 1915–2005, surgeon, Ferguson Clinic, Grand Rapids, MI, USA.
Antonio Longo, contemporary, surgeon, Sicily, Italy.

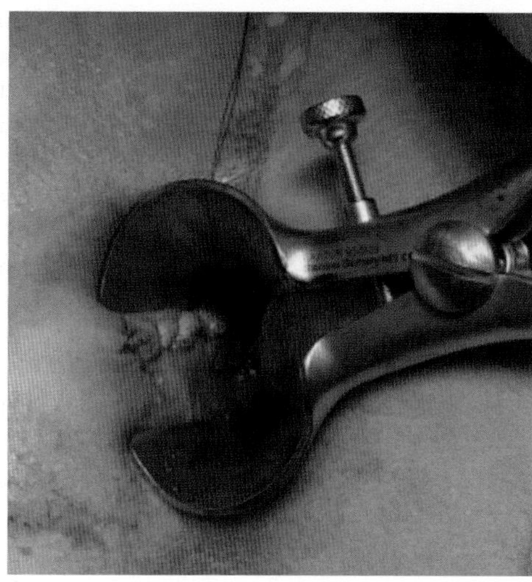

Figure 80.24 Closed technique: the haemorrhoidectomy wound has been closed with a continuous suture.

must be taken to ensure the staple line is above the dentate line and that the posterior vaginal wall is not accidently included. The procedure is less painful than conventional haemorrhoidectomy and is associated with quicker recovery. However, recurrence rates are higher than following conventional haemorrhoidectomy and external haemorrhoids may persist. Moreover, stapled haemorrhoidopexy has the potential for serious morbidity (staple line dehiscence, infection, rectovaginal fistula) and distressing new symptoms such as tenesmus (related to mucosal stimulation by the staples) may require reoperation and staple removal. Counselling and shared decision making is important such that the patient can weigh the short-term benefits against higher recurrence rates.

- **Transanal haemorrhoidal ligation (HAL)**. Transanal Doppler-guided ligation of those vessels feeding the haemorrhoidal masses with or without suture 'mucopexy' can be used to treat second- and third-degree haemorrhoids. The HubBLe trial, which compared HAL with rubber band ligation, found that the recurrence rate following HAL was significantly lower, but HAL was less cost-effective. The complication rate and postoperative pain scores are better after HAL than with conventional surgery.

Summary box 80.8

Treatment of haemorrhoids

- Symptomatic – advice about defecatory habits, stool softeners and bulking agents
- Injection of sclerosant
- Rubber banding
- HAL/stapled haemorrhoidopexy
- Haemorrhoidectomy

Postoperative care

In many countries, haemorrhoidectomy is performed on a day-case basis. The patient is instructed to take two warm baths each day and is given a bulk laxative to take twice daily, together with appropriate analgesia. A 5-day course of oral metronidazole may reduce pain. Dry dressings are applied as necessary, a sterile sanitary towel usually being ideal. The patient is seen again 3–4 weeks after discharge and a rectal examination is performed. If there is evidence of stenosis, the patient is encouraged to use an anal dilator.

Postoperative complications

Postoperative complications may be early or late.

Early complications include:

- **Pain**. Opiate analgesia, local anaesthetic agents, GTN and calcium channel blockers, together with botulinum toxin are useful postoperative adjuncts for postoperative pain.

(a)

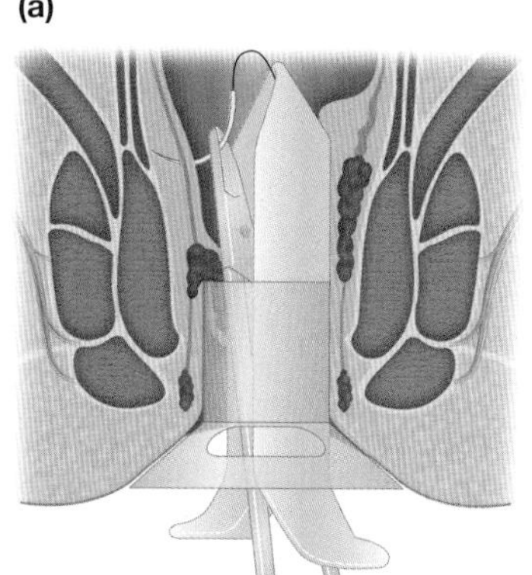

(b)

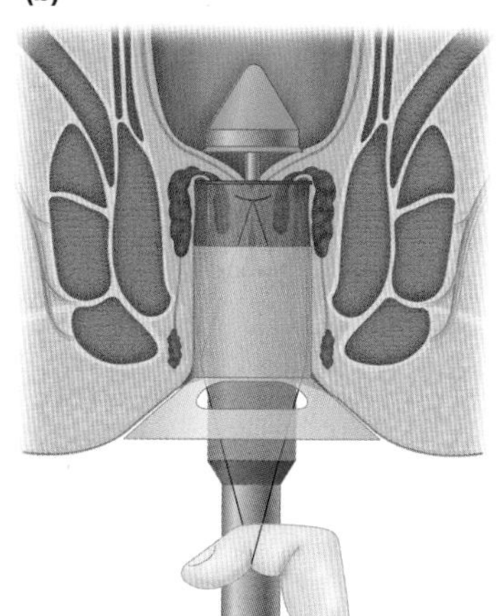

(c)

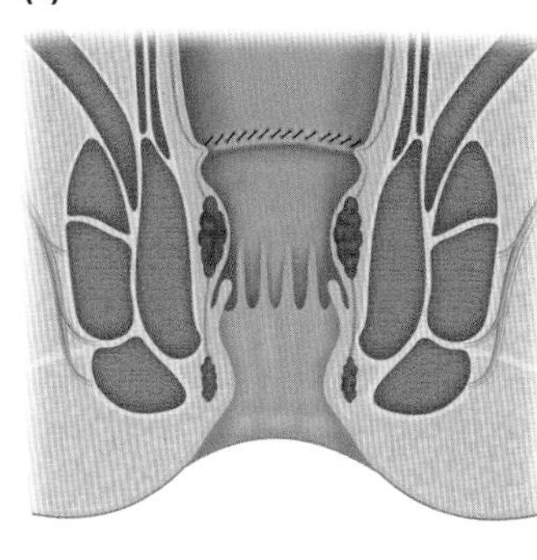

Figure 80.25 Stapled haemorrhoidectomy: (a) the purse-string suture is placed several centimetres above the dentate line; (b) the anvil of the fully opened stapling gun is inserted endoanally so that it is above the purse-string suture, which is then tied around the shaft of the gun. The gun is closed and fired; (c) after firing, a 3- to 4-cm strip of mucosa and submucosa containing the haemorrhoids is excised and the mucosal edges are simultaneously stapled together.

Christian Johann Doppler, 1803–1853, Professor of Experimental Physics, Vienna, Austria, enunciated the 'Doppler principle' in 1842.

- **Retention of urine**. This occurs especially in men, and may need relief by catheterisation.
- **Reactionary haemorrhage**. This is much more common than secondary haemorrhage. The haemorrhage may be mainly or entirely concealed but will become evident on examining the rectum. If persistent following adequate analgesia, the patient must be taken to the operating theatre and the bleeding point secured by careful diathermy or under-running with a ligature on a needle, care being taken to avoid damage to the internal sphincter. Should a definite bleeding point not be found, the anal canal and rectum should be packed to ensure haemostasis and the area re-examined under anaesthesia on removal of the packs.

Late postoperative complications include:

- **Secondary haemorrhage**. This is uncommon, occurring about the seventh or eighth day after operation. If severe, the bleeding will need to be controlled under general anaesthesia.
- **Anal stricture**. This must be prevented at all costs. A rectal examination at the postoperative review will indicate whether it may be necessary to dilate the anal canal under general anaesthetic. Daily use of a dilator should give a satisfactory result.
- **Anal fissures and submucous abscesses**.
- **Incontinence**. This occurs if there has been inadvertent damage to the underlying internal sphincter.

Summary box 80.9

Complications of haemorrhoidectomy

Early	Late
• Pain	• Secondary haemorrhage
• Acute retention of urine	• Anal stricture
• Reactionary haemorrhage	• Anal fissure
	• Incontinence

External haemorrhoids

A thrombosed external haemorrhoid relates anatomically to the veins of the superficial or external haemorrhoidal plexus and is commonly termed a perianal haematoma. It presents as a sudden onset, olive-shaped, painful blue subcutaneous swelling at the anal margin and is usually consequent upon straining at stool, coughing or lifting a heavy weight. The thrombosis is usually situated in a lateral region of the anal margin. If the patient presents within the first 48 hours, the clot may be evacuated under local anaesthesia. Untreated it may resolve, suppurate, fibrose and give rise to a cutaneous tag, burst and the clot extrude (*Figure 80.26*) or continue bleeding. In the majority of cases, resolution or fibrosis occurs.

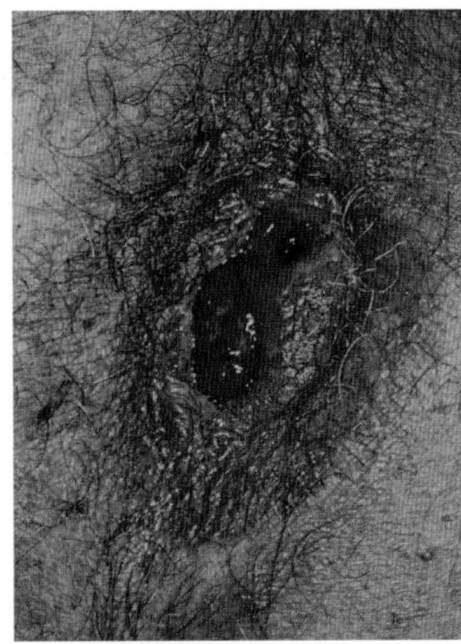

Figure 80.26 A thrombosed external haemorrhoid that has spontaneously ruptured. Most of the underlying blood clot has extruded. There is also a mucosal prolapse, which is separate from the cutaneous lesion.

PRURITUS ANI

This is intractable itching around the anus, a common and embarrassing condition. Usually, the skin is reddened and hyperkeratotic and it may become cracked and moist. The causes are numerous but most commonly relate to poor or excessive hygiene, moist discharge secondary to other anorectal conditions, parasitic causes, especially threadworms (*Enterobius vermicularis*), and dermatological conditions (allergy, psoriasis, lichen planus). Care must be taken not to miss neoplastic changes such as anal SCC, malignant melanoma, Bowen's disease and extramammary Paget's disease.

Treatment

Symptomatic treatment begins with dietary measures to ensure a soft, formed stool. For hygiene, cotton wool or moist tissue should be substituted for toilet paper. Soap is avoided and replaced by water alone, and the area pat-dried rather than rubbed. These measures, combined with wearing cotton underwear and the application of calamine lotion or zinc oxide barrier cream, are sufficient in many cases. In patients with dermatitis topical application of 0.5% or 1% hydrocortisone cream is beneficial.

Summary box 80.10

Pruritus ani

- Common
- Numerous causes, including skin diseases, parasites (threadworm), anal discharge, allergies, diabetes
- Treat the cause if possible
- Symptomatic treatment is the mainstay

John Templeton Bowen, 1857–1941, Professor of Dermatology, Harvard University Medical School, Boston, MA, USA, described this intradermal precancerous skin lesion in 1912.

Sir James Paget, 1814–1899, surgeon, St Bartholomew's Hospital, London, UK, described this disease in 1874.

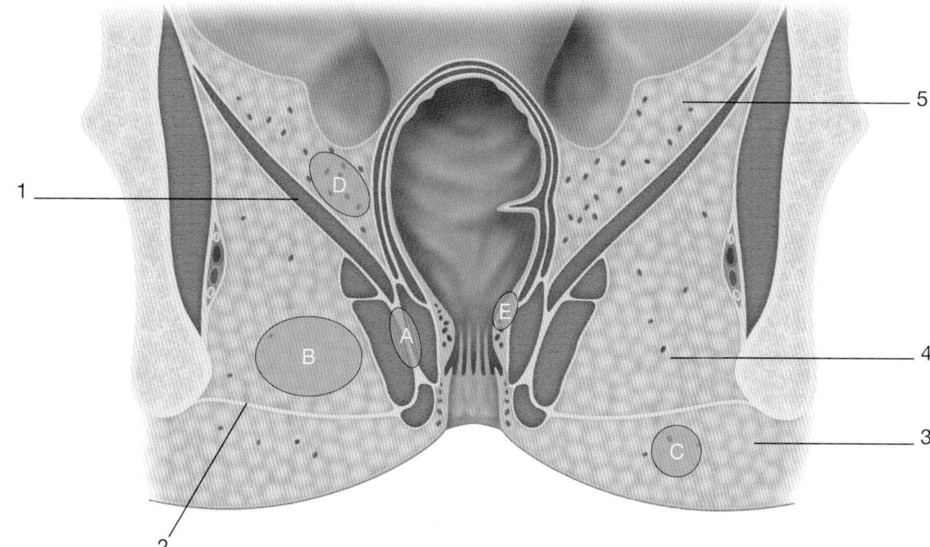

Figure 80.27 Coronal section of pelvis showing the anatomy relevant to anorectal infection and sites of abscess formation. 1, Levator ani muscle; 2, superficial perineal fascia; 3, superficial perianal space; 4, ischiorectal space; 5, supralevator space. A, Intersphincteric; B, ischiorectal; C, superficial perianal; D, supralevator; E, submucosal.

ANORECTAL ABSCESSES

Aetiology

Acute sepsis in the region of the anus is common, more in men than women, although perianal infections with skin-type organisms (and thus unrelated to fistula) are evenly distributed. The cryptoglandular theory of intersphincteric anal gland infection (Parks) holds that pus, which travels along the path of least resistance, may spread caudally to present as a perianal abscess, laterally across the external sphincter to form an ischiorectal abscess or, rarely, superiorly above the anorectal junction to form a supralevator intermuscular or pararectal abscess (depending on its relation to the longitudinal muscle) (***Figure 80.27***), as well as circumferentially in any of the three planes: intersphincteric/intermuscular, ischiorectal or pararectal supralevator (***Figure 80.28***). Sepsis unrelated to anal gland infection may occur at other sites, including submucosal abscess (following haemorrhoidal sclerotherapy, which usually resolves spontaneously), mucocutaneous or marginal abscess (infected haematoma), ischiorectal abscess (foreign body, trauma, deep skin-related infection) and pelvirectal supralevator sepsis originating from pelvic disease. Underlying rectal disease, such as neoplasm and particularly Crohn's disease, may be the cause. Immunosuppressed patients or those with diabetes or acquired immunodeficiency syndrome (AIDS) may present with perianal or pelvirectal sepsis that may run an aggressive course.

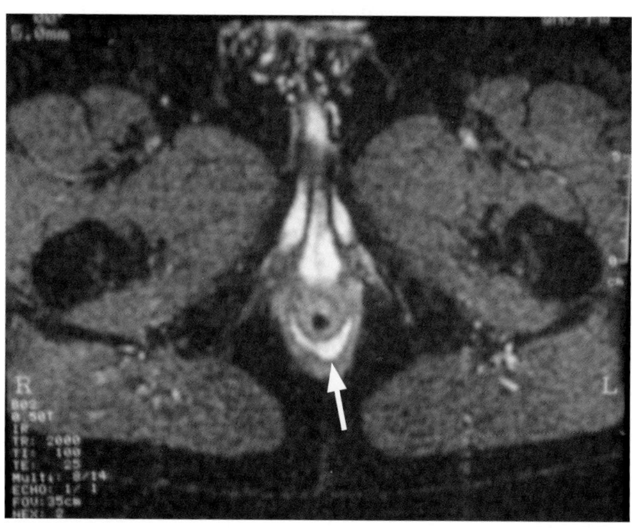

Figure 80.28 Axial magnetic resonance imaging scan (short tau inversion recovery [STIR] sequence) showing posterior horseshoe spread of sepsis within the intersphincteric space (arrow).

Presentation

A perianal abscess, confined by the terminal extensions of the longitudinal muscle, is usually associated with a short (2–3 day) history of increasingly severe, well-localised pain and a palpable tender lump at the anal margin. Examination reveals an indurated hot, tender perianal swelling. Patients with infection in the larger fatty-filled ischiorectal space, in which tissue tension is much lower, usually present later, with less well-localised symptoms but more constitutional upset and fever. On examination, the affected buttock is diffusely swollen with widespread induration and deep tenderness. If sepsis is higher, deep rectal pain, fever and sometimes disturbed micturition may be the only features, with nothing evident on external examination but tender supralevator induration palpable on digital examination above the anorectal junction.

Differential diagnosis

The only conditions with which an anorectal abscess is likely to be confused are abscesses connected with a pilonidal sinus, Bartholin's gland or Cowper's gland.

Caspar Bartholin (Secundus), 1655–1709, Professor of Medicine, Anatomy and Physics, Copenhagen, Denmark, described these glands in 1677.
William Cowper, 1666–1709, surgeon, London, UK, described these glands in 1697.

Management

Management of acute anorectal sepsis is primarily surgical, including careful examination under anaesthesia, sigmoidoscopy and proctoscopy, and adequate drainage of the pus. For perianal and ischiorectal sepsis (with an incidence of 60% and 30%, respectively), drainage is through the perineal skin. Traditionally this has been through a cruciate incision over the most fluctuant point, with excision of the skin edges to deroof the abscess; however, although drainage must be ensured, skin preservation is important and wide excision of otherwise healthy tissue should be avoided. A gentle search may be made for an underlying fistula if the surgeon is experienced; if obvious, a loose draining seton may be passed. Injudicious probing in the acute stage is, however, potentially dangerous and may lead to a much more difficult situation. Unless by highly experienced hands, immediate fistulotomy should not be performed. Despite lack of evidence, the practice of packing the abscess cavity is commonplace.

The management of supralevator sepsis is dependent upon its origin. Sepsis originating in pelvic disease necessitates appropriate management of the underlying cause (appendiceal, gynaecological, diverticular, Crohn's disease, malignancy), although intrarectal drainage may be appropriate to avoid creation of an extrasphincteric fistula.

Summary box 80.11

Anorectal abscess

- Presents as a painful, throbbing swelling in the anal region with associated pyrexia
- Classified according to anatomical site
- Treatment is drainage of pus and appropriate systemic antibiotics
- Consider underlying diagnosis: fistula-*in-ano*, Crohn's disease, diabetes, immunosuppression

FISTULA-*IN-ANO*

Aetiology

A fistula-*in-ano*, or anal fistula, is a chronic abnormal communication extending from the anorectal lumen (the internal opening) to an external opening on the skin of the perineum or buttock (or rarely, in women, to the vagina). The majority are idiopathic or cryptoglandular and are lined by granulation tissue. Anal fistulae may be found in association with Crohn's disease, tuberculosis, lymphogranuloma venereum, actinomycosis, rectal duplication, foreign body and malignancy (which may also very rarely arise within a longstanding fistula).

Presentation

Patients usually complain of intermittent purulent discharge (which may be bloody) and discomfort, which increases until temporary relief occurs when the pus discharges. There is often a history of anorectal sepsis. The passage of flatus or faeces through the external opening is suggestive of a rectal rather than an anal internal opening.

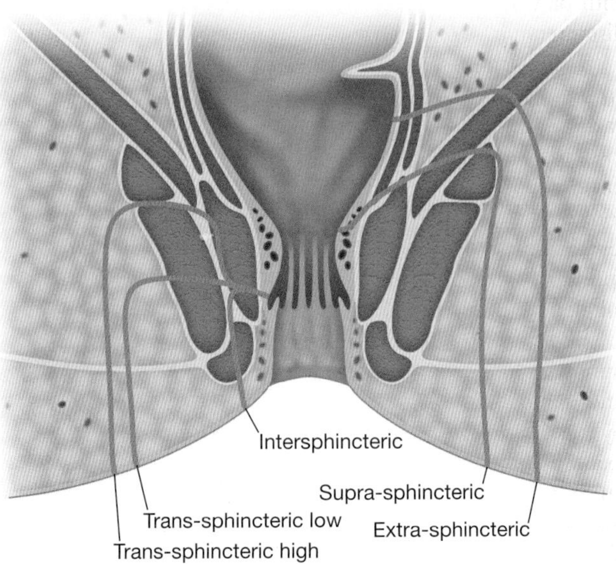

Figure 80.29 Coronal section of pelvis showing Parks' classification of anal fistula tracts.

Classification

The most widely used classification of anal fistulae (Parks') is based on anal gland sepsis in the intersphincteric space (the internal opening is at the dentate line); this results in a primary track whose relation to the external sphincter defines the type of fistula, which influences management (***Figure 80.29***).

The vast majority of fistulae are intersphincteric or trans-sphincteric. The American Gastroenterology Association classification (***Table 80.2***), which condenses the Parks' classification into simple and complex fistula, is helpful in the decision to operate on clinical findings, investigate further or refer for specialist opinion.

TABLE 80.2 American Gastroenterology Association classification of anal fistula.

Simple fistula
• Low (superficial or low inter- or low trans-sphincteric tract)
• Single external opening
Complex fistula
• High (high inter- or trans-sphincteric tract)
• Extra- or suprasphincteric tract
• Presence of abscess or collection
• Ano-vaginal fistula
• Anal stricture

Intersphincteric fistulae (45%) do not cross the external sphincter (bar, for the purist, the most medial subcutaneous fibres running below the distal border of the internal sphincter); most commonly they run directly from the internal to the external openings across the distal internal sphincter but may extend proximally in the intersphincteric plane to end blindly with or without an abscess or enter the upper anal canal or distal rectum at a second internal opening.

Trans-sphincteric fistulae (40%) have a primary track that crosses both internal and external sphincters (the latter at a variable level) and that then passes through the ischiorectal fossa to reach the skin of the buttock. The primary track may have secondary tracks arising from it, which often reach the roof of the ischiorectal fossa; they may rarely pass through the levator muscle to reach the pelvis. Circumferential (horseshoe) spread of sepsis may occur in the intersphincteric and pararectal planes, as well as in the ischiorectal plane.

Suprasphincteric fistulae (10%) run up to a level above the puborectalis and then curl downwards through the levators and ischioanal fossa to reach the skin. They are often caused by excessive probing of an abscess cavity or fistula tract during examination under anaesthesia. They are difficult to distinguish from high-level trans-sphincteric tracks; however, the management strategies are similar. Extrasphincteric fistulae (5%) run without specific relation to the sphincters and usually result from pelvic disease or trauma.

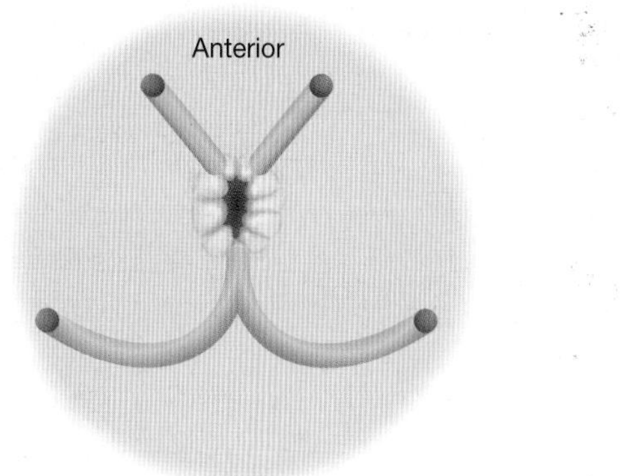

Figure 80.30 Goodsall's rule.

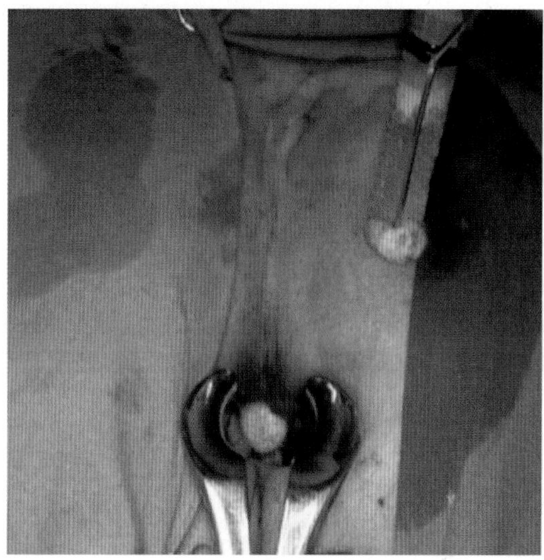

Figure 80.31 Injection of dilute hydrogen peroxide through the external fistula opening identifies the position of the internal opening at the dentate line.

Clinical assessment

A full medical (including obstetric, gastrointestinal, anal surgical and continence) history and proctosigmoidoscopy are necessary to gain information about sphincter strength and to exclude associated conditions. The key points to determine by clinical assessment of the fistula involve the following essential points:

- the site of the internal opening;
- the site of the external opening(s);
- the course of the primary track;
- the presence of secondary extensions; and
- the presence of other conditions complicating the fistula.

Palpable induration between the external opening and the anal margin suggests a relatively superficial track, whereas supralevator induration suggests a primary track above the levators or high in the roof of the ischiorectal fossa, or a high secondary extension. Intersphincteric fistulae usually have an external opening close to the anal verge. Goodsall's rule (***Figure 80.30***), used to indicate the likely position of the internal opening according to the position of the external opening(s), is helpful; however, the majority of internal openings are midline in both the anterior and posterior planes. The site of the internal opening may be felt as a point of induration or seen as an enlarged papilla. Dilute hydrogen peroxide, instilled via the external opening, can demonstrate the site of the internal opening (***Figure 80.31***); gentle use of probes (***Figure 80.32***) and a finger in the anorectum usually delineates primary and secondary tracks and their relations to the sphincters. Any concerns about fistula topography at clinical examination or examination under anaesthesia (more common after previous unsuccessful surgery) should prompt further investigations before surgical intervention.

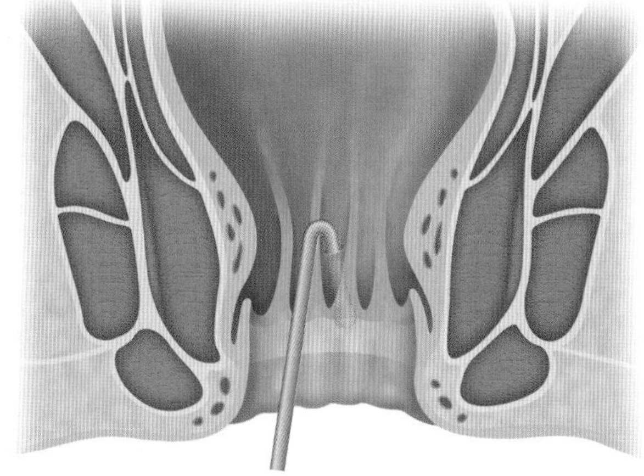

Figure 80.32 Retrograde probing of an anal canal sometimes reveals the internal orifice of the fistula.

David Henry Goodsall, 1843–1906, surgeon, St Mark's Hospital, London, UK.

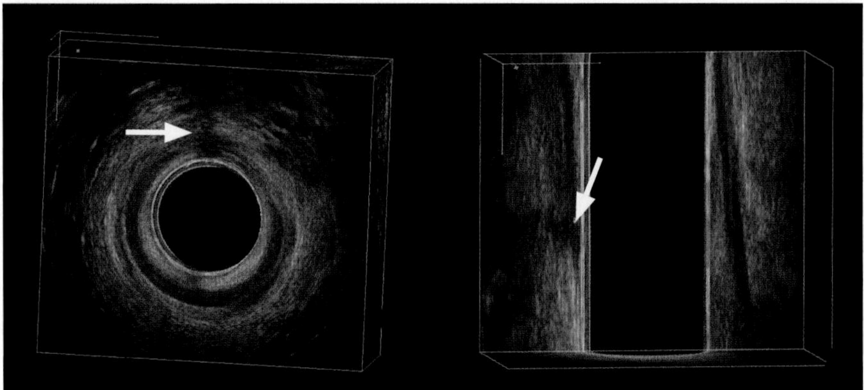

Figure 80.33 Three-dimensional endoanal ultrasonography images in the axial and sagittal plane showing an ano-vagina fistula (arrows) tracking from 12 o'clock towards the posterior vaginal wall at the lower canal level (courtesy of Dr Alison Corr, Consultant Radiologist, St Mark's Hospital, London, UK).

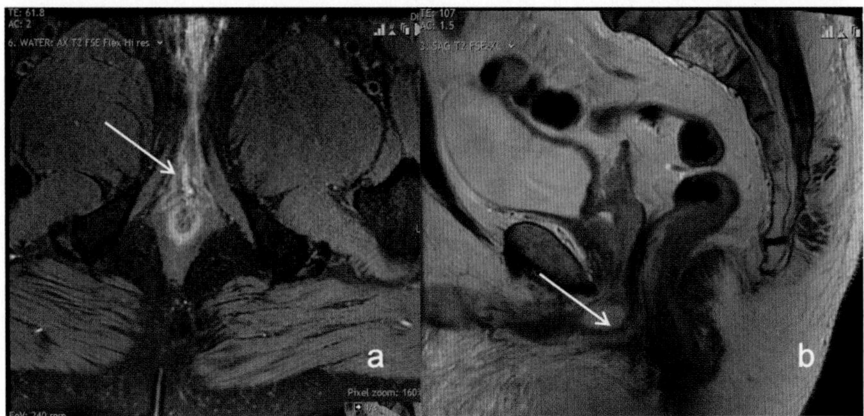

Figure 80.34 Axial T1-weighted post-contrast **(a)** and sagittal T2-weighted **(b)** magnetic resonance imaging sequences demonstrating an anterior fistula tract (arrow) traversing the perineal body to track under the base of the penis towards the scrotum (courtesy of Dr Alison Corr, Consultant Radiologist, St Mark's Hospital, London, UK).

Special investigations

A successful outcome after fistula surgery requires careful assessment of the fistula tract, sphincter integrity and function and patient expectations (especially in terms of risk to continence). Clinical examination will give some indication of functional anal sphincter length, resting tone and voluntary squeeze; these may be more objectively assessed by manometry, whereas EAUS gives useful information about sphincter integrity – the knowledge so gained may well influence surgical strategy. EAUS, especially with hydrogen peroxide instilled through the external opening, is more accurate than clinical examination and is useful to determine whether a fistula is simple or complex (***Figure 80.33***).

MRI is the 'gold standard' for fistula imaging. Short tau inversion recovery (STIR) sequencing (a fat-suppression technique) to highlight the presence of pus and granulation tissue without the need for contrast medium has been revolutionary (***Figure 80.34***). The great advantage of MRI is its ability to demonstrate secondary extensions, which may be missed at surgery and cause persistence (***Figure 80.35***). Fistulography and computed tomography (CT) are useful if an extrasphincteric fistula is suspected.

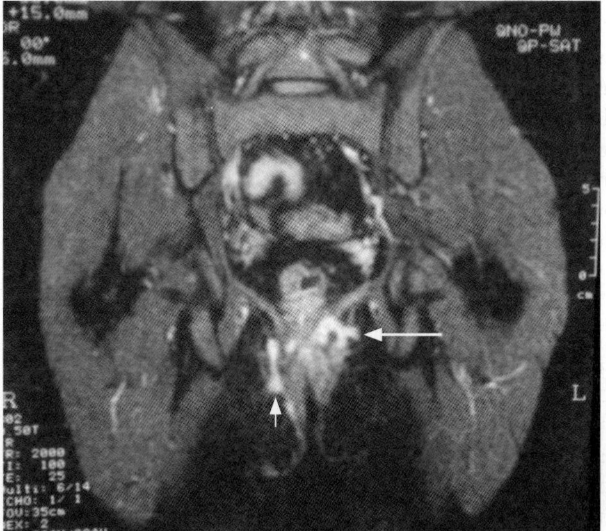

Figure 80.35 Coronal magnetic resonance imaging scan (short tau inversion recovery [STIR] sequence) demonstrating a primary track in the right ischiorectal space (short arrow) that crosses the sphincters to open into the anal canal just below the puborectalis. A blind secondary extension (long arrow) passing to the contralateral side in the roof of the left ischiorectal fossa was the cause of fistula persistence.

Principles of fistula surgery

The aim of surgery is to keep the patient continent and comfortable and whenever possible to eradicate the fistula. Fistulotomy, or laying the fistula tract open and allowing it to heal by secondary intention, has been practised for centuries and was beautifully described by John of Arderne in his *De Arte*

John of Arderne, 1307–1390, was the first English surgeon of note. He practised at Newark-on-Trent, and, from 1370, in London, UK. He described his operation for the treatment of fistulae in about 1376.

Phisicali et de Cirurgia. The use of a seton (from the Latin *seta*, meaning a bristle) to drain fistula tracts and gradually deliver the tract to the surface has a long history, most famously used by Charles Felix to treat French King Louis XIV.

Patients with minimal symptoms may be managed expectantly. Fistula eradication requires surgery, the extent of which must be balanced with the need to preserve continence. Division of any component of the sphincter mechanism carries some risk to continence. The most important determinant of function after fistulotomy is the amount of muscle left behind rather than that divided. In the presence of a normal bowel habit, continence is usually maintained as long as a minimum length of external sphincter is retained (2 cm as a rule but less in some cases).

Most fistulae are simple; however, a significant minority are complex (***Table 80.2***) and warrant specialist referral. The multitude of strategies advocated attests to these difficult situations; comparisons between techniques are difficult because of the heterogeneity of patient groups, the variability in classification, the inapplicability of certain techniques in some situations, inadequate reporting of functional outcomes, inadequate follow-up and surgeon preference over-riding entry into prospective randomised trials.

Track preparation

Tract preparation is an increasingly accepted concept in fistula surgery. It assumes that healing is prevented by epithelialisation of the track or that a secondary extension or undrained collection will induce early recurrence. Thus, a period of loose seton drainage followed by thorough debridement of the fistula track should improve healing rates. Some techniques, such as fistula plug, 'ligation of the intersphincteric fistula tract' (LIFT) (Rojanasakul) or 'fistula tract laser closure' (FiLaC™), require a particular track anatomy – such as a single straight trans-sphincteric tract – to be successful. In these cases, track preparation will facilitate healing of secondary tracks before definitive surgery.

Fistulotomy

Fistulotomy involves division of all structures lying between the external and internal openings. It is therefore applied mainly to intersphincteric fistulae and trans-sphincteric fistulae involving less than 30% of the external sphincter (but not anterior fistulae in women). After full examination under anaesthesia in the lithotomy or prone jack-knife position, during which the internal opening is identified, a grooved fistula probe is passed from the external to the internal opening (***Figure 80.36***), the amount of sphincter below and above the probe is noted and, if indicated, the track is laid open over the probe. Granulation tissue is curetted and sent for histological appraisal and the wound edges are trimmed. Secondary tracks, often identified as granulation tissue that persists despite curettage, should be laid open or drained. Marsupialisation reduces wound size and speeds up healing. Primary tracks crossing the external sphincter more deeply have been managed with good outcomes by fistulotomy and immediate reconstitution of the divided muscle – failure to eradicate all sepsis and subsequent breakdown of the repair can be problematic. Alternatively, a staged fistulotomy may be carried out in which secondary tracks are laid open and only part of the sphincter enclosed by the primary track is divided, with the remainder encircled by a loose seton. After sufficient time for healing of the wound and fibrosis, the seton-enclosed track is divided at a second stage.

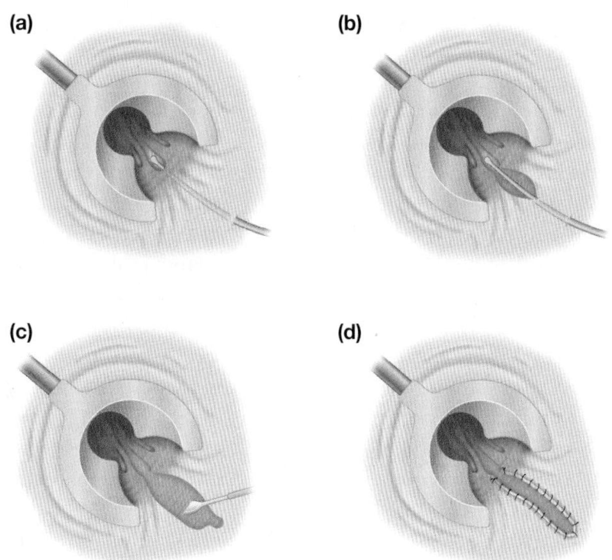

Figure 80.36 Fistulotomy. A grooved probe is passed from the external to internal openings (a) and the track laid open over the probe (b). The track is curetted to remove granulation tissue (c), the edges of the wound are trimmed and the wound may then be marsupialised (d). (Redrawn with permission from Nicholls RJ, Dozois RR. *Surgery of the colon and rectum*. Edinburgh: Churchill Livingstone, 1997.)

Fistulectomy

This technique involves coring out of the fistula, usually by diathermy cautery; it allows better definition of fistula anatomy than fistulotomy, especially the level at which the track crosses the sphincters and the presence of secondary extensions. If the sphincteric component of the fistula is deemed low enough to allow safe fistulotomy, then this may proceed (at the expense of longer healing times than conventional fistulotomy). If laying open is not advisable, the sphincteric component can be managed by another method.

Setons

Setons have been used in a variety of ways in fistula surgery and it is important for surgeons to be clear about what they are trying to achieve in a particular situation. Loose setons are tied such that there is no tension upon the encircled tissue; there is no intent to cut the tissue. A variety of materials have been used but the seton should be non-absorbable, non-degenerative and comfortable. Tight or cutting setons are placed with the intention of cutting through the enclosed muscle.

Loose setons are most commonly used before 'advanced' techniques (fistulectomy, advancement flap, cutting seton)

Charles Felix de Tassy, 1635–1703, on 18 November 1686 operated on Louis XIV, inserting a seton.
Arun Rojanasakul, contemporary, Professor of Surgery, Chulalongkorn University, Bangkok, Thailand.

while sepsis resolves and secondary extensions heal as part of a staged fistulotomy. Such a staged approach is valuable in treating secondary (horseshoe) tracks in the ischiorectal fossa, where the primary track crosses the external sphincter to reach the deep postanal space (Hanley). The internal sphincter is laid open to the level of the internal opening (or higher if there is a cephalad intersphincteric extension) to eradicate the presumed source and the sepsis in the intersphincteric space. A seton is then passed along the residual track around the denuded external sphincter and tied loosely, and the wounds are dressed. The seton is left in place for 3 months and either simply removed or replaced by a cutting seton to complete the fistulotomy.

Loose setons are also used for long-term palliation to avoid septic and painful exacerbations by establishing effective drainage, most often in Crohn's disease and in those with problematic fistulae not wishing to countenance the possibility of incontinence (***Figure 80.37***).

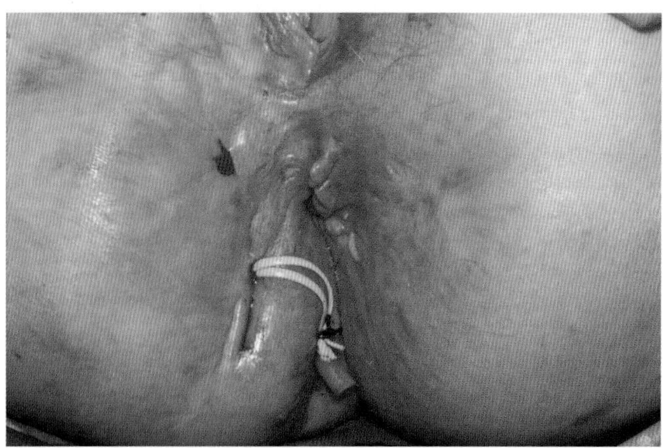

Figure 80.37 Complex horseshoe fistula-*in-ano* in Crohn's disease with healed ischiorectal sepsis, a loose seton in the residual tract and a draining 12 FG Malecot catheter to the deep postanal space.

Cutting setons aim to achieve the high fistula eradication rates associated with fistulotomy but without the degree of functional impairment endowed by division of the sphincters at a single stage. The enclosed muscle is gradually severed ('cheese wiring'), such that the divided muscles do not spring apart, and the site of the fistula track is replaced by a thin line of fibrosis. Some recommend prior internal sphincter division; others recommend incorporation of the internal sphincter within the cutting seton. A variety of seton material has been used, either elastic and 'self-cutting' or non-elastic and tightened at intervals, with the sphincter being divided at varying speeds. The same aim has been achieved by chemical cautery using an Ayurvedic method known in India as *ksharasootra*, in which a specially prepared seton thread burns through the enclosed tissue. This outpatient method has been shown to be equivalent to one-stage fistulotomy in patients with intersphincteric and distal trans-sphincteric fistulae.

Ligation of intersphincteric fistula tract

LIFT involves disconnection of the internal opening from the fistula tract at the level of the intersphincteric plane and removal of the residual infected glands without dividing any part of the sphincter complex. The tract is then ligated and divided, the internal part is removed and the external part of the track is curetted and drained (***Figure 80.38***). Hence it is a sphincter-preserving procedure, thereby maintaining continence. Systematic reviews report healing rates of 75% with little or no impairment of continence.

Advancement flaps

When the sphincter complex is not too indurated and adequate intra-anal access can be obtained, an advancement flap technique can be employed; this aims to preserve both anatomy and function. Ideally sepsis and secondary tracks have healed, leaving a direct track that can be cored. The internal opening is then closed with a broad-based, well-vascularised flap of anorectal mucosa and the internal sphincter is sutured without tension to the anoderm below the dentate line.

Biological agents

The functional consequences of fistulotomy have led to a search for agents that seal the fistula track and allow ingrowth of healthy tissue to replace it. Intuitively, success must depend on the biomaterial itself and the environment into which it is placed. Many agents have been tried with moderate success. These include fibrin glue, cross-linked porcine dermal collagen and more recently mesenchymal stem cells. Antibiotics, particularly metronidazole and ciprofloxacin, are of value in treating fistula-associated sepsis and many have immune-modulating effects of value in Crohn's disease. Patients must be warned of potential side effects of prolonged therapy, including peripheral neuropathy (metronidazole) and tendinopathy (ciprofloxacin). Biological therapies, including the anti-tumour necrosis factor drug vedolizumab and ciclosporin, are of value as part of multimodality treatment of perianal Crohn's disease (***Chapter 75***).

Other techniques

Video-assisted anal fistula treatment (VAAFT) involves the introduction of a rigid fistuloscope into the tract through the external opening. The scope has a channel to accommodate a forceps, brush or diathermy. The scope is passed into accessible tracks to allow lavage, curettage, cautery or the introduction of setons. VAAFT represents a form of advanced track identification and preparation before a definitive technique is performed. Fistula tract laser closure (FiLaC) uses radial emitting laser to obliterate the luminal aspect of the fistula to a known depth, throughout its length. An over-the-scope clip (OTSC) involves closing the internal opening using a nitinol clip, disconnecting the external tract. Clip migration and elective removal because of pain are the main complications. The FISCLOSE trial is currently recruiting.

Patrick H Hanley, 1909–1994, surgeon, Ochsner Clinic, New Orleans, LA, USA.
Achille Etienne Malecot, 1852–?, urologist, Paris, France, described a self-retaining catheter in 1895.

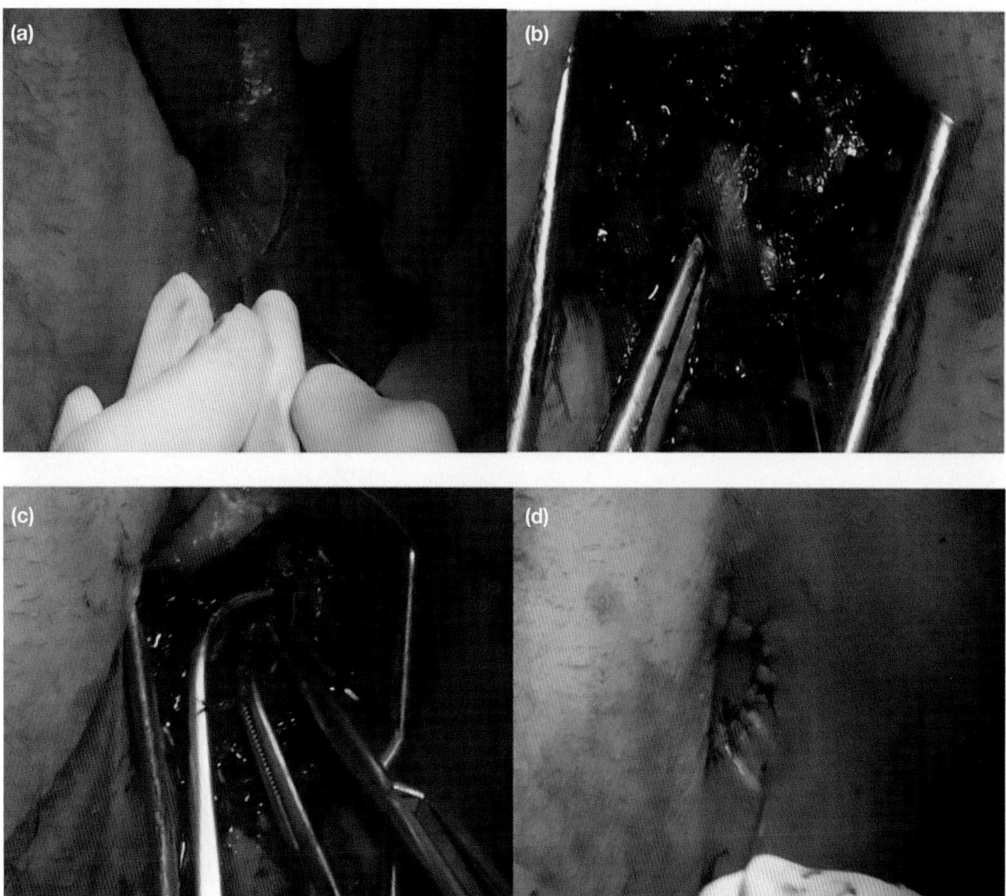

Figure 80.38 Ligation of an intersphincteric fistula tract. (a) A curved incision is made over the intersphincteric groove. (b) The fistula tract is identified in the intersphincteric space. (c) The fistula tract is divided between right-angled forceps and transfixed with 2/0 vicryl sutures. (d) Wound closure and intact tract ligation is confirmed with a probe (courtesy of Mr Rory Kennelly, FRCSI, Dublin, Ireland).

Summary box 80.12

Anorectal fistulae

- Are classified according to the relationship to the anal sphincters
- The majority are simple and may be safely treated by fistulotomy
- Complex fistulae require detailed anatomical assessment that may include MRI
- Staged treatment including use of setons should be considered
- LIFT, flap advancement, VAAFT, FiLaC and OTSC allow sphincter preservation
- Biological therapy is used in multimodality treatment of fistulae associated with Crohn's disease

HIDRADENITIS SUPPURATIVA

HA is a chronic suppurative condition of apocrine gland-bearing skin found in the axillae, submammary regions, nape of the neck, groin, mons pubis, inner thighs and sides of the scrotum, as well as the perineum and buttocks. It is a source of considerable physical and psychological morbidity. There is no confirmatory test or specific characteristic for diagnosis, which makes definition difficult. Acne, pilonidal sinus and chronic scalp folliculitis may coexist.

Pathology

Occlusion of gland ducts leads to bacterial proliferation, gland rupture and the spread of infection and epithelial components into the surrounding soft tissue and to adjacent glands. Secondary infection causes further local extension, skin damage and deformity, with multiple communicating subcutaneous sinus tracts. There is some evidence that the disease may be related to a relative androgen excess.

Presentation

The condition is not seen before puberty and rarely presents after the fourth decade of life. Overall, it is three times more common in women than in men, although anogenital disease is more common in men. Obesity is a common association. When affecting the perineum, lesions begin as multiple raised boils, with recurrent lesions within the same vicinity leading to sinus tract formation, bridged scarring and multiple points of discharge. Rarely, it may involve the anal canal anoderm, but it does not extend above the dentate line or involve the sphincter muscle.

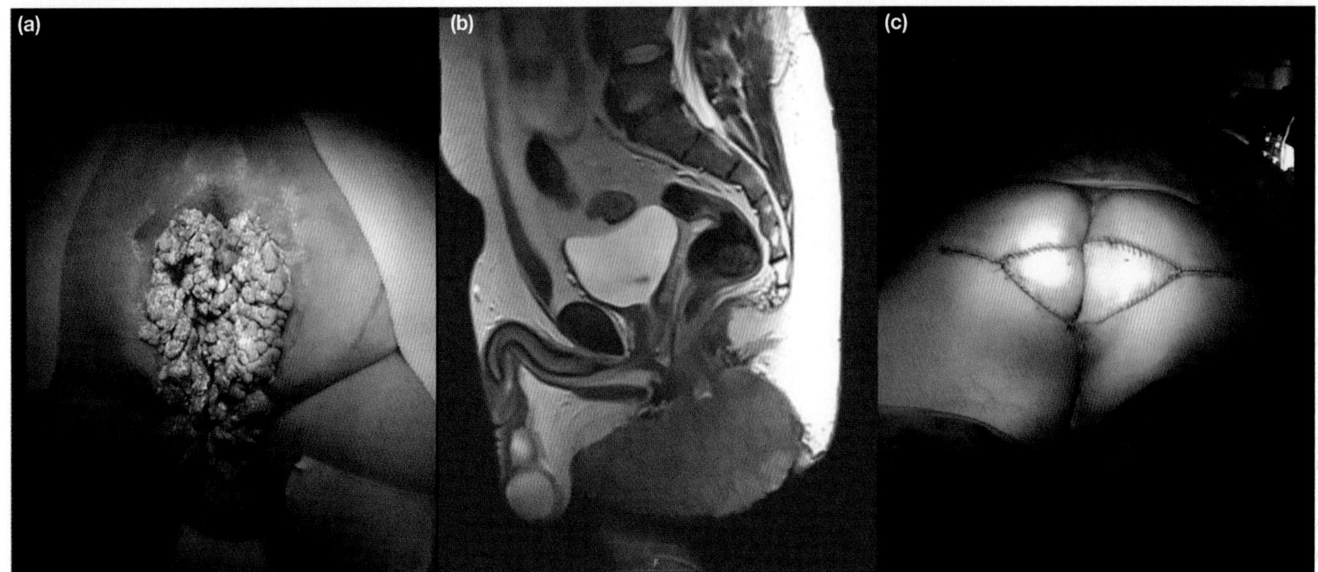

Figure 80.39 Preoperative image (a) of a giant condyloma acuminatum (Buschke–Löwenstein tumour) with sagittal T2-weighted magnetic resonance imaging (b) demonstrating the large exophytic frond-like mass protruding from the anal verge. Bilateral inferior gluteal artery perforator (I-GAP) flap reconstruction following perineal resection (c) (courtesy of Mr Anthony Antoniou, Consultant Colorectal Surgeon, St Mark's Hospital, London, UK).

Differential diagnosis

In the early stages, distinction from furunculosis can be difficult. Crohn's disease, cryptoglandular fistula, pilonidal sinus, tuberculosis, actinomycosis, lymphogranuloma venereum and granuloma inguinale must be considered when later stages present.

Treatment

In the early stages, general measures, including weight reduction and antiseptic soaps, may be helpful. Antibiotics may induce remission but often the disease relapses and progresses, at which point surgery is indicated. Inadequate treatment may lead to prolonged morbidity, but any surgery should be less debilitating than the condition. Surgical intervention ranges from simple incision and drainage of acute sepsis to radical excision of all apocrine gland-bearing skin. Careful laying open of all tracts, possibly as a staged procedure according to anatomical location, is an option that appeals to many patients. Radical excision requires closure by skin graft or rotation flap and, occasionally, a defunctioning colostomy to allow healing.

CONDYLOMATA ACUMINATA (ANAL WARTS)

There is increasing evidence that sexually transmitted infection with human papillomavirus (HPV) forms the aetiological basis of anal and perianal warts, anal intraepithelial neoplasia (AIN) and SCC of the anus. In areas of the world where sexual promiscuity (especially anal intercourse) is more common, and in immunocompromised individuals (HIV-infected individuals and transplant recipients), there have been dramatic increases in the incidence of these conditions over the last 30 years, most importantly of AIN and anal cancers. Similar virally induced changes have been noted in the genital tracts of women (vulval intraepithelial neoplasia [VIN], cervical intraepithelial neoplasia [CIN] and cancers). It is essential to examine all areas of the genitalia and perineum in an affected person as there is often a field change with the virus affecting any squamous epithelium in that area. There are over 170 subtypes of HPV, but certain subtypes (16, 18, 31, 33) are associated with a greater risk of progression to dysplasia and malignancy. SCC is associated with HPV (especially subtypes 16, 18, 31 or 33). Associated warts on the penis and the female genital tract are common.

Presentation

Many are asymptomatic but pruritus, discharge, bleeding and pain are usual presenting complaints. In the early stages, examination reveals separate pinkish-white warts close to the anal margin and also often on the anoderm within the distal anal canal. Later, the warts enlarge, coalesce and carpet the skin. Rarely, relentless growth results in giant condylomata (Buschke–Löwenstein tumour), which may obliterate the anal orifice (***Figure 80.39***). The diagnosis is aided by aceto-whitening on application of acetic acid but confirmed by biopsy, which will also indicate the presence or absence of dysplasia.

Treatment

Because of the field effect endowed by viral skin infection, long-term resolution can be problematic. Careful serial application of 25% podophyllin to discrete warts on the perianal skin is

Abraham Buschke, 1868–1943, Chief of Dermatology, Rudolf Virchow Hospital, Berlin, Germany.
Ludwig W Löwenstein, 1895–1959, pathologist, Berlin, Germany, later New York Post-Graduate Medical School, NY, USA, described this condition in 1925.

often used; however, it cannot be used intra-anally. Surgical excision under local, regional or general anaesthesia involves raising and separating the lesions with local infiltration of dilute adrenaline, which allows more accurate scissor or electrocautery excision to maximise the preservation of normal skin.

ANAL INTRAEPITHELIAL NEOPLASIA

AIN is a multifocal virally induced dysplasia of the perianal or intra-anal epidermis associated with HPV. Subtypes 6 and 11 are most often associated with warts and early AIN, whereas subtypes 16 and 18 account for more than 75% of anal cancers. The prevalence is <1% of the population with a rising incidence, especially in those areas where ano-receptive intercourse and HIV are prevalent. At-risk groups include patients with HIV as well as immunocompromised patients, women with a history of other genital intraepithelial neoplasia (VIN and CIN) and patients with extensive anogenital condylomata. Patients may be asymptomatic and the diagnosis is often a histological surprise, although increasing numbers in high-risk groups are picked up on anal cytology. It is classified according to the degree of dysplasia on biopsy into AIN I, AIN II and AIN III, according to the lack of keratocyte maturation and extension of the proliferative zone from the lower third (AIN I) to the full thickness of the epithelium (AIN III), in the same manner as cervical or vulval dysplasia. The natural history is uncertain but progression from AIN II to AIN III to invasive carcinoma has been observed, notably in the immunocompromised. The term Bowen's disease is no longer used.

Presentation

Around 10% of AIN lesions are diagnosed by the pathologist after excision of abnormal skin lesions. Low-grade lesions may be raised and similar to anal condylomata; however, high-grade AIN III lesions may be characterised by hyperkeratosis or by changes in the pigmentation of the epithelium, so this may appear white, red or brown with the pigmentation commonly being irregular. The lesions may be flat or raised, but ulceration is suggestive of invasive disease. It is important that any suspicious areas are biopsied and examined histologically.

Patients' symptoms include pruritus, pain, bleeding and discharge. AIN is present in 28–35% of excised anal warts. Approximately 10% of AIN III lesions will progress to anal carcinoma at 5 years. Regression of AIN III rarely occurs, but AIN I and AIN II may regress. The association between AIN III and carcinoma is strengthened by the findings of AIN III in 80% of anal cancer biopsies.

Diagnosis and management

A high index of suspicion and targeted biopsy yields the diagnosis, whereas multiple (mapping) biopsies give an indication of the extent and overall severity of the disease. AIN III should be regularly monitored clinically and, if necessary, by repeat biopsy to exclude invasive disease. Specialised centres may offer colposcopy of the anus (anoscopy), utilising 5% acetic acid with Lugol's iodine to assess *in vivo* the dysplastic areas of the anus. The affected areas show up white and can be biopsied. Focal disease may be excised and local excision is effective for lesions <30% of the circumference of the anus. More widespread disease can be dealt with surgically by wide local excision and closure of the resultant defect by flap or skin graft, with or without covering colostomy (especially if there is intra-anal disease). However, for a condition with uncertain malignant potential, this approach should be used with caution as it carries with it significant morbidity. Anal mapping uses a 3-mm corneal punch biopsy, and a total of 8–12 biopsies allows for adequate mapping of most disease. An operative map or photograph is helpful. Examination of the vulva, vagina and cervix is also needed as female patients are at risk of other anogenital intraepithelial neoplasia; it is recommended that those with AIN III have a yearly cervical smear test. The grade and extent of anal disease determines management. Localised or focal AIN is defined as <30% of the anal circumference, whereas extensive AIN involves more than 30% of the circumference. Lesions involving <30% of the anal circumference can be simply excised with the resulting wound left to granulate or closed as appropriate. AIN III lesions involving >30% of the anal margin or canal cannot be excised as the risk of severe anal stenosis is significant. The remaining areas are regularly observed at 6-monthly intervals. AIN I/II and AIN III have differing natural histories.

Topical imiquimod (5%) or oral retinoids have some effect on the progression of dysplasia and can cause regression by at least two histological grades. Other newer options may include anti-HPV treatment; vaccination may reduce the incidence in the long term.

AIN I/II has an indolent course except in immunocompetent patients, for whom 12-monthly anoscopy is recommended. Patients with AIN III and multicentric intraepithelial neoplasia should be managed by clinicians with an interest in this disease and require a multidisciplinary approach involving gynaecological specialists. Immuno-incompetent patients (including those with HIV) are considered separately in view of the higher progression rates and poorer results, with higher recurrence rates after surgery compared with immunocompetent patients. These require extended follow-up with 6-monthly anoscopy.

MALIGNANT TUMOURS

Malignant lesions of the anus and anal canal

Anal malignancy is rare and accounts for less than 2% of all large bowel cancers; however, the incidence is rising, with a direct association with HPV infection, AIN and immunosuppression. The crude incidence rate is 0.65 per 100 000 in the UK. The male-to-female ratio is approximately 1:2. The great majority are SCCs. Those arising below the dentate line are usually keratinising, whereas those above

Jean Lugol, 1786–1851, French physician, Lugol's iodine was first made in 1829.

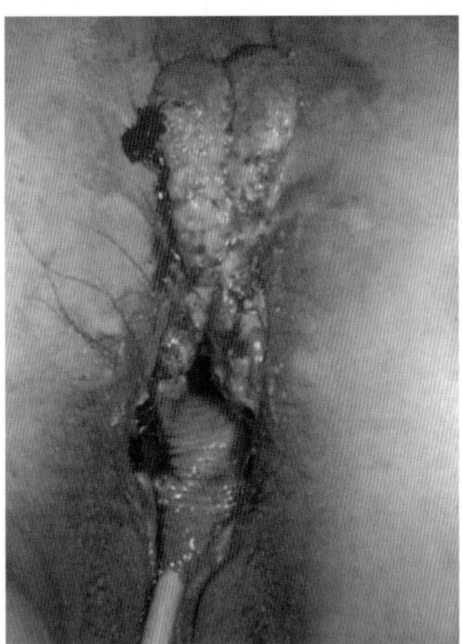

Figure 80.40 Anus squamous cell carcinoma.

are non-keratinising squamous, variously termed basaloid, cloacogenic or transitional. There is now broad consensus that both are similar in their presentation and response to treatment and should be treated as carcinomas whether keratinising or not. Adenocarcinomas are the next most common and are thought to arise from anal glands. Other tumours include melanoma, lymphoma, sarcoma and tumours of perianal skin.

Squamous cell carcinoma

Anal SCC usually presents with pain and bleeding, thus it is often initially misdiagnosed as a benign condition, highlighting the need for a level of suspicion and adequate examination. A mass, pruritus or discharge is less common. Advanced tumours may cause faecal incontinence by invasion of the sphincters and, in women, anterior extension may result in anovaginal fistulation. On examination, anal margin tumours look like malignant ulcers, with raised indurated edges (***Figure 80.40***). There may be associated HPV lesions. Anal canal tumours are palpable as irregular indurated tender ulceration. Sphincter involvement may be evident. Involvement of perirectal and groin lymph nodes may be palpable on examination.

Investigation

An examination under anaesthetic allows detailed assessment of the tumour size, involvement of regional nodes and adjacent structures and the opportunity to obtain a biopsy for histological examination.

Management

MRI scanning of the pelvis and CT of the chest, abdomen and pelvis allows locoregional and distant staging. Positron emission tomography (PET)-CT is increasingly used and may help in equivocal inguinal node assessment.

Historically anal cancer was treated by abdominoperineal resection; however, since the late 1970s chemoradiotherapy (Nigro) has become the primary treatment. The UK Coordinating Committee on Cancer Research (UKCCCR) Anal Cancer Trial (ACT I) found that chemoradiation with radiotherapy (50.5 Gy) gave superior local control compared with radiotherapy alone while the ACT II trial found similar outcomes when chemoradiotherapy using cisplatin/5-fluorouracil (5-FU) was compared with mitomycin/5-FU. The longer infusion time required to administer cisplatin/5-FU has led to the preferred use of the mitomycin/5-FU combination. Current trials (ACT III, ACT IV and ACT V) are investigating more personalised treatment protocols, including local excision only for small tumours and a combination of excision along with varying radiotherapy regimes for other tumours.

Radical surgical excision by abdominoperineal resection is indicated in those with residual tumour, complications of treatment, incontinence or fistula after tumour resolution and recurrent disease. Despite good results with chemoradiotherapy, 20–25% of patients will have an incomplete tumour response or local disease recurrence. After thorough assessment, these patients may require radical abdominoperineal resection as a salvage procedure. Locally extensive disease may require pelvic exenterative procedures that usually entail perineal reconstruction using a myocutaneous flap.

Enlarged regional inguinal lymph nodes are common and may be secondary to inflammation rather than malignancy. Histological/cytological confirmation is mandatory. Positive nodes are treated by chemoradiotherapy. Radial groin dissection has a high morbidity.

Other anal malignancies

Adenocarcinoma within the anal canal is usually an extension of a distal rectal cancer. Rarely, adenocarcinoma may arise from anal glandular epithelium or develop within a longstanding (usually complex) anal fistula, hence the need to biopsy non-healing fistula-*in-ano*. The treatment is as for low rectal cancers (i.e. abdominoperineal excision of the rectum with or without neoadjuvant chemoradiotherapy, ***Chapter 79***). Malignant melanoma of the anus is very rare and usually presents as a bluish-black soft mass that may mimic a thrombosed external pile, although it may be amelanotic. The prognosis, irrespective of treatment, is extremely poor. Perianal Paget's disease is exceedingly rare.

Summary box 80.13

Anal cancer

- Uncommon, usually squamous cell
- Associated with HPV, HIV and immunosuppression
- Lymphatic spread is to the inguinal lymph nodes
- Treatment is by chemoradiotherapy in the first instance
- Major ablative surgery is required for salvage

Norman D Nigro, 1912–2009, surgeon, Wayne State University, Detroit, MI, USA.

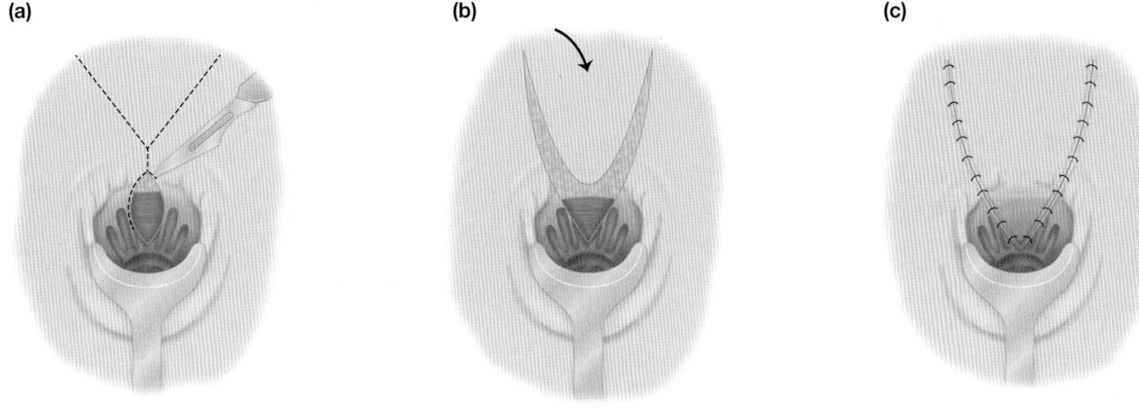

Figure 80.41 Y–V advancement flap for anal stenosis.

NON-MALIGNANT STRICTURES: ANAL STENOSIS

Anal stenosis is a rare but serious complication of anorectal surgery. Removal of excess anoderm and mucosa without adequate skin bridges during haemorrhoidectomy can lead to scarring and stricturing. Stenosis can also occur after stapled haemorrhoidopexy and coloanal anastomoses. Other causes include trauma, postradiation fibrosis, tuberculosis and fibrosing skin conditions, e.g. scleroderma. Lymphogranuloma inguinale may cause an inflammatory stricture of the rectum.

Inflammatory bowel disease

Stricture of the anorectum may complicate Crohn's disease and, in this instance, the stricture is annular. These stenoses are characterised by transmural scarring and inflammation. Occasionally, an anal stricture may occur in ulcerative colitis. Until a biopsy is obtained, a carcinoma should be suspected.

Endometriosis

Endometriosis of the rectovaginal septum may present as a stricture. There is usually a history of frequent menstrual periods with severe pain during the first 2 days of the menstrual flow.

Clinical features

Increasing difficulty in defecation is the leading symptom. The patient finds that increasingly large doses of aperients are required and, if the stools are formed, they are 'pipe-stem' in shape. In cases of inflammatory stricture, tenesmus, bleeding and the passage of mucopus are superadded. Sometimes the patient comes under observation only when subacute or acute intestinal obstruction has supervened.

Rectal examination

The finger encounters a sharply defined shelf-like interruption of the lumen. If the calibre is large enough to admit the finger, it should be noted whether the stricture is annular or tubular. Sometimes this point can be determined only after dilatation. A biopsy of the stricture must be taken. Often the examination will be painful and needs to be performed under general anaesthesia when biopsies and gentle, graduated dilatation may be undertaken.

Treatment

Non-operative treatment is recommended for mild stenosis. The use of stool softeners and fibre supplements helps aid the passage of stools.

Dilatation

Anal dilatation can be performed under general anaesthesia and then by the patient, using an anal dilator. For anal and many rectal strictures, dilatation at regular intervals is all that is required.

Anoplasty

For severe anal stenosis, an anoplasty is used to replace loss of anal tissue. The stricture is incised and a rotation or advancement flap of skin and subcutaneous tissue replaces the defect and enlarges the anal orifice (***Figure 80.41***). This technique is particularly useful for postoperative strictures.

Colostomy

Colostomy must be undertaken when a stricture is causing intestinal obstruction and in advanced cases of stricture complicated by fistulae-*in-ano*. In selected cases, this can be followed by restorative resection of the stricture-bearing area. If this step is anticipated, a loop ileostomy is constructed.

Rectal excision and coloanal anastomosis

Rectal excision is required when the strictures are at, or just above, the anorectal junction and are associated with a normal anal canal, but irreversible changes necessitate removal of the area. Coloanal anastomosis can restore function but is contraindicated in Crohn's disease.

Summary box 80.14

Benign anal stricture

- May be iatrogenic, e.g. after haemorrhoidectomy
- Biopsy must be taken to rule out malignancy
- Can usually be managed by regular dilatation
- Severe anal stenosis may require an anoplasty

FURTHER READING

Chu CS, Pfister DG. Opportunities and challenges: human papillomavirus and cancer. *J Natl Compr Canc Netw* 2017; **15**(5S): 726–9.

Cross KL, Massey EJ, Fowler AL *et al.* The management of anal fissure: ACPGBI position statement. *Colorectal Dis* 2008; **10**(Suppl 3): 1–7.

Geh I, Gollins S, Renehan A *et al.* Association of Coloproctology of Great Britain & Ireland (ACPGBI): guidelines for the management of cancer of the colon, rectum and anus (2017) – anal cancer. *Colorectal Dis* 2017; **19**(Suppl 1): 82–97.

Keighley MRB, Williams NS. *Surgery of the anus, rectum and colon*, 3rd edn. Philadelphia: Saunders, 2008.

Nordon IM, Senapati A, Cripps NP. A prospective randomized controlled trial of simple Bascom's technique versus Bascom's cleft closure for the treatment of chronic pilonidal disease. *Am J Surg* 2009; **197**: 189–92.

Scholefield JH, Harris D, Radcliffe A. Guidelines for management of anal intraepithelial neoplasia. *Colorectal Dis* 2011; **13**(Suppl 1): 3–10.

Williams G, Williams A, Tozer P *et al.* The treatment of anal fistula: second ACPGBI position statement - 2018. *Colorectal Dis* 2018; 20 (Suppl 3): 5-31.

PART 12 | Genitourinary

CHAPTER 81 Urinary symptoms and investigations

Learning objectives

To understand:
- The significance of pain relating to urinary tract pathology
- The difference between renal pain and ureteric colic
- The definitions of common lower urinary tract symptoms

To be able to:
- Select the appropriate diagnostic tests

PAIN

Pain is a common urological symptom. Pain while passing urine is called dysuria and refers to discomfort experienced during voiding – typically described as a sensation akin to passing razor blades or glass. Most commonly, dysuria is due to an infection in the lower urinary tract but can rarely be due to carcinoma *in situ* (CIS) of the bladder, especially in an older male smoker with haematuria.

Renal pain is usually caused by distension of the renal capsule and is felt as a constant, gnawing pain in the loin/renal angle. Ureteric colic (often incorrectly referred to as renal colic) is different from renal pain and is typified by the lateralised, colicky pain experienced by someone with a ureteric calculus. Ureteric colic can radiate to the groin or to the testicle/labium but does not radiate to the back of the leg. Ureteric colic can also, rarely, be caused by a blood clot or a sloughed renal papilla in the ureter. Some patients simultaneously experience both ureteric colic and renal pain.

Summary box 81.1

Pain from the urinary tract
- Renal colic is a misnomer and should be referred to as ureteric colic
- Renal pain can be distinguished from ureteric colic by careful history taking
- Renal pain and ureteric colic may be experienced simultaneously
- Ureteric colic may radiate to the groin/testicle/labium
- Ureteric colic does not radiate to the chest or the back of the leg

Infection or inflammation of the bladder can produce suprapubic pain. Suprapubic pain that is experienced when the bladder is full and is relieved by micturition is typical of interstitial cystitis, an idiopathic inflammatory disorder of the bladder typically seen in middle-aged women.

Testicular pain is a common symptom in boys and young men. Sudden, severe testicular pain should be treated as a medical emergency to rule out a diagnosis of acute testicular torsion. Hydroceles and epididymal cysts usually do not cause significant pain but can have an increasing pressure effect as they enlarge. A dragging sensation in the scrotum that gets worse towards the end of the day is characteristic of a varicocele. Testicular tumours in young men are not usually associated with significant pain. Investigation of testicular pain in the young adult male/middle-aged male is frequently negative, resulting in a highly unsatisfactory diagnostic label of 'idiopathic testicular pain' or 'chronic orchialgia'. Patients undergoing vasectomy are routinely counselled about the approximately 10% risk of testicular pain in the short term following surgery and, more importantly, the 1% chance of chronic testicular pain in the longer term.

Perineal pain is often a feature of a complex of symptoms typically seen in middle-aged men who, by a process of exclusion, are diagnosed as having acute or chronic prostatitis. With prostatitis, perineal pain may be accompanied by suprapubic pain, low back pain that radiates to the legs and penile pain as well as frequency of micturition and dysuria. In the absence of the specific features that are required to diagnose prostatitis, these patients should be considered to have chronic pelvic pain syndrome (CPPS) and not prostatitis. Perineal pain is an ominous symptom after previous treatment for a pelvic malignancy, often signifying recurrent pelvic disease.

LOWER URINARY TRACT SYMPTOMS

A normal micturition cycle consists of two phases: storage and voiding. During the storage phase, the bladder holds urine at low pressures and the urethral sphincter is closed. During voiding, the bladder contracts to expel urine and the voluntary urethral sphincter relaxes to allow its passage. In addition, the urethral lumen must be patent to allow voiding to occur. Disruption of these processes results in lower urinary tract symptoms (LUTS). In general terms, LUTS are classified as either storage LUTS (frequency, nocturia, urgency and urinary incontinence); voiding LUTS (hesitancy, a reduced stream, straining); or postmicturition LUTS (incomplete emptying and postmicturition dribble). Storage LUTS result from failure of the bladder to act as a functioning reservoir and are commonly seen in patients with an overactive bladder or a bladder neuropathy. Voiding and postmicturition LUTS are commonly seen in men with bladder outlet obstruction (BOO) or an underactive bladder; however, a man with BOO may also have storage LUTS. BOO is also reported in women and may be caused by urethral stenosis, strictures or a hypocontractile bladder.

The term 'prostatism' is obsolete. It was used to describe a combination of LUTS in men who were presumed to have an enlarged prostate or benign prostatic hyperplasia (BPH). However, the symptoms are not specific to BPH and may occur in several other conditions, including urinary tract infections (UTIs), urethral stricture, overactive bladder, CIS of the bladder, etc. Further, not all symptoms may be present in every patient and most patients have a variable degree of different symptoms. Thus, the term LUTS is now used to describe all such symptoms. It may not always be possible to identify the aetiology of LUTS and additional investigations with urodynamics (see *Urodynamics*) may occasionally be required.

The International Continence Society provides the internationally accepted definitions for symptoms relating to lower urinary tract function.

- **Frequency** – the patient considers that they void too often during the day.
- **Nocturia** – the individual wakes at night at least once to void.
- **Strangury** – a sensation of constantly needing to void. Typically, the patient describes having to stand/sit for long periods with the sensation that micturition is imminent.
- **Urgency** – a sudden compelling desire to pass urine that is difficult to defer.
- **Urge incontinence** – involuntary urinary leakage, often a large volume, immediately preceded by the sensation of urgency.
- **Stress incontinence** – involuntary urinary leakage that occurs when the intra-abdominal pressure rises during coughing, laughing, sneezing or exercising.
- **Nocturnal enuresis** – involuntary loss of urine during sleep.
- **Hesitancy** – when an individual has difficulty initiating micturition, resulting in a delay in the onset of voiding.
- **Reduced urinary stream** – usually reported compared with previous performance or in comparison with the performance of others.
- **Intermittency** – when urine flow stops and starts, on one or more occasions.
- **Straining** – the muscular effort used in order to initiate, maintain or improve the urinary stream.
- **Incomplete emptying** – the sensation that, at the end of micturition, bladder fullness persists.
- **Postmicturition dribble** – when involuntary loss of urine occurs immediately after the individual has finished passing urine.

Summary box 81.2

Lower urinary tract symptoms (LUTS)

- LUTS are classified as storage, voiding or post micturition
- Storage LUTS are typical of an overactive bladder
- Voiding LUTS are typical of BOO
- Some patients have storage and voiding LUTS in combination
- LUTS are sometimes investigated with urodynamics

HAEMATURIA

Haematuria occurs when there is blood in the urine. This is now classified as visible haematuria (VH) or non-visible haematuria (NVH). Enquiry should be made about the timing of the blood in relation to the urinary stream – initial (urethral pathology), throughout the stream (bladder or upper tracts) or terminal (bladder neck or prostatic pathology) – as well as the degree of haematuria and its frequency. A patient with haematuria should be investigated regardless of whether they are taking anticoagulant therapy. The concern is that the haematuria, especially if painless, may be due to an underlying neoplasm, usually a bladder or renal tumour. Causes of haematuria include trauma (**T**), infection (**I**) and neoplasm (**N**) anywhere in the urinary tract. Haematuria in association with loin pain and a palpable loin mass defines the classic triad of symptoms and signs of a renal tumour, although this triad is seen in less than 10% of these patients. In countries with endemic tuberculosis (TB) or filarial disease, haematuria is also seen in patients with these genitourinary infections. In genitourinary TB, haematuria is usually associated with dysuria and frequency due to bladder infection. In patients with filarial involvement of the retroperitoneal lymphatics, haematuria is intermittent, often lasting months or years, and is associated with 'milky' or cloudy urine, a condition called chyluria.

Haematuria requires detailed investigation in almost all cases except young women with a proven UTI. Investigations include an ultrasound scan (USS) of the kidneys–ureters–bladder (KUB) and additional contrast imaging if needed. If no aetiology can be identified on laboratory and imaging studies, cystoscopy is mandatory. Although BPH can cause haematuria in older men, this diagnosis should be considered after exclusion of all other causes. The cancer detection rate depends on the degree of haematuria, being approximately 20% in those patients with VH but very much lower in those with NVH (<5%).

Summary box 81.3

Haematuria

- Classified as VH or NVH
- A list of potential causes for haematuria can be rapidly generated by considering trauma (T), infection (I) and neoplasm (N) anywhere in the urinary tract
- Haematuria requires detailed investigation in nearly all cases

Discoloration of the urine

Many drugs and foodstuffs have been reported to produce abnormal discoloration of the urine. Most colours have been reported but the most frequently encountered clinically are red/orange and brown. Apart from haematuria, the presence of haem in the urine also produces red discoloration and generates a positive dipstick test. Red urine discoloration due to haemoglobinuria may present in haemolytic disorders such as 'march haematuria', classically seen in dehydrated soldiers after prolonged marching. Likewise, myoglobinuria due to myocyte destruction, e.g. caused by rhabdomyolysis after crush injury or compartment syndrome, can also result in red discoloration of the urine. Disordered haem production, seen in porphyria, can result in red discoloration that may change to brown or purple with exposure to sunlight. Several medications can cause red/orange discoloration of the urine, most commonly rifampicin, isoniazid or phenazopyridine. Others include chlorpromazine, thioridazine, senna and laxatives containing a phenolphthalein component. Consumption of large quantities of beetroot can result in red discoloration of the urine. This discoloration is due to the excretion of betalain (betacyanin) pigments such as betanin. The commonly used antibiotics nitrofurantoin and metronidazole can lead to brown urine. Brown urine due to high levels of circulating bilirubin is a feature of obstructive jaundice.

Uraemia

Rarely, the initial symptoms of urological disease may be those of severe renal dysfunction or uraemia. In infants and children, this may manifest as failure to thrive as well as anorexia, vomiting and altered sensorium due to encephalopathy.

LESS COMMON URINARY SYMPTOMS

Haematospermia

This refers to blood, which can be bright red or a brown colour, in semen. It is most commonly due to benign inflammatory change in the prostate or TB. A digital rectal examination (DRE) should be performed alongside a prostate-specific antigen (PSA) test. A transrectal ultrasound (TRUS) or magnetic resonance imaging (MRI) of the prostate should be considered. In most cases, haematospermia is self-limiting.

Pneumaturia

This is gas in the urine. Patients typically describe frothy urine, bubbles in the urine or a stream that intermittently stops and starts. The commonest cause is an underlying colovesical fistula, usually due to primary pathology in the rectum or sigmoid colon.

'White urine'

White urine is a complaint seen in two distinct conditions. One is in young men who may report the presence of a white substance in urine. This substance is usually semen and requires no treatment other than reassurance. The second condition is chyluria where lymphatic fluid, from channels obstructed by filarial inflammation, leaks into the renal pelvicalyceal system. This condition requires investigation for confirmation of the diagnosis.

SYMPTOMS RELATED TO THE EXTERNAL GENITALIA

Testis

A testis may be absent from the scrotum in patients with undescended or ectopic testes.

In boys <5 years, a common cause of testicular pain and swelling is torsion of a hydatid of Morgagni (appendix testis). In a young male suspected of having a testicular torsion, examination of the normal, i.e. contralateral, testis may reveal a horizontal lie or 'clapper bell testis', raising the level of clinical suspicion. If torsion is suspected, immediate testicular exploration is mandatory and, if confirmed, bilateral testicular fixation is performed. A Doppler USS may aid in the diagnosis.

Patients with Klinefelter's syndrome have bilateral small, firm testes in addition to the other signs typical of this condition.

A hydrocele is an accumulation of fluid between the testis and the tunica vaginalis; in the younger male it can be associated with a patent processus vaginalis. The hydrocele fluid is typically a yellow colour. A testis that cannot be felt in a tense hydrocele, in the age groups at risk of testicular cancer, needs to be assessed by USS.

Epididymis

Epididymal pathology is rare in prepubertal males. In sexually active males, acute epididymitis (often due to *Chlamydia*) with significant pain and swelling needs to be distinguished from acute testicular torsion. A Doppler USS may help differentiate between the two conditions: in epididymitis it shows an increased blood flow into the inflamed epididymis, whereas in torsion it shows decreased or complete lack of blood flow to the testis. If there is any doubt, scrotal exploration is undertaken.

Epididymal cysts can form similar scrotal swellings to hydroceles but can be distinguished by the fact that the testis can often be felt separately. They contain clear or white fluid. Both hydroceles and epididymal cysts transilluminate on clinical examination.

Genitourinary TB can result in bilateral nodular induration of the epididymis and nodularity of the vas deferens. It may also result in scrotal abscesses that, unlike pyogenic abscesses,

---

Giovanni Battista Morgagni, 1682–1771, Professor of Anatomy, University of Padua, Italy.
Christian Johann Doppler, 1803–1853, Professor of Experimental Physics, Vienna, Austria, enunciated the 'Doppler principle' in 1842.
Harry Fitch Klinefelter, 1912–1990, American rheumatologist and endocrinologist, first described Klinefelter's syndrome in 1942.

are chronic, painless and not warm to touch ('cold abscess') (*Figure 81.1*).

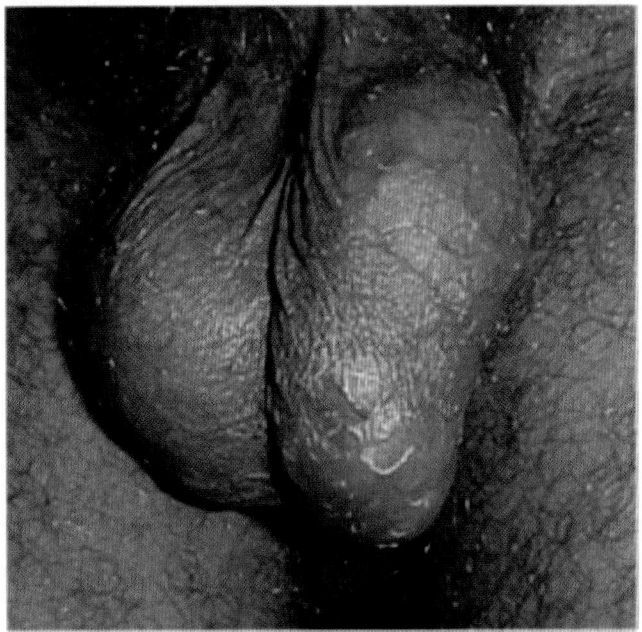

Figure 81.1 Cold abscess of the left scrotum. (Reproduced with permission from Kumar R. Reproductive tract tuberculosis and male infertility. *Indian J Urol* 2008; **24**: 392–5.)

Spermatic cord

Ten per cent of males have a left-sided varicocele and a smaller left testis. Masses are occasionally found associated with the spermatic cord, which on removal are found to be lipomas, mesotheliomas or sarcomas.

Prepuce (foreskin)

Phimosis occurs when the distal foreskin is tight and will not retract. Paraphimosis occurs when a poorly retractile foreskin becomes trapped in the retracted state and cannot be replaced. Significant oedema of the foreskin results, making replacement of the foreskin increasingly difficult. Depigmentation and scarring of the distal prepuce occurs in balanitis xerotica obliterans (BXO).

Penis

Peyronie's disease is an idiopathic condition in which fibrosis develops in the corpora cavernosa of the penis. The 'plaque' of Peyronie's fibrosis is usually palpable in the midline anywhere from the base of the penis to just behind the corona. It gives rise to painful angulation of the penis on erection.

Penile fracture occurs when there is trauma to the erect penis. Classically, there is an audible crack during sexual intercourse or forceful masturbation that is followed by immediate penile detumescence. The patient presents with gross bruising of the penile shaft skin.

Glans penis

In the younger male, genitourinary warts due to human papillomavirus (HPV) infection may be observed. In the older male, red raised patches on the glans penis or the inner aspect of the prepuce due to Zoon's balanitis or CIS (also known as erythroplasia of Queyrat or Bowen's disease) are distinguished only on penile biopsy.

Urethra

Hypospadias occurs when there is failure of the urethra to completely close on the ventral aspect and epispadias occurs when there is failure of closure on the dorsal surface. A urethral diverticulum in a female can be a cause for recurrent UTIs and is notable for its capacity to fill and empty at cystoscopy. A urethral caruncle is a minor prolapse of the urethral mucosa in a female and usually requires no treatment.

INVESTIGATION OF URINARY SYMPTOMS

Blood tests

Blood counts and chemistry

Initial blood tests in suspected urological pathologies include a full blood count, urea, creatinine and electrolytes. Creatinine, a surrogate marker for renal function (glomerular filtration), is an end product of muscle catabolism and may be unchanged despite a wide variation in estimated glomerular filtration rate (eGFR). eGFR is recommended as the optimal method of reporting renal function in many countries.

Patients with calculous disease routinely have serum calcium, uric acid and parathyroid hormone levels checked to rule out a metabolic predisposition to stone formation.

Serum alkaline phosphatase may be elevated in patients with bone metastases due to a urological malignancy and is commonly seen in men with disseminated prostate cancer.

Summary box 81.4

Biochemical assessment of renal function

- eGFR is increasingly reported along with urea and creatinine as it is more informative of true renal function
- With both kidneys functioning normally, an individual has approximately six times the renal function needed to remain off dialysis
- Serum creatinine will remain normal with unilateral renal pathology but a normally functioning contralateral kidney

François Gigot de la Peyronie, 1678–1747, French surgeon.
Johannes Jacobus Zoon, 1902–1958, Professor of Dermatology, University of Utrecht, The Netherlands, described Zoon's balanitis in 1952.
Louis Auguste Queyrat, 1856–1933, French dermatologist, described erythroplasia of Queyrat in 1911.
John Templeton Bowen, 1857–1940, American dermatologist, described Bowen's disease.

Tumour markers

Serum tumour markers are utilised in patients with prostate and testicular cancer. Currently no serum tumour markers exist in routine clinical practice for renal or bladder cancer.

Prostate-specific antigen

PSA is a glycoprotein produced by prostatic epithelial cells. Altered architecture of the prostate in conditions such as BPH, prostatitis and prostate cancer allows PSA to enter the bloodstream and be detected by a blood test. The commonly used PSA assays measure the total amount of PSA (tPSA). PSA levels can be influenced by certain drugs, most notably 5α-reductase inhibitors used to treat men with LUTS, but also by aspirin, statins and thiazide diuretics. The PSA test can be significantly influenced by a recent UTI and the true PSA level only returns to baseline 6 weeks after eradication of an infection.

Summary box 81.5

Prostate-specific antigen

- Is not significantly altered by DRE
- Can be significantly altered by a UTI
- After an infective episode, takes 6 weeks to return to baseline values
- Is artificially lowered, up to two times, in men taking 5α-reductase inhibitors (finasteride, dutasteride)

PSA values in a population of men form a continuum with no clear abnormal threshold. The value of PSA that triggers a biopsy is variable and is influenced by age, ethnicity, family history and findings on DRE.

The benefits of screening asymptomatic men for prostate cancer using PSA testing are controversial and a large UK-based clinical study (ProtecT trial) found that at a median of 10 years very few patients died of prostate cancer irrespective of treatment or surveillance. At present, PSA-based screening for prostate cancer is not routinely performed in the UK but men interested in having a PSA test can request this from their family practitioners. A similar practice is followed in many countries.

Risk prediction models have been developed in recent years to assist clinicians and patients in predicting prostate cancer diagnosis, stage and prognosis. A number of these risk assessment tools are available online as a decision aid for an individual man to evaluate his own risk of prostate cancer. These include the Prostate Cancer Prevention Trial (PCPT) Risk Calculator and the European Randomized Study of Screening for Prostate Cancer (ERSPC) Risk Calculator.

For men newly diagnosed with prostate cancer, PSA assists with risk (of disease progression) stratification. It is also a useful marker of response to treatment and of disease recurrence after treatment.

Prostate-specific antigen derivatives and kinetics

Since PSA may be elevated in non-malignant conditions, PSA derivatives/kinetics have been used to improve the specificity of testing. Some of the derivatives include free PSA (fPSA), complexed PSA (cPSA) and free/total PSA ratio (f/tPSA). Since BPH tissue within the prostate also contributes to tPSA, PSA density (PSAD) factors in the volume of the prostate by dividing tPSA by prostate volume. A high PSAD increases the likelihood that the elevated PSA is due to malignancy and not due to the large gland alone. PSA kinetics involve measurement of the rate of change of various forms of PSA based on the premise that a rapid increase or change may be more predictive of cancer. PSA velocity is the annual absolute increase in tPSA and a value >0.75 ng/mL per year compared with baseline has been considered suspicious. PSA doubling time is the number of months it takes for a baseline PSA to double.

Testis tumour markers

Serum tumour markers routinely used in the management of men with suspected testicular cancer are alpha-fetoprotein (αFP), beta-human chorionic gonadotropin (βHCG) and lactate dehydrogenase (LDH). These markers sometimes provide insight into the likely diagnosis, histological subtype of germ cell tumour present, success of treatment and recurrence. They also contribute to the stratification of patients with testicular cancer into prognostic categories using a classification devised by the International Germ Cell Cancer Collaborative Group.

Urine-based tests

Urinalysis

In a urine dipstick test, used to screen for significant disease, urine is dipped with a stick on which there is a series of small chemical-containing pads designed to detect, typically, glucose, bilirubin, ketones, the specific gravity, blood, pH, protein, urobilinogen, nitrites and leukocyte esterase through colour changes. A similar test may be performed using reagents in a laboratory.

Midstream specimen of urine or urine culture

A midstream specimen of urine (MSU) or urine culture is used to establish the diagnosis of a UTI and allows identification of the urinary pathogen and selection of the most appropriate antibiotic. Most MSUs will be processed in two stages, with initial urine microscopy followed by urine culture only if appropriate. Normal urine contains small numbers of white blood cells, red blood cells and epithelial cells as indicated in *Table 81.1*.

Early-morning urine

Early-morning urine (EMU) samples are sent on three consecutive days for Ziehl–Neelsen staining and culture for acid-fast bacilli if genitourinary TB is suspected. Staining results are

Franz Ziehl, 1859–1926, German bacteriologist and a professor in Lübeck, Germany.
Friedrich Carl Adolf Neelsen, 1854–1898, German pathologist and professor at the Institute of Pathology, University of Rostock, Germany.

TABLE 81.1 Cells in normal urine.	
White blood cells	3–5 per high-power field
Epithelial cells	<10–15 per high-power field
Red blood cells	0–2 per high-power field

available within a day but culture results take 6 weeks. Nucleic acid amplification tests based on polymerase chain reaction (PCR), such as GeneXpert® and TruNAAT®, are frequently used for rapid detection of a small amount of bacterial DNA. An early-morning sample is preferred since it is expected that overnight shedding of bacilli will increase detection rates.

Voided urine cytology

Voided urine cytology is performed when a urothelial carcinoma is suspected. The test has the disadvantage of a high false-negative rate. Approximately 15% of low-grade transitional cell carcinomas produce positive voided urine cytology compared with approximately 50% of high-grade transitional cell tumours.

Urine for chyle

Testing urine for chyle is performed in specific situations where the suspicion for chyluria is high. This is restricted to certain endemic regions of the world. A high-fat diet is administered the night prior to collection of a morning sample of urine. The urine may visibly appear milky white (*Figures 81.2 and 81.3*).

Endoscopy

Cystoscopy

To further evaluate urinary symptoms, the entire lining of the urinary tract can be directly visualised from the urethra and bladder (using a cystoscope) to the ureter and renal pelvis (using a semirigid ureteroscope), and finally the renal calyces (using a flexible ureteroscope). Cystoscopy can be undertaken either as flexible cystoscopy (*Figure 81.4*), using local anaesthesia, or as rigid cystoscopy (*Figure 81.5*), preferably under a general anaesthetic. Telescopes with different fields of view are available (0°, 12°, 30° and 70° lenses are commonly used). In the operating theatre, most endoscopic procedures, including cystoscopy, require a urology stack consisting of a camera, monitor, light source, electrocautery and insufflator for laparoscopy procedures (*Figure 81.6*).

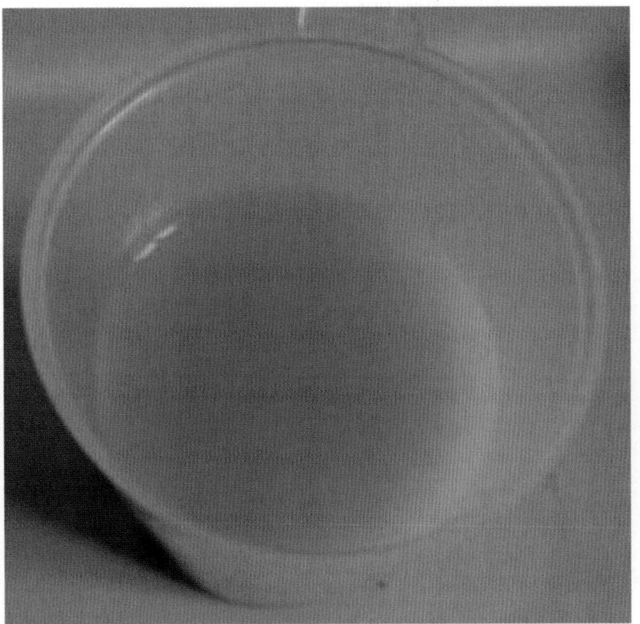

Figure 81.2 White urine seen in chyluria (courtesy of Dr TC Goel, Emeritus Professor of Surgery, King George's Medical University, Lucknow, India).

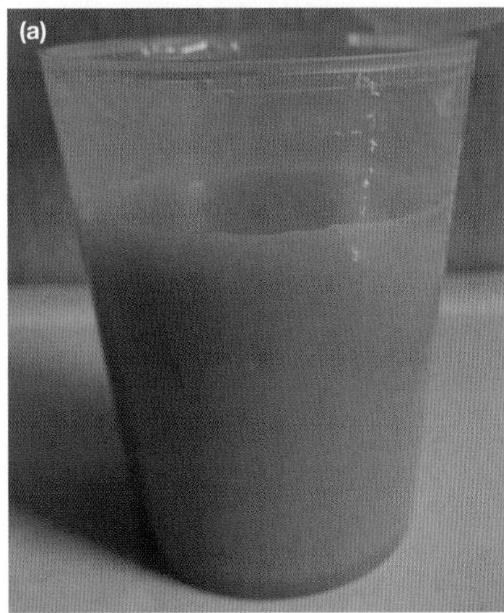

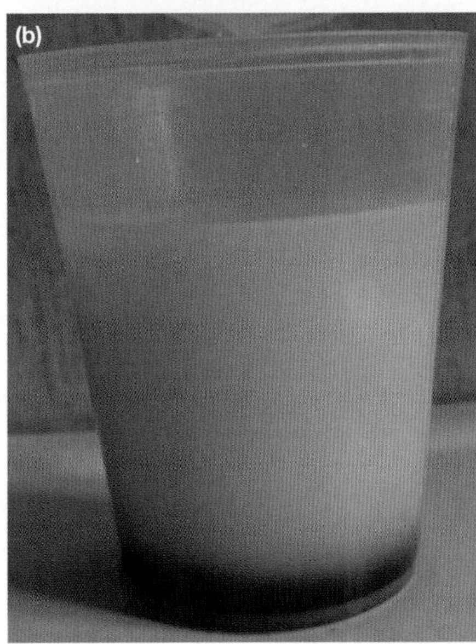

Figure 81.3 Haematochyluria with milky-red urine (a); the blood settles after some time, leaving chyluria above (b) (courtesy of Dr TC Goel).

The male urethra is longer than the female urethra and is angulated at the level of the symphysis pubis (*Figures 81.7–81.12*). Flexible cystoscopy is thus relatively poorly tolerated in young males, in whom it may be uncomfortable. It is principally a diagnostic tool but a few minor procedures can be

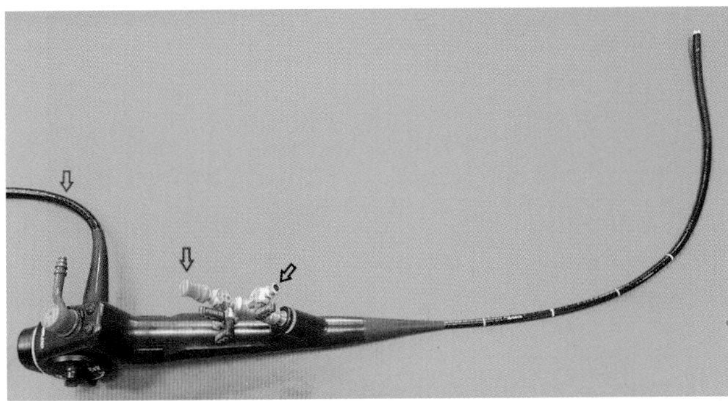

Figure 81.4 Flexible cystoscope with attachments for irrigating fluid (black arrow), instruments (red arrow), and connection to video equipment (blue arrow).

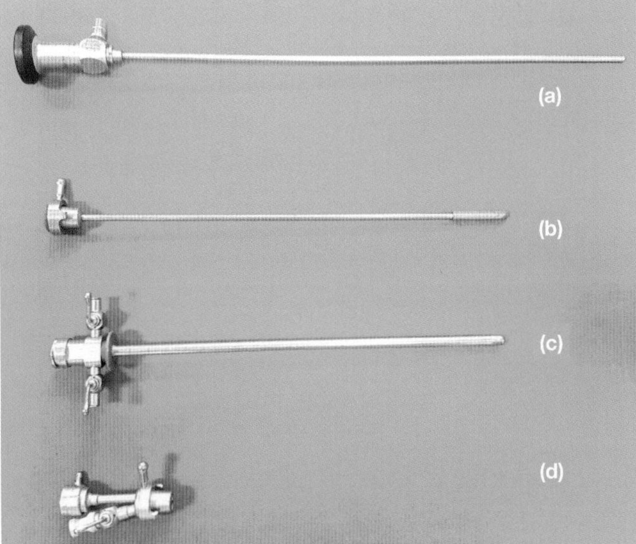

Figure 81.5 Parts of a rigid cystoscope. Telescope (a), obturator (b), sheath (c) and bridge (d). The obturator is inserted into the outer sheath for blind insertion of the cystoscope sheath – usually in females. The light cable and camera are attached to the telescope, which replaces the obturator in blind insertions. In males, the bridge is attached to the sheath to provide additional length and the telescope is placed through the bridge for insertion of the cystoscope under vision.

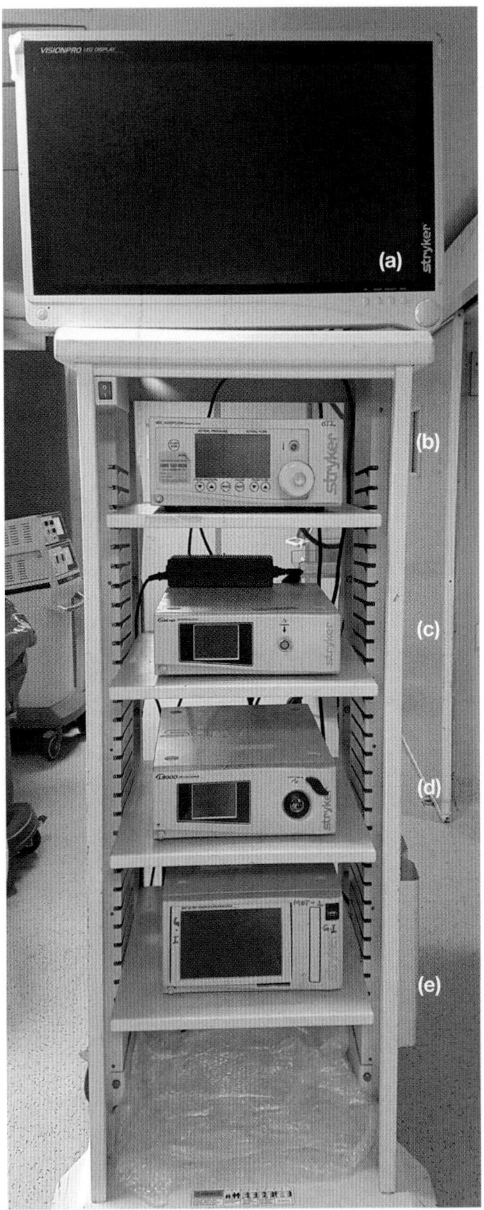

Figure 81.6 The urology stack. In this stack, from top down, are the monitor (a), insufflator for carbon dioxide for laparoscopy (b), camera connector (c), light source (d) and a video recording device (e).

accomplished using the flexible cystoscope, such as insertion/removal of ureteric stents, small biopsies and diathermy/laser of small bladder lesions. More can be achieved with a rigid cystoscope under general anaesthesia, especially in relation to instrumentation of the ureters.

Summary box 81.6

Cystoscopy

- Can be performed with either a rigid cystoscope under general anaesthesia or a flexible cystoscope under local anaesthesia
- Flexible cystoscopy is principally a diagnostic procedure
- Rigid cystoscopy allows more procedures to be performed

Ureteroscopy

Ureteroscopy can be performed as both a diagnostic and a therapeutic procedure. A rigid or semirigid ureteroscope can be used in the ureter as far as the renal pelvis, but to inspect or operate on the renal pelvis or renal calyces a flexible ureteroscope is, generally, needed (*Figure 81.13*). The procedure is most often performed when pathology, commonly stones, strictures or tumours, of the ureter is suspected.

Radiology

Urinary tract ultrasound scan

USS (*Figure 81.14*) can characterise pathologies of the kidney, bladder, prostate and testis very well but is not very good for

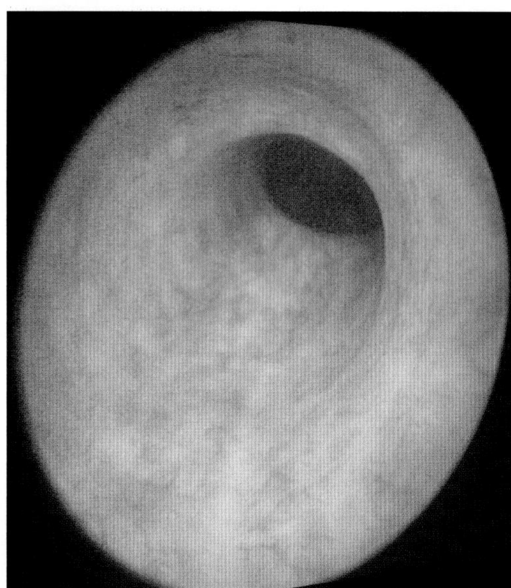

Figure 81.7 A normal urethra on urethroscopy.

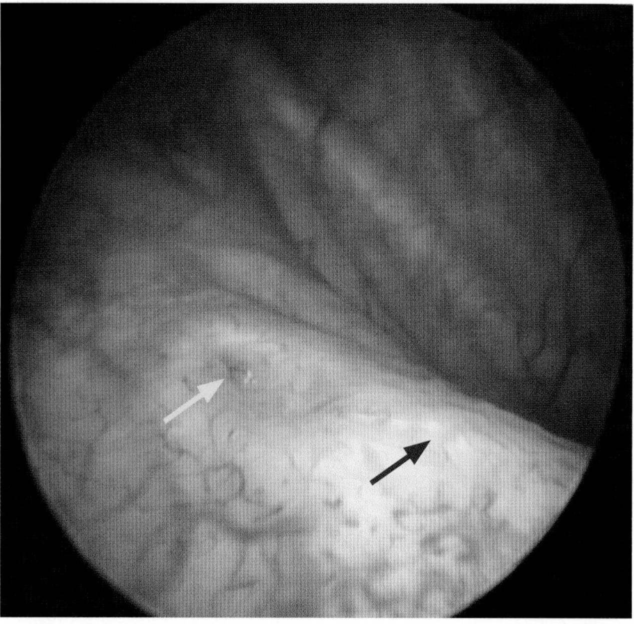

Figure 81.8 The appearance of normal bladder mucosa on cystoscopy: a normal right ureteric orifice (yellow arrow) at the end of the interureteric bar (red arrow).

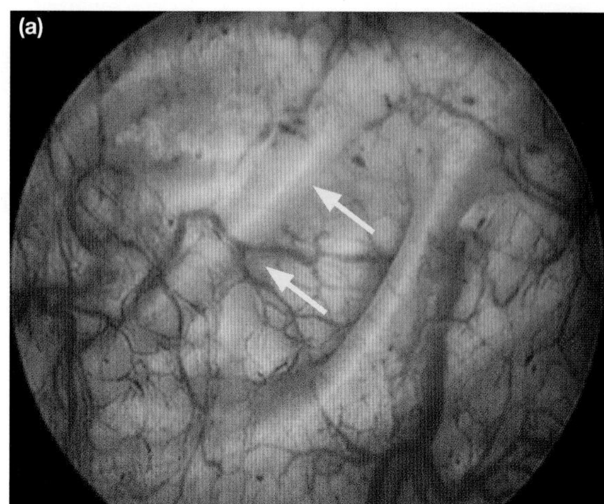

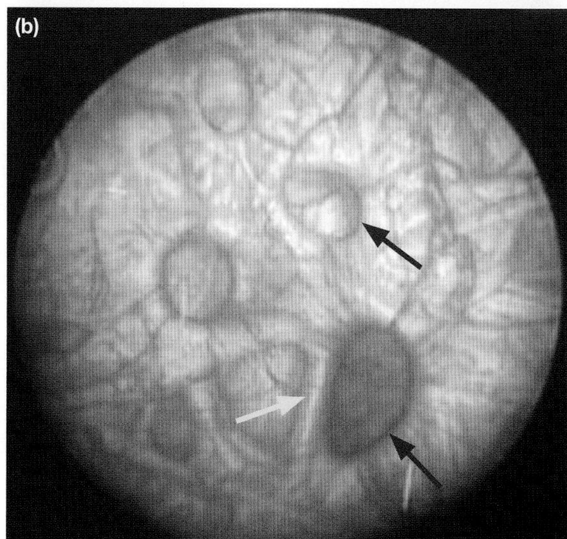

Figure 81.9 (a, b) Bladder wall trabeculation (yellow arrows) and saccules (red arrows) seen on cystoscopy. (Image (a) courtesy of The Center for Reconstructive Urology, CA, USA.)

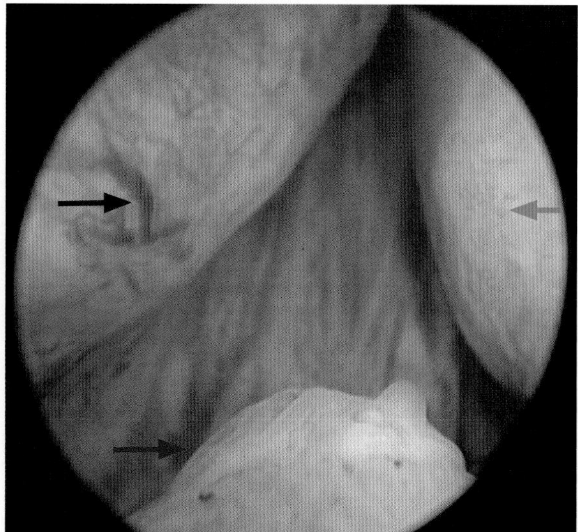

Figure 81.10 An endoscopic view of the prostatic urethra with the verumontanum at 6 o'clock (red arrow) and the bulging right (black arrow) and left (blue arrow) lobes of the prostate.

assessing the ureters unless they are significantly dilated or have sizeable pathology. The lack of radiation and contrast exposure coupled with portability and availability make USS the first imaging investigation in urological diseases. It is extremely useful in the detection of hydronephrosis (even at the bedside in an emergency), renal cysts, tumours, scarring and stones. Stones classically produce an acoustic shadow, but USS is not the most sensitive imaging modality for detecting renal stones. USS is extensively used for the insertion of a percutaneous nephrostomy (PCN) to drain an obstructed renal collecting system. It is sometimes used to further characterise renal lesions detected by other modalities such as computed

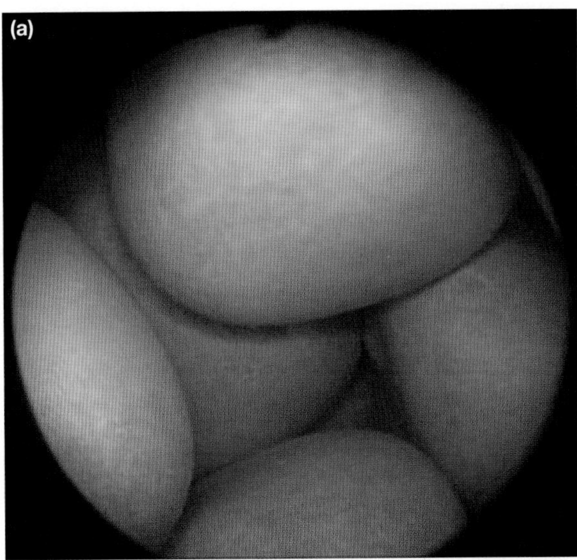

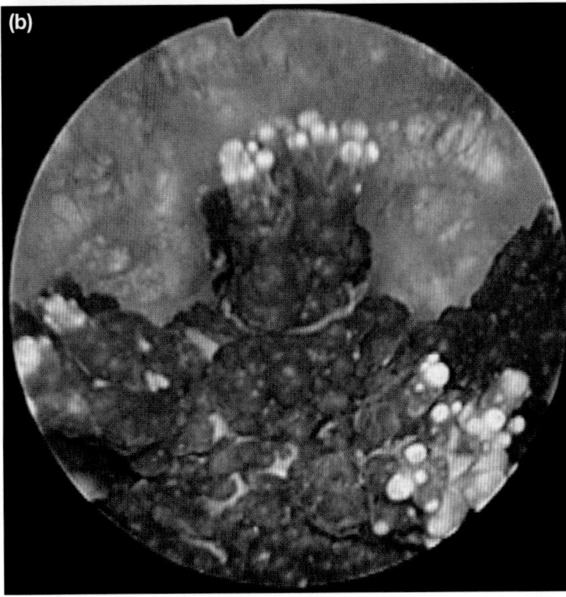

Figure 81.11 Bladder calculi seen on cystoscopy. Stones may be multiple (a) or single (b). The stone in (b) has a characteristic shape and is referred to as a 'jack' stone. (Image (b) reprinted with permission from Medscape Drugs & Diseases (http://emedicine.medscape.com/), 2017, available at: http://emedicine.medscape.com/article/2120102-overview).

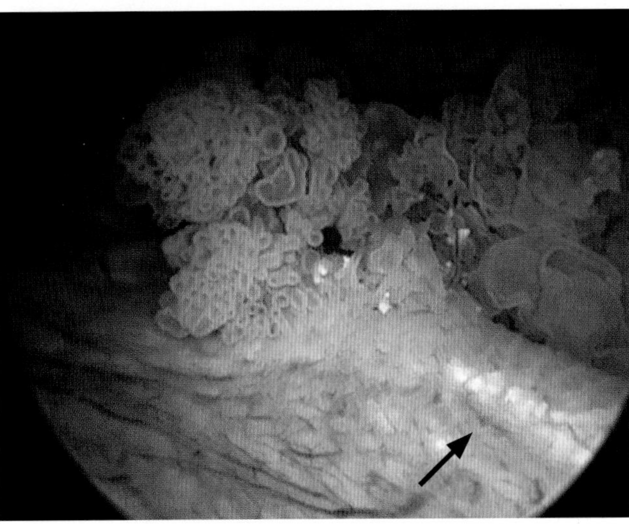

Figure 81.12 Papillary bladder tumours seen at cystoscopy near the right ureteric orifice (arrow) (courtesy of Tim Nathan).

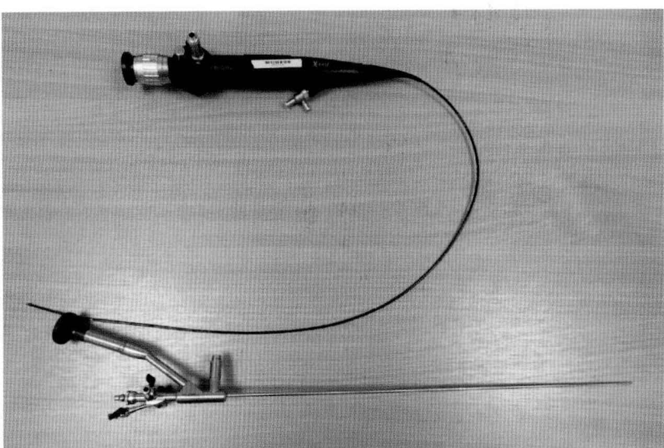

Figure 81.13 A flexible ureteroscope (top) and a semirigid ureteroscope (bottom).

tomography (CT) or MRI, particularly for haemorrhagic cysts versus solid lesions. USS can detect bladder tumours, calculi, a thickened, trabeculated bladder wall in patients with BOO and large bladder diverticula. It can also be used to determine the residual urine after micturition.

In addition, USS is frequently employed to investigate men with scrotal swellings and has a role to play in the assessment of urethral stricture disease.

Summary box 81.7

Ultrasound scan

- Frequently used to screen patients with suspected urological pathology
- Frequently part of a haematuria clinic protocol
- An excellent method to detect hydronephrosis
- Can be performed at the bedside in critically ill patients
- Recently has been combined with contrast enhancement in certain settings, such as in the assessment of renal cysts

Transrectal ultrasound scan

TRUS is often performed in conjunction with biopsy of the prostate. It requires the use of a special probe (*Figure 81.15*) that provides transverse as well as sagittal views of the prostate (*Figure 81.16*). TRUS is most often used to guide a prostate biopsy in men suspected to have prostate cancer. The classic abnormality associated with prostate cancer is a hypoechoic area in the peripheral zone but this is rarely found in the absence of a palpable abnormality on DRE. Typically, 12 or more systematic biopsies are taken using a biopsy device such as that shown in *Figure 81.17*. Additional biopsies may be taken from areas that are suspected to be malignant.

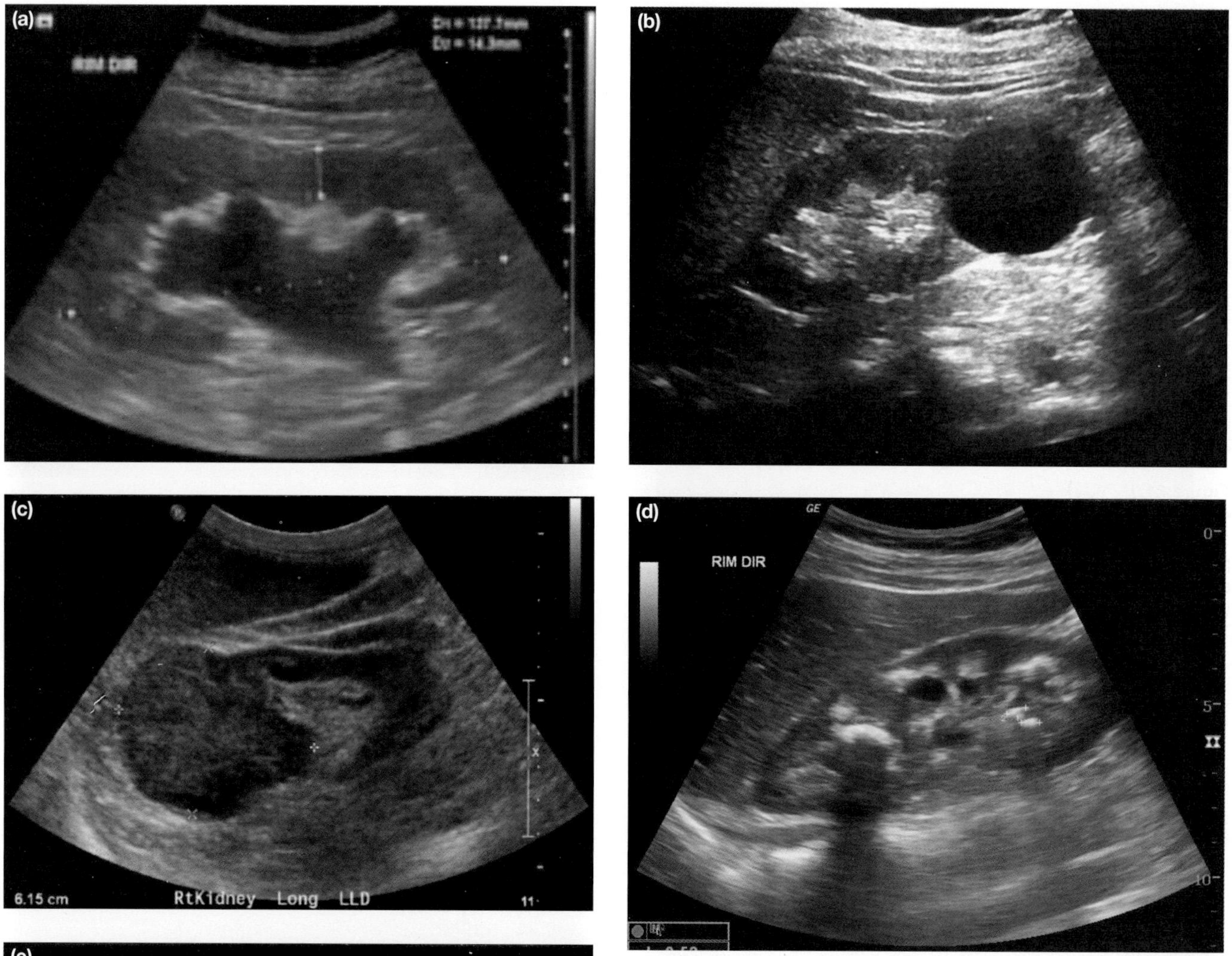

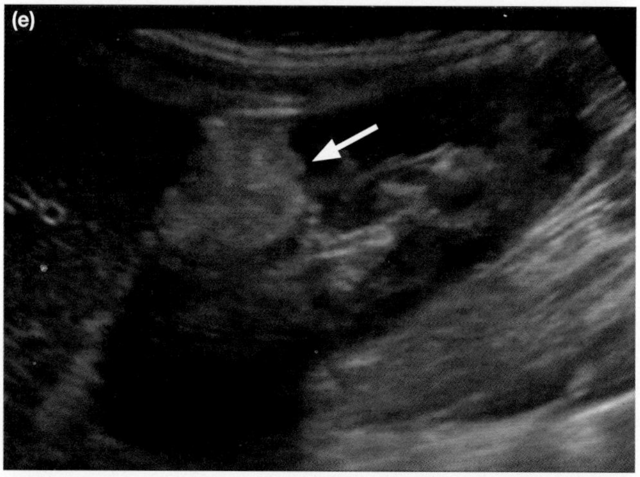

Figure 81.14 Ultrasound scan showing: (a) hydronephrosis (courtesy of Dr Bruno Di Muzio, Radiopaedia.org, rID: 21885); (b) renal cyst (courtesy of Dr Ian Bickle, Radiopaedia.org, rID: 21139); (c) renal tumour (courtesy of Wendy Boller); (d) medullary sponge kidney with renal calculi – note the stone gives rise to an acoustic window (courtesy of Dr Bruno Di Muzio, Radiopaedia.org, rID: 12141); (e) angiomyolipoma (arrow).

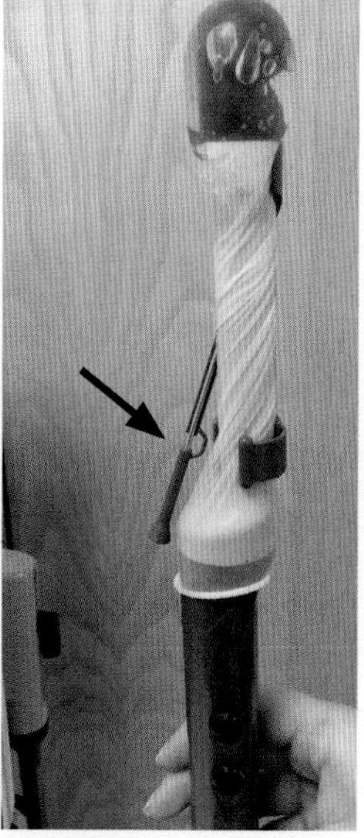

Figure 81.15 Transrectal probe demonstrating the diagonal channel for the biopsy needle (arrow).

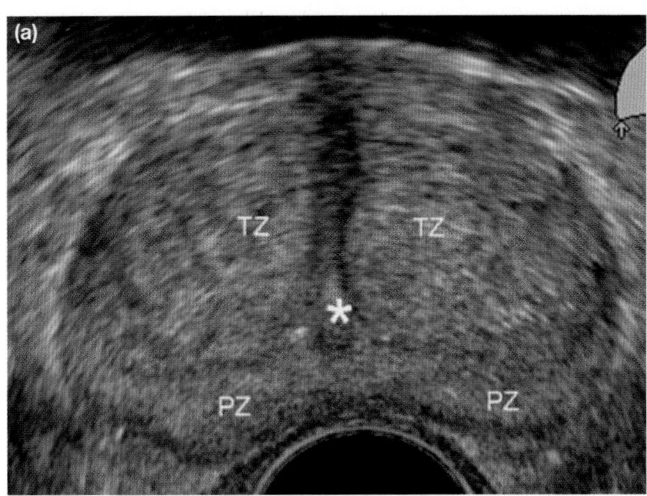

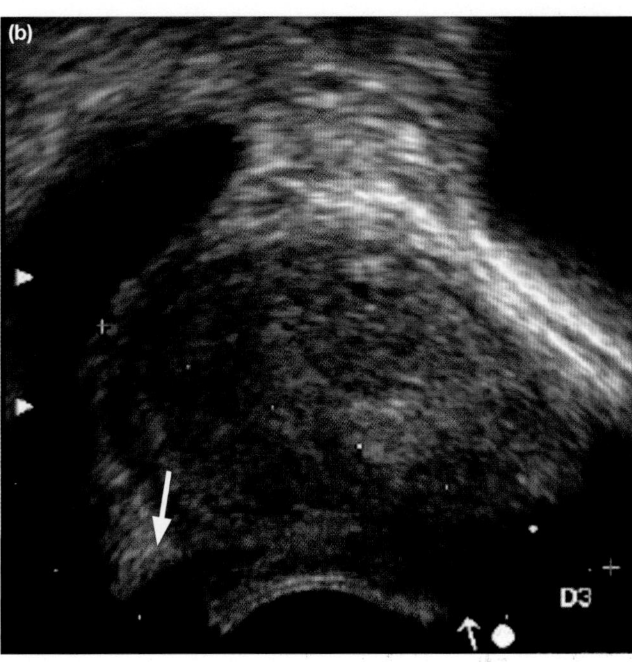

Figure 81.16 Views of the prostate on a transrectal ultrasound scan. (a) On the transverse image, the normal prostate demonstrates an anterior transition zone (TZ) and a posterior (cow-horn-shaped) peripheral zone (PZ). Asterisk indicates the verumontanum. (b) On the sagittal image the bladder is seen above the prostate (arrowheads) as well as the seminal vesicles (arrow).

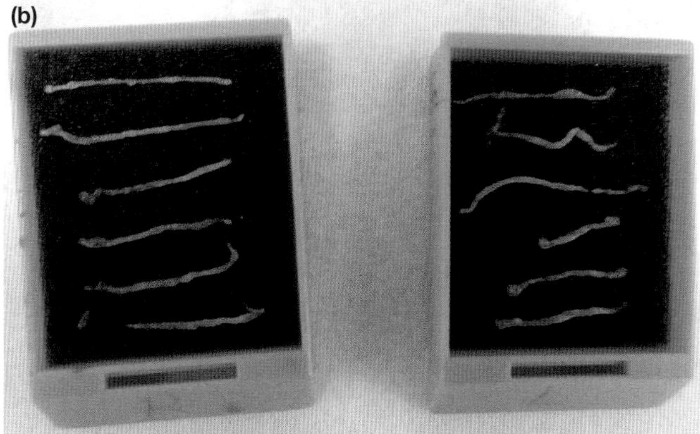

Figure 81.17 (a) A biopsy device used for prostatic biopsy. (b) Biopsy cores taken from the right and left prostatic lobes during transrectal ultrasound scanning.

Transperineal template biopsies of the prostate

Transperineal template biopsies of the prostate (TPTBP) are increasingly used clinically and may replace TRUS-guided prostate biopsies as a first-line test. Currently, TPTBP are used to further evaluate men with a negative TRUS-guided prostate biopsy in whom the PSA trend remains suspicious, or younger men for whom a diagnosis of low-risk prostate cancer has been made and in whom it is important to exclude more significant disease in other parts of the prostate (most notably in the anterior aspects of the gland) not easily accessible via the transrectal route. TPTBP are usually performed under local anaesthetic and have a much lower risk of sepsis than TRUS-guided biopsies.

Summary box 81.8

Prostate biopsies

- TRUS has been the traditional method of guiding prostate biopsies
- TPTBP are becoming increasingly popular
- TPTBP have a much lower sepsis risk than TRUS biopsies

Kidneys-ureters-bladder radiograph

A plain radiograph of the abdomen and pelvis that includes the regions of the body occupied by the KUB is frequently called an x-ray KUB (*Figure 81.18*). In the normal setting, soft-tissue outlines of the kidneys are commonly seen but normal ureters and bladder will not be seen. The commonest indication for a KUB radiograph is to screen patients for the presence of urinary tract calculi. Patients who have had a CT scan resulting in the diagnosis of a urinary tract calculus often have a supplementary KUB radiograph to determine if a plain radiograph can be used in the subsequent follow-up of the patient. Phleboliths (thrombosed, calcified veins in the pelvis) can easily be mistaken for distal ureteric stones. Finally, a KUB radiograph is often used to check for correct positioning of a ureteric stent.

Intravenous urography

Intravenous urography (IVU) continues to be frequently used in the evaluation and management of patients with urinary

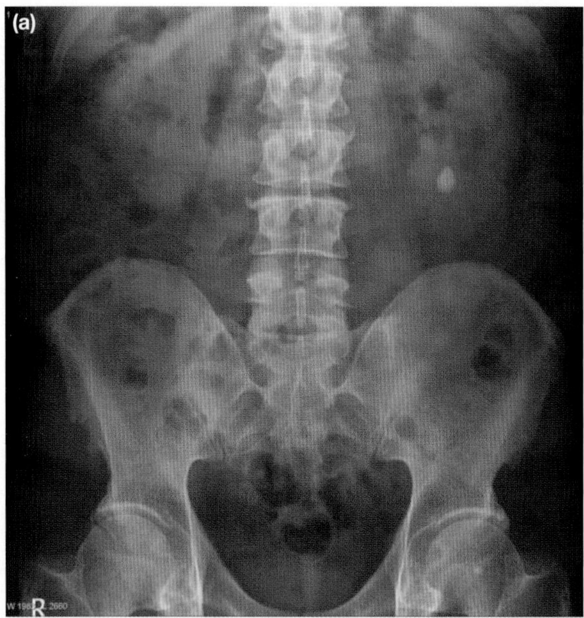

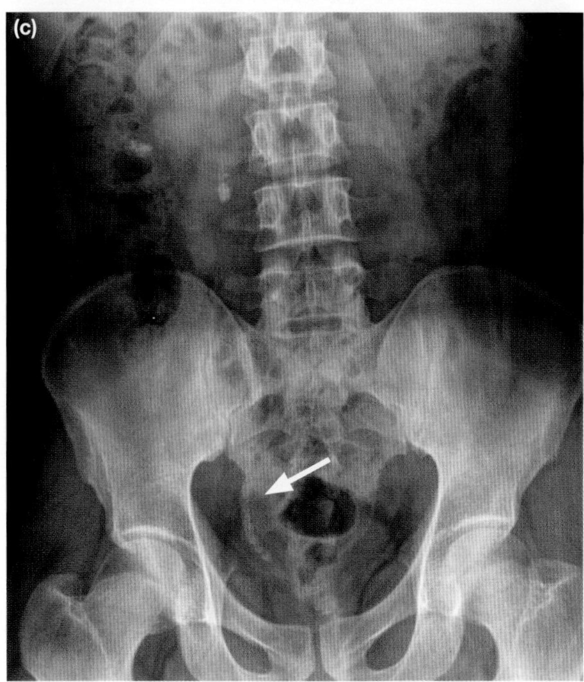

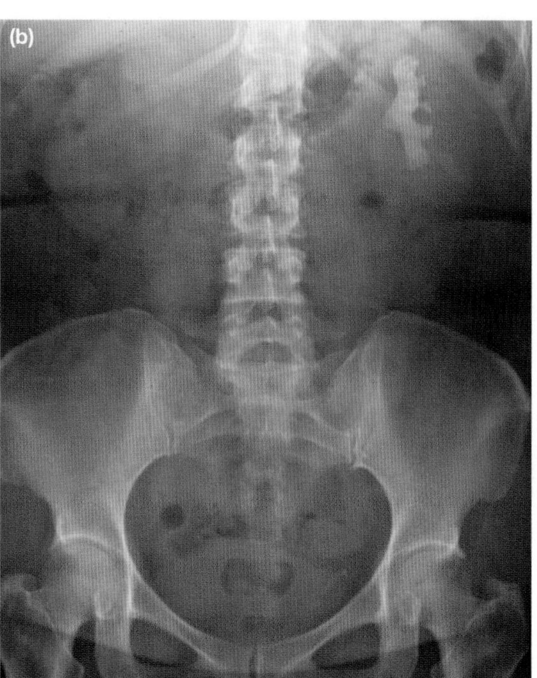

Figure 81.18 (a) Left lower pole renal stone on a plain kidneys–ureters–bladder radiograph (courtesy of Professor Frank Gaillard, Radiopaedia.org, rID: 12555). (b) A staghorn calculus in the left kidney (courtesy of Dr Natalie Yang, Radiopaedia.org, rID: 9733). (c) Right lower pole calculi and steinstrasse (multiple stone fragments from shock-wave lithotripsy to break the kidney stone), leading to the formation of a 'stone street or steinstrasse' in the distal right ureter (arrow) (courtesy of Dr Ali Abougazia, Radiopaedia.org).

stones and urinary TB in many parts of the world, even though it provides less information than a CT scan. This is primarily due to its wider availability, lower cost and lower radiation exposure (*Figure 81.19*).

Retrograde urethrogram and voiding cystourethrogram

During a retrograde urethrogram (RGU), radiocontrast material is gently instilled into the urethra to delineate its anatomy. The investigation is primarily used to identify urethral strictures in men. Radiocontrast material is instilled into the bladder, through either a urethral catheter or a suprapubic tube for a voiding cystourethrogram (VCUG). VCUGs are used to identify reflux into the ureter, usually in children, and for delineation of the proximal urethra in men with complete urethral strictures. They may also help in assessing bladder capacity in TB (*Figure 81.20*).

Computed tomography scan

A non-contrast CT scan is the imaging modality of choice in the investigation of a patient with suspected urinary tract calculi (*Figure 81.21*). This investigation is quick, often taking less than 2 minutes to perform, picks up most calculi and can be tailored to deliver low radiation doses. Other variations of the CT scan include a contrast CT, which can be tailored to acquire images in multiple phases (triple phase for renal tumours) and a urographic phase for urothelial tumours.

A contrast CT scan of the chest, abdomen and pelvis is frequently used to stage patients with renal tumours (*Figure 81.22*), muscle-invasive bladder cancer and young men with testicular cancer. CT is less frequently used in men with prostate cancer but does have a role to play when lymph node disease is being assessed prior to treatment.

Cysts are a frequent incidental finding on USS and CT scans of the kidneys. In 1986, a classification of renal cysts based on CT criteria, known as the Bosniak classification, was devised. This classification can also be applied to MRI.

Morton A Bosniak, 1929–2016, Professor of Radiology, New York University (NYU) Langone School of Medicine, New York, NY, USA.

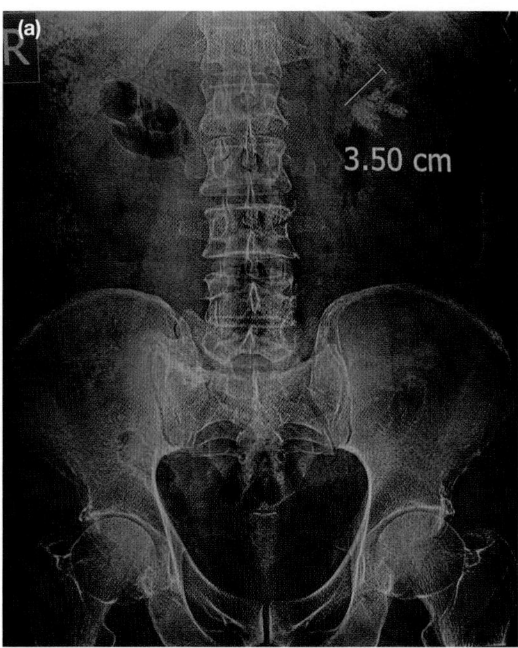

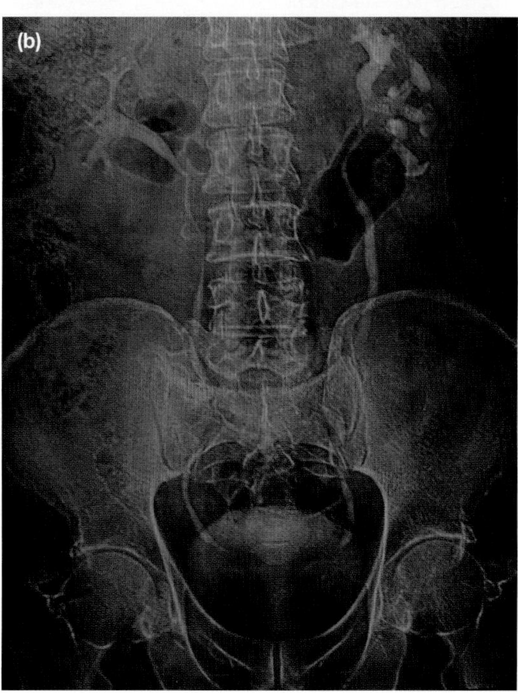

Figure 81.19 Intravenous urogram plain (a) and 5-minute (b) films, demonstrating a partial staghorn stone in the left kidney. The right kidney is normal. A 5-minute film shows contrast entering the pelvicalyceal system and helps in identifying the location of the stone.

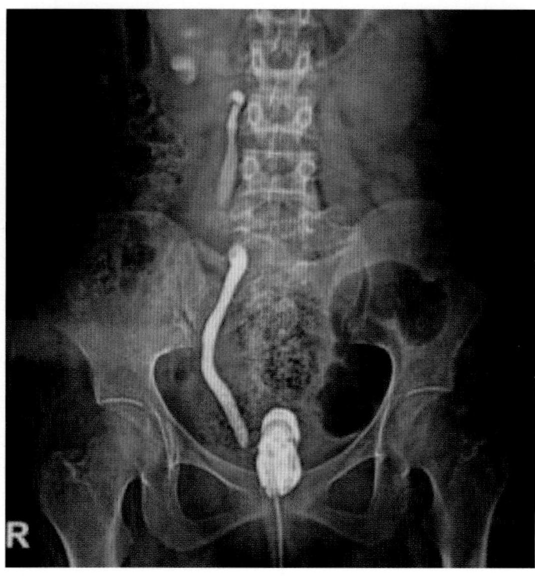

Figure 81.20 Cystogram in a patient with tuberculosis, demonstrating a small 'thimble' bladder and reflux into the right kidney.

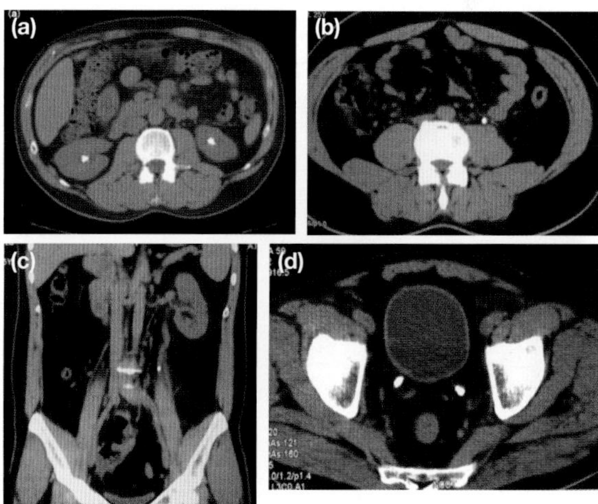

Figure 81.21 (a) A non-contrast computed tomography scan demonstrating bilateral renal calculi (courtesy of Dr Jeremy Jones, Radiopaedia.org, rID: 6211); (b, c) left ureteric calculus in the axial and coronal reconstructions (courtesy of Dr Raju Sharma and Dr Ankur Goyal); (d) bilateral lower ureteric calculi (courtesy of Dr Raju Sharma and Dr Ankur Goyal).

It is used to predict the likelihood of malignancy in the lesion. Based on this classification (*Figures 81.23 and 81.24*), the majority of cysts are category I and II and do not require treatment or follow-up imaging. Category IIF ('F' indicating the need for follow-up) cysts do require further imaging but the duration of this is uncertain. Category III cysts have a risk of malignancy of 30–100% and should undergo a biopsy to identify those patients requiring surgery. Category IV 'cysts' have an incidence of malignancy of 67–100% and surgical removal should be considered.

Magnetic resonance imaging

MRI scanning has a significant role to play, either on its own or as an adjunct to other cross-sectional imaging modalities, in the staging of a number of urological cancers, particularly prostate cancer. Modern MRI techniques utilise both anatomical and

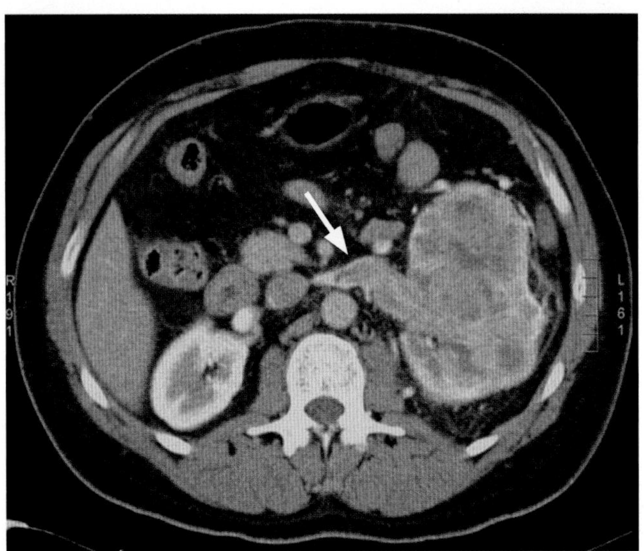

Figure 81.22 Computed tomography scan demonstrating a large left renal tumour with involvement of the left renal vein (arrow) (courtesy of Dr Laughlin Dawes, Radiopaedia.org, rID: 35937).

functional imaging and are known as multiparametric MRI (mpMRI). Anatomical imaging is based on standard MRI techniques (T1- and T2-weighted images) and functional imaging is based on diffusion-weighted imaging (DWI) (for water molecule motion assessment) and dynamic contrast-enhanced (DCE) imaging (for tissue perfusion assessment after intravenous contrast administration) (*Figure 81.25*). The multiple parameters assessed in the scan are combined in a five-point scoring system, called PI-RADS (Prostate Imaging – Reporting and Data System), to assign a likelihood (from 1, benign to 5, highly suspicious) that prostate cancer is present within the abnormality detected on mpMRI of the prostate. The lesions identified on mpMRI can be specifically targeted for biopsy using novel technologies. MRI images can be fused with real-time TRUS-USS images to guide the biopsies to these abnormal areas in a similar manner to TRUS biopsy. Such 'fusion' biopsies require specialised workstations. Similar scoring systems are being used to assess bladder cancer.

Summary box 81.9

Magnetic resonance imaging

- Used to stage many urological cancers
- mpMRI has a significant role in the assessment of men with suspected prostate cancer
- mpMRI is increasingly used prior to prostate biopsy. Prebiopsy MRI permits selection of biopsy technique (TRUS versus TPTBP)
- Prebiopsy MRI assists with targeting of biopsies

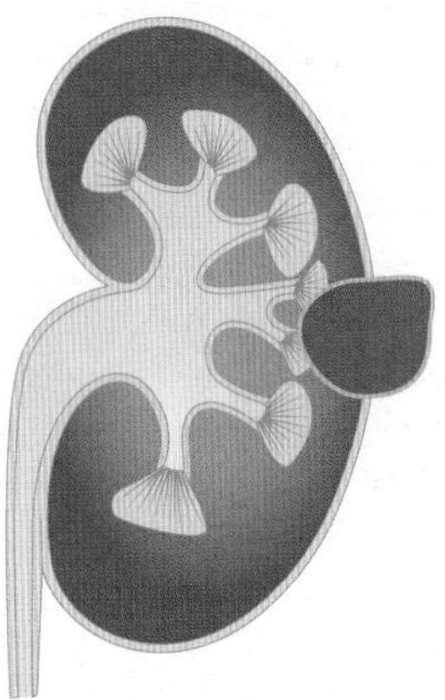

I ~0% are malignant

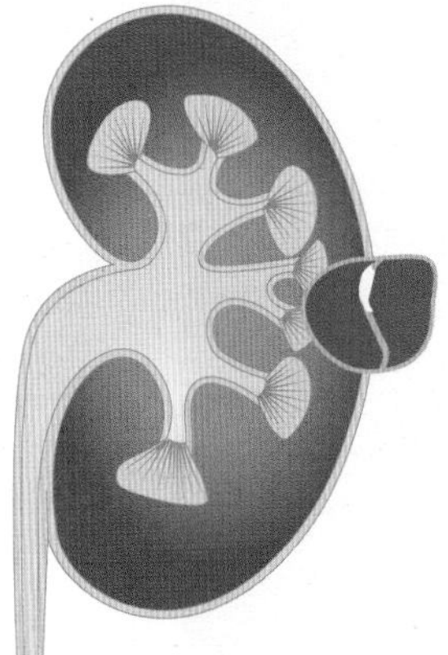

II ~0% are malignant

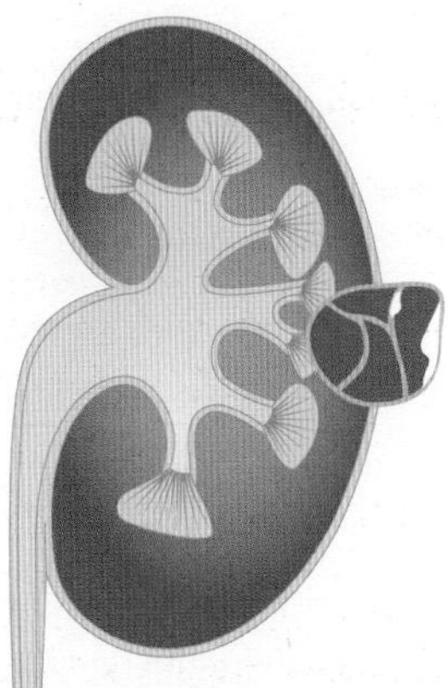

IIF ~5% are malignant

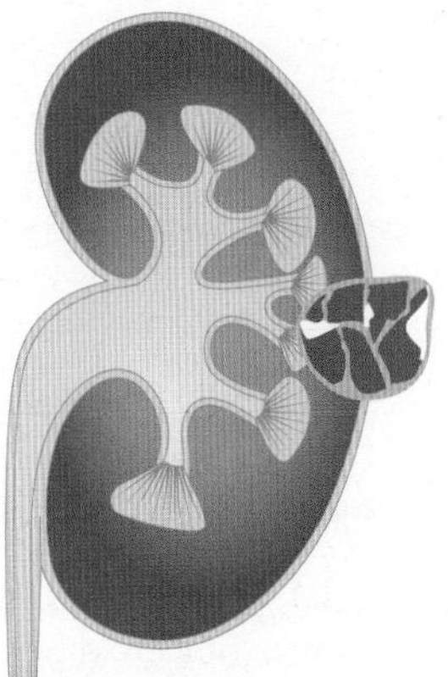

III ~50% are malignant

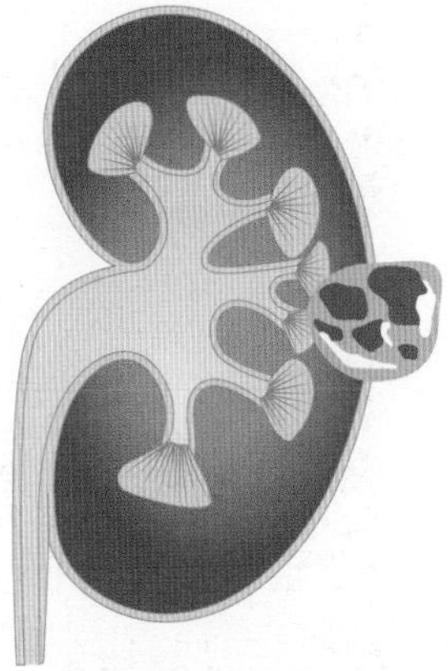

IV ~100% are malignant

Figure 81.23 Bosniak classification of renal cysts. The classification depends on the characteristics of the cyst wall, septae, solid component and enhancement on contrast administration.

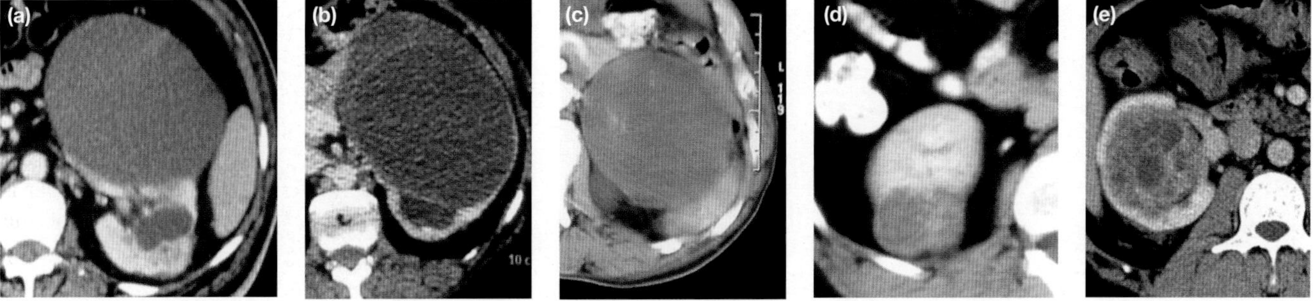

Figure 81.24 Computed tomography scans showing cysts of various categories: (a) Bosniak I cyst; (b) Bosniak II cyst; (c) Bosniak IIF cyst; (d) Bosniak III cyst; (e) Bosniak IV cyst (courtesy of Dr Raju Sharma and Dr Ankur Goyal).

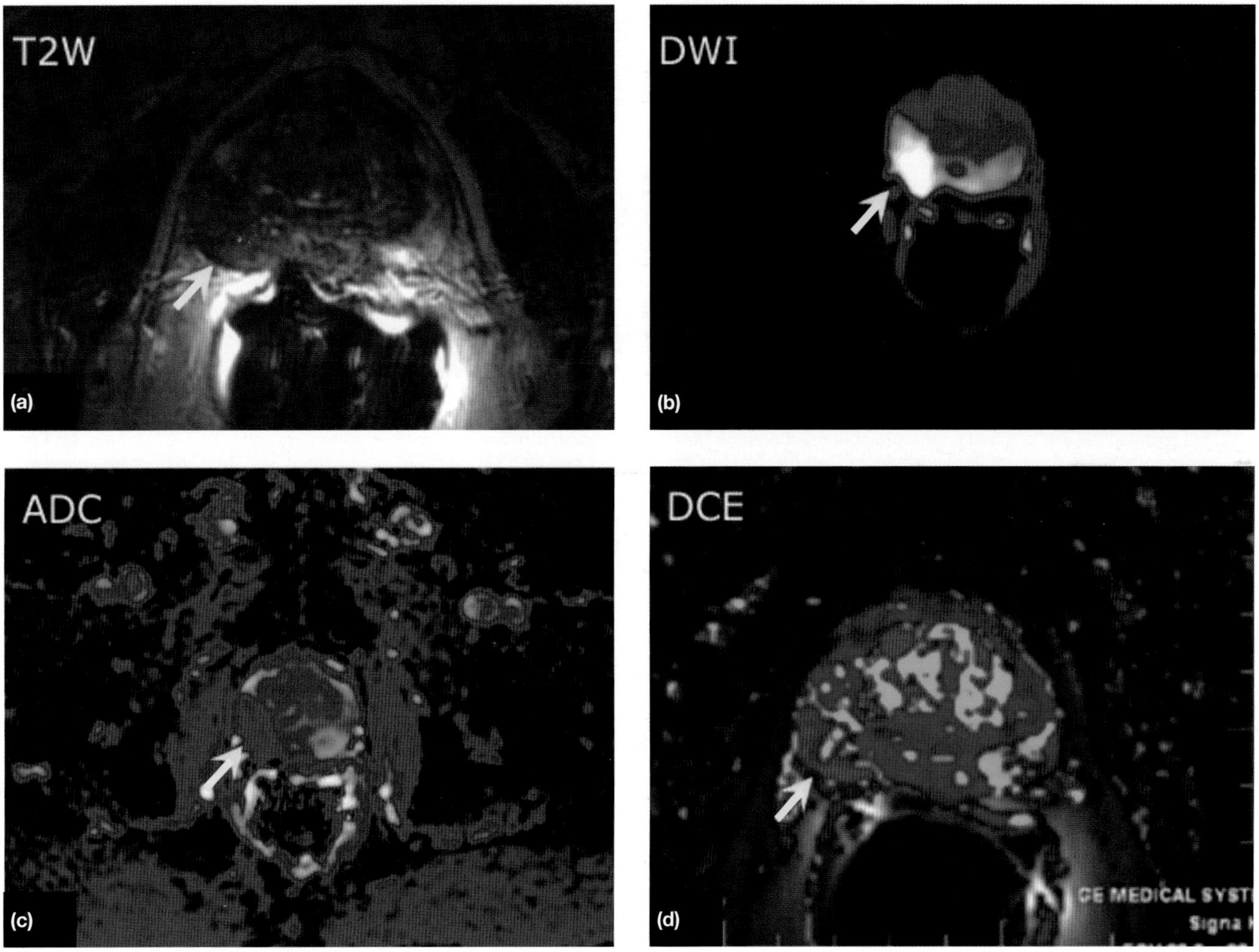

Figure 81.25 Multiparametric magnetic resonance images of a patient with prostate cancer. (a) T2 weighted. (b) Diffusion weighted (DWI). (c) Apparent diffusion coefficient (ADC). (d) Dynamic contrast enhanced (DCE). The tumour appears dark on the axial T2-weighted image (arrow); the corresponding area shows restricted diffusion on the DWI and ADC images as well as abnormal contrast enhancement on the DCE axial image (within the prostate, the red colour denotes abnormal areas that are possibly malignant) (courtesy of Janet Cochrane Miller, Radiology Rounds, Massachusetts General Hospital).

SPECT/CT and PET/CT

Single photon emission computed tomography (SPECT) and positron emission tomography (PET) are nuclear medicine imaging techniques that provide metabolic and functional information, unlike CT and MRI. They have both been combined with CT and MRI to provide detailed anatomical and metabolic information.

PET/CT looks promising as a tool for the detection of distant metastases in bladder cancer. To date, the technique has not been used extensively in patients with renal cancer. In men with testicular cancer, it is recommended in the

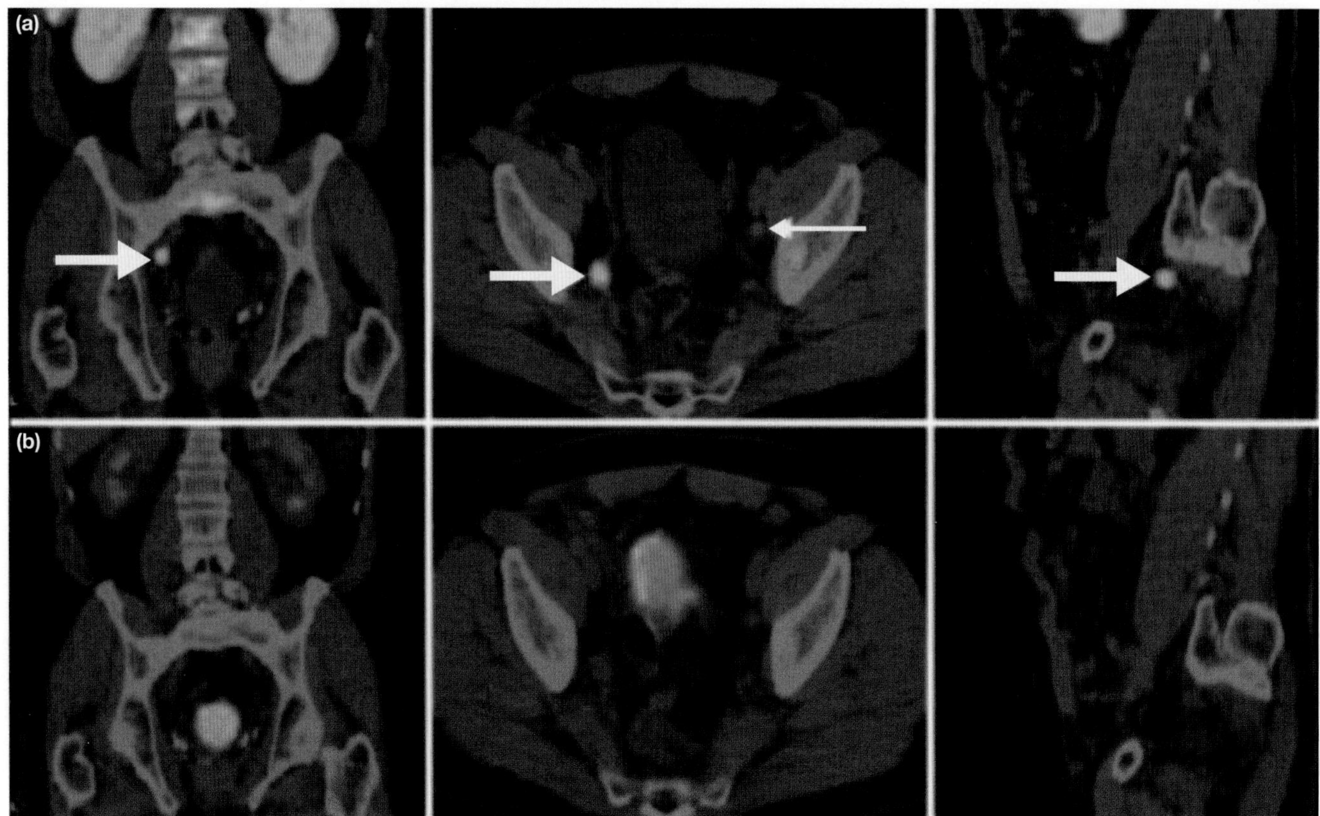

Figure 81.26 A 55-year-old patient with an increasing prostate-specific antigen level 27 months after radical prostatectomy. Coronal (left), axial (middle) and sagittal (right) fused image projections of choline positron emission tomography/computed tomography (PET/CT) scans. (a) Focal ^{11}C-choline uptake in the right (large arrow) and left (thin arrow) iliac regions revealed lymph node involvement. (b) This was not observed with 18F-fluorodeoxyglucose PET (courtesy of Hussein Farghaly).

follow-up of patients with seminoma with any residual mass. PET/CT may use a number of different radiotracers, including ^{11}C-choline, ^{18}F-choline (*Figure 81.26*), ^{18}F-fluciclovine and the newer gallium-68 (^{68}GA)-labelled antibodies targeting prostate-specific membrane antigen (PSMA) for the detection and staging of prostate cancer and its recurrence after initial definitive therapy.

Bone scan

A bone scan is most frequently used when bone metastases are suspected based on symptoms or other investigations. It is also used in the routine staging of patients with high-risk prostate cancer, although there is a <5% chance of a bone scan being positive until the PSA is >40 ng/mL.

Dimercaptosuccinic acid renogram

^{99m}Tc dimercaptosuccinic acid (DMSA) is a technetium radiopharmaceutical used in renal imaging to evaluate renal structure, especially in the paediatric population, where it is used to detect renal scarring (*Figure 81.27*).

Diethylenetriaminepenta-acetate renogram

^{99m}Tc diethylenetriaminepenta-acetate (DTPA) is another technetium radiopharmaceutical used in renal imaging. Previously it was used frequently in patients suspected of having ureteropelvic junction (UPJ) obstruction but it has largely been superseded by the mercaptoacetyltriglycine (MAG3) renogram in such cases.

Mercaptoacetyltriglycine renogram

^{99m}Tc Mercaptoacetyltriglycine (MAG3) is now the radiopharmaceutical of choice used in the assessment of patients with suspected upper urinary tract obstruction such as UPJ obstruction.

The shape of the renogram curve (following subtraction of background activity) is dependent, first, on MAG3 uptake from the circulation to the kidney and, second, on MAG3 elimination from the kidney into the bladder.

Classically, the normal MAG3 renogram curve has three phases (*Figure 81.28*):

1 The curve rises steeply upwards following intravenous tracer injection. This is indicative of the speed of tracer injection and its delivery to the kidneys (i.e. renal vascular supply).
2 A more gradual slope that represents renal handling of MAG3 (renal uptake by tubular secretion and glomerular filtration) and peaks between 2 and 5 minutes. The time taken for the curve to peak following tracer injection is referred to as T_{max}. This may be delayed in patients with renovascular insufficiency, renal failure and obstruction.
3 Commences after the peak. It is associated with the

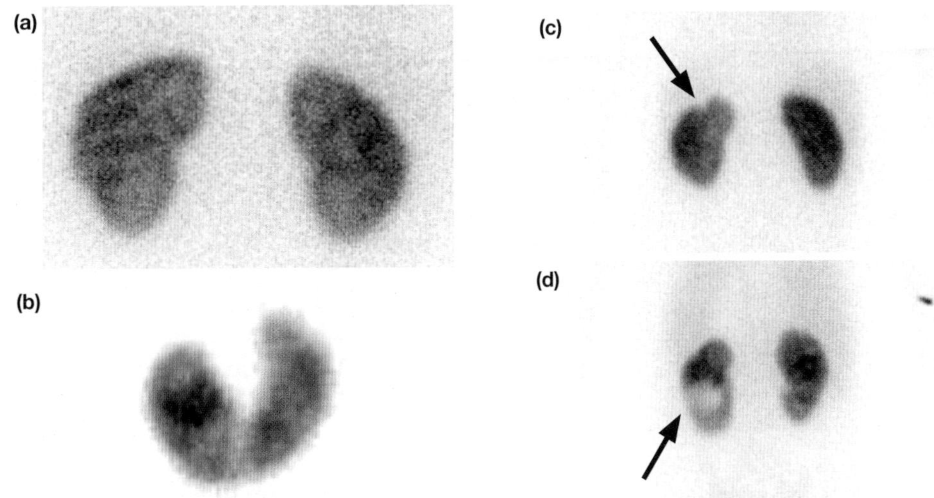

Figure 81.27 Dimercaptosuccinic acid scans. (a) Normal kidneys; (b) horseshoe kidney; (c) focal renal scarring (arrow); (d) renal tumour (arrow).

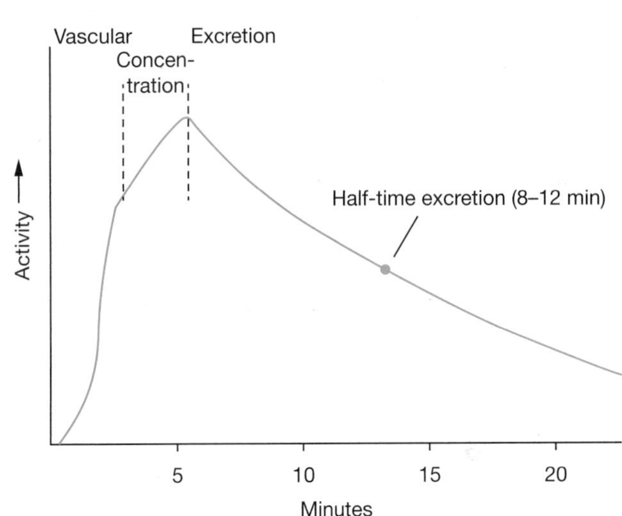

Figure 81.28 Diagrammatic representation of the three principal phases (vascular, concentration and excretion) of a mercaptoacetyltriglycine renogram curve. The time taken for the activity to become half of the peak level is called the half-time excretion and is used to determine the presence or absence of obstruction to urine outflow. Increased half-time suggests obstruction.

emergence of tracer in the bladder and represents elimination (but also delivery) of tracer from the kidney.

After 3 minutes, both elimination and uptake are in competition, but the former subsequently dominates. It is this elimination curve that is dependent on the upper tract urodynamics. Renogram curves of a number of normal and pathological conditions are shown in *Figure 81.29*.

Bladder function assessment

Flow rate and ultrasound scan residual urine

Men with LUTS and women with recurrent UTIs or LUTS are frequently investigated with a flow rate and a USS residual urine at the first clinic appointment (*Figures 81.30–81.32*). A peak flow rate (Q_{max}) in excess of 15 mL/s suggests that significant BOO is not present, whereas a flow rate of <10 mL/s suggests that BOO is present. A very low flow rate with a very protracted pattern of voiding is suggestive of a urethral stricture. Caution is required when interpreting the significance of a single high USS residual volume; repeated tests often give a more representative picture of the degree of bladder emptying.

Urodynamics

A urodynamic evaluation provides information about bladder pressure and urine flow and has been referred to as a pressure–flow study. The test is performed to investigate patients with unexplained or complicated LUTS or incontinence. It is also commonly used in patients with a suspected bladder neuropathy. A device for urodynamic assessment is shown in *Figure 81.33*. During urodynamics, fine catheters (or a dual-lumen catheter) are inserted through the urethra into the bladder to allow bladder filling and to record the intravesical pressure. Involuntary rises in the intravesical (detrusor) pressure during the filling phase, with or without a desire to void, are a classical sign of an overactive bladder. High intravesical pressure during voiding with a reduced flow rate is typically seen with BOO. An atonic bladder (no detrusor activity) is seen in diabetic neuropathy and in some patients following abdominoperineal excision of the rectum when damage to the pelvic nerve

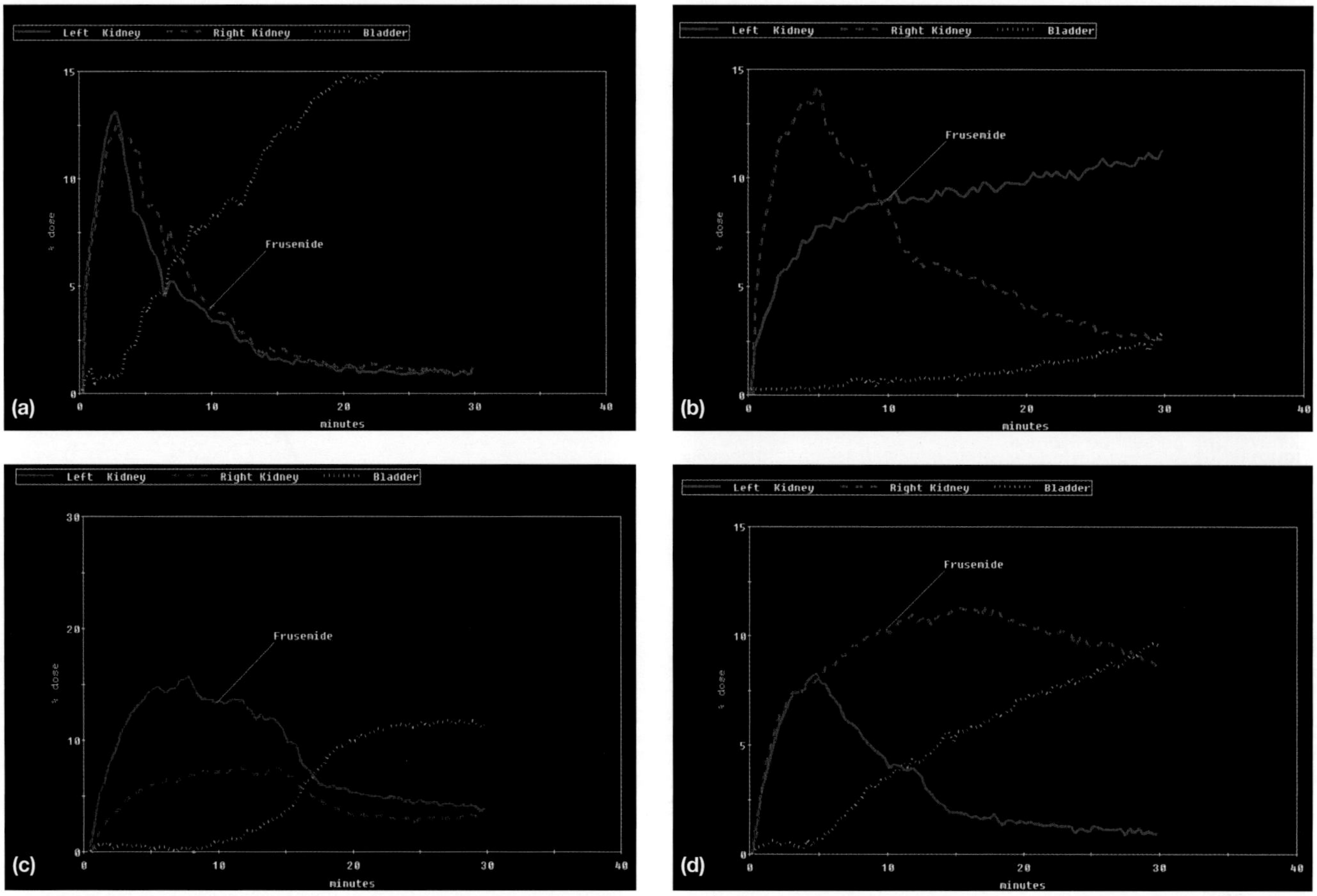

Figure 81.29 Curves from a series of mercaptoacetyltriglycine renograms (red line for right kidney; blue line for left kidney). (a) Normal excretion. (b) The left kidney graph does not go downwards, suggesting accumulation of radiotracer in the kidney – a sign of outflow obstruction. (c) Both the graphs show prolonged plateau phases, suggesting slow drainage from the kidneys – suggestive of bilateral dilated non-obstructed systems. (d) The right kidney shows a plateau phase with a delayed decline in the curve, suggesting a partially obstructed right system.

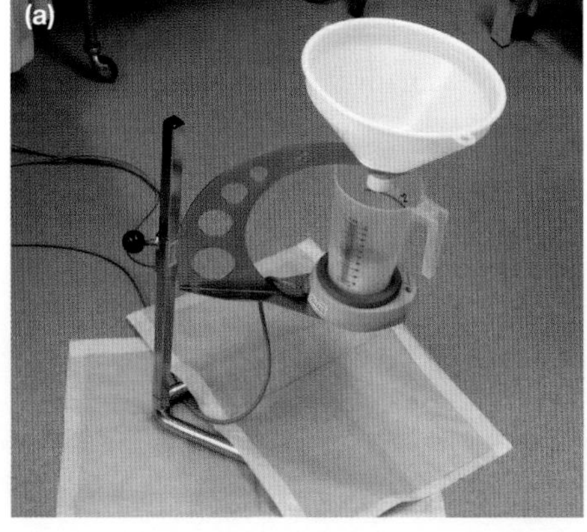

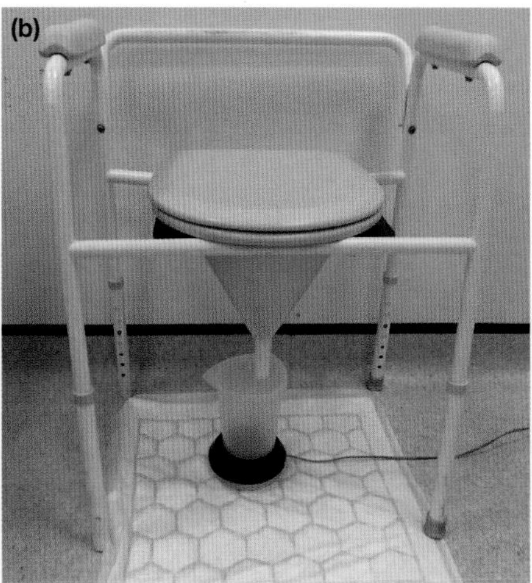

Figure 81.30 (a) A flow meter for use in males. (b) A flow meter for females

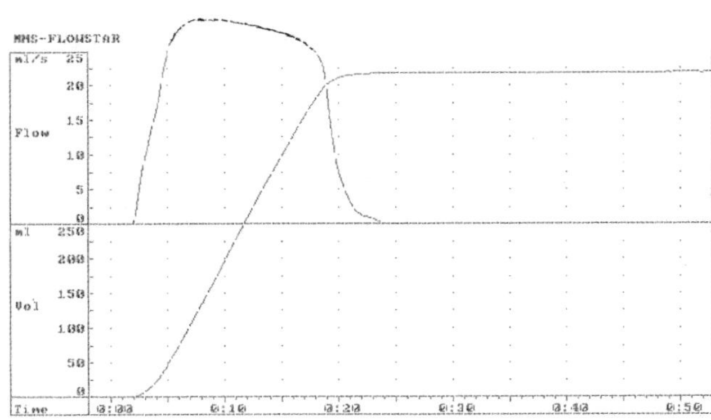

Figure 81.31 A flow study from a young healthy male patient showing a high-volume rapid void with an excellent peak flow of 32 mL/s. The upper curve shows the flow rate of urine while the lower graph shows total urine voided.

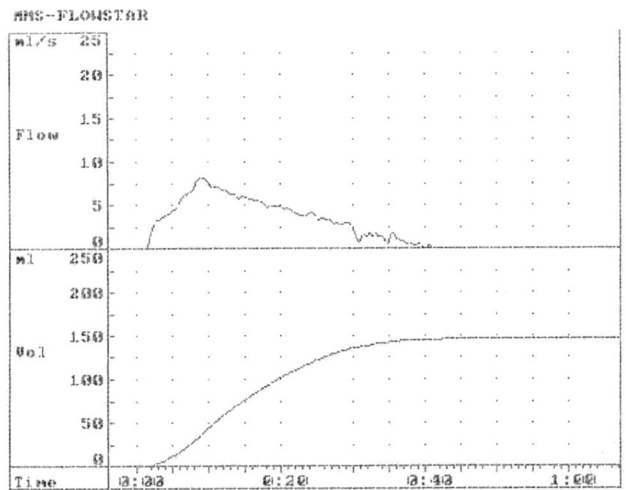

Figure 81.32 A flow study performed by a patient with bladder outlet obstruction showing a reduced peak flow of urine (8.1 mL/s).

plexus has occurred. Detrusor–sphincter dyssynergia – when coordinated contraction of the detrusor muscle in conjunction with relaxation of the external sphincter, necessary to permit normal voiding, is lost – is often seen in neurological conditions such as multiple sclerosis.

Summary box 81.10

Assessment of bladder function

- Simple tests are a flow rate and a USS residual urine estimation
- Urodynamics provides a pressure–flow profile
- Urodynamics requires fine catheters to be inserted into the bladder and usually the rectum
- A non-invasive technique in males using a penile cuff has a limited clinical role

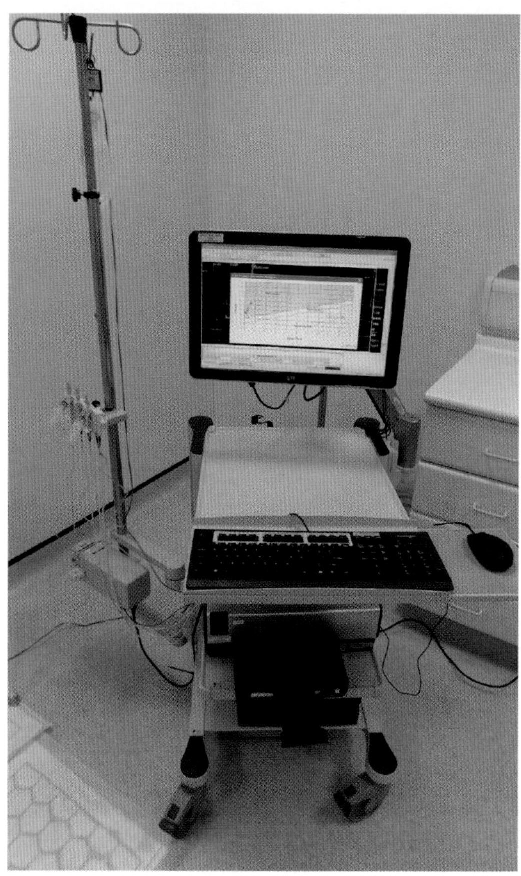

Figure 81.33 A modern urodynamic machine.

FURTHER READING

Dalkin BL, Ahmann FR, Kopp JB. Prostate specific antigen levels in men older than 50 years without clinical evidence of prostatic carcinoma. *J Urol* 1993; **150**(6): 1837–9.

DeAntoni EP, Crawford ED, Oesterling JE *et al.* Age- and race-specific reference ranges for prostate-specific antigen from a large community-based study. *Urology* 1996; **48**(2): 234–9.

European Randomized Study of Screening for Prostate Cancer (ERSPC) Risk Calculator. Available from http://www.prostatecancer-riskcalculator.com/seven-prostate-cancer-risk-calculators.

Hamdy FC, Donovan JL, Lane JA *et al.* 10-year outcomes after monitoring, surgery, or radiotherapy for localized prostate cancer. *N Engl J Med* 2016; **375**(15): 1415–24.

Kaisary AV, Ballaro A, Pigott K. *Urology: lecture notes*, 7th edn. Hoboken, NJ: Wiley-Blackwell, 2016.

McAninch JW, Lue TF. *Smith & Tanagho's general urology*, 18th edn. New York: Lange, 2012.

Oesterling JE, Jacobsen SJ, Chute CG *et al.* Serum prostate-specific antigen in a community-based population of healthy men. Establishment of age-specific reference ranges. *JAMA* 1993; **270**(7): 860–4.

Prostate Cancer Prevention Trial Risk Calculator Version 2.0. Available from https://riskcalc.org/PCPTRC/.

Wein AJ, Kavoussi LR, Partin AW, Peters CA. *Campbell–Walsh urology*, 12th edn. Amsterdam: Elsevier, 2020.

CHAPTER 82 The kidney and ureter

Learning objectives

To know:

- Congenital anomalies of the kidney and ureter
- Classification of renal cysts
- Classification, definitions, pathogenesis and management of urinary tract infections
- The pathophysiology and management of renal and ureteric stone disease
- Trauma to the kidney and ureter
- Presentation and management of renal neoplasms

CONGENITAL DISEASES

Renal agenesis

Complete absence of one kidney occurs in 1 in 3000 live births. The other formed kidney is usually hypertrophic. Reproductive tract anomalies are common in females with unilateral renal agenesis.

Bilateral renal agenesis is incompatible with life.

Ectopic kidney

This occurs when the mature kidney fails to reach its normal location in the lumbar region. The incidence is 1 in 500–1200. An ectopic kidney (*Figure 82.1*) may be found anywhere along the path of ascent: pelvic, iliac, abdominal and rarely thoracic. When the ectopic kidney is located on the contralateral side to its ureteric insertion, it is called crossed ectopia. Renal ectopia may be associated with reflux in the ectopic or orthotopic kidney and with pelviureteric junction (PUJ) and ureterovesical junction (UVJ) obstruction.

Horseshoe kidney

This is the most common renal fusion anomaly, occurring in about1 in 400 live births with a male predominance. The isthmus lies at the level of the fourth to fifth lumbar vertebrae (fused lower poles). This causes failure to ascend and rotate so that the renal pelvis faces anteriorly and vertically with the malrotated calyces pointing posteromedially (*Figure 82.2*). The vascular supply is variable and the ureter may insert high on the renal pelvis. Most horseshoe kidneys (HSKs) are asymptomatic but they are associated with an increased incidence of genital anomalies, PUJ obstruction (PUJO) and stone formation. The incidence of Wilms' tumour is higher in HSK.

Multicystic dysplastic kidney

Multicystic dysplastic kidney (MCDK) is the second most common cause of an abdominal mass in newborns after hydronephrosis due to PUJO. The unilateral incidence is 1 in 1000–4000 live births. It has a 'bunch of grapes' appearance

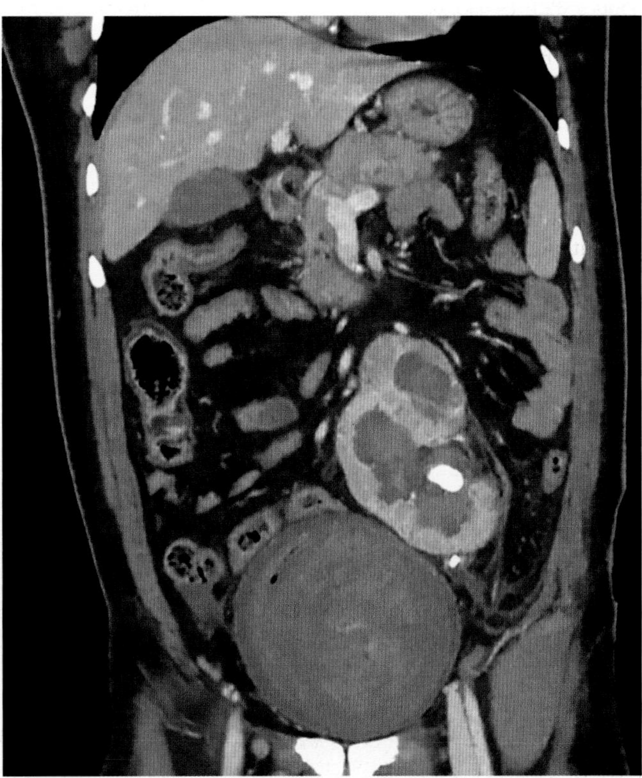

Figure 82.1 Computed tomography scan showing a pelvic kidney with calculus.

Carl Max Wilhelm Wilms, 1867–1918, German surgeon, described Wilms' tumour in 1899.

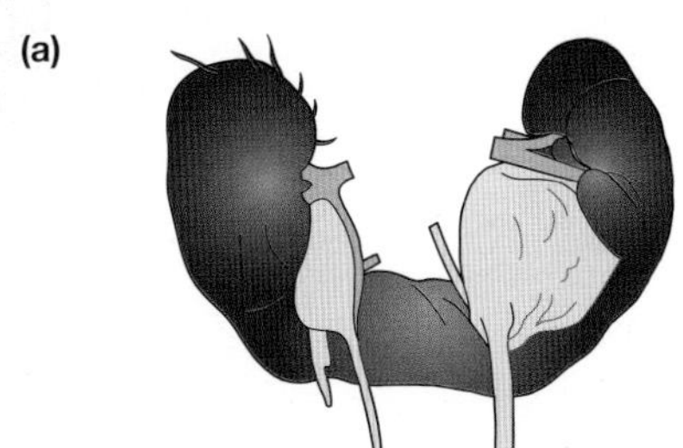

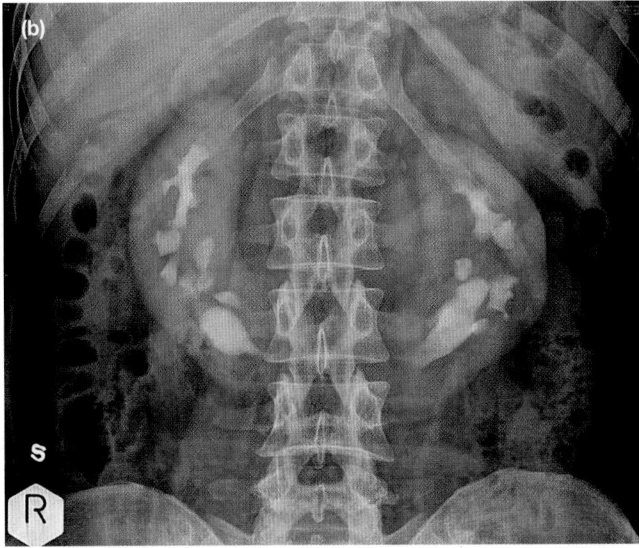

Figure 82.2 (a) Horseshoe kidney (courtesy of Nivedita Kekre and Dr Madhuri Sadanala). (b) Intravenous urogram image at 5 minutes, showing horseshoe kidney and posterior orientation of the calyces (courtesy of Department of Urology, Christian Medical College, Vellore, India).

with multiple non-communicating cysts of varying sizes without identifiable renal parenchyma. MCDKs can be diagnosed on antenatal ultrasound (US), with multiple cysts being evident as early as 15 weeks' gestation. Isotope renal scan will show a photopenic area in the renal fossa with surrounding background activity. Newborns may present with a palpable renal mass but nephrectomy is not necessary as the majority undergo involution within 5 years. Bilateral MCKD is incompatible with life.

Ureteral duplication

Duplication of the ureter (*Figure 82.3*) and renal pelvis is a common anomaly, with an incidence of approximately 1 in 150 births. Unilateral duplication is six times more common than bilateral. It is more common in females. The duplication may be incomplete (Y-shaped ureter) or complete. It is associated with vesicoureteric reflux (VUR), PUJO and ureterocele. Incomplete duplex ureters with a 'Y' ureter arise when the ureteric bud bifurcates after its initial development from the Wolffian duct. Complete ureteric duplication occurs when there are two separate ureteric buds that develop into two separate ureters, which drain the upper and lower kidney moieties separately. The lower moiety ureter has a shorter submucosal tunnel and is prone to VUR. PUJO is more common with the upper moiety. The upper moiety ureter may be ectopic and is often associated with a concomitant ureterocele. The upper moiety of the kidney is often dysplastic.

Ectopic ureters

An ectopic ureter is one that drains to regions other than the bladder. Ectopic ureters are almost always associated with ureteric duplication and are bilateral in 10%. The female-to-male ratio is 7:1. In females, the ectopic ureter opens either into the urethra below the sphincter or into the vagina (*Figure 82.3*). Such a child would complain of incontinence of urine despite normal voiding. In contrast, the male child is always continent as the ureter opens above the external urethral sphincter. Computed tomo-urography (CTU) or magnetic resonance urography (MRU) is diagnostic.

Ureterocele

Ureterocele is a cystic enlargement of the intramural ureter, which probably occurs as a result of atresia of the ureteric orifice. It has a female-to-male ratio of 4:1 and occurs bilaterally in 10%. Similar to ectopic ureters, ectopic ureteroceles frequently drain the upper pole and are often associated with dysplastic or non-functional renal tissue. In childhood, they usually present with infection. When large, they can obstruct the bladder neck or even the contralateral ureteric orifice. The classic feature of a ureterocele on an intravenous urogram (IVU) is the 'cobra head' sign. The treatment of simple ureteroceles is surgical excision with reimplantation of the ureter. Endoscopic incision of a ureterocele is the preferred treatment method for simple ureteroceles in infants and small children, but may result in subsequent ureteric reflux. A non-functioning kidney may need nephrectomy.

Congenital megaureter

The normal ureteric diameter in children up to 16 years is 0.50–0.65 mm. If the ureter is dilated by more than 7 mm, it is classed as a dilated or megaureter. This may occur with or without obstruction or reflux. Most cases of megaureter with obstruction present in childhood with severe infections. Renal stones can form easily in the dilated systems. Surgical correction is indicated in symptomatic patients who have recurrent urinary tract infections (UTIs), progressive dilation on US and differential renal function of less than 40%. Surgery involves excision of the stenosed distal ureter and non-refluxing ureteric reimplantation.

Retrocaval ureter

This is due to anomalous development of the inferior vena cava (IVC) with persistence of the posterior subcardinal vein. The right ureter passes behind the IVC rather than lying on its right side and may lead to ureteric obstruction, hydronephrosis and calculi. Most cases remain asymptomatic. Contrast imaging with IVU, CTU, MRU and diuretic renogram aid the diagnosis. The classic sign of a dilated upper ureter at L3/L4 with proximal hydronephrosis and the ureter passing

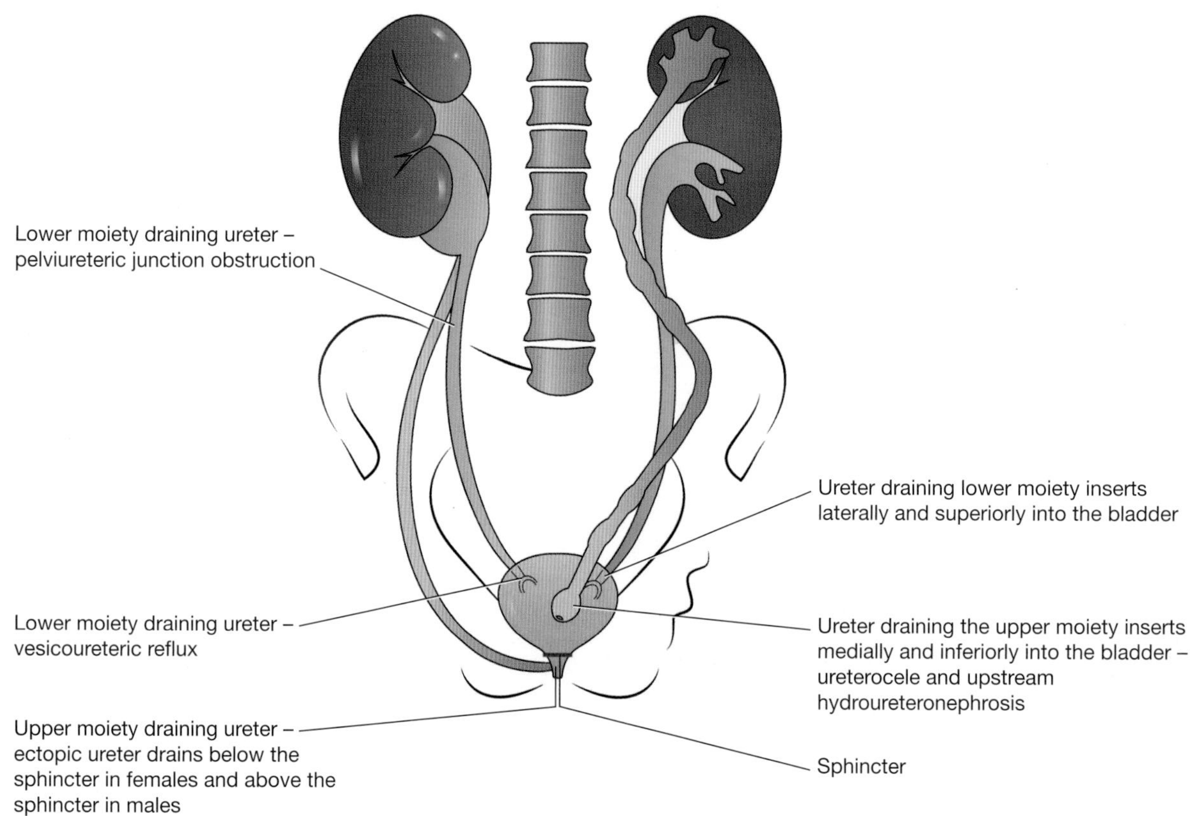

Figure 82.3 Complete duplication of the ureter and associated anomalies (courtesy of Nivedita Kekre and Dr Madhuri Sadanala).

medially behind the IVC is described as the reverse 'J' sign (*Figure 82.4*). Surgical correction is indicated in symptomatic patients with ureteroureterostomy or pyeloplasty depending on the level of obstruction.

Antenatal hydronephrosis

The prevalence of antenatal hydronephrosis (ANH) ranges from 0.6% to 5.4%. The majority of cases of ANH are transient and resolve after birth. The optimal timing of postnatal US in patients with ANH is at least 48 hours after birth. Diuretic renography can be performed after 4–6 weeks of life. ANH is classified into low, intermediate and high risk. A voiding cystourethrogram (VCUG), antibiotic prophylaxis and functional scan are recommended for high-risk infants along with monthly follow-up, whereas 1- to 3-monthly follow-up with US may suffice in low-risk infants.

Congenital pelviureteric junction obstruction

Congenital PUJO is the most common cause of unilateral hydronephrosis with an incidence of 1 in 500 live births. It may result from intrinsic obstruction secondary to an aperistaltic segment at the PUJ due to muscular hypoplasia. Other causes include a high insertion of the ureter into the pelvis and the presence of crossing aberrant vessels at the PUJ. It is more

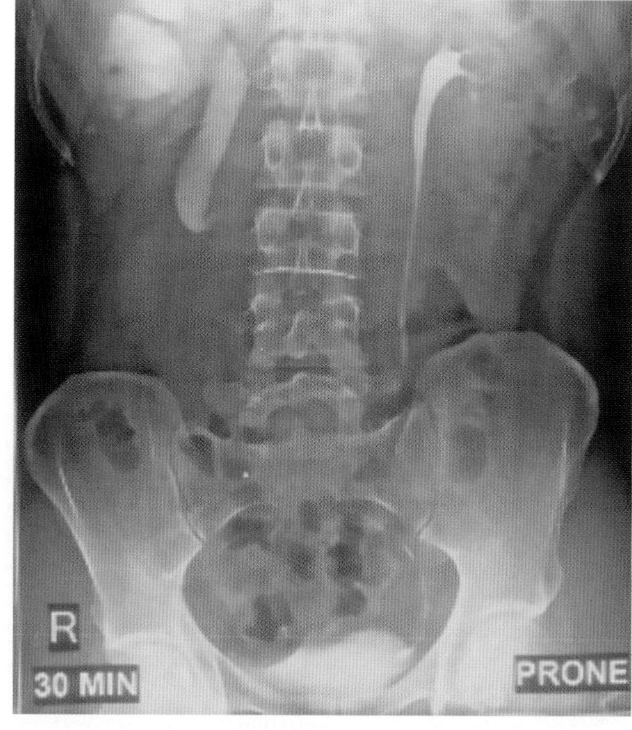

Figure 82.4 Retrocaval ureter with a classic 'reverse J' sign seen on intravenous urogram (courtesy of Department of Urology, Christian Medical College, Vellore, India).

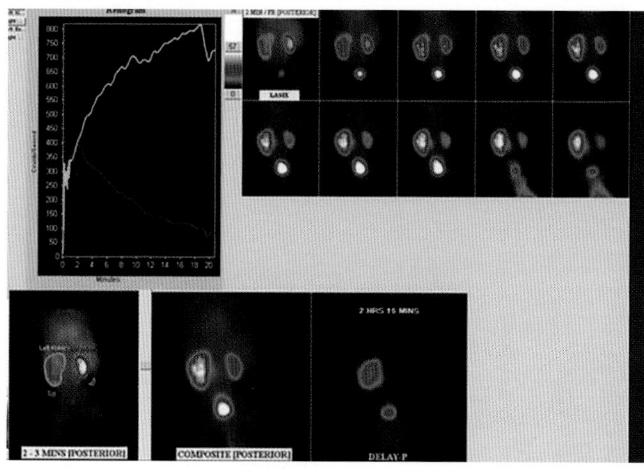

Figure 82.5 Isotope renal scan using diethylenetriaminepenta-acetate showing an obstructive pattern on the time–activity graph with hold-up of contrast of up to 2 hours. This finding is consistent with pelviureteric junction obstruction (courtesy of Department of Urology, Christian Medical College, Vellore, India).

common in males and on the left side. Bilateral obstruction occurs in 10% of cases. Historically, PUJO presented as a palpable flank mass in an infant or a child, but most are now detected before birth with antenatal US. Older children may present with intermittent flank pain, UTI or a flank mass. Adults present with back or flank pain or recurrent pyelonephritis. Rarely, a patient may present with a history of severe flank pain following ingestion of large amounts of fluid, which is relieved after passing a large amount of urine (**Dietl's crisis**).

US may show symmetrical hydronephrosis and a dilated renal pelvis and can provide information on the severity of obstruction by measuring the degree of dilatation, parenchymal thickness and cortical echogenicity. Isotope diuretic renography is the current investigation of choice. Isotope uptake and washout of the isotope can be followed with time to produce a renogram curve. Usually, half of the peak isotope activity is cleared within 10–15 minutes ($T_{1/2max}$). A rising curve following administration of furosemide, a $T_{1/2max}$ of greater than 20 minutes and a differential function of less than 40% on the affected side is suggestive of significant obstruction and is an indication for surgical intervention (*Figure 82.5*). CTU or MRU may also be used in the evaluation of PUJO.

The Anderson–Hynes dismembered pyeloplasty is the procedure of choice with a wide funnelled, dependent anastomosis, maintaining good vascularity of the upper ureter and pelvis and excision of the redundant pelvis (*Figure 82.6*). The indications for pyeloplasty are persistent pain, hypertension, haematuria, secondary renal calculi and recurrent UTIs. Endoscopic management in the form of endopyelotomy is reserved for post-pyeloplasty strictures.

Summary box 82.1

Congenital anomalies

- Congenital anomalies are usually detected incidentally and often only manifest when effected by pathology such as stone disease or malignancy
- Ectopic ureter should be suspected in a female child who presents with continuous incontinence of urine and also voids normally
- **Weigert–Meyer rule**
  - The ureter that drains the upper moiety is at a more inferior and medial position and is prone to obstruction and dysplasia
  - The ureter that drains the lower moiety is at a more superior and lateral position and is prone to VUR
- Most cases of ANH are transient and resolve after birth

RENAL CYSTS

Renal cysts can be broadly classified into sporadic, acquired and genetic causes.

Sporadic renal cysts

Sporadic renal cysts are usually benign. Cysts with thin, sharply defined walls and clear fluid content are known as simple renal cysts. This category of cysts may be diagnosed with certainty by US. Apart from a few thin septa, any variation in the nature of the fluid, thickness of the cyst wall or septa or the presence of either calcification or a solid nodule would require further imaging with either computed tomography (CT) scan or magnetic resonance imaging (MRI) to rule out cystic renal cell carcinoma (RCC). Bosniak proposed a four-tiered classification of the malignant potential of cystic renal lesions. Category I cysts represent benign lesions that require no further follow-up, whereas categories III and IV have a higher probability of malignancy and require surgical excision. Category II cysts can be safely followed up.

Acquired renal cystic disease

Most patients on haemodialysis develop bilateral renal cysts after 10 years. On follow-up one-fifth of these patients with acquired renal cystic disease (ARCD) develop renal cancers.

Genetic renal cysts

These cystic renal lesions have a known genetic inheritance. They are usually accompanied by involvement of other organ systems and present earlier in life than sporadic renal cysts.

Dietl's crisis, first reported by **Josef Dietl**, 1804–1878, in 1864, an Austrian doctor and pathologist known for his work on floating kidneys.
James Christie Anderson, 1899–1984, urologist, Royal Hallamshire Hospital, Sheffield, UK.
Wilfred Hynes, 1903–1991, plastic surgeon, The Plastic and Jaw Department, The Royal Hospital, Sheffield, UK. Anderson and Hynes devised the operation in 1949.
Carl Weigert, 1845–1904, German pathologist and anatomist known for work on cellular staining.
Robert Meyer, 1864–1947, German pathologist and gynaecologist in Berlin, removed from his position for being Jewish, emigrated in 1939 to Minneapolis, MN, USA.
Morton A Bosniak, 1929–2016, Professor of Radiology, New York University (NYU) Langone School of Medicine, New York, NY, USA.

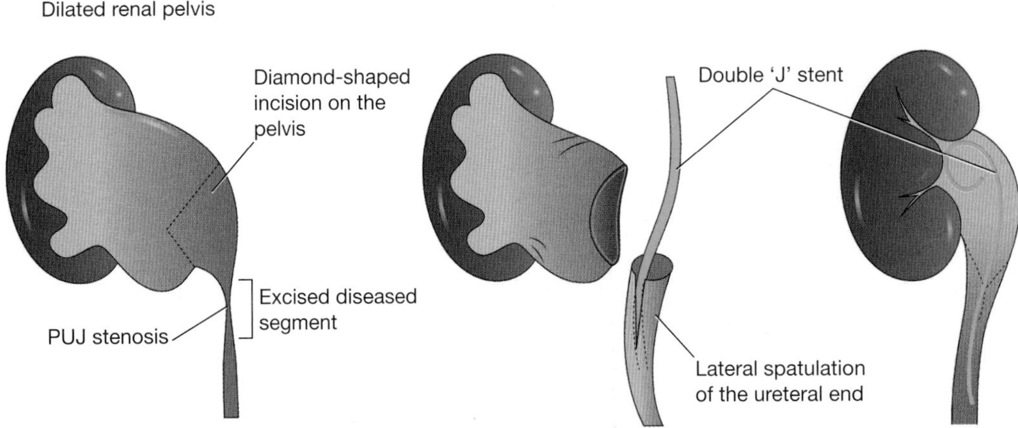

Figure 82.6 Steps of open dismembered pyeloplasty (courtesy of Nivedita Kekre and Dr Madhuri Sadanala). PUJ, pelviureteric junction.

Autosomal dominant polycystic kidney disease

Autosomal dominant polycystic kidney disease (ADPKD) is the most common autosomal dominant genetic cystic renal disease causing chronic renal failure requiring dialysis and renal transplantation. It occurs as a result of mutation in one of two genes (*PKD1* on chromosome 16 and *PKD2* on chromosome 4). ADPKD gene loci can be identified in individuals with a family history before the development of cysts begins; this is helpful in screening a potential sibling for kidney donation. ADPKD has variable penetration and approximately 50% of affected individuals eventually develop end-stage renal disease (ESRD). Risk factors for the development of ESRD are:

- early age of presentation;
- hypertension;
- male sex;
- ADPKD gene 1;
- African ethnic group.

ADPKD is associated with cysts in other organs, such as the liver, pancreas, arachnoid membranes and seminal vesicles. It does not usually manifest before the age of 30 years and in some patients it is never diagnosed. Renal symptoms include abdominal pain, haematuria or a palpable mass. Most patients older than 20 years are hypertensive and good control of blood pressure can delay progression to renal failure. Novel agents such as vasopressin antagonists (tolvaptan), somatostatin analogues and mammalian target of rapamycin (mTOR) inhibitors have shown potential to prevent cystogenesis, cyst expansion and declining renal function. Intracranial aneurysms occur in approximately 10–30% of patients with ADPKD and subarachnoid haemorrhage may cause sudden death in young adults.

Summary box 82.2

Renal cystic disease

- Bosniak renal cyst classification is used to grade cysts and probability of malignancy
- ADPKD – autosomal dominant, systemic disease:
  - Rarely manifests before the fourth decade
  - Hypertension, abdominal pain, haematuria or a palpable flank mass are common presentations
  - Control of hypertension can delay progression

INFECTIONS

UTI is very common and affects all ages and both sexes. It can cause significant morbidity and is a rare cause of mortality in patients with serious comorbidities or in patients with urinary tract obstruction. Recurrent UTI is more common in women, affecting 30–40% in the sexually active age group. It can be defined as an inflammatory response of the urothelium (host) to invading bacteria. Asymptomatic colonisation or bacteriuria (ABU) is also common and can be differentiated from a UTI by the absence of symptoms and pyuria (leukocytes in urine).

Classification

UTI is classified as uncomplicated when it occurs in an immunocompetent host with an anatomically normal and functional urinary tract. UTIs may also be classified on their site of origin as pyelonephritis (kidney), cystitis (bladder), urethritis or prostatitis. While acute pyelonephritis indicates an acute infection of the kidney, **chronic pyelonephritis** is only a morphological description of previous infection-related sequelae such as scarring in the kidney as seen on radiological or nuclear imaging.

Acute pyelonephritis

This commonly occurs as a result of ascending infection from organisms in the lower tract, usually caused by Gram-negative bacteria. Haematogenous spread may be seen in patients with diabetes and in immunocompromised hosts, people who inject drugs and patients with bacterial endocarditis. It is more common in females, especially during childhood, at puberty, after intercourse and during pregnancy. Acute pyelonephritis usually presents with fever, chills, flank pain, nausea and vomiting. Loin tenderness may be present. Symptoms may vary from mild to severe illness with septic shock and renal failure. Pyuria is almost always present and its absence in a patient with pyelonephritis may point towards an obstructed urinary tract. Urine and blood should be collected for culture. *Escherichia coli* and other Gram-negative organisms are commonly responsible. Imaging is necessary when the patient is not responding to antibiotics to rule out pyonephrosis, renal abscess and obstruction. Renal US is often the first imaging modality used. Contrast-enhanced CT (CECT) typically shows decreased patchy opacification of the affected parenchyma.

Pyelonephritis complicating pregnancy

The relaxing effect of progesterone during pregnancy causes ureteral smooth muscle relaxation and dilatation, presumably predisposing pregnant women to ascending upper tract infections. It is associated with fetal growth retardation and preterm delivery. Therefore, all pregnant women must be screened in the first trimester for ABU because, untreated, a third of these patients will develop UTI. Lower tract UTI typically occurs in the first trimester whereas pyelonephritis most often presents in the second or third trimester with acute abdominal pain or premature labour. Pyelonephritis is more common in pregnant women with an underlying urological abnormality or diabetes. A renal US is indicated if response to treatment is poor. Antibiotic use during pregnancy is tailored to avoid fetal harm and typically includes fosfomycin, penicillins or cephalosporins.

Renal and perirenal abscess

A renal abscess results from an ascending UTI in association with an underlying urinary tract abnormality such as obstructive uropathy or VUR. It is usually caused by common uropathogens such as *E. coli* and other Gram-negative bacilli. Renal abscesses may extend and perforate the renal capsule to form a perirenal abscess. Multiple renal abscesses may conglomerate into a solitary suppurative lesion called a renal carbuncle. This is usually caused by *Staphylococcus aureus*, which reaches the kidney by haematogenous spread.

The clinical presentation may be insidious and non-specific but patients usually present with persistent fever, back pain, abdominal pain and costovertebral tenderness. Urine examination may be normal if the abscess does not communicate with the collecting system. CECT scan is the investigation of choice to establish the diagnosis.

Treatment with antibiotics without drainage may be effective in carefully selected patients when the abscess is small (<3 cm) or in a stable patient (up to 5 cm). Empiric antibiotic therapy should be broad spectrum and should cover *S. aureus* and other uropathogens causing complicated UTI. Culture-directed antibiotics may be needed for 2 weeks or longer depending on response.

Percutaneous aspiration or drainage of pus is indicated in abscesses >5 cm and in patients not responding to antibiotics. Open surgical drainage is indicated when percutaneous drainage is inadequate.

Emphysematous pyelonephritis

This is an acute-onset, rapidly progressive, possibly lethal form of pyelonephritis characterised by parenchymal necrosis and gas formation, caused by organisms including *E. coli*, *Klebsiella pneumoniae*, *Pseudomonas aeruginosa* and *Proteus mirabilis*. Most patients have diabetes (up to 90%) and they may have obstruction secondary to calculi or papillary necrosis. Increased glucose levels in those with diabetes may provide a substrate for carbon dioxide production from fermentation. Symptoms are suggestive of pyelonephritis and an abdominal mass may be palpable. CECT of the abdomen is diagnostic and shows gas in the renal parenchyma, collecting system or both, along with other features of infection such as abscess, obstruction and perinephric stranding. Early diagnosis, intravenous broad-spectrum antibiotics and percutaneous drainage of the abscess and obstructed kidneys have improved outcomes in these patients. Emergency nephrectomy is rarely required and is reserved for patients who do not respond to the described measures.

Xanthogranulomatous pyelonephritis

Xanthogranulomatous pyelonephritis (XGP) occurs with severe renal infection in an obstructed kidney and is usually associated with calculi, causing loss of function and parenchymal destruction. Pathological examination typically shows accumulation of lipid-laden foamy macrophages. Patients may present with flank pain, fever with chills, persistent bacteriuria and a flank mass. A history of stone disease may be present. It is usually unilateral. CECT of the abdomen is diagnostic and shows a non-functioning enlarged hydronephrotic kidney around a shrunken pelvis with a calculus, also known as the **bear's paw sign** (*Figure 82.7*). Nephrectomy is the definitive treatment.

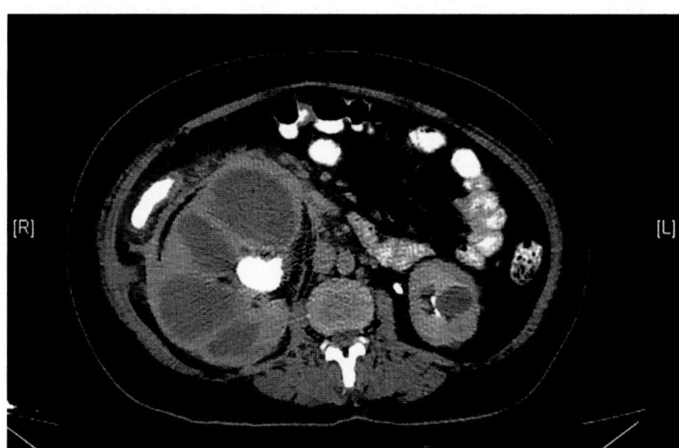

Figure 82.7 Xanthogranulomatous pyelonephritis with the 'bear's paw sign'.

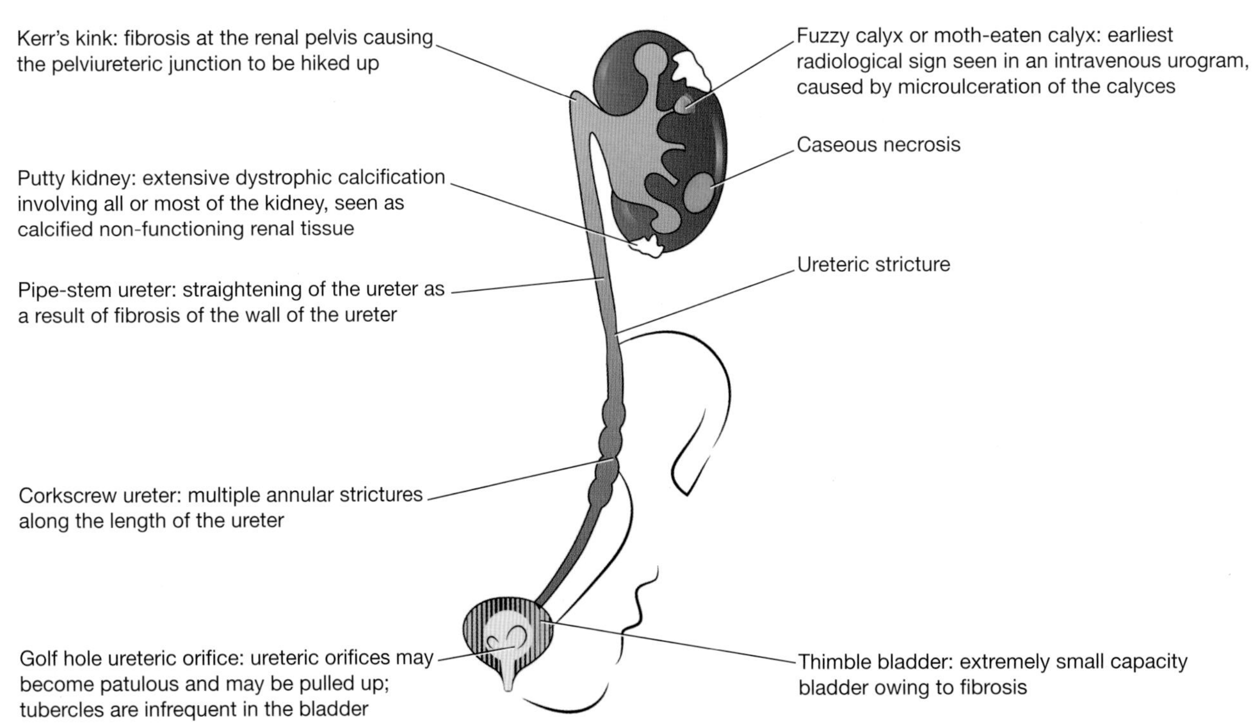

Figure 82.8 Schematic illustration showing the sequelae of urinary tuberculosis (courtesy of Nivedita Kekre and Dr Madhuri Sadanala).

Tuberculosis of the urinary tract

Genitourinary tuberculosis (GUTB) accounts for 15–20% of extrapulmonary cases of TB. It is secondary and caused by haematogenous spread of tubercle bacilli from the thoracic lymph nodes or the lungs. GUTB occurs as a result of either reinfection or reactivation of old TB granulomas. Blood-borne organisms are deposited close to the glomeruli, causing an inflammatory reaction. Macrophages react and granulomas are formed. If bacterial multiplication goes unchecked, caseous necrosis results in the formation of tubercles. Multiple tubercles coalesce and rupture into the collecting system, causing intermittent tuberculous bacilluria and pyuria. The disease spreads through the collecting system with ulceration initially. When bacterial multiplication is halted by the immune system, sequelae due to fibrosis appear (*Figure 82.8*). Tubercular obstructing or destructive lesions in the kidneys and ureters are responsible for renal function loss. Involvement of the bladder is secondary to renal disease. The disease gradually involves the bladder musculature, which is replaced by fibrous tissue, causing a decrease in the size and capacity of the bladder ('thimble' bladder). Urinary bladder involvement is responsible for urinary frequency, which is the most common symptom of GUTB.

Epididymal tuberculosis presents as a painless epididymal nodule, usually involving the tail of the epididymis, or a chronic discharging sinus in the posterior scrotal wall. Patients may present with urinary frequency, colicky flank pain, haematuria and, rarely, fever and constitutional symptoms. They may also present with symptoms suggestive of recurrent UTIs and, rarely, calcified tubercular lesions may be misdiagnosed as urinary tract calculi.

For microbiological confirmation, at least three consecutive early-morning specimens of urine are examined for acid-fast bacilli. The gold standard for microbiological diagnosis is urine culture. Nucleic acid amplification tests (NAATs) provide rapid diagnosis (within hours). When the diagnosis remains uncertain, bladder biopsy, tissue culture and tissue NAATs may be required. Imaging with CTU may also help and can show early signs such as calyceal distortion and papillary necrosis, hydronephrosis, poor function of renal segments secondary to parenchymal destruction, fibrosis and chronic obstruction. Ureteric strictures and proximal dilatation may also be seen. IVU can pick up the earliest signs of disease activity, such as calyceal distortion.

Treatment involves short-course antituberculous therapy (ATT). Rifampicin, isoniazid and pyrazinamide are used sometimes with ethambutol as first-line drugs.

The primary aim of therapy is preservation of renal function and avoidance of fibrotic sequelae. Ureteric strictures may require double J (DJ) stenting to preserve function until definitive reconstruction is attempted. Percutaneous nephrostomy (PCN) is recommended in obliterative strictures to achieve prompt decompression. Definitive surgery is usually done 3–6 weeks after starting ATT. The choice of reconstructive procedure depends on the type and location of sequelae.

Open surgical repair is generally superior to balloon dilatation for tubercular ureteric strictures. Augmentation enterocystoplasty (usually using ileum) for small-capacity bladders,

William 'Bill' K Kerr, a Canadian urologist, described his eponymous sign in 1967.

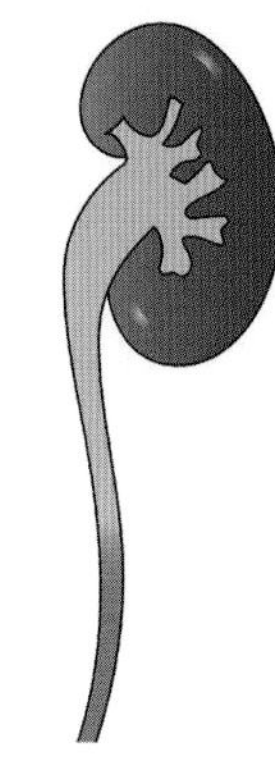
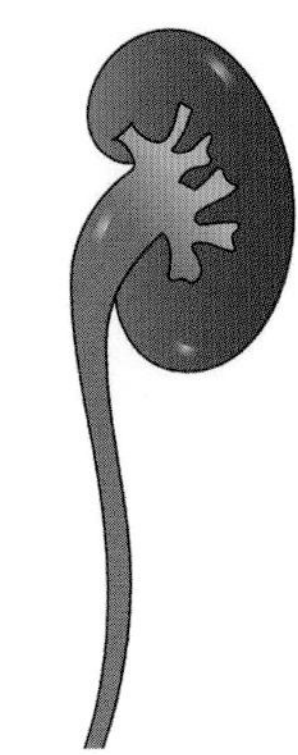
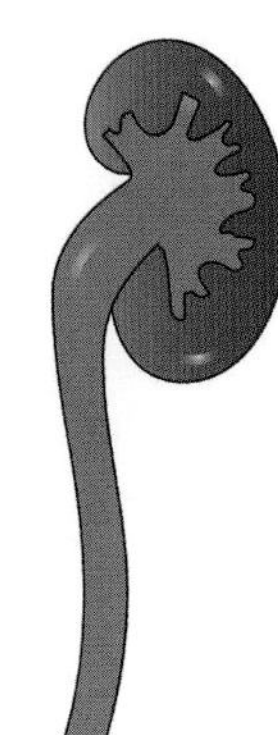
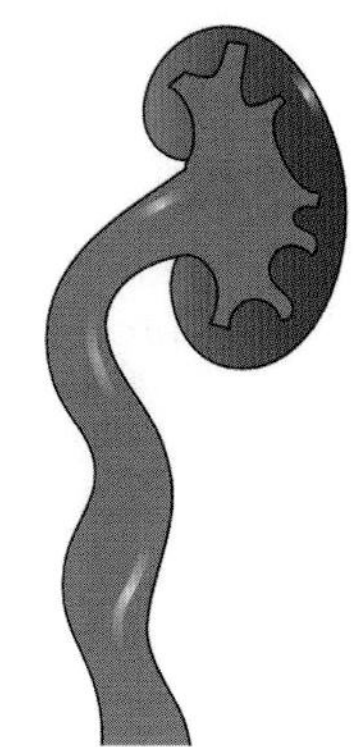
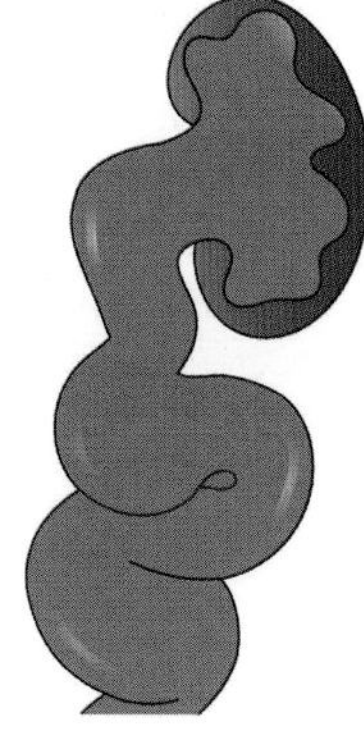

Figure 82.9 Grades of vesicoureteric reflux (courtesy of Nivedita Kekre and Dr Madhuri Sadanala).

ureteric reimplantation with or without a Boari flap (bladder tube) for lower ureteric stricture and ileal replacement of the ureter for multiple long ureteric strictures may be required. Nephrectomy is done for major renal lesions with a poorly functioning kidney.

Urinary infection in childhood and vesicoureteric reflux

All children with UTI must be evaluated for underlying predisposing conditions as recurrent pyelonephritis can cause renal scarring and loss of renal function. UTIs account for 7% of childhood febrile illness. In the age group <3 months, it is more common in males and in the age group >1 year, it is more common in females. Structural and functional abnormalities of the urinary tract such as VUR and posterior urethral valves predispose to UTI. Reflux is considered primary when it is due to an incompetent UVJ and secondary when it is due to increased bladder pressure or outlet obstruction. Presenting symptoms in neonates and infants include febrile illness or sepsis and may not be localised to the urinary tract. The method of urine sampling, especially before toilet training, is crucial and may involve suprapubic aspiration or per urethral catheter collection. A bacterial count of 50 000 colony-forming units per millilitre is generally considered a positive culture result in children, although a lower count from a suprapubic aspirate in a symptomatic child is significant. The most important complication of UTI in a child is renal scarring secondary to renal parenchymal inflammation. US should be performed in all children, and children with recurrent UTIs or a first time UTI with pyelonephritis should be evaluated further. VCUG is the investigation of choice to diagnose reflux and should be performed in high-risk children. ^{99m}Tc dimercaptosuccinic acid (DMSA) radionuclide cortical scan is the best modality to detect parenchymal lesions. VUR is present in approximately 30% of children with UTI and in up to 90% of children with renal scarring. Renal scarring may cause hypertension in up to 20% and is an important cause of renal failure. The grades of VUR are summarised in *Figure 82.9*, with grades I–III generally resolving spontaneously.

Low-dose nocturnal antibiotic prophylaxis to prevent scar-inducing pyelonephritis is the mainstay of treatment as the majority of reflux cases resolve with time. However, surgery (ureteric reimplantation, periureteric injections of Teflon or collagen) should be considered if episodes of acute pyelonephritis recur despite antibiotic therapy or if severe reflux is accompanied by a surgically correctable malformation such as a paraureteric bladder diverticulum.

Summary box 82.3

Infections

- UTI: inflammatory response of the urothelium (host) to invading bacteria
- ABU: colonisation of urine with bacteria with no evidence of inflammation
- All pregnant women must be screened in the first trimester for ABU because, untreated, one-third of these patients will develop UTI
- GUTB:
  - Always due to either reinfection or reactivation of old tuberculosis
  - Urine examination: sterile pyuria in acidic urine
  - Close monitoring of upper tract during the initial phase of ATT and timely urological intervention may prevent renal loss
- UTI in children:
  - More common in girls after 1 year of age
  - Sample collection method is important to avoid contamination
  - VUR occurs in 30% of children with a UTI
  - Renal scarring is a possible long-term consequence

Achille Boari, nineteenth century urological surgeon from Ferrara, Italy, described the technique of a bladder flap in dogs in 1894; it was first performed in a patient in 1936.

UROLITHIASIS

Urolithiasis is as old as mankind. The first documented cystolithotomy was described by Sushruta, an ancient Indian surgeon in almost 600 BCE. The development of shockwave lithotripsy (SWL) and endourological procedures with multiple efficient energy-generating devices (such as US, pneumatic, electrohydraulic) for stone fragmentation have revolutionised the management of stone disease. Although the incidence of bladder stones has declined progressively owing to the alleviation of poverty and the improvement in basic nutrition, the modern world is witnessing a steady increase in the incidence of renal calculi.

Epidemiology

The lifetime prevalence varies from 1% to 20% and the causes are multifactorial. Recurrence of stone disease is high, with 50% having recurrence within the first decade of diagnosis.

Non-modifiable factors associated with stone formation

- **Age**. The adult peak incidence in men is the fourth to sixth decade; women have a bimodal peak in incidence in the third decade and the postmenopausal period.
- **Gender**. Men are twice as likely to form stones.
- **Ethnic origin**. White people have a higher risk of stone disease than other ethnic groups. Recent evidence suggests that environmental and dietary factors may be more important than ethnic origin.
- **Family history**. Patients with a family history of stone disease are 2.5 times more likely to develop stone disease themselves. Examples of hereditary forms of stone disease include cystinuria, type I renal tubular acidosis (RTA) and primary hyperoxaluria.

Modifiable factors associated with stone formation

- **Environmental factors**. People living in hot and arid regions such as the desert or tropical areas have a higher incidence of stone disease owing to increased perspiratory fluid loss.
- **Drugs**. Drugs can predispose to stone formation through metabolic effects (e.g. corticosteroids, chemotherapeutic agents).

Pathogenesis

Stone formation results from a cascade of events that occur during and after urine formation.

When the concentration of culprit salts such as calcium and oxalate overwhelm inhibitory factors (e.g. citrate, potassium, magnesium, Tamm–Horsfall mucoproteins, pH changes), they precipitate into crystals. These crystal nuclei may be washed off with the flow of urine or they may anchor onto sites like renal papillae to form Randall's plaques. Variations in the pH of urine may also facilitate or inhibit stone growth; acidic pH precipitates the formation of uric acid stones and alkaline pH precipitates the formation of calcium phosphate stones. Hence, the manipulation of pH through medication can help in preventing new stone formation.

Stasis of urine also promotes stone formation. Stasis stones are usually multiple, round and have a smooth surface. These are called 'milk of calcium stones'.

Types of stones

Calcium oxalate stones

This is the most common type of stone, constituting 60–85% of all stones. Hypercalciuria, hypercalcaemia, hyperoxaluria, hyperuricosuria and hypocitraturia are known metabolic abnormalities that can predispose to its formation. Hypercalciuria is the most common metabolic abnormality and occurs as a result of dysregulation of transport at various sites, including the intestine, bone or kidney.

Primary hyperparathyroidism is the most common disease associated with hypercalcaemia and stone disease. Increased parathyroid hormone causes increased bone resorption and increased synthesis of 1,25-dihydroxyvitamin D3. This causes increased intestinal absorption of calcium, leading to hypercalcaemia and hypercalciuria.

Hyperuricosuria causes uric acid crystal formation, especially in association with acidic urine, over which calcium oxalate crystals aggregate.

Calcium phosphate stones

Pure calcium phosphate stones are rare. Common forms seen are apatite and brushite stones. Apatite is seen with infection and brushite stones are usually seen with distal RTA.

Uric acid stones

Hyperuricosuria promotes the formation of both calcium oxalate and uric acid stones. Uric acid precipitates into crystals in acidic urine and remains soluble in alkaline urine. Conditions that can cause hyperuricosuria are gout and myeloproliferative disorders after cytotoxic treatment.

Infection stones

These are struvite and apatite stones. They form as a result of urease-producing bacterial infections, such as those caused by *Proteus*, *Klebsiella*, *Serratia* or *Enterobacter*. Alkalinisation of urine takes place as urease hydrolyses urea to carbon dioxide and ammonium.

Staghorn calculi are infection stones that grow in a branching pattern, taking the form of the pelvicalyceal system.

Sushruta, 600 BCE, authored Suśruta-saṃhitā, considered the father of plastic surgery.

Igor Tamm, 1922–1995, an outstanding cytologist, virologist and biochemist, pioneer in the study of viral replication, professor at the Rockefeller Institute for Medical Research, New York, NY, USA.

Frank Lappin Horsfall Jr, 1906–1971, American microbiologist specialising in pathology, worked at the Rockefeller Institute, New York, NY, USA. The Tamm–Horsfall protein was first purified in 1952 during his work with Igor Tamm.

Alexander Randall, 1883–1951, American urologist, first described the plaques in 1937 as part of a postmortem case series using a hand lens.

They can grow very large before clinical detection and cause significant morbidity, which includes loss of renal function owing to chronic infection and obstructive uropathy. Complete clearance of a staghorn calculus is necessary, as residual fragments after treatment can cause rapid recurrence and persistence of bacteriuria. Long-term chemoprophylaxis is mandatory for a few months after successful removal of infection calculus.

Cystine stones

Cystine stones constitute approximately 1% of stones. Cystinuria is an autosomal recessive inherited disease that causes decreased reabsorption of cystine from the intestine and the proximal tubule of the kidney. Cystine is insoluble even at physiological pH and worsens with increasing acidity. Cystine stones are very hard stones as a result of disulphide bonds and do not fragment with SWL.

Clinical presentation

Incidentally detected asymptomatic stones are increasingly diagnosed because of the widespread use of imaging. The presenting symptoms depend on the location of the stone, the size and type of stone, underlying infections and complications related to stone disease. Haematuria may be gross or microscopic, especially during episodes of renal colic. Calculuria is described as sand or gravel accompanying urine. Ureteric colic is acute abdominal pain caused by hyperperistalsis of the ureteric musculature against the obstructing stone. It manifests as sudden-onset excruciating pain in the flank that can radiate to the groin, scrotum or labia. Lower ureteric stones close to or lodged at the UVJ can cause symptoms of urgency and frequency. Malaise and weight loss can occur in longstanding infection stones or as a manifestation of renal failure. High-grade fever with chills suggests an underlying UTI and should be considered an emergency. During history taking, information about risk factors such as diet, physical activity, fluid intake, history of urinary tract infections, gastrointestinal symptoms, previous surgical history, family history and previous treatment for stone disease should be enquired about.

Complications

Renal and ureteric stones can lead to significant morbidity owing to urinary tract obstruction, infectious complications and loss of renal function. Bilateral obstructing ureteric stones or ureteric calculi in a solitary kidney can present with anuria (calculous anuria). Infectious complications include pyelonephritis, pyonephrosis, renal abscess or septicaemia. Uncommon but serious complications include XGP and pyeloenteric or cutaneous fistulae in neglected cases. Nephron loss can occur as a result of recurrent episodes of infection and obstruction, causing chronic renal failure.

Diagnosis

The diagnostic approach can be classified into investigations done in the emergency setting and those done in the non-emergency setting.

Approach to ureteric colic

The most common acute presentation of stone disease is 'ureteric colic'. Small 3- to 5-mm calculi are usually responsible for ureteric colic and commonly lodge at the UVJ. Non-steroidal anti-inflammatory drugs and paracetamol are effective. Antispasmodic medications are not necessary to alleviate pain. Abdominal examination may reveal renal angle tenderness. Pelvic examination is especially important in women to exclude tubo-ovarian pathology such as an ectopic pregnancy or twisted ovarian cyst. *Table 82.1* lists the differential diagnoses.

TABLE 82.1 Differential diagnoses for ureteric colic.

Urinary tract

• Clot colic
  ◦ Anticoagulation therapy, haemophilia, vascular tumours
• Papillary necrosis
  ◦ Diabetes, NSAIDs, sickle cell disease

Other organs
• Acute appendicitis • Ectopic pregnancy • Ovarian torsion • Acute intestinal obstruction • Abdominal aortic aneurysm • Malingering

NSAID, non-steroidal anti-inflammatory drug.

Investigations include urinary examination, blood examination and diagnostic imaging. The majority have microscopic haematuria and pyuria. Pyuria may be sterile pyuria or due to infection. An elevated leukocyte count suggests infection and may be an indication for starting antibiotics.

Pregnancy should be ruled out.

A radiograph of the kidneys, ureters and bladder and US are good first-line tests. Non-contrast CT (NCCT) is the investigation of choice for the diagnosis of stones. It allows for diagnosis of both radio-opaque and radiolucent stones with the exception of indinavir stones. Most patients respond to medication to alleviate pain. However, if the pain does not reduce with analgesics, or if the patient shows features of sepsis or urinary obstruction, emergency urinary decompression should be planned. Blood and urine should be cultured in patients suspected of sepsis, and empirical broad-spectrum antibiotics should be initiated. If the patient is clinically unstable, initial stabilisation in critical care may be warranted. Emergency urinary decompression may be done either with ureteric stenting or with PCN. However, in the absence of infection, in a certain select group of symptomatic but surgically fit patients, removal of stones may be possible by ureteroscopy.

Metabolic evaluation

The extent of metabolic evaluation depends on the risk associated with the recurrence of stone formation.

Urinary examination is done to look at crystals and pH in the non-emergency setting. Urine culture is performed if definitive management is planned. Blood chemistry for serum levels of calcium, phosphorus and uric acid are done to rule out hypercalcaemia, hypophosphataemia and hyperuricaemia.

Further detailed metabolic work-up should be done for high-risk patients.

Non-surgical management of stone disease

This involves watchful waiting, medical expulsive therapy, SWL and stone dissolution therapy.

Watchful waiting

Patients with small (<5 mm), non-obstructive, asymptomatic, lower pole renal calculi with preserved renal function may be kept on follow-up. Up to 90% of 4-mm stones and 50% of 6- to 10-mm stones pass spontaneously.

Medical expulsive therapy

Tamsulosin is an α_1-adrenergic adrenoreceptor blocker (α-blocker) that causes smooth muscle relaxation of the distal ureteric muscle. It can be used for distal ureteric stones larger than 5 mm and to assist passage of fragments following SWL.

Extracorporeal shockwave lithotripsy

SWL is a non-invasive method introduced in 1980 by Christian Chaussy that allowed stones to be treated on an outpatient basis.

Mechanism of action

The stone is localised using either fluoroscopy or US or both. Then acoustic pulse waves are generated and focused on the stone. Stone fragmentation occurs as a result of mechanical stress caused directly by the energy transmitted by the incident shockwave and indirectly by the collapse of bubbles. The efficacy of SWL reduces with an increasing number of stones and volume of stone burden.

Steinstrasse is a German word meaning 'street of stones'. It describes a row of closely gathered stone fragments that line the distal end of the ureter (*Figure 82.10*). This occurs when the stone burden is high or when the stones are hard. These stones are usually asymptomatic and pass spontaneously; however, they may cause obstruction, requiring surgical intervention. 'Clinically insignificant residual fragments' are residual stone fragments of 4 mm in size or less after treatment that are expected to pass spontaneously. However, 20–40% of these fragments may not clear and form a nidus for stone regrowth.

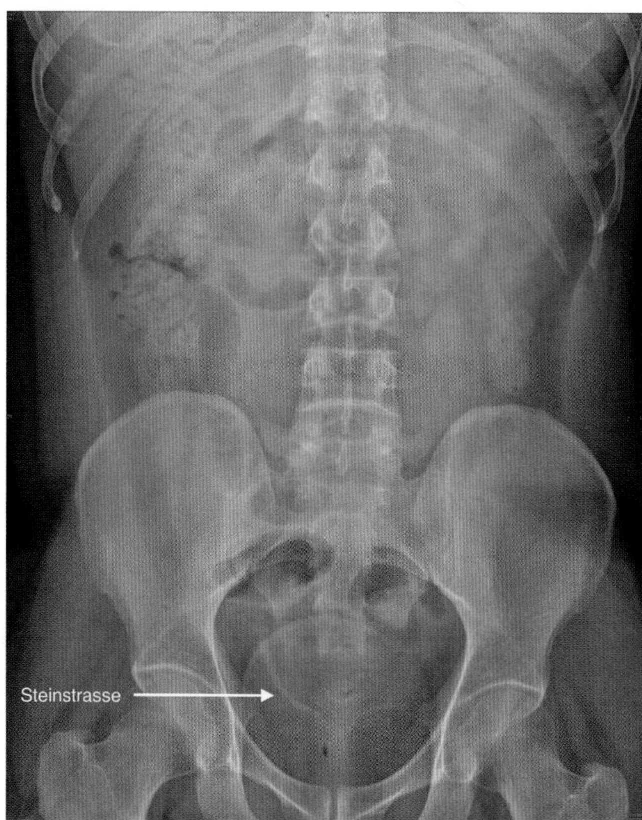

Figure 82.10 Steinstrasse formation after extracorporeal shock wave lithotripsy at the right distal ureter (courtesy of Department of Urology, Christian Medical College, Vellore, India).

Surgical management

Indications for surgical intervention

- Failure of medical management.
- Impaired renal function.
- Chronic infection – staghorn calculi, matrix calculi.
- High-risk occupation or geographical location – pilots, long-distance locomotive drivers, sailors.
- Patient's preference.

The choice of therapy depends on multiple factors such as surgical fitness, body habitus and stone characteristics. The general principle is to choose the least invasive method possible for that particular stone.

Endourology

Endourological procedures are the current preferred mode of treatment owing to their minimal invasive nature, technological advancements in instrumentation and more efficient energy sources for stone fragmentation. Current energy sources are pneumatic, US or laser lithotripsy. The type of energy source depends on the type of surgery and stone characteristics. Laser energy can be delivered via flexible instruments.

Ureterorenoscopy

Ureterorenoscopes (URSs) are long thin scopes that are used to remove ureteric and renal stones. They have working channels that allow for the introduction of energy sources, graspers and baskets. Current models are either semirigid or flexible scopes. A semirigid URS is usually used with a pneumatic lithotripter or laser energy device. Complications include ureteric perforation, avulsion and retropulsion. Ureteric avulsion can be avoided by careful use of baskets under vision. URSs can also be used in patients with bleeding disorders, with a moderate increase in complications.

Christian G Chaussy, b. 1945, German urologist.

Retrograde intrarenal surgery

A slimmer and more flexible URS with active deflection of the tip and laser technology with thinner fibres allows for retrograde access to the kidney via the ureteric orifice. This procedure avoids the morbidity associated with percutaneous nephrolithotomy (PCNL). Laser is used as an energy source for stone fragmentation.

Indications for retrograde intrarenal surgery (RIRS)

- Renal stones <2 cm.
- Lower pole calculi.
- Obesity.
- Musculoskeletal deformities (e.g. kyphoscoliosis) and renal anomalies (HSK or pelvic kidney).
- Bleeding diathesis.

Percutaneous nephrolithotomy

PCNL involves removal of renal stones by creating a track between the skin and the pelvicalyceal system. Typically, this procedure is done in the prone position. Fluoroscopy or US is used for localisation. The posterolateral calyx is commonly chosen for entry. US in conjunction with pneumatic and laser lithotripsy is the most common energy source used. Complications include bleeding, infection and pleural violation in cases of supracostal puncture. Severe bleeding may require selective angioembolisation.

Indications for percutaneous nephrolithotomy

- Renal stones >2 cm.
- Lower pole renal stones with anatomy that is unfavourable for SWL.
- Failed SWL or RIRS for renal calculi.
- Staghorn calculi.

Contraindications to percutaneous nephrolithotomy

- Pregnancy.
- Untreated UTI.
- Bleeding diathesis.
- Current anticoagulation.

Miniaturised percutaneous nephrolithotomy

Miniaturised PCNL (e.g. mini-perc) involves the use of smaller access tracks. The standard PCNL access track is >28Fr compared with miniaturised versions using <22Fr tracks. Miniaturised PCNL is most useful in patients with a smaller stone burden and in children.

Lateral and supine PCNL are associated with fewer anaesthetic complications. Moreover, concomitant flexible ureteroscopy for endoscopic combined intrarenal surgery can be done to address complex renal stones, multiple stones or stones in challenging locations.

Non-endourological surgical management

Open surgery such as pyelolithotomy and anatrophic nephrolithotomy is reserved for complex and infected stones with anatomical abnormalities.

Prevention of recurrent stone disease

High-risk stone formers should be advised to follow preventive measures to reduce recurrence. General measures advised to all patients include:

- fluid intake of more than 2.5 litres per day;
- dietary calcium should not be restricted; supplemental calcium, if necessary, should be taken at meal times;
- reduce intake of animal protein and salt.

Pregnancy

Renal colic is the leading cause of non-obstetric hospital admission in pregnancy.

The physiological changes that take place during pregnancy include an increase in glomerular filtration rate by 50%; increased excretion of calcium, uric acid and sodium; and increased excretion of inhibitors of crystallisation such as citrate and magnesium. Urine pH is alkaline and so the predominant stone type seen in pregnancy is calcium phosphate stones.

US is the primary mode of investigation for renal colic. MRI can be used as a second-line investigation to define the level of obstruction.

Most stones pass spontaneously. However, stones can cause loss of pregnancy and premature labour. Hence, emergency ureteroscopy is a reasonable first-line option in well-selected distal ureteric stones. Internal stenting or PCN can be used in the interim and a definitive procedure can be planned following childbirth. Pregnancy is an absolute contraindication to SWL.

Children

See also *Chapter 20*.

Stones are rare in children. Childhood urolithiasis is more common in males in the first decade and in young adolescent females. Calcium oxalate stones are the most common variety. Genetic disorders are seen in 17% of children with stones. They may be asymptomatic or may present with non-specific symptoms such as crying, irritability and vomiting. Diagnosis and treatment should be planned such that ionising radiation is kept to a minimum. Indications for various modes of treatment are similar to those for adults.

Summary box 82.4

Urolithiasis

- Causes of stone formation are multifactorial, including age, gender, ethnic origin, family history, environmental factors, geography and diet
- Ureteric colic is the most common acute presentation. NCCT is the investigation of choice
- Decreased animal protein intake, decreased salt intake and adequate fluid intake are necessary to prevent recurrence
- Complete removal and long-term antibiotics are important to prevent recurrence of infection stones

TRAUMA TO KIDNEYS AND URETERS

Renal trauma

Kidneys are retroperitoneal structures; they are relatively fixed by their vascular pedicles and are well protected by perinephric fat, strong posterior abdominal wall muscles and the lower rib cage. Renal trauma is usually a part of polytrauma and is present in only 5% of all trauma cases.

Mechanism of injury

Trauma may be penetrating or blunt, the latter being far more common. Common modes of injuries are head-on collisions in road traffic accidents, falls from height and contact sports. Sudden, rapid deceleration can cause avulsion injury to the ureters at the PUJ or renal pedicle. Penetrating injuries cause direct tissue disruption and are usually associated with adjacent organ injuries.

Presentation

Patients with polytrauma may present with loss of consciousness and haemodynamic shock because of associated injuries. Haematuria – gross or microscopic – is pathognomonic of renal trauma; however, its absence does not exclude serious renal trauma. Similarly, the severity of renal trauma does not correlate with the degree of haematuria. Trauma causing lower rib fractures with or without vertebral fractures and abdominal pain with flank contusions should raise suspicion about the underlying renal injury and should be evaluated further.

Management

CECT of the abdomen is necessary to delineate the type and extent of renal injury. It provides information about the presence of parenchymal laceration, its depth, extension into the pelvicalyceal system and the extent of urinary extravasation (*Figure 82.11*). It also provides valuable information about other abdominal injuries and the status of the contralateral kidney. Based on the CECT, renal injuries are classified according to the renal injury scale of the American Association for the Surgery of Trauma (*Figure 82.12*).

Common indications for CECT in abdominal trauma include:

- abdominal trauma with gross haematuria;
- microscopic haematuria with hypotension (systolic <90 mmHg);
- rapid deceleration injury;
- children with microscopic haematuria (>5 red blood cells [RBCs]);
- all penetrating injuries.

Conservative management with close surveillance is sufficient in the majority of cases of isolated renal trauma. Lower grade injuries, sometimes including grade IV, can be managed conservatively with bed rest, antibiotics in case of penetrating injuries and serial haemoglobin estimation. Reimaging is usually done after 2–4 days in cases of falling haemoglobin levels, fever or expanding flank mass. Persistent urinary leak can be managed with an internal DJ stent or PCN.

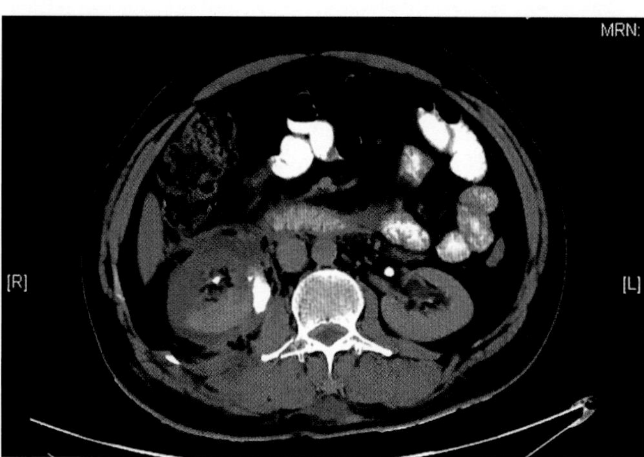

Figure 82.11 Axial image showing pelviureteric injury with contrast in the peripelvic region (courtesy of Department of Urology, Christian Medical College, Vellore, India).

Indications for emergency surgical exploration are:

- expanding or pulsatile retroperitoneal haematoma;
- PUJ avulsion;
- renal pedicle injury;
- haemodynamic instability.

Ureteral trauma

Most ureteral injuries are iatrogenic and occur during surgery near the ureter. Gunshot or penetrating injuries to the abdomen can cause ureteric injury. Management of ureteral injuries as a result of external trauma is dictated by the severity of trauma and associated visceral injuries.

Iatrogenic ureteral injury

The overall incidence of iatrogenic ureteral injury varies between 0.5% and 1.0%. Hysterectomy accounts for most of these cases, followed by ureteroscopy. Common sites of injuries to the pelvic ureter are at the pelvic brim, where it might be injured while ligating the infundibulopelvic ligament; at the bifurcation of the common iliac artery, while ligating the internal iliac artery; or at the paracervical region, while developing the ureteric tunnel or while clamping and dividing the upper vagina.

During open surgery, ureteral injury may be identified intraoperatively. However, most injuries (70–80%) are identified postoperatively. The postoperative course of these patients can be difficult and presentation may include abdominal pain, fever or sepsis. It is not uncommon to miss ureteric injuries; if left unrecognised, they can lead to significant morbidity, such as formation of urinoma, abscess, ureteral stricture and urinary fistula.

Management of iatrogenic ureteral injury

Triphasic abdomen and pelvic CECT is the imaging modality of choice. The choice of treatment is based on the location, type, extent and timing of presentation. If an injury is recognised intraoperatively or in the immediate postoperative period, it should be surgically repaired immediately. The viability of the

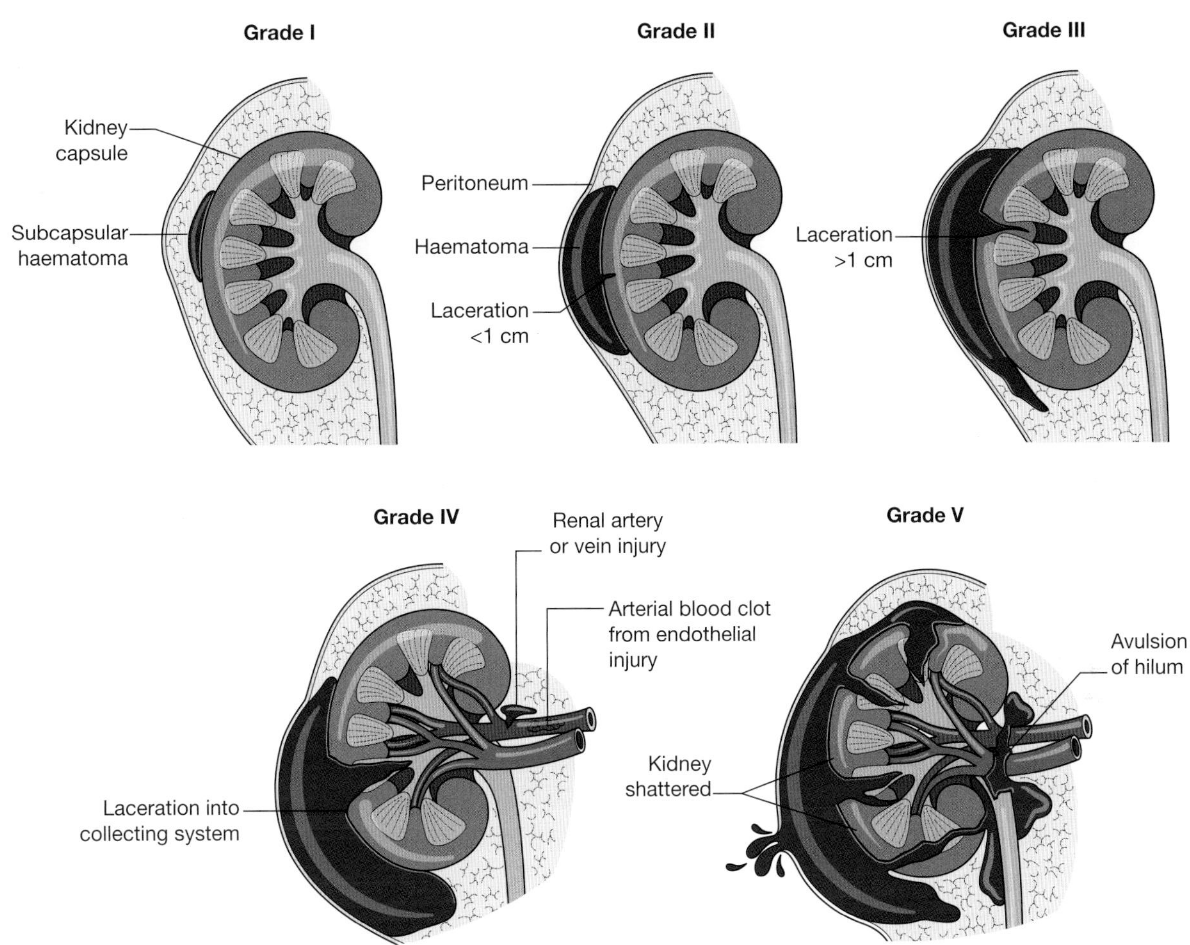

Figure 82.12 Classification of renal trauma.

ureter must be assessed. In cases of contusion, DJ stenting must be performed. In cases of partial transection, primary repair over a DJ stent may be performed. A tension-free spatulated ureteric anastomosis using fine absorbable sutures can be done for short segment loss. This is usually done in upper ureteric injuries (*Figure 82.13*). Longer segment loss, especially in the pelvic ureter, is managed by ureteroneocystostomy with or without a Boari flap. Longer defects up to 15 cm can be repaired by mobilising and hitching the bladder to the psoas major muscle (psoas hitch) with a Boari flap (*Figure 82.14*). Transureteroureterostomy (anastomosing the injured ureter to the contralateral ureter) can be an option in selected situations.

Delay in diagnosis would result in late presentation and delay the definite repair by 2–3 months to allow resolution of urinoma and periureteric inflammation. In such situations an initial endourological approach either with a retrograde ureteric stent or with PCN would decrease the morbidity associated with urinoma and help to preserve renal function.

Summary box 82.5

Urinary tract trauma

- Suspect renal injury in abdominal trauma in adults with modes of injury such as sudden deceleration, penetrating injury directed towards the renal bed, hypotension and haematuria and in children
- Triphasic (arterial, nephrogenic and delayed phase) CT is the investigation of choice to diagnose and grade urinary tract injury in a haemodynamically stable patient
- Most grade I–IV renal trauma (including penetrating injuries) can be managed conservatively
- Most ureteric injuries are iatrogenic and prompt diagnosis will prevent morbidity

TUMOURS OF THE KIDNEYS AND URETERS

Upper tract urothelial cancer

Primary urothelial neoplasms of the renal pelvis and ureter are rare. They account for less than 10% of all urothelial tumours. They are more common in adult men. Important risk factors are tobacco consumption, occupations in the dye, petrochemicals and rubber industries, analgesic abuse, high arsenic content in drinking water, exposure to cyclophosphamide and the presence of chronic inflammation. Chronic inflammatory conditions are also associated with squamous cell carcinoma.

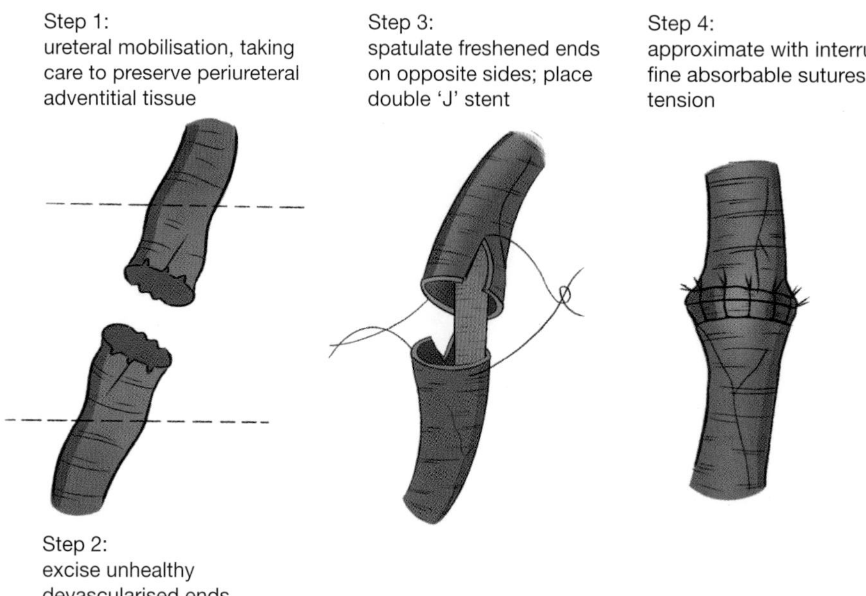

Figure 82.13 Technique for upper ureteric injury repair. Steps 1 and 2: freshen the devascularised edges. Step 3: spatulate both ends and place an internal double J stent. Step 4: approximate both ends with interrupted absorbable sutures (courtesy of Nivedita Kekre and Dr Madhuri Sadanala).

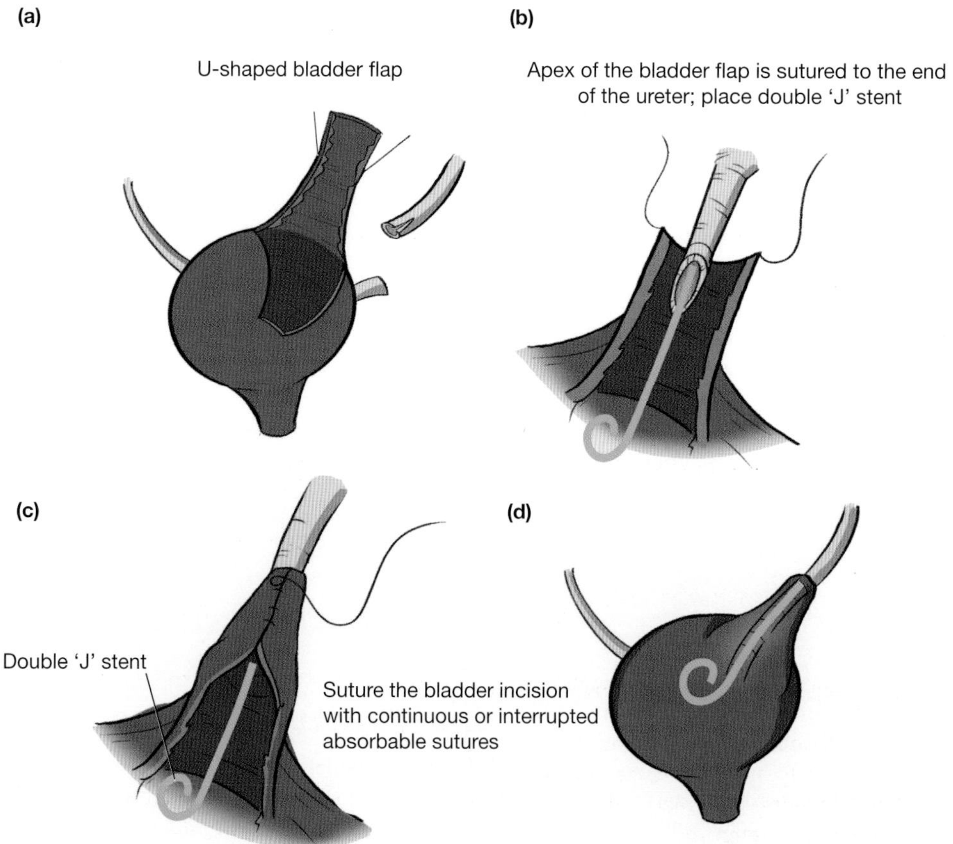

Figure 82.14 Steps of Boari flap creation. (a) U-shaped bladder flap. (b, c) The apex of the bladder flap is sutured to the ureteric end and an internal DJ stent is placed in the ureter with a distal loop in the bladder. (d) Suture the bladder incision with absorbable sutures (courtesy of Nivedita Kekre and Dr Madhuri Sadanala).

Presentation

Patients commonly present with gross haematuria, with or without flank pain and occasionally clot colic. Passage of long, slender, worm-like clots is suggestive of upper tract involvement. Patients with known bladder tumours should always be screened for upper tract tumours. Very few present with advanced constitutional symptoms and a palpable mass. Microscopic haematuria should be evaluated to exclude urothelial malignancy in the high-risk adult (chronic smokers, occupational exposure, older age) population.

Pathology

Both the PCS and the ureter have a thinner muscular layer than the bladder. Therefore, aggressive tumours of the upper tract can easily invade the muscle layers; hence, the prognosis is poor. Most of these tumours are caused by a field change; hence, tumours tend to be multifocal and may be associated with carcinoma *in situ* (CIS) in normal-looking urothelium. This also explains the higher incidence of recurrence of tumours in the bladder after successful treatment of upper tract disease. Therefore, long-term bladder follow-up with cytology and cystoscopy is necessary.

Histological grading is of great prognostic significance. Low-grade tumours follow a relatively benign course with multiple recurrences. High-grade tumours are potentially invasive with a poor prognosis. Histological variants, such as micropapillary, neuroendocrine, sarcomatoid and squamous tumours, have a worse prognosis.

Urothelial tumours can invade surrounding tissues, metastasise to regional lymph nodes and spread haematogenously to lungs, liver and bones.

Squamous cell and adenocarcinoma are rare non-urothelial malignancies involving the upper tract. They usually present at an advanced state and have a very poor prognosis. Squamous cell carcinoma occurs predominantly in the renal pelvis.

Diagnosis

Urinalysis may reveal numerous RBCs and white blood cells. Urine cytology should be obtained. The presence of atypical or malignant cells in a freshly voided sample has a high specificity for urothelial malignancies. CTU, cystoscopy, retrograde pyelogram and flexible ureterorenoscopy are required for diagnosis.

CTU is the investigation of choice. Findings suggestive of urothelial carcinoma are radiolucent filling defects, incomplete visualisation of calyces and the presence of hydronephrosis. CT also provides important staging information about local spread and lymph node involvement. Flexible ureterorenoscopy may be used to visualise the ureter, renal pelvis and collecting system and to biopsy suspicious lesions. URS biopsies can determine tumour grade and help in planning treatment. Incorporation of narrow-band imaging and blue light have improved the diagnostic capability of ureterorenoscopy.

Staging

Staging of upper tract urothelial cancer is similar to that for urothelial bladder cancer by the TNM system.

Prognostic factors

Unifocal, small (<1 cm), low-grade disease with no evidence of invasion on CTU is characterised as a low-risk tumour. Upper tract urothelial cancers that invade the muscle wall usually have poor prognosis. The 5-year survival is <50% and <10% for pathologically proven T2/T3 and T4 tumours, respectively.

Management

The management depends upon the stage, grade and risk stratification.

Low-risk localised tumours may be managed with endoscopic ablation or segmental excision. Kidney-sparing surgery is important in patients with solitary kidney, renal insufficiency and synchronous bilateral tumours.

High-risk tumours warrant radical nephroureterectomy with bladder cuff resection with or without lymphadenectomy.

Locally advanced disease is usually treated with cisplatinum-based neoadjuvant chemotherapy to downstage the disease prior to surgical ablation. Adjuvant chemotherapy has been shown to improve survival.

Benign renal tumours

Incidental detection of renal lesions has increased owing to the widespread use of abdominal imaging. The lesions may be cystic or solid. Solid renal tumours should be considered malignant unless proven otherwise.

Renal oncocytoma

This derives its name from its cellular appearance on histopathology, where uniformly highly granular eosinophilic cytoplasm owing to abundant mitochondria (oncocyte) is seen. It accounts for around 5% of renal tumours. It appears as an enhancing mass on cross-sectional imaging and is difficult to differentiate from RCC. Both RCC and oncocytoma present at around the seventh decade and have a male preponderance. It coexists with RCC in approximately 10% of cases.

The characteristic radiological features on axial imaging are the presence of central stellate scarring and a spoke wheel appearance in the angiographic phase. Nephron-sparing surgery, such as partial nephrectomy, should be the preferred option, whenever feasible. The diagnosis is usually confirmed after removal. Histologically, it can be confused with chromophobe RCC, particularly the eosinophilic variant. They may be differentiated by the use of immunohistochemistry staining, where chromophobe RCC stains positive for cytokeratin-7.

Renal angiomyolipoma

Angiomyolipoma comprises a composite mix of fat tissue with dysmorphic blood vessels and smooth muscle. It is most often detected incidentally and has a female preponderance. Angiomyolipoma may be associated with syndromes such as the tuberous sclerosis complex or it may be sporadic in nature. Spontaneous acute haemorrhage into the mass can present with loin pain. Pregnancy is a potential risk factor for bleeding.

US shows a bright echogenic mass lesion on account of the high fat content. CT scan shows an intralesional fat density of –15 to –20 Hounsfield units (HU) within the mass, which is the hallmark of an angiomyolipoma radiological diagnosis. Management depends upon the size of the tumour, the risk of haemorrhage and the symptoms. Tumours <4 cm can be followed up. Nephron-sparing surgery such as partial nephrectomy is the preferred option. Angioembolisation is the preferred modality of choice in the setting of acute haemorrhage. Drugs that inhibit this pathway (mTOR pathway), such as everolimus and sirolimus, have recently been shown to have excellent response rates in this subgroup of patients with the tuberous sclerosis complex who have activation of the tumorigenic mTOR pathway.

Juxtaglomerular cell tumour

These are extremely rare tumours that occur at a young age, often presenting with hypertension and hypokalaemia with high renin levels. These tumours are unique in that hypertension resolves with surgery.

Renal cell carcinoma

RCC is the most common solid neoplasm of the kidney. It accounts for around 90% of renal tumours and constitutes 2–5% of all cancers in adult men and 1–3% in adult women. There has been a recent steady increase in the incidence of RCC. It may be sporadic or familial.

Familial renal cell carcinoma

von Hippel–Lindau (VHL) syndrome is the most common familial syndrome associated with RCC.

VHL disease is a rare autosomal dominant disorder that is characterised by multiple pathologies, including clear-cell RCC (ccRCC), phaeochromocytoma, retinal angiomas and haemangioblastomas of the brainstem, cerebellum or spinal cord.

Aetiology

Cigarette smoking, obesity and hypertension are the major risk factors associated with RCC. Others include diuretics, occupational exposure to petrochemicals and dyes and ARCD in patients on long-term haemodialysis.

Clinical presentation

The classic triad of flank pain, haematuria and a palpable mass is now uncommon as most renal masses are detected incidentally. Symptoms and signs may be non-specific. The most common presenting symptom is haematuria. Patients may have constitutional symptoms such as fever, malaise and weight loss in advanced disease. Advanced disease can present with bilateral lower limb oedema or recent-onset non-reducing right-sided varicocele owing to thrombus in the IVC.

Paraneoplastic syndromes (PNSs) are found in up to one-third of patients with RCC. The most common PNS is an elevated erythrocyte sedimentation rate (ESR) followed by hypertension, anaemia and hypercalcaemia. Up to a quarter of the patients may have evidence of metastatic disease on presentation. The most common site of metastasis is the lung and is classically described as **cannon ball** metastases. Metastases may occasionally present as pathological fractures.

Pathology

ccRCC is histologically an adenocarcinoma arising from the proximal renal tubular epithelium. They are slow growing and bulge out of the renal contour (*Figure 82.15*). Most are solitary, but bilateral and multiple tumours are found in familial RCC. The prognosis of ccRCC varies depending on various histopathological features, such as nuclear grading. Other histological variants are papillary RCC, chromophobe RCC and, rarely, collecting duct carcinoma and renal medullary carcinoma. *Table 82.2* summarises the salient features of subtypes of RCC.

The tumour can spread directly, invading the perinephric tissue through the capsule or at times directly extending into the renal vein as a tumour thrombus. Vein wall invasion is associated with poor prognosis.

Diagnosis

Laboratory findings

Evaluation should include blood count, ESR, serum creatinine, liver function tests, lactate dehydrogenase (LDH), corrected serum calcium, coagulation markers and urine analysis. Increased alkaline phosphatase should prompt further investigation to rule out liver and skeletal metastases. LDH is useful in risk stratification of metastatic disease.

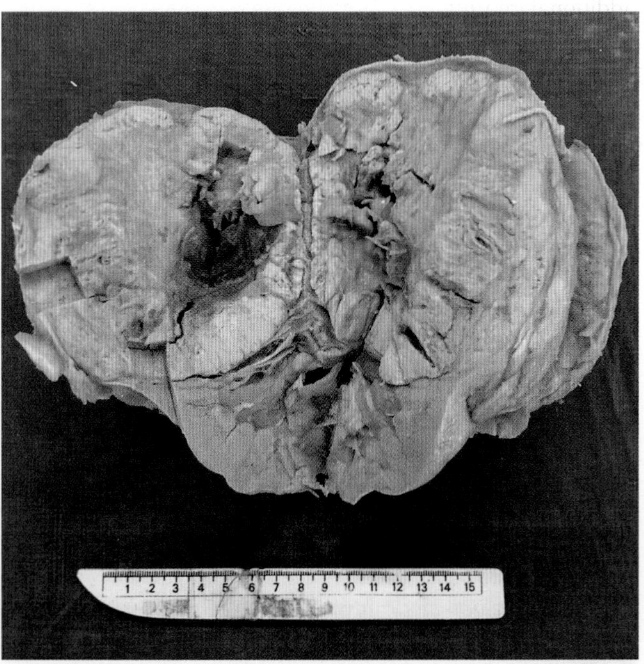

Figure 82.15 Cut surface of a kidney showing a large, well-demarcated clear-cell renal cell carcinoma in the upper pole with foci of yellowish areas signifying the lipid content of the tumour (courtesy of Dr Vikram Raj Gopinathan, Department of Pathology; photo credit: Sekhar, Christian Medical College, Vellore, India).

Eugen von Hippel, 1867–1939, Professor of Ophthalmology, Göttingen, Germany, first described angiomas in the eye in 1904.
Arvid Vilhelm Lindau, 1892–1958, Swedish pathologist, described angiomas of the cerebellum and spine in 1927.

TABLE 82.2 Classification and salient features of subtypes of renal cell carcinoma (RCC).

RCC subtype	Salient features
Clear-cell RCC	• Most common subtype • Usually sporadic • May be associated with loss of chromosome 3p and a mutated von Hippel–Lindau gene
Papillary (type I and II) RCC	• Second most common • Usually sporadic but may be familial • Type 1 tumour has a better prognosis than type 2
Chromophobe RCC	• Usually sporadic but may be familial • Good prognosis
Collecting duct carcinoma	• Uncommon (1–2%) • Aggressive tumour • Arises from the renal medulla, hence centrally located tumour
Renal medullary carcinoma	• Rare (<0.5%) • Very aggressive • Associated with a younger age and sickle cell trait • Centrally located tumour

Radiological investigations

Although US can diagnose the tumour, triphasic CECT is the investigation of choice for diagnosis and staging. RCC typically shows contrast enhancement after contrast injection (a change of >15 HU is considered significant). The CT also provides additional information on the function of the opposite kidney, primary tumour extension, venous involvement, enlargement of regional lymph nodes, the status of the adrenal glands and intra-abdominal metastatic disease (*Figure 82.16*). MRI provides similar information to CT, but can be superior at detecting tumour infiltration into the vein wall and the level of thrombus.

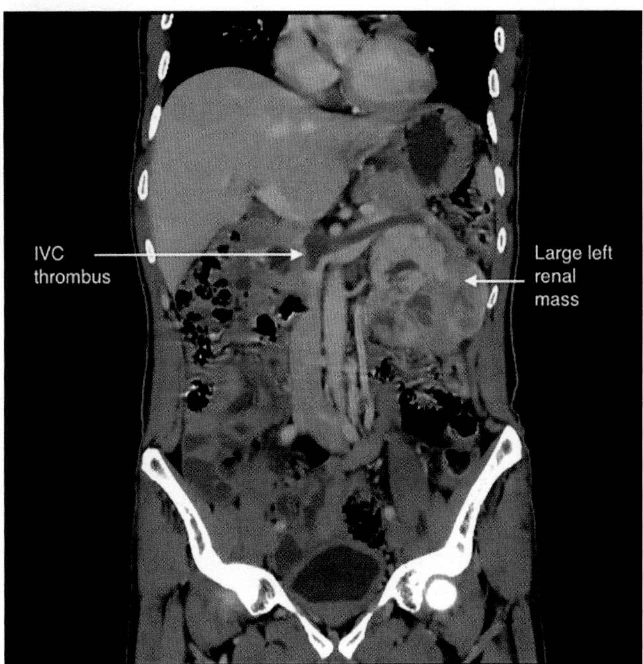

Figure 82.16 Contrast-enhanced computed tomogram showing a left renal mass with left renal vein thrombus extending into the inferior vena cava (IVC) (hypoattenuated linear area within the IVC) (courtesy of Department of Urology, Christian Medical College, Vellore, India).

A chest radiograph should be obtained in all cases. A bone scan is necessary in a patient with elevated alkaline phosphatase, bone pain or hypercalcaemia.

Tumour staging

The treatment and prognosis of RCC depends on its pathological staging. The most important factors are the size of the tumour and whether it is confined within the renal capsule and Gerota's fascia. Involvement of the lymph nodes, renal sinus and vein wall are associated with a poorer prognosis than the presence of tumour thrombus in the renal vein or IVC. Currently the most commonly used system for staging RCC is the TNM classification (*Figure 82.17*).

Prognostic factors

Currently, the grading system proposed by the International Society of Urological Pathology (WHO/ISUP) is used for grading renal cancer. Anatomical factors such as tumour size, venous invasion, renal capsular invasion and adrenal involvement herald a poorer prognosis. Certain histological types, e.g. sarcomatoid, have a worse prognosis.

Management

Nephron-sparing surgery

Radical nephrectomy remains the gold standard treatment for localised disease. However, with the recent increase in incidental detection of small renal masses (tumours <4 cm), more nephron-sparing surgery is being performed. Partial nephrectomy should be the treatment of choice in tumours less than 4 cm, in well-selected tumours between 4 and 7 cm, in bilateral tumours, in tumours in solitary kidneys and in patients with pre-existing renal dysfunction. Minimally invasive techniques by laparoscopy or robots have reduced postoperative morbidity. Because of the limitation of ischaemia time, minimally invasive techniques should be reserved for tumours with non-complex anatomy, as predicted by nephrometry scores.

Alternative techniques such as surveillance, cryoablation or radiofrequency ablation of small renal tumours may be offered in patients with high surgical risk (e.g. elderly patients, patients with multiple comorbidities). Active surveillance is based on the fact that most incidental tumours detected in the elderly grow slowly and have a low chance of local invasion or metastasis.

Radical nephrectomy

Classically, radical nephrectomy involved removal of the entire kidney enclosed in Gerota's fascia with the ipsilateral adrenal gland and regional lymphadenectomy. Most are now performed laparoscopically and the adrenal is spared if there is no involvement on CT/MRI. Lymphadenectomy is indicated only in high-risk patients with large primary tumours and enlarged lymph nodes.

Dimitrie D Gerota, 1867–1939, Romanian anatomist, physician and radiologist.

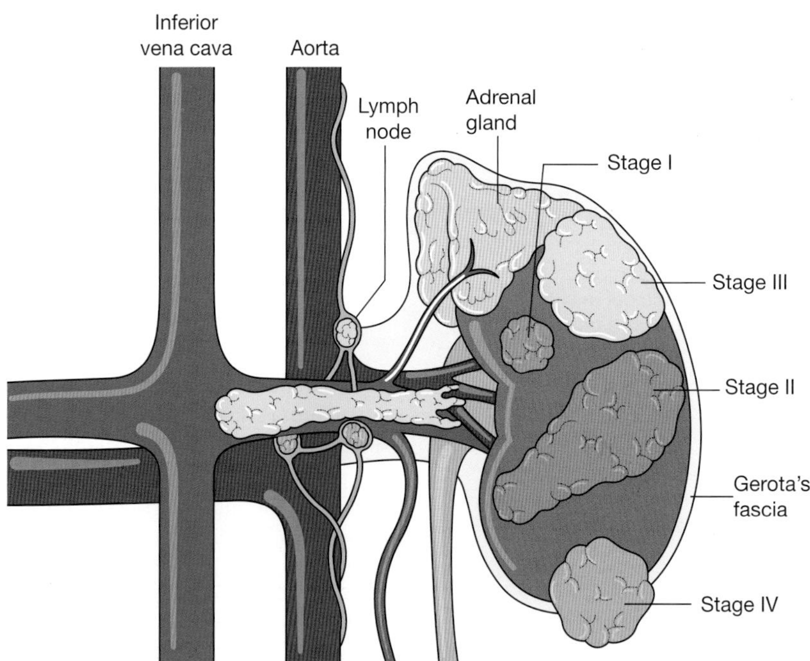

Figure 82.17 Staging of renal cell carcinoma is based on size, position and lymph node involvement:
Stage I: tumour <7 cm in the largest dimension, limited to the kidney.
Stage II: tumour >7 cm in the largest dimension, limited to the kidney.
Stage III: tumour in the major veins or adrenal gland with intact Gerota's fascia, or regional lymph nodes involved.
Stage IV: tumour beyond Gerota's fascia.

Surgical management of inferior vena cava thrombus

Renal tumours are associated with IVC tumour thrombus in 5–10% of cases. Tumour thrombus may extend as far as the right atrium. Thrombus extending to the retrohepatic or suprahepatic segment of the IVC requires full mobilisation of the liver, and thrombus extending to the right atrium may require cardiopulmonary bypass and circulatory arrest.

Management of metastatic renal cell carcinoma

Up to one-third of patients with RCC will present with disseminated disease. The International Metastatic Renal Cell Carcinoma Database Consortium risk stratification classifies a patient with metastases into risk groups based on performance status, time from diagnosis to systemic therapy, haemoglobin levels, calcium levels and platelet and neutrophil counts. The median survival of the good risk group is little more than 3.5 years, compared with just under 2 years in the intermediate-risk group. The expected median survival of the poor risk group is just over 7 months.

Tyrosine kinase inhibitors inhibit vascular endothelial growth factor (e.g. sunitinib, pazopanib) and these drugs have improved survival in metastatic ccRCC. RCC is an immunogenic tumour and responds to immunotherapy. The first generation of agents were interleukins and interferons. More recently, targeted therapy in the form of immune checkpoint inhibitors and anti-programmed death 1/programmed death ligand-1 inhibitors have been used.

Cytoreductive nephrectomy may be beneficial in good and intermediate-risk patients. Palliative nephrectomy may be considered for intractable haematuria, pain and symptomatic PNS. Angioembolisation of renal tumour can be performed in medically unfit patients with intractable haematuria.

Wilms' tumour

See also *Chapter 17*.

This is the most common tumour of childhood, accounting for 5% of all childhood cancers. They are bilateral in 5% of cases and familial in 1%. The tumour has mixed elements derived from the embryonic nephrogenic tissue, namely blastemal or undifferentiated tissue, epithelial tubules and stroma. The typical presentation is a child aged between 1 and 4 years of either gender with a large, palpable abdominal mass that may cross the midline. It may also be associated with haematuria, hypertension, fever and weight loss. Pain is relatively uncommon. The large tumour can rupture and present as an acute abdomen. Other causes of renal masses include neuroblastoma, congenital mesoblastic nephroma, RCC, clear-cell sarcoma and rhabdoid tumour.

US can confirm the renal origin and solid nature of the mass. Further definitive imaging with either CECT or MRI is necessary to stage the disease. Up to 13% of patients have bilateral tumours. The tumours usually infiltrate the kidneys and normal renal parenchyma is compressed at the periphery around the tumour (**claw sign**). A CT of the chest should be obtained as the lung is the most common site of distant metastasis. Current treatment is nephrectomy with pre- or postoperative chemotherapy. Both regimes have a comparable survival of ~90%.

Summary box 82.6

Tumours of the kidney and ureters

- Rule out urothelial malignancy in high-risk adults (chronic smokers, occupational exposure, older age) with microscopic haematuria
- Nephron-sparing surgery should be considered in small renal masses to preserve renal function, more so in patients with compromised renal function
- PNSs are found in up to 30% and IVC tumour thrombus in 5–10% of patients with RCC
- Targeted therapy and immunotherapy have improved survival in metastatic RCC
- Wilms' tumour is the most common renal tumour in children <15 years old and should be treated in a multidisciplinary setting

FURTHER READING

Brierley JD, Gospodarowicz MK, Wittekind C (eds). *TNM classification of malignant tumours*, 8th edn. Oxford: Wiley, 2016. Available from https://www.uicc.org/8th-edition-uicc-tnm-classification-malignant-tumors-published/.

Khan F, Ahmed K, Lee N *et al.* Management of ureteropelvic junction obstruction in adults. *Nature Rev Urol* 2014; **11**(11): 629–38.

Moore EE, Shackford SR, Pachter HL *et al.* Organ injury scaling: spleen, liver, and kidney. *J Trauma* 1989; **29**(12): 1664–6.

CHAPTER 83 The urinary bladder

Learning objectives

To describe:

- The anatomical, embryological and pharmacological features of the bladder
- The physiology of micturition and the neurological basis of lower urinary tract function
- The clinical features, investigations and principles of management of congenital anomalies of the bladder
- The clinical features, investigation and principles of management of urinary incontinence
- The principles of management of acute and chronic retention of urine
- The indications and technique of urethral and suprapubic bladder catheterisation
- The causes, investigations and principles of management of bladder diverticula and bladder stones
- The clinical features, investigations and principles of management of urinary tract infections and chronic inflammatory bladder diseases
- The causes, investigations and principles of management of haematuria
- The clinical features, investigations and principles of management of bladder cancer
- The clinical features, investigations and principles of management of bladder trauma

To describe and distinguish:

- Based on the clinical presentation, the types of bladder dysfunction associated with diseases of the central nervous system

APPLIED ANATOMY OF THE BLADDER

Arterial supply

- Superior vesical artery (from the umbilical artery, which arises from the internal iliac artery).
- Inferior vesical artery (directly from the anterior division of the internal iliac artery, or in females from the vaginal artery, which arises from the internal iliac artery).
- Division of the contralateral superior vesical pedicle can aid cephalad mobilisation of the bladder for psoas hitch procedures.

Venous drainage

Vesical plexuses on the lateral and inferior surfaces of the bladder drain into the internal iliac vein (the prostatic plexus in males and the vaginal plexus in females are continuous with the vesical plexus).

Lymphatics

- Internal iliac, hypogastric, obturator and external iliac chain of nodes.
- Pelvic lymphadenectomy for bladder cancer should include complete clearance of all these nodes.

Fascia and ligamentous supports

- At the posterolateral bladder neck, condensations of fascia pass forward medially and laterally to the ureter to join with the prostatic fascia; this fascia needs to be divided during cystectomy.
- The puboprostatic ligaments are well-defined condensations of the anterior endopelvic fascia; they stretch from the front of the prostate to the periosteum of the pubis and lie lateral to the dorsal vein complex.
- The urachus and obliterated hypogastric arteries, together with the folds of peritoneum overlying them, are called the median and lateral umbilical ligaments.
- Condensations of fascia also occur around the superior and inferior vascular pedicles.
- The pelvic floor organs are supported by the pelvic floor muscles, which predominantly consist of the levator ani group of muscles. The muscles are covered by endopelvic fascia, which attaches the vagina to the pelvic sidewall and is thickened laterally as the arcus tendineus fascia pelvis (ATFP). The ATFP lies medial to the obturator internus and is an important landmark into which sutures are placed for pelvic organ prolapse surgery.

Bladder

The urinary bladder is a hollow muscular organ that consists of three principal layers: lamina propria, smooth muscle and

TABLE 83.1 Spinal and peripheral innervation of the lower urinary tract.

Nervous system	Origin	Course	Neurotransmitter	Receptor	Action on bladder	Action on bladder outlet
Sympathetic	T10–L2 (thoracolumbar cord)	Hypogastric nerve	Noradrenaline (norepinephrine)	• β3-adrenergic (bladder)	• Relaxation of detrusor smooth muscle	Contraction of smooth muscle of urethra and bladder base
				• α_1-adrenergic (urethra and bladder neck)	• Inhibition of parasympathetic ganglia, thereby inhibiting detrusor contraction	
Parasympathetic	S2–4 (sacral cord 'spinal micturition centre')	Pelvic nerve	Acetylcholine	M3 (smooth muscle of bladder)	Contraction of the detrusor smooth muscle	None
Somatic	S2–4 (sacral cord 'Onuf's nucleus')	Pudendal nerve	Acetylcholine	Nicotinic (striated muscle of external urethral sphincter)	Afferent sensory nerves (stretch, temperature and pain)	Contraction of external urethral sphincter

urothelium. The lamina propria contains a rich plexus of vessels, nerves and lymphatics. The detrusor is made up of a complex haphazard arrangement of smooth muscle, which acts as functional syncytium, and elastic connective tissue, which gives the bladder its viscoelastic properties. The urothelium is an active layer that not only acts as a barrier to protect underlying stroma from irritant urinary toxins and bacteria but also has a role in afferent signalling within the bladder; defects in the urothelial lining are thought to lead to several chronic benign bladder conditions.

The bladder is made up of the bladder body (the area above the level of the ureteric orifices), the bladder base/trigone (the area below the level of the ureteric orifices) and the bladder neck smooth muscle.

INNERVATION OF THE BLADDER

The lower urinary tract (LUT) is innervated by sympathetic, parasympathetic and somatic afferent and efferent nerves, under higher control from the cerebral cortex and pontine micturition centre (PMC). The actions of the spinal and peripheral nerves on the LUT are summarised in *Table 83.1*.

Coordination of the micturition process is performed by the PMC in the brainstem and is under the control of higher centres in the cortex, thalamus and hypothalamus, which play an important role in delaying voiding until it is socially convenient.

APPLIED PHARMACOLOGY OF THE BLADDER

The two predominant neurotransmitters controlling LUT function are acetylcholine and noradrenaline (norepinephrine). Acetylcholine from the somatic nervous system causes contraction of striated muscle by activating nicotinic receptors, whereas acetylcholine from parasympathetic nerves causes detrusor smooth muscle contraction by activating muscarinic receptors. Noradrenaline is released from the sympathetic nervous system and activates β_3-adrenergic receptors on the smooth muscle of the detrusor to cause relaxation and α_1-adrenergic receptors on the smooth muscle of the bladder base and urethra to cause contraction. The underlying second-messenger mechanisms by which smooth muscle contraction and relaxation occur are shown in *Figure 83.1*. Smooth muscle contraction is dependent on calcium influx causing contraction via actin and myosin. Smooth muscle relaxation is dependent on calcium efflux back into the sarcoplasmic reticulum, mediated by the cyclic adenosine monophosphate and cyclic guanosine monophosphate pathways.

The commonly used agents, their principal actions and their side effects are summarised in *Table 83.2*.

Antimuscarinics

There are five types of muscarinic receptor, M1–5, in various organs in the human body (heart, brain, salivary glands, eye, smooth muscle). Although the M2 receptor is most abundant in the bladder, it is the M3 receptor that binds acetylcholine to cause detrusor contraction. The most widely used pharmacological agents to improve bladder function in patients with neurogenic LUT dysfunction or idiopathic overactive bladder are muscarinic receptor antagonists (antimuscarinics).

Mechanism of action

Antimuscarinics reduce bladder storage pressures, treat detrusor overactivity and improve overactive bladder symptoms. Although commonly thought to exert their effect during the voiding phase by antagonising acetylcholine released from parasympathetic nerves and thereby reducing detrusor contraction, they are now thought to exert their primary effects

Onuf's nucleus refers to a group of motor neurones located in the anterior horn of the sacral (predominantly S2) spinal cord; it is named after Bronislaw Onuf-Onufrowicz, 1863–1928, who discovered this group of cells in 1899.

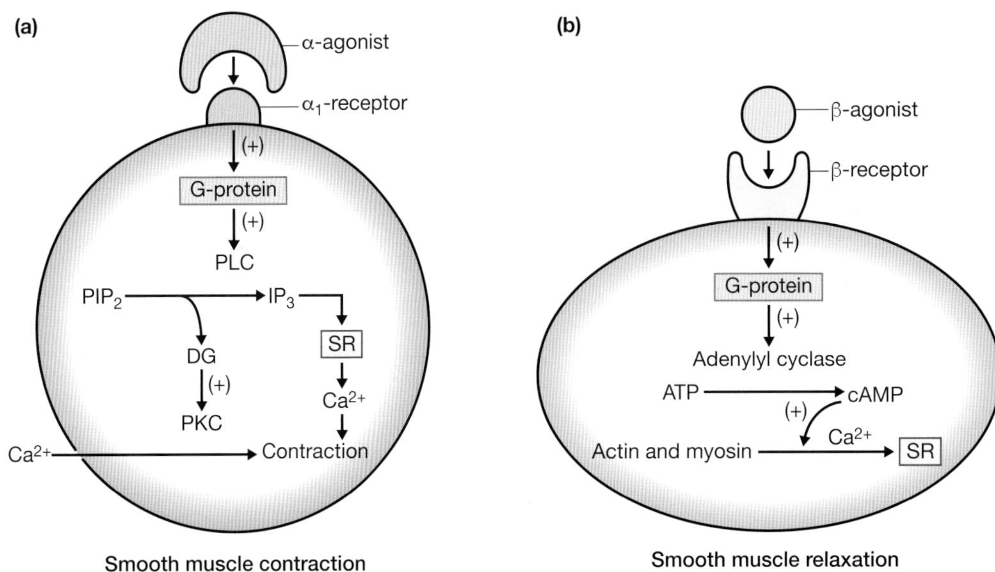

Figure 83.1 Second-messenger systems involved in (a) smooth muscle contraction and (b) smooth muscle relaxation. ATP, adenosine triphosphate; cAMP, cyclic AMP; DG, diacylglycerol; IP_3, inositol 1,4,5-trisphosphate; PIP_2, phosphatidylinositol 4,5-bisphosphate; PKC, protein kinase C; PLC, phospholipase C; SR, sarcoplasmic reticulum.

TABLE 83.2 Actions and side effects of commonly used pharmacological agents for the bladder.

Class	Examples	Action	Common side effects
Antimuscarinics	• Solifenacin • Oxybutynin • Tolterodine • Fesoterodine • Darifenacin • Trospium	• Reduce bladder storage pressure • Reduce detrusor overactivity • Improve functional bladder capacity	• Dry mouth • Dry eyes • Blurred vision • Constipation • Cognitive decline • Dizziness (postural hypotension) • Cardiac arrhythmia
β_3-agonists	• Mirabegron • Vibegron	• Reduce bladder storage pressure • Reduce detrusor overactivity • Improve functional bladder capacity	• Increased blood pressure • Headaches • Urinary tract infection • Nasal congestion
α_1-antagonists	• Tamsulosin • Alfuzosin • Doxazosin	• Reduce bladder outlet resistance from bladder neck and proximal/ prostatic urethra	• Dizziness (postural hypotension) • Ejaculatory dysfunction • Headache • Nasal congestion

in the storage phase of the micturition cycle. During the storage phase they act as antagonists of acetylcholine released from the urothelium, thereby decreasing activity in bladder afferent nerves and suppressing involuntary detrusor contractions and the sensation of urgency.

β_3-adrenoceptor agonists

β_3-adrenoceptor agonists are relatively new pharmacological agents that are used for the treatment of overactive bladder and neurogenic LUT dysfunction.

Mechanism of action

Similar to antimuscarinics, the β_3-agonists are thought to exert their principal effects during the storage phase of the micturition cycle by reducing bladder afferent activity. It is also thought that activation of β_3-adrenoceptors may downregulate acetylcholine release, resulting in inhibition of parasympathetic activity.

α_1-adrenoceptor antagonists

The α_1-adrenoceptor antagonists are commonly used to improve voiding lower urinary tract symptoms (LUTS) in men.

Mechanism of action

The α_1-receptors are densely prevalent at the bladder base, bladder neck and proximal urethra in males, and antagonism of these receptors inhibits sympathetic-mediated contraction of the bladder outlet, thereby reducing outlet resistance.

APPLIED PHYSIOLOGY OF THE BLADDER

The LUT consists of the bladder and urethra, and its two functions are urinary storage and urinary emptying. These functions depend on coordinated activity between the smooth and striated muscles of the bladder and the outlet (consisting of the bladder neck, urethral smooth muscle, external urethral sphincter and pelvic floor muscles), which is mediated by a complex of neural circuits in the central and peripheral nervous systems.

The micturition cycle

The key characteristics of the two phases of the micturition cycle are (*Figure 83.2*):

1 Urinary storage (filling):
- low pressure (normal compliance) – dependent on viscoelastic properties of the bladder wall and lack of parasympathetic input to the detrusor;
- normal sensation (absence of pain or urgency);
- absence of involuntary contractions (detrusor overactivity);
- a closed bladder outlet to enable continence – dependent on the sympathetic reflex, which increases outlet resistance (α-adrenergic stimulation), inhibits detrusor contractility (through inhibitory effect on parasympathetic ganglia) and reduces bladder smooth muscle tension (β_3-adrenergic stimulation).

2 Urinary emptying (voiding):
- coordinated detrusor contraction of appropriate strength and duration to enable complete bladder emptying – dependent on inhibition of the spinal sympathetic reflexes and activation of parasympathetic efferent pathways to the bladder;
- relaxation of the bladder neck and external urethral sphincter – dependent on inhibition of spinal sympathetic reflexes.

Disorders of the LUT can therefore be related to failure to store urine (due to the bladder or the outlet) or failure to empty (due to the bladder or the outlet).

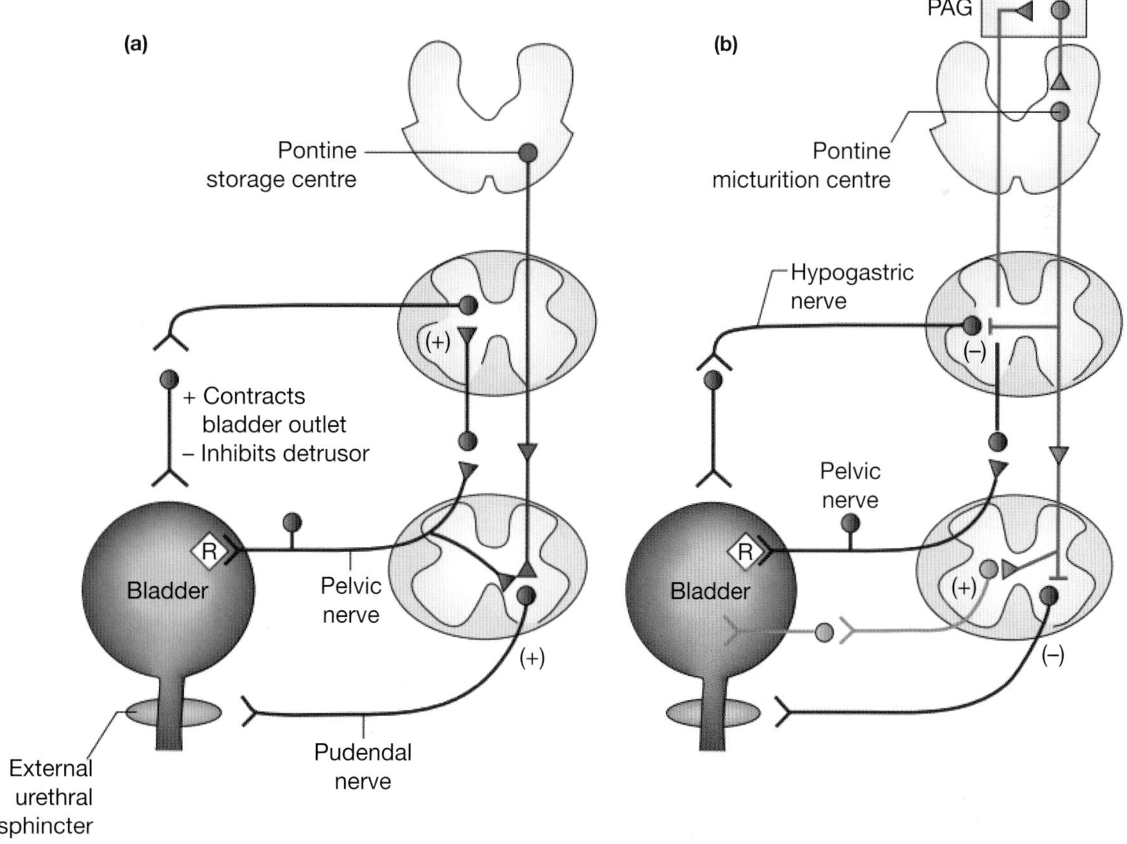

Figure 83.2 The micturition cycle and its neurological control. (a) Urine storage reflexes. During bladder filling, increased sympathetic nervous system and pudendal nerve activity leads to contraction of the bladder neck and external sphincter, and relaxation of the detrusor muscle. (b) Urine voiding reflexes. During voiding, the pontine micturition centre stimulates detrusor contraction through activation of the parasympathetic outflow to the bladder, with inhibition of sympathetic outflow to the bladder neck and external urethral sphincter. PAG, periaqueductal grey; R, receptor. (Reproduced with permission from Fowler CJ, Griffiths D, de Groat WC. The neural control of micturition. *Nat Rev Neurosci* 2008; **9**(6): 453–66.)

Neural control during the micturition cycle

Storage phase

The storage phase of the micturition cycle requires relaxation of the detrusor to ensure low-pressure filling, and contraction of the smooth and striated muscle of the bladder neck, urethra and external urethral sphincter to ensure continence. The higher centres in the cortex receive low-intensity afferent signals during bladder filling, which in turn induces the PMC to inhibit micturition by inhibiting parasympathetic innervation (resulting in detrusor relaxation) and activating somatic innervation (resulting in closure of the bladder outlet). Glutamate is the principal efferent neurotransmitter involved in activating the pudendal nerve through Onuf's nucleus. Detrusor relaxation and bladder outlet contraction are achieved through sympathetic β_3-noradrenergic activity, resulting in direct relaxation of the detrusor smooth muscle; inhibition of parasympathetic ganglia, resulting in indirect relaxation of the detrusor smooth muscle; and α_1-noradrenergic activity, resulting in contraction of the smooth muscle of the bladder neck and urethra. Furthermore, somatic cholinergic activity results in contraction of the striated external urethral sphincter.

Voiding phase

The voiding phase of the micturition cycle requires coordinated detrusor contraction and relaxation of the bladder outlet to ensure complete bladder emptying. When the desire to void is strong enough, the higher centres in the cortex receive high-intensity afferent signals from the bladder, which in turn switches the PMC to 'voiding' mode. The PMC then activates micturition by activating parasympathetic nerves and inhibiting somatic nerves (by cessation of the glutamate effect on Onuf's nucleus). This is achieved through parasympathetic cholinergic activity via M3 receptors, resulting in detrusor contraction, and central inhibition of somatic and sympathetic nerves, resulting in relaxation of the bladder outlet.

APPLIED EMBRYOLOGY OF THE BLADDER

The bladder originally develops from the cloaca, the endodermis-lined hindgut structure that is the common opening for the urinary, genital and gastrointestinal tracts. Between weeks 4 and 7 of gestation, the cloaca is partitioned into a ventral urogenital tract (the primitive urogenital sinus) and a dorsal anorectal tract by the urorectal septum (***Figure 83.3***). The portion of the primitive urogenital sinus that lies above the entry point of the mesonephric ducts becomes the vesicourethral canal, which gives rise to the bladder and pelvic urethra, whereas the portion of the urogenital sinus caudal to this entry point forms the bulbar and penile urethra in males and the vaginal vestibule in females. Initially, the superior end of the lumen of the bladder is continuous with the allantois, a sac-like structure that is responsible for embryonic nutrition and waste excretion. Between the fifth and seventh week of gestation the allantois is obliterated and becomes a fibrous cord, the urachus, which runs within the umbilical cord and drains the fetal urinary bladder. As the bladder descends into the pelvis during development, this fibrous cord elongates. Postnatally, this obliterated fibrous cord extends from the apex of the bladder to the umbilicus as the median umbilical ligament. The urachus acts as a landmark during radical cystectomy and can be traced to the apex of the bladder; identification of this structure can prevent early entry into a high-riding bladder, and the urachus is then removed en bloc with the bladder specimen.

CONGENITAL BLADDER ANOMALIES

Most congenital bladder anomalies can be detected on antenatal ultrasound after 10–13 weeks' gestation, when the bladder should be visualised in the majority of cases.

Congenital and acquired bladder diverticula

Bladder diverticula can be congenital or acquired (secondary to infravesical bladder outlet obstruction). Acquired bladder diverticula are most commonly seen in adult men with benign prostatic obstruction; acquired diverticula can less commonly be seen in children with infravesical obstruction (e.g. secondary to posterior urethral valves) or in children with neurogenic bladder associated with detrusor–sphincter dyssynergia (DSD).

Primary congenital bladder diverticula develop as a herniation of bladder mucosa through a congenital muscular defect between the intravesical ureter and the roof of the ureteral hiatus, the so-called 'Hutch' diverticulum. Congenital diverticula are therefore typically located in the vicinity of the ureteric orifice and may be associated with vesicoureteric reflux (VUR), both of which are thought to occur as a result of inadequate development of the musculature of the bladder wall or Waldeyer's fascia around the portion of the intravesical ureter, at

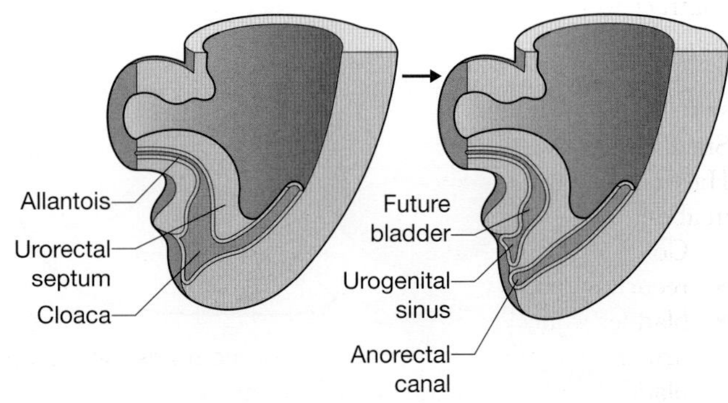

Figure 83.3 Partitioning of the cloaca to form the urogenital sinus and anorectal canal. (Redrawn with permission from Wein AJ, Kavoussi LR, Partin AW, Peters CA. *Campbell-Walsh urology*, 11th edn. Philadelphia, PA: Elsevier, 2016: 2834.)

John Hutch, 1922–1972, American urologist, described paraureteric bladder diverticula in 1961.
Heinrich Wilhelm Gottfried Waldeyer-Hartz, 1836–1921, Professor of Pathological Anatomy, Berlin, Germany. Waldeyer's fascia is a layer of fascia that divides the retrorectal space into superior and inferior compartments; it was described by Waldeyer in 1899.

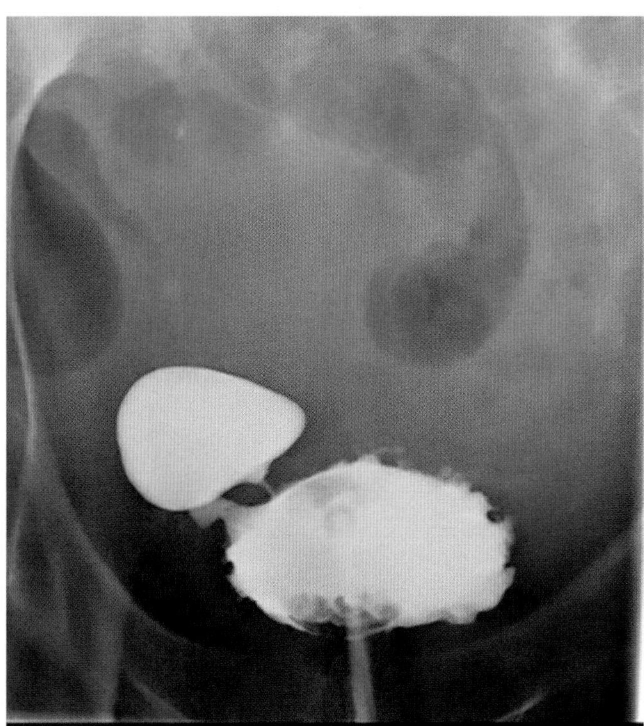

Figure 83.4 Cystogram showing a large bladder diverticulum.

the embryological junction of the ureteric bud and urogenital sinus. As opposed to acquired diverticula, intravesical pressures in those with congenital diverticula are not elevated and so the bladder is generally thin walled, without trabeculation or multiple diverticula. In adults with acquired diverticula, the intravesical pressures are often elevated, and the bladder is thick walled with trabeculations and multiple diverticula. The raised intravesical pressure causes the lining between the inner layer of hypertrophied muscle to protrude, forming multiple saccules. If a saccule is forced through the bladder wall, it becomes a diverticulum. The diverticulum is made up of mucosa with very few, if any, muscle fibre coverings. As a result, it does not contract to empty and therefore holds residual urine, which can lead to the complications described below (*Figure 83.4*).

Clinical features

Small congenital bladder diverticula are often asymptomatic. Haematuria (due to infection, stone or tumour) is a symptom in about 30%.

Common symptoms or complications include:

- recurrent urinary tract infections (UTIs);
- bladder stones (*Figure 83.5*);
- urinary retention – due to extrinsic compression of the bladder outlet by a large diverticulum;
- hydronephrosis – due to extrinsic ureteral compression by a large diverticulum;
- neoplasm (*Figure 83.6*) – account for 1% of all bladder tumours; the lack of a muscular layer to the diverticulum affects pathological staging of bladder tumours as there is, by definition, no T2 stage. Therefore, any invasion beyond the lamina propria in a bladder diverticular tumour should be staged as T3.

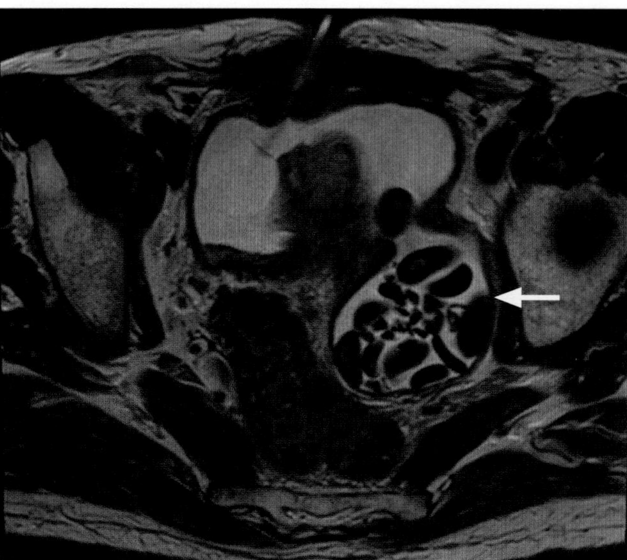

Figure 83.5 Magnetic resonance imaging scan showing a large left-sided bladder diverticulum containing stones (arrow).

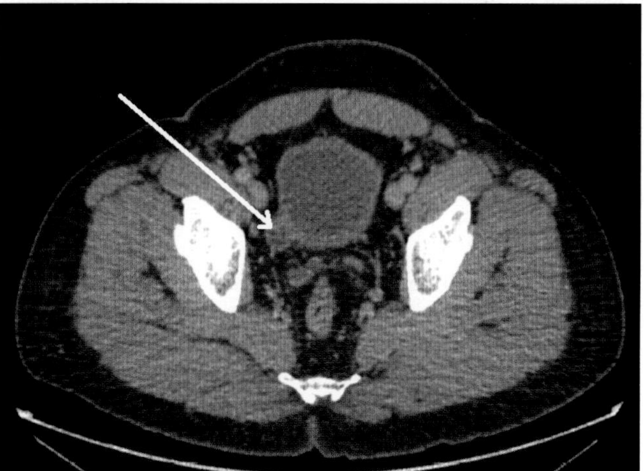

Figure 83.6 Computed tomography scan showing a bladder diverticulum containing soft-tissue material consistent with tumour (arrow).

Investigation

The diagnosis is made on imaging (ultrasound, computed tomography [CT], magnetic resonance imaging [MRI] or cystogram) or through direct vision at cystoscopy (*Figure 83.7*). Bladder outlet obstruction should be confirmed with urodynamics if suspected.

Surgical treatment of bladder diverticula

Congenital bladder diverticula should only be treated if symptomatic, or if there is concern regarding malignant transformation. Bladder outlet obstruction should be excluded by flow rate or urodynamic studies prior to any surgical intervention, and this should be treated prior to consideration of bladder diverticulectomy. Even large diverticula do not require treatment if there is no evidence of bladder outlet obstruction and the patient is asymptomatic with none of the above complicating factors.

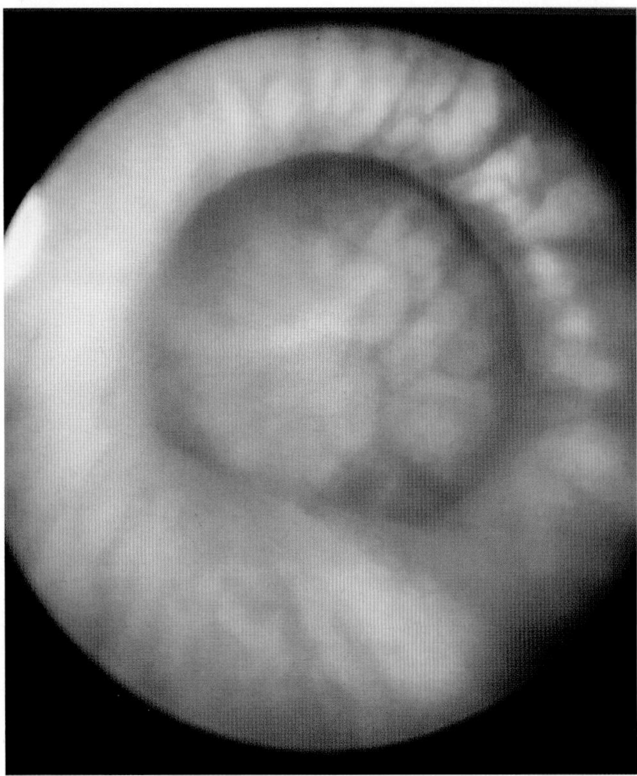

Figure 83.7 Bladder diverticulum seen cystoscopically.

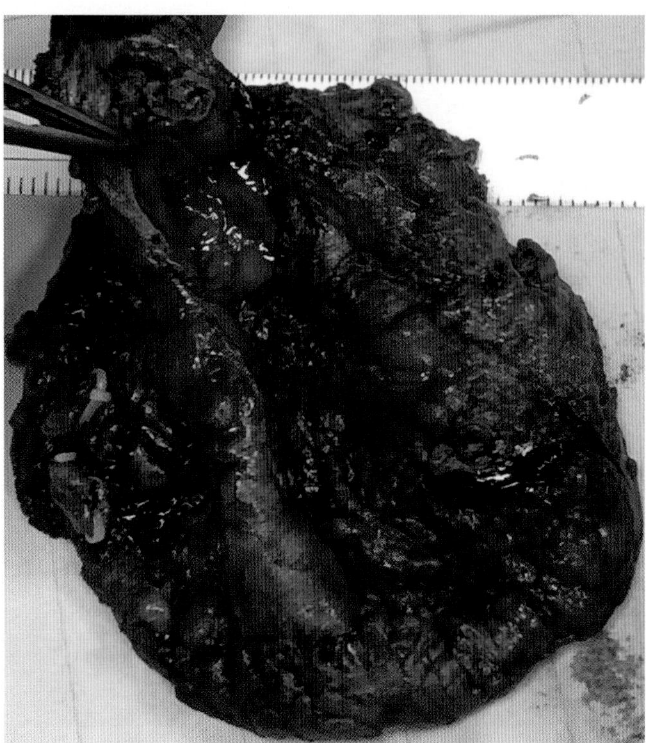

Figure 83.8 Bladder diverticulum following excision.

Surgical excision of a bladder diverticulum can be performed through an open approach (Pfannenstiel or low midline abdominal incision) or through minimally invasive (laparoscopic or robotic) techniques. Depending on the proximity of the neck of the diverticulum to the ureteric orifice, patients should be counselled about the possible need for concomitant ureteric reimplantation. Repair can be performed purely extravesically, or through a combined extravesical and intravesical approach (*Figure 83.8*).

Summary box 83.1

Bladder diverticula

- Can be congenital or acquired
- Complications include infection, stones, renal obstruction and rarely malignancy
- Bladder outlet obstruction should be identified and, if present, treated prior to bladder diverticulectomy

Bladder exstrophy

Bladder exstrophy is a congenital disorder in which failure of development of the lower abdominal wall leads to an abdominal wall defect through which the bladder is exposed (*Figure 83.9*). Diastasis of the pubic symphysis and an anterior opening of the urethra (epispadias) can coexist. The condition forms part of a spectrum of conditions ranging from epispadias to bladder exstrophy or to more severe cloacal exstrophy, the so-called exstrophy–epispadias complex. During development, mesenchymal ingrowth between the ectodermal and endodermal layers of the cloacal membrane leads to formation of the lower abdominal wall muscles and pelvic bones. However, failure of this mesodermal ingrowth leads to premature rupture of the cloacal membrane and results in epispadias, bladder exstrophy or cloacal exstrophy depending on the developmental stage at which rupture occurs. The incidence of bladder exstrophy is approximately 1 in 46 000 live births, with a male-to-female ratio of 2.3:1.

Clinical features

Exstrophy of the bladder can be associated with a spectrum of anomalies affecting the external genitalia, urinary system, bony pelvis, abdominal wall, rectum and anus.

Male external genitalia

Shortened penis due to diastasis of the pubic symphysis resulting in wide separation of the crural attachments, and congenital deficiency of the corporeal tissue.

Female external genitalia

- Shortened, stenotic and anteriorly displaced vagina.
- Bifid clitoris.

Hermann Johann Pfannenstiel, 1862–1909, gynaecologist, Breslau, Germany (now Wrocław, Poland), described this 'bikini-line' suprapubic horizontal incision in 1900.

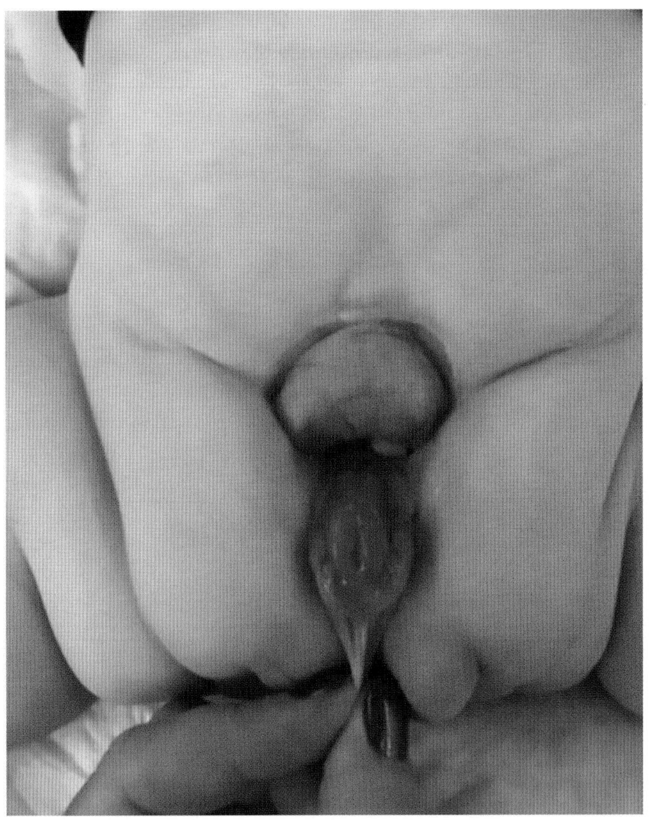

Figure 83.9 Bladder exstrophy. (Reproduced with permission from Wein AJ, Kavoussi LR, Partin AW, Peters CA. *Campbell-Walsh urology*, 11th edn. Philadelphia, PA: Elsevier, 2016: 2424.)

Urinary system

- Incompetent bladder neck continence mechanism.
- VUR due to lack of obliquity of the vesicoureteric junction.

Bony pelvis

- Widening (diastasis) of the pubic bones due to malrotation of the innominate bones, leading to a waddling gait.
- External rotation of the anterior and posterior segments of the bony pelvis, leading to outward rotation of the lower limbs.

Abdominal wall

- Low-set umbilicus with a triangular-shaped fascial defect of the lower abdominal wall.
- Higher incidence of indirect inguinal hernia owing to the lack of oblique muscle fibres of the inguinal canal and large internal and external inguinal rings.

Anorectum

- Shortened perineum and anteriorly displaced anus.
- Imperforate anus (absence of the normal anal opening) or rectal stenosis.
- Rectal prolapse.

Surgical treatment of bladder exstrophy

The aim of surgical treatment is to preserve renal function, achieve urinary continence and create functional and cosmetically acceptable external genitalia. The modern staged repair of exstrophy consists of bilateral iliac osteotomies with bladder exstrophy and abdominal wall closure in the neonatal period, followed by epispadias repair and phallic reconstruction at 6 months to 1 year of age, and finally bladder neck reconstruction and bilateral ureteric reimplantation (to treat VUR) at age 5–7 years. More recently, complete primary repair of exstrophy in the neonatal period has been advocated in an attempt to optimise outcomes with fewer procedures and without a formal bladder neck closure procedure.

Congenital neuropathic bladder

Neurogenic lower urinary tract dysfunction (NLUTD) refers to the spectrum of bladder dysfunction that can arise from congenital or acquired abnormalities of those parts of the nervous system that are responsible for normal bladder function (*Table 83.3*).

The most common congenital cause of NLUTD is abnormal development of the spinal canal (neural tube defects). The neural tube develops in early gestation (closure of the spinal canal is complete by day 35) and maternal folic acid deficiency is one of the primary risk factors for incomplete closure. Spina bifida, the most common neural tube defect, ranges in severity from mild (spina bifida occulta), in which there is only mild separation of the spinal vertebrae but no neurological involvement, to severe (myelomeningocele), in

TABLE 83.3 Common congenital and acquired causes of neurogenic lower urinary tract dysfunction.

Congenital	Acquired
• Neural tube defects • Sacral agenesis • Anorectal malformations (e.g. VACTERL syndrome) • Central nervous system tumours • Transverse myelitis	• Central nervous system tumours • Inflammatory/infective conditions of the central nervous system (encephalitis, transverse myelitis) • Vascular conditions affecting the central nervous system (infarct, haemorrhage) • Spinal cord injury • Neurodegenerative and demyelinating diseases (e.g. multiple sclerosis, Parkinson's disease) • Other encephalopathy (e.g. cerebral palsy) • Iatrogenic – pelvic/spinal/cerebral surgery • Lesions of the peripheral nervous system (e.g. diabetes)

VACTERL, vertebral defects, anal atresia, cardiac defects, tracheo-oesophageal fistula, renal anomalies and limb abnormalities.

James Parkinson, 1755–1824, general practitioner of Shoreditch, London, UK, published *An essay on the shaking palsy* in 1817.

which the neural elements and meningocele sac are everted and exposed onto the skin of the lower back.

Clinical features

The clinical features of myelomeningocele can be variable, depending on which nerves have been everted in the meningocele sac. Infants will have a visible cutaneous abnormality overlying the lower spine. In cases of spina bifida occulta, any suspicion of lower spinal cutaneous abnormality warrants further investigation with spinal ultrasound or MRI. In some cases, cutaneous lesions may be absent and, as the child grows with increasing age, tethering of the cord (fixation of the lower spinal cord due to scarring from surgery, lipoma or deep skin dimples, leading to stretching of the cord with growth of the child) can lead to the development of symptoms. Therefore, spinal investigation should be considered in any infant presenting with bladder or bowel dysfunction, failure to toilet train or lower extremity weakness, as this may be a sign of occult spinal dysraphism.

An associated Arnold–Chiari malformation with hydrocephalus is commonly seen with myelomeningocele, resulting in developmental brain abnormalities. Infants may develop urinary infections, dribbling of urine and incomplete bladder emptying.

End-stage renal disease (ESRD) is the commonest cause of death in infants with spina bifida and so early identification, surveillance and treatment of those at risk for ESRD is the cornerstone of management.

Investigation

Myelomeningocele requires surgical closure of the spinal defect immediately after birth, and so urological investigations are delayed until the patient has recovered from surgery.

- Renal tract ultrasound and postvoid residual urine measurement are required.
- Video urodynamics should be performed as soon as feasible (usually in the first 2–3 months of life) to assess bladder function.
- In the presence of VUR, a dimercaptosuccinic acid (DMSA) renal scan is recommended at 3 months to provide accurate measurement of renal function.
- In those with risk factors for renal deterioration (hydronephrosis, elevated postvoid residual, poor compliance, detrusor overactivity and DSD) early treatment should be initiated. All infants should undergo lifelong surveillance, initially with 6-monthly renal tract ultrasound and postvoid residual, and yearly urodynamics for the first 2 years to detect any deterioration in renal drainage and bladder function.

Treatment

Bladder management aims to prevent deterioration in renal function. This is dependent on achieving low-pressure storage and voiding, with complete bladder emptying.

Treatment of NLUTD depends on the baseline urodynamic findings (***Table 83.4***). The management of incomplete bladder emptying, high-pressure storage, detrusor overactivity and high-pressure voiding is centred around clean intermittent self-catheterisation (CISC) in combination with antimuscarinic therapy to reduce bladder pressure. If this fails, then intravesical botulinum toxin A (BTX-A) is injected into the bladder wall. Augmentation enterocystoplasty, in which the bladder is bivalved and enlarged using a segment of ileum, is reserved for those with ongoing risk factors for renal deterioration despite the above treatments. Patients, or parents, who are unable to perform urethral CISC should be considered for a continent urinary diversion with appendicovesicostomy, in which the appendix is used as a channel to connect the bladder with the skin of the umbilicus through which the patient can perform self-catheterisation. These management options are discussed in more detail later in this chapter.

Disorders that cause NLUTD often also lead to neuropathic bowel dysfunction (constipation or faecal incontinence) and so this should also be addressed in all children presenting with NLUTD.

Summary box 83.2

Congenital neuropathic bladder

- The pattern of NLUTD depends on the site, severity and type of neurological lesion
- The bladder and sphincter may be overactive, normoactive or underactive
- The combination of an overactive bladder and overactive sphincter represents the highest risk of renal deterioration
- An overactive bladder is treated with pharmacotherapy, intravesical BTX-A, sacral neuromodulation or augmentation enterocystoplasty
- An underactive bladder is managed primarily with CISC, or if urethral catheterisation cannot be performed, then appendicovesicostomy
- An overactive sphincter is primarily treated with intrasphincteric BTX-A or sacral neuromodulation
- Bladder and bowel dysfunction often coexist and should be addressed together

Enuresis

Enuresis, or bedwetting, describes urinary incontinence during sleep in any child over the age of 5 years, in the absence of congenital or acquired neurological disorders. Monosymptomatic enuresis (MSE) is defined as enuresis without any other urinary symptoms; primary MSE describes those who have never achieved night-time continence, whereas secondary MSE refers to those who develop enuresis after a dry period of at least 6 months. Enuresis with any daytime LUTS is defined as non-monosymptomatic enuresis (NMSE).

By 15 years of age 1–2% will suffer from enuresis and the prevalence in adults is 0.5%.

Julius Arnold, 1835–1915, Professor of Pathological Anatomy, the University of Heidelberg, Heidelberg, Germany, described this condition in 1894.

Hans Chiari, 1851–1916, Austrian, Professor of Pathological Anatomy, Strasbourg, Germany (Strasbourg was returned to France in 1918 after the end of the First World War), gave his account of this condition in 1891. The Arnold–Chiari malformation refers to a structural defect in the cerebellum characterised by ventral herniation of the cerebellar tonsils through the foramen magnum of the skull.

TABLE 83.4 Management of neurogenic lower urinary tract dysfunction.

Storage-phase disorder	Treatment options

Low compliance/ detrusor overactivity/low capacity[a]	• CISC
	• Overnight catheter drainage
	• Pharmacological therapy
	  ◦ Antimuscarinic
	  ◦ β_3-agonist
	• Minimally invasive therapy
	  ◦ Intravesical BTX-A
	• Surgical therapy
	  ◦ Augmentation cystoplasty
	  ◦ Urinary diversion

Low outlet resistance	• Bladder neck bulking agent injection • Bladder neck sling or bladder neck reconstruction • Artificial urinary sphincter
Voiding-phase disorder	

Detrusor–sphincter dyssynergia[a]	• CISC
	• Overnight catheter drainage
	• Pharmacological therapy
	  ◦ Antimuscarinic
	  ◦ β_3-agonist
	• Minimally invasive therapy
	  ◦ Intravesical and intrasphincteric BTX-A
	  ◦ Neuromodulation
	• Surgical therapy
	  ◦ Augmentation cystoplasty
	• Urinary diversion

Detrusor underactivity	• CISC • Overnight catheter drainage • Neuromodulation

BTX-A, botulinum toxin A; CISC, clean intermittent self-catheterisation.

[a]Risk of renal function deterioration.

Investigation

Three underlying pathophysiological mechanisms are predominantly implicated in enuresis and should be evaluated clinically.

1. **Nocturnal detrusor overactivity and reduced nocturnal bladder capacity**. Up to half of all children with enuresis are found to have isolated nocturnal detrusor overactivity or reduced functional capacity, in the absence of nocturnal polyuria. Patients should be investigated initially with a bladder diary to assess daytime and night-time frequency and incontinence episodes, as well as to assess functional capacity. Urodynamics should be reserved for those who fail initial therapy; if detrusor overactivity is present then patients should be managed with antimuscarinics or β_3-agonists.
2. **Nocturnal polyuria**. Increased nocturnal urine production (defined as a nocturnal urine output exceeding 130% of expected bladder capacity for age), which may be due to increased intake or underlying medical conditions, should be identified on a bladder diary and investigated further if present (e.g. diabetes insipidus, obstructive sleep apnoea).
3. **Arousal and sleep disorders**. Children with enuresis are typically unable to wake from sleep to void, and it is thought that arousal disorders may account for part of the pathogenesis of this condition. Evaluation by a sleep specialist should be considered as part of the management strategy for children in whom sleep disorders are suspected.

Treatment

The treatment of enuresis consists initially of behavioural management techniques. These include fluid modification (night-time fluid restriction, reducing sugary, caffeinated and fizzy drink intake), bedwetting alarms, star charts and rewards systems, and maintaining regular bowel habits.

If this fails to improve symptoms and the child is experiencing distress from these symptoms, pharmacological therapy should be considered. Desmopressin, a synthetic analogue of antidiuretic hormone, is best suited for those with nocturnal polyuria with normal bladder function, whereas antimuscarinics and β_3-agonists should be considered for those with low functional capacity or those who have failed to respond to desmopressin.

Urachal anomalies

Urachal anomalies are often detected after birth with symptoms of umbilical discharge or bleeding (*Figure 83.10*). However, asymptomatic urachal anomalies may be incidentally found on abdominal imaging in adults. There are four principal

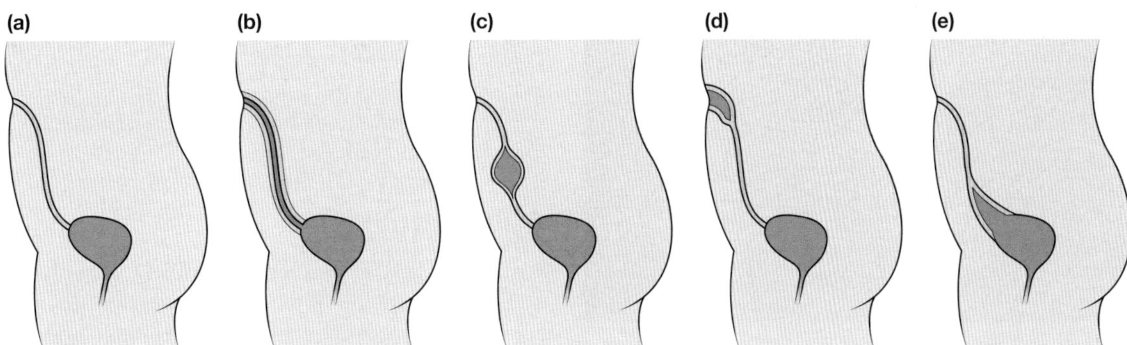

Figure 83.10 Urachal anomalies. (a) Normal; (b) patent urachus; (c) urachal cyst; (d) urachal sinus; (e) urachal diverticulum.

anomalies. A patent urachus is the result of failure of obliteration of the urachus, resulting in a connection between the bladder and umbilicus. A urachal cyst occurs when a portion of the urachus does not obliterate but there is no connection between the bladder and umbilicus. A urachal sinus occurs when the urachus fails to obliterate close to the umbilicus, resulting in a blind-ending tract from the umbilicus into the urachus. A urachal diverticulum occurs when the urachus fails to obliterate close to the bladder, resulting in a blind-ending tract from the bladder into the urachus.

Clinical features

Depending on the anomaly, symptoms include:

- umbilical discharge or bleeding;
- enlarged or oedematous umbilicus;
- lower abdominal pain;
- UTI;
- haematuria.

Investigation

In children, ultrasound or micturating cystography will demonstrate a patent urachus. In adolescents and adults, MRI will clearly demonstrate the anomaly (*Figure 83.11*). If patients present with UTIs or haematuria, thorough investigation with renal tract imaging, cystoscopy and postvoid residual measurement should be performed to exclude other more common causes for these symptoms.

Treatment

Urachal anomalies have a small risk of malignant transformation to adenocarcinoma, with high mortality rates. Complete surgical excision is therefore recommended for both symptomatic and asymptomatic cases. Surgical excision can be performed through open or minimally invasive (laparoscopic or robotic) approaches. Cystoscopy and insertion of a small catheter into the patent urachal tract can aid identification during surgery. The principle is to excise the urachus with a wide bladder cuff. The bladder is then closed in two layers. The urachus can be circumscribed and removed at the umbilicus, leaving the umbilicus intact for optimal cosmesis.

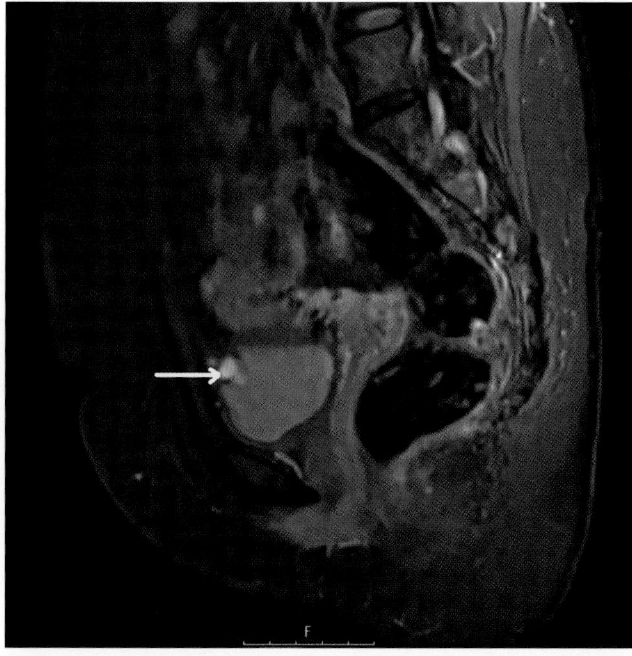

Figure 83.11 Magnetic resonance imaging scan showing a urachal cyst (arrow).

URINARY INCONTINENCE

Urinary incontinence refers to the involuntary leakage of urine. It can be classified into several different subtypes based on the circumstances leading to episodes of leakage.

- **Stress urinary incontinence (SUI)** refers to involuntary leakage on effort or exertion, or on sneezing or coughing.
- **Urgency urinary incontinence (UUI)** refers to involuntary leakage accompanied by or immediately preceded by urgency (a sudden compelling desire to pass urine which is difficult to defer).
- **Mixed urinary incontinence (MUI)** refers to involuntary leakage associated with urgency and also with exertion, effort, sneezing or coughing.
- **Continuous urinary incontinence** refers to the continuous involuntary loss of urine (this warrants investigation for anatomical pathology such as ectopic ureter or fistula from the ureter, bladder or urethra to the vagina).
- **Nocturnal enuresis** refers to involuntary leakage during sleep.
- **Incontinence associated with chronic urinary retention** refers to leakage in conditions where the bladder does not empty completely.
- **Functional incontinence** refers to leakage that results from an inability to reach the toilet because of cognitive, functional or mobility impairments in the presence of an intact LUT system.
- **Overactive bladder (OAB)** refers to symptoms of urgency with or without UUI, usually with frequency and nocturia. It can be neurogenic (secondary to a neurological condition) or idiopathic (without identifiable cause).

Urinary incontinence can occur in isolation, but more commonly is associated with other LUTS. The International Continence Society classifies LUTS based on the phase of the micturition cycle in which they occur, as storage (frequency, urgency, nocturia), voiding (hesitancy, slow stream, intermittency, straining to void, splitting of the stream, terminal dribble) and post micturition (feeling of incomplete emptying, postmicturition dribble).

Epidemiology

Urinary incontinence is highly prevalent, affecting 25–45% of men and women, and this increases with age. In men, the most common cause of SUI is radical prostatectomy for prostate cancer, with prevalence estimates of 5% at 24–36 months after surgery.

Pathogenesis

Continence is primarily dependent on normal bladder compliance, an intact urethral sphincter, strong urethral support by the pelvic floor and a leakproof mucosal seal.

Compliance is the ability of the bladder to expand in volume without any significant rise in pressure, and during the normal storage phase the bladder pressure remains low until maximum capacity is reached. This enables normal renal drainage and is dependent on the viscoelastic properties of the bladder wall (low collagen levels). However, detrusor overactivity during the storage phase, bladder muscle hypertrophy or increased levels of bladder wall collagen (e.g. due to fibrosis) can all reduce compliance and lead to incontinence and deterioration in renal drainage. This may occur as a result of pelvic surgery, irradiation, neurological conditions, chronic inflammatory bladder conditions leading to bladder fibrosis or longstanding bladder outlet obstruction.

Deficiencies in the active urethral sphincter mechanism, the urethral mucosal seal and the pelvic floor support contribute to varying degrees of SUI. Hypermobility of the bladder base and proximal urethra due to laxity of the usual supporting 'hammock', consisting of endopelvic and pubocervical fascia attached to the ATFP and levator ani, is thought to lead to displacement of the urethra out of the pelvis. As a result, during stress manoeuvres the raised intra-abdominal pressure is not transmitted to the urethra and so incontinence occurs. Laxity of the vaginal wall and pubourethral ligaments is thought to contribute to this deficiency in urethral support. These theories are the basis for retropubic suspension and mid-urethral sling procedures to treat SUI. Intrinsic sphincter deficiency occurs when the normal submucosal vascularity of the urethra and sphincter muscle tone are deficient. This may occur as a result of previous surgery, causing fibrosis, irradiation and nerve injury, or loss of oestrogenisation. Hypermobility and intrinsic sphincter deficiency exist on a spectrum and most women with SUI have elements of both.

TABLE 83.5 Predisposing and exacerbating factors for urinary incontinence (UI)

Predisposing	Exacerbating
• Familial (increased risk in those with family history of UI) • Congenital or acquired anatomical abnormalities (e.g. ectopic ureter, urinary tract fistulae, urethral diverticulum) • Neurological conditions (e.g. spina bifida, spinal cord injury, Parkinson's disease, stroke, multiple sclerosis) • Pregnancy and childbirth • Pelvic surgery • Pelvic radiotherapy • Chronic inflammatory conditions resulting in bladder fibrosis (tuberculous cystitis, ketamine cystitis, interstitial cystitis)	• Age • Obesity • Increased intra-abdominal pressure (chronic cough, straining due to constipation, exercise) • Cognitive impairment • Restricted mobility • Urinary tract infection • Drugs (e.g. diuretics) • Menopause causing atrophic vaginitis • Fluid intake (e.g. excess caffeine)

Evaluation

When evaluating patients with urinary incontinence, the history should ascertain whether symptoms are predominantly SUI, UUI or MUI, and should assess their impact on the patient's quality of life. Predisposing and exacerbating factors should be treated where possible (*Table 83.5*). The body mass index (BMI) should be noted and patients advised to lose weight if this is elevated. Abdominal examination to identify a palpable bladder suggestive of chronic urinary retention, and vaginal examination to assess pelvic floor tone and oestrogenisation status and to identify pelvic organ prolapse, should also be performed. Neurological examination to assess anal tone and sensation and lower limb function will aid identification of a neurological lesion.

Investigation

Investigation should aim to identify predisposing or exacerbating factors for urinary incontinence, as well as any features that may have a detrimental outcome on treatment (e.g. BMI). The following investigations are recommended:

1 Urinalysis – to identify UTI.
2 Flow rate and postvoid residual measurement – to identify voiding dysfunction or urinary retention.
3 Three-day bladder diary – to assess daytime and night-time frequency episodes, polyuria (the production of >2.8 litres of urine in 24 hours in adults), nocturnal polyuria (>20–33% of urine production occurs at night), functional capacity (based on voided volumes) and incontinence episode frequency.

The following investigations should be considered if conservative and pharmacological measures have failed to improve symptoms, if there is suspicion of underlying anatomical or neurological pathology based on the history and examination or in cases of recurrent urinary incontinence after previous surgery.

1 CT urogram or MRI will identify an ectopic ureter or ureterovaginal or vesicovaginal fistula (VVF). MRI should be performed if there is suspicion of a urethral diverticulum.
2 Cystourethroscopy in cases where fistula or iatrogenic bladder or urethral pathology is suspected (e.g. following previous incontinence surgery).
3 Urodynamics/video urodynamics – this test is used to assess the pressure–volume relationship of the bladder during the storage and voiding phases of the micturition cycle. In the investigation of urinary incontinence, urodynamics is recommended in the following situations:
   - MUI (SUI with UUI or overactive bladder symptoms);
   - suspicion of voiding dysfunction or neurological LUT dysfunction;
   - previous failed anti-incontinence surgery;
   - prior to invasive treatment.

Urodynamics (filling and voiding cystometry)

Urodynamic investigation is used to measure the detrusor pressure during filling and voiding. The detrusor pressure cannot

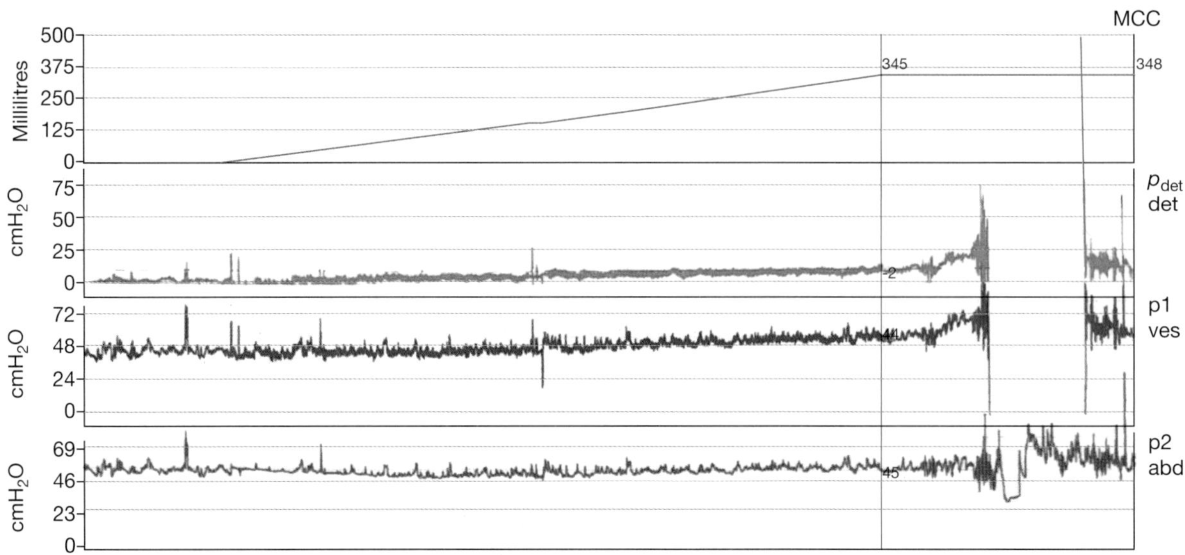

Figure 83.12 Urodynamic trace showing normal bladder storage and voiding. The red line represents intra-abdominal pressure (p_{abd}) and the blue line intravesical pressure (p_{ves}). The subtracted pressure – the detrusor pressure (p_{det}) – is shown by the orange line. During filling, there is no rise in p_{det}, which represents a normal bladder storage phase. abd, intra-abdominal; det, detrusor; MCC, maximum cystometric capacity; p1, pressure 1; p2, pressure 2; ves, intravesical.

be measured directly and so it is derived from subtracting the intra-abdominal pressure from the intravesical pressure (*Figure 83.12*).

- **Technique**. A 6Fr or 8Fr transurethral pressure-measuring catheter is inserted into the bladder to measure the intravesical pressure (p_{ves}), and another is inserted into the rectum (or vagina) to measure the intra-abdominal pressure (p_{abd}). The detrusor pressure (p_{det}) can then be derived by subtracting intra-abdominal pressure from intravesical pressure.
- **Storage phase**. The bladder is filled with saline through the transurethral catheter at a steady rate (usually 50 mL/min in non-neurogenic patients) and the following observations are recorded: cystometric capacity, compliance of the bladder (the relationship between the change in bladder volume and the change in detrusor pressure), bladder sensations and the presence of phasic rises in detrusor pressure (detrusor overactivity) (*Figure 83.13*). Any incontinence associated with phasic rises in detrusor pressure represents UUI. Stress tests (e.g. cough) are also performed throughout the filling phase and any leakage associated with increases in intra-abdominal pressure, in the absence of an increase in detrusor pressure, represents SUI.
- **Voiding phase**. When the patient has reached a strong desire to pass urine, bladder filling is stopped and the patient is asked to void. During voiding, a high detrusor pressure with corresponding low flow rate represents bladder outlet obstruction (*Figure 83.14*). Several nomograms to identify bladder outlet obstruction based on pressure–flow criteria exist for men and women.
- **Video urodynamics**. The addition of fluoroscopic imaging enables the diagnosis of VUR and anatomical abnormalities (bladder or urethral diverticula or fistulae) and can classify the type of SUI (*Table 83.6*). In this case, the bladder is filled with radiographic contrast.

TABLE 83.6 Blaivas–Olsson classification of stress urinary incontinence.

Type	At rest	On stress
0	• Bladder neck closed • Situated above the superior margin of the pubic symphysis	Rotational descent, bladder neck open, but no leak demonstrated
I	• Bladder neck closed • Situated above the inferior margin of the pubic symphysis	Descent less than 2 cm, bladder neck open and leak seen. No cystocele
IIA	• Bladder neck closed • Situated above the inferior margin of the pubic symphysis	Descent more than 2 cm, bladder neck open and leak seen. Cystocele seen
IIB	• Bladder neck closed • Situated below the inferior margin of the pubic symphysis	May or may not be further descent, but bladder neck opens and leak seen
3	• Bladder neck and proximal urethra open at rest (in the absence of a detrusor contraction)	Obvious gravitational incontinence in the absence of significant mobility

Positions at rest and on stress refer to the bladder neck and proximal urethra.

Jerry G Blaivas, b. 1943, American urologist.
Carl A Olsson, contemporary, American urologist, with Jerry G Blavias described the radiographic classification of stress urinary incontinence in 1988.

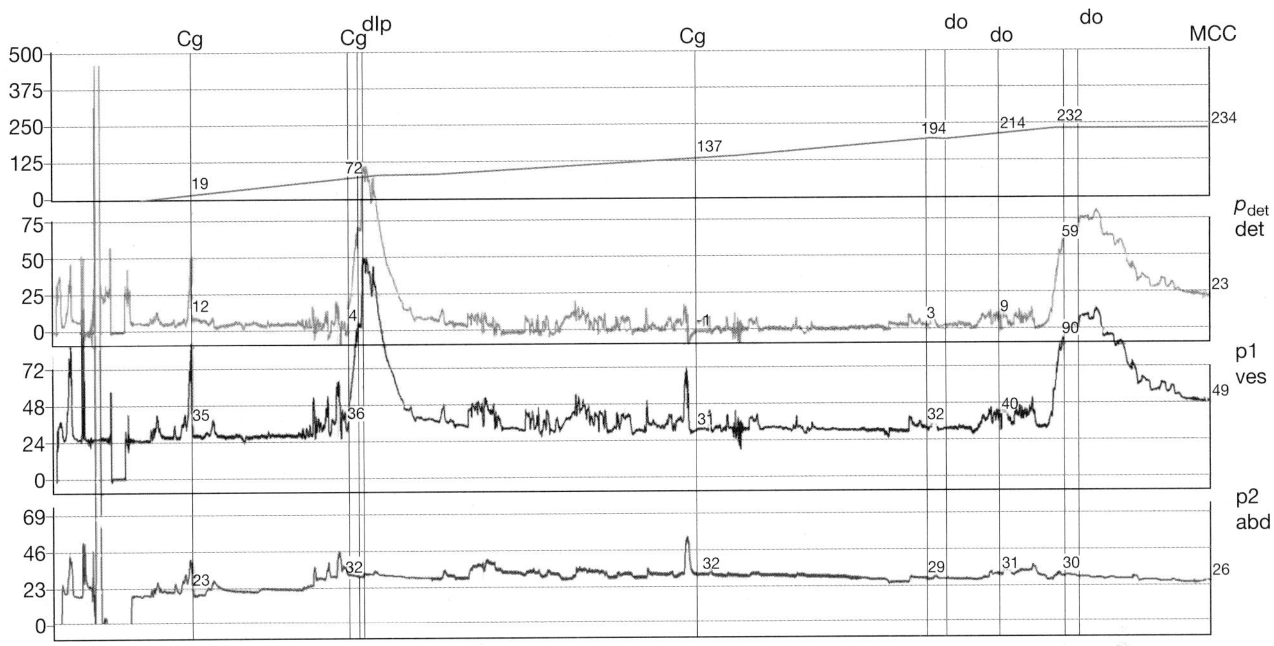

Figure 83.13 Urodynamic trace showing detrusor overactivity (phasic rises in intravesical pressure [p_{ves}] and detrusor pressure [p_{det}] without a corresponding rise in intra-abdominal pressure [p_{abd}]). abd, intra-abdominal; Cg, cough; det, detrusor; dlp, detrusor leak point; do, detrusor overactivity; MCC, maximum cystometric capacity; p1, pressure 1; p2, pressure 2; ves, intravesical.

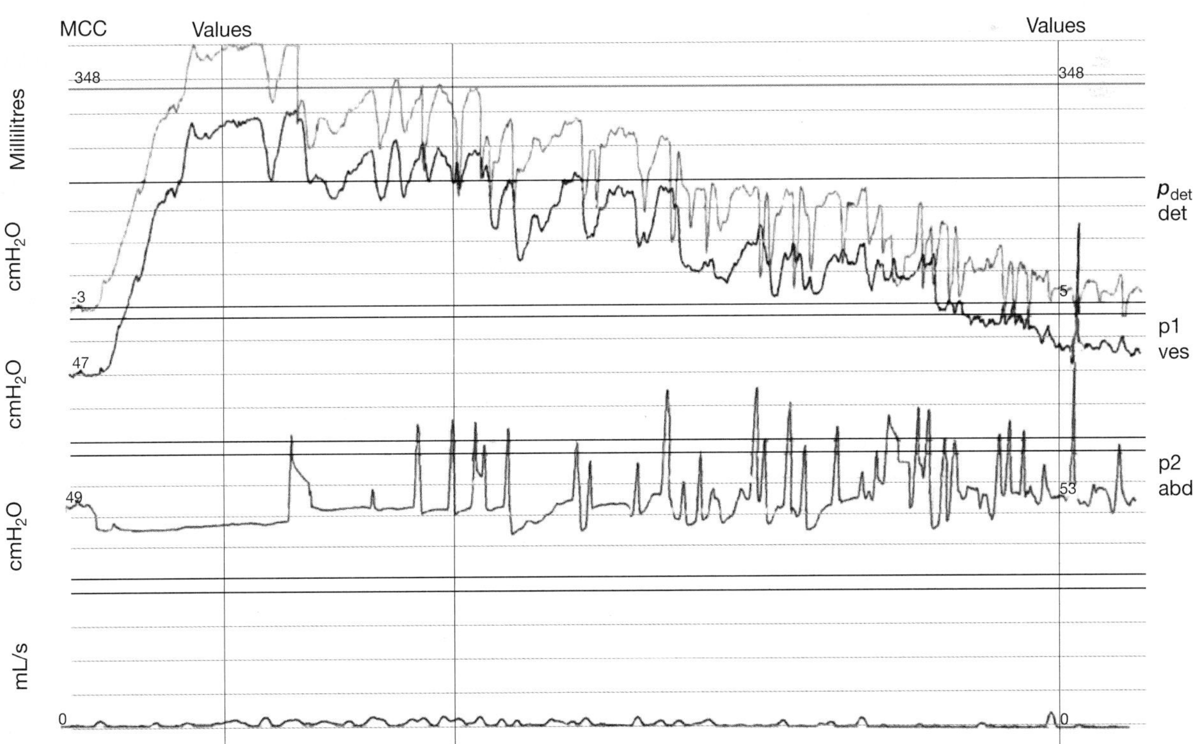

Figure 83.14 Urodynamic trace showing bladder outlet obstruction (very high intravesical pressure [p_{ves}] and detrusor pressure [p_{det}] with the low flow rate represented by the lowest trace). abd, intra-abdominal; det, detrusor; MCC, maximum cystometric capacity; p1, pressure 1; p2, pressure 2; ves, intravesical.

Treatment

Conservative

The recommended initial treatment for urinary incontinence consists of lifestyle interventions (weight loss, fluid modification, smoking cessation, treat constipation), behavioural therapy (timed voiding and bladder training) and pelvic floor muscle training.

Pharmacological therapy

Pharmacotherapy with antimuscarinics and β_3-agonists is the mainstay of management. Antimuscarinics should be used with caution in the elderly or in those who take multiple medications with antimuscarinic activity owing to the association with dementia with long-term use.

The aim of pharmacological treatment of SUI is to increase the urethral closure pressure by increasing smooth and striated muscle tone. Duloxetine, a selective serotonin and noradrenaline reuptake inhibitor, has been shown to increase sphincteric muscle activity and therefore improve urinary incontinence. However, pharmacological treatment for SUI is less commonly used than for OAB because of high discontinuation rates and reports of serious adverse events, such as mental health disorders and suicide, with duloxetine.

Invasive treatment of stress urinary incontinence in women

Several surgical options for the treatment of SUI are available, and the choice of therapy depends upon the pathophysiology of the incontinence (relative degree of hypermobility and intrinsic sphincter deficiency) and individual patient preferences.

Intraurethral injection therapy

The least invasive surgical option for the treatment of SUI is the injection of bulking agent into the urethral submucosa to improve the urethral closure mechanism and hence restore continence. This is particularly beneficial for those with a greater degree of intrinsic sphincter deficiency (type 3 SUI) rather than those with predominant hypermobility.

The procedure can be performed as an outpatient and involves injecting bulking agent into different aspects of the urethra, at the level of the bladder neck or mid-urethra, in order to obtain visual urethral coaptation (*Figure 83.15*).

Although less invasive than other surgical treatments, success rates are generally lower, with patient-reported improvement rates of approximately 60% in the short term; repeat injections are often required.

Synthetic mid-urethral sling

The synthetic mid-urethral sling has been the most commonly performed surgical procedure for SUI over the past three decades. Its less invasive nature compared with the autologous sling and retropubic suspension procedures in addition to its relative ease of insertion have contributed to its popularity. Synthetic slings are made of type 1 macroporous polypropylene mesh and can be inserted through the retropubic or transobturator routes.

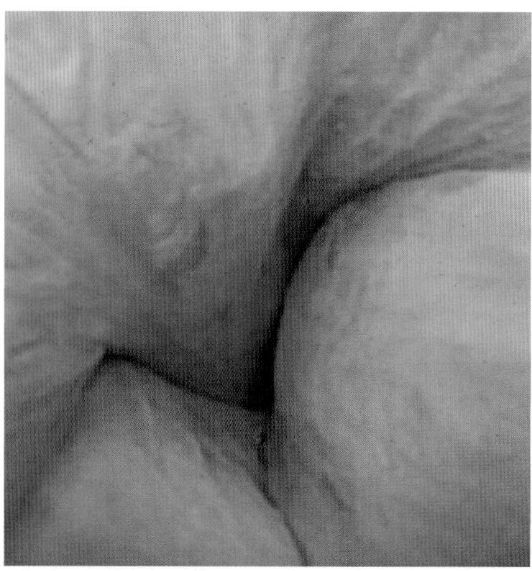

Figure 83.15 Urethral mucosal coaptation following intraurethral injection of bulking agent. The urethral mucosa can be seen to be bulging at the site of bulking agent injection, thereby occluding the urethral lumen.

A 1-cm incision in the anterior vaginal wall at the level of the mid-urethra is made, and the paraurethral space is dissected bilaterally to the pubic bone. With an empty bladder, the sling is placed through the retropubic space, exiting on the lower abdominal wall approximately 2–3 cm lateral to the midline bilaterally. Cystoscopy should be performed after sling placement to ensure that the mesh has not perforated the bladder or urethra. The sling is placed without tension. The transobturator sling is placed in a similar manner, but the sling is placed through the obturator foramen, exiting in the groin crease at the level of the clitoris.

Success rates are high with an almost 90% cure rate at 17-year follow-up, and efficacy is similar between retropubic and transobturator slings. However, increasing concerns about serious long-term mesh-related complications (erosion; chronic pelvic, groin, perineal and vaginal pain; sexual dysfunction) have led surgeons in many countries to abandon the use of these devices.

Retropubic suspension procedures

Colposuspension aims to restore the bladder neck and proximal urethra to their normal intra-abdominal position, thereby allowing equal pressure transmission to the bladder and proximal urethra at times of raised intra-abdominal pressure, and so improve SUI by augmenting the urethral closure pressure. It is recommended for those with demonstrable hypermobility and concomitant cystocele.

The procedure is traditionally performed through a Pfannenstiel incision, although minimally invasive approaches (laparoscopic, robot assisted) have been described in recent years in an attempt to reduce morbidity. The procedure involves dissection of the retropubic space (space of Retzius), the relatively avascular space between the pubic symphysis and

Anders Retzius, 1796–1860, Swedish anatomist.

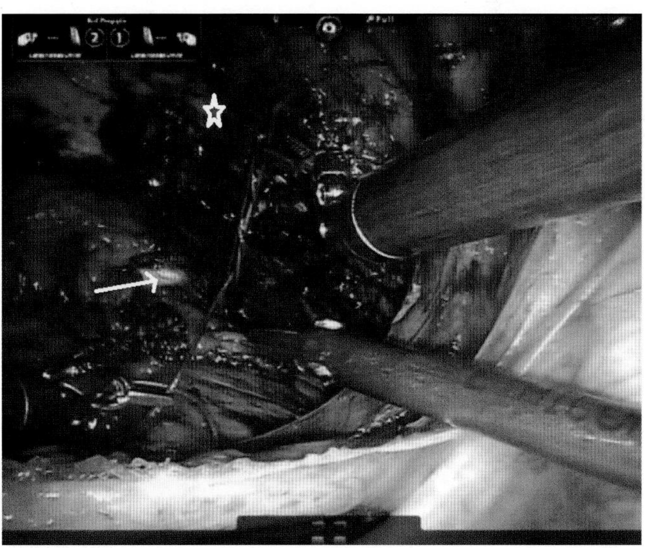

Figure 83.16 Burch colposuspension showing the suture position from the vaginal fascia (arrow) to the iliopectineal (Cooper's) ligament (star).

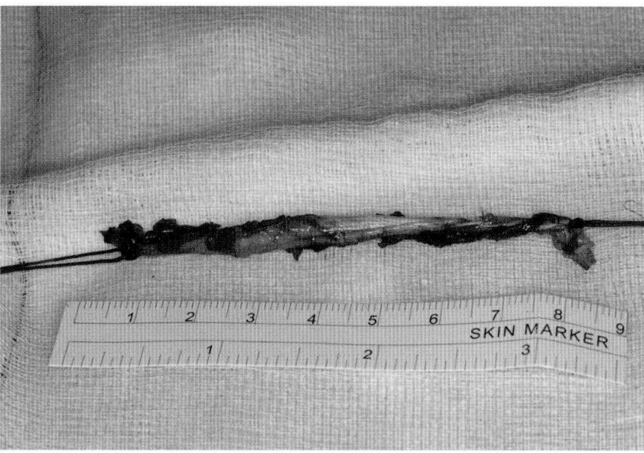

Figure 83.17 Autologous rectus fascial sling harvested and attached to non-absorbable sutures ('sling on a string').

bladder. The vaginal fascia at the level of the bladder neck and proximal urethra is exposed bilaterally and two to four non-absorbable sutures are placed 2–3 cm lateral to the bladder neck (proximal suture) and proximal urethra (distal suture) on each side. These sutures are then attached to the iliopectineal ligament (Cooper's ligament) and the knots tied gently in order to achieve elevation without tension (*Figure 83.16*). Cystoscopy should be performed following the procedure to ensure that the sutures have not been passed through the bladder.

The Burch colposuspension has good long-term efficacy with cure rates of 70–90% at 5-year follow-up. However, risks of posterior pelvic organ prolapse are higher than with sling procedures.

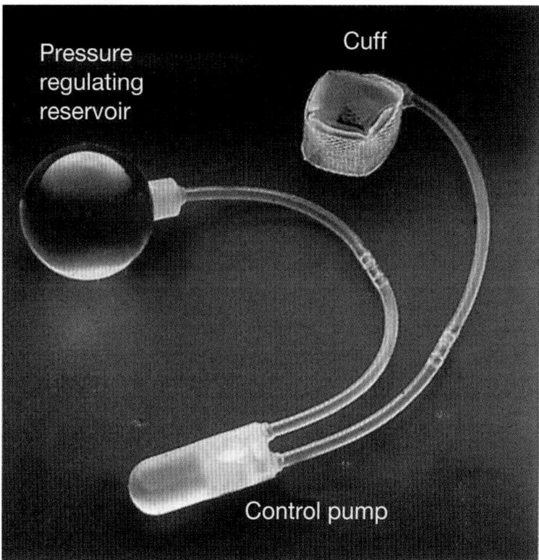

Figure 83.18 The AMS 800 Artificial Urinary Sphincter.

Autologous fascial sling

The autologous pubovaginal sling aims to improve SUI by adding strength to the mid-urethral posterior supporting 'hammock'. It is an effective and durable treatment for SUI and can be inserted 'tension-free', similar to the synthetic mid-urethral sling, or can be inserted under tension in order to provide a compressive effect on the urethra for those with intrinsic sphincter deficiency. As this sling is not a foreign body, there is very low risk of urethral erosion.

Most commonly, a strip of rectus fascia (8 × 2 cm) is harvested through a small Pfannenstiel incision, although if this cannot be used then fascia lata can be harvested from the leg using a fascial stripper. The sling is then attached to a 0 polydioxanone (PDS) suture on each side (*Figure 83.17*) and passed into the retropubic space in a similar manner to the synthetic mid-urethral sling. In patients with a greater degree of intrinsic sphincter deficiency the sling can be inserted under a greater degree of tension.

Success rates of 75% at 10-year follow-up are reported. The pubovaginal sling is a suitable option for those who have failed previous SUI surgery, irradiated patients or those with urethral fibrosis from previous urethral pathology (e.g. urethral diverticulum, fistula, mesh erosion). However, there is a higher risk of voiding dysfunction requiring CISC with this technique, as well as new onset OAB symptoms.

Artificial urinary sphincter

The artificial urinary sphincter (AUS) is considered for women with severe recurrent SUI due to intrinsic sphincter deficiency that has failed to improve after previous surgical intervention. This three-piece device consists of a cuff that is placed around the urethra at the level of the bladder neck, a pressure-regulating balloon placed in the extraperitoneal space and a control pump placed in the labia majora (*Figure 83.18*). Recent advances in minimally invasive surgery have reduced the morbidity associated with the traditional open approach,

Sir Astley Paston Cooper, 1768–1841, surgeon, Guy's Hospital, London, UK, described the ligament that runs on the pectineal line of the pubic bone in 1804.
John C Burch, 1900–1977, gynaecologist, Vanderbilt University, Nashville, TN, USA.

but the technique still requires long-term evaluation of efficacy and safety in randomised trials.

Evidence of efficacy is limited to case series from specialist centres. One of the largest series of 376 AUS implantations reported a cure rate of 85.6% at a mean of 9.6 years of follow-up, but this was at the expense of a 10-year revision rate of 30%.

TABLE 83.7 Factors contributing to post-prostatectomy incontinence.

Patient factors	Surgical factors
• BMI • Age • Prostate size • Membranous urethra length • Pre-existing LUTS • Previous TURP • Previous radiotherapy	• Fibrosis • Urethral stricture • Technique of prostatectomy (non-nerve-sparing) • Laxity of posterior support • Neurovascular bundle damage • Devascularisation

BMI, body mass index; LUTS, lower urinary tract symptom; TURP, transurethral resection of the prostate.

Invasive treatment of stress urinary incontinence in men

Post-prostatectomy incontinence is the commonest cause of SUI in men. Several factors may contribute (***Table 83.7***).

Pharmacological treatment with duloxetine has a limited role; the mainstay of treatment is surgical, with the male suburethral sling or the AUS.

The male transobturator suburethral sling is recommended for men with mild to moderate SUI and those who have not had prior radiotherapy. In cases of severe SUI or recurrent SUI or in those who have had prior radiotherapy, the AUS is the gold standard treatment. The male sling repositions the bulb of the urethra in a retrourethral position, providing additional support to the existing sphincter without causing obstruction. The AUS is occlusive. Both approaches require a midline perineal incision through the bulbospongiosus muscle. For placement of the male suburethral sling, a helical trocar is used to pass the polypropylene mesh through the obturator foramina bilaterally. Placement of the AUS requires circumferential mobilisation of the proximal bulbar urethra for insertion of the cuff, and a separate inguinal incision for insertion of the pressure-regulating balloon into the extraperitoneal space (***Figure 83.19***). The control pump is connected and inserted into a subdartos pouch in the scrotum through this inguinal incision.

The transobturator suburethral sling has reported cure rates of 66% at 3-year follow-up whereas the AUS has long-term satisfaction rates of 80–90%. Reoperation with the AUS is required in 26% in the long term for infection, erosion or mechanical failure.

Invasive treatment of overactive bladder and urgency urinary incontinence

If pharmacological therapy for idiopathic or neurogenic OAB fails, intravesical injection of BTX-A and sacral nerve stimulation (SNS) have demonstrated high efficacy in randomised trials. For those who prefer a less invasive alternative, percutaneous tibial nerve stimulation (PTNS) may be useful. Failure to respond to these minimally invasive treatments often leads to surgical treatment with augmentation enterocystoplasty or urinary diversion for end-stage incontinence.

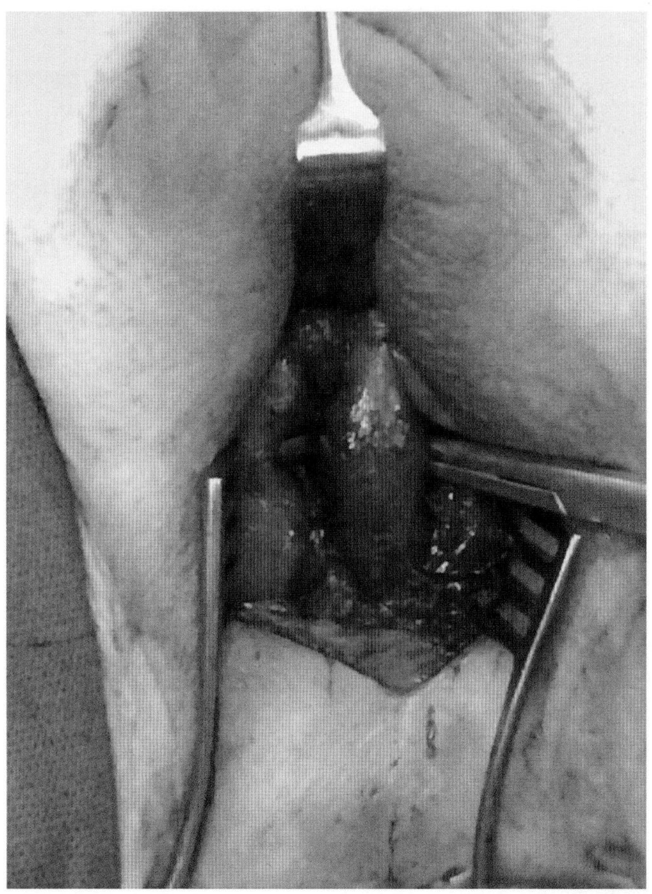

Figure 83.19 Perineal approach demonstrating exposure of the corpus spongiosum.

Intravesical injection of botulinum toxin A

BTX-A is a neurotoxin produced by the anaerobic bacterium *Clostridium botulinum*. There are seven subtypes (A–G) and type A is most clinically useful because of its longer duration of action. It is thought to have both afferent and efferent mechanisms of action.

The procedure is performed under local anaesthesia with a flexible cystoscope. Risks include UTI and voiding dysfunction requiring CISC in approximately 10%. Furthermore, symptoms typically return after around 6 months owing to regeneration of new nerve terminals, so the treatment needs to be repeated at regular intervals.

High-quality randomised trials have demonstrated the efficacy of BTX-A for both idiopathic OAB and neurogenic detrusor overactivity, with success rates of approximately 60–90%.

Sacral nerve stimulation

This treatment involves implantation of an electrical pulse generator to stimulate the S3 sacral nerve root, thereby improving OAB symptoms. The mechanism of action is not

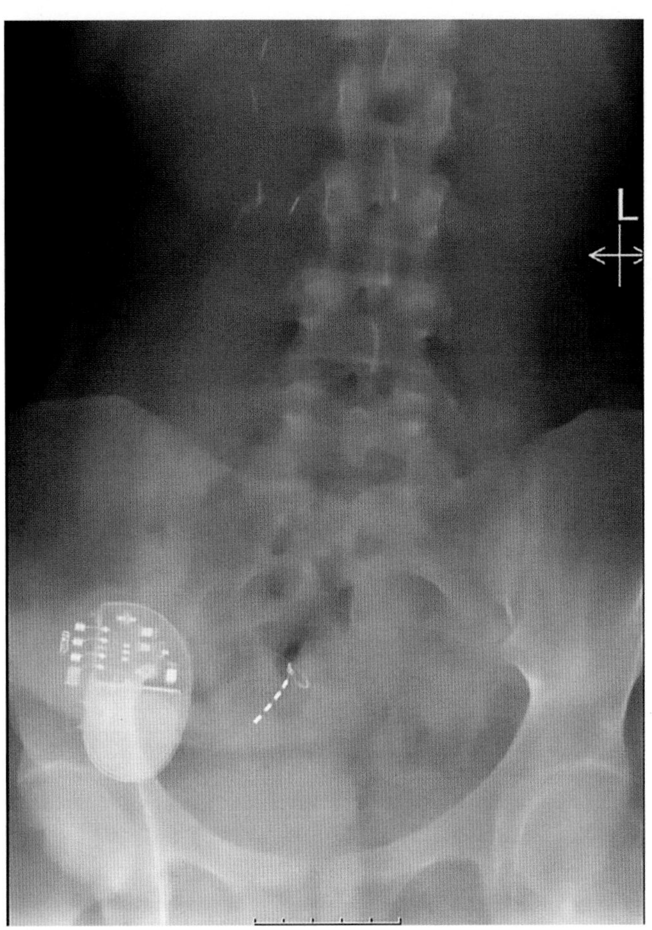

Figure 83.20 Radiograph demonstrating correct lead placement of the tined lead in the S3 foramen and the implant in the buttock.

completely understood but it is thought that afferent stimulation modulates reflex pathways involved in the micturition cycle.

The procedure is typically performed in two stages. The first, known as the 'first stage tined lead', involves insertion of a lead with four electrodes percutaneously, under fluoroscopic guidance, to the S3 foramen via a posterior approach. Electrical current is then applied to achieve stimulation of the sacral nerve, and correct lead placement is identified by the typical motor responses of plantarflexion of the great toe and inward movement of the intergluteal fold due to contraction of the levator ani (anal reflex). This lead is then kept in place for approximately 2 weeks; if clinical efficacy (based on at least 50% improvement in bladder diary parameters) has been achieved then the second stage involves insertion of a permanent implant (*Figure 83.20*).

Efficacy rates of 70–80% have been reported with this technique for both idiopathic OAB and NLUTD, and there is no significant difference in terms of efficacy between BTX-A and SNS. Complications include lead migration, device infection and implant site pain.

Percutaneous tibial nerve stimulation

PTNS is a minimally invasive form of peripheral neuromodulation that is recommended for patients who are unsuitable for, or who decline, intravesical BTX-A injections or SNS. It is thought to improve symptoms of idiopathic OAB through stimulation of the sacral plexus S2–4, indirectly via the tibial nerve. Success rates are lower than those reported for BTX-A and SNS (approximately 50%), and patients require weekly treatment sessions over 12 weeks. However, there are no significant side effects related to this treatment.

Augmentation enterocystoplasty

Augmentation enterocystoplasty is reserved for those with high-pressure detrusor overactivity, poor compliance and reduced bladder capacity who have failed to respond to the above treatments. It is recommended for patients with both idiopathic and neurogenic bladder dysfunction. The aim is to create a low-pressure reservoir with increased functional capacity, thereby preserving renal function.

The procedure can be performed through a Pfannenstiel or lower midline abdominal incision with an extraperitoneal approach to mobilise the bladder from the peritoneum. The bladder is then bivalved in the coronal plane to a point 1 cm anterior to the ureteric orifices bilaterally. Although several gastrointestinal segments have been used, ileocystoplasty is the most common. A 25-cm segment of ileum is isolated, opened along its antimesenteric border and attached to the bivalved bladder, thereby increasing the bladder capacity (*Figure 83.21*). A suprapubic catheter is placed, and the patient undergoes a cystogram 3 weeks after surgery to ensure that the enterocystoplasty segment has completely healed prior to catheter removal.

Augmentation cystoplasty is an effective option with continence and satisfaction rates of over 90%, as well as considerable improvements in urodynamic parameters (detrusor overactivity, compliance, maximum detrusor pressure). However, this is a major surgical undertaking with risks of UTI, need for CISC, metabolic disturbances, mucus and stone formation, spontaneous perforation and possibly a small long-term risk of malignancy.

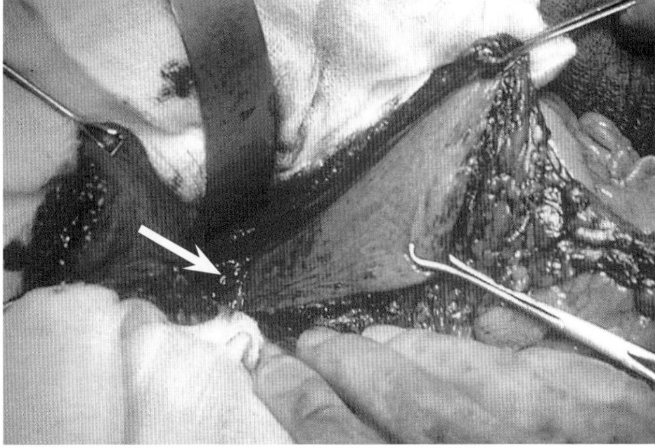

Figure 83.21 Augmentation ileocystoplasty. One of the ureteric orifices can be seen with the interureteric bar (arrow).

Urinary diversion

In those with so-called 'end-stage' incontinence that has failed to respond to the above measures, urinary diversion remains a last resort to improve quality of life. Ileal conduit urinary diversion, with or without cystectomy, is most commonly performed. When performed for benign indications, overall revision rates approach 40% (incisional or parastomal hernia, stomal complications, ureteroileal anastomosis revision or secondary cystectomy for refractory pyocystis).

Summary box 83.3

Urinary incontinence

- Urinary incontinence should be classified as UUI, SUI or MUI
- Initial management for urinary incontinence of any type is with behavioural modification, bladder training and pelvic floor muscle training
- OAB and UUI can be managed in a stepwise manner with pharmacotherapy, intravesical BTX-A, SNS or augmentation enterocystoplasty
- SUI in women is initially managed with bulking agents, mid-urethral slings (synthetic or autologous) or colposuspension
- SUI in men is managed with the suburethral sling or AUS
- Urinary diversion is a last-resort option for those with end-stage urinary incontinence

NEUROGENIC LOWER URINARY TRACT DYSFUNCTION

NLUTD refers to bladder and/or urethral sphincteric disorders that result from neurological lesions. Discrete neurological lesions will affect LUT storage and voiding in a consistent manner depending on the site of the lesion, the nature of the lesion (destructive, inflammatory, irritative) and the extent of the lesion (complete or incomplete). Neurological lesions can be classified based on location as suprapontine, spinal (infrapontine–suprasacral) and sacral/infrasacral. Each has characteristic clinical and urodynamic features (*Figure 83.22*). Suprapontine lesions (e.g. cerebrovascular accident, Parkinson's disease, brain injury) lead to storage LUTS owing to loss of inhibition from higher brain centres. This results in neurogenic detrusor overactivity, but since local sacral micturition refluxes are preserved the voiding phase is intact. Spinal lesions (e.g. spinal cord injury [SCI], myelitis, disc herniation) can have the most serious impact as they can lead to both detrusor overactivity and sphincteric overactivity (DSD), resulting in high-pressure voiding, which risks deterioration in renal function. Furthermore, patients with spinal lesions above the T6 spinal cord level are at risk of developing autonomic dysreflexia (see *Autonomic dysreflexia*). Sacral and infrasacral lesions are relatively safe as they result in low-pressure underactive bladder and/or sphincter function. Patients predominantly

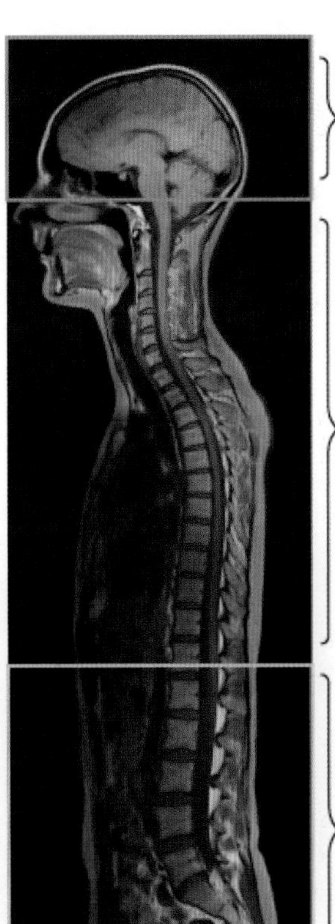

Suprapontine lesion
- **History**: predominantly storage problems
- **Ultrasound**: insignificant PVR urine volume
- **Urodynamics**: detrusor overactivity

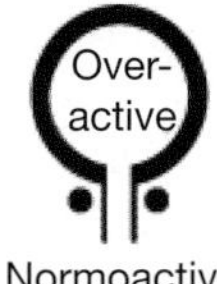

Spinal (infrapontine–suprasacral) lesion
- **History**: both storage and voiding problems
- **Ultrasound**: PVR urine volume usually raised
- **Urodynamics**: detrusor overactivity, detrusor–sphincter dyssynergia

Sacral/infrasacral lesion
- **History**: predominantly voiding symptoms
- **Ultrasound**: PVR urine volume raised
- **Urodynamics**: hypocontractile or acontractile detrusor

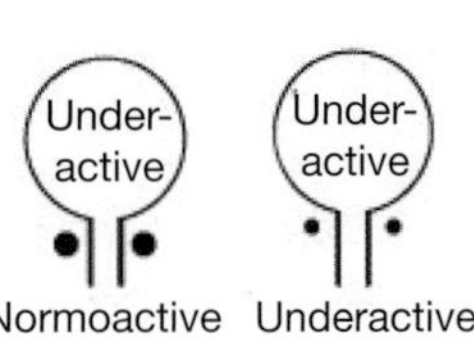

Figure 83.22 Characteristic lower urinary tract disorders arising from neurological disease. (Reproduced with permission from Panicker JN, Fowler CJ, Kessler TM. Lower urinary tract dysfunction in the neurological patient: clinical assessment and management. *Lancet Neurol* 2015; **14**(7): 720–32.)

suffer from voiding symptoms (reduced flow, incomplete bladder emptying) and SUI.

The aims of treatment in NLUTD are to:

1 preserve renal function by ensuring low-pressure storage and voiding;
2 achieve continence;
3 prevent UTI.

Treatment of detrusor overactivity and poor compliance in order to attain low-pressure storage is achieved through the conservative, medical and surgical treatment pathways outlined above for the treatment of UUI. Treatment of sphincteric overactivity or DSD to attain low-pressure voiding is typically achieved by CISC, although sphincteric overactivity can be treated with intrasphincteric BTX-A, sacral neuromodulation, SNS or direct sphincterotomy. If these methods are ineffective or unsuitable for the patient, continent diversion (appendicovesicostomy) can be performed to prevent high-pressure voiding. Detrusor underactivity is managed with CISC and sphincteric underactivity is treated as described above for SUI. Several factors should be considered when managing patients with NLUTD. These relate to patient factors (body habitus, hand function, motivation and level of compliance, mental status, values and preferences, support network) and neurological disease factors (prognosis).

Spinal cord injury

SCI often results in significant LUT dysfunction with a high risk of UTI/sepsis, renal function deterioration, renal and bladder calculi and autonomic dysreflexia. Urinary tract complications and renal failure were the leading causes of death in this population, but thorough evaluation and early definitive management have considerably improved urinary tract outcomes in patients with SCI.

Immediately after SCI, a period of 'spinal shock' occurs in which there is a marked reduction in all spinal reflex activity below the level of the lesion. This results in an areflexic and acontractile bladder; urinary retention lasts 6–12 weeks in complete SCI but may be shorter in incomplete lesions. Patients are managed with indwelling catheterisation or CISC during this phase. Return of function is characterised by spasticity (detrusor overactivity and DSD) and should be managed as described under ***Urinary incontinence, Treatment***.

Autonomic dysreflexia

Autonomic dysreflexia is a sudden and exaggerated autonomic (primarily sympathetic) response to various stimuli in patients with SCI or spinal dysfunction above the cord level of T6–8 (the sympathetic outflow). Stimuli below the level of the lesion (commonly a distended bladder or rectum) lead to symptoms of headache, hypertension (varying from mild headache to seizures or cerebral haemorrhage) and flushing or sweating of the face and body above the level of the lesion.

Autonomic dysreflexia is thought to occur as a result of an unopposed sympathetic response to noxious stimuli. Nociceptive afferents elicit reflex sympathetic outflow, resulting in piloerection, sweating and arteriolar vasoconstriction, leading to hypertension. The peripheral vasoconstriction activates baroreceptors, which results in a parasympathetic surge originating in the central nervous system to counteract the sympathetic outflow. The resulting vagal outflow causes bradycardia, but this parasympathetic signal is unable to transmit below the level of the spinal cord lesion. This leads to bradycardia, vasodilatation and flushing above the level of the lesion, but hypertension and pale, cold skin due to ongoing vasoconstriction below the level of the lesion.

Initial treatment involves sitting the patient upright, removing any constricting clothing and identifying and removing the source of stimulation (urinary retention, blocked catheter, loaded rectum). Regular blood pressure monitoring should be performed; if the systolic blood pressure remains elevated (>150 mmHg), patients should be treated with fast-acting antihypertensives such as sublingual nifedipine or glyceryl trinitrate.

URINARY TRACT FISTULAE

A fistula is an abnormal or surgically made passage between a hollow or tubular organ and the body surface, or between two hollow or tubular organs. The most common cause of urinary tract fistulae in less economically developed countries is traumatic labour; in well-resourced countries, fistulae are most commonly iatrogenic, resulting from pelvic surgery (hysterectomy accounts for the majority) or radiotherapy, or they can be due to advanced pelvic malignancy, inflammatory conditions (e.g. tuberculosis [TB]), congenital disorders or foreign body erosion.

Vesicovaginal fistulae

VVF is the most common urinary tract fistula. In developing countries, obstetric fistula account for the majority of cases. Lack of adequate prenatal care, younger age at first marriage, short stature, low socioeconomic status and illiteracy are risk factors for developing obstetric fistulae. These fistulae are due to prolonged obstructed labour resulting in ischaemic pressure necrosis to the anterior vaginal wall, bladder and urethra, and large areas of the bladder neck and urethra may be involved. Concomitant rectovaginal fistulae may also be present, making these fistulae very complex to manage. In developed countries, iatrogenic VVF most commonly occurs after hysterectomy, usually thought to be due to an unrecognised bladder injury near the vaginal cuff. Other mechanisms include diathermy injury resulting in delayed tissue necrosis or a suture placed through the bladder and vaginal wall during closure of the vaginal cuff. Abdominal hysterectomy is three times more likely to result in fistula than vaginal hysterectomy, although the overall rate of VVF after hysterectomy is low at 0.1–4%.

Clinical features

The most common presenting symptom is constant urinary leak from the vagina. This may be intermittent in cases of very small fistulae, and so other causes of urinary incontinence (SUI, UUI) must be excluded. Post-hysterectomy VVF may be recognised in the first few days after surgery, or 1–3 weeks later after catheter removal. Post-irradiation VVF may not manifest until years later.

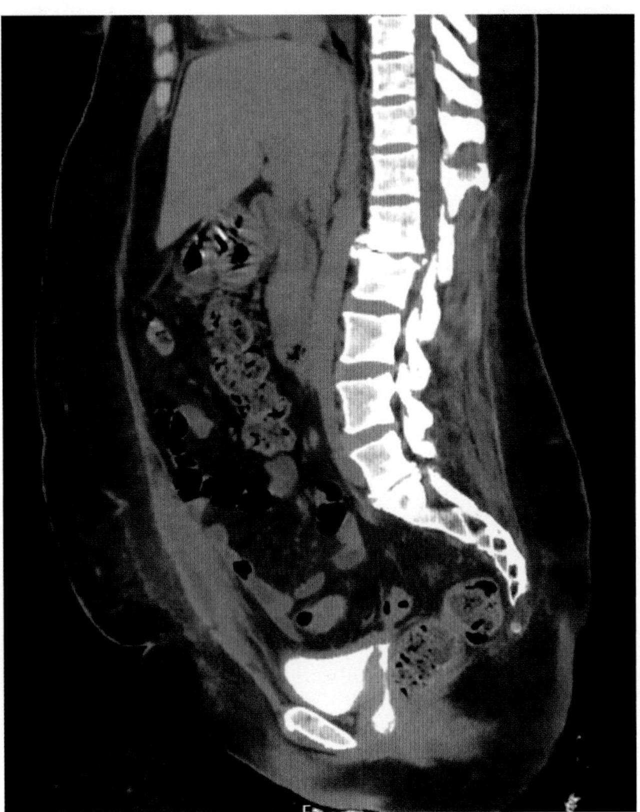

Figure 83.23 Computed tomography scan showing a vesicovaginal fistula from the posterior wall of the bladder to the vagina.

Physical examination may demonstrate the fistula site, typically on the anterior vaginal wall at the vaginal cuff, and leakage of urine may be seen. Instillation of blue dye into the bladder may aid visual identification of the fistula site.

Investigation

1. **Cross-sectional imaging** with CT urogram, MRI with gadolinium contrast or cystogram will aid diagnosis of the fistulous tract and exclude concomitant ureteric injury (*Figure 83.23*).
2. **Cystoscopy**, bilateral retrograde ureteropyelography and examination under anaesthesia should be performed to assess the fistula site, location, size, proximity to ureteric orifices, vaginal size, depth and mobility. This will aid surgical planning and help to determine whether an abdominal or vaginal approach will be most suitable. Furthermore, biopsy of the fistula tract to exclude recurrent malignancy can be performed in cases of prior history of pelvic malignancy.
3. **'Three-swab' test**. This investigation can be performed in cases where fistula is suspected but cannot be identified on the investigations above. Three numbered gauze swabs are placed into the vagina, with swab number 1 placed most proximally, swab number 2 in the middle and swab number 3 most distal in the vagina. A blue dye is then instilled into the bladder through a catheter, and the catheter removed. Blue staining of swab 1 or 2 suggests VVF whereas blue staining of swab 3 suggests a urethra–vaginal fistula or SUI. If swab 1 is wet but not stained blue, this suggests the presence of a ureterovaginal fistula.

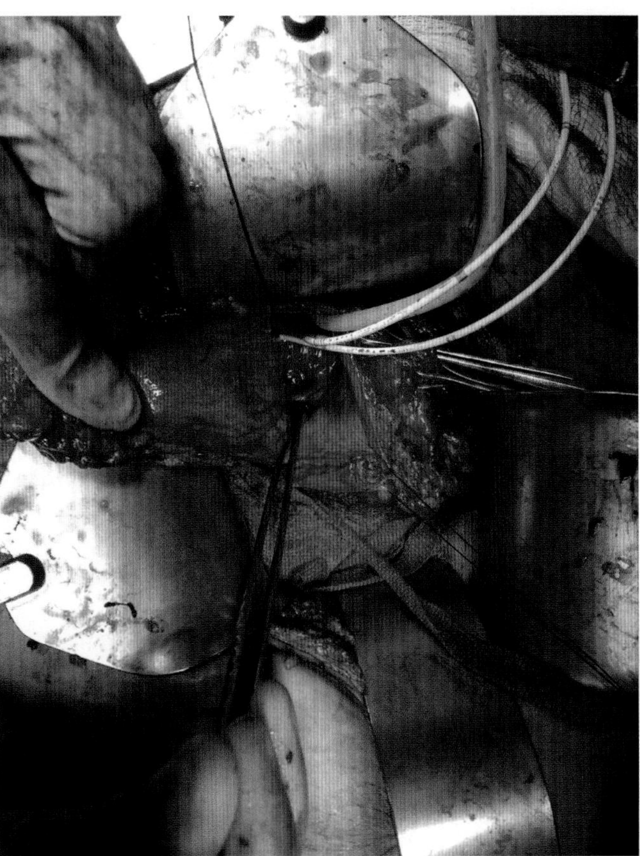

Figure 83.24 Transabdominal approach showing a vesicovaginal fistula (VVF) on the posterior wall (forceps in VVF). White ureteric catheters have been inserted into the ureteric orifices and there is a catheter in the urethra.

TABLE 83.8 Principles of surgical repair of a vesicovaginal fistula.

- Adequate exposure of the fistula tract and debridement of ischaemic tissue
- Adequate separation of involved organs
- Watertight closure, multilayer closure, tension-free, non-overlapping suture lines
- Use of well-vascularised tissue flaps (omentum, peritoneum, Martius labial fat pad)
- Adequate postoperative urinary drainage
- Treatment and prevention of infection
- Meticulous haemostasis

Treatment

Conservative treatment with urethral catheter drainage is rarely successful, but in certain situations (e.g. very small VVF in the absence of radiotherapy) may be warranted for an initial 2- to 6-week period. If this fails to heal the fistula surgical treatment is required. The approach can be vaginal, transabdominal (open or minimally invasive) or a combination of both (*Figure 83.24*). Principles of surgical repair are shown in *Table 83.8*. Vaginal repair relies on adequate exposure of the fistulous opening. The fistula is circumscribed, and the bladder

TABLE 83.9 Causes of urinary retention in men and women

Mechanism	Men	Women

Anatomical bladder outlet obstruction	• Benign prostatic obstruction
	• Malignant enlargement of prostate
	• Bladder neck obstruction
	• Urethral stricture
	• Urethral rupture (e.g. following pelvic fracture)
		• Urethral
		  ◦ Stricture
		  ◦ Diverticulum
		  ◦ Meatal stenosis
		  ◦ Carcinoma
		• Prolapse
		• Extrinsic compression
		  ◦ Paraurethral cyst
		  ◦ Pelvic mass (e.g. large fibroids)
		  ◦ Gynaecological malignancy
		• Iatrogenic
		  ◦ Anti-incontinence surgery
		  ◦ Urethral reconstruction

Functional bladder outlet obstruction	• Idiopathic high-tone non-relaxing external urethral sphincter	• Idiopathic high-tone non-relaxing external urethral sphincter (Fowler's syndrome) • Dysfunctional voiding • Primary bladder neck obstruction
Detrusor underactivity	• Pelvic surgery • Peripheral neuropathy • Diabetic cystopathy • Secondary to longstanding bladder outlet obstruction	
Neurological disease	• Detrusor–sphincter dyssynergia (any cause of suprasacral spinal cord disease) causing obstructed voiding • Sacral nerve lesion or cauda equina causing detrusor underactivity	
Drugs	• Antimuscarinics or β_3-agonists • Sympathomimetic drugs • Anaesthetic agents • Opioids	
Transient causes	• Following spinal or general anaesthesia • Pain • Faecal impaction due to constipation • Blood clot secondary to haematuria	

side is adequately separated from the vaginal side. The bladder is closed in two layers and a Martius labial fat pad is then harvested to cover the fistula. The vaginal wall is then closed, and a labial drain is placed for 1–2 days. Abdominal repair is typically performed transvesically. The bladder is opened, and the fistulous site identified and circumscribed to separate it from the vaginal wall. If the ureteric orifices are in close proximity, then ureteric catheters are placed intraoperatively. The vaginal wall is closed and then the bladder is closed in two layers after insertion of omentum or peritoneum between the fistula margins. The patient is discharged with a urethral catheter *in situ*; this is typically removed 3 weeks later after a pericatheter urethrogram confirms absence of leak.

URINARY RETENTION

Urinary retention is defined as the inability to pass urine despite persistent effort. It can be classified as acute (painful inability to pass urine with relief of pain on catheterisation) or chronic (painless, elevated residual volume after passing urine).

The causes of urinary retention in men and women are given in *Table 83.9*.

Summary box 83.4

Urinary tract fistulae

The principles of surgical repair of VVF are:

- Adequate exposure of the fistula tract
- Tension-free, watertight, multilayer closure with non-overlapping suture lines
- Interposition with a well-vascularised flap
- Urinary tract drainage postoperatively to allow healing

Catheterisation

The immediate treatment for urinary retention of any cause is urethral catheterisation. Other indications for catheterisation are shown in *Table 83.10*. In chronic urinary retention, patients may have a postobstructive diuresis producing >200 mL of urine per hour for three consecutive hours. If this is the case, patients should be managed with strict fluid balance monitoring, postural blood pressure checks to detect postural hypotension and daily serum electrolyte monitoring

Heinrich Martius, 1885–1965, German surgeon, described a labial flap of bulbocavernosus muscle (Martius modified labial fat pad) in 1928.
Clare Juliet Fowler, contemporary, Professor of Uroneurology, National Hospital for Neurology and Neurosurgery, London, UK.

TABLE 83.10 Indications for catheterisation.	
Drainage	• Urinary retention (acute and chronic) • Fluid management/monitoring in critically unwell patients • Palliative management for urinary incontinence where other measures have failed or are unsuitable • Following urological surgery to allow healing of the bladder or urethra
Therapeutic drug delivery	• Non-muscle-invasive bladder cancer (e.g. mitomycin C, gemcitabine, BCG) • Chronic cystitis such as UTI and interstitial cystitis (e.g. GAG-layer replacement therapies, antibiotics)
Diagnostic	• Micturating cystourethrogram • Urodynamics • To obtain a catheter specimen of urine for analysis

BCG, bacillus Calmette–Guérin; GAG, glycosaminoglycan; UTI, urinary tract infection.

and occasionally may require intravenous fluid replacement to match the loss if the patient is unable to take enough orally.

Types of catheter

Catheters can be classified based on their size (French scale), number of channels or composition (latex-coated or silicone) (*Figure 83.25*).

Size

The French scale refers to the external diameter of the catheter, and 1Fr is 0.3 mm in diameter. The standard catheter size for uncomplicated urethral catheterisation in women is 12Fr or 14Fr, and in men 16Fr. In patients with urethral stricture, a smaller size catheter should be considered. In cases of haematuria with 'clot retention', a 22Fr catheter is typically used to aid drainage of thick clots. Coudé tip catheters have a curved tip to allow easier passage past an enlarged prostate.

Number of channels

Single-channel catheters consist of a single drainage channel only and are used for CISC as these catheters do not require an indwelling retention mechanism. The Foley catheter consists of two channels – a drainage channel and a channel for inflation of a balloon at the tip, which allows the catheter to be retained in the bladder. This is the standard catheter used for uncomplicated cases of urinary retention. The 'three-way' catheter has an additional channel for bladder irrigation and is used for patients with haematuria and 'clot retention' and following transurethral prostate or bladder surgery.

Urethral catheterisation

1. Aseptic technique – handwashing, sterile gloves, sterile catheter pack.
2. Clean urethral meatus with antiseptic solution.
3. Instil lidocaine gel into the urethra and hold for 2–3 minutes. In men, the penis should be held perpendicular and taught. In women, the labia should be held apart to provide adequate exposure of the urethral meatus.
4. The catheter should be inserted as far as the 'hilt' of the catheter and should pass freely (the type of catheter is dependent on the indication). If there is any resistance catheterisation should be stopped and assistance sought. The patient may require a coudé tip catheter if the obstruction is thought to be a large prostate, or a cystoscopy to negotiate a false passage or stricture.
5. The position in the bladder is confirmed with the drainage of clear urine and the balloon should be inflated with 10 mL of sterile water. The catheter bag should then be attached.
6. Details regarding the type and size of catheter, and residual volume, should be clearly recorded.

Suprapubic catheterisation

Suprapubic catheterisation (SPC) carries a small but significant risk of bowel injury, especially in those who have undergone previous abdominal or pelvic surgery, and so should be performed under ultrasound and cystoscopic guidance. SPC should be considered for those who require long-term catheterisation, as it is often more comfortable with no risk of urethral trauma compared with long-term urethral catheterisation, as well as for those in whom urethral catheterisation is not suitable or possible. Contraindications to SPC insertion include known or suspected bladder carcinoma, abdominal wall infection at

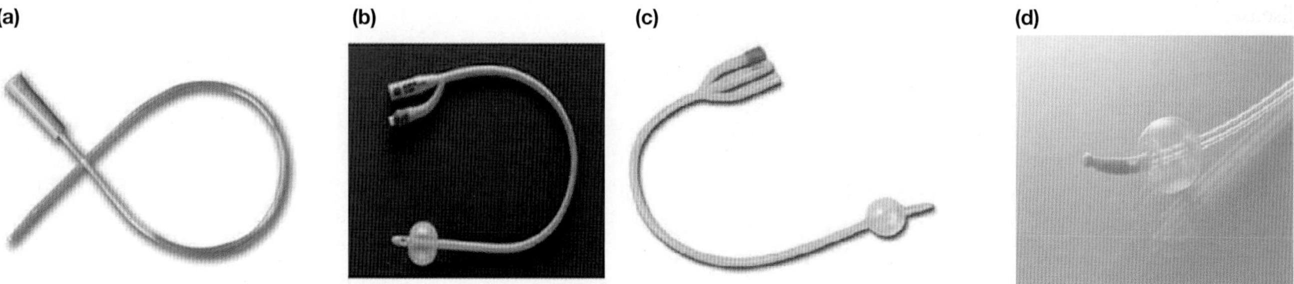

Figure 83.25 Types of urethral catheter. (a) Single-lumen catheter used for self-catheterisation; (b) standard urethral catheter with an inflatable balloon retention mechanism; (c) a three-way catheter with an extra channel for irrigation; (d) coudé tip catheter.

Frederic Eugene Basil Foley, 1891–1966, urologist, Anker Hospital, St Paul, MN, USA.

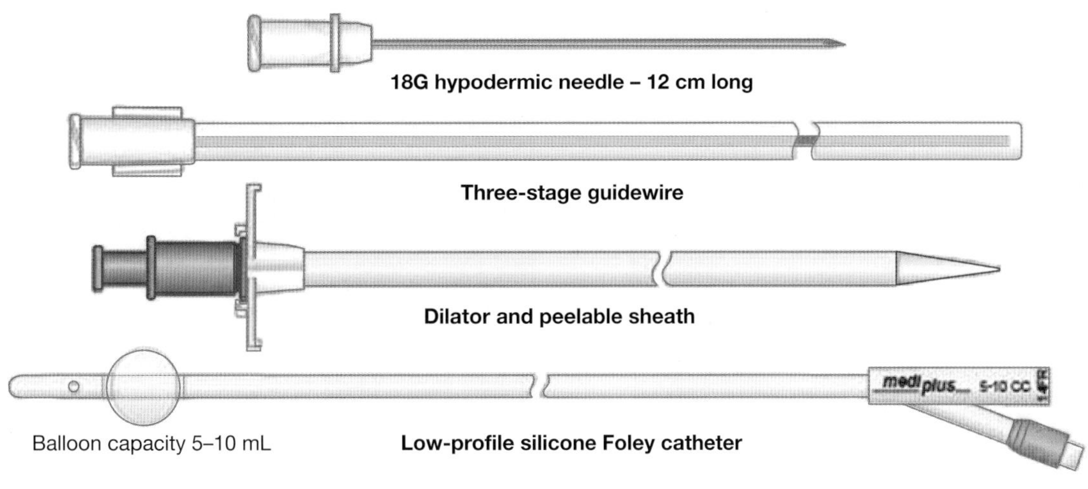

Figure 83.26 A suprapubic 'Seldinger' catheter kit.

the site of insertion, uncorrected coagulopathy or the presence of a vascular graft in the suprapubic region.

The procedure requires infiltration of local anaesthesia (1% lidocaine) to the skin and fascia of the suprapubic region, two fingerbreadths above the pubic symphysis in the midline. This procedure should only be performed in those with a palpable bladder. A Seldinger technique of insertion is the safest for percutaneous insertion (*Figure 83.26*). A long needle is inserted in a perpendicular direction into the bladder and aspiration of clear urine confirms correct entry. A guidewire is placed through the needle, and the needle removed. A small skin incision at the site of the guidewire allows a trocar to pass over the guidewire and into the bladder, thereby dilating the tract. Through this trocar, a 16Fr catheter is placed and the balloon inflated. The trocar is removed and the catheter bag attached. If the bladder cannot be confidently identified, or in those with extensive abdominal or pelvic surgery, an open cystotomy should be performed to safely enter the bladder and ensure that there is no bowel in the path of the catheter.

BLADDER STONES

Bladder stones account for 5% of all urinary tract stone disease. They can be classified as primary (without underlying urinary tract pathology) or secondary (due to underlying renal tract pathology). Primary bladder stones are commonly seen in children in the developing world and are due to nutritional deficiency in vitamins A and B6, magnesium and phosphate and a reduced protein–carbohydrate ratio. Secondary bladder stones are most commonly related to urinary stasis from elevated postvoid residual volume due to bladder outlet obstruction (*Table 83.11*).

TABLE 83.11 Aetiology of bladder stones.

Primary	• Nutritional deficiency
Secondary	
• Urinary stasis (elevated residual volume)	• Bladder outlet obstruction • Detrusor underactivity • Bladder augmentation or substitution • Neurogenic lower urinary tract dysfunction
• Foreign body	• Suture or mesh from previous prolapse/ continence/pelvic surgery • Stone from upper tract • Indwelling catheter or ureteric stent • Migrated intrauterine devices
• Infection	
• Drugs	• Indinavir • Triamterene

Composition

Primary endemic bladder stones in children are usually composed of ammonium urate and calcium oxalate. Secondary stones due to bladder outlet obstruction are typically smooth and yellow-brown in colour and are composed of uric acid. Infection-related stones tend to be triple phosphate (magnesium ammonium phosphate) and are white in colour (*Figure 83.27*).

Clinical features

- May be asymptomatic.
- Haematuria.
- Dysuria.
- Frequency and urgency.
- Suprapubic pain.
- Hesitancy and intermittency.

Sven Ivar Seldinger, 1921–1998, Swedish radiologist, introduced this technique in 1953.

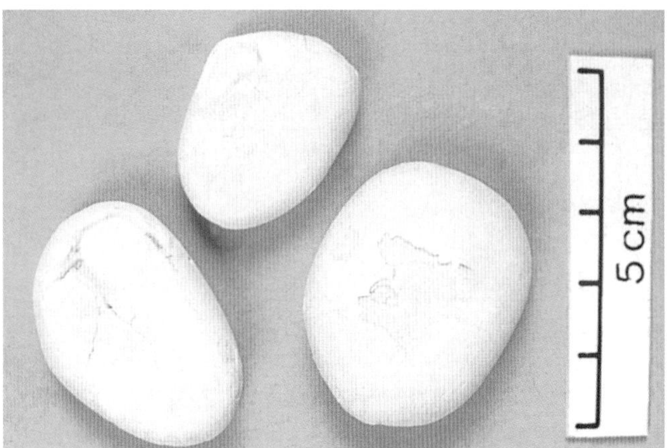

Figure 83.27 Smooth uric acid bladder stones.

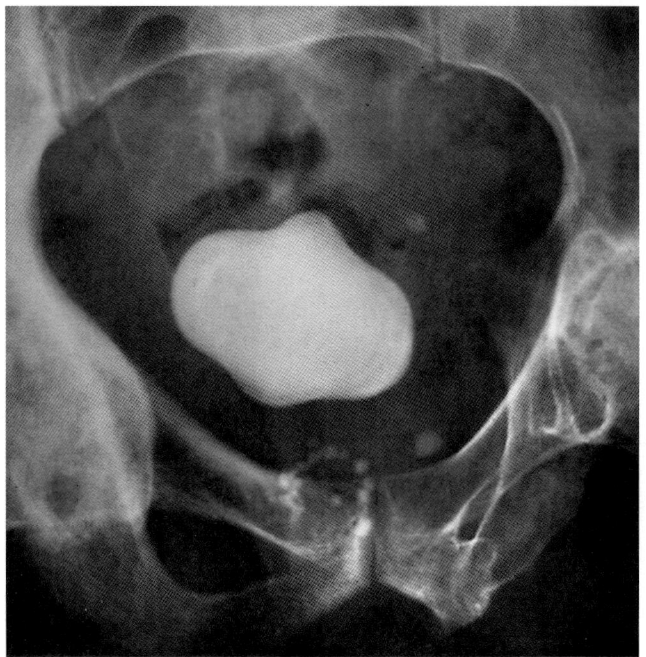

Figure 83.28 Radiograph showing a vesical calculus (no contrast has been used).

Investigation

Plain radiograph of the bladder, renal tract ultrasound or CT will confirm the diagnosis and provide an estimation of size to aid treatment planning (*Figure 83.28*).

Treatment

The cause of the stone should be sought and treated; this may include bladder outlet obstruction, incomplete bladder emptying in patients with neurogenic bladder dysfunction or the presence of a foreign body that should be excised simultaneously (*Figure 83.29*).

The majority of stones can be managed endoscopically with a stone punch, ultrasound lithotripsy or holmium laser lithotripsy (*Figure 83.30*). In those in whom urethral access is

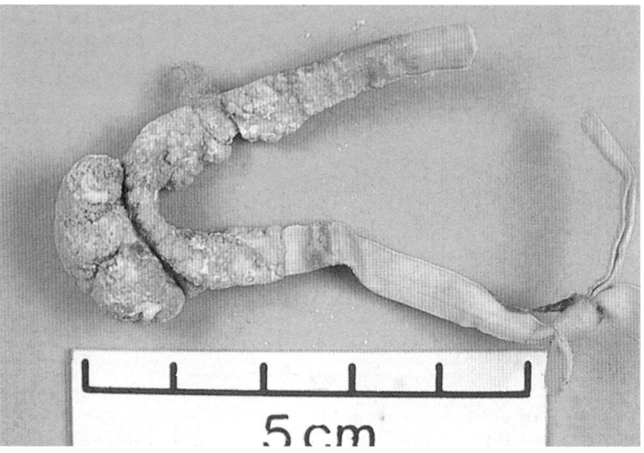

Figure 83.29 Stone on a vaginal sling that had eroded into the bladder.

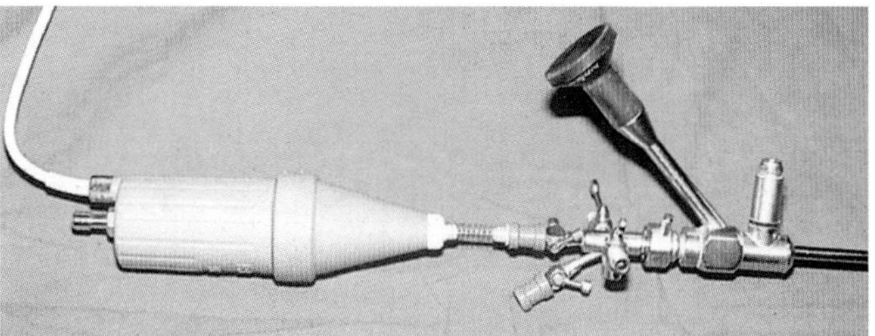

Figure 83.30 An endoscopic ultrasound probe, which is used to fragment bladder or kidney stones.

not possible (e.g. reconstructed LUT), percutaneous cystolithotomy can be performed using a similar technique to percutaneous nephrolithotomy.

The open approach (open cystolithotomy) is reserved for those with very large bladder stones that cannot be treated with endoscopic means.

URINARY TRACT INFECTION

UTI is the inflammatory response of the urothelium to bacterial invasion, usually associated with bacteriuria (the presence of bacteria in the urine) and pyuria (the presence of white blood cells in the urine). Pyuria in the absence of bacteriuria (sterile pyuria) indicates an inflammatory response that may still be related to UTI or that may be a response to another pathology such as fastidious organisms (e.g. TB, gonorrhoea), carcinoma *in situ* (CIS) bladder stones or other inflammatory conditions. UTIs can be classified as **uncomplicated** (occurring in a healthy patient with a structurally and functionally normal urinary tract) or **complicated** (occurring in a patient with an anatomical or functional urinary tract abnormality, in an immunocompromised patient or with more virulent or resistant bacteria). Factors that suggest a complicated UTI are shown in *Table 83.12*. An **isolated** UTI is one in which there has been an interval of at least 6 months between infections. A **recurrent** UTI (rUTI) is defined as ≥2 episodes in 6 months or ≥3 episodes in 12 months. Infections can also be classified based on their site (urethritis, prostatitis, cystitis, pyelonephritis). This chapter focuses on cystitis.

TABLE 83.12 Factors that suggest a complicated urinary tract infection.

Patient factors	• Functional or anatomical abnormality of the urinary tract • Sex (male gender) • Age (postmenopausal) • Pregnant • Immunosuppressed (e.g. diabetes, transplant, steroids) • Indwelling catheter
Bacterial factors	• Increased virulence (hospital-acquired infection) • Antimicrobial resistance (recent antibiotic use)

Half of all women have been estimated to experience a UTI in their lifetime, and up to 50% of these will have recurrent infection within the following 6-month period.

Pathogenesis

The most common route of infection is ascending UTI; contamination of the vaginal and periurethral area with uropathogenic organisms originating from the gastrointestinal tract leads to adherence and migration of bacteria into the urethra and bladder. Once in the bladder, adherence of the bacteria to the urothelium triggers a process of bacterial internalisation into the urothelial cell and the subsequent formation of intracellular bacterial communities (IBCs) and quiescent intracellular reservoirs (QIRs), which may remain viable for months and act as a source of rUTI. These IBCs and QIRs act in a similar way to a biofilm, protecting bacteria from the host immune response and from the action of antimicrobial agents.

Less common routes of infection include haematogenous spread (seen with *Staphylococcus aureus* and fungal infections) or direct infection from retroperitoneal abscess or inflammatory bowel disease.

The commonest organisms implicated in uncomplicated UTI are *Escherichia coli* (85%), *Staphylococcus saprophyticus, Enterococcus faecalis, Proteus* and *Klebsiella*. Complicated UTIs are caused by *E. coli* (50%), enterococci, *S. aureus* and *Pseudomonas*.

Successful infection depends on the bacterial virulence relative to the host defence mechanisms. The common bacterial virulence factors and host defence mechanisms are shown in *Table 83.13*.

Clinical features

The classic symptoms of UTI include dysuria, suprapubic pain, urinary frequency and urgency. Patients may also present with haematuria, loin pain, fevers, nausea and vomiting. A physical examination should be performed to check for a palpable bladder, for renal angle tenderness and for evidence of pelvic organ prolapse, urethral diverticulum and atrophic vaginitis.

TABLE 83.13 Bacterial virulence factors and host defence mechanisms.

Bacterial virulence factors	Host defence mechanisms
• Adherence mechanisms (fimbrial and afimbrial) • Immune evasion (lipopolysaccharide O, capsule K) • Anti-IgA proteases, toxin production, β-lactamase • Resistance to antimicrobial bactericidal activity (alteration of antimicrobial binding sites) • Iron acquisition	• Commensal organisms (lactobacilli) • Mechanical integrity of mucous membranes • Antibacterial secretions (lysozyme, lactoferrin, IgA) • Antegrade flow of urine causing flushing effect • Tamm–Horsfall protein (binds to bacterial adhesion molecules) • Composition of urine (low pH, high urea) • Immune system integrity

IgA, immunoglobulin A.

Investigation

Initial investigation is with urinalysis (a dipstick test checks for the presence of red cells, white cells and nitrites), urine microscopy, culture and sensitivity, flow rate assessment and measurement of postvoid residual volume. In those with rUTI, renal tract ultrasound to exclude anatomical pathology should be performed; cystoscopy is reserved for those with atypical symptoms, haematuria or other features that raise suspicion of underlying pathology (e.g. bladder cancer, stones, urinary tract fistula).

Current methods of microbiological UTI diagnosis are based on the identification of a 'significant' pure growth of a known uropathogen in the urine. A cut-off of $\geq 10^3$ colony-forming units/mL is commonly used to diagnose acute uncomplicated cystitis in women, but it is becoming increasingly clear that patients can develop symptoms of UTI with much lower concentrations of urinary bacteria; the minimum concentration required to cause UTI or rUTI has not yet been defined.

Treatment

Acute UTI should be treated with an appropriate antimicrobial agent based on local antibiograms and resistance patterns. Following treatment of an acute UTI, non-antimicrobial measures to prevent future UTI should be considered (e.g. increasing fluid intake, probiotics, methenamine hippurate, d-mannose, vaginal oestrogen therapy for postmenopausal women). Episodes of rUTI can be treated with antimicrobial prophylaxis, postcoital antimicrobial use for those with sex-linked infections or intermittent self-start antimicrobial therapy.

Theodor Albrecht Edwin Klebs, 1834–1913, Professor of Bacteriology successively at Prague, Czechoslovakia, Zurich, Switzerland, and the Rush Medical College, Chicago, IL, USA.
Igor Tamm, 1922–1995, American virologist.
Frank Horsfall, 1906–1971, American microbiologist, together with Igor Tamm first purified the Tamm–Horsfall protein in 1952.

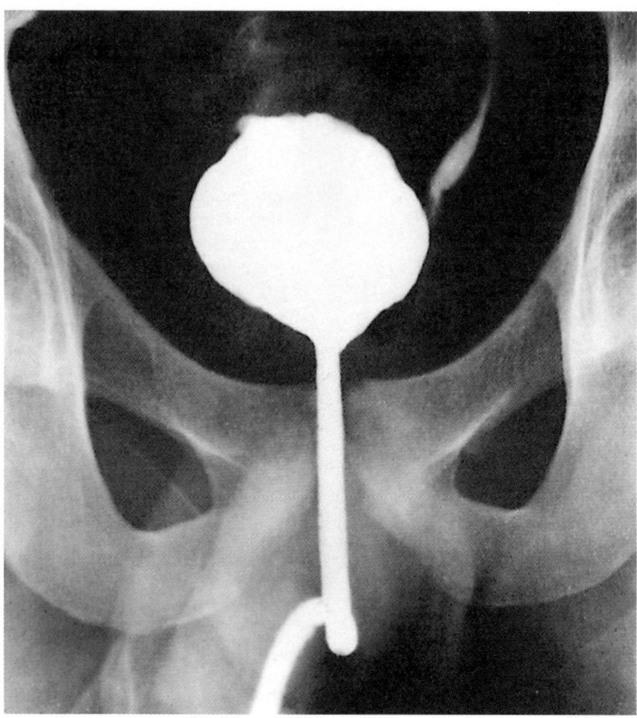

Figure 83.31 Retrograde cystography showing a small 'thimble' bladder due to tuberculosis.

Special cases

Genitourinary tuberculosis

Genitourinary tuberculosis (GU-TB) caused by *Mycobacterium tuberculosis* can affect any part of the urinary tract. Renal calcification and ureteric strictures are typical in the upper urinary tract. In the bladder, initial manifestations include a red, oedematous bladder wall with ulceration and visible tubercles (yellow lesions with a red halo). This typically starts around the ureteric orifices and trigone. As the disease progresses, fibrosis and contraction of the bladder occur ('thimble bladder'), as well as calcification and fistula formation (***Figure 83.31***).

Patients may present with fevers, weight loss, night sweats, UTI symptoms or haematuria. Investigation may reveal a sterile pyuria, and cystoscopy with biopsy will confirm the diagnosis. Three early morning urine samples for acid-fast bacilli or polymerase chain reaction of the urine can be used for diagnosis of TB infection. Cross-sectional imaging with a CT urogram should be performed to evaluate the kidneys and ureters as they are likely to also be affected.

Treatment consists of antituberculous therapy with isoniazid, rifampicin, pyrazinamide and ethambutol. Severe bladder disease may require surgical treatment following completion of antituberculous therapy. Options include augmentation enterocystoplasty, cystectomy and orthotopic bladder substitution, or ileal conduit urinary diversion. However, the choice of treatment will depend upon the concomitant upper tract involvement and patient preferences.

Schistosomiasis

Parasitic infection with the trematode *Schistosoma haematobium* originates from infection with freshwater snails. The disease is endemic in Egypt, parts of Africa, Israel, Syria, Saudi Arabia, Iran, Iraq and the shores of China's great lakes. The parasite penetrates the skin and travels to the liver (as schistosomules), where it matures. Adult trematodes migrate to vesical veins and lay eggs (containing miracidium larvae), which leave the body by penetrating the bladder and entering the urine. The active phase is when eggs are actively being laid, whereas the inactive phase is when the adult has died but there is an ongoing reaction to the remaining eggs.

At the time of infection, a local inflammatory response leads to irritation of the skin ('swimmer's itch'). Acute fever (Katayama fever) may ensue at the onset of egg laying (3 weeks to 4 months after infection) with fever, lymphadenopathy, splenomegaly and eosinophilia. When the eggs are deposited in the bladder, the typical bladder symptoms of intermittent painless haematuria and terminal dysuria occur. Chronic infection can lead to a small, contracted, fibrotic bladder similar to that seen with tuberculous cystitis. Patients are at increased risk of developing ureteric strictures, urethral strictures and squamous cell carcinoma of the bladder.

Investigation with midday (to coincide with the time of maximum egg shedding) urine microscopy may show characteristic eggs with terminal spines (***Figure 83.32***). Cystoscopy may show characteristic 'sandy patches' at the trigone (due to calcified dead ova with degeneration of the overlying urothelium), ulceration or papillomas. In advanced cases, carcinoma may be present. Bladder or rectal biopsies may identify eggs.

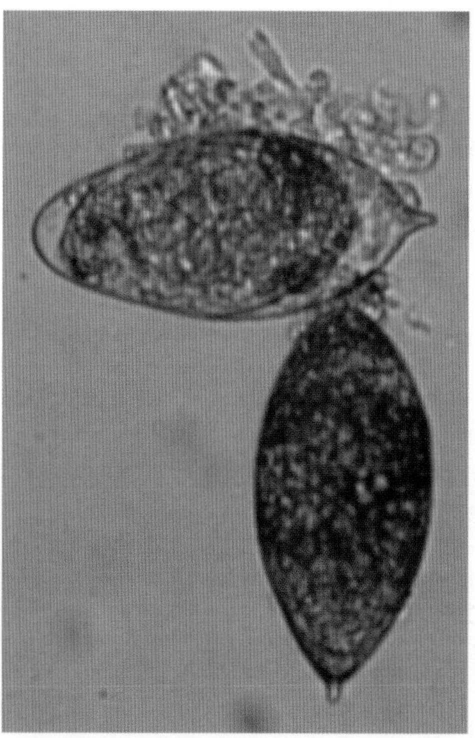

Figure 83.32 *Schistosoma haematobium* eggs with terminal spines. (Reproduced with permission from Ray D, Nelson TA, Fu CL *et al.* Transcriptional profiling of the bladder in urogenital schistosomiasis reveals pathways of inflammatory fibrosis and urothelial compromise. *PLoS Negl Trop Dis* 2012; **6**(11): e1912.)

In cases where suspicion remains high but eggs have not been identified, serology (enzyme-linked immunosorbent assay [ELISA]) has high sensitivity and specificity. A CT urogram should be performed to assess for obstructive uropathy secondary to a scarred, contracted bladder.

Treatment is with praziquantel 20 mg/kg in two divided doses 4–6 hours apart. A small, contracted bladder may require reconstruction with augmentation enterocystoplasty, cystectomy and orthotopic bladder substitution, or ileal conduit urinary diversion.

Summary box 83.5

Urinary tract infections

- UTIs can be classified as uncomplicated or complicated
- Patients should undergo evaluation for TB and schistosomiasis if suspected based on the history or presence of persistent sterile pyuria

CHRONIC INFLAMMATORY CONDITIONS OF THE BLADDER

Chronic inflammatory conditions of the bladder are of multifactorial aetiology but present with a similar clinical picture of urinary frequency, urgency and pain, with or without haematuria (*Table 83.14*). The principles of management are to exclude a malignant cause for the symptoms, to preserve upper tract function and to improve symptoms and quality of life.

TABLE 83.14 Common chronic inflammatory bladder diseases.

Idiopathic	Interstitial cystitis
Infective	• Chronic bacterial UTI • Fastidious organisms and parasites (*Chlamydia*, *Gonorrhoea*, tuberculosis, schistosomiasis)
Radiation therapy	Radiation cystitis
Drugs	• Ketamine cystitis • Cyclophosphamide cystitis
Iatrogenic	BCG cystitis
Autoimmune	Lupus cystitis

BCG, bacillus Calmette–Guérin; UTI, urinary tract infection.

Bladder pain syndrome/interstitial cystitis

Bladder pain syndrome (BPS) is a chronic condition characterised by pelvic pain or pressure that is perceived to be originating from the bladder, accompanied by one or more urinary symptoms, including frequency, urgency and nocturia. The diagnosis is made once other confusable diseases that could cause similar symptoms have been excluded. The term interstitial cystitis (IC) is often used interchangeably with BPS but represents a distinctive bladder organ-specific phenotype with characteristic cystoscopic and histopathological features as opposed to the systemic phenotype of BPS. The precise aetiology of BPS/IC is unknown.

Clinical features

Patients present with disabling bladder or pelvic pain, urinary urgency and severe urinary frequency and nocturia. Those with BPS may have other associated chronic medical conditions (e.g. fibromyalgia, irritable bowel syndrome, migraines).

Investigation

Urine analysis and culture, testing for sexually transmitted infections and urine cytology should be performed to exclude an infective or malignant cause for symptoms. Pelvic imaging should be performed if an alternative diagnosis, such as endometriosis, is suspected. Cystoscopy should be performed to exclude other pathology and also to aid accurate phenotyping of BPS (bladder capacity, presence of Hunner lesions). The aim of phenotyping is to separate those with clear bladder pathology (small capacity, Hunner lesions, chronic inflammation) from those with anatomically normal bladders as treatment options vary. In those with Hunner lesions, bladder biopsy shows a chronic pancystitis, often with marked infiltration with lymphocytes and macrophages and mast cell infiltration. The 'INPUT' classification system allows patients' symptoms to be described in five different clinical domains in order to guide multimodal therapy: Infection, Neurological/systemic, Psychosocial, Ulcers and Tenderness of muscles. The aim of the evaluation is to assess the relative contribution of each of these factors to the patient's symptoms.

Treatment

Treatment of BPS/IC consists of conservative, pharmacological, intravesical and surgical options.

Conservative

Patient education about the chronicity of the condition, behavioural modification (timed voiding, bladder training), stress reduction, dietary alteration (avoidance of caffeine and spicy and acidic foods) and physical therapy should be the initial management for all patients.

Pharmacological

Several pharmacological therapies have been studied for BPS/IC, all with variable efficacy. Neuropathic analgesics (e.g. amitriptyline, pregabalin) are used for those with a significant pain component, whereas antimuscarinics and β_3-agonists are used for frequency, nocturia and urgency symptoms. Oral pentosan polysulphate (Elmiron), a glycosaminoglycan (GAG) layer replacement treatment, has demonstrated efficacy in pain and urinary symptoms but recent reports of ophthalmic adverse events with long-term exposure may limit its use. Evidence for other oral therapies (e.g. antihistamines and immunosuppressants) is mixed.

Guy Hunner, 1868–1957, American surgeon, first described the characteristic inflammatory lesions of the bladder in 1915.

Intravesical

Direct instillation of GAG layer replacement therapies are thought to repair the defective GAG layer, which may be part of the pathophysiology of BPS/IC. Although the evidence base is weak, they are widely used with satisfactory outcomes in some patients without the side effects seen with oral therapies. Intravesical 'cocktails' with combinations of alkalinised local anaesthetic, steroid and GAG layer therapies may be useful for acute flares.

Surgical

Several surgical options have been studied. For those with Hunner lesions, fulguration or laser to these lesions can be beneficial. Cystodistension as a treatment has variable evidence for success. Minimally invasive treatment with intravesical BTX-A or SNS should be offered after the above measures have failed. If these options fail to improve symptoms major surgical reconstruction can be considered in selected cases. This is more suitable for those with clear evidence of bladder pathology (small capacity, fibrotic, ulcerated bladder). The aim is to increase the capacity of the bladder or divert the urinary stream, with options including bladder augmentation cystoplasty, cystoplasty with or without subtrigonal resection or urinary diversion with or without cystectomy. It is generally thought that cystectomy with orthotopic bladder reconstruction or ileal conduit urinary diversion is the best option as any form of bladder preservation risks ongoing pain in the remnant bladder segment with requirement for secondary cystectomy in up to 65%.

Radiation cystitis

Radiation cystitis is a common complication of pelvic radiotherapy with incidence rates ranging from 23% to 80%. Radiation treatment causes endothelial cell damage and perivascular fibrosis, resulting in ischaemia and obliterative endarteritis. Haematuria is more pronounced than that seen in BPS/IC. The end stage is a small, fibrotic bladder with poor compliance and a risk of upper tract compromise, as for other chronic inflammatory bladder diseases.

Emergency admission with haematuria requires resuscitation, catheterisation and bladder washout and blood transfusion as required. Cystoscopic management with fulguration or laser to bleeding vessels should be performed initially to stop bleeding. Intravesical GAG layer replacement therapies can be considered, and hyperbaric oxygen therapy has shown benefit in severe, refractory cases of haemorrhagic cystitis. Radiological arterial embolisation can also be considered for refractory cases, but ischaemic complications occur in 10–63% (e.g. skin or bladder necrosis, gluteal paresis, perineal or buttock pain). Finally, urinary diversion with or without cystectomy can be performed for end-stage cases, but perioperative morbidity is almost 50% and mortality is 16%.

Ketamine cystitis

Ketamine is an *N*-methyl-d-aspartate (NMDA) antagonist. It has been used for decades as an anaesthetic agent but has become increasingly popular as a recreational 'street drug' because of its euphoric and psychedelic effects. As a result of long-term ketamine abuse, up to 30% develop the condition of ketamine cystitis – a chronic inflammatory bladder condition characterised by a small, contracted, inflamed bladder with ureteric stricture and hydronephrosis in advanced cases. The severity of the inflammatory effect is related to the duration of abuse.

The clinical presentation is very similar to that of BPS/IC and investigation with cystoscopy, bladder biopsy and CT urogram should be performed to exclude other inflammatory or infective conditions (e.g. TB, schistosomiasis) and to evaluate the effect on the upper urinary tract (***Figure 83.33***).

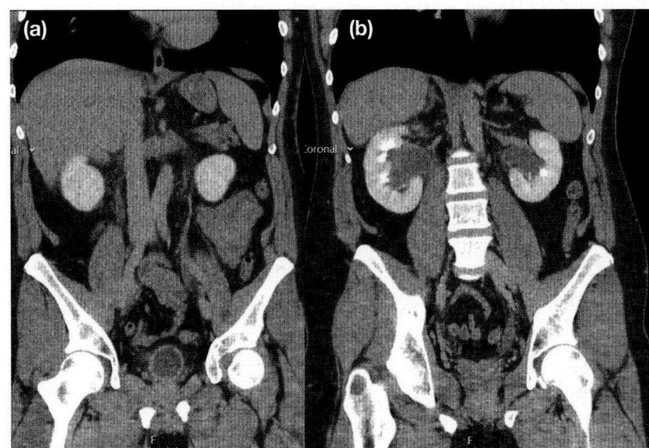

Figure 83.33 Computed tomography showing a thickened bladder (a) and bilateral hydroureteronephrosis (b) secondary to ketamine cystitis.

Initial management is centred around the cessation of ketamine use as surgical intervention should not be performed in those continuing to use ketamine. If patients have upper tract obstruction due to ureteric involvement in the inflammatory process, renal drainage with stent or nephrostomy will be required as a temporising measure to preserve renal function. Management of LUTS and pain follows the same pathway of oral and intravesical therapies as for BPS/IC, although regimes for analgesia consisting of co-codamol, amitriptyline and buprenorphine patches have proved particularly beneficial in this condition.

Surgical approaches are similar to those for the other chronic inflammatory conditions, namely augmentation enterocystoplasty, supratrigonal cystectomy and ureteric reimplantation, total cystectomy with orthotopic neobladder, heterotopic neobladder with appendicovesicostomy or urinary diversion with or without a cystectomy. However, the rate of perioperative complications with major reconstructive surgery in this population is high; those with upper tract involvement at presentation are likely be at higher risk of postoperative complications.

Summary box 83.6

Chronic inflammatory conditions of the bladder

- Patients with chronic inflammatory bladder conditions should have a bladder biopsy to identify a treatable cause (e.g. TB)
- Upper tracts should be evaluated with cross-sectional imaging to identify renal obstruction due to a high-pressure bladder
- Management is aimed at symptomatic improvement and maintaining low bladder pressure

HAEMATURIA

Haematuria is the presence of blood in the urine. It can be classified as visible (VH, or macroscopic) and non-visible (NVH, microscopic or dipstick). Microscopic haematuria is defined as the presence of red blood cells (RBCs) on microscopic examination of the urine and is variably defined as three or more or five or more RBCs per high-power field. A few RBCs can be found in the urine of healthy people, especially after rigorous exercise, sexual intercourse or from menstrual contamination, with an upper limit of 1 million RBCs per 24 hours considered normal. Overall, 30–60% of patients with NVH are found to have an underlying cause, depending upon the age and risk factors of the population studied and the type of investigation performed, but the rate of malignancy is around 5% for those with NVH compared with almost 20% for those with VH.

Both VH and NVH can arise from anywhere in the renal tract, including renal parenchyma, renal pelvis, ureter, bladder, prostate and urethra. Certain diseases outside the renal tract may also lead to haematuria (*Table 83.15*).

There is a lack of consensus between national guidelines regarding who should be investigated for haematuria. However, all patients should have a digital rectal examination to evaluate prostate size and consistency, urine culture to exclude infection and urine cytology to aid diagnosis of urothelial malignancy in those at higher risk (smokers, occupational history, family history, elderly). Serum estimated glomerular filtration rate (eGFR) should be assessed, and prostate-specific antigen (PSA) testing should be discussed in men with a 10- to 15-year life expectancy to assess prostate cancer risk. Those with visible haematuria should undergo evaluation of the LUT with cystoscopy and upper urinary tract with CT urogram. Patients with NVH should have the urine microscopy repeated on three occasions, and only be investigated if the haematuria is persistent. Patients with NVH who are over 40 years old should also undergo evaluation with flexible cystoscopy and renal tract imaging (ultrasound or CT urogram), but investigations could be rationalised to flexible cystoscopy and renal tract ultrasound in younger patients deemed to be at low risk of urothelial malignancy. In those with NVH and proteinuria, where the above urological investigations are negative, nephrological causes should be sought.

Summary box 83.7

Haematuria

- Patients with haematuria require upper tract investigation with CT urogram and lower tract investigation with cystoscopy

TABLE 83.15 Common causes of haematuria.

Site	Cause
Kidney	• Cancer (renal cell, urothelial, squamous cell, adenocarcinoma) • Stones • Infection • Trauma • Cystic diseases (e.g. medullary sponge kidney, polycystic kidney disease) • Vascular disorder (e.g. vascular malformations, renal vein thrombosis) • Nephrological causes (IgA nephropathy, glomerulonephritis, vasculitis, Henoch–Schönlein purpura) • Papillary necrosis
Ureter	• Cancer (urothelial) • Stones • Infection • Trauma • Benign diseases (PUJ obstruction, stricture)
Bladder	• Cancer (urothelial, squamous cell, adenocarcinoma) • Stones • Infection (bacterial, TB, schistosomiasis) • Trauma • Chronic inflammatory conditions (IC, radiation cystitis, ketamine cystitis, cyclophosphamide cystitis)
Prostate	• Cancer • Benign prostatic enlargement • Infection
Medical	• Bleeding disorders (e.g. sickle cell, thrombophilia) • Anticoagulation therapy
Iatrogenic	• Urethral instrumentation • Nephrostomy

IC, interstitial cystitis; IgA, immunoglobulin A; PUJ, pelviureteric junction; TB, tuberculosis.

BLADDER CANCER

Bladder cancer is a highly prevalent disease with 540 000 cases worldwide and 188 000 deaths reported in 2015. Risk factors for developing bladder cancer are shown in *Table 83.16*.

Pathology

The commonest type of bladder cancer is transitional cell (urothelial) carcinoma (*Table 83.17*). Squamous cell carcinoma occurs secondary to chronic inflammation (e.g. indwelling catheter, stone, schistosomiasis), and primary adenocarcinoma usually originates in the urachus (dome of the bladder) or in

Eduard Heinrich Henoch, 1820–1910, Professor of Diseases of Children, Berlin, Germany, described this form of purpura in 1868.
Johann Lucas Schönlein, 1793–1864, Professor of Medicine, Berlin, Germany, published his description of this form of purpura in 1837.

TABLE 83.16 Risk factors for bladder cancer.

Smoking	2–5 times increased risk
Occupational exposure (aromatic hydrocarbons)	• Tanner • Rubber • Paint and dyes • Gas and tar • Hairdressers • Plumbers • Painters
Environmental carcinogens	Arsenic in drinking water
Chronic inflammation of bladder	• Indwelling catheter • Stones • Schistosomiasis (predisposes to squamous cell carcinoma) • Recurrent infections leading to keratinising squamous metaplasia
Drugs	• Phenacetin • Cyclophosphamide
Pelvic radiotherapy	

those with bowel in the urinary tract (augmentation enterocystoplasty, bladder exstrophy repair). Histological variants (e.g. micropapillary, sarcomatoid, plasmacytoid, nested variant) can coexist with urothelial carcinoma and generally signify aggressive tumours with poorer prognosis than pure urothelial carcinoma.

TABLE 83.17 Common histological subtypes of bladder cancer.

Type	Frequency
Transitional cell carcinoma	>90%
Squamous cell carcinoma	1–7%
Adenocarcinoma	2%
Rare: Melanoma, lymphoma, sarcoma, small cell carcinoma, phaeochromocytoma	<1%
Metastatic adenocarcinoma (colorectal, prostate, kidney, ovary)	<1%

Grading and staging

Bladder cancer is graded as well differentiated (G1), moderately differentiated (G2) and poorly differentiated (G3). Stages Tis, Ta and T1 are non-muscle-invasive (NMIBC) and stages T2, T3 and T4 are muscle-invasive (MIBC) or locally advanced (*Figure 83.34*). Approximately 70% of tumours are NMIBC at presentation, whereas 30% are MIBC or metastatic.

Presentation

Patients most commonly present with painless haematuria (in 85%). Storage LUTS of frequency, urgency, dysuria and recurrent UTI may be present. Rarely, patients may present

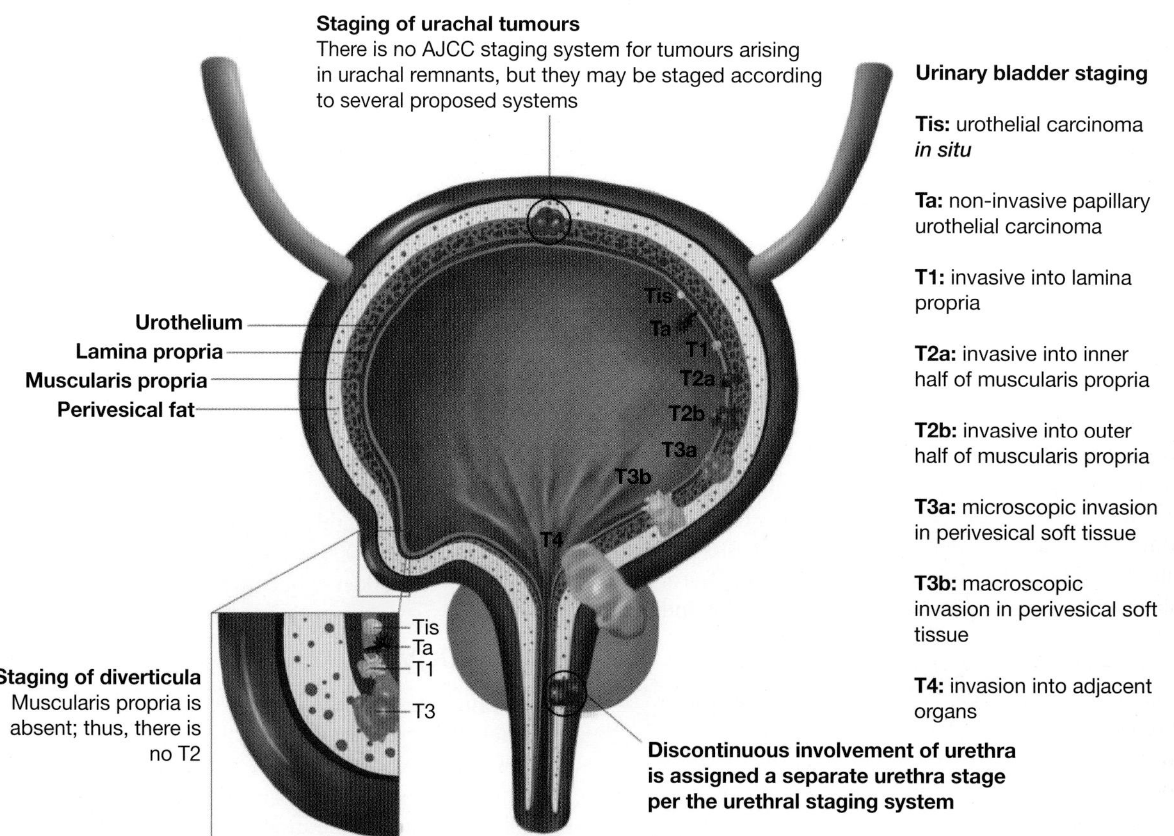

Figure 83.34 Staging of the primary tumour in bladder cancer. (Reproduced with permission from Magers MJ, Lopez-Beltran A, Montironi R *et al*. Staging of bladder cancer. *Histopathology* 2019; **74**(1): 112–34.)

with flank pain, weight loss, pelvic or bone pain and lower limb oedema in advanced cases.

Investigation

Urine

Urine should be cultured and examined cytologically for malignant cells. An increasing number of urinary biomarkers based on panels of epigenetic markers are being studied, but none has been shown to surpass the accuracy of cystoscopy and so are not routinely used.

Cross-sectional imaging: CT urography and MRI of the bladder

CT urogram is the gold standard evaluation for upper tract disease (including hydronephrosis) and assessment of nodal metastases (*Figure 83.35*). MRI of the bladder can be useful in staging of the primary tumour. Imaging should ideally be performed prior to transurethral resection of the bladder tumour (TURBT) as false-positive T3 disease can be diagnosed if cross-sectional imaging is carried out too soon after TURBT. CT of the chest should be performed in confirmed bladder cancer cases for complete staging.

Cystourethroscopy

Flexible cystourethroscopy under local anaesthetic is the mainstay of diagnosis and should always be performed on patients with haematuria (*Figure 83.36*). The diagnostic accuracy of conventional 'white' light cystoscopy has been improved by optical enhancement techniques such as narrow-band imaging (NBI) and photodynamic 'blue' light cystoscopy (PDD), which relies on the photosensitiser hexaminolevulinate. These techniques are recommended in patients with a high suspicion of cancer and negative initial findings, or in those with positive cytology but negative 'white' light cystoscopy.

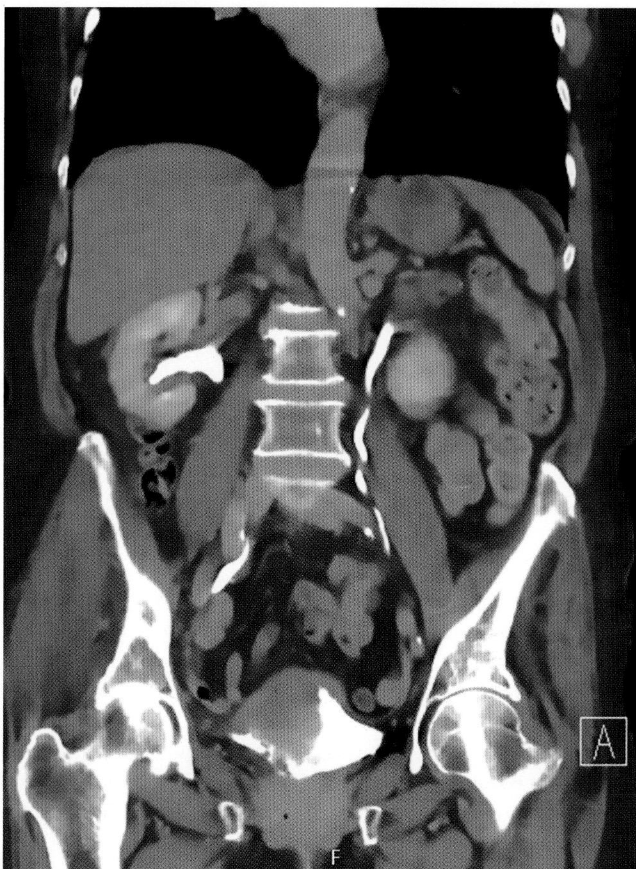

Figure 83.35 Computed tomography showing a large right-sided bladder tumour.

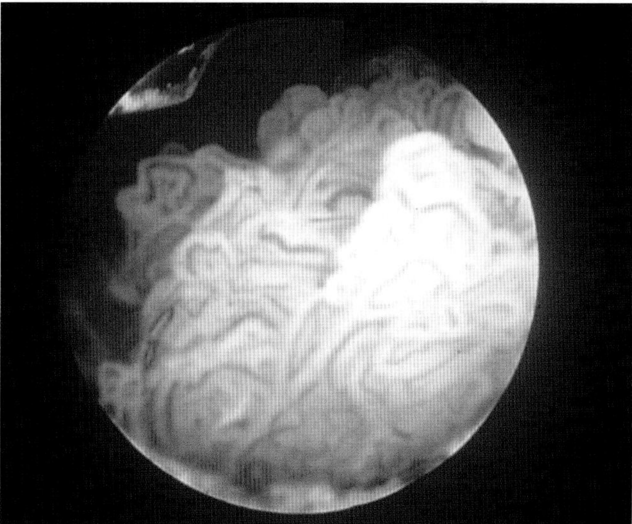

Figure 83.36 Cystoscopic appearance of a papillary bladder tumour.

Non-muscle-invasive bladder cancer

The aim of managing patients with NMIBC is to reduce the risk of tumour recurrence and progression to MIBC.

Transurethral resection

The initial management of bladder tumours consists of TURBT for accurate staging purposes. This is performed with a rigid cystoscope under general anaesthesia. A bimanual examination should be performed prior to resection to determine whether a mass is palpable and, if so, whether it is mobile or fixed. This should be repeated following resection. For large tumours, a standard fractionated resection of the entire tumour, including the tumour base with deep muscle, is performed. For smaller (<3 cm) solitary tumours, en bloc resection of the entire tumour can be performed and may reduce the risk of tumour recurrence by preventing the spread of tumour cells and subsequent implantation across the bladder. The following details should be recorded to enable accurate risk stratification: the size of the primary tumour, the number of tumours, the nodular or papillary features, concern for the presence of CIS and completeness of visual resection.

Mapping biopsies from the trigone, bladder dome and the right, left, anterior and posterior bladder wall should be taken if CIS is suspected.

Postoperative mitomycin C instillation

Approximately 30% of patients with NMIBC will experience early recurrence following initial TURBT and so an immediate post-TURBT dose of mitomycin C should be instilled into the bladder. This has been shown to reduce the risk of tumour recurrence by 12%.

Risk stratification

Based on the final histological grade and stage, the patient can be risk stratified. Those with multifocal high-grade T1 tumours with CIS are at highest risk of disease recurrence and progression to MIBC. For these patients, early radical cystectomy should be discussed as they are at high risk of tumour progression. An alternative is intravesical bacillus Calmette–Guérin (BCG) to reduce the risk of tumour progression. Those with solitary low-grade Ta tumours have the lowest risk of recurrence and progression and so the management of this group consists of regular cystoscopic surveillance alone. For intermediate-risk tumours, a 6-week course of intravesical mitomycin C can be considered to reduce the risk of recurrence.

Repeat TURBT

For those with high-grade or T1 tumours, a repeat TURBT 2–6 weeks after initial TURBT should be performed to identify any residual tumour. Upstaging to MIBC is found in up to 40%.

Intravesical BCG

For high-risk tumours, intravesical treatment with immunotherapy (BCG) has been shown to reduce the risk of progression to MIBC. The treatment is given weekly for 6 weeks, followed by a 3-weekly treatment every 6 months for 3 years. Side effects include transient fever, dysuria, rarely BCG sepsis and BCG cystitis necessitating cystectomy.

Muscle-invasive bladder cancer

The two primary radical treatment options for MIBC are radical cystectomy with urinary diversion or chemoradiotherapy. Whichever modality is employed, 5-year survival rates are approximately 60%. There is a move towards primary surgical treatment in most centres. The use of systemic chemotherapy given before (neoadjuvant) radical cystectomy has been shown to improve survival by about 5–7%. Newer immunotherapy approaches are being evaluated in the neoadjuvant and adjuvant setting; in particular, immune-checkpoint inhibitors with antibodies targeting the programmed cell death ligand 1 (PDL1) pathway are demonstrating promising results.

Radical cystectomy and ileal conduit urinary diversion

Those with poor bladder function, significant haematuria, upper tract obstruction, widespread CIS or factors that affect successful radiotherapy (e.g. bilateral hip replacements, inflammatory bowel disease) are more suitable for radical cystectomy and pelvic lymphadenectomy. This is major surgery with a perioperative morbidity rate of up to 50%, and so patients should undergo anaesthetic assessment to assess suitability for surgery.

Alternative drainage for urine is necessary after removal of the bladder. The standard procedure is to perform an ileal conduit diversion. Male patients should be counselled about the onset of erectile dysfunction and anejaculation after the operation, although in some cases the nerve supply for erectile function can be preserved through careful dissection; they should also be told about alternative forms of urinary diversion, which include continent urinary diversions and orthotopic bladder replacement.

Patients should be seen by a stoma care therapist, who will ensure that the correct stoma site is chosen, avoiding skin creases to prevent leakage from the ileostomy.

The abdomen is opened through a lower midline incision from the umbilicus to pubic symphysis. The liver and the retroperitoneum are checked for evidence of metastases and the operability of the bladder is assessed. A bilateral pelvic lymphadenectomy is performed, removing external iliac nodes, internal iliac nodes and the nodes in the obturator fossae. The vessels passing to the bladder from the side wall of the pelvis are ligated and divided; the ureters are then divided. The posterior ligaments extending from the pararectal area to the back of the bladder are ligated and divided, and the layer posterior to Denonvilliers' fascia is opened. The endopelvic fascia is then divided on each side and the puboprostatic ligaments are divided. The dorsal venous complex is divided, and the urethra is then mobilised and divided. The ligaments lateral to the prostate are divided and the bladder is removed. In women, the uterus and anterior vaginal wall need to be included. Women must be counselled about the loss of ovarian and uterine function. Laparoscopic and robotic cystectomy are increasingly becoming the standard of care with the aim of minimising perioperative morbidity, but evidence for superiority of these techniques over the traditional open approach is awaited.

An isolated loop of ileum is then prepared on its own mesentery, and continuity of the small bowel restored. The ureters are then implanted into the bowel either separately (Bricker) or as one plate (Wallace) and the ileostomy is created. Meticulous care must be taken to close all mesenteric windows, thus avoiding internal hernias (*Figure 83.37*).

Alternative techniques of urinary diversion

Alternative forms of diversion are most suitable for highly motivated patients with adequate renal and liver function who wish to avoid an external collection device.

Orthotopic bladder

An orthotopic bladder is the creation of a pouch (typically using small or large bowel) that is then anastomosed to the patient's urethra. Contraindications to an orthotopic bladder include widespread CIS and tumour in the prostatic urethra. Many different types of orthotopic bladder have been described but

---

Charles Pierre Denonvilliers, 1808–1872, Professor of Anatomy and later of Surgery, Paris, France. Denonvilliers' fascia is the fascial layer that separates the prostate and bladder from the rectum.

Eugene Bricker, 1908–2000, American surgeon, described the separate anastomosis of each ureter to the ileal segment.

David Mitchell Wallace, 1913–1992, urologist, St Peter's Hospital, London, UK, described the anastomosis of both ureters together followed by anastomosis to the ileal segment in one plate in 1966.

the Studer pouch is widely performed. The aim is to achieve a large-capacity, low-pressure reservoir. A pouch is made from 57 cm of detubularised ileum. The ureters are implanted into a proximal 'chimney' that acts as an antireflux mechanism, and the pouch is anastomosed to the urethra (*Figure 83.37*). Patients can void by relaxing the pelvic floor and straining, but CISC may be required to completely empty the pouch in 15–30%.

Continent cutaneous diversion (heterotopic bladder substitute)

For those who require urethrectomy, or in whom the urethra is non-functional, a continent cutaneous diversion can be performed. A Studer pouch can be made as described above. The appendix, or a separate section of ileum if the appendix is not available, is then anastomosed from the bladder to the umbilicus or right iliac fossa. The patient can then intermittently catheterise this channel to drain the pouch.

Ureterosigmoidostomy (Mainz II pouch)

This option is popular in developing countries as there is no requirement for an external appliance or catheters. Patients require good anal sphincteric function. The sigmoid colon is detubularised and refashioned into a pouch into which the ureters are inserted (*Figure 83.37*). However, high rates of ascending UTI and increased risk of malignancy (associated with mixing of faecal and urinary streams), bowel frequency and urge incontinence have limited its use.

Complications of urinary diversion

The ileal conduit urinary diversion has the lowest rate of complications of all forms of urinary diversion. Risks include ureteroileal leak or stricture (5%), stomal complications such as stenosis or hernia (20%), upper tract dilatation (30%), recurrent UTIs and rarely metabolic complications (hyperchloraemic metabolic acidosis).

Summary box 83.8

Bladder cancer

- The commonest presenting symptom of bladder cancer is haematuria
- Smoking and occupational exposure to certain chemicals are the commonest risk factors
- Bladder cancer can be non-muscle-invasive or muscle-invasive
- The management of NMIBC is TURBT, followed by intravesical mitomycin C or BCG depending on the risk stratification
- The management of MIBC is neoadjuvant chemotherapy followed by radical cystectomy
- Options for urinary diversion include ileal conduit, orthotopic bladder substitute, heterotopic bladder substitute or ureterosigmoidostomy
- The choice of diversion is dependent on patient factors, tumour factors and surgeon experience

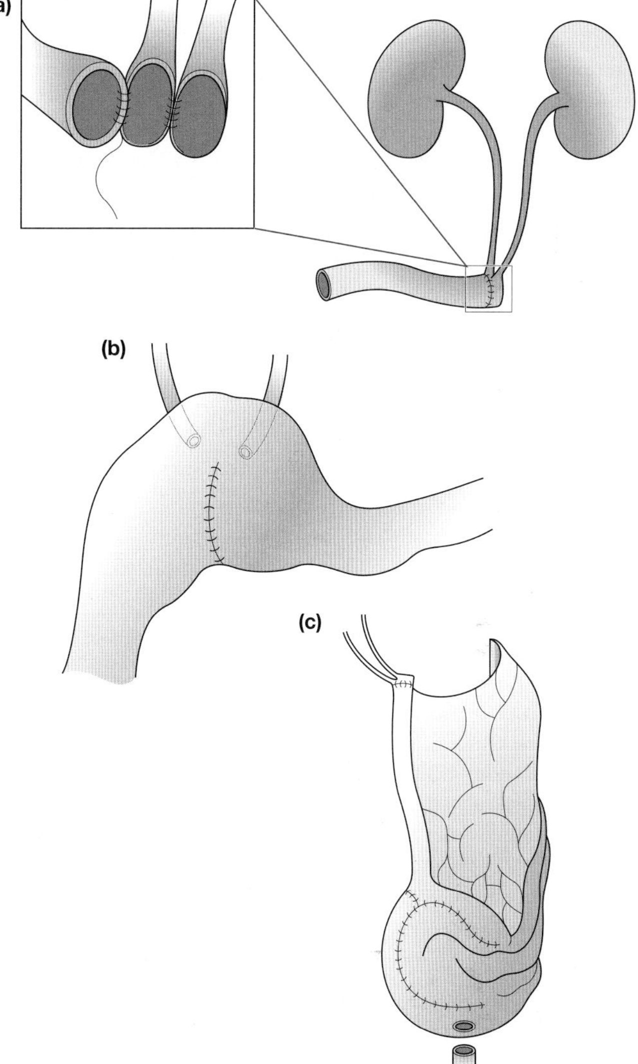

Figure 83.37 Techniques of urinary diversion of urine. (a) Ileal conduit; the ureters are spatulated and anastomosed to ileum; (b) ureterosigmoidostomy; (c) ileal neobladder with an antireflux long afferent limb.

Complications of orthotopic or continent pouches include ureteroileal leak or stricture, urinary leak from the pouch, stone formation, UTIs, metabolic complications (hyperchloraemic metabolic acidosis) and rarely adenocarcinoma (5%). Stenosis and incontinence are the main complications of appendicovesicostomy and up to 50% may require some form of revision surgery to the channel over a 5-year period.

Radical external beam radiotherapy

Radical radiotherapy is an option for very elderly or unfit patients who are unsuitable for radical cystectomy. Typically, treatment with 66 Gy is administered in 30 fractions over 6 weeks. However, long-term urinary and bowel side effects can impair quality of life and there is a risk of secondary malignancy and fistula.

Urs Studer, contemporary, Swiss urologist, described a neobladder pouch that is made of ileum.
The **Mainz II** pouch describes the formation of a low-pressure sigmoid colon pouch into which both ureters are anastomosed. It is named after the city where the inventors of this technique worked.

Bladder preservation with radical TURBT, neoadjuvant chemotherapy and then chemoradiotherapy is being studied as an option for those with very localised MIBC, but this remains an option for only a very select group.

BLADDER TRAUMA

Bladder trauma can be classified as iatrogenic or non-iatrogenic (blunt or penetrating). Of non-iatrogenic causes, abdominal trauma and pelvic fracture are the most common, with bladder injury reported in 10% of cases. Iatrogenic injury is most commonly the result of TURBT, anti-incontinence surgery or pelvic surgery (e.g. hysterectomy, caesarean section, colorectal surgery). Rarely, spontaneous rupture can occur after bladder augmentation without any history of trauma. This is due to overdistension in those with limited bladder sensation (e.g. SCI), and often presents with vague abdominal pain, fever or sepsis. A high index of suspicion of bladder rupture in patients with a history of bladder augmentation is required.

Classification

Bladder injuries can be either extraperitoneal (the peritoneum is intact and urine extravasates into the retropubic space but not into the peritoneal cavity), intraperitoneal (the peritoneum over the bladder is injured and urine extravasates into the peritoneal cavity) or mixed (*Table 83.18*). Intraperitoneal ruptures are associated with a risk of urinary peritonitis and ileus, and so are more significant than extraperitoneal ruptures.

Clinical features

If iatrogenic, the injury may be recognised at the time. If perforation during transurethral surgery is noted, the procedure should be stopped, haemostasis should be achieved and the patient should be catheterised. In cases of trauma, patients typically present with suprapubic pain, difficulty or inability to pass urine, haematuria and abdominal distension.

Investigation

Retrograde cystogram or CT cystogram confirms the diagnosis and identifies whether the injury is intraperitoneal or extraperitoneal (*Figure 83.38*). Postdrainage views should be obtained as a small amount of contrast extravasation may be missed with a full bladder. With intraperitoneal perforation, contrast is seen to outline loops of bowel.

Extraperitoneal injury

The management of extraperitoneal rupture consists of urethral catheterisation with free bladder drainage for 10–14 days, followed by a cystogram to ensure that the injury has healed prior to removal of the catheter. If the extraperitoneal injury is iatrogenic and recognised at the time of open or laparoscopic surgery, it can be repaired at the time in two layers with 2/0 Vicryl absorbable suture. If the bladder injury is associated with a pelvic fracture and the patient is undergoing surgery for open fixation, or repair of a rectal or vaginal perforation, the bladder should be repaired at the same time.

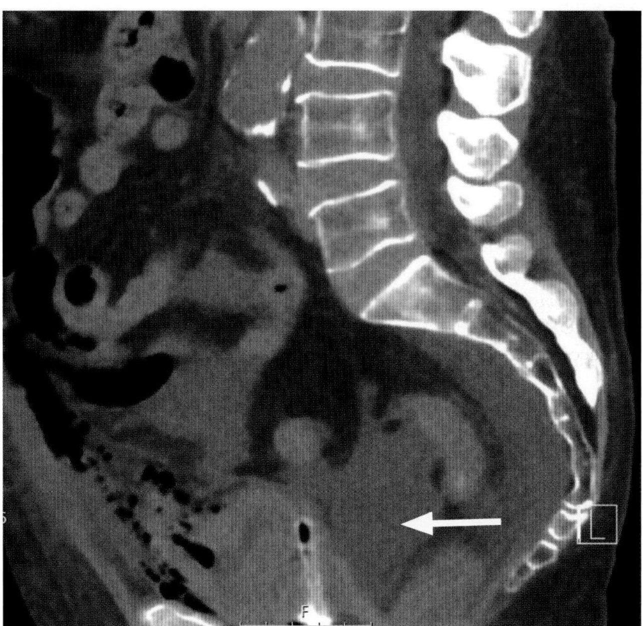

Figure 83.38 Computed tomography showing intraperitoneal bladder injury after transurethral resection of the bladder tumour (arrow pointing to intraperitoneal urinary extravasation).

TABLE 83.18 Grading of bladder trauma.

Grade	Injury	Description
I	Haematoma	Contusion, intramural haematoma
	Laceration	Partial thickness
II	Laceration	Extraperitoneal bladder wall laceration <2 cm
III	Laceration	Extraperitoneal ≥2 cm or intraperitoneal <2 cm bladder wall laceration
IV	Laceration	Intraperitoneal bladder wall laceration ≥2 cm
V	Laceration	Laceration extending into the bladder neck or ureteral orifice (trigone)

Intraperitoneal injury

Intraperitoneal injuries usually require open surgical repair to reduce the risks of urinary contamination of the peritoneal space. If the injury is small without significant fluid extravasation, a period of catheterisation can be attempted in clinically well patients, but close monitoring is required and a cystogram at 2 weeks should confirm complete healing prior to removal of the catheter. If it has not healed, open repair will be required.

Summary box 83.9

Bladder trauma

- Bladder trauma can be extraperitoneal or intraperitoneal
- Extraperitoneal injury can be managed with indwelling catheterisation for 10–14 days
- Intraperitoneal injury most often requires laparotomy and repair of the bladder defect

FURTHER READING

Abrams P, Andersson KE, Birder L *et al.* Fourth International Consultation on Incontinence Recommendations of the International Scientific Committee: evaluation and treatment of urinary incontinence, pelvic organ prolapse, and fecal incontinence. *Neurourol Urodyn* 2010; **29**(1): 213–40.

Babjuk M, Burger M, Compérat EM. European Association of Urology guidelines on non-muscle-invasive bladder cancer (TaT1 and carcinoma in situ) – 2019 update. *Eur Urol* 2019; **76**: 639–57.

Bonkat G, Bartoletti R, Bruyere F *et al. EAU guidelines on urological infections*. Available from https://uroweb.org/wp-content/uploads/EAU-Guidelines-on-Urological-Infections-2018-large-text.pdf (accessed 29 August 2020).

Fowler CJ, Griffiths D, de Groat WC. The neural control of micturition. *Nat Rev Neurosci* 2008; **9**(6): 453–66.

Malde S, Palmisani S, Al-Kaisy A, Sahai A. Guideline of guidelines: bladder pain syndrome. *BJU Int* 2018; **122**(5): 729–43.

Partin AW, Peters CA, Kavoussi LR, Dmochowksi RR, Wein AJ. *Campbell–Walsh–Wein urology*, 12th edn. Philadelphia, PA: Elsevier, 2021.

Witjes JA, Bruins HM, Cathomas R *et al.* European Association of Urology guidelines on muscle-invasive and metastatic bladder cancer: summary of the 2020 guidelines. *Eur Urol* 2021; **79**(1): 82–104.

CHAPTER

84 The prostate and seminal vesicles

Learning objectives

To understand:

- The relationship of anatomical structure and biochemical function to the development and treatment of benign and malignant disease of the prostate
- The terminology used to describe lower urinary tract symptoms and to know their causes as well as the treatment options available
- Which investigations are appropriate for benign and malignant conditions of the prostate
- Clinical staging of carcinoma of the prostate and how staging contributes to the complex decision making

BENIGN PROSTATIC HYPERPLASIA

Aetiology

Hormones

Serum testosterone levels slowly but significantly decrease with advancing age; however, levels of oestrogenic steroids are not decreased equally. According to this theory, the prostate enlarges because of increased oestrogenic effects. It is likely that the secretion of intermediate peptide growth factors plays a part in the development of **benign prostatic hyperplasia** (BPH). Metabolic syndrome and hereditary factors have also been implicated in its development.

Summary box 84.1

Benign prostatic hyperplasia (BPH)

- Occurs in men over 50 years of age; by the age of 60 years, 50% of men have histological evidence of BPH
- It is a common cause of significant lower urinary tract symptoms (LUTS) in men and the most common cause of bladder outflow obstruction (BOO) in men >70 years of age

Pathology

BPH affects both glandular epithelium and connective tissue stroma to variable degrees. BPH typically affects the submucous group of glands in the transitional zone, forming a nodular enlargement. Eventually, this overgrowth compresses the peripheral zone glands into a false capsule and causes the appearance of the typical 'lateral' lobes.

When BPH affects the central zone glands, a 'middle' lobe develops that projects up into the bladder within the internal sphincter (*Figure 84.1*).

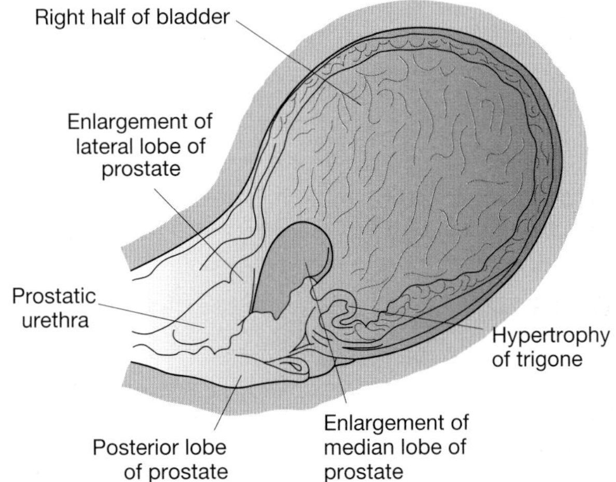

Figure 84.1 Diagram of late-stage bladder outflow obstruction showing enlargement of the prostate from benign prostatic hyperplasia, trabeculation of the bladder with smooth muscle hypertrophy and fibrosis.

Effects of benign prostatic hyperplasia

It is important to realise that the relationship between anatomical prostatic enlargement, LUTS and urodynamic evidence of BOO is complex (*Figure 84.2*).

Summary box 84.2

Consequences of BPH

- No symptoms, no BOO
- No symptoms, but urodynamic evidence of BOO
- LUTS, no evidence of BOO
- LUTS and BOO
- Others (acute/chronic retention, haematuria, urinary infection and stone formation)

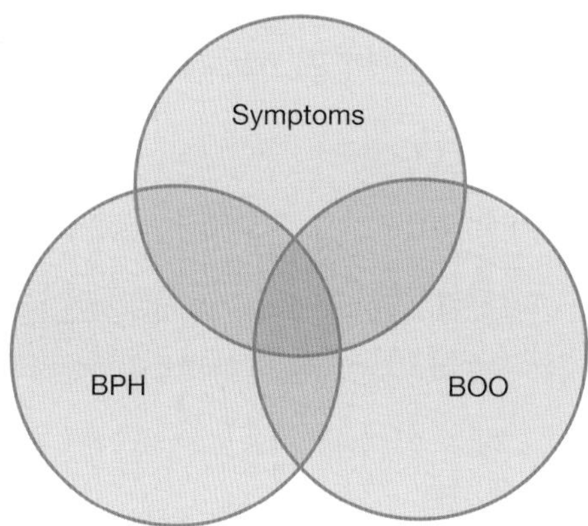

Figure 84.2 Diagrammatic representation of the relation between symptoms of prostatism, benign prostate hyperplasia (BPH) and urodynamically proven bladder outflow obstruction (BOO).

Anatomically, the effects are as follows:

- **Urethra**. The prostatic urethra is lengthened, sometimes to twice its normal length, but it is not narrowed anatomically. The normal posterior curve may be so exaggerated that it requires a curved catheter to negotiate it. When only one lateral lobe is enlarged, distortion of the prostatic urethra occurs.
- **Bladder**. If BPH causes BOO, the musculature of the bladder hypertrophies to overcome the obstruction and appears trabeculated (*Figure 84.3*). Significant BPH is associated with increased blood flow, and the resultant veins at the base of the bladder are apt to cause haematuria.

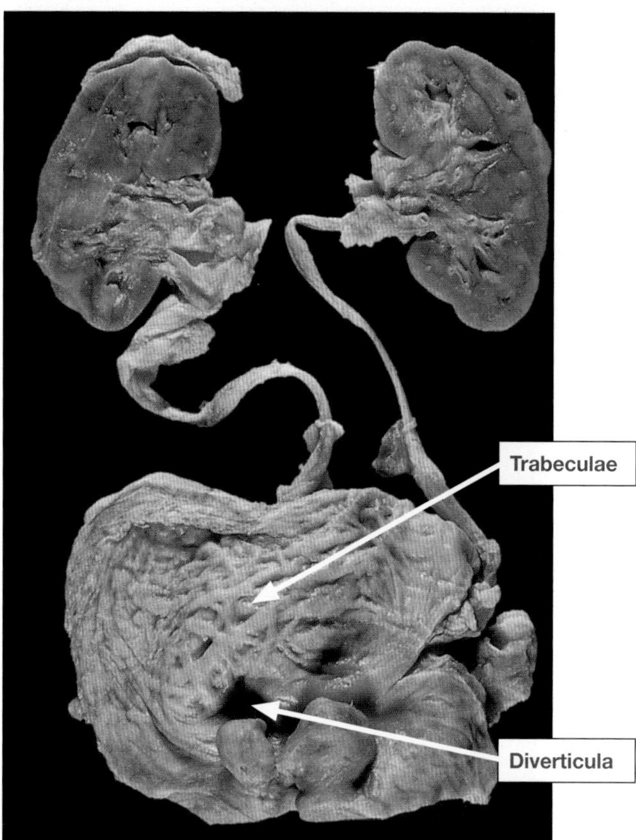

Figure 84.3 Pathological specimen of bladder and kidneys in a case of bladder outflow obstruction caused by benign prostatic hyperplasia. Bladder trabeculation, bilateral hydroureter and hydronephrosis can be seen.

Lower urinary tract symptoms

In both sexes, non-specific symptoms of bladder dysfunction become more common with age, probably owing to impairment of smooth muscle function and neurovesical coordination. Not all symptoms of disturbed voiding in ageing men should therefore be attributed to BPH causing BOO. Urologists prefer the term LUTS and discourage the use of the descriptive term 'prostatism'.

The following conditions can coexist with BOO, leading to difficulty in diagnosis and in predicting the outcome of treatment:

- idiopathic detrusor overactivity (see *Chapter 83*);
- neuropathic bladder dysfunction as a result of diabetes, stroke, Alzheimer's disease or Parkinson's disease (see *Chapter 83*); degeneration of bladder smooth muscle giving rise to impaired voiding and detrusor instability;
- BOO due to BPH.

LUTS can be described as:

- Voiding:
  - hesitancy (worsened if the bladder is very full);
  - poor flow (unimproved by straining);
  - intermittent stream – stops and starts;
  - dribbling (including after micturition);
  - sensation of poor bladder emptying;
  - episodes of near retention.
- Storage:
  - frequency;
  - nocturia;
  - urgency;
  - urge incontinence;
  - nocturnal incontinence (enuresis).

LUTS are usually assessed by means of scoring systems, which give a semiobjective measure of severity and may be helpful in assessing the outcome of the therapy.

Severe irritative symptoms are usually associated with detrusor instability. Postmicturition dribbling is now known not to be a consequence of BOO and is not usually improved by prostatectomy. It is due to retained urine in the urethra.

Bladder outflow obstruction

This is a urodynamic concept based on the combination of low flow rates in the presence of high voiding pressures. It can

Alois Alzheimer, 1864–1915, neurologist, worked at Heidelberg and Munich before being appointed Professor of Psychiatry at Breslau, Germany (now Wrocław, Poland).
James Parkinson, 1755–1824, general practitioner of Shoreditch, London, UK, published *An essay on the shaking palsy* in 1817.

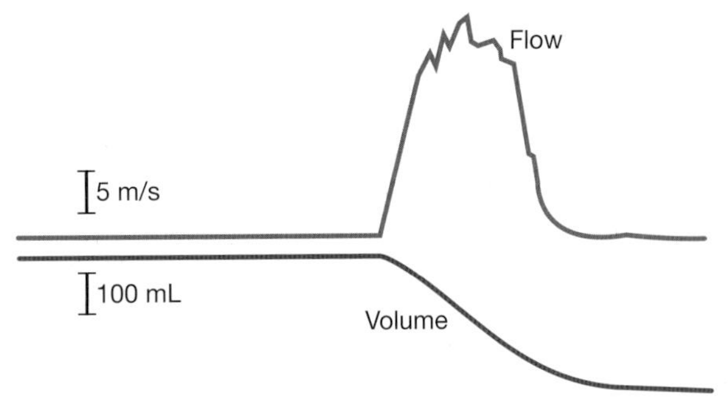

Figure 84.4 Normal flow rate. The voided volume is well in excess of 350 mL, and the maximum flow rate is in excess of 25 mL/s.

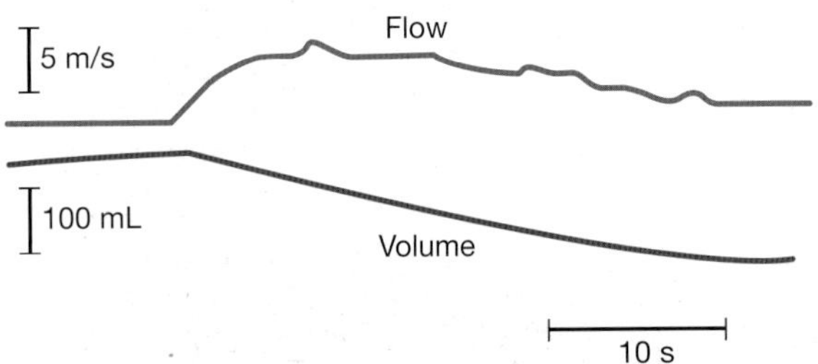

Figure 84.5 Diagram of a low flow rate showing a rather low voided volume of about 200 mL, but with a markedly decreased flow rate. Such a flow rate could be caused by a urethral stricture, bladder outflow obstruction or a weak detrusor.

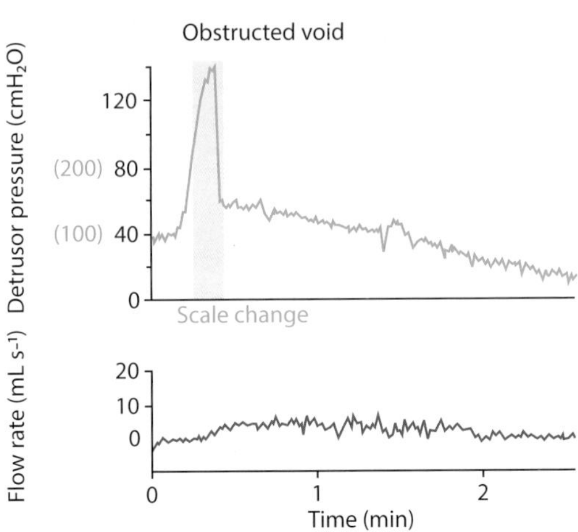

Figure 84.6 Conventional urodynamic trace showing detrusor pressure during voiding (voided volume 340 mL). There has been a change in scale because the pressure was so high; voiding pressures are increased with a low flow rate. This is diagnostic of bladder outflow obstruction.

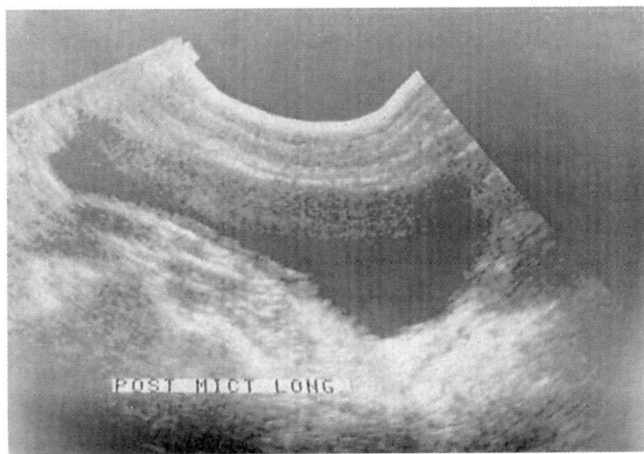

Figure 84.7 An ultrasonogram showing a large postvoid residual urine.

be diagnosed definitively only by pressure–flow studies. This is because symptoms are relatively non-specific and can result from detrusor instability, neurological dysfunction and weak bladder contraction. Even low measured peak flow rates (<10–12 mL/s) are not absolutely diagnostic because, in addition to BOO, weak detrusor contractions or low voided volumes (owing to instability) can be the cause. Nonetheless, flow rates provide a useful guide for everyday clinical management.

Urodynamically proven BOO may result from:

- BPH;
- bladder neck stenosis;
- bladder neck dyssynergia or functional bladder neck obstruction;
- bladder neck hypertrophy;
- prostate cancer;
- urethral stricture;
- functional obstruction due to neuropathic conditions.

The primary effects of BOO on the bladder are as follows:

- **Urinary flow rates decrease**: for a voided volume >200 mL, a peak flow rate of >15 mL/s is normal (*Figure 84.4*); one of 10–15 mL/s is equivocal; and one <10 mL/s is low (*Figure 84.5*).
- **Voiding pressures increase**: pressures >80 cmH_2O are high (*Figure 84.6*); pressures between 60 and 80 cmH_2O are equivocal; and pressures <60 cmH_2O are normal.

The long-term effects of BOO are as follows:

- The bladder may decompensate so that detrusor contraction becomes progressively less efficient and a residual urine develops, leading to chronic retention.
- The bladder may become more irritable during filling with a decrease in functional capacity partly caused by detrusor overactivity (see *Chapter 83*), which may also be caused by neurological dysfunction or ageing, or may be idiopathic.

Aside from symptoms, the complications of BOO are as follows:

- Acute retention of urine is sometimes the first symptom of BOO.
- Chronic retention. In patients in whom the residual volume is >250 mL or so (*Figure 84.7*), the tension in the bladder wall increases owing to the combination of a large volume of residual urine and increased resting and filling bladder pressures (a condition known as high-pressure chronic retention). The increased intramural tension results in functional obstruction of the upper urinary

tract with the development of bilateral hydronephrosis (*Figures 84.8–84.10*). As a result, upper tract infection and renal impairment may develop. Such men may present with overflow incontinence, enuresis and renal insufficiency. These symptoms should alert the doctor to the presence of this condition.

- Impaired bladder emptying. If the bladder decompensates with the development of a large volume of residual urine, urinary infection and calculi are prone to develop.
- Development of storage bladder symptoms secondary to BOO that can be irreversible if BOO is not treated.
- Haematuria. This may be a complication of BPH. Other causes must be excluded by carrying out urine culture, cytology, computed tomography (CT) urography and cystoscopy.

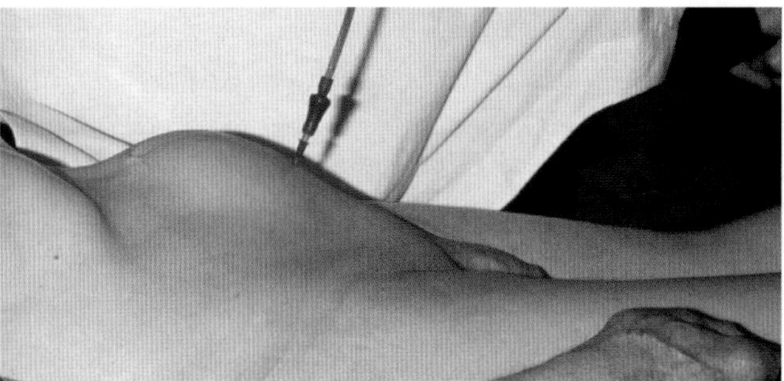

Figure 84.8 An abdomen with high-pressure urinary retention.

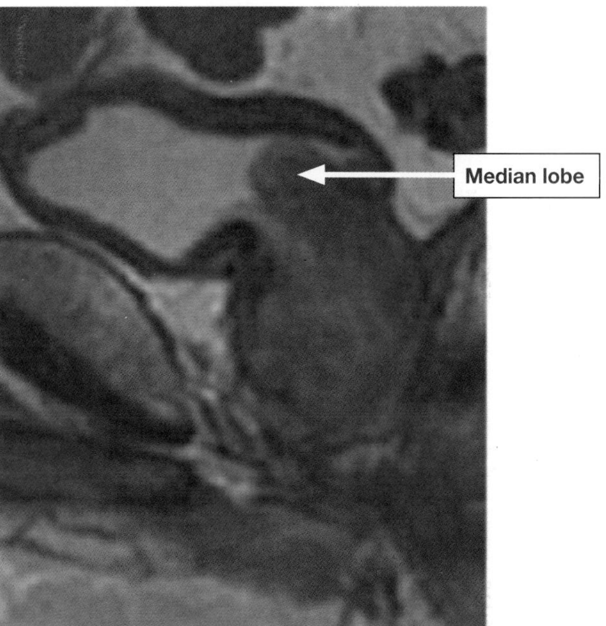

Figure 84.9 Magnetic resonance image showing an enlarged prostate and a median lobe projecting into the bladder and causing bladder outflow obstruction.

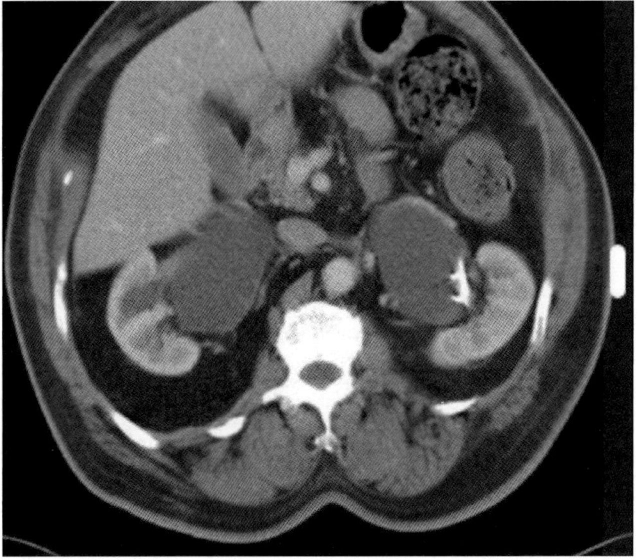

Figure 84.10 Computed tomography scan showing bilateral hydronephrosis as a result of bladder outflow obstruction.

ASSESSMENT OF THE PATIENT WITH LOWER URINARY TRACT SYMPTOMS

History

Symptom score sheets such as the International Prostate Symptom Score (IPSS) assign a score that gives information regarding the severity of symptoms at the outset and changes over time and following intervention. The IPSS assessment should include an assessment of quality of life, which is a reflection of the degree of 'bother' caused by a patient's symptoms. In addition to the IPSS, a frequency–volume diary completed by the patient before attending the clinic is invaluable in revealing fluid intake habits, diurnal variation in outputs and low-volume, frequent voiding.

Summary box 84.3

Investigations of men with LUTS

Essential investigations

- Urine analysis by dipstick for blood, leukocyte esterase, glucose and protein
- Urine culture for infection
- Serum creatinine
- Urinary flow rate and residual volume measurement

Additional investigations

- PSA if indicated
- Pressure–flow studies

Abdominal examination

Abdominal examination is usually normal. In patients with chronic retention, a distended bladder will be found on palpation, on percussion and sometimes on inspection with loss of the transverse suprapubic skin crease. General physical examination may demonstrate signs of chronic renal impairment with anaemia, pedal oedema and dehydration. The external urinary meatus should be examined to exclude stenosis and the epididymides are palpated for signs of inflammation.

Rectal examination

In benign enlargement, the posterior surface of the prostate is smooth, convex and typically elastic, but the fibrous element may give the prostate a firm consistency. The rectal mucosa can be made to move over the prostate. It should be noted that, if there is a considerable amount of residual urine present, it pushes the prostate downwards, making it appear larger than it is. It is not always possible to examine the cranial extreme of the very large prostate per rectum. An inability to get to the prostate base implies a volume of at least 50 mL.

The nervous system

The nervous system is examined to eliminate a neurological lesion. Diabetes mellitus, tabes dorsalis, disseminated sclerosis, cervical spondylosis, Parkinson's disease and other neurological states may mimic prostatic obstruction. If these are suspected, then a pressure–flow urodynamic study should be carried out to diagnose BOO. Examination of perianal sensation and anal tone is useful in detection of an S2–4 cauda equina lesion.

Serum prostate-specific antigen

After suitable counselling, measurement of serum PSA may be helpful. Men in whom a diagnosis of early prostate cancer might influence treatment option (such as those under 70 years or those with a positive family history who might be offered radical treatment) should be offered a PSA measurement. If the PSA range is 4–10 ng/L, a free-to-total PSA ratio of less than 15% should be suspicious of malignancy. Multiparametric magnetic resonance imaging (mpMRI) should be done, which may show a suspicious index lesion. In this situation, transrectal ultrasound (TRUS)-guided or transperineal biopsies should be considered.

Flow rate measurement

For this to be meaningful, two or three voids should be recorded using a special flow meter, usually found in urology outpatient clinics; the voided volume should be in excess of 150–200 mL. A typical history and a flow rate <10 mL/s (for a voided volume of >200 mL; *Figure 84.5*) will be sufficient for most urologists to recommend treatment. Usually, a flow rate measurement will be coupled with ultrasound measurement of postvoid residual urine.

There are pitfalls in the measurement of flow rates. The machine must be accurately calibrated. The patient must void volumes in excess of 150 mL and two or three recordings are needed to obtain a representative measurement. Decreased flow rates and LUTS may be seen in:

- BOO;
- low voided volumes (characteristically in men with detrusor instability);
- men with weak bladder contractions (low pressure–flow voiding), also known as underactive detrusor.

Pressure-flow urodynamic studies

Details of these studies are outlined in *Chapter 81*. They should be performed on the following patients:

- men with suspected neuropathy (Parkinson's disease, dementia, longstanding diabetes, previous strokes, multiple sclerosis);
- men with a dominant history of irritative symptoms and men with lifelong urgency and frequency;
- men with a doubtful history and those with flow rates in the near normal range (~ or >15 mL/s);
- men with invalid flow rate measurements (because of low voided volumes);
- high residual/chronic retention;
- men with recurrence of LUTS after previous BPH surgery (in the absence of urethral or bladder pathology);
- young men (<50 years) and older men (>80 years) with LUTS.

Blood tests

Serum creatinine, electrolytes and haemoglobin should be measured.

Examination of urine

The urine is examined for glucose, leukocyte esterase and blood; a midstream specimen should be sent for bacteriological examination and cytological examination may be carried out if carcinoma *in situ* is thought possible.

Upper tract imaging

Most urologists no longer carry out imaging of the upper tract in men with straightforward symptoms. Obviously, if infection or haematuria is present, then the upper tract should be imaged by means of intravenous urogram/CT urography or ultrasound scan.

Cystourethroscopy

Inspection of the urethra, the prostate and the urothelium of the bladder should be done immediately prior to prostatectomy to exclude a urethral stricture, a bladder carcinoma and the occasional non-opaque vesical calculus. This should be based on the patient's symptoms, signs and investigations. Direct inspection of the prostate is not used as an indicator to establish the presence of BOO and the need for surgery.

MANAGEMENT OF MEN WITH BENIGN PROSTATIC HYPERPLASIA OR BLADDER OUTFLOW OBSTRUCTION

Strong indications for treatment (usually prostatectomy) include:

- **Acute retention** (see *Chapter 83*) in fit men with no other cause for retention (drugs, constipation, recent operation, etc.) (accounts for 25% of prostatectomies).

- **Chronic retention and renal impairment**: a residual urine of 200 mL or more, hydroureter or hydronephrosis demonstrated on ultrasound, uraemic manifestations and abnormal renal function (accounts for 15% of prostatectomies).
- **Complications of BOO**: stone, infection and diverticulum formation.
- **Haemorrhage**: these patients present with recurrent haematuria with no obvious cause and a very vascular prostate can be seen on cystoscopy.
- **Elective prostatectomy for severe symptoms**: this accounts for about 60% of prostatectomies. Frequency alone is not a strong indication for prostatectomy. The natural progression of outflow obstruction is variable and rarely gets worse after 10 years. Severe symptoms not responding to drug therapy, a low maximum flow rate (<10 mL/s) and an increased residual volume of urine (100–250 mL) are relatively strong indications for operative treatment.

Summary box 84.4

Options for treatment of LUTS secondary to BPH

- Conservative measures include watchful waiting in conjunction with fluid manipulation (avoid fluid binge and late night intake) and a reduction in caffeinated and alcoholic drinks
- Drug therapy is with α-blockers or, in men with a large prostate, a 5α-reductase inhibitor, or both; combination therapy has a better outcome in glands bigger than 35 g
- Interventional measures include transurethral resection of the prostate (TURP), which remains the gold standard; consider HOLEP (holmium laser enucleation of the prostate), open/robotic simple prostatectomy for large glands; new minimally invasive treatment options that are available to patients include prostate artery embolisation (PAE), water vapour prostate treatment (Rezūm), prostatic urethral lift (Urolift) and water jet treatment (Aquablation)

Acute retention

The management of retention is discussed in detail in *Chapter 83*. Once the bladder has been drained by means of a catheter, the patient's fitness for treatment is determined. If retention was not caused by drugs or constipation, then prostatectomy would usually be the correct management. Unfit men or those with dementia may be treated by means of an indwelling urethral or suprapubic catheter. The role of α-adrenergic drugs followed by a trial of a catheter has been tested and found to be successful in certain groups with a short history and a low residual volume of urine, but the recurrence rate becomes cumulatively high. 5α-reductase is given to prevent progression of symptoms in men with large (>35–40 mL) prostates. Combination therapy (α-blocker and 5α-reductase) is better for the larger gland. Patients who develop renal impairment and/or hydronephrosis after urinary retention will need to keep the catheter until definitive surgical treatment is provided, usually not less than 6 weeks afterwards to allow renal function recovery.

Special problems in the management of chronic retention

Men with chronic retention who have relatively low volumes of residual urine and who do not have symptoms suggestive of coexisting infection and with good renal function do not necessarily require catheterisation before proceeding to prostatectomy on the next available list. For those who are uraemic, urgent catheterisation is mandatory to allow renal function to recover and stabilise. Haematuria often occurs following catheterisation owing to collapse of the distended bladder and upper tract, but settles within a couple of days.

Uraemic patients with chronic retention are often dehydrated at the time of admission. Owing to the chronic back pressure on the distal tubules within the kidney, there is loss of the ability to reabsorb salts and water. The result, following release of this pressure, may be an enormous outflow of salts and water, which is known as postobstructive diuresis. It is for this reason that a careful fluid chart, daily measurements of the patient's weight and serial estimations of creatinine and electrolytes are essential. Intravenous fluid replacement is required if the patient is unable to keep up with this fluid loss. These patients are often anaemic and may require a blood transfusion once fluid balance is stabilised (if haemoglobin is <9 g/L).

Considerations for elective treatment in men with LUTS secondary to BPH

The following questions should be answered before considering a surgical treatment:

- Have they failed a preliminary trial of medical therapy? Commonly, men will have been treated with α-blockers or 5α-reductase inhibitors and will have failed treatment.
- Is BOO present? In many cases, the findings of significant symptoms (assessed by symptom scoring) and a benign enlarged prostate supplemented by the finding of a low maximum flow rate (<10–12 mL/s for a good voided volume [>150–200 mL]) – will suffice to make a reasonable working diagnosis of BOO.
- How severe are the symptoms and what are the risks of doing nothing? Severe symptoms and a large residual volume of urine will usually require treatment. Men with mild symptoms, good flow rates (>15 mL/s) and good bladder emptying (residual urine <100 mL) may be safely managed by reassurance and review; such patients rarely develop severe complications such as retention in the long term.
- Is the man fit for operative treatment?
- What treatments are available, what are the outcomes and do the side effects justify treatment?

Treatment

Men with symptoms attending for elective treatment (excluding acute and chronic retention)

Conservative treatment

It is in men with relatively mild symptoms, reasonable flow rates (>10–15 mL/s) and good bladder emptying (residual urine <100 mL) that careful discussion over the merits and side effects of operative treatment is warranted. Waiting for a period of 6 months after careful discussion of the diagnosis is indicated. After this, a repeat assessment of symptoms and flow rates and an ultrasound scan are helpful; many men with stable symptoms will elect to leave matters be.

Drugs

In men who are very concerned about the development of sexual dysfunction after TURP, the use of drugs may be helpful. Two classes of drug have been used in the treatment of men with BOO. α-adrenergic blocking agents inhibit the contraction of smooth muscle that is found in the prostate. The other class of drug is the 5α-reductase inhibitors, which inhibit the conversion of testosterone to 1,5-dihydrotestosterone (DHT), the most active form of androgen. These drugs, when taken for a year, result in a 25% reduction in the size of the prostate gland. Both groups of drugs are effective; however, α-blockers work more quickly and although the 5α-reductase inhibitors have fewer side effects they need to be taken for at least 6 months and their effect is greatest in patients with large (>40 g) glands. Drug therapy results in improvements in maximum flow rates by about 2 mL/s more than placebo and results in a mild (20%) improvement in symptom scores. Another drug class that has improved patients' symptom scores but not their maximum flow rate are the phosphodiesterase 5 inhibitors, which reduce smooth muscle tone and possibly the inflammation in the prostate gland. These drugs are particularly useful if patients have concomitant erectile dysfunction. TURP, however, results in improvements in maximum flow rates from 9 to 18 mL/s and a 75% improvement in symptom scores. These drugs are expensive in comparison with their effectiveness, and a significant proportion of men who try these drugs will subsequently undergo surgical treatment.

Operative treatment

Apart from the strong indications for operative treatment mentioned above, the most common reason for TURP is a combination of severe symptoms and a low flow rate of <12 mL/s. The key is to assess the symptoms carefully and to counsel men about side effects and likely outcome before advising operative treatment.

Counselling men undergoing prostatectomy

Men undergoing prostatectomy need to be advised about the following:

- **Retrograde ejaculation or anejaculation**. This occurs in about 65–85% of men after prostatectomy.
- **Erectile dysfunction**. This occurs in about 5–10% of men, usually in those whose potency is waning.
- **Success rate**. On the whole, men with acute and chronic retention do well from the symptomatic point of view. Ninety per cent of men undergoing elective operation for severe symptoms and urodynamically proven BOO do well in terms of symptoms and flow rates. Only about 65% of those with mild symptoms or those with weak bladder contraction as the cause of their symptoms do well. Men who are unobstructed and have detrusor instability do not respond well to TURP; in fact, their storage symptoms could accentuate postoperatively. Patients who have concomitant BOO and secondary detrusor overactivity may need an anticholinergic drug for a few months if they have persistent irritative symptoms.
- **Risk of reoperation**. After TURP, this is about 15% after 8–10 years.
- **Morbidity rate**. Death after TURP is infrequent (<0.5%); severe sepsis is found in about 6%; and severe haematuria requiring transfusion of more than 2 units of blood occurs in about 3%. After discharge, about 15–20% of men subsequently require antibiotic treatment for symptoms of urinary infection.
- **Incontinence**. Although the risk is rare and is about 1%, the risk is higher in older patients and those with a very large prostate.

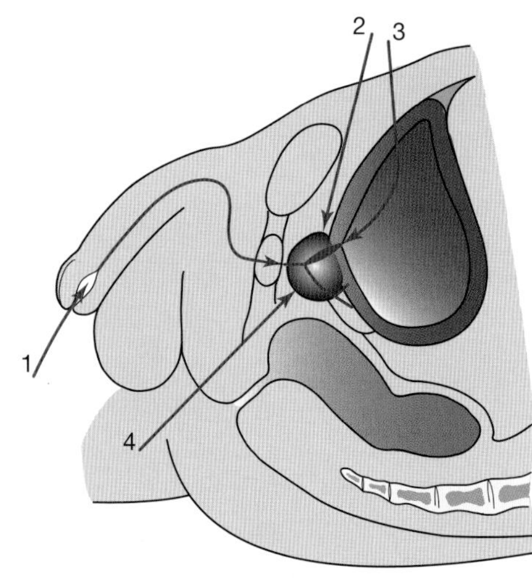

Figure 84.11 The surgical approaches to the prostate. (For key see text.)

Methods of performing prostatectomy

The prostate can be approached (1) transurethrally (TURP); (2) retropubically (RPP); (3) through the bladder (transvesically; TVP); or (4) from the perineum (*Figure 84.11*).

Transurethral prostate surgery

Transurethral resection of the prostate

TURP remains the most commonly performed procedure for the surgical correction of BOO. Perhaps the greatest advance in the history of transurethral surgery was marked by the development of the rigid lens system of Professor Harold

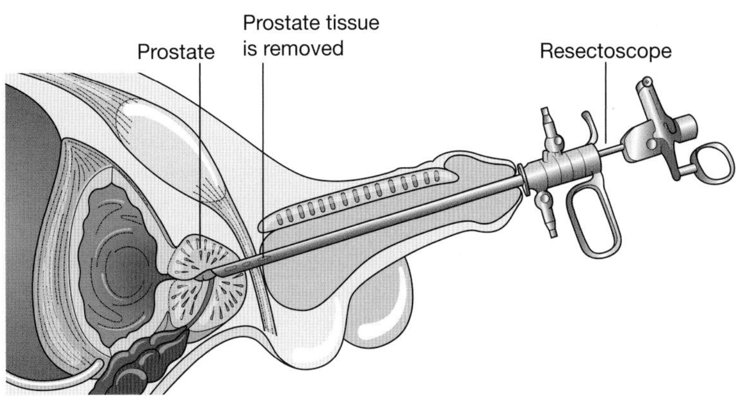

Figure 84.12 For transurethral resection of the prostate the resectoscope is inserted transurethrally. Electric current is passed through a diathermy loop at the end of the instrument. The surgeon moves this back and forth to create a cavity using diathermy to cauterise as they go. The resultant chips are washed out of the bladder intermittently throughout the procedure. A visual image of the operative field is transmitted through lenses running in the middle of the resectoscope. Around this lens, irrigating fluid is instilled and flows out, washing blood away from the operative field. The procedure is complete when an adequate channel has been created through the prostate.

Hopkins. His lenses, illuminated by a fibreoptic light source, permit unparalleled visualisation of the working field. Men with indwelling catheters, those with recent urinary infection, those with chronic retention or those with prosthetic material or heart valves benefit from prophylactic antibiotics in addition to the standard for clean surgery at induction of anaesthesia.

Strips of tissue are cut from the bladder neck down to the level of the verumontanum (*Figure 84.12*). Cutting is performed by a high-frequency diathermy current, which is applied across a loop mounted on the hand-held trigger of the resectoscope. Coagulation of bleeding points can be accurately achieved. The 'chips' of prostate are then removed from the bladder using an Ellik evacuator. Resection proceeds at 1 g/minute in experienced hands. The duration of resection for monopolar TURP is limited to 1 hour due to the risk of resorption of water if 1% glycine is used as an irrigant. The advent of bipolar TURP where normal saline is used as an irrigant permits resection of larger prostates. Following TURP, careful haemostasis is performed, and a three-way, self-retaining catheter irrigated with isotonic saline is introduced into the bladder to prevent any further bleeding from forming blood clots. Irrigation is continued until the outflow is pale pink, and the catheter is usually removed on the second or third postoperative day. In men with small prostates or bladder neck dyssynergia or stenosis, it is better to divide the bladder neck and prostatic urethra with a Collins knife or laser.

Laser prostatectomy

Laser can be used to ablate or vaporise (e.g. green light laser) or enucleate (e.g. HOLEP) the prostate. Photoselective vaporisation of the prostate or green light laser has the advantage that vaporisation is haemostatic and this procedure can be performed even while patients are anticoagulated; however, it is unsuitable for a very large gland. In holmium laser enucleation of the prostate (HOLEP), laser is used to cut all the attachments of the adenoma to the false capsule and simultaneously coagulate any of the small vessels crossing the relatively avascular plane between the peripheral and transitional zones of the prostate while the tip of the cystoscope is used, much like the surgeon's finger in Millin's prostatectomy, to enucleate the transitional zone adenoma. The enucleated adenoma is pushed into the bladder, where it is morcellated and extracted via the cystoscope. Damage to the external sphincter is avoided provided the verumontanum is used as a guide to the most distal point of the resection/vaporisation/enucleation.

Complications of prostatectomy

Local

Haemorrhage is a major risk following prostatectomy whatever the surgical approach. Care should be taken in applying diathermy to arterial bleeding points after TURP, and to any bleeding vessels at the bladder neck; they are often better seen when the rate of inflow of fluid is decreased. Some of the venous bleeding due to deep resection can only be stopped by gentle traction via a Foley catheter balloon inflated to 30–40 mL and kept in the bladder. Sustained traction is applied by taping the catheter to the anterior abdominal wall or thigh for 12–24 hours. This causes compression of the prostatic tissue and veins and thus stops the bleeding. In the recovery room, one should check that the bladder is draining adequately; if it is not, this may indicate that a clot is blocking the eye of the catheter. The bladder should be promptly washed out using a strict aseptic technique. The catheter should be changed by the surgeon. Only rarely is it necessary to return the patient to the operating room.

Secondary haemorrhage tends to occur several days after the patient has been discharged. All men should be warned about this possibility and given appropriate advice to rest and to have a high fluid intake. It is usually minor in degree but if

Harold Horace Hopkins, 1918–1994, Professor of Applied Optics, University of Reading, Reading, UK, invented the rigid rod endoscope (Hopkins' rod, 1954) and contributed to the development of the fibres for flexible endoscopes.

Milo Ellik, 1905–1975, American urologist, developed the Ellik evacuator in 1937.

Terence John Millin, 1903–1980, surgeon, Westminster Hospital, London, UK, and honorary surgeon, All Saints' Hospital for Genitourinary Diseases, London, UK, described the operation of retropubic prostatectomy in 1945. He was regarded as 'the greatest of Irish urologists' and 'the pioneer of the retropubic space'. To facilitate his operation, he devised a self-retaining retractor that goes by his name and the 'boomerang' needle to close the prostatic capsule. He used to be invited all over the world to operate on VIPs. He was a former President of the Royal College of Surgeons in Ireland. He gave up operating at the age of 57 to enjoy his farm in County Wicklow, where he died of laryngeal carcinoma. He played international rugby for Ireland.

Frederic Eugene Basil Foley, 1891–1966, urologist, Ancker Hospital, St Paul, MN, USA.

clot retention occurs the patient will need to be readmitted, a catheter passed and the bladder washed out.

Perforation of the bladder or the prostatic capsule can occur at the time of transurethral surgery. This usually occurs from a combination of inexperience in association with a large prostate or heavy blood loss. If the field of vision becomes obscured by heavy blood loss, it is often prudent to achieve adequate haemostasis and abandon the operation, swallowing one's pride on the understanding that a second attempt may be necessary. A large perforation with marked extravasation may require the insertion of a small suprapubic drain. Rectal perforation should be extremely rare.

Sepsis

Bacteraemia is common even in men with sterile urine and occurs in over 50% of men with infected urine, prolonged catheterisation or chronic retention. Sepsis can occur in these patients shortly after operation or when the catheter is removed. Routine use of prophylactic antibiotics is recommended based on local antimicrobial sensitivity profiles. The most worrying aspect of infection is the early rigor following surgery. If left undetected and untreated, this may progress to septic shock with profound hypotension. A blood culture should be taken and antibiotics given parenterally (e.g. amoxicillin plus cefuroxime, or gentamicin).

Incontinence

Incontinence is rare after BPH surgery; however, it is inevitable if the external sphincter mechanism is damaged. The bladder neck is rendered incompetent by any prostatectomy and, therefore, an intact distal sphincter mechanism is essential for continence. The verumontanum marks the proximal margin of the external sphincter. In some patients, detrusor instability contributes to the incontinence. The use of anticholinergic agents such as mirabegron/solifenacin/tolterodine may help. Mild degrees of stress incontinence usually recover in a few days to a few weeks. If physiotherapy is ineffective, then full assessment with cystoscopy and pressure studies including video urodynamics should be carried out before proceeding with offering the patient the insertion of an artificial urinary sphincter or a sling to increase the resistance of the urethra. One should usually wait for 6 months to 1 year before any sling or sphincter is implanted.

Retrograde ejaculation and erectile dysfunction

Men with prior good sexual function are less likely to have erectile dysfunction following BPH surgery, but retrograde ejaculation occurs commonly (>75%) because of disruption to the bladder neck mechanism; occasionally, anejaculation can occur as a result of disruption of the ejaculatory ducts. This should be discussed with all men before the surgery.

Urethral stricture

This may be secondary to prolonged catheterisation, the use of an unnecessarily large catheter, clumsy instrumentation or the presence of the resectoscope in the urethra for too long a period. These strictures arise either just inside the meatus or in the bulbar urethra. An early stricture can usually be managed by simple dilatation or urethrotomy if dense fibrosis is present. If the stricture recurs then urethroplasty is considered. The use of an Otis urethrotomy in the tight urethra prior to TURP can reduce the incidence of postoperative stricture.

Bladder neck contracture

Occasionally, a dense fibrotic stenosis of the bladder neck occurs following overaggressive resection of a small prostate. It may be due to the overuse of coagulating diathermy. This usually happens in the early postoperative period. Transurethral incision of the scar tissue is necessary using laser or diathermy.

General complications

Death occurs in about 0.2–0.3% of men undergoing elective prostatectomy. In very elderly men, in men with prostate cancer admitted as an emergency with acute or chronic retention or in those with very large prostates, the 30-day death rate may be of the order of 1%.

Cardiovascular

Pulmonary atelectasis, pneumonia, myocardial infarction, congestive cardiac failure and deep venous thrombosis are all potentially life-threatening conditions that can affect this elderly and often frail group of men.

Water intoxication

Absorption of water into the circulation at the time of transurethral resection can give rise to congestive cardiac failure, hyponatraemia and haemolysis. Accompanying this, there is frequently confusion and other cerebral events often mimicking a stroke. The incidence of this condition has been reduced since the introduction of isotonic glycine for irrigating during resection, and further still with the development of bipolar TURP where saline is used as an irrigant. The treatment consists of fluid restriction.

BLADDER OUTFLOW OBSTRUCTION CAUSED BY THE BLADDER NECK

Aetiology

This condition usually occurs in men but can rarely affect children of both sexes and women. It may be due to muscular hypertrophy or fibrosis of the tissues at the bladder neck following TURP.

Clinical syndromes

Owing to muscle hypertrophy or dyssynergia

Marion described a series of cases in which muscular hypertrophy of the internal sphincter in a young person had resulted in the development of a vesical diverticulum or hydro-

Fessenden Nott Otis, 1825–1900, nineteenth century American urologist.
Jean Baptiste Camile Marion, 1869–1932, Professor of Urology, The Faculty of Medicine, Paris, France.

nephrosis (Marion's disease or 'prostatism sans prostate'). It is thought that dyssynergic contraction of the smooth muscle of the bladder neck (bladder neck dyssynergia) may account for some cases of BOO. It is also known as functional bladder neck obstruction.

Owing to fibrosis

The symptoms are similar to those of prostatic enlargement but are a consequence of scarring after TURP or radical prostatectomy (usually compounded by external beam radiotherapy [EBRT]).

Treatment

The management of these patients depends on achieving an accurate diagnosis. For this, urodynamic investigation is often necessary, which should demonstrate raised voiding pressures and diminished flow rate.

Drugs

The presence of α-adrenergic receptors in the region of the bladder neck and prostatic urethra allows pharmacological manipulation of the outflow to the bladder.

α-blocking drugs

Alfuzosin (10 mg once daily), tamsulosin (0.4 mg once daily), doxazosin (1 mg at night, up to a maximum of 8 mg/day), indoramin (20 mg twice daily, increased to a total maximum of 100 mg/day in divided doses), prazosin (2.5 mg twice daily, maintenance up to 2 mg/day) terazosin (1 mg at night, to a total maximum of 10 mg/day) and Silodosin (4 to 8 mg once a day) can be very useful, causing relaxation of the bladder neck. These drugs are not target specific, and patients must be warned of the possibility of postural hypotension, which is usually limited to the first few doses.

Transurethral incision

Transurethral incision of the bladder neck is the operation of choice. Sometimes symptoms recur, but this is usually due to inadequate division of the fibres of the bladder neck.

Congenital valves of the prostatic urethra

See *Chapter 85*.

PROSTATIC CALCULI

Prostatic calculi are of two varieties: endogenous, which are common, and exogenous, which are comparatively rare. An exogenous prostatic calculus is a urinary (commonly ureteric) calculus that becomes arrested in the prostatic urethra. Endogenous prostatic calculi are usually composed of calcium phosphate combined with about 20% organic material.

Clinical features

Prostatic calculi are usually symptomless, being discovered on TRUS, on radiography of the pelvis, during prostatectomy or associated with carcinoma of the prostate or chronic prostatitis. In cases associated with severe chronic prostatic infection, the associated fibrosis and nodularity are difficult to differentiate from carcinoma. On radiographs or ultrasound scans, these stones are often seen to form a horseshoe (*Figure 84.13*) or a circle. It is postulated that they are associated with BOO.

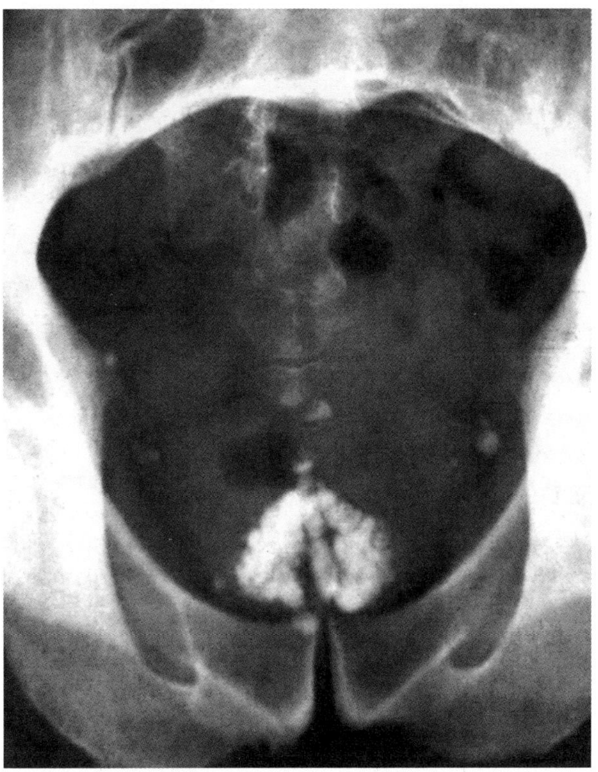

Figure 84.13 Endogenous prostatic calculi.

Treatment of prostatic calculi

Prostatic calculi usually require no treatment.

Conservative measures

Associated chronic prostatic infection may be treated by means of ciprofloxacin or trimethoprim.

Transurethral resection

Transurethral resection will often release small calculi as the strips of prostatic tissue are excised. Others are passed through the urethra at a later date. Any associated benign prostatic enlargement is treated in the same sitting with TURP.

Corpora amylaceae

Corpora amylaceae are tiny calcified lamellated bodies found in the glandular alveoli of the prostates of elderly men and apes, but not in the prostates of animals lower in the phylogenetic scale than anthropoids. Corpora amylaceae are probably the forerunners of endogenous prostatic calculi.

CARCINOMA OF THE PROSTATE

Carcinoma of the prostate is the most common malignant tumour in men over the age of 65 years. In the UK in 2017, more than 48 000 men were diagnosed with, and more than

11 800 died from, prostate carcinoma; the corresponding figures in the USA were 190 000 and 33 000, respectively. If histological section of prostates at autopsy is performed, increasingly frequent foci of microscopic prostate cancers are found with increasing age. These foci of prostate cancer have variable potential for progressing clinically to metastatic disease. About 10–15% of younger men who develop prostate cancer have a positive family history of the disease, but the aetiology is unclear. Throughout the world, rates of microscopic foci of prostate cancer are constant, but rates of clinically evident disease are low in men in Japan, China and India. Carcinoma of the prostate usually originates in the peripheral zone of the prostate, so 'prostatectomy' for benign enlargement of the gland confers no protection from subsequent carcinoma.

Pathology

Serial sections of prostates obtained at routine necropsy demonstrate prostate carcinoma in 25% of men between 50 and 65 years of age. The incidence in men over 80 years is in the region of 70%. Most of these neoplasms are tiny and (if life had continued) might have remained latent for years. Most men die with the prostate cancer rather than because of cancer.

The following types of prostate cancer occur:

- microscopic latent cancer found on autopsy or at cysto-prostatectomy;
- tumours found incidentally during TURP (T1a and T1b) or following screening by PSA measurement (T1c);
- early, localised prostate cancer (T2);
- locally advanced and high-risk prostate cancer (T3 and T4);
- metastatic disease, which may arise from a clinically evident tumour (T2, T3 or T4) or from an apparently benign gland (T0, T1) (i.e. occult prostate cancer).

It should be noted that only the last two groups cause symptoms, and such tumours are not curable. Only screening or the treatment of incidentally found tumours or early prostate cancer (T1 and T2) can result in cure of the disease. The problem is that many such tumours would never progress during the patient's lifetime and only a few will grow and metastasise; herein lies the problem with prostate cancer.

Screening for prostate cancer

Prostate cancer screening with PSA is controversial and the test does not fulfil the World Health Organization's (WHO) criteria for an adequate screening programme. Screening trials are limited by contamination of patients who have already had prior PSA tests, and most include mainly white men. Most screening trials do not include high-risk groups of men (family history of prostate cancer, Africans) and screening can lead to overdiagnosis of insignificant disease. The four largest randomised trials include in total around 700 000 patients; they have shown that screening did not improve overall mortality, but there is a small improvement in prostate cancer-specific mortality. However, screening increased prostate cancer detection in 18 men per 1000 men screened, increased complications from prostate biopsies and can lead to overdiagnosis.

Summary box 84.5

Screening for prostate cancer

The results of several large-scale randomised clinical trials evaluating the role of PSA screening for prostate cancer suggest that, at present, screening the entire population with serum PSA is not cost-effective as a large number of men must be screened, biopsied and treated in order to prevent each death from prostate cancer

Local spread

Locally advanced tumours tend to grow upwards to involve the seminal vesicles, the bladder neck and trigone and, later, the tumours tend to spread distally to involve the distal sphincter mechanism. Further upward extension obstructs the lower end of one or both ureters, with obstruction of both resulting in anuria. The rectum may become stenosed by tumour infiltrating around it, but direct involvement is rare.

Spread by the bloodstream

Spread by the bloodstream occurs particularly to bone; indeed, the prostate is the most common site of origin for skeletal metastases, followed in turn by the breast, the kidney, the bronchus and the thyroid gland. The bones involved most frequently by carcinoma of the prostate are the pelvic bones and the lower lumbar vertebrae. The femoral head, ribcage and skull are other common sites.

Lymphatic spread

Lymphatic spread may occur via (i) lymphatic vessels passing to the obturator fossa or along the sides of the rectum to the lymph nodes beside the internal iliac vein and in the hollow of the sacrum and (ii) lymphatics that pass over the seminal vesicles and follow the vas deferens for a short distance to drain into the external iliac lymph nodes. From retroperitoneal lymph nodes, the mediastinal nodes and occasionally the supraclavicular nodes may become implicated.

Staging using the tumour-node-metastasis (TNM) system

The TNM staging system for prostate cancer is shown in *Figure 84.14*.

- **T1a, T1b and T1c**. These are incidentally found tumours in a clinically benign gland after histological examination of a prostatectomy specimen. T1a is a tumour involving less than 5% of the resected specimen; these tumours are usually well or moderately well differentiated. T1b is a tumour involving >5% of the resected specimen. T1c tumours are impalpable tumours found following investigation of a raised PSA.
- **T2a** disease presents as a suspicious nodule (*Figure 84.15*) on rectal examination that is confined within the prostate capsule and involves one lobe.

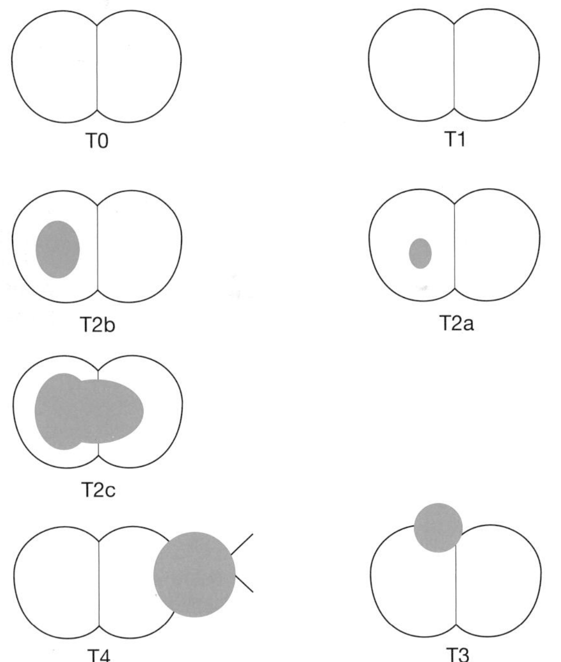

Figure 84.14 Tumour–node–metastasis staging system for prostate cancer.

- **T2b** means that the cancer is in more than half of one side of the prostate gland, but not both sides.
- **T2c** means that the cancer is in both sides but is still inside the prostate gland.
- **T3** tumour extends through the capsule:
  - T3a, uni- or bilateral extension;
  - T3b, seminal vesical extension.
- **T4** is a tumour that is fixed or invading adjacent structures other than seminal vesicles – levator muscles, external sphincter, rectum or pelvic side wall.

Summary box 84.6

The natural history of prostate cancer

This depends on the stage and grade of disease:

- T1 and T2
  - The progression rate of well-differentiated T1a prostate cancer is very low: 10–14% after 8 years. For moderately differentiated tumours, the rate is about 20%. For T1b and T2 tumours, the rate is in excess of 35%
- T3 and T4 (M0)
  - About 50% progress to bony metastases after 3–5 years
- M1
  - The median survival of men with metastatic disease is about 3 years

Clinical features

Only advanced disease gives rise to symptoms, but even advanced disease may be asymptomatic. Symptoms of advanced disease include:

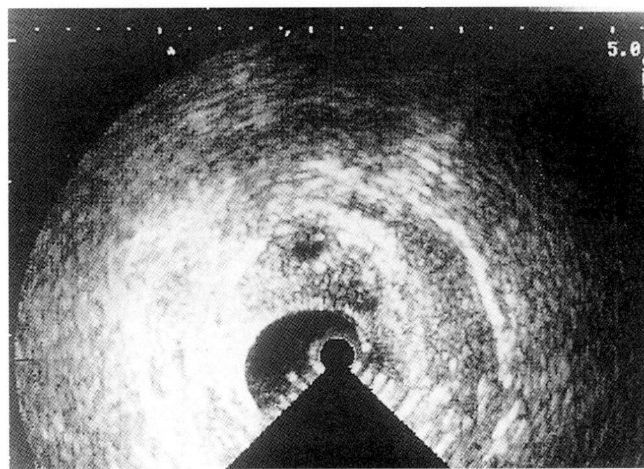

Figure 84.15 Transrectal ultrasound scan of a T2 nodule in the prostate.

- BOO;
- pelvic pain and haematuria;
- bone pain, malaise, 'arthritis', anaemia or pancytopenia;
- renal failure;
- locally advanced disease or even asymptomatic metastases, which may be found incidentally on investigation of other symptoms.

Early prostate cancer is asymptomatic and may be found:

- incidentally following TURP for clinically benign disease (T1a and b);
- T1c – because of serum PSA screening;
- as a nodule (T2) on rectal examination.

Summary box 84.7

The presentation of men with prostate cancer

- Often men are asymptomatic and detection is by opportunistic PSA testing
- Cancer is detected in men describing LUTS or may present with symptoms of metastatic disease

Rectal examination

Rectal examination can detect nodules within the prostate and advanced disease. Irregular induration, characteristically stony hard in part or in the whole of the gland (with obliteration of the median sulcus), suggests carcinoma. Extension beyond the capsule up into the bladder base and vesicles (*Figure 84.16*) is diagnostic, as is local extension through the capsule (*Figure 84.17*).

Multiparametric magnetic resonance imaging

mpMRI is an investigation to diagnose an early prostate cancer that might reduce overdiagnosis of insignificant prostate cancer. Here dynamic contrast is given and should have four sequences: T1-weighted imaging, T2-weighted imaging,

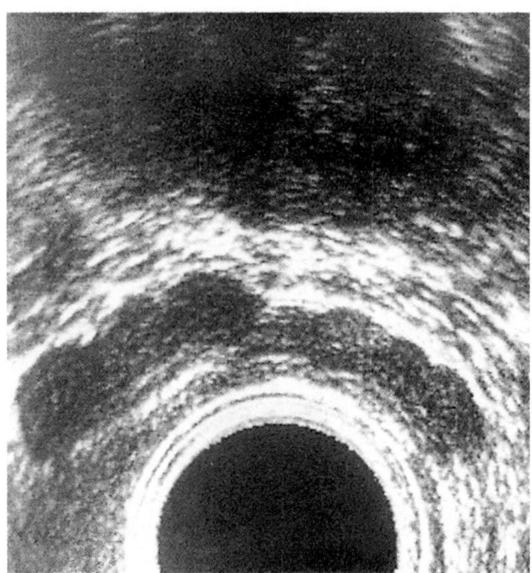

Figure 84.16 Transrectal ultrasound scan showing normal seminal vesicles.

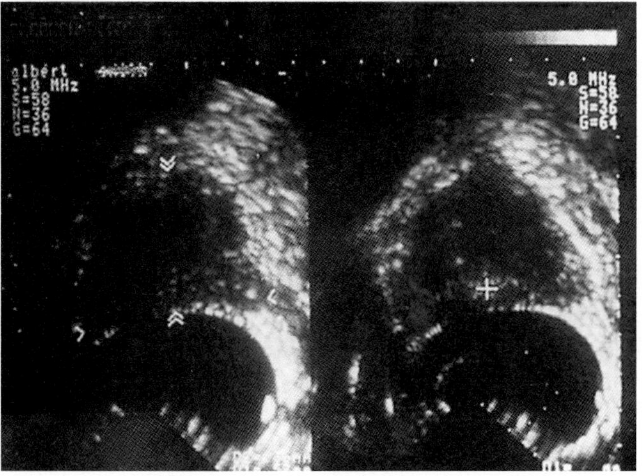

Figure 84.17 Transrectal ultrasound scan showing local extension of a T3 prostate cancer.

diffusion-weighted imaging and dynamic contrast-enhanced imaging and spectroscopic imaging. The accuracy of mpMRI in localising and staging prostate cancer shows a high degree of variation between reporting radiologists. Interpretation and reporting of mpMRI must be carried out following standardised scoring systems (such as Prostate Imaging Reporting and Data System [PI-RADS] v.2). A score of 3 or above is indicative of malignancy.

Prostatic biopsy

If there is suspicion of prostate cancer, because of local findings, a raised PSA or metastatic disease, then a prostate biopsy using an automated gun under TRUS guidance is recommended (***Figure 84.18***). This is usually performed

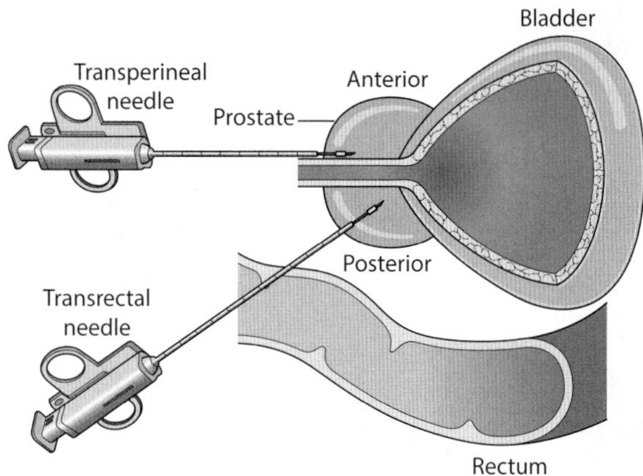

Figure 84.18 The prostate is commonly biopsied by two routes. The biopsy needle can be inserted through the skin between the scrotum and anus (perineum) or through the rectum. In both cases the passage of the needle is usually guided to the correct place with transrectal ultrasound. Transrectal ultrasound is not good for sampling the anterior prostate, particularly when the prostate is large. Transperineal biopsy is gaining popularity as an alternative to conventional transrectal biopsy.

transrectally, although increasingly the transperineal approach is being used. Broad-spectrum antibiotic cover is given to all patients to reduce the incidence of sepsis, which is greater with transrectal than with transperineal biopsy. Transperineal biopsy usually involves sedation or general anaesthetic while transrectal biopsy can be performed under local anaesthetic. Increasingly, areas appearing suspicious for prostate cancer on mpMRI can be targeted for biopsy to increase the diagnostic yield. Nowadays, fusion biopsy is becoming popular; this is where mpMRI and TRUS images are fused with the help of software and a biopsy is taken very accurately from the index lesion.

Histological appearances

The prostate is a glandular structure consisting of ducts and acini; thus, the histological pattern is one of an adenocarcinoma. The prostatic glands are surrounded by a layer of myoepithelial cells. The first change associated with carcinoma is the loss of the basement membrane, with glands appearing to be in confluence. As the cell type becomes less differentiated, more solid sheets of carcinoma cells are seen. A classification of the histological pattern based on the degree of glandular dedifferentiation and its relation to stroma has been devised by Gleason. Prostate cancers exhibit heterogeneity within tissue, and so two histological areas of prostate are each scored between 3 and 5. Grades 1 and 2 are now not reported as their outcome is similar to grade 3. Grade 3 cancers almost never metastasise. The scores are added to give an overall Gleason score of between 6 and 10; this (and the volume of the cancer) appears to correlate well with the likelihood of spread and the prognosis. The International Society of Urological Pathology (ISUP) and WHO have recommended a simplified grading system composed of five prognostic grade groups. Each group

Donald F Gleason, 1920–2008, pathologist, University of Minnesota, Minneapolis, MN, USA, published the Gleason System in 1966. He spent his last 20 years sailing, baking bread and playing bridge.

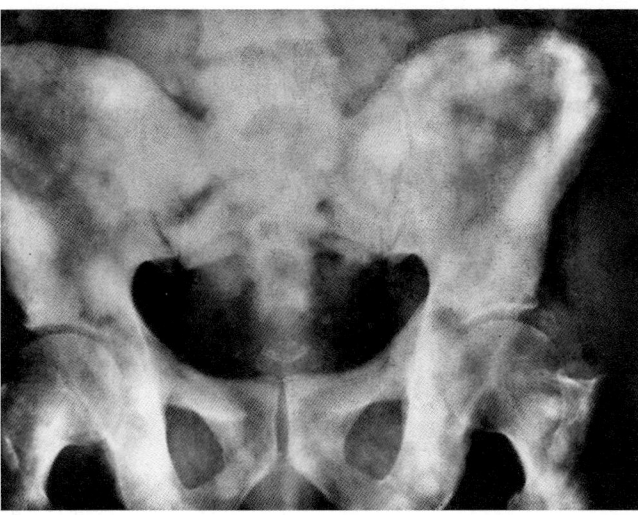

Figure 84.19 Osseous metastases of the pelvic bones in carcinoma of the prostate (courtesy of LN Pyrah, Leeds, UK).

has prognostic significance and a higher grade group has a poorer prognosis.

Grade groups are as follows:

- 1 = Gleason score 3 + 3 = 6
- 2 = Gleason score 3 + 4 = 7
- 3 = Gleason score 4 + 3 = 7
- 4 = Gleason score 8 (4 + 4 = 8, 3 + 5 = 8, 5 + 3 = 8)
- 5 = Gleason score ≥9 (4 + 5 = 9, 5 + 4 = 9, 5 + 5 = 10)

General blood tests

These are normal in early disease but, in metastatic disease, there may be leukoerythroblastic anaemia secondary to extensive marrow invasion, or anaemia may be secondary to renal failure. There may be thrombocytopenia and evidence of disseminated intravascular coagulopathy with increased fibrinogen degradation products.

Liver function tests

These will be abnormal if there is extensive metastatic invasion of the liver. Alkaline phosphatase may be raised from either hepatic involvement or secondaries in the bone. These can be distinguished by measurement of isoenzymes or gamma-glutamyltransferase.

Prostate-specific antigen

This is discussed earlier in this chapter. It is good at following the course of advanced disease; however, it is lacking in sensitivity and specificity in the diagnosis of early localised prostate cancer. Nevertheless, the finding of a PSA >10 ng/mL is suggestive of cancer and >35 ng/mL is almost diagnostic of advanced prostate cancer, in the absence of active urinary tract infection. A decrease in PSA to the normal range following hormonal ablation is a good prognostic sign. Following radical prostatectomy the serum PSA should fall to undetectable levels (the limit for detection for modern supersensitive assays is <0.03 ng/mL).

Radiological examination

Radiographs of the chest may reveal metastases in either the lung fields or the ribs. An abdominal radiograph may show the characteristic sclerotic metastases in lumbar vertebrae and pelvic bones (*Figure 84.19*). The bone appears dense and coarse, and it is sometimes difficult to distinguish the change from that in Paget's disease of bone. Nevertheless, osteolytic metastases are very common in prostate cancer and may coexist with sclerotic ones.

Cross-sectional imaging with magnetic resonance imaging and transrectal ultrasound

MRI with a high-tesla magnet (1.5–3 T) is the most accurate method of staging local disease. mpMRI is used preoperatively to assess pelvic lymph nodes as well as local stage, although the sensitivity of mpMRI to detect small areas of capsular spread is limited, even in the best hands. As well as preoperative staging, mpMRI plays an important role in active surveillance and localisation of recurrent prostate cancer after surgery. Low-grade tumours are frequently not seen on MRI and are often clinically insignificant.

TRUS scanning can also be used to stage prostate cancer. Locally extensive disease (T2) can be diagnosed with increased sensitivity by TRUS (*Figure 84.15*) compared with rectal examination, but many tumours will still be missed. This problem remains a real one in screening for early prostate cancer; in comparison with breast cancer, with mammography detecting 70–80% of tumours, TRUS plus rectal examination and measurement of PSA will detect only 30–50% of cancers that are known to be present on autopsy studies (although it may detect the larger, more significant cancers).

Bone scan

Once the diagnosis has been established, if metastatic spread is suspected (on the basis of a high PSA [>10 ng/mL], locally advanced disease or presence of Gleason 7 or higher) a bone scan should be carried out. If, however, the PSA is <10 ng/mL, then a bone scan would be performed only on clinical indications. The bone scan is performed by the injection of technetium-99m, which is then monitored using a gamma camera. It is more sensitive in the diagnosis of metastases (*Figure 84.20*) than a skeletal survey, but false positives occur in areas of arthritis, osteomyelitis or a healing fracture.

Positron emission tomography scan

In prostate cancer gallium-labelled prostate-specific membrane antigen (PSMA) has been increasingly used in positron

Sir James Paget, 1814–1899, English surgeon and pathologist, best known for his description of Paget's disease of the bone.

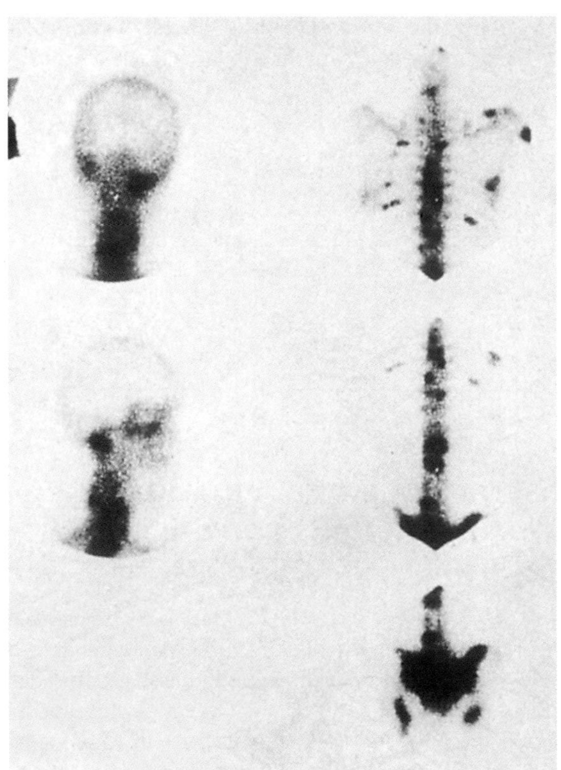

Figure 84.20 Bone scan showing multiple hot spots suggestive of metastatic disease in a man with prostate cancer.

emission tomography (PET) scans. It is sensitive in detecting lymph node metastasis and may be superior to MRI; however, smaller lymph nodes can be missed on PSMA-PET. If available, this test offers an additional and highly sensitive modality for detecting metastasis prior to offering treatment. It also has an increasing role in restaging after treatment relapse.

Treatment

Patients are counselled on their treatment options based on an estimated risk of a localised cancer spreading and causing death. The patient's life expectancy and comorbidities should be taken into consideration. The strongest risk factors for metastasis are PSA level, Gleason grade and clinical stage. Tables and nomograms are available using these three parameters to predict lymph node involvement and risk of metastasis.

Early disease

Curative treatment can only be offered to patients with early disease. Low-risk prostate cancer (low PSA, small foci of Gleason 6 disease) can be managed by active surveillance. Here, with 3-to 6-monthly digital rectal examination (DRE) and PSA measurement, mpMRI yearly or 2-yearly and repeated prostate biopsy, a proportion can safely avoid the toxicity of radical treatment. However, one-third of patients embarking on this approach will require radical treatment within a few years. The options available for T1, T2 or some T3 disease need to take into account the patient's age, performance status and lifestyle preferences. The treatment of patients with advanced disease (T4 or any nodal or distant metastases) is only palliative.

Summary box 84.8

Treatment and stage

- Treatment options for prostate cancer depend on stage of disease, life expectancy of the patient and patient preference
- PSA, DRE and biopsy Gleason grade are used to predict pathological stage
- Localised cancers can be treated by radical prostatectomy, radiation therapy and active monitoring (surveillance)
- Treatment of advanced disease is palliative, and hormone ablation remains the first-line therapy; once it starts failing, chemotherapy is used with short-term success

Summary of treatment for carcinoma of the prostate

- **Low-risk disease**. For men in their seventies, conservative treatment would usually be the correct approach. Radical surgical treatment might be considered in younger (<70 years) men with this form of the disease and/or with a family history, although, even in this group, some men will elect to pursue a conservative course (active surveillance) when counselled about risks versus benefits (impotence/incontinence).
- **Intermediate-risk disease**. In younger (<70 years), fitter men, this may be treated by radical prostatectomy or radical radiotherapy. Active monitoring remains an option, particularly for more elderly patients towards the lower end of the risk spectrum. In elderly patients with outflow obstruction, transurethral resection with or without hormone therapy is indicated. The benefit of radical treatment over a conservative approach is likely to be about 25%, given that progression to metastatic disease is of this order of magnitude after 10 years.
- **High-risk disease**. These patients are at significant risk of disease progression. They need multimodal therapy. Early androgen ablation is favoured if close follow-up is not possible. For the sexually active, a careful conservative approach with the adoption of androgen ablation when symptoms arise is reasonable. Androgen ablation coupled with radiotherapy, perhaps with surgery (radical prostatectomy plus salvage radiotherapy) as part of a multimodal approach, is standard treatment for younger men with T3 disease.
- **Metastatic disease**. Once metastases have developed, the outlook is poor. For patients with symptoms, there is no dilemma; androgen ablation will provide symptomatic relief in over two-thirds of patients. For patients with asymptomatic metastases, the timing of treatment is less clear. Systemic chemotherapy with docetaxel should be considered in younger, fitter men.

PROSTATITIS

In both acute and chronic prostatitis, the seminal vesicles and posterior urethra are usually also involved.

Acute prostatitis

Aetiology

Acute prostatitis is common, but underdiagnosed. The usual organism responsible is *Escherichia coli*, but *Staphylococcus aureus*, *Staphylococcus albus*, *Streptococcus faecalis*, *Neisseria gonorrhoeae* or *Chlamydia* may be responsible. The infection may be haematogenous from a distant focus or it may be secondary to acute urinary infection.

Clinical features

General manifestations overshadow the local: the patient feels ill, shivers, may have a rigor, has 'aches' all over, especially in the back, and may easily be diagnosed as having influenza. The temperature may be up to 39°C. Pain on micturition is usual, but not invariable. The urine contains threads in the initial voided sample, which should be cultured. Perineal heaviness, rectal irritation and pain on defecation can occur; a urethral discharge is rare. Frequency occurs when the infection involves the bladder. Rectal examination reveals a tender prostate; one lobe may be swollen more than the other, and the seminal vesicles may be involved. A frankly fluctuant abscess is uncommon.

Treatment

Treatment must be rigorous and prolonged or the infection will not be eradicated and recurrent attacks may ensue. Spread of infection to the epididymides and testes may occur. Prolonged treatment with an antibiotic that penetrates the prostate wall is indicated (trimethoprim, ciprofloxacin or aminoglycoside).

Prostatic abscess

In addition to the foregoing symptoms and signs, the advent of a prostatic abscess is heralded by the temperature rising steeply with rigors. Antibiotics disguise these features. Severe, unremitting perineal and rectal pain with occasional tenesmus often cause the condition to be confused with an anorectal abscess. Nevertheless, if a rectal examination is performed, the prostate will be felt to be enlarged, hot, extremely tender and perhaps fluctuant. TRUS or MRI may aid diagnosis. Retention of urine is likely to occur and, in such men, suprapubic catheterisation is best.

Treatment

The abscess should be drained without delay by transurethral resection (unroofing the whole cavity) or using a needle via the transrectal or perineal route. Injectable antibiotics such as aminoglycoside or a third-generation cephalosporin is often required for a week.

Chronic prostatitis

Many urologists find the diagnosis of chronic prostatitis and 'prostatodynia' very difficult as many men present with perigenital pain, testicular pain, prostatic pain exacerbated by sexual intercourse or pain that apparently renders sexual intercourse out of the question. Psychosexual dysfunction in such patients may be the underlying problem. The diagnosis of chronic prostatitis has to be based on:

- persistent threads in voided urine;
- prostatic massage showing pus cells with or without bacteria in the absence of urinary infection.

Aetiology

This is thought to be the sequela of inadequately treated acute prostatitis. While pus is present in the prostatic secretion, the responsible organism is often difficult to find. Other organisms such as *Chlamydia* species may be responsible for chronic abacterial prostatitis.

Clinical features

The clinical features are extremely varied. Only men with symptoms of posterior urethritis, prostatic pain and perigenital pain accompanied by intermittent fever and pus cells or bacteria in the postprostatic massage specimen should be diagnosed as having chronic prostatitis.

Diagnosis

The three-glass urine test is valuable. If the first glass with the initial voided sample is clear and the second and third glasses show urine containing prostatic threads and leukocytes, prostatitis is present. Rectal examination of the prostate may be normal or may show a soft, boggy and tender prostate. Examination of the prostatic fluid obtained by prostatic massage should show pus cells and bacteria. Urethroscopy may reveal inflammation of the prostatic urethra, and pus may be seen exuding from the prostatic ducts. The verumontanum is likely to be enlarged and oedematous. In many men with the symptoms described above, all investigations are normal.

Treatment

Antibiotic therapy should be administered only in accordance with bacteriological sensitivity tests. Trimethoprim or ciprofloxacin penetrate well into the prostate. If *Trichomonas* or anaerobes are the responsible agent, a rapid response is obtained from administration of metronidazole (200 mg three times daily for 7 days to both partners). If *Chlamydia* is suspected, doxycycline is the antibiotic treatment of choice. α-blockers and anti-inflammatory drugs have been used with some success. There is little evidence that prostatic massage helps in eradicating the infection.

Prostatodynia

This diagnosis is made by the presence of perigenital pain in the absence of any objective evidence of prostatic inflammation. Whether the syndrome has any relationship with the prostate is unclear. The syndrome is part of the chronic pelvic pain syndrome spectrum and often has psychological and stress components.

FURTHER READING

Mundy AR, Fitzpatrick J, Neal DE, George NJ (eds). *The scientific basis of urology*, 3rd edn. London: Informa Healthcare, 2010.

Partin AW, Peters CA, Kavoussi LR, Dmochowksi RR, Wein AJ. *Campbell–Walsh–Wein urology*, 12th edn. Philadelphia, PA: Elsevier, 2021.

Scardino PT, Linehan WM, Zelefsky MJ, Vogelzang NJ. *Comprehensive textbook of genitourinary oncology*, 4th edn. Philadelphia, PA: Lippincott Williams & Wilkins, 2012.

CHAPTER 85 The urethra and penis

Learning objectives

To recognise and understand:

- The common congenital anomalies of the urethra
- The diagnosis and treatment of urethral trauma
- The diagnosis and treatment of urethral stricture
- The diagnosis and treatment of phimosis
- The diagnosis and treatment of erectile dysfunction
- The common diseases of the penis and urethra and the principles of their surgical management

THE MALE URETHRA

Anatomy

The male urethra is a fibromuscular tube that extends from the bladder neck to the meatus. Functionally the urethra allows transport of urine from the bladder and semen from the ejaculatory ducts through the penis. The male urethra is subdivided into the following parts. The meatus is a vertical slit-like opening at the tip of the glans penis. The glandular part of the urethra is called the fossa navicularis. The penile urethra extends from the meatus to the penoscrotal junction. The bulbar urethra extends from the penoscrotal junction to the bulbomembranous junction. The penile urethra and bulbar urethra are surrounded by corpora spongiosa. The membranous urethra extends from the bulbomembranous junction to the verumontanum. It is surrounded by the voluntary external sphincter, which consists of both the smooth muscle external sphincter and the striated rhabdosphincter. It is innervated by the pudendal nerve, originating from spinal segments S2–4. The prostatic urethra extends from the bladder neck to the verumontanum and is surrounded by the prostate. The bladder neck contributes to the maintenance of continence in the male. Its main role is to act as a genital sphincter that closes at the time of ejaculation. The bladder neck and external sphincter can independently maintain continence in men. The urethral lining changes from transitional cell epithelium proximally to stratified squamous cell epithelium distally.

Congenital anomalies

Posterior urethral valves

The incidence of posterior urethral valves is around 1 in 8000 live male births. The valves are membranes that have a small posterior slit within them. They typically lie just distal to the verumontanum and cause obstruction to the urethra. They function as flap valves; although they are obstructive to antegrade urinary flow, a urethral catheter can be passed retrogradely without any difficulty. Posterior urethral valves need to be detected and treated as early as possible to minimise the degree of renal failure.

Diagnosis

Antenatal ultrasound shows a distended bladder, dilated prostatic urethra and hydroureteronephrosis. The presentation varies according to the severity of the obstruction. The more severe the obstruction, the earlier the presentation. If the diagnosis is not made antenatally, babies typically are presented by parents because of voiding complaints and urinary tract infection (UTI). Rarely the valves are incomplete, and the patient may present in adolescence or adulthood.

Impaired renal function is assessed by ultrasound to check renal cortical thickness and by nuclear renography to check for differential renal function. Investigations include a voiding cystourethrogram (VCUG), which shows a dilated posterior (prostatic) urethra (***Figure 85.1***). The bladder is hypertrophied and often shows diverticula. Typically, there may be vesicoureteral reflux.

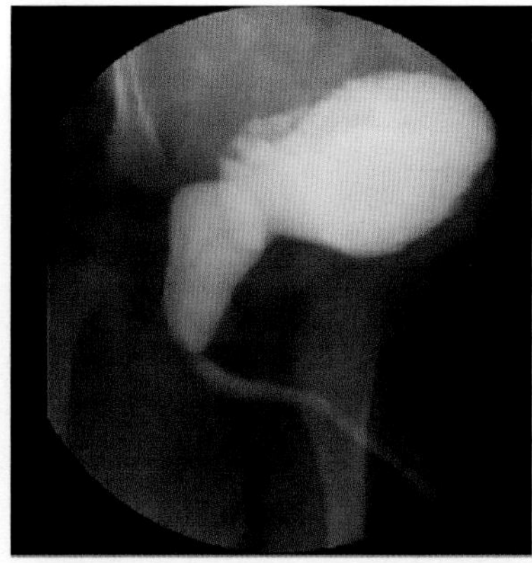

Figure 85.1 A voiding cystourethrogram showing a dilated bladder with a dilated prostatic urethra above an obstruction at the level of the posterior urethral valves (courtesy of Dr Shashank Shrotriya, Pune, India).

Treatment

Initial treatment is by catheterisation to drain the urine and decompress the bladder and upper urinary tracts. The valves themselves can be difficult to see on urethroscopy because the flow of irrigant sweeps them into the open position.

Definitive treatment is by endoscopic ablation of the valves. Long-term follow-up is required in view of the associated vesicoureteral reflux, bladder dysfunction and renal impairment.

> **Summary box 85.1**
>
> **Posterior urethral valves**
>
> - Posterior urethral valves are congenital membranes that cause obstruction to the urinary tract in the male
> - Antenatal ultrasound typically shows a distended bladder, dilated prostatic urethra and hydroureteronephrosis
> - Treatment is by endoscopic valve ablation
> - Patients need long-term follow-up in view of recurrent UTI, bladder dysfunction and renal impairment

Hypospadias

The incidence of hypospadias is around 1 in 300 male live births. It is the most common congenital abnormality of the urethra. Diagnosis is made on physical examination. There are three characteristic features, including an ectopic ventrally located urethral meatus; usually a ventral penile curvature (chordee); and an incomplete dorsal hood prepuce.

Hypospadias is classified according to the position of the meatus (*Figure 85.2a–d*).

- Glanular hypospadias: the ectopic meatus is placed on the glans penis, but proximal to the normal site of the external meatus, which is marked by a blind pit.
- Coronal hypospadias: the meatus is placed at the level of the coronal sulcus.
- Penile hypospadias: the meatus is on the underside of the penile shaft.
- Penoscrotal hypospadias: the meatus is at the level of the penoscrotal junction.
- Perineal hypospadias: this is a rare and severe abnormality. The scrotum is bifid, and the urethra opens between

(a)
Hooded foreskin
Glanular
Coronal
Penoscrotal
Perineal

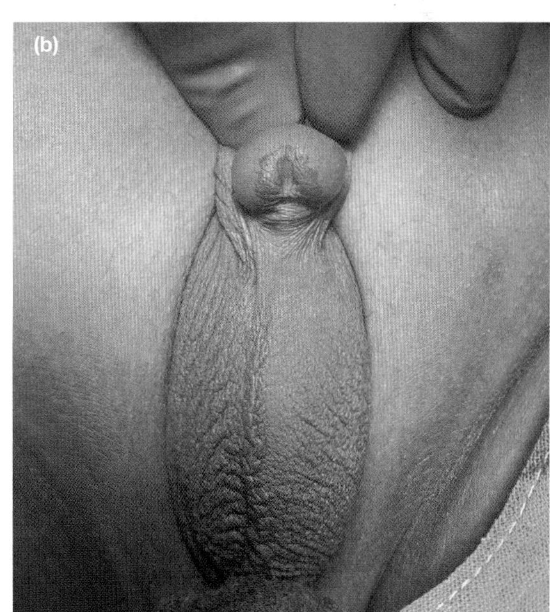

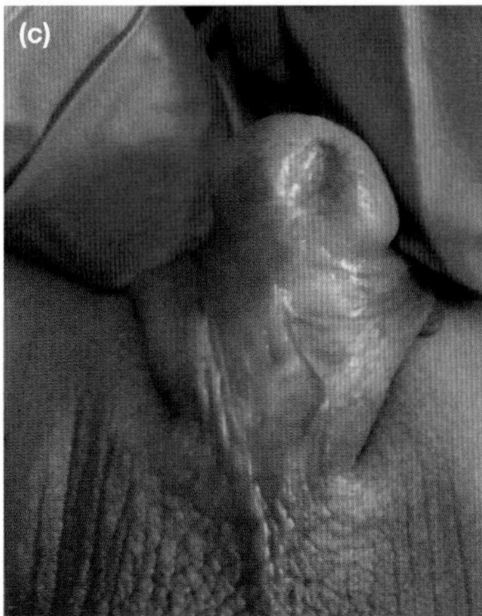

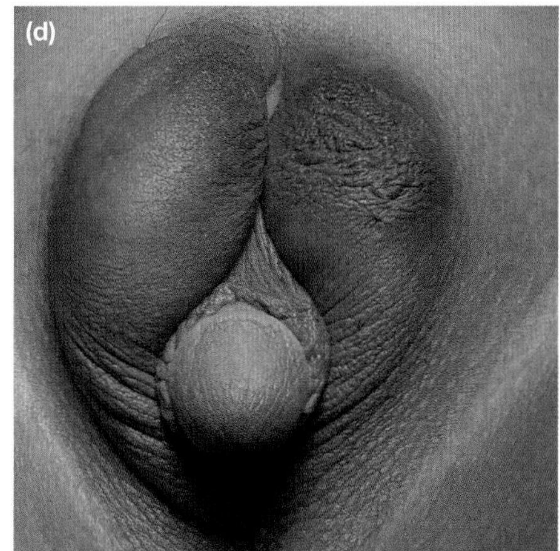

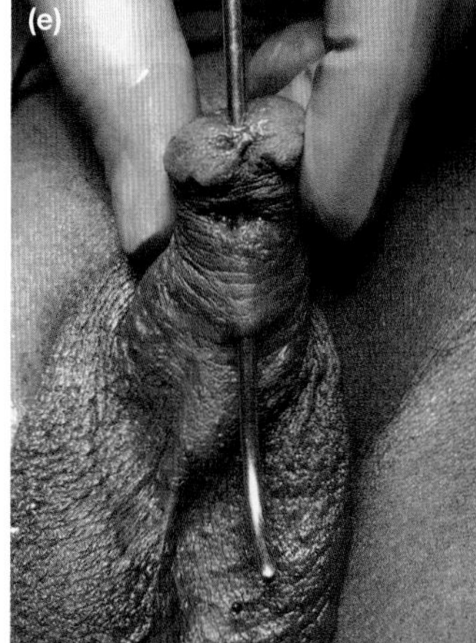

Figure 85.2 (a) Hypospadias classification. (b) Coronal hypospadias. (c) Midpenile hypospadias. (d) Hypospadias with penoscrotal transposition in which the scrotum is placed superior and anterior to the penis. (e) Urethrocutaneous fistula seen in multiple failed hypospadias surgeries.

its two halves. In children with severe hypospadias it is important to consider disorders of sexual development, which are usually associated with undescended testes, hernia and micropenis.

Treatment

Surgery for distal hypospadias is often for cosmetic reasons. This is usually treated by a tubularised incised plate urethroplasty. Proximal hypospadias with chordee needs surgical correction and may involve a two-stage repair. The first stage corrects the penile curvature and the second stage repairs the urethra. Circumcision should be avoided as preputial skin may be required for future repairs or revisions. Surgery for hypospadias is best performed by experts in hypospadias surgery and is typically undertaken before the age of 18 months. Failed hypospadias repair can present as urethrocutaneous fistula (*Figure 85.2e*).

Epispadias

Epispadias is very rare. In penile epispadias, the urethral opening is on the dorsum of the penis and is associated with an upward curvature of the erect penis (*Figure 85.3*). Epispadias often coexists with bladder exstrophy and other severe developmental defects.

Summary box 85.2

Hypospadias

- Hypospadias is diagnosed clinically by a ventrally placed urethral meatus, a hooded foreskin and penile curvature
- In severe cases with coexisting testicular maldescent and micropenis, consider disorders of sexual development as a diagnosis
- Avoid circumcision as the prepuce may be used in procedures to correct the abnormality
- Surgical treatment should be undertaken by experts

Urethral diverticulum

Congenital urethral diverticulum is rare. It is commonly seen post urethroplasty where genital skin is used for augmentation (*Figure 85.4*). Typically, patients present with postmicturition dribble. Diagnosis is made by urethrography and the diverticulum is repaired by surgery.

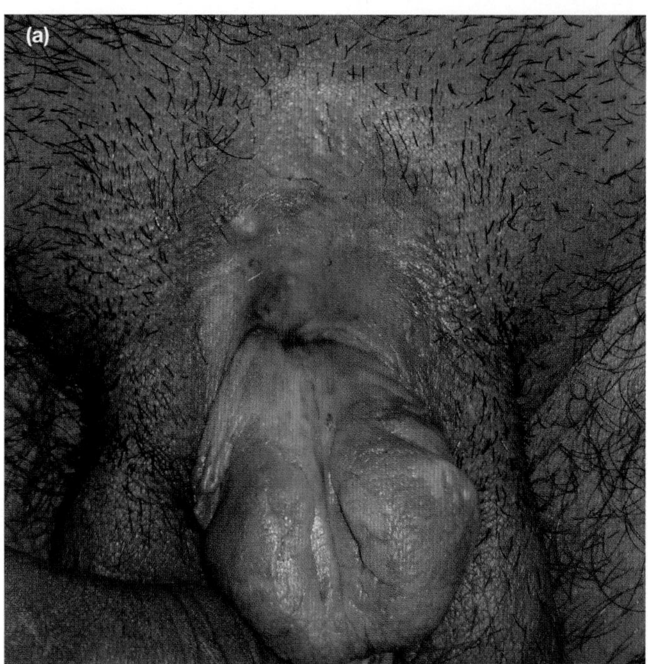

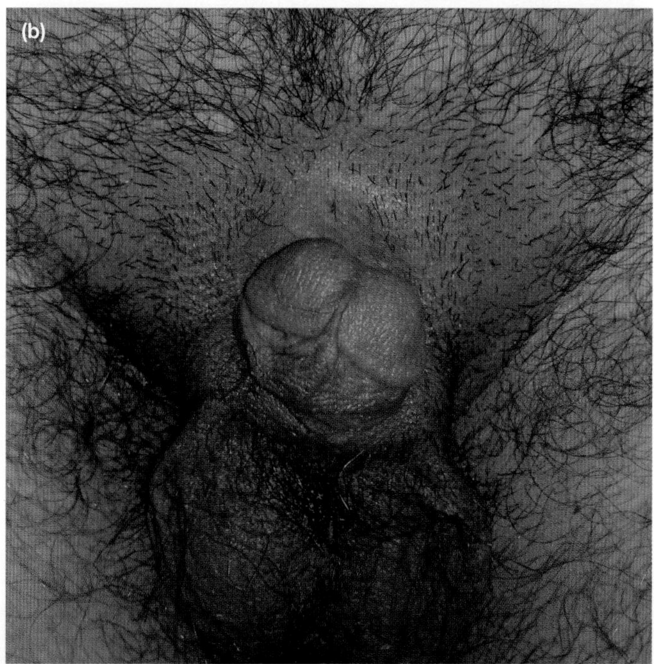

Figure 85.3 (a) Epispadias in an adult showing a dorsal urethral plate that is open and the meatus opened at the penopubic junction. (b) Dorsal chordee in a patient with epispadias (courtesy of Dr GV Datar, Pune, India).

Injuries to the male urethra

Bulbar urethral trauma

The patient usually gives a history of a falling-astride injury, leading to blunt trauma of the perineum. Other common causes include falling from a tree, cycling, skating and industrial accidents. The bulbar urethra is crushed upwards onto the pubic bone, typically with significant bruising.

Clinical features

The signs of a ruptured bulbar urethra are perineal bruising and haematoma, typically with a butterfly distribution. There is usually bleeding from the urethral meatus and retention of urine.

Management

Investigations include a retrograde urethrogram (RGU). A gentle attempt at catheterisation may be made. If the catheter fails to drain urine, a suprapubic cystostomy is performed (*Figure 85.5*).

Delayed anastomotic urethroplasty is performed after 3 months with excellent success rates.

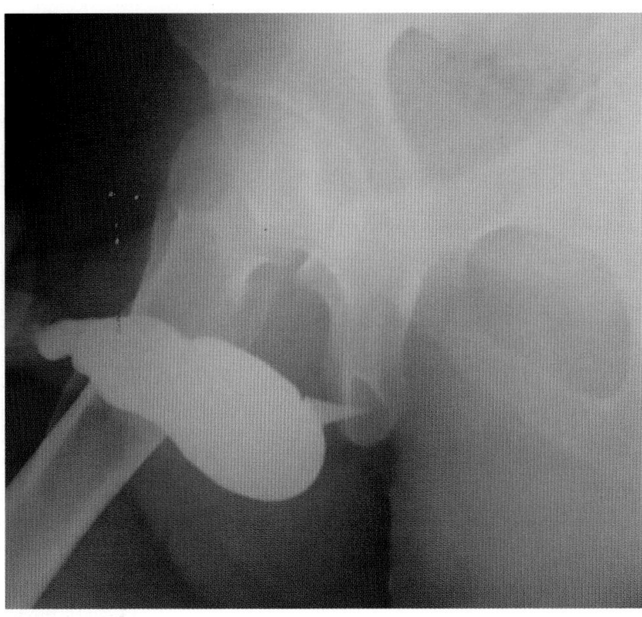

Figure 85.4 Urethrogram showing a urethral diverticulum in the penile urethra.

Summary box 85.3

Bulbar urethral trauma

- The aetiology is usually blunt injury to the perineum
- Diagnosis is made by urethrography
- If a catheter fails to drain, suprapubic cystostomy is performed
- Delayed urethroplasty is the surgical treatment of choice

Pelvic fractures and urethral injuries

The incidence of posterior urethral injury in pelvic fracture is approximately 10%. These are crush injuries. They are most commonly seen after road traffic accidents.

The site of injury is usually the bulbomembranous junction. The bladder with the prostate and membranous urethra is disrupted from the bulbar urethra. The displacement can be both posterior and superior (***Figure 85.6***). The injury can be partial or complete. Occasionally the injury is complex with bladder neck disruption and rectourethral fistula.

Clinical features

Initial treatment includes resuscitation and haemodynamic stabilisation of the patient.

Clinical features include blood at the meatus and urinary retention. The injury is usually diagnosed on the ultrasound or computed tomography (CT) scan done as part of trauma management (Focused Assessment with Sonography in Trauma [FAST]). To confirm the diagnosis an RGU is performed (***Figure 85.6***). If the tear is partial a gentle attempt at catheterisation is made. If urine does not drain, a suprapubic cystostomy (percutaneous or open) is performed. Complex patients may need evaluation with a three-dimensional CT or magnetic resonance imaging (MRI) scan of the pelvis. Emergency laparotomy is required for bladder rupture and bladder neck injuries. A diverting colostomy is performed in associated rectal injuries.

Treatment

In some centres, early endoscopic realignment is attempted. Once the patient is stable, endoscopy is performed from a suprapubic cystostomy. A guidewire is passed from the urethral

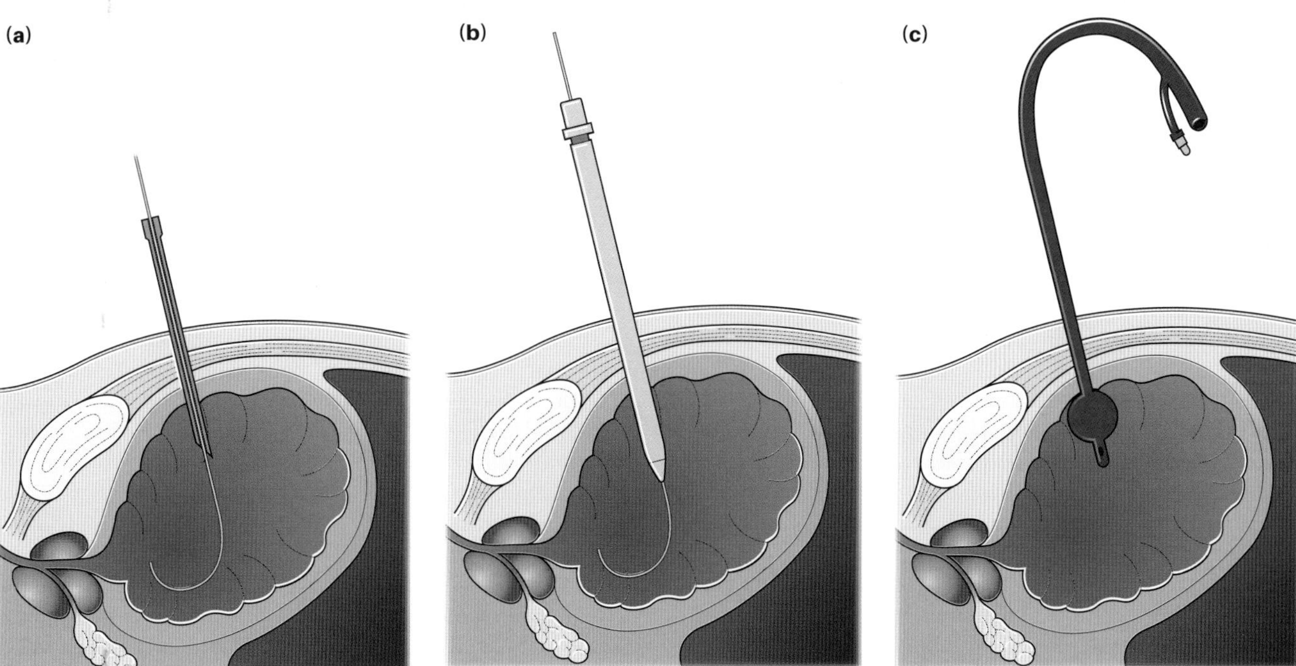

Figure 85.5 (a) Percutaneous puncture of the bladder with passage of a guidewire into the bladder followed by dilatation of the track over the guidewire (b), thereby allowing placement of a catheter into the bladder (c).

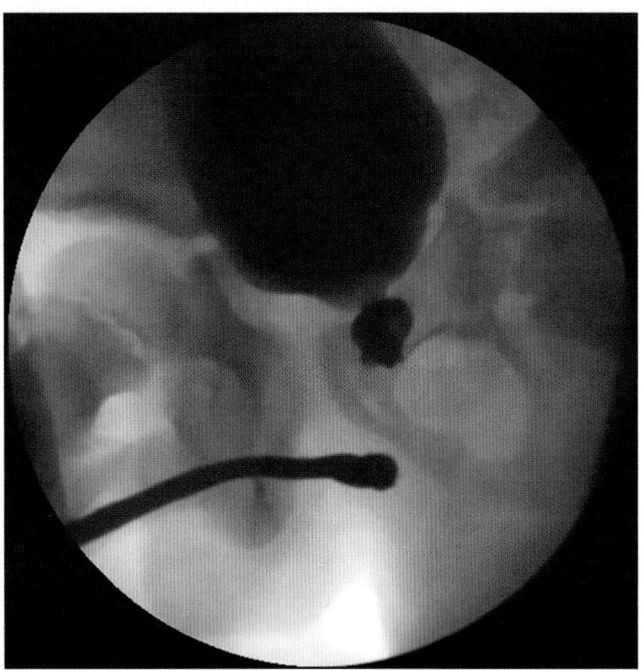

Figure 85.6 A retrograde urethrogram and voiding cystourethrogram in a patient with a pelvic fracture urethral injury showing the gap. The bladder along with the prostate is displaced upwards and there is a gap between the bulbar urethra and membranous urethra.

meatus and pulled up into the bladder through the haematoma. A Foley catheter is passed over the guidewire. This procedure is challenging and is not always successful. There is an increased risk of infection of the haematoma. If endoscopic realignment is successful, some patients may not need further surgery. Even if it fails, the gap may become shorter and easier to manage with urethroplasty. Delayed anastomotic urethroplasty is the treatment of choice and is performed after 3–6 months. It is a highly challenging procedure and should be undertaken at specialist centres where the surgery has higher success rates.

Complications

Erectile dysfunction (ED). This is common after pelvic fracture with urethral injury. It can be vasculogenic (damage to dorsal arteries) or neurogenic (damage to cavernosal nerves). The erectile function is evaluated by penile Doppler ultrasound. Usually, an intracavernosal injection of a vasoactive agent (papaverine) is given prior to Doppler evaluation. Penile Doppler ultrasound is used to evaluate the velocity of blood flow in the cavernosal and dorsal penile arteries. Patients often recover from ED over a period of time (up to 1 year). Those who fail may require further treatment with oral agents such as sildenafil. If this fails they are treated with self-intracavernosal injection of vasoactive agents, a vacuum device or a penile implant.

Urinary incontinence. Incontinence is rare. In complex cases, the injury may affect the prostate–membranous urethra with a bladder neck tear. These patients have a higher risk of incontinence.

Orthopaedic injuries. Stabilisation of the fractured pelvis may be performed by the orthopaedic team by either external or internal fixation.

Summary box 85.4

Pelvic fractures and urethral injury

- Suspect a pelvic fracture and associated urethral injury if there is retention of urine or blood at the meatus
- Diagnostic RGU is performed
- Partial tears can be treated with a single gentle attempt at catheterisation
- Initial management is insertion of a suprapubic catheter
- Delayed anastomotic urethroplasty has a high success rate in specialised centres

Penile and bulbar urethral stricture

Aetiology

The common causes of urethral stricture are:

- lichen sclerosus (LS);
- iatrogenic (post catheter and/or instrumentation);
- sexually transmitted diseases (gonorrhoea);
- post radiation;
- traumatic;
- idiopathic;
- congenital.

Pathophysiology

Postinflammatory strictures are less common since the introduction of effective antibiotic treatment of gonorrhoea. The stricture is commonly seen in the bulbar urethra. There is infection in the periurethral glands, which persists after inadequately treated gonorrhoea. The infection spreads to cause a periurethritis, which heals by fibrosis. Most strictures appear within 1 year of infection but may not cause difficulty in micturition until later.

LS (previously known as balanitis xerotica obliterans [BXO]) is a condition characterised by fibrosis of the foreskin, resulting in phimosis. The glans may be involved and it presents as white patches. There can be a meatal stenosis and penile urethral stricture. The cause of the condition is unknown. The majority of studies suggest that it is an autoimmune condition or caused by infection. LS is usually diagnosed by visual inspection but a biopsy will confirm the diagnosis. It is seen in two forms: active and burnt out. Patients usually present with poor flow. A uroflowmetry study followed by RGU and VCUG can help in making the diagnosis of stricture.

The strictures produced are typically long and difficult to treat. Common sites of stricture in LS are penile or panurethral. However, isolated bulbar urethral strictures are also seen in LS.

Frederic Eugene Basil Foley, 1891–1966, urologist, Ancker Hospital, St Paul, MN, USA.
Christian Johann Doppler, 1803–1853, Professor of Experimental Physics, Vienna, Austria, enunciated the 'Doppler principle' in 1842.

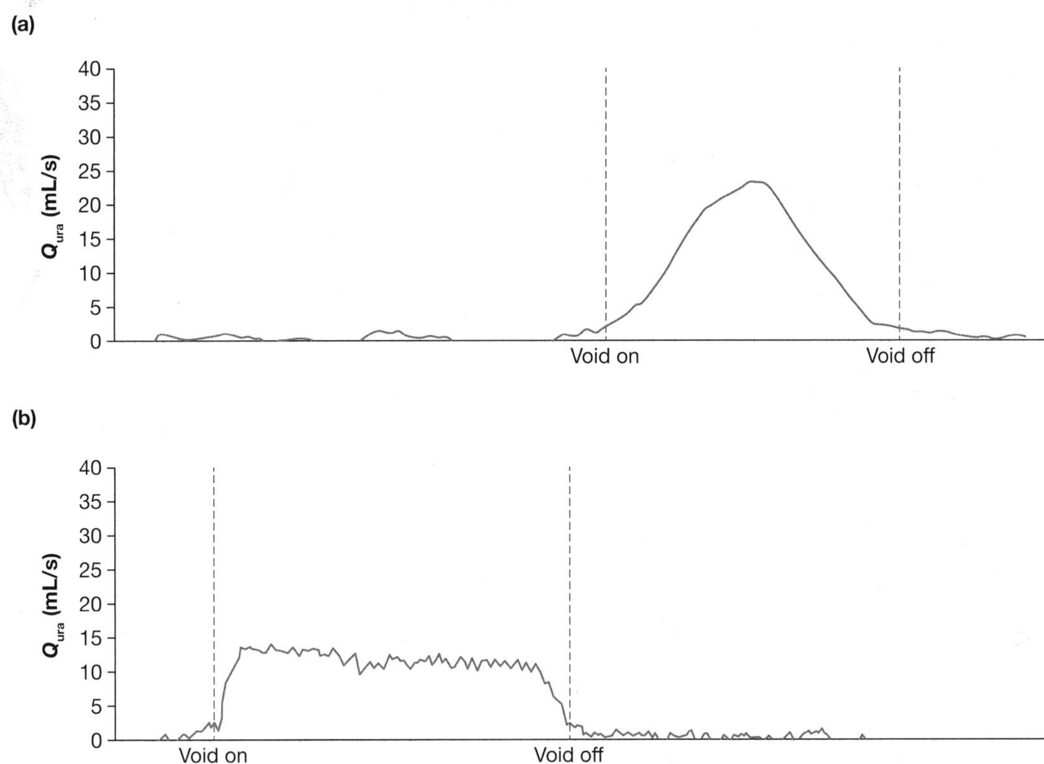

Figure 85.7 (a) A normal uroflow pattern. Normal flow is a bell-shaped curve with a maximum flow rate of more than 15 mL/s. (b) A urinary flow rate trace from a patient with a urethral stricture. Note the prolonged flow with the typical box pattern (the vertical lines depict the start and end of micturition).

Postinstrumentation strictures following an endoscopy or catheterisation may affect any part of the urethra. Post-transurethral resection of prostate (TURP) strictures are seen in the submeatal area, the bulbar urethra or penoscrotal junction. Bladder neck stenosis can occur following TURP and following radical prostatectomy for the treatment of prostate cancer.

Clinical features

Symptoms are usually hesitancy, poor flow and prolonged voiding time. The patients may complain of recurrent UTIs. Occasionally patients present with urinary retention. Investigations include uroflowmetry, urethroscopy, urethrography and ultrasound scanning to assess bladder emptying and to detect any upper tract dilatation. The urinary flow rate is typically prolonged and shows a box pattern (*Figure 85.7*). RGU and VCUG using a water-soluble contrast medium are performed (*Figures 85.8 and 85.9*). Urethroscopy is used to assess the stricture intraoperatively (*Figure 85.10*).

Complications

These include recurrent UTI, retention of urine, upper tract dilatation, bladder stones and periurethral abscess.

Treatment

The management of urethral strictures has changed considerably over the past 25 years. Urethral dilatation is one of the oldest surgical procedures and has been performed for 5000 years. In the past, serial metal dilators were used under local anaesthesia. The complications include pain, fever, bleeding and false passage creation. Nowadays, dilatation is performed over a guidewire using serial plastic dilators. Dilatation is particularly effective for soft and short strictures. It is also indicated for unfit patients, patients refusing urethroplasty or those with multiple failed urethroplasties. Urethral dilatation rarely cures stricture and most patients require repeated dilations.

Direct visual internal urethrotomy (DVIU). DVIU is performed using an optical urethrotome. The stricture is incised under visual control using a cold knife passed through the sheath of a rigid urethrotome.

Alternatively, a laser fibre (holmium/thulium) can be used. DVIU is indicated for short, non-traumatic bulbar strictures but should not be used in the penile urethra or the sphincter active membranous urethra.

Self-dilatation/clean intermittent catheterisation. In self-dilatation, the patient inserts a small-calibre (12/14Fr), usually disposable catheter into the urethra at regular intervals. Thus, the patient dilates his own stricture, but this is not a curative option. Patients who are not willing to undergo urethroplasty may choose the option of self-dilatation.

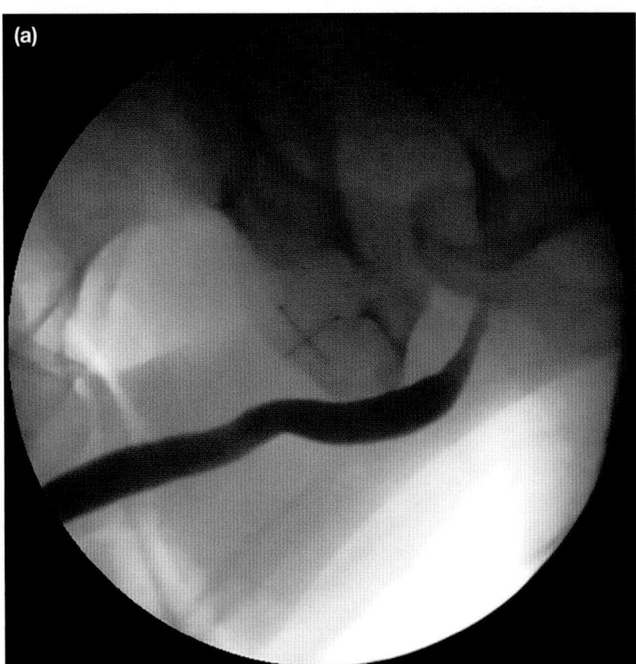

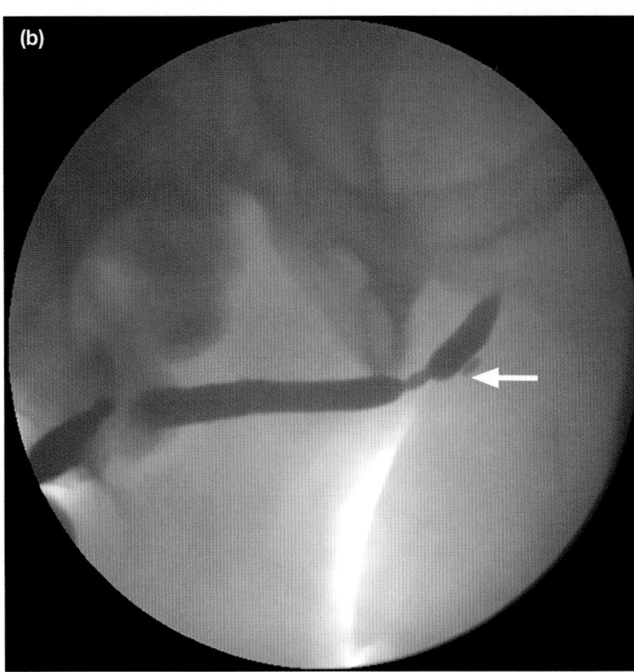

Figure 85.8 (a) A normal urethrogram. (b) An ascending urethrogram showing urethral stricture of the bulbar urethra (arrow).

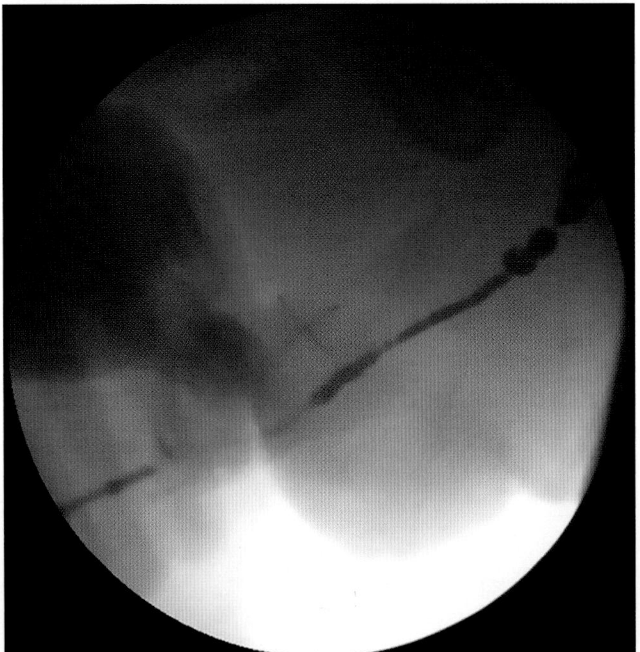

Figure 85.9 Panurethral stricture.

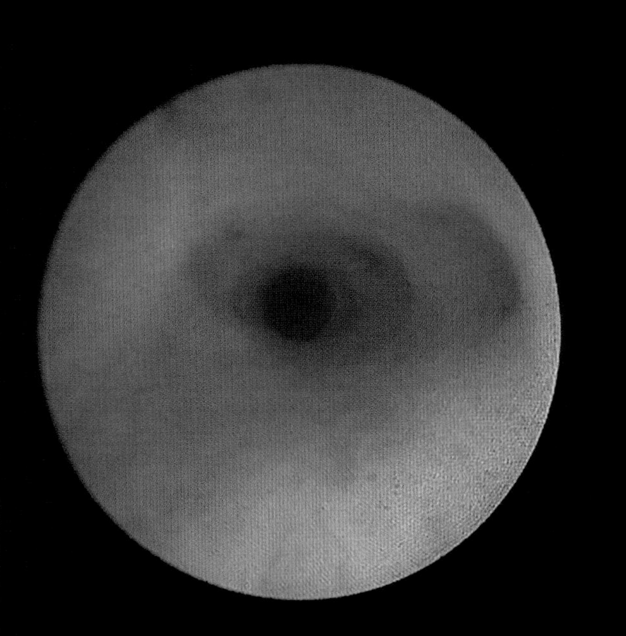

Figure 85.10 Endoscopic appearance of a urethral stricture with a fibreoptic endoscope.

Urethroplasty. There are two types of urethroplasty: anastomotic and augmentation. Anastomotic urethroplasty is performed for bulbar urethral traumatic strictures where there is a gap in the urethra. This involves dissection of the two ends of the urethra, spatulation and anastomosis. Augmentation urethroplasty is performed for non-traumatic and long strictures. In this type of urethroplasty the structured segment of urethra is incised and augmented with a patch (graft). The usual choice of patch material for augmentation urethroplasty is buccal mucosa. If required, lingual grafts can be harvested from the undersurface of the tongue. The techniques include dorsal onlay augmentation, dorsal inlay or ventral onlay.

Panurethral stricture

This is a long urethral stricture (*Figure 85.9*). The aetiology includes LS and iatrogenic causes. The treatment is by urethroplasty. A perineal incision is made and the penis is invaginated. The urethra is dissected along the full length on one side and a dorsal onlay buccal mucosa urethroplasty is performed.

Use of flaps

Preputial and penile fasciocutaneous flaps with their own vascular pedicle can be utilised for complex posterior urethroplasty to bridge long gaps in the urethra and postradiation strictures.

Summary box 85.5

Treatment of urethral strictures

- A newly diagnosed short bulbar stricture is best treated initially by DVIU
- Traumatic strictures need anastomotic urethroplasty
- Long non-traumatic strictures are treated by augmentation urethroplasty
- Anastomotic urethroplasty has a success rate of around 90%, while augmentation urethroplasty has a success rate of 85% over 10 years. Long-term follow-up is required

Other conditions of the urethra

Urethral fistula

This is seen after failed hypospadias surgery (*Figure 85.2e*). Tight strictures with periurethral abscess can present as multiple fistulae (watering-can perineum).

Urethral calculi

Urethral calculi can arise primarily behind a stricture or in an infected urethral diverticulum. More commonly, the stone is a renal calculus that has migrated to the urethra via the bladder.

Clinical features

Urethral calculi present as episodes of retention, pain or haematuria.

Treatment

A stone lodged within the prostatic urethra should be displaced back into the bladder and treated by laser or pneumatic fragmentation. Calculi in more distal parts of the urethra are fragmented *in situ* by a holmium/thulium laser. Open removal is indicated in large or multiple calculi inside a urethral diverticulum.

Neoplasms

Bloody urethral discharge without infection should raise suspicion that the patient has a urethral tumour, although such tumours are rare. Multifocal transitional cell cancer of the bladder is sometimes associated with tumours in the prostatic urethra and occasionally more distally. They can be treated by local laser ablation but are associated with a tendency to distant spread. Squamous carcinoma may develop in an area of squamous metaplasia in patients with LS. It is treated by radical surgery and carries a poor prognosis.

THE FEMALE URETHRA

Anatomy

The female urethra is around 4 cm long, extending from the bladder neck to the meatus. The entire length of female urethra is sphincter active. There is extra support from the surrounding pelvic floor musculature.

Abnormalities of the female urethra include:

- caruncle;
- stricture;
- diverticulum;
- papillomas;
- carcinoma.

Caruncle

This is seen in elderly women. It presents as a soft, raspberry-like mass about the size of a pea. It is actually the prolapsed urethral mucosa at the 6 o'clock position (*Figure 85.11*). Occasionally, there is bleeding. If required it is treated by excision and diathermy coagulation of the base of the stalk.

Stricture

Urethral stricture is uncommon in women. The aetiology includes urethritis, trauma associated with a prolonged or difficult labour or instrumentation. Urinary retention is an occasional consequence and is usually chronic. The stricture is initially managed by urethral dilatation. Urethroplasty with buccal mucosa augmentation is advocated for recurrent strictures.

Diverticulum

A female urethral diverticulum may be congenital or caused by rupture of a distended and infected paraurethral gland or by injury of the urethra during childbirth. Urine within the diverticulum becomes infected, causing local pain and repeated bouts of cystitis. Purulent urine is discharged if the urethra is compressed with a finger placed in the vagina. Diagnosis is by MRI or by transvaginal ultrasound. Excision of

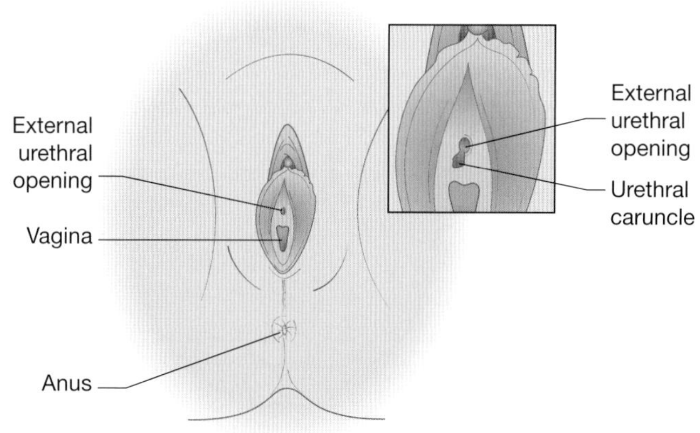

Figure 85.11 A urethral caruncle.

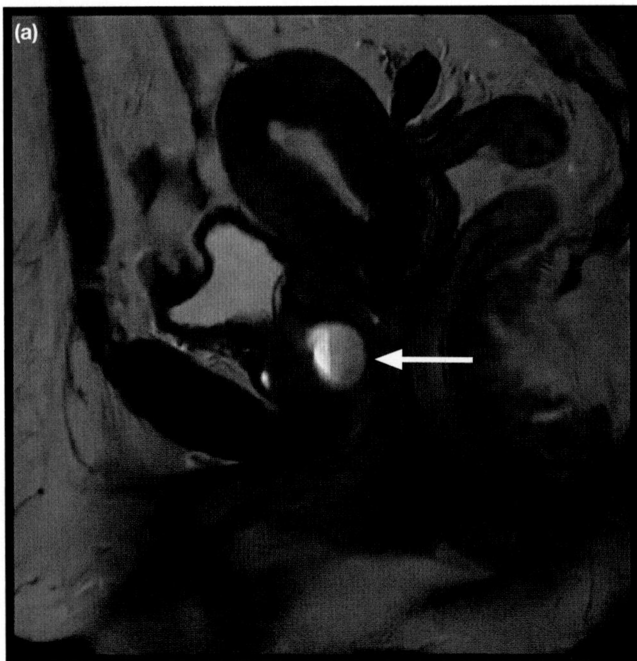

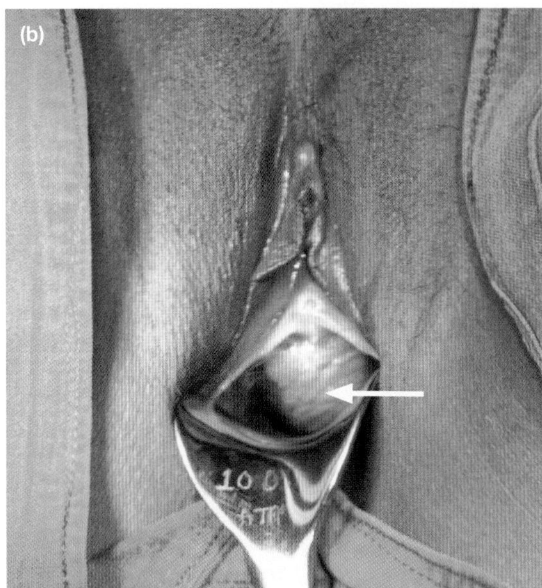

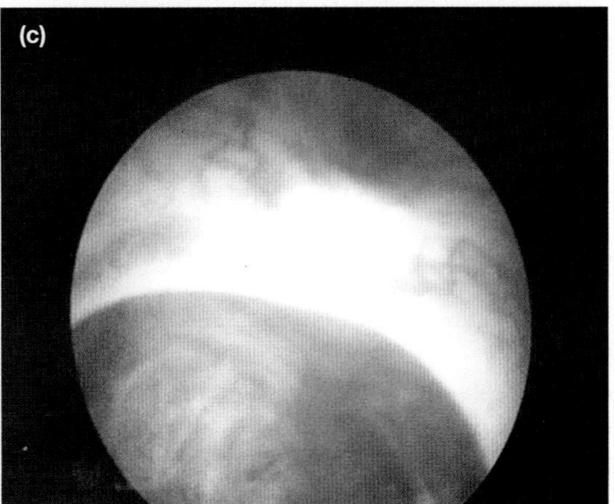

Figure 85.12 (a) Magnetic resonance imaging showing a diverticulum arising from the posterior wall of the urethra. It appears bright owing to accumulated urine and infected material (arrow). (b) Intraoperative picture of a urethral diverticulum in a female (arrow). (c) Endoscopic view of the diverticulum.

the diverticulum through the anterior vaginal wall is effective, but care must be taken not to damage the urethral sphincter (*Figure 85.12*).

Papillomas/condyloma acuminata

Condyloma acuminata (also known as anogenital warts) are a common sexually transmitted disease caused by human papillomavirus (HPV) types 6 and 11. Warts are small, skin-coloured or pink growths and may be smooth and flat or raised with a rough texture. They are usually located on the labia, at the opening of the vagina or around or inside the anus. Most women with warts do not have any symptoms at all. Less commonly, there may be itching, burning or tenderness in the genital area.

The treatment options vary depending on the size. They include local application of podophyllotoxin or imiquimod; surgical treatments include cryotherapy, electrocautery, excision and laser therapy.

Carcinoma of the urethra

This occurs twice as often in women as in men. Whether a caruncle can become malignant is disputed, but caruncles and tumours often occur close together. Malignant swellings of the urethra feel harder than benign ones. Treatment is by radiotherapy or radical surgery. The overall prognosis is poor.

THE PENIS

Anatomy

The penis is a sexual organ and composed of three tubular structures. The two dorsal structures, the corpora cavernosa, provide erectile function and are anchored posteriorly onto the pubic rami. The ventral tubular structure is the corpus spongiosum, which surrounds the urethra. It expands distally to form the glans penis.

The corpora cavernosa have an outer tough covering of tunica albuginea. There is a septum between them. The tunica albuginea encloses the erectile tissue, which has a trabecular structure with a network of sinusoidal spaces lined by endothelium within which blood pools during erection. The central arterial blood supply (cavernosal artery) is a branch of the internal pudendal artery. Sacral parasympathetic nerves are responsible for erection. They cause smooth muscle relaxation

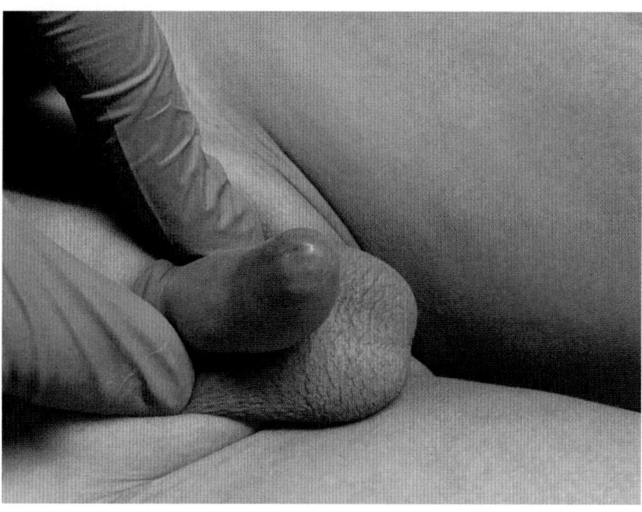

Figure 85.13 Phimosis in a child with inability to retract the prepuce.

with increased arterial inflow, dilatation of the sinusoids and blood accumulation within the trabecular spaces. Simultaneously there is venous outflow occlusion by the coverings of the corpora cavernosa.

DISEASES OF THE FORESKIN

Phimosis

There are physiological adhesions between the foreskin and the glans penis at birth. They begin to disappear around the age of 2 years and may persist until 6 years of age or later, giving the false impression that the prepuce will not retract. This condition (sometimes known as physiological phimosis) should not be confused with true phimosis in young boys.

Phimosis in boys

In true phimosis the prepuce does not retract (*Figure 85.13*). This may result in ballooning of the foreskin during micturition and may also result in infection (balanoposthitis).

Phimosis in adults

Scarring in adults occurs as a result of balanitis (inflammation of the glans penis), posthitis (inflammation of the foreskin) or LS. In LS (*Figures 85.14 and 85.15*) the normal pliant foreskin becomes thickened, typically whitish in appearance and forms a constricting band that prevents retraction. As a consequence, it is difficult to keep the penis clean and there may be recurrent attacks of balanitis.

Treatment

In physiological phimosis, no treatment is necessary or appropriate. True phimosis causing symptoms requires circumcision. In emergency situations, such as when catheterisation is required, a dorsal slit under local anaesthesia may be required.

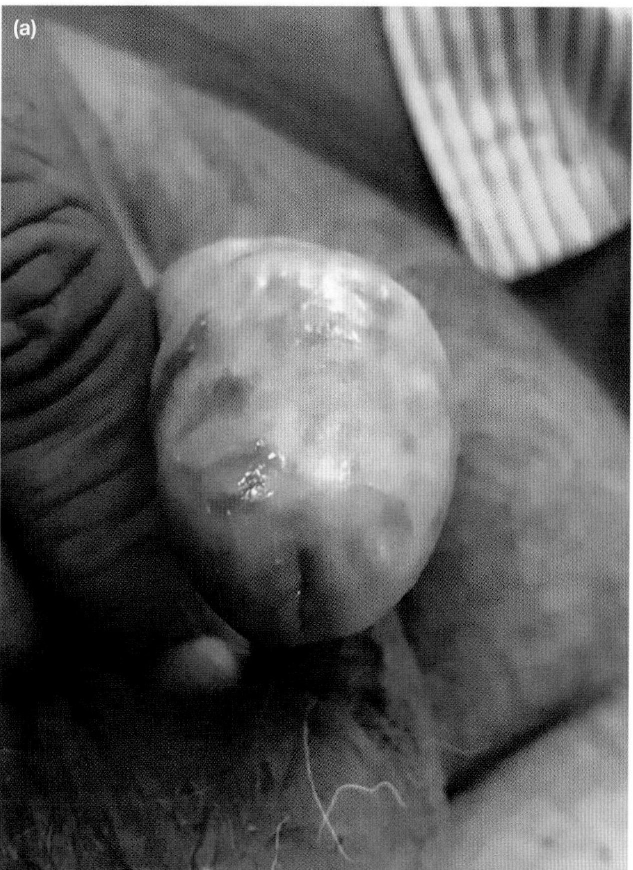

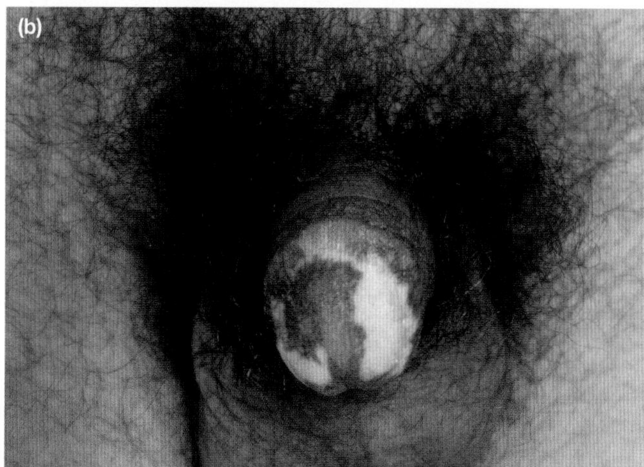

Figure 85.14 (a) Active phase of lichen sclerosus (LS). (b) Burnt-out phase of LS.

Circumcision

Circumcision has been practised since as early as 4000 BCE. Circumcision should not be performed in the presence of hypospadias, penile curvature or buried penis.

Indications. In infants and young boys, circumcision is usually performed at the request of the parents for social or religious reasons. Medical indications for circumcision in boys include true phimosis, LS (rare under the age of 5 years), recurrent

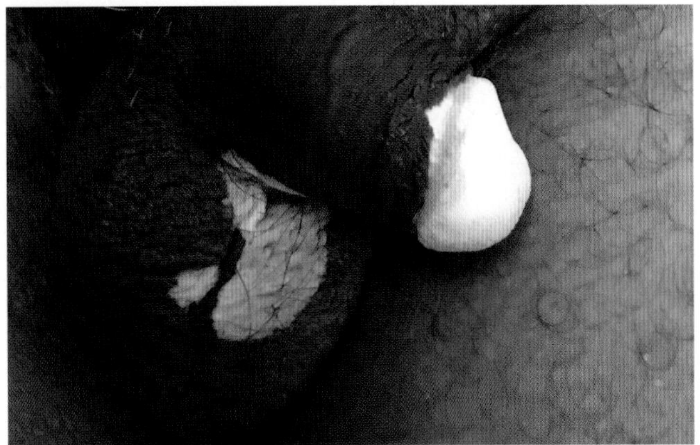

Figure 85.15 Lichen sclerosus is a genital skin disease and can involve the skin of the genitalia.

attacks of balanoposthitis and recurrent UTIs with abnormalities such as high-grade vesicoureteral reflux.

In adults, circumcision is indicated when there is inability to retract the foreskin for intercourse, for splitting of an abnormally tight frenulum or for recurrent balanitis.

Recently, evidence has emerged that circumcision protects against the spread of human immunodeficiency virus (HIV). The virus dies quickly on a dry penis. A large-scale programme of adolescent circumcision under the auspices of the World Health Organization is ongoing in some African countries.

Technique. Under anaesthesia the prepuce is held in artery forceps and put on a gentle stretch. A circumferential incision in the penile skin is made at the level of the corona using a knife. The prepuce is then slit dorsally in the midline to within 1 cm of the corona. (An alternative technique slits the prepuce first.) This converts the foreskin into two flaps.

When the undersurface of the prepuce has been separated from the glans, the inner layer of each flap is again marked with a pen and then incised with a second circumferential incision, leaving about 0.5 cm of the inner layer of the preputial skin. Cutting the remaining connective tissue completes the excision (*Figure 85.16*). Vessels should be preferably secured with bipolar diathermy or with absorbable sutures. The cut edges of the skin are approximated using interrupted sutures, making certain that the frenular vessels are ligated.

In LS, the separation of prepuce from foreskin is at times difficult. The excised skin should be sent for histology.

Summary box 85.6

Circumcision

- Commonly performed for religious and cultural reasons
- Physiological phimosis does not need circumcision
- Symptomatic phimosis is treated by circumcision

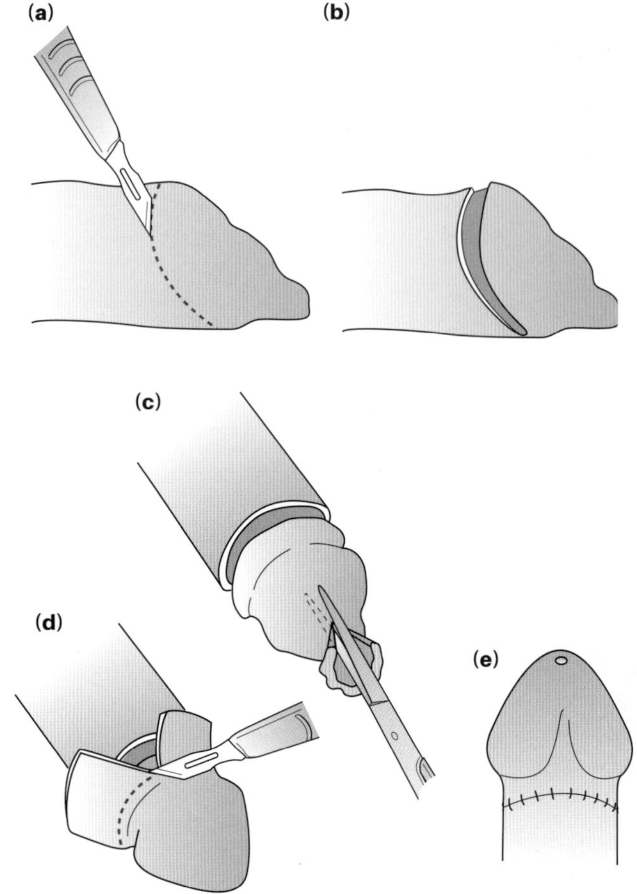

Figure 85.16 (a–e) Stages in circumcision.

Short frenulum

Phimosis should not be confused with the condition where the frenulum is short. It causes pain when the foreskin is retracted. Another possible presentation is tearing of the frenulum during sexual activity. Treatment is by frenuloplasty, which utilises the Heineke–Mikulicz principle to lengthen the frenulum.

Paraphimosis

A tight foreskin once retracted may be difficult to return and a paraphimosis results. In this condition, the venous and lymphatic return from the glans and distal foreskin is obstructed and these structures become oedematous, causing even more pressure within the obstructing ring of prepuce (*Figure 85.17*). Gentle manual compression and injection of a solution of hyaluronidase in normal saline may help to reduce the swelling. A dorsal slit of the prepuce under local anaesthesia may be enough in an emergency. These patients can be treated by circumcision if careful manipulation fails.

Walter Hermann von Heineke, 1834–1901, surgeon and Professor of Surgery in Erlangen, Germany.
Jan Mikulicz-Radecki, 1850–1905, surgeon and Director of Surgery in Krakow and Wrocław, Poland.

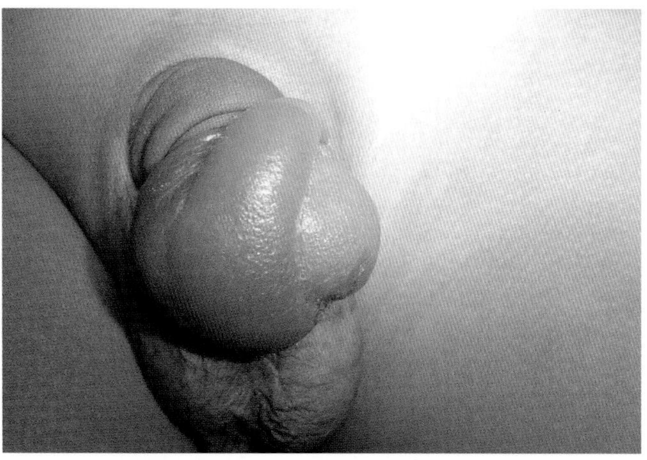

Figure 85.17 Paraphimosis.

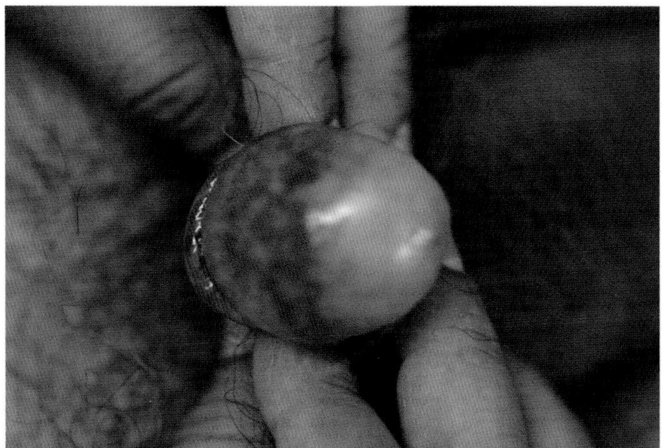

Figure 85.18 Balanoposthitis.

Balanoposthitis

Inflammation of the prepuce is known as posthitis; inflammation of the glans is balanitis. The opposing surfaces of the two structures are often involved, hence the term balanoposthitis (*Figure 85.18*). In mild cases, the only symptoms are itching and some discharge. In more severe inflammation, the glans and foreskin are red-raw and pus exudes. Treatment is by broad-spectrum antibiotics and local hygiene measures. Balanoposthitis is common in patients with diabetes. Recurrent balanoposthitis requires circumcision.

INJURIES OF THE PENIS

Avulsion of the skin of the penis

Entanglement of clothing in rotating machinery and zip injuries are the usual causes. Partial injury to the penile skin can be repaired. Complete avulsion is treated by a two-stage procedure. Burying the penis in the scrotum is the first stage and lifting it is the second stage. The scrotal skin now forms the covering of the penis. An alternative approach is initial debridement with skin grafting later.

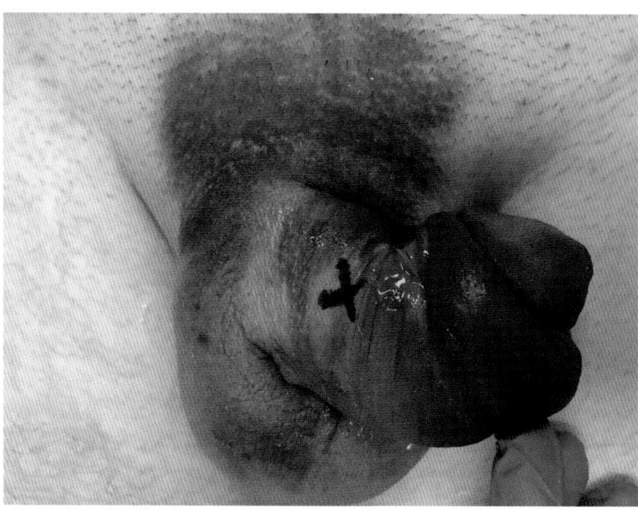

Figure 85.19 Penile fracture. Note the extensive bruising of the penis and scrotum.

Fracture of the penis

Fracture of the penis usually occurs when the erect penis is bent suddenly. It leads to rupture of the tunica albuginea with extravasation of blood from within the penis. Usually the patient feels a cracking or popping sound. It is associated with pain and detumescence. Clinically there is bruising and penile haematoma (*Figure 85.19*). There may occasionally be an associated urethral injury.

Investigations include ultrasound and MRI. Surgical management involves early exploration of the penis with surgical repair of the ruptured tunica albuginea.

Strangulation of the penis

Strangulation of the penis is caused by rings placed on the penis, usually for sexual pleasure. It can cause venous engorgement, which prevents their removal. The ring must be cut off with a ring cutter.

Other abnormalities of the penis

Erectile dysfunction

ED is failure to attain or maintain an erection. It can arise as a consequence of psychological issues, but the commonest cause is vascular disease affecting the penile arterial blood flow; as such, ED is associated with diabetes, hypertension, dyslipidaemia and smoking. Other rarer causes include endocrine disease (hypogonadism and prolactin-secreting pituitary tumours), neurological disease (multiple sclerosis, spinal cord injury and prolapsed intervertebral disc), iatrogenic damage to the cavernosal nerves owing to radical pelvic surgery (e.g. radical prostatectomy, abdominoperineal excision of the rectum and radical cystectomy), neuropathy secondary to pelvic radiotherapy and drug-induced causes (including antihypertensive agents, antidepressants and antipsychotics). ED may be a marker of cardiovascular disease.

Physical examination of the genitalia, measurement of the blood pressure and assessment of the secondary sexual characteristics is required; biochemical assessment of the blood sugar, the serum lipid profile and the serum testosterone is necessary in all cases. Penile Doppler ultrasound is performed with the use of intracavernosal vasoactive agents such as papaverine. Initially the ED is treated with phosphodiesterase type 5 inhibitors (such as sildenafil).

A few patients need treatment with self-intracavernosal injection of vasoactive agents. Vacuum erection devices are a non-invasive alternative. Penile implants are broadly of two types: semirigid and inflatable. Their use is becoming increasingly popular.

Summary box 85.7

Erectile dysfunction

- Appropriate investigation involves identification of vascular risk factors
- Phosphodiesterase inhibitors are the first-line treatment
- Penile implants are becoming popular for management of ED

Peyronie's disease

Peyronie's disease (PD) is characterised by penile deformity (*Figure 85.20*), palpable penile plaques inside the penis, ED and pain on erection. The cause is unknown, but probably involves minor injury to the erect penis with secondary microhaemorrhage beneath the tunica albuginea and fibrosis. The latter results in the palpable plaques that can be identified on examination. The plaques may rarely be calcified (*Figure 85.21*). The presence of these relatively inelastic plaques causes the erect penis to bend towards the side of the plaque. The deformity is commonly dorsal (towards the abdomen) and the deformity may prevent penetrative sexual intercourse.

While the aetiology is uncertain, there is an association with Dupuytren's contracture. The natural history of the condition is that it typically progresses for 18–24 months before stabilising. During this active phase of the disease, surgery is not indicated; a variety of medical treatments have been tried, although none with any good evidence of benefit.

The diagnosis is usually made on clinical examination but MRI may be helpful.

Newer treatments include intralesional injections of collagenase clostridium histolyticum (Xiaflex).

Surgical correction can be performed in two ways. If the penis is of adequate length, it is possible to plicate the tunica albuginea on the side opposite to the maximum curvature. The plication can be done by Nesbit's technique or a 16-dot technique. The second option involves incision of the plaque and a bovine pericardial patch.

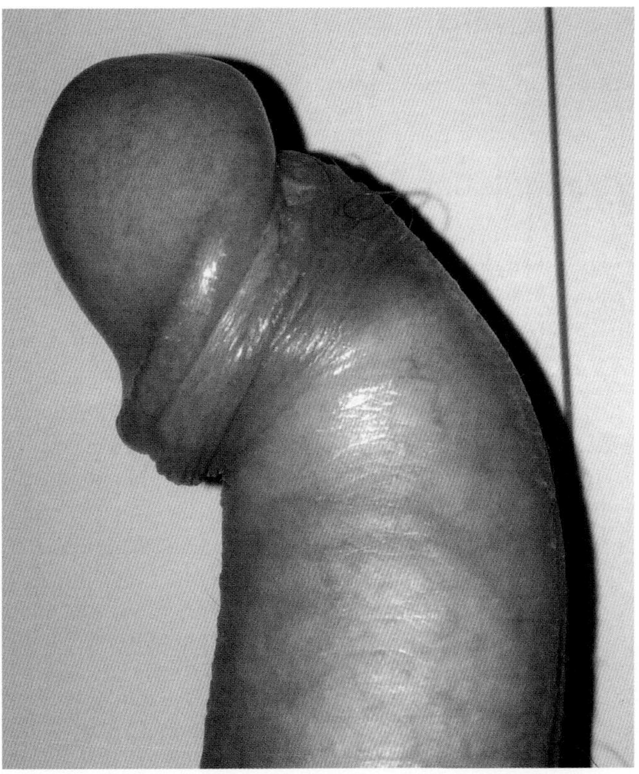

Figure 85.20 Dorsal deformity of the erect penis that is typical of Peyronie's disease.

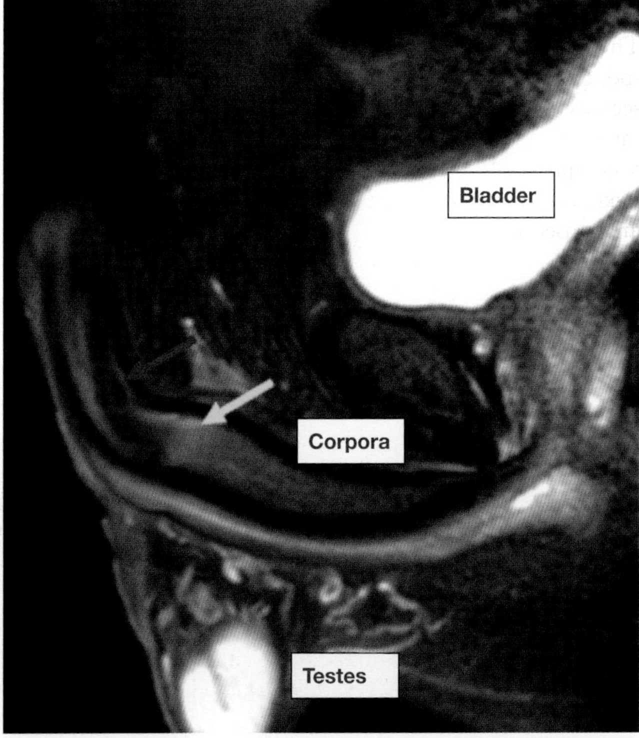

Figure 85.21 Magnetic resonance imaging in Peyronie's disease showing plaque. The yellow arrow shows calcified plaque; the red arrow shows active disease on the dorsal wall of the penis.

Francois de la Peyronie, 1678–1747, surgeon to King Louis XIV of France and founder of the Royal Academy of Surgery, Paris, France.
Baron Guillaume Dupuytren, 1777–1835, surgeon, Hôtel Dieu, Paris, France, described this condition in 1831.
Reed Miller Nesbit, 1898–1979, urologist, University of Michigan Medical School, Ann Arbor, MI, USA. Nesbit was a pioneer of transurethral resection of the prostate.

Summary box 85.8

Peyronie's disease

- The disease has two phases: an initial active phase and a later stable phase
- There is no effective treatment in the active phase
- Surgery may be indicated in the chronic phase to correct deformity that interferes with sexual activity

Congenital curvature of the penis

This penile deformity is similar and analogous to Peyronie's disease and is occasionally seen in young men (*Figure 85.22*). In congenital curvature of the penis, the urethral length is normal and it typically results in a ventral deformity of the erect penis. If the deformity interferes with sexual activity, then surgery, usually a Nesbit procedure, will straighten the erect penis.

Priapism

Priapism means a persistent erection lasting longer than 4 hours; it is a surgical emergency. There are two main types of priapism: ischaemic and non-ischaemic.

Ischaemic priapism

Ischaemic or veno-occlusive priapism is the more common. It is due to venous congestion, with consequent thrombosis and ischaemia. The penis remains erect and becomes painful. This is a pathological erection and the glans penis and corpus spongiosum are not involved. The condition is most commonly seen as a side effect of medication, most notably antipsychotic medication and intracavernosal injections. It can also arise as a complication of hypercoagulable blood disorders such as sickle cell disease or leukaemia. A small proportion of cases are caused by malignant disease in the corpora cavernosa or the pelvis.

Blood taken from the penis shows hypoxia, hypercapnia and acidosis, while Doppler scanning shows an absence of blood flow within the penis.

An underlying cause should be excluded and the patient should be referred for specialist urological care. The condition is an emergency since delay beyond 6 hours results in progressive, irreversible damage to the corpora cavernosa tissue with subsequent fibrosis and ED. Aspiration of the sludged blood in the corpora cavernosa is the first-line therapy; if this fails, intracavernosal injection of phenylephrine (an α-adrenoceptor agonist) is the next line of therapy. If that proves ineffective, it may be necessary to decompress the penis by creating a shunt between the corpus cavernosum and either the glans penis or the corpus spongiosum. Treatment initiated after 24–36 hours rarely restores normal erectile function. Recurrent ischaemic (stuttering) priapism is seen in sickle cell disease.

Non-ischaemic priapism

This rarer form of priapism arises as a consequence of traumatic damage to the central penile artery, usually as a consequence of blunt perineal trauma. A fistula develops between the artery and the sinusoidal space, which results in a persistent erection that is painless, in contrast to ischaemic priapism. This is a high-flow priapism. Blood gas analysis shows the characteristics of arterial blood and Doppler scanning and selective arteriography will demonstrate the fistula. Treatment involves androgen ablation therapy. If medical therapy fails, selective arterial embolisation is performed.

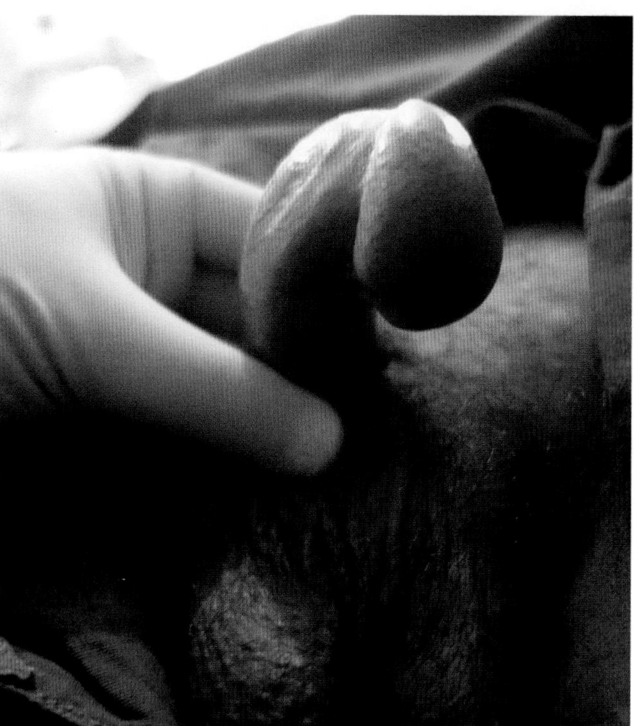

Figure 85.22 Congenital curvature of the penis.

Summary box 85.9

Ischaemic priapism

- The characteristic clinical features are a painful erection not involving the glans penis
- Blood gas analysis from the penis shows hypoxia, hypercapnia and acidosis
- Detumescence should be ideally achieved within 6 hours to avoid long-term ED

CARCINOMA OF THE PENIS

Aetiology

Circumcision soon after birth confers immunity against carcinoma of the penis. Later circumcision does not seem to have the same benefit, with the assumption that smegma is in some way carcinogenic. Infection with HPV types 16 and 18 is a risk factor, as are LS (*Figure 85.23*) and smoking. Phimosis and chronic balanoposthitis are known to be contributory factors and there are definite *precancerous* states including leukoplakia of the glans, which is similar to the condition seen on the tongue, and penile intraepithelial neoplasia (PeIN).

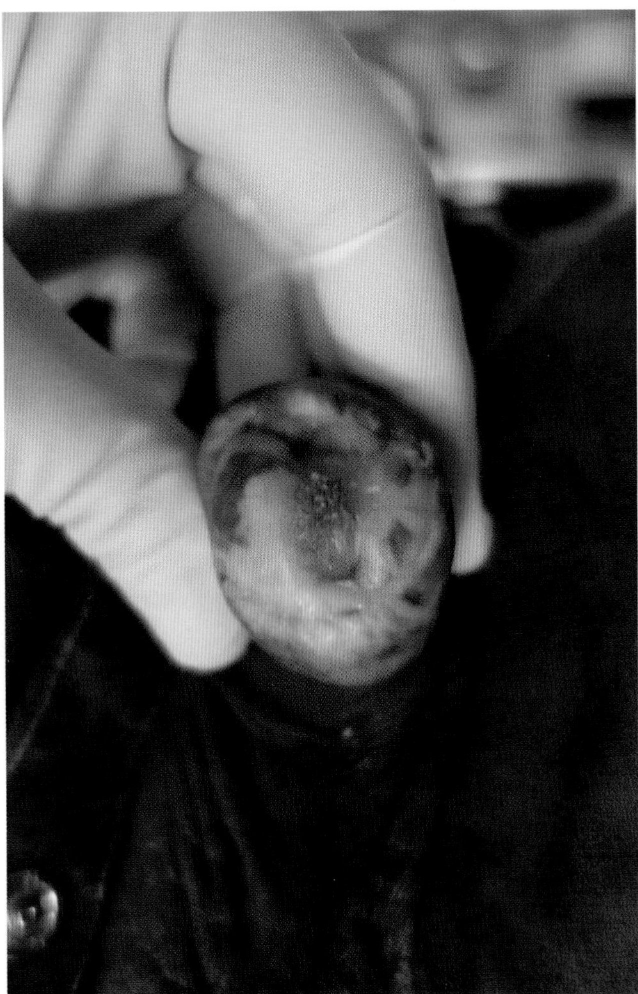

Figure 85.23 Early penile cancer seen in a patient with lichen sclerosus.

Investigations

A biopsy should be performed. MRI is performed for local staging. Assessment of locoregional lymph node status is essential.

Penile intraepithelial neoplasia (carcinoma *in situ* of the penis, Bowen's disease, erythroplasia of Queyrat)

PeIN is typically seen as a red cutaneous patch on the penis. When it occurs on the glans penis, it is known as erythroplasia of Queyrat; when it occurs on the shaft of the penis, it is called Bowen's disease. There are several other benign causes of red patches on the penis; when there is clinical doubt as to the underlying diagnosis a biopsy is indicated. When the diagnosis of carcinoma *in situ* is confirmed, treatment is by means of topical 5-fluorouracil cream, CO_2 laser ablation or surgical excision.

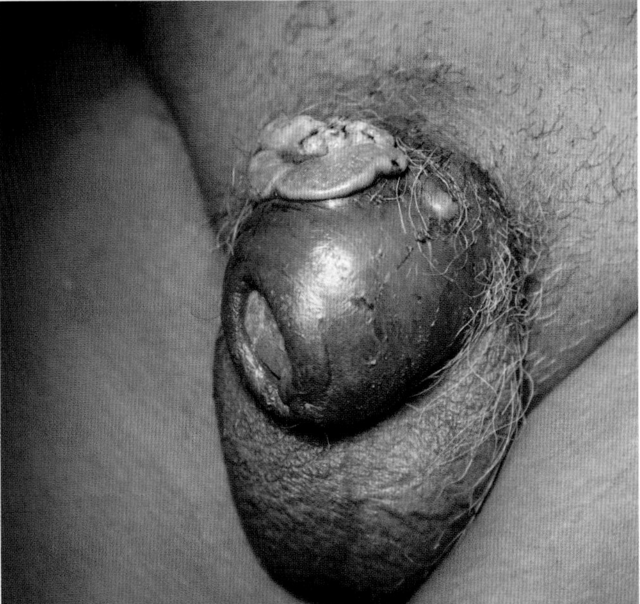

Figure 85.24 A squamous cell cancer of the penis.

Pathology

Carcinoma of the penis is most typically a squamous cell carcinoma arising in the skin of the glans penis or the prepuce. It may be flat and infiltrating or warty in appearance. The former often starts as leukoplakia or PeIN; the latter results from an existing papilloma. Local growth continues for months or years. T1 tumours are confined to the skin, with T2 tumours invading the corpus spongiosum or the corpus cavernosum. T3 tumours invade the urethra and T4 tumours invade adjacent structures. The earliest lymphatic spread is to the inguinal nodes (N1 and N2 disease) and then to the iliac nodes (N3 disease). Distant metastatic deposits are infrequent.

Clinical features

Many patients present late as a fungating/ulcerative growth (***Figure 85.24***), either because of embarrassment or because of misdiagnosis. About 10% of patients are under 40 years of age. By the time the patient presents, the growth is often large and secondary infection causes a foul, bloody discharge. There is typically little or no pain.

Around 50% have inguinal lymph node enlargement at presentation but the nodal enlargement often reflects infection. In many, the prepuce is non-retractile and must be split to view the lesion. A biopsy should be performed to make the diagnosis. Untreated, the whole glans may be replaced by a fungating offensive mass. Later, the inguinal nodes can erode the skin of the groin and, in rare cases, death of the patient can result from erosion of the femoral or external iliac vessels.

Treatment

Management is divided into treatment of the primary tumour and treatment of the inguinal nodes. Patients with small lesions

John Templeton Bowen, 1857–1940, American dermatologist, described this condition in 1912.
Louis Auguste Queyrat, 1856–1933, French dermatologist, described this condition in 1911.

of low grade and low stage are treated with organ-preserving surgery, such as limited excision, Mohs' surgery or laser ablation. Mohs' micrographic surgery is based on sequential tissue excision under repeat microscopic control. This helps in accurately identifying the tumour margin and maximally preserves the uninvolved tissues. For most primary tumours surgical excision is the mainstay of treatment, with the traditional view that a 2-cm margin of normal tissue be removed being superseded by a more recent, more conservative view, such that penis-preserving surgery with excision of much lower margins of normal tissue is now accepted. Tumours affecting the glans penis require glansectomy, with more advanced tumours requiring partial penectomy. In advanced cases, total penectomy is required with the formation of a perineal urethrostomy. These techniques are indicated even in advanced metastatic disease for reasons of local control.

Treatment of any associated enlarged inguinal lymph nodes should be delayed until at least 3 weeks after local treatment of the primary lesion. Enlargement caused by infection will usually show signs of subsiding with antibiotic treatment. For palpable nodes, ultrasound-guided fine-needle aspiration will confirm the diagnosis and a block dissection of both groins should be undertaken. The management of patients where the nodes are not palpable involves the use of sentinel lymph node biopsy (SLNB) followed by inguinal node dissection if the SLNB is positive.

Management of the pelvic nodes is controversial. When they are involved on CT scanning, surgery probably has little role; however, when the iliac nodes are not enlarged in the presence of N2 disease, the options are observation, pelvic lymphadenectomy or radiotherapy. Chemotherapy is relatively ineffective and currently is reserved for palliation in those with metastatic disease. The prognosis for tumours confined to the penis is good with 5-year survival rates in excess of 80%. With nodal involvement the 5-year survival rate falls to around 40%.

Summary box 85.10

Carcinoma of the penis

- Enlargement of superficial inguinal lymph nodes may be caused by infection or metastatic spread
- Surgery is the mainstay of treatment
- Nodal involvement indicates a poor prognosis

Buschke-Löwenstein tumour

The Buschke–Löwenstein tumour is uncommon. It has the histological pattern of a verrucous carcinoma. It is locally destructive and invasive but appears not to spread to lymph nodes or to metastasise. Treatment is by surgical excision.

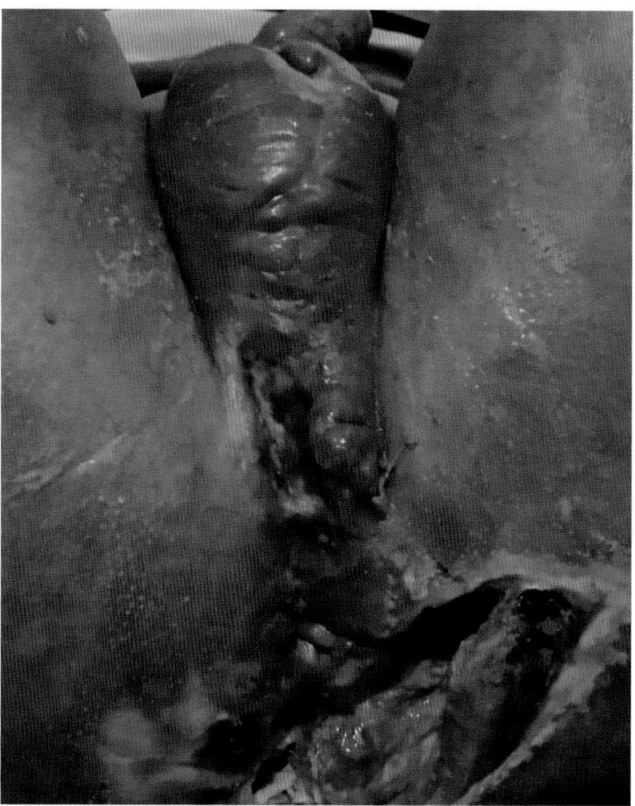

Figure 85.25 Fournier's gangrene.

Malignant melanoma of the penis

This is an uncommon tumour with the principles of management being the same as for squamous cell carcinoma. Blood-borne metastatic disease is, however, more common.

INFECTION AND INFLAMMATION OF THE PENIS AND URETHRA

Fournier's gangrene

This is progressive infection of the genitalia and perineum (***Figure 85.25***). It is usually caused by mixed bacterial flora (*Escherichia coli*, *Bacteroides* spp., *Streptococcus pyogenes*, *Staphylococcus aureus*). It may be associated with diabetes, cancer, malnutrition, recent urogenital or colorectal instrumentation or trauma. The hallmark is rapid progression from symptoms and signs of cellulitis. There is erythema, swelling, pain and blister formation with ultimately foul-smelling necrotic lesions. It is a surgical emergency. Progression from genitalia to perineum to

Frederic E Mohs, 1910–2002, twentieth century American physician and general surgeon, University of Wisconsin, Madison, WI, USA, developed the Mohs' micrographic surgical technique in 1938 for cutaneous malignant lesions.
Abraham Buschke, 1868–1943, dermatologist, Berlin, Germany.
Ludwig Löwenstein, 1885–1959, dermatologist, Berlin, Germany.
Jean Alfred Fournier, 1832–1915, French syphilologist and founder of the Venereal and Dermatological Clinic, Hôpital St Louis, Paris, France.

abdominal wall occurs extremely rapidly. There is an increased risk of bacterial septicaemia. It will lead to death if untreated.

Treatment involves a combination of broad-spectrum antibiotics and extensive surgical debridement.

Urethral discharge

The commonest cause of urethral discharge in men is urethritis; the two commonest causes of urethritis are non-specific urethritis (NSU) and gonococcal urethritis. Other related symptoms include dysuria and urethral pruritus while epididymitis can also be present. A sexual history should be sought, particularly a history of unprotected intercourse, oral sex and anal intercourse. A routine investigative screen includes a Gram stain of the discharge, dipstick testing and culture of a urine specimen as well as nucleic acid amplification testing (NAAT) of either a urine specimen or a urethral swab. If relevant, the same techniques can be used for vaginal, endocervical, anal and pharyngeal swabs. NAAT is a sensitive way of identifying both gonococcal and chlamydial urethritis. As with all sexually transmitted infections (STIs) the possibility of other infections (such as HIV) should always be borne in mind and, where appropriate, tested for.

Non-specific urethritis (synonym: non-gonococcal urethritis)

NSU is an STI that is the commonest cause of urethritis in the western world. In around 40% of cases it is due to *Chlamydia trachomatis*, with other cases being caused by *Ureaplasma urealyticum*, *Trichomonas vaginalis* or *Mycoplasma genitalium*. The causative agent in up to 50% of cases is unknown.

NSU can affect both men and women and asymptomatic infection is common in both. In men, dysuria and a white mucopurulent urethral discharge appear up to 6 weeks after sexual intercourse. Dysuria is usual. The urine appears to be clear but may contain 'threads' or pus cells. Epididymitis is common and urethral stricture is a potential late complication. In women, the condition is usually asymptomatic, although it can present as vaginal discharge or as a form of urethrotrigonitis. It may result in cervicitis or pelvic inflammatory disease.

Exclusion of gonorrhoeal infection is important. The diagnostic test of choice is NAAT: in men either a first-catch urine specimen or a urethral swab can be used; in women urine, endocervical or vaginal swabs can be used. If testing is positive, then partners should be screened.

The standard treatment regimens are azithromycin as a single dose (1 g) or doxycycline (100 mg orally twice daily) for 7 days. Treatment is usually effective, although relapse is common, especially in men, in whom the prostate may act as a reservoir of infection. It is important to treat both partners as reinfection is probable if this is not done; retesting of both partners at 3 months is recommended.

Gonorrhoeal urethritis

Gonorrhoea is a sexually transmitted disease caused by *Neisseria gonorrhoeae* (gonococcus), a Gram-negative kidney-shaped diplococcus that infects the anterior urethra in men, the urethra and cervix in women and the oropharynx, rectum and anal canal in both sexes, but especially men. It is transmitted by unprotected sexual intercourse and is the second commonest cause of urethritis in western countries.

Most men have symptoms of urethral discomfort and urethral discharge within a few days of infection. There is often scalding dysuria. In women it is often asymptomatic. There can be mild dysuria or slight urethral discharge, which can go unnoticed by the patient. Cervicitis can occur with about 10% suffering from pelvic inflammatory disease (salpingitis), which, if bilateral, may lead to infertility. A mother may transmit gonorrhoea to her newborn during childbirth, with the risk that blindness of the child can result. In addition, in both men and women exposed orally or anally, gonococcal infections can cause a predominantly asymptomatic pharyngitis or proctitis.

Traditionally, the diagnosis was made by identification of pus and gonococci in a Gram-stained urethral smear with subsequent culture. However, more recently, NAAT, which is more sensitive, has become the norm.

Complications are prevented by effective early treatment. In men complications include posterior urethritis, prostatitis (acute or chronic), acute epididymo-orchitis, periurethral abscess and urethral stricture. Gonococcal arthritis, iridocyclitis, septicaemia and endocarditis are unusual.

Treatment is with antibiotics. Ceftriaxone (250 mg intramuscularly) and azithromycin (1 g orally) are currently the treatment of choice. There is increasing antibiotic resistance to more traditional antibiotics such as ciprofloxacin or penicillin. Contact tracing is important in controlling the spread of the disease and management is usually by a genitourinary physician. Failure to respond to first-line treatment should raise the possibility of antibiotic resistance or co-infection with *Chlamydia*.

Reiter's disease (synonym: sexually acquired reactive arthritis)

Reiter's disease is an autoimmune disease characterised by the triad of urethritis, conjunctivitis and polyarthritis. Common triggers include chlamydial urethritis, less commonly gonococcal urethritis and diarrhoea secondary to *Salmonella*, *Shigella* or *Campylobacter*. It is an HLA-B27-associated condition. The conjunctivitis (present in around 50%) and arthritis typically occur 1–3 weeks after the primary infection. Diagnosis is made on clinical grounds and treatment is largely symptomatic, although antibiotic treatment of the precipitating infection is important. The urethritis and conjunctivitis frequently subside

---

Hans Christian Joachim Gram, 1853–1938, Professor of Pharmacology (1891–1900) and of Medicine (1900–1923), Copenhagen, Denmark, described this method of staining bacteria in 1884.

Albert Ludwig Siegmund Neisser, 1855–1916, Director of the Dermatological Institute, Breslau, Germany (now Wroclaw, Poland).

Hans Conrad Julius Reiter, 1881–1969, President of the Health Service and Honorary Professor of Hygiene, Berlin, Germany, described this condition in 1916. He was subsequently convicted of war crimes as a consequence of his involvement in the death of hundreds of inmates in Buchenwald.

Daniel Elmer Salmon, 1850–1914, veterinary pathologist, Chief of the Bureau of Animal Industry, Washington, DC, USA.

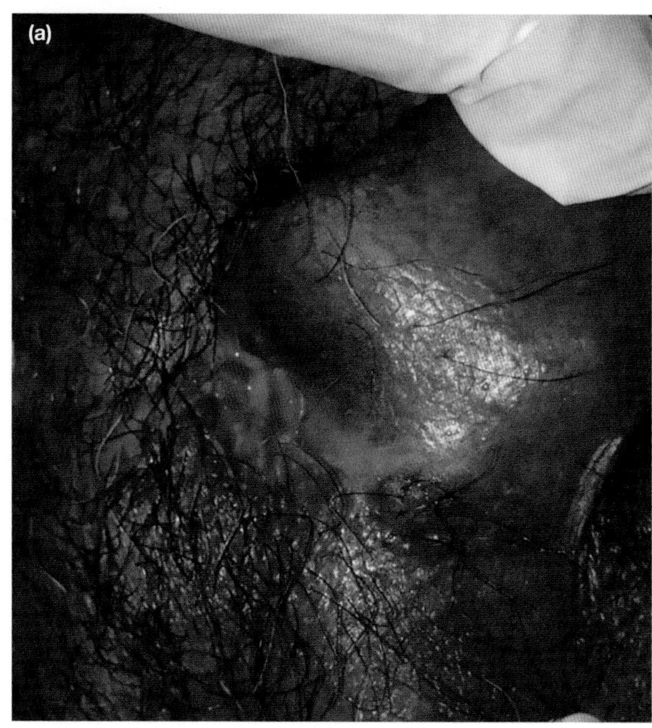

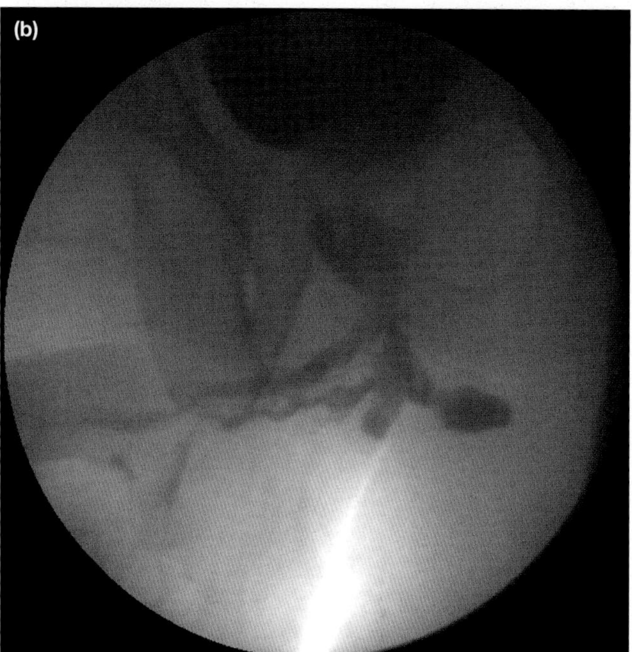

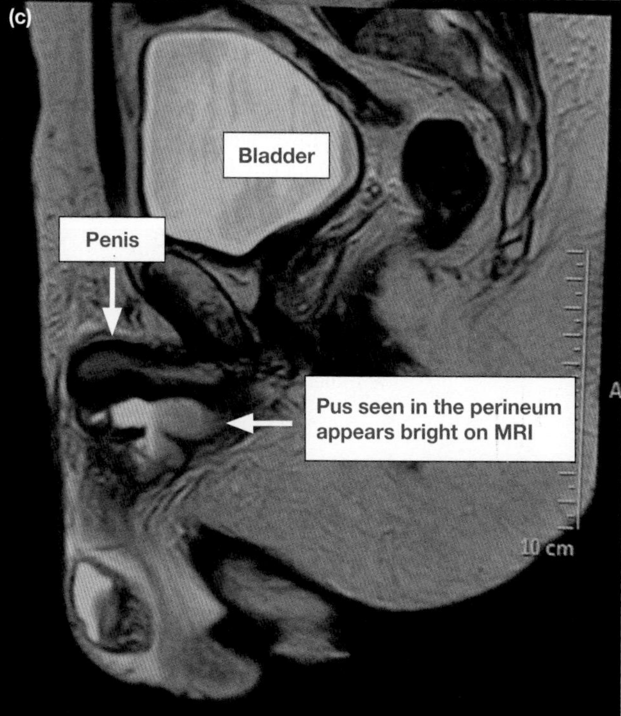

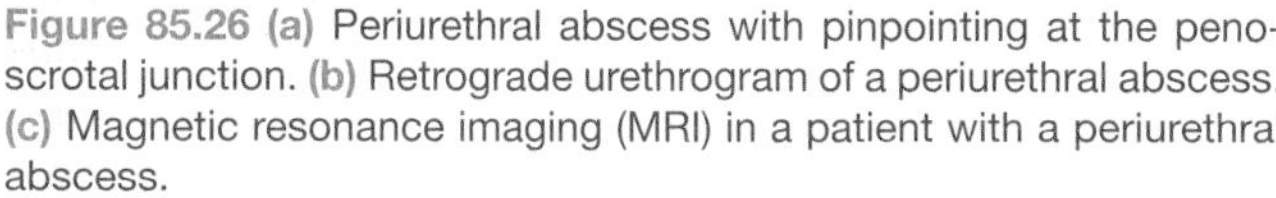
Figure 85.26 (a) Periurethral abscess with pinpointing at the penoscrotal junction. (b) Retrograde urethrogram of a periurethral abscess. (c) Magnetic resonance imaging (MRI) in a patient with a periurethral abscess.

after a few weeks, but the arthritis may persist for months. Severe anterior uveitis and frequently recurrent attacks suggest a poor outlook.

Periurethral abscess

Periurethral abscesses were once common with high morbidity but are now rare. Clinical presentation is varied but may include fever, dysuria, urethral discharge and swelling of the penis or scrotum. In untreated cases urethral fistulation and occasionally extensive cellulitis or necrotising fasciitis can occur.

A penile periurethral abscess arises following a gonococcal or chlamydial infection of one of the glands of Littre. There can be a coexisting urethral stricture. There is usually penile swelling with tender induration felt on the underside of the penis, which, if left untreated, may discharge externally, often leaving a fistula. Diagnosis can be helped by ultrasound of the urethra. Treatment should include both antibiotic treatment, as for urethritis, and surgical drainage into the urethra.

A periurethral abscess in relation to the bulbar urethra is even more uncommon. It may be associated with a urethral stricture, urethral trauma or, rarely, a urethral cancer. The infecting organisms are varied and can include both streptococci and anaerobic organisms. Extravasation of urine is not unusual. There is perineal pain with pyrexia, rigors and tachycardia. Tenderness and swelling rapidly spread from the perineum to the penis and the anterior abdominal wall. Ultrasound scanning and MRI are useful diagnostic aids and treatment with antibiotics is essential. Collections of pus should be drained and the urine should be diverted by a suprapubic urinary catheter.

A chronic periurethral abscess sometimes results from a longstanding urethral stricture (*Figure 85.26*). The multiple loculi of pus should be drained and the stricture treated. Urethral fistula occurs either spontaneously or as a result of incision of the abscess.

Alexis Littre, 1658–1726, surgeon and lecturer in anatomy, Paris, France.

Genital ulcers

The commonest cause of a genital ulcer is genital herpes. Other less common causes include syphilis and chancroid. As with all STIs, the possibility of other infections (such as HIV) should always be borne in mind and, where appropriate, tested for.

Genital herpes

Genital herpes is caused by sexual transmission of the herpes simplex virus (usually HSV-2, occasionally HSV-1). Infection is lifelong with recurrent symptomatic attacks occurring in 50% or more of cases. Pain along the distribution of the sensory nerve, usually the genitofemoral nerve, precedes the eruption by 2 days and may be particularly severe around the anus. A group of tiny vesicles rapidly erodes to form shallow ulcers, which are painful (***Figure 85.27a***). The first attack occurs around 4 days after exposure and is typically accompanied by fever, myalgia and inguinal lymphadenopathy. In female patients, the ulcers often spread onto the thighs during the attack. Involvement of the urethra may cause retention of urine, which may persist for up to 14 days if there is radiculitis of the S2 and S3 nerve roots.

Diagnosis is made clinically or, when there is doubt, by either cell culture or polymerase chain reaction (PCR)-based techniques. All primary infections should be treated by oral antiviral agents such as aciclovir (400 mg three times a day for 7–10 days), valaciclovir (1 g orally twice a day for 7–10 days) or famciclovir (250 mg three times a day for 7–10 days).

A child born to a mother with active infection is susceptible to a fatal generalised herpes infection in the neonatal period. Caesarean section should be considered in these circumstances. There is an increased risk of carcinoma of the cervix and annual cytology for life is recommended.

Syphilis

Syphilitic ulcers are typically painless, rubbery and indurated. Caused by the spirochaete *Treponema pallidum*, diagnosis was traditionally achieved by dark-field microscopy, but modern serological techniques are nowadays more appropriate. The incidence of syphilis is increasing since the advent of the retroviral drugs used to treat HIV in the mid-1990s. Treatment is with long-acting penicillin.

Tropical sexually transmitted infections

Lymphogranuloma venereum

Lymphogranuloma venereum is a sexually transmitted disease caused by *C. trachomatis* (chlamydia A) types L1–L3 and is primarily an infection of the lymphatics and lymph nodes. It can affect both sexes. While it was considered rare in resource-rich countries, some recent outbreaks in Europe have occurred, usually in conjunction with HIV.

The primary lesion is a fleeting, painless, genital papule or ulcer that develops 1–4 weeks after infection and is often unnoticed by the patient. The inguinal glands become enlarged and painful around 2–6 weeks after the primary lesion. The masses

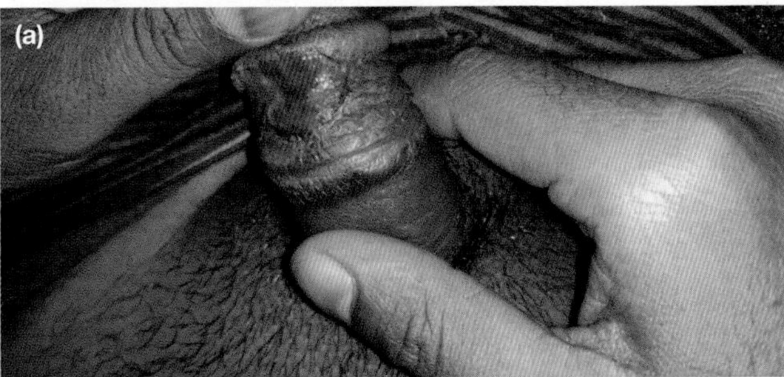

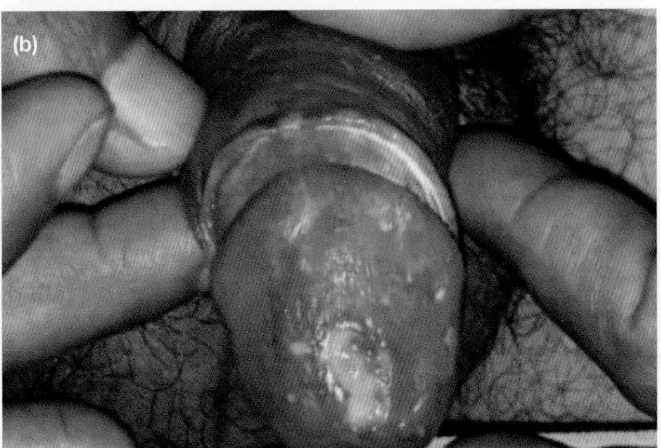

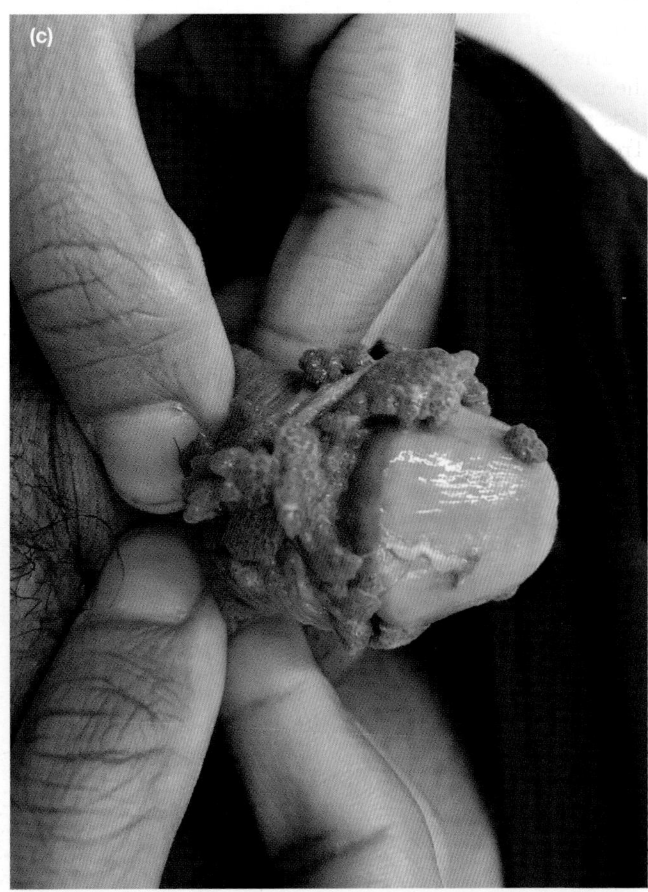

Figure 85.27 (a) Genital herpes. (b) Ulcer seen in chancroid. (c) Genital warts affecting the prepuce and glans (courtesy of Dr Narendra Patwardhan, dermatologist, Pune, India).

of nodes mat together above and below the inguinal ligament to give the 'sign of the groove'. The overlying skin reddens, there may be fluctuance and the mass occasionally ruptures. There may be a proctitis, which can go on to produce a rectal stricture if untreated. Lymphatic obstruction leads to lymphoedema in the perineum and, occasionally, the lower limbs. Urethritis and urethral stricture occur in men.

Diagnosis is confirmed clinically and by the detection of antibodies against the organism. Culture, direct immunofluorescence and NAAT can be performed. Treatment is by a combination of antibiotics, which may include doxycycline, azithromycin, erythromycin and ciprofloxacin. The multilocular lymphatic masses should not be incised, although aspiration is permissible to reduce discomfort.

Lymphogranuloma inguinale

This is a chronic and slowly progressive ulcerative tropical disease affecting the genitals and surrounding tissue, but occasionally occurring elsewhere in the body. It is usually sexually transmitted and is caused by *Klebsiella granulomatis*; it is most commonly seen among socially deprived people. The incubation period varies greatly but is typically between 7 and 30 days.

A painless vesicle or indurated papule, usually on the external genitals but occasionally elsewhere on the skin, gradually erodes into a slowly extending ulcer with a beefy-red, granulomatous base. More chronic lesions may become greyish, especially at the edges, where, after months or years, malignant change may develop. The ulcerated area may bleed if touched but is usually surprisingly painless. Without treatment healing is only partial and keloid is common.

Diagnosis is by microscopy of material from the edges of the ulcer, which shows the presence of short Gram-negative rods within the cytoplasm of the large mononuclear cells. Treatment is with azithromycin, although doxycycline, erythromycin, trimethoprim–sulfamethoxazole and gentamicin are alternatives.

Chancroid

Chancroid is a sexually transmitted, acute, ulcerative disease caused by *Haemophilus ducreyi*, a Gram-negative facultative anaerobe. Following an incubation period of 3–10 days, a soft painful penile ulcer (*Figure 85.27b*) appears and is commonly followed by the development of inguinal lymphadenopathy. Diagnosis is by bacterial culture or PCR techniques. Antibiotic treatment with ceftriaxone or azithromycin is usually effective therapy.

Condylomata acuminata (synonym: genital warts)

Genital warts are caused by infection with HPV and are sexually transmitted. Infection is very common, with only a small proportion of infected patients actually having visible warts.

Most commonly due to HPV types 6 and 11, these viruses do not cause cervical cancer. Ordinary skin warts can occur on the genitals by direct contact with a finger lesion, but they are less moist and soft and less often pedunculated than the genital variety. The lesions most commonly occur under the prepuce in the coronal sulcus but may be found elsewhere, including inside the urinary meatus and on the outer prepuce (*Figure 85.27c*). In women, genital warts are most commonly found on the vulva, but they may line the vagina and occur on the cervix. Perianal warts are common.

Other associated sexually transmitted diseases should be excluded: in women mainly candidiasis and *Trichomonas* infection and in men syphilis or gonorrhoea. Genital warts may complicate HIV infection.

Treatment is by chemical or physical means. Podophyllin is often effective as a topical application. It is applied to the wart, taking great care to avoid the surrounding skin, and washed off after 6 hours or so. An alternative agent is imiquimod. If chemical methods fail, the warts can be excised or they can be ablated with cryosurgery, electrosurgery or laser. Circumcision is sometimes advised if there are florid lesions under the foreskin.

ACKNOWLEDGEMENT

The author is grateful to Pankaj M Joshi MBBS, MS, DNB Urology (Gold Medal), Reconstructive Urologist, Kulkarni Reconstructive Urology Center, India, for his input to this chapter.

FURTHER READING

Kaisary AV, Ballaro A, Pigott K. *Urology: lecture notes*, 7th edn. Hoboken, NJ: Wiley-Blackwell, 2016.

Wein AJ, Kavoussi LR, Partin AW, Peters CA. *Campbell–Walsh urology*, 12th edn. Amsterdam: Elsevier, 2020.

Theodor Albrecht Edwin Klebs, 1834–1913, Professor of Bacteriology successively at Prague, Czechoslovakia, Zurich, Switzerland and Rush Medical College, Chicago, IL, USA.

CHAPTER 86 The testis and scrotum

Learning objectives

To diagnose and manage:
- Testicular maldescent
- Testicular torsion
- Common scrotal swellings (varicocele, hydrocele and epididymal cysts)
- Testicular and scrotal infections
- Testicular tumours
- Male factor infertility
- Testicular trauma

INCOMPLETE DESCENT OF THE TESTIS

Definition

Incomplete descent of the testis, also known as cryptorchidism, occurs when one or both testes are arrested at some point in the normal path to the scrotum. An ectopic testis is a testis that is abnormally placed outside this path (*Figure 86.1*).

Incidence

About 3% of full-term and 30% of premature male infants are born with one or both testes undescended. About two-thirds of these reach the scrotum during the first 3 months of life, but full descent after that is uncommon. The incidence of testicular maldescent at the age of 1 year is around 1%. The condition is sometimes missed in the neonatal period and only discovered later in life. The presence of a hernia, testicular pain or acute torsion may direct attention to the abnormality. Cryptorchidism occurs in approximately 1.5–4% of fathers and 6% of brothers of individuals with cryptorchidism.

Pathology

The condition is more common on the right and is bilateral in 20% of cases. In adults, secondary sexual characteristics are typically normal.

The testis may be:

- intra-abdominal; usually extraperitoneal just inside the internal inguinal ring;
- within the inguinal canal; it may not be palpable (*Figure 86.2*);
- extracanalicular; usually at the scrotal neck (high scrotal);

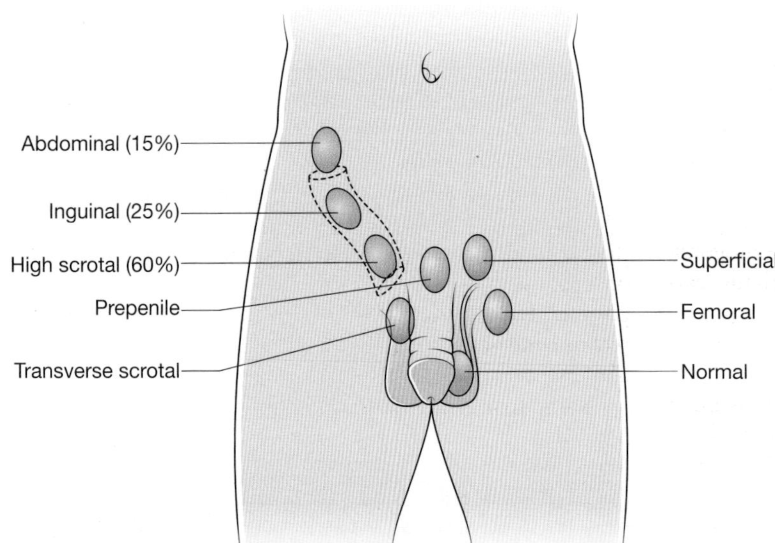

Figure 86.1 The path of descent of the testis from the abdomen (retroperitoneal) down the inguinal canal to the scrotum. Descent can be arrested at any stage with the majority in the high scrotal area. Rarely, the testis occupies a more ectopic position outside the normal path of descent (courtesy of Dr Mohan Gundeti).

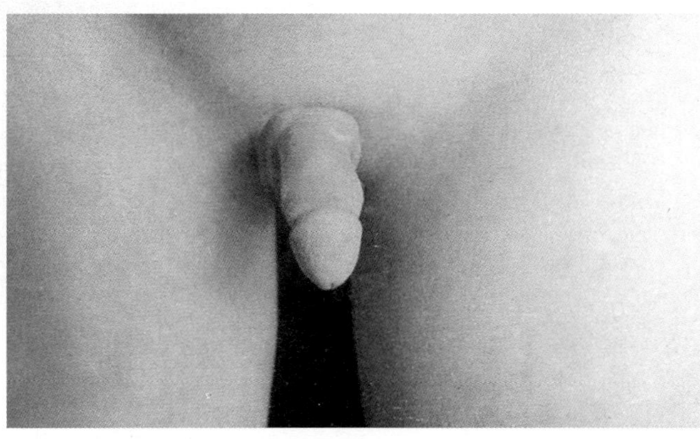

Figure 86.2 Undescended testes in a boy aged 12 years. Note the bilateral undescended testes with the underdeveloped scrotum. In cases of retractile testis, the scrotum is relatively well developed.

- ectopic; an ectopic testis is one that has ended up away from the normal path of descent. The commonest site is the superficial inguinal pouch, just inferior and medial to the superficial inguinal ring. Other rarer ectopic sites include the femoral triangle, root of the penis and perineum.

Incompletely descended testes are often macroscopically normal in early childhood, but by puberty the testis is typically smaller than its intrascrotal counterpart. Microscopic changes are apparent from 1–2 years, including loss of Leydig cells, degeneration of Sertoli cells and decreased spermatogenesis. The higher the testis, the greater the degree of histological change.

Consequences

Infertility

Men with undescended testes may have reduced fertility, even after orchidopexy.

- The infertility rate for unilateral cases is not believed to be very different from the general population.
- The fertility reduction after orchidopexy for bilateral cryptorchidism is about 38%.
- Patients with bilateral undescended testes who receive orchidopexies as adults are almost always infertile and azoospermic; but there are reports of pregnancies achieved through sperm retrieval and assisted reproduction in this group.
- The recommendation for early surgery is due to degeneration of spermatogenic tissue and reduced spermatogonia counts after the second year of life in patients with untreated undescended testes.

Malignancy

Overall, the risk of testicular cancer if orchidopexy is done before puberty is around two to three times that of the general population. It is five to six times higher when orchidopexy is done after puberty. The risk of cancer does not seem to be different when orchidopexy is done early in infancy compared with later in childhood.

- The most common type of testicular cancer in untreated undescended testes is seminoma.
- The peak age range for this tumour is 15–45 years.
- In contrast, after orchidopexy, seminomas represent only 30% of testicular tumours in previously undescended testes.
- It is treatable if caught early, so boys who had an orchidopexy as infants should be taught testicular self-examination.

Hernia

Around 90% of boys with an undescended testis have a patent processus vaginalis although the incidence of a clinically apparent hernia is much lower.

Testicular torsion

The undescended testis is more prone to testicular torsion, largely as a consequence of a developmental abnormality between the testis and its mesentery.

Summary box 86.1

Undescended testis

- Testes that are absent from the scrotum after 3 months of age are unlikely to descend
- Histological changes in the testis can be seen from 1 year of age
- An incompletely descended testis tends to atrophy as puberty approaches
- Boys with undescended testes are at greater risk of infertility, testicular malignancy, hernia and torsion

Clinical features

When assessing a child with suspected testicular maldescent, it is helpful to have the boy as relaxed as possible in a warm room, usually in a supine position. The important differential diagnosis is the so-called 'retractile testis'. During childhood the testes are mobile and the cremasteric reflex is active, so that, in some boys, any stimulation of the skin of the scrotum or thigh causes the testis to ascend and to temporarily disappear into the inguinal canal. When the cremaster relaxes, the testis reappears only to vanish when the scrotal skin is touched again.

In comparison with a true undescended testis, the scrotum in the retractile testis is normal as opposed to underdeveloped, and the retractile testis can be gently milked from its position in the inguinal region to the bottom of the scrotum. A diagnosis of true incomplete descent should be made only if this is not possible. For retractile testes, a yearly physical examination is recommended because of the 2–50% reported risk of a retractile testis becoming an acquired undescended testis.

More than 70% of cryptorchid testes are palpable by physical examination. In the remaining 30% of cases with a non-palpable testis, the challenge is to confirm the absence or presence of the testis and to identify the location of the viable non-palpable testis. Ultrasound has a high positive predictive value for inguinal located testes, but only 45% sensitivity in

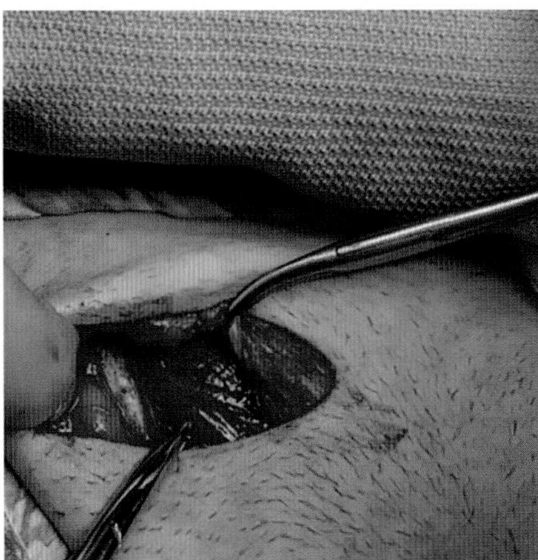
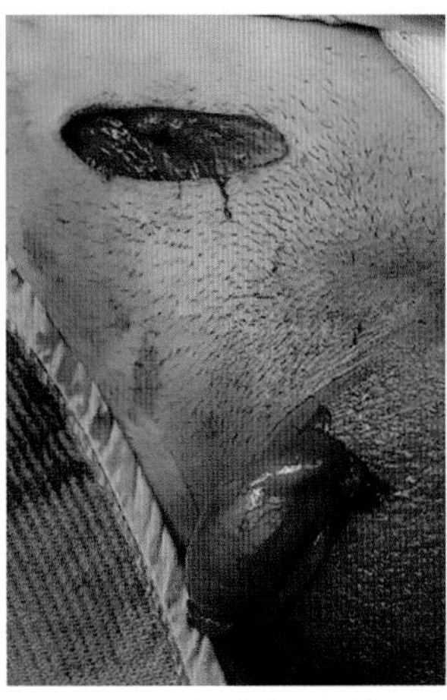
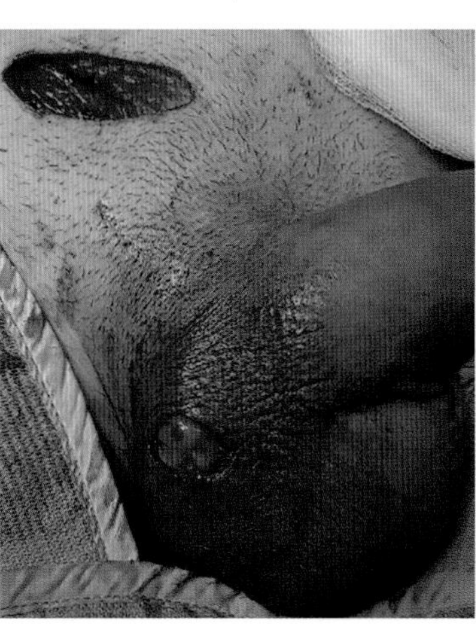

Figure 86.3 Adult undescended testis. The undescended inguinal testis is mobilised and retained in a pouch constructed between the dartos muscle and skin (courtesy of the author and Dr Mohamed Abdellatif).

localising all non-palpable testes. The cost and ionising radiation exposure associated with computed tomography (CT) scanning preclude its use. Magnetic resonance imaging (MRI) has been more widely used with greater sensitivity and specificity but has cost and availability issues, and may require anaesthesia in the paediatric population. At this time, there is no radiological test that can conclude with 100% accuracy that a testis is absent. Instead, laparoscopy has become the gold standard diagnostic method for a non-palpable testis. In addition, laparoscopy provides an option for treatment of this condition.

Summary box 86.2

Retractile testis

- Retractile testes should be differentiated from true undescended testes
- This is most easily done with the child relaxed in a warm room
- Retractile testes are more common than true undescended testes
- Retractile testes require no treatment but should be monitored

Medical treatment

There is little evidence currently for hormonal therapy to induce testicular descent, with low response rates (equivalent to placebo) and a lack of long-term efficacy.

Surgical treatment

Orchidopexy

Orchidopexy is usually performed between 6 and 18 months of age in an attempt to prevent the consequences described earlier. For premature babies, corrected age is used to determine surgery timing. The testis and spermatic cord are mobilised and the testis is repositioned in the scrotum. The operation is performed through a short incision over the deep inguinal ring. The inguinal canal is exposed by division of the external oblique aponeurosis in the direction of its fibres.

Three manoeuvres help to gain the length required to bring the testis down into the bottom of the scrotum. First, the patent processus vaginalis should be identified, separated and ligated. Second, the coverings of the spermatic cord (including the cremasteric muscle) should be divided and, third, lateral fibrous bands just inside the internal inguinal ring should be divided. Although these techniques are usually effective, the tiny vas and testicular vessels are vulnerable to injury. The empty hemiscrotum is stretched with a finger passed into it through the inguinal incision to give enough room for the testis, which is placed in a pouch constructed between the dartos muscle and the skin (*Figure 86.3*).

Orchidectomy should be considered if the incompletely descended testis is atrophic and/or there is a suspicion of malignancy, particularly in the postpubertal boy if the other testis is normal.

Impalpable testis

For non-palpable testes under anaesthesia, diagnostic laparoscopy is recommended. If a testis is found during laparoscopy, the options are:

1 Laparoscopic orchidopexy preserving the vessels: the testis is dissected off a triangular pedicle containing the testicular vessels and the vas.
2 Laparoscopic one-stage Fowler–Stephens orchidopexy: vessels are divided and the testis is dissected off a pedicle of the vas and brought down in one stage.
3 Laparoscopic two-stage Fowler–Stephens orchidopexy: vessels are divided with clips but dissection of the testis is postponed for 6 months to allow for optimal development of collaterals.

Robert Fowler Jr, b. 1928, paediatric surgeon, Royal Children's Hospital, Melbourne, Australia.
Frank Douglas Stephens, 1913–2011, paediatric surgeon, Royal Children's Hospital, Melbourne, Australia, published a landmark paper with Robert Fowler in 1959 that described the surgical management of high undescended testes by dividing the testicular vessels high from the testis to maintain a collateral blood supply.

If no testis is found during exploratory laparoscopy, one has to determine the presence of either blind-ending vessels or a testicular nubbin to completely rule out a missing testis. The vas can be dissociated from the testis and thus is not always a good guide to find the gonad.

If the internal ring is closed but vessels are going into it, a scrotal exploration usually will find a testicular nubbin. If vessels are going into an open inguinal ring, one can usually push the testis into the abdomen; if not, an inguinal or scrotal exploration would be warranted.

Absent testis

'Vanishing' testis describes a condition in which a testis develops but disappears before birth. The most likely cause for this is prenatal torsion. True agenesis of the testis is rarer. Laparoscopy is useful in distinguishing these causes of clinically absent testis from intra-abdominal maldescent.

TORSION OF THE TESTIS

Definition

Testicular torsion is the twisting of the spermatic cord and its contents such that the testicular blood supply becomes compromised. If left untreated the blood flow to the testicle ceases and the testicle dies. Testicular torsion is therefore a surgical emergency and the earlier the surgery to untwist the testis can be undertaken the better the outcome.

Incidence

Testicular torsion affects 3.8 per 100 000 males younger than 18 years annually. It accounts for 10–15% of acute scrotal disease in children.

Pathophysiology

Torsion of the testis is uncommon because the normal testis is anchored and cannot rotate. Extravaginal torsion is seen almost exclusively in neonates because of the increased mobility of the testicle before the descent into the scrotum when attached to the scrotal wall via the tunica vaginalis. Beyond this age, intravaginal torsion occurs as a result of a combination of:

- High investment of the tunica vaginalis, causing the testis to hang within the tunica like a clapper in a bell (*Figure 86.4*). This is the most common cause in adolescents and is typically a bilateral abnormality.
- Inversion of the testis: the testis is rotated so that it lies transversely or upside down.
- Separation of the epididymis from the body of the testis, permitting torsion of the testis on the pedicle that connects the testis with the epididymis (*Figure 86.4*).

Normally, when there is a contraction of the abdominal muscles, the cremaster contracts as well. In the presence of one of the abnormalities described above, the spiral attachment of the cremaster favours rotation of the testis around the vertical axis. Sudden contraction of the cremasteric muscle, which may be a response to mechanical, sexual or thermic stimulation, may cause a rotational effect on the testis as it is pulled upward. Accordingly, straining at stool, lifting of a heavy weight, sexual activity and sport can all precipitate an episode.

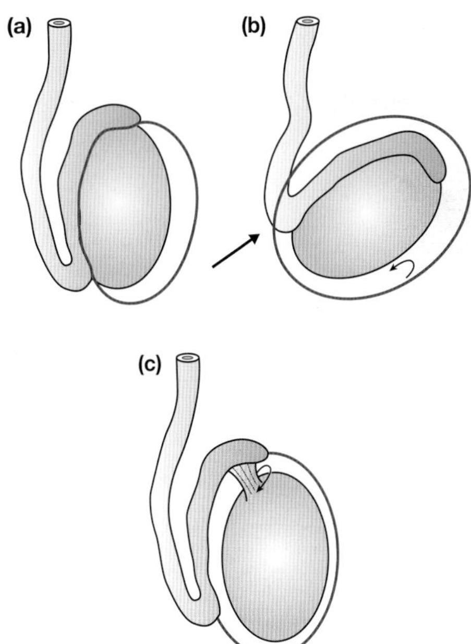

Figure 86.4 Testicular torsion. (a) Normal attachment. (b) An abnormally high attachment (arrow) of the tunica vaginalis predisposes to torsion – the 'bell-clapper'. (c) Separation of the testis from the epididymis – torsion about the pedicle between them.

The two main factors determining damage to the testis are the extent of the twist and the duration of the episode. Twists of 720° cause more rapid ischaemia than twists of 360° or less, and if the testis can be untwisted within 6 hours of the torsion taking place there is nearly a 100% chance of testicular salvage compared with a 20% salvage rate if the surgery is delayed for 24 hours.

Occasionally the testis untwists spontaneously without surgical treatment and 'intermittent' testicular torsion should be considered as a cause of testicular pain in adolescents.

Clinical features

Testicular torsion is most common between 10 and 25 years of age, although a few cases occur outside this age range. Typically there is sudden severe pain in the groin and the lower abdomen and the patient feels nauseated and may vomit. The scrotum is swollen and tender, while the skin is usually not erythematous initially (although it may become so with a prolonged history) and the patient is apyrexial. The testis itself is swollen and tender and seems high within the scrotum, while the tender twisted cord can often be palpated above it. The cremasteric reflex is lost.

Differential diagnosis

Skin redness and mild pyrexia may result in the condition being confused with epididymo-orchitis in the older patient; however,

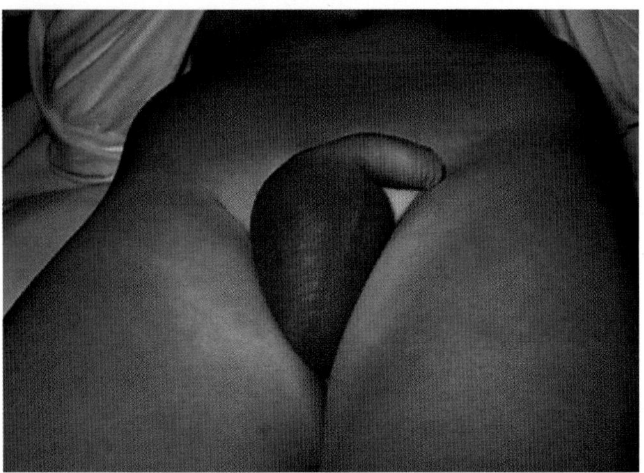

Figure 86.5 Idiopathic oedema of the scrotum.

there will usually be dysuria associated with an accompanying urinary infection. Elevation of the testis reduces the pain in epididymo-orchitis but makes it worse in torsion.

Torsion of a testicular appendage cannot always be distinguished with certainty from testicular torsion. The most common structure to twist is the appendix of the testis (the hydatid of Morgagni), which is sometimes visible through the scrotal wall as a small dark spot. If the diagnosis is made clinically, conservative management is possible; if in doubt, surgical exploration should be undertaken with removal of the twisted appendage.

In mumps orchitis, the cord is not particularly thickened and the condition is often bilateral.

Idiopathic scrotal oedema is an oddity that occurs between the age of 4 and 12 years and must be differentiated from torsion. The scrotum is very swollen but there is little pain or tenderness. The swelling is usually bilateral and may extend into the perineum, groin and penis. It is thought to be an allergic phenomenon and occasionally there is eosinophilia. The swelling subsides after a day or so but may recur (*Figure 86.5*).

Very occasionally, torsion can be convincingly mimicked by a small tense strangulated inguinal hernia compressing the cord and causing compression of the pampiniform plexus.

Management

The management of the case should be determined primarily on clinical grounds. While Doppler ultrasound scanning (*Figure 86.6*) can confirm the absence of the blood supply to the affected testis, false-positive results can be seen so it is not routinely recommended. If there is any doubt as to the diagnosis, then urgent scrotal exploration is indicated. The typical window of opportunity for surgical intervention and testicular salvage is 6 hours from onset of pain. Therefore, early urological surgery consultation upon presentation may be critical even in the absence of confirmatory testing.

Exploration for torsion can be performed through a transverse or midline scrotal incision. If the testis is viable when the cord is untwisted, it should be prevented from twisting again by fixation with three non-absorbable sutures between the tunica albuginea of the testis and the scrotal raphe. The use of absorbable sutures risks the possibility of recurrent torsion at some time in the future. The other testis should also be fixed because the anatomical predisposition is likely to be bilateral. If there is clinical doubt as to testicular viability after detorsion of the testis, then it should be wrapped in a warm swab and observed over a few minutes. If a small incision in the tunica albuginea demonstrates bright red arterial bleeding then the testis may survive. An infarcted testis should be removed – the patient can be counselled later about a prosthetic replacement.

In cases where there is a history of pain for several days, the affected testis will be dead. It is not possible to recover such a testis and, although little is gained (other than pain relief) by immediate exploration, it is necessary to fix the contralateral testis.

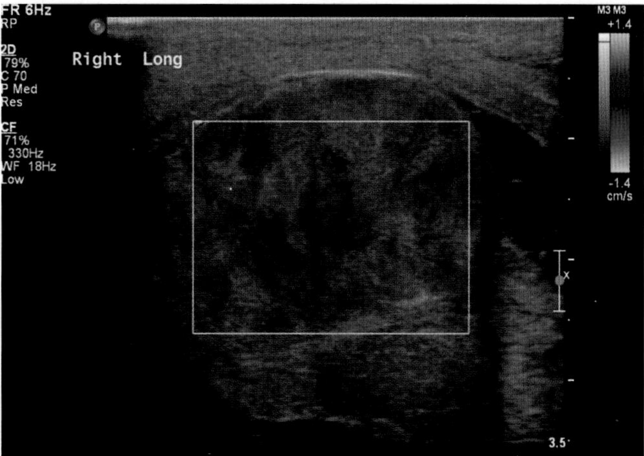

Figure 86.6 Doppler ultrasound scanning of a torted right testis showing the absence of blood flow and heterogeneous architecture indicating late necrosis (courtesy of Dr Davide Prezzi).

Summary box 86.3

Testicular torsion

- If the diagnosis of testicular torsion is possible, then surgical exploration is indicated
- Prompt exploration, untwisting and fixation is the only way to save the torted testis
- The patient should be counselled and consented for orchidectomy before exploration
- The anatomical abnormality is bilateral and the contralateral testis should also be fixed
- Non-absorbable sutures should be used for the fixation of each testis

Giovanni Battista Morgagni, 1682–1771, Professor of Anatomy, University of Padua, Padua, Italy, is associated with a number of eponymous structures, including the aortic sinus, the appendix testis, the anal columns and the sternocostal triangles. He is regarded as the 'father of morbid anatomy'.

Christian Johann Doppler, 1803–1853, Professor of Experimental Physics, Vienna, Austria, enunciated the 'Doppler principle' in 1842.

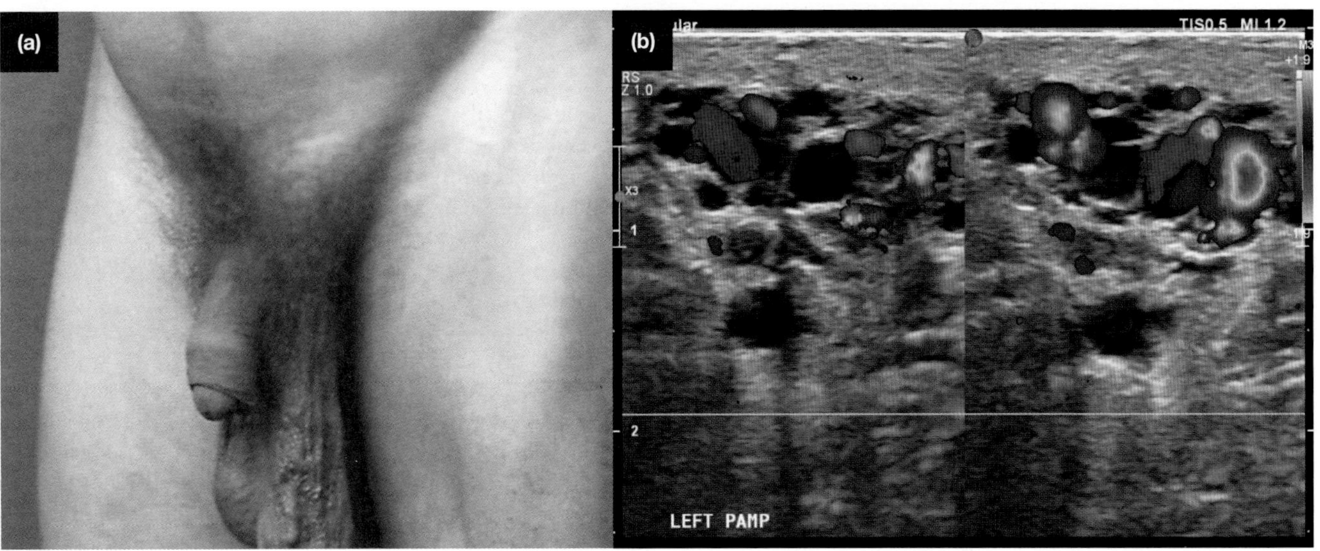

Figure 86.7 (a) Large varicocele in a pendulous scrotum. Note the left inguinal hernia. (b) Doppler ultrasound of a left varicocele (courtesy of Dr Davide Prezzi).

VARICOCELE

Definition

A varicocele is an abnormal dilatation and enlargement of the scrotal venous plexus draining the testis.

Incidence

Varicoceles are common, affecting 10–20% of adult males. About 90% are left sided, reflecting the proximal venous anatomy – the left testicular vein empties into the relatively high-pressure left renal vein while the right empties into the low-pressure inferior vena cava below the right renal vein. If a left varicocele is identified, there is a 30–40% probability that it is a bilateral condition.

They are unusual in boys and typically develop during late childhood and adolescence. Varicoceles occur in around 15–20% of all males but are found in about 40% of infertile males.

Pathophysiology

The veins draining the testis and the epididymis form the pampiniform plexus. The veins gradually join each other as they traverse the inguinal canal and at, or near, the inguinal ring there are only one or two testicular veins, which pass upwards within the retroperitoneum. The left testicular vein empties into the left renal vein while the right empties into the inferior vena cava below the right renal vein. There is an alternative (collateral) venous return from the testes through the cremasteric veins, which drain mainly into the inferior epigastric veins.

There are three theories as to the cause of varicoceles:

1 The absence or failure of the antireflux valve usually located where the testicular vein joins the left renal vein or the inferior vena cava on the right. This causes reflux and retrograde flow in the testicular vein.
2 The 'nutcracker' effect that occurs when the left testicular vein gets trapped between the superior mesenteric artery and the aorta. This causes venous compression and testicular vein obstruction.
3 Angulation at the junction of the left testicular vein and the left renal vein.

In some cases, the dilated vessels are cremasteric veins and not part of the pampiniform plexus. While most varicoceles are idiopathic, obstruction of the testicular vein by a renal tumour or nephrectomy is a cause of varicocele in later life; characteristically, in such cases the varicocele does not decompress in the supine position. The presence of an isolated right-sided varicocele is extremely rare. Hence, imaging should be considered to exclude a retroperitoneal mass in such cases. Rarer causes include deep vein thrombosis, renal arteriovenous malformations and thrombosis of the pampiniform plexus.

Clinical features

While most varicoceles are asymptomatic, those that are symptomatic tend to present in adolescence or early adulthood, when there may be a dragging discomfort that is worse on standing at the end of the day. When examined in the erect position, the scrotum on the affected side often hangs lower than normal (***Figure 86.7a***); on palpation, with the patient standing, the varicose plexus feels like a bag of worms. There may be a cough impulse. If the patient lies down the veins empty by gravity and this provides an opportunity to ensure that the underlying testis is normal to palpation. In longstanding cases the affected testis is smaller and softer than the opposite side owing to atrophy.

Ultrasound can be helpful in the diagnosis of small varicoceles (***Figure 86.7b***), and in the less common right/bilateral varicoceles (and older men with an apparently recent onset of varicocele), ultrasound of the kidneys is important in excluding a renal tumour.

The following classification of varicocele is useful in clinical practice:

- subclinical: not palpable or visible at rest or during a Valsalva manoeuvre, but can be shown by special tests (Doppler ultrasound studies);
- grade 1: palpable during Valsalva manoeuvre, but not otherwise;
- grade 2: palpable at rest, but not visible;
- grade 3: visible and palpable at rest.

Varicoceles and infertility

Varicoceles are present in 10–20% of adult men and in over 25% of men with abnormal semen analysis. The exact association between reduced male fertility and varicocele is unknown. The most accepted theory is that increased blood flow leads to higher intratesticular temperatures, which are the main cause of impaired sperm in varicoceles.

Large varicoceles may eventually cause testicular failure, ultimately resulting possibly in lower testosterone production, low sperm count and quality and testicular atrophy. Varicoceles can also decrease sperm nuclear DNA integrity, which has been linked to poor sperm motility, viability, counts and morphology.

A Cochrane review from 2012 concluded that there is some evidence to suggest that treatment of a varicocele in men from couples with otherwise unexplained subfertility may improve a couple's chance of spontaneous pregnancies. However, varicocele repair in men with a subclinical varicocele or normal semen parameters is considered ineffective for increasing the chances of spontaneous pregnancies. Varicocelectomy may also improve outcomes following assisted reproductive techniques in men with abnormal sperm parameters.

Treatment

Varicocele repair can be effective in men with a low sperm count, a clinical varicocele and otherwise unexplained infertility. However, treatment of varicocele in adolescents poses a risk of overtreatment: most boys with a varicocele will have no fertility problems later in life.

When the discomfort is significant, then percutaneous embolisation of the gonadal veins is the usual first-line intervention. If this is not possible, or if the varicocele recurs (as it does in around 20% after embolisation), surgical ligation of the testicular veins is the appropriate treatment, although recurrence can occur even after such surgery. Current evidence indicates that microsurgical varicocelectomy is the most effective method among the different surgical varicocelectomy techniques, with fewer complications and lower recurrence rates.

Summary box 86.4

Varicocele

- Varicocele is a common condition and 90% are left sided
- The presence of varicocele in some men is associated with progressive testicular damage from adolescence onwards and a consequent reduction in fertility
- Varicocele repair can be effective in men with a low sperm count, a clinical varicocele and otherwise unexplained infertility

HYDROCELE

Definition

A hydrocele is an abnormal collection of serous fluid in a part of the processus vaginalis, usually the tunica vaginalis around the testis and occasionally along the spermatic cord. Acquired hydroceles are primary or idiopathic, or secondary to epididymal or testicular disease.

Incidence

Hydroceles affect an estimated 1% of adult men. More than 80% of newborn boys have a patent processus vaginalis, but most close spontaneously within 18 months of age.

Pathophysiology

Embryologically, the processus vaginalis is a diverticulum of the peritoneal cavity. It descends with the testes into the scrotum via the inguinal canal around the 28th week of gestation with gradual closure through infancy and childhood.

Structurally, hydroceles are classified into three key types:

1. Communicating (congenital) hydrocele: a patent processus vaginalis permits flow of peritoneal fluid into the scrotum (tunica vaginalis); associated with indirect inguinal hernias (*Figure 86.8a*).
2. Non-communicating (vaginal) hydrocele: the processus vaginalis is closed with no communication with the peritoneal cavity. Instead, fluid accumulation can be due to excessive production and/or defective absorption by the tunica vaginalis, primarily because of disruption to the lymphatic drainage of scrotal structures (*Figure 86.8b*). If idiopathic, these are called 'primary' hydroceles.
3. The distal end of the processus vaginalis closes correctly, but the mid-portion of the processus remains patent. The proximal end may be open and communicating with the tunica vaginalis, resulting in an 'infantile' hydrocele' (*Figure 86.8c*), or closed, resulting in a hydrocele of the cord (*Figure 86.8d*).

Non-communicating primary hydroceles are the most common type of hydrocele globally. 'Secondary' hydroceles usually occur in men >40 years and may present acutely from local injury (including torsion), infection, neoplasm or radiotherapy. If a tumour is suspected, the hydrocele should not be punctured (risk of malignant needle-track implantation).

Antonio Maria Valsalva, 1666–1723, Italian physician and anatomist.

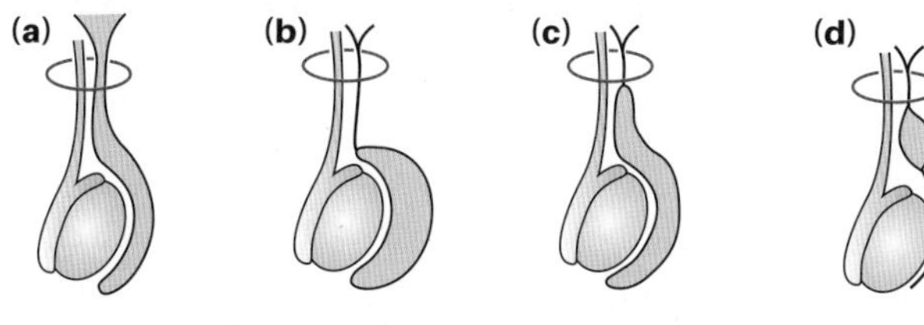

Figure 86.8 (a) Vaginal hydrocele (very common); (b) 'infantile' hydrocele; (c) congenital hydrocele; (d) hydrocele of the cord.

Clinical features

Examination of a scrotal swelling should be undertaken in both the upright and supine position. The examiner should ask:

1 Is it possible to get above the swelling to palpate a normal cord? If not the swelling may represent an inguinal hernia that has entered the scrotum.
2 Is the testicle or epididymis palpable or is the swelling enclosing both of those structures? A hydrocele encloses the testis and epididymis such that they may be impalpable, and it is possible to get 'above' it to palpate a normal spermatic cord.
3 Does the swelling transilluminate? Hydroceles are typically translucent.

In almost all cases of scrotal swelling an ultrasound is a useful adjunct to clarify the nature of the swelling and assess whether the testis itself is diseased.

A primary hydrocele (*Figure 86.9*) is seen most commonly in middle and later life, but can also occur in older children. Because the swelling is usually painless it may reach a significant size before the patient presents for treatment. Be wary of an acute hydrocele in a young man since there may be a testicular tumour.

In congenital hydrocele, the processus vaginalis – the communication with the peritoneal cavity – is usually too small to allow herniation of intra-abdominal contents. Pressure on the hydrocele does not always empty it but the hydrocele fluid may drain into the peritoneal cavity when the child is lying down; thus, the hydrocele may be intermittent. Ascites should be checked for if the swellings are bilateral.

A hydrocele of the cord is a smooth oval swelling that lies above the testis near the spermatic cord, which is liable to be mistaken for an inguinal hernia. The swelling moves downwards and becomes less mobile if the testis is pulled gently downwards. Hydrocele of the canal of Nuck is a similar condition in females. The cyst lies in relation to the round ligament and is always at least partially within the inguinal canal.

Treatment

Congenital hydroceles are treated by ligation of the patent processus vaginalis (herniotomy) if they do not resolve spontaneously.

Small hydroceles do not need treatment. If they are sizeable and bothersome for the patient, then surgical treatment is indicated. Established acquired hydroceles often have thick walls. There are three main surgical techniques for hydroceles:

1 **Plication**. Lord's operation is suitable when the sac is reasonably thin walled (*Figure 86.10*). There is minimal dissection and the risk of haematoma is reduced.
2 **Eversion**. The sac is opened and everted behind the testis, with placement of the testis in a pouch prepared by dissection in the fascial planes of the scrotum (Jaboulay's procedure) (*Figure 86.10*).

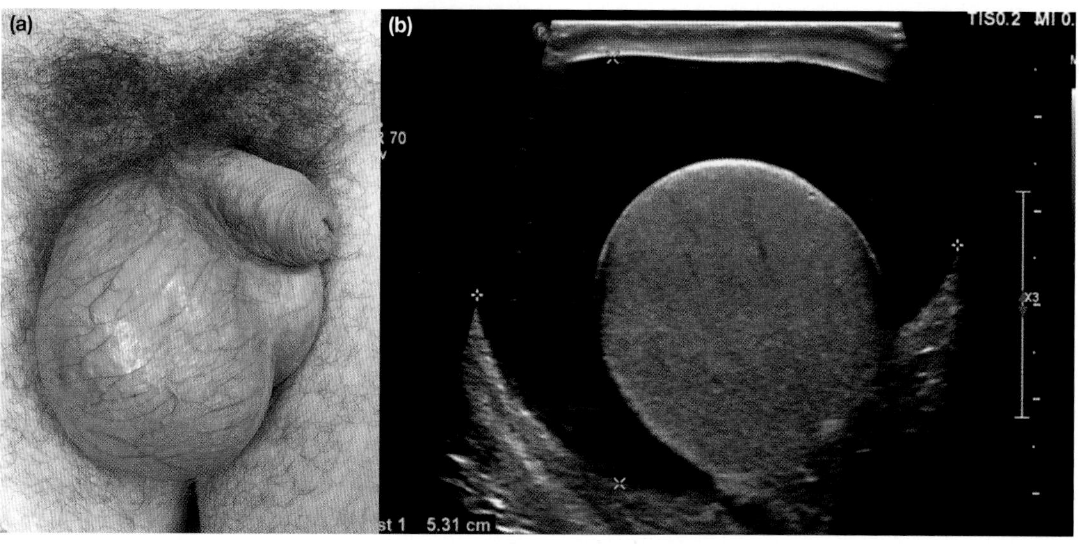

Figure 86.9 A right-sided hydrocele (a). Ultrasound image (b) (courtesy of Dr Davide Prezzi).

Anton Nuck, 1650–1692, Professor of Anatomy and Medicine, Leiden, The Netherlands.
Peter Herent Lord, contemporary, formerly surgeon, Wycombe General Hospital, High Wycombe, UK.
Mathieu Jaboulay, 1860–1913, Professor of Surgery, Lyons, France.

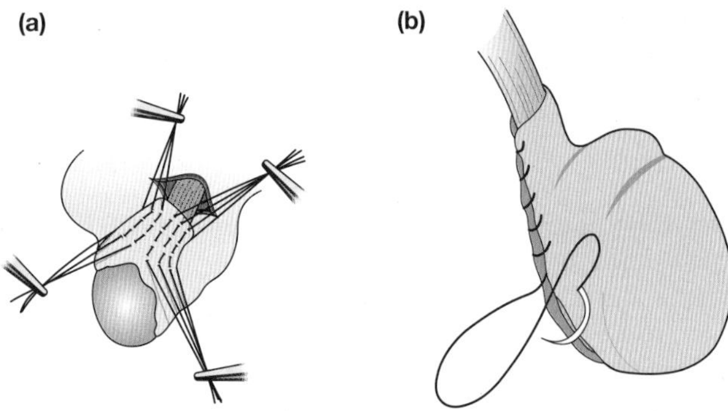

Figure 86.10 Lord's operation (a). A series of interrupted absorbable sutures is used to plicate the redundant tunica vaginalis. When these are tied, the tunica bunches at its attachment to the testis. Jaboulay's procedure (b). The hydrocele sac is everted and anchored with sutures. Unless great care is taken to stop bleeding after excision of the wall, haemorrhage from the cut edge is liable to cause a large scrotal haematoma. Overrunning stitches at the cut edge can be used to reduce this risk.

3 **Aspiration** of the hydrocele fluid is simple, but the fluid always reaccumulates within a week or so. It may be suitable for men who are unfit for scrotal surgery, although hydrocele surgery can be undertaken under local anaesthetic. Aspiration can result in bleeding into the hydrocele sac and haematocele formation. Injection of a sclerosant, such as tetracycline, can be effective but painful.

Summary box 86.5

Hydrocele

- A hydrocele is a collection of fluid within the tunica vaginalis
- Hydroceles surround the testis and transilluminate brightly
- Ultrasound examination is valuable, especially when the testis and epididymis are impalpable
- Hydroceles can be treated conservatively unless they are large and symptomatic
- Surgery is the mainstay of treatment
- Testicular malignancy is an uncommon cause of hydrocele that can be excluded by ultrasound examination

Filarial hydroceles and chyloceles

Filarial hydroceles and chyloceles account for up to 80% of hydroceles in tropical countries, where the parasite *Wuchereria bancrofti* is endemic. Filarial hydroceles follow repeated attacks of filarial epididymo-orchitis. Occasionally, the fluid contains liquid fat, which is rich in cholesterol. This is caused by rupture of a lymphatic varix with discharge of chyle into the hydrocele. In longstanding chyloceles, there are dense adhesions between the scrotum and its contents. Filarial elephantiasis supervenes in a small number of cases. Treatment is by rest and aspiration with chronic cases treated by excision of the sac.

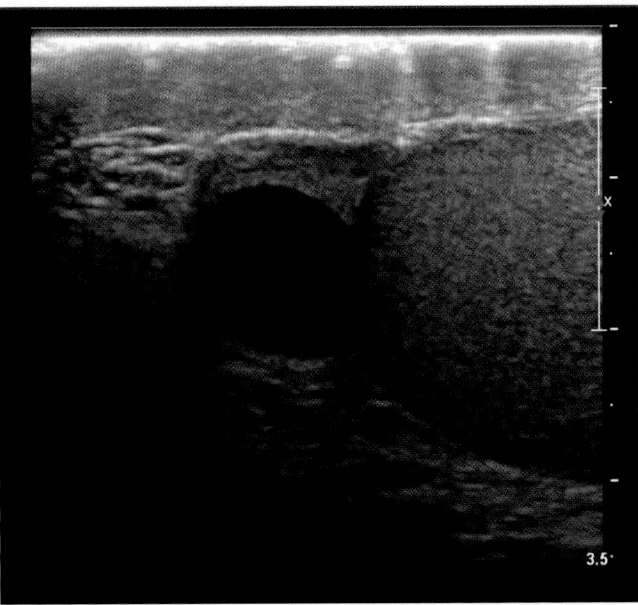

Figure 86.11 Ultrasound image of an epididymal cyst (courtesy of Dr Davide Prezzi).

CYSTS ASSOCIATED WITH THE EPIDIDYMIS

There are several types of cyst associated with the epididymis, including epididymal cysts and spermatoceles.

Epididymal cysts

These are filled with a clear fluid. They are very common, usually multiple and vary in size at presentation. They represent cystic degeneration of the epididymis. Cysts of the epididymis are usually found in middle age and are often bilateral. The clusters of tense cysts feel like tiny bunches of grapes that lie posterior to, and quite separate from, the testis. They should transilluminate. The diagnosis can by confirmed by ultrasound (*Figure 86.11*).

Aspiration is ineffective because the cysts are usually multilocular. If they are causing discomfort they should be excised. While single large cysts can be excised separately, recurrent or multilocular cysts usually require partial or total epididymectomy. Excision should be expected to interfere with the transportation of sperm from the testis on that side and young men should be counselled regarding this.

Spermatocele

This is a unilocular retention cyst derived from a portion of the sperm-conducting mechanism of the epididymis. A spermatocele typically lies in the epididymal head above and behind the upper pole of the testis. It is usually softer and laxer than other cystic lesions in the scrotum but, like them, it transilluminates. The fluid contains spermatozoa and resembles barley water in

Otto Eduard Heinrich Wucherer, 1820–1873, German physician who practised in Brazil.
Joseph Bancroft, 1836–1894, English physician working in Australia.

appearance. Spermatoceles are usually small. Small spermatoceles can be ignored. Larger ones can be excised.

Summary box 86.6

Cysts associated with the epididymis

- Lie posterior to and separate from the testis and they transilluminate
- Diagnosis can be confirmed by ultrasound examination
- Can be treated conservatively unless they are large or uncomfortable

INFECTIONS OF THE TESTIS AND EPIDIDYMIS

Epididymo-orchitis

Definition

Inflammation confined to the epididymis is epididymitis; if this inflammation, usually due to infection, involves the testis it is called epididymo-orchitis.

Incidence

Epididymitis, commonly preceding epididymo-orchitis, occurs in about 1 in 1000 men annually. Acute epididymitis most commonly occurs in men aged 20–59 years (43% in men aged 20–39 years and 29% in men aged 40–59 years). Childhood (prepubertal) epididymitis is rare; torsion is more common in this age group. Forty-seven per cent of prepubertal boys with epididymitis have associated urogenital abnormalities, including ectopic vas deferens or ureters, and urethral abnormalities.

Pathophysiology

Infection reaches the epididymis via the vas from a primary infection of the urethra, prostate or seminal vesicles. A general rule is that epididymitis arises in sexually active young men from a sexually transmitted genital infection, while in older men it more usually arises from a urinary infection or may be secondary to an indwelling urethral catheter.

In young sexually active men, the most common cause of epididymitis is now *Chlamydia trachomatis*, but gonococcal epididymitis is still occasionally seen. In older men with bladder outflow obstruction, epididymitis may result from a urinary infection – it is proposed that a high pressure in the prostatic urethra might cause reflux of infected urine up the vasa. Blood-borne infections of the epididymis are less common but may be suspected when there is epididymal infection without evidence of urinary infection; it is presumably the only possible mechanism in men who have previously undergone a vasectomy. Acute epididymo-orchitis can follow any form of urethral instrumentation and it is particularly common when an indwelling catheter is associated with infection of the prostate.

Infection usually starts in the tail of the epididymis and spreads to the rest of the epididymis and occasionally to the testis. Complications include abscess formation, testicular infarction, testicular atrophy, chronic induration and inflammation and infertility.

Clinical features

While there may be initial symptoms of a urinary or a genital infection, such symptoms are not always seen. The development of an ache in the groin and a fever can herald the onset of epididymitis. The epididymis and testis swell and become painful. The scrotal wall, at first red, oedematous and shiny, may become adherent to the epididymis.

Investigation should include a urethral swab, a urine specimen for culture, nucleic acid amplification testing (NAAT) of either a urine specimen or a urethral swab and scrotal ultrasound. Urinalysis will usually show leukocytes and may show a formal urinary tract infection. NAAT is a sensitive way of identifying both gonococcal and chlamydial urethritis. Ultrasound is useful in the initial assessment of epididymitis (*Figure 86.12*) and will identify abscess formation.

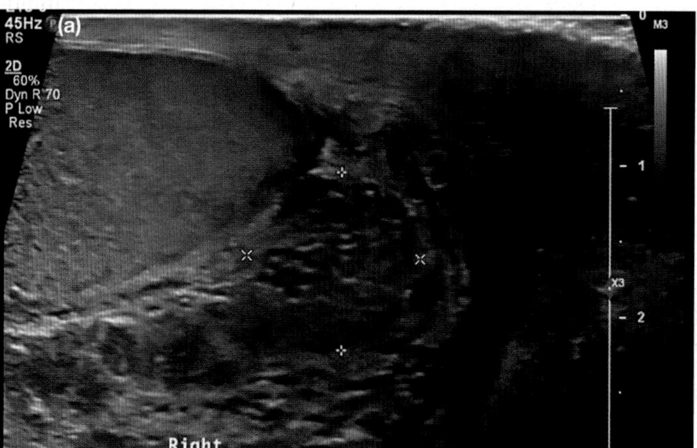

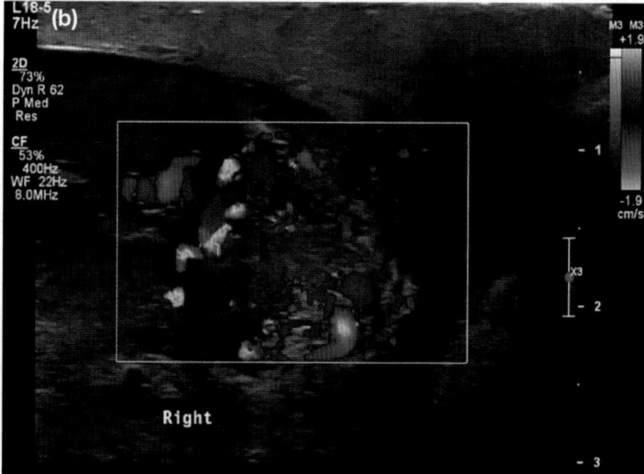

Figure 86.12 Ultrasound findings in epididymitis. Enlarged epididymis with a heterogeneous echotexture (grey-scale ultrasonography) (a) and increased blood flow (Doppler ultrasonography) (b) (courtesy of Dr Davide Prezzi).

In adolescents, the differential diagnosis is testicular torsion; if there is any clinical doubt as to the diagnosis then testicular exploration should always be performed.

Treatment

To prevent complications and transmission of sexually transmitted infections, presumptive therapy is indicated at the time of the visit before all laboratory test results are available.

Presumptive therapy is based on risk for chlamydia and gonorrhoea (usually younger men) and/or gut organisms (usually older men). The aims of treatment of acute epididymitis are (i) cure of infection, (ii) improvement of signs and symptoms, (iii) prevention of transmission of chlamydia and gonorrhoea to others, and (iv) a decrease in potential epididymitis complications (e.g. infertility and chronic pain). Local sensitivities do change with increasing antibiotic resistance. Examples of regimens are shown below from the 2021 Sexually Transmitted Infections Treatment Guidelines from the US Centers for Disease Control and Prevention (https://www.cdc.gov/std/treatment-guidelines/STI-Guidelines-2021.pdf).

- For acute epididymitis most likely caused by sexually transmitted chlamydia and gonorrhoea:
  - Ceftriaxone intramuscularly (IM) single dose and oral doxycycline for 10 days.
- For acute epididymitis most likely caused by sexually transmitted and enteric organisms (men who practise insertive anal sex):
  - Ceftriaxone IM single dose and levofloxacin for 10 days.
- For acute epididymitis most likely caused by enteric organisms:
  - Levofloxacin for 10 days.
- There should be contact tracing of the partner and treatment if necessary.

In older men, quinolones are the usual initial treatment; however, if there is evidence of systemic sepsis, intravenous antibiotics may be valuable. If an organism is isolated from the urine, this simplifies the choice of antibiotic.

Local measures including scrotal support and analgesia are helpful. Oral antibiotic treatment should continue for at least 10 days or until the inflammation has subsided. If abscess formation occurs, drainage is necessary.

Chronic disease

Chronic non-tuberculous epididymitis usually follows the failure of resolution of an acute episode of epididymitis. Patients typically complain of intermittent episodes of discomfort and the epididymis feels thickened and tender. Treatment involves use of antibiotics (usually quinolones or doxycycline) and anti-inflammatory agents for 4–6 weeks. Epididymectomy or orchidectomy can be considered if there is no resolution, although up to 50% of patients continue to have pain despite such surgery.

Summary box 86.7

Acute epididymo-orchitis

- In young men usually arises secondary to a sexually transmitted genital infection
- In older men usually arises secondary to urinary infection
- May be a complication of catheterisation or instrumentation of the urinary tract
- May need aggressive treatment with parenteral antibiotics

Tuberculous epididymo-orchitis

Chronic tuberculous epididymo-orchitis usually begins insidiously. The frequency with which the lower pole of the epididymis is involved first indicates that the infection is usually retrograde from a tuberculous focus in the seminal vesicles.

Clinical features

Typically, there is a firm, uncomfortable discrete swelling of the lower pole of the epididymis. The disease progresses until the whole epididymis is firm and craggy behind a normal-feeling testis. There is a lax secondary hydrocele in 30% of cases, and a characteristic beading of the vas may be apparent as a result of subepithelial tubercles. The seminal vesicles feel indurated and swollen. In neglected cases, a tuberculous 'cold' abscess forms, which may discharge. The body of the testis may be uninvolved for years but the contralateral epididymis often becomes diseased. In two-thirds of cases there is evidence of renal tuberculosis or previous disease. Otherwise, patients typically appear healthy.

The urine and semen should be examined repeatedly for tubercle bacilli in all patients with chronic epididymo-orchitis. Imaging of the chest and upper urinary tract should be performed. Ultrasound will demonstrate a thickened epididymis.

Treatment

Secondary tuberculous epididymitis may resolve when the primary focus is treated. Treatment with antituberculous drugs is less effective in genital tuberculosis than in urinary tuberculosis. If resolution does not occur within 2 months, epididymectomy or orchidectomy is advisable. A course of antituberculous chemotherapy should be completed even if there is no evidence of disease elsewhere.

Other common forms of orchitis

Mumps orchitis, which is the most common form of orchitis, develops in 20–30% of postpubertal patients with a mumps virus infection and it usually develops as the parotid swelling is waning. Evidence of immunoglobulin M antibodies in the serum supports the diagnosis. The main complication is testicular atrophy, which may cause infertility if the condition is bilateral. Partial testicular atrophy is associated with persistent testicular pain.

Syphilitic orchitis is now uncommon. It can cause bilateral orchitis (which is a feature of congenital syphilis), interstitial fibrosis (which causes painless destruction of the testis) or, rarely, a gumma of the testis (which presents as a unilateral slowly growing painless swelling). The last presentation may be difficult to distinguish from a neoplasm without surgical exploration. Diagnosis is confirmed by serology.

TUMOURS OF THE TESTES

Incidence

Testicular cancer represents around 1–1.5% of male neoplasms and there is clear evidence of an increased incidence of these tumours in the past 30 years with 3–10 new cases per 100 000 males/per year in western societies. The predominant histology is germ cell tumours (GCTs) (90–95% of cases). The peak incidence of seminomas is in the fourth decade of life, with the non-seminomatous germ cell tumours (NSGCT) being more common in the third decade of life. They are the commonest form of tumour in young men. A specific genetic marker – an isochromosome of the short arm of chromosome 12 (i12p) – is pathognomonic of all types of adult GCTs as well as germ cell neoplasia *in situ* (GCNIS). Epidemiological risk factors include cryptorchidism, male factor infertility (including Klinefelter syndrome), familial history of testicular tumours among first-grade relatives and the presence of a contralateral tumour or GCNIS.

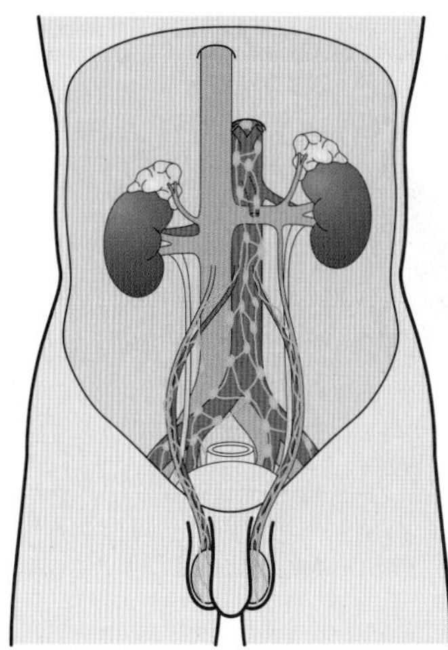

Figure 86.14 Lymphatic drainage of the testes to para-aortic lymph nodes.

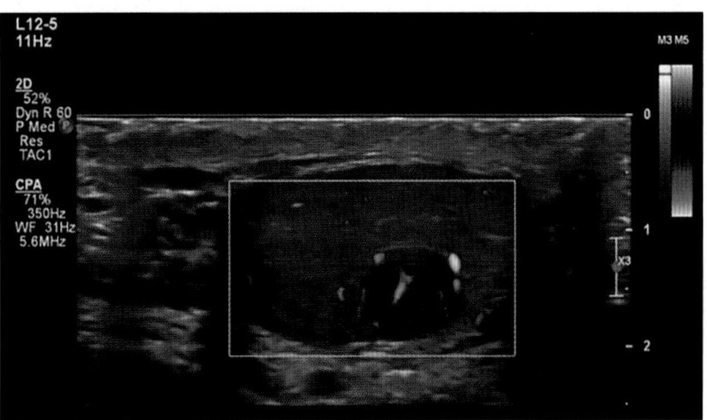

Figure 86.15 Ultrasound of a small seminoma with minimal distortion of the tunica albuginea (courtesy of Dr Davide Prezzi).

Classification and pathology

Tumours of the testis are classified according to their predominant cellular type:

- **GCTs** (90–95%): these include seminoma, embryonal cell carcinoma, yolk sac tumour, teratoma and choriocarcinoma;
- **sex cord–stromal tumours** (1–2%): these include Leydig cell tumours;
- **lymphoma** (3–7%);
- **other tumours** (1–2%).

Seminoma

A seminoma typically has a cut surface that is homogeneous and pinkish cream in colour. It appears to compress neighbouring testicular tissue (***Figure 86.13***). It consists of oval cells with clear cytoplasm and large, rounded nuclei with prominent acidophilic nucleoli. Sheets of cells resembling spermatocytes are separated by a fine fibrous stroma. Active lymphocytic infiltration of the tumour suggests a good host response and a better prognosis. Seminoma accounts for 50% of all testicular germinal cell tumours. They seldom occur in childhood, in young adults or in patients over 70 years of age.

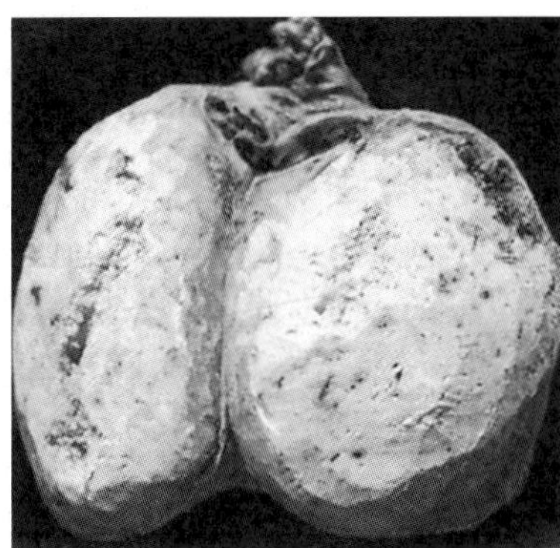

Figure 86.13 Seminoma of the testis.

Seminomas metastasise mainly via the lymphatics (***Figure 86.14***) and haematogenous spread is uncommon. The lymphatic drainage of the testes is to the para-aortic lymph nodes near the origin of the gonadal vessels. The contralateral para-aortic lymph nodes are sometimes involved by tumour spread, but the inguinal lymph nodes are affected only if the scrotal skin is involved. Ultrasound is the first-line investigation (***Figure 86.15***).

Non-seminomatous germ cell tumours

There are a number of histological types of NSGCT, which may coexist within a single tumour:

- **Embryonal carcinoma** (***Figure 86.16***). Highly malignant tumours that occasionally invade cord structures.
- **Yolk sac tumour**. Usually present with a loose stroma and a component similar to embryonal carcinoma, sometimes with liver and intestinal tissue differentiation. It appears as a single tumour type in children and part of a

Harry Fitch Klinefelter Jr, 1912–1990, physician of Baltimore, MD, USA, described this syndrome in 1942.

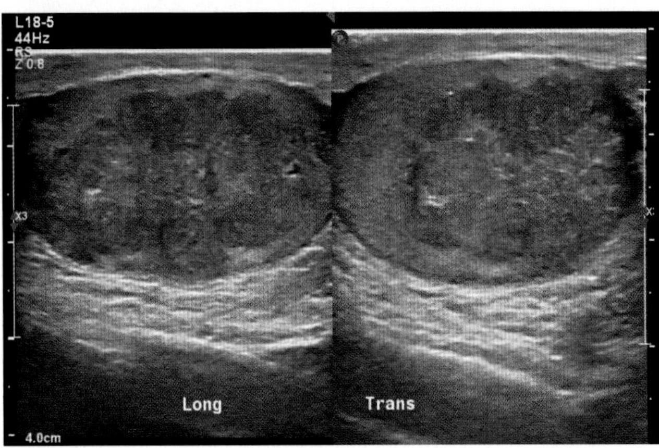

Figure 86.16 Ultrasound of a large embryonal carcinoma occupying nearly the whole testis; long, longitudinal view; trans, transverse view (courtesy of Dr Davide Prezzi).

mixed tumour in adults. They produce alpha-fetoprotein (AFP), which can be measured in serum.

- **Teratoma** (*Figure 86.17*). Teratomas consist of different tissues derived from ectoderm, endoderm and mesoderm. Immature components are often neuroectodermal or mesenchymal tissue, while more mature tissue is often cystic with epithelial differentiation or consists of smooth muscle, connective tissue or cartilage. Since most teratomas consist of a mixture of tissues, the old separation into mature and immature types has been abandoned. All can metastasise.
- **Choriocarcinoma**. This is part of a testicular GCT in 25% of tumours in adults. It very seldom appears as the single tumour component. Choriocarcinoma is almost never seen in childhood. This tumour produces human chorionic gonadotropin (HCG), which can be detected in blood. This is a highly malignant tumour that metastasises early via both the lymphatics and the bloodstream.

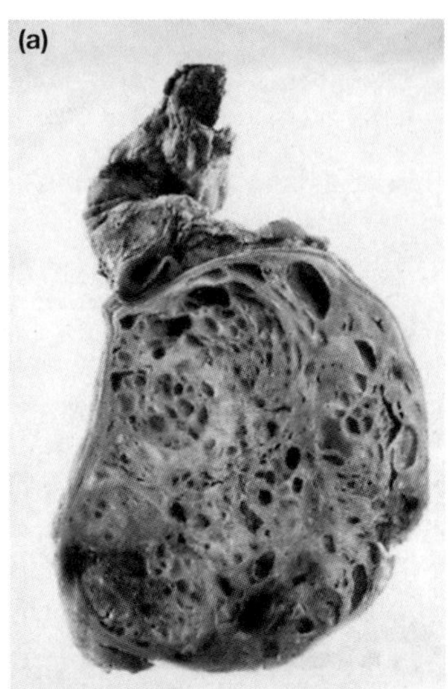

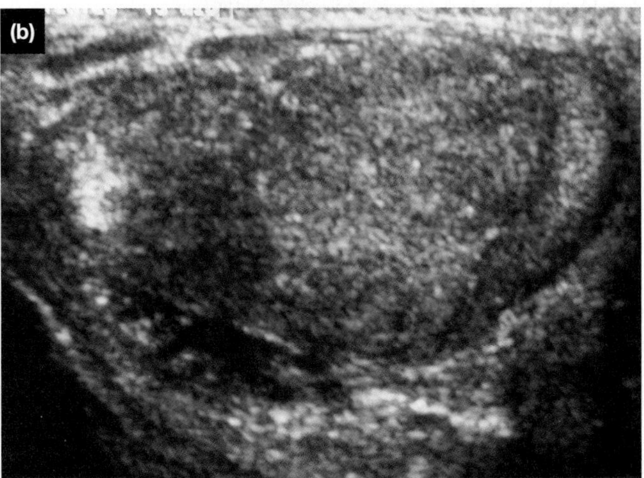

Figure 86.17 Teratoma of the testis specimen (a). Note the solid and cystic areas (courtesy of Dr Keith Simpson, London, UK). Testicular ultrasound (b). The homogeneous tissue of the testicular teratoma on the left of the image produces multiple ultrasound reflections.

Spermatocytic seminoma

This tumour was earlier believed to be a variant of seminoma, but is now considered to be a separate tumour type, accounting for 1–2% of all GCTs of the testis. Only seen in adult men usually >50 years old, they rarely metastasise; therefore, an orchidectomy is the only necessary treatment, even in large tumours. Development of sarcomas has been reported when left untreated for long time.

Sex cord-stromal tumours

Sex cord–stromal tumours are rare and constitute less than 5% of testicular neoplasms.

Leydig cell tumour

Leydig cell tumours are the most common type of sex cord–stromal tumours, constituting 1–3% of adult testicular tumours and 3% of testicular tumours in infants and children. These tumours occur in about 8% of patients with Klinefelter's syndrome. They are well delineated on histology and usually up to 5 cm in diameter. They are solid, yellow to tan in colour with haemorrhage and/or necrosis in 30% of cases. Most of these tumours are benign. Malignant transformation occurs in 10% and is related to increased size (>5 cm), increased cellular atypia, increased cell proliferation, necrosis, vessel invasion and DNA aneuploidy.

Sertoli cell tumour

Sertoli cell tumours account for less than 1% of testicular tumours, and the mean age at diagnosis is around 45 years, with sporadic cases under 20 years of age. Rarely, these occur in patients with androgen insensitivity syndrome and Peutz–Jeghers syndrome. The rate of malignancy ranges between 10% and 22%.

John Law Augustine Peutz, 1886–1968, Chief Specialist for Internal Medicine, St John's Hospital, The Hague, The Netherlands.
Harold Joseph Jeghers, 1904–1990, Professor of Internal Medicine, New Jersey College of Medicine and Dentistry, Jersey City, NJ, USA.

Granulosa cell tumour

Granulosa cell tumours of the testis are extremely rare in adult men, but a juvenile type accounts for 6% of testis tumours in childhood.

Mixed germ cell/sex cord tumour: gonadoblastoma

This tumour consists of two cell types: large germinal cell-like seminoma cells and small granulosa-like or Sertoli cells or rarely Leydig/luteinised cells. Gonadoblastoma is seen in individuals with mixed gonadal dysgenesis (risk 15–25%), which is associated with cryptorchidism, hypospadias, gynaecomastia or female internal genitalia. It seldom occurs in phenotypical and genotypical males.

Clinical features

Usually the patient presents with a painless testicular lump. A sensation of heaviness can occur if large, but few patients experience pain. Occasionally, an episode of trauma calls attention to the swelling. Some cases may simulate epididymo-orchitis and, rarely, acute painful enlargement of the testis occurs because of haemorrhage into the tumour, which can mimic testicular torsion.

Rarely, the predominant symptoms are those of metastatic disease. Intra-abdominal disease may cause abdominal or lumbar pain. Lung metastases are usually silent, but they can cause chest pain, dyspnoea and haemoptysis in the later stages of the disease. The primary tumour may not have been noticed by the patient, and indeed may be detected only by ultrasound (*Figure 86.15*).

On examination there is an intratesticular solid mass. A secondary hydrocele may be present. The epididymis can become more difficult to feel. Around 5% of cases have gynaecomastia (mainly NSGCT). Metastatic disease is rarely apparent clinically and is more usually identified by formal staging investigations. In 1–2% of cases the tumour is bilateral at diagnosis.

Investigation and staging

The diagnosis is confirmed by ultrasound scanning of the testis (*Figure 86.16*), which is also able to assess the contralateral testis. It is a mandatory test in all suspected cases of testicular tumour.

In confirmed cases, staging is an essential step in planning treatment. Blood is taken prior to orchidectomy to measure the levels of tumour markers, which are raised in around 50% of cases. A rise in AFP is seen in around 50–70% of NSGCTs and a rise in HCG is seen in 40–60% of NSGCTs and around 30% of seminomas. Lactate dehydrogenase (LDH) is expressed on chromosome 12p, which is often amplified in testis cancer cells. LDH is less specific for testis cancer than HCG or AFP. However, elevated LDH levels are associated with high tumour burden in seminoma and recurrence in NSGCT.

When raised, these markers are used to monitor the response to treatment. The mean serum half-lives of AFP and HCG are 5–7 days and 2–3 days, respectively, and reassessment of the markers following orchidectomy can indicate whether all the tumour tissue has been removed.

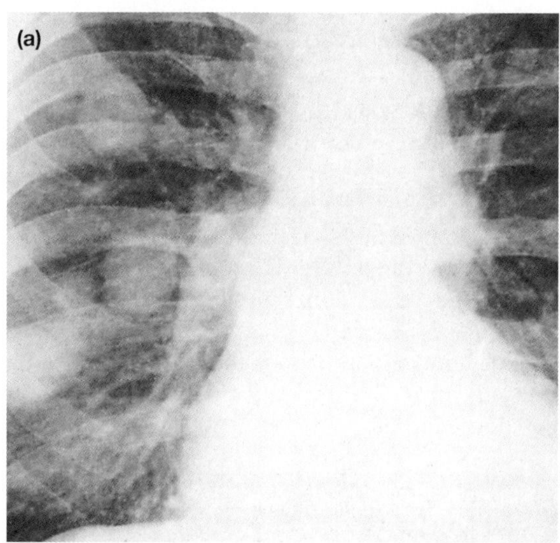

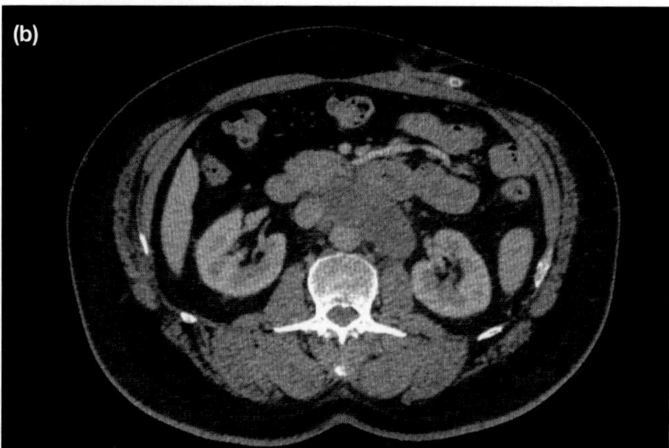

Figure 86.18 (a) Chest radiograph showing cannonball metastases from carcinoma of the testis and (b) computed tomography showing large para-aortic lymph node metastasis from carcinoma of the testis resulting in retroperitoneal mass (courtesy of Dr Davide Prezzi).

While a chest radiograph can show the 'classical' cannonball metastases (*Figure 86.18a*) CT scanning of the chest, abdomen and pelvis has taken over as the most useful means of detecting metastases and monitoring the response to therapy (*Figure 86.18b*).

Summary box 86.8

Testicular tumours

- A solid testicular lump that cannot be felt separately from the testis may be a malignant tumour
- Lymphatic spread is to the para-aortic lymph nodes
- Ultrasound is a mandatory investigation in all cases of suspected testicular tumour
- Tumour markers (AFP, HCG and LDH) should be measured prior to orchidectomy

Treatment

Men should be offered semen analysis and sperm banking prior to interventions such as surgery and chemotherapy that may render them infertile.

Surgery: radical orchidectomy

The orchidectomy is undertaken via an inguinal incision. The spermatic cord is displayed by dividing the external oblique aponeurosis and a soft clamp is placed across the cord to stop dissemination of malignant cells as the testis is mobilised into the wound. If there is a tumour the cord should be double transfixed and divided at the level of the internal inguinal ring and the testis removed.

Management by staging and histological diagnosis (after orchidectomy)

The treatment of patients with GCTs of the testis is usually successful, even in advanced cases. This largely reflects the excellent response of these tumours to chemotherapy and (for seminomatous tumours) to radiotherapy. Prognostic groups can be defined according to non-metastatic (stage I) and metastatic disease (lymph node metastasis – stage II; distant metastasis or nodal metastasis with elevated tumour markers – stage III). (The exact classification details can be found in the *TNM Classification of Malignant Tumours*, 8th edn; see **Further reading**.) Between 75% and 80% of patients with seminoma and about 55–64% of patients with NSGCT have stage I disease at diagnosis.

The management strategies below are adapted from the European Association of Urology's current guidelines.

Non-metastatic disease (stage I)

Seminoma. About 15% of patients with clinical stage I (CSI) seminoma have subclinical metastatic disease, usually in the retroperitoneum, and will relapse after orchidectomy alone.

Surveillance. Recurrence rates of 6% have been described in patients with low-risk features, including tumours size <4 cm and no stromal rete testis invasion with cancer-specific survival rate reported with surveillance at >95%. The main limitation of surveillance is the need for intensive follow-up.

Adjuvant chemotherapy. One course of adjuvant carboplatin therapy compared with radiotherapy shows no significant difference in recurrence rate, time to recurrence and survival after a median follow-up of 4 years.

Adjuvant radiotherapy. Seminomas are radiosensitive. Radiotherapy to a para-aortic field or to para-aortic and ipsilateral iliac nodes reduces the relapse rate to 1–3%. The rate of severe radiation toxicity is <2%. The main concern is the long-term risk of secondary malignancies.

NSGCT. Up to 50% of patients with NSGCT with CSI disease have subclinical metastases and will relapse during surveillance.

- *Surveillance.* 14–48% of CSI-NSGCT patients undergoing surveillance have recurrence within 2 years of orchidectomy. Careful surveillance can be an option for compliant, risk-stratified (based on the presence of lymphovascular invasion) patients who are well informed about the expected recurrence rate as well as the salvage treatment.
- *Adjuvant chemotherapy*. One cycle of bleomycin–etoposide–cisplatin (BEP) is now the recommended strategy with recurrence rates of around 3%. The very long-term side effects, particularly cardiovascular, remain to be ascertained.
- *Retroperitoneal lymph node dissection (RPLND).* The role of this surgery has now decreased with 2-year recurrence-free survival with adjuvant BEP × 1 versus RPLND favouring chemotherapy with recurrence-free survival of 99.5% versus 91%.

Metastatic disease (stages II and III)

Treatment for metastatic testicular cancer is chemotherapy. Previously, radiotherapy was often used for early stage II seminoma but the cardiovascular and second malignancy risks have led to chemotherapy (three cycles of BEP or four cycles of etoposide and cisplatin [EP]) being the preferred alternative. Both are similarly effective, with a trend towards greater efficacy for chemotherapy in stage IIB seminoma. The initial treatment is chemotherapy (BEP) in all advanced cases of NSGCT except postpubertal teratoma without elevated tumour markers, which can be managed by RPLND surgery.

Sex cord-stromal tumours

Most of these tumours are benign (around 80%), so conservative treatment of small lesions with organ-sparing surgery is feasible, if the diagnosis is considered. For larger tumours, orchidectomy is necessary with multimodality treatment for those with the rare malignant forms of these tumours.

Summary box 86.9

Testis tumour staging and treatment

- Tumour markers (AFP, HCG and LDH) help to make the diagnosis and to follow the response to treatment
- CT scanning of chest, abdomen and pelvis is central to the staging of testicular tumours
- Testicular tumours are extremely sensitive to platinum-based chemotherapy
- Prognosis is excellent when the patient is treated with combination chemotherapy in a cancer centre

Testicular tumours in children

Paediatric testicular tumours are distinct from adult testicular tumours. GCTs in adults represent about 95% of all testicular tumours but only 60–75% in children. The most common malignant tumour in children is the yolk sac tumour, which is very rare in its pure form in adults. Surgical treatment usually begins with radical orchidectomy, which is often recommended whenever the AFP level is elevated (suggesting the presence of a yolk sac tumour at age >1 year). A normal AFP level in children suggests a strong likelihood of a benign tumour. For such tumours, as in cases of epidermoid cysts, testis-sparing surgery of the mass rather than radical orchidectomy can be considered.

TUMOURS OF THE EPIDIDYMIS

Paratesticular tumours are rare and account for about 5% of all intrascrotal tumours. Between 70% and 80% of all these tumours are benign and 30% of these occur in the epididymis. Epididymis tumours are commonly soft tissue or mesothelial neoplasm in origin. Benign cystadenomas, papillary tumours and adenomatoid tumours are the most common, although malignant sarcoma or secondary metastasis from a carcinoma may also occur. They are extremely rare.

THE SCROTUM

Fournier's gangrene

Fournier's gangrene is an uncommon and nasty condition (*Figure 86.19*) characterised by a polymicrobial infection of the soft tissues of the perineum, external genitalia and perianal region. It is a form of necrotising fasciitis. There is rapid onset of gangrene leading to exposure of the scrotal contents. Although it can occur in conjunction with sepsis of the testis, epididymis or perianal region, an obvious cause is absent in over half the cases. It can arise following minor injuries or procedures in the perineal area, such as a bruise, scratch, urethral dilatation, injection of haemorrhoids or opening of a periurethral abscess. Many patients have concurrent illnesses that diminish their defences, most notably diabetes mellitus and alcoholism.

There is a mixed infection of aerobic and anaerobic bacteria in a fulminating inflammation of the subcutaneous tissues, which results in an obliterative arteritis of the arterioles to the scrotal skin that in turn results in gangrene. The condition can spread rapidly to involve the fascia and skin of the penis, perineum and abdominal wall.

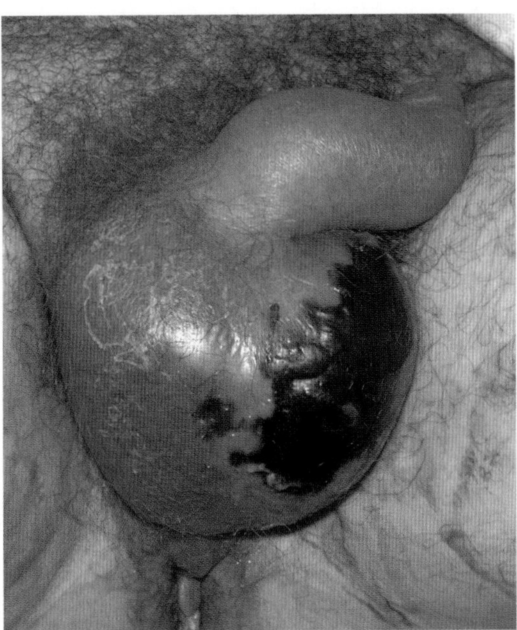

Figure 86.19 Fournier's gangrene with an area of necrotic skin overlying an area of scrotal inflammation.

Clinical features

The hallmark of Fournier's gangrene is intense pain and tenderness in the genitalia. The clinical course usually progresses through the following phases:

1. prodromal symptoms of fever and lethargy for 2–7 days;
2. intense genital pain usually associated with oedema of the overlying skin; pruritus may be present;
3. increasing genital pain with progressive erythema of the overlying skin;
4. dusky appearance of the overlying skin; subcutaneous crepitation;
5. obvious gangrene of part of the genitalia; purulent discharge from wounds.

Early on, pain may be out of proportion to the physical findings. As gangrene develops, pain may subside as nerve tissue becomes necrotic. Systemic effects of this process vary from local tenderness to massive septic shock, with the greater the necrosis the more severe the systemic effects.

Treatment

Treatment of a case of Fournier's gangrene is a surgical emergency. Initial management involves intravenous fluid resuscitation and broad-spectrum intravenous antibiotics. Urgent wide surgical excision of the dead and infected tissue is essential and the extent of the internal necrosis is typically much greater than the external appearances suggest, with extensive debridement often necessary. Urinary and faecal diversion may be necessary. Supportive care is essential because patients often become severely septic.

Early review of the wounds is helpful to confirm that all dead tissue has been removed; when the infection has been controlled, vacuum-assisted dressing is helpful, if it is available. If the patient survives the acute episode, skin grafting is often necessary. Despite best therapy, mortality rates as high as 50% are often reported.

Summary box 86.10

Fournier's gangrene

- Fournier's gangrene requires early and aggressive treatment if the patient is to survive
- Treatment involves urgent surgical debridement of necrotic tissue in combination with early use of intravenous broad-spectrum antibiotics

Jean Alfred Fournier, 1832–1915, syphilologist, founder of the Venereal and Dermatological Clinic, Hôpital St Louis, Paris, France.

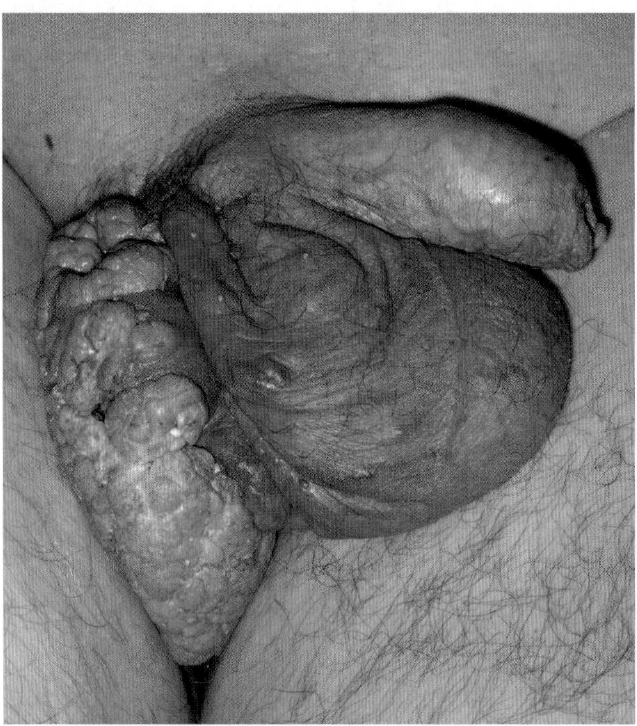

Figure 86.20 Scrotal cancer.

Carcinoma of the scrotum

'Chimney sweep's cancer' was the first reported occupational cancer (described by Percival Pott in 1775). It is a rare cancer that has also been seen in other workers who come into contact with oil and coal products. Animal studies suggest that aromatic cyclic hydrocarbons are the aetiological factor. Nowadays, this tumour is rarely associated with any obvious aetiological factor.

The growth starts as a wart or ulcer (*Figure 86.20*); as it grows it may involve the testis. The tumour should be excised with a margin of healthy skin. The management of the inguinal nodes parallels the management of penile cancer, and nodal assessment, either with sentinel node biopsies or bilateral groin dissections, is indicated.

TRAUMA TO THE TESTIS

The testis can be damaged either by blunt or by penetrating trauma. Injuries can range from simple bruising, through significant intratesticular haematomas to rupture of the tunica albuginea, with very significant collections of blood within the tunica vaginalis (haematocele) (*Figure 86.21*). If the tunica ruptures, the blood can track into the groin and perineum.

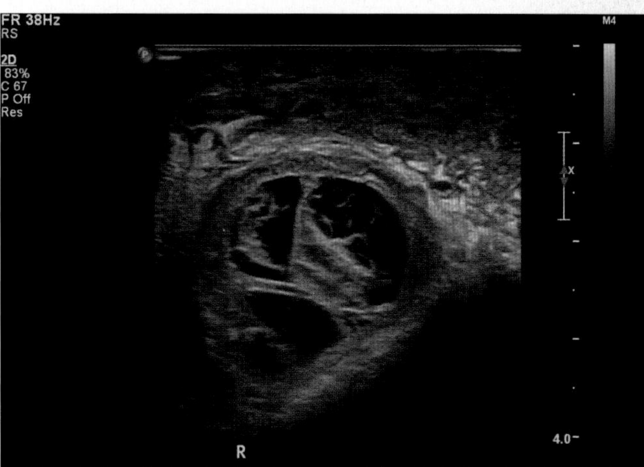

Figure 86.21 Ultrasound of a ruptured testicle with a haematocele (courtesy of Dr Davide Prezzi).

Careful clinical assessment, together with the use of ultrasound examination, is central to the management of men with a scrotal injury. Ultrasound has excellent sensitivity and specificity in the diagnosis of testicular rupture. If there is testicular rupture, there is good evidence that early surgical exploration, with debridement and repair of the tunica albuginea, is more likely to preserve useful testicular function. Also, early intervention results in orchidectomy in less than 10% compared with the 50% rate in delayed surgery.

Summary box 86.11

Scrotal trauma

- In cases of scrotal trauma, surgical exploration is indicated when there is testicular rupture or when there is a rapidly expanding scrotal haematoma
- Ultrasound is important in the assessment of the injury

FURTHER READING

Brierley JD, Gospodarowicz MK, Wittekind C (eds). *TNM classification of malignant tumours*, 8th edn. Oxford: Wiley Blackwell/Union for International Cancer Control, 2017.

Laguna MP, Albers P, Algaba F *et al. EAU guidelines on testicular cancer*. Arnhem, The Netherlands: EAU Guidelines Office, 2020. Available from https://uroweb.org/wp-content/uploads/EAU-Guidelines-on-Testicular-Cancer-2020.pdf.

Percival Pott, 1714–1788, surgeon, St Bartholomew's Hospital, London, UK, described chimney sweep's cancer of the scrotum in 1775. In those days the chimney sweep's apprentice climbed up inside the chimney.

CHAPTER 87 Gynaecology

Learning objectives

To understand:

- Pelvic anatomy
- Early pregnancy complications (ectopic pregnancy)
- Common causes of an acute abdomen and chronic abdominal pain
- Causes of abnormal uterine bleeding in the non-pregnant state
- Surgical management of endometriosis, adenomyosis, uterine fibroids, uterovaginal prolapse and ovarian tumours

ANATOMY

The reproductive structures of the dividing embryo differentiate after the seventh week of development. The gonads and internal and external genitalia constitute the sex organs. In the female, the Müllerian ducts develop into the uterus, fallopian tubes, cervix and upper third of the vagina. The urogenital sinus in turn forms the lower two-thirds of the vagina.

The female external genitalia are described as the vulva, which is bordered by the mons pubis anteriorly and the labiocrural folds posterolaterally. The opposing skin that covers the introitus is known as the labia majora. The labia minora are folds of skin that fuse anteriorly around the clitoris, which contains erectile tissue similar to the penis in the male. The posterior part of the introitus is referred to as the fourchette and this stretches considerably during childbirth to allow delivery of the baby.

The vagina is an elastic, distensible tube, approximately 6–7 cm long, passing upwards and backwards from the introitus. The cervix protrudes into the vault of the vagina, dividing it into the anterior, posterior and lateral fornices. Pelvic structures can be felt in the posterior and lateral fornices on bimanual examination, as the vaginal vault sits just below the pouch of Douglas (the area at the bottom of the pelvic cavity bordered by the uterus anteriorly and rectum posteriorly). The urethra and bladder neck sit above the anterior wall of the vagina; the perineal body and rectum behind the posterior wall (*Figure 87.1*).

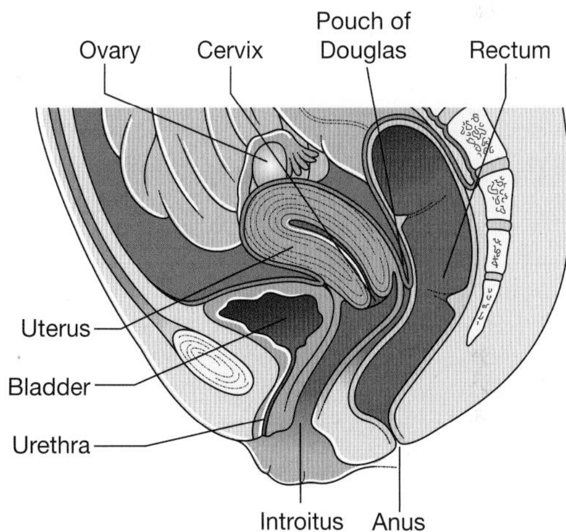

Figure 87.1 Female anatomy.

The uterus consists of a body and a cervix (neck of the uterus) and is an upside-down pear-shaped structure that is flattened anteroposteriorly, giving its cavity a flat, triangular shape. The uterus is supported partly by ligaments attached to the cervix (transverse cervical, pubocervical and uterosacral) that consist of condensed connective tissue. The cervix is a canal, approximately 2–3 cm long in the non-pregnant woman, connecting the external os, which can be seen on speculum examination, to the internal os, where the cervix enters the uterine cavity. The uterine cavity to cervical length ratio varies through hormonal influences and developmental phases, with the uterine body increasing in size as puberty progresses.

The cervical canal is located within the centre of the bony cavity of the pelvis, with the uterus pivoted around this point. It is more commonly angled forwards (anteverted) relative to the vagina. It is usually freely mobile, with filling of the bladder

Johannes Peter Müller, 1801–1858, Professor of Anatomy and Physiology, Berlin, Germany, described the paramesonephric duct in 1825.

James Douglas, 1675–1742, anatomist, midwife and physician to Queen Caroline, London, UK, helped expose the fraudulent claims of Mary Toft, who, in 1726, famously tricked a number of doctors into believing that she had given birth to rabbits.

Gabriele Falloppio (Fallopius), 1523–1563, Professor of Anatomy, Surgery and Botany, Padua, Italy. He carried out what may have been the first clinical trial in over 1000 men of the use of condoms to prevent transmission of syphilis.

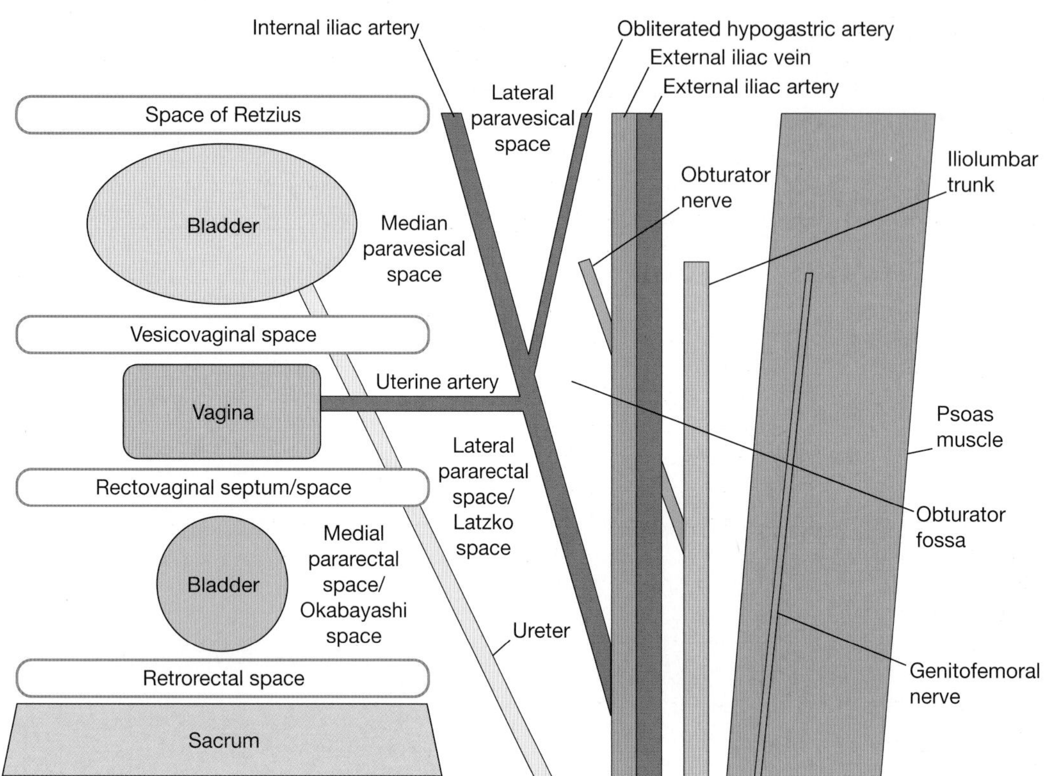

Figure 87.2 Surgical anatomy of the pelvis, including the key surgical spaces, vessels and nerves in relation to the pelvic organs (illustrative representation of anatomical spaces by PR Supramaniam).

or changes in position rotating it backwards. In others, it can be retroverted, a variation of normal, or secondary to weak ligaments or because it becomes adherent as the result of a disease process such as endometriosis. The uterus may also be angled forwards (anteflexed) relative to the cervix or backwards (retroflexed), which can be determined through bimanual examination.

The uterine walls are 1–2 cm thick and composed of smooth muscular tissue (myometrium). The uterine cavity is lined with endometrium, a tissue that undergoes cyclical changes in response to ovarian hormones. The endometrium has both a basal and functional layer. The basal layer lies adjacent to the myometrium and from it develops the functional layer. The basal layer is not shed during menstruation, unlike the functional layer. The functional layer is influenced by oestrogen and progesterone, which thicken it, preparing the lining for implantation. This layer is completely shed during menstruation should conception not occur.

In the lean patient, the uterine size can be estimated on palpation. This is usually a subjective assessment outside of imaging modalities. The most common cause of an enlarged uterus, apart from pregnancy, is fibroids (benign tumours of the myometrium) growing inside or outside of the uterus. In the presence of fibroids or other conditions causing enlargement of the uterus, the uterine size is often described in terms of the number of weeks' gestation it approximates to, were the woman pregnant.

At the uterine fundus, on either side, are the cornua, which connect the uterus to the fallopian tubes. These are thin, muscular tubes, approximately 10 cm long. They are divided into four parts: intramural, isthmus, ampulla and the fimbriated opening, which picks up the oocyte following its release at the time of ovulation. The tubes are very narrow in the isthmic and intramural parts but widen at the ampullary region. Each tube is contained within the upper part of the broad ligament, a fold of peritoneum on either side of the uterus, which also contains blood vessels as well as the round and ovarian ligaments. The fimbriated opening and part of the ampulla, however, are free and closely associated with the ovary on either side. The ovaries are flattened, ovoid structures, approximately 3–4 cm in dimension, suspended from the back of the broad ligament on either side of the pelvic side wall by the ovarian ligament, which originates from the uterine body. The ovarian blood vessels are contained within the infundibulopelvic ligaments, which are continuations of the broad ligament to the pelvic brim on either side.

A sound understanding of pelvic anatomy is key to surgical excellence and safety (***Figure 87.2***).

The sacral promontory is considered a crucial landmark and the summit of the pelvis. While pelvic pathology may reach into the abdominal cavity, the origin is always below the sacral promontory. The sacrum is a bony prominence that is used as a point of reference in surgery and in surgical anatomy. The sacral promontory is the level at which the common iliac vessels bifurcate into the external and internal iliac vessels, and the level at which the ureter transverses from the lateral to medial side. Another key structure at this level is the superior hypogastric nerve plexus (autonomic nerve plexus), which is formed from the convergence of the right and left hypogastric nerves.

The aorta bifurcates at the level of the L4 vertebral body, where it forms the right and left common iliac vessels. The common iliac vessel then further bifurcates as described above at the level of the sacral promontory. The external iliac artery mainly supplies the lower limbs and has one anterior branch known as the inferior epigastric artery. Note should be made of the position of this artery when determining placement of lateral ports during laparoscopy, to avoid vascular injury. The internal iliac artery divides further into the anterior and posterior divisions. The anterior division is the main blood supply to the vital organs of the pelvis. The posterior division mainly supplies the gluteal region. The anterior division travels parallel to the ureter and gives off its first branch, the uterine artery, followed by the superior vesical artery, and continues as the obliterated umbilical artery. There is often a 5- to 6-cm distance from the origin of the anterior division prior to the first branch. This is often the level at which surgeons perform internal iliac artery ligation to manage cases of massive haemorrhage during obstetric surgery and prophylactically in pelvic exenteration surgery.

The pelvic structures are supplied by the autonomic nervous system. The inferior hypogastric nerve (T10–L2) provides sympathetic fibres and the pelvic splanchnic nerve provides parasympathetic fibres. These fibres merge to supply both the ureter and urinary bladder and can often be injured in complex pelvic surgery, leading to complications of residual bladder dysfunction and sexual dysfunction.

Pelvic spaces have recently featured in surgical anatomy as a key learning point to aid surgeons in performing safe surgery. The retroperitoneal spaces are divided into those that are present bilaterally (pararectal and paravesical spaces) and those that are present in the midline (space of Retzius, rectovaginal space and the retrorectal space). The pararectal space is bound medially by the rectum and laterally by the internal iliac artery. The posterior leaf of the broad ligament forms the roof and the levator ani muscle forms the floor. Cranially, the space is bordered by the uterine artery. The pararectal space is further divided into medial and lateral spaces by the ureter, with the medial pararectal space also known as the Okabayashi space and the lateral pararectal space called the Latzko space.

The paravesical space is a retroperitoneal space that is lateral to the urinary bladder. Medially it is bound by the urinary bladder, laterally by the pelvic walls and inferiorly by the uterine artery. The paravesical space is further divided into medial and lateral spaces by the obliterated hypogastric artery. The floor of the medial paravesical space is formed by the levator ani muscle. The obturator and pelvic lymph nodes are contained in the lateral paravesical space, important during a radical hysterectomy, and the limit of dissection is bounded by the posterior limit of the obturator nerve.

The space of Retzius is the midline retroperitoneal space between the bladder and the anterior abdominal wall. It is connected to the paravesical space and is enclosed laterally by the obliterated hypogastric artery. This space is often used in urogynaecological procedures as the bladder neck is exposed, aiding surgery performed for incontinence. It is also used in deep endometriosis surgery during management of bladder nodules to aid in tension-free closure of the cystotomy.

The rectovaginal space refers to the posterior retroperitoneal space that is formed by the uterus anteriorly and the rectum posteriorly. The lateral borders of this space are provided by the uterosacral ligament. This space is often explored to aid in radical hysterectomy and deep endometriosis surgery.

The retrorectal space is a retroperitoneal space that is bound by the rectum anteriorly. It is often explored in complex pelvic surgery and deep endometriosis surgery associated with excision of the rectum. The presacral vein that lies posterior to Waldeyer's fascia is often an area of concern because, if not carefully dissected, it can lead to severe uncontrollable haemorrhage.

EARLY PREGNANCY COMPLICATIONS

Ectopic pregnancy

An ectopic pregnancy refers to a pregnancy that grows outside of the uterine cavity, most commonly within the fallopian tube. To facilitate management of an ectopic pregnancy it is important to be able to describe the location of the pregnancy as accurately as possible. The newly agreed terminology broadly divides ectopic pregnancies into uterine (defined by evidence of trophoblast invasion beyond the endometrial–myometrial junction, but not outside the uterine visceral/broad ligament peritoneum) and extrauterine ectopic pregnancies (***Table 87.1***). They are further described as being complete (solely confined to the myometrium) or partial (involving both the myometrium and the uterine cavity).

Additional variations include rudimentary horn pregnancies. These are rare, with a reported incidence of 1 in 75 000–150 000 pregnancies. They are able to develop into the second trimester if not diagnosed early through the identification of a single interstitial portion of the fallopian tube attached to the main unicornuate uterine body, with products of conception completely surrounded by myometrium, presenting with severe pain and uterine rupture.

A residual ectopic pregnancy refers to an ectopic pregnancy that remains visible on ultrasound scan 3 months after a negative urinary pregnancy test and serum beta-human chorionic gonadotropin (βHCG) level of <20 IU/L.

As the ectopic pregnancy grows, the placental tissue can infiltrate the blood vessels surrounding the fallopian tube, leading to bleeding within the tube and into the peritoneal cavity. Further growth of the ectopic pregnancy can rupture the fallopian tube, causing significant intraperitoneal blood

Anders Retzius, 1796–1860, Swedish anatomist.
Hidekazu Okabayashi, 1884–1953, Japanese gynaecologist, demonstrated the first nerve-sparing radical hysterectomy in Kyoto Imperial University Hospital, Kyoto, Japan, 1921.
Wilhelm Latzko, 1863–1945, Austrian gynaecologist, described a technique for vaginal closure of vesicovaginal fistula following a hysterectomy, 1914.
Heinrich Wilhelm Gottfried Waldeyer-Hartz, 1836–1921, Professor of Pathological Anatomy, Berlin, Germany.

TABLE 87.1 Examples of uterine and extrauterine ectopic pregnancies.

Uterine ectopic pregnancies	Extrauterine ectopic pregnancies
• Cervical (the gestational sac is present below the level of the internal os with absence of the 'sliding sign' and evidence of blood flow around the gestational sac using colour Doppler) • Caesarean scar (the gestational sac is located low in the uterus, close to the internal os with trophoblast invading into the anterior myometrium) (*Figure 87.3*) • Intramural (located above the level of the internal os)	• Tubal (*Figure 87.4*) (further divided into interstitial [*Figure 87.5*], isthmic and ampullary) • Ovarian (colour Doppler can help identify an area of increased vascularity within the ovary that is representative of peritrophoblastic blood flow separate from that of the corpus luteum) (*Figure 87.6*) • Abdominal (commonly the broad ligament, pouch of Douglas, uterovesical pouch and surfaces of the tubes and uterus)

loss. This constitutes a gynaecological emergency. An ectopic pregnancy occurs in 11 per 1000 pregnancies, and there is a maternal mortality rate of 0.2 per 1000 estimated ectopic pregnancies. The major risk factors for an ectopic pregnancy are shown in *Summary box 87.1*.

Summary box 87.1

Risk factors for an ectopic pregnancy

- Previous pelvic inflammatory disease (PID)
- Smoking
- History of infertility
- Use of an intrauterine contraceptive device (IUCD)
- Previous ectopic pregnancy
- Previous abdominal/pelvic surgery, e.g. myomectomy, hysteroscopic resection
- Previous tubal surgery, e.g. sterilisation, salpingostomy, tuboplasty
- Endometriosis

An ectopic pregnancy may be suspected on clinical grounds, but making the diagnosis can be difficult (*Table 87.2*).

TABLE 87.2 Symptoms and signs of an ectopic pregnancy.

Symptoms	Signs
• Abdominal or pelvic pain • Amenorrhoea or missed period • Vaginal bleeding • Breast tenderness • Gastrointestinal symptoms • Dizziness, fainting, syncope • Shoulder tip pain • Rectal pressure or pain on defecation • Asymptomatic	• Pelvic, abdominal and/or adnexal tenderness or fullness • Signs of peritonism • Pallor • Abdominal distension • Cervical motion tenderness (pain on moving the cervix) • Enlarged uterus • Tachycardia, hypotension • Shock, collapse • Orthostatic hypotension

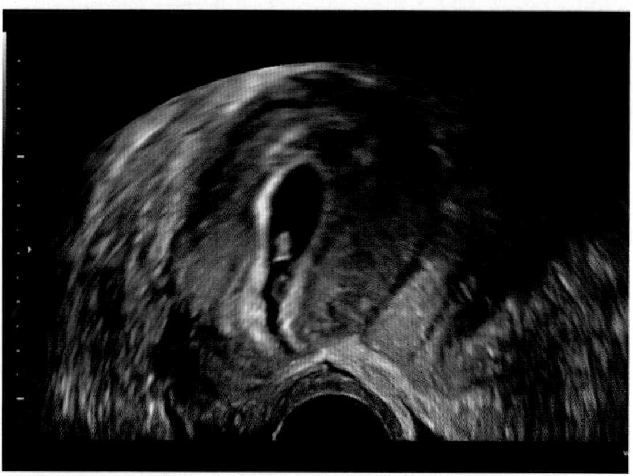

Figure 87.3 Ultrasound image of a caesarean scar ectopic pregnancy.

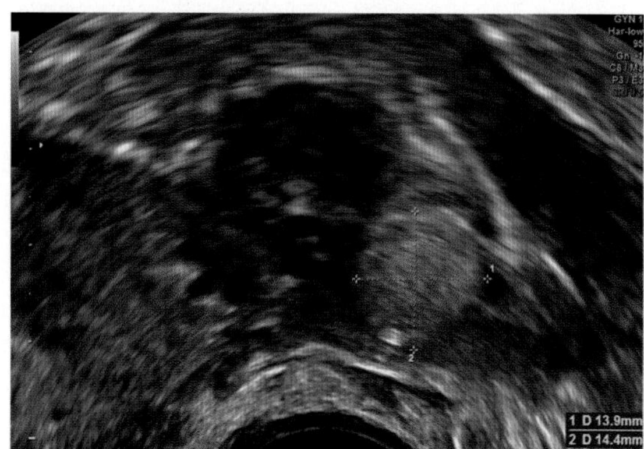

Figure 87.4 Ultrasound image of a tubal ectopic pregnancy.

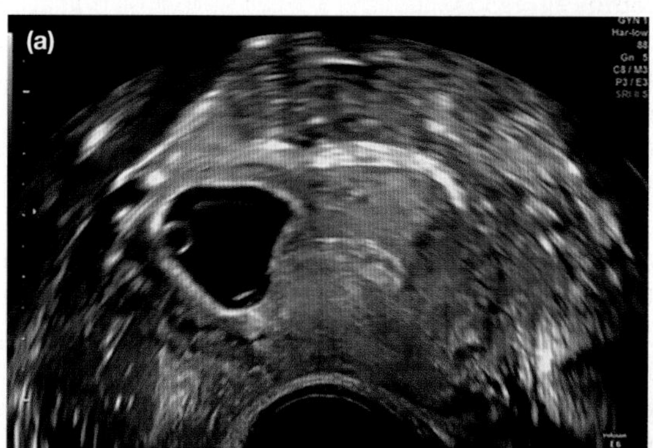

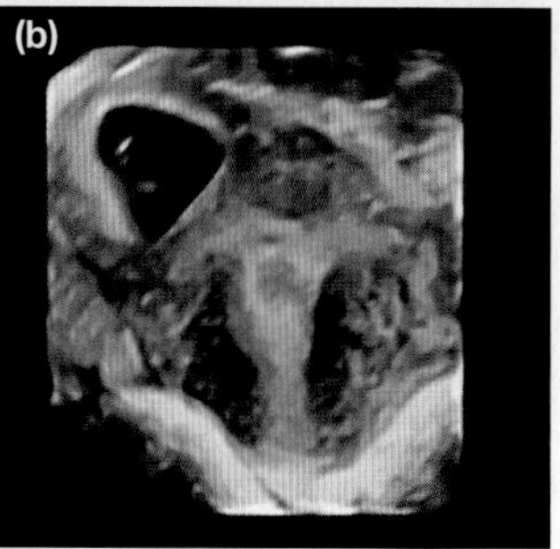

Figure 87.5 (a, b) Ultrasound images of an interstitial ectopic pregnancy.

Christian Johann Doppler, 1803–1853, Professor of Experimental Physics, Vienna, Austria, enunciated the 'Doppler principle' in 1842.

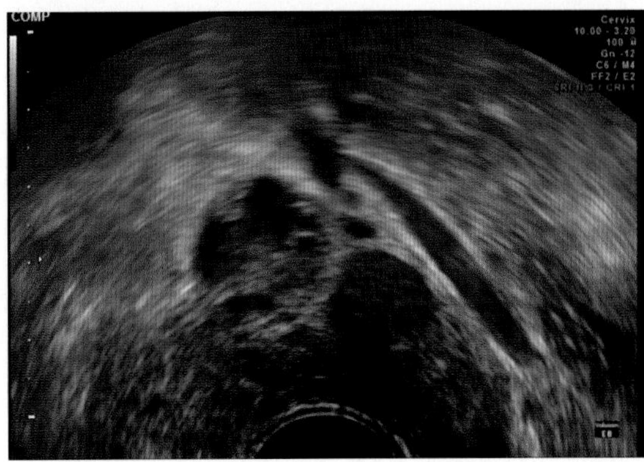

Figure 87.6 Ultrasound image of an ovarian ectopic pregnancy.

The presentation of an ectopic pregnancy is variable and the differential diagnoses include:

- miscarriage;
- urinary tract infection;
- ovarian cyst accident;
- appendicitis.

A transvaginal ultrasound scan should be performed if the diagnosis is suspected (see *Table 87.1* for the defining ultrasound characteristics of uterine and extrauterine ectopic pregnancies). The complete absence of an intrauterine gestational sac with a positive pregnancy test increases the probability of an ectopic pregnancy unless the pregnancy is not sufficiently advanced for the sac to be seen on ultrasound scan. An ectopic pregnancy is more likely if free fluid is seen in the pouch of Douglas or an adnexal mass is identified on ultrasound scan.

In equivocal cases, serial measurements of serum βHCG levels, 48 hours apart, can help to establish the diagnosis. A rise in the βHCG level by at least 63% is more indicative of a viable intrauterine pregnancy and an ultrasound scan should be offered between 7 and 14 days. Levels that halve when taken 48 hours apart are more suggestive of a failing pregnancy and a urinary pregnancy test should be repeated after 14 days. Levels that remain static or show a suboptimal increase or decrease over a 48-hour period are more likely to be representative of an ectopic pregnancy. Furthermore, a single level above approximately 1500 IU/L, in association with an empty uterus on ultrasound scan, in the absence of a heavy bleed, is suggestive of an ectopic pregnancy. Laparoscopy can also be used as a diagnostic tool (*Figure 87.7*); occasionally, however, a false-negative diagnosis is obtained when the pregnancy is not sufficiently advanced and is, therefore, too small to be seen within the fallopian tube.

Management of an ectopic pregnancy can be divided into expectant, medical (methotrexate) or surgical treatment. The choice of treatment is dependent on: the haemodynamic stability of the patient; ultrasound features of the ectopic pregnancy (presence of free fluid, presence or absence of fetal cardiac activity); serum βHCG level; and the patient's understanding of the diagnosis, commitment to follow-up and choice.

Expectant management and medical management in the form of methotrexate can be offered to women who are clinically stable and pain free, who have a serum βHCG level

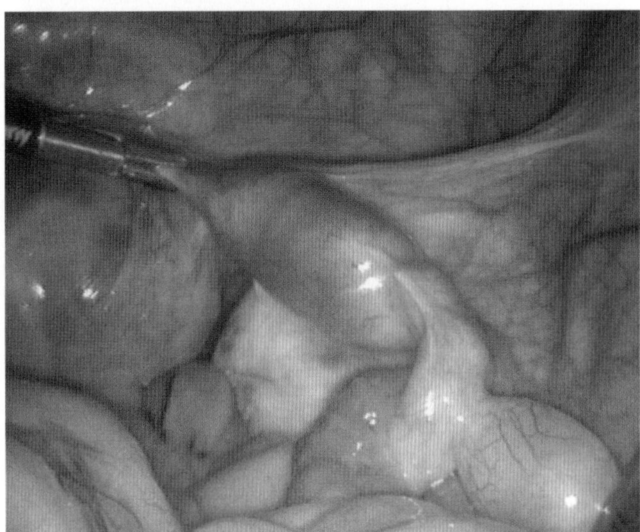

Figure 87.7 Laparoscopic image of a tubal ectopic pregnancy.

<1500 IU/L for expectant management and between 1500 and <5000 IU/L for medical management, who are committed to the follow-up protocol and where the ectopic pregnancy is not alive and measures <35 mm. In these circumstances, repeat serum βHCG levels are recommended on days 4 and 7. A fall of ≥15% is considered reassuring and should be repeated weekly thereafter until <20 IU/L. If the levels deviate from this, then the patient should be reviewed further to plan ongoing management. Women should be advised of the risk of rupture and the need for additional/alternative treatment if the situation should change.

Methotrexate is a folic acid antagonist that interferes with DNA synthesis. Significant side effects include hepatotoxicity. Further pregnancies should be avoided for a minimum of 3 months following treatment with methotrexate. Careful patient selection is vital. Furthermore, some patients fail to respond to this medication and will require surgical management.

Surgical management should be offered to women who prefer to have surgery or those who are unable to commit to follow-up as well as those with significant pain, those who have a rising serum βHCG level of ≥5000 IU/L and/or those in whom the ectopic pregnancy is considered to be live and measures ≥35 mm.

Surgical options include a salpingectomy (removal of the fallopian tube) or salpingostomy (opening of the fallopian tube and extraction of the pregnancy tissue) (*Figure 87.8*). This is ideally performed laparoscopically in a stable patient as it

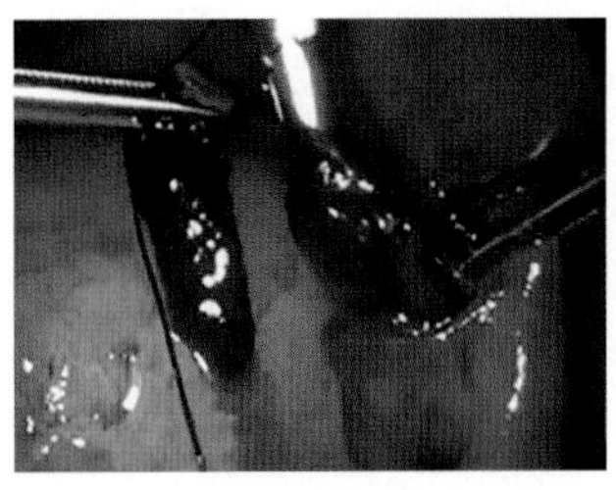

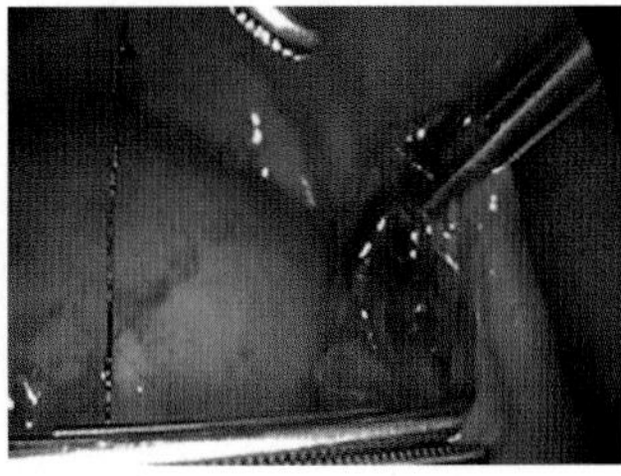

Figure 87.8 Laparoscopic salpingostomy.

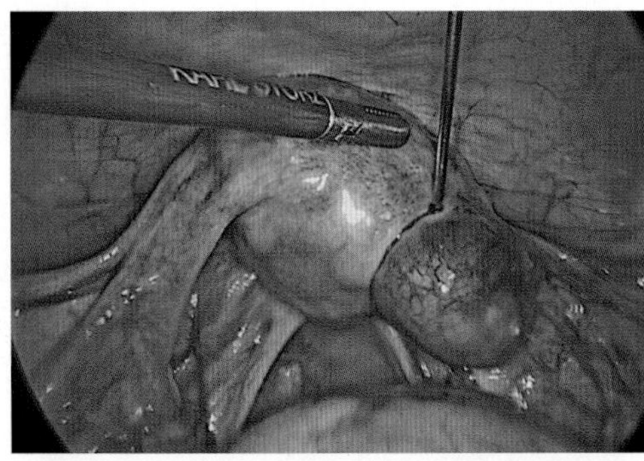
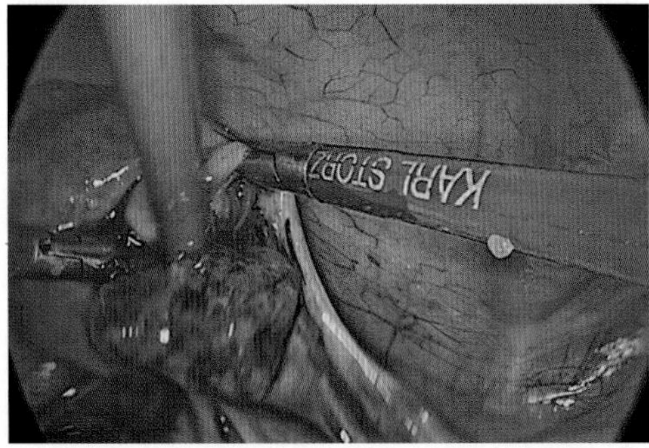

Figure 87.9 Laparoscopy of an interstitial ectopic pregnancy.

is associated with shorter operative times, less intraoperative blood loss, shorter hospital stays and similar subsequent intrauterine pregnancy rates. A laparotomy may be required if the woman is haemodynamically unstable. A salpingectomy is the preferred technique in the presence of a contralateral healthy fallopian tube. A salpingostomy is associated with an 8% risk of persistent trophoblastic tissue, intra-abdominal bleeding and an increased risk of a repeat ectopic pregnancy. These patients are subsequently followed up with serial serum βHCG levels until a negative result is obtained to exclude the presence of residual trophoblastic tissue. If a further ectopic pregnancy occurs within the same fallopian tube, then a salpingectomy is recommended regardless of the condition of the contralateral fallopian tube.

The management of non-tubal ectopic pregnancies (e.g. interstitial ectopic pregnancies [*Figure 87.9*], caesarean section scar ectopic pregnancies) can be complex and associated with more significant complications, such as bleeding, leading to an increased risk of a hysterectomy. These cases are best managed in tertiary centres. The management plan will be guided by the haemodynamic stability of the patient and the location of the ectopic pregnancy, including the expertise of the clinician managing the case.

These patients should be counselled regarding their increased risk of further ectopic pregnancies in subsequent conceptions. In view of this, they are encouraged to present as early as possible in any subsequent pregnancy to establish its location. Anti-D immunoglobin should be administered to non-sensitised rhesus (Rh)-negative women.

ACUTE ABDOMEN

Abdominal pain is one of the most challenging presenting complaints in the emergency department. Common causes of acute lower abdominal pain in the non-pregnant woman include:

- adnexal torsion;
- ovarian cyst accident, e.g. rupture;
- PID;
- endometriosis;
- appendicitis;
- bowel obstruction.

Adnexal torsion

An adnexal torsion is commonly the result of an ovary, and occasionally a fallopian tube, twisting along its pedicle and interrupting its arterial supply, leading to ischaemia. Rapid identification and intervention are necessary to preserve ovarian function. *Table 87.3* lists the presenting characteristics, recommended investigations and management options of an ovarian torsion.

TABLE 87.3 Presenting characteristics, recommended investigations and management options of an ovarian torsion.

Characteristics	
Symptoms and signs	• Abdominal pain (sudden onset) • Nausea/vomiting • Diarrhoea • Abdominal/pelvic tenderness • Palpable adnexal mass • Signs of peritonism • Non-specific and, therefore, a high clinical suspicion is necessary
Risk factors	• Enlarged ovary, e.g. cyst • Para-ovarian cyst • Hydrosalpinx • Previous torsion
Investigations	
Ultrasound	• Unilateral ovarian enlargement and ovarian tissue oedema, with less defined borders. Comparison with the contralateral ovary will show a distinct difference • Peripheral displacement of follicles; follicular ring sign • Central placement of the ovarian/adnexal mass in the suprapubic region • The affected ovary may appear as a solid mass with hypo- and hyperechoic areas, in keeping with haemorrhage and necrosis • The pedicle that is twisted may be seen as a 'whirlpool' that is visible both in grey-scale and on colour Doppler • Abnormal Doppler signals, e.g. coiling of the ovarian vessels (early/subacute), complete absence of perfusion (late) • Free fluid in the pelvis
Bloods	• Raised inflammatory markers (can also be normal)
Management	
Laparoscopy (*Figure 87.10*)	• Detorsion • Ovarian cystectomy to be performed at the same time or at a later date once the ovary is reperfused and the degree of oedema has diminished to reduce the likelihood of an oophorectomy

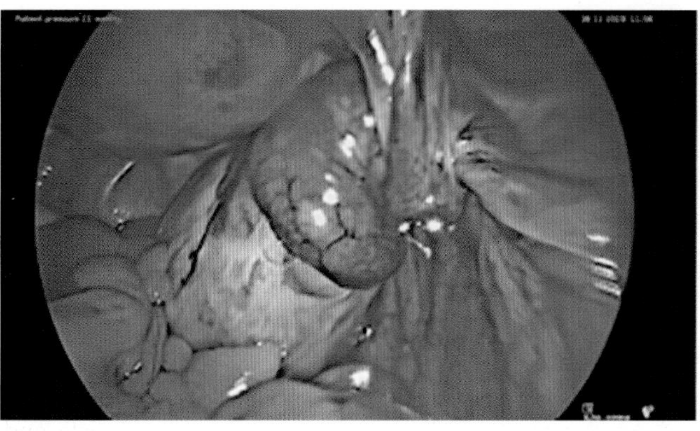

Figure 87.10 Laparoscopic image of ovarian torsion.

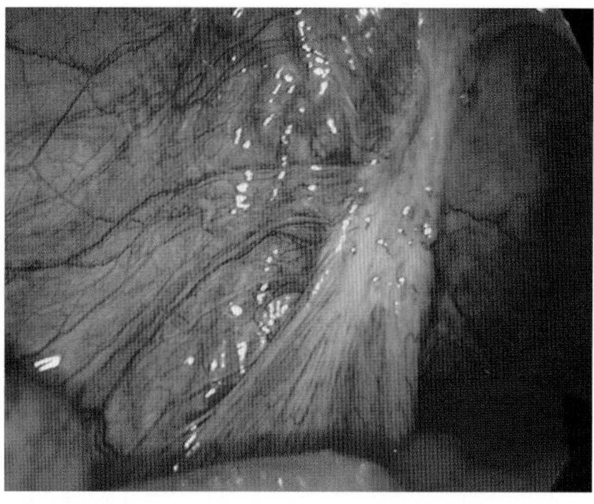

Figure 87.12 Endometriosis seen on the uterosacral ligament.

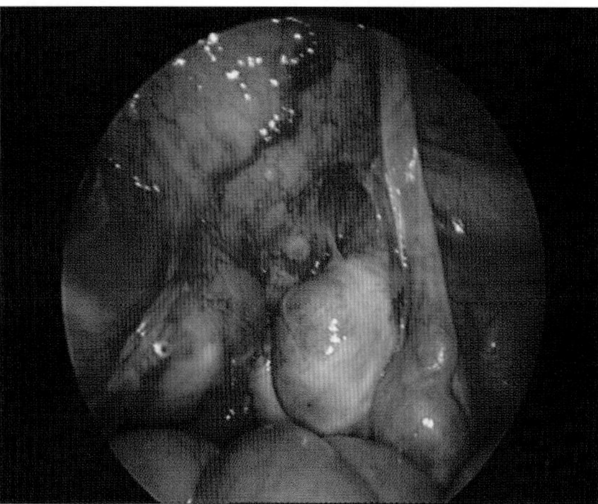

Figure 87.13 Bilateral ovarian endometriosis with pelvic adhesions.

CHRONIC ABDOMINAL PAIN

Endometriosis

Endometriosis is a common inflammatory condition and is diagnosed by the presence of endometrium-like tissue in extrauterine sites. The most commonly affected sites are the pelvic organs and peritoneum, although distant sites such as the lungs are occasionally affected (resulting in symptoms such as recurrent haemoptysis at the time of menstruation or recurrent pneumothoraces) (*Figure 87.11*). The exact pathognomonic mechanism remains elusive, but it is widely believed that most endometriotic lesions develop from retrograde menstruation. It is estimated to affect 5–10% of women, mainly of reproductive age, with the incidence reported to be higher in certain subgroups, e.g. women with a history of infertility. Endometriosis may be associated with a number of symptoms, but the predictive value of any one symptom or set of symptoms remains uncertain as each can have other causes (e.g. irritable bowel syndrome or interstitial cystitis), with a significant proportion of affected women remaining asymptomatic. The most common symptom is pain. Other symptoms include: cyclical and non-cyclical pain; dysmenorrhoea (pain related to menstruation); deep dyspareunia (pain during intercourse); dyschezia (pain on opening the bowels); and dysuria. Many women also suffer from fatigue, haematuria, chronic pelvic pain, infertility and rectal bleeding (haematochezia).

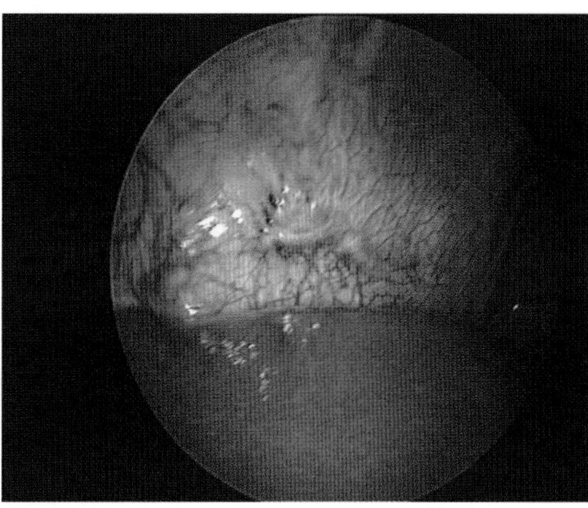

Figure 87.11 Endometriosis seen on the peritoneal surface of the diaphragm.

The extent of the disease varies from a few small peritoneal lesions on otherwise normal pelvic organs to deep endometriosis and large ovarian endometriotic cysts (endometriomas). The identification of endometriomas has been synonymous with deep disease. There can be extensive fibrosis in structures such as the uterosacral ligaments (*Figure 87.12*), and adhesion formation causing marked distortion of the pelvic anatomy (*Figure 87.13*). Disease severity can be assessed by describing the operative findings, or quantitatively using various classification systems, but there is little correlation between such systems and the type or severity of symptoms experienced.

Endometriosis typically appears as superficial 'powder burn' or 'gunshot' lesions on the ovaries, serosal surfaces and peritoneum – black, dark brown or bluish puckered lesions, nodules or small cysts containing old haemorrhage surrounded by a variable extent of fibrosis. Atypical or 'subtle' lesions are also common, including red implants (petechial, vesicular, polypoid, haemorrhagic, red flame-like) and serous or clear vesicles. Other appearances include white plaques or scarring and yellow-brown discoloration of the peritoneum. Ovarian endometriomas usually contain thick fluid-like tar and have been reported in 17–44% of women with endometriosis. They are distinguishable from simple haemorrhagic ovarian cysts because typically they are densely adherent to the peritoneum of the ovarian fossa, fallopian tube and posterolateral aspect of the uterus. The surrounding fibrosis may also involve the bowel. Deep endometriosis represents another disease type. This is defined by the presence of endometrium-like tissue 5 mm beneath the peritoneum, with growth seen in the utero-sacral ligaments, vagina, bowel, bladder or ureters; when such lesions grow into the vagina they may be visible on speculum examination as 'blue-domed' cystic lesions in the posterior fornix. Lesions infiltrating the bowel may mimic cancer in their presentation.

The gold standard for making a diagnosis of endometriosis is through laparoscopy with histological confirmation; non-invasive diagnostic tools, such as ultrasound scanning (transvaginal and transrectal), can reliably detect only severe forms of the disease, i.e. endometriomas or deep endometriosis of the pelvis. MRI can detect haemosiderin deposits in abdominal organs to suggest deep endometriosis. A sigmoidoscopy may also provide additional information on the level of disease involvement in cases of deep endometriosis involving the bowel. The distance between the inferior border of a bowel lesion and anal verge can impact on the proposed surgical intervention and degree of associated risks. Excision of low rectal lesions (5–8 cm from the anal verge) has been associated with a higher risk of anastomotic leaks and transient neurogenic bladder dysfunction.

Finding pelvic tenderness, a fixed retroverted uterus, tender uterosacral ligaments or enlarged ovaries on examination is suggestive of endometriosis. The diagnosis is more certain if deeply infiltrating nodules are found on the uterosacral ligaments or in the pouch of Douglas and/or visible lesions are seen in the vagina or on the cervix. A digital rectal examination should also be conducted to assess for disease involving the rectosigmoid area, as well as lateral and dorsal extension of the disease suggesting involvement of the hypogastric vessels and/or nerves. The findings may, however, be normal.

The treatment options are limited because the cause is uncertain. These include: conservative management; medical management (simple analgesia or hormonal drugs to suppress ovarian function [progestogens, the levonorgestrel intrauterine system, gonadotropin-releasing hormone agonists in conjunction with add-back hormone replacement therapy]); and surgical management (ablation or excision of endometriotic lesions). Women may require multiple admissions for surgery and/or prolonged treatment with costly drugs that can have problematic side effects. Surgical planning needs to be aware of the proximity of the disease to the ureter and the risk of ureteric stricture leading to hydronephrosis and renal dysfunction. The surgical risks include those for any laparoscopic procedure, including damage to the bowel, bladder and ureters (2 in 1000 women); the risks are increased if deep endometriosis is present secondary to anatomical displacement of structures such as the ureter, as well as in repeat surgical cases where repeated ureterolysis can increase the risk of ureteral ischaemia and repeated bowel shavings can reduce the integrity of the bowel wall increasing the risk of fistula formation. Bowel resection or injury increases the risk of faecal peritonitis. Bowel integrity can be assessed by stretching the bowel over a rectal manipulator to identify thinned areas, filling the pelvis with fluid and then pushing air into the rectal lumen whilst looking for bubbles or injecting methylene blue in the rectum and looking for leaks. Consideration should be given to ureteral stent insertion in cases of bladder endometriosis close to the trigonum which can usually be removed after approximately 6 weeks. A catheter will be needed for 8–10 days postoperatively, followed by a cystogram checking for suture integrity prior to removal. Rarely, infection in an endometrioma will result in the formation of a tubo-ovarian abscess.

For a woman who has completed her family, hysterectomy plus bilateral salpingo-oophorectomy with total excision of endometriotic disease offers a good chance of cure. Surgical treatment, however, in a woman who wishes to retain her fertility needs to be as conservative as possible, ensuring that ovarian function is preserved. The aim is to remove the endometriotic tissue while restoring the pelvic anatomy. The preferential method to retain ovarian function is ovarian drainage with directed spot ablation (electrocoagulation, thermal coagulation, laser or plasma energy) over cystectomy. Counselling needs to include the increased risk of recurrence with cyst drainage versus a cystectomy, as well as consideration for preoperative oocyte cryopreservation, especially in the presence of bilateral ovarian disease. Furthermore, bowel shaving versus bowel resection is associated with the risk of incomplete disease resection.

Several classification and staging systems have been proposed for the diagnosis, management and prognosis of endometriosis. Currently, there is a need for an internationally accepted system. The endometriosis fertility index has demonstrated good predictive value in the determination of fecundity after endometriosis surgery. Endometriosis is also associated with an increased risk of ovarian cancer (endometrioid and clear-cell types) and non-Hodgkin's lymphoma, adding to the burden of the disease.

Adenomyosis

Adenomyosis is a benign uterine disorder characterised by the presence of ectopic endometrium or endometrium-like structures within the myometrium accompanied by smooth muscle hypertrophy or hyperplasia. The ectopic endometrium can be present either diffusely or focally within the myometrium. The complexity of the condition is contributed to by its variable presentation and difficulty in making an accurate diagnosis, and, subsequently, its management. The true prevalence of the condition is unknown because of variable diagnostic criteria, and ranges from 1% to 70%. ***Table 87.4*** outlines the presenting characteristics, recommended investigations and management options.

Thomas Hodgkin, 1798–1866, curator of the museum and demonstrator of morbid anatomy, Guy's Hospital, London, UK.

TABLE 87.4 Presenting characteristics, recommended investigations and management options for adenomyosis.	
Presenting characteristics	
Symptoms	• Non-specific • Dysmenorrhoea • Abnormal uterine bleeding • Chronic pelvic pain • Subfertility • Presentation in the fourth and fifth decades of life • Asymptomatic • Dyspareunia
Signs	• Uterine enlargement • Uterine tenderness • Abnormalities identified at hysteroscopy (irregular endometrium with endometrial defects, cystic haemorrhagic lesions, altered vascularisation)
Risk factors	• Increased/longer oestrogen exposure (early menarche [≤10 years of age], short menstrual cycles [≤24 days in length], elevated body mass index, oral contraceptive use, increasing age, tamoxifen use) • Spontaneous miscarriage and multiple pregnancies • Increasing parity • Uterine instrumentation/incision (caesarean sections, surgical termination of pregnancy, SMM, endometrial curettage) • Endometrial hyperplasia • Leiomyomas that breach the endometrial–myometrial interface • Endometriosis • Smoking
Diagnosis	
Ultrasound	• The Morphological Uterus Sonographic Assessment (MUSA) group recommends commenting on eight morphological features in its classification of adenomyosis (presence, location, differentiation, cystic or non-cystic, myometrial layer, the extent of disease, size of the lesion and vascularity). Typical features include an enlarged globular uterus with asymmetrical thickening of the myometrium, myometrial cysts, echogenic subendometrial lesions, hyperechogenic islands, fan-shaped shadowing, an irregular junctional zone and vascularity on colour Doppler (*Figures 87.14–87.17*) • Three or more sonographic criteria are usually required to make a diagnosis of adenomyosis
Magnetic resonance imaging	• Can help differentiate an adenomyoma from fibroids
Histology	• Historically obtained at the time of hysterectomy; considered the gold standard • Limited in those wishing to preserve their fertility
Management	
Medical management	• Analgesia (i.e. NSAIDs) • Hormonal preparations (i.e. levonorgestrel IUS [off-label use]; combined oral contraceptive pill; progestogens, i.e. dienogest; GnRH agonists and antagonists; danazol; aromatase inhibitors, i.e. letrozole; selective progesterone receptor modulators)
Radiological interventions/ minimally invasive treatment options	• HIFU or MRgFUS: adverse effects include abdominal pain, skin burns and leg pain secondary to thermal injury of the sciatic nerve, intestinal perforation and temporary acute renal failure • UAE: postembolisation syndrome is reported, which consists of pelvic pain, nausea, fever secondary to necrosis and haematoma formation at the femoral artery puncture site. In addition, complications such as those associated with radiation exposure, haemorrhage, unplanned surgery, infections and an age-related impairment of ovarian reserve have also been reported
Surgical management (uterus preserving) (adenomyomectomy)	Different techniques: • Non-excisional surgical techniques (thermal coagulation of diseased myometrium) • Partial reduction surgeries (i.e. for diffuse adenomyosis including wedge resections, wedge-shaped uterine wall removal, modified reductive surgery and transverse H incisions) • Complete adenomyotic excision (i.e. for focal adenomyosis including the double- or triple-flap method and asymmetric dissection method)
Surgical management (non-uterine preserving)	• Hysterectomy: a total hysterectomy is preferred over a subtotal procedure as recurrence of the disease has been reported within the cervical stump and rectovaginal septum • Endometrial ablation/resection
Postoperative complications	• Uterine rupture (6% [>1% following an adenomyomectomy versus 0.26% following a myomectomy]), silent uterine rupture • Higher incidence of placenta accreta, increta and percreta compared with caesarean sections and myomectomies • Asherman's syndrome • Disease recurrence

GnRH, gonadotropin-releasing hormone; HIFU, high-intensity focused ultrasound; IUS, intrauterine system; MRgFUS, magnetic resonance-guided focused ultrasound; NSAID, non-steroidal anti-inflammatory drug; SMM, surgical management of miscarriage; UAE, uterine artery embolisation.

Joseph (Gustav) Asherman, 1889–1968, Czech–Israeli gynaecologist. This syndrome was first described by Heinrich Fritsch in 1894, Asherman further characterised it in 1948.

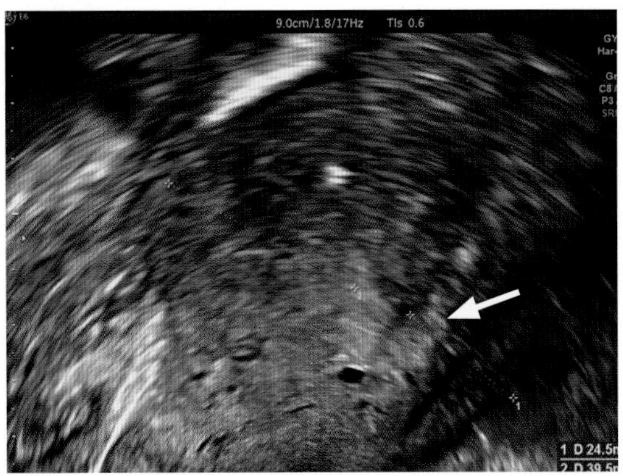

Figure 87.14 Ultrasound features of adenomyosis. Asymmetry between the anterior and posterior uterine wall and hyperechoic islands (arrow).

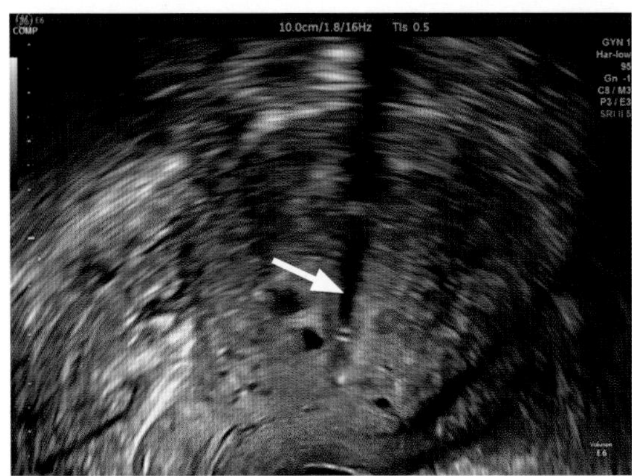

Figure 87.16 Ultrasound features of adenomyosis. Anechogenic myometrial tissue with acoustic shadowing posterior to it (arrow).

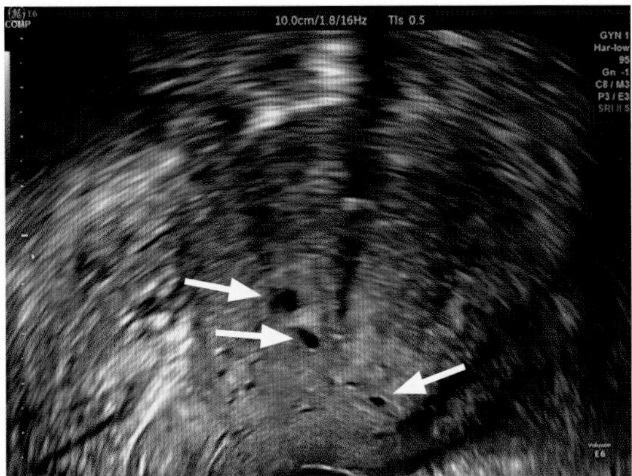

Figure 87.15 Ultrasound features of adenomyosis. Myometrial cysts (arrows).

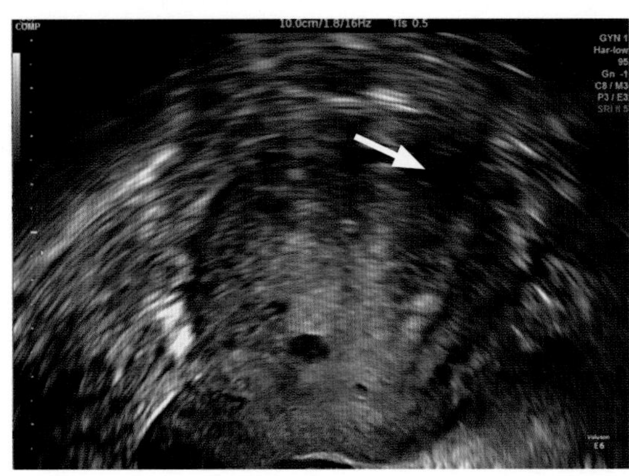

Figure 87.17 Ultrasound features of adenomyosis. Fan-shaped shadowing (arrow).

ABNORMAL UTERINE BLEEDING IN THE NON-PREGNANT STATE

Bleeding in the non-pregnant state may occur at the time of an expected menstrual period, between periods (intermenstrual bleeding; IMB), after intercourse (postcoital bleeding; PCB) or following the menopause (postmenopausal bleeding; PMB). Menopause is diagnosed in women who have not had a menstrual period after 12 months without the use of hormonal contraception. Vaginal bleeding may also occur after surgical instrumentation of the uterus and/or cervix, including insertion of an IUCD. The principal causes of uterine and vaginal bleeding in the non-pregnant state can be divided into structural and non-structural causes (*Table 87.5*) and their relationship to menses or coitus (*Table 87.6*).

The mainstay of management is to identify and treat the associated pathology. Investigations include a pregnancy test and ultrasound assessment of the pelvic anatomy (two-dimensional/three-dimensional ultrasound scan or saline sonogram) as well as an endometrial biopsy of the uterine cavity, performed either under direct vision at hysteroscopy or blindly with a Pipelle® biopsy. Hysteroscopy combined with endometrial biopsy improves the sensitivity and specificity for detection of endometrial pathology compared with either performed alone (*Figure 87.18*). The indications for undertaking an endometrial biopsy are shown in *Summary box 87.2*. A colonoscopy may also be indicated to exclude colorectal pathology as a potential cause for the bleeding.

Women taking tamoxifen, a selective oestrogen receptor modulator used in the treatment of breast cancer, represent a special group as the drug can induce uterine abnormalities in 10–40% of women, such as the development of endometrial polyps, hyperplasia, cancer and, rarely, uterine sarcomas, which are much more aggressive. Tamoxifen treatment results in a doubling of the risk of endometrial cancer after 1–2 years and has a quadrupling effect after 5 years. The relationship is time dependent but dose independent. The risk does not decrease on cessation of treatment. There is no consensus regarding the need for screening and which method to use; the alternative, more common approach is to investigate only those women who develop abnormal uterine bleeding with tamoxifen use. Aromatase inhibitors such as anastrozole, letrozole and exemestane are also used in the treatment of breast cancer, but their effects are not mediated via the oestrogen receptor so they have been associated with less endometrial pathology than tamoxifen. They may also reverse abnormalities induced by tamoxifen use.

TABLE 87.5 Structural and non-structural causes of uterine and vaginal bleeding.

Structural	• Endometrial or endocervical polyp • Fibroids (leiomyoma) • Endometrial hyperplasia • Malignancy of the genital tract
Non-structural	• Endometriosis • Adenomyosis • Coagulopathy, e.g. thrombocytopenia, von Willebrand's disease • Ovulatory dysfunction, e.g. polycystic ovary syndrome • Endometrial, e.g. endometritis • Iatrogenic, e.g. exogenous sex steroid administration, IUCD, hormonal contraceptive use • Other, e.g. arteriovenous malformations, chronic renal/hepatic disease

IUCD, intrauterine contraceptive device.

TABLE 87.6 Uterine and vaginal bleeding in the non-pregnant state in relation to menstrual bleeding.

Menstrual	• Endometrial polyp/malignancy[a] • Fibroids
Intermenstrual	• Vaginal trauma/malignancy[a] • Cervical polyp/malignancy • Endometrial polyp/malignancy[a]
Postcoital	• Vaginal malignancy[a] • Cervical ectropion/polyp/malignancy

[a]These cancers occur principally in postmenopausal women.

Summary box 87.2

Indications for an endometrial biopsy

Endometrial biopsy should be considered in the following cases:

- Women with suspected endometrial pathology
- All women >45 years old in whom medical treatment has been unsuccessful
- Women with persistent intermenstrual bleeding
- Endometrial thickness >4 mm in postmenopausal women or persistently thickened or abnormal appearance of the endometrium in premenopausal women and endometrial thickness >7 mm in women with known polycystic ovarian syndrome
- Irregular or unscheduled bleeding while on hormone replacement therapy after the initial 3 months
- Younger women with major risk factors for endometrial hyperplasia/cancer:
  - Polycystic ovarian syndrome
  - Obesity
  - Treatment with tamoxifen
- Irregular bleeding while on unopposed oestrogen
- Irregular bleeding in high-risk populations, such as family history of endometrial/colon cancer, especially hereditary non-polyposis colorectal cancer

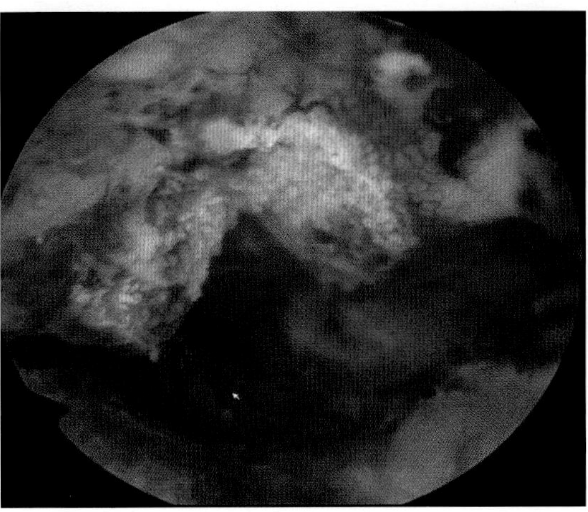

Figure 87.18 Hysteroscopic biopsy of endometrial cancer (cystic endometrium is visible at hysteroscopy).

Women known to have Lynch syndrome (hereditary non-polyposis colorectal cancer) and those considered at risk of inheriting a mismatch repair gene abnormality are another special group, as their lifetime risk of developing endometrial cancer is as high as 60%. Unlike sporadic cases of endometrial cancer, which are usually diagnosed during the sixth and seventh decades, the mean age at diagnosis in Lynch syndrome is the fifth decade. However, it appears that the 5-year survival rate in patients with Lynch syndrome-associated endometrial cancer is similar to that in women with sporadic disease. International guidelines suggest that these women should be screened annually from the age of 35 years with transvaginal ultrasound to measure the endometrial thickness and an endometrial biopsy.

Abnormal bleeding can also be caused by invasive carcinoma of the cervix, the incidence of which has been reduced by screening programmes that aim to detect the precancerous state, cervical intraepithelial neoplasia (CIN), using cervical cytology. The sample is checked for high-risk serotypes of human papillomavirus (HPV) (16, 18, 31 and 33) that can cause changes to the cervical cells. If these types of HPV are not identified on the sample, then no further action is required. If, however, these high-risk HPV serotypes are identified, the sample is checked for cervical cell changes, with the aim of treating these before they get a chance to turn into cervical cancer. In the UK, this is carried out every 3 years in women aged 25–49 years, and every 5 years in women aged 50–64 years. In women aged 65 years or older, a cervical screen will be conducted if one of the last three tests was abnormal or no test had been performed since the age of 50 years. Abnormalities in cervical cytology are followed up by microscopic examination of the cervix (colposcopy). CIN may be treated with local ablation (cryocautery, cold coagulation, electrocoagulation or laser) or excision (large loop excision of the transformation zone [LLETZ]).

Erik Adolf von Willebrand, 1870–1949, physician, Helsinki, Finland.
Henry T Lynch, 1928–2019, Professor of Preventative Medicine, Creighton University, Omaha, NE, USA, discovered familial susceptibility to certain kinds of cancer.

TABLE 87.7 Investigation and management of heavy menstrual bleeding.

Investigations	
Radiological imaging	TVUS has high sensitivity and specificity; MRI may be indicated if the women declines a TVUS or the findings are unclear. Identification of potential pathology such as polyps, fibroids
Hysteroscopy and histology	Direct visualisation of pathology with guided samples taken for histopathology
Management	
Medical management	• Tranexamic acid, NSAIDs (off-label use) • Oestrogen suppression with hormonal treatments (i.e. levonorgestrel IUS [after 1 year of use, there is a 71–95% reduction in menstrual blood loss with approximately 50% of women becoming amenorrhoeic], combined oral contraceptive pill [off-label use], progestogens, i.e. desogestrel [off-label use], GnRH agonists with or without add-back hormone replacement therapy) • GnRH agonists aim to shrink fibroids by inducing a hypo-oestrogenic state. This class of drug, however, is limited by its association with a loss in bone mineral density; in addition, fibroids tend to regrow to their original size when treatment is discontinued • Ulipristal acetate (Esmya®), an SPRM, is only licensed for use in premenopausal women in whom surgical procedures (including uterine fibroid embolisation) are not appropriate or have not worked. This drug should be used with caution as it has been associated with severe liver injury and liver function should be monitored during its use
Radiological interventions/minimally invasive treatment options	• HIFU or MRgFUS: adverse effects include abdominal pain, skin burns and leg pain secondary to thermal injury of the sciatic nerve, intestinal perforation and temporary acute renal failure • UAE involves blocking the blood supply to the fibroids using a technique in which particles are embolised into each uterine artery via an angiographic catheter (*Figure 87.19*). This technique has shown more value in the presence of a single large fibroid than in a multifibroid uterus. Postembolisation syndrome is reported, which consists of pelvic pain as a result of uterine ischaemia, nausea, fever secondary to necrosis and haematoma formation at the femoral artery puncture site. In addition, complications such as those associated with radiation exposure, haemorrhage, unplanned surgery, infection, thrombosis and an age-related impairment of ovarian reserve have also been reported
Surgical management (uterus preserving)	• Hysteroscopic polypectomy (risks include uterine perforation; damage to surrounding organs) • Transcervical resection of fibroids (complications include hyponatraemic fluid overload and thermal injury to surrounding structures) • Myomectomy (open or laparoscopic [*Figure 87.20*]). Surgical complications include bleeding and damage to surrounding structures, with the risk of conversion to a hysterectomy <1% secondary to excessive bleeding. Morcellation is described in further detail in *Uterine fibroids (leiomyoma)*
Surgical management (non-uterine preserving)	• Endometrial ablation/resection (risks include thermal injury to surrounding organs and fluid overload; not recommended in women wishing to retain their fertility). The aim of ablative methods is to reduce the menstrual bleeding by ablating the endometrium down to the basalis layer using electrical, thermal or laser energy. More than 90% of women report a reduction in menstrual blood loss without the need for further treatment at 2 years of follow-up, with 25–35% experiencing amenorrhoea. The criteria for endometrial ablation are described in *Table 87.8* • Hysterectomy: a total hysterectomy is preferred over a subtotal procedure as persistence of symptoms is reported within the cervical stump (risks include damage to surrounding organs and fistula formation)

GnRH, gonadotropin-releasing hormone; HIFU, high-intensity focused ultrasound; IUS, intrauterine system; MRgFUS, magnetic resonance-guided focused ultrasound; MRI, magnetic resonance imaging; NSAID, non-steroidal anti-inflammatory drug; SPRM, selective progesterone receptor modulator; TVUS, transvaginal ultrasound scan; UAE, uterine artery embolisation.

Cervical cancer is one of the leading causes of mortality in the world. To improve the uptake of the cervical screening programme, testing for HPV in the comfort of a woman's own home is being investigated.

Current vaccination programmes against HPV serotypes are aimed at reducing the incidence of cervical carcinoma. In the UK, the vaccination is currently offered to girls and boys aged 12–13 years with a repeat dose offered 6–24 months later, prior to becoming sexually active. The vaccine helps protect against mouth, throat, anal and genital cancers as well cervical cancer.

Menstrual bleeding may be excessively heavy, irregular or frequent in the absence of pathology; this is known as dysfunctional uterine bleeding. NICE guidance in the UK has suggested a three-step hierarchal treatment approach to the management of heavy menstrual bleeding (***Table 87.7***).

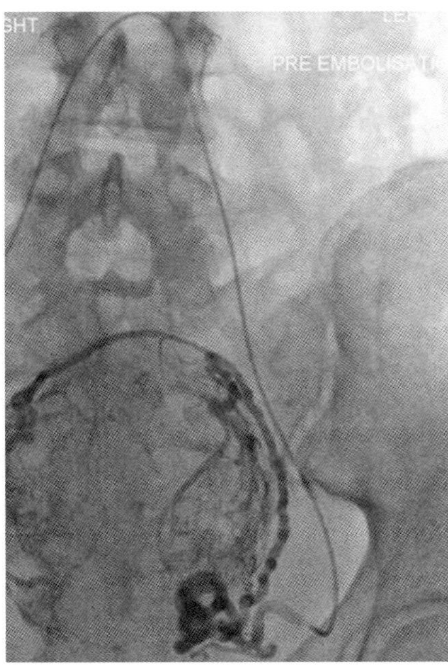

Figure 87.19 Pre-embolisation angiogram showing catheterisation of the left uterine artery and blood supply to a large fundal fibroid (courtesy of Dr Mark Bratby, Consultant Vascular and Interventional Radiologist, John Radcliffe Hospital, Oxford, UK).

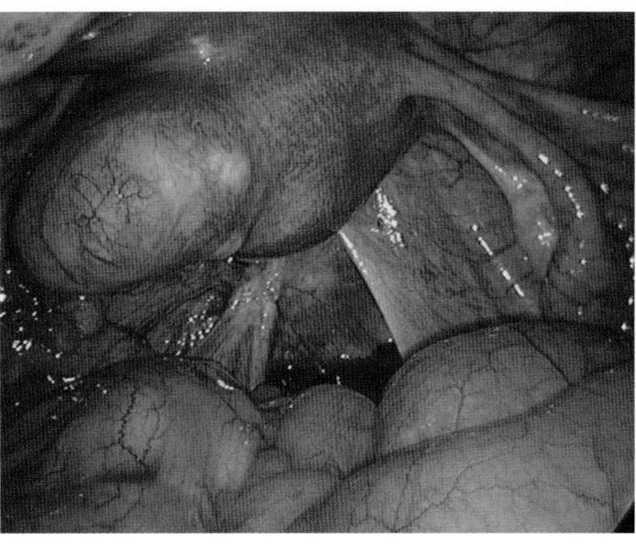

Figure 87.20 Laparoscopic view of a uterine fundal fibroid.

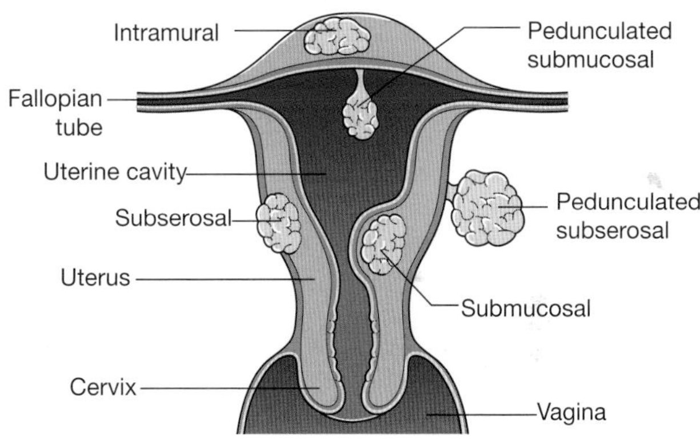

Figure 87.21 Uterine fibroids.

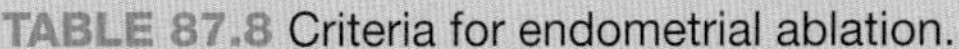

TABLE 87.8 Criteria for endometrial ablation.

- Uterus <10 cm in length
- Absence of major intrauterine pathology that would distort the uterine cavity
- No history of previous endometrial ablation procedures
- No evidence of endometritis
- Family is complete

The management plans are individualised for the patient, taking into account concomitant symptoms and fertility requirements.

A hysterectomy can be carried out by three different routes: vaginally, abdominally or laparoscopically. The route of entry is dependent on a number of factors, including: uterine size; presence of other pathology; mobility and descent of the uterus; history of previous surgery; and skill of the operating surgeon. No difference in prolapse symptoms, sexual satisfaction or pelvic pain has been reported between a total or subtotal (conservation of the cervix) hysterectomy. Furthermore, it is now recommended that the fallopian tubes are removed in conjunction with the uterine body, whether the ovaries are conserved or not. The fallopian tubes have no continued functionality following a hysterectomy but can be a potential source of malignancy if retained. Conservation or removal of the ovaries is dependent on the woman's age, presence of coexisting pathology and/or risk factors for malignancy.

Uterine fibroids (leiomyoma)

Fibroids are usually benign, well-circumscribed, smooth muscle tumours of the uterus. Less than 1% of fibroids undergo malignant transformation (leiomyosarcoma). They are more common in certain populations (African–Caribbean women) and vary in size and number. They are typically found in the following locations (***Figure 87.21***):

- Subserosal: may cause pressure-type symptoms; if pedunculated, they can be difficult to distinguish from an ovarian tumour.
- Intramural: may similarly cause pressure-type symptoms; can be associated with infertility and heavy periods if they lead to endometrial distortion.
- Submucosal: associated with infertility, recurrent pregnancy loss and heavy periods; if pedunculated, they may occasionally extrude through the cervical os.
- Rare: sites include the broad ligament and cervix.

Women with uterine fibroids may present with heavy and/or irregular menstrual bleeding, anaemia, pressure-type symptoms or infertility, especially if the fibroid is distorting the uterine cavity. The pressure-type symptoms can include pelvic discomfort, urinary incontinence, frequency and retention, constipation and backache. When large fibroids are present, back pressure may cause or exacerbate varicosities. Although these symptoms are common, it is important to note that some women with fibroids are asymptomatic. Rarely, women may present acutely with pain arising from torsion of a pedunculated fibroid or red degeneration, especially in pregnancy.

A diagnosis can usually be made on bimanual and/or abdominal examination, in the presence of an enlarged uterus with attached swellings. The principal differential diagnosis is an ovarian tumour; in general, if an ovarian tumour is present, the uterus is felt separately on vaginal examination, although not if the structures are adherent to each other. A pelvic ultrasound scan is the first-line investigation with high sensitivity and specificity. An MRI can be performed if an ultrasound is declined by the patient or is inconclusive (***Figure 87.22***).

Treatment can be divided into: conservative if the woman is asymptomatic; medical to reduce the quantity of menstrual bleeding; hormonal manipulation to control menstrual bleeding or to shrink the fibroids; or surgical (uterus-preserving or non-uterus-preserving methodologies) (***Table 87.7***). The choice of treatment depends upon the woman's age and fertility intentions, the size and number of fibroids as well as their location. Emergency surgical treatment is only required if there is substantial menstrual bleeding or uncontrollable pain; these are rare events.

Morcellation

This is the process whereby larger tissue is broken down into smaller pieces, facilitating their removal through smaller incisions in the abdomen. In gynaecology, this is usually offered in the context of a laparoscopic myomectomy to remove fibroids or a laparoscopic subtotal hysterectomy to remove the body of the uterus. This procedure is undertaken with an instrument called a morcellator. The risks associated with morcellation include parasitic spread of tissue where the cut tissue deposits itself elsewhere and grows (1:120 to 1:1200) and the upstaging of previously undiagnosed malignancies (noting that this is also considered a risk during an open myomectomy if the fibroid capsule is breached), as well as missed malignancies owing to lost anatomy. Retrieval bags have been proposed to prevent dissemination of the tissue but the evidence regarding their use is currently awaited. In view of this, careful case selection is important. The risk of an uterine sarcoma increases as age increases, in the perimenopausal and postmenopausal stages of life, in the presence of *BRCA* mutations and Lynch syndrome, and in the context of rapidly growing fibroids non-responsive to oestrogen deprivation.

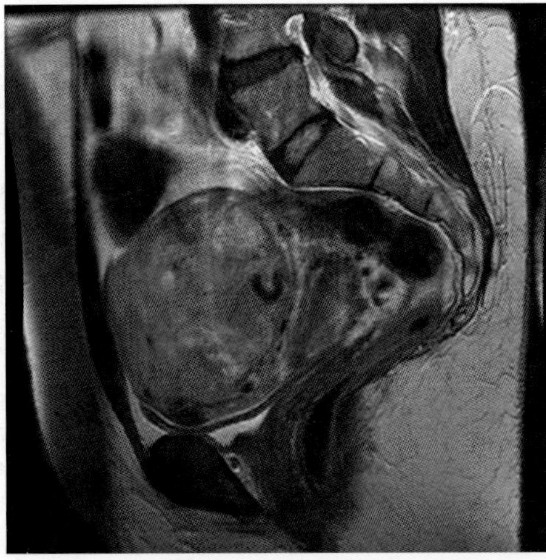

Figure 87.22 Magnetic resonance imaging of uterine fibroids.

UROGYNAECOLOGY

Urinary incontinence

Urinary incontinence is defined as the involuntary leakage of urine. It is said to affect approximately 30% of women, with a higher prevalence seen in older age groups. It can have a significant impact on quality of life.

Incontinence can be classified into:

- stress urinary incontinence (SUI) (involuntary leakage of urine secondary to increased intra-abdominal pressure, e.g. coughing, sneezing);
- overactive bladder (OAB); urinary urgency, usually with urinary frequency and nocturia, with or without urinary incontinence;
- mixed urinary incontinence (combination of both OAB and SUI).

It can result from both functional and anatomical causes, including:

- multiparity;
- childbirth complications and vaginal delivery;
- risng female age - menopause;
- fistulae;
- urethral diverticulum/congenital anomalies, e.g. ectopic ureters;
- immobility, constipation or urinary tract infection;
- chronic medical conditions, e.g. congestive heart failure, diabetes mellitus, multiple sclerosis;
- medications, e.g. loop diuretics;
- secondary to pelvic masses;
- obesity and weight gain.

Common symptoms and complaints include:

- storage symptoms:
  - frequency (increased frequency of more than eight times during the day)
  - urgency
  - nocturia (increased frequency of voiding more than once a night)
- emptying symptoms:
  - hesitancy
  - slow stream
  - incomplete emptying
  - straining to urinate
- urinary leakage with exertion/coughing

- haematuria (in women >40 years of age, additional investigations should be performed to rule out malignancy).

Investigations include:

- urinary incontinence-specific symptom and quality of life questionnaire, including a bladder diary;
- digital examination;
- urine analysis and a midstream urine sample for microscopy, culture and sensitivity;
- urodynamics, including an assessment of postvoid residual volumes – if conservative measures have failed, the type of incontinence is unclear or there is a recurrence of symptoms following surgical intervention;
- ultrasound of the kidneys, ureters and bladder in patients with recurrent urinary tract infections/haematuria;
- cystoscopy if pathology is suspected.

Management can be divided into conservative methods, medical therapy or surgical intervention (*Tables 87.9–87.11*). The treatment of choice is dependent on the underlying cause.

Treatments can be combined and are individualised for the patient. Should initial therapy be unsuccessful or repeat procedures be required, then the patients should be discussed within a multidisciplinary team (MDT) setting.

TABLE 87.9 Management options for overactive bladder (OAB).

Conservative	• Lifestyle changes (i.e. limit fluid intake, avoid diuretics such as tea/coffee, weight loss) • Behavioural modification (e.g. bladder drills) for a minimum of 6 weeks • Review of coexistent medications (e.g. diuretics) • Pelvic floor training (physiotherapy) for at least 3 months, comprising at least eight contractions three times per day • Bladder catheterisation-intermittent self catheterisation if increased post void residuals
Medical therapy	• Anticholinergics (e.g. oxybutynin [avoid in elderly frail women at risk of cognitive impairment], tolterodine); side effects include a dry mouth and constipation • Selective β_3-adrenoreceptor agonist (e.g. mirabegron) for the management of urge incontinence • Desmopressin specifically used to treat symptoms of nocturia
Surgical	• Intravesical botulinum toxin A • Neuromodulation (tibial nerve stimulation or sacral neuromodulation) • Bladder reconstruction (augmentation cystoplasty – risks include bowel disturbance, metabolic acidosis, mucus production and/or retention in the bladder, urinary tract infection, urinary retention and malignancy) • Urinary diversion only when non-surgical management has failed and if botulinum toxin type A, percutaneous sacral nerve stimulation and augmentation cystoplasty are not appropriate or are unacceptable

TABLE 87.10 Management options for stress urinary incontinence (SUI).

Conservative	• Pelvic floor training (physiotherapy) for at least 3 months, comprising at least eight contractions three times per day • Management of a persistent cough • Bladder catheterisation-intermittent self catheterisation if increased post void residuals
Medical therapy	• Serotonin and noradrenaline (norepinephrine) reuptake inhibitors (e.g. duloxetine) (can be used when conservative measures have failed and surgical treatment is contraindicated or declined)
Surgical	• Colposuspension (bladder neck suspension) • Autologous rectus fascial sling procedures and retropubic midurethral mesh slings • Periurethral bulking agents • Artificial urinary sphincter • Do not offer: anterior colporrhaphy; needle suspension; paravaginal defect repair; porcine dermis sling; the Marshall–Marchetti–Krantz procedure

TABLE 87.11 Management options for specific conditions causing urinary incontinence.

Pelvic masses	• Surgical approach, e.g. myomectomy or hysterectomy
Recurrent urinary tract infections	• Antibiotics – treatment, low dose prophylaxis, rescue course • 3 month course of vaginal oestrogen in post menopausal women
Fistulae or ectopic ureters	• Surgical correction

Uterovaginal prolapse

Pelvic organ prolapse refers to the protrusion or displacement of the pelvic organs from their normal anatomical position into or through the vagina to varying degrees (*Figure 87.23*). It is said to affect up to 40% of women at some point in their lifetime. A prolapse can have a detrimental impact on normal organ performance, including anorectal, urinary and sexual function.

A prolapse is more common in certain groups, including:

- older women;
- parous women, increased parity, prolonged labours, vaginal deliveries;
- obese women;
- women who have chronic constipation;
- women with occupations that involve heavy lifting;
- women with oestrogen deficiency;
- women with a family history or genetic risk;
- women with connective tissue disorders, e.g. Ehlers–Danlos syndrome, Marfan syndrome.

Edvard Laurits Ehlers, 1863–1937, dermatologist, Copenhagen, Denmark.
Henri-Alexandre Danlos, 1844–1912, dermatologist, Paris, France.
Antoine Bernard-Jean Marfan, 1858–1942, paediatrician, Paris, France.

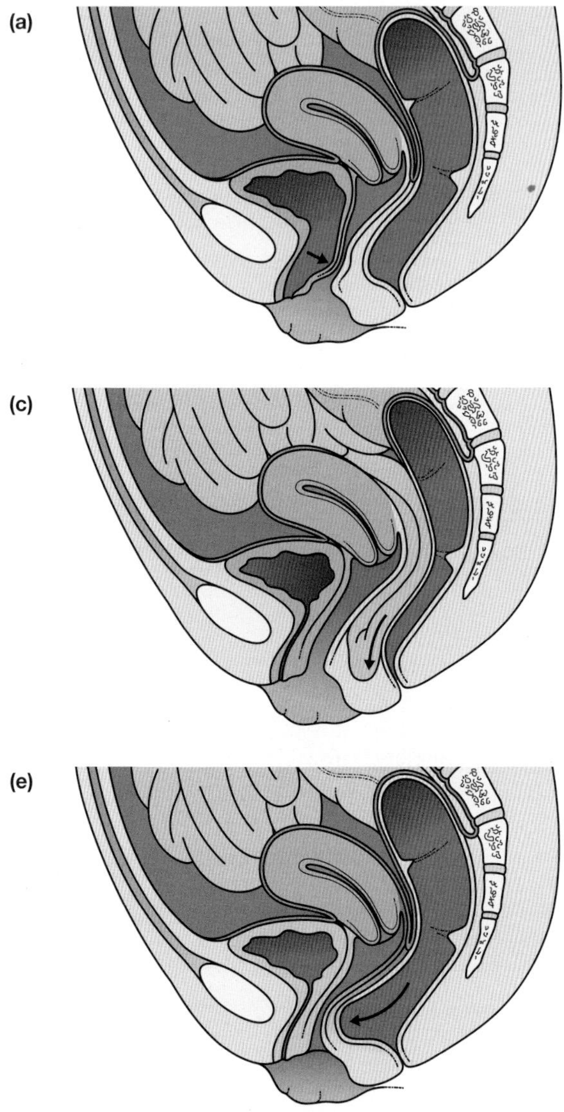

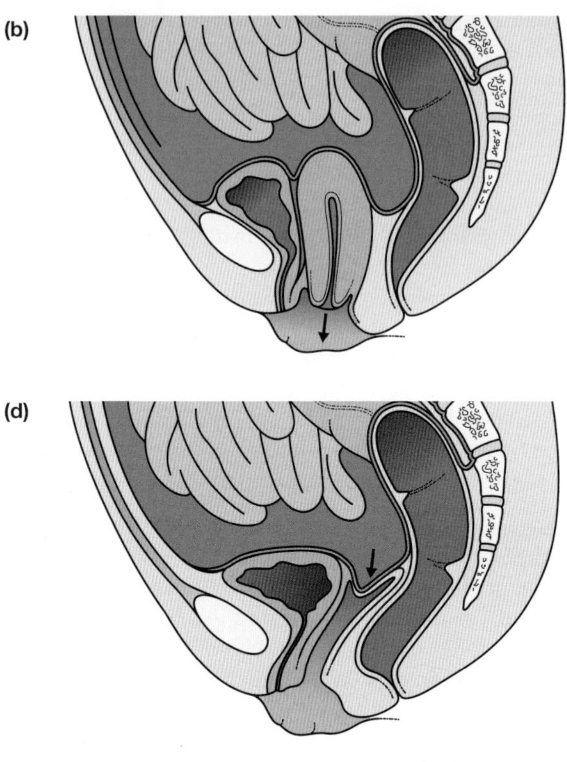

Figure 87.23 Uterovaginal prolapse: (a) urethrocele/cystocele (arrow); (b) uterine prolapse (arrow); (c) enterocele (arrow); (d) vaginal vault prolapse (arrow); (e) rectocele (arrow).

Women with minor prolapses may be asymptomatic, but those with more significant degrees may present with a sensation of 'something coming down'. A cystocele (bladder prolapse) and a cystourethrocele (prolapse of the bladder and urethra) can lead to the sensation of a lump in the vagina and may be associated with urinary urgency (OAB symptoms) and recurrent urinary tract infections. Uterine descent can lead to a lump in the vagina or a dragging sensation; with complete prolapse of the uterus (procidentia) there may be associated vaginal discharge, ulceration of the vaginal mucosa and bleeding. A rectocele (prolapse of the rectum into the vagina) may cause difficulties with defecation or a sensation of incomplete emptying, which can be relieved by digital reduction of the prolapse.

The degree of prolapse is graded in terms of descent. Currently, the commonly used grading system is the Pelvic Organ Prolapse Quantification System (POP-Q):

- grade 0: no prolapse is demonstrated;
- grade 1: the most distal portion of the prolapse is >1 cm above the level of the hymen;
- grade 2: the most distal portion of the prolapse is ≤1 cm above or below the level of the hymen;
- grade 3: the most distal portion of the prolapse is >1 cm below the level of the hymen but 2 cm less than the total vaginal length;
- grade 4: maximal descent.

Non-surgical management of a uterovaginal prolapse includes: lifestyle changes (avoidance of constipation); physiotherapy to help strengthen the pelvic floor muscles for at least 16 weeks for those with grade 1 or 2 organ prolapse; topical oestrogen replacement for oestrogen deficiency to help increase tissue strength and elasticity; and vaginal pessaries. There are a number of different pessaries available and they are replaced every 3–6 months, with the ring pessary being the most frequently used. It is inserted between the posterior fornix and the pubic bone. The main complications are of vaginal ulceration and infection leading to discharge and bleeding; it is advisable, therefore, to replace the ring frequently.

Surgical management aims to correct the prolapse. The surgical procedures are intended to restore the uterovaginal anatomy and position. They may be carried out using a vaginal or abdominal (open or laparoscopic) approach (*Table 87.12*).

TABLE 87.12 Surgical treatments for uterovaginal prolapse.

Condition	Treatment	Complications
Urethrocele/cystocele (*Figure 87.23a*)	• An anterior vaginal wall repair (anterior colporrhaphy) without the use of mesh	• Bleeding • Infection • Fistula formation • Voiding dysfunction • Unmasking of occult SUI • Failure • Recurrence
Uterine prolapse (*Figure 87.23b*)	• If the patient's family is complete, a vaginal hysterectomy with or without vaginal sacrospinous fixation can be performed • Uterus-preserving surgery includes: amputation of the cervix with suturing of the transverse cervical ligaments vaginally (Manchester repair); laparoscopic plication of the uterosacral ligaments (McCall suture); or hysteropexy, which may be vaginal (attaching the cervix to the sacrospinous ligaments using non-absorbable sutures) or laparoscopic/abdominal (sacrohysteropexy using a polypropylene mesh to suspend the uterus to the sacral promontory) • A colpocleisis can be considered in women who no longer wish to have penetrative intercourse	• Bleeding • Infection • Injury to the bladder, bowel or ureters • Voiding dysfunction • Dyspareunia • Failure • Recurrence • Conversion to a laparotomy • A Manchester repair can specifically be associated with infertility, miscarriage and dystocia
Enterocele (*Figure 87.23c*)	• A similar technique to repair of a hernia is used. The vaginal mucosa is opened and the hernial sac repaired	• Bleeding • Infection • Rectal or small bowel injury (fistula formation) • Dyspareunia • Failure • Recurrence
Vaginal vault prolapse (*Figure 87.23d*)	• Sacrospinous fixation performed vaginally: the vault is attached to the right sacrospinous ligament using a non-absorbable suture/mesh, avoiding the rectosigmoid colon on the left • Sacrocolpopexy performed abdominally or laparoscopically: the vaginal vault is attached to the sacral promontory using a mesh • A colpocleisis can be considered in women who no longer wish to have penetrative intercourse	• Bleeding • Infection • Injury to the bowel or ureter • Unmasking of occult SUI • Right buttock pain • Sexual dysfunction
Rectocele (*Figure 87.23e*)	• Posterior colpoperineorrhaphy without mesh: the posterior vaginal wall is opened, the rectum returned to its normal position and redundant vaginal mucosa excised	• Bleeding • Infection • Rectal or small bowel injury (fistula formation) • Dyspareunia • Failure • Recurrence

SUI, stress urinary incontinence.

Approximately 30% of women in their lifetime report a recurrence of their symptoms following surgical treatment. This figure increases with subsequent procedures.

Mesh

In the UK, mesh-related surgery is considered to be a high-vigilance operation, whereby use of synthetic mesh to treat SUI or urogynaecological prolapse has been restricted nationally secondary to a number of safety concerns that have been raised:

- pain or sensory change in the back, abdomen, vagina, pelvis, leg, groin and/or perineum;
- vaginal problems, including discharge, bleeding, dyspareunia, penile trauma or pain in sexual partners;
- urinary problems, including recurrent infections, incontinence, retention, difficulty or pain during voiding;
- bowel problems, including difficulty or pain on defecation, faecal incontinence, rectal bleeding or passage of mucus.

In view of this, an MDT approach is recommended to manage complex pelvic floor dysfunction and mesh-related problems. For women with a confirmed mesh-related complication or unexplained symptoms after a mesh procedure, referral should be made to regional centres specialising in the diagnosis and management of mesh-related complications. Continence surgery requiring mesh usage such as transvaginal tapes and

The **Manchester repair** was introduced at St Mary's Hospital for Women and Children, Manchester, UK.
Milton Lawrence McCall, 1911–1963, obstetrician, Magee-Women's Hospital, Pittsburgh, PA, USA.

transobturator tapes has been replaced by open/laparoscopic continence surgery in the form of colposuspension or insertion of an autologous fascial sling. Uterine prolapse and vaginal vault prolapse surgery requiring the use of mesh during hysteropexy and sacrocolpopexy procedures can be undertaken following detailed counselling and MDT agreement.

TUMOURS

Benign ovarian tumours and cysts

Overall, 90% of ovarian tumours are benign, with an increased risk of malignancy in older women: the malignant potential of an ovarian cyst in a premenopausal woman is 1:1000, increasing to 3:1000 at the age of 50 years. Ovarian tumours are subdivided into five main categories according to the World Health Organization's classification system (*Table 87.13*).

TABLE 87.13 Classification of ovarian tumours.

Surface epithelial tumours	• Represent approximately 65% of all ovarian tumours and 90% of ovarian malignancies • Further classified by cell type (serous, mucinous, endometrioid, clear cell, transitional cell, epithelial–stromal [undifferentiated]) and atypia (benign, borderline or malignant)
Germ cell tumours	• Represent approximately 15% of all ovarian neoplasms • Mature teratomas are the most common type of ovarian germ cell tumour (benign), often called a dermoid cyst. They most commonly occur in women of reproductive age and contain a variety of tissues, including skin, hair follicles, sweat glands, bone and teeth • Malignant germ cell tumours include immature teratomas, dysgerminomas, yolk sac tumours, choriocarcinomas and embryonal carcinomas
Sex cord–stromal tumours	• Represent approximately 10% of all ovarian neoplasms
Metastatic tumours	• Represent approximately 5% of ovarian malignancies; usually arise from breast, colon, endometrium, stomach and cervical cancers
Other/miscellaneous	• A small number of other types of neoplasms, which develop from ovarian soft tissue or non-neoplastic processes

Benign ovarian tumours are often asymptomatic and may present incidentally, for example when an abdominal radiograph reveals the appearance of a tooth in the abdomen or pelvis. Conversely, they may present with pain, abdominal swelling, pressure-type symptoms, nausea or vomiting. Sudden-onset pain with vomiting and raised inflammatory markers can be more diagnostic of ovarian torsion (see *Adnexal torsion*).

Management will depend on the age of the woman and the characteristics of the cyst (*Summary box 87.3*). In older women, a conservative approach is only reasonable if the risk of malignancy is low (see *Ovarian cancer*). In perimenopausal women, the cyst can be followed by serial ultrasound scanning as many will regress. If there is uncontrollable pain, haemodynamic compromise, suspicion of torsion or the cyst does not regress, then surgical management is advised. In most cases this would involve a laparoscopic ovarian cystectomy with conservation of ovarian tissue as the treatment of choice. As the vast majority of oocytes lie within 5 mm of the surface of the ovary, a carefully carried out cystectomy can leave a normally functioning ovary (*Figure 87.24*).

Summary box 87.3

Management of benign ovarian cysts

- Commonly, an incidental finding, but may be suggested by symptoms and signs
- A pregnancy test should be performed to exclude an ectopic pregnancy (however, it is important to note that HCG can also be positive in dysgerminomas and choriocarcinomas)
- TVUS is the mainstay diagnostic tool with high sensitivity and specificity in being able to differentiate a benign mass from a malignant one (*Table 87.14*). If the results are indeterminate, an MRI or CT scan may help; an MRI is more useful than a CT scan for the assessment of complex cysts/endometriosis. Masses with radiographic characteristics of cancer (e.g. cystic and solid components, surface excrescences, multilocular appearance, irregular shape) require removal
- Tumour markers may help in the diagnosis of specific masses (see *Ovarian cancer*)
- In women of reproductive age, simple, thin-walled cystic adnexal masses of a maximum diameter of 50 mm without characteristics of cancer do not require further investigation unless they persist for >3 months. A follow-up scan can be arranged after 4 months to check for resolution. In postmenopausal women, this is conducted every 4 months in conjunction with a serum blood test for the cancer antigen 125 (CA-125) for a duration of 1 year; if no change is detected, the women can be discharged
- Perimenopausal women with simple cysts measuring 50–70 mm in diameter should undergo annual ultrasound follow-up
- Women with larger cysts (>70 mm) or persistent cysts may benefit from an MRI scan or surgical intervention
- Cyst removal (ovarian cystectomy) is preferably performed laparoscopically. Cyst aspiration is associated with a high risk of recurrence but can be considered after detailed counselling if the woman wishes to retain her fertility. Bilateral salpingo-oophorectomy is preferable for postmenopausal women if surgery is indicated
- An oophorectomy may become necessary if the cyst cannot be surgically removed from the ovary

TABLE 87.14 International Ovarian Tumor Analysis (IOTA) group classification for the ultrasound assessment of ovarian cysts.

Benign features (B-rules)	Malignant features (M-rules)
• Unilocular cysts • Solid components, the largest of which is <7 mm • Acoustic shadowing • Smooth multilocular tumour <100 mm • No blood flow	• Irregular solid tumour • Ascites • Minimum of four papillary structures • Irregular multilocular tumour ≥100 mm • Blood flow

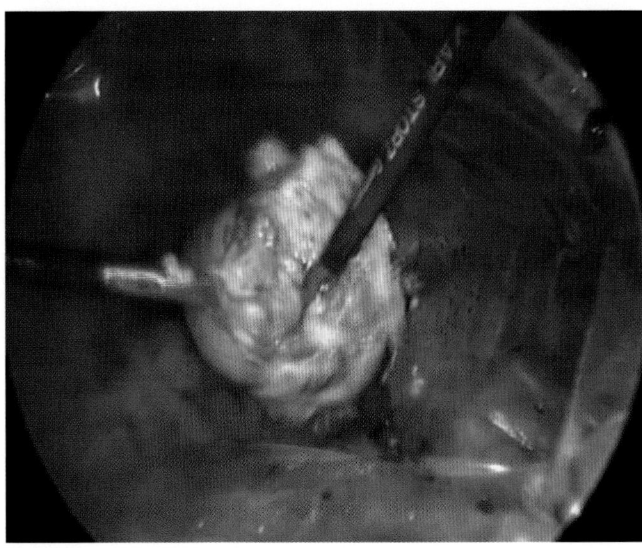

Figure 87.24 Ovarian cystectomy.

Ovarian cancer

Ovarian cancer is the sixth most common malignancy in women, behind breast, lung, bowel, uterine cancer and malignant melanoma. In the UK, over 7000 women are diagnosed with ovarian cancer each year. Over 90% of cancers arise from the surface epithelium of the ovary (which has the same embryological origins as the peritoneum); the majority arise sporadically rather than secondary to inheritance. The peak incidence is in the age range 65–69 years. The overall 5-year survival rate is <50% because approximately two-thirds of women present with advanced disease.

The common presenting symptoms are:

- abdominal distension and/or pain;
- change in appetite;
- weight gain and increased girth (ascites);
- urinary obstruction.

Over half of all women, however, present initially to a speciality other than gynaecology, with often vague symptoms caused by metastatic disease, e.g. shortness of breath, gastrointestinal disturbance or a change in bowel habit. Consequently, it is important to include ovarian cancer in the differential diagnosis of any woman presenting with a recent onset of persistent, non-specific, abdominal symptoms (including those whose abdomen and pelvis appear normal on clinical examination). A pelvic mass in conjunction with ascites usually indicates ovarian cancer but may also be indicative of Meigs' syndrome (a benign fibroma with ascites and the presence of a pleural effusion). *Summary box 87.4* addresses the basic tests that can be conducted to diagnose ovarian malignancy.

CA-125 is a glycoprotein expressed on tissue derived from coelomic and Müllerian epithelia; the normal cut-off value is 35 U/mL. Elevated levels are found in 50% of patients with stage I disease and >90% of those with advanced disease. It primarily detects epithelial ovarian cancers. However, CA-125 is a non-specific marker with raised levels also seen in other cancers, e.g. pancreatic, breast, lung and colon. Levels may also be increased during menstruation; in benign conditions such as endometriosis, PID and liver disease; if ascites or other effusions are present; and after a recent laparotomy. Combining menopausal status, ultrasound features and CA-125 measurements using the risk of malignancy index (RMI) algorithm (*Summary box 87.5*) can help guide management and identify those who require an onward referral to a gynaecological oncologist in a cancer centre.

Summary box 87.4

Basic tests on suspicion of ovarian malignancy

- Ultrasound scan is considered the first-line investigation (*Table 87.12*)
- A staging CT or MRI is carried out prior to surgery to determine the extent of disease
- Tumour markers, including βHCG, lactate dehydrogenase, alpha-fetoprotein (αFP), CA-125, CA-19-9 and carcinoembryonic antigen (CEA), should be measured. Lactate dehydrogenase, αFP, inhibin and βHCG are particularly recommended in women <40 years old with a suspected complex ovarian mass, to exclude germ cell tumours

Summary box 87.5

Risk of malignancy index (RMI)

- RMI = U × M × CA-125

  U, ultrasound features scoring 1 for each malignant feature (multilocular, solid components, metastases, ascites, bilateral lesions); M, menopausal status with 1 for premenopausal and 3 for postmenopausal; CA-125, CA-125 level in U/mL

There is currently no national screening programme for ovarian cancer in the UK (including for women at high risk of the disease) because no test has been identified to reliably pick up ovarian cancer at an early stage. The UK Collaborative Trial of Ovarian Cancer Screening aimed to establish the effect of early detection of the disease by screening on ovarian cancer mortality. The preliminary study recruited over 200 000 women aged between 50 and 74 years and randomised them to either a control arm or one of two screening strategies: primary screening using measurement of serum CA-125 levels followed by TVUS as a second-line test; or TVUS alone. The two screening procedures were found to be similar in terms of sensitivity for all primary ovarian and fallopian tube cancers, but specificity was higher with combined screening.

Some genetic mutations are known to predispose women to ovarian cancer, e.g. *BRCA1* and *BRCA2* and the mismatch repair genes associated with Lynch syndrome families. *BRCA1* mutations confer a 39% lifetime risk of ovarian cancer up to the age of 70 years; this is 11–17% for *BRCA2* mutations up to the age of 70 years. The mismatch repair genes confer an increased lifetime risk of ovarian cancer of 9–12% in addition to the increased risk of endometrial cancer. Referral to a specialist cancer genetics service is advisable. Women at high risk of ovarian cancer may be offered risk-reducing surgery in the form of prophylactic bilateral salpingo-oophorectomy,

Joe Vincent Meigs, 1892–1964, gynaecological surgeon, Massachusetts General Hospital, Boston, MA, USA.

especially as they may also be at increased risk of breast cancer with some evidence suggesting that an oophorectomy can reduce the risk of breast cancer in these women.

Surgical staging of ovarian cancer (*Table 87.15*) is performed at laparotomy via a midline incision if disease is suspected preoperatively by:

- careful evaluation of all peritoneal surfaces;
- four washings of the peritoneal cavity: diaphragm, right and left abdomen, pelvis;
- infracolic omentectomy;
- selected lymphadenectomy of the pelvic and para-aortic lymph nodes;
- biopsy and/or resection of suspicious lesions, masses and adhesions;
- random blind biopsies of normal peritoneal surfaces, including that from the undersurface of the right hemidiaphragm, bladder reflection, cul-de-sac, right and left paracolic recesses and both pelvic side walls;
- total abdominal hysterectomy and bilateral salpingo-oophorectomy;
- appendicectomy for mucinous tumours; if a routine appendicectomy results in an intraoperative suspicion of a mucinous tumour, the surgeon should take washings and a biopsy from suspicious area(s).

TABLE 87.15 Condensed staging of ovarian cancer.

Stage I	Growth limited to the ovaries
Stage II	Growth involving one or both ovaries with pelvic extension (uterus, bladder, sigmoid colon, rectum) or primary peritoneal cancer but not including the lymph nodes
Stage III	Tumour involving one or both ovaries with histologically confirmed peritoneal implants outside of the pelvis including spread to retroperitoneal lymph nodes (pelvic and/or para-aortic) only
Stage IV	Growth involving one or both ovaries with distant metastases

The general principle is cytoreductive surgery followed by combination chemotherapy; only a minority of patients with ovarian cancer require a bowel resection during the primary procedure or surgery for recurrent disease. The only exception to this rule is a young woman with stage I disease or a borderline tumour who requests a unilateral oophorectomy to conserve her fertility.

Fertility preservation in the form of controlled ovarian stimulation with oocyte or embryo cryopreservation has been undertaken in patients with low-grade tumours (grade IA/B) who wish to preserve their fertility; however, the effect of this on the underlying disease process is not known, with the additional risk of seeding the cancer during oocyte retrieval. This must, therefore, be carried out with caution and under the guidance of oncological specialists. Ovarian tissue cryopreservation at the time of cytoreductive surgery has also been undertaken, holding the promise for *in vitro* maturation of oocytes in the future. Autologous transplantation would be contraindicated as it has the risk of cancer recurrence.

FURTHER READING

British Association for Sexual Health and HIV. *UK national guideline for the management of pelvic inflammatory disease.* Macclesfield, UK: BASHH, 2011. Available from https://www.bashh.org/documents/3572.pdf.

European Society of Human Reproduction and Embryology (ESHRE). Guideline on the management of women with endometriosis. Available from https://www.eshre.eu/Guidelines-and-Legal/Guidelines/Endometriosis-guideline.aspx.

National Institute for Health and Care Excellence. *Guidance on ectopic pregnancy and miscarriage: diagnosis and initial management.* NICE Guideline 126. London: NICE, last updated, 2021. Available from https://www.nice.org.uk/guidance/ng126.

National Institute for Health and Care Excellence. *Guidance on heavy menstrual bleeding: assessment and management.* NICE Guideline 88. London: NICE, last updated, 2021. Available from https://www.nice.org.uk/guidance/ng88.

NHS Cervical Screening Programme. Available from https://www.gov.uk/guidance/cervical-screening-programme-overview.

Prat J, FIGO Committee on Gynaecologic Oncology. Staging classification for cancer of the ovary, fallopian tube, and peritoneum. *Int J Gynaecol Obstet* 2014; **124**(1): 1–5.

Royal College of Obstetricians and Gynaecologists. *Green-top guidelines on ovarian cysts in postmenopausal women.* Green-top Guideline no. 34. London: RCOG, 2017. Available from http://www.rcog.org.uk/en/guidelines-research-services/guidelines/gtg34/.

Royal College of Obstetricians and Gynaecologists. *Green-top guidelines on management of suspected ovarian masses in premenopausal women.* Green-top Guideline no. 62. London: RCOG, 2014. Available from http://www.rcog.org.uk/en/guidelines-research-services/guidelines/gtg62/.

Scottish Intercollegiate Guidelines Network. *Management of epithelial ovarian cancer.* SIGN 135. Edinburgh: SIGN, 2018. Available from https://www.sign.ac.uk/media/1073/sign135_oct2018.pdf.

CHAPTER 88 Kidney transplantation and the principles of transplantation

Learning objectives

To recognise and understand:

- The immunological basis of allograft rejection
- The principles of immunosuppressive therapy
- The side effects of immunosuppressive therapy
- The major issues concerning organ donation
- The main indications for organ transplantation
- The surgical principles of organ transplantation
- The expected outcomes after transplantation
- The potential future developments in transplantation

INTRODUCTION

Successful solid organ transplantation represents one of the great medical advances of the twentieth century. The field continues to be an exciting and fast-moving one. Unfortunately, there continues to be a shortage of suitable donor organs for transplantation. In the UK there are approximately 4000 patients waiting for a kidney but only 3750 transplants are performed annually. This has led to a median waiting time for transplantation of around 3 years. Similar shortages exist for heart, lung, liver and pancreas transplantation across the world. Most transplant organs are from deceased donors, of which there are two types: donation after brainstem death (DBD) and donation after circulatory death (DCD). Living donation is limited to kidney, liver and lung transplantation.

ORGAN DONATION

Donation after brainstem death

Brainstem death occurs after severe brain injury as a result of either trauma or a cerebrovascular accident. Potential DBD donors are in an apnoeic coma that requires mechanical ventilation on the intensive care unit (ICU). There must be a known cause of irreversible brain damage demonstrated by a computerised tomography (CT) scan. Brainstem death is defined as the permanent loss of the capacity for consciousness and spontaneous breathing. These two essential functions are controlled by the brainstem. The reticular activating formation controls consciousness and is diffuse throughout the brainstem; the respiratory centre is in the medulla oblongata.

In this situation the circulation can be maintained for a period of time after death and DBD donors were formerly called heart-beating donors. In most countries it is accepted that brainstem death equates in medical, legal and religious terms to the death of the patient.

Before brainstem death testing can be considered, all reversible causes of coma must be excluded. These include: hypothermia, muscle relaxants, drugs with central nervous system depressive effects, alcohol intoxication, hypothyroidism, uraemic encephalopathy, hepatic encephalopathy, hypoglycaemia and hyponatraemia. When these preconditions are met then formal brainstem death testing can be undertaken (***Table 88.1***).

The UK guidelines state that the tests should be performed twice by two clinicians who are independent of the transplant team. One of them should be a consultant and the other must have been registered with the General Medical Council for at least 5 years.

TABLE 88.1 Clinical testing for brainstem death.

Cranial nerve reflexes	**1.** Pupillary reflex (cranial nerves II and III) **2.** Corneal reflex (cranial nerves V_1 and VII) **3.** Oculocephalic (doll's eyes movements – cranial nerves III, IV and VI) **4.** Vestibulo-ocular (cranial nerves VIII, III and VI) **5.** Cough/gag reflex (cranial nerves IX and X) **6.** It is not possible to test cranial nerves I and XII in unconscious individuals
Motor response	Absence of cranial nerve motor response to supraorbital pressure (cranial nerves V and VII) and absence of motor response in the cranial nerve distribution to adequate stimulation of any somatic area (commonly nail-bed pressure)
Apnoea test	After preoxygenation with 100% oxygen the patient is disconnected from the ventilator for >5 minutes in order to achieve a $PaCO_2$ ≥6.0 kPa (and pH<7.4). If there are no respiratory movements in response to the progressive hypercarbia then the test confirms that the brainstem respiratory centre has been destroyed. To prevent hypoxia during the apnoeic period, O_2 (6 L/min) is delivered via an endotracheal catheter

$PaCO_2$, partial pressure of carbon dioxide.

In DBD donors the organs continue to be perfused with oxygenated blood during the procurement surgery. The thoracic and abdominal organs are accessed through a median sternotomy and a midline laparotomy incision and their inflow vessels are cannulated. The organs to be recovered are usually dissected and mobilised with the heart beating. Ice-cold cardioplegia solution is then perfused into the coronary arteries via a cannula in the ascending aorta to stop the heart. At the same time the abdominal organs are perfused with ice-cold preservation solution via cannulae in the abdominal aorta and the portal vein. Each organ is removed and stored in fresh preservation solution and then packed in crushed ice for transport.

Donation after circulatory death

Donation after circulatory death describes the recovery of organs for transplantation after death confirmed by circulatory criteria. These donors were formerly called asystolic or non-heart-beating donors. There have been very significant increases in DCD programmes in many countries over the last decade. The modified Maastricht classification is widely used to categorise DCD (***Table 88.2***). Organ donation after unexpected and irreversible cardiac arrest is referred to as uncontrolled DCD. Donation after death resulting from the planned withdrawal of life-sustaining cardiorespiratory support is called controlled DCD.

In DCD donors cardiorespiratory arrest occurs prior to starting organ retrieval. The organs are therefore warm but not being perfused with oxygenated blood for a period of time before they are flushed with cold preservation solution. This warm ischaemia period should be limited as much as possible.

Controlled DCD donors are ICU-based and have suffered massive and irreversible cerebral damage but have an intact brainstem so that they are self-ventilating. In a situation where further attempts at treatment would be futile, the withdrawal of supportive treatment inevitably leads to cardiorespiratory arrest, and this usually occurs within a short time. In the UK, after cardiac arrest there is a mandatory 'no-touch' period of 5 minutes. This is deemed to be the time beyond which there is irreversible loss of cardiac and cerebral function. The donor is transferred from ICU to the operating department and a rapid median sternotomy and midline laparotomy are performed. The ascending aorta and abdominal aorta are cannulated and the organs are perfused with ice-cold preservation fluid *in situ* without any initial dissection. The warm ischaemic period is usually less than 10 minutes. Organ procurement is then carried out in standard fashion.

Uncontrolled DCD donors have usually suffered an unexpected and irrecoverable cardiac event either outside or inside hospital. After a period of attempted, but failed, cardiopulmonary resuscitation (CPR) and observation of the 5-minute rule, CPR with administration of high-concentration oxygen is recommenced, often using a mechanical resuscitation device. *In situ* renal cooling is performed by placing a double-balloon, triple-lumen perfusion catheter into the aorta via a femoral artery cut-down (***Figure 88.1***). The donor can then be transferred to the operating theatre and the kidneys are removed using standard techniques. Uncontrolled DCD donation is usually reserved for the kidneys only as they are able to recover from warm ischaemic periods of up to 45 minutes.

TABLE 88.2 Modified Maastricht classification of donation after circulatory death (DCD).

Category	Description	Type of DCD	Location
I	Dead on arrival at hospital	Uncontrolled	ED
II	Unsuccessful resuscitation after cardiac arrest	Uncontrolled	ED
III	Anticipated cardiac arrest after withdrawal of support	Controlled	ICU
IV	Cardiac arrest in brain-dead donor	Controlled	ICU
V	Unexpected cardiac arrest in ICU	Uncontrolled	ICU

ED, emergency department; ICU, intensive care unit.

Evaluation of the deceased donor

The absolute contraindications to organ donation include active systemic sepsis and transmissible infection. Malignancy within the last 5 years is also an absolute contraindication with the exception of tumours that do not metastasise (primary brain tumours, non-melanotic skin cancer and *in situ* carcinoma of the cervix). However, there is now evidence that organs from high-risk donors can be transplanted safely and

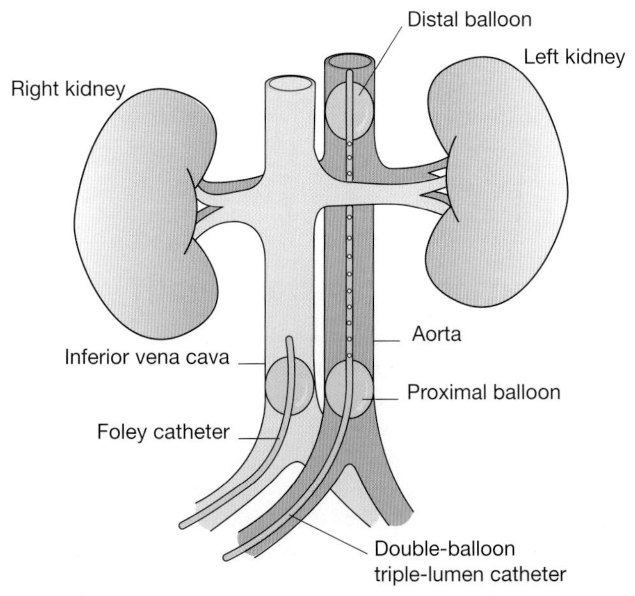

Figure 88.1 *In situ* perfusion of kidneys in a non-heart-beating donor (donation after circulatory death [DCD]). A double-balloon aortic catheter is introduced through a groin incision and 10–15 litres of chilled preservation solution is administered. The perfusate is vented through a Foley catheter introduced into the femoral vein.

Frederic Eugene Basil Foley, 1891–1966, urologist, Ancker Hospital, St Paul, MN, USA.

yield transplant outcomes that are equivalent to those from conventional donors. Thus, as a further response to the organ donor shortage, organs are now being transplanted from donors with meningitis/encephalitis, human immunodeficiency virus (HIV), hepatitis B and C and high-risk behaviour with the potential for blood-borne infection.

Living donation

Living kidney donation is possible because most individuals have two healthy kidneys and it is possible to live a normal life with a single kidney. Parts of non-paired organs can also be removed from live donors; these include liver and lung lobes, the tail of the pancreas and segments of small intestine.

The majority of liver transplants performed in India are from live donors and the number of programmes has expanded rapidly in recent years. The liver has the capacity to regenerate following resection of a segment or lobe. The growth of new liver tissue happens quickly and the liver returns to its pre-resectional mass. Liver resection is difficult because of the complex segmental anatomy (***Figure 88.2***). In children, the left lateral segment (segments II and III) of an adult provides enough liver function and this is a relatively straightforward procedure. In adult-to-adult live donor liver transplantation the whole right lobe of the liver is removed from the donor (segments V–VIII). This is a more complex operation and the risk of donor mortality is 0.5–1%.

Transplants from live donors have a number of advantages over deceased donor organs. Live donor organs are from healthy individuals without the comorbidities commonly seen in deceased donors. In the agonal period before death deceased donors exhibit marked changes in physiology related to a catecholamine storm and this can cause organ dysfunction. Clearly, live donor organs are not subjected to this insult. Potential live donors undergo a rigorous assessment process that includes imaging of the relevant vasculature by CT or magnetic resonance angiography (MRA) and tests of organ functional capacity. The operations are planned elective procedures undertaken in daylight hours and often adjacent theatres so that the cold ischaemia time is very short. It is usual for live donor organs to function immediately after transplantation and this is essential for liver and lung transplants. As a result of these advantages the long-term outcomes of live donor transplantation are superior to deceased donor outcomes.

Set against these advantages for the recipient is the fact that the live donor is subjected to a major operation that they do not need. All live donor operations have uncommon but potentially life-threatening morbidity rates and there is a small risk of death. The ethical issues raised by live donation are understandably complex.

ORGAN PRESERVATION

Transplant organs need to be stored and preserved in the period between procurement from the donor and transplantation into the recipient. Static cold storage is the traditional method of organ preservation, but more recently there have been developments in preservation by machine perfusion.

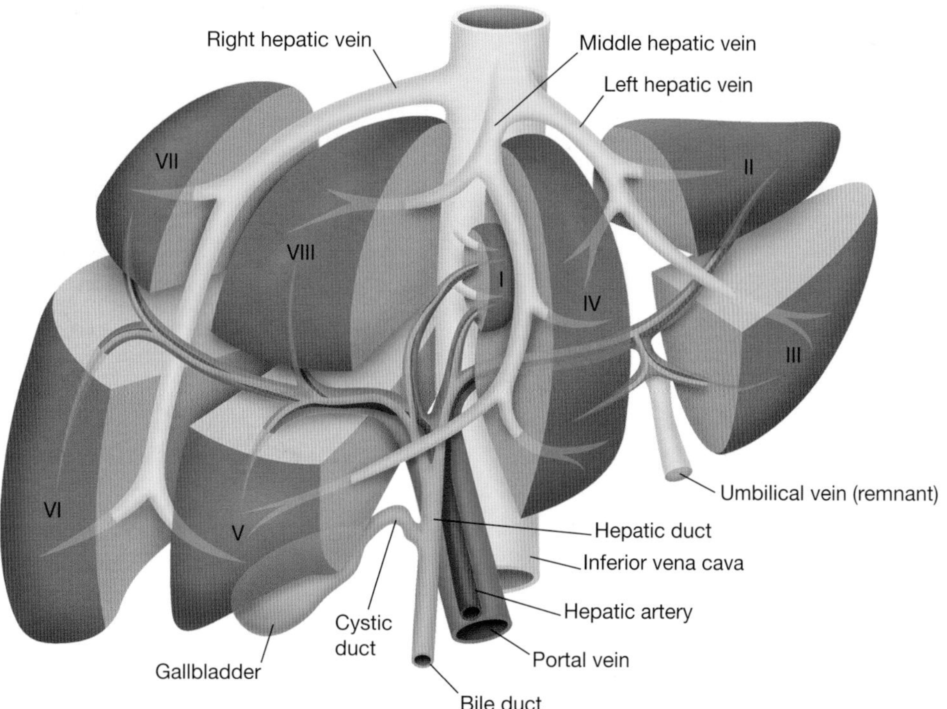

Figure 88.2 Segmental anatomy of the liver (Couinaud segments).

Claude Couinaud, 1922–2008, French surgeon and anatomist, described the segmental anatomy of the liver in his seminal book *Le Foie: Études anatomiques et chirurgicales*.

Pathophysiology of ischaemia

In the absence of oxygen, organs switch from aerobic to anaerobic metabolism. The mitochondrial electron transport chain cannot function without oxygen as the final electron acceptor. Oxidative phosphorylation ceases and, in consequence, so does the tricarboxylic acid (Krebs) cycle and the link reaction (conversion of pyruvate to acetyl coenzyme A). This leaves glycolysis as the only source of adenosine triphosphate (ATP). Anaerobic metabolism of one glucose molecule produces only two ATP molecules compared with the 36 ATP molecules that are produced during aerobic metabolism. Consumption of ATP rapidly exceeds production, leading to depletion of cellular ATP. Na^+/K^+ ATPase pumps are disabled and this leads to an influx of Na^+ ions into the cell down their concentration gradient. Na^+ ions are followed by H_2O by osmosis and this causes swelling and disruption of membrane-bound intracellular organelles and lysis of the cell membrane. Anaerobic glycolysis generates lactate and promotes intracellular acidosis. At low pH phospholipase and protease enzymes are activated and cause lysosomal damage and eventually cell death. ATP-dependent active transport of calcium out of cells is impeded, leading to the intracellular accumulation of Ca^{2+} ions and activation of the calcium-dependent processes. This leads to breakdown of the cytoskeleton and loss of cell structure.

Static cold storage

Hypothermia suppresses metabolism to maintain organ viability. The first requirement is to flush the donor organs with an appropriate preservation solution at a temperature of approximately 4°C (***Figure 88.3***). This is normally done *in situ* via cannulae placed in the donor aorta and portal vein. This process has three effects: (i) it flushes blood out of the microcirculation to prevent thrombosis; (ii) it cools the organs to a temperature of <5°C and so reduces tissue oxygen requirements; (iii) it replaces the normal extracellular fluid with the preservation fluid.

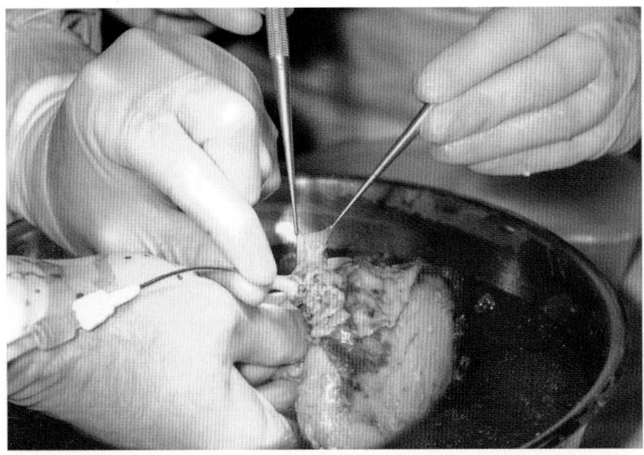

Figure 88.3 After removal from the donor, the kidney is flushed with chilled organ preservation solution and, if necessary, stored briefly on ice until transplanted into the recipient.

Preservation solutions have three main components: electrolytes, an impermeant and a buffer. In general, the electrolyte composition mimics the high K^+ ion concentration and low Na^+ ion concentration of intracellular fluid. This eliminates ionic fluxes, and therefore the movement of H_2O across cell membranes. Impermeants such as mannitol, lactobionate and raffinose are large osmotically active molecules. They cannot pass through the cell membrane and remain in the extracellular space. Here, they prevent cellular swelling by counteracting the osmotic force from intracellular proteins. The buffer component of preservation fluids is based on either HCO_3^- or PO_4^{3-} and acts to maintain a stable physiological pH in the extracellular space. A number of different preservation solutions are available, but the University of Wisconsin (UW) solution is widely regarded as the current gold standard.

Hypothermic machine perfusion

The transplant organ is placed in a sterile chamber and cold preservation fluid is continually recirculated through the vasculature at low temperature and pressure (30 mmHg) (***Figure 88.4***). The perfusion fluid is based on UW solution and some systems include oxygenation. This technique flushes the microcirculation more effectively. There are trial and meta-analysis data showing that hypothermic machine perfusion reduces the rate of delayed graft function (DGF) in renal transplantation, but the effect size is small.

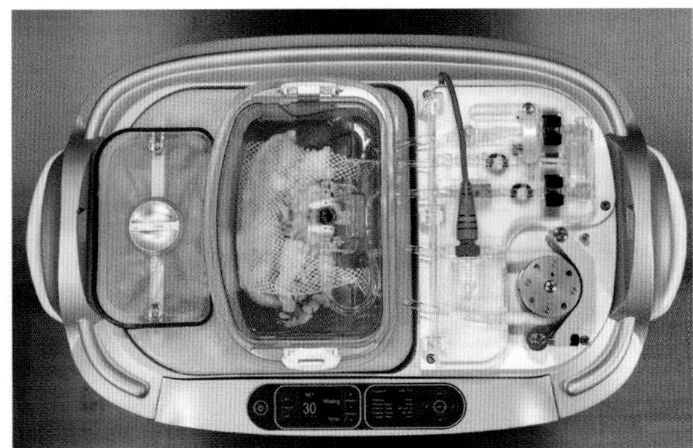

Figure 88.4 The LifePort® hypothermic perfusion machine (LifePort® Kidney Transporter courtesy of Organ Recovery Systems).

Normothermic machine perfusion

Normothermic machine perfusion (NMP) utilises the principles of cardiopulmonary bypass technology and has been used for heart, lung, liver and kidney preservation. Warmed and oxygenated red blood cell-based perfusate is circulated through the donor organ (***Figure 88.5***). This provides a more physiological environment that restores graft function *ex vivo* and replenishes depleted ATP levels. NMP restores organ function *ex vivo* and this allows for assessment of allograft quality and viability. This has led to increased utility of marginal organs that would previously have been discarded on the basis of adverse clinical parameters. NMP may also improve early

Sir Hans Adolf Krebs, 1900–1981, Professor of Biochemistry, University of Oxford, Oxford, UK.

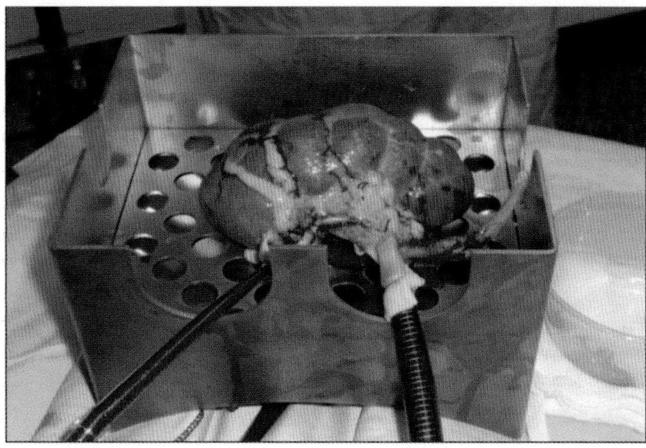

Figure 88.5 Donor kidney undergoing normothermic machine perfusion.

allograft function and is being developed as a platform for the delivery of pretransplant therapies.

Normothermic regional perfusion

This technique has been developed for donation after circulatory arrest. A cardiopulmonary bypass system is used to recirculate the donor's own blood through the thoracic and abdominal organs for 2 hours. The underlying principle is to avoid early cold ischaemia injury. The early experience of normothermic regional perfusion in DCD liver preservation and transplantation shows reduced rates of early allograft dysfunction.

IMMUNOLOGY OF TRANSPLANT REJECTION

ABO blood groups

ABO blood group antigens are glycoproteins with different carbohydrate components. ABO antigens are expressed not only on the surface of red blood cells but also on endothelial cells. In all organ transplants there must therefore be ABO blood group compatibility between the recipient and the donor organ, using the same rules for blood transfusion (***Table 88.3***).

TABLE 88.3 Blood group compatibility.

Donor blood group	Permissible recipients
O (universal donor)	O, A, B and AB
A	A and AB
B	B and AB
AB (universal recipient)	AB

HLA matching

Allograft rejection is directed against human leukocyte antigens (HLAs). These are a group of cell surface glycoprotein molecules. HLA molecules are divided into class I (A, B and C) and class II (DR, DP and DQ). Class I molecules are expressed on the surface of all nucleated cells, but class II are only expressed by antigen-presenting cells (APCs) such as dendritic cells and B lymphocytes. HLA molecules are encoded for in the major histocompatibility complex (MHC) on chromosome 6. They are highly polymorphic, i.e. their amino acid sequences differ widely between individuals. To give an example, there are >1000 variants of the HLA-B gene. This genetic variability means that most transplant donors and recipients have different HLA profiles. Donors and transplant recipients are HLA-typed using DNA sequencing. The antigens at HLA-A, -B and -DR are together described as the tissue type.

The level of mismatch between the HLA molecules determines the strength of the immune response. Every individual has two copies of each HLA gene and so for each locus (A, B or DR) it is possible to have 0, 1 or 2 mismatched genes. As the number of mismatches increases so does the chance of immune recognition and rejection. The best matched grafts are described as having a mismatch of 0–0–0, i.e. no mismatches at A, B or DR, respectively. A completely mismatched graft would be annotated as a 2–2–2 mismatch. The effects of the different HLA antigens are not uniform. DR mismatches have a more powerful effect than B mismatches, and A mismatches are the least important. The tissue types of potential renal transplant recipients are held by national organisations, such as NHS Blood and Transplant in the UK, and used to allocate donor organs to patients with the lowest level of HLA mismatch.

The immune response to a transplanted organ

The main immune cells involved in transplant immunology are APCs and T and B lymphocytes. These cell types interact by a series of specific surface molecules that are designated by CD (cluster of differentiation) numbers. Cell surface receptors can only interact if they have the correct complementary three-dimensional structures.

The immune response to an allograft is orchestrated by T lymphocytes. When T cells encounter foreign transplant HLA antigens they become activated and then proliferate into clones of cells that attack the allograft. Full T-cell activation requires a number of signals (***Figure 88.6***). Transplant antigen

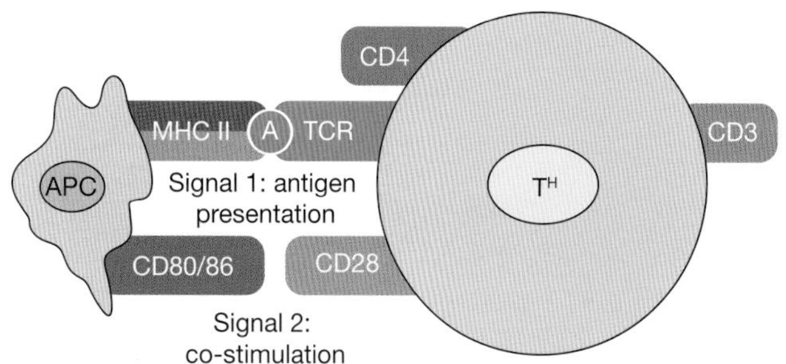

Figure 88.6 Interaction between an antigen-presenting cell and a CD4+ T-helper cell. A, antigen; APC, antigen-presenting cell; CD, cluster of differentiation; MHC II, major histocompatibility complex class II; TCR, T-cell receptor; T^H, T-helper cell. (Adapted with permission from Clatworthy M, Watson C, Allison M, Dark J. *Transplantation at a glance*. John Wiley and Sons Ltd, 2012.)

is presented to T-helper cells (CD4+) on self-MHC class II molecules by specialised APCs. The class II/peptide antigen complex is recognised by the T-cell receptor (signal 1). CD4+ T-helper cell activation also requires a co-stimulatory signal involving the interaction of pairs of molecules, one on the surface of the T cell and the other on the surface of the APC (signal 2). An example of signal 2 is the interaction of T-cell CD28 with CD80 on the APC. When both signal 1 and signal 2 are received the CD4+ T-helper cell will upregulate expression of the interleukin-2 (IL-2) receptor (CD25) on its cell surface. Binding of IL-2 to its receptor causes further activation of the T cell (signal 3). The T cell will then proliferate and release more IL-2, which, in turn, leads to activation and clonal proliferation of T-killer cells (CD8+). These cytotoxic killer cells infiltrate the allograft and cause cell death by the release of molecules called perforin and granzyme. Perforin punches holes in the target cell membrane and this allows passive diffusion of granzyme into the cell, where it activates caspase enzymes and causes cell death by apoptosis.

Antigen presentation in transplantation

There are two main types of antigen presentation to T lymphocytes (*Figure 88.7*). Direct antigen presentation involves donor APCs showing intact and unprocessed donor HLA (class I or class II) molecules on their cell surface to recipient T cells. In contrast, indirect presentation is performed by recipient APCs. These internalise foreign donor HLA molecules from the graft, process them into short peptide fragments and then load them into the peptide groove of recipient (self) HLA class II molecules. The donor peptide–recipient HLA class II complex is then expressed on the cell surface and presented to recipient T cells. Direct antigen presentation only occurs for the first 6–12 weeks after transplantation because this is the lifespan of the donor passenger APCs that are present in the allograft. As indirect presentation involves recipient APCs it is a long-lived response.

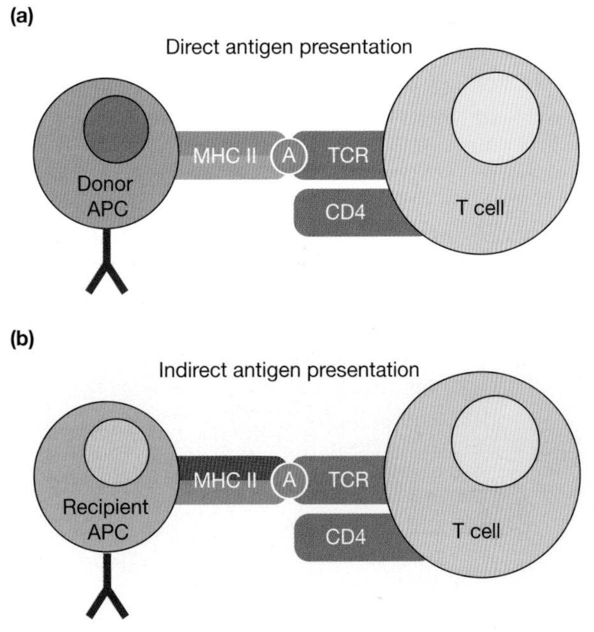

Figure 88.7 Direct (a) and indirect (b) antigen presentation. A, antigen; APC, antigen-presenting cell; CD, cluster of differentiation; MHC II, major histocompatibility complex class II; TCR, T-cell receptor. (Adapted with permission from Clatworthy M, Watson C, Allison M, Dark J. *Transplantation at a glance*. John Wiley and Sons Ltd, 2012.)

TRANSPLANT REJECTION

Allograft rejection can be divided into distinct types.

Hyperacute rejection

Hyperacute rejection is extremely rare. It can result from an inadvertent ABO blood group-incompatible transplantation after a clerical error in recording blood groups. It may also occur when there are preformed circulating donor-specific HLA antibodies (DSA) or ABO antibodies. In either case, immediately after revascularisation of the transplant antibodies will bind to ABO or HLA antigens on the surface of the graft vascular endothelial cells. The antibodies are complement fixing and this leads to activation of the complement cascade and phagocytes. This leads to endothelial damage with release of tissue factor and activation of the clotting cascade. Widespread intravascular thrombosis causes infarction of the allograft within minutes or hours. This is untreatable and inevitably results in graft loss.

Acute cell-mediated rejection

In the era of modern immunosuppressive drugs, the incidence of acute cell-mediated rejection (CMR) is only 10–20%. Acute CMR is largely mediated by direct antigen presentation. As donor APCs in the allograft have a lifespan of only a few weeks, the peak incidence of acute CMR is in the first 3 months post transplantation. The characteristic biopsy finding of acute CMR is a marked interstitial lymphocytic infiltrate (*Figure 88.8*). In the kidney, the presence of lymphocytes inside the basement membrane of the renal tubular epithelium is referred to as tubulitis and is diagnostic of acute CMR. Initial treatment is by high-dose pulsed intravenous steroids (methylprednisolone 0.5 g intravenously for 3 days), which is

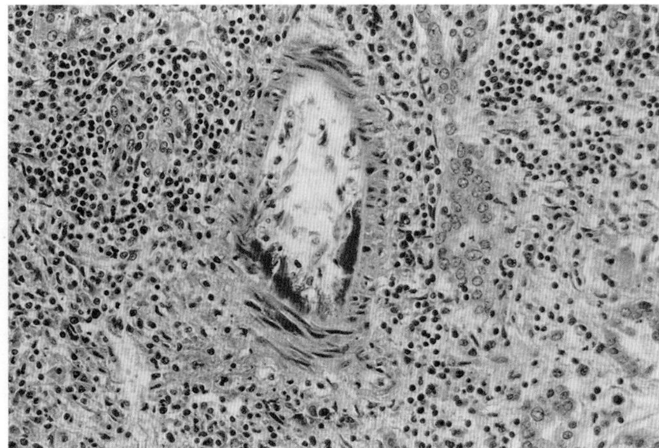

Figure 88.8 Severe acute renal allograft rejection with a heavy mononuclear cell infiltrate and intimal arteritis.

successful in up to 90% of cases. Severe or steroid-resistant rejection is treated with lymphocyte-depleting intravenous antithymocyte globulin (ATG).

Acute antibody-mediated rejection

Acute antibody-mediated rejection (AMR) occurs in <5% of renal transplants but is more serious and more difficult to treat than cell-mediated rejection. It is caused by HLA DSA, which are produced by a sensitising episode from a previous transplant, a blood transfusion or pregnancy. Binding of DSA to mismatched HLA antigens on the surface of allograft endothelial cells leads to activation of the complement system and tissue injury. In the kidney, transplant biopsy will show inflammation of the vessels (vasculitis) and deposition of the complement component C4d in the peritubular capillaries (***Figure 88.9***). Treatment is by plasma exchange to remove circulating antibodies. Rituximab, an anti-CD20 monoclonal antibody, can also be used to destroy B cells and prevent further production of DSA.

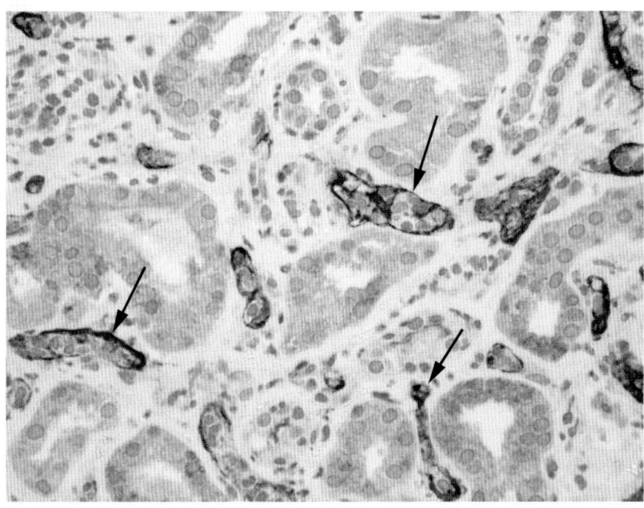

Figure 88.9 Acute antibody-mediated renal allograft rejection. There is widespread staining for the complement component C4d within the peritubular capillaries (arrows), which indicates alloantibody binding to the graft vasculature.

Chronic antibody-mediated rejection

The pathophysiology is not well understood but the long-lived indirect antigen presentation pathway is likely to be important. CD4 T-cell activation also promotes donor-specific alloantibody production, and this causes ongoing allograft damage.

IMMUNOSUPPRESSION

Modern immunosuppression is so effective that acute rejection rates of 10–20% can be achieved in all types of solid organ transplantation. The challenge is to deliver sufficient immunosuppression to prevent rejection while minimising drug side effects. Immunosuppression also increases the risk of both infection and malignancy. This is a non-specific effect related to the total burden of immunosuppression rather than agent-specific side effects.

The mechanisms of action of current immunosuppressive drugs depend on anti-inflammatory effects and the prevention of lymphocyte activation and proliferation (***Figure 88.10***). Lymphocytes are some of the most rapidly dividing cells in the body and their activation and clonal expansion forms the immunological basis of acute allograft rejection.

Immunosuppression for transplantation has two phases: induction and maintenance. Induction therapy commonly consists of a combination of high-dose intravenous steroids and the anti-CD25 monoclonal antibody basiliximab, which blocks IL-2 receptors. Other induction agents for high-risk cases are ATG and the monoclonal antibody alemtuzumab (Campath).

The commonest maintenance immunosuppressive regimen for solid organ transplants consists of triple therapy with a calcineurin inhibitor (ciclosporin or tacrolimus), an antiproliferative agent (azathioprine or mycophenolic acid) and steroids.

Calcineurin inhibitors (ciclosporin and tacrolimus)

The calcineurin inhibitors (CNIs) are the mainstay of modern immunosuppressive regimens. CNIs prevent transcription of the IL-2 gene in T cells. As IL-2 is the main T-cell growth factor, inhibition of its production prevents T-cell proliferation.

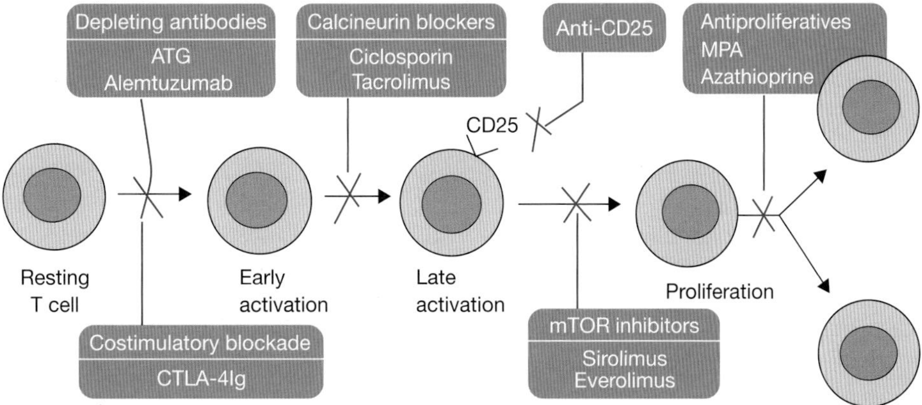

Figure 88.10 Site of action of immunosuppressive agents on T cell. ATG, antithymocyte globulin; CTLA-4Ig, cytotoxic T-lymphocyte-associated protein 4 immunoglobulin; MPA, mycophenolic acid derivatives; mTOR, mammalian target of rapamycin.

The main side effect of both ciclosporin and tacrolimus is nephrotoxicity. CNIs have a narrow therapeutic index (a small difference between the minimum effective concentration and the minimum toxic concentration). CNI dosage must therefore be guided by monitoring drug blood levels.

Antiproliferative agents (azathioprine and mycophenolic acid)

These drugs are antiproliferative agents. Their mechanism of action is to block purine nucleotide synthesis. This prevents replication of DNA and thus interferes with lymphocyte proliferation. The main side effects of both drugs are bone marrow suppression (anaemia, leukopenia, thrombocytopenia) and gastrointestinal symptoms (nausea, vomiting and diarrhoea).

Corticosteroids

These are potent anti-inflammatory agents that have wide-ranging effects on the immune system. Prolonged exposure to steroids causes numerous potential side effects, including: a Cushingoid appearance with a moon face, central obesity, abdominal striae and proximal myopathy; thin skin that bruises easily; hypertension; glucose intolerance that may lead to new-onset diabetes mellitus; osteoporosis; and peptic ulcer disease. These may be minimised by rapid reduction or withdrawal of steroids.

Mammalian target of rapamycin (mTOR) inhibitors

The mTOR inhibitors rapamycin and everolimus act by binding to and inhibiting a cytoplasmic kinase enzyme complex called mTOR. This prevents intracellular signalling from the IL-2 receptor. The downstream effect is arrest of T-cell division at the G1–S phase. The cell cycle effects of mTOR inhibitors are not limited to lymphocytes and their side-effect profile includes severe mouth ulceration, poor wound healing and lymphocele formation. This limits the use of mTOR inhibitors in the first few weeks post transplantation. However, mTOR inhibitors are not nephrotoxic and they may be used 3 months or more after transplantation as an alternative to CNIs to minimise CNI-associated renal dysfunction.

KIDNEY TRANSPLANTATION

End-stage renal disease

The incidence of end-stage renal disease (ESRD) in the UK is approximately 120 per million population and around 8000 people require renal replacement therapy annually. The leading causes of ESRD are diabetes, hypertension and chronic glomerulonephritis (*Summary box 88.1*). ESRD is largely a disease of older adults with the mean age at commencement of renal replacement therapy being 64 years.

Summary box 88.1

Common causes of ESRD

- Chronic glomerulonephritis
- Diabetic nephropathy
- Hypertension
- Renal vascular disease
- Polycystic kidney disease
- Chronic pyelonephritis
- Obstructive uropathy

Rationale for kidney transplantation

Kidney transplantation improves life expectancy and quality of life when compared with dialysis. However, only approximately one-third of patients with ESRD are fit enough to withstand transplant surgery and long-term immunosuppression. Successful transplantation frees patients from the rigors of dialysis and eliminates uraemic symptoms. Transplant kidneys produce normal levels of erythropoietin and this reverses the anaemia of chronic renal disease. Transplant patients therefore have more energy and better exercise capacity than patients on dialysis. There are also no fluid or dietary restrictions after transplantation. Importantly, for women of child-bearing age pregnancy is also possible after a successful kidney transplant. Life expectancy is higher in the transplant population with 5-year survival of >85% compared with <50% for patients on dialysis. However, these figures cannot be directly compared as there is selection bias because only relatively fit patients are offered transplantation.

Selection of patients for transplantation

Potential transplant recipients undergo a rigorous work-up process to identify major comorbidities that would preclude transplant surgery. Age per se is not a contraindication to renal transplantation and it is now common to transplant patients in their seventies as long as they have the necessary cardiovascular fitness. Uncontrolled infection and most malignancies are contraindications to transplantation. Patients with ESRD have a greatly increased risk of cardiovascular disease and require a chest radiograph, electrocardiogram (ECG) and, if indicated, an echocardiogram. Patients with a history of diabetes or ischaemic heart disease should undergo a stress echocardiogram and sometimes coronary angiography.

There are a number of technical considerations before a patient is deemed suitable for transplantation. The iliac blood vessels must be suitable for anastomosis and there must be a means of draining the transplant ureter. In patients with a history of vascular disease or deep venous thrombosis, the iliac arterial and venous system should be assessed by Doppler ultrasound scanning and possibly also MRA or CT angiography. Patients who have been anuric for a number of years may have a small non-compliant bladder and this should be assessed by urodynamics. In patients with polycystic kidney disease, the size of the native kidneys should be assessed clinically to make sure that there is sufficient room for a kidney

Harvey Williams Cushing, 1869–1939, Professor of Surgery, Harvard University Medical School, Boston, MA, USA.
Christian Johann Doppler, 1803–1853, Professor of Experimental Physics, Vienna, Austria, enunciated the Doppler principle in 1842.

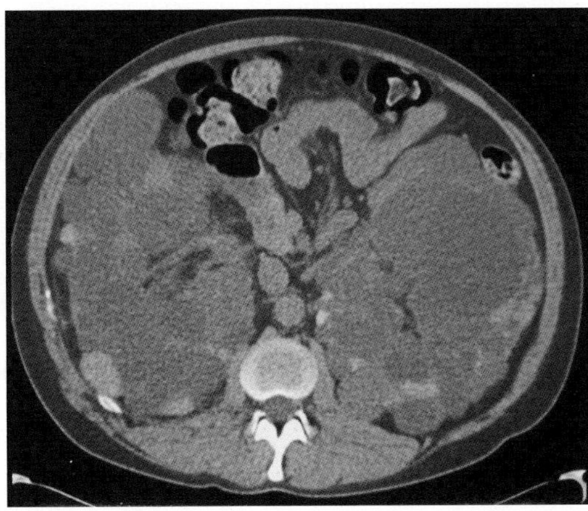

Figure 88.11 Computed tomography scan of a patient with very large polycystic kidneys that extend well into both iliac fossae. The patient requires removal of one of the polycystic kidneys to make room for a subsequent renal transplant. Nephrectomy should be performed several weeks before transplantation.

transplant in at least one iliac fossa. If there is inadequate space on both sides, then a pretransplant native nephrectomy will be necessary (*Figure 88.11*). With the exclusion of non-melanotic skin cancer, patients who have had a malignant disease should be deferred for a disease-free period of at least 2 years. Where possible patients should be listed for transplantation pre-emptively when they are within 6 months of requiring dialysis. This equates to an estimated glomerular filtration rate (eGFR) of 10–15 mL/min/1.73m^2.

RENAL TRANSPLANT SURGERY

Preparation of the donor kidney

The donor kidney must be examined and prepared on the back-table in order to check that it is suitable to be transplanted. Multiple renal arteries are present in up to 25% of kidneys and, if present, may require reconstructive bench surgery to simplify implantation. The renal arteries are end arteries, so it is important whenever possible to preserve all branches (*Figure 88.12*).

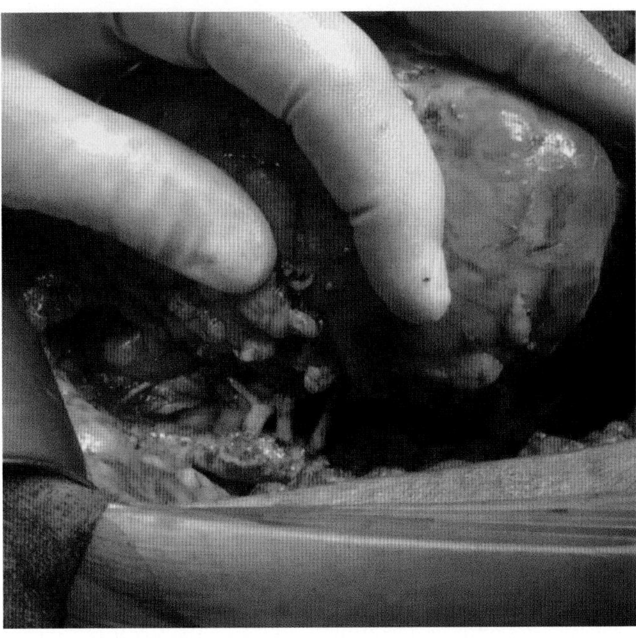

Figure 88.12 Deceased donor renal transplant with three arteries that have been reconstructed using a patch of donor aorta and anastomosed to the external iliac artery.

Renal transplant operative technique

The donor kidney is transplanted heterotopically into one of the iliac fossae via a curvilinear incision. The peritoneum should be kept intact and swept upwards to reveal the iliac vasculature. The transplant renal vein is anastomosed end to side to the external or common iliac vein. The renal artery is anastomosed either end to side to the external or common iliac artery or end to end to the divided internal iliac artery (*Figure 88.13*). The internal iliac artery is used more commonly for live donor kidneys because of the lack of an aortic patch. There are several

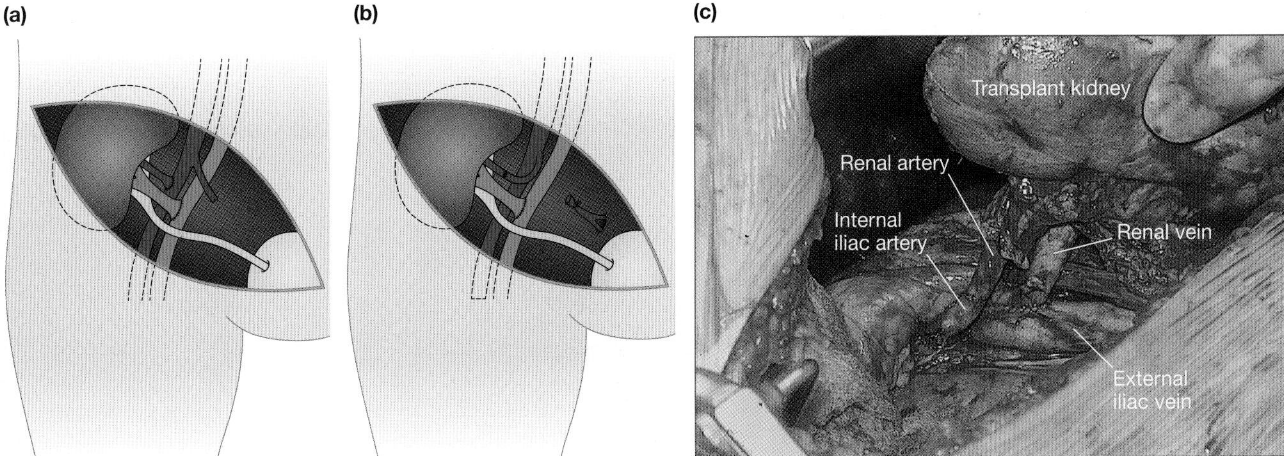

Figure 88.13 Renal allograft implantation techniques. (a) Anastomosis of the renal artery on a donor aortic patch end to side to the external iliac artery. (b) Anastomosis of the renal artery end to end to the divided internal iliac artery. (c) Operative photograph of anastomosis of the renal artery end to end to the internal iliac artery and the renal vein end to side to the external iliac vein.

techniques for anastomosing live donor kidneys with multiple arteries, but it is best to minimise the number of anastomoses by careful bench surgery. For example, equal-sized arteries can be 'trousered' to create a single ostium for anastomosis. Upper or lower polar arteries may also be anastomosed to the divided inferior epigastric artery. It is especially important to anastomose lower polar arteries as these may provide the only blood supply to the ureter. After revascularisation of the transplant kidney the ureter is anastomosed to the bladder as an extravesical onlay (the Lich–Grégoir technique) (*Figure 88.14*). It is now routine practice to place a double-J stent across the ureteric anastomosis. The stent is removed by flexible cystoscopy under local anaesthesia after a few weeks. Before closing the wound it is important to ensure that the kidney is lying in a satisfactory position without kinking of the renal blood vessels.

Dual kidney transplantation

This involves the transplantation of a pair of marginal quality kidneys from the same donor into one recipient in order to provide adequate nephron mass. Both kidneys can be placed in the same iliac fossa. This approach is used for kidneys from elderly DCD donors and so-called expanded criteria donors, which are defined by age >60 years or age >50 years with at least two of the following: hypertension; terminal creatinine >133 μmol/L; death from stroke.

Renal transplantation in children

In children with established renal failure, kidney transplantation facilitates their growth and development and markedly improves the quality of life of the child and their parents. In young children there is often a size mismatch between the donor kidney, which may be from an adult, and the recipient. In this case the kidney is transplanted intraperitoneally with anastomosis of the renal artery to the distal aorta and the renal vein to the inferior vena cava or common iliac vein.

Living donor kidney transplantation

This accounts for approximately 1000 kidney transplants annually in the UK, which is approximately one-third of the total renal transplant programme. Living donors may be related, unrelated, altruistic or part of a donor exchange scheme (for ABO blood group or HLA incompatibility). Potential live donors undergo extensive assessment that includes urine and blood screening tests, chest radiograph, ECG, echocardiography (if indicated) and CT angiography or MRA for the assessment of renal vascular anatomy. Renal function is measured by an accurate isotope GFR technique and must be above evidence-based age- and gender-specific safety thresholds for donation. Following unilateral nephrectomy, there is considerable compensation by the remaining kidney and donors are usually left with 70% of their predonation GFR. The mortality from donor nephrectomy is approximately 1:3000 and major morbidity occurs in <5%. Donation increases the risks of hypertension, renal failure and pregnancy-related complications.

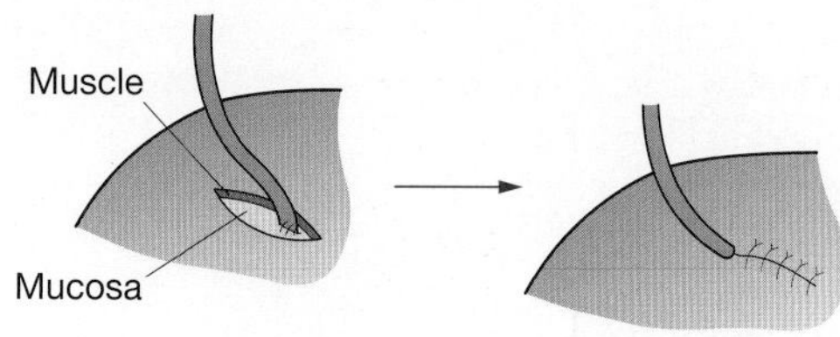

Figure 88.14 Ureteric implantation by direct anastomosis to a small cystotomy: Lich–Grégoir technique.

Minimally invasive donor nephrectomy

Laparoscopic surgery is now widely established and there are a number of techniques. After a fully laparoscopic transperitoneal dissection (*Figure 88.15*), the kidney is removed through a small retrieval incision. Hand-assisted laparoscopic nephrectomy is also used widely. A hand port is used to aid the dissection and for extraction of the kidney. This technique is easier to learn and can be safely performed by surgeons with less laparoscopic experience.

Immunosuppressive regimen for renal transplantation

Immunosuppression for renal transplantation generally comprises induction therapy with the anti-CD25 monoclonal antibody basiliximab followed by a maintenance regimen of a calcineurin inhibitor (most usually tacrolimus), an antiproliferative agent (usually mycophenolic acid) and corticosteroid (prednisolone). The anti-CD52 monoclonal antibody alemtuzumab can be used for induction instead of basiliximab for

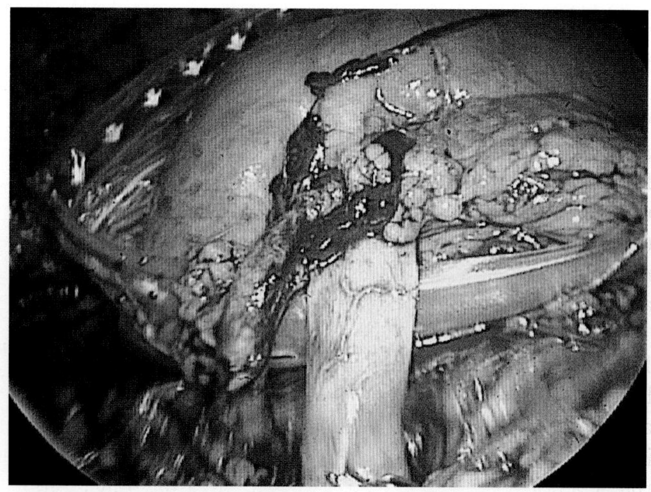

Figure 88.15 Completed laparoscopic dissection of the left kidney, which is ready for stapling of the vessels and removal in an Endocatch bag.

Robert Lich Jr, urologist, Louisville, KY, USA.
Willy Grégoir, Chef de Clinique Urologique, Brussels, Belgium (1962–1987).

patients at high risk of allograft rejection or as part of a steroid avoidance strategy in patients at high risk of developing diabetes post transplantation.

Early postoperative course

Accurate fluid and electrolyte balance are maintained with the help of central venous pressure monitoring. Hyperkalaemia is common in the early post-transplant period, especially in patients with DGF. This should be managed initially with intravenous glucose and insulin but early dialysis is often required. Recovery is straightforward in the majority of renal transplant patients. The bladder catheter is removed on postoperative day 5 and most patients can be discharged on day 6.

Delayed renal allograft function

DGF is defined as the need for dialysis in the first 7 days post transplant. The patient will be oliguric or anuric and the serum creatinine will fail to fall in the early postoperative period. DGF is usually the clinical consequence of acute tubular necrosis related to ischaemia–reperfusion injury. It occurs in around 30% of DBD kidneys and 60% of DCD kidneys because of the significantly longer warm ischaemic period prior to *in situ* organ cooling. In contrast, DGF occurs in <5% of live donor kidneys because of the short cold ischaemic time. An early Doppler ultrasound study should be performed in all patients with DGF to check that the graft is well vascularised. The management of DGF is supportive with haemodialysis, careful fluid balance and avoidance of CNI toxicity. Graft function usually recovers within a few days, but it may take several weeks. Primary non-function is the term used for grafts that never work. This occurs in <5% of renal transplants as a result of either vascular thrombosis or irreversible ischaemic injury leading to cortical necrosis.

Surgical complications of renal transplantation

Haemorrhage

A haematoma may develop in the transplant bed in the first few postoperative days. This is often due to bleeding from small unsecured vessels in the renal hilum that were not apparent at the time of surgery. In this situation the patient is haemodynamically stable and can be investigated by CT angiography and subsequently re-explored to remove the haematoma.

Anastomotic haemorrhage can also occur but is very rare. It presents as haemorrhagic shock associated with a fall in the haemoglobin to <50 g/L. This is a life-threatening situation and the patient should be returned to the operating theatre immediately. It may be possible to repair a defect in an arterial or venous anastomosis but transplant nephrectomy is often required.

Late anastomotic haemorrhage can also occur after some weeks or months owing to the development of a mycotic aneurysm. The commonest causative organism is donor-derived *Candida albicans*. A ruptured mycotic aneurysm requires an immediate graft nephrectomy and has a significant mortality.

Renal artery thrombosis

Although this occurs in <1% of renal transplants, the most common outcome is loss of the allograft. Most cases are due to technical complications at the arterial anastomosis. The usual presentation of renal artery thrombosis is sudden anuria and a rapid decline in renal function. The diagnosis may be missed in patients who have DGF or a normal urine output from their native kidneys. An urgent Doppler ultrasound scan will show an absence of perfusion to the graft. The patient must be returned to the operating theatre immediately to attempt thrombectomy, but most grafts will already be infarcted and transplant nephrectomy will be required.

Renal vein thrombosis

Renal vein thrombosis occurs in 1–5% of transplants. It may be due to a technical error such as kinking or torsion of the venous anastomosis, but many cases are idiopathic. The peak incidence occurs at postoperative days 3–7. The presentation is distinctive with sudden pain over the renal transplant associated with frank haematuria. In early cases with partial thrombosis, Doppler ultrasound scanning may demonstrate reversal of arterial blood flow in diastole. In an established renal vein thrombosis Doppler scanning will demonstrate marked swelling of the renal allograft, often with a significant surrounding haematoma due to rupture of the renal capsule. Re-exploration to attempt a thrombectomy is rarely successful and the vast majority of cases lead to graft loss.

Urological complications

Urological complications occur in approximately 5% of renal transplants but they rarely result in graft loss. After dissection of the ureters at organ retrieval, only the ureteric blood supply from the renal artery is preserved. In consequence, the blood supply of the distal transplant ureter can be poor.

Urinary leak

Urinary leaks can occur in any part of the urinary drainage system but are commonly due to ischaemic necrosis of the distal ureter. The peak incidence is at the time of urinary catheter removal (day 5) but leaks can be delayed for a few weeks. In early leaks clear fluid discharges through the wound or collects in the drains. Biochemical analysis will show that the fluid is urine (creatinine in the millimolar range) rather than lymph (creatinine in the micromolar range and equal to the serum level). Leaks presenting later on when the wound is fully healed present as a peritransplant fluid collection.

Initial management is bladder catheterisation and cystography to confirm the diagnosis. The anatomical site and extent of the leak can be determined by inserting a percutaneous nephrostomy and performing antegrade pyelography. It is sometimes possible to place a double-J stent across the leakage point using an antegrade approach. If there has been significant ischaemic necrosis of the distal transplant ureter the leak will not resolve and surgery will be required. There are a number of alternatives for reconstructing the urinary drainage system. If there is a sufficient length of transplant ureter after excision of the necrotic segment, the ureter can be reimplanted directly into the bladder over a new double-J stent. If the healthy section of the transplant ureter is too short, a native-to-transplant ureteroureterostomy or ureteropyelostomy can be performed. Finally, if the ipsilateral native ureter is absent, because of a previous nephrectomy, a Boari bladder flap can be fashioned to drain the transplant kidney.

Ureteric obstruction

This can occur at any time after transplantation (days to years). Early obstruction is usually due to a technical error in the bladder anastomosis. Obstruction occurring after 3 months is invariably due to an ischaemic stricture. BK polyomavirus infection is also a cause of ureteric stricture. Patients present with renal dysfunction and investigation by ultrasound scanning reveals hydronephrosis. The initial management of choice is to place a percutaneous nephrostomy. An antegrade pyelogram can then be performed to define the site and extent of the stricture. Short strictures may be treated by interventional radiology with antegrade balloon dilatation and placement of a double-J stent across the stricture. Long, tight strictures require surgery and the options for reconstruction are the same as those for a urine leak.

Lymphocele

The incidence of significant lymphoceles (>3 cm) that cause complications and need treatment is around 5%. Small lymphoceles (<3 cm) are more common but asymptomatic and resolve spontaneously. The usual source of a lymph leak is from lymphatics that are divided during dissection of the iliac vessels. Lymph accumulates as a collection because of the extraperitoneal position of the kidney. Large lymphoceles can compress surrounding structures and, in some cases, cause renal vein thrombosis or ureteric obstruction.

All large peritransplant collections should be aspirated under ultrasound to exclude a urinary leak. Lymph is characterised by having the same biochemical profile as serum. Percutaneous drainage, sometimes on a number of occasions, leads to resolution of most lymphoceles. If this fails surgical drainage is required. This is usually performed laparoscopically and involves creating a fenestration in the wall of the lymphocele so that it drains into the peritoneal cavity.

Transplant renal artery stenosis

The incidence of transplant renal artery stenosis (TRAS) is approximately 5%. The usual presentation is refractory hypertension associated with allograft dysfunction at 3–6 months post transplant. TRAS activates the renin–angiotensin–aldosterone system and may become evident by a sudden increase in serum creatinine after prescribing an angiotensin-converting enzyme inhibitor.

Doppler scanning is suggestive of TRAS when the arterial peak systolic velocity is >250 cm/s and the waveform may have the characteristic tardus parvus (Latin for late and small) pattern. MRA or CT angiography are useful for anatomical definition. Percutaneous transluminal angioplasty with or without stenting is the preferred treatment.

Acute renal allograft dysfunction

This can be defined as a rise in serum creatinine of >10% from baseline or an absolute rise of ≥20 μmol/L. Common causes are listed in ***Summary box 88.2***. Allograft dysfunction should be investigated by urinalysis and culture to exclude urinary tract infection, CNI blood levels for drug-mediated nephrotoxicity and Doppler ultrasound scanning to check for arterial perfusion, venous drainage and hydronephrosis due to urinary obstruction. If there is uncertainty about the cause of graft dysfunction, a percutaneous needle-core transplant biopsy should be performed to establish whether allograft rejection is present.

Summary box 88.2

Causes of early graft dysfunction

Any rise in serum creatinine of >10% of baseline or ≥20 μmol/L should be considered as acute allograft dysfunction that requires investigation. Possible causes are:

- Acute rejection (antibody mediated or cell mediated)
- Calcineurin inhibitor toxicity
- Dehydration
- Urinary tract infection or pyelonephritis
- Any other source of sepsis
- Renal vein or renal artery thrombosis
- Ureteric obstruction or urine leak

Long-term allograft dysfunction

There are immunological and non-immunological causes for a progressive decline in renal allograft function over a period of months or years (***Summary box 88.3***). The commonest cause of long-term renal allograft damage and subsequent loss is chronic AMR. This is often related to inadequate compliance with immunosuppressive medication. There is no proven treatment for chronic AMR.

Non-immunological causes are also significant risk factors for chronic allograft damage. Irrespective of the cause, chronic transplant injury leads to interstitial fibrosis and tubular atrophy. Once established these changes are irreversible and will eventually lead to failure of the transplant.

The two most important factors in maintaining good long-term allograft function are meticulous adherence to immunosuppressive medication and good blood pressure control (<130/80 mmHg).

Outcomes after renal transplantation

Patient and graft survivals vary according to donor type and are presented in ***Table 88.4***. Overall, kidney transplantation is a highly successful treatment for ESRD. Living donor transplants yield better results than deceased donor transplants.

Achille Boari, nineteenth century Italian urological surgeon from Ferrara, described the technique of a bladder flap in dogs in 1894; it was first performed in a patient in 1936.

Summary box 88.3

Causes of long-term graft dysfunction

- Immunological
  - Chronic AMR
  - Acute CMR or AMR, which can occur at any time
- Non-immunological
  - Pre-existing damage in the donor kidney (especially relevant to DCD and extended criteria donor kidneys)
  - Early ischaemia–reperfusion injury
  - Chronic calcineurin nephrotoxicity
  - Ureteric or bladder outflow obstruction
  - Recurrent urinary tract infection or pyelonephritis
  - BK polyomavirus nephropathy
  - Recurrent native disease: glomerulonephritis; focal segmental glomerulosclerosis; immunoglobulin A nephropathy
  - Renal artery stenosis
  - Poorly controlled hypertension
  - Dyslipidaemia

DBD and DCD kidney transplants have comparable patient and graft survival.

Although these survival analyses are helpful, most patients want to know how long their transplant can be expected to last. This is best expressed by graft half-life ($t_{1/2}$) data (median graft survival). The current overall $t_{1/2}$ for live donor transplants is approximately 25 years and for deceased donor transplants approximately 15 years.

For all types of kidney, increasing donor age is the most important risk factor for poorer graft survival. Long cold ischaemic time (>12 hours for DCD kidneys and >24 hours for DBD kidneys) is also associated with reduced graft survival. Graft survival also decreases as the number of HLA mismatches increases.

TABLE 88.4 Patient and graft survival after renal transplantation.

Type of allograft (donor source)	5-year patient survival	10-year patient survival	5-year graft survival	10-year graft survival
Live donor	95%	90%	90%	80%
Deceased donor	90%	80%	85%	75%

Deceased donor includes both DBD and DCD results, which are comparable.

FURTHER READING

Bolton EM, Bradley JA. Principles of transplant immunology and immunosuppressive therapy. In: Thomas WEG, Reed MWR, Wyatt MG (eds). *Oxford textbook of fundamentals of surgery*. Oxford: Oxford University Press, 2016: 767–71.

Bradley JA, Nicholson M. Kidney transplantation. In: Thomas WEG, Reed MWR, Wyatt MG (eds). *Oxford textbook of fundamentals of surgery*. Oxford: Oxford University Press, 2016: 772–7.

Casey JJ. Pancreas and islet transplantation. In: Thomas WEG, Reed MWR, Wyatt MG (eds). *Oxford textbook of fundamentals of surgery*. Oxford: Oxford University Press, 2016: 778–80.

Chandak P, Callaghan CJ. Organ donation. In: Thomas WEG, Reed MWR, Wyatt MG (eds). *Oxford textbook of fundamentals of surgery*. Oxford: Oxford University Press, 2016: 761–6.

Clatworthy M, Watson C, Allison M, Dark J. *Transplantation at a glance*. Oxford: Wiley-Blackwell, 2012.

Harper S, Praseedom RK. Liver transplantation. In: Thomas WEG, Reed MWR, Wyatt MG (eds). *Oxford textbook of fundamentals of surgery*. Oxford: Oxford University Press, 2016: 781–3.

Knechtle S, Marson L, Morris P. *Kidney transplantation – principles and practice*, 8th edn. Philadelphia, PA: Elsevier, 2019.

PART 13 | Transplantation

CHAPTER 89 Liver transplantation

Learning objectives

To know:

- The surgical principles of liver transplantation
- Potential future developments in liver transplantation

To understand:

- The main indications and patient selection for liver transplantation
- The complications after liver transplantation
- Living donor and paediatric liver transplantation
- The causes of liver graft dysfunction
- Liver graft preservation techniques

INDICATIONS AND PATIENT SELECTION

The indications for liver transplantation (LT) fall into four groups:

1. chronic liver disease (CLD);
2. acute liver failure (ALF);
3. metabolic liver disease (including liver-based inborn errors of metabolism);
4. primary hepatic malignancy (hepatocellular carcinoma [HCC], hepatoblastoma).

The most common indication for LT is decompensated CLD (***Table 89.1***). In adults the most common causes are alcoholic liver disease, non-alcoholic fatty liver disease (NAFLD), chronic viral hepatitis (hepatitis B virus [HBV] and hepatitis C virus [HCV]), autoimmune liver diseases (primary biliary cirrhosis, primary sclerosing cholangitis, autoimmune hepatitis and overlap syndromes) and cirrhotic metabolic liver diseases (Wilson's disease). The specific frequencies of these aetiologies depend on geographical variations. In the last two decades hepatitis-related CLD (HBV and HCV) was the most common indication for LT. However, with universal vaccination for HBV and newer treatment options for HCV and with increasing obesity in affluent countries, NAFLD is projected to become the most common indication for LT in the future. In children, who account for around 10–15% of all LTs, biliary atresia is the most common indication for transplantation. ALF requiring transplantation on an urgent basis accounts for approximately 10% of LT activity and is usually drug induced or viral (e.g. paracetamol overdose in the UK). There are a variety of non-cirrhotic metabolic diseases for which transplantation offers the prospect of cure, including urea cycle defect, oxalosis and familial hypercholesterolaemia. Primary hepatic malignancy is more common in patients with cirrhosis, especially viral-induced liver disease and NAFLD, and may be best treated by transplantation when advanced liver disease precludes liver resection because of the risk of postoperative liver failure or when the tumour is multifocal as a result of field changes in the cirrhotic liver that predispose to recurrence or further primary malignancies.

LTs are usually performed between ABO blood group-compatible donor–recipient pairs. Histocompatibility matching, as in kidney transplantation, has not been necessary in LT as the liver is considered a more immunologically privileged organ. In countries where living donor liver transplantations (LDLTs) are performed in large numbers because of a lack of deceased donor organs, there has been a recent increase in the number of ABO-incompatible LTs when there is no blood group-compatible donor available. However, there is an increased risk of infection owing to a higher immunosuppression protocol and a higher incidence of antibody-mediated rejection with this type of transplantation.

Potential candidates undergo a comprehensive multidisciplinary assessment, including hepatologists, transplant surgeons, anaesthetists, specialist nurses in LT, drug and alcohol rehabilitation services, dietician, psychologists and specialists from other clinical disciplines where indicated. Three underlying principles dictate which patients should be referred for, and potentially undergo, LT. First, the recipient should have irreversible liver disease (acute or chronic) that is expected to be fatal without transplantation. Second, the patient should have sufficient reserve to survive the operative and perioperative period. Finally, the candidate should be expected to have significant survival (>50% at 5 years) and quality of life benefit from LT.

Samuel Alexander Kinnier Wilson, 1878–1937, Professor of Neurology at King's College Hospital, London, UK. He described hepatolenticular degeneration in his gold medal winning MD dissertation of 1912 titled 'Progressive lenticular degeneration', which led the disease to be named after him as Wilson's disease.

TABLE 89.1 Conditions that are considered for liver transplantation in adults and children.

	Aetiology in adult	Aetiology in children
Acute liver failure (severe acute impairment of liver function with encephalopathy that occurs within 8 weeks of the onset of symptoms and no recognised underlying chronic liver disease)	• Drugs (paracetamol overdose) • Hepatitis A and E • Acute Wilson's disease • Autoimmune hepatitis • Acute fatty liver of pregnancy	• Drugs and toxins • Hepatitis A and E • Acute Wilson's disease
Chronic liver disease (any diseases that cause cirrhosis and its associated complications)	• Fatty liver disease: alcohol or non-alcohol related • Chronic viral hepatitis B, C, D • Autoimmune liver diseases: primary biliary cirrhosis, primary sclerosing cholangitis, overlap syndromes • Genetic haemochromatosis • Wilson's disease • α_1-antitrypsin deficiency • Secondary biliary cirrhosis	• Biliary atresia • α_1-antitrypsin deficiency • Autoimmune hepatitis • Sclerosing cholangitis • Caroli's syndrome • Wilson's disease • Cystic fibrosis • Progressive familial intrahepatic cholestasis • Alagille's syndrome • Glycogen storage disease (types 3 and 4) • Tyrosinaemia type 1 • Budd–Chiari syndrome • Any aetiology leading to hepatopulmonary syndrome or portopulmonary hypertension
Variant syndromes (metabolic liver disease with life-threatening extrahepatic complications in children)	• Intractable pruritus • Hepatopulmonary syndrome • Familial amyloidosis • Primary hypercholesterolaemia • Hepatic epithelioid haemangioendothelioma • Recurrent cholangitis • Nodular regenerative hyperplasia • Hereditary haemorrhagic telangiectasia • Glycogen storage disease • Ornithine transcarbamylase deficiency • Primary hyperoxaluria • Maple syrup urine disease • Porphyria • Amyloidosis	• Crigler–Najjar syndrome • Urea cycle defects • Hypercholesterolaemia • Organic acidaemias • Glycogen storage disease type 1 • Maple syrup urine disease • Porphyria
Liver tumours	• Hepatocellular carcinoma • Rarely – cholangiocarcinoma, neuroendocrine tumours, colorectal liver metastasis	• Unresectable hepatoblastoma (without active extrahepatic disease) • Unresectable benign liver tumours with disabling symptoms

LIVER TRANSPLANTATION FOR HEPATIC MALIGNANCY

As a general rule, malignancy in a solid organ is not an indication for transplantation. This is because of the risk of recurrence with immunosuppression post transplant; immunosuppression suppresses not only the host's immunity preventing rejection of the transplanted graft but also the host's immunity against cancer, which may cause rapid progression of disease after transplantation. However, LT is one area where a total hepatectomy in selected patients can remove the entire disease en bloc and give patients a full chance of cure. LT is widely indicated as a curative treatment for selected patients with HCC, haemangioendothelioma and hepatoblastoma. Because of its association with CLD, up to 25% of LTs in the UK are in patients with HCC. Using the size and number of HCCs on pretransplant imaging, there are a number of criteria that aim to select patients who have HCC with favourable tumour biology and hence a good outcome following LT. The two main staging criteria of HCC for the indication of LT are the Milan and the University of California San Francisco (UCSF) criteria.

With recent advances in diagnostic modalities and chemotherapeutic agents, LT has been carefully expanded to patients

---

Jacques Caroli, 1902–1979, Professor of Medicine, St Antoine Hospital, Paris, France, described the disease in 1958.
Daniel Alagille, 1925–2005, Eminent Professor of Paediatric Hepatology, Hôpital Bicêtre, Paris, France, first described this condition in 1969.
George Budd, 1808–1882, Professor of Medicine, King's College Hospital, London, UK, described this syndrome in 1845.
Hans Chiari, 1851–1916, Professor of Pathological Anatomy, Strasbourg, Germany (Strasbourg was returned to France after the end of the First World War, in 1918), gave his account of this condition in 1898.
John Fielding Crigler, 1919–2018, American pediatrician, described the rare inherited disorder Crigler–Najjar syndrome in 1952.
Victor Assad Najjar, 1914–2002, Lebanese–American pediatrician and microbiologist, described the rare inherited disorder Crigler–Najjar syndrome in 1952.

Summary box 89.1

Evaluation of potential recipients for LT

- Evaluation is undertaken by a multidisciplinary team, including a transplant surgeon and hepatologist
- Determine the presence of physical and mental health comorbidities
- Exclude malignancy and systemic sepsis
- Determine any contraindications
- Determine if the patient will benefit from LT with an acceptable quality of life
- Determine if the disease is sufficiently advanced to meet the minimal listing criteria for LT (e.g. UK end-stage liver disease [UKELD] score 49 or more)
- Determine the availability of family or social support and probable ability to cope psychologically with LT and comply with immunosuppression
- Optimise recipient condition before LT

with other primary or secondary malignancies of the liver. Cholangiocarcinoma (CCA) has been an uncommon indication for LT for nearly three decades. Recently there has been more interest with wider adaptation of the Mayo protocol, which involves strict patient selection, intensive pre-LT chemoradiation therapy, staging laparoscopy to assess tumour spread and then transplantation. Five-year survival has been reported in the range of 55–65% for hilar CCA in patients with primary sclerosing cholangitis (PSC), who get these cancers more commonly than *de novo* CCAs.

Summary box 89.2

LT for hepatic malignancy

- LT for HCC simultaneously treats the tumour and the underlying liver disease
- LT for HCC represents 15–50% of all transplants performed in most centres
- Milan criteria allow selection of HCC patients for LT, with improved overall and disease-free survival
- Milan criteria (one lesion ≤5 cm, or three or fewer lesions ≤3 cm each)
- UCSF criteria (one lesion ≤6.5 cm, or three or fewer lesions ≤4.5 cm each, with a total tumour diameter ≤8 cm)
- UK HCC criteria (one lesion <5 cm, or five or fewer lesions all ≤3 cm, or a single tumour >5 cm and ≤7 cm in diameter with no evidence of progression over a 6-month period)
- Tumour recurrence after LT for HCC ranges between 8% and 20% depending upon the criteria followed
- Primary malignant liver tumours constitute just over 1% of all childhood cancers
- The most common tumours that require LT in children are hepatoblastoma and HCC
- CCA, colorectal and neuroendocrine liver metastases are among the new indications for LT

LISTING FOR LIVER TRANSPLANTATION

The allocation of liver grafts to patients with end-stage liver disease is dominated by three ethical principles: equity (need), utility (usefulness) and transplant benefit. The equity model gives prioritisation for sickest first, the utility prioritises the patient with the best expected outcome from transplantation and transplant benefit prioritises the patient with the greatest difference in expected survival with and without transplantation. The last balances both equity and utility and is expected to minimise mortality and maximise survival for the overall patients listed for transplant.

TECHNIQUE OF LIVER TRANSPLANTATION

Deceased donor liver transplantation

A reverse-L or a Mercedes-Benz (transverse abdominal incision with a midline extension) incision is usually made and the diseased liver is mobilised. As a result of portal hypertension, the recipient hepatectomy (removal of damaged liver) is often the most difficult part of the operation, especially if there has been previous upper abdominal surgery. The common bile duct is divided, as are the hepatic arteries. The inferior vena cava is mobilised above and below the liver; the portal vein is clamped and divided, and the vena cava is divided above and below, allowing the recipient liver to be removed. This 'classical' technique (***Figure 89.1a***) allows quick removal of the recipient liver without the need to free the liver from the cava by tying all the short and named hepatic veins (i.e. caval 'preservation' technique). Occlusion of the vena cava and portal vein results in a reduction in cardiac output and may necessitate the use of venovenous bypass, albeit not commonly. The bypass circuit delivers blood from the inferior vena cava and/or portal vein, back to the heart via a cannula inserted into the internal jugular vein. This improves venous return to the heart and provides haemodynamic stability during the operation. The portal limb of the bypass also reduces portal hypertension and congestion of the bowel during the implantation phase and potentially can reduce blood loss.

After total hepatectomy the implantation starts by placing the liver graft in the orthotopic position. The supra- and infrahepatic caval anastomoses are the first to be performed. The liver is flushed through the portal vein with normal saline at room temperature to remove the preservative solution with the effluent draining out through the lower caval anastomosis, which is left incomplete until the flushing. The portal vein anastomosis is then completed and the graft is reperfused. The hepatic artery anastomosis can sometimes be done first to reperfuse the liver with arterial blood followed by the portal vein anastomosis. ***Figure 89.2*** shows a cirrhotic liver and the deceased donor liver after transplantation. Finally, biliary drainage is re-established usually by a duct-to-duct anastomosis

The Mercedes-Benz sign takes its name from the insignia displayed on the bonnet of a Mercedes-Benz car.

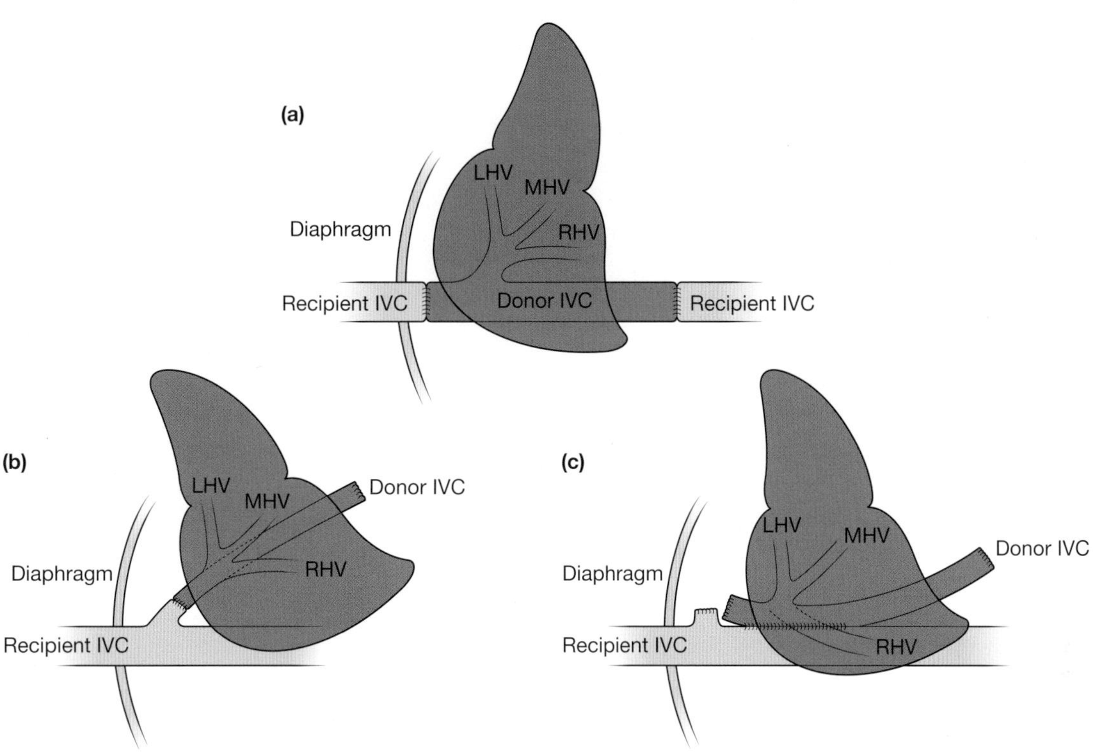

Figure 89.1 Pictorial representation of inferior vena cava (IVC) reconstruction in a deceased donor live transplantation. (a) A 'classical' caval replacement technique in which the recipient's retrohepatic IVC is replaced with donor IVC. (b) A 'piggyback' technique in which the confluence of the three hepatic veins in the recipient is used to anastomose with the top end of the donor IVC. (c) 'Side-to-side cavo-cavoplasty' in which the side of the donor IVC is joined with the side of the recipient IVC. LHV, left hepatic vein; MHV, middle hepatic vein; RHV, right hepatic vein.

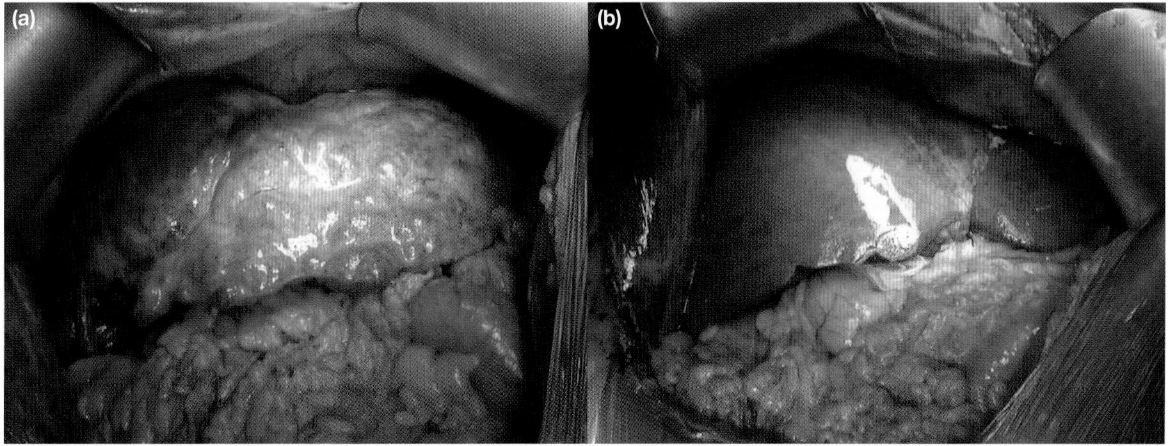

Figure 89.2 Adult deceased donor liver transplantation. (a) Recipient cirrhotic liver; (b) whole liver graft after reperfusion with the portal vein and hepatic artery.

(*Figure 89.3a*). In recipients with biliary atresia where the bile duct is absent or in those with PSC where the bile duct is diseased, the donor bile duct is reconstructed through a Roux-en-Y hepaticojejunostomy (*Figure 89.3b*).

An alternative and more commonly performed technique is the 'caval preservation' technique, which allows the recipient liver to be removed without cross-clamping the vena cava, thus avoiding venovenous bypass. The donor liver here is implanted using a 'piggyback' technique onto the confluence of the three hepatic veins in the recipient (*Figure 89.1b*) or using a side-to-side cavo-cavoplasty (joining donor and recipient cava side to side) (*Figure 89.1c*).

Optimal perioperative management is crucial to a successful outcome and presents a major challenge. These patients are often very sick preoperatively, especially those transplanted for ALF. Blood loss during and after the transplantation procedure can be very considerable, and management of coagulopathy is particularly important. Coagulation is assessed repeatedly

Cesar Roux, 1857–1934, Professor of Surgery and Gynaecology, Lausanne, Switzerland, described this method of forming a jejunal conduit in 1908.

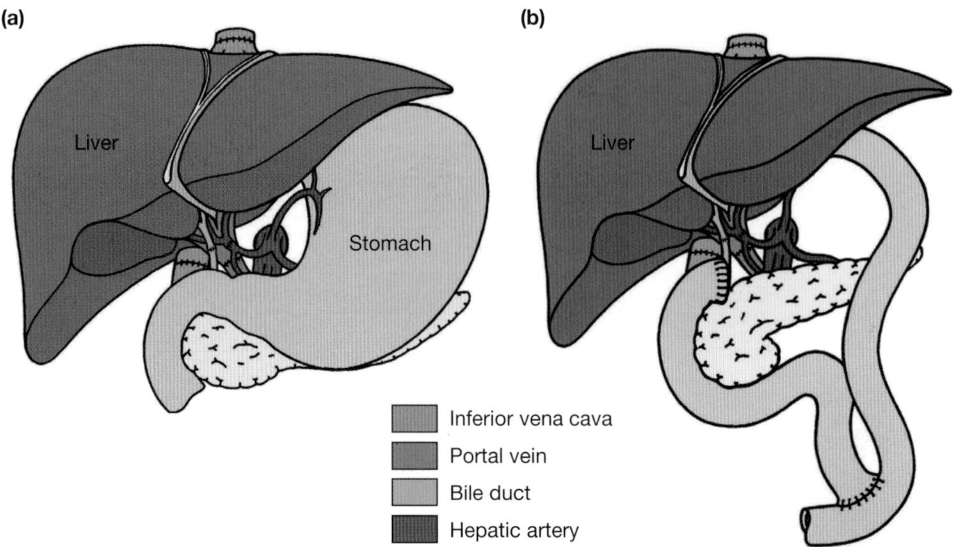

Figure 89.3 Pictorial representation of the standard deceased donor liver transplant with a 'classical' caval replacement technique. (a) A liver graft after completion of all anastomoses, in order of performance: (1) suprahepatic cava; (2) infrahepatic cava; (3) portal vein; (4) hepatic artery; (5) bile duct. (b) A Roux-en-Y reconstruction where the donor bile duct is anastomosed to the loop of jejunum. The rest of the anastomoses and order of performance are the same.

throughout the transplantation period and corrected with appropriate clotting factors, if required. Many centres routinely use point-of-care 'viscoelastic monitoring' such as thromboelastography (TEG) or rotational thromboelastometry (ROTEM) to perform dynamic assessment of coagulation.

The deceased donor liver transplant (DDLT) grafts come from either donation after brain death (DBD) donors or donation after circulatory death (DCD) donors. The latter are considered 'extended criteria' donors owing to greater ischaemia associated with donor hypoxia/death, higher risk of graft dysfunction, higher risk of vascular and biliary complications and poor long-term outcomes. Although LT has established itself as a life-saving treatment, the limited availability of deceased donor liver grafts has urged the transplant community to devise newer techniques and strategies to reduce the gap between organ demand and supply. The various options to increase organ availability are: LDLT, split and reduced-size LT, use of extended criteria donors (ECDs), auxiliary LT, domino LT and the paired-exchange programme.

Summary box 89.3

Types of LT (based on source of liver allograft)

- DDLT, which includes DBD (70–80%) and DCD (20–30%)
- LDLT – this can be adult to adult or adult to child
- Split and reduced-size LT
- ECDs
- Auxiliary LT
- Domino LT
- Paired-exchange programme

Living donor liver transplantation

In 1988, Silvano Raia in Sao Paolo, Brazil, was the first to introduce the concept of LDLT in a child. Although unsuccessful, this was followed by a report of a successful outcome in paediatric LDLT by Russell Strong in Brisbane, Australia. The expansion of LDLT to the adult population began in 1993, when the Shinshu group in Tokyo performed the first successful adult-to-adult LDLT. However, adult-to-adult LDLT is not without risks to the donor, with the global mortality risk quoted at 1 in 300–500 for adult donors. Right lobe, left lobe or left lateral segments can be used as grafts depending on the size requirement for the recipient. Right lobe grafts, which account for 60–70% of the total liver volume, are the most commonly used grafts for adult LDLT (***Figure 89.4***). The required graft volume is measured by either the graft weight to recipient weight ratio (GRWR) or the ratio of graft volume relative to the standard liver volume of the recipient (GV/SLV). An ideal GRWR must be >0.8% and/or GV/SLV >35%. The assessment of volume of the graft in the donor is measured by marking the boundaries of the liver lobe on the donor computed tomography (CT) scan manually, but this can also be done more accurately using complex three-dimensional software such as MeVis (HepaVision®, Bremen, Germany). The remnant liver mass in the donor must be kept to >30% of the whole liver, which allows for safe regeneration and prevents the risk of liver insufficiency in the donor.

LDLT is now undertaken in a number of transplant centres worldwide and is relatively common practice in some countries where deceased donation is not practised for cultural or religious reasons, notably in the Far East and South Asia. Over 90% of

Silvano Raia, b. 1930, Emeritus Professor at the Faculty of Medicine, Sao Paulo, Brazil, performed the first living donor liver transplantation in a child.
Russell Strong, contemporary, Emeritus Professor of Surgery, University of Queensland, Princess Alexandra Hospital, Australia. He successfully performed a living donor liver transplant of the left lateral segment of a Japanese mother's liver into her 18-month-old son in 1989. Both were alive and well 27 years later (2016); the recipient graduated and is practising as a physiotherapist.

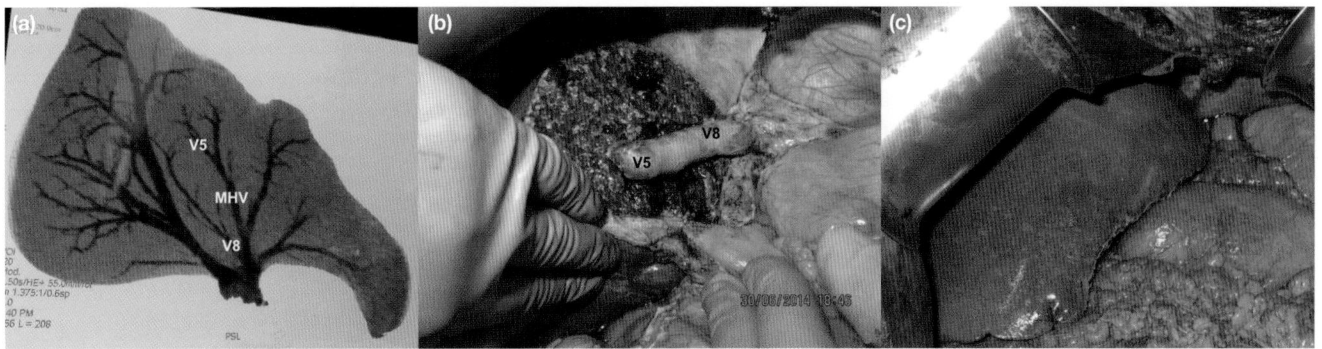

Figure 89.4 Adult right lobe living donor liver transplantation (LDLT). (a) Hepatic vein cuts showing the segment 5 vein (V5) and segment 8 vein (V8) draining into the middle hepatic vein (MHV). (b) A right lobe LDLT graft after implantation showing the reconstructed V5 and V8 using a deceased donor iliac vein graft. (c) A well-perfused right lobe liver graft.

transplants in the East come from LDLT, whereas in the West over 90% of all LTs are DDLT. With increasing experience and innovation, the graft and recipient survival of adult-to-adult LDLT now compare favourably with those of DDLT.

If the recipient size is large, a right liver LDLT graft might not give an adequate GRWR. Similarly, if the donor remnant is small, it is not safe for the donation to proceed. To tackle the problem of inadequate graft size in LDLT one innovative approach is 'dual-graft liver transplantation', done mostly in Korea and rarely in other LDLT countries; this approach is to transplant the recipient with two left lobe grafts or one right lobe and one left lobe graft from two living donors. With this approach, donor safety is maintained and the recipient is transplanted with adequate graft volume. The procedure is technically very demanding and requires massive infrastructure where two donor hepatectomies and recipient LT surgery have to take place all at the same time. However, the ethical issue of putting two donors at risk simultaneously for one recipient's benefit is contentious.

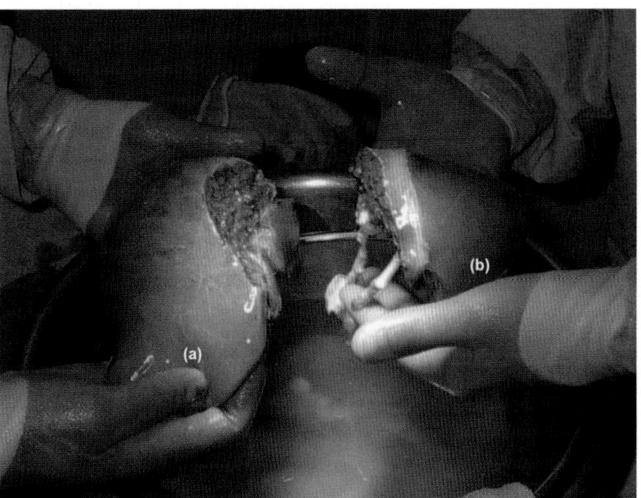

Figure 89.5 *Ex situ* splitting of a donation after brain death liver. (a) Extended right lobe liver graft (Couinaud's segments I and IV–VIII) prepared for implantation into an adult recipient; (b) left lateral segment graft (Couinaud's segments II and III) prepared for implantation into a paediatric recipient.

Split and reduced-size liver transplantation

Split LT is a valuable option for making the best use of good-quality deceased donor liver grafts, by splitting the graft into a left lateral segment (segments II and III) for a paediatric recipient and an extended right liver lobe (segments I and IV–VIII) for an adult recipient. Not so commonly, the whole liver can be split as anatomical right and left lobes, the latter being used for a larger child or a smaller adult. The splitting procedure can be done *ex situ*, where the whole organ is retrieved and split on the back-bench along the anatomical planes, so as to preserve the inflow and outflow vessels to both grafts (***Figure 89.5***). In *in situ* splitting, liver transection is performed during the donor procedure, similar to procuring a living liver donor graft. The major advantage of *in situ* splitting in contrast to *ex situ* bench splitting is that haemostasis on the cut surface can be obtained during the donor procedure with less blood loss from the cut surface during reperfusion in the recipient. *In situ* splitting also facilitates prompt transportation of the liver to transplant centres if the two split lobes are to be used in two different centres far away from each other, thereby reducing the cold ischaemic times for both organs.

Although technically demanding, split LT is a safe procedure resulting in an increased number of LTs, increased feasibility of LT in children and a reduced waitlist mortality. Short- and long-term outcomes and survival with these grafts are similar to those with whole-graft LT. Reduced-size LT is the forerunner of split LT and involves *ex vivo* resection of a full liver into an appropriate size liver to fit a small adult, with the rest of the reduced-size portion being discarded. Reduced-size LT, unlike a split technique, does not produce an additional graft. It is therefore not widely practised and is reserved for situations where a small adult or adolescent patient requires an urgent transplant and a whole liver or an extended right lobe is too large for the abdominal cavity.

Claude Couinaud, 1922–2008, French surgeon and anatomist, described the segmental anatomy of the liver in his seminal book *Le Foie: Études anatomiques et chirurgicales*.

Extended criteria donors

Using grafts from ECDs is a strategy to address organ shortage in LT. An ECD graft has been described as an organ with an increased risk of poor graft function (liver from older donors or fatty livers) and/or transmission of disease (i.e. infection or malignancy) to the recipient because of unfavourable donor characteristics (*Table 89.2*). In comparison with DBD, DCD LTs have been associated with higher rates of biliary complications and graft loss, historically limiting their use. Worldwide, there is considerable variation in the contributions that DCD makes to deceased donation overall. While some countries have no DCD programmes whatsoever (such as India, where it is illegal to procure a DCD organ), in countries like the UK and Australia DCD accounts for 20–30% of all LTs. DCD livers reduce waiting list mortality (i.e. by taking patients off the LT waiting list) and there is survival advantage in accepting a DCD offer than waiting for a 'better' DBD liver, which is more pronounced in patients with advanced liver disease. Outcomes with ECD organs can be improved with careful recipient selection and possibly with machine perfusion of the donor liver, so as to assess its function and quality, prior to transplantation.

Auxiliary liver transplantation

Auxiliary LT involves implanting a healthy liver graft placed either heterotopically or orthotopically while leaving all or part of the native liver intact. Auxiliary heterotopic LT, where the graft is implanted below the native liver, was proposed as an alternative to orthotopic LT in the early era of transplantation when recipient hepatectomy was associated with massive blood loss and transfusion requirements. But the technique was marred with failures due to the heterotopic position of the graft resulting in poor venous drainage. More recently there has been a renewed interest in auxiliary LT for ALF and certain metabolic liver diseases. To overcome the previous technical difficulties, the procedure is now performed with a partial graft placed in an orthotopic position following a recipient partial hepatectomy to create space for the graft (*Figure 89.6*). The procedure is therefore termed auxiliary partial orthotopic liver transplantation (APOLT). It is a technically

TABLE 89.2 Extended criteria donors in liver transplantation.

Type of extended criteria donor	Primary risk to the recipient
Advanced donor age	Delayed graft function
Macrovesicular steatosis	Delayed graft function
Donation after circulatory death organs	Biliary complication
Organ dysfunction at procurement: • ICU stay >7 days • Hypernatraemia >165 mmol/L • Bilirubin >51 μmol/L • Elevated liver enzymes (AST, ALT) • Vasopressor use	Delayed graft function, primary non-function
Cause of death: anoxia, cerebrovascular accident	Delayed graft function, biliary complication
Disease transmission: • Hepatitis B core antibody-positive donor • Hepatitis B surface antigen-positive donor • Hepatitis C virus-positive donor • HIV-positive donor • High-risk history (active drug abuser, etc.) • Extrahepatic malignancy	Infectious risk
Cold ischaemia time >12 hours (long storage of organ after procurement)	Delayed graft function, primary non-function

ALT, alanine aminotransferase; AST, aspartate aminotransferase; HIV, human immunodeficiency virus; ICU, intensive care unit.

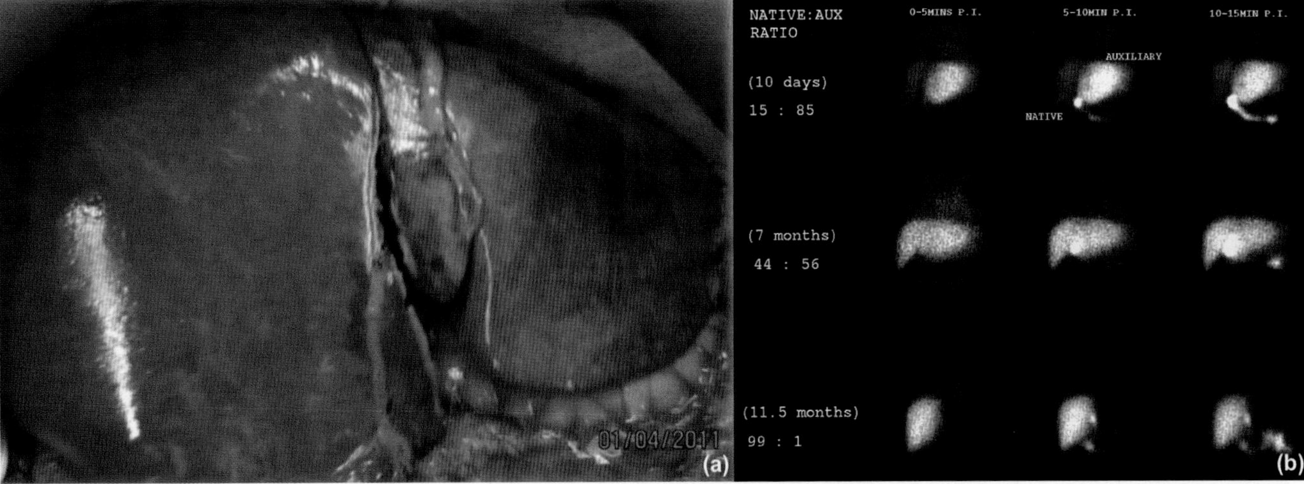

Figure 89.6 Right lobe auxiliary partial orthotopic liver transplantation (APOLT) for acute liver failure due to yellow phosphorus poisoning. **(a)** Recipient left lateral section of the liver looking pale and fatty owing to yellow phosphorus poisoning; right lobe graft from the donor implanted into the orthotopic position. **(b)** Hepatobiliary iminodiacetic acid (HIDA) scans done over the first year after transplant in a left lobe APOLT. The scans show regression of the left lobe auxiliary graft and functioning native liver.

complex procedure and has gained acceptance as a bridge to native liver regeneration in ALF. The most important benefit of APOLT is the potential for immunosuppression withdrawal when the native liver fully regenerates, although outcomes have been suboptimal in less experienced hands. In metabolic liver diseases in children, APOLT is performed with the intention of keeping part of the native liver for future gene therapy.

Domino liver transplantation

Domino LT involves transplanting a liver from a patient with metabolic disease who needs LT into a patient with end-stage liver disease with the expectation that the recipient will not develop the metabolic syndrome or the recurrent syndrome will have minimal effect. Several hereditary metabolic diseases such as familial amyloid polyneuropathy (FAP), maple syrup urine disease and familial hypercholesterolaemia are caused by aberrant or deficient protein production in the liver, and these conditions can be cured with an orthotopic LT. Although their native livers eventually caused severe systemic disease in these patients, these livers are otherwise structurally and functionally normal, and hence used as domino into those with end-stage liver failure. A typical example of domino LT is the use of a liver from a patient with FAP to a patient who is outside transplant criteria for liver malignancy. Even if they develop amyloidosis, it would take 10–20 years for the disease to become symptomatic in these recipients. If they have no recurrence of tumour and become symptomatic from FAP in the future they can be offered a retransplant without the risk of recurrence of malignancy.

Paired-exchange programmes

Liver paired exchange (LPE) allows liver donors and their intended incompatible recipients to exchange livers with another donor–recipient pair so that a compatible transplant can be performed. The advantage is that it allows the two transplant recipients to be removed from the deceased donor waiting list, thereby shortening the waiting for other patients who remain on the list, decreasing waiting list mortality. ABO blood group incompatibility, size incompatibility (small donor liver into large recipient or vice versa) or anatomical considerations (multiple arteries or bile ducts to reconstruct) are common reasons for non-acceptance of otherwise suitable donors in LDLT. In all these circumstances, donor and recipient pairs who are not optimally matched might benefit from a better match through LPE. At times, these LPEs can be initiated by a non-directed anonymous living donor (i.e. a domino paired exchange), where a person effectively donates a portion of their liver to the pool of patients on the deceased donor transplant waiting list. Compared with kidney paired exchange, LPE is inherently more complex owing to the greater morbidity and mortality risks to the donor and to the logistics involved, hence it is not widely practised.

Summary box 89.4

Strategies to overcome the shortage of livers for transplantation

- Increasing the donor pool
  - Implementing an organ donation opt-out system (introduced in the UK in Wales – December 2015; England – May 2020; Scotland – March 2021)
  - Use of marginal DBD deceased donors
  - Use of DCD deceased donors
  - Increased use of split LT
  - Increased living donor LT
  - Use of HCV-positive donor grafts
- Improve the preservation and assessment of quality of donor grafts
  - Use of machine perfusion systems (normothermic/hypothermic machine perfusion)
- Maximise post-transplant long-term survival
  - Reduce or avoid immunosuppression after LT to minimise side effects

IMMEDIATE POST-TRANSPLANT CARE

Following LT, patients are monitored in an intensive care unit (ICU) and maintained on a ventilator, usually for less than 24 hours. If haemodynamically stable and awake with good early liver graft function and renal function they are extubated. Spontaneous correction of lactic acidosis and correction of coagulopathy (falling international normalised ratio [INR]) and low serum transaminases are indicators of good early graft function. A Doppler ultrasound is also performed prior to extubation to assess the patency of blood supply to the liver. Most patients with an uncomplicated postoperative course get moved to the high-dependency unit or ward after 2 days. During the ICU stay, there is close management of fluid and electrolytes, which could be significantly abnormal as a result of the prolonged operation and massive fluid shifts. Following transfer to the transplant wards, the patient is closely monitored by the transplant surgical and medical (hepatology) team, as well as by pharmacists, nutritionists and physiotherapists. The liver and kidney function, the coagulation parameters and full blood count are monitored daily. Doppler ultrasound scans are performed at regular intervals to ensure that the blood vessels are patent and there are no other abnormalities. Dosages of immunosuppressive agents are adjusted according to blood levels and organ function during this period. Antibacterial, antiviral and antifungal prophylaxis are given to prevent infections, including those from opportunistic organisms, such as cytomegalovirus (CMV) and *Pneumocystis carinii*.

Christian Johann Doppler, 1803–1853, Professor of Experimental Physics, Vienna, Austria, enunciated the Doppler principle in 1842.

Summary box 89.5

Factors determining graft function after LT

- Donor characteristics
  - Advanced donor age
  - DCD donors
  - Steatotic livers
  - Small graft size in LDLT ('small for size syndrome')
- Procurement-related factors
  - Warm ischaemic time
  - Type of preservation solution
  - Cold ischaemic time
- Recipient-related factor
  - High MELD or UKELD score
  - Severe portal hypertension
  - Technical factors relating to implantation
  - Haemodynamic and metabolic stability
  - Massive transfusion of blood and blood-related products
  - Immunological factors

IMMUNOSUPPRESSION FOLLOWING LIVER TRANSPLANTATION

Liver is considered to be an 'immunoregulatory' solid organ with specialised venous endothelial turnover, a high number of extramedullary haematopoietic stem cells and the ability to produce numerous immunoregulatory substances. The privileged state of liver in transplantation is highlighted by the relatively lower need for human leukocyte antigen (HLA) or blood-group matching. Compared with other organs, such as kidneys and lungs, the liver allograft has the advantage of demonstrating lower rates of acute and chronic rejection, a resistance to antibody-mediated rejection and a higher likelihood of developing spontaneous tolerance. Induction agents such as antithymocyte globulin (ATG), CD25 monoclonal antibodies (basiliximab and daclizumab) or cluster of differentiation (CD)52 monoclonal antibodies (alemtuzumab; Campath-1H), which routinely form part of kidney, pancreas and other organ transplants, are rarely used in LT. They are only considered in selected patients with a high immunological risk or renal compromise, in the latter case to delay the introduction of calcineurin inhibitors (CNIs). CNIs (tacrolimus and ciclosporin) are the mainstay of LT maintenance immunosuppression, with mycophenolate mofetil (MMF), azathioprine and corticosteroids considered as the essential adjuncts to CNIs (***Table 89.3***). Mammalian target of rapamycin inhibitors (mTORi) such as sirolimus and everolimus have established roles in patients with worsening renal function and in those with LT for HCCs and incidental cancers on explant. The side effects of prolonged immunosuppression are one of the limitations of long-term survival among LT recipients, especially those due to immunosuppression-induced metabolic syndrome, cardiovascular disease, renal impairment and malignancy. Several studies have shown that 20% of LT patients can achieve operational tolerance, whereby there is long-term survival of the allograft in the absence of immunosuppression. However, there is a need for more research to understand this better and to identify the group of patients who will benefit from withdrawal of immunosuppression.

POST-LIVER TRANSPLANT COMPLICATIONS

Primary non-function

Primary non-function (PNF) is one of the most serious and life-threatening conditions in the immediate post-transplant period. It is defined as an aggravated form of reperfusion injury resulting in irreversible graft failure without detectable

TABLE 89.3 Common immunosuppression medications after liver transplant.

Drug	Mechanism of action	Major side effects	Monitoring
Calcineurin inhibitors (tacrolimus, ciclosporin)	Inhibit T-cell signalling, prevent lymphocyte activation and block cytokine transcription	• Nephrotoxicity • Hypertension • Diabetogenic (tacrolimus) • Gingival hypertrophy/hirsutism (ciclosporin) • Increased susceptibility to infection	Blood trough levels
Mycophenolate mofetil	Inhibits T-cell and B-cell proliferation	• Leukopenia • Increased susceptibility to infection and cancers	No monitoring
Azathioprine	Purine analogue, impedes DNA and RNA synthesis	Bone marrow suppression with cytopenias, pancreatitis	No monitoring
Corticosteroids	• Decrease cytokine production • Decrease lymphocyte activation and proliferation • Decrease antibody production • Decrease phagocytosis and release of proteolytic enzymes	Steroid excess (Cushing's syndrome)	No monitoring
mTORi (sirolimus/everolimus)	Mammalian target of rapamycin inhibitor	Impaired wound healing, hyperlipidaemia, proteinuria, hepatic artery thrombosis	Blood trough levels

Harvey Williams Cushing, 1869–1939, Professor of Surgery, Harvard University Medical School, Boston, MA, USA.

technical or immunological problems. The reported incidence is 4–8% and this is the most common indication for retransplantation after LT. It is almost always a problem associated with DDLT, but can present in LDLT as well.

Haemorrhage

Portal hypertension and coagulopathy of CLD are important causes of bleeding that are unique to LT procedures. A study of more than 12 000 LTs showed 12.5% needing re-explorations during the same hospitalisation, of which 68% were for bleeding. Meticulous haemostasis during the transplantation operation is important in order to minimise the risk of early haemorrhage. Excessive haemorrhage is also common if the graft has sustained a severe reperfusion injury or if a marginal graft is used and the early graft function is poor. *Ex situ* split LT can also have a high blood loss from the cut surface of the liver. This is not the case in *in situ* split LT and LDLT partial grafts where haemostasis is secured during the donor operation.

It is standard practice to place two large drains behind the right and left lobes of the liver to monitor for bleeding and bile leak. It may be necessary, occasionally, to pack the peritransplant area for 24–48 hours to achieve adequate haemostasis when there is diffuse oozing despite correction of coagulopathy. Evacuation of an extensive perihepatic haematoma may be required to avoid secondary infection.

Vascular complications

Hepatic artery thrombosis (HAT) is one of the most dreaded complications after LT, and may occur spontaneously or as a result of acute rejection; it is more common in children and in adults with PSC. The incidence of HAT has been reported to be in the range of 1–10% after LT. Anatomical variant grafts such as split, reduced and LDLT grafts have a higher risk of HAT when compared with whole-organ LT. Early HAT (within 4 weeks of LT) may present as a rise in serum transaminase levels, unexplained fever or bile leak. The risk factors for early HAT are not only related to technical factors such as vessel kinking, stenotic anastomosis and intimal dissection, but also to other factors such as elderly donors with calcified vessels, a hypercoagulable state in the recipient and rejection episodes. Doppler ultrasound or CT angiography is used to confirm the diagnosis, and urgent retransplantation is usually required. Endovascular interventions and thrombolysis are rarely successful. The UK super-urgent liver scheme allows listing of those patients who develop early HAT, up to 21 days after transplantation. Late HAT (after 4 weeks of LT) usually has an insidious course and can present as asymptomatic elevation of liver enzymes, bile duct strictures or liver abscess. The bile ducts suffer the most ischaemic insult as they primarily depend on arterial blood supply with no portal venous blood supply. Retransplantation is usually reserved for those with severe biliary complications.

Portal vein thrombosis and stenosis are rare and can present with features of portal hypertension. The management usually involves endovascular interventions such as balloon dilatation or stent insertion, surgical bypass or retransplantation. Late portal vein thrombosis/stenosis manifests as portal hypertension without graft dysfunction. Most can be managed conservatively without risk of graft loss.

Hepatic venous outflow obstruction often presents with increasing ascitic fluid losses over the postoperative period. A cavogram with hepatic vein pressure studies should be undertaken to confirm the diagnosis, and insertion of vascular stents, surgical correction or retransplantation may be required to treat the problem.

Biliary complications

The biliary complications usually present as bile leak, biliary anastomotic stricture (AS), biliary non-anastomotic stricture (NAS), bile duct sludge/stone/casts, biloma and duct loss (ductopenia) in patients with chronic rejection. Biliary complications following LT can be caused by the vulnerable vascular supply to the biliary tree (supplied by hepatic artery alone), the biliary epithelium being more liable to ischaemic injury than hepatocytes, suboptimal preservation of the peribiliary plexus

Summary box 89.6

Complications after LT

Early complications (within 6 months)

- Graft
  - Primary non-function
  - Delayed graft function
- Surgical
  - Bleeding
  - Hepatic artery thrombosis
  - Portal vein thrombosis
  - Hepatic venous outflow obstruction
  - Bile leak
  - Biliary anastomotic stricture
- Medical
  - Infections (bacterial, viral, fungal)
  - Rejections
  - Acute kidney injury

Late complications (after 6 months)

- Graft
  - Ischaemic cholangiopathy (non-anastomotic biliary strictures)
- Surgical
  - Vascular stenosis (hepatic artery, portal vein or hepatic vein)
  - Late HAT
  - Biliary AS
  - Incisional hernia
- Medical
  - Infections (bacterial, viral, fungal)
  - Rejections/chronic rejection leading to graft failure
  - Renal impairment
  - Disease recurrence
  - Cardiovascular disease
  - Metabolic and bone diseases
  - Malignancy

during organ procurement and storage and ischaemia–reperfusion injury. The incidence of biliary complications is higher in LDLT and other anatomical variant grafts than in whole-graft LT. This is because of the small size of the ducts, multiple duct anastomoses and also cut surface leaks. Due to the morbidity involved with biliary complications, bile duct anastomosis is considered the Achilles' heel of LT. The management of bile leaks usually involves bile duct reconstruction with Roux-en-Y hepaticojejunostomy in the immediate post-transplant period or endoscopic decompression of the bile duct and percutaneous drain insertion. For AS, the management involves endoscopic dilatation, stent insertion or surgical revision. The NAS or ischaemic-type biliary lesions (ITBL) are the most severe form of biliary strictures, where there is widespread desquamation of biliary epithelial cells with formation of biliary casts, multiple segmental stenosis and a picture similar to PSC. This can happen within a few weeks, months or years after transplantation and the incidence is 25–30% with DCD grafts but is less common in DBD grafts. The management will include imaging to rule out HAT or stenosis, dilatation of dominant strictures, ursodeoxycholic acid to increase bile flow and lower the lithogenicity and antibiotic maintenance therapy to prevent recurrent episodes of cholangitis. Eventually most patients will require retransplantation.

CAUSES OF ALLOGRAFT DYSFUNCTION

Liver graft dysfunction can happen any time after transplantation; if not identified early and treated promptly, it can lead to graft loss. The most common presentation is an asymptomatic elevation of liver enzyme levels. Early after LT, acute cellular rejection is the most common cause of graft dysfunction and is usually treated by increasing the dose of immunosuppression, which includes pulsed-steroid therapy for 3 days or more depending on the degree of rejection. The other common reasons for graft dysfunction are the vascular complications, bile leak or bile duct obstruction, post-transplant infections and drug toxicity. Even if rejection is suspected, it is important to rule out any vascular or biliary complications by performing a Doppler ultrasound scan and, if there is any doubt, a contrast-enhanced CT scan. Liver biopsy is usually performed through a percutaneous route, but a coagulopathic patient might need transjugular liver biopsy.

LT patients are followed up more frequently in the first 3 months after transplant, as this is the time when presentation with graft-related issues is most common and also when monitoring and optimisation of immunosuppression are crucial. The follow-up protocol varies between LT centres, but mostly includes once a week for the first 6 weeks after transplant and then once a fortnight for another 6 weeks, before reducing the frequency of appointment. Late graft dysfunction is usually due to acute/chronic rejection, vascular issues such as hepatic artery stenosis or venous outflow obstruction, biliary obstruction, recurrence of primary disease such as hepatitis C (rare nowadays owing to viral clearance prior to transplant), autoimmune diseases or NAFLD, and other opportunistic infections such as CMV or herpes simplex hepatitis.

DISEASE RECURRENCE AFTER LIVER TRANSPLANTATION

Disease recurrence after LT has increased over the past decade, as many more patients are living more than 15–20 years with their liver graft. Disease recurrence after LT can be divided into four main groups: (i) malignant disease, (ii) viral disease, (iii) autoimmune diseases such as primary biliary cholangitis (PBC) and PSC, and (iv) lifestyle-related diseases such as NAFLD and alcoholic liver disease. The severity of recurrence varies from mild to the development of progressive allograft failure.

Despite strict morphological criteria in selecting patients with HCC for LT, tumour recurrence still occurs in 8–20% of cases, being associated with a median survival of 7–16 months after recurrence. The risk factors for tumour recurrence are larger tumour burden (beyond the Milan criteria), poor tumour biology, microvascular invasion, higher AFP levels, viral aetiology and obesity in the recipient, percutaneous biopsy of the tumour leading to spillage of cells, longer waiting time to transplant, higher donor age, DCD transplants and higher burden of immunosuppression in the post-transplant period. HBV recurrence has been reported in 10% of patients after LT. However, new combinations of post-LT prophylaxis, including hepatitis B immunoglobulin and nucleos(t)ide analogues such as lamivudine, have reduced the recurrence rates and are part of most LT guidelines. HCV recurrence post LT leads to accelerated liver disease and cirrhosis, with reduced graft and patient survival. Factors associated with increased HCV risk or severity of recurrence after LT include older age, immunosuppression, HCV genotype 1 and high viral load at LT. The introduction of protease inhibitors in 2011 and direct-acting antiviral agents in 2013 has led to the reduction both of HCV complications requiring LT and of the consequences of recurrent HCV infection after LT. Autoimmune diseases commonly recur after LT and may need retransplantation. This usually happens when corticosteroids are withdrawn, but patients usually respond rapidly to the reintroduction of steroids with no adverse long-term impact. PBC and PSC can recur in 20% of patients at 5 years, some of which can be *de novo* secondary disease. Resumption of alcohol use post LT leads to recurrent ALD and has an overall poor outcome. NAFLD can recur in patients with metabolic syndrome who continue with poor dietary habits post LT, leading to fibrosis in the graft and eventually needing retransplantation. Prothrombotic conditions such as Budd–Chiari syndrome can recur in the transplanted liver, requiring retransplantation, but with dismal outcomes.

Summary box 89.7

Diseases that recur after LT

- Chronic hepatitis B and C
- PBC
- PSC
- Autoimmune hepatitis
- Alcoholic liver disease (recurrence alcohol consumption)
- NAFLD
- Budd–Chiari syndrome
- Malignant tumours (HCC, hepatoblastoma)

OUTCOMES AFTER LIVER TRANSPLANTATION

The outcomes after LT depend on the underlying liver disease; the best results are seen in patients with CLD. Patients undergoing transplantation as a result of ALF have a higher mortality in the early post-transplantation period because of multiorgan failure, but those who make a satisfactory recovery have very good long-term liver allograft survival. In the UK, unadjusted 1-, 5- and 10-year patient survival for adult patients receiving their first elective transplant is 94%, 84% and 72%, respectively. For super-urgent transplant, the survival is less: 90%, 82% and 70%, respectively (NHSBT Annual Report September 2020). Conversely, patients transplanted for tumour have a very good early outcome but ultimately fare less well because of recurrent malignancy. As with other solid organ transplants, chronic immunosuppression has its effect on the LT recipient with increased risk of infections, metabolic syndrome and cancers. The common causes of death in post-LT recipients after 3 years of transplant are mostly non-transplant related, such as malignancy or cardiovascular disease, and are less due to chronic rejection and recurrent primary liver disease.

PAEDIATRIC LIVER TRANSPLANTATION

Paediatric LT has now been carried out for more than three decades and enjoys excellent success with good long-term outcomes. Split LT and LDLT have contributed to reduced waiting times in these children with improved outcomes (***Figure 89.7***). Contraindications to LT in children are uncommon, and usually include: (i) non-resectable extrahepatic malignant tumour; (ii) concomitant end-stage organ failure that cannot be corrected by a combined transplant; (iii) uncontrolled sepsis; and (iv) irreversible neurological damage. Left lateral segment grafts usually suffice for small children, but larger children will need left lobe or right lobe grafts. The left lateral segment graft donor operation involves removal of around 20–25% of the liver; this is associated with a low and acceptable risk of donor complications. Monosegment grafts (transplanting isolated liver segments such as segment II or segment III for an infant) for small children (less than 5 kg) is a norm in experienced centres and can solve the problem of 'large for size' grafts in this age group.

CHALLENGES AND POTENTIAL FUTURE DEVELOPMENTS IN LIVER TRANSPLANTATION

Donor shortage is the key issue in LT. The biggest challenge ahead for the LT community will be to implement strategies that will overcome donor organ shortage, but at the same time maximise the long-term outcomes of the grafts transplanted. Reducing the waiting list mortality will involve bridging the gap between the demand and availability. Optimising the organ quality using newer technologies such as machine perfusion and 'growing livers in the lab' are exciting prospects that could overcome the chronic organ shortage.

Machine perfusion

With the advances and improvements in outcomes in LT over the last four decades, there has been a focus on expanding deceased donor organs. Static cold storage (SCS) remains the standard-of-care preservation method in LT. This is achieved by cooling the liver to 4°C with preservation solution; this decreases cellular energy consumption by reducing the metabolic demand of the tissue. However, when these SCS organs are reperfused, there is a higher ischaemia–reperfusion injury owing to efflux of accumulated metabolic products formed during cold storage, resulting in a profound inflammatory immune response and causing damage to the hepatocytes and cholangiocytes, thereby leading to poor short- and long-term outcomes. One of the ways of reducing ischaemia–reperfusion injury is to perfuse the liver with cold solution (hypothermic machine perfusion; HMP) or warm blood (normothermic

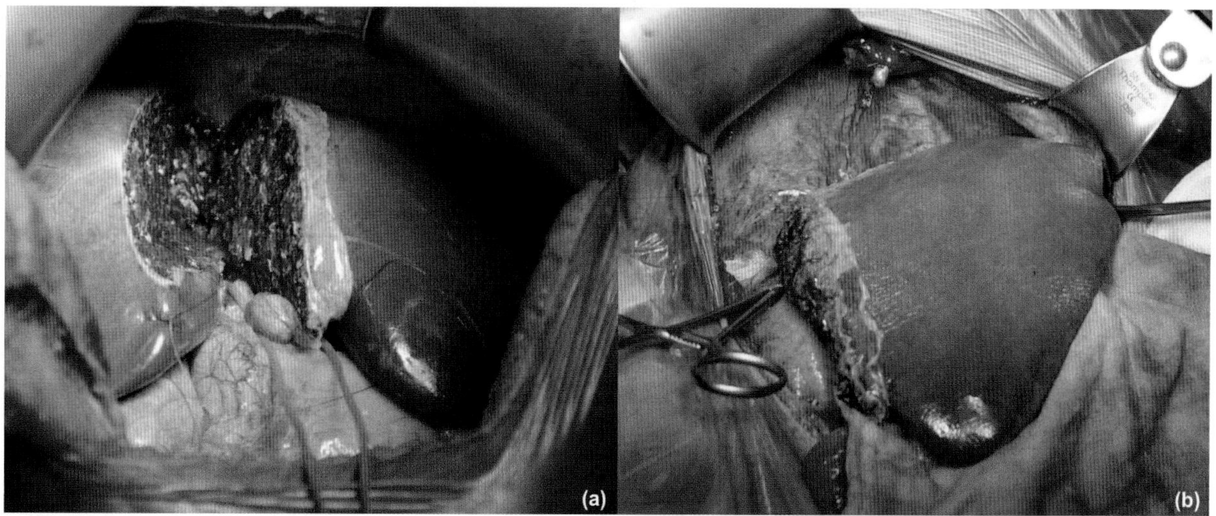

Figure 89.7 Paediatric living donor liver transplantation. **(a)** Donor left lateral segmentectomy where the parenchymal transection is completed and the graft is ready to be taken out; **(b)** the left lateral segment graft implanted into a paediatric recipient.

machine perfusion; NMP) with the aim of maintaining a healthy endothelium, replenishing adenosine triphosphate (ATP) and thereby improving quality. This allows the organs to be preserved for a longer period prior to transplantation, thereby addressing the logistics of LT. Further studies will be needed to explore the ideal perfusion method with the aim of improving longer term outcomes and avoiding biliary complications such as ischaemic cholangiopathy and to study viability markers to identify livers that will not function in the recipient, allowing liver-directed therapeutic interventions on the machine. In other exciting technology – *in situ* normothermic regional perfusion (NRP) – the blood supply to the abdominal organs after death is restored using extracorporeal circulation for a limited period before organ recovery. This leads to superior liver outcomes in DCD livers compared with conventional organ recovery, and may be an answer to the problem of ischaemic cholangiopathy.

Liver support devices

ALF has a high mortality in the range of 50–80%. Extracorporeal liver support systems have the potential to provide temporary support to bridge patients with ALF to LT or spontaneous recovery.

Artificial liver support devices function as 'dialysis' machines, which filter and adsorb toxic substances such as bilirubin, bile acids, metabolites of aromatic amino acids, medium-chain fatty acids and cytokines without significant loss of albumin from the circulation. Some examples of commonly available artificial liver support systems are the Molecular Adsorbent Recirculating System (MARS®; Gambro, Stockholm, Sweden) and Hepa Wash® (Hepa Wash GmbH, Munich, Germany). Biological liver support uses whole animal or human liver, and the liver support–detoxification is achieved by portal and/or artery perfusion. Some examples of commonly available biological liver support systems are the Extracorporeal Liver Assist Device (ELAD®; Vital Therapies Inc., San Diego, CA, USA) and the HepatAssist® system (Alliqua Inc., Langhorne, PA, USA).

Summary box 89.8

Definitions

- Acute liver failure: complex multisystem illness that evolves quickly after a catastrophic insult to the liver, leading to coagulopathy and encephalopathy; based on onset of encephalopathy – hyperacute (within 7 days), acute (8–28 days), subacute (>28 days)
- Allograft: an organ or tissue transplanted from one individual to another
- Chronic liver disease: progressive deterioration of liver functions for more than 6 months, with inflammation, destruction and regeneration of liver parenchyma, leading to fibrosis and cirrhosis
- Heterotopic graft: a graft placed in a site different from that where the organ is normally located
- HLA: human leukocyte antigen, the main trigger to graft rejection
- MELD score: model for end-stage liver disease score; predicts prognosis in patients with chronic liver disease and is used to allocate liver for transplant
- NAFLD: non-alcoholic fatty liver disease; associated with metabolic syndrome (obesity, hyperlipidaemia and diabetes mellitus). Some patients develop non-alcoholic steatohepatitis (NASH), which leads to fibrosis and cirrhosis
- Orthotopic graft: a graft placed in its normal anatomical site
- UKELD score: United Kingdom model for end-stage liver disease score; predicts survival of patients listed for LT in the UK

FURTHER READING

Busuttil R, Klinymalm G (eds). *Transplantation of the liver*, 3rd edn. Philadelphia, PA: Elsevier-Saunders, 2015.

Clavien P, Trotter J (eds). *Medical care of the liver transplant patient*, 4th edn. Oxford: Wiley-Blackwell, 2012.

Croome K, Muiesan P, Taner B (eds). *Donation after circulatory death (DCD) liver transplantation: a practical guide*. Springer, 2020.

Fan ST (ed.). *Living donor liver transplantation*, 2nd edn. Singapore: World Scientific, 2011.

Hadzic N, Baumann U, McLin V. *Pediatric liver transplantation: a clinical guide*. Philadelphia, PA: Elsevier, 2021.

Hricik D (ed.). *Primer on transplantation*, 3rd edn. Oxford: Wiley-Blackwell, 2011.

Garden OJ, Parks RW, Wigmore SJ (eds). *Principles and practice of surgery*, 8th edn. Elsevier, 2022.

Oniscu G, Forsythe J, Fung J (eds). *Abdominal organ retrieval and transplantation bench surgery*. Oxford: Wiley-Blackwell, 2013.

Sutcliffe R, Antoniades C, Deshpande R *et al. Liver and pancreatobiliary surgery: with liver transplantation*. Oxford: Oxford University Press, 2009.

USEFUL WEBSITES IN LIVER TRANSPLANTATION

- www.bts.org.uk
- www.odt.nhs.uk
- www.nhsbt.nhs.uk
- www.bsg.org.uk
- www.esot.org
- www.ilts.org
- www.ltsi.org.in
- www.eltr.org
- www.unos.org
- www.ctstransplant.org
- www.scandiatransplant.org
- www.iltr.org

CHAPTER

90 Pancreas transplantation

Learning objectives

To understand:
- The indications and patient selection for solid organ pancreas transplant
- The different types of pancreas transplant and the respective surgical techniques
- The principles of immunosuppression
- The common surgical and long-term complications of solid organ pancreas transplant and their principles of management

To appreciate:
- The principles of pancreas retrieval and preservation

INTRODUCTION

Current World Health Organization estimates are that about 9% of the global population have diabetes. This translates to over 600 000 000 people living with diabetes, with a significant proportion of these patients requiring insulin: approximately 10% of this population has type 1 diabetes. The aims of pancreas transplantation are to restore normoglycaemia, with freedom from insulin therapy, and to limit the progression of complications associated with diabetes. Pancreas transplantation is most commonly (but not exclusively) performed in individuals with type 1 diabetes with end-stage renal disease. In certain diabetic patients without renal insufficiency, pancreas transplantation alone can be performed to avert life-threatening complications of hypoglycaemia and to prevent the progression of diabetic complications. Unlike cardiac, lung and liver transplant, pancreas transplantation is not an immediately life-saving procedure, although it significantly improves not only quality of life but also life expectancy. Despite successful outcomes in the majority of patients following transplant, particularly for combined kidney–pancreas transplant, there is significant morbidity and mortality associated with the procedure. These factors, including the complications of long-term immunosuppression, must be carefully weighed against any potential benefit prior to patient listing. Current data indicate that more than 42 000 pancreas transplants have been performed worldwide, with the majority having been in the USA.

BACKGROUND AND INDICATIONS

History

Kelly, Lillehei and colleagues performed the first successful pancreas transplant in a human at the University of Minnesota, USA, in 1966. Initial results were poor, with high mortality associated with sepsis, rejection and other complications, but over the subsequent 30 years there was a steady increase in the numbers of pancreas transplants and an improvement in outcomes. Important factors in this improvement were changes in surgical techniques and the introduction of the immunosuppressive agent ciclosporin in the mid-1980s: this reduced both the need for steroids and the incidence of rejection. By 1996 patient survival and pancreas graft survival were 91% and 72% at 1 year and 84% and 62% at 3 years, respectively. The introduction of tacrolimus and mycophenolate mofetil as maintenance immunosuppression and the use of T-cell-depleting agents such as rabbit antithymocyte globulin (ATG) and alemtuzumab in the 1990s and 2000s resulted in further reductions in cellular rejection rates and improved graft survival. Continued refinement of surgical technique, organ preservation and postoperative care have led to steady improvements in outcomes of all types of pancreas transplant.

Types of solid organ pancreas transplant

1 **Simultaneous pancreas–kidney transplant (SPK)**. Both organs come from the same deceased donor. This is the commonest type of pancreas transplant and is indicated in patients with chronic renal failure (on or close to requiring dialysis) secondary to diabetes.
2 **Pancreas transplant alone (PTA)**. Primarily for patients with type 1 diabetes who have repeated episodes of hypoglycaemia associated with unawareness (i.e. patients develop hypoglycaemic coma without warning). This is a life-threatening situation and such patients are

William D Kelly, 1922–2006, led the surgical team at University of Minnesota, Minneapolis, MN, USA, that performed the first pancreas transplant.
Clarence W Lillehei, 1918–1999, part of the surgical team at University of Minnesota, Minneapolis, MN, USA, that performed the first pancreas transplant, subsequently went on to pioneer open heart surgery.

often unable to live independently or carry out normal employment.

3 **Pancreas-after-kidney transplant (PAK).** Deceased donor pancreas transplantation is performed after a previous kidney transplant, from either a living or deceased donor.
4 **Simultaneous deceased donor pancreas and live donor kidney transplant.** This option may shorten waiting times but is logistically very challenging and rarely performed.

Transplantation of the islets of Langerhans (islet cell transplant) is an alternative to pancreas transplant alone for patients with hypoglycaemic unawareness. This is not a solid organ transplant and therefore not detailed in this chapter, but a brief description follows. After pancreas retrieval, islets are isolated, prepared and delivered into the portal vein (PV) of the recipient, usually via a percutaneous transhepatic radiologically guided procedure. Early results demonstrated that the presence of functioning islets appeared to protect against refractory hypoglycaemia and improve glycaemic control but with a low incidence of insulin independence. However, success rates have improved in the last decade with some series showing 50% of patients remaining insulin independent at 5 years. Immunosuppression is required for islet transplantation and the associated long-term risks need to be balanced with the treatment benefits.

Indications

The indications for pancreas transplant can be split into those for patients with concomitant renal failure and those without. SPK is the most frequently performed procedure for patients with type 1 diabetes and renal failure due to diabetic nephropathy. There is a small population of patients with type 1 diabetes with renal failure due to primary renal disease or non-diabetic causes and they are also included in this group. The organs are almost exclusively from the same deceased donor, although there are rare examples of organs from living donors (LDs); however, LD pancreas transplantation has not been widely accepted and carries significant risk to the donor.

In patients with type 1 diabetes and the option of an LD kidney the possibilities are to undergo an LD kidney transplantation followed by either a PAK or an SPK. The decision is not clear-cut: although pancreas graft survival was historically superior in SPK, PAK results have improved over recent years and the outcomes of the two procedures are now similar. If the patient presents late and has already accrued time on dialysis, the high morbidity and mortality associated with dialysis (30% mortality at 5 years) renders LD kidney transplantation followed by PAK somewhat more desirable. The policy regarding SPK or LD kidney transplantation followed by PAK is dependent on many factors, particularly the expected waiting time for an SPK.

SPK indications as defined by the NHS Blood and Transplant Pancreatic Advisory Group (NHSBT PAG) include type 1 diabetes with end-stage renal failure requiring dialysis or dialysis predicted within 6 months (glomerular filtration rate [GFR] <20 mL/min). Patients with type 1 diabetes without renal failure but with life-threatening hypoglycaemic unawareness are potential candidates of solid organ PTA or islet transplantation. The annual mortality rate of patients with insulin-induced hypoglycaemic unawareness is estimated to be between 3% and 6% – a major risk for this group of typically young patients. In patients with early diabetic nephropathy the risk of repeated acute kidney injury (AKI) needs to be considered prior to PTA to minimise the chance of accelerating renal failure, and a baseline GFR of 80–100 mL/min/1.73m^2 means the patient is unlikely to need a kidney transplant.

Patients with type 2 diabetes can also be considered for SPK, although after careful selection: many obese patients with type 2 diabetes are better managed with diet and/or bariatric surgery. Suitable candidates are non-morbidly obese patients, typically with insulin requirements of less than <1 unit/kg body weight in 24 hours (to exclude patients with insulin resistance). When selected in this way, the results of SPK in these patients are similar to those in patients with type 1 diabetes.

Patient selection

Once the indication for pancreas transplantation is satisfied the patient needs a comprehensive assessment of cardiovascular and surgical fitness. An anaesthetic review, echocardiogram and assessment of inducible cardiac ischaemia using dynamic imaging such as a myocardial perfusion scan or stress echocardiogram should be performed. If cardiac assessment demonstrates occult ischaemic heart disease (IHD) then angiography and revascularisation via angioplasty or bypass surgery may be needed prior to wait-listing. Patients with diabetic nephropathy usually have other manifestations of secondary diabetic complications, including sensory neuropathy, retinopathy, gastropathy, peripheral vascular disease, foot ulcers and autonomic neuropathy leading to postural hypotension. These complications should be sought and discussed prior to listing as they can have an impact on whether a pancreas transplant is appropriate and may alter the surgical strategy. For example, the significant anticoagulation required post transplant can lead to retinal haemorrhage; in a patient with severe retinopathy, this can lead to a deterioration in vision and even blindness. Patients with severe gastropathy may require a feeding jejunostomy at the time of transplant surgery, as gastropathy and bowel dysfunction are frequently exacerbated by surgery, which can lead to vomiting, difficulties absorbing immunosuppressants and malnutrition. The overall risks of this major surgery and immunosuppression in a patient with advanced diabetic complications have to be balanced with the likely benefits in severely overweight patients: most transplant centres have a body mass index (BMI) cut-off (e.g. <32 kg/m^2).

Paul Langerhans, 1847–1888, German pathologist, physiologist and biologist credited with the discovery of the 'islets of Langerhans', the cells that secrete insulin in the pancreas.

Summary box 90.1

Types of transplant and patient selection

- There are three main types of solid organ pancreas transplant: SPK; PTA; PAK
- The most common indication for pancreas transplant is type 1 diabetes with diabetic nephropathy
- Hypoglycaemic unawareness and life-limiting complications from insulin therapy are indications for pancreas transplant alone
- A comprehensive preoperative assessment of surgical fitness and occult cardiac disease is essential prior to wait-listing

ORGAN DONATION AND PRESERVATION

Organ retrieval

Pancreas organ retrieval is standardised in the UK and is carried out by dedicated abdominal organ retrieval teams. Donation after brain death (DBD) donors constitute 75% of all pancreas donors with donation after circulatory death (DCD) donors making up 25%. The pancreas can be retrieved either alone or en bloc with the liver. If the liver and pancreas are retrieved en bloc the retrieval surgeon separates the organs, ensuring that there is 10 mm of PV and an adequate length of splenic artery (SA) and superior mesenteric artery (SMA) for reconstruction. The bifurcation of the iliac vessels is sent with the pancreas to facilitate a vascular Y-graft construction (***Figure 90.1***), creating a single arterial inflow. Only around 50% of pancreases that are retrieved with the intention of transplantation are actually transplanted; this is a much higher discard rate than occurs in other abdominal organs and is for a number of reasons. The condition of the pancreas is frequently suboptimal owing to fatty infiltration or fibrosis, features that are associated with a poorer outcome. Also, injury to the pancreas during retrieval is much more common than in other organs: it is easily damaged and the consequences of even a relatively minor parenchymal injury can be severe, with postoperative leakage of exocrine secretions. Acceptance criteria for pancreases varies between centres and is usually related to donor age, BMI, alcohol intake and lifestyle factors. Other adverse donor and retrieval features that impact acceptance rates include: a prolonged agonal phase in DCD donors, evidence of hepatic or pancreatic ischaemic injury (raised transaminases, amylase and lipase) and complex vascular anatomy.

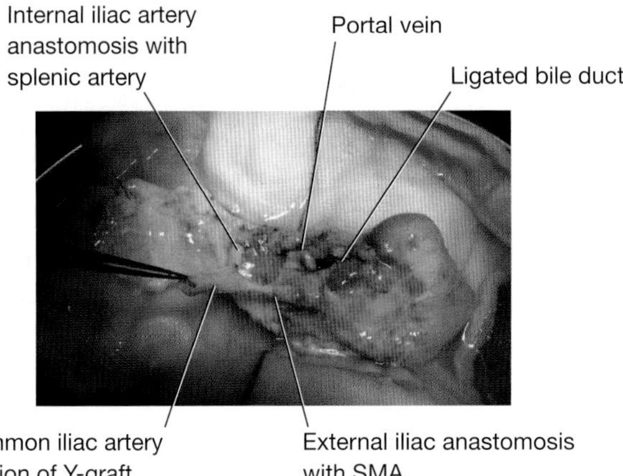

Figure 90.1 The inferior border of the donor pancreas prepared for implantation demonstrating a completed vascular reconstruction. The surgical forceps are holding the cut end of the donor common iliac artery and the completed anastomoses between the donor external iliac artery and the superior mesenteric artery (SMA) and the donor interior iliac artery with the splenic artery are demonstrated (blue vascular suture).

Organ preservation

Static cold storage (SCS) has remained the gold standard preservation method for the pancreas graft since the first transplantation was performed in 1966. SCS is the most common preservation method for organs after retrieval because of its simplicity, relative effectiveness for many organs and low cost. Hypothermic preservation is based on the principle that cooling an organ reduces the metabolic rate and the demand for adenosine triphosphate (ATP). The pancreas is extremely sensitive to both warm and cold ischaemia, which has a significant impact on preservation. Once retrieved from the donor, the pancreas is inspected for any damage and for adequacy of perfusion and then submerged in preservation solution within an organ bag and placed in an icebox for transport to the transplant centre. Unlike other organs the pancreas is not flushed following retrieval in order to minimise endothelial damage and (supposedly) to reduce the risk of early graft pancreatitis and thrombosis. Early pancreas transplants suffered from a significant thrombosis rate of up to 25%. For this reason, in 1986 Belzer and Southard set out to redefine the needs of pancreas preservation by developing a new preservation solution. This new solution – University of Wisconsin (UW) solution – was first successfully applied in experimental pancreas transplantation; this study was published by Wahlberg, who was a member of the Wisconsin group. The colloid constituent, hydroxyethyl starch (HES), was particularly important in the pancreas, especially in suboptimal organs and those with longer cold ischaemia times. Translation to clinical use of the UW solution led to a significant improvement in the results of pancreas transplantation and a marked reduction in pancreatitis and thrombosis of the grafts.

There have been studies in experimental pancreas preservation using hypothermic machine perfusion; in these studies the organ is continuously pumped with a cooled solution, but this has yet to translate into clinical practice, although recent results are promising. Normothermic machine perfusion of pancreases has been performed on animal and discarded human organs but led to organ injury, possibly because of

Folkert O Belzer, 1930–1995, pioneering transplant surgeon who was Chairman of the Department of Surgery, University of Wisconsin, USA, along with Jan Wahlberg (Uppsala, Sweden) and Rutger Ploeg (Leiden, the Netherlands) developed University of Wisconsin solution.

James H Southard, contemporary, Emeritus Professor, Department of Surgery, University of Wisconsin, USA, co-inventor of the University of Wisconsin solution with Belzer.

high concentrations of autolytic enzymes (amylase and lipase). Normothermic regional perfusion is a technique in which, following cessation of circulation in a DCD organ donor, the donor blood is warmed, oxygenated and then pumped back around the abdominal organs. This appears to be beneficial in the context of the liver, but has yet to show convincing data in pancreas transplantation – the numbers studied are small and the technique is still in its infancy.

Summary box 90.2

Organ donation and preservation

- The majority of pancreas transplants (75%) are from DBD donors
- The pancreas is the most frequently damaged organ during retrieval, which can impact on clinical outcomes
- SCS remains the gold standard of preservation, although research into machine perfusion is gaining momentum

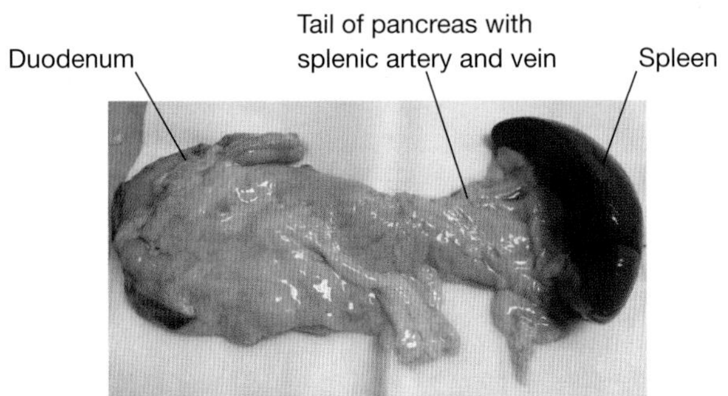

Figure 90.2 A healthy donor pancreas prior to preparation for surgical implantation. The pancreas is lying in its anatomical position with the head of the pancreas beneath omental fat encircled by the duodenum and the tail within the hilum of the spleen.

SURGICAL TECHNIQUES

Preparation for transplant

Once the organ has been inspected and is deemed suitable for transplant it needs to be prepared for implantation. This is a crucial step and meticulous attention to detail and a systematic approach are vital to minimise bleeding and complications after reperfusion. The pancreas is retrieved with the spleen attached, a length of duodenum and the cut ends of the SMA, SA and PV (***Figure 90.2***). The splenic vessels are ligated and the spleen removed; the duodenum is shortened, stapled and the staple lines buried with a suture. Excess fat and omentum are removed, and the cut end of the inferior mesenteric vein ligated. An arterial 'Y-graft' is usually fashioned between the SMA and SA of the pancreas using donor iliac vessels, so that the end of the common iliac artery (CIA) can be used for a single arterial anastomosis (***Figure 90.1***).

Transplantation procedure

Pancreas transplant can be performed as an intraperitoneal or extraperitoneal procedure and the exocrine drainage of the pancreas can be managed by connection to the small intestine or urinary bladder (***Figure 90.3***). The majority of surgeons favour an intraperitoneal approach as the peritoneal cavity has an excellent capacity for containing and reabsorbing fluid generated as a result of reperfusion pancreatitis. The steps of the surgical procedure are as follows. A midline laparotomy is performed and the retroperitoneum is exposed. The inferior vena cava (IVC) and CIA are dissected and controlled. In the enteric drainage procedure (donor duodenum anastomosed to recipient jejunum) the organ is positioned with the head of the pancreas towards the liver and the tail towards the pelvis. However, for bladder drainage (donor duodenum anastomosed to recipient urinary bladder) the organ is positioned with the head facing towards the pelvis and tail towards the liver. A side-biting vascular clamp is used to partially occlude the IVC and the PV is anastomosed end to side to the IVC. Whether performing a single arterial anastomosis or separate SMA and SA anastomoses, the right CIA is most frequently used. Heparin is administered prior to clamping the CIA and the arterial anastomosis is performed. The organ is reperfused and haemostasis is ensured before performing the duodenal anastomosis (this renders the organ less mobile and more difficult to access). For enteric drainage, the jejunum is identified as close as convenient to the duodenojejunal flexure and anastomosed side to side to the duodenum in two layers. This can be performed by passing the duodenum through a window in the colonic mesentery, using a Roux-en-Y technique or with the two sections of bowel lying adjacent underneath the colon (***Figure 90.3***). The Roux-en-Y technique creates a blind-ending loop of bowel; if severe complications develop and the pancreas needs to be removed, then separation from the main enteric flow is straightforward and the need for a defunctioning stoma is avoided. In the bladder drainage technique, the anastomosis to the bladder is also performed in two layers and a urinary catheter is kept in place for 7–10 days to reduce the chance of anastomotic leak.

Enteric conversion

Bladder drainage of the exocrine secretions is associated with complications that may require conversion to enteric drainage. Enteric conversion is performed in patients to eliminate these complications of bladder drainage (see ***Postoperative management, Complications***). It is usually delayed until 1 year post transplant but can be performed sooner if indicated. A lower midline laparotomy is performed and the urinary bladder is filled and the transplant duodenum is identified. The transplant duodenum is disconnected from the bladder and the bladder is closed in two layers. An adjacent section of small bowel is identified and a longitudinal enterotomy is performed on the antimesenteric border; the anastomosis to the duodenum is completed in two layers. Surgical drains are placed adjacent to the anastomoses and a urinary catheter is usually kept in place for 14 days.

César Roux, 1857–1934, Professor of Surgery and Gynaecology, Lausanne, Switzerland. Described the Roux-en-Y loop in 1908.

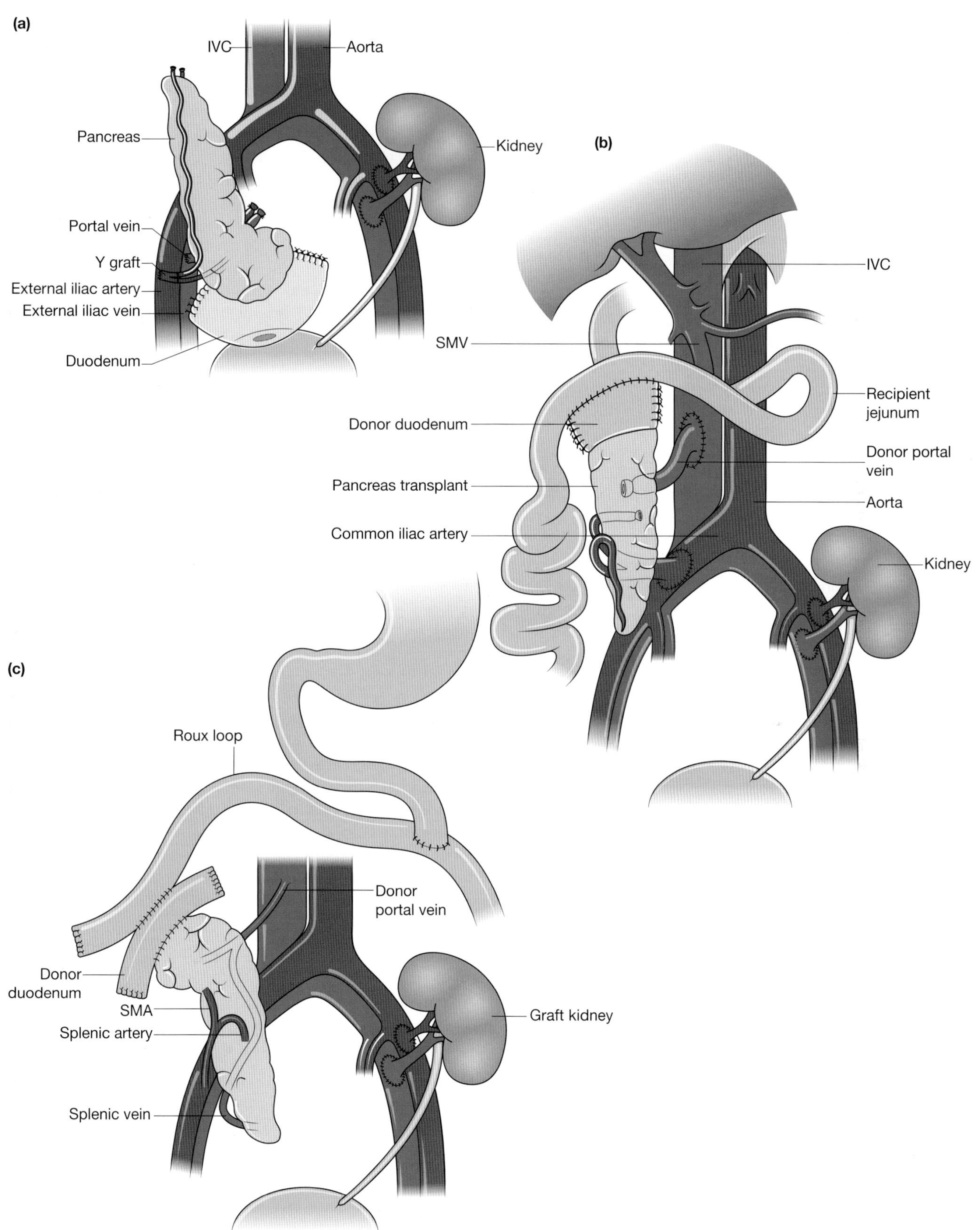

Figure 90.3 Illustration of the organ positions in a simultaneous kidney–pancreas transplant and the options for management of the exocrine secretions. **(a)** Transplanted pancreas positioned head-down with the duodenum anastomosed to the urinary bladder. **(b)** Transplanted pancreas positioned head-up with the duodenum anastomosed to the jejunum. **(c)** The donor duodenum anastomosed to the Roux limb of the Roux-en-Y construction. IVC, inferior vena cava; SMA, superior mesenteric artery; SMV, superior mesenteric vein.

Summary box 90.3

Surgical techniques

- Careful inspection and preparation of the pancreas is essential and involves the construction of a Y-graft between donor iliac vessels and the SA and SMA to aid arterial anastomosis
- The pancreas is usually transplanted intraperitoneally with the PV anastomosed to the IVC and the Y-graft anastomosed to the CIA
- Drainage of enteric secretions is performed by anastomosis to the bowel, although bladder drainage can also be performed

POSTOPERATIVE MANAGEMENT

Anticoagulation

To minimise the risk of graft thrombosis in the early postoperative period anticoagulation is indicated for all patients. Every centre has its specific protocol: the exact details are less important than the balance between adequate anticoagulation to minimise thrombosis and over-anticoagulation leading to bleeding and the need for further surgery. Intravenous unfractionated heparin, dextran or epoprostenol are examples of preparations used; monitoring of their effect can be achieved by measuring prothrombin time (PT) and/or thromboelastography (TEG). TEG is a real-time bedside test that gives a numerical value for overall coagulation. The heparin dose or infusion rate of therapy can be amended according to the TEG or PT results. TEG has an advantage over PT as the result is immediate and analysis incorporates the entire clotting cascade and platelet function. Patients usually require 24–48 hours of high-dependency care (high-dependency unit or intensive care unit) and close blood glucose monitoring is essential. Insulin secreted by the transplant pancreas drains directly into the IVC and straight into the systemic circulation without passing through the liver, thereby avoiding first-pass metabolism. This is unlike normal physiology where insulin drains via the portal vein through the liver. As a result of high systemic insulin levels the patient may require intravenous glucose supplementation to maintain blood glucose levels. This phenomenon usually accommodates within 48 hours. If blood glucose levels rise above 8 mmol/L, then cross-sectional imaging with arterial phase contrast is usually performed to assess for thrombosis. The presence of a small volume of thrombus in the distal ligated end of the SMA is considered normal. However, thrombus propagating from the stump into the SMA, SA thrombus or PV thrombus should be treated with full anticoagulation. The indication for surgery is limited to complete thrombosis of the arterial inflow or PV; thrombectomy usually fails, resulting in graft pancreatectomy.

Complications

Major abdominal surgery carries a number of general risks which are well detailed elsewhere; for the sake of brevity, they will not be discussed here. Pancreas transplant patients are assessed preoperatively to rule out significant cardiac disease and to ensure that they are suitable for major surgery. Despite this, longstanding diabetes means that complications are common and potentially serious. Intraoperative complications such as bleeding following reperfusion can lead to the need for blood transfusion and inotropic support. Up to one in three patients require further surgery postoperatively. This may be due to reperfusion pancreatitis or bleeding. Reperfusion pancreatitis (a manifestation of ischaemia–reperfusion-related injury) can result in an amylase-rich transudate around the pancreas and in the abdominal cavity. Drainage may be necessary to aid recovery: in patients with an ongoing inflammatory state clinicians have a low threshold to return to the operating theatre for washout and debridement of peripancreatic necrosis. Thrombosis affects up to 8% of patients and this may result in early graft loss or β-cell dysfunction. Anastomotic leaks, particularly from the duodenum, are rare but difficult to manage; they can be controlled with direct drainage, such as a Foley catheter within the duodenum. However, such complications may necessitate surgical revision or, in extreme cases, graft pancreatectomy.

Bladder-drained pancreases can cause cystitis from pancreatic enzyme secretion and electrolyte disturbance, acidosis and dehydration from the loss of bicarbonate. Up to 50% of patients with bladder-drained pancreas transplants require enteric conversion (where the transplant duodenum is surgically detached from the bladder and reconnected to the small bowel) within the first year following transplant. This usually follows recurrent hospital admissions for acidosis and is performed to mitigate the risk of acute kidney injury. Also, the indication for conversion may be driven by patient choice because of symptoms from chemical cystitis, urinary tract infection (UTI) and the need for high-dose oral sodium bicarbonate. Late complications of pancreas transplantation include pseudoaneurysm formation, which may result from fungal infection or a vascular anastomosis, and highlights the importance of culturing the preservation fluid at the time of transplant and treating any cultured microorganisms.

A full list of complications following pancreas transplantation is given in ***Table 90.1***

IMMUNOSUPPRESSION AND FOLLOW-UP

Long-term monitoring

Blood glucose monitoring is reassuring for the patient but, once glucose levels are raised as a result of graft rejection, it is usually too late to reverse. Haemoglobin A1c (HbA1c) levels are an independent predictor of long-term graft function and oral glucose tolerance testing can also be used to assess organ dysfunction and aid management. Fasting C-peptide and insulin levels can also give an idea of pancreatic function. Cellular rejection is difficult to diagnose owing to the absence of a biomarker: in patients who have undergone SPK, serum creatinine can be used as a surrogate marker and renal biopsy

Frederic Eugene Basil Foley, 1891–1966, urologist, Ancker Hospital, St Paul, MN, USA.

TABLE 90.1 Complications following pancreas transplantation.

Generic complications	Enteric drainage	Bladder drainage
• Bleeding • Reperfusion pancreatitis • Thrombosis • Paralytic ileus • Rejection • Infection – e.g. CMV, candida • Retinal haemorrhage and worsening of vision • Limb ischaemia	• Anastomotic leak • Stoma formation • Exacerbation of gastropathy and malnutrition	• Loss of sodium bicarbonate and acidosis/ extracellular volume depletion • Chemical cystitis • Urethritis • Bladder leak • Reflux pancreatitis • Recurrent UTIs • Bladder stones[a] • Urethral strictures[b] • Urethral irritation[b] • Epididymitis[b] • Prostatitis and prostatic abscess[b]

CMV, cytomegalovirus.
[a]Linked to duration of transplant.
[b]Documented complications but very rare.

performed, although discordant rejection of kidney and pancreas is a well-recognised event. However, if the pancreas rejects but not the kidney, the diagnosis is much more difficult and relies on cross-sectional imaging (to exclude vascular complications) and a high level of clinical suspicion. In PTA, the exocrine secretions can be managed by anastomosis with the urinary bladder, which means that urinary amylase can be measured sequentially and used as a biomarker of pancreatic function and a surrogate for rejection. A reduction in levels of urinary amylase may indicate rejection. Cystoscopic duodenal biopsy can be performed but the histology is often difficult to interpret and the presence of lymphocytes may not necessarily indicate rejection. Computed tomography angiography may show peripancreatic inflammation, which would be consistent with rejection and be an indication for rescue therapy.

Outcomes

There are no randomised controlled trials that compare the outcome of SPK transplantation with kidney transplantation alone, so best practice has mostly been determined from registry analyses and single-centre experiences. The major limitation of comparing SPK with deceased donor kidney transplantation is the inherent selection bias that patients who are suitable for SPK are fit enough to undergo major abdominal surgery and those undergoing deceased donor kidney transplant may not be. However, registry analyses show a clear survival benefit of SPK compared with deceased donor transplant. Adjusted 10-year patient survival rates were 67% for SPK recipients, 65% for LD kidney recipients and 46% for deceased donor kidney recipients. In the UK, 1- and 5-year pancreas graft survival for patients undergoing their first SPK is 90% and 81%, respectively. Patient survival is 98% and 89% at 1 and 5 years, respectively. PTA has the poorest long-term survival because of high rates of early thrombosis and cellular rejection but provides exogenous insulin production to treat the complications detailed above. For pancreas alone transplants the outcomes are still inferior with 1- and 5-year pancreas graft survival of 82% and 54%, respectively. In the USA, the data are similar with 5-year pancreas graft survival currently 73% for SPK, 65% for PAK and 53% for PTA; 5-year patient survival rates are 93% for SPK, 91% for PAK and 78% for PTA recipients, respectively.

Immunosuppression

Immunosuppression is split into induction (immediate post transplant) and maintenance (long term) therapy. Induction therapies include non-depleting antilymphocyte antibodies that cause T-cell inactivation, such as basiliximab, which blocks the interleukin-2 receptor and inhibits T-cell expansion. T-cell-depleting antibodies have largely replaced non-depleting therapies as a more effective way of suppressing lymphocytes. These include polyclonal ATG and the monoclonal antibody alemtuzumab (Sanofi). The use of T-cell-depleting antibody therapy has reduced rejection levels but without a corresponding effect on graft or patient survival. Alemtuzumab is easier to administer and is associated with lower rates of viral infection than ATG, so is preferred by some transplant units. Maintenance immunosuppression has evolved from triple therapy with ciclosporin, azathioprine and steroid to current practice with tacrolimus and mycophenolate mofetil. Steroid-free regimes are aimed at minimising insulin resistance and wound infection and are favoured by some centres. Comparison of ciclosporin with tacrolimus in combination with mycophenolate mofetil (MMF) and steroid, plus induction with ATG, in the EUROSPK 001 trial showed a reduction in the rates of severe rejection, with lower rates of pancreas graft loss at 3 years in the tacrolimus combination group.

Summary box 90.4

Immunosuppression and follow-up

- Pancreas rejection is challenging to diagnose and once glucose levels rise it is usually too late to reverse
- Outcomes from SPK and LD kidney transplant are similar and both options offer a survival advantage compared with deceased donor transplant
- Induction therapy with lymphocyte-depleting antibodies (alemtuzumab, ATG) has reduced rejection rates without changing graft and patient survival

FUTURE WORK

The major limiting factor in pancreas transplantation is greater morbidity compared with kidney transplantation alone. This is largely a function of the immediate reperfusion pancreatitis that is a common sequel to implantation. A second limitation is the very poor utilisation of donor organs: in the UK, only 25% of organs that are offered are actually transplanted. The risk profile of the organ donor population is increasing (largely because of age) and this increases the need to develop a means of preservation and organ assessment that gives clinicians the confidence that organs are suitable for transplant.

The development of novel preservation methods, such as machine perfusion, has been successful in other organs, but there has been no such advance in pancreas transplantation – this is largely a function of the relatively small numbers of patients undergoing this procedure. New methods of graft surveillance to detect rejection or other complications at a much earlier stage are also needed. International collaboration and multicentre clinical trials are needed to advance practice. If it were possible to reduce the morbidity and improve the survival of pancreas transplants to the same level as kidney transplants, the indications for this procedure would expand, possibly allowing patients to benefit before developing kidney failure.

ACKNOWLEDGEMENT

Our sincere thanks to Mr James Gilbert for supplying the photographic images.

FURTHER READING

Al-Qaoud TM, Kaufman DB, Odorico JS, Friend PJ. Pancreas and kidney transplantation for diabetic nephropathy. In: Knechtle SJ, Marson LP, Morris PJ (eds). *Kidney transplantation, principles and practice*, 8th edn. Philadelphia, PA; Elsevier, 2020: 608–32.

Dean PG, Kukla A, Stegall MD, Kudva YC. Pancreas transplantation. *BMJ* 2017; **357**: j1321.

White SA, Shaw JA, Sutherland DE. Pancreas transplantation. *Lancet* 2009; **373**(9677): 1808–17.

CHAPTER 91 Intestinal and multivisceral transplantation

Learning objectives

To understand:

- The indications for intestinal transplantation
- The assessment process for intestinal transplantation
- The different transplant types
- Both the medical and surgical complications associated with intestinal transplantation
- The outcomes associated with intestinal transplantation

BACKGROUND

Intestinal and multivisceral transplantation can be a life-saving therapy for patients with complications from the treatment of intestinal failure. Indications for this highly specialised type of transplant are broadening to include acute vascular catastrophes and some otherwise irresectable intra-abdominal tumours (e.g. desmoids and pseudomyxoma peritonei). Since the first successful multivisceral transplant in the late 1980s, more than 4000 transplants have taken place worldwide and outcomes continue to improve. Intestinal transplantation is the most challenging area of abdominal transplantation, with higher rates of complications than other transplant groups. These complications include rejection, sepsis, post-transplant lymphoproliferative disease (PTLD) and graft-versus-host disease (GVHD).

Graft and patient outcomes for isolated intestinal transplants are close to those for long-term parenteral nutrition (PN). The role of intestinal transplantation may be changing with earlier referral to try to avoid the complications of long-term PN, including intestinal failure-associated liver disease (IFALD).

INTRODUCTION

The first reported intestine-containing transplant in humans was performed in 1966, when a short segment of duodenum was included in a pancreas transplant. This was followed by attempts to transplant more substantial amounts of intestine, but these did not result in long-term survival. It was not until 1988 that the first 'successful' intestine-containing transplant was reported.

At this time intestinal transplants were a rarity but with increasing experience (both surgical and immunological) outcomes have improved, making intestinal transplantation a relatively routine procedure.

Changes in immunosuppression regimes (depleting antibodies and tacrolimus) have improved rates of rejection, a complication that is difficult to control and can be life-threatening.

In 1996 the International Intestinal Transplant Registry was established and reported a total of 180 transplants performed in 25 centres worldwide. By 2019 this number was over 4100, with almost double the number of active centres. The majority of transplants have been performed in the USA and Europe, with the most prolific units performing over 10 adult transplants per year.

With improvements in the management of paediatric intestinal failure the number of multivisceral and intestinal transplants in this group has fallen.

INDICATIONS FOR TRANSPLANTATION

Complications from PN for irreversible intestinal failure are the most well-established indications for intestinal transplantation (***Table 91.1***). Short bowel syndrome (SBS) is the most frequent cause for the need for PN. The aetiologies of SBS vary between the adult and paediatric population.

The most common causes for SBS in the paediatric population are volvulus, gastroschisis, necrotising enterocolitis and intestinal dysmotility or pseudo-obstruction. The last two result in functional SBS.

The most common causes for SBS in adults result from bowel resections owing to mesenteric ischaemia, inflammatory bowel disease (most commonly Crohn's disease), benign tumour resection and dysmotility or pseudo-obstruction.

Until recently, intestinal transplantation was only considered for patients with complications of PN, including loss of vascular access, recurrent life-threatening line infections (especially fungal infections) and IFALD. Increasingly patients are being transplanted for quality-of-life indications, although this remains controversial.

Burrill Bernard Crohn, 1884–1983, gastroenterologist, Mount Sinai Hospital, New York, NY, USA, described regional ileitis in 1932.

TABLE 91.1 Current indications for intestinal transplantation in the UK.

1. Life-threatening complications of parenteral nutrition a. Progressive IFALD or non-IFALD • Assessed by biochemistry and biopsy • Combined intestinal and liver transplant is best considered in the presence of advanced liver disease (portal hypertension or advanced fibrosis)
b. Severe sepsis • More than one life-threatening episode of catheter-related sepsis for which no remediable cause can be identified • Endocarditis or other metastatic infection
c. Limited central venous access • Venous access limited to three major conventional sites in adults (above and below the diaphragm) and two major conventional sites above the diaphragm in children • Conventional central venous sites are defined as internal jugular, subclavian and femoral veins
2. Very poor quality of life thought likely to be correctable by transplantation
3. Surgery to remove a large proportion of the abdominal viscera considered untenable without associated multivisceral transplantation (e.g. extensive desmoid disease, extensive critical mesenteric arterial disease)
4. Localised malignancy considered amenable to curative resection requiring extensive evisceration (e.g. localised neuroendocrine tumours). Particular caution should be exercised in this group and patients should be discussed in a multidisciplinary multicentre forum (e.g. National Adult Small Intestinal Transplant [NASIT] forum)
5. Where the transplantation procedure is expected to preclude the possibility of future intestinal transplantation (e.g. loss of venous access or further human leukocyte antigen sensitisation)
6. Where the need for subsequent intestinal transplantation is considered likely and the risk of death is increased by excluding the intestine from the graft *Examples include predictable problems related to administering immunosuppression (e.g. line sepsis), or continuing severe intestinal disease such as diabetic visceral neuropathy, or ultra-short bowel syndrome, which may cause fluid, electrolyte and acid–base balance problems that would damage an existing or planned renal graft*
7. Transplantation of additional organs for feasibility reasons a. Renal transplantation b. Adults and children with corrected GFR of <45 mL/min/m^2 are evaluated for the possibility of simultaneous renal transplantation

GFR, glomerular filtration rate; IFALD, intestinal failure-associated liver disease.
Adapted from NHS Blood and Transplant (https://www.odt.nhs.uk/transplantation/small-bowel/).

If the indication for transplant is IFALD, the degree of liver impairment influences the organs required at transplant. Mild to moderate liver fibrosis may allow an isolated intestinal transplant to be undertaken. This results in improved patient outcomes, better organ utilisation and reversal of liver fibrosis with discontinuation of PN. Severe liver fibrosis or cirrhosis will necessitate a liver-containing graft.

Indications for intestinal transplantation continue to change and now include to facilitate the resection of some tumours (desmoids and pseudomyxoma peritonei). In this situation, without intestinal transplantation, extensive evisceration would render the patient dependent on PN. Hepatic cirrhosis with extensive portomesenteric thrombosis may make isolated liver transplantation technically impossible, so multivisceral transplantation may be considered for some individuals.

Acute widespread splanchnic ischaemia (arterial and venous) is a rare but growing indication for super-urgent intestinal and multivisceral transplantation as well as other acute abdominal catastrophes.

ASSESSMENT FOR TRANSPLANTATION

Assessment for a multivisceral/intestinal transplant requires a multidisciplinary approach, including:

- transplant surgeons;
- intestinal failure physicians;
- transplant anaesthetists;
- hepatologists;
- psychiatrists and/or psychologists;
- radiologists;
- infectious disease physicians;
- transplant specialist nurses;
- dieticians.

Assessment of venous access and the degree of liver fibrosis is critical. Patients on PN for a substantial time or who have ultra-short gut are at high risk of developing IFALD. They will need a liver biopsy as part of the assessment process. Detailed venous mapping is essential in all candidates.

Appropriate assessment of the cardiovascular and respiratory systems is necessary. Upper and lower gastrointestinal endoscopies may be necessary.

Cross-sectional imaging of the abdomen to assess the abdominal anatomy is central to operative planning.

Significant renal impairment may result in the need to consider inclusion of a kidney at the time of transplant.

Patients should have anaesthetic and psychiatric assessment and dietetic review.

TYPES OF TRANSPLANT

Multivisceral or intestinal transplant covers a number of different 'cluster' transplants, as shown in ***Table 91.2*** and ***Figure 91.1***.

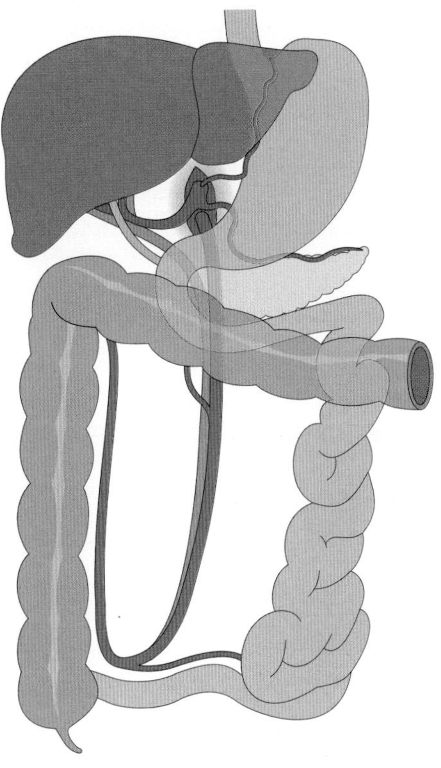
Full multivisceral transplant

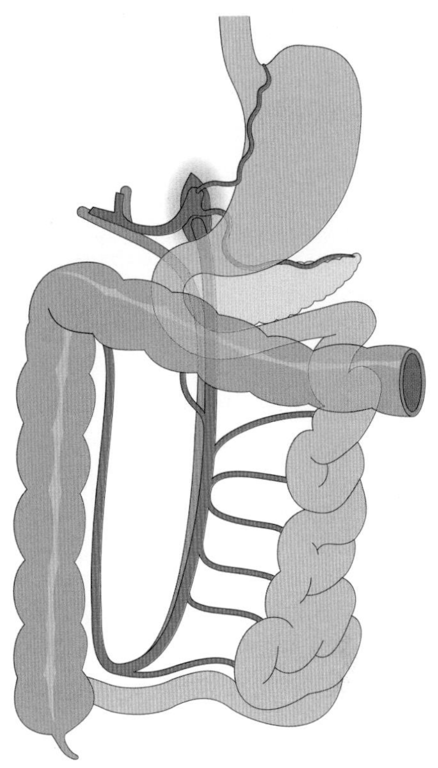
Modified multivisceral transplant

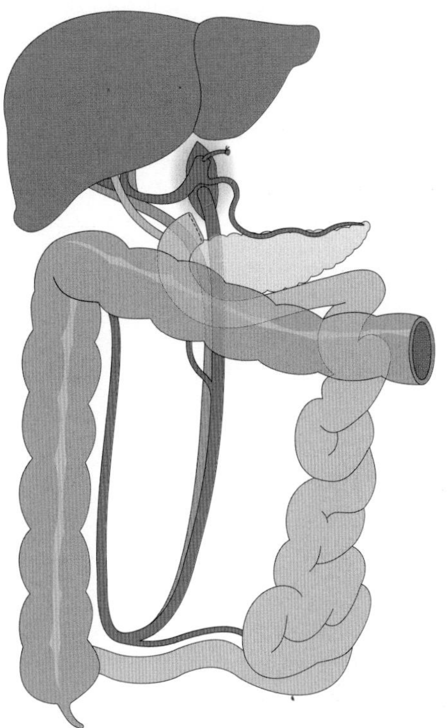
Liver and small bowel transplant

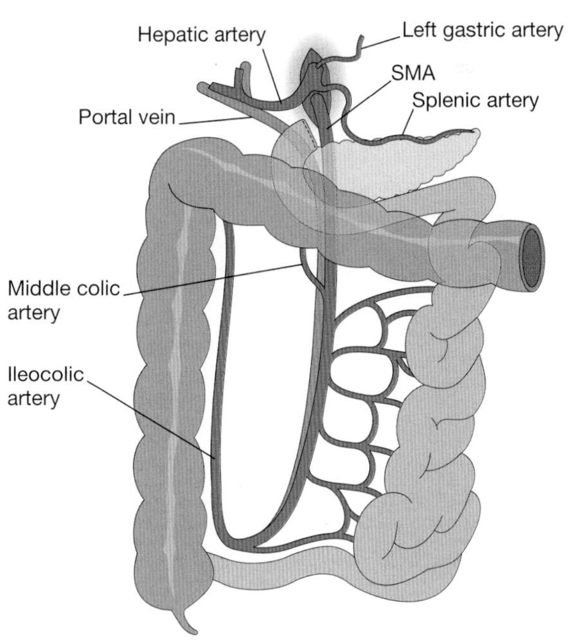

Small bowel, pancreas and colon transplant

Figure 91.1 Types of intestinal transplant. SMA, superior mesenteric artery.

TABLE 91.2 'Cluster' transplants.

Transplant	Organs included	Extent of resection	Proximal enteric anastomosis
Small intestinal and colon transplant	Small intestine and colon (with/without pancreas)	Small intestine and part of colon	Duodenum or proximal jejunum
Modified multivisceral transplant	Stomach, pancreas, small intestine and colon	Stomach, pancreas, spleen, small intestine and part of colon	Proximal stomach or oesophagus
Liver and small bowel transplant	Liver, pancreas, small intestine and colon	Liver, small intestine and part of colon	Duodenum or proximal jejunum
Multivisceral transplant	Liver, stomach, pancreas, small intestine and colon	Liver, stomach, pancreas, spleen, small intestine and part of colon	Proximal stomach or oesophagus

PREOPERATIVE PLANNING

The decision regarding the type of transplant to be performed is dependent on a variety of patient factors. Intraoperative flexibility is necessary and may change the type of transplant undertaken.

A robust plan for adequate venous access is necessary and may require pretransplant venous reconstruction by the interventional radiology team or surgical reconstruction.

If substantial intraoperative blood loss is predicted, selective arterial embolisation may be considered. Commonly this will involve the superior mesenteric artery and coeliac axis, but more selective embolisation can be undertaken if preservation of the stomach or the pancreaticoduodenal complex is planned.

THE TRANSPLANT

Multivisceral/intestinal transplants are almost invariably performed with organs donated from deceased brain dead donors. A small number of living donor intestinal transplants have been performed.

In intestinal and multivisceral transplant procedures the donor and recipient operations occur simultaneously; this is not the case for liver and kidney transplantation. This is to minimise cold ischaemia time (the intestine is intolerant of ischaemia and ideally cold ischaemia times of less than 6 hours are required).

The recipient operation is often complex and technically challenging. Portal hypertension, extensive adhesions and distorted anatomy all result in these patients having surgically hostile abdomens, making the explant challenging. Substantial blood loss and transfusion may result in severe coagulopathy. Preoperative embolisation can reduce blood loss significantly. The extent of the explant is dependent on what transplant is required, a full multivisceral being the most extreme (***Figure 91.2***).

At retrieval the organs are retrieved en bloc (***Figure 91.3***), with the vascular inflow coming from the coeliac axis and superior mesenteric artery (SMA) and the venous outflow from either the portal vein (in a non-liver-containing graft) or the vena cava when a liver is implanted. This technique was first described by Starzl in the 1990s.

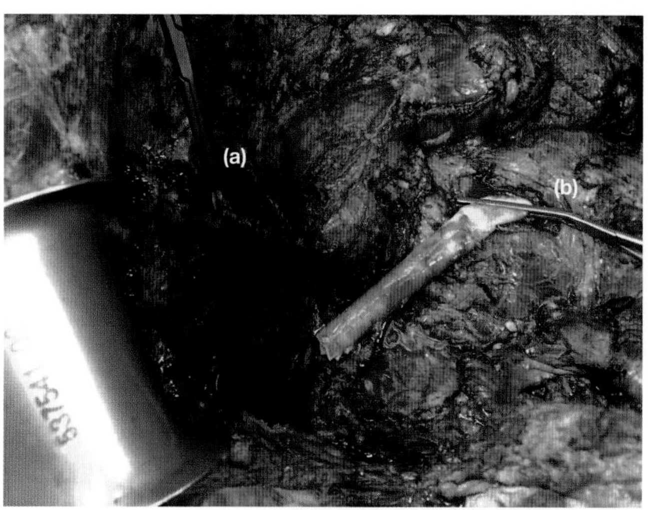

Figure 91.2 Intraoperative picture following exenteration. (a) Clamp on the retrohepatic cava in preparation for caval anastomosis (venous outflow for the multivisceral graft). (b) Clamp on the donor thoracic aorta anastomosed to the infrarenal aorta of the recipient (arterial inflow to the multivisceral graft).

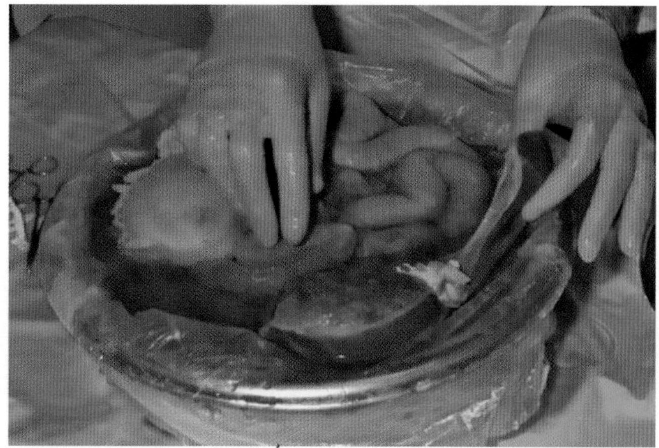

Figure 91.3 Intraoperative picture following exenteration. Multivisceral graft (stomach, small bowel, pancreas and liver) immediately prior to implantation. The graft is preserved using University of Wisconsin solution.

Thomas Earl Starzl, 1926–2017, Distinguished Professor of Surgery, University of Pittsburgh School of Medicine, Pittsburgh, PA, USA. Referred to as 'the father of modern transplantation'. He was awarded the USA's highest honour for scientific achievement, the Medal of Science, in 2005.

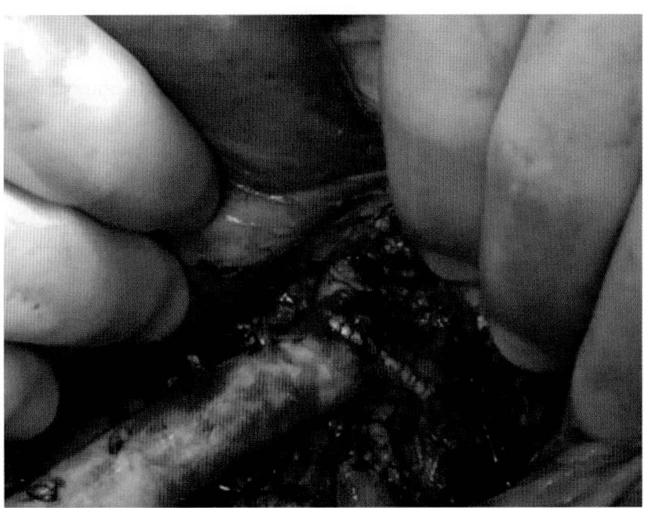

Figure 91.4 Intraoperative picture following exenteration. A Carrel patch (donor superior mesenteric artery and coeliac artery) onto an aortic conduit constituting the arterial inflow to the multivisceral block.

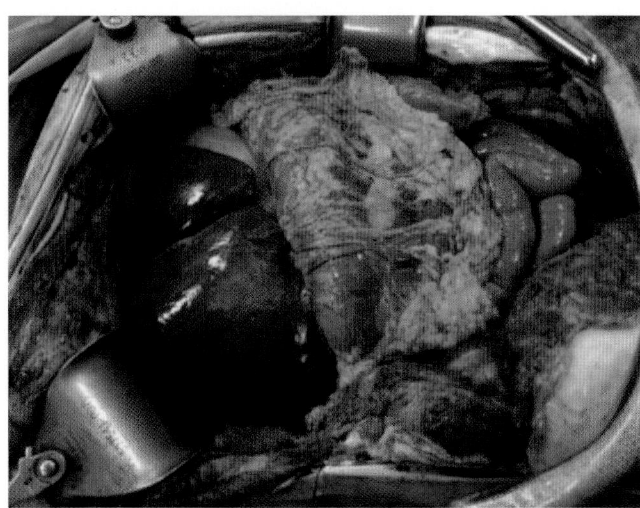

Figure 91.5 Intraoperative picture following exenteration. Intraoperative photograph of a multivisceral block (stomach, liver, small bowel, pancreas and colon) following reperfusion.

Arterial inflow to the graft is usually achieved from the infrarenal aorta. Commonly a section of donor thoracic aorta is used as an arterial conduit, onto which the donor aortic patch containing SMA and coeliac artery is anastomosed (***Figure 91.4***). In intestine-only grafts (not including the pancreas) the inflow is the SMA, which is either anastomosed directly to the aorta (as a Carrel patch) or the recipient SMA or a conduit can be fashioned from donor iliac vessels.

When undertaking a liver-containing graft, venous outflow from the whole graft is via the hepatic veins and inferior vena cava (IVC). For non-liver-containing grafts the venous outflow is via the portal vein. This can be drained either systematically via the IVC or into the portal circulation.

Following reperfusion of the graft (***Figure 91.5***) the enteric anastomoses are performed. This requires a proximal enteric anastomosis and a distal stoma or anastomosis. In some circumstances (modified multivisceral transplant) a biliary anastomosis may be required.

The proximal bowel anastomosis may be either oesophagogastric, oesophagojejunal, gastrogastric, gastrojejunal or jejunojejunal. If an oesophagogastric or gastrogastric anastomosis is performed, then a pyloroplasty is necessary (the block lacking vagal innervation).

An end stoma is the simplest option distally, but, where safe, a primary distal anastomosis can be considered. In most circumstances a covering ileostomy is performed. This allows ready access to the graft for endoscopic surveillance.

ABDOMINAL CLOSURE

One of the most challenging parts of a multivisceral/intestinal transplant is achieving abdominal closure. Multiple previous laparotomies and enterocutaneous fistulae can result in a rigid abdominal wall and loss of the abdominal domain owing to extensive bowel resections. Many techniques to achieve primary closure under these circumstances have been developed. These include preoperative tissue expansion, the use of biological meshes and plastic surgery techniques (e.g. vascularised pedicle flaps).

Transplantation allows novel techniques to be used, including transplantation of part or all of the abdominal wall from a donor. The rectus sheath from the donor can be used as a non-vascularised sheet of fascia. Prior to implantation the muscle and fat are removed from the rectus abdominis graft, leaving the fascial and peritoneal components. This can then be used as a biological 'mesh'. Unlike other biological mesh it vascularises rapidly. Skin coverage is achieved by mobilisation of the recipient's skin and subcutaneous tissues, although rarely a skin graft is needed.

Vascularised abdominal wall grafts can also be used where the anterior abdominal wall with its over lying subcutaneous fat and skin is transplanted using the inferior epigastric arteries and veins as the vascular inflow and outflow.

POST-TRANSPLANT COMPLICATIONS

With the complexity of multivisceral/intestinal transplantation complications are common (***Table 91.3***).

Early postoperative

Many patients considered for multivisceral/intestinal transplantation have underlying prothrombotic tendencies. A defined prothrombotic disease may be characterised but a history of multiple previous thrombotic episodes without a specific diagnosis necessitates a need for anticoagulation after transplantation. Balancing the risks of bleeding and thrombosis after transplant is challenging.

Enteric anastomotic leaks can occur after transplantation, most commonly if an oesophagogastric anastomosis is

Alexis Carrel, 1873–1944, French surgeon, received the Nobel Prize in Physiology or Medicine in 1912 for developing a method of suturing blood vessels.

TABLE 91.3 Early and late complications in multivisceral/intestinal transplantation.

	Surgical	Medical
Early	• Vascular (thrombosis, bleeding, secondary haemorrhage, mycotic aneurysm) • Enteric leak (anastomotic or non-anastomotic) • Abdominal collections (chylous, pancreatic, infected) • Pancreatitis (graft or native) • Stomal complications	• Renal impairment • Drug related (PRES, TMA, pancreatitis) • Infections (viral, bacterial, fungal) • GVHD • PTLD • Acute cellular rejection
Late	• Thrombosis • Mycotic aneurysm • Hernias • Stomal complications	• Renal impairment • Acute cellular rejection • Chronic rejection • PTLD • Immunosuppression-related malignancy

GVHD, graft-versus-host disease; PRES, posterior reversible encephalopathy syndrome; PTLD, post-transplant lymphoproliferative disease; TMA, thrombotic microangiopathy.

undertaken. Given that the enteric anastomoses are performed on previously ischaemic bowel, often under circumstances where inotrope requirements are substantial, the rate of anastomotic leaks is surprisingly low.

When an enteric leak does occur, the immunosuppressed state of the patient can result in an atypical presentation. Therefore, a high index of suspicion is needed should a patient fail to progress as expected postoperatively.

Proximal enteric anastomotic leaks, especially involving the oesophagus, are the most challenging to deal with. Oesophagogastric anastomotic leaks have a significant morbidity and mortality in the general population and are even more challenging to manage in an immunosuppressed patient. The use of an EndoVac® has improved management of these patients. A vacuum (vac) sponge fixed to a nasogastric tube is placed endoscopically in the cavity at the site of the leak. This controls the leak and facilitates healing without operative intervention.

Intra-abdominal collections are common and should be treated by aggressive radiological drainage where possible. These collections may be chylous and may require nutritional modifications, either PN or (if the patient is enterally fed) a medium-chain triglyceride diet should be adopted.

Immunosuppression and rejection

The rate of acute cellular rejection for intestinal grafts is higher than for any other abdominal organ. This is reflected in the magnitude of immunosuppression required. As with other solid organ transplants acute cellular rejection is most common in the first few months after transplantation, although it can occur at any time.

Multivisceral/intestinal transplant immunosuppression regimens commonly utilise an induction agent, usually a lymphocyte-depleting antibody such as antithymocyte globulin (ATG) or alemtuzumab. Paediatric regimens commonly use non-depleting antibody induction. Maintenance immunosuppression comprises a calcineurin inhibitor (most commonly tacrolimus), an antimetabolite (mycophenolate or azathioprine) and prednisolone. In addition, some programmes supplement this with early addition of an mTOR (mammalian target of rapamycin) inhibitor (sirolimus or everolimus).

Acute cellular rejection is usually initially manifested in the terminal ileum. Rarely other organs (liver/pancreas) may be affected without intestinal rejection.

Rejection most commonly presents with increased stoma output or diarrhoea, sometimes with an associated fever. Severe (exfoliative) acute cellular rejection with loss of intestinal mucosa results in rapid bacterial translocation and sepsis. In any intestinal transplant recipient presenting with sepsis or septic shock, a diagnosis of rejection needs to be considered.

Endoscopic assessment and biopsy of the graft are required for the diagnosis and assessment of the severity of acute cellular rejection. Graft surveillance in a protocolised manner is performed in some programmes; others respond to symptoms suggestive of rejection (i.e. an increase in stoma output).

At endoscopy, rejection can range from mild, with some erythema of the mucosa, to moderate, with some ulceration, to severe, with confluent loss of mucosa. At biopsy, salient features of rejection are an inflammatory infiltrate in the lamina propria, crypt loss and ulceration and an increase in apoptotic bodies in the base of the crypts.

Rejection is treated primarily with high-dose intravenous pulsed steroids. If the rejection is steroid resistant then further lymphocyte depletion may be needed with either ATG or alemtuzumab.

Infectious complications

Infection is the leading cause of death in multivisceral/intestinal transplant recipients. This is as a consequence of the degree of immunosuppression and also the potential for bacterial translocation across the graft mucosa. Opportunistic infections, common to all solid organ transplant recipients, such as cytomegalovirus (CMV), *Pneumocystis jirovecii* (PJP), adenovirus, Epstein–Barr virus (EBV) and fungal infections, are all more common following intestinal transplantation. Appropriate prophylaxis with antiviral (valganciclovir or aciclovir), antifungal (fluconazole) and anti-PJP (co-trimoxazole) agents is critical.

Infective enteritis is common among transplant recipients and can mimic rejection, thus it is important to send stool for culture and viral polymerase chain reaction when a patient presents with a high-output stoma or diarrhoea. Rejection triggered by infection is possible and a high index of suspicion and early repeat endoscopy are important if clinical improvement does not occur.

Michael Anthony Epstein, b. 1921, Professor of Pathology, University of Bristol, Bristol, UK.
Yvonne Barr, 1931–2016, virologist who emigrated to Australia. Epstein and Barr discovered this virus in 1964.

Long-term complications

PTLD is a potential complication of immunosuppression for any patient after transplant. The incidence in intestinal transplant recipients is higher than for other solid organ transplant recipients – up to 17% in some series. This is likely to be due to both the level of immunosuppression and the amount of lymphoid tissue associated with an intestinal-containing graft. PTLD should be considered if there is a persistent positive EBV viraemia or B symptoms such as night sweats, unexplained fevers and weight loss. If diagnosed with PTLD the first-line treatment is usually with rituximab and immunosuppression reduction. This has to be done with great caution in multivisceral/intestinal transplant recipients because of the risk of rejection and the consequences thereof.

The extent of lymphoid tissue associated with the multivisceral/intestinal graft increases the risk of GVHD. Outcomes from GVHD in this patient group can be very poor. The most common presenting symptoms of GVHD are a rash, fever and bone marrow suppression. Optimal management of GVHD is unclear and proposed strategies include both enhancement and also reduction of immunosuppression. Management is guided by the level of peripheral T-cell chimerism. There is an increasing trend towards withdrawing immunosuppression initially to rebalance the equilibrium between the host and donor immune systems. Bone marrow involvement and ultimately failure is almost universally fatal.

Deterioration in renal function is common to all solid organ transplant groups but is most marked following multivisceral/intestinal transplantation. The cause of this is multifactorial but is likely to include contributions from the physiological insult of surgery, the use of nephrotoxic medication (e.g. tacrolimus) and fluid losses associated with the stoma. It is imperative to maintain good hydration postoperatively and home intravenous fluids may be needed initially post discharge. Immunosuppression modifications including conversion from calcineurin inhibitor-based protocols to mTOR inhibitors may prevent further deterioration of renal function. These interventions need to be undertaken with caution as they may precipitate an episode of acute cellular rejection.

OUTCOMES

Graft and patient outcomes vary depending on the type of transplant undertaken with survival post-multivisceral transplant being markedly poorer than isolated small intestinal transplant. As with many transplant groups, outcomes are improving over time and the outcomes in the last published Intestinal Transplant Registry report in 2015 showed continued improvement in both 1- and 5-year patient survival. In 2019 the overall 1-year patient survival for intestinal-only grafts was >80% and for liver-containing grafts was >70%. A decade ago the 1-year patient survival for *all* intestinal transplant recipients (intestine only and multivisceral grafts) was 70%. Five-year survival rates have also improved and the long-term results of intestinal-only transplants are now comparable to those of long-term PN. Intestinal transplantation may have progressed to the stage at which it may be offered to patients on PN to improve their quality of life rather than just for those with life-threatening complications of PN.

SUMMARY

Multivisceral and intestinal transplantation remains a complex and uncommon treatment, however it can be life-saving. The risks are high but with improvements in surgical techniques, especially the introduction of preoperative embolisation, the intraoperative risks have improved. With this and a better understanding of how to manage the varied and complex postoperative complications, outcomes continue to improve.

Intestinal transplantation for patients on PN was previously reserved for those with life-threatening complications of this treatment. Outcomes have improved such that, in certain circumstances, it can now be offered to improve quality of life.

With time, improvement in patient management may allow intestinal transplantation to fulfil the same role for patients on PN as kidney transplantation currently offers those on dialysis: to improve both quality and length of life.

The need for liver-containing grafts will always remain for those who require a liver transplant but are unable to have a single-organ transplant for anatomical reasons. With improvements in liver functional assessment and increasing awareness of the possibility of earlier intestinal transplantation, it may be possible to reduce and hopefully eliminate the need for liver transplantation for IFALD. The benefits for the individual in terms of improved survival and also the population with better organ utilisation are substantial.

The main cause of death in multivisceral and intestinal transplant recipients remains sepsis. This is frequently associated with a preceding episode of severe acute cellular rejection and so further developments in immunosuppression regimens will be necessary to continue to improve patient outcomes.

FURTHER READING

Abu-Elmagd K, Mazariegos G, Armanyous S *et al.* Five hundred patients with gut malrotation: thirty years of experience with the introduction of a new surgical procedure. *Ann Surg* 2021; **274**(4): 581–96.

Matsumoto CS, Subramanian S, Fishbein TM. Adult intestinal transplantation. *Gastroenterol Clin North Am* 2018; **47**(2): 341–54.

Tzakis AG, Kato T, Levi DM *et al.* 100 multivisceral transplants at a single center. *Ann Surg* 2005; **242**(4): 480–90; discussion 491–3.

CHAPTER 92 Heart and lung transplantation

Learning objectives

To recognise and understand:

- The indications and contraindications to transplantation of the heart and lungs
- The selection of recipients
- Heart and lung donation
- The technique for heart and lung transplantation
- Early postoperative complications
- Long-term outcomes

HEART TRANSPLANTATION

The incidence of heart failure is increasing as the population ages and coronary artery disease, hypertension and obesity rise. Current medical therapy, including resynchronisation pacemakers and implantable defibrillators, is effective in improving symptoms and survival but many will develop end-stage disease for which heart transplantation remains the gold standard surgical treatment.

Experimental procedures by Demikhov in the 1940s and the xenotransplantation of a chimpanzee heart into a patient with intracardiac thrombus by Hardy in 1964 led Lower and Shumway at Stanford University, CA, USA, to demonstrate that the circulation could be maintained entirely by an orthotopically transplanted heart. The first clinical heart transplant was undertaken in 1967 by the South African Christian Barnard, but mortality remained very high until the advent of modern immunosuppressants.

Heterotopic heart transplantation, in which a donor heart is transplanted as a biological biventricular assist with the native heart remaining in place, was first used clinically in 1974 but is now seldom used as long-term survival is poor.

Recipient selection

The primary indication for transplantation is prolonged advanced heart failure despite optimal medical management, often typified by repeated admissions or acute deterioration. The decision to transplant must take into account the patient's ability to withstand surgery and adhere to long-term treatment.

The most frequent indications for heart transplantation in adults are dilated and ischaemic cardiomyopathy. An increasing number of patients with adult congenital heart disease (ACHD) are now considered but need more complex surgery (abnormal anatomy, previous operations) and may have elevated pulmonary vascular resistance and immune sensitisation. There are higher early mortality results after transplantation although the long-term outcome in survivors is excellent.

Patients should be within the 'transplant window', being robust enough to survive the operation but their condition and prognosis should warrant the risks involved. As advanced failure can increase risk through the dysfunction of other organs (e.g. cardiorenal syndrome, liver dysfunction) reversible issues that can resolve with the improved cardiac output that transplantation will bring must be identified.

Elevated pulmonary vascular resistance (>5 Wood units and a transpulmonary gradient >15 mmHg) is associated with an increased risk of right ventricular failure and mortality after heart transplantation; if irreversible despite vasodilators, this resistance is a contraindication.

Age and previous cardiac surgery do not preclude transplantation and neither does diabetes if controlled with an absence of microvascular complications. A body mass index (BMI) >30 kg/m^2 has been associated with a worse outcome and weight loss is required before listing. Active infection is an absolute contraindication. Patients with chronic infections

---

Vladimir Demikhov, 1916–1998, Russian pioneer of organ transplantation, performed heart and heart–lung transplantation in animals between 1940 and 1950.
James Hardy, 1918–2003, performed the world's first lung transplant in 1963, undertook the world's first heart transplant attempt when he transplanted the heart of a chimpanzee into a dying patient in 1964.
Richard Lower, 1929–2008, American pioneer of heart transplantation who, with Shumway, developed many of the techniques required, including the use of hypothermia and the orthotopic technique in Stanford, CA, USA. Instrumental in the use of ciclosporin and in developing techniques of myocardial biopsy to monitor rejection.
Norman Shumway, 1923–2006, American pioneer of heart transplantation who, with Lower, developed many of the techniques required, including the use of hypothermia and the orthotopic technique in Stanford, CA, USA. Performed his first human heart transplant in 1968.
Christiaan Barnard, 1922–2001, performed the world's first successful heart transplant in 1967 after studying the techniques used by Lower and Shumway.

should have these eradicated by appropriate antimicrobial and surgical therapy. Malignancy, other than localised non-melanoma skin cancer, precludes transplantation but patients who have achieved sustained remission following cancer therapy may become candidates.

The presence of circulating antibodies against the allograft (allosensitisation) owing to pregnancy, blood transfusion, previous transplantation and the use of ventricular assist devices (VADs) is associated with worse outcomes and candidates are likely to have an extended waiting time to find a compatible donor. Screening for anti-human leukocyte antigen (HLA) antibodies is routine for all heart transplantation candidates.

Psychosocial factors such as substance abuse (including tobacco, alcohol) is a relative contraindication. Relapse of smoking has been associated with a poor outcome after cardiac transplantation.

Summary box 92.1

Criteria for heart transplantation

1. Impaired left ventricular systolic function
2. New York Heart Association III (e.g. patient cannot climb one flight of stairs without symptoms)
3. Receiving optimal medical therapy (maximum tolerated doses of β-adrenergic antagonists, angiotensin-converting enzyme inhibitors, aldosterone antagonists)
4. Resynchronisation pacing or implantable defibrillator device inserted (if indicated)
5. Evidence of a poor prognosis, e.g.
   a. Exercise testing (O_2 max <12 mL/kg/min if on β-blockade)
   b. Elevated B-type natriuretic peptide serum levels
   c. Calculated Seattle Heart Failure score indicating >20% 1-year mortality

Summary box 92.2

Factors considered in heart allocation

- Biological matching
  - Blood group compatibility
  - Appropriate size matching (accounting for recipient sex and pulmonary hypertension)
  - Need to avoid specific donor HLA antigens in sensitised recipients
- Clinical need
  - Severity of heart failure
  - Prognosis
- Logistic factors influencing ischaemia time
  - Distance of donor from the recipient centre
  - Prior surgery in the recipient (multiple sternotomies)
  - Surgical complexity (e.g. prior VAD, ACHD)
- Fairness
  - Time on the waiting list

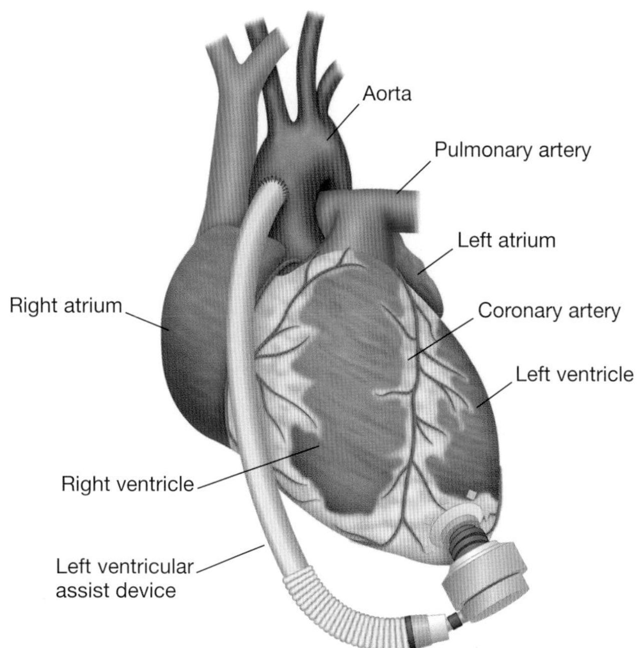

Figure 92.1 Typical implantable left ventricular assist device that takes blood from the apex of the left ventricle and passes it through a rotor to a graft anastomosed to the aorta. A driveline crosses the skin to a controller and battery pack providing electrical power.

Ventricular assist devices

VADs have had a significant impact. They may be used as a bridge to transplantation, a bridge to recovery (where the device is explanted if the patient's cardiac function improves) or as long-term durable destination therapy.

The first total artificial heart implant was performed by Cooley in Houston, Texas, USA, in 1969 with the patient subsequently undergoing heart transplantation 48 hours later. In 1966, DeBakey utilised a left VAD in a patient unable to wean from cardiopulmonary bypass after valve surgery.

Current generation devices use continuous non-pulsatile flow technology, which permits small device size, has the rotor as the only moving part and uses electrical rather than the more bulky pneumatic power delivery (***Figure 92.1***).

Patients can now remain on device support for years if necessary, although complications from anticoagulation (stroke, device thrombosis, gastrointestinal bleeding), right ventricular failure, aortic valve regurgitation and driveline infection are common; hospital readmission is frequent. Early mortality is akin to heart transplantation but long-term survival is inferior with 50% survival at 5 years.

Given the shortage of suitable donor organs, VAD implantation is an increasingly common approach for those deteriorating on the waiting list to gain time for a suitable donor heart to be become available. Future technology improvements are

Denton Cooley, 1920–2016, American surgeon, performed the first implantation of a total artificial heart and made major contributions to all aspects of cardiac surgery.
Michael DeBakey, 1908–2008, American cardiovascular surgeon, undertook the first surgery to implant an external ventricular assist device for heart failure and developed a classification of aortic dissection.

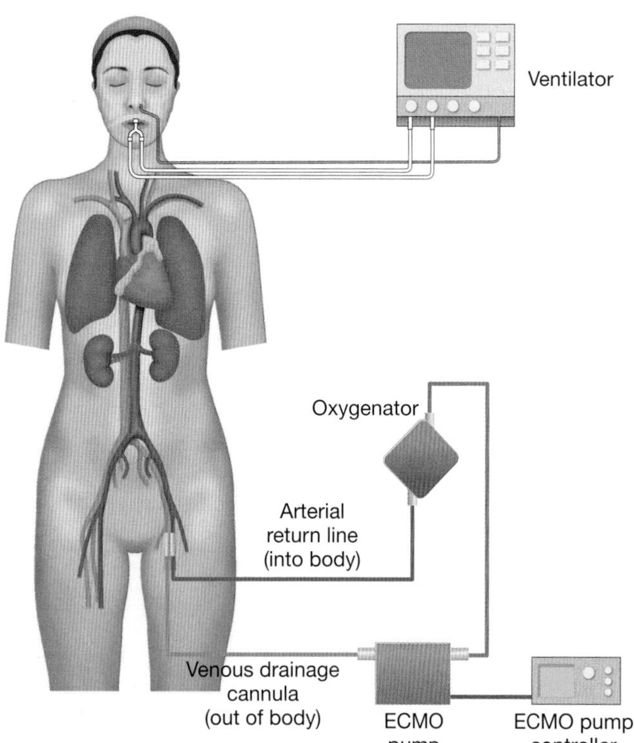

Figure 92.2 Extracorporeal membrane oxygenation (ECMO), which can be used for cardiorespiratory support before or after heart and lung transplantation. Blood is drained from the right atrium via the femoral vein, oxygenated and pumped back to the arterial circulation. In a variation where respiratory and not circulatory support is needed (venovenous ECMO) oxygenated blood is returned to the right atrium via the other femoral vein or jugular vein.

focused on increased biocompatibility, artificially generated pulsatility and avoidance of drivelines.

Among patients admitted in cardiogenic shock, venoarterial extracorporeal membrane oxygenation (ECMO) can be used to restore perfusion rapidly via the peripheral femoral artery and vein cannulation and permit urgent heart transplantation to be carried out within days, although the results are inferior (***Figure** 92.2*).

Summary box 92.3

Complications associated with VADs

- Anticoagulation
  - Bleeding – gastrointestinal tract, intracerebral, subarachnoid, extradural
- Thrombosis
  - Pump obstruction
- Device failure
- Infection
  - Driveline, systemic sepsis
- Structural
  - Aortic regurgitation, tricuspid regurgitation
- Right ventricular failure
- Higher risks at transplantation
  - Adhesions, infection, vasoplegia

Donor selection and organ preservation

At the time of heart procurement from brainstem dead (donation after brainstem death [DBD]) donors, the heart must be arrested and explanted prior to transportation. There follows a period of ischaemia until the heart is reperfused in the recipient. Allograft ischaemic time is a strong risk factor for post-transplant mortality, especially when it exceeds 3–4 hours, so every effort must be made to keep this time period as short as possible. At retrieval cardioplegic solutions that inhibit the Na^+/K^+ ATPase cell membrane pump or lead to cellular depolarisation and diastolic cardiac arrest are infused into the aortic root to rapidly arrest and uniformly cool the heart.

Continuous heart perfusion is an alternative but more expensive and complex method of preservation. This is typified by the widely used Transmedics Organ Care System (***Figure** 92.3*). Rather than being stored in an arrested and hypothermic state, the heart is kept warm and beating. It can be managed with inotropes and monitored through lactate assays, permitting longer transport times. Trials have shown that 30-day post-transplant survival is similar to standard preservation. There is some evidence to suggest that machine perfusion reduces mortality in higher risk donors and recipients and opens the potential for organ modification and improvement. Other systems that utilise cold oxygenated continuous perfusion of a still heart are under investigation.

To expand the current donor pool hearts may be retrieved from patients suffering circulatory arrest (donation after circulatory death [DCD]) after the withdrawal of life-sustaining care and proclamation of death (***Figure** 92.3*). The heart is then rapidly retrieved and reperfused in an organ care system before transport and transplantation. Clinical results appear equivalent to conventional donation and this has been a major advance.

Heart retrieval

After exposing the heart by median sternotomy and opening the pericardium the organ is thoroughly inspected for contractility and coronary artery disease. Heparin is administered (300 U/kg) and a cannula placed into the aorta. The venae cavae are then occluded, the aorta cross-clamped and cardioplegia administered to arrest and cool the heart. The inferior vena cava (IVC) is vented.

When the lungs are retrieved the pulmonary artery will also have been cannulated and the left atrial appendage incised.

Cardiectomy is then carried out by dividing the superior vena cava (SVC), removing the cross-clamp and dividing the aorta and pulmonary artery at the bifurcation. The inferior vena caval incision is completed and the heart lifted to expose the inferior wall of the left atrium, which is then circumferentially incised to explant the heart. The interatrial septum is inspected to rule out a patent foramen ovale and all valves are carefully examined.

The heart is then placed in a bag filled with cardioplegia solution at 4°C. Two additional sterile bags are wrapped around it. These bags are then placed in a sterile container and then in a cooler for transport.

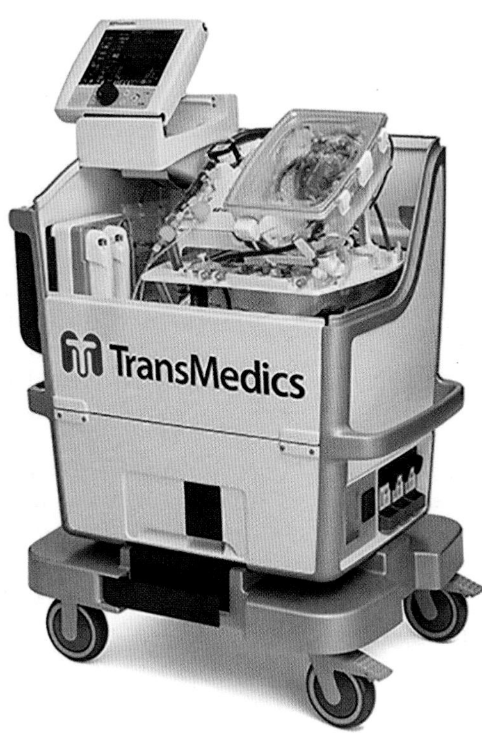

Figure 92.3 An organ care system that allows retrieved hearts to be perfused with warm oxygenated blood and remain beating during transportation to the recipient hospital. Devices can shorten ischaemic time and may be beneficial in higher risk patients. They have facilitated highly successful donor circulatory arrest heart donation to expand the donor pool.

Operative technique

Coordination between the retrieval team and the implanting team is of paramount importance to minimise ischaemic time and the duration of cardiopulmonary bypass.

A median sternotomy incision is performed and the aorta, SVC and IVC are encircled. After heparin administration the ascending aorta, SVC and IVC are all cannulated in sequence to establish cardiopulmonary bypass. Blood is drained from the cavae into a reservoir, then oxygenated, cooled to 32°C and returned via a roller pump to the ascending aorta to perfuse the body while the heart is excised and the transplant performed (*Figure 92.4*). Carbon dioxide is insufflated into the pericardial cavity to reduce the risk of air embolism.

When the donor heart arrives in the operating theatre, the recipient aorta is cross-clamped and the heart excised by dividing the SVC, IVC, aorta and pulmonary artery. The left atrium is incised, leaving a cuff of atrium into which the four pulmonary veins drain.

After administering a dose of cardioplegia to the donor heart, the left atrial cuff is anastomosed, followed by the pulmonary artery, aorta and both cavae. Donor and recipient vessels are trimmed to obtain a perfect match in terms of length and width.

A vent is placed in the ascending aorta for de-airing and the cross-clamp is removed, allowing reperfusion of the heart (*Figure 92.5*). Steroids are usually administered to reduce rejection.

Sinus rhythm is usually restored but temporary pacing wires are sutured to the heart for heart rate control. After a period of reperfusion (20 minutes for each hour of ischaemic time) to allow myocardial recovery, the new heart can be separated from cardiopulmonary bypass gradually, until it has taken over the circulation. Nitric oxide is useful at this stage to reduce pulmonary vascular resistance and protect the right ventricle from dysfunction. Isoprenaline is commonly infused.

A transoesophageal echocardiogram can help to assess biventricular function and valvular competence.

Outcomes and complications

Survival has dramatically improved with advances in immunosuppression and perioperative care, with 1-year post-transplant survival of over 90% and a median post-transplant survival of

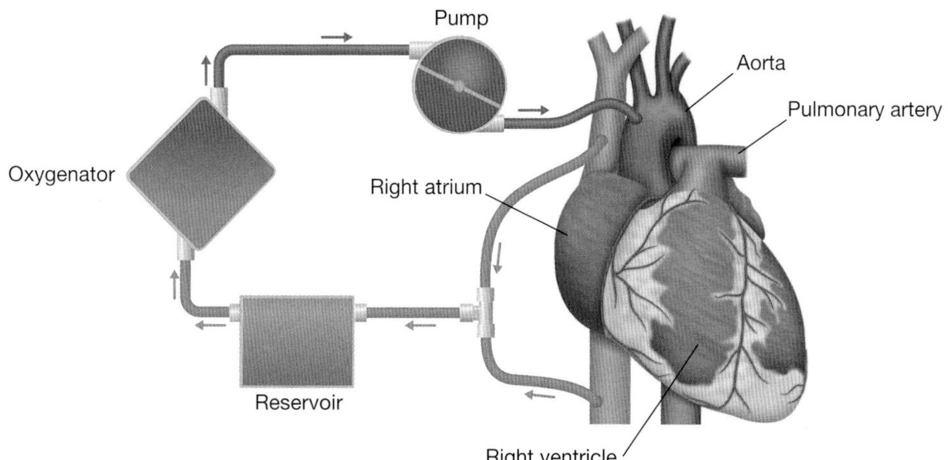

Figure 92.4 Cardiopulmonary bypass is used in heart transplantation and sometimes in lung transplantation. Blood is drained from cannulae in the superior and inferior venae cavae to a reservoir, then oxygenated in a membrane oxygenator before return to the ascending aorta via a roller or centrifugal pump. The patient can have their circulation maintained with oxygenated blood while the heart or lungs are explanted during transplantation.

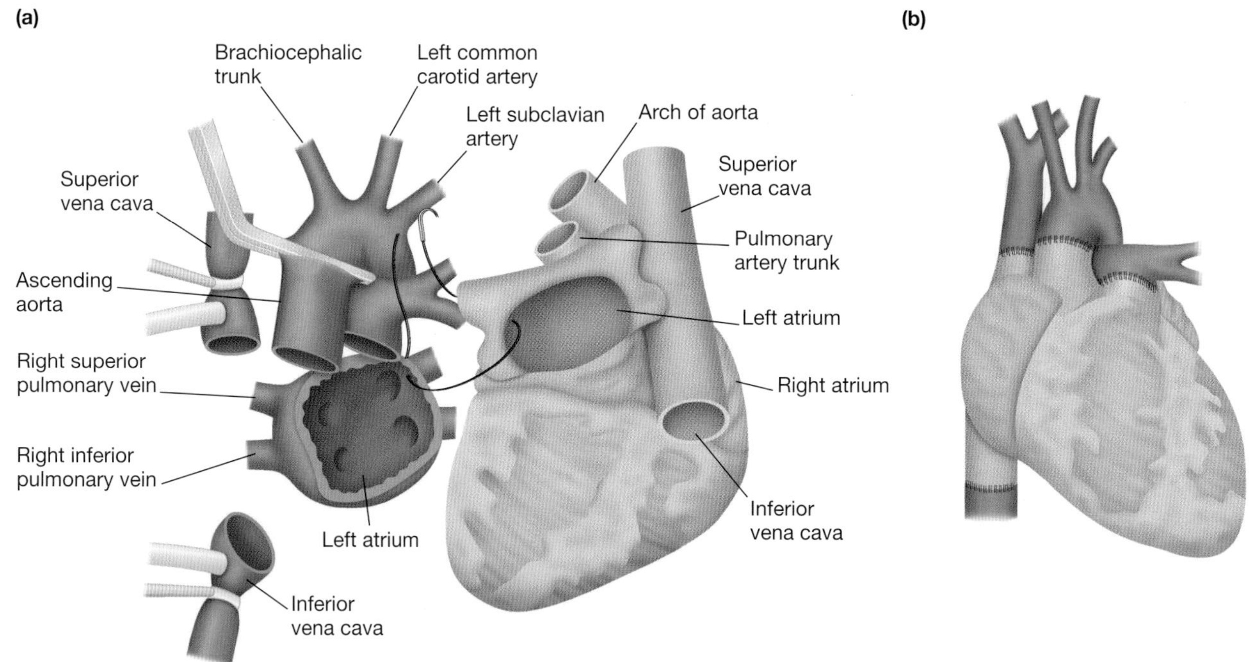

Figure 92.5 Cardiac transplantation. (a) A left atrial cuff is fashioned, into which the four pulmonary veins drain. This is anastomosed to a cuff of left atrium on the donor heart followed by anastomosis of the pulmonary artery, aorta and both venae cavae to complete the implant (b).

approximately 12 years anticipated. Early mortality is 5–10% at 30 days but often higher in those who have a VAD implanted as the device must be explanted with the recipient's heart, increasing the complexity of surgery owing to adhesions and vasoplegia from long-term non-pulsatile flow or infection often being encountered.

After surgery most patients do not require rehospitalisation and functional status is good, with many returning to work and having a greatly improved health-related quality of life. Denervation of the heart is an unavoidable consequence of transplantation but, despite this, baseline cardiac function is preserved and increases in cardiac output are mediated by circulating catecholamines and stretch receptors responding to increased venous return with exercise.

Early after transplantation, the main causes of mortality include primary graft dysfunction, rejection and infection. Long-term survival is dictated by the development of chronic allograft vasculopathy (CAV) and immunosuppression-related malignancy, diabetes, infection and renal dysfunction.

Primary graft dysfunction occurs soon after implantation in around 10% of cases and is the leading cause of death. Low cardiac output and uni- or biventricular failure secondary to ischaemia–reperfusion injury occurs and is associated with older donor or recipient age, female-to-male donation, prolonged ischaemic time (>240 minutes) and donor-to-recipient size mismatch. Escalating inotropic support is needed, sometimes culminating in the institution of ECMO for circulatory support until the recovery of heart function.

Isolated acute right ventricular failure may occur secondary to prolonged ischaemic time, elevated pulmonary vascular resistance, volume overload or donor size mismatch. The use of inotropes and nitric oxide and the optimisation of volume and mechanical support may be required.

Three types of rejection can occur after heart transplantation: hyperacute rejection, acute cellular rejection and antibody-mediated rejection. Hyperacute rejection occurs intraoperatively immediately after reperfusion. Cross-matching of blood type and panel reactive antibodies has rendered this very unlikely.

Lifelong immunosuppression is required, balancing prevention of rejection but avoiding the adverse effects of malignancy, infection, renal dysfunction, hypertension, diabetes and hyperlipidaemia. Most patients are prescribed triple therapy, consisting of a calcineurin inhibitor (e.g. ciclosporin, tacrolimus), an antimetabolite (e.g. azathioprine) and a tapering dose of steroids. Induction therapy with antithymocyte globulin or interleukin-2 receptor antagonists (basiliximab) is sometimes used but this may increase the risk of infection and malignancy with no survival benefit.

The risk of acute rejection is highest in the first 6 months and a regime of routine surveillance cardiac biopsies obtained from the right ventricle via a bioptome inserted through the internal jugular vein are carried out. Alternatives to biopsy have been explored, especially the modalities of cardiac imaging, but they have been associated with low accuracy. Gene expression profiling of blood mononuclear cells is under investigation and may be promising in the future. Free DNA of donor origin in the recipient's blood has also been tested as a means to predict rejection in the transplanted heart.

Acute cellular rejection is a T-cell reaction to the donor's HLA molecules that occurs in 20–40% of patients, most commonly during the first 12 months. It is classified based on the severity of lymphocytic infiltrates and myocyte damage and is treated with high-dose corticosteroids. With modern immunosuppression and the low risk of late cellular rejection, biopsies are often ceased after 3 years.

Antibody-mediated rejection is seen in 10–20% of patients and has a mortality rate of 8%. Donor antigens and recipient antibodies form an antigen–antibody membrane attack complex that leads to endothelial injury. The diagnosis of antibody-mediated rejection is confirmed by the presence of circulating donor-specific antibodies (DSAs) with evidence of complement activation. This is treated with intravenous immunoglobulin, plasmapheresis, antilymphocyte antibodies and high-dose steroids.

CAV is a frequent long-term complication of heart transplantation and the leading cause of late mortality. It has an incidence of 30% at 5 years with a complex pathogenesis involving immunological factors and ischaemia–reperfusion all implicated. Diffuse thickening of coronary arterial intima occurs, often affecting the entire length of the epicardial vessels and typically extending to the microvasculature. As the heart is denervated recipients do not experience ischaemic chest pain. By the time the patient presents with declining left ventricular function and heart failure, the prognosis is poor. CAV surveillance by serial coronary angiography often combined with intravascular ultrasound can reliably detect intimal changes early to allow for treatment modification or consideration of retransplantation.

Future perspectives

Contemporary immunosuppressive therapies and modern surgical and perioperative techniques have all contributed to improved outcomes. The principal innovations being investigated for the future are aimed at increasing donor availability and improving the long-term survival.

Xenotransplantation has been extensively investigated with the use of transgenic pig hearts. In 1964, Hardy performed a xenotransplant using a chimpanzee heart that beat for 90 minutes before failing, and in 1984 infant Stephanie Fae Beauclair (often referred to as Baby Fae) famously lived for 21 days after receiving a baboon heart. Gene-editing techniques that allow modification of antigen expression are among the biggest technological breakthroughs to support the resurgence of xenotransplantation. Knockout pigs that lack swine leukocyte antigens to reduce organ immunogenicity have led to pig-to-primate allograft survival of up to 945 days. Despite the technical and scientific challenges the first contemporary pig-to-human transplant was undertaken in 2022 at the University of Maryland, USA, with good early clinical xenograft function using a pig heart with 10 genetic modifications, including four knockouts (three responsible for rapid antibody-mediated rejection of pig organ and one to prevent excessive growth) and six human genes added to increase the likelihood of acceptance. Rejection in the medium and long term and the hazard of infection transmission with porcine retroviruses remain of concern.

The problems faced by xenotransplantation could be overcome by organ engineering. Decellularised extracellular matrix scaffolds of hearts can be created by removing cellular tissue then repopulating with autologous cardiac cells. Automatic contractility has been demonstrated.

In addition to finding new sources of donor organs, improvement of long-term survival remains a priority. New agents to provide better immunosuppression with less rejection and a more favourable side-effect profile remain under investigation. The induction of tolerance of the recipient immune system to donor antigens has promise and T-cell co-stimulation blockade, mixed chimerism (recipient bone marrow engraftment with donor bone marrow cells) and regulatory T-cell infusions are being studied. Personalisation of current immunosuppressants to individual patients may allow for adjustments based on molecular diagnostic techniques to increase efficacy and reduce side effects.

LUNG TRANSPLANTATION

Pulmonary transplantation has made significant advances since the first human lung transplant performed by James Hardy in 1963 in Mississippi, USA. Mortality and morbidity remain high, in part because lungs remain exposed to the environment through the airway.

For patients with end-stage pulmonary disease, lung transplantation can significantly improve both survival and quality of life. Approximately 80% of lung transplants are bilateral, with single-lung transplants and living related lobar transplants undertaken less often. Long-term outcomes for all recipient pathologies are superior with bilateral lung transplantation. Single-lung transplantation cannot be used in diseases where infection may remain in the other lung, such as in cystic fibrosis (CF) or bronchiectasis.

Recipient selection

Candidates have advanced lung disease with shortened life expectancy and poor quality of life owing to breathlessness and oxygen dependency. The most common indications are chronic obstructive pulmonary disease (COPD), CF, pulmonary arterial hypertension (PAH) and interstitial lung disease (ILD). Organ allocation schemes recognise the last as associated with rapid decline and poor prognosis. Their prioritisation has led to shorter waiting times and a 20–40% reduction in death on the waiting list. The lung allocation score (LAS) is a useful tool to select those most in need of a particular donor lung. Risks are calculated using a set of 17 patient-related variables,

Summary box 92.4

Pulmonary diseases and type of transplant

- Cystic fibrosis
  - Bilateral and living related (or cadaveric lobar transplants in small highly selected recipients in experienced centres)
- Interstitial (fibrotic) lung disease
  - Bilateral or single (but associated with poorer long-term survival)
- Emphysema/COPD
  - Bilateral or single (but associated with poorer long-term survival)
- Pulmonary hypertension
  - Bilateral (or rarely combined heart–lung transplantation especially if associated with congenital heart disease)

including age, BMI, underlying diagnosis group, presence of pulmonary hypertension and the 6-minute walk distance.

In deteriorating patients more conventional treatments can be used in some groups before transplant assessment. In COPD endoscopic lung volume reduction is increasingly recognised as a treatment option. Transmembrane conductance regulator modulators have improved outcomes for patients with CF with a reduction in exacerbation frequency and an improvement in quality of life and prognosis. This has resulted in a recent fall in transplantation for CF.

In idiopathic pulmonary fibrosis, antifibrotic drugs (e.g. nintedanib, pirfenidone) have slowed the rate of functional decline, but the clinical course remains progressive and unpredictable.

Although age should not be considered a contraindication to transplantation it is associated with comorbid conditions that may need to be taken into account. It is unusual to transplant patients over 70 years of age.

Previous surgery, such as lobectomy, lung volume reduction or pleurodesis, is not a contraindication to lung transplantation, although inevitably it makes the transplantation operation more challenging with a greater risk of bleeding, phrenic nerve injury, chylothorax and renal dysfunction. A pneumothorax occurring in a waiting-list patient can be managed as required as the choice of intervention is unlikely to affect future acceptance.

Untreatable major organ dysfunction, severe atherosclerosis, bleeding diathesis, high or low BMI, severe osteoporosis and chronic infection are all contraindications. In particular, infection with *Burkholderia cenocepacia*, *Burkholderia gladioli* and *Mycobacterium abscessus* can be associated with very poor post-transplant outcomes. For patients infected with hepatitis B and/or C, surgery can occur provided cirrhosis or portal hypertension are absent. Controlled human immunodeficiency virus (HIV) disease with undetectable HIV RNA, and compliance with antiretroviral therapy, allows transplantation to occur.

For those with a history of malignancy a low predicted risk of recurrence and a 5-year period of remission are required.

With regard to coronary artery disease, percutaneous coronary intervention may be undertaken ahead of transplantation or coronary artery bypass grafting when lung transplantation occurs. The degree of coronary artery disease deemed acceptable will vary but good results have been achieved.

In rapidly deteriorating patients who are otherwise excellent candidates a bridge to lung transplantation may be undertaken using ECMO support. This permits ongoing rehabilitation while awaiting a suitable organ and is preferable to ventilation, which is usually a contraindication to pulmonary transplantation as physiotherapy is more difficult, deconditioning likely and the onset of pneumonia and barotrauma more common. Venovenous ECMO can be used in patients with severe hypoxia whereas venoarterial ECMO is used for patients with both hypoxia and haemodynamic instability or pulmonary hypertension. Instituting ECMO, however, is associated with serious and potentially fatal complications, such as bleeding, infection and thromboembolism. Recent series have shown that outcomes from bridging to transplantation can be similar to those transplanted electively despite being far sicker.

Donor selection and organ preservation

More than 80% of potential lung grafts are declined because of concerns over donor history, chest trauma, pneumonia or aspiration. Ideally lung donors should demonstrate standard criteria but in reality only 20% of donors actually meet these values. Those outside of the standard criteria are called extended criteria donors. Experience has shown that these organs can be safely transplanted without detrimental effects on survival or longer term outcome. When oxygenation of donor lungs falls below the standard criterion of 300 mmHg aggressive donor management with alveolar recruitment, ventilatory optimisation, bronchoscopy and diuretics can lead to improvements.

Additionally the opiate abuse epidemic in the USA has led to a significant rise in the number of organ donors but with a concomitant increase in hepatitis C infection. Antiviral therapies, however, may enable widespread use of such donors in hepatitis C-negative recipients.

Summary box 92.5

Standard criteria lung donors

- Investigations
  - Clear chest radiograph
  - Negative Gram stain of bronchial secretions or purulent secretions
  - Arterial oxygen tension >300 mmHg (inspired oxygen fraction of 100% and positive end-expiratory pressure 5 cmH_2O)
- History
  - Age <55 years
  - Smoking <20 pack-years
  - No chest trauma
  - No aspiration
  - No pneumonia

Outcomes are adversely affected by a donor smoking history of an increasing number of pack-years. Recipients of donor lungs from smokers have a higher 3-year mortality and prolonged hospital stay after adjusting for age and oxygenation but this is not a consistent finding and there remains an overall survival benefit to using lungs from heavy smoking donors to reduce waiting-list mortality.

Lungs from older donors (>55 years) can be safely used to 70 years old and short-term outcomes of older donors are similar in well-selected cases. A history of cancer in the donor does not automatically preclude lung donation. Those with a history of skin cancer, as well as certain low-grade central nervous system tumours, can be used with minimal risk.

Lung retrieval

Flexible bronchoscopy is first performed to clear mucopurulent secretions or aspiration. After median sternotomy and exposure of the lungs in each pleural space, detailed inspection is carried out for masses, consolidation or contusion. Uniform lung inflation must be observed with resolution of any areas of atelectasis. Lung compliance is also assessed by observing lung deflation when disconnected from the ventilator.

Heparin is administered and the main pulmonary artery cannulated. Prostaglandin E (500 μg) is then injected to induce pulmonary vasodilatation and 3 litres of a cold pulmoplegia preservative infusion is initiated. The left atrial appendage is incised to vent the effluent while the lungs are also topically cooled with saline. Lung ventilation continues during flushing to improve fluid distribution and prevent atelectasis.

The pulmonary artery is then divided proximal to the bifurcation and the left atrium is incised to create a cuff of left atrium on each side, into which the two pulmonary veins drain. Division of the pulmonary ligament on each side allows the lungs to be removed after inflating them to 25 mmHg and stapling the trachea, the lungs remaining inflated for transportation.

A 500-mL retrograde pulmoplegia infusion is carried out into each pulmonary vein to augment preservation and flush out clots from the vasculature.

The lungs are then placed into a bag containing pulmoplegia and double-bagged for transport within an ice-packed cooler.

Lungs are more resistant to warm and cold ischaemic times and safe transplantation can be undertaken with preservation times of 6–12 hours.

As in heart transplantation the use of DCD donors has expanded the donor pool. After the declaration of death the lungs are rapidly retrieved. Lungs are resistant to the effects of warm ischaemia much more so than the heart and outcomes are equal to those obtained with DBD donors. The avoidance of the catecholamine storm and associated inflammation associated with brain death may be particularly advantageous in these cases.

The technique for DCD lung retrieval is somewhat different. Five minutes after the declaration of death, bronchoscopy is performed and the lungs inflated. After rapid chest entry the pulmonary artery is quickly cannulated, the left atrial appendage is incised and pulmoplegia is started. The lungs are quickly inspected for abnormalities and topical hypothermia is accomplished with ice slush to limit the warm ischaemic time.

Most donors involve controlled withdrawal of treatment (Maastricht 3) but uncontrolled DCD (Maastricht 2) donation where failed resuscitation from unexpected cardiac arrest with a declaration of death is followed by heparinisation, the insertion of chest drains with *in situ* cooling of the lungs and consent for donation and organ retrieval has been shown to be efficacious in Spain. The use of *ex vivo* lung perfusion (EVLP) is recommended to allow for assessment.

Ex vivo lung perfusion

This technique involves placing donor lungs into a machine at the recipient centre; the lungs are ventilated and perfused with an electrolyte and protein solution for 2–4 hours, sometimes longer. This permits the reconditioning and evaluation of lungs that may not appear to be useable for transplantation in the first instance. Treatments may be administered that can optimise graft function, such as antibiotics, steroids and immunomodulatory drugs, and biomarkers for poor outcomes can be detected. EVLP may be used for logistic reasons to reduce ischaemic time and in the future it may permit *ex vivo* therapeutic interventions such as gene therapy. By using perfusates with an optimised colloid osmotic pressure, pulmonary oedema can be reduced, thereby improving gas exchange. The lungs can be monitored on the device for the development of changes in compliance, airway pressure, pulmonary vascular resistance and perfusate oxygenation. Bronchoscopy can be performed to resolve areas of atelectasis (***Figures 92.6 and 92.7***).

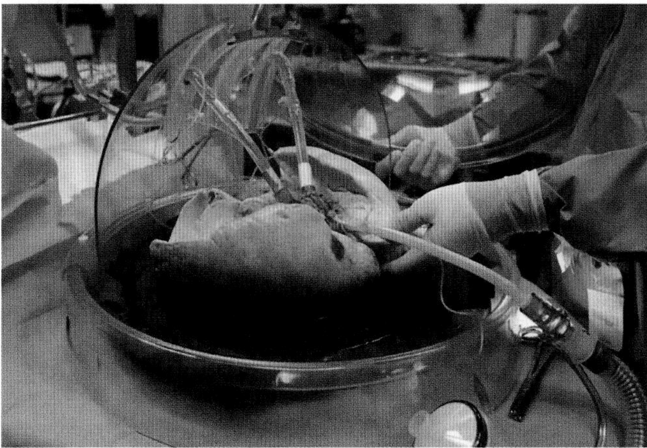

Figure 92.6 *Ex vivo* lung perfusion. The lungs have been explanted from the donor but may be borderline for acceptance for transplantation. Perfusion, bronchoscopy and ventilation in the system can recondition lungs to a useable state to permit the transplant to proceed.

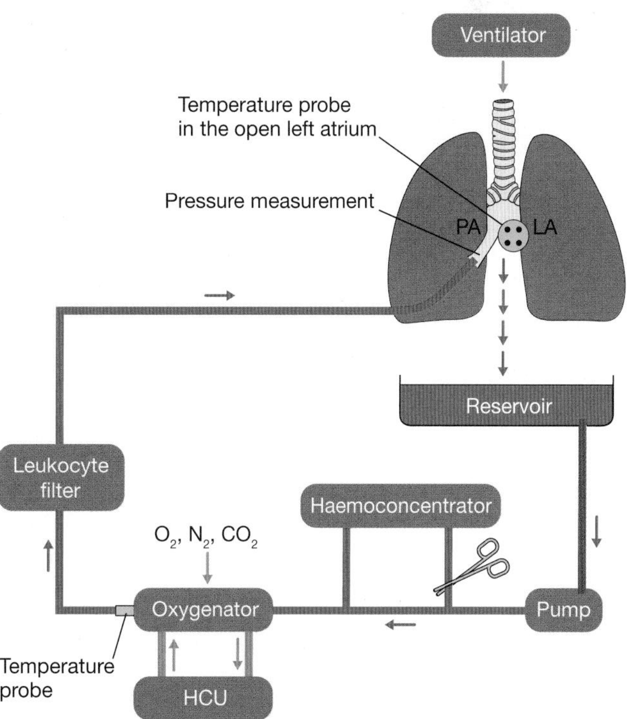

Figure 92.7 Schematic of a typical *ex vivo* lung perfusion circuit. HCU, heater–cooler unit; LA, left atrium; PA, pulmonary artery.

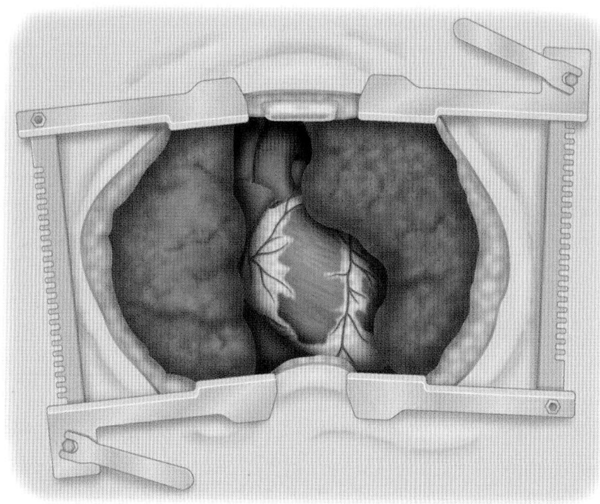

Figure 92.8 The clamshell thoracotomy commonly used for bilateral lung transplantation. Bilateral anterior thoracotomies through the fourth or fifth intercostal space are connected by division of the sternum. This facilitates excellent visualisation of the thorax

With this technique, lungs can be evaluated for function and quality between donation and transplantation with 35–97% of initially unacceptable lungs being used successfully with 5-year mortality rates equivalent to those of conventional transplantation, although some studies have suggested an increase in postoperative ECMO requirements and longer intensive care unit stays.

A different EVLP system that involves a portable organ preservation system taken to the donor hospital rather than the recipient hospital has also been shown to have favourable safety and efficacy.

Trials have been completed in which EVLP was used in standard criteria donors to assess whether this would lead to improved outcomes but no benefit was demonstrated.

Operative technique

The decision as to whether to use extracorporeal support during the transplant in the form of cardiopulmonary bypass or ECMO during bilateral lung transplantation varies with institutional experience, intraoperative stability and patient selection. Cannulation can be achieved either within the thorax or peripherally via the femoral vessels.

A clamshell thoracotomy incision (*Figure 92.8*) through the fourth or fifth intercostal space is often favoured with division of the sternum, but the procedure may also be performed using separate bilateral sternum-sparing anterior thoracotomies or via median sternotomy.

After opening both pleurae the pericardium is opened in preparation for central cannulation and to aid with hilar dissection and retraction of the heart. There are often significant adhesions in the pleural spaces that need dissection, although care not to injure the phrenic or vagus nerves should be exercised.

If an elective decision is made for cardiopulmonary bypass or ECMO, heparin is administered and aortic/femoral artery cannulation is performed for oxygenated blood return with right atrial (direct or via the femoral vein) cannulation for venous drainage. Extracorporeal support is generally avoided where possible owing to increased bleeding and an association with ischaemia–reperfusion injury.

After releasing the inferior pulmonary ligament, hilar dissection is carried out and pneumonectomy performed by division of the bronchus, pulmonary artery and both pulmonary veins. A large Satinsky clamp is placed across the left atrium and the individual pulmonary veins are opened and connected, creating a recipient cuff for anastomosis.

Recipient lung bronchial secretions are sent for microbiology and the hilum is prepared by circumferentially opening the pericardium to mobilise the left atrium and pulmonary artery. Mediastinal lymph nodes may need excision to facilitate the transplant. Bronchial arteries are ligated to prevent significant bleeding. Denudation of the recipient bronchus should be avoided to limit local ischaemia at the site of the anastomosis. The pleural space is then liberally irrigated with antibiotic or aseptic solutions.

The donor lungs are prepared for implantation by obtaining bronchial cultures for microbiology and dissecting the bronchus, pulmonary arteries and the left atrial cuff, into which the two pulmonary veins drain. Importantly the donor bronchus should be cut short just one or two rings from the bifurcation into the upper and lower lobe bronchi to minimise ischaemia at the anastomosis.

The implantation is then conducted by sequentially creating anastomoses between the bronchus, the left atrial cuff of the donor lung and the left atrium of the recipient and the pulmonary artery (*Figure 92.9*). Prior to reperfusion, 500 mg of intravenous methylprednisolone is administered.

The pulmonary artery clamp is removed slowly to lessen reperfusion injury and blood is permitted to escape from the left atrial suture line to de-air the vasculature before the left atrial clamp is opened.

After a period of ventilation on a low inspired oxygen concentration to reduce oxygen free radical release, the patient is ventilated and weaned from cardiopulmonary bypass or

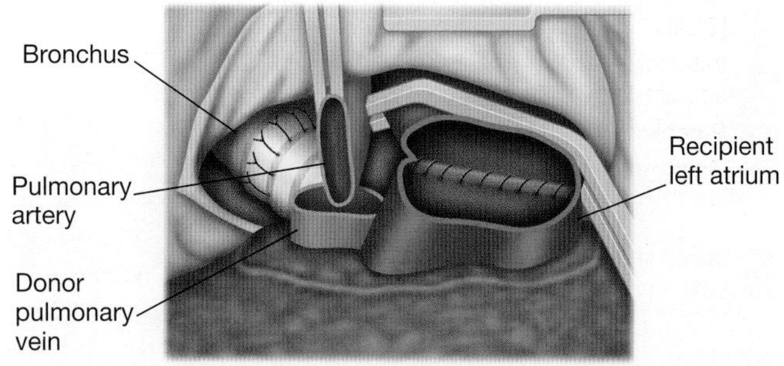

Figure 92.9 Hilum of the lung during lung transplantation. A left atrial cuff is fashioned into which the donor pulmonary veins drain. This is anastomosed to the left atrium of the recipient. The bronchus has been anastomosed already and the pulmonary artery is to be connected next.

Victor Satinsky, 1912–1997, American cardiovascular surgeon and co-creator of coronary bypass surgery.

ECMO if this has been used. Intraoperative echocardiography is used to check de-airing and the patency of the vascular anastomoses.

There has been a growing trend in the use of living related lobar lung transplantation for small recipients, especially in restrictive lung disease with low intrathoracic lung volume with two relatives each undergoing lower lobectomy. Results in a limited number of centres have been good but must be balanced against the risk of complications or death in the two donors.

Alternatively larger donor lungs can be reduced in size through multiple wedge resections and right middle lobectomy. With this technique, variable outcomes have been reported when using oversized donor lungs with donor–recipient size mismatch.

Outcomes and complications

Current median survival after pulmonary transplantation is 6.2 years. In recipients who survive the first year the median survival is 8.3 years and this is associated with a significant improvement in quality of life.

The main cause of postoperative mortality is primary graft dysfunction in which florid pulmonary oedema occurs with diffuse alveolar damage resulting from ischaemia–reperfusion injury. In survivors this is also associated with later dysfunction of the graft in the form of bronchiolitis obliterans syndrome (BOS). The pathogenesis is highly complex and involves acute-phase cytokines that are involved in inflammation that are upregulated or augmented in response to ischaemia or reperfusion and donor-specific characteristics such as infection, transfusion, barotrauma or smoking.

Summary box 92.6

Complications of lung transplantation

- Primary graft dysfunction
- Bleeding
- Parenchymal and pleural infection
- Bronchial anastomotic dehiscence or stenosis
- Vascular anastomotic stenosis or kinking
- Rejection – acute or chronic (chronic lung allograft dysfunction [CLAD])
- Infection – bacterial, viral or fungal – donor or recipient acquired
- Phrenic nerve palsy
- Gastro-oesophageal reflux

Summary box 92.7

Immunosuppression after heart and/or lung transplantation

- Induction (if used)
  - Antithymocyte globulin/interleukin-2 receptor antagonists (basiliximab)
- Maintenance
  - Ciclosporin, azathioprine, methylprednisolone

Primary graft dysfunction is treated with optimised ventilation, nitric oxide to improve ventilation–perfusion mismatch and diuresis. Support with ECMO is highly beneficial to allow for lung protective ventilation with eventual weaning when the lung injury recovers.

Infections are the second highest cause of mortality within 30 days. Most centres use broad-spectrum antibiotics in the postoperative period based on bronchoalveolar lavage specimens from both the donor and recipient lungs. Using donor lungs from hepatitis B core-positive donors is feasible with a low risk of transmission.

Rejection commonly occurs after lung transplantation. Immunosuppression is used postoperatively to prevent acute rejection as well as CLAD by inhibiting T- and B-cell proliferation and activation. Agents similar to those used after heart transplantation are commonly utilised but generally greater immunosuppression is needed compared with other organs because of the increased susceptibility of the lungs to rejection, and this significantly increases the risks of drug toxicity such as renal failure, diabetes and hypertension. Induction therapy may be given as in heart transplants but is not universally applied and side effects such as major infection and malignancies limit its use despite evidence of a survival benefit.

Acute cellular rejection occurs in around 30% of patients in the first year and is characterised by an acute decline in pulmonary graft function without any other cause. Diagnosis is confirmed histologically using scheduled transbronchial biopsies and is based on the presence of perivascular and interstitial mononuclear cell infiltrates. Pulsed high-dose steroid therapy is the mainstay of treatment with modified or augmented immunosuppression in resistant cases.

Antibody-mediated rejection is a separate entity in which DSAs directed towards donor HLA are present with neutrophil margination, arteritis and evidence of complement activation (C4d) present on histology. Treatment strategies focus on using plasmapheresis to deplete circulating DSAs, intravenous immunoglobulin and rituximab. Despite this a poor outcome is expected with a 1-year survival of less than 50%.

CLAD (which includes BOS) limits long-term survival after lung transplantation and has a prevalence of 50% at 5 years. It leads to a significant fall in lung function and treatment options are limited but may include extracorporeal photopheresis combined with augmented immunosuppressive regimens and total lymphoid irradiation. Pirfenidone is being investigated as a possible option. In advanced CLAD, retransplantation can be considered.

Gastro-oesophageal reflux disease is very common after pulmonary transplantation and has a strong association with the development of CLAD. Intraoperative vagal nerve injury, loss of cough reflex, impaired mucociliary clearance and immunosuppression-related gastroparesis may all be implicated. Early fundoplication has been suggested as an option.

The bronchial anastomosis is a common site of complications with dehiscence occurring from local ischaemia or infection and stenosis occurring longer term in 5% of cases. Reoperation to cover a defect with an intercostal muscle flap or endobronchial stent insertion for narrowed anastomoses is effective.

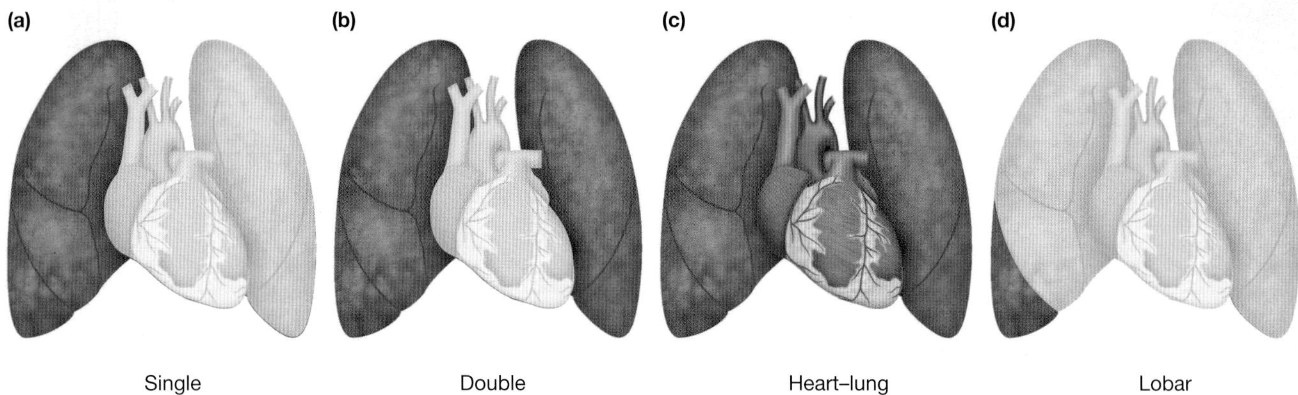

Figure 92.10 Types of lung transplant. Heart–lung combined transplantation is now rarely performed and is reserved mainly for congenital heart disease associated with pulmonary hypertension. Bilateral lung transplantation is the commonest option and accounts for 80% of pulmonary transplants performed. Single-lung transplantation can be used in cases where retention of the other lung will not pose a risk from infection, such as fibrotic lung disease or emphysema. Using this option in cystic fibrosis, for example, would be contraindicated. Single-lung transplantation is associated with inferior survival. Lobar transplantation is rarely performed but in experienced centres can provide good results in highly selected patients. In living related donation relatives would donate a lower lobe but risk complications.

Heart-lung transplantation

Combined heart–lung transplantation is an excellent treatment for PAH (***Figure 92.10***). However resolution of right ventricular dysfunction has been observed consistently after bilateral lung transplantation, making it the favoured option in the vast majority of patients, Currently, the main indication is in congenital heart disease with pulmonary hypertension. Early post-transplant survival remains lower than after lung transplantation. After a peak of activity in the late 1980s, the number of procedures has steadily declined to less than 100 per annum. Organ allocation systems are weighted towards directing hearts and lungs separately to urgently listed patients, making combined heart–lung donor blocks a rarity for these patients.

Future perspectives

Bioengineered artificial lung technology using recipient cells grown onto a decellularised lung scaffold is under development and will avoid an immune response; however, it remains a long way from clinical reality. Success would permit lung transplantation without the need for immunosuppression, waiting lists or rejection.

Artificial lungs, mimicking the success of VADs in heart transplantation, remain elusive. The physical volume of membrane oxygenators is too great for implantation within the thorax and devices are not durable, lasting weeks rather than months or years. Membranes are thrombogenic and high levels of anticoagulation would be required.

SUMMARY

As the population ages and coronary artery disease, hypertension and obesity increase in prevalence the incidence of heart failure continues to rise. Current medical therapy is effective in improving symptoms and survival but many continue to develop end-stage syndromes. The most critical issue is the growing number of patients on the waiting list and the relatively static donor pool. VADs have emerged as a strategy to bridge patients to cardiac transplantation if they are deteriorating or as durable destination therapy. However complications such as stroke, pump thrombosis and poorer long-term survival remain a challenge. Cardiac transplantation remains the gold standard for the treatment of end-stage heart failure and is associated with excellent outcomes for patients, but it is limited by chronic rejection and the side effects of immunosuppression.

Lung donor availability and increased waiting-list mortality are major challenges in pulmonary transplantation, but extended criteria donors can be safely used with good results. The use of DCD lungs and organs reconditioned with *ex vivo* lung perfusion has further expanded the donor pool, the latter technique showing promise for therapeutic interventions in due course.

Bridging patients with ECMO rather than ventilation to lung transplantation is successful for those most in need and new allocation systems have been implemented that have led to decreased waiting list mortality, especially in those with fibrotic ILD.

Overcoming primary graft dysfunction in the early postoperative period and chronic lung allograft dysfunction in the longer term are the main targets of ongoing research to improve outcomes for lung transplant recipients.

FURTHER READING

Miller L, Birks E, Guglin M *et al.* Use of ventricular assist devices and heart transplantation for advanced heart failure. *Circ Res* 2019; **124**(11): 1658–78.

Vieira JL, Mehra MR. Heart transplantation candidacy. *Curr Opin Organ Transplant* 2021; **26**(1): 69–76.

Young KA, Dilling DF. The future of lung transplantation. *Chest* 2019; **155**(3): 465–73.

Index

Note: page numbers in *italics* indicate figures, tables and boxes.